## CEREBROSPINAL FLUID NORMAL VALUES

| | |
|---|---|
| Bilirubin | 0 |
| Cells | 0-5/mm$^3$, all lymphocytes |
| Chloride | 110-129 mEq/L |
| Glucose | 48-86 mg/dl or ≥60% of serum glucose |
| pH | 7.34-7.43 |
| Pressure | 7-20 cm water |
| Protein, lumbar | 15-45 mg/dl |
| Albumin | 58% |
| $\alpha_1$-globulins | 9% |
| $\alpha_2$-globulins | 8% |
| β-globulins | 10% |
| γ-globulins | 10 (5-12)% |
| Protein, cisternal | 15-25 mg/dl |
| Protein, ventricular | 5-15 mg/dl |

## ENDOCRINOLOGIC NORMAL VALUES
### Hormone and Metabolite Normal Values

| | |
|---|---|
| Adrenocorticotropin (ACTH), serum | 15-100 pg/ml |
| Aldosterone (mean ± standard deviation) | |
| Serum | |
| 210 mEq/day sodium diet | |
| Supine | 48 ± 29 pg/ml |
| Upright (2 hr) | 65 ± 23 pg/ml |
| 110 mEq/day sodium diet | |
| Supine | 107 ± 45 pg/ml |
| Upright (2 hr) | 532 ± 228 pg/ml |
| Urine | 5-19 μg/24 hr |
| Calcitonin, serum | |
| Basal | 0.15-0.35 ng/ml |
| Stimulated | <0.6 ng/ml |
| Catecholamines, free urinary | <110 μg/24 hr |
| Chorionic gonadotropin, serum | |
| Pregnancy | |
| First month | 10-10,000 mIU/ml |
| Second and third months | 10,000-100,000 mIU/ml |
| Second trimester | 10,000-30,000 mIU/ml |
| Third trimester | 5000–15,000 mIU/ml |
| Nonpregnant | <3 mIU/ml |
| Cortisol | |
| Serum | |
| 8 AM | 5-25 μg/dl |
| 8 PM | <10 μg/dl |
| Cosyntropin stimulation (30-90 min after 0.25 mg cosyntropin intramuscularly or intravenously) | >10 μg/dl rise over baseline |
| Overnight suppression (8 AM serum cortisol after 1 mg dexamethasone orally at 11 PM) | ≤5 μg/dl |
| Urine | 20-70 μg/24 hr |
| C-peptide, serum | 0.28-0.63 pmol/ml |
| 11-Deoxycortisol, serum | |
| Basal | 0-1.4 μg/dl |
| Metyrapone stimulation (30 mg/kg orally 8 hr prior to level) | >7.5 μg/dl |
| Epinephrine, plasma | <35 pg/ml |
| Estradiol, serum | |
| Male | 20-50 pg/ml |
| Female | 25-200 pg/ml |

| Estrogens, urine (increased during pregnancy; decreased after menopause) | *Male* | *Female* |
|---|---|---|
| Total | 4-25 μg/24 hr | 5-100 μg/24 hr |
| Estriol | 1-11 μg/24 hr | 0-65 μg/24 hr |
| Estradiol | 0-6 μg/24 hr | 0-14 μg/24 hr |
| Estrone | 3-8 μg/24 hr | 4-31 μg/24 hr |

| | |
|---|---|
| Etiocholanolone, serum | <1.2 μg/dl |
| Follicle-stimulating hormone, serum | |
| Male | 2-18 mIU/ml |
| Female | |
| Follicular phase | 5-20 mIU/ml |
| Peak midcycle | 30-50 mIU/ml |
| Luteal phase | 5-15 mIU/ml |
| Postmenopausal | >50 mIU/ml |
| Free thyroxine index, serum | 1-4 ng/dl |
| Gastrin, serum (fasting) | 30-200 pg/ml |
| Growth hormone, serum | |
| Adult, fasting | <5 ng/ml |
| Glucose load (100 g orally) | <5 ng/ml |
| Levodopa stimulation (500 mg orally in a fasting state) | >5 ng/ml rise over baseline within 2 hr |
| 17-Hydroxycorticosteroids, urine | |
| Male | 2-12 mg/24 hr |
| Female | 2-8 mg/24 hr |
| 5′-Hydroxyindoleacetic acid (5′-HIAA), urine | 2-9 mg/24 hr |
| Insulin, plasma | |
| Fasting | 6-20 μU/ml |
| Hypoglycemia (serum glucose <50 mg/dl) | <5 μU/ml |
| 17-Ketosteroids, urine | |
| Under 8 years old | 0-2 mg/24 hr |
| Adolescent | 0-18 mg/24 hr |
| Adult | |
| Male | 8-18 mg/24 hr |
| Female | 5-15 mg/24 hr |
| Luteinizing hormone, serum | |
| Male adult | 2-18 mIU/ml |
| Female adult | |
| Basal | 5-22 mIU/ml |
| Ovulation | 30-250 mIU/ml |
| Postmenopausal | >30 mIU/ml |
| Metanephrines, urine | <1.3 mg/24 hr |
| Norepinephrine | |
| Plasma | 150-450 pg/ml |
| Urine | <100 μg/24 hr |
| Parathyroid hormone, serum | |
| C-terminal | 150-350 pg/ml |
| N-terminal | 230-630 pg/ml |
| Pregnanediol, urine | |
| Female | |
| Follicular phase | <1.5 mg/24 hr |
| Luteal phase | 2.0-4.2 mg/24 hr |
| Postmenopausal | 0.2-1.0 mg/24 hr |
| Male | <1.5 mg/24 hr |
| Progesterone, serum | |
| Female | |
| Follicular phase | 0.02-0.9 ng/ml |
| Luteal phase | 6-30 ng/ml |
| Male | <2 ng/ml |
| Prolactin, serum | |
| Nonpregnant | |
| Day | 5-25 ng/ml |
| Night | 20-40 ng/ml |
| Pregnant | 150-200 ng/ml |
| Radioactive iodine ($^{131}$I) uptake (RAIU) | 5%-25% at 24 hr (varies with iodine intake) |
| Renin activity, plasma (mean ± standard deviation) | |
| Normal diet | |
| Supine | 1.1 ± 0.8 ng/ml/hr |
| Upright | 1.9 ± 1.7 ng/ml/hr |
| Low-sodium diet | |
| Supine | 2.7 ± 1.8 ng/ml/hr |
| Upright | 6.6 ± 2.5 ng/ml/hr |
| Diuretics and low-sodium diet | 10.0 ± 3.7 ng/ml/hr |
| Testosterone, total plasma | |
| Bound | |
| Adolescent male | <100 ng/dl |
| Adult male | 300-1100 ng/dl |
| Female | 25-90 ng/dl |
| Unbound | |
| Adult male | 3-24 ng/dl |
| Female | 0.09-1.30 ng/dl |
| Thyroid-stimulating hormone, serum | <10 μU/ml |
| Thyroxine ($T_4$), serum | |
| Total | 4-11 μg/dl |
| Free | 0.8-2.4 ng/dl |
| Thyroxine-binding globulin capacity, serum | 15-25 μg $T_4$/dl |
| Thyroxine index, free | 1-4 ng/dl |
| Tri-iodothyronine ($T_3$), serum | 70-190 ng/dl |
| $T_3$ resin uptake | 25%-45% |
| Vanillylmandelic acid (VMA), urine | 1-8 mg/24 hr |

## Endocrine Function Tests

| | |
|---|---|
| **Adrenal gland** | |
| Glucocorticoid suppression: overnight dexamethasone suppression test (8 AM serum cortisol after 1 mg dexamethasone orally at 11 PM) | ≤5 µg/dl |
| Glucocorticoid stimulation: cosyntropin stimulation test (serum cortisol 30-90 min after 0.25 mg cosyntropin intramuscularly or intravenously) | >10 µg/ml more than baseline serum cortisol |
| Metyrapone test, single dose (8 AM serum deoxycortisol after 30 mg/kg metyrapone orally at midnight) | >7.5 µg/dl |
| Aldosterone suppression: sodium depletion test (urine aldosterone collected on day 3 of 200 mEq day/sodium diet) | <20 µg/24 hr |
| **Pancreas** | |
| Glucose tolerance test* serum glucose after 100 g glucose orally) | |
| 60 min after ingestion | <180 mg/dl |
| 90 min after ingestion | <160 mg/dl |
| 120 min after ingestion | <125 mg/dl |
| **Pituitary gland** | |
| Adrenocorticotropic hormone (ACTH) stimulation. See Adrenal gland, Metyrapone test | |
| Growth hormone stimulation: insulin tolerance test (serum growth hormone after 0.1 U/kg regular insulin intravenously after an overnight fast to induce a 50% fall in serum glucose concentration or symptomatic hypoglycemia) | >5 ng/ml rise over baseline |
| Levodopa test (serum growth hormone after 0.5 g levodopa orally while fasting) | >5 ng/ml rise over baseline within 2 hr |
| Growth hormone suppression: glucose tolerance test (serum growth hormone after 100 g glucose orally after 8 hr fast) | <5 ng/ml within 2 hr |
| Luteinizing hormone (LH) stimulation: gonadotropin-releasing hormone (GnRH) test (serum LH after 100 µg GnRH intravenously or intramuscularly) | 4- to 6-fold rise over baseline |
| Thyroid-stimulating hormone (TSH) stimulation: thyrotropin-releasing hormone (TRH) stimulation test (serum TSH after 400 µg TRH intraveneously) | >2-fold rise over baseline within 2 hr |
| **Thyroid gland** | |
| Radioactive iodine uptake (RAIU) suppression test (RAIU on day 7 after 25 µg tri-iodothyronine orally 4 times daily) | <10% to <50% baseline |
| Thyrotropin-releasing hormone (TRH) stimulation test. See Pituitary gland, Thyroid-stimulating hormone (TSH) stimulation | |

*Add 10 mg/dl for each decade over 50 years of age.

## HEMATOLOGIC NORMAL VALUES

**Table 2.** Differential cell count of bone marrow

| | |
|---|---|
| Myeloid cells | |
| Neutrophilic series | |
| Myeloblasts | 0.3%-5.0% |
| Promyelocytes | 1%-8% |
| Myelocytes | 5%-19% |
| Metamyelocytes | 9%-24% |
| Bands | 9%-15% |
| Segmented cells | 7%-30% |
| Eosinophil precursors | 0.5%-3.0% |
| Eosinophils | 0.5%-4.0% |
| Basophilic series | 0.2%-0.7% |
| Erythroid cells | |
| Pronormoblasts | 1%-8% |
| Basophilic normoblasts | |
| Polychromatophilic normoblasts | 7%-32% |
| Orthochromatic normoblasts | |
| Megakaryocytes | 0.1% |
| Lymphoreticular cells | |
| Lymphocytes | 3%-17% |
| Plasma cells | 0%-2% |
| Reticulum cells | 0.1%-2.0% |
| Monocytes | 0.5%-5.0% |
| Myeloid/erythroid ratio | 0.6-2.7 |

TEXTBOOK OF

# PRIMARY CARE MEDICINE

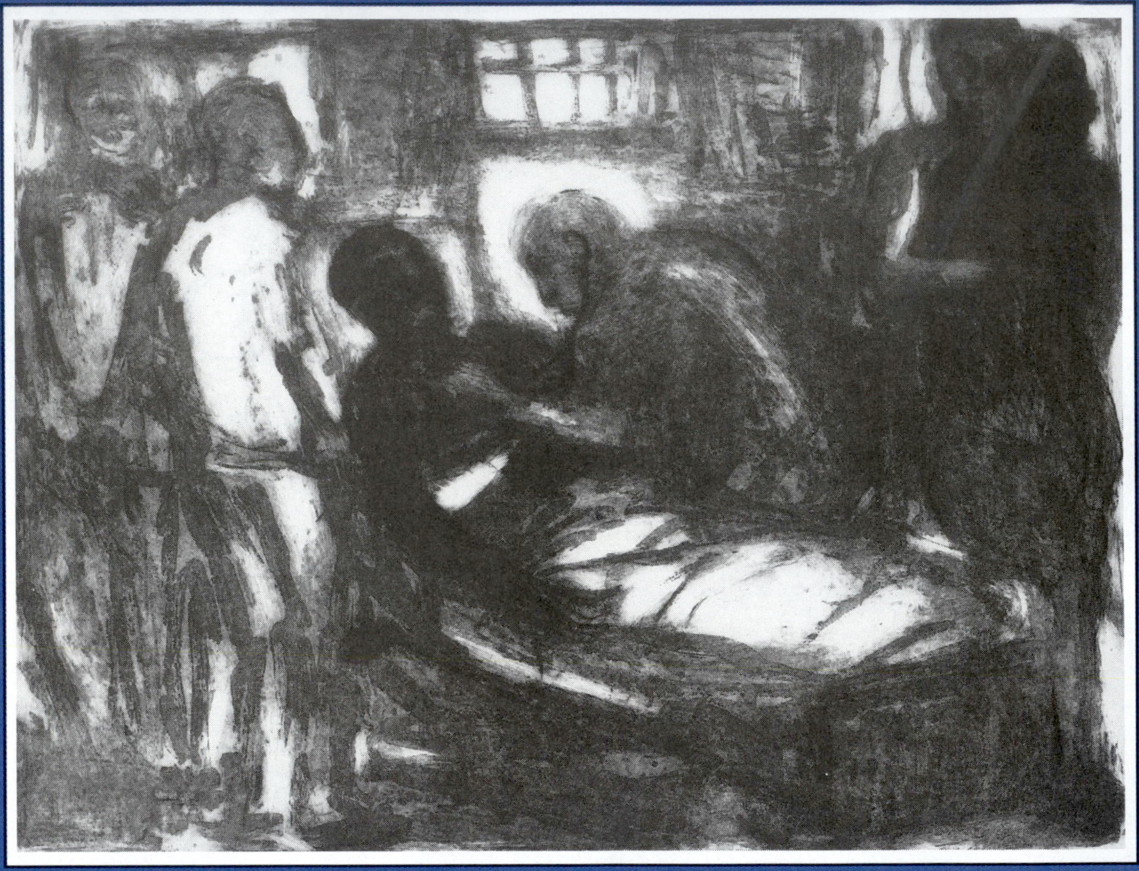

Courtesy May H. Lesser

SECOND EDITION

# TEXTBOOK OF PRIMARY CARE MEDICINE


EDITOR-IN-CHIEF

**JOHN NOBLE, M.D.**
*Professor of Medicine*
*Boston University School of Medicine*
*Chief, Section of General Internal Medicine*
*Boston City Hospital*
*Boston, Massachusetts*

SENIOR EDITORS

**HARRY L. GREENE II, M.D.**
*Executive Vice President*
*Massachusetts Medical Society*
*Waltham, Massachusetts*

**WENDY LEVINSON, M.D.**
*Professor of Medicine*
*Department of Medicine*
*Oregon Health Sciences University*
*Assistant Chief of Medicine*
*Good Samaritan Hospital*
*Portland, Oregon*

**GEOFFREY A. MODEST, M.D.**
*Associate Clinical Professor of Medicine*
*Boston University School of Medicine*
*Medical Director*
*Upham's Corner Health Center*
*Boston, Massachusetts*

**MARK J. YOUNG, M.D.**
*Associate Chairman*
*Department of Internal Medicine*
*Henry Ford Health Sciences Center*
*Detroit, Michigan*



Mosby

St. Louis Baltimore Boston Carlsbad Chicago Naples New York Philadelphia Portland
London Madrid Mexico City Singapore Sydney Tokyo Toronto Wiesbaden

Mosby
Dedicated to Publishing Excellence

A Times Mirror
Company

*Editor:* Stephanie Manning
*Developmental Editors:* Carolyn Malik, Laura DeYoung
*Project Manager:* Carol Sullivan Weis
*Production Editor:* David Stein
*Designer:* Sheilah Barrett
*Manufacturing Supervisor:* David Graybill
*Logo Calligraphy:* Charles Mullen
*Artist:* May H. Lesser

SECOND EDITION



Printed in the United States of America
Composition by Graphic World, Inc.
Printing/binding by Rand McNally

Mosby–Year Book, Inc.
11830 Westline Industrial Drive
St. Louis, Missouri 63146

**International Standard Book Number 0-8016-7841-2**

95 96 97 98 99 / 9 8 7 6 5 4 3 2 1

# Contributors

**Nezam H. Afdhal,** M.D.
Chief, Section of Gastroenterology/Hepatology, Boston City Hospital, Associate Professor of Medicine, Boston University School of Medicine, Boston, Massachusetts

**Joseph S. Alpert,** M.D.
Robert S. and Irene P. Flinn Professor of Medicine, Head, Department of Medicine, University of Arizona Health Sciences Center, Tucson, Arizona

**Jack E. Ansell,** M.D.
Vice Chairman, Department of Medicine, Boston University School of Medicine, Boston, Massachusetts

***Richard K. Babayan,** M.D.
Professor, Department of Urology, Boston University School of Medicine, Boston, Massachusetts

***Brian N. Bachynski,** M.D.
Director of Pediatric Ophthalmology, Department of Ophthalmology, Henry Ford Health Sciences Center, Detroit, Michigan

**Ann Sullivan Baker,** M.D.
Associate Professor of Medicine, Harvard Medical School, Physician, Massachusetts General Hospital, Boston, Massachusetts

**Daniel T. Baran,** M.D.
Professor of Orthopedics and Medicine, Department of Orthopedics, University of Massachusetts Medical Center, Worcester, Massachusetts

**Patricia P. Barry,** M.P.S.
Associate Professor of Medicine, Director, Gerontology Center, Boston University, Boston, Massachusetts

**Nesli Basgoz,** M.D.
Assistant in Medicine, Massachusetts General Hospital, Instructor, Harvard Medical School, Division of Infectious Diseases, Boston, Massachusetts

**Bahar Bastani,** M.D.
Assistant Professor, Department of Internal Medicine, Division of Nephrology, St. Louis University Health Sciences Center, St. Louis, Missouri

**Kenneth L. Baughman,** M.D.
Director, Cardiology Division, Professor of Medicine, Division of Cardiology, The Johns Hopkins University School of Medicine, Baltimore, Maryland

**Michael S. Benninger,** M.D.
Chairman, Department of Otolaryngology, Head and Neck Surgery, Henry Ford Health Sciences Center, Detroit, Michigan

**Peter R. Bergethon,** M.D.
Assistant Professor in Neurology, Research Assistant Professor in Biochemistry, Departments of Neurology and Biochemistry, Boston University School of Medicine, Boston, Massachusetts

**Sheilah A. Bernard,** M.D.
Associate Clinical Professor of Medicine, Director, Clinical Cardiology, Boston City Hospital, Boston, Massachusetts

**Barry M. Bernstein,** M.D.
Associate Professor, Medical College of Wisconsin, Division of Infectious Diseases, Milwaukee, Wisconsin

***Julie A. Biller,** M.D.
Pulmonary and Critical Care Section, Zablocki VA Medical Center Milwaukee, Wisconsin

**Desmond H. Birkett,** M.D., FACS
Professor of Surgery, Department of Surgery, Chief, Gastrointestinal Surgery and Surgical Endoscopy, Boston University School of Medicine, Boston, Massachusetts

**John H. Bland,** M.D.
Professor of Medicine—Rheumatology Emeritus, Department of Rheumatology and Clinical Immunology Unit, University of Vermont College of Medicine, Burlington, Vermont

***C. Michael Bliss,** M.D.
Associate Professor of Medicine, Gastroenterology Section, Boston University School of Medicine, Boston, Massachusetts

**David D. Bogorad,** M.D., FACS
Division Head, West Bloomfield Eye Care Services, Department of Ophthalmology, Henry Ford Health Sciences Center, Detroit, Michigan

**Robert V. Brody,** M.D.
Professor of Medicine and Family and Community Medicine, University of California, San Francisco, San Francisco General Hospital, San Francisco, California

**Frank W. Brown,** M.D.
Assistant Professor, Department of Psychiatry and Behavioral Sciences, Emory University School of Medicine, Atlanta, Georgia

**Melanie J. Brunt,** M.D.
Assistant Professor of Medicine, Department of Medicine, Section of Endocrinology, Boston University School of Medicine, Assistant Director, Diabetes Clinic, Boston City Hospital, Boston, Massachusetts

**Robert Burakoff,** M.D.
Professor of Medicine, School of Medicine, Health Sciences Center, State University of New York at Stony Brook, Stony Brook, New York, Chief, Division of Gastroenterology, Hepatology, and Nutrition, Department of Medicine, Winthrop-University Hospital, Mineola, New York

**Denise Ann Burke,** M.D.
Department of Dermatology, Oregon Health Sciences University, Portland, Oregon

**John McVey Burket,** M.D.
Clinical Professor, Department of Dermatology, Oregon Health Sciences University, Portland, Oregon

---

*Author of a chapter in Noble: *Primary Care Medicine* CD-ROM, an expanded electronic version of *Textbook of Primary Care Medicine.*

**Robert E. Burr,** M.D.
Medical Advisor, U.S. Army Research Institute of Environmental Medicine, Natick, Massachusetts, Attending Physician, Boston City Hospital, Boston, Massachusetts

***John W. Burress,** M.D., M.P.H.
Department of Occupational Health, Harvard School of Public Health, Boston, Massachusetts

**Thomas J. Byrd,** M.D.
Director, Cornea Service, Department of Ophthalmology, Henry Ford Health Sciences Center, Detroit, Michigan

**Lisa Rowland Callahan,** M.D.
Clinical Instructor, Team Physician, Stanford University Soccer Teams, Associate Team Physician, San Jose State University, Division of Family Medicine, Stanford University, Palo Alto, California

**Thomas L. Campbell,** M.D.
Associate Professor of Family Medicine and Psychiatry, Highland Hospital Primary Care Institute, University of Rochester School of Medicine & Dentistry, Rochester, New York

***David Canavan,** M.D.
Medical Director, Physicians' Health Program, Medical Society of New Jersey, Lawrenceville, New Jersey

**Juan J. Canoso,** M.D.
Adjunct Professor of Medicine, New England Medical Center (Medicine), Tufts University, Boston, Massachusetts

***J. David Carey,** M.D.
Vice Chairman, Department of Ophthalmology, Henry Ford Health Sciences Center, Detroit, Michigan

***Darrell L. Carter,** M.D., FAAFP, DABFP
Clinical Associate Professor, Department of Family Practice and Community Health, University of Minnesota Medical School, Minneapolis, Minnesota, Rural Family Practitioner, Granite Falls, Minnesota

**Anthony C. Caruso,** M.D.
Clinical Assistant Professor, Cardiology Section, Department of Medicine, Arizona Health Science Center, Tucson, Arizona

**Marc Cendron,** M.D.
Assistant Professor of Urology and Pediatrics, Department of Surgery—Urology, Dartmouth University, Lebanon, New Hampshire

**Joseph T. Chambers,** Ph.D., M.D.
Associate Professor, Division of Gynecologic Oncology, Department of Obstetrics and Gynecology, Associate Director, Gynecologic Oncology, Yale University School of Medicine, New Haven, Connecticut

**Setsuko K. Chambers,** M.D.
Associate Professor, Division of Gynecologic Oncology, Department of Obstetrics and Gynecology, Yale University School of Medicine, New Haven, Connecticut

**Stuart R. Chipkin,** M.D.
Associate Professor of Medicine and Physiology, Boston University School of Medicine, Boston, Massachusetts

***David C. Christiani,** M.D., M.P.H., M.S.
Associate Professor of Occupational Medicine, Department of Environmental Health, Occupational Health Program, Harvard School of Public Health, Associate Professor of Medicine, Harvard Medical School, Boston, Massachusetts

**Murray D. Christianson,** M.D.
Department of Ophthalmology, Henry Ford Hospital, Detroit, Michigan

**Matthew M. Clark,** Ph.D.
Clinical Assistant Professor, Department of Psychiatry and Human Behavior, Brown University School of Medicine, Providence, Rhode Island

**William D. Clark,** M.D.
Medical Director, Addiction Resource Center, Bath, Maine, Lecturer in Medicine, Harvard Medical School, Boston, Massachusetts

**Clifton R. Cleaveland,** M.D., M.A.C.P.
Clinical Professor, Department of Medicine, Chattanooga Unit of the College of Medicine, University of Tennessee, Chattanooga, Tennessee

**Michael J. Clement,** M.D.
Assistant Clinical Professor of Medicine, University of California, San Francisco, San Francisco, California, Department of Medicine, Oakland Kaiser Hospital, Oakland, California

**Jay D. Coffman,** M.D.
Professor of Medicine, Chief, Peripheral Vascular Section, Department of Medicine, Boston University School of Medicine, Boston, Massachusetts

**Steven A. Cole,** M.D.
Professor of Psychiatry, Albert Einstein School of Medicine, Director of Managed Care, Hillside Hospital, Glen Oaks, New York

**Joshua A. Copel,** M.D.
Professor of Obstetrics and Gynecology, Section Head, Maternal-Fetal Medicine, Department of Obstetrics and Gynecology, Yale University School of Medicine, New Haven, Connecticut

**Robert B. Copeland,** M.D., M.A.C.P.
Clinical Professor of Medicine, University of Alabama at Birmingham, Birmingham, Alabama, Director, Georgia Heart Clinic, La Grange, Georgia

**James M. Coumas,** M.D.
Carolinas Medical Center, Charlotte Radiology, Charlotte, North Carolina

**Jennifer S. Daly,** M.D.
Associate Professor of Medicine, Division of Infectious Diseases, The Medical Center of Central Massachusetts, University of Massachusetts Medical School, Worcester, Massachusetts

**Deborah A. Darnley-Fisch,** M.D.
Bloomfield Village, Michigan

**James A. Delmez,** M.D.
Professor of Medicine, Medical Director, Chromalloy American Kidney Center, Renal Division, Washington University School of Medicine, St. Louis, Missouri

**Alfred DeMaria, Jr.,** M.D.
Assistant Commissioner of Public Health, State Epidemiologist, Bureau of Communicable Disease Control, Massachusetts Department of Public Health, Boston, Massachusetts

***Patrick J. Dennehy,** M.D.
Henry Ford Hospital, Department of Ophthalmology, Detroit, Michigan

**Richard A. DeRemee,** M.D.
Professor of Medicine, Mayo Medical School, Pulmonary Division, Mayo Clinic, Rochester, Minnesota

---

*Author of a chapter in Noble: *Primary Care Medicine* CD-ROM, an expanded electronic version of *Textbook of Primary Care Medicine.*

**Uday R. Desai,** M.D.
Department of Ophthalmology, Henry Ford Hospital, Detroit, Michigan

**Michael F. Dillingham,** M.D.
Department of Functional Restoration, Clinical Professor, Department of Orthopedics and Rehabilitation Medicine, Director, Musculoskeletal Medicine Sports Medicine Program, Stanford University, Stanford, California, Team Orthopedic Surgeon, San Francisco 49ers, Team Physician, Santa Clara University Sports Program, Santa Clara, California

**Roger R. Dmochowski,** M.D.
Assistant Professor of Urology, Chief, Division of Neurology, Department of Urology, University of Tennessee, Memphis, Tennessee

**Michael J. Droller,** M.D.
Department of Urology, Mt. Sinai Medical Center, New York, New York

**Douglas A. Drossman,** M.D.
Professor of Medicine and Psychiatry, Department of Medicine, Division of Digestive Diseases, University of North Carolina at Chapel Hill, Chapel Hill, North Carolina

***Marshall B. Dunning III,** Ph.D.
Assistant Professor and Director, Pulmonary Diagnostic Laboratory, Froedtert Memorial Lutheran Hospital, Milwaukee, Wisconsin

**Margaret Durkin,** M.D.
Clinical Assistant Professor of Medicine, Brown University School of Medicine, Providence, Rhode Island

**Susana A. Ebner,** M.D.
Assistant Professor of Medicine, Department of Endocrinology, Boston University School of Medicine, Boston, Massachusetts

**Linda D. Eckert,** M.D.
Acting Assistant Professor, Department of Obstetrics and Gynecology, University of Washington, Seattle, Washington

**Kathryn L. Edmiston,** M.D.
Assistant Professor of Medicine, Department of Hematology/ Oncology, University of Massachusetts Medical Center, Worcester, Massachusetts

**Richard M. Effros,** M.D.
Professor of Medicine, Chief, Division of Pulmonary and Critical Care Medicine, Department of Medicine, Medical College of Wisconsin, Milwaukee, Wisconsin

**Sherman Eisenthal,** Ph.D.
Associate Professor Psychology, Harvard Medical School, Psychologist, Department of Psychiatry, Massachusetts General Hospital, Boston, Massachusetts

**Charles C. Engel, Jr.,** M.D., M.P.H.
Director, Mental Health Services Research, Tripler Army Medical Center, Research Associate, Hawaii Medical Treatment Effectiveness Program, Pacific Health Research Institute, Honolulu, Hawaii

**Arthur H. Eskew,** M.D.
Assistant Professor of Medicine, Boston City Hospital, Boston University School of Medicine, Boston, Massachusetts

***Ann E. Eyler,** M.D., M.P.H.
Clinical Assistant Professor, Department of Family Practice, University of Michigan Medical School and Department of Health Management and Policy, University of Michigan School of Public Health, Ann Arbor, Michigan

*Author of a chapter in Noble: *Primary Care Medicine* CD-ROM, an expanded electronic version of *Textbook of Primary Care Medicine*.

**Alan P. Farwell,** M.D., FACP
Assistant Professor of Medicine, Department of Medicine, Division of Endocrinology, University of Massachusetts Medical Center, Worcester, Massachusetts

**Mark Feldman,** M.D.
Professor and Vice Chairman, Chief, Dallas VA Medical Service, Department of Internal Medicine, University of Texas Southwestern Medical School at Dallas, Dallas, Texas

**Joseph T. Ferrucci,** M.D.
Chairman and Professor, Department of Radiology, Boston University School of Medicine, Boston, Massachusetts

***Kenneth L. Fox, Jr.,** M.D.
Instructor, Department of Social Medicine, Harvard Medical School, Boston, Massachusetts

**Robert G. Frykberg,** DPM, M.P.H.
Clinical Instructor in Surgery, Harvard Medical School, New England Deaconess Hospital, Department of Surgery, Division of Podiatry, Harvard Medical School, Boston, Massachusetts

**Akira Funahashi,** M.D., Ph.D
Professor of Medicine, Department of Medicine, Medical College of Wisconsin, Milwaukee, Wisconsin

**Laurence Fuortes,** M.D., M.S.
Assistant Professor, Departments of Preventive Medicine and Environmental Health and Internal Medicine, The University of Iowa, Iowa City, Iowa

**Joel E. Gallant,** M.D., M.P.H.
Assistant Professor of Medicine, Director, HIV Clinic, Division of Infectious Diseases, Department of Medicine, Johns Hopkins University School of Medicine, Baltimore, Maryland

**Nelson M. Gantz,** M.D., FACP
Clinical Professor of Medicine, Pennsylvania State University College of Medicine, Hershey, Pennsylvania, Chairman of Medicine, Department of Medicine, Chief, Division of Infectious Diseases, Polyclinic Medical Center, Harrisburg, Pennsylvania

**David F. Giansiracusa,** M.D.
Professor, Department of Medicine, Division of Rheumatology, Associate Chairman, Department of Medicine, University of Massachusetts Medical Center, Worcester, Massachusetts

***Matthew W. Gillman,** M.D., S.M.
Assistant Professor of Medicine, Pediatrics, and Public Health, Evans Section of Preventive Medicine & Epidemiology, Boston University School of Medicine, Boston, Massachusetts

**Marianne E. Giuffra,** M.D.
Assistant Professor of Neurology, Boston City Hospital, Neurological Unit, Boston University, Boston, Massachusetts

**Richard H. Glew,** M.D.
Professor of Medicine, Molecular Genetics and Microbiology (UMMS), Chairman, Department of Medicine, The Medical Center of Central Massachusetts, University of Massachusetts Medical School, Worcester, Massachusetts

**Eliot W. Godofsky,** M.D.
Assistant Professor of Medicine, Department of Infectious Diseases, University of South Florida-Tampa, Bradenton, Florida

**Erika Goldstein,** M.D.
Assistant Professor, Department of Medicine, University of Washington School of Medicine, Seattle, Washington

**Irwin Goldstein,** M.D.
Professor of Urology, Department of Urology, Boston University School of Medicine, Boston, Massachusetts

**Michael G. Goldstein,** M.D.
Associate Professor of Psychiatry and Human Behavior, Department of Psychiatry and Human Behavior, Brown University School of Medicine, Providence, Rhode Island

**Peter A. Gottlieb,** M.D.
Assistant Professor—Pediatrics and Medicine, Barbara Davis Center for Childhood Diabetes, University of Colorado Health Sciences Center, Denver, Colorado

**The Late John R. Graham,** M.D.
Professor of Medicine, Tufts University School of Medicine, Former Chief of Medicine and Founder of the John R. Graham Headache Institute at Faulkner Hospital, Jamaica Plain, Massachusetts

**Norton J. Greenberger,** M.D., M.A.C.P.
Professor and Chairman, Department of Internal Medicine, University of Kansas Medical Center, Kansas City, Kansas

**Harry L. Greene II,** M.D.
Executive Vice-President, Massachusetts Medical Society, Waltham, Massachusetts

**Jerry M. Greene,** M.D.
Instructor in Medicine, Harvard Medical School, Chief, Rheumatology Section, Medical Service, West Roxbury/Brockton VA Medical Center, Boston, Massachusetts

**Elzbieta B. Griffiths,** M.D.
Chief Resident, Clinical Pathology, Department of Pathology, University of Massachusetts, Worcester, Massachusetts

**Barrie J. Guise,** Ph.D.
Coordinator of Behavioral Medicine, Department of Medicine, Lenox Hill Hospital, New York, New York

**Carolyn I. Hale,** M.D.
Clinical Instructor of Dermatology, Department of Dermatology, Oregon Health Sciences University, Portland, Oregon

***John M. Harris, Jr.,** M.D.
Medical Director, CA Care, Woodland Hills, California

**Florence P. Haseltine,** Ph.D., M.D.
Director, Center for Population Research, NICHD, National Institutes of Health, Bethesda, Maryland

**James J. Heffernan,** M.D., M.P.H.
Associate Professor of Medicine, Boston University School of Medicine, Boston City Hospital, Boston, Massachusetts

***Robert C. Hendel,** M.D.
Assistant Professor of Medicine, Divisions of Cardiology and Critical Care Medicine, Northwestern University Medical School, Chicago, Illinois

**Janet B. Henrich,** M.D.
Associate Professor of Medicine, Department of Internal Medicine, Yale University School of Medicine, New Haven, Connecticut

**Ahvie Herskowitz,** M.D.
Division of Cardiology, Johns Hopkins University School of Medicine, Baltimore, Maryland

***W. Ladson Hinton IV,** M.D.
Lecturer, Department of Social Medicine, Harvard Medical School, Boston, Massachusetts

**Erwin F. Hirsch,** M.D., FACS
Chief, General Surgery, Boston City Hospital, Boston University Medical Center Hospital, Boston, Massachusetts

*Author of a chapter in Noble: *Primary Care Medicine* CD-ROM, an expanded electronic version of *Textbook of Primary Care Medicine.*

**Eleanor T. Hobbs,** M.D.
Instructor in Medicine, Harvard Medical School, Medical Director, Emergency Services, Deaconess Hospital, Boston, Massachusetts

**Richard M. Hoffman,** M.D., M.P.H.
Staff Physician, Primary Care, VA Medical Center, Albuquerque, New Mexico

**Michael F. Holick,** Ph.D., M.D.
Professor of Medicine, Chief of Endocrinology, Endocrine Section, Department of Medicine, Boston University Medical Center, Boston, Massachusetts

**Howard R. Horn,** M.D.
The L. W. Diggs Professor of Medicine and Chair of Excellence in Medical Education, Department of Medicine/Cardiology, University of Tennessee, Memphis, Memphis, Tennessee

**Charles S. Houston,** M.D.
Professor of Medicine and Environmental Health (Emeritus), University of Vermont, Burlington, Vermont

**Brian A. Howard,** M.D.
Osteoradiologist, Department of Radiology, Carolina Medical Centre, Charlotte, North Carolina

**Kinan K. Hreib,** M.D., Ph.D.
Director of Stroke Service, Department of Neurology, Lahey Hitchock Clinic, Burlington, Massachusetts

**Robin R. Ingalls,** M.D.
Clinical Instructor in Medicine, Department of Medicine, Division of Infectious Diseases, Boston University Medical Center, Boston City Hospital, Boston, Massachusetts

**Joseph A. Ingelfinger,** M.D.
Medical Director, Bowdoin Street Community Health Center, Boston, Massachusetts

**Richard J. Iseke,** M.D.
Assistant Professor of Emergency Medicine, University of Massachusetts Medical School, Director Emergency Services, Lawrence General Hospital, Worcester, Massachusetts

**Eric W. Jacobson,** M.D.
Assistant Professor of Medicine, Director, Clerkship in Internal Medicine, Department of Medicine, Division of Rheumatology, University of Massachusetts Medical School, Worcester, Massachusetts

**Manoj Jain,** M.D., M.P.H.
Fellow in Infectious Disease, Geographic Medicine and Infectious Diseases, Tufts University School of Medicine, Boston, Massachusetts

**Leon G. Josephs,** M.D.
Assistant Professor, Director, Minimal Access Surgery Center, Boston University Medical Center, Department of Surgery, Boston University School of Medicine, Boston, Massachusetts

**Leslie E. Kahl,** M.D.
Associate Professor of Medicine, Associate Dean for Student Affairs, Department of Internal Medicine, Washington University, St. Louis, Missouri

**Wishwa N. Kapoor,** M.D., M.P.H.
Falk Professor of Medicine, Chief, Division of General Medicine, Department of Medicine, University of Pittsburgh, Pittsburgh, Pennsylvania

**Michael S. Karasik,** M.D.
Assistant Professor of Medicine, Boston University School of Medicine, Director of Endoscopy, Section of Gastroenterology/Hepatology, Boston City Hospital, Boston, Massachusetts

**Edward K. Kasper,** M.D.
Assistant Professor of Medicine, Director, Cardiomyopathy and Heart Transplant Service, Department of Medicine, Johns Hopkins University School of Medicine, Baltimore, Maryland

**Wayne J. Katon,** M.D.
Professor, Chief, Division of Consultation-Liaison Psychiatry, Department of Psychiatry and Behavioral Sciences, University of Washington School of Medicine, Seattle, Washington

**Jack Kaufman,** M.D.
Professor, General Internal Medicine, John L. Doyne Hospital, Milwaukee, Wisconsin

**Julie Kaufmann,** M.D., Ph.D.
Assistant Clinical Professor, Boston University School of Medicine, General Internist, Dorchester House Community Health Center and Section of General Internal Medicine, Boston City Hospital, Boston, Massachusetts

**David L. Keefe,** M.D.
Assistant Professor, Director, Reproductive Aging Unit, Division of Reproductive Medicine, Department of Obstetrics and Gynecology, Yale University School of Medicine, New Haven, Connecticut

**Mumtaz J. Khan,** M.D.
Department of Otolaryngology, Henry Ford Hospital, Detroit, Michigan

**Saulo Klahr,** M.D.
Simon Professor of Medicine, Co-Chairman, Department of Medicine, Washington University School of Medicine, Physician-in-Chief, The Jewish Hospital of St. Louis, Department of Medicine, Washington University School of Medicine, St. Louis, Missouri

***Arthur Kleinman,** M.D.
Professor of Psychiatry and Presley Professor of Medical Anthropology, Chairman, Department of Social Medicine, Harvard Medical School, Professor of Social Anthropology, Harvard University, Boston, Massachusetts

**Raymond S. Koff,** M.D.
Professor of Medicine, Department of Medicine, University of Massachusetts Medical School, Chairman, Department of Medicine, Metrowest Medical Center, Worcester, Massachusetts

**Robert J. Krane,** M.D.
Professor and Chairman, Department of Urology, Boston University School of Medicine, Boston, Massachusetts

**Dennis H. Kraus,** M.D.
Assistant Professor Otolaryngology, Cornell University Medical Center, Assistant Attending Surgeon, Head and Neck Service, Director, Speech, Hearing and Rehabilitation Center, Memorial Sloan-Kettering Cancer Center, New York, New York

**Talya H. Kupin,** M.D.
Senior Staff Ophthalmologist, Glaucoma Service, Department of Ophthalmology, Henry Ford Hospital, Detroit, Michigan

**Edward V. Lally,** M.D.
Associate Professor of Medicine, Director, Division of Rheumatology, Department of Medicine, Brown University School of Medicine, Providence, Rhode Island

**J. Thomas LaMont,** M.D.
Professor of Medicine, Chief Section of Gastroenterology, Department of Medicine/Gastroenterology, Boston University Medical Center, Boston, Massachusetts

**Gary E. Leach,** M.D.
Associate Clinical Professor of Urology, University of California, Chief of Urology, Kaiser Permanente Medical Center, Los Angeles, California

**Joseph M. Lenehan,** M.D.
Plastic and Reconstructive Surgery, Department of Surgery, Boston University Medical School, Boston, Massachusetts

**Herbert Lepor,** M.D.
Department of Urology, Medical College of Wisconsin, Milwaukee, Wisconsin

**Robert H. Lerman,** M.D., Ph.D.
Associate Clinical Professor of Medicine, Boston University School of Medicine, Director of Clinical Nutrition, Boston University Medical Center Hospital, Jewish Memorial Hospital and Rehabilitation Center, Medical Director, Evans Nutrition Group, Boston, Massachusetts

**G. Robert Lesser,** M.D.
Director, Glaucoma Service, Department of Ophthalmology, Henry Ford Health Sciences Center, Detroit, Michigan

**Claire A. Levesque,** M.D.
Assistant Professor of Neurology, Director of Geriatric Neurology, Boston City Hospital, Neurological Unit, Boston University, Boston, Massachusetts

**Sharon A. Levine,** M.D.
Assistant Professor of Medicine, Director, Geriatric Assessment Center, Boston University Medical Center and Boston City Hospital, Director, Geriatric Education, Geriatrics Section, Boston University School of Medicine, Boston, Massachusetts

**Wendy Levinson,** M.D.
Professor of Medicine, Department of Medicine, Oregon Health Sciences University, Assistant Chief of Medicine, Good Samaritan Hospital, Portland, Oregon

**Howard Libman,** M.D.
Assistant Professor of Medicine, Harvard Medical School, Division of General Medicine Primary Care, Department of Medicine, Beth Israel Hospital, Boston, Massachusetts

**Leonard S. Lilly,** M.D.
Assistant Professor of Medicine, Harvard Medical School, Staff Cardiologist, Brigham and Women's Hospital, Boston, Massachusetts

**Randolph J. Lipchik,** M.D.
Assistant Professor of Medicine, Pulmonary and Critical Care Medicine, Department of Medicine, Medical College of Wisconsin, Milwaukee, Wisconsin

**Mack Lipkin, Jr.,** M.D.
Associate Professor of Clinical Medicine, Director, Primary Care, New York University Medical Center, President, American Academy on Physicians and Patient, New York, New York

**Martin R. Lipp,** M.D.
Associate Clinical Professor, University of California at San Francisco, San Francisco, California, Short-Term Director, Board of Directors, The Permanente Medical Group, Oakland, California

**Nancy Y.N. Liu,** M.D.
Assistant Professor of Medicine, Department of Medicine, University of Massachusetts Medical School, Worcester, Massachusetts

***Farrell J. Lloyd,** M.D., M.P.H.
Assistant Professor of Clinical Medicine, Section of General Internal Medicine, Department of Medicine, University of Arizona, Tucson, Arizona

*Author of a chapter in Noble: *Primary Care Medicine* CD-ROM, an expanded electronic version of *Textbook of Primary Care Medicine.*

**Ana Maria Lopez,** M.D., M.P.H.
Assistant Professor of Medicine, Hematology/Oncology Section, Department of Medicine, University of Arizona, Tucson, Arizona

**Philip A. Lowry,** M.D.
Assistant Professor of Medicine, Division of Hematology/Oncology, University of Massachusetts Medical Center, Worcester, Massachusetts

**Debra M. Lundquist,** M.S.N., RN, CS, OCN
Clinical Nurse Specialist/Nurse Practitioner, Division of Hematology/Oncology, University of Massachusetts Medical Center, Worcester, Massachusetts

**Urania Magriples,** M.D.
Assistant Professor, Department of Obstetrics and Gynecology, Yale University School of Medicine, New Haven, Connecticut

**Kevin J. Martin,** M.B., B.Ch.
Professor of Internal Medicine, Director Division of Nephrology, Department of Internal Medicine, St. Louis University School of Medicine, St. Louis, Missouri

**Elcinda L. McCrone,** M.D.
Director of Infectious Diseases, Morton Hospital and Medical Center, Taunton, Massachusetts

**Susan H. McDaniel,** Ph.D.
Associate Professor of Psychiatry and Family Medicine, Highland Hospital Primary Care Institute, University of Rochester School of Medicine & Dentistry, Rochester, New York

**James L. McGuire,** M.D.
Associate Professor of Medicine, Associate Dean for Graduate Medical Education, Department of Medicine, Stanford University School of Medicine, Stanford, California

**Margaret McHugh,** M.D.
Clinical Associate Professor, Pediatrics, Director, Child Protection Team, Bellevue Hospital, Department of Pediatrics, New York University, New York, New York

**W. Paul McKinney,** M.D.
Associate Professor of Medicine, University of Texas Southwestern Medical School, Chief, Section of General Internal Medicine, Dallas Veterans Administration Medical Center, Department of Internal Medicine, Dallas, Texas

**James C. Melby,** M.D.
Professor of Medicine and Physiology, Boston University School of Medicine, Boston, Massachusetts

**Samuel A. Mickelson,** M.D., FACS
Residency Training Program Director, Department of Otolaryngology—Head and Neck Surgery, Henry Ford Health Sciences Center, Detroit, Michigan

**Geoffrey A. Modest,** M.D.
Associate Clinical Professor of Medicine, Boston University School of Medicine, Medical Director, Upham's Corner Health Center, Boston, Massachusetts

**Elinor A. Mody,** M.D.
Clinical Fellow in Rheumatology, Brigham and Women's Hospital, Arthritis Center, BWH, Boston, Massachusetts

**Lynne H. Morrison,** M.D.
Assistant Professor of Dermatology, Department of Dermatology, Oregon Health Sciences University, Portland, Oregon

**Ronald A. Morton,** M.D.
Assistant Professor, Scott Department of Urology, Baylor College of Medicine, Houston, Texas

**Mark Murphy,** M.D.
Division of Digestive Diseases, Department of Medicine, The University of North Carolina at Chapel Hill, Chapel Hill, North Carolina

**Katherine Murray-Leisure,** M.D.
Persian Gulf Coordinator, Infectious Diseases and Epidemiology, Good Samaritan Hospital and Lebanon VA Medical Center, Lebanon, Pennsylvania

**John Noble,** M.D.
Professor of Medicine, Boston University School of Medicine, Chief, Section of General Internal Medicine, Boston City Hospital, Boston, Massachusetts

**Julian J. Nussbaum,** M.D.
Chairman, Department of Ophthalmology, Henry Ford Health Sciences Center, Detroit, Michigan

**Robert D. Oates,** M.D.
Associate Professor, Department of Urology, Boston University, Boston, Massachusetts

**Nsidinanya Okike,** M.D.
Professor, Cardiac and Thoracic Surgery, Vice Chair, Division of Thoracic and Cardiac Surgery, Department of Surgery, University of Massachusetts, Worcester, Massachusetts

***David M. Ozonoff,** M.D., M.P.H.
Professor of Public Health, Department Head of Environmental Health, School of Public Health—Environmental Health, Boston University School of Medicine, Boston, Massachusetts

**Ann L. Parke,** M.D.
Professor of Medicine, Department of Medicine, Division of Rheumatic Disease, University of Connecticut Health Center, Farmington, Connecticut

**Frank Parker,** M.D.
Professor of Dermatology, Department of Dermatology, Oregon Health Sciences University, Portland, Oregon

**Liberto Pechet,** M.D.
Professor Emeritus in Medicine & Pathology, Division of Hematology/Oncology, University of Massachusetts Medical Center, Worcester, Massachusetts

***Lewis Pepper,** M.D.
Department of Environmental Health, Boston University School of Public Health, Boston, Massachusetts

**Marguerite Perikles,** B.S.
National Cancer Institute, National Institutes of Health, Bethesda, Maryland

**Kathryn M. Peuvrelle,** M.A.
Consultant, Sports Medicine & Rheumatology, Health Counselor; Figure Skating Coach, Stanford University, Stanford, California

***John-Henry Pfifferling,** Ph.D.
Clinical Associate Professor, Post Doctorate, Director, Center for Professional Well-Being, University of North Carolina at Chapel Hill, Chapel Hill, North Carolina

**David G. Pfister,** M.D.
Assistant Professor of Medicine—Cornell University Medical College, Department of Medicine, Memorial Sloan-Kettering Cancer Center, Cornell University Medical College, Assistant Attending Physician—Memorial Hospital, New York, New York

*Author of a chapter in Noble: *Primary Care Medicine* CD-ROM, an expanded electronic version of *Textbook of Primary Care Medicine.*

**Glenn M. Preminger,** M.D.

Professor of Urologic Surgery, Director, Duke Comprehensive Kidney Stone Center, Department of Urology, Duke University Medical Center, Durham, North Carolina

**Kenneth W. Presberg,** M.D.

Assistant Professor of Medicine, Co-director of Medical Intensive Care, Pulmonary and Critical Care Division, Department of Medicine, Medical College of Wisconsin, Milwaukee, Wisconsin

**David W. Puett,** M.D.

Carolina Arthritis Associates, Wilmington, North Carolina

**Timothy E. Quill,** M.D.

Professor of Medicine and Psychiatry, University of Rochester School of Medicine and Dentistry, Associate Chief of Medicine, The Genesee Hospital, Rochester, New York

**Kodangudi B. Ramanathan,** M.D., M.R.C.P. (U.K.)

Professor of Medicine, Chief of Cardiology, Veteran's Administration Medical Center, Associate Chief of Cardiology, Department of Medicine/Cardiology, University of Tennessee, Memphis, Memphis, Tennessee

**Andrea J. Rapkin,** M.D.

Department of Obstetrics and Gynecology, University of California, Los Angeles Medical Center, Los Angeles, California

**Lynn F. Reinke,** RN, M.S.N.

Veterans Affairs Medical Center, Pulmonary and Critical Care Medicine, Milwaukee, Wisconsin

**Michael Reiss,** M.D.

Associate Professor of Medicine, Director, Breast Cancer Research Program, Yale Cancer Center, Section of Medical Oncology, Department of Medicine, Yale University, New Haven, Connecticut

**Peter A. Rice,** M.D.

Professor of Medicine, Boston University School of Medicine, Chief, Section of Infectious Diseases, Department of Infectious Diseases, Boston University School of Medicine, Boston, Massachusetts

**John A. Rich,** M.D., M.P.H.

Assistant Professor of Medicine, Director, Young Men's Health Clinic, Boston City Hospital, Section of General Internal Medicine, Boston University School of Medicine, Boston, Massachusetts

**Phoebe Rich,** M.D.

Clinical Instructor, Department of Dermatology, Oregon Health Sciences University, Portland, Oregon

**Janet L. Roberts,** M.D.

Clinical Professor, Department of Dermatology, Oregon Health Sciences University, Portland, Oregon

**Margaret Hewitt Robertson,** M.D.

Associate Clinical Professor, Oregon Health Sciences University, Lake Oswego, Oregon

**David Rosenzweig,** M.D.

Associate Professor, Pulmonary and Critical Care Division, Department of Medicine, Medical College of Wisconsin, Milwaukee, Wisconsin

**Neil W. Ross,** M.A.

Marine Recreation Specialist, Kingston, Rhode Island

**Richard I. Rothstein,** M.D.

Associate Professor, Section of Gastroenterology, Department of Medicine, Dartmouth Medical School, Hanover, New Hampshire

**Thomas D. Sabin,** M.D.

Professor of Neurology and Psychiatry, Boston University School of Medicine, Director, Neurological Unit, Boston City Hospital, Boston, Massachusetts

**Carol Mahon Salazar,** M.D.

Clinical Instructor, Department of Medicine, New York University, New York, New York

**Grannum R. Sant,** M.D.

Professor and Vice-Chairman, Department of Urology, Tufts University School of Medicine/New England Medical Center, Boston, Massachusetts

**Diane Savarese,** M.D.

Assistant Professor, Department of Medicine, Division of Hematology/Oncology, University of Massachusetts Medical Center, Worcester, Massachusetts

**Ralph M. Schapira,** M.D.

Assistant Professor, The Clement J. Zablocki Veterans Affairs Medical Center, Pulmonary and Critical Care, The Medical College of Wisconsin, Milwaukee, Wisconsin

**Edgar C. Schick, Jr.,** M.D.

Director, Echocardiography Laboratory, Lahey Clinic Medical Center, Burlington, Massachusetts

**Harold B. Schiff,** M.D.

Assistant Professor, Department of Neurology, Tufts Medical School, Boston, Massachusetts

**Rhett M. Schiffman,** M.D., M.S.

Associate Director of Research, Department of Ophthalmology, Henry Ford Hospital, Detroit, Michigan

**Donald P. Schlueter,** M.D.

Professor, Medical College of Wisconsin, Pulmonary and Critical Care Medicine, Pulmonary Diagnostic Laboratory, Froedtert Memorial Lutheran Hospital, Milwaukee, Wisconsin

**Jeremy D. Schmahmann,** M.D.

Assistant Professor of Neurology, Department of Neurology, Massachusetts General Hospital, Harvard Medical School, Boston, Massachusetts

**Paul G. Schmitz,** M.D.

Assistant Professor of Medicine, Department of Internal Medicine, Division of Nephrology, St. Louis University School of Medicine, St. Louis, Missouri

**David J. Schoetz, Jr.,** M.D.

Associate Clinical Professor of Surgery, Boston University School of Medicine, Boston, Massachusetts, Chairman, Department of Colon and Rectal Surgery, Lahey Clinic Medical Center, Burlington, Massachusetts

**Paul C. Schroy III,** M.D.

Assistant Professor of Medicine, Department of Medicine, Section of Gastroenterology, Boston University School of Medicine, Boston, Massachusetts

**Michelle Z. Schultz,** M.D.

Assistant Professor of Medicine, Division of Medical Oncology, Washington University School of Medicine, St. Louis VA Medical Center, St. Louis, Missouri

**David A. Schwartz,** M.D.

Associate Professor of Medicine, Director of Occupational Medicine, Department of Internal Medicine, University of Iowa, Iowa City, Iowa

*Author of a chapter in Noble: *Primary Care Medicine* CD-ROM, an expanded electronic version of *Textbook of Primary Care Medicine.*

**Vanessa Gayl Schweitzer,** M.D., FACS
Clinical Professor, Department of Otolaryngology—Head and Neck Surgery, University of Michigan, Ann Arbor, Michigan, Attending Senior Staff and Division Head, Department of Otolaryngology—Head and Neck Surgery, Henry Ford Health Sciences Center, Detroit, Michigan

***David B. Seaburn,** M.S.
Assistant Professor of Psychiatry and Family Medicine, Department of Family Medicine, University of Rochester School of Medicine & Dentistry, Rochester, New York

**Michael D. Seidman,** M.D.
Assistant Clinical Professor, Department of Otolaryngology—Head and Neck Surgery, Wayne State University, Attending Physician, Department of Otolaryngology—Head and Neck Surgery, Division of Otology/Neurotology, Henry Ford Health Sciences Center, Detroit, Michigan

**Jay R. Seltzer,** M.D.
Assistant Professor of Medicine, Washington University School of Medicine, Clinical Director—Renal Stone Center, Jewish Hospital, Department of Medicine, Renal Division, Washington University School of Medicine, St. Louis, Missouri

**John S. Sergent,** M.D.
Chief Medical Officer, Vanderbilt University Medical Center, Nashville, Tennessee

**Paul A. Severson,** M.D., FACS
Clinical Assistant Professor, University of Minnesota—Duluth, Rural Physician Associate Program, Crosby, Minnesota

**Fereydoun Shahrokhi,** M.D.
Associate Clinical Professor, Department of Neurology, Boston University School of Medicine, Boston, Massachusetts

**James C. Shaw,** M.D.
Clinical Associate Professor, Department of Dermatology, Oregon Health Sciences University, Portland, Oregon

**Daniel Shine,** M.D.
Assistant Professor of Medicine, Director of Medicine, Vice Chair of Medicine, The New York Medical College, New York, New York

**Tammi L. Shlotzhauer,** M.D.
Instructor, University of Rochester, Rochester, New York

**George T. Simpson II,** M.D.
Chairman, Department of Otolaryngology, State University of New York at Buffalo, Buffalo, New York

***Mike B. Siroky,** M.D.
Professor, Department of Urology, Boston University, Boston, Massachusetts

**Barry Skarf,** Ph.D., M.D.
Director, Neuro-ophthalmology Unit, Department of Ophthalmology, Henry Ford Health Sciences Center, Detroit, Michigan

***Mindy A. Smith,** M.D., M.S.
Associate Professor, Department of Family Practice, University of Michigan, Ann Arbor, Michigan

**Leon Speroff,** M.D.
Professor, Department of Obstetrics and Gynecology, Oregon Health Sciences University, Portland, Oregon

*Author of a chapter in Noble: *Primary Care Medicine* CD-ROM, an expanded electronic version of *Textbook of Primary Care Medicine.*

**Virginia D. Steen,** M.D.
Professor of Medicine, Department of Medicine/Rheumatology, University of Georgetown, Washington, D.C.

**David W. Stepnick,** M.D.
Assistant Professor, Department of Otolaryngology—Head and Neck Surgery, Case Western Reserve University, Cleveland, Ohio

**John D. Stoeckle,** M.D.
Professor of Medicine Emeritus, Harvard Medical School, Boston, Massachusetts

**Elizabeth Gardner Stratte,** M.D.
Department of Dermatology, Oregon Health Sciences University, Portland, Oregon

**Linda M. Sutton,** M.D.
Assistant Professor of Medicine, Associate Director, Duke Oncology Outreach Service, Department of Medicine, Division of Hematology/Oncology, Duke University Medical Center, Durham, North Carolina

**Irma O. Szymanski,** M.D.
Professor of Pathology & Medicine, University of Massachusetts Medical Center, Medical Director, Blood Bank, Worcester, Massachusetts

**Bert G. Tavelli,** M.D.
Clinical Assistant Professor, Department of Dermatology, Oregon Health Sciences University, Portland, Oregon

**Michael Thane,** M.D.
Assistant Professor, Department of Medicine, Boston University School of Medicine, Boston, Massachusetts

**Ronald W. Thebarge,** Ph.D.
Clinical Assistant Professor, Department of Psychiatry and Human Behavior, Brown University School of Medicine, Providence, Rhode Island

**Basil Varkey,** M.D.
Professor of Medicine, The Medical College of Wisconsin, Chief, Pulmonary and Critical Care Section, Zablocki Veterans Affairs Medical Center, Milwaukee, Wisconsin

**Nagagopal Venna,** M.D.
Associate Professor of Neurology, Department of Neurology, Boston University School of Medicine, Director, Clinical Neurology, Neurological Unit, Boston City Hospital, Boston, Massachusetts

**Pantel S. Vokonas,** M.D.
Professor of Medicine and Public Health, Boston University School of Medicine, Boston, Massachusetts

**Barbara A. Ward,** M.D.
Assistant Professor, Director, Yale Breast Center, Department of Surgery, Yale University School of Medicine, New Haven, Connecticut

**Bruce R. Weinstein,** M.D.
Assistant Professor of Medicine, Division of Primary Care, General Medicine and Geriatrics, University of Massachusetts Medical Center, Worcester, Massachusetts

**Michael A. Werner,** M.D.
Attending, Department of Urology, White Plains Hospital, White Plains, New York

**Jocelyn C. White,** M.D.
Assistant Professor of Medicine, Department of Medicine, Legacy Good Samaritan Hospital, Oregon Health Sciences University, Portland, Oregon

**Cynthia J. Whitener,** M.D.

Assistant Professor of Medicine, Infectious Diseases, Department of Medicine, Milton S. Hershey Medical Center, Hershey, Pennsylvania

***David W. Windus,** M.D.

Associate Professor, Department of Medicine, Renal Division, Washington University School of Medicine, St. Louis, Missouri

**Lorentz E. Wittmers, Jr.,** Ph.D.

Associate Professor, Department of Medical and Molecular Physiology, University of Minnesota, Duluth, Duluth, Minnesota

***Adel S. Yaacoub,** M.D.

Fellow, Division of Cardiology, Department of Medicine, Northwestern University Medical School, Chicago, Illinois

*Author of a chapter in Noble: *Primary Care Medicine* CD-ROM, an expanded electronic version of *Textbook of Primary Care Medicine.*

**Mark J. Young,** M.D.

Associate Chairman, Department of Internal Medicine, Henry Ford Health Sciences Center, Detroit, Michigan

**Steven R. Ytterberg,** M.D.

Staff Physician, VA Medical Center, Department of Medicine, University of Minnesota, Minneapolis, Minnesota

**Bernard Zimmermann III,** M.D.

Assistant Professor of Medicine, Division of Rheumatology, Department of Medicine, Brown University School of Medicine, Providence, Rhode Island

**John J. Zurlo,** M.D.

Assistant Professor of Medicine, Department of Medicine, Pennsylvania State University, Milton S. Hershey Medical Center, Hershey, Pennsylvania

# Advisory Board

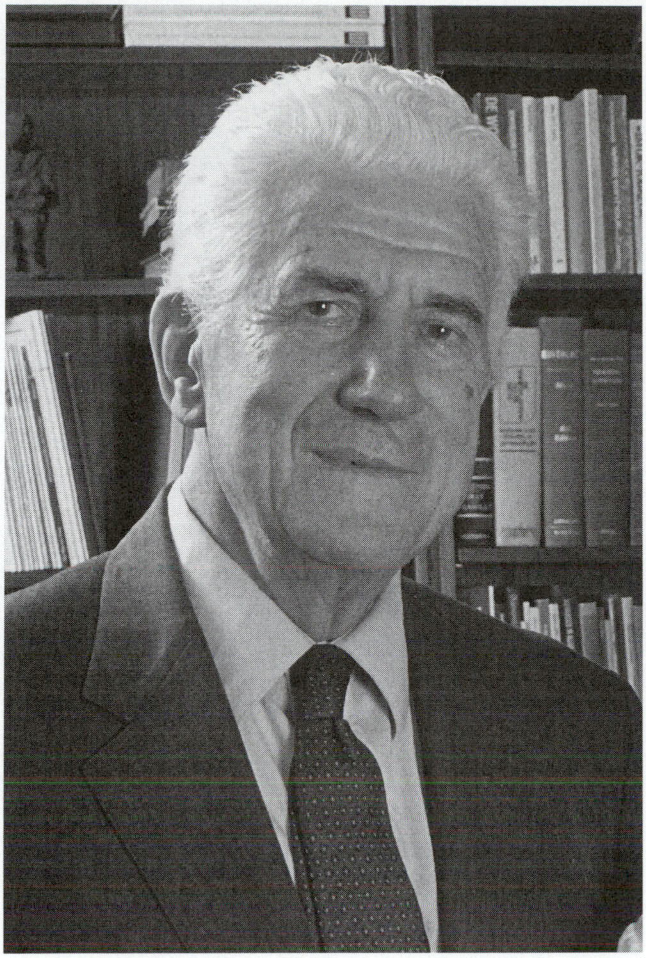

*John Ruskin Graham*

1909-1992

Masterful clinician, teacher, and friend,
*Jack Graham* was both an expert generalist
and a generalist's expert in the
evaluation and treatment of headache.
With his vast knowledge, keen sense of humor,
compassion, and caring,
he was a superb mentor and role model of the
compleat physician.

# Preface

A busy day with patients in the office brought many questions. All too often, discovering the answers was difficult, whether I found myself in a rural practice or at a major teaching hospital. I realized that there was no effective reference text to support the modern practicing primary care physician, be he or she an internist, family practitioner, surgeon, or specialist by training. I decided to record my cases and experiences, in the tradition of John Fry and Keith Hodgkin, and use them as the organizational basis for a textbook of general and primary care medicine.

Three myths perpetuated in academic centers distort the concept of primary care practice. These myths suggest that (1) most of the very sick patients are treated in major teaching hospitals; (2) only specialists see really interesting and rare diseases; and (3) primary care physicians are not knowledgeable like specialists. These myths were rapidly dispelled for me and my colleagues by our years in rural primary care, where practice required broad and thorough knowledge; where an ever-changing array of patients with common, uncommon, and rare conditions came to see us every day; and where very sick patients needed all the resources that we could mobilize for their relief.

The clinical presentation and management of the illnesses and problems of primary care as it is actually practiced, therefore, have served as the major focus for this text. The principles to be followed and pitfalls to be avoided in diagnosis and treatment are stressed.

*Textbook of Primary Care Medicine* is a state-of-the-art medical information system comprised of a comprehensive clinical text and a CD-ROM designed for today's busy primary care physician. This edition has been completely reorganized and rewritten to provide up-to-date information on the broad field of primary care medicine. The text has become a truly national work with distinguished senior editors and authors from all parts of the nation who are leaders in their fields. It presents up-to-date Managed Care Guides for the diagnosis and treatment of patients in this managed care era.

The new section on women's health provides comprehensive information (in nine chapters) on the special health problems of women, as well as the many common diseases that affect women differently than men. Special chapters on fever of unknown origin and on fever with rash provide up-to-date, detailed information on these challenging problems in primary care. The musculoskeletal diseases section is expanded to present extensive reference information on sports injuries, repetitive motion, and specific joint related problems that commonly present to the busy practitioner.

Psychosocial and behavioral medicine are masterfully presented in fifteen chapters by authors who are the founders of the internationally acclaimed Academy of the Doctor and Patient. Medical interviewing, counseling of couples and families, eating disorders, death and dying, and the health problems of gay men and lesbian women are a sample of subjects covered. Patient centered care, family dynamics, the human life cycle, and occupational and environmental health are featured on the CD, as well as the cardinal manifestations of common diseases. Nationally acclaimed authors have contributed to every section of the text and to the CD-ROM to form a comprehensive primary care information system.

This *Textbook of Primary Care Medicine* is intended to serve as a valuable reference in the office, the clinic, and the emergency room. The information that it contains reflects the commonality of medical experience shared by generalists and specialists. To capture the traditions and the essence of primary care we have incorporated a few pictures of doctors and their patients and original figures that still accurately describe clinical conditions. My colleagues and I have sought to create an extensive source of knowledge and experience to aid all physicians in the practice of general medicine and primary care.

**JOHN NOBLE**

# Acknowledgments

The *Textbook of Primary Care Medicine* is the product of careful planning and the scholarship of all of our contributors: authors, section editors, senior editors, the advisory board, and publishers. The enthusiastic support of Stephanie Manning, Medical Editor of Mosby, in expanding the original text to include a CD-ROM has enabled us to create this primary care information system. We greatly appreciate her vision and guidance, as well as the invaluable assistance of Carolyn Malik, Laura DeYoung, David Stein, Carol Weis, Sheilah Barrett, and their colleagues at Mosby.

In this second edition, we have established the *Textbook of Primary Care Medicine* as a truly national work by appointing outstanding educators as Senior Editors and expanding authorship to include leading authorities from all regions of the country. We greatly appreciate the enthusiastic support that our medical artist, May H. Lesser, has given to this work.

There are many individuals who have helped our editors. Special acknowledgments are extended to Dr. Stephen R. Jones for his support of Wendy Levinson, in all of her professional activities, as well as to James Shaw, her spouse and editor and major contributor to the Dermatology Section. For Harry Greene, special thanks are given to his wife, Linda; his children, Harry III, Michele, and Jennifer; and his parents, Harry and Helen Greene. Dr. Greene also acknowledges his student support group at the University of Arizona. Geoffrey Modest acknowledges the extra support of Julie Kaufmann, his spouse and contributor; to their sons, Zachary, Jacob, and Nicholas; and to our colleagues, Arthur Eskew and Leonor Fernandez. Mark Young gives special thanks to Ellen Bishop, and Erica and Suzanne Young. Finally, Ewa Kuligowska-Noble, spouse and radiologic consultant, has greatly assisted the Editor-in-Chief.

**JOHN NOBLE**

# Contents

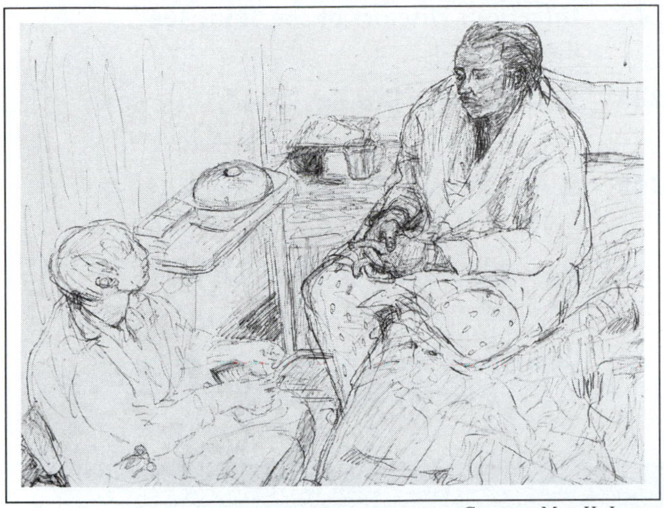

Courtesy May H. Lesser

PART ONE

## Special Topics in Primary Care

John Noble, Geoffrey A. Modest, Senior Editors;
John Noble, Section Editor



PART TWO

## Systemic Disease in Primary Care

### CARDIOVASCULAR DISEASE I

Harry L. Greene II, Senior Editor;
Joseph S. Alpert, Section Editor

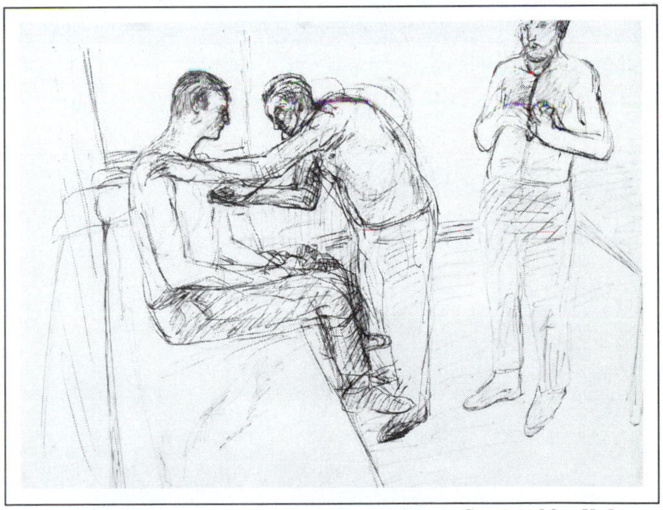

Courtesy May H. Lesser

## II DERMATOLOGY

Wendy Levinson, Senior Editor;
Frank Parker, James C. Shaw, Section Editors

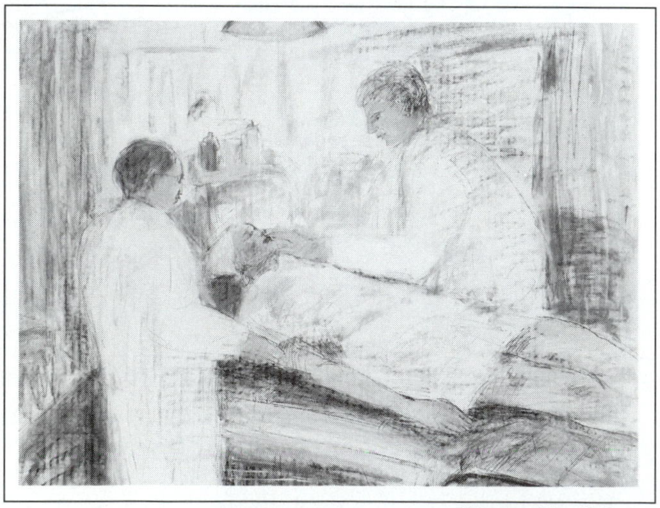

Courtesy May H. Lesser



## EAR, NOSE, AND THROAT III

Mark J. Young, Senior Editor;
Michael S. Benninger, Section Editor

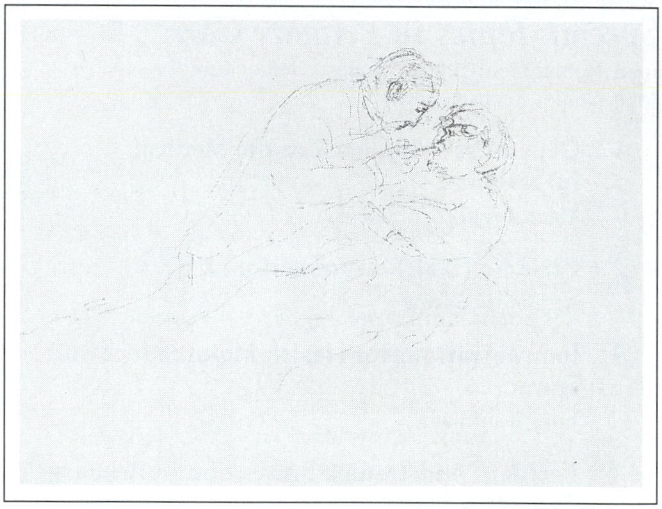

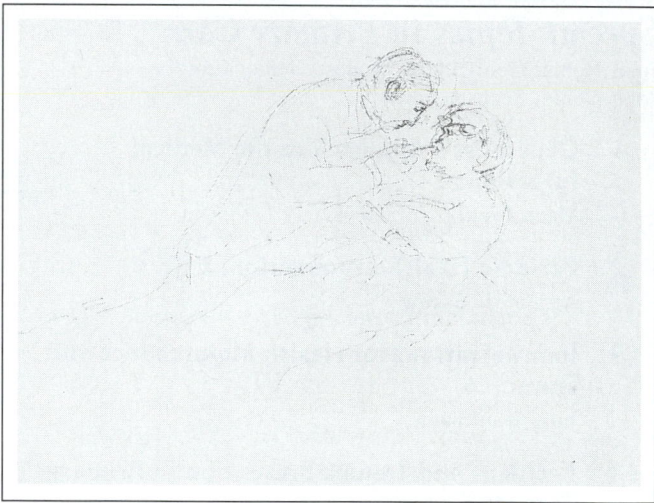

Courtesy May H. Lesser

## IV ENDOCRINE, DIABETES, AND METABOLISM

Geoffrey A. Modest, Senior Editor;
Stuart R. Chipkin, Section Editor

Courtesy May H. Lesser



## GASTROINTESTINAL DISEASE V

John Noble, Senior Editor; J. Thomas LaMont, Section Editor

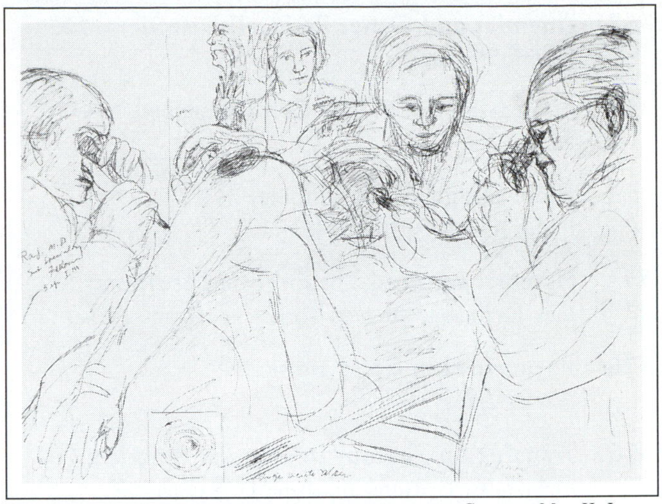

Courtesy May H. Lesser

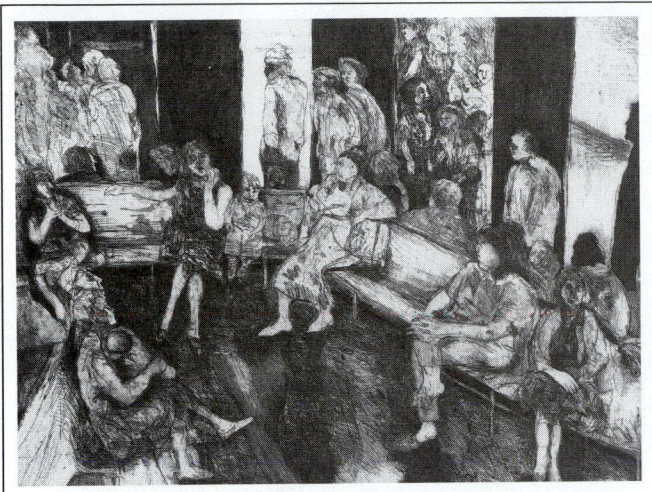

## VI HEMATOLOGY/ONCOLOGY

Harry L. Greene II, Senior Editor;
Jack E. Ansell, Section Editor



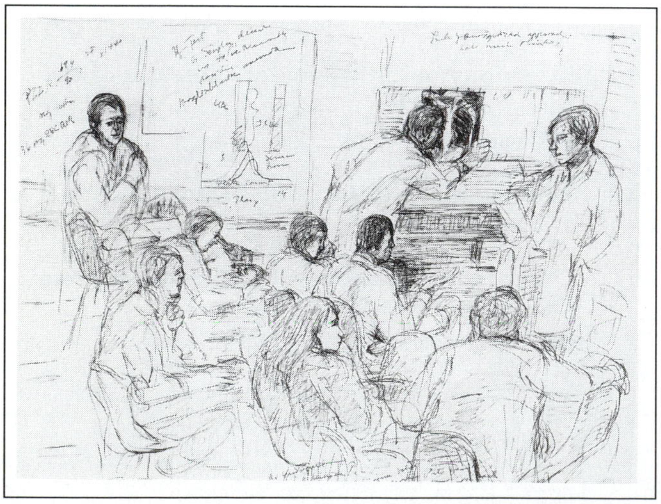

Courtesy May H. Lesser

## INFECTIOUS DISEASE VII

Mark J. Young, Senior Editor;
Nelson M. Gantz, Section Editor

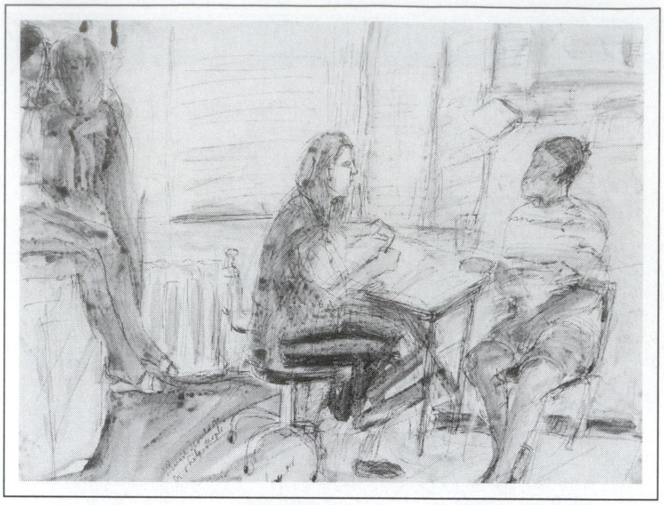

Courtesy May H. Lesser



## MUSCULOSKELETAL VIII

Harry L. Greene II, Senior Editor;
David F. Giansiracusa, Section Editor

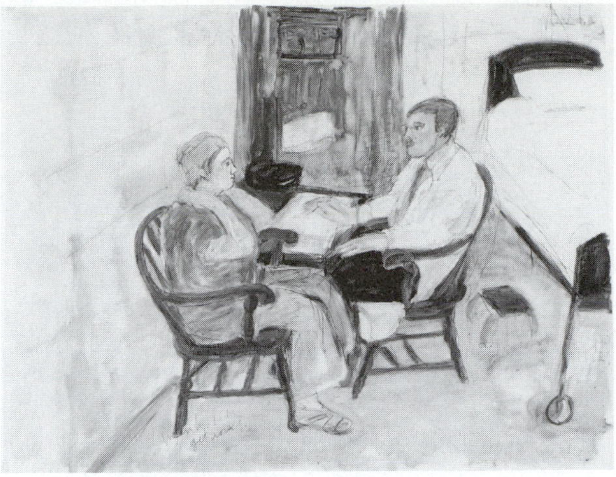

Courtesy May H. Lesser



## NEPHROLOGY IX

Geoffrey A. Modest, Senior Editor;
Saulo Klahr, Section Editor

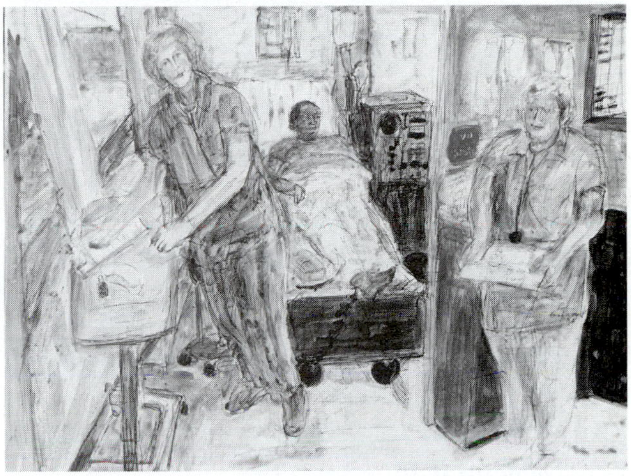

Courtesy May H. Lesser

## X NEUROLOGY

John Noble, Senior Editor; Thomas D. Sabin, Section Editor

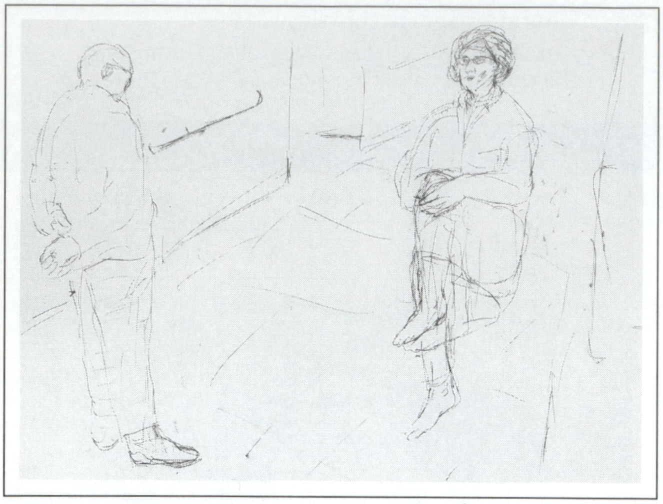

Courtesy May H. Lesser



## XI OPHTHALMOLOGY

Mark J. Young, Senior Editor;
Julian J. Nussbaum, Section Editor



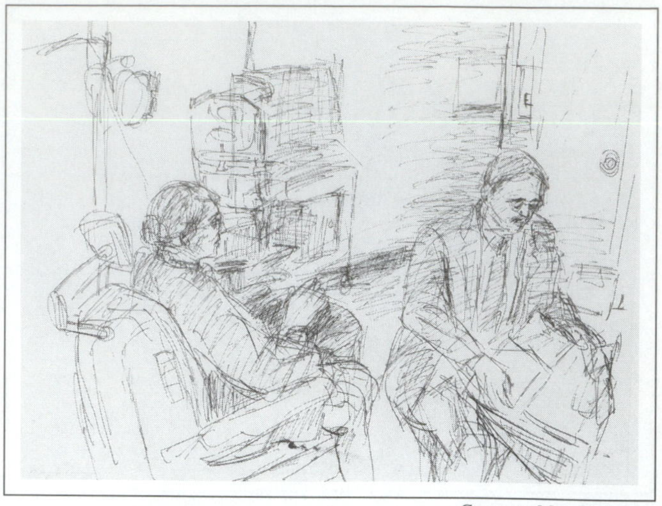

Courtesy May H. Lesser



## PULMONARY DISEASE XII

Mark J. Young, Senior Editor;
Richard M. Effros, Section Editor

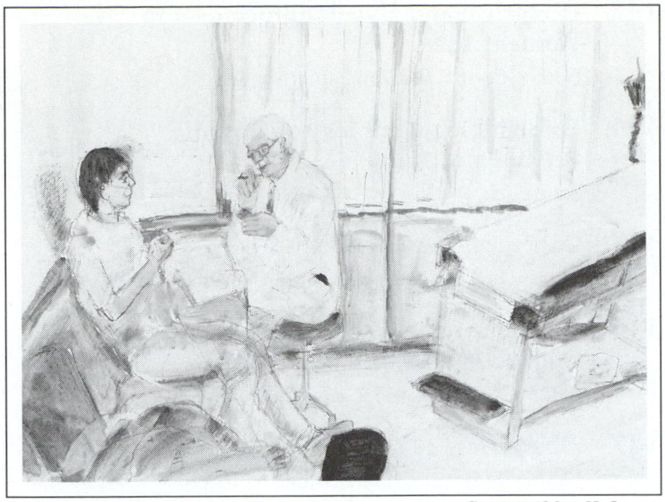

Courtesy May H. Lesser



## XIII PSYCHOSOCIAL AND BEHAVIORAL ISSUES

Wendy Levinson, Senior Editor;
Mack Lipkin, Jr., Section Editor

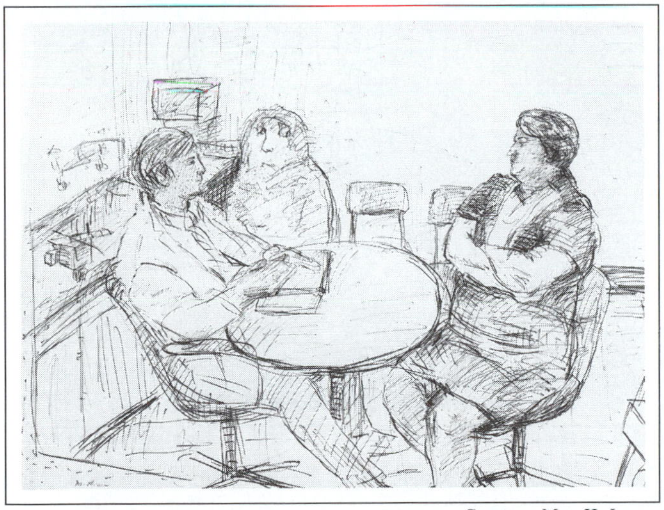

Courtesy May H. Lesser



## UROLOGY XIV

John Noble, Senior Editor; Robert J. Krane, Section Editor

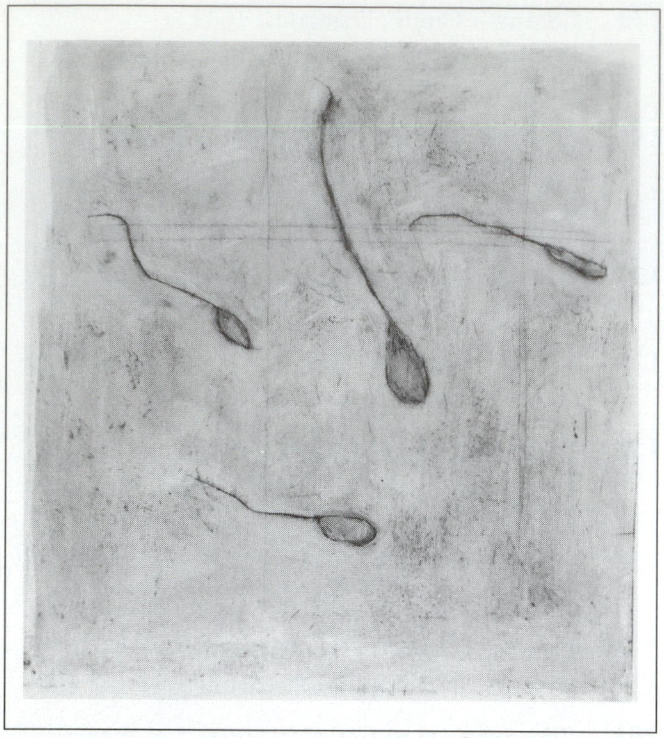

Courtesy May H. Lesser



## XV WOMEN'S HEALTH

Wendy Levinson, Senior Editor;
Janet B. Henrich, Section Editor



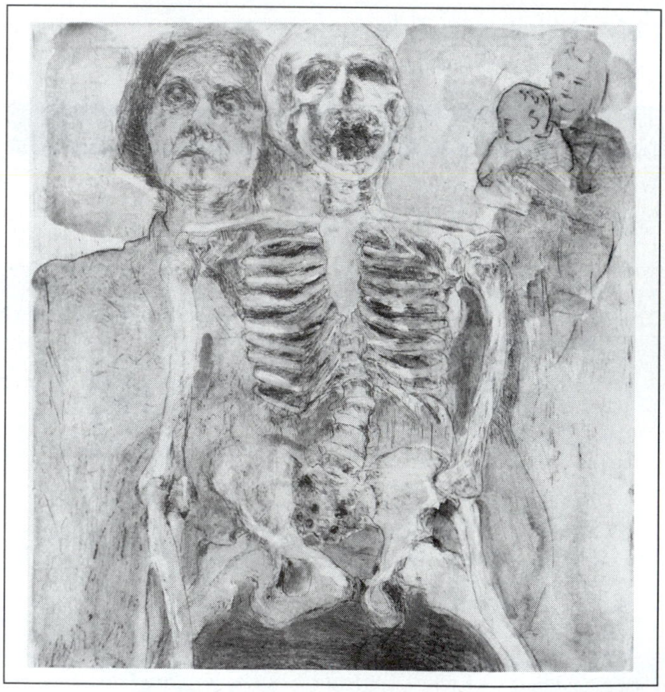

Courtesy May H. Lesser

# Chapters Found Exclusively in the CD ROM Version

# Introduction

## On Entering the Practice of Medicine: A Guide to Transition

John Noble
Clifton R. Cleaveland
Robert B. Copeland

Medicine and the health care industry are in the midst of major changes in 1995. They include fiscal constraint and cost reductions, quality improvement, and workforce reform. Despite the uncertainties caused by these actions, applications to medical school are at an all time high and physicians still occupy a respected role in society. Since earliest recorded history the practice of medicine has been a challenging and rewarding career. Medical diagnosis and treatment remain one of the most exciting and potentially satisfying careers. While treating the problems described in this text, physicians must continually make decisions that bear on their clinical practice, their families, and their own personal lives. The wisdom and appropriateness of these decisions will not only shape their lives but may also determine the success of their careers.

The demands of clinical practice are of such magnitude that it is essential that career goals and the tasks of practice be viewed from a healthy perspective. The double task of the physician as a clinician was well described by Dana Atchley in 1954:

> It is thus apparent that the physician of today, at his or her best, represents a fusion of the healer and the scientist.

This fusion of precise scientific knowledge and compassionate understanding leads to the highly personal relationships that develop between patients and physicians as they work together over time. It is from these relationships that the unique rewards of medical practice are derived. Although the rewards of practice are great, they are not easily attained unless careful planning and preparation are done before heavy commitments of service and time are made.

This introduction reviews a few basic principles of planning and preparing for practice. It is our goal to alert the reader, the physician already in or contemplating primary care practice, to some of the pitfalls and complications of practice.

### EVOLUTIONARY CHANGES IN MEDICAL PRACTICE

Physicians have traditionally attached high value to autonomy. This autonomy was reflected until recently in the prevalence of solo or small group practices as the dominant arrangement for clinical practice. Two forces have stimulated consolidation of practices into larger entities in recent years. By pooling resources, larger groups of physicians can offer broader diagnostic and therapeutic services. In addition, administrative overhead can often be more effectively controlled in a larger practice setting.

Although large single specialty and multispecialty group practices have thrived in various settings across America, the stimulus toward consolidation has intensified through pressure from the health insurance industry. New practice entities representing a veritable alphabet soup of organizations (IPAs, PPOs, PHOs, HMOs) have developed in response to business and industrial desires to control health care expenditures. The guiding principle of these

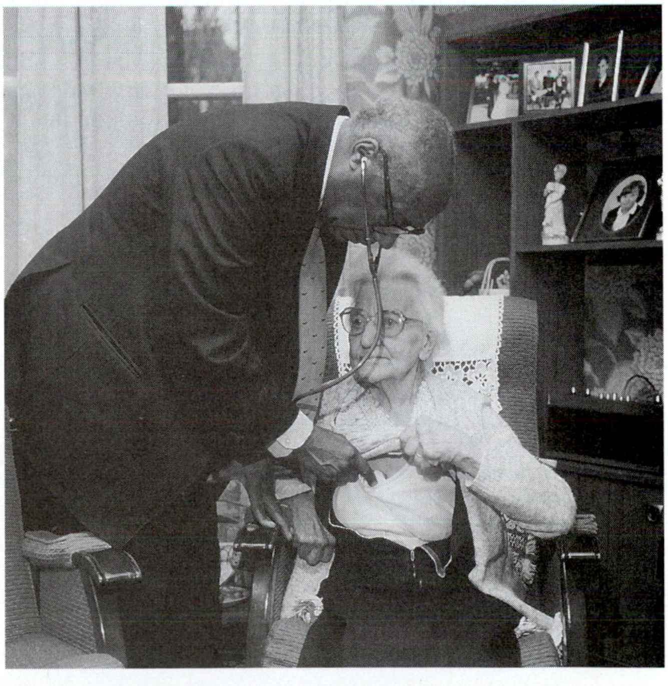

**Fig. 1.** Male general practice doctor using a stethoscope to examine an elderly woman patient's chest. (From St. Bartholomew's Hospital/Science Photo Library.)

organizations is a contractual relationship through which physicians discount their traditional fees and agree to administrative oversight in exchange for access to a defined group of patients. In its simplest form, such managed care arrangements involve a discount of traditional fee for service. In its most complex form, physicians are salaried by a health maintenance organization, which provides comprehensive health care services at a fixed price to its clients.

The traditional solo practice or small group practice may participate as an independent contractor in several managed care plans. Alternatively, the practice may be owned by a large health management system that will determine the market to be served. In the most complex systems, the physician may be part of a vertically integrated health care network that will involve a complete array of inpatient and outpatient clinical services. Typically, such a network will include preventive and rehabilitative services, as well as long-term care. Physicians may work in such structures with a variety of health care professionals, including traditional nurses, physician assistants, nurse practitioners, clinical psychologists, and social workers.

Ferment and experimentation characterize clinical practice in the final decade of the century.

## PREPARATION FOR PRACTICE

Knowledge of self is fundamentally important in making the decision to begin clinical practice in a particular location. This understanding should be based on a realistic appraisal of personal motivation, ambition, strengths and weaknesses, needs, and experiences. It is important to consider the special attributes of mentors, teachers, and role models when assessing one's goals. The careers of these men and women are the standards beside which the physician will measure his or her own success in the future.

One needs to hold opinions not only about one's professional capability but also about what one stands for and wants to be thought of by peers and family. Without effective consideration of these simple-sounding but often elusive principles, entering the practice of medicine is unnecessarily precarious.

The attributes of an able clinician entering clinical practice were described by David Seegal as follows:

- Good training maintained by continuing scholarship
- A sense of value that distinguishes the important from the unimportant
- Appropriate and efficient patient management
- Interest in people and communications
- Knowledge of both the patient and the case
- Ability to work hard, not dictated by the clock
- Punctuality
- Knowledge of limitations and willingness to seek help
- Pride in work well done
- Ability to pace oneself
- Commitment to the Golden Rule when making difficult decisions
- Ability to bring out the best and to inspire confidence in contemporaries
- A demeanor of enthusiasm and equanimity.

These attributes are magnificent professional goals: they are also consistent with and descriptive of many attributes of an ideal spouse, parent, and person.

Self-knowledge and an assessment of one's values and desires are a guide to the next stage: planning for practice. It is important to clarify one's preferences for lifestyle, geography, type of practice, and size of community. Cultural, ethnic, and religious orientation should be considered, as well as the needs of one's spouse and children.

## HOW TO SELECT A PRACTICE

Practice planning ideally should be conducted throughout training and should involve one's spouse from the beginning. Plans should be made to explore potential practice opportunities. In addition to the professional features of a given practice location, one must consider the geographic area as a place to live. Are ample educational, religious, and cultural resources available? Are the recreational opportunities appealing? Is there an employment opportunity for one's spouse? Special education and child-rearing resources? Can family ties be maintained from this location, and is the community one to be happy with?

The physician entering practice in the late 1990s will most likely be a part of a group practice. Because of the time spent with practice colleagues and because of the trust that must permeate a practice, great care is required in evaluating and selecting potential partners. The practice can work only if there are shared values that relate to such key issues as quality of patient care, postgraduate continuing medical education, and reimbursement. If the physician is to join an established practice, he must learn how that practice is regarded by the local medical community, the local medical society, the leadership of affiliated hospitals, and civic and business leaders, as well as how physicians in other practices and other disciplines regard the practice.

## VISITING A PRACTICE

Visiting a prospective practice and community is a crucial step in the decision-making process. While seeking answers to the aforementioned questions and concerns, it is important to meet not only with physicians but also with hospital administrators, nurses, community leaders, and local citizens. These individuals may provide valuable insight and information. Such meetings also afford them an opportunity to meet and form opinions about the prospective physician. Important future relationships may develop from these initial encounters. Disparagement or an apparent lack of respect, even if unintended, may be long remembered by the people visited. Each person met during an evaluation site visit is a potential friend, patient, and source of referrals.

The larger medical community requires careful scrutiny as well. Hospitals with which the potential practice is affiliated deserve an unhurried visit to meet with the CEO, laboratory, and x-ray heads and other staff leaders. Does the hospital offer programs in continuing education? Is the library up-to-date, and does it offer electronic information retrieval services? Are the patient care areas, intensive care units, and emergency room facilities appropriately staffed and equipped? The reputation of the practice can be no better than that of its inpatient partner.

The importance of a personal, carefully planned evaluation of a practice and community during multiple visits cannot be overemphasized. There is simply no satisfactory substitute for getting to know the people with whom one will be personally involved and on whom one will have to depend for many years. Getting to know the physicians in a practice ideally should include working with them in their offices, as well as visiting with them socially. One should start the search for a practice location at least 12 months before finishing residency or fellowship training in order to have adequate time for careful evaluation.

Beyond the immediate office and hospital environment, the larger professional community merits scrutiny. Is the medical community collegial, or is it characterized by factionalism and in-fighting? What are the relationships of the practice to the other offices and disciplines within the community? What subspecialists are available for consultation, and how well trained are they? The primary care physician depends crucially upon a team approach in caring for his patients, and thus it is appropriate to know just who those teammates will be.

Since the knowledge base for clinical practice evolves so rapidly, the opportunities for continuing education must be a part of the new practice environment. These educational needs will require access to formal programs as well as the time necessary for participation, study, and reflection. Perhaps no single factor defines a potential medical community better than the value it attaches to continued professional and intellectual growth.

It is best to be circumspect and to seek a variety of opinions, not only about the quality of the practice being considered, but also about realtors, banks, school districts, and other aspects of the greater community. Hasty decisions that result in poor choices may prove to be difficult, time-consuming, and expensive to rectify. The aphorism "Never fall in love with something until you own it and never fall out of love with it until you sell it" applies to practice selection. Falling in love with one feature of a potential site and failing to determine, or ignoring, major problems is a common mistake. A mistake in practice selection can be ill afforded when one considers the wrenching effect on oneself and one's family and the monetary cost of relocating to another practice. Recognizing what one does not know and applying principles of problem solving is just as important when starting up a practice as it is, subsequently, in diagnosing and treating a clinical problem.

For the married physician, the selection of a practice site and arrangement is necessarily a marital decision. The physician can be happy only if the community offers the potential for happiness and fulfillment for spouse and children alike.

## CONTRACT ANALYSIS

Typically, medical contracts are lengthy and filled with arcane terminology. No contract should be signed until analyzed by both an independent attorney and accountant. The cost involved in this analysis is trivial compared to the financial implications of the contractual document. Following are key revisions to consider:

1. Length of service required to become a full partner.
2. Amount of stock or accounts receivable that must be purchased to become a full partner.
3. Division of clinical and administrative responsibilities among all of the physicians in the practice.
4. Conditions under which a new physician may be dismissed from the practice.
5. Sickness, disability, and vacation benefits.
6. Presence of any no-compete clauses in the event the physician leaves the practice.

The contract represents an important guarantee of rights at the same time it details responsibilities. The contract must not be treated casually.

## TRANSITION TO PRACTICE

The transition from trainee to practicing physician or from a practice in one community to a practice in a new community demands a great amount of time and attention. During this period, many other transitions are also taking place of which the physician must be aware. The establishment of new relationships for the entire family—physician, spouse, and children—throughout the community is time-consuming and can be stressful. During this time many unfamiliar demands will be made on the physician's time, energy, and judgment. While working industriously to establish the practice, the physician will want to ensure that all members of the family make a happy and healthy adjustment to the new community.

## MANAGEMENT OF TIME

From the very beginning of medical practice attention must be paid to the management of time. Unfortunately, many physicians become very busy before they have clearly established their goals and defined their plans for practice. The pressure of their increasingly busy business life may lead them to devote less time to organizing their practice and their lives. The longer one proceeds with a poorly understood and disorganized work activity, the harder it is to change to a more satisfactory mode of practice. Limits must be set to ensure that there is time to provide excellent care to individual patients, to relate effectively with colleagues, and to interact with one's family. During this period of transition it is essential to maintain an openness to suggestions, learning from one's colleagues, and others who live in the community, about ways to cope with professional, personal, and family needs. From the outset, one must design a balanced daily routine. Mealtimes in the evening with the family should be protected, and there should be time for rest and recreation. On-call systems must be arranged to provide protected time and peace of mind.

Such a healthy balance in one's total life may make it easier to carry the heavy responsibilities that are inherent in a physician's practice. These responsibilities were well described by Albert Schweitzer during his first months at the mission hospital in Lambarene-Gabon:

> The actual work, heavy as it was, I found a lighter burden than the care and responsibility which came with it. I belong unfortunately to the number of those medical men who have not the robust temperament which is desirable in that calling, and are so consumed with unceasing anxiety about the condition of their severe cases and of those on whom they have operated. In vain have I tried to train myself to that equanimity which makes it possible for a doctor, in spite of all his sympathy with the sufferings of his patients, to husband, as is desirable, his spiritual and nervous energy.

Daumier depicted these same worries and concerns almost 100 years earlier.

The concern engendered by the care of sick patients is an unending reality in primary care and many other forms

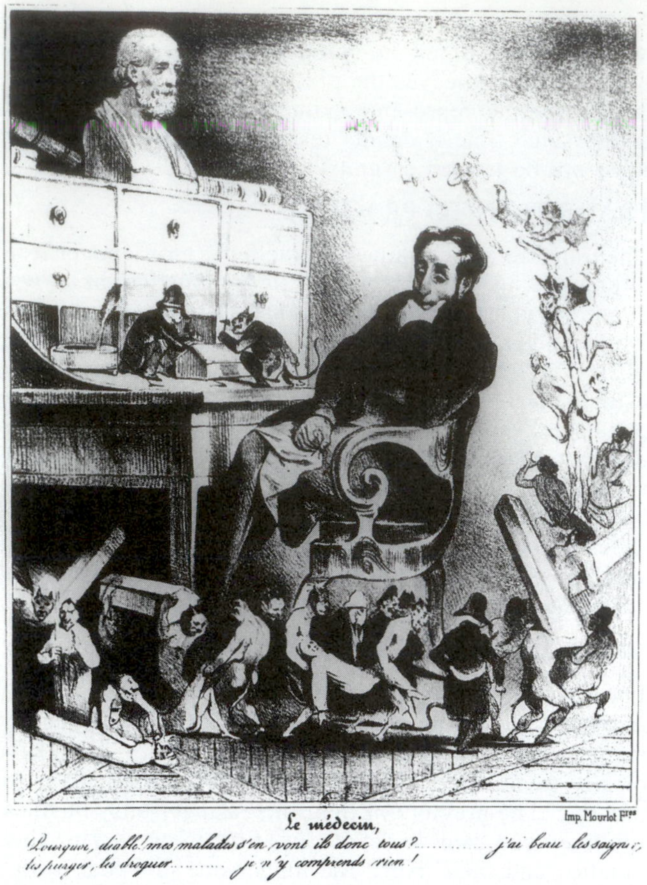
Le médecin,
Pourquoi, diable! mes malades s'en vont ils donc tous? .......... j'ai beau les saigner,
les purger, les droguer ......... je n'y comprends rien!
Imp. Mourlot Frès

**Fig. 2.** The Doctor: "How the devil does it happen that all my patients succumb . . . yet I bleed them, I physic them, I drug them . . . I simply can't understand." (Honoré Daumier, August 19, 1833.)

of medical practice. When the burden becomes unduly heavy, it is time to get help through appropriate and effective consultation and the sharing of responsibility with physicians and other allied health professionals.

## SATISFACTIONS OF PRACTICE

The satisfactions of primary medical care often are diluted by the constant responsibility and the less than successful outcomes that are inevitably true of some cases. In the midst of a busy practice it is easy to overlook successes and to dwell extensively on problems that have been resolved less happily or not at all.

During a transition into a new practice it is very helpful to maintain a list of three types of outcome. The first list should tally all instances of a particularly good outcome. Cures, early and prompt diagnoses, successful treatment, and effective management of complex problems should be noted briefly in a practice ledger.

It is equally important to list problems that could have been avoided or might have been solved if a diagnosis had been made earlier or if a different diagnostic test or therapy had been used. E. A. Codman stated in 1900 that it was the *end result* in medicine that counted the most, not the great diagnosis, the successful operation, or the special treatment. The second list is an excellent way to learn from one's experience and to prevent technical and systems problems from undermining the quality of care—e.g., misfiled lab reports, inappropriately handled telephone messages, and interruptions that lessen one's sensitivity to a patient's history. With such an inventory of relative wins and losses the physician maintains an internal check on his or her own effectiveness and is able to review those cases in which clinical knowledge and practice proved adequate and those in which a more desirable end result might have been achieved.

On a third sheet, a list should be kept of all expected and unexpected deaths that occur in the practice. Sudden death is often preceded by a visit to the physician. A review of the records of these patients may uncover clues that will make an earlier diagnosis possible in the future, or lead to the prevention and/or treatment of a problem.

## SUMMARY

Medical practice is a challenging proposition that offers many rewards. Success is dependent on professional excellence, effective communication, and good planning. Good planning must be a continuing process, directed by the input and feedback of information, data, and the outcomes of practice. It begins with a knowledge of self and extends to knowledge of opportunities, practice sites, and communities. Good planning must continue throughout the entire course of a career in practice. It determines the success of a career to the same degree that effective education ensures continued professional excellence.

With a foundation of solid planning the practitioner will find that no career is more satisfying, nor blessed with greater opportunity, variety, or responsibility, than that of being a successful physician in community practice. The clinical practice of primary care medicine remains a thrilling endeavor. Continuing care of patients who present with the widest variety of physical and psychological complaints stretches the intellect and broadens the sympathies as no other profession. The doctor/patient relationship, in essence, is the partnership which will define, inform, and enrich the life of the practitioner.

## BIBLIOGRAPHY


Atchley DW: The healer and the scientist, *Saturday Review* January 9, 1954.

Brent RL, Brent LH: Medicine: an excuse from living, *Res Staff Phys* 24(12):61, 1978.

Codman EA: *A study in hospital efficiency,* Boston, 1916, Thomas Todd.

Duffy JC: *Emotional issues in the lives of physicians,* Springfield, IL, 1970, Thomas.

Fine C: *Married to medicine: an intimate portrait of doctors' wives,* New York, 1981, Atheneum.

Hippocrates: Aphorisms. In *The genuine works of Hippocrates,* translated from the Greek by Francis Adams. New York, 1849, William Wood & Co.

Hippocrates: The Oath. In *The genuine works of Hippocrates,* translated from the Greek by Francis Adams. New York, 1849, William Wood & Co.

Jackson J: *Letters to a young physician just entering upon practice,* Boston, 1855, Hobart & Robins.

*Life,* October 1959. Quoted in Dubos R: *Man adapting,* New Haven, 1965, Yale University Press.

McCue JD: *Private practice: surviving the first year,* Lexington, Ma, 1982, Collamore Press.

Modlin HC, Montes A: Narcotic addiction in physicians, *Am J Psychiatry* 121:358, 1964.

Osler W: *Aequanimitas,* Philadelphia, 1914, P. Blakiston's Son & Co.

Ross M: Suicide among physicians, *Psychiatry Med* 2:189, 1971.

Schweitzer A: *Out of my life and thought,* C.T. Campion, translator. New York, 1949, Henry Holt.

Seegal D: Never a dull day for the compleat physician, *Pharos* 26:7, 1963.

Sox HC, Margulies I, Sox CH: Psychologically mediated effects of diagnostic tests, *Ann Intern Med* 95:680, 1982.

Thomas RB, Luber SA, Smith JA: A survey of alcohol and drug use in medical students, *Dis Nerv Syst* 38:41, 1977.

# TEXTBOOK OF PRIMARY CARE MEDICINE

# PART ONE

# Special Topics in Primary Care

CHAPTER

# 1 Generalist's Approach to the Medical Interview

**Mack Lipkin, Jr.**
**Wendy Levinson**

The medical interview is the primary care physician's most powerful and efficient tool. It is also the most utilized. A full-time generalist practitioner conducts at least 160,000 interviews in the course of a 40-year career. Among other things, the interview determines the set of problems worked on, the accuracy and completeness of the data used in clinical reasoning, the satisfaction of both patient and physician, the nature of the physician-patient relationship, and the degree of compliance achieved in the care process. It determines how well one knows one's patient and how fully one understands the context of the illness and the patient's views and attitudes about it. Each of these is crucial to effective and satisfying care.

## WHAT MAKES AN INTERVIEW EFFICIENT?

Several factors make the interview and patient care process efficient. Most important among these are getting the problem straight to begin with, listening and observing actively at several levels simultaneously (e.g., the story, how it is told, affect, and mental status), detecting and correcting barriers to communication (e.g., patient deafness, delirium), creating an efficient structure, completing the three functions of the interview, and using correct technique. In this chapter we present the interview as having structure and functions. The interview's 10 structural elements and three functions are shown in the box below. Table 1-1 shows some common errors leading to inefficiency and possible solutions.

### Structure and functions of the interview

**Structural elements**

Preparing
  Self
  Office environment
Opening
Setting the agenda for the visit
Assessing a problem
Allowing patients to tell the story in their own words; establishing narrative thread
Using open to closed cones of questions
Understanding the patient as a person
Understanding the setting of the illness
Eliciting patients' beliefs about the problem
Closure

**Functions**

Gathering information
Developing and maintaining a relationship
Communicating information and patient education

**Table 1-1.** Common practices leading to inefficiency

| | Problem | Potential solution |
|---|---|---|
| **Early part of interview** | Being distracted by other patient concerns | Take a moment to get prepared, hand off beeper, take no calls |
| | Keeping patient waiting | Inform patients about delays and apologize to them |
| | Lacking medical data (e.g., lab) | Review relevant data beforehand |
| | Not knowing patient's name | Check beforehand |
| | Overlooking patient discomfort or distress | Observe and address directly |
| | Premature interruptions | Allow time for patient to complete opening statement |
| | Not eliciting all reasons for visit early on | Ask "What else?" |
| | Imposing own agenda | Negotiate |
| **Middle of interview** | Long lists of close-ended questions | Open-ended questions; use open to closed cone |
| | Delaying social history until after history of present problem | Interweave social history naturally |
| | Interrupting patient story and directing conversation | Allow patient to tell story; build narrative thread |
| **End of interview** | Assuming patient can remember everything | Write instructions<br>Give pamphlets on diseases |
| | Failing to check patient beliefs about diagnosis | Ask what patient thinks |
| | Not checking for patient questions | Ask if patient has questions |
| | Assuming patient agrees with treatment | Elicit patient opinion |
| | Assuming patient can implement | Ask what parts will be difficult |
| | Giving too much treatment advice at once | Simplify; write it down; give patient pamphlets about problem |

## STRUCTURE

### Preparing self and environment

Effective preparation of the office environment, the medical data, and oneself can make the interview more efficient and effective. Usually patients first come in contact with the office by phone and then by interacting with office staff in the reception area or waiting room. The quality of all these initial interactions can have a significant effect on patients before they even meet the physician. Patients who have waited for a long time without explanation or who have had negative interactions with the office staff may be irritated, making a barrier to effective communication (Fig. 1-1). The environment of the consultation or examination room may also be important to the interview. Ensuring privacy, avoiding unnecessary distractions, and creating a comfortable seating environment for patients indicate concern and readiness on the part of the physician to address patient needs.

Preparation of the medical data can significantly increase the efficiency of the interview. Use of structured questionnaires that patients complete before meeting with the physician may provide clues about issues patients want to discuss. These forms can be particularly useful with new patients for efficient collection of data related to family history, allergies, and pertinent social history, but they generate many false positives and negatives. For return patients, reviewing recent laboratory data, x-ray reports, and other results before the interview can help the physician maximize use of the interview time. Review of pertinent medical data before the visit also indicates that the physician has been thoughtful about the patient's problem since the last visit. This communicates the physician's concern for the patient and may enhance the sense of trust.

In addition to preparing the environment and the data, the physician is well advised to take a moment for self-preparation. There are many distractions in a busy day, and taking a moment on the threshold of the consultation room to look at the chart, take a deep breath, and prepare psychologically to work with the next patient increases effectiveness by focusing attention on the present task.

### The opening

The opening moments of the interview are critical in the relationship between the physician and patient and the effectiveness of the visit. From the moment the examination room door opens, the physician starts learning about the patient by actively observing mood, grooming, style of dress, and other nonverbal factors. These clues help in understanding the patient. The physician can use these initial nonverbal clues to make the patient more comfortable (e.g., "You look like you are in some discomfort. Can I help to make you more comfortable before we begin?").

The physician starts the visit by greeting the patient and introducing himself or herself to new patients. These greetings set the tone, helping the patient to feel welcome. Asking patients what they prefer to be called (Ms., Mr., Dr., John, Jack), communicates respect for patient preferences.

After introductions, we usually begin by eliciting the reason for the visit with open-ended questions like, "What is the problem that brings you here today?" or "What concerns have led to your visit today?" Studies support the importance of letting patients complete the opening statement about their concerns uninterrupted. Interrupting the patient before completion of the initial statement may be interpreted as a lack of interest or a lack of time. Furthermore, interrupting early in the interview may lead the patient to delay expressing real concerns until late in the visit or not at all. Although physicians often worry that the patient will take too long, most patients complete their opening statement within 90 seconds and provide important historic details.

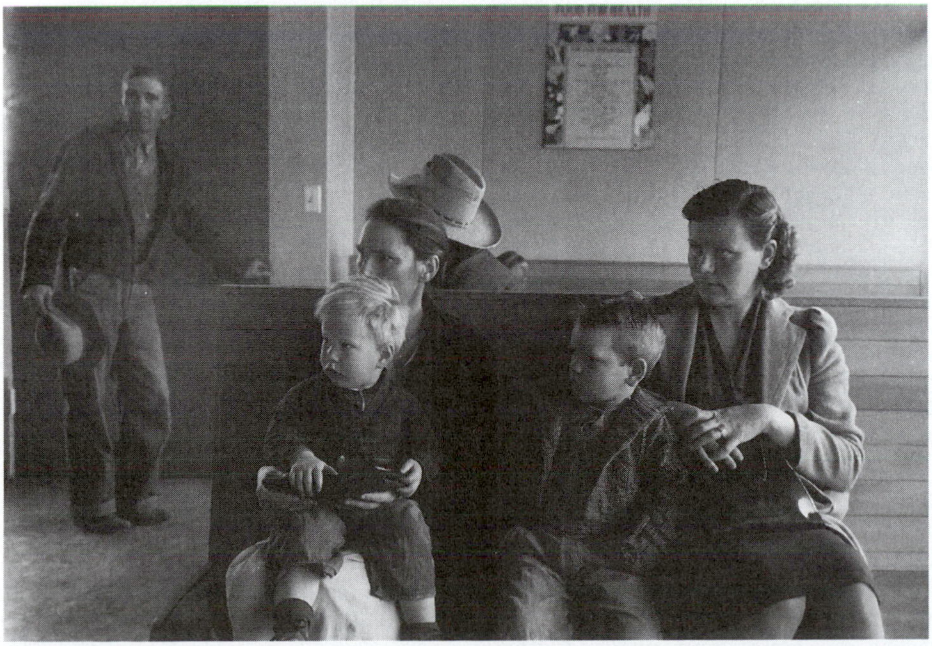

**Fig. 1-1.** Patients in waiting room. (From the Collections of the Library of Congress.)

After the patient has explained the initial concern, it is effective to ask the patient, "What else concerns you?" This is important, since on average patients have three problems at a first visit, and often the concern mentioned initially is not the most important. Allowing the patient to express all concerns at the beginning of the interview enhances efficiency: (1) it allows the physician to know all of the problems that the patient is hoping to cover in the visit, instead of discovering them at the end of the visit; last-minute problems ("Oh by the way!") can be particularly frustrating to the physician; (2) allowing the patient to state all concerns in the early phase of the interview can remind the patient of concerns that may have been forgotten initially; (3) this strategy allows the physician to prepare to negotiate with the patient about what concerns can be covered in this visit and what will be dealt with at a later time. After eliciting all the patient's concerns, the physician can summarize before proceeding to in-depth questioning about any one of the problems. This communicates to the patient that the physician has listened attentively and allows the physician a moment to organize the problem list mentally.

### Setting the agenda for the visit

Once the physician knows all of the patient's concerns, it may be necessary to work with the patient to negotiate the priorities for the visit. Particular concerns may be a high priority for the patient and must be addressed during that visit for the patient to feel the time was well spent. The physician may have other concerns, particularly about urgent medical problems. A typical sequence of dialogue follows:

*Physician:* So I understand that there are four concerns you would like to address today: your headache, shoulder pain, heart palpitations, and constipation. In the time we have available today, we may not be able to cover all of these. Which is most important to address today?

*Patient:* I would like to make sure we talk about my headaches.

*Physician:* That's fine. I'd be happy to address that. In addition, I want to discuss your heart palpitations just to be sure that everything is okay there. Why don't we start with those two and plan to address the shoulder pain and constipation at a follow-up visit if we don't have time today? Would that be all right?

*Patient:* That sounds fine as long as you can help me get an appointment about the other problems within a few weeks.

*Physician:* I think we can arrange that before you leave.

Negotiation allows the physician and patient to plan together how to use the time available. In this manner the patient is assured that the important problems will be addressed and the physician is assured that there is adequate time for investigation of medical concerns.

### Assessing a problem

After a mutually agreeable negotiation, the task for the physician is to work together with the patient to provide an adequate assessment of the priority problem: *Work together* because only the patient has the information needed and because the physician needs the patient to provide that information with as much clarity and completeness as possible; *adequate* because in practice one needs to know only what is necessary, not everything there is to know about a problem. The idea of a "complete" history is an unobtainable and undesirable myth. To facilitate this shared work, the physician needs to make it clear to the patient what he or she wants to happen and to train the patient if necessary to provide the information at the necessary level of detail and thoroughness.

### Allowing the patient to tell story in own words

Allowing the patient to tell the story of the illness in his or her own words is the most efficient and comfortable way to begin to assess a problem. The patient frames what he or she perceives as relevant, revealing personal views of cause and effect. The patient mentions details and facts a physician would not think to ask about. While the patient is talking, the physician can be thinking about what is said and developing hypotheses about the nature of the problem and approaches to ruling in and ruling out these hypotheses. Inviting the patient to tell the story of the illness also reveals the context of the illness—the nature of the patient's work, the home in its complexity, and important relationships. This understanding is needed in planning approaches to care. Telling a story also improves patient recall because it places their attention in a remembered context, where the fine details are accessible to recall.

This story telling is initiated by asking the patient, "So, tell me what happened," or "Let's go back to the beginning and tell me the story of your problem." This creates a *narrative thread* that organizes the interview. Once the patient is telling the story, the physician can quietly ask for elaboration on points about the person, the context, and relationships, learn as much as needed ("Tell me more about your husband"), and then return to the narrative thread by asking, "And then what happened?"

### Using open to closed cones of questions

Note that the above questions begin with "Tell me" and little else. This is because it is more efficient and more thorough to begin each line of inquiry with an open-ended question, which invites a free-form response to a query rather than a short specific answer (e.g., "Tell me about your chest pain" rather than "Where does it hurt?"). Studies have documented that open-ended questions produce more information, more efficiently, with greater satisfaction by both physician and patient. In addition, the patient includes unanticipated information and connections. Initially the advantages of open-ended questions seemed counterintuitive to us, but our experience has borne them out. Once the patient has responded, the physician can then begin to focus on smaller aspects of the situations. Once the open-ended approach has been exhausted (often quickly), one then can ask close-ended questions about facts not covered (Table 1-2).

### Understanding the patient as a person

Although the importance of understanding the patient as a person in the process of assessing the problem cannot be overstated, the process of acquiring that understanding can be highly efficient and minimalistic. The opening observation often reveals ethnicity, style, socioeconomic status, and sometimes work and marital status. The content and presentation of speech and information show how the patient reasons and believes. The affect shown, a frown or sadness, shows feelings about the subject, as does

**Table 1-2.** Screening questions for patients with suspected disorders

| Condition | Specific questions | Indicator |
|---|---|---|
| Alcohol | CAGE:<br>Have you even tried to *C*ut down on your drinking?<br>Are you ever *A*nnoyed when people comment on your drinking?<br>Have you even felt *G*uilty about something you've done after drinking?<br>Do you ever have an *E*ye opener? | Screen all *new* patients |
| Sexual preference | Are you sexually active? Is this with men, women, *or both*? | All new patients |
| Domestic violence | Does your partner (or other name) ever threaten to hurt you?<br>Has anyone ever hit you or injured you? | Female patients with recurrent trauma |

gesturing—covering the face, looking down and away, suddenly brightening.

## Understanding the setting of the illness

One cannot be sure in advance what aspects of the illness setting will be crucial or contributory. Several dimensions are usually relevant in most patients. First is social setting—who is at home (if there is a home), who is close or painfully distant, what are the supports. Environmental features may be critical, such as type of work, location of home or work (e.g., isolated in the country, a fifth floor walk-up, a violent neighborhood with strong pressures to drink or use drugs). Ethnic and cultural background may determine health care–seeking behavior, adherence to agreed plans, or use of dangerous remedies.

Although discussion of the "activated patient" is increasing in the literature, there is still relatively little about the "activated physician," our notion of a physician actively mining every aspect of each moment with a patient for the gold of information, suggestion, and implication. This is known as active listening. It means that, as well as hearing the strictly factual content of what is being said, the physician also hears subtle facets of the communication—the tone, what is not said, the way in which the framing of an answer or description provides insight into the patient's modes of thinking or beliefs. Every moment of each interview is laden with information. More experienced, alert, and mentally active physicians can absorb and process more of this. This, together with pattern recognition, underlies the precise diagnostic ability, insight, and effectiveness of some excellent clinicians. This is not only a matter of talent, sensitivity, and intelligence; it can be practiced and learned.

## Eliciting the patient's beliefs about the problem

The patient's beliefs about the problem, health care in general, and how to relate to physicians can be crucial to the outcomes of care. If the patient believes the problem is due to an excess of hot or cold humors—as some Puerto Ricans believe—then prescribing the wrong remedy (e.g., a hot remedy for a hot disease, such as orange juice with potassium supplementation for hypertensives on diuretics) leads to total noncompliance. Therefore it is necessary to check, probably several times, to what the patient attributes the problem. Similarly, if the patient believes that physicians are judgmental, are not to be trusted, or are out to do things only for money, they will reveal less and cooperate less. If the patient's culture dictates that seeking care is shameful, he or she will not come for care soon enough, even for emergencies. If the patient believes that the physician should not be upset, the difficult facts will be hidden (e.g., by many persons of orthodox or authoritarian background, by some traditional Chinese).

This method deviates from the idea that one should collect the social history separately. This is because when social and personal information are collected simultaneously with biomedical information more is revealed, patient recall is improved, and the process proves more efficient. One can always complete information not elicited later.

## Other factors

*Dealing with the secondary problems.* After having elicited what is needed concerning the priority problem, the physician should turn to the patient's secondary problems or to other problems the physician wishes to address. These are dealt with in the same way. One starts with an open-ended invitation to tell the story, elaborates when appropriate, and moves from open to closed types of questions.

*Physical examination.* Should the interview continue during the physical? Does this common practice enhance time efficiency or does it breed error? No one really knows, although both are likely to some extent. The argument against talking during the physical examination is that it distracts the examiner, thereby decreasing sensitivity and causing him or her to miss physical findings, especially on auscultation and palpation.

The reality, however, is that most physicians do talk before and during the examination. It is very helpful to the patient to have the examination introduced and to explain what is being done, especially if painful, unusual, or in difficult areas (rectal and genital examinations). Clearly the physician's perceptions should be directed toward the examination. Social talk, chatting, or pursuing a review of systems will distract unduly.

*Laying on of hands.* Should a physical examination always be done? Obviously, there are some follow-up visits that do not require a physical reexamination. But there are several reasons to err on the side of examining. First, things change, sometimes unexpectedly. Second, it has become very clear that the act of physical touch has a reassuring, calming, and perhaps healing effect. It also, done gently and caringly, improves the physician-patient relationship and rapport. Third, patients expect to be examined. Failure to do so when the patient expects it leads to loss of trust in the physician's caring or competence, unless explained effectively. This then affects healing, comfort, and satisfaction. Many patients find the absence of physical examination unacceptable regardless of explanation.

***Summary of thoughts and findings.*** The end of the physical examination is a pivotal point in most interviews. The patient feels increasingly vulnerable, since the physician now has information he or she does not—information the patient fears may be bad news. At this point plans must be created and negotiated with the patient. Therefore it is always important at this stage to summarize thoughts, findings, and preliminary ideas about the next steps in discussion and planning.

After the physician presents ideas and thoughts about the patient's diagnosis, it is important to check the patient's feelings and reactions. The patient may have beliefs about the nature of the illness that either fit or are in disagreement with the physician's opinion. To explore the patient's reactions and beliefs, the physician might ask a sequence of questions:

*Physician:* I've explained to you that I think your symptoms may be due to a peptic ulcer. How does that fit with your ideas about your stomach pain?

*Patient:* I'm a bit uncertain; I thought that ulcers only occurred when people were stressed and I feel like everything is going well in my life. How could I have an ulcer?

*Physician:* That's a good question, since lots of people believe that stress and ulcers are related. In fact, a number of factors contribute to the formation of ulcers, such as fatigue, a genetic disposition, and a stomach infection. So people commonly develop ulcers even without stress.

A simple explanation helps the patient accept the physician's diagnosis and be more prepared to work with the physician to plan the treatment course. In other cases it is necessary to integrate the patient's beliefs into the diagnostic explanation, even if the patient's ideas come from a different frame of reference than the physician's. For example, patients may have beliefs about illnesses due to certain food substances that do not fit with the physician's scientific approach to the nature of the illness. Where possible, if the physician can accept the patient's beliefs as possible and integrate these beliefs with a scientific explanation, the patient may be more likely to collaborate in the treatment plan.

***Planning.*** Like the presentation of the diagnosis, the physician often presents the options for treatment. It is essential to involve the patient in the planning process. If a patient does not believe that the treatment plan is likely to succeed or does not understand the details of the treatment, follow-through is unlikely. It is important for the physician to check the patient's beliefs and feelings about the treatment plan just as he or she checked beliefs about the diagnosis. Then the physician can engage in a dialogue with the patient about the suggested treatment.

*Physician:* I've suggested that you use these pills to treat your peptic ulcer disease. What do you think of that?

*Patient:* It seems reasonable to me, although I've always heard that diet is important for ulcer treatment. Couldn't I treat this by avoiding certain foods and not use the pills?

By probing the patient's beliefs, the physician can identify barriers that might lead the patient to leave the physician's office without intending to fill the prescription or follow the treatment plan.

If the patient and physician are in agreement about the treatment, it is useful to help the patient anticipate the problems in implementing the treatment.

*Physician:* It's difficult to remember pills three times a day. What do you think the hard part of this will be for you? How might you provide reminders to yourself?

This gives the patient permission to express the possibility of forgetting the pills and allows an opportunity for the doctor and patient to discuss ways to help the patient remember.

Other simple strategies can help the patient in the planning phase, including writing down instructions, referring patients to educational programs available in the health care facility or in public, giving the patient educational pamphlets pertinent to the illness, and sending a visiting nurse to follow up (e.g., with a new diabetic).

It is essential to ask the patient whether there are questions and to have the patient review the main points before moving to the closing phase of the interview. By having the patient reiterate and the physician clarify before ending the interview, the physician can increase the likelihood that the patient will understand and comply with the treatment planned. Ultimately this makes the physician's work much more efficient by avoiding unnecessary treatment failures.

### Closure

After the educational phase of the interview, the final few moments are spent in closure. During closure the physician reviews the immediate next steps: "Now I'd like you to go to the reception desk with this laboratory slip. Ms. Cruz will direct you to the laboratory." The physician also can reiterate the plan for the timing of the next visit, checking with the patient about whether that seems appropriate ("Perhaps we can see each other in approximately 4 weeks. Does that seem about the right length of time from your perspective?") The physician can outline the plan for contact in the interim between visits if this is appropriate. Understanding how to reach the physician in an emergency or how to get the results of pertinent laboratory tests can save time-consuming phone calls to the office. Finally, in saying goodbye to the patient the physician often sets the tone for the next visit and can do some planning: "I look forward to seeing you in a month and will be eager to see your headache diary so we can explore this problem further."

## FUNCTIONS

The broad functions of the interview fall into three categories: gathering data, developing a relationship and dealing with patient feelings, and educating the patient about diagnosis and treatment. The process of data collection has been described in the previous section.

### Developing and maintaining a relationship

Patients seeking care from their primary care physician often are worried about their health problems or have emotional distress about issues in their personal lives. They may come to the appointment feeling sadness, anger, frustration, or anxiety. To build trust and make the interview most effective, the physician must recognize and address patient feelings. This may be the most challenging task for the physician. It is often neglected.

When patients are experiencing strong emotions, the physician may fear that discussing these emotions directly will slow the interview down by "opening a can of worms." What to do if the patient expresses deep feelings of loneliness and the physician cannot fix the situation or make the patient feel better? What if the patient is angry and directs this at the physician? Often a physician's personal feelings or worries serve as barriers to discussing these emotional issues. In fact, studies show that talking to patients about their feelings and understanding their emotional experience is therapeutic and builds the relationship between patients and physicians.

It is best to address feelings when they first appear in the interview. This can be accomplished by first commenting directly on the feelings and then making a statement that indicates understanding the patient's experience.

> *Physician:* You seem pretty sad about these recent events.
> *Patient:* Yes, I feel so terrible. I had hoped this would never happen.
> *Physician:* I can understand feeling like that. It must feel so disappointing to you to have it turn out this way.

Such brief comments by the physician indicate recognition of the patient's pain and an understanding about the life experience of the patient. Furthermore, if appropriate, the physician can make a further statement of empathy, such as "I would feel the same way in your position" or "Many people would feel as you do in this situation." These statements are appropriate only if genuine. Even if the physician disagrees with the patient's point of view, certain statements indicate understanding, for example, "I can understand your feeling frustrated or angry if you have felt that I have not been taking your complaints seriously" or "I can understand feeling angry with the delay in getting an appointment when you were worried there was something seriously wrong with your health." In these examples the physician accepts how the patient feels even though he or she would not have had the same reaction as the patient in a similar situation or believes the patient's response is unreasonable.

In addition to direct discussion of patient feelings, physicians can indicate their acceptance of patients by echoing the patient's words or reiterating what a patient has said. Brief phrases can indicate attention and caring. For example, the physician listening to a patient's worries about an episode of shortness of breath can say "Sounds like it was frightening for you."

Nonverbal indicators of concern can also be powerful in building the relationship with the patient. This can include maintaining a relaxed and nondefensive posture when a patient is expressing anger directly at the physician. Body posture may indicate acceptance. Also, touching the patient as an expression of caring, for example, a patient who is crying, is often a strong statement of a physical and psychologic connection.

### Communicating information and patient education

One of the most challenging tasks for the physician, and sometimes the most frustrating, is helping patients to change a strong behavior, like smoking. Sometimes it seems like the physician is working harder than the patient to come up with solutions to the patient's problem. The key to helping patients with behavior change most effectively is ensuring that the discussion is collaborative. It is essential that patients first clarify whether they are truly interested in making behavior change; they should consider what might be most effective for them personally. Patients are their own best resource in understanding what strategies are most useful for them and in anticipating the potential difficulties.

The sequence of questions listed below can be an efficient strategy in helping patients with any behavior change (weight reduction, smoking, cholesterol-lowering diet).

| Physician question | Task |
|---|---|
| What do you *feel* about your high cholesterol? | Understand patient concerns and motivation for change. |
| What do you *know* about the effects of high cholesterol on your health? | Clarify any misconceptions. |
| What do you *want to do* at this time? | Assess motivation and patient ideas about strategies for change. |
| What or who might *help you* make these changes? (What helped in prior attempts to change?) | Explore patient ideas about strategies. |
| What will be the *difficult times?* How can you handle them? | Anticipate barriers and plan for them. |
| What are your *plans now?* | Review plans; write contract if appropriate. |

This series of questions allows the physician to assess the motivation of the patient for change, clarify any important information about the health reasons for change, and facilitate the patient developing a personal plan. This plan makes the patient responsible for planning and draws on the patient's personal strengths.

If the patient is not prepared to make a change in the behavior at a particular time, it can be inefficient to try to proceed into details of planning. Rather, it can be more effective to help "plant the seeds" and suggest that the patient start to contemplate a future change in the behavior. Strategies to help patients with behavior change are discussed in detail in Chapter 124.

## SPECIAL INTERVIEW SITUATIONS

This section highlights several series of questions that can be useful in special interviews. Details about the relevant conditions are elucidated in other sections of this book.

### Breaking sad or bad news

Broken insensitively, bad news can have a negative impact on giver and recipient. For the recipient especially the effect can be longlasting and can include unnecessary pain and suffering, misunderstanding or inadequate understanding of the condition, compromised decision making, and worse outcomes of care or quality of life. For the physician ineffective or damaging provision of bad news can be traumatic and lead to decreased personal and professional satisfaction and the propensity to avoid such situations, even when necessary.

In contrast, when done well, giving bad news can be a satisfying experience for both patient and physician (see the box below). Not that it may be painless or easy, but the patient may then clearly understand what to expect, know what to hope for or focus on, and feel cared for and supported. The patient knows he or she will not have to go through the subsequent difficulties alone. Likewise, the physician may feel considerable personal and professional satisfaction in a difficult job well done.

### Adolescent patients

Talking with adolescent patients is often a challenge. They may not be seeking treatment voluntarily; they may be embarrassed or ashamed to be talking to a stranger about themselves and about their condition; they may be in an antiauthority phase. The key to effectiveness is recognizing what barriers the particular adolescent has brought in and then adapting appropriately. In most cases three physician actions are effective: (1) it helps to be easy, relaxed, and not in a hurry or overly professional, although being falsely chummy will be spotted and rejected instantly; (2) at the outset the physician must assure the patient of *confidentiality* and mean it; (3) once sincerity is shown through action and demeanor, the physician should emphasize to the adolescent that the alliance is between the physician and the patient and not between the physician and the parents. These things may be circumstantially difficult or impossible to do or say, but when and if possible they help.

#### When breaking bad news

- Make preparations as fully as possible (e.g., checking notes, test results, and time arranged for follow-up investigations or admission in hand).
- Break bad news in a suitable room, perhaps with a nurse present. Arrange furniture appropriately and ensure privacy with no interruptions.
- Allow enough time.
- Make sure patients and relatives know who you are and the purpose of the consultation.
- Remember that what is hopeful news for you might still be bad news for the patient depending on circumstances, and vice versa.
- Do not assume that someone else has handled important parts of the information giving process. Check patient's understanding.
- Do not be falsely reassuring, but give as much positive practical support and information as possible.
- Ensure that the patient has enough time to let the news sink in; check understanding before patient leaves.
- Offer follow-up appointment, number to call, or addresses of other helpful agencies.
- Check your own feelings before seeing another patient.
- Remember, a shocked person may hear nothing or only one or two things. Give the essential points, and review and expand at the next visit—soon.

Modified from Fallowfield LS, Lipkin M. In Lipkin M, Putnam SA, Lazare A, editors: *The medical interview: clinical care, education, and research,* New York, 1995, Springer-Verlag.

### Elderly patients

Data show that primary care physicians like to work with older patients, and older patients like their physicians more than other age groups do. The stereotypes about the elderly are often triggered by one limitation, such as deafness, which is then generalized into the misconception that the patient is generally incompetent. Physicians should assume that patients have significant and even surprising areas of competence.

The elderly have barriers to communication more frequently than do other adults. It is critical to calibrate the interview early by checking for such barriers. All too often inexperienced physicians spend a great deal of well-intentioned time talking in detail when the patient suffers from delirium and cannot cooperate accurately or effectively. Frequently, the patient hears only a portion of what is said and covers with generalities, niceties, and evasion. This is particularly damaging in the patient education phase, when the patient may not adequately know what is planned or what to do, with possible serious sequelae. Dementia can be subtle and even cleverly hidden. This can be assessed easily and nonconfrontationally in the process of the interview by asking the patient a question that requires addition or subtraction (e.g., "So your arthritis began when you were 59. What year was that?"), by introducing a fact or name ("My partner is Dr. Geoff Gordon and he will be cross covering with me") and later ("I want to be sure you are not surprised if you call me at night and another doctor answers. Do you recall my partner's name?"), checking its recall shortly, or by asking the patient a question that calls for abstract thinking in response ("If you were to move in with your daughter's family, what would happen?"). If still in doubt, one can use the more sensitive but also more upsetting Mini-Mental Status Test.

CHAPTER

# 2 Periodic Health Examination

Arthur H. Eskew

The "checkup" remains one of the most common reasons cited for visits to primary care providers (Fig. 2-1). While once advocated as the mainstay of preventive care, the comprehensive annual physical examination has largely been replaced by a different approach in which preventive health counseling and procedures are integrated into symptom-related episodic visits. This new approach places the onus on providers to organize their practice and patient encounters to ensure that periodic health examination is effectively implemented and that any given patient receives an appropriate array of preventive health services, in addition to symptom-related care. The complete physical examination is not eliminated but rather becomes a tool in the preventive care strategy.

The recent increase in available information regarding a broad spectrum of preventive health procedures, largely attributable to the work of the Canadian Task Force on the Periodic Health Examination and the US Preventive Services Task Force (USPSTF), makes it possible for providers and patients to make more informed decisions regarding the risks and benefits of many procedures. While the benefit of many other commonly recommended screening and preventive procedures remains unproven, the clinician has a wealth of expert consensus on which to draw in designing a screening strategy (Fig. 2-2).

This chapter on periodic health examination outlines an approach to evaluating various preventive procedures by discussing barriers and suggesting strategies to ensure that the clinician achieves a high rate of compliance with these procedures. Tables summarize recommended procedures in an age-specific format. Rather than advocating a "cookbook" approach, emphasis is placed on a practice-specific, patient-specific strategy. Important issues and areas in which clinicians can provide support and anticipatory guidance are discussed.

## DEFINITION

Even though the concept of prevention is inherent throughout medical care, it has traditionally focused on tertiary prevention in individuals with symptomatic illness. The periodic health examination emphasizes primary and secondary prevention. It involves the performance of tasks that include history and physical examination, laboratory and other tests, and procedures designed to determine an individual's risk for certain preventable conditions and provide guidance to reduce or avoid additional risk or to diagnose those conditions in an early, presymptomatic state in the hope of reducing morbidity and mortality.

## THE PERIODIC HEALTH EXAMINATION VS. THE COMPLETE PHYSICAL EXAMINATION

The periodic health examination is distinct from the routine or annual physical examination in that it involves the delivery of specific services and procedures based on an individual's age, sex, and estimated risk for disease. It is a process of collecting data, estimating risks and determining specific diseases and conditions for which a patient is at risk, and focusing clinical, cognitive, and diagnostic resources in a fashion that would provide most benefit. The complete history and physical examination should be done when a patient is first encountered and periodically updated. The history and examination provide both the foundation of data on which the preventive care strategy is based and the opportunity to carry out some of that care.

## PREVENTIVE CARE

Prevention in the primary care setting refers to care that is directed at preserving the health of an individual patient and the community in which the provider practices. The importance and potential effect of preventive care is evident, given the estimate that as much as 50% of the mortality from the 10 leading causes of death in the United States is attributable to potentially modifiable lifestyle

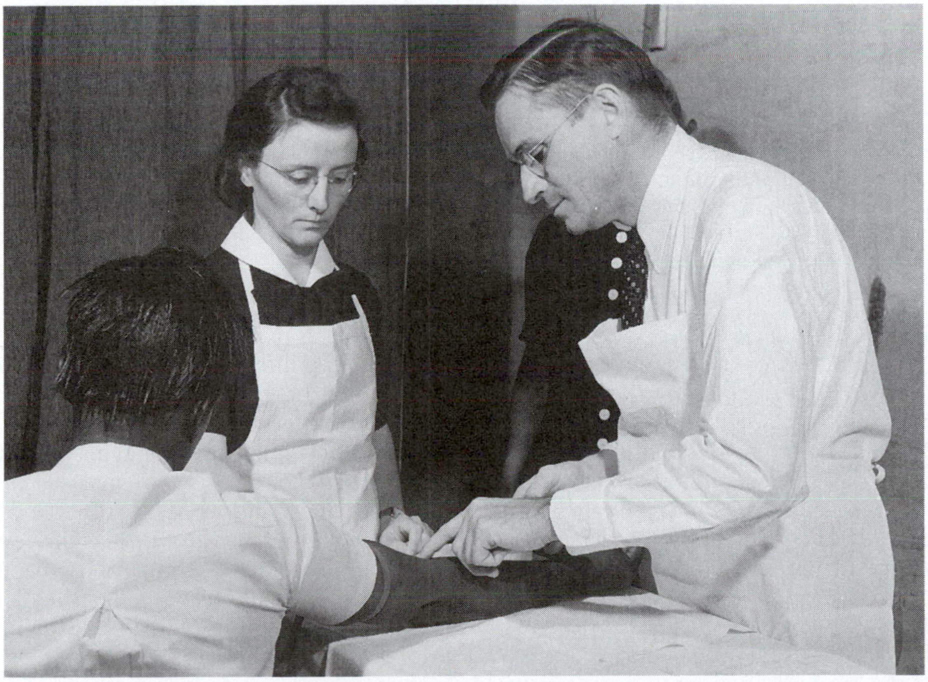

**Fig. 2-1.** The health clinic, 1941. Courtesy Library of Congress.

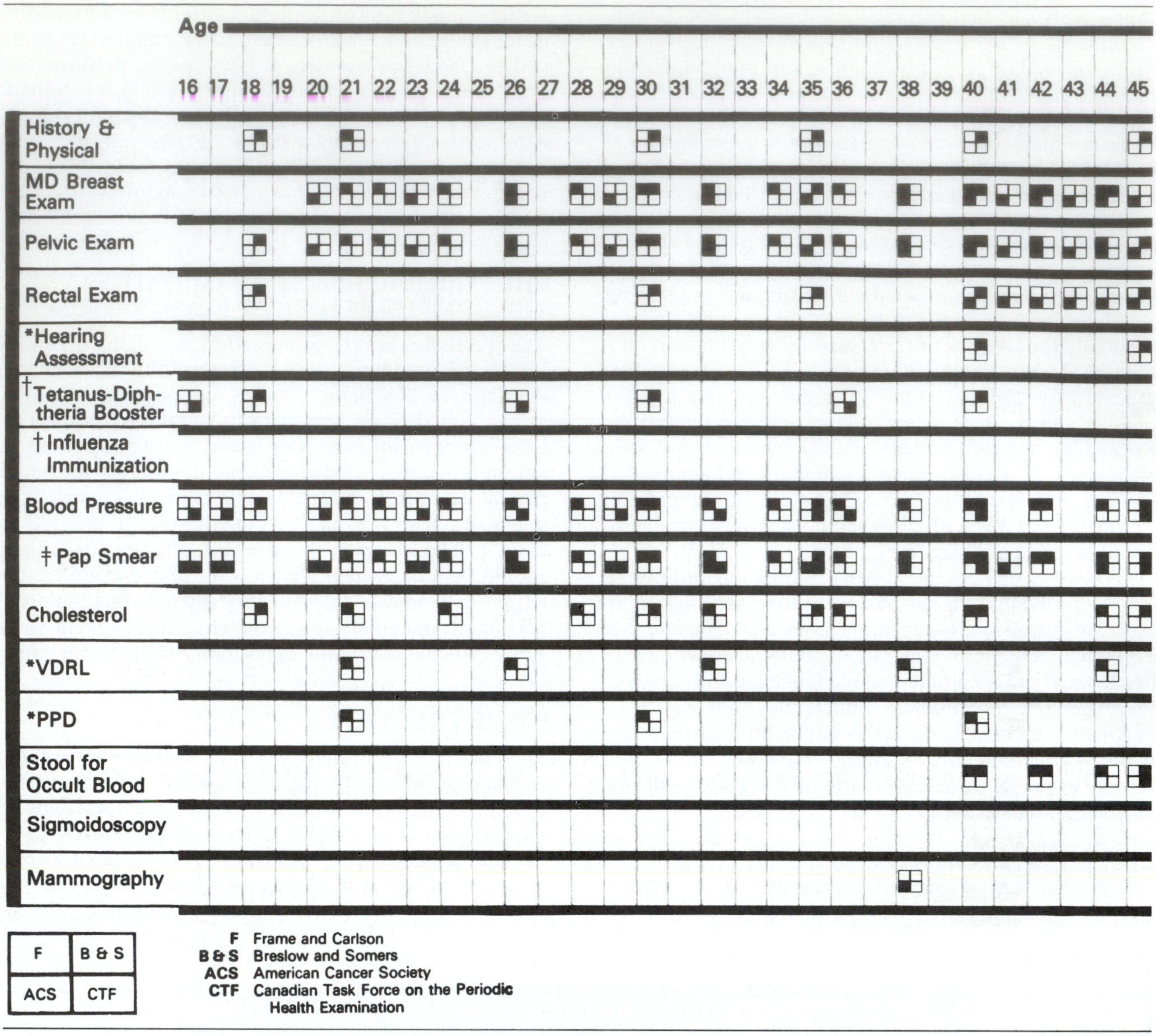


**Fig. 2-2.** Summary of recommendations of the four major studies. *Canadian Task Force recommends that this be done on the basis of clinical judgment. †Centers for Disease Control recommends that at first visit physician check immunization history for rubella, mumps, poliomyelitis, diphtheria/tetanus toxoids, and pertussis. ‡If sexually active. A blackened square indicates that a study has considered the maneuver and recommended it. Empty squares indicate that the study was either not considered or considered but not recommended. (From Hayward RA et al. *Ann Intern Med* 114:758, 1991.)

factors. The proficient performance of preventive health care requires the clinician to possess a firm understanding of clinical epidemiology, the performance characteristics of a broad array of tests and procedures, and clinical decision making. Also necessary is a detailed understanding of an individual's risks, their social situation, values and preferences, and the incidence and prevalence of conditions and diseases, which are important causes of morbidity and mortality in the surrounding community.

## Types of prevention

Prevention can be divided into several categories, each of which is familiar to the primary care provider. *Primary prevention* refers to services directed at the prevention of disease before its onset. Examples include immunizations to prevent infectious diseases or counseling to prevent unwanted pregnancy in teenagers. *Secondary prevention* would involve maneuvers designed to detect diseases at an earlier, presymptomatic stage, so as to decrease morbidity and mortality. The use of mammography to detect early breast cancer before it is palpable or metastasizes is an example. *Tertiary prevention* is the care directly associated with preventing complications or undue morbidity in persons with established symptomatic chronic disease, for example, using angiotensin converting enzyme inhibitors to reduce symptoms and prolong survival in chronic congestive heart failure patients. The goal is to provide primary prevention whenever practical or possible, and to

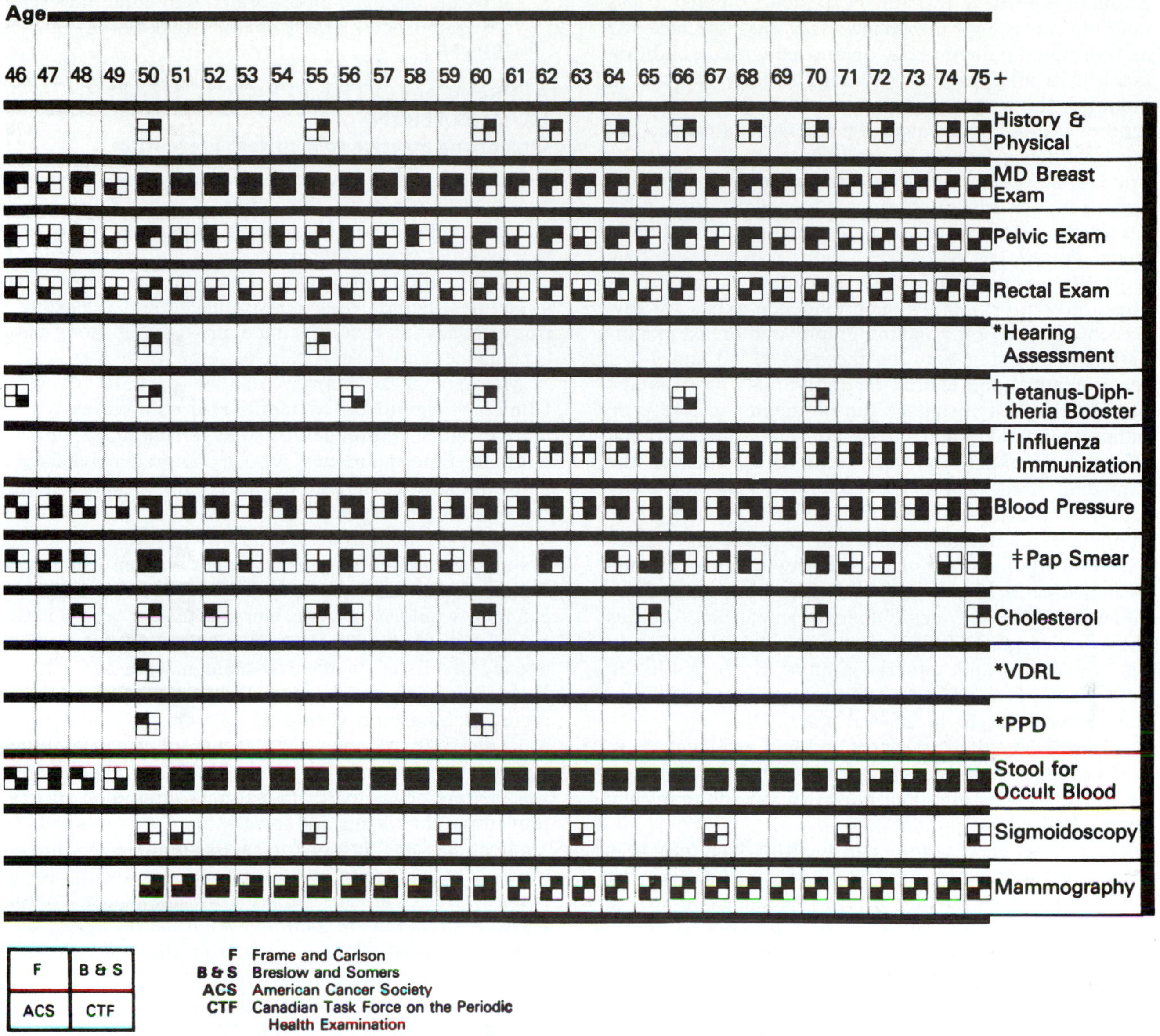


fall back on secondary preventive care when it is not. Tertiary prevention is employed when both primary and secondary preventive care for a given condition are either not available, have not been done, or have failed.

## Deciding which preventive services to provide

In approaching the provision of comprehensive preventive care, the clinician is faced with selecting from a large number of screening and early detection strategies for a large number of important conditions and diseases. For those conditions that are potentially amenable to screening, early detection, or anticipatory guidance, the following criteria need to be met:

1. The condition should be an important cause of morbidity and mortality in the screened population.
2. The condition should have a high enough prevalence so as to be suitable for screening. This criterion is important because prevalence will determine the number of false positives and false negatives (and hence the positive and negative predictive values) for any given screening test for that procedure. Rare conditions will yield higher false positive rates on screening tests, regardless of the characteristics of those tests. This is undesirable if an individual with a positive screening test must undergo risky or expensive confirmatory procedures.
3. An effective screening test or procedure must exist for the condition. This test should be sensitive enough to detect most cases and specific enough to keep the number of individuals misdiagnosed with the condition to a minimum. Ideally, the test should be demonstrated to be effective in controlled clinical trials and in practice situations.
4. The screening test should be low risk and acceptable to individuals undergoing the procedure. The risks attendant to screening can include the direct physical risk of the screening procedure or of subsequent procedures that are performed as a result of a positive screening test (such as the risk of bowel perforation with sigmoidoscopy or with colonoscopy performed to

evaluate a positive test for fecal occult blood) or less tangible risks, e.g., the unnecessary anxiety caused if an individual is incorrectly diagnosed with a condition (such as a malignancy). Although usually difficult to quantify, the risk of false reassurance (e.g., a patient ignores symptoms because of a recent negative screening test) also needs to be considered.

5. There should be a benefit to early intervention for the condition. The most definitive evidence of efficacy for a screening procedure comes from controlled clinical trials demonstrating a reduction in cause-specific mortality resulting from the screening procedure in question. Unfortunately, such evidence exists for few screening tests (e.g., mammography and breast examination for women between the ages of 50 and 74 or fecal occult blood testing for individuals past the age of 50). In most instances the clinician must rely on indirect evidence, such as case-control or observational studies and expert opinion. Authorities, such as the Canadian Task Force on Preventive Services, the USPSTF, and the American College of Physicians, have published recommendations and practice guidelines based on rigorous and methodical review of published evidence on a broad variety of screening procedures and preventive services. Other organizations, such as the American Cancer Society, have relied more heavily on consensus and expert opinion. Such published guidelines form the foundation for the provision of preventive services in general practice.

   In considering the quality of indirect evidence from observational studies and consensus, the clinician must be aware of the following biases in studies involving screening and early detection:
   - *Lead time bias* occurs when early detection at a preclinical stage only results in more time knowing of the presence of the disease rather than improved survival. If a condition has a long preclinical phase, then individuals who are detected by screening will automatically appear to have longer survival than individuals who present with symptoms, even when there is no benefit.
   - *Length time bias* refers to bias introduced if a condition such as a malignancy has a variable biologic behavior and exists in rapidly progressive and more indolent forms. At any given point in time, the more indolent form has a longer preclinical phase and is more likely to exist in asymptomatic individuals and is therefore more likely to be detected by screening in comparison with the rapidly progressive disease. Cases detected by screening in this situation will appear to have more favorable survival than cases in the general population.
   - *Overdetection (Overdiagnosis) bias* occurs when screening detects an inordinate number of early insignificant lesions that were never destined to cause clinical illness or that in some instances would have regressed. Such screen-detected cases also will appear to have more favorable survival in comparison with symptomatic cases, even in the absence of true benefit.

6. The screening test or procedure should be affordable and/or cost-effective. Such information is rarely available directly but has been estimated for many procedures and has been incorporated into guidelines such as those published by the Canadian Task Force (CTF) and USPSTF.

## APPROACH TO THE PERIODIC HEALTH EXAMINATION

### Organizing practice to facilitate prevention

Despite a growing body of evidence, expert opinion, and consensus concerning the value of many routine health maintenance procedures, generalists perform rather poorly in providing preventive procedures and counseling. The commonly cited reasons for poor adherence to published guidelines include time constraints, doubt regarding the true efficacy of recommended procedures, poor patient acceptance, and lack of reimbursement.

Many of these barriers can be partially overcome. Clinicians should try to familiarize themselves with the more established procedures so as to best judge which are worth the time and money. Also, a comprehensive database helps pinpoint those patients at risk for certain conditions who should be targeted for all levels of prevention.

Many studies have established the utility of using a system of reminders to prompt the clinician when certain indicated periodic preventive procedures are due. An example would be a paper spreadsheet in which patient-specific preventive health procedures and proposed frequency are listed in the left-hand margin and dates are listed across the top. As procedures are performed they are recorded, thus providing a prompt to perform that procedure after a specified amount of time has elapsed since last performed (Fig. 2-3). An effective strategy is to send letters or postcards to patients reminding them that preventive care is due and to call for an appointment. Such applications are perfect for small computers, which can track dates and provide automatic reminders to both patients and clinicians. A growing number of computer software products are available to assist in this endeavor.

Regardless of whether a paper or an electronic system is used to keep track of preventive health care, certain characteristics are essential for success. The reminder should be readily available at the point of patient encounter, and the clinician should have the ability to instantaneously update the patient's prevention database. The prevention profile should be customized for each patient with the clinician having the option to suppress reminders when they are no longer warranted. The clinician should be able to derive summary statistics so as to gauge overall performance. Peer review mechanisms can be devised within a practice to ensure maximum compliance with previously established guidelines.

Most routine prevention can be organized or carried out by office staff or midlevel practitioners and thus incorporated into waiting time or an exit interview with a nurse. Literature and pamphlets emphasizing the importance of preventive care is often effective in increasing patient awareness and interest and can be prominently displayed in the waiting area and examining rooms.

***Building the database.*** One of the most important aspects of providing effective preventive care during the periodic health examination is a complete and comprehensive clinical database, one used to assess risk of disease and direct anticipatory guidance and screening procedures.

## PRIMARY CARE CENTER GUIDELINES FOR ROUTINE HEALTH MAINTENANCE

Record Date and Results

|  |  | | | | | | | | | | | | | | | | | | |
|---|---|---|---|---|---|---|---|---|---|---|---|---|---|---|---|---|---|---|---|
| SCREENING | Weight: Q2 years | | | | | | | | | | | | | | | | | | |
| | Blood Pressure: Yearly | | | | | | | | | | | | | | | | | | |
| | Stool for Blood Yearly after age 50 | | | | | | | | | | | | | | | | | | |
| | Rectal: Optional yearly after age 40 | | | | | | | | | | | | | | | | | | |
| | PPD: Q3-5 years until age 35 | | | | | | | | | | | | | | | | | | |
| | Breast Exam: Yearly | | | | | | | | | | | | | | | | | | |
| | Mammograms: Yearly between ages 50-75 | | | | | | | | | | | | | | | | | | |
| | Pelvic & Pap: Yearly 18-70; optional s/p hst. | | | | | | | | | | | | | | | | | | |

| IMMUNIZATION | | | | | |
|---|---|---|---|---|---|
| Tet/Diph Q10 years | | | | | |
| Flu Vaccine yearly after age 65 | | | | | |
| Pneumovax once, as indicated | | | | | |
| Rubella Screen once | | | | | |

| OTHER | | | | | |
|---|---|---|---|---|---|
| Hearing | | | | | |
| Oral Exam | | | | | |
| Tonometry | | | | | |
| | | | | | |

| LAB SCREEN | | | | | | | | |
|---|---|---|---|---|---|---|---|---|
| Hct | | | | | | | | |
| Bun | | | | | | | | |
| Glucose | | | | | | | | |
| VDRL once | | | | | | | | |

| TEACHING | | | | | | |
|---|---|---|---|---|---|---|
| Breast Self Exam | | | | | | |
| Seat Belt | | | | | | |
| Smoking | | | | | | |
| Alcohol | | | | | | |
| Exercise | | | | | | |
| Nutrition: salt/weight | | | | | | |
| Other | | | | | | |

| RISK FACTORS | |
|---|---|
| Family History | |
| Occupational History | |
| Life Style | |

Comments:

Medical Records Copy

**Fig. 2-3.** Primary care center guidelines for routine health maintenance.

| | |
|---|---|
| PATIENT'S NAME | MEDICAL RECORD NUMBER |
| HOME PHONE | FAMILY |
| WORK PHONE | PHONE NUMBER |

*PROBLEM LIST*

| | |
|---|---|
| 1. | 11. |
| 2. | 12. |
| 3. | 13. |
| 4. | 14. |
| 5. | 15. |
| 6. | 16. |
| 7. | 17. |
| 8. | 18. |
| 9. | 19. |
| 10. | 20. |

| | CURRENT AND ACTIVE PROBLEMS | DATE | | INACTIVE PROBLEMS OR RESOLVED |
|---|---|---|---|---|
| | | First noted or change of title. | Resolved or date of past problem. | INCLUDE major past illnesses, operations. DO NOT INCLUDE problems for which you will provide active care. |
| | | | | |
| | | | | |
| | | | | |
| | | | | |
| | | | | |
| | | | | |
| | | | | |
| | | | | |
| | | | | |
| | | | | |
| | | | | |
| | | | | |

**Fig. 2-4.** Problem list format.

Collecting data can be a time-consuming task, part of which the clinician may want to delegate to the patient or to office staff through the use of self-completed history forms or questionnaires. They can be completed before the appointment or while the patient is in the waiting room. The form should then be reviewed and clarified with the patient during their examination. The self-completed history form also may alert the clinician to a patient's limited English proficiency or illiteracy.

**Medical history.** Perhaps the most central part of any medical database involves the collection of information regarding previous medical diagnoses, their treatment and response to treatment, current and previous medications and allergies, history of immunizations and childhood illnesses, and prior surgical history including response to anesthesia. This is generally accomplished through patient interview, review of immediately available medical records, and by formally requesting medical records from previous providers or hospitals at which the patient was treated. The information obtained should be recorded on a problem list, which is generally organized into active and inactive problems, and prominently located in the patient's office chart (Fig. 2-4).

**Family history.** A detailed family history is essential for gauging patient's susceptibility to a variety of important and potentially preventable conditions, and thus determines the primary and secondary preventive efforts. The box below contains a partial list of conditions in which family history influences risk of infection.

**Social history.** Providing individualized and attentive health care depends upon thorough knowledge of the patients and their circumstances. It is also increasingly recognized that there is a correlation between socioeconomic conditions and the risk of cardiovascular disease, cancer, substance abuse, and violence. In addition to occupation, the clinician should inquire about education, military service, marital status, relationships, household members, leisure activities, and travel. Any use of alcohol, tobacco, and other psychoactive substances also should be noted.

**Occupational and environmental history.** Although it has been estimated recently that 390,000 cases of occupation-related illnesses and 100,000 occupational illness–related deaths occur in the United States annually, only a small percentage of the illnesses responsible for those deaths are recognized as being related to workplace exposures, since the clinical presentation is rarely diagnostic of occupational disease. Primary care providers should take an occupational history of each patient as part of a general physical examination, concentrating on both present and any previous long-term jobs. Efforts should be made to determine the exact nature of the patient's job and to specifically ask about exposure to dust, fumes, solvents or chemicals, noise, vibration, or repetitive motion. The clinician should consider the possibility of an occupational cause of illness in patients with dermatologic problems, respiratory illnesses, cardiovascular diseases, emotional disturbances, musculoskeletal pains, malignancies, neurologic problems, hearing losses, traumatic injuries, and certain infectious diseases, such as hepatitis or HIV. The National Institute for Occupational Safety and Health (NIOSH) has listed the top 10 categories of work-related health problems (see box below).

Many patients are concerned about the role of their environment in causing disease. An environmental cause is often suggested by an abnormal geographic clustering of disease. In addition, many specific environmental exposures have been linked to disease, such as radon exposure, lead exposure, and proximity to toxic waste dump sites. It is therefore reasonable for the clinician to ask patients if they feel that something in the environment may be contributing to their medical problems.

Awareness of the protean manifestations of occupational-related diseases, as well as the spectrum of industry in the surrounding community, should lead to earlier recognition and treatment. Furthermore, it should position the clinician as an advocate for improved workplace procedures and other public health measures designed to protect workers and their households.

**The sexual history.** The sexual history of a patient is an essential part of the physical examination. A large number of medical, social, and psychiatric conditions can manifest themselves as sexual problems or dysfunction through the life cycle, and yet patients usually will not volunteer such information. The clinician who cares for adolescents realizes that sexuality is a central focus for them and that the opportunity to offer preventive guidance against sexually transmitted diseases (e.g., HIV), unwanted pregnancy, and sexual abuse depends on the clinician establishing an atmosphere in which sexual problems, concerns, and questions can be openly discussed. Sexual dysfunction is a problem in the elderly, and an often overlooked yet treatable cause of a decreased quality of life.

### Common conditions in which family history contributes to risk

Cancer, especially breast, colon, and prostate
Hypertension
Diabetes
Hyperlipidemia, atherosclerosis, coronary artery disease
Alcoholism
Mental illness (e.g., bipolar disorder)
Autoimmune disease

### Top 10 categories of work-related health problems

1. Occupational lung disease
2. Musculoskeletal injuries
3. Occupational cancers
4. Severe occupational trauma
5. Cardiovascular disease
6. Disorders of reproduction
7. Neurotoxic disorders
8. Noise-induced loss of hearing
9. Dermatologic conditions
10. Psychologic disorders

It is not possible to design a cookbook method for asking patients about sexual function and orientation. Clinicians should develop their own style, one tempered by their familiarity with each individual patient. Questions should be asked in a neutral, nonjudgmental fashion, unencumbered by medical jargon and colloquialisms. The subject should be introduced by letting the patient know that sex is a normal body function of equal concern to the clinician as are other physiologic functions. Structuring questions with phrases such as "It is common for most people to have difficulty with . . . Have you ever had such a difficulty?" is effective in that it lets the patient know that their possible difficulties are not odd or unique and that the clinician is willing to help with them. The provider should reassure the patient that the interview will remain confidential. Directness is important, otherwise questions may be misunderstood or the clinician may convey discomfort by being oblique.

With the advent of the AIDS epidemic, it is crucial that the clinician ask not only about sexual function but also about sexual orientation and behavior. An effective approach might be to begin a general discussion about high-risk behaviors with all or selected patients and then afford the opportunity for the patient to ask questions. The clinician may appropriately choose to collect sensitive information and counsel the patient at follow-up visits rather than at the first encounter, unless a specific complaint dictates otherwise. Although it is common for patients to be reticent regarding their reproductive health concerns most open up later if the provider establishes that such concerns are welcomed for discussion.

**Laboratory testing.** Most clinicians consider it prudent to perform baseline or periodic laboratory and other diagnostic testing on patients during a general physical examination. Although the value of such a practice is difficult to analyze if one employs the principles of evaluating screening tests or test performances, the rationale might include the establishment of a baseline study for comparison at a later time should symptoms arise or the detection of unsuspected illness, particularly ones unamenable to or unevaluated for screening efforts. The baseline electrocardiogram (ECG) is a case in point. Although no organization suggests routine ECGs, in elderly people with a high prevalence of cardiovascular disease, some studies have found the existence of a baseline ECG to alter diagnostic assessments in 22% and management plans (including decisions to admit the patients) by 14%. The clinician will wish to tailor the "standard" laboratory panel according to a patient's age, sex, identifiable chronic conditions, and presenting complaints. In addition, if there are no well-established guidelines, the clinician's knowledge of the patient's community and its demographics and epidemiology will determine an appropriate laboratory database and which tests to order periodically.

Many clinicians, for example, feel that obtaining routine CBCs are indicated in premenopausal women, since as many as 30% may be iron deficient. Similarly, although the prevalence of both subclinical and overt hypothyroidism varies markedly among studies, up to 10% of women greater than 40 years old may be subclinically hypothyroid and 1% to 2% may be overtly hypothyroid. Some clinicians therefore routinely assess thyroid-stimulating hormone (TSH) levels on women over 40 years of age. Routine urinalysis, although not rigorously evaluated and not recommended by the USPSTF, is performed by some clinicians in hopes of detecting early renal and bladder malignancies. Most clinicians obtain a rapid plasma reagin test (RPR) or veneral disease research laboratories test (VDRL) at least once on adults, and periodically if the patients engage in high-risk sexual practices, have a history of sexually transmitted disease, or reside in urban areas. It is also important not to discount either common perception on the part of many patients that bloodwork is an important part of a complete checkup or the reassurance that may come from knowing that things are "all right."

***Anticipatory guidance***

**Counseling on diet and exercise.** During periodic health examinations, the clinician should take the opportunity to provide advice regarding proper nutrition, weight maintenance, and aerobic exercise.

Proper diet is being increasingly recognized as central to any preventive strategy. Dietary fat and cholesterol play a major causal role in atherogenesis, and saturated fat intake has been implicated in increasing the risk of colon and breast cancer. Severe obesity (30% above ideal body weight) is a risk factor for increased mortality, largely through an increase in cardiovascular and cerebrovascular disease.

The clinician should include a baseline dietary assessment in each patient's database. Dietary guidelines appropriate for the general population should be promulgated (e.g., the American Heart Association Step I diet) (see Chapter 40). Most patients can be advised to cut down on fatty meats by substituting chicken, fish, and lean meats, to select more fruits and vegetables, and to substitute low or nonfat dairy products for whole ones. The maintenance of body weight in the basal state requires approximately 1500 to 1800 calories per day. Patients should reach and maintain their approximate ideal body weight by adjusting intake according to their activity level.

Aerobic exercise is beneficial in reducing cardiovascular risk and helps to reduce stress and promote a sense of well-being. In postmenopausal women, weightbearing aerobic exercise can aid in preventing the loss of bone mineral density. Spending as little as 15 minutes a day 3 days a week on modest aerobic exercise such as brisk walking may be beneficial and can be recommended to most patients.

**Alcohol and other chemical dependence.** When one considers the prevalence of alcohol, nicotine, other chemical dependence, and their propensity to predispose to serious health problems (e.g., trauma, liver disease, cancer, heart disease), it is not so difficult to accept that substance abuse is a major contributor to death and morbidity in the United States.

***Alcohol.*** The primary care provider must be aware of not only the high prevalence of alcohol abuse in his or her practice but also of the highly variable and frequently subtle presentation. Alcohol is toxic to virtually every organ system in the body and can result in a multitude of health effects. The provider should be alert to the potential role of serious alcohol abuse in patients presenting with the following:

- Excitability or anxiety

- Gastrointestinal tract complaints, such as dyspepsia, heartburn, or recurrent diarrhea
- Hypertension (especially with poor response to treatment)
- Arrhythmias (especially atrial fibrillation), palpitations, or cardiomyopathy
- Depression
- Sleep disturbances
- Sexual dysfunction
- Recurrent major or minor trauma
- Multiple somatic complaints
- Absenteeism, interpersonal problems, or marital difficulties

Since an individual's alcohol abuse frequently affects the family, the primary care provider may receive the first hints of a problem from the presenting complaints, often subtle, of those nearest the patient.

There are varying definitions of alcohol abuse and dependency. All of them emphasize the consequences of the individual's alcohol intake rather than the frequency or amount of intake and include some requirement of loss of control over drinking despite these adverse consequences. Denial is prevalent, and patients usually will not attribute their problems to a continued use of alcohol, despite overwhelming evidence to the contrary. Adult and adolescent patients should be asked about their use of alcoholic beverages. Those who respond positively should have a more in-depth history taken, one that focuses on the association between alcohol consumption and other events, such as injuries, traffic violations or accidents, arguments, interpersonal conflicts or marital problems, and school or job problems (e.g., absenteeism). In addition, a number of instruments such as the CAGE questionnaire (see box below) or the longer Michigan Alcohol Screening Test (MAST) are available to clinicians to screen for dysfunctional alcohol use. The CAGE is popular because of its brevity, the ease with which it can be memorized, and the reasonably good sensitivity and specificity when two positive responses are elicited. One positive response also may indicate a significant alcohol abuse problem and is worthy of further investigation. Those patients with a family history of alcoholism, particularly in one or both parents, are at higher risk of becoming alcoholic and should be periodically rescreened (see Chapter 130).

Although the diagnosis of alcohol abuse or dependency is largely made by history, there are a number of supportive diagnostic tests that can be used to define the extent of physiologic damage and the urgency of intervention. Many consider a measurable blood alcohol level (BAL) during a routine office visit to be virtually diagnostic. In addition, a BAL of 0.10% or more in the absence of overt symptoms of intoxication is a good indication of physiologic dependence. Abnormalities in a number of routine laboratory tests, although lacking the sensitivity or specificity to be useful as screening tests, may be indicative of heavy, consistent alcohol use, such as an elevation in the mean corpuscular volume (MCV) to greater than 100, with or without anemia or multiple old rib fractures on a chest x-ray. An elevation in the aspartate aminotransferase (AST) or a rise in the AST/alanine aminotransferase (ALT) ratio should suggest early liver damage from alcohol. The γ-glutamyltransferase (GGT) is perhaps the most sensitive serum test for heavy alcohol use and frequently will be the only abnormal serum test in an individual with heavy intake. The provider should be cautioned, however, that abnormalities in these tests generally occur with heavy, consistent use (e.g., more than 60 to 80 grams or four or more drinks per day) and patients may experience significant difficulties with much lower or less frequent intake and normal laboratory tests.

### The CAGE Questionnaire

C: "Have you ever felt the need to *C*ut down on drinking?"
A: "Have people *A*nnoyed you by criticizing your drinking?"
G: "Have you ever felt bad or *G*uilty about your drinking?"
E: "Have you ever had a drink first thing in the morning to steady your nerves or get rid of a hangover? (*E*ye-opener)"

***Tobacco (nicotine) dependency.*** Despite increasing public knowledge about the adverse consequences of tobacco use, smoking continues to contribute to an enormous burden of suffering in the United States (see Chapters 7 and 124). It is important that the primary care provider ask all patients regularly about tobacco use. Those who do smoke should be educated about both its adverse effects, and the health and economic benefits of quitting (e.g., a one pack-per-day smoker now spends about $1000 a year on cigarettes), and be advised to quit. A small but significant number of patients quit simply because their physician advised them to do so. See Chapter 124 for smoking cessation techniques.

***Other substances.*** The clinical presentation of the abuse of substances other than alcohol varies with the chemical in question, but abuse syndromes share a common ground of social and relationship dysfunction, financial problems, and trauma (see Chapter 131). Cocaine use can cause catastrophic cardiovascular and neurologic events, as well as depression and panic disorder. Marijuana smoking can lead to chronic lung disease. Injection drug use is a leading cause of HIV infection, hepatitis, endocarditis, and local infectious complications.

As with alcohol, the primary care provider should ask about other substance use to take a more in-depth history of those patients responding affirmatively. Treatment referral should be offered to patients who continue their abuse. Patients who use a substance despite evidence of significant medical or social consequences or whose history suggests a loss of control over the substance should be strongly urged to seek treatment.

**Domestic violence.** Domestic violence traditionally has been an underreported and underrecognized problem in primary care populations. Although as many as 2 to 4 million women are battered by their husbands or significant others, only about 1 in 20 is diagnosed with the battering syndrome by their physician, since few women disclose abuse, despite the fact that many consider their physician as a source of help. Homes in which domestic violence is perpetrated by men against women (the vast majority of domestic violence) are far more likely to include abused and neglected children, and those children are apt to grow up to abuse their spouses and children.

Domestic violence is a major cause of suicide among women and homicide committed by women against their husbands or significant others. There is a strong association between domestic violence and alcohol and substance abuse, both on the part of the perpetrator and the victim (see Chapter 127).

Victims of battering occasionally present with recurring physical evidence of trauma but more commonly present with nonspecific constellations of symptoms, such as depression, fatigue, unexplained abdominal or pelvic pain, or multiple somatic complaints that are frequently atypical. The prevalence of physical, emotional, or sexual abuse in these patients may be as high as 45%.

The most effective strategy for detecting domestic violence is to ask, since patients rarely volunteer the information. Statements such as "Marriages (or relationships) are frequently very difficult" and "Does your husband (or partner) ever strike you or make you feel badly about yourself?" convey a message of concern, letting the patient know that the provider is willing to discuss such subjects. Surveys on the issue indicate that most patients not only do not mind being asked but actually expect the inquiry. It is important to assure patients about the confidentiality of the conversation, since they may fear reprisal. Younger women who are beginning the coupling process should be asked in a neutral fashion if they have been coerced into performing sexual acts through intimidation or physical violence. Children and adolescents should be asked about arguments at home and their consequences, as well as about their parents' usual methods of punishment.

Although it is tempting to do so, the primary care physician should avoid the urge to rescue the victim. The provider's main role is that of counselor and supporter. The victim should receive the message that violence is wrong and illegal and that there are laws offering protection. Careful documentation of the history and physical findings, as well as x-rays done to evaluate injuries, may assist the patient in pursuing legal protection later. The physician should at least provide the phone number to a local violence hotline or battered women's shelter. If the situation is more urgent, the patient should be encouraged to notify the local authorities. In some instances the actions taken by the clinician are governed by local mandated reporting laws, such as in cases of suspected abuse of a minor or an older adult. The treatment of victims with severe physical and psychologic sequelae should be referred to providers experienced in the management of domestic violence. See Chapter 127 for further discussion.

**Adolescent health issues.** Adolescence is a time of rapid emotional and physical change, when many lifestyle factors that are likely to influence long-term health are established. Health issues of particular salience to adolescents include teenage pregnancy; sexually transmitted diseases (STDs); violence and injuries; substance abuse, including alcohol and tobacco; physical and sexual abuse; depression and suicide; eating disorders and proper nutrition; and exercise. Despite the apparent opportunity for meaningful primary prevention, adolescents remain medically underserved. Young men, in particular, are unlikely to see physicians except for sporadic, symptom-related care, while young women may be seen annually on routine gynecologic visits. These occasions should be viewed as an opportunity to ask about concerns, to screen for possible problems, and to provide appropriate anticipatory guidance and referral as necessary. The primary care provider should be familiar with and comfortable asking about these issues. Participation in school-based programs and clinics such as those providing presports participation physicals may afford the opportunity to intervene with a broader sample of the adolescent population in a community.

***Teenage pregnancy and STD prevention.*** Unwanted teenage pregnancy is occurring in truly epidemic proportions. Forty percent of young women in the United States become pregnant by the time they are 19 years old, 20% become mothers, and 15% have therapeutic abortions. The teenage abortion rate in the United States exceeds the teenage pregnancy rate in other western countries (e.g., in Sweden, a young woman is half as likely to become pregnant despite a sexual activity rate 50% higher than that of adolescent women in the United States). This statistic has been attributed to the greater availability and acceptance of contraceptives in the European teenage population. The potential for increasing contraceptive use is apparent when one considers that 51% of American teenagers do not use contraception on first intercourse, and 20% of the young women who become pregnant do so within one month of first intercourse.

The primary care physician may wish to become active on a community-wide basis by advocating school-based educational programs, and by breaking down barriers that inhibit the availability of contraceptives for teens. In the absence of such programs the providers themselves are the major source of contraceptive information for teens. Unfortunately teens are unlikely to initiate a discussion about sexual concerns, leaving it to the provider to inquire in a neutral, nonthreatening fashion at unrelated visits, e.g., a routine gynecologic appointment. Phrasing questions such as "Many women (or men) your age have questions about sex and avoiding pregnancy. I would be happy to answer any questions you have today or in the future if you would like" creates an atmosphere in which the teen can feel that the subject of sexuality is fair territory for discussion, and that their provider is an ally. Toward this end, the provider should stress the confidentiality of the discussion and avoid adopting a judgmental or moralizing attitude. Providers should familiarize themselves with state laws regarding the treatment of minors, but in general it is unlikely that a provider will be subject to legal recourse for prescribing birth control to a teen who requests it. Federally funded facilities are required to provide birth control to a minor who requests it, and although individual providers have the right to refuse, they are required to provide referral to a facility or provider who will.

Primary and secondary prevention of both teenage pregnancy and STDs should include a discussion about the physiology of reproduction, transmission of STDs, and information about behaviors and contraceptives. Oral contraceptives, although effective at preventing conception, may not be an ideal method for teens, in that they require advanced planning and strict compliance, and provide no protection against STDs. Barrier methods, particularly condoms, are better in the latter regard, but less effective in the former. Therefore, condoms plus another method, such as OCPs, should be recommended for adolescents who choose to remain sexually active. The provider should stress that no contraceptive method other than abstinence is 100% effective in preventing HIV transmission; should discuss the intense social, emotional, and physical impact of becoming sexually aware; and should educate teens on the potential advantage of postponing sexual intimacy until later in adulthood.

***Violence, risk-taking behavior, and injury prevention.*** Homicide is the third leading cause of death among 15-to 24-year-old men in the United States and is now recognized as a major health problem. Providers should routinely ask about fighting and injuries, and the circumstances under which they occur. The possibility of substance abuse and its relationship to fighting or injuries should be explored, and the connection emphasized to the patient. The association of substance abuse with domestic violence must be kept in mind, and patients should be routinely questioned regarding their homelife and their parents' attitudes toward punishment. The teen with a history of violence should be warned about the risk of death and/or serious injury, and given general advice regarding nonviolent techniques for resolving conflicts. Those with a history of alcohol or drug use should be offered referral for treatment.

Injuries are the leading cause of death in persons 1 to 44 years old, and automobile-related accidents are the most important source of injury. Providers should routinely point out the effectiveness of seatbelts, especially those with shoulder restraints, and encourage their use even for brief trips. The use of child restraint seats should be encouraged, since an unrestrained child is 11 times more likely to die in an accident than a restrained one. Fortunately, the provider is assisted in these endeavors as more and more states invoke mandatory seatbelt and child restraint laws. Alcohol use is at the root of approximately 50% of all traffic fatalities, and adolescents should be advised against drinking and driving.

Providers also should promote the use of other appropriate protective equipment (e.g., head, wrist, elbow, and knee protection during in-line skating, and bicycle and motorcycle helmets).

***Depression and suicide.*** Suicide is the second leading cause of death among persons 15 to 24 years old. Young women attempt suicide more frequently than young men; however, men are more likely to succeed, and, therefore, account for the vast majority of suicide-related deaths in this group. Clinicians should be aware of the association between an adolescent's suicidal behavior and major life stressors, such as school difficulties, domestic discord and abuse, parental divorce, and relationship problems. Additional factors include substance abuse, antisocial behavior, homosexuality, and major depression. The history of prior suicide attempts is a strong risk factor, although none of the above factors alone or in combination have been found to have value in defining a high-risk individual. The periodic health examination of the adolescent should include routine questioning about social functioning, home life, and mood, as well as screening questions for the vegetative signs of depression. Those who report serious suicidal ideation should be further assessed for the "lethality" of their plan (e.g., having a specific method in mind, having already obtained the planned means, etc.). Those who are determined to act must be hospitalized; those less intent can be managed as outpatients. The complexity of the average teenager's social and maturational hurdles, as well as the frequent need to include parents and other family members in the treatment plan, makes referral to a provider skilled in this area almost always a necessity.

***Eating disorders.*** As a result of definitional and reporting problems, the exact incidence of eating disorders is unknown; however, it is believed to have increased dramatically in the past two decades. The reasons for this are unclear but are felt to be associated with the current trend equating thinness with beauty. Women outnumber men with these disorders by as much as 25 to 1. Anorexia Nervosa and Bulimia Nervosa may present quite overtly in their severe forms or subtly with minor degrees of severity. The routine care of the adolescent should include a dietary history, not only to provide anticipatory guidance regarding nutritional habits, but also to screen for unusual attitudes and obsessions about food, eating, distorted body image, or inappropriate self-perception that the adolescent is overweight. Adolescents with eating disorders frequently present with depressed mood and/or anxiety and hyperactivity. They often experience problems at home, in school, and at work and may be socially isolated. Any of these signs should raise suspicion. Additionally, the clinician should be aware of the possibility of an eating disorder in an adolescent who presents with unexplained electrolyte abnormalities, especially hypokalemia, who is remarkably underweight (more than 15% below ideal body weight [IBW]); shows a delay or plateau in the development of secondary sex characteristics; has primary or secondary amenorrhea; displays severe periodontal disease, (a result of habitual purging of stomach contents); or has difficulty adjusting socially. Patients with Bulimia Nervosa may show wide swings in body weight over months or years, but most often present at or near their IBW. Bulimics suffer the most severe metabolic derangements, which are frequently life-threatening. Hospitalization for fluid and electrolyte replacement is indicated in extreme cases, even without the patient's consent if their refusal constitutes an immediate threat to survival. Management of less severe cases can be done on an outpatient basis, though referral to a clinician experienced in these disorders (usually a psychiatrist, psychiatric nurse, or psychologist) is wise. See Chapter 126 for more information on the diagnosis and treatment of eating disorders.

**Special issues in the elderly**

***Prevention in the elderly.*** Prevention in the elderly should generally be focused on attempts to deter frailty and functional decline. The causal factors behind loss of vitality in the elderly include the realms of lifestyle, social factors, and the accumulation of chronic illness, in addition to the loss of physiologic reserve that is part of normative aging. Early research suggests that attention to modifiable factors such as proper diet, exercise, and avoidance of tobacco and alcohol, as well as attention to such common geriatric problems as sensory loss, social isolation, and depression, may go far in improving the aging process. Many of the topics touched upon in this chapter are discussed more fully in the section on geriatric medicine, Chapter 6.

***Hearing impairment.*** More than one third of all individuals over the age of 65 have audiometrically detectable hearing loss, and a substantial proportion report a significant decrease in the quality of their lives as a result. There is evidence linking hearing loss to social isolation, and possibly to depression and cognitive decline.

Given this significant burden of suffering, efforts at screening and detection seem advisable. However, such common bedside examination techniques as the whisper test, the finger rub test, and the tuning fork test are unlikely to be either sensitive or specific enough to serve as reliable screening tests. There is good evidence that a hand held audioscope performs very well in this regard, provided it is combined with visual inspection of the auditory canals and removal of any obstructing earwax. In addition, standardized questionnaires have been developed that focus on social or communication impairment as a result of hearing loss, (e.g., the Hearing Handicap Inventory for the Elderly-Screening [HHIE-S] version in the box below). For each of the questions, a "no" response scores a 0, a "sometimes" 2, and a "yes" 4. Total scores less than 10 are indicative of no impairment, scores of 24 to 40 indicate moderate-to-severe impairment.

Once a potential hearing problem is uncovered through the use of a screening tool, formal audiologic evaluation should be arranged. Despite the real concerns about hearing aid compliance and the cost of these devices in the absence of medicare reimbursement, many patients benefit greatly.

***Visual impairment.*** The suffering from visual impairment in older individuals is probably similar to that from hearing impairment; however, the fact that glasses are less socially stigmatizing than hearing aids, and that decreasing visual acuity interferes more with important activities like reading and driving, leads many persons to seek eye examinations and corrective prescriptions from ophthalmologists and optometrists directly.

The major causes of visual decline in the elderly, other than refractive error, include glaucoma, senile macular degeneration, cataracts, and diabetic retinopathy. There is probably benefit to early detection of glaucoma, although the primary care clinician is relatively limited in screening options. Schiotz tonometry is not widely recommended for screening, a result of its relative difficulty, operator dependency, and questionable reliability. Thus, screening still lies in the hands of the ophthalmologist. As there is no effective treatment for senile macular degeneration, screening for this disease is probably unwarranted. Laser therapy for early proliferative diabetic retinopathy is effective in reducing the incidence of severe visual loss by as much as 50%; however, routine funduscopic examination is not sensitive enough to detect most instances of this disease in its early stages, before visual acuity is lost. Cataracts are readily detectable on routine ophthalmoscopic examination, but determining the amount of visual impairment attributable to them requires sophisticated methods, and there is probably no benefit to early treatment.

This is not to imply that primary care clinicians should not routinely ask about or examine their elderly patients' vision. Visual loss that has developed gradually may go unnoticed or unreported, or the patient may accept it as part of being old. Visual loss may be an important, yet reversible factor in patients presenting with depression, cognitive decline, falls and injuries, or other functional decline. Visual acuity is readily testable using a Snellen wall chart or pocket visual screener. Patients with best corrected vision less than 20/40 or with decline since their last examination should be referred for further evaluation.

All patients older than 40 should have a routine eye examination by an ophthalmologist, with a follow-up examination at least every several years for patients with no problems uncovered. Patients with diabetes should have annual eye examinations by an ophthalmologist to screen for proliferative diabetic retinopathy and also in light of the higher incidence of glaucoma.

***Screening for cognitive impairment.*** Recent studies have suggested that approximately 10% of all individuals over the age of 65 have dementia. That prevalence may increase to almost 50% in individuals over the age of 85. The vast majority of these individuals have Alzheimer's disease or other primary degenerative dementia; however, a substantial minority have a vascular cause. Despite the staggering prevalence, in most instances mild degrees of cognitive impairment go unrecognized by clinicians. Most likely this is because the usual screening questions about orientation to person, place, and time, although meaningful when they are abnormal, lack sufficient sensitivity to detect most cases.

A number of brief, simple instruments are available to screen for dementia. One of the most widely used and best validated is the Folstein Mini Mental Status Examination (MMSE). It consists of 11 questions and tasks with a total possible score of 30. Scores greater than 24 are considered normal, while scores less than 24 are indicative of dementia and usually warrant further evaluation. The

**The hearing handicap inventory for the elderly-screening version (HHIE-s). Score: Yes = 4; Sometimes = 0; No = 0.**

1. Does a hearing problem cause you to feel embarrassed when you meet new people? ______
2. Does a hearing problem cause you to feel frustrated when talking to members of your family? ______
3. Do you have difficulty hearing when someone speaks in a whisper? ______
4. Do you feel handicapped by a hearing problem? ______
5. Does a hearing problem cause you difficulty when visiting friends, relatives, or neighbors? ______
6. Does a hearing problem cause you to attend religious services less often than you would like? ______
7. Does a hearing problem cause you to have arguments with family members? ______
8. Does a hearing problem cause you to have difficulty when listening to television or radio? ______
9. Do you feel that any difficulty with your hearing limits/hampers your personal or social life? ______
10. Does a hearing problem cause you difficulty when in a restaurant with relatives or friends? ______

A score of 10 or less is normal. Scores of 24 to 40 are indicative of moderate to severe impairment.

From *ASHA* 31(8):59, 1989.

MMSE is relatively insensitive to the early loss of higher executive function, especially in individuals with a high educational background (see Chapters 6 and 97).

The value of early detection of dementia lies in the fact that a small number (perhaps 1 in 10 in some instances) are the result of reversible causes, e.g., vitamin B12 deficiency or thyroid disease, and may become irreversible if not recognized early. Vascular dementias may stabilize with aggressive control of cardiovascular risk factors, especially cigarette smoking and hypertension. The clinician should always pay careful attention to potentially offending drugs, including alcohol. Even with an Alzehimer's-type dementia, in which no effective treatment of the underlying process exists, early diagnosis may lead to the prevention of unnecessary comorbidity and caregiver stress, through early referral to community-based services and home-care services.

***Depression.*** Although no major authority recommends routine screening for depression in asymptomatic individuals, depression in the elderly may be quite subtle, making recognition and diagnosis difficult. It should be recognized that the elderly, particularly men, account for a disproportionate number of suicides, the majority of which are associated with depression and/or anxiety. Depression is commonly associated with early dementia where it serves to increase the severity of symptoms, and, in general, is a common concomitant or cause of functional decline. Depression itself may present as cognitive decline, which may be erroneously attributed to a primary dementia. This pseudodementia, as it is commonly called, is an important cause of reversible dementia. Depression is extremely common following stroke in the elderly, in which case it may impede or prevent maximal recovery.

For all of these reasons, the clinician should consider screening elderly patients for depressive symptoms. A simple, validated questionnaire, e.g., the geriatric depression scale, is useful in this regard. Once diagnosed, depression is readily treatable in the primary care setting, with referral or hospitalization reserved for patients who represent diagnostic or management dilemmas or who are actively suicidal. See Chapters 132 and 133 for a complete discussion of depression and its management.

***Falls.*** Falls are a major cause of morbidity and mortality in community-dwelling elderly. One in three persons over the age of 75 falls each year, one fourth of those will suffer a serious injury, and one twentieth will suffer a fracture. The highest risk exists in patients with a history of falling. Other important risk factors include the use of sedative medication, cognitive impairment, abnormalities of balance and gait, and urinary incontinence. Environmental hazards such as poor lighting, loose rugs, extension cords, and low furniture also frequently play a role.

Although there may be some overlap, fall syndromes should be distinguished from syncope, which has its own differential diagnosis and should prompt hospitalization in most instances. Clinicians should ask older patients about falls routinely, and follow up positive responses with questions designed to accurately characterize the event, keeping in mind that patients often give nonspecific answers, e.g., "I must have slipped."

The primary and secondary prevention of falls includes a routine history and physical with attention paid to excluding previously unrecognized acute illness, and evaluating and simplifying the patient's medication regimen, eliminating sedatives whenever possible. Orthostatic hypotension, which can be caused by a variety of medications and medical conditions, should be sought out and offending agents or conditions removed or treated. Vision, hearing, and cognitive status should be evaluated, and intervention or referral carried out when appropriate. Physical therapy or an exercise program may be of benefit in improving strength, gait, and balance. Patients should be counseled about the value of improving lighting, removing low furniture, and taping down loose rugs and lamp cords. The clinician should consider the potential benefit of a home visit by the clinician, or a home evaluation from a certified home health agency (see Chapter 6 for a more detailed discussion).

***Urinary incontinence.*** The prevalence of urinary incontinence rises steadily with age, and women are more frequently affected than men. Urinary incontinence is the single most common factor precipitating institutionalization in the elderly. Other important impairments and morbidity that can result from established urinary incontinence include social isolation, depression, and falls.

Urinary incontinence is a distressing and embarrassing problem that frequently is not volunteered by the patient. The clinician should routinely ask in a neutral and direct fashion about difficulty with bladder control, paying attention to timing (diurnal vs. nocturnal), amount voided, dribbling, and any association between coughing or laughing and dribbling. A history of urgency or dysuria is also important to consider. Often, the office history and physical examination lead to a diagnosis and effective intervention without referral. For a more detailed discussion of the evaluation and treatment of urinary incontinence, see Chapters 6 and 137.

***Cancer screening in the elderly.*** One of the most difficult questions primary care clinicians face is, "which screening procedures should I perform on or recommend to my older patients?" This question becomes more difficult when the procedure recommended is difficult, expensive, or invasive. The elderly bear a disproportionate amount of cancer in society, if incidence alone is considered, which would seem to make continued cancer surveillance at least attractive.

A large part of the problem is that the reports on the more common cancer screening studies either do not include or underrepresent the elderly in their study groups. The fact that a particular procedure is demonstrated to be beneficial in a younger study population should not be taken as evidence that the same strategy will prove beneficial in a frail, elderly population under normal practice conditions. Compliance with screening procedures is generally less satisfactory in the elderly, and medicare reimbursement for many of these procedures, e.g., flexible sigmoidoscopy, is lacking. The elderly are usually more concerned with preventing pain and disability in their later years, rather than simply living longer, and the main goal of geriatric medicine is improving functional survival rather than just overall survival.

The decision about which health maintenance procedures to offer, therefore, depends on a patient's preexisting functional status, preexisting illness and life expectancy, attitudes and desires about preventive care, and the time course of a given strategy's possible benefit. Thus an 80-year-old woman in relatively good health, with a life expectancy of about 7 years, is likely to benefit from continued screening mammography, which has been demonstrated in studies to result in a significant decrease in mortality of about 40% within 5 years. The same is clearly not true of an 80-year-old woman confined to a nursing home because of end-stage Alzheimer's disease. Pap smears may be beneficial in preventing invasive cervical cancer in older women who have not received prior screening but probably offer little to those who have been screened regularly up to the age of 65. The decision to continue stool guaiac testing into a patient's later years is more difficult, given the fact that the benefit is smaller and takes much longer to be realized. In addition, the high rate of false-positive results that involve uncomfortable and risky subsequent work-up needs to be considered.

## Immunizations and chemoprophylaxis

Providing immunizations is one of the most important functions of the primary care clinician. This important topic is addressed fully in Chapter 3 as well as travel-related immunization procedures and chemoprophylaxis.

In light of the recent increase in incidence of tuberculosis, purified protein derivative (PPD) testing is an important preventive procedure both for certain individuals and for the community at large. Persons with known exposures, who are employed in health care-related fields or who have immigrated from endemic areas, should be screened and considered for appropriate chemoprophylaxis if positive. Nursing home residents should be screened with a two-step procedure on admission and annually. For a full discussion see Chapter 114.

## Screening tests

*Colorectal cancer screening.* Colon cancer is the second most common lethal cancer in the United States, affecting both men and women equally. Lifetime incidence for persons of average risk is approximately 6%, but is 2 to 3 times higher for persons with an affected first-degree relative. Patients with a familial polyposis syndrome have a risk 20 to 30 times higher, virtually a 100% lifetime risk. Persons with ulcerative or Crohn's colitis also have a greatly increased risk, as much as 5- to 6-fold lifetime risk.

There is mounting evidence that colorectal cancer may be linked to certain dietary factors and therefore may be somewhat preventable. Treatment of advanced disease remains unsatisfactory, placing an emphasis on screening to detect early, potentially curable disease.

The clinician has a relatively wide array of useful screening procedures that vary dramatically in terms of availability, acceptability, efficacy, and cost. For most of these procedures, controlled, prospective data demonstrating a reduction in mortality from colorectal cancer are lacking. Therefore, a screening strategy must be chosen based on a patient's estimated risk and preferences.

**Digital rectal examination.** The digital rectal examination (DRE), in which the examiner inserts a gloved finger into the rectum to detect palpable neoplasia, is probably of minimal efficacy, since only about 10% of lesions arise within 7 cm of the anal verge. The main utilities are that the DRE allows direct palpation of the prostate gland in men and can be combined with office stool guaiac testing.

**Stool guaiac testing.** Stool guaiac testing is based on the detection of peroxidase-like activity in the stool, a result of the presence of occult blood (see Chapter 45 for a detailed discussion). Procedurally, the patient is instructed to test three consecutive stools by sampling two different areas of each stool using a wooden spatula or similar implement and applying it to the two slide windows of a guaiac testing card. One card is needed for each of the three bowel movements. The cards are subsequently developed by placing a few drops of a hydrogen peroxide solution onto them. A test is positive when any of the six slide windows turns blue, denoting the presence of heme. One week before testing it is recommended that the patient be placed on a meat-free diet that also omits foods high in peroxidase, e.g., horseradish and cauliflower. To minimize the false-negative rate, the cards should be developed within 1 week of sampling. Controversy has surrounded rehydrating the slides by placing a drop of deionized water on the slide before adding the developer solution. This increases the sensitivity of the test but also raises the false-positive rate and lowers the positive predictive value. However, a recent study by Mandel and colleagues, showing a 33% reduction in cause-specific mortality through annual stool guaiac testing, supports the use of rehydration before developing the cards. Stool guaiac testing has an approximate sensitivity of 50% to 60% for malignancy (lower for polyps), and a positive test has a 5% to 10% positive predictive value for malignancy and 15% to 45% for polyps. Any patient with a positive result should be further investigated with colonoscopy or air-contrast barium enema.

**Sigmoidoscopy.** The use of sigmoidoscopy to screen for colorectal cancer is being reevaluated. The American Cancer Society recommends flexible sigmoidoscopy every 3 to 5 years following two negative examinations 1 year apart for persons of usual risk over the age of 50, based on data from uncontrolled, observational studies. The USPSTF and National Cancer Institute have not recommended routine sigmoidoscopy, citing a lack of evidence of efficacy (see Chapter 45). The theoretic advantage and intuitive appeal of sigmoidoscopy stem from the well-accepted natural history of colorectal cancer, in which most invasive cancers arise from premalignant, adenomatous polyps, a process that is felt to take an average of 7 years. Using a sigmoidoscope, the examiner can identify, biopsy, and/or remove suspicious lesions within reach of the instrument. Sigmoidoscopy can be considered therefore to be virtually 100% sensitive and specific within its reach, and 60% of all potential cancers arise within reach of a 65 cm flexible sigmoidoscope. Although there are no prospective controlled studies demonstrating that screening with sigmoidoscopy reduces mortality from colorectal cancer, studies do demonstrate that malignant lesions discovered during sigmoidoscopic screening are less advanced (Dukes' A and B) than lesions that present with symptoms, a trend also demonstrated with stool guaiac screening, which has now been shown to reduce mortality from colon cancer. If one accepts this shift toward less advanced lesions as a surrogate endpoint, then the evidence strongly supports the use of sigmoidoscopy for screening. Indeed, it is anticipated that the USPSTF will soon update its recommendations so as to be more in favor of screening both by stool guaiacs and sigmoidoscopy.

Weighed against the use of sigmoidoscopy are its relatively low availability (though this procedure is well within the purview of the generalist), its significant cost, greater discomfort, and the risk of bleeding or perforation from the procedure. If performed, the sigmoidoscopy should be combined with annual DRE and stool guaiac testing.

**Colonoscopy.** The use of colonoscopy to screen for colorectal cancer offers the advantage of direct visualization of the entire colon from rectum to cecum, with the removal or biopsy of all suspicious lesions. This is achieved through greater discomfort, a more difficult bowel preparation, much greater cost, and higher risk of perforation. Furthermore, it is estimated that the increase in efficacy over a program of stool guaiacs, DRE, and sigmoidoscopy is marginal. For all of these reasons colonoscopy is rarely used purely for screening in persons of usual risk, but is quite reasonable and frequently recommended for persons at much greater risk, e.g., first-degree relative with colon cancer, familial polyposis syndromes, or inflammatory bowel disease (IBD).

*Cervical cancer screening.* A woman of average risk in the United States has an approximately 0.7% cumulative lifetime risk of developing invasive carcinoma of the uterine cervix, and a 2% lifetime risk of carcinoma in situ. While these risks are relatively low in comparison with other important malignancies, they are heavily affected by screening, and, according to estimates, would be 2 to 3 times higher in an unscreened population. The risk is increased in African-Americans and Hispanics, as well as with early age of first intercourse, multiple sexual partners, cigarette smoking, and oral contraceptive use.

Based on a wealth of empiric evidence, the efficacy of cervical cancer screening using the Pap smear is widely accepted. Numerous population-based reports looking at the effects of widespread screening studies have demonstrated a dramatic impact on the incidence of invasive cervical carcinoma and carcinoma in situ.

Some controversy remains regarding the age to begin screening, the age to end screening, and the optimal frequency at which to screen. It appears that to maintain most of its efficacy, screening should begin in a patient's early 20s at the latest and continue until the age of 65. Beginning at age 17 or continuing until age 75 results in only marginal gains at a substantial cost, if considered on a population-wide basis. Notably, the efficacy of screening from age 65 to 75 or later is much higher if the woman has not had a prior Pap smear. Likewise, screening annually rather than every 3 years results in marginal benefit. At intervals greater than every 3 years the benefit falls off significantly, but screening still retains approximately 65% efficacy at an interval of every 10 years. Ultimately, decisions regarding the age to begin screening and the interval at which to screen should be based on the patient's preferences, as well as on an assessment of their baseline risk. Current recommendations are for screenings to begin at age 18 or at the beginning of sexual activity, with annual examinations through the age of 65. This protocol is estimated to reduce invasive cervical cancer by more than 90%.

*Breast cancer screening.* Breast cancer is currently the second most common cause of cancer death among women. At present, a woman of average risk has a one in nine cumulative lifetime risk of developing breast cancer, with the risk increasing two to three times in those who have a first-degree relative afflicted. Of those who develop breast cancer, approximately one half will die from the disease. In the absence of knowledge regarding effective primary prevention, the primary care provider must emphasize early detection and cure. Fortunately, effective screening strategies exist that utilize one- and two-view mammography, singularly and in combination with clinician-performed breast examination. However, many unanswered questions and controversies remain.

The efficacy of mammography with and without clinician-performed breast palpation in lowering breast cancer-related mortality for women between the ages of 50 and 74 has been demonstrated by several large prospective studies and is accepted by most authorities. The magnitude of this reduction ranges from approximately 15% to 30% and may be higher for women in the 50- to 60-year-old age group. Standard recommendations for women of average risk include annual two-view mammography in combination with at least annual clinician-performed breast palpation beginning at age 50. Although of unproven benefit, a baseline mammogram is commonly performed between the ages of 40 and 50 to improve the diagnostic accuracy of subsequent mammograms. If annual screenings are planned beginning at age 40, then a baseline mammogram at age 35 is customary.

*Controversies in breast cancer screening*

**Screening in younger women.** No study has definitively demonstrated a benefit of mammography with or without breast palpation in the 40- to 49-year-old age bracket, although late follow-up from one study has strongly suggested an emerging trend. Factors contributing to a lesser efficacy of screening in this cohort include a lower incidence of breast cancer in younger women, radiographically denser breasts that may conceal important mammographic abnormalities, and the detection of tumors that may be less amenable to therapy. Factors that further weigh against mammographic screening in this age group include potentially higher risk of radiation-induced breast cancer, both through higher sensitivity of the breast tissue and through a longer period of time over which a woman will be exposed. Despite these reservations, the American Cancer Society recommends mammography in the 40- to 49-year age group.

**Screening in older women.** Most available studies address the use of breast palpation and mammography in women 40 to 75 years old. Evidence suggests that women between the ages of 50 and 69 derive the majority of mammography's benefit. A possible reason for a lack of efficacy for mammography in older women is the tendency for postmenopausal breast cancer to behave in a less aggressive manner and to respond readily to hormonal therapy. The use of mammography in women over the age of 75 should therefore be individualized. Most authorities recommend the continued use of clinician performed breast palpation with or without breast self-examination in women older than 75.

**Breast self-examination.** Although widely recommended and taught, Breast Self-Examination (BSE) has not been subjected to enough scientific study to allow specific recommendations regarding its use. It is likely that efficacy is linked to technique, method of instruction, and reinforcement. The most favorable estimates place sensitivity at approximately 25%, in comparison to the approximately 50% sensitivity for both mammography and clinician-performed breast examination. Since the false positive rate, and hence specificity, is unknown, its value as a screening procedure, either alone or in combination with other modalities, cannot be determined.

However, BSE may have higher sensitivity in younger women for whom mammography may be less desirable. If employed, it is best used either as a sole screening strategy when other modalities are unavailable or impractical, or in combination with mammography and clinician-performed breast examination, where it has the potential to detect interval tumors (cancers which become manifest between screening visits).

**Frequency of screening.** The optimal frequency of screening is unknown, but data from several studies suggest that the mortality reduction increases as the interval between screenings decreases. Annual mammography is most widely recommended, BSE is generally recommended at monthly intervals, and a clinician-performed breast palpation should be done at least annually.

***Prostate cancer.*** Prostate cancer is currently the most common malignancy, and the second most common cause of cancer-related death, in men in the United States (see Chapter 138 for a detailed discussion). The incidence of prostate cancer increases steadily with advancing age, and may approach 100% in men past 90, if one includes small microscopic foci of disease. Since effective primary prevention is unclear, early diagnosis in the hopes of curative therapy has been emphasized as an effective strategy to combat this disease, which accounts for more than 35,000 deaths in the United States annually. The lifetime cumulative risk of developing prostate cancer is approximately 10% in men of average risk. Risk doubles for men who have a first-degree relative affected by prostate cancer, and the risk redoubles for each additional first-degree relative affected. For reasons which are not understood, African-Americans have a 50% increased risk of developing prostate cancer.

Despite the significant burden of disease from prostate cancer, poor knowledge regarding natural history and prognostic factors, as well as a lack of prospectively determined proof of the efficacy of screening in terms of disease-specific mortality reduction, poses significant decision-making difficulties for the clinician regarding the potential benefit of screening. Therefore, the standard screening modalities are discussed in terms of their characteristics and potential efficacy, and remaining controversies and limitations are emphasized.

**Digital rectal examination.** An annual DRE is recommended for men over the age of 40 by the American Cancer Society, both to detect prostate cancer and to act as part of a screening strategy for colorectal cancer. Early studies suggested benefit for populations screened by this method based on survival comparisons with historic controls. Furthermore, there seems to be a shift toward the detection of disease confined to the gland in serially screened patients. Although the sensitivity, specificity, and positive predictive values of DRE have been estimated (Table 2-1), they are likely to be overestimates. Tumors arising in the medial lobe and transitional zones (approximately 30% of significant tumors) are not readily detectable. The DRE's ability to detect disease confined to the gland is apparently limited, as approximately 50% of tumors detected by DRE that have clinically limited-stage disease (stages A and B) are found to have more advanced disease after surgical staging. Despite this, 30% of significant prostate cancers are potentially detectable at a curable stage by DRE.

**Table 2-1.** Representative sensitivity, specificity, positive predictive value, and detection rates of DRE, PSA, and TRUS in the evaluation for prostate cancer

| Method | Sensitivity (%) | Specificity (%) | Positive predictive value (%) | Detection rate (%) |
|---|---|---|---|---|
| DRE | 69-89 | 84-98 | 26-35 | 1.3-1.7 |
| PSA | 57-79 | 59-68 | 40-49 | 2.2-2.6 |
| TRUS | 36-85 | 41-79 | 27-36 | 2.6 |

From *Mayo Clin Proc* 68:300 1993.

*DRE*, digital rectal examination; *PSA*, prostate-specific antigen; *TRUS*, transrectal ultrasonography.

**Prostate-specific antigen.** The prostate-specific antigen (PSA) is a serine protease produced only in the prostate gland and detectable in the serum. Because both normal and malignant prostatic cells produce PSA, it can be elevated in a variety of prostate disorders, most commonly BPH. Although the degree of elevation is generally higher with prostate cancer, there is enough overlap between benign and malignant disease, particularly early malignant disease, to necessitate further investigation. Values between 0 and 4 ng/ml are considered normal, although they are not inconsistent with early cancer. Values greater than 10 are highly specific for prostate cancer, although many patients with values in this range already have incurable disease. In the range from 4 to 10 ng/ml, the PSA levels generated by most curable prostate cancers, there is maximal overlap between benign and malignant disease, making interpretation difficult. Thus, PSA has neither a sufficient sensitivity or specificity to be useful as a sole screening method. PSA's abilities to distinguish benign from malignant prostatic disease may be improved substantially by relating the PSA to a transrectal ultrasound-determined prostate volume to yield a PSA Density (PSAD). This method relies on the observation that for an equal volume of prostate tissue, malignant tissue produces a greater elevation in serum PSA. Although promising, this method has not been subjected to prospective clinical validation. Measuring the rate of change of the PSA over time, especially at lower serum values, may improve the specificity when a cutoff threshold of 0.75 ng/ml/year is used, but again this has not been adequately studied.

**Transrectal ultrasound.** Like DRE and PSA, transrectal ultrasound (TRUS) lacks the adequate sensitivity and specificity to be used as a sole screening method, especially considering its cost and lesser acceptability. Although it has the ability to detect many tumors missed

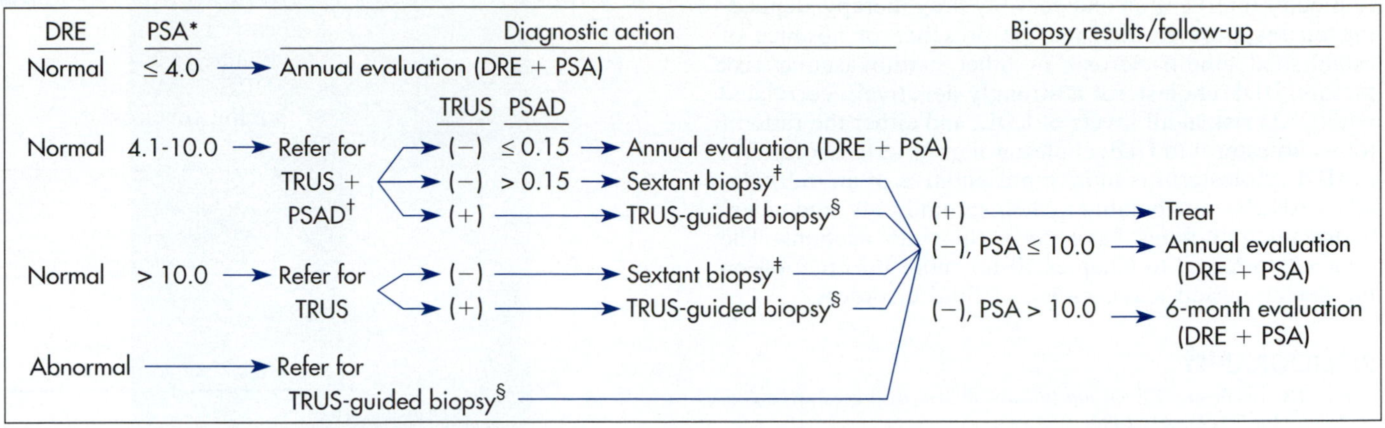


**Fig. 2-5.** Algorithm for the use of digital rectal examination (DRE), prostate-specific antigen (PSA) value, and transrectal ultrasonography (TRUS) in early detection of significant prostate cancer. *, Tandem-R PSA assay, ng/ml; †, PSA density (serum PSA concentration/prostate volume); ‡, three cores from each side of the prostate (base, middle, and apex); §, single or multiple cores from lesion identified by TRUS. (From *Mayo Clin Proc* 68:304, 1993.)

by DRE, TRUS adds little when both the DRE and PSA are normal. At present, the main role of TRUS is in the further evaluation of an abnormal DRE or PSA, and in guiding biopsies.

**Combined use of DRE, PSA, and TRUS.** Although PSA and DRE have comparable abilities to detect early prostate cancer, they do not always detect the same tumors and are therefore complementary in terms of diagnostic accuracy. Fig. 2-5 gives an example of a diagnostic strategy for the early detection of prostate cancer. It is based on the use of DRE and PSA as screening modalities, with TRUS (and PSAD) reserved for patients with abnormal results.

Despite the rational appeal of such algorithms, no prospective study exists that demonstrates a benefit of prostate cancer screening in terms of a reduced disease-specific mortality. Furthermore, much of what is known about the performance of DRE, PSA, and TRUS has been determined from studies involving self-referred subjects or patients referred for the evaluation of early obstructive symptoms. The results for the general population could be radically different. Because of a variable, but frequently indolent natural history for untreated early prostate cancer, the benefits of screening may be less for older men despite a higher prevalence of disease.

The NCI has recently begun a prospective study of screening involving the use of DRE and PSA, but results are still many years away. Despite the controversy, the American Cancer Society continues to recommend an annual DRE for men over the age of 50 and recently has joined several other authorities in embracing the PSA on an annual basis for the early detection of prostate cancer. The NCI and USPSTF do not recommend PSA for screening asymptomatic patients. The clinician is therefore left to devise an appropriate protocol based on the available information as well as patient risks and preferences regarding cancer screening.

***Screening for CHD risk with serum cholesterol.*** Coronary heart disease (CHD) is the most common cause of death in the United States and in many western countries and causes a large amount of morbidity. The established risk factors for CHD include male sex, family history of premature CHD, hypertension, cigarette smoking, sedentary lifestyle, obesity, diabetes, and elevated serum cholesterol.

In recent years, screening for elevated serum cholesterol has become a central focus of the periodic health examination. This is a result of the importance of CHD in the population; the establishment of a causal link between elevated serum cholesterol (specifically the LDL fraction) and CHD; the synergy with and interplay between elevated serum cholesterol and other modifiable cardiovascular risk factors; the availability of management strategies that can significantly lower total and LDL cholesterol; and the growing amount of experimental evidence that interventions lowering serum total and LDL cholesterol result in a reduced risk of CHD and CHD-related mortality. See Chapter 7 for a detailed discussion of cardiovascular risk factors, including serum cholesterol.

The National Cholesterol Education Program of the National Heart, Blood, and Lung Institute has issued guidelines for routine screening, detection, and follow-up and treatment of persons with elevated serum (LDL) cholesterol. Although the optimal interval is not firmly established, screenings are recommended at least every 5 years for all adults over the age of 20, regardless of other cardiovascular risk factors. Screening is accomplished through the measurement of a random total serum cholesterol. Individuals with a total serum cholesterol under 200 mg% are considered to have a desirable cholesterol. Total serum cholesterols between 200 and 239 mg% are considered borderline, and a total serum cholesterol of 240 mg% or more is considered to be elevated.

For individuals with either a borderline or elevated total serum cholesterol, further investigation with a fasting lipoprotein electrophoresis and triglyceride is recommended, in order to determine the LDL cholesterol and HDL cholesterol. LDL values less than 130 are desirable and do not warrant further specific intervention. Individuals with either borderline (130 to 159 mg%) or elevated (greater than 160 mg%) are candidates for varying degrees of dietary intervention and possibly drug therapy, depending on response to diet and the presence or absence of established atherosclerosis or other cardiovascular risk factors. HDL cholesterol is strongly negatively correlated with CAD risk at all levels of LDL, and either the ratio of total cholesterol to HDL cholesterol or of LDL cholesterol to HDL cholesterol is more representative of an individual's CAD risk attributable to their serum lipids, and newer treatment guidelines have taken this into account. The reader is referred to Chapter 40 for more information on the detection and management of lipid disorders.

## BIBLIOGRAPHY

Baker DB, Landrigan PJ: Occupationally related disorders, *Med Clin North Am* 74 (2):441, 1990.

Eddy DM: Screening for cervical cancer, *Ann Intern Med* 113:214, 1990.

Eddy DM: Screening for colorectal cancer, *Ann Intern Med* 113:373, 1990.

Fletcher SW, Siscovick DS, Inui TS: Research of the periodic health examination: opportunities for the general internist, *J Gen Intern Med* 1 (Suppl):S45, 1986.

Frame PS: Can computerized reminder systems have an impact on preventive services in practice?, *J Gen Intern Med* 5 (Suppl):S112, 1990.

Hayward RS et al: Preventive care guidelines: 1991, *Ann Intern Med* 114:758, 1991.

Hurley SF, Kaldor JM: The benefits and risks of mammographic screening for breast cancer, *Epidemiol Rev* 14:101, 1992.

Kramer BS et al: Prostate cancer screening: what we know and what we need to know, *Ann Intern Med* 119:914, 1993.

Lowenstein SR, Hunt D: Injury prevention in primary care, *Ann Intern Med* 113(4):261, 1990.

Morrison AS: Screening for cancer of the breast, *Epidemiol Rev* 15(1):244, 1993.

O'Malley MS, Fletcher SW: Screening for breast cancer with breast self-examination: a critical review, *JAMA* 257:2196, 1987.

Polen MR, Friedman GD: United States Preventive Services Task Force. Automobile injury—selected risk factors and prevention in the health care setting, *JAMA* 259(1):76, 1988.

Sassetti MR: Domestic violence, *Prim Care,* 20(2):289, 1993.

Slap GB: The periodic health examination and adolescent pregnancy: 1988, *Ann Intern Med* 109(9):692, 1988.

Stringham P, Weitzman M: Violence counseling in the routine health care of adolescents, *J Adolesc Health Care* 9:389, 1988.

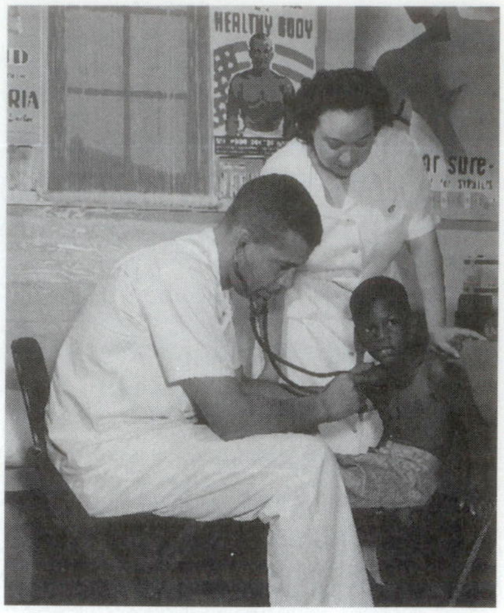


**Fig. 3-1.** Courtesy the Library of Congress.

CHAPTER

# 3 Immunizations for Health Maintenance and Travel

**Julie Kaufmann**

Immunizations are one of the most cost-effective medical interventions for public health. The widespread use of immunizations in pediatric practices has greatly reduced the incidence of vaccine-preventable diseases in children. Unfortunately, immunizations are not a part of routine care in many adult medicine practices. As a result, a substantial proportion of the morbidity and the overwhelming majority of the mortality from vaccine-preventable diseases occur in older adolescents and adults. Improvements in adult immunization practices are needed to continue the beneficial impact that has resulted from vaccination. The primary care practitioner is in a unique position to assess the need for and to administer vaccines on a regular basis to their older adolescent and adult patients. To ensure patients' optimal protection against vaccine-preventable illnesses, practitioners must learn to evaluate patients according to their age criteria and their individual risk for specific vaccine-preventable illnesses. These risks include concomitant medical illnesses, lifestyle, occupational and environmental exposures, nationality, and travel plans.

## GENERAL CONSIDERATIONS

One of the more readily achieved goals of vaccination is the prevention of disease in an individual. The ultimate goal is the elimination of disease by maintaining a high level of immunity in the population. The recommendations for vaccinations in this country come from the Advisory Committee on Immunization Practices (ACIP). The American College of Physicians also publishes guidelines. These recommendations are based on an individual's risk of exposure to the disease, susceptibility to the disease, and the risk of transmitting the disease to others. The characteristics of the immunobiologic (vaccine or immune globulin), scientific knowledge about the principles of immunization, and the risk, benefit, and cost of the immunobiologic are also considered.

Most vaccine-preventable illnesses and disease exposures requiring postexposure prophylaxis must be reported to the local or state health department. Public health officials rely on the reporting of vaccine-preventable illnesses to evaluate and plan prevention strategies on a local level. In addition, the data are used to evaluate national policies, practices, and strategies for future vaccination programs.

The Vaccine Adverse Event Reporting System (VAERS) is a reporting system for monitoring serious adverse reactions to immunobiologics (see the box at right). The reported information helps to both improve the general knowledge about adverse reactions, since these

## Agencies and abbreviations

**Agencies**

US Department of Health and Human Services
Public Health Service
Centers for Disease Control
National Center for Prevention Services
Division of Quarantine
Atlanta, GA 30333
1-404-639-3311

Traveler's Hotline: Centers for Disease Control
1-404-332-4559

Vaccine Adverse Event Reporting System (VAERS)
PO Box 1100
Rockville, MD 20849-1100
1-800-822-7967

**Abbreviations**

**Td:** tetanus diphtheria vaccine
**MMR:** measles, mumps, rubella vaccine
**IPV:** inactivated poliovirus vaccine
**OPV:** oral polio vaccine
**HBV:** hepatitis B vaccine
**HbCV:** hemophilus influenza b conjugate vaccine
**ACIP:** Advisory Committee on Immunization Practices
**VAERS:** Vaccine Adverse Event Reporting System
**IG:** immune globulin
**HBIG:** hepatitis B IG
**VZIG:** varicella-zoster IG
**TIG:** tetanus IG
**HRIG:** human rabies IG

reactions are indeed rare, and provide a database for reactions to newer vaccines. It is also used to stimulate research to confirm a causal association and to identify risk factors for adverse events.

### Principles of vaccination

Active immunization is achieved by using immunogens to simulate a natural infection which results in an antitoxic, antiinvasive, or neutralizing activity in the recipient. Such immunogens include live attenuated virus, inactivated virus, and bacterial proteins or polysaccharides. Some agents induce lifelong protection, some provide partial protection, and some must be readministered for continued effectiveness. The efficacy of the vaccine is defined by the protection against natural disease. The antibody response is an indirect measure of protection because in some instances the immunologic reaction responsible for protection is poorly understood; in these instances the serum antibody concentrations are not always predictive of protection.

Passive immunization with immune globulin is used to provide immediate antibody levels for individuals who have recently been exposed or who soon may be exposed to a disease. Passive immunization is also used to provide antibody for individuals who are immunocompromised and would be expected to have a poor immunogenic response to an illness exposure or to a previous active immunization. It is used therapeutically when a disease is already present and the antibody may help to suppress the effects of a toxin (see Immune Globulins).

### Records, route, site, and dosage

Physicians should maintain a permanent vaccination record for each patient as required by law. This record should include the type of immunization, the site of vaccination, the lot number, and the date given. Patients should be given information on the risks and benefits of immunization and their own vaccination record for future reference.

The route of immunization is important for each individual vaccine. Vaccines developed for intramuscular use should not be given subcutaneously because the immune response may be decreased, and there is a risk of local irritation, inflammation, and necrosis from the adjuvant present in the vaccine. The preferred site for intramuscular injections in adults is the deltoid muscle where the risk of vascular or neural injury is low. The buttock should not be used routinely as a site for intramuscular injection because of the proximity of the sciatic nerve and because the depth of fat may make performing a true intramuscular injection difficult. If the buttock must be used to accommodate large volume injections, such as IG or multiple doses of vaccines, the upper outer quadrant is preferred. In general, no more than 5 ml should be given at one site. It is preferable to avoid giving two intramuscular injections in the same limb, especially if one is known to commonly cause a local reaction. If it is necessary to give more than one vaccine in a limb, the vaccine sites should be at least 1 to 2 inches apart. Whenever administering any vaccine and immune globulin, the sites chosen should be remote from each other (e.g., the deltoid for the vaccine and the buttock for the immune globulin). In adults, a 20 to 25 gauge 1- to 1½-inch needle is used for intramuscular injections (care should be taken to perform a true intramuscular injection in an obese patient), a 23 to 25 gauge ⅝- to ¾-inch needle for subcutaneous injections, and a 25 to 27 gauge ⅜- to ¾-inch needle for intradermal injections.

### Vaccine schedules and missed doses

The recommendations for the dosage of vaccines are derived from clinical experience, experimental trials, and theoretic considerations. Adherence to the recommended schedules provides the most predictable outcome in terms of side effects and clinical efficacy. If during the course of a vaccination series a dose is delayed, it is recommended that the schedule be continued and not restarted, since this does not generally lead to a decline in final antibody levels. Giving doses at less than the recommended interval, however, should be avoided because it may weaken the immune response, and some vaccines are more likely to produce local or systemic symptoms if given this way. If a vaccine is given at less than the recommended time interval it should not be considered part of a series. Minor illness with or without fever is not a contraindication to receiving a vaccine, especially if poor compliance is a concern. Moderate or severe illness with or without fever is a contraindication. Vaccination should be delayed if possible, so that symptoms of the illness are not mistaken for side effects of the vaccine, and to ensure an optimum immune response to the vaccine.

**Table 3-1.** Administration of multiple vaccines and immune globulins

| Vaccine combination | Recommended minimum interval between doses |
|---|---|
| ≥2 Killed vaccines | None. May be administered simultaneously or at any interval between doses. (If possible, cholera, parenteral typhoid, and plague vaccines should be given on separate occasions to avoid accentuating their side effects.) |
| Killed and live vaccines | None. May be administered simultaneously or at any interval between doses. (Cholera vaccine with yellow fever vaccine is the exception. These vaccines should be given separately at least 3 weeks apart; otherwise the antibody response to each may be suboptimal.) |
| ≥2 Live vaccines | May be administered simultaneously. If given separately, there must be an interval at least 4 weeks between them. However, OPV can be administered at any time before, with, or after an MMR or oral typhoid, if indicated. |
| Live vaccine and PPD | May be administered simultaneously. If given separately, the PPD should be given 4 to 6 weeks after the live vaccine. |
| Immune globulin and killed vaccine | None. May be administered simultaneously or at any interval between doses. |
| Immune globulin and live vaccine | Should not be given together. The live vaccine should be given a minimum of two weeks before the immune globulin. If the live vaccine is to be given after the immune globulin, the minimum time that should elapse between administration is dose dependent and is outlined in Table 3-1A. Of note, OPV, oral typhoid, and yellow fever are exceptions to these recommendations and can be given any time before, during, or after an immune globulin-containing product. |

Modified from *MMWR* 43 (RR-1): 15 and 16, 1994.

**Table 3-1A.** Suggested time intervals between administration of immune globulin-containing products for various indications and vaccines containing live measles virus*

| Indication | Dose (including mg IgG/kg) | Suggested interval before measles vaccination (months) |
|---|---|---|
| Tetanus (TIG) | 250 units (10 mg IgG/kg) IM | 3 |
| Hepatitis A (IG) | | |
| Contact prophylaxis | 0.02 ml/kg (3.3 mg IgG/kg) IM | 3 |
| International travel | 0.06 ml/kg (10 mg IgG/kg) IM | 3 |
| Hepatitis B prophylaxis (HBIG) | 0.06 ml/kg (10 mg IgG/kg) IM | 3 |
| Rabies prophylaxis (HRIG) | 20 IU/kg (22 mg IgG/kg) IM | 4 |
| Varicella prophylaxis (VZIG) | 125 units/10 kg (20-40 mg IgG/kg) IM (maximum 625 units) | 5 |
| Measles prophylaxis (IG) | | |
| Normal contact | 0.25 ml/kg (40 mg IgG/kg) IM | 5 |
| Immunocompromised contact | 0.50 ml/kg (80 mg IgG/kg) IM | 6 |
| Blood transfusion | | |
| Red blood cells (RBCs), washed | 10 ml/kg (negligible IgG/kg) IV | 0 |
| RBCs, adenine-saline added | 10 ml/kg (10 mg IgG/kg) IV | 3 |
| Packed RBCs (Hct 65%)† | 10 ml/kg (60 mg IgG/kg) IV | 6 |
| Whole blood (Hct 35%-50%)† | 10 ml/kg (80-100 mg IgG/kg) IV | 6 |
| Plasma/platelet products | 10 ml/kg (160 mg IgG/kg) IV | 7 |
| Replacement of humoral immune deficiencies | 300-400 mg/kg IV (as IGIV) | 8 |
| Treatment of: | | |
| ITP‡ | 400 mg/kg IV (as IGIV) | 8 |
| ITP‡ | 1000 mg/kg IV (as IGIV) | 10 |
| Kawasaki disease | 2 grams/kg IV (as IGIV) | 11 |

From *MMWR* 43 (No. RR-1): 17, 1994.

*This table is not intended for determining the correct indications and dosage for the use of immune globulin preparations. Unvaccinated persons may not be fully protected against measles during the entire suggested interval and additional doses of immune globulin and/or measles vaccine may be indicated following measles exposure. The concentration of measles antibody in a particular immune globulin preparation can vary by lot. The rate of antibody clearance following receipt of an immune globulin preparation can also vary. The recommended intervals are extrapolated from an estimated half-life of 30 days for passively acquired antibody and an observed interference with the immune response to measles vaccine for 5 months following a dose of 80 mg IgG/kg.

†Assumes a serum IgG concentration of 16 mg/ml.

‡Immune (formally, idiopathic) thrombocytopenic purpura.

### Hypersensitivity and local reactions

Some vaccines contain antibiotics and animal protein that may induce hypersensitivity reactions. Influenza, the MMR, and yellow fever vaccines are prepared in chicken embryos. Any person with an anaphylactic response to chicken eggs should not receive these vaccines; rubella vaccine grown in human diploid cell cultures is available and safe for these patients. OPV and IPV contain small amounts of streptomycin, and IPV contains small amounts of polymyxin B. The MMR vaccines and their individual components, as well as OPV and IPV vaccines, contain small amounts of neomycin. Anyone with an anaphylactic response to the antibiotic in a vaccine should not receive the vaccine. Most often the allergy to neomycin is not an anaphylactic response but a contact dermatitis. This cell-mediated response is not a contraindication for these vaccines. Some vaccines such as cholera, Td, plague, and parenteral typhoid commonly cause fever, local redness, and soreness. These reactions appear to be toxic rather than hypersensitive. If an urticarial reaction to any vaccine is noted or if a person has a history of a hypersensitivity reaction to a vaccine component, the recipient should have skin testing before a decision is made to discontinue the vaccine altogether. Any unusual or severe reaction should be reported to VAERS.

### Administration of multiple vaccines and immune globulins

The administration of multiple vaccines is often desirable to minimize patient visits for vaccination and increase compliance, especially if there is uncertainty of patient follow-up. It may also be necessary if several vaccinations are needed in a short time in preparation for travel abroad. In general, any combination of inactivated vaccines, or inactivated vaccines and a live vaccine, can be given simultaneously or at any interval between doses without interfering with the immune response or side effect profile. A notable exception is the combination of cholera and yellow fever vaccines, because their simultaneous administration blunts the immune response to both. Ideally, they should be spaced at least 3 weeks apart. In addition, some inactivated vaccines such as cholera, parenteral typhoid, and plague commonly cause local or systemic reactions; therefore, simultaneous administration of these vaccines should be avoided if possible. Any combination of live vaccines can be administered on the same day. If live vaccines are to be given at separate times, they should be given at least 1 month apart to ensure adequate antibody response. If the time interval is less, serologic testing should be performed or the second vaccine should be repeated after the 1-month interval. A notable exception is that, if necessary, OPV can be given any time before or after either an MMR or oral typhoid vaccine, because the immune responses to the vaccines are not affected. The response to purified protein derivative (PPD) may be blunted because of a developing immune response to a live vaccine. A PPD may be administered on the same day as the live vaccine or 4 to 6 weeks later (Table 3-1).

Immune globulin preparations and other antibody-containing blood products do not interfere with the immune response to inactivated vaccines. Immune globulin preparations do interfere with the antibody response to live vaccines, with the exception of OPV, oral typhoid, and yellow fever. Since the immune response to a live vaccine occurs 1 to 2 weeks postvaccination, any immune globulin-containing product should be given at least 2 weeks after a live vaccine. If the time interval is less, serologic testing should be performed or the vaccination repeated after the 2-week interval. The time interval between administering immune globulin–containing product and then a live vaccine appears to be dose dependent and is shown in Table 3-1A. The suggested intervals are based on the estimated half-life of 30 days for passively acquired antibody and the immune response to measles vaccine administered after 80 mg IG/kg. Despite these recommendations, one should not miss the opportunity to vaccinate a postpartum woman who needs an MMR, even if she has received anti-Rho-IG or any IG-containing products. If it is necessary to administer a live vaccine within the recommended time interval, serologic testing should be performed to ensure an adequate response or the vaccination should be repeated after the appropriate interval.

## GENERAL RECOMMENDATIONS

Childhood vaccination in the United States is one of the mainstays of disease prevention. Diseases for which childhood vaccination is recommended include tetanus, diphtheria, pertussis, measles, mumps, rubella, polio, hemophilus influenza type b, and hepatitis B (Table 3-2). In addition, varicella and hepatitis A vaccines were recently approved by the Food and Drug Administration.

*Text continued on p. 34.*

**Table 3-2.** Immunizations for children in the United States*

| Vaccine | Birth | 2 Months | 4 Months | 6 Months | 6-18 Months | 15 Months | 4-6 Years | 11-12 Years | 14-16 Years |
|---|---|---|---|---|---|---|---|---|---|
| DPT | | X | X | X | | X | X | | as Td |
| OPV | | X | X | X | | | X | | |
| MMR | | | | | | X | X | | |
| HbCV | | X | X | X | | | | | |
| HBV | X | X | | | X | | | X† | |

*A representative and commonly used schedule. Consult a pediatric text for specific details and other schedule options. Varicella vaccine was recently approved, although recommendations are pending.

*DPT*, Diphtheria, tetanus, and pertussis; *OPV*, oral polio vaccine; *MMR*, measles, mumps, rubella vaccine; *HbCV*, hemophilus influenza b conjugate vaccine; *HBV*, hepatitis B vaccine; *Td*, tetanus diptheria vaccine.

†Adolescents at risk who were not vaccinated previously should be given the series.

**Table 3-3.** Immunizations for adults in the United States ≥18 years of age*

| Name | Primary schedule and booster(s) | Indications | Side effects |
|---|---|---|---|
| Tetanus/diphtheria adsorbed toxoid (Td) | Two 0.5 ml IM doses 1 month apart and third dose 6-12 months after the second; booster every 10 years; (see Table 3-6 for post-exposure prophylaxis). | All adults; check for receipt of primary series in refugees, immigrants, foreign born. | Local erythema and pain; rarely anaphylaxis, neuropathy, encephalopathy. |
| Measles (as MMR) live virus | One 0.5 ml SC dose; second dose at least 1 month later (or immunity by antibody titers or physician-diagnosed measles). | Adults born after 1956 need one dose; an additional dose is given upon entering school, a long-term correctional facility, health-care work, during outbreaks, and for foreign travel; adults born before 1957 are considered immune, but giving one dose to health-care workers at risk of exposure may be prudent. | Local erythema and pain, low grade fever, rash, arthralgias from 1 to 21 days postvaccination; rarely, high fever from 5 to 21 days postvaccination. |
| Mumps (as MMR) live virus | One 0.5 ml SC dose (or immunity by antibody titers or physician-diagnosed mumps). | All adults born after 1956; adults born before 1957 are considered immune. | As for measles. |
| Rubella (as MMR) live virus | One 0.5 ml SC dose (or immunity by antibody titers). | All adults. | As for measles. |
| Polio (OPV), live virus, oral; (IPV), inactivated virus | IPV preferred for primary vaccination. Two 0.5 ml SC doses 1 to 2 months apart and third dose 6-12 months after the second; one booster dose for travelers. | Adults generally considered immune; indicated for health-care workers exposed to the virus, unimmunized persons whose children receive OPV, travelers to high-risk countries (see Table 3-7). | Rarely poliomyelitis (OPV); local pain and erythema, rarely fever (IPV). |
| Hepatitis B, recombinant DNA–derived surface antigen particles | Two IM doses 1 month apart and third dose 5 months after the second; higher dose and more frequent schedule for persons with chronic renal failure approaching dialysis; check postvaccination antibody titers in health-care workers, immunocompromised, HIV-infected and persons with chronic renal failure; yearly titers with boosters as needed for persons on dialysis (see Tables 3-4 and 3-5 for post-exposure prophylaxis). | Persons with multiple sex partners or sexually transmitted diseases, male homosexuals, injection drug users, persons whose sex partner is in a high-risk group, frequent recipients of blood products, persons on hemodialysis, Native Alaskans, health-care or public safety workers with frequent blood or body fluid exposures, institutionalized developmentally disabled and their staff, household and sexual contacts of chronically infected carriers (for contacts of acutely infected persons see Table 3-4); consider for persons from an endemic area residing in a similar cultural community in the U.S.; certain travelers to high risk areas (see Table 3-7). | Local erythema and pain; rarely fever |

Modified from *MMWR* 40 (RR-12): 60, 82, 1991 and *MMWR* 42 (RR-4): 16, 1993.

*See text for detailed information on individual vaccines.

**If able, it is prudent to wait to vaccinate until after the first trimester to minimize any concern about teratogenicity. "Pregnancy" as a contraindication also includes the time 3 months before conception.

| Contraindications | Pregnancy** | HIV infection | Severe immunocompromise† |
|---|---|---|---|
| Neurologic or anaphylactic reation to a previous dose (can be given TIG for post-exposure prophylaxis). | Recommended; no confirmed risk to fetus. | Recommended. | Recommended. |
| Anaphylaxis to chicken eggs or neomycin (contact dermatitis to neomycin is not a contraindication); severe reaction to a previous dose. | Contraindicated; no confirmed risk to fetus; vaccination of susceptible women should be part of postpartum care. | Recommended/considered (see text). | Contraindicated. |
| As for measles. | As for measles. | As for measles. | As for measles. |
| As for measles; rubella vaccine from human diploid cells can be given to persons with anaphylaxis to chicken eggs. | As for measles. | As for measles. | As for measles. |
| Anaphylactic reaction to a previous dose, to neomycin or streptomycin (and for IPV, polymyxin B) (contact dermatitis to these antibiotics is not a contraindication); household contacts and close nursing personnel of immunocompromised persons should be given IPV, not OPV. | Use IPV; if immediate protection in less than 4 weeks is needed, then use OPV (see text); no confirmed risk to fetus. | Use IPV; OPV contraindicated. | Use IPV; OPV contraindicated. |
| Anaphylactic reaction to common baker's yeast. | Use if indicated; no reported risk to fetus. | Use if indicated (check postvaccination antibody titer). | Use if indicated (check postvaccination antibody titer). |

*Continued.*

†Includes persons with congenital immunodeficiency, leukemia, lymphoma, generalized malignancy receiving chemotherapy or radiation, persons on high dose steroids or receiving immunosuppressive therapy for any reason; does not include persons with functional or anatomic asplenia or complement component deficiency.
*IM*, Intramuscular; *SC*, subcutaneous; *ID*, intradermal..

**Table 3-3.** Immunizations for adults in the United States ≥18 years of age—cont'd

| Name | Primary schedule and booster(s) | Indications | Side effects |
|---|---|---|---|
| Pneumococcal bacterial polysaccharide | One 0.5 ml IM or SC dose; consider revaccination after 6 years for persons at highest risk of fatal disease (splenic dysfunction or anatomic asplenia) or declining antibody levels (nephrotic, chronic renal failure, transplant recipients). | Adults over 65 years; persons with chronic pulmonary disease, cardiovascular disease, diabetes, alcoholism, cirrhosis, chronic renal failure, nephrotic syndrome, organ transplantation, functional or anatomic asplenia, or immunocompromise for any reason; homeless persons and Native Alaskans. | Local erythema and pain; low grade fever. |
| Influenza inactivated virus | One 0.5 ml IM dose, seasonally. | As for pneumococcal vaccine with the exception of some Native Alaskans; caregivers and household contacts of persons for whom the vaccine is indicated, health-care workers and visiting nurses, travelers to the tropics or southern hemisphere who are at risk of poor outcome if infected (see Table 3-7). | Local erythema and pain, malaise, low grade fever, headache. |
| Hemophilus influenza type b (HbCV) bacterial polysaccharide, conjugated | Dose for adults has not been determined; generally one 0.5 ml IM dose is used. | Adults at highest theoretic risk; functional or anatomic asplenia, severe non-HIV immunocompromise; consider in HIV infected persons. | Local erythema and pain, malaise, fever. |
| Meningococcal bacterial polysaccharide (serogroups A, C, W135, and Y) | One 0.5 ml SC dose; duration of immunity unknown. | Adults with functional or anatomic asplenia or with terminal complement component deficiency; prophylaxis during outbreaks if serogroup represented in the vaccine; travelers to endemic areas (see Table 3-7). | |
| Rabies human diploid cell vaccine (HDCV), rabies vaccine adsorbed (RVA) | Preexposure prophylaxis: 1.0 ml IM doses (HDCV or RVA) on days 0, 7, and 28; or 0.1 ml ID doses (HDCV) on days 0, 7, and 21 or 28; one booster dose or check antibody titers every 2 years; chloroquine can interfere with immunity, see text for vaccine schedule for travelers taking chloroquine. | Veterinarians, animal handlers, certain lab workers, travelers for greater than one month to countries where rabies is endemic in domesticated animals (see Table 3-7). | Local erythema and pain (in 75%), malaise, fever, headache, abdominal pain, myalgias, dizziness (in 5%-40%), anaphylaxis (in 0.1%); mild immune complex hypersensitivity reaction in persons given a booster (in 6%). |
| | Postexposure prophylaxis: wound care first, then: if received appropriate preexposure prophylaxis or previous postexposure prophylaxis—two 1.0 ml IM doses (HDCV or RVA) on days 0 and 3. All other persons—HRIG (20 IU/kg) half dose to infiltrate the wound and half the dose IM, with five 0.1 ml IM doses (HDCV or RVA) on days 0, 3, 7, 14, and 28 | Any significant exposure. | |

| Contraindications | Pregnancy** | HIV infection | Severe immunocompromise† |
|---|---|---|---|
| More severe local reactions in persons revaccinated in less than 14 months. | Use if indicated; unknown risk to fetus. | Recommended. | Recommended. |
| Severe reaction to a previous dose; anaphylaxis to chicken eggs. | Use if indicated; do not delay if influenza season imminent; no confirmed risk to fetus. | Recommended. | Recommended. |
| Hypersensitivity reaction to the conjugated protein carriers. | Use if high risk of infection; unknown risk to fetus. | Consider (see text). | Recommended. |
| None to date. | Use if high risk of infection; unknown risk to fetus. | Use if indicated. | Use if indicated. |
| Severe reaction to a previous dose; consult public health department if postexposure prophylaxis is needed. | Use if indicated; unknown risk to fetus. | Use if indicated (check postvaccination antibody titer). | Use if indicated (check postvaccination antibody titer). |

*Continued.*

**Table 3-3.** Immunizations for adults in the United States ≥18 years of age—cont'd

| Name | Primary schedule and booster(s) | Indications | Side effects |
|---|---|---|---|
| Hepatitis A inactivated virus | 1.0 ml dose; booster in 6 months. | Certain travelers to high risk areas (see Table 3-7); certain occupations at risk. | Local erythema and pain. |
| Yellow fever live virus | One 0.5 ml SC dose 10 days to 10 years before travel; booster dose every ten years; avoid mosquitoes; space three weeks from cholera vaccine. | Certain travelers to areas where yellow fever is endemic (see Table 3-7). | Low grade fever, headache, myalgias (in 2%-5%), encephalitis (extremely rare). |
| Japanese encephalitis inactivated virus | Three 0.5 cc SC doses on days 0, 7, and 30; last dose to precede travel by ten days; need for boosters unknown; avoid mosquitoes. | Certain travelers to areas where Japanese encephalitis is endemic (see Table 3-7). | Local erythema and pain, fever, malaise, nausea, abdominal discomfort; anaphylaxis precautions. |
| Cholera inactivated bacteria | Two 0.5 ml IM or SC doses; or two 0.2 ml ID doses given 1 to 4 weeks apart; booster dose every 6 months; careful food and water selection; space 3 weeks from yellow fever vaccine. | Travelers to areas that require vaccination or certain travelers at high risk (see Table 3-7). | Local erythema and pain, fever, malaise. |
| Typhoid live bacteria, oral; inactivated bacteria, parenteral | Four oral doses on days 0, 2, 4, and 6 with the series repeated every 5 years; or two 0.5 ml SC doses 4 weeks apart or three SC doses at weekly intervals with a 0.5 ml SC or 0.1 ml ID booster every 3 years; careful food and water selection. | Certain travelers to high risk areas (see Table 3-7), certain lab workers, household contacts of a chronic carrier. | Live—nausea, abdominal discomfort, rash; inactivated—local pain and erythema, rare fever, malaise, headache. |
| Plague infected bacteria | One 1.0 ml IM dose followed by a 0.2 ml dose at 1 month and another 3 to 6 months after the second; if the exposure is ongoing six months later, give two 0.2 ml doses six months apart then a dose every 1 to 2 years. | Certain laboratory workers and certain travelers to high risk areas (see Table 3-7). | Local erythema and pain, fever, malaise, headache (in 10%). |
| Anthrax inactivated bacteria | Six SC doses, three given at 2-week intervals and three given at 6-month intervals; yearly booster. | Persons working with imported animal hides. | Local erythema and pain. |

To reduce the morbidity and mortality of vaccine-preventable illnesses, vaccination surveillance should continue throughout adolescence and adulthood. See Table 3-3 for adult vaccines and individual vaccines for further information.

Children are given a primary series of tetanus, diphtheria, and pertussis toxoids and are given a Td booster in adolescence. All adults should have received a primary tetanus and diphtheria toxoid series and should be given a booster every 10 years; Td should be used. Some authorities recommend a primary series, a booster in adolescence, and a single Td booster at age 50. If the primary series status is unknown, vaccine series as outlined for adults is recommended. The whole-cell pertussis vaccine is not given to adults because of the high frequency of adverse side effects. An acellular vaccine is being studied in hopes of reducing the spread of the disease by asymptomatic adult carriers.

Adults born before 1957 can be considered immune to measles and mumps and do not need to be vaccinated unless they are in a high-risk setting for measles exposure (e.g., health-care workers at risk for occupational exposure, when giving one dose of vaccine to persons in this age group may be prudent). They should be tested for rubella antibody and if not immune should be vaccinated. Persons born after 1956 should have been given one dose of measles, mumps, and rubella vaccine in childhood at or after 15 months of age as an MMR or have laboratory evidence of immunity. For measles and mumps but not rubella, a physician-diagnosed case may also serve as evidence for immunity. People born after 1956 who find themselves in a high-risk setting for measles exposure, such as students at school, health-care employees, inmates of long-term correctional facilities, travelers abroad, or those caught in an outbreak, should be given two doses of an MMR. Since 1990 it has been recommended that all

| Contraindications | Pregnancy** | HIV infection | Severe immunocompromise† |
|---|---|---|---|
| Severe reaction to a previous dose. | No data; unknown risk to fetus. | Use if indicated; pooled-IG may be preferred. | Use if indicated; pooled-IG may be preferred. |
| Severe reaction to a previous dose; anaphylaxis to chicken eggs. | Postponement of travel is preferable; vaccinate if at high risk; attempt waiver if at low risk; unknown risk to fetus. | Contraindicated if HIV is symptomatic; weigh risk vs benefit if HIV is asymptomatic. | Contraindicated. |
| Severe reaction to a previous dose; persons with atopy are at risk of severe reactions. | Weigh risk vs benefit; unknown risk to fetus. | Weigh risk vs benefit. | Weigh risk vs benefit. |
| Severe reaction to a previous dose. | Use if high risk of infection; unknown risk to fetus. | Use if indicated. | Use if indicated. |
| None to date. | Use if high risk of infection; no confirmed risk to fetus. | Use parenteral if at high risk; oral is contraindicated. | Use parenteral if at high risk; oral is contraindicated. |
| Hypersensitivity to casein, beef protein, soya, phenol, or formaldehyde. | Use if high risk of infection; no reported risk to fetus. | Use if indicated. | Use if indicated. |
| Severe reaction to a previous dose. | No data; unknown risk to fetus. | Use if indicated. | Use if indicated. |

children be given a second MMR either before entry into school or in their midteens.

Adults who are 65 years or older should receive a single dose of pneumococcal vaccine and a yearly influenza vaccine. Their caregivers and household and close family members should be given influenza vaccine as well. Routine immunization of adults for other illnesses is not recommended unless there is an indication.

## SPECIAL RECOMMENDATIONS

Certain vaccines may be recommended for persons with particular medical conditions, living situations, or lifestyles. Other vaccines are to be avoided (see Table 3-3 for individual vaccine doses).

### Pregnancy and breast-feeding

Since many young women receive care in obstetrics and gynecology practices or family-planning practices, health-care providers in these settings should be well-versed in vaccination principles and strategies. As part of ongoing preventive health, all women should be evaluated for their risk of vaccine-preventable illnesses and updated on their immunizations. In addition to any other vaccines that are indicated, women of childbearing age in particular should be given an MMR if they are not current for measles, mumps, or rubella vaccination recommendations. Natural rubella infection in a nonimmune pregnant woman results in an extremely high rate of fetal malformations and defects, up to 80% if infected during the first trimester. Natural measles infection during pregnancy can result in spontaneous abortion, premature labor, and low birth weight. Although malformations have been reported in association with measles infection, no specific syndrome has been described.

Pregnant women should be tested for hepatitis B infection, and if they are infected, the newborn and household and sexual contacts should be evaluated and treated appropriately.

Pregnant women or women planning to become pregnant within 3 months should not receive live vaccines. Household contacts of pregnant woman can receive live vaccines. The inadvertent administration of an MMR to a pregnant woman has not as yet been associated with congenital rubella syndrome but there is an increased risk of spontaneous abortion in the first trimester. A pregnant woman who needs measles, mumps, or rubella vaccination because of general recommendations or who lacks rubella immunity should receive an MMR immediately after delivery. This should be given even if she has received anti-Rho-IG or any IG-containing products, so that the opportunity for vaccination is not lost. In this instance, serologic testing should be performed to ensure adequate immune response or the vaccination repeated at the appropriate time interval (see Administration of Multiple Vaccines and Immune Globulins). For the discussion on administering the live vaccines yellow fever, OPV, and oral typhoid during pregnancy see the section on individual vaccines.

If any inactivated virus, bacterial vaccine, or toxoid is to be given to a pregnant woman, it is prudent to wait until the second trimester to reduce the theoretic risk of teratogenicity. Vaccination should not be delayed, however, if there is a risk of developing the vaccine-preventable illnesses during the first trimester. Pregnant women should be both evaluated for and given a Td during the second trimester if it is indicated. Furthermore, if they are at risk for other vaccine-preventable illnesses (e.g., hepatitis B or influenza), they should be vaccinated against them as long as the vaccines are not live.

There is no known risk to the fetus from passive immunization of the mother with any immune globulin preparation; passive immunization should be used as in other healthy adults. Natural measles infection in a pregnant woman can be life-threatening for the fetus. Thus special consideration should be given to the administration of pooled-IG to susceptible (nonimmune) pregnant women exposed to measles. There is no known benefit from giving pooled-IG for preventing the congenital rubella syndrome. Varicella-zoster infection in a woman during the first half of pregnancy can result in embryopathy in 2% to 3% of cases. The incidence is less in later pregnancy. Varicella infection in women 5 days before and up to 2 days after delivery can result in disease in 50% of newborns. Often the illness is severe with a case fatality rate of up to 5%. Pregnant women exposed to varicella zoster should be evaluated for VZIG. (See Accidental or Unavoidable Exposures for postexposure prophylaxis recommendations for individual diseases.)

Inactivated vaccines pose no special risk to breast-feeding mothers or their infants. Live vaccines multiply in the body but most are not excreted in breast milk. Although rubella may be excreted in breast milk, the virus usually does not affect the infant and if it does the infection is well-tolerated. There is no contraindication to giving yellow fever vaccine or OPV to a breast-feeding woman.

### Immunocompromise and other high risk medical conditions

Immunocompromise may be the result of infection with HIV, hematologic or generalized malignancies, chemotherapeutic or immunosuppresive agents, radiation, steroids, functional or anatomic asplenia, and complement or immune globulin deficiencies. Certain medical conditions are associated with defects in host defense, and therefore are associated with a higher incidence of illness or increased morbidity and mortality from illness because of poor physiologic reserve. The degree of immunocompromise can vary with stage of disease and treatment and should be determined on an individual basis. In general the patients can be divided into those with HIV, those with severe immunocompromise not resulting from HIV, and those whose illness does not dictate the avoidance of any vaccine but does necessitate additional vaccines not given to healthy adults.

***Human immunodeficiency virus (HIV)-infected persons.*** Persons with HIV should be evaluated for their vaccination history and their risk of vaccine-preventable illnesses as outlined for all adults. Any needed immunization should be given early in the course of the disease rather than later when the immune response may be suboptimal. In theory, people who do not respond adequately to initial vaccination may respond to higher doses of vaccine or to additional doses, but this has not been rigorously studied. The need for booster doses of any vaccine has not been studied in these patients.

Inactivated virus, bacterial vaccines, or toxoids can be given to people with HIV. These individuals should be updated on their Td booster or given a primary series if indicated. In general, HIV-infected individuals should not be given live virus vaccines because of the risk of uncontrolled viral replication. However, an MMR is recommended for individuals with asymptomatic HIV infection and should be considered for symptomatic individuals, if it is otherwise indicated, because of high risk exposure to measles. Measles infection in these patients can be serious, and in limited studies the vaccine has been safe (see the individual vaccine for relative and absolute contraindications to giving other live vaccines).

People with HIV are at increased risk for pneumococcal disease and severe influenza. They should be given a pneumococcal vaccine and considered for revaccination in 6 years. A yearly influenza vaccine is recommended for them as well as for their caregivers and household members. HIV-infected people may also benefit from HbCV if their risk of disease is high.

Since the risk factors for HIV and hepatitis B often overlap, patients with HIV should be evaluated for hepatitis B immunity and infection. If they are not already immune or infected and are at risk of ongoing exposure, they should be vaccinated. Their antibody response to the vaccination series should be tested, and if it is inadequate, additional doses can be given in an attempt to stimulate an antibody response.

Household contacts and close nursing attendants of HIV-infected people should not be given live OPV because of the risk of viral shedding; however, they can be given the inactivated vaccine IPV. If a household contact or attendant is inadvertently given OPV, exposure to this person should be avoided for at least 6 to 8 weeks.

Regardless of previous vaccination status, symptomatic HIV-infected people should be given pooled-IG after measles exposure. They should then be given an MMR 6 months later. HIV-infected patients who are susceptible to varicella zoster and have a significant exposure to chicken pox or zoster should be considered for VZIG. Some experts recommend that persons with HIV be given a Td for any wound and a TIG regardless of vaccination status if they sustain any wound other than a clean, minor one; however, this is not part of the current ACIP guidelines.

***Severely immunocompromised, non-HIV-infected individuals.*** Individuals can be severely immunocompromised as a result of hematologic or general malignancy, chemotherapy, radiation therapy, high doses of steroids (generally the equivalent of 20 mg/day prednisone for greater than 2 weeks), or other immunosuppressive therapies. The degree of immunocompromise should be evaluated on an individual basis. Steroids given for less than 2 weeks; alternate day therapy with short-acting, low dose preparations; physiologic replacement doses; topical preparations used for either skin, eye, or lung; or injections into joints are not considered immunosuppressive for the purpose of vaccination decisions.

Inactivated virus, bacterial vaccines, or toxoids are safe for all of these individuals. Live vaccines are contraindicated in this group of patients; however live vaccines can be given to patients with leukemia in remission who have not received chemotherapy for 3 months. A vaccine should be given early in the course of a disease rather than later when the immune response may be suboptimal. Ideally vaccination should precede chemotherapy or radiation therapy by more than 2 weeks and should be avoided during chemotherapy because of a potential suboptimal response. The efficacy of vaccination after chemotherapy is variable; vaccine should be given at least 3 months after chemotherapy. The ability to mount an immune response may be compromised for up to a year after chemotherapy. If there is doubt regarding the strength of the immune response, antibody titers can be tested or vaccination repeated.

Individuals with immunocompromise should be evaluated for their vaccination history and their risk of vaccine-preventable illnesses as outlined for all adults. They should be updated on their Td booster or given a primary series, if indicated. In addition people with immunocompromise are at increased risk for pneumococcal disease and severe influenza, and should be given a pneumococcal vaccine and considered for revaccination in 6 years. A yearly influenza vaccine is advised for them, their caregivers, and household members. In addition, the ACIP recommends that HbCV be given to the severely immunocompromised because of increased risk of infection, although there are no data showing efficacy.

Household contacts and close nursing attendants of immunocompromised patients should not be given live OPV because of the risk of viral shedding; however, they can receive the inactivated IPV. If a household contact or attendant is inadvertently given OPV, exposure to this person should be avoided for 6 to 8 weeks.

Immunocompromised patients exposed to measles should be given pooled-IG, followed by an MMR 6 months later if they are in a high risk exposure setting and if it is not contraindicated because of persistent immunocompromise. Also, immunocompromised patients susceptible to varicella zoster who have a significant exposure to chicken pox or zoster should be considered for VZIG.

***Medical conditions with special indications for vaccines.*** There is a group of medical illnesses that are considered to be special indications for additional vaccines. People with these illnesses should be evaluated for their vaccination history and their risk of vaccine-preventable illnesses and given any needed vaccines as outlined for all adults.

People with either functional or anatomic asplenia should be considered for hemophilus influenza type b vaccine, meningococcal vaccine, and pneumococcal vaccine. These vaccines must be given at least 2 weeks in advance of an elective splenectomy. HbCV is immunogenic in 87% of splenectomized adults. It is recommended that revaccination with pneumococcal vaccine be considered at 6 years because of the higher fatality rate from infection. Meningococcal vaccine is advised for individuals with deficiencies of terminal complement components. Hemophiliacs should be evaluated for hepatitis B vaccine because the multiple doses of blood products that they may receive puts them at risk for the disease.

Chronic renal failure patients are candidates for the pneumococcal vaccine because of increased risk of disease. There is evidence that the antibody response to pneumococcal vaccine may be diminished in patients with uremia and especially in those on dialysis. Therefore vaccination strategies should be formulated early in the illness. Antibody levels may decline at a higher rate in those individuals with nephrotic syndrome, chronic renal failure, or a renal transplant. Revaccination with pneumococcal vaccine is recommended at least every 6 years. Because of their increased morbidity from influenza, individuals with chronic renal disease and renal transplants, as well as their caregivers and household members, should be immunized yearly with influenza vaccine. Patients who may soon need or are already receiving long-term hemodialysis should be given hepatitis B vaccine at higher doses than used for healthy adults. They should have antibody titers checked postvaccination and at yearly intervals.

Individuals with congenital or acquired pulmonary or cardiovascular disease should be given pneumococcal and influenza vaccine because of increased morbidity and mortality from these diseases. People with diabetes should also receive pneumococcal vaccine and influenza vaccine because long-standing diabetes can lead to renal and cardiovascular dysfunction. Since alcoholism is associated with increased risk of pneumonia, alcoholics should be vaccinated for pneumococcal disease as well as influenza. In addition any caregiver or household member of these persons should be given influenza vaccine.

### Lifestyle and environmental risk

Homosexual men and injection drug users are at increased risk for hepatitis B infection (between 35% and 80% have serologic evidence of exposure). They should be screened for hepatitis B exposure, and if not already immune or infected they should be vaccinated. People should be evaluated early, since continued exposure increases the chance of infection (between 10% and 20% of homosexual men are infected with hepatitis B each year). HBV is also recommended for prostitutes, heterosexuals with multiple sex partners, and individuals with sexually transmitted diseases. They should also be evaluated for hepatitis C, HIV, and other sexually transmitted diseases because of concomitant risk. HIV-infected individuals may not respond as well to the HBV and should have an antibody titer measured after receiving the vaccine series. If it is inadequate, an additional dose can be given in an attempt to stimulate an antibody response. Injection drug users have an increased incidence of tetanus; providers should be diligent in giving a Td to these patients.

Inmates of long-term correctional facilities have a high prevalence of hepatitis B (ranging from 10% to 80%), largely because of injection drug use and male homosexual activity. They should be considered for hepatitis B vaccination and evaluated as other high risk populations. In addition, measles and rubella outbreaks have occurred in long-term correctional facilities, and all inmates should be evaluated for immunity or vaccinated as appropriate for persons at increased risk.

The prevalence of hepatitis B in residents of institutions for the developmentally disabled is between 35% and 80%. The virus may be transmitted through bites or contact with blood, saliva, skin lesions, or other infectious secretions. Residents should be screened for hepatitis B exposure, and if not already immune or infected, they should be vaccinated. Newly admitted persons should be vaccinated for hepatitis B. All residents should be given yearly influenza vaccine because some residents may have medical illnesses that make influenza more serious. The staff should also be given HBV and influenza vaccine.

The homeless are at risk for pneumococcal disease and influenza and should be vaccinated. Shelter staff should also be given influenza vaccine. The homeless may also be at risk for hepatitis B through lifestyle habits and should be evaluated individually. Alaskan native populations are at increased risk for pneumococcal disease and should be vaccinated. There is also a high prevalence of hepatitis B in the Alaskan native population. These individuals should be screened for hepatitis B exposure, and if not already immune or infected, they should be vaccinated.

### Occupational risk

Health-care workers are not only at increased risk of exposure and illness; they can transmit the illness to susceptible patients. Regardless of age, support staff and health-care personnel in a health-care facility that services or employs women of childbearing age should have serologic evidence of rubella immunity or should have been vaccinated at least once. Measles and mumps immunity should also be evaluated in health-care staff who have any patient contact as follows. If they were born after 1956, they should have been vaccinated twice with measles vaccine and once with mumps vaccine on or after their first birthday, have had physician-diagnosed measles and mumps, or have laboratory immunity. Adults born before 1957 are generally considered immune to measles and mumps by virtue of natural immunity. Some health-care workers are at increased risk of exposure, however, and if infected, they can transmit the virus to others. Health-care facilities should therefore consider requiring one dose of measles vaccine for these employees unless they have serologic proof of measles immunity or have had physician-diagnosed measles. An MMR is the vaccine of choice for any of these indications because it provides additional protection against two other illnesses.

All health-care workers and support staff who have patient contact should also be given a yearly influenza vaccine. OPV is a live virus vaccine and should not be given to health-care workers because they may excrete the virus and inadvertently transmit it to susceptible patients.

People with direct patient contact and laboratory personnel working with blood or body fluids should be immunized for hepatitis B. Individuals with frequent exposure to blood in this setting have a prevalence of hepatitis B infection of between 15% and 30%, compared to less than 5% in the general population. An antibody titer should be measured after the vaccine series because it is useful in determining postexposure prophylaxis.

Hepatitis B vaccine is recommended for public safety personnel (e.g., police, firefighters, and emergency medical technicians) who may be exposed to blood and secretions. It is also recommended for the staff of institutions for the developmentally disabled because of the high prevalence of hepatitis B in the clients and the risk of exposure through bites or contact with blood, saliva, skin lesions, or other infectious secretions. These staff workers should also be given a yearly influenza vaccine.

Preexposure rabies vaccine should be given to laboratory workers who handle the virus, to veterinarians, and to animal handlers and field personnel who work with dogs, cats, raccoons, bats, and skunks. Those with avocations that bring them into contact with potentially rabid animals should be considered for immunization. Preexposure vaccination eliminates the need for postexposure HRIG and reduces the number of rabies vaccines needed.

Laboratory personnel who may handle specimens containing the polio virus, small pox virus, *Yersinia pestis,* or *Bacillus anthracis* should be vaccinated for these illnesses. Anyone working with imported hides, furs, wools, and animal hair should receive anthrax vaccine. Field personnel dealing with rodents, rabbits, or their fleas should receive plague vaccine.

### Students

Students in colleges, universities, or other postgraduate institutions should be evaluated on entry for any needed vaccination as outlined for adults. Foreign students should provide documentation of prior vaccination or be considered unvaccinated. Students born after 1956 should have been given two doses of measles vaccine on or after their first birthday, have had physician-diagnosed measles, or have serologic evidence of immunity. They also should have one dose of mumps vaccine, have had a physician-diagnosed illness, or have serologic evidence of immunity. Students born before 1957 can be considered immune to measles and mumps. All students should either receive one dose of rubella vaccine or provide serologic evidence of immunity. An MMR is the vaccine of choice for any of these indications because it provides additional protection against two other illnesses.

### Immigrants and refugees

In many countries, routine vaccines are not given. Foreigners entering this country should provide documentation or receive vaccinations appropriate to their age and concomitant risk. For some vaccines this may require a primary series. People from endemic areas of hepatitis B (see Table 3-7) should be screened for the virus, and if they are carriers, susceptible household members and sexual partners should be evaluated for HBV. Individuals from countries with endemic hepatitis B who reside in a similar cultural community in the United States should be given HBV if they are not already immune or infected.

## VACCINES, IMMUNE GLOBULINS, AND THE EPIDEMIOLOGY OF VACCINE-PREVENTABLE ILLNESSES

The following sections discuss vaccines individually. See Table 3-2 for a summary of vaccines and dosing schedules used in childhood and Table 3-3 for a summary of vaccines, dose schedules, indications, contraindications, and side effects for adults.

### Tetanus and diphtheria vaccine

Tetanus vaccine became available in the United States in the middle-to-late 1940s. Its use has contributed largely to a 90% reduction in the incidence of tetanus morbidity and mortality. The shift in population from rural to urban areas (resulting in a decreased exposure to spores), improved wound care, and postexposure prophylaxis have also contributed to this phenomenon. Vaccination of school-age children is required in 47 states, and since 1980 more than 95% of students have received a primary series. Vaccination of adults is much more sporadic. Between 31% and 71% of older adults lack antibody to tetanus. Of the 50 to 100 cases of tetanus in the United States reported annually, 94% occur in adults over 20 years old and 70% occur in adults 50 years or older. Many of these individuals were born outside of the United States and have never had a primary immunization series. Of the cases with a known vaccination history, 93% had not received a primary series or booster dose. The case fatality rate is approximately 25% and increases with age; all of the recently reported deaths have occurred in adults older than 40 years. Most individuals with reported tetanus had an identifiable acute injury: puncture, laceration, abrasion, bite, or scratch. Other sources of entry included chronic ulceration, abscess, or history of IV drug use. Only one third of those with tetanus sought medical care after an injury; of these, three quarters were not appropriately managed according to current recommendations.

The vaccine is recommended for all adults. Immigrants, refugees, and foreign students should be evaluated to ensure that they received the primary series. If the primary series status is unknown or in doubt, a primary series should be given and a booster dose given every 10 years.

Diphtheria is rare in the United States. Until recently, an average of only two cases per year have been reported, the majority in persons older than 20 years. Between 40% and 80% of adults older than 60 years lack protective antibody.

Td, a combined preparation of adsorbed tetanus toxoid derived from the bacterium, *Clostridium tetani,* and diphtheria toxoid derived from *Corynebacterium diphtheriae,* is recommended for adults. It contains tetanus toxoid and 25% less diphtheria toxoid than the childhood immunization to reduce side effects (the childhood vaccine is denoted DT). The vaccine is nearly 100% effective in preventing tetanus and 85% effective in preventing diphtheria. The vaccine does not contain any pertussis immunogens because the current whole-cell preparation has an unacceptably high frequency of side effects. An acellular preparation of *Bordetella pertussis* is being studied in an effort to cut down the spread of the disease by asymptomatic adult carriers. A fluid tetanus vaccine is no longer available in the United States because of its poor immunogenicity. It may still be used in other countries; this is important to note when providing postexposure prophylaxis because recipients of this vaccine are regarded as less immune. People who develop urticaria or anaphylaxis to the vaccine should be allergy tested before it is deemed that they should never receive further doses. If an acute exposure occurs in these individuals, TIG should be given. Postexposure prophylaxis for tetanus is discussed in Accidental or Unavoidable Exposures.

### Measles, mumps, and rubella vaccine

***Measles.*** Measles vaccine became available in the United States in 1963. The cases of measles declined by 99% to a low of 3,600 in 1988. In 1989 and 1990, outbreaks of measles occurred and the reported cases rose to 28,000. Two major types of outbreaks were noted, one among unvaccinated school-age children, including those younger than the recommended age for vaccination (less than 15 months) and another among vaccinated school-age children. Also, in 1989 a substantial number of cases occurred among students and personnel on college campuses. In response to these outbreaks, it was recommended that all children receive two doses of measles vaccine, one at 15 months (or at 12 months if in an endemic area) and the other at school entry. Adults and adolescents born after 1956 and in high risk groups were also to be given a second dose. Subsequently the number of measles cases declined to 175 in the first 6 months of 1993. Of note, a similar 2-dose regimen used in Finland for 12 years has virtually eliminated the disease in that country. Encephalitis or death from measles occurs in one per 1000 cases. Measles infection during pregnancy can result in spontaneous abortion, premature labor, and low birth weight. Although malformations have been reported in association with measles infection, no specific syndrome has been described.

Adults born after 1956 should have received one dose of measles vaccine after their first birthday (usually at 15 months), have serologic evidence of immunity, or have had physician-diagnosed measles. One dose of the measles vaccine is clinically effective in 95% of the recipients; however, in settings where large numbers of young adults congregate or where there is high risk of exposure this may not prevent epidemics. Thus those individuals born after 1956 and in high risk settings should be given two doses of vaccine. Since 1990, it has been recommended that all children be given a second MMR either before entry into school or in their mid-teens. (Of note, a relatively ineffective, killed measles vaccine was available from 1963 to 1967; recipients of either this vaccine or one of unknown type should be considered unvaccinated.) An MMR is less efficacious if it is given before 12 months of age, presumably because maternal antibody may persist and interfere with the immune response to the vaccine. Anyone receiving the vaccine before 12 months of age should be considered unvaccinated.

In general, persons born before 1957 are considered naturally exposed and immune to measles. However, during the measles outbreaks in 1989 and 1990 serologic testing of hospital workers revealed that 9% born before 1957 were not immune, while 29% of the health-care workers who developed measles between 1985 and 1990 were born before 1957. It may be prudent to give one dose of measles vaccine to health-care workers born before 1957 and at risk for exposure. Postexposure prophylaxis for measles is discussed in Accidental or Unavoidable Exposures.

***Mumps.*** Live mumps vaccine was available in 1967, but because of cost it was not routinely used until 1977. The number of reported cases of mumps declined from 185,000 in 1967 to 2000 in 1985, but rose in 1987 to 12,000 because of an unvaccinated cohort of young adults. The number of cases has been declining since then. The mumps vaccine is 75% to 95% effective in preventing disease. Mumps is generally a self-limiting illness, and although orchitis can occur in postpubertal males, sterility is rare.

Adults born after 1956 should receive one dose of mumps vaccine after their first birthday, have serologic evidence of mumps immunity, or have had physician-diagnosed mumps. A killed mumps vaccine was available from 1950 to 1978, and those who received it may benefit from revaccination. Individuals born before 1957 are considered naturally exposed and immune to mumps. Although a second mumps vaccine is not currently recommended, it may be important because mumps outbreaks can also occur in highly vaccinated populations in high-risk settings.

***Rubella.*** The live rubella vaccine was licensed in the United States in 1969. The incidence of rubella infection declined from 56,000 cases in 1969 to 225 in 1988 but rose to 930 cases in 1990. It is estimated that 6% to 11% of young adults are susceptible to rubella. The goal of vaccination is to prevent fetal infection and congenital rubella syndrome (CRS). The rubella vaccine is 95% effective in preventing clinical disease. Twenty-five percent of infants infected during the first trimester will develop CRS that is recognizable at birth, while another 55% will have more mild debilitating defects. Defects are rare when infections occur beyond 20 weeks' gestation. Pooled-IG given as postexposure prophylaxis has no proven benefit in preventing fetal malformations.

The rubella vaccine is indicated for all adults, especially women, if they have not received the vaccine on or after their first birthday or have no serologic evidence of immunity. This is especially important in health-care settings, schools and universities, or other places where women of childbearing age congregate, and in travel abroad where the prevalence of rubella may be higher.

***The trivalent vaccine.*** Whenever there is an indication for measles, mumps, or rubella vaccine, the live trivalent vaccine that contains all three immunogens (prepared in chicken embryos) should be used because it provides additional protection against two other diseases. A single dose of an MMR provides long-lasting immunity for each of the viral infections in 90% to 95% of recipients. As discussed, certain individuals should have two doses to prevent measles infection. There is some evidence to suggest that administration of the vaccine during an upper respiratory illness may diminish the immune response; however, one must weigh this against the lost opportunity for vaccination. Therefore it is recommended that vaccination not be postponed because of minor illness. It may be postponed, however, because of severe febrile illness. Of note, rubella vaccine grown in human diploid cell cultures rather than chicken embryos is available and safe for those people with anaphylactic reactions to chicken eggs who need the rubella vaccine. Because it is a live virus vaccine, certain principles apply to giving an MMR and other live vaccines or immune globulins (see the section on administration of multiple vaccines and immune globulins) to pregnant or immunocompromised persons (see Special Recommendations).

### Poliomyelitis vaccine

In the United States, the incidence of poliomyelitis is low because of the maintenance of very high vaccination rates since the vaccine became available in the mid-1950s and early 1960s. The last polio epidemic occurred in 1979 in a group who refused vaccination. Since that time the only cases of poliomyelitis in the United States (about ten per year) have been vaccine associated. Likewise in other parts of the western hemisphere, except for Colombia and Peru, there have been no reports of wild poliovirus infection since 1991. In 1988 the World Health Organization (WHO) embarked on a campaign to eradicate polio from the world, particularly outside the western hemisphere; but its efforts are only beginning. In most developing countries, poliomyelitis is much more prevalent. In temperate areas poliomyelitis occurs mostly during summer and fall, but in the tropics it can occur at any time.

In the United States the vaccine is given during childhood as a primary series. Unfortunately, in recent years the vaccination rate of children under 2 years has declined precipitously and dangerously to 50%, probably as a response to the low incidence of disease. The vaccine generally is not recommended for adults in the United States even if they were never immunized as children because most adults are immune. However, the vaccine is recommended for adults who were not vaccinated during childhood if they are at high risk of exposure. Health-care or laboratory workers having contact with either patients who may excrete poliovirus or specimens that may contain wild poliovirus should be given a primary series. Adults who are traveling to areas where poliomyelitis is endemic should be vaccinated or given a booster (see Table 3-7). The vaccine series is 95% effective.

OPV is a live virus vaccine and should not be given to health-care workers because they may excrete the virus and inadvertently transmit it to susceptible patients. It should not be given to immunocompromised patients; nor should it be given to their household contacts and nursing personnel. IPV can be used, although its immunogenicity in immunocompromised individuals is unknown. If OPV is inadvertently given to a household member or close nursing attendant, this person should avoid contact with the susceptible immunocompromised patient for 6 to 8 weeks. Unimmunized healthy household contacts of OPV recipients have a small risk of paralysis, which occurs in 1 in 1.2 million persons after the first dose, and 1 in 116.5 million persons after subsequent doses. Childhood vaccination should not be delayed because of an unimmunized household contact. Rather, the responsible adult should be informed of the risk, and fecal-oral contact during activities such as diaper changing should be avoided.

Because it is a live vaccine, OPV should not be given to pregnant women or women planning to become pregnant within 3 months. If a pregnant woman going abroad has not received a primary series of polio vaccine, IPV should be used if at least two doses 1 month apart can be given before travel. However, if travel to a high risk area cannot be avoided and protection in less than 4 weeks is needed, one dose of OPV is preferred. Since the immune response develops more rapidly to OPV than to IPV, the risk of acquiring vaccine associated poliomyelitis is presumed to be less than that from the upcoming exposure, and there is no evidence of increased adverse effects on the fetus from OPV.

The polio vaccine is available as either a live trivalent virus vaccine containing virus types 1, 2, and 3 (OPV) or as an inactivated trivalent virus vaccine (IPV). Because adults given OPV have a higher but still rare incidence of vaccine-associated paralysis compared to children (one in 1.0 million adults after the first dose and one in 25.9 million after subsequent doses), IPV rather than OPV is used in adults. The paralysis generally occurs after the first dose of vaccine; therefore an adult who has received either OPV or IPV in the past can be given OPV if necessary. In adults the primary series of IPV is three doses. If time does not allow for three doses as specified, the vaccine should be given as a series of three doses each a month apart. If time does not permit for at least two doses of IPV and protection is needed in less than 4 weeks, one dose of OPV is preferred because of more rapid immune response compared with IPV, and the risk of vaccine-associated paralysis is assumed to be less than that from the upcoming exposure. The primary series should then be completed when it is possible. If travelers have already received a primary series, they should be given a booster dose.

Because OPV is a live virus vaccine there are certain principles that apply to giving it and other live vaccines that do not apply to the attenuated vaccine IPV (see Administration of Multiple Vaccines and Immune Globulins).

### Hepatitis B vaccine

In certain areas of the world, such as Southeast Asia, the Middle East (except Israel), Africa, the Amazon basin, Haiti, the Dominican Republic, and parts of Alaska, hepatitis B is endemic, with the virus predominantly transmitted perinatally and during childhood. In the United States most afflicted people acquire hepatitis B infection during young adulthood or late adolescence (more than 89% of the cases occur in individuals older than 20 years) through body secretions or blood exposure. The lifetime risk of developing hepatitis B in the United States is less than 5% for the general population. In high risk groups, such as injection drug users, it can approach 80%. Approximately 300,000 cases of acute hepatitis B infections occur each year in the United States, resulting in 10,000 hospitalizations and 250 deaths. The rate at which persons become chronic carriers is age-dependent; infection in adults is associated with a 6% to 10% chronic carrier rate, infection in childhood with a rate as high as 60%, and perinatal infection with a rate as high as 90%. Each year in the United States, 4000 people die of cirrhosis and 800 people die of liver cancer related to hepatitis B infection.

Previously, high risk groups were targeted for vaccination in an effort to decrease the incidence of disease, but the incidence continued to rise. Because Native Alaskans have a high incidence of hepatitis B, they were the subject of a perinatal and adult vaccination program in 1982. The incidence of acute hepatitis B was reduced by 99%. Since 1990 it is recommended that all newborns in the United States be given hepatitis B vaccine. The vaccine also is recommended for adults who are in or entering into certain high risk groups (see Table 3-3) and for certain travelers (see Table 3-7). Travelers to countries where hepatitis B is endemic can minimize exposure by avoiding intimate contact with the native population, especially contact involving blood and sex and prolonged household contact.

Prevaccination screening may be cost effective in high risk groups such as homosexual men, intravenous drug users, anyone receiving hemodialysis, recipients of multiple infusions of clotting factor concentrates or whole blood, and immigrants from high risk countries. More importantly, prevaccination screening can identify people who are infected and who may benefit from treatment, as well as their household and sexual contacts who are at risk. Using any one serologic marker for screening is imperfect. Screening for hepatitis B surface antigen alone would identify those who are currently infected, but not those who are immune and do not require vaccination. Screening for hepatitis B surface antibody alone would identify most of those who are immune, but not those who are infected for whom treatment and evaluation of sexual or household contacts is important. Screening for hepatitis B core antibody alone identifies anyone infected but does not differentiate between carriers and noncarriers. Hepatitis B core antibody should be tested if the goal of screening is to eliminate individuals who do not require vaccination. However, this is problematic because people who have core antibody alone cannot necessarily be considered immune. In a study of United States blood donors (with a relatively low incidence of hepatitis B) one-quarter of patients who had isolated hepatitis B core antibody alone were shown to have a false positive test. In several studies of populations with endemic hepatitis B, people with hepatitis B core antibody alone that was persistent and reproducible had a variable response to vaccination. Less than 20% had an anamnestic response, suggesting that more than 80% were not immune. In addition, between 10% and 40% had no response to a full series, suggesting a low-level carrier state. These studies suggest that people with hepatitis B core antibody alone should be included in vaccination programs targeting high risk groups.

The vaccine used in the United States today contains purified hepatitis B surface antigen made with recombinant DNA technology. In adults the vaccine series is greater than 90% effective. In some studies the antibody response to vaccination is reduced in older adults and in those individuals who smoke or who are obese (perhaps a function of inadequate intramuscular injection). If doses are missed, the second and third doses should be given at least 2 months apart. Higher doses of HBV are available for persons with chronic renal failure who are approaching or receiving hemodialysis because these patients have a poor antibody response to the usual doses. Because only 60% of hemodialysis patients and a slightly higher proportion of patients with chronic renal failure develop protective antibody, the antibody response to the vaccine series should be measured. Additional doses can be given if needed.

Yearly antibody titers should be measured in patients on hemodialysis because of the rapid decline in their antibody titers. A booster should be given if the antibody titer falls below 10 U/ml. Immunocompromised individuals may also have a poor response to the vaccine. Their antibody response should be measured postvaccination; if it is inadequate they can be given additional doses, although this has not been studied. Postvaccination antibody testing is also recommended for anyone at occupational risk to aid in deciding postexposure prophylaxis. If indicated, postvaccination titers should be evaluated from at least one month after the series is completed. In one study of those who did not respond to the vaccine series, 15% to 25% developed an adequate antibody titer to one additional dose. An additional 30% to 50% developed an adequate antibody response to another series. Revaccination with one or more doses should be considered for nonresponders. In healthy individuals, immunologic memory seems to persist for up to 9 years despite low antibody titers, as demonstrated by the absence of clinical disease and hepatitis B surface antigen in the serum during this time period. Currently, booster doses are not recommended for healthy individuals, although this may change in the future. Postexposure prophylaxis for hepatitis B is discussed in Accidental or Unavoidable Exposures.

Some people at risk for hepatitis B may be at risk for other illnesses such as hepatitis C, HIV, and sexually transmitted diseases, and these people should be evaluated individually.

### Pneumococcal vaccine

The incidence of pneumococcal disease in the United States is difficult to determine because it is so common. Estimates suggest that annually it causes between 150,000 to 570,000 cases of pneumonia, 2600 to 6200 cases of meningitis, and about 40,000 deaths. The mortality is highest in people with meningitis, bacteremia, or other medical illnesses, and in the elderly. Up to two thirds of patients hospitalized with serious pneumococcal disease have been hospitalized in the previous 5 years and have not been vaccinated as recommended. The pneumococcal vaccine is estimated to be at least 60% effective in preventing disease in immunocompetent adults older than 65 years. This degree of efficacy has been shown using cohort analysis for persons with diabetes, congestive heart failure, coronary vascular disease, and asplenia. Efficacy data for immunocompromised people and those with alcoholism or cirrhosis are lacking. The vaccine is currently recommended for adults 65 years or older and for other high risk groups (see Table 3-3).

The pneumococcal vaccine contains capsular antigens of the 23 types of *Streptococcus pneumoniae* that cause 88% of pneumococcal bacteremia. Although there is little information on the need for revaccination, it should be considered after 6 years for those who are most susceptible to a fatal disease, such as individuals with functional or anatomic asplenia, or for those whose antibody levels decline at a rapid rate, such as individuals with chronic renal failure or nephrotic syndrome or who have had transplants. Some authorities recommend that all adults be revaccinated after 6 years. Severe local reactions have been reported in people vaccinated twice within 14 months. Such reactions have not occurred when the revaccination is done after 4 or more years.

### Influenza vaccine

Influenza infection causes serious morbidity and mortality in the United States, especially in the elderly and in people with underlying medical illnesses. During influenza season there is an increased incidence of hospitalization for comorbid conditions and an increased number of cardiopulmonary deaths exacerbated by influenza and concomitant pneumonia. The average number of deaths attributable to influenza is estimated to be 10,000 per year and the number of hospitalizations to be 170,000. The attributable deaths are as high as 40,000 during years with severe epidemics. The efficacy of the influenza vaccine varies. In young healthy adults it is up to 90% effective in preventing disease. In the elderly or those with chronic illnesses the antibody response can be much lower. In these individuals the vaccine is more effective in preventing lower tract disease and disease severity, rather than preventing the disease altogether. It is 75% effective in reducing deaths in the institutionalized elderly. The vaccine is recommended for adults 65 years or older and for other high risk groups, caregivers and household contacts of susceptible individuals, health-care workers, and certain travelers (see Tables 3-3 and 3-7).

Influenza A and B viruses are classified into subtypes according to two surface antigens: neuraminidase and hemagglutinin. Immunity to one subtype confers little or no protection against viruses of another subtype. Furthermore, antigenic variation within a subtype may occur so that vaccination with one strain may not protect against another distantly-related strain of the same subtype. Influenza season is from April to September in the southern hemisphere and all year long in the tropics. Worldwide surveillance and antigenic characterization of the circulating strains of influenza provide the basis for predicting which viral strains are most likely to cause illness in the United States in a given year. The inactivated vaccine, derived from two strains of influenza A and one strain of influenza B, contains either whole virus, viral antigen, or split virus (treated with lipid solvents) all initially grown in chicken embryos. The whole virus vaccine causes more febrile reactions in children and therefore is not recommended for them. In adults, the side effect profile and efficacy are no different from the other vaccine preparations. Since influenza season in the United States typically begins in December and peaks in January and February, the vaccine is usually given in November. The vaccine can be used as long as influenza is documented in a community and can be used as late as April. Antibodies to the influenza vaccine develop within 2 weeks with immunity lasting up to 6 months; however, it may last considerably less time in the elderly. Because immunity to the vaccine is short-lived and because strains of the virus in circulation may change, an annual vaccination is recommended. Unlike the 1976 swine flu vaccine, there is no clear association between any subsequent influenza A and B vaccine and the Guillain-Barré syndrome. For the treatment of susceptible individuals exposed to influenza A see Chapter 111.

### Hemophilus influenza b vaccine

Invasive disease caused by hemophilus influenza type b occurs mostly in childhood, with 85% of the cases occurring in children under the age of 5 years. The vaccine is given routinely in pediatric practice. Invasive hemophilus influenza disease is rare in adults and occurs predominantly in those with conditions that predispose them to infection with encapsulated organisms. Even so, less than half of the invasive disease in these individuals is caused by the type b bacteria from which the vaccine is derived. The ACIP recommends vaccination for anyone at high risk of infection with encapsulated organisms, such as those with functional or anatomic asplenia or with severe immunocompromise. Although the ACIP does not include those with HIV, there may be people in this group at increased risk who should be considered for vaccination. The clinical efficacy and optimum dose in adults is not known and the need for boosters has not been established.

The vaccine is derived from a type b capsular polysaccharide of hemophilus influenza type b. It is conjugated to protein carriers to induce a greater immune response. The protein carriers include diphtheria toxoid or the outer membrane protein complex of *Neisseria meningitidis.* For the postexposure prophylaxis of hemophilus influenza type b see Chapter 64.

### Meningococcal vaccine

In the United States, meningococcal disease occurs mostly in children under the age of 5 years with the peak incidence between the ages of 6 and 12 months. One third of the cases, however, occur in persons older than 20 years. The vaccine is recommended for adults with functional or anatomic asplenia or with terminal complement component deficiency. It can be used to reduce the number of secondary cases during outbreaks if the responsible serogroups in the index case are represented by the vaccine. In the United States, serogroups B and C cause the majority of the cases and serotypes Y and W135 cause most of the rest. The vaccine should also be given to travelers entering areas with endemic disease. It is not required by any country, but is required for pilgrims to Mecca, Saudia Arabia, during the annual hajj (see Table 3-7).

The vaccine contains polysaccharides of *Neisseria meningitidis* serotypes A, C, Y, and W135. The need for booster doses has not been studied, and the duration of protection is probably variable for the individual serotypes. For postexposure prophylaxis of *Neisseria meningitidis* see Chapter 64 and 69.

### Rabies vaccine

While rabies infection is almost uniformly fatal, it rarely affects humans in the United States. Since rabies in domesticated animals was controlled in the 1940s and 1950s, only two to three cases of human rabies are reported each year. An epidemic of rabies infection in certain wild animals has spread to many parts of the United States in recent years, and there are many instances in which postexposure prophylaxis is appropriately sought (see section on Accidental or Unavoidable Exposures). Preexposure prophylaxis with the vaccine is recommended for animal handlers, laboratory workers exposed to the virus, field personnel, individuals whose avocations bring them into contact with potentially rabid animals, and anyone traveling for greater than one month to countries where rabies is common in domesticated animals or for shorter periods when risks of exposure are higher (see Table 3-7).

In all states but Michigan the vaccine contains an inactivated virus that was grown in human diploid cells (HDCV). In the state of Michigan the vaccine is derived from rabies virus grown in rhesus lung cell culture (RVA). Immunocompromised individuals who receive preexposure prophylaxis should have an antibody titer checked one month after the series is given. Anaphylaxis occurs in 0.1% of recipients and is a reason to discontinue the primary series. If postexposure prophylaxis is indicated, the health department should be contacted to determine the course of action and to report the exposure. Chloroquine and similar compounds such as mefloquine can interfere with the immune response to rabies vaccine when it is given intradermally. Travelers planning to take these antimalarials should receive at least three doses of the intradermal vaccine before taking the medication. If this cannot be accomplished, then the intramuscular route should be used giving as much of the series as is possible.

### Yellow fever vaccine

Yellow fever has been reported in central Africa in the forest and savannah zones and in northern and central South America, and is probably underreported in these areas. The virus is transmitted by mosquito vector. Vaccination is recommended for anyone living in or traveling to these areas and for laboratory personnel working with the virus. In addition, some countries in Africa not in the yellow fever zone, as well as countries in Asia and the Middle East, require the vaccine for travelers coming from infected areas (see Table 3-7). The vaccine is available only at an approved Yellow Fever Vaccination Center, which can be located by contacting the local health department. Anyone vaccinated should receive a validated International Certificate of Vaccination. Failure to document prior vaccination may result in revaccination, quarantine, or refusal of entry.

If a pregnant woman or a woman planning to become pregnant within 3 months plans to travel to endemic areas, yellow fever vaccine can be given if travel plans cannot be delayed and exposure is imminent. Even though it is a live vaccine, there is no known risk to the fetus and disease in the mother has serious morbidity and mortality. Yellow fever vaccine should not be given to anyone who is immunocompromised or who has symptomatic HIV infection, although there are no data on adverse reactions. If the risk of yellow fever is high, asymptomatic HIV-infected individuals should be advised of the risk vs. benefit of vaccination and given the choice of vaccination.

The vaccine is an attenuated live virus vaccine grown in chicken embryos. Booster doses are recommended every ten years, although recent evidence suggests that serologic immunity lasts for at least 30 years. People should also be educated as to the means to avoid mosquito bites (see Chapter 66). Since yellow fever vaccine is a live virus vaccine, certain principles apply to giving it and other live vaccines. Also, yellow fever vaccine and cholera vaccine can interfere with the immune response to each other (see Administration of Multiple Vaccines and Immune Globulins).

### Japanese encephalitis virus vaccine

The mosquito-borne Japanese encephalitis virus is the leading cause of viral encephalitis in Asia. This encephalitis also occurs in the Indian subcontinent and in Oceania. The viral infection appears most commonly in native populations and leads to encephalitis in 1 out of 20 to 1000 cases, with death occurring in 25% of those infected and neurologic sequelae occurring in 30%. By adulthood, nearly everyone in endemic countries has serologic evidence of exposure. The virus is transmitted seasonally in temperate regions, mostly during summer and early fall. In tropical areas transmission can be year-round. The risk of acquiring infection is low for most travelers to these areas. However, the vaccine is recommended for travelers spending at least a month during the transmission season, especially if traveling in rural areas, and for those spending less time but most of it outdoors in rural areas (see Table 3-7). The vaccine is also recommended for immigrants to endemic areas and for laboratory workers handling the virus. The vaccine is 80% to 90% effective in preventing encephalitis.

The vaccine is composed of inactivated virus that is derived from virus-infected mouse brain. It has become available only recently in the United States. If there are time constraints and the recommended series cannot be completed, the vaccine can be given on days 0, 7, and 14. The last dose should precede travel by 10 days. The need for booster doses is unknown, but immunity appears to last for at least two years. Travelers should also be educated as to the means to avoid mosquito bites (see Chapter 66). A serious reaction to the vaccine consists of generalized urticaria and angioedema which can occur up to two weeks postvaccination and at a rate of 5:1000. Medications to treat anaphylaxis should be on hand at the time of vaccination and the recipient should be observed for 30 minutes. Recipients should be warned of the symptoms of anaphylaxis and advised to seek medical attention if any occur in the ensuing weeks. Individuals with a history of hypersensitivity phenomena appear to be at increased risk. Vaccine-associated encephalitis is extremely rare; only one to two cases per million vaccines have been documented.

### Cholera vaccine

Cholera is a risk to travelers in out-of-the-way areas of Africa, Asia, and Latin America, although recent epidemics have occurred more broadly. The vaccine series is recommended for travelers to these countries who are at high risk (see Table 3-7). While no country currently requires the vaccine, some local authorities may (see Table 3-7). The current vaccine series is only 50% effective in preventing clinical illness for 3 to 6 months.

The vaccine is derived from the inactivated bacterium, *Vibrio cholerae*. A single dose satisfies most area requirements. However, if a person is at high risk, the series should be given. People should also be educated to avoid exposure through careful food and water selection (see Chapter 66). Yellow fever and cholera vaccines should be given at least three weeks apart; if given together the antibody response to both vaccines can be diminished. In addition, some inactivated vaccines such as cholera, parenteral typhoid, and plague commonly cause local or systemic reactions; therefore the simultaneous administration of these vaccines should be avoided if possible.

### Typhoid vaccine

In the United States approximately 450 cases of typhoid fever occur annually. Seventy percent of these are acquired through foreign travel. Typhoid vaccine is recommended for certain travelers (see Table 3-7). The vaccine is also recommended for anyone having continued household contact with a known carrier, or for laboratory workers handling the bacterium. The vaccine series is 70% to 90% effective.

There are several preparations of the vaccine derived from the bacterium *Salmonella typhi*. There are no data on the safety of any of the vaccines during pregnancy. The oral live vaccine should not be given to immunocompromised people, but the inactivated vaccine can theoretically be considered safe. People should be educated to avoid exposure through careful food and water selection (see Chapter 66). Because the oral typhoid vaccine is a live vaccine, certain principles apply to giving it and other vaccines and immune globulins. Parenteral typhoid should not be given with certain other vaccines because of its local and systemic side effects (see section on administration of multiple vaccines and immune globulins). The antimalarial mefloquine may interfere with the immune response to oral typhoid; therefore the vaccine should be given 24 hours before or after a dose of the antimalarial.

### Immune globulins

Passive immunization with immune globulins (IG) is used to provide immediate antibody levels for individuals who recently have been exposed or soon may be exposed to a disease. It is used therapeutically when a disease is already present and the antibody may help to suppress the effects of a toxin. Immune globulins are also used to provide antibody for individuals who are immunocompromised and would be expected to have a poor immunogenic response to an illness exposure or to a previous active immunization. Pooled-IG is derived from a large pool of donors so it is likely to contain antibodies to hepatitis A and to measles. The disease-specific immune globulins, HBIG, TIG, HRIG, and VZIG (see the box on p. 27) are all derived from selected donor pools with high titers of the desired antibody. None of these products has been associated with the transmission of hepatitis B or HIV. Recently, however, pooled-IG from one manufacturer was taken off the market because it was associated with hepatitis C transmission. Subsequently, the manufacturing process has been changed to further inactivate contaminating viruses and the IG should pose no further risk of hepatitis C. There is no known risk to the fetus from passive immunization with immune globulins; they are safe to give in pregnancy and should be used as indicated.

The various intramuscular preparations and doses of the immune globulins are discussed individually in detail (see Accidental or Unavoidable Exposures). In general, the upper outer quadrant of the buttock is the site of administration because of the large volumes given. No more than 5 ml should be given at one site. Side effects are rare. They include minor reactions such as headache, chills, flushing and nausea, and a pyogenic reaction with high fever. On rare occasions a hypersensitivity reaction can occur, most commonly in people with IgA deficiency. When pooled-IG is indicated and there is a contraindication to intramuscular injections, such as in someone with severe thrombocytopenia or a coagulation disorder, an intravenous preparation can be used at a dose of 110 mg/kg. These intravenous immune globulin preparations are used for the treatment of immune deficiency and certain autoimmune diseases. They are derived from smaller donor pools and may not be as effective for hepatitis A or measles prophylaxis, and their efficacy for these purposes is unknown. Certain principles apply to administering immune globulins with vaccines (see Administration of Multiple Vaccines and Immune Globulins).

## ACCIDENTAL OR UNAVOIDABLE EXPOSURES

### Hepatitis B

The recommendations for postexposure management of hepatitis B are summarized in Tables 3-4 and 3-5. Sexual and household contacts of a person with chronic hepatitis B should be evaluated for immunity and infection; if they have neither they should receive hepatitis B vaccine. Sexual contacts of someone with acute hepatitis B should receive HBIG as soon as possible and within two weeks of the last exposure; this is 75% effective in preventing disease. Contacts can be tested for an already acquired infection if testing will not delay giving HBIG or HBV beyond two weeks. HBIG should be given with HBV and the series of HBV completed if sexual contact is likely to continue. Alternatively, HBIG can be given (adding one dose of HBV may increase effectiveness) and the index person retested in three months. If the index person is not still infectious, nothing further is needed. If sexual contact is not likely to continue and the exposed person is otherwise at low risk for exposure to hepatitis B in the future, one dose of HBIG is sufficient (adding one dose of HBV may increase effectiveness). If the index person is still infectious, then a second HBIG should be given and the series of HBV started in the partner. If HBIG and HBV are to be given, separate sites should be used. Household contacts of someone with acute hepatitis B, who have a known exposure such as blood contact through toothbrushes or razors, should be treated similarly to those with sexual exposure.

The treatment for percutaneous (needle-stick, laceration, or bite) or permucosal (ocular or mucous membrane) exposure to hepatitis B depends on the exposed person's and source person's status. The evaluation should include whether the source of the blood is available and can be

**Table 3-4.** Postexposure immunoprophylaxis for hepatitis B virus following a sexual or household exposure

| Index person | Exposure type | Immunoprophylaxis |
|---|---|---|
| Chronically infected | Household | Vaccination series* |
| Chronically infected | Sexual | Vaccination series* |
| Acutely infected | Household | None unless known exposure |
| Acutely infected | Household: known blood exposure | HBIG with or without vaccination series* |
| Acutely infected | Sexual | HBIG with or without vaccination series* |
| Either† | Percutaneous/permucosal | Vaccination series with or without HBIG† |

Modified from *MMWR* 40 (RR-13): 9, 1991.
*See text.
†See text and Table 3-5 for further details.
*HBIG*, Hepatitis B immune globulin (0.06 ml/kg intramuscularly) and Hepatitis B vaccine (For the dose see Table 3-3).

**Table 3-5.** Immunoprophylaxis for hepatitis B virus following a percutaneous or permucosal exposure

| | Treatment, when source is found to be | | |
|---|---|---|---|
| **Exposed person** | **HBsAg positive** | **HBsAg negative** | **Unknown** |
| Unvaccinated | HBIG and vaccination series | Vaccination series | Vaccination series |
| Previously vaccinated | | | |
| Known responder | Test exposed person for anti-HBs titer<br>1. If adequate, none<br>2. If inadequate, give vaccine booster | None | None |
| Known nonresponder* | HBIG and vaccine booster (check anti-HBs titer at one month) *or* HBIG at 0 and 1 month* | None | If high risk source, treat as HBsAg positive source |
| Response unknown | Test exposed person for anti-HBs titer<br>1. If adequate, none<br>2. If inadequate, HBIG and vaccine booster | Test exposed person for anti-HBs titer for future exposure management | Test exposed person for anti-HBs titer<br>1. If adequate, none<br>2. If inadequate, vaccine booster<br>3. Consider checking anti-HBs titer at one month*. |

Modified from *MMWR* 40 (RR-13): 22, 1991.
*See text for further details.
*HBsAg*, Hepatitis B surface antigen; *anti-HBs*, hepatitis B surface antibody; adequate anti-HBs titer is >10 mIU; *HBIG*, hepatitis B immune globulin (0.06 cc/kg intramuscularly); *Hepatitis B Vaccine* (as soon as possible and within 1 week of exposure, for dose see Table 3-3).

tested for hepatitis B antigen, and whether the exposed person has been vaccinated and has developed antibody to hepatitis B. The recommended management is summarized in Table 3-5. If HBIG or HBV is needed, they should be given as soon as possible. In this setting the utility of giving them beyond one week of the exposure is not known. If HBIG and HBV are to be given, separate sites should be used.

Individuals with hepatitis B and their contacts should also be evaluated for hepatitis C and, HIV if there is concomitant risk, and other sexually transmitted diseases in the case of sexual exposures. The source person in a needle-stick injury should be evaluated for hepatitis C and/or abnormal liver function and HIV, especially if he or she is at high risk for these illnesses. The use of giving pooled-IG to prevent hepatitis C transmission is unknown. Postexposure prophylaxis for HIV infection is discussed in Chapter 68. Health-care providers should also review and update patients with respect to other vaccines, such as a Td and an MMR. (If HBIG is given, ideally an MMR should not be given until 3 months later.)

### Hepatitis A

Pooled-IG is used for the postexposure prophylaxis of hepatitis A. To be effective, pooled-IG (0.02 ml/kg intramuscularly) should be given as soon as possible and within two weeks of exposure. Close household or sexual contacts of a person with acute hepatitis A should be given pooled-IG. If a custodial institution has an outbreak of hepatitis A, selected staff with close contact to the index patient and clients should be given pooled-IG. Coworkers of food handlers with hepatitis A should be given pooled-IG. Any food handler with active disease should be excluded from working until one week after the onset of symptoms or until the jaundice disappears, whichever is longer. If a day-care center has an outbreak of hepatitis A, the staff and children and household contacts of diapered children should be given pooled-IG. Any person with active disease should be excluded from attending until 1 week after the onset of symptoms or until the jaundice disappears, whichever is longer.

Pooled-IG is used for preexposure prophylaxis of hepatitis A in travelers to developing countries where exposure to contaminated food and water is unavoidable. For anyone traveling for 2 to 3 months, a single dose (0.02 ml/kg intramuscularly) is recommended. If travel time is longer, a higher dose (0.06 ml/kg intramuscularly) given every five months is recommended. Hepatitis A vaccine has recently been licensed for preexposure prophylaxis. The first dose should be given at least 2 weeks before travel/exposure. For prolonged travel/exposure, a booster dose should be given at 6 months. People should also be educated to avoid exposure through careful food and water selection and preparation (see Chapter 66). An antibody titer should be measured in frequent travelers because if they are immune the need for pooled-IG prophylaxis is eliminated. Approximately 30% of the adult United States population is immune.

Health-care providers should also take the opportunity to review and update patients with respect to other vaccines, such as a Td and an MMR. (If pooled-IG is given for hepatitis A prophylaxis, an MMR should not be given until 3 months later.)

### Measles

Measles illness may be modified in susceptible contacts by giving an MMR within 72 hours of exposure. Giving an MMR has the advantage of providing protection against subsequent measles infection. If giving an MMR is contraindicated (pregnant women or individuals with non-HIV immunocompromise) or if the person is unlikely to mount an adequate immune response (individuals with symptomatic HIV infection and those with non-HIV immunocompromise) pooled-IG should be given within 6 days of exposure. Special consideration should be given for pooled-IG administration to susceptible (nonimmune) pregnant women exposed to measles. Measles infection in a nonimmune pregnant woman is associated with spontaneous abortion, preterm labor, and low birth weight. Malformation has been reported but no specific syndrome has been described. Pooled-IG administered within 6 days of measles exposure may be of some benefit, although this is unproved.

The dose of pooled-IG for measles exposure in a healthy adult is 0.25 ml/kg to a maximum of 15 cc intramuscularly. Immunocompromised individuals and those who are symptomatic HIV-infected should receive pooled-IG regardless of their vaccination history at twice the dose given to healthy people (0.50 ml/kg to a maximum of 15 ml intramuscularly). If an immunocompromised person was receiving a standard dose (100 to 400 mg/kg) of intravenous IG for other reasons at regular intervals and the last dose was given within 3 weeks of the measles exposure, this may be sufficient to prevent measles. However, these intravenous immune-globulin preparations are derived from smaller donor pools and in theory may not be as effective for measles prophylaxis.

The disease is transmitted by direct contact with infectious droplets and less commonly by airborne spread. The incubation period after exposure is generally 8 to 12 days. People are contagious for 1 to 2 days before the onset of symptoms (3 to 5 days before the rash) and up to 4 days after the appearance of the rash. Susceptible individuals exposed to measles should avoid contact with health-care workers, patients, those who are immunocompromised, and pregnant women for 5 to 21 days after the exposure regardless of postexposure prophylaxis. People who are ill with measles should avoid such contact for 7 days after they have developed the rash.

If pooled-IG is used for measles prophylaxis, an MMR should be given to healthy people after five months and to immunocompromised or symptomatic HIV-infected people after six months if it is not contraindicated at that time. If intravenous IG was used, an MMR should not be given until after 8 months later. A second MMR dose may be indicated for those born after 1956 if they are at high risk of subsequent measles exposure (see Table 3-3). Health-care providers should take the opportunity to review and update patients with respect to other vaccines when they seek advice after measles exposure.

### Varicella-zoster

The decision to administer VZIG is based on the likelihood that an individual is susceptible to varicella, the probability that a given exposure will result in infection, and whether a person will develop complications of varicella if infected.

Chicken pox is a very common childhood illness. Serologic evidence of immunity is present in 85% to 95% of adults who give no clear history of previous illness. The percentage may be less for those living in remote or tropical areas. Susceptibility to the illness needs to be evaluated on an individual basis. Elder siblings in large families, parents whose children have had chicken pox, or those who have had other significant exposure to chicken pox are probably immune.

The morbidity and mortality from varicella infection is higher in adults than in children and likely to be much higher in immunocompromised adults. If a person has a serum varicella antibody and is currently receiving immunosuppressive therapy, he or she may still be susceptible to infection. Susceptible pregnant women infected in the first half of pregnancy may have a malformed fetus in up to 2% to 3% of cases. The incidence is less in the later stages of pregnancy. Even if IG aborts clinical disease in the mother, it is not known whether this protects the infant from infection and malformation. Varicella infection in women five days before delivery and up to two days after delivery can result in disease in half of the newborns. Often the illness in newborns is severe with a fatality rate of up to 5%.

A significant exposure to a person with chicken pox includes household contact, close indoor contact greater than an hour, sharing a hospital room, or prolonged direct face-to-face contact (e.g., provider and patient). The period of highest risk of contagion is 1 to 2 days before the onset of the rash and until the last eruptions form a crust, which may take as long as 5 days after the rash appears. Immunocompromised people may have an extended period of new eruptions and therefore are contagious longer. A significant exposure to a person with shingles results from direct contact with uncovered lesions; airborne spread is rare. An immunocompromised person with shingles, however, may shed a large viral load that can be aerosolized; in this setting, a significant exposure as described for chicken pox may therefore be operable.

Anyone susceptible to varicella-zoster who has a significant exposure to chicken pox or zoster, and a high likelihood of developing complications from the infection should be given VZIG. It is preferable to measure a varicella antibody titer in people with an unknown susceptibility to determine their immune status, if this will not delay the administration of VZIG beyond 96 hours. The dose is 12.5 U/kg to a maximum of 625 U (the ideal dose has not been determined for immunocompromised individuals) given within 48 hours of exposure and preferably not beyond 96 hours. VZIG prophylaxis in this setting may last up to 2 weeks. If clinical disease does not develop and there is a new exposure after this time, another dose should be given. People who receive VZIG and who do not develop clinical disease may develop serologic immunity, but it is not known whether this is protective against future exposures.

Anyone with varicella should avoid contact with susceptible people for at least five days after the onset of the rash and for the duration of any new eruptions or until all the lesions have crusted over, whichever is longer. The incubation period is generally 14 to 16 days but can be anywhere from 11 to 20 days. Exposed, susceptible people should avoid other susceptible people for 10 to 21 days after the development of the rash in the index patient. Those who receive VZIG for postexposure prophylaxis should avoid contact with susceptible individuals for 28 days because VZIG may prolong the incubation period of clinical disease. A new varicella vaccine has been recently licensed by the Food and Drug Administration, although the indications have not been determined.

Health care providers should also take the opportunity to review and update patients with respect to other vaccines, such as a Td and an MMR. (If VZIG is given, ideally an MMR should not be given until 5 months later.)

## Tetanus

Tetanus is uncommon in the United States, but it can be fatal. It is preventable through vaccination and wound prophylaxis. The management of wound prophylaxis is summarized in Table 3-6. Local wound care is important. The need for a Td and TIG depends on the vaccination status of the patient and the type of injury sustained. The provider needs to elicit exactly how many doses of vaccine a patient has received in the past. In particular, immigrants, refugees, and foreign students should be evaluated to ensure that they received the primary series (often not routinely given in childhood in other countries). If receipt of a full primary series is uncertain, the patient should be managed as if they are unvaccinated. If a person has had a primary series, evaluating the date of the last dose given is important. A fluid tetanus vaccine previously available in the United States is no longer used because of its poor immunogenicity. It may still be used in other countries, which is important to note when providing postexposure prophylaxis because anyone who received it is considered less immune. Some experts recommend that individuals with HIV be given a Td for any wound and be given TIG regardless of vaccination status if they sustain any wound other than a clean minor one, although this is not part of the current ACIP guidelines.

The incubation period for clinical disease in the majority of cases is three days to three weeks, the average being eight days. Immune prophylaxis should be administered as soon as possible and ideally within three days, but can be given later if it is unavoidable. If a Td is indicated after an exposure but it is contraindicated

**Table 3-6.** Postexposure immunoprophylaxis for *clostridium tetani*

| Tetanus vaccine doses | Clean, minor wounds | | All other wounds* | |
|---|---|---|---|---|
| | Td | TIG | Td | TIG |
| Uncertain or <3† | Yes | No | Yes | Yes |
| >/=3‡ | No§ | No | No‖ | No |

Modified from *MMWR,* 40 (RR-12): 70, 1991.

*All other wounds—such as but not limited to wounds contaminated with dirt, feces, soil, or saliva, as well as puncture wounds, avulsions, or wounds resulting from missiles, crushing, burns, or frostbite.

†Follow-up arrangements should be made to complete the primary series.

‡If only three doses of a fluid toxoid have been received, a fourth dose of adsorbed tetanus toxoid should be given regardless of the type of wound (see text).

§Yes, if more than 10 years since last dose.

‖Yes, if more than 5 years since last dose.

*TIG,* Tetanus Immune Globulin (250 U intramuscularly) as soon as possible and preferably within 3 days; *Td,* adsorbed tetanus/diphtheria toxoid for adult use (for dose see Table 3-3) as soon as possible and preferably within 3 days.

**Table 3-7.** Travel

| Disease* | Areas affected† | Prophylaxis recommended‡ |
|---|---|---|
| Tetanus | All | All travelers: vaccine series/booster |
| Measles | All | Born after 1956: ensure immunity by antibody titer, diagnosed measles, or two doses of vaccine |
| Rubella | All | All travelers: ensure immunity by antibody titer or vaccine |
| Mumps | All | Born after 1956: ensure immunity by antibody titer, diagnosed mumps, or one dose of vaccine |
| Poliomyelitis | Developing countries not in the western hemisphere but including Peru and Colombia; tropics at risk all year; temperate zones have increased cases in summer and fall | All travelers: vaccine series/booster |
| Hepatitis B | 5%-20% population are carriers—Africa, Middle East except Israel, all Southeast Asia, Amazon basin, Haiti, Dominican Republic; 1%-5% population are carriers—South Central and Southwest Asia, Israel, Japan, the Americas, Russia, eastern and southern Europe | Travelers for more than 6 months and having close contact with the population or staying less time but having higher risk activities (sex, close household contact, seeking dental or medical care): vaccine series |
| Hepatitis A | Developing countries (see Chapter 66 on how to limit exposure) | Travelers to rural areas, eating and drinking in settings of poor sanitation: hepatitis A vaccine or pooled-IG prophylaxis |
| Influenza | Tropics throughout the year; southern hemisphere April to September | Travelers for whom vaccine is otherwise indicated: give the current vaccine and revaccinate in fall as usual |
| Meningococcus* | Tanzania, Kenya, sub-Saharan Africa from Mali to Ethiopia; required for pilgrims to Mecca, Saudi Arabia, during the hajj | All travelers: vaccine |
| Rabies | Endemic dog rabies exist in parts of Mexico, El Salvador, Guatemala, Peru, Colombia, Ecuador, India, Nepal, Philippines, Sri Lanka, Thailand, Viet Nam | Travelers staying for more than 30 days or at high risk of exposure: vaccine series/booster |
| Yellow Fever* | North and central South America, forest-savannah zones of Africa, some countries in Africa, Asia and Middle East require travelers from endemic areas to be vaccinated. | All travelers: vaccine/booster at approved Yellow Fever Vaccination Center. (see Chapter 66 on how to limit mosquito exposure) |
| Japanese Encephalitis | Seasonally in most areas of Asia; in temperate zones the incidence is increased in summer and early fall; in the tropics occurs all year | Travelers to high risk rural areas, staying outdoors or during the transmission season: vaccine series. (see Chapter 66 on how to limit mosquito exposure) |
| Cholera* | Certain undeveloped countries. (see Chapter 66 on how to limit exposure) | If required by local authorities, one dose usually suffices. Primary series only for those living in high-risk areas under poor sanitary conditions or those with compromised gastric defense mechanisms (achlorhydria, antacid therapy or previous ulcer surgery): booster every 6 months |
| Typhoid Fever | Many countries of Asia, Africa, Central and South America. (see Chapter 66 on how to limit exposure) | Travelers with prolonged stay in rural areas with poor sanitation: vaccine series/booster |
| Plague | Africa, Asia, Americas in rural mountainous or upland areas | Travelers with research or field activities that bring them in contact with rodents: vaccine series/booster. Consider taking tetracycline (500 mg qid) for chemoprophylaxis (inferred from clinical experience in treating plague) |

*Only yellow fever vaccine is required for entry by any country, cholera vaccine may be required by some local authorities, and meningococcus vaccine is only required for pilgrims to Mecca, Saudi Arabia, during the hajj. However, it is important to follow the recommendations for other vaccines for disease prevention. If a required vaccine is contraindicated or withheld for any reason attempts should be made to obtain a waiver from the country's consulate or embassy.

†Because areas affected can change, and for more specific details, consult the CDC's traveler's hotline 1-401-332-4559 or the most recent edition of *Health Information for the International Traveler.*

‡For detailed information concerning the administration of individual vaccines, consult the text under each vaccine and Table 3-3, for hepatitis A additional information is found in Accidental or Unavoidable Exposure.

because of a previous severe reaction, TIG should be given instead. If TIG (250 U intramuscularly) is to be given with a Td, separate sites should be used. Arrangements should be made to have patients complete a primary series if they have not done so previously. During this time, patients should be evaluated and updated for any other vaccines that they require, such as an MMR. (If TIG is given, ideally an MMR should not be given until 3 months later.)

### Rabies

Although rabies infection is almost uniformly fatal, it rarely affects humans in the United States. See above and Table 3-3 for specifics of the vaccine. See Chapter 4G for discussion of postexposure prophylaxis.

## TRAVEL

The WHO and the CDC publish disease surveillance data regularly, but the data are based on information that generally underestimates the incidence of disease. There is underreporting in many countries for a variety of reasons: the countries themselves may have no mechanism for reporting and recording cases, medical personnel may not always report cases, infected individuals do not always come to medical attention and lastly there may be no medical personnel in the area. In underdeveloped countries, poor living conditions and sanitation, lack of hygiene, and nonavailability of vaccines may result in a higher prevalence of some diseases. The risk of infection varies considerably within countries.

Many of the recommendations for vaccinating and educating travelers are not required by other countries, but are advisable to prevent illness. It is important for travelers to get the recommended immunizations for their age and any special recommendations that may apply to them, since the prevalence of these vaccine-preventable illnesses is higher in many other countries than in the United States. The majority of travelers do not need additional vaccines. In some countries where the prevalence of hepatitis A and B, polio, measles, mumps, rubella, yellow fever, cholera, rabies (carried by domesticated animals), typhoid, Japanese encephalitis, or meningococcal meningitis is high, special vaccines are recommended. The vaccines and immune globulins recommended for travelers are listed in Table 3-7 (see Table 3-3 for the specific doses). Table 3-7 is a general one because recommendations change periodically according to disease surveillance. Health care providers should consult the CDC's *Health Information for the International Traveler* or call the CDC's traveler's hotline for up-to-date information on vaccine-preventable illnesses in a specific area (see the box on p. 27).

International travelers should be evaluated at least 6 weeks before departure to obtain health information on the countries they plan to visit and any recommended vaccinations. If a vaccine is contraindicated or withheld for any reason and the country requires a vaccination certificate or the local authorities require documentation of the vaccine, attempts should be made to obtain a waiver from the country's embassy or consulate. Noncompliance with these requirements can result in quarantine on arrival. In many instances travelers can minimize disease exposure. See Chapter 66 for suggestions on how to avoid mosquito-borne illnesses and illnesses associated with an infected water supply, and for other advice to the traveler.

## BIBLIOGRAPHY

American Academy of Pediatrics Committee on Infectious Diseases: *Report of the committee on infectious diseases,* ed 22, Elk Grove Village, Ill, 1991, The Academy.

American College of Physicians TaskForce on Adult Immunization, Infectious Diseases Society of North America. *Guide for adult immunization,* ed 3, Philadelphia, 1994, The American College of Physicians.

CDC: General recommendations on immunization. Recommendations of the ACIP, *MMWR,* 43 (RR-1):1, 1994.

CDC: Recommendations of the ACIP: Use of vaccines and immune globulins in persons with altered immunocompetence, *MMWR,* 42, (RR-4):1, 1993.

CDC: Update on adult immunization: recommendations of the ACIP, *MMWR* 40 (RR-12):1, 1991.

Hepatitis B virus: a comprehensive strategy for eliminating transmission in the United States through universal childhood vaccination. Recommendations of the ACIP, *MMWR* 40 (RR-13):1, 1991.

Onorato IM, Markowitz LE: Immunizations and vaccine-preventable diseases, and HIV infection. In Wormser GP, editor: *AIDS and other manifestations of HIV infection,* New York, 1992, Raven Press.

US Department of Health and Human Services, Centers for Disease Control: *Health information for international travel 1994,* Washington, DC, 1994, Publication no. (CDC) 94-8280, US Government Printing Office.

CHAPTER

# 4A Accident and Trauma Prevention in Primary Care

**Paul A. Severson**

Injury has become the most important health problem in the United States. The dramatic impact of injury has resulted in a growing national effort to not only treat injuries more effectively, but to prevent them.

When the word "injury" is heard by Americans, physicians included, it is immediately associate with emergency rooms, and a focus on treatment rather than on prevention. In recent years, increasing attention has been given to the prevention of chronic diseases, such as heart disease and hypertension. Discussions between doctor and patient regarding diet, exercise, weight loss, and stress reduction are commonplace. It is time for the primary care physicians to consider injury prevention as equally important and to inform their patients how to prevent or at least reduce this leading cause of death among our young people. It is time that all physicians help direct the nation's attention to this ongoing tragedy that suddenly takes away loved ones,

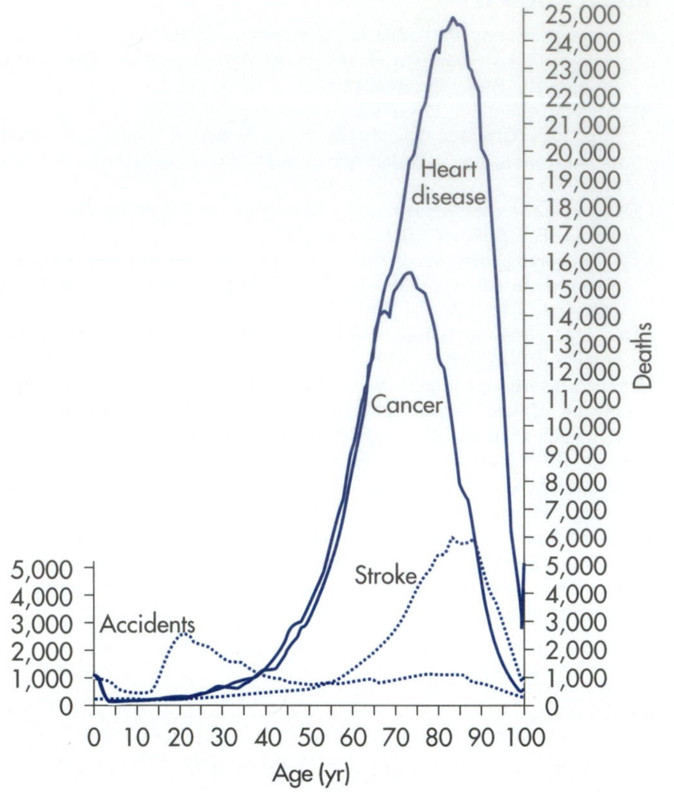


Fig. 4A-1. Leading causes of death by age in 1986. (From National Safety Council: *Accident facts,* 1989.)

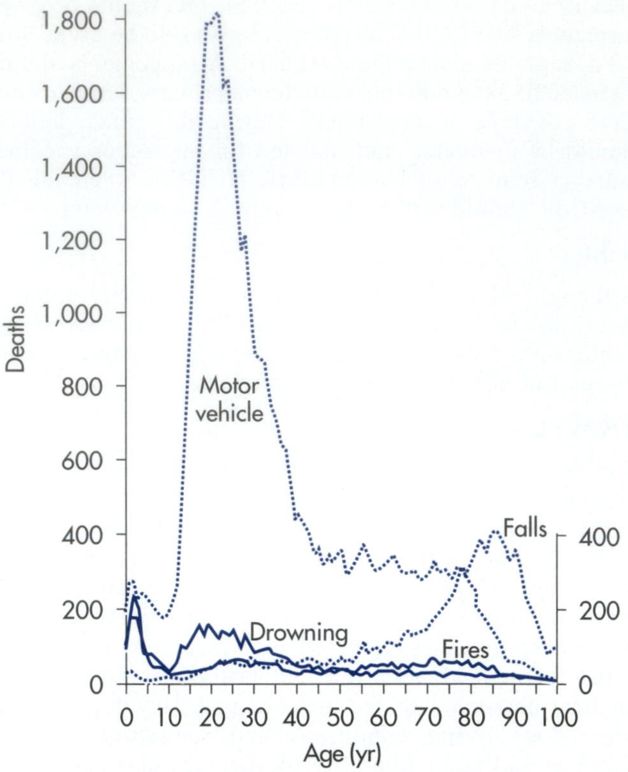


Fig. 4A-2. Leading causes of accidental death by age in 1986. (From National Safety Council: *Accident facts,* 1989.)

steals workers from the economy, and leaves millions unable to live a normal life.

## EPIDEMIOLOGY

### Incidence of trauma

Trauma is the most serious health problem facing the United States, whether measured in dollars, premature deaths, physician contacts, or lost productive years of life. Of 70 million injuries each year, 10 million are disabling. Injury annually claims the lives of approximately 150,000 Americans.

Injury is the fourth leading cause of death, exceeded only by cardiovascular disease, cancer, and stroke (Fig. 4A-1). Since it is by far the leading cause of death for those under age 44, injury accounts for more years of life lost than cancer and heart disease combined. In 1990, an estimated $200 billion was spent to treat injuries in the United States, far exceeding money spent on all other disease categories (including heart disease and cancer).

Injuries are of special concern to pediatricians. They are the most frequent cause of death during childhood, accounting for more fatalities than the next six most frequent causes combined, and costing the nation an estimated $107.3 billion. Nonfatal injuries occur at least 1300 times more frequently than fatal injuries, with one in five children needing medical attention each year. It is estimated that 8.7 million injuries occur annually to children. The underlying conditions surrounding the injury are different in children, accounting for the preponderance of pedestrian and bicycle accidents, drownings, burns, playground injuries, and poisonings.

### Causes of accidental death

Motor vehicle accidents, falls, drownings, and burns are the leading causes of accidental death. Motor vehicle accidents are the leading cause of death (nearly half), with a dramatic increase in incidence between ages 14 and 21 (Fig. 4A-2). More people are killed on the highways each year than during the entire Vietnam war. More than half of the fatalities are alcohol-related. Ironically, the nation's best trauma systems have been developed in urban areas, whereas 70% of the fatalities occur in rural areas.

Falls are the second most common cause of accidental death (first for adults past age 79). Drowning is third and has its peak incidence in one-year-olds. In many southern states, drowning is the leading cause of death for children under 5 years of age. Burns, the fourth leading cause, also peak at one year of age. Increasingly prevalent causes of death in the United States are homicide and suicide, especially between ages 15 and 24.

Trauma deaths occur at three distinct time periods following the injury (Fig. 4A-3). The first peak of fatalities occurs immediately after the injury. The victims suffer severe, often massive injuries resulting in death within seconds or minutes. Their injuries are typified by lacerations to the brain or brainstem, high cervical spinal cord, great vessels, or heart. The second peak occurs within the first few hours of injury. The injuries are typified by

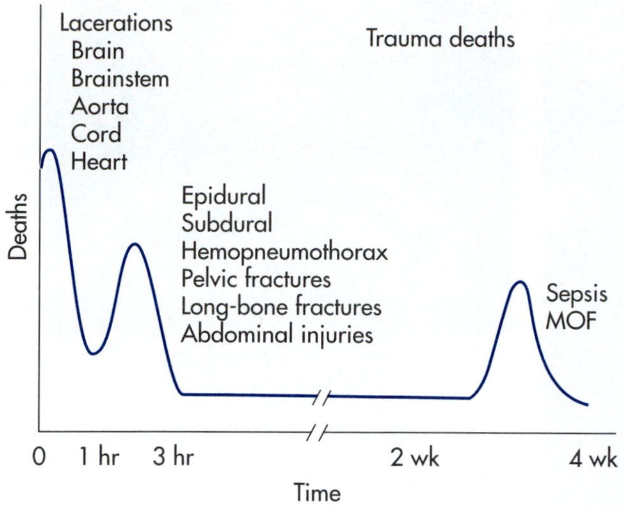


**Fig. 4A-3.** The trimodal distribution of death from trauma. (MOF = multisystem organ failure.) (This figure was prepared by Donald D. Trunkey, Chairman of the Department of Surgery, Oregon Health Sciences University, Portland, OR, and is used with his kind permission.)

subdural and epidural hematomas, hemothorax, pneumothorax, ruptured spleen, liver lacerations, fractured pelvis, or multiple injuries with cumulative blood loss. The third peak is a delayed phenomenon, occurring days to weeks after the injury. Death nearly always results from sepsis and multisystem organ failure.

Death is frequently an unavoidable result during the second and third peaks. However, many studies have shown that large numbers of the victims might have been saved with appropriate and timely trauma management. The landmark study, "Accidental Death and Disability: The Neglected Disease of Modern Society," first exposed several glaring problems:

(1) lack of public awareness
(2) neglect of prehospital emergency medical services
(3) inadequate medical facilities for trauma care
(4) lack of research and funding

While some improvements have been made, it is estimated that only 25% of the U.S. population has access to an effective trauma system.

## PREVENTION

Despite increasing attention in recent years, progress in the prevention of injuries has been minimal. Not only is the public poorly informed and the government slow to enact responsible legislation, but also primary care physicians are not cognizant of their important role in the prevention of trauma. Only a small percentage of pediatricians, family practitioners, and general internists provide prevention counseling.

There is a growing consensus that trauma should no longer be categorized as a behavioral malady with all its associated connotations of chance, unexpectedness, and blame. Instead, it should be addressed as a disease entity amenable to scientific, research-based strategies similar to those that have been developed to eliminate communicable infectious diseases. While progress in the management of trauma has resulted in the saving of many lives, virtually no reduction in the incidence of serious injuries has been observed. In fact, many types of injuries are becoming more frequent. Prevention is still the best cure, and yet too little emphasis is placed on instituting preventive measures, and available means for preventing injuries are too often ignored.

One retrospective review of pediatric trauma deaths showed that only 5% could have been avoided with better postinjury care, but 47% could have been prevented altogether.

Preventive measures that provide automatic protection (e.g., air bags, helmets) have been found to be more effective than those requiring individual action. To date, no effective educational campaigns have addressed these issues adequately, excepting possibly the recent campaign against drunk driving.

An injury prevention campaign was instituted in two communities in Norway, and after two years of public education the injury rate declined 29%. A study of a childhood-injury prevention program in suburban Massachusetts showed a 15.3% decrease in injury rates. Physician counseling took place within a context of community education efforts.

To reduce the devastating toll of traumatic death and disability, there must be an increase in the allocation of resources to further develop and disseminate information regarding prevention. In addition to advocating a comprehensive public health strategy that emphasizes technology, legislation, and education, primary care physicians should make office-based safety education a prominent part of their practice.

### Farm injuries

Although farming injuries account for a small number of fatalities each year, 44 farmworkers per 100,000 are killed, compared to 9 workers per 100,000 in industry. Farming is one of the most dangerous occupations in the United States. 4400 serious injuries per 100,000 farmworkers occurred in 1991. One in every five farm families has someone seriously injured annually. Children are disproportionately injured. In Washington State, 36% of injured-worker claims for minors under 14 were farm-related.

Many reasons have been cited for the high injury rate. First, farm equipment is inherently dangerous. Second, long working hours during planting and harvesting may result in worker fatigue. Third, children on family farms help with chores, frequently using dangerous machinery. Fourth, the working environment may be harsh because of weather (e.g., rain, thunderstorms, heat, humidity, cold, or darkness). Lastly, and perhaps most importantly, farmers frequently modify equipment to make it easier to use (e.g., they remove safety guards) (Fig. 4A-4).

Farm injuries are unique in that they frequently occur while the farmer is working alone in a remote field where notification and access are problematic. The injury often involves limb entrapment in machinery requiring challenging extrication techniques. Ambulance response times

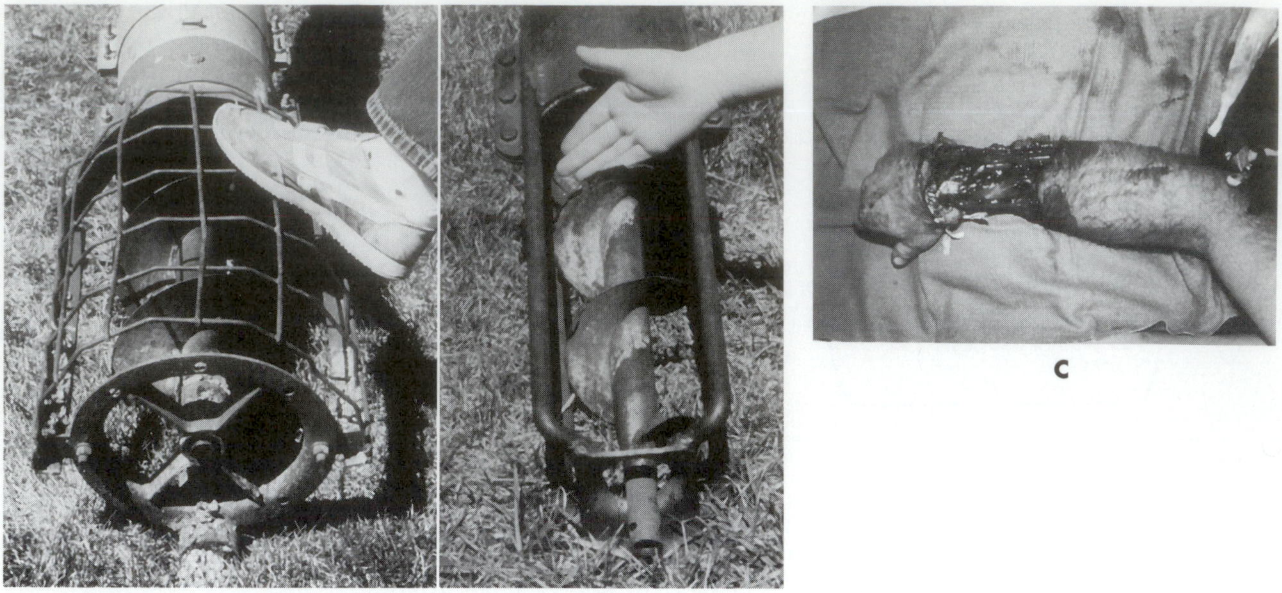

C

A B

**Fig. 4A-4.** **A**, The power takeoff is always manufactured with a protective guard. Farmers frequently remove the guard to allow more rapid access to the moving parts. **B**, Removal of protective guards continues to be the leading cause of limb-threatening farm injuries. **C**, Loss of limb injury resulting from mangling in farm machinery.

are usually prolonged, and served by Basic Life Support EMT's or local volunteers. While the prehospital care may be satisfactory, response time is slow and treatment often delayed. For this reason, "First Care" programs have been developed in farming states, such as Minnesota and North Dakota. They train all members of farm families in emergency medical care. The courses are usually provided free of charge by the Farm Bureau. Participants receive first-aid kits and instruction in the "Ten Steps to First Care" (see the box at right).

Prevention of injury is stressed by warning of the dangers of power take offs, leaving equipment safety guards in place, arranging regular time checks on farmers working alone, and keeping children away from potentially dangerous machinery.

### "Ten steps to first care"

Don't panic
Shut off equipment
Check airway
Check breathing
Check circulation
Stop bleeding
Check spine
Splint fractures
Notify neighbor
Transport

## Motor vehicle accidents

Motor vehicle accidents account for the majority of traumatic deaths in the United States. Because all the other causes of accidental death combined do not begin to approach the massive toll on U.S. highways, most efforts for prevention should be concentrated on the automobile and its driver. Even though there is no evidence that clinically-based efforts are effective long-term, physicians are urged to promote both clinical and nonclinical automobile-injury prevention measures because of the enormous social and economic costs of automobile injury (see the box on p. 54).

Head injury is the most common cause of death and disability in motor vehicle crashes. In addition, over half of all brain trauma result from auto accidents. Prevention strategies proven effective in other countries have not yet been universally applied in the United States. The most effective measures involve legislation, technology, and design changes rather than behavior modification.

Roadway design improvements are instrumental in reducing accidents and injuries. These include widening roadside recovery zones, removing fixed objects from roadsides, and installing breakaway utility poles and dividers between opposing lanes.

The National Highway Traffic Safety Administration now regulates vehicle design and has been helpful in improving safety features. Design requirements that have demonstrated efficacy include lap and shoulder belts in the front seat, automatic safety belts, air bags, head restraints, reinforced side and roof beams, and, most recently, the rear-window center-mounted brake light. Many authors agree that the next major advance will be mandatory provisions of full front-seat air bags in all vehicles. It is estimated that one fourth of brain trauma could be prevented or reduced in severity by this measure alone. Additional safety features that should be required by auto manufacturers include rear-seat restraints, antilock brakes, roof padding, and vehicle-rollover standards.

Measures already proven beneficial include the safety belt–use laws, license suspension for intoxicated drivers, 21-year-old legal drinking age, driving curfews for youthful drivers, and postponement of licensure for teenagers. Further research is needed in developing prevention techniques for the older impaired driver.

### Alcohol and driving

Drunken driving is the most important issue in all of trauma prevention. It leads to more loss of human life than any other preventable cause of death in the United States. While drunken driving accounted for nearly half of all traffic fatalities a decade ago, modest improvements have been made as a result of widespread public outcry.

Beginning in 1980, drunken driving became widely recognized as a serious social problem. Perhaps the most effective citizen-activist group, Mothers Against Drunk Driving (MADD), formed local chapters throughout the country. Between 1980 and 1985, considerable progress was made in reducing drunken driving and highway fatalities. The efforts of over 400 citizens' groups brought about a fiftyfold increase in media coverage. More than 500 legislative reforms were enacted. All states adopted a legal drinking age of 21. Some states passed criminal and "administrative per se" laws and increased penalties for drunken driving. Then in 1985 the number of fatalities fell to 39,168 from 45,284 in 1980, a decrease of 16%. After 1984, public interest and media attention declined, and in 1986 the number of fatal crashes rose 5% and has stabilized without further significant declines. As the years progressed, MADD chapter leaders shifted their emphasis toward strong legal penalties and strict enforcement of DWI laws, considering them more effective than other prevention and treatment measures.

The three types of drinking-driving laws that were developed are called "per se" laws. The first of these defines DUI (driving under the influence) by using blood alcohol–concentration (BAC) thresholds (usually 100 milligrams per deciliter). The second type calls for administrative license suspension prior to conviction for DUI ("administrative per se" laws). The third type of law mandates jail sentence or community service for first convictions. It is estimated that if all 48 contiguous states adopted these laws, another 2000 fatalities could be prevented each year. License suspension appears to be most effective (9% reduction compared to 6% reductions for both of the other types).

It is important that the primary care physician understand that counseling and education in the clinical setting are unlikely to have much impact on the prevention of auto crashes. It is more important that physicians become vocal and involved in the crusade to eliminate drunken driving by becoming acutely aware of legislative proposals.

***Efforts outside the United States.*** Random breath testing was first introduced in Finland in 1977. Since then, the rate of drinking and driving has been halved and dramatic reductions in death and injury rates have been observed. The results of Finnish studies show that random breath testing deters social drinkers and detects problem drinkers.

Problem drinkers are detected easiest in morning traffic, and random breath testing was shown to be the most effective police intervention. Random breath testing has not only saved countless lives, it has considerably cut the amount spent on health services as well. The other Nordic countries have adopted similar breath testing programs with great success.

In addition to proposing a random breath testing program, Great Britain has introduced legislation to revise the legal BAC downwards. Whereas many states have chosen legal limits of 100 mg/dl, the legal limit in Britain has always been 80 mg/dl. Based on results of recent research and favorable changes in public opinion, it has been suggested that the legal limit be lowered to 50 mg/dl, and a zero limit instituted for learner, first-year, and youthful drivers. These high-risk groups are more likely to crash with or without the influence of alcohol.

Australia accomplished a remarkable two-thirds reduction in fatalities since 1970. The United States needs only to emulate the demonstrated success of the Australian program and enact similar legislation despite the objections of private interest groups. Legislation for compulsory seat-belt wearing reduced the Australian fatality rate for crashes by one third. Tough countermeasures against drunken driving accounted for another one-third reduction. The Australians adopted the 50 mg/dl legal limit, random breath testing, mandatory license suspension, compulsory blood alcohol tests on all crash victims, and a zero BAC limit for learner and probationary drivers as well as motorcyclists. Motorcyclists are required to wear helmets and are restricted to an engine capacity of less than 260 cc. There has been a steady reduction in motor vehicle fatalities and injuries since 1977, including a dramatic reduction in injurious motorcycle accidents.

***Efforts in the United States.*** In response to the extraordinary success of the grassroots movement in the United States to fight drunken driving, the federal government created the Presidential Commission on Drunk Driving. The 1985 report supported the development of programs involving education, deterrence, treatment, and publicity campaigns. It was heavily criticized for failing to recognize that these strategies have minimal long-term impact. Newer research on environmental factors such as alcohol availability, server-intervention programs, price and tax policies, alcohol advertising, and transportation policies should be part of a comprehensive prevention program. These factors need to be considered as well as those individual behavior-changing strategies suggested in the Presidential Commission report.

The "designated driver" concept in preventing drunken driving has come under attack recently. The alcohol industry, the media, and various public-service groups have focused so much attention here that other alcohol-related problems accounting for the vast majority of deaths and injuries have been somewhat ignored. Policy makers should not be distracted from the more momentous task of increasing public awareness of environmental, social, and economic factors that influence alcohol consumption. They should promote debate on legislative proposals and other public policy solutions with a comprehensive strategy that includes "sobriety checkpoints," strict enforcement of laws forbidding alcohol sales to minors, alcohol advertising reform, and increased excise taxes. These additional measures will curb underage and heavy alcohol consumption, creating a legal and social environment that could eliminate drunken driving. Alternative strategies should include, but not be limited to, the use of designated drivers.

A field evaluation of a server-intervention program in 1987 concluded that trained servers initiated more interventions than untrained and consistently kept the BACs of bar patrons lower. This study suggests that server-intervention programs could reduce drunken driving by lowering the exit BACs of bar patrons. Other studies have confirmed the benefit of server liability since then.

***Physician responsibility.*** It is time that physicians act responsibly when admitting injured drivers who are intoxicated. Few patients are referred either to alcoholism rehabilitation programs or to the courts for prosecution. Society has the right to protect innocent people from intoxicated drivers, but current medical and legal practices do not serve the innocent victims or the drunken drivers. Physicians can do their part by referring all injured patients with illegal BACs to an alcohol rehabilitation program. The injury should be a reportable condition. Furthermore, blood alcohol measurements taken for normal clinical reasons should be routinely used by authorities to aid in prosecuting anyone driving under the influence. Juveniles found guilty of driving under the influence should be required to attend an educational program before license reinstatement. Participants of these programs have been shown to have a significantly lower number of repeat offenses.

Primary care physicians have an important role to play in bringing about a reduction in alcohol-related motor vehicle fatalities (see the box at right). They must educate families, reinforce public campaign efforts, and act as leaders in supporting legislation reforms if the bloodshed on the nation's highways is to be eliminated.

### Motor vehicles

- Never drink and drive
- Never allow anyone else to drink and drive
- Always wear your seat belt (lap and shoulder) even if you have an air bag
- Always protect every child with child-restraint devices and use the back seat
- Drive cars with air bags and antilock brakes
- Avoid driving late at night or on holiday weekends
- Explore alternative transportation for commuting to work or school
- Never speed and obey all traffic laws
- Avoid the use of radar detectors-they increase your risk for an accident
- Keep teenage drivers off the roads late at night
- Never drink and ride a motorcycle
- Always wear a helmet if riding a motorcycle

## Pedestrian injuries

Motor vehicle injuries are the leading cause of death and disability in children older than 1 year.

Each year, more than 50,000 child pedestrians are injured, 1800 die, 18,000 are admitted to hospitals, and 5000 are disabled.

Educational and preventive efforts by physicians and policy makers have dealt primarily with the occupants of motor vehicles. However, more preschool- and school-aged children die as pedestrians than as vehicle occupants. The prevention of pedestrian injuries has not yet been adequately addressed. Despite its importance, the pedestrian safety issue is often neglected in reports on vehicular injury.

Childhood pedestrian injuries usually take place in residential areas close to home, and commonly occur while the child is playing. The highest risk groups are boys ranging in age from 5 to 9 and children of lower socioeconomic classes. The most common type of accident is the midblock dart-out.

Analysis of recent programs to modify both pedestrian and driver behavior demonstrates only marginal success. Parents of 5 to 8 year olds consistently overestimate their child's pedestrian skills. This fact is important because unrealistic expectations of these skills may lead to premature traffic exposure. School training programs in pedestrian skills are essential and demonstrate improved skills over time. An eight-session program by a single teacher with cross-age teaching, videotape feedback, and parent-child activity workbooks was found to be effective in Seattle. In Montreal, simulation games, including role-playing, group dynamics, and modeling were shown to be effective in both changing attitudes and improving pedestrian skills. Since many children are still injured despite school training, additional preventive measures must be explored. Urban designers and traffic engineers and architects in Europe have been somewhat successful in preventing injuries by redesigning traffic flow through high-risk areas.

Greater understanding of how and why pedestrian accidents occur is needed, as well as a multifaceted prevention effort that addresses the role of environmental, psychosocial, and behavioral factors in these injuries. School training for pedestrian-skill development should be mandated and parental education secured. New legislation, environmental modifications, and vehicle design changes are areas for future study. Pediatricians and family practitioners can focus attention on this area of trauma neglected by researchers and policy makers.

## Burns

In 1985, fire and burn injuries killed 1461 children in the United States. It cost $3.5 billion to treat 440,000 burns and hospitalize 23,638 children. Young children accounted for 47% of the deaths. The next most frequently injured age group are the elderly. The majority of burns in these two groups are preventable and result from scalding by tap water or spilled liquids and ignition of fabrics by cigarettes or faulty heaters. More than 40% of the elderly victims have a permanent change in health status because of the burns; burn prevention could significantly improve the morbidity of aging.

A recent study showed that 37% of an outpatient clinic population did not have smoke detectors. Although the physicians were knowledgeable regarding injuries, 62% "never" and 23% "seldom" counseled patients about smoke detectors.

The mentally and physically handicapped are another group vulnerable to burns, especially scalding from hot tap water. This common type of burn injury is almost totally preventable by lowering water heater thermostats to 49° C (120° F). Legislation to mandate this change has proven effective in reducing the frequency, morbidity, and mortality of tap-water burn injuries. Lower water heater settings proved to be acceptable to consumers.

In addition to counseling families with children and the elderly about the importance of lowering hot water temperature, physicians should support legislation that would accomplish this end. In states without legislation, the use of facilitating devices such as a liquid crystal thermometer in combination with instruction at the doctor's office can improve compliance.

Antiscald devices or thermoscopic mixing valves can totally eliminate the possibility of tap water burns. Antiscald devices installed at the bathtub faucet are effective but unfortunately are frequently removed because of sediment accumulation. Better technology is needed. Another study concludes that wider provision of bathing aids to the elderly, a nationwide program to update inefficient immersion heaters and gas-boiler central heating systems, and public education campaigns would eliminate many of these burn injuries.

Hot oil and grease burns account for about 5% of burn injuries but deserve special attention because of the high morbidity associated with them. The high boiling point, high viscosity, and combustibility of oil increase the soft tissue damaged compared to scald burns from hot water. Seventy-eight percent of these burns occur in the home and 34% occur in children less than 8 years old. The most common scenario encountered is that of a child grabbing the handle or electric cord of a frying pan and pulling the hot oil down onto themself. Prevention of these injuries is possible through public education regarding the serious nature of these burns, the dangers of transporting hot oil, and the need to supervise children while cooking. Management of grease fires should be taught as well.

Gasoline burns account for about 15% of burn admissions, and occur largely in young men. It is estimated that at least 60% of these burns are preventable because they result from the inappropriate or unsupervised use of gasoline. Public education is essential because many young people are unaware of the dangers of gasoline.

Preventive efforts to reduce burn injuries have proven successful (see the box above). In the late 1970s, a statewide system for burn prevention and treatment was established in Maine. The annual number of deaths per million people declined from 41 before the program to 25 after the program's inception. This was a significantly greater decrease than for the United States as a whole. Despite some reported successes with public campaigns, worldwide burn mortality has not decreased. Burn prevention campaigns have had disappointingly little impact, suggesting that although education increases knowledge, it does not often lead to behavioral or lifestyle changes. Consequently, a restructuring of burn prevention programs is needed. Emphasis should be placed on technology development such as self-extinguishing or fire-safe cigarettes, residential sprinklers, child-resistant lighters, and antiscald devices. Legislation should mandate fire safety standards as well as product safety. Modern motivational theory must be incorporated in campaigns to promote public concern, and it must be effective enough to change individual behavior.

### Burns

- Install smoke detectors and check monthly
- Lower hot water thermostat to 49° C (120° F)
- Check tap water temperature with a liquid crystal thermometer to assess thermostat
- Install antiscald device or thermoscopic mixing valve at faucet if water temperature cannot be lowered
- Never ignite gasoline; it is a dangerous explosive
- Supervise children while cooking with hot oil or grease; keep cords and handles inaccessible
- Do not transport hot oil or grease; wait for it to cool
- Do not allow smoking in bed
- Have periodic inspections of heating units to ensure good working conditions
- Have complete home fire-safety programs

## Drowning

Drowning is defined as death from asphyxia occurring within 24 hours after fluid submersion. Annually, 8000 people drown in the United States, 150,000 worldwide. Near-drowning is defined as survival for at least 24 hours after submersion-immersion event and occurs much more frequently than drowning; there are nearly 500,000 in the United States annually.

Drowning is the third most common cause of death in infants and children; in ten states it is the leading cause. Residential swimming pools are the most common site of drowning in preschool children, with bathtubs the most common site for infants. Child abuse must be suspected in infant bathtub submersions. Epilepsy is frequently the etiology for drowning in older children. Adolescents frequently drown in lakes, rivers, or oceans; are often engaged in water sports at the time, such as diving, waterskiing, or surfing; and in 25% to 50% of the cases, have traces of alcohol or drugs. Absence of supervision is a prelude to most drownings.

While most studies of drownings deal primarily with children, and prevention measures are easily recognized, the epidemiology of adult drowning is quite different and prevention is problematic. Drowning rates are highest in men 20 to 29 years of age and in blacks. Swimmers, boaters, and motor vehicle occupants are most frequently involved. Alcohol use is involved in 48% of all cases and 77% of drownings involving motor vehicle occupants. Prevention of drowning in adults needs to focus on the elimination of alcohol use. Enactment and enforcement of "Boating While Intoxicated" laws, avoidance of swimming and water sports by epileptics, and public education efforts for boating and water safety are recommended as preventive measures.

Prevention of childhood drownings can be most easily implemented by legislation. Nations with mandatory fencing of all swimming pools have seen dramatic reductions in drownings in preschool children. A retrospective review of drowning deaths in New Zealand after passage of the 1987 "Fencing of Swimming Pools Act" concluded that 80% of the drownings would have been prevented by the legislation alone. Examination of the circumstances of the drownings shows that other alternatives to the fencing law, such as teaching water skills to infants, fencing property boundaries, and use of pool covers, are unlikely to have been as effective.

After legislation, parental education is the key factor in the prevention of childhood drownings. The primary care physician caring for children needs to communicate vital information about water safety to parents during the child's first year of life (see the box below). Designated teaching nurses and safety checklists should be considered to impart the information regarding barriers and fencing, supervision, and emergency procedures. Every physician should recommend CPR certification to the parents and explain how it can be obtained.

In order to decrease the mortality of near-drowning, immediate, good-quality onsite cardiopulmonary resuscitation is the most crucial factor. This must be initiated onsite, and continued during transport and in the emergency room, where evaluation, stabilization, and definitive care can be delivered. Early and effective intervention is the best predictor of survival.

## Bicycle injuries

There are over 100 million bicycle riders in America. About 1.2 million injuries are reported annually and 77% of these occur in children under 15 years of age. The large majority of deaths are the result of head injury. Only 3% of children wear helmets when riding even though helmets reduce the risk of serious head injury by 85% and brain injury by 88%.

Contrary to popular belief, most bicycle accidents do not involve collisions with motor vehicles. More injuries occur when people fall off bicycles, crash into fixed objects, or lose control. While motor vehicle collisions only account for about one third of injuries, a recent coroner's review showed 96% of the deaths occurred as a result of motor vehicle collisions. No victim was wearing a helmet at the time of injury. In 70% of the deaths, the cyclist caused the collision, either because of a road traffic violation or poor road sense.

### Drowning

Residential swimming pools must be completely fenced in and locked while not in use
Never leave a small child unsupervised in a bathtub
Never leave outdoor play pools or large buckets of water unattended in the presence of toddlers
Epileptics should shower (*not bathe*), and need restricted swimming privileges
Parents, pool owners, and other adult supervisors of swimmers should be capable of lifesaving skills, knowledgeable in water safety, and certified in CPR
Alcohol consumption should be avoided during water sports and boating activities

The following conclusions have been synthesized from the medical literature (see the box below):

(1) Children under 8 years old should not be allowed to ride bicycles on public roads.
(2) Older children should be allowed on the roads only after formal training.
(3) Bicycle safety should be a mandatory part of the school curriculum.
(4) Public campaigns are needed to increase the awareness of motorists toward cyclists.
(5) Bicyclists should be separated from road traffic by designated bicycle paths.
(6) Legislation requiring helmet use should be considered.
(7) Health-care workers could play an important role in campaigns promoting helmet use.
(8) Cyclists should wear protective gear.
(9) Children should wear helmets from the time of their first ride, and parents should always wear helmets to both protect themselves and teach their children.

## Motorized sports

***All-terrain vehicles.*** In 1991, it was reported that All-Terrain Vehicles (ATVs) have resulted in over 1400 deaths and 400,000 injuries in the United States since their introduction in the 1970s. Three-wheel ATVs have been declared illegal, but four-wheelers are still potentially dangerous.

Approximately one half of injuries occur in children. The majority of accidents typically involve vehicle overturns, whether occurring on slopes or on level ground. Half the time the vehicle turns on the side. A total of 27% fall backwards and 19% flip forward. ATVs present a danger whether used by a child or an adult, experienced or inexperienced (see box on ATVs on p. 57). The average casual user may not be aware that ATVs demand considerable skill and caution. Although a majority of the fatalities result from alcohol use, carelessness and youthful impetuosity, many occur during occupational use with experienced riders. Poor terrain contributes to many of the accidents.

Several injury control strategies have been proposed:

(1) requiring users to be at least 16 years old (licensure)
(2) requiring safety helmets
(3) requiring a safety course for youthful drivers
(4) increasing vehicular visibility through devices such as flags
(5) making engineering designs to prevent turnovers
(6) making technical improvements in leg room, footboards, and protective roll bar

Statewide legislative reform to enact these safety guidelines is recommended.

### Bicycles

Always wear your helmet (ANSI or Snell-approved)
Obey traffic laws
Ride on designated bicycle paths apart from road traffic
Keep smaller children off public roads

***Snowmobiles.*** While snowmobiling has become increasingly popular in recent years, injuries and deaths resulting from this motorized sport have also increased. Unlike ATVs, the snowmobile is not inherently dangerous in its design (it is hard to tip it over). However, manufacturers have steadily raised the engine's horsepower and improved the suspension and handling, encouraging drivers to reach ever-increasing speeds. The majority of injuries occur to males, three fourths to those less than 30 years old. Drivers are the injured party 57% of the time and passengers 43%. Falling off the machine and collisions account for 60% of the injuries. Only 3% of the injuries are the result of mechanical failure.

Suggestions to prevent injury include enforcement of existing laws such as speed limits and registration. Snowmobiles should be allowed only on designated trails. Legislation to place a zero limit on blood alcohol concentration should be introduced and random breath testing instituted. Educational programs have been required for children in some states and should be extended to adults before licensure (see the box below). Young children should be restricted from using a snowmobile. Penalties should be assessed for not wearing a helmet. A majority of the deaths occur as a result of alcohol intoxication and "overdriving the headlights" at night. Night driving should be avoided. Responsible legislation and enforcement by the Department of Natural Resources should eliminate a majority of the fatalities and many of the injuries.

## Falls

Falls among the elderly are covered in detail in Chapter 6. Falls in children deserve special consideration. Accidents on playgrounds, whether home or public, account for more than 150,000 injuries each year. Falls to the ground account for many injuries in addition to those specifically occurring on playground apparatuses, such as swings, gliders, and slides. The Consumer Product Safety Commission has developed voluntary safety standards for playgrounds. Absorbent surfaces other than asphalt (e.g., sand) are recommended to reduce injury. The height of a playground's climbing apparatuses should be kept to a minimum. Safety standards should be mandatory for home as well as public playgrounds.

Young children also fall off bunk beds, and infants down stairs. These injuries are common enough to have been studied and the Consumer Product Safety Commission has published standards. Children 6 and under should not use a bunk bed. Falling from the top bunk can result in serious fractures and even fatal head injuries; if a bunk bed is used, side rails should be mandatory for the top bed. Children also should be discouraged from using the bed for play. All stairways should be secured from toddlers, and walking devices that can roll down stairs should be avoided. Primary care physicians need to discuss the potential injuries resulting from falls with young mothers and also with older patients as they are largely avoidable (see the box below for patient education suggestions).

## Injuries from violence

Violence has permeated American culture so deeply that virtually no citizen is immune to its threat. It has become a major public concern, fueling media attention and even political debate over crime and gun control. Injuries resulting from violence encompass child, elder, and spouse abuse; sexual abuse; assault; suicide; and homicide. In addition, political violence is the greatest health threat in many countries.

### All-terrain vehicles

Do not allow children under 16 years of age to drive ATVs
Always wear a safety helmet
Wear stiff high boots
Never drink and drive
Avoid dangerous conditions, steep slopes, and poor terrain

### Snowmobiles

Never drink and drive
Always wear a Snell-approved helmet
Always wear warm close-fitting protective clothing
Avoid excessive speed
Always keep to the right side of trails and take great caution at turns
Avoid night driving completely
Always ride on designated snowmobile trails

### Falls

**Elderly**

Avoid alcohol—injury might result from impaired balance
Make sure railings are present for all stairs, always use them, and exercise special caution
Remove all rugs and objects from floors to avoid tripping
Avoid deeply-padded and thick carpets
Avoid high-heeled shoes
Do not walk in the dark
If your balance is impaired, a cane or walker prescribed by your doctor should be used
Never walk on slippery surfaces such as ice, snow, or water
See your doctor promptly for dizziness, lightheadedness, or fainting

**Children**

Avoid purchasing walking devices that roll for infants; secure all stairways
Keep children six and under out of bunk beds
Always keep side rails on the upper bunk
Discourage children from using beds for play
Supervise children when they use playground equipment and instruct in how to avoid injury
Do not allow children to play on climbing apparatuses that overlie concrete or asphalt or seem excessively high off the ground

Suicide, the eighth leading cause of death, accounts for 20% of all injury-related deaths. Trends in rates of violent death closely correlate with the use of firearms. Some 61% of homicides and 59% of suicides involve firearms. In 1991, 38,317 Americans were killed from firearms. Only 4% of these were unintentional shootings. Young African-American men are particularly vulnerable, with homicide rates increasing dramatically since 1984. The rate of suicide resulting from firearms more than doubled between the years 1982 and 1987. Most firearm deaths occurred by handguns (76%). In many states, firearm deaths now exceed motor vehicle fatalities.

This country's problem of homicide as a result of handgun injuries is staggering compared to other industrialized nations. In 1990, 22 handgun murders occurred in Great Britain, 68 in Canada, 87 in Japan, and 10,567 in the United States. This is sixty times the rate of all the other countries combined.

Since the start of this century, more than 1.3 million civilians have been killed by bullets. This number exceeds the total military casualties suffered by our armed forces throughout all of American history. More Americans are slain at home every two years than were killed in combat during the entire Vietnam War.

Between 1979 and 1988, 26,865 teenagers between 15 and 19 years old died from firearm injuries. These teenagers represent 15 to 19 years of private and public human capital investment costing this society $426.2 billion. While families and communities experience the grief and tragedy, society experiences not only the loss of this investment, but a very significant loss of future returns. Yet public policy has not adequately addressed gun control, especially among youth. Violence prevention programs are desperately needed.

While it is clear that violence is a problem of critical and international importance, there is no uniform consensus about its etiologic fators. We know that minority and disadvantaged populations have a much higher incidence, but this has been repeatedly demonstrated to be secondary to low socioeconomic status. Those involved in illicit drug trafficking or who have low self-esteem are more likely to be victims of violence. Some investigators attribute the skyrocketing incidence of violence to violence in the media, while others point to a decline in moral values and a breakdown of family life (see Chapter 127 on domestic violence). Despite the complex nature of etiology, violence prevention experts agree that organized medicine, through its resources and infrastructure, can play a key role in mobilizing physicians to help solve the problem (see the box at right).

Although handgun violence is only a part of the problem, the alarming statistics mandate that public health officials carefully study the problem of firearm accessibility; assess the risks, costs, and benefits of firearms; and evaluate policy initiatives, including gun control and prevention programs.

The financial costs to society are deeply disturbing. In 1985, the nation's bill for firearm injuries was estimated to be $14.4 billion. One study showed that 86% of the hospital costs from nonfatal injuries were paid by taxes.

Handguns are usually purchased for protection; however, several studies conclude that firearms in the home are far more likely to claim the life of a household member than of an intruder. Surprisingly, each year about 80,000 U.S. citizens defend themselves with firearms against assault, robbery, rape, or burglary. However, 800,000 violent crimes are committed with guns each year. Access to firearms in the home increases the risk for suicide nearly fivefold. One study showed that of 398 firearm deaths occurring in gun owners' homes over a six year period, only nine of the deaths were justifiable homicide (2.3%), 12 were accidental (3%), 41 were homicide (10.3%), and 333 were suicides (83.6%). The probability of using a gun to kill oneself or a friend or relative was markedly greater than the incidence of justifiable homicide.

***Gun control.*** Gun control laws attack the very last link in the chain of events leading to firearm injuries. They do not address the problem of violence and aggression, and certainly do nothing to prevent homicide and suicide from other weapons. However, the international experience and regional observations clearly show that gun control works. In Washington, D.C., a 25% drop in homicide and suicide by firearms abruptly occurred after stricter licensing laws were enacted. Seattle's homicide rate is 65% higher than Vancouver, British Columbia, where gun control regulations exist. Handgun-related homicide is five times higher in Seattle, despite the two cities' comparable economic and social conditions, as well as their equal rates of burglary, robbery, assault, and law enforcement. Canada's experience with strict gun control is one of many international lessons available to Americans looking for answers to the rising death toll. In fact, the United States is the only industrialized nation without effective regulation of private firearm ownership. Canada responded to a school massacre in Montreal by instituting gun control in 1892 and enacting stricter control through a series of regulations between 1989 and 1992. National Canadian standards now exist for all phases of firearm management, including age, licensure, screening, safe storage, safety training, banned and restricted weapons, and penalties.

***A national violence-prevention program.*** The National Center for Injury Control has recommendations for prevention of violence. These are summarized below:

(1) Develop and implement a broad, comprehensive foundation for violence prevention. This requires the cooperation of organizations in public health, education, mental health, social services, and law-enforcement to empower communities to de-

### Violent injuries

Keep firearms out of the home
Teenagers should avoid associating with gangs
Avoid people who carry handguns
Avoid high-risk public locations, such as bars, late at night
If you live in a home with firearms, know where the gun is, keep the bullets separate, and if you feel threatened by a household member just leave
Always seek professional help if you or someone you know is a victim of verbal, physical, or sexual abuse

velop their own violence prevention programs, especially in areas that have high rates of violent injury.

(2) Minimize ready access to firearms. Effective, less lethal means of providing security against assailants and intruders should be developed. Technologies to prevent firearms in high-risk settings should be studied (e.g., metal detectors in schools and bars). Law enforcement agencies should be given broad authority to regulate the design and manufacture of firearms and ammunition, as well as to commit resources to the prosecution of illegal trafficking of firearms. A national registration system for all handguns is essential with possession of unregistered handguns an enforceable criminal offense. A national waiting period for all purchases coupled with a mandatory criminal-record background check is recommended. Restricted licensing of handguns and an excise tax on firearms and ammunition sufficient to cover the cost of injuries are also recommended.

(3) Improve the identification, referral, and treatment of individuals at high risk of violent behavior because of alcohol and drug use.

(4) Develop programs to reduce childhood violence, especially among abused and neglected children. Education for children and parents to resolve conflicts without violence should be implemented.

(5) Improve efforts to identify and treat people at risk for mental and addictive disorders associated with suicide.

**Table 4A-1.** Poisonings by nonpharmaceutical agents in children under 6 years old*

| Agent | No. | % |
|---|---|---|
| Cleaning products and deodorizers | 81,075 | 17.7 |
| Cosmetics/personal-care products | 79,592 | 17.4 |
| Plants | 74,874 | 16.3 |
| Foreign bodies and toys | 31,844 | 7.0 |
| Other/unknown | 24,261 | 5.3 |
| Hydrocarbons | 23,689 | 5.2 |
| Herbicides/fungicides/pesticides | 21,933 | 4.8 |
| Art, crafts, office, photographic supplies | 17,135 | 3.7 |
| Alcohols | 13,710 | 3.0 |
| Adhesives and glues | 13,632 | 3.0 |
| Chemicals | 12,694 | 2.8 |
| Bites and envenomations | 9,842 | 2.2 |
| Food poisoning | 9,498 | 2.1 |
| Stripping agents and paints | 9,345 | 2.0 |
| Rodenticides | 8,651 | 2.0 |
| Tobacco | 7,414 | 1.6 |
| Mushrooms | 5,807 | 1.3 |
| Moth repellents | 3,867 | 0.8 |
| Batteries | 2,732 | 0.6 |
| Matches and fireworks | 2,508 | 0.5 |
| Heavy metals | 2,382 | 0.5 |
| Fumes and gases | 1,532 | 0.3 |
| Total | 458,017 | 100.1 |

*Reported to 63 poison centers in the United States in 1987.
Modified from Litovitz TL et al: *Am J Emerg Med* 6:497, 1988.

With violence rapidly becoming the world's greatest health threat, physicians need to assess the risk of violence in their patients. The most important step is to ask questions during the initial history and during subsequent visits. Just asking whether there is a gun in the house could help prevent an unintentional shooting or a suicide. Patients usually respond favorably when physicians initiate discussions on the risks of violence. One study demonstrated that patients recalled counseling on firearms more than any other topic, including sex.

Society looks to its physicians for health maintenance, life preservation, and death prevention. Primary care physicians have a responsibility to the patients, families, and communities they serve. Consequently, physicians should speak out vigorously against violence, call for action, back responsible legislation, and educate the public in a widespread effort to stop the senseless carnage in our streets and homes.

## Poisoning

Poisoning is one of the most common emergencies in the United States. Over 1.5 million poisonings are reported to poison centers each year, with 60% occurring in children less than 5 years old. Most childhood poisonings are minor, but over 100,000 are admitted to hospitals each year. While few children die from poisoning, adult poisonings frequently result in serious morbidity and mortality. Over 12,000 deaths occur annually, 6000 resulting from intentional adult self-poisonings.

The peak age for childhood poisoning is between 18 and 36 months. These children are in the oral stage of development and have become accomplished in fine motor skills but haven't yet developed sufficient judgment in protecting their own safety.

Children often ingest anything within reach, and Tables 4A-1 and 4A-2 show the most common toxic exposures. Childhood poisonings occur when children are ignored,

**Table 4A-2.** Poisonings by pharmaceutical agents in children under 6 years old*

| Agent | No. | % |
|---|---|---|
| Analgesics (includes narcotics) | 60,352 | 21.1 |
| Cold and cough preparations | 48,055 | 16.8 |
| Topicals | 33,517 | 11.7 |
| Vitamins | 26,651 | 9.3 |
| Antimicrobials | 23,522 | 8.2 |
| Gastrointestinal preparations | 18,999 | 6.7 |
| Other/unknown | 17,100 | 6.0 |
| Hormones | 12,286 | 4.3 |
| Electrolytes/minerals | 8,058 | 2.8 |
| Cardiovascular agents | 7,225 | 2.5 |
| Antihistamines | 7,068 | 2.5 |
| Sedatives/hypnotics/antipsychotics | 6,434 | 2.3 |
| Eye, ear, nose, throat preparations | 6,173 | 2.2 |
| Stimulants and street drugs | 4,140 | 1.5 |
| Asthma therapies | 3,836 | 1.3 |
| Antidepressants | 2,262 | 0.8 |
| Total | 285,688 | 100.0 |

*Reported to 63 poison centers in the United States in 1987.
Modified from Litovitz TL et al: *Am J Emerg Med* 6:501, 1988.

## Commonly ingested nontoxic substances

| | |
|---|---|
| Antacids | Magic Markers |
| Baby product cosmetics | Magnesium silicate |
| Ballpoint pen inks | Makeup (hypoallergenic) |
| Bathtub floating toys | Modeling clay |
| Birth-control pills (without iron) | Paint (Latex) |
| Bubble-bath soap | Pastes |
| Calamine lotion | Pencil |
| Candles (beeswax or paraffin) | Petroleum jelly (Vaseline) |
| Carboxymethylcellulose | Play-Doh |
| Chalk | Porous-tip marking pens |
| Crayons marked AP or CP | Putty |
| Crepe paper | Sachets |
| Dehumidifying packets (silica gel) | Shampoos |
| Deodorants | Shaving cream |
| Deodorizer sprays | Shaving gels |
| Elmer's Glue | Silly Putty |
| Etch-A-Sketch | Soap |
| Fishbowl additives | Spackle |
| Fish foods | Suntan preparations (watch alcohol contents) |
| Glycerol | Sweeteners |
| Golf balls | Teething rings |
| Gums | Thermometers |
| Hand lotion | Titanium oxide |
| Hydrogen peroxide (3%) | Toothpaste |
| Incense | Toy-gun caps |
| Indelible markers | Toys with "snow" inside |
| Ink (blue, black) | Watercolor paints |
| Lanolin | Zinc oxide |
| Linseed oil | Zirconium oxide |
| Lipstick | |

especially during mealtimes, on weekends and holidays, and when parents are entertaining. Thirty-six percent occur in the homes of grandparents, where "childproofing" hasn't been considered. In addition, grandparents usually do not purchase child-resistant containers from their pharmacists, making ingestion a serious threat to their grandchildren. One study suggests that if all pharmacists targeted poison control education to the elderly, childhood poisonings could be reduced by one third.

A child who has ingested a poison is likely to attempt it again. These repeaters have been characterized as more daring, aggressive, demanding, and active. Parents of repeaters have more poorly-developed parenting skills and are more socially isolated. These families are more frequently torn by divorce, alcoholism, or mental illness. Their homes have been found to be less safe.

***Prehospital care.*** Most childhood poisonings are minor and can be confidently managed by telephone advice. The most important principle in dealing with a frantic, emotionally distraught parent is to obtain a careful accurate history. The clinician should ask the following:

(1) Who are the witnesses?
(2) What are the suspected poisons?
(3) When did the poisoning occur?
(4) How much poison was taken?
(5) What is the patient profile (age, weight, underlying conditions, allergies)?
(6) Are symptoms present, and if so, is the condition changing?

A Physician's Desk Reference (PDR), Poisindex, or Regional Poison Control Center can be used to provide specific guidelines for management.

Most ingestions are of nontoxic substances (see the box above). Home observation can be recommended for these. If a toxic substance is suspected, the clinician must advise the parent to either take syrup of ipecac at home or proceed directly to the emergency room where specific and definitive care can be initiated.

***Prevention.*** Education remains the hallmark of poisoning prevention efforts. The primary care physician assumes the roles of teacher and counselor for families who have young children. They must guide parents in "poison-proofing" their homes, help them identify toxic substances, and prescribe drugs with great care, explaining any adverse side effects or any overdose risks (see the box at right). Toxic drugs and household agents need to be locked into overhead cabinets. Any unnecessary toxic substances should be removed from the home. Physicians should prepare each family by ensuring that syrup of ipecac is in the home and by making sure that the regional poison-center telephone number is next to the family's telephone. The astute clinician needs to be vigilant in assessing the need for psychiatric intervention in teenagers and adults if intentional poisonings are to be reduced.

The Poison Prevention Packaging Act of 1970 required

## Poisoning

Keep drugs and chemicals locked up or out of reach
Drain cleaners, furniture polish, and insecticides should be placed in overhead cupboards
Beware of the dangers of alcoholic beverages and mouthwash (10% to 25% alcohol)
Always keep the safety caps on new medicines, recheck dosage before giving to a child
Don't leave drugs (including aspirin and vitamins) on countertops or in a purse
Remove poisonous plants from the house, learn the names of any plants you do have. Teach children never to put any plant parts into the mouth
Don't ever put chemicals or kerosene in soft-drink bottles
Check older homes for lead-paint flakes and keep children away from lead-painted rooms
Keep syrup of ipecac and the Poison Control Center telephone number readily available

child-resistant packaging and resulting in a significant reduction in childhood poisonings. Improved packaging technology, such as unit-dose containers and reduction of the number of tablets per bottle, also continue to help reduce poisonings.

A well-developed, regionalized poison-center system has emerged throughout the country. Consequently, more efficient triage and management has lowered morbidity and mortality. Primary care physicians can now confidently manage poisonings in concert with the expert guidance of toxicologists in their regional poison center.

## MANAGEMENT

### History

Following the identification of trauma as a serious public health issue in 1966, federal legislation in 1973 mandated the development of comprehensive emergency medical service (EMS) systems.

A trauma system has four components:
(1) access to care
(2) prehospital care
(3) hospital care
(4) rehabilitation

Prevention of the injury is not an integral part of the current trauma system, which concerns itself with the already-injured patient.

The American College of Surgeons has been providing leadership in many areas of trauma management. While prevention is the best cure, many positive changes have occurred in the last decade to lower the incidence of preventable deaths once injury has occurred.

Access to the trauma system has been improved significantly by the introduction of "911." As communications improve in rural areas, universal access to the dispatch of emergency response teams should become a reality. Even with good prehospital care available, access problems still result in the loss of many lives in remote areas because of late discovery and limited availability of a telephone. Furthermore, once access has been achieved, dispatch may be delayed. Greater distances to the scene result in additional delays.

Prehospital care involves the "first responder" network, education and certification of Basic and Advanced Life Support personnel, communication systems allowing an organized rapid response to the scene, certified transport vehicles and equipment, protocols for medical management at the scene, and predetermined destination hospitals.

Hospital care involves the emergency room stabilization of the traumatized patient, triage and transport mechanisms, and definitive care in an operating room, intensive care unit, or hospital bed.

Several studies between 1967 and 1977 demonstrated serious deficiencies in hospital trauma care resulting in the death of as many as 50% of potential survivors. In particular, management of rural trauma has been shown to be well below the nationally accepted standards. Since 70% of the deaths from vehicular accidents occur in rural areas, primary care physicians need to evaluate and manage injuries in accordance with the American College of Surgeons' standards as taught in Advanced Trauma Life Support (ATLS) courses. It has been suggested that all physicians caring for emergency room patients be required to hold ATLS certification.

### The rural physician

Most primary care physicians who find themselves caring for major trauma patients in an emergency room setting are located in rural areas at level III trauma centers or undesignated small hospitals.

The small rural hospital has a unique set of problems frequently overlooked by educators and planners who largely work in levels I and II urban facilities. First, major trauma cases are an infrequent occurrence for most primary physicians in rural areas. While on emergency call, the physician is usually not at the hospital, but at a home or in the office. Consequently, the hospital has no immediately available physician. Second, the emergency room may be seriously understaffed or not staffed at all. Nurses may be called from inpatient duties to initiate care for the emergency patient. Third, many small hospitals have no laboratory or x-ray personnel after daytime hours. Therefore, extremely long delays in the treatment of critically injured patients may occur simply because needed personnel are unavailable.

Frequently, the rural physician does not assume responsibility for the trauma management of their hospital. The physician may be untrained or poorly trained in trauma management. Many ATLS-certified physicians may lack "hands-on" experience. Residency-training programs frequently exclude primary care physicians from trauma management, preparing only emergency physicians and general surgeons in these skills.

In addition to the possibility of having inadequately trained or unskilled physicians, many small hospitals have no surgeon, or a surgeon not immediately available. Additional delays in definitive care occur when the surgeon requests operating room personnel late in the course of emergency room management.

Despite these dilemmas, many physicians in small hospitals have not developed an organized approach to trauma management. These factors have contributed to the higher preventable death rate of major trauma in rural areas.

## THE PRIMARY CARE PHYSICIAN'S ROLE IN TRAUMA

Since direct transport to regional trauma centers without stabilization in the rural hospital results in higher mortality, it is essential that rural physicians be trained to resuscitate and stabilize trauma victims before transport. Despite the widespread availability of helicopter transport with trained medical flight teams, studies indicate that major delays prior to definitive care frequently occur, and a lack of appropriate management before transfer increases morbidity and mortality. The delays result from the physician's failure to examine, stabilize, and provide life-saving emergency procedures before the flight team's arrival.

First and foremost the rural physician must invest the time and effort into trauma education and develop a trauma protocol. The physician should start by becoming certified in Advanced Trauma Life Support. The nursing staff should attend conferences on trauma management at a nearby regional trauma center. Prehospital personnel should continually be instructed and drilled by regional EMS educators and should participate in mock disaster drills.

Organization of the emergency room with a special cubical designated for resuscitation of the critical patient is recommended. Storage of essential, ready-to-use trays in well-labeled, easily visible, and readily accessible areas minimizes confusion during resuscitation. All nursing personnel should be knowledgeable as to their location.

The physician in charge should then develop a trauma team. The trauma team might consist of the following personnel:

- Two physicians (surgeon if available)
- Two nurses
- Laboratory technician
- X-ray technician
- Anesthetist or respiratory therapist
- Recorder (extra nurse or ward clerk)
- Chaplain or social worker
- Surgery personnel on standby

The initiation of the "trauma code" should take place from the scene by the EMT or paramedic based on criteria consisting of the following:

(1) Unstable patient
  (a) Shock (e.g., BP $< 80$, P $> 120$)
  (b) Respiratory distress
  (c) Altered level of consciousness
(2) Potentially unstable patient, because of mechanism of injury

Radio communication with the hospital allows immediate assembly of the trauma team. Planned assembly of the trauma team before the arrival of the severely injured patient makes a dramatic difference in the rapidity of trauma care delivery.

Each team member has assigned responsibilities to allow for an orderly evaluation and resuscitation. The physician team leader is responsible for the overall care, performs the primary and secondary surveys, and decides on the disposition as soon as possible. The second physician performs the procedures ordered by the team leader. One nurse exposes the patient and places the monitors and Foley catheter, while the other manages IV solutions and medications and provides needed trays and equipment. The laboratory technician uses standing orders for CBC, chemistry panel, type and crossmatch, alcohol level, cardiac enzymes, urinalysis, and arterial blood gases. The standard protocol for x-ray is to proceed with lateral C-spine, then chest x-ray,and finally AP pelvis. The anesthetist assists with airway management, while the reocrder maintains a trauma flow sheet documenting the details of the resuscitation. This is useful to the regional trauma center, since transport usually occurs before the physician and nurse complete reports. All additional data and reports should then be baxed to the regional trauma center. The chaplain or social worker helsp by managing the family of the trauma victim.

Finally, the rural physician should establish a case conference to review each trauma code. Careful analysis of each case results in meaningful discussion as to how the delivery of care may be improved in the future. Physicians from nearby regional trauma centers should periodically be invited to attend these conferences to give follow-up informatin and to provide guidance and further education.

If the primary care physician is successful in implementing a trauma protocol for the small rural hospital, early stabilization and rapid transport will result in the salvaging of many lives.

## BIBLIOGRAPHY


Adleson L: The gun and the sanctity of human life; or the bullet as pathogen, *Arch Surg* 127(6):659, 1992.

Brunette D: Going after guns, *Minn Med* 77:25, 1994.

Cales RH, Trunkey DD: Preventable trauma deaths: a review of trauma care system development, *JAMA* 254:1059, 1985.

Carethers M: Health promotion in the elderly, *Am Fam Physician* 45(5):2253, 1992.

Certo TF, Rogers FB, Pilcher DB: Review of care of fatally injured patients in a rural state: 5 year followup, *J Trauma* 23:559, 1983.

Coffman SP: Parent education for drowning prevention, *J Pediatric Health Care* 5(3):141, 1991.

Eastman AB: Blood in our streets, *Arch Surg* 127(6):677, 1992.

Hamdy CR, et al: Snowmobile injuries in northern Newfoundland and Labrador: an 18 year review, *J Trauma* 28(8):1232, 1988.

Hargarten SW: All-terrain vehicle mortality in Wisconsin: a case study in injury control, *Am J Emerg Med* 9(2):149, 1991.

Injury Control in the 1990's: *A National Plan for Action.* Second World Conference on Injury Control, May 1993.

Jagger J: Prevention of brain trauma by legislation, regulation, and improved technology: a focus on motor vehicles, *J Neurotrauma* 9 (Suppl 1): S313, 1992.

Leicht MJ, Dula DJ et al: Rural interhospital helicopter transport of motor vehicle trauma victims: causes for delays and recommendations, *Am Emerg Med* 15:450, 1986.

Malek M, Guyer B, Lescohier I: The epidemiology and prevention of child pedestrian injury, *Accid Anal Prev* 22(1):301, 1990.

McLoughlin G, McGuire A: The causes, cost, and prevention of childhood burn injuries, *Am J Dis Child* 144(6):677, 1990.

Petro JA et al: Burn accidents and the elderly: what is happening and how to prevent it, *Geriatrics* 44(3):26, 1988.

Quan L et al: Ten-year study of pediatric drownings and near-drownings in King County, Washington: lessons in injury prevention, *Pediatrics* 83(6):1035, 1989.

Simpson AH, Mineiro J: Prevention of bicycle accidents, *Injury* 23(3):171, 1992.

Smith GS: The physician's role in injury prevention: beyond the U.S. Preventive Services Task Force report, *J Gen Intern Med* 5(5):567, 1990.

CHAPTER

# 4B Heat-Related Illnesses

Richard J. Iseke

The popularity of physical fitness has led to an interest in heat-related illnesses. Several clinical syndromes can result from exposure to excessive heat and can affect athletes, the elderly, infants, and patients with chronic illnesses or on certain medications.

## MECHANISMS OF HEAT DISSIPATION

To arrive at an understanding of the pathophysiology of the heat-related illnesses, we shall review the physiology of thermoregulation. The body is able to generate energy through metabolism, and this metabolism results in the production of heat. During exercise even more heat is generated. In order to maintain body temperature within a narrowly defined range, any excess heat must be dissipated. Conduction, convection, and radiation account for the major losses. Perspiration accounts for the rest. Breathing produces a minute amount. The rate of heat dissipation through these various mechanisms depends on the rate of perspiration and extent of cutaneous vasodilatation, all factors controlled by the hypothalamus and mediated through the cholinergic system.

As environmental temperatures approach body temperature, less heat can be lost through conduction, convection, and radiation, and perspiration must assume a greater role. As the relative humidity rises, the effectiveness of heat loss through perspiration diminishes. If heat production overwhelms heat dissipation, body temperature then begins to rise.

This imbalance is reached faster in certain individuals. Individuals exercising have a higher degree of heat generation and overwhelm the body's rate of heat loss quicker than sedentary individuals, especially if they are not acclimatized to the heat. The elderly have impaired heat dissipation mechanisms, as do individuals who are on medications that curb their ability to perspire. Dehydration and cardiovascular insufficiency reduce the effectiveness of peripheral vasodilatation in dissipating heat. Therefore individuals who suffer from heart disease or are dehydrated from drinking alcohol or using diuretics are also at high risk of developing hyperpyrexia. Finally in children the heat-losing mechanism is quickly overwhelmed because their greater ratio of surface area to body mass makes them absorb heat more rapidly, their rate of sweating is less than adults, and the temperature at which they initiate sweating is higher than in adults.

## HEAT CRAMPS

Heat cramps are characterized by painful muscle spasms, usually of the lower extremities. They most commonly occur in poorly-conditioned individuals who have been exercising in unaccustomed hot, humid weather. The diagnosis is usually made from a history of cramps in the large muscle groups, usually the quadriceps, hamstrings, or soleus muscles. Such cramps are prevalent during the early weeks of warm weather.

Immediate therapy consists of ceasing the exercise, rehydration, massaging of the affected muscles, and applying ice packs to those muscles.

Some authors have speculated that the cramps may result from diminished circulation to muscles secondary to the dehydration that can occur with excessive sweating while exercising in the heat.

There is no evidence that salt deficiency is the reason for the cramps. Therefore the use of supplemental salt by exercising individuals on hot days serves no purpose. Normal use of salt at meals should provide adequate sodium during summer workouts. Individuals who suffer from heat cramps should be warned to exercise carefully in warm weather, starting at reduced levels of exertion and building up gradually to maximum effort over 7 to 10 daily sessions. Weekend athletes, such as joggers and tennis players, should remember that when the weather turns warm, they should take several weeks of early conditioning and stretching exercises before going out and strenuously exercising.

## HEAT SYNCOPE

Heat syncope refers to the very common occurrence of fainting on hot days, especially by individuals who have been standing in one place for a very long time. Everyone is familiar with this condition, especially at sporting events and military marches. The syncope is due to hypotension, which is caused by peripheral vasodilatation from the heat. This leads to a shift in blood volume from the arterial circulation, with subsequent venous pooling in the extremities. There may also be a vasovagal contribution to the syncope. The patient should be removed to a cool place in the shade, kept in a recumbent position, and have cold compresses placed on the forehead. These individuals are usually not truly hypovolemic but may feel better if they can drink some cool liquid. Their core body temperature is normal, and they usually recover without any difficulty.

## HEAT EXHAUSTION

The human body dissipates its excessive heat through peripheral vasodilatation and sweating. If a person is exposed to high environmental temperatures and generates excessive heat through exercise, then sweating results in order to dissipate the heat. If the excessive fluid loss cannot be replaced through increased fluid intake, hypovolemia may result. If the hypovolemia is severe enough, it will lead to heat exhaustion.

Patients suffering from heat exhaustion present with fatigue, nausea, vomiting, and lightheadedness. Physical examination reveals a cold, clammy, diaphoretic skin; weakness; muscle cramps; orthostatic hypotension, and a weak but rapid pulse. Core body temperature is usually normal, although it can increase to as high as 100°F.

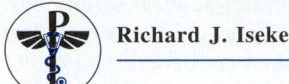

Patients with heat exhaustion should be placed in a recumbent position in a cool area. If they are not vomiting and have an intact gag reflex, they should have their fluid losses replaced by oral fluids. Oral fluids can be in the form of water, juice, or any hypotonic beverage. Affected individuals are usually not salt-depleted and therefore do not need hypertonic solutions. Severely hypotensive patients with mental clouding or severe nausea or vomiting require intravenous administration of Ringer lactate or normal saline. Recovery is usually quite rapid, although some patients may need to be hospitalized if their hypotension has been severe enough to affect perfusion to critical organs such as the brain, heart, or kidneys. Elderly patients especially should be closely monitored during volume replacement, so that heart failure resulting from volume overload is avoided.

## HEAT STROKE

When an individual is exposed to high environmental temperatures and generates excessive internal heat, the human body dissipates this heat through peripheral vasodilatation and perspiration. Internal body temperature can rise to dangerous levels whenever the amount of heat generated overwhelms the body's systems for heat dissipation. It usually occurs in situations of high environmental temperature and humidity or in clinical settings where drugs or illness has impaired the ability of the body to accelerate heat loss. When internal core body temperature rises to levels of 105° to 106°F, the risk of suffering from heat stroke is high.

### Clinical syndrome of heat stroke

Heat stroke is characterized by elevated body temperature in the range of 105° to 106° F, central nervous system dysfunction, and anhidrosis. The central nervous system manifestations can range from slight alterations in the mental status of the patient to delirium, seizures, and coma. Lack of perspiration is usually the rule, although in exercising athletes one may observe the development of heat stroke in the presence of active diaphoresis. The body temperature can rise above 106°F. Patients suffering from heat stroke may also develop a variety of complications, including disseminated intravascular coagulation, renal failure, jaundice, and myocardial failure because of petechial hemorrhages in the myocardium.

### Management

***Immediate cooling.*** Treatment of heat stroke should be initiated as soon as the diagnosis is considered. The longer the delay in lowering the temperature, the greater the morbidity and mortality. Cooling should be started in the field as soon as heat stroke is suspected. The patient should be put in the shade and an ambulance called. In the ambulance vital signs should be checked as soon as possible and ice packs or cold wet compresses placed on the neck, groin, axillae, and other body parts. One should make sure that the patient's airway is secure; if there is any question about it, the patient should be intubated. Intravenous lines should be started and 500 to 1000 ml of normal saline infused immediately. An ampule of 50% dextrose in water should also be infused in order to make sure that any alteration in mental status is not because of hypoglycemia. If the ambulance has fans in it, they should be turned on and directed at the patient. Oxygen should be administered to the patient en route to the hospital.

Once the patient arrives in the emergency department, the cooling process should be continued. Three cooling techniques are classically used in the treatment of heat stroke: (1) an ice water bath; (2) a stretcher packed with ice cubes; and (3) a spray of lukewarm water blown over the patient by a fan, resulting in heat loss through evaporation. The ice water bath has several disadvantages. It makes monitoring of the patient's temperature through rectal probes awkward. It makes it difficult to protect the airway should the patient begin to have seizures or vomit. Should the patient experience a cardiopulmonary arrest, defibrillation may be delayed until the patient is removed from the water. Finally, an ice water bath may interfere with control of the shivering that often starts during the cooling process. Shivering can be violent and lead to increases in body temperature. Intravenous chlorpromazine, occasionally used to control this shivering, may result in hypotension, which can be difficult to treat in an ice water bath.

A simpler method is to place the patient on a stretcher and pack ice cubes around the body, while rubbing it with cool, moist compresses. The ice cubes produce peripheral vasoconstriction and may impede heat loss. Rubbing is theoretically intended to counteract this.

In the most efficient cooling technique a fine mist of warm water is sprinkled over the patient while a fan blows a steady stream of air across the body. The warm mist keeps the skin's blood vessels dilated, and the moving air dissipates the heat by evaporation. It is the fastest method of treatment for heat stroke, but it requires special equipment.

At a body temperature of 101° to 102° F the cooling process should be stopped, since the patient can develop clinical hypothermia. Stopping cooling at this temperature is particularly important in the case of patients who are on phenothiazines and have an altered thermoregulatory process. Once the cooling process is begun and the airway is protected, any hypotension must be treated.

***Treatment of hypotension.*** The cause of the hypotension can be either hypovolemia or myocardial failure secondary to heat-induced damages to the myocardium. Treatment should always start with fluid challenge of a crystalloid solution such as normal saline, and the initial amount should not be greater than 250 to 500 ml. Hypovolemia should be suspected as the cause of the hypotension if neck veins are flat, lung sounds are clear, no third heart sound is present during cardiac auscultation, and clear lung fields are seen on the chest x-ray. Hypovolemia is also probable if the blood pressure rises after crystalloid infusion. Subsequent fluid challenges should be undertaken until the blood pressure rises to normal levels.

Primary cardiac failure is the likely cause if the neck veins are elevated, a third heart sound is audible on cardiac auscultation, bilateral rales are heard during examination of the lungs, and the chest x-ray reveals pulmonary congestion. In such circumstances a fluid challenge rarely leads to a rise in blood pressure. Sometimes it is extremely difficult to differentiate between the causes of hypotension, and it may be necessary to insert a Swan-Ganz catheter. Once a diagnosis of cardiac failure is made, further treatment requires administration of intravenous isoproterenol, dopamine, or dobutamine. One should avoid epinephrine or other strong alpha-agonist medications because of their tendency to constrict peripheral blood vessels and inhibit heat loss.

***Complications.*** Initial laboratory studies (see the box below) in all cases of heat stroke include a complete blood count (CBC), platelet count, prothrombin time, partial thromboplastin time, electrolytes, blood urea nitrogen (BUN), creatinine, and glucose. Disseminated intravascular coagulation (DIC) can be a complication in severe cases of heat stroke; treatment consists of fresh frozen plasma, platelets, and consultation with a hematologist. Although there is some evidence that low dose heparin helps control life-threatening bleeding secondary to DIC, it should be given only after consultation with an experienced hematologist. Electrolytes may be altered because of hypovolemia. Elevated BUN and creatinine levels may signal renal failure.

Renal failure is multifactorial, stemming from direct damage from hyperpyrexia as well as acute tubular necrosis from a combination of hypotension and myoglobinuria. Urinalysis should allow detection of significant myoglobinuria. Some experts advocate the use of intravenous mannitol and bicarbonate in addition to volume infusions, if gross myoglobinuria is present. These medications should be given cautiously, since patients may have underlying cardiac failure, and large amounts of bicarbonate may precipitate pulmonary edema. During the first few days of hospitalization, it is very common for a person with severe heat stroke to exhibit jaundice and elevations of liver enzymes as a result of central lobular necrosis.

The severity of central nervous system manifestations depends on individual host factors, such as age and underlying illnesses, as well as on the severity of heat-induced damages on the brain. Brain damage can be caused by the high temperature or can be secondary to petechial hemorrhages. Hyperpyrexia by itself does not lead to central nervous system aberrations and may not warrant a diagnosis of heat stroke.

### Differential diagnosis

It is worthwhile to review the differential diagnosis of hyperpyrexia (see the box at right) in order to exclude other entities that may contribute to heat stroke. Hyperpyrexia can develop through three basic mechanisms: heat gain from the environment, usually in the setting of some impairment of the body's heat dissipation system; increased heat production, as seen in infectious states, hyperthyroidism, drugs, and exercise; and decreased heat dissipation. Environmental heat stroke is usually easy to diagnose from the presenting history. In some cases an underlying medical disorder or drug use must be considered. Such cases usually involve individuals who are brought in comatose and hyperpyrexic without a clear history of exertion. A toxic screen for drugs as well as a search for an infectious etiology through blood cultures and lumbar puncture is certainly appropriate. As with other conditions, it should be ascertained that there is little likelihood of a space-occupying brain lesion prior to the lumbar puncture.

### Mortality

Mortality of heat stroke ranges from 6% to 50%, depending on the patient's age, underlying illnesses such as diabetes and cardiovascular disease, magnitude and duration of the peak temperature in the patient, initial blood pressure, and development of jaundice or coma. Health care professionals can influence the mortality of heat stroke through early diagnosis, rapid lowering of the temperature, and competent management of the varied complications as they are manifested.

## PREVENTION

Physicians should warn their patients with chronic ailments, and any patients taking psychotropic medications, about the special hazards high environmental temperatures may pose for them. Any elderly patients who suddenly develop mental disturbances during a heat wave should be examined promptly for evidence of a heat-related illness. This is especially true for patients in nursing homes if there is a malfunction of the air conditioning or a series of hot days. The provision of extra beverages and cooling fans usually suffices; however, close monitoring of patient temperatures is essential.

Physicians who are asked to cover sporting events should alert the sponsors to possible hazards of heat to contestants. The American College of Sports Medicine has developed guidelines that present their recommendations for precautions that need to be taken during road races, including adequacy of water supplies and equipment and organization of medical stations. They have also developed a heat index that helps sports organizers decide on whether an event should take place and if so, the support systems and precautions necessary. This index, which uses a wet-bulb-globe temperature (WBGT), is based on several measurements such as ambient air temperature, humidity, and radiant heat load.

#### Laboratory studies appropriate for heat stroke victims

CBC
Platelets, PT, PTT
Electrolytes
BUN, creatinine
Blood sugar
Urinalysis
Liver function tests

#### Differential diagnosis of heat stroke

Increased heat production
- Infection (sepsis, meningitis)
- Metabolic (thyroid storm)
- Drugs (sympathomimetics, antidepressants)

Decreased heat dissipation
- Disorder of skin or sweat glands
- Central nervous system disorders (subarachnoid hemorrhage)
- Drugs (anticholinergics, psychotropic agents)

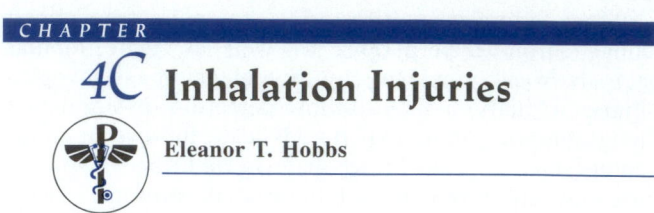

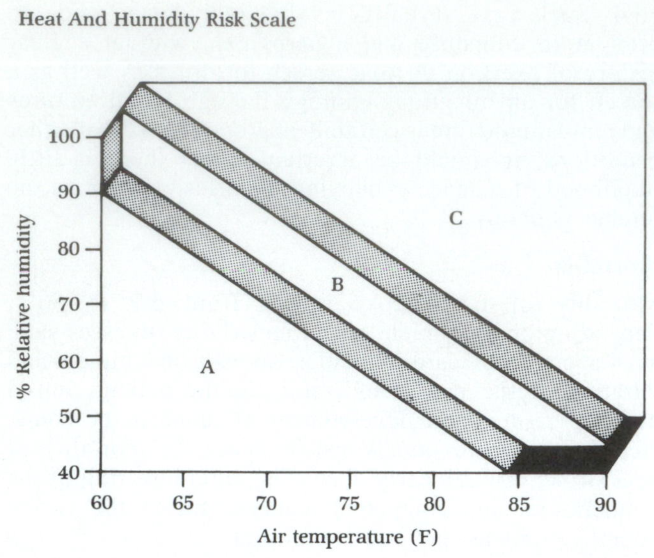


**Fig. 4B-1.** This graph, based on studies of football players and Marine recruits, shows the relative safety of exercise at different temperatures. A = safe, B = caution, C = danger.

This index can be calculated using a WBGT or deriving it through the following formula: WBGT = (0.567* DBT) + (0.393*Pa) + 3.94. DBT is the dry-bulb temperature, and Pa is the environmental water vapor pressure. These can be obtained from local weather stations. Based on the WBGT, one can assess the risk of heat injury as low, moderate, or high risk. The risk of heat injury is possible and high for WBGT greater than 73° F, moderate for temperatures greater than 65° F, and low for temperatures less than 65° F.

Since these can be cumbersome to calculate, rough guidelines can be used for less formal events (Fig. 4B-1). Prolonged strenuous exercise is generally safe when temperatures are below 65° F and relative humidity is below 40%. Risk increases as temperature or humidity rises, and cancellation of physical activity should be seriously considered when the temperature rises above 80° F and relative humidity is greater than 70%. Participants should be warned of the dangers of using certain medications, such as anticholinergics, and of competing without adequate preparation.

There should be adequate observation and monitoring of sports participants, including water stations and frequent water breaks. Running events should have aid stations stocked with medical supplies and water every 2 to 3 km for races longer than 10 km and run in warm weather. Shorter races should have such a station at the halfway point. Finally, the best prevention is to have athletes achieve adequate conditioning and acclimatization to the heat before competing.

Since former heat stroke patients may be predisposed to hyperpyrexia on repeat exposure to a hot environment while exercising, it is important that their return to exercising under adverse conditions be done only in very closely supervised settings.

## BIBLIOGRAPHY

American College of Sports Medicine position stand on the prevention of thermal injuries during distance running, *Med Sci Sports Exerc* 19(5):529, 1987.

Clowes GHA, O'Donnell TF: Heat stroke, *N Engl J Med* 291:564, 1974.

Heat illness. Fluid and electrolyte issues for pediatric and adolescent athletes, *Pediatr Clin North Am* 37(5):1085, 1990.

Iseke RJ: Danger: summer heat illness, *Diagnosis* 96, July, 1983.

O'Donnell TF: Acute heat stroke, *JAMA* 234:824, 1975.

Shapiro Y, Magazanik H, Udassin R: Heat intolerance in former heat stroke patients, *Ann Intern Med* 90:913, 1979.

Stine RJ: Heat illness, *JACEP* 8:154, 1979.

CHAPTER

# 4C Inhalation Injuries

Eleanor T. Hobbs

## DROWNING AND NEAR-DROWNING

There are at least 8000 deaths from drowning in the United States each year and many additional near-drownings. About 40% of the deaths are in children under age 4.

### Definitions

Drowning is defined as asphyxia and death within 24 hours of submersion in a fluid medium; near-drowning is survival for at least 24 hours after asphyxia resulting from submersion. Two other mechanisms of submersion injury are immersion hypothermia, which may occur with or without drowning, and the rare immersion syndrome, in which ventricular fibrillation is precipitated by a sudden plunge into icy water. Some individuals, particularly young children, may be transiently protected from cerebral hypoxia by an active diving reflex. Here, immersion in cold water produces bradycardia and intense vasoconstriction of all but coronary and cerebral blood vessels, temporarily preserving blood flow to the heart and brain despite the absence of respiration (see Chapter 4E).

Two types of pathophysiologic mechanisms have been observed in drownings. Some 10% to 20% are *dry drownings,* in which laryngospasm results in asphyxia, and the glottis relaxes only after respiratory efforts have ceased; thus, no fluid is aspirated. The majority, however, are *wet drownings,* in which variable amounts of fluid are aspirated. The term secondary drowning refers broadly to the development of respiratory distress syndrome after surviving submersion and may begin 1 to 72 hours later.

### Mechanisms of injury

***Asphyxia.*** The immediate result of submersion is asphyxia; $Po_2$ rapidly falls, $Pco_2$ rises, and a combined metabolic and respiratory acidosis develops. Much has been made of the differences between freshwater and salt water drownings, but the amount of fluid aspirated is rarely enough to cause clinically significant abnormalities in electrolytes or intravascular volume.

Despite differing mechanisms of lung injury from impurities, particulate matter, freshwater, or salt water, the net result is ventilation-perfusion mismatch, intrapulmonary shunting, and hypoxemia.

***Metabolic alteration.*** In the rare cases where a large amount of freshwater is aspirated (greater than 22 ml/kg), the metabolic abnormalities that may occur include a lowering of serum sodium, chloride, calcium, and magnesium; volume overload; intravascular hemolysis leading to hyperkalemia, hemoglobinemia, and hemoglobinuria with potential hemoglobinuric renal failure; and disseminated intravascular coagulation. With salt water aspiration hemoconcentration and hypovolemia may be seen.

***Anoxia.*** Aside from the direct lung damage from fluid aspiration and the occasional metabolic abnormalities, the effects of drowning on the heart, kidney, and brain are those of anoxia. The two most important prognostic factors for survival with good neurologic function are the duration of the anoxic episode (length of submersion plus time until effective cardiopulmonary resuscitation [CPR] begins) and the water temperature.

In warm water drownings the following factors have been found to indicate a poor prognosis: submersion for more than 5 minutes, no CPR for 10 minutes, a pH of less than 7.10 on arrival at the hospital, a continuing need for CPR in the emergency department, the presence of deep coma, and especially the presence of fixed dilatated pupils. Cold water drowning is reviewed in Chapter 4E.

***Complicating factors.*** An integral part of the assessment of a drowning victim includes the consideration of possible predisposing factors, such as cervical spine injury, alcohol or drug intoxication, seizure disorder, arrhythmia, suicide attempt, and child abuse.

## Treatment

Emergency treatment (see the box at right) should begin with mouth-to-mouth breathing as soon as the rescuer reaches the victim, even before removal from the water. If there is any suspicion of a neck injury, the cervical spine should be immobilized. CPR and advanced cardiopulmonary life support (ACLS) should be instituted at the scene and continued on route if possible. Once in the emergency department, vital signs should be checked, including temperature and pupil size. If the patient is in cardiopulmonary arrest, the usual ACLS protocol should be instituted with the addition of rewarming if hypothermia is present (see Chapter 4E).

***Endotracheal intubation.*** The indications for endotracheal intubation of a drowning victim who has regained spontaneous respirations include coma with inability to protect the airway, the presence of copious secretions or gross aspiration of particulate matter, and a $Pco_2$ greater than 45 torr or a $Po_2$ less than 80 to 90 torr on 40% oxygen by mask. Intubated patients should be maintained on a volume ventilator with positive end-expiratory pressure (PEEP) (the amount titrated for each patient); if they have spontaneous respirations, intermittent mandatory ventilation with continuous positive airway pressure (CPAP) may

### Protocol for managing the drowned or near-drowned patient

Check airway, breathing, and circulation, and begin CPR as needed (CPR, ACLS)
Provide supplemental oxygen. Airway maintenance and intubation/ventilation as needed
Check for hypothermia and begin rewarming if present
Obtain ABGs, CBC, electrolytes, BUN, creatinine, Ca, Mg, PT, PTT, urinalysis, ECG
Insert nasogastric tube
Chest x-ray
Adjunctive pulmonary therapy
- Ventilation with PEEP if necessary to maintain $PO_2$
- Bronchodilators: inhaled β-adrenergic agents for wheezing
- Pulmonary toilet, chest physical therapy, suctioning as needed
- Bronchoscopy for gross aspiration of particulate matter
- Prophylactic antibiotics and/or steroids are *not* generally indicated

Correct fluid and electrolyte abnormalities
Insert Foley catheter, if indicated
Consider early transfer for intensive cerebral resuscitation
Admit and observe all patients with a significant history of submersion and aspiration

be tried, adjusting the $FIO_2$ to maintain an adequate $Po_2$. An awake, cooperative patient with borderline blood gases may be given CPAP with a tight-fitting mask in an attempt to avoid intubation. A nasogastric tube should be placed, as a large amount of water and air is often swallowed that can further compromise respiration and provide potential for vomiting and aspiration. Blood should be obtained for CBC, electrolytes, BUN, creatinine, calcium, magnesium, PT, PTT, platelets, and urinalysis for hemoglobin. A chest x-ray should be obtained, recognizing that in 25% of patients with significant pulmonary problems the initial chest x-ray is normal. The majority of patients have radiographic evidence of perihilar or generalized pulmonary edema early on, with later evolution to focal areas of atelectasis or infiltrates (Fig. 4C-1).

Once the airway and adequate ventilation are assured, adjunctive therapy should be instituted to further improve gas exchange. This includes standard doses of inhaled β-adrenergic agents for treatment of bronchospasm. Chest physical therapy and suctioning may need to be frequently performed, and early therapeutic bronchoscopy should be considered when the aspiration of particulate matter such as vomitus or mud is suspected. There is general agreement that neither prophylactic antibiotics nor prophylactic steroids are beneficial in treating pulmonary complications of near-drowning.

***Intensive resuscitation.*** The prognosis for meaningful recovery after near-drowning has improved in recent years

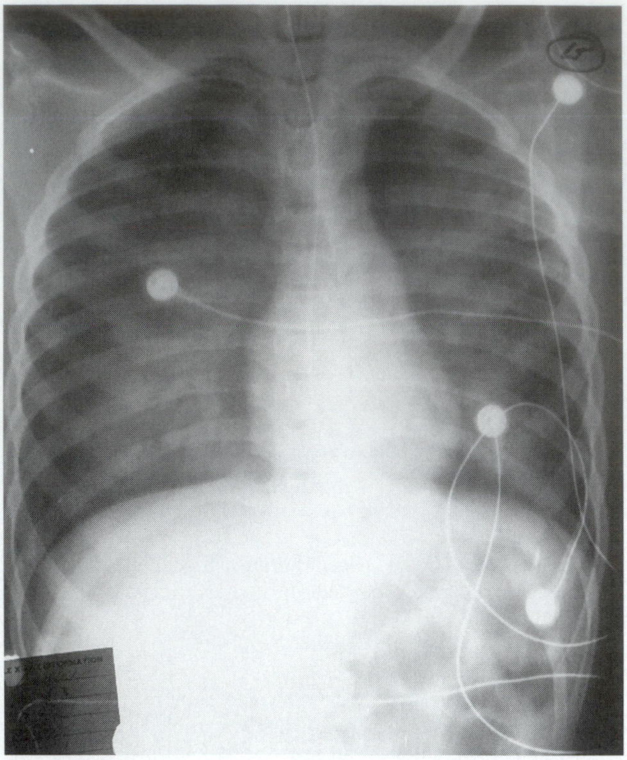

**Fig. 4C-1.** Generalized pulmonary edema in an 8-year-old boy several hours after resuscitation from drowning.

because of the increasing availability of centers equipped for intensive cerebral resuscitative measures, including intracranial pressure monitoring and fluid and pharmacologic intervention tailored to maximize intracranial perfusion pressure.

Because it often takes hours for the pulmonary complications of fluid aspiration to develop, patients with a history of a significant episode of submersion and aspiration should be under medical observation for at least 24 hours.

## SMOKE INHALATION

Pulmonary complications of smoke inhalation usually are associated with body burns but may occur in isolation. It is estimated that half the deaths resulting from fire are attributable to smoke inhalation.

### Pathophysiologic mechanisms

Six mechanisms of respiratory compromise may be seen in victims of fire. (1) Death by asphyxiation is the result of breathing smoke, a gas with a variably reduced concentration of oxygen and increased concentrations of carbon dioxide and carbon monoxide. (2) Upper airway obstruction may develop within hours of exposure, as heat and noxious particulate matter and gases incite pharyngeal and laryngeal edema. (3) Circumferential thoracic burns can produce severe ventilatory restriction, which must be relieved by escharotomies. (4) Carbon monoxide poisoning is frequently associated with smoke inhalation and contributes to morbidity. (5) Inhalation injury, which in its narrower sense refers to chemical tracheobronchitis and/or injury to small airways and alveoli as a result of smoke exposure, may lead to progressive respiratory compromise. (6) This serves as a substrate for late pulmonary infection, often the cause of death in burn victims.

Three components of smoke, which account for different aspects of the pulmonary pathophysiology, are present to a varying degree in different fires. (1) Heat and steam cause direct thermal injury usually confined to the supraglottic region and produce pharyngeal and laryngeal edema, erythema, and blistering. (2) Particles consisting of carbonaceous material coated with organic acids and aldehydes are damaging to the tracheobronchial mucosa. (3) Among the products of combustion and pyrolysis are gases such as chlorine, phosgene, nitrogen dioxide, sulfur dioxide, ammonia, and hydrochloric acid; they cause a marked inflammatory response in the lung. Pulmonary capillary permeability is increased, with leakage of protein-rich fluid into the alveoli and loss of lung surfactant, resulting in pulmonary edema, focal atelectasis, and intrapulmonary shunting.

### Clinical assessment

***History.*** Certain factors in the history suggest that a victim is at high risk for having sustained a significant inhalation injury. Patients exposed to smoke in a closed space, patients with impaired ability to protect themselves (infants, the elderly, the infirm, drug- or alcohol-intoxicated individuals, and those with head injuries or loss of consciousness), and patients with previous lung disease are all at high risk. Certain types of smoke and fumes are especially noxious, particularly those liberated by the burning or thermal degradation of polyvinylchloride (PVC), a substance present in plastics, telephone and electric cables, and much upholstery.

The patient may complain of a sore throat or substernal burning (a prominent symptom in fires involving PVC). Hoarseness or stridor indicates upper airway edema and potential obstruction. Face and neck burns and singed nasal hairs or mustache are frequently associated with an inhalation injury. Positive findings on physical examination include tachypnea and tachycardia; low $O_2$ saturation by pulse oximetry; erythema, edema, and blistering of the oropharynx; and wheezing, rales, and cough productive of carbonaceous sputum. It is important to remember that some patients with normal findings on initial examination may develop significant inhalation injuries (see the box at right).

***Diagnostic tests.*** Certain laboratory and diagnostic tests help in evaluating the presence, extent, and anatomic level of an inhalation injury. Pulse oximetry and early blood gas measurements on breathing of room air can be falsely reassuring, showing mild to moderate hypoxemia or even a normal $PO_2$. The $PCO_2$ is usually low but may be normal or high. The calculation of an alveolar-arterial oxygen gradient on room air

$$P_{AO_2} - Pa_{O_2} = A - a \text{ gradient}$$

$$\text{where } P_{AO_2} = 150 - 1.25 \times Pa_{CO_2}$$

$$\text{and } Pa_{O_2} \text{ is that measured}$$

reflects intrapulmonary shunting and increases the sensitivity of room-air arterial blood gas measurements. A normal gradient is about 8 torr; a gradient of over 28 torr has been found to be well-correlated with inhalation injury documented by other means. The initial carboxyhemoglobin level is probably a better indicator of the severity of exposure than initial room-air gas measurements. The measurement of the A-a gradient on an $FIO_2$ of 100% increases the sensitivity of blood gases even further. A $PAO_2$ less than 250 torr on 100% oxygen or an A-a gradient increasing over time is highly predictive of significant pulmonary injury, as is falling $O_2$ saturation by pulse oximetry.

The initial chest x-ray is usually normal, but within 24 to 48 hours pulmonary edema and focal atelectasis or infiltrates may be seen (see the box at right). Three additional diagnostic modalities have been used to further evaluate the presence and extent of pulmonary injury. Fiberoptic bronchoscopy, which can be performed transnasally at the bedside under local anesthesia, is helpful in assessing both upper and lower airway injury. Positive findings include mucosal erythema, edema, ulceration, and hemorrhage; carbonaceous sputum; and bronchorrhea.

Xenon 133 ventilation lung scanning has been advocated for assessing injury to small airways and alveoli, and when positive shows a delay in clearance and/or an inequality of clearance of the isotope from the lungs. A scan done within the first hour or two of exposure may prove a false negative, as it often takes several hours for the pulmonary reaction to develop. False positives are seen in patients with preexisting obstructive lung disease.

The most useful pulmonary function test in assessing pulmonary injury is analysis of the maximum expiratory flow volume (MEFV) curve. An expiratory flow rate at 50% of vital capacity, which is less than 50% of predicted, has a high correlation with other evidence of pulmonary injury. MEFV curve analysis can also be used to follow response to therapy. Conventional spirometric measurements may be abnormal but are less specific.

### Therapy

Treatment begins with immediate attention to the upper airway. Experts differ on the timing of intubation of patients whose airways are initially patent but who have signs of upper airway injury and are at risk for developing later obstruction. Some favor early prophylactic intubation; others favor waiting until signs of early obstruction develop. Watchful waiting should only be employed in settings where experienced personnel are continuously available to manage difficult intubations. Definite indications for intubation are upper airway obstruction, impaired consciousness with inability to protect the airway, elevated $PCO_2$, and hypoxia despite supplemental oxygen by mask. Nasotracheal intubation is the preferred method; tracheostomy should be avoided, especially in patients with coexisting body burns. If a patient is to be transferred for definitive care and has evidence of upper airway injury, it is imperative to intubate before transportation (after consultation with the receiving facility). All patients, intubated or not, should initially be put on as high a concentration of humidified oxygen as possible to treat potential carbon monoxide poisoning. Ventilated patients should be maintained on PEEP or CPAP to prevent terminal airway closure. Patients should be encouraged to cough and breathe deeply by using incentive spirometry; suctioning is to be avoided unless absolutely necessary, as it adds to the potential for infection. Therapeutic bronchoscopy may be helpful to patients with copious bronchorrhea and carbonaceous sputum. Inhaled β-adrenergic agents are useful in treating associated bronchospasm. The current consensus is that neither prophylactic antibiotics nor prophylactic steroids are indicated in the management of inhalation injuries; steroids may actually increase mor-

### Protocol for management of victims of smoke inhalation

**All cases**

Take a history focusing on risk factors, length of exposure, and symptoms. Perform physical examination that includes vital signs, body burns, nasal and oropharyngeal examinations, and chest examination. Categorize the case as one of the following:

**Trivial exposure:**

Very low-risk history, no symptoms or signs of inhalation, normal vital signs. Short emergency room observation and discharge

**Probable mild exposure:**

Some risk by history, minimal if any symptoms, normal physical examination

(1) Measure room-air ABGs and carboxyhemoglobin levels
(2) Give humidified 100% $O_2$ via facemask
(3) Obtain ECG
(4) Obtain chest x-ray
(5) Observe for 4 hours from time of exposure. If no signs or symptoms develop, and ABGs and CO levels are satisfactory, discharge with warning about possible late complications
(6) If patient develops signs or symptoms, designate as moderate exposure

**Moderate exposure:**

Moderate-risk history, symptoms, and/or signs such as singed nasal hairs, carbonaceous sputum, cough

(1) Follow first three steps for "Probable mild exposure"
(2) Obtain chest x-ray
(3) Admit and observe
(4) Perform pulmonary toilet; encourage coughing but avoid suctioning
(5) Treat bronchospasm, if it occurs
(6) Consider further diagnostic workup to assess extent of injury: A-a gradient, fiberoptic bronchoscopy, Xenon 133 scanning

**Severe exposure:**

High-risk history, multiplicity of signs and symptoms of upper and/or lower airway injury

(1) Decide about early intubation
(2) Measure ABGs, CO level; give/obtain 100% humidified $O_2$; ECG, chest x-ray
(3) Volume ventilator with PEEP
(4) Bronchodilators as needed
(5) Consider further diagnostic and therapeutic modalities outlined in text

Modified from Wilkins EW, editor: *MGH Textbook of Emergency Medicine*, ed 2, Baltimore, 1983, Williams & Wilkins.

bidity and mortality. Adjunctive measures include the placement of a nasogastric tube, the prophylactic use of $H_2$-blockers to protect against gastric ulceration, and avoidance of fluid overload.

The decision regarding admission and length of observation can be difficult; some general guidelines are presented in the box on p. 69, but each case needs to be individualized.

## CARBON MONOXIDE POISONING

Acute carbon monoxide poisoning accounts for about 3500 deaths annually in the United States and contributes to morbidity and mortality in countless cases of burns and smoke inhalation.

### Pathophysiologic mechanisms

Because carbon monoxide (CO) is a colorless, odorless, nonirritating gas it has been called a "silent killer." It is produced by the incomplete combustion of organic materials and is present in most fires, motor vehicle exhaust, and many factories. With an affinity for hemoglobin about 240 times higher than that of oxygen, CO rapidly binds to hemoglobin, forming carboxyhemoglobin (COHb). As COHb levels rise, oxyhemoglobin ($O_2$Hb) falls proportionately, thus impairing oxygen transport. In addition COHb shifts the $O_2$Hb dissociation curve to the left, so that the oxygen bound to hemoglobin is less rapidly released to the tissues. At the cellular level the use of oxygen is impaired, as CO binds to the iron-containing molecules of the cytochrome system. Organs with the most active cellular metabolism, such as heart and brain, are the most susceptible to injury.

### Clinical manifestations

The symptoms of CO poisoning are those of hypoxia, which are nonspecific. At low levels of COHb the only symptoms may be dyspnea on exertion or a tightness across the head. With COHb levels between 20% and 30%, patients complain increasingly of headache, nausea, fatigue, dyspnea, dizziness, or dimmed vision. As COHb levels rise, these symptoms become more pronounced, and patients may exhibit vomiting, confusion, or syncope. Finally there is loss of consciousness, seizures, and respiratory arrest (Table 4C-1). Patients with coronary artery disease may present with angina or arrhythmias even at low COHb levels.

The COHb level measured in the emergency department can be considerably lower than the patient's peak COHb level if sufficient time has elapsed since exposure, or if oxygen has been administered at the scene or during transport. As it is the peak level that carries prognostic significance, some attempt should be made to estimate it, if possible.

On physical examination the patient usually is tachycardic and may be tachypneic. The classic "cherry red" hue of the patient's lips and skin is not a reliable sign; more often the patient appears pale. Because of the nonspecific and protean manifestations of CO poisoning, the physician must be careful to avoid missing the diagnosis. Some unusual presentations include multiple family members with what appears to be the simultaneous onset of food poisoning or gastroenteritis, patients appearing intoxicated, and firefighters with angina. CO poisoning should always be assumed to be present in victims of smoke inhalation and patients with major body burns. Treatment should begin presumptively with a high concentration of oxygen, while the results of blood gas and COHb-level measurements are awaited. Blood gases usually show a normal $PO_2$, a low $PCO_2$, and a lower pH than would be predicted by the $PCO_2$; that is, a combined respiratory alkalosis and metabolic acidosis. In most hospital laboratories the $O_2$Hb saturation reported with the blood gas is calculated from the $PO_2$ and thus is grossly inaccurate in the presence of an elevated COHb level. An electrocardiogram should be obtained and may show ischemic changes or ventricular arrhythmias, even when the patient has no cardiac symptoms.

**Table 4C-1.** Symptoms of carbon monoxide poisoning

| COHb level | Symptoms* |
|---|---|
| ≤10% | Usually none; dyspnea on extreme exertion |
| 10%-20% | Bandlike or throbbing headache, dyspnea on moderate exertion |
| 20%-30% | More severe headache; throbbing temples, dyspnea on mild exertion, nausea |
| 30%-40% | All of above plus visual dimming, dizziness, irritability, vomiting, tachycardia |
| 40%-50% | All of above plus tachypnea, dyspnea at rest, syncope |
| >50% | Coma, seizures, cardiorespiratory depression, death |

*Patients with coronary artery disease may have angina at any level.

**Table 4C-2.** Half-life of carboxyhemoglobin by treatment with room air, oxygen, and hyperbaric oxygen

| $F_IO_2$ | $PO_2$ (torr) | t½ of COHb | $O_2$ dissolved (vol. per ml) |
|---|---|---|---|
| 21% (room air) | 160 | 5-6 h | 0.3 |
| 100% at 1 ATA (sea level) | 760 | 80 min | 2.09 |
| 100% at 3 ATA (hyperbaric chamber) | 2280 | 25 min | 6.9 |

### Treatment

Oxygen is the mainstay of treatment. The two major decisions are which patients to intubate and when to employ hyperbaric oxygen therapy. Hyperbaric oxygen has two major beneficial effects. First, it greatly speeds the rate of CO elimination, reducing the t½ for COHb from 5 to 6 hours on room air to a t½ of about 25 minutes on 100% oxygen at 3 atmospheres (3 ATA) (Table 4C-2). Second, breathing of 100% oxygen at 2.5 to 3 ATA results in a dissolved oxygen content in plasma of 5.6 to 6.9 vol/dl, which is approximately the amount of $O_2$, extracted by the body under normal conditions (the normal A-V $O_2$ content difference is 5 to 6 vol/dl). Patients with COHb levels over 15% to 20% should be treated with hyperbaric oxygen. Clinical parameters such as neuropsychiatric and cardiac symptoms are more important indicators of the need for hyperbaric oxygen treatment than any absolute level. Patients who are comatose, uncooperative, or hypoventilating or who have a COHb level over 40% require intubation and ventilation on 100% oxygen and expeditious transfer to a chamber for hyperbaric oxygen therapy. The actual administration of hyperbaric oxygen should be done only by experienced personnel and is beyond the scope of this chapter. Regardless of the method of oxygen administration, treatment should be continued until COHb levels are less than 10%, and clinical symptoms have resolved.

In addition to provision of oxygen, an attempt should be made to reduce oxygen demand by keeping the patient at rest. Cardiac monitoring should be done. Further experimental measures advocated to reduce oxygen demand and decrease cerebral edema in severe cases include controlled hypothermia, steroids, and fluid restriction.

Complications of CO poisoning include late neurologic sequelae and, rarely, rhabdomyolysis, with or without myoglobinuric renal failure, as a result of either pressure myonecrosis or generalized muscle hypoxia.

## BIBLIOGRAPHY

Agree RN et al: Use of Xenon 133 in early diagnosis of inhalation injury, *J Trauma* 16:217, 1976.

Bartlett RH et al: Consensus report on smoke inhalation, *J Trauma* 19:913, 1979.

Dyer RF et al: Polyvinyl chloride toxicity in fires, *JAMA* 235:393, 1976.

Hunt JL et al: Fiberoptic bronchoscopy in acute inhalation injury, *J Trauma* 15:641, 1975.

Luce EA et al: Alveolar-arterial oxygen gradient in the burn patient, *J Trauma* 16:212, 1976.

Moylan JA: Inhalation injury, an increasing problem, *Ann Surg* 188:34, 1978.

Petroff PA et al: Pulmonary function studies after smoke inhalation, *Am J Surg* 132:346, 1976.

Pruitt BA et al: Progressive pulmonary insufficiency and other pulmonary complications of thermal injury, *J Trauma* 15:369, 1975.

Tomaszewski CA et al: Use of hyperbaric oxygen in toxicology, *Emerg Med Clin North Am* 12(2):437, 1994.

Zawacki BE: Smoke, burns, and the natural history of inhalation injury in fire victims, *Ann Surg* 185:100, 1977.

CHAPTER

# 4D Burns and Nuclear

**Erwin F. Hirsch**

Thermal injuries commonly occur around the home, at work, or in vehicular accidents. Although most medical attention and resources are directed toward the severely injured, countless patients are seen in physicians' offices and emergency rooms with thermal-burn injuries not requiring hospitalization. These injuries may not be life-threatening, but they may produce functional or cosmetic defects if not cared for properly. This chapter describes the evaluation and management of a subgroup of burn patients who can be treated in the primary care setting by physicians who, during their training or professional life, have been exposed to thermal injuries.

## CASUALTY EVALUATION

A burn patient should receive the same care at the scene of the fire as in any other accident. Burning clothes should be removed immediately and the victim taken from the area. Inhalation injuries and carbon monoxide intoxication are common results of fires in closed environments. These injuries often may be present in the absence of cutaneous thermal lesions and should be recognized and treated (see Chapter 4C). If the patient has sustained an inhalation injury, care should be directed by a physician with expertise in acute pulmonary diseases (Fig. 4D-1).

## BURN WOUND EVALUATION

The extent and depth of a burn injury must be determined quickly and an optimal plan made for its management. The extent of the wound is usually overestimated and the depth underestimated. Tables 4D-1 and 4D-2 show the methods

**Table 4D-1.** Rule of nines

| Area | %* |
|---|---|
| Head and neck | 9 |
| Right upper extremity | 9 |
| Left upper extremity | 9 |
| Anterior chest and abdomen | 18 |
| Posterior chest and abdomen | 18 |
| Genitals | 1 |
| Right lower extremity | 18 |
| Left lower extremity | 18 |
| Total | 100 |

*The percentages are added to determine the extent of burn injury in the patient.

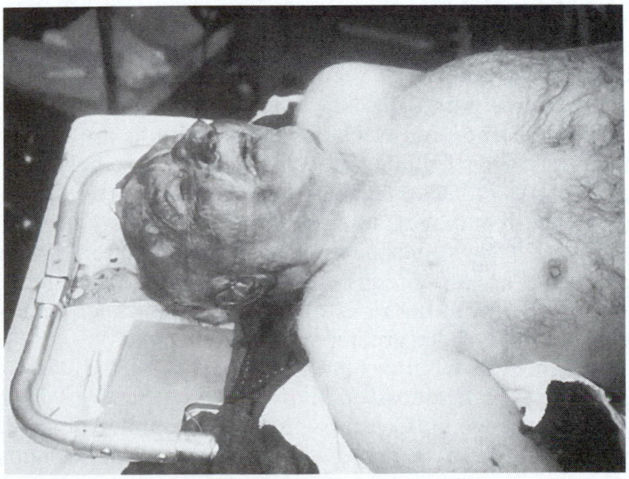

**Fig. 4D-1.** Smoke inhalation and second-degree burn to face.

**Table 4D-2.** Lund-Browder chart for burn estimate (percentage of body surface area)

| Area | Age (yr) 0-1 | 1-4 | 5-9 | 10-15 | Adult |
|---|---|---|---|---|---|
| Head | 19 | 17 | 13 | 10 | 7 |
| Neck | 2 | 2 | 2 | 2 | 2 |
| Anterior trunk | 13 | 17 | 13 | 13 | 13 |
| Posterior trunk | 13 | 13 | 13 | 13 | 13 |
| Right buttock | 2½ | 2½ | 2½ | 2½ | 2½ |
| Left buttock | 2½ | 2½ | 2½ | 2½ | 2½ |
| Genitalia | 1 | 1 | 1 | 1 | 1 |
| Right upper arm | 4 | 4 | 4 | 4 | 4 |
| Left upper arm | 4 | 4 | 4 | 4 | 4 |
| Right lower arm | 3 | 3 | 3 | 3 | 3 |
| Left lower arm | 3 | 3 | 3 | 3 | 3 |
| Right hand | 2½ | 2½ | 2½ | 2½ | 2½ |
| Left hand | 2½ | 2½ | 2½ | 2½ | 2½ |
| Right thigh | 5½ | 6½ | 8½ | 8½ | 9½ |
| Left thigh | 5½ | 6½ | 8½ | 8½ | 9½ |
| Right leg | 5 | 5 | 5½ | 6 | 7 |
| Left leg | 5 | 5 | 5½ | 6 | 7 |
| Right foot | 3½ | 3½ | 3½ | 3½ | 3½ |
| Left foot | 3½ | 3½ | 3½ | 3½ | 3½ |

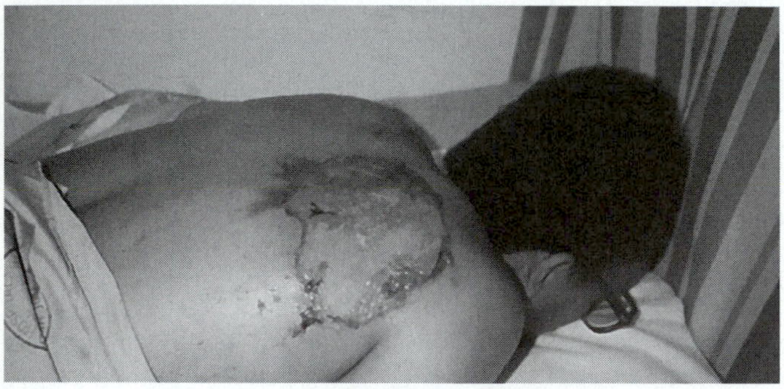

**Fig. 4D-2.** Second-degree burn from water.

by which the extent of the burn wound can be determined in adults and children. The mechanism of injury is important in evaluating the burn, since different modalities can produce injuries of greater or lesser depth.

Superficial partial-thickness burns heal spontaneously if they don't become infected. These wounds are usually moist, have hair follicles present, and are extremely painful (Fig. 4D-2). Deep partial-thickness burns are less sensitive. The skin may be less erythematous, but not leathery in texture. The wounds heal without surgical intervention; however, the healing requires a much longer time period (3 to 5 weeks). Both the risks of infection and functional or cosmetic deficits are greater with these wounds.

Full-thickness burns involve all layers of the dermis, epidermis, and, occasionally, deeper structures (Fig. 4D-3). These wounds are brownish-yellow and leathery. In most cases, pain is not associated with these wounds. Patients with or suspected of having full-thickness wounds should be referred to an experienced surgeon.

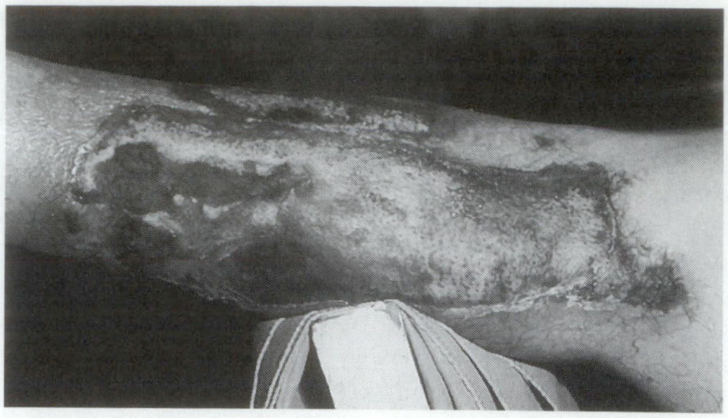

**Fig. 4D-3.** Third-degree burn.

During burn wound evaluation, the primary care physician must keep in mind the likelihood of local edema occurring, and must evaluate the circulatory status of the involved area. Objects, garments, and dressings that may compromise the adequacy of the circulation should be removed.

## CRITERIA FOR PRIMARY CARE MANAGEMENT

Patients suffering superficial partial-thickness burns without significant comorbid factors can be cared for by primary care providers. The management of patients with deep partial-thickness burns of anatomic areas not at risk for functional or cosmetic deficits can also be undertaken by primary care providers, if burn areas are small in size. All patients with deep partial-thickness burns, full-thickness burns, or injuries involving the face, neck, shoulders, elbows, hands, perineum, popliteal fossa, ankles, or feet require a surgical specialist with knowledge and interest in such problems.

## MANAGEMENT OF THE BURN WOUND BY PRIMARY CARE PROVIDER

The final goal of burn wound management is restoration of functional and normal cosmetic appearance. Burn wound management needs to be addressed after the patient's evaluation is completed. During this time the involved area needs to be cooled with either cold water or ice. The cooling of the wound has an anesthetic effect and limits the amount of tissue damage produced by the heat exposure. Gentle debridement and cleansing of the wound should be carried out using a mild detergent. Pain should be controlled with oral analgesics during and after the procedure. Intravenous pain medication should be used only for major injuries outside the scope of primary care. Intramuscular or subcutaneous pain control in burn patients is not indicated.

Blisters should be opened and devitalized skin excised. Following debridement and cleansing, the wound should be covered with a bacteriostatic ointment to prevent infection. The most commonly used ointments are sulfadiazine (Silvadine) or povidone-iodine (Betadine). A bulky, soft dressing should be applied ensuring that space is available to accept the edema that follows burn wounds. The patient should be seen 72 hours after the injury for a wound check, and every 5 to 7 days thereafter, until the wound is healed. Dressing changes should be carried out at least twice a day by the patient, a relative, a companion, or a visiting nurse.

The patient's tetanus prophylaxis should be reviewed and updated if necessary. Systematic antibiotics are not indicated. Referral to a physical therapy department for evaluation and therapy depends on the size and location of the wound. Such referral should be carried out early in the postburn period.

## PROBLEMS AND COMPLICATIONS

Excessive swelling may occur during the early management of the burn wound. It is imperative that the circulation be assessed in these cases. If there is no threat present, elevation of the involved area is sufficient. In questionable cases a surgical consultation is mandatory to evaluate the wound and the possibility of a compartment syndrome. Wounds that initially appear superficial may convert to full thickness over time. In these instances immediate surgical consultation is advisable.

Superficial infection of these wounds is not uncommon, particularly if the patient avoids medical attention for a few days after the injury. In such cases a wound culture and sensitivity should be obtained. In the absence of systemic signs of sepsis (i.e., fever, leukocytosis, or extensive erythema), the local wound should be managed aggressively. The patient should be placed on appropriate systemic antibiotics as indicated by the culture and antibiotic sensitivity reports.

The presence of swelling and erythema requires elevation and warm, moist dressings. Functional disability should be prevented with an active program in physical therapy. If the program proves unsuccessful, early consultation with a reconstructive surgical specialist is necessary. Significant itching is common during the healing process; application of a moisturizing cream in the involved area usually handles the problem.

## MANAGEMENT OF CHEMICAL BURNS

Immediate and aggressive action must be taken with chemical burns to prevent extension of the injury. The magnitude of a chemical burn is related to the concentration of the caustic substance and contact time. Therefore removal of all clothing and copious irrigation with water to the involved areas and in particular to the eyes is urgent and mandatory. Abundant irrigation with water is acceptable and in most instances sufficient. For a more specific irrigant, however, the nearest poison center should be called once the patient arrives in the emergency room.

## MANAGEMENT OF ELECTRICAL INJURIES

High tension electrical injuries occur most often during industrial accidents or sporting events, or when unsupervised children trespass into restricted areas. These injuries continue to occur despite training and safety programs.

Electrical burns have pathophysiologic characteristics different from those of thermal or chemical burns. The damage that high voltage electric current produces in the body is dependent on six factors: (1) resistance, (2) type of current, (3) amperage, (4) voltage, (5) duration, and (6) pathway. Dry skin offers a significant impediment to the flow of electric current, whereas moisture or blistering decreases resistance significantly. The relative internal resistance of tissue is least in nerves, blood, and muscle and greater in skin, fat, and bone. Electricity tends to travel along the paths of least resistance. The neurovascular bundles and the muscles therefore are the tissues that in most instances sustain the greatest damage.

Cardiorespiratory arrest is common in patients with high voltage electrical injuries. Cardiopulmonary resuscitation and advanced cardiac life support should be instituted immediately after extrication of a victim and continued until the victim is resuscitated. Electrocardiographic and enzymatic changes (elevation of $CPK_2$) are often observed in these patients even in the absence of an acute cardiac emergency.

The current of injury is most intense at the port of entry and exit and produces characteristic lesions. Entrance wounds are usually charred and depressed, whereas exit wounds may have the appearance of a blast injury. Significant injuries may be present in other anatomic areas. After cardiopulmonary and hemodynamic resuscitation, early decompressive fasciotomies and debridement may be needed to assess the extent of the tissue damage. The incidence of major amputation in these injuries is 33%. Muscle destruction may be responsible for significant myoglobulinuria, in which case the judicious use of an osmotic diuretic to promote diuresis is indicated.

All severe high voltage electrical injuries should be transferred to specialized centers for wound management as soon as the patient has been medically stabilized.

## NUCLEAR RADIATION

As radioactive materials are used with ever greater frequency, accidental contamination from a transportation accident, an industrial accident, or accidental exposure in a radiation therapy facility has become a distinct possibility. This section describes the principles of management that can be used by primary care physicians and other medical professionals in case of emergency radioactive contamination.

According to data from the U.S. Radiation Accident Registry and from foreign countries, most radiation accidents have caused isolated instances of focal radiation burns, commonly on the hand. Some 46 such mishaps, involving 76 individuals, were reported worldwide from 1948 to 1980. During this period a total of 93 radiation accidents were registered in the United States, affecting more than 500 people, including the 390 who were exposed to fallout at the Marshall Islands in 1954. Only 16 fatalities from radiation injury have been reported to the U.S. Radiation Accident Registry. One area in which increased radiation accidents are being observed is the pipeline construction industry where accidents are resulting in part from poor safety checks and personal negligence. The integrity of welded seams in the construction of pipelines is determined with cesium. The shiny, small devices containing the cesium have occasionally been left unattended or carried with no shield, causing severe radiation injuries.

During the meltdown in the nuclear power station at Chernobyl, Ukraine, on April 26, 1986, many people were seriously exposed to irradiation and required medical care from area physicians and health care professionals.

**Table 4D-3.** Relationship of dose of ionizing radiation to symptoms of acute radiation syndrome

| Syndrome | Dose (in rad) | Symptoms and signs | Prognosis |
|---|---|---|---|
| No acute disease | <200 | Nausea and vomiting | Excellent |
| Acute radiation syndrome | | | |
| Hematopoietic effects | 200-1000 | Prodromal phase of anorexia, nausea, vomiting, pancytopenia, and bone marrow suppression | Good to poor |
| Gastrointestinal effects | 1000-5000 | Intractable nausea, vomiting, diarrhea, bowel necrosis, and bone marrow suppression | Hopeless |
| Neurovascular effects | ≥5000 | Prodromal phase of nausea, vomiting and listlessness, tremors, convulsions, ataxia | Hopeless |

### Managed Care Guide
### Radiation Emergency Assistance Center, Oakridge, TN

The Radiation Emergency Assistance Center/Training Site (REAC/TS) provides worldwide assistance and information 24 hours a day. Call REAC/TS at Oakridge Hospital, Oakridge, TN (615-481-1000).

Most recently a large number of victims, including four fatalities, were exposed internally and externally to Cesium 137 after the dismantling of a radiotherapy unit in Goiania, Brazil, and to Cobalt 60 (2 fatalities) in two accidents involving sterilizing plants. The symptoms of acute radiation sickness and a protocol for decontamination are described in this chapter.

## Acute radiation syndrome

The acute radiation syndrome comprises the physiologic changes that occur after a substantial dose of ionizing radiation. Four systems are affected: the hematopoietic, gastrointestinal, cardiovascular, and nervous (Table 4D-3). Significant hematopoietic changes occur with doses of 200 rad or more. Gastrointestinal changes occur with doses closer to 1000 rad, while cardiovascular and central nervous system changes rarely occur unless exposure is in excess of 5000 rad. Patients exposed to significant, but not immediately lethal, doses of radiation progress through four clinical periods: an initial toxic period, a latent period, a period of manifest disease, and finally a period of late or delayed effects.

***Initial toxic period.*** The initial toxic period is characterized by prodromal symptoms such as nausea, vomiting, diarrhea, headaches, malaise, and, at times, erythema with itching. The time interval from accident to appearance of these symptoms and the duration of this period give an indication of the dose that was absorbed. Doses of less than 50 rad rarely produce prodromal symptoms: doses greater than 400 rad almost always do. The appearance of these symptoms in less than 2 hours usually indicates a dose of greater than 200 rad. If the height of the symptoms occurs in 6 to 8 hours and disappears within 48 hours, the dose absorbed is probably less than 400 rad. A toxic period lasting more than 72 hours is usually indicative of more than 400 rad, and if the patient is exposed to more than 600 rad, the toxic period usually merges with the following period of manifest disease.

***Latent period.*** There are no symptoms during the latent period. If the initial injury is less than 400 rad, this time period will last between 2 and 3 weeks. If the dose was 600 rad or greater, the symptom-free interval or latent period is usually less than a week.

***Period of manifest disease.*** The radiosensitivity of human cells is related to their mitotic activity and metabolic rates; therefore, depending on the dose, dose rate, and quality of radiation (proton, electron, neutron) to which a system is exposed, certain changes may be expected in certain organs. Some of these changes may be transient and others may result in late permanent changes or death. Cellular changes require a certain amount of time to become clinically apparent. Loss of hair rarely occurs with doses of less than 350 rad. Permanent hair loss will result from a dose exceeding 700 rad. Skin changes typical of first-degree burns are seen with doses of 100 rad or less. Partial-thickness burn type lesions usually result when the doses exceed 300 rad. During this period the effects of radiation on the bone marrow, lymph nodes, and spleen also become apparent. Red cell precursors are the most sensitive, followed by white cells and, finally, platelets, resulting in pancytopenia.

***Hematopoietic changes.*** Figs. 4D-4 and 4D-5 show hypothetical blood counts according to radiation dose. Symptoms are related to increasing degrees of pancytopenia and include malaise, fever, headaches, susceptibility to infection, pneumonia, skin ulceration, diarrhea, bleeding, and hemorrhage. Chronic anemia occurs later, when red cells formed before radiation exposure have died and are not replaced.

Treatment of the hematopoietic syndrome is symptomatic initially. If the granulocyte count drops below 1000 cells per cubic millimeter, the patient should be given trimethoprimsulfamethoxazole (Bactrim, Septra), two tablets twice daily, plus 1 million U nystatin every 4 hours.

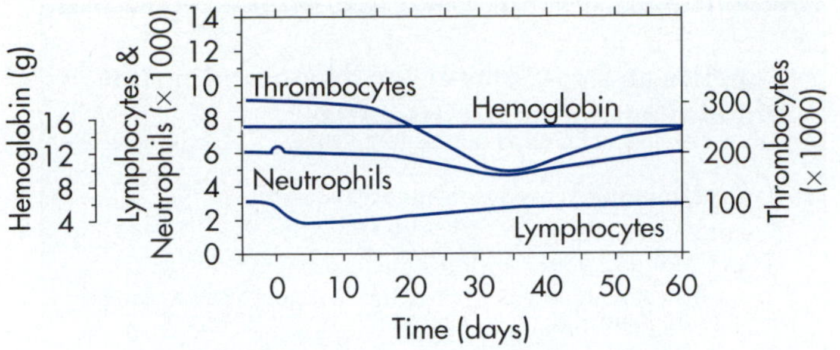


**Fig. 4D-4.** Hematologic response to 100 rad whole-body exposure. (Courtesy the Armed Forces Radiobiology Research Institute.)

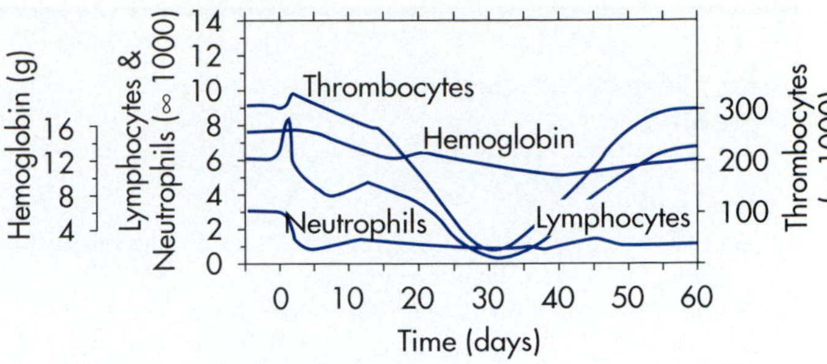


**Fig. 4D-5.** Hematologic response to 300 rad whole-body exposure. (Courtesy the Armed Forces Radiobiology Research Institute.)

This therapy reduces the chance of fever and bacteremia. Reverse isolation or a "life-island" system such as that used for immunosuppressed patients also helps lessen the opportunity for infection. The prognosis varies from good to poor, since the median lethal dose ($LD_{50}$) of radiation for humans is 650 rad. Exposure to doses in the range of 650 to 1000 rad usually result in death from the complications of bone marrow suppression.

*Gastrointestinal changes.* Gastrointestinal symptoms are primarily associated with changes in the small bowel. The epithelium of the small intestine is almost as radiosensitive as the bone marrow, whereas the stomach and colon are less sensitive. Clinical symptoms do not usually occur unless exposure is greater than 500 rad. The pathologic findings are characterized by markedly decreased cell production in the mucosal crypts, which leads to the destruction of mucosal cells and villi. Vomiting, diarrhea, malabsorption, and bacterial contamination result. Symptoms appear in two stages. Watery and often bloody diarrhea occurs during the initial toxic period and lasts for approximately 2 weeks. The diarrhea is followed by absence of peristalsis and a resulting paralytic ileus. Dehydration and electrolyte imbalance occur and often result in hemodynamic instability and renal failure. In severe cases, particularly if complicated by pancytopenia, the patient dies in 1 or 2 weeks. If the patient is treated with fluids and electrolytes and the radiation dose was less than 1300 rad, the small bowel reconstitutes its mucosa in approximately 6 days.

*Cardiovascular and central nervous system changes.* With doses greater than 1300 rad mucosal regeneration is poor or nonexistent. With doses in excess of 2000 to 3000 rad there is cardiovascular and central nervous system involvement and death within days.

## Patient decontamination

Radiation casualties should be treated at medical facilities without fear of serious risk to the facility or staff. Guidelines delineating appropriate procedures for treating a patient who has received ionizing radiation should be followed carefully and should cover the following:

(1) Begin appropriate life support procedures.
(2) Do not panic.
(3) If possible, excuse personnel who are pregnant or of childbearing potential.

**Table 4D-4.** Lymphocyte count in response to radiation exposure

| Lymphocyte count per mm³ at 48 h | Degree of radiation exposure |
|---|---|
| 1500 or more | Mild |
| 1000-1500 | Moderate |
| 500-1000 | Severe |
| 100-500 | Very severe |
| 0-100 | Lethal |

(4) Promptly remove patient's outer clothing (most of the contamination is removed upon removal of clothing). Removal should be carried out expeditiously, and all clothing should be appropriately bagged and tagged.
(5) Perform all procedures in as small an area as possible to facilitate housekeeping chores.
(6) Use standard sterile techniques. They are sufficient to meet all decontamination standards.
(7) Obtain blood samples, primarily for lymphocyte count (Table 4D-4).
(8) Establish patient and staff flow according to guidelines by controlling access to, egress from, and movement of patients. If monitoring equipment is not readily available, restrict exit from the patient area. All personnel should strip off all clothing and shower prior to exit.
(9) After removal of all clothing and physiologic stabilization of the patient has occurred, decontamination to remove radioactive material requires vigorous washing with progressively stronger detergents or, rarely, debridement. Decontamination should continue until safe levels of radiation are determined (see the box on p. 76). The supplies and equipment for decontamination of radiological accident casualties are summarized in the box at right.

## Evaluation of the radiated patient

The initial evaluation of a patient exposed, or possibly exposed, to ionizing radiation should include the following:

### Procedures for specific decontamination problems

**Total body**

Take shower or sponge bath using Betadine (or equivalent), household bleach, laundry detergent
Avoid contaminating any body openings

**Skin**

Cover adjacent areas with plastic taped down at edges
Apply agents listed in the box at right
If not effective, cover with a clean dressing and evaluate necessity of using more stringent techniques. Normal epithelial sluffing transfers contamination to dressing and increases efficacy of washing at a later time

**Eyes**

Irrigate with water or normal saline
Wash from inner angle toward outer angle
Monitor waste fluid to verify decontamination

**Ears**

Irrigate with water or normal saline
Dry with cotton swabs

**Mouth**

Brush teeth and rinse with 3% hydrogen peroxide

**Miscellaneous body openings**

Decontaminate around opening, using agents listed in the box at right
Cleanse opening gently with moistened gauze
Repeat as required
Cover with sterile dressing
Consult health physicist and physician to determine need for surgical decontamination

### Supplies and equipment for decontamination of radiologic accident casualties

**Radiation monitoring instruments**

Scintillation counter
Geiger-Müller counter with handheld probe
(If no instruments are available, the location of the nearest source should be identified)

**Radiation dosimeters**
*Protective clothing*

Coveralls
Shoe covers
Head covers
Surgical gowns or suits
Rubber gloves
Rubber aprons

**Decontamination supplies**

Absorbent (ABD) pads
Culture swabs
Gauze pads
Plastic bags (small and large)
Forceps
Masking tape
Sponges
Scissors
Basins
Irrigation sets
Betadine (or equivalent)
Household bleach
Laundry detergent
Cornmeal
Sterile water
Sterile sheets
Waste drums
1- to 2-gallon liquid waste containers
Waterless hand cleaner

**Miscellaneous**

Patient identification tags
Writing materials
Warning signs
Barrier rope
Small plastic bags for blood smears
Timers

(1) Address immediately life-threatening injuries by
 (a) Management of airway
 (b) Maintenance of circulation
 (c) Control of hemorrhage
(2) Assess magnitude of distribution of exposure by
 (a) Available information
 (b) Radiation safety officer
(3) If the information and officer are not available, document the characteristics of the initial blood samples. In addition to the characteristics of the initial toxic period, the lymphocyte count is most valuable in determining radiation dose. A 50% drop in lymphocyte count in the initial 48 hours or a lymphocyte count of less than 1000 is indication of severe exposure.
(4) Decontaminate patient.

## Treatment

Internal decontamination is carried out by encouraging the patient to cough, blow his nose, and not to swallow saliva, and by the careful use of laxatives and blocking agents. Hospitalization is mandatory for patients if the dose is known to have exceeded 100 rad, if there is a significant prodromal period, or if the lymphocyte count falls more than 50% within 2 days. During this period of time in the hospital, symptomatic treatment is indicated: sedatives, antiemetics, fluid and electrolyte management, and nutrition. If the severity of the prodromal period indicates that the manifest illness stage will be significant, the patient should be located at a medical facility with a full range of hematologic services, infection control systems, and other support services.

After the most recent accident a significant addition to the therapeutic armamentarium is the introduction of cytokines, specifically GM-CSF G CSF, to restore bone marrow function. Recovery begins usually at 6 to 8 weeks. Patients may feel ill for prolonged periods of time, however, and the late effects of radiation may develop years later.

CHAPTER

# 4E Cold

Lorentz E. Wittmers, Jr.

## ACCIDENTAL HYPOTHERMIA

Hypothermia is generally defined as a decrease in deep body or "core" temperature to 35° C or less. Accidental hypothermia implies an *unintentional* lowering of the body temperature, in contrast to hypothermia induced for medical or surgical reasons. Although most cases of hypothermia occur in the winter, a substantial number of cases can be found during the summer and in relatively warm climates. Environmental and physiologic conditions that may contribute to the development of hypothermia are prolonged exposure to cold air; exposure to moderately cold-wet (rain) conditions in combination with exercise-exhaustion (hikers' hypothermia); immersion in cold water; pathologic states that may predispose the patient to heat loss; and drugs, especially alcohol and barbiturates, that may alter temperature regulation as well as mental status, resulting in poor judgment and inappropriate or dangerous behavior, such as sitting in a snowdrift to take a nap.

### Thermoregulation

Heat production by the body can be divided into three types: (1) *basal metabolic rate*—even at rest the body produces a given amount of heat as the byproduct of metabolic processes; (2) *exercise*—muscle activity produces heat (as a metabolic byproduct and by friction) that can be conserved to maintain core temperature under cold stress; and (3) *shivering*—an involuntary response to cold in which muscle fiber groups undergo random contractions that do little except produce heat. The heat produced by maximal shivering can be nearly four times that produced by basal metabolic rate, about 50% of maximal oxygen consumption.

There are two ways heat is conserved under cold stress conditions. The first, and most important, is behavior adjustment. With the development of effective shelters and proper clothing people are able to live in cold climates. The importance of this is underscored by the prevalence of hypothermia in moderate climates where knowledge of coping with the cold is absent, or in conditions where people on fixed incomes reduce home heating to save money (urban hypothermia). The latter example is extremely distressing because the elderly, many of whom are on fixed incomes, often have reduced physiologic mechanisms regulating their body temperature.

The use of appropriate clothing to provide extra insulation limits heat loss. Effective garments, whether composed of natural or synthetic material, trap heated air close to the body and minimize heat loss by conduction and convection. Wetting of the garments either from the outside (e.g., rain, snow) or from the inside (e.g., sweat) increases their heat conductivity and decreases their insulating ability. Certain fabrics with low absorption characteristics retain their insulating value, even when wetted, by maintaining dead air space. These fabrics include wool and several synthetic materials (e.g., polypropylene and Thermax Hollofil). They are preferred by cold-weather athletes and outdoor workers.

Skin and subcutaneous tissue function as insulating material and are the second defense against heat loss. The amount of heat lost depends to a great extent on the blood flow to these tissues. Heat produced throughout the body is carried to the periphery as a function of blood flow. Temperature sensors in the skin and core provide information to the central nervous system via the posterior hypothalamus. This input is analyzed and, if heat conservation is necessary, efferent impulses are transmitted via the sympathetic nervous system producing vasoconstriction. The vasoconstriction effectively increases the layer of insulation surrounding the core by reducing its conductivity. In addition, the central nervous system responds to cold by inhibiting sweating and initiating shivering.

### Underlying conditions

Although all age groups are susceptible to accidental hypothermia, the very young and people over age 65 are at greater risk. The newborn has an incomplete nervous system that cannot respond effectively to the stresses of temperature. A small individual also has a very large surface area to volume ratio, and loses heat rapidly when a significant temperature gradient is imposed.

The development of hypothermia depends on the magnitude and duration of cold exposure in a normal individual. However, there are numerous conditions that can lead to or accelerate the development of hypothermic state. These conditions may be divided as follows:

1. Deficits in heat production
   (a) Malnutrition
   (b) Muscular inactivity
   (c) Hypoglycemia
   (d) Hypothyroidism
   (e) Hypopituitarism
2. Defects in thermoregulation
   (a) Age (very young and over age 65)
   (b) Nervous system disorders (localized central lesions, peripheral sensory loss, psychiatric disturbances)
   (c) Drugs (alcohol, barbiturates, phenothiazine etc.)

3. Associated injuries
4. Other diseases such as cardiovascular problems that limit the body's ability to maintain temperature

## Clinical features

*Measuring Core Temperature.* In general a patient with a core temperature below 35° C is considered to be in a hypothermic state. If the core temperature is defined as the temperature of the heart, then the best measurement is a myocardial temperature, which is impossible. A temperature taken in the lower third of the esophagus has been shown to be a close approximation to myocardial temperature. These measurements are not usually available; therefore other estimates of core must be considered. The most acceptable estimate is a rectal temperature taken 3 inches (8 cm) past the anus. This estimate may be in error if the patient's temperature is changing rapidly or if there is severe peripheral cooling (e.g., a patient found lying in a snowbank or submerged in water). Tympanic temperature has become widely used as the easiest measure of core temperature. Although there is some question as to its reliability, the procedure, if performed appropriately and if the external auditory canal is occluded, yields recordings adequate for assessing the temperature in hypothermic patients. Oral and axillary temperatures should not be used as estimate's of core temperature since they are greatly affected by air temperature and skin perfusion.

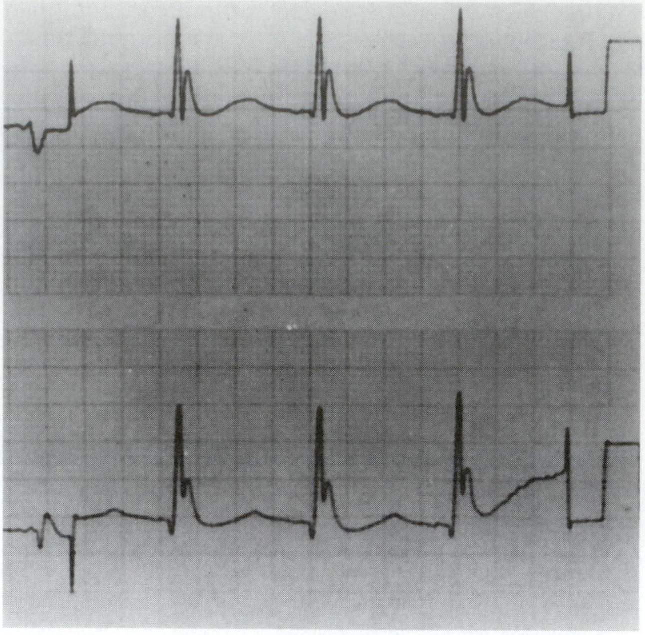

**Fig. 4E-1.** Pathognomonic j (Osborn) wave occurring with hypothermia following the QRS complex. (From Reuler JR, Jones SR, Giraud DE: Hypothermia in the erythroderma syndrome, *West J Med* 127:243, 1977.)

## Pathophysiology

*Central nervous system.* A fall in body temperature is accompanied by a decrease in metabolism of the brain and other organs (decreased oxygen consumption). The depression of central nervous system (CNS) metabolism is an approximately 6% to 7% per degree centigrade drop in core temperature over the range of 35° to 25° C. Around 32° C mental function begins to deteriorate, and clouding of sensorium, confusion, and drowsiness occur. The electroencephalogram (EEG) resembles light sleep or early stages of anesthesia. The individual becomes unconscious at about 30° to 32° C. The EEG becomes flat at about 20° C.

Muscle activity (shivering) producing heat stops at about 32° C. The absence of shivering in individuals exposed to cold for extended periods indicates a worsening of their condition. Below 30° C muscles become stiff, resulting in rigidity in the neck and extremities. Below 27° C muscles become flaccid.

## Cardiovascular system

*Rate and rhythm.* Early in the development of hypothermia the heart rate increases followed by a progressive fall. In contrast to the bradycardia seen at normal temperatures, the hypothermic heart shows a prolongation of systole greater than diastole. Additional changes in the ECG include prolonged PR, QRS and QT intervals, as well as ST segment and t-wave alterations.

In approximately one third of the patients with core temperatures below 32° C, the j (Osborn) wave can be seen in the ECG. The configuration of the j wave is usually a positive (upward) deflection at the junction of the QRS complex and the segment (Fig. 4E-1). Both the magnitude and lead location of the j wave are a function of the depth of the temperature depression.

As the myocardium continues to cool below 32° C all atrial and ventricular arrhythmias have been observed. The end result is either asystole or ventricular fibrillation.

*Peripheral vascular response.* In the early stages of hypothermia, blood pressure is probably elevated, although measurement by the auscultatory method is often difficult to obtain because of intense peripheral vasoconstriction. At core temperatures below 30° C, plasma levels of epinephrine and norepinephrine decrease, possibly contributing to depressed cardiovascular function. The intense peripheral vasoconstriction results in pallor and sometimes cyanosis. A characteristic puffiness of the face develops from subcutaneous edema resulting from increased capillary permeability.

*Respiratory system.* Early in the development of hypothermia the respirations increase, after which there is a progressive decrease in respiratory minute volume as metabolism falls coincident with the depression of core temperature. As severe hypothermia ensues carbon dioxide retention results in respiratory acidosis. In addition the functions of the airway mucosa are impaired, ciliary motility decreases, and mucous viscosity and volume increase. Alterations in capillary function may result in pulmonary edema.

*Body fluid.* Individuals exposed to cold stress undergo body fluid shifts between the fluid compartments, as well as an overall dehydration. They often curtail their fluid intake, partly the result of discomfort felt when consuming cold liquids. Peripheral vascular constriction tends to shift water out of the plasma, bringing about an increased hematocrit along with a decrease in plasma volume. Cold

**Table 4E-1.** Symptoms and physiologic landmarks during progressive hypothermia

| Core temperature °C | Observation |
|---|---|
| 37 | Normal rectal temperature |
| 36 | Increased metabolic rate—shivering |
| 35 | Maximum shivering thermogenesis |
| 34 | Judgment problems, dysarthria, amnesia, decreased fine motor movements |
| 33 | Ataxia, apathy |
| 32 | Stupor, decreased oxygen consumption |
| 31 | Shivering stops |
| 30 | Onset of cardiac arrhythmias, heart rate and cardiac output decrease |
| 29 | Decrease in level of consciousness, pulse, and respirations; pupils dilated |
| 27 | Loss of reflexes and voluntary motion |
| 25 | Significant depression of cerebral blood flow and cardiac output, possible onset of pulmonary edema |
| 24 | Significant hypotension |
| 23 | No corneal or oculocephalic reflexes |
| 22 | Maximum risk of ventricular fibrillation |
| 19 | Flat EEG |
| 18 | Asystole |
| 16 | Lowest adult accidental hypothermia survival |
| 15 | Lowest infant accidental hypothermia survival |

exposure also induces a diuresis resulting in increased water loss. This diuresis is caused by depression in the secretion of antidiuretic hormone. If the victim is immersed in cold water, the immersion itself increases urine flow and augments fluid loss. The consumption of alcohol by the subject further stimulates the diuresis. The physician must be aware of the possibility of volume depletion and the necessity of fluid replacement during rewarming treatment.

Table 4E-1 summarizes the signs, symptoms, and physiologic changes that occur as the patient's core temperature decreases.

## Treatment

***Prehospital management.*** Anyone suffering from mild to severe hypothermia should be evaluated at a medical facility immediately. Even mild cases of hypothermia may be associated with other medical conditions that could surface during an evaluation of the patient's presenting condition. The severely hypothermic patient may appear dead, rigid, cold, and cyanotic, with fixed, dilated pupils and no detectable heartbeat or respirations. A logical approach is to minimize further cooling and transport the patient to a treatment facility. When hypothermia can be considered a possible etiology for the patient's condition, it is safest to consider that "no one is dead until warm and dead." The diagnosis of death can be made only if the hypothermia is irreversible or the cardiovascular system is unresponsive after rewarming to 32° C.

### Prehospital evaluation of the hypothermic patient

**Victim responsive: YES or NO but with respirations**

Passive external rewarming (add heated humidified air or oxygen if available)
Intravenous fluids (D5 NS)
Cardiac monitoring
Gentle evacuation
Emergency room assessment

**Victim responsive: NO and NO respirations**

Tracheal intubation
Passive external rewarming (add heated humidified air or oxygen if available)
Cardiac monitoring

***If cardiac arrest present - CPR - evacuation***

Nonarrest rhythm

***If no central pulse - CPR - evacuation***

Central pulse present, continue on
Gentle evacuation
Emergency room assessment

Modified from Danzl D, Pozos RS, Hamlet MP. In Auerbach PS, Geehr EC, editors: *Management of wilderness and environmental emergencies,* ed 2, St. Louis, 1989, Mosby.

The hypothermic patient should be transported to a treatment facility immediately. Before or during transport any wet clothing should be removed, passive rewarming should be initiated by wrapping the patient in blankets, and the patient should be sheltered from the wind. These efforts minimize heat loss and initiate rewarming if shivering is present. Active methods of rewarming in the field may be detrimental; warming the skin or administering warm fluids may result in suppression of shivering and peripheral vasodilation, and actually produce an increase in heat loss. (Note: very little heat can be added by a few cups of warm fluid.)

Under field conditions, active external rewarming is not recommended. The one exception is inhalation therapy with warm humidified air or oxygen. This not only provides heat but prevents respiratory heat loss, a significant factor as the patient's core temperature falls.

The evacuation of a hypothermic patient should always be a gentle process. Responsive patients should not exercise, since muscular activity may result in cold blood—trapped in the extremities by vasoconstriction—returning to the core. This cold blood causes a further decrease in core temperature (afterdrop). In the nonresponsive patient, undue agitation may induce ventricular fibrillation. If cardiopulmonary arrest occurs, cardiopulmonary resuscitation (CPR) should be initiated. Without a cardiac monitor, assessing the myocardial rhythm may be difficult. CPR should not be initiated unless ventricular fibrillation or asystole is present because CPR in the hypothermic victim may induce ventricular fibrillation.

In summary, prehospital management of the hypothermic victim is outlined in the box above.

***Hospital management.*** After assessing vital signs in the emergency room, an accurate estimate of core temperature should be obtained. Rectal temperature measurements are the most common but may be inaccurate if the feces are excessively cold since the body is not in a steady state. The esophageal temperature gives an estimate of core temperature as long as heated inspired gas is not being used as a treatment modality. Tympanic temperatures are increasingly used in the emergency room as a measure but as previously noted, the accuracy of these measurements is in question.

Hospital treatment of the hypothermic patient depends on the evaluation of the following parameters:

1. Primary considerations for hypothermia
   (a) Magnitude of core temperature drop
   (b) Neurologic status - consciousness
   (c) Cardiovascular-respiratory status
   (d) Metabolic status
2. Associated considerations
   (a) Trauma
   (b) Coexisting pathology
   (c) Etiology of hypothermia
   (d) Duration of hypothermia

Treatment is determined by the severity of the parameters present.

Initial rewarming should consist of passive external methods with the addition of warm humidified air or oxygen if available. An intravenous line should be placed and cardiac monitoring initiated. Central venous pressure and pulmonary catheters should be avoided unless absolutely necessary; placement of such catheters may induce cardiac arrhythmias. If the core temperature is below 32° C, arrhythmias, including ventricular fibrillation, are a possibility. The *cold heart* may be refractory to antiarrhythmic drugs, regaining its responsiveness upon rewarming. Excessive use of these agents during hypothermia may lead to drug toxicity upon rewarming.

Almost all atrial arrhythmias convert to normal sinus rhythm upon rewarming; therefore treatment is unnecessary unless there is preexisting cardiac disease. Ventricular arrhythmias, on the other hand, must be treated immediately. The pharmacology of the drugs employed in this treatment is not well-defined under hypothermic conditions. Doses employed are usually the same as those used for patients having normal core temperatures.

Laboratory tests cannot in themselves assess the severity of the hypothermia; however, they can evaluate associated abnormalities and possibly preexisting pathology important in planning effective treatment. In all cases of hypothermia, with the exception of very mild core temperature drops, a blood chemistry profile is needed that includes: electrolytes, complete blood count, blood sugar, BUN, creatinine, calcium, magnesium, and amylase. A urinalysis should also be obtained. In the more severely hypothermic patient, laboratory analysis should be expanded to include a coagulation screen and an arterial blood gas in order to evaluate the patient's acid-base status. A toxicology screen may be indicated because hypothermia can be associated with or precipitated by drug ingestion (including alcohol).

Abnormalities in acid-base status occur frequently in the hypothermic patient. The most frequent problem is metabolic acidosis; however, mixed acidosis and even alkalosis may occur. As pointed out by Hofstrand there is an ongoing debate in the literature as to how arterial blood gas values should be interpreted. It is current practice to analyze the specimen without warming it and to interpret the result in relationship to the hypothermic patient.

### Rewarming

The methods employed to rewarm a hypothermic victim depend on the magnitude of the core temperature drop and on the facilities and expertise of the treatment personnel. Much controversy exists over the best way to rewarm a hypothermic victim. Complications of rewarming include core temperature afterdrop and rewarming shock. As the patient is rewarmed, vasodilation occurs. Since the vascular volume is decreased and the cardiac output is low, a shock condition may develop. Cooled blood from the skin, subcutaneous tissue, and muscles is also released into the central circulation, causing a further (transitory) drop in core temperature. The release of stagnant blood with a high concentration of metabolites can add to the acid-base imbalance.

Rewarming strategies are divided into three groups: passive external rewarming, active external rewarming, and active core rewarming. When passive external rewarming (PER) is used, the patient is stripped of all wet clothing and insulated with dry blankets or clothing to minimize loss of heat to the environment (at a suggested ambient temperature between 25° and 30° C) The heat generated by the patient's basal metabolic processes and/or shivering thermogenesis is conserved by the insulation and increases the core temperature. Under these conditions peripheral vasoconstriction is maintained and the probability of afterdrop and rewarming shock are decreased. Passive external rewarming is usually the method of choice for patients with mild to moderate hypothermia and a core temperature greater than 32° C, and for those patients in a stable cardiovascular-respiratory state.

At a core temperature below 32° C metabolic heat production is severely depressed and shivering stops. Under these conditions PER is not an effective method of rewarming. This necessitates the implementation of an active heat transfer to the patient either externally or directly to the core. The first level of active external rewarming (AER) is the delivery of heat to the skin. This is done with heated blankets; hot-water bottles; garments containing circulating tubing (plumbed garments); radiant heat; warm, circulating air; and immersion in warm water. When using AER the temperature of the heat source must be below a level that could result in tissue damage. Most recommendations put this temperature around 42° C, with the temperature not to exceed 45° C.

The most effective method of AER is warm water immersion. The patient is placed in a tub with arms and legs excluded from the warm water in an attempt to minimize afterdrop and rewarming shock. If electrical monitoring equipment is to be employed (e.g., ECG, recording temperature probes) it should be either battery driven or have the appropriate electrical isolation to prevent accidents. The water temperature should be monitored and held constant. This method of rewarming limits access to the patient and may make certain procedures difficult. If CPR becomes necessary, the patient must be removed from the tub. At a core temperature of 33° C consciousness should return and the patient can be removed from the tub and rewarming continued passively.

If the patient is in a state of moderate to severe hypothermia (core temperature less than 32° C) and in unstable cardiovascular status, active core rewarming (ACR) should be considered. Theoretically, ACR increases the temperature of the core and periphery simultaneously, reducing the amount of vasodilation that causes afterdrop and rewarming shock. The method chosen depends on the overall severity of the situation and the facilities available. Numerous methods can be employed to actively deliver heat to the core: (1) One method is the use of heated intravenous fluids (warmed to 40° to 42° C). In a 70 kg person with a core temperature of 28° C, the administration of 1 L of warm fluid (42° C) increases the core temperature 1/3 ° C. The actual benefit of warm IV fluids depends on the amount of fluid that can be tolerated. In any case, if fluids and blood are administered they should be warmed. (2) Gastric lavage has been employed in rewarming but it has numerous disadvantages including small surface area for heat exchange, possibilities of fluid and electrolyte shifts, and regurgitation with aspiration. A safer method employs a double-lumen intragastric balloon. (3) Colonic irrigation may suffer from limited surface area for heat transfer. (4) Peritoneal lavage is a rapid and available technique for core rewarming. The temperature of the inflowing fluid should be monitored. The procedure should be discontinued at a core temperature of 35° C to avoid "overshoot." This technique, however, is more invasive than those previously considered and may result in injury, infection, and fluid and electrolyte shifts. It does, however, allow good access to the patient and can be used along with other rewarming strategies. (5) Airway rewarming has been discussed earlier as a method employed in the field and emergency room to minimize the loss of heat via the respiratory system and, in addition, add heat to the core. The administered gas (oxygen) must be humidified at a temperature between 40° and 45° C; if dry gas is employed the patient's respiratory tract is forced to humidify it, resulting in heat loss caused by the latent heat of vaporization. The water condensing from the administered gas subsequently delivers heat to the respiratory airways and eventually to the core. In general, airway rewarming is considered safe and can be easily employed under most conditions. (6) Extracorporeal rewarming. In cases of extreme hypothermia that are refractory to the rewarming methods discussed above, the use of extracorporeal systems to effect rewarming should be considered, if the appropriate expertise is available. Cardiopulmonary bypass equipment with a heat exchanger can be employed to deliver warm blood to the patient. The rate of rewarming depends on the magnitude of the blood flow through the system. An additional advantage to this technique is the maintenance of circulation under conditions in which the heart becomes nonfunctional.

### Outcome

The magnitude and duration of hypothermia is directly correlated to mortality. However, estimates of this mortality cannot be based on temperature alone; the final outcome may be affected by associated injuries and underlying pathology. The available data seem to indicate that a core temperature of 32° C is a critical point. A series of patients presenting with core temperatures between 30 and 32° C show mortality rates as high as 33%. Core temperatures below 30° C have mortality rates as high as 70%. Patients with core temperatures above 32° C have a mortality rate as low as 4%. Certain conditions are associated with a poorer outcome: cardiac arrest occurring before arrival at the hospital, a low or absent presenting blood pressure, elevated BUN, and a need for endotracheal or nasogastric intubation in the emergency room.

## PERIPHERAL COLD INJURIES

Cold injuries have been reported throughout history especially in association with military operations. One dramatic example was the devastation of Napoleon's army in its retreat from Russia. Additional examples include World War II, the Korean conflict, and, more recently, the operations in the Falkland Islands.

### Classification and associated factors

Tissue injury resulting from cold exposure can be divided into freezing and nonfreezing. The type and magnitude of cold injury depends on several factors associated with the individual and the environment.

*Primary environmental factors* are the ambient temperature and the duration of exposure.

*Secondary host factors:* (1) Underlying pathology (e.g., diabetes, atherosclerosis, Raynaud's disease, previous frostbite) that results in decreased peripheral blood flow reduces the rate of heat delivered to the tissue, increasing the possibility and rapidness of cold injury; (2) poor physical conditioning and exhaustion; (3) previous exposure to cold resulting in injury; (4) drug and alcohol use that may depress perception of cold and therefore impair judgment leading to overexposure; (5) tobacco (nicotine) use producing peripheral vasoconstriction and a decrease in heat delivery.

*Secondary environmental factors:* (1) The wind chill factor relates wind velocity and temperature with respect to cold injuries. In order for freezing injuries to occur, the ambient temperature must be below freezing; however, the increasing movement of air at the skin replaces the warm air layer with cold air, increasing heat loss. The relationship between air velocity, ambient temperature, and tissue injury is summarized in Table 4E-2; (2) moisture on the skin or in the subject's clothing accelerates heat loss by both conduction and evaporation; (3) contact with cold objects such as metal surfaces also increases heat loss (4) exposure to cold at high altitudes results in decreased plasma volume and oxygen levels. The reduction of peripheral oxygen delivery may also accelerate tissue damage.

***Nonfreezing injuries.*** The group of nonfreezing injuries includes chilblain, trench foot, and immersion foot. Chilblain is an abnormal, peripheral vasoconstrictor response to cold exposure seen in susceptible individuals. Under normal conditions the vasoconstriction induced by cold exposure is relieved periodically by vasodilation, resulting in heat delivery to the tissue and protection against cold injury. In chilblain the vasoconstriction is

**Table 4E-2.** Equivalent chill temperature

| | Cooling power of wind expressed as equivalent chill temperature | | | | | | | | | | | |
|---|---|---|---|---|---|---|---|---|---|---|---|---|
| **Wind speed (MPH)** | **Temperature (°F)** | | | | | | | | | | | |
| **Calm** | **30** | **25** | **20** | **15** | **10** | **5** | **0** | **25** | **210** | **215** | **220** | **225** |
| | **Equivalent chill temperature** | | | | | | | | | | | |
| 5 | 25 | 20 | 15 | 10 | 5 | 0 | −5 | −10 | −15 | −20 | −25 | −30 |
| 10 | 15 | 10 | 5 | 0 | −10 | −15 | −20 | −25 | −35 | −40 | −45 | −50 |
| 15 | 10 | 0 | −5 | −10 | −20 | −25 | −30 | −40 | −45 | −50 | −60 | −65 |
| 20 | 5 | 0 | −10 | −15 | −25 | −30 | −35 | −45 | −50 | −60 | −65 | −75 |
| 25 | 0 | −5 | −15 | −20 | −30 | −35 | −45 | −50 | −60 | −65 | −75 | −80 |
| 30 | 0 | −10 | −20 | −25 | −30 | −40 | −50 | −55 | −65 | −70 | −80 | −85 |
| 35 | −5 | −10 | −20 | −30 | −35 | −40 | −50 | −60 | −65 | −75 | −80 | −90 |
| 40 | −5 | −15 | −20 | −30 | −35 | −45 | −55 | −60 | −70 | −75 | −85 | −95 |
| Winds above 40 mph have little additional effect | *Little Danger | | | *Increasing Danger (flesh may freeze within 1 minute) | | | | | | *Great Danger (flesh may freeze within 30 seconds) | | |

Modified from United States Air Force Survival Manual 64-3.
*Danger of Freezing Exposed Flesh for Properly Clothed Persons

prolonged, in some cases beyond the cold exposure, and causes tissue ischemia and edema. The areas most commonly affected are the distal portions of the body, along with regions most often exposed to the cold. Certain vascular conditions, such as Raynaud's disease, predispose an individual to chilblain. Since treatment for chilblain is ineffective, prevention by proper clothing, controlled environment, and stimulation of peripheral circulation is most important.

Trench foot (wearing cold/wet footwear) and immersion foot (feet actually immersed in cold water) combined with prolonged hours of exposure to temperatures at or below 50° F (10 ° C) (but not below freezing) results in tissue injuries. The injuries can be divided into three stages: (1) *ischemic* or prehyperemic (hours to days). Feet are cold, swollen, and discolored, and pulses and sensations are decreased or absent; (2) *hyperemic* (days to weeks). Feet are hot with pulses (sometimes exaggerated), and pain, blisters, and ulcerations may occur; and (3) *recovery* or posthyperemic (weeks to months). Tissue and pulses return to normal; however, cold sensitivity may persist. As in chilblain, prevention is the key; the treatment is basically supportive.

***Freezing injury.*** Frostbite is the actual freezing of tissue leading to tissue injury and/or death. Two pathophysiologic processes are responsible for the tissue damage: (1) Ice crystal formation, in which the crystals themselves may disrupt cellular and subcellular anatomy. In addition, crystal formation in the extracellular fluid results in an increase in osmolarity, which draws water out of the cells. This cell water loss may bring the concentration of intracellular components to toxic levels. (2) Vascular stasis. As the tissue freezes, vasoconstriction, increased viscosity, and the freezing itself decrease the blood supply to the tissue. The capillary permeability is increased, with subsequent fluid leakage—edema formation. On rewarming, obstruction of the vasculature occurs with arteriovenous shunting. The tissue is destroyed by either direct effects of freezing or the subsequent disruption of nutritive blood flow.

## Clinical manifestations

***Frostnip.*** The earliest stage of a freezing injury is frostnip. The patient feels cold in the affected region along with pain and numbness (total loss of sensation does not occur). Upon rewarming, the tissue returns to normal. The frostnip injury may be effectively treated in the field, if care is taken to prevent reinjury.

***Superficial frostbite.*** In superficial frostbite freezing is limited to the skin and subcutaneous tissue. There is no pain or sensation while the area is frozen. The skin appears paraffin-like (waxy), and minimal to no capillary refilling occurs. Upon rewarming, pain begins and progressively worsens. The tissue becomes edematous and the skin color is reddish, purplish, or mottled. Blisters are usually clear, resolving, and possibly leaving an eschar. The eschar may turn black and be mistaken as gangrene.

***Deep frostbite.*** In deep frostbite, tissues below the subcutaneous layer (e.g., muscle, tendon) are frozen. There is no pain while the tissue is frozen and sensation does not return upon rewarming if the sensory nerves were damaged. The skin remains cold after rewarming and the color does not return; it remains grayish. Blisters are not common and if they develop are often hemorrhagic.

## Treatment

Thawing should begin when refreezing of the frozen tissue cannot occur and other medical emergencies (e.g., trauma, hypothermia) have been addressed. Rapid thawing in a whirlpool bath, water temperature between 38° and 43° C (100° to 110° F) is recommended. Water temperature should be continuously monitored. Nonsterile conditions can be used initially but subsequent treatment should be aseptic. Care should be taken to not inflict any additional trauma on the tissue being thawed.

Depending on the depth of freezing, the thawing process should take between 20 and 30 minutes if superficial structures were frozen and up to 60 minutes if deep structures were involved. The skin becomes soft and there should be some evidence of blood flow, which may be temporary. Intense pain may require treatment. Continued support and treatment can be patterned after that employed with burn victims.

## COLD WATER NEAR-DROWNING

The growing popularity of outdoor recreation on or near water increases the probability of cold water submersion. A general discussion of drowning is covered in Chapter 4C. The special case of cold water submersion is discussed in this section.

In near-drowning a victim has been submerged in water for an extended period of time but is successfully resuscitated, at least for 24 hours. In the most dramatic near-drowning situations the victims are usually children, the water is very cold (near freezing), and the immersion may be as lengthy as 45 minutes. These cases often result in remarkable recovery after resuscitation.

### Mechanisms prolonging life

Two possible factors that may explain the survival after prolonged submersion are the diving reflex and rapid body cooling upon submersion.

The diving reflex is the response of certain diving mammals to submersion. The physiologic adjustments include apnea, vasoconstriction in tissues that are not acutely necessary for life (i.e., skin, muscle, gastrointestinal tract, kidneys), and a decrease in heart rate (minimizing the work of the heart and therefore the oxygen consumption of the myocardium). The result of these adjustments conserves the oxygen carried in the blood and to some extent the oxygen stored in the tissues for use by the heart and brain (critical organ systems). The diving reflex is vestigial in humans, and its magnitude is a function of age, being more prominent in children. Many adults do not exhibit a diving reflex when attempts are made to elicit it by cooling the face.

Immersion in cold water eventually results in cooling of the body core temperature. In addition, upon submersion the victim may aspirate cold water. If this is freshwater, it is rapidly transported across the blood gas barrier in the lungs, contributing to the cooling of the blood and eventually the core. The aspirated cold water may initiate early cerebral cooling and therefore protect against the decrease in available oxygen.

The cold water environment (see Accidental Hypothermia) will extracts heat from the body and decreases the core temperature. The rate of core temperature decrease depends on the water temperature and the surface area/body mass ratio of the victim. As the core temperature drops, metabolic processes are depressed and the need for oxygen supply decreases.

Young children benefit the most from the diving reflex and the fact that they have a large surface area/body mass ratio promoting heat loss and a decrease in core temperature. Under these conditions, the body is conserving oxygen for the vital organs and the decreased core temperature is depressing oxygen demand. The result is an extended submersion time and the possibility of successful resuscitation. Cases of an adult and a child immersed simultaneously in cold water have shown successful resuscitation of the child but failure to save the adult.

The term near-drowning denotes a positive outcome from the submersion. Victims not successfully resuscitated are placed in the drowned category and do not make the national media coverage. However, the history of successful resuscitation of children indicates that aggressive treatment of such victims is indicated.

## BIBLIOGRAPHY


Clark RC, Edholm OG: *Man and his thermal environment,* London, 1984, Edward Arnold.

Danzl D, Pozos RS, Hamlet MP: Accidental hypothermia. In Auerbach PS, Geehr EC, editors: *Management of wilderness and environmental emergencies,* ed 2, St Louis, 1989, Mosby.

Hales JRS, editor: *Thermal physiology,* New York, 1984, Raven Press.

Hamlet M: Human cold injuries. In Pandolf KB, Sawka MN, Gonzalez RR, editors: *Human performance physiology and environmental medicine at terrestrial extremes,* Indianapolis, 1988, Benchmark Press.

Hofstrand HT: Accidental hypothermia and frostbite. In Barkin R, editor: *Pediatric emergency medicine: concepts in clinical practice,* St Louis, 1992, Mosby.

Mills WJ: Accidental hypothermia. In Pozos RS, Wittmers LE, editors: *The nature and treatment of hypothermia,* Minneapolis, 1983, University of Minnesota Press.

Modell JH, Grave SA, Ketover A: Clinical course of 91 consecutive near-drownings: the protective effect of the diving reflex, Am Rev Respir Dis 115(4):145, 1976.

Nelson RN: Accidental hypothermia. In Nelson RN, Rund DA, Keller MD, editors: *Environmental emergencies,* Philadelphia, 1985, WB Saunders.

Nelson RN: Drowning and near-drowning. In Nelson RN, Rund DA, Keller MD, editors: *Environmental emergencies,* Philadelphia, 1985, WB Saunders.

Nelson RN: Peripheral cold injury. In Nelson RN, Rund DA, Keller MD, editors: *Environmental emergencies,* Philadelphia, 1985, WB Saunders.

Nemiroff M: Submersion hypothermia and acid base balance. In Larson GA, Pozos RS, Hempel FG, editors: *Human performance in the cold,* Bethesda, Md, 1984, Undersea Medical Society.

Paton B: Accidental hypothermia. In *International encyclopedia of pharmacology and therapeutics. Thermoregulation: pathology, pharmacology and therapy,* New York, 1991, Pergamon Press.

Tabeling BB: Near-drowning and its treatment. In Pozos RS, Wittmers LE, editors: *The nature and treatment of hypothermia,* Minneapolis, 1983, University of Minnesota Press.


CHAPTER

# 4F Altitude Illnesses

**Charles S. Houston**

More and more men and women of all ages are visiting the mountains for work or recreation. Others trek in the ranges of Asia or South America, and some climb the highest mountains. Many ask their physicians for advice, but the family physician may be unaware of how altitude affects people, particularly those with heart or lung problems, and is unable to advise them properly. The physician practicing in a mountain environment may not be familiar with all aspects of mountain sickness. Cardiac and pulmonary specialists often do not consider mountain sickness important. Despite much study for many decades, altitude illnesses are still not widely appreciated and only partly understood.

Altitude means one thing to the Himalayan climber, another to the resort skier. In general, *moderate* suggests altitudes up to 12,000 feet, *high* would be 12,000 to 20,000 feet, and *extreme* is usually reserved for anything above this. Because barometric pressure decreases while the percentage of oxygen in air remains constant, less oxygen is available in the atmosphere as one goes higher. The resulting hypoxia, rather than the decreased pressure, is the principal and probably the only cause of mountain sickness. It can be devastating.

A 45-year-old airline pilot drove to 9000 feet to ski. The next day he had a headache but continued to ski. On the third day after arrival, he stumbled and fell frequently and said he had "flu"; his wife and friends persuaded him to go home to bed. He appeared to be sleeping when they returned, but early next morning he could not be roused. He was resuscitated, flown to hospital, but died 10 days later of massive cerebral and pulmonary edema complicated by pneumonia.

## CLASSIFICATION

The box below lists the most common forms of altitude sickness. These may appear separately or together. Indeed, altitude illnesses are considered to be a continuum or spectrum with one, then another form predominating. The common signs and symptoms suggest that this is primarily a central nervous system (CNS) disorder, with many manifestations caused by lack of oxygen.

Several more altitude-related syndromes have been described recently and are listed in the box at right.

### Acute mountain sickness (AMS)

Most cases of AMS develop within 48 hours after the person arrives. The incidence of AMS is determined by speed of ascent, altitude reached, length of stay, and individual characteristics. Approximately one quarter of all visitors at 8000 to 9000 feet experience AMS. The number increases to 50% at 10,000 feet. Men may be somewhat more susceptible than women, and children more than older persons.

Headache is the most common symptom, sometimes severe and unrelieved by analgesics. Easy fatigability, difficulty concentrating, increased exertional dyspnea, anorexia, nausea, and vomiting occur less frequently. Insomnia or broken restless sleep is more frequent than increased somnolence. Remember that other illnesses, such as pneumonia, meningitis, gastroenteritis, or flu, may also occur and be mistaken for altitude sickness.

### High-altitude pulmonary edema (HAPE)

Most individuals going rapidly from low to moderate altitude accumulate some fluid in the pulmonary interstitial space; usually this is quickly reabsorbed. In perhaps one tenth of 1% of visitors, the fluid seeps into and accumulates in the alveoli, causing more severe dyspnea, productive cough, and weakness. HAPE may become rapidly life-threatening unless recognized and treated promptly.

### High-altitude cerebral edema (HACE)

In rare instances the CNS signs dominate; gait ataxia is an early sign, and severe headache, confusion, and hallucinations are typical. Evidence of AMS or HAPE may also be present. The person is likely to lapse into coma and die within hours without emergency care. Judgment may be impaired early, and unrecognized HACE prevents persons from perceiving their plight.

A fit, experienced skier drove to 8400 feet and easily skied to 9800 feet. Next day he had a mild headache and trouble keeping up; the party climbed only 400 feet. On the third day, at 10,100 feet, his headache was severe, and he could barely stand. During the night he became irrational. When a rescue helicopter arrived on the fifth morning, he was near death. At the hospital he had fluid in his lungs and alarming evidence of brain damage. He remained comatose for 48 hours but recovered and was discharged well.

This nearly fatal case exemplifies the merging and progression of several forms of altitude illness, as well as the dangerous impact of altitude on judgment. Both he and his companions failed to realize how rapidly dangerous signs and symptoms were progressing. Similar errors have killed mountaineers on very high mountains.

### Common forms and manifestations of mountain sickness

Acute mountain sickness (AMS): headache, nausea, vomiting, fatigue, sleep disturbance, seldom serious, self-limited
High-altitude pulmonary edema (HAPE): dyspnea, cough (productive), headache, fatigue, malaise, cyanosis, may be serious
High-altitude cerebral edema (HACE): ataxia, headache, confusion, hallucinations, coma, very serious if untreated
High-altitude retinal hemorrhage (HARH): no symptoms, common above 14,000 feet, may occur in other sites, self-limited
High-altitude edema (HAE): peripheral and facial edema, common above 10,000 feet, benign, self-limited
High-altitude syncope (HAS): sudden fainting soon after arrival at 8000 to 9000 feet, brief, rarely significant

### Less common altitude illnesses

Acute hypoxia
Migraine formes frustes
Transient cortical blindness (TCB)
Sickle cell crisis
Cerebrovascular accident (CVA [stroke], thrombosis, hemorrhage)
Chronic mountain sickness (polycythemia) (CMS or CMP)
Adult subacute mountain sickness (ASMS)
Infantile subacute mountain sickness (ISMS)
Altitude edema

### High-altitude retinal hemorrhage (HARH)

Many persons going to 14,000 feet or higher develop retinal vascular engorgement and hemorrhages. These are usually asymptomatic and disappear in 10 to 14 days even at altitude. Rarely, a small hemorrhage at or near the macula leaves a persistent visual defect. Similar small hemorrhages found elsewhere, in the kidney or beneath the nails suggest they may also occur in the brain. Although sometimes HARH seems alarming, most cases leave no residual effects. Rarely, cotton wool exudates occur and take longer to resolve. If papilledema is observed, HACE is likely and the patient should descend at once.

### Acute hypoxia

Acute hypoxia, inaccurately called "asphyxia," involves abrupt interruption of the normal oxygen supply, which causes desperate effects: unconsciousness, seizures, and death within 6 minutes if interruption is complete. Persons rapidly exposed to extreme altitude (in ½ hour or less) quickly lose consciousness and may die. The time of useful consciousness depends mainly on the speed and severity of exposure; individual characteristics intervene. Acute hypoxia is not a problem for altitude sojourners, although it may be critical in aviation and elsewhere.

> A teenager climbed down into a deep, dry well and became unconscious before anything wrong was suspected. He was dead when rescuers reached him. Marsh gas and carbon dioxide had accumulated to a lethal level in the bottom of the well.

Other causes of acute hypoxia are not so dramatic; they include carbon monoxide poisoning, failure of an oxygen delivery system, suffocation, and choking.

### High-altitude syncope (HAS)

Several recent reports have described sudden fainting in visitors soon after arrival at altitude. Most episodes are very brief and come without warning, often after a few drinks or a hearty meal. Recovery is almost immediate, and no pathology is found. These are attributed to brief vasovagal overload.

### Migraine formes frustes

Migraine may be precipitated by altitude with or without other stress. Prodromata and headache may be characteristic, but both may be absent.

> An experienced mountaineer began to develop blurred vision while on rock climbs. Over time the episodes became more frequent and severe, accompanied by weakness and finally paralysis of legs and arms. All symptoms disappeared with descent. Thorough neurologic studies were normal. A consultant suggested migraine and advised one aspirin daily as prophylaxis. No episodes occurred for several years with this program, but they recurred when aspirin was stopped.

This individual was a senior scientist, and the account of his experience is difficult to challenge; he had no history of migraine.

### Cortical blindness

Several visual effects caused by altitude have been described, usually above 14,000 feet. These range from scotomata, blurred or distorted vision, to "blindness" (although light reflexes are unimpaired). They have been attributed to hypoxia and disappear promptly with descent or with supplemental oxygen. Whether they are atypical migraine or result from transitory vascular changes in the visual cortex is unknown.

### Sickle cell disease (sickle cell anemia, sickle cell trait, thalassemia)

This genetic defect is present in 5% to 10% of Americans of African or Mediterranean ancestry that may be remote and unsuspected. In sickle disease the red blood cells (RBCs) are deformed. During hypoxia from any cause, they deform further, becoming stiff and rigid. The deformed cells stick in capillaries, leading to thrombosis and infarction in many parts of the body, often in the spleen.

> A young white male flew to 7000 feet and in a few hours was hospitalized with severe abdominal pain that, over the next few days, settled in the left upper quadrant. Surgery showed massive splenic infarction, and sickle cell crisis was diagnosed. His father flew to visit him and experienced the identical problem. A remote African ancestor was identified from the family history.

### Cerebrovascular accident (CVA [stroke], thrombosis, hemorrhage)

Vascular accidents are rare but serious and usually occur above 16,000 feet. They are caused by a combination of dehydration, excessive RBC formation from acclimatization, and changes in blood coagulability at altitude. Warning signs may appear and may be mistaken for HACE before the neurologic changes clarify the diagnosis.

> A 60-year-old physician rode a cable car and then climbed higher to 14,000 feet, where he was too tired to descend. During the night he became disoriented, hallucinated, and was incontinent. On waking he was ataxic and disoriented and was evacuated by helicopter. He became asymptomatic and refused hospitalization. On returning home, he showed right-sided facial and upper extremity weakness; studies showed an area of brain infarction.

Similar episodes have happened to mountaineers on high Himalayan peaks. Peripheral venous thromboses with pulmonary emboli may occur. Below 12,000 to 14,000 feet, these vascular problems are usually not attributable to altitude and are more likely caused by preexisting vascular disease.

### Chronic mountain sickness (polycythemia) (CMS or CMP)

After months or years of residence, usually above 11,000 feet, some individuals (usually natives and less often long-term visitors), develop overexuberant RBC formation and polycythemia. The person tires easily and has multiple nonspecific pains, emotional problems, dyspnea, plethoric cyanosis, and thrombophlebitis. If untreated, right-sided heart failure develops from pulmonary artery hypertension. Descent to sea level brings slow recovery, but reascent leads to recurrence. This is more common in the Andes but is also seen in the Himalayas. To diagnose in miners, it is necessary to exclude pneumoconioses.

### Adult subacute mountain sickness (ASMS)

First noted 35 years ago, ASMS became important during recent border conflicts in Asia. About 10% of troops stationed at 18,000 to 20,000 feet for many weeks or months did not acclimatize but developed congestive heart failure (CHF) with dilated right ventricles, hydrothorax, and edema caused by pulmonary hypertension. Descent to low altitude and treatment for CHF brought slow and complete recovery. The condition is similar to brisket disease in certain strains of cattle taken from low to moderate elevations.

### Infantile subacute mountain sickness (ISMS)

Many months after being taken from low to moderate altitude, some infants develop CHF similar to that described in adults. The condition has only been described so far in Han (Chinese) infants taken from lowlands to the Tibetan plateau and has not been seen in other ethnic groups. This may be a demographic coincidence. The cause is unknown; therapy consists of descent.

### Altitude edema

Many and perhaps most persons going to altitude shift water from the intravascular to the extravascular space for a short time; this is manifested as peripheral or facial edema. In part, this results from the impact of hypoxia on hormone complexes. However, strenuous exertion even at low altitude causes similar fluid shifts and edema, an effect that cannot be separated from that of altitude in mountain trekkers and climbers.

## PHYSIOLOGY

A complex transport system ensures delivery of oxygen throughout the body, since oxygen is neither manufactured nor stored. Lungs, heart, blood, and blood vessels are the main parts of the system providing oxygen to all living cells. Failure in this transport system is the cause of altitude illnesses. Their coordinated function is necessary to maintain what Claude Bernard called "the constancy of the internal environment."

Hypobaric hypoxia of altitude and some causes of oxygen deficiency at sea level provoke the same responses, which, although protective, may exacerbate the symptoms. The box at right lists the normal responses to a lack of oxygen.

### Normal responses to oxygen lack

**Primary responses**

Hyperventilation: raises alveolar $PO_2$ but lowers $PCO_2$
Hemoconcentration: increases oxygen-carrying capacity
Increased EPO release: increases RBC production
Increased cardiac output: increases distribution of oxygen
Capillary recruitment: improves tissue oxygenation

**Secondary responses**

Respiratory alkalosis: shifts hemoglobin curve to left; stimulates bicarbonate excretion; decreases cerebral blood flow
Increased autonomic nervous system response: increases vasoconstriction and raises blood pressure
Hormonal stimulation: complex interplay causes fluid and electrolyte shifts

**Tertiary response**

Blood buffers depleted: increased reaction to lactic and other acid formation

**Cellular response**

Changes in size or position of mitochondria

### Normal responses to hypobaric hypoxia

The first and most powerful response to hypoxia is an increase in rate and/or depth of breathing, increasing alveolar oxygen while washing out carbon dioxide and initiating respiratory alkalosis. The hypoxic ventilatory response (HVR) differs among individuals and changes under different circumstances.

Hypoxia increases pulse rate and both systolic and diastolic blood pressure because of an increase in circulating catecholamines. Both normotensive and hypertensive individuals show this increase. Pulmonary arterial pressure rises even more, proportionately. The elevated blood pressure and pulse rate increase the work of the heart; all return nearly to sea level values after several days or weeks at altitude.

Another normal physiologic response to altitude is salt and water diuresis, opposing the abnormal fluid retention noted later. This causes contraction of both plasma and an extracellular volumes, resulting in an apparent increase in circulating RBCs. It does not change the oxygen content or carrying capacity of circulating blood because blood volume is decreased. Within 1 hour of exposure, erythropoietin is increased, stimulating formation of new RBCs, and as these mature, they increase the oxygen-carrying capacity of blood. Circulating aldosterone is decreased, but atrial natriuretic peptide (ANP), which produces vasodilation, is slightly increased.

Recruitment of inactive tissue capillaries occurs later, improving delivery to tissues. No immediate changes occur within cells, but as acclimatization matures, important adjustments occur.

## PATHOPHYSIOLOGY

The sensitivity of the HVR is the main determinant of ventilation at altitude; individuals with a blunted response are more prone to altitude illnesses, although exceptions exist. The HVR usually becomes more sensitive during a stay at altitude but may be blunted by severe stresses such as starvation and exhaustion.

Periodic, or Cheyne-Stokes, breathing, which reflects a "searching" by the respiratory control system, is common and not abnormal at altitude. At sea level the frequency and depth of ventilation are dictated primarily in the medulla by arterial carbon dioxide pressure ($PaCO_2$) and pH and less strongly by the carotid bodies responsive to arterial oxygen pressure ($PaO_2$). At altitude the roles are reversed: as $PaO_2$ falls, the carotid bodies take control and increase respiration, then, as $PaCO_2$ drops, the medullary centers override and dictate a decrease. During sleep, these swings are prominent, and since desaturation is more pronounced during the apneic periods, periodic breathing is thought to explain why AMS is often worse on wakening. The broken sleep is often troublesome, and periodic breathing is eliminated by acetazolamide (see later discussion).

Pulmonary artery pressure (PAP) rises immediately on exposure to hypoxia, proportionately more than systemic pressure, and remains high. The increased PAP extends to the alveolar capillaries but no further; left atrial pressure is normal. Alveolar fluid obtained by bronchial lavage in patients with HAPE is similar to that seen in adult respiratory distress syndrome (ARDS), containing increased high-molecular-weight protein, increased leukocytes, and other indicators of inflammation.

The elevated PAP is accompanied by or causes other changes. The capillary endothelial cells are stressed, the normally tight intercellular junctions are stretched and may rupture, and leakage from capillary into interstitium and alveoli results. Endothelial stress causes release of a series of kinins (the arachidonic cascade) into the pulmonary circulation. Some of these cause vasoconstriction; others cause vasodilation. Some increase platelet aggregation; others suppress it. It is postulated that whichever of these complex interactions prevails will determine whether alveolar edema increases or whether it disappears.

Both increased PAP and increased capillary permeability are necessary for the development of HAPE; neither alone produces this clinical picture.

Chest x-ray films in HAPE is distinctive: fluffy scattered areas of increased density are peripheral rather than hilar and more in the right than left lung; they are thought to indicate areas of overperfusion.

Individuals with congenital absence of a pulmonary artery develop HAPE as low as 6000 feet. HAPE has also occurred in persons with a history of pulmonary emboli or scattered alveolar damage. Such cases support the hypothesis of perfusion/ventilation inequity. Some individuals have repeated episodes of HAPE without adequate explanation. Some altitude residents returning after a brief stay at sea level are at risk of "reentry HAPE." Even a mild "cold" or "influenza" seems to increase the risk of HAPE.

Altitude edema is caused by abnormal antidiuresis, sodium retention, increased plasma and extracellular volumes, and increased aldosterone. ANP may be slightly increased and contribute to edema formation by direct action on transcapillary fluid exchange. Both renal blood flow and glomerular filtration rate are decreased. Such changes are opposite to the normal response to hypoxia but similar to those caused by strenuous exertion at sea level. By contrast, polyuria ("hohendiuresen") is favorable at altitude; this has led to the exhortation to "drink more water, till the urine is gin clear."

It is tempting to blame failure of the sodium pump for the fluid and electrolyte shifts characteristic of altitude illness, since the sodium pump is a high-energy, oxygen-dependent system. But no solid evidence supports this theory.

Headache is difficult to explain. Cerebral blood vessels are quickly responsive to changes in $PaCO_2$ or $PaO_2$, dilating from hypoxia and constricting with hypocapnia. One theory is that changes in tension on the sensitive membranes covering these vessels and the brain causes headache. In severe cases of HACE, edema has been demonstrated in the corpus callosum by magnetic resonance imaging (MRI). Thirty years ago, increased spinal fluid pressure was found in a few soldiers with severe altitude illnesses; a recent study at simulated altitude has confirmed this. At autopsy, victims of HACE show petechial hemorrhages and generalized edema.

The impact of hypoxia on higher mental functions such as judgment is similar to that of alcohol. Veteran mountaineers believe alcohol has added effect at altitude: "One drink does the work of two," but limited studies do not support this belief. Alcohol does not increase AMS, although AMS does resemble a bad hangover.

## Age and preexisting illnesses

Practitioners are often asked how age affects tolerance for altitude. Several studies have shown that the incidence of AMS (and presumably of other forms as well) decreases linearly with increasing age; children are more susceptible than their grandparents. Age alone is not a contraindication to going to moderate elevation, and men and women over 70 have climbed higher than 20,000 feet.

Persons with coronary artery disease (CAD) require individual evaluation. A study of 97 men and women ages 65 to 83, a third of whom had proven CAD, found that persons who were asymptomatic at sea level tolerated 8000 feet well. In another study, older men showed no cardiac changes while skiing at 9000 to 10,000 feet. Many individuals have gone to moderate altitude after coronary bypass surgery, and some have climbed much higher. Morbidity and mortality reports from the Himalayas and the Alps show surprisingly few adverse incidents among many thousand visitors of all ages.

Similar conclusions apply to persons with chronic pulmonary problems (asthma, chronic obstructive pulmonary disease, [COPD], bronchitis): if asymptomatic at sea level, these individuals tolerate moderate altitude well. Again, each patient needs individual consideration.

Systolic and diastolic blood pressure increase normally during the first days or weeks at altitude; is this a problem for the hypertensive person? Existing data are not conclusive. In general, patients who are well controlled by medication appear to tolerate altitude well, although some may require readjustment of medication. Those with hypertension that is poorly controlled may be at greater risk at altitude than at sea level.

## Other contraindications

Any condition that interferes with oxygen transport may increase the likelihood of altitude illness. These include diffuse pulmonary disease (fibrosis, sarcoid), obstructive disease (severe asthma or COPD), CHF, anemia, abnormal hemoglobin (sickle cell disease), extensive vascular disease, obesity, oral contraceptives, and abnormal clotting mechanisms. Diabetic persons may require extra attention to insulin and diet. The exercise of climbing or skiing often reduces a disbetic's insulin requirement significantly. Epilepsy or psychosis may also endanger the individual. Neonatal birth weights are lower after pregnancy at altitude, but the added risk to infant or mother at altitude is not great. All these conditions require careful individual evaluation of their impact on oxygen transport and delivery, as well as consideration of the benefits from the beauty and majesty of the mountain environment.

## PREVENTION

The best and most effective prevention of altitude illness is to allow time for the body to adjust. By ascending slowly, the protective mechanisms come into play, and all parts of the oxygen transport system contribute to maintain oxygen to the tissues near normal levels. Just how slow is slow enough is an individual matter. Conventional wisdom suggests ascending at 1000 feet per day above 5000 to 6000 feet, but few persons will take time and need to do this. Those who have experienced AMS before will recognize the symptoms; they are advised to stop and wait a day before proceeding. Others have no difficulty going to moderate altitude in a few hours. The only reliable rule is to take as much time as the most susceptible member of the party may need and, above all, if symptoms increase or become alarming, to go down.

Medication is effective. Acetazolamide (Diamox) prevents AMS in most people. The preferred dose is 125 mg morning and night, starting on the day the ascent starts and continuing for a day or two after arrival. Some people may need twice that amount. Delayed-action tablets are available but have not been adequately evaluated. Acetazolamide is effective not so much for its mild diuretic effect as for its inhibition of carbonic anhydrase, thus enhancing the excretion of bicarbonate in urine and hastening acclimatization.

Dexamethasone (Decadron) is also helpful, probably for its stabilizing effect on fluid shifts. It is not as effective as acetazolamide, and the two may be used together in highly susceptible persons. The recommended dose is 4 mg twice daily.

Individuals who have had one or more episodes of HAPE may be advised to take a calcium channel blocker (nifedipine [Procardia]) to decrease pulmonary hypertension. This is effective either as 20 mg every 4 hours or in a delayed-action form twice daily. This may lower systemic pressure as well, and orthostatic hypotension may occasionally result.

Migraine attacks at altitude may be forestalled by one aspirin tablet daily. Migraine is an unusual altitude problem, however, and this preventive measure is not clearly established.

The altitude at which one sleeps is more important than how high one goes during the day, thus the advice to "sleep low and climb high." Although drinking more water is good advice to prevent dehydration, no verified proof indicates that it prevents mountain sickness. Avoiding salt decreases the tendency to develop edema. In theory a very high carbohydrate diet improves oxygen tolerance, but research data are lacking, and the diet is not palatable for long. Small, frequent snacks during the day and a light meal at night are reasonable measures.

*The most important advice a practitioner can give patients is to understand the problem, to recognize early danger signs, and to turn back before these signs worsen.*

## TREATMENT

Minor signs and symptoms improve in a few days, but if the patient's condition is worsening, the cardinal treatment is descent. Breathing supplemental oxygen improves all symptoms and may be sufficient while the body adjusts. However, oxygen is only a temporizing measure: descent is mandatory for severe cases. Placing the patient in a pressurizing bag provides temporary relief, but symptoms soon return after the treatment; this is most valuable high on a mountain when descent is impossible and oxygen unavailable.

Medication relieves many symptoms of AMS. Increasing the dose of acetazolamide to 250 or even 500 mg twice daily or adding 4 mg of dexamethasone every 4 hours is safe and often sufficient. Nifedipine (20 to 40 mg) brings prompt improvement in HAPE, although persons with severe conditions should descend. Once HACE is obvious, immediate descent is mandatory because the hallucinations, ataxia, and confusion may progress rapidly to coma. Intravenous dexamethasone (4 to 6 mg) should be given but requires several hours to be effective. Oxygen is not sufficient. Patients with HACE improve during descent but do so more slowly than those with HAPE.

Cortical blindness, migraine equivalents, and other rare forms of altitude illness are usually relieved dramatically by descending a few thousand feet. Retinal hemorrhages require no treatment and heal spontaneously.

## ACCLIMATIZATION

Although acclimatization is not relevant to most of the advice practitioners may give their patients who plan to go to mountain resorts, some persons have higher ambitions and will ask about this. Acclimatization is an intricate process involving all parts of the oxygen transport system. Small changes can be detected as low as 6000 feet. Acclimatization takes time to evolve, and no medications have been found to hasten the process. Current practice on very high mountains is to climb slowly, setting the pace to avoid symptoms, to 17,000 to 18,000 feet. From this base camp, short day climbs to neighboring peaks are made for a few weeks. By then, one may be able to rush a much higher summit and return safely (unless a storm or accident delays descent). Such alpine-style mountaineering is probably safer and less costly and avoids altitude deterioration, which is now widely recognized after longer stays above 20,000 to 22,000 feet.

Humans can acclimatize to extreme altitude so well that more than 30 men and women have climbed Mt. Everest breathing only the thin air about them, which contains less than one-third the oxygen pressure at sea level. Sudden exposure to this altitude causes unconsciousness in 4 or 5 minutes and death soon afterward.

## SUMMARY

Altitude illnesses are physiologic disturbances caused by lack of oxygen in the ambient air. They are readily preventable and treatable. At the same time they cause significant emotional and economic distress to travelers and others and, not infrequently, death to careless and uninformed persons.

## BIBLIOGRAPHY

Grissom CK: Acetazolamide in the treatment of acute mountain sickness: clinical efficay and effect on gas exchange, *Ann Intern Med* 116:461, 1992.

Grover RF: Speculations on the pathogenesis of high-altitude pulmonary edema, *Adv Cardiol* 27:1, 1980.

Hackett PH, Rennie ID, Levine HD: The incidence, importance, and prophylaxis of acute mountain sickness, *Lancet* 2(7995):1149, 1976.

Hackett PH, Roach RC, Sutton JR: Medical problems of high altitude. In Auerbach PS, Geehr E, editors: *Management of wilderness and environmental emergencies,* St Louis, 1988, Mosby.
Halhuber MJ, Humpeler KI, Jungmann H: Does altitude cause exhaustion of the heart and circulatory system? *Med Sports Sci* 19:192, 1985.
Houston CS: Trekking at high altitudes: how safe is it for your patients? *Postgrad Med* 88(1):56, 1990.

CHAPTER

# 4G Bites/Stings Irritation

Nesli Basgoz
Ann Sullivan Baker
Neil W. Ross

## BITES AND STINGS

### Animal and human bites

More than 500,000 animal bites are reported yearly in the United States. Dog bites constitute the largest group. The human victim is usually a 7- to 9-year-old boy, often teasing or playing with a dog. The biting dog is usually 6 to 12 months old, is often female, and is usually a working dog, such as a boxer, collie, German shepherd, Great Dane, or Saint Bernard, or a sporting dog, such as a pointer, setter, or retriever. Hounds are relatively safe.

The evaluation and treatment of all bites is based on a careful history, including the type of animal, the site of the bite, and the geographic setting. Hand and puncture wounds most often become infected. Most bites should be cultured and a Gram stain prepared; they should then be washed, irrigated well, and left open. Selection of an antibiotic depends on the bite history and Gram stain results. Most patients with deep cat bites, deep cat scratches, and sutured wounds should be treated with penicillin or tetracycline because they are at increased risk of *Pasteurella multocida* infection. All splenectomized patients with dog bites should be treated with penicillin to prevent *Capnocytophaga canimorsus* (formerly known as DF-2) bacteremia. Tetanus immune status should be evaluated, and rabies immunization should be considered.

Human bites and monkey bites deserve special mention, since 30% become infected with aerobic or anaerobic mouth organisms. Anaerobic infection may spread through the metacarpophalangeal space and cause severe damage as described in Chapter 72. The same procedure should be followed with other animal bites, i.e., culture and Gram stain, thorough washing, and wide dissection. Wounds should be left open, if possible, especially hand wounds and followed closely. Patients with human bites should be treated with penicillin for 7 to 10 days. Clenched fist injuries should be evaluated by a hand surgeon because of the possibility of deep space or joint infection (see Chapter 72).

***Bacterial infections pasteurella multocida.*** A common organism infecting bite wounds is *P. multocida.* It is present in the nasopharynx of 50% of dogs and 75% of cats. Most infections in humans fall into one of three clinical patterns:

1. The most common pattern is that of local infection with adenitis after a dog or cat bite or scratch. In cases of cat bite, it may then progress to tenosynovitis or osteomyelitis, which is due to inoculation of the organism into the periosteum by the long, sharp tooth of the animal. Canine teeth are more blunt and less likely to penetrate the periosteum.
2. Chronic pulmonary infection may be caused by *P. multocida* as the primary pathogen or in association with other organisms. Bacteria may enter through the respiratory tract by inhalation of barn dust or infectious droplets sprayed by the sneeze of an animal. In such cases the bacteria probably colonize the respiratory tract and lie dormant in the patient with chronic lung disease. Acute infection occurs only after trauma to the bronchial tree. Bronchiectasis, emphysema, peritonsillar abscess, and sinusitis have all been described with this organism.
3. Systemic infection with bacteremia or meningitis sometimes occurs, particularly in patients with other underlying medical problems.

*P. multocida* is a small, gram-negative, ovoid bacillus that grows well on blood agar but does not grow on gram-negative media such as MacConkey agar. Because of its superficial resemblance to *Haemophilus influenzae* and *Neisseria* organisms, infection with *P. multocida* in the respiratory tract and central nervous system may initially be misdiagnosed. Failure of growth on routine gram-negative media is an important clue.

Treatment of the patient with presumptive *P. multocida* infection (that is, any patient with a deep cat bite or scratch or a deep dog bite) should include careful washing and an attempt to leave the wound open. The antibiotic of choice is penicillin, taken for 8 to 10 days orally. Ampicillin, tetracycline, and quinolones are alternatives.

***Plague.*** Infection with *Yersinia pestis* usually results from a flea bite. Urban plague from *Y. pestis* is seen today as an important cycle only in devastated and impoverished cities. Sylvatic plague is the major cycle in the United States and is endemic in the southwest. The infected flea vector enters a community of susceptible rodents, such as ground squirrels, prairie dogs, marmots, wood rats, and rabbits, and transmits the bacteria. Mortality is high, and transmission to humans has recently been reported to be increased in New Mexico, California, Arizona, Colorado, and Utah.

Human plague occurs most often when an individual in a rural area is bitten by an infected flea. Infection may also occur through handling the carcasses of small mammals or by transfer of the vector from a domestic pet. Direct skin contact with an infected mammal (as when skinning rabbits) may also result in infection.

*Y. pestis* is a gram-negative bacillus that grows well in ordinary broth and agar. Bacteria usually are transmitted by the rat flea from the infected rodent. Immune rodents and humans maintain the organism in local vesicles. In less resistant hosts it spreads to lymph nodes and the bloodstream.

The incubation period is 2 to 6 days. Tender lymphadenitis and a local bubo (painful lymph node) then develop.

Systemic onset is abrupt, with high fever. Bacteremia and shock follow in 3 to 5 days.

Diagnosis is made by Gram stain and culture of the aspirate of a bubo and by blood culture. Other means include inoculation of the organism into mice or guinea pigs. Sera from patients in acute and convalescent stages of the disease may be obtained for serologic confirmation of the diagnosis.

All patients with plague should be isolated for the first 48 hours until secondary plague pneumonia can be ruled out. Lymph nodes should not be incised and drained until the patient has been treated with antibiotics. Oral tetracycline is effective early in the course of illness. Streptomycin, 30 mg/kg/day intramuscularly in two divided doses for 10 days, is the preferred agent for inpatient therapy. Alternative antibiotics include tetracycline and chloramphenicol.

Patients with plague pneumonia should be isolated, and all contacts should be quarantined and treated with tetracycline for 10 days.

Preventive measures include education, avoidance of sick or dead rodents and rabbits, and defleaing of pets.

***Tularemia.*** Tularemia has been reported from all states, but four (Arkansas, Louisiana, Oklahoma, and Texas) have had particularly high rates of infection. *Francisella tularensis,* a gram-negative pleomorphic coccobacillus, is the offending agent. Although the peak seasonal incidence varies with the climate, tick-borne tularemia is generally most common in summer, whereas in winter, contact with wild mammals (mainly rabbits during the hunting season) is most frequently the cause of disease.

Although infection with *F. tularensis* has been proved in at least 100 different species of mammals, wild rodents, especially cottontail rabbits, are the principal reservoir. Since transovarial passage occurs in ticks, ticks may serve as both reservoir and vector.

There are three main types of human infection:

1. Cutaneous lesions (ulceroglandular). This form is most common, and often occurs either after skinning or dressing rabbits or deer or after a tick bite. Tularemia is an occupational hazard for hunters, butchers, sheepshearers, and felt hat manufacturers.
   The typical lesion is macular and pruritic and ulcerates within 2 days (Fig. 4G-1). Regional lymph nodes then enlarge, become tender, and drain, with accompanying high fever (104 to 106° F, or 40 to 41° C). The tick bite is not always easy to find. A recent episode affected a 5-year-old boy from the Massachusetts coast, who developed fever and occipital lymphadenopathy. After a long search, repeated careful scalp examination revealed an engorged tick.
2. Tularemic pneumonia. This form is much less common, but may occur after inhalation of large amounts of infected particles; one example was a patient who had skinned and eviscerated six rabbits. Tularemic pneumonia also broke out in a family vacationing on Martha's Vineyard in August 1978. Mice were found inside the cottage and rabbits and ticks outside. The conclusion was that dogs may have mangled infected rabbits and then transmitted the bacteria via aerosol of saliva.
3. Typhoidal tularemia. This form occurs after ingestion of raw or improperly cooked meat. Symptoms include abdominal pain, diarrhea, fever, and bacteremia. A recent case occurred in a man from New Mexico who ate prairie dog meat cooked for only 2 minutes.

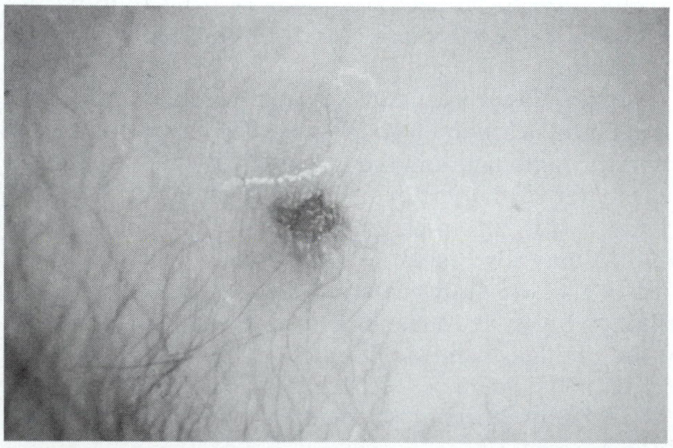

**Fig. 4G-1.** Cutaneous papule of tularemia after either a tick bite or the skinning or dressing of a rabbit or deer.

The diagnosis of tularemia is made based on a compatible history of exposure and clinical syndrome. Specific cysteine-dextrose blood agar is required for growth of the organism, but because laboratory propagation is potentially hazardous, culture should not be attempted. When cultured, the organism may require 10 days for growth. Diagnosis may be confirmed by a fluorescent antibody test or by development of an elevated serum antibody titer of 1:640 or greater within a week of onset of symptoms.

Treatment is with streptomycin, 1 g every 12 hours for 3 days, then 1 g/day. Tetracycline may be used alternatively.

***Rat-bite fever.*** Two bacteria that may cause disease after a rat bite are *Streptobacillus moniliformis* and *Spirillum minor.* Table 4G-1 gives the differences between the two diseases.

***Cat-scratch disease.*** Cat-scratch disease (CSD) is a bacterial infection that typically occurs in children or adolescents, often in the early fall to late winter. Over 90% of patients have a history of some contact with cats, commonly a scratch or a bite. However, the disease may follow other trauma, such as a dog or monkey bite or scratch or even a scratch from a rose thorn or porcupine quill. Cats only act as vectors; they do not become ill themselves.

The incubation period is 3 to 10 days, and the primary lesion is a tender papule (Fig. 4G-2). Lymphadenopathy then develops within 5 days to 2 months and is usually unilateral. The lymph node is tender, there may be overlying erythema, and 10% to 20% of nodes suppurate and drain. Systemic symptoms may include fever, headache, and malaise. Rarely, encephalopathy, radiculopathy, or oculoglandular disease (Parinaud syndrome) may be seen. Even more unusual cases have involved widespread dissemination to bone, liver and spleen, and lungs.

In the past diagnosis has relied on clinical and histologic criteria. These included a history of cat contact, sometimes with a primary lesion as well as regional adenopathy, with negative evaluation for other causes of lymphadenopathy. At one time, skin testing with a preparation made from tissues of CSD patients was also used. Node biopsy revealing the typical histologic lesion of CSD (stellate abscess) and a pleomorphic small gram-negative rod seen on Warthin-Starry silver staining or electron microscopy was confirmatory. It was not until 1988 that a group at the Armed Forces Institute of Pathology isolated the putative CSD bacillus, which they called *Afipia felis*. In some patients, culture of nodes as well as serologic testing with antibodies against *Afipia felis* suggested this was indeed the etiologic agent. However, since then, despite attempts by many investigators, these observations have not been reproduced in any other CSD patients.

Recently, an association between many cases of CSD and the organisms seen in Bacillary angiomatosis (BA) was noted. BA is a disease usually seen in patients infected with the human immunodeficiency virus (HIV), and is characterized by vascular lesions caused by infection with small gram-negative organisms of the genus *Rochalimaea*. Two species, *Rochalimaea henselae* and *Rochalimaea quintana* (the agent of trench fever) were described in BA lesions. In addition, these agents were found to cause a vascular abnormality of the liver called Bacillary peliosis (BP) as well as bacteremia without any cutaneous or visceral angiogenic lesions. Recently, based on further genetic analysis, the genus Rochalimaea has been unified with the genus *Bartonella*. While *Bartonella* is phylogenetically related to *Afipia,* they are distinct.

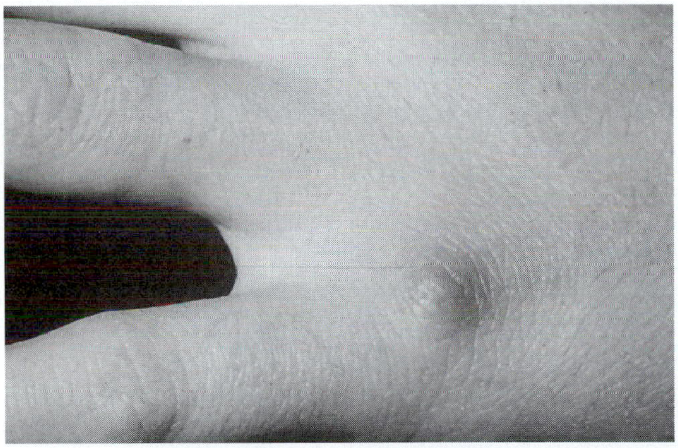

**Fig. 4G-2.** Primary lesion of cat scratch disease is a tender papule occurring 3 to 10 days after a scratch.

Multiple lines of evidence now support the *Bartonella* species as the cause of the majority of cases of CSD. A recent study found 41% of cats had asymptomatic bacteremia with *Bartonella henselae,* and the bacterium was also detected in their fleas. Characteristics of bacilli revealed by Warthin-Starry staining of tissues from patients with BA/BP and CSD are identical. Strong serologic responses to *Bartonella* have been detected in many patients with CSD. PCR (polymerase chain reaction) studies of multiple skin test antigens shown to be clinically useful in the diagnosis of CSD revealed *Bartonella* species and not *Afipia.* Similar studies of tissues from patients themselves are underway.

Thus it appears that domestic cats are a reservoir for zoonoses caused by *Bartonella* species, and that the organisms may cause a wide spectrum of disease, from CSD to BA or BP to bacteremia, depending on the characteristics of the host and perhaps other factors which have yet to be understood.

Treatment of CSD has been symptomatic in mild cases. Antibiotics that have been used successfully for treatment have included erythromycin, aminoglycosides (sometimes in combination), tetracyline and doxycycline or possibly Ciprofloxacin, although experience is limited.

### Viral infections

***Rabies.*** The most notorious viral disease caused by an animal bite is rabies. The epidemiology of rabies differs markedly between North America and Western Europe, where domestic animal rabies has been controlled since the 1950s, and the rest of the world, where it has not. Dogs account for the majority of cases worldwide, whereas sylvatic animals such as skunks, raccoons, wolves, bats (from bites or rarely aerosols), woodchucks, and foxes account for more than 90% of cases of animal rabies in North America. Dogs and cats are potentially rabid if they come into contact with these other animals. Although cases have been diagnosed in livestock, no cow-to-human transmission has ever been documented. Recent years have seen a raccoon rabies epizootic spread from the southern United States to the mid-Atlantic states and now to New England, with more cats than dogs becoming infected.

**Table 4G-1.** Rat-bite fever

| Differentiating characteristics | Streptobacillary fever | Spirillar fever |
|---|---|---|
| Organism | *Streptobacillus moniliformis* | *Spirillum* minor |
| Epidemiology | Bite, food | Bite |
| Incubation | <1 week | 1-3 weeks |
| Bite site | Prompt healing | Healing, then reactivation at the bite site |
| Rash | + | + |
| Arthralgia | + | – |
| Diagnosis | Culture, titer | Smear, dark field |
| Treatment | Penicillin, 1.5 g per day, for 10 days | Penicillin, 1.5 g per day for 10 days |

This points out the critical importance of knowing the epidemiology of rabies in one's region, information that is available from the Department of Public Health.

Human rabies is a rare disease in the United States with 18 cases reported between 1980 and 1993; three cases were diagnosed in 1993. Since monoclonal antibody typing of rabies strains can determine the regional and animal source, it is known that most of the United States' cases were acquired in countries where dog rabies is endemic. However, locally acquired cases do occur, and since 1980, seven of the nine patients known to have acquired rabies in the United States had bat-associated viruses. History of bat exposure, through spelunking was elicited in four of these seven cases.

**Mechanism.** Live virus is introduced into nerve tissue at the time of the bite. The virus persists 96 hours at the site and then spreads to the central nervous system. It replicates in gray matter and spreads along autonomic nerves to the salivary glands (Fig. 4G-3), adrenal glands, and the heart. The incubation period varies with the site of the bite from 10 days to, on rare occasions, as long as years.

**Clinical features.** Clinical features include a prodromal period of 1 to 4 days followed by high fever, headache, and malaise. Paresthesia at the site of inoculation occurs in 80% of patients. The rest of the sequence of events is familiar: agitation, hyperesthesia, dysphagia, paralysis, and death.

**Diagnosis.** In patients, no test is reliably positive before the onset of symptoms. Indirect fluorescent antibody (IFA) for virus is positive in biopsies of the brain or full-thickness skin in densely innervated areas, such as the nape of the neck. Brain biopsies are similarly positive in the affected animal. Cultures of these sites or of saliva is also diagnostic. Neutralizing antibodies are always detectable once clinical illness is present.

***Management of the patient with clinical rabies.*** When the rare patient is admitted with the clinical diagnosis of rabies, several steps should be taken quickly.

*Diagnosis.* The diagnosis must be made rapidly by fluorescent antibody staining of tissues as well as by mouse inoculation of the animal's brain tissue. Elevated antibody titers in the absence of immunization are clear evidence of infection. The first signs of clinical rabies are usually non-specific, such as malaise, anorexia, fatigue, headache, and fever. The acute neurologic illness that follows is most commonly characterized by intermittent episodes of hyperactivity. In some cases, however, there is progressive paralysis. The usual period of onset of symptoms to onset of coma is 10 days.

*Prevention of complications.* Basic clinical management consists of anticipating and preventing all treatable complications of the rabies infection.* Pulmonary hypoxia should be prevented by tracheostomy at the first sign of respiratory difficulty, monitoring of actual $Po_2$, and use of supplemental oxygen.

Anticonvulsant therapy should also be instituted. Extreme increases in intracranial pressure may be prevented by insertion of a CSF reservoir connected to the lateral ventricle, allowing withdrawal of the intraventricular fluid and measurement of intracranial pressure.

Cardiac arrhythmias may be anticipated by careful monitoring.

*Rabies prophylaxis information can be obtained by first contacting your local or state laboratory; and if needed Centers for Disease Control, 1600 Clifton Road, Atlanta, GA 30333 (404-639-3311, 24 hours a day).

A

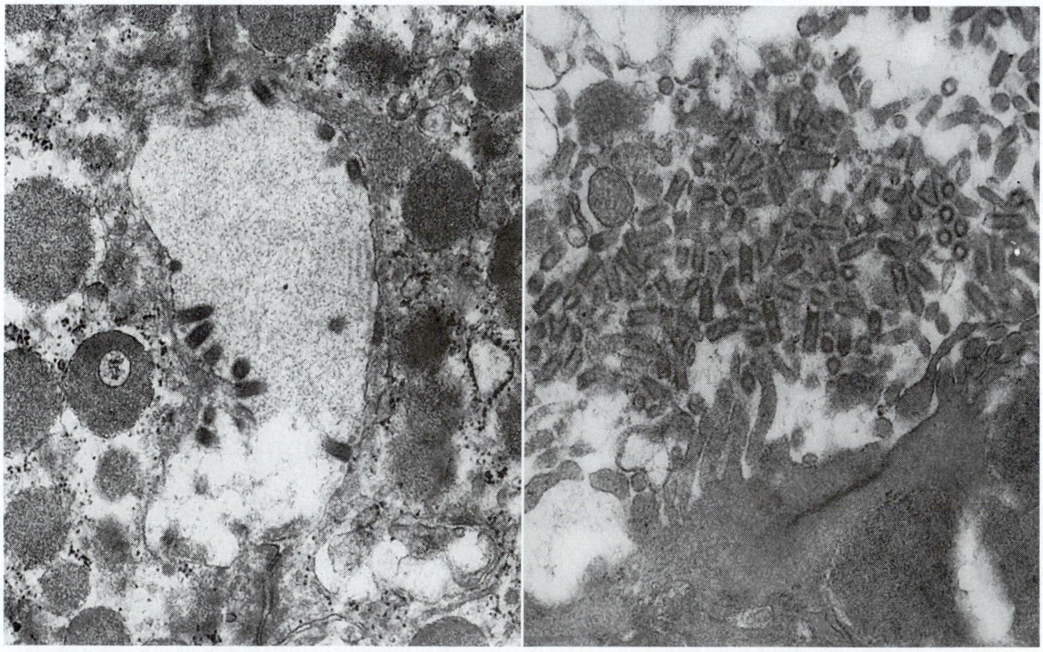

B

**Fig. 4G-3.** Rabies virus proliferates abundantly in the salivary glands of infected animals. Bullet-shaped rabies virions can be seen budding through the plasma membrane (**A**) and extracellular to the acinar cells (**B**). (Courtesy Frederick A. Murphy and Alyne K. Harrison, Viral Pathology Branch, Centers for Disease Control.)

Risk of exposure of hospital staff includes contamination of open wounds or mucous membranes with saliva or other potentially infectious material, such as neurologic tissue, spinal fluid, and urine. Blood, serum, and stool are not considered infectious.

Unfortunately there is no specific antiviral treatment for rabies, and the disease has been regarded as uniformly fatal. There now have been several cases of survival with prolonged cardiorespiratory support. It is certainly worth taking an aggressive approach to the patient with known rabies infection.

***Lymphocytic choriomeningitis.*** Lymphocytic choriomeningitis (LCM) virus is an infectious agent common to the house mouse but rarely transmitted to humans. Outbreaks of LCM virus infection in the United States recently have been traced to pet hamsters. Hamsters may excrete LCM virus for several months and, like many mice, may become lifelong carriers.

Three major forms of the illness in humans are a grippe-like illness, meningitis, or encephalitis. CSF usually reveals an increased mononuclear leukocyte count and hypoglycorrhachia. Symptomatic therapy is all that is available.

***Simian herpes B virus.*** Simian herpes B virus is found in old-world monkeys, especially rhesus and cynomolgus species. Infection occurs usually through a bite and less commonly after inhalation of monkey saliva or contact with infected monkey cell cultures. A vesicular lesion develops at the wound site, and there is progressive lymphangitis and fever. Confusion, reduced tendon reflexes in lower extremities, and respiratory paralysis may follow.

Diagnosis depends on viral isolation or the demonstration of intranuclear inclusion bodies in lymph nodes or in a brain biopsy specimen from the patient or animal, or on observation of a rise in neutralizing antibody titer to simian herpes B virus. Treatment includes Acyclovir and supportive care.

***Orf (contagious ecthyma).*** Orf is an endemic viral disease of sheep and goats. The disease in humans is contracted through direct cutaneous transmission. A nodular, vesicular, or pustular lesion develops at the site of contact, regional lymphadenopathy follows, and the lesions may progress to diffuse vesiculopapular rash which then subsides after 2 to 6 weeks.

## Managed Care Guide
## Bite Wounds

### Treatment

*Preexposure prophylaxis*

Preexposure prophylaxis is important for spelunkers, veterinarians, and virologists. Human diploid vaccine should be given. The neutralizing antibody titer should be followed to assure immunity in high-risk or exposed individuals.

*Postexposure prophylaxis*

After exposure the following questions must be asked:

1. What is the status of animal rabies in the locale where the exposure took place? (This may require a call to your public health department.)
2. Was the attack provoked or unprovoked?
3. Of what species was the animal?
4. What was the state of health of the animal?

Most animals transmit rabies virus in saliva only a few days before becoming ill themselves (dog and skunk, 5 days; fox, 3 days; cat, 1 day); bats, however, may harbor the virus for many months.

*Bites by household pets.* If the dog or cat is healthy and available for observation for 10 days, do not treat the patient unless the animal develops rabies. An exception to this rule is bites to the head, where an incubation period of 4 days has been reported and prophylaxis should begin immediately. At the first sign of rabies in the animal, treat the patient with rabies immune globulin (RIG) and human diploid cell vaccine (HDCV) (see Chapter 3). The symptomatic animal should be killed and tested as soon as possible.

If the pet is rabid or suspected to be rabid, or a pet from outside the US (especially Latin America, Africa, and most of Asia), treat with RIG and HDCV.

*Bites by wild animals.* All skunks, bats, foxes, coyotes, raccoons, bobcats, and other carnivores should be regarded as rabid unless laboratory tests prove negative. Treat the patient with RIG and HDCV.

*Bites by other animals.* Consider other animals (e.g., livestock, rodents, lagomorphs) individually. Local and state public health officials should be consulted on the need for prophylaxis. Bites by the following almost never call for antirabies prophylaxis: squirrels, hamsters, guinea pigs, gerbils, chipmunks, rats, mice and other rodents, rabbits, and hares.

### Specifics of treatment

1. The most important step is to cleanse the wound immediately and with a brush and soap to remove as much virus as possible. Rinse well, then perform a second scrub with soap or alcohol, **which is rabicidal**. This reduces the risk of rabies by as much as 90%.
2. If vaccine treatment is indicated, both RIG and human diploid cell rabies vaccine should be given as soon as possible, regardless of interval after exposure.

The administration of RIG is the more urgent procedure. If HDCV is not immediately available, start RIG and give HDCV as soon as it is obtained. RIG is given at a total dose of 20 IU/kg, with half infiltrated at the wound site and half IM in the arm or thigh. This passive immunization results in the early appearance of antibody but also inhibits the development of the active antibody from the human diploid vaccine: thus, the reason for prolonged dosage of the vaccines.

Active immunization is accomplished with the HDCV. It is given intramuscularly for a total of five doses, on days 0, 3, 7, 14, and 28. Serum for rabies antibody testing should be collected 2 weeks after the fifth dose. If there is no antibody response, give an additional booster.

Diagnosis is made by a complement fixation titer of more than 1:8 or isolation of virus on ovine kidney cell culture. Treatment is supportive.

## Arthropods: ticks

See Tularemia under Bacterial Infections and Lyme disease under Spirochetal Infections also.

### *Rickettsial infections*

**Rocky mountain spotted fever.** There are two principal tick vectors of Rocky Mountain spotted fever in the United States. *Dermacentor andersoni,* the wood tick, is distributed in the Rocky Mountain states and is active in the spring and early summer. *D. variabilis,* the dog tick, is found mainly in the eastern half of the United States, especially in the southern portion, extending from Oklahoma to Tennessee and northeast to Long Island and southern New England.

The clinical syndrome includes severe headache, then myalgia, followed by a maculopapular rash 2 or 3 days later. The rash typically starts on the wrists and ankles, extends to palms and soles, and then becomes central. If allowed to progress without treatment, the rash may become petechial.

Complement fixation (CF), indirect fluorescent antibody (IFA), indirect hemagglutination (IHA), latex agglutination (LA), and microagglutination (MA) studies are now available. These tests are more specific and more sensitive than the Weil-Felix (Proteus OX-19 or OX-2) titers.

Treatment for probable Rocky Mountain spotted fever is chloramphenicol, 2 or 3 g per day, or tetracycline, 2 g per day for 10 to 14 days, in adults. Prevention includes protective clothing, insecticides such as deet, inspection after possible tick exposure, and slow and steady tick removal with tweezers. Removal should be followed by careful washing of the site of attachment.

### *Parasitic infections*

**Babesiosis.** Babesiosis, a disease caused by the intracellular red blood cell parasite *Babesia microti* (Fig. 4G-4), is also transmitted by ticks. The parasite is transmitted by the larvae of the deer tick, *Ixodes dammini.*

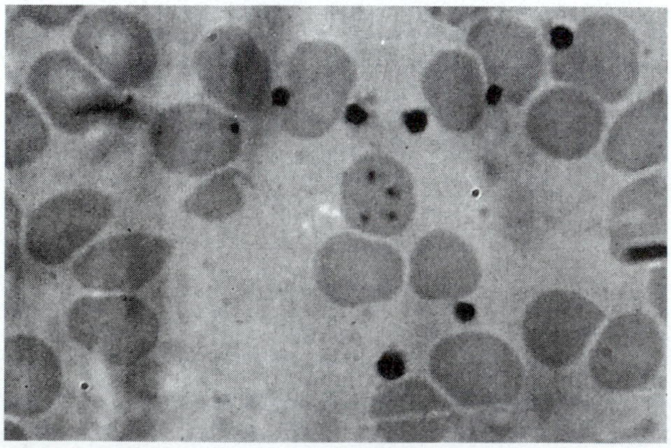

**Fig. 4G-4.** The location of babesiosis in red blood cells is evident in this peripheral blood smear.

The larvae overwinter, and the disease is spread by the nymph from May through July. The nymphs are tiny (1 mm) and usually not recognized. Eastern Long Island and Martha's Vineyard and Nantucket are the major endemic areas.

There is an increased risk in patients with T-lymphocyte depression or after splenectomy, but several cases have occurred in normal hosts. Symptoms of babesiosis include fever, drenching sweats, myalgia, and hemolytic anemia. Diagnosis is made by observation of the intracellular red blood cell parasite on a Giemsa-stained smear. The tetrads may be confused with the findings in falciparum malaria, but the epidemiology is usually distinct, and *Babesia*-infected red blood cells do not have pigment granules. Antibody titers are also helpful in making the diagnosis.

Treatment of mild infection is symptomatic. The combination of oral clindamycin, 600 mg, and quinine, 650 mg t.i.d., is effective. In splenectomized patients or other patients with high-grade parasitemia, exchange transfusion may be required.

### *Spirochetal infections*

**Lyme disease.** Lyme disease is caused by a spirochete, *Borrelia burgdorferi,* transmitted by *Ixodes dammini* or related ixodid ticks (see Chapter 87).

### *Toxin*

**Tick paralysis.** Tick paralysis may be caused by 43 different species of ticks, but most human cases in the United States arise from *Dermacentor* species. The paralysis is thought to be caused by a toxin secreted in the saliva of the tick that affects central as well as peripheral nerves. Typically the tick is attached from 4 to 7 days before the onset of symptoms. The presentation is an ascending flaccid paralysis, acute ataxia, or a combination of the two. Diagnosis depends on careful search of the scalp and body for the attached tick. Treatment consists of removing the tick after which improvement is seen within a few hours.

See Table 4G-2 for a complete listing of vectors, agents, and tick-transmitted disease.

## Arthropods: spiders, scorpions, and hymenoptera

***Spider bites.*** Although more than 100,000 species of spiders use venom to kill their prey, humans are sensitive to only a few of these toxins and death from spider envenomization is rare (Table 4G-3). Physicians should be aware of two spiders in particular in the United States, the black widow and the brown recluse.

**Black widow.** The black widow spider, *Latrodectus mactans* (4G-5), may be found in basements and backyards throughout the United States, especially in the South and in western Ohio. The female is venomous and aggressive. The spider is jet black and globular, with a red mark shaped like an hourglass on the abdomen. The venom causes central and peripheral nervous system excitement, autonomic activity, muscle spasms, hypertension, and vasoconstriction.

Sharp pain occurs at the site of the bite and is followed in about an hour by cramping pain locally, which spreads to the skeletal muscles of the extremities and the trunk. Severe abdominal pain may occur, causing a boardlike abdomen that is rigid but not tender. This is an important

**Table 4G-2.** Human diseases transmitted by ticks (United States)

| Disease | Etiologic agent | Vector |
|---|---|---|
| Colorado tick fever | Virus | *Dermacentor andersoni* |
| Human babesiosis | *Babesia* sp. (protozoon) | *Dermacentor variabilis Ixodes* sp. |
| Powassan encephalitis | Virus | *Ixodes cookei* |
| Q fever | *Coxiella burnetii* (rickettsia) | *Dermacentor andersoni*<br>*Amblyomma americanum*<br>*Octobius megnini** |
| Relapsing fever | *Borrelia* sp. (bacterium) | *Ornithodoros* sp. |
| Rocky Mountain spotted fever | *Rickettsia rickettsii* (rickettsia) | *Dermacentor andersoni*<br>*Dermacentor variabilis*<br>*Dermacentor occidentalis*<br>*Amblyomma americanum*<br>*Haemaphysalis leporispalustris*† |
| Tick paralysis | Salivary neurotoxin | *Dermacentor andersoni*<br>*Dermacentor variabilis* |
| *Borrelia burgdorferi*, Tularemia | *Francisella tularensis* (bacterium) | *Dermacentor andersoni*<br>*Dermacentor variabilis*<br>*Haemaphysalis leporispalustris*†<br>*Amblyomma americanum* |

*Found infected in nature, but transmission to man has not been reported.
†Transmits disease among rabbits.
Source: From HEW Publication No. (CDC) 79-8142, 1978.

**Table 4G-3.** Classification of poisonous spiders

| Family | Common name | Distribution |
|---|---|---|
| Theraphosidae | Tarantula | Worldwide |
| Dipluridae | Funnel-web spider | Australia |
| Heteropodidae | Banana spider | Tropics |
| Lycosidae | Wolf spider | South America |
| Ctenidae | Wandering spider | North America<br>Africa<br>South America<br>Middle East |
| Loxoscelidae | Recluse spider<br>Band-spinning spider | United States<br>South America |

From Pence HL: Sting, *Primary Care* 6:587, 1979.

differentiating point on examination. Ascending motor paralysis and hyperreflexia may also be present. A fatal outcome is rare. Treatment is usually supportive only; antivenin may be needed for children or the elderly.

**Brown recluse.** The brown recluse, *Loxosceles reclusus* (see Fig. 4G-5), prefers dark, undisturbed places like old sofas and old fur coats. Commonly found in the Missouri valley, it is 1.5 cm long and 0.6 cm wide, with a dark-brown, violin-shaped marking on the dorsal thorax. The brown recluse never attacks unless threatened. After the bite there is immediate local pain. The venom is cytotoxic and hematoxic, initiating tissue necrosis. Extensive extravasation of blood may occur at the site in the next 24 hours. The area of the bite may become necrotic, with ulceration extending down to the muscles 1 to 2 days later. Rarely, there is systemic toxicity with malaise, chills, nausea, and generalized rash. Treatment is supportive; no antiserum is available. Some surgeons suggest early excision of the bite site to prevent severe ulceration.

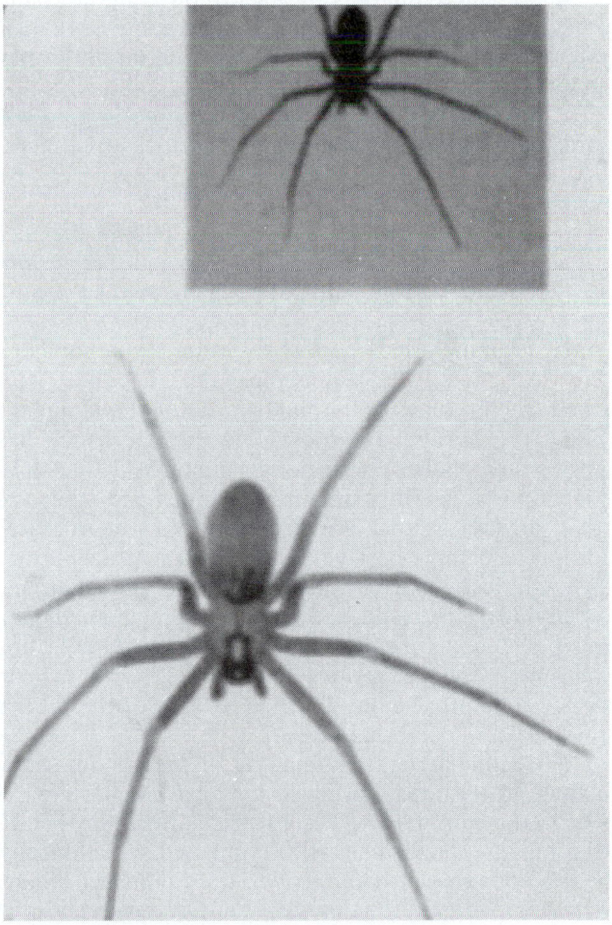

**Fig. 4G-5.** Brown recluse and black widow spiders may produce extensive tissue necrosis and ulceration.

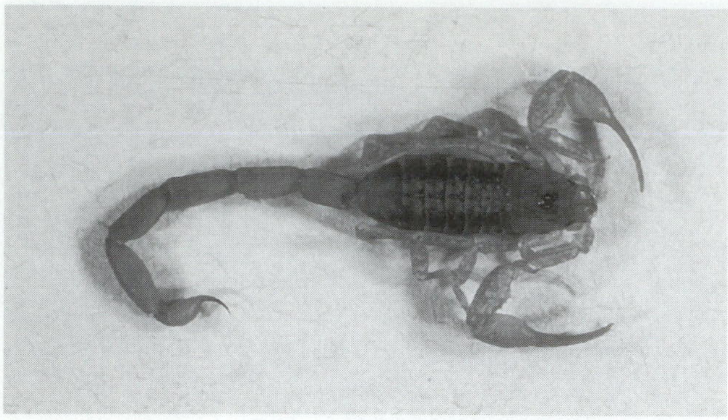

**Fig. 4G-6.** Scorpion.

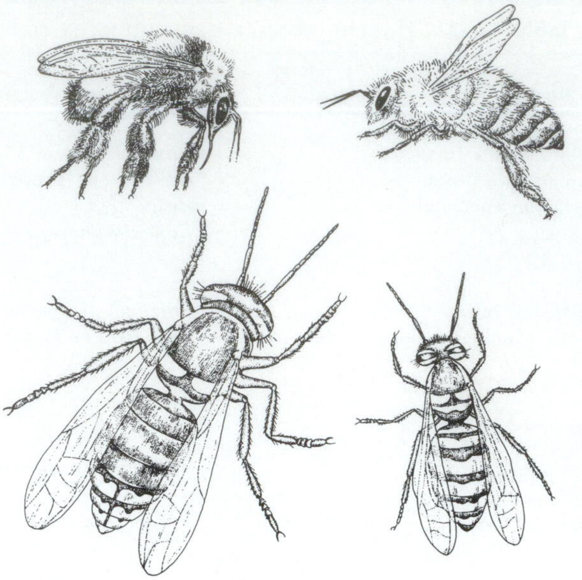


**Fig. 4G-7.** Hymenoptera stinging insects. (**A**) *Boribus sonorus,* the bumblebee. (**B**) *Apix mellifera,* the honeybee. (**C**) *Vespula maculata,* the white-faced wasp. (**D**) *Vespula maculifrous,* the yellow jacket. (From Lichenstein LM: *Hospital Practice* 10; No. 3, 1975. Drawing by Nancy Lou Makris.)

***Scorpion stings.*** The scorpion is an arthropod of 1 to 8 cm in length. It has an exoskeleton, a pair of pinching claws, and a tail with poison gland and stinger (Fig. 4G-6). There are about 650 species of scorpions, approximately 40 of which are found in the United States; most are not venomous. The venomous scorpions belong to the family Buthidae. Particularly dangerous species include *Centruroides sculpturatus* and *Centruroides gertschi,* which are found in the southwestern United States.

The clinical symptoms of a scorpion sting are painful burning and/or localized numbness at the site of the sting. Systemic manifestations such as tachycardia, high blood pressure, and respiratory impairment occur rarely.

Therapy includes immersion of the limb in cold water and a tourniquet about the limb, as well as treatment of symptoms.*

***Hymenoptera stings.*** Twice as many people die in the United States from Hymenoptera stings as from snake bites. Hymenoptera include bees, wasps, hornets, and fire ants.

Four prominent members of the order Hymenoptera are easily recognized: the bumblebee; the honeybee, with a barbed stinger, fuzzy body, and brown, blunt abdomen; the white-faced hornet; and the yellow jacket, which has a black shiny thorax with long antennae (Fig. 4G-7). Hymenoptera venoms contain histamines and other vasoactive substances that are hemolytic and neurotoxic in addition to being effective hypersensitizing agents.

The clinical syndrome after a sting includes sharp pain, a local wheal, erythema, and intense itching and edema. In the 1% of the population who are hypersensitive, a single sting may produce serious anaphylaxis with urticaria, nausea, abdominal pain, dypsnea, edema of the face and glottis, hypertension, and death.

The treatment requires removal of the venom sac and washing of the area, followed by local supportive care, such as cool compresses. The allergic patient may need 0.3 to 0.5 ml of epinephrine (1:1000) injected subcutaneously. The major factor in the consideration of insect stings in hypersensitive people is prevention. Desensitization with venom rather than with whole-body extract is now possible. The hypersensitive patient should have available an insect sting kit, such as that made by Hollister-Stier, containing medihaler epinephrine and chlorpheniramine maleate (Chlor-Trimeton).

***Insect sting allergies.*** Among the acute allergic reactions of greatest concern to primary care physicians are those due to insect stings. It is estimaged that 40 deaths occur each year due to anaphylaxis following insect stings. Acute nonfatal reactions following insect stings are fairly common and may occur as often as ten times each year for every 100,000 population. The stinging Hymenoptera, which includes bees, wasps, hornets, and yellow jackets, are the culprits. Except in beekeepers, the most common cause of such reactions is the yellow jacket, but most patients cannot identify the insect by which they were stung.

Based on the premise that patients who have had a systemic reaction are at substantial risk for another and that reactions tend to get worse, preventive measures were advocated beginning about 25 years ago. Patients who suffered only increasingly large local reactions were given immunotherapy at that time with extracts made from the entire bee bodies (whole body extract). Over a period of 15 years, thousands of patients were given immunotherapy with wholebody extract and seemed to do very well. Subsequently, a study done in beekeepers compared treatment with bee venom extract, whole-body extract, and placebo. Patients were then challenged by a deliberate bee sting. Venom therapy was shown to be effective, and treatment with whole-body extract was indistinguishable from placebo. If treatment with whole-body extract is relatively ineffective, then the favorable experience in the 15-year period in which it was used with apparent success suggests that the risk of a second life-threatening reaction following an acute systemic reaction is not great.

*Antivenin is obtainable from the Arizona State University Antivenom Laboratory (602-965-3116).

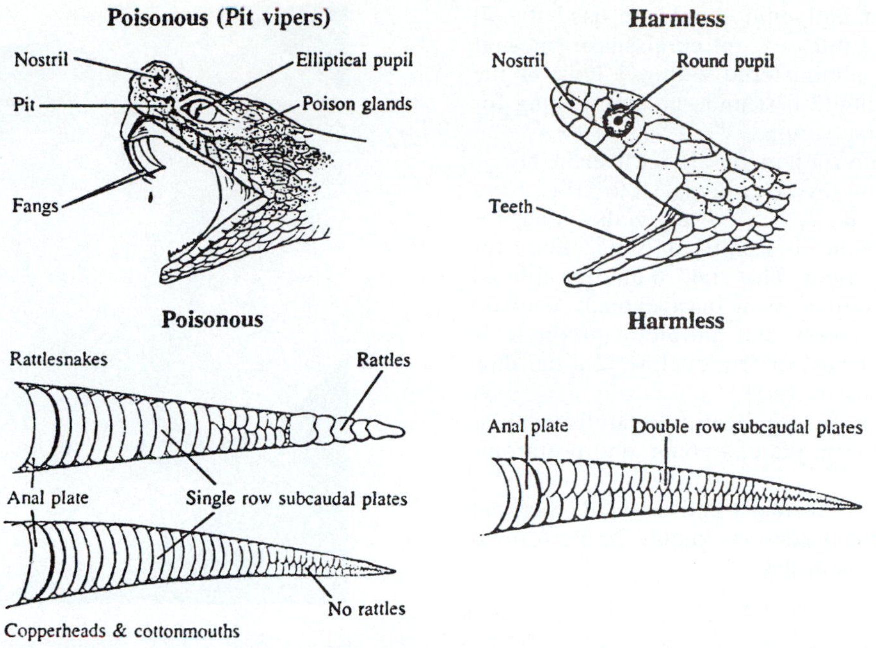


**Fig. 4G-8.** The differentiation of poisonous from harmless snakes. (From Wingert WA, and Wainschel J: *Resident and Staff Physician* 23:56, 1977.)

Venom extracts are now available for testing and treatment. Testing can identify those who have a high degree of IgE sensitivity to specific venoms. It would be imprudent not to recommend immunotherapy to those who have had either a drop in blood pressure, collapse, or respiratory difficulty after an insect sting and who have a high degree of skin sensitivity to one or more venoms. Since testing with venom extracts requires great care and freshly made extracts, it should be left to the expert. In addition, the primary care physician should immediately instruct the patient in the self-administration of epinephrine and provide the patient with an insect sting kit or its equivalent. Kits contain a preloaded syringe with epinephrine, antihistaminic tablets, and a tourniquet. The tourniquet is to be placed above the site of the sting if the sting is on an extremity. It is important to adequately instruct the patient or the parent in the technique of injection and, if possible, to have the patient or parent demonstrate that they have learned it. Patients should be told to take the antihistaminic immediately on being stung and to head for the nearest local emergency medical facility. They should inject epinephrine only if they feel a reaction coming on. Skin testing with venoms is not reliable if done shortly after a sting and should not be scheduled for three or four weeks after the sting has occurred.

## Snake bites

The two major poisonous snakes in the Americas are the pit viper and the coral snake. The coral snake belongs to the family Elapidae. The remainder of all poisonous snakes in the Western Hemisphere belong to the family Viperidae. The subfamily of pit vipers includes the rattlesnake, water moccasin, and copperhead.

About 7000 poisonous snakebites are reported in the United States annually. The largest number occur in the southwestern and Gulf states. Two poisonous snakes are native to New England. The northern copperhead, also called the highland moccasin, is pink or reddish-brown and is marked with large barrels of chestnut brown resembling dumbbells or hourglasses. The bite is painful but rarely fatal. The timber rattler is dark brown with chevrons of black and brown. The rattle on the tail buzzes when the snake is disturbed.

***Clinical signs.*** The degree of toxicity of a snakebite depends on the potency of the venom, the amount injected, the size and condition of the snake, and the size of the person bitten. The pit viper bite has instant clinical manifestations. There is a painful wheal at the site of the bite, with local edema, numbness, and within moments ecchymosis and painful lymphadenopathy. Nausea, vomiting, sweating, fever, drowsiness, and slurred speech may then develop. Bleeding of the gums and hematemesis are common hemorrhagic manifestations.

To ensure proper treatment, it is extremely important to establish that the bite is from a poisonous snake, i.e., that there are distinct fang punctures and immediate local pain, followed by edema and discoloration within 30 minutes. It is helpful to inspect the snake, since those that are poisonous may be distinguished by the presence of fangs and the shape of the pupils (Fig. 4G-8).

***Treatment.*** The limb should be immobilized and a ligature applied proximal to the wound. The ligature should be released for 90 seconds every 15 minutes. The physician should make two longitudinal incisions through the fang marks and apply suction intermittently for the first hour. An attempt should be made to neutralize the venom with immune serum.* A photograph of snakes common to the geographic area is important for the emergency ward.

*Emergency information and specific immune serum can be obtained from the Oklahoma City Poison Control Center (405-271-5454, 24 hours a day); Wyeth Laboratory (antivenom) (215-688-4400, days; local Wyeth number, nights).

Polyvalent pit viper antivenin should be used for all severe American snake bites except coral snake bites. If possible it should be administered within 1 hour of the bite, and the patient should first undergo skin testing for hypersensitivity to horse serum.

The dose of antivenin for a moderate rattlesnake bite is 4 to 7 μ (vials), and for severe cases is 15 to 20 μ; for a water moccasin bite, it is 1 to 4 μ (vials); and for copperhead bites, antivenin is usually only necessary for a child or an elderly patient. The vials should be diluted in 500 ml of normal saline given intravenously over 30 minutes. Antitetanus therapy and antibiotic prophylaxis with penicillin, 2 g per day, or tetracycline, 2 g per day, should be started for severe bites.

Supportive treatment (hospitalization), careful evaluation of baseline hematocrit, platelet count, and prothrombin time are important.

The wound should be cleansed and covered. Surgical debridement of superficial necrosis should be performed between the third and tenth days.

## Marine diseases

***Erysipeloid.*** Erysipeloid is an acute infection of traumatized skin, usually affecting fishermen, butchers, and those handling raw fish, poultry, or meat produce. *Erysipelothrix rhusiopathiae* is a gram-positive bacillus found in the mouth of fish, swine, and poultry.

The initial symptom after a bite or injury, is burning pain at the site. This is followed by a warm, tender, raised, violaceous, or wine-colored area often associated with lymphangitis. As infection advances, the central lesion clears.

The antibiotic of choice is oral penicillin (1 to 2 g per day) for 10 days, with immobilization and soaking of the limb for 2 or 3 days.

***Seal bite.*** Normally seal bite is on the finger of a trainer or a seal hunter, thus the term *seal finger* or *Spaek finger* (Fig. 4G-9). The etiologic agent is unclear; the Canadian government is now subsidizing a study in an attempt to isolate the organism.

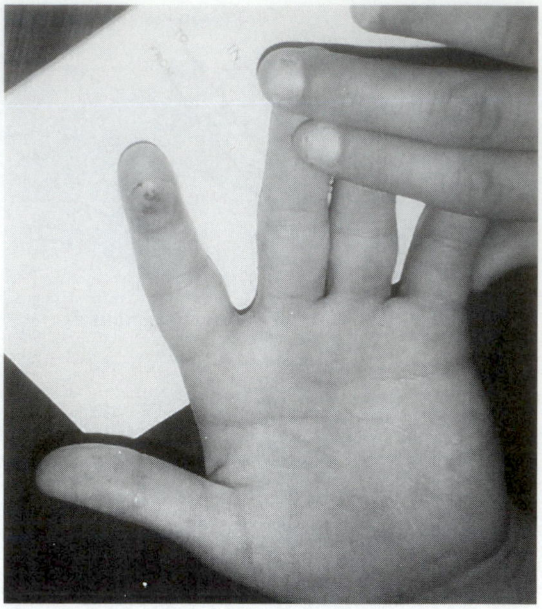

**Fig. 4G-9.** "Seal finger," a bite injury that may produce cellulitis, tenosynovitis, and progressive arthritis.

The incubation period is 4 to 8 days and is followed by throbbing pain, erythema at the site, and swelling of the joint proximal to the bite. Untreated, Spaek finger produces cellulitis, tenosynovitis, and progressive arthritis. The treatment before antibiotics was amputation of the affected finger to relieve the severe pain and deformity. Tetracycline, 500 mg orally q.i.d. for 10 days, is now the antibiotic of choice. It is also helpful to immobilize and elevate the finger, as well as to soak it several times a day.

***Jellyfish sting.*** Venom is discharged from nematocysts in the tentacles of the larger jellyfish. Stings are characterized by instant burning pain where the tentacles contact the skin, followed by the development of red, elevated, linear lesions. In more severe cases the victim experiences nausea, vomiting, abdominal and generalized muscular cramps, and difficulty in breathing. Stings of the sea wasps *Chironex fleckeri* and *Chiropsalmus* are extremely severe.

Several species of the most common poisonous jellyfish have a red, yellow, or brownish color when they attain a medium to large size. The sea nettle *(Chyrsaora quinqecirrha)* is one of the most common of these jellyfish along the Atlantic and Gulf coasts (Fig. 4G-10). Its close relative, the lined sea nettle, is commonly encountered along the Alaska and California coasts. Contact with a sea nettle usually produces a mild pruritic rash. Extensive contact may produce a systemic reaction including severe cramps and respiratory difficulty.

Highly toxic reactions may result from contact with two common, large jellyfish. The first, the Portuguese man-of-war *(Physalia physalis),* is a jellyfish that floats on the surface by means of a gas-filled float that changes shape to catch the prevailing wind. Its tentacles contain an extremely toxic poison that can produce severe burns and blisters even when the jellyfish is dead and has washed up on the beach.

The lion's mane *(Cyanea capillata)* is the other highly toxic jellyfish. It is prevalent along the Pacific, Atlantic, and Gulf coasts (see Plate I-8). This jellyfish has a bell-like saucer shape and develops a reddish-brown color as it grows larger. It has 16 marginal lobes and shaggy clusters of more than 150 tentacles below. Lion's mane is the largest jellyfish in the world, sometimes attaining a diameter of 8 feet. Its tentacles produce severe burning and blistering and severe exposure may cause muscle cramps and respiratory difficulty. In Sir Arthur Conan Doyle's story "The Adventure of the Lion's Mane," Sherlock Holmes solves a homicide caused by contact between the victim and this medusae in a tidepool. For further information, see the *Audubon Society Field Guide to North American Seashore Creatures* and other sources listed in the Bibliography.

On-site resuscitation must be the first priority. A swimmer who sustains major contact with any poisonous jellyfish should be brought aboard a boat or assisted to the beach. Pour ocean water over the wound; do not rub with sand, as this will fire the nematocysts that have *not*

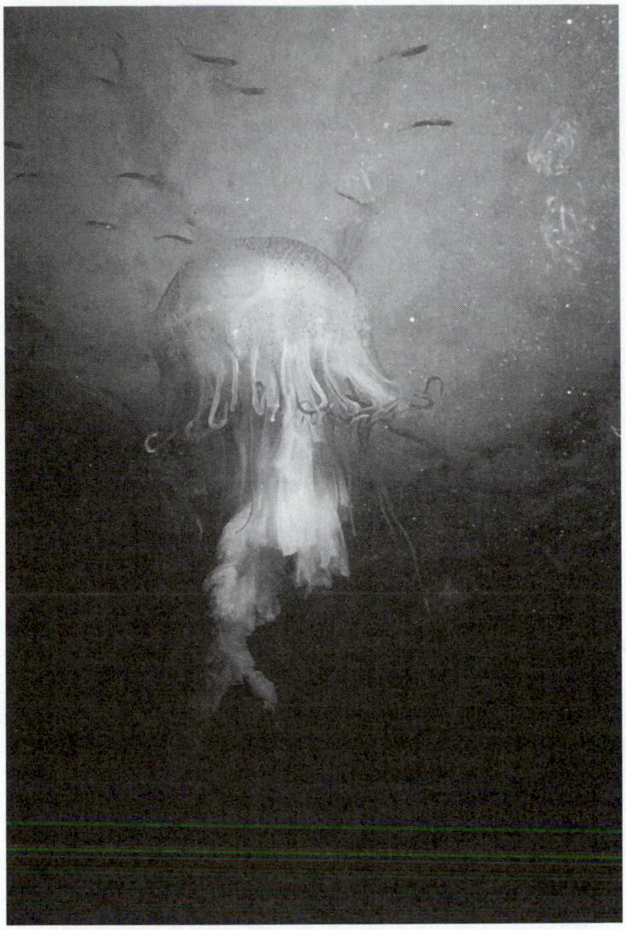

**Fig. 4G-10.** Sea nettle, a common toxic jellyfish along the Atlantic and Gulf coasts. This specimen was photographed in Block Island Sound, Rhode Island. (Courtesy Harold Wes Pratt.)

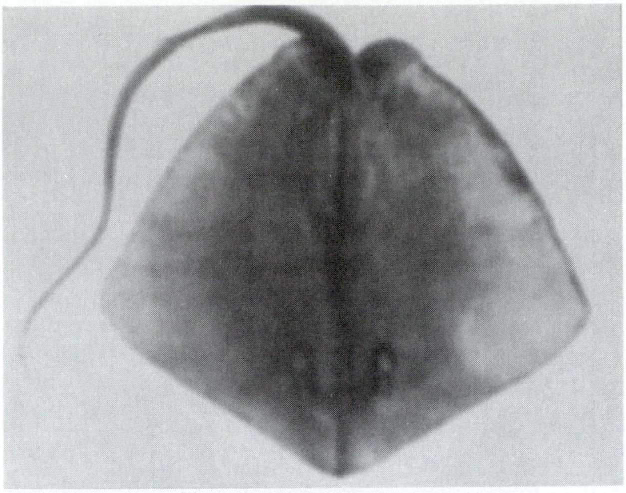

**Fig. 4G-11.** Stingray, commonly found along the southern California and south Atlantic coasts.

discharged. Attempt to remove tentacles with gloves. Alcohol or acetic acid (or vinegar) then inactivates the penetrating nematocysts. An effective first line treatment is to cover affected areas of skin with meat tenderizer. The papain present in most of these preparations digests the nematocysts and tentacles, and alleviates the discomfort. Meat tenderizer should be applied gently and generously. Hot water should not be used on coelenterate stings; it may also cause firing of the nematocysts.

***Stingray sting.*** On the North American coast several spiny groups of fish contain poison: the stingray, scorpion, catfish, certain sea urchins, and one shellfish, *Conus californicus*.

Stingrays abound off the coast of southern California, the south Atlantic states, and the Gulf Coast. The body is flattened and the pectoral fins broadened laterally so that they present a flat disk. The tail is long and equipped with barbs (Fig. 4G-11). The barb penetrates a foot, releases venom, and lacerates tissue on coming out. The pain is sharp and immediate. The jagged wound bleeds and may contain torn integumentary sheath. The leg becomes edematous, and if a large amount of venom is inoculated, systemic symptoms may also occur.

Treatment starts with immediate and thorough irrigation of the wound with salt water to remove venom and act as a vasoconstrictor. Then the wound is immersed in hot water for at least one-half to one hour. The heat will neutralize the toxin. Finally, remaining pieces of sheath should be searched for. Tetanus toxoid and antibiotics may also be necessary.

***Sea urchin injuries.*** A whorl or broken spine from some varieties of sea urchin may cause a granulomatous reaction several days to weeks later. Gross evidence of foreign material should be removed with tweezers when these injuries occur. The area should also be x-rayed if irritation persists.

***Coral cuts.*** Coral cuts may produce chronic ulcers if not treated; fragments of calcareous material and animal protein may be left behind. First aid should include thorough cleansing with a soft brush and soapy water, then an alcohol rinse, followed by peroxide to remove bacteria and fine material.

Fire coral is a highly toxic species that is found throughout the Caribbean and Gulf Coast (Fig. 4G-12). It has an upright, branching or platelike structure. It is brown to creamy yellow and is covered with tiny pores occupied by white polyps. This coral can produce a severe burning sensation and bullous dermatitis. Many other corals may produce skin irritation and mild rashes when touched. Treatment is symptomatic.

## Red tide

Red tides occur naturally along many parts of the North American coasts and are caused by a population explosion of a reddish brown phytoplankton. These microscopic algae thrive in low turbulence, estuarine, or coastal water. Most species are harmless, but some are indirectly poisonous to man. Shellfish that feed on the posionous species accumulate high concentrations of any toxins that may be present. These toxins may produce paralytic shellfish poisoning (PSP), diarrheic shellfish poisoning

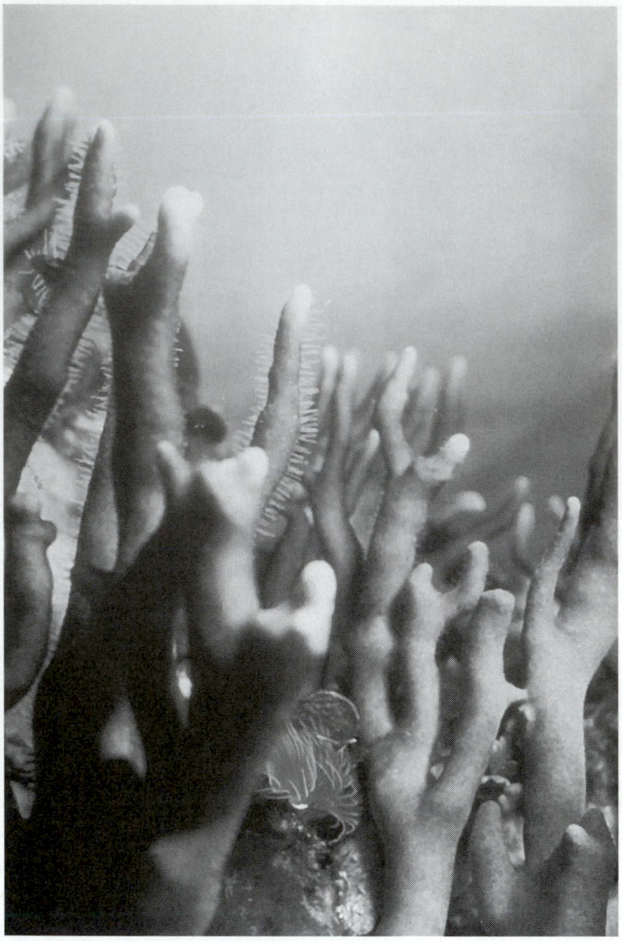

Fig. 4G-12. Fire coral is found in large branching or platelike configurations along the Florida coast and in the West Indies. (Courtesy Harold Wes Pratt.)

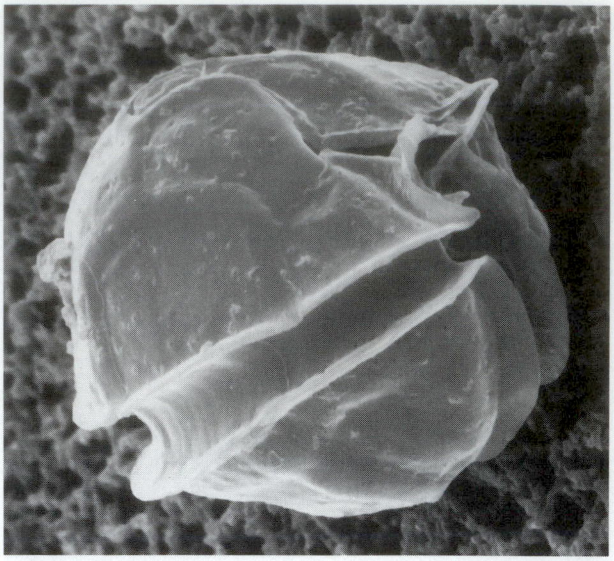

Fig. 4G-13. Electron microscopic photograph of PSP causing *Gonyaulax tamarensises* plankton. (From the University of Rhode Island.)

(DSP), and neurotoxic shellfish poisoning (NSP) when ingested by people.

***Occurrence in North America.*** Red tides occur in many parts of the world and were mentioned in the Bible. In North America they are found along the Atlantic coast, off Florida, and along the Pacific coast into Alaska. In New England toxic red tide first became a problem in 1972 when population blooms of toxic *Gonyaulax* (Fig. 4G-13) appeared from Maine to Cape Cod. Approximately thirty cases of illness were reported during this tide, with no fatalities. Official bans on shellfish shipments controlled spread of PSP, but the public overreacted by not eating many other seafoods that were safe. The "Florida red tide" (*Gymnodinium breve* or *Ptychodiscus brevis*), found in the Gulf of Mexico where it causes massive fish kills, makes shellfish mildly toxic. It is also associated with the respiratory problems affecting some people in coastal areas from wind-borne surf spray.

Public health surveillance has successfully protected most individuals in the United States from eating shellfish that have been contaminated by red tide toxins. "However, recreational boaters cruising from Southern New England to Canada may be unknowingly exposed to paralytic shellfish poisoning. 'Picking up a bucket of clams for a chowder' is a tradition of cruising and boating people. Frequently they dig clams or mussels in remote coves or on ledges where there is no posting. They may not be aware that a local shellfish bed is closed because of red tide." Because of unfamiliarity with local conditions, therefore, people who gather shellfish recreationally have higher chances of being at risk than does the public, which consumes commercially harvested clams, oysters, and mussels.

***The toxic phytoplankton.*** Red tide is caused by at least 60 different species of phytoplankton; of these, only four or five have been identified as a toxic Saxitoxin (Fig. 4G-14) and its closely related analogs are the most common of the neurotoxins elaborated by these phytoplankton. These toxins are paralytic poisions that block nerve transmission and skeletal muscle contraction. The toxins appear to inhibit sodium influx specifically without changing other ionic potentials within a cell. The muscles of the diaphragm are particularly sensitive to saxitoxin, and death usually results from respiratory failure. Many people also suffer from transient gastrointestinal reactions after eating shellfish from areas with large populations of diarrhetic shellfish-toxin–producing dinoflagellates. *Dinophysis* and *Prorocentrum* spp. are suspected to be the cause of DSP.

Shellfish, including clams, quahogs, scallops, mussels, oysters, and other bivalves, which survive by filter feeding, siphon large volumes of water each day. A single large oyster has the capability of filtering up to 7 gallons of water an hour. When red tide is present, vast numbers of toxin-bearing plankton may be filtered by shellfish, remaining in their stomachs. Other types of seafood, such as finfish, lobsters, and crabs, which are eaten without stomachs, are safe when fresh, even when caught in red tide waters. (Scallops, although filter feeders, are not considered to be a high red tide risk, since only the muscle

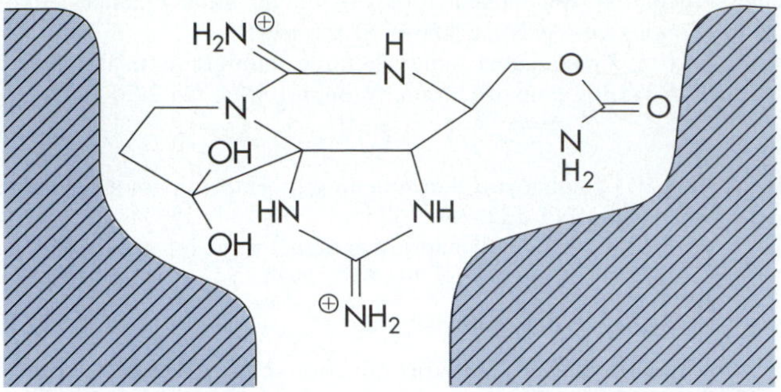


**Fig. 4G-14.** Hypothetic plugging model for saxitoxin-sodium channel mteraction. (From Hille B: *Biophys J* 15:615, 1975.)

is consumed, not the stomach, as is the case with all other shellfish.) Shellfish, on the other hand, may remain contaminated long after the red tide appears to have subsided. It takes at least several weeks of flushing with clean water to purge shellfish of the phytoplankton and its saxitoxin before they become safe to eat.

The concentration of toxin in three contaminated clams may be enough to make a person ill. The toxin attacks the human nervous system within 3 minutes, producing symptoms that include numbness of the lips, tingling of the extremities, and loss of coordination. Speech may become incoherent, and the patient may complain of lightheadedness and nausea. Symptoms of paralytic shellfish poisoning may be mistaken for drunkenness. Eventually, if large amounts of toxin have been ingested, respiratory paralysis may occur. There is no known antidote for the toxin. Artificial ventilation may provide support for a patient during the acute phases of poisoning. When substantial doses of poison have been ingested, however, fatal outcomes have been recorded.

In addition to saxitoxin, eleven other toxins have been isolated: gonyautoxin I through VII, neosaxitoxin, and epigonyautoxin VIII, C3, and C4. "The toxicity of paralytic shellfish toxins is traditionally expressed in mouse units (mu), where one mouse unit is defined as the amount required to kill a 20 g mouse within 15 minutes by intraperitoneal injection." Table 4G-4 compares selected toxicities to the strength of saxitoxin.

***Precautions.*** During the spring, later summer, and fall many types of microscopic algae mass together and bloom or proliferate. During these times, they may color the water reddish, yellow, or green. No single factor is known to cause these population explosions of algae. In New England increased rainfall with inceased stream discharges followed by days with cloudless and bright weather usually precipitate one. The red tide may appear in localized patches or as longshore streamers. The red color suddenly disappears after a few days or weeks. Discoloration of the water, however, does not necessarily accompany the presence of phytoplankton blooms, which may be contaminated with saxitoxin. This is particularly true in northern Maine and off the Canadian seacoast. Some organisms that may produce the red tide emit a bluish green bioluminescence that can make the waves glow at night. Travelers along coastal areas of the United States and Canada should be alert for warnings about red

**Table 4G-4.** Specific and relative toxicities of paralytic shellfish poisons

| Toxin | Specific toxicity (mu/mole) | Relative toxicity |
|---|---|---|
| Saxitoxin | 2045 | 1 |
| Neosaxitoxin | 1038 | 0.50 |
| Gonyautoxin-I | 1638 | 0.80 |
| Gonyautoxin-II | 793 | 0.39 |
| Gonyautoxin-III | 2234 | 1.09 |
| Gonyautoxin IV | 673 | 0.33 |
| Gonyautoxin-V | 354 | 0.17 |
| Gonyautoxin-VI | 180 | 0.09 |
| Gonyautoxin-VIII | 280 | 0.14 |
| 11-Epigonyautoxin-VIII | 17 | $8.3 \times 10^{-3}$ |

tide and should inquire about the safety of shellfish. Cooking of shellfish, while it kills bacteria, does not destroy the toxins that cause PSP. It is advisable to enjoy those other types of seafood that are entirely safe, even when caught in red tide waters.

## BIBLIOGRAPHY


### General

Berzon DR et al: Animal bites in a large city—a report on Baltimore, Maryland, *Am J Public Health* 62:422, 1972.

Elliot DL et al: Pet associated illness, *N Engl J Med* 313:985, 1985.

Hubbert WT et al: *Diseases transmitted from animal to man,* Springfield, Ill, 1975, Charles C Thomas.

Kahrs RF et al: Diseases transmitted from pets to man: an evolving concern for veterinarians, *Cornell Vet* 68:442, 1978.

Steele JH: A bookshelf on veterinary public health, *Am J Public Health* 63:291, 1973.

Strassburg MA et al: Animal bites: Patterns of treatment, *Ann Emerg Med* 10:193, 1981.

### Dog Bites

Callaham M: Prophylactic antibiotics in common dog bite wounds: a controlled study, *Ann Emerg Med* 9:410, 1980.

Kalb R et al: Cutaneous infection at dog bite wounds associated with fulminant DF-2 septicemia, *Am J Med* 78:687, 1985.

Klein D: Friendly dog syndrome, *N Y State J Med* 66:2306, 1966.

Parris HM et al: Epidemiology of dog bites, *Public Health Rep* 74:891, 1959.

### Human Bites

Goldstein EJC: Role of anaerobic bacteria in bite-wound infections, *Rev Infect Dis* 6(Suppl I):S177, 1984.

Mann R et al: Human bites of the hand: twenty years of experience, *J Hand Surg* 77, 1977.

Peeples E et al: Wounds of the hand contaminated by human or animal saliva, *J Trauma* 20:383, 1980.

### Pasteurella Multocida

Gump GW, Holden RA: Endocarditis caused by a new species of Pasteurella, *Ann Intern Med* 76:275, 1972.

Hubbert WT et al: *Pasteurella multocida* infection due to animal bite, *Am J Public Health* 60:1103, 1970.

Jarvis WR et al: *Pasteurella multocida* osteomyelitis following dog bites, *Am J Dis Child* 135:625, 1981.

Lucas GL, Bartlett DH: *Pasteurella multocida* infection in the hand, *Plast Reconstr Surg* 67:49, 1981.

Stevens DL: Antibiotics susceptibilities of human isolates of *Pasteurella multocida, Antimicrob Agents Chemother* 16:322, 1979.

Swartz MN, Kunz LF: *Pasteurella multocida* infection in man, *N Engl J Med* 261:889, 1959.

Weber DJ et al: *Pasteurella multocida* infections. Report of 34 cases and review of the literature, *Medicine* 63:133, 1984.

### Plague

Butler T et al: *Yersinia pestis* infections in Vietnam, *J Infect Dis* 133:493, 1976.
Finegold KJ: Pathogenesis of plague, *Am J Med* 45:549, 1968.
Kaufmann AF et al: Trends in human plague in the US, *J Infect Dis* 141:522, 1980.
Reed WP et al: Bubonic plague in southwestern United States, *Medicine* 49:465, 1970.
von Reyn CF et al: Epidemiologic and clinical features of an outbreak of bubonic plague in New Mexico, *J Infect Dis* 136:489, 1977.
Weninger BG et al: Human bubonic plague transmitted by a domestic cat scratch, *JAMA* 251:927, 1984.

### Tularemia

Guerrant RL: Tick-borne oculo-glandular tularemia, *Arch Intern Med* 136:811, 1976.
Kloch CE et al: Tularemia epidemic associated with the deerfly, *JAMA* 266:149, 1973.
Markowitz LE: Tick-borne tularemia: An outbreak of lymphadenopathy in children, *JAMA* 254:2922, 1985.
Roueche B: Annals of Medicine, *The New Yorker* pp 49-57, August, 1980.
Teutsch SM et al: Pneumonic tularemia on Martha's Vineyard, *N Engl J Med* 301:824, 1979.
Young LS et al: Tularemia epidemic: Vermont 1968. Forty-seven cases limited to contact with muskrats, *N Engl J Med* 280:1253, 1969.

### Rat-Bite Fever

Cole JS et al: Rat-bite fever, *Ann Intern Med* 71:979, 1969.
Rogosa M: *Streptobacillus moniliformis* and *Spirillum minor.* Lennette EH et al, editors: *Manual of Clinical Microbiology,* American Society of Microbiology, 1974.
Roughgarden JW: Antimicrobial therapy of rat-bite fever: a review, *Arch Intern Med* 116:39, 1975.

### Cat-Scratch Disease

Brenner DJ et al: Proposal of *Afipia* gen nov, with *Afipia felis* sp nov (formerly the cat scratch disease bacillus), *Afipia clevelandensis* sp nov (formerly the Cleveland Clinic Foundation strain), *Afipia broomeae* sp nov, and three unnamed genospecies, *J Clin Microbiol* 29:2450, 1991.
Carithers HA et al: Cat scratch disease. Its natural history, *JAMA* 207:312, 1969.
English CK et al: Cat scratch disease: isolation and culture of the bacterial agent, *JAMA* 259:1347, 1988.
Gerber MA et al: The aetiological agent of cat scratch disease, *Lancet* 1:1236, 1985.
Koehler JE et al: *Rochalimaea henselae* infection. A new zoonosis with the domestic cat as reservoir, *JAMA* 271:531, 1994.
Koehler JE, Tappero JW: Bacillary angiomatosis and bacillary peliosis in patients infected with human immunodeficiency virus, *Clin Infect Dis* 17:612, 1993.
Margileth AM: Cat scratch disease: Non-bacterial regional lymphadenitis. The study of 145 patients and a review of the literature, *Pediatrics* 42:803, 1968.
Regnery RL et al: Serological response to *Rochalimaea henselae* antigen in suspected cat-scratch disease, *Lancet* 339:1443, 1992.
Warwick WJ: The cat scratch syndrome, many diseases or one disease? *Prog Med Virol* 9:256, 1967.
Wear DJ et al: Cat scratch disease: a bacterial infection, *Science* 221:1403, 1983.

### Rabies

Anderson LJ et al: Postexposure trial of human diploid cell strain, *J Infect Dis* 142:133, 1980.
Fishbein DB: Rabies, *Infect Dis Clin North Am* 5:53, 1991.
Hough SA et al: Human to human transmission of rabies virus by a corneal transplant, *N Engl J Med* 300:603, 1979.
Meyer HW: Rabies vaccine, *J Infect Dis* 2:287, 1980.
Porras C et al: Recovery from rabies in man, *Ann Intern Med* 85:44, 1976.
Rabies Prevention: Recommendation of Immunization Practices Advisory Committee (ACIP), *MMWR* 40:86, 1991.
Smith JS et al: Unexplained rabies in three immigrants in the United States. A virologic investigation, *N Engl J Med* 324:205, 1991.

### LCM

Biggar RJ et al: Lymphocytic choriomeningitis outbreak associated with pet hamsters, *JAMA* 232:494, 1975.
Hirsch MS et al: Lymphocytic choriomeningitis virus infection traced to a pet hamster, *N Engl J Med* 291:610, 1974.

### Simian Herpes B Virus

Davidson WF, Hummeier R: B virus infection in man, *Ann N Y Acad Sci* 85:970, 1968.
Holmes GP et al: B virus *(Herpesvirus simae)* infection in humans: epidemiologic investigation of a cluster, *Ann Intern Med* 112:833, 1990.

### Arthropods
### Rocky Mountain Spotted Fever

Hazard GW: Rocky Mountain spotted fever in the eastern United States, *N Engl J Med* 380:57, 1969.
Hilmick CG et al: Rocky Mountain spotted fever: clinical, laboratory and epidemiologic features of 262 cases, *J Infect Dis* 150:480, 1984.
Kaplowitz LG et al: Rocky Mountain spotted fever: a clinical dilemma, *Curr Clin Top Infect Dis* 2:89, 1981.
Rocky Mountain spotted fever—United States, 1982, *MMWR* 32(17): 229, 1983.

### Babesiosis

Jacoby GA et al: Treatment of transfusion-transmitted babesiosis by exchange transfusion, *N Engl J Med* 303:1098, 1980.
Ruebush TK et al: Human babesiosis on Nantucket Island, *Ann Intern Med* 86:6, 1976.
Ruebush TK, Spielman A: Human babesiosis in the United States, *Ann Intern Med* 88:263, 1978.
Wittner M: Successful chemotherapy of transfusion babesiosis, *Ann Intern Med* 96:601, 1982.

### Tick Paralysis

Centers for Disease Control: *Ticks: of public health importance and their control.* HEW Publication No. (CDC) 79-8142, 1978.
Gothe R et al: The mechanisms of pathogenicity in the tick paralysis, *J Med Entomol* 16:357, 1979.
Tick paralysis, *MMWR* 30(18):217, 1981.

### Spider Bites

Editorial: Spider bites, *Lancet* 2:509, 1969.
Gorham JR: The brown recluse spider, *Ioxosceles reclusa* and necrotic spider bite—a new public health problem in the U.S., *J Environ Health* 31:138, 1968.
Hunt GP: Bites and stings of uncommon arthropods. 1. Spiders, *Postgrad Med* 70:91, 1981.
Pence HL: Stinging insect allergy, *Prim Care* 6:587, 1979.
Rees RS: Do brown recluse spider bites induce pyoderma gangrenosum? *South Med J* 78:2837, 1985.

### Scorpion Stings

Horen WP: Insect and scorpion stings, *JAMA* 221:894, 1972.
Hunt GR: Bites and stings of uncommon arthropods. *Postgrad Med* 70:107, 1981.
Kizer KW et al: Scorpaenidae envenomation. A five-year poison center experience, *JAMA* 253:807, 1985.
Rimsza ME et al: Scorpion envomization, *Pediatrics* 66:299, 1980.
Stahnke HL: Arizona's lethal scorpion, *Arizona Med* 39:490, 1972.

### Hymenoptera Stings

Emergency treatment of insect sting allergy, *JAMA* 240:27, 1978.
Golden DB et al: Regimens of hymenoptera venom immuno therapy, *Ann Intern Med* 92:620, 1980.
Hunt KJ et al: Diagnosis of allergy to stinging insects by skin testing with hymenoptera venoms, *Ann Intern Med* 85:56, 1976.

Lichtenstein LM et al: A case for venom treatment in anaphylactic sensitivity to hymenoptera sting, *N Engl J Med* 290:1223, 1974.

### Snake Bites

Garlin SR et al: Role of surgical decompression in treatment of rattlesnake bites, *Surg Forum* 30:502, 1979.
Glass TG: Early debridement in pit viper bites, *JAMA* 235:2513, 1976.
Goldstine EJC: Bacteriology of rattlesnake venom and implications for therapy, *J Infect Dis* 140:818, 1979.
Grace TG et al: The management of upper extremity pit viper wounds. *J Hand Surg* 2:168, 1980.
Parrish HM et al: Poisonous snake bites in New England, *N Engl J Med* 263:788, 1960.
Russell F: Jaws that bite, *Emerg Med* 25:40, 1978.
Russell F et al: Snake venom poisoning in the United States, *JAMA* 233:341, 1975.
Sutherland SK et al: Early management of bites by the eastern diamond back rattlesnake, *Am J Trop Med Hyg* 30:497, 1981.

### Marine Diseases (General)

Halstead BW: *Poisonous and Venomous Marine Animals of the World.* Vols. 1 and 2. Washington DC: 1965, 1967. US Government Printing Office.

### Erysipeloid

Arndt K: *Erysipelothrix rhusiopathiae* septicemia, *N Engl J Med* 298:957, 1978.
Grieco MH, Sheldon C: *Erysipelothrix rhusiopathiae, Ann N Y Acad Sci* 174:523, 1970.
Klanden J: Erysipeloid as an occupational disease, *JAMA* 111:1345, 1938.
Nelson E: Five hundred cases of erysipeloid, *Rocky Mountain Med J* 52:40, 1955.
Price J, Bennett W: The erysipeloid of Rosenbach, *BMJ* 2:1060, 1951.

### Red Tide

Halstead BW: *Poisonous and venomous marine animals of the world,* Princeton, NJ, 1978, Darwin.
Morris PD et al: Clinical and epidemiological features of neurotoxic shellfish poisoning in North Carolina, *Am J Public Health* 81(4): 471, 1991.
Ross NW: *Red tide*, University of Rhode Island Marine Advisory Service, Narragansett, July 1979. Fact sheet.
Schantz EJ: Seafood toxicants. In *Toxicants occurring naturally in foods,* ed 2, Washington, DC, 1973, *National Academy of Sciences.*
Shimizu Y: Paralytic shellfish poisons. In *Progress in the chemistry of organic natural products, 45* New York, 1984, Wien/Springer-Verlag.
Shimizu Y: Personal communication, 1986.
Shimizu Y: Survey of diarrhetic shellfish poisons in United States coasts. University of Rhode Island, Kingston, Sea Grant Project Summary (study in progress 1983-1985), 1984.
Wang JL, Oesterlin R, Raproport H: Structure of saxotoxin, *J Am Chem Soc* 93:7344, 1971.

### Seal Bite

Beck B, Smith TG: Seal finger: An unsolved medical problem in Canada. Technical report of the Fisheries Research Board of Canada. No 625. Arctic Biological Station, Fisheries and Marine Service. (Quebec: Ste. Anne de Bellevue), 1976.
Hillenbrand FKM: Whale finger and seal finger, *Lancet* 2:680, 1953.
Markham RB, Polk F: Seal finger, *J Infect Dis* 1:567, 1979.

### Coelenterata

Drury JK et al: Jelly fish sting with serious hand complications, *Injury* 12:66, 1980.
Hartwick R et al: Disarming the box-jelly fish: Nemocyst inhibition in *Chironex fleckeri, Med J Aust* 1:15, 1980.
Meinkoth NA: *Audubon Society Field Guide to North American Seashore Creatures,* New York, 1981, Knopf.

CHAPTER

# 4H Pesticides

**Laurence Fuortes**
**David A. Schwartz**

## EPIDEMIOLOGY

Pesticide poisoning is a major public health problem globally. The World Health Organization (WHO) estimates that there are 3 million severe acute pesticide poisonings yearly, with approximately 220,000 resultant deaths. Most of these poisonings occur in developing countries. Globally, as well as in the United States, approximately 50% of severe pesticide poisonings are occupational and the rest intentional or via environmental contamination. No accurate, comprehensive statistics are available in the United States on the incidence of pesticide poisoning. The Environmental Protection Agency (EPA) estimates that there are approximately 3000 hospital admissions for pesticide poisoning yearly and 20,000 emergency room visits for suspected pesticide exposure in the United States. Each year, 30 to 40 people die from pesticide poisoning. Based on a national household pesticide use survey in 1977, the EPA estimated that 2.5 million symptomatic pesticide exposures occurred in the home yearly. Many of those affected, particularly in occupational settings, never see a physician and never are diagnosed (Fig. 4H-1).

**Fig. 4H-1.** Workers handling pesticides may be exposed during preparation for field application.

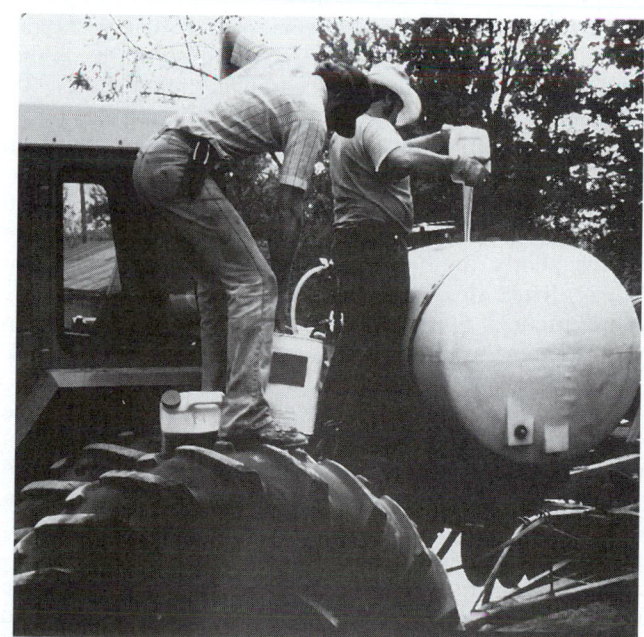

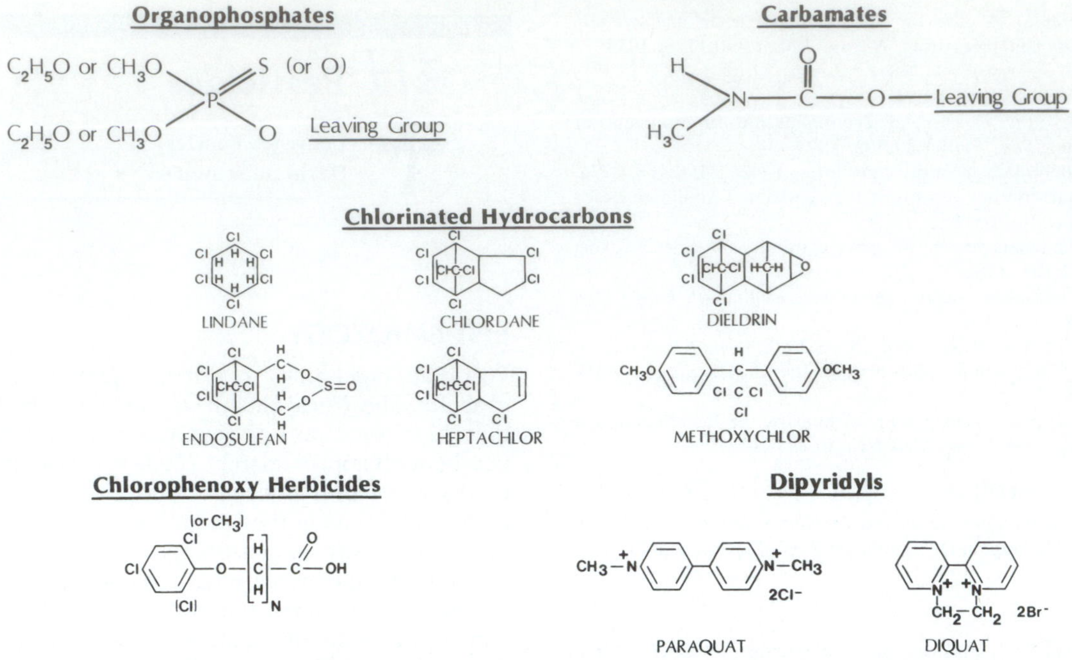


**Fig. 4H-2.** Chemical structures of pesticides.

Pesticides can be defined loosely as agents used to control undesirable animals and plants (insecticides, fungicides, rodenticides, molluscacides, algicides, herbicides). This chapter focuses primarily on insecticides and herbicides, delineating their acute and chronic effects as well as recommended management and prevention of exposure. Before World War II, pesticides were generally not effective (except sulfur, copper, mercury, and arsenicals), and crop spraying was not a common practice in farming. With the development of DDT in the early 1940s and organophosphates a short time later, pesticide use in agriculture and in disease control has been steadily increasing. In 1987, approximately 5 billion pounds of active pesticides were used worldwide. Most pesticides used in the United States are in agriculture, which accounted for 77% of the 1.08 billion pounds used in 1985. Currently, approximately 600 active pesticides are registered with the EPA and used primarily in agriculture. In general, these active pesticides are marketed in combination with "inert" ingredients in approximately 45,000 separate formulations or products. These inert ingredients are frequently toxic in and of themselves but are not always listed by name on the pesticide packaging. Approximately 60% to 70% of the pesticides used in agriculture in the United States are herbicides, 25% to 30% insecticides, and 10% to 15% fungicides.

The occupational groups at greatest risk for pesticide poisonings include pesticide formulators and manufacturers, the nearly 2 million U.S. farmers and additional 6 million farm family members, the estimated 2.5 million seasonal and migrant workers and their families, veterinary workers, gardeners, and commercial pesticide applicators. It is estimated that 25% of migrant workers are under 16 years of age. Cultural, economic, linguistic, and educational differences place this group at increased risk of pesticide exposure, and these same factors result in suboptimal access to health care and worker's compensation. The widespread use of aerial spraying places the surrounding community at risk of contamination. Home use (garden and indoor pest control) accounts for 20% of all pesticide sales. Pesticides are also used in vector control (mosquitoes); securing the right of way for highways, telephone lines, and railroad beds (major uses of herbicides); consumer products (paints, soaps, food processing, and fabrics); and, unfortunately, warfare. Pesticides are therefore pervasive in rural and urban environments as well as in agrarian occupations.

Skin contamination is the most important route of pesticide exposure in the occupational setting. Field studies indicate that 95% of absorbed pesticide during agricultural work is via the dermal route. Farm workers have been poisoned from dermal contact with pesticide residues on plants sprayed several days earlier. Similarly, several cases of severe poisonings and fatalities have occurred from pesticide residues spilled on clothing or fabric surfaces. Ingestion is the major route of exposure from either intentional poisoning or environmental contamination. In general, when dealing with such toxic substances, less toxic alternatives should always be sought and safety measures should be periodically tested and updated. Both workers and the community should be informed of the inherent toxicity of potentially dangerous chemicals.

Modern agriculture uses five categories of pesticides (Fig. 4H-2). Nationwide the majority of pesticides used are herbicides. The organophosphate and carbamate (cholinesterase-inhibiting) insecticides account for 80% of insecticide use, while the chlorinated hydrocarbons, pyrethroids and biologic derivatives make up the remainder. Pesticide use differs from one crop to the next and from area to area. An understanding of the types of pesticides used with each crop from season to season allows the physician to make an educated guess when confronted with a poorly informed agricultural worker exposed to a pesticide (Table 4H-1). This information generally can be supplied by the local agricultural extension agent.

**Table 4H-1.** Pesticide usage in Imperial County, California

| *Cotton* pesticide generic name | Common name | Class | Pounds | Season |
|---|---|---|---|---|
| Monocrotophos | Azodrin | Organophosphate | 176,151 | April, July-September |
| Methomyl | Lannate, Nudrin | Carbamate | 113,002 | March-October |
| Methyl Parathion | Azophos | Organophosphate | 63,234 | April-October |
| Parathion | — | Organophosphate | 47,339 | April-June |
| Dicrotophos | Bidrin | Organophosphate | 36,591 | April |
| Aldicarb | Temik | Carbamate | 23,924 | April |
| Azinphos-Methyl | Guthion | Organophosphate | 22,673 | June-August |
| Carbaryl | Sevin | Carbamate | 11,648 | April-July |
| Methamidophos | Monitor | Organophosphate | 11,412 | Variable use |
| Disulfoton | Di-syston | Organophosphate | 8,002 | March-June |
| Paraquat | Paraquat | Dipyridyl herbicide | 1,463 | September-November |
| Endosulfan | Thiodan | Organochlorine | 1,021 | Variable use |
| Toxaphene | — | Organochlorine | 880 | Variable use |
| Phorate | Thimet | Organophosphate | 779 | March-June |
| Methidathion | Supracide | Organophosphate | 562 | April-September |
| Strychnine | — | Vertebrate poison | 42 | Variable use |
| Aluminum | Phostoxin | Fumigant | 7 | Variable use |

Source: Newsum LA, Prieto F, Schwartz DA: *Health handbook on pesticides: Imperial County Component*, NTIS (PB83-162685), 1983.

## PATHOPHYSIOLOGY

Before turning to the specific categories of pesticides, it is important to note some observations regarding the general health hazards of pesticides for humans. The statistics for pesticide poisoning reflect only the reported cases and are undoubtedly an underestimation of total pesticide-related events. It is even harder to obtain data on chronic health effects of pesticide exposure. The latency between exposure and chronic effects, as well as multiple causes of chronic diseases, makes risk assessment for chronic outcomes harder to evaluate than acute effects. In several studies individuals chronically exposed to low doses of pesticides were discovered to have significant increases in nausea, eye and skin irritations, and chronic headaches. Recent studies have shown that both acute and chronic exposure to a variety of pesticides may result in previously unrecognized chronic neurotoxicity. These data are most consistent for the organophosphates and carbamates. The possible carcinogenicity, mutagenicity, and teratogenicity of several pesticides are still not settled. Pesticides have been found to cause cancer in laboratory animals; moreover, epidemiologic data among exposed populations supports human carcinogenic potential. Worldwide occupational studies have documented consistently increasing rates of non-Hodgkin lymphoma, leukemia, soft tissue sarcoma, and skin, lip, brain, stomach, and prostate cancer among farmers. In addition, several studies from the United States and China have reported increased risk of childhood leukemia associated with parental pesticide exposure. These cancer studies have implicated DDT, organophosphates, and the phenoxy acid herbicides, such as 2,4-D. Similarly, various other pesticides have been found to be mutagenic and teratogenic in animal systems but data are less clear in humans. Adverse reproductive outcomes include infertility, intrauterine growth retardation, spontaneous abortion, and limb-reduction defects. Pesticides suspected of causing adverse birth outcomes include DDT, chlordecone, lindane, dibromochloropropane, ethylene dibromide, triazines, carbaryl, and organophosphates. While these health issues remain controversial, concerns about possible toxic side effects will be raised by patients. Health care providers need to be knowledgeable regarding the type and amount of pesticide exposure one has, potential toxicities, and means of limiting exposure.

### Occupational and environmental history

List subject's present and previous residences and include information regarding neighboring factories or waste sites.
List subject's present and previous jobs with job title as well as description of actual task.
List present and previous jobs of subject's spouse.
List subject's hobbies.
Ascertain relation of symptoms to work day, weekend, and vacations.
Determine the presence of similar symptoms in other workers or neighbors.

This chapter examines each major type of pesticide: organophosphates and carbamates, organochlorines, chlorophenoxy herbicides, and dipyridyls, and briefly outlines the toxicology of each agent and the symptom complex of acute poisonings, with particular attention paid to the available laboratory tests and specific treatment modalities. To diagnose pesticide poisoning, physicians must maintain a high degree of suspicion and obtain environmental and occupational histories (see the box above). General guidelines regarding the treatment of all pesticide exposures are outlined in the box on p. 106 (see Chapter 4A for further information on the management of poisoning).

### General guidelines of management for pesticide exposures

Bathe the patient.
Identify the pesticide.
Change the patient's clothing.
Empty the stomach if the pesticide was ingested. (Do not do if the pesticide is mixed with a hydrocarbon solvent; chlorinated hydrocarbons usually are.)
Report the incident to the local health department.

## ORGANOPHOSPHATES

Common examples of organophosphates are Chlorpyrifos, Diazinon, Dicathon, dimethoate, Dursban, ethion, Fenthion, Gardona, malathion, and parathion (see Fig. 4H-2).

The organophosphates are the most common pesticides worldwide. They are used primarily as insecticides and nematocides. The organophosphates have largely replaced the chlorinated hydrocarbons, such as DDT, because they do not bioaccumulate in the environment. However, these substances are far more acutely toxic than the chlorinated hydrocarbons. Their major use is in the control of agricultural pests; they are used to a lesser degree in residential settings.

### Toxicology

Organophosphates bind to the acetylcholinesterase enzyme, allowing acetylcholine to accumulate at the cholinergic neuroeffector junctions (muscarinic effects), at the skeletal muscle myoneural junctions, at the autonomic ganglia (nicotinic effects), and in the central nervous system (CNS). The organophosphates can produce the following acute effects.

(1) Cholinomimetic actions of the muscarinic type at the autonomic effector organs (parasympathetic effects)
(2) Stimulation, followed by depression or paralysis, of autonomic ganglia and skeletal muscles (nicotinic actions)
(3) Stimulation with subsequent depression at cholinoceptive sites in the CNS.

Mortality from organophosphates results from respiratory compromise and is attributable to all three types of receptor overstimulation. Bronchoconstriction, pulmonary secretions, and pulmonary edema result from muscarinic activity; respiratory muscle failure results from nicotinic activity; and decreased respiratory drive results from CNS toxicity.

Relative toxicity among the organophosphates depends on the persistence of the organophosphate-acetylcholinesterase bond and on the lipid solubility of the particular pesticide (allowing for penetration through the skin and the gastrointestinal (GI) and respiratory tracts, for passage into the CNS, and for storage in adipose tissue). Chronic exposure to several organophosphorous compounds can produce a particular syndrome of neuronal degeneration associated with demyelinization and characterized by peripheral neuropathy. The chronic neurotoxic potential of organophosphates is exemplified by the story of Jamaica ginger or ginger-jake paralysis. During Prohibition, a popular medicinal tonic of Jamaica ginger in 70% to 80% ethanol solution was widely marketed. The high concentration of actual ginger being unpalatable in larger dosages led one bootlegger in 1930 to adulterate ethanol with Lyndol, an oil substance containing the organophosphate triorthocresyl phosphate, and marketing this as gingertonic. The ingested organophosphate resulted in an epidemic of peripheral neuropathy from axonal degeneration. Between 20,000 and 100,000 people were said to be permanently affected by ginger-jake paralysis.

### Symptomatology

The clinical presentation should be viewed through the pathophysiologic mechanisms outlined above. The muscarinic effects include miosis, (pinpoint pupils), increased gastrointestinal motility (diarrhea, abdominal cramps), increased secretion of gastric acid with nausea and vomiting, increased salivation, bronchoconstriction with increased respiratory secretions, bradycardia with decreased cardiac output and hypotension, and involuntary defecation and urination.

The nicotinic effects include fatigue, muscle fasciculations, and generalized weakness followed by paralysis.

General CNS symptomatology may include confusion, ataxia, slurred speech, loss of reflexes, convulsions, and coma. There is increasing evidence that the neurotoxic effects of organophosphate exposure may result in chronic neurotoxicity manifested by mood and memory dysfunction.

### Laboratory studies

When acute or chronic intoxication is suspected, it is often possible to establish the diagnosis by determining the plasma and erythrocyte (red blood cell) cholinesterase activity levels. Erythrocyte cholinesterase activity is more specific for organophosphate exposure. Under ideal circumstances a comparison of the test sample with the preexposure value offers the best confirmation of organophosphate absorption; a depression in activity of 25% or more is strong evidence of excessive absorption, indicating a need to modify work practices or personal protective measures in order to prevent toxicity. Ordinarily, clinical symptoms do not occur until the red blood cell cholinesterase level decreases by more than 50% of the baseline value. The development of signs and symptoms of toxicity is related more to the rate of decline in enzyme activity than to the absolute enzyme activity levels. If a baseline value is not available, serial erythrocyte cholinesterase levels should be obtained for several weeks after the exposure to document substantial improvement in the postexposure level. The diagnosis of acute intoxication should be made on clinical grounds; however, erythrocyte cholinesterase levels can confirm the diagnosis. Plasma cholinesterase levels are available at most hospitals.

Plasma or pseudocholinesterase activity is a reasonable screening tool for evaluating suspected organophosphate poisoning. However, plasma cholinesterase may be markedly depressed from other causes, including liver disease, pregnancy, mercury, or carbon disulfide exposure. It must be remembered that up to 3% of the general population have markedly depressed plasma cholinesterase activity on a genetic basis. These individuals are dramatically hypersusceptible to the effects of succinylcholine and may also be hypersusceptible to the effects of organophosphates. Urinary metabolites (alkyl phosphates) may be measured for many organophosphates. These extremely sensitive assays are useful for identifying agents in cases of poisoning and for monitoring absorption in occupationally exposed workers. This monitoring may help assess the adequacy of personal protective measures.

### Management

(1) Establish a clear airway, remove clothing, and decontaminate skin, hair, GI tract, and eyes as indicated. Supplemental oxygen and/or artificial ventilation may be indicated.

(2) Atropine sulfate antagonizes the action of acetylcholine both at muscarinic effector sites and in the CNS. Dosage for adults is between 0.5 and 2.0 mg intravenously repeated every 15 to 30 minutes as needed. Dosage for children under 12 years of age is 0.05 mg/kg of body weight. Continuous infusion may be considered in severe poisonings. Note that atropine dosages used for organophosphate poisoning are considerably higher than cardiac dosages for bradycardia. Hundreds of milligrams of atropine may be needed over a 24-hour period. Atropine should be used only as symptoms or signs or organophosphate poisoning emerge. The effects of atropine may wear off before the toxicity of organophosphates resolves. Patients requiring atropine should be hospitalized and observed for recurrence. The dose of atropine must be titrated to the patient's physical signs of toxicity (bradycardia, rales, and state of consciousness). Adequacy of atropinization may be monitored by the drying up of secretions, clearance of rales, tachycardia, and dilated pupils. Signs of atropine poisoning are fever, muscle fibrillation, and delirium. The prophylactic use of atropine in the occupational setting is contraindicated.

(3) Pralidoxime (2-PAM) reactivates acetylcholinesterase by displacing phosphate from the cholinesterase enzyme and reverses the peripheral neuromuscular paralysis. Furthermore, pralidoxime has some intrinsic atropinic activity and can bind to and inactivate unbound organophosphate in the bloodstream. Early treatment is essential and should be initiated at the same time as atropine. Dosage for adults is 1 g given intravenously no faster than 0.5 g per minute. Dosage for children under 12 is 20 to 40 mg/kg given intravenously, at no more than half the total dose per minute. The adult dose should be repeated every 20 to 60 minutes if symptoms persist or reappear; the child's dose should be repeated every 3 to 12 hours, as needed. Pralidoxime is relatively nontoxic although it may cause labile blood pressure.

(4) Convulsions can usually be controlled with diazepam.

(5) Observation for at least 24 hours is needed to be sure that symptoms do not recur as effects of antidotal treatment wear off.

(6) The patient should be removed from all possible sources of exposure until the red blood cell cholinesterase activity is greater than 80% of baseline; this may take several weeks.

## N-METHYL CARBAMATE INSECTICIDES

Common examples of carbamate insecticides are Propoxur (Baygon), Carbaryl (Sevin), Methomyl (Lannate), and Carbofuran (Furadan) (see Fig 4H-2). These substances are widely used in agriculture, by hobby gardeners, as flea powder, in flea collars, or in "flea bombs."

### Toxicology

Like organophosphates, carbamates bind to the acetylcholinesterase enzyme, allowing acetylcholine to accumulate primarily at the cholinergic neuroeffector junctions (muscarinic effects). No significant nicotinic effects occur as a result of carbamate exposure. Carbamates produce acute symptoms identical to those of organophosphates. These pesticides are highly lipid-soluble, quickly absorbed via all routes, and readily cross the skin. In addition, there have been numerous reports of translocation of Aldicarb, a particularly toxic carbamate, into cucumbers or watermelons resulting in outbreaks of carbamate poisoning. Compared to organophosphates, carbamates produce much more short-lived acute toxicity because of the spontaneous reversible bond between the carbamate and acetylcholinesterase. Episodes of neurotoxicity have been reported after exposure to "flea bombs" in residential settings. In addition to carbamate insecticides there are carbamate fungicides and herbicides. These have no anticholinesterase effect. The carbamate herbicides are dermal irritants and the carbamate fungicides (Thiram) have an Antabuse-like effect resulting in severe reactions upon exposure to alcohol.

### Symptomatology

The symptoms are identical to those of organophosphate poisoning, with the exception that nicotinic activity (fasciculation and muscular weakness) is minimal.

### Laboratory studies

Upon evaluation of a carbamate exposure it is important to obtain the chemical name to confirm its being an *insecticide, herbicide,* or *fungicide* (Table 4H-2). Although the symptoms of carbamate intoxication may persist for days, the cholinesterase activity (both plasma and erythrocyte) commonly reverts to normal within hours of intoxication (a result of the reversible nature of the carbamate-acetylcholinesterase bond). Therefore the laboratory cholinesterase values may be misleading unless measured within one or two hours after exposure. The diagnosis of acute or chronic intoxication should be made on clinical grounds, with cholinesterase levels used to confirm but not rule out the diagnosis. Urinary metabolite analysis is an extremely sensitive means of confirming carbamate exposure and can be used clinically or as a way of monitoring worker's exposure.

### Management

Management is identical to acute organophosphate poisoning, frequently requiring high doses of atropine.

**Table 4H-2.** Carbamate pesticides

| Class | Chemicals | Brand names | Toxicity |
|---|---|---|---|
| Insecticides | Aldicarb<br>Carbofuran<br>Methomyl<br>Propoxur<br>Carbaryl | Temik<br>Furadan<br>Lanox<br>Baygon<br>Sevin | Reversible carbamation of acetyl-cholinesterase enzyme |
| Herbicides | Butylate<br>EPTC | Sutan<br>Eradicane | Primarily mucosal irritants |
| Fungicides | Thiram<br>Metham-sodium<br>Ziram<br>Maneb, mancozeb | AAtack<br>Busan<br>Dithane<br>Dithane | Potential Antabuse or disulfiram reactions |

However, pralidoxime is of no value and should not be used.

## CHLORINATED HYDROCARBONS (ORGANOCHLORINES)

Examples of organochlorines include chlordane, DDT, Dicofol, dieldrin, aldrin, endrin, Kepone, heptachlor, lindane, mirex, hexachlorobenzene, endosulfan, and toxaphene (see Fig. 4H-2).

The organochlorine compounds are used as insecticides and acaricides in agricultural and public health settings. These agents have successfully controlled such vector-borne diseases as malaria, and are still used in many developing countries. The best known organochlorine, DDT, has been banned or restricted in many countries based on ecologic considerations of persistence and bioaccumulation. Chlordane, dieldrin, aldrin, Kepone, and heptachlor have been banned or severely restricted because of potential human health effects.

### Toxicology

Organochlorines interfere with axonal transmission of nerve impulses (altering sodium and potassium transport), causing either stimulation or depression of the central nervous system. This results in behavior changes, sensory and equilibrium disturbances, involuntary muscular activity (myoclonus), and depression of medullary function. Massive exposures can increase myocardial irritability and cause degenerative changes in the liver and kidneys. Symptoms and signs vary with particular agents but may occur within 30 minutes of massive exposure. Seizures have resulted in children treated repeatedly with lindane for louse or scabies infestation. These agents are highly lipid-soluble, and exposed individuals have much higher levels of chlorinated hydrocarbons in body fat (as well as in breast milk) than the nonexposed population. When body fat is mobilized by dieting or serious illness, these individuals may develop signs of acute intoxication. Some of these compounds are stable expoxides, and toxicologic and epidemiologic studies suggest that they may be associated with an increased risk of certain hematologic disorders and cancers. Because of its bioaccumulation up the food chain and devastating effect upon certain raptor birds, DDT was banned in the United States in the 1970s. Hexachlorobenzene, an organochlorine fungicide has caused episodes of porphyria cutanea tarda but is not particularly neurotoxic. The chief excretory route of organochlorines is biliary. Enterohepatic recirculation frequently occurs retarding excretion.

### Symptomatology

Exposure to toxic levels of chlorinated hydrocarbons can result in nausea, vomiting, rapid heart rate, respiratory depression, headache, miosis, vertigo, paresthesias, fasciculations, tremors, ataxia, hyperexcitability, disorientation, seizure activity and, in rare cases, coma. Children may be hypersusceptible to the effects.

### Laboratory studies

Organochlorine and/or metabolites can usually be identified by gas-liquid chromatography in blood and urine samples taken within 72 hours of exposure, although some of these substances (DDT, dieldrin, mirex, heptachlor, and chlordecone), persist in tissues and blood for months. These tests are not readily available in most medical centers, and a history of exposure with consistent symptomatology should serve as sufficient evidence for diagnosis.

### Management

(1) Supportive therapy is important.
(2) Seizure activity should be controlled with diazepam, phenobarbital, or Dilantin.
(3) Because the organochlorines are frequently myocardial irritants, sympathomimetic agents (epinephrine) should be avoided.
(4) In many cases the chlorinated hydrocarbons are mixed with hydrocarbon solvents; thus, emesis is contraindicated. Gastric lavage with protection of the airway is preferable. Administration of activated charcoal or cholestyramine resin interrupts the cycle of enterohepatic recirculation, dramatically enhancing biliary-fecal excretion. Prolonged treatment for several weeks may be necessary.

## CHLOROPHENOXY HERBICIDES

Common examples of chlorophenoxy herbicides are 2,4-D, MCPA, Dicamba, and 2,4,5-T (see Fig. 4H-2). 2,4,5-T was banned in 1978 because of concerns regarding teratogenicity and carcinogenicity purportedly associated with contamination with dioxin.

Chlorophenoxy compounds are used as agricultural herbicides for control of broad-leaved weeds and as growth regulators to increase citrus fruit size.

### Toxicology

The chlorophenoxy herbicides are absorbed readily from the skin, GI tract, and lungs. These agents irritate epithelial tissues of the skin, eye, and respiratory and GI tracts. Although these herbicides act as growth hormone inhibitors in plants, they have no hormonal action in animals, and how they exert their toxic action is poorly understood. Humans demonstrate an unusually high tolerance to these agents; one individual consumed 500 mg per day of 2,4-D for 3 weeks without developing any symptoms or signs of illness. Excretion of the parent compound occurs via the urine and is nearly complete within 2 to 5 days; no significant storage occurs inside the fat cells.

### Symptomatology

Several chlorophenoxy compounds are irritating to skin and mucous membranes. Some individuals suffer localized depigmentation after prolonged dermal contact. Exposure to chlorophenoxy herbicides causes skin irritation, burning in the throat, cough, nausea and vomiting, esophagitis, and, with intense exposure, fasciculations, peripheral neuropathy, and myopathy. There are case reports of peripheral neuropathy developing after dermal exposure to 2,4-D. Seizures, coma, fever, and metabolic acidosis have been reported. Several of these substances have been implicated as potential causes of non-Hodgkin lymphoma and soft tissue sarcoma among farmers.

### Laboratory studies

Gas-liquid chromatography is available through reference laboratories for testing of these compounds in the patient's urine.

### Management

(1) Use of supportive measures is usually adequate.
(2) Follow general guidelines for all pesticide exposures, including decontamination of skin and gut.
(3) Alkalinization of urine by administration of sodium bicarbonate to maintain urine pH greater than 7.5 may enhance excretion.

## DIPYRIDYLS

Common examples of dipyridyls are paraquat and diquat (see Fig. 4H-2). These nonselective contact herbicides are applied as liquid sprays.

They kill broad-leaved and grassy weeds on contact and are used as defoliants on certain crops, such as potatoes, cotton, and sugarcane. At higher concentrations they are used to maintain railway lines and roadsides.

### Toxicology

The dipyridyl substances are caustic, resulting in contact dermatitis, burns, and ulceration. These compounds bind to and cause proliferative changes in the epithelial tissues of the skin, nails, nose, mouth, eyes, and respiratory and GI tracts. Diquat predominantly affects the skin, GI mucosa, and kidney, and is much less toxic than Paraquat, which can cause fatal liver, kidney, and lung lesions. Three clinical stages occur after the ingestion of paraquat. They are characterized by potentially reversible central hepatic and renal tubular necrosis, and then by intraalveolar hemorrhage with rapid proliferation of bronchial epithelium, loss of surfactant, and progressive pulmonary fibrosis. The pathophysiologic mechanism for injury is thought to be superoxide radical formation resulting in peroxidation of alveolar membrane lipids. The mortality of paraquat ingestion is as high as 65%; as little as one ounce may prove fatal. Absorption across the skin is minimal; however, fibrotic lung disease and fatalities have been reported after extensive dermal exposure. Additionally, there is some concern regarding the potential for neurotoxicity from occupational exposure to paraquat.

### Symptomatology

The symptoms caused by exposure to toxic levels of dipyridyls are best viewed chronologically:

(1) Early symptoms are a result of direct mucosal irritation and include burning in the mouth and throat, epistaxis, emesis, and diarrhea.
(2) Two to three days after ingestion, evidence of renal and hepatic damage appears. Abnormal urinary sediments with elevations in BUN and creatinine along with elevations in liver function tests (bilirubin, SGOT, SGPT, LDH, and alkaline phosphatase) are consistent with the central hepatic necrosis and renal tubular necrosis, both of which are generally reversible.
(3) Three to fourteen days after ingestion, cough, dyspnea, and tachypnea may progress to a diffuse pneumonitis with adult respiratory distress syndrome. This clinical presentation is a manifestation of intraalveolar edema and hemorrhage along with impaired production of surfactant. It is followed by alveolar fibroblastic proliferation with irreversible pulmonary fibrosis. In most cases, pulmonary disease leads to death resulting from extensive pulmonary edema and fibrosis.

### Laboratory studies

Quantitative and qualitative measures of these agents in the blood and urine are available through reference laboratories. Plasma concentrations can be used for prognostic purposes and to follow treatment.

### Management

(1) Treatment should be aimed at limiting absorption and increasing excretion. Considering the inherent toxicity of paraquat, these measures should be taken in all cases regardless of the quantity ingested.
  (a) GI lavage with normal saline or 5% sodium bicarbonate solution should be carried out and 8 ounces of an absorbent (made up of Fuller Earth, 30% suspension, and bentonite 7% suspension) should be administered. These agents bind dipyridyls in the gut. One hour following the administration of the absorbent, administer a cathartic (sorbitol) and repeat every 4 hours for at least 12 complete doses.
  (b) Contaminated skin and eyes must be flushed with large amounts of water or saline. All patients with eye contamination should be seen by an ophthalmologist.
(2) Forced diuresis by the infusion of large amounts of saline with furosemide is indicated. If this is not possible, peritoneal dialysis should be substituted.
(3) Supplemental oxygen may worsen the pulmonary lesions and should be avoided, if oxygenation can otherwise be maintained at 90% saturation. There may be some benefit from relative oxygen deprivation although this is clearly experimental and cannot be recommended at this time.

(4) Theoretically a person who can be hemoperfused within 10 hours of paraquat ingestion may derive some marginal benefit. Unfortunately relatively little paraquat is carried in the circulation within a few hours after ingestion. Aside from the efforts to remove dipyridyls from the blood, dialysis may be necessary in order to treat acute renal failure.

(5) Corticosteroids, azathioprine, dextro-protopropranolol, and superoxide dismutase have been used by some researchers but at this point there is no evidence for their clinical efficacy.

## SUMMARY

In summary, the practitioner must understand that pesticides are classified according to their chemical class and target species. One must be able to identify the specific exposure in order to anticipate the symptoms and signs and be prepared to manage toxicity. In addition, a practitioner working in an agrarian community should know the major crops and local uses of pesticides. This information assists in determining exposure in a poorly informed patient. Obtaining pesticide containers in order to confirm their contents through labels or laboratory analysis is critical. As with other toxic exposures collection of blood, urine, and gastric contents for toxicologic analysis should be routine.

A discussion of pesticides would not be complete without a word about prevention. The incidence of reported deaths caused by acute pesticide exposure was diminished by 60% simply by instituting reentry waiting periods for workers after a field had been sprayed. Other means of minimizing exposure include (1) protective personal clothing, in particular impermeable gloves, hats, and long-sleeved work clothes; (2) education of those working with pesticides; (3) proper disposal of pesticide containers; and (4) proper storage and labeling of pesticides. Finally, efforts must be made to replace the more toxic pesticides with less toxic alternatives.

## BIBLIOGRAPHY

Davis KJ, Fitzhugh OG: Tumorigenic potential of aldrin and dieldrin for mice, *Toxicol Appl Pharmacol* 4:187, 1962.

Epstein SS, Legator MS, editors: *Mutagenicity of Pesticides: Concepts and Evaluation,* Cambridge, MA, 1900, MIT Press.

Fasal E, Jackson EW, Klauber MR: Leukemia and lymphoma mortality and farm residence, *Am J Epidemiol* 87:267, 1968.

Hayes WJ, Vaughan WK: Mortality from pesticides in the United States in 1973 and 1974, *Toxicol Appl Pharmacol* 42:235, 1977.

Kahn E: Pesticide-related illness in California farm workers, *J Occup Med* 18:693, 1976.

Khera KS, Clegg DJ: Perinatal toxicity of pesticides, *Can Med Assoc J* 100:167, 1969.

Milby TH: Prevention and management of organophosphate poisoning, *JAMA* 216:2131, 1971.

Moses M: Pesticides. In Rom WN, editor: *Environmental and occupational Medicine,* Boston, 1983, Little, Brown.

Newsum LA, Prieto F, Schwartz DA: *Health handbook on pesticides: Imperial County Component,* NTIS (PB83-162685), 1983.

Rappolt RT: Kern County pesticide study, *Indiana Med* 39:40, 1970.

Ridgway RL et al: Pesticide use in agriculture, *Environ Health Perspect* 27:103, 1978.

Sandifer SH et al: Pesticide effects on occupationally exposed workers, *Int Med* 41:9, 1972.

Schwartz DA, Newsum LA, Heifetz RM: Parental occupation and birth outcome in an agricultural community, *Scand J Work Environ Health* 12:1251, 1986.

Senanayake N, Johnson MK: Acute polyneuropathy after poisoning by a new organophosphate insecticide, *N Engl J Med* 306:155, 1982.

Wang HH, MacMahon B: Mortality of pesticide applicators, *J Occup Med* 21:741, 1979.

World Health Organization (Vector Biology & Control): *The present place of DDT in world operations.* Presented at conference: Impact of pesticides on the environment, Corvallis, Oregon, August 18-20, 1969.

Wyckoff DW et al: Diagnostic and therapeutic problems of parathion poisonings, *Ann Intern Med* 68:875, 1968.

CHAPTER

# 5 Consultation Medicine

James J. Heffernan
Robert A. Witzburg

Consultation practice is an important component of many physicians' professional activity (Fig. 5-1). Up to 30% of the clinical activity of general internists and up to 50% of the patient care activities of selected medical subspecialists may be devoted to consultation. It is likely that the continued growth of managed care will increase the role of primary care physicians on surgical services. Denial of preoperative hospital days by health insurers has already

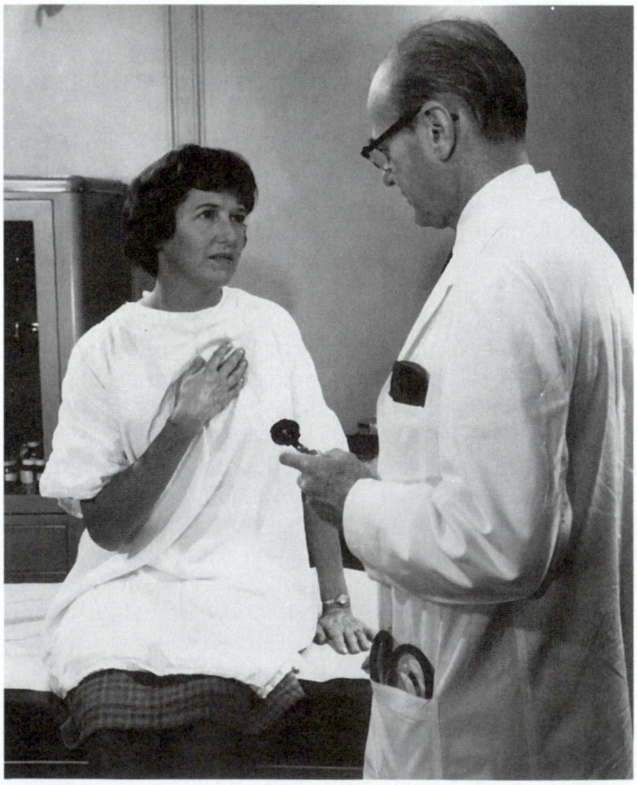

**Fig. 5-1.** Portrait of an internist. (From American College of Physicians Archives.)

shifted preoperative evaluation of patients undergoing elective surgery to the outpatient setting, sometimes to specialized preoperative clinics and sometimes to the clinical practice sites of primary care physicians.

Effective interaction with colleagues in other specialties requires a thorough grounding in the language and science of these other disciplines, as well as an awareness of basic guidelines for consultation (see the box below). The consultant's role in perioperative care is focused on those medical factors which may increase the risks of anesthesia and surgery, with the formulation of a management plan to minimize risk.

Continued advances in the techniques of anesthesia and surgery have made surgical death very uncommon. In the United States expected perioperative mortality (during surgery or within the first 48 hours postoperatively) is less than 0.01% in healthy adults younger than 70 years undergoing elective surgery. Of all perioperative deaths 10% to 15% occur during anesthesia induction, 30% to 40% during surgery, and the remaining 45% to 60% during the subsequent 48 hours. This broad temporal distribution of perioperative mortality dictates the need for medical vigilance well into the recovery phase.

### Guidelines for consultation practice

- Complete a prompt, thorough, generalist-oriented evaluation.
- Respond specifically to the question(s) posed.
- Indicate clearly the perioperative importance of any observations and recommendations outside the area of initial concern.
- Provide focused, detailed, and precise diagnostic and therapeutic guidance.
- Communicate verbally with the anesthesiologist and surgeon, particularly to resolve complex issues.
- Avoid chart notations that unnecessarily create or exacerbate regulatory or medicolegal risk.
- Employ frequent follow-up visits in difficult cases to monitor clinical status and compliance with recommendations.

Modified from Witzburg RA. In *Medical knowledge self-assessment program IX,* Philadelphia, 1991, American College of Physicians.

Systematic assessment of surgical risk requires the identification of anesthesia-specific, procedure-specific, practitioner-specific, and especially patient-specific factors. No one method of anesthesia appropriate for major procedures is inherently safer than another. The selection of anesthetic technique for a given patient, procedure, surgeon, and anesthetist is highly individualized and remains the primary responsibility of the anesthesiologist rather than that of the consultant.

Certain procedures are associated with a higher risk, such as craniotomy and cardiovascular surgery, whereas others, such as herniorrhaphy, cystoscopy, cervical dilatation and curettage, and ophthalmologic surgery, carry a lower risk. The importance of comorbid disease in determining surgical risk may outweigh the nature of the procedure in predicting outcome. Any procedure conducted as an emergency carries an increased risk—as much as twice the expected mortality for similar surgery performed electively.

Several protocols have been developed for estimating an overall, integrated risk profile for patients subjected to general anesthesia and surgery. None has a clear advantage over the traditional and widely utilized classification system of the American Society of Anesthesiologists (ASA), which can assist in risk stratification (Table 5-1). This schema is predicated on a global assessment of the patient's medical problems and functional status. Clinical studies have demonstrated that a patient's functional status, especially exercise capacity, is an excellent and independent predictor of surgical outcome, most likely as a reflection of overall cardiopulmonary reserve. Patients in higher risk classes generally require more intensive preoperative evaluation and more vigilant perioperative management.

## PREOPERATIVE LABORATORY EVALUATION

### Screening blood tests

Medical reasons for ordering preoperative tests include detection of unsuspected conditions, sometimes unmodifiable, that may alter assessment of surgical risk, detection

**Table 5-1.** Physical status scale of the American Society of Anesthesiologists (ASA)

| Class | Physical status | Cardiac complications | Life-threatening | Cardiac death |
|---|---|---|---|---|
| I | Normal healthy person under age 80 | 0% | 0% | 0% |
| II | Mild systemic disease or healthy person over age 80 | 3% | 2% | 1% |
| III | Severe but not incapacitating systemic disease | 6% | 4% | 2% |
| IV | Incapacitating systemic disease that is a constant threat to life | 22% | 17% | 5% |
| V | Moribund patient not expected to survive 24 hours despite surgery | | | |
| E | Suffix to any class indicating emergency surgery | Increased | Increased | Increased |

Modified from Tantrum KR. In Kammerer WS, Gross RJ, editors: *Medical consultation: the internist on surgical, obstetric, and psychiatric services,* ed 2, Baltimore, 1990, Williams & Wilkins; and Merli GJ, Weitz HH, editors: *Medical management of the surgical patient,* Philadelphia, 1992, WB Saunders.

of unsuspected conditions for which intervention may lower surgical risk, and acquisition of baseline results that may assist surgical and postoperative management. Nonmedical reasons for ordering preoperative tests include institutional requirement, habit, unrelated screening, and medicolegal concerns.

There is no proven utility, although there is enormous expense, associated with routine preoperative blood testing. Much of the cost is that of the tests themselves, but other significant expense arises from secondary costs associated with pursuing false positive or inconsequential abnormal results. Most truly abnormal findings occur among tests anticipated to be abnormal on the basis of a history of underlying clinical conditions. Among healthy patients (ASA class 1) undergoing elective surgery who have routine preoperative lab screening, only 4% demonstrate significantly abnormal results, generally involving hepatic transaminases, glucose, potassium, platelet count, or hemoglobin. The abnormalities noted rarely require treatment and generally neither delay surgery nor result in adverse outcomes. There are no data to support obtaining coagulation studies routinely in the preoperative setting. Rather, preoperative laboratory screening should be driven by the history of underlying illness, with directed laboratory evaluation in the setting of known or suspected renal impairment, liver disease, metabolic disease, especially diabetes mellitus, hemorrhagic or thromboembolic diatheses, or treatment with medications known to cause metabolic derangements, especially diuretics. Results of tests performed in the preceding year may be safely substituted for preoperative screening tests if the previous results are normal and there is no obvious clinical indication for retesting.

### Electrocardiogram

There is likewise no clearly demonstrated utility in obtaining routine preoperative electrocardiograms (ECGs). Abnormal preoperative ECGs are associated with higher rates of adverse outcomes in patients undergoing surgery, but the ECG is generally not an independent predictor of such adverse outcomes; among ambulatory surgery patients abnormal ECGs have been associated with older age, higher ASA class, and obesity. The limited available data suggest the reasonable criteria for ordering preoperative ECGs listed in the Managed Care Guide.

### Chest radiograph

Chest radiographs are frequently abnormal, especially among older patients. The reported rates of abnormal preoperative chest radiographs vary greatly, from 1.2% to 52.9% among patients in different clinical series. Management changes on the basis of an abnormal chest radiograph alone are uncommon, and prospectively obtained data assessing the utility of preoperative chest radiographs do not exist. Recent data suggest that an abnormal chest radiograph in a patient with known or suspected chronic obstructive pulmonary disease (COPD) is a factor associated with a higher likelihood of postoperative complications. Reasonable criteria for obtaining a preoperative chest radiograph include age greater than 60 years and suspicion of cardiac or pulmonary disease on the basis of history and examination.

### Managed Care Guide
### Clinical indications for selective ordering of preoperative ECGs

- Men older than 45 years; women older than 55 years
- History of clinically important heart disease, including dysrhythmias
- Conditions associated with heart disease, especially peripheral vascular disease
- Conditions predisposing to heart disease, such as diabetes mellitus
- Potentially cardiotoxic medications
- Intrathoracic, intraperitoneal, aortic, and/or emergency surgery
- Predisposition toward electrolyte disturbances

Modified from Goldberger AL, O'Konski M: *Ann Intern Med* 105:552, 1986.

### Pulmonary function testing

Minor postoperative pulmonary complications, such as microatalectasis, atalectasis, and bronchospasm, are quite common among patients with and without COPD; the frequency of such minor complications does not differ significantly between those with mild to moderate and those with severe COPD. Severe postoperative pulmonary complications, such as pneumonia, reintubation, and ventilatory failure, are correlated with the severity of underlying COPD and may occur in up to 25% of patients with severe COPD undergoing major surgery. Death and cardiac complications are also more common among patients with severe COPD and are strikingly more frequent among such patients who undergo coronary artery bypass surgery or major abdominal procedures, or who have longer operative times. Traditionally, spirometric values have been cited as predictors of increased postoperative risk: forced expiratory volume in 1 second ($FEV_1$) under 1.2 L or less than 50% predicted; forced vital capacity (FVC) under 2.0 L or less than 50% predicted; $FEV_1$/FVC less than 70%; or maximal voluntary ventilation less than 50% predicted. Prospective, controlled studies assessing the utility of preoperative pulmonary function testing in predicting postoperative complications do not exist. Recent data suggest no independent predictive value of routine spirometry, whereas the clinical variables of higher ASA class, increasing age, abnormal chest radiograph, and preoperative bronchodilator use are significantly associated with postoperative complication rates. In general, patients with better exercise tolerance or better cardiovascular classification experience fewer pulmonary complications. It is most reasonable to consider obtaining preoperative spirometry in patients with a history of tobacco use, regular sputum production, wheezing, asthma, older age, or obesity only if they are undergoing major abdominal or cardiac surgery. Those with abnormal spirometric results should undergo sampling of arterial blood gases, since a preoperative $Paco_2$ greater than 45 mm Hg predicts increased surgical mortality and morbidity.

## CARDIOVASCULAR RISK ASSESSMENT AND MODIFICATION

An estimate of the cardiac risks of noncardiac surgery can be based on a clinical assessment of ventricular function, the presence of certain arrhythmias, recent history of myocardial infarction or unstable angina, the presence of aortic stenosis, the patient's general medical condition and age, and the nature of anticipated surgery. In 1977 Goldman and colleagues published the first objective scale for quantification of cardiac risk associated with noncardiac surgery. This scale, prospectively validated and widely utilized, has formed the backbone of preoperative cardiac evaluation (Tables 5-2 and 5-3). More recently, however, it has become clear that this cardiac risk index tends to underestimate complications in patients undergoing major intrathoracic, upper abdominal, or great vessel procedures. In addition, clinical findings of left ventricular dysfunction, such as pulmonary edema, jugular venous distention, a ventricular gallop, and frequent ventricular ectopic beats, provide only an indirect and imprecise appraisal of myocardial function. Analysis of the Coronary Artery Surgery Study (CASS) experience suggests that the degree of objectively defined left ventricular dysfunction may be the single most important predictor of perioperative cardiac morbidity and mortality. Similarly, studies of preoperative exercise testing indicate that the functional limitations associated with left ventricular dysfunction have important implications for surgical risk. The demonstration of adequate exercise capacity correlates strongly with low operative risk.

A thorough history and physical examination, supported in appropriate instances by the chest x-ray and ECG, remain the mainstays of cardiovascular risk assessment. Patients with no clinical evidence of ischemic heart disease need not undergo any further cardiac diagnostic evaluation before general noncardiac surgery. Similarly, stable patients with New York Heart Association (NYHA) functional class I or II angina do not routinely require additional preoperative testing. However, such patients about to undergo a high-risk procedure, especially central vascular surgery, or who also have diabetes or left ventricular dysfunction should be considered for preoperative exercise testing or dipyridamole radionuclide (or dobutamine echocardiography) imaging if unable to exercise. Such imaging studies have demonstrated good discriminatory power in predicting complications among vascular surgery patients with intermediate clinical risk profiles who are scheduled to undergo major procedures; those with a low estimated risk on the basis of readily available clinical parameters generally do well without further testing, whereas those felt to be at high risk should probably undergo coronary arteriography and, if indicated, coronary revascularization before major peripheral vascular surgery. Patients with more severe functional limitations (NYHA class III or IV) or unstable angina are not appropriate candidates for elective surgery and may require coronary arteriography and therapeutic intervention before noncardiac surgery. Patients with a history of recent myocardial infarction, cardiomyopathy, or hemodynamically significant valvular disease and signs or symptoms of congestive heart failure should undergo preoperative noninvasive assessment of left ventricular function; hemodynamic monitoring throughout surgery and the immediate perioperative period is generally indicated in such patients.

**Table 5-2.** Cardiac risk index in noncardiac surgery

| Clinical variable | Point assignment |
|---|---|
| **History** | |
| Age >70 years | 5 |
| Recent myocardial infarction (≤6 months) | 10 |
| **Physical examination** | |
| Ventricular gallop or venous pressure ≥12 cm water | 11 |
| Significant valvular aortic stenosis | 3 |
| **Electrocardiogram** | |
| Rhythm other than sinus, or atrial ectopy on preoperative tracing | 7 |
| More than 5 ectopic ventricular beats per minute on any tracing before surgery | 7 |
| **Poor general medical condition (any factor)** | 3 |
| $Pa_{O_2}$ <60 mm Hg or $Pa_{CO_2}$ >50 mm Hg | |
| $K^+$ <3.0 mEq/L or $HCO_3$ <20 mEq/L | |
| BUN >50 mg/dl or creatinine >3.0 mg/dl | |
| Chronic liver disease | |
| Noncardiac debilitation | |
| **Surgical procedure** | |
| Intraperitoneal, intrathoracic, aortic | 3 |
| Emergency | 4 |
| MAXIMUM SCORE | 53 |

Modified from Goldman L et al: *N Engl J Med* 297:845, 1977.

**Table 5-3.** Perioperative cardiac complications stratified by Goldman risk index

| Risk index class | Point score | No or minimal complications (%) | Severe complications (%) | Cardiac death (%) |
|---|---|---|---|---|
| I | 0-5 | 99 | 0.6 | 0.2 |
| II | 6-12 | 96 | 3 | 1 |
| III | 13-25 | 86 | 11 | 3 |
| IV | ≥26 | 49 | 12 | 39 |

Modified from Weitz HH, Goldman L: *Med Clin North Am* 71:413, 1987.

## Endocarditis prophylaxis guidelines*

**Cardiac condition**

*Prophylaxis recommended*

Prosthetic cardiac valves
Previous bacterial endocarditis
Most congenital cardiac malformations
Rheumatic and other acquired valvular dysfunction
Hypertrophic cardiomyopathy
Mitral valve prolapse with regurgitation

*Prophylaxis not recommended*

Isolated secundum atrial septal defect
Surgical repair without residua beyond 6 months of secundum atrial septal defect, ventricular septal defect, or patent ductus arteriosus
Previous coronary artery bypass graft surgery
Mitral valve prolapse without regurgitation†
Physiologic or functional heart murmurs
Previous Kawasaki disease without valvular dysfunction
Previous rheumatic fever without valvular dysfunction
Cardiac pacemakers and implanted defibrillators

**Dental or surgical procedure ‡**

*Prophylaxis recommended*

Dental procedures known to induce gingival or mucosal bleeding, including professional cleaning
Tonsillectomy/adenoidectomy
Surgery involving intestinal or respiratory mucosae
Bronchoscopy with rigid bronchoscope
Sclerotherapy for esophageal varices
Esophageal dilatation
Gallbladder surgery

**Dental or surgical procedure—cont'd**

Cystoscopy
Urethral dilatation
Urethral catheterization if urinary tract infection present
Urinary tract surgery if infection is present
Prostatic surgery
Incision and drainage of infected tissue
Vaginal hysterectomy
Vaginal delivery in setting of infection

*Prophylaxis not recommended*

Dental procedures not likely to promote gingival bleeding
Injection of local intraoral anesthetic (except intraligamentary injections)
Shedding of primary teeth
Tympanostomy tube insertion
Endotracheal intubation
Bronchoscopy with flexible bronchoscope, with or without biopsy
Cardiac catheterization
Endoscopy with or without biopsy
Cesarean section
In the absence of infection—
 Urethral catheterization
 Dilatation and curettage
 Uncomplicated vaginal delivery
 Therapeutic abortion
 Sterilization procedures
 Insertion/removal of intrauterine devices

Modified from Dajani AS et al: *JAMA* 264: 2919, 1990.

*Selected cardiac conditions and procedures listed; table not intended to be all inclusive.

†Consider prophylaxis if mitral valve prolapse is associated with thickening and/or redundancy of valve leaflets, especially in men who are 45 years of age or older.

‡In patients with prosthetic heart valves, a history of endocarditis, or surgically constructed systemic-pulmonary shunts or conduits, physicians may reasonably choose to administer prophylactic antibiotics.

Patients with clinical evidence of significant valvular heart disease or of hypertrophic cardiomyopathy should undergo echocardiographic evaluation before all but the most emergent surgery. Hemodynamic management of the patient with an important valvular or subvalvular lesion requires cooperation between the internist and anesthesiologist. Recent experience suggests that even patients with severe aortic stenosis can undergo anesthesia and surgery relatively safely when carefully managed.

## PREVENTION OF BACTERIAL ENDOCARDITIS

Patients with valvular heart disease, hypertrophic cardiomyopathy, most congenital cardiac lesions, and systemic-pulmonary shunts should receive endocarditis prophylaxis before certain surgical or dental procedures. The risk of endocarditis in a given patient depends on the type and severity of the underlying cardiac condition, the specific nature of the surgical or dental procedure to be performed, and its association, if any, with bacteremia (see the box above). α-Hemolytic streptococci *(Streptococcus viridans)* and related organisms are the leading cause of endocarditis following dental and respiratory tract procedures, whereas enterococci pose the greatest risk of endocarditis in patients undergoing genitourinary, gynecologic, or gastrointestinal procedures. The standard of care has shifted toward a single preoperative dose of one or two clinically appropriate antibiotics followed by, at most, one postoperative dose (Table 5-4).

## HEMODYNAMIC MONITORING

Substantial reductions in perioperative cardiovascular complications and mortality have been noted among patients undergoing noncardiac surgery over the past 40 years: perioperative mortality among patients over 80 years of age has dropped from 20% in 1960 to approximately 6%, and perioperative cardiac reinfarction within 3 months of initial myocardial infarction has dropped from 30% to 5.8%. These reductions are probably due in part to pulmonary artery catheter monitoring, although there are no prospective, randomized trials assessing the benefit of pulmonary artery catheter monitoring among general surgery patients. Several trials have demonstrated signifi-

**Table 5-4.** Endocarditis prophylaxis regimens

| Clinical setting | Regimen | Antibiotics and dosages |
|---|---|---|
| Dental, oral, and upper respiratory tract procedures (standard) | Standard | Amoxicillin, 3 gm PO 1 hr before procedure; then 1.5 g 6 hr after initial dose |
| | β-Lactam–allergic patients | Erythromycin ethylsuccinate, 800 mg, or erythromycin stearate, 1 g PO 2 hr before procedure; then half the dose 6 hr after initial dose<br>or<br>Clindamycin, 300 mg PO 1 hr before procedure and 150 mg 6 hr after initial dose |
| Dental, oral, and upper respiratory tract procedures (alternative) | Unable to take oral medication | Ampicillin, 2 g IV/IM 30 min before procedure; then 1 g IV/IM, or amoxicillin, 1.5 g PO, 6 hr after initial dose |
| | β-Lactam–allergic patients unable to take oral medication | Clindamycin, 300 mg IV 30 min before procedure and 150 mg IV/PO 6 hr after initial dose |
| | Patients considered high risk and not candidates for standard regimen | Ampicillin, 2 g IV/IM, plus gentamicin, 1.5 mg/kg (not to exceed 80 mg) IV/IM 30 min before procedure; then amoxicillin, 1.5 g PO 6 hr after procedure, or parenteral regimen may be repeated 8 hr after initial dose |
| | β-Lactam–allergic patients considered high risk | Vancomycin, 1 g over 1 hr, starting 1 hr before procedure; no subsequent dose necessary |
| Genitourinary/gastrointestinal procedures | Standard | Ampicillin, 2 g IV/IM, plus gentamicin, 1.5 mg/kg (not to exceed 80 mg) IV/IM 30 min before procedure; then amoxicillin, 1.5 g PO 6 hr after procedure, or parenteral regimen may be repeated 8 hr after initial dose |
| | β-Lactam–allergic patients | Vancomycin, 1 g over 1 hr, and gentamicin, 1.5 mg/kg (not to exceed 80 mg), 1 hr before procedure; may repeat once 8 hr after initial dose |
| | Alternate low-risk patient regimen | Amoxicillin, 3 gm PO 1 hr before procedure; then 1.5 g 6 hr after initial dose |

Modified from Dajani AS et al: *JAMA* 264:2919, 1990.

cant benefit among peripheral vascular surgery patients. Criteria for selecting patients in whom perioperative central hemodynamic monitoring appears warranted are listed in the box at right.

## PERIOPERATIVE DRUG THERAPY

Questions regarding the manipulation of ongoing drug treatment comprise some of the most common and difficult issues in perioperative consultation. Often, the literature does not support clear, forceful articulation of guidelines, and the internist must tailor management to individual circumstances. In general, three factors must be considered in managing each situation: (1) Have the indications and dosages for the specific drug been clearly defined? (2) What are the likely anesthetic and surgical complications/interactions? (3) Is a clinically important withdrawal syndrome likely, and how can it be safely managed?

### Indications for perioperative pulmonary artery catheter monitoring

- Recent (within 6 months) myocardial infarction
- Clinically apparent congestive heart failure
- Suspected congestive heart failure in patient requiring emergent surgery
- Coronary artery bypass graft patients with any of the following:
  - Poor left ventricular function
  - Recent myocardial infarction
  - Severe/unstable angina
  - High-grade left main coronary artery stenosis
- Severe aortic or mitral stenosis
- Major vascular procedure in setting of coronary heart disease
- Pulmonary edema of unknown etiology

**Table 5-5.** Perioperative pharmacologic management

| Drug | Management | Commentary |
|---|---|---|
| **Anticoagulant** | | |
| Warfarin | *High risk*: stop and substitute heparin<br>*Low risk*: stop before surgery and restart postoperatively | Major surgery may be performed safely in anticoagulated patients; bleeding risk may prohibit perioperative anticoagulation with certain procedures |
| Heparin | *High risk*: continue adjusted dosage subcutaneous, low molecular weight heparin subcutaneous or intravenous infusion<br>*Low risk*: stop day of surgery and restart 1-2 d postoperatively | |
| **Anticonvulsant** | Continue maintenance | Short-acting oral agents may require substitutes |
| **Antiinflammatory** | | |
| Aspirin | Stop 1-3 wk preoperatively | Consider bleeding time before neurosurgery or cardiothoracic surgery |
| Nonsteroidal antiinflammatory drugs | Stop 1-3 d preoperatively | |
| **Cardiac** | | |
| Digitalis | Continue maintenance | Avoid preoperative digitalization |
| Antidysrhythmic medicines | Continue maintenance; prophylactic lidocaine for symptomatic ventricular tachycardia or fibrillation | Check serum concentrations; short-acting oral agents may require substitutes |
| Diuretics | Individualize fluid management | Hemodynamic monitoring may be indicated |
| β-Blockers | Continue or substitute | Avoid withdrawal |
| Calcium channel blockers | Continue maintenance | Parenteral substitute may be necessary |
| Nitrates | Continue or substitute | |
| **Antihypertensive** | | |
| Diuretics | Individualize fluid management | May stop 2 d preoperatively |
| Other agents | Continue or substitute | Avoid withdrawal symptoms |
| **Endocrine** | | |
| Diabetes mellitus | | |
| Oral agents | *Chlorpropamide*: stop 3 d preoperatively<br>*Glyburide*: stop 2 d preoperatively<br>*Others*: stop 1 d preoperatively | Monitor metabolic status<br>Start insulin by appropriate route for blood glucose >250 mg/dl or for incipient diabetic ketoacidosis |
| Insulin | *Minor procedure*: ½ to ⅔ usual dose of intermediate insulin<br>*Major procedure or ketoacidosis*: insulin infusion at 0.5-4.0 U/hr | Provide substrate—glucose @ 100 mg/kg/h |
| Estrogen | | |
| Contraceptive uses | Stop 3-4 wk preoperatively | Appropriate deep vein thrombosis prophylaxis |
| Replacement | Continue or hold | |
| Thyroid | | |
| Replacement | Continue maintenance or hold up to 1 wk | Urgent surgery may be safely performed in untreated hypothyroidism |
| Suppression | Continue or initiate therapy | Establish adequate suppression preoperatively |
| **Pulmonary** | Continue or substitute | Check levels (theophylline) |
| **Psychotropic** | | |
| Tricyclic antidepressants | Stop 1 wk preoperatively | Altered response to anesthetics and drug interactions |
| Tranquilizers | Stop or taper preoperatively, if feasible | Anticipate withdrawal reactions |
| Lithium | Stop or taper preoperatively | Metabolic disturbances |

Modified from Cygan R, Waitzkin H: *J Gen Intern Med* 2:270, 1987.

Most drugs used in the management of chronic medical illness should be continued through the perioperative period. For minor procedures the patient can receive an oral dose with sips of water on the morning of surgery and another dose later in the day as indicated. For more difficult surgery with a prolonged recovery period, long-acting or parenteral substitutes for chronic therapy may be needed. Table 5-5 provides summary recommendations for commonly used therapeutic agents.

## PROPHYLACTIC ANTIMICROBIAL THERAPY

Elective surgery should be delayed until preexisting bacterial infections are treated. Bacterial colonization or infection of the urinary tract is relatively common, especially among individuals with a history of urinary tract infection, in those with indwelling catheters, in those with atonic bladders or obstructive uropathy, and among the elderly. A preoperative screening urinalysis and, when the urinalysis is abnormal, a culture with antibiotic sensitivities, is appropriate in such patients. To reduce the likelihood of perioperative urosepsis, treatment should be initiated with an appropriate antibiotic before surgery in patients with evidence of bacterial colonization or infection of the urinary tract, especially if urinary tract instrumentation is necessary.

Acute exacerbations of chronic bronchitis should be treated to the point of resolution or substantial improvement before surgery. Subsequent perioperative flares must be assumed to be caused by bacteria resistant to whatever antibiotic might have been employed preoperatively.

Antimicrobial agents may be given perioperatively to prevent infection of normally sterile tissues by direct contamination during a surgical procedure. Such therapy is appropriate when the likelihood of infection is great or the sequelae of infection are severe, when relatively well-tolerated drugs are effective against the likely organisms, and when available evidence demonstrates a reduction in perioperative morbidity as a result of prophylaxis.

Most clinical trials have focused on clean-contaminated procedures such as vaginal hysterectomy and colorectal surgery or unusual and extensive clean surgery such as cardiothoracic procedures and hip arthroplasty. However, limited recent data suggest that antibiotic prophylaxis may also be cost effective for some commonly performed, relatively simple clean procedures such as inguinal herniorrhaphy and certain types of breast surgery. Recent trials have also highlighted the efficacy of very short courses of therapy; a single dose of antibiotic immediately before surgery, followed by no more than one dose postoperatively, is as effective as longer regimens and less likely to be associated with toxicity or the development of resistant organisms.

Table 5-6 lists the common surgical procedures for which antibiotic prophylaxis is recommended. The specific regimen must be individualized to the patient and the local microbial environment.

**Table 5-6.** Perioperative wound infection prophylaxis

| Procedure | Regimen |
|---|---|
| **Cardiothoracic and vascular** | 1 |
| Median sternotomy | |
| Coronary artery bypass* | |
| Prosthetic valve | |
| Pacemaker insertion | |
| Lobectomy/pneumonectomy | |
| Peripheral vascular | |
| **General surgery** | |
| Breast surgery† | 3 |
| Colorectal procedures | 4 or 5 |
| Biliary tract‡ | 1 |
| Herniorrhaphy† | 3 |
| Appendectomy (primary) | 5 |
| Gastroduodenal/small bowel‡ | 1 |
| Penetrating abdominal trauma | 5 |
| **Gynecologic surgery** | 1 |
| Cesarean section§ | |
| Hysterectomy | |
| **Orthopedic surgery** | 1 or 2 |
| Arthroplasty/joint replacement | |
| Internal fixation | |
| Amputation of lower limb | |
| **Neurosurgery** | |
| Craniotomy‖ | 6 or 7 |
| Cerebrospinal fluid shunt¶ | 8 |
| **Head and neck surgery** | |
| Mucous membranes crossed | 1 |

*1*, Cefazolin, 1 g IM or IV immediately before surgery and 6-8 hr later; *2*, vancomycin, 1 g IV immediately before surgery; *3*, cefonicid, 1 g IV immediately before surgery; *4*, neomycin and erythromycin, 1 g each by mouth at 1 PM, 2 PM, and 11 PM the day before surgery, with mechanical bowel preparation; *5*, cefoxitin, 2 g IV immediately before surgery; *6*, clindamycin, 300 mg IV immediately before surgery and 4 hr after; *7*, vancomycin, 1 g IV, and gentamicin, 80 mg IV, immediately before surgery; *8*, trimethoprim, 160 mg, sulfamethoxazole, 800 mg, IV immediately before surgery and every 12 hr for three doses.

*Poorly substantiated by literature, but the standard practice.

†Based on recent data; no uniform practice yet established.

‡High risk; advanced age, infection or inflammation, biliary tract obstruction, jaundice.

§High risk; emergency, premature rupture of membranes, obesity.

‖High risk; open wound, reexploration, microsurgery.

¶May be beneficial in centers with high infection rates.

## THROMBOEMBOLISM PROPHYLAXIS

The surgical environment often presents circumstances that fulfill Virchow's triad: stasis, intimal injury, and a hypercoagulable state. However, some patients and procedures present a particularly high risk. Specific factors predisposing patients to thromboembolic complications include advanced age, prolonged anesthesia or surgery, extended perioperative immobilization, paralysis, malignancy, history of venous disease or thromboembolism, and premenopausal exogenous estrogen use (Table 5-7).

There is general agreement that patients at moderate or high risk for perioperative thromboembolism should receive prophylaxis. Available data from a number of well-conducted clinical studies have demonstrated substantial reductions in thromboembolic complications with a variety of regimens in different surgical settings. The box on p. 118 presents guidelines, by category of surgery and perceived underlying risk, for thromboembolism prophylaxis in the surgical patient.

**Table 5-7.** Postoperative venous thromboembolism risk classification

| Risk categories | Calf deep vein thrombosis | Proximal deep vein thrombosis | Pulmonary embolism |
|---|---|---|---|
| **High risk** | 40%-80% | 10%-20% | 1%-5% |
| Age >40 years | | | |
| Surgery >30 minutes | | | |
| Orthopedic surgery | | | |
| Pelvic or abdominal cancer surgery | | | |
| Previous deep vein thrombosis or pulmonary embolism | | | |
| Secondary risk factors* | | | |
| Hereditary or acquired coagulopathies† | | | |
| **Moderate risk** | 10%-40% | 2%-10% | 0.1%-0.7% |
| Age >40 years | | | |
| Other surgery >30 minutes | | | |
| Secondary risk factors* | | | |
| **Low risk** | <10% | <1% | <0.01% |
| Age < 40 years, or >40 years and surgery <30 minutes | | | |
| No secondary risk factors | | | |

Modified from Hull et al: *Chest* 85:379, 1986.
*Obesity, immobilization, malignancy, varicose veins, estrogen use, paralysis.
†Especially protein C, S, antithrombin III deficiency, anticardiolipin antibodies.

## Recommended venous thromboembolism (VTE) prophylaxis for patients undergoing surgery

### General surgery

Low-risk patients: early ambulation
Moderate-risk patients: elastic stockings and low-dose heparin
High-risk patients: low-dose heparin (3500-5000 U q8h) or low molecular weight heparin
Higher risk patients prone to wound complications: dextran or intermittent pneumatic compression
Very high risk patients:low-dose heparin, low molecular weight heparin, or dextran *and* intermittent pneumatic compression
Selected high-risk patients: warfarin (titrated to INR of 2.0-3.0)
Aspirin should not be used for VTE prophylaxis in general surgery patients

### Orthopedic patients

Patients undergoing elective total hip replacement: warfarin, low molecular weight heparin, or adjusted dose heparin
Patients with hip fractures: warfarin or low molecular weight heparin
Knee surgery patients: intermittent pneumatic compression

### Neurosurgery

Patients undergoing intracranial neurosurgery: intermittent pneumatic compression
Patients with spinal cord injuries with paralysis: adjusted dose heparin or low molecular weight heparin; warfarin or intermittent pneumatic compression may also be effective

### Other

Multiple trauma patients: intermittent pneumatic compression, warfarin, or low molecular weight heparin, when feasible
Selected high-risk orthopedic/multiple trauma patients: placement of inferior vena cava filter when other forms of prophylaxis contraindicated or ineffective
Patients with indwelling central venous catheters for more than several days: warfarin, 1 mg PO qd, to prevent axillary-subclavian venous thrombosis

Modified from Clagett et al: *Chest* 102:391S, 1992.

## MANAGEMENT OF SELECTED CLINICAL PROBLEMS IN PATIENTS UNDERGOING SURGERY

### Hypertension

Patients with hypertension experience greater blood pressure lability during anesthesia, surgery, and the perioperative period than do normotensive individuals. This lability manifests primarily in hypertensive episodes, although interventions to support blood pressure (fluid challenge or adrenergic agents) are more common among hypertensive patients than those with normal blood pressure taking no medications. Among hypertensives this lability is largely independent of preoperative blood pressure control and appears to be mediated primarily by transient sympathetic overactivity following noxious stimuli, such as laryngoscopy before endotracheal intubation. Perioperative hemorrhagic complications, generally within the operative field, are more common among patients with poor preoperative blood pressure control (diastolic blood pressure 110 mm Hg or higher).

#### Managed Care Guide

- Maintain usual antihypertensive medications throughout surgery and the perioperative period in the patient whose blood pressure is in reasonable control.
  1. Administer with a sip of water on the morning of surgery; continue usual regimen postoperatively.
  2. For a patient unable to take oral medications postoperatively, substitute appropriate parenteral forms of β-blockers, methyldopa, enalaprilat, calcium blockers, or diuretics.
  3. To preclude rebound hypertension, substitute methyldopa or a β-blocker for clonidine preoperatively for a patient expected to be unable to take oral medications postoperatively.

- For a newly identified hypertensive patient who requires surgery, consider a sympatholytic agent if preoperative treatment is necessary.
  1. Avoid new use of diuretics in the several weeks before surgery to preclude volume depletion and electrolyte disturbances.
- Elevated blood pressure in the postoperative period often responds to analgesia or optimization of respiratory status and oxygenation.
  1. Persistent moderate or severe elevation of blood pressure, without evidence of acute end-organ damage, generally responds to initiation of a maintenance dose of an oral agent (or the appropriate parenteral form in patients unable to take oral medications).
- Because of the documented risk of extreme blood pressure lability, worsening tachycardia, and cardiac ischemic events, sublingual nifedipine should not be used to treat perioperative hypertension.
- True perioperative hypertensive crises (defined by end-organ damage) should be treated with appropriate parenteral agents, generally sodium nitroprusside or labetolol.

### Diabetes mellitus

Diabetes mellitus is the most common endocrine problem encountered among surgical patients. Patients with diabetes require surgery more often than do nondiabetic individuals, and surgery among diabetic patients is more often associated with complications, especially adverse cardiovascular events and perioperative infections. As many as half the diabetic individuals in the United States are undiagnosed, and it is not uncommon for a patient's diabetes to first come to medical attention when he or she presents for evaluation of a surgical problem. Although surgical and perioperative mortality and morbidity are increased in patients with diabetes, most such patients fare extremely well when appropriately supported through surgery. Several clinical series have demonstrated a modest advantage of intravenously infused insulin over the use of intermediate-acting insulin injected subcutaneously in patients undergoing surgery. In practice, insulin infusion is generally reserved for surgical patients perceived to be at unusually high risk or those who are in ketoacidosis and require emergent surgery. Diabetic patients undergoing coronary artery bypass surgery, however, generally require an insulin infusion to achieve reasonable glucose control intraoperatively and in the immediate postoperative period.

Objectives in the management of the diabetic patient undergoing surgery include (1) characterization of the status of the patient's diabetes, (2) preoperative optimization of glucose control, (3) identification of preexisting complications, treating those amenable to immediate intervention and anticipating problems with others, (4) provision of adequate insulin and substrate for cellular function during surgery, striving for smooth, moderate blood glucose control (150 to 250 mg/dl) and avoiding hypoglycemic and hyperglycemic peaks and ketoacidosis, (5) resumption of appropriate diabetic maintenance therapy and nutritional support postoperatively, and (6) aggressive postoperative monitoring of potential problems arising from the chronic complications of diabetes.

#### Managed Care Guide

- Diabetic patients should have a preoperative determination of serum creatinine and a urinalysis to exclude pyuria, bacteriuria, and substantial proteinuria.
- All adult diabetic patients should have an ECG preoperatively, in the immediate postoperative period, and, if still hospitalized, on the third postoperative day, as well as for any episode of global deterioration.
- Diabetic patients who are maintained on diet with moderate or tight glycemic control may be managed operatively without insulin and with non–dextrose-containing intravenous fluids.
  1. Close monitoring of blood glucose and acid-base status is necessary.
  2. Insulin therapy should be initiated for blood glucose values over 250 mg/dl or for incipient ketoacidosis.
  3. Operative and postoperative patients who are receiving no alimentation may develop ketoacidosis at low blood glucose levels and may require concurrent glucose and insulin infusions.
- Diabetic patients maintained on oral hypoglycemic agents should hold these medications for 24 hours (tolbutamide or glipizide) or 48 to 72 hours (tolazamide, glyburide, or chlorpropamide) preoperatively.
  1. Operative management is as described for the diet-maintained diabetic patient, with very close

monitoring of blood glucose, especially in patients who had been using long-acting oral hypoglycemic agents.

- Patients maintained preoperatively on insulin with good glycemic control can generally be managed throughout surgery with half to two thirds of their usual intermediate-acting insulin administered subcutaneously *and* provision of adequate substrate, generally 100 mg glucose per kilogram of body weight per hour (equivalent to a 5% dextrose-containing intravenous infusate at 2 ml/kg/hour).
  1. Where close operative glucose monitoring is available, insulin infusion to start at 1 to 2 U per hour, concurrent with adequate substrate delivery as above, is an appropriate alternative and should be employed as a routine for coronary artery bypass surgery in insulin-requiring diabetic patients.
- Patients in diabetic ketoacidosis who require emergent surgery should receive aggressive volume resuscitation, intravenous insulin (bolus followed by infusion), and correction of major metabolic derangements in whatever preoperative period is available.
- Postoperative screening of the surgical wound, vascular access sites, and the urinary tract is essential to identify incipient infection.

### Asthma/chronic obstructive pulmonary disease

Patients with reactive airways disease are at substantially increased risk of postoperative pulmonary complications but can generally be supported through surgery with little or no excessive morbidity. Special risk groups and the preoperative evaluation of the patient with known or suspected reactive airways disease are described above. The patient who smokes is at special risk of postoperative infection. Cessation of smoking can reduce this risk, but available data suggest that 6 to 8 weeks of smoking abstinence may be necessary to realize measurable reductions of postoperative respiratory infections. Elective surgery in the patient with an active clinical exacerbation of reactive airways disease should be delayed at least 2 weeks.

Halogenated hydrocarbon anesthetic agents are bronchodilatory, but adjunctive agents often employed during surgery, such as esmolol and parenteral narcotics, are frank or potential bronchoconstrictors (as is the combination of cyclopropane and thiopental, which is rarely if ever employed). D-Tubocurarine possesses histamine-like effects. Maintenance bronchodilator drugs, especially theophylline preparations and β-sympathomimetics, may also interact with anesthetic agents to enhance the likelihood of dysrhythmias. A history of corticosteroid use, parenteral, oral, and/or inhaled, should always be sought from a patient with reactive airways disease; the possibility of adrenal suppression must be considered. Close preoperative cooperation between the anesthesiologist and medical consultant minimizes such preventable complications.

### Managed Care Guide

- Delay elective surgery for at least 2 weeks in patients with an active episode of bronchospasm or bronchitis.
- Maintain usual inhaled bronchodilators until surgery and in the postoperative period.
- Oral theophylline preparations with long half-lives may be maintained up to the morning of surgery in patients who have shown benefit from them.
  1. Check and achieve therapeutic level preoperatively.
  2. Usual oral dosage or substitution of intravenous infusion may result in higher than anticipated level on the basis of unpredictable hepatic blood flow during surgery.
  3. Consider reducing or holding the dose on the morning of surgery.
     a. Immediate preoperative level will decay slowly ($t_{1/2} > 4$ to 6 hours generally among adults).
- Anticipate adrenal suppression in patients previously maintained on oral prednisone equivalent (more than 40 mg/day for over 1 week) or inhaled beclomethasone equivalent (over 1500 μg/day for more than 6 months) in the preceding year, and treat expectantly with stress dose corticosteroids (see below).
- For patients taking maintenance corticosteroids, boost the dosage to counter the stress of surgery (see below).
- For patients with an acute exacerbation of reactive airways disease who require urgent or emergent surgery, administer parenteral corticosteroids (more than 60 mg methylprednisolone IV every 6 hours, preferably starting 6 to 12 hours before surgery), and nebulized β-sympathomimetics.
- Anticipate delayed weaning from ventilatory support in patients with impaired pulmonary function and/or preoperative hypercarbia.
- Institute preoperative instruction in deep breathing exercises and incentive spirometry and continue postoperatively.

### Thyroid disease

Hypothyroidism is quite prevalent in the general population, especially among older individuals. Patients who are euthyroid when taking replacement L-thyroxine are at no increased surgical risk. Patients with mild to moderate hypothyroidism who have not been treated should generally be made euthyroid before elective surgery. These patients, however, and even those who are severely myxedematous, can be safely managed throughout urgently required surgery. Special attention must be paid to (1) the mode and rate of treatment of the underlying hypothyroidism, (2) monitoring for hypoglycemia and hyponatremia, (3) exaggerated responses to anesthetic and other agents in the setting of an often profound hypometabolic rate, (4) avoidance of cold stress and hypothermia in the operative and postoperative setting, and (5) anticipated hypoventilation and its implications for assisted ventilation.

Untreated hyperthyroidism poses a more serious risk to the operative patient than does either treated or untreated hypothyroidism. The predominant risks of general anesthesia and surgery in thyrotoxic patients are (1) the predisposition toward dysrhythmias and high-output cardiac failure engendered by striking increases in metabolic rate, (2) the unpredictable level and duration of response to various medications, including anesthetic agents, and (3) the induction of thyroid storm, with its substantial associated morbidity and 5% to 10% mortality. While the symptoms and signs of hyperthyroidism can be ameliorated in thyrotoxic patients, thyroid storm cannot be prevented until the patient is rendered euthyroid for several months. Indeed, in older clinical reviews surgery was the most common precipitant of this endocrine emergency. Accordingly, elective surgery should be postponed until a known hyperthyroid patient has been made and maintained euthyroid for 3 months.

Thyrotoxic patients who need urgent or emergent surgery require extremely close monitoring and aggressive management. A combination of thyroid-blocking agents, sympatholytics, and stress-dose corticosteroids is generally employed.

### Managed Care Guide

- Hypothyroid and hyperthyroid patients should be rendered euthyroid before elective surgery.
  1. The effects of hypothyroidism can be largely corrected over a period of 3 to 4 weeks.
  2. Hyperthyroidism generally requires several months to achieve control.
- Hypothyroid patients who require urgent or emergent surgery may be managed safely with special attention to the following:
  1. Propensity to develop hypoglycemia and hyponatremia
  2. Exaggerated response to anesthetics and other medications
  3. Sensitivity to cold stress
  4. Hypoventilation
- Thyroid replacement therapy should be initiated as soon as possible in hypothyroid patients who need urgent or emergent surgery with the exception of those undergoing coronary revascularization.
- Thyrotoxic patients who need urgent or emergent surgery require close preoperative, intraoperative, and postoperative monitoring and management, consisting of the following:
  1. Intensive care unit level of monitoring
  2. Initiation of thyroid blockade, preferably with propylthiouracil, 100 to 300 mg orally or per nasogastric tube every 8 hours
     a. Methimazole may be employed alternatively (at a dosage of 30 to 60 mg daily) but does not block peripheral conversion of thyroxine ($T_4$) to triiodothyronine ($T_3$).
  3. Sodium iodide (250 mg intravenously every 6 hours or 500 to 1000 mg intravenously every 12 hours) may be an appropriate adjunct to block thyroid hormone secretion and reduce gland vascularity.
  4. Sympathetic overactivity may be controlled with propranolol (initial dosage 10 to 40 mg orally or 1 to 2 mg intravenously every 4 to 6 hours) titrated to achieve a pulse less than 90.
     a. Parenteral esmolol or labetolol may be substituted, especially in refractory cases.
- Patients with significant hyperthyroidism or hypothyroidism who require emergent or urgent surgery should receive stress-dose steroid coverage (see below).

### The patient taking corticosteroids

Primary adrenal insufficiency (Addison disease) is quite uncommon, as is secondary adrenal insufficiency on the basis of an intrinsic deficit of corticotropin. Adrenal suppression by exogenous corticosteroid administration is, on the other hand, quite prevalent. Patients who receive potentially suppressive doses of exogenous corticosteroids are most often those with severe dermatoses, inflammatory rheumatologic conditions, hematologic or lymphoproliferative disorders, or those with asthma or other forms of COPD. Individuals who have received more than 40 mg prednisone per day, or its equivalent, for more than 1 week in the preceding year are at risk of adrenal suppression. Smaller doses of oral corticosteroids administered for longer periods, and even the inhaled corticosteroids employed now as mainline therapy in the management of reactive airways disease, may also result in adrenal suppression. Alternate day administration of relatively low doses of oral corticosteroids (less than 20 mg prednisone equivalent) reduces the risk of suppression. Long-term treatment with very low doses of corticosteroids (less than 5 mg per day prednisone equivalent) is also associated with a low likelihood of adrenal suppression.

The goal of perioperative management for patients with known or suspected adrenal suppression is the provision of sufficient exogenous corticosteroid to match the maximal physiologic output caused by the stress of surgery and anesthesia. This has been established at 300 to 400 mg cortisol equivalent in the first 24 hours after general anesthesia and major surgery. Hydrocortisone sodium succinate or hydrocortisone sodium phosphate should be employed preferentially to achieve combined glucocorticoid and mineralocorticoid effects. Protocols using the intramuscular route of administration have demonstrated variable effectiveness. Repeated intravenous boluses or combined bolus and infusion protocols are the most reliable means of supporting patients through surgery. Up to 40% of bolus-administered hydrocortisone may be lost in the urine.

### Managed Care Guide

- Suspected adrenal suppression may be excluded by a normal response to a cosyntropin stimulation test performed preoperatively.
- If adrenal suppression is confirmed or is suspected in a patient who requires surgery urgently or in whom a cosyntropin stimulation test has not been performed, the following apply:
  1. When possible, a priming dose of hydrocortisone (100 mg) may be administered orally, intramuscularly, or intravenously at midnight before the patient's surgery.
  2. Administer hydrocortisone sodium succinate or hydrocortisone sodium phosphate, 100 mg, intravenously on call to the operating room and every 6 to 8 hours thereafter for 24 hours.
     a. After initial bolus, an infusion of hydrocortisone at 10 mg per hour may be substituted for repeated boluses.
  3. After complicated or prolonged surgery, consider extending stress-dose steroid coverage.
     a. Hydrocortisone, 50 mg every 6 to 8 hours on postoperative day 1
     b. Hydrocortisone, 25 mg every 6 to 8 hours on postoperative day 2
  4. For intraoperative or postoperative hypotension include intravenous bolus administration of hydrocortisone, 50 to 100 mg, in the treatment regimen.

### The elderly patient

Changing demographics combined with advances in anesthetic and surgical technique have led to a steady increase in minor and major surgery for elderly patients. Although the elderly currently comprise less than 15% of the population, they account for 20% to 40% of all surgery, 50% of emergency procedures, and 75% of overall surgical mortality. Age itself appears to account for little, if any, of the excess mortality seen in elderly surgical patients. More important variables include the nature and severity of underlying disease(s), and the type of surgery, especially if performed as an emergency procedure. Age is, however, an independent risk factor for cardiovascular morbidity, including congestive heart failure, myocardial infarction, and stroke. Therefore the commonly utilized schema for quantifying perioperative risk, described earlier, includes an adjustment for age alone. There are no data to support the routine use of perioperative invasive hemodynamic monitoring in the elderly, although such monitoring can be carried out safely when indicated on the basis of underlying disease. As in younger patients, an inadequate cardiovascular response to exercise is an important predictor of risk and constitutes an indication for additional evaluation, aggressive perioperative management, and/or reconsideration of the surgical decision.

#### Managed Care Guide

- Preoperative evaluation should include explicit estimation of functional status and rehabilitation goals.
- History and physical examination should be supplemented with baseline renal function tests, glucose determination, a screening test for thyroid function, and other studies as indicated clinically.
- In cases where cardiovascular reserve is uncertain, and in patients undergoing high risk procedures, preoperative exercise testing or dipyridamole radionuclide imaging may provide guidance.
- Meticulous attention to drug selection and dosing is necessary.
- Resuscitation wishes and a health care proxy should be established preoperatively in all patients, including elderly operative candidates.

### Liver disease

Patients with serious underlying liver disease tolerate general anesthesia and surgery poorly. All anesthetic regimens, including epidural and spinal anesthesia, reduce hepatic blood flow. Older halogenated hydrocarbon anesthetic gases (halothane and methoxyflurane) carry an independent risk of hepatic toxicity. Isoflurane, in wide use at present, is not a direct hepatotoxin but does cause systemic vasodilatation and a reduction in cardiac output with resultant risk of impaired hepatic blood flow.

The quantifiable risk of surgery in patients with underlying liver disease correlates with the extent of hepatic functional impairment. This is generally manifested by readily identifiable factors: encephalopathy, cutaneous stigmata of chronic hepatic dysfunction, the presence and severity of ascites, elevation in serum bilirubin, hypoalbuminemia, and coagulopathy. Hepatic synthetic dysfunction may complicate acute processes (viral, alcoholic, or drug-induced hepatitis, shock liver) or chronic liver diseases (cirrhosis, chronic viral or autoimmune hepatitis). Surgical and perioperative mortality among patients with cirrhosis undergoing major vascular surgery (excluding portal-systemic shunt surgery) ranges from less than 10% in those with well-compensated livers to greater than 75% in those with evidence of severe derangements in hepatic function. Elevations in hepatic transaminases alone do not predict an adverse outcome from anesthesia and surgery, but must be interpreted in context, and may be an early marker of severe hepatic injury after shock, trauma, toxic insult, or in severe viral hepatitis.

Preoperative efforts for a patient with evidence of hepatic dysfunction must be directed at optimizing nutritional and volume status, including reduction of significant ascites, correcting coagulopathy, anticipating and treating encephalopathy, and correcting electrolyte disturbances. Common operative complications include excessive hemorrhage and exaggerated responses to sedatives, narcotic analgesics, intravenous induction agents, and neuromuscular blocking agents. Postoperative complications include worsening of hepatic function, hemorrhage in the operative field and from the gastrointestinal tract, encephalopathy, impaired wound healing, pneumonia, volume and electrolyte derangements, acute tubular necrosis, and hepatorenal syndrome.

#### Managed Care Guide

- Quantify risk by profiling clinical features (encephalopathy, ascites, cutaneous stigmata) and biochemical markers (albumin, bilirubin, coagulation studies) of hepatic dysfunction in patients with known or suspected liver disease.
- Perform noninvasive imaging studies preoperatively to identify an obstructive basis for jaundice.
- Consider alternatives to surgery for patients with severe, irremediable hepatic dysfunction.
- Temporize to allow correction of remediable derangements in patients where surgery is necessary.
- Administer vitamin K, fresh frozen plasma, and occasionally plasmapheresis combined with plasma infusion for coagulopathy.
- Manage edema/ascites with the following:
  1. Bed rest in lateral decubitus position and lower extremity elevation
  2. Rigid salt restriction (250 to 500 mg sodium per day) and moderate fluid restriction (less than 1.5 L per day)
  3. Escalating doses of aldactone, beginning at 100 mg per day, increasing by 100 mg per day every 3 days, to a total of 600 mg per day, in divided doses, monitoring serum potassium, BUN, and creatinine closely
  4. Occasional supplementation with a loop diuretic, beginning at furosemide, 40 mg per day, or equivalent
  5. Large-volume paracenteses (up to 5 L), generally with intravenous albumin infusion, to achieve control of refractory ascites
- Treat or prevent hepatic encephalopathy with dietary protein restriction and lactulose (30 ml three times daily).

### Renal disease

Special precautions are necessary in patients with acute renal failure (ARF), chronic renal failure (CRF), or the nephrotic syndrome. Among such patients physiologic derangements relevant to surgery include impairment of fluid and electrolyte balance, acidosis, increased risk from hypotension and potential nephrotoxins, exaggerated responses to neuromuscular blocking agents eliminated through renal means, anemia, a hemorrhagic diathesis from platelet dysfunction, hypercoagulability in the setting of the nephrotic syndrome, increased risk of infection, and impaired wound healing.

Azotemic patients handle volume loads poorly, and such patients are at risk for both dehydration and volume overload with perioperative stresses that would be well compensated in individuals with normal renal function. Volume overload, in particular, may result in the rapid development of hypertension, pulmonary edema, or peripheral edema despite normal cardiac function. Hypoalbuminemia from the nephrotic syndrome enhances the risk of total body volume overload and confounds estimation of intravascular volume status.

Potassium handling is impaired in patients with severe renal dysfunction but may also be quite deranged among those with only modest degrees of azotemia in the clinical setting of distal tubulointerstitial disease or the hyporenin-hypoaldosterone syndrome, most commonly noted in diabetic patients. Operative stresses, muscle injuries, burns, gastrointestinal or traumatic hemorrhage, and perioperative infections markedly enhance catabolism, with the production of enormous endogenous potassium loads, whereas transfused blood contributes an added exogenous potassium burden. Metabolic acidoses and further derangements in calcium-phosphate balance may also be engendered by the same processes that promote perioperative hyperkalemia.

A variety of diagnostic pharmaceuticals and medications may compound preexisting renal abnormalities in the perioperative setting. Those which pose the greatest risk to azotemic surgical patients include iodinated radiocontrast agents and aminoglycoside antibiotics. Other medications that carry substantial nephrotoxic risk, but which are less often indicated perioperatively, include nonsteroidal antiinflammatory drugs, chemotherapeutic agents, amphotericin B, and angiotensin converting enzyme inhibitors. Substitution of interventions with less potential nephrotoxicity should be considered when feasible; if a potential nephrotoxin is strongly indicated on clinical grounds, pretreatment optimization of volume status and close monitoring of renal function are necessary.

Human recombinant erythropoietin improves the anemia associated with renal failure, but in the setting of surgery such patients often require transfusion to achieve or maintain an optimal hematocrit, generally above 30%. Dialysis itself may also improve the anemia somewhat. Clinically significant platelet dysfunction associated with uremia is generally manifested by an abnormal bleeding time. This disorder often does not fully correct despite dialysis but generally responds promptly to some combination of arginine vasopressin, cryoprecipitate, and red cell transfusion. Estrogens have also been found to be effective in controlling the bleeding that is associated with uremia.

Hemodialysis provides the means of optimizing volume, electrolyte balance, acid-base status, and to some extent the hemostasis defect associated with renal failure. Dialysis is generally best timed to occur on the days preceding and following surgery. Patients with the nephrotic syndrome have an increased risk of venous thromboembolism, which is compounded by surgery, and require appropriate prophylaxis (see the box on p. 118).

#### Managed Care Guide

- Where hemodialysis is indicated to correct volume, electrolyte, acid-base, and hemostasis defects, perform preferentially at least 12 hours before and 12 to 24 hours after planned surgery.
- For a patient not on dialysis, salt and fluid requirements may be estimated from results of a 24-hour urine collection when patient is in balance.
  1. Mild overhydration may be corrected by fluid restriction and administration of loop diuretics.
- Hemodynamic monitoring may be indicated to determine intravascular volume status in patients with severe renal failure with or without hypoalbuminuria and pulmonary edema.
  1. Emergency dialysis may be necessary to correct serious refractory volume derangements.
- Clinically significant hyperkalemia (generally over 6 mEq/L with ECG abnormalities) should be treated emergently with calcium chloride, dextrose and insulin infusion, and/or sodium bicarbonate infusion (see Chapter 90).
  1. Definitive treatment generally requires diuresis, generally effective only in the setting of mild renal dysfunction, ion exchange resins, or dialysis.
- Pretreatment with volume expansion followed by mannitol or a loop diuretic should accompany iodinated radiocontrast administration in the setting of renal failure.
- Atracurium or vercuronium should be employed preferentially to achieve operative neuromuscular blockade.
- Use of aminoglycoside antibiotics, nonsteroidal antiinflammatory drugs, angiotensin converting enzyme inhibitors, and other potential nephrotoxins should be restricted or, when strongly indicated, monitored closely in the perioperative setting.
- Dialysis, recombinant erythropoietin, and transfusion should be employed to achieve and maintain hematocrit at 30% or greater.
- Defects in hemostasis should be corrected with dialysis, arginine vasopressin, cryoprecipitate, or red cell infusion.

### The pregnant patient

Pregnant women generally tolerate nonobstetric surgery without significantly increased morbidity or mortality. Putative risks from exposure of the fetus to general anesthetic agents can be minimized by avoiding all but emergent surgery during the periods of organogenesis (first trimester) and central nervous system myelination (third trimester); indeed, the risk to the fetus of nonemergent maternal surgery performed in the second trimester has been shown to be extremely low. The risk of fetal loss or of premature delivery increases substantially with increasing severity of the underlying surgical problem, with intraoperative shock, hypoxemia, or acidosis, and with postoperative complications. Trauma and acute abdominal processes, such as appendicitis and cholecystitis, are the most common clinical conditions necessitating urgent or emergent surgery among pregnant women. Abdominal processes may confound or be confounded by obstetric complications. The possibility of pregnancy must be considered in any woman of childbearing potential who requires surgery.

Evaluation and management of the pregnant woman undergoing nonobstetric surgery require knowledge of the major physiologic changes associated with pregnancy. Blood pressure drops in early to midgestation; relatively modest blood pressure elevations near term, especially after the twenty-eigth week, may presage the obstetric emergency of preeclampsia. Dyspnea, pedal edema, and a third heart sound are common findings in late stages of normal pregnancies. Also late in gestation, uterine compression of the vena cava and aorta may compromise both maternal cardiac output and placental perfusion when a pregnant woman is maintained in supine recumbency, a position also associated with arterial hypoxemia. The normal respiratory pattern of pregnancy is one of hyperventilation ($Pco_2$ 25 to 30 mm Hg) with metabolic compensation ($HCO_3$ 17 to 22 mEq/L), factors that must be considered in pregnant patients who require intubation and mechanical ventilation. In normal pregnancies blood and plasma volumes increase substantially, generally with little clinical consequence, although the volume of distribution of many medications may be affected. Venous stasis, from increased filling of capacitance vessels and extrinsic compression of pelvic veins by the uterine contents, and the hypercoagulability associated with pregnancy result in a marked increase in the risk of thromboembolic disease, a situation compounded by trauma or surgery. Delayed gastric emptying and relaxation of the lower esophageal sphincter during pregnancy lead to an increased perioperative risk of aspiration pneumonitis. Dilatation of the urinary collecting system predisposes to retention, bacterial colonization, and infection. The glomerular filtration rate increases 30% to 50% in normal pregnancies, with an associated increase in the clearance of many drugs.

Pregnant women undergoing nonobstetric surgery often require adjunctive medications, such as antibiotics, in the perioperative period. Many medications can be safely administered to a pregnant woman without adversely affecting the fetus: heparin, most β-lactam antibiotics, erythromycin, methyldopa, hydralazine, most asthma medications, and others. In many instances, especially with newer drugs, the fetal risk is unknown. A moderate number of common medications are known to be fetotoxic or result in malformations; these should be employed during pregnancy only when strongly indicated and when suitable alternatives do not exist or cannot be used because of other reasons, such as drug allergy. Medications that are problematic in pregnancy include aminoglycosides, tetracycline, quinolone, and sulfonamide antimicrobials; warfarin; angiotensin converting enzyme inhibitors; phenytoin; barbiturates; high-dose aspirin; histamine-$_2$ blockers; and a wide range of chemotherapeutic agents.

### Managed Care Guide

- Avoid all but urgent or emergent surgery during pregnancy.
- Optimal time for *necessary* surgery is second trimester.
- Limit adjunctive medication usage to agents that are safe in pregnancy and clearly indicated on strong clinical grounds (see above).
  1. Anticipate increased volume of distribution and accelerated renal excretion of medications.
- Position the pregnant patient who requires surgery in lateral decubitus position or supine with the right hip tilted up at least 15 degrees from the horizontal.
- For patients who require ventilatory support, maintain $Pco_2$ in range normal for pregnant state (30 mm Hg).
- Anticipate increased risk of aspiration of gastric contents and treat expectantly by delay of procedures after feedings, head-of-bed elevation, and antacids.
- Survey for urinary retention and infection.
- Conduct aggressive prophylaxis and treatment for thromboembolic disease for with an appropriate heparin regimen supplemented by venous compression (see Chapter 119).

## Seizure disorders

New-onset seizures in the perioperative setting generally relate to metabolic derangements, such as hypoglycemia, severe hyponatremia, and malignant hyperthermia; unanticipated alcohol or sedative-hypnotic withdrawal; toxic medication effects, as with enflurane, high doses of local anesthetic agents, or meperidine against a backdrop of monoamine oxidase inhibitor use; or a structural problem, such as an intracranial tumor or abscess, but especially after trauma, with central nervous system hemorrhage, cerebral contusion, or penetrating brain injury. Patients with established seizure disorders that are well-controlled with anticonvulsant medications generally tolerate surgery well, without neurologic sequelae. Indeed, although inhalation induction of anesthesia and emergence are risk periods for increased seizure activity, barbiturate coma and general anesthesia are accepted therapies for refractory status epilepticus. Maintenance of oral anticonvulsant therapy in the perioperative period may not be possible, and alternate dosage forms or different agents may be necessary. Prophylaxis of seizure activity in the neurologically injured patient is somewhat controversial, although there is consensus on treating certain categories of such patients (see below).

### Managed Care Guide

- Delay elective surgery until clinical control of underlying epilepsy is achieved and appropriate blood levels of anticonvulsants are confirmed.
- Maintain phenytoin (orally or intravenously) or phenobarbital (orally, intramuscularly, or intravenously) through the perioperative period.
- Substitute phenytoin or phenobarbital for carbamazepine in patients unable to receive medications enterally in the perioperative period who require maintenance therapy.
- Valproic acid syrup may be administered rectally in special situations, but substitution of phenytoin or

phenobarbital, as for carbamazepine, is generally more appropriate in patients unable to continue oral valproate.
- Identify metabolic, toxic, withdrawal, and anatomic causes of new-onset seizures in perioperative patients and treat accordingly.
- Consider seizure prophylaxis in patients with the following:
  1. Intracranial abscess or subdural empyema
  2. Intracranial trauma patients with a history of acute hematoma, early posttraumatic seizures, penetrating head wounds, or depressed skull fractures
  3. Tumors at or near the motor cortex
  4. Planned surgery where seizure activity would be catastrophic

### The alcoholic patient

There are 10 to 20 million alcoholics and problem drinkers in the United States. These individuals require surgery at a greater rate than the nondrinking public on the basis of the medical complications of alcohol (and usually concurrent tobacco abuse), but especially as a result of trauma associated with alcohol use—motor vehicle and other accidents, burns, and interpersonal violence. Complications of surgery in alcohol-abusing patients may relate to (1) metabolic derangements, especially of intermediary metabolism and of potassium, calcium, and magnesium homeostasis, (2) organ system dysfunction, especially of the cardiac, hematologic, hepatic, and central nervous systems, and (3) the withdrawal state. Treatment is predicated on rapid identification and treatment of correctable derangements and anticipatory treatment of alcohol withdrawal states.

#### Managed Care Guide

- Elicit history of alcohol, tobacco, and other drug use in all preoperative patients.
  1. Use CAGE questionnaire or an alternative in alcohol-using patients to further estimate severity of use (see Chapter 130).
- Preoperative examination should include testing for fecal blood loss.
- For patients suspected of significant recent or sustained alcohol use, preoperative laboratory screen should include complete blood count, glucose, sodium, bicarbonate, potassium, magnesium, BUN, creatinine, calcium, phosphate, bilirubin, albumin, transaminases, prothrombin and partial thromboplastin times, and urine dipstick for ketones.
- Thiamine, 100 mg intravenously or intramuscularly, should be administered to all acutely ill alcoholic patients undergoing urgent surgery.
- Alcohol-induced thrombocytopenia is rarely profound and generally responds to abstinence with appropriate vitamin supplementation, especially folate.
- Alcoholic ketoacidosis generally responds promptly to dextrose infusion.
- One should anticipate a drop in serum phosphate with dextrose administration and treat severe hypophosphatemia (less than 1 mg/dl) cautiously with intravenous potassium phosphate.
- Modest elevations in serum transaminases among alcoholics are common and do not carry an independent risk of adverse outcome but may serve as markers of a higher likelihood of alcohol withdrawal.
- Hepatic synthetic dysfunction, manifested by encephalopathy, physical stigmata of chronic liver disease (e.g., ascites, spider angiomata, palmar erythema), coagulopathy, hyperbilirubinemia, and hypoalbuminemia, presages significant surgical mortality.
  1. All but life-saving emergent surgery should be delayed until remediable defects are corrected.
  2. Coagulopathy rarely responds to vitamin K and often requires support with plasma or clotting factor concentrates.
- Early symptoms of alcohol withdrawal should be treated aggressively to minimize the likelihood of progression in perioperative patients.
  1. Diazepam, 20 mg orally every hour for 3 to 6 hours or until control of symptoms in patients able to take oral medication with mild to moderate withdrawal symptoms
  2. Lorazepam, 1 to 4 mg intramuscularly every 1 or 2 hours in patients unable to use the alimentary tract with symptoms of mild to moderate withdrawal
  3. β-Blockers are reasonable adjuncts for patients with uncontrolled tachycardia or hypertension, if benzodiazepine administration does not result in acceptable control.
  4. Intravenous diazepam should be employed in a monitored setting for patients in frank delirium tremens.
  5. Intravenous haloperidol is a reasonable adjunct for patients whose alcoholic delirium or hallucinosis fails to respond fully to benzodiazepines.

### Narcotic-, sedative-hypnotic-, and cocaine-addicted patients

Patients addicted to narcotics require special attention to analgesics and other medications in the perioperative period. Narcotic tolerance and metabolism are generally enhanced in such patients. Those addicted at the time of surgery require administration of narcotic agents sufficient to suppress withdrawal and control pain, most often achieved by the administration of an appropriate methadone regimen to suppress withdrawal supplemented by appropriate narcotic agonists. Narcotic antagonists and mixed agonist-antagonists must be avoided to preclude precipitating acute narcotic withdrawal. Coordination of this aspect of care with the anesthesiologist is clearly important, since administration of narcotic antagonists and mixed agonist-antagonists in the operative setting is common. Narcotic-addicted patients scheduled to undergo elective surgery may be offered a withdrawal regimen before surgery.

Patients who have been maintained on long-term sedative hypnotics, most commonly benzodiazepines, may experience a withdrawal reaction similar to that associated with withdrawal from alcohol, including seizures and frank delirium, in the postoperative setting. Onset of symptoms may be quite delayed in patients addicted to agents with longer half-lives. Treatment is predicated on identification of the risk of withdrawal, observation for minor symptoms, and administration of appropriate cross-tolerant agents.

Cocaine-addicted individuals carry to surgery an enhanced risk of cardiovascular complications, including blood pressure lability, cardiac ischemic events, dysrhythmias, stroke, and vascular compromise of other organs. This risk appears to persist for at least 2 weeks after last use of cocaine. Elective surgery should be delayed accordingly. Optimum prophylaxis and treatment of these complications in cocaine-addicted individuals who require emergency surgery are not known, but α- and β-adrenergic blockers, labetolol, and chlorpromazine have been used in individual cases. Individuals abusing amphetamines in the preoperative period may experience reactions similar to those associated with cocaine as well as frank psychosis perioperatively.

### Managed Care Guide

- Offer addicted individuals the opportunity for detoxification, whenever possible, before elective surgery.
- For a patient maintained on methadone up to the time of surgery, administer the usual oral dose daily and provide appropriate analgesia with narcotic agonists or nonsteroidal antiinflammatory drugs as clinically indicated.
  1. Intramuscular or subcutaneous methadone, two thirds the usual oral maintenance dose every 12 hours, may be substituted for oral methadone in patients unable to take oral medications in the perioperative period.
- For a narcotic-addicted patient who requires surgery and is not on a methadone maintenance regimen, achieve immediate analgesia and suppression of withdrawal with an appropriate potent narcotic agonist.
  1. In the postoperative period titrate a methadone maintenance regimen or withdrawal regimen as wished by the patient.
- Coordinate perioperative analgesic use with the anesthesiologist.
  1. Consider epidural or other regional analgesic techniques.
  2. Avoid narcotic antagonists or mixed agonist-antagonists.
- Anticipate shorter duration of action of narcotic analgesics among narcotic addicts than among nonaddicted patients with similar surgical pain.
- Anticipate a withdrawal reaction in patients habituated to sedative-hypnotic drugs.
  1. Observe for symptoms similar to those seen with alcohol withdrawal.
  2. Provide patient's maintenance medication or an appropriate cross-tolerant agent (e.g., clonazepam or diazepam orally or lorazepam intramuscularly) to suppress withdrawal.
- Defer surgery, when possible, until 2 weeks after last cocaine or amphetamine use.
- Treat cocaine-associated cardiovascular instability with standard agents but with a preference for labetolol.

## BIBLIOGRAPHY


Caputo GM, Gross RJ: Medical consultation on surgical services: an annotated bibliography, *Ann Intern Med* 118:290, 1993.

Clagett GP et al: Prevention of venous thromboembolism, *Chest* 102:391S, 1992.

Classen DC et al: The timing of prophylactic administration of antibiotics and the risk of surgical-wound infection, *N Engl J Med* 326:281, 1992.

Dajani AS et al: Prevention of bacterial endocarditis: recommendations by the American Heart Association, *JAMA* 264:2919, 1990.

Djokovic JL, Hedley-White J: Prediction of outcome of surgery and anesthesia in patients over 80, *JAMA* 242:2301, 1979.

Goldman L et al: Multifactorial index of cardiac risk in noncardiac surgical procedures, *N Engl J Med* 297:843, 1977.

Johnson WP, Lloyd F: Perioperative evaluation. In Greene HL, Johnson WP, Maricic MJ, editors: *Decision making in medicine,* St. Louis, 1993, Mosby.

Kammerer WS, Gross RJ, editors: *Medical consultation: the internist on surgical, obstetric, and psychiatric services,* Baltimore, 1990, Williams & Wilkins.

Keating HJ: Perioperative care of the older patient, *Clin Geriatr Med* 6:459, 1990.

Kroenke K et al: Postoperative complications after thoracic and major abdominal surgery in patients with and without obstructive lung disease, *Chest* 104:1445, 1993.

Merli GJ, Weitz HH, editors: *Medical management of the surgical patient,* Philadelphia, 1992, WB Saunders.

Merli GJ, Weitz HH, Lubin MF: Medical consultation, *Med Clin North Am* 77:289, 1993.

Nelson ER: Medical problems in pregnancy, *Med Clin North Am* 73:517, 1989.

Wong T, Detsky AS: Preoperative cardiac risk assessment for patients having peripheral vascular surgery, *Ann Intern Med* 116:743, 1992.


CHAPTER

# 6 The Geriatric Patient


**Sharon A. Levine**
**Patricia P. Barry**
**Arthur H. Eskew**


## DEMOGRAPHICS

In 1900 3.1 million Americans—about 4% of the population—were 65 or older. At present the number is more than 31 million, or 12.5% of the population. By 2030 the group is projected to grow to 65.6 million, some 22% of the population, largely due to improved life expectancy in the United States and the effect of the "baby boom" cohort. The oldest old, those 85 years and older, are the fastest growing population segment. Centenarians, 100 years and older, are expected to increase in number dramatically from 32,000 in 1982 to 597,000 in 2040. The ranks of the elderly are therefore increasing both in absolute terms and relative to the population (Fig. 6-2).

The great improvements in life expectancy during the 20th century in the United States can be attributed largely to decreases in deaths from acute illness, infectious disease, and accidents and better prevention of chronic disease. A person who turned 65 in 1900 had a life expectancy of 76.9 years; a 65-year-old in 1991 had a life expectancy of 82.4 years. Whites are expected to outlive African-Americans by an average of 7 years: life expectancy in 1991 was 79.6 years for white women, 73.8 for African-American women, 72.9 for white men, and 64.6 for African-American men.

Women are expected to outlive men by 6.9 years. The gender gap in life expectancy means a preponderance of women among the elderly. The sex ratio for elders—the number of men per 100 women—has been dropping over recent decades. It also decreases dramatically with age. As

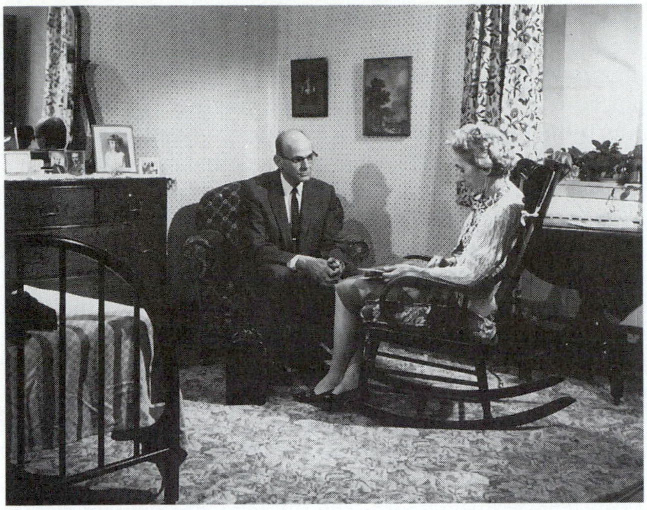

Fig. 6-1. House call. (From American College of Physicians Archives.)

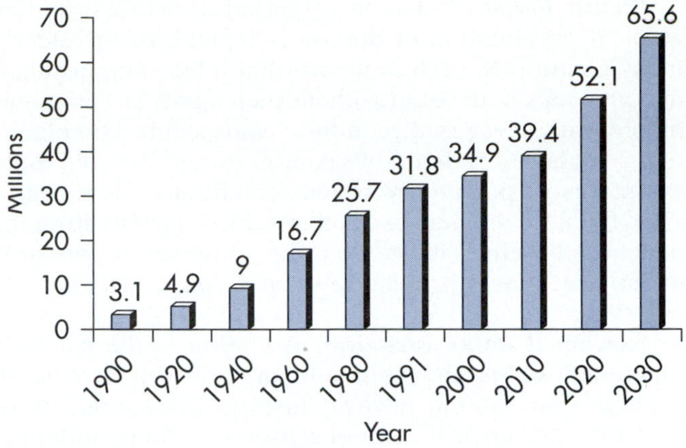


Fig. 6-2. Number (in millions) of persons 65 years of age and older from 1900 to 2030, based on data from the US Bureau of the Census. Note that increments in years are uneven.

a result, elderly women are more likely than men to be living alone and to be dependent on nonspousal family or formal supports for care.

Despite decreased mortality and longer life, chronic illnesses continue to have a major impact on the elderly. Chronic conditions such as arthritis, hypertension, hearing impairments, and heart disease represent 60% of ailments plaguing community-dwelling elderly. In addition to addressing the three major causes of death in older Americans—cardiovascular disease, cancer, and stroke (which account for nearly 80% of deaths among the elderly)—the primary care physicians of the 21st century will have to confront issues of dependency and functional impairment in an older, sicker patient population with a multitude of coincident problems. Even without providing cures for chronic illnesses, a clinician who improves sight, hearing, ambulation, or continence may enable a patient to remain in the community and avoid long-term institutionalization.

Many functionally impaired elderly currently reside in the community and are in need of primary care: only 5% of people over 65 are in nursing homes, and most of these are older than 85. Although the majority of noninstitutionalized elderly function well physically, dependency needs do increase with age. Long-term care survey data indicate that 4.6 million elderly living in the community have limitations in their activities of daily living (ADLs), which include bathing, toileting, feeding, and dressing, and instrumental activities of daily living (IADLs), which enable elders to live independently in the community and include managing finances, taking medications, preparing meals, housekeeping, and shopping.

For those who are 65 to 74 only 6.7% depend on others for care. At 85 or older that number soars to 44%. In this age group personal care assistance is required by 9.6% of those living alone, 18.8% of those who live with a spouse, and 25% of those who live with others. Caregiver stress among family members on whom these elders depend has been well documented. Spouses often are elderly and disabled themselves, and children juggle work and childrearing with providing care for aging parents. The primary care clinician must be sensitive to the burdens placed on family and friends. Additionally, the clinician should function as a resource for community services and exploration of possible long-term institutionalization.

## APPROACH TO THE ELDERLY PATIENT

### Environment

The environment where the history and physical examination take place should be adapted for the elderly patient. Rooms should be warm so that patients can comfortably disrobe. Lighting should be adequate, with minimal shadows and glare, to maximize sight for visually impaired patients. Rooms should be located away from noisy corridors and have adequate sound insulation so that hearing-impaired patients are not at a disadvantage. Doorways should be wide enough to accommodate adaptive devices such as wheelchairs. Chairs should have firm backs, high seats, and arms that make sitting and rising easy, especially for patients with arthritis or proximal lower extremity muscle weakness. Examination tables should be low enough for patients to mount and dismount safely. Pillows can be used to elevate the heads of patients with kyphoscoliosis.

Patients should be encouraged to wear eyeglasses and hearing aids. Amplification aids can be kept in the office for hearing-impaired patients. The use of adaptive aids such as walkers, canes, and wheelchairs should be encouraged and provided for those who need them.

### Eliciting the history

The examiner must speak slowly and clearly. Providers with high-pitched voices should be aware that high-frequency hearing loss is common among the elderly and should lower their voice accordingly. History taking can be time consuming. The patient should first be interviewed alone to allow an opportunity for discussion of private matters. Well-meaning family members may try to answer questions posed to cognitively impaired or frail patients, but an attempt should be made to use the patient as a primary source when possible. It is also important, however, to gather data from medical records, family members, friends, and formal caregivers. Family observations are particularly significant, and when cognitive impairment is present, they may be far more sensitive than rough screens for intellectual function.

***Present illness.*** A maxim of geriatric medicine is that atypical presentation of disease is typical. In the elderly many conditions, such as myocardial infarction, pneumonia, and sepsis, develop without their familiar symptoms or present as vague discomfort. Nonspecific complaints (e.g., malaise, fatigue, weakness) often are the only symptoms of potentially serious conditions. New confusion, falls, incontinence, or other subtle changes from the patient's baseline must alert the clinician to possible underlying illness presenting in an atypical fashion.

***Functional status assessment.*** Attention to the patient's functional status and ability to provide self-care is an essential part of the medical history. Measurements of ADLs include critical items of self-care: bathing, toileting, feeding, dressing, and transferring or ambulating. In community-dwelling elderly, assessment of IADLs, which require a higher level of function, may identify impairment at an earlier stage. IADLs usually include managing finances, managing medication, preparing meals, housekeeping, shopping, using a telephone, and arranging transportation. However, IADLs are biased toward activities performed by women and may overestimate deficiencies in men who cannot adequately prepare meals or keep house due to lack of familiarity with such tasks. Although the most accurate evaluations of function probably come from direct observation, useful information may be reported by the patient or described by the family.

To determine which services are needed for assistance, patients may be graded into three levels, based on performance of ADLs and IADLs: (1) independent, including those who need mechanical aids but do not require caregiver assistance, (2) in need of some caregiver assistance, and (3) unable to perform, even with assistance.

***Social history.*** The clinician should take a more detailed social history than for younger adults, including information about the patient's family, friends, living arrangements, pets, religious community, ability to drive, financial status, and caregiving responsibilities (see the box below). The responses may shed light on various issues: whether the patient has the resources to remain safely in the community; which supports would be needed to maximize the patient's functional status at home; whether placement in a long-term care facility is warranted. Nutrition history, including appetite changes and information on who buys and prepares meals, can uncover poverty and functional disabilities and may provide clues to managing conditions such as deficiencies in vitamins $B_{12}$ and D, congestive heart failure, diabetes, and hypertension. Immunization status for pneumococcal infections, influenza, and tetanus should be obtained (see Chapter 3). Family history is of lesser importance, except in the case of the onset of Alzheimer's disease in a younger patient.

During the history and physical the patient's values and advance directives regarding end-of-life decisions can be elicited and documented by the physician (see Chapter 128). These discussions should take place over several visits once the clinician has established a relationship with the patient.

Instruments have been developed to assess both well-being and social resources. Concepts of well-being are not easily defined and are heavily influenced by cultural factors and individual value systems. Clinicians should be careful not to project their own values, particularly with regard to quality of life, onto their patients. Social resources are more easily determined and are especially important for appropriate clinical care. Identification of caregivers who are available to provide help, their willingness and ability to do so, their sources of stress and support, and the strengths of interpersonal relationships is critical.

The clinician should take note of community resources such as day care, respite care, home health care, and homemakers. Information about financial resources is necessary to determine eligibility for programs such as Medicaid and to assess the patient's ability to pay for services not funded by outside sources.

***Medications.*** Medication review of indications, dosage, dosage schedule, and untoward effects of all over-the-counter and prescription drugs is mandatory, with a brown bag review (i.e., review of the actual containers or dispensers) providing the most accurate information. The best place to obtain a medication review is in the home, where errors of omission or duplication are often discovered.

***Review of systems.*** In addition to conducting a routine review of systems (e.g., cardiovascular, respiratory, gastrointestinal), the clinician should inquire specifically about near and far vision, including ability to read, drive, and watch television, and hearing loss. Arthritis, incontinence, falls, memory impairment, behavior changes, depression, and abuse, if suspected, should all be addressed. Sexual and substance abuse history should not be omitted simply because of age.

Affect measurement usually attempts to identify depression, which is common, treatable, and an important cause of dysfunction in the elderly. The geriatric depression scale (GDS) (Fig. 6-3) has been validated in the clinical setting and was developed specifically for use with the elderly.

### Adaptation of the medical history

- Expanded social history including family, friends, caregivers, living arrangements, pets, religious community involvement, driving, caregiving responsibilities, financial status, substance abuse, elder abuse
- Activities of daily living and instrumental activities of daily living
- Nutrition
- "Brown bag" (examination of containers/dispensers) or home medication review including indication, dosage, dosage schedule, untoward effects
- Immunizations
- Targeted review of systems to include near and far vision, hearing, incontinence, sexual dysfunction, falls, memory problems, mood changes, mobility, and gait problems

**Geriatric Depression Scale (GDS)**

Forced Y/N Choice

1. Are you basically satisfied with your life? N = 1
2. Have you dropped any of your activities or interests? Y = 1
3. Do you feel that your life is empty? Y = 1
4. Do you often get bored? Y = 1
5. Are you hopeful about the future? N = 1
6. Are you bothered by thoughts you can't get out of your head? Y = 1
7. Are you in good spirits most of the time? N = 1
8. Are you afraid that something bad is going to happen to you? Y = 1
9. Do you feel happy most of the time? N = 1
10. Do you often feel helpless? Y = 1
11. Do you often get restless and fidgety? Y = 1
12. Do you prefer to stay at home, rather than going out and doing new things? Y = 1
13. Do you frequently worry about the future? Y = 1
14. Do you feel you have more problems with memory than most? Y = 1
15. Do you think it is wonderful to be alive now? N = 1
16. Do you often feel downhearted and blue? Y = 1
17. Do you feel pretty worthless the way you are now? Y = 1
18. Do you worry a lot about the past? Y = 1
19. Do you find life very exciting? N = 1
20. Is it hard for you to get started on new projects? Y = 1
21. Do you feel full of energy? N = 1
22. Do you feel that your situation is hopeless? Y = 1
23. Do you think that most people are better off than you are? Y = 1
24. Do you frequently get upset over little things? Y = 1
25. Do you frequently feel like crying? Y = 1
26. Do you have trouble concentrating? Y = 1
27. Do you enjoy getting up in the morning? N = 1
28. Do you prefer to avoid social gatherings? Y = 1
29. Is it easy for you to make decisions? N = 1
30. Is your mind as clear as it used to be? N = 1

A score of 11 has been shown to be useful in the diagnosis of depression.

**Fig. 6-3.** Geriatric depression scale. (Adapted from Yesavage JA et al: *J Psychiatr Res* 17:37, 1982.)

## Focused physical examination

- General: hygiene, mood
- Height and weight
- Vital signs: pulse and postural blood pressure, supine to standing
- Eyes: visual acuity, visual fields, ectropion, entropion, cataracts, increased cup-to-disc ratio, retinopathy
- Ears: audioscopy or whisper test, cerumen
- Oropharynx (with and without dentures): teeth, denture fit, exudates, lesions, gum disease
- Neck: range of motion, thyroid nodules or enlargement
- Chest: breasts, intertriginous areas, kyphoscoliosis, tenderness of vertebral spines
- Cardiac: murmurs
- Abdomen: scars, masses including aneurysms, bladder palpation, hernias
- Rectal: prostate examination, impaction, hemorrhoids, masses, fecal occult blood testing
- Pelvic: atrophic vaginitis, cystocele, urethrocele, rectocele, uterine prolapse, Pap smear, bimanual examination (ovaries should be nonpalpable)
- Extremities (with and without shoes): range of motion, deformities, venous stasis disease, peripheral pulses, edema, corns, calluses, bunions, hammertoes, warts, fungal infection, toenails, shoe fit
- Neurologic: mental status screen, sensorimotor examination, reflexes, gait
- Performance-oriented tests of gait and balance: Get Up and Go Test, Tinetti Performance-Oriented Assessment of Gait and Balance
- Skin: ulcers, stasis changes, cellulitis, actinic keratoses, basal cell carcinoma, malignant melanoma, pressure sores

### Physical examination

The examiner should note the patient's personal hygiene and mood, which can provide clues to overall functional status (see the box above).

Height and weight should be recorded at the first visit, and weight thereafter, to uncover problems with nutrition and to monitor fluid overload or overdiuresis in patients with congestive heart failure. Unintentional weight loss may indicate abuse, neglect, underlying malignancy, thyroid disease, or depression.

Postural blood pressure and pulse are noted. Postural hypotension, although present in 10% of healthy community-dwelling elderly, may indicate changes in volume status or medication side effects, both of which may predispose the patient to falls. Orthostatic hypotension is defined as a 20 mm Hg decrease in systolic pressure or a 10 mm Hg decrease in diastolic pressure 3 minutes after the patient has risen from supine to standing. Systolic hypertension is a systolic blood pressure of 160 or greater; diastolic hypertension is 90 or above. Stiff, atherosclerotic brachial arteries may give elevated blood pressure measurements—pseudohypertension—even when intraarterial measurements are normal. The Osler maneuver should be employed when there is a suspicion of pseudohypertension. To perform the maneuver, the cuff should be inflated above the first Korotkoff sound. If the radial or brachial artery does not collapse and is still palpable, this may indicate rigid arteries mimicking hypertension. This maneuver is especially helpful in a patient who has absence of retinal findings or cardiac changes suggestive of long-standing hypertension.

Visual acuity should be assessed with a Snellen eye chart. The prevalence of cataracts, glaucoma, macular degeneration, and refractive errors increases with age. Examination of gross visual fields by confrontation may reveal deficits due to glaucoma, cerebrovascular events, or mass lesions. Ectropion (eversion of the eyelid) or entropion (inversion of the eyelid) may be present. Arcus senilis (depigmentation of the iris) occurs with normal aging. Dilated funduscopic examination may reveal increased cup-to-disc ratios associated with glaucoma or retinopathy due to diabetes or hypertension. Schiotz tonometry is an unreliable office maneuver, and patients should be referred to an ophthalmologist for measurement of intraocular pressures.

Hearing can be assessed by whisper test or a hand-held audioscope, which has excellent specificity and sensitivity; external auditory canals should be examined for cerumen impaction. Inspection and palpation of the oral cavity include evaluation of dentition and detection of gum disease, ill-fitting dentures, and abnormal lesions or masses.

Examination of the neck includes range of motion, which is important for driving skills and may give clues to vertebrobasilar insufficiency in patients with falls or near syncope. The thyroid should be inspected and palpated for nodules or goiter. Auscultation of the carotids can reveal bruits or radiation of cardiac murmurs. The presence of asymptomatic carotid bruits is not in itself a risk for death from cerebrovascular disease but can imply atherosclerotic disease elsewhere.

Because of the increasing incidence of breast cancer with age, yearly breast examinations for elderly women are important. Intertriginous areas also should be inspected for dermatitis or fungal infection.

Chest examination includes inspection for kyphosis and scoliosis and palpation of vertebral spines for tenderness. Otherwise the examination is the same as for younger adults.

The cardiac examination commonly reveals systolic murmurs, which occur in 30% to 80% of patients 65 and older. The differential diagnosis includes aortic sclerosis, aortic stenosis, idiopathic hypertrophic subaortic stenosis, and mitral regurgitation. Aortic sclerosis usually has an early peaking systolic murmur that may radiate to the carotids. The murmur of aortic stenosis is late peaking, radiates to the carotids, and may be associated with delayed carotid upstroke and an $S_4$. Delayed upstroke suggests significant aortic stenosis and should be documented promptly by echocardiography, since advanced age is not a contraindication to aortic valve replacement. However, in the elderly the carotid upstroke may be brisker than expected because of stiff arteries, and significant aortic stenosis may be associated with an apparently normal carotid upstroke. An $S_4$ is commonly found in healthy elderly and is due to decreased ventricular compliance. For a patient who is unable to squat, the clinician can simply raise the patient's lower extremities to increase venous return as a way of determining the characteristics of a murmur. Diastolic murmurs are never considered normal in the elderly.

The abdomen should be inspected for scars, which may indicate surgery that the patient has neglected to mention. An aortic aneurysm can be detected as a pulsatile mass greater than 3 cm, often with an associated bruit. The bladder can be palpated to assess for urinary retention when the history points in this direction. Inguinal canals and femoral triangles should be examined for hernias. Yearly digital rectal examinations (DRE), which can be comfortably performed with the patient in the left lateral decubitus position, are essential to screen for prostate nodules and hyperplasia in men and for fecal impaction, rectal masses, and occult blood in all elderly patients. It should be noted that pathology in the prostate's median lobe, which is not accessible to the examining finger, may be missed on DRE. Prostate size on DRE does not correlate with outlet obstruction.

The gynecologic examination continues to remain part of the routine evaluation of the elderly woman. For a patient with kyphosis a pillow under the head and neck makes the examination more comfortable. Patients with degenerative disease at the hips or knees can be examined in the dorsal lithotomy position with the use of extenders on the leg rests. For patients who cannot tolerate this position, the left lateral decubitus position is helpful. The patient should be examined for the presence of atrophic vaginitis, cystocele, rectocele, urethrocele, and uterine

## Mini-Mental State

**Orientation (maximum score 10)**

"What is the _______?" Date (1)
Month (1)
Day (1)
Season (1)
Year (1)
"What is the name of this hospital?" (1)
"What floor are we on?" (1)
"What town (or city) are we in?" (1)
"What county are we in?" (1)
"What state are we in?" (1)

**Registration (maximum score 3)**

Say *ball, flag,* and *tree* clearly and slowly, about 1 second for each. After you have said all three words, ask the patient to repeat them. This determines the score (1-3). Keep repeating the words (up to six trials) until the patient can repeat all three. If all three are not learned, recall cannot be meaningfully tested.

Ball (1) Flag (1) Tree (1)

**Attention and calculation (maximum score 5)**

Ask the patient to begin at 100 and count backward by 7, stopping after 5 subtractions. Score one point for each.

93 (1) 86 (1) 79 (1) 72 (1) 65 (1)

If the patient cannot or will not perform this task, ask him or her to spell *world* backward (D-L-R-O-W). The score is one point for each correctly placed letter.

D (1) L (1) R (1) O (1) W (1)

**Recall (maximum score 3)**

Ask the patient to recall the three words you previously asked him or her to remember.

Ball (1) Flag (1) Tree (1)

**Language (maximum score 9)**

***Naming***

Show the subject a wristwatch and a pencil, asking in turn, "What is this?" Score one point for each item.

Watch (1) Pencil (1)

***Repetition***

Ask the patient to repeat "No ifs, ands, or buts." Score one point if correct.

Repetition (1)

***Three-stage command***

Give the subject a piece of blank paper and say, "Take the paper in your right hand, fold it in half, and put in on the floor." Score one point for each action performed correctly.

Takes in right hand (1) Folds in half (1) Puts on floor (1)

***Reading***

On a blank piece of paper, print the sentence "Close your eyes" in large letters. Ask the patient to read it and do what it says. Score if he or she actually closes the eyes.

Closes eyes (1)

***Writing***

Give the patient a blank piece of paper and ask him or her to write a sentence. It must contain a subject and a verb and make sense. Ignore grammar, spelling, and punctuation.

Writes sentence (1)

***Copying***

On a clean piece of paper, draw intersecting pentagons, each side about 1 inch, and ask patient to copy it exactly as it is. All 10 angles must be present, and two must intersect to score 1 point.

Draws pentagons (1)

**Total score**

Thirty points are possible. A score of 23 or less correlates well with moderate or worse cognitive function.

Modified from Folstein MF, Folstein ME, McHugh PR: *J Psychiatr Res* 12:189, 1975.

prolapse. All women should have speculum examinations even if they have undergone hysterectomies, since in the past many hysterectomies were performed as supracervical procedures, leaving an intact cervix in which a carcinoma may develop. Frequency of Pap smears is discussed in Chapter 2. In a normal elderly woman the ovaries should be nonpalpable; if appreciated on bimanual examination, there may be ovarian malignancy.

Extremities should be inspected and joints put through active and passive range of motion. Common skin findings such as venous stasis changes, including hyperpigmentation and stasis ulcers, may be noted. Peripheral pulses should be assessed and, if absent, the distal extremity should be examined for signs of arterial insufficiency such as pallor, dependent rubor, or coolness. Pitting edema below the knees may indicate right-sided heart failure, venous stasis, or diseases associated with hypoalbuminemia. The podiatric examination includes evaluation for corns, calluses, bunions, hammertoes, plantar warts, tinea pedis, and nails that are affected by fungus or simply overgrown. Determining the condition of the feet is essential in the evaluation of falls and gait disturbances. In addition, diabetic patients and others with peripheral neuropathies may be unaware of potentially dangerous foot ulcers or sores. Patients should be examined with and without shoes to ensure that the shoes fit properly and are in good repair.

The neurologic examination should include an office assessment of mental status such as the Folstein Mini-Mental State Examination (see the box on p. 131), during which subtle well-compensated dementia can be unmasked and severe memory impairment recognized and quantified. Such instruments enable the clinician to establish a baseline and follow cognitive function objectively over time. The cranial nerve, sensorimotor, and reflex examinations are performed as usual. Common findings in healthy elderly include primitive reflexes such as the snout, glabellar and palmomental reflexes, which in the absence of other findings are nonpathologic, and symmetrically diminished vibratory sense and ankle jerks. Cranial nerve changes include diminished accommodation, pupillary response to light, and upward gaze.

Although motor strength is decreased in the elderly, this finding should not have clinical manifestations unless the patient has joint pain, decreased range of motion, or weakness. It has been documented that the neuromuscular examination may be normal in patients who have functional limitations. For instance, hip and knee flexors may be entirely normal in patients who have difficulty sitting down. For this reason it is imperative to use performance-based assessments in trying to identify patients with functional disability, especially those who fall or have gait and balance problems. The Tinetti Performance-Oriented Assessment of Gait and Balance can easily be performed during an office evaluation with little time added to the visit (see the section on Falls).

Skin should be inspected for xerosis, cellulitis, stasis dermatitis and ulcers, actinic keratoses, basal cell carcinomas, malignant melanoma, and pressure sores.

## ASSESSMENT OF GERIATRIC CONDITIONS

Because of the complexity of problems facing elderly patients, a diagnosis-oriented approach may be inadequate for assessing and maintaining overall health and functional status. Many older patients suffer from multiple disabilities and illnesses. The clinician needs information not only about individual ailments, but also about their interwoven physical, mental, and social aspects. To answer that need, a coordinated multidisciplinary approach has evolved, known as geriatric assessment, which typically involves a physician, nurse, and social worker. Information is obtained and organized regarding five basic domains: physical health, performance of ADLs, (basic and instrumental), mental health, socioeconomic resources, and the patient's environment, with special emphasis on the relationships between the factors. The assessment of physical health, functional status, mental health, and socioeconomic resources are as outlined above, although the full geriatric assessment is more thorough with the multidisciplinary approach.

The environmental assessment covers factors such as the convenience, safety, and availability of services and social supports. A home visit by the physician or other health care professional often provides essential information regarding the need for specific interventions, including physical equipment (ramps, grab bars), special services (homemakers, meals), and increased social activity (visitors, day care) (see Home Care section below).

Well-designed studies have demonstrated the value of assessment by multidisciplinary teams—usually with follow-up management—in improving diagnostic and therapeutic outcomes in settings such as geriatric inpatient and outpatient units. Although several studies have demonstrated that geriatric assessment in the office and hospital practice of the individual physician can identify previously unsuspected problems, the impact on outcome depends on the ability to target appropriate patients and to identify resources and services necessary for follow-up care.

In 1988 the National Institutes of Health sponsored the Consensus Development Conference on Geriatric Assessment Methods for Clinical Decision-Making. The consensus statement issued by the conference noted that the goals of assessment often are interdependent; diagnostic accuracy leads to appropriate interventions and better use of available services, resulting in improved function and optimal placement for the patient. Geriatric assessment can and should be performed in many different clinical settings, both institutional and community. The consensus statement pointed out that two aspects of geriatric assessment are particularly important: (1) targeting patients most likely to benefit, especially those who are frail but not terminally ill and those at critical transition points (e.g., change in living situation, loss of a loved one or caregiver), and (2) linking assessment with care management and follow-up services to implement the recommendations resulting from assessment. Geriatric assessment is thus a *process* involving referral, collection of information, assessment, and development and implementation of a care plan, with periodic reassessment and modification of that plan.

Certain conditions and problems are commonly seen during geriatric assessment. Falls, incontinence, and adverse drug reactions collectively take an enormous toll on the physical well-being and social functioning of the aged population. These problems are amenable to relatively simple, low-tech interventions. But, because patients may not volunteer the relevant information, the practitioner may have to delve deeply into the medical and social history.

Additional geriatric syndromes, including dementia, delirium, hearing loss, visual impairment, osteoporosis, and osteomalacia, as well as issues surrounding death and dying are covered in other chapters. Problems such as pressure sores and the inappropriate use of restraints, which are more commonly found in institutionalized or acutely hospitalized patients, are outside the scope of this text.

### Predisposing and risk factors for falls

- Sensory deficits: vision, hearing, proprioception, vibration, vestibular function
- Orthostatic hypotension
- Gait and balance changes
- Musculoskeletal changes
- Cognitive impairment
- Medications
- Environmental hazards

## FALLS

Falls are a common and morbid problem among both community-dwelling and institutionalized elderly. They can result in minor to severe acute injuries, prolonged physical and psychologic disability, institutionalization, and death. As with many geriatric conditions, their causes are often multifactorial and reversible with intervention. The tendency to fall represents a confluence of factors, including physical illness, disability, medications, and environmental hazards, often with a minor event tipping the balance. Most recent geriatrics literature uses the Kellogg International Work Group definition, in which the term *falls* excludes incidents resulting from instrinsic factors, such as syncope and stroke, or sequelae of violent acts, such as blows to the head (see Chapter 4A).

### Epidemiology

Worldwide, approximately one third of community-dwelling elderly over the age of 65 fall each year. That percentage rises with advancing age; the rate approaches 50% for those 80 and older. The number also rises with institutionalization: elders in institutions have an average of 1.6 to 2.0 falls per year. Women fall more often than men until age 75, when the frequencies become the same, but men die more often from their falls. Half of those who fall do so more than once. Falls precipitate most injuries in people over 65, an age group for which injuries are the sixth leading cause of death.

About 5% to 10% of falls lead to serious soft tissue injury such as bruises, lacerations, hematomas, sprains, and joint dislocations. Some 5% of falls result in fractures, usually of the hip, pelvis, wrist, or humerus. One in 100 falls results in a hip fracture, with this morbid and sometimes fatal complication occurring in one in 10 elderly over the age of 80 who fall.

Perhaps as devastating as the physical injuries and disabilities caused by falls are the psychologic and social sequelae. Fear of falling develops in almost 50% of those who have fallen, and 26% curtail their activities due to fear. Elders withdraw from activities, thereby losing functional ability, becoming further deconditioned and increasing their risk of falling. This cycle can be a contributing factor in the ultimate institutionalization of a patient.

### Pathophysiology and risk factors

Falls often are due to a complex interaction of intrinsic age- and disease-related changes in the patient and extrinsic or environmental factors (see the box above). Gait, balance, and the capacity to avoid a fall by regaining stability are affected by interrelated changes in the visual, neurosensory, and musculoskeletal systems. Gait changes include short steps, decreased velocity, decreased step height, and decreased arm swing. A senile gait is described as small stepped and wide based, with decreased arm swing and stooped posture; hips and knees are flexed; there is uncertainty and stiffness in turning and sometimes difficulty initiating steps; there is a tendency to fall without a clear reason.

Aging results in increased sway and decreased balance on one leg, but conditions such as Parkinson's disease, hemiplegia, neuropathies, myelopathies, and severe orthopedic deformities of feet, knees, and hips also affect gait. There is a 20% to 40% decrease in isometric strength for ages 60 to 80.

Changes that occur in vision due to normal aging include decreased accommodation, acuity, contrast sensitivity, and adaptation to dark as well as glare intolerance. This situation is worsened by pathologic conditions commonly found in the elderly, such as presbyopia, cataracts, macular degeneration, retinopathy, and glaucoma. Vestibular function may decline from age-related changes such as disruption of vestibuloocular reflexes. Vestibulospinal function may be altered in patients with peripheral and central lesions from vestibulotoxins, including furosemide, aminoglycosides, aspirin, quinine, and ethanol. Proprioception may be affected by loss of proprioceptors in cervical or weight-bearing joints. Older peripheral nervous systems have delayed motor and sensory nerve conduction velocities in comparison to those in young people. The same is true of somatosensory evoked potentials. Decreased vibration in toes and ankles has been documented. However, peripheral neuropathies due to vitamin $B_{12}$ deficiency, diabetes, alcoholism, and syphilis are common in the elderly and may contribute to problems with gait and balance.

Cognitive impairment can lead to loss of awareness of the environment and predispose people to falls. Falls occur three times more frequently in patients with senile dementia of the Alzheimer type (SDAT) than in healthy elderly.

Orthostatic hypotension occurs in 10% of community-dwelling elderly and is associated with 2% to 15% of falls. Causes of postural hypotension include autonomic dysfunction due to age, central nervous system damage, diabetes mellitus, hypovolemia, and decreased cardiac output. Metabolic and endocrine disorders, including

Addison's disease, can cause orthostasis. Age-related physiologic changes, such as decreased renin-angiotensin response and decreased baroreceptor sensitivity, may contribute. Postprandial hypotension has been well documented. Drop attacks, which have been reported to be associated with up to 10% of falls, result in sudden falls while walking or standing, without loss of consciousness. These may be due to vertebral artery insufficiency secondary to atherosclerosis or compression by cervical spondylosis.

Several medications have been implicated in falls (see the box below): benzodiazepines, particularly if long-acting; tricyclic antidepressants, because of postural hypotension; and antihypertensives, including diuretics, calcium channel blockers, α-blockers, central α-adrenergic agents, and major tranquilizers. Phenothiazines, benzodiazepines, and tricyclic antidepressants have been implicated independent of other risk factors, including dementia and depression, for which they are often prescribed. The risk of falls increases with the number of medications taken. Diuretics may cause volume loss, orthostatic hypotension, and electrolyte abnormalities. Sedatives and hypnotics may cause fatigue and disorientation. Antihypertensives may cause sedation and orthostatic changes.

Some 40% to 50% of accidental falls are related to environmental hazards. Furthermore, falls resulting in injury are more often related to environmental causes than are those that do not produce injury, particularly in younger and more active patients. Environmental factors include stairs (descent is especially hazardous where edges of steps are unclear); slippery, icy, uneven, or wet surfaces; poor lighting; unexpected obstacles such as children, toys, and pets; ill-fitting footwear and trousers; low beds, chairs, and toilets; loose rugs; wire; and clutter.

However, falls are usually due to the combined effects of many factors. It has been found that sedatives, cognitive impairment, disability to the lower extremities, presence of a palmomental reflex, abnormalities of gait and balance, and foot problems pose the greatest risks. In addition, the risk of falling increases linearly with the number of these risk factors: it goes from 8% in patients with none to more than 78% in patients with four or more.

### History

Questions about falls should be part of a routine history in patients 65 and older. A detailed history, including the what, when, where, and why of a fall, can reveal high-risk conditions or behaviors as well as patterns for recurrent problems. Open-ended questions such as "Tell me about this fall and others you have had," may be very revealing. It is helpful to ask for a demonstration of the patient's positions before, during, and after a fall. The examiner also should ask about problems with gait, balance, or walking secondary to joint or foot conditions. Premonitory symptoms such as dizziness, light-headedness, and vertigo can indicate hypotension, vestibular problems, hypoglycemia, or drug side effects. Incontinence causes falls by creating slippery surfaces. Chest pain associated with arrhythmias or ischemia can cause hypotension. Questions about eyesight, hearing, sensation, memory problems, and depression also are relevant. If a patient is too cognitively impaired to give a meaningful history, information should be obtained from family, friends, and caregivers. Review of all over-the-counter and prescription drugs is essential. Questions about recreational drugs and alcohol are important. A medical history covering all medical and surgical conditions may identify patients who are at high risk.

### Physical examination

Supine-to-standing blood pressure after a 3-minute interval should be obtained to rule out postural hypotension. Skin examination for turgor, pallor, and trauma is necessary. The head examination should include tests for visual acuity and fields, gaze preferences, nystagmus, and hearing loss. During the neck examination the clinician should listen for carotid bruits and check for range of motion at the cervical spine. Pulmonary status can be assessed by listening for rales or egophony. The cardiac examination includes appreciation of murmurs, especially aortic stenosis, arrhythmias, and gallops. Extremities should be evaluated for joint deformities, range of motion, corns, calluses, ulcers, bunions, long toenails, ill-fitting shoes, and signs of fractures. Range of motion and stability of the thoracic and lumbar spine also are important.

A neurologic evaluation for mental status, focal motor deficits, paresis, tremor, rigidity, decreased proprioception, and vibration should be carefully performed, although it has been shown that the standard neuromuscular examination may not reveal functional impairments. For instance, knee and hip flexion may be normal most of the time, even when a patient remains functionally impaired and has difficulty sitting or standing. It is therefore important to perform functional assessments of gait and balance required for daily activities. In the Get Up and Go test the patient is instructed to arise from a chair without using the hands, walk 15 to 30 m, return, stand still, and then sit down. This test or the Tinetti Performance-Oriented Assessment of Gait and Balance can be performed easily in a few minutes during a home or office evaluation. (See boxes at right).

### Environmental assessment

Because the majority of falls in community-dwelling elderly occur at home during normal activities of daily living and because 40% to 50% of accidental falls are related to environmental hazards, a home evaluation by a physician, nurse, or physical therapist is essential in the workup of falls.

#### Medications implicated in falls

- Narcotics
- Hypnotics
- Benzodiazepines (especially long acting)
- Phenothiazines
- Tricyclic antidepressants
- Diuretics
- Vasodilators
- Alcohol

From Kellogg International Work Group: *Dan Med Bull* 34(Suppl 4):1, 1987.

## Performance-oriented assessment of balance

- Sitting balance
- Arising from chair
- Immediate standing balance within 5 seconds
- Prolonged standing balance with eyes closed and feet close together
- Turning balance (360 degrees)
- Sternal nudge
- Neck turning side to side
- One leg standing balance
- Back extension
- Reaching up as if retrieving object from high shelf
- Bending down as if to pick up object from floor
- Sitting down

Modified from Tinetti ME, Ginter SF: *J Am Geriatr Soc* 34:119, 1986.

## Performance-oriented assessment of gait

- Initiation of gait
- Step height
- Step length
- Step symmetry
- Step continuity
- Path deviation
- Trunk stability
- Walk stance
- Turning while walking

Modified from Tinetti ME, Ginter SF: *J Am Geriatr Soc* 34:119, 1986.

Falls by healthier older adults often are associated with environmental factors. What is more, this group of elders has a higher frequency of falls that lead to injuries. Environmental checklists have been designed to evaluate the home for safety hazards (see the box at top right).

### Laboratory tests and diagnostic evaluation

The diagnostic workup should be guided by the history and physical examination (see the box at bottom right). Electrolytes and the ratio of blood urea nitrogen (BUN) to creatinine can be used to assess volume status. Complete blood count (CBC) is helpful in assessment of infection and anemias, particularly for a patient with hypotensive symptoms. In cases of muscle weakness tests for creatine phosphokinase, thyroid function, and potassium, phosphate, calcium, and magnesium levels are helpful. Serum glucose should be measured to screen for diabetes and hypoglycemia. Urinalysis should be performed in cases of suspected urinary tract infection. Vitamin $B_{12}$ levels and syphilis serology should be done for patients with peripheral neuropathy. Substance abuse is not uncommon in the elderly, and therefore a blood and urine toxicology screen should be done and ethanol levels determined if indicated by history, physical, or mental status. Chest x-ray can be ordered if history, signs, or symptoms suggest congestive heart failure, pneumonia, or other cardiopulmonary problems. Electrocardiogram (ECG) is indicated if the history and examination suggest myocardial infarction or arrhythmias. Holter monitoring has not been shown to be useful in the routine evaluation of nonsyncopal episodes without cardiac symptoms, since there is a high incidence of ventricular and supraventricular arrhythmias in both fallers and nonfallers, and treatment of unclear value is fraught with side effects that can lead to falls. Computerized tomographic (CT) scan of the head can be

## Environmental safety checklist

**Home**

- Ensure adequate lighting, especially of stairs, walkways, door thresholds and bathrooms.
- Remove clutter, toys, low furniture.
- Secure carpet and tile edges.
- Remove throw rugs.
- Clearly mark or remove door thresholds.
- Remove cords and wires from floors.
- Avoid floor wax.
- Install grab bars in tub and shower and by toilet.
- Use rubber tub mats.
- Ensure that steps are even and edges are clearly marked.

**Institution**

- Adjust beds, chairs, and toilets to appropriate height.
- Provide adequate lighting of bathrooms and hallways.
- Ensure nonskid footwear that fits.

**Outside**

- Repair uneven, cracked, or broken sidewalks and steps.
- Cut back overgrown shrubbery blocking walkways.
- Provide handrails on steps.
- Ensure adequate illumination of walkways and steps.

Modified from Rubenstein LZ et al: *J Am Geriatr Soc,* 36:266, 1988.

## Laboratory and diagnostic workup after a fall

- CBC: infection, anemia
- Electrolytes, BUN, creatinine: volume status
- Glucose: diabetes, hypoglycemia
- Calcium: delirium
- Vitamin $B_{12}$: peripheral neuropathy, dementia
- Thyroid function tests: hypothyroidism, hyperthyroidism
- Urinalysis: infection if indicated by history or physical examination
- Electrocardiogram: arrhythmia, myocardial infarction
- Chest x-ray: congestive heart failure, pneumonia
- CT or MRI of head: subdural hematoma, hydrocephalus, tumor
- Toxicology screen and ethanol level
- Echocardiogram: valvular lesion

performed to rule out subdural hematoma, stroke, and normal pressure hydrocephalus. Echocardiography is indicated if there is evidence of aortic stenosis or near syncope. Stool for occult blood should be obtained in patients with premonitory symptoms.

### Management and interventions

Those patients who are considered to be at high risk for falls because of their physical or mental status or environmental factors should have their charts flagged for intervention. When prescribing medications, the physician should weigh the benefits of treatment with possible reactions affecting gait, balance, and mental status and should adjust dosages based on age-related changes in drug metabolism (see further). Carefully review all over-the-counter, recreational, and prescribed drugs.

Patients who fall should also be evaluated and treated for underlying arrhythmias clearly associated with the fall, heart block, volume loss, and Parkinson's disease. Patients with orthostatic hypotension should receive education about raising the head of the bed to decrease the incidence of hypotensive falls on standing. These patients may find it helpful to wear graded pressure stockings to decrease venous pooling, to sit at the edge of the bed before standing, and to liberalize dietary salt. Sometimes mineralocorticoids are helpful. Drop attacks due to vertebrobasilar insufficiency may be helped by a cervical collar. Glasses, hearing aids, new shoes, and assistive devices should be supplied when necessary.

Education regarding community services such as adult day care and social senior centers where patients can be more closely supervised, transportation, medical alert devices, and nutrition and alcohol counseling should be initiated. Physical or occupational therapy and specific strength and balance training, though not proven to decrease falls, may be beneficial. The patient should be instructed in how to arise from a fall. Finally, a careful home assessment for environmental hazards is very important.

## URINARY INCONTINENCE

### Epidemiology

Urinary incontinence represents a major cause of disability, social isolation and institutionalization in the elderly. It affects 5% to 15% of those over the age of 65 living in the community and 50% or more of those living in long-term care facilities. Neurologic impairment, immobility, and female sex are the major independent risk factors. Some 40% of hospitalized elderly are reported to be incontinent; much of this is transient and reversible if recognized and appropriately evaluated. Urinary incontinence is frequently cited by families as the major factor leading to the decision to place an elder in a nursing home. Institutionalized patients who are incontinent are much more expensive to care for than patients who are continent, owing to increased secondary problems such as falls and skin breakdown as well as expanded nursing care needs.

### Pathophysiology

Continence requires structurally intact and functional detrusor and sphincter muscles, as well as the reflexes that coordinate them. The onset of urinary incontinence is not part of normal aging, but there are age-related physiologic changes that may predispose to it:

- Decreased bladder capacity
- Decreased ability to postpone voiding
- Decreased urethral and bladder compliance
- Decreased maximal urethral closing pressure
- Decreased urinary flow rate
- Increased postvoid residual (PVR)
- Increased uninhibited detrusor contractions

Any of these in combination with another medical or physiologic insult may result in incontinence.

Proper function of the lower urinary tract is heavily dependent on normal function of the autonomic nervous system. The detrusor and sphincter are innervated by parasympathetic cholinergic fibers that emerge from the spinal cord at the S2-S4 level and travel via the pelvic splanchnic nerves, as well as sympathetic noradrenergic fibers via the paraaortic sympathetic chain. Parasympathetic influence results in detrusor contraction, sphincter relaxation, and voiding. Sympathetic stimulation inhibits detrusor contractions and increases the tone of the involuntary sphincter, thus promoting the storage of urine. The balance between the two sides of the autonomic nervous system and thus the control of the micturition reflex is mediated by several micturition centers located in the lower spinal cord, brainstem and cerebral cortex. The cerebral cortex is the site of voluntary control and exerts an inhibitory influence on voiding. Injury, disease, or pharmacologic side effects at any point in the neurologic circuit can result in a disorder of either the storage or voiding of urine and therefore result in incontinence.

### History and physical examination

The initial evaluation of the elderly incontinent patient includes a thorough history and physical examination, which often includes obtaining information from family members. The history should focus on the frequency, timing (diurnal versus nocturnal), volume, and symptoms associated with incontinence episodes. An incontinence chart or diary can be useful diagnostically and in the development of a treatment plan (Fig. 6-4).

Urinary incontinence can be triggered or perpetuated by a broad variety of medical and psychologic illnesses, most of which are not directly related to the function of the lower urinary tract itself. However, because local structural and neurologic abnormalities frequently coexist with and contribute to incontinence, the clinician should be particularly attentive to certain aspects of the neurologic and abdominopelvic examination. Sacral levels 2 through 4, which carry parasympathetic fibers to the detrusor and sphincter, can be examined by assessing rectal tone, perianal sensation, and the bulbocavernosis reflex. Abnormalities suggest significant spinal cord or cauda equina pathology. The abdomen should be carefully palpated and percussed for a suprapubic mass suggestive of a distended bladder. The rectal, and in women pelvic, examination is essential in excluding causes such as fecal impaction, rectal or pelvic masses, pelvic floor abnormalities such as uterine prolapse, and cystocele or urethrocele. Vaginal infection should be excluded or treated and atrophic changes noted. Laboratory evaluation should include urinalysis and culture as appropriate. Chemistries to evaluate the patient's metabolic status and renal function are important.

Careful review of medications and their indications is essential to any initial evaluation. Many prescription and over-the-counter drugs affect detrusor and sphincter function and may cause subtle degrees of delirium and cognitive dysfunction. Antihypertensives, which can affect the autonomic nervous system or smooth muscle tone directly, and patent cold medications, which usually contain sympathomimetics or antihistamines with significant anticholinergic effects, are most often the cause. Diuretics contribute by overwhelming an elderly person's limited storage capacity. Topical ophthalmologic agents such as β-blockers and cholinergics used in the treatment of glaucoma can be absorbed in sufficient quantity to have systemic effects. The box at top right lists some general categories of drugs and the mechanisms by which they can interfere with continence.

## Classification and etiology

*Transient incontinence* accounts for approximately 75% of new-onset incontinence and is most likely to have a reversible cause. The etiology usually is not readily referrable to the urinary tract, with the notable exception of urinary tract infection. Transient incontinence is common in elderly hospitalized patients. The DIAPPERS mnemonic helps in recalling the common causes of transient incontinence (see the box at bottom right).

*Established incontinence* refers to chronic incontinence caused by dysfunction of the detrusor, the outlet, or the neurologic pathways controlling them. Established incontinence is commonly divided into four general clinical syndromes to provide a framework for diagnosis and management.

Incontinence that is potentially transient can become established if not promptly identified and managed, or if it is assumed to be established from the outset. Established incontinence is less likely to be completely reversible, though management can ameliorate symptoms and reduce social impairment.

***Urge incontinence.*** Urge incontinence represents the most common clinical incontinence syndrome. The history reveals a warning sensation occurring seconds to minutes before the involuntary voiding of moderate to large volumes of urine. Increased urinary frequency and nocturnal incontinence are common features. The PVR is typically low, and cystometry demonstrates contraction at low bladder volumes. There may be no objective neurologic findings, although this clinical pattern of incontinence is commonly associated with an underlying neurologic problem.

The cause of urge incontinence is usually detrusor hyperreflexia, either primary or secondary. Primary detrusor hyperreflexia is properly referred to as detrusor instability. The differential diagnosis of secondary detrusor hyperreflexia includes stroke, Alzheimer's disease, parkinsonism, central nervous system tumors, and early outlet obstruction. The evaluation of a patient with urge incontinence begins with a routine urinalysis and, if indicated, urine culture. The evaluation of women includes a pelvic examination with attention paid to contributory

### Medications that can cause incontinence

**Antihypertensives**

***Antiadrenergics***

Clonidine, α-methyldopa, β-blockers: decreased sphincter tone, cognitive dysfunction, depression

***Calcium channel blockers***

Verapamil, nifedipine, diltiazem, others: decreased detrusor contractility, constipation and fecal impaction

***ACE inhibitors***

Captopril, others: drug-induced cough

**Diuretics**

Hydrochlorothiazide, furosemide, others: increased urine production, glucose intolerance

**Sedative-hypnotics**

Benzodiazepines, chloral hydrate, antihistamines (e.g., diphenhydramine): cognitive dysfunction (delirium), anticholinergic effects

**Antidepressants**

Tricyclic agents (e.g., amitriptyline, others): anticholinergic side effects, cognitive dysfunction

**Neuroleptics**

Haloperidol, others: cognitive dysfunction, Parkinson's syndrome, anticholinergic effects, especially in low potency neuroleptics (e.g., thioridazine [Mellaril])

**Narcotic analgesics**

Various: cognitive dysfunction

**Ethanol**

Cognitive, motor dysfunction, increased urine production

**Decongestants**

Ephedrine, pseudoephedrine, phenylpropanolamine: sphincter dysfunction, decreased detrusor contractility

**Antihistamines**

Diphenhydramine, chlorpheniramine, many others: anticholinergic effects

***ACE*, Angiotensin converting enzyme.**

### Common causes of transient incontinence

*D*-Delirium
*I*-Infection
*A*-Atrophic vaginitis
*P*-Pharmacy (drugs)
*P*-Psychologic (e.g., depression)
*E*-Endocrine
*R*-Restricted mobility
*S*-Stool (fecal) impaction

From Resnick NM, Yalla SV: *N Engl J Med* 313:800, 1985.

conditions such as infectious or atrophic vaginitis. When infection or atrophy is diagnosed and treated, resolution or marked improvement in incontinence can occur. For men a DRE with careful palpation of the prostate gland is essential. Although the size of the prostate gland correlates poorly with the presence or absence of outlet obstruction, the finding of a very large gland is usually meaningful. In addition, any finding of asymmetry, nodularity or stony hardness warrants further investigation with prostate-specific antigen (PSA) testing and possible referral for transrectal ultrasound (TRU) and/or biopsy.

In most instances the initial evaluation of urge incontinence also should include a PVR volume determination. Volumes greater than 100 ml can indicate an emptying problem and hyperreflexia or instability (either obstruction or poor detrusor contractility) and should prompt consideration of further investigation (e.g., bedside urodynamics) or referral. An empiric pharmacologic trial in such a setting carries a high risk of inducing urinary retention and is probably best avoided. The finding of a normal PVR (less than 50 ml) is reassuring but does not exclude the possibility that urinary retention will occur, especially in men, where a normal PVR can be seen with significant prostate enlargement. Devices that measure urine flow during voiding can be used to screen for male patients with significant mechanical obstruction before a drug trial. When such measurements are not possible, men should be referred for cystoscopy and urodynamics before any pharmacologic intervention.

A bedside urodynamics test involves inserting a Foley catheter in the patient's bladder. The catheter attaches to a 1-L irrigation bag of sterile normal saline, which is hung on an IV pole. Saline is slowly run into the bladder. Using a manometer, the physician notes the volume and pressure at which the patient first notices the urge to void and then the volume and pressure at which the patient does void. If bladder capacitance is normal there should be minimal rise in bladder pressure (i.e., filling should occur at pressures less than 15 cm of water. Additionally, the patient should be able to postpone voiding until the bladder capacity reaches at least 600 ml. Patients with detrusor instability or hyperreflexia have normal PVRs but experience the urge to void at low bladder volumes (less than 300 ml), demonstrate intermittent rises in the manometry column, or demonstrate a decreased ability to postpone voiding. Because bedside studies are not an exact science, a negative study does not exclude the diagnosis, but such studies may be of some benefit for a patient who is unable to provide a detailed history of symptoms or complete an incontinence chart. Patients for whom diagnostic uncertainty remains should be referred for formal testing.

The management of urge incontinence is aimed at treating underlying predisposing conditions when possible or appropriate; otherwise, treatment is aimed at managing symptoms. Assistive devices such as bedside commodes and urinals can be great helps in managing nocturnal symptoms. Toileting regimens that are based on the completion of an incontinence chart often are effective for patients who can cooperate (see Fig. 6-4). Instructing patients to limit fluids in the evening or before car or bus trips can restore control and confidence. Diuretic use should be avoided or minimized.

A logical clinical approach can lead to the satisfactory management of most patients without referral and the appropriate referral of a subset of patients who need further investigation. Empiric pharmacologic intervention can be very effective in urge incontinence if implemented with appropriate caution (see the box at right). Therapy is aimed at decreasing the contractility and suppressing spontaneous contractions of the detrusor and can be accomplished with the use of drugs such as oxybutynin, anticholinergics, and tricyclic agents such as imipramine.

**BLADDER RECORD**

Name ______________________ Week Starting ______ / ______ / ______
Month Day Year

Instructions:

Mark **D** for **"Dry"** each time urination occurs without leakage

Mark **W** for **"Wet"** each time leakage occurs
(If you cannot tell when the leakage occurred, mark **W** at the time closest to when you find the wetness.)

| | 7am | 8am | 9am | 10am | 11am | 12n. | 1pm | 2pm | 3pm | 4pm | 5pm | 6pm | 7pm | 8pm | 9pm | 10pm | 11pm | 12am | 1am | 2am | 3am | 4am | 5am | 6am |
|---|---|---|---|---|---|---|---|---|---|---|---|---|---|---|---|---|---|---|---|---|---|---|---|---|
| Mon | | | | | | | | | | | | | | | | | | | | | | | | |
| Tues | | | | | | | | | | | | | | | | | | | | | | | | |
| Wed | | | | | | | | | | | | | | | | | | | | | | | | |
| Thur | | | | | | | | | | | | | | | | | | | | | | | | |
| Fri | | | | | | | | | | | | | | | | | | | | | | | | |
| Sat | | | | | | | | | | | | | | | | | | | | | | | | |
| Sun | | | | | | | | | | | | | | | | | | | | | | | | |
| | Morning | | | | | Afternoon | | | | | | Evening | | | | | Night | | | | | | | |

**Fig. 6-4.** Example of a bladder record for outpatient settings.

The selection of an agent depends on consideration of side effects and cost, as well as comorbid conditions. Dosing should be initiated at the lower end of the stated range for each agent until symptoms are ameliorated, side effects are encountered, or the upper end of the dosage range is reached without discernible effect.

The use of calcium channel blockers such as nifedipine and verapamil has been advocated by many clinicians but must be considered investigational at this time. The incontinent patient with angina or hypertension, however, might best be treated with a calcium channel blocker, which may also help the incontinence.

*Reflex incontinence.* Reflex incontinence is similar in presentation to urge incontinence except that patients receive no warning before voiding. This situation occurs when the lower spinal micturition center is cut off from brainstem and cortical centers and usually is seen in the setting of severe spinal cord disease or injury. Because there is no signal before voiding, behavioral management and assistive devices are less effective. Pharmacologic management is similar to that for urge incontinence but is more problematic. Fortunately this pattern of incontinence is rare in ambulatory geriatric populations.

*Stress incontinence.* Stress incontinence is a common presenting pattern of urinary incontinence in women. It is relatively uncommon in men, unless there has been traumatic or surgical damage to the urinary sphincter. Patients complain of intermittent leakage of small amounts of urine associated with laughing, coughing, or lifting heavy objects. The cause is usually related to the postmenopausal decrease in estrogen with subsequent atrophy and thinning of the urinary sphincter and pelvic floor muscles. The bladder neck and sphincter, which are normally located within the pelvis and are therefore intraabdominal, can actually descend out of the pelvis. In this situation transient increases in intraabdominal pressure, rather than reinforcing the resting tone of the urinary sphincter instead overwhelm it, resulting in the expulsion of urine. Another variant of stress incontinence is stress-induced detrusor instability, in which coughing, laughing, lifting, or other maneuvers that produce a sudden rise in intraabdominal pressure result in an uninhibited contraction of the bladder. Several features distinguish this condition from simple stress incontinence: the volume leaked is moderate to large, nighttime incontinence is more common, there may be a brief but detectable delay between the stress-inducing maneuver and the passage of urine, and the patient may experience urgency.

The diagnosis of stress incontinence is based largely on history and physical examination. Pelvic and rectal examinations are indicated to detect evidence of estrogen deficiency and to exclude anatomic problems such as urethrocele or vesicocele, which might warrant surgical intervention. During the examination the patient should be asked to strain or cough, and the leakage of any urine should be noted. The patient then can be asked to repeat the maneuver after the examiner has inserted a finger in the vagina and elevated the bladder neck by exerting gentle pressure anteriorly. In a positive test, the leakage of urine is corrected by the elevation of the bladder.

The management of stress incontinence depends on the underlying cause, and the majority of patients respond to conservative therapy. Weight loss is indicated in obese patients and result in decreased pressure on the pelvic floor. The patient should be taught Kegel exercises, which involve isometric contraction of the pelvic sling muscles and can increase the strength and resting tone of the urinary sphincter. Estrogen therapy, either topical or systemic, is sometimes effective, especially for women with clinical evidence of estrogen deficiency such as atrophic vaginitis and hot flashes. In patients who do not respond to these therapies a trial of an adrenergic agent such as pseudoephedrine, phenylpropanolamine, or imipramine can be given (see the box below); however, the side effects of these agents in the elderly can be considerable.

A variety of surgical procedures are available for selected patients who fail medical management. When surgery is not possible, a vaginal pessary or penile clamp may restore continence.

The clinician should be aware of the existence of mixed stress-urge incontinence, in which a sudden rise in intraabdominal pressure triggers detrusor contractions. The management is essentially the same as for urge incontinence, although the diagnosis is frequently difficult to make clinically. This is because the delay between the stress and detrusor contraction may be extremely brief, although the volume voided usually is larger than with pure stress incontinence. Imipramine may be the drug of choice in the treatment of stress-induced detrusor instability, since it combines sympathomimetic effects on the urinary sphincter and anticholinergic effects on the detrusor.

*Overflow incontinence.* Overflow incontinence refers to incontinence that occurs in the setting of abnormally high

### Drugs used in the management of urge incontinence

Oxybutynin: 2.5-5 mg tid
Propantheline: 15-30 mg tid
Imipramine: 25-50 mg tid*
Dicyclomine: 10-20 mg tid

*Should be begun at lower dosages (e.g., 10-25 mg qd) and gradually titrated upward. Can cause serious cardiac conduction problems.

### α-Adrenergic agents used in the treatment of stress incontinence

Pseudoephedrine: 15-30 mg tid
Phenylpropanolamine: 75 mg bid
Imipramine: 25-50 mg tid*

*Should be gradually titrated up to this dosage, starting with 10-25 mg qd.

bladder volumes and incomplete emptying. The most common underlying conditions are mechanical outlet obstruction (usually benign prostatic hypertrophy in men) and neurologic lesions. The PVR is by definition high, and patients report constant or frequent dribbling, which may be exacerbated by stress, and decreased force of urinary stream. Patients also may report the sensation of incomplete bladder emptying and the need to strain to void. Physical findings may include a palpable bladder or suprapubic dullness to percussion in addition to any underlying neurologic deficits. Prostate size as determined by DRE correlates very poorly with the presence of outlet obstruction.

The performance of urodynamics is particularly important in suspected overflow incontinence. Cystoscopy is necessary to determine the presence and site of a mechanical obstruction. Management includes relief of mechanical obstruction followed by intermittent catheterization until the bladder regains contractility. If the bladder does not regain contractility, continued catheterization may be necessary. Management also may include the use of cholinergic agents to increase bladder contractility and α-adrenergic blockers to decrease resting sphincter tone. When employed, pharmacologic agents are rarely of long-term utility.

***Functional incontinence.*** Functional incontinence refers to incontinence that occurs because an individual has lost the capacity to move to an appropriate place to void in a timely manner. This definition incorporates both individuals with normally functioning urinary tracts and those with impaired function. An obvious example would be a patient who is hospitalized with a hip fracture and is placed in traction with an intravenous infusion. The patient is likely to become incontinent unless supplied with aids such as a bedside urinal or bedpan, prompt assistance from hospital staff, and aggressive restorative services such as physical and occupational therapy. Although usually less overt, global functional problems such as visual and auditory impairment, mobility problems, and deconditioning are frequently contributory factors in both transient and established incontinence. Identification and management of these functional difficulties are essential.

### Use of assistive devices

As previously discussed, the use of assistive devices such as a bedside commode or urinal can be an indispensable part of the management plan, particularly for a patient with a component of nocturnal urge incontinence. In the daytime a regular toileting schedule (based on the patient's incontinence chart) can preempt inadequate warning time before voiding and can be effective even in patients with moderate cognitive impairment. Patients should modify their fluid intake so that most of it takes place at times when appropriate facilities are nearby. Avoiding fluid intake in the evening may reduce nocturia and incontinence.

The judicious use of adult incontinence briefs can provide substantial independence and prevent homeboundedness, functional decline, and institutionalization. Overuse can lead to skin maceration and breakdown, along with urinary and vaginal infections. The use of an indwelling or suprapubic Foley catheter should be reserved for instances when all other approaches have failed or are unacceptable to the patient. For those with hypocontractile bladders and retention as a cause of their incontinence, intermittent self-catheterization is a preferred method with a lower infection rate.

Given the potential complications and loss of dignity, the use of Foley catheters and adult incontinence garments in acutely ill patients with transient incontinence is rarely appropriate, since the risk usually outweighs the benefit. Such management should not be invoked for the convenience of the hospital or nursing home staff alone.

## PRESSURE SORES

The pressure sore is one of the most difficult management problems encountered in elderly patients and is always best dealt with by prevention rather than cure. Recent advances have improved our understanding of the epidemiology, pathophysiology, and principles of management of this condition. Surveys of general hospitals indicate that from 3% to 11% of hospitalized patients bring pressure sores into the hospital and that between 1 and 5% of newly admitted patients develop pressure sores during hospitalization. The mortality associated with pressure sores in some studies leads to a fourfold increased risk of dying in those patients coming from nursing home environments. The elderly are most likely to develop this condition. Risk factors for the development of pressure sores have been identified for hospitalized patients and include fecal incontinence, fractures, and hypoalbuminemia. Nursing instruments such as the Norton Scale have been developed to predict which patients are at greatest risk for the development of decubitus ulcers and therefore require assiduous attention to ameliorating those risks and treating underlying disease.

Pressure sores occur over bony prominences with 65% being found in the pelvic area and 30% on the lower extremities. Four critical factors have been proposed to explain the pathophysiology of decubiti: pressure, shearing forces, friction, and moisture. Prolonged direct pressure above 32 mmHg produces tissue anoxia with subsequent necrosis of epidermis and superficial dermis. When supine, 70 mmHg of pressure may be generated at sacrum, and 45 mmHg is generated at the heels. It is not surprising, then, that pressure sores may arise in less than an hour of total immobility.

In addition, the elderly have less subcutaneous fat and therefore less "cushioning" as well as a higher likelihood of diseases that reduce cutaneous blood flow, such as congestive heart failure, atherosclerosis and dehydration. Shearing forces result from the relative displacement of tissues and occur, for example, when the head of the bed is raised and the torso slides down. In this case the skin is fixed to the sheets but the subcutaneous tissue is stretched, resulting in angulated blood vessels and thrombosis in the underlying dermis.

Friction results when two surfaces in contact move across each other, as when a patient is dragged across a sheet. Moisture results from fecal and urinary incontinence, drainage from tubes, food, and sweat leading to skin maceration and breakdown.

The differential diagnosis of the pressure sore is made substantially by location of the lesion. Early ischiorectal abscesses, vasculitis, deep mycosis, and necrotic malignancies should be considered if the location and features are suggestive. There is a high rate of complications from pressure sores. Osteomyelitis and sepsis carry a high mortality, approaching 50%. Appropriate radiographic evaluation and sinography should be undertaken to define the extent of any complicated pressure ulcer.

The primary approach to management is in prevention, with an eye to the four factors noted above. Pressure can be relieved by turning the patients every 2 hours. Alternating air mattresses and water beds have been shown in European trials to prevent decubiti. Sheepskin and eggcrate mattresses do not lower pressure enough. Donuts are undesirable because they occlude blood vessels and delay healing. Shearing can be prevented by not raising the head of the bed for more than 2 hours and getting a footboard to avoid slipping. Excess moisture may be avoided by careful attention to skin care, preventing leakage, and using true sheepskin to absorb moisture. Finally, friction can be decreased by using loose fitting sheets, clearing the bed of crumbs, and not dragging the patient across the sheets.

Once an ulcer forms its size, location, and stage should be documented. Conditions affecting healing, such as malnutrition, underlying disease, and dehydration, should be addressed. Infection must be treated with broad spectrum antibiotics, since 20% to 38% of patients with bacteremia have polymicrobial sepsis and require coverage for gram-positive and gram-negative, as well as anaerobic, bacteria.

Specialized beds have been investigated and a randomized controlled trial comparing an airfluidized (e.g., Clinitron) vs. an alternating air mattress has shown that healing is greater for those on the air-fluidized mattress, especially for patients with large decubiti. Complications of air-fluidized mattresses include heat and water loss, deranged electrolytes, sensory deprivation, and problems with nursing tasks such as feeding and positioning. Local wound care is aimed at removing devitalized tissue in order to promote wound healing and lower bacterial counts. Several options are available for stage I and II ulcers and include wet-to-dry saline povidone dressings qid. Povidone iodine and $H_2O_2$ should be avoided because they are cytotoxic and impair wound healing. Topical antibiotics such as silver sulfadiazine and gentamicin have been used to lower bacterial counts. Enzymatic debridement with collagenase or elastase can also be accomplished with care to avoid damaging regenerating borders. Biologic dressings have been popular because they have been shown to speed epithelialization, keep out bacteria, and absorb wound fluids. They may be of the hydrocolloid type that are oxygen impermeable (e.g., Duoderm and Restore) or oxygen permeable (e.g., Opsite or Tegaderm) and have a polyurethane film with an adhesive. Calcium alginate, a seaweed derivative, has been used because it is highly osmotic and is good for exudative wounds. There are no well-done studies comparing all the local therapies. For stage I and II pressure sores local wound care can be tailored depending on how clean the base of the wound is and the evaluation of nursing or caregiving resources. For example, wet-to-dry dressings qid may accomplish the same healing as biologic dressing once per week with less nursing care involved.

### The staging classification by Shea used to describe pressure ulcers

Stage I-Acute inflammatory response, which involves the epidermis with edema, swelling, heat, erythema, and induration.

State II-Ulceration extends through the dermis to the subcutaneous tissue.

State III-Extends into the subcutaneous tissue with extensive undermining and is a full thickness defect. If eschar is present it is at least a stage III.

Stage IV-Involves deep fascia muscle and bone.

From Shea JD: *Clin Orthop* 112:89, 1975.

## DRUG PRESCRIBING FOR THE ELDERLY

The primary provider caring for the elderly is likely to confront problems of adverse drug reactions (ADRs) and polypharmacy, in part because the elderly use a disproportionate volume of medications. The 13% of the US population that is elderly consumes about 30% of all prescription drugs. Cross-sectional studies have shown that the average elderly patient takes 1.7 to 2.7 prescription drugs and one over-the-counter medication, and the number of drugs used increases with age.

Although there is a greater probability of ADRs in old age, the risk of adverse reactions appears to depend on number of medications taken rather than on age alone. Information on the subject is relatively scarce; data on drug effects in the elderly are limited because most drug trials have often excluded women and the elderly. Also, since the majority of studies have surveyed hospital admissions or inpatient populations, there is limited information on ADRs in outpatients. Elderly outpatients have been reported to have increased likelihood of noncompliance with drug regimens, but this may be an effect of numbers of medications and complexity of schedules rather than patient age. Another area where data are limited is in nursing home patients: although frail institutionalized elderly have the highest use of medications, prevention of ADRs in this population has not been adequately studied.

Idiosyncratic and allergic reactions appear to occur with the same frequency in elderly as in younger adult patients. Toxicity and side effects, on the other hand, are more common in the elderly. Several factors appear to be significant: (1) some elderly patients have diminished-physiologic reserves, secondary to disease, leading to decreased ability to tolerate stress and to respond appropriately to medications; (2) disease is more prevalent in the elderly, resulting in the need for more therapeutic interventions; and (3) deficits in memory, sensation, and function increase the likelihood that patients will make medication errors. Certain illnesses appear to increase the risk of ADRs, including sensory loss, cognitive dysfunction, and diseases of the kidneys, liver and heart.

Polypharmacy adds another dimension to the problem of drug reactions. First, it increases the risk of individual ADRs. It also increases the likelihood of drug-drug interactions. If multiple drugs are prescribed and regimens are complex, prescribing errors such as incorrect dosages

## Physiologic changes of aging

**Body composition**
Water: decreased
Fat: increased
Muscle mass: decreased

**Hepatic function**
Microsomal enzyme activity: decreased
Blood flow: decreased

**Renal function**
Glomerular filtration: decreased
Blood flow: decreased

## Useful guidelines in prescribing for the elderly

- Take a thorough medication history.
- Prescribe only when necessary; consider alternatives to medications whenever possible.
- Choose carefully, considering toxicity, drug and disease interactions, compliance, and cost.
- Give careful instructions, both verbal and written.
- Initiate therapy one drug at a time.
- Titrate dosage carefully (i.e., start low, go slow).
- Monitor effects and toxicity closely; monitor serum levels when appropriate.
- Stop nonessential medications.
- Review indications for all drugs.
- Review evidence of efficacy.
- Always consider drugs as a cause of morbidity and toxicity.

are also more likely to occur, and patients have more difficulty with compliance.

Drug reactions are influenced by the common physiologic effects of aging (see the box on p. 142). These physiologic changes may also result in altered pharmacokinetics. Since most drugs are absorbed by passive diffusion, absorption is generally unchanged, but many poorly absorbed drugs have not been studied. Changes in body composition may affect drug distribution: lipid-soluble drugs may have a larger volume of distribution and thus a prolonged duration of action; water-soluble drugs may have a decreased volume of distribution, resulting in higher concentrations at standard dosages. Decreased phase I hepatic metabolism has variable effects and is influenced by other factors such as smoking and alcohol consumption, but it may result in prolonged clearance of active forms of many drugs. Phase II metabolism, such as conjugation, shows little or no change with aging. Renal elimination, correlated with creatinine clearance, may be decreased.

Pharmacodynamic effects depend on drug action at the receptor site and have not been well studied in the elderly. In general, most drug effects are similar to or greater than those in younger patients; effects may be magnified when disease states are present that further alter drug elimination or response. Although cardiovascular β-adrenergic receptors appear to be less responsive, central nervous system receptors may be more sensitive, especially in patients with dementia.

Sedation and confusion are common drug complications in the elderly, especially from medications such as anticholinergics and sedative-hypnotics that affect the central nervous system. Other disturbances that suggest adverse reactions include orthostasis, falls, depression, urinary retention or incontinence, constipation, anorexia, and metabolic abnormalities such as hypoglycemia, hypokalemia or hyperkalemia, hyponatremia or hypernatremia, and azotemia.

Guidelines useful in prescribing for the elderly are listed in the box at bottom left.

## HOME CARE

Until the 1940s primary care was often delivered in the home. As medical technology grew more complex and patients became more mobile, care switched to hospitals, clinics, and offices; the prevalence of house calls gradually diminished. But with prospective payment systems now encouraging early discharge and Medicare allowing home-care services without prior hospitalization, the provision of home care is rising meteorically. The home-care industry is growing at 20% per year, 10 times the growth in the number of nursing home beds. At the same time, because of a demographic increase in the number of elderly, more functionally impaired elders are residing in the community. Some 4.6 million elderly people with limitations in their ADLs are currently noninstitutionalized. Survey data show that these elders and their families prefer the home as the primary site for care.

Home care is the provision of a wide range of services and equipment to the patient in the home for the purpose of restoring and maintaining the maximal level of comfort, function, and health. Homebound patients are community-dwelling individuals who depend on the assistance of others to perform some ADLs because of acute or chronic medical conditions or disabilities. In the absence of this help, they would be at high risk of institutionalization.

An impressive array of professional, ancillary, and diagnostic services can be provided in the home, as can advanced technology (see the box at right). Funding for these services comes from a variety of sources, including federal and state governments (e.g., Medicare, Medicaid, Title XX of the Social Security Act, Title III of the Older Americans Act, the Veterans Administration, and research and demonstration grants), charities, Blue Cross and other commercial carriers, and private out-of-pocket payments (see the box at far right).

Indications for a home care referral include advanced age and frailty, multiple comorbidities, recurrent and frequent admissions, homeboundedness, and impaired psychosocial or functional status. Often the first sign of decline in status is the inability to keep scheduled office or clinic appointments. A house call as part of comprehensive geriatric assessment helps to identify medical, psychosocial, and environmental factors that affect functional ability. Problems identifiable by house calls include alcoholism (finding bottles or cans), incontinence (by odor), sensory impairment, pain, medical noncompliance, falls (with special attention to environmental factors), and

### Services available in the home

**Professional**
- Physician
- Nurse
- Dentist
- Podiatrist
- Optometrist
- Rehabilitation therapists: occupational, physical, speech, respiratory
- Psychologist
- Dietitian
- Pharmacist
- Social worker

**Ancillary/supportive**
- Home health aides
- Personal care assistants
- Homemakers
- Chore aides
- Volunteers
- Home-delivered meals

**Diagnostics**
- Phlebotomy
- X-rays
- Electrocardiograms
- Holter monitoring
- Oximetry
- Blood cultures

**Medical equipment**
- Intravenous infusion for chemotherapy, blood transfusion, antibiotics, total parenteral nutrition, pain management and other medications
- Ventilators
- Hemodialysis
- Medical alert devices
- Glucometers

### Services covered by Medicare

**Part A (100%)**
- Home health aide
- Visiting nurse: RN observation/assessment, management, and evaluation of care plan
- Social service
- Physical therapy, occupational therapy, speech therapy if accompanied by skilled nursing need

**Part B (20% copayment)**
- Physician visit
- Certain durable medical equipment
- Some diagnostic tests, electrocardiography, and x-rays

### Problems identified by house calls

**Medical**
- Alcoholism
- Incontinence
- Sensory impairment
- Pain
- Compliance and medication errors
- Falls
- Depression

**Other**
- Safety/environmental
- Psychobehavioral
- Caregiver stress
- Elder abuse and neglect
- Nutrition
- Finances
- Limitations in ADLs/IADLs

depression (see the box at right). In one study of 200 patients, the home visit revealed an average of two new problems per patient and from one to eight new recommendations for the treatment plan, when compared with office-based assessment. About 23% of the newly diagnosed problems indicated extreme morbidity and were potentially life-threatening. The house call can be used for diagnostic purposes, for emergency evaluations that otherwise would require a trip to the emergency department, or for ongoing primary care of the truly homebound population.

The home is the ideal nonthreatening location to identify the elder's strengths, abilities, and supports, both formal and informal. These factors are important in developing a care plan that can be put into operation realistically and complies with the patient's and family's wishes. A team approach and the use of a home care coordinator for case management are essential in implementing complex plans that may include numerous referrals and services as well as education for the patient and family. They also allow continuous assessment of outcomes over time so that the plan can be revised as the patient's needs and health status change.

## ELDER ABUSE AND NEGLECT

### Epidemiology and definition

Mistreatment of the elderly is found among all racial, ethnic, and socioeconomic groups, and it occurs in both the community and institutions. Incidence and prevalence rates in the community vary, largely because of the lack of uniform definitions of elder abuse and neglect, particularly among states and municipalities where reporting is mandatory. Lack of awareness or denial of this problem on the part of the public and health care professionals themselves can result in underreporting of suspected cases of mistreatment. Victims who require heavy care may not report abuse or neglect for fear that they will hasten their placement in nursing homes, or they may be embarrassed to admit to mistreatment. Studies indicate that between 1 and 2 million elderly people per year are victims of abuse—physical, psychological, financial—or neglect. Inclusion of elders who are receiving inadequate care, which is a less restrictive definition, expands these numbers substantially.

Abuse or neglect can be active, as in the conscious withholding of food, clothing, shelter, or medicine, or passive, perhaps because the caregiver is unable to bathe, dress, or feed the patient. Fullmer and O'Malley suggest the less judgmental approach of regarding the situation as a mismatch between the person's care needs and the services he or she receives. The problem of inadequate care must be dealt with, however, irrespective of cause.

### Etiology

There are several theories to explain abuse and neglect. The dependency theory says that the more physically and mentally impaired the patient, the greater the risk for abuse, though dependency alone is an insufficient cause. The stressed caregiver theory proposes that a threshold is exceeded by care needs, and this triggers abusive behavior. Superimposed external stresses, such as job loss or illness, exacerbate these caregiving burdens to the point where abusive behavior is triggered. The transgenerational family violence theory holds that children who are abused learn violence as a behavior and abuse their own children and elderly parents. Social isolation can set the stage, since patients have little access to social supports or confidants. The pathologic abuser theory states that the psychopathology of the abuser is the etiology of family violence, especially where alcohol, substance abuse, or psychiatric illness is involved.

There is no difference between the incidence in women and that in men, nor do age and level of cognition appear to be factors. The most significant risk factors are a history of previous family violence and evidence of substance abuse in the perpetrator. These risk factors, superimposed on an elder with heavy care needs, limited family resources, and stresses due to juggling job and care for the elder, can lead to a multifactorial etiology for the abuse.

### History

Several historical clues may be of help in the diagnosis of elder abuse and neglect. Inconsistent or implausible explanations for disease or injury should alert the astute clinician to possible elder mistreatment. Several hospital admissions or emergency room visits (often to different facilities) for illness or trauma, with explanations such as that the elder is accident prone, should raise a red flag. The caregiver's insistence on providing history or refusal to leave the room also should arouse suspicion. Functional status of the patient in terms of ADLs and IADLs is important. Recent family stresses, such as loss of a loved one or job, the presence of family violence, and substance abuse, again point to high-risk patients.

The patient should be interviewed in private so that he or she will not be intimidated by possibly abusive caregivers. Specific questions should be asked about being hit, kicked, restrained, unfed, or left in soiled clothes. A sexual history, including questions about rape and incest, also should be elicited.

A nonjudgmental, nonaccusatory interview with the suspected abuser should take place in private. It is important to know if the alleged abuser is the patient's caregiver. The health care provider should determine the degree of the elder's dependence on the care provider, as well as whether there is a fiduciary relationship (i.e., whether the provider is reimbursed for care or depends on the income of the elder).

### Signs of abuse, neglect, and inadequate care

Contusions
Lacerations
Abrasions
Fractures
Sprains
Dislocations
Burns
Oversedation
Anxiety
Over- or undermedication
Decubiti
Untreated but previously diagnosed problems
Dehydration
Misuse of medications
Malnutrition
Hypothermia or hyperthermia
Poor hygiene
Depression

Modified from O'Malley TA et al: *Ann Intern Med* 98:998, 1983.

### Physical examination

Careful documentation of injuries and appearance should be recorded with narrative, drawings, or photographs. Dementia or delirium should be determined by mental status examination at the outset with an instrument such as the Folstein Mini-Mental State Exam (see the box on p. 131). Signs of abuse are listed in the box above.

### Intervention and treatment

The approach to elder abuse, neglect, and inadequate care usually involves a multidisciplinary team, including the skills of physicians, nurses, and social workers. Health professionals are mandated to report suspected cases of mistreatment in most states. State agencies often support elderly protective service programs that employ workers to make home assessments. These visits can be made under the guise of assessing care needs that may be met by outside agencies. If needs are not being met and the competent patient wants to be relocated or separated from an abuser, arrangements can be made to find alternate living situations or to remove the perpetrator. If the patient is competent and resists intervention (which is often the case), then it is incumbent upon the health care provider to inform the elder that he or she need not remain in such an environment and that help can be provided. This help can be in the form of home care services such as home health aides, visiting nurses, or delivered meals, or it can involve respite, counseling, and education for the caregiver. If the patient does not have the mental capacity for decision making, a court-appointed guardian or conservator may be necessary. Often education, counseling, and support services for a stressed caregiver, even one who cares for a severely demented patient, can end the cycle of abuse. In the case of an elder who lives with a pathologic abuser, interventions aimed at the abuser such as counseling, job training, or the order to evacuate may be necessary. Many complex ethical issues raised in the evaluation and treatment of elder abuse have to do with the patient's autonomy and right to refuse treatment as well as the confidentiality of the physician-patient relationship.

## BIBLIOGRAPHY

Allman RM: Pressure ulcers among the elderly, *N Engl J Med* 320:850, 1989.

Applegate WB, Blass JB, Williams TF: Instruments for the functional assessment of older patients, *N Engl J Med* 322:1207, 1990.

Consensus Development Panel: National Institutes of Health consensus development conference statement: geriatric assessment methods for clinical decision-making, *J Am Geriatr Soc* 36:342, 1988.

Council on Scientific Affairs: Home care in the 1990s, *JAMA* 263:1241, 1990.

Fields SD: Special considerations in the physical exam of older patients, *Geriatrics* 46:39, 1991.

Fowles DG: *A profile of older Americans: 1992,* Washington, DC, 1992, American Association of Retired Persons and the Administration on Aging, US Department of Health and Human Services.

Gurwitz JH, Avorn J: The ambiguous relation between aging and adverse drug reactions, *Ann Intern Med* 114:956, 1991.

Kellogg International Work Group on the Prevention of Falls by the Elderly: The prevention of falls in later life, *Dan Med Bull* 34(suppl 4):1, 1987.

Lachs MS, Fulmer T: Recognizing elder abuse and neglect, *Clin Geriatr Med* 9:665, 1993.

Montamat SC, Cusack BJ, Vestal RE: Management of drug therapy in the elderly, *N Engl J Med* 321:303, 1989.

Nelson RC, Amin MA: Falls in the elderly, *Emerg Med Clin North Am* 8:309, 1990.

Ouslander JG: Diagnostic evaluation of geriatric urinary incontinence, *Clin Geriatr Med* 2:715, 1986.

Ouslander JG, Seir HC: Drug therapy for urinary incontinence, *Clin Geriatr Med* 2:789, 1986.

Resnick NM, Yalla SV: The pathophysiology of urinary incontinence among institutionalized elderly persons, *N Engl J Med* 320:1, 1989.

Soldo BJ, Manton KG: Demography: characteristics and implications of an aging population. In Rowe WJ, Besdine RW editors: *Geriatric Medicine,* Boston, 1988, Little, Brown.

Steel K: Home care for the elderly—the new institution, *Arch Intern Med* 151:439, 1991.

Tinetti ME, Speechley M: Prevention of falls among the elderly, *N Engl J Med* 320:1055, 1989.

# PART TWO

# *Systemic Disease in Primary Care*

# I Cardiovascular Disease

CHAPTER

# 7 Cardiovascular Risk Factors: Social Determinants of Cardiovascular Disease

**Geoffrey A. Modest**

Don't crowd diseases (epidemics) point everywhere to deficiencies of society?

**Virchow, 1879***

Many of the risk factors for atherosclerotic cardiovascular disease (ASCVD) are interrelated. For ease of discussion, the risk factors are discussed individually, although unifying hypotheses will be presented as they have evolved in the literature.

Many of these risk factors, including hypercholesterolemia, hypertension, smoking, and stress, have strong social components; they derive from social and cultural environments. The major disease-related components for an individual are diet, occupation, air and water quality, housing conditions, various stressors, and the social support network.

To be an effective clinician, it is important to assess an individual's disease in the context of this broader social framework. For example, one must understand the occupational components of disease to intervene in the occupational environment. In addition, if the causes of disease are predominantly in the social, economic, and political arenas, disease prevention requires involvement on a broader scale that may involve family, community, and regional or national interventions. Health professionals must understand the links between society and disease and can therefore play an extremely important role in helping change the underlying social causes.

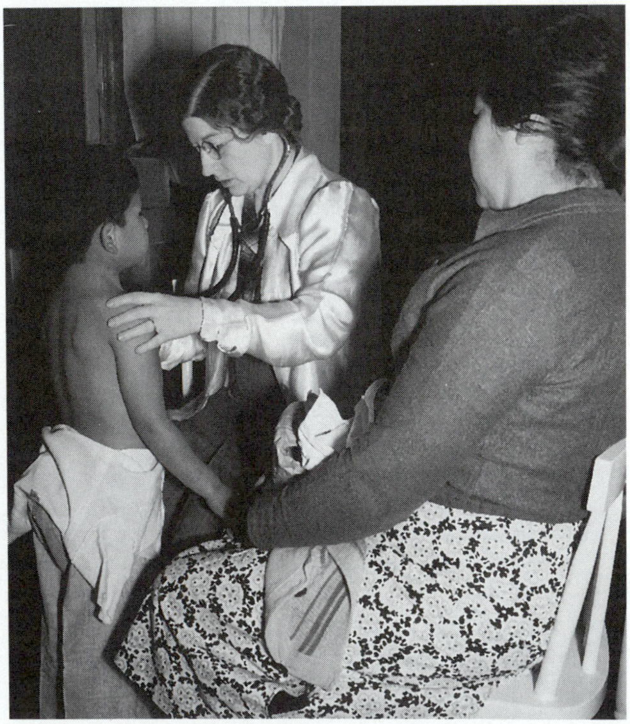

**Fig. 7-1.** From the Collection of the Library of Congress.

## CHOLESTEROL

Serum cholesterol has been generally accepted as one of the most important ASCVD risk factors. In fact, in countries where ASCVD is rare, serum cholesterol levels stay in the 120 to 160 mg/dl range. In the United States, at least 25% of people have serum cholesterol levels greater than 250 mg/dl. Cholesterol levels tend to increase with age.

The relationship between serum cholesterol and ASCVD is continuous (Fig. 7-2), with no evidence of a critical level that separates high from low risk. The pooled results of five large longitudinal epidemiologic investigations on the risk factors for ASCVD in middle-aged white men found a doubling of the rate of ASCVD when serum cholesterol levels are above 250 mg/dl and a tripling when they are above 300 mg/dl. The data in women are somewhat less clear, in part because there have been fewer studies involving women. The age-adjusted incidence of ASCVD is lower in women than men for the same total cholesterol level, with no increase in ASCVD until levels are 265 mg/dl or more. Large observational studies do not support a strong relationship between cholesterol levels and the new development of ASCVD in people over 70 years old.

Over the past several years it has been repeatedly shown that low-density lipoprotein (LDL) cholesterol is athero-

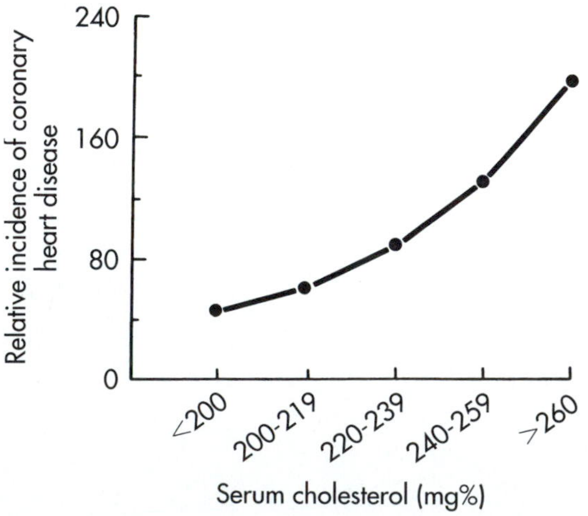


**Fig. 7-2.** Relative incidence rate of ASCVD of white men classified by entry level of serum cholesterol, as pooled from three large U.S. studies (Framingham, Albany, and Minneapolis). (From Connor WE, Connor SL: *Prev Med* 1:49, 1977.)

*From E.H. Ackerknecht, *Rudolf Virchow: Doctor, Statesman, Anthropologist.* Madison: University of Wisconsin Press, 1953.

genic and that high-density lipoprotein (HDL) cholesterol is protective. In fact, HDL is at least as cardioprotective as the LDL is injurious, and the ratio of LDL to HDL is significantly more predictive of an ASCVD event than the total cholesterol level (Fig. 7-3). For men, each 1 mg/dl increase in HDL is associated with a 2% to 3% decrease in ASCVD risk, and each 1 mg/dl increase in LDL confers a 1% increase in ASCVD risk.

HDL cholesterol seems to be especially important in women. The Lipid Research Clinics found that HDL cholesterol was strongly, inversely related to ASCVD mortality. In their 14-year follow-up of 1405 women aged 50 to 69 there was a relative risk of 1.74 for an HDL level less than 50 mg/dl, adjusting for other risk factors. Total cholesterol and LDL cholesterol levels had poor predictive value. In both the Lipid Research Clinics and Framingham Studies, there were 5% reductions in ASCVD risk associated with a 1 mg/dl increase in HDL cholesterol in women.

HDL is cardioprotective presumably through its role in the reverse transport of cholesterol, although the details are poorly understood. HDL is probably directly antiatherogenic, because infusion of HDL in rabbits results in reversal of established ASCVD. HDL cholesterol is composed of several different subfractions. Although some studies suggest that $HDL_2$ is the most cardioprotective, others have not. The prospective Physicians' Health Study found that assessment of HDL subfractions did not provide further utility than the total HDL measurement. The relationship of HDL cholesterol to other risk factors is shown in Table 7-1.

LDL is better understood biochemically than HDL. LDL receptors on a variety of cells affect the cellular uptake of LDL. Defects in the number or function of these receptors cause a decrease in LDL clearance from the plasma, which occurs largely in the liver, and an increase in serum levels of LDL cholesterol. LDL cholesterol levels are related to other ASCVD risk factors (see Table 7-1).

Although the HDL and LDL cholesterol levels explain most of the variance in cholesterol-associated ASCVD risk, other factors may also be involved. For example, the respective apolipoproteins associated with HDL and LDL seem to be even more related to cardioprotection and ASCVD than HDL or LDL cholesterol. Perhaps the most important role of apolipoproteins is that of ligands that bind to the appropriate receptors. In general, there is a strong correlation between apolipoprotein B (apo B) and LDL cholesterol levels and between apolipoprotein A (apo A) and HDL. However, some patients with hypertriglyceridemia who have minimally elevated or even normal LDL cholesterol levels and high levels of apo B seem to be at high risk of ASCVD. Still others have normal triglyceride and cholesterol levels and have high apo B levels with increased ASCVD. It seems that some of these patients have small, dense LDL particles, and because there is only one apolipoprotein molecule per LDL particle, they have higher ratios of apo B to LDL cholesterol. In most cases, small LDL particles are associated with high triglyceride and low HDL levels. Some clinical studies suggest that these small LDL particles are highly atherogenic. For unknown reasons, people with diabetes tend to have small, dense LDL particles, as do people on β-blockers, sedentary individuals, and those with central obesity. Also, part of the reason that LDL cholesterol is much less predictive of ASCVD in women than in men may be that women may have less dense LDL particles. Similarly, studies suggest that apo A is more cardioprotective than HDL cholesterol; however, in the cases of apo A and B, the studies are mostly retrospective and done in people with established ASCVD.

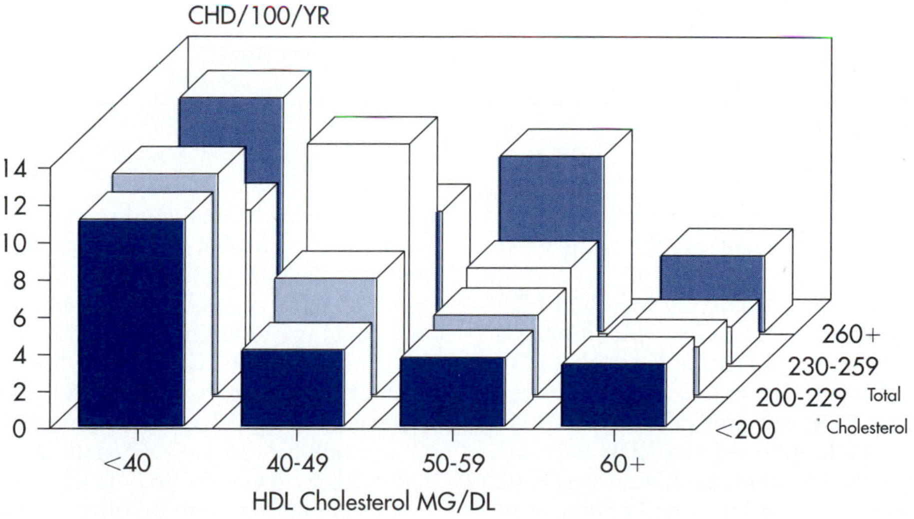


**Fig. 7-3.** Four-year rate of ASCVD of men and women aged 50 to 79 who were initially free of ASCVD, according to distribution of HDL and total cholesterol levels. Note that the negative correlation between HDL cholesterol levels and ASCVD is stronger than the positive correlation between LDL cholesterol levels and ASCVD, which is especially true in women (see text). Also, the ASCVD risk is high even in people with low total cholesterol levels who have very low HDL cholesterol levels. *CHD,* Coronary heart disease (ASCVD). (From Castelli WP, Garrison RJ, Wilson PWF et al: *JAMA* 256:2835, 1986.)

**Table 7-1.** Influences on cholesterol

| Risk factor | Associations | Comments |
|---|---|---|
| ↓HDL cholesterol | Smoking* | |
| | Central obesity* | One third of interindividual HDL variation explained by waist-to-hip ratios |
| | Diabetes* | Especially if fasting hyperinsulinemia, also with poorer glycemic control |
| | Medications | Especially β-blockers; anabolic steroids decrease HDL 50% |
| | Menopause | Improves with estrogen replacement |
| | Diet | |
| ↑HDL cholesterol | Exercise | |
| | Alcohol consumption | |
| | Medications | Examples: Chromium supplement, α-blockers |
| | Menstruation | |
| | African-American race | |
| | Higher education levels | ? Related to associated lifestyles |
| | Diet | |
| | ↓Platelet aggregation | |
| ↑LDL cholesterol | Smoking* | |
| | Central obesity* | |
| | Diabetes* | More atherogenic, dense LDL (see text) |
| | Psychosocial stressors | |
| | Menopause | Improves with estrogen replacement |
| | Coffee consumption | If prepared by boiling instead of filtering |
| | Medications | Especially thiazide diuretics |
| | Diet | See later section on Diet and Cholesterol |
| | ↑Platelet activation | Also, ↑ thromboxane released |
| | Medical conditions | Examples: nephrotic syndrome, hypothyroidism, Cushing's syndrome, dysproteinemia, hypogonadism in men |
| | Genetic factors | |
| | Age | |
| ↑Lipoprotein(a) [Lp(a)] | Genetic factors | Not much relation to dietary intake |
| | Diabetes* | Especially if nephropathy |
| | Nephrotic syndrome* | |
| | Renal failure | Especially if on hemodialysis |
| | Menopause | Improves with estrogen replacement |
| | African-American race | |
| | Inflammation | Acute phase reactant |
| ↓Lipoprotein(a) [Lp(a)] | Vigorous exercise | |
| | Alcohol ingestion | |
| | Niacin | Especially in high doses |
| | Asian race | |

*Reversing the association ameliorates the lipid risk factor.

At this point, it is difficult to obtain accurate, readily available apolipoprotein measurements, so the clinical use of apolipoproteins remains to be determined.

New studies suggest that an oxidatively modified LDL may be the most atherogenic LDL moiety. Macrophages have receptors only for oxidized LDL and not native LDL and can form foam cells only by the uptake of this oxidized LDL. Unlike the regular LDL receptor pathway on other cells, the macrophage uptake of oxidized LDL does not exhibit feedback inhibition. The oxidized LDL is cytotoxic to endothelial cells unlike native LDL. One hypothesis of atherogenesis is that high concentrations of plasma LDL lead to higher levels of oxidized LDL within the artery wall. Oxidized LDL is a chemoattractant for monocytes, which become macrophages and then foam cells. The oxidized LDL also causes endothelial injury, thereby attracting platelets and platelet-derived growth factors that promote smooth muscle cell proliferation and ultimately atherogenesis. Animal studies suggest that strong antioxidants, such as probucol, interfere with LDL oxidation and decrease the rate of atherogenesis even more than effective lipid-lowering medications. Human studies with probucol are ongoing. Vitamin E, a potent antioxidant, increases LDL resistance to oxidation. Observational studies have found that men and women with higher intakes of vitamin E have about a 40% decrease in ASCVD. In men, vitamin C has not proved to be beneficial. β-Carotene, another antioxidant, seems to be beneficial in men who smoke in some studies but not in others. Some early data from randomized studies suggest benefit in men with histories of ASCVD. In the absence of large, randomized primary or secondary prevention studies, antioxidant therapy via supplements, however, cannot be recommended.

There has recently been a resurgence of interest in lipoprotein(a), or Lp(a), as a major and independent ASCVD risk factor. Structurally, Lp(a) is an LDL-like particle—containing cholesterol, phospholipid, and apo B—covalently linked with apolipoprotein(a), which is structurally homologous to plasminogen. Large accumulations of Lp(a) are found in human atherosclerotic coronary artery lesions, the extent of which parallels the serum Lp(a) level. Epidemiologically, case-controlled and prospective studies have suggested a major role for Lp(a) in men and women. For example, a study of 776 men aged 50 who were followed prospectively for 6 years found that those with the highest level of Lp(a) had an increased incidence of myocardial infarctions; 27% of the infarctions were directly attributable to high LP(a) levels, controlling for cholesterol, smoking, hypertension, fibrinogen, diabetes, and family history. The Lipid Research Clinics also found an independent role for Lp(a), although the Physician's Health Study did not. The region of Lp(a) homologous to plasminogen inhibits plasminogen activation, interfering with fibrinolysis. As with LDL, Lp(a) can become oxidized, and oxidized Lp(a) is taken up by macrophages at a dramatically increased rate over native Lp(a), leading to increased macrophage cholesterol content. Oxidized Lp(a) is also a stronger antagonist of plasminogen activity and is more thrombogenic than native Lp(a). Thus Lp(a) provides a direct link between the atherosclerotic and thrombotic mechanisms of ASCVD. However, although the data are impressive for a strong role of Lp(a) in ASCVD, no data show that a decreasing Lp(a) level has any effect on clinical outcome.

### Diet and cholesterol

The relationship between dietary intake and serum cholesterol levels is also generally accepted, although it is less clear-cut. Many animal and human studies confirm the basic hypothesis that increased consumption of cholesterol and certain types of fats results in increased serum cholesterol levels. This relationship, however, seems to have some genetic variance.

The relationship between dietary fats and serum cholesterol levels is complex and somewhat contradictory. In general, saturated fats are associated with higher cholesterol levels; for a 1% increase in calories from saturated fats, there is an approximately 2.7 mg/dl increase in serum cholesterol. Although the precise mechanism is unclear, it seems that saturated fats cause a decrease in the number of LDL receptors, resulting in higher serum cholesterol levels. Polyunsaturated fats decrease cholesterol levels by decreasing both the LDL and HDL cholesterol levels, so there may be no cardioprotection as predicted by the model previously described. Monounsaturated fats (e.g., canola and olive oils) decrease LDL cholesterol levels without lowering levels of HDL and therefore should be the most cardioprotective. *Trans*-fatty acids caused by hydrogenating unsaturated fatty acids (e.g., as in margarine) and also found in the fat of ruminants (e.g., as in cow's milk) increase LDL cholesterol levels. Unfortunately, many people substitute margarine for saturated fats in attempting to lower cholesterol levels. LDL cholesterol levels are lowered by increasing the amount of fiber in the diet. People on psyllium, 5.1g twice a day, independent of their fat intake, had a 5% decrease in total cholesterol levels and a 7% decrease in LDL levels. Garlic decreases cholesterol levels 9%. Although the general relationship between dietary intake and serum cholesterol levels holds true for men and women, data suggest that women have less serum response to changes in dietary cholesterol or fats than men and that at least part of this difference is mediated by hormones. Changes in diet are associated with changes in the serum cholesterol levels and ASCVD. For example, Seventh Day Adventist men in the United States have lower cholesterol diets than the U.S. average, lower serum cholesterol levels, and approximatley 40% less ASCVD.

### Stress and cholesterol

A positive association between stress and cholesterol levels has been found in most studies. Tax accountants evaluated at the time of the April tax-return deadline had a rise in serum cholesterol levels from 210 to 252 mg/dl, with no significant changes in diet, exercise, or weight. Fig. 7-4 displays the results of a study in which a small number of individuals were kept on the metabolic unit of a hospital for up to 5 months. Marked increases in serum cholesterol levels correlated with the "normal," day-to-day stresses of the hospital (e.g., stressful interactions with other patients or staff). Other studies have found the cholesterol elevations to be in the LDL fraction, and that these increases were most significant in people with little emotional support.

The mechanism by which stress can cause cholesterol elevations remains unclear. Epinephrine-induced lipolysis may stimulate increased hepatic synthesis of cholesterol. Adrenergic $\alpha_1$-inhibitors, which antagonize some of the catecholamine effects, lower cholesterol levels. Epinephrine activates hepatic 3-hydroxy-3-methylglutaryl CoA reductase, the rate-limiting enzyme in cholesterol synthesis, and may also decrease receptor-mediated cellular binding and uptake of LDL. Other animal studies suggest that the catecholamine-induced increases in cholesterol may be secondary to decreased cholesterol excretion.

Concern has been raised that low cholesterol levels themselves might have adverse psychologic effects. This concern has been inspired by the finding of increased violent deaths and accidents in several but not all of the cholesterol-lowering trials. Animal studies have demonstrated that dietary fat changes are associated with changes in the lipid composition of neuronal cell membranes, the postulated site of mental processes, and that animals fed low-cholesterol foods following the American Heart Association recommendations had more aggressive behavior. Low-cholesterol diets are associated with changes in pain threshold, learning ability, and physical activity in animals. The link in humans is less clear. The Family Heart Study in Oregon, a 5-year dietary intervention study to lower cholesterol levels, found that those who consumed low-fat foods and had a 3% reduction in cholesterol levels also had a significant decrease in depression and aggressive hostility. Several recent large prospective epidemiologic and intervention studies did not find any relation between serum cholesterol levels and accidents or violence. It is important to recognize that in general the long-term change in ASCVD mortality associated with cholesterol lowering probably far surpasses the increase in deaths from violent causes. An additional concern is that given the belief about the deleterious effects of hypercholesterolemia, people with this condition may take on a "sick role."

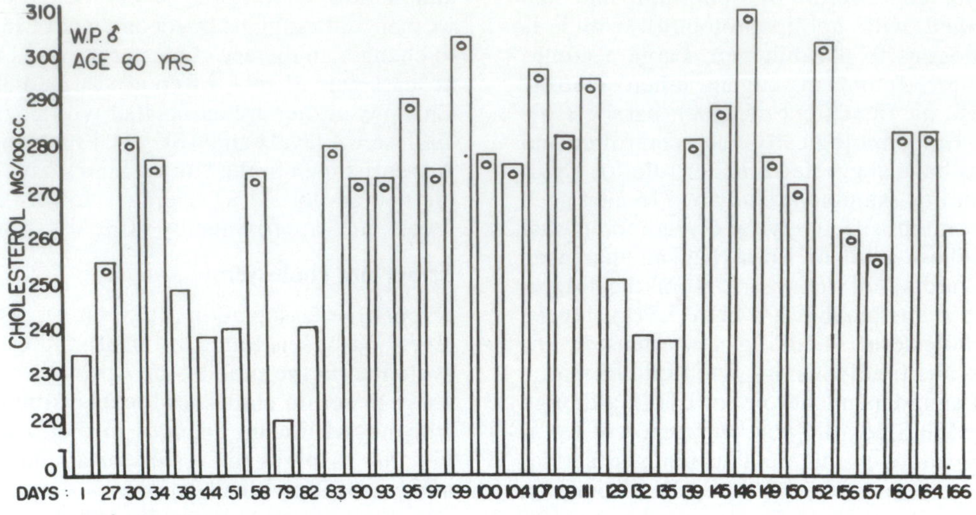


**Fig. 7-4.** Changes in serum cholesterol levels in one individual during several months of constant diet and exercise. The mean cholesterol level on stressful days was 283 ± 12.5 mg/dl and on nonstressful days 212 ± 10.3 mg/dl. (From Wolf S, McCabe WR, Yamamoto J et al: *Circulation* 26:379, 1962.)

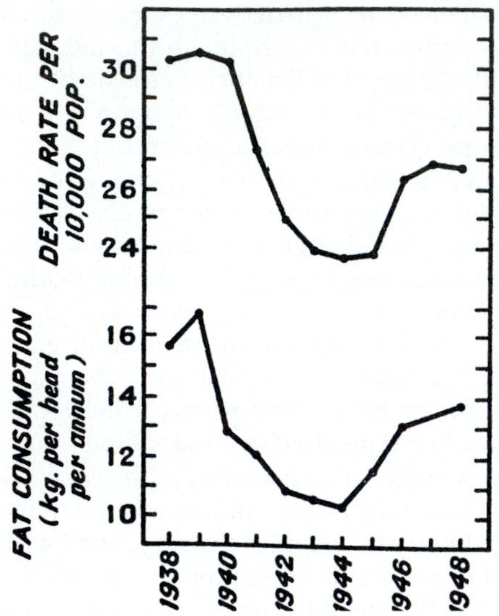


**Fig. 7-5.** Mortality from circulatory diseases in Norway during World War II. Note the parallel decline in the mortality rate with changes in fat consumption. Fat consumption was determined from per capita consumption of butter, milk, cheese, and eggs. (From Strøm A, Jensen RA: *Lancet* 1:126, 1951.)

## Effect of lowering serum cholesterol

Decreasing serum cholesterol levels is associated with decreased ASCVD mortality rates. Several historical observational studies have confirmed this relationship. Changes in ASCVD mortality rates in World War II paralleled the dietary changes of the people and were independent of war-related stresses. In Norway, which had a very high prevalence of ASCVD, war-related deprivation of high-fat foods led to a dramatic decrease in the ASCVD mortality rate after about 2 years (Fig. 7-5). In England, the consumption of fats remained unchanged, as did the ASCVD incidence. In the United States, both the fat consumption and ASCVD incidence increased. Recent U.S. history suggests that the marked decrease in the ASCVD mortality rate since 1970 parallels the decrease in consumption of dairy products (see section on Decline in ASCVD Mortality).

Several dietary intervention studies have confirmed the effect of decreasing dietary fats on ASCVD mortality rates. Prison studies have corroborated that serum cholesterol levels correlate with dietary cholesterol levels, with a 1- to 2-week lag. An increase in serum cholesterol of approximately 12 mg/dl was found with each dietary increment of 100 mg of cholesterol per 1000 kcal. On the basis of extensive metabolic ward studies, mathematic models that can accurately predict changes in serum cholesterol levels from dietary changes have been developed.

A few dietary intervention studies have been performed on people without known preexisting ASCVD (primary prevention). For example, an 8-year prospective study of 850 domiciled residents over 55 years old had a 12.7% decrease in serum cholesterol levels in the low-cholesterol diet group and a significant decrease in the total ASCVD morbidity and mortality rates. There was an increase in cancer and traumatic deaths in the study group, however. A 12-year prospective crossover dietary intervention program in two mental hospitals in Finland, effecting a 10% to 15% change in serum cholesterol levels associated with a low-cholesterol diet, found a significant 47% reduction in the ASCVD mortality rate for men. The rates for total mortality for men and the rates for ASCVD and total mortality for women were decreased but did not achieve statistical significance.

The role of reducing serum cholesterol medically in the primary prevention of ASCVD has been studied. The Lipid Research Clinics Coronary Primary Prevention Trial followed 3800 men who initially free of known heart disease for more than 7 years. One group received cholestyramine; the other was given placebo. The study group achieved a

13.4% decrease in serum cholesterol levels, a 24% decrease in ASCVD mortality, a 19% decrease in nonfatal infarctions, and a 20% to 25% decrease in new-onset angina and new exercise stress tests with positive results. Subgroup analysis revealed a dose-response curve: men who achieved a 25% decrease in serum cholesterol levels had half the ASCVD incidence. In general, a 1% reduction in cholesterol levels was associated with a 2% reduction in ASCVD risk.

Reducing serum cholesterol levels in people who already have ASCVD (secondary prevention) is also beneficial. A controlled study in Oslo of 412 patients after myocardial infarction who were followed for 5 years found a significant reduction in subsequent ASCVD symptoms in patients on low-cholesterol diets. These dieters were able to achieve a 31% decrease in their serum cholesterol levels from an initial average of 296 mg/dl. In addition, dieters who had recurrent symptoms had higher serum cholesterol levels than dieters whose conditions remained asymptomatic. These findings were significant only for people under 60 years of age.

Since the efficacy of cholesterol-lowering treatments has been established through studies mostly of middle-aged men, concern has been raised about the applicability of the results to other age groups and to women. The relative risk of ASCVD attributable to cholesterol is in fact higher in younger people than older ones. Because the incidence of ASCVD is higher among the elderly, even the lower relative risk indicates that more elderly people are likely to benefit from lowering cholesterol levels than younger ones. Since there does not appear to be a significant relationship between cholesterol levels and the new development of ASCVD in the elderly, especially in women, it may not be appropriate to screen or provide primary prevention for those over 70 years old. A recent Scandinavian trial using simvastatin in 4444 patients with ASCVD followed 5 years found a dramatic 42% reduction in cardiac deaths and a 30% reduction in total mortality. These benefits applied to both genders and to both younger and older (60 to 70 years old) individuals. There are essentially no data on primary prevention in women, although as previously noted, cholesterol is at least as strong an ASCVD risk factor in women as in men. Women do get ASCVD at rates even higher than men but with a 10-year lag, and ASCVD is the most common cause of death in elderly women. A few secondary prevention trials in women suggest benefit from therapy, although more data are clearly necessary.

Several studies have assessed angiographically proven regression of atherosclerotic lesions. In general, whether serum cholesterol levels are lowered by diet, medications, or surgery, it has been shown repeatedly that atherosclerotic lesions—once thought to be fixed, permanent defects—can regress. The Familial Atherosclerosis Treatment Study, for example, found that intensive medical anticholesterol therapy led to regression of atherosclerosis in 32% to 39% vs. 11% of controls and progression in 21% to 25% vs. 46% of controls.

### Weight reduction and serum cholesterol

Weight reduction by itself lowers serum cholesterol levels. A prospective noninterventional, 20-year study of 1900 middle-aged men at Western Electric showed a correlation between dietary cholesterol and serum cholesterol levels at the beginning of the study, changes in diet and changes in serum cholesterol levels, the 19-year ASCVD mortality rate and dietary cholesterol intake as well as serum cholesterol level, and weight changes of 1 kg/m$^2$ and serum cholesterol changes of 5.5 mg/dl independent of cholesterol or dietary fat intake. The Framingham Study also found a linear relationship between naturally occurring weight change and the serum cholesterol level.

### Genetic factors and hypercholesterolemia

It is difficult to assess accurately the frequency of genetic hypercholesterolemia in the United States because of the pervasiveness of high-cholesterol diets and familial influences on diet. Higher cholesterol levels are found more often in people with type A blood than in those with type O. Overall, high estimates suggest that up to 3% of the population have autosomal dominant hypercholesterolemia and 5% have a poorly defined "polygenic" variety. In these cases, diet is still effective in lowering the cholesterol level, although medications are usually also necessary.

### Comments

The Consensus Conference sponsored by the National Heart, Lung, and Blood Institute felt that sufficient evidence exists to conclude that dietary cholesterol consumption is related to serum cholesterol level, elevated serum cholesterol is "a major cause of coronary artery disease," and lowering serum cholesterol helps prevent the development of ASCVD (see Chapter 40 for details of the recommendations). A recent update of the recommendations includes measuring HDL levels. The arguments (see Fig. 7-3) support including HDL in the risk profile. Data on women suggest that HDL cholesterol is the single most important lipid to measure.

One of the implications of this discussion is that there is an inherent problem in defining a "normal" serum cholesterol level. Some laboratories report it as a broad range (e.g., 130 to 200 or 240 mg/dl), perhaps increasing with advancing age. However, these values apply to a society in which the "normal" person is more likely to die of ASCVD than of any other single cause. In societies where ASCVD is unusual, serum cholesterol levels tend to be in the 120 to 160 mg/dl range and do not increase with age.

## HYPERTENSION

Hypertension is a major risk factor for ASCVD as well as for stroke and chronic renal failure. Overall, 20% of people in the United States are hypertensive; 90% of these have hypertension of unknown etiology, or "essential" hypertension. The prevalence of hypertension increases with age, from 5% of 20 year olds to 50% of those aged 70. In this chapter *hypertension* is defined as a diastolic blood pressure greater than 90 mm Hg or a systolic blood pressure greater than 140 mm Hg. Hypertension is further described in Chapter 8.

### Hypertension and ASCVD

One methodologic problem when assessing the role of hypertension in ASCVD is the wide fluctuation of pressure found in normotensive and hypertensive individuals (see

Chapter 8). Routine 24-hour ambulatory blood pressure monitoring reveals systolic variations of up to 16 mm Hg and diastolic variations of 12 mm Hg, often associated with stressors (e.g., "white-coat" hypertension).

There is evidence that hypertension is associated with ASCVD. The huge Pooling Project combined the results of six major 10-year prospective studies on cardiovascular risk factors. This compilation found the relationship between hypertension and ASCVD deaths to be continuous, with an increasing number of deaths associated with increasing blood pressures. Table 7-2 displays this finding for five of the largest prospective studies, showing a remarkable uniformity of results. The relationship to ASCVD holds for diastolic or systolic blood pressure. Hypertension is related to the development of angina pectoris as well as to ASCVD mortality.

**Table 7-2.** Blood pressure and ASCVD incidence

| Quintile | Systolic blood pressure | Standardized incidence ratio |
|---|---|---|
| All | All | 100 |
| I | <120 | 70 |
| II | 120-130 | 86 |
| III | 130-138 | 87 |
| IV | 138-150 | 102 |
| V | >150 | 150 |
| Risk ratio: V/(I + II) | | 1.9 |
| 95% confidence level | | |
| Low | | 1.6 |
| High | | 2.4 |

Incidence of first ASCVD events correlated to quintile of systolic blood pressure. Data pooled from several studies, including Albany Study, Chicago Gas Company Study, Chicago Firemen, Framingham Study, and Tecumseh Study. Pooled data represent 8381 men at risk for total of 71,757 person-years, developing total of 658 first ASCVD events. Risk ratio is computed for most vs. least severe systolic blood pressure elevations. Similar relationships apply to diastolic blood pressure. Studies that include women have similar results. Adapted from Pooling Project Research Group: *J Chronic Dis* 31:201, 1978.

## Etiology

The etiologies of hypertension are discussed in Chapter 8. There are several interrelations between hypertension and other ASCVD risk factors (Table 7-3), some of which are synergistic.

Many stressors appear to be associated with the development of hypertension. These include stressors related to the perceived quality of community life, to migration, to external crises, and to aspects of employment or unemployment. These stressors derive from common areas of our social environment and affect large numbers of people. (See the section on Occupational Exposures for the relationships between specific occupational exposures and hypertension.) Obesity and hypertension as well as exercise and hypertension are discussed in Chapter 8.

***Sodium.*** There is a general relationship between sodium intake and hypertension in most studies. Part of the problem in defining this relationship precisely is that there is so much intraindividual variation in sodium intake that even a 24-hour urinary sodium excretion may not reflect true sodium intake over time.

Many studies done on populations with a consistently low sodium intake reveal a very low incidence of hypertension. Subgroups of a single population who have consumed less sodium have a lower incidence of hypertension than those on a high-sodium diet. However, there are conflicting results. For example, there is a low incidence of hypertension in some economically less developed countries where sodium intake is high. There may well be a genetic link between hypertension and sodium; first-degree relatives of hypertensive persons, who are themselves at increased risk of developing hypertension, often have a decreased ability to excrete sodium. The effects of sodium restriction in hypertensive individuals is discussed in Chapter 8.

There are important inconsistencies in the sodium-hypertension link. For example, in a study of 80

**Table 7-3.** Influences on hypertension

| Risk factor | Associations | Comments |
|---|---|---|
| ↑Blood pressure | Sodium consumption* | See text; association only in some individuals |
| | Alcohol* | May account for 5% to 7% of prevalence of hypertension. Blood pressure increases with daily consumption of 3 drinks or more. |
| | Genetic factors | |
| | Stress | See text; includes migration to nonsupportive areas, environmental stressors, occupational stressors, job loss, status incongruity |
| | Obesity* | 1% ↓ in weight associated with 2 mm ↓ in systolic and 1 mm ↓ in diastolic blood pressure. |
| | Psychologic factors | See text; especially suppressed hostility and anxiety |
| | Smoking* | May be synergistic with stress |
| | Caffeine* | Stimulates renin and corticosterone release, a short-term effect |
| | Diabetes | See text |
| | ↑Thrombotic factors | ↑Platelet aggregability, ↑platelet-derived growth factor, ↑inhibitor to tissue plaminogen activator (PAI-1), ↑fibrinogen |
| | Age | |
| ↓Blood pressure | Diet | Especially high-potassium, high-calcium, or high-fiber diets |
| | Exercise | |

*Reversing the association ameliorates the hypertension.

schoolchildren with borderline hypertension followed for 1 year, there was no significant decrease in blood pressure with documented salt restriction. There seem to be two subpopulations of hypertensive persons: salt-sensitive and non-salt-sensitive. People in the salt-sensitive group have a more dramatic blood pressure variation when on a low- vs. high-sodium diet than people in the non-salt-sensitive group. In addition, persons in the salt-sensitive group excrete less sodium during both sodium loading and sodium depletion and are therefore more sodium avid. This heterogeneity in responsiveness may explain why, even in the studies in which salt depletion or diuretics are effective, there is a large group of hypertensive patients who do not respond to treatment. The effects of other dietary factors (e.g., potassium, calcium, magnesium, chloride, fiber) on hypertension are given in Chapter 8.

*Alcohol.* The relationship between alcohol and hypertension is discussed in Chapter 8.

*Genetic factors.* There is a well-documented tendency for hypertension to run in families and even to begin at an early age. Interfamily blood pressure variance far exceeds intrafamily differences. Monozygotic twins have a significantly higher concordance for hypertension than dizygotic twins, further suggesting the role of genetics in hypertension. Genetics may play a role in terms of sympathetic responsiveness to stress or renal salt handling. The majority of epidemiologic studies, however, point against genetics being a determinant, although it is perhaps a "predisposing" factor.

Migration studies suggest a relatively minor role for heredity. In several Pacific Islanders, the average systolic and diastolic blood pressures increase in parallel with the degree of Westernization. In general, studies of essentially every racial group show members in different environments with high or low incidences of hypertension (Fig. 7-6). Modernization and hypertension are especially linked among individuals who actively strive for a Western, high-material-consumption lifestyle with little chance of success in achieving it, more so than in those whose aspirations and resources are more matched. These migration studies support a role of stress in hypertension.

*Stress.* Many types of stressors have been associated with hypertension. Animal studies have confirmed a relationship between psychosocial stress and the development of hypertension. Hypertension immediately follows external threat from a predator, disruption of social relationships, simultaneously presented excitatory and inhibitory conditioned stimuli, and other stressful tasks. Interestingly, animals under a series of short-term stresses for a long time can develop persistent blood pressure elevations, even in the subsequent absence of further stress. A study of air traffic controllers revealed that high work-related cardiovascular reactivity predicted the development of sustained hypertension over 1 to 3 years of follow-up, although most human experiments revealed that

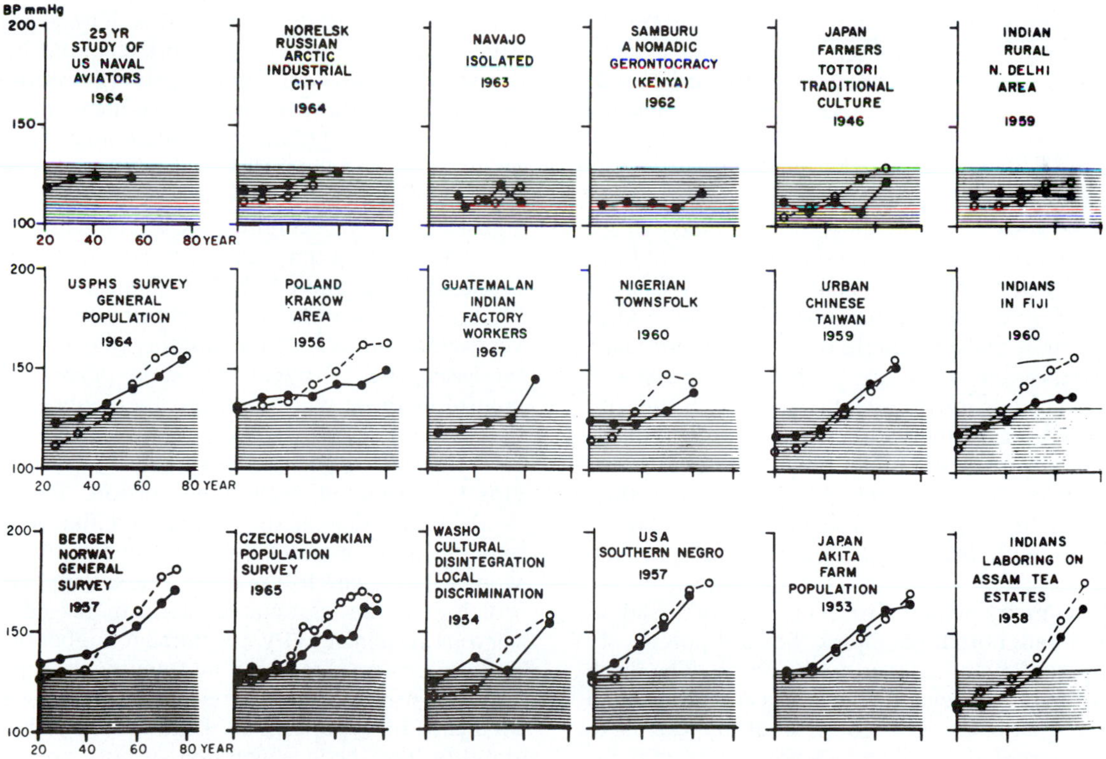


**Fig. 7-6.** Contrasting rates of change of blood pressure with age can be found in all races. Vertical sets of graphs represent people of presumably similar racial and genetic backgrounds. In general, blood pressure is lower where the culture is stable, traditional forms are honored, and the group members are secure in their roles and adapted to them by early experience. *Open circles,* Women; *closed circles,* men. (From Henry JP, Cassel JC: *Am J Epidemiol* 90:171, 1969.)

repeated stress-induced hypertension is usually followed by a return to baseline blood pressure.

Epidemiologic studies suggest an important role for stress in the development of human hypertension. One of the most striking findings in the United States is the disproportionately higher incidence of hypertension in the African-American population. As the fourth column of Fig. 7-6 suggests, the prevalence of hypertension among rural Africans is extremely low, increases some in urban Africans, and is very high in African-Americans. In the highly stressful environment of South Africa, however, the Bantu and "coloured races" have an increased incidence of hypertension; as in the United States, this increase progresses with age so that there is a 16.1% incidence in those age 60 and over.

Several studies in the United States have assessed possible social causes of racial differences in hypertension. African-American immigrants in a needy section of Chicago had higher blood pressure if they thought their neighborhood was undesirable than if they had more positive feelings, further confirming the migration studies noted in the section on Genetic Factors. Another study in Detroit assessed high- and low-stress environments, taking into account factors such as crime, population density, and socioeconomic status (SES). There proved to be significantly higher blood pressure in the African-American high-stress areas. In low-stress areas, there was no significant difference in blood pressures between African-American and white people. The Hypertension Detection and Follow-up Program found a strong inverse correlation between the amount of education, which roughly parallels the SES, and the prevalence of hypertension in African-American and white people. There was an approximate 40% decreased prevalence in both racial groups when comparing college-educated individuals with those with fewer than 10 years of school; however, the African-American:white ratio of hypertension prevalence was 2:1 within each educational category.

Other stressors have been associated with hypertension. External crises, such as explosions or war, have been associated with increased blood pressure, even in children. Prisoners in crowded cells, especially in the setting of unwanted social interactions, have significantly higher blood pressure than those in single rooms. Difficult tasks that are not impossible to do are related to increases in blood pressure, according to several studies. Similarly, working-class African-American men with low educational levels and high expectations to succeed (a form of "status incongruity") have higher blood pressures than those with either low educational levels and low expectations or those with high education and high or low expectations.

The mechanism by which different stressors lead to hypertension is undoubtedly complex. Several potentially relevant hormonal events occur with stress. The high catecholamine levels associated with stress are often found in hypertensive patients; 25% to 40% of hypertensive patients have increased basal catecholamine levels, increased sympathetic reactivity in response to postural changes or to psychologic stressors, and dramatic antihypertensive responses to β-blockers. In addition, brachial arteries in hypertensive individuals are hyperreactive to many different vasoconstrictive stimuli. Cortisol, another stress hormone, potentiates the effects of catecholamines by sensitizing β-receptors.

Mental stress leads to decreased sodium excretion, and in animals, stress is associated with increased salt appetite. Salt may cause hypertension by increasing sympathetic neurotransmitter release. Studies support synergism between stress and salt in hypertension development.

One hypothesis is that stress-related catecholamines have direct effects on the heart (increased pulse and force of contraction and the development of left ventricular hypertrophy), on the vasculature (often, increased peripheral resistance), and indirect effects largely mediated through renin release. Renin stimulates the generation of angiotensin, which leads to further vasoconstriction, and which may also have direct vasculotoxic effects and stimulate smooth muscle cell hyperplasia. The formation of angiotension also leads to the generation of aldosterone, which is associated with salt and water retention. In addition, stress is associated with increased secretion of antidiuretic hormone, which with aldosterone increases sodium retention and intravascular volume and further promotes hypertension. Individuals predisposed to having hypertensive responses to stress may, through unknown mechanisms, develop chronic hypertension.

***Work.*** Stressors related to employment have also been associated with hypertension. Persons with less secure jobs, especially those with lower levels of education in the same job as their peers (another form of status incongruity), have increased blood pressure. A case-controlled study of 215 employed men in seven urban worksites assessed the relationship between job strain and hypertension. Work with high strain was defined as having high psychologic demands (e.g., work fast and hard) but low decision latitude (e.g., noncreative, repetitive jobs with little ability of the worker to make decisions or give input into the work process). Ambulatory blood pressure monitoring confirmed that men with high-strain jobs had more hypertension, with an odds ratio of 3:1 after adjusting for age, weight, type A behavior, 24-hour urine sodium excretion, physical demands of the job, education level, smoking, and alcohol consumption. In addition, the 30 to 40 year olds had a significant increase in left ventricular mass. Other studies have also found an increased risk of hypertension in people with low job control or those who have lost their jobs.

***Psychologic correlates.*** Several psychologic factors are closely correlated with hypertension. The Framingham Study found that anxiety predicted the development of hypertension in initially normotensive men (but not women) who were followed 18 years. Suppressed hostility, which may be associated with increased sympathetic nervous system activity, is related to higher blood pressure in both African-American and white subjects. A relationship has also been found between submissiveness and the incidence of hypertension. Emotional and blood pressure stability have been correlated in both normotensive and hypertensive people. The relationship between the intense, type A personality and hypertension is inconclusive. However, several studies have found that type A individuals performing stressful tasks have amplified sympathetic and blood pressure responses.

The diagnosis of hypertension itself is associated with adverse psychologic effects. Hypertensive employees have twice the number of sick days as non-hypertensive employees. One workplace program found that detection of hypertension was associated with an 80% increase in work absenteeism compared with the same individuals during the year before its detection; the absenteeism was independent of the level of hypertension, the use of medication, or the degree of blood pressure control achieved.

### Effects of treatment and unifying theories

Hypertension is clearly a major ASCVD risk factor. Therapy for moderate or severe hypertension is definitely beneficial. Therapy for mild hypertension leads to well-documented benefits in decreased mortality and morbidity from strokes and congestive heart failure. It is striking, however, that the benefit in ASCVD reduction by treating mild hypertension is much less impressive, both when done as sole therapy and as part of multiple risk-factor interventions. In fact, most studies show no benefit in treating diastolic blood pressures below 95 to 100 mm Hg. These results seem to contradict the epidemiologic data suggesting that the lower the diastolic pressure, the lower the ASCVD morbidity and mortality rate; fewer events occur in people with diastolic blood pressures of 70 mm Hg than in people with diastolic blood pressures of 80 mm Hg, for example. Many reasons may explain this discrepancy.

First, almost all of the intervention studies last fewer than 9 years; most are only 5 years, and perhaps intervention needs to be early or long term to benefit hypertension, a frequently lifelong process. An argument supporting early treatment is that hypertension may cause vascular changes early, which makes later treatment ineffective. For example, several intervention studies suggest that there is a J-curve in hypertension therapy; increased mortality rates are associated with diastolic blood pressures below 85 to 90 mm Hg, which may in turn be related to hypertension-induced changes in vascular compliance and function. Longer studies may be beneficial: the Multiple Risk Factor Intervention Trial began to see an advantage of treating mild hypertension but only after more than 10 years of follow-up.

Second, the thiazides and β-blockers used in the trials may adversely affect other ASCVD risk factors such as cholesterol or blood glucose levels (note in the section on Diabetes that even mild hyperglycemia can be associated with increased ASCVD risk). The use of such drugs may also increase platelet aggregability (especially β-blockers). Therapy with some of the newer agents, such as calcium channel blockers or angiotensin-converting enzyme inhibitors, which do not adversely affect these other risk factors, may prove more beneficial.

Third, three intriguing "innocent-bystander" theories hypothesize that the association between mild hypertension and ASCVD is not causal but that mild hypertension is a marker of another pathologic process. One theory is that the culprit is a cellular defect in lithium-sodium countertransport, which is typically found in people with clinical hypertension or a predisposition to hypertension. Although weight loss is associated with a normalization of this defect, medications are not. According to this theory, the medication trials are unable to decrease ASCVD because ASCVD is a consequence of defective lithium-sodium countertransport and not of hypertension.

Another innocent-bystander theory relates to a primary role for hyperinsulinemia in hypertension, with hyperinsulinemia having the real association with ASCVD (see section on Diabetes). In nondiabetic hypertensive persons, there is a close correlation between the increase in blood pressure and the severity of insulin resistance; this correlation is independent of obesity. Insulin resistance is found in children of hypertensive parents and antedates the development of hypertension in genetically predisposed individuals. This insulin resistance and the resultant hyperinsulinemia are associated with activation of the sympathetic nervous system and cortisol secretion, enhanced sodium and water reabsorption, altered intracellular electrolyte regulation associated with hypertension (e.g., increased sodium-hydrogen pump and decreased Ca-ATPase activity), and stimulation of arterial smooth muscle proliferation. In obese adolescents, hyperinsulinemia is also associated with increased sodium sensitivity. Therefore according to this theory, the hyperinsulinemia that confers increased ASCVD risk causes mild hypertension coincidentally. Unfortunately, vasoconstrictors such as β-blockers increase insulin resistance and may further compound ASCVD. In association with its antihypertensive effects, physical training also decreases insulin resistance.

High sympathetic activity, which is perhaps related to stress, is the third innocent-bystander theory. Patients with hypertension as a group have increased sympathoadrenal response to stress. In this regard, mildly hypertensive patients with left ventricular hypertrophy (especially if it is concentric) and those with high renin profiles have many times the number of myocardial infarctions as those without these findings. Increased catecholamine secretion is in fact associated with increased left ventricular mass and increased renin release. In addition, stress, which is usually mediated by increased levels of catecholamines or cortisol, is associated with increased platelet aggregability, insulin resistance, abnormal lipid levels (arterial epinephrine levels correlate with non-HDL cholesterol in hypertensive but not normotensive individuals), and even increased cigarette consumption by smokers, as well as increased risk of coronary vasoconstriction and ventricular arrhythmias. According to this theory, hypertension is largely a marker for individuals with increased sympathetic responsiveness. Further empiric support is that people with the greatest daily variability of blood pressures (such as those with marked "white-coat hypertension"), which is largely related to catecholamine secretion, seem to have more left ventricular hypertrophy than others with similar blood pressures.

## SMOKING

Cigarette smoking is generally considered one of the major risk factors for the development of ASCVD: Roughly 200,000 cardiovascular deaths in 1988 were attributable to smoking. Smoking is strongly associated with accelerated atherosclerosis of the abdominal aorta and peripheral arteries, moderately associated with that of the coronary arteries, and minimally associated with that of the cerebral arteries. Air pollution is also associated strongly with heart disease mortality rates, with a dramatic increase in smokers.

The relationship between smoking and ASCVD is strongest for sudden cardiac death, is somewhat weaker for fatal and nonfatal myocardial infarctions, and is negligible for chronic angina pectoris. Autopsy studies show a direct relationship between the extent of smoking and the degree of atherosclerosis. However, the marked increase in ASCVD mortality noted later is out of proportion to the mild to moderate increased atherogenesis found in these autopsy studies. The large U.S. Veterans Study (Fig. 7-7) found increasing ASCVD mortality with increasing cigarette consumption. A pronounced, increased ASCVD risk from smoking was found in young individuals. The Framingham Study and others have found that smoking confers a 2-fold to 3-fold risk of ASCVD mortality for men and a 1.5-fold to 3-fold risk for women. Some studies have suggested that smoking is atherogenic only in the presence of hyperlipidemia. Smoking may be the dominant ASCVD risk factor for women under 50, especially those who use oral contraceptives or have high cholesterol levels; it is also a major risk factor for men under the age of 36 who sustain myocardial infarctions.

The documentation of a dose-response curve provides strong support for the relationship between smoking and ASCVD (see Fig. 7-7). This dose-response curve also confirms that no level of cigarette smoking can be considered safe. Death rates also increase relative to the self-reported degree of inhalation. The use of low-tar, low-nicotine cigarettes may not lower the risk of ASCVD, since the levels of carbon monoxide in alveolar air and nicotine in plasma do not significantly decrease with these cigarettes. One study in women under 65 years old found no difference in the risk of nonfatal myocardial infarctions in women who smoked low-tar, low-nicotine cigarettes compared with those who smoked the higher-yield brands. In addition, there is evidence accumulating that even nonsmokers exposed to smoke are adversely affected. For example, nonsmokers with angina pectoris have noted aggravation of their symptoms through "passive smoking." ASCVD mortality is increased in nonsmoking spouses of smokers compared with those of nonsmokers, with a relative risk between 1.25 and 2, resulting in an excess of 35,000 to 40,000 deaths from ASCVD annually. Pipe and cigar smokers have increased ASCVD mortality, but this is less than with cigarette smokers. Data on smokeless tobacco are insufficient to show an association with ASCVD, although systemic absorption has been documented.

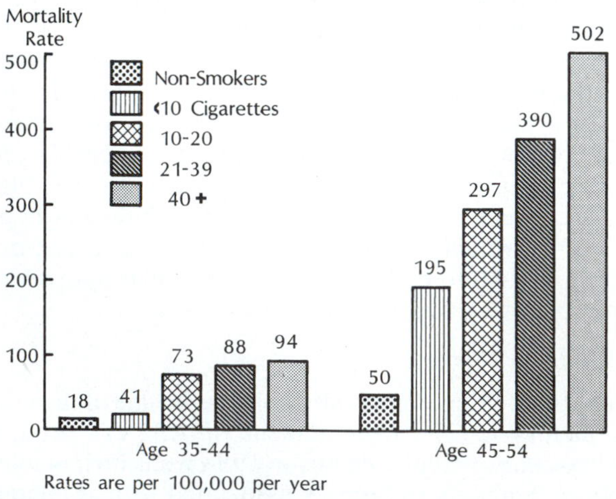


**Fig. 7-7.** ASCVD mortality rates by number of cigarettes smoked per day by men aged 35 to 54. Similar results were found in older age groups, although these results are less dramatic. (From Stamler J: *Bull N Y Acad Med* 44:1476, 1968.)

Smoking cessation causes a decrease of ASCVD risk to near nonsmoker levels in 1 to 2 years, although there is some residual increased risk. The Framingham Study showed that if men under 65 years of age quit smoking, the risk of death and myocardial infarction is half the rate of those who continue to smoke. Several other observational studies have found a 40% to 60% ASCVD mortality reduction by smoking cessation.

The exact mechanisms by which smoking causes ASCVD mortality remain unclear. Part of the problem stems from the fact that cigarette smoke has over 4000 components. Much of the attributable risk of ASCVD conferred by cigarette smoking is related to its effects on other known risk factors (Table 7-4).

Smoking affects the heart in several ways. First, and what seems to be the most important, is its hemostatic effects. Smoking is prothrombotic through its effects on fibrinogen and platelet aggregability. Its strong association with myocardial infarction and unstable angina, which are linked to the development of thrombi, more than its association with chronic angina, suggests a substantial thrombotic role. Also, that smoking may have a primary effect on thrombosis is suggested because the ASCVD risk conferred by smoking decreases so rapidly after smoking cessation. Smoking's effects on increasing blood viscosity (largely through its effects on fibrinogen) and erythrocytosis would also tend to increase the likelihood of thrombosis. Second, smoking has a direct atherosclerotic effect. Smoking is associated with endothelial injury, probably the inciting event of ASCVD, and autopsy and angiographic studies suggest accelerated atherosclerosis. The fact that the atherosclerotic risk after smoking cessation does not return completely to nonsmoker levels suggests residual increased atherosclerosis. Third, smoking is proarrhythmic and induces vasospasm. Smoking lowers the ventricular fibrillation threshold in animals in a dose-dependent fashion. In addition, smoking and infusions of nicotine are associated with arrhythmias, perhaps because of their effect on sympathoadrenal stimulation and catecholamine release. Also, smokers have abnormal endothelial function, and stimuli that cause coronary vasodilatation in nonsmokers (e.g., acetylcholine) cause vasoconstriction in smokers. In fact, coronary blood flow does not increase acutely with smoking, even though the heart rate increases by 20% to 30% and the blood pressure by 5% to 10%, perhaps explaining why the symptoms of angina increase in people with established ASCVD who smoke. Cigarette smoking also increases arterial wall stiffness. Fourth, smoking's mutagenic effects on cells may play a role. Some researchers have observed that human fibrous plaques are often monoclonal, suggesting that they develop from a single transformed smooth muscle cell and that the mutagenic effects of smoking might accelerate this transformation.

**Table 7-4.** Associations with smoking

| Associations | Comments |
|---|---|
| ↑Fibrinogen levels* | Smoking is the major determinant of elevated fibrinogen; up to 50% of attributable risk of ASCVD in smokers is through fibrinogen |
| ↓HDL cholesterol levels* | Most impressive lipid abnormality |
| ↑LDL cholesterol levels* | |
| ↑Triglyceride levels* | |
| ↑Platelet aggregability* | |
| ↑White blood cell counts* | |
| ↑Red blood cell counts* | |
| ↑Carboxyhemoglobin | See section on occupational exposures |
| ↑Blood pressure* | Smoking is associated with sympathoadrenal activation and catecholamine release |
| Hyperinsulinemia | Perhaps mediated through vasoconstriction/reduced skeletal muscle blood flow |
| Genetics | Possible genetic role in smoking addiction |
| Stress | Increases cigarette consumption in smokers |

*Smoking cessation ameliorates the association.

### Changing smoking patterns

In the United States the demographic pattern of cigarette use has changed dramatically over the past 20 years. Since 1974, the prevalence of smoking by men has decreased by about 1% per year to 28.1% in 1991 and by women by 0.33% per year to 23.5%. Smoking initiation decreased among young men by 1% per year but remained the same in young women. Still, in the early 1980s, approximately 1 million new young people per year became regular smokers, and as of 1990, 46 million people in the United States continue to smoke. The most dramatic change may be that smoking is more prevalent now among less-educated people and is decreasing 5 times more slowly among them than more-educated people. Until 1987, less-educated young women were the only group with increasing smoking initiation, although this also changed in 1987. The rate of smoking declined more for African-Americans (0.75% per year to 35.6% in 1985) than for whites (0.57% per year to 29.4%). Overall, from 1974 to 1991, approximately 2.5% of U.S. smokers permanently quit smoking each year.

Given the intensity of the physiologic and psychologic addiction frequently associated with cigarette smoking, the primary social goal is to prevent people from starting to smoke. An analysis of cigarette use from 1960 to 1973 suggests strongly the role of cigarette advertising on cigarette consumption. The downturns in cigarette consumption during the mid-1960s and 1970s corresponded directly to the Surgeon General's report on smoking and to massive antismoking campaigns by the American Heart Association. Increases in smoking have been temporally related to extensive advertising by the tobacco industry. By 1988, total cigarette advertising and promotional expenses reached $3.27 billion, a 3-fold increase over 1975, adjusting for inflation. Many smoking-cessation programs have confirmed a relationship between the extensiveness and intensiveness of antismoking mass media advertising and short- and long-term smoking cessation. In all, mass media advertising is an effective tool for smoking promotion and cessation, and the relative strength of prosmoking and antismoking advertising affects smoking consumption accordingly.

Advertising has been increasingly targeted to specific groups, especially women (the "slim" brands), African-Americans, Latinos, and blue-collar workers. Unfortunately, one clear audience is adolescents and children; 90% of 6 year olds are as able to identify The Disney Channel's logo of Mickey Mouse as Camel cigarettes' logo of Old Joe the Camel. By targeting adolescents, this approach reaches out to the segment of society that is most influenced by peer pressure, that takes the most risks (and who has distorted feelings of invulnerability), and that is therefore most susceptible to developing lifelong addictions. In addition, much of the advertising is associated with unwarranted prohealth messages (e.g., cigarette promotion of sports events, which also gives cigarette manufacturers access to television, or logos such as "alive with pleasure"). Cigarette companies have also advertised the low-tar, low-nicotine cigarettes aggressively, and many smokers erroneously believe that these cigarettes are less hazardous. With the decreased cigarette consumption in the United States, there has been a dramatic shift in promoting overseas cigarette sales, which have increased 75% over the past 2 decades.

Cigarette smoking is an important and modifiable ASCVD risk factor. There is substantial evidence that smoking can decrease on a national scale through effective mass media education. However, large-scale tobacco company advertising can effectively counteract this positive effect, especially if antismoking education is comparatively poorly funded. The only way to effectively decrease smoking on a society-wide basis may be to eliminate the double messages to the public.

## DIABETES/INSULIN

The overall prevalence of diabetes mellitus in the United States is roughly 7%. There are dramatic ethnic group differences within the United States, with a higher incidence in Native American and Latino populations. Epidemiologic studies have generally found that diabetes is independently associated with an increase in the incidence and severity of ASCVD. Analysis of the Framingham Study data suggests that diabetic persons have higher lipid values, more hypertension, and more obesity than controls but that there still is an independent contribution of diabetes to the development of ASCVD. Subgroup analysis of the Framingham data has further shown that diabetes is an especially important risk factor for women, including premenopausal women, who would otherwise have a substantially reduced risk of ASCVD. In 3390 people followed 12 years in Busselton, Australia, a blood glucose level greater than 200 mg/dl after a 50-g glucose load was significantly associated with ASCVD in men (risk ratio, 2.2) and women (risk ratio, 2.6). The Multiple Risk Factor Intervention Trial followed over 350,000 men for 12 years and found that diabetes was a strong and independent ASCVD risk factor. The addition of another risk factor or of multiple risk factors led to a more dramatic increase in ASCVD deaths (Fig. 7-8). The Nurses' Health Study of over 100,000 middle-aged women followed prospectively for 8 years also found that diabetes was a strong and independent ASCVD risk factor and that the absolute increase in risk was even more dramatic in the presence of other risk factors. Even "high normal" blood glucose levels may be deleterious. The Honolulu Heart Program study of 6394 nondiabetic Japanese men aged 45 to 70 and followed for 12 years found that those with blood glucose levels even in the "normal" 157 to 189 mg/dl range 1 hour after a 50-g glucose load had twice the risk of fatal ASCVD events and that in general there was a continuous risk gradient between the glucose level and the ASCVD risk. The Whitehall Study of 18,403 male civil servants also found a doubling of ASCVD mortality after 7½ years in men whose postchallenge blood glucose levels exceeded 96 mg/dl, controlling for cholesterol, systolic blood pressure, and body mass index; the relationship was not linear.

Insulin seems to play a very important and probably direct role in atherogenesis. Hyperinsulinemia may be more atherogenic than hyperglycemia. A prospective 9½ year study of 982 Helsinki policemen aged 35 to 64 found that plasma insulin levels were independently associated with the development of ASCVD, more than cholesterol levels, smoking, blood pressure, or glucose levels. The Busselton, Australia, study found that men in the upper range of insulin levels after a 50-g glucose load had 2.3 times the 12-year ASCVD mortality rate. No association was found in women. The 5- and 11-year follow-ups of a prospective study of 7246 male nondiabetic Parisian civil servants aged 43 to 54 found that high fasting insulin levels was an independent ASCVD risk factor, controlling for cholesterol levels, blood pressure, smoking, obesity, and blood glucose levels; the role of insulin seemed to attenuate some at the 15-year follow-up. None of these studies assessed cholesterol subfractions, and HDL cholesterol is inversely related to fasting insulin levels.

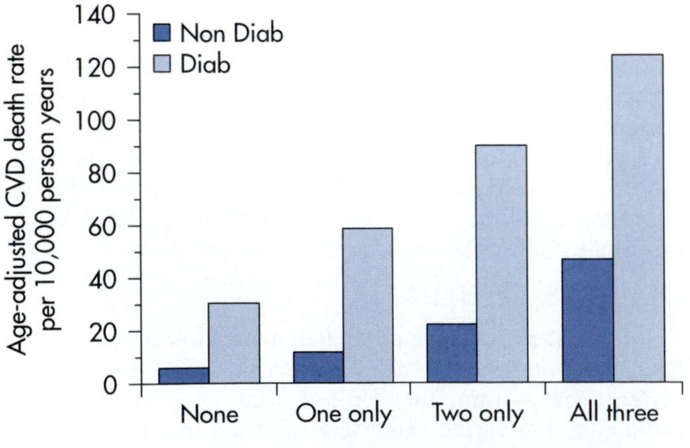


**Fig. 7-8.** Age-adjusted ASCVD death rates by presence of number of risk factors for men screened for Multiple Risk Factor Intervention Trial, with and without diabetes at baseline. *CVD,* Cardiovascular disease. (From Stamler J, Vaccaro O, Neaton JD et al: *Diabetes Care* 16:434, 1993.)

Both hyperglycemia and hyperinsulinemia are integrally interrelated with other cardiovascular risk factors (Table 7-5). The most evident interrelation is between hyperglycemia and hyperinsulinemia. For example, people destined to develop non-insulin-dependent diabetes (NIDDM) have hyperinsulinemia 10 to 20 years before hyperglycemia. In fact, the best predictor of NIDDM in adulthood is the presence of hyperinsulinemia in childhood. There is a circular relationship between insulin resistance and hyperinsulinemia in which hyperinsulinemia leads to down-regulation of insulin receptors, which leads to decreased muscle glucose utilization and to increased production of insulin to compensate. NIDDM can develop over time if the pancreas is unable to compensate adequately with increased insulin production. Obesity itself is associated with insulin resistance, although to a lesser degree than in obese or nonobese people with NIDDM. In NIDDM the major site of insulin resistance is in the muscle cells, and insulin resistance leads to decreased muscle glucose use, which leads to enhanced glucose uptake by adipocytes and further propagates obesity. In addition, hyperinsulinism from insulin resistance stimulates the ventromedial thalamic satiety center and stimulates the appetite, again leading to more obesity and more insulin resistance.

There has been intensive research into how hyperglycemia or hyperinsulinemia can lead to ASCVD independent of their effects on other cardiovascular risk factors. Hyperglycemia is associated with glycosylation of LDL molecules. These altered structures do not bind normally to LDL receptors and through decreased clearance lead to higher plasma LDL levels. This glycosylated LDL, similar to the oxidized LDL mentioned in the section on Cholesterol, may be taken up even more rapidly by macrophages than native LDL. In addition, prolonged exposure of LDL to high glucose concentrations leads to the generation of advanced glycosylation end-products, which are taken up by macrophages. Through both of these mechanisms, the macrophage uptake of LDL may lead to enhanced formation of foam cells. Diabetic persons with nephropathy are at increased risk of ASCVD, with perhaps a 30-fold increase in ASCVD compared with that in diabetic persons without nephropathy. Part of this risk is because of the association of nephropathy with higher blood pressure and higher total cholesterol, lower HDL cholesterol, and increased Lp(a) levels. Complement complexes are also found in atherosclerotic plaques, and diabetes is associated with increased activation of the complement system, increasingly so with increasing renal involvement. Insulin by itself has several effects that promote ASCVD. For example, chickens fed an atherogenic diet and subsequently changed to a low-fat diet had reversal of their

**Table 7-5.** Influences on diabetes/hyperinsulinism

| Risk factor | Associations | Comments |
|---|---|---|
| ↑Insulin levels or insulin resistance | Diabetes* | See text |
| | Obesity* | See text; also associated with increased appetite |
| | ↓HDL cholesterol levels* | |
| | ↑Blood pressure | Correlates with degree of insulin resistance; insulin resistance found in prehypertensive persons |
| | PAI-1† | Insulin is main regulator |
| | Anabolic steroids | |
| | Smoking | |
| | Genetics | |
| | Race | Higher in some Native Americans |
| Diabetes | ↑LDL cholesterol levels* | Especially in women; more atherogenic small, dense LDL variant |
| | ↓HDL cholesterol levels* | |
| | ↑Triglyceride levels* | |
| | ?Stress | Infusions of epinephrine cause glucose intolerance |
| | ↑Platelet aggregability | |
| | ↑Fibrinogen levels | |
| | Genetics | |
| | Race | Higher in Latinos, Native Americans |
| | Age | |

*Reversing the association ameliorates the risk factor.
†*PAI-1*, tissue plasminogen activator inhibitor

lipid deposition. However, the lipid deposition of those simultaneously given insulin did not. Also, insulin given to chickens was able to override the protective effect of estrogens. Other animal studies show that local infusion of insulin leads to local atherosclerotic changes. In vitro experiments show that insulin stimulates smooth muscle growth and proliferation, stimulates macrophage proliferation, stimulates LDL receptor activity, augments cholesterol synthesis within arterial smooth muscle cells (insulin stimulates the activity of 3-hydroxy-3 methylglutaryl coenzyme A [HMG-CoA] reductase, the rate-limiting enzyme in cholesterol synthesis), promotes collagen synthesis, and stimulates the formation of other growth factors, such as insulin-like growth factor-1 and some platelet-derived growth factors, which further stimulate smooth muscle proliferation.

In summary, hyperglycemia and hyperinsulinemia/insulin resistance are major ASCVD risk factors. In addition, there is an extensive network of interrelationships between glucose and insulin with other ASCVD risk factors. In this regard, it is notable that two primary therapies for diabetes—diet and exercise—have important ripple effects through many of these interrelated risk factors. Australian aborigines given a high-calorie diet with refined carbohydrates and low-fiber and decreasing physical activity developed obesity, NIDDM, hypertension, hyperinsulinemia, and high triglyceride levels, which all improved after a reversion to a traditional hunter-gatherer diet and lifestyle. Weight loss of 10 kg in moderately obese individuals leads to a 37% increase in insulin sensitivity, regardless of whether the weight loss was from, for example, 108 to 97 kg or from 86 to 75 kg. This benefit therefore occurs even without attaining ideal body weight. Weight loss also leads to decreased sympathetic activity, decreased hypertension, improved lipid profiles, and improved antithrombotic factors as outlined in the section on Obesity. Eating multiple small meals daily, instead of fewer and larger meals, decreases insulin levels and improves lipid profiles in nondiabetic persons. A diet with increased complex carbohydrates and decreased fat augments insulin sensitivity, leading to improved glucose tolerance. Exercising 1 hour with a bicycle leads to a 30% increase in insulin-mediated glucose uptake, suggesting decreased insulin resistance. Exercise is also associated with a reduced occurrence of NIDDM, especially in people otherwise at high risk of developing this condition. Minimizing the level of endogenous insulin in patients on medications may be beneficial. For example, the majority of diabetic patients treated with insulin or oral hypoglycemic agents have chronically elevated peripheral insulin levels. Some improvements have been found when administration of exogenous injected insulin is decreased or some of the newer oral agents are used. However, the prescription for exercise and weight loss when indicated remains of paramount importance.

## LIFE STRESSES AND ASCVD

Many animal studies have confirmed increased atherogenesis associated with stress. For example cynomolgous monkeys placed in unstable social environments have extensive ASCVD that is independent of other risk factors. There is a dramatic synergistic effect of an atherogenic diet and stress in the development and extent of ASCVD in monkeys.

Many human studies have found a relationship between significant life changes (e.g., death of close relative, job change, moving) and ASCVD. For example, several retrospective analyses that reviewed the 6-month period before myocardial infarction have shown a dramatically increased number of life changes in those sustaining a myocardial infarction compared with age-matched controls and an increased incidence of people who suffered sudden death compared with those who had nonfatal myocardial infarctions. Twins selected for discordance of ASCVD found that the twin with the highest "life dissatisfaction" and least leisure time had more severe ASCVD. There is a general relationship between life changes and ASCVD; however, the data are not conclusive because of failure to control for other risk factors and the retrospective nature of most of the studies. People with known ASCVD who were under the emotional stress of public speaking had ischemic wall-motion abnormalities on echocardiography similar to those who were under vigorous physical exertion; these abnormalities were frequently asymptomatic.

There is a roughly 40% increase in mortality in widowers in the 6-month period after the death of their wives, mostly from ASCVD. Studies are less consistent for widows, with some showing little if any increase after the deaths of their husbands.

Emotional support tends to negate many of the stress-related increases in other ASCVD risk factors. In addition, social support may be important in moderating ASCVD itself; there is increased ASCVD in people with low social support. For example, a 9-year study of 6928 men and women in Alameda County, California, found twice the ASCVD mortality in those with fewer social connections. A study of Italian-American communities in Pennsylvania found that the ASCVD mortality rate was less than half in one community, Roseto, than in other communities in the study. Roseto was noted for its close family and community ties, respect for the elderly, and general adherence to traditional values. All of the communities were similar in terms of other ASCVD risk factors. Over time, as Rosetans abandoned their traditional family and community structures, their ASCVD mortality rates equaled that of their neighbors. Several migration studies (see section on Hypertension) have confirmed increased ASCVD related to the degree of Westernization. Only part of this increased ASCVD risk is attributable to changes in the traditional risk factors, further suggesting a direct role of psychosocial factors related to migration.

Social support affects ASCVD mortality in people with established ASCVD. One prospective population-based study of elderly men and women found that of 194 patients after myocardial infarction, lack of emotional support was associated with a 3-fold increase in the 6-month mortality rate, controlling for the major risk factors except for cholesterol levels. The β-Blocker Heart Attack Trial found that the 3-year mortality rate of 2320 male survivors of myocardial infarctions was 4 times higher in those who were socially isolated and had high levels of stress; there was a roughly equal contribution of each of these psychosocial factors to that mortality rate. Widowers who remarry have much lower mortality rates than those who remain single.

### Socioeconomic status

Socioeconomic status (SES) has been assessed in several ways to elicit a relationship with ASCVD, although the results have been inconsistent. Most studies have found a relationship between markers of low social status (e.g., income levels, educational levels, occupational status) and ASCVD.

Status incongruity, which occurs when a person has simultaneous characteristics of different social classes (e.g., discrepancies in education, occupation, income, housing quality) also seems to be associated with ASCVD. For example, the 5-year prospective Western Electric study of 1472 healthy men found 2.3 times the incidence of ASCVD in the subgroup in which either the man or his wife were from a different social class than their present one.

### Work stress

Occupational stressors are associated with various aspects of the work environment and the development of ASCVD. For example, there are significantly more sudden cardiac deaths on Mondays, "back-to-work" days, even in men with no known history of ASCVD. Shift work is associated with a 40% increase in ASCVD: the longer the exposure, the higher the risk.

Workload and job stress are associated with ASCVD. For example, a prospective study of 5187 healthy construction workers followed for 2 years showed a significant relationship between workload and the incidence of myocardial infarction. This study, as well as another 5-year study of 10,000 men, also found that the development of myocardial infarction (in the first study) and angina pectoris (in the second) was significantly related to co-worker problems. A study of professionals found an increasing prevalence of ASCVD as their self-assessed job stress increased. This gradient was statistically significant within each professional job category. A person's perception of job stress is modified in part by the extent of social support networks on the job and at home.

A two-dimensional model of occupational characteristics was devised to refine the definition of job stress, taking into account the psychologic demands of the job and the degree of job decision latitude or job autonomy. In a prospective study done in Sweden, ASCVD symptoms and these job stress parameters were assessed for all men aged 15 to 75 born on the fifteenth day of each month. Over a 6-year period the development of ASCVD symptoms correlated independently with both job demands and lack of job decision latitude. The correlation with ASCVD symptoms was impressive (Fig. 7-9), suggesting that in demanding work situations the workers' flexibility in how to respond to the demands (autonomy) may be an important factor in the development of ASCVD. Data from the large U.S. Health and Nutrition Examination Survey (HANES) on a sample of 2190 white men found similar results. The Framingham Study assessed 876 employed men and women over a 10-year period using a similar two-dimensional model and found a 3-fold increase in ASCVD in women who reported having high-demand, low-control jobs over those reporting low-demand, high-control jobs. In clerical workers the relative risk was a remarkable 5.2, controlling for other ASCVD risk factors. The increased ASCVD risk among female clerical workers was especially pronounced in those with nonsupportive bosses. A crude analysis of job titles, without assessment of individuals in those jobs, found a 1.5 times increase in

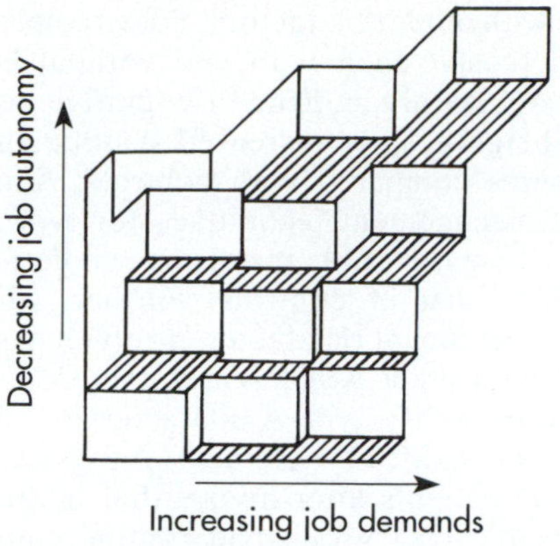


**Fig. 7-9.** Cross-sectional prevalence of ASCVD symptoms among asymptomatic respondents 6 years previously, by job characteristics. The proportions of employed men with the symptoms are displayed as a vertical bar on the grid of job demands and job decision latitude. (From Karasek R, Baker D, Marxer R: *Am J Public Health* 71:694, 1981.)

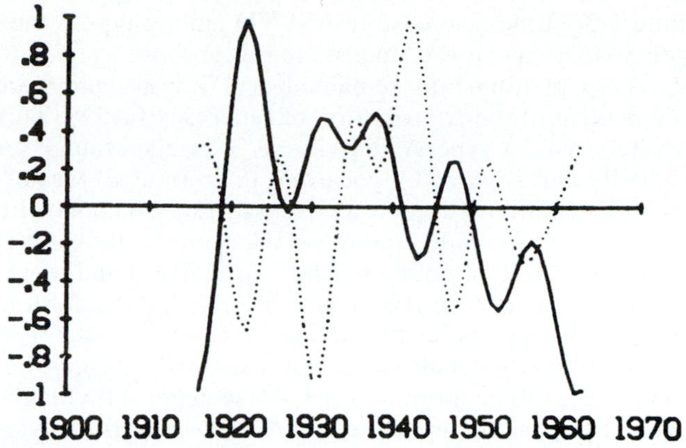


**Fig. 7-10.** Heart disease mortality rate *(solid line)* in New York State, moved forward 2 years to represent a 2-year lag. The dotted line represents the employment index of New York State. Note the inverse correlation between employment levels and heart disease mortality over this 50-year period. (From Brenner MH: *Am J Public Health* 61:606, 1971.)

ASCVD in men and women in the high-demand, low-control jobs.

Job reorganization can significantly affect ASCVD status. A Swedish study evaluated 1937 white-collar workers who experienced a major job reorganization. As anticipated, the job change itself was associated with an increase in ASCVD symptoms. Two years later, however, except for women under the age of 40 (a low-risk group for ASCVD), people who received jobs with greater job decision latitude had significantly fewer ASCVD symptoms. This group had roughly half the ASCVD symptoms and half the incidence of depression as the group with less job control.

The implications of this information are profound. Job-related parameters, such as heavy workloads and evidence of a nonsupportive work environment, seem to be related to ASCVD. In addition, the amount of control a worker has over a job situation substantially modulates the ASCVD risk. Job reorganization to increase worker control seems to decrease ASCVD symptoms.

## Mobility

The relationship between mobility and ASCVD is not clear-cut. A 5-year prospective study of 270,000 Bell system employees found no relation to job transfers. However, a 5-year prospective study of 10,000 Israeli men showed geographic mobility to be associated with an increased incidence of new-onset angina since beginning work. Geographic or occupational mobility may be associated with a higher ASCVD rate. The implication of these conflicting results is that mobility may not be an ASCVD risk factor by itself but perhaps is for only some subgroups, such as those moving for less desirable jobs or with less social support; it may be a cofactor with another risk factor.

## Unemployment

Several studies on unemployment have shown a relationship to ASCVD. One retrospective study compared the employment index (the inverse of which approximates the unemployment index) and heart disease mortality data in New York State from 1915 to 1967. A striking inverse correlation was found between the unemployment levels and heart disease mortality rate, with an approximately 2-year lag period (Fig. 7-10).

## Psychologic factors

On prospective evaluation, ASCVD seems to be related to depression, hysteria, and hypochondriasis. For example, a 14-year prospective study found a significant correlation between hypochondriasis and the development of ASCVD in men. A 5-year prospective study of 10,000 men found that of the major ASCVD risk factors, anxiety and family problems were independently the strongest predictors for the development of angina. Social support from a spouse proved to be particularly beneficial. These psychosocial correlates, however, applied only to angina, and there may have been increased reporting of chest pain unrelated to actual ASCVD among these individuals. There also seems to be an increased ASCVD incidence in people who see their environments as more conflict laden or who are less secure about the results of their actions.

Sleep difficulties have also been related to ASCVD. Difficulty getting to sleep, frequently a manifestation of psychic disturbance, is associated with the later development of angina and myocardial infarction.

***Type A personality.*** Much has been written about the relationship between type A behavior and ASCVD. Type A, or coronary-prone, behavior is a behavior pattern characterized by aggressiveness, heightened competitive drive, impatience, sense of time urgency, and preoccupation with deadlines. Type A people are more likely to work excessive hours, be "work addicts" with great devotion to their jobs and less able to relax away from their jobs, and be perfectionists unsatisfied with their work. There seems to be a familial aggregation of this behavior type.

The prospective Western Collaborative Group Study of 3400 men who initially had no evidence of ASCVD focused specifically on behavior type. After 4½ years, they found a 2.7 times increase in ASCVD among type A men aged 39 to 49 and a 1.4 times increase for those aged 50 to 59. These relationships remained at 8½ years and were independent of the contribution of other risk factors. This elevated risk in type A individuals was also found for clinically unrecognized myocardial infarctions. It was estimated that elimination of the excess risk associated with type A behavior would lead to a 31% decrease in ASCVD incidence. The Framingham Study similarly found an independent role of type A behavior in ASCVD. In addition, type A behavior has been found to be a valid predictor of angiographically documented atherosclerosis. Type A behavior seems to be more of a risk for younger individuals, especially those under 50 years old. Subsequent analysis by the Western Collaborative Group, however, found that recurrent ASCVD events were actually less common in type A men than their type B counterparts. Several other prospective and angiographic studies have also not found a relationship between type A behavior and ASCVD, especially studies of people already at high risk of ASCVD or who already have ASCVD.

It is difficult to determine the exact role of type A behavior and ASCVD, given the conflicting findings previously noted. Some observers feel that there may be some important interaction with other factors that may increase ASCVD, such as young age. Others feel that the problem is in the definition of type A behavior, that the full definition includes many components, and that perhaps only some of the components are associated with ASCVD. In this case, different populations studied might have different predominating components of type A behavior and therefore have different degrees of ASCVD on that basis. Some studies, for example, have found that over 70% of individuals fit the "global" definition of type A behavior.

Hostility and anger are likely to increase ASCVD risk. In a large angiographic study at Duke University, although a significant relation between hostility (and the tendency to hold anger in) and ASCVD was found, the study did not associate type A behavior with the presence of ASCVD. The 20-year observational Western Electric Study found a significant relationship between hostility and the total mortality rate. The Framingham Study noted that the increased incidence of ASCVD among female clerical workers was particularly profound in the subgroup with suppressed hostility. Patients who have had myocardial infarctions and who have separation anxiety and a tendency to direct hostility inward were found to have more cardiac arrhythmias. Two long-term studies on physicians undergoing psychologic testing in medical school found that the 25-year subsequent ASCVD mortality rate was increased 4 to 5 times in those with high hostility scores in one study and no different in the other. Overall, studies suggest that hostility and anger may be related to ASCVD and all-cause mortality, especially with an individual who directs anger inward and in individuals who are self-involved, cynical, and distrustful.

**Behavior-modification studies.** Because type A behavior encompasses many different and independent behavioral aspects, it is difficult to determine the most effective type of intervention. In addition, a problem in assessing behavior modification is that even though type A behavior may be independently associated with ASCVD, it is also interrelated with other risk factors. For example, in a study of 58 normotensive men with and without evidence of ASCVD who were given difficult cognitive tasks, type A subjects had significantly increased systolic and diastolic blood pressures compared with controls. Another study using stress-management techniques for type A subjects showed a 21 mg/dl fall in serum cholesterol levels compared with that of controls. Further, when type A behavior is a significant risk factor, its effect has been most pronounced with other ASCVD risk factors.

Attempts to modify type A characteristics have had a positive effect on ASCVD outcomes. A 3-year prospective study of 1000 patients after myocardial infarction found dramatic results. One group had routine counseling for reduction of ASCVD risk factors and occasional psychiatric counseling for anxiety, depression, and phobias. A second group had additional psychiatric counseling focused on type A behavior. Persons in the second group had significantly fewer recurrent ASCVD events than those in the first group (7.2% vs. 13.0%). In the subjects who exhibited a significant reduction of type A behavior, 36% of the study group, the recurrent cardiovascular event rate was one fourth of those without type A behavior reduction.

Several conclusions can be made from these data. First, some type A personality characteristics are probably independently associated with ASCVD risk. Second, even though there is familial aggregation of type A behavior, behavior modification can successfully reduce type A characteristics in many people. Third, individuals who are capable of changing their type A characteristics seem to decrease their risk of recurrent ASCVD events.

### Physiologic basis

Stress has been repeatedly shown to elevate catecholamine levels, which in different situations can be predominantly norepinephrine or epinephrine; serum cortisol levels have also been elevated. A variety of stressors have been involved, including public speaking, impending unemployment, the performance of a complex task quickly and with little control by the subjects, and significant life changes. In this last instance, men with strong psychologic defenses and therefore less subjective perceptions of the stresses had lesser catecholamine increases. Indeed, people with ASCVD have a markedly increased adrenergic response to mental and physical stressors, suggesting that individuals who are most predisposed to the physiologic stress response are also those at highest risk of ASCVD.

Stress is associated with other physiologic responses that may increase ASCVD risk. Tax accountants have accelerated blood-clotting times associated with work stress. Stress is associated with increased platelet aggregation. There may also be neural consequences of stress. For example, one study showed significant ST-segment changes and ventricular ectopic beats when ASCVD patients drove their cars in city traffic; these changes were independent of a measurable change in catecholamine secretion. In addition, stress leads indirectly to increased ASCVD through its effect on other risk factors. It leads to increases in serum cholesterol levels and blood pressure as well as to increased cigarette use in smokers. Stress also leads to decreased muscle perfusion through catecholamine-induced, α-mediated vasoconstriction, leading to increased insulin resistance. Stress can impair ovarian function in menstruating women. Chronic stress-induced ovarian dysfunction in monkeys eliminates the protective cardiovascular effect found in premenopausal women.

The mechanism by which stress could directly cause ASCVD is undoubtedly multifactorial. First, the central nervous system clearly plays a role. For example, hypothalamic lesions from subarachnoid hemorrhage are frequently associated with arrhythmias and necrotic myocardial lesions, and these cardiac lesions can be prevented with α- and β-blockers, demonstrating that central events can cause cardiac effects. Indeed, stimulation of the ventromedial hypothalamus produces increased catecholamine secretion and ventricular arrhythmias. In addition, dramatic increases in arrhythmias are noted clinically in the 3-day period after a stroke. Second, circulating stress hormones directly and indirectly affect the heart. Stress in animals is associated with direct catecholamine-induced acute myofibrillar degeneration (also called *contraction band necrosis*), ST-segment changes, and arrhythmias. Myocardial sensitivity to catecholamines is enhanced in the presence of increases in adrenocorticotropic hormone and cortisol, other stress-related hormones. An angiographic study found that high cortisol levels are associated with increased ASCVD. Increased cortisol levels are also associated with insulin resistance, glucose intolerance, dyslipidemia, hypertension, and abdominal obesity. These associations are evident in diseased states with sustained hypercortisolism (e.g., Cushing's syndrome) and may play a role in intermittent, stress-related increases in cortisol. Norepinephrine markedly reduces the ventricular fibrillation threshold in dogs and stimulates cellular growth, a component of the atherosclerotic process. In animals, catecholamines can cause endothelial injury, and regenerated endothelial cells have an increased permeability to LDLs; these findings might explain the synergy found between stress and high cholesterol levels in animals. A human angiographic study found that mental stress led to higher cardiac workload (blood pressure–heart rate product), higher catecholamine levels (especially norepinephrine), but differing coronary artery responses. In normal coronary arteries, there was stress-induced vasodilatation; in atherosclerotic coronary arteries, there was paradoxic vasoconstriction. Presumably, in coronary arteries with intact endothelium, the vasoconstrictive response to catecholamines is overcome by the endothelium-derived relaxing factor (probably nitric oxide). In patients with ASCVD, there is endothelial disruption and dysfunction, leading to a deficiency in endothelium-derived relaxing factor, and unopposed catecholamine-induced vasoconstriction. A combination of direct and indirect cytotoxic effects of stress hormones, coronary vasospasm, and neural effects may be important mechanisms of stress-induced ASCVD morbidity and mortality.

### Perspective on stress

The existence of stress-related diseases in society relates to the discordance between the slow evolution of stress-coping mechanisms and the extremely rapid rate of societal change. The basic physiologic response to stress is similar in all animals and reflects the ancient response necessary for the survival of the species (the "defense reaction"). The nature of human stress, however, has changed phenomenally in the past 150 years, since the development of the "machine age" and the dramatic shift of stressors to the mental and emotional arena. Historically, the response to stress was appropriate to support upcoming physical exertion (fight or flight): increased blood flow to the muscles supported by increased blood pressure, increased pulse (central suppression of vagal activity), decreased blood flow to the viscera (kidneys, splanchnic blood flow, skin), increased central blood volume (through peripheral vasoconstriction and increased blood volume by renin release and decreased salt excretion), as well as increased fuel for the muscles (largely through catecholamine-induced increases in lipids). Through the evolution of an advanced neocortex, human beings are able to learn how to cope with mental stressors. One of these coping mechanisms is to internalize feelings. This suppression of feelings is often not reflected in a suppression of the physiologic response. Without having the outlet of physical exertion, there is less muscle vasodilation (leading to higher peripheral resistance and blood pressure), decreased use of fuel (leading to an increased blood lipid levels), and through internalization of problems, a prolonged stressful experience. Exercise probably also helps deal with the negative emotional experience through endorphin release. In addition, frequent stress may lead to structural changes in the cardiovascular system. Low levels of catecholamines can lead to smooth muscle cell growth in animals. Sustained renin release and sympathetic stimulation may be associated with left ventricular hypertrophy. Cortisol is also related to adverse ASCVD risk factors, including increased abdominal obesity, insulin resistance, hypertension, hyperlipidemia, sodium retention, and increased sensitivity of arterioles to catecholamines.

## HEREDITY

A family history of ASCVD is independently associated with the development of ASCVD in offspring. As mentioned in the sections on individual risk factors, there are clear genetic links for many of them. There are also familial links through common lifestyles, which often combine with genetic factors. High cholesterol levels frequently run in families, probably largely through common dietary preferences but sometimes through genetic factors such as the function of LDL receptors. Smoking is also largely a learned behavior but may have a genetic component as an addictive behavior. However, in spite of all of the familial and genetic interactions of the known risk factors, there still seems to be an independent contribution of parental ASCVD to an individual's risk. It should be noted that several studies have called into question the accuracy of family histories. For example, the Framingham Study, which has accurate records of parental medical histories for many of their subjects, found that 17% of the family histories obtained were discordant with the actual medical records. Other studies have suggested even higher levels of inaccuracy, in the 35% to 40% range.

A relationship exists between the development of ASCVD and parental ASCVD before age 50 or 60. The Framingham Study found that a family history increased the risk of ASCVD by 29%; this increased risk was similar to that of the other major risk factors. Division of subjects

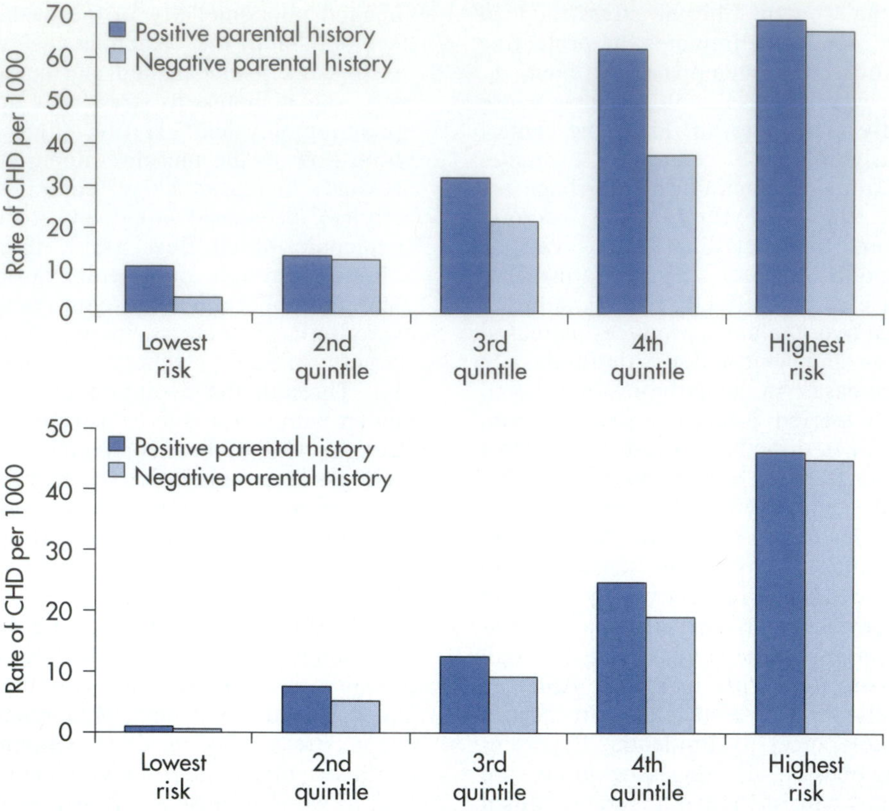


**Fig. 7-11.** Relation between parental history of ASCVD death and personal risk for men *(top)* and women *(bottom)* per quintile of multivariate risk. For men, the increase is significant in the lowest and fourth quintiles. For women, the risk is most evident in the middle three quintiles of risk. *CHD,* Coronary heart disease. (From Myers RH, Kiely DK, Cupples LA et al: *Am Heart J* 120:963, 1990.)

into quintiles of multivariate risk showed a significant additive effect of parental history in most quintiles in men and women (Fig. 7-11).

Further analysis from the Framingham Study found that the relative risk of ASCVD, adjusted for other risk factors, was 1.4 if either parent died of ASCVD before age 65 and 1.3 if either parent died of ASCVD after age 65, a small difference. The adjusted relative risk was higher if a man's mother died than if his father died of ASCVD (1.4 vs. 1.2); for a woman the risk was similar for either parent (1.3). Independent of the age at which the parent had ASCVD, a positive parental history could predict the onset of ASCVD at an age younger than 60 years in offspring (adjusted relative risk of 1.5). However, there was also an increased risk of ASCVD at an older age (adjusted relative risk of 1.2)

## OBESITY

In the United States, the overall prevalence of obesity in adults is 30%, ranging from 5% in 20 year olds to 50% in 70 year olds. Among high school students, 44% of girls and 15% of boys were attempting to lose weight. Some 25% of American women aged 35 to 64 have body mass indexes (BMIs) in the "excessively obese" category. Overweight is more prevalent among African-Americans and Latinos than whites. In this weight-conscious society, the problem of overweight continues to get worse. Between 1960 and 1980, the prevalence of overweight increased 3% and 6% for white women and men and 7% and 28% for African-American women and men. Among people aged 25 to 34, 3.9% of men and 8.4% of women followed 10 years had a weight gain (increase of BMI of more than 5 $kg/m^2$). Also, 13% to 16% of those not overweight at baseline became overweight.

Older epidemiologic studies have found minimal or no independent contribution of obesity to ASCVD, although obesity was associated with adverse effects on other ASCVD risk factors such as cholesterol, hypertension, and diabetes. However, assessment of the regional distribution of obesity does seem to impart an independent risk for ASCVD. In general, obese men typically have a central, or abdominal, fat distribution, and obese women typically have a peripheral, or gluteofemoral, distribution. In most studies, general obesity is measured as BMI, a calculation of weight/height$^2$. Central obesity is measured by the waist-to-hip ratio (WHR), a variety of skinfold ratios, or computerized tomographic indices of intraabdominal fat distribution. In obese subjects the WHR correlates best with the computerized tomographic index of visceral fat, and both of these measures most closely correlate with the metabolic abnormalities later noted. Nonobese people can have an increased WHR; however, in lean subjects the WHR does not correlate with increased visceral fat, and its role as an ASCVD risk factor is unclear.

**Table 7-6.** Influences on obesity

| Risk factor | Associations | Comments |
|---|---|---|
| BMI | ↑Insulin levels | |
| | ↑Triglyceride levels | |
| | ↑Blood pressure | |
| | Genetic factors | |
| | Age | |
| WHR | ↑Insulin levels* | Stronger correlation than with BMI |
| | ↑Triglyceride levels* | Stronger correlation than with BMI |
| | ↑Blood pressure* | Stronger correlation than with BMI |
| | ↑Glucose intolerance* | |
| | ↑Total cholesterol level | |
| | ↑LDL cholesterol level* | |
| | ↑Apolipoprotein B* | |
| | ↓HDL cholesterol level | 32% of variance of $HDL_2$ levels explained by WHR |
| | ↑Fibrinogen | |
| | Male gender | WHR more common in men |
| | Genetic factors | |
| | Age | |
| Obesity | ↑Left ventricular mass* | |
| | ↑Factor VII* | Prothrombotic factor |
| | ↓Fibrinolytic activity* | Prothrombotic factor |

*Weight loss and/or exercise ameliorates the associated risk factor.

The association between central obesity in men and ASCVD events is generally consistent. The 6-year Paris Prospective Study of 6718 men aged 42 to 53 found that men in the highest quintile of central obesity as determined by skinfold measurements had 2.4 times the ASCVD risk as those in the lowest quintile, controlling for the degree of obesity and the standard risk factors. The 12-year Honolulu Heart Program study of 7692 men found that the relative risk of ASCVD for those in the upper tertile as determined by subscapular skinfold measurements compared with those in the lower tertile was 1.5, after controlling for BMI and ASCVD risk factors. Long-term follow-up of the Study of Men Born in 1913 did not find an independent contribution of central obesity.

There are fewer studies in women. The 12-year Göteborg study of 1462 women is the only prospective study to assess the regional pattern of obesity and ASCVD. Multivariate analysis controlling for age, BMI, smoking, cholesterol and triglyceride levels, and blood pressure confirmed an independent role of WHR for myocardial infarction. BMI was not an independent risk factor.

Obesity is associated with several other ASCVD risk factors, and the atherogenic effects of obesity are in part mediated through these other risk factors (Table 7-6). Adverse ASCVD risk factors are found in obese men more than in obese women for the same degree of obesity, but the male pattern of risk factors prevails in women with central obesity. Children and young adults have the same ASCVD risk factor association of obesity as older adults, whether measured via BMI or subscapular skinfold. Studies of twins suggest a strong genetic component in the tendency to obesity and in the regional distribution of fat associated with overeating. Genetic factors contribute 25% to the distribution of fat, and studies of overfeeding suggest that over 50% of the distribution of additional fat is genetically determined.

Exercise is associated preferentially with decreasing abdominal obesity in men and parallel changes in ASCVD risk factors (see Table 7-6). In women with central obesity, exercise seems to be less effective in reducing body fat stores, although the changes ASCVD risk factors are found. There is no significant correlation between these changes and changes in BMI.

The mechanism by which obesity confers increased ASCVD risk remains speculative. Adipocytes in central obesity have higher rates of lipolysis, increased free fatty acids, and consequent insulin resistance. High androgen levels, which are found in women with central obesity, parallel changes in plasma glucose and insulin levels and can augment lipolysis directly. Visceral obesity is associated with other abnormalities, including increased cortisol secretion and blunting of the dexamethasone suppression test, which also lead to more insulin resistance and more abdominal fat accumulation and visceral obesity. Catecholamine levels, which are increased in overeating and stress, can also increase lipase activity, insulin resistance, and associated adverse lipid profiles. Weight loss decreases sympathetic activity.

Weight loss has become a national obsession. At any time 25% to 50% of adult Americans are on diets to lose weight. Diets with moderate or severe caloric restriction can be effective, resulting in weight losses of 20 to 45 pounds in 3 to 4 months. Unfortunately, a third to half of the lost weight is usually regained in 1 year, with slow increases afterward. Appetite-suppressant drugs are widely used and are effective only for a short time; lost weight is regained with cessation of the medication. The most effective approach to weight loss is long-term behavior modification involving decreased caloric intake and an exercise program.

No study has been done to show that changes in central obesity through weight loss results in decreased ASCVD events. The Framingham Study and the Multiple Risk Factor Intervention Trial found increased mortality associated with weight loss, although neither study assessed whether the weight loss was voluntary, since weight loss is often associated with increased cigarette consumption. In addition, ineffective weight loss may be harmful. For example, the 32-year follow-up of the Framingham Study found that total mortality as well as ASCVD mortality in men and women increased with fluctuations in body weight, independent of the actual weight of the person. The Western Electric Study found higher mortality rates in men whose weight cycled. This finding could prove to be significant, because repeated cycles of weight loss and weight gain are particularly common; the average weight loss attempt is for only 5 to 6 months.

## HORMONES AND ORAL CONTRACEPTIVES

Oral contraceptives (OCs) are the most frequent method of prescribed birth control. In general, there is a consistent relationship between the use of OCs and ASCVD, although most of these data derive from the use of OCs with at least 50 mcg of estrogen and the data are from observational, not randomized, controlled studies. There is an approximately 3-fold increase in myocardial infarction in women aged 30 to 39 (from 4 to 11/100,000 women-years, an increase of 7/100,000 women-years) and a 4-fold increase in those aged 40 to 44 (from 22 to 89/100,000 women-years, an increase of 67/100,000 women-years). This increased risk is especially pronounced among smokers. The Nurses' Health Study found an age-adjusted relative risk of 2.5 in current OC users, also with a concentration of the excess risk among smokers. These increases in ASCVD must be viewed in perspective because the actual incidence of ASCVD is low in premenopausal women. Most studies have found that the excess risk of ASCVD conferred by OCs returns rapidly to baseline with cessation of OC use. For example, the Nurses' Health Study found that even with prolonged prior use of OCs, there was no increase in ASCVD events in the group that had used OCs compared with the group who had never used OCs.

OC use is associated with several changes in ASCVD risk factors (Table 7-7). Most OCs combine the estrogen ethinyl estradiol, typically in concentrations of 30 to 35 mcg, with differing amounts of different progestins. The lipid changes from OCs depend on the relative strength of the estrogen/progestin balance, as well as the type of progestin used. The estrogen component raises the HDL cholesterol level and decreases the LDL cholesterol level. Progestins in general do the opposite, although this is much more marked by progestins with androgenic activity, such as levonorgestrel, and change much less with norethindrone. The fact that the ASCVD risk returns to baseline with cessation of OC use suggests that much of the increased risk of OC use relates to changes in the thrombotic factors.

Many studies have found a cardioprotective effect of postmenopausal estrogen use. This is not surprising, since premenopausal women have a much reduced ASCVD incidence compared to age-matched men, which increases significantly with menopause. The Lipid Research Clinics found no deaths from ASCVD after 8.5 years among women under 50. Several different meta-analyses of estrogens and ASCVD have found a 40% to 50% decrease in ASCVD in women on estrogen therapy. However, these studies have been observational and may be subject to bias. The observed decrease in ASCVD also applies for women with established disease. In a retrospective study of 2268 women with angiographically documented ASCVD, the 10-year survival rate of those with mild to moderate stenosis was 95.6% in those who had used estrogens and 85% in those who had never used them. In women with severe stenosis, the 10-year survival rate was 97% in

**Table 7-7.** Influences on hormones

| Risk factor | Associations | Comments |
|---|---|---|
| Oral contraceptives* | Cholesterol levels | Relative estrogen/progesterone strength determines relative change in HDL and LDL cholesterol levels |
| | ↑Triglyceride levels | |
| | ↑Glucose intolerance | |
| | ↑Insulin levels and ↑insulin resistance | |
| | ↑Blood pressure | In less than 5%, usually remits with discontinuing pills |
| | ↑Platelet aggregability | |
| | ↑Fibrinogen levels | |
| | ↑Clotting factors II, VII, IX, X, XII, and XIII | |
| | ↓Antithrombin III | |
| | Fibrinolytic activity, PAI-1 | Mixed effects in different studies |
| | ↑White blood cell count | |
| Hormone replacement* | ↑HDL cholesterol levels, ↑ Apo A | See text |
| | ↓LDL cholesterol levels, ↓ Apo B | See text |
| | ↓Lp(a) levels | |
| | ↓Platelet adhesiveness | |
| | ↓ Fibrinogen | |
| | ↓Blood pressure | Paradoxical increase in 5% |
| | ↓ Insulin levels | |
| | ↓ Antithrombin III | |

*All of these associations are reversed by eliminating hormone therapy.

women who had used estrogens vs. 60% in those who had never used them. A total of 25% to 50% of the cardioprotective effect of estrogens is explained by change in lipids. Conjugated estrogens at the standard dose of 0.625 mg/day leads to a 15% decrease in LDL cholesterol levels and a 16% increase in HDL cholesterol levels. Ovariectomized cynomolgus monkeys who have ASCVD and who have been given the endothelium-dependent dilator acetylcholine have paradoxical vasoconstriction. The monkeys given estrogens had vasodilatation, suggesting that estrogens have a direct vasomotor effect and decrease the incidence of ASCVD. Estrogen therapy also seems to inhibit the oxidation of LDL cholesterol. Many women with intact uteri are given combined estrogen and progesterone therapy to decrease the likelihood of endometrial carcinoma. As expected, the lipid changes are less favorable. For example, with the continuous regimen of 0.625 mg of conjugated estrogens and 2.5 mg of medroxyprogesterone, the LDL cholesterol level decreases 7.6%, and the HDL cholesterol level increases 4.5%. However, cynomolgus monkeys on bihormonal therapy have no decrease in cardioprotection compared with those on estrogens alone. Preliminary results of a Swedish study suggest that a decrease in ASCVD from the combination of estrogens and norgestrel was also roughly 50%, no different from estrogen alone.

Postmenopausal hormone and OC replacement therapy are associated with opposite ASCVD risks. There are important differences between these therapies. First, the estrogens used in women on OCs are high-potency, synthetic estrogens compared with the natural estrogens used in women on postmenopausal hormone replacement therapy; these natural estrogens have roughly one tenth the potency of OC estrogens. Second, in menopause, there is a natural increase in antithrombin III levels. This increase in antithrombin III activity might compensate for the addition of exogenous, low-dose estrogens and the attendant increases in factor VII and some other clotting factors. In addition, fibrinogen levels are higher in women, increase further with OC use, increase also with menopause, but decrease with postmenopausal estrogen administration.

In men, increased testosterone levels are associated with decreased HDL cholesterol levels. Levels of dehydroepiandosterone (DHEA) and its sulfate ester, dehydroepiandrosterone sulfate (DHEA-S), the major secretory products of the adrenal gland, may be inversely related to ASCVD. A 12-year study of 242 men aged 50 to 79 using a single baseline measurement of DHEA-S found that a 100 mcg/dl increase in the DHEA-S level was associated with a 48% decrease in ASCVD mortality, controlling for age, systolic blood pressure, cholesterol, obesity, fasting blood glucose levels, and cigarette smoking; a baseline measurement below 140 mcg/dl was associated with an age-adjusted relative risk of ASCVD death of 3.2. DHEA-S levels tend to decrease with age, in diabetes, with hyperinsulinemia (insulin inhibits DHEA-S formation), and with hypercholesterolemia and tend to increase with weight loss and a low-fat vegetarian diet. Further studies are necessary to confirm low levels of DHEA-S as a significant ASCVD risk factor.

A major part of the different prevalence of ASCVD between men and women is undoubtedly related to hormones. The actual lifetime incidence of ASCVD is higher in women than in men, but women tend to acquire ASCVD approximately 10 years later than men. This gender difference is most prominent in white people. Arterial smooth muscle contains receptors for androgens, estrogens, and progestins, and these hormones have direct effects on the arterial wall.

## OCCUPATIONAL EXPOSURES

Several occupational chemical exposures have been linked to ASCVD, either directly or indirectly through their effects on other ASCVD risk factors.

Carbon disulfide is a solvent used primarily in the production of viscose rayon but is also used as a solvent for rubber, chemicals, oils, and resins. Workers exposed to carbon disulfide have a 2.5-5-fold increase in ASCVD mortality. This increased risk can be eliminated through workplace interventions that decrease exposure. In addition, after 2 years without exposure, workers' ASCVD risk returns to baseline. Carbon disulfide is associated with increased blood pressure and an increased serum LDL/HDL cholesterol ratio; however, increased ASCVD risk persists after controlling for these variables. The exact mechanism is unclear.

Carbon monoxide, often related to exposure to products of combustion, is associated with impaired exercise tolerance, the development of angina and ST-segment changes at lower exercise thresholds in people with preexisting ASCVD, and a decreased ventricular fibrillation threshold. Animals exposed to carbon monoxide in association with hypercholesterolemia have accelerated atherosclerosis, which can be inhibited by the use of inhaled oxygen. There is some evidence that carbon monoxide exposure is associated with increased cholesterol levels, increased permeability of arterial walls to cholesterol, and enhanced platelet aggregation.

Lead exposure is most consistently associated with hypertension and thereby indirectly with ASCVD. There may be an increased incidence of strokes in lead-exposed workers and decreased incidence after workplace improvements in which lead exposure has been lowered. In some of the studies, lead exposure is associated with elevations in serum cholesterol levels. Arsenic or arsine gas exposure may increase ASCVD, with one case-controlled study finding a 2.8-fold increase in workers with the heaviest chronic arsenic exposure.

Other occupational exposures are associated with increased ASCVD mortality through indirect mechanisms. For example, workers chronically exposed to organic nitrates have a 2.5-fold increased risk of cardiovascular mortality, typically after a 36- to 72-hour withdrawal from exposure ("Monday morning angina"). Presumably, these workers develop compensatory vasoconstriction from the nitrate exposure that is unopposed after the exposure ends, putting them at risk for coronary vasospasm. Organic solvents, chlorophenoxy-based pesticides, chronic benzene exposure (especially in people with benzene-induced hepatic damage), mercury and cadmium are associated with hypertension. Workers exposed to high levels of noise or whole-body vibration at work may have increased blood pressure and ASCVD. Residents living in areas with high levels of airport noise have higher levels of hypertension. Excessive heat and cold have also been associated with acute cardiovascular events. Occupational stress and physical inactivity, both associated with ASCVD, are discussed in the sections on Stress and Exercise, respectively.

## THROMBOTIC FACTORS AND FIBRINOGEN

Analysis suggests that ASCVD results from the complex and interrelated effects of atherosclerotic and thrombotic events. The best studied thrombotic factor is fibrinogen. When the fibrinogen level has been assessed prospectively, it has been a consistent and sometimes the strongest predictor of ASCVD events. A 12-year follow-up of 1315 people in the Framingham Study, for example, found that controlling for the standard cardiac risk factors, elevated fibrinogen levels were associated with ASCVD to approximately the same degree as age, systolic blood pressure, hypercholesterolemia, and glucose intolerance. This increased risk held for both genders, although it was more pronounced in men. In women only, the risk conferred by fibrinogen decreased with age, so that by age 70 there was no increased risk. In the Northwick Park Heart Study of 1511 white men aged 40 to 64 at the 5- and 10-year follow-up, the fibrinogen level surpassed the cholesterol level and systolic blood pressure as an independent risk factor for ASCVD morbidity and mortality. After 5 years, a 1 standard-deviation increase in the fibrinogen level increased the risk of an ASCVD event by 84%, whereas a 1 standard-deviation increase in the cholesterol level was associated with a 43% increase in ASCVD events. A recent meta-analysis of many prospective epidemiologic studies confirmed the consistency and strength of the independent relationship between fibrinogen and ASCVD, with an odds ratio of 2.3 comparing those with fibrinogen levels in the upper vs. lower tertiles.

Other hematologic risk factors have also been independently associated with ASCVD. Several studies have found factor VII coagulant activity to have an independent role in atherogenesis. The Northwick Park study found factor VII coagulant activity to be more significant than either cholesterol levels or systolic blood pressure in their 5-year data, with a 1 standard-deviation increase in factor VII activity associated with a 62% increased risk of ASCVD; the effect of factor VII activity diminished over time. Reduced fibrinolytic activity is also associated independently with ASCVD. Specifically, low levels of tissue plasminogen activator inhibitor (PAI-1) has been associated with the occurrence and recurrence of myocardial infarctions. Platelets have been identified as a possible major risk factor. Patients with atherosclerotic disease have increased platelet adhesiveness, decreased platelet survival, and increased platelet turnover when compared with controls. In fact, in survivors of myocardial infarction, the presence of spontaneous platelet aggregation is a useful biologic marker for subsequent cardiac events. The protective role of aspirin in primary and secondary prevention of ASCVD events further supports a role of platelets. Also, the major cardioprotective effect of fish oils may be mediated through their incorporation into platelets, with significant decreases in platelet aggregability. It is perhaps surprising that thrombocytosis itself, either reactive or essential, is not clearly associated with ASCVD, although the key factor may be increased platelet aggregability and not simply increased numbers of platelets. Antithrombin III may have protective effects against ASCVD. Antithrombin III levels are low in premenopausal women but increase with OC use and in menopause.

Although the thrombotic factors are independent ASCVD risk factors as determined through multiple regression analysis, they are interrelated with other risk factors (Table 7-8). Cigarette smoking is the most potent determinant known for fibrinogen; the Framingham Study found that 50% of the ASCVD risk conferred by cigarette smoking is mediated through its effects on fibrinogen. A cross-sectional study of English civil servants found that controlling for traditional ASCVD risk factors, serum fibrinogen levels correlated with social class. In this study, in which ASCVD is 3 times higher in civil servants working in the lowest grade of employment, fibrinogen levels were 15% higher in the lowest-grade employment group. Within both the lowest- and highest-grade employment groups, there was a strong, significant, and continuous trend in fibrinogen levels between men who described high job stress compared with those who described low job stress. There was no relationship between fibrinogen and type A personality.

The strongest association for factor VII activity is with triglyceride levels, with changes in triglyceride levels followed in 3 hours by changes in factor VII activity levels. Impaired fibrinolytic activity in general and increased PAI-1 specifically are associated with several risk factors; insulin is fibrinogen's major known regulator. Medically lowering triglyceride levels with gemfibrozil is associated with reduced factor VII activity and PAI-1 levels. Platelet aggregability is associated with several other risk factors. For example, there are LDL and HDL receptors on platelets; increased serum LDL cholesterol levels and especially oxidized LDL levels stimulate platelet aggregability, whereas HDL levels decrease it. Increased platelet aggregability occurs with stress, presumably mediated through increased sympathetic activity. Several food additives, including mo-er (a tree fungus used in Chinese cooking), onion, garlic, and ginger, decrease platelet aggregability. Caffeine also lowers platelet aggregability. The "French paradox" of very low ASCVD incidence, yet high saturated fat and cholesterol intake and high serum cholesterol/HDL ratios may be largely mediated by alcohol-associated decreased platelet aggregability and perhaps by the ability of alcohol to increase endogenous tissue plasminogen activator levels.

Physiologic evidence supports a direct role of hematologic factors in several aspects of the atherosclerotic process. High concentrations of fibrinogen are incorporated into developing atherosclerotic lesions. Within the atheroma, fibrinogen binds to LDLs, which sequester additional fibrinogen into the plaque. Fibrinogen also stimulates smooth muscle proliferation and migration, another component of the atheroma. In addition, fibrinogen has direct effects on blood flow. It is the principal determinant of blood viscosity that has been found in some studies to be associated with ASCVD; it also induces red blood cell aggregation and decreased red cell distortability. Fibrinogen might then reduce blood flow in advanced atherosclerotic lesions, in which blood flow is already marginal. In addition, fibrinogen and the other prothrombotic factors (factor VII, PAI-1, platelets, antithrombin III) play a pivotal role in thrombosis. The increased role of factor VII activity noted early in the follow-up period in the North-

**Table 7-8.** Influences on thrombotic factors

| Risk factor | Associations | Comments |
|---|---|---|
| ↑Fibrinogen | Smoking*† | Greater risk factor in men |
| | Diabetes and ↑insulin levels | Correlates with microvascular complications |
| | ↑Blood pressure | |
| | ↑LDL cholesterol levels | |
| | ↑Triglyceride levels | |
| | ↑Lp(a) | |
| | Race | African-Americans |
| | Female gender | |
| | Age | |
| | OC use† | |
| | Menopause | Decreases with estrogen therapy |
| | Central obesity | |
| | Sedentary lifestyle | |
| | Stress | |
| | ↓Socioeconimic status | See text |
| | ↑Carbohydrate diet | |
| | ↑Leukocyte count | |
| | Genetic factors | |
| ↓Fibrinogen | Alcohol consumption | Also, decreases platelet aggregability and increases tissue plasminogen activator levels |
| | Exercise | |
| | ↑HDL cholesterol levels | |
| ↑Factor VII activity | ↑Triglycerides in diet*† | |
| | Menopause | Decreases with estrogen therapy |
| | OC and estrogen use† | |
| | Obesity† | |
| | ↑Alcohol | |
| | White race | |
| ↑PAI-1 and ↓ fibrinolytic activity | ↑Insulin levels* | |
| | Obesity† | |
| | ↑Triglycerides in diet† | |
| | Smoking | |
| | ↑Lp(a) | |
| ↑Platelet aggregability | Stress and ↑sympathetic tone | |
| | ↑Fibrinogen | |
| | ↑LDL cholesterol levels | See text |
| | ↑Saturated-fat diets | |
| | ↑Insulin levels | |
| | Diabetes | |
| | ↑Blood pressure | |
| | Smoking | |
| ↓Antithrombin III | Premenopausal women | |

*Major known regulator.
†Reversing risk factor ameliorates the level of thrombotic factor.

wick Park study supports the thrombotic role of factor VII activity in advanced atherosclerotic lesions and is supported by the observation that the development of acute coronary syndromes, including myocardial infarction, is through thrombus formation and resultant arterial occlusion. Fibrinogen also directly affects platelet aggregation by binding on platelet membrane receptors. It should be noted that early atherosclerosis has an inflammatory component; therefore some of the elevated serum fibrinogen found with ASCVD may reflect its action as an acute-phase reactant. Platelet thrombi are integrated into the atherosclerotic plaque and are associated with acute coronary syndromes. Platelet-derived growth factor released from platelets is a potent stimulus for arterial smooth muscle proliferation and migration. These data suggest that hematologic factors play an important role in ASCVD. The best documented is fibrinogen, although there is a complex interplay between the different procoagulant and anticoagulant factors and the resulting thrombotic tendency relates to the relative strengths of these factors. There are also remarkable interconnections between these hematologic factors and other ASCVD risk factors.

## EXERCISE

There is the general perception in the United States that exercise is "good for the heart." However, of 87,433 adults surveyed in 1990, nearly 60% had sedentary lifestyles. The percentages were essentially the same for men and women and increased from 55% in the 18 to 34 year old group to 62% for those older than 55. In general, there is abundant epidemiologic data that supports a positive relationship between exercise and cardioprotection, although there are serious methodologic flaws in this data.

Several studies quantitate the relationship between the amount of exercise and subsequent ASCVD events. A recent meta-analysis that reviewed 27 studies of over 700,000 people confirmed the general relationship between exercise and the primary prevention of ASCVD. This relationship displays an inverse dose-response curve. In addition, the better the quality of the study, the more impressive the relationship. Overall, moderate exertion was associated with a roughly 50% decrease in ASCVD outcomes (including death, myocardial infarction, angina, congestive heart failure, and sudden death). There are two very important methodologic flaws in all of these studies. First, very few of the studies controlled for other ASCVD risk factors except age. Indeed, there may be a tendency for those with sedentary jobs to have diets richer in animal fats. Also, much of the benefit of the exercise might be mediated by its effect on other cardiac risk factors. For example, exercise is associated with lowering blood pressure, increasing HDL cholesterol levels, and decreasing insulin resistance. There may even be important different ways that people do vigorous leisure time exercise, with some people approaching the exercise in a much more intensive, hard-driving, type A manner than others and conceivably having a different degree of cardioprotection. Second, none of the studies were randomized. Therefore even though people were followed prospectively in many studies, there was a probable selection bias because people with high risks of heart disease and decreased exercise tolerance may gravitate to more sedentary jobs and lifestyles. Smokers, for example, may select less vigorous occupations and exercise.

The best of these epidemiologic studies assess both leisure time and work-related exertion. In 5000 men and women in the Framingham Study, for example, total physical activity was inversely associated with subsequent fatal myocardial infarction. This relationship was independent of the other ASCVD risk factors, although less clinically significant. Large prospective studies done in Israel and in East Finland, controlling for other ASCVD risk factors, found that the cardioprotective effect of physical activity at work was more profound than leisure time exertion.

The other type of epidemiologic study that confirms a beneficial effect of exercise assesses the relationship between physical fitness and ASCVD, with people who were the most physically fit having the least ASCVD. For example, a Norwegian study of 2000 men found that those who performed best on a bicycle ergometer test had less than half the cardiovascular mortality of those who performed worst. Again, these studies are flawed by preselection bias as well as the fact that approximately 40% of physical fitness is genetic, as shown in studies of twins.

The benefit of exercise for patients who already have ASCVD is clearer. Meta-analysis of prospective randomized studies suggests that there is a 20% decrease in overall and ASCVD mortality in patients randomized to a structured exercise program. These results are evident after 1 year and persist throughout a 3-year follow-up. Most of these studies modified several different risk factors, so it was difficult in the meta-analysis to isolate a specific benefit of exercise.

There is concern that exercise might acutely increase the incidence of ASCVD deaths. One community-based study of 133 men without known heart disease who suffered primary cardiac arrest found that although exercise did in fact transiently increase the incidence of sudden death at the time of exercise, the overall risk of sudden death in habitually exercising men was only 40% that of sedentary men. The meta-analysis cited above, however, found that even sudden death was also reduced in people with known ASCVD. Although acute myocardial infarctions may occur more commonly in people while performing strenuous physical exertion, these acute effects of exercise are profoundly higher in sedentary people than in those who exercise regularly.

There is good physiologic support for an overall cardioprotective effect of exercise. Monkeys on atherogenic diets and moderate exercise programs, when compared with those on atherogenic diets alone, had wider coronary arteries and substantially less atherosclerosis. Human studies have demonstrated that exercise positively affects many of the ASCVD risk factors (Table 7-9).

**Table 7-9.** Beneficial effects of exercise

| Associated changes | Comments |
|---|---|
| ↓Cholesterol | Especially if the patient also loses weight |
| ↓LDL cholesterol levels | Especially if the patient also loses weight |
| ↑HDL cholesterol levels | Especially if the patient also loses weight |
| ↓Carbon monoxide levels | Decreases serum half-life (see section Occupational Exposures) |
| ↓Platelet aggregability | Strenuous exercise can increase platelet aggregability but only in sedentary people |
| ↓Stress response | Lower catecholamine response to physical and mental tasks |
| ↓Blood pressure | |
| ↓Diabetes | Improves diabetic control |
| ↓Insulin resistance | |
| ↓Central obesity | |
| ↓Fibrinogen levels | |
| ↑Fibrinolysis | |
| ↓Ventricular fibrillation | Lowers ventricular fibrillation threshold in animals |
| ↓Coronary spasm | Decreases drug-induced spasm in animals |

## TRIGLYCERIDES

Early studies suggested that serum triglyceride concentrations were related to the development of ASCVD. However, subsequent analysis controlling for other risk factors have suggested a minimal independent role in atherogenesis.

The most significant interrelation between triglyceride levels and ASCVD risk factors is the impressive inverse relation with HDL cholesterol levels. In fact, simply controlling for HDL cholesterol in the large majority of epidemiologic studies eliminates an independent role for triglycerides. Triglyceride levels appear to be an independent ASCVD risk factor in women. Both the Framingham and Lipid Research Clinics studies found that especially in women with low HDL cholesterol levels, there was an independent relationship between triglyceride levels and ASCVD. As noted in the section on Cholesterol, some people, especially diabetics, have apparent hypertriglyceridemia and normal cholesterol levels; yet they have accelerated ASCVD. Many of these people have high apo B levels, which may be an independent finding or may be associated with the highly atherogenic small, dense LDL cholesterol particles. High triglyceride levels are typically found in diabetic persons, as well as in people with hyperinsulinemia and insulin resistance. Also, factor VII activity is strongly associated with triglyceride levels; significant decreases occur in factor VII activity accompanying medical reduction in triglyceride levels, such as with gemfibrozil.

## LEFT VENTRICULAR HYPERTROPHY

The Framingham Study found echocardiographically determined left ventricular hypertrophy (LVH) in 16% of men and 19% of women; the prevalence increases dramatically with age, so that LVH is present by age 70 in 33% of men and 49% of women.

The independent risk factors associated with LVH include age, blood pressure, obesity, valvular heart disease, and history of a myocardial infarction. Fig. 7-12 displays the relationship among systolic blood pressure, BMI, and the prevalence of LVH. Weight reduction results in a concomitant decrease in LVH, independent of changes in blood pressure. Antihypertensive therapy can also decrease LVH, especially with the use of β-blockers, calcium channel blockers, and angiotensin-converting enzyme inhibitors.

There also seems to be an independent role for stress in LVH. Both animal and human studies demonstrate that sympathetic stimulation can cause LVH, independent of hypertension. A study of 215 employed men found a significant relationship between job strain and increased left ventricular mass (LVM). Another study of 100 men and women, using 24-hour ambulatory blood pressure monitoring, found that echocardiographic LVM correlated best with hypertension associated with recurring work stress and only weakly with hypertension at home.

LVH is an independent risk factor for ASCVD. Older studies have found that electrocardiographic determination of LVH is independently associated with ASCVD. Newer studies using echocardiography have confirmed and extended this finding. The Framingham Study found that echocardiographically determined increased LVM was associated with an increased 4-year mortality rate in their predominantly white population, independent of age, blood pressure, cigarette smoking, diabetes, obesity, and the ratio of total to HDL cholesterol. For each increment in LVM/height of 50 g/m there was an associated increase in ASCVD incidence (relative risk of 1.5 in men and women), ASCVD mortality (relative risk of 1.7 in men and 2.1 in women), and total mortality (relative risk of 1.5 in men and 2 in women); this relationship also applied to people over 60 years old (relative risk of 1.6 in men and women). Indeed, some studies have found echocardiographically determined LVH to be a stronger risk factor for ASCVD than blood pressure, smoking, or total cholesterol level. In inner-city African-Americans, all-cause mortality was increased in people with echocardiographically determined LVH, both in those with angiographically documented ASCVD (relative risk of 2.1) and in those angiographically free of ASCVD (relative risk of 4.1).

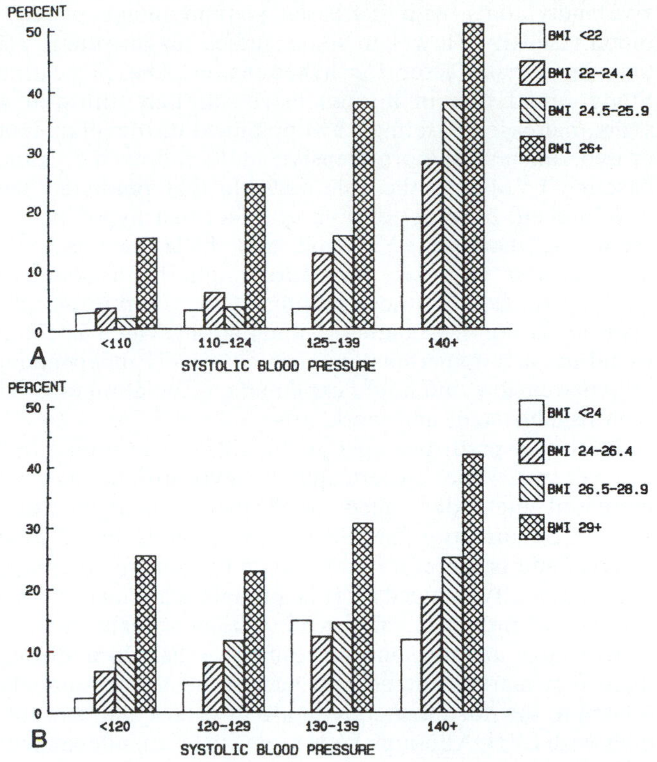


**Fig. 7-12.** Age-adjusted prevalence of LVH (rate/100) according to approximate quartiles of systolic blood pressure and BMI in women *(top)* and men *(bottom)*. BMI is measured in kilograms per meters squared. (From Levy D, Anderson KM, Savage DD et al: *Ann Intern Med* 108:7, 1988.)

The pattern of LVH seems to be important. Echocardiographic LVH was found in one study in 27% of 280 hypertensive patients. After 10 years of follow-up, the incidence of ASCVD events correlated with the pattern of LVH; a total of 11% of patients with ASCVD events had normal echocardiograms, 23% had eccentric ventricular hypertrophy, and 31% had concentric hypertrophy.

The relationship between hypertension and LVH is intriguing. Hypertension is certainly an important risk factor for LVH. Some 20% to 40% of hypertensive individuals have LVH on echocardiography, which is much more sensitive than the 3% to 8% found by electrocardiography. LVH is more prevalent in hypertensive individuals with increased sodium intake or high blood viscosity. However, some studies suggest that LVH may be a risk factor for hypertension. The Muscatine Study found that in normotensive children followed 4 years, increased baseline LVM predicted the development of hypertension. In normotensive adults followed 5 years, baseline LVM was the sole variable that predicted the development of hypertension. The fact that hypertension seems to increase LVH and that LVH can precede hypertension suggests that there might be a common etiology for both of these findings. One possible mechanism is through sympathetic stimulation, which is often found in early hypertension, can cause LVH independent of hypertension, and might explain the association of LVH with psychosocial and work stressors.

LVH may predispose people to ASCVD through a few mechanisms. The hypertrophied myocardium has an increased metabolic need, with increased myocardial oxygen consumption and decreased coronary blood flow reserve, and is therefore more prone to ischemic damage. Experimentally induced LVH in animals is associated with myocardial infarctions that tend to be more extensive, to evolve more rapidly, and to be more lethal. In addition, there is a marked increase in sudden death, presumably related to the documented increase in ventricular arrhythmias with LVH. Although LVH seems to be an independent ASCVD risk factor and LVH can be reversed through therapy for hypertension and obesity, no data show that LVH regression is associated with decreased ASCVD incidence.

## OTHER RISK FACTORS

A literature review identified 246 risk factors for ASCVD. One of the obvious problems in identifying risk factors is the complex interrelation among them. It is impossible to perform long-term prospective studies on this many variables. In this section, several other possible ASCVD risk factors are reviewed.

### Coffee

Eleven prospective studies, including over 100,000 people, have assessed the relationship between coffee consumption and ASCVD. Although some studies have found positive correlations between the amount of coffee consumed and ASCVD, a huge meta-analysis failed to confirm any association, even without adjusting for other risk factors.

There seems to be a relationship between coffee consumption and cholesterol levels, especially if the coffee is brewed by boiling instead of filtering. In one study, filtered coffee had no significant effect on cholesterol, but boiled coffee increased total cholesterol levels by almost 19 mg/dl and LDL cholesterol levels by 15 mg/dl. Another study, however, found that consuming 24 ounces of filtered coffee increased both the LDL and HDL cholesterol levels by 6 mg/dl and 3 mg/dl, respectively, which would translate to minimal anticipated change in ASCVD risk.

### Anemia and iron

Anemia and a low-iron state may be protective from ASCVD. In animals, deferoxamine, an iron chelator, significantly limits injury and improves recovery in myocardium exposed to an ischemic insult. A study of 1931 men in Eastern Finland found that acute myocardial infarctions were 2.2-fold as frequent in men with serum ferritin levels greater than 220 mcg/L, controlling for age, smoking, blood pressure, white blood cell count, glucose level, and several lipid levels. This association was even higher in men who also had high LDL cholesterol levels.

However, a recent analysis of the National Health and Nutrition Examination Survey after 15 years of follow-up found a somewhat decreased risk of cardiovascular death in men and women with higher transferrin saturation. Overall, there is not enough evidence to implicate iron or hemoglobin in as major ASCVD risk factors.

### White blood cells

A few studies have found a relationship between the total white blood cell count and ASCVD. The National Health and Nutritional Examination Survey followed people aged 45 to 74; in people with white blood cell counts of over 8100 cells/$mm^3$ compared with those with counts below 6600 cells/$mm^3$, there was a relative risk of ASCVD in white men and women of 1.31, independent of age, smoking, blood pressure, cholesterol levels, diabetes, hemoglobin levels, BMI, and education. For unclear reasons, in this study but not in the Framingham Offspring Study, the relationship with high white blood cell counts did not hold for men who never smoked. There was a nonsignificant increase in ASCVD in African-American men and women with counts over 7100 cells/$mm^3$. The Paris Prospective Study found a marked increase in ASCVD events in men aged 29 to 52 that was associated with high monocyte counts. Although no relationship existed between total white blood cell count and ASCVD, a comparison of men with monocyte counts greater than 500 cells/$mm^3$ with those with counts below 500 cells/$mm^3$ showed a relative risk of ASCVD of 4.6, controlling for age, smoking, BMI, cholesterol levels, and blood pressure. Although the white blood cell count may be a marker of the inflammation found early in ASCVD, white blood cells may also have a role in producing free radicals that might have a role in oxidizing lipids, injuring endothelial cells through release of proteolytic enzymes, and activating platelets. Monocytes, which migrate into the arteries and become macrophages, are the principal cells that transform into foam cells early in the ASCVD process.

### Phenacetin

A 20-year prospective Swiss study of 623 healthy working women aged 30 to 49 who used phenacetin chronically found an increased incidence of ASCVD, with a relative risk of 1.8. In the group of women who used high doses of phenacetin, there was a higher incidence of hypertension, but only half of the excess risk of ASCVD was attributable to hypertension. Since this study did not control for other ASCVD risk factors, further study is warranted.

### Homocysteinuria

Homocysteinuria is an autosomal recessive condition usually caused by a deficiency of the enzyme cystathionine β-synthase, which leads to the inability to break down homocysteine from dietary methionine into cystathionine.

Persons with homozygous homocysteinuria are at a markedly increased risk of ASCVD and venous thrombosis. People with higher-than-normal serum levels of homocysteine, most of whom are heterozygous for homocysteinuria, also seem to be at increased risk of early ASCVD. It is possible that homocysteinuria is a significant risk factor for ASCVD, since heterozygous homocysteinuria has an estimated prevalence of 1% to 2% of the population. Homocysteine is associated with ASCVD probably because it is directly toxic to vascular endothelium and can augment the oxidation of LDL cholesterol (see section on Cholesterol). In addition, platelets may have a role, since ASCVD can be prevented in baboons with homocysteinemia by platelet inhibitors.

### *Chlamydia pneumoniae*

A few studies have suggested that infection with *Chlamydia pneumoniae* (formerly called *TWAR,*) a common cause of respiratory infections, is associated with ASCVD. In comparing men with ASCVD with controls, the 5-year Helsinki Heart Study found the odds ratio for developing ASCVD to be more than 2 if there was serologic evidence of *Chlamydia pneumoniae,* controlling for age, hypertension, smoking, and cholesterol levels. There are several proposed mechanisms. Chlamydial lipopolysaccharide can bind to HDL and LDL. Modified LDL, as oxidized LDL, can be taken up by macrophages and form foam cells (see section on Cholesterol). Lipopolysaccharide also has direct effects on vascular permeability and can affect the clotting mechanism. The development of immune complexes can also be directly cytotoxic.

### Endothelin

The plasma concentration of endothelin, an endothelium-derived contracting protein, correlates with the extent of ASCVD. Endothelin levels tend to be increased in hypertension or congestive heart failure and in men. In ASCVD the increased endothelin levels may be secondary to endothelial disruption and may therefore be a marker of the extent of ASCVD. However, evidence suggests that endothelin may have a role in potentiating the atherosclerotic process. Unlike normal arteries, atherosclerotic arteries have endothelin in their smooth muscle cells. Endothelin stimulates synthesis of smooth muscle cells, and in the presence of endothelial dysfunction caused by ASCVD, endothelin causes enhanced vasoconstriction.

### Miscellaneous risk factors

Case-controlled studies have found that male pattern baldness is associated with ASCVD in men under 55 years old. There seems to be a dose-response curve, with the greatest degree of vertex baldness associated with the greatest increment of ASCVD (relative risk of 3), independent of smoking, hypertension, cholesterol levels, or family history of ASCVD. The mechanism is unclear, although there may be some role of dihydrotestosterone, the principal androgen associated with male pattern baldness.

Corneal arcus has been associated with an increase in ASCVD in several studies. Although arcus increases in frequency with hyperlipidemia and with age, the Lipid Research Clinics found that it was associated with ASCVD, with a relative risk of 3.7 in men under 50 years old, controlling for cholesterol levels and smoking. The Western Collaborative Group Study also found an association of arcus with ASCVD in men under 50. No increased risk was found in older men or in women.

A vertical or diagonal earlobe crease has been associated with a relative risk of ASCVD of 1.5 to 2 in a few prospective studies; increased risk exists in people with and without known preexisting ASCVD. The presence of ear-canal hair may also be associated with ASCVD, perhaps mediated through androgens.

## CIRCADIAN RHYTHM

It is generally accepted that there is an association between circadian rhythm and ASCVD; in fact, ASCVD increases early in the morning. One study of 2999 patients with acute myocardial infarction found a roughly 2-fold increase in the frequency of the onset of symptoms between the peak time interval (6 AM until noon) compared with the trough (4 PM until midnight). This effect was not observed in people who were on β-blockers. Other studies have confirmed that the frequency of symptomatic and asymptomatic myocardial ischemia is maximal in the morning.

Several physiologic phenomena are affected by circadian rhythms. In the early morning, there are increases in systemic blood pressure, platelet aggregability, plasma norepinephrine and epinephrine levels, plasma renin activity, cortisol secretion, and levels of atrial natriuretic factor and decreases in blood fibrinolytic activity. Basal forearm vascular resistance is 50% higher in the morning, an effect that can be negated through α-blockade. This constellation of prothrombotic effects and increased vascular tone might explain the morning increase in acute myocardial infarctions in people with established ASCVD.

## DECLINE IN ASCVD MORTALITY

There has been a steady, dramatic decline in the age-adjusted ASCVD mortality rate in the United States; this decline began in the mid-1960's and has continued to the present. In fact, life expectancy in the United States increased more significantly during this period than during the time when antibiotics were developed. Ironically, one of the major reasons that studies such as the Multiple Risk Factor Intervention Trial (see section on Combination of Risk Factors) took so long to find improvements in ASCVD was that the control group had such an unexpected decrease in ASCVD, with only two thirds of the anticipated ASCVD events, resulting in a loss of statistical power. In spite of the improvements, however, ASCVD is still the most common cause of death in men and women.

By 1968 ASCVD mortality was clearly decreasing. From 1968 to 1976, there was a 21% decrease. From 1979 to 1988, there was an additional 17% decrease. A decline was found in all ages (greater in the younger group), all major ethnic and racial groups (greater in nonwhites), in both sexes (although more in women), and in all areas of the country (greater in the West).

Analyses have assessed the reasons for the decrease, focusing on the relative effects of medical interventions vs. lifestyle changes. Based on conservative assumptions from generalizing the medical literature, it seems that improved therapy in the cardiac care unit might account for up to 13.5% of the decline; prehospital basic and advanced life-support systems, 4%; coronary artery bypass surgery, less than 4%; and improved medical therapy, 10%; these figures add up to a roughly 30% decrease through medical interventions directed specifically at ASCVD. Other medical interventions such as the use of aspirin and newer techniques that have allowed earlier detection of ASCVD have probably contributed additional decreases in ASCVD mortality.

ASCVD risk factor reductions have probably contributed much of the other 70%. The effect of hypertension therapy is difficult to assess, given the wide range of efficacies found in the literature. An average estimate of the benefit of hypertension therapy would explain 8.5% of the decline in ASCVD.

The major effect on ASCVD mortality has been through dietary changes. Cholesterol consumption in the United States was at its peak in 1959, and cholesterol and saturated fat consumption have decreased considerably since then. The Framingham Study found a general decrease in total cholesterol levels of 10.3 mg/dl from 1966 to 1975. Nationally, the percentage of people with high cholesterol levels decreased from about 27% in 1960 to 1962 to 23% in 1971 to 1974. The National Health and Nutrition Examination Survey found a decrease of 6.5 to 7 mg/dl among men and women from 1960 to 1962 to 1971 to 1974. Cholesterol consumption continues to fall. Consumption of beef has fallen consistently from 1976 peak of 88.8 pounds per person to 62.8 pounds per person in 1992. Chicken, turkey, and fish consumption have increased. Vegetable and fruit consumption rose 10% from 1980 to 1990. Overall, over 30% of the decline in ASCVD can be attributed to dietary changes.

Reduction in smoking has also been dramatic (see section on Smoking). Since smoking cessation leads to rapid reversal in ASCVD risk, it is likely that the decrease in smoking initiation and increase in cessation led to another 24% decrease in ASCVD mortality. In general, there has been some worsening of the prevalence of obesity in the population. Exercise has increased overall since the 1960s; however, its effect is difficult to measure. Other changes in risk factors, such as stress, have little generalizable data.

In summary, there seems to be a great decrease in the ASCVD mortality rate. This decrease is largely accounted for by changes in the social environment, including diet, decreased smoking, hypertension detection and control, and reduction in risk factor profiles.

## COMBINATION OF RISK FACTORS

It is common for individuals to have several ASCVD risk factors. The effect of these combinations is a geometric increase in ASCVD risk. Risk factor reduction in such people requires multiple lifestyle changes.

Several studies have assessed the risk of ASCVD in patients possessing more than one risk factor. Fig. 7-7 shows the synergistic effect of diabetes with other risk factors. The National Cooperative Pooling Project of the American Heart Association found that a combination of serum cholesterol levels greater than 250 mg/dl, diastolic blood pressure greater than 90 mm Hg, and smoking cigarettes led to an 8-fold increase in ASCVD. The Framingham Study similarly showed a greatly increased ASCVD mortality rate with multiple risk factors (Fig. 7-13). The combination of risk factors led to an ASCVD

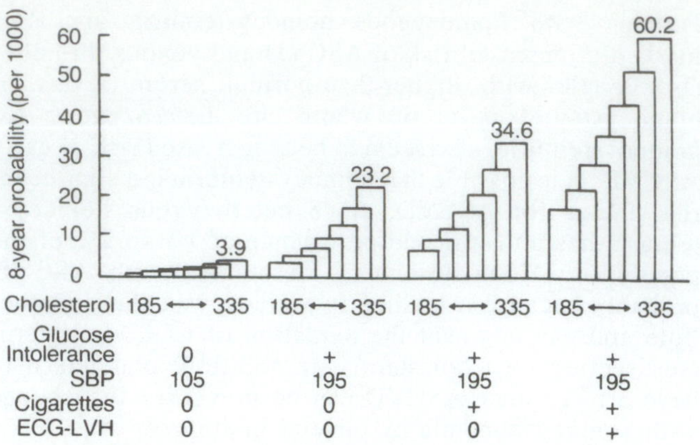


**Fig. 7-13.** Risk of ASCVD according to serum cholesterol at specified levels of other risk factors in men 35 years old. From the Framingham Study, after 18-year follow-up. *ECG-LVH,* Electrocardiographic evidence of LVH; *SBP,* systolic blood pressure. (From Kannel WB: *Am J Cardiol* 52:9B, 1983.)

incidence in men 30-fold and in women 70-fold higher than in patients without those risk factors. Another study of angina in 10,000 Israeli men found prospectively that anxiety and family problems were independently the most significant of the standard risk factors and, taken together, conferred about 3 times the independent risk of these two factors separately.

As mentioned previously, interrelations exist among individual risk factors. The Prospective Cardiovascular Münster study followed 4043 men and 1333 women aged 50 to 65 and found that more than 50% of all diabetic persons were hypertensive, that diabetic persons had hypercholesterolemia 2 to 3 times more than nondiabetic persons, and that hypertensive patients had 1.5 times the incidence of high cholesterol and high triglyceride levels. The San Antonio Heart Study of 2930 subjects also found that with the exception of obesity, it was extremely unusual to find other risk factors (diabetes, hypertension, high triglyceride levels, high cholesterol levels) as single conditions.

### Multiple risk-factor reduction programs

A few studies have addressed the benefits of reducing several ASCVD risk factors simultaneously. Most of these studies approached risk-factor reduction through the use of educational techniques. The risk factors addressed in most of these studies included hypertension, hyperlipidemia, and smoking and did not include stress reduction, for example.

The Oslo Study Group focused on hypercholesterolemia (serum cholesterol levels of 290 to 380 mg/dl) and cigarette smoking in normotensive men. Through education and support, the study group achieved a mean serum cholesterol reduction of 13% and a 45% decrease in cigarette consumption. There was a 55% decrease in ASCVD mortality in the intervention group; total mortality was lowered by 33%, which did not reach statistical significance, related in part to an increase in cancer mortality in the intervention group.

The randomized Multiple Risk Factor Intervention Trial studied 12,866 high-risk men for 7 years; these men received counseling for hypercholesterolemia, smoking, and hypertension and antihypertensive therapy as needed. Reductions in total cholesterol levels (5 mg/dl, mostly in LDL), smoking (50%, vs. 30% in controls), and diastolic blood pressure (3 mm Hg) were achieved, but after the 7-year intervention, no significant reduction in ASCVD or total mortality was realized. Important benefits were found for treating high cholesterol levels and smoking, but there was an unexpected 15% trend toward decreased survival in men with mild hypertension. However, at 10.5 years, 3.5 years after the study was stopped, there were improvements in the incidence of ASCVD (10.6%) and the total mortality rate (7.7%) and a statistically significant 24% decrease in the incidence of acute myocardial infarctions. The principle factor that caused the continuing improvement in ASCVD was treatment of hypertension. For men with diastolic blood pressures of at least 100 mm Hg who were not on antihypertensive therapy at baseline, the total mortality rate decreased 50%, and ASCVD mortality decreased by 35%. For men with diastolic blood pressures in the 90 to 99 mm Hg range, the ASCVD mortality reversed directions, with an improvement of 13%. These findings were true regardless of the presence of electrocardiographic abnormalities at rest. The reasons for these changes are not entirely clear. One explanation is simply that the positive effects of therapy for hypertension require a longer intervention than that for cholesterol or smoking because the changes induced by even mild hypertension take longer to reverse. Another explanation is that late in the study, because of the decreased survival trend found for hypertensive men randomized specifically to receive hydrochlorothiazide, all men on diuretics were changed to the diuretic chlorthalidone. For unknown reasons, perhaps chlorthalidone decreases ASCVD more than hydrochlorothiazide.

In an area of East Finland where ASCVD mortality is exceptionally high, one of two neighboring cities had an intensive 5-year education program involving media, public campaigns, and increased community services and support to modify cigarette smoking, cholesterol and animal fat intake, and hypertension; the other city, with similar ASCVD rates, served as the control. Smoking decreased in both communities, with a trend toward a further decrease in the experimental community. In the experimental city serum cholesterol levels were significantly decreased in men (11.1 mg/dl), and there was a trend to lower levels in women. Systolic blood pressure decreased significantly for men and women. Definite myocardial infarctions and strokes were statistically reduced for men and women in the experimental community. Overall ASCVD rates showed a statistically significant 17% reduction only in men over the 5-year period in the experimental community. The reductions found were more marked for young subjects. There was a greater decrease in recurrent infarctions compared with first infarctions, suggesting a beneficial role in secondary as well as primary prevention.

A 2-year study was done in California to assess the feasibility of risk-factor reduction. Two roughly similar small towns were chosen. One served as a control, and one had mass media education about smoking, diet, and exercise that focused on education and behavior-modification techniques. For the intervention group there was a significant decrease in saturated fat intake (25% vs. 5%), cigarette smoking (15% vs. 3%), systolic blood pressure (5% vs. 1%), and plasma cholesterol levels (2% vs. 1%). These changes found after the first year of the program and continued or improved over the second year.

In conclusion, there is a marked increase in ASCVD in patients possessing more than one risk factor. However, effective programs can be developed to simultaneously lower several risk factors. It is significant that these risk factors can be successfully reduced on a large scale through mass education techniques.

## IMPLICATIONS AND APPROACHES TO CARE

There is an intricate web of interactions among the different identified ASCVD risk factors, which is sometimes referred to as the *metabolic cardiovascular syndrome, atherothrombogenic syndrome,* or *insulin-resistance syndrome.* Fig. 7-14 displays many of the interactions documented in the medical literature. A brief review of this figure suggests that the traditional view of individual risk factors is simplistic at best.

One implication of this web of interactions is that it is difficult to assess a risk factor in isolation or assess its true significance. No studies have the database or statistical power to control for each of these ASCVD risk factors and to decide which are truly independent. This makes it difficult for clinicians to know which potential risk factors should be evaluated and followed. Given the complexity of risk factor interactions (see Fig. 7-14), clinicians must be careful in assuming that the identification of a risk factor implies that the amelioration of that risk factor is beneficial in reducing ASCVD. One example is hyperten-

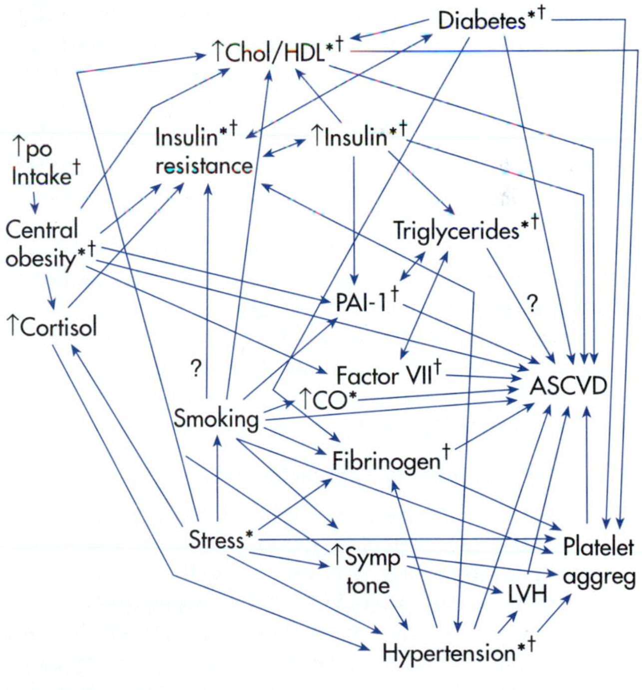


**Fig. 7-14.** Most of the identified major ASCVD risk factors, with their predominant interrelations. *, Exercise helps; †, diet helps ?, scant data; *po intake,* increased eating; *chol/HDL,* total cholesterol/HDL cholesterol ratio; *PAI-1,* tissue plasminogen activator inhibitor; *CO,* carbon monoxide; *symp tone,* sympathetic tone; *LVH,* left ventricular hypertrophy; *platelet aggreg,* platelet aggregability.

sion, in which there is definite epidemiologic evidence that even low levels of mild hypertension are associated with increased ASCVD, yet therapy is of equivocal significance in reducing the ASCVD. According to Fig. 7-14, hypertension is integrally related directly to at least seven other risk factors and indirectly to the rest. It would not be surprising if the ASCVD risk associated with hypertension were conferred in large part by one or more of these other factors, with hypertension being a marker for the more causal factors.

Another implication is that even without knowing which risk factors are the most pivotal, improving the correctable single risk factors may still be critical. For example, one of the important risk factors is smoking. The fact that the relationship between smoking and ASCVD is complex and mediated largely through other risk factors (e.g., fibrinogen levels) does not negate the primary importance of smoking cessation to its documented effect in ASCVD reduction.

Lastly, there may be instances where focusing on a single risk factor may have dramatic ripple effects on other risk factors. Stress is a good example of this. Different individuals respond differently to similar stressors, and some individuals seem to have an "exaggerated" physiologic stress response. This stress response is associated independently with hypertension, LVH, glucose intolerance, abnormal lipid level, insulin resistance, increased fibrinogen levels, increased platelet aggregability, possible increases in compulsive eating and central obesity (and even an increase in consumption of fast foods and their attendant risks), and increased cigarette consumption by smokers. The existence of significant amounts of ASCVD correlates with modernization. The age-old stress response, similar in all animals, evolved as the fight-or-flight response. However, this stress response may be harmful in the context of the present-day high-stress society, in which the predominant stressors are emotional and mental and a major coping mechanism is through internalization. However, many of the risk factors in Fig. 7-14 are improved by exercise (which is the standard response of an animal to the stress of a predator, for example).

The social environment significantly influences ASCVD risk factors. A review of essentially all risk factors reveals the predominance of social links. Most ASCVD risk factors are directly affected by diet, exercise, stress, smoking, the work environment, and the individual's social network. This observation emphasizes the role of intervention into the social sphere.

## Family and community approaches to care

Much of the reduction of cardiovascular risk factors requires individual behavior modification. To achieve effective risk reduction it is important for the individual and the primary care provider to keep a broad perspective. It is too easy to focus on blaming the patient: it is the patient's "fault" because of smoking cigarettes or eating unhealthy fast foods. The issues are more complex. Advertising of cigarettes and fast foods is a proven effective way to create popular consumption of these items and is promoted by our society. Some of these unhealthy items, such as cigarettes, are addictive once begun and are typically begun during adolescence when people feel immortal. To make matters worse, cigarette advertisers specifically target this group. Others factors, such as fast foods, are reinforced by a society of two working parents or single parents and a fast-paced, over-committed lifestyle, with the outlet of low-cost, convenient, and good-tasting (albeit unhealthy) foods. As most clinicians know, changing an individual's behavior is a challenging and difficult task. Given this context, the family and community take on even larger roles in behavior modification.

There is abundant evidence cited throughout this chapter that social support networks are important. Many studies in the literature have found that people with social supports have decreased physiologic responses to stress, have increased survival after a myocardial infarction, and in general, live longer. Therefore an important part of caring for the individual is to assess the support network and, where it is lacking, make referrals to available resources.

It is necessary for the family to support the individual at risk. The whole family must eat healthily for an individual to do so, because few families make different meals for different family members. Family members need to support people trying to quit smoking cigarettes, neither ignoring the problem nor subtly encouraging it (co-dependence) but also not blaming the victim. The ability of a person to exercise would likely be enhanced if family members understood its importance, allowed the time for the individual to exercise, encouraged the person, and exercised with the person. In these regards, it is particularly useful for the primary care provider to meet with the family members and the patient to discuss these issues openly. In addition, the disease of an individual or even threat of a disease because of elevated risk factors has a ripple effect throughout the family, disturbing the usual social relations that existed. For example, the long-standing pillar of the family may now be seen as vulnerable or may require a role reversal, with others needing to take care of him or her. It is important to assess the coping skills of the family to help the family unit function positively, both for itself and for the individual.

The major community issue is to figure out ways to act on local and national levels to address the broader issues. Even in highly motivated and informed experimental subjects the achieved reduction in risk factors is small. For example, the Multiple Risk Factor Intervention Trial achieved only a 3 mm Hg reduction in diastolic blood pressure and a 5 mg/dl decrease in cholesterol levels. There has to be a global approach to care to achieve greater changes in risk factors and decreases in ASCVD.

Through collective action, several communities have eliminated advertising billboards that promote unhealthy behavior (e.g., alcohol, cigarettes). Communities can create collective healthy actions (e.g., sports activities in which participants have running competitions, smoking-cessation support groups, classes focusing on cooking healthy food). Through such community action, larger changes in behavior can be achieved.

Nationally, many issues affect the health of people. Economic factors are associated with an increased incidence of many diseases. Unemployment, as well as employment in occupations with high levels of job strain, are associated with ASCVD. In fact, the very existence of major shifts in employment associated with economic cycles is unhealthy. Job reorganizations that increase workers' control over their work lives seem to be health promoting. Another evident change necessary to improve the health of the nation is to have accessible health care, especially preventive care, for all people. In this way adverse risk factors can be determined early and corrective action attempted before the onset of disease. The political agenda has to be changed to support health. It is certainly counterproductive for health professionals to condemn cigarette smoking when tobacco growers, with economic support from the government, create a prosmoking ideologic environment.

Health care providers have a unique and important role, in conjunction with citizen groups, in leading the fight to eliminate unhealthy lifestyles (e.g., smoking) and promoting healthy ones (e.g., exercise breaks in workplaces). Clinicians are in a key position to understand the links between society and disease and are therefore well situated to help spearhead the necessary social and political changes to positively affect people's health nationally.

To be effective, disease prevention must be approached at all three levels: the individual and family, the local community, and the national level. With such an orientation, dramatic decreases in morbidity and mortality and improvements in the quantity and quality of life of people can be achieved.

## BIBLIOGRAPHY


Arnesen H, editor: The metabolic cardiovascular syndrome, *J Cardiovasc Pharm* 20(suppl 8):S1-S53, 1992.

Austin MA: Plasma triglyceride as a risk factor for coronary heart disease: the epidemiologic evidence and beyond, *Am J Epidemiol* 129:249-259, 1989.

Benowitz NL: Cardiotoxicity in the workplace, *Occupational Med* 7(3):465-478, 1992.

Björntorp P, Smith U, Lonnroth P, editors: Health implications of regional obesity, *Acta Med Scand Suppl* 723:1-236, 1988.

Bush TL, Fried LP, Barrett-Connor E: Cholesterol, lipoproteins, and coronary heart disease in women, *Clin Chem* 34(8B):B60-70, 1988.

Criqui MH: Cholesterol, primary and secondary prevention, and all-cause mortality, *Ann Intern Med* 115:973-976, 1991.

Denke MA, Grundy SM: Hypercholesterolemia in elderly persons: resolving the treatment dilemma, *Ann Intern Med* 112:780-792, 1990.

Diana JN, editor: Tobacco smoking and atherosclerosis: pathogenesis and cellular mechanisms, *Adv Exper Med Biol* 273:1-380, 1990.

Ernst E, Resch KL: Fibrinogen as a cardiovascular risk factor: a meta-analysis and review of the literature, *Ann Intern Med* 118:956-963, 1993.

Grady D, Rubin SM, Petitti DB et al: Hormone therapy to prevent disease and prolong life in postmenopausal women, *Ann Intern Med* 117:1016-1037, 1992.

Higgins M, Thom T: Trends in CHD in the United States, *Int J Epidemiol* 18(suppl 1):S58-S66, 1989.

Levy D, Garrison RJ, Savage DD et al: Prognostic implications of echocardiographically determined left ventricular mass in the Framingham Heart Study, *N Engl J Med* 322:1561-1566, 1990.

Multiple Risk Factor Intervention Group: Mortality after 10 years for hypertensive participants in the Multiple Risk Factor Intervention Trial, *Circulation* 82:1616-1628, 1990.

Prichard BNC, editor: Insulin sensitivity: cardioprotection vs metabolic disorders, *J Cardiovasc Pharm* 20(suppl 11):S1-S84, 1992.

Shepherd JT, Weiss SM, editors: Conference on behavioral medicine and cardiovascular disease, *Circulation monograph,* No 6, 76(suppl 1):1-227, 1987.

Stolar MW: Atherosclerosis in diabetes: the role of hyperinsulinemia, *Metabolism* 37(suppl 1):1-9, 1988.


CHAPTER

# 8 Hypertension


**Harry L. Greene II**
**Richard M. Hoffman**
**Joseph A. Ingelfinger**


Nearly 60 million Americans have high blood pressure or are being treated with antihypertensive medications. The annual cost for hypertension, including medications, office visits, and laboratory visits, is estimated to be more than $10 billion. Although these direct costs alone are substantial, hypertension also contributes to nearly 800,000 premature deaths each year, and is a leading risk factor for congestive heart failure, renal failure, stroke, coronary artery disease, and retinopathy.

Recognition of the public health burden from high blood pressure led to the creation of the National High Blood Pressure Education Program in 1972. Ongoing educational efforts, including publication of consensus guidelines, have led to considerable progress in detecting, treating, and controlling hypertension. In 1972, only half of hypertensives were aware of their condition and only one in six cases were adequately controlled. By 1991, more than 80% of hypertensives were aware of their high blood pressure and more than half of all cases were adequately controlled. Following a discussion of the

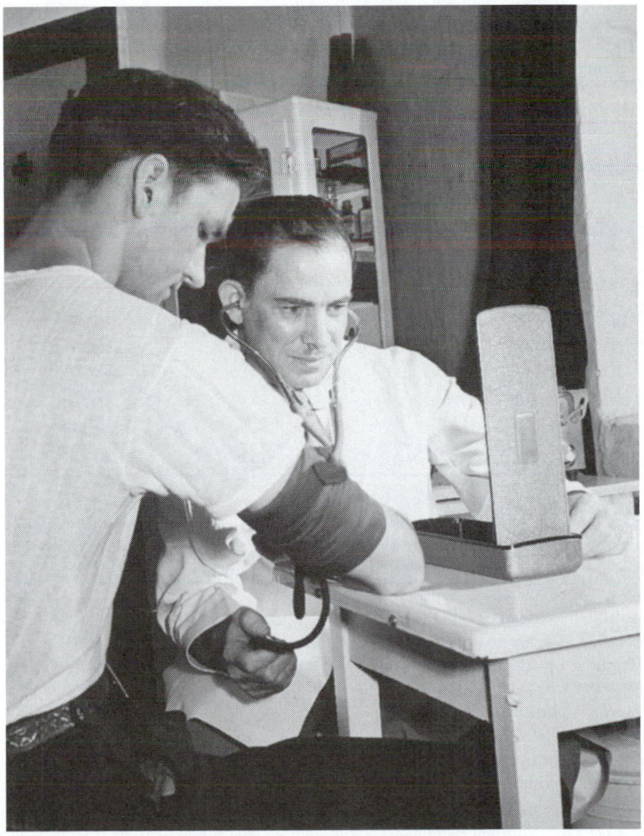

**Fig. 8-1.** Blood pressure determination. (From the collection of the Library of Congress).

epidemiology and pathophysiology of hypertension, this chapter focuses on the evaluation and management of high blood pressure.

## DEFINITION

The upper limit of normal adult blood pressure has been defined as 140/90 mm Hg. All levels of higher blood pressure are associated with an increased risk of cardiovascular disease. The Joint National Committee (JNC-V) on Detection, Evaluation, and Treatment of High Blood Pressure further classifies hypertension by stages based on systolic and diastolic blood pressures (Table 8-1).

## EPIDEMIOLOGY

The prevalence of hypertension increases progressively with age, as shown in Fig. 8-2. Hypertension is found more frequently in African-Americans than in whites, and is more prevalent among less educated and lower socioeconomic classes. Most hypertension develops in the second and third decades, although it can occur at any age. In young adulthood and early middle-age, hypertension is more prevalent in men than in women, but this reverses after age 60. Isolated systolic hypertension is seen most often in the elderly.

The risk for cardiovascular morbidity and mortality increases with higher levels of systolic and diastolic pressures, although Framingham data has shown that systolic hypertension is a better risk predictor. The risk of cardiovascular disease for any level of high blood pressure is considerably increased for persons with target-organ damage, including cardiovascular disease, nephropathy, and retinopathy (see box at right). Hypertension interacts greatly with other independent cardiovascular risk factors. Framingham data showed that the eight-year cardiovascular risk from hypertension for 40-year-old men increases tenfold in the presence of high cholesterol, cigarette smoking, and diabetes.

Between 1972 and 1990, age-adjusted mortality from coronary heart disease decreased approximately 50%, and mortality from stroke decreased by 57%. These declines have been observed for men and women, and for African-Americans and whites. Part of the decline is attributable to decreases in cigarette smoking and fat

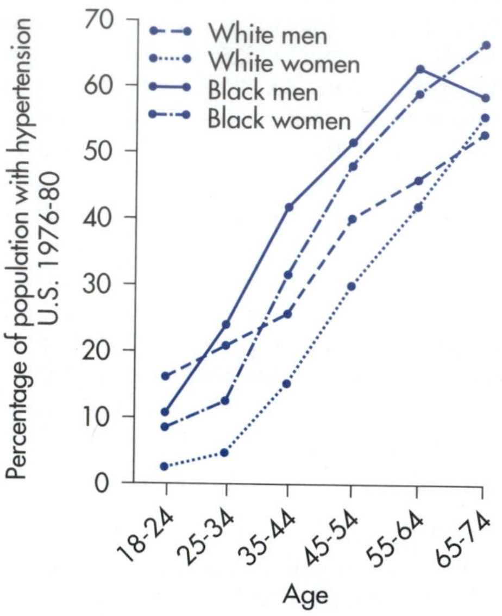


**Fig. 8-2.** The prevalence of hypertension among white and African-American men and women in the United States defined as systolic of 140 mm Hg and/or diastolic of 90 mm Hg or higher. (From Rowland M, Roberts J: Health and Nutrition Examination Survey II. Advance data, vital and health statistics of the National Center for Health Statistics. No. 84, October 8, 1982.)

**Table 8-1.** Classification of blood pressure for adults age 18 years and older*

| Category | Systolic (mm Hg) | Diastolic (mm Hg) |
|---|---|---|
| Normal† | <130 | <85 |
| High normal | 130-139 | 85-89 |
| Hypertension‡ | | |
| Stage 1 (mild) | 140-159 | 90-99 |
| Stage 2 (moderate) | 160-179 | 100-109 |
| Stage 3 (severe) | 180-209 | 110-119 |
| Stage 4 (very severe) | ≥210 | ≥120 |

From *Arch Intern Med:* 153:154, 1993.

*Not taking antihypertensive drugs and not acutely ill. When systolic and diastolic pressures fall into different categories, the higher category should be selected to classify the individual's blood pressure status. For instance, 160/92 mm Hg should be classified as stage 2, and 180/120 mm Hg should be classified as stage 4. Isolated systolic hypertension (ISH) is defined as SBP ≥ 140 mm Hg and DBP <90 mm Hg and staged appropriately (e.g., 170/85 mm Hg is defined as stage 2 ISH).

†Optimal blood pressure with respect to cardiovascular risk is SBP <120 mm Hg and DBP <80 mm Hg. However, unusually low readings should be evaluated for clinical significance.

‡Based on the average of two or more readings taken at each of two or more visits following an initial screening.

NOTE: In addition to classifying stages of hypertension based on average blood pressure levels, the physician should specify the presence or absence of target-organ disease and additional risk factors. For example, a patient with diabetes and a blood pressure of 142/94 mm Hg plus left ventricular hypertrophy should be classified as stage 1 hypertension with target-organ disease (left ventricular hypertrophy) and with another major risk factor (diabetes). This specificity is important for risk classification and management.

### Target-organ damage

**Cardiovascular**

Atherosclerosis
Myocardial infarction
Left-ventricular hypertrophy
Congestive heart failure
Transient ischemic attacks
Cerebrovascular accidents (hemorrhagic/thromboembolic)
Aortic dissection
Abdominal aortic aneurysms

**Kidney**

Renal insufficiency
Proteinuria
Microalbuminuria

**Retina**

Hemorrhage
Exudate
Infarction
Papilledema

intake, but improved control of high blood pressure has also been an important factor. There is convincing evidence from randomized, placebo-controlled intervention trials that antihypertensive therapy reduces the risk of cardiovascular disease. A consistent finding has been a dramatic decrease in the risk of stroke with a more modest effect on coronary artery disease. Collins' metaanalyses of 14 placebo-controlled trials estimated a 42% reduction in the incidence of strokes and a 14% decrease in the incidence of myocardial infarction.

## PHYSIOLOGY

The search for the etiology of hypertension is an exciting area of physiology. Although the exact mechanism remains elusive, many steps in the regulation of blood pressure have been discovered and a number of pathogenic mechanisms have been suggested.

Blood pressure (BP) is related to cardiac output (CO) and peripheral vascular resistance (PVR). Cardiac output, in turn, is related to stroke volume and heart rate. These formulas are shown below.

BP = CO × PVR

CO = Stroke Volume × Heart Rate

Stroke volume is largely related to the venous return of blood to the heart and to cardiac contractility. The factors that interact to control blood pressure are shown in Fig. 8-3. As shown in Fig. 8-4, there are a number of other organs that interact through feedback loops to maintain an adequate blood pressure. Any change in blood pressure is sensed by baroreceptors located throughout the circulatory system. The receptors send efferent signals to the central nervous system (CNS), which sends efferent output to the adrenal glands that is relayed through the autonomic nervous system to the heart and blood vessels. These feedback mechanisms can increase or decrease heart rate. Catecholamine secretion may increase or decrease, leading to either vasoconstriction or vasodilatation.

Additionally, the renin-angiotensin-aldosterone system allows the kidney to play a major role in blood pressure control. Renin is a proteolytic enzyme produced by smooth muscle cells in the juxtaglomerular apparatus of the afferent arteriole in the kidney. These smooth muscle cells are innervated by renal nerves and release renin in response to decreased renal perfusion pressures, low sodium concentration, and β-adrenergic stimulation.

In the liver, an α-globulin, called renin substrate, is synthesized and released into the circulation. Renin acts on this substrate to produce a decapeptide called angiotensin

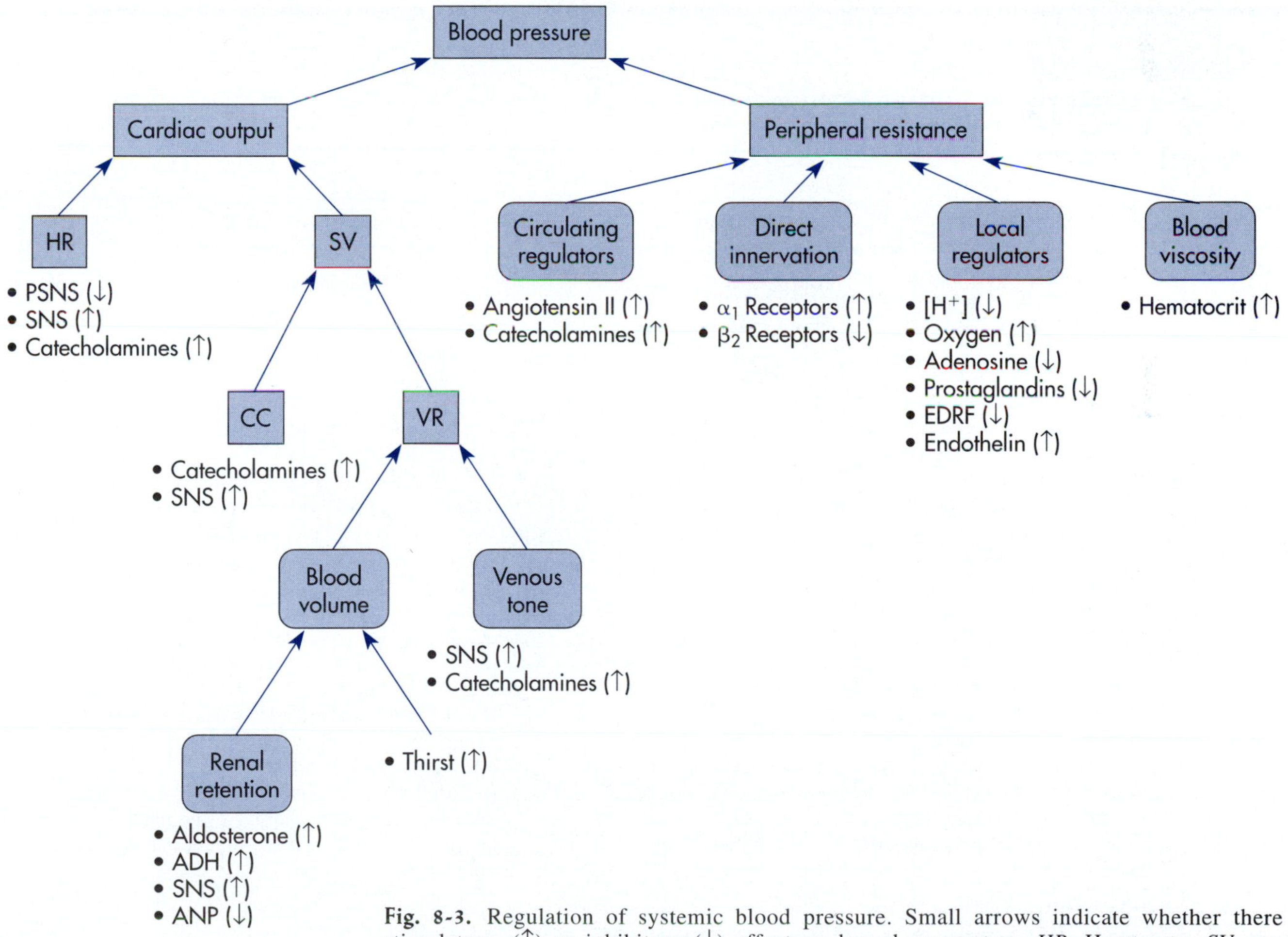


**Fig. 8-3.** Regulation of systemic blood pressure. Small arrows indicate whether there is stimulatory (↑) or inhibitory (↓) effect on boxed parameters. *HR*, Heart rate; *SV*, stroke volume; *PSNS*, parasympathetic nervous system; *SNS*, sympathetic nervous system; *CC*, cardiac contractility; *VR*, venous return; *EDRF*, endothelium-derived relaxing factor; *ADH*, antidiuretic hormone; *ANP*, atrial natriuretic peptide. (Redrawn from Mangrulkar RS, Nigrovic PA, Moore TJ: Hypertension. In Lilly LS, editor: *Hypertension in pathophysiology of heart disease,* Philadelphia, 1993, Lea & Febiger.)

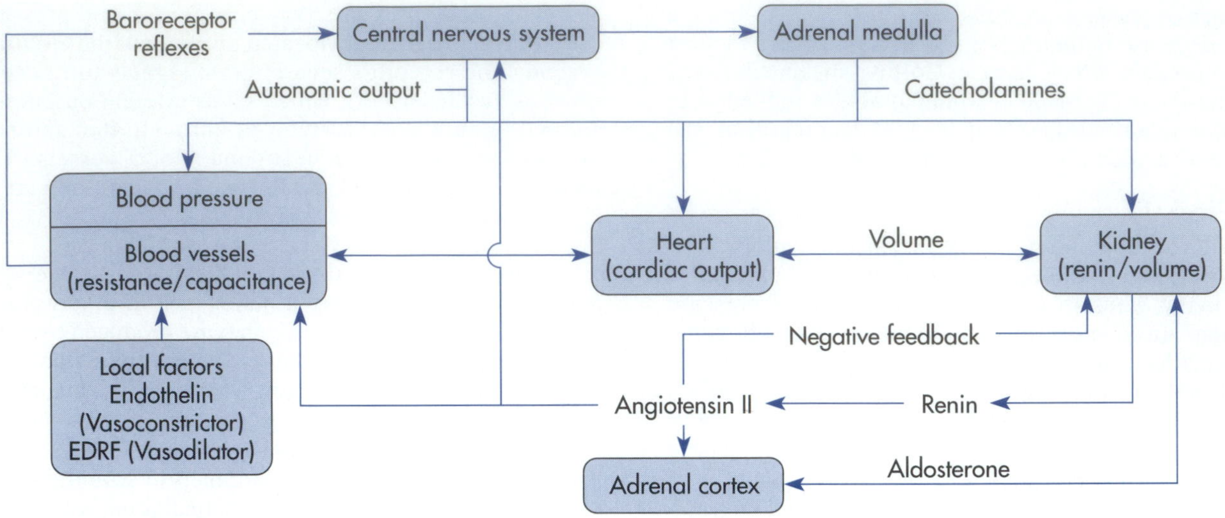


**Fig. 8-4.** A series of feedback loops (of which the major ones are shown) regulate blood pressure. (Redrawn from McCarron DA, Haber E, Slater E: *Sci Am* 64:1, 1990.)

## Managed Care Guide
## Guidelines for measuring blood pressure

I. Conditions for the patient
  A. Posture
    1. Some prefer readings after the patient has been supine for five minutes. Sitting pressures are usually adequate.
    2. Patient should sit quietly with back supported for five minutes and the arm supported at the level of the heart.
    3. For patients who are over age 65, diabetic, or receiving antihypertensive therapy, check for postural changes by taking readings immediately and two minutes after the patient stands.
  B. Circumstances
    1. No caffeine for the preceding hour.
    2. No smoking for the preceding 15 minutes.
    3. No exogenous adrenergic stimulants, for example, phenylephrine in nasal decongestants or eyedrops for pupillary dilation.
    4. A quiet, warm setting.
    5. Home readings taken under varying circumstances: 24-hour ambulatory recordings may be preferable and more accurate in predicting subsequent cardiovascular disease.

II. Equipment
  A. Cuff size: The bladder should encircle and cover two thirds of the length of the arm; if not, place the bladder over the brachial artery; if the bladder is too small, spuriously high readings may result.
  B. Manometer: Aneroid gauges should be calibrated every six months against a mercury manometer.
  C. For infants, use equipment employing ultrasound, for example, the Doppler method.

III. Technique
  A. Number of readings
    1. On each occasion, take at least two readings, separated by as much time as is practical. If readings vary by more than 5 mm Hg, take additional readings until two are close.
    2. For diagnosis, obtain three sets of readings at least a week apart.
    3. Initially, take pressure in both arms; if pressure differs, use arm with higher pressure.
    4. If arm pressure is elevated, take pressure in one leg, particularly in patients below age 30.
  B. Performance
    1. Inflate the bladder quickly to a pressure of 20 mm Hg above the systolic, as recognized by the disappearance of the radial pulse.
    2. Deflate the bladder 3 mg Hg every second.
    3. Record the Korotkoff phase V (disappearance) except in children, in whom use of phase IV (muffling) is advocated.
    4. If Korotkoff sounds are weak, have the patient raise the arm, open and close the hand five to ten times, after which the bladder should be inflated quickly.

From Kaplan NM: Arterial hypertension. In Stein JH et al, editors: *Internal medicine,* ed 4, St. Louis, 1994, Mosby–Year Book.

I, which, after exposure to a converting enzyme in the lungs, is converted to angiotensin II. Angiotensin II regulates renal sodium uptake, acts as a powerful vasoconstrictor, and stimulates the adrenal cortex to produce aldosterone. Aldosterone acts on the renal tubules to promote the reabsorption of sodium and water. Plasma volume is increased through this reabsorption, thus increasing cardiac output. The combination of aldosterone (increasing volume) and angiotensin II (producing vasoconstriction) increases blood pressure. This process is turned off when the juxtaglomerular apparatus in the kidney decreases renin production after fluid volume, blood pressure, and angiotensin II reach threshold levels.

A number of other factors that affect blood pressure have been identified, including factors from vascular endothelial cells, the atrial natriuretic factor, calcium-regulating hormones, the kallikrein system, and vasopressin. Vascular endothelial cells produce both endothelin, a vasoconstrictor, and endothelium-derived relaxing factor (now known to be nitrous oxide), a relaxing factor. The interplay of these substances may control vascular pressure at the local level. Another peptide, atrial natriuretic factor, is produced by atrial tissue in response to atrial dilatation. This hormone causes vasodilatation, increases the glomerular filtration rate, and enhances sodium excretion. Atrial natriuretic factor release is associated with decreased renin and aldosterone secretion.

Kininogen is a plasma substrate synthesized in the liver and acted on by kallikrien (from the kidney) to produce bradykinin. One of bradykinin's degradation products is the converting enzyme that produces angiotensin II. The calcium-controlling hormones, calcitriol (vasocontrictor) and parathyroid hormone (vasodilator), also have vascular effects on blood pressure. Finally, antidiuretic hormone (ADH), or vasopressin, is produced by the pituitary and released in response to major hemorrhage, severe stress, or head injury. ADH is a potent vasoconstrictor and causes increased sodium and water reabsorption.

## DETECTING HYPERTENSION

Hypertension control begins by detecting and confirming high blood pressure. In the office, three separate readings should be taken and averaged. Kaplan has provided useful guidelines for measuring blood pressure (see box at left). The patient should be comfortable and relaxed before pressures are taken. Sitting pressures are usually adequate. The upper arm is bare and free of tight sleeves, with the arm supported at the level of the heart. Patients should avoid caffeine or tobacco products for 30 minutes before recordings and should not be taking exogenous adrenergic stimulants. Patients who are over 65 years old, diabetic, or taking antihypertensive medications should have pressures measured sitting and two minutes after standing.

Blood pressures can be measured with either a mercury or aneroid type sphygmomanometer. The inflatable rubber bladder should encircle two thirds of the upper arm length, and the width of the cuff should equal 1.2 to 1.5 times the arm diameter. The lower edge of the cuff should be 1″ above the antecubital fossa with the bladder over the brachial artery. The cuff is quickly inflated to 20 to 30 mm Hg above the point at which the radial pulse is no longer palpable, and then slowly deflated (2 to 5 mm/sec). The systolic pressure is the point at which sound is first heard. The diastolic pressure is the point at which sound disappears, not the point at which sound changes.

Hypertension should not be diagnosed or treated on the basis of initial readings unless the patient has evidence of acute target-organ damage (hypertensive crisis or urgency). Subjects with stage 3 blood pressures (Table 8-1) should be further evaluated or referred to a source of care within one week, stage 2 within one month. Stage 1 blood pressures should be confirmed within two months, and pressures in the normal range can be rechecked in one year.

Ambulatory readings may help to assess blood pressure. "White-coat" hypertension is a common problem; an estimated 10% to 25% of subjects have been misdiagnosed as hypertensive based on falsely elevated office readings. Studies have shown that ambulatory blood pressures correlate better with target-organ damage, particularly left ventricular hypertrophy, and with cardiovascular complications. Regression to the mean also occurs in measuring blood pressure; high pressures tend to be lower when repeated. Readings taken during emergency room visits for trauma or painful complaints should be interpreted cautiously since they are known to be misleadingly high. Conversely, hypertensive patients hospitalized with bed rest often have misleadingly low pressures. These patients may be discharged without adequate blood pressure medication, only to remanifest their hypertension soon after leaving the hospital.

Physicians should also be aware of pseudohypertension. Some elderly patients have very stiff, atheromatous arteries that cannot be occluded without very high sphygmomanometric pressures, falsely elevating blood pressure readings. In these patients, an intraarterial pressure reading is the only way to truly determine the blood pressure. This invasive measurement is impractical for most patients. Pseudohypertension should be suspected in elderly patients with chronically elevated blood pressures, widened pulse pressures, orthostatic hypotension on medication, and no evidence of target-organ damage.

## EVALUATING HYPERTENSION

The evaluation of the hypertensive patient should address the following three issues:

1. Is there evidence of target-organ damage?
2. Are there additional cardiovascular risk factors?
3. Does the patient have primary or secondary hypertension?

### History

Hypertension is a disease with a long asymptomatic period, usually 10 to 20 years, and is often detected only during routine screening. Patients with elevated pressures should be questioned about their personal history; symptoms of cardiovascular, cerebrovascular, and renal disease; and family history of high blood pressure, cardiovascular disease, or diabetes. If hypertension has already been diagnosed, the patient should be asked about the duration and levels of blood pressure, any complications of hypertension, and the types and results of previous treatments. The history should also identify other cardiovascular risk factors, such as smoking, hyperlipidemia, inactivity, obesity, and diabetes. Additional important factors to ask about include dietary intake of salt, cholesterol, and saturated fats; drug use, especially

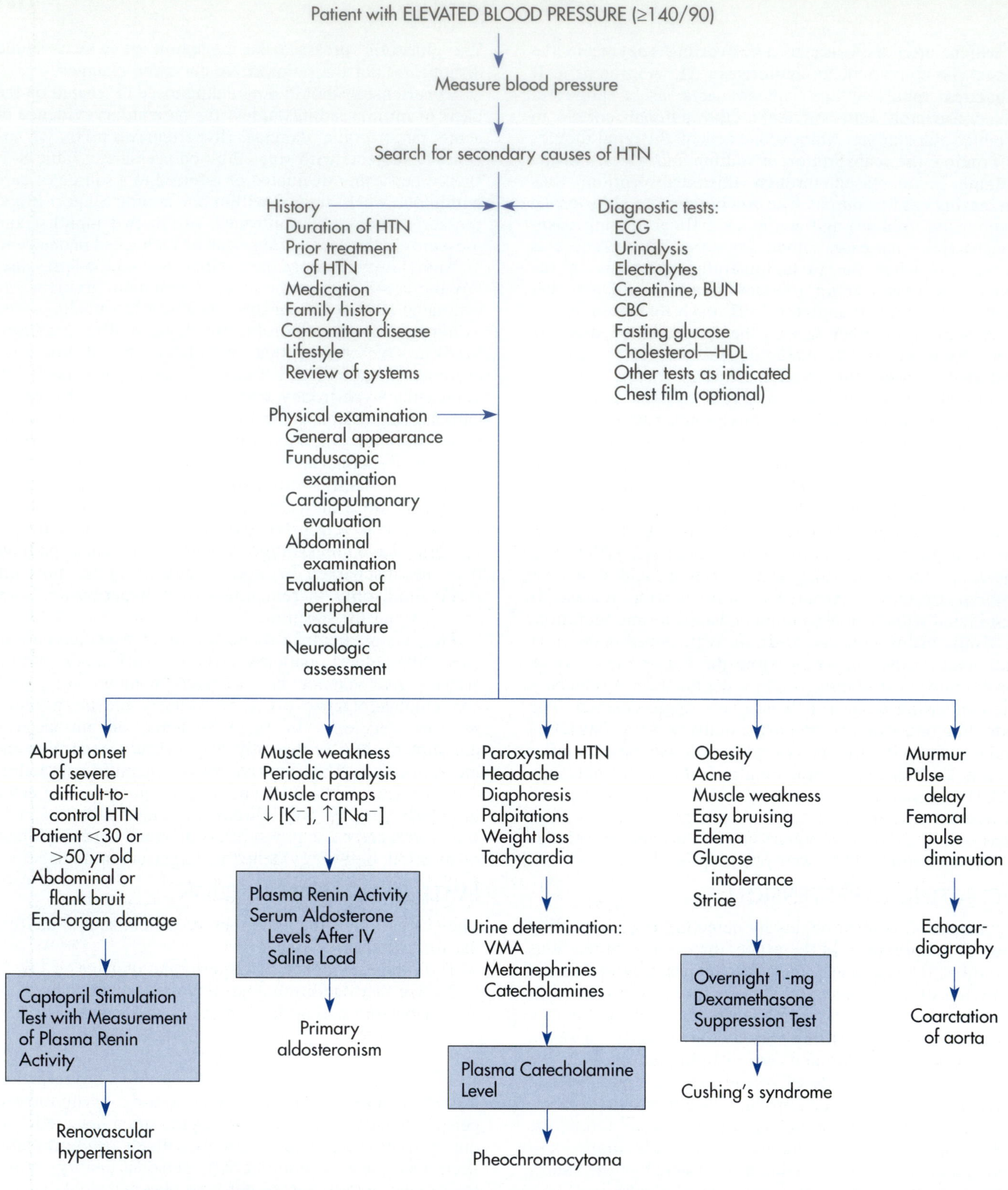


**Fig. 8-5.** Algorithm for the evaluation of hypertension. (From Greene HL, Johnson WP, Maricic MJ, editors: *Decision making in medicine,* St. Louis, 1993, Mosby.)

alcohol, steroids, nonsteroidal antiinflammatory drugs (NSAIDs), cold or allergy medications, estrogen, oral contraceptives, thyroid hormone, diet pills, amphetamines, and cocaine.

A careful review of systems may reveal possible causes of secondary hypertension. Suggestive symptom clusters include episodic headaches, palpitations, orthostatic hypotension, pallor and sweating (pheochromocytoma); weight gain, central obesity, striae, hirsutism, myopathy, and amenorrhea (Cushing syndrome); muscle cramps, weakness, and polyuria (hyperaldosteronism); and leg claudication (coarctation of the aorta).

### Physical examination

The physical examination should include checking for evidence of target-organ damage and secondary causes of hypertension. Blood pressure should be measured in both arms, and radial and femoral pulses should be palpated simultaneously. Diminished or delayed peripheral pulses or decreased lower extremity blood pressures suggest coarctation. The initial examination should include measuring weight and height and examining the optic fundus, thyroid, heart, lungs, and peripheral vasculature. Severe acute hypertension can cause retinal changes, including hemorrhages, exudation of plasma lipids, and areas of infarction. Malignant hypertension can cause high intracranial pressures, leading to papilledema or swelling of the optic disk. Retinopathy from chronic hypertension develops gradually and is characterized first by arteriolar narrowing, then by areas of nicking, where the hypertensive arteries cross the veins. In cases of more severe chronic hypertension, arterial sclerosis occurs and the vessels take on the appearance of copper electrical wires.

The neck should be examined for bruits, elevated jugular venous pressures, and thyroid abnormalities, including goiters, tenderness, or nodules. The heart should be carefully auscultated for tachycardia, arrhythmias, gallops, and murmurs. An infrascapular murmur may indicate aortic coarctation. Ischemic changes of the extremities should be noted, such as hair loss, cyanosis, and digital ischemia. Abdominal bruits, especially lateralizing types or those with a diastolic component, are associated with renovascular disease. Palpation of the liver to determine size and consistency may suggest chronic alcoholism; enlarged kidneys suggest polycystic renal disease; and an abdominal aortic aneurysm may be palpable. Skin findings may suggest secondary causes, including striae (Cushing syndrome), neurofibromas (neurofibromatosis), and pruritic areas (renal failure). A thorough neurologic examination is also important to assess target-organ damage.

## Laboratory Evaluation

Because secondary hypertension is uncommon, laboratory testing should be used judiciously. The practice of ruling out all causes of hypertension is no longer tenable. A baseline laboratory evaluation should include urinalysis (U/A), complete blood count (CBC), fasting blood sugar, potassium, urea nitrogen, creatinine, uric acid, cholesterol, triglycerides, and an electrocardiogram (ECG). The ECG, U/A and renal panel help to determine the extent of hypertensive target-organ damage; fasting blood sugar and lipids identify other cardiovascular risk factors, and potassium and uric acid levels provide baseline values for following the biochemical effects of therapy. This workup is shown in Fig. 8-5.

## Differential Diagnosis (see box on p. 186)

***Essential hypertension.*** Essential (primary) hypertension affects more than 90% of hypertensives and has no identifiable cause. The diagnosis of essential hypertension is one of exclusion, reached when the physician has ruled out secondary causes for hypertension (see below).

***Secondary hypertension.*** Secondary hypertension, by definition, has an identifiable underlying cause. Secondary hypertension should be suspected in patients who present with sudden onset or worsening of hypertension, refractory hypertension, onset before age 20 or after age 50, malignant or accelerated hypertension, or suggestive features on initial clinical examination. Although less than 5% of hypertensive patients have secondary hypertension, this accounts for nearly 3 million people in the United States. Searching for a secondary cause is important because the hypertension may be curable.

The most common cause of secondary hypertension is renal parenchymal disease, which is responsible for 2% to 3% of all hypertension. The diagnosis is based on finding elevated blood urea nitrogen (BUN) and creatinine, decreased creatinine clearance, and an abnormal U/A.

Renovascular disease (RVD) accounts for approximately 1% of hypertension and is suggested by severe hypertension (diastolic blood pressure greater than or equal to 125 mm Hg), an abdominal bruit (up to 50% of RVD patients in contrast to 9% of those with essential hypertension), worsening renal function, and occurrence in younger women or older men. Although renal vascular disease can be caused by cholesterol or clot emboli, aortic dissection, compression of the arteries, or vasculitis, the most frequent etiologies are fibromuscular hyperplasia and atherosclerosis. Fibromuscular hyperplasia occurs principally in young, white women, whereas the more common atherosclerosis is often seen in elderly males. The screening evaluation for this disorder should be either a renal scintigraphy or a plasma renin activity; both are measured before and one hour after a 50-mg dose of captopril. A decrease in renal blood flow or an elevation of venous plasma renin activity are abnormal responses. Angiography and plasma renal vein renin assays confirm the diagnosis; the renal vein plasma renin activity from the stenotic artery should be increased by at least 1.5. During the workup for renovascular hypertension, rare causes of hypertension, including Wilm tumors or renal malignancies (renin secreting), may also be found.

The various medullary and cortical adrenal hyperfunctions account for approximately 0.5% of hypertension. Pheochromocytoma is associated with sustained or intermittent episodes of tachycardia, tremor, sweating, pallor, headache, and orthostatic hypotension. A spot urine test for metanephrine is the initial screening test. Values greater than 1 mg per mg of creatinine should be followed by a 24-hour urine collection for vanillylmandelic acid, metanephrines, and catecholamines.

Nearly 80% of patients with Cushing syndrome have elevated blood pressure because the high levels of cortisol have mineralocorticoid activity. Cushing syndrome is suggested by moon facies, truncal obesity, proximal muscle weakness, and hirsutism. The initial diagnostic test is a morning plasma cortisol after suppression with 1 mg of dexamethasone at bedtime the night before. A cortisol level under 5 μg/dl excludes Cushing syndrome with 98% certainty.

Hyperaldosteronism induces hypertension and potassium wasting, although hypokalemia is not always present. Patients with unprovoked hypokalemia or those who become severely hypokalemic on minimal diuretic therapy may have hyperaldosteronism. Screening tests for hyperaldosteronism include measuring the plasma aldosterone/renin ratio (greater than 20:1 suggests primary hyperaldosteronism) or a stimulated plasma renin determination, which yields a very low response in primary hyperaldosteronism. Other abnormal laboratory screening tests

### Classification of hypertension

I. Systolic and diastolic hypertension
  A. Primary, essential, or idiopathic
  B. Secondary
    1. Renal
      a. Renal parenchymal disease
        (1) Acute glomerulonephritis
        (2) Chronic nephritis
        (3) Polycystic disease
        (4) Connective tissue diseases
        (5) Diabetic nephropathy
        (6) Hydronephrosis
      b. Renovascular
      c. Renin-producing tumors
      d. Renoprival
      e. Primary sodium retention (Liddle syndrome, Gordon syndrome)
    2. Endocrine
      a. Acromegaly
      b. Hypothyroidism
      c. Hyperthyroidism
      d. Hypercalcemia (hyperparathyroidism)
      e. Adrenal
        (1) Cortical
          (a) Cushing syndrome
          (b) Primary aldosteronism
          (c) Congenital adrenal hyperplasia
        (2) Medullary: pheochromocytoma
      f. Extraadrenal chromaffin tumors
      g. Carcinoid
      h. Exogenous hormones
        (1) Estrogen
        (2) Glucocorticoids
        (3) Mineralocorticoids: licorice
        (4) Sympathomimetics
        (5) Tyramine-containing foods and monoamine oxidase inhibitors
    3. Coarctation of the aorta
    4. Pregnancy-induced hypertension
    5. Neurologic disorders
      a. Increased intracranial pressure
        (1) Brain tumor
        (2) Encephalitis
        (3) Respiratory acidosis
      b. Sleep apnea
      c. Quadriplegia
      d. Acute porphyria
      e. Familial dysautonomia
      f. Lead poisoning
      g. Guillain-Barré syndrome
    6. Acute stress, including surgery
      a. Psychogenic hyperventilation
      b. Hypoglycemia
      c. Burns
      d. Pancreatitis
      e. Alcohol withdrawal
      f. Sickle cell crisis
      g. Postresuscitation
      h. Postoperative
    7. Increased intravascular volume
    8. Alcohol, drugs, etc.
II. Systolic hypertension
  A. Increased cardiac output
    1. Aortic valvular regurgitation
    2. Arteriovenous fistula, patent ductus
    3. Thyrotoxicosis
    4. Paget disease of bone
    5. Beriberi
    6. Hyperkinetic circulation
  B. Rigidity of aorta

From Kaplan NM: Arterial hypertension. In Stein JH et al, editors: *Internal medicine,* ed 4, St. Louis, 1994, Mosby–Year Book.

include a 24-hour urine potassium level exceeding 30 mEq, in spite of hypokalemia, and nonsuppressible plasma adosterone levels following a 25-mg dose of captopril. Plasma and urine aldosterone levels should be determined only after adequate potassium replacement, and plasma levels should be measured at 8:00 A.M. If hyperaldosteronism is suspected, computed tomography (CT) scanning and adrenal venous sampling can localize pathology. Bilaterally elevated aldosterone levels suggest idiopathic hyperaldosteronism, whereas Conn syndrome is characterized by a unilateral elevation of aldosterone and an adrenal adenoma. Other endocrine causes of secondary hypertension include acromegaly, hypothyroidism, hyperthyroidism, and hypercalcemia (hyperparathyroidism). These diagnosis are suggested by characteristic clinical findings (gigantism, thyromegaly or thyroid nodules) or abnormal laboratory studies (serum calcium, thyroid function tests).

Coarctation of the aorta is suggested by delayed or absent femoral pulses and decreased lower extremity blood pressure. A chest x-ray may show the "E" sign, formed by the abnormal contour of the aortic knob and the uppermost portion of the descending aorta. Notching of rib may be noted. An aortogram confirms the diagnosis, but coarctation may also be demonstrated on CT scan or magnetic resonance imaging (MRI).

Other miscellaneous causes of hypertension are shown in the box above. A number of exogenous drugs and chemicals can lead to hypertension. Physicians should always query patients about using nasal decongestants, which contain sympathomimetics, and NSAIDs, which cause fluid retention and interfere with antihypertensive agents. Most women who take oral contraceptives have an increase in blood pressure, usually within the normal range. After prescribing birth control pills, the physician should recheck the blood pressure within the first two to four weeks and at three-month to six-month intervals thereafter. Low-dose postmenopausal hormone replacement is not a cause of hypertension.

## MANAGEMENT

Antihypertensive therapy has been proven to decrease cardiovascular morbidity and mortality in a number of long-term clinical trials. Randomized controlled trials have convincingly shown that drug therapy for mild to severe hypertension (systolic and diastolic) and for isolated systolic hypertension can prevent strokes, congestive heart failure, renal failure, and ischemic heart disease. One landmark trial, the first Veterans Administration (VA) Cooperative Study Group, showed that treating severe hypertension (diastolic blood pressure 115 to 129 mm Hg) with hydralazine, reserpine, and hydrochlorothiazide significantly reduced morbidity from congestive heart failure, renal failure, stroke, and myocardial infarction. A second VA cooperative study found that antihypertensive therapy reduced the incidence of morbid events in men with diastolic pressures from 90 to 114 mm Hg. Treatment was most effective in men with a diastolic blood pressure greater than or equal to 105, who were over 50, and who had evidence of baseline target-organ damage.

Several large placebo-controlled trials have demonstrated benefits from treating patients with a diastolic blood pressure 90 to 104 mm Hg. The Australian National Blood Pressure Study and the Medical Research Counsel trial showed a significant decrease in the incidence of cerebrovascular events and cardiovascular mortality. There was a trend toward reduction of coronary events in the treatment groups. Two community-based studies compared stepped-care drug treatment and risk-factor counseling with usual care. In the Multiple Risk Factor Intervention Trial (MRFIT), the intervention reduced coronary heart disease mortality by 7.1%, but the difference was not significant. The Hypertension Detection and Follow-up Program (HDFP) found that the intervention led to a significant 17% decrease in the 5-year, all-cause mortality rate. There was a trend toward fewer deaths from stroke and myocardial infarction in the intervention group; the effect was greatest in patients who have a diastolic blood pressure between 90 and 104 mm Hg. Neither study was placebo controlled, and it was unclear which component(s) of the interventions affected survival.

The Systolic Hypertension in the Elderly Program provided the first evidence that treating isolated systolic hypertension significantly reduces cardiovascular complications. The incidence of stroke was reduced by 36% and the combined endpoint of nonfatal myocardial infarction plus coronary death was reduced by 27%. Results from the Swedish Trial in Old Patients with Hypertension (STOP-Hypertension), the Medical Research Council (MRC) trial of treatment of hypertension in older adults, and the European Working Party on High Blood Pressure in the Elderly Trial (EWPHE) further supported the benefit of treating hypertension in the elderly. The STOP-Hypertension study enrolled subjects who were 70 to 84 years old and randomized one of three β-blockers, a diuretic, or a placebo. Active treatment reduced total mortality by 43%, the incident of fatal myocardial infarctions by 25%, and the incident of strokes by 47%. The MRC trial enrolled subjects who were 65 to 74 years old. Actively treated subjects who received diuretics or β-blockers had a 25% reduction in strokes and a 19% reduction in coronary events. The EWPHE, which used diuretics and/or methyldopa, showed a 29% decrease in total cardiovascular events for subjects aged 60 to 80 years.

Two recent trials, the Treatment of Mild Hypertension Study and the VA Cooperative Study Group on Antihypertensive Agents demonstrated that other drug classes, including angiotensin converting enzyme (ACE) inhibitors, calcium blockers, α-β-blockers, $\alpha_1$ antagonists, and central $\alpha_2$ agonists, are well tolerated and just as effective in lowering blood pressure. However, there are no data demonstrating that any of these agents reduces long-term cardiovascular morbidity and mortality. Only β-blockers and diuretics have been proven effective in controlled clinical trials, and the JNC V recommends these agents for initial drug therapy.

### Nonpharmacologic Therapy

Numerous studies have shown that lifestyle changes, such as weight reduction, salt restriction, regular aerobic exercise, and decreased alcohol consumption, can lower blood pressure. Although there are no long-term studies to prove that using these modalities prevents the morbidity and mortality of hypertension, the interventions are harmless, may reduce other risk factors for cardiovascular disease, and avoid the costs and side effects of medication. Behavioral science studies show that a physician's advice alone can affect behavior, but the chance of bringing about a true life-style change is greatly increased by combining frequent follow-up visits with client-centered counseling, contracting, and setting achievable goals.

***Weight reduction.*** Weight gain is associated with hypertension and weight loss of 1 kg leads to a 1 to 2 mm Hg fall in blood pressure. The effect of weight loss is independent of sodium restriction or increased exercise. Weight loss, however, is one of the most difficult life-style changes to sustain. Thus, if blood pressure control is achieved using this modality, follow-up visits are encouraged to help maintain the weight loss.

***Diet.*** Aside from causing weight loss with decreased caloric intake, the composition of diet may be important. Adequate amounts of calcium, magnesium, and potassium have all been shown to have a modest effect in lowering blood pressure. Supplements are usually unnecessary for a patient with an adequate diet. Saturated fat increases blood pressure, independent of obesity, and a switch to polyunsaturated and monounsaturated fats moderately reduces pressure. This dietary change can have an impact on two cardiovascular risks, hypertension and cholesterol. Daily alcohol consumption greater than 2 oz is associated with hypertension. Alcohol use is the most common cause of secondary hypertension and is often a major factor in hypertension that is difficult to control. Suspected hypertensive patients should refrain from alcohol completely to determine if the elevated readings are alcohol related. The risks of alcohol-related morbidity and mortality for abusers far outweigh any benefit from high-density lipoprotein (HDL) rise and decreased risk of coronary heart disease.

***Sodium restriction.*** Limiting sodium intake to less than 2.3 g per day has been shown to lower blood pressure in most patients, with substantial lowering in the 5% to 10% of patients with salt-sensitive hypertension. Patients must refrain from salting food at the table and while cooking and should avoid processed foods with a high salt content. For all dietary interventions, patients should be encouraged to read food labels.

*Exercise.* Exercising aerobically at least three times a week for 30 to 45 minutes has been shown to lower blood pressure and prolong life. Exercise is also a valuable adjunct to weight control. The key is to begin gradually with a realistic program that fits the patient's life-style. A useful start may be a simple walking program, which is easily achievable and has minimal risk of injury. Isometric exercise has some potential risk for stroke because it elevates intracranial pressure; therefore, it has no place in the therapy of hypertension.

*Stress reduction.* Blood pressure can be lowered using stress reduction techniques, meditation, and biofeedback. Benefits have been shown in those who achieve the relaxation response through a program of regular, daily sessions.

*Smoking cessation.* Although smoking is not directly associated with hypertension, smoking cessation is strongly encouraged because it is a major risk factor for cardiovascular disease that interacts synergistically with hypertension (see Chapter 124).

### Pharmacologic Therapy

The drug treatment of hypertension is the single greatest indication for medication use in the United States. A vast array of drugs are available: diuretics, sympatholytics, ACE inhibitors, peripheral inhibitors, calcium channel blockers, and vasodilators. With this plethora of medication, virtually all patients with hypertension can be adequately treated. Although the previous recommendation of the JNC suggested a stepped-care approach in which additional medications are sequentially added to obtain blood pressure control, experience has shown this to be generally unnecessary. Indeed, the JNC currently advocates a customized approach using a single agent that is selected on the basis of the patient's age, race, comorbidity, possible etiologies for the hypertension, and lifestyle. This single drug is then increased until blood pressure is controlled unless side effects or drug intolerance dictate changing to a new agent. Antihypertensive medications, their representative trade names, initial and maximal dosages, dosing frequency, and average cost per month are given in Table 8-2.

*Diuretics.* A decade ago diuretics were the first-line drug choice in the stepped-care management of hypertension. This is no longer the case. Although diuretics can lower blood pressure, they tend to produce effects that may increase cardiovascular risk (e.g., hypokalemia, hyperglycemia, and hypercholesterolemia).

Diuretics are believed to lower blood pressure by decreasing plasma volume and, perhaps, through a direct effect on arterial smooth muscle. There is more clinical trial experience with diuretics than with any other medication. Diuretics are inexpensive, can be given once a day, and can be expected to control blood pressure in approximately 50% of patients with mild hypertension (diastolic 90 to 105 mm Hg). African-Americans are more responsive to diuretics than are whites. The maximum effect may take 2 to 4 weeks to develop. Moderate salt restriction can enhance the effect. Regardless of the severity of hypertension, diuretics are often used with other agents to counteract the sodium-retaining properties of nondiuretics and antihypertensive drugs.

**Thiazides.** Thiazide diuretics cause a slight fall in serum potassium in most patients. Only a few develop symptoms of severe hypokalemia. The importance of diuretic-induced hypokalemia is controversial. For patients on digitalis (where hypokalemia may exacerbate toxicity) or patients with a history of ischemic heart disease or ventricular arrhythmias, the serum potassium is closely monitored and the potassium is replaced if hypokalemia develops. Some physicians monitor potassium soon after instituting diuretic therapy in all patients and follow the serum potassium every six to 12 months.

Hypokalemia can be treated with potassium replacement or with the addition of a potassium-sparing diuretic. Longer acting diuretics, such as chlorthalidone and metolazone, may produce more severe hypokalemia. They do not appear to be more effective antihypertensive agents.

Thiazide diuretics cause glucose intolerance and may precipitate clinical diabetes mellitus. They are best avoided in patients with a history of glucose intolerance or diet-controlled diabetes. The diabetogenic properties of indapamide and metolazone are unclear.

Serum uric acid increases approximately 1 mg/dl in all patients started on diuretics. Unless clinical gout develops, modest hyperuricemia need not be treated. If diuretic therapy is essential for the patient with frequent gouty attacks, a uric acid-lowering agent may be added.

Sexual dysfunction, particularly impotence in men, is a relatively frequent side effect of thiazide (and perhaps all diuretic agents). Patients should be warned and questioned specifically about impotence on follow-up visits.

**Loop diuretics: ethacrynic acid, furosemide, bumetanide.** Ethacrynic acid and furosemide block sodium absorption in the loop of Henle. These short-acting agents, which need to be administered twice daily, are more potent diuretics than the thiazides but have no greater antihypertensive effect. Because loop diuretics are more expensive than thiazides and have a propensity for causing wide fluid shifts, they should be used as second-line drugs. In general, they are used for patients with renal failure (serum creatinine greater than 2.5 mg/dl) or for patients with fluid retention and congestive heart failure (metolazone may potentiate the effect in patients with renal insufficiency). Ethacrynic acid and furosemide may cause less glucose intolerance or sexual dysfunction than thiazides.

**Potassium-sparing diuretics: triamterene, amiloride, spinolactone.** Potassium-sparing diuretics promote sodium excretion and potassium retention by preventing sodium/potassium exchange in the distal nephron. These drugs are rarely used as the sole diuretic for treating hypertension unless the patient has thiazide sensitivity, diet-controlled glucose intolerance, or gout. They are particularly useful in combination with other diuretics for patients at risk for hypokalemia. Because these drugs can cause hyperkalemia, they are best avoided for patients with impaired renal function, diabetics with type IV renal tubular acidosis, or those receiving a converting enzyme inhibitor. They should be used cautiously in the elderly.

**Table 8-2.** Antihypertensive drugs

| Generic name | Brand name | Initial dose | Maintenance dosage | Cost per month | Adverse effects |
|---|---|---|---|---|---|
| **Diuretics: thiazide type** | | | | | |
| Hydrochlorothiazide | Esidrix, HydroDIURIL, others | 25 mg qd | 12.5-25 mg qd | $ 7.50 | Hyperuricemia, hypokalemia, hypomagnesemia, hyperglycemia, hyponatremia, hypercalcemia, hypercholesterolemia, hypertriglyceridemia, pancreatitis, rashes, weakness, sexual dysfunction |
| Chlorthalidone | Hygroton, others | 25 mg qd | 12.5-50 mg qd | $22.94 | |
| Indapamide | Lozol | 2.5 mg qd | 2.5-5 mg qd | $25.98 | |
| Metolazone | Zaroxolyn, others | 2.5 mg qd | 2.5-20 mg qd | $ 8.18 | |
| **Diuretics: loop** | | | | | |
| Bumetanide | Bumex, others | 0.5-2 mg qd | 0.5-5 mg qd-bid | $10.11 (0.5 mg) | Dehydration, circulatory collapse, hypokalemia, hyponatremia, hypomagnesemia, hypocalcemia, hyperglycemia, metabolic alkalosis, hyperuricemia, blood dycrasias, rashes, lipid changes as with thiazide diuretics |
| Ethacrynic acid | Edecrin | 12.5-50 mg qd | 12.5-100 mg qd-bid | $ 6.29 (12.5 mg) | |
| Furosemide | Lasix | 20-40 mg qd-bid | 20-320 mg qd-bid | $ 3.75 (20 mg) | |
| **Diuretics: potassium sparing** | | | | | |
| Amiloride | Midamor, others | 5 mg qd | 5-10 mg qd-bid | $15.08 | Amiloride: hyperkalemia, gastrointestinal (GI) disturbances, rash, headache, Spironolactone: hyperkalemia, hyponatremia, mastodynia, gynecomastia, agranulocytosis, menstrual abnormalities, GI disturbances, rash, Triamterene: hyperkalemia, GI disturbances, nephrolithiasis |
| Spironolactone | Aldactone, others | 25-50 mg qd-bid | 25-100 mg qd-bid | $ 3.75 (25 mg qd) | |
| Triamterene | Dyrenium, others | 50-100 mg qd-bid | 50-150 mg qd-bid | $10.21 (50 mg qd) | |
| **Diuretics: combination** | | | | | |
| HCTZ 25 or 50 mg, spironolactone 25 or 50 mg | Aldactazide, others | 1 tab qd | 1 tab qd | $11.57 (AWP) | Same as individual components |
| HCTZ 25 mg, triamterene 50 mg | Dyazide, Maxzide | 1 cap qd | 1 or 2 cap qd | $ 9.27 | |
| HCTZ 25 or 50 mg, triamterene 37.5 or 50 mg | Maxzide | 1 tab qd | 1 tab qd | $12.52 | |
| HCTZ 50 mg, amiloride 5 mg | Moduretic | ½-1 tab qd | ½-1 tab qd | $12.68 | |

*HCTZ,* Hydrochlorothiazide; *AWP,* average wholesale price.

*Continued.*

**Table 8-2.** Antihypertensive drugs—cont'd

| Generic name | Brand name | Initial dosage | Maintenance dosage | Cost per month | Adverse effects |
|---|---|---|---|---|---|
| **β-Adrenergic blocking drugs** | | | | | |
| Atenolol | Tenormin | 25-50 mg qd | 25-100 mg qd | $23.22 (25 mg) | Fatigue, depression, bradycardia, decreased exercise tolerance, congestive heart failure, aggravation of peripheral arterial insufficiency, GI disturbances, bronchospasm, masking of symptoms of hypoglycemia, Raynaud phenomenon, insomnia, vivid dreams or hallucinations, organic brain syndrome, rare blood dyscrasias and other allergic disorders, increased serum triglycerides, decreased HDL cholesterol, generalized pustular psoriasis, transient hearing loss, sudden withdrawal can lead to exacerbation of angina and myocardial infarction |
| Betaxolol | Kerlone, others | 5-10 mg qd | 5-40 mg qd | $12.02 (5 mg) | |
| Metoprolol | Lopressor, Toprol XL | 50-100 mg qd-bid | 50-200 mg qd-bid | $14.78 (50 mg) | |
| Nadolol | Corgard, Corzide | 20-40 mg qd | 20-240 mg qd | $32.76 (40 mg) | |
| Propranolol | Inderal, others | 40 mg bid | 40-240 mg qd-bid | $9.10 | |
| Timolol | Blocadren, others | 10 mg bid | 10-40 mg bid | $14.35 (AWP) | |
| **β-Blocking drugs with intrinsic sympathomimetic activity** | | | | | |
| Acebutolol | Sectral | 200-400 mg qd-bid | 200-1200 mg qd-bid | $23.07 | Similar to other β-adrenergic blocking drugs but with less bradycardia and lipid changes; acebutolol is cardioselective at low dosages and can be associated with a positive antinuclear antibody test and occasional drug-induced lupus |
| Pindolol | Visken | 5 mg bid | 10-60 mg bid | $43.83 | |
| **α-β Blocker** | | | | | |
| Labetalol | Trandate, Normodyne | 100-200 mg qd-bid | 200-1200 mg qd-bid | $18.62 (200 mg) | Similar to other β-adrenergic drugs but has intrinsic sympathomimetic activity and more orthostatic hypotension, fever, and hepatotoxicity |
| **α-Adrenergic blockers** | | | | | |
| Prazosin | Minipress | 1 mg qhs | 1-20 mg bid | $ 9.23 | Prazosin, terazosin: syncope with first dose, dizziness and vertigo, palpitations, fluid retention, headache, drowsiness, weakness, anticholinergic effects, priaprism, urinary incontinence. Doxazosin: similar to prazosin and terazosin but with less hypotension after the first dose |
| Terazosin | Hytrin | 1 mg qhs | 1-20 mg qd (2 mg) | $37.96 (2 mg) | |
| Doxazosin | Cardura | 1 mg qhs | 1-16 mg qd (2 mg) | $28.72 (2 mg) | |
| **Peripheral adrenergic neuron antagonists** | | | | | |
| Guanethidine | Ismelin, Esimil | 10 mg qd | 10-100 mg qd | $16.90 | Guanethidine: orthostatic hypotension, exercise hypotension, diarrhea, may aggravate bronchial asthma, bradycardia, sodium and water retention, retrograde ejaculation. Reserpine: psychic depression, nightmares, nasal stuffiness, drowsiness, GI disturbances, bradycardia |
| Guanadrel | Hylorel | 10 mg qd | 10-75 mg qd | | |
| Reserpine | Serapasil | .05-0.1 mg qd | 0.5-0.1 mg qd | $ 7.50 | |

| | | | | | |
|---|---|---|---|---|---|
| **Central sympatholytic drugs** | | | | | |
| Clonidine | Catapres, others | 0.1-0.2 mg bid | 0.1-0.6 mg bid | $ 3.75 (0.1 mg) | Clonidine: CNS reactions similar to methyldopa but more sedation and dry mouth, bradycardia, heart block, rebound hypertension. Guanabenz: similar to clonidine. Guanfacine: similar to clonidine but milder. Methyldopa: drowsiness, sedation, dry mouth, fatigue, orthostatic hypotension, bradycardia, heart block, GI disorders including colitis, hepatitis, cirrhosis, hepatic necrosis, fever, Coombs positive hemolytic anemia, lupuslike syndrome, immune thrombocytopenia, red cell aplasia |
| Guanabenz | Wytensin | 4 mg bid | 4-64 mg bid | $20.77 | |
| Guanfacine | Tenex | 1 mg qd | 1-3 mg qd | $24.20 | |
| Methyldopa | Aldomet, others | 250 mg bid | 250-2 gm bid | $ 6.01 | |
| **Angiotensin converting enzyme (ACE) inhibitors** | | | | | |
| Benazepril | Lotensin | 10 mg qd | 10-40 mg qd-bid | $21.09 | Cough, hypotension, particularly with a diuretic or volume depletion; loss of taste with anorexia; rash; acute renal failure with bilateral renal artery stenosis or stenosis of the artery to a solitary kidney; cholestatic jaundice; pancreatitis; angioedema, hyperkalemia; blood dyscrasias and renal damage, except in patients with renal dysfunction; may increase fetal mortality and should not be used during second and third trimesters of pregnancy |
| Captopril | Capoten | 12.5-25 mg bid-tid | 12.5-150 mg bid-tid | $20.35 | |
| Enalapril | Vasotec | 2.5-5 mg qd-bid | 2.5-40 mg qd-bid | $22.82 (2.5 mg) | |
| Fosinopril | Monopril | 10 mg qd | 10-40 mg qd-bid | $21.26 | |
| Lisinopril | Prinivil, Zestril, others | 5-10 mg qd | 5-40 mg qd | $24.64 (5 mg) | |
| Quinapril | Accupril | 5-10 mg qd | 5-80 mg qd-bid | $24.97 (AWP) | |
| Ramipril | Altace | 1.25-2.5 mg qd | 1.25-20 mg qd-bid | $17.72 (AWP) | |
| **Calcium channel blockers** | | | | | |
| Diltiazem | Cardizem SR | 60-120 mg bid | 120-360 mg bid | $48.14 (60 mg) | Diltiazem, verapamil: dizziness, headache, edema, constipation (especially verapamil), AV block, bradycardia, heart failure, gingival hyperplasia. Dihydropyridines: dizziness, headache, peripheral edema (more than with verapamil), flushing, tachycardia, rash, gingival hyperplasia |
| Diltiazem | Cardizem CD | 120-240 mg qd | 120-360 mg qd | $32.00 (120 mg) | |
| Verapamil | Calan, others | 120-240 mg bid-tid | 120-480 mg bid-tid | $39.88 (120 mg) | |
| Verapamil | Calan SR | 120 mg qd | 120-480 mg qd-bid | $26.76 | |
| Amlodipine | Norvasc | 2.5 mg qd | 2.5-10 mg qd | $36.86 | |
| Felodipine | Plendil | 5 mg qd | 5-20 mg qd | $28.06 | |
| Isradipine | DynaCirc | 5 mg qd | 5-10 mg qd-bid | $37.85 | |
| Nicardipine | Cardene | 20 mg tid | 60-120 mg tid | $37.26 | |
| Nifedipine | Procardia XL, others | 30 mg qd | 30-90 mg qd | $27.23 | |
| **Direct vasodilators** | | | | | |
| Hydralazine | Apresoline, others | 25 mg bid | 40-200 mg qd-qid | $ 4.40 | GI disturbances, tachycardia, aggravation of angina, headache and dizziness, fluid retention, nasal congestion, rashes and other allergic reactions, lupuslike syndrome, hepatitis |
| Minoxidil | Loniten, others | 5 mg qd | 5-40 mg qd | | Tachycardia, aggravation or angina-marked fluid retention, possible pericardial effusion, hirsutism, thromboarterpenia, leukopenia |

Courtesy Michael Katz.

*Sympatholytic agents.* Sympatholytic agents include β-blockers, α-blockers and α- and β-adrenergic blockers. Next to diuretics, the β-adenergic blocking agents have been the most extensively studied antihypertensives and have been shown to lower morbidity and mortality from cardiovascular disease. Blood pressure is lowered through β-adrenergic blockade and, at higher dosages, through a CNS mechanism. The majority of younger patients with hypertension respond to these agents, but the response rate decreases with advancing age. β-blockers are ideal for hypertensive patients with angina, myocardial infarction, migraine headaches, and essential tremor. Although there are many β-blocking agents, if one β-blocker is ineffective in lowering blood pressure, substituting another β-blocker is futile. However, if a noncardioselective β-blocker is discontinued because of side effects, a selective $\beta_1$ antagonist might be substituted. Response to β-blockers is seen over a wide dosage range; for example, the effective daily dose of propranolol varies between 80 and 480 mg. Because of the broad dosage response range, β-blockers often require frequent visits until the dosage is adequately adjusted.

β-Blockers exacerbate congestive heart failure, asthma, second-degree or third-degree heart block, ischemic peripheral vascular disease, male sexual dysfunction, and may mask hypoglycemic symptoms in type I diabetics. β-blockers may interfere with weight loss through inhibition of lipid mobility and may increase levels of plasma triglycerides while reducing HDL levels. Athletes who depend on an increased heart rate to boost performance may not tolerate β-blockers.

There are a large number of β-blockers available. From a pharmacologic standpoint, these agents can be grouped into the nonspecific β-antagonists, the selective $\beta_1$-antagonists, and those with and without intrinsic sympathomimetic activity (ISA). At low dosages, $\beta_1$-blockers, such as acebutolol, atenolol, and metoprolol, should not induce brochospasm in patients with reactive airway disease. Agents like acebutolol and pindolol have intrinsic sympathomimetic activity and may not lower the heart rate as much as agents without sympathomimetic activity. Lipid soluble β-blockers (e.g., metoprolol, propranolol) may have greater CNS effects and may make it more difficult to sustain therapeutic blood levels.

*Central inhibition of sympathetic drive*

**Clonidine, guanabenz, and guanfacine.** Clonidine, guanabenz, and guanfacine are centrally acting adrenergic depressants. These agents are central $\alpha_2$-adrenergic agonists and decrease sympathetic output in the CNS. There is moderate clinical experience with clonidine, whereas guanabenz and guanfacine have only recently been approved for use in the United States. Clonidine is usually added to a diuretic or another agent when single therapy proves unsatisfactory. Occasionally, clonidine is a useful single-drug treatment for patients who cannot be managed with diuretics or β-blockers, but it should be given twice daily.

Rebound hypertension, often accompanied by tachycardia, may occur with sudden withdrawal of clonidine or guanabenz. Readministration of the drug is usually sufficient treatment. Patients should be advised not to run out of medicine and doses should tapered over two or three weeks when stopping the drug. These drugs should probably be avoided in patients with a history of intermittent or poor compliance.

**Methyldopa.** Methyldopa is also a central-acting adrenergic antagonist. It may act by a mechanism that is similar to clonidine or by forming a false neurotransmitter. Methyldopa has been used safely for more than 20 years in the treatment of mild to moderate hypertension, usually in combination with a diuretic and/or other therapeutic agents. Some clinicians believe that methyldopa's side effects, such as drowsiness, fatigue, and impotence, may limit its effectiveness.

*α-Blocking agents.* Prazosin, terazosin, and doxazosin block the smooth muscle postsynaptic $\alpha_1$-receptors, dilating arteries without causing reflex tachycardia. In general, α-blockers are not used as initial therapy, but are used in combination with a diuretic or another sympatholytic medication. α-blockers may be particularly beneficial for hypertensive patients with peripheral arterial disease or with congestive heart failure. Terazosin relaxes smooth muscle in prostatic tissues and effectively relieves symptoms of prostatism in men with prostatic hypertrophy.

*Combination α- and β-blockers.* Labetalol, a relatively new drug in the United States, has both α-blocking and β-blocking properties, with the α effect being roughly one third of the β effect. Clinical investigation has shown it to lower blood pressure effectively. Labetalol causes some slowing of the heart rate; however, in contrast to pure β-blockers, it does not decrease cardiac output or increase peripheral vascular resistance. For these reasons, labetalol offers some theoretic advantages over β-blockers, but its current place in the treatment of hypertension has not been clearly defined. The drug is relatively expensive and requires dosing twice daily. The starting dose is 200 mg per day.

*Vasodilating agents.* Under the stepped-care approach to hypertension, a direct-acting vasodilator was added as a third drug for the small percentage of patients who could not be controlled with two drugs. The medications available in this class are hydralazine and minoxidil.

Hydralazine is a direct-acting vasodilator that causes decreased arterial resistance, a reflex increase in heart rate, and a secondary increase in plasma renin. It has been used for years in the therapy of hypertension. Because hydralazine induces reflex tachycardia and fluid retention, it is most often used in combination with a diuretic and a β-blocker or reserpine. Hydralazine is an effective antihypertensive agent with proven ability to lower morbidity and mortality, as well as to lower blood pressure. The drug is relatively inexpensive, with few side effects and no adverse CNS effects. Lupus syndrome is rare with dosages of 200 mg or less per day. The starting dosage for hydrazaline is 50 mg per day given in two divided doses.

Minoxidil is a direct-acting vasodilator that also causes reflex tachycardia and fluid retention. It is a potent antihypertensive agent used in severe resistant hypertension and may be especially effective for patients with renal failure. Cardiovascular side effects, including congestive heart failure, hypotension, and angina, can be severe, and its associated hypertrichosis and coarsening of facial features may be unacceptable to women and adolescents, although balding men may be pleased. The initial dose for minoxidil is 5 mg given once daily.

***Angiotensin converting enzyme (ACE) inhibitors.*** These agents inhibit the enzyme that converts angiotensin I (inactive) to angiotensin II, a potent vasoconstrictor that causes aldosterone secretion from the adrenal gland. The ACE inhibitors have become the first-line therapy because they effectively lower blood pressure in most patients and have minimal side effects. Peripheral resistance is lowered without decreasing cardiac output or decreasing the glomerular filtration rate. ACE inhibitors reduce mortality for patients who have congestive heart failure and slow the progression of renal failure in diabetics. The starting doses and costs of the ACE inhibitors are shown in Table 8-2.

Because ACE inhibitors can cause hyperkalemia, they should not be used concomitantly with potassium-sparing agents or for patients with diabetes and a tendency toward potassium retention. They produce an intermittent cough productive of excess mucous in about 30% of patients. This symptom tends to decrease and may be less on a different ACE inhibitor. ACE inhibitors can cause serious nephrotoxicity in patients with bilateral renal artery stenosis or unilateral stenosis with a solitary kidney by dramatically decreasing renal blood flow.

***Calcium channel blockers.*** Calcium is essential for muscle contraction and increased levels of calcium may play a role in the development, if not the maintenance, of hypertension. By excluding the influx of calcium into smooth muscle cells, blood pressure can be reduced. From a functional standpoint, calcium channel blockers act as vasodilators. They come in two chemical forms: (1) the dihydropyridines (e.g., nifedipine, amlodipine, felodipine, isradipine, and nicardipine); and (2) the nondihydropyridines (e.g., verapamil and diltiazem). Although both classes of drugs lower blood pressure, verapamil and diltiazem have a substantial negative chronotropic effect and need to be used carefully in patients using β-blockers or with conduction defects. Although initially given three times per day, these drugs have now been formulated for daily or twice daily dosing. The starting dose is 60 mg for diltiazem, 30 mg for nifedipine, and 120 mg for verapamil.

## HYPERTENSIVE EMERGENCIES

### Malignant hypertension

Malignant hypertension is a syndrome of markedly elevated diastolic pressure—always greater than 110 mm Hg and usually greater than 130 mm Hg—that is accompanied by signs or symptoms of acute cardiac, renal, or CNS damage. Malignant hypertension occurs in less than 1% of hypertensive patients. Patients are usually symptomatic with a headache, blurred vision, or dyspnea. Funduscopic examination reveals grade 3 or 4 retinopathy. Acute renal damage is manifested by rising BUN, proteinuria, and/or hematuria. CNS findings include focal neurologic deficits or hypertensive encephalopathy. Some patients complain predominantly of dyspnea and have acute left ventricular failure and pulmonary edema. A characteristic pathologic lesion of malignant hypertension is fibrinoid necrosis of small arterioles. A list of hypertensive emergencies is given in the above box.

#### Hypertensive emergencies

Aortic aneurysm: leaking or dissection
Unstable angina
Myocardial infarction
Eclampsia
Encephalopathy (hypertensive)
Malignant hypertension with CNS or systemic effects
Pheochromocytoma
Pulmonary edema
Subarachnoid or intracranial bleeding
Surgical or postoperative bleeding due to severe hypertension

Malignant hypertension is a medical emergency. Patients with any of the above syndromes require hospitalization and treatment with parenteral antihypertensive agents to rapidly lower blood pressure and relieve symptoms. Patients with diastolic blood pressures greater than 130 mm Hg, but without symptoms of acute target-organ damage, are also candidates for hospitalization and rapid management of their elevated pressure. Hypertensive patients who have been noncompliant sometimes have similar marked elevations of diastolic pressure without evidence of malignant hypertension. It is often possible to restart drug therapy for these patients and follow them closely every day or two on an outpatient basis.

Drug therapy for malignant hypertension is administered to lower the diastolic pressure below 105 mm Hg and resolve the symptoms of target-organ damage. Renal failure may sometimes worsen following abrupt blood pressure lowering, and urine output and renal function need to be monitored. In some cases, acute renal failure must be tolerated and treated with dialysis if symptoms of encephalopathy or congestive heart failure resolve only when blood pressure is lowered to a point that compromises renal function. Sodium nitroprusside, diazoxide, and hydralazine are commonly used in the treatment of malignant hypertension. Sodium nitroprusside is a direct-acting vasodilator that is administered as an intravenous infusion. The initial dose is 25 to 50 μg per minute; the maximum dose is 200 to 300 μg per minute. The dose is titrated to blood pressure and the drug must be administered in an intensive care unit where the patient can be constantly monitored.

Sodium nitroprusside is the drug of choice for patients with ischemic heart disease and malignant hypertension. Side effects include hypotension; cyanide toxicity manifested by headache, hyperpnea, acidosis, and cyanosis; and thiocyanate toxicity manifested by nausea, vomiting, muscle cramps, and altered mental functioning. Thiocyanate levels are therefore determined every 24 to 48 hours, particularly during prolonged use.

Diazoxide is also a direct-acting vasodilator. It can be given in repeated boluses of 50 to 150 mg every five minutes for rapid blood pressure control or as an infusion.

Overshoot hypotension occurs, particularly with patients already on other (nondiuretic) antihypertensive agents. Diazoxide causes reflex tachycardia and an increase in cardiac output that may aggravate ischemic heart disease. Fluid retention and hyperglycemia are also frequent side effects. Because diazoxide has a duration of action ranging from two to 12 hours, it should be avoided when overshoot hypotension might have serious consequences; for example, angina, myocardial infarction, hypertensive encephalopathy, stroke (either hemorrhagic or thrombotic), eclampsia, or a leaking or dissecting aortic aneurysm.

Hydralazine is administered intramuscularly or intravenously in dosages of 10 to 15 mg every four to six hours as needed. Hydralazine relaxes arterial smooth muscle and has an onset of action within 15 to 30 minutes. Reflex tachycardia and increased cardiac output may worsen ischemic heart disease. Hydralazine is useful in the treatment of eclampsia (see below). Dosages should be adjusted downward for elderly patients.

Oral antihypertensive agents are instituted as soon as the patient can be weaned from parenteral therapy.

### Hypertension in patients with other medical emergencies

***Acute pulmonary edema.*** Hypertension often accompanies pulmonary edema and usually resolves with the standard treatment (e.g., diuretics and digitalis). If hypertension persists despite treatment for pulmonary edema, nitroprusside is an appropriate, rapidly acting antihypertensive agent.

***Acute myocardial infarction.*** β-blockers and calcium channel blockers have been used to reduce blood pressure in patients with acute myocardial infarction and hypertension. Some patients with hypertension and myocardial infarction may respond to intravenous nitroglycerin. Nitroglycerin has venodilating properties at low dosages and arteriolar dilating properties at high dosages, with rapid onset and rapid cessation of action. Nitroprusside may be the drug of choice when myocardial infarction is complicated by left ventricular failure.

***Dissecting aortic aneurysm.*** Medical therapy of acute dissecting aneurysm is directed toward lowering blood pressure and reducing myocardial contractility. Sodium nitroprusside is often used in combination with propranolol. Nitroprusside causes vasodilatation; propranolol blocks the reflex tachycardia, slows myocardial contractility, and decreases cardiac output. Both agents are given intravenously after a pulmonary arterial catheter has been placed to monitor pressure changes. For patients who cannot tolerate nitroprusside or who do not respond to it, trimethaphan camsylate may be used. It is a short-acting ganglionic blocker that has rapid onset and rapid cessation of action. Trimethaphan has significant side effects, including urinary obstruction and paralytic ileus.

***Acute cerebrovascular accidents.*** Hypertension due to intracranial bleeding usually cannot be effectively treated with antihypertensive drugs. Hypertensive patients who experience subarachnoid hemorrhage or thrombotic or embolic stroke can usually be managed with cautious administration of oral agents to slowly reduce blood pressure. Nifedipine is currently the agent of choice, with a starting dose of 30 mg. If vasodilators are used, β-blockers should be administered as well. Nitroprusside has been used to treat hypertensive emergencies in patients with acute cerebral events.

***Pheochromocytoma.*** The drug of choice for a pheochromocytoma hypertensive crisis is phentolamine, an α-blocking agent, administered intravenously at doses of 2 to 5 mg every five minutes. Once the α effects (lowering of pressure) are evident, propranolol may be used to block the reflex tachycardia and increase cardiac output. Alternatively, nitroprusside and β-blockers may be used.

***Drug-induced catecholamine excess state.*** Patients taking monoamine oxidase inhibiting medications who ingest tyramine can have a severe hypertensive response like that seen with pheochromocytoma. A similar problem can occur after the sudden withdrawal of clonidine. Both situations can be managed using a β-blocker with phentolamine or nitroprusside.

***Toxemia of pregnancy.*** The American College of Obstetricians and Gynecologists divides hypertension in pregnancy into four categories: preeclampsia/eclampsia, chronic hypertension, preexisting hypertension complicated by preeclampsia, and late transient hypertension. The emergency states are discussed first, and the remaining conditions are covered later in this chapter.

Preeclampsia and eclampsia are the most emergent hypertensive conditions in pregnancy, presenting with elevated pressure, proteinuria, edema, signs of intravascular hemolysis or coagulopathy, liver transaminase abnormalities, and seizures (eclampsia). Preeclampsia syndrome occurs more often in nulliparous patients between the 20th week and term and can rapidly progress to seizures after a brief period of symptoms, such as headache, abdominal or epigastric pain, and signs of hyperreflexia. Because preeclampsia and eclampsia are aggravated by continuing pregnancy, the best treatment is to terminate the pregnancy, preferably after establishing fetal viability. Lowering blood pressure may lead to fetal compromise if done too vigorously. While preparing for delivery, physicians should keep diastolic pressure below 105 mm Hg. Hydralazine given intravenously in 5-mg doses at five-minute intervals is effective for control of eclampsia. An intravenous infusion of 1 to 2 g per hour of magnesium sulfate is also given after a loading dose of 2 g given over five to 10 minutes. The infusion should be continued for the first 24 hours after parturition.

Women who are hypertensive before pregnancy comprise one third of all preeclampsia (discussed later in this chapter). Whether these women are successfully able to deliver a viable baby depends on the extent of organ damage before pregnancy (renal function, cardiac states). Although most women without significant comorbidity do well, those with polyarteritis and scleroderma do not. Many experts advocate that these women avoid pregnancy and that any pregnancy should be managed in close collaboration with a rheumatologist and an obstetrician.

There is a final group of women who become hypertensive later in pregnancy or just before delivery but have no findings to suggest preeclampsia. These women are managed as though preeclamptic and generally do very well. Late gestational hypertension, which corrects post partum, may be a harbinger of essential hypertension later in life. Some studies suggest that increased calcium (2 g per day calcium carbonate) may decrease the risk of both gestational hypertension and preeclampsia/eclampsia. Other studies show that a low dosage of aspirin (60 mg per day) given in the second and third trimester of high-risk pregnancies may lessen the development of preeclampsia/eclampsia. Neither of these chemicals was reported to cause any damage to mother or baby.

## SPECIAL CONSIDERATIONS IN THERAPY

### Resistant hypertension

Almost all patients with hypertension can achieve good blood pressure control with minimal side effects, although a few patients may persistently have unacceptably high diastolic pressures (diastolic blood pressure greater than 105 mm Hg). For these patients, consider the following:

1. *Poor adherence to drug regimen.* Nonadherence to drug therapy is probably the major cause of poor blood pressure control. An estimated 50% of patients take less than 80% of their prescribed antihypertensive pills (see below).
2. *Sodium retention.* Patients who take one or more nondiuretic antihypertensive agents often have reflex sodium retention. Adding a diuretic (or using a more potent one) and reemphasizing the need for a low-sodium diet may improve blood pressure control.
3. *Excessive alcohol intake.* If the hypertensive patient has a substantial alcohol intake, physicians should encourage total abstention from alcohol for four to six weeks while monitoring changes in blood pressure.
4. *Secondary hypertension.* Refer to the previous section on secondary hypertension for screening evaluations.
5. *Other drugs.* The patient's use of prescription and nonprescription medications should be carefully reviewed. Corticosteroids, amphetamines, sympathomimetics, and birth control pills may exacerbate hypertension. *NSAIDs* may promote sodium retention and blunt the antihypertensive effect of diuretics. Tricyclic antidepressants interact with a number of antihypertensive agents to reduce their potency.
6. *Inadequate drug dosage.* Most drugs (except reserpine) can be prescribed in dosages greater than those outlined in Table 8-2 without intolerable side effects. Consider increasing the dosage of a drug that has caused some blood pressure lowering.
7. *Substitute more potent antihypertensive agents.* For example, substitute minoxidil or an ACE inhibitor for hydralazine.

Side effects are sometimes unavoidable. Physicians should negotiate with patients, choosing a combination of drugs that is effective but that minimizes bothersome side effects. Patients should understand that some side effects (e.g., postural hypotension) are not serious and can be minimized by standing up slowly.

Close observation is essential for patients with resistant hypertension. Physicians should evaluate these patients for causes of secondary hypertension and carefully monitor the drug regimen and diet. Some patients require hospitalization to control their blood pressure. Most patients experience a fall of 5 to 15 mm Hg in diastolic blood pressure during hospitalization, but this does not necessarily reflect increased drug effect. Occasionally, poor adherence can be diagnosed if there is a substantial blood pressure fall to almost hypotensive levels when the patient is hospitalized and continued on the prescribed medication.

## NONCOMPLIANCE WITH TREATMENT

Diagnosing poor compliance can be difficult and requires a frank, nonjudgmental exploration with the patient about pill-taking habits. Physicians may preface this discussion by acknowledging that pills are expensive, symbolic of illness, sometimes accompanied by unpleasant side effects, and, for many people, including physicians, difficult to take as prescribed. Another helpful approach is to identify the time of day when the patient takes medications and to review the exact number of pills taken during the previous 24 hours.

Compliance may be assessed clinically or biochemically because some antihypertensive agents cause predictable physiologic effects. For example, β-blockers consistently decrease pulse, and thiazide diuretics consistently increase uric acid and usually decrease serum potassium. When a patient is taking one of these agents, compliance can be assessed by these secondary effects. Occasionally, measuring serum (propranolol) or urine (methyldopa) drug levels can be used to diagnose adherence.

The following are methods to improve adherence for noncompliant patients.

1. *Encourage the patient to report side effects.* Acknowledge that unpleasant side effects can occur during drug therapy and select an acceptable treatment regimen. Ask patients specifically about side effects they may be reluctant to voluntarily discuss, such as sexual dysfunction or the expense of treatment.
2. *Simplify the drug regimen.* Ask if once-a-day therapy would be easier than twice-a-day treatment. Be satisfied with adequate blood pressure control with a simple regimen rather than perfect control with a complex regimen.
3. *Try to give consistent, unchanging drug treatment.* Frequent changes of dosage and/or medicine may confuse and frustrate the patient.
4. *Provide simple, written instructions about dosage and side effects.* Review pill-taking habits with the patient. Recommend keeping pill bottles in a convenient location and emphasize the need to take pills at set times.
5. *Educate patients.* Discuss in a nonthreatening way the consequences of high blood pressure and the benefits of treatment. Emphasize that treating high blood pressure does not generally make patients feel better but, rather, is designed to prevent morbidity and mortality.
6. *Improve the convenience of office visits.* Sending appointment reminders, having flexible scheduling hours, and contacting patients who have missed appointments helps to improve adherence. However,

it is important to emphasize to patients that high blood pressure may be a lifelong problem and that they are responsible for returning for follow-up appointments and promptly refilling their medication. The physician's task is to be available with advice and assistance. Giving the patient responsibility for treatment is better than the physician cajoling or scolding the patient into complying with antihypertensive therapy.

## SYSTOLIC HYPERTENSION

The JNC defines isolated systolic hypertension as a systolic pressure greater than 160 mm Hg when diastolic pressure is less than 90 mm Hg. Isolated systolic hypertension is clearly a risk for morbidity and mortality. Isolated systolic hypertension in a young person is often seen in the setting of a hyperkinetic circulation with a rapid heart rate, increased cardiac output, and normal peripheral vascular resistance. Nonpharmacologic therapy, including diet, exercise, and stress reduction, is used as the first approach to treatment. Home measurement of blood pressure may show normal systolic readings, in contrast with measurement during office visits. Treatment is indicated for those who fit the criteria of Table 8-3. If systolic hypertension persists, diuretics or β-blockers may be given. Treating isolated systolic hypertension is inappropriate for patients who have a physiologic cause for high stroke volume. For example, patients with chronic anemia or aortic insufficiency should not be treated for systolic hypertension.

The prevalence of isolated systolic hypertension is greater in the elderly, approaching 25% in patients over 75 years of age. Low dosages of diuretics and clonidine, hydralazine, or methyldopa can be used to reduce systolic pressure with few side effects. The treatment goal for systolic hypertension is a 10% reduction in systolic blood pressure with therapy adjusted to minimize side effects.

## HYPERTENSION IN OLDER PATIENTS

Hypertension in older patients can be classified as either systolic hypertension (systolic blood pressure greater than or equal to 140 mm Hg, diastolic blood pressure less than 90 mm Hg) or diastolic hypertension (diastolic blood pressure greater than or equal to 90 mm Hg). The elderly patient with systolic hypertension usually has decreased vascular elasticity, lower cardiac output, lower ejection fraction, lower plasma volume, and increased peripheral vascular resistance compared with normotensive, age-matched subjects. Older patients with diastolic hypertension are similar to their younger counterparts with essential hypertension, but are more prone to atherosclerosis and renal artery stenosis.

Several studies show a benefit to treating hypertension in the elderly, including the Systolic Hypertension in the Elderly Program (SHEP), STOP-Hypertension, and the EWPHE (see Epidemiology). Many studies report that older patients tolerate antihypertensive therapy with minimal side effects. Orthostatic hypotension increases with age, so elderly patients on antihypertensive therapy should be monitored with supine and standing pressures and questioned about positional symptoms. Additionally, there is a high prevalence of subclinical congestive heart failure and chronic lung disease in elderly patients, making the use of β-blockers potentially risky. Because slight changes in function and mentation can produce substantial changes in the elderly patient's quality of life, side effects of antihypertensive therapy must be monitored very closely. A goal diastolic blood pressure of 95 to 100 mm Hg is often acceptable, especially if further therapy produces side effects. Drugs are started at very low dosages and titrated slowly until a stable dosage is reached.

Although many of the studies of hypertension in the elderly have used diuretics, there are other effective agents. The once-a-day calcium antagonists (although expensive) have limited side effects and may have additional advantages for hypertensive patients with cardiac hypertrophy. ACE inhibitors may be somewhat less effective than diuretics and calcium channel blockers (Table 8-4).

**Table 8-3.** Hypertension criteria

| Blood pressure (mm Hg) | Category |
|---|---|
| **Diastolic** | |
| <85 | Normal |
| 85-89 | High normal |
| 90-104 | Mild hypertension |
| 105-114 | Moderate hypertension |
| >114 | Severe hypertension |
| **If diastolic is <90 mm Hg** | |
| **Systolic** | |
| <140 | Normal |
| 140-159 | Borderline systolic hypertension |
| >160 | Isolated systolic hypertension |

Modified from *Hypertension* 7:460, 1985.

## HYPERTENSION IN PATIENTS WITH OTHER MEDICAL CONDITIONS

### Cerebrovascular disease

Therapy for high blood pressure in patients with a history of cerebrovascular disease reduces the incidence of initial and recurrent stroke and decreases the morbidity and mortality from other complications of hypertension. The presence of cerebrovascular disease is not a contraindication to antihypertensive therapy.

The cerebral blood vessels are acutely responsive to pressure changes and can adjust, through autoregulation, down to a mean pressure level of 60 mm Hg. Below this level, cerebral flow decreases and the brain is exposed to hypoxia. When diastolic blood pressure exceeds an upper threshold of 140 mm Hg, cerebral blood flow increases and may progress to hypertensive encephalopathy.

The chronically hypertensive patient develops increased resistance to autoregulation and may manifest symptoms at mean pressures above 60 mm Hg. Autoregulation is believed to readapt over time when the hypertension is treated. In light of these findings, the goal of treatment is unchanged, but therapy is instituted slowly, with particular attention to avoiding orthostatic hypotension.

**Table 8-4.** Treatment for subsets of hypertension

| Patient group | Recommended drugs | Alternative drugs | Contraindicated relative or absolute |
|---|---|---|---|
| Elderly | Calcium blockers<br>Diuretics<br>Clonidine | ACE inhibitors<br>Hydralazine<br>Aldomet | α-β-blocker<br>Guanethidine<br>$\alpha_1$-receptor blockers |
| Race: African-American | Diuretics<br>Calcium blockers<br>Clonidine<br>α-β-blocker<br>$\alpha_1$-receptor blockers | Methyldopa<br>Reserpine<br>Vasodilators<br>ACE inhibitors | |
| Coronary artery disease | β-blockers (avoid ISA)<br>Calcium blockers<br>Clonidine | ACE inhibitors<br>Diuretics<br>Methyldopa<br>$\alpha_1$-receptor blockers | Hydralazine<br>Minoxidil<br>Guanethidine |
| Congestive heart failure | ACE inhibitors<br>Diuretics<br>Hydralazine<br>$\alpha_1$-receptor blockers | Nifedipine<br>Diltiazem<br>Central $\alpha_2$ agonists | Verapamil<br>β-blockers<br>Reserpine<br>Guanethidine |
| Peripheral vascular disease | Calcium blockers<br>ACE inhibitors<br>Vasodilators<br>$\alpha_1$-receptor blockers | Diuretics<br>Central $\alpha_2$ agonists<br>Reserpine | β-blockers |
| Chronic renal insufficiency | Diuretics (loop)<br>ACE inhibitors<br>Central $\alpha_2$ agonists | Vasodilators<br>$\alpha_1$-receptor blockers | Diuretics (potassium sparing) |
| Diabetes | ACE inhibitors<br>Clonidine | Calcium blockers<br>Vasodilators | β-blockers<br>Diuretics<br>$\alpha_1$-receptor blockers |
| Dyslipidemia | $\alpha_1$-receptor blockers<br>Central $\alpha_2$ agonists | Calcium blockers<br>ACE inhibitors | Diuretics<br>β-blockers |
| Chronic airway disease | | | β-blockers<br>α-β-blocker |
| Gout | | | Diuretics |
| Pregnancy | Hydralazine<br>Thiazides<br>Methyldopa<br>β-blockers<br>β-blockers | | ACE inhibitors |
| Lactation | Propranolol<br>Timolol<br>ACE inhibitors | | Diuretics |
| Hypertrophic cardiomyopathy | β-blockers<br>Calcium blockers | | ACE inhibitors<br>Vasodilators<br>$\alpha_1$-receptor blockers<br>Diuretics |

### Left ventricular hypertrophy

These patients frequently have diastolic dysfunction and may benefit from a calcium channel blocker. They need to be closely monitored for signs of congestive heart failure and renal failure.

### Diabetes mellitus

Patients with diabetes mellitus and high blood pressure are at substantial risk for the macrovascular complications of high blood pressure and the microvascular complications of diabetes. Even mild hypertension is treated aggressively in patients with diabetes.

ACE inhibitors are now emerging as the initial therapy because they may reverse or improve diabetic nephropathy. When using ACE inhibitors, proteinuria and creatinine clearance should be carefully monitored following any change in therapy.

Diuretics may exacerbate glucose intolerance in diabetic patients who are controlled with diet or oral agents. β-blockers may interfere with counterregulatory responses to hypoglycemia and mask or prolong hypoglycemic attacks. β-blockers also aggravate the symptoms of peripheral vascular disease. Nevertheless, diuretics and β-blockers are frequently used with great caution for patients with diabetes.

### Renal disease

Hypertension in patients with renal disease is often very responsive to sodium intake and volume status. For patients with a creatinine greater than 2.5 mg/dl or a creatinine clearance less than 30 ml/min, thiazide diuretics may not induce sufficient diuresis to lower blood pressure. A more potent loop diuretic, such as furosemide, bumetanide, ethacrynic acid, or metolazone is usually needed. Overdiuresis may worsen azotemia, although lowering blood pressure to less than 90 mm Hg does not usually exacerbate renal failure. The usual antihypertensive agents are effective in treating high blood pressure for patients with renal disease. Those with renal disease and severe hypertension may need minoxidil if they are unresponsive to hydralazine. As renal failure worsens, a multiple-drug regimen is often needed to control hypertension.

Hypertension is a significant factor in the further decline of renal function in those with existing renal disease. Adequate control of hypertension slows the rate of decline in renal function and prevents its secondary manifestations.

### Dialysis patients

Eighty percent of hypertensive renal patients who undergo dialysis have a decreased need for antihypertensive medication. In the remainder, blood pressure control may remain difficult to achieve. More frequent dialysis or an increase in ultrafiltration may help, but medication often must be increased. A rare patient may require nephrectomy due to poor blood pressure control.

### Renal transplantation

Controlling hypertension in a renal-transplant patient is imperative and often difficult. Regulating volume status and secondary medication effects (e.g., those from prednisone and cyclosporine) can be challenging. Removing the native kidneys may help to control blood pressure. In addition to carefully adjusting steroid and cyclosporine dosages, diuretics may help to restore pressure to normal. Persistent high pressure may indicate arterial stenosis in the transplant. ACE inhibitors should probably be avoided in this setting due to the risk of reducing renal perfusion pressures.

### Surgery

Surgery is usually safe and need not be postponed for patients with hypertension (see detailed review in Chapter 5).

### Pregnancy

Thiazide diuretics, methyldopa, and hydralazine have been widely used to treat hypertension during pregnancy. More recent experience with propranolol and labetalol shows that they are probably also well tolerated. They have no serious adverse effects on the fetus, although there is a concern about decreasing placental blood flow. Hypertensive patients who wish to become pregnant should probably be treated with the above agents. Antihypertensive agents that have not been approved for pregnancy should be avoided. New drugs, such as ACE inhibitors and calcium channel blockers, should not be used because their effects on the human fetus are unknown and animal data show fetal deaths.

Blood pressure during early pregnancy is normally low, often less than 110/75 mm Hg. Blood pressures greater than 140/90 mm Hg that develop after 26 weeks of pregnancy and are accompanied by edema and proteinuria indicate preeclampsia (see Chapter 147). Treatment includes bed rest, hospitalization, and, if necessary, drug therapy (diuretics and salt restriction are best avoided). Elevations of blood pressure that occur earlier in pregnancy may represent an exacerbation of previously undiagnosed essential hypertension or another underlying illness. The physician should search for acute illness, such as glomerulonephritis. Treatment includes bed rest, antihypertensive drug therapy, and hospitalization. (Preeclampsia/eclampsia and hypertension that complicate pregnancy are discussed in Chapter 147.)

***Lactation.*** Choosing a postpartum antihypertensive drug depends on whether the woman wishes to breastfeed. There are limited data on the appearance of medication in breast milk, but propranolol, timolol, and captopril seem to be safe. Diuretics should be avoided because they decrease the production of breast milk.

## BIBLIOGRAPHY

Amery A et al: Mortality and morbidity results from the European Working Party on High Blood Pressure in the Elderly trial, *Lancet* 1:1349, 1985.

Collins R et al: Blood pressure, stroke, and coronary heart disease. Part 2, short-term reductions in blood pressure: overview of randomised drug trials in their epidemiologic context, *Lancet* 335:827, 1990.

Dahlöf B et al: Morbidity and mortality in the Swedish trial in old patients with hypertension (STOP-Hypertension), *Lancet* 338:1281, 1991.

Davis PJ: Hypertension. In Greene HL, Johnson WP, Maricic MJ, editors: Decision making in medicine, St. Louis, 1993, Mosby–Year Book.

High blood pressure in medicine. In Rubenstein, Federman, editors: *Scientific American,* 1, 1993.

Hypertension Detection and Follow-up Program Cooperative Group: Five-year findings of the Hypertension Detection and Follow-up Program. I. Reduction in mortality of persons with high blood pressure, including mild hypertension, *JAMA* 242:2562, 1979.

Lilly LS, editor: *Hypertension in pathophysiology of heart disease.* Philadelphia, 1993, Lea & Febiger.

Kaplan NM: Arterial hypertension. In Stein JH et al, editors: *Internal Medicine,* ed 4, St. Louis, 1994, Mosby–Year Book.

The Management Committee: Australian therapeutic trial in mild hypertension, *Lancet* 1:1261, 1980.

Mangrulkar RS, Nigrovic PA, Moore TJ: Hypertension. In Lilly LS, editor: *Hypertension in pathophysiology of heart disease,* Philadelphia, 1993, Lea & Febiger.

Materson BJ et al: Single-drug therapy for hypertension in men. A comparison of six antihypertensive agents with placebo, *N Engl J Med* 328:914, 1993.

Medical Research Council Working Party: MRC trial of treatment of mild hypertension: principal results, *Br Med J* 291:97, 1985.

Medical Research Council Working Party: Medical Research Council trial of treatment of hypertension in older adults: principal results, *Br Med J* 304:405, 1992.

Multiple Risk Factor Intervention Trial Research Group: Multiple risk factor intervention trial. Risk factor changes and mortality results, *JAMA* 248:1465, 1982.

National High Blood Pressure Education Program: The fifth report of the Joint National Committee on Detection, Evaluation, and Treatment of High Blood Pressure, *Arch Intern Med* 153:154, 1993.

Neaton JD et al: Treatment of mild hypertension study. Final results, *JAMA* 270:713, 1993.

SHEP Cooperative Research Group: Prevention of stroke by antihypertensive drug treatment in older persons with isolated systolic hypertension. Final results of the systolic hypertension in the elderly program (SHEP), *JAMA* 265:3255, 1991.

Veterans Administration Cooperative Study Group on Antihypertensive Agents: Effects of treatment on morbidity in hypertension. Results in patients with diastolic blood pressure averaging 115 through 129 mm Hg, *JAMA* 202:116, 1967.

Veterans Administration Cooperative Study Group on Antihypertensive Agents: Effects of treatment on morbidity in hypertension. II. Results in patients with diastolic blood pressure averaging 90 through 114 mm Hg, *JAMA* 213:1143, 1970.

CHAPTER

# 9 Arrhythmias

**Anthony C. Caruso**

The prompt diagnosis and proper management of cardiac arrhythmias require a thorough history and physical examination as well as careful attention to the clinical electrocardiogram (ECG). The presenting symptom or chief complaint of a patient's arrhythmia may be palpitations, chest discomfort, dyspnea, some dizziness, or syncope. Some patients may suffer sudden cardiac death. In the patient who has palpitations or a feeling of cardiac irregularity it is essential that a careful history be obtained, including evaluation of chest pains, dyspnea, and other symptoms of myocardial ischemia. The circumstances surrounding the events and whether these events are predictable should be determined. A thorough assessment of the patient's intake of caffeine and other stimulant beverages, alcohol, and nonprescription drugs is very important. A careful family history regarding cardiac disease, endocrine disorders, and sudden death is indicated. The review of systems should include careful assessment for pulmonary disease as well as endocrine disorders, especially thyroid dysfunction.

In patients with a history of hypertension, anxiety, or flushing, pheochromocytoma should be considered. In patients who experience palpitations that are not associated with dizziness or hemodynamic compromise, an outpatient evaluation beginning with a Holter monitor is reasonable. In patients with known coronary artery disease or structural heart disease who have symptoms of hemodynamic instability, an inpatient evaluation is often prudent. Physical examination of patients with heart rhythm disturbances should include orthostatic vital signs, careful thyroid examination, and close attention to the cardiopulmonary examination. The evaluation is completed by review of ancillary tests, which must always include a 12-lead ECG. Baseline chemistries and an assessment of thyroid function are part of the workup. Data regarding the presence or absence of structural heart disease are helpful, and an echocardiogram is reasonable.

Holter monitoring is quite helpful when the patient's rhythm disturbance occurs frequently or is predictable. It is extremely important to emphasize that the patient use the diary that accompanies this device. The value of correlating the patient's symptoms with the subsequent recordings cannot be overemphasized. In those patients whose symptoms are infrequent and not predictable, the use of an event monitor is appropriate.

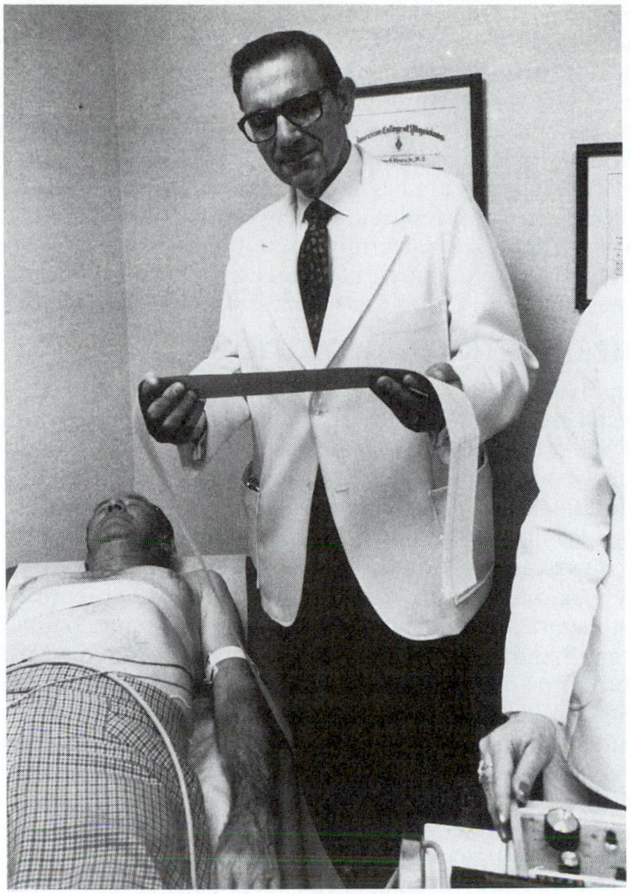

**Fig. 9-1.** From ACP Archives.

Although a detailed review of the mechanisms of rhythm disturbances is beyond the scope of this discussion, it is appropriate to review some general principles. Almost all rhythm disturbances are a function of enhanced automaticity, reentry, or combination of these two phenomena. Ectopic atrial tachycardia, multifocal atrial tachycardia, and accelerated junctional rhythm are all examples of abnormal automaticity. These rhythm disturbances involve activation of latent pacemaker cells in various regions of the heart. These regions typically include the inferior right atrium at the junction with the inferior vena cava, the atrioventricular (AV) junction, the His bundle and the Purkinje fibers, and the ventricle. The reentrant supraventricular tachycardias (AV nodal reentrant tachycardia, Wolff-Parkinson-White [WPW] syndrome) and ventricular tachycardia are typical examples of reentrant phenomena. In ventricular tachycardia the myocardium adjacent to the area of the scar allows the action potential to pass through slowly. This area of slow conduction permits the action potential to escape back in to depolarized myocardium, which can then accept the action potential and complete the reentry circuit. Antiarrhythmic therapy is aimed at suppressing the abnormal focus or changing the relationship between the area of normal conduction. Understanding the components of the reentry loop allows for more precise therapies, such as in catheter-directed ablation of WPW syndrome. Each of the important rhythm disturbances to be described is accompanied by recommendations for acute and long-term therapy with the mechanisms of each of these dysrhythmias kept clearly in mind.

To facilitate diagnosis and proper management of patients with cardiac arrhythmias, this discussion is divided into three areas: obvious supraventricular tachycardias, obvious ventricular tachycardias, and wide QRS tachycardias of undetermined etiology. Common tachycardias in each of these categories are discussed along with their acute and chronic management.

## SUPRAVENTRICULAR TACHYCARDIAS

Supraventricular tachycardias are a diverse group of tachycardias including everything from sinus tachycardia to WPW syndrome. These usually benign rhythm disturbances occasionally can be associated with hemodynamic consequences and in rare cases may be life threatening (e.g., atrial fibrillation in WPW syndrome).

Supraventricular tachycardias can be divided into those tachycardias that are regular, of which reentrant paroxysmal supraventricular tachycardias are the predominant group, and those that are irregular, of which atrial fibrillation is clearly the most common. Irregularity of the tachycardia is often very useful in therapy triage for a patient with narrow complex tachycardia. Once the irregularity or its absence is determined, careful analysis of atrial activity usually clarifies the etiology of most narrow QRS complex tachycardias. If careful analysis of the 12-lead ECG fails to characterize the rhythm disturbance, the use of vagal maneuvers can be very useful. Table 9-1 provides a summary of regular tachycardias that can be discriminated by the surface ECG. The use of an esophageal probe is often helpful in determining atrial activity, and this can usually be accomplished quickly even in the patient in whom a supraventricular etiology is suspected with wide QRS complex tachycardia.

### Regular supraventricular tachycardias

***AV nodal reentrant tachycardia.*** Paroxysmal supraventricular tachycardia is a narrow complex tachycardia in which P waves, if at all visible, follow the QRS complex rather than precede it. AV nodal reentrant tachycardia is the most common form of paroxysmal supraventricular tachycardia in the older population. When atrial fibrillation and atrial flutter are excluded, this form of supraventricular tachycardia represents about 50% of all described supraventricular rhythm disturbances. Dual AV node conduction is necessary for AV nodal reentrant tachycardia. The mechanism of this rhythm disturbance has in the past been simplified to imply a slow and a fast pathway within the confines of the AV node. Recent data suggest that this is not the case and that the slow and fast pathways include not only AV nodal tissue but also adjacent perinodal atrial tissue. In either model the AV node is an integral part of the reentry circuit and provides an important key to the treatment of this rhythm disturbance. AV nodal reentrant tachycardia is of two types, the slow-fast sequence being more common and occurring in 90% of patients. In this situation electrical impulses are conducted from the atrium to the ventricle via a slow pathway and return via the AV node to the atrium over a fast pathway. In the second form or uncommon type of AV node reentrant tachycardia, conduction from the atrium to the ventricle occurs over the fast AV nodal pathway with reentry to the atrium by way of the slow pathway. The reentrant rhythm can be initiated by an atrial or ventricular premature complex, which results in a reentry loop involving the AV node and the perinodal atrial tissue (Fig. 9-2). Therapy of this rhythm disturbance is primarily via AV node blocking agents such as digitalis, calcium channel blockers (verapamil), β-blockers, and class I antiarrhythmic agents. At this time flecainide is the only agent approved for treatment of paroxysmal supraventricular tachycardias in patients without evidence of structural heart disease. As with accessory pathway–mediated tachycardias (to be discussed later), AV nodal reentrant tachycardia is amenable to catheter-directed ablative therapy. In women of childbearing years or in patients who have had unsuccessful trials of antiarrhythmic therapy, catheter-directed modification of the slow pathway is indicated. This procedure carries a 1% to 8%

**Table 9-1.** Electrocardiographic clues to differentiation of supraventricular tachycardia

| Classification | QRS complex | Rate (beats/min) | Configuration P wave in lead II | Comments |
|---|---|---|---|---|
| Sinus nodal reentrant tachycardia | Narrow | 100-160 | Precedes QRS; same morphology as in sinus rhythm | Differentiated from sinus tachycardia by abrupt onset and termination |
| Ectopic atrial tachycardia | Narrow | 100-180 | Precedes QRS; upright or inverted; gradual increase in rate | Onset with premature atrial beat late in diastole |
| AV nodal reentrant tachycardia (common type) | Narrow | 140-220 | Inverted; usually not seen on ECG | May terminate with CSM |
| AV nodal reentrant tachycardia (uncommon type) | Narrow | 100-250 | Inverted; appears late with long R-P interval | May terminate with CSM |
| Orthodromic reciprocating AV tachycardia | Narrow | 150-240 | Inverted; appears after QRS complex, with short R-P interval | AV block excludes this diagnosis |

*CSM*, Carotid sinus massage; *ECG*, electrocardiogram; *AV*, atrioventricular.

risk of complete heart block with an overall success rate of over 90%.

A sequella of supraventricular tachycardia may be the post-tachycardia T-wave syndrome (Fig. 9-3).

The acute treatment of AV nodal reentrant tachycardia and WPW syndrome is similar. Vagal maneuvers such as carotid sinus massage and Valsalva's maneuver are often successful in terminating either of these causes of paroxysmal supraventricular tachycardia. When these approaches fail, the use of verapamil or adenosine is the next logical step. Both agents are equally efficacious. Adenosine has a much shorter half-life and is the preferred therapy for this reason. Of particular concern is the use of verapamil in patients with a history of atrial fibrillation and WPW syndrome or in a situation where wide QRS complex tachycardia is found and presumed to be of supraventricular origin. Because of the hypotension due to the negative inotropic effects of verapamil and its half-life of 4 to 7 hours when administered intravenously, the use of this agent in wide QRS complex tachycardias of undetermined origin is contraindicated. The administration of verapamil to patients with a suspected supraventricular etiology for a wide QRS complex tachycardia can be catastrophic.

Adenosine is a naturally occurring substance with numerous cardiac effects. It is rapidly metabolized by blood elements and vascular endothelium, with rapid cellular uptake and subsequent conversion to an inactive metabolite. Adenosine has a half-life of less than 1 second in whole blood and is completely cleared from the plasma within 30 seconds. Although adverse effects from adenosine are relatively common, they are minor and transient. Flushing, dyspnea, and chest discomfort are the most common adverse effects. Of note is the interaction of adenosine with theophylline and other methyl xanthines that competitively bind the same receptor used by adenosine. Consequently, higher doses of adenosine are necessary in patients on chronic theophylline or methylxanthine therapy. Conversely a reduced dose may be necessary in patients receiving dipyridamole, an agent that inhibits the metabolism of adenosine.

***WPW syndrome and accessory pathway-mediated tachycardias.*** WPW syndrome (Fig. 9-4) is characterized by a short PR interval with preexcitation in the form of a delta wave, a wide QRS, and associated T wave abnormalities (repolarization changes) in a patient with symptomatic palpitations. Many patients with AV nodal reentrant tachycardia have what is called concealed conduction; nevertheless, they use an accessory pathway as the retrograde limb of the reentry circuit. Orthodromic AV nodal reentrant tachycardia is the cause of supraventricular tachycardia in about 50% of our younger patients. In orthodromic AV nodal reentrant tachycardia the reentrant circuit consists of the atrium, the AV node, the His-Purkinje system, the ventricle, and the accessory pathway. In the past, accessory pathways were thought to represent specialized conduction tissue, but this is not the case. The accessory pathway represents the absence of the normal fibrocartilaginous skeleton of the AV ring and in essence represents the absence of the normal insulation between the atrium and the ventricle. In patients with a preexcitation (delta wave), antegrade conduction exists that allows a portion of the ventricle to depolarize prematurely. The larger the area of early activation, the more dramatic is the delta wave.

In patients with a concealed accessory pathway there is only retrograde conduction across the accessory pathway; there is no delta wave, and the resting ECG is usually completely normal. In this setting the etiology of paroxysmal supraventricular tachycardia may be confused with

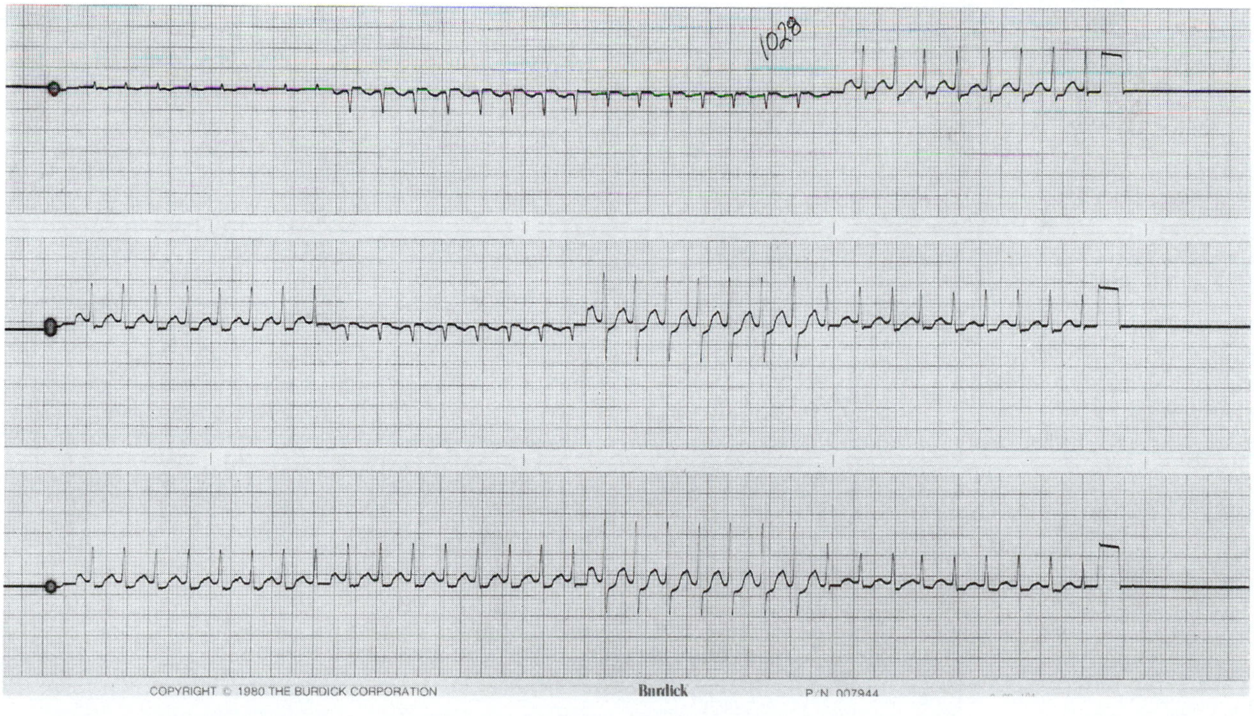


**Fig. 9-2.** Paroxysmal supraventricular tachycardia resulting from a concealed left-sided accessory pathway in a 32-year-old woman.

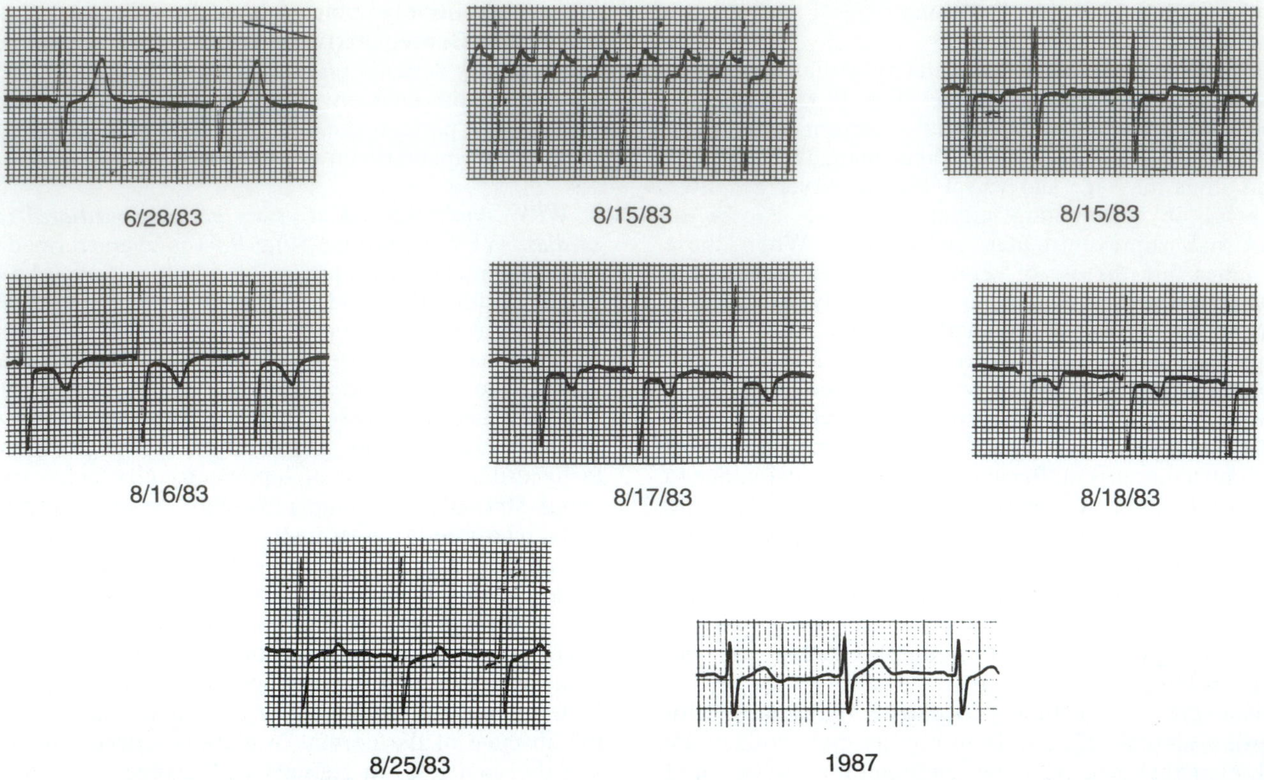


**Fig. 9-3.** Post-tachycardia T-Wave syndrome. Serial ECGS (lead $V_4$) in 67-year-old man taking digoxin for PSVT. An ECG obtained on June 28, 1983, showed no abnormalities. About 6 weeks later on August 15, while awaiting surgery for peripheral vascular disease, patient had episode of PSVT (first ECG in second row) that responded to carotid-sinus massage. ECG shortly after conversion to sinus rhythm showed atrial premature beats and minor T-wave inversions (second ECG in second row), which became deeper over the next 24 hours (third ECG in second row). Patient was given verapamil 80 mg four times daily. Because of persistent T-wave inversions (recorded on August 17 and 18) he underwent cardiac catheterization and angiography, which revealed normal coronary arteries and normal left ventricular function. The T-wave abnormalities, which are those classically seen in the post-tachycardia syndrome, had decreased by August 25, and he underwent successful femoral-artery bypass surgery. Four years later, in 1987, his ECG had returned to normal. (From Katz AM: *Images in Clinical Medicine* 332(3):161, 1995.)

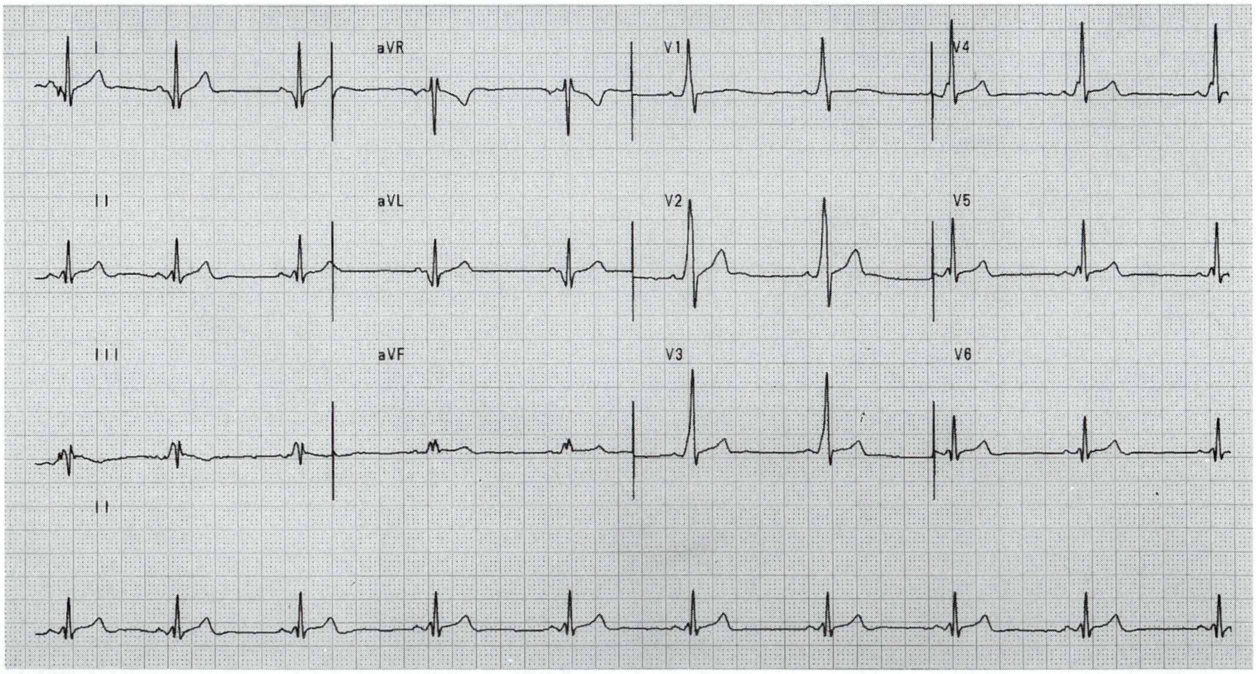


**Fig. 9-4.** Wolff-Parkinson-White syndrome. 17-year-old boy with history of syncope and classic preexcitation over a left-sided accessory pathway.

AV node reentry. Invasive electrophysiology studies are helpful in this regard but should be pursued only if the patient is being considered for ablation therapy. The medical therapy for AV nodal reentrant tachycardia is identical to that for the patient with concealed conduction over an accessory pathway. Clearly, fluctuations in autonomic tone can increase or decrease the amount of preexcitation. When a delta wave is suspected, the use of adenosine can transiently depress AV node conduction and allow greater excitation of the ventricle by way of the accessory pathway, thus accentuating the delta wave. As in AV nodal reentrant tachycardia, AV node depressing agents can be useful, but they can also be hazardous. If AV node suppression is induced and atrial fibrillation occurs, a 1:1 conduction across the accessory pathway can lead to ventricular fibrillation. This is the great risk for patients with antegrade conduction across an accessory pathway and why there is concern regarding sudden death in patients with WPW syndrome. To protect against this catastrophe the use of agents such as digitalis and verapamil is contraindicated in the presence of antegrade conduction in a patient with a history of atrial fibrillation. Many of the agents described for AV nodal reentrant tachycardia, such as β-blockers and class I agents (flecainide) can be used for the treatment of accessory pathway–mediated tachycardias.

Recent advances in catheter technology have permitted success in closed chested catheter ablation of the accessory pathway. Catheter ablation utilizing radiofrequency energy is relatively safe, efficacious, and cost effective, and it is now reasonable to consider catheter-directed therapy as the first-line approach to patients with symptomatic accessory pathway–mediated rhythm disturbances. This is especially true in women of childbearing years due to the potentially serious adverse effects of medical therapy to the unborn child as well as the hemodynamic consequences of rapid reentrant tachycardia.

***Atrial flutter.*** Although atrial flutter may present as an irregular tachycardia, it more commonly presents as a regular narrow QRS complex tachycardia. When a narrow QRS complex tachycardia at 150 beats/min is encountered, atrial flutter should always be considered. The classic sawtooth flutter waves are best observed in lead II, but in 2:1 flutter may be obscured by the T waves. Vagal maneuvers to slow ventricular response will unmask the flutter waves and allow for easy diagnosis.

Although carotid sinus massage and Valsalva's maneuver are traditionally used, an adjunct to unmasking flutter is the use of adenosine, which transiently depresses AV node conduction (Fig. 9-5). Acute therapy of atrial flutter utilizing β-blockers or verapamil is superior to digitalis therapy, since these agents may permit conversion to sinus rhythm in addition to slowing ventricular response. The use of AV node blocking agents should precede the initiation of class I agents. As in atrial fibrillation, DC cardioversion using synchronized shock may be performed. This therapy is usually effective, requires lower energy (25 to 50 J), and has a low risk of embolic stroke.

Atrial flutter is a complex rhythm disturbance with characteristics more consistent with intraatrial reentry than atrial fibrillation (Fig. 9-6). Consequently, in addition to the use of class I and class II antiarrhythmic agents, antitachycardia pacing has been demonstrated to be effective in the treatment of atrial flutter. In the acute setting transesophageal atrial pacing may be employed as an alternative to transvenous pacing. Indwelling permanent pacemakers with antitachycardia pacing capability (Intertach II) have been shown to be effective long-term therapy.

Recent advances in catheter-directed therapy have made atrial flutter amenable to treatment. Although investigational at this time, the use of radiofrequency ablation is likely to become a first line therapy. The acute therapy of atrial flutter involves the use of AV node depressing agents to control ventricular response. Of special concern with atrial flutter is the use of class I agents, which may slow the atrial rate, thus permitting 2:1 or 1:1 AV conduction and potentially leading to hemodynamic collapse. It is traditionally taught that drugs such as quinidine should not be initiated without first instituting digitalis or other AV node depressant therapy. This is also true of the class IC agents such as propafenone and flecainide. As in other atrial tachycardias, amiodarone is very effective in suppressing atrial flutter, but for this indication this drug is not approved by the FDA.

***Accelerated junctional rhythm.*** Accelerated junctional rhythm is a narrow complex tachycardia varying between 70 and 130 beats/min. This regular tachycardia is frequently seen following cardiovascular surgery, inferior myocardial infarction, digitalis intoxication, and myocarditis (Fig. 9-7). Therapy of this rhythm disturbance is directed at the underlying etiology; DC cardioversion has no benefit and should not be attempted.

***Ectopic atrial tachycardia.*** Ectopic atrial tachycardia is a narrow complex tachycardia in which a P wave precedes each QRS complex. This P wave is morphologically distinct from sinus P waves; however, each P wave is identical to those preceding and following it. The etiology of this rhythm disturbance is a competing ectopic focus within the atrium. Consequently, maneuvers that would depress the sinus or AV node are rarely successful in disrupting this rhythm disturbance. Verapamil and β-blockers are used acutely as well as long term. The chronic inhibition of this automatic focus may be achieved by class I antiarrhythmic agents. Although usually paroxysmal, ectopic atrial tachycardia may be chronic and is associated with the development of a cardiomyopathy. In recent years attempts at catheter ablation have shown promise, but this remains an investigational form of therapy.

***Sinus nodal reentrant tachycardia.*** Sinus nodal reentrant tachycardia is often indistinguishable from sinus tachycardia. This rhythm disturbance is due to reentry phenomena within the sinus node producing a rapid narrow complex tachycardia with P waves preceding each QRS. Each P wave is identical to the P waves of sinus nodal rhythm. The onset is abrupt, as is the termination, and this represents the key to its diagnosis. Verapamil and β-blockade represent the mainstays of both acute and long-term therapy, with class I antiarrhythmic agents being helpful when calcium channel blockers or β-blockers are unsuccessful. As in ectopic atrial tachycardia, catheter-directed therapies remain investigational for this rhythm disturbance.

A

B

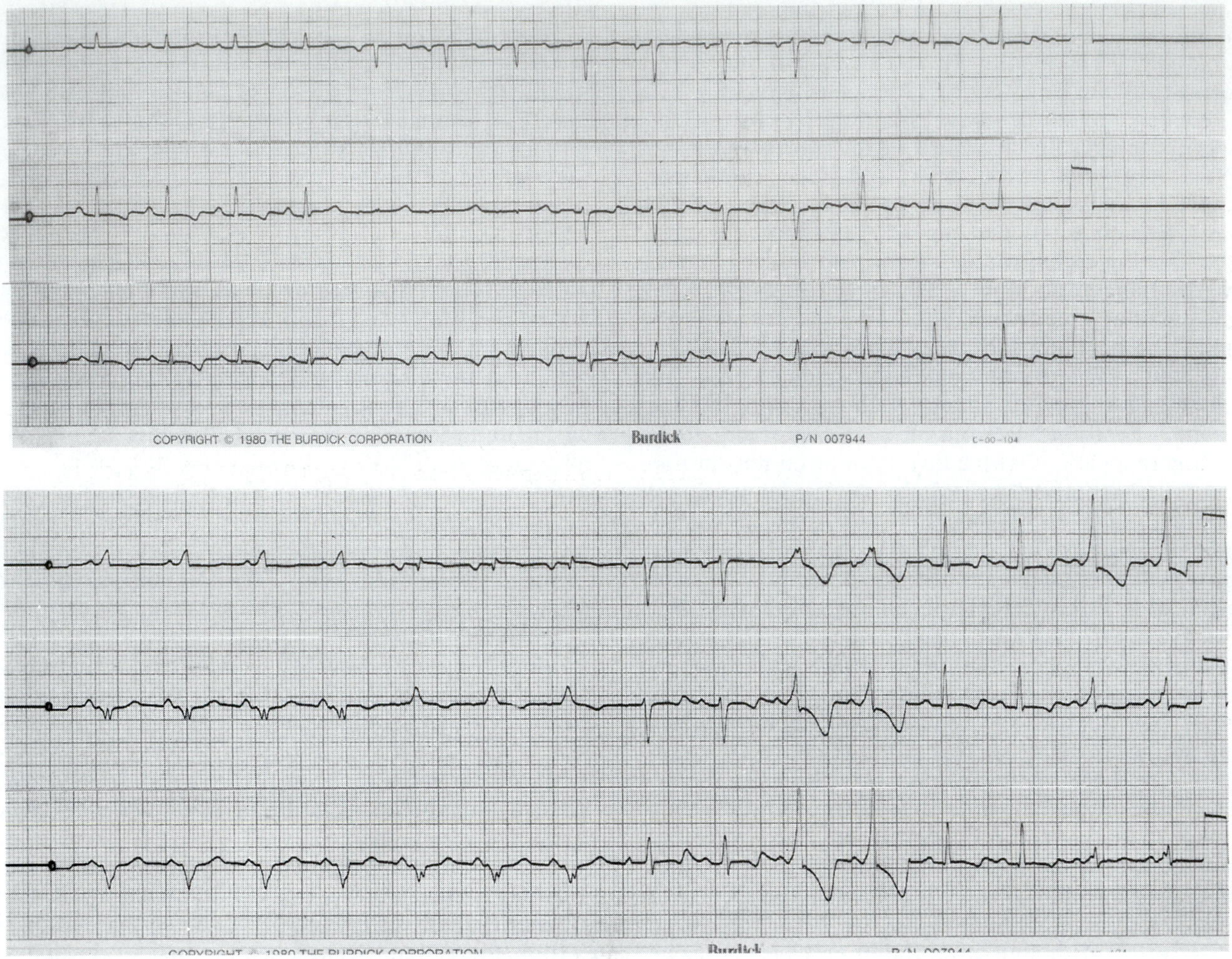


**Fig. 9-5. A,** Resting ECG of a 30-year-old woman with history of symptomatic narrow complex tachycardia. **B,** ECG of the same woman following administration of 6 mg adenosine, which unmasks a left posteroseptal accessory pathway.

## Irregular narrow complex tachycardias

***Atrial fibrillation.*** The irregular narrow QRS complex of atrial fibrillation is one of the most common rhythm disturbances seen in clinical practice. Atrial fibrillation occurs in 2% of patients over the age of 60, and in over 10% of patients age 70 and older. Though relatively common, atrial fibrillation is associated with significant morbidity even in the absence of valvular heart disease. Data from the Framingham study showed a fivefold increase in stroke and twofold increase in death. The etiologies of atrial fibrillation include hypertension, diabetes mellitus, coronary artery disease, and valvular heart disease, with mitral stenosis secondary to rheumatic fever being the most common coexistent valvular abnormality historically. Thyroid dysfunction should always be suspected, since 13% of patients with hyperthyroidism have lone atrial fibrillation. The acute therapy of atrial fibrillation involves control of ventricular response via digoxin, β-blockers, or calcium channel blocking agents. Hemodynamic instability due to rapid ventricular response should warrant prompt DC cardioversion (200 J). Digoxin is the most common method of controlling ventricular response. Adequate doses of this drug are often not utilized, resulting in a prolonged time between initiation of therapy and satisfactory rate control. Recommended management of acute atrial fibrillation with digoxin via an oral load is 9 µg/kg (lean body weight) with half the dose given initially, one fourth the dose given 4 to 6 hours later, and the remaining one fourth 6 to 12 hours later. Intravenous dosing is approximately 75% of the oral dosage, but the short-acting β-blockers and intravenous diltiazem are preferred.

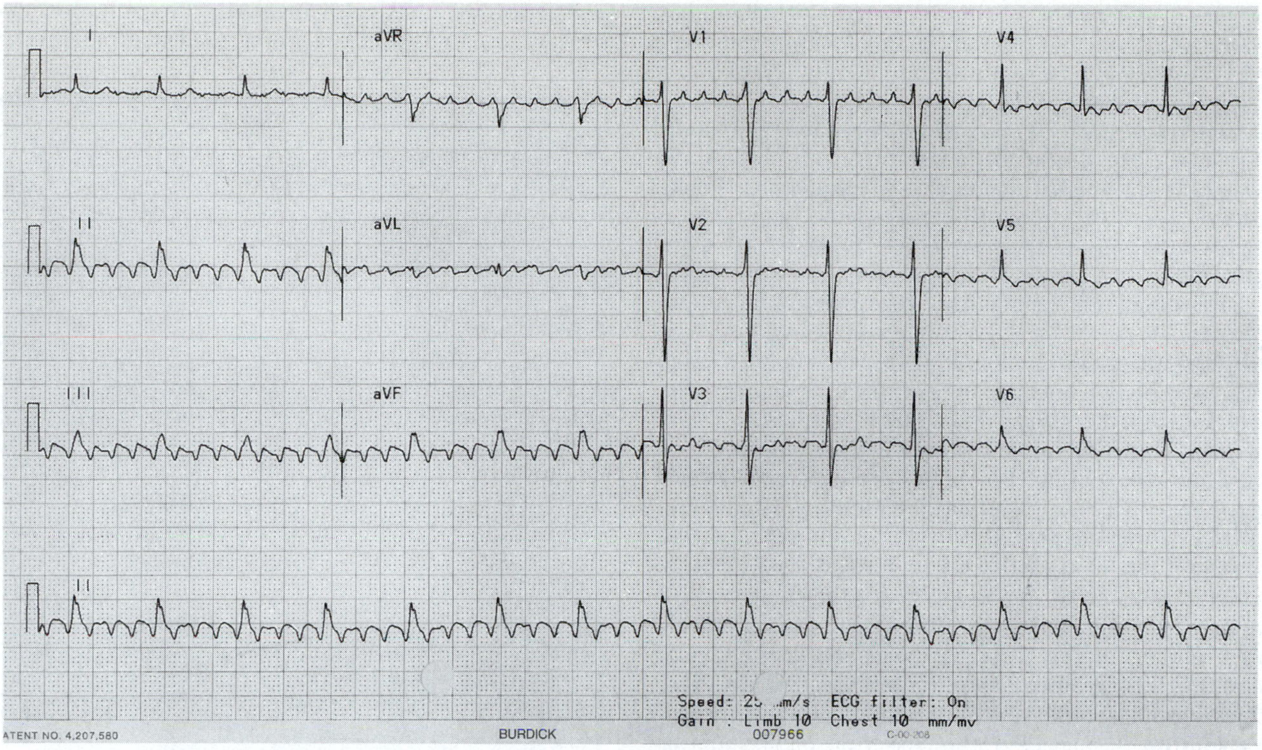


**Fig. 9-6.** Atrial flutter in a 50-year-old man with 4:1 AV conduction.

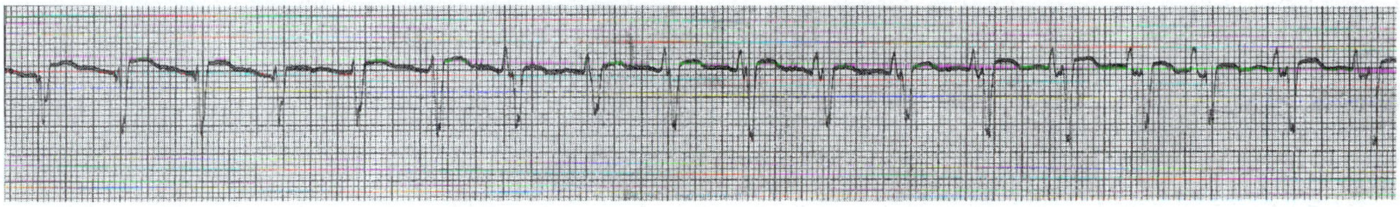

**Fig. 9-7.** Nonparoxysmal junctional tachycardia due to digoxin toxicity. The rate (105 beats/minute) approximates that of the sinus rate, and AV dissociation is initially present. In the latter half of the tracing, sinus rhythm emerges.

Although digitalis is useful in controlling ventricular response, it does not hasten the restoration of sinus rhythm and may actually prolong the episode of atrial fibrillation. The use of esmolol or other short-acting β-blockers is an effective management of rapid ventricular response to atrial fibrillation. The onset of action of esmolol is short; this allows easy titration due to its half-life of 9 minutes. Hypotension is predictably the most common adverse effect. Significant hypotension can be avoided by careful hemodynamic monitoring during intravenous administration. An alternative to esmolol is intravenous diltiazem, a short-acting agent with AV node blocking ability but without the undue hypotension associated with the agent esmolol.

An increased incidence of stroke and a progression to congestive heart failure is associated with chronic atrial fibrillation. An effort to restore sinus rhythm should be made in patients presenting with their first episode of atrial fibrillation. Due to the increased risk of an embolic event at the time of elective cardioversion we strongly recommend that patients undergo oral warfarin therapy for 2 to 3 weeks before and after elective cardioversion (INR 2.0-3.0). In dilated cardiomyopathy (Fig. 9-8) and left atrial enlargement greater than 4.5 cm only approximately 50% of patients remain in sinus rhythm 6 months after cardioversion when treated conventionally; however, more potent antiarrhythmic agents such as amiodarone significantly increase the number of patients who remain in sinus rhythm over time. The decision to utilize antiarrhythmic therapy for the maintenance of sinus rhythm must be made with the consideration of the possible proarrhythmic effect of the agent to be used. Coplen assessed six major trials involving 808 patients treated with quinidine for the maintenance of sinus rhythm after cardioversion. Although quinidine was clearly effective in maintaining sinus rhythm, it was associated with an increased total mortality. Criticism of this study has been made based on the fact that it was a retrospective analysis of a heterogeneous group of trials, many of which included uncontrolled digitalis use concurrent with the use of quinidine. Nevertheless, the risk of proarrhythmia is clearly present with the use of class I agents, and a careful risk/benefit assessment is warranted in each patient. Proarrhythmia is lowest in those patients without structural heart disease. All drugs that prolong the QT, including amiodarone and sotalol, carry the risk of proarrhythmia; however, this risk can be minimized by follow-up of electrolytes and avoidance of digitalis toxicity.

It is generally accepted that efforts to reduce the risk of embolic stroke are warranted in patients with chronic or paroxysmal atrial fibrillation. In patients under the age of 70 who are free from structural heart disease, aspirin is a reasonable alternative to coumadin. In patients with structural heart disease (e.g., mitral stenosis) anticoagulation with coumadin remains the therapy of choice.

*Multifocal atrial tachycardia.* Multifocal atrial tachycardia (Fig. 9-9) is an irregular supraventricular tachycardia characterized by the presence of three or more P wave morphologies with PP intervals that vary irregularly. This rhythm occurs most often in patients with chronic obstructive pulmonary disease or elderly patients treated with digoxin. In patients treated with digoxin multifocal atrial tachycardia is due to digoxin toxicity unless proven otherwise. In the absence of digoxin toxicity the treatment of the underlying pulmonary condition often is the most effective form of therapy. Verapamil may be given to patients with chronic obstructive pulmonary disease and multifocal atrial tachycardia. For patients in whom digoxin overdose is suspected, the cessation of digitalis is often all that is necessary, though use of Digibind may be helpful.

## WIDE QRS COMPLEX TACHYCARDIA

Wide QRS tachycardia represents one of the most challenging rhythm disturbances for the clinician. This rhythm disturbance may be either supraventricular with aberration or ventricular in origin. Preexcitation may be present. It is generally recommended that patients with a

### Classification of antiarrhythmic drugs

**Class I (block fast sodium channel)**

IA: Quinidine
Procanimide
Disopyramide
IB: Tocainide
Mexiletine
Phenytoin
IC: Flecainide
Propafenone

**Class II (block beta-adrenergic receptors)**

Propanolol
Metoprolol
Atenolol
Others

**Class III (block potassium channels and prolong repolarization)**

Bretylium
Amiodarone
Sotalol
NAPA

**Class IV (block slow calcium channel)**

Verapamil
Diltiazem

Adapted from Williams ES, Fisch C: Cardiac arrhythmias. In Stein JH, editor: *Internal medicine*, ed 4, St. Louis, 1994, Mosby.

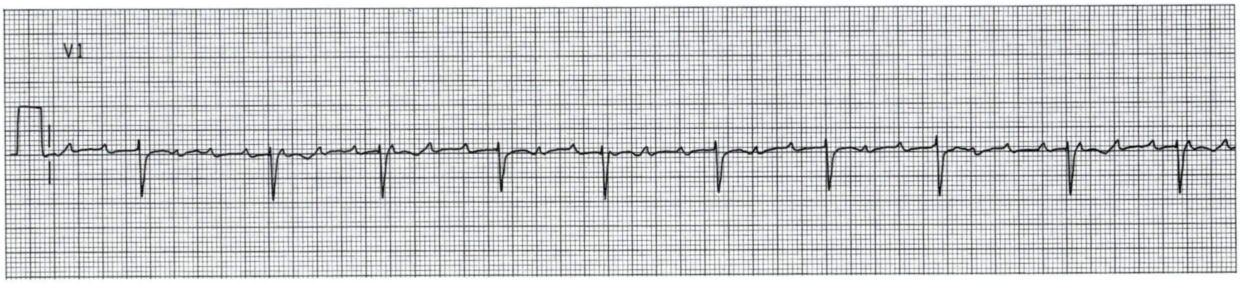


**Fig. 9-8.** Paroxysmal atrial tachycardia with variable block in a patient with dilated cardiomyopathy. The atrial rate is 200 beats/minute with a variable ventricular rate of 60 to 70 beats/minute.

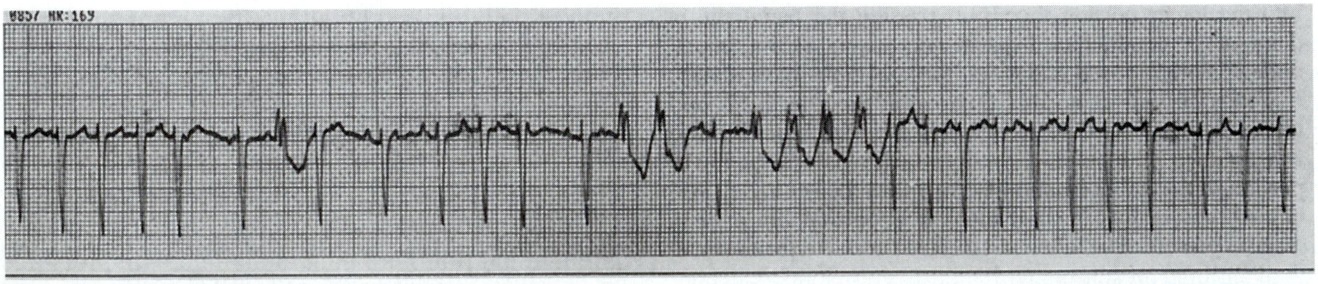

**Fig. 9-9.** Multifocal atrial tachycardia. Lead V1. There is an irregular rapid rhythm, suggesting atrial fibrillation. However, on close examination, P waves of differing morphology are seen to precede each QRS. Several beats are conducted aberrantly with a right bundle branch block configuration.

history of coronary artery disease and wide QRS tachycardia be considered to have ventricular tachycardia until proven otherwise. With that said and with the understanding that none of the ECG criteria commonly enjoy 100% specificity, there are some useful criteria to differentiate supraventricular tachycardia with aberration from a tachycardia of ventricular origin. Clearly, the most specific findings for ventricular tachycardia are the presence of capture beats or fusion beats. AV dissociation is also a strong marker for ventricular tachycardia, as is marked left axis deviation and QRS duration greater than 140 msec. The morphology in $V_1$ is also helpful. The monomorphic right bundle branch block QRS in $V_1$ almost always represents ventricular tachycardia. A small qR, QR, RS right bundle branch block pattern in $V_1$ is highly suggestive of ventricular tachycardia. The presence of either positive or negative QRS concordance is highly suggestive of ventricular tachycardia, though positive concordance can be seen in WPW syndrome with antidromic AV reciprocating tachycardia. In the presence of a left bundle branch block the QRS with an R wave of 45 msec or longer and a prominent notch in the downward stroke in $V_1$ with a QR or QS pattern in $V_6$ is highly suggestive of ventricular tachycardia. Hemodynamic stability of the rhythm disturbance in no way assists in determining its etiology. As stated previously, the presence of coronary artery disease should represent a contraindication to the use of verapamil for termination of a wide QRS tachycardia due to the serious potential for hemodynamic collapse in this setting.

## VENTRICULAR TACHYARRHYTHMIAS

Sudden cardiac death affects up to 400,000 patients each year with ventricular tachycardia/ventricular fibrillation as the likely etiology in the vast majority. The therapy of ventricular arrhythmias may be divided into four categories: pharmacologic therapy, the use of antitachycardia devices, surgical intervention, and the investigational use of closed chest ablation technology. The arrhythmias may be divided into three categories based on the gravity of their prognosis: benign rhythm disturbances such as premature ventricular contractions (PVCs), malignant rhythm disturbances such as nonsustained ventricular tachycardia, and those of intermediate severity which are not sustained ventricular tachycardia. In terms of this discussion sustained ventricular tachycardia is defined as ventricular tachycardia of 30 seconds or more or a ventricular tachycardia that degenerates to ventricular fibrillation. Nonsustained ventricular tachycardia is defined as a ventricular tachycardia of less than 30 seconds. Both nonsustained and sustained ventricular tachycardia may be associated with hemodynamic compromise. The decision of when and in what manner to initiate therapy in each of these categories is discussed below.

### Premature ventricular contractions

In asymptomatic patients with no evidence of structural heart disease or known coronary artery disease there is no indication for therapy. Numerous studies have shown that PVCs in the absence of heart disease do not present an increased risk for sudden cardiac death. A long-term follow-up study of patients who had frequent and complex ventricular ectopy demonstrated no increased risk of cardiac death. In the period between 1973 and 1983, 73 asymptomatic patients were found to have an average of 72 PVCs per hour. The death rate for this group was less than that predicted for age when tested against historical controls. There was only one episode of sudden cardiac death in the group. In the absence of structural heart disease and coronary artery disease, reassurance is clearly the best medicine for this patient group. In symptomatic patients it is recommended that a correlation of the patient's symptoms and the rhythm disturbance be made before initiating therapy. The use of an ambulatory 24-hour Holter monitor is recommended if the symptoms presumed secondary to a dysrhythmia are frequent. The importance of correlating symptoms with a specific rhythm disturbance cannot be overemphasized. Using the diary provided with the Holter assists enormously in this regard. For patients who experience infrequent but disturbing symptoms an event recorder, which may be activated at the time symptoms are present, is advisable. If PVCs can be reasonably associated with the patient's symptoms, the patient should be counseled to avoid caffeine-containing products, tobacco, and alcohol. Consideration of thyroid dysfunction with appropriate testing (TSH) should be made at this time if not previously assessed. If the patient remains symptomatic following these measures, a trial of a β-adrenergic blocking agent is recommended as the initial pharmacologic therapy. β-Adrenergic blocking agents have the most favorable risk benefit profile and are usually well tolerated. Class I antiarrhythmic agents should be used only after a careful risk/benefit analysis is applied to the patient at hand.

The presence of PVCs in patients with known coronary artery disease or cardiomyopathy represents an independent risk factor for subsequent mortality. Although β-blockade following myocardial infarction has been shown to reduce both overall cardiac mortality and sudden death, there is no body of data to support the empiric use of class I antiarrhythmic agents to suppress asymptomatic PVCs in these groups. The cardiac arrhythmia suppression trial (CAST) provided the best support for avoiding prophylactic therapy of asymptomatic PVCs in patients with coronary artery disease. The CAST study was based on the PVC hypothesis, which stated that, if PVCs were associated with increased mortality, then suppression of PVCs via antiarrhythmic agents would improve survival due to a reduction in arrhythmic death. Patients with frequent PVCs or nonsustained ventricular tachycardia were randomly placed in placebo or treatment limbs, with those in the treatment limb receiving the potent PVC suppressors encainide, flecainide, or moricizine. The trial was abruptly halted in those patients receiving encainide or flecainide when these groups were found to have a higher mortality than the placebo group (Table 9-2). The trial continued as CAST II with comparison of moricizine to placebo until it became clear there was not benefit to moricizine and there was a nonstatistically significant trend toward higher mortality in the moricizine-treated group. Although some have restricted the CAST results to the class IC agents, many extend the concern about proarrhythmia to all Class I agents (see box).

Recent metaanalyses suggest amiodarone is beneficial in reducing sudden death in the year following myocardial infarction. Entry of the majority of these patients into the

**Table 9-2.** CAST mortality in 1455 patients randomly assigned to encainide, flecainide, or placebo groups*

| | Encainide/Flecainide ($n$ = 730) | Placebo ($n$ = 725) |
|---|---|---|
| Arrhythmic death | 33 (4.5%) | 9 (1.2%) |
| Nonarrhythmic cardiac death | 14 (1.9%) | 6 (0.8%) |
| Noncardiac or unclassified death or cardiac arrest | 9 (1.2%) | 7 (1.0%) |
| Total deaths or cardiac arrest | 56 (7.6%) | 22 (3.0%) |

*Difference in values for total deaths between drug and placebo groups is statistically significant with a $p$ value of .003.

placebo-controlled studies was not determined by any frequency of PVCs. A treatment period of 1 year seems most appropriate based on long-term observation from the BASIS trial. The approach clearly associated with less morbidity is β-blockade, and it is unclear whether amiodarone provides greater protection than the use of this more benign therapy.

### Nonsustained ventricular tachycardia

As in the case of asymptomatic PVCs, the presence of nonsustained ventricular tachycardia unassociated with hemodynamic compromise in patients with preserved left ventricular function and without evidence of coronary artery disease raises the low risk for sudden cardiac death. In those patients with depressed left ventricular function, nonsustained ventricular tachycardia is clearly an indicator of increased morbidity and mortality. The severity of left ventricular dysfunction clearly remains the most significant prognostic factor, with left ventricular ejection fraction of less than 30% representing patients at high risk of sudden cardiac death. For patients with left ventricular dysfunction, a history of coronary artery disease, and nonsustained ventricular tachycardia it is recommended that programed electrical stimulation be performed. Over 40% of the patients with nonsustained ventricular tachycardia and left ventricular dysfunction have been shown to have inducible sustained ventricular tachycardia and represent a high-risk group for subsequent arrhythmic events.

The signal-averaged ECG (SAECG) represents another means of triaging patients with nonsustained ventricular tachycardia to either high- or low-risk groups for sudden cardiac death. Although a "positive" SAECG does not markedly increase the risk of sudden death in this group, the absence of late potentials places the patient in a group with considerably better prognosis and thus obviates the need for invasive electrophysiology study. As with PVCs, empiric therapy for nonsustained ventricular tachycardias is discouraged based on the CAST data. For patients with sustained ventricular tachycardia, either clinical or inducible at electrophysiologic study, options for therapy should include empiric therapy with β-blockers or amiodarone as well as electrophysiologically guided therapy or Holter-guided therapy with a class III agent such as sotalol or amiodarone. The use of antitachycardiac devices (AICD, PCD, Cadence) implanted via a transvenous approach is becoming increasingly attractive. Closed chest catheter ablation or open chest surgical excision of the ectopic focus is usually reserved for refractory tachycardias. Class IC agents in patients with coronary artery disease are discouraged.

### Sustained ventricular tachycardia

Sustained ventricular tachycardia (Fig. 9-10) associated with hemodynamic compromise should warrant prompt synchronized DC cardioversion. In patients who are hemodynamically stable, initial therapy should include the utilization of a lidocaine bolus similar to that described for the treatment of ventricular tachycardia in the setting of acute myocardial infarction. In the event that lidocaine does not terminate the rhythm disturbance, procainamide should be instituted. Should the patient have persistent hemodynamically stable ventricular tachycardia following the administration of an appropriate procainamide loading dose with a constant maintenance infusion of 3 mg/min, the addition of bretylium tosylate at 5 mg/kg with careful hemodynamic monitoring would be the next pharmacologic intervention. In many centers intravenous amiodarone is available on protocol, and this should be considered in instances of recurrent sustained ventricular tachycardia or in tachycardia refractory to conventional measures. As stated previously, hemodynamic compromise warrants prompt DC cardioversion, and this intervention should not be delayed while pharmacologic interventions are attempted.

Following return to sinus rhythm, a decision regarding long-term therapy should be made based on the circumstances in which ventricular tachycardia occurs. In the setting of acute myocardial infarction there may be no need for long-term therapy; however, in many patients long-term therapy is required, and appropriate consultation by a cardiologist is recommended. Options for long-term therapy include empiric β-blockade or amiodarone, electrophysiologically or Holter-guided antiarrhythmic therapy using class I or class III antiarrhythmic agents, antitachycardia devices either via a transvenous approach or the more conventional thoracotomy, or median sternotomy approach, as well as aneurysm resection and surgical excision of the reentry circuit at specialized surgical centers. In patients with a left bundle branch block pattern to their ventricular tachycardia, consideration should be given to bundle branch reentry. This tachycardia is responsive to verapamil; however, careful electrophysiologic study is required to confirm this diagnosis and emperic verapamil therapy should never be attempted without the careful guidance of an electrophysiologist if bundle branch reentry is suspected.

### Ventricular tachycardia in the setting of acute myocardial infarction

In the setting of suspected or confirmed acute myocardial infarction complicated by ventricular tachycardia, lidocaine remains the standard antiarrhythmic treatment in most coronary care units. Although several protocols have been proposed to facilitate a rapid administration of therapeutic doses of lidocaine, the protocol originally

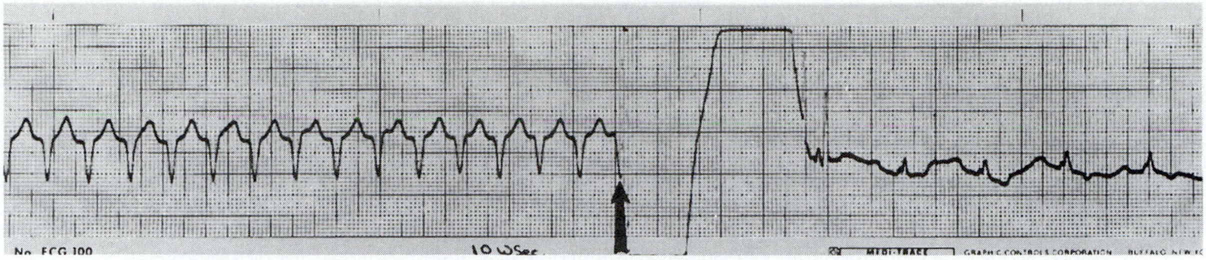

**Fig. 9-10.** Ventricular tachycardia at 150 beats/minute. A DC shock at 10 watt-seconds (*arrow*) converts the arrhythmia to normal sinus rhythm.

**Table 9-3.** Lidocaine loading and maintenance

| | Time | | | |
|---|---|---|---|---|
| | **0** | **8 min** | **16 min** | **24 min** |
| **Lidocaine loading for average patient** | | | | |
| Normal patient | 100 mg | 50 mg | 50 mg | 50 mg |
| Patient with CHF | 50 mg | 25 mg | 25 mg | 25 mg |
| **Lidocaine Maintenance Therapy for Average Patients** | | | | |
| Normal | 2-3 mg/min | | | |
| Heart failure | 1-3 mg/min | | | |
| Liver disease | 0.5-1 mg/min | | | |

described by Benowitz is recommended (Table 9-3). This regimen reliably establishes a therapeutic blood level in patients. The lidocaine levels recommended as the therapeutic window for this therapy are quite narrow, especially in the elderly. Reduction of both the loading and maintenance infusion should be made in patients with heart failure. The loading dose remains unchanged for patients with hepatic dysfunction, but the maintenance dose is reduced. The appearance of bradycardia, heart block, hypotension, or neurologic disturbance should result in cessation of therapy. In the event that ventricular tachydysrhythmias persist on therapeutic lidocaine levels, it is advisable to add procainamide rather than increase the lidocaine dose to potentially toxic levels. Procainamide is administered in an initial dose of 15 mg/kg no faster than 50 mg/min followed by a maintenance infusion of 3 mg/min. Blood levels of both procainamide and NAPA are followed with an optimal combined level of 15 mg/dl. Other intravenous agents have been investigated. Intravenous quinidine is limited by profound peripheral vasodilatation. The use of disopyramide in patients with acute myocardial infarction has shown no reduction in the incidence of ventricular fibrillation or mortality. Intravenous amiodarone remains an option only in referral centers that have this available to them under investigational protocol. Although the recurrence of ventricular tachycardia/ventricular fibrillation during the first few hours of acute myocardial infarction is clearly associated with increased in-hospital mortality, there is no evidence that patients who have experienced serious ventricular dysrhythmias during the first 24 hours following a myocardial infarction are at greater long-term risk of serious cardiac dysrhythmias or sudden death than those patients who have experienced an uncomplicated myocardial infarction. The use of a β-blocker in the year following infarction is strongly recommended for either group.

In recent years the role of prophylactic lidocaine has undergone reevaluation, and following recent metaanalysis it has fallen out of favor as a prophylactic agent. Magnesium sulfate may soon emerge as the prophylactic drug of choice. Recent metaanalysis by McMann and Hines showed no evidence of any beneficial effect on early mortality in patients with uncomplicated acute myocardial infarction when patients receive prophylactic lidocaine. Bradycardia as a result of sinus node dysfunction or AV block, confusion, tremors, and seizures are often serious complications of lidocaine toxicity, especially in the elderly. The use of prophylactic lidocaine in patients with high risk of ventricular fibrillation or sudden death remains appropriate, and current recommendations by the joint American College of Cardiology–American Heart Association task force on the early management of acute myocardial infarction recommends the use of prophylactic lidocaine in patients with acute myocardial ischemia or infarction in which PVCs are either frequent (better than 6 PVCs per minute), closely coupled, or multiform. The patients with ventricular tachycardia or ventricular fibrillation are candidates for intravenous lidocaine.

Data from the second Leicester Intravenous Magnesium Intervention Trial (LIMIT 2) suggested that intravenous magnesium sulfate is a simple, safe, and effective empiric prophylaxis for life-threatening rhythm disturbances. This therapy is generally well tolerated, although flushing and occasional nausea and local discomfort are reported. These adverse effects are usually limited to the initial bolus and are transient despite the maintenance of a high serum magnesium level by a 24-hour continuous infusion.

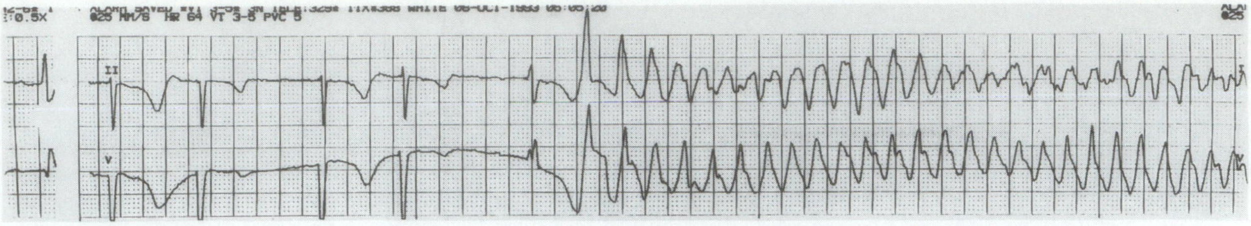

**Fig. 9-11.** Torsades de pointes in a 62-year-old man with a history of atrial fibrillation treated with Solatol. Superfically resembling ventricular tachycardia, it is rapid ventricular arrhythmia often caused by hypokalemia or drug overdose with varying QRS height and frequent changes in polarity that may either revert to normal sinus rhythm or cause sudden death.

Although no contraindications are present to the use of magnesium, the presence of moderate to severe renal insufficiency warrants appropriate adjustment of the magnesium infusion to avoid toxicity.

In addition to intravenous magnesium and lidocaine, the early use of β-blockers has been shown to reduce the risk of sudden cardiac death secondary to life-threatening arrhythmias. Metoprolol, propranolol, and atenolol have all been approved to treat tachyarrhythmias and prevent sudden cardiac death following myocardial infarction. Each of these agents, when titrated to the proper dose, is effective in reducing the incidence of sudden cardiac death. We recommend that metoprolol (or other approved β-blocker) be administered in the absence of contraindications in all patients admitted for myocardial infarction.

## The long QT syndromes

Torsades de pointes (Fig. 9-11) (prolonged QT in association with polymorphic ventricular tachycardia) represents a unique variant of ventricular tachycardia. Congenitally prolonged QT associated with deafness (Romano-Ward syndrome) or as an isolated abnormality (Lange-Nielson syndrome) is associated with a high risk of sudden death. Ventricular tachycardia is often initiated with an R-on-T phenomenon in patients with a QT of 0.56 second or greater. All class IA agents prolong QRS (depolarization) and QT (repolarization) through sodium channel blockade and therefore all are potentially associated with torsades. It is conventionally taught that patients receiving a Class IA agent (e.g., quinidine) who have a QT greater than 600 msec have an increased incidence of torsades. There are no data to support this, since there is no distinction between a therapeutically prolonged QT and one associated with proarrhythmia. Class III agents such as sotalol and amiodarone cause no appreciable prolongation of the QRS yet significantly prolong QT and have been associated with torsades. Many antidepressants have class IA characteristics that prolong QT and hence pose a risk of polymorphic ventricular tachycardia. Therapy for torsades de pointes should include a bolus of 2 to 4 g of magnesium sulfate over 5 to 15 minutes. Traditional approaches using an isoproterenol infusion (or overdrive pacing) to hasten repolarization and shorten the QT are often effective and should be utilized until the drug effect wanes and QT returns to normal. Correction of electrolyte abnormalities and cessation of agents that may prolong the QT are essential. Terfenadine (Seldane), erythromycin, and thioridazine are agents that prolong QT.

Prevention of sudden death in patients with the prolonged QT syndrome emphasizes manipulations of the autonomic nervous system. Traditional electrophysiologically guided therapy is not effective, and electrophysiologic studies are not clinically indicated. Empiric use of β-blockade is not only for the symptomatic patient but also for affected family members. High thoracic left sympathectomy to restore appropriate autonomic balance to the heart has been effective. This requires a specialized referral center, since success is clearly operator dependent. The use of an internal cardioverter defibrillator is an alternative strategy.

## Ventricular fibrillation

Ventricular fibrillation is the most lethal of ventricular rhythm disturbances and is commonly associated with acute myocardial infarction or end-stage cardiomyopathy. It can also occur in the setting of earlier stages of hypertrophic cardiomyopathy and rarely in mitral valve prolapse. Ventricular fibrillation in association with ischemia may be the cause of sudden death in the year following myocardial infarction. The only treatment for ventricular fibrillation is prompt defibrillation. Prophylaxis of this rhythm disturbance may be achieved by β-blockers or other antiarrhythmic agents. For the patient with a history of ventricular fibrillation consideration of an internal cardioverter defibrillator is strongly recommended. The transvenous lead systems now available allow lower perioperative mortality while providing reasonable efficacy compared to the more traditional surgical approaches (thoracotomy, median sternotomy).

## BIBLIOGRAPHY


ACC/AHA Task Force: Guidelines for the early management of patients with acute myocardial infarction, *Circulation* 82:664, 1990.

Akhtar M et al: Wide QRS complex tachycardia: reappraisal of a common clinical problem, *Ann Intern Med* 109:905, 1988.

DiMarco JP et al: Adenosine for paroxysmal supraventricular tachycardia: dose ranging and comparison with verapamil. Assessment in placebo-controlled, multicenter trials, *Ann Intern Med* 113(2):104, 1990 (erratum, Ann Intern Med 1990, Dec 15).

Echt DS et al: Mortality and morbidity in patients receiving encainide, flecainide, or placebo. The Cardiac Arrhythmia Suppression Trial, *N Engl J Med* 324:781, 1991.

Ewy GA, Caruso A, Marcus FI: Supraventricular tachycardias: recognition and management. In Ewy GA, Bressler R, editors: *Cardiovascular drugs and the management of heart disease,* ed 2, New York, 1992, Raven.

Jackman WM et al: The long QT syndromes: a critical review, new clinical observations, and a unifying hypothesis, *Prog Cardiovasc Dis* 31:115, 1988.

Jackman WM et al: Catheter ablation of accessory atrioventricular pathways (Wolff-Parkinson-White syndrome) by radiofrequency current, *N Engl J Med* 324:1605, 1991.

Jackman WM et al: Treatment of supraventricular tachycardia due to atrioventricular nodal reentry by radiofrequency catheter ablation of slow-pathway conduction, *N Engl J Med* 372:313, 1992.

McGovern B, Garan H, Ruskin JN: Precipitation of cardiac arrest by verapamil in patients with Wolff-Parkinson-White syndrome, *Ann Intern Med* 104(6):791, 1986.

Porterfield JG et al: Experience with three different third generation cardioverter defibrillators in patients with coronary artery disease or cardiomyopathy, *Am J Cardiol* 72:301, 1993.

Pritchett ELC: Management of atrial fibrillation, *N Engl J Med* 326:1264, 1992.

Cascade Investigators: Randomized antiarrhythmic drug therapy in survivors of cardiac arrest (the Cascade Study), *Am J Cardiol* 72:280, 1993.

Wilber DJ et al: Electrophysiological testing and nonsustained ventricular tachycardia. Use and limitations in patients with coronary artery disease and impaired ventricular function, *Circulation* 82:350, 1990.

Woods KL et al: Intravenous magnesium sulphate in suspected acute myocardial infarction: results of the second Leicester Intravenous Magnesium Intervention Trial (LIMIT 2), *Lancet* 339:1553, 1992.

Zarembski DG et al: Empiric long-term amiodarone prophylaxis following myocardial infarction: a metaanalysis, *Arch Intern Med* 1993.

CHAPTER

# 10 Syncope

**Wishwa N. Kapoor**

## EPIDEMIOLOGY/ETIOLOGY

Syncope is defined as a sudden transient loss of consciousness associated with loss of postural tone with spontaneous recovery not requiring cardioversion. Syncope must be separated from seizures and other states of altered consciousness such as dizziness, vertigo, coma, and narcolepsy. See Chapter 134 for dizziness.

Syncope is a common problem. Loss of consciousness is reported by 12% to 30% of young adults. This symptom accounts for 1% to 6% of hospital admissions and up to 3% of emergency department visits. Syncope is also common in the elderly. In one study of residents of a long-term care institution (older than 75 years of age), the annual incidence was 6%, and 23% had previous lifetime episodes.

Syncope can be a prelude to sudden death in certain subgroups. The 1-year mortality of patients with a cardiac cause of syncope is consistently high in all of the recent studies, ranging between 18% and 33%. These rates have been higher than those in patients with noncardiac cause (up to 12%) or patients with unknown cause (6%). One-year incidence of sudden death was 24% in patients with a cardiac cause as compared to 3% to 4% in the other two groups. Even when adjustments for differences in baseline comorbidity were made, cardiac syncope was still an independent predictor of mortality and sudden death.

### Etiologies of syncope

**Vasomotor instability and hypotension**

Vasovagal
Situational
- -Micturition
- -Cough
- -Swallow
- -Defecation

Orthostasis
Postprandial hypotension
Drugs
Neuralgias
Psychiatric illness

**Focal decreased cerebral blood flow**

**TIA**

**Decreased cardiac output**

Obstruction to LV outflow
- -Aortic stenosis, IHSS
- -Mitral stenosis, myxoma

Obstruction to RV outflow
- -Pulmonic stenosis
- -PE, pulmonary hypertension
- -Myxoma

Pump failure
- -MI, CAD, coronary spasm

Tamponade, dissection
Arrhythmias

*TIA*, Transient ischemic attack; *IHSS*, idiopathic hypertrophic subaortic stenosis; *LV*, left ventricle; *RV*, right ventricle; *PE*, pulmonary embolism; *MI*, myocardial infarction; *CAD*, coronary artery disease.

Syncope has a large differential diagnosis from benign problems to life-threatening illnesses (see the box above). A detailed description of these entities is beyond the scope of this review; see bibliography for references.

In studies that evaluated patients presenting with syncope, there has been a wide variation in the proportion of patients diagnosed with various etiologies. This variation is largely due to patient selection (differences ranging from emergency room to ICU patients) and lack of uniform criteria for assigning causes of syncope. The most common etiologies were vasovagal syncope (1% to 29%), situational syncope (1% to 8%), orthostatic hypotension (4% to 12%), and drug-induced syncope (2% to 9%). Causes due to organic cardiac diseases were found in 3% to 11% and arrhythmias in 5% to 30%. Each of the remaining etiologies were reported in less than 5% of patients with 38% to 47% having no etiology identified.

One study reported a 13% rate of syncope of unknown etiology, but about one third of patients had well-recognized seizure at presentation, which may partially explain this low rate. Three types of etiology may account for a large proportion of unexplained syncope.

### Vasovagal syncope

Vasovagal syncope generally has been diagnosed on a clinical basis such as syncope in the setting of various precipitating factors (e.g., pain and instrumentation) or using associated autonomic symptoms. Recent studies using upright tilt testing to provoke vasovagal syncope have shown that, in 26% to 87% of selected patients with unexplained syncope, symptoms can be induced on tilt testing, suggesting that vasovagal syncope may be a common cause of syncope.

### Psychiatric disorders

A subgroup of patients with unexplained syncope may have psychiatric diseases (15% to 20%) that are not recognized as a possible cause of syncope. These illnesses include generalized anxiety disorder, panic disorder, major depression, and somatization disorder.

### Miscellaneous disorders

A third group of patients are those in whom new diagnoses, which caused their initial syncopal episode, become apparent in follow-up. This group comprises less than 5% of patients with unexplained syncope and includes patients with arrhythmias (e.g., supraventricular tachycardia) and seizures.

## PATHOPHYSIOLOGY

The vast majority of causes of syncope result from transient reduction of cerebral blood flow to those parts of the brain subserving consciousness (brainstem, reticular activating system). There are four broad categories of mechanisms that may result in sudden decrease in cerebral blood flow (box on p. 211): (1) vasomotor instability associated with disorders that decrease systemic vascular resistance or venous return or both, (2) severe reduction of cardiac output due to obstruction of blood flow within the heart or pulmonary circulation, (3) cardiac arrhythmias leading to transient decline in cardiac output, and (4) transient ischemia due to cerebrovascular disease with focal or generalized decreased cerebral perfusion.

Rarely, normal or even increased cerebral blood flow may be associated with loss or alteration of consciousness because of a lack of essential nutrients necessary for cerebral metabolism. These states include hypoglycemia and hypoxemia; however, these disorders more frequently lead to somnolence and coma than syncope. Additionally, seizures may present as syncope; in this instance cerebral blood flow is generally normal.

## HISTORY

The evaluation of syncope begins with defining the episode and associated symptoms. Once the patient is found to have had syncope, a workup can be initiated to determine the etiology.

A detailed history of the episode (from the patient and a witness, if present) is needed to separate syncope from other states of altered consciousness such as dizziness, vertigo, drop attacks, coma, and seizure. A particularly difficult distinction is between syncope and seizure. A study comparing the symptoms of syncope and seizure showed that seizures were associated with blue face (or not pale), frothing at the mouth, tongue biting, disorientation, aching muscles, sleepiness after the event, and duration of unconsciousness of more than 5 minutes. On the other hand, symptoms associated with syncope were sweating or nausea before the event and being oriented after the event. The best discriminatory symptom is disorientation after the episode, which often signifies a seizure.

Once it has been determined that the patient had syncope, a history is crucial in choosing diagnostic tests selectively to arrive at an etiology. Emphasis is placed on the details of the events leading to the episode, the characteristics of the loss of consciousness, and symptoms immediately after the patient regains consciousness (Table 10-1). For example, in diagnosing vasovagal syncope a history of a particular precipitating factor or the presence of autonomic symptoms is useful. Micturition, cough, defecation, and swallowing may be associated with sudden loss of consciousness. These disorders, termed situational syncope, are diagnosed by history from the patient. Brainstem ischemia due to transient ischemic attacks, basilar artery migraines, and subclavian steal syndrome

**Table 10-1.** Clinical features suggestive of specific causes

| Symptom or finding | Diagnostic consideration |
|---|---|
| After sudden unexpected pain, unpleasant sight, sound, or smell | Vasovagal syncope |
| During or immediately after micturition, cough, swallow, or defecation | Situational syncope |
| With neuralgia (glossopharyngeal or trigeminal) | Bradycardia or vasodepressor reaction |
| Upon standing | Orthostatic hypotension |
| Prolonged standing at attention | Vasovagal |
| Well-trained athlete after exertion | Vasovagal |
| Changing position (from sitting to lying, bending, turning over in bed) | Atrial myxoma, thrombus |
| Syncope with exertion | Aortic stenosis, pulmonary hypertension, mitral stenosis, IHSS, coronary artery disease |
| With head rotation, pressure on carotid sinus (as in tumors, shaving, tight collars) | Carotid sinus syncope |
| Associated with vertigo, dysarthria, diplopia, and other motor and sensory symptoms of brainstem ischemia | TIA, subclavian steal |
| With arm exercise | Subclavian steal |

*IHSS*, Idiopathic hypertrophic subaortic stenosis; *TIA*, transient ischemic attack.

may lead to drop attacks or syncope, but loss of consciousness is generally associated with other neurologic symptoms and signs referable to the brainstem. A detailed drug history may uncover a potential etiology for syncope. The most common drugs causing syncope include nitrates, vasodilators, and β-blockers (see the box below).

History may suggest specific entities that can be further evaluated by directed testing (see Table 10-1). For example, syncope with arm exercise suggests subclavian steal syndrome; loss of consciousness in a deaf child with effort or emotional distress may be due to ventricular tachyarrhythmias associated with congenital long QT syndromes; and fainting in a patient with flushing and itching may be a manifestation of systemic mastocytosis. A description of these entities can be found elsewhere. The box on p. 211 shows specific features from the history that suggest various diagnoses.

## PHYSICAL EXAMINATION

A detailed physical examination may provide information needed to establish specific entities as a cause of syncope and exclude others. Findings on examination of particular importance are orthostatic hypotension, cardiovascular abnormalities, and neurologic signs.

### Common drugs causing syncope

**Vasodilators**
- Nitrates
- Calcium channel blockers
- ACE inhibitors
- Others (e.g., prazosin, hydralazine)

**Drugs associated with torsades de pointes**
- Quinidine
- Procainamide
- Disopyramide
- Flecainide
- Encainide
- Amiodarone
- Satolol

**Diuretics**

**Psychoactive drugs**
- Phenothiazines
- Antidepressants (e.g., tricyclic agents, MAO inhibitors)
- CNS depressants (e.g., barbiturates)

**β-Blockers**

**Other mechanisms**
- Vincristine and other neuropathic drugs
- Digitalis
- Insulin
- Marijuana
- Alcohol
- Cocaine

Reprinted from Kapoor WN: Diagnostic evaluation of syncope, *Am J Med* 90:91-106, 1991.

*ACE,* Angiotensin-converting enzyme; *CNS,* central nervous system; *MAO,* monoamine oxidase.

Syncope due to orthostatic hypotension can be difficult to diagnose, since 5% to 55% of patients with other etiologies of syncope have orthostatic hypotension (defined as a systolic blood pressure decline of 20 mm Hg or more), and postural hypotension is reported in up to 24% of the elderly. Thus the development of syncope or presyncope upon standing, in association with orthostatic blood pressure decline, is important in the diagnosis of etiology of loss of consciousness. Blood pressure measurements should be performed upon standing after a supine period of 5 to 10 minutes. Lack of a blood pressure drop upon sitting does not exclude orthostatic hypotension. Several blood pressure determinations upon standing during a 2-minute period are sufficient to detect orthostatic hypotension in most patients. Repeated orthostatic blood pressure measurements are needed when there is high clinical suspicion for orthostatic hypotension, since postural hypotension can be episodic. Orthostatic hypotension may be worse upon arising in the morning or after meals.

Cardiovascular findings may be important clues to the etiology of syncope. For example, aortic dissection and subclavian steal syndrome are associated with differences in the pulse intensity and blood pressure (generally less than 20 mm Hg) in the two arms. Many organic heart diseases that cause syncope have specific cardiovascular findings. These entities include aortic stenosis, idiopathic hypertrophic subaortic stenosis, pulmonary hypertension, myxomas, and aortic dissection.

When a cause of syncope can be found, the history and physical examination lead to the etiology in 56% to 85% of patients. Furthermore, organic cardiac diseases and neurologic diseases (e.g., subclavian steal syndrome) are strongly suspected by the history and physical examination. Testing for these diseases should be selective and based on findings from the history and physical examination. In our experience suggestive findings on the history and physical examination were helpful in assigning the ultimate cause of syncope by directed testing in 8% of additional patients.

## DIAGNOSTIC TESTING

Results of blood tests are generally not helpful in assigning an etiology for syncope. Hypoglycemia, hyponatremia, hypocalcemia, and renal failure have been found in 2% to 3% of patients, but primarily in those with seizures. These disorders were often clinically suspected; in one study only one unexpected finding was discovered (hyponatremia with seizures). Syncope due to bleeding has been diagnosed clinically with confirmation by hemoccult tests or complete blood counts.

In patients in whom a history and physical examination do not lead to an etiology or provide clues for directed testing, further evaluation focuses on arrhythmia detection, search for vasovagal syncope, and less commonly on psychiatric illnesses.

### Arrhythmia detection

Arrhythmias are primarily of concern in patients with structural heart disease or abnormal electrocardiogram (ECG). If symptoms are consistent with arrhythmic syncope, efforts should be directed first to rule out arrhythmias as the cause of syncope. The following means are available for diagnosis of arrhythmias.

*ECG/rhythm strip.* An ECG or a rhythm strip is useful in three ways. First, an ECG may show severe abnormalities that are diagnostic of the cause of syncope (2% to 11% of patients). Examples include complete heart block, symptomatic supraventricular tachyarrhythmias, and ventricular tachycardias. Second, an ECG may show abnormalities that increase the likelihood of arrhythmic syncope but are not diagnostic of the cause of syncope (e.g., bundle branch block, Wolff-Parkinson-White syndrome). Third, an ECG may be normal, which markedly decreases the probability of arrhythmias as the cause of syncope.

Treadmill testing can be used to provoke exercise-induced tachyarrhythmias when they are suspected clinically (e.g., patients with exertional syncope) or to look for ischemia. However, this test is rarely useful in establishing a cause of syncope.

*Carotid massage.* Less than 1% of patients presenting with syncope are assigned the diagnosis of carotid sinus syncope. Carotid sinus hypersensitivity is found in 5% to 25% of asymptomatic populations, but only 5% to 20% of these individuals have spontaneous symptoms consistent with carotid sinus syncope. Consider carotid sinus syncope in (1) those who have spontaneous symptoms suggestive of carotid sinus syncope (e.g., syncope while shaving, wearing tight collars, or turning the head) and (2) in elderly patients with recurrent syncope with a negative diagnostic evaluation. To diagnose carotid hypersensitivity, carotid massage can be performed for 5 to 15 seconds on each side with concurrent ECG and blood pressure monitoring. A cardioinhibitory response is defined as a cardiac asystole of greater than 3 seconds. A vasodepressor response is diagnosed when there is a systolic blood pressure decline of 50 mm Hg or more that is not associated with bradycardia or after bradycardia has been abolished with atropine or atrioventricular sequential pacing.

*Prolonged ECG monitoring.* The sensitivity and specificity of ECG monitoring for diagnosis of arrhythmic syncope are not known because of the lack of criteria for abnormal results or a gold standard that is independent of arrhythmias diagnosed by monitoring. The only certain means of diagnosing arrhythmias as a cause of syncope is to document arrhythmias at the time of symptoms. The results of ambulatory monitoring have been disappointing, since symptom correlation is found in only 4% of patients. In an additional 17% no arrhythmias are found during symptoms, thus potentially excluding arrhythmias as the etiology. In the remaining patients (approximately 80%) either asymptomatic arrhythmias or no arrhythmias are found. Since arrhythmias may be episodic, finding asymptomatic brief arrhythmias or no arrhythmias does not exclude a rhythm disturbance as a cause of syncope.

Monitoring longer than 24 hours is not likely to increase the yield of symptomatic arrhythmias. In one study, although there was an increased yield of brief arrhythmias after the first 24 hours (14.7% were abnormal during the first 24 hours, 11% during the second 24 hours, and 4.2% during the third 24 hours), none of the arrhythmias during the second and third 24 hours were associated with symptoms.

More prolonged monitoring for weeks to months is also possible using patient-activated intermittent loop recorders. This type of recorder can capture arrhythmias during a syncopal episode if the patient activates it after regaining consciousness. Experience with this recorder has been limited, and technical problems exist (18 of 57 patients). In one study of patients with multiple recurrences of syncope (median of 10 episodes), seven of the 57 patients had an arrhythmia found with recurrent symptoms of which three were due to neurally mediated syncope. Seven others had negative findings, therefore excluding arrhythmias as a cause of syncope. Thus patient-activated loop monitors are useful only in a small subset of patients who have had multiple recurrences of syncope.

*Electrophysiologic studies.* In patients with structural heart disease or abnormal ECG (e.g., bundle branch block, accessory pathway, old myocardial infarction), electrophysiologic studies (EPS) should be considered if arrhythmias are not excluded by noninvasive tests (ECG and ambulatory or loop monitoring). These tests are generally not indicated in patients without heart disease and normal ECG.

Some centers have used the detection of low-amplitude signals in the terminal portion of QRS complex by signal-averaged ECG as a screening test for selecting patients for EPS. The sensitivity of low-amplitude signals (late potentials) is reported to be 73% to 89% with a specificity of 89% to 100% for detection of inducible sustained ventricular tachycardia in patients with syncope. However, this test is not generally useful to eliminate further consideration of EPS; complete studies are often needed in patients with organic heart disease and syncope because other abnormalities (conduction system disease and supraventricular tachycardia) as well as multiple abnormalities are relatively common findings on these tests.

### Upright tilt testing

Vasovagal syncope (also termed neurally mediated or neurocardiogenic syncope) can be induced by keeping susceptible individuals upright on a tilt table with or without stimulation with adrenergic agents such as isoproterenol (Table 10-2). The mechanism of tilt-induced syncope is not entirely understood (Fig. 10-1). Inhibitory reflexes originating from the heart are widely believed to be responsible for this type of syncope. This reflex originates in the cardiac sensory receptors (mechanoreceptors) located primarily in the inferior and posterior wall of the left ventricle. These receptors may be stimulated by stretch, cardiac distention, forceful, rapid systolic contraction, or chemical substances. The stimulation of receptors leads to increased neural discharges through unmyelinated C fibers to the medulla (vasomotor center), leading to enhanced parasympathetic and decreased sympathetic activity. The result is sudden hypotension and/or bradycardia.

Upright posture leads to pooling of blood in the lower limbs, resulting in decreased venous return (see Fig. 10-1). Normal compensatory response to orthostatic stress is reflex tachycardia, more forceful contraction of the ventricles, and vasoconstriction. However, in individuals

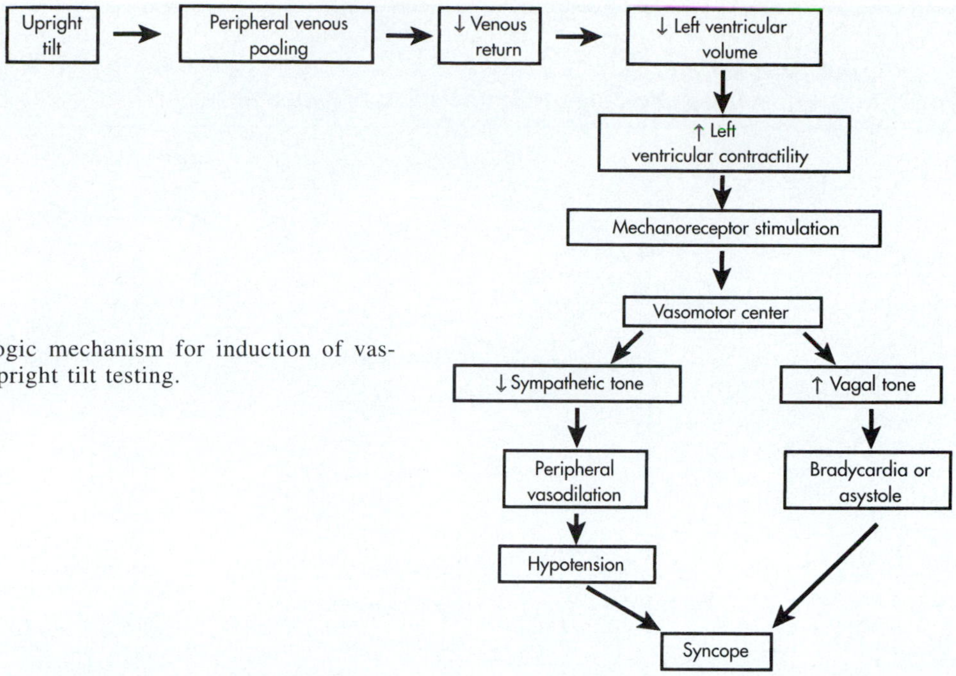


**Fig. 10-1.** Pathophysiologic mechanism for induction of vasovagal syncope during upright tilt testing.

**Table 10-2.** Positive responses to upright tilt testing

| | Total subjects | No. positive | % positive | Positive range |
|---|---|---|---|---|
| Passive tilt only | 372 | 181 | 49 | 26-90 |
| Isoproterenol tilt | | | | |
| Passive phase | 473 | 107 | 23 | 0-57 |
| Isoproterenol phase | 366 | 181 | 49 | 12-81 |
| Overall | 473 | 313* | 66 | 39-87 |

*These 313 patients include 25 positive patients from one study, which did not specify whether those patients were positive during the isoproterenol phase or the passive phase.

susceptible to vasovagal syncope, this forceful ventricular contraction, in the setting of a relatively empty ventricle, may activate the cardiac mechanoreceptors triggering reflex hypotension and/or bradycardia. Catecholamine release (as may occur with anxiety, fear, and panic), by increasing ventricular contraction, may also activate the nerve endings responsible for triggering this reflex.

What is the role of tilt table testing in evaluating syncope? In patients without heart disease in whom the history, physical examination, and initial ECG do not lead to an etiology of syncope, upright tilt testing may define a potential diagnosis. Furthermore, in patients who have underlying heart disease and do not have evidence of arrhythmias based on ECG monitoring and EPS, this test may provide a specific diagnosis. However, because of problems with the specificity of the test, only symptom reproduction during testing should be considered a positive response. Furthermore, tilt testing should generally be limited to patients who have had multiple recurrences of syncope, since treatment is the major issue in this group.

## Psychiatric assessment

Several psychiatric illnesses can result in syncope. Generalized anxiety disorder may produce hyperventilation and vasodepressor reaction. In panic disorder up to 9% of the patients have faintness as a somatic complaint. Patients with somatization disorder have multiple physical symptoms including loss of consciousness, which is reported in 4.5% of patients with this disorder. Medical patients with major depression often have nonspecific physical complaints, and syncope may be one of the manifestations. Patients with syncope due to psychiatric disorders are generally younger and have multiple episodes. They have lower prevalence of heart disease and may have other nonspecific complaints associated with syncope such as headache, fatigue, dizziness, and palpitations.

## Low-yield tests

Other tests are rarely helpful in assigning an etiology for syncope. Skull films, lumbar puncture, radionuclide brain scan, and cerebral angiography have not yielded diagnostic information for a cause of syncope in the absence of clinical findings suggestive of a specific neurologic process. Glucose tolerance testing has not led to a diagnosis of hypoglycemia in patients with syncope. Studies of electroencephalogram (EEG) in syncope have shown that in 1% of patients an epileptiform abnormality is found; almost all of these were suspected clinically. Head CT scans are rarely useful to assign an etiology but are needed if subdural bleeding due to head injury is suspected or for patients in whom seizure is suspected as the cause of loss of consciousness.

## Summary of diagnostic approach

The Managed Care Guide is a flow diagram that summarizes the diagnostic approach to syncope. A detailed clini-

**Managed Care Guide**
**Algorithm summarizing the diagnostic approach to syncope**

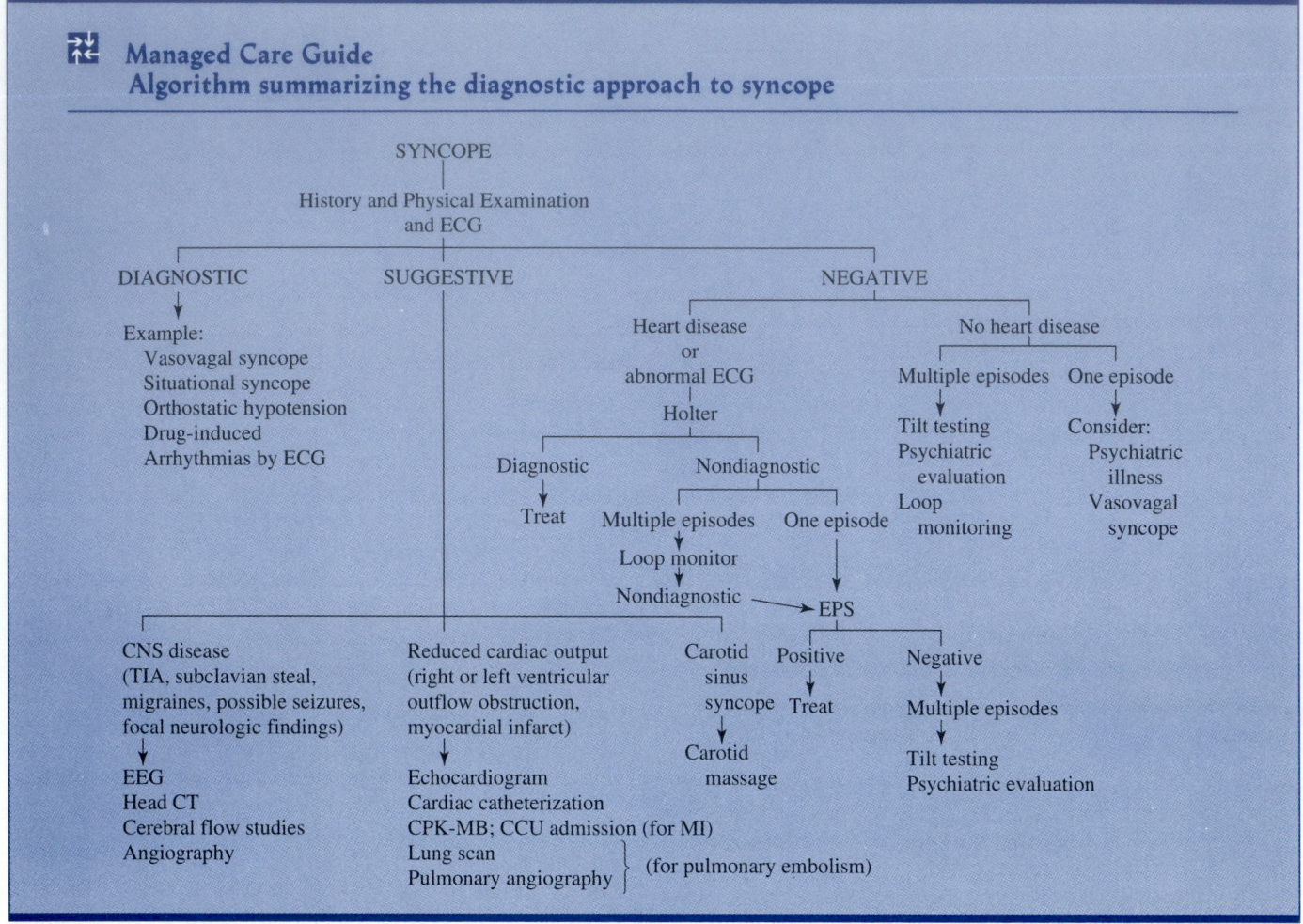

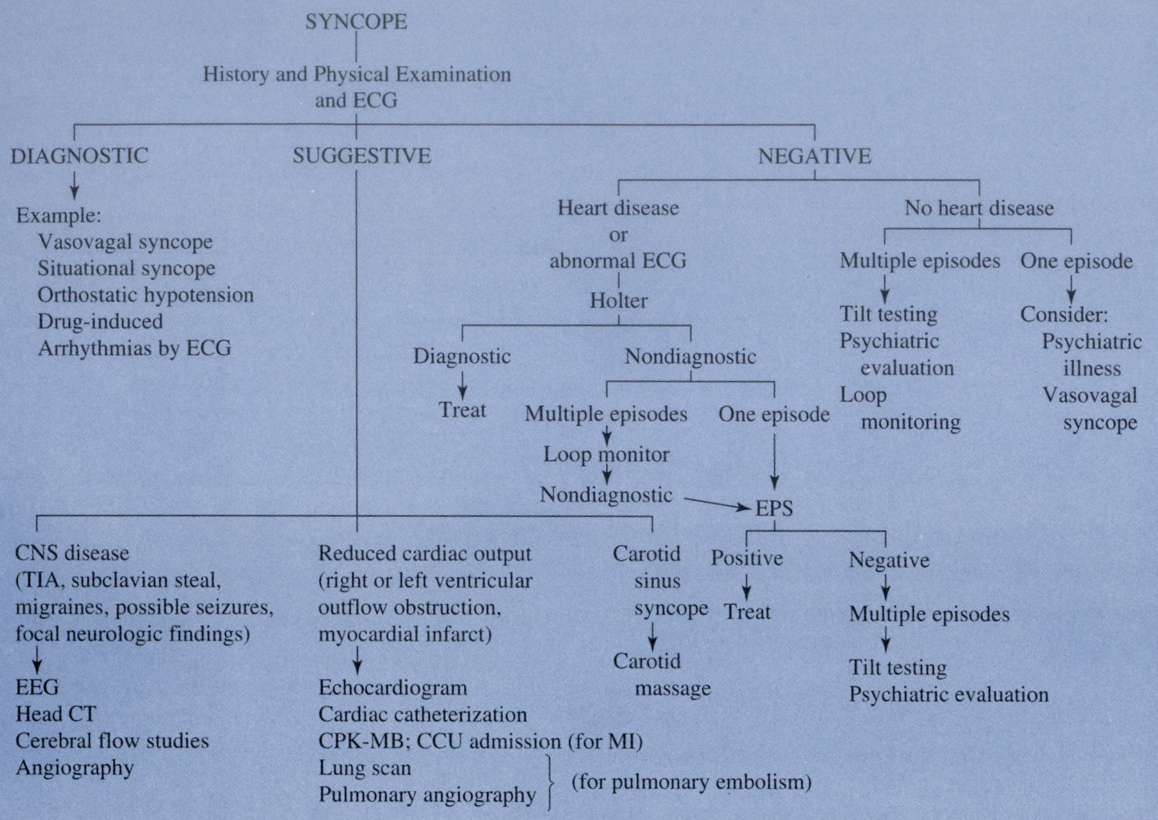


cal assessment (by history and physical examination) of patients with syncope is crucial and leads to the assignment of the vast majority of the causes of syncope. Additionally, in a smaller proportion of patients, clinical assessment suggests specific entities such as aortic stenosis or neurologic signs and symptoms suggestive of a seizure disorder. These findings should be used to guide further testing to arrive at a diagnosis and initiate treatment.

An ECG is needed in most patients with syncope, except when the etiology by the history and physical examination is clearly not cardiac. As noted previously, a normal ECG may help decrease the probability of cardiac etiologies.

When a cause of syncope is not established by the history, physical examination, and initial ECG, the following approach can be used to proceed with the diagnostic evaluation.

***Tests for arrhythmia detection.*** Arrhythmic syncope is a major concern in patients with structural heart disease or abnormal ECG. The first step in the evaluation of these patients is prolonged ECG monitoring, since this is a noninvasive test. If a diagnosis is made by finding arrhythmias and correlating symptoms, invasive tests such as EPS may be avoided. In patients with negative or unclear findings on ECG monitoring (e.g., asymptomatic brief nonsustained ventricular tachycardia) who have recurrent syncope, event recorders are recommended. If ambulatory and event recorders are nondiagnostic, EPS should be considered for selection of therapy.

Since the prognosis of patients with negative EPS is favorable, empiric therapy (with a pacemaker or antiarrhythmic drugs) is not justified. Upright tilt testing is recommended in patients with recurrent or disabling symptoms who have negative EPS to define a potential etiology and initiate treatment.

***Patients without heart disease.*** Prognosis of syncope patients without heart disease is excellent with regard to the outcome of mortality. In young patients with a normal ECG the likelihood of arrhythmias is low. In this group prolonged ECG monitoring or EPS is generally negative and not needed. Vasovagal syncope and psychiatric disorders are the major diagnostic considerations and should be pursued as the initial step in the evaluation. A similar diagnostic approach can be taken with older patients without heart disease and normal ECG, but further studies are needed to better define the role of prolonged ECG monitoring in these patients. The yield of EPS is low in this group, and so it is not justified in the vast majority of the patients.

***Recurrent syncope.*** In patients with recurrent syncope (five or more in the last year) the diagnostic considerations are large, but these patients are less likely to have arrhythmias and are more likely to have psychiatric illnesses and vasovagal syncope. The initial approach to diagnostic testing should be based on the presence or absence of heart disease (as noted above). In this group of patients, if a cause of syncope is not established, patient-activated intermittent ECG loop recorders may be useful for the evaluation of brief episodic arrhythmias.

Although studies in the 1980s have shown that a cause of syncope was not established in up to 45% of patients, by using the approach outlined here with the availability of newer diagnostic modalities a cause of syncope can be assigned in the vast majority of patients presenting with this symptom. Patients without a diagnosis have a low incidence of mortality and sudden death but should be followed closely and reevaluated upon recurrence.

**Table 10-3.** Commonly used therapies for recurrent vasovagal syncope

| Therapies | Dosage |
|---|---|
| β-Blockers | |
| Atenolol | 25-200 mg/day |
| Metoprolol | 50-200 mg/day |
| Propranolol | 40-160 mg/day |
| Disopyramide | 200-600 mg/day |
| Fludrocortisone | 0.1-1 mg/day |
| Fluoxetine | 40 mg/day |
| Scopolamine patch | 1 patch every 2-3 days |
| Theophylline | 6-12 mg/kg/day |

## MANAGEMENT

Treatment decisions are based on the etiology of syncope. A detailed discussion of the treatments of all of the etiologies is covered in specific chapters. General considerations for treatments are as follows.

### Vasovagal syncope

The severity and natural history of vasovagal syncope are variable. Patients may have a large number of events at one time that diminish or resolve spontaneously. There are rare patients who continue to have episodes over many years. Thus the frequency and severity of events are important in devising treatment plans for the patient. Because treatments may have potential side effects, they should be reserved for patients who have frequent or disabling symptoms. Treatment should be avoided in those with one or rare lifetime episodes.

Many patients with vasovagal syncope have precipitating factors or situations. These should be identified by a careful history and the patient should be instructed to avoid these situations. Common triggers include prolonged standing, venipuncture, large meals, and heat (such as hot baths or sunbathing). Additionally fasting, lack of sleep, and alcohol intake may predispose to vasovagal syncope and should be avoided. Since psychiatric illnesses probably lead to vasovagal reactions, screening for the psychiatric illnesses noted above should be performed. Treatment of the psychiatric illness often resolves the recurrent syncope.

Several types of drug therapies have been tried for patients with vasovagal syncope (Table 10-3). β-Blockers (e.g., metoprolol, atenolol) are the most commonly used drugs. The mechanism of action of β-blockers is not fully understood, but they can diminish cardiac contractility, inhibiting the activation of cardiac mechanoreceptors. Anticholinergic agents such as transdermal scopolamine (one patch every 3 days) are particularly useful in patients with profound bradycardia during upright tilt testing. Disopyramide has also been reported to decrease recurrence of syncope. This drug has anticholinergic and negative inotropic effects, which may inhibit activation of cardiac mechanoreceptors. Theophylline has rarely been used at doses as low as 6 to 12 mg/kg/day. The mechanism of action of theophylline in the treatment of vasovagal syncope is not known, but a blockade of the effects of adenosine, which has vasodilatory effects, is postulated. Measures to expand volume have been used and include increased salt intake, custom fitted counterpressure support garments from ankle to waist, and fludrocortisone acetate. Potential side effects include recumbent hypertension, hypokalemia, fluid retention, and congestive heart failure. Finally, atrioventricular pacing may be considered in patients with significant bradycardia in response to upright tilt testing. Even in these patients, the initial treatment of choice is pharmacologic. Pacemaker therapy should be reserved for those who have disabling symptoms and fail drug therapy.

### Orthostatic hypotension

The initial approach to treatment of orthostatic hypotension is to ensure adequate salt and volume intake and to avoid or discontinue drugs that cause orthostatic hypotension. Patients with orthostatic hypotension should be advised to raise the head of the bed at night, to rise from bed or chair slowly, and to avoid prolonged standing. Compressive stockings applied up to thigh levels may help decrease venous pooling. Frequent small feedings may be helpful in patients with marked postprandial orthostatic hypotension.

Pharmacologic agents of potential benefit include fludrocortisone (0.1 to 1 mg/day) in conjunction with increased salt intake. Various adrenergic agents have been used, including ephedrine, phenylephrine, and others. A more detailed discussion of pharmacologic treatment of orthostatic hypotension is found elsewhere.

### Syncope in the elderly

The elderly often have multiple chronic diseases and physiologic impairments that can predispose to syncope. Thus in the elderly several seemingly mild abnormalities may contribute to a sudden reduction of cerebral blood flow and syncope. As an example, mild volume depletion with upper respiratory tract infection in a patient with chronic renal insufficiency and systolic hypertension may be sufficient to cause syncope, whereas any one problem alone is not severe enough to cause loss of consciousness.

The initial approach to the management of the elderly should be to search for a single disease as a cause of syncope. If a single disease is found (such as severe aortic stenosis, symptomatic bradycardia, or symptomatic orthostatic hypotension), treatment of that disease can be planned. However, a single disease as the cause of syncope is often not apparent. In these patients, inability to compensate for common situational stresses may be a factor in the setting of multiple medical problems, medications, and physiologic impairments. A careful assessment of the effect of underlying pathologic conditions and medications is important to determine whether multiple pathologic processes could have led to syncope. Once these potential processes are identified, treatment should be directed to correcting these factors. As an example, consider an elderly patient presenting with syncope, who has taken enalapril, 10 mg/day and has anemia (hemoglobin 9.0), mild orthostatic hypotension, and a recent upper respiratory tract infection. In this patient, if no other etiology of syncope is apparent based on clinical findings and selective use of laboratory tests, volume repletion, treatment of anemia, and adjustment or change of antihypertensive medication may help prevent further episodes of syncope.

## BIBLIOGRAPHY

Abboud FM: Neurocardiogenic syncope, *N Engl J Med* 328:1117, 1993.

Day SC et al: Evaluation and outcome of emergency room patients with transient loss of consciousness, *Am J Med* 73:15, 1982.

DiMarco JP: Electrophysiologic studies in patients with unexplained syncope, *Circulation* 75(suppl III):140, 1987.

DiMarco JP, Philbrick JT: Use of ambulatory electrocardiographic (Holter) monitoring, *Ann Intern Med* 113:53, 1990.

Kapoor WN: Evaluation and management of the patients with syncope, *JAMA* 268(18):2553, 1992.

Kapoor WN: Evaluation and outcome of patients with syncope, *Medicine* 69:160, 1990.

Kapoor WN: Hypotension and syncope. In Braunwald E, editor: *Heart disease: a textbook of cardiovascular medicine,* Philadelphia, 1991, WB Saunders.

Kapoor WN, Brant NL: Evaluation of syncope by upright tilt testing with isoproterenol: a nonspecific test, *Ann Intern Med* 116:358, 1992.

Linzer M et al: Incremental diagnostic yield of loop electrocardiographic recorders in unexplained syncope, *Am J Cardiol* 66:214, 1990.

Lipsitz L: Orthostatic hypotension in the elderly, *N Engl J Med* 321:952, 1989.

McAnulty JH: Syncope of unknown origin: the role of electrophysiologic studies, *Circulation* 75(suppl III):144, 1987.

Ross RT: *Syncope,* London, 1988, WB Saunders.

CHAPTER

# 11 Ischemic Heart Disease

**Leonard S. Lilly**

Ischemic heart disease (IHD) is the leading cause of mortality in industrialized societies. It is estimated that this condition afflicts 7 million individuals in the United States and is responsible for more than 500,000 deaths annually. Despite these daunting numbers, during the past three decades there has been a gradual decline in IHD-related deaths, which likely reflects recognition and correction of cardiac risk factors and dramatic improvements in medical and surgical therapies. To a great extent the primary care physician plays a pivotal role in the prevention, diagnosis, and long-term management of individuals with this condition.

The clinical presentation of patients with IHD is highly variable (Table 11-1). It may be manifest by classic exertional angina, but in other cases myocardial ischemia may occur without any symptoms (silent ischemia). Sometimes the first manifestation is an acute myocardial infarction (MI) or sudden death.

## PATHOPHYSIOLOGY OF MYOCARDIAL ISCHEMIA

Myocardial ischemia results when there is an imbalance between myocardial oxygen supply and demand. This most often occurs because of the presence of atherosclerotic plaque within one or more coronary arteries, which limits the normal rise in coronary blood flow in response to increases in myocardial oxygen demand.

The major determinants of myocardial oxygen demand are heart rate, the force of ventricular contraction, and ventricular wall tension. The latter is proportional to ventricular volume and pressure. Conditions that increase myocardial oxygen consumption, such as physical exertion and emotional stress, would be expected to result in myocardial ischemia unless there is a concomitant rise in oxygen supply.

Myocardial oxygen supply depends on the oxygen-carrying capacity of the blood, coronary blood flow, and the ability of the heart muscle to extract oxygen from circulating blood. The oxygen-carrying capacity relates to the content of hemoglobin and systemic $Po_2$, and in the absence of anemia or lung disease it is fairly constant. Unlike other organs, the extraction of oxygen from the blood by heart muscle is nearly maximal in the resting state and cannot be significantly increased during periods of increased demand. Therefore it is primarily the increase in coronary blood flow that maintains myocardial supply when oxygen demands increase. During periods of increased myocardial work, the local accumulation of vasoactive metabolites stimulates local coronary arteriolar dilatation and causes the coronary blood flow to rise several-fold. However, when atherosclerotic disease is present, the artery lumen is narrowed and vasodilatation is impaired, such that coronary blood flow cannot increase in the face of increased demands, and ischemia may result. When ischemia occurs, it is frequently accompanied by the chest discomfort known as angina pectoris. The predictable pattern of intermittent symptoms of myocardial ischemia during exertion or emotional stress is known as *chronic stable angina.*

The degree of narrowing in an atherosclerotic vessel is not constant; it can vary from moment to moment because of superimposed spasm of the artery, which further reduces coronary blood flow. The mechanism of coronary vasospasm is not known but may relate to endothelial dysfunction in the setting of atherosclerotic disease. In some patients alterations of vascular tone play a minor role in narrowing the coronary lumen, but in other individuals the degree of vasospasm may be even more important than the degree of fixed atherosclerotic stenosis itself. In the majority of patients with angina the development of myocardial ischemia results from a combination of fixed

**Table 11-1.** Clinical definitions

| Syndrome | Description |
|---|---|
| Ischemic heart disease | Condition in which an imbalance between myocardial oxygen supply and demand results in myocardial hypoxia and accumulation of waste metabolites; most often due to atherosclerotic disease of the coronary arteries |
| Angina pectoris | Uncomfortable sensation in the chest or neighboring anatomic structures produced by myocardial ischemia |
| Stable angina | Chronic pattern of transient angina pectoris, precipitated by physical activity or emotional upset, relieved by rest within a few minutes; episodes often associated with temporary depression of the ST segment, but permanent myocardial damage does not result |
| Variant angina | Typical anginal discomfort, usually *at rest*, which develops because of coronary artery spasm, rather than an increase of myocardial oxygen demand; episodes often associated with transient shifts of the ST segment (usually ST elevation) |
| Unstable angina | Pattern of increased frequency and duration of angina episodes, produced by less exertion, or at rest; high frequency of progression to myocardial infarction if untreated |
| Silent ischemia | Asymptomatic episodes of myocardial ischemia; can be detected by ECG and other laboratory techniques |
| Myocardial infarction | Region of myocardial necrosis due to prolonged cessation of blood supply; most often results from acute thrombus at site of coronary atherosclerotic stenosis; may be first clinical manifestation of ischemic heart disease, or there may be a history of angina pectoris |

Modified from Lilly LS, editor: *Pathophysiology of heart disease*, Philadelphia, 1993, Lea & Febiger.

and vasospastic stenosis. The variation in vascular tone may explain the variable threshold of angina: one day exertion might not produce any angina at all, but on another day similar effort does result in symptoms of ischemia.

A small number of patients experience episodes of intense focal coronary artery spasm in the absence of underlying atherosclerotic disease. In that situation angina can occur at rest (i.e., not provoked by increased myocardial oxygen demand) because of the marked reduction in coronary blood flow. This form of ischemia, known as *variant* or *Prinzmetal angina,* is rare.

In addition to coronary atherosclerotic disease, other conditions may upset the balance between myocardial oxygen supply and demand and result in ischemia. For example, decreased perfusion pressure into the coronaries can occur during systemic hypotension, and severe anemia can result in a marked decrease in the oxygen-carrying capacity of blood. Such reductions in myocardial oxygen supply may cause angina even in the absence of atherosclerotic coronary artery disease (CAD). Similarly, conditions that markedly increase myocardial oxygen demand, such as severe aortic stenosis and hypertrophic cardiomyopathy, can also upset the supply-demand balance and result in ischemia.

A patient with chronic stable angina may develop a sudden increase in the frequency and duration of ischemic episodes, occurring at lower workloads than previously or even at rest. This acceleration is known as *unstable angina,* and up to 20% of such patients sustain an MI over the ensuing 3 months. Although the majority of such patients have severe atherosclerotic coronary disease, unstable angina can also arise in patients with only mildly obstructive coronary lesions. Catheterization and angioscopy studies have shown that the pathogenesis of unstable angina is multifactorial, often involving rupture of an atherosclerotic plaque with subsequent platelet aggregation and local thrombus formation. In other cases transient periods of intense coronary vasospasm at sites of atherosclerotic plaque play a role. Similar mechanisms also appear responsible for the development of MI: more than 85% of acute MIs result from an acute thrombus obstructing a coronary artery with resultant prolonged ischemia and tissue necrosis.

**Major risk factors for coronary artery disease**

- Hypercholesterolemia (↑ LDL, ↓ HDL)
- Hypertension
- Cigarette smoking
- Diabetes mellitus
- Advanced age
- Male sex
- Family history of premature CAD

*LDL,* Low-density lipoprotein; *HDL,* high-density lipoprotein.

This summary of the pathogenesis of IHD has therapeutic consequences: the treatment of chronic angina is directed at minimizing myocardial oxygen demand and increasing coronary flow, whereas in the acute syndromes of unstable angina or MI primary therapy is also directed against platelet aggregation and thrombosis.

## EPIDEMIOLOGY OF ISCHEMIC HEART DISEASE

Many large epidemiologic studies have implicated certain habits and predisposing conditions that correlate with the development of atherosclerosis and IHD. The Framingham Heart Study, for example, identified four major potentially modifiable risk factors: hyperlipidemia (elevated low-density lipoprotein [LDL] cholesterol and low high-density lipoprotein [HDL] cholesterol [see Chapter 40]), hypertension, cigarette smoking, and diabetes mellitus (see the box above). Several nonmodifiable risk factors include advanced age, male sex, and a family history of premature coronary disease (i.e., coronary disease in related males age 55 or less or females age 65 or less). Other potential risk factors of unproven magnitude include obesity, a sedentary lifestyle, and stressful emotional states.

Correction of the modifiable risk factors are critical to the long-term management of IHD to prevent disease progression and resulting complications. For example, emerging data suggest that strict control of serum cholesterol (achieving LDL cholesterol of 100 mg/dl or less) can substantially slow, and possibly reverse, the development of atherosclerotic plaque.

## CLINICAL FEATURES OF ANGINA PECTORIS

### History

> There is a disorder of the breast marked with strong and peculiar symptoms, considerable for the kind of danger belonging to it, and not extremely rare, which deserves to be mentioned more at length. The seat of it, and sense of strangling, and anxiety with which it is attended, may make it not improperly be called angina pectoris.
>
> They who are afflicted with it, are seized while they are walking, (more especially if it be up hill, and soon after eating) with a painful and most disagreeable sensation in the breast, which seems as if it would extinguish life, if it were to increase or continue; but the moment they stand still, all this uneasiness vanishes.
>
> **William Heberden, 1768**

The most common manifestation of myocardial ischemia is the intermittent discomfort of angina pectoris. Although many laboratory tests can identify the presence of ischemia, the most important aspect of the clinical evaluation remains a careful history to evaluate for anginal symptoms. Several characteristics derived from the history can aid in the differentiation between myocardial ischemia and other causes of chest discomfort (Table 11-2). Features of angina relate to the quality of the discomfort, its location and radiation, precipitating factors, and frequency.

**Table 11-2.** Differential diagnosis of recurrent chest pain

| Condition | Helpful distinguishing features |
|---|---|
| Myocardial ischemia | Diffuse tightness/constriction/heaviness; not sharp or pleuritic<br>Brought on by exertion or emotional upset |
| Pericarditis | Sharp, pleuritic, positional<br>Friction rub<br>Diffuse ST elevation, PR depression on ECG |
| Chest wall pain | Sharp, localized pain<br>Reproduced by palpation over painful area |
| Cervical or thoracic spine pain | Shooting pains or ache worsened by movement of neck or back<br>Pain may be in dermatomal distribution |
| Esophageal or gastric pains | Nonexertional pains<br>Often associated with dysphagia or gastric reflux<br>Worsened by certain foods, aspirin, lying supine<br>May be relieved by antacids |
| Biliary pain | Right upper quadrant tenderness<br>Fatty food intolerance |

***Quality of discomfort.*** Most often angina is described as a tightness, squeezing, heaviness, pressure, burning, indigestion, or aching sensation. It is only rarely described as a pain, and patients sometimes correct the physician who refers to it as such. It is never sharp, stabbing, prickly, spasmodic, or pleuritic. It is usually a steady discomfort that lasts a few minutes, rarely more than 10, unless unstable angina or an MI is evolving. It always lasts more than a few seconds, which helps differentiate it from some types of musculoskeletal pain. Angina is usually relieved quickly by sublingual nitroglycerin (in less than 5 minutes), which can be a useful distinguishing feature. Sometimes, while describing angina, a patient raises a clenched fist to the sternum (Levine sign) as if to indicate the constrictive sensation by that tight grip.

Symptoms that frequently accompany angina include dyspnea, diaphoresis, and nausea, which resolve quickly along with the chest discomfort.

***Location and radiation.*** Angina is usually a diffuse sensation rather than located at a discrete spot. If the patient can localize the discomfort with a single finger, myocardial ischemia is an unlikely cause. Generally, the discomfort is most intense retrosternally or in the anterior left chest but may occur anywhere between the jaw and the upper abdomen. It frequently radiates to the shoulders, upper back, neck, or inner aspect of the arms, particularly on the left side. Although the location of angina may vary between individuals, it is usually the same sensation in a given patient with each attack, unless an MI is in progress, at which time it is generally more diffuse and severe.

***Precipitants.*** Angina, except when due to pure vasospasm, is caused by factors that increase myocardial demand. Typically it is provoked by exertion, such as climbing stairs, walking up an inclined surface, vigorous work using the arms, or sexual activity. Other factors that increase myocardial oxygen demand and can result in angina include emotional excitement, eating a large meal, and physical activities in cold weather. The latter results in vasoconstriction of the extremities, an increase in systemic vascular resistance, and therefore an increase in myocardial wall tension and oxygen requirements. In addition, myocardial ischemia displays a circadian rhythm, such that the threshold for angina is usually lower in the morning hours.

Patients who primarily experience coronary vasospasm most often have symptoms at rest, independent of activities that increase myocardial oxygen demand. Chest discomfort that awakens a patient from sleep may be precipitated by this mechanism, or because of the emotional stress (and therefore increased myocardial oxygen demand) of a bad dream.

***Frequency.*** For an individual with IHD the level of exertion needed to precipitate angina and therefore its frequency remains fairly constant (depending on superimposed vascular tone). However, the patient may quickly realize what activities produce angina and avoid them.

Therefore it is important to ask about recent reduction in activities when taking the history.

### Physical examination

The general examination of patients with suspected IHD should address the manifestations of atherosclerosis as well as transient findings during episodes of angina. External signs of hypercholesterolemia may be present, including arcus senilis and tendinous xanthomas. Funduscopic examination may show evidence of chronic hypertension or diabetes. Also look for signs of hyperthyroidism, which can contribute to increased myocardial oxygen demand.

A general vascular examination should assess for the equality of blood pressure between the two arms (to rule out atherosclerotic narrowings), as well as palpation and auscultation of the carotid and peripheral arteries and examination of the abdomen for evidence of an aortic aneurysm.

On cardiac examination an $S_4$ is common in patients with CAD because of atrial contraction into a "stiffened" left ventricle. This sign is not diagnostic for IHD, however, since it is present in many healthy elderly patients. The cardiac examination may be otherwise normal while the patient is asymptomatic, but during an episode of angina, several transient physical findings may appear. Increased sympathetic tone during chest pain may result in an increase in heart rate and blood pressure. Myocardial ischemia may result in papillary muscle dysfunction with a transient systolic murmur of mitral regurgitation. Ischemia-induced left ventricular wall motion abnormalities may be detected as an abnormal precordial bulge on chest palpation. A transient $S_3$ gallop and pulmonary rales may appear if ischemia-induced left ventricular dysfunction occurs.

## DIAGNOSTIC TESTS

Blood tests to evaluate for underlying risk factors include measurement of the serum lipids (see Chapter 40) and fasting serum glucose. The hematocrit and thyroid function tests should be measured if clinically appropriate, since anemia and hyperthyroidism can exacerbate myocardial ischemia.

Noninvasive cardiac testing is useful to confirm the diagnosis of IHD, to help stratify patients into categories of risk, and to guide therapy. Many of these tests are expensive, and it is therefore important to choose the appropriate study for each patient. Beyond the resting electrocardiogram (ECG) they include exercise testing, with or without nuclear scintigraphy, exercise radionuclide ventriculography or echocardiography, pharmacologic stress testing, and ambulatory ECG monitoring.

### Resting ECG

Many patients with CAD have normal baseline ECGs, or may demonstrate pathologic Q waves indicative of previous infarction. In many patients minor ST and T wave abnormalities are present but are not specific for CAD. However, the ECG can be diagnostically useful if recorded during an episode of chest pain, whereupon ischemia often results in transient horizontal or downsloping ST segments or T wave inversions, which normalize following resolution of the pain. Less often, transient ST *elevation* may be observed, which suggests severe transmural ischemia or coronary artery spasm.

### Exercise stress testing

The most useful noninvasive tests in the evaluation of angina involve exercise testing. In patients without resting ST or T wave abnormalities the standard treadmill (or bicycle) exercise test, without additional imaging modalities, should be the initial procedure, since it is the most convenient and cost effective. For patients whose presentation strongly suggests myocardial ischemia, the exercise test has a sensitivity and specificity greater than 85%. However, when the probability of significant coronary disease is low (e.g., a young woman with prickly chest pains), the test is less specific, and false positive results are more common.

Exercise testing is most commonly used (1) to confirm the diagnosis of angina, (2) to identify IHD patients at high risk of complications, (3) to assess the response of antianginal therapy, and (4) as a screening procedure for certain asymptomatic populations, such as individuals with strong cardiac risk factors, older patients about to begin exercise programs, and individuals whose well-being could affect public safety (e.g., airline pilots).

Different protocols may be used for exercise testing, but in each the intensity of exercise is incrementally augmented (e.g., increased grade and speed on the treadmill) to raise myocardial oxygen consumption. During the test the ECG and heart rate are monitored continuously and the blood pressure measured every few minutes. The product of heart rate and systolic blood pressure (known as the double product) correlates with myocardial oxygen demand and is useful in describing a patient's anginal threshold.

Exercise is continued until a target heart rate (usually 85% of the maximal predicted heart rate based on the patient's age) or symptom-limited end points (e.g., precipitation of anginal pain) are achieved. However, the test should be terminated immediately if hypotension, high-grade ventricular arrhythmias, or more than 3 mm ST segment depression develop. The complications of exercise testing are few, and death and MI are extremely uncommon. However, the risks are increased and the test should not be performed in individuals with unstable angina or suspected advanced aortic stenosis.

Exercise testing suggests the presence of IHD if the patient's typical chest discomfort is reproduced, or if specific ECG abnormalities develop (see the box on p. 222). The ECG criteria for a positive test is 1 mm (0.1 mV) horizontal or downsloping ST depression, measured 0.08 second after the termination of the QRS complex. The degree and location of ST segment abnormalities are not always a reliable indication of the extent and anatomic localization of CAD. However, taken together, the magnitude, time of onset, duration, and number of ECG leads that develop abnormal ST segments can predict the severity of CAD. For example, individuals who develop ST depression in multiple leads during the first 3 minutes of exercise are very likely to have left main or severe three-vessel disease. Other criteria for a markedly positive test, which are indicative of such severe coronary artery disease and a poor cardiac prognosis, are listed in the box on p. 222.

### Interpretation of exercise treadmill test

*Positive test*

- Reproduction of chest pain
- ST depression (horizontal or downsloping at 0.08 second after termination of QRS)

*Markedly positive test (predictors of severe coronary disease)*

- Chest pain or ST changes in first 3 minutes of test
- ≥ 3 mm ST depression during test
- Persistence of ST changes > 5 minutes after exercise stopped
- Decline in systolic BP during test
- Multifocal ventricular ectopy or ventricular tachycardia during or after exercise, if accompanied by ST segment changes
- Poor duration of exercise (≤ 2 minutes) due to cardiopulmonary limitations

### Commonly used forms of stress testing

*Standard tests*

- Exercise treadmill
- Stationary bicycle
- Arm ergometry (if arms are better conditioned than legs)

*If baseline ECG precludes interpretation of exercise-induced ischemia, or if greater sensitivity and specificity required**

- Exercise perfusion scintigraphy ($^{201}$Tl or other radionuclides)
- Exercise radionuclide ventriculogram ($^{99m}$Tc)
- Exercise echocardiography

*If unable to exercise**

- Dipyridamole (or adenosine) perfusion scintigraphy ($^{201}$Tl or other radionuclides)
- Dipyridamole or dobutamine echocardiography

*Choice of study should be dictated by local expertise.

Conversely a negative test or one that becomes positive only after 9 minutes of exercise or at a heart rate greater than 160 beats/min correlates with a very optimistic prognosis, even if angina or ST segment depressions develop during the test.

The diagnostic value of an exercise test may be limited by medications, especially β-blockers, which can blunt the achieved heart rate or rise in blood pressure. If the purpose of the stress test is to confirm the presence of angina, such medications should be withheld for 1 to 2 days before the test, and if necessary sublingual nitroglycerin can be used as needed during that time. However, if the purpose is to judge the effects of and gauge medical therapy, then the usual drug regimen should be continued on the day of testing.

## Radionuclide studies

Two types of nuclear studies are used to enhance the diagnostic value of standard exercise tests: myocardial perfusion imaging and radionuclide ventriculography. These tests can provide additional information regarding the location and extent of CAD, and their interpretations are not hampered by resting ECG abnormalities. However, they are more expensive than standard treadmill tests and should be used judiciously (see the box at right).

***Myocardial perfusion scintigraphy.*** This test is generally more sensitive and specific than conventional stress testing. During this test a radionuclide (e.g., $^{201}$Tl or $^{99m}$Tc sestamibi) is used, which after peripheral venous injection distributes to the myocardium in proportion to coronary blood flow. The radionuclide is injected at peak exercise, and immediate imaging is performed. Perfusion defects (cold spots) indicate regions of prior infarction or exercise-induced ischemia. Repeat imaging at rest several hours later shows filling in of the zones that were ischemic, differentiating them from regions of previous infarction. The location of perfusion abnormalities correlates with coronary disease in the respective territory (e.g., left anterior descending artery disease results in perfusion abnormalities within the anterior wall). Multiple large perfusion defects correlate with left main or severe three-vessel disease. A recent enhancement of the radionuclide studies is single photon emission computed tomography (SPECT), which creates a three-dimensional view of the myocardium with improved image resolution.

Because of its added expense, perfusion scintigraphy should be performed in place of a standard exercise test only in certain circumstances (see the box at right).

In experienced departments of nuclear medicine thallium scintigraphy has a sensitivity of 75% to 90% but may be positive in up to 20% of normal individuals. In females attenuation due to breast tissue artifact is a common cause of false positive studies. In addition to previous MIs, other conditions that may produce persistent myocardial defects include infiltrative disease (e.g., sarcoidosis) and dilated cardiomyopathy.

For patients who are unable to exercise, pharmacologic stress testing in conjunction with myocardial perfusion imaging can be undertaken. IV dipyridamole (or adenosine) produces vasodilatation and increases flow to the myocardium perfused by healthy coronaries. This effect steals blood away from stenotic coronaries, creating regional ischemia that can be detected following injection of radionuclides such as $^{201}$Tl. This type of nonexercise stress test has proven useful in predicting cardiac ischemic events in patients with chronic stable angina and in those about to undergo noncardiac surgery.

***Exercise radionuclide ventriculography.*** This test entails imaging blood flow through the left ventricle during the cardiac cycle at rest and then with exercise. Two commonly used techniques are (1) the first-pass technique, in which a large bolus of radionuclide (e.g., $^{99m}$Tc) is injected and the tracer is imaged as it flows through the heart as it is quickly cleared from the circulation; and (2) the multigated equilibrium technique (MUGA) in which red blood cells are labeled and several minutes of transventricular flow are analyzed as a composite image.

In normal individuals contractile function of the left ventricle increases with exercise (the ejection fraction

### Criteria for use of perfusion scintigraphy

- An abnormal baseline ECG that precludes interpretation of the standard ETT (left bundle branch block, baseline ST-T wave abnormalities, WPW syndrome)
- To confirm exercise test results that conflict with the clinical impression (unexpected ST shifts during exercise in an asymptomatic patient)
- To increase the sensitivity of CAD detection in an individual with a negative exercise test, but strongly suspected coronary disease
- To localize regions of ischemia (to identify culprit lesions responsible for ischemia in patients with multivessel CAD).

*ETT,* Exercise tolerance test; *WPW,* Wolff-Parkinson-White.

should increase more than 5%). Myocardial ischemia is suggested if the ejection fraction falls with exercise or if segmental left ventricular wall motion abnormalities develop. Exercise radionuclide ventriculography has a sensitivity similar to that of $^{201}$Tl perfusion imaging, but it is less specific because other etiologies of left ventricular dysfunction can produce similar results.

## Echocardiography

Imaging of the left ventricle by ultrasound can reveal segmental wall motion abnormalities indicative of ischemia or previous infarction. In exercise echocardiography left ventricular function is assessed before and during vigorous exercise (supine bicycle or treadmill); exercise-induced segmental regional wall motion abnormalities are an indication of ischemia. Exercise echocardiography is therefore analogous to exercise radionuclide ventriculography and has similar sensitivity and specificity for the presence of significant coronary disease. Proper interpretation of exercise echocardiography requires a great deal of experience, and the choice between nuclear studies and exercise echocardiography should ultimately be dictated by the local departmental expertise in these sophisticated modalities.

For patients who are unable to exercise, pharmacologic stress testing with echocardiography can be performed in one of two fashions: (1) using potent vasodilators such as dipyridamole or adenosine (analogous to dipyridamole $^{201}$Tl scintigraphy described above), or (2) using an adrenergic stimulating drug (e.g., dobutamine) which increases the heart rate and systolic blood pressure. Either of these techniques signifies the presence of myocardial ischemia by drug-induced left ventricular wall motion abnormalities.

## Ambulatory ECG monitoring

Frequency-modulated ambulatory ECG monitors can detect shifts in the ST segments indicative of ischemia. Approximately 40% of patients with known stable CAD display such transient shifts, and in most cases, asymptomatic silent episodes (described below) are even more common than symptomatic events. The role of this technique in documenting the presence of CAD has not yet been defined; however, some studies have shown its usefulness as a prognostic guide. For example, the absence of ST segment shifts on ambulatory monitoring predicts a low risk of cardiac complications in patients undergoing noncardiac surgery.

### Common indications for coronary arteriography in ambulatory patients

- Chronic angina with limiting symptoms refractory to medical therapy
- Markedly positive exercise test
- Chronic angina with left ventricular dysfunction (ejection fraction less than 40%)
- Angina soon after myocardial infarction (spontaneous or exercise test induced)
- Cardiomyopathy in which coronary disease is suspected cause
- Patients with chest pain who are diagnostic dilemmas

## Coronary arteriography

Coronary arteriography allows selective visualization of the coronary arteries and their major branches and is the most accurate means to detect the presence and extent of CAD. In experienced laboratories it is performed with low mortality (approximately 0.2%) or severe vascular complications (0.7%). However, this technique is costly, is not risk free, and is seldom needed to simply establish the diagnosis of significant coronary disease. The decision to proceed with arteriography should be dictated by the patient's clinical presentation and only when a change in therapeutic plan is under consideration. Commonly accepted indications for coronary angiography are indicated in the box above and the Managed Care Guide on p. 224.

Note that an individual with mild to moderate angina that is reasonably controlled with medical therapy does not generally require cardiac catheterization, since the long-term prognosis and quality of life may not be significantly affected. However, if that individual has other markers of a poor prognosis by exercise testing or impaired left ventricular function, then catheterization should be performed (see the Managed Care Guide on p. 224). If left main or three-vessel disease is identified, mechanical revascularization would likely be indicated.

At catheterization, coronary narrowings of greater than 70% are significant (i.e., the ones most likely to produce clinical ischemia). Natural history studies have shown that the mortality of patients with CAD correlates with the number of significantly narrowed vessels, and those with left main disease (greater than 50% stenosis) have the highest mortality. Outcomes are correspondingly worse in patients with decreased left ventricular contractile function.

Left ventriculography can be performed at the time of cardiac catheterization to measure global and regional left ventricular function and assess the presence of mitral regurgitation. However, such information can usually be derived by noninvasive techniques (echocardiography or radionuclide ventriculography), sparing the patient from additional intravenous contrast material.

## Managed Care Guide
### Suggested approach to patients with suspected angina

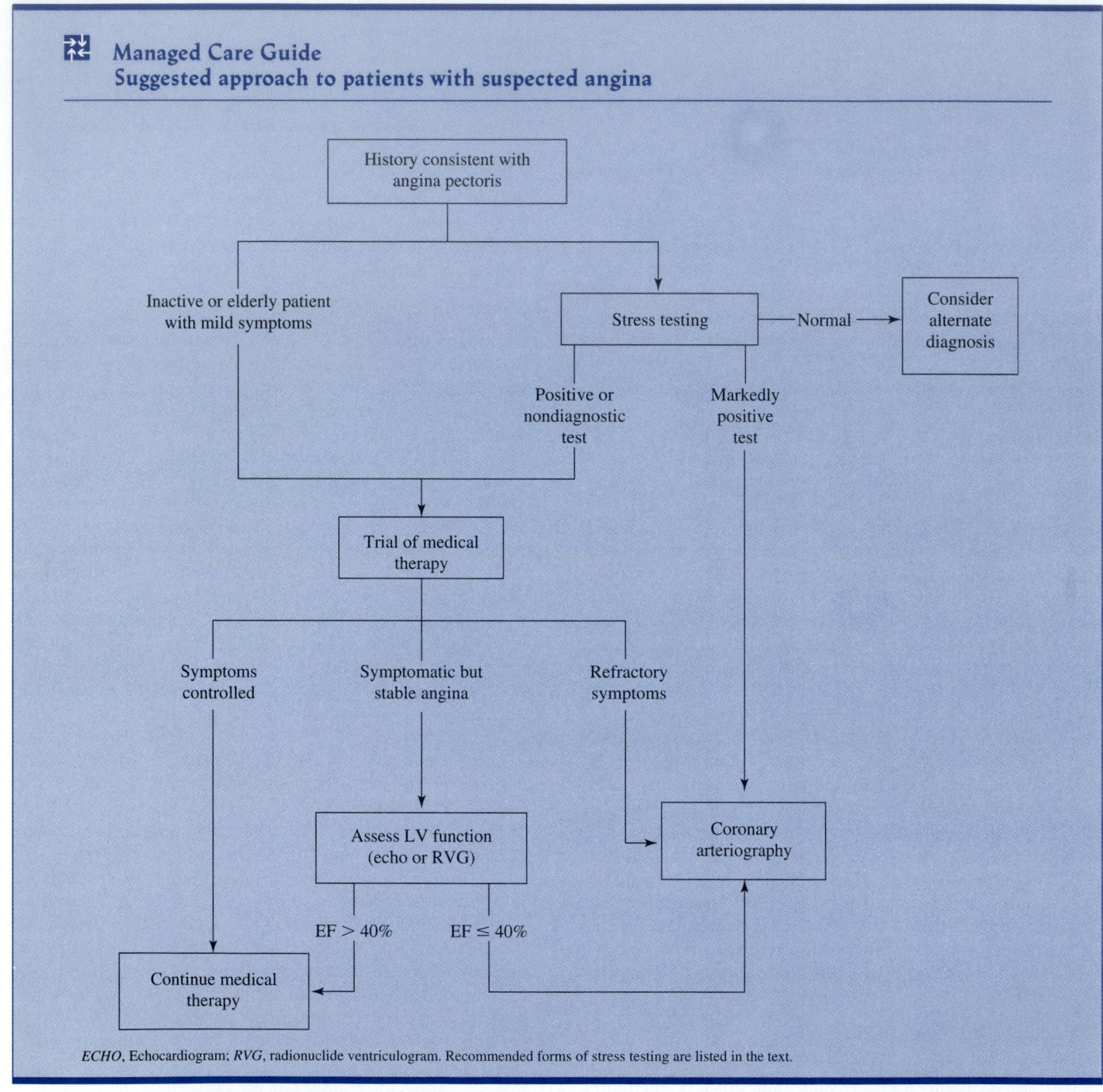

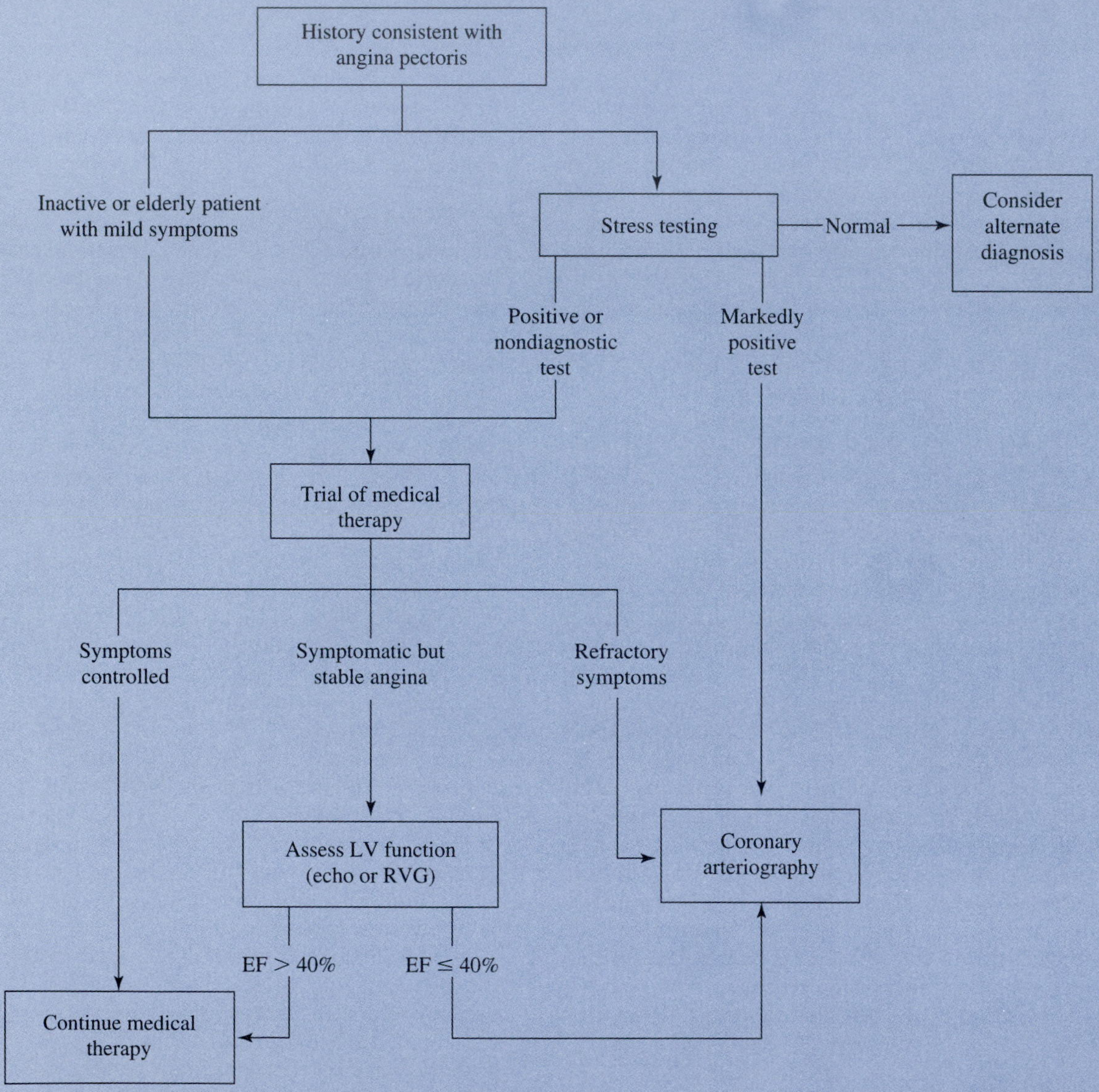


*ECHO*, Echocardiogram; *RVG*, radionuclide ventriculogram. Recommended forms of stress testing are listed in the text.

## MANAGEMENT OF PATIENTS WITH SUSPECTED ANGINA

### General principles

The Managed Care Guide on p. 224 summarizes the approach to the evaluation and management of patients with suspected IHD. Once angina is suggested by the clinical history, stress testing is useful to confirm the diagnosis and stratify patients into high- and low-risk groups. The standard form of stress testing is the graded treadmill test, but for those patients with abnormal baseline ECGs or those unable to exercise, the alternative forms of testing are appropriate. Patients with markedly positive stress tests should undergo coronary arteriography because of the high likelihood of left main or three-vessel coronary disease, conditions that could warrant mechanical revascularization. For patients with only mildly positive stress tests or those with nondiagnostic studies, a trial of pharmacologic management is recommended, with further evaluation dictated by the response to therapy. An alternative approach in inactive or elderly patients is to begin a trial of medical therapy based on the clinical history of angina, without stress testing. The early response to therapy would then dictate further evaluation.

The management goals for IHD are to reduce anginal symptoms, prevent complications such as MI, and prolong life. General measures begin with a discussion of the disease and the importance of eliminating risk factors that have led to it. Patients should be encouraged to stop smoking, lose excess weight, and control hypertension, hyperlipidemia, and diabetes.

There are often psychosocial issues faced by individuals who are diagnosed with angina for the first time. Many patients may be unnecessarily pessimistic about their prognosis, so a frank discussion should stress the common nature of IHD and the advanced therapeutic options available that often allow the quality of life to be unimpaired. Similarly, it is important to inform the patient that transient anginal attacks do not result in permanent heart damage.

Angina is particularly likely to occur during bursts of activity, particularly after periods of rest (e.g., walking up a flight of stairs after watching TV for several hours). Therefore a period of warming up (e.g., walking around the house a few times before mowing the lawn) is often a useful way to prevent angina. In addition, the prophylactic use of nitroglycerin should be encouraged before activities likely to bring on chest discomfort. Angina often exhibits a circadian pattern, with episodes more common in the hours shortly after arising, so the use of prophylactic nitroglycerin before dressing and shaving can be particularly beneficial. If a patient notes that angina is frequently precipitated by emotional upset, attempts should be made to minimize these; counseling or antianxiety medications may be useful.

Patients with stable angina should be encouraged to participate in a regular exercise program, most often walking. Such activity can have a beneficial conditioning effect on skeletal muscles and may contribute to raising the anginal threshold. Patients who exercise are also less likely to smoke and more likely to watch their diet and weight.

### Pharmacologic therapy

In the prevention or treatment of angina, pharmacologic therapy is aimed at restoring the balance between myocardial oxygen supply and demand. The agents most useful in this regard are the nitrates, β-blockers, and calcium channel blockers.

*Nitrates.* The major antianginal effect of nitrates is to reduce myocardial oxygen demand. These agents relax vascular smooth muscle, particularly in the venous circulation at usual dosages. Since this action reduces venous return to the heart, there is a corresponding decline in left ventricular volume (a determinant of wall stress), which causes myocardial oxygen consumption to fall. To a lesser extent the nitrates act as arteriolar dilators, an action that beneficially reduces the resistance against which the left ventricle contracts, further reducing wall tension and oxygen demand. A third action of the nitrates is to dilate the coronary arteries with augmentation of coronary blood flow. This action increases myocardial oxygen supply and may be particularly important in the prevention and treatment of coronary artery vasospasm.

Rapidly acting nitroglycerin remains the drug of choice to treat acute anginal attacks. Sublingual or aerosol nitroglycerin spray (Table 11-3) typically relieves angina in less than 5 minutes, although sometimes repeated doses are necessary, and can be administered at 5-minute intervals.

Some clinical tips on the use of nitroglycerin are indicated in the box below. For many patients the use of nitrates is accompanied by a feeling of generalized warmth and a transient throbbing headache or lightheadedness. This can be quite frightening if not expected, and patients should be warned about these effects. Even better is to stand by as the patient administers the first nitroglycerin

#### Clinical tips for successful nitroglycerin (TNG) use

1. Observe patient in your office during first test dose of sublingual TNG and guide through expected reaction: burning under tongue, diffuse warmth or flushing, brief head-throbbing.
2. Instruct patient to sit down when using TNG for first few times to avoid hypotension.
3. Teach prophylactic use of TNG before activities likely to precipitate angina.
4. Usual dose is 0.3 or 0.4 mg sublingual, but elderly patients may not tolerate more than 0.15 mg.
5. After a bottle of TNG is opened, it should be discarded after 6 months, since potency wanes after exposure to air (patient may notice lack of sublingual burning during use). TNG spray does not have this limitation and may be preferred for patients who have only occasional angina.
6. Assure patient that TNG has no long-term side effects, and liberal use should be encouraged.
7. If angina persists longer than 20 minutes or after three tablets taken 5 minutes apart, MI may be in progress, and patient should proceed to closest emergency ward.

**Table 11-3.** Commonly used nitrates

| | Usual dosage | Onset of action (min) | Duration of action | Recommended dosing frequency |
|---|---|---|---|---|
| **Short-acting agents** | | | | |
| Sublingual TNG | 0.15-0.6 mg (usual dose 0.4 mg) | 2-5 | 10-30 min | As needed |
| Aerosol TNG | 0.4 mg (1 inhalation) | 2-5 | 10-30 min | As needed |
| Sublingual ISDN | 2.5-10 mg | 5-20 | 1-2 hr | As needed |
| **Long-acting agents** | | | | |
| Oral ISDN | 5-30 mg | 15-30 | 4-6 hr | tid (mealtimes) |
| Sustained-action | 40 mg | 30-60 | 6-10 hr | bid (once in AM, then 7 hours later) |
| Oral PET | 10-40 mg | 30-60 | 3-6 hr | tid (mealtimes) |
| Sustained-action | 30-80 mg | slow | 6-10 hr | bid (once in AM, then 7 hours later) |
| TNG ointment (2%) | 0.5-2 in | 15-60 | 3-8 hr | qid (with one 7- to 10-hr nitrate-free interval) |
| TNG skin patches | 0.1-0.6 mg/hr | 30-60 | up to 24 hr | Apply in morning, remove in evening |
| ISMO | 20-40 mg | 30-60 | 12-14 hr | bid (once in AM, then 7 hours later) |

*TNG*, Nitroglycerin; *ISDN*, isosorbide dinitrate; *PET*, pentaerythritol tetranitrate; *ISMO*, isosorbide mononitrate.

in your office, so as to explain these reactions and instill confidence. The patient should also be instructed to sit down before using nitroglycerin the first few times, to avoid the potential of symptomatic hypotension. In addition, advice should be given that, if an anginal episode persists more than 20 minutes or is unresponsive to three or more nitroglycerin tablets, then the appropriate course is to proceed to the closest emergency ward for evaluation of possible unstable angina or MI.

Long-acting nitrates (see Table 11-3) are useful in the chronic prevention of anginal episodes and are available in oral and transdermal preparations. Low initial dosages should be used to avoid headache and lightheadedness and can be augmented over time. Side effects are similar to but often less pronounced than those associated with rapidly acting nitroglycerin administration. If a headache occurs, acetaminophen can be prescribed concurrently during the first few days of therapy, after which side effect tends to wane. An important problem associated with chronic nitrate therapy is the development of drug tolerance (i.e., continued administration of the drug leads to decreased effectiveness over time). It can be prevented by allowing an 8- to 10-hour nitrate-free interval each day, and effective dosage schedules to accomplish this are indicated in Table 11-3.

For elderly or inactive patients long-acting nitrates may alone suffice as chronic antianginal therapy. However, for many physically active individuals additional drugs are usually required.

***β-Blockers.*** β-Adrenergic antagonists have become the mainstay of therapy to prevent effort-induced angina and also have been shown to reduce mortality following MI. The main antianginal effect of β-blockers is to reduce myocardial oxygen demand by slowing the heart rate, reducing the force of ventricular contraction, and lowering blood pressure (thereby decreasing left ventricular wall tension). In the United States only a handful of β-blockers have been approved for the treatment of angina, although all are probably effective and have been used for this

**Table 11-4.** β-Blockers approved for use in the United States

| | Usual oral dosage | β-Agonist activity |
|---|---|---|
| **Nonselective agents** | | |
| Carteolol | 2.5-10 mg qd | + |
| Labetolol* | 100-600 mg bid | |
| Nadolol† | 40-80 mg qd | |
| Penbutolol | 20 mg qd | + |
| Pindolol | 5-30 mg bid | + |
| Propranolol† | 20-60 mg qid | |
| Sustained-action† | 80-160 mg qd | |
| Timolol† | 20 mg bid | |
| **$\beta_1$-selective agents** | | |
| Acebutolol | 200-1200 mg qd | + |
| Atenolol† | 50-100 mg qd | |
| Betaxolol | 10-20 mg qd | |
| Metoprolol† | 50-100 mg bid | |
| Sustained-action† | 50-100 mg qd | |
| Esmolol | 50-200 μg/kg/min IV | |

*Also has $\alpha_1$-blocking properties.
†Approved by FDA for use in coronary artery disease.

purpose (Table 11-4). β-Blockers differ from one another by several properties that influence their choice in certain patient groups, based on their duration of action, selectivity for the $\beta_1$-receptor, partial β-agonist activity, and α-adrenergic blocking properties. The goal of $\beta_1$-selectivity is to block myocardial receptors with less effect on bronchial and vascular smooth muscle, of theoretical benefit to those with asthma or intermittent claudication. However, at the high doses used to treat angina, $\beta_1$-selectivity is often lost.

β-Blockers with partial β-agonist activity (also termed intrinsic sympathomimetic activity [ISA]) have the un-

**Table 11-5.** Calcium channel antagonists

| | Usual oral dose | Vasodilatation | ↓ Inotropy | ↓ Heart rate and AV conduction | Adverse effects |
|---|---|---|---|---|---|
| Verapamil* | 40-120 mg tid-qid | Moderate | ↓↓↓ | ↓↓↓ | Hypotension<br>Bradycardia |
| SR formulation | 120-240 mg qd-bid | | | | AV block<br>Heart failure<br>Constipation |
| Diltiazem* | 30-120 mg tid-qid | Moderate | ↓↓ | ↓↓ | Hypotension<br>Peripheral edema |
| SR formulation | 60-180 mg bid | | | | Bradycardia |
| CD formulation | 180-360 mg qd | | | | AV block<br>Heart failure |
| **Dihydropyridines** | | Marked | 0 to ↓ | 0 | Hypotension |
| Nifedipine* | 10-30 mg tid-qid | | | | Peripheral edema |
| XL formulation* | 30-120 mg qd | | | | Headache |
| Nicardipine* | 20-40 mg tid | | † | | Flushing |
| SR formulation | 30-60 mg bid | | † | | |
| Isradipine | 2.5-10 mg bid | | † | | |
| Felodipine | 5-20 mg qd | | † | | |
| Amlodipine* | 2.5-10 mg qd | | † | | |

*Approved by FDA for use in coronary artery disease.
†Least negatively inotropic agents.

usual property of mild direct stimulation of the β-receptor while blocking the receptor against circulating catecholamines. Thus the resting heart rate tends not to fall as much as with other drugs of this class, but the chronotropic response to exercise is blunted. Agents with ISA may be less desirable in patients with angina, since the comparatively higher heart rates during their use may exacerbate angina, and, unlike β-blockers without this property, they have not reliably reduced mortality following acute MI.

The duration of action of β-blockers largely depends on their lipid solubility and accounts for the different dosage schedules listed in Table 11-4. Esmolol is a very short-acting agent administered intravenously. Its effectiveness and any adverse reactions disappear within minutes of its discontinuation; thus it can be used to test the tolerability of β-blockade. It is used most commonly in the treatment of acute tachyarrhythmias and as a continuous infusion in unstable angina.

Several randomized trials have shown that, following MI, cardiovascular mortality and nonfatal secondary MIs are reduced by β-blocker therapy (with the possible exception of those with ISA). There is also evidence that they may reduce the incidence of first MIs among patients with hypertension. These attributes, combined with the β-blockers' ability to raise the anginal threshold at least as well as other antianginal drugs, place them at the forefront of chronic antianginal therapy.

Contraindications to the use of β-blockers include symptomatic congestive heart failure, a history of bronchospasm, marked resting bradycardia or AV block, and peripheral vascular disease with symptoms of claudication. In patients without such contraindications, β-blockers are started at the lower range of doses listed in Table 11-4 and advanced until the resting heart rate falls to 50 to 60 beats/min (or heart rate with exercise does not exceed 90 to 100 beats/min) or side effects occur.

Common side effects of the β-blockers include bronchoconstriction in patients with reactive airways disease, the precipitation of congestive heart failure, depression, sexual dysfunction, AV block, exacerbation of claudication, and potential masking of hypoglycemia in insulin-dependent diabetic patients. Rarely, the abrupt cessation of β-blocker therapy can lead to tachycardia, angina, or MI. In addition, β-blockers have the theoretical potential of decreasing coronary blood flow in patients with predominant coronary artery vasospasm (by inhibiting vasodilatory $\beta_2$-receptors) and should be avoided in such patients. Another long-term adverse effect of β-blocker therapy relates to the serum lipids, since they may result in the reduction of HDL cholesterol and an increase in triglycerides. These values should be monitored in patients with adverse baseline lipid profiles. This effect does not occur with β-blockers that have β-agonist activity (see Table 11-4) or α-blocking properties (i.e., labetolol).

***Calcium channel blockers.*** The calcium channel blockers are effective antianginal agents when used alone or in combination with β-blockers or nitrates. They can prevent exertional angina and are also helpful in patients with episodes of coronary vasospasm. Each drug in this class can reduce myocardial oxygen requirements and increase myocardial oxygen supply through coronary vasodilatation. However, the available agents (Table 11-5) differ in their structure and specific actions. Nifedipine and the other dihydropyridine calcium blockers are potent arterial vasodilators that reduce systemic vascular resistance, blood pressure, and therefore left ventricular wall stress with a decrease in myocardial oxygen consumption. The resultant fall in blood pressure may trigger an increase in the heart rate, an undesired effect that can be blunted by concomitant use of a β-blocker. Diltiazem and verapamil are also arteriolar dilators but are less potent than the dihydropyridines. However, they demonstrate additional properties that decrease myocardial oxygen demand: they slow the resting heart rate and decrease the left ventricular force of contraction, so concomitant β-blocker therapy is not necessary and in many cases is not desirable. Bepridil is a new calcium channel blocker that also has antiarrhythmic properties. Its place in antianginal management has not yet been defined, as its side-effect profile includes possible precipitation of ventricular arrhythmias in association with prolongation of the QT interval.

All of the calcium channel blockers have the potential to adversely reduce left ventricular contractility and should be used cautiously in patients with underlying left ventricular dysfunction. Newer dihydropyridines (e.g., nicardipine, isradipine, felodipine, and amlodipine) have the least negative inotropic effects, but their safety in patients with congestive heart failure has not been firmly established. Other common side effects of the calcium channel blockers are listed in Table 11-5.

***Antiplatelet therapy.*** Coronary thrombosis has been implicated in the majority of patients with MIs and in unstable angina. Aspirin, as an antiplatelet antithrombotic agent, has been demonstrated in primary prevention studies in men to reduce the incidence of MI, especially in individuals over age 50, and to reduce the likelihood of death or progression to MI in patients with unstable angina. In the absence of contraindications (bleeding, gastritis, or drug allergy) aspirin (80 to 325 mg every day) is recommended as part of the routine antianginal regimen.

***Antioxidant therapy.*** LDL cholesterol undergoes oxidation in proximity to the arterial wall and in that form is particularly prone to contribute to the atherosclerotic process. Recently the antioxidant vitamin E, when taken in doses of at least 100 IU per day, was shown to have reduced the incidence of primary MI in both men and women. The optimal dosage and long-term side effects of vitamin E therapy are not yet known, but in combination with other antioxidants such as vitamin C or β-carotene, it may become recommended as routine prophylaxis in patients prone to coronary disease.

## Approach to antianginal drug selection

The use of the above antianginal drugs alone, or in combination, depends on the severity of symptoms, concomitant illnesses, and the patient's activity level (see the box at right). All patients with angina should be taught the proper use of nitroglycerin for acute attacks. For chronic suppression of angina in elderly or inactive patients one can choose a long-acting nitrate (e.g., isosorbide dinitrate, 10 mg, three times daily with meals, or nitroglycerin patch 0.2 to 0.4 mg/hour, removed at bedtime, plus aspirin, 80 to 325 mg daily).

For active individuals with chronic stable exertional angina consider a β-blocker (e.g., nadolol, 40 mg daily), and if symptoms persist add a long-acting nitrate or a calcium channel blocker (not verapamil, to avoid the additive bradycardic effect), or both. For those with contraindications to β-blockade, a calcium channel blocker is recommended. If the contraindication to β-blockade is the presence of bronchospasm, insulin-dependent diabetes, or claudication, any of the calcium channel blockers approved for angina is appropriate. However, verapamil or diltiazem is preferred because of the effect on slowing the heart rate. For patients with resting bradycardia or AV block, the dihydropyridine calcium blockers (e.g., nifedipine, nicardipine, amlodipine) are better choices. In patients with congestive heart failure nitrates are the preferred initial agents; if additional therapy is needed, nicardipine or amlodipine should be considered, since they have less negative inotropic effect than other calcium channel blockers.

### Medical management of chronic stable angina

1. Correct cardiac risk factors.
2. Identify reversible contributors (e.g., anemia, hyperthyroidism, hypertension).
3. Initiate pharmacologic therapy.
   a. Nitroglycerin (sublingual, spray) as needed
   b. Aspirin, 80-325 mg/day
   c. Long-acting agents (consider concomitant diseases):
      (1) Sedentary, elderly patients: long-acting nitrates (Table 31-3)
      (2) Active, otherwise healthy patients: β-blocker (or verapamil or diltiazem)
      (3) Bronchospastic disease: calcium channel blocker* or nitrates
      (4) Insulin-dependent diabetes: calcium channel blocker* or nitrates
      (5) Intermittent claudication: calcium channel blocker* or nitrates
      (6) Resting bradycardia or AV block: calcium channel blocker (***not*** verapamil or diltiazem) or nitrates
      (7) CHF: nitrates ± dihydropyridine calcium channel blocker (especially nicardipine or amlodipine)
      (8) Atrial fibrillation: β-blocker, verapamil, or diltiazem

*Verapamil or diltiazem preferred for negative chronotropic effect, especially if combined with nitrates.

Patients suspected of having primarily coronary vasospasm should not be treated with β-blockers, which could aggravate coronary constriction; rather nitrates and calcium channel blockers are preferred. In patients with concomitant hypertension, β-blocker or calcium channel blockers are useful in treating both conditions. Similarly, patients with IHD and atrial fibrillation would benefit from a β-blocker, verapamil, or diltiazem, each of which can slow the ventricular rate.

For patients who do not respond to initial antianginal therapy, the drug dosages should be increased unless side effects occur. Combination therapy often allows the successful use of lower dosages of nitrates with or without a β-blocker with or without a calcium channel blocker while minimizing the individual drug side effects. Typical beneficial combinations include the following:

1. A nitrate plus a β-blocker, as the latter blunts the nitrate-associated tachycardia.

2. A nitrate plus verapamil or diltiazem for similar reasons.
3. A dihydropyridine calcium channel blocker plus a β-blocker is similarly beneficial, but a dihydropyridine plus nitrate is often not tolerated without concomitant β-blockade because of marked vasodilatation, with resultant headache and increased heart rate. As indicated above, a β-blocker should be combined only very cautiously with verapamil or diltiazem because of the potential of excessive bradycardia or precipitation of congestive heart failure in patients with left ventricular dysfunction.

As illustrated in the Managed Care Guide on p. 224, patients with angina who become asymptomatic on medical therapy can be followed clinically without additional interventions. Those individuals with frequent angina refractory to multidrug therapy should be referred for cardiac catheterization and consideration of mechanical revascularization. The approach to patients with diminished but persistant symptoms on medical therapy depends on whether left ventricular contractile function is compromised. Many studies indicate that patients with impaired left ventricular function (e.g., ejection fraction less than 40%) have a worse cardiac prognosis than those with similar coronary disease but preserved left ventricular function. Therefore our policy in patients with even mildly persistent angina is to obtain an assessment of left ventricular function (echocardiography or radionuclide ventriculography); if the ejection fraction is less than 40%, the patient is considered for coronary arteriography to identify those whose prognosis would improve by mechanical revascularization.

### Mechanical revascularization

As indicated above, many patients with chronic stable angina can be successfully managed by pharmacologic therapy alone. However, for those with refractory symptoms or in certain high-risk subgroups, revascularization procedures, including coronary artery bypass graft surgery (CABG) and percutaneous transluminal coronary angioplasty (PTCA), are recommended.

***Coronary artery bypass graft surgery.*** CABG consists of suturing segments of saphenous vein between the ascending aorta and to the coronary arteries distal to their stenotic narrowings. At present, in most routine cases surgeons attempt to bypass at least one diseased vessel (normally the left anterior descending coronary artery [LAD]) with an internal mammary artery, since the latter results in a higher long-term patency rate (80% to 90% at 10 years) compared to venous bypasses (10% occlusion in the first year, 2% per year for the next 6 years, 5% per year for the next 5 years). Antiplatelet therapy with aspirin has been shown to improve long-term graft patency rates.

After CABG anginal symptoms usually are relieved, exercise capacity is improved, and the need for pharmacologic therapy diminishes. The mortality of CABG is low (1% to 3% in otherwise healthy individuals) with an incidence of perioperative MI of 2% to 6%. The risk increases in patients with impaired left ventricular function, those requiring other cardiac procedures (e.g., valve replacement), in elderly patients, and those undergoing repeat CABG. In addition the recuperation of elderly or frail patients can be quite slow and accompanied by postoperative reductions of cognitive function. Therefore it is incumbent upon the physician to weigh the potential benefits of surgery against the risks of the procedure and its impact on a patient's total quality of life before recommending bypass surgery. The insight of the patient's long-term primary care physician is of great importance in rendering this decision.

CABG has been shown to prolong survival in patients with (1) greater than 50% obstruction of the left main coronary artery and (2) in patients with three-vessel disease and impaired left ventricular contractile function (ejection fraction less than 40%). Patients with one- or two-vessel disease could be expected to have symptomatic improvement with CABG but no increase in longevity compared with medical therapy alone, and revascularization for such patients should be performed only if symptoms refractory to antianginal drug therapy are present. Many patients with one- or two-vessel disease refractory to medical therapy can be managed by PTCA. In patients with three-vessel disease and preserved left ventricular function the evidence for improved survival with CABG is less clear, and we operate on such patients only if they display persistent symptoms while undergoing medical therapy, have severe proximal disease (especially of the LAD), or if extensive ischemia is demonstrated by noninvasive testing.

***Percutaneous transluminal coronary angioplasty.*** With increased experience and improved technology the range of coronary lesions amenable to PTCA has expanded over recent years. It can now be successfully performed in multivessel coronary disease as well as in stenoses of coronary bypass grafts. The lesions most likely to benefit are short and are located proximally within a coronary artery away from vessel branch points. The major complication of the procedure is dissection of the vessel intima with subsequent occlusion of the vessel requiring repeat PTCA or emergent coronary bypass graft surgery. Even after successful PTCA approximately one third of dilated vessels redevelop significant stenosis within the following 6 months. The mechanism of this complication is not known, nor have successful regimens been developed to prevent it. Fortunately, restenosis is often amenable to a repeat balloon dilatation procedure.

Patients who undergo PTCA have much shorter hospital stays and easier recuperation compared with those who undergo CABG. This has contributed to the explosive popularity of this technique, but there is concern about its overuse. Although one study has shown that PTCA is superior to medical therapy for symptomatic relief of angina, it did not reduce the risk of infarction or mortality. Large controlled studies of PTCA versus medical or coronary bypass surgery are needed to clarify the proper role of this technique, but at present the most widely accepted indication is in the treatment of angina refractory to medical therapy in the presence of suitable coronary stenoses.

In addition to balloon catheter PTCA, investigational angioplasty techniques have included laser and atherectomy devices and the placement of intracoronary stents. The early success and restenosis rates of these techniques have not proved superior to balloon angioplasty.

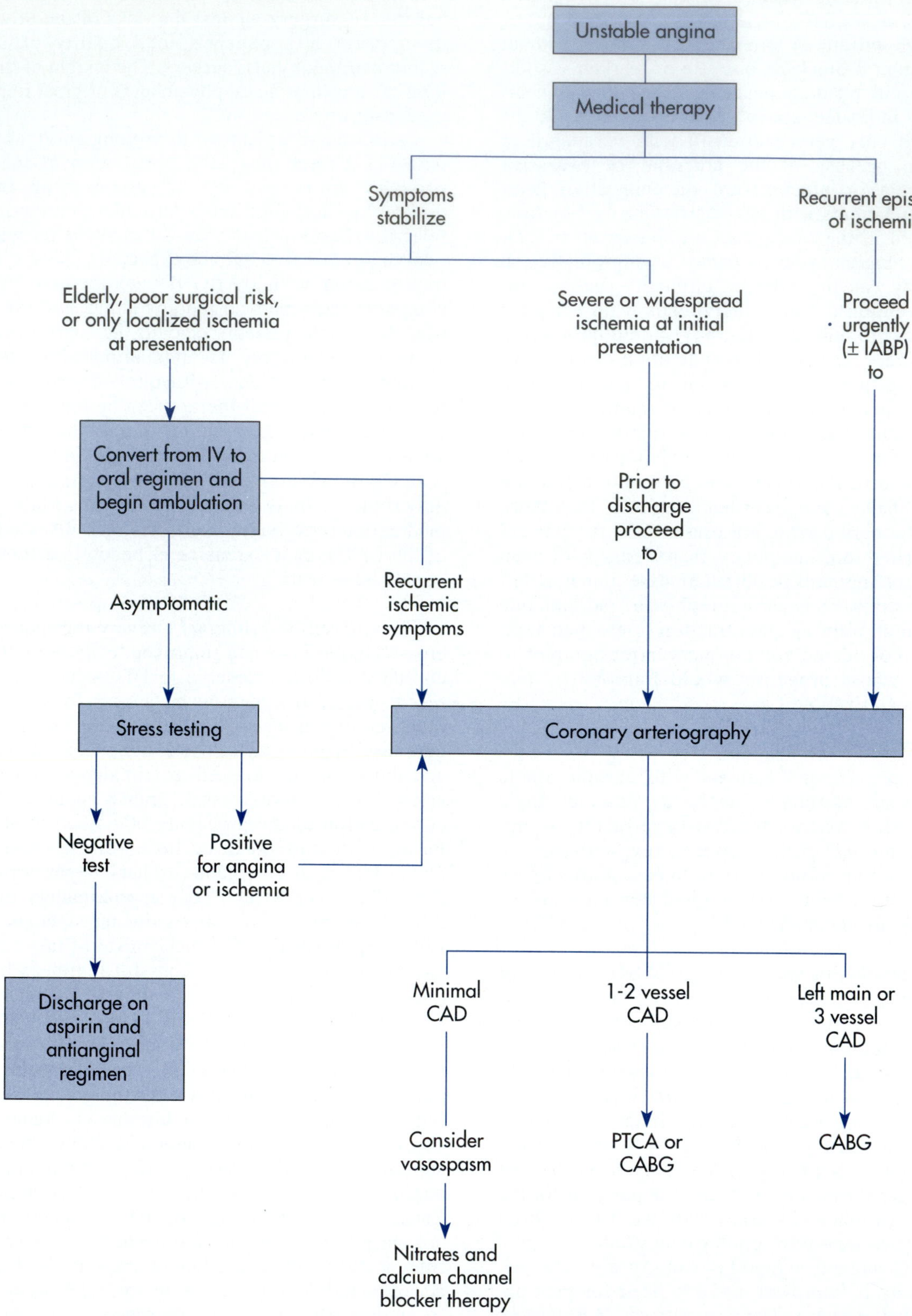


**Fig. 11-1.** Management decisions in unstable angina. *IABP,* intra-aortic balloon pump; *CAD,* coronary artery disease; *PTCA,* percutaneous transluminal coronary angioplasty; *CABG,* coronary artery bypass graft surgery.

## UNSTABLE ANGINA

Patients with coronary artery disease may show a stable pattern of symptoms for many years. However, unstable angina refers to an acceleration of symptoms in which ischemic episodes occur more frequently, are more intense, last longer, and are precipitated by less activity than previously, or even by rest. A large number of such patients progress to acute MI due to the presence of complicated coronary lesions with ulceration, hemorrhage, or thrombosis at the site of atherosclerotic plaque. In other cases the lesions responsible for unstable angina may heal and the patient's symptoms return to a more stable pattern.

Unstable angina is a medical emergency. The patient should be hospitalized in an ECG-monitored unit and confined to bed (see the box at right). During episodes of angina transient ST segment shifts or T wave flattening or inversion is likely. In addition, signs of left ventricular dysfunction (pulmonary rales, $S_3$, mitral regurgitation) may accompany ischemic episodes. Contributing factors to the imbalance between myocardial oxygen supply and demand should be considered and corrected, including hypoxemia, anemia, hypertension, thyrotoxicosis, and tachyarrhythmias.

Therapy of unstable angina consists of measures to reduce myocardial oxygen demand and increase coronary flow. In addition, since intravascular thrombosis appears to play such an important role in the pathogenesis of unstable angina, antiplatelet and anticoagulant agents are a mainstay of therapy. Both aspirin and intravenous heparin have been shown to decrease the incidence of MI and cardiac death in unstable angina, whether used alone or together. Our policy is to begin aspirin (160 to 325 mg daily) immediately upon presentation (the oral antiplatelet drug ticlopidine has also been shown to reduce complications of unstable angina and is a reasonable alternative in aspirin-intolerant individuals). For patients with recurrent bouts of ischemia, full-dose intravenous heparin is added to achieve an activated partial thromboplastin time (PTT) of two times control for several days. Studies thus far have not shown thrombolytic therapy to reduce morbidity or mortality in the setting of unstable angina without acute MI.

For patients who are refractory to medical therapy, coronary arteriography should be performed urgently (Fig. 11-1) followed by mechanical revascularization (CABG in those with left main or three-vessel disease; PTCA may be possible in those with one- or two-vessel disease). If facilities for these procedures are not available, it is recommended that an intraaortic balloon pump be placed to improve diastolic perfusion of coronary arteries and to provide afterload reduction to the left ventricle (to reduce wall tension and myocardial oxygen consumption) while the patient is transferred to an institution where revascularization procedures can be undertaken.

For patients who do stabilize on medical therapy, there remains a risk of recurrent unstable angina or MI, and additional evaluation is necessary (see Fig. 11-1). For active patients who were admitted to the hospital with severe symptoms and marked, diffuse ECG evidence of ischemia, elective cardiac catheterization is recommended before discharge to determine whether revascularization procedures are warranted. In selected patients, such as the elderly, those at poor surgical risk, or those with less severe presentations and more limited ECG evidence of ischemia, a less invasive approach is reasonable. That is, after 2 to 3 days, if symptoms of angina have responded to therapy, the intravenous heparin and antianginal agents can be replaced by oral drugs and gentle ambulation begun. Before discharge exercise or pharmacologic (e.g., dipyridamole) stress testing should be performed. If spontaneous or exercise-induced ischemia is demonstrated, coronary angiography would be recommended. However, those who do well on exercise testing could be discharged on the oral antianginal regimen with further interventions guided by their symptoms.

Sometimes the recent onset of angina in a previously asymptomatic individual is also termed unstable angina. However, if symptoms occur only on exertion and are quickly relieved by rest or medical therapy, the need for hospitalization and the aggressive therapy indicated in the box above are often not necessary.

### Initial management of unstable angina

1. Admit to monitored bed, prescribe supplemental oxygen, mild sedation
2. Consider contributing factors: anemia, hypoxemia, hypertension, thyrotoxicosis
3. Anticoagulant and antiplatelet therapy:
   a. Aspirin, 160-325 mg on admission, then daily
   b. IV heparin to maintain a PTT at two times control for several days
4. Nitrates: oral, transcutaneous paste, or IV (start at 10 μg/min and titrate upward)
5. β-Blocker (to attain heart rate 60-70), e.g., IV metoprolol, 5 mg every 5 minutes for 3 doses, then switch to oral
6. If symptoms persist, add calcium channel blocker (if β-blocker contraindicated, use verapamil or diltiazem; if added in conjunction with β-blocker, use nifedipine or other dihydropyridine calcium channel blocker)

## TYPICAL ANGINA PECTORIS WITH NORMAL CORONARY ARTERIOGRAM

This condition, often referred to as *syndrome X,* is characterized by classic exertional angina in individuals found to have no significant coronary stenoses at cardiac catheterization. Yet such patients may have convincing evidence of myocardial ischemia at exercise testing and nuclear scintigraphy. Some of these patients have coronary artery spasm, but most do not. Rather, many patients with this syndrome have evidence of inadequate coronary vasodilator reserve: small branches of the coronaries (the resistance vessels not visible by angiography) do not dilate appropriately during periods of increased myocardial oxygen demand, resulting in ischemia. The underlying mechanism is unknown, but the prognosis of such patients is excellent. Symptoms usually respond to nitrate or calcium channel blocker therapy.

This syndrome is to be distinguished from other forms of cardiac pathology that produce ischemia in the absence of coronary disease, due to increased myocardial oxygen demand, such as advanced aortic stenosis. In addition, some patients with classic symptoms of angina and normal coronary arteries do not have organic illness at all. They have no evidence of ischemia by exercise scintigraphy or other testing and may suffer from anxiety disorders. An understanding attitude by the physician, reassurance of an excellent prognosis, and psychologic counseling may be of great benefit.

## SILENT ISCHEMIA

When patients with chronic stable angina undergo ambulatory ECG monitoring, ST segment shifts usually occur during anginal episodes. But many patients demonstrate similar ischemic ST shifts during the day in the absence of symptoms, and this is termed silent, or painless, ischemia. Why some episodes are symptomatic and others silent is not known, but the presence of ST shifts on ambulatory monitoring, whether accompanied by symptoms or not, portends increased risk of MI and cardiac death.

In addition, among patients with severe coronary artery disease there is a subset who demonstrate ST shifts with activity, but *never* experience the pain of angina. Such individuals have abnormal ST shifts during exercise tests but no accompanying chest pain. These patients are believed to have a defective anginal warning system, the mechanism of which is not known, but this syndrome is more common in diabetic individuals. Despite the lack of symptoms, patients with totally silent ischemia are at risk for acute MI or cardiac death. Indeed, it is estimated that approximately 20% of acute MIs are clinically silent.

The proper management of patients with silent ischemia is under debate. While the incidence of asymptomatic shifts can be reduced by antianginal medical therapy, PTCA, or CABG, it has not been shown that such treatment alters a patient's prognosis. Thus the management of patients with silent ischemia remains individualized. Our policy is that patients with severe or diffuse ischemia on exercise or pharmacologic stress testing are given antianginal medications (e.g., a β-blocker or calcium channel blocker plus aspirin) and undergo cardiac catheterization. If left main or three-vessel disease with left ventricular dysfunction is demonstrated, CABG is usually recommended.

## ACUTE MYOCARDIAL INFARCTION

Acute MI is one of the most feared outcomes of IHD. Nearly 1.5 million people sustain an MI in the United States each year, with a mortality rate of 25%. Sixty percent of MI-related deaths occur before medical facilities are reached, and even though survival after hospitalization has been steadily improving, an additional 10% die during the following year. The location and extent of myocardial damage determine the acute presentation as well as early and long-term complications of MI. As such, limiting the size of an acute infarct is the subject of intense investigative efforts.

### Etiology

MI is the result of prolonged myocardial ischemia that leads to irreversible necrosis of heart muscle. In more than 90% of cases the causal event is the development of an acute thrombus at the site of underlying coronary atherosclerosis. Although the exact mechanism is not known, such thrombosis appears to be the result of interactions between the atherosclerotic plaque, the coronary endothelium, circulating platelets, and dynamic vasomotor tone of the coronary arterial wall.

Rarely, MI may be due to nonatherosclerotic causes, examples of which are indicated in the box below. These should be suspected particularly in young individuals and those without underlying coronary risk factors. Cocaine use is a rare and unfortunate cause of infarction. It is likely due to the ability of cocaine to increase myocardial oxygen demand, induce coronary vasospasm, and promote coronary thrombosis, in association with platelet activation and endothelial cell dysfunction.

### Clinical presentation

The initial diagnosis of MI relies on the presenting history, physical examination, and ECG. The most common symptom is severe crushing chest pain, the location of which may be similar to previous angina, but it lasts longer, is more intense, and is often accompanied by nausea, diaphoresis, dyspnea, and the feeling of impending doom. There is a circadian variability to the development of MI, occurring most commonly in the morning hours, soon after awakening. Symptoms of MI usually begin while at rest, and only occasionally are brought on by physical exertion that may have resulted in anginal episodes previously. Rather than severe chest pain, some patients with acute MI present with less pronounced symptoms, including generalized weakness, dyspnea, and indigestion. In up to 20% of cases an acute MI is free of *any* symptoms and is detected only in retrospect by changes on a routine ECG.

Common physical findings in MI (see the box at right) relate to impaired left ventricular systolic and diastolic function, associated inflammatory responses, and stimulation of the sympathetic and parasympathetic nervous systems.

#### Nonatherosclerotic causes of myocardial infarction

- Coronary emboli
  - Endocarditis
  - Prosthetic heart valve thromboemboli
- Congenital anomalies
  - Abnormal origin of the left anterior descending coronary artery, allowing it to be physically compressed
- Acquired coronary abnormalities
  - Coronary artery aneurysm or dissection
- Severe coronary artery spasm
  - Prinzmetal
  - Cocaine-induced
- Vasculitis
  - Systemic lupus erythematosus
  - Takayasu arteritis
- Increased blood viscosity
  - Polycythemia vera
  - Thrombocytosis
- Marked increase in myocardial oxygen demand
  - Severe aortic stenosis

Certain other causes of substernal chest pain may resemble that of acute MI (Table 11-6) and must be considered to avoid inappropriate initial therapy. In particular, aortic dissection or pulmonary emboli may be fatal if not quickly recognized. If confused with MI, inappropriate administration of thrombolytic therapy to patients with pericarditis or aortic dissection could result in severe complications or death.

## Electrocardiogram

Typically, ECG changes occur during an acute MI in a characteristic, sequential fashion. As shown in Fig. 11-2, in *Q wave infarctions* (formally termed transmural infarctions), initial hyperacute T waves and ST elevation are present in the leads overlying the involved myocardium. Over the next several hours, as cell death occurs, there is loss of the R wave and progressive Q wave development. The T wave begins to invert, followed by return of the ST segment to its baseline over subsequent days. The T wave may remain inverted for weeks to months before returning to its baseline, but the new Q wave persists as a permanent marker of the infarction. The anatomic site of infarction is determined by the ECG leads affected by these sequential changes (Table 11-7). Note that posterior wall infarctions produce a mirror image pattern in the anterior chest leads, with initial T wave inversion, ST segment depression, and development of tall R waves in leads $V_1$ and $V_2$.

In *non–Q wave infarction* (formally termed nontransmural MI), the ECG evolution is more subtle: new ST depression and/or T wave inversions persist for 48 hours, or longer, in the leads overlying the infarcting segments. The ST segments later normalize, but pathologic Q waves

### Major physical signs in acute myocardial infarction

General appearance
- Diaphoresis, anxious
- Cool, clammy skin

Vital signs
- Mild tachycardia and hypertension frequent, but bradycardia and hypotension common in inferior wall MI (increased vagal tone)

Jugular veins
- Distended if biventricular heart failure or right ventricular infarction present

Pulmonary
- Rales if LV heart failure present

Cardiac
- Precordial bulge if large anterior MI
- $S_4$ common, also $S_3$ if heart failure present
- Mitral regurgitation murmur if papillary muscle ischemia/infarction present

**Table 11-6.** Conditions that may mimic pain of acute myocardial infarction

| Condition | Clues to diagnosis | Confirmatory studies |
|---|---|---|
| Aortic dissection | Sharp, ripping pain that migrates<br>Asymmetry of arterial pulses | Transesophageal echo, MRI, CT, angiography |
| Acute pericarditis | Sharp, pleuritic, positional pain<br>Pericardial friction rub<br>Diffuse ST elevation on ECG | Pericardial effusion on echocardiogram |
| Pulmonary embolism | Dyspnea, pleuritic chest pain<br>Predisposing factors for venous thrombosis | Ventilation/perfusion scan<br>Pulmonary angiography |
| Pneumothorax | Sudden dyspnea, very sharp pain<br>Absent breath sounds over affected region | Chest x-ray |
| Esophageal spasm | Worse upon swallowing<br>History of dysphagia, especially to cold liquids | Barium swallow<br>Esophageal manometry |
| Acute cholecystitis | Right upper quadrant tenderness<br>Nausea, vomiting<br>History of fatty food intolerance | Abdominal ultrasound |

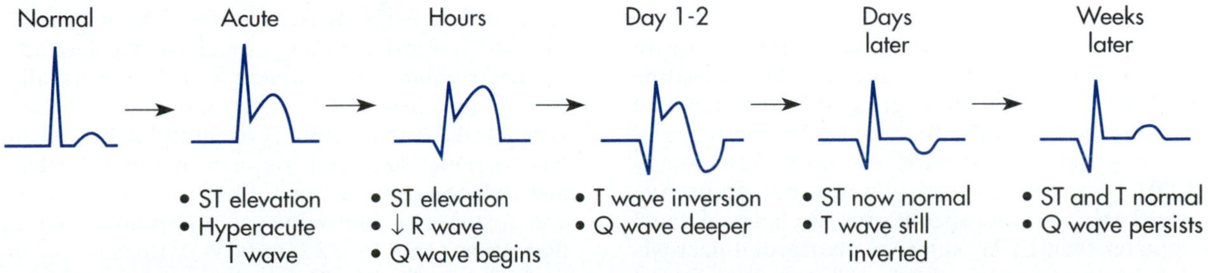


**Fig. 11-2.** ECG evolution of acute Q wave infarction. (Modified from Lilly LS, editor: *Pathophysiology of heart disease,* Philadelphia, 1993, Lea & Febiger.)

**Table 11-7.** Myocardial infarction localization

| Anatomic site | Leads with acute changes | Coronary artery likely involved |
|---|---|---|
| Inferior | II, III, aVF | RCA |
| Anteroseptal | $V_1$-$V_2$ | LAD (proximal) |
| Anteroapical | $V_3$-$V_4$ | LAD or its branches |
| Anterolateral | $V_5$-$V_6$, I, aVL | Mid-LAD or CFX |
| High lateral | I, aVL | CFX |
| Extensive anterior | $V_1$-$V_6$ | LAD (proximal) |
| Posterior | $V_1$-$V_2$* | PDA |

*RCA*, Right coronary; *LAD*, left anterior descending; *CFX*, left circumflex; *PDA*, posterior descending.

*Mirror-image changes in these leads (i.e., ST depression and tall R waves in Q wave posterior MI).

do not appear. Such patients may have otherwise typical symptoms and enzyme abnormalities indicative of acute MI, and the natural history and therapeutic implications of this type of infarct are described below.

In patients with markedly abnormal baseline ECGs (e.g., left bundle branch block) diagnostic ECG evolution may not occur, and the diagnosis of MI relies on the serum enzymes and other laboratory modalities.

### Serum enzymes

Certain enzymes are released into the circulation in a predictable temporal fashion during acute MI, and are therefore diagnostically helpful.

Creatine kinase (CK) rises in the plasma within 6 to 8 hours, peaks at 24 hours, and returns to normal by 48 to 72 hours. The peak rise is greater and occurs earlier (less than 12 hours) following thrombolytic therapy. The total CK can also rise after skeletal muscle trauma, intramuscular injections, and in hypothyroidism. The CK-MB isoenzyme should be measured on admission, then 12 and 24 hours later in the diagnostic evaluation of an acute MI.

CK-MB is the most important enzymatic measurement in the diagnosis of acute MI. It is present in only tiny quantities in noncardiac tissues and is not influenced by skeletal muscle injuries. The serum CK-MB rises and peaks slightly earlier than the total CK and returns to normal within 36 to 72 hours. Generally, in MI, the CK-MB is greater than 5% of the total serum CK. Serum CK-MB levels may be elevated in other conditions such as myocarditis, following cardiac surgery, after repetitive cardioversions, and in hypothyroidism. However, in these conditions the temporal sequence of release seen in MI does not occur.

Lactate dehydrogenase (LDH) rises within 24 to 48 hours of MI, peaks at 3 to 5 days, and returns to baseline by 7 to 10 days. Its usefulness is greatest in patients who are admitted to the hospital 2 to 3 days after the onset of symptoms, at which time the CK evolution has already passed. LDH is present in many tissues, but of its five isoenzymes, $LDH_1$ is most specific for the heart. A level of $LDH_1$ greater than $LDH_2$ suggests myocardial necrosis in the appropriate clinical setting.

Other enzymatic markers to aid in the diagnosis of MI are under investigation. For example, serum myoglobin rises quickly during an MI (less than 3 hours) and may have a role in early diagnosis, but it is also elevated following skeletal muscle injury.

### Other laboratory studies

In some cases the history, ECG, and cardiac enzymes are not sufficient to confirm the diagnosis of MI, and other laboratory tests can be useful. For example, acute infarct scintigraphy using $^{99m}$Tc pyrophosphate is highly sensitive for imaging large transmural infarcts. This type of hot spot scan is positive 2 to 7 days after MI, so is most useful for patients who are seen a few days after the onset of symptoms. In addition, echocardiography and radionuclide ventriculography can identify wall motion abnormalities indicative of infarction, but unless a previous study is available, they cannot indicate when the injury occurred.

## Management

The in-hospital mortality for acute MI has fallen substantially in the past 30 years thanks to marked improvements in therapy. The primary goals of hospitalization are to limit the size of the infarct and promptly recognize and treat complications.

***Thrombolytic therapy.*** As indicated above, most cases of MI are due to the formation of an acute thrombus that obstructs a coronary artery. Pharmacologic activation of the natural fibrinolytic system, to dissolve that thrombus, successfully restores flow in 60% to 90% of patients. Such therapy has been conclusively demonstrated to reduce mortality and improve recovery of left ventricular function following acute MI. The benefit of thrombolysis relies on early and sustained patency of the obstructed coronary artery.

**Thrombolytic agents.** The commonly used agents are streptokinase (SK), anisoylated plasminogen-SK activator complex (APSAC), and tissue plasminogen activator (t-PA). Each of these results in the conversion of the proenzyme plasminogen to active plasmin, which dissolves fibrin clots. However, different mechanisms of action and pharmacology of these drugs result in varying specificity for the thrombus responsible for the MI (Table 11-8). For example, t-PA attaches preferentially to a formed thrombus and lyses it without substantially activating fibrinolysis in the general circulation, in contrast to streptokinase. Nonetheless, bleeding is the most important risk of each of these agents and their adjunctive therapies.

Successful reperfusion is heralded by the relief of chest pain, and an early peak of serum CK (within 12 hours). Reperfusion arrhythmias, especially accelerated idioventricular rhythm, are common and do not usually require therapy (see below). To maintain patency of the coronary vessel following thrombolysis, antiplatelet and anticoagulant therapies are used. Aspirin inhibits platelet function and reduces reocclusion following thrombolysis, so it is administered at the time of admission, and each day thereafter (160 to 325 mg/day). Because of the short half-life of t-PA, intravenous heparin is needed to maintain vessel patency after initial thrombolysis. Intravenous heparin may also be beneficial in patients receiving

**Table 11-8.** Thrombolytic agents

| | Streptokinase | APSAC | t-PA |
|---|---|---|---|
| Fibrin clot specificity | None | Mild | Moderate |
| Initial reperfusion rate | 50%-60% | 60% | 75%-85% |
| Early reocclusion rate | 5%-20% | 10%-20% | 10%-20% |
| Major advantage | Least expensive | Ease of administration | Limited systemic lytic state<br>Small survival advantage in certain subgroups |
| Major complications | Bleeding and antigenic reactions | Bleeding and antigenic reactions | Bleeding |
| Dose | 1.5 million units IV over 1 hour | 30 units IV over 5 minutes | 10 mg bolus, then 50 mg over 1 hour, then 40 mg over next 2 hours<br>Accelerated regimen preferred by some centers, but not yet approved by FDA: 15 mg bolus, then 50 mg over 30 minutes, then 35 mg over 60 minutes |
| Approximate cost ($) | 500 | 1500 | 2200 |

*APSAC*, Anisoylated plasminogen-streptokinase activator complex; *t-PA*, tissue plasminogen activator.

streptokinase, but this indication has not yet been conclusively demonstrated, and subcutaneous heparin may be as effective. At present our policy is to use intravenous heparin following administration of all currently used thrombolytic agents, to achieve an activated PTT of two times control, for 2 to 3 days.

Several trials have compared the efficacy of the available thrombolytic agents. The large GISSI-2 and ISIS-3 trials published in 1990 and 1992, respectively, showed no survival advantage of one agent over the others. However, in 1993 the early results of the international GUSTO trial found a small survival advantage for t-PA (mortality 6.3%) compared with streptokinase (mortality 7.3%) at 30 days following MI. In that study the additional benefit of t-PA may have related to treatment strategies in which the drug was administered in an accelerated fashion (see Table 11-8) and intravenous heparin was used as adjunctive therapy, which had not been the routine policy in previous studies. Long-term results from this trial are not available as of this writing, and it is not yet clear whether the initial small survival benefit of t-PA will be sustained or apply only to certain patient subsets. Given the high cost of t-PA, clearly superior outcomes would be necessary to justify its widespread use.

The most important message of the recent thrombolytic trials is that early and sustained patency of an infarct-related coronary artery improves survival. It is crucial that patients receive thrombolysis as quickly as possible, and at this time the choice of which thrombolytic agent is used is less critical.

**Patient selection.** The usual criteria for selecting patients for thrombolytic therapy include evidence of an evolving Q wave MI and the ability to administer the thrombolytic drug within a period likely to result in an improved outcome (Fig. 11-3). The greatest survival benefit occurs when thrombolytic therapy is administered less than 6 hours after the onset of symptoms. Nonetheless, several studies have shown that treatment as late as 24 hours into the course of an MI can reduce the mortality rate. Therefore in certain situations, such as a stuttering course of chest pain during an evolving MI, it is reasonable to undertake thrombolytic therapy up to 24 hours after the onset of symptoms.

The major contraindications to thrombolytic therapy are situations that increase the likelihood of bleeding (see Fig. 11-3). In addition, patients who have received streptokinase or APSAC previously should not be rechallenged with either agent because of the potential of allergic reactions. Advanced age is not a contraindication to thrombolytic therapy; although most often administered to those under 75 years old, it should also be considered in older patients who are otherwise healthy and do not have specific contraindications.

When thrombolytic therapy *is* contraindicated (e.g., following recent surgery), an equally effective approach to restore coronary blood flow is to refer the patient to a cardiologist for emergent PTCA, if facilities are available and can be rapidly mobilized.

Recent studies have shown that routine coronary angiography and revascularization following successful thrombolytic therapy is not mandatory, but should be performed promptly in patients with recurrent spontaneous ischemia, or if ischemia is provoked by a predischarge exercise test (see below).

***Routine MI management.*** Whether or not thrombolytic therapy is administered, routine MI management is aimed at restoring the balance between myocardial oxygen demand and supply and at relieving ischemic pain (see the box on p. 238 and the Managed Care Guides on p. 237).

**General measures.** The patient should be admitted to a monitored coronary care unit bed for 24 to 48 hours where activities should be minimized, mild sedation administered, a soft diet and stool softener prescribed, and an intravenous line placed for emergency access, should a

**General selection criteria**

1. Chest pain consistent with MI of ≥ 30 minutes duration
2. Electrocardiographic evidence of acute Q wave MI:
   - ST elevation (≥0.1 mV) in at least 2 leads in anterior, inferior, or lateral locations
   - Acute ST depression with prominent R wave in leads $V_1$-$V_2$ (posterior MI)
   - New left bundle branch block
3. Time since symptoms began:
   < 6 hours: greatest benefit
   > 12 hours: less benefit, but still useful if chest pain continues

↓

**Exclusion criteria**

- Major surgery or trauma in preceding 6 weeks
- Gastrointestinal or genitourinary bleeding within 6 months
- Systemic bleeding disorder
- Acute pericarditis or aortic dissection
- Cardiopulmonary resuscitation for > 10 minutes
- Intracranial tumor or previous intracranial surgery
- Cerebrovascular accident within previous 6 months
- Severe hypertension (> 200/120)
- Pregnancy

↓

**Administer**
**streptokinase** or **APSAC** or **t-PA**
**with adjunctive therapy:**

1. Heparin to maintain aPTT = 2 × control for 2-3 days
2. Aspirin 160-325 mg po qd

↓

**Subsequent coronary arteriography reserved for:**

- Spontaneous recurrent ischemia
- Positive exercise test before discharge

**Fig. 11-3.** Approach to thrombolytic therapy in acute Q wave MI.

## Managed Care Guide
## Acute myocardial infarction: practice guidelines*

1. Confirm discharge diagnosis of acute MI (by CPK, LDH isoenzymes, ECG)
2. Use thrombolytics (for >30 minutes pain, ST elevation on ECG, age <80, onset <6 hours, usual exclusions)
3. Give aspirin (except for usual exclusions including platelets <100K, Hgb <10, creat >3)
4. Use (low dose) heparin (>4000 U/24 hours, usual exclusions including PT >16)
5. IV NTG for persistant chest pain
6. Give thrombolytics early (log time from hopital arrival until drug administration)
7. Give aspirin early (log time in days from hospital arrival until ASA administration)
8. Aspirin at discharge (usual exclusions, similar to no. 3)
9. β-Blockers at discharge (EF >35%, no pulmonary edema, CHF, hypotension, or shock during hospitalization, BPs >100, P >50 at discharge, other usual exclusions including also very low risk for recurrent MI)
10. ACE at discharge for EF <40% (except with BPs <100, AS, creat ≥2)
11. No calcium blocker at discharge if poor ventricular function (EF <40%, CHF, pulmonary edema or shock during hospitalization)
12. Advice or counseling at discharge on smoking cessation

*National Cooperative Cardiovascular Project (HCFA + PROs): Quality improvement project starting nationwide January 1, 1995. (From American Heart Association.)

## Managed Care Guide
## Generally accepted eligibility/exclusion criteria: thrombolytic therapy for AMI

**1. Eligibility criteria**

***Clinical***

Chest pain or chest-pain–equivalent syndrome consistent with AMI ≤12 hours from symptom onset with:

***ECG***

- ≥1 mm ST elevation in ≥2 contiguous limb leads
- ≥2 mm ST elevation in ≥2 contiguous precordial leads
- New bundle branch block

***Cardiogenic shock***

Emergency catheterization and revascularization if possible; consider thrombolysis if catheterization not immediately available

**2. Contraindications**

***Absolute contraindications: require consideration of other reperfusion strategy, such as PTCA or CABG***

- Altered consciousness
- Active internal bleeding
- Known spinal cord or cerebral arteriovenous malformation or tumor
- Recent head trauma
- Known previous hemorrhagic cerebrovascular accident
- Intracranial or intraspinal surgery within 2 months
- Trauma or surgery within 2 weeks, which could result in bleeding into a closed space
- Persistent blood pressure >200/120 mm HG
- Known bleeding disorder
- Pregnancy
- Suspected aortic dissection
- Previous allergy to a streptokinase product (but not a contraindication to use of other thrombolytic agents)

***Relative contraindications:***

- Active peptic ulcer disease
- History of ischemic or embolic cerebrovascular accident (CVA)
- Current use of oral anticoagulants
- Major trauma or surgery >2 weeks, <2 months
- History of chronic, uncontrolled hypertension (diastolic >100 mmHG), treated or untreated
- Subclavian or internal jugular venous cannulation

(From American Heart Association.)

### Initial routine management of acute myocardial infarction

Admit to monitored bed, supplemental oxygen, soft diet, mild sedation
Pain relief:
Nitroglycerin, 0.4 mg sublingual every 5 minutes for 3 doses (if not hypotensive)
Morphine sulfate, 1-4 mg IV every 5 to 10 minutes
IV nitroglycerin, start at 10 μg/min (see text)
β-Blocker (e.g., metoprolol, 5 mg IV every 2 to 5 minutes for 3 doses)
Aspirin, 160-325 mg (chewed or swallowed) on admission and every day thereafter
Heparin:
Administer IV (to achieve a PTT 2 times control) if patient receives thrombolytic therapy or has large akinetic segment or intraventricular thrombus
OTHERWISE
5000 U subcutaneous every 8 to 12 hours

sudden arrhythmia appear. Supplemental oxygen (2 to 4 L/min via nasal cannula) is recommended, since mild hypoxemia is common in acute MI. The hemoglobin oxygen saturation can be measured noninvasively by pulse oximetry and should be maintained at greater than 90%.

**Pain relief.** Sublingual nitroglycerin (0.3 to 0.4 mg) can be administered every 5 minutes in the absence of hypotension. If pain persists for more than three doses, morphine sulphate should be used, 1 to 4 mg every 5 to 10 minutes. Side effects of morphine include nausea, dizziness, hypotension, and respiratory depression (reversible by naloxone, 0.4 mg IV). Morphine may also produce bradycardia via a vagal effect, which responds to atropine (0.6 to 1.0 mg IV). Intravenous nitroglycerin should be reserved for patients with severe hypertension or recurrent chest pain unresponsive to β-blockers. Although early intravenous nitroglycerin may have a beneficial effect on limitation of infarct size in selected patients, it may also result in detrimental excess hypotension or reflex tachycardia, and its routine use is not recommended.

**β-Blockers.** These have been shown to reduce myocardial infarct size and post MI mortality, and are routinely administered if contraindications (i.e., heart rate under 55, systolic blood pressure under 100 mm Hg, bronchospasm, congestive heart failure, advanced AV block) are absent. β-Blockers are particularly useful in patients with sympathetic hyperactivity manifest as hypertension or tachycardia to reduce myocardial oxygen demand. Our standard regimen is to administer three doses of metoprolol, 5 mg IV, 2 to 5 minutes apart, followed by oral doses of 50 to 100 mg every 12 hours. For patients at potential risk of β-blocker complications, the ultra–short-acting agent esmolol HCl is preferred, since its side effects resolve quickly upon its discontinuation. It is administered as a 250- to 500-μg/kg bolus over 1 minute, followed by 50 μg/kg/min titrated to a heart rate of 55 to 60 beats/min.

**Aspirin.** This has been shown to decrease mortality following MI. In the absence of contraindications, 160 to 325 mg should be administered at the time of admission and each day thereafter.

**Heparin.** Heparin is administered intravenously to patients who receive thrombolytic therapy, for 2 to 3 days as indicated above. Patients with large akinetic segments (e.g., in association with a large anterior MI) or intraventricular thrombus formation should also receive intravenous heparin, followed by oral warfarin for 3 to 6 months to prevent peripheral thromboemboli. Patients who do not receive intravenous anticoagulation should be maintained on low-dose heparin, 5000 units subcutaneously every 8 to 12 hours to prevent deep venous thrombosis.

**Magnesium.** Administered intravenously during the early phase of MI, magnesium has been shown to reduce mortality in retrospective and small prospective randomized studies. A large trial known as ISIS-4 is prospectively investigating the role of IV magnesium in the setting of acute MI and will likely resolve whether such therapy should be routine. At present we administer magnesium sulfate (2 g IV over 30 minutes) at the time of admission for acute MI, with an additional 18 g IV over the next 24 hours, if renal function is not impaired.

***Recognition and treatment of complications.*** The recognition and prompt resolution of complications following MI is critical for short- and long-term survival. Most of these complications are best approached in consultation with a cardiologist.

**Recurrent ischemia and reinfarction.** Approximately 30% of patients develop recurrent ischemia during the early phase of hospitalization, which is associated with increased mortality. Prompt referral for coronary arteriography should be performed to assess which patients would benefit from PTCA or CABG. If cardiac catheterization facilities are not immediately available, aggressive therapy with nitrates, β-blockade, and intravenous heparin should be undertaken as arrangements are made to transfer the patient to an institution where such procedures can be performed.

**Arrhythmias.** These are common in the acute MI period and usually require immediate attention. Potential contributors to the development of arrhythmias include electrolyte disorders (hypokalemia, hypomagnesemia), hypoxemia, acidosis, congestive heart failure, and certain drugs (e.g., digitalis, dopamine). Table 11-9 lists the most common rhythm disturbances following MI, their likely causes, and recommended initial therapies.

The prophylactic use of lidocaine is not generally recommended because ventricular arrhythmias can be rapidly recognized and treated in coronary care units, and potential side effects of lidocaine administration include respiratory arrest, seizures, and suppression of sinus node activity. When lidocaine is used, dosage should be reduced in the elderly and those with congestive heart failure or hepatic disease, since these conditions can slow the drug's metabolism and increase its toxicity.

**Conduction blocks.** Atrioventricular block is common during acute MI. First-degree AV block does not require therapy. Second-degree block is most often of the Wenckebach type (Mobitz type I) and requires treatment only if it results in a symptomatically slow heart rate. If so, it usually responds to atropine, 0.6 to 1.0 mg IV.

**Table 11-9.** Common rhythm disorders in acute myocardial infarction

| Disorder | Etiology | Initial treatment |
|---|---|---|
| Sinus bradycardia | Increased vagal tone | Atropine 0.6-1.0 mg IV<br>Temporary pacemaker rarely needed |
| | Effects of drugs (β-blockers, verapamil, diltiazem) | Reduce dosage |
| Sinus tachycardia | Pain, anxiety, fever, anemia, hypovolemia, congestive heart failure | Correct underlying cause<br>Treat hypovolemia and congestive heart failure (see Tables 11-10 and 11-11) |
| Supraventricular premature beats | Metabolic (hypoxia, hypokalemia, hypomagnesemia) | Correct underlying disorder |
| Atrial fibrillation | Congestive heart failure or atrial ischemia | If unstable: cardioversion<br>If no CHF: slow rate with diltiazem, verapamil, or β-blocker<br>If congestive heart failure present: slow rate with digoxin |
| Ventricular premature beats (VPBs) | Ischemia, congestive heart failure, or metabolic (hypoxia, hypokalemia, hypomagnesemia) | Treat underlying cause<br>If ≥6 VPBs/min, couplets, or R-on-T VPBs: IV lidocaine* or procainamide†<br>If no congestive heart failure: consider β-blocker therapy |
| Ventricular tachycardia (VT) | Same as for VPBs | If unstable: defibrillation<br>If stable: IV lidocaine* or procainamide†<br>For refractory VT: bretylium‡ |
| Ventricular fibrillation | Same as for VPBs | Defibrillation |
| Accelerated idioventricular rhythm | Often benign rhythm during acute MI<br>Common reperfusion rhythm after thrombolytic therapy | No therapy usually needed<br>If symptomatic: atropine 0.6-1.0 mg IV |

*IV lidocaine 1 mg/kg bolus, then 2-4 mg/min (a second bolus, 0.5 mg/kg 10 min, after the first is recommended).
†IV procainamide 500-1000 mg load (no faster than 50 mg/min), then 2-5 mg/min.
‡IV bretylium tosylate 5 mg/kg over 5 min, then 1-2 mg/min.

The prognostic significance of third-degree (complete) AV block depends on whether it occurs in the setting of an acute inferior (IMI) or anterior (AMI) infarction. In IMI complete heart block is usually transient and occurs because of heightened vagal tone or temporary ischemia of the AV node. The ventricular escape rhythm usually consists of narrow (i.e., normal) QRS complexes, since the block is high within the conduction system. Often AV conduction can be restored in this situation by IV atropine (0.6 to 1 mg), but if not, a temporary pacemaker is required.

Conversely, when AV block develops in the setting of an acute AMI, the site of block is usually more distal and widespread within the conduction pathway, due to extensive tissue destruction. Mobitz type II, or complete, heart block in AMI are ominous prognostic signs, and emergency placement of a temporary pacemaker is required, followed by permanent pacemaker placement later. Patients who develop complete heart block in the setting of AMI have a high mortality rate due to the severe underlying myocardial damage.

Other conduction defects that portend progression to complete heart block include (1) new left bundle branch block and (2) new right bundle branch block with left anterior or left posterior hemiblock. Prophylactic transvenous pacemakers should generally be placed in such individuals. The advent of external temporary pacing units may reduce the need for prophylactic transvenous pacing in these settings but are currently useful only for short periods because of the discomfort associated with their use.

**Hypertension.** During an acute MI hypertension (blood pressure over 160/100) may result from chest pain or anxiety or reflect chronic blood pressure elevation. It often improves with routine MI management, resolution of pain, and mild sedation. However, persistent hypertension can be deleterious since it increases the afterload against which the left ventricle contracts and can increase myocardial oxygen demand. Several therapeutic options exist, including (1) mild diuresis with IV furosemide if congestive heart failure is also present, (2) transcutaneous or oral nitrates (see Table 11-3); (3) IV or oral β-blockers (see Table 11-4), and (4) for severe hypertension IV nitroprusside or nitroglycerin (see below). If intravenous therapy is used, an arterial line should be placed for careful blood pressure monitoring.

**Hemodynamic complications.** These include the development of congestive heart failure, hypotension, and shock. Left ventricular failure in the setting of an MI is due to both reduced systolic contractile function and decreased diastolic compliance of the myocardium. The severity of congestive heart failure depends on the extent of infarcted tissue and whether superimposed mechanical complications (described below) have occurred.

Mild congestive heart failure, manifest by basilar rales and a cardiac third heart sound is very common during

**Table 11-10.** Hemodynamic categories in acute myocardial infarction

| Condition | Cardiac index ($L/min/m^2$) | PCWP (mm Hg) | Systolic BP (mm Hg) | Treatment |
|---|---|---|---|---|
| Normal in acute MI | >2.5 | ≤18 | >100 | |
| Hypovolemia | <2.5 | <15 | <100 | Successive boluses of 100 ml normal saline<br>If inferior MI in evolution and right atrial pressure >10: consider RV infarction |
| Volume overload | >2.5 | >18 | >100 | Diuretic (e.g., furosemide 10-20 mg IV)<br>Nitroglycerine, topical paste or IV (see Table 11-3) |
| LV failure | <2.5 | >18 | >100 | Diuretic (e.g., furosemide 10-20 mg IV)<br>IV nitroglycerine, or if markedly hypertensive use IV sodium nitroprusside |
| Severe LV failure | <2.5 | >18 | <100 | If BP ≥90: IV dobutamine ± IV nitroglycerin or sodium nitroprusside<br>If BP <90: IV dopamine<br>If accompanied by pulmonary edema: attempt diuresis with IV furosemide; may be limited by hypotension<br>May require intraaortic balloon pump |
| Cardiogenic shock | <1.8 | >18 | <90 with oliguria and confusion | IV dopamine<br>Intraaortic balloon pump<br>Emergency coronary angioplasty may be life-saving |

*PCWP*, Pulmonary artery wedge pressure; *RV*, right ventricle; *LV*, left ventricle.

early hospitalization. Therapy is similar to congestive heart failure in other conditions, with the exception that digitalis is not usually effective. Most patients respond to diuresis (e.g., furosemide, 10 to 20 mg IV), which should be administered cautiously to avoid hypovolemia and hypotension. In addition, vasodilators may be beneficial, such as topical nitroglycerin ointment (see Table 11-3).

In patients with more advanced heart failure or those with hypotension that does not quickly respond to fluid administration, invasive hemodynamic monitoring (with a balloon-tipped pulmonary artery catheter and arterial line) can greatly aid in diagnosis and therapy. Measurements of pulmonary capillary wedge pressure and the cardiac index can categorize the hemodynamic abnormality and guide an appropriate course of action (Table 11-10). Because the left ventricle is often stiff due to diminished compliance in the setting of a large MI, the desired pulmonary capillary wedge pressure is higher than normal, at approximately 15 to 18 mm Hg. Echocardiography is very useful in the evaluation of patients with congestive heart failure or hypotension in acute MI, to determine the degree of contractile dysfunction and to assess for complications such as mitral regurgitation, ventricular septal defect, cardiac tamponade, or right ventricular infarction (Table 11-11).

Right ventricular infarction should be considered when a patient with an IMI shows signs of diminished cardiac output and jugular venous distention out of proportion to left ventricular failure. The pulmonary capillary wedge pressure is commonly low in this situation, but the right atrial pressure is elevated (greater than 10 mm Hg). The diagnosis is further suggested by the presence of ST segment elevation in ECG leads placed over the right parasternal region, and right ventricular dysfunction can be confirmed by echocardiography. As a result of impeded flow through the poorly contractile right ventricle, hypotension may result and can be worsened by diuretic therapy (which further reduces filling of the heart and cardiac output). Appropriate therapy of right ventricular infarction consists of fluid administration to achieve a pulmonary capillary wedge pressure of 15 to 18 mm Hg, to ensure optimal left ventricular filling.

**Mechanical defects.** These include full or partial *rupture of a papillary muscle* and the development of a *ventricular septal defect* (VSD) due to focal weakening of the infarcting myocardium. Although these complications occur rarely, they may result in pulmonary edema, cardiogenic shock, or death. They typically occur 3 to 7 days following acute AMI or IMI, and both result in new systolic murmurs. The location of the murmur is at the cardiac apex in mitral regurgitation and at the left parasternal region in the case of a VSD. Both conditions can be readily identified by Doppler echocardiography. Invasive hemodynamic monitoring confirms the presence of a VSD by demonstrating a rise in the oxygen saturation in the pulmonary artery compared with blood in the right atrium. In acute mitral regurgitation, the pulmonary capillary wedge tracing show a large systolic v wave, although that sign is not specific for this disorder. The initial treatment of these mechanical defects includes IV vasodilators (nitroprusside or nitroglycerin) (Table 11-12), inotropic support (dobutamine or dopamine), and if cardiogenic shock supervenes, the placement of an intraaortic balloon pump. Unstable patients require urgent surgical repair.

*Rupture of the left ventricular free wall* due to ischemic necrosis occurs in less than 1% of acute MIs and is nearly always fatal because of the development of cardiac

**Table 11-11.** Differential diagnosis of hemodynamic complications following myocardial infarction

| Complication | Clinical findings | Doppler echocardiography | Right heart catheter findings |
|---|---|---|---|
| Hypovolemia | Hypotension without jugular venous distention<br>Absence of pulmonary rales | LV contractile dysfunction not sufficiently severe to explain hypotension | PCWP ≤18 mm Hg |
| Severe LV contractile dysfunction | Left and right-sided CHF; pulmonary rales, $S_3$ jugular venous distention | Marked LV contractile dysfunction | PCWP >18 mm Hg |
| Cardiac tamponade (due to pericarditis of LV free-wall rupture) | Hypotension with pulsus paradoxus<br>Jugular venous distention<br>Pericardial rub | Pericardial effusion with right-sided chamber compression | Elevated and equal PCWP and RA pressures |
| Mitral regurgitation | New apical systolic murmur<br>Acute pulmonary edema common | Abnormal systolic blood flow from LV into LA | Large v wave on PCWP tracing |
| Ventricular septal defect | New left parasternal systolic murmur<br>Acute pulmonary edema common | Abnormal systolic blood flow from LV into RV | Increased oxygen saturation in pulmonary artery compared with RA |
| Right ventricular infarction | In setting of inferior MI<br>Jugular venous distention without pulmonary rales<br>ST elevation in *right* parasternal chest leads | RV contractile dysfunction with relatively preserved LV contraction | Elevated RA pressure (>10 mm Hg) but usually normal PCWP (<18 mm Hg) |

*LV*, Left ventricle; *RV*, right ventricle; *RA*, right atrium; *LA*, left atrium; *PCWP*, pulmonary capillary wedge pressure; *CHF*, congestive heart failure.

**Table 11-12.** Intravenous vasodilators and inotropic drugs used in acute myocardial infarction

| Drug | Starting dose | Dosage range | Comment |
|---|---|---|---|
| Nitroglycerin | 10 μg/min | Up to 10 μg/kg/min | May improve coronary blood flow to ischemic myocardium |
| Sodium nitroprusside | 0.25 μg/kg/min | Up to 10 μg/kg/min | More potent vasodilator than nitroglycerin; less beneficial for improving coronary blood flow<br>Thiocyanate toxicity (blurred vision, tinnitus, delirium) can occur during prolonged therapy or in renal failure |
| Dobutamine | 2.5 μg/kg/min | Up to 20 μg/kg/min | Promotes ↑ cardiac output, ↓ PCWP, but does not raise blood pressure |
| Dopamine | 2 μg/kg/min | 10 μg/kg/min or higher | More useful than dobutamine if hypotensive<br>Effects vary by dosage:<br><5 μg/kg/min ↑ renal blood flow<br>2.5-10 μg/kg/min positive inotrope<br>>10 μg/kg/min vasoconstriction |
| Amrinone | 0.75 mg/kg bolus then 5 μg/kg/min | Up to 10 μg/kg/min | Positive inotrope and vasodilator<br>Can combine with dopamine or dobutamine<br>Long duration of action limits flexibility<br>May cause thrombocytopenia |

tamponade and shock. It occurs within the first week following MI and is most common in older women, those with a history of hypertension, and patients treated in the early postinfarct period with steroids or nonsteroidal antiinflammatory drugs. If the rupture is incomplete, the leak may seal itself off with thrombus material within the pericardium. This unstable condition is termed a *pseudoaneurysm.* If detected (usually by echocardiography), surgical repair is indicated to prevent delayed rupture.

A *true left ventricular aneurysm* is a late complication of Q wave infarctions and consists of a scarred area of myocardium that bulges outward during systole. It can be suspected clinically by persistent ST elevation on the patient's ECG many weeks following an acute MI and can be confirmed by echocardiography or left ventricular angiography. This type of aneurysm does not usually rupture, but it can lead to heart failure, ventricular arrhythmias, or thromboemboli. Surgical repair of the aneurysm is indicated if these complications are refractory to standard medical therapy.

**Pericarditis.** Manifest by pleuritic chest pain, low-grade fever, and a pericardial friction rub, pericarditis occurs in 10% to 15% of patients within the first week following MI. Aspirin (up to 650 mg every 4 to 6 hours) is the recommended therapy for pain relief, but steroids and nonsteroidal antiinflammatory agents should be avoided as they can delay healing of the infarcting myocardium. Anticoagulation with heparin or coumadin is relatively contraindicated in patients with pericarditis to avoid hemorrhagic tamponade.

A late form of pericarditis occurring 2 to 10 weeks following MI is known as Dressler's syndrome. It develops in less than 5% of post-MI patients and is thought to be of autoimmune origin. It, too, responds to aspirin, but since the myocardium has already substantially healed by the time of its occurrence, other nonsteroidal antiinflammatory agents could also be used. Glucocorticoids (prednisone, 1 mg/kg/day) should be considered only as a last resort, since such therapy can be very difficult to taper without recurrence of pain and long-term steroid dependence may result.

## REHABILITATION, RISK STRATIFICATION, AND SECONDARY PREVENTION OF RECURRENT MI

The length of hospitalization for uncomplicated MIs in the 1990s is typically 5 to 8 days but can be prolonged by the superimposed conditions described above. The patient usually remains in the coronary care unit for 24 to 48 hours. Activities are limited to near total bed rest on day 1, but progress to sitting in a chair for 30 minutes at a time, with use of the bedside commode on day 2. By day 3 the patient is usually allowed to walk within the hospital room and may shower if stable. By day 5 patients who have no complications may fully ambulate on the hospital floor.

Following discharge from the hospital, the patient can perform limited activities at home but should avoid isometric activities such as lifting objects heavier than 10 pounds. Two to 6 weeks after discharge, patients should walk ½ to 1½ miles a day, depending on the results of exercise testing; normal sexual activity can resume during this time. Additional activities can be gauged by supervised rehabilitation programs, and most patients can return to work 4 to 12 weeks following discharge. It is an important role of the patient's primary care physician to reinforce a positive outlook during this period and encourage progressive activity to aid in the rehabilitation process. The emotional stress and uncertainties that follow an MI can weigh heavily on the patient and the family. An understanding, compassionate attitude by the physicians and other health care providers can greatly facilitate emotional recuperation.

The long-term prognosis following acute MI depends on three main factors: the degree of residual myocardium at ischemic risk, the extent of left ventricular dysfunction, and the presence of ventricular arrhythmias. Assessment of these variables should be part of routine post-MI management (Table 11-13). A submaximal exercise test, aiming for 70% of the maximal predicted heart rate (with radionuclide perfusion scintigraphy if needed for accurate interpretation, or a dipyridamole-thallium study if the patient is unable to exercise) should be performed before or soon after discharge. This level of exercise exceeds the energy expended in climbing a flight of stairs and is useful to gauge activities at home. Patients with positive stress tests (development of angina, ST segment shifts, or hypotension) should undergo cardiac catheterization to assess subsequent prognosis and need for revascularization. Standard exercise testing, achieving 85% of the maximal predicted heart rate, can be performed 4 to 6 weeks after MI and is useful to guide further physical activities in the rehabilitation process.

**Table 11-13.** Evaluation and long-term therapy after myocardial infarction

| Therapy or procedure | Comments |
|---|---|
| Submaximal exercise test | Target heart rate = 70% maximal, using low-level protocol<br>If positive for angina or evidence of ischemia then proceed to cardiac catheterization<br>If negative, prescribe medical therapy as indicated below and perform full exercise test (85% maximal heart rate) 4-6 weeks post-MI |
| Evaluate left ventricular contractile function (echocardiography or radionuclide ventriculography) | If LV ejection fraction ≤40%, add ACE inhibitor (e.g., captopril titrated to 50 mg po tid)<br>If intraventricular thrombus or large anterior akinetic segment present (by echo), prescribe warfarin for 3-6 months (achieve INR 2-3), then replace with aspirin |
| Ambulatory ECG monitoring | Not recommended for patients without symptomatic arrhythmias<br>If symptomatic ventricular arrhythmias present, add β-blocker as indicated below, and obtain cardiology consultation to determine whether electrophysiologic testing or empiric antiarrhythmic therapy appropriate |
| β-Blocker | If no contraindications (e.g., timolol 10 mg bid or metoprolol 50-100 mg bid)<br>If β-blocker contraindicated (e.g., asthma) and no evidence of CHF, consider verapamil<br>In non–Q wave infarction without CHF consider diltiazem in place of β-blocker |
| Aspirin | 160-325 mg po qd (withhold if on warfarin therapy) |
| Correct predisposing risk factors | Target LDL cholesterol ≤100 mg/dl<br>Control hypertension, diabetes<br>Eliminate cigarette smoking |

*LV*, Left ventricular; *ACE*, angiotensin converting enzyme; *CHF*, congestive heart failure; *LDL*, low-density lipoprotein.

Assessment of left ventricular function by echocardiography or radionuclide ventriculography is also recommended before or soon after discharge. Recent studies have shown that patients with left ventricular ejection fractions less than 40% soon after benefit from long-term angiotensin converting enzyme inhibitor therapy (e.g., captopril, gradually titrated to 50 mg three times a day), even if such a patient is free of congestive heart failure symptoms. Study patients showed a significant decline in mortality, development of congestive heart failure, or reinfarction on such therapy when followed for an average of 3.5 years after MI.

The presence of ventricular arrhythmias (more than 10 ventricular premature beats per hour or repetitive forms) correlates with decreased survival following MI. However, routine ambulatory ECG monitoring and signal averaged ECG measurements are not recommended, because recent studies of antiarrhythmic therapy for *asymptomatic* ventricular ectopy following an MI has not been shown to reduce, and in some cases has increased, post-MI mortality. Patients with *symptomatic* ventricular arrhythmias do require interventions, however, and should be referred to a cardiologist to determine whether invasive electrophysiologic testing or a trial of antiarrhythmic drug therapy is appropriate.

Routine pharmacologic therapy following hospital discharge for acute MI includes aspirin (*if* not on warfarin) and β-blocker therapy. Aspirin, in dosages of 325 mg daily or less, has been shown to reduce post-MI mortality and reinfarction rates. β-blockers (those without intrinsic sympathomimetic activity) also reduce mortality and reinfarction, and in the absence of contraindications typical regimens include the following: timolol, 10 mg twice a day; atenolol, 50 to 100 mg daily; or metoprolol, 50 to 100 mg twice a day. If β-blockers are contraindicated (e.g., bronchospasm), verapamil may be a reasonable alternative, since limited data have shown it to reduce death and reinfarction rates in patients *without significant left ventricular dysfunction* after MI.

Patients who have sustained a non–Q wave infarction need to be considered separately. This type of infarct represents an incomplete process such that viable myocardium often remains at ischemic risk. Although the early prognosis in non–Q wave MI is good, subsequent reinfarction and the need for mechanical revascularization *exceeds* that of Q wave infarcts. In studies following non–Q wave MI, β-blockers have not consistently reduced cardiac morbidity. However, the calcium channel blocker diltiazem (approximately 240 mg daily) has been shown to reduce the rate of reinfarction in this setting, *if* there is no evidence of congestive heart failure. Therefore our approach to patients following non–Q wave MI is to proceed with exercise testing; if ischemia is induced, cardiac catheterization is undertaken. Otherwise, aspirin and diltiazem (if congestive heart failure is absent) are prescribed.

Finally, the risk factors that led to the development of atherosclerosis should be corrected because of the belief that such an approach can reduce the progression, or potentially promote the regression, of atherosclerosis. The goal for serum LDL cholesterol levels is under 100 mg/dl by dietary or pharmacologic means (see Chapter 40). Cessation of cigarette smoking and treatment of hypertension and diabetes should also be strongly reinforced by the patient's primary care physician and cardiologist.

## ISCHEMIC HEART DISEASE IN WOMEN

Coronary artery disease has historically been considered to be a disease of men, but the magnitude of this condition and its complications in women has become increasingly clear. IHD accounts for 23% of mortality among women and is the leading cause of death in women over the age of 50, resulting in 250,000 deaths per year in the United States. The manifestations of coronary disease in women may differ from those in men, in terms of its onset and outcome. For example, on average, women develop symptoms of coronary disease 10 years later than men, after the menopause, associated with the fall in serum estrogen levels. Although the rate of CAD-related mortality in men is constant after age 60, it continues to rise in women until age 70. Furthermore, women experience a greater proportion of silent MIs than men, and when an MI is symptomatic, women generally come to the hospital after a greater time delay than men with comparable symptoms. In the setting of an acute MI, the outcome of women is worse than male counterparts: there are more complications, longer hospital stays, and a greater likelihood of mortality during hospitalization and during the first post-MI year.

Nonetheless, studies have shown that the evaluation of chest pain, invasive testing, CABG, and PTCA are all performed less often in women than in men with similar symptoms. When they are referred for revascularization procedures, women are usually at more advanced stages of disease, when morbidity and mortality would be expected to be greater.

It is not known whether the comparably adverse outcome in women reflects their older age at presentation, more severe concurrent illnesses, or less intensive therapies prescribed by physicians. However, chest pain symptoms in a woman should not be downplayed, and female patients with documented angina should be educated to respond promptly to symptoms of MI to increase the likelihood of receiving beneficial early interventions.

As in men, it is crucial to reduce risk factors for coronary disease in the female population, particularly cigarette smoking, hypertension, hypercholesterolemia, and diabetes. However, in women postmenopausal hormone administration also plays an important role. There is a decreased risk of coronary disease and its associated mortality among such women who receive estrogen therapy. The combination of estrogens plus progestin is appropriate in women who have not undergone hysterectomy, to blunt the risk of endometrial cancer; the addition of progestin does not appear to prevent the beneficial cardiovascular effect of estrogen. The decision to prescribe hormonal therapy to postmenopausal women requires careful consideration by the primary care physician, who must weigh the beneficial effects of this therapy on coronary disease, osteoporosis, and menopausal symptoms versus the potential risks of uterine and breast cancer.

Pooled analysis of secondary prevention studies following an MI have shown that aspirin reduces mortality, reinfarction rates, and stroke significantly in women, similar to the results in men. β-Blockers also have comparable effectiveness in both sexes in preventing reinfarction.

As indicated above, primary prevention of MI has been demonstrated in men receiving aspirin. However, in women, primary prevention studies have been limited to observational data rather than randomized, prospective trials, and the results have been mixed. For example, in the Nurses' Health Study, women who used one to six aspirins per week had a 25% reduction in the incidence of MI compared with those who did not use aspirin. However, no benefit was seen in those taking more than seven aspirins per week. A large randomized study is needed for clarification, and it is clear that future research of IHD and its complications must address outcomes in both women and men.

## BIBLIOGRAPHY

Abrams J, editor: Angina pectoris: mechanisms, diagnosis, and therapy, *Cardiol Clin* 9:1, 1991.

American College of Cardiology/American Heart Association Task Force Report: Guidelines and indications for coronary artery bypass graft surgery, *J Am Coll Cardiol* 17:543, 1991.

Anderson HV, Willerson JT: Current concepts: thrombolysis in acute myocardial infarction, *N Engl J Med* 329:703, 1993.

Cairns JA et al: Antithrombotic agents in coronary artery disease, *Chest Suppl* 102:456S, 1992.

Elkayam U: Tolerance to organic nitrates: evidence, mechanisms, clinical relevance, and strategies for prevention, *Ann Intern Med* 14:667, 1991.

Francis GS, Alpert JS, editors: *Modern coronary care,* Boston, 1990, Little, Brown.

Guidelines for the early management of patients with acute myocardial infarction: a report of the American College of Cardiology/American Heart Association Task Force on Assessment of Diagnostic and Therapeutic Cardiovascular Procedures, *J Am Coll Cardiol* 16:249, 1990.

Pfeffer M et al: Effect of captopril on mortality and morbidity in patients with left ventricular dysfunction after myocardial infarction, *N Engl J Med* 327:669, 1992.

Wenger NK et al: Cardiovascular health and disease in women, *N Engl J Med* 329:247, 1993.

Zaret BL, Wackers FJ: Medical progress: nuclear cardiology, *N Engl J Med* 329:775; 855, 1993.

CHAPTER

# 12 Myocardial Revascularization

Nsidinanya Okike

Of the current United States population of 250 million, more than 70 million suffer from cardiovascular disease. In 1990 diseases of the heart and blood vessels were responsible for over 930,000 deaths. Consequently, knowledge of diagnostic and therapeutic modalities available for the management of coronary artery disease is important to primary care physicians.

## HISTORIC PERSPECTIVE

Many advances, including the development of coronary cinearteriography by Sones and Shirley, early experimental vascular surgery, the development of cardiopulmonary bypass by Gibbon, and direct implantation of the internal mammary artery into the myocardium by Vineberg and Miller, set the stage for the emergence of current methods of myocardial revascularization. Although Sabiston and Garret and DeBakey performed aortosaphenous vein coronary artery bypass in 1962 and 1964, respectively, Favoloro and Effler established this procedure as a reliable and effective treatment for patients with severe coronary atherosclerosis. In 1968 Green used the left internal mammary artery to bypass the left anterior descending coronary artery. Thus the foundation for the two major techniques for coronary revascularization was laid and they are now employed in many surgical centers.

## CHANGING PATIENT POPULATION

In contrast to patients undergoing bypass surgery before 1976, the current patient population is older, consists of more women, and is more likely to have severe three-vessel disease, left main coronary disease, impaired left ventricular function, diabetes mellitus, hypertension, and severe peripheral vascular disease. This new cohort of patients is also more likely to have undergone percutaneous transluminal coronary angioplasty (PTCA) or previous coronary bypass surgery.

Multiple factors have contributed to the significant increase of the elderly patients undergoing coronary bypass surgery. The average life expectancy of individuals in the United States population is increasing. Also, surgeons have eliminated the age criterion for invasive treatment of coronary artery disease. Finally, elderly patients reject the concept that they are too old to undergo cardiac operations.

The preponderance of high-risk patients undergoing coronary bypass operations is due to the recognition by surgeons and cardiologists that this procedure provides the greatest benefit in survival and relief of symptoms in patients with left main coronary artery disease and in those with severe triple vessel coronary artery disease and impaired left ventricular function.

## CORONARY ATHEROSCLEROSIS

### Morphology

Atherosclerosis of the coronary artery is a progressive disease characterized by deposition of fatty substances, cholesterol, complex mucopolysaccharides, fibrin, and calcium in the subintimal surface. Fibromuscular and fibrolipid lesions consisting of smooth muscle cells and collagen surrounding multiple lipid cores are eventually converted into atherosclerotic plaques. Microthrombi in different stages of fibrotic organization are also associated with the formation of atherosclerotic plaques.

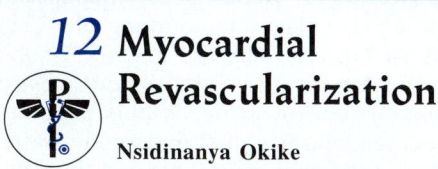

These subintimal plaques compromise the lumen of the vessel by development of new layers and hemorrhage from small blood vessels around or within the atheroma. Sudden hemorrhage associated with disruption of the atherosclerotic plaque and formation of occlusive thrombus is the morphologic substrate for unstable angina and acute myocardial infarction. Platelet aggregation alone or in combination with platelet-derived vasoactive substances (thromboxane $A_2$ and platelet-derived growth factor) may induce atheroma formation, vasospasm, and vessel occlusion. Focal involvement of the proximal segment of the coronary arteries is generally the rule. In accordance with the response-to-injury hypothesis developed by Ross, sites of branching that are subjected to turbulence are particularly prone to atherosclerosis. Muscle bridging may occasionally lead to hemodynamically significant stenosis. This segment of the artery is almost always devoid of atheroma.

### Clinical manifestations

Angina pectoris, the classic symptom of ischemic heart disease, is not always present in patients with significant coronary artery stenosis. In a report from Harper and associates only 48% of 577 patients presenting to the hospital with an acute myocardial infarction had a history of angina pectoris. Angina equivalents (i.e., symptoms of myocardial ischemia other than angina) such as abnormal exertional dyspnea, faintness, fatigue, and eructations may be the only symptoms. The usefulness of angina as an indicator of coronary artery disease is further limited by the fact that 10% of patients who present with classic angina symptoms have normal coronary arteries on cardiac catheterization. Furthermore, approximately 1 million patients with significant myocardial ischemia are asymptomatic. Hence, the emphasis should be placed on the diagnosis of myocardial ischemia that angina only in part represents.

### Diagnosis

***Noninvasive testing.*** The *noninvasive testing* that is currently used to identify and quantitate coronary artery disease includes chest x-ray, resting and exercise electrocardiogram (ECG), resting and stress radioisotope imaging, positron emission tomography (PET), magnetic resonance imaging (MRI), computerized tomography (CT), and stress echocardiogram. These methods are discussed in detail in related chapters.

***Coronary arteriography.*** From a surgical standpoint properly performed coronary arteriography remains the definitive diagnostic procedure. Coronary angiography is indicated in patients with the following:

1. Unstable angina pectoris and documented myocardial ischemia
2. Recent myocardial infarction and documented postinfarction myocardial ischemia
3. Medically refractory angina pectoris
4. Chest pain of unclear etiology
5. Significant valvular disease presenting with angina or with myocardial ischemia during noninvasive testing

Furthermore, coronary angiography is indicated in patients who are over the age of 40 years and are undergoing cardiac catheterization for surgically treatable cardiac disease. The angiogram should visualize the left main, the right and left coronary artery systems. Although coronary angiography is considered the gold standard for evaluation of coronary anatomy, it may underestimate the severity of coronary atherosclerosis. Left ventriculography provides accurate assessment of left ventricular function. Significant coronary artery stenosis compromises 50% of the diameter of the vessel, or 75% of its cross-sectional area. Multiple sequential stenotic lesions, although individually less than 50% stenosis, can together produce marked impairment of regional blood flow. Stenosis of the left main coronary artery is the most serious of all coronary lesions, and its recognition in coronary angiography is of singular importance. Left main coronary artery stenosis is best visualized on either a direct frontal projection or by the use of the sagittal angulated views. Myocardial bridging occurs in 5% to 12% of humans and is almost exclusively confined to the left anterior descending artery. Significant systolic narrowing caused by myocardial bridging can lead to myocardial ischemia during tachycardia. Eccentric stenoses and slitlike atherosclerotic narrowings can remain unrecognized unless coronary arteries are viewed in at least two projections that are separated by 90 degrees. Evaluation of *systolic left ventricular function* is essential because it is a major risk factor in the surgical outcome. An ejection fraction of 35% or more is generally associated with good surgical results. Conversely, an ejection fraction of 20% or less, especially when accompanied by left ventricular enlargement, often leads to poor surgical results. Abnormalities in the *left ventricular diastolic function* generally occur in patients with extensive coronary artery disease. Because ischemia impairs the rate of relaxation of myocardial fibers, there is reduction in the peak rate of left ventricular filling as well as an increase in the time required to achieve peak filling rate. When systolic and diastolic function are significantly impaired, they can lead to a significant elevation in left ventricular end diastolic pressure with exercise.

## INDICATIONS FOR MYOCARDIAL REVASCULARIZATION

Myocardial revascularization can be accomplished by coronary artery bypass surgery and PTCA. The indications for *coronary bypass surgery* in patients with severe angina pectoris can be best understood in the context of natural history of coronary artery disease (no treatment) and the results of other competing treating modalities (medical therapy and PTCA). The severity of the symptoms, the amount of myocardium at risk, the age of the patient, and the presence of other medical problems may affect the decision to recommend coronary bypass surgery. Specific indications follow:

1. Left main coronary artery stenosis (over 50%)
2. Critical stenosis (over 70%) involving three major arteries in the presence of moderate to severe left ventricular dysfunction
3. Critical stenosis (over 70%) of the proximal left anterior descending coronary artery in association with a severe obstruction of a second major coronary artery
4. Severe disabling angina pectoris that is unresponsive to maximum medical therapy
5. Myocardial infarction with hemodynamic deterioration
6. Acute complications of PTCA
7. Ischemic events after previous coronary bypass operation
8. Combined procedure during other cardiac operations

### Left main coronary artery disease

Medical treatment of left main artery stenosis of at least 50% is associated with 22% to 44% mortality in 1 year and 40% to 50% mortality in 3 years. This high mortality rate persists even when the patients are asymptomatic. PTCA is contraindicated because of high complication and mortality rates. Coronary bypass surgery for left main coronary artery disease is associated with operative mortality between 1.4% and 1.6%. Thus coronary bypass surgery is the treatment of choice for significant left main coronary artery disease.

### Three-vessel disease

In the presence of good left ventricular function coronary artery bypass surgery generally does not provide better survival for patients with three-vessel disease and severe angina pectoris. Exceptions occur if one or more of the stenoses are proximally located and especially if the proximal left anterior descending coronary artery is involved. If, however, moderate to severe left ventricular dysfunction is present, the 1-year survival for medically and surgically treated patients is 62% and 90%, respectively. PTCA has not been shown to prolong life in patients with three-vessel disease and impaired left ventricular function. Consequently, coronary artery bypass surgery is indicated in patients with severe three-vessel disease if there is moderate to severe left ventricular dysfunction and there are stenoses involving the proximal left anterior descending artery and other major vessels.

### Two-vessel disease

The Coronary Artery Surgery Study (CASS) has shown that the results of medical treatment in patients with chronic stable angina and two-vessel coronary artery disease are comparable to those obtained after coronary bypass surgery. If the patient has medically refractory angina, PTCA appears to offer effective therapy provided none of the vessels has total chronic occlusion. When such a patient has total occlusion of the proximal left anterior descending artery and the left ventricular function is impaired, then coronary bypass surgery is indicated.

### Single-vessel disease

PTCA and medical therapy generally provide good results in patients with single-vessel disease. Thus coronary bypass surgery is rarely indicated for single-vessel coronary artery disease. Exceptions may be patients with proximal total occlusion of the left anterior descending artery, a patent distal vessel, and large ischemic territory.

### Unstable angina pectoris

Unstable angina is defined as crescendo angina of recent onset that may be superimposed on a preexisting stable angina pattern and is in most cases associated with ECG changes.

The initial treatment for unstable angina pectoris consists of intensive medical therapy (see the Managed Care Guides). An intraaortic balloon is placed if unstable angina is not relieved with the maximum tolerated medical treatment. Following cardiac catheterization the nature and urgency of further treatment depend on the coronary anatomy, left ventricular function, and condition of the patient. Surgery appears to be the treatment of choice for patients with unstable angina pectoris, left ventricular dysfunction, and extensive coronary artery disease.

### Myocardial infarction with hemodynamic deterioration

Early reperfusion of the injured myocardium reduces infarct size, improves myocardial function, and enhances survival. Streptokinase, recombinant tissue plasminogen activator (rt-PA), and anisoylated plasminogen streptokinase activator complex (APSAC) have been found to reopen the infarct-related artery in 60%, 75%, and 60% of the patients, respectively. Emergency PTCA in hemodynamically unstable patients and in whom thrombolytic therapy fails to achieve reperfusion can be effective in 75% of the cases. Reperfusion of ischemic myocardium with unmodified blood has been shown to have a deleterious effect on myocardial recovery. Consequently, surgical myocardial protection in the clinical setting of cardiogenic shock following myocardial infarction consists of (1) induction with warm aspartate glutamate–enriched cardioplegic solution, (2) introduction of cold blood cardioplegic solution as the first medium that perfuses the ischemic territory following completion of the distal anastomoses, and (3) administration of warm blood cardioplegia immediately before release of the cross-clamp. Thus the injured myocardium is allowed to replenish its energy stores, encourage the sequestration of cystosolic calcium, and reduce the production of oxygen-free radicals during the period of electromechanical quiescence. Patients who have coronary artery bypass surgery within 6 hours of acute myocardial infarction and in whom modified myocardial protection technique is used have a 9% operative mortality. Emergency PTCA in the clinical setting of cardiogenic shock is associated with an operative mortality of 50%.

### Acute complications of PTCA

Emergency coronary artery bypass surgery for abrupt closure of the dilated vessel associated with clinical and ECG evidence of myocardial ischemia is required for 2.5% to 4% of patients who undergo PTCA. Such life-threatening complications mandate that PTCA be performed only in institutions with a well-trained cardiac surgery team. Insertion of the intraaortic balloon or institution of percutaneous partial cardiopulmonary bypass is necessary to reduce the severity of myocardial ischemia. The operative mortality and incidence of perioperative myocardial infarction in surgically managed patients are 6.6% and 41%, respectively. The optimal surgical results are obtained when (1) the surgical team is notified immediately following the PTCA failure, (2) there is no further manipulation of the damaged vessel, (3) the surgery is performed promptly, and (4) special myocardial protection techniques are used during the operation.

### Ischemic events after previous coronary bypass operation

Occlusion of vein grafts in the early or late postoperative period can lead to reemergence of myocardial ischemia. Furthermore, progression of disease in the native coronary arteries predisposes to recurrence of myocardial ischemia. The role of suction arthrectomy in the management of vein graft occlusion is not clearly defined. PTCA is associated with dislodgement and embolization of graft debris into

## Managed Care Guide
## Pointers for management of patients with moderate and unstable angina pectoris

### Moderate angina

1. Resting LV function determined with two-dimensional echocardiogram or RVG has prognostic significance on the severity of the underlying coronary artery disease.
2. Thallium and treadmill ETT should be performed when LV function is normal at rest.
3. Cardiac catheterization is indicated when there is evidence of either significant exercise-induced LV dysfunction or ischemia.
4. Medical therapy is recommended when the stress test achieves the equivalent of stage IV Bruce protocol without evidence of ischemia.
5. Cardiac catheterization is indicated when LV function is abnormal at rest.

### Therapeutic recommendations based on the results of cardiac catheterization

1. Coronary artery bypass grafting (CABG) is recommended for patients with significant left main stenosis, severe three-vessel disease (3VD) and impaired LV function (EF<40%), severe double-vessel disease (2VD), LV dysfunction (EF<40%), and significant (>70%) LAD stenosis.
2. The decision for medical therapy or PTCA or coronary bypass grafting should be individualized in patients with single-vessel (1VD) or double-vessel disease (2VD) and normal LV function.

### Unstable angina

1. The life-threatening nature should always be borne in mind.
2. If the patient has abnormal ECG at rest or uncontrolled angina, intensive medical therapy and intraaortic ballon (when necessary) are used to stabilize the patient before proceeding with cardiac catheterization.
3. If resting ECG (after bedrest and medical therapy) is negative for ischemia, careful ambulation is started.
4. If the patient develops effort-induced ischemia, cardiac catheterization is performed.
5. If the patient remains asymptomatic with ambulation, stress test is performed under very careful conditions.
6. If the patient develops LV dysfunction or stress-induced ischemia, cardiac catheterization is performed.

### Therapeutic choices

1. Although the therapeutic choices are the same as in patients with moderate angina, the patients with unstable angina are approached with a greater sense of urgency.

**Managed Care Guide**
**Algorithm comparing treatment for moderate and unstable angina**

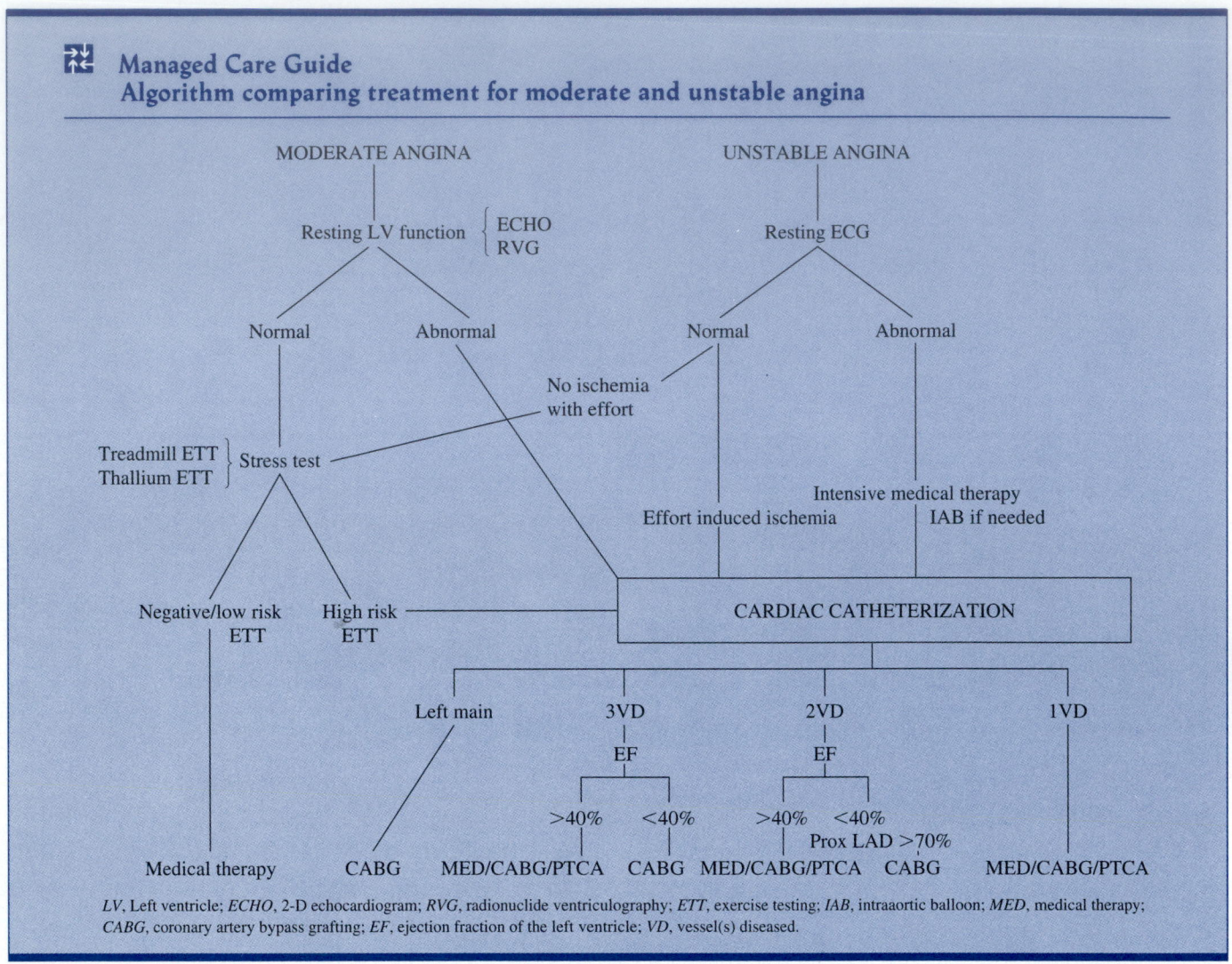

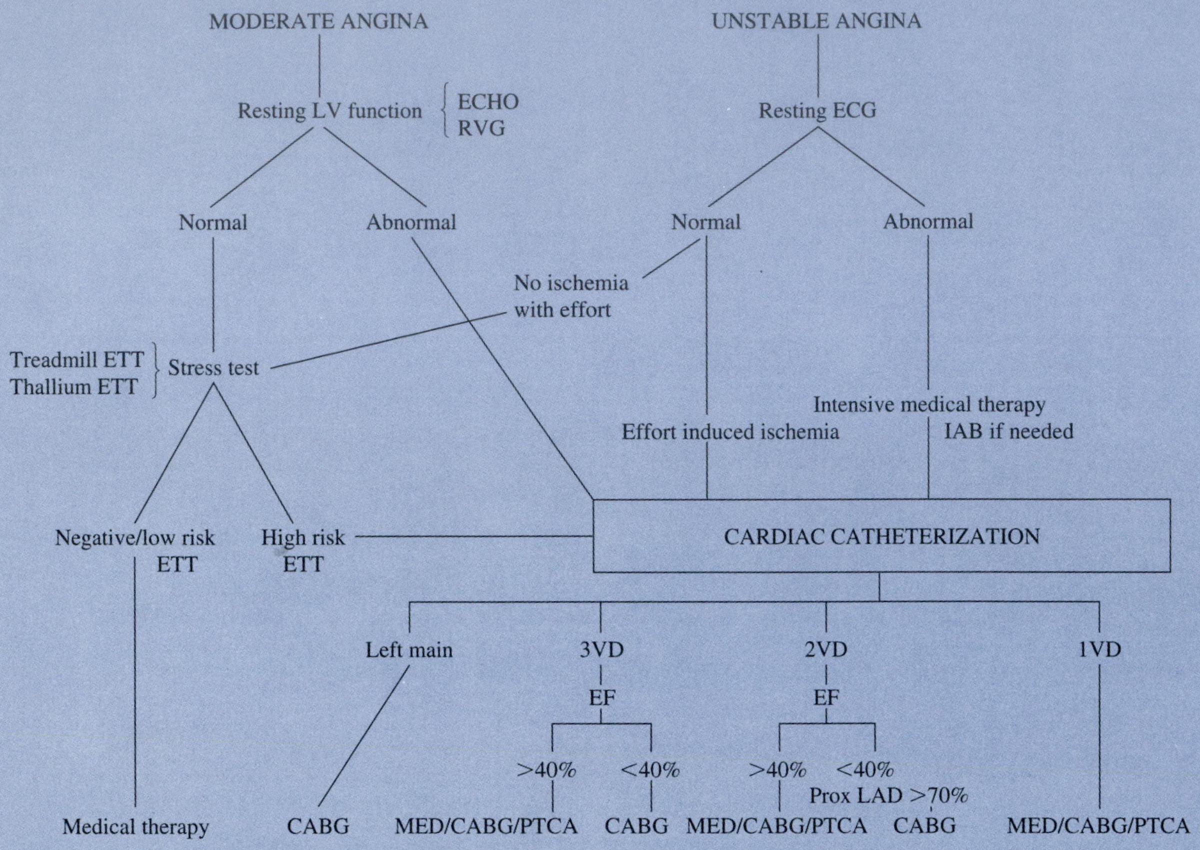


*LV*, Left ventricle; *ECHO*, 2-D echocardiogram; *RVG*, radionuclide ventriculography; *ETT*, exercise testing; *IAB*, intraaortic balloon; *MED*, medical therapy; *CABG*, coronary artery bypass grafting; *EF*, ejection fraction of the left ventricle; *VD*, vessel(s) diseased.

the myocardium. Reoperation is therefore indicated if the patient has a bypassable distal coronary artery.

### Combined procedure during other cardiac operations

Acute mitral regurgitation, postinfarction ventricular septal defect, and left ventricular aneurysm are complications of myocardial ischemia and infarction. If preoperative cardiac catheterization documents the presence of critically stenotic coronary vessels, concomitant coronary artery bypass surgery should be performed. This is particularly true if there is evidence of myocardial ischemia. In the presence of left ventricular aneurysm and severe coronary artery disease, long-term survival is enhanced by coronary artery bypass performed during the left ventricular aneurysm repair. Valvular heart disease is frequently associated with coronary disease in patients over the age of 40 years. Consequently, coronary angiography is routinely performed in this subgroup of patients even in the absence of symptoms indicative of myocardial ischemia. Concomitant coronary artery bypass and aortic valve replacement are associated with operative mortality varying between 3% and 15%. The operative mortality for combined mitral replacement and coronary artery bypass is 8% to 12%.

## CHOICE AND FATE OF BYPASS CONDUITS

Conduit selection is determined by the clinical setting (emergency or elective), conduit availability, surgeon's preference, and experience. Although the internal mammary artery and saphenous veins are the most important conduits used for myocardial revascularization, they differ significantly in their biocharacteristics. Other alternative conduits have also been used with varying success rates (Table 12-1).

The superior long-term patency rate of the internal mammary artery and documented improved survival in patients who received internal mammary artery graft should encourage its use in all patients.

**Table 12-1.** Comparison of coronary bypass conduits

| Conduit | Advantages | Disadvantages | Patency rates (%) 1 Year | 5 Years | 10 Years |
|---|---|---|---|---|---|
| Internal mammary artery (IMA) | Devoid of atherosclerosis<br>Intimal hyperplasia rarely develops<br>High content of endothelium-derived relaxing factor (EDRF) and prostacyclin militate against vasoconstriction and occlusion<br>Enormous flow reserve | Intrathoracic harvesting<br>Sternal wound complications in diabetics | 98 | 96 | 94 |
| Saphenous vein | Subcutaneous location promotes easy harvesting<br>Long segments of vein readily available | Undergoes extensive and complex changes after bypass grafting: endothelial loss, intimal hyperplasia, formation of fibrous plaques and atherosclerosis | 87 | 78 | 70 |
| Right gastroepiploic artery | Rarely develops intimal hyperplasia or atherosclerosis | Requires abdominal exploration | 80-85 | | |
| Radial artery | Muscular wall makes suturing more secure<br>Superficial position facilitates harvesting<br>Large caliber and regular lumen<br>Rarely atherosclerotic changes | Potential intimal hyperplasia<br>Sensitive to spasm | 35 | | |
| Splenic artery | Basically same as IMA | Difficulties in harvesting<br>Tortuous course<br>Possibility of splenectomy | 90* | | |
| Upper extremity vein | Superficial location<br>Easy harvesting | Thin and friable<br>May be associated with perioperative bleeding<br>Tortuous and aneurysmal changes after grafting<br>Undergoes rapid complex changes leading to early occlusion | 60 | 20 | |
| Cryopreserved allograft veins | Commercially available<br>Preserves cellular viability and structural integrity<br>Possible decrease in immunologic response | Freezing destroys cellular elements | 85 | | |
| Synthetic graft—polytetrafluoroethylene | Readily available | Early occlusion in small sizes<br>Stimulates foreign body reaction<br>Pseudointimal thickening and bridge formation | 64 | | |
| Bovine internal mammary artery | Commercially available | Lack of endothelium in the intima<br>Very thrombogenic surface | 85† | | |

*1-2 years.
†6 months.

## ENDARTERECTOMY

Endarterectomy is used in patients with diffuse coronary artery disease that precludes safe insertion of the internal mammary artery or vein as bypass grafts. Endarterectomy is most easily performed on the right coronary artery because of its location and size. The patency of vein grafts to an endarterectomized right coronary artery in 1 year is 72%, in contrast to 94% for vein grafts to an unendarterectomized distal right coronary artery. Brenowitz, Kayser, and Johnson reported on 1246 patients who underwent endarterectomies. The operative risk and perioperative myocardial infarction rates were 10.4% and 13.1%, respectively, for multiple endarterectomies, 6.3% and 6.5% for single vessel endarterectomy, and 4.0% and 5.6% for patients managed with bypass grafting without endarterectomy.

## POSTOPERATIVE MANAGEMENT

### Early postoperative care

An uneventful postoperative course begins with preoperative training and coaching of patients in effective deep breathing and coughing. The importance of early ambulation is also emphasized.

Most patients are extubated and transferred from the intensive care unit to the telemetry ward on the following morning. The majority of patients are discharged to home on the sixth or seventh postoperative day. Arrangements are made for home care nurses to visit the patients and monitor their postoperative recovery. Events that prolong the in-hospital postoperative course, such as bleeding and supraventricular arrhythmias, are mitigated by complete rewarming of the patient, meticulous hemostasis, and prophylactic administration of β-adrenergic receptor blockers. Aspirin (325 mg) is administered daily starting on the first postoperative day. Aspirin is not given to patients with gastrointestinal bleeding or a history of ulcer diathesis. The prophylaxis for gastrointestinal complications consists of ranitidine (Zantac) and metoclopramide (Reglan). Zantac, 50 mg, is administered intravenously every 8 hours until the patient is extubated. Thereafter Zantac 150 mg is given orally twice daily. Reglan, 10 mg, is administered intravenously every 8 hours and continued orally at 10 mg every 8 hours after extubation. Zantac and Reglan are discontinued when the patient is discharged from the hospital.

### Late postoperative care

*Early return to an active life and employment.* Patients are encouraged to carry out the exercise program that was initiated by the rehabilitation nurse in the hospital. This program consists of daily walks and specific exercises for the patient's different muscle groups. Patients are enrolled in rehabilitation programs when they are able to fully participate in rigorous exercises. Those patients who were employed before the coronary bypass operation are urged to return to work after they have fully recovered.

*Modification of risk factors for atherosclerosis.* Patients are instructed in eating a prudent or vegetarian diet. Lipid-lowering medication may be needed for patients who have an elevated lipid profile despite an altered diet. Smoking must be stopped and hypertension controlled with medications. Control of risk factors for atherosclerosis and administration of aspirin, 325 mg daily, promote the long-term patency of the vein grafts.

*Evaluation of efficacy of myocardial revascularization.* Patients generally undergo a stress exercise test 8 to 12 weeks after the operation. This stress test serves as a baseline for subsequent yearly exercise-tolerance tests (ETT).

## PROGNOSIS

### Operative mortality

The hospital mortality for isolated coronary artery bypass operation has risen from 1% in 1980 to 3% in 1990 in most university hospitals. This rise in operative mortality is attributed to the changes in patient population over the past 6 years. Kirklin and others have outlined the risk factors for death after coronary artery bypass operation. They include (1) presence of left main coronary artery stenosis, (2) preoperative biologic factors (diabetes mellitus, old age, small body size), (3) severe or unstable angina pectoris, recent myocardial infarction, and left ventricular dysfunction, (4) intraoperative myocardial injury and failure to use the internal mammary artery, and (5) environmental factors that include the institution and the surgeon.

With growing indications for PTCA, surgeons are operating on sicker, older patients with left ventricular dysfunction. Cosgrove's analysis of patients who underwent primary isolated coronary artery bypass in 1980 to 1982 identified emergency operation, advanced age, female gender, and clinical congestive heart failure as the persistent risk factors.

### Relief of angina

Freedom from angina in the early postoperative period is achieved in 90% of the patients who receive complete revascularization. An additional 3% to 5% of patients show significant improvement in their angina pattern. The early peak in the return of angina occurs at about 3 months and is caused by early graft occlusion. Thus mitigation of angina symptoms is related to adequacy of revascularization and to graft patency. It has been observed that a major risk factor for the early return of angina pectoris is failure to use the internal mammary artery.

### Perioperative myocardial infarction

Perioperative myocardial infarction is defined by the appearance of a new Q wave on ECG, elevation of the MB fraction of creatine kinase enzyme, and new wall motion abnormality on the echocardiogram. Despite advances in myocardial protection, 6.4% of the patients sustained myocardial infarction in the CASS trial. Factors that may lead to perioperative myocardial infarction are incomplete revascularization, embolization of atheromatous debris from diseased vein grafts, technical errors in performance of anastomosis, endarterectomy of diffusely diseased coronary arteries, and spasm of the coronary arteries of the internal mammary artery. Patients who sustain perioperative myocardial infarctions exhibit a higher mortality rate.

### Neurologic dysfunction

Neurologic dysfunction includes changes in memory, concentration, and visual motor skills and stroke, which might result from the coronary artery bypass operation. Changes in cognitive function may be so subtle that only specific neurologic tests will detect them. The incidence of stroke has been shown to be directly related to the age of the patient and the diffuseness of atherosclerosis. The incidence is less than 1% in young patients but increases significantly to 6% to 8% in patients over the age of 70 years. The mechanisms of cerebral injury include (1) embolism of gas, aggregates of blood cells, platelets, or fibrin and particles from the polyvinyl tubing, (2) hypoperfusion of the brain due to nonpulsatile blood flow and low systemic pressure, and (3) atheromatous debris from the cannulation or cross-clamp sites on the ascending aorta. Intraoperative scanning of the ascending aorta with a surgeon-held Doppler ultrasound probe led to an altered surgical strategy in 12% to 25% of the patients. The alterations included changes in sites of cannulation, cross-clamping, proximal anastomosis, and the insertion of the cardioplegia catheter. The insertion of appropriate filters in the arterial arm of the extracorporeal circuit can minimize the embolization of debris from the pump oxygenator.

### Bleeding complications

Reoperations for excessive bleeding are performed in 2% to 5% of patients after coronary artery bypass surgery. Bleeding is caused by the interaction of blood constituents and the extracorporeal circuit, hypothermia, circulating heparin, and hemodilution of plasma proteins. Interaction of platelets with a synthetic surface leads to platelet activation, aggregation, degranulation, and irreversible loss. Qualitative dysfunction of circulating platelets is caused by heparin and hypothermia. Although the concentration of the coagulation proteins decreases during cardiopulmonary bypass, it rarely falls into a range where hemostasis would be compromised. In contrast, fibrinolysis seems to play an important role in postoperative bleeding. Meticulous surgical technique and hemostasis, complete rewarming of the patient to 37°C, and adequate reversal of heparin are necessary for reduction of postoperative blood loss. When postoperative bleeding is suspected to have surgical causes, the patient is promptly reexplored and the bleeding controlled. Diffuse, nonsurgical bleeding can be managed pharmacologically by administration of protamine, *E*-amino caproic acid in large doses (25 to 30 g), tranexamic acid, and aprotinin. Intravenous desmopressin acetate (DDAVP) may be useful for patients with renal failure.

### Wound complications

There is a 1.1% incidence of major wound infection (mediastinitis) after coronary artery bypass operations. The risk factors for postoperative wound infection are obesity, number of units of transfused blood, and increased operating time. Bilateral internal mammary artery grafting in diabetic patients is associated with fivefold increase in wound complications. When wound complications occur, the hospital stay is significantly prolonged, hospital charges are markedly increased, and 14% of the patients die in the hospital. Mediastinitis is managed by prompt recognition, sternal debridement, and evacuation of the infected thrombus and tissues from the mediastinum. In the majority of patients the sternum is closed and the mediastinum irrigated with 0.1% povidone-iodine solution. The remainder of the patients will require debridement, open packing of the wound, and delayed closure with omentum, pectoralis, and rectus muscle flaps. Measures that we have instituted to reduce wound infection include preoperative shower with disinfectant, administration of antibiotics on arrival in the operating room, avoidance of closure of the leg wounds before the reversal of heparin, and sparing use of cautery in the leg wound. Antibiotic paste made from vancomycin, thrombin and Gelfoam is used to seal the sternal marrow.

## LATE RESULTS

### Late mortality

Kirklin and colleagues in the American College of Cardiology/American Heart Association (ACC/AHA) task force cited the late survival rate of 92% in 5 years and 81% in 10 years for a heterogeneous group of patients undergoing coronary artery bypass operation. They also found that 55% of the deaths had cardiac causes. The incremental risk factors that affect late survival after coronary artery bypass are advancing age, poor left ventricular function, failure to use the internal mammary artery, smoking, severe three vessel coronary artery disease, left main coronary artery disease, and incomplete revascularization. The rate of progression of atherosclerosis in the native vessels and bypass grafts as well as other noncardiac conditions affect the long-term survival. The ACC/AHA task force further confirmed that, in patients with chronic stable angina, coronary artery bypass surgery prolongs the survival if the patients have left main or severe three vessel coronary artery disease with moderate to severe impairment of left ventricular function. Furthermore, surgery provides better survival in patients with severe three vessel coronary artery disease and normal left ventricular function if two of the stenoses are in the proximal segments of the arteries and one of the arteries is the left anterior descending. Patients with two vessel coronary artery disease that includes the proximal left anterior descending and impaired left ventricular function have better survival with coronary artery bypass surgery. Patients with single-vessel coronary artery disease are rarely offered surgery as initial treatment because of the excellent survival with medical therapy. The exception may occur in patients with proximal total occlusion of the left anterior descending artery, a patent distal vessel, and large ischemic territory.

### Late return of angina

Campeau's review of a heterogeneous group of patients showed that only 60% are free from angina after 10 years. Kirklin and colleagues found that probability of freedom from return of angina was 83% at 5 years and 63% at 10 years after coronary artery bypass surgery. The reasons for return of angina are deterioration and occlusion of vein grafts, progression of disease in the native coronary arteries, not using the internal mammary artery, and incomplete revascularization. The increasing use of arte-

### Criteria for successful reoperation

- Avoid injury to the right ventricle, anteriorly located grafts to the RCA or LAD, and IMA grafts during reentry by using the oscillating saw and employing diligent and careful dissection.
- Prevent embolization of atheromatous debris from the vein grafts into the myocardium by ligating the diseased grafts after the first dose of cold antegrade cardioplegia.
- Provide adequate myocardial protection by occluding the IMA graft and using combined antegrade and retrograde cold cardioplegia.
- Aim at complete revascularization and the use of IMA if it was not used during the primary operation.

*RCA*, Right coronary artery; *LAD*, left anterior descending artery; *IMA*, internal mammary artery.

rial grafts (internal mammary, gastroepiploic artery) for coronary bypass will have a positive impact on the late angina-free status of patients.

### Reoperation

About 10% to 20% of all isolated coronary artery bypass operations that are currently performed in large institutions are reoperations. Young age, good left ventricular function, incomplete revascularization at primary operation, and nonuse of the internal mammary artery increase the risk of reoperation. In a review of Cleveland Clinic series of 1009 reoperations performed between 1985 and 1987 the following data emerged: the mean age at reoperation was 61 years; and angiographic indications for reoperations were graft failure in 25% of patients, progression of disease in native vessels in 15% of patients, and combination of graft failure and progression of disease in native vessels in 60% of the patients. The mean interval between primary operation and reoperation was 83 months.

The operative mortality for first reoperation ranged from 2% to 10%; 50% of patients experienced return of angina symptoms 5 years after the first reoperation. Late survival for patients following reoperation was 85% to 90% at 5 years and 69% at 10 years.

The box above shows criteria for successful reoperation.

## CONTROVERSIES AND SPECIAL TOPICS

### PTCA or coronary bypass surgery

The introduction of steerable, over-the-wire systems in 1982 has greatly increased the number of patients in whom angioplasty can be performed and has also increased the primary success rate of this procedure. It is generally accepted that, in patients with chronic stable angina unresponsive to medical therapy and unstable angina, PTCA is indicated for single- and two-vessel disease if the left ventricular function is normal or mildly reduced. Conversely, patients with left main coronary artery disease, three-vessel disease, and moderate to severe left ventricular dysfunction should be offered a coronary bypass operation. Furthermore, symptomatic patients with prior bypass grafts should undergo reoperation. Although there are controversies about the appropriate management of many patients, there is agreement that the following questions should be asked before performing any PTCA: (1) Does the team performing PTCA have adequate experience and is there backup by an experienced surgical team? (2) Does the target vessel have an easily dilated lesion? (3) If the myocardium was previously acutely ischemic, will reperfusion with unmodified blood cause reperfusion injury? (4) Will an abrupt closure of the dilated vessel carry disastrous consequences for the patient? (5) Will PTCA, under the most favorable conditions, provide complete revascularization?

The Randomized Intervention Treatment of Angina (RITA) trial compared long-term effects of PTCA and CABG in 1011 patients with one-, two-, or three-vessel coronary artery disease. After 2 years 19% of PTCA patients required CABG. There was higher prevalence of angina in PTCA patients (32% vs. 11% at 6 months and 31% vs. 22% after 2 years); 62% of the PTCA patients and 89% of the CABG patients remained free from all major cardiac events and interventions. There was, however, no statistically significant difference in risk of death and myocardial infarction between the two groups after 2 years. The results of the Bypass Angioplasty Research Investigation (BARI) trials will soon be published. This prospective, randomized, multiinstitutional study should further provide excellent knowledge for choosing appropriate revascularization strategy for a given clinical condition.

### Combined carotid and coronary artery disease

The prevalence of significant stenosis (over 50% of the luminal diameter) of one internal carotid artery in patients 65 years and over undergoing coronary artery bypass operation is 17%. Furthermore, 6% of patients of the same cohort have greater than 80% stenosis in one internal carotid artery. Patients who have both significant coronary artery and carotid artery disease are elderly and have severe angina, a high prevalence of left main and three-vessel coronary artery disease, and abnormal left ventricular function. Thus operations on these patients result in high operative mortality and morbidity irrespective of the strategies adopted in the management of both the carotid and coronary artery disease.

### Coronary artery disease in women

Coronary heart disease accounts for 250,000 deaths (one third of all female deaths) each year in women in the United States. About 39% of women who have myocardial infarctions die within a year, compared with 31% in men. From ages 35 to 74 years the death rate from myocardial infarctions for African-American women is about twice that of white women and three times that of women of other races. These data support the existence of gender and racial difference in the course of coronary heart disease. The National Heart, Lung, and Blood Institute (NHLBI) Registry's data indicate that PTCA in women was associated with lower initial success rate (60.3% vs. 66.2%; $p<.01$), less favorable short-term outcome (56.5% vs. 62.2%; $p<.01$) and higher in-hospital mortality rate (1.8% vs. 0.7%; $p<.01$) than in men. The incidence of acute complication in patients undergoing coronary atherectomy is significantly higher in women than in men (6.2% vs.

1.4%; $p<.016$). Following coronary artery bypass surgery, women have higher operative mortality (2.9% vs. 1.4%), lower graft patency rate (72.8% vs. 79.2%), and a lower percentage of asymptomatic patients (53% vs. 71%) than men. Investigators have attempted to elucidate the reason for these differences. CASS suggested that it was primarily a result of differences in coronary artery size rather than gender. Other observations indicate that the difference might be linked to sicker clinical profile of women, suggesting delayed referral and treatment. Further studies are needed to determine unique clinical approaches to the female patient with coronary heart disease.

## BIBLIOGRAPHY


Barzilai B, et al: Avoidance of embolic complications by ultrasonic characterization of the ascending aorta, *Circulation* 80(suppl I):275, 1989.

Brenowitz JB, Kayser KL, Johnson WD: Results of coronary artery endarterectomy and reconstruction, *J Thorac Cardiovasc Surg* 95:1, 1988.

CASS Principal Investigators and Their Associates: Coronary artery surgery study (CASS): a randomized trial of coronary artery bypass surgery—survival data, *Circulation* 68:939, 1983.

Cowley MJ, et al: Emergency coronary artery bypass surgery after coronary angioplasty: The National Heart, Lung and Blood Institute's Percutaneous Transluminal Coronary Angioplasty Registry experience, *Am J Cardiol* 53:22C, 1984.

Cowley MJ, et al: Sex differences in early and long-term results of coronary angioplasty in the NHLBI PTCA Registry, *Circulation* 71:90, 1985.

Favaloro RG: Saphenous vein autograft replacement of severe segmental coronary artery occlusion: operative technique, *Ann Thorac Surg* 5:334, 1968.

Fuster V, et al: The pathogenesis of coronary artery disease and acute coronary syndromes, *N Engl J Med* 326:242, 1992.

Harper RW et al: The incidence and pattern of angina prior to acute myocardial infarction: a study of 577 cases, *Am Heart J* 97:178, 1979.

Khuri SF, Michelson AD, Valeri CR: The effect of cardiopulmonary bypass on hemostasis and coagulation. In Loscalzo J, Schafer Al, editors: *Thrombosis and hemorrhage,* Cambridge, Mass, 1993, Blackwell.

Kirklin JW et al: Summary of a consensus concerning death and ischemic events after coronary artery bypass grafting, *Circulation* 79 (suppl 1):81, 1989.

Kirklin JW et al: ACC/AHA task force report: guidelines and indications for coronary artery bypass graft surgery, *J Am Coll Cardiol* 17:543, 1991.

Lytle BW, Cosgrove DM: Coronary artery bypass surgery, *Curr Probl Surg* 29:792, 1992.

McConahay DR et al: Coronary artery bypass surgery for left main coronary artery disease, *Am J Cardiol* 37:885, 1976.

RITA Trial Participants: Coronary angioplasty versus coronary artery bypass surgery: the randomized intervention treatment of angina (RITA) trial, *Lancet* 341:573, 1993.

Rosenkranz ER et al: Warm induction of cardioplegia with glutamate-enriched blood in coronary patients with cardiogenic shock who are dependent on inotropic drugs and intra-aortic balloon support, *J Thorac Cardiovasc Surg* 86:507, 1983.

Ross R: The pathogenesis of atherosclerosis—an update, *N Engl J Med* 314:488, 1986.

Sones FM Jr, Shirley EK: Cine coronary arteriography, *Mod Concepts Cardiovasc Dis* 31:735, 1962.

Talano JV et al: Influence of surgery on survival in 145 patients with left main coronary artery disease, *Circulation* 52 (suppl I):105, 1975.

Varnauskas E, European Coronary Surgery Study Group: Survival, myocardial infarction, and employment status in a prospective, randomized study of coronary bypass surgery, *Circulation* 72 (suppl V):90, 1985.


CHAPTER

# 13 Congestive Heart Failure


**Kodangudi B. Ramanathan**
**Pantel S. Vokonas**
**Howard R. Horn**


## EPIDEMIOLOGY

Congestive heart failure (CHF) remains a major cause of disability and morbidity in the United States. Unlike other disease states, the incidence and prevalence of CHF has been increasing, especially in the elderly population; it afflicts at least 4 million Americans. Each year, 400,000 people develop heart failure for the first time. CHF is diagnosed in 10% of the population by the age of 75. It is the most common discharge diagnosis in patients over 65.

Although the cardiovascular mortality rate has declined during the past 3 decades, mortality resulting from CHF has not declined at least until 1988. Once CHF is diagnosed, the prognosis is poor. The 5-year survival rate for those with severe CHF is about 50%, and the annual mortality rate is as high as 60%. The prognosis for CHF is worse than for most forms of cancer. In spite of the advances in the management of this disorder, the mortality rate remains around 40% in the first 4 years. In the United States alone, about 200,000 patients die of heart failure each year. Recent data from the Framingham study showed a median survival time of 1.7 years in men and 3.2 years in women with CHF. The 5-year survival rate for men with CHF is 25% and women 38%.

## DEFINITION

CHF is a syndrome characterized by clinical evidence of pulmonary and/or systemic venous congestion at rest or on exercise and that results from an abnormality in the systolic and/or diastolic performance of the heart. Defined in pathophysiologic terms, CHF is a state in which the heart is unable to pump an adequate amount of blood to meet the metabolic body's demands, or can do so only from an abnormally elevated filling pressure at rest or on exercise. Myocardial failure leads to heart failure; the converse is not true. The contractile performance of the heart may be preserved when impairment of cardiac filling or emptying, as in valvular abnormalities, leads to symptoms and signs of heart failure. Circulatory failure is not synonymous with heart failure, since a variety of noncardiac conditions, such as hemorrhagic shock, can lead to circulatory collapse while cardiac pumping is preserved.

## PATHOPHYSIOLOGY

During the past 3 decades, our understanding of the pathophysiology of CHF has changed considerably. The heart is a muscular pump, and the clinical manifestations of heart failure to a large extent are related to failure of hemodynamic adaptations to the failing pump. However, the heart has other adaptive mechanisms, neural and humoral adaptations. Neural adaptation involves the autonomic nervous system. The major humoral adaptation involves activation of the renin-angiotensin system and augmented release of vasopressin. The heart, especially the atria, also produces a hormone called *atrial natriuretic peptide* that may have a role in heart failure. Finally, it is becoming increasingly apparent that diastolic dysfunction is indeed an essential component of heart failure. To a large extent the syndrome of CHF encompasses systolic and diastolic abnormalities, yet clinical manifestations of heart failure occur with normal systolic function.

For the heart to eject a volume of blood during a single heart beat (stroke volume), it initially needs to fill by venous return during diastole (preload) and contract forcefully during systole (contractility), overcoming the impedance imposed by peripheral vascular resistance (afterload). Thus the determinants of ventricular performance as measured by stroke volume are preload, afterload, and the contractile state of the myocardium.

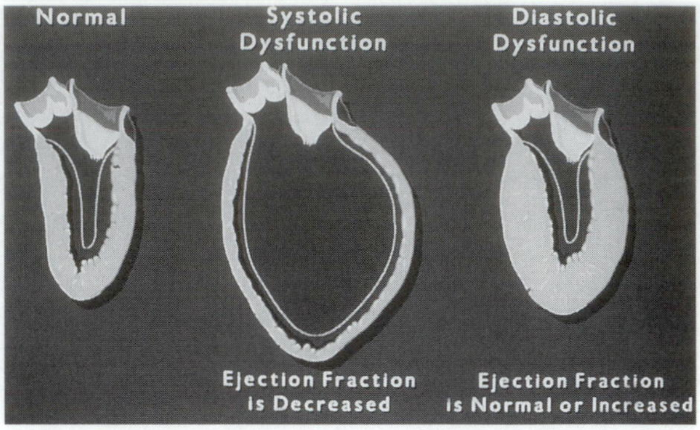


**Fig. 13-1.** Systolic and diastolic LV dysfunction. Dashed lines indicate the extent of contraction.

## Systolic and diastolic dysfunction

Systolic dysfunction is characterized by a reduced extent of contraction, a decreased ejection fraction, and LV dilation. Diastolic dysfunction occurs when hearts with systolic dysfunction reach their limit of dilation and distensibility and resistance to diastolic filling increases. Thus, many patients have both systolic and diastolic dysfunction (Fig. 13-1).

Diastolic dysfunction can also occur in a "pure" form, without systolic dysfunction, although this is very rare. Such primary diastolic dysfunction is often associated with left ventricular hypertrophy (LVH) and a normal or supernormal extent of contraction and ejection fraction. An increased resistance to diastolic filling results from the increased LV mass itself and also from interstitial fibrosis and subendocardial ischemia, which is often present with LVH. Diastolic dysfunction can occur in the absence of LVH with myocardial infiltrative disease. The increased resistance to filling results in an elevated LV diastolic (filling) pressure, which, transmitted to the pulmonary capillaries, causes pulmonary congestion.

## Preload

*Preload* refers to the passive stretch of myocardial fibers or diastolic muscle length. In the intact heart, this is approximated by end-diastolic volume, which is closely related to end-diastolic ventricular filling pressure. In the clinical setting, left ventricular end-diastolic pressure is closely approximated by pulmonary capillary wedge pressure. Filling pressure in the right ventricle is reflected by central venous pressure. The determinants of preload are venous return, total blood volume and its distribution, and the atrial transport mechanism. When heart failure develops, diastolic filling increases because of an increase in venous return secondary to sympathoadrenal stimulation or because of the expansion of blood volume resulting from renal conservation of salt and water.

## Afterload

*Afterload* refers to the resistance (or impedance) to ejection of blood by the ventricles. The major determinant of left ventricular afterload is systemic vascular resistance. Arterial blood pressure, which is related to the product of cardiac output and systemic vascular resistance, generally reflects left ventricular afterload. Afterload is typically increased in systemic hypertension, aortic valvular stenosis, and coarctation of the aorta.

## Contractility

The contractile performance of the myocardium clinically is poorly defined. "Improvement" in myocardial performance may not involve myocardial contractility but may be related to changes in preload and afterload. True myocardial contractility or inotropic state reflects the force velocity relationship of myocardial fibers. Contractility is altered by sympathetic stimulation or administration of positive or negative inotropic agents. Cardiac contractility is difficult to measure in the clinical setting, since it requires maintaining constant loading conditions.

In the clinical setting the tests commonly used to determine myocardial performance are measurement of cardiac output in the intensive care setting and measurement of ejection fraction (EF) invasively in the cardiac catheterization laboratory or noninvasively using echocardiography or nuclear angiography (multiple-gated acquisition [MUGA] analysis). Isovolumic indices of cardiac performance, such as the rate of rise of intraventricular pressure (dp/dt) determined by electronic differentiation of the left ventricular pressure signal to yield the first derivative, are no longer used because they are difficult to measure and are highly variable. Recently, the use of pressure-volume relationship, especially the ratio of peak systolic pressure to end-systolic volume, a noninvasive measure, has been suggested to determine myocardial contractility independent of loading conditions.

## Renin-angiotensin-aldosterone system

Excess salt and water retention during heart failure is due to diminished renal perfusion that results in activation of the renin-angiotensin-aldosterone system. This activation occurs with activation of the sympathetic nervous system, and the two complement one another's activity. Diminished renal perfusion and enhanced sympathetic activity result in enhanced renin release. This results in increased levels of angiotensin II, which is a potent peripheral vasoconstrictor that helps maintain blood pressure. Release of angiotensin leads to an increase in the levels of aldosterone, which has potent sodium-retaining properties. This results in expansion of the intravascular volume, which again may aid in maintaining cardiac output by the Frank-Starling mechanism but also promotes edema formation in the lungs and periphery, accounting for many of the clinical manifestations of CHF (Fig. 13-2).

### Arginine vasopressin

Arginine vasopressin is another potent vasoconstrictor that is released to maintain systemic blood pressure with falling cardiac output in CHF. The mechanism of release is probably related to decreased sensitivity of the atrial stretch receptors in heart failure; this decreased sensitivity normally inhibits the release of arginine vasopressin. An increase in arginine vasopressin levels is probably responsible for hyponatremia in advanced CHF.

### Atrial natriuretic peptide

Unlike vasopressin, norepinephrine, and angiotensin, atrial natriuretic peptide is not a vasoconstrictor but a vasodilator. Unlike aldosterone, it promotes renal excretion of salt and water. This peptide does not cause sympathetic stimulation that promotes an increase in heart rate; it reduces heart rate by modulating baroceptor function. Thus it is a counter-regulatory hormone whose function appears to balance and negate excessive action of the neurohormonal compensation. All compensatory mechanisms in heart failure become self-perpetuating; control of these factors has become the goal of treatment.

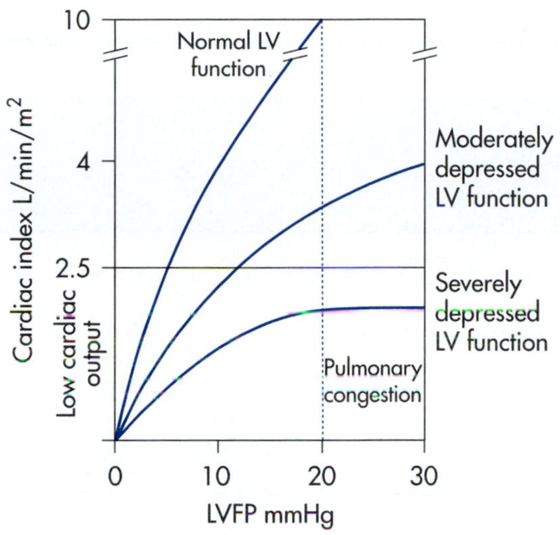


**Fig. 13-2.** Ventricular function curves depicting the relation between left ventricular filling pressure *(LVFP)* and cardiac index based on the Frank-Starling mechanism for normal and moderately and severely decompensated hearts. Values for cardiac index below 2.5 L/min/$m^2$ are associated with low cardiac output and diminished tissue perfusion. Values for LVFP greater than 20 mm Hg are associated with pulmonary congestion.

## FORMS OF HEART FAILURE

Heart failure has been described by various terms. Some terms such as *backward* or *forward heart failure,* although originally intended to describe underlying pathophysiology, have only a historical significance. Other terms, including *acute* or *chronic heart failure, low-output* or *high-output heart failure, left-sided* or *right-sided heart failure,* and *systolic* or *diastolic heart failure,* try to describe a pathophysiologic state.

### Acute vs. chronic heart failure

The syndrome of CHF usually describes the chronic form in which cardiac decompensation takes place after years of attempted compensation for the underlying cardiac disorder. Chronic heart failure, as in cardiomyopathy or rheumatic valvular disease, demonstrates a gradual progression of symptoms and signs that are characteristic of CHF. On the other hand, acute heart failure presents as acute pulmonary edema (Table 13-1).

### Low-output vs. high-output heart failure

In most instances of chronic CHF, cardiac output is low at rest or fails to rise adequately on exercise. Sometimes, manifestations of CHF occur in spite of marked elevations in cardiac output. In the commonly encountered low-output CHF the extremities tend to be cold, pale, and sometimes cyanotic, reflecting peripheral vasoconstriction. In high-output failure the extremities remain warm and flushed, reflecting peripheral vasodilatation. Frequent causes of high-output failure are listed in Table 13-1.

**Table 13-1.** Special forms of heart failure

| Type | Etiology | Manifestation |
|---|---|---|
| Acute heart failure | Acute myocardial infarction<br>Ventricular septal rupture<br>Papillary muscle rupture<br>Rupture of chordae tendineae<br>Perforated aortic cup resulting from bacterial endocarditis | Acute pulmonary edema |
| High-output heart failure | Anemia<br>Beriberi<br>Atrioventricular fistula<br>Hyperthyroidism<br>Paget's disease<br>Heart disease during pregnancy | Right- and left-sided heart failure |
| Right-sided heart failure | Pulmonary hypertension<br>Chronic lung disease<br>Multiple pulmonary emboli | Right-sided heart failure |
| Diastolic heart failure | Hypertrophic cardiomyopathy<br>Amyloidosis<br>Hemachromatosis<br>Left ventricular hypertrophy<br>Constrictive pericarditis | Right- and/or left-sided heart failure |

**Table 13-2.** Features of LV systolic and diastolic dysfunction

| | Pure systolic dysfunction | Pure diastolic dysfunction | Combined dysfunction |
|---|---|---|---|
| Pulmonary congestion | No | Yes | Yes |
| Cardiac output | ↓ | Normal | ↓ |
| Ejection fraction | ↓ | Normal | ↓ |
| LV dilation | Usually | Rarely | Usually |
| Inotropic agents | Yes | No | Yes |
| Preload reduction | No | Yes | Yes |
| Afterload reduction | Yes | No | Yes |
| Diuretic agents | No | Yes | Yes |

**Table 13-3.** Etiology of heart failure

| | | | Impaired filling | | |
|---|---|---|---|---|---|
| **Contractile dysfunction** | **Pressure overload** | **Volume overload** | **Valvular disease** | **Diastolic dysfunction** | **Increased demand** |
| Myocarditis | Hypertension | Aortic insufficiency | Mitral stenosis | Hypertrophic cardiomyopathy | Anemia |
| Cardiomyopathy | Aortic stenosis | Mitral insufficiency | Tricuspid stenosis | Amyloidosis | Thyrotoxicosis |
| Coronary artery disease | Coarctation of the aorta | Tricuspid regurgitation | | | Beriberi |
| | | Left-to-right shunt | | | Atrioventricular fistula |

### Left-sided vs. right-sided heart failure

Chronic CHF commonly presents with symptoms and signs of right-sided and left-sided heart failure. Left-sided heart failure leads to pulmonary venous congestion, and this in turn leads to pulmonary hypertension and subsequent right-sided heart failure. Thus chronic CHF in general represents biventricular failure. However, isolated right-sided heart failure related to pulmonary hypertension that is primary or secondary to lung disease does not affect the left ventricle. Clinical manifestations are limited to right-sided heart failure with jugular venous distension, edema, and congestive hepatomegaly. The symptoms of left-sided heart failure, such as orthopnea and signs of pulmonary venous congestion, are generally absent.

### Systolic vs. diastolic failure

For the heart to eject blood commensurate with the metabolic requirements during systole, it first has to receive blood during diastole. Heart failure is deemed to be present if the heart is unable to receive blood without unduly elevating the filling pressure in the ventricles. Symptoms and signs of systemic or pulmonary venous congestion generally result from diastolic impairment (Table 13-2). Symptoms of systolic impairment generally result from inadequate cardiac output with weakness, fatigue, and other symptoms of hypoperfusion. Although isolated diastolic dysfunction is being increasingly recognized as the cause of heart failure with normal systolic function, in chronic CHF, both forms of failure coexist. Table 13-1 lists the causes of isolated diastolic dysfunction.

## ETIOLOGY

Heart failure is caused by underlying structural disease states and precipitating or aggravating factors. Structural disease states can be classified into those due to loss of contractility of the cardiac muscle, resulting from volume or pressure overload, with abnormality in cardiac filling because of valvular disease or diastolic dysfunction, and with increased metabolic demand (Table 13-3).

Many changes have occurred in the past 30 years in the etiologic factors in heart failure. Rheumatic heart disease has become infrequent; in fact, ischemic heart disease has become more frequent. In the Framingham study and in the Studies of Left Ventricular Dysfunction (SOLVD) registry, hypertension and coronary disease have been the most frequent causes of heart failure. In the Framingham study, hypertension was the most frequent cause, but in the SOLVD registry, coronary disease was more frequent.

### Precipitating or aggravating factors

Although the primary disease states noted in the previous section are responsible for the structural changes leading to CHF, decompensation often occurs because of certain aggravating factors. They can be divided into patient-related factors, physician-related factors, heart failure–related disease states, and unrelated causes. It is important to recognize these factors because the patient's condition could be returned to baseline if they are corrected promptly. Inability to correct these factors may lead to persistence of heart failure in spite of adequate treatment.

***Patient-related factors***
1. Change in prescribed activity
2. Change in diet, especially salt intake
3. Noncompliance/alteration in prescribed medication
4. Excessive consumption of alcohol

***Physician-related factors***
1. Use of therapeutic agents that retain salt and water: estrogens, steroids, or nonsteroidal antiinflammatory agents
2. Use of negative inotropic agents: β-blockers, calcium channel blockers, disopyramide, and doxorubicin (adriamycin)

***Heart failure–related disease states***
1. Uncontrolled hypertension
2. Unstable angina or acute myocardial infarction
3. Atrial or ventricular arrhythmias
4. Pulmonary emboli
5. Systemic infection
6. Bacterial endocarditis

***Unrelated disease states***
1. High-output states
2. Renal or hepatic failure

## HISTORY

### Symptoms of left-sided heart failure

Left-sided heart failure causes dyspnea related to pulmonary congestion. Dyspnea is a subjective difficulty in breathing. In the early stages of heart failure, dyspnea occurs primarily on effort. As the disease progresses, the extent of effort required to provoke dyspnea decreases. Finally, the patient becomes dyspneic at rest. Since activity levels vary between individuals, it is necessary to categorize patients based on activity levels. The New York Heart Association classification helps in the follow-up of patients regarding the progression of disease or improvement with drug treatment (see box at right).

**New York Heart Association classification**

*Class I:* No limitations of physical activity. Ordinary physical activity does not cause undue fatigue, dyspnea, palpitations, or angina.
*Class II:* Slight limitation of physical activity. Such patients are comfortable at rest. Ordinary physical activity may result in fatigue, dyspnea, palpitation's, or angina.
*Class III:* Marked limitation of physical activity. These patients are fairly comfortable at rest. Less than ordinary physical activity will lead to symptoms.
*Class IV:* Inability to carry on any physical activity without discomfort. Symptoms of heart failure or angina are present even at rest. If any physical activity is undertaken, increased discomfort is experienced.

From New York Heart Association.

***Orthopnea.*** *Orthopnea* refers to dyspnea that manifests or is aggravated when the patient is in the recumbent position. Orthopnea is due to redistribution of fluid from the abdomen and the lower body into the chest during recumbency, an increase in the work of breathing when a patient with decreased lung compliance lies flat, and an elevation of the diaphragm by ascites and hepatomegaly.

The presence of orthopnea should be related to the patient's normal habits. In the initial stages breathing is eased by using more pillows during sleep. As the disease progresses the patient has to sit to sleep.

Two symptoms related to orthopnea are a nocturnal cough and dyspnea in the left lateral decubitus position. Nocturnal cough is related to orthopnea in the early stages of CHF. When the head slips off the pillows, the patient is awakened with a coughing bout that is relieved by sitting. Dyspnea in the left lateral decubitus position occurs when the patient has dyspnea after turning on the left side. The exact rationale for this symptom is unclear but may be related to alterations in the coronary perfusion pressure. These symptoms may not seem to be related to heart failure, but their origin becomes clear when heart failure is first diagnosed. With advanced biventricular failure, orthopnea diminishes with tricuspid insufficiency.

***Paroxysmal nocturnal dyspnea.*** Paroxysmal nocturnal dyspnea is an extension of orthopnea, with further progression of left ventricular failure. Similar to orthopnea, the patient wakes up in the night and has to sit. Unlike orthopnea, it occurs after prolonged recumbency and is unpredictable in its occurrence, and sitting provides only partial relief. The episodes are accompanied by coughing and wheezing and are frightening to the patient and family.

The factors responsible for orthopnea also contribute to paroxysmal nocturnal dyspnea. In addition, reduced ventilatory drive because of depression of the respiratory center and impairment of left ventricular function related to reduced adrenergic stimulation may have a role in the pathogenesis of this symptom.

When significant wheezing is associated with paroxysmal nocturnal dyspnea, it resembles an acute asthmatic attack and is therefore called *cardiac asthma.* Acute pulmonary edema can be a further extension of paroxysmal nocturnal dyspnea. Alternatively, often referred to as "flash" pulmonary edema it can occur de novo as the primary symptom with acute myocardial infarction or accelerated hypertension before CHF becomes established. Untreated, it can be fatal. The patient is extremely short of breath and coughs up pink, frothy sputum. Acute pulmonary edema occurs when there is significant elevation of the pulmonary capillary wedge pressure leading to alveolar edema.

***Cheyne-Stokes respiration.*** Cheyne-Stokes respiration is also called *periodic* or *cyclical respiration.* In this symptom complex, periods of hyperpnea alternate with periods of apnea. This symptom is probably caused by prolonged circulation time from the heart to the brain, which affects the normal regulation of breathing. Further, there is diminished sensitivity of the respiratory center to the arterial carbon dioxide pressure, which waxes and wanes during periods of hyperpnea and apnea (see Chapter 96). The fall in oxygen pressure and rise in carbon dioxide pressure during the apneic phase stimulates the respiratory center and results in hyperpnea, and the cycle continues.

This symptom complex is common among the elderly who have left ventricular failure and usually occurs among patients with hypertensive heart failure and heart failure resulting from coronary disease. The presence of cerebral arteriosclerosis and use of hypnotics such as barbiturates may be partly responsible for this symptom. The patient is generally unaware of the alteration in breathing pattern, but the spouse or members of the family notice it with alarm. Insomnia may be caused by the patient waking up during the hyperpneic phase. Alternatively, hyperpnea may be a forerunner of paroxysmal nocturnal dyspnea.

### Symptoms of right-sided heart failure

Whereas symptoms of left-sided heart failure are related to fluid accumulation in the lungs, symptoms of right-sided heart failure result in edema or fluid accumulation in the left side of the heart.

Perhaps the earliest symptoms may be an inappropriate weight gain. This is followed by ankle swelling by the end of the day, which is noticed by pitting depressions noted in the legs when the shoes or garters are removed. Edema in the lower part of the body is due to extravascular fluid accumulation because of elevated hydrostatic pressure in the dependent portions of the body. Transient edema in the ankles becomes persistent edema with the progression of heart failure. In patients who are immobilized because of heart failure, dependent edema is noticed not in the legs, but in the presacral region.

As heart failure progresses, fluid accumulation involves other parts of the body. Massive edema involving the entire body and all the serous cavities is termed *anasarca.* Ascites is an increase in abdominal girth. In biventricular failure, hydrothorax makes the patient more breathless.

Besides fluid accumulation in the extracellular compartment, there is also congestion of fluid in the liver and intestines. Stretching of capsule of the liver results in abdominal pain in the right upper quadrant, and the patient often complains of pain on exertion in this region. Congestion of fluid in the intestines leads to anorexia, nausea, and vomiting.

Oliguria and nocturia are common kidney-related symptoms. The relative oliguria results from renal vasoconstriction during activity in the daytime. Improved cardiac output and renal vasodilatation results in nocturia. This again causes insomnia. In patients with biventricular failure the insomnia associated with pulmonary congestion of left-sided heart failure is aggravated by the nocturia associated with right-sided heart failure.

### Symptoms related to diminished cardiac output

Symptoms related to diminished cardiac output can occur with right- or left-sided heart failure but in general are noticed in patients with long-standing biventricular failure. They are fatigability, lethargy, confusion, and loss of memory. The cerebral symptoms generally occur among older patients, and cerebral arteriosclerosis is commonly associated with diminished cardiac output. Criteria for identifying CHF developed for the Framingham Study are presented in the box at right.

Cardiac cachexia occurs late during biventricular failure and is due to persistent low cardiac output and a congested and poorly functioning gastrointestinal system. Late in the course of the disease, nocturia is replaced by persistent oliguria, which indicates end-stage heart failure.

### Criteria for CHF

**Major criteria**

Paroxysmal nocturnal dyspnea
Neck vein distention
Rales
Radiographic cardiomegaly (increasing heart size on chart x-ray film)
Acute pulmonary edema
Third-sound gallop
Increased central venous pressure (more than 16 cm of water at right atrium)
Circulation time of at least 255
Hepatojugular reflux
Pulmonary edema, visceral congestion of cardiomyopathy at autopsy
Weight loss of at least 4.5 kg in 5 days in response to treatment of CHF

**Minor criteria**

Bilateral ankle edema
Nocturnal cough
Dyspnea on ordinary exertion
Hepatomegaly
Pleural effusion
Decrease in vital capacity by 33% from maximum value recorded
Tachycardia (rate of at least 20 beats/min)

From Ho KK et al: The epidemiology of heart failure: The Framingham Study, *J Am Coll Cardiol* 22(4 suppl A):6A, 1993.

## PHYSICAL EXAMINATION

The physical signs of CHF can again be divided into those that pertain to left ventricular failure and those that primarily result from right ventricular failure. Signs of left ventricular failure relate to pulmonary venous congestion, and signs of right-sided heart failure relate to systemic venous congestion. These signs all relate to systolic dysfunction. There are no typical physical signs of diastolic dysfunction per se.

Since physical examination is better conducted in an organized sequence and since most patients have some degree of biventricular failure, the signs are described starting with the patient's general appearance, the jugular venous pulse, the peripheral pulse, and examination of the heart, lungs, and abdomen.

### General appearance

Patients with compensated or mildly decompensated CHF can look deceptively normal. Those with acute onset of heart failure have orthopnea and may be unable to lie down for examination. As stated, chronic biventricular failure can lead to cardiac cachexia.

In severe heart failure, there is some peripheral cyanosis resulting from low cardiac output and increased peripheral vasoconstriction. In these situations, the extremities are often cold and sweaty, with a tinge of cyanosis. A low-grade fever may also occur.

In severe right-sided heart failure, hepatic congestion can lead to some jaundice. Sometimes the clinician may have to seek peripheral pitting edema. In patients on bed rest who may be unaware of the existence of edema, presacral edema may be found.

### Jugular venous pulse

Elevation of the jugular venous pressure is a hallmark of elevated systemic venous pressure resulting from right-sided heart failure. Under normal conditions with the patient in a semirecumbent position, the upper level of pulsation of the internal jugular veins is no higher than about 1 cm above the clavicles, corresponding to right atrial pressure of 5 to 10 cm of water. Higher levels of venous pulsation, approaching the angle at the jaw even in the upright position, are common in many instances of right-sided failure. The a and the v waves of jugular venous pulse are elevated in patients whose hearts have a normal sinus rhythm. With the development of tricuspid insufficiency in severe right-sided heart failure, the descending limb of the a wave is attenuated, and the v wave increases with a rapid y-wave descent. Rarely, it is possible to demonstrate increased venous pressure in the veins in the arm or under the tongue.

When jugular venous distention is not apparent, hepatojugular reflux may be elicited by applying gentle but firm manual pressure over the liver for 1 minute while observing the neck veins. Normally, abdominal or hepatic compression leads to a transient increase in jugular venous pressure. The normal right ventricle compensates for the increase in venous return, and the venous pressure returns to normal in spite of continued abdominal pressure. The abnormal right ventricle in CHF is unable to accept an increase in venous return, and there is a persistent rise in jugular venous pressure. The patient must breathe normally and not strain during this maneuver. Elevated jugular venous pressure at rest or after hepatic or abdominal compression is a highly sensitive and specific marker of increased pulmonary capillary wedge pressure.

### Arterial pulse

Mild tachycardia is common. It reflects a compensatory phenomenon in which a higher heart rate is required to maintain adequate cardiac output in reduced stroke volume. In mild heart failure the heart rate at rest may be normal, but it increases excessively with exercise and fails to normalize with rest for a prolonged period.

*Pulsus alternans* implies severe left ventricular dysfunction. It occurs in CHF resulting from increased resistance to left ventricular ejection such as in aortic stenosis or hypertensive heart failure. Clinically, strong and weak beats alternate. They are detected by palpation of the pulse or determined with the sphygmomanometer. The cause is depletion in the number of contracting cells in every other cycle because of incomplete recovery leading to alteration in the stroke volume. The weaker beats may fail to open the semilunar valves, resulting in halving of the pulse rate. This is termed *total alternans*.

### Examination of the heart

***Precordial palpation.*** CHF is accompanied by cardiac enlargement, which is denoted by a lateral and downward shift in the apical impulse. In severe heart failure the third sound can be palpated. In biventricular or severe right-sided heart failure, a right ventricular impulse can be felt in the lower sternal edge or in the subxyphoid area.

***Auscultation.*** The presence of a third heart sound (gallop rhythm) generally implies ventricular dysfunction in adults over the age of 40 years. This protodiastolic sound is heard normally in children and young adults. Excessive flow into the left ventricle associated with mitral or tricuspid regurgitation and left-to-right shunts can also cause a third heart sound without ventricular dysfunction. In CHF the presence of a third heart sound is probably related to a sudden deceleration of ventricular inflow that takes place after the early filling phase accompanied by closure of the atrioventricular valves. Compliance abnormality or diastolic dysfunction also may play a part in the genesis of the gallop rhythm. A left-sided third heart sound is located at the apex and is louder after inspiration, whereas a right-sided third heart sound becomes louder during inspiration.

Alteration in ventricular geometry that accompanies cardiac enlargement in CHF causes incompetence of the atrioventricular valves. Thus murmurs of mitral or tricuspid regurgitation are common in CHF without structural disease involving these valves. The murmurs diminish or disappear after successful treatment of heart failure.

In biventricular failure or isolated right-sided heart failure, pulmonary hypertension develops, and the pulmonary component of the second heart sound becomes louder.

### Examination of the lungs

The major finding is rales. Generally, they are heard at the bases, but depending on the severity of heart failure, they may be heard all over the lungs. Wheezing can occur with congestion of the bronchial mucosa. In biventricular failure, bilateral pleural effusions can occur. When the rales or pleural effusion is limited to one side, the left lung seems to be spared. When effusion or rales occurs on the left side, the clinician should suspect pulmonary infarction.

### Examination of the abdomen

The two major findings in the abdomen are hepatomegaly and ascites. Hepatomegaly is an early sign of systemic venous congestion. In the early stages of failure the liver is tender, but with progression into the chronic state, tenderness may disappear. With the onset of tricuspid regurgitation, the v wave can be transmitted to the liver with systolic pulsation. Long-standing hepatic congestion may lead to cardiac cirrhosis with portal hypertension and congestive splenomegaly.

Ascites tends to be minimal in most patients with CHF. With massive ascites the clinician should suspect pericardial constriction.

## LABORATORY STUDIES AND DIAGNOSTIC PROCEDURES

Approaches to the diagnosis of suspected CHF are presented in Fig. 13-3 and Table 13-4.

### CBC

Although it is not a diagnostic indicator of heart failure, severe anemia is associated with high-output heart failure.

### Erythrocyte sedimentation rate

The erythrocyte sedimentation rate decreases in heart failure because of impaired fibrinogen synthesis and decreased fibrinogen concentration. If the sedimentation rate is increased, the causes of elevation are sought.

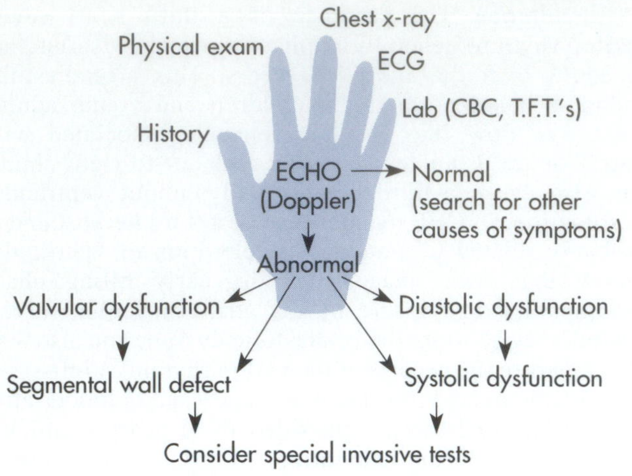


**Fig. 13-3.** Approaches to the diagnosis of suspected CHF. (From Noble J: Speakers forum on congestive heart failure, 1989, Burroughs Wellcome Co.)

## Electrolyte levels

Hyponatremia is common in severe heart failure and is the result of prolonged sodium restriction, diuretic therapy, and expansion of extracellular volume causing dilutional hyponatremia. An alteration in the neurohumoral axis caused by an elevation of circulating vasopressin levels can also be responsible for hyponatremia. Hyponatremia is an adverse prognostic factor for long-term survival in patients with CHF.

Hypokalemia is usually caused by diuretic therapy without oral supplement of potassium salts. Hypokalemia may also result from activation of the renin-angiotensin-aldosterone axis. It may lead to ventricular arrhythmias, especially after digitalis administration.

Hyperkalemia can occur when cardiac failure leads to renal failure, especially when excessive potassium supplementation has occurred or potassium-retaining diuretics or ACE converting enzyme inhibitors are used.

**Table 13-4.** Algorithm for the work-up of patients with congestive heart failure

| Work-up | Comment |
|---|---|
| History | Define nature of preexisting heart disease such as hypertension or coronary artery disease.<br>Exclude reversible causes such as alcoholism or substance abuse (cocaine). |
| Physical examination | Exclude correctible causes such as primary valvular heart disease or congenital heart disease. |
| Laboratory | |
| Complete blood count | Exclude anemia. |
| Hypokalemia | Secondary to diuretic therapy. |
| Hyponatremia | Indicator of poor prognosis. |
| Bun/creatinine ratio | Differentiation of primary renal disease from prerenal azotemia results from diminished cardiac output. |
| Liver function test | Elevated hepatic enzyme levels secondary to passive congestion. Persistent abnormality that may indicate cardiac cirrhosis. |
| Hypophosphatemia | Cause of reversible cardiac failure. |
| Urinalysis | |
| Glycosuria | Diabetes mellitus. |
| Albuminuria | Long-standing hypertension or diabetes. |
| Hematuria | Microscopic hematuria that may suggest bacterial endocarditis. |
| Chest x-ray | Generalized cardiomegaly with pulmonary venous hypertension. Classical CHF with systolic dysfunction.<br>Small heart with pulmonary venous hypertension, which may be indicative of primary diastolic heart failure. |
| Electrocardiogram | |
| Left ventricular hypertrophy | Preexisting systemic hypertension, aortic valve disease, or hypertrophic cardiomyopathy. |
| Right ventricular hypertrophy | Pulmonary hypertension primary or secondary to congenital heart disease or chronic lung disease. |
| Pathologic Q-waves | Previous myocardial infarction. |
| Low voltage with left axis deviation | Amyloidosis. |
| Biatrial enlargement | Chronic CHF. |
| Echocardiogram (indicated in all cases) | Exclude primary valvular or congenital heart disease.<br>Determine left ventricular function.<br>Determine nature of chamber enlargement.<br>Determine wall-motion abnormalities to distinguish ischemic from idiopathic cardiomyopathy.<br>Exclude ventricular aneurysm with or without thrombus formation. |
| Radionuclide ventriculography (indications) | Used to evaluate left ventricular function when echocardiogram cannot be performed because of poor acoustic window. Used to follow-up left ventricular function in treated patients. |
| Cardiac catheterization (indications) | In congenital or primary valvular disease to determine suitability for surgical correction.<br>In coronary disease when angina accompanies symptoms and signs of CHF to determine suitability for revascularization.<br>Echocardiogram or nuclear angiogram demonstrates asynergic left ventricle suggestive of underlying correctible coronary disease. |
| Endomyocardial biopsy (indications) | Congestive cardiomyopathy after a viral infection suggestive of myocarditis.<br>History of clinical features are suggestive of amyloidosis, hemochromatosis, or sarcoidosis. |

Hypophosphatemia can lead to a reversible form of cardiomyopathy that is treatable with phosphate supplements. This occurs in alcoholic persons and in patients who have consumed large amounts of antacids.

Hypomagnesemia also occurs in persons who have chronic alcoholism with cardiomyopathy. Changes in the magnesium level parallel potassium level changes, and hypomagnesemia is also arrhythmogenic.

### Blood urea nitrogen and creatinine levels

The blood urea nitrogen and creatinine levels are moderately elevated in severe CHF because of a reduction in renal blood flow and the glomerular filtration rate.

### Liver function tests

Chronic right-sided heart failure leads to abnormal liver function. Serum bilirubin and alkaline phosphatase levels are elevated; prothrombin time is rarely prolonged.

### Arterial blood gas levels

Arterial blood gas tests are useful especially in acute pulmonary edema; in this condition, improvement in oxygenation can be quantitated with therapy. In cor pulmonale, carbon dioxide retention can be measured, and oxygen administration can be controlled.

### Electrocardiography

No specific electrocardiographic pattern is diagnostic for congestive cardiac failure. However, the electrocardiogram may provide important information relevant to the nature of underlying cardiac disease. Electrocardiographic evidence of left ventricular hypertrophy and left atrial enlargement may suggest left-sided heart failure resulting from antecedent hypertension, cardiomyopathy, or a specific valvular lesion such as aortic stenosis. The presence of pathologic Q waves in ischemic heart disease indicates the presence and location of myocardial infarction. Abnormalities of rhythm such as atrial fibrillation may be secondary to failure or may represent inadequacy of therapy if the ventricular response is uncontrolled. If present, ventricular ectopy may represent inadequate treatment or overtreatment with digoxin. Adrenergic stimulation with elevation of norepinephrine levels also can be responsible for ventricular arrhythmias.

### Chest radiography

The two basic abnormalities in the chest x-ray film are an alteration in the cardiac silhouette and pulmonary venous congestion. Change in cardiac size and the cardiothoracic ratio are often used to decide improvement with therapy. Specific chamber enlargement helps determine the etiology of heart failure.

The degree of pulmonary venous congestion often parallels increases in the pulmonary capillary wedge pressure. When the wedge pressure is 20 to 25 mm Hg, interstitial pulmonary edema exists. Early radiologic signs of pulmonary venous hypertension and interstitial edema include distention of the pulmonary veins extending upward from the hila, loss of definition of pulmonary vascular markings, haziness of hilar shadows, and thickening of interlobular septa (Kerley's B lines). Pleural effusions of varying size and distribution may also be present. When the pulmonary capillary wedge pressure exceeds 25 mm Hg, alveolar edema is manifested by a radiographic pattern of diffuse haziness extending downward toward the lower portions of one lung field; more common, both lung fields are involved, causing the so-called butterfly pattern.

### Noninvasive studies

The two noninvasive techniques commonly used in the evaluation of CHF are echocardiography and radionuclide angiography. Neither of these tests are diagnostic for CHF.

Two-dimensional echocardiography is useful for three reasons: It can determine the nature of underlying structural defect, especially valvular disease; it can predictably determine the extent of systolic dysfunction; and it is very useful in measuring wall thickness. With the advent of Doppler studies, echocardiography can reliably estimate the nature and extent of diastolic dysfunction. The advent of transesophageal echocardiography has made it possible to obtain reliable information even when there is no adequate window to perform transthoracic studies.

Radionuclide angiography, commonly designated as MUGA, is superior to echocardiography in determining the EF more accurately. It can characterize wall-motion abnormalities especially in ischemic heart disease.

### Invasive studies

Right heart catheterization (Swan-Ganz catheterization) is mandatory when doubt exists about whether acute pulmonary edema is cardiac or noncardiac. The test is used primarily to determine response to therapy in severe heart failure, with sequential values for right and left ventricular filling pressures (right atrial and pulmonary wedge pressures), cardiac output, and systemic and pulmonary vascular resistances. This is true in the intensive care setting where treatment with vasodilators, inotropic agents, and/or intraaortic balloon pumping occurs.

### Left heart catheterization, left ventriculography, and coronary arteriography

Left heart catheterization, left ventriculography, and coronary arteriography have no role in establishing the presence of heart failure. Yet the presence of CHF implies a dismal, long-term prognosis, and the clinician must be sure that surgically remediable causes such as coronary, valvular, or congenital heart disease are ruled out. Cardiac catheterization and angiographic studies are usually planned electively after adequate medical management of CHF. However, the clinician must watch for certain cardiac lesions, initially seen as acute or severe cardiac failure, in which emergent invasive study and surgical intervention save the patient's life. Three such lesions are massive mitral regurgitation resulting from ruptured chordae tendineae, massive aortic regurgitation secondary to bacterial endocarditis, and perforation of the interventricular septum or (partial) papillary muscle rupture with acute myocardial infarction. It has become apparent that LV dysfunction may be due to a prolonged low flow state as a result of coronary obstruction that improves with revascularization. This is termed *hibernating myocardium.*

### Transmyocardial biopsy

Biopsy is useful for the diagnosis of myocarditis, especially in young individuals with antecedent viral infection and in patients with idiopathic congestive cardiomyopathy. It is useful in differentiating restrictive cardiomyopathy related to amyloidosis from constrictive pericarditis.

## DIFFERENTIAL DIAGNOSIS

Many symptoms and physical findings suggesting heart failure may be caused by other conditions (Table 13-5).

In a patient who has dyspnea, the clinician must distinguish cardiac from pulmonary causes. Sometimes, this differentiation is difficult. For example, orthopnea may be a well-established symptom in some patients with severe chronic obstructive lung disease. Patients with underlying pulmonary disease also may experience episodic dyspnea that mimics paroxysmal nocturnal dyspnea during sleep. In pulmonary disease, this is usually due to accumulation of tracheobronchial secretions and is relieved by coughing and expectorating the sputum, but in cardiac disease the patient has to sit upright and open the windows. Wheezing caused by bronchoconstriction may be a prominent symptom when left-sided heart failure supervenes in individuals with reactive airway disease (bronchial asthma or chronic bronchitis). Patients with cardiac asthma more frequently exhibit diaphoresis and varying degrees of cyanosis than those with bronchial asthma. Differentiating dyspnea related to heart disease from that related to pulmonary disease is more difficult when the diseases coexist, a situation common in some chronically ill elderly patients. Pulmonary function studies may help delineate whether pulmonary or cardiac disease is the predominant condition causing dyspnea.

## MANAGEMENT

Management of CHF has changed considerably during the past 3 decades. Years ago the most frequent cause was rheumatic valvular disease, which has become rare. Today the most frequent cause of chronic CHF is left ventricular dysfunction resulting from coronary artery disease. Rheumatic valvular disease was a slowly progressive disease, so the heart was able to compensate for valvular dysfunction for many years before symptoms of heart failure became prominent. With coronary disease, such progression can be rapid, occurring in a matter of weeks rather than years. In the past, major problems that confronted physicians were peripheral and pulmonary edema; with the advent of potent diuretics, the treatment of refractory edema is no longer a major problem. Now the significant problem is effort intolerance.

Three closely related therapeutic objectives for managing CHF are identifying and treating precipitating or aggravating factors, recognizing and treating underlying cardiac disease, and managing heart failure.

**Table 13-5.** Differential diagnosis

| Symptom | Differential diagnosis |
|---|---|
| Dyspnea | Anxiety neurosis, lung disease |
| Edema | Venous insufficiency, nephrotic syndrome |
| Ascites | Hepatic cirrhosis |
| Distended neck veins | Superior vena cava syndrome, constrictive pericarditis, pericardial effusion |

The management of heart failure also has three related components: diminution of the workload of the heart, control of excessive salt and water retention, and improvement of cardiac pump performance. Diminution of cardiac workload is achieved by rest and the use of vasodilators. Control of edema is achieved by restriction of dietary salt, use of diuretics, and when necessary, mechanical removal of edema fluid. Therapeutic measures to improve cardiac performance include administration of digitalis glycosides and when necessary, certain inotropic agents such as dopamine, dobutamine, or amrinone.

The onset and progression of CHF are highly variable and may differ greatly among patients. Thus selection of appropriate therapeutic measures for individuals depends primarily on the underlying causes of heart failure, the severity of functional impairment, and the response to measures already instituted. Effective management must also consider the patient's age, occupation, lifestyle, and family setting, as well as presence of associated illness. The patient's ability and motivation to cooperate with planned therapeutic measures must also be considered.

An initial period of hospitalization is required when patients present for the first time in acute heart failure. The duration of hospitalization is variable, but in most patients, stabilization can be achieved in a week. Subsequent care is undertaken as on outpatient basis. With the advent of ACE inhibitors, it has become possible to prevent exacerbations of heart failure in most patients.

Follow-up is generally for life unless the cause of CHF can be cured (e.g., surgery for valvular disease). The frequency of follow-up depends on the nature of heart disease, but the patient usually needs to be seen by the primary physician every 3 months. In the early stages, monthly follow-up is essential, and in patients receiving long-term warfarin sodium (Coumadin) therapy, frequency is dictated by the adequacy and stability of anticoagulation. The prothrombin time is checked at least every 6 weeks to prevent iatrogenic complications.

The prognosis of heart failure depends on the etiology. Unless a correctable factor is identified, the long-term prognosis is poor, varying from 6 months to 5 years depending on the severity of heart failure.

### Nonpharmacologic therapy

***Rest.*** Appropriate restriction of physical activity is essential in the treatment of most patients with CHF. Physical rest reduces metabolic demands and thus the overall work required of the failing heart. Bed rest in the hospital is usually necessary in the management of acute cardiac failure and other forms of severe cardiac decompensation. In the absence of hypotension, the patient is positioned in bed in a semirecumbent or upright posture to help alleviate respiratory distress. Elevation of the legs during rest, passive leg exercises, and elastic stockings are used to reduce the risk of venous thrombosis and pulmonary embolism. If there are no significant contraindications, minidose heparin therapy (5000 USP units every 12 h) is given, especially to patients with massive peripheral edema in whom prolonged immobilization is likely and to those with prior thromboembolic disease. Progressive mobilization is initiated when the patient's condition permits and is encouraged as further clinical improvement results. Explicit instructions regarding physical activity and rest are discussed before discharge.

Emotional rest is also essential in the management of heart failure. Reassurance and careful explanation of procedures and therapeutic measures often allay patient anxiety. Sometimes, mild tranquilization with diazepam (Valium) may help.

Reduction of physical activity is also important when managing milder forms of heart failure. In general, physical activities that can be performed below the patient's limits of fatigue and dyspnea are encouraged. Periods of physical activity are alternated with specified periods of rest, such as taking a nap in the early afternoon or minimizing physical activity on weekends. Adjustment in work schedules may be necessary to accommodate these restrictions if the patient is to remain employed.

*Diet.* Reduction of the dietary intake of sodium is an important measure in counteracting the pronounced tendency toward the salt and water retention of heart failure. However, with the widespread use of effective diuretic therapy, severe restriction of dietary salt is no longer as critically necessary as it once was in the management of CHF.

The average American diet without salt restriction contains as much as 10 g/day of salt. Prohibiting the addition of salt to cooked food and eliminating some salty foods (e.g., potato chips, salted nuts) often reduces salt intake to about 4 to 5 g/day. A salt substitute (potassium chloride) or herbs and spices may be used to flavor food. Removal of salt from cooking reduces intake to about 2 g of salt per day but often results in unpalatable food and poor compliance. This degree of salt restriction is often unnecessary unless edema persists after vigorous diuretic therapy. Further reduction of salt intake, when necessary, requires elimination of most processed foods and when possible, substitution with low-sodium foods (e.g., fresh vegetables; low-sodium milk, cheese, and bread).

In the obese patient with heart failure, weight reduction by dietary means is of critical importance in reducing the workload of the heart. Specific dietary advice regarding caloric restriction is given, and the therapeutic goal of weight reduction is reinforced during follow-up.

## Pharmacologic therapy

The combination of an inotropic agent and vasodilator with or without a diuretic achieves a more normal left ventricular function than does the single administration of an inotropic agent, vasodilator, or diuretic (Fig. 13-4).

The goal of combination drug therapy is to maximally restore a normal relationship between stroke volume and left ventricular filling pressure (the Starling curve).

*Diuretics.* Diuretic therapy is an important element in the treatment of edema associated with heart failure. When used with rest, salt restriction, and digitalis, diuretics often improve many symptoms and signs of CHF. Diuretics can be classified into the following categories:

1. Thiazide and related compounds
2. Carbonic anhydrase inhibitors
3. Osmotic diuretics
4. Loop diuretics
5. Potassium-sparing diuretics

In the treatment of CHF, commonly used diuretics are thiazides, loop diuretics, and potassium-sparing diuretics (Table 13-6).

**Thiazides and related drugs.** Thiazides exert their diuretic effects primarily by inhibiting sodium and chloride reabsorption in the distal convoluted tubule of the kidney. They are well absorbed orally and are usually well tolerated and thus are useful in the treatment of milder forms of CHF. However, thiazides usually lose their diuretic potency when glomerular filtration rates fall below 30 ml/min. Because these diuretics also enhance the secretion of potassium, significant hypokalemia and potassium depletion can follow prolonged therapy. Metabolic alkalosis, hyperglycemia, hyperuricemia, and dilutional hyponatremia are other complications of thiazide therapy.

Chlorothiazide and hydrochlorothiazide are the thiazides most commonly used in clinical practice.

Although chemically different from thiazides, chlorthalidone, metolazone, and indapamide are considered here because they have similar sites of action and potency. Metolazone has a long duration of action (24 to 48 h) because of serum protein binding and retains its diuretic properties even when renal function is compromised. Indapamide has vasodilatory and diuretic effects; its advantage is negligible alteration in serum cholesterol and triglyceride levels that supposedly accompanies its use.

**Loop diuretics.** Furosemide, ethacrynic acid, and bumetanide are potent diuretic agents that can be administered either orally or intravenously. These agents inhibit the tubular reabsorption of sodium and chloride in the ascending limb of the loop of Henle. Because their initial action augments renal blood flow, these drugs, unlike the thiazides, generally retain their diuretic potency when glomerular filtration rates are diminished.

Loop diuretics are useful in the management of more severe forms of CHF, especially acute pulmonary edema, for which they are usually administered intravenously. Because of potent diuretic effects, injudicious use may result in a severe reduction in intravascular volume and hypotension. Other side effects include hypokalemia, azotemia, metabolic alkalosis, hyperglycemia, hyperuricemia, and ototoxicity (particularly with ethacrynic acid).

**Potassium-sparing agents.** The potassium-sparing drugs include spironolactone, triamterene, and amiloride. All three have relatively mild diuretic potency when used alone. When used with a thiazide or a loop diuretic, however, they enhance sodium excretion and counteract the potassium-wasting properties of these drugs. Potassium-sparing diuretics are contraindicated in renal failure because they may result in life-threatening hyperkalemia.

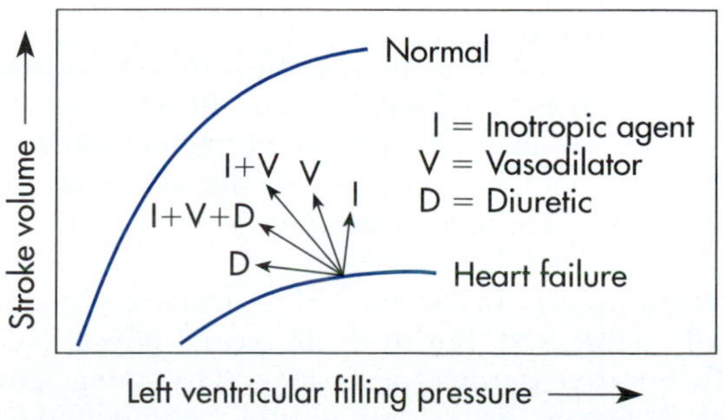


**Fig. 13-4.** Directional shifts in the relationship between left ventricular filling pressure *(LVFP)* and stroke volume produced by various pharmacologic interventions designed to reduce preload and/or afterload or to increase cardiac contractility in the severely decompensated heart. Endpoints indicate improved hemodynamic status.

**Table 13-6.** Dosages of diuretic agents used in heart failure

| Generic name | Trade names | Usual oral dose | Duration of action (h) |
|---|---|---|---|
| **Thiazides and related drugs** | | | |
| Chlorothiazide | Diuril | 500-100 mg/day | 6-12 |
| Hydrochlorothiazide | Hydrodiuril | 50-100 mg/day | >12 |
| Trichloromethiazide | Metahydrin, Naqua | 4-8 mg/day | 24 |
| Chlorthalidone | Hygroton | 100 mg/day | 24 |
| Metolazone | Zaroxolyn | 5-10 mg/day | 24-48 |
| Indapamide | Lozol | 1.25-5 mg/day | 24 |
| **Loop diuretics** | | | |
| Furosemide | Lasix | 40-160 mg/day<br>10-80 mg/IV | 6-8 (po) |
| Ethacrynic acid | Sodium Edecrin | 50-150 mg/day<br>50-100 mg/IV | 6-8 (po) |
| Bumetanide | Bumex | 0.5-4.0 mg/day<br>0.5-2.0 mg/IV | 4-6 (po) |
| **Potassium-sparing agents** | | | |
| Spironolactone | Aldactone | 100 mg/day | 3 days after starting therapy |
| Triamterene | Dyrenium | 100-200 mg/day | 12-16 |
| Amiloride | Midamor | 5-10 mg/day | 24 |

*po*, By mouth; *IV*, intravenously.

**Therapeutic effects and precautions.** The dosage of diuretics should be carefully titrated and then the patient monitored throughout treatment for problems related to diuretic therapy. Potential complications follow:

1. Intravascular volume depletion and hypotension from overly vigorous diuresis.
2. Hyponatremia, often resulting from prolonged diuretic therapy with inadequate sodium intake or excess water intake.
3. Extracellular or intracellular magnesium depletion from the use of diuretics. Magnesium and potassium deficits often coexist; correction of hypomagnesemia may be a prerequisite for treating hypokalemia.
4. Hypokalemia from thiazides or loop diuretics, or both, with inadequate potassium supplementation.
5. Hyperkalemia from potassium-sparing diuretic administration and potassium supplements.
6. Metabolic alkalosis, with or without potassium depletion.
7. Hyperuricemia secondary to thiazide or loop diuretic administration.
8. Reduced carbohydrate tolerance from thiazides and, to a lesser extent, loop diuretics. Preexisting diabetic conditions may be aggravated or unmasked.

Patients should be treated with the smallest possible dose to get the desired effects.

***Inotropic agents.*** In chronic CHF, cardiac contractility is generally depressed. For over 200 years, physicians have tried to improve cardiac performance by using inotropic agents. However, except for digitalis compounds, these drugs have not proved effective in the long-term treatment of heart failure. Inotropic agents can be classified into β-adrenergic receptor agonists, phosphodiasterase inhibitors, and digitalis glycosides.

**β-Adrenergic receptor agonists.** β-Adrenergic receptor agonists augment cardiac contractility by promoting the synthesis of cyclic adenosine monophosphate (AMP). Cyclic AMP enhances the entry of calcium into the cell by activating membrane-bound calcium channels. One of the most commonly used β-adrenergic receptor agonists is dobutamine, which must be infused intravenously. In severe heart failure, patients are admitted to the hospital, and dobutamine infusions are undertaken as a temporizing measure. Pumps to infuse dobutamine have also been developed as bridges to patients with severe heart failure waiting for cardiac transplantation. However, a randomized trial of intermittent infusion was halted because it appeared to significantly increase the mortality rate.

**Phosphodiesterase inhibitors.** Phosphodiesterase inhibitors increase intracellular cyclic AMP by preventing the degradation of the nucleotide. In addition to inotropic properties, these drugs function as vasodilators. The commonly known phosphodiesterase inhibitors are amrinone and milrinone. A recent placebo-controlled multicenter trial using milrinone demonstrated a higher mortality rate among those randomized to the drug.

Recently vesnarinone, a phosphodiesterase inhibitor with possible antiarrhythmic effect because of its action on the sodium channel, has been shown to have remarkable effect on survival in patients with CHF. This was true, however, only when the drug was used in smaller doses; higher doses actually increased the mortality rate.

**Digitalis glycosides.** Although digitalis glycosides have been used to treat heart failure since 1785, controversy continues concerning their utility, especially in patients with heart failure whose hearts remain in sinus rhythm. Recent multicenter trials have established beyond doubt the positive role of digitalis in improving symptoms of heart failure (see Table 13-8). However, its role in improving survival remains to be established; such studies are under way.

Digitalis augments the force of cardiac contraction, which in turn increases cardiac output, promotes diuresis, and reduces filling pressures in both ventricles, thus promoting relief of pulmonary congestion. Thus digitalis may benefit patients with CHF associated with pressure or volume overload or chronic ischemic heart disease.

Besides its inotropic properties, the negative chronotropic effects of digitalis result in prolongation of the refractory period of the atrioventricular (AV) node. This effect is particularly useful for treating heart failure in patients with atrial fibrillation or flutter with rapid ventricular rates. Further, digitalis counterbalances the neurohumoral activation in CHF by its action on cardiac baroceptors.

It is used with caution in older persons in whom lower doses are used to compensate for slower renal excretion of the drug; digitalis is used with great caution in patients with acute myocardial infarction, renal insufficiency, hypoxemia, myocarditis, and hypothyroidism. It is contraindicated in second- or third-degree AV block unless a temporary electrical pacemaker has been inserted.

Several digitalis glycosides are available for clinical use. Digoxin is the agent most frequently used in clinical practice. It has an intermediate action time, can be used for most clinical situations in which digitalis therapy is indicated, and may be administered intravenously or orally, depending on the rapidity of drug action desired.

***Methods of administration.*** When a rapid therapeutic effect is not required, such as in the treatment of mild heart failure in the outpatient setting, the oral maintenance therapy of digoxin, 0.125 to 0.25 mg per day (i.e., no loading dose), is started. In the presence of normal renal function, full digitalization occurs within approximately 1 week. To achieve more rapid digitalization (within 24 to 48 h) in a patient who has not previously taken digitalis, an oral loading dose of 1.0 to 1.5 mg is given in divided doses over 24 h: 0.5 mg initially followed by 0.25 to 0.5 mg every 6 to 8 h until the loading dose is reached.

If rapid digitalization is required, an initial dose of 0.25 to 0.5 mg digoxin is given intravenously, followed by 0.125 to 0.25 mg every 2 to 4 h as indicated until a total digitalizing dose of approximately 1.0 mg is reached. The peak effect is usually achieved between 1.5 and 6 h. Electrocardiographic monitoring during rapid digitalization is essential to avoid drug toxicity.

***Therapeutic effects and precautions.*** Commonly observed therapeutic effects of digitalis therapy include slowing of the heart rate (disappearance of the disparity between apical and radial pulse rates in atrial fibrillation), improvement in symptoms and signs of pulmonary congestion, diuresis, and weight loss. Later, a decrease in heart size may be evident on the chest roentgenogram or may be documented by echocardiography. Some electrocardiographic changes may reflect the effects of digitalis and should not be construed as evidence for drug toxicity; these changes include lengthening of the PR interval, shortening of the QT interval, depression of the ST segment, and flattening or inversion of the T wave.

Hypokalemia, renal insufficiency, and hypoxia commonly predispose individuals to the toxic effects of digitalis. Therefore careful attention is given to each patient's electrolyte balance, renal function, and arterial blood gas status before therapy is initiated and when questions regarding possible toxicity arise. Serum glycoside levels are useful guides to therapy, particularly in patients in whom drug toxicity is likely to be encountered (e.g., those with advanced age, compromised renal function, and hypothyroidism) or in whom compliance to therapy is uncertain. Concomitant treatment with quinidine or verapamil often increases serum digoxin levels.

***Digitalis toxicity.*** Toxic manifestations of digitalis include a wide range of cardiac arrhythmias as well as anorexia, nausea, vomiting, and visual disturbances (blurred vision or xanthopsia). The new occurrence of ventricular premature beats and a significant increase in their frequency are probably the most common rhythm disturbances related to digitalis excess. Other cardiac arrhythmias include second-degree Wenkebach-type AV block, paroxysmal atrial tachycardia with block, and nonparoxysmal AV junctional tachycardia. Ventricular tachycardia and fibrillation are the most life-threatening arrhythmias associated with toxicity.

Digitalis toxicity is usually reversed by simply withdrawing the drug. Hypokalemia, if present, is corrected by careful administration of potassium; potassium is not given intravenously when significant degrees of AV block are present. High-grade AV blocks with very slow heart rates may require insertion of temporary electrical pacemakers. Significant ventricular arrhythmias associated with digitalis toxicity are treated with appropriate antiarrhythmic drugs, including lidocaine, phenytoin, and propranolol (small, incremental doses). Severe digoxin toxicity associated with recurrent ventricular arrhythmias, as might occur with massive overdosing, has been successfully treated using purified Fab fragments of digoxin-specific antibodies. The glycoside antibody complex is gradually excreted in the urine.

***Vasodilators.*** It is apparent from the therapies listed in Table 13-7 that ACE inhibition can postpone the development of heart failure in patients with asymptomatic left ventricular dysfunction. Further, in patients with myocardial infarction, these agents can prevent changes in myocardial structure and mechanics that may facilitate progression of left ventricular dysfunction. Finally, recent trials have established that improvement with ACE inhibitors is a group effect and not limited to one or two of the drugs used in the earlier trials (see Table 13-9).

Vasodilators can exert their effects by several mechanisms: (1) preferentially altering vascular tone in capacitance vessels of the venous bed (e.g., nitrates), thereby reducing right and left ventricular filling pressures (preload); (2) preferentially dilating arteriolar resistance vessels, thereby reducing afterload (e.g., hydralazine); (3) exerting balanced dilating effects on arteriolar and venous vessels (e.g., prazosin); (4) blocking the renin-angiotensin system by converting enzyme inhibition (e.g., ACE inhibitors). These effects counteract many of the neurohumoral changes in congestive heart failure that enhance vasoconstriction. The dosage and characteristics of vasodilators commonly used in the treatment of heart failure are shown in Table 13-7.

Furthermore, phosphodiesterase inhibitors combine vasodilatation with inotropic properties and are sometimes called *inodilators.* β-Blockers with α-blocking properties (e.g., carvedilol) combine β-blockade with vasodilatation and are termed *vasodilating β-blockers.* Dihydropyridine calcium blockers (e.g., nifedipine, amlodipine) have calcium blocking and vasodilating properties. In the

**Table 13-7.** Vasodilator therapy in congestive heart failure

| Generic name | Trade names | Route of administration | Usual dose | Principal sites of dilating action |
|---|---|---|---|---|
| **Nitrates** | | | | |
| Nitroglycerin | Nitrostat and others | Sublingual | 0.3-0.4 mg (initial) | Venous |
| Nitroglycerin | NitroBid and others | Topical | 1-2 inches every 4-6 h | Venous |
| Nitroglycerin | Tridil, Nitrostat IV | Intravenous | 5 μg/min (initial) | Venous |
| Isosorbide dinitrate | Isordil and others | Sublingual | 5-10 mg every 2-4 h | Venous |
| Isosorbide dinitrate | Isordil and others | Oral | 20-100 mg every 6 h | Venous |
| **Other agents** | | | | |
| Hydralazine | Apresoline | Oral | 25-100 mg every 6 h | Arteriolar |
| Prazosin | Minipress | Oral | 1-5 mg every 6 h | Arteriolar and venous |
| Nitroprusside | Nipride | Intravenous | 10-20 μg/min (initial) | Arteriolar and venous |
| Captopril | Capoten | Oral | 6.25-25 mg every 6 h | Arteriolar and venous |
| Enalapril | Vasotec | Oral | 2.5 to 15 mg po bid | Arteriolar and venous |
| Lisinopril | Zestril, Prinivil | Oral | 5-40 mg po daily | Arteriolar and venous |

*po*, By mouth; *bid*, twice a day.

treatment of CHF, survival benefits have been demonstrated only for the ACE inhibitors and hydralazine-nitrate combination. Trials are underway with β-blockers (e.g., metoprolol and carvedilol) and calcium blockers (e.g., amlodipine).

**ACE inhibitors.** The renin-angiotensin system is often activated in individuals with CHF, resulting in increased circulating levels of angiotensin II. This substance is a potent vasoconstrictor that increases systemic vascular resistance and thus afterload. Because it also causes the release of aldosterone, salt and water retention is enhanced, ultimately increasing preload. By inhibiting the enzyme that converts angiotensin I to angiotensin II, ACE inhibitors have a balanced effect on hemodynamics, reducing preload and afterload. ACE inhibitors also prevent the breakdown of bradykinin, which is a vasodilator; decrease circulating catecholamine levels at rest and on exercise; and may restore downregulated β-adrenergic receptors in chronic CHF. Tissue angiotensin may not be blocked by some ACE inhibitors.

With the demonstration of survival benefits, ACE inhibitors have become standard in the treatment of CHF related to systolic dysfunction, unless they are contraindicated. Most studies were done using captopril and enalapril. Recently, similar benefits have been demonstrated for other drugs in the group such as lisinopril and ramipril. The choice of ACE inhibitor may soon be dictated by its cost and convenience of administration. Table 13-7 describes most ACE inhibitors.

Hypotension is a prominent side effect of ACE inhibitors. The best way to avoid hypotension is to stop diuretic therapy on the first day of treatment. Hyperkalemia is common with ACE inhibitors, and the potassium supplementation required for concomitant diuretic therapy should be carefully monitored. The use of potassium-sparing diuretics is generally avoided. The minor side effect in about 30% of patients is a dry cough and tenacious sputum. Major side effects include renal failure in bilateral renal artery stenosis, angioedema, and neutropenia. ACE inhibitors are contraindicated in pregnancy.

When the use of ACE inhibitors is contraindicated, the best alternative is a hydralazine-nitrate combination. Because of their preferential venodilator effects, nitrates tend to reduce ventricular filling pressures and therefore aid in the relief of pulmonary congestion without significantly affecting cardiac output or arterial blood pressure. Nitrates can be administered via several routes: Nitroglycerin can be given sublingually, applied topically as an ointment, or administered intravenously. (Intravenous use of nitroglycerin and other vasodilators is discussed in the section on treatment of acute pulmonary edema.) Isosorbide dinitrate is usually given orally, 20 to 60 mg every 4 h.

Hydralazine reduces systemic vascular resistance by preferentially dilating arterioles. A common effect in individuals without cardiomegaly, reflex tachycardia, occurs somewhat infrequently in patients with CHF. In contrast to the effects of nitrates, with hydralazine, the ventricular filling pressure (preload) is only slightly reduced.

Treatment with hydralazine is started with 25 mg by mouth every 6 h and gradually increased over a period of days to weeks. Usually, doses of 200 mg/day or greater are necessary to achieve a beneficial effect. Side effects are flushing, headaches, and gastrointestinal upset. Many individuals, especially those requiring large doses for prolonged periods, develop positive titers of antinuclear antibodies. A smaller number of people develop a systemic lupus erythematosus–like syndrome, which usually resolves after discontinuation of the drug. Because of their differential hemodynamic properties on preload and afterload, nitrates (e.g., isosorbide dinitrate) and hydralazine are used in combination in an effort to enhance the limited beneficial effects that either drug achieves alone.

When ACE inhibitors and the hydralazine-nitrate combination are contraindicated, the best afterload-reducing agent may be prazosin. Prazosin is an α-adrenergic receptor blocking drug that exerts balanced arteriolar and venous dilating effects, resulting in intermediate hemodynamic changes between those of nitrates and hydralazine. A problematic side effect of prazosin is postural hypotension or syncope after the initial dose. Other side effects include headache, gastrointestinal upset, and salt and water retention that must be countered by increasing the dosage of diuretic. Treatment is initiated with 1 mg orally at bedtime, and the dosage is adjusted upward to achieve a desirable response. Total dosage should not exceed 20 mg/day. Early effects often subside with prolonged use.

### Other therapeutic modalities

In patients with massive edema, cautious mechanical removal of fluid from large accumulations in the pericardial, pleural or peritoneal spaces occasionally results in marked improvement of symptoms. Peritoneal dialysis may be used to remove excess fluid in individuals with severely compromised renal function. In selected patients with profound anemia, sequential phlebotomy and plasmapheresis with retransfusion of the patient's red blood cells may prove extremely effective in managing heart failure. In severe hypoalbuminemia, the cautious administration of salt-free albumin may be of additional benefit.

Severe bradycardia complicating CHF may be treated with atropine, isoproterenol (for brief periods), or preferably, insertion of an electrical pacemaker. If preservation of atrial transport function is deemed essential a sequential AV pacemaker may be used.

Circulatory-assist devices (e.g., intraaortic balloon counterpulsation) are reserved for patients with severe heart failure. Cardiac transplantation is considered.

## MANAGEMENT OF ACUTE PULMONARY EDEMA

Acute pulmonary edema secondary to cardiac disease is a life-threatening medical emergency that requires prompt identification and decisive treatment. Critical goals of therapy are the improvement and maintenance of adequate tissue oxygenation and prompt reduction in the workload of the heart (i.e., reducing circulatory demands by decreasing venous return [preload] and systemic vascular resistance [afterload]). General measures often effective in the treatment of acute pulmonary edema follow:

1. The patient is placed in an upright, sitting position.
2. Oxygen is administered by a well-fitted face mask (Venturi or reservoir bag). A concentration of 100% oxygen may be given initially; however, after blood gas determinations are made, inspired concentrations and flow rates are adjusted to achieve an arterial oxygen tension of at least 60 to 70 mm Hg.
3. Morphine sulfate, 3 to 5 mg, is given intravenously. If necessary the dose can be repeated in approximately 15 minutes. A specific morphine antagonist such as naloxone hydrochloride (Narcan) should be available in case respiratory depression occurs. A critical effect of morphine sulfate is venodilatation resulting in decreased venous return and preload.
4. A rapidly acting diuretic such as furosemide (Lasix), 20 to 40 mg, or bumetanide, 1 to 2 mg, is given intravenously.
5. Vasodilators are of additional benefit if the arterial blood pressure is normal or elevated. Either nitroglycerin (a venodilator) or sodium nitroprusside (a balanced dilator) can be given intravenously, depending on the hemodynamic response desired (i.e., predominant reduction in preload or reduction in preload and afterload). Nitroglycerin is administered intravenously using a low-flow constant-infusion pump at an initial rate of 5 mcg/min, which is increased by increments of 5 mcg/min every 5 to 10 minutes until pulmonary edema is relieved or arterial systolic blood pressure falls below 100 mm Hg. Intravenous vasodilators are administered only when the following are continuously monitored: Swan-Ganz catheterization to measure pulmonary capillary wedge pressures, cardiac output determination by thermodilution, and when necessary, direct arterial cannulation for precise systemic pressure.
6. In patients with bronchospasm, aminophylline, 250 to 500 mg, may be given intravenously. Aminophylline relieves bronchoconstriction, has a direct vasodilating effect, promotes diuresis, and may improve cardiac contractility.
7. Venous return to the heart may be further reduced by the application of tourniquets to three extremities. Tourniquets are rotated every 15 minutes and removed sequentially when no longer needed. If reduction in venous return using this method is inadequate, particularly in the presence of marked venous distention, phlebotomy with the removal of 300 to 500 ml of blood is considered.
8. Digitalis, given intravenously, may be of benefit, particularly in patients with atrial flutter or fibrillation associated with rapid ventricular rates. However, in the treatment of acute cardiac failure, digitalis is generally considered a secondary or ancillary measure compared with the rapid effectiveness of measures already outlined.
9. When a critically ill patient with acute pulmonary edema fails to respond to these measures and when arterial blood gas levels suggest rapidly progressive deterioration (severe hypoxia and hypercapnia), endotracheal intubation is performed, and continuous positive-pressure ventilation is applied. Further improvement in arterial oxygenation can be achieved, if necessary, by the application of positive and expiratory pressure. This must be undertaken with caution because reduction in venous return can be dramatic and results in a markedly diminished cardiac output and hypotension. Under conditions of controlled, assisted ventilation, administration of larger incremental doses of intravenous morphine sulfate is possible and frequently reverses even the most severe forms of acute pulmonary edema.

### Refractory heart failure

Heart failure is refractory when its symptoms and signs persist or even worsen despite intensive therapy that includes digoxin, diuretics, and vasodilators. This usually occurs in the late stages of heart failure; workup for transplantation ought to be undertaken before it is too late.

Frequently the term *intractable* or *refractory failure* is loosely applied when the treatment is inappropriate or inadequate. Inappropriate treatment is the result of excessive diuresis or digitalis toxicity. These conditions should be recognized and corrected.

CHF is a chronic disease, and noncompliance with the diet or treatment sometimes occurs. Alcohol is a myocardial toxin; excessive consumption can interfere with the treatment of heart failure.

Patients with chronic CHF are prone to venous thrombosis and pulmonary emboli that are clinically silent. Such patients may require long-term anticoagulation with warfarin sodium (Coumadin). The congested lung in heart failure is prone to infection, which should be assiduously treated. Patients with valvular heart disease are prone to bacterial endocarditis, which if unrecognized can lead to persistent heart failure. Other disease states

## Managed Care Guide
## Treatment of CHF due to pure LV diastolic dysfunction

- Treat pulmonary congestion (diuretics, venodilation, preload reduction)
- Avoid excess preload reduction
- Anti-ischemic therapy
- Heart rate control; maintain sinus rhythm
- Blood pressure control
- LVH regression
- Calcium channel blockers may reduce symptoms of CHF due to lusitropic action
- Inotropic agents probably not useful if EF is normal

From Noble J: Speaker's forum on congestive heart failure, 1989, Burroughs Wellcome Co.

## Etiology of heart failure among adolescents

Rheumatic fever
Acute hypertension (glomerulonephritis)
Viral myocarditis
Thyrotoxicosis
Hemochromatosis, hemosiderosis
Cancer chemotherapy (radiation, doxorubicin [Adriamycin])
Sickle cell anemia
Endocarditis
Cor pulmonale (cystic fibrosis)
Cardiomyopathy (hypertrophic, dilated, postviral)

Adapted from Behrman RE, editor: *Nelson textbook of pediatrics*, Philadelphia, 1992, WB Saunders.

such as hypothyroidism or hyperthyroidism and drugs that retain fluid such as corticosteroids, nonsteroidal antiinflammatory agents, and negative inotropes such as verapamil, disopyramide, or propranolol may complicate treatment of heart failure.

Occasionally, refractory failure occurs when all these causes are ruled out. This is generally demonstrated by persistent pulmonary congestion, hypoperfusion manifested by hypotension, and marked hyponatremia secondary to neurohormonal activation leading to mental confusion. Vasodilator and diuretic therapy become difficult to control. Such patients require admission to the critical care unit, where with the help of hemodynamic monitoring, treatment is instituted with a combination of an inotrope such as dobutamine (a dobutamine "sprint") or amrinone and a vasodilator such as nitroglycerin or nitroprusside. Once preload and afterload are controlled, oral treatment with diuretics and ACE inhibitors is optimized while being supported by intravenous agents. It has become possible to control most cases of refractory heart failure with such intermittent intensive therapy and close monitoring of the patient at home, using daily weight as an indicator for titrating diuretics. Intermittent metolazone is particularly useful as an adjunct diuretic for this purpose.

### Diastolic heart failure

The management of diastolic dysfunction and congestive heart failure differs from that of systolic dysfunction.

Patients with primary LV diastolic dysfunction often have current or previous hypertension and LVH and can present with pulmonary congestion or edema despite a normal ejection fraction.

The pulmonary congestion usually responds rapidly to preload reduction. Because of the increased myocardial stiffness, a small decrease in plasma and LV volume can cause a precipitous decrease in LV filling pressure, stroke volume, and cardiac output. It is critical to avoid excessive preload reduction, which can rapidly cause hypotension.

Patients with LVH are especially prone to subendocardial ischemia, even in the absence of coronary atherosclerosis. Such ischemia increases myocardial diastolic stiffness and exacerbates diastolic dysfunction.

Heart rate control is important to provide adequate subendocardial perfusion. Most coronary flow occurs in diastole; tachycardia compromises myocardial perfusion because diastole is shortened and the time available for coronary flow is reduced. Calcium channel blockers (e.g., verapamil and diltiazem) and β-adrenergic blockers are useful for control of heart rate.

Because of their increased LV diastolic stiffness, patients with diastolic dysfunction have reduced passive LV filling in early and mid-diastole and particularly depend on an active atrial contribution to late ventricular filling. Thus maintenance of sinus rhythm is important for achieving adequate stroke volume and cardiac output.

Blood pressure control is important in hypertensive patients to prevent progression of LVH and possibly to promote its regression. Hypertensive pressures in the coronary arteries may directly contribute to increased diastolic chamber stiffness by an increase in coronary turgor. Good control of blood pressure may improve diastolic filling properties, relieve the load on the left atrium, and help preserve sinus rhythm. Poor blood pressure control can result in progressive LVH. Effective hypertensive therapy is associated with LVH regression and potential reversal of the pathophysiology associated with LVH.

Calcium channel blockers may reduce symptoms of CHF because of their lusitropic action. Verapamil can inhibit tachycardia, reduce hypertension, increase coronary vasodilation, and possibly improve myocyte calcium metabolism to improve relaxation directly. A placebo-controlled, blinded trial of verapamil in patients with primary diastolic dysfunction demonstrated a marked improvement in exercise tolerance and diastolic filling rate with this drug. There is no evidence that calcium channel blockers improve survival in diastolic dysfunction.

### Heart failure in special situations

***Heart failure among adolescents.*** CHF resulting from congenital or acquired heart disease is uncommon among adolescents. The box above lists causes. Treatment of heart failure is unchanged among adolescents. In cancer chemotherapy, the dose of doxorubicin (Adriamycin) should be carefully controlled to prevent cardiotoxicity. If myocarditis or cardiomyopathy leads to end-stage heart failure, cardiac transplantation remains a viable option.

***Heart failure among older patients.*** As stated, the prevalence of heart failure increases in old age. Some 75% of ambulatory patients with heart failure are 60 years of age or older. However, the underlying causes of heart failure are similar to those found among middle-aged individuals. Aging in itself is not responsible for heart failure. The incidence of diastolic heart failure with hypercontractile left ventricle may be higher among elderly women. In the geriatric population, an echocardiogram should help the clinician distinguish between diastolic and systolic dysfunction. In the former, calcium blockers or β-blockers may help improve diastolic relaxation; in the latter, treatment remains the same as in other age groups. The dose of digoxin needs to be carefully adjusted because the creatinine clearance is often greatly diminished in this age group. On the other hand, the use of ACE inhibitors remains useful, since enalapril reduces the fatality rate by 27% among patients with severe heart failure who have a mean age of 70 years.

*Heart failure during pregnancy.* Pregnancy leads to a high-output state, so preexisting heart disease may cause decompensation as the pregnancy advances. Rheumatic heart disease with mitral stenosis was once the most dreaded complication of pregnancy. Now, the only cause of heart failure peculiar to pregnancy is peripartum cardiomyopathy. This condition is characterized by the occurrence of heart failure without any apparent etiology during the last month of gestation or immediately after the birth. The disorder is more common among women who have had twins, who are older than 30 years, who are black, or who are multiparous.

The incidence of myocarditis may be higher among pregnant women with cardiomyopathy. The condition is reversible in about half of patients after the peripartum period. Subsequent pregnancy is complicated by recurrence among those who demonstrate persistent left ventricular dysfunction. Treatment of peripartum heart failure that generally manifests as biventricular failure consists of rest, digoxin, and diuretics. Use of hydralazine for afterload reduction, especially among women with pregnancy-induced or preexisting hypertension, is indicated because hydralazine increases uterine blood flow. On the other hand, ACE inhibitors can affect fetal renal function and are therefore contraindicated during pregnancy.

*Perioperative heart failure.* See Chapter 5.

### *Family and community-centered approaches to diagnosis and management*

**Genetics.** Except for hypertrophic cardiomyopathy, which may lead to heart failure in the late stages, the role of genetic influences on the diagnosis or treatment of heart failure is negligible. However, hypertrophy often precedes the development of failure. The technique of molecular biology and recombinant DNA have now provided the molecular basis for exploring cardiac growth and hypertrophy. They further allow us study of gene expressions in the failing heart. It is hoped that these techniques will allow greater understanding of the heart's function, which in turn may provide better tools to investigate and treat heart failure. Preliminary experimental observations indicate the possibility of genetic transfer of beta receptors to improve the failing heart.

**Psychosocial aspects of heart failure.** The term *heart failure* carries a different connotation from diseases of other organ systems of the body. Not only does the heart symbolize love and affection, but in most cultures and health beliefs, it also represents the center of one's entire being. Furthermore, the patient and family think of imminent death when heart failure is mentioned. Cultural myths surrounding the heart make the person suffering from a chronic heart ailment seem different than before. The patient is generally viewed as an invalid incapable of participating in normal activities, including sex. This generally leads to depression and loss of self-respect. The physician should allay such anxiety and involve the spouse in discussions relating to physical and sexual activity. Although rest is essential in acute heart failure, it is becoming apparent that prolonged bed rest in chronic heart failure may lead to deconditioning changes in the skeletal muscle and peripheral circulation and exercise intolerance. Sexual activity may not be physically possible in severe heart failure. Some medications such as β-blockers and tranquilizers may affect sexual activity. In compensated chronic CHF, sexual activity does not have to be unnecessarily forbidden. When undertaken, sex should be limited to the usual partner and carried out in the most comfortable position. It should not be undertaken immediately after a heavy meal, and it should be relaxed and unhurried. Prophylactic nitroglycerin may help, but if intercourse leads to angina, persistent tachycardia, or extreme fatigue, it should be postponed until the patient's cardiac status improves.

## CASE STUDIES IN THE MANAGEMENT OF CONGESTIVE HEART FAILURE*

**Patient with "holiday heart" syndrome** A 50-year-old man was seen in the emergency ward after a long holiday weekend. He was a heavy smoker, obese, and had a history of episodic alcohol abuse. During the holiday he had imbibed and eaten more than usual. His medical history included arthritis, treated with ibuprofen, and hypertension for which he had refused medication because of side effects.

He sought medical attention because of rapid heartbeat, marked shortness of breath, orthopnea, and weakness that had started the night before. He did not have chest pains. Swelling of his feet had been noted before the onset of these symptoms.

On physical examination, the patient was dyspneic and slightly diaphoretic. Apical pulse was approximately 180 bpm and irregular. Blood pressure was 180/95 mm Hg. Heart sounds were largely obscured by loud rhonchi, rales, and wheezes. Both feet showed pitting edema. Neck veins could not be adequately evaluated because of his short neck and obesity. Blood chemistry studies showed abnormal liver enzymes and elevated lipids but were otherwise within normal limits. The ECG showed atrial fibrillation with rapid ventricular rate. Chest x-ray revealed mild cardiomegaly and pulmonary venous redistribution. There was no evidence of pulmonary infiltrates or masses.

Initial treatment of CHF in this and all patients with pulmonary edema should include oxygen, morphine, and a loop diuretic. After aggressive treatment, auscultation of the patient's lungs revealed marked improvement. A basal II/VI systolic murmur was apparent. Blood pressure remained moderately elevated. An echocardiogram/Doppler study was undertaken to investigate the murmur. The study revealed a bicuspid aortic valve with mild aortic stenosis and symmetrical left ventricular hypertrophy. Ejection fraction was 45%. A thallium stress test revealed no evidence of ischemia and no exercise-related arrhythmias.

The patient was discharged in stable condition. Because of the presence of a bicuspid aortic valve, he was placed on bacterial endocarditis prophylaxis. In addition to appropriate

*Case studies are provided by Sheilah A. Bernard and John Noble.

## Managed Care Guide
## For congestive heart failure

From Konstam M et al: *Heart failure: management of patients with left-ventricular systolic dysfunction. Quick reference guide for clinicians No. 11.* AHCPR Publication No. 94-0613, Rockville, MD: Agency for Health Care Policy and Research, Public Health Service, U.S. Department of Health and Human Services. June 1994.

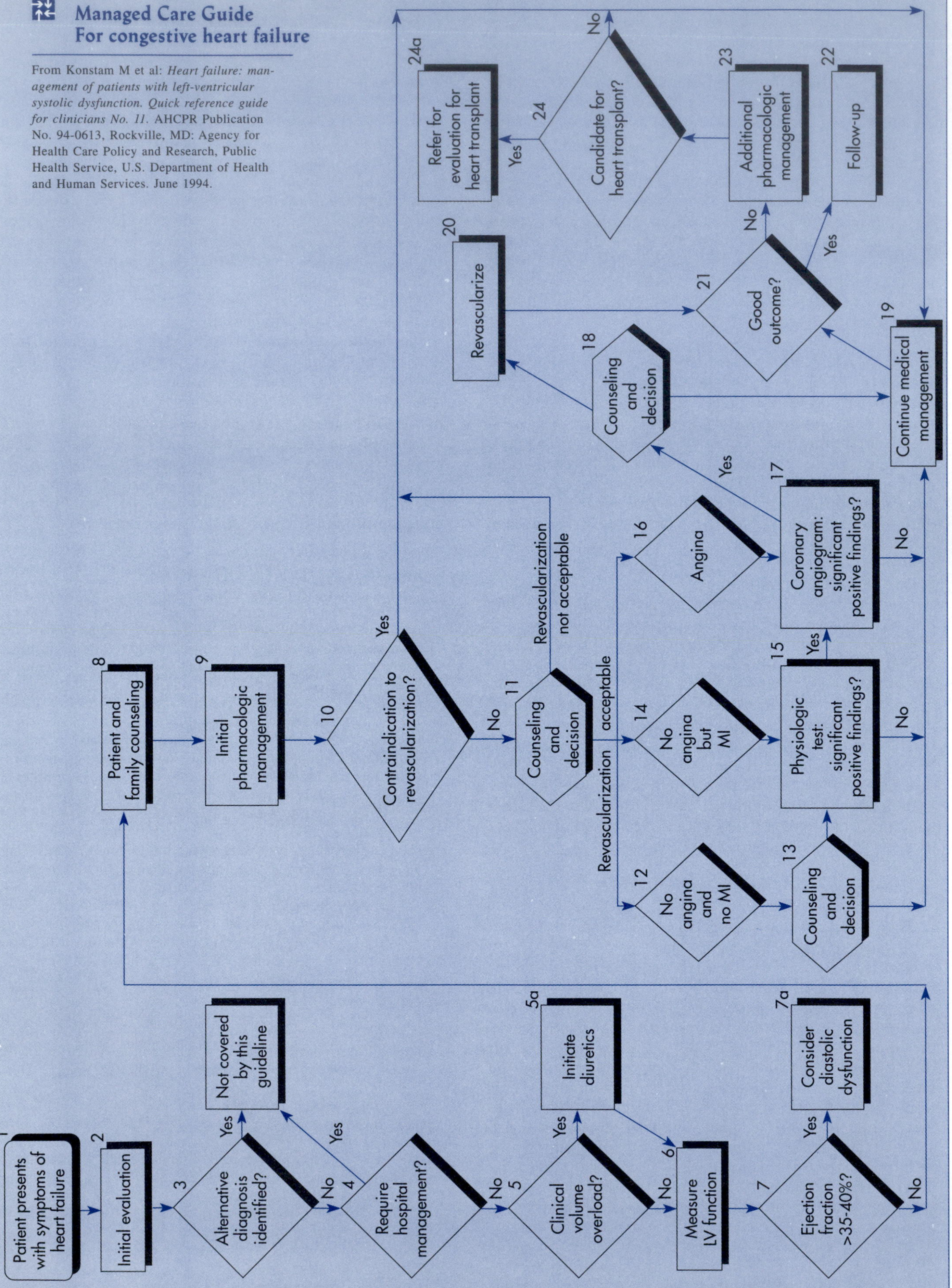

## Managed Care Guide
## "Holiday Heart" Syndrome

Atrial fibrillation with a rapid ventricular response is likely to be responsible for his acute decompensation, although he had evidence of right heart failure (peripheral edema) preceding this arrhythmia. The initial approach to management of this arrhythmia is to slow the rate; this results with appropriate treatment for congestive heart failure, which lowers sympathetic drive. Pharmacologic agents such as digitalis, intravenous calcium antagonists (diltiazem, verapamil), or β-blockers also quickly reduce the ventricular response and are appropriate if the rapid response is thought to be causing the CHF. The latter two classes of medication must be used cautiously if a patient is suspected of having systolic impairment.

Once the heart rate is slowed and congestive heart failure is treated, cardioversion to sinus rhythm is recommended. Approximately one half of patients with atrial fibrillation resulting from alcohol ingestion spontaneously revert to normal sinus rhythm within 24 hours of the above treatment. If the onset can be accurately timed to less than 24 hours, anticoagulation is not necessary before cardioversion. However, some physicians use heparin empirically during this time period to prevent embolization. If the atrial fibrillation persists for at least 72 hours, the consensus is that the patient be anticoagulated before cardioversion, with either transesophageal echo to exclude left atrial appendage thrombosis before chemical or electrical cardioversion or an empiric three-week course of anticoagulation before cardioversion. Studies are under way to determine the cost benefit ratio of these two approaches. Pharmacologic conversion is usually performed with a 1A agent (quinidine, procainamide, disopyramide). For a first episode of atrial fibrillation, long-term therapy is not indicated.

Diuretics are appropriate for treatment of the example patient's elevated blood pressure and dyspnea. Discontinuation of alcohol consumption may result in normalization of blood pressure without further therapy in some patients. Afterload-reducing drugs may be appropriate, especially if a favorable response with diuretics is not prompt.

Nitrates may not be the first drug of choice in the absence of angina or other indications of ischemia; however, they are highly effective in reducing preload acutely in pulmonary edema.

A risk-factor–reduction program must be developed with this patient and his family. It should include the following:

(1) stopping excess alcohol consumption
(2) quitting smoking; consider clonidine or nicotine patches to help decrease craving for tobacco
(3) treating hypertension
(4) commencing a conditioning exercise program using results of the exercise tolerance test to assess presence of significant ischemic disease
(5) teaching low cholesterol, cardiac-prudent diet

### BIBLIOGRAPHY

Manning WJ, et al: Cardioversion from atrial fibrillation without prolonged anticoagulation with use of transesophageal echocardiography to exclude the presence of atrial thrombus, *N Engl J Med* 328:750, 1993.

medication, treatment for his hypertension included counseling for lifestyle changes—principally abstinence from alcohol and cigarettes—and dietary modifications including salt, calorie, and lipid restriction. Regular recreational exercise was advised. Periodic follow-up of his blood pressure and heart murmur was scheduled.

**Patient with diastolic dysfunction and pulmonary edema** A 72-year-old diabetic, hypertensive, African-American woman was well until 2 months before admission, when she first noticed dyspnea on exertion and loss of energy. On the morning of admission, she experienced sudden shortness of breath and came promptly to the emergency room. She had nocturia four times a night for the past month but denied chest pain, palpitations, nausea, pedal edema, or a change in weight. Medications included hydrochlorothiazide 50 mg/d, glyburide 5 mg/d, ibuprofen 600 mg/d.

On physical examination, she was moderately obese and in mild respiratory distress. Blood pressure was 210/110 mm Hg and her pulse was 100 bpm. The carotid pulses were full, equal, and had a brisk upstroke. The jugular veins were distended sitting upright. The PMI was forceful and sustained. There was a loud $S_4$ and a III/VI systolic ejection murmur at the aortic area radiating to the neck. There were bibasilar rales, diffuse expiratory wheezes and no pedal edema.

Clinically, the patient has acute pulmonary edema, a hyperdynamic left ventricle, an aortic stenosis murmur, and lung findings suggestive of pulmonary congestion. She has an aortic stenosis or sclerosis murmur. She may have left ventricular failure from either hypertensive heart disease or from aortic stenosis, and occult coronary artery disease cannot be excluded.

The patient was treated for hypertension and acute pulmonary edema with diuretics and afterload reduction; improvement was rapid.

Furosemide, in addition to diuresis, produces a dilation of the venous system, thus reducing the preload and further alleviating pulmonary edema. It is important to note, however, that furosemide must be used with caution to prevent too great a reduction in preload and a concomitant

## Managed Care Guide
## The treatment of diastolic dysfunction

Recognition of diastolic dysfunction is critical because of different management strategies. Current experience suggests that afterload-reducing agents can be helpful. β-Blockers and calcium antagonists, although usually contraindicated in patients with heart failure, may have a role in treating these patients. The ACE inhibitors slow the development of diabetic nephropathy in addition to reducing afterload. There is also evidence that they alter excessive collagen matrix deposition in left ventricular hypertrophy, thereby changing left ventricular stiffness and local ischemia. Chronic use of digitalis and diuretics is usually not helpful. Diuretics may even be harmful by excessively reducing the preload; salt and fluid intake should be mildly restricted.

While optimal treatment is as yet undetermined in patients with diastolic dysfunction, the calcium channel blocker verapamil has been reported to improve exercise tolerance and diastolic function.

### BIBLIOGRAPHY

Bonow RO, Udelson JE: Left ventricular diastolic dysfunction as a cause of congestive heart failure, *Ann Intern Med* 117:502, 1992.

reduction to cardiac output. Blood pressure was controlled with intravenous nitroprusside. Intravenous nitroglycerin could also be used acutely for preload reduction or suspected ischemia. At higher doses, nitroglycerin also reduces afterload. In patients with LVH and high left ventricular diastolic pressures resulting from hypertension or aortic stenosis, the subendocardial vessels are compressed. Reduction of preload and LV diastolic pressures may improve subendocardial perfusion and reduce ischemia. Diabetes mellitus can cause microvascular changes as well, contributing to an ischemic presentation of heart disease.

The laboratory examination shows a reduced sodium to 132 mEq/L. The potassium is reduced to 3.1 mEq/L, probably reflecting chronic hydrochlorothiazide use. The glucose is elevated to 285 mg/dL because of diabetes mellitus. The creatinine is high normal. However, for a woman of her age and weight, this value probably represents some renal insufficiency. The slightly elevated BUN bolsters this impression. The proteinuria indicates hypertensive renal disease, and the glycosuria indicates diabetes.

The hemoglobin is slightly reduced. Initial arterial blood gases show an acute respiratory acidosis and hypoxemia, even on oxygen at 5 L/min.

The ECG confirms the x-ray impression by showing left ventricular hypertrophy with left atrial enlargement, probably a result of the hypertension. The sinus tachycardia is a manifestation of left ventricular failure. The chest x-ray shows pulmonary congestion, as expected from the physical examination, but the heart is only slightly enlarged. This unexpected finding suggests that the left ventricle has not dilated and, in turn, may signal a stiff left ventricle producing diastolic dysfunction.

Findings from the echocardiogram establish the impression gleaned from the chest x-ray and ECG. There is no evidence of focal wall motion abnormality, ruling out infarction as a cause of the sudden left ventricular dysfunction. It shows the hypertrophied left ventricle and normal systolic function but also a small, nondilated left ventricular chamber. This implies hypertension and diastolic dysfunction. The echocardiogram confirms that the murmur is due to aortic stenosis.

**Patient with left ventricular systolic dysfunction with borderline renal function** An 82-year-old man was evaluated with increasing shortness of breath and orthopnea over 3 months. He denied any recent chest pain.

The patient had a history of systemic hypertension for 20 years and mild renal insufficiency. He was hospitalized one year ago with an anterior myocardial infarction. Because of poorly controlled hypertension and continued angina, the patient was started on diltiazem and isosorbide dinitrate. His hypertension and angina were controlled at subsequent 3-month–interval visits prior to his presenting symptoms.

Medication at the time of evaluation included furosemide 20 mg/qd, isosorbide dinitrate 60 mg/tid, and diltiazem 90 mg/tid. Physical examination and laboratory findings are shown below:

Physical Examination
- HR: 100 bpm
- BP: 140/80 mm Hg
- Respiratory rate: 20/min
- Jugular venous pressure: 12 cm
- Rales one third of the way up both lungs
- Cardiac impulse displaced laterally
- Normal $S_1$ and $S_2$; $S_3$ gallop
- Gr II/VI HSM LLSB to axilla
- Liver not enlarged; no HJ reflex
- edema of ankles and feet

Laboratory Findings

| | |
|---|---|
| Na: 138 | Creatinine: 2.0 |
| $K^+$: 4.0 | BUN: 26 |

The ECG showed regular sinus rhythm. The mean QRS axis was −30 degrees and the mean T wave axis was +105 degrees. There were voltage criteria for left ventricular hypertrophy. T waves were inverted in leads I and an AVL. The ECG was compatible with an old anterior myocardial infarction.

Chest x-ray showed mild cardiomegaly with a calculated cardiothoracic ratio of 0.5. There was some pulmonary venous congestion. The echocardiogram confirmed left ventricular dilatation with severe wall motion abnormalities and poor systolic function. The diagnosis at this time was systemic hypertension, which was well controlled with antihypertensive therapy, and chronic renal failure.

The patient was believed to have worsening CHF secondary to hypertension and prior anterior myocardial infarction. This elderly patient had an echocardiogram consistent with heart failure because of his prior infarction and was not receptive to any invasive intervention. Therefore cardiac catheterization was not indicated and maximization of medical therapy was planned. Because of evidence of fluid overload, initial treatment was directed at diuresis, with increase in his furosemide dose to 40 mg/d. The patient was instructed to check his weight daily and to call if symptoms worsened.

In 2 days, his weight had decreased by four pounds; he had less orthopnea and dyspnea on exertion (DOE) and his physical examination revealed a jugular venous pressure of 8 cm, crackles were present only at the bases, and his pedal edema was decreased to 1+.

By day 6 he had lost seven pounds. Evidence of CHF was linked to an $S_3$ on physical examination and significant dyspnea on exertion after walking one block. He was given a test dose of captopril 6.25 mg in the office without developing orthostatic hypotension. Captopril was then prescribed initially at 6.25 mg/tid/PO and increased after 3 days to 12.5 mg/tid.

One week later, the patient's examination was stable, as was his weight, and he had less dyspnea on exertion. However, his creatinine was elevated to 3.2, BUN 70, and $K^+$ 5.1. The captopril was discontinued and furosemide was decreased to 20 mg/d. Digoxin 0.125 mg/d/PO was begun to improve cardiac output.

One week later, his clinical examination was stable and his left ventricular ejection fraction had increased to 39% on the echocardiogram. His blood chemistry studies revealed a digoxin level of 1.3, creatinine 1.9, BUN 36 and $K^+$ 4.1.

## Managed Care Guide
## Systolic dysfunction and CHF

The case presentation does not demonstrate how this patient necessarily should have been managed.

Digoxin was introduced only after captopril had produced an increased impairment of renal function. Digoxin should have been introduced as first-line therapy along with the initial medications given his CHF and $S_3$ gallop (Table 13-8).

Combined treatment including an inotropic agent (cardiac glycoside) and vasodilator (nitrate, ACE inhibitor, or hydralazine) with or without a diuretic results in better left ventricular function than one agent alone (Table 13-9). The complementary effects of these various classes of drugs produce optimum cardiovascular results at lower doses, thus minimizing side effects. The newer generation calcium antagonists (amlodipine, felodipine) have less negative inotropic effects and may be better tolerated than diltiazem in this patient with heart failure. Aspirin should also be used for secondary MI prevention.

**Table 13-8.** Prospective, randomized, placebo-controlled trials of oral positive inotropic agents that included patients with dilated cardiomyopathy

| Study | Drug studied | Number enrolled | NYHA class (%) | Patients with IDC (%) | Key findings |
|---|---|---|---|---|---|
| Captopril-Digoxin Multicenter Research Trial | Captopril, digoxin | 300 | I (26)<br>II (50)<br>III (24) | 32 | Digoxin decreased hospitalizations for heart failure. |
| Multicenter Enoximone Trial | Enoximone | 102 | II (35)<br>III (65) | 50 | Enoximone failed to improve symptoms or exercise capacity. |
| PROMISE Trial | Milrinone | 1088 | III (58)<br>IV (42) | 40 | Milrinone failed to improve symptoms and increased cardiovascular mortality. |
| Xamoterol in Severe Heart Failure Trial | Xamoterol | 516 | III (75)<br>IV (25) | 31 | Xamoterol failed to improve symptoms or exercise capacity and increased cardiovascular mortality. |
| Pimobendan Multicenter Research Trial | Pimobendan | 198 | III (96)<br>IV (4) | 40 | Pimobendan improved symptoms and exercise capacity. |
| Multicenter Vesnarinone Trial | Vesnarinone | 564 | III (60)<br>IV (10) | 48 | Moderate-dose vesnarinone (60 mg/day) decreased hospitalizations for heart failure and cardiovascular mortality; high-dose vesnarinone (120 mg/day) increased cardiovascular mortality. |
| RADIANCE Trial | Digoxin | 178 | III (60)<br>IV (25) | 28 | Digoxin withdrawal resulted in worsening symptoms and exercise capacity despite the concomitant use of an ACE inhibitor. |

From Dec WG, Fuster V: *N Engl J Med* 331:1564, 1994.
*RADIANCE*, Randomized Assessment of [the effect of] Digoxin on Inhibitors of the Angiotensin-Converting Enzyme.

**Table 13-9.** Prospective, randomized trials of vasodilators in heart failure that included patients with dilated cardiomyopathy

| Study | Drug studied | Number enrolled | NYHA class (%) | Patients with IDC (%) | Key findings |
|---|---|---|---|---|---|
| CONSENSUS I | Enalapril | 253 | IV (100) | 15 | Enalapril reduced symptoms and mortality in severe heart failure. |
| V-HeFT I | Hydralazine plus isosorbide dinitrate, prazosin | 642 | II (NA)<br>III (NA) | 15 | Hydralazine–isosorbide reduced mortality in moderate heart failure. |
| Captopril–Digoxin Multicenter Research Trial | Captopril, digoxin | 300 | I (26)<br>II (50)<br>III (24) | 32 | Captopril improved symptoms and exercise tolerance in mild-to-moderate heart failure. |
| V-HeFT II | Hydralazine plus isosorbide dinitrate, enalapril | 804 | II (51)<br>III (43) | 11 | Enalapril was superior to hydralazine–isosorbide in reducing mortality in moderate heart failure. |
| SOLVD Treatment Trial | Enalapril | 2569 | II (57)<br>III (30) | 18 | Enalapril reduced mortality and hospitalizations in moderate heart failure. |
| SOLVD Prevention Trial | Enalapril | 4228 | I (67)<br>II (33) | 9.5 | Enalapril reduced heart failure and hospitalizations among patients with asymptomatic left ventricular dysfunction. |
| Munich Mild Heart Failure Trial | Captopril | 170 | I (5)<br>II (82)<br>III (13) | 32 | Captopril slowed the progression of heart-failure symptoms in mild-to-moderate heart failure. |

From Dec WG, Fuster V: *N Engl J Med* 331:1564, 1994.
*NA*, Not available.

## Managed Care Guide
## Severe CHF with systolic dysfunction

In the patient with congestive heart failure, a careful search for correctable factors that may worsen heart failure (such as hypertension, anemia, thyroid disease, and valvular heart disease) must be undertaken at the onset of symptoms and when symptoms increase during therapy. Attention should be paid to the possible presence of arrhythmias or thromboembolic problems. Electrolytes ($K^+$, $Mg^+$) must be repleted.

Depending on the severity of left ventricular dysfunction and ischemic phenomena, an imaged stress test or coronary arteriography may be considered now or earlier in the course of the illness, in light of the evidence that patients with triple-vessel coronary artery disease and left ventricular dysfunction (with ejection fractions between 35% and 50%) show improved survival after coronary artery bypass.

His age of 62 is a relative contraindication for cardiac transplantation. He has no absolute contraindications, however, including active infection, positive HIV serology, malignancy, peptic ulcer disease, a long history of noncompliance, or other life-limiting illness. Hemodynamic evaluation must be performed to include the assessment of elevated pulmonary vascular resistance (>5 wood units).

The use of β-blocking agents remains investigational, but preliminary studies demonstrate improvement in symptoms, exercise capacity, and ejection fraction in patients with severe refractory congestive heart failure. There is a trend of long-term survival after the use of these agents, most notably in patients with excessive sympathetic tone.

On stable doses of digitalis and ACE inhibitor, the physician and patient are left with the challenge of balancing diet, furosemide, and supplemental diuretics (metolazone) with intermittent parenteral dobutamine to maximize cardiac function and the quality of his remaining life.

It is often necessary to hospitalize patients with severe CHF to adjust volume status and vasodilation. In addition to intravenous therapy with nitroprusside sodium (Nipride, Nitropress) and/or nitroglycerin (Nitro-Bid IV, Tridil), combined with intravenous diuretics, it may be necessary to add infusions of dobutamine (Dobutrex) or dopamine hydrochloride (Dopastat, Intropin).

After 48 to 72 hours of intravenous therapy, most patients can be weaned onto oral vasodilators and eventually discharged. In patients needing further escalation of therapies first intravenous amrinone lactate (Inocor) or milrinone lactate (Primacor) may be added, and then epinephrine or, rarely, norepinephrine (Levophed). Steps beyond that include a trial of intraaortic balloon counterpulsation, implantation of a mechanical assist device, or use of an external centrifugal pump. Cardiac transplantation is indicated for a patient in critical or unstable condition who has no contraindications to the procedure. The patient's profile for compliance must be carefully evaluated. Reform of the selection process is needed to identify patients who, though not critically ill, will not survive without early transplantation.

**Patient with coronary heart disease and myocardial infarction as the cause of congestive heart failure** A 55-year-old postman has a history of hypertension and mild CHF with LVH on ECG. He responded to treatment with a β-blocker and isosorbide dinitrate.

Five years later, the patient developed nausea and severe retrosternal chest discomfort. Ten hours after the onset of pain, he presented to an emergency room with mild dyspnea and bibasilar rales. A diagnosis of acute anterior myocardial infarction was made. His rales cleared promptly after treatment with morphine sulfate and furosemide; his myocardial infarction was otherwise uncomplicated. The predischarge chest x-ray showed a normal heart size and clear lung fields. After convalescence, he was able to return to a less physically demanding job at the post office.

One year after his myocardial infarction, he developed increasing dyspnea on mild exertion, unaccompanied by chest pressure. The dyspnea was sufficiently disabling to interfere with his ability to carry out his job responsibilities in moving mailbags. He now experiences occasional episodes of paroxysmal nocturnal dyspnea and requires two pillows to sleep comfortably. His only medications are a β-blocker, isosorbide dinitrate, and timoptic for glaucoma.

Physical examination reveals BP of 110/80 mm Hg and a pulse rate of 55. Auscultation reveals that the apical impulse is displaced to the left and has a dyskinetic quality. Bibasilar inspiratory rales and a soft $S_3$ heart sound are also present.

The abdomen is distended; abdominal ultrasound examination reveals mild ascites. There is 4+ edema to the knees.

The patient has now developed biventricular systolic dysfunction. Initial therapy should include withdrawal of the β-blocking agent, with careful attention to symptoms suggesting active ischemia. Limitation of dietary sodium and a further decrease in physical activity are advisable.

The patient responds partially to sodium restriction and discontinuation of the β-blocker but continues to have dyspnea on mild exertion. Digoxin and a mild diuretic are added, and an ACE inhibitor is added to isosorbide dinitrate.

An intermittent cough is bothersome to the patient. Chest x-ray suggests moderate cardiac enlargement and pulmonary vascular congestion.

The ACE inhibitor is discontinued for 2 weeks. However, the cough persists and CHF worsens. Therefore the ACE inhibitor is restarted and the cough responds to Robitussin AC. The patient's ophthalmologist substitutes pilocarpine for the timoptic to minimize sodium retention. Sodium intake is restricted to less than 4 grams daily and free water is limited.

On a maximal regimen of digoxin, an ACE inhibitor, nitrates, and diuretics, the patient remains in severe CHF. LVEF measured on echocardiography is 20% with 2+ mitral regurgitation. He can walk short distances but feels tired most of the time. Paroxysmal nocturnal dyspnea interferes with sleep and peripheral edema reaccumulates rapidly after 6 weeks at home.

The patient is admitted with severe congestive heart failure after gaining 25 pounds. Intravenous dobutamine is administered in a monitored unit; symptoms improve and weight decreases. The blood pressure, however, remains between 90 mm Hg/70 mm Hg and 105 mm Hg/70 mm Hg. Reduction of the vasodilator dose produces greater paroxysmal nocturnal dyspnea. Increased doses result in dizziness. Digoxin serum levels are maintained at 1.7 ng/mL.

## BIBLIOGRAPHY


Braunwald E, Grossman W: Clinical aspects of heart failure. In Braunwald E, editor: *A textbook of cardiovascular medicine,* Philadelphia, 1992, WB Saunders.

Braunwald E, Ross J Jr, Sonnenblick EH: *Mechanism of contraction of the normal and failing heart,* ed 2, Boston, 1976, Little, Brown.

Brutsaert DL, Sys SU, Gillebert TC: Diastolic failure: pathophysiology and therapeutic implications, *J Am Coll Cardiol* 22:318, 1993.

Cohn J: *Drug treatment of heart failure,* ed 2, Secaucus, NJ, 1988, Advanced Therapeutic Communications International.

Francis GS, Cohn JN: Heart failure: mechanisms of cardiac and vascular dysfunction and the rationale for pharmacologic intervention, *FASEB J* 4:3068, 1990.

Garg R et al: Mechanisms and management of heart failure: implications of clinical trials for clinical practice, *J Am Coll Cardiol* 4(suppl A):1A, 1993.

Gillum RF: Epidemiology of heart failure in the United States, *Am Heart J* 126:1042, 1993.

Konstam M et al: *Heart failure: evaluation and care of patients with left-ventricular systolic dysfunction. Clinical Practice Guideline No. 11.* AHCPR Publication No. 94-0612. Rockville, MD: Agency for Health Care Policy and Research, Public Health Service, U.S. Department of Health and Human Services, June 1994.

Mudge GH et al: 24th Bethesda conference: Cardiac transplantation. Task Force 3: Recipient guidelines/prioritization, *J Am Coll Cardiol* 22(1):21, 1993.

Packer M: The neurohormonal hypothesis: a theory to explain the mechanism of disease progression in heart failure, *J Am Coll Cardiol* 20:248, 1992.

Packer M et al: Effect of milrinone on mortality in severe heart failure, *N Engl J Med* 325:1468, 1991.

Packer M, et al: Withdrawal of digoxin from patients with chronic heart failure treated with angiotensin-converting enzyme inhibitors, *N Engl J Med* 329:1, 1993.

Perloff JK: The clinical manifestation of cardiac failure in adults. In Braunwald E, Selwyn A, editors: *Myocardial failure and infarction,* New York, 1974, HP Publishing.

Rizzuto C: Psychosocial problems in congestive heart failure: health care implications. In Michaelson, editor: *Congestive heart failure,* St Louis, 1983, Mosby.

Smith TW, Braunwald E, Kelly RA: The management of heart failure. In Braunwald E, editor: *A textbook of cardiovascular medicine,* ed 4, Philadelphia, 1992, WB Saunders.

Stevenson LW: Selection and management of patients for cardiac transplantation, *Curr Opin Cardiol* 9(3):315, 1994.

Uretsky BF et al: Randomized study assessing the effect of digoxin withdrawal in patients with mild to moderate chronic congestive heart failure: results of the PROVED trial, *J Am Coll Cardiol* 22:955, 1993.


CHAPTER

# 14 Valvular Heart Disease

**Edgar C. Schick, Jr.**

Significant valvular heart disease is likely to be found in only a small proportion of patients in the average primary care practice. The primary practitioner, however, has a large measure to contribute to the detection of valvular disease and the initial management of these patients. Despite the growth of noninvasive diagnostic technology, the answers to many important questions about possible valvular pathology remain the prerogative of the bedside physician. Diligent auscultatory characterization of heart murmurs and pursuit of cogent ancillary physical findings often provide adequate basis for a diagnosis and obviate the need for additional, more expensive studies. Evaluation of the patient with valvular disease offers the clinician a gratifying opportunity to exercise cardiovascular diagnostic skills but also poses challenging questions related to such matters as drug therapy, referral for a cardiologist's opinion, cardiac catheterization, anticoagulation, and prophylactic antibiotic use. This chapter focuses specifically on these aspects and attempts to provide the busy practitioner with a capsular overview of management for the valvular heart disease patient.

## AORTIC STENOSIS

Fifty years ago, commenting on aortic stenosis, the eminent British cardiologist Sir Thomas Lewis wrote, "It is a sound rule to rarely diagnose conditions that occur rarely." The use of penicillin in the treatment of syphilitic and rheumatic disease as well as the ever-lengthening life expectancy have drastically altered this perspective. Aortic stenosis is now the most common acquired valvular disease among adults and is preponderantly an affliction of older men.

After adolescence but before the eighth decade, stenosis of the aortic orifice occurs as a poorly elucidated consequence of congenital bicuspid valvular anatomy in two of every three cases. Sclerocalcific degeneration of an ostensibly normal tricuspid aortic valve predominates among older patients. Rheumatic fever may also cause aortic stenosis but seldom without evidence of other valvular involvement, usually the mitral valve.

### Innocent murmur

Aortic flow murmurs are very common among adolescents and young adults. These murmurs are usually harsh in quality, crescendo-decrescendo in profile, and best appreciated along the middle to lower left sternal border. Uncertainty about the significance of murmurs with these tonal and temporal aspects presents a common clinical problem. How can the so-called innocent, functional, or normal flow murmur be distinguished from that which either connotes the presence or portends the development of important valvular pathology?

***Pathophysiology.*** When the stenotic process has contracted the aortic orifice, normally between 2 and 4 $cm^2$, by about half (Fig. 14-1), the left ventricle is presented with a progressively increasing pressure burden. This challenge is adaptively matched by ventricular hypertrophy, which maintains the systolic stress on the myocardium within the normal range; resting cardiac output is usually normal as well. Significant ventricular dilatation is not a feature of uncomplicated aortic stenosis; when present it indicates failure of the primary compensatory mechanism. Systolic wall stress increases as a result, and the ejection fraction declines. In the majority of patients these adjustments are reversible after surgery. Ventricular wall thickness and dilatation recede, and depressed ejection fractions improve after surgery, but these indices may not normalize fully.

***History and physical examination.*** Patients with aortic stenosis may remain free of symptoms for extended periods. The average age at the onset of the classic

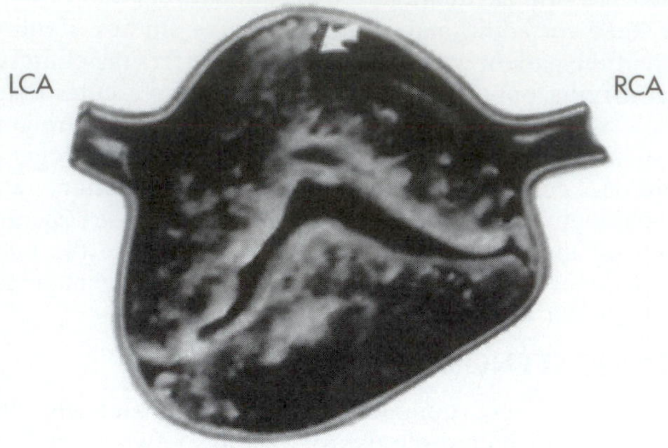


**Fig. 14-1.** Calcific stenosis of a congenitally bicuspid aortic valve. The effective orifice is reduced to a V-shaped slit, less than 10% of the area available for opening under normal circumstances. The arrow points to a raphe at the site of what would have been the commissure between the right and left coronary cusps. *RCA,* Right coronary artery, *LCA,* left coronary artery. (From Edwards JE: *Pract Cardiol* 8:117, 1982.)

symptoms of dyspnea, angina, and syncope is about 60 years. Dyspnea reflects the development of abnormal compliance in the hypertrophied ventricle. Despite maintenance of normal diastolic volumes, and ostensibly ejection fraction, resting diastolic pressures become elevated and may rise drastically during exercise. Exertional angina may occur in the presence of angiographically normal coronary arteries, but it is impossible to exclude concomitant coronary disease clinically. Significant coronary lesions are seldom present in patients with significant aortic stenosis without angina and occur in about 50% of patients with angina. Ischemic symptoms in the remaining patients apparently result from insufficient coronary flow to meet demand. The traditional teaching that syncope in aortic stenosis develops as a consequence of exertional muscular vasodilation in the presence of a cardiac output response that is limited by the stenosis seems at best only a partial explanation. Abnormal peripheral vasomotor responses to exercise and transient arrhythmias, either supraventricular or ventricular, are more likely possibilities.

Although the individual symptoms carry slightly different prognostic implications, it is the presence of *any* cardiac symptom in conjunction with physical evidence of aortic stenosis that is of paramount importance. Coincident with the advent of symptoms is a sharp downward turn in life expectancy with an average survival thereafter of approximately 3 years. Thus the occurrence of angina, syncope, or congestive heart failure in the presence of a reasonable suspicion of aortic stenosis should always prompt referral for specialized evaluation.

Although a completely satisfactory distinction cannot always be made, several features of the examination may be helpful in distinguishing the functional from the pathologic murmur. Typically, aortic murmurs radiate to the right base in contrast to the innocent pulmonic flow murmur, which, although often prominent along the lower sternal margin, radiates to the upper left parasternal region. Pulmonic flow murmurs are characteristically associated with high-output states (e.g., pregnancy, fever, or anemia), although similar conditions may induce or augment aortic murmurs as well. Innocent flow murmurs are generally grade II/VI or less in intensity, reach their peak amplitude during early systole, and are relatively brief and diminish greatly in prominence or disappear altogether during the strain phase of the Valsalva maneuver.

It must be emphasized that an aortic murmur with these characteristics may bespeak a completely normal valve in the adolescent, and may also represent hemodynamically inconsequential aortic sclerosis; however, it may be consequential in the middle-aged adult. Findings that may be dismissed as innocuous in the young assume a different significance if discovered for the first time in an adult, particularly during the fifth and sixth decades. Several studies have demonstrated that, once established, the stenotic process may progress rapidly from insignificant to a severe degree over spans as brief as 2 years.

Other innocent murmurs audible in the parasternal area include the mammary souffle, to be considered especially in the pregnant or lactating patient, and a systolic subclavian murmur that radiates downward. The latter, which may be entirely "normal," can also denote vascular tortuosity, compression, or intrinsic disease. Careful localization by auscultation and attenuation of the murmur with shoulder maneuvers (e.g., hyperextension) clarifies the nature of this bruit.

The peripheral manifestations of critical aortic stenosis are a reduced pulse volume and delayed upstroke, usually best appreciated on carotid artery palpation, which may also reveal systolic vibration or shudder (Fig. 14-2). The cardiac apex impulse is not displaced in uncomplicated aortic stenosis but is forceful and sustained. An exaggerated presystolic excursion somewhat medial to the apex may represent exaggerated atrial kick. A systolic thrill is often palpable at the base. A normal first sound is followed, usually after a brief gap, by a late-peaking, harsh, but occasionally musical murmur with radiational features already mentioned above. The second heart sound is most often single in older adults, the result of attenuation of $A_2$ by the immobility of the rigid aortic cusps. Paradoxical splitting of $S_2$ may reflect delayed ventricular emptying in adolescents and young adults.

Milder degrees of aortic stenosis are indicated by an earlier peak of the systolic murmur and preservation of the aortic closure sound in the adult. A systolic ejection click is the hallmark of the bicuspid aortic valve, but this may be absent with advanced scarring and calcification of the leaflets. Aortic ejection sounds may indicate bicuspid valvular anatomy even in the absence of a systolic murmur.

***Diagnostic studies.*** Further evaluation of a basal ejection murmur is obligatory whenever aortic valve pathology is suggested. This applies to all adults with ejection murmurs of grade III/VI or greater intensity, particularly when accompanied by any additional signs of significant stenosis. Adolescents or adults with less prominent murmurs are referred for noninvasive study if an early systolic sound compatible with an aortic ejection click is

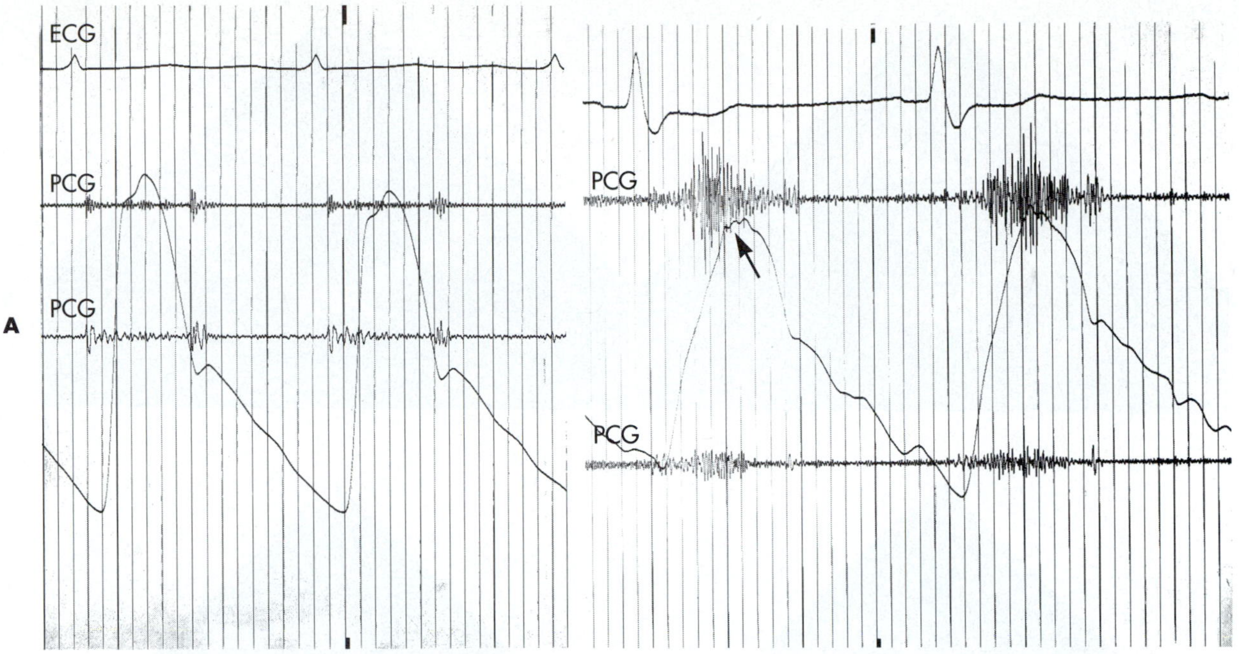


**Fig. 14-2.** Comparison of a normal carotid pulse **(A)** and the pulse tracing of a patient with aortic stenosis **(B).** Note the delay in upstroke with aortic stenosis and the vibration or shudder evident at the pulse peak *(arrow)*. A prominent systolic murmur, which peaks in midsystole, is evident on the phonocardiogram *(PCG)*.

detected. Although it is true that confirmation of an abnormal aortic valve may not lead to immediate corrective therapy, the noninvasive studies may prove very useful in reassuring patients in whom valvular disease can be excluded, identifying individuals who are at risk and require closer follow-up, and establishing the diagnosis of bicuspid valvular anatomy, which has other therapeutic implications.

The noninvasive studies are also helpful in distinguishing the discrete membranous and muscular subvalvular variants of left ventricular outflow obstruction, which are the most common entities to be differentiated from valvular stenosis in the adult. Membranous subaortic stenosis may be impossible to distinguish from valvular disease on examination, but a characteristic aortic motion pattern may be seen on M-mode echo, and direct visualization of the subvalvular membrane is possible with two-dimensional echocardiography or MRI.

The electrocardiogram (ECG) and chest film may contribute to the assessment of an aortic murmur by providing evidence of either left ventricular hypertrophy with strain or valvular calcification. However, hypertrophy by ECG criteria may be lacking in up to 20% of patients with significant aortic stenosis, and routine radiography is insensitive in that only advanced calcification is apparent on plain chest films. Fluoroscopy remains very useful, and fluoroscopic demonstration of dense circumferential valvular calcification strongly supports the clinical suspicion of aortic stenosis. Noninvasive techniques including echo modalities, Doppler flowmetry, and MRI have proved effective in establishing or excluding the presence of critical stenosis in selected patients referred to major centers for evaluation of this possibility. There are shortcomings with each of these techniques, however, and catheterization provides the authoritative answer when suggestive signs and symptoms are met with equivocal noninvasive results.

***Management.*** In general, although there has been an upsurge in the opinion that aortic valve replacement may be safely accomplished without the need of catheterization in adolescents and young adults, there is a reluctance on the part of surgeons to undertake surgery without the complete characterization of valvular and ventricular function afforded by hemodynamic and angiographic study. This applies especially to middle-aged and older patients, in whom coronary artery disease may coexist. Theoretical considerations related to myocardial preservation suggest that an improved outcome of aortic valve replacement with stenosis may be expected if diseased coronaries are also bypassed routinely. Although it remains an issue for the individual surgeon to resolve, there is no dispute that knowledge of the presence and extent of coronary disease may be crucial in the setting of ventricular dysfunction that prevents withdrawal from cardiopulmonary bypass. Mixed valvular disease unquestionably mandates catheterization. Thus the majority of patients with aortic stenosis will continue to require cardiac catheterization for the foreseeable future.

Successful surgery has largely supplanted medical therapy for aortic stenosis. However, some patients may present with advanced congestive failure that requires treatment before catheterization and surgery can be undertaken. Conventional measures, diuretics, and possibly digitalis usually suffice. Diuretics are administered cautiously, since many of these patients require high ventricular filling pressures to sustain an adequate cardiac

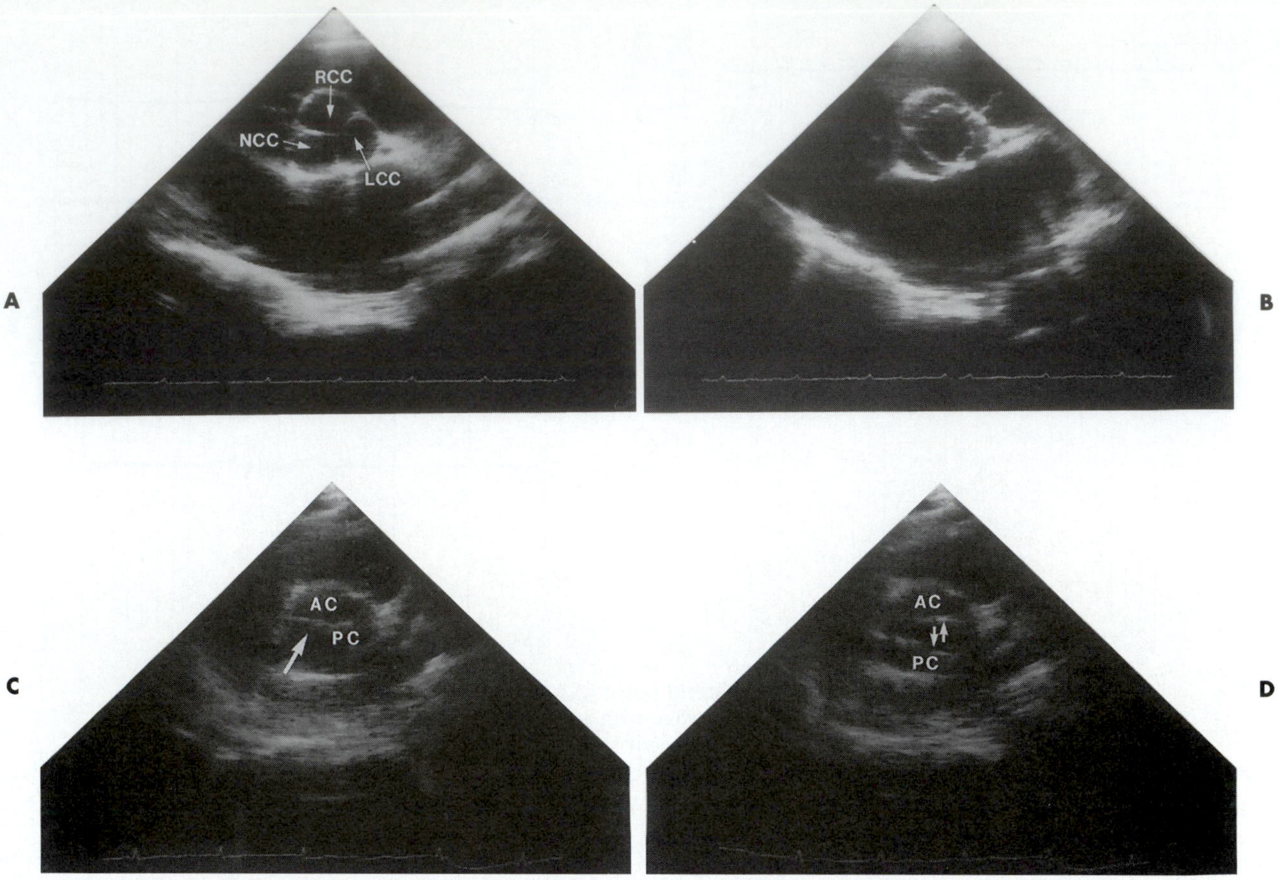


**Fig. 14-3.** Two-dimensional echocardiogram of a normal tricuspid aortic valve (**A, B**) and a bicuspid valve (**C, D**). Diastole is to the left and systole to the right. Three aortic cusps are clearly seen in the normal recording. A single horizontal commissure is evident during diastole in the bicuspid valve *(arrow)* with restricted opening during systole *(arrow). RCC,* Right coronary cusp; *LCC,* left coronary cusp; *NCC,* noncoronary cusp; *AC,* anterior cusp; *PC,* posterior cusp.

output. For similar reasons vasodilators, including nitrates, to which some patients with aortic stenosis and angina respond favorably, are used with discretion. Exercise testing is usually contraindicated.

The natural course of the bicuspid aortic valve is not entirely clear, since there has been no basis for prospective follow-up until recently. Pathology studies suggest, however, that about two thirds of these patients eventually develop clinical evidence of some degree of aortic stenosis or insufficiency beyond age 40. Pathologic evidence of significant aortic stenosis actually occurs in slightly less than one third, and the percentage in whom symptoms might warrant valve replacement is certainly lower still.

Of much greater importance is the propensity for the bicuspid aortic valve to provide a nidus for endocarditis, a risk that has been unquestionably established. In studies of the bicuspid aortic valve the majority of patients with aortic incompetence develop it *after* an episode of endocarditis. Thus antibiotic prophylaxis is a foremost consideration in the management of these cases, and for this reason young patients with aortic ejection sounds and murmurs should undergo echocardiography (Fig. 14-3) to elucidate aortic valve anatomy. Older patients with a murmur and evidence of aortic valvular calcification also require prophylaxis in the asymptomatic stage.

## AORTIC REGURGITATION

Aortic regurgitation as it is encountered in clinical practice can be divided into two chronologic categories, acute and chronic. This distinction reflects differences in the response to the rate at which the valvular incompetence develops. The hemodynamic differences are summarized in Fig. 14-4.

### Chronic aortic regurgitation

Although the etiologic list is long, the most likely basis for chronic aortic regurgitation is a congenitally bicuspid aortic valve. In the past, aortic regurgitation was frequently attributed to rheumatic fever, but the occurrence of isolated rheumatic aortic regurgitation is now thought to be unusual. Other causes include connective tissue disorders, e.g., the Marfan and Ehlers-Danlos syndromes, aortic aneurysm, myxomatous valvular degeneration, syphilis, and aortic involvement by rheumatoid arthritis or one of its variants.

***History and physical examination.*** Most often, patients with chronic aortic regurgitation are asymptomatic except for manifestations of any predisposing disorder at the time of diagnosis. The essential features of the physical examination are the bounding, collapsing peripheral

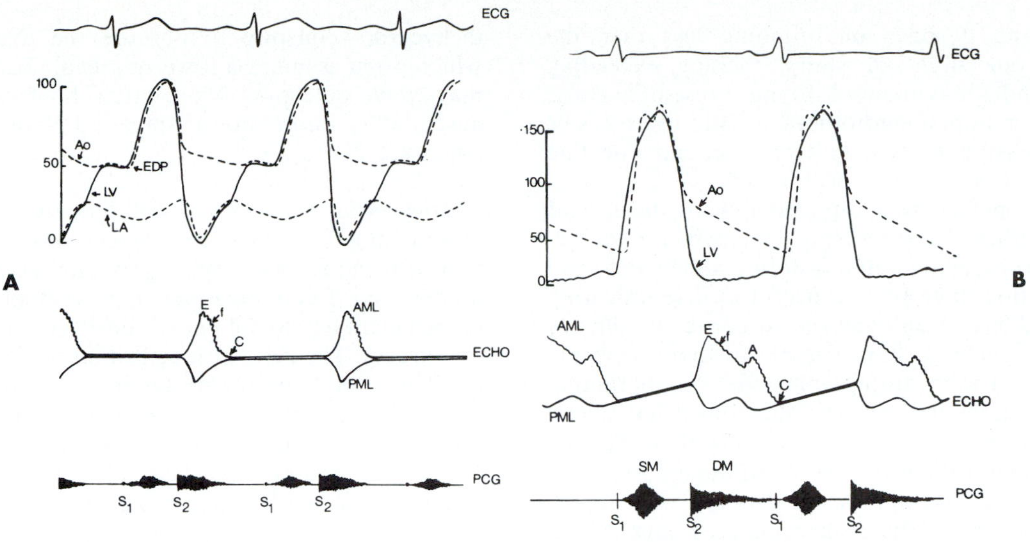


**Fig. 14-4.** Hemodynamic, echocardiographic *(ECHO),* and phonocardiographic *(PCG)* differences between acute severe **(A)** and chronic severe **(B)** aortic regurgitation. Left ventricular end diastolic pressure *(EDP)* is much higher in **A** with a narrower pulse pressure and preclosure of the mitral valve. *Ao,* Aorta; *LV,* left ventricle; *LA,* left atrium; *AML,* anterior mitral leaflet; *PML,* posterior mitral leaflet; *f,* flutter of the anterior mitral leaflet; *C,* mitral closure; *SM,* systolic murmur; *DM,* diastolic murmur. (From Morganroth J et al: *Ann Intern Med* 87:223, 1977.)

pulses, a downward, laterally displaced, hyperdynamic apex impulse, and the characteristic murmur. The high-pitched, blowing diastolic murmur is usually best heard along the left sternal margin; audibility to the right of the sternum suggests a syphilitic basis or an aortic aneurysm. A plethora of eponymic designations have been attached to the many peripheral manifestations caused by the rapid ejection of the abnormally large stroke volume, but few of these are actually valuable in assessing the severity of regurgitation. One possible exception to this is the Hill sign, the difference in systolic blood pressure between simultaneous supine measurements in the arm and the leg. Normally, there is no difference. Correlation with angiographic quantitation of regurgitation has suggested that a difference of 20 mm Hg or less indicates mild incompetence, 20 to 40 mm Hg moderate disease, and above 60 mm Hg severe regurgitation. These guidelines serve as a rough index in the asymptomatic patient but should not be relied on too heavily, particularly in patients with congestive failure in whom an underestimation of the severity of regurgitation may result.

***Management.*** Although severe aortic regurgitation can be tolerated for many years without symptoms, the adaptive reserve of the left ventricle is eventually exhausted. Ventricular function begins to decline, precipitously in some instances, and eventually culminates in symptoms of congestive heart failure or angina. The latter symptom has been related to the increased left ventricular muscle mass and low diastolic (coronary perfusion) pressure in the presence of aortic regurgitation. The advent of moderate to severe symptoms is a definite indication to refer for a cardiologist's evaluation and possible surgical intervention. Many patients with chronic aortic regurgitation, however, manifest mild to moderate exertional dyspnea which may remain stable for extended intervals or improve after the administration of digitalis and diuretics. Thus the mere appearance of congestive symptoms, particularly when satisfactorily controlled by minimal therapy, should not be the sole determinant of the need for valve replacement. Oral vasodilators have been demonstrated to relieve symptoms, reduce ventricular dilatation, and improve ventricular function in patients with aortic regurgitation. However, it is not clear that these agents materially alter the natural course of aortic regurgitation, particularly after the appearance of symptoms. Because ventricular dysfunction may progress despite an apparent clinical response, vasodilator therapy in symptomatic patients is done only with a consulting cardiologist.

Ventricular dilatation and hypertrophy regress rapidly in most symptomatic patients after valve replacement, but a number of studies have demonstrated that patients with ventricular dysfunction before surgery often remain in advanced congestive failure despite a technically successful operation. These patients have a much higher mortality rate over the first 2 to 5 postoperative years. For this reason, there have been many attempts to define the subgroup at risk for symptomatic deterioration and to identify characteristics that augur an unfavorable response to surgery.

The combination of a systolic blood pressure above 140 mm Hg or a diastolic pressure below 40 mm Hg, cardiomegaly on plain chest film, and left ventricular hypertrophy with strain has been found to confer a high risk for the development of symptoms. Two thirds of patients with aortic regurgitation manifesting all these features develop congestive failure or angina, or die within 3 years. One study found a higher operative mortality and probability of late myocardial death associated with many factors, including dyspnea on climbing less than the equivalent of one flight of stairs, therapy exceeding digitalization and a maximum of 40 mg furosemide daily, rales and an $S_3$ gallop, a cardiothoracic ratio in excess of 0.64 or a progressive increase in heart size, and a decline in the serially measured ejection fraction.

Much attention has been directed toward the use of noninvasive studies for projecting the response to surgery. Echocardiographic end-systolic dimension and shortening fraction have proved useful in discriminating between favorable and unfavorable responses to surgery in symptomatic patients. For example, patients with the combination of an echocardiographic systolic shortening fraction below 29% and end-systolic dimension above 55 mm fared much worse postoperatively than patients with more normal values in one often-quoted study. It was suggested that asymptomatic patients who reproducibly manifest one of these abnormalities have a high likelihood of developing symptoms mandating surgery within 3 years, but the validity of these criteria has not been proved. Others have found the combination of ejection fraction under 50% and class III-IV symptoms as reliable predictors of unfavorable long-term outcome. Thus it seems reasonable to obtain a baseline echocardiogram on all patients with evidence of significant aortic regurgitation. The echocardiogram may then be repeated at yearly intervals to detect signs of declining systolic function which, if apparent, may be confirmed by exercise radioventriculography gated scan. Asymptomatic patients who demonstrate clinical features indicating a high probability of symptomatic deterioration or a less favorable surgical outcome, or whose echocardiographic values approach or exceed those cited above, are referred for surgical consideration.

### Acute aortic regurgitation

***Pathophysiology.*** Acute aortic regurgitation is most commonly related to infective endocarditis. It is occasionally the result of aortic trauma, prolapse, or rupture of a myxomatous valve, aortic dissection, or rupture of one of the sinuses of Valsalva, which usually results in regurgitation into the right heart. In contrast to the slow, insidiously progressive type of regurgitation dealt with above, which permits the left ventricle to mount an adaptive response, effective compensation is not possible in the face of sudden, massive aortic valvular incompetence. In the former situation, the left ventricle gradually dilates to accommodate the necessarily larger end-diastolic volume while maintaining a normal end-diastolic pressure, i.e., improved compliance. Contractility is enhanced with an increase in the rate of ventricular ejection. Acute aortic regurgitation, however, precludes such a response. The abrupt increase in diastolic volume produces a sharp increase in end-diastolic pressure, and the contractile response is inadequate, resulting in a decreased stroke volume. Increases in left atrial pressure and pulmonary arterial pressure ensue, aggravated by tachycardia and partial closure of the mitral valve by the impinging regurgitant jet.

***Physical examination.*** The characteristic bounding pulse and low diastolic pressure of the chronic counterpart are usually absent. Furthermore, lowered aortic pressure and tachycardia conspire to obscure the diastolic murmur, which often assumes a lower-pitched, coarser quality and may evade detection. More often, however, a to-and-fro auscultatory impression is imparted along the left sternal edge (see Fig. 14-4).

***Diagnostic testing.*** Echocardiography may be useful in establishing the presence of vegetations larger than 2 to 3 mm with endocarditis. When present, vegetations confer a higher risk of complications and eventual need for valve replacement but do not per se constitute sufficient grounds for surgery. The echo also contributes to the evaluation of the degree of acute regurgitation. In addition to diastolic mitral fluttering, severe acute regurgitation produces mitral valve closure before the onset of systole (see Fig. 14-4); this finding may help identify patients who are candidates for early valve replacement.

***Management.*** Severe regurgitation of this type, apart from considerations pertinent to the primary cause (e.g., aortic dissection), is best managed by prompt replacement of the aortic valve. Interim support is frequently necessary, since these patients often verge on shock. Infusion of isoproterenol (Isuprel), which combines inotropic stimulation with peripheral vasodilatation, produces dramatic, albeit temporary, improvement in many cases. Alternatively, a combination of dobutamine and a vasodilator may be effective, particularly if ventricular ectopy is present. In less extreme circumstances a more tempered approach is possible, but the need for surgery remains urgent.

An aggressive surgical attack on endocarditis has been advocated by some, consisting of valve replacement within the first week after diagnosis of staphylococcal endocarditis and urgent surgery in the presence of moderate to severe congestive failure. This approach has been followed by surprisingly few instances of prosthetic endocarditis, despite the brevity of preoperative antibiotic therapy. Certainly, the hemodynamic state is a major determinant of outcome, and early surgery is unquestionably beneficial in the presence of advanced failure. Until further confirmation of the superiority of early surgery to medical therapy in staphylococcal endocarditis is available, however, it seems prudent to base decisions about surgery on the hemodynamic picture.

## MITRAL STENOSIS

### Pathophysiology

Mitral stenosis in the adult is almost invariably the consequence of rheumatic endocarditis, although only about half the patients with this condition, two thirds of whom are women, can provide a history of acute rheumatic fever. Restriction of the mitral orifice may rarely be congenital or may be physiologically simulated by an atrial tumor or a supravalvular membrane (cor triatriatum). Increased attention has been directed to extensive calcification of the mitral annulus as the basis for mitral stenosis in the elderly.

### History and physical examination

The prototypic chronicle of rheumatic mitral stenosis, as elucidated by the now classic observations of Wood, includes a prolonged asymptomatic latency, a span approaching 20 years after the episode of rheumatic fever. More than a decade may lapse before there is diagnostic evidence on physical examination. Typically, an otherwise asymptomatic course is punctuated by symptoms during periods of cardiovascular stress, particularly pregnancy, before sustained manifestations materialize. Once established, symptoms progress to disabling proportion within about 7 years. This capsulized history, although conceptually useful, is subject to wide individual variability. Although progression of stenosis usually leads to symptoms during the fourth and fifth decades, a significant proportion of patients remain asymptomatic for much longer periods, some for a lifetime. The factors governing the development and the rate of progression of orificial cicatrization are poorly understood.

When the original mitral valve orifice has been reduced by about half, atrial pressure must increase to maintain normal diastolic flow into the left ventricle; conversely, higher flow requires higher atrial pressures. Atrial pressures reach 20 to 25 mm Hg at rest when the orifice is reduced to about 1 $cm^2$ or during exertion with less severe stenosis. This pressure is transmitted to the pulmonary capillary bed, where disruption of the normal transcapillary balance fosters extrusion of lymph into the interstitium. These abnormalities are counterpoised to some extent by the development of pulmonary arteriolar vasoconstriction, pulmonary hypertension, and the decline in cardiac output which is so characteristic of mitral stenosis.

From these hemodynamic considerations the primacy of dyspnea as a manifestation of mitral stenosis as well as the basis for the exacerbations of pulmonary congestion that accompany febrile conditions, anemia, and pregnancy is readily apparent. Asymptomatic or mildly symptomatic patients may decompensate precipitously with the onset of atrial fibrillation, which occasions an abrupt rise in left atrial pressure. When querying patients with mitral stenosis, it is important to consider the dilatory pace of the symptoms, which affords the opportunity for both physiologic and psychologic adaptation. Chronic accommodation by unwitting restriction of activity may largely obviate symptoms, and responses to routine daily tasks and abstinence from exertional recreation should be specifically sought.

Other symptoms typical of mitral stenosis may include ease of fatigue and palpitations related to paroxysmal atrial arrhythmias. Hemoptysis is related to hypertension in the bronchial veins, which empty into the pulmonary veins. This seems to occur less frequently now than the older literature implied. Chest pain, noted by about 10% of patients and usually atypical of angina, has been imputed to pulmonary hypertension; a typical history of angina pectoris, more common in older patients, implies the presence of obstructive coronary disease.

On examination the patient with isolated mitral stenosis may be expected to manifest a reduced volume of the carotid pulse, which is variable if atrial fibrillation is present. The left ventricular apex impulse, which may elude palpation because of posterior rotation by an enlarged right ventricle, is normal in diameter, tapping, and nearly always accompanied by a systolic lift along the lower sternal edge.

Emblematic of mitral stenosis is the accentuation of $S_1$, which is often palpable. The opening snap, a high frequency sound heard during early diastole and widely transmitted across the precordium, denotes the abrupt halting of anterior movement of the pliable though tethered anterior mitral leaflet and imparts a characteristic auscultatory cadence (Fig. 14-5). The third cardinal feature on auscultation, the low-pitched diastolic rumble, may be audible only in a circumscribed area over the apex or, as underscored by Sir William Osler, "may be concealed under a quarter of a dollar." It is thus essential to listen with the bell of the stethoscope applied immediately superjacent to the apex impulse. In the presence of the distinctive cadence, the presence of a diastolic rumble should not be dismissed without efforts at

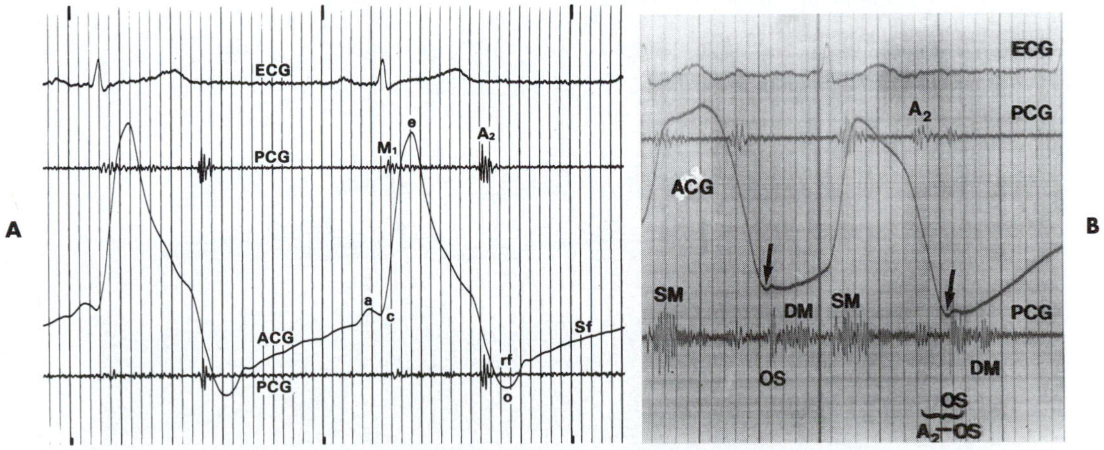


**Fig. 14-5.** A normal apexcardiogram *(ACG)* and phonocardiogram *(PCG)* **(A)** contrasted with that from a patient with mild mitral stenosis in atrial fibrillation **(B)**. A mitral opening snap *(OS)* occurs shortly after the O point and is followed by a murmur *(DM)* that extends through only half of diastole with longer cycles. The $A_2$-OS stenosis interval of 125 ms is consistent with mild mitral stenosis. The rapid filling deflection *(rf)*, normally corresponding to rapid early diastolic filling, is notably attenuated *(arrow)*. A brief systolic murmur *(SM)* is also present. The normal a wave (a) is absent with atrial fibrillation. $A_2$ Aortic second sound.

provocation. Several situps are usually sufficient to evoke a nascent murmur. The pulmonic component of the second heart sound is accentuated, and narrow inspiratory splitting is preserved.

The interval $A_2$–opening snap ($A_2$-OS) provides a rough clue to the severity of mitral stenosis. The more stenotic the valve, the higher is the left atrial pressure; this displaces the atrioventricular (AV) pressure crossover upward on the descending limb of the ventricular pressure curve and results in earlier opening of the mitral valve (Fig. 14-6). When gauging $A_2$-OS, a useful comparison is normal splitting of the second sound, ordinarily about 0.04 second. Generally, an $A_2$-OS interval of 0.08 second or less indicates moderate to severe stenosis. Unfortunately, a number of other factors (e.g., cardiac output, heart rate, and ventricular diastolic pressure) also influence atrial pressure and limit the correlation of $A_2$-OS with measured valve area.

### Diagnostic testing

A straightened left heart border on chest film is a manifestation of left atrial enlargement, as is the appearance of a "double density" and a bulge high along the posterior cardiac margin on the lateral view. Vascular redistribution to the upper lung fields is also characteristic of mitral stenosis. Although broad-notched P waves in lead II of the ECG (P-mitrale) may be present, a more typical pattern is atrial fibrillation and right axis deviation, a concurrence which always suggests mitral stenosis. A frontal plain QRS axis to the right of +60 degrees suggests moderate to severe disease.

Mitral stenosis transforms the diastolic motion pattern of the mitral leaflets and inscribes a distinctive diagnostic echocardiographic signature (see Fig. 14-6). Commissural leaflet fusion precludes the normal contrary excursion of the anterior and posterior leaflets, and both leaflets move anteriorly in concordance during diastole. Other typical findings include dense mitral echoes generated by leaflet thickening, reduced leaflet excursion, and flattening of the E-F slope. Enthusiasm about the correlation of a reduced E-F slope with the severity of stenosis proved premature, but two-dimensional echocardiography has supplanted this indirect index with the capability to directly visualize and measure the actual valve orifice in many patients.

## Management

Mindful of the tendency for these patients to view behavioral adjustments, restrictions, and omissions as normal, symptoms that limit routine daily activities should prompt referral for evaluation and possible surgical intervention. Atrial fibrillation, which ultimately develops in the majority of patients with mitral stenosis, is not an indication for immediate surgical referral, although it often marks the onset of the progressive symptomatic phase. The ventricular response rate usually slows satisfactorily after digitalization, but some patients display a resistance to digitalis. In these instances, addition of low-dose verapamil or propranolol may be necessary. It is probably worth emphasis here that digitalis has no role in the management of congestive pulmonary symptoms in the presence of sinus rhythm. Some have advocated the use of

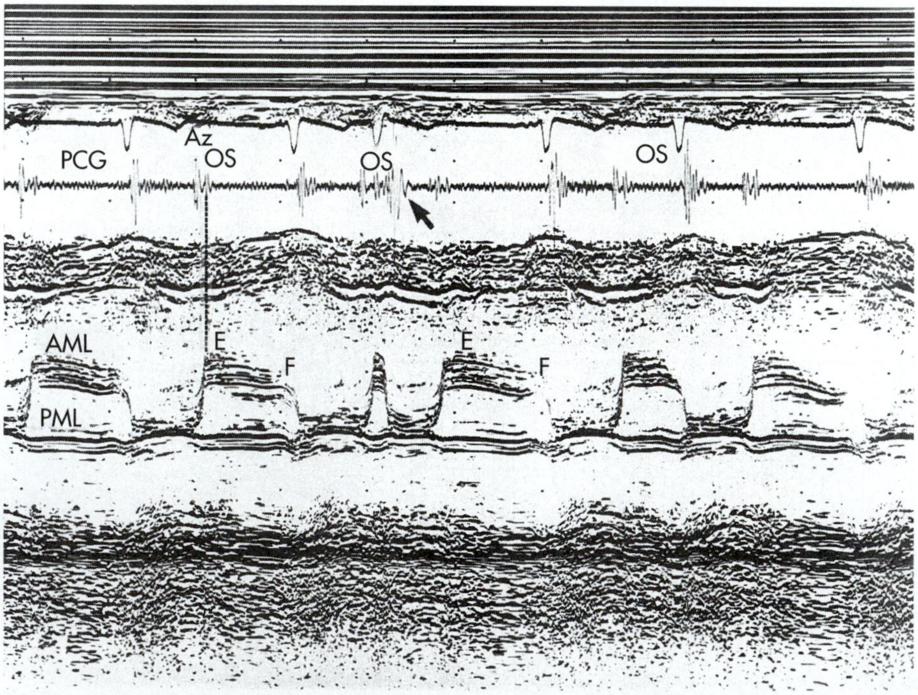


**Fig. 14-6.** M-mode echocardiographic tracing and phonocardiogram *(PCG)* from a patient with mitral stenosis. The mitral leaflets are markedly thickened with restricted motion (contrast to Fig. 14-9) and reduced E to F slope. The opening snap *(OS)* corresponds to the peak excursion *(E)* of the anterior mitral leaflet *(AML)*. Accentuation of $M_1$ is particularly prominent after a short diastolic interval *(arrow)*. *PML,* Posterior mitral leaflet; $A_2$, Aortic closure.

propranolol to eliminate the tachycardia-related exertional dyspnea and thus minimize symptoms in patients with sinus rhythm. This has not been useful in our experience, since β-blockade seems to intensify symptoms related to low cardiac output.

Systemic embolism, most commonly cerebral, complicates the course of mitral stenosis in about 10% to 20% of cases and is usually associated with atrial fibrillation. Embolization may occur in sinus rhythm, but the rate, estimated to be slightly less than 1% per patient-year, is exceeded by the risks of anticoagulation. Patients with atrial fibrillation who have experienced an embolism but are otherwise asymptomatic are probably best managed by anticoagulation alone, since there is no evidence that surgery under these circumstances reduces the subsequent risk of embolization. Embolization in the presence of other symptoms and a mitral valve area of 1.5 $cm^2$ or less is an indication for valve surgery.

Subacute bacterial endocarditis is seldom encountered as a complication of pure mitral stenosis. Nevertheless, antibiotic prophylaxis is recommended for dental and other procedures in the presence of rheumatic valvular disease.

When symptoms have progressed to the moderate range or beyond in the presence of moderate to severe stenosis (mitral valve area of less than 1.5 $cm^2$), surgery or catheter balloon valvuloplasty is usually recommended. If the patient is young and the physical findings are unmistakably those of isolated mitral stenosis and can be corroborated by two-dimensional or Doppler echocardiography, cardiac catheterization is probably unnecessary. However, catheterization is essential if there is any uncertainty about the severity of stenosis or accompanying mitral regurgitation, if there is any question of associated valvular disease, or if there is any reason to suspect coronary artery disease. Mitral valvuloplasty is preferred whenever possible. Mitral valve replacement is necessary if the dense valvular calcification precludes satisfactory valvuloplasty or if significant mitral incompetence is present.

## MITRAL REGURGITATION

### Pathophysiology and natural history

Competence of the mitral valve during ventricular systole requires precisely coordinated interaction of the principal components of the mitral valve complex: valve leaflets, chordae tendineae, papillary muscles, and mitral annulus. The insights afforded by angiography and echocardiography over the past two decades have expanded the understanding of the etiologic basis for mitral regurgitation to include dysfunction of any of these components. As a result, it is now recognized that rheumatic disease, once considered responsible for most cases of mitral regurgitation, accounts for fewer than half. Other common primary causes of mitral incompetence are mitral valve prolapse (myxomatous degeneration of the mitral valve), ruptured chordae tendineae, papillary muscle ischemia or infarction, tissue erosion related to endocarditis, and calcification of the mitral annulus. Mitral regurgitation may also occur as a consequence of any process that results in dilatation of the left ventricle, or "functional" mitral regurgitation.

The natural history of this disorder is highly variable and depends on the etiology, the severity of the regurgitation, and the ability to mount and sustain an adaptive response. As an extreme example, the severe acute mitral regurgitation occasioned by papillary muscle rupture or endocarditic valvular disruption is immediately associated with pulmonary edema and often rapidly fatal if uncorrected. On the other hand, reports indicate that some patients with clinically severe rheumatic mitral regurgitation may maintain functional class I status for over 20 years, some as long as 65 years. A broad spectrum of subacute to chronic mitral regurgitation spans these extreme poles, and in the individual instance it is difficult to project the clinical course accurately.

The left ventricle's ability to withstand the often massive volume overload imposed by mitral incompetence apparently results from the rapid decline in systolic wall tension (related to the product of systolic pressure and radius) permitted by the presence of a left atrial "vent." Ventricular radius shortens more rapidly than normal in the presence of regurgitation. Because development of tension is a much more important determinant of myocardial oxygen demand than an actual decrease in muscle length, this compensation limits the energy cost and allows prolonged stability. The left atrium also contributes importantly to the adaptive response. In chronic mitral regurgitation the left atrium dilates and may provide a cushion for the pulmonary circuit by absorbing a huge regurgitant volume with minimal increases in pressure. Massive acute regurgitation into a small, noncompliant atrium, however, often results in marked pulmonary venous hypertension and pulmonary edema (Fig. 14-7).

Because there is no obstruction to ventricular filling in pure mitral regurgitation, left atrial pressure elevation is not an obligatory response to a shortened diastole as with mitral stenosis. Thus exertional dyspnea is not prominent with compensated volume overload of mitral origin, and pulmonary edema, even after the development of atrial fibrillation, is less common. Despite the compensatory mechanisms outlined above, ventricular adaptability may eventually be exhausted; elevated diastolic pressures and prominent congestive symptoms follow. Hemoptysis and chest pain are not associated with mitral regurgitation, but systemic embolization apparently occurs at about the same rate as mitral stenosis, particularly after age 35 in the presence of atrial fibrillation.

### Physical examination

The physical examination in severe mitral regurgitation usually discloses a briskly rising and somewhat collapsing arterial pulse; hence the designation "little water hammer," an allusion to similar but much more pronounced findings in aortic regurgitation. The apex impulse is enlarged, is displaced downward to the left, and is a rapidly retracted or dynamic impulse. A systolic lift appreciated along the lower left sternal edge may suggest right ventricular overload but is as likely to reflect anterior displacement of the entire heart by left atrial expansion in systole. An attenuated $S_1$ coincides with the onset of a high-pitched, holosystolic murmur, which typically radiates to the axilla and may extend beyond $A_2$. Because $A_2$ occurs prematurely due to the inability to sustain ventricular pressure, splitting of the second sound often widens. Rapid, early diastolic filling of the left ventricle produces a prominent $S_3$ gallop, which frequently corre-

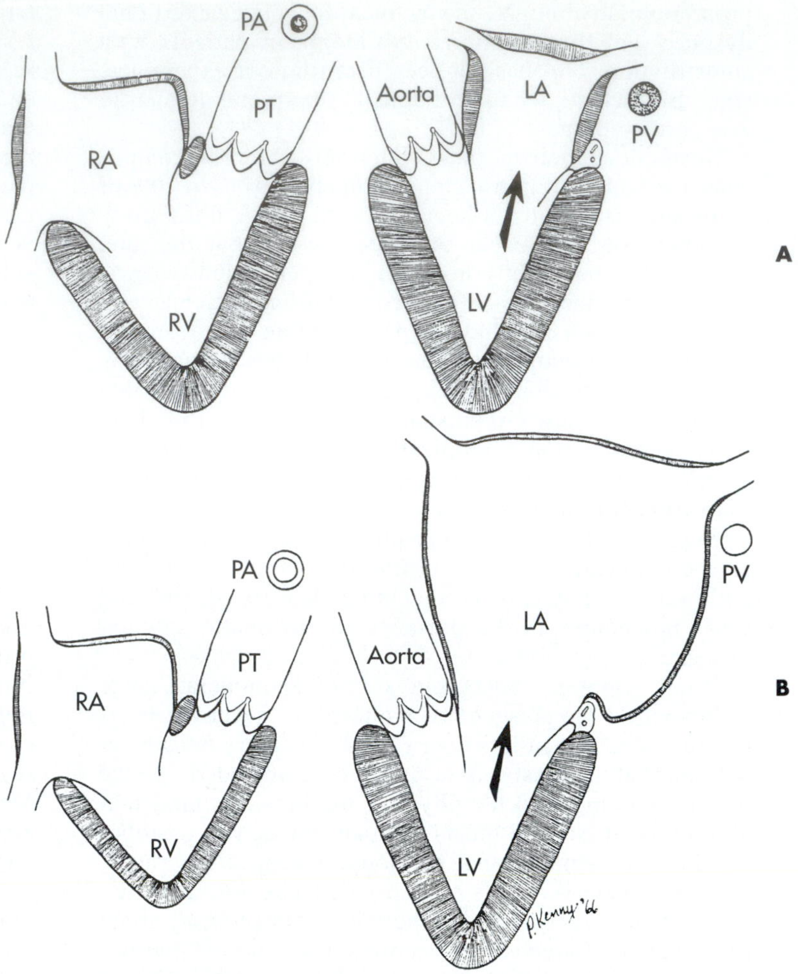


**Fig. 14-7.** The two extremes of pure mitral regurgitation *(MR)*. **A,** In acute severe MR, the left atrium *(LA)* is small and not compliant. As a result, high pressures are transmitted to the pulmonary venous *(PV)* and arterial *(PA)* system resulting in medial hypertrophy in these vessels as well as hypertrophy of the right ventricle *(RV)*. **B,** With chronic severe MR, the LA dilates and is able to "absorb" regurgitant volume without marked pressure elevation, thereby sparing the pulmonary circulation. *PT,* Pulmonary trunk; *RA,* right atrium, *LV,* left ventricle. (From Roberts WC, Perloff JK: *Ann Intern Med* 77:939, 1972.)

sponds to a palpable filling wave and may be followed by a brief flow rumble. The presence of an $S_4$ gallop or palpable presystolic apical excursion is indicative of a small, noncompliant, forcefully contracting left atrium and implies recent onset (within approximately 18 months), e.g., chordal rupture.

It is difficult to distinguish among the various causes of pure mitral regurgitation at the bedside. Although the murmur is typically described as holosystolic in rheumatic disease, it may assume many configurations, including a crescendo-decrescendo profile. Transmission to the axilla and failure of the murmur to increase following a premature ventricular contraction (PVC) or to diminish in response to the Valsalva maneuver usually allow distinction from ejection murmurs. The presence of coronary disease or a nonejection systolic click may suggest other etiologies. Another easily confused murmur, that of obstructive hypertrophic myopathy, is dissimilar in response to provocative maneuvers, although often accompanied by mitral regurgitation.

## Management

Digitalis, diuretics, and vasodilators constitute the mainstays of therapy in the presence of atrial fibrillation and congestive symptoms. In addition to factors previously mentioned, the volume of mitral regurgitation is a dynamic function of peripheral resistance. Agents that lower systemic arterial resistance (e.g., nitroprusside or hydralazine) decrease regurgitation, reduce left atrial pressure, and enhance cardiac output. Although vasodilators are clearly beneficial in acute situations, their influence on the chronic course is undefined.

Asymptomatic patients with evidence of severe mitral regurgitation are followed expectantly without specific therapy beyond endocarditis prophylaxis. Echocardiography, particularly two-dimensional study, allows serial evaluation of left ventricular and left atrial dimensions as well as ventricular function, and it occasionally helps establish a definite etiology, although this is often not possible. Mild to moderate symptoms may be managed medically as outlined above, but their appearance probably warrants referral for a cardiology evaluation. More severe symptoms constitute a clear indication for surgical intervention. Cardiac catheterization is essential to define the degree of regurgitation angiographically, evaluate the possibility of other valvular disease, and assess any contribution of coronary disease.

Despite successful surgical elimination of mitral regurgitation, some patients fail to improve postoperatively. Removal of the systolic vent into the atrium restores full aortic impedance to left ventricular ejection; thus the ejection fraction almost invariably declines after surgical correction. In patients with mild to moderate preoperative ventricular dilatation, the lower postoperative value usually remains within the normal range. Patients with markedly dilated ventricles, however, or those with impaired systolic function preoperatively may deteriorate further afterward. Although it is probable that the majority of patients in these categories will manifest advanced symptoms, it is essential that they be promptly referred to ensure maximum restitution of ventricular function.

## MITRAL VALVE PROLAPSE

The observations of Reid and Barlow just over two decades ago established the relationship between systolic prolapse of the mitral valve leaflets and the auscultatory findings of midsystolic click with or without a late systolic murmur. Facilitated by the development of echocardiography, this disorder has now emerged as one of the most prevalent and problematic concerns of the medical practitioner. Approximately 5% of the general population display some evidence of this disorder. Prolapse is encountered at all ages, and, contrary to popular belief, involvement appears to be approximately equal in men and women.

### Pathophysiology

The term *primary mitral prolapse* has been applied to distinguish inherent abnormalities in the mitral valve apparatus from prolapse secondary to other problems, e.g., coronary artery disease and mitral valvuloplasty. The most important primary abnormality is the disruption of normal connective tissue components, the valve, the chordae, and in some instances the annulus as well by so-called myxomatous degeneration. Myxomatous tissue, consisting of a relative dearth of collagen fibers haphazardly arrayed within an abundant mucopolysaccharide matrix, proliferates and sunders the normal valvular support architecture. Ultimately, this process is responsible for the characteristic redundancy or hooding of the valve leaflets on gross inspection and for the propensity to chordal rupture associated with mitral prolapse. It is speculated that primary prolapse has a hereditary basis and may be transmitted as an autosomal dominant trait with variable expression. The causes of secondary mitral prolapse are numerous, but connective tissue disorders, notably Marfan's syndrome and secundum atrial septal defect, are commonly cited in addition to those previously mentioned.

### History and physical examination

Although the available literature indicates a rather high prevalence of symptoms among patients with mitral prolapse, these observations are slanted by the identification of patients through symptoms. It seems clear that the majority of affected individuals are asymptomatic. Furthermore, several of the symptoms associated with prolapse, e.g., dyspnea in the absence of significant mitral regurgitation, fatigue, dizziness, syncope, and neurosis, seem to bear no direct relation to the valvular abnormality and may be only coincidentally associated. However, similar symptoms have been ascribed to the vaguely defined disorder vasoregulatory asthenia in the past, and there may be some parallel, if not identity, between this entity and the abnormal sympathetic vasomotor responses that have been noted in patients with mitral valve prolapse.

The two most common complaints from patients with mitral prolapse are chest pain and palpitations. The prepectoral pain usually differs from typical angina in several respects; specifically, the character is usually sharp or stabbing, the duration is often protracted, a relationship to exertion is absent, and nitroglycerin seldom affords relief. Very rarely, the pain closely mimics angina. Theories advanced to account for the pain have included excessive traction exerted on the papillary muscles by the prolapsing leaflets, but the precise mechanisms await definition. Palpitations have been noted in about half of patients with prolapse.

Except for thoracic cage abnormalities such as pectus excavatum and straight back or features of a related disorder, the extracardiac physical examination is usually unremarkable. Cardiac examination, auscultatory aspects aside, is noteworthy only insofar as it reflects any significant degree of mitral regurgitation. The hallmark of prolapse is the midsystolic to late systolic click, which is the only detectable manifestation in more than half the cases. Aortic or pulmonic ejection clicks are frequently mistaken as indicators of prolapse but are distinguishable by their timing with the upstroke of the carotid pulse and by typical respiratory variation in the case of the pulmonic click. Rarely, a prolapsing mitral leaflet generates an early systolic click. Estimates vary, but in approximately 15% of cases the click is followed by a brief midsystolic or late systolic murmur. Occasionally the murmur is pansystolic in duration or honking in quality.

The timing of mitral prolapse has been demonstrated to occur reproducibly at a critical systolic volume, thereby accounting for the effects of various maneuvers in evoking characteristic responses in this condition (Fig. 14-8).

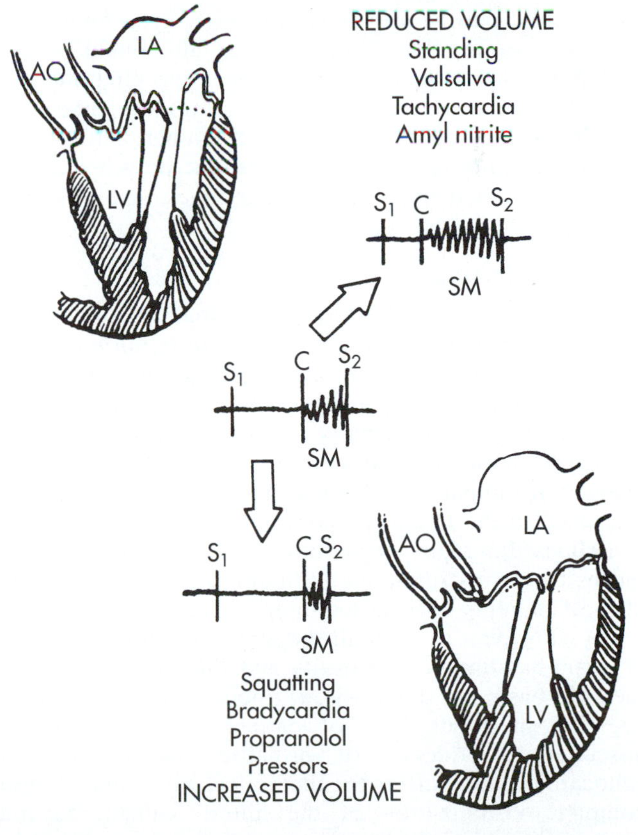


**Fig. 14-8.** Effects of various maneuvers that influence diastolic ventricular volume on the timing of the click (*C*) and murmur (*SM*) in mitral valve prolapse. *AO*, Aorta; *LA*, left atrium, *LV*, left ventricle. (From Devereux RB et al: *Circulation* 54:3, 1976.)

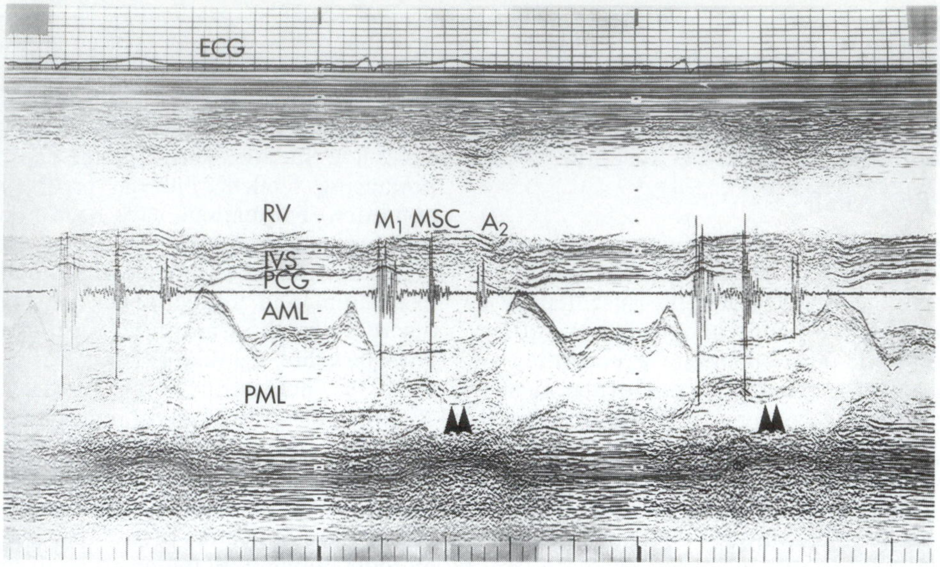


**Fig. 14-9.** Echocardiogram and phonocardiogram *(PCG)* from a patient with mitral valve prolapse. A prominent midsystolic click *(MSC)* coincides with posterior buckling of the mitral valve leaflets *(arrowheads).* The anterior mitral leaflet *(AML)* is also slightly thickened, a finding consistent with myxomatous degeneration. $M_1$, Mitral closure; $A_2$, aortic closure; *PML,* posterior mitral leaflet; *IVS,* interventricular septum; *RV,* right ventricle.

Measures that decrease cardiac filling, e.g., standing, Valsalva strain, and amyl nitrite administration, reduce ventricular end-diastolic volume. As a result the critical systolic volume and the click/murmur occur earlier. Conversely, passive leg elevation or a deep knee bend increases ventricular filling, delays attainment of the prolapse volume, and either displaces the click/murmur into later systole or eradicates the findings altogether. The variability in auscultation from one examination to another may be striking. Some patients exhibit only a click on occasion, no evidence of prolapse at times, and both click and murmur in other instances.

## Diagnostic testing

The chest x-ray may highlight abnormalities of thoracic development, but the cardiac silhouette is normal in the absence of significant mitral regurgitation. Somewhat more than one third of patients display ECG repolarization abnormalities. These usually consist in T-wave flattening or inversion in the inferior leads. Variable ST-segment changes accompany the T-wave changes, which frequently are noted in the lateral precordial leads as well.

Echocardiography provides a simple noninvasive means to corroborate clinical findings and to identify the 20% of patients with auscultatorily silent prolapse (Fig. 14-9). However, as with all diagnostic tests, the echocardiogram has limited sensitivity and should not constitute the sole basis for diagnosis. M-mode echoes are falsely negative in about 15% of patients with unequivocal auscultatory evidence of prolapse. Two-dimensional echocardiography offers the theoretical advantage of more complete visualization of the mitral leaflets, but the various diagnostic criteria proposed are not universally accepted and the lack of any reference standard hinders accurate appraisal of sensitivity and specificity.

## Management

The outlook in patients with mitral prolapse, although still incompletely defined, is generally favorable, and it is this aspect that deserves strongest emphasis in discussions of this diagnosis with patients. In recognition of the preponderantly benign prognosis, the term *normal mitral prolapse* has been proposed to describe the majority of affected patients. An awareness that the medical literature includes a disproportion of symptomatic patients complicates extrapolation of the incidence of progression to chordal rupture or significant mitral regurgitation, reported at about 15%, to the asymptomatic patient seen in the office. The presence of a systolic murmur at diagnosis seems to confer a higher risk for subsequent complications, and these individuals probably warrant more cautious observation. As a rule, biennial follow-up with echocardiograms to follow chamber dimensions is sufficient. Significant mitral regurgitation is managed as previously outlined.

Controversy pervades considerations of endocarditis with prolapse. Although it is widely conceded that prolapse poses a hazard for endocarditis in patients with a systolic murmur, there is no firm evidence that an isolated click imparts the same liability. As a result, most authorities recommend that antibiotic prophylaxis be reserved for patients with a murmur or thickening of the valve on echocardiographic examination.

All varieties of arrhythmia have been associated with mitral prolapse, but the 75% to 80% figure detected by Holter monitor in patients referred to university centers undoubtedly overestimates the actual prevalence. In addition to the mechanisms described elsewhere, supraventricular premature beats and tachyarrhythmias in mitral valve prolapse may be caused by depolarization of smooth muscle cells that have been identified in mitral valve tissue. Alternatively, concealed AV nodal bypass tracts, so called because they permit any retrograde conduction (ventricle to atrium), may foster reentry. Regardless of the substrate, therapy is necessary only for symptomatic and distressing arrhythmias, and a β-blocker is a good first choice.

Similarly, symptomatic ventricular arrhythmias may require treatment. Evidence favoring suppressive therapy for frequent but asymptomatic PVCs however, is less compelling. Although there is no doubt that sudden death occurs in a small proportion of patients with prolapse, only 25 cases could be culled from the literature in a comprehensive 1979 review. These patients were women, age 40 or older, usually with evidence of mitral regurgitation. Ventricular ectopy was evident in more than three fourths of those for whom the information was available, and more than half of those reported in sufficient detail had previously experienced syncope. These features are not exclusive but should be factored into the therapeutic balance when antiarrhythmic therapy is being considered.

Both transient and permanent neurologic impairments have been reported in patients with mitral valve prolapse. An excessive prevalence of mitral prolapse has also been noted among patients under 40 years of age who incur a stroke. The inference that cerebral embolism explains these observations derives from the identification of macroscopic coalescence of platelets and fibrin on the atrial surface of the abnormal mitral leaflets in some patients. Attractive as this hypothesis may seem, it is far from firmly established. The role played by atrial rhythm disturbances requires further clarification, and an association of migraine headache with prolapse suggests another possible basis, i.e., vasospasm. Convincing evidence in support of anticoagulant or antiplatelet therapy in these patients is unavailable.

## TRICUSPID VALVE DISEASE

### Tricuspid stenosis

Tricuspid stenosis is nearly always a consequence of rheumatic fever and is almost invariably accompanied at least by mitral valve disease and often aortic valve disease as well. The pathology is similar to that described in mitral stenosis. Fatigue, a consequence of low cardiac output, is a prominent symptom, as are the other signs of right atrial hypertension including edema or anasarca, ascites, and hepatomegaly. A clinical maxim suggests that tricuspid stenosis be considered in mitral stenosis when peripheral edema is disproportionate to dyspnea, an expression of the concept that a protective effect on the pulmonary circuit conferred by right ventricular inflow obstruction reduces the incidence of pulmonary congestion.

Diagnostic physical findings include large jugular a waves with sinus rhythm and sluggish y descent, which may be more palpable than visible if atrial fibrillation is present. The most helpful auscultatory finding is the diastolic decrescendo murmur to the left of the lower sternum, which is relatively high pitched and easily misconstrued by the neophyte as evidence for aortic regurgitation. Electrocardiographically the high voltage of right atrial enlargement may be superimposed on P mitrale with sinus rhythm. The echocardiographic pattern of tricuspid stenosis is similar to mitral stenosis.

### Tricuspid regurgitation

Tricuspid regurgitation is also a frequent component of a multivalvular rheumatic disease picture. However, conditions such as left ventricular failure, regardless of etiology, or atrial septal defect, which impose chronic pressure or volume overload on the right ventricle with subsequent dilatation, may induce secondary or "functional" tricuspid incompetence. The majority of patients with tricuspid regurgitation are numbered in this category. Tricuspid stenosis usually coincides to some degree if the regurgitation results from primary rheumatic valvular involvement. Other primary causes of tricuspid regurgitation include trauma, carcinoid syndrome, endocarditis, and myxomatous degeneration.

***History and physical examination.*** Primary tricuspid regurgitation may be tolerated well for an indefinite period in the absence of pulmonary hypertension. Secondary regurgitation, however, serves only to exacerbate the manifestations of right ventricular failure. In addition to complaints related to the prime etiology and systemic venous hypertension, patients may become aware of venous throbbing in the neck. Specific support for tricuspid regurgitation on examination is conveyed by the observation of sustained ascent instead of descent of the jugular meniscus during systole and palpable hepatic pulsation. A parasternal decrescendo murmur of variable intensity and a right ventricular $S_3$ gallop may be appreciated when tricuspid regurgitation is the sole abnormality, but these findings are often obscured by manifestations of concomitant valvular disease.

The echocardiographic findings of right ventricular volume overload, right atrial and ventricular enlargement, and paradoxical septal motion are confirmatory of suspected tricuspid regurgitation. A two-dimensional study may also elucidate the etiology by defining either associated valvular disease or intrinsic tricuspid abnormalities such as chordal rupture, vegetations, or the thickening and immobility characteristic of carcinoid. Studies have also demonstrated a role for contrast echocardiography in assessing the severity of tricuspid regurgitation.

***Management.*** Secondary tricuspid regurgitation usually responds to therapeutic measures directed at the principal offender, i.e., digitalis, diuretics, and vasodilators in left ventricular failure, surgical correction of aortic or mitral valve disease, and measures intended to lower pulmonary pressures in the presence of lung disease. Indications for referral to a cardiologist include those previously indicated for any associated valvular disease, symptomatic primary tricuspid regurgitation, or recalcitrance to the medical therapy. Cardiac catheterization is often required to clarify the severity of combined valvular lesions, the nature of other primary causes, and the degree of tricuspid involvement.

Surgery for tricuspid stenosis is usually undertaken simultaneously with correction of the mitral and aortic valve abnormalities and most often consists of valve replacement, preferably with a tissue prosthesis. Selected patients may be candidates for commissurotomy.

Considerations in tricuspid regurgitation are more complex, since secondary regurgitation often improves substantially or resolves completely when right ventricular overload is relieved by replacement of a diseased mitral valve and abatement of pulmonary hypertension. Tricuspid annuloplasty, either by suture techniques or insertion of a prosthetic ring, has gained increasing acceptance as an effective means of alleviating tricuspid regurgitation. Valve replacement remains a necessary treatment in circumstances in which satisfactory annular plication cannot be achieved.

## ENDOCARDITIS

Patients with infective endocarditis present a variety of symptoms in primary care practice. Although the onset of acute endocarditis can be abrupt and the course fulminating, subacute endocarditis may present with subtle clinical symptoms and signs. For further discussion see Chapter 17.

### Acute infective bacterial endocarditis

High fever, shaking chills, and congestive heart failure often occur at the onset of acute endocarditis. Patients may have had a staphylococcal skin infection, a pneumonia, or have injected drugs intravenously. Valvular and perivalvular tissues may be rapidly destroyed by the infecting organism, resulting in hemodynamic regurgitation. Left-sided lesions result in aortic or mitral regurgitation, pulmonary congestion, and symptoms of left-sided congestive heart failure (dyspnea, orthopnea, and paroxysmal nocturnal dyspnea). Right-sided lesions may produce tricuspid regurgitation and embolization of septic material to the lung. Cough, pleurisy, and dyspnea may be noted along with multiple pulmonary infiltrates and/or abscesses on chest x-ray). Acute endocarditis may be relatively silent in elderly patients, who may present with vague changes in mental status, are afebrile, have a new regurgitant murmur and a normal white count with increased immature band forms.

Systemic embolization occurs often in acute endocarditis. Infective thromboemboli may produce abscesses in the brain, kidneys, coronary arteries, or bowel. Large bulky emboli characteristic of candidal endocarditis may actually occlude large arteries. Cerebral embolization occurs in approximately 20% of patients with left-sided staphylococcal endocarditis. Seizures, confusion, and focal neurologic deficits often occur after multiple small emboli, while major stroke syndromes are caused by large ones.

The physical examination may reveal tachycardia, fever, and rigors. The murmur of regurgitation may not be loud, but $S_3$ and $S_4$ sounds are often present. The clinical findings of subacute bacterial endocarditis—Osler's nodes, splinter hemorrhages, Janeway spots, petechiae, and Roth's spots—are not present in acute endocarditis.

***Diagnostic testing.*** Laboratory tests may reveal a leukocytosis with increased bands, microscopic hematuria, and normal hemoglobin. Pulmonary congestion, pleural effusion, and patchy infiltrates may be noted on the chest x-ray depending on whether a left- or right-sided infection is present. Cardiac size and electrocardiogram are usually normal in the acutely ill patient due to the short duration of illness. Echocardiography defines the presence of vegetation and ventricular function.

The organisms that commonly produce acute endocarditis are invasive and not part of the normal flora. They include *Staphylococcus aureus, Streptococcus pneumoniae, Neisseria gonorrhoeae,* gram-negative rods, and *Candida.* The causal organism is related in part to the source of infection (Table 14-1).

***Management.*** Complications include those mentioned above and myocardial abscess, which may produce conduction abnormalities, or an abscess of the sinus of Valsalva, which may rupture into the right atrium or ventricle and produce a left-to-right shunt acutely.

The treatment of acute endocarditis requires prompt, early diagnosis, immediate consultation with a cardiologist, and transfer of the patient to a hospital where a comprehensive evaluation is possible and emergency valve replacement may be carried out if needed. While medical therapy alone (intravenous oxacillin or nafcillin for *Staphylococcus aureus*) may cure tricuspid valve infection, valve replacement is recommended if patients with aortic lesions show signs of hemodynamic decompensation.

### Endocarditis in intravenous drug abuse

Cellulitis or infective material injected intravenously often causes endocarditis in intravenous drug abusers. Puffy hands and the other stigmata of drug abuse may be present. Patients who present with exquisitely tender feet or hands and a history of drug abuse may have Osler-like nodes distal to an infected valve, mycotic arterial lesion, or recent intraarterial injection of drugs. *Staphylococcus aureus* is present in more than 50% of these patients. *Candida* and gram-negative organisms, especially *Pseudomonas,* are also commonly isolated. Due to the fact that these patients usually continue intravenous drug use dur-

**Table 14-1.** Sources of organisms leading to infective endocarditis

| Source | Infecting organism |
|---|---|
| Oral cavity (tooth brushing, dental extractions, preexisting pyorrhea) | *Streptococcus viridans*<br>Anaerobic streptococci<br>*Staphylococcus epidermidis* |
| Upper airway (bronchoscopy, intubation) | *Streptococcus* species<br>*Staphylococcus epidermidis*<br>*Streptococcus pneumoniae* |
| Genitourinary tract (pyelonephritis, instrumentation) | Gram-negative rods<br>Enterococci |
| Gastrointestinal tract (sigmoidoscopy, barium enema, invasive percutaneous procedures) | Gram-negative rods<br>*Streptococcus bovis*<br>Enterococci |
| Indwelling IV catheters, hemodialysis access sites, hyperalimentation catheters | *Staphylococcus* species<br>*Candida* species |
| Skin infections, burns | *Staphylococcus* species |
| Pneumonia | *Streptococcus pneumoniae*<br>*Haemophilus influenzae* |

Modified from Lilly LS, Kloner RA. In Kloner RA, editor: *The guide to cardiology,* New York, 1984, Wiley.

ing and after treatment, they may develop a syndrome that includes some of the features of both acute and subacute endocarditis. Although right-sided lesions involving the tricuspid valve are classically described, left-sided lesions are also very common in intravenous drug abusers.

### Subacute infective endocarditis

The symptoms of subacute endocarditis may present as a nonspecific illness. It usually occurs in the presence of a preexisting valvular or congenital heart lesion. The streptococcus is the most common infecting organism; however, a wide range of other organisms may also produce this infection. They include gram-positive organisms, *Streptococcus viridans,* microaerophilic streptococci, β-hemolytic streptococci, pneumococcus, gram-negative organisms, *Pseudomonas, Escherichia coli,* gonococci, *Salmonella,* fungi, and *Candida.*

The clinical symptoms of subacute endocarditis are produced by the toxicity of infection, embolization from vegetations, and valve destruction. Heart murmurs are present in 90% of patients. These may be difficult to differentiate from possible flow murmurs of concomitant anemia. The classic cutaneous and ocular signs of subacute endocarditis are presented in Table 14-2. Other symptoms include fever, chills, low back pain, anorexia, weight loss, and weakness. Splenomegaly and pain related to embolic infarct in various organs may occur along with clubbing of the fingers.

Laboratory studies usually reveal a mild anemia, leukocytosis with a dominance of polymorphonuclear leukocytes and microscopic hematuria in more than 50% of patients. This is caused by immune complexes that deposit in tissues and in the kidneys, where they may cause an autoimmune glomerulonephritis. The ECG and the chest x-ray may reflect the underlying heart disease, and vegetations larger than 2 mm in diameter may be visualized on the valve leaflets by echocardiography. Three sets of blood cultures should be drawn, spread over 24 hours. The causative organism will be isolated in 95% to 99% of cases. If blood cultures are negative, treatment should be given if subacute endocarditis is suspected.

Subacute endocarditis can be cured if treated with a long course (4 to 6 weeks) of intravenous antibiotics to which the infecting organism is sensitive. High dose penicillin is the drug of choice for *Streptococcus viridans.* Other antibiotics may be appropriate. Cardiologic and infectious disease consultations should be obtained to participate in the assessment and to ensure that peak and trough levels of antibiotic are effective.

**Table 14-2.** Cutaneous and ocular signs of subacute endocarditis

| Sign | Site and appearance |
|---|---|
| Petechiae | Conjunctiva, oral cavity, skin |
| Splinter hemorrhages | Linear subungual hemorrhages that do not reach the distal nail bed |
| Osler's nodes | Small painful red nodules in the distal phalanges |
| Janeway lesions | Small erythematous nontender macules on the palms and soles |
| Roth spots | Small white retinal infarcts surrounded by hemorrhage |

Modified from Lilly LS, Kloner RA. In Kloner RA, editor: *The guide to cardiology,* New York, 1984, Wiley.

### Prophylaxis

Patients with structural abnormalities of the heart have an increased risk of developing infective endocarditis from transient bacteremias that may be produced by invasive procedures. Dental care and procedures, bronchoscopy, cytoscopy, septic abortion, and needle biopsy procedures all may cause bacteremia. The Committee on Prevention of Bacterial Endocarditis of the American Heart Association recommends the prophylactic antibiotic regimens listed in Tables 14-3, 14-4, and 14-5. The major targets of these regimens are *Streptococcus viridans,* which is found in the upper respiratory tract and mouth, and enterococci from the gastrointestinal and genitourinary tracts. Prophylaxis is extremely important for the management of patients with prosthetic valves who must undergo invasive procedures. Antibiotic prophylaxis is not usually necessary for normal vaginal delivery, dilatation and curettage of the uterus, barium enema, sigmoidoscopy, and fiberoptic gastroscopy without biopsy.

## POSTOPERATIVE VALVULAR PATIENTS

Inaugurated by the pioneering ventures of Harken and Starr in 1960, surgical valve replacement rapidly burgeoned and completely transformed the approach to patients with valvular heart disease. Current estimates place the number of valve operations between 15,000 and 20,000 annually, which cumulatively projects to a large population of patients who require vigilant follow-up care. Obviously, it is impractical to expect the practitioner to command the minute details of individual artificial valves,

**Table 14-3.** Recommended standard prophylactic regimen for dental, oral, or upper respiratory tract procedures in patients at risk for subacute bacterial endocarditis*

| Drug | Dosing regimen† |
|---|---|
| **Standard regimen** | |
| Amoxicillin | 3.0 g orally 1 hr before procedure; then 1.5 g 6 hr after initial dose |
| **Amoxicillin/penicillin–allergic patients** | |
| Erythromycin | Erythromycin ethylsuccinate, 800 mg, or erythromycin stearate 1.0 g, orally 2 hr before procedure; then half the dose 6 hr after initial dose |
| or | |
| Clindamycin | 300 mg orally 1 hr before procedure and 150 mg 6 hr after initial dose |

*Includes those with prosthetic heart valves and other high-risk patients.

†Initial pediatric doses are as follows: amoxicillin, 50 mg/kg; erythromycin ethylsuccinate or erythromycin stearate, 20 mg/kg; and clindamycin, 10 mg/kg. Follow-up doses should be one half the initial dose. Total pediatric dose should not exceed total adult dose. The following weight ranges may also be used for the initial pediatric dose of amoxicillin: <15 kg, 750 mg; 15 to 30 kg, 1500 mg; and >30 kg, 3000 mg (full adult dose).

**Table 14-4.** Alternate prophylactic regimens for dental, oral, or upper respiratory tract procedures in patients at risk for subacute bacterial endocarditis

| Drug | Dosing regimen* |
|---|---|
| **Patients unable to take oral medications** | |
| Ampicillin | Intravenous or intramuscular administration of ampicillin, 2.0 g, 30 min before procedure; then intravenous or intramuscular administration of ampicillin, 1.0 g, or oral administration of amoxicillin, 1.5 g, 6 hr after initial dose |
| **Ampicillin/amoxicillin/penicillin–allergic patients unable to take oral medications** | |
| Clindamycin | Intravenous administration of 300 mg 30 min before procedure and an intravenous or oral administration of 150 mg 6 hr after initial dose |
| **Patients considered high risk and not candidates for standard regimen** | |
| Ampicillin, gentamicin, and amoxicillin | Intravenous or intramuscular administration of ampicillin, 2.0 g, plus gentamicin, 1.5 mg/kg (not to exceed 80 mg), 30 min before procedure; followed by amoxicillin, 1.5 g, orally 6 hr after initial dose; alternatively, the parenteral regimen may be repeated 6 hr after initial dose |
| **Ampicillin/amoxicillin/penicillin–allergic patients considered high risk** | |
| Vancomycin | Intravenous administration of 1.0 g over 1 hr, starting 1 hr before procedure; no repeated dose necessary |

*Initial pediatric doses are as follows: ampicillin, 50 mg/kg; clindamycin, 10 mg/kg; gentamycin, 2.0 mg/kg; and vancomycin, 20 mg/kg. Follow-up doses should be one half the initial dose. Total pediatric dose should not exceed total adult dose. No initial dose is recommended in this table for amoxicillin (25 mg/kg is the follow-up dose).

**Table 14-5.** Regimens for genitourinary/gastrointestinal procedures in patients at risk for subacute bacterial endocarditis

| Drug | Dosage regimen* |
|---|---|
| **Standard regimen** | |
| Ampicillin, gentamycin, and amoxicillin | Intravenous or intramuscular administration of ampicillin, 2.0 g, plus gentamicin, 1.5 mg/kg (not to exceed 80 mg), 30 min before procedure; followed by amoxicillin, 1.5 g, orally 6 hr after initial dose; alternatively, the parenteral regimen may be repeated once 6 hr after initial dose |
| **Ampicillin/amoxicillin/penicillin–allergic patient regimen** | |
| Vancomycin and gentamicin | Intravenous administration of vancomycin, 1.0 g, over 1 hr, plus intravenous or intramuscular administration of gentamicin, 1.5 mg/kg (not to exceed 80 mg), 1 hr before procedure; may be repeated once 8 hr after initial dose |
| **Alternate low-risk patient regimen** | |
| Amoxicillin | 3.0 g orally 1 hr before procedure; then 1.5 g 6 hr after initial dose |

*Initial pediatric doses are as follows: ampicillin, 50 mg/kg; amoxicillin, 50 mg/kg; gentamycin, 2.0 mg/kg; and vancomycin, 20 mg/kg. Follow-up doses should be half the initial dose. Total pediatric dose should not exceed total adult dose.

but design similarities allow manageable grouping, and the long-term complications remain the common denominator of all prostheses. Familiarity with these fundamental aspects is essential, considering the high probability that postoperative valvular patients are eventually encountered in any practice.

As a rule of thumb, operative mortality for the replacement of either aortic or mitral valve is about 3% to 5% and is approximately twice this figure for the double valve replacement. Similarly, the late postoperative mortality rate for a prosthesis in either the aortic or the mitral position is roughly 4% per year. After successful surgery, complications may be grouped into three major categories: (1) prosthetic valve failure, (2) thromboembolism and the hazards of anticoagulation, and (3) prosthetic endocarditis.

### Prosthetic valve failure

The majority of commonly implanted prostheses are assigned to one of four classes: (1) caged ball prostheses, epitomized by the Starr-Edwards valve, (2) caged disk prostheses, exemplified by the Beall-Surgitool valve, (3) tilting disk valves, of which the Bjork-Shiley is most common, and (4) bioprostheses.

Prosthetic valve dysfunction is usually not a consequence of structural failure of a mechanical prosthesis; problems such as poppet variance and disk erosion have been essentially eliminated by changes in components and design. Thus the term most often implies prosthetic obstruction or regurgitation; the former usually results from pannus ingrowth or thrombosis, and the latter is actually periprosthetic. Bioprosthetic tissue is obviously subject to dysfunction by erosion or scarring. The current

**Table 14-6.** Summary of auscultatory findings for the generic types of prosthetic valves in the aortic and mitral position

| | Mitral prosthesis | | Aortic prosthesis | |
|---|---|---|---|---|
| **Prosthesis type** | **Form** | **Acoustic characteristics** | **Form** | **Acoustic characteristics** |
| Ball valves | 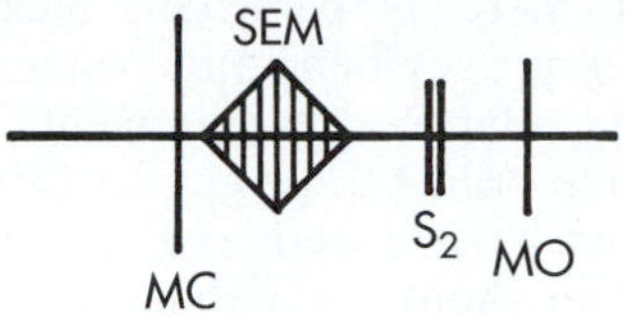  | $A_2$–MO interval<br>0.07–0.11 sec<br>MO > MC<br>II-III/VI SEM<br>No diastolic murmur | 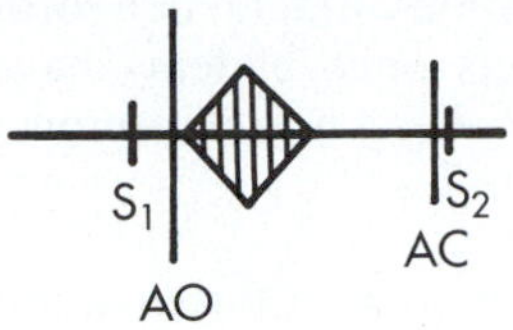  | $S_1$–AO interval 0.07 sec<br>AO > AC<br>II/VI harsh SEM<br>No diastolic murmur |
| Disk valves* | 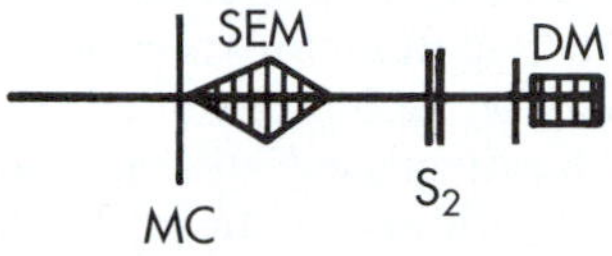  | $A_2$–MO interval<br>0.05–0.09 sec<br>MO rarely heard<br>II/VI SEM usually heard<br>I-II/VI diastolic rumble<br>heard occasionally | 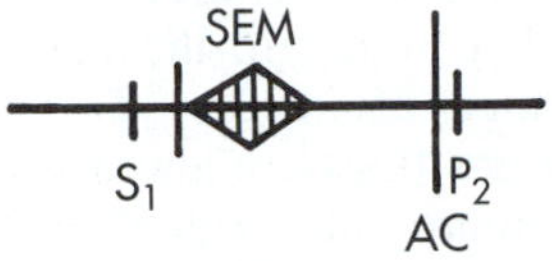  | $S_1$–AO interval 0.04 sec<br>AO uncommonly heard,<br>AC usually heard<br>II/VI SEM usually heard<br>No diastolic murmur |
| Porcine valves | 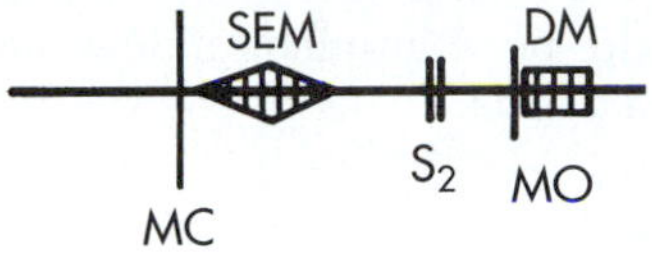  | $A_2$–MO interval 0.1 sec<br>MO audible 50%<br>I-II/VI apical SEM 50%<br>Diastolic rumble ½–⅔ | 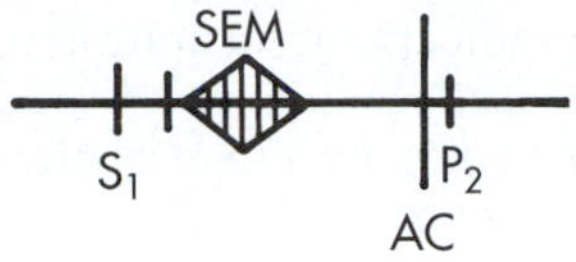  | $S_1$–AO interval 0.03–<br>0.08 sec<br>AO uncommonly heard,<br>AC usually heard<br>II/VI SEM in most<br>No diastolic murmur |

*SEM,* Systolic ejection murmur; *DM,* diastolic murmur; $S_1$, first heart sound; $S_2$, second heart sound; $P_2$, pulmonary second sound; *AO,* aortic opening sound; *AC,* aortic closure sound; *MO,* mitral opening sound; *MC,* mitral closure sound.
*The opening click of caged disk prostheses is usually prominent in contrast to the diagram, which applies to tilting disk valves.
Adapted from Smith ND, Raizda V, Abrams J: *Ann Intern Med* 95:594, 1981.

literature suggests an annual failure rate of about 1% over the first 5 years. Thereafter, a higher incidence of dysfunction seems to apply, but precise figures await longer follow-up.

***Physical examination.*** Auscultatory expectations vary with the type of prosthesis and are summarized in Table 14-6. The caged ball prostheses generate prominent opening and closure clicks. In the aortic position, multiple systolic clicks superimposed on a harsh ejection murmur result from the bounce of the ball in the cage. A systolic murmur with this valve in the mitral position is related to ventricular outflow turbulence created by the cage and need not imply mitral regurgitation. Caged disk prostheses are usually used in the mitral position and produce soft opening and louder closure clicks, both of which are less prominent than the caged ball sounds. Opening clicks with the tilting disk valves are faint and very often inaudible, but a distinct closure sound is present. Systolic murmurs may be associated with normal tilting disk valves in the aortic or mitral position, as well as a brief diastolic murmur in the aortic position. A diastolic mitral murmur may occur with high flow rates across the mitral valve, but prosthetic dysfunction should be considered. Mitral bioprostheses may normally impart an opening snap and a brief diastolic rumble. An ejection murmur with normal intensity of the closure sound is typical of the aortic bioprosthesis.

It is important to establish a reference baseline by meticulous examination soon after valve replacement. More important than the results of a given examination are changes from the baseline that cannot be accounted for by changes in hemodynamic state, such as variable intensity of opening and closure sounds with atrial fibrillation or enhancement of murmurs by anemia. Disappearance of a previously audible opening or closure click alerts the examiner to possible prosthetic dysfunction, although it is well recognized that even severe prosthetic abnormalities may develop without detectable auscultatory evidence. Beat-to-beat alteration in prosthetic sound intensity always suggests dysfunction. Any suggestion of prosthetic failure is a basis for urgent referral.

Recurrence of symptoms after surgery need not necessarily imply prosthetic malfunction. Congestive symptoms may, for example, relate to persistence of preoperative ventricular dysfunction, impaired ventricular function acquired during surgery, or the mismatch of valve to patient. Evaluation of such symptoms always requires some assessment of ventricular function in addition to studies focused primarily on valve function. Symptoms of valve dysfunction may be cataclysmic, such as acute valvular thrombosis, but are more often indolent. Progressive fatigue, dyspnea, dizziness, syncope, angina, or transient neurologic symptoms are regarded with a high index of suspicion in patients with artificial valves.

Noninvasive studies have a role in detecting prosthetic valve dysfunction. M-mode echo alone is insensitive in directly identifying prosthetic abnormalities, but transesophageal echocardiography is often useful. A variety of other echo findings provide indirect evidence of abnormal valve function. Baseline evaluation at 6 to 8 weeks after surgery provides a basis for future comparison and resolves confusion about whether findings such as a soft murmur of aortic insufficiency detected at late follow-up represent new problems or have simply been undetectable by stethoscope. Echocardiography is the modality of choice in evaluation of bioprostheses. Cinefluoroscopy is also helpful in experienced hands. In selected instances strong noninvasive evidence favoring prosthetic dysfunction is sufficient grounds for reoperation without catheterization.

Although some hemolysis occurs with all mechanical prostheses, an increase in the degree of hemolysis suggests valve dysfunction. Determination of lactic dehydrogenase (LDH) and haptoglobin levels once patients have fully recovered from surgery establishes a useful reference base.

### Thromboembolism

For anticoagulated patients, the risk of thromboembolism from a mechanical aortic prosthesis averages 2% per year or less. The risk is somewhat higher in the case of the mitral prosthesis, approximately 5%. Figures for bioprostheses in the corresponding positions are about the same, but few of these patients require anticoagulation beyond the immediate postoperative period. This is the major advantage of these valves. Atrial fibrillation and marked left atrial enlargement are indications for long-term anticoagulation with bioprostheses. Estimates of significant hemorrhage in anticoagulated patients range as high as 6% to 8% annually with severe episodes in 2% and related fatality in about 0.5%. An isolated thromboembolic event should not occasion extensive evaluation in the absence of other suggestions of valve dysfunction. Recurrent embolization within a short time span may be managed by addition of aspirin and dipyridamole (Persantine) to a demonstrably adequate coumadin regimen and consideration of replacement of a mechanical valve with a bioprosthesis.

Anticoagulation should probably be temporarily withheld following embolic stroke until the possibility of a hemorrhagic component can be clarified. For major surgery, dental extractions, gynecologic procedures, or diagnostic procedures that may eventuate in surgery, anticoagulation is usually discontinued 1 to 3 days beforehand.

The administration of vitamin K is discouraged. The literature provides no support for the interim use of heparin in most circumstances, and oral anticoagulation may be safely restarted as soon as is feasible after surgery. The Bjork-Shiley prosthesis is an apparent exception to this general rule, and heparinization except for the period of highest risk of hemorrhage is advisable. The potential for developmental defects during the first trimester and the unpredictable need for restitution of normal coagulation at delivery provides the rationale for the substitution of twice daily subcutaneous heparin for coumadin during the first 3 months and again for the last 2 or 3 weeks before term in pregnant women with prostheses.

### Prosthetic endocarditis

Prosthetic valve infection occurs at a rate of about 1% annually. Endocarditis manifesting within 2 months of surgery is most often caused by *Staphylococcus epidermidis, Staphylococcus aureus,* or gram-negative bacilli. The mortality rate, despite effective antibiotic therapy, remains at about 50% to 75%. Because infection with mechanical prostheses is paravalvular, which reduces the likelihood of successful eradication with antibiotics alone, many favor obligatory operation as part of the treatment program, usually after a period of 1 to 2 weeks of drug therapy. Infection of tissue valves may be confined to the leaflets, which portends a favorable response to antibiotics.

Late endocarditis is more often of streptococcal etiology and carries a lower mortality risk, usually in the range of 40% to 50%. Removal of an infected prosthesis is indicated if there is persistent bacteremia despite appropriate therapy, evidence of valve dehiscence or dysfunction, and relapse after treatment.

There are three points to be emphasized. Patients with prosthetic valves have a high risk of endocarditis with bacteremia and so should be imbued with a strong sense of the need for antibiotic prophylaxis during dental and other procedures; parenteral regimens are preferred. Embolization may be an indication of prosthetic infection and should not be dismissed without some evaluation in this regard. The limited data available suggest that cerebrovascular morbidity is higher if anticoagulation is stopped during the course of prosthetic endocarditis; thus coumadin should be continued unless another specific contraindication arises.

## BIBLIOGRAPHY

Assey ME, Spann JF: Indications for heart valve replacement, *Clin Cardiol* 13:81, 1990.

Braunwald E: Mitral regurgitation: physiologic clinical and surgical considerations, *N Engl J Med* 281:425, 1969.

Dalen JE, Alpert JS: *Valvular heart disease,* ed 2, Boston, 1987, Little, Brown.

Devereux RB et al: Mitral valve prolapse, *Circulation* 54:3, 1976.

Kennedy JW, Doces J, Stewart DK: Left ventricular function before and following aortic valve replacement, *Circulation* 56:944, 1977.

Lilly LS, Kloner RA: Infective endocarditis. In Kloner RA, editor: *The guide to cardiology,* New York, 1984, Wiley.

Morganroth J: Acute severe aortic regurgitation: pathophysiology, clinical recognition and management, *Ann Intern Med* 87:223, 1977.

Rahimtoola SH: Perspective on valvular heart disease: an update, *J Am Coll Cardiol* 14:1, 1989.

Rapaport E: Natural history of aortic and mitral valve disease, *Am J Cardiol* 35:221, 1975.

Samuels DA et al: Valve replacement for aortic regurgitation: long-term followup with factors influencing the results, *Circulation* 60:647, 1979.

Schuler G et al: Temporal response of left ventricular performance to mitral valve surgery, *Circulation* 59:1218, 1979.

Wood P: An appreciation of mitral stenosis. Part I. Clinical features, *Br Med J* 1:1051, 1954; Part II. Investigation and results, *Br Med J* 1:1113, 1954.

CHAPTER

# 15 Adult Manifestations of Congenital Heart Disease

**Edgar C. Schick, Jr.**

The adult practitioner is likely to confront a considerably narrower spectrum of congenital heart disease than the pediatrician. Even among major adult referral centers, congenital defects seldom constitute more than 5% of all cases; of those, atrial septal defects account for about half, with coarctation of aorta, patent ductus arteriosus, and pulmonic stenosis comprising the bulk of the remainder. Unmodified cyanotic congenital disease, in which surgical correction or palliation has not been attempted, has essentially vanished from adult practice and has been supplanted by either long-term surgical survivors with persistent intracardiac shunts or those with irremediable pulmonary hypertension resulting from congenital shunt—patients who are no longer candidates for primary correction.

Despite this restricted purview, some contact with congenital heart patients, whether undiagnosed, corrected (with or without residua), or palliated, is virtually certain in any practice, particularly as more subjects of corrective surgery survive beyond childhood. The incidence of congenital defects in the United States is approximately 1% of all live births, and it is estimated that at least 8500 individuals who have undergone repair reach adulthood annually. By the late 1990s, projections indicate that the population of adult survivors of congenital heart disease will reach 500,000. Although patients with the more complex and esoteric disorders are customarily followed at specialized centers, the growing number of survivors guarantees at least limited encounters with congenital cardiac patients and mandates some familiarity with the fundamental and modified pathophysiology of the more common conditions.

## CLASSIFICATION

Several systems for classifying congenital disease have been derived from anatomic, physiologic, and even radiographic perspectives, but no single schema is entirely satisfactory and utility is often lost in detail. Fundamentally, congenital defects dichotomize into the cyanotic or acyanotic category. The acyanotic group is further divided by the presence of either left-to-right shunting of blood via some systemic-to-pulmonary connection producing increased pulmonary blood flow or valvular and other abnormalities in the absence of a shunt. Cyanotic congenital disease can be subcategorized according to whether there is obstruction to right heart flow at any level from the pulmonary arterioles (Eisenmenger syndrome) to the tricuspid valve with decreased pulmonary blood flow as a result, intracardiac lesions that allow arteriovenous admixture, or the presence of abnormal relationships between the great vessels.

## ACYANOTIC CONGENITAL DISEASE WITHOUT SHUNT

### Pulmonic stenosis

Most commonly, pulmonic stenosis narrows the semilunar valve proper, but, as with left ventricular outflow obstruction, the subvalvular and supravalvular counterparts also occur. The former is usually muscular and involves the infundibulum, whereas the latter may involve the main pulmonary arteries or smaller peripheral branches. Pulmonic stenosis imposes a systolic pressure burden on the right ventricle that stimulates right ventricular hypertrophy. Symptoms in this disorder reflect an inability to increase cardiac output because of the systolic afterload imposed on the right ventricle and the right heart failure that may ensue. Exertional fatigue and dyspnea are common complaints; chest pain and syncope are encountered less frequently. Patients with mild-to-moderate degrees of obstruction, usually defined as a peak transvalvular gradient of 80 mm Hg or less, may remain asymptomatic well into adult life. More severe obstruction, with gradients exceeding 80 mm Hg, portends a less favorable course and warrants early intervention.

The clinical findings generally correlate well with the results of catheterization. Mild pulmonic stenosis is implied by a crescendo-decrescendo murmur at the upper left sternal edge that ends well before aortic valve closure (Fig. 15-1). A prolonged systolic murmur, which may extend beyond and obscure the sound of aortic closure, suggests more severe obstruction. The pulmonic component of the second heart sound becomes muffled or absent because of valvular thickening; when it is audible, the second sound is widely split. A pulmonic ejection click is typically present, and with increasingly severe stenosis the click migrates toward the first heart sound. Further markers of severe stenosis include a prominent jugular "a" wave, signifying a hypertrophic and relatively noncompliant right ventricle, a right ventricular lift, a systolic thrill along the left sternal edge, and an $S_4$ gallop that intensifies on inspiration. Mild cyanosis may develop

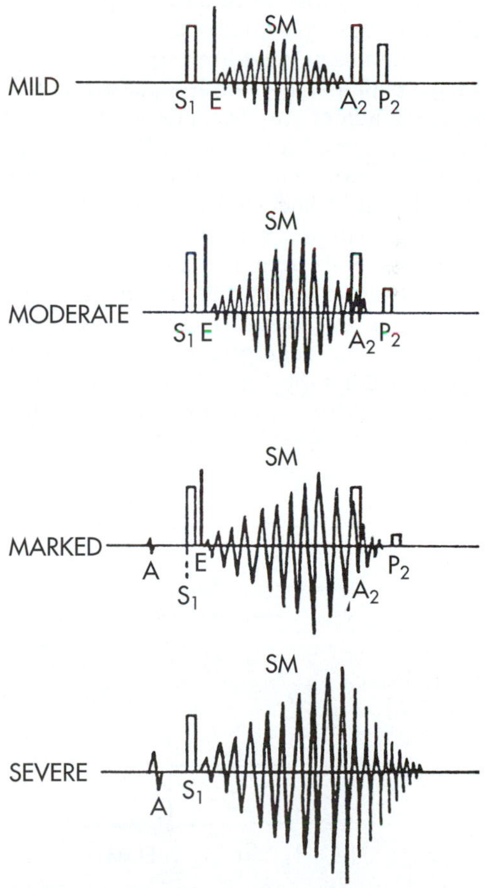


**Fig. 15-1.** Auscultatory findings in congenital pulmonic stenosis. With increasing severity, the duration of the murmur *(SM)* is prolonged and the intensity of the pulmonic closure *($P_2$)* diminishes. *$S_1$*, First heart sound; *E*, pulmonic ejection click; *$A_2$*, aortic closure. (From Perloff JK: The clinical recognition of congenital heart disease, Philadelphia, 1970, Saunders.)

if a patent foramen ovale is present, permitting some degree of right-to-left shunting at the atrial level.

The electrocardiogram (ECG) is usually normal with mild pulmonic stenosis and exhibits evidence of right ventricular hypertrophy and right atrial enlargement with increasing severity. The x-ray may show so-called post-stenotic dilatation of the main pulmonary artery as the only abnormality. This finding confirms suspected valvular stenosis, but does not correlate with the level of the gradient. Right ventricular and right atrial prominence imply more severe outflow obstruction. Echocardiography affords direct visualization of not only the pulmonic valve but the ventricular outflow tract and the proximal pulmonary artery as well. This allows both precise identification of the level of obstruction and assessment of right ventricular wall thickness and function. Doppler flow measurements usually provide accurate derivation of the stenotic pressure gradient.

Mild pulmonary stenosis carries an excellent prognosis. Patients with evidence of mild stenosis during adolescence are unlikely to develop problems later. However, severe stenosis provides grounds for intervention, and patients with findings suggesting this possibility require cardiology evaluation. Patients in whom the measured gradient falls in the moderate range, i.e., between 50 and 80 mm Hg, may do well for extended periods; but natural history studies indicate that the majority eventually require intervention and merit cardiology consultation.

Balloon pulmonary valvuloplasty, the procedure of choice in most patients, has a high success rate in reducing the valvular gradient to acceptable levels. Surgical valvulotomy is reserved for those with suboptimal results. The pulmonic insufficiency resulting from these procedures is usually mild and well-tolerated, particularly by younger patients. Adults, who tolerate regurgitation less well, may infrequently require valve replacement. Post-operatively, a systolic murmur almost invariably persists, although with a decreased intensity. A low-pitched, rumbling pulmonary regurgitant murmur is common. Periodic echocardiography is useful early after valvuloplasty to assess stability of the result. Serial echocardiography is not indicated in patients with mild stenosis because of the extremely low probability of progressive worsening of the stenosis.

### Aortic stenosis

Aortic stenosis is discussed in detail in Chapter 14.

### Coarctation of aorta

Coarctation, a narrowing of the aorta by a fibrous dorsal invagination usually at or just beyond the origin of the left subclavian artery, is one of the correctable causes of hypertension. Coarctation is more common in male subjects and is occasionally associated with Turner syndrome. As a result of the excessive afterload imposed by the coarctation, heart failure may occur during infancy; however, the condition is frequently well-tolerated into adult life. Beyond age 40, however, symptoms of congestive failure become the rule. There is a relatively high coincidence of other abnormalities in infants, particularly patent ductus arteriosus, ventricular septal defect, and defects of the mitral valve. In those individuals undetected until adulthood, the most common associated abnormality is a bicuspid aortic valve (see Chapter 14). Complications encountered with coarctation include bacterial endarteritis at the site of the coarctation or endocarditis involving the bicuspid aortic valve, stroke from cerebral aneurysms, aortic dissection, and rupture.

Most patients with coarctation display evidence of upper torso hypertension; however, this may be undetected in the left arm if the left subclavian artery is involved in the narrowed segment.

On rare occasions arm hypertension may be absent altogether in the case of aberrant origin of the right subclavian artery distal to the coarctation. The carotid pulses are bounding, and a prominent suprasternal pulse may be present. Palpation may disclose a damped or even absent femoral pulse, but delayed arrival of the femoral pulse compared to the radial artery is a more diagnostically specific characteristic. Additional systolic or diastolic murmurs arising from associated aortic valve disease are common (Fig. 15-2).

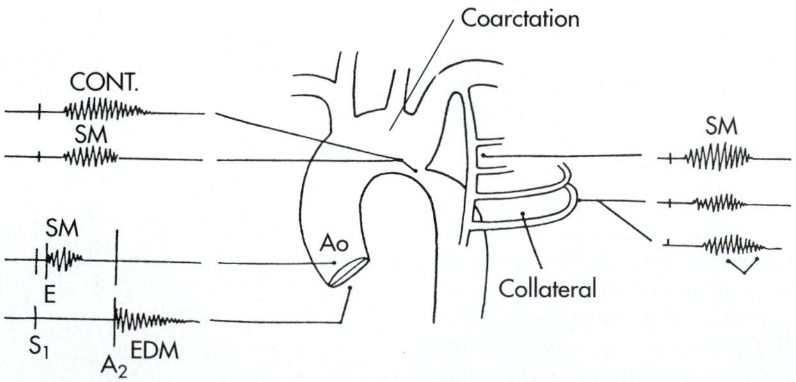


**Fig. 15-2.** Auscultatory findings in aortic coarctation. The click *(E)*, systolic murmur, and early diastolic murmur *(EDM)* at the base are related to the associated bicuspid aortic valve. A continuous murmur may be audible along the upper left sternum in the region of the coarctation, and a murmur may also be audible in more lateral and posterior intercostal spaces as a result of turbulent collateral flow. (From Perloff JK: The clinical recognition of congenital heart disease, Philadelphia, 1970, Saunders.)

The ECG, often unremarkable in the early stages, is likely to manifest evidence of left ventricular hypertrophy in adults. The chest x-ray usually displays normal heart size. A dilated transverse aorta and the poststenotic dilatation of the descending aorta may create a "figure-three" sign along the upper left cardiac margin (Fig. 15-3). Rib notching is related to intercostal collateral development, and when evident, becomes apparent after childhood, usually involving the third to eighth ribs posteriorly. Echocardiography from the suprasternal area provides direct visualization of the coarctated segment, particularly in younger patients, as well as estimation of the pressure gradient by Doppler velocimetry, even when the coarctation is not imaged clearly; ultrasound also effectively characterizes associated cardiac abnormalities.

Referral for cardiologic evaluation is recommended in all instances of suspected coarctation. Uncorrected, this anomaly shortens expected life span; in older series nearly 90% of the patients succumbed before age 50. Aortography to delineate the coarctation site and the degree of collateralization is indicated in all cases (Fig. 15-4). Surgical repair during childhood remains the preferred treatment. Operative approaches devised to eliminate the coarctation include resection and primary reanastomosis, ligation of the subclavian artery and conversion of its proximal segment into a plicating flap, patch aortoplasty, and prosthetic grafts, either interposed at the coarctation site or bypassing it. Previous reports suggested a high rate of recoarctation when repair was undertaken during infancy, but improved surgical technique appears to have eliminated the problem. Considerable enthusiasm greeted early reports of balloon catheter dilatation of coarctation. Although several centers report excellent initial results compared to surgery, debate continues over the long-term outcome, specifically focusing on residual gradients and aneurysm formation at the dilatation site; surgery is preferred in most centers.

After childhood, the earlier the correction the more favorable the results. This is primarily because of a progressive increase in the incidence of postoperative hypertension with age. Disregarding acute postoperative hypertensive crisis, which is seldom a serious problem with modern pharmacotherapy, data suggest a 25% incidence of hypertension after correction if surgery is performed before age 10 and about 50% thereafter. There is a small risk of paraplegia because of spinal cord ischemia during surgical repair. Despite corrective surgery, coarctation patients remain subject to such problems as cerebral aneurysm rupture, progression of aortic valve disease, and infective endocarditis. Available studies suggest that a majority of patients display some evidence of persistent cardiovascular abnormality at late follow-up after coarctation repair.

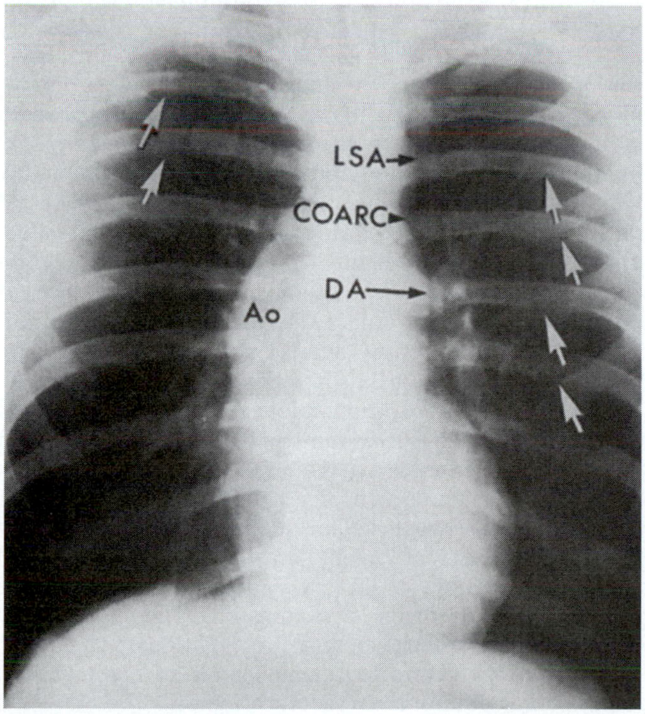


**Fig. 15-3.** Chest film from a patient with aortic coarctation illustrating the components that contribute to the "figure-three" sign. The convexity of the left subclavian artery *(LSA)* and the descending aorta *(DA)* separated by the indentation of the coarctation create the "3." The dilated ascending aorta *(Ao)* is also notable, as well as rib notching *(arrows)*. (From Perloff JK: The clinical recognition of congenital heart disease, 1970, Saunders.)

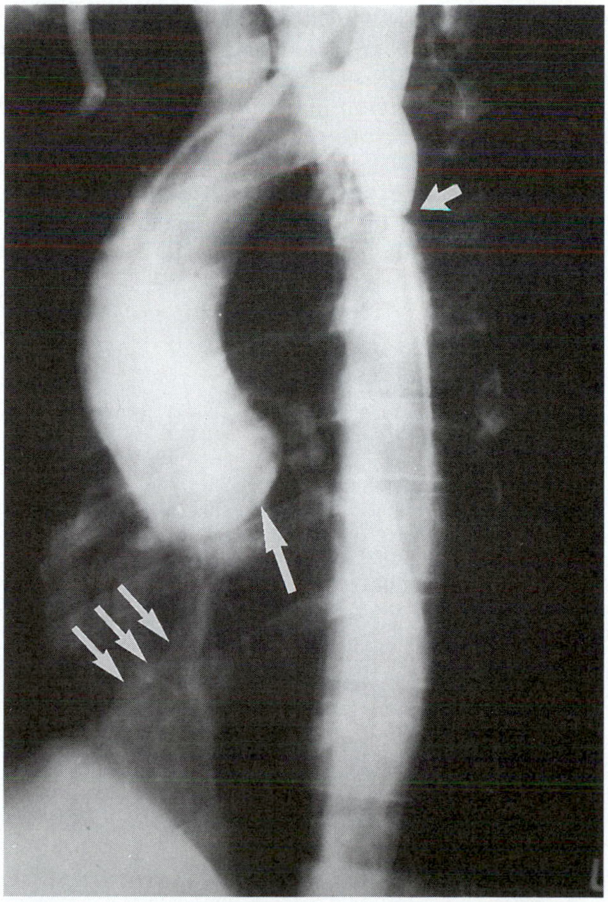

**Fig. 15-4.** Aortogram from a patient with coarctation. The coarctation is well visualized *(upper arrow)* beyond the origin of the left subclavian artery. A bicuspid aortic valve is also present *(lower arrow)* with a faint blush of aortic regurgitation *(arrows)*.

## ACYANOTIC CONGENITAL DISEASE WITH SHUNT

### Atrial septal defect

Atrial septal defect (ASD), the most common intracardiac shunt diagnosed in the adult, frequently eludes early detection because its characteristic features are absent at birth and may be subtle enough to escape recognition in childhood. Symptoms frequently do not emerge until midlife or late adult life. Defects of the atrial septum occur more frequently in women, and may be hereditary in some instances, notably in conjunction with hypoplastic abnormalities of the thumb and forearm as part of Holt-Oram syndrome.

Of the several types of ASD, the septum secundum defect is most common (Fig. 15-5). It is located in the midatrial septum, circumscribing the usual site of the fossa ovalis, the landmark corresponding to the fetal foramen ovale. Even in the absence of detectable shunting, the limbs of the foramen frequently fail to fuse and may provide a potential interatrial communication in up to 30% of adults. Less common septal defects involve other portions of the atrial septum. Defects in the low atrial septum are septum primum defects, and are usually accompanied by clefts in the atrioventricular valves. Communications located high in the atrial septum are sinus venosus defects and are often associated with both anomalous pulmonary venous return to the right atrium and abnormalities of the sinus node. Rarely, defects involve the posterior atrial septum, accompanied by absence of the coronary sinus and persistence of a left superior vena cava.

Diversion of flow from the left to the right atrium via the ASD occurs because the more compliant right ventricle offers less resistance to diastolic flow. The result is volume overload of the right heart and the pulmonary circuit. Commensurate with the course of other chronic volume overload states, this burden is usually well-tolerated

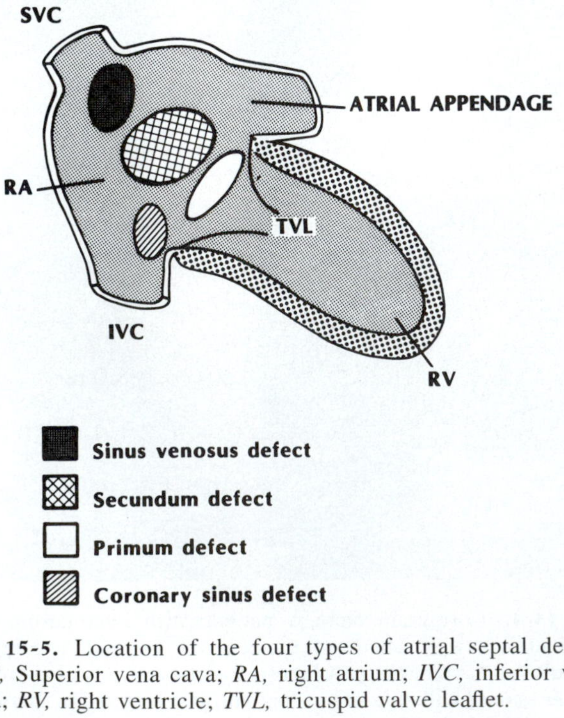


**Fig. 15-5.** Location of the four types of atrial septal defect. *SVC,* Superior vena cava; *RA,* right atrium; *IVC,* inferior vena cava; *RV,* right ventricle; *TVL,* tricuspid valve leaflet.

throughout young adult life, but thereafter complications begin to appear. Symptoms predominantly reflect right ventricular decompensation, and are occasionally abetted by development of pulmonary hypertension. Left-to-right shunting may actually increase with age, particularly if superimposed processes, such as hypertension or coronary disease, produce elevation of filling pressures in the left heart. Supraventricular arrhythmias, facilitated by atrial enlargement (most importantly atrial fibrillation), contribute substantially to morbidity.

Exertional dyspnea, probably caused by the increased lung blood volume, is a frequent complaint of patients with ASD. Overt right heart failure begins to appear after age 30. Although the incidence of pulmonary hypertension increases with age, obliterative pulmonary vascular disease sufficient to result in shunt reversal (Eisenmenger syndrome) develops in fewer than 5% of patients. The association between secundum ASD and mitral valve prolapse has received considerable attention, with an incidence in excess of 50% reported in some series. Mitral regurgitation severe enough to warrant consideration of valve repair or replacement is, however, unusual.

On physical examination, a dynamic systolic impulse immediately to the left of the sternum should direct attention to the possibility of increased volume flow through the right heart. A brief, flow-related systolic ejection murmur is usually audible in the pulmonic area. The two components of the second heart sound are widely split during expiration with imperceptible variation on inspiration. This phenomenon, referred to as fixed splitting, constitutes the single most important and most frequently overlooked or misinterpreted clue to the presence of a shunt. Wide, fixed splitting of $S_2$, a nearly universal finding with ASD in younger patients, may become less consistent in older adults and when pulmonary hypertension develops. However, any expiratory splitting of the second sound in adults unexplained by right bundle branch block should bring suspicion of ASD to the fore. An audible diastolic rumble at the lower left sternal edge, created by torrential flow across the tricuspid valve, almost invariably indicates a significant left-to-right shunt. A midsystolic click may be audible over the apex if mitral valve prolapse coincides, and a murmur of mitral regurgitation may represent either mitral prolapse or a mitral valve cleft in the case of an ostium primum defect.

The ECG pattern of incomplete right bundle branch is present in about 90% of patients with ASD. Associated left axis deviation connotes a defect of the endocardial cushion and predicts the presence of a primum ASD. An abnormally leftward P-wave vector suggests the possibility of sinus venosus defect, which may disrupt normal atrial activation. Marked right axis deviation implies the presence of pulmonary hypertension. The chest x-ray reveals variable enlargement of the right heart chambers, dilatation of the central pulmonary arteries, and a pattern of peripheral pulmonary vascular plethora (Fig. 15-6).

Thanks to recent advances in color flow and transesophageal imaging, echocardiography provides for complete anatomic and physiologic characterization of ASD in most patients. Not only can available techniques define the presence of interatrial communication by indirect means (Fig. 15-7) and delineate associated abnormalities in great detail, they can also directly visualize and size the defect from the esophageal approach, and estimate shunt flow and pulmonary artery pressure with reasonable accuracy. These advances have eliminated the need for catheterization in most younger patients with a straightforward anomaly.

To deter late complications of ASD, repair is recommended for all patients with evidence of a physiologically significant shunt, e.g., right atrial and right ventricular enlargement or (in more traditional terms) calculated pulmonary to systemic flow ratios of 1.5:1 or more. Although older literature suggests a significant increase in the risk of surgical closure in the presence of increased pulmonary arteriolar resistance and pulmonary hypertension, recent series indicate that ASDs may be safely corrected even in patients over age 60 with markedly elevated pulmonary resistance, as long as a net left-to-right shunt is present. Shunt reversal, however, precludes surgical closure. Despite evidence that normal function is unlikely to be fully restored, overt right ventricular failure should not deter surgery, which arrests an otherwise progressive process. Promising reports of transvenous closure of secundum defects by catheter deployment of a double umbrella-like device have appeared, but these devices are not yet available for widespread clinical application.

Postoperatively, evidence of volume overload regresses, but wide, fixed splitting of the second heart sound, as well as complete right bundle branch block and x-ray evidence of pulmonary plethora, may persist indefinitely. Antibiotic prophylaxis is not recommended for the uncomplicated secundum ASD, but is necessary both preoperatively and postoperatively with a primum defect or when mitral valve prolapse with mitral regurgitation coexists.

## Ventricular septal defect

Ventricular septal defects (VSDs) are currently categorized according to a four component model of the interventricular septum (Fig. 15-8). Defects tend to occur along the boundaries of these segments. Perimembranous septal defects involving or immediately adjacent to the membranous septum are by far the most common. They are found at the base of the interventricular septum immediately behind the septal leaflet of the tricuspid valve and below the crista supraventricularis, a muscular bar that separates the right ventricular inflow and outflow tracts. Typically, these defects lie subjacent to the right coronary

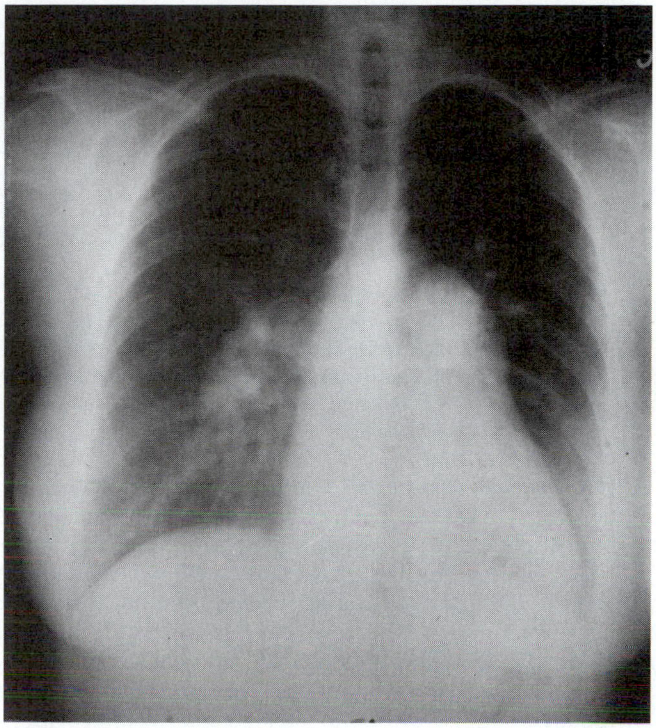

**Fig. 15-6.** Posteroanterior chest film from a patient with a secundum atrial septal defect (3.7:1 pulmonary-systemic flow ratio) and normal pulmonary artery pressures. Note the dilatation of the main pulmonary artery segment, which obscures the left pulmonary artery, and the prominent right pulmonary artery and branches.

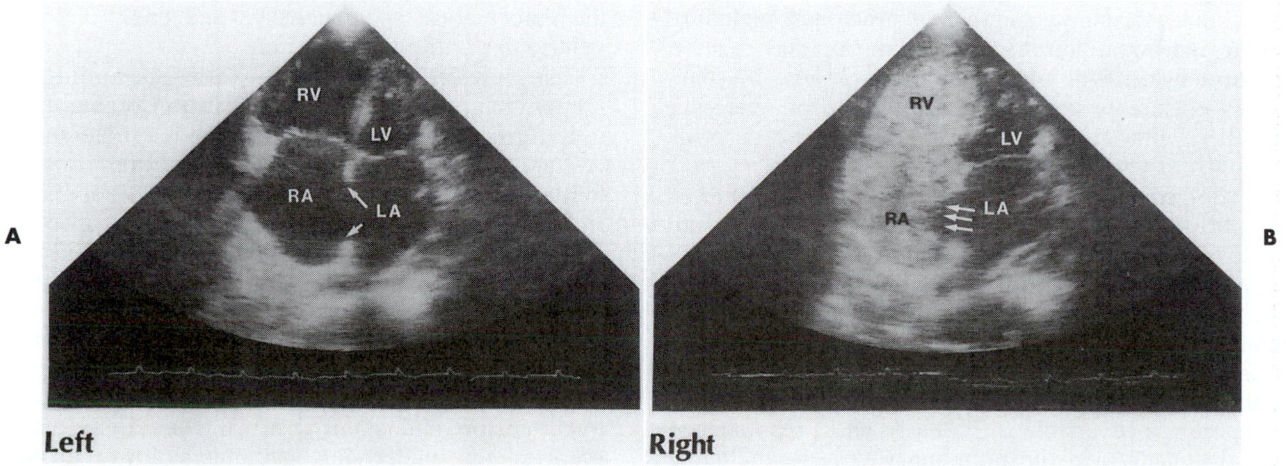


**Fig. 15-7.** Two-dimensional contrast echocardiogram from the apex in a patient with a secundum atrial septal defect. Baseline (**A**) shows enlargement of the right atrium *(RA)* and ventricle *(RV)*. Apparent discontinuity of the interatrial septum is evident *(arrows)* but is not diagnostic of ASD. Echo contrast injected from an antecubital vein (**B**) has now completely opacified the right atrium and ventricle. The dark area extending into the RA across the atrial septum *(arrows)* is created by left-to-right flow of contrast-free blood across a spetal defect and confirms the diagnosis. *LA*, Left atrium; *LV*, left ventricle.

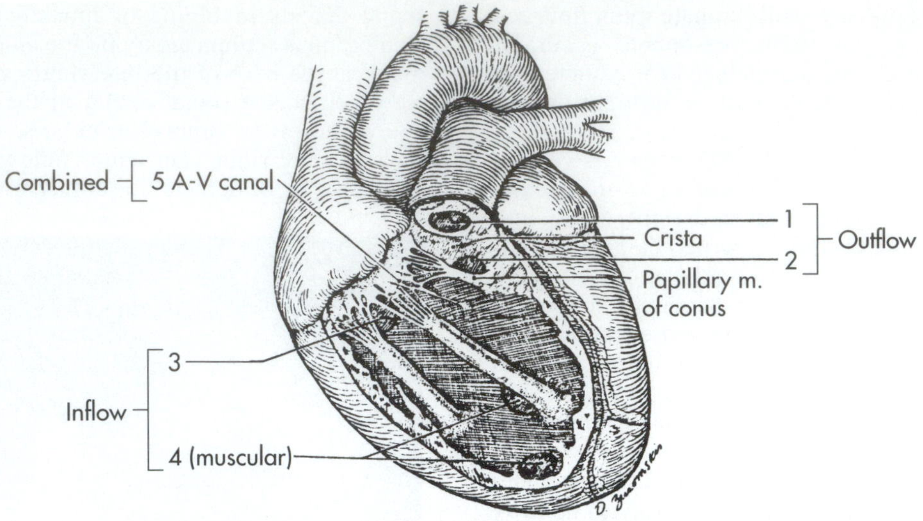


**Fig. 15-8.** Most common locations of ventricular septal defects seen through the right ventricle. Inflow and outflow tracts are indicated as well as the position of supracristal (1) and infracristal (2) defects. The AV canal defect is a variety of endocardial cushion defect and lies behind the tricuspid valve as indicated. (From Nadas AS, Flyer DC: *Pediatric cardiology,* Philadelphia, 1972, WB Saunders)

cusp on the left side of the septum. Muscular defects, the second most common VSD, may involve any of the other three segments and are often multiple.

A spectrum of physiologic derangement is possible with a defect in the interventricular septum, ranging from pure volume overload of both ventricles to pure pressure overload of the right ventricle (Eisenmenger syndrome). The governing features are the size of the defect and pulmonary outflow (vascular) resistance. Volume effects predominate when large defects concur with low pulmonary resistance, whereas both pressure and volume overload of the right ventricle ensue if pulmonary resistance increases.

VSDs are more common in infants and children than in adults, since about 30% of these defects close spontaneously during childhood. Spontaneous closure of the defects occurs through a number of processes, including muscular ingrowth, fibrous encroachment, and relative diminution by growth of surrounding tissues. In some instances closure is secondary to adhesion of overlying tricuspid valvular tissue, prolapse of an aortic cusp, or formation of a ventricular septal aneurysm.

Of major concern is the potential for development of irreversible pulmonary vascular disease, which may preclude surgical correction. Pulmonary vascular resistance, normally high at birth, decreases over the first few weeks of life. Pressure and volume overload of the pulmonary circulation may prevent or reverse this process with persistence or reappearance of elevated pulmonary resistance and pulmonary pressures. Although this abnormal response is reversible in its early phases, associated pathologic changes in the pulmonary vessels, including thickened arterial media and intima, may eventuate in irreversible pulmonary hypertension. Ultimately, pulmonary resistance may rise to levels that reverse the direction of net interventricular shunting; at this point, surgical intervention is no longer feasible. Since irreversible changes may develop within the first 2 years of life, infants with evidence of a significant VSD are carefully observed. It is now unusual to be confronted by an uncorrected, large VSD with pulmonary hypertension in adults.

Irreversible, obliterative pulmonary vascular disease evolves only in patients with large shunts and significantly elevated pulmonary artery pressures. Small VSDs increase pulmonary flow only slightly; patients with those defects, the so-called maladie de Roger, are not liable to this complication. Serial catheterizations demonstrate hemodynamic stability or a reduction in shunt magnitude and pulmonary resistance in most patients with VSD. Occasionally muscular hypertrophy of the infundibulum develops, producing a degree of right ventricular outflow obstruction (Fig. 15-9) that elevates right ventricular pressures and lessens the shunt. One study indicated that of every ten VSD patients observed with serial catheterization, seven show no change in hemodynamics, two have the defect close spontaneously, and one develops right ventricular outflow obstruction.

The physical examination varies according to the predominant physiologic abnormality. Commonly, a systolic thrill is palpable along the lower left sternal border. A loud, harsh, often pansystolic murmur, one that is loudest along the left sternal border and radiating to the right, is characteristic. Absent at birth because of high pulmonary resistance in the neonatal period, the murmur gradually becomes evident during the first several weeks of life as the high resistance regresses, allowing increased left-to-right flow across the defect. Later the murmur may shorten in duration and disappear altogether because of either spontaneous closure or the advent of pulmonary hypertension and shunt reversal. The ECG accurately predicts the underlying pathophysiology, manifesting evidence of left atrial and left ventricular enlargement in the presence of predominant volume overload, right ventricular hypertrophy with increased pulmonary pressure, or both with balanced lesions. Chest roentgenographic findings similarly vary. Echocardiography, particularly color flow imaging, provides excellent anatomic localization of VSDs, estimation of shunt magnitude, and

A

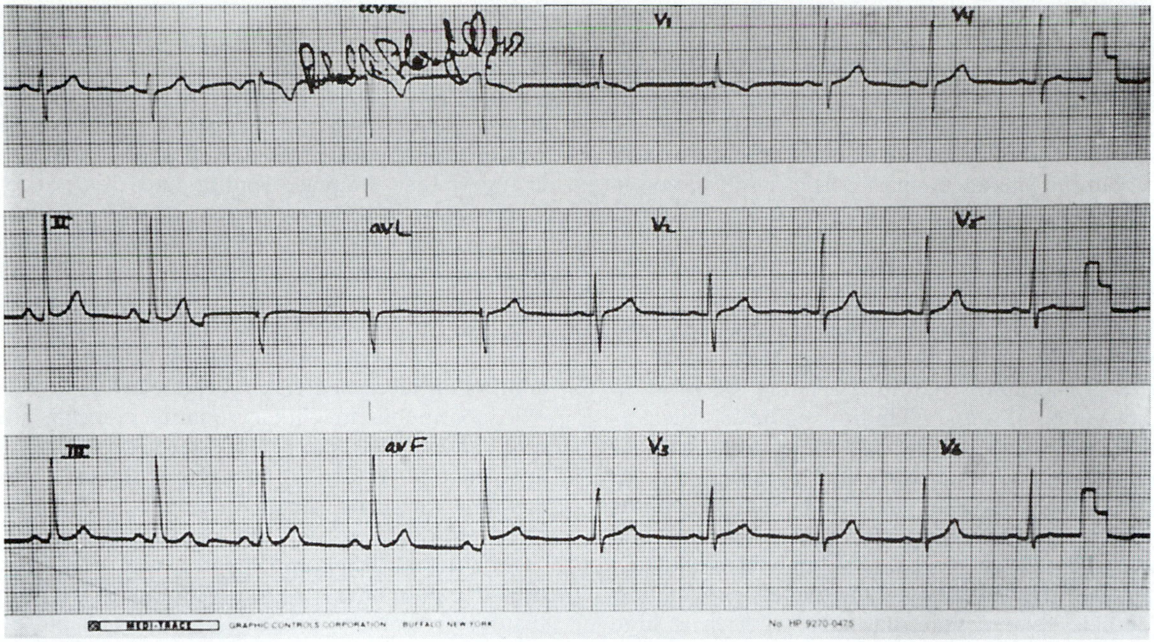


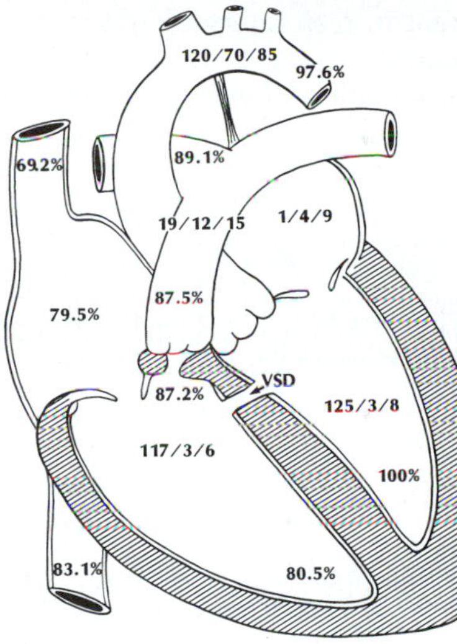


B

**Fig. 15-9. A,** ECG from a 28-year-old man with a childhood history of CHF and a holosystolic murmur consistent with VSD. There is right axis deviation with prominent R waves in lead $V_1$ indicative of right ventricular hypertrophy. **B,** Catheterization results demonstrate a VSD with an oxygen step-up at the right ventricular outflow level and a 100 mm Hg subvalvular gradient in the right ventricular outflow tract. These findings are consistent with acquired right ventricular outflow obstruction (Gasul phenomenon).

derivation of right ventricular and pulmonary artery systolic pressures.

The patient with the murmur of VSD without symptoms, evidence of significant volume overload, or pulmonary hypertension requires only endocarditis prophylaxis. The risk of endocarditis is low, as indicated by the 1.9 cases per 1000 patient years found in a large cooperative study. Congestive failure, usually occurring during infancy, or other suggestion of a significant shunt is usually evaluated with catheterization. Early surgical closure is recommended for left-to-right shunts of more than 2:1 or in the presence of mild-to-moderate pulmonary hypertension. Correction of smaller shunts without evidence of reactive pulmonary hypertension may be deferred until preschool age. Nonsurgical closure of selected muscular defects with a double umbrella-like device deployed by catheter holds future promise but is not yet widely available. The need for antibiotic prophylaxis continues beyond surgery, as a significant proportion of patients exhibit persistent, though minor, shunting and remain at risk for endocarditis.

ECG abnormalities are common after VSD repair. Complete heart block, once a frequent manifestation of surgical trauma to the conduction system, which courses in proximity to the inferior margins of the perimembranous defect, now occurs only rarely. Right bundle branch block is common following right ventriculotomy for surgical closure and is less common following repair via the right atrium, which is the preferred approach in many centers. Ventricular arrhythmias, which are evident in 40% to 50% of patients after surgical repair, are also somewhat more likely after ventriculotomy. Late sudden death occurs in approximately 4% of the patients, but electrophysiologic study has proved nonpredictive, and drug therapy is discouraged in the absence of major symptoms.

It should also be noted that about 5% of VSD patients develop aortic regurgitation, partly because of abnormal tissue support for the aortic cusps. The regurgitation may progress irrespective of VSD closure; in fact, the regurgitation may first appear after repair of the defect. Successful aortic valvuloplasty has been combined with VSD repair, but the management of aortic regurgitation in combination with a small VSD is the same as aortic regurgitation alone.

## Patent ductus arteriosus

The ductus arteriosus, which shunts blood from the pulmonary to the systemic circuit during fetal development, closes functionally within 24 hours of birth in patients. Inhibitors of prostaglandin synthesis, such as indomethacin, enhance this process, whereas prostaglandin infusion delays ductal closure and at times may be useful in sustaining arterial oxygenation. Anatomic obliteration usually follows within the first 2 months, and patency of the ductus beyond this is abnormal. Several factors increase the likelihood of ductal persistence, including female gender, maternal rubella, birth at high altitude, and neonatal hypoxemia, as exemplified by the premature infant in respiratory distress.

As with ventricular septal defect, two features dictate the clinical presentation of ductal patency: the size of the defect and the level of pulmonary vascular resistance. Large defects in the presence of low pulmonary vascular resistance result in volume overload of both the lungs and the left heart. Transmission of aortic pressure to the pulmonary arteries also occurs, and the combination of pressure and volume overload may stimulate arteriolar changes that increase pulmonary resistance. In this instance, pulmonary hypertension may eventually supervene and culminate in reversal of the shunt. Older studies indicated a progression to Eisenmenger syndrome in about 5% of patients with patent ductus arteriosus (PDA). In addition to left ventricular volume overload, which may result in congestive failure during infancy, ductal patency confers an increased risk of endocarditis.

A continuous machinery quality murmur, most prominent along the upper left sternum is the distinctive auscultatory feature of the patent ductus. This murmur envelops the second heart sound and is often accompanied by a palpable thrill (Fig. 15-10, *A*). The large left ventricular stroke volume and rapid runoff into the low pressure pulmonary system (similar to an arteriovenous fistula) frequently produce a widened pulse pressure. Other findings are variable and depend on the precedence of left ventricular volume overload or right ventricular pressure overload. Shunt reversal, if it occurs, produces a characteristic pattern referred to as differential cyanosis:

A
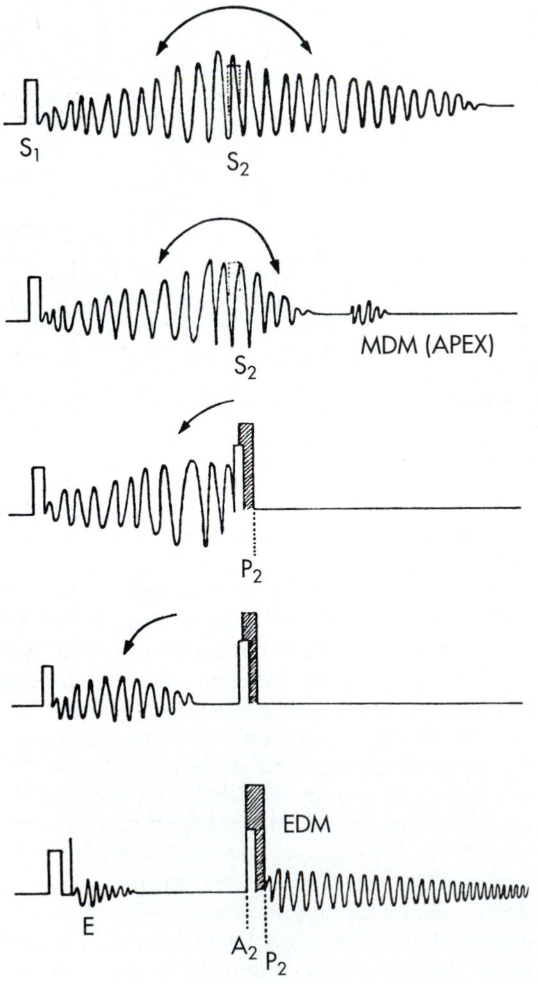


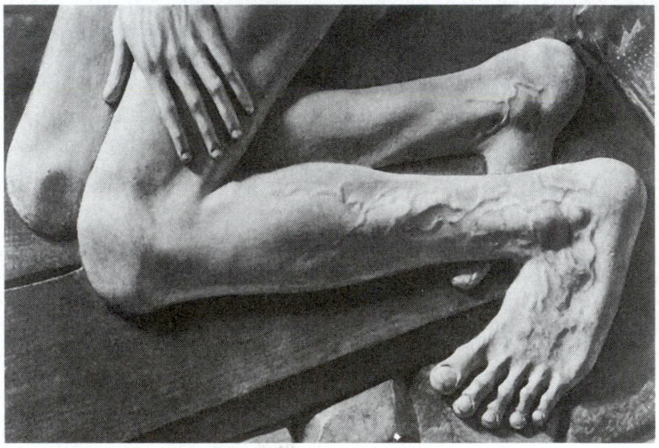
B

**Fig. 15-10. A,** Auscultatory findings in patent ductus arteriosus with progressively increasing levels of pulmonary vascular resistance. With large volume ductus flow and low pulmonary resistance *(top),* the continuous (Gibson) murmur extends uninterruptedly through the second sound ($S_2$). Increases in pulmonary resistance attentuate the diastolic murmur at first and the systolic murmur later as pulmonary pressures rise to systemic levels. Ultimately, reversed ductal flow produces no murmur *(bottom),* and the findings may include a pulmonic ejection click *(E),* a brief pulmonic ejection murmur, a loud pulmonic closure ($P_2$) sound, and a diastolic murmur *(EDM)* of pulmonic insufficiency. *MDM,* Middiastolic murmur. **B,** Clubbed toe deformity of a supplicant suggesting a reversed shunt from PDA. (**A,** From Perloff JK: *Prog Cardiovasc Dis* 9:303, 1967. **B,** carved by Wit Stwosz, from altar in Cathedral of Krakow, Poland, 1465.)

evidence of hemoglobin desaturation is confined to the lower body as unoxygenated blood is shunted from right to left directly into the descending aorta, whereas the upper body, which receives its perfusion proximal to the ductus, is spared (Fig. 15-10, *B*). The diastolic portion of the murmur abbreviates progressively as pulmonary hypertension worsens, and late in the course only a brief systolic murmur may remain.

Pulmonary shunt vascularity with left ventricular prominence is typical of the chest film of PDA. In older patients the aorta may also be somewhat enlarged, and calcification of the ductus occasionally projects in the area between the aortic and pulmonary convexities on the posteroanterior firm. With a large shunt the ECG demonstrates evidence of left atrial enlargement, and first-degree atrioventricular block is common. Prominent QRS voltage in the lateral precordial leads reflects left ventricular volume overload. Evidence of biventricular overload develops with the advent of pulmonary hypertension. Abnormal flow from a patent ductus into the pulmonary artery is easily detected by echocardiography, which also provides pertinent information about left heart chamber sizes and pulmonary artery pressure. In uncomplicated young patients, an adequate echocardiographic study may obviate catheterization.

All patients suspected of having a patent ductus should be referred for cardiology evaluation. Closure, increasingly accomplished by catheter introduction of a polyurethane double-umbrella occluder or similarly conceived device, is the preferred treatment of PDA, regardless of shunt magnitude. The exception to this is when the patient has a tiny flow jet consistent with ductal patency on echocardiography and no corresponding physical findings. This incident, only recently detectable, probably requires simply endocarditis prophylaxis. Advanced age may also temper the therapeutic approach to the asymptomatic patient with a small shunt in whom ductal tortuosity and calcification may increase the technical difficulty and risks of catheter closure or ligation; preprocedural angiographic definition is a must in these cases. Antibiotic prophylaxis is not required after closure if there is no echocardiographic evidence of a shunt.

## BIBLIOGRAPHY

Kirklin JW et al: Clinical outcomes after the arterial switch operation for transposition. Patient, support, procedural, and institutional risk factors. Congenital Heart Surgeons Society, *Circulation* 1501, 1992.

Murphy JG et al: Long-term outcome in patients undergoing surgical repair of tetralogy of Fallot, *New Engl J Med* 329:593, 1993.

O'Fallon WM, Weidman WH, editors: Long-term follow-up of congenital aortic stenosis, pulmonary stenosis, and ventricular septal defect. Report from the Second Joint Study on the Natural History of Congenital Heart Defects (NHS-2), *Circulation* 87 (suppl I):I1, 1993.

Rao PS: Transcatheter treatment of pulmonary outflow tract obstruction: a review, *Prog Cardiovasc Dis* 35:119, 1992.

St. John Sutton MG, Tajik A, McGoon DC: Atrial septal defect in patients ages 60 years and older: operative results and long-term postoperative followup, *Circulation* 64:402, 1981.

Stewart AB et al: Coarctation of the aorta life and health 20-44 years after surgical correction, *British Heart J* 69:65, 1993.

Transcatheter occlusion of persistent arterial duct. Report of the European Registry, *Lancet* 340:1062, 1992.

CHAPTER

# 16 Myocardial and Pericardial Disease

**Kenneth L. Baughman**
**Edward K. Kasper**
**Ahvie Herskowitz**

## EPIDEMIOLOGY AND ETIOLOGY

Congestive heart failure is one of the most frequently made diagnoses in general medical practice. It is important to recognize not only the entity of heart failure itself, but also its diverse causes. This chapter addresses causes of heart failure related to myocardial and pericardial disease.

The prevalence of congestive heart failure varies by the method of assessment. Whereas death certificates would suggest a rate of 0.1 per thousand U.S. population, community surveys rate the true prevalence at 13 patients per thousand. Approximately 3.8 to 5 new cases per thousand are diagnosed each year. Both the prevalence and incidence of congestive heart failure doubled between 1968 and 1983. Males are more frequently affected than females, and older patients more than younger. Although individuals in urban environments are more frequently affected than those in rural areas, the gap is closing. Regardless of the etiology, the prognosis is poor for patients who have heart failure. The anticipated 5-year mortality rate for men is over 60% and for women over 40%.

Cardiomyopathy implies an abnormality of the heart muscle itself as the cause of congestive heart failure. There are three types of cardiomyopathy: dilated, hypertrophic, and restrictive. Of these, over 95% of patients develop the dilated form of heart muscle disorder, 4% have hypertrophic cardiomyopathy, and only 1% or fewer have a restrictive cardiomyopathy. Reliable incidence and prevalence data on hypertrophic and restrictive cardiomyopathy do not exist. The incidence of dilated cardiomyopathy in 1984 was judged to be 7.9 per 100,000 person-years in a discrete, well-defined population. As with heart failure, the prevalence of dilated cardiomyopathy increases with age and is more common in males.

A partial listing of the etiology of dilated cardiomyopathy is reviewed in the box on p. 302. In evaluating patients with dilated cardiomyopathy, one must exclude "look-alikes" not due to primary muscle disease, including focal coronary artery disease (left ventricular aneurysm), primary valvular disease (aortic stenosis and aortic or mitral regurgitation), and pericardial disease (pericardial effusion or tamponade). The etiologies of dilated cardiomyopathy that can be reversible include myocarditis, metabolic disorders (thyroid disease or pheochromocytoma), toxicity (alcohol or drugs), tachycardia-induced dysfunction, infiltrative diseases (hemochromatosis or sarcoidosis), septic shock, carnitine deficiency, and postpartum cardiomyopathy. Patients with a history of asthma, hypertension, and dilated cardiomyopathy in a first-degree

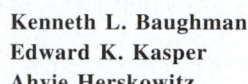

### Etiology of dilated cardiomyopathy

Idiopathic
Ischemic
Inflammatory
  Infectious: Chagas disease, myocarditis
  Collagen vascular: systemic lupus erythematosus
Metabolic
  Thyroid disease
  Pheochromocytoma
  Thiamine deficiency
Toxic
  Alcohol
  Adriamycin
  Cocaine
Drug reaction
  Sulfa
  Penicillin
Infiltrative
  Amyloidosis
  Hemochromatosis
Neuromuscular
  Duchenne muscular dystrophy
  Becker muscular dystrophy
Physical agents
  Heat
  Cold
  Radiation
Hematologic
  Thrombotic thrombocytopenic purpura
  Sickle cell anemia

relative may be predisposed to develop dilated cardiomyopathy themselves.

Hypertrophic cardiomyopathy is the result of a genetic abnormality in the myosin heavy chain gene. The inheritance pattern is dominant, and 50% of those at risk are probably affected. Familial hypertrophic cardiomyopathy may not express itself until puberty. Some patients present with hypertrophic cardiomyopathy but have no family history due to variable penetrance or single mutations. Patients with hypertension may develop a nongenetic hypertensive hypertrophic cardiomyopathy. These patients, presumably in response to long-standing hypertension, develop significant hypertrophy of the myocardium. Patients with hypertensive hypertrophic cardiomyopathy never display asymmetric hypertrophy, but this is not uncommon in patients with the inherited form.

Restrictive cardiomyopathy is due to the infiltration of a foreign substance in or around the myocardial cells. Etiologies include amyloidosis, hemochromatosis, and sarcoidosis. Virtually all patients with these disorders display evidence of systemic illness, making diagnosis more obvious.

Pericardial disease may cause congestive heart failure due to its influence on the myocardium and the diastolic pressures within the heart chambers. Potential forms of involvement include pericardial effusions, pericardial constriction, and effusive-constrictive pericarditis. Viral or tuberculous pericarditis may cause acute pericarditis, tamponade, effusive-constrictive pericarditis, and constrictive pericarditis. Some etiologies, such as trauma, myocardial perforation, and malignancy, do not result in effusive-constrictive or constrictive pericarditis.

## PATHOPHYSIOLOGY

Dilated cardiomyopathy is initiated by an insult that decreases left ventricular contractility. This may be a viral illness, alcohol, or the toxic effect of some medication. The decrease in contractility reduces the cardiac output, which stimulates the juxtaglomerular apparatus in the kidney, resulting in an activation of the renin-angiotensin system and the subsequent retention of salt and water. This fluid retention increases ventricular volume (preload) and causes dilatation of the left ventricle. Either due to progressive left ventricular dilatation or to hypertrophy and fibrosis of the heart muscle, the chamber stiffens (becomes less compliant). Increased volume in a noncompliant ventricle increases the end-diastolic pressure, which increases left atrial and pulmonary venous pressures, causing pulmonary congestion. Decreased coronary blood *supply* (due to the low cardiac output), in association with increased *demand* for myocardial oxygen (due to an increase in heart rate, contractility, and wall stress), leads to subendocardial ischemia. Prolonged global ischemia may result in interstitial fibrosis. The interstitial fibrosis associated with individual cellular hypertrophy further worsens diastolic compliance and ultimately decreases contractility. A vicious cycle is created, resulting in high filling pressures and low cardiac output.

Although an abnormality in the genetic locus responsible for myosin heavy chain is associated with hypertrophic cardiomyopathy, the pathophysiology is unknown. Some evidence has indicated that there is also an increase in the number of calcium receptors in the myocardium and that the myofilaments may be excessively responsive to sympathetic stimulation. The result of these abnormalities is a ventricle characterized by increased contractility with a hyperdynamic ejection of ventricular contents. Because of the dramatic muscle hypertrophy, the left ventricular cavity is small and the diastolic filling pressures in the heart are elevated. Although the antithesis of dilated cardiomyopathy, the end result is the same, with elevated filling pressures and a low cardiac output.

Restrictive cardiomyopathy is characterized by an infiltration in and around the myocardial cells of a substance that alters the cell's ability to contract and relax. The influence is to alter diastolic compliance much more dramatically than systolic contractility until late in the course. Patients therefore have markedly elevated filling pressures, which are usually equal in both the left and right ventricles. Only late in the course is contractility negatively influenced.

Pericardial disease is initiated by injury, infection, or inflammation in the pericardial space. This results in a fluid accumulation. If the fluid accumulates rapidly, even small amounts may dramatically alter ventricular function due to the inability of the pericardium to stretch abruptly with the accumulation of fluid and the subsequent compression of the heart. Pericardial effusions accumulated over long periods, however, may result in massive accumulations of fluid before pericardial compliance is altered. As the pericardium surrounds the right and left

**Table 16-1.** Dilated cardiomyopathy (DCM) survival

| Author (*n*) | DCM type | 1 Year* | 2 Year† | 3 Year‡ |
|---|---|---|---|---|
| Field (36) | No CAD | 69% | 50% | 33% |
| Roberts (152) | No CAD | 75% | 59% | 48% |
| Cohn (139) | | 76% | 54% | 41% |
| Unverferth (69) | No CAD | 65% | | |
| Franciosa (182) | | 66% | 41% | 24% |
| (95) | CAD | 54% | 31% | |
| (87) | No CAD | 77% | 52% | |
| Keogh (79) | IDCM | 75% | 59% | |
| (232) | | 68% | 56% | 41% |
| Consensus (253) (placebo) | | 48% | | |
| VA (642) (placebo) | | | 66% | 53% |

*CAD*, Coronary artery disease; *IDCM*, idiopathic dilated cardiomyopathy; *VA*, Veterans Administration.
*$x$ + SD = 68% ± 9%.
†$x$ + SD = 55% ± 8%.
‡$x$ + SD = 40% ± 10%.

ventricle, pressure achieved in the pericardial space is equally distributed to those ventricles. Therefore pressure elevations due to fluid, constriction, or an admixture of both may adversely influence left ventricular and right ventricular end-diastolic pressures. Therefore, when the pressure in the pericardial space is higher than the intrinsic left ventricular pressure, the diastolic ventricular pressures are equal to the pericardial pressure. Additionally, pericardial fluid or constriction may limit the amount of volume that the left ventricle can accept. The volume of blood in the ventricle in patients with pericardial disease is usually small. When the mitral and tricuspid valves are open, diastolic pressures in all chambers of the heart are equivalent and are also equal to the pericardial pressure. As with dilated and restrictive cardiomyopathies, the end result of pericardial disease is an increase in diastolic filling pressures and a decrease in cardiac output.

Since all forms of myocardial and pericardial disease may have the same result of increased diastolic pressures and low cardiac output, it is exceedingly important that the entity responsible for congestive heart failure and its pathophysiology be recognized so the appropriate long-term treatment can be initiated.

## NATURAL HISTORY

Dilated cardiomyopathy, as with heart failure itself, is associated with a poor prognosis (Table 16-1).

Considering patients with ischemic and idiopathic dilated cardiomyopathy, the average 1-year survival is approximately 70%, 2-year survival 55%, and 3-year survival only 40%. Patients have symptoms of low cardiac output including weakness, fatigability, malaise, and angina. They may also display left-heart pulmonary and right-heart venous congestion. About 15% of patients with dilated cardiomyopathy not on anticoagulants may have symptomatic embolic events during the course of their illnesses. Additionally, patients may develop atrial or ventricular arrhythmias, the latter increasing the risk for sudden death. Patients with dilated cardiomyopathy die from progressive congestive heart failure (60%) or sudden death (40%). Poor prognostic features are demonstrated in the box at right.

### Poor prognostic features of dilated cardiomyopathy

- Advanced functional class: New York Heart Association III-IV
- Age: greater than 55 years
- Gender: male.
- Examination: $S_3$
- Etiology: ischemic
- Electrocardiogram: interventricular conduction delay
- Chest x-ray: cardiothoracic ratio greater than 0.55
- Ejection fraction: below 10%
- Wall thickness by echocardiogram: <0.9 cm
- Metabolic exercise stress test: oxygen consumption below 12 ml/kg/min
- Holter monitor: ventricular tachycardia
- Elevated filling pressures: pulmonary capillary wedge pressure > 20 mm Hg
- Elevated plasma norepinephrine

The prognosis for patients with dilated cardiomyopathy has been demonstrably improved with the use of angiotensin-converting enzyme inhibitors.

The natural history of hypertrophic cardiomyopathy is variable. Affected patients may be asymptomatic. Sudden death may be the first clinical manifestation of the disease. More characteristically the patient shows symptoms of congestive heart failure, low cardiac output, chest pain, and/or syncope. Although treatment with β-blockers or calcium blockers may improve the patient's symptoms, there is no evidence as yet that the patient's prognosis is favorably affected by this treatment.

Even though the natural history of patients with restrictive cardiomyopathy is influenced by the etiology of the restrictive cardiomyopathy, once cardiac involvement is present, the prognosis is exceedingly poor. Treatment of the symptoms of heart failure is extraordinarily difficult in this group of patients, since renal underperfusion is common with levels of diuresis that afford some relief from congestive symptoms. Treatment of the primary disorder associated with restrictive cardiomyopathy only rarely improves the patient's overall prognosis by reversing the accumulation of the infiltrative agent.

The natural history of pericardial disease is progressive cardiac compromise. However, all forms of pericardial disease are treatable and, in fact, virtually curable. The primary mission of the primary care physician is to differentiate pericardial disease, which is curable, from restrictive disease, which is terminal. Pericardial effusions can be drained, regardless of their etiology, and the patient's hemodynamics normalized. Pericardial constriction can be prevented by appropriately treating the cause of the fluid accumulation in patients with pericardial effusions or effusive-constrictive states. Pericardial constriction demands surgical pericardiectomy, which universally improves the patient's hemodynamics and functional capacity.

## HISTORY

All patients with myocardial or pericardial disease may present with congestive heart failure. Criteria for heart failure (major and minor) are listed in the box below. The signs and symptoms of these disorders result in congestion and low output, as noted in Table 16-2.

In addition, patients with congestive heart failure and dilated cardiomyopathy may have embolic events originating from any of the cardiac chambers. Patients with any form of cardiomyopathy may also have symptomatic systemic emboli due to supraventricular arrhythmias, particularly atrial fibrillation. Arrhythmias are common in all patients who have cardiomyopathy and may include supraventricular or ventricular arrhythmias with lightheadedness, dizziness, presyncope, or syncope.

Some specific historical features can help distinguish the form of cardiomyopathy present. Patients with hypertrophic cardiomyopathy more frequently complain of ischemic chest pain and often have dizziness following exercise or with Valsalva's maneuver. Restrictive cardiomyopathy patients and patients with pericardial disease display right-sided signs and symptoms of congestion much in excess of left-sided signs and symptoms. In both of these etiologies the diastolic pressures in the left and right ventricles are elevated and equal. Whereas a left ventricular end-diastolic pressure of 20 mm Hg may cause pulmonary congestion from left-sided involvement, it results in a dramatic elevation of the right atrial pressure, causing massive jugular venous distention, hepatomegaly, and possible ascites. These right-sided signs and symptoms are much in excess of those signs of congestion associated with the left-sided elevation.

Patients may present with cardiomyopathy or pericardial disease and still be totally asymptomatic. Their pericardial or myocardial abnormalities may have been discovered by routine chest x-ray, electrocardiogram (ECG), or echocardiogram performed for other reasons. The most frequent "error" in the management of patients is the early misdiagnosis of a young patient presenting with cough, congestion, and breathlessness. Such patients are usually thought to have bronchitis and are treated with antibiotics before the myocardial or pericardial etiology is recognized. All patients with a family history of hypertrophic cardiomyopathy should be screened for the disorder. Similarly, all patients with hypertrophic cardiomyopathy should have their immediate families and first-degree relatives screened for myocardial involvement. Patients with restrictive cardiomyopathy more frequently display a pseudoinfarct pattern by ECG, making differentiation of ischemic disease difficult.

Patients with pericardial effusion or constriction often

### Criteria for heart failure

**Major**

Paroxysms of nocturnal dyspnea
Orthopnea
Neck vein distention
Hepatojugular reflux
Central venous pressure >16 cm $H_2O$
Rales
Pulmonary edema
Cardiomegaly
$S_3$ gallop

**Minor**

Ankle edema
Night cough
Dyspnea on exertion
Hepatomegaly
Pleural effusions
Decreased vital capacity (1/3)
Heart rate >120 beats/min

**Major or minor**

Weight loss >4.5 kg/5 days

From McKee PA et al: The natural history of congestive heart failure: the Framingham study, *N Eng J Med* 285 (26): 1441, 1971. Used with permission.

**Table 16-2.** Signs and symptoms of heart failure

| Result | Signs | Symptoms |
|---|---|---|
| Right heart congestion | Elevated venous pressure<br>Hepatomegaly<br>Ascites<br>Peripheral edema | Lower extremity swelling<br>Early satiety<br>Right upper quadrant pain |
| Left heart congestion | Rales<br>Wheezing | Dyspnea on exertion<br>Shortness of breath<br>Asthma<br>Orthopnea<br>Paroxysmal nocturnal dyspnea |
| Right and left congestion | Pleural effusion | |
| Low output | Peripheral cyanosis<br>Low blood pressure<br>Tachycardia<br>Sympathetic discharge | Fatigue<br>Malaise<br>Weakness<br>Low energy<br>Angina |

begin their pericardial involvement with acute pericarditis. These patients present with precordial discomfort, which is usually more omnipresent than angina and is position dependent, being more symptomatic lying down. The pericardial involvement may be associated with pleural inflammation as well as a pleuropericardial syndrome. These symptoms may be confused with the symptoms of myocardial infarction, pulmonary emboli, or dissection.

Mistakes can be avoided by obtaining a chest x-ray early for patients who present with bibasilar rales as opposed to unilateral findings of pneumonitis. Additionally, patients with persistent cough or wheezing should have a careful examination and chest x-ray to rule out myocardial disease. Similarly, patients with suspected myocardial or pericardial disease are easily and definitively diagnosed with an echocardiogram acquired at an appropriate time during their examination.

## PHYSICAL EXAMINATION

The physical examination of the cardiovascular patient can be dissected into several parts. Each of these may provide clues as to the presence and etiology of heart failure.

### Jugular venous pressure

Patients with congestive heart failure have elevations of the right atrial pressure and therefore distended jugular veins. Patients with dilated cardiomyopathy have modest distention of the jugular veins and often dominant v waves due to tricuspid regurgitation. In these cases the regurgitation is due to dilatation of the tricuspid annulus secondary to myocardial disease. Patients with hypertrophic cardiomyopathy display prominent A waves in the venous pulse. This is due to the increased atrial pressure necessary to force blood into the stiff right ventricle. Patients with restrictive cardiomyopathy display even greater elevations of the A waves for similar reasons. Patients with pericardial disease display dramatic abnormalities of the venous pressure. These patients have equally prominent A and v waves. Patients with pericardial constriction have dominant x and y descents after the A and v waves, whereas patients with pericardial tamponade display only a prominent x descent.

### Carotids

In dilated and restrictive cardiomyopathy, and pericardial disease the carotid volumes are diminished due to the low stroke volume of the left ventricle. In dilated cardiomyopathy the rate of rise of the carotid pulse is diminished. The carotid pulse upstroke in patients with restrictive cardiomyopathy is usually maintained until late in the course. In pericardial disease the carotid upstroke is normal, although decreased in volume. Patients with a hypertrophic cardiomyopathy have a hyperdynamic carotid upstroke due to the ejection of blood from the ventricle. There is often a bifid nature to the carotid upstroke associated with hypertrophic cardiomyopathy due to the early rapid ejection of blood from the ventricle followed by a later secondary peak of ejection. The peripheral pulses are relatively indistinguishable in these disorders, with the exception of pericardial disease. With pericardial tamponade, inspiration results in a more significant decrease in the pulse pressure than normal (paradoxical pulse).

### Lung examination

When the left ventricular end-diastolic and left atrial pressures are elevated, these elevations are transmitted to the pulmonary veins. This may result in exudation of fluid into the lungs, producing rales or, when associated with right-heart failure, pleural effusions. Patients may also have peribronchial edema, resulting in wheezing. Not infrequently, patients with severe disease have absolutely clear lung fields, particularly if the elevation of end-diastolic pressure has occurred over a long period. Patients with restrictive cardiomyopathy may display lung involvement with a primary process such as sarcoidosis or amyloidosis.

### Heart

The point of maximal impulse in patients with dilated cardiomyopathy is markedly displaced and weak, with a palpable $S_3$ gallop. Patients with hypertrophic cardiomyopathy have a dynamic, forceful, heaving left-ventricular point of maximal impulse. Restrictive cardiomyopathy patients have a weakened but usually minimally displaced point of maximal impulse. Patients with pericardial disease are remarkable for their quiet precordium and percussion of a cardiac silhouette much beyond the point of maximal cardiac pulsation. Heart sounds are also variable. Patients with dilated cardiomyopathy usually have $S_3$ gallops. Hypertrophic cardiomyopathies usually have $S_4$ gallops, depending on the degree of compliance abnormality in the left ventricle and the rate of deceleration of blood entering the cavity. Restrictive cardiomyopathy patients often have $S_4$ gallops. Patients with pericardial effusions may display in early diastole a pericardial knock, which must be differentiated from an $S_3$ gallop.

Patients with dilated cardiomyopathy develop murmurs of mitral and tricuspid regurgitation as a result of annular dilatation and malalignment of the chordae tendineae. Patients with hypertrophic cardiomyopathy usually have an outflow murmur. If there is asymmetric septal hypertrophy, these patients display a harsh murmur in the aortic outflow region that sounds like aortic stenosis with a blowing character at the base more compatible with mitral regurgitation. Restrictive cardiomyopathy patients frequently have no murmurs whatsoever. Patients with pericardial disease, in addition to their pericardial knocks, may display a one-, two-, or three-component friction rub.

### Abdomen

The liver may be enlarged in any patient with elevation of right atrial pressures. Since pericardial and restrictive diseases more often have higher elevations of right-sided pressures than dilated or hypertrophic cardiomyopathy, the liver is frequently more engorged in these diseases. Similarly, the liver may be involved in certain of the primary etiologies of restrictive or constrictive disease. Ascites is much more common in patients with restrictive or constrictive heart disease due to the dramatic elevations of right atrial pressures in excess of the diminution in cardiac output. This causes weeping of edema fluid from the liver well before there is generalized salt and water retention due to low cardiac output and its compensatory renal effect.

### Extremities

Patients with pericardial, restrictive, and hypertrophic disease have less edema than patients with dilated cardiomyopathy, probably due to the lower cardiac output found early in patients with dilated cardiomyopathy.

### Subtle or misleading findings

Often the jugular venous pressure elevation is not appreciated. This is due to the dramatic distention in the veins when the patient is supine. The patient's head and upper body must be raised until a meniscus is evident in the vein to judge the height of the venous pressure. If venous pressure is seen, often the A and v waves are not appreciated, nor are the x and y descents.

Carotid pulsations are often mistaken for venous pulsations in patients with dramatic elevation of their venous pressure. The carotid pulse is medial to the venous pulse and protected by the strap muscles.

The point of maximal impulse can be frequently missed due to the patient's habitus and should be felt for in the left lateral decubitus position if not apparent with the patient supine.

The differentiation of a pericardial knock from an $S_3$ gallop is difficult in timing but straightforward by the nature of the sound produced. Patients with midsystolic clicks are often diagnosed mistakenly as having a pericardial knock or an $S_3$ gallop. The finding of a crisp third sound with a normal point of maximal impulse should suggest a midsystolic click. Rubs and murmurs may be misinterpreted.

### Classic signs lacking

Often with a very low cardiac output, murmurs may be inapparent. This can include aortic stenosis and hemodynamically significant mitral regurgitation. Patients with massive obesity display many signs and symptoms expected in the cardiac disorders noted above. Patients may have chronic obstructive pulmonary disease or intrinsic asthma that mimics cardiac disease, and when both cardiac and pulmonary diseases are present, differentiation may be difficult. Finally, palpation or auscultation of the left heart may be difficult in women with large breasts.

## LABORATORY STUDIES

### Diagnosis

The transthoracic echocardiogram is the single most useful procedure to diagnose myocardial and pericardial disease. The test carries the highest sensitivity and specificity, is noninvasive, and is only moderately expensive. Patients with dilated cardiomyopathy characteristically have thin left ventricular walls, a dilated left ventricular internal diastolic dimension (greater than 2.7 cm/m$^2$ body area), and poor contractility. Patients with hypertrophic cardiomyopathy have markedly thickened left ventricular walls, often asymmetric, small left ventricular cavities, and hyperdynamic contractility. Patients with restrictive cardiomyopathy have normal or slightly thickened walls, a normal ventricular cavity, and, late in their course, diminished contractility. Patients with amyloidosis, hemochromatosis, or interstitial fibrosis may display a speckled pattern in the left ventricular myocardium, which is strongly suggestive of an infiltrative process. Patients with pericardial effusions are easily diagnosed with echocardiography. An echocardiogram may detect as little as 10 ml of pericardial fluid and can easily distinguish large pericardial from large pleural effusions. Thickening of the pericardium, compatible with constrictive pericarditis, is more difficult to assess, but patients have normal left ventricular wall thickness and contractility. Patients with pericardial disease display rapid diastolic relaxation as opposed to patients with hypertrophic and restrictive cardiomyopathy, where the rate of relaxation is slow. Echocardiography allows determination of the size of each chamber within the heart. It also allows a noninvasive assessment of the presence or absence of valvular disease and its etiology (secondary or primary).

Chest x-ray may determine that the patient has cardiomegaly and suggest chamber enlargement. These findings are not as sensitive or as specific as those obtained by echocardiography. Pericardial calcification by x-ray hints strongly at the possibility of pericardial constriction.

### Etiology

A number of studies can be performed to determine the etiology of the condition identified as being abnormal. These include blood and urine studies and an array of noninvasive and invasive techniques.

#### *Diagnostic laboratory studies*

**Dilated cardiomyopathy.** Antinuclear antibody, thyroid function, and urine for vanillylmandelic acid (VMA) excretion are tested in patients with dilated cardiomyopathy of unknown etiology. Antinuclear antibody tests serve to rule out connective tissue abnormalities. Thyroid function tests and VMA tests rule out endocrinopathies, particularly hyperthyroidism and hypothyroidism, as well as pheochromocytoma. Patients with advanced cardiomyopathy display signs and symptoms compatible with the presence of each of these disorders, and the distinguishing features may be obscured by the primary cardiac illness.

**Hypertrophic cardiomyopathy.** Routine genetic screening to identify defects in the myosin heavy chain are not yet available to screen patients with hypertrophic cardiomyopathy.

**Restrictive cardiomyopathy.** Specific studies may be performed to identify the potential etiology of restrictive cardiomyopathy. Iron, ferritin, iron-binding capacity, and percent saturation studies are helpful in evaluating hemochromatosis. Patients with suspected amyloidosis, particularly those associated with multiple myeloma, should have serum and urinary protein electrophoresis performed to characterize protein abnormalities. Some patients with hypereosinophilia may develop a restrictive-like cardiomyopathy due to endocardial fibrosis (Löffler's syndrome). Obviously, a differential white blood cell count is beneficial. Patients with suspected myeloma should have long bone series performed to identify foci of abnormalities and bone marrow aspirates to identify the excess of plasma cells responsible. Patients with constrictive pericarditis have no distinguishing blood laboratory studies. Patients with pericardial effusions may have laboratory values that reflect the inflammatory nature of this process. Only with a suppurative infective pericarditis would blood cultures identify the etiology.

***Electrocardiogram.*** Patients with dilated cardiomyopathy often display abnormalities due to atrial enlargement, low voltage, and poor R wave progression, often in a pseudoinfarct pattern. Patients with a hypertrophic cardiomyopathy, on the other hand, have a dramatic increase in voltage and may display ventricular hypertrophy and strain pattern in addition to atrial enlargement. Restrictive cardiomyopathy patients display a dramatic decrease in voltage and are notorious for the pseudoinfarct pattern of Q wave development in the inferior or anterior leads. Patients with pericardial effusions similarly display low voltage. Acute pericarditis is characterized by PR segment depression and ST segment elevation. The differentiation between pericardial inflammation and ischemia is often difficult in patients with ST segment elevation. Patients with pericarditis always have a return of their ST segments to baseline before inverting their T waves, whereas patients with ischemia often have persistent ST elevation while T waves are inverted. Patients with any form of myocardial or pericardial disease may display nonspecific ST-T wave changes and supraventricular or ventricular arrhythmias.

*Chest x-ray.* Patients with dilated cardiomyopathy have enlargement of their cardiac silhouette usually with evidence of four-chamber involvement by chest x-ray. Patients with hypertrophic cardiomyopathy have less robust enlargement of their ventricular silhouettes and tend to have less right ventricular prominence. Restrictive cardiomyopathy patients often have normal-appearing cardiac silhouettes despite an increase in pulmonary vascularity. Patients with pericardial disease may display pericardial calcification but almost always have normal heart size unless they have significant pericardial effusion where the cardiac silhouette appears enlarged. Pericardial calcification hints at pericardial constriction. A chest x-ray in pericardial constriction may also demonstrate evidence of prior tuberculosis, which may be etiologic for the pericardial process.

*Cardiac catheterization.* Coronary arteriography should be performed in patients over 35 years of age with dilated cardiomyopathy in whom no other etiology for the muscle disorder is apparent. The finding of more than 50% narrowing in any coronary artery results in the diagnosis of ischemic cardiomyopathy. Often, however, the left ventricular dysfunction is far in excess of that which could be attributable to the degree of coronary artery disease. Left ventriculography performed as part of cardiac catheterization allows determination of the degree of mitral regurgitation. This should be performed only in patients where the mitral regurgitation is felt to be etiologic. Determining the degree and significance of mitral regurgitation is difficult, since gradual dilatation of the left ventricular cavity results in progressive mitral regurgitation in all patients with dilated cardiomyopathy. Supravalvular aortic injection allows the clinician to judge the degree of aortic reflux where this is suspected to be etiologic. Aortic stenosis can be judged by the pressure gradient and associated cardiac output across the aortic valve. For clinical purposes the degree of aortic and mitral valve disease can usually be adequately judged by echocardiography using Doppler techniques.

Only in patients considered to be operative candidates should more invasive investigation of valvular disease be performed. Catheterization may be of benefit in patients with hypertrophic cardiomyopathy to rule out associated coronary artery disease and to assess the degree of apparent outflow obstruction. This is performed by measuring intercavitary and aortic pressures while ensuring that there is no valvular component to the pressure gradient. Patients with constrictive and restrictive heart disease do not usually benefit from dye studies. Their diastolic pressures display a characteristic pattern of filling in which the left and right ventricular end-diastolic pressures are elevated, and the early diastolic pressure displays a square root configuration due to the rapid influx and achievement of maximal cavity volumes early in the course of filling. Additionally, patients with significant constrictive and restrictive heart disease have equalization of the diastolic pressures, including the pulmonary capillary wedge pressure (left atrial pressure), pulmonary artery diastolic pressure, right ventricular end-diastolic pressure, and right atrial pressure. Some patients who have undergone diuresis do not display this equalization until challenged with additional hydration. Patients with restrictive disease are more likely to have a higher left ventricular than right ventricular end-diastolic pressure and often display higher pulmonary artery pressures.

*Endomyocardial biopsy.* Endomyocardial biopsy may be performed in patients with dilated or restrictive cardiomyopathy. Listed in Table 16-3 are the final diagnoses reached after performance of history, physical examination, routine blood work, endomyocardial biopsy, and coronary angiography, when necessary, in 673 patients at The Johns Hopkins Hospital.

**Table 16-3.** Etiology of cardiomyopathy

| Diagnosis | Frequency | Percent (%) |
|---|---|---|
| Idiopathic dilated | 313 | 46.5 |
| Idiopathic myocarditis | 81 | 12.0 |
| Coronary artery disease | 74 | 11.0 |
| HIV | 33 | 4.9 |
| Peripartum | 33 | 4.9 |
| Chronic alcohol abuse | 23 | 3.4 |
| Drug-induced | 21 | 3.1 |
| Connective tissue diseases | 15 | 2.2 |
| Amyloidosis | 14 | 2.1 |
| Hypertension | 14 | 2.1 |
| Familial | 12 | 1.8 |
| Metabolic | 10 | 1.5 |
| Valvular myopathy | 10 | 1.5 |
| Congenital heart disease | 4 | 0.6 |
| Neuromuscular diseases | 4 | 0.6 |
| Postcoronary bypass surgery | 4 | 0.6 |
| Sarcoidosis | 4 | 0.6 |
| Atrial fibrillation | 1 | 0.1 |
| Endomyocardial fibroelastosis | 1 | 0.1 |
| Histiocylosis X | 1 | 0.1 |
| Thorabotic thrombocytopenic purpura | 1 | 0.1 |
| TOTAL | 673 | 99.8 |

From Kasper EK et al: The causes of dilated cardiomyopathy: a clinicopathologic review of 673 consecutive patients, *J Am Coll Cardiol* 23:586, 1994.

As noted, many of these diagnoses are tissue diagnoses, including postviral myocarditis, myocarditis associated with peripartum and HIV, amyloidosis, sarcoidosis, hemochromatosis, ischemia, adriamycin toxicity, histiocytosis X, and connective tissue diseases including scleroderma and thrombotic thrombocytopenic purpura (TTP). Utilizing this approach, only 50% of patients with dilated cardiomyopathy have no etiology identified and are considered idiopathic. Patients with new-onset dilated cardiomyopathy of less than 6 months' duration and those who are young or potential transplant candidates should be considered for heart biopsy. Biopsy is of even greater benefit for patients with restrictive cardiomyopathy. The etiology can virtually always be established by endomyocardial biopsy in view of the causes of restrictive cardiomyopathy including hemochromatosis, amyloidosis, sarcoidosis, and interstitial fibrosis. The biopsy is particularly beneficial for patients with constrictive-restrictive hemodynamics, since it is less risky to perform an endomyocardial biopsy to rule out infiltrative disease than to submit the patient to an exploratory pericardiectomy to rule out constrictive pericarditis. Biopsy of patients with hypertrophic cardiomyopathy is rarely warranted. The typical fiber disarray and interstitial fibrosis seen in patients with hypertrophic cardiomyopathy may also be seen in patients with hypertensive hypertrophic disease, particularly if the biopsy specimen is taken near the papillary muscle base.

### Differential diagnosis

**Dilated cardiomyopathy**

Focal coronary artery disease
- Left ventricular aneurysm
- Left ventricular pseudoaneurysm

Valvular disease
- Aortic stenosis
- Aortic regurgitation
- Mitral stenosis
- Mitral regurgitation

Pericardial disease
- Effusion
- Effusive constriction

**Hypertrophic cardiomyopathy**

Hypertensive hypertrophic cardiomyopathy
Aortic stenosis
Subaortic stenosis
Infiltrative cardiomyopathy

**Restrictive cardiomyopathy**

Hypertensive hypertrophic cardiomyopathy
Hypertrophic cardiomyopathy
Normal heart
Pericardial disease
- Constriction

## DIFFERENTIAL DIAGNOSIS

See the box at right.

### Dilated cardiomyopathy

*Focal coronary artery disease*

**Left ventricular aneurysm.** Patients with a proximal left anterior descending obstruction may develop massive degrees of dilatation and dyskinesis of the anterior wall. This can produce a markedly enlarged cardiac silhouette and a falsely low ejection fraction by gated blood pool scanning. Echocardiography or ventriculography demonstrates active inferior and lateral walls as well as the focal nature of the left ventricular aneurysm.

**Left ventricular pseudoaneurysm.** Patients may experience a rupture of the anterior wall confined in the pericardial space, which is adherent to the anterior wall due to focal pericardial inflammation. Such patients similarly show an enlargement of the left ventricular silhouette in noninvasive studies.

*Primary valvular disease*

**Aortic stenosis.** Patients with end-stage aortic stenosis may develop significant ventricular dilatation and hypofunction. Due to the low cardiac output generated by the failing heart, murmurs of aortic stenosis are markedly diminished in intensity.

**Aortic regurgitation.** Regurgitant lesions of the aortic and mitral valve result in a volume challenge to the left ventricle. This volume challenge is handled extraordinarily well until late in the course of decompensation. Because of the low aortic diastolic pressure and high left ventricular end-diastolic pressure, the diastolic pressure gradient is low and results in a barely audible murmur. Patients usually still have the peripheral stigmata of significant aortic regurgitation, including more bounding pulses than anticipated for the degree of ventricular enlargement, a lower diastolic blood pressure than expected, and the Quincke sign or Duroziez murmur.

**Mitral regurgitation.** Of all the valvular lesions, mitral regurgitation is the most difficult to distinguish, since patients with dilated cardiomyopathy develop this murmur due to annular dilatation and papillary muscle malalignment. A prior history of mitral regurgitation and the finding of moderate to severe regurgitation by noninvasive or invasive studies, as well as a finding of primary valvular pathology by echocardiography, suggest that the mitral regurgitation caused the dilated cardiomyopathy.

**Mitral stenosis.** Rarely, patients with severe mitral stenosis and pulmonary hypertension and right heart failure develop massive enlargement of the right ventricle. This may result in a huge heart by chest x-ray and palpable gallops in the usual position for the point of maximal impulse of the left ventricle.

*Pericardial disease.* Pericardial effusions may produce marked cardiac silhouette enlargement and heart failure, while ventricular function remains entirely normal. This is the most important of the lesions in differential diagnosis in view of the treatability of the disorder.

### Hypertrophic cardiomyopathy

*Hypertensive hypertrophic cardiomyopathy.* Patients with long-standing hypertension may develop left ventricular thickening in congestive heart failure.

*Valvular aortic stenosis.* Aortic stenosis results in a significant obstruction to flow through the aortic valve as the stenosis progresses. Patients develop progressive myocardial hypertrophy in response to this increased workload, resulting in myocardial thickness. Contractility is increased in aortic stenosis until such time as the ventricle decompensates.

***Subaortic stenosis.*** Rarely, patients may present with discrete subaortic rings simulating hypertrophic subaortic stenosis and aortic stenosis.

***Infiltrative disorders.*** Patients with amyloidosis and other infiltrative disorders may appear to have significant ventricular hypertrophy with normal or enhanced contractility until such time as the disease progresses.

### Restrictive cardiomyopathy

***Hypertrophic cardiomyopathy.*** See text.

***Hypertensive hypertrophic cardiomyopathy.*** See text.

***Normal heart size and function.*** Some patients with restrictive cardiomyopathy appear to have normal ventricular wall thickness and contractility early in their course, only to have wall thickness increase and contractility diminish over time.

***Pericardial disease.*** A pericardial effusion can be mistaken for any of the generalized causes of cardiomegaly noted above.

Pericardial constriction may be mistaken for restrictive cardiomyopathy.

## MANAGEMENT

The primary tenet in the management of all of these patients is to treat the primary cause of the muscle disorder if it is identified and if treatment is appropriate. For example, patients with hypothyroidism or other endocrinopathies should be treated. Patients with regurgitant or stenotic valvular lesions may be candidates for surgical correction of their valvular lesions. Similarly, patients with coronary artery disease may be appropriate for revascularization.

### Medical management

All of the pericardial and myocardial diseases noted above can cause significant congestive heart failure. Heart failure is treated with preload reduction, afterload reduction, and/or agents to affect contractility. The general usefulness of these agents in each of the categories is listed in Table 16-4.

Simple measures and general treatment should not be forgotten. These include a low-sodium diet, bed rest, oxygen, and water restriction.

***Diuretics.*** Following are diuretic action and equivalent potency by weight:

*Proximal tubular diuretic:* acetazolamide

*Loop diuretics:* furosemide (40 mg), bumetanide (1 mg), ethacrynic acid (50mg)

*Early distal tubular diuretics:* hydrochlorothiazide (50 mg), metolazone (2.5 mg)

*Late distal tubular diuretics:* spironolactone (100 mg), triamterene (100 mg), amiloride (5 mg)

It is important to match the power of the diuretics to the clinical need. Loop diuretics are much more powerful than other diuretic agents. Diuretics should be given no more frequently than twice per day unless the patient is in extremis. This prevents excessive diuretic-induced electrolyte or volume abnormalities. Combination therapy is occasionally necessary in patients refractory to standard diuretic therapy. Only one agent effective in each site of action should be used. Patients should be initiated on a loop diuretic. When the equivalent of 80 mg of furosemide is given twice daily, a potassium-sparing diuretic should be added, which saves potassium and magnesium. If additional diuresis is needed, an early distal tubular diuretic agent can be administered. Of the early distal tubular diuretic agents only metolazone is active in patients with a diminished creatinine clearance. The addition of potassium-sparing diuretics must result in a decreased need for supplemental potassium replacement and must be used with caution in patients taking angiotensin-converting enzyme inhibitors. Similarly, angiotensin-converting enzyme inhibitors diminish the aldosterone present in the kidney, making spironolactone less effective as a potassium-sparing agent.

Diuretics may be harmful to individuals with small or fixed stroke volumes. This is the case for patients with hypertrophic cardiomyopathy, restrictive cardiomyopathy, and pericardial effusion with tamponade and constrictive pericarditis. Careful attention to excessive diuresis characterized by decreased cerebral or renal perfusion must be shown. Diuretics can be used in all forms of congestive heart failure in which the patient has a dramatic excess of fluid and pulmonary or hepatic venous congestion. The extent to which diuretics can be used depends on the

**Table 16-4.** The usefulness of agents in treating heart failure associated with cardiomyopathy

| | Restrictive-constrictive cardiomyopathy | Hypertrophic cardiomyopathy | Dilated cardiomyopathy |
|---|---|---|---|
| Preload reduction | 2 | 3 | 1 |
| Afterload reduction | 3 | 3 | 1 |
| Inotropic positive | 2 | 3 | 2 |
| Inotropic negative | 2 | 1 | 3 |
| Antiarrhythmic | 2 | 2 | 2 |

*1*, Benefit; *2*, ± benefit; *3*, harmful.

pathophysiology of the condition as noted in earlier sections of this chapter.

***Afterload-reducing agents.*** Afterload-reducing agents are beneficial in patients with dilated cardiomyopathy but are of no benefit to patients with pericardial disease and may be harmful to patients with restrictive cardiomyopathy or hypertrophic cardiomyopathy. In dilated cardiomyopathy patients often have an excessive increase in systemic vascular resistance associated with a decrease in cardiac output. Lowering the systemic vascular resistance may allow an increase in the cardiac output and minimal change in the patient's perfusion pressure. Agents that have been demonstrated to improve symptoms, filling pressures, exercise capacity, and survival include nitrates combined with hydralazine, angiotensin-converting enzyme inhibitors, and in some patients β-blockers. The starting dose of all agents must be small and increased progressively over time. Patients receiving less than 40 mg of isordil four times a day with less than 50 mg of hydralazine four times a day are probably not being appropriately vasodilated. Angiotensin-converting enzyme inhibitors must be initiated at a low dose because of the first-dose response, which is characterized by a dramatic fall in blood pressure associated with the first, but not subsequent, dose of these agents. The dosage of afterload-reducing agents should be increased until the patient is significantly improved with regard to symptoms or until symptomatic hypotension is present.

Afterload-reducing agents are potentially dangerous to patients with hypertrophic cardiomyopathy, restrictive cardiomyopathy, or pericardial disease. Afterload-reducing agents reduce the blood pressure in these categories. Since the heart's stroke volume is fixed, the only mechanism by which patients could increase cardiac output is to increase heart rate. The heart rate increase is usually inadequate, and since cardiac output is the product of heart rate times stroke volume, patients develop a lower cardiac output with the use of these medications. This is particularly the case with hypertrophic cardiomyopathy, in which afterload reduction may exacerbate the hyperdynamic contractility and associated predisposition toward syncope or presyncope.

***Positive inotropic agents.*** Positive inotropic agents are of benefit to patients with dilated cardiomyopathy and of limited benefit to those with restrictive cardiomyopathy or constrictive pericarditis. Positive inotropic agents are contraindicated for patients with hypertrophic cardiomyopathy where hypercontractility already characterizes the condition. The only exceptions are in patients with atrial fibrillation and hypertrophic cardiomyopathy, where digoxin may be utilized for rate control and in advanced decompensated states of the condition, where patients develop a more dilated and hypofunctional heart muscle.

Positive inotropic agents include the sodium potassium ATPase inhibitor (digitalis), adrenergic agonist (dopamine and dobutamine), phosphodiesterase inhibitors (amrinone, caffeine, theophylline), and others (vesnarinone). Digoxin is effective in patients with dilated cardiomyopathy who have chronic heart failure and persistent signs and symptoms of dysfunction despite diuretics and afterload reduction. Dopamine in low doses stimulates the β-receptor and myocardial contractility as well as the dopaminergic receptor with dilatation of the coronary, cerebral, and renal vascular systems. The latter may allow dramatic improvement in renal perfusion and urinary output in patients who are refractory to standard diuretics. Doses of dopamine above 5 μ/kg/min may increase blood pressure through the peripheral α-receptor stimulation effect. Dobutamine stimulates the $\beta_1$-receptor in the heart, causing an increase in heart rate and contractility. In the arterial circulation, dobutamine stimulates the $\beta_2$-receptor, causing vasodilatation in the α-receptor and constriction with a net result of no significant vascular effect.

Dobutamine may cause some preload reduction. Phosphodiesterase inhibitors may be given intravenously to patients in moribund heart failure for no more than 48 hours. Phosphodiesterase inhibitors are mild inotropes and vasodilators and are as effective acutely as dobutamine in patients with refractory heart failure. Dopamine, dobutamine, and amrinone should not be used as initial therapy of heart failure unless the patient is in extremis. Experience has taught us that low doses of inotropic agents are somewhat less effective acutely but have better long-term potential for improvement in symptoms and prolongation of life. High-dose inotropes improve symptoms but worsen life expectancy.

Patients with dilated cardiomyopathy are at risk for developing systemic emboli. Patients with any form of myocardial or pericardial disease may develop atrial fibrillation and may similarly be at risk, particularly if they have heart failure. Therefore, patients with myocardial disease and atrial fibrillation or dilated cardiomyopathy with an ejection fraction below 30% should receive anticoagulants to prevent systemic embolization unless there is a contraindication.

Arrhythmias are common in patients with myocardial and pericardial disease. Patients from all categories are prone to atrial fibrillation. Patients with myocardial disease who develop atrial fibrillation have a significant decrease in their cardiac output due to the increased heart rate, decreased diastolic filling time, and lack of atrial systole preloading the ventricle before contraction. Control of the rapid ventricular response in atrial fibrillation and conversion to sinus rhythm are important objectives for patients with myocardial or pericardial disease and atrial fibrillation. Those with myocardial diseases, particularly dilated cardiomyopathy and hypertrophic cardiomyopathy, are markedly prone to ventricular arrhythmias, including ventricular tachycardia, and are at risk for sudden death. There is as yet no convincing study to indicate that treatment of ventricular arrhythmias prolongs survival in patients with dilated, hypertrophic, restrictive, or pericardial disease. Nonetheless, in patients with symptomatic ventricular tachycardia, treatment is initiated with medicines or an automatic implantable defibrillator. For patients with ventricular tachycardia in excess of 10 beats in duration, serious consideration must be given to prophylactic treatment with drugs or devices. Of the agents available, β-blockers and amiodarone appear to be the most efficacious and least risky. Antiarrhythmic agents in patients with ischemic cardiomyopathy are particularly fraught with prorhythmic hazard and an increased risk of sudden death.

Specific treatment of the etiologies of causes of dilated and restrictive cardiomyopathies is beyond the scope of this chapter. Careful consideration must be given to the pros and cons of treatment of disorders such as myocarditis or ischemic cardiomyopathy. Consultation with a cardiologist is appropriate.

***Negative inotropic agents.*** Negative inotropic agents include β-blockers, calcium blockers, and disopyramide. Patients with dilated cardiomyopathy tolerate negative inotropic agents poorly; therefore these agents are generally contraindicated in these patients. β-Blockers may be an exception but are considered *experimental.* β-Blockers may protect the β-receptor in patients with dilated cardiomyopathy from excessive catecholamine stimulation. The norepinephrine spillover from sympathetic stimulation increases with worsening heart failure and is associated with a poor prognosis. β-Blockade allows the β-receptor to upregulate. This has been demonstrated in some patients to improve contractility, symptoms, and perhaps survival. Unfortunately, it is not yet clear which group of patients tolerates this medication, and until further evidence is forthcoming, agents should not be administered except under experimental conditions. Negative inotropic agents will be of no benefit to patients with restrictive cardiomyopathy or pericardial disease. In fact, these agents may be harmful due to depression of the contractility necessary to maintain reasonable forward perfusion.

Patients with hypertrophic cardiomyopathy are significantly improved with the use of β-blockers or calcium channel blockers. Both agents decrease intrinsic heart rate, allowing greater ventricular filling before contraction and improved stroke volume. Calcium blockers may additionally improve calcium overload of the myocardium, which has been associated with a hypertrophic cardiomyopathic state. β-Blockers and calcium blockers decrease the hypercontractility characteristic of this disorder, which may diminish chest pain, presyncope, syncope, and excessive fatigability.

## Pacing

Patients with dilated cardiomyopathy are currently being investigated to determine whether pacing with a short PR interval or biapical ventricular pacing may improve signs and symptoms of congestive heart failure. Similarly, patients with hypertrophic cardiomyopathy are being investigated to determine whether AV sequential pacing or pacing from a hypertrophic, hyperdynamic septum may improve symptoms and outflow gradients.

## Surgical therapy

***Pericardial disease.*** Pericardial effusion can be drained percutaneously or surgically. Drainage of a significant pericardial effusion associated with tamponade immediately and dramatically improves the patient's hemodynamics and returns the patient to a normal state of well-being, assuming there is no associated myocardial dysfunction. The fluid removed from the pericardial sac must be carefully examined to determine the etiology of the effusion so that it may be appropriately treated and prevented from recurring. If no etiology is identified, antiinflammatory medications may be of benefit.

Pericardial constriction is treatable with surgical intervention. The surgery for pericardial constriction is virtually always of benefit. The degree of benefit depends on the magnitude of adherence of the pericardial surface to the epicardial surface. Some pericardial constrictions are as easy to remove as an orange peel, whereas others must be painstakingly chiseled from the anterior heart wall. One must remember that a pericardiectomy is, in fact, only a release of the anterior pericardium between the vagus nerves, since the posterior pericardium cannot be reached.

***Dilated cardiomyopathy.*** Patients with dilated cardiomyopathy may improve with the use of dynamic cardiomyoplasty or heart transplantation. Dynamic cardiomyoplasty is experimental and utilizes the latissimus dorsi wrapped around the heart muscle in a complicated surgical technique. The latissimus is then stimulated by a pacemaker to contract in conjunction with the myocardium and, by its presence around the myocardium, to prevent further myocardial dilatation. Cardiac transplantation is not available to all patients with dilated cardiomyopathy. Significant limitations due to age, pulmonary vascular resistance, diabetes, excessive obesity, extracardiac vascular disease, other comorbidities, or psychosocial factors govern its utilization. Cardiac transplantation results in the replacement of an end-stage, life-threatening heart condition with a multitude of posttransplant medical problems associated with immunosuppressive drugs and their side effects. These are significant and include glucocorticoid-induced weight gain, peptic ulceration, hypertension, bone disease, and glucose intolerance. Azathioprine may induce fevers, nausea, and a decrease in white blood cell count. Cyclosporin results in hirsutism and is associated with hypertension. The agents together cause a dramatic increase in cholesterol.

***Hypertrophic cardiomyopathy.*** Patients with hypertrophic cardiomyopathy and an outflow gradient that is not relieved by medical or pacing therapy may be submitted to septal myectomy. This surgical procedure is characterized by the removal of a slice of the ventricular septum approximately the size of the distal portion of the fifth finger. This does decrease the outflow gradient, and there has been no regrowth of this tissue demonstrated over time. Patients with hypertrophic cardiomyopathy have been submitted to mitral valve replacement. This likewise significantly alters septal contractility and clearly prevents mitral regurgitation or the anterior movement of the mitral leaflet to oppose the septum.

In conclusion, it is important to recognize that all forms of myocardial and pericardial disease may present with similar symptoms of congestive heart failure. Only by determining the etiology of the heart failure can an appropriate understanding of the pathophysiology be reached and appropriate treatment rendered.

## BIBLIOGRAPHY

Captopril Multicenter Research Group: A placebo-controlled trial of captopril in refractory chronic congestive heart failure, *J Am Coll Cardiol* 2(4):755, 1983.

Cohn JN et al: Effect of vasodilator therapy on mortality in chronic congestive heart failure, *N Engl J Med* 314(24):1547, 1986.

Cohn JN et al: A comparison of enalapril with hydralazine-isosorbide dinitrate in the treatment of chronic congestive heart failure, *N Engl J Med* 325(5):303, 1991.

Consensus Trial Study Group: Effects of enalapril on mortality in severe congestive heart failure, *N Engl J Med* 316(23):1429, 1987.

Franciosa JA et al: Survival in men with severe chronic left ventricular failure due to either coronary heart disease or idiopathic dilated cardiomyopathy, *Am J Cardiol* 51:831, 1983.

McKee PA et al: The natural history of congestive heart failure: the Framingham study, *N Eng J Med* 285(26):1441, 1971.

Report of the WHO/ISFC task force on the definition and classification of cardiomyopathies, *Br Heart J* 44:672, 1980.

Smith WM: Epidemiology of congestive heart failure, *Am J Cardiol* 55:3A, 1985.

SOLVD Investigators: Effect of enalapril on survival in patients with reduced left ventricular ejection fractions and congestive heart failure, *N Engl J Med* 325(5):293, 1991.

CHAPTER

# 17 Endocarditis

**Nelson M. Gantz**
**Katherine Murray-Leisure**

## ETIOLOGY AND EPIDEMIOLOGY

Infective endocarditis is a microbial infection of one or more heart valves or, less commonly, infection of the endomyocardial wall of the heart. When infective endocarditis presents as a subacute bacterial infection of the heart valves, it is called subacute bacterial endocarditis (SBE). Infective endocarditis, however, is a more general term that includes those endocardial infections caused by fungi, rickettsia, and *Chlamydia* species.

SBE presents insidiously with gradual onset. The illness may have begun 3 to 6 weeks before diagnosis. Most cases of SBE are caused by relatively avirulent bacteria that attach to abnormal or defective heart valves, including prosthetic valves. Gram-positive cocci such as viridans streptococci (nongroupable) species, microaerophilic streptococci, β-hemolytic streptococci, enterococci, and *Streptococcus* (*Diplococcus*) *pneumoniae* cause SBE most frequently (Fig. 17-1). Septicemia or endocarditis due to *Streptococcus bovis* is associated frequently with colonic malignancy, polyps, and other gastrointestinal illness. Less frequently, gram-negative bacteria, including those from the HACEK group (*Haemophilus aphrophilus, Haemophilus paraphrophilus, Actinobacillus actinomycetemcomitans, Cardiobacterium hominis,* and *Kingella kingae*), and *Neisseria gonorrhoeae* can cause SBE. Unfortunately, all these otherwise fastidious and relatively avirulent bacteria, once attached to the heart valve, can cause progressive valvular destruction, form valvular vegetations, and cause systemic embolization.

Acute bacterial endocarditis is infective endocarditis of less than 6 weeks' duration. Typically, acute bacterial endocarditis is caused by virulent and invasive microorganisms that attack normal heart valves in addition to damaged cardiac tissues. Hospital- or procedure-associated cases occur with intravascular catheters, intrathoracic or intravascular monitors, and after angioplasty or cardiothoracic surgery. Intravenous or injection drug abuse can also precipitate acute bacterial endocarditis. In addition to streptococcal species, acute bacterial endocarditis is caused by *Staphylococcus aureus, Staphylococcus epidermidis, Pseudomonas aeruginosa, Salmonella* species, other enteric gram-negative Enterobacteriaceae species, and fungi such as *Candida albicans.* Cardiologic aspects of endocarditis are presented on pp. 288-290.

## PATHOPHYSIOLOGY

Congenital bicuspid aortic valves, rheumatic mitral and aortic valves, and otherwise diseased, calcified, stenotic, prolapsed, or regurgitant heart valves predispose to the

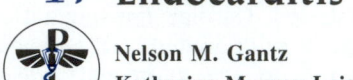

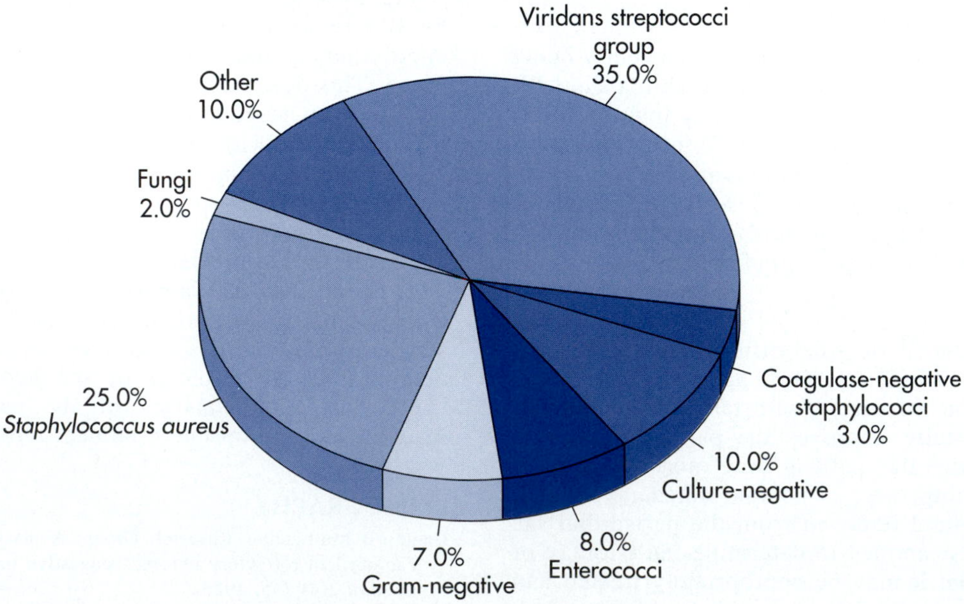


**Fig. 17-1.** Microbiology of infective endocarditis.

development of SBE (see the box below). The left heart, a higher pressure system, is affected more frequently than the right, and the mitral valve is infected more frequently than the aortic valve. Right-sided endocarditis occurs rarely, mostly with injection drug abuse or central vein catheterization into the superior vena cava. Deposits of platelets and fibrin form a fibrin clot wherever there is hemodynamic turbulence or a foreign body. Microorganisms adhere to the valve or fibrin clot during a transient bacteremia. Organisms multiply and form friable vegetations, aggregates of microbes and fibrin, on the valves. Vegetations may subsequently break off and, as systemic emboli, cause infarction in the brain, kidneys, spleen, or other tissues. Locally, bacteria may invade the endomyocardium and the His-Purkinje conduction fibers of the septum, resulting in dysrhythmias or heart block. Eventually, after the valve is destroyed and incompetent, heart failure ensues. Death due to SBE occurs with either overwhelming septic shock, complications from embolization, or congestive heart failure.

In the laboratory, rats develop endocarditis with a central venous plastic catheter in the right heart and small bacterial inocula, especially after trauma or disturbance instituted by the catheter. This is a good animal model for acute bacterial endocarditis. In humans any foreign material, as is seen with drug addicts or central vascular catheters inserted either into the superior vena cava or retrograde into the aorta and coronary arteries, can precipitate acute bacterial endocarditis with a relatively small inoculum of virulent organisms. *S. aureus* is a frequent cause of acute bacterial endocarditis. Acute bacterial endocarditis can involve normal, native valves, defective valves, or prosthetic valves.

Mechanical and bioprosthetic (porcine) valves are also prone to infection, chiefly with *S. epidermidis* and other coagulase-negative staphylococci. In the acute postoperative period infection due to coagulase-negative staphylococci, diptheroids (from the skin), gram-negative bacilli, and fungi including *Aspergillus* may be seen. Some cases of nosocomial prosthetic valve endocarditis due to *Legionella* species have also been reported. In late prosthetic valve endocarditis over 12 months after valve replacement, however, the microbiology approaches that of native valve endocarditis, with viridans streptococci, enterococci, and the HACEK group of organisms causing infection as frequently as *S. epidermidis* and *S. aureus*. Infection of prosthetic heart valves not only threatens the prosthesis but it may also invade the perivalvular tissues, cause necrosis of the annulus with subsequent ring abscesses, and cause dissection into the myocardium.

### Cardiac lesions predisposing to infective endocarditis

**Congenital**

Bicuspid aortic valve
Mitral valve prolapse with insufficiency
Patent ductus arteriosus
Ventricular septal defect
Atrial septal defect, ostium primum type
Tetralogy of Fallot
Pulmonic stenosis
Marfan syndrome (aortic valve)
Asymmetric septal hypertrophy/idiopathic hypertrophic subaortic stenosis

**Acquired or degenerative**

Rheumatic mitral and/or aortic valves
Calcific mitral or aortic stenosis, calcified mitral annulus
Atherosclerotic, calcified nodularities
Regurgitant or stenotic valves
Postinfarction thrombus
Syphilitic or luetic aortitis

**Postoperative, posttraumatic, or foreign body**

Intracardiac prostheses
Cardiac pacemaker wires
Intravascular (venous or arterial) catheters
Injection drug abuse
Mechanical or bioprosthetic heart valves
Orthotopic cardiac transplant

## HISTORY AND PHYSICAL FINDINGS

SBE presents insidiously with weeks or months of malaise, weakness, intermittent fevers, sweats, myalgias, and arthralgias, especially low back or flank pains (Table 17-1). Patients might also have anorexia, cough, and upper respiratory tract infection, palpitations, or an unexplained embolic cerebrovascular accident. Most of these symptoms disappear with appropriate antibiotic therapy. Acute bacterial endocarditis presents more suddenly with acute fevers, toxic symptoms, encephalopathy, and septicemia with sustained bacteremias. This is commonly seen in nosocomial cases where patients have undergone invasive procedures or intravascular manipulation. *S. aureus* is a common pathogen.

**Table 17-1.** Clinical findings in infective endocarditis

| Finding | Incidence % |
|---|---|
| **Symptoms** | |
| Fevers | 85 |
| Chills, sweats | 40 |
| Weakness | 40 |
| Dyspnea | 40 |
| Anorexia | 40 |
| Cough | 25 |
| Headache | 20 |
| Nausea, vomiting | 20 |
| Skin lesions | 20 |
| Stroke | 20 |
| Chest pains | 15 |
| Back pains | 10 |
| **Signs** | |
| Fevers | 90 |
| Heart murmur(s) | 85 |
| Petechiae | 28 |
| Conjunctival hemorrhage | 20 |
| Splenomegaly | 25 |
| Renal failure | 15 |
| Splenic abscess | 8 |

### Laboratory findings in infective endocarditis

Leukocytosis
Anemia
Azotemia
Microscopic hematuria
Significant microbial growth in blood cultures

Medical history is important for noting any prior rheumatic fever, valvular heart disease, the patient's most recent operative procedures and postoperative convalescence from each procedure, recent dental procedures and dental care, skin or soft tissue infections, insulin-dependent diabetes mellitus, injecting drug abuse, and any antibiotics taken recently. A portal of entry from a prior tonsillectomy, dental extraction, cystoscopy, rectal surgery, skin or foot infection, or recent cardiac catheterization or angioplasty may be ascertained.

Physical examination reveals sustained low- or high-grade fevers, tachycardia, and weight loss if the patient is anorectic. Facial and conjunctival pallor are consistent with anemia. Conjunctival and palatal petechiae may be present, even after starting antibiotic therapy. Petechial or flame-shaped hemorrhages of the retina may have oval white central areas on funduscopic exam (Roth spots). Lung findings may be consistent with early heart failure. Cardiac murmurs are present in at least two thirds of cases and are especially noteworthy if documented to have changed over time. Prosthetic valve dysfunction is detected by a new or changing murmur or by a muffling of the opening or closing valve clicks or sounds. Splenomegaly or at least a tender, palpable spleen tip is present in some cases. Vertebral tenderness and low back pains may be present acutely, mimicking vertebral osteomyelitis or pyelonephritis. On the skin of the lower extremities petechiae may persist for a few weeks into the course of appropriate antibiotic therapy. Linear subungual splinter hemorrhages of the fingernails and small, slightly nodular or hemorrhagic papules on the palms or soles (Janeway lesions) are usually nontender. Rarely, painful nodules on the fingertips may be present; these nodules are called Osler nodes.

Laboratory findings include anemia, leukocytosis, azotemia, and microscopic hematuria (see the box above). The erythrocyte sedimentation rate is elevated, and in some subacute or chronic cases the rheumatoid factor may be reactive. Three or more sets of blood cultures, with 10 ml of adult blood inoculated into aerobic and anaerobic media for each set, should be taken minutes or hours apart in time before starting antibiotics. Blood cultures taken before the initiation of therapy should all grow the causative microorganism, reflecting a sustained bacteremia or fungemia. Negative blood cultures in the presence of active infective endocarditis reflect the presence of a fastidious microorganism, the use of antibiotics (anytime up to 10 days before blood culture collections), or, rarely, right-sided endocarditis due to a fastidious microorganism.

## DIAGNOSIS

The blood culture is the key test in the diagnosis of endocarditis. Patients with infective endocarditis have a sustained bacteremia or fungemia. In native valve endocarditis blood cultures are positive in 85% to 90% of patients. Blood cultures are positive in 90% to 95% of those with prosthetic valve endocarditis. Factors that are responsible for some patients to have culture-negative endocarditis include prior antibiotic use, uremia, and infection caused by fastidious pathogens. The major cause of negative blood cultures in patients with infective endocarditis is the administration of antibiotics before obtaining blood cultures. The use of blood cultures that contain resins to remove antimicrobial agents may help detect the organism in a patient receiving an antibiotic. The presence of a fastidious organism that fails to grow on routine media may be responsible for a patient having negative blood cultures. Examples of fastidious organisms are members of the HACEK group, small pleomorphic gram-negative rods. Other organisms that are difficult to isolate using standard blood culture techniques include nutritionally deficient streptococci, *Legionella* species, *Neisseria* species, anaerobes, *Chlamydia* species, fungi and *Coxiella burnetti,* the cause of Q fever. Studies show that generally three sets of blood cultures are sufficient to establish the diagnosis. Usually all blood cultures with infective endocarditis are positive, and intermittently positive blood cultures are uncommon. In adults 20 ml of blood should be taken per set of blood cultures and divided between an aerobic and anaerobic bottle. In patients with suspected acute endocarditis three sets of blood cultures should be obtained within 1 hour and antimicrobial therapy instituted. In patients with suspected SBE blood cultures should be drawn over 24 hours, since there is no urgency to begin therapy. Blood cultures should always be obtained from different venipuncture sites using sterile technique to avoid contamination.

When laboratory reports indicate sterile blood cultures in patients with suspected endocarditis, it is important to alert the microbiologist to this diagnosis so that special measures can be used to detect a fastidious organism. Nutritionally deficient streptococci may require the addition of pyridoxine to the media for detection. Other organisms such as fungi and *Brucella* species are slow growing and require incubating the blood culture bottles longer than 7 days. Fungi should be suspected in intravenous drug users, and their isolation can be facilitated by using the lysis centrifugation technique and biphasic blood culture bottles, which contain both solid and liquid media.

Other strategies may also be useful to establish a diagnosis in a patient with suspected endocarditis and sterile blood cultures. Serologic methods that show a fourfold rise in antibodies in the patient's serum may be helpful in the diagnosis of endocarditis caused by *Chlamydia* species or *C. burnetti.* Certain organisms such as fungi or *Haemophilus* species are prone to produce a presentation of SBE with large emboli. Examination of emboli using histologic techniques as well as culture may be helpful in establishing an etiologic diagnosis. Examination of a bone marrow aspirate using special stains and cultures can be helpful in the diagnosis of endocarditis.

Noninfectious causes of endocarditis such as atrial myxoma or marantic endocarditis can mimic the clinical presentation of culture-negative infective endocarditis.

In addition to obtaining blood cultures, electrocardiography, and echocardiography are important in the diagnosis and management of patients with suspected endocarditis. The electrocardiogram (ECG) may reveal conduction abnormalities secondary to inflammation or abscess formation of the His-Purkinje and other myocardial conduction fibers. Approximately 10% of patients with endocarditis have dysrhythmias, heart block, or other conduction abnormalities that may be due to abscess formation, myocarditis, and the use of digitalis or other drugs. However, a normal ECG does not exclude the presence of an abscess. A baseline ECG is always indicated in a patient with suspected endocarditis.

Echocardiography can provide valuable information with respect to the presence of valvular heart disease and whether there are vegetations. Two-dimensional transthoracic echocardiography (TTE) was developed in the 1970s. The TTE has a sensitivity of about 50% to 60% in detecting the presence of vegetations. The demonstration of left-sided vegetations by TTE is associated with an increased frequency of systemic large vessel emboli, congestive heart failure, and valve disruption. There is also an increased mortality in patients with large right-sided vegetations demonstrated by TTE. In the late 1980s transesophageal echocardiography (TEE) was developed with markedly improved visualization of left-sided vegetations and the mitral valve. The technique of TEE involves placing a transducer on the end of a gastroscope and passing the scope into the esophagus to view the heart. TEE is superior to TTE for viewing prosthetic valves and for detecting vegetations smaller than 5 mm in diameter. The sensitivity of TEE in detecting valvular vegetations in patients with endocarditis is about 90%. Thus repeated negative TEE studies provide strong evidence against the diagnosis of infective endocarditis.

## MANAGEMENT

### Antibiotic therapy

The vegetation that contains the infecting organism in patients with endocarditis is relatively protected on the valve leaflet from host defenses. Consequently, antimicrobial therapy for patients with endocarditis should be bactericidal rather than bacteriostatic. Examples of bactericidal antimicrobials are the penicillins, cephalosporins, aminoglycosides, and vancomycin. Clindamycin, tetracycline, and chloramphenicol are bacteriostatic. Parenteral therapy, particularly via the intravenous route, is preferred over oral therapy, since higher and more predictable serum levels can be achieved. Table 17-2 lists various regimens used to treat patients with endocarditis based on identification of the causative organism. Antibiotics are usually administered for 4 to 6 weeks. In patients with culture-negative endocarditis, a combination of high-dose penicillin (24 million units/day) plus gentamicin is used in those with infected native valves. In the penicillin-allergic patient with native valve endocarditis, vancomycin can be substituted for penicillin. In patients with culture-negative prosthetic valve endocarditis a combination of vancomycin plus gentamicin is recommended to cover organisms such as coagulase-negative staphylococci.

### Monitoring therapy

Antimicrobial therapy should be monitored by repeating the blood cultures to demonstrate sterility of the blood after therapy is initiated. The adequacy of therapy should also be monitored by observing the clinical course of the illness. Clinical defervescence should occur within 10 days after starting antibiotics. Persistent fever is always a concern. Fever may be due to (1) inadequate antimicrobial therapy, (2) sterile or infected emboli, (3) splenic, renal, or other systemic abscess, (4) drug fever, or (5) thrombophlebitis secondary to an intravenous line.

The serum bactericidal, or Schlichter, test is used to predict outcome in patients receiving antimicrobial agents for endocarditis. This test involves determining the highest dilution of the patient's serum that kills an inoculum of the patient's organism in vitro. The serum is obtained while the patient is receiving antimicrobial therapy and is drawn at the times when the antibiotic is at the peak and trough levels. However, the clinical interpretation of the serum bactericidal titer is unclear. Some experts suggest that a peak serum bactericidal titer of a 1:8 dilution or greater is desirable. It is not mandatory that a serum bactericidal titer be obtained. The test is useful in monitoring therapy only when the clinical response is suboptimal. Response may also be followed by measuring the erythrocyte sedimentation rate and noting a decrease at the end of therapy. Finally, blood cultures should be repeated within 1 month of completing therapy to detect a relapse.

### Surgery

Medical therapy with at least 4 weeks of antibiotics is effective for most patients with infective endocarditis. However, moderate to severe congestive heart failure is an indication for surgery. Persistent bacteremia, despite appropriate antibiotic therapy, is another indication for valve replacement cardiac surgery. Blood cultures should become sterile within 5 to 7 days after the institution of appropriate antibiotic therapy. A prosthetic valve can be inserted safely in the site of active infection while the patient is receiving appropriate antibiotics. Patients with valvular obstruction or a myocardial abscess also require surgery for cure, as do patients with fungal endocarditis. In addition to the above absolute indications for surgery in patients with either native or prosthetic valve endocarditis, patients with an unstable prosthesis also require surgery. Patients with two or more major systemic emboli may also be candidates for surgery. However, the decision for surgery in patients with a relative indication such as multiple systemic emboli should be individualized based on a careful clinical assessment. It is important to emphasize that, once surgery is indicated, the decision should not be delayed.

## PROPHYLAXIS

Patients with certain underlying cardiac lesions should receive prophylactic antibiotics just before undergoing procedures that might cause a bacteremia resulting in endocarditis. Although use of prophylactic antibiotics to prevent endocarditis is the standard of care, there are no studies to prove the efficacy of this practice. The current guidelines for prophylaxis of endocarditis are based on recommendations from the American Heart Association (AHA) and the Working Party of the British Society for Antimicrobial Chemotherapy. Adherence to these regimens by practicing dentists is often faulty.

A key factor in the pathogenesis of infective endocarditis is the occurrence of a transient bacteremia. When bacteria invade the bloodstream, persons who have rheumatic heart disease, congenital heart disease, a prosthetic heart valve, mitral valve prolapse, or other cardiovascular diseases are at risk of developing infective endocarditis.

Transient bacteremias occur commonly. They may occur spontaneously, such as when chewing food. They may result from many procedures, such as dental extractions and urethral catheterizations, that traumatize mucous membranes with an indigenous microbial flora. Bacteremias following procedures resulting from mucosal trauma are asymptomatic and last only for 15 to 30 minutes. Transient bacteremias can also occur from incision and drainage of a local abscess or manipulation of the urinary tract in a patient with asymptomatic bacteriuria.

A history of a predisposing event can at times be elicited from a patient with endocarditis. From 4% to 20% of patients with nonenterococcal streptococcal endocarditis recall a preceding dental procedure; a preceding genitourinary tract procedure has been reported in up to 42% of patients with enterococcal endocarditis; 35% of patients with staphylococcal endocarditis have had a preceding infection of the skin or soft tissue. However,

**Table 17-2.** Endocarditis treatment regimens (adult doses)

| Regimen | Antibiotic dosage and duration options |
|---|---|
| Highly penicillin-susceptible streptococci (penicillin MIC ≤ 0.1 μg/ml) | Aqueous penicillin G, 12 million U daily IV for 4 weeks |
| | Aqueous penicillin G, 12 million U daily IV for 4 weeks; plus gentamicin, 1 mg/kg (maximum 80 mg) q8h IV for 2 weeks |
| Highly penicillin-susceptible streptococci in penicillin-allergic patients | Cefazolin 1 g q8h IV |
| Enterococci or other streptococci (penicillin MIC ≥ 0.1 μg/ml) | Aqueous penicillin G, 24 million U daily IV for 4-6 weeks; plus gentamicin, 1 mg/kg (maximum 80 mg) q8h IV |
| | Ampicillin, 12 g daily IV for 4-6 weeks; plus gentamicin, 1 mg/kg (maximum 80 mg) q8h IV/IM |
| Enterococci or other streptococci in penicillin-allergic patient (MIC ≥ 0.1 mg/ml) | Vancomycin, 30 mg/kg daily (maximum 2 g/day unless serum levels are monitored) divided q6h or q12h IV; plus gentamicin, 1 mg/kg (maximum 80 mg) q8h IV/IM |
| Methicillin-susceptible staphylococci | Nafcillin or oxacillin, 2 g q4h IV for 4-6 weeks; plus gentamicin, 1 mg/kg (maximum 80 mg) q8h IV for first 3-5 days |
| Methicillin-susceptible staphylococci in penicillin-allergic patients | Cefazolin, 2 g q8h IV, with or without gentamicin, 1 mg/kg (maximum 80 mg) q8h IV for first 3-5 days |
| | Vancomycin, 30 mg/kg daily (maximum 2 g/day unless serum levels are monitored) divided q6h or q12h IV for 4-6 weeks |
| Methicillin-resistant staphylococci | Vancomycin, 30 mg/kg daily (maximum 2 g/day unless serum levels are monitored) divided q6h or q12h IV for 4-6 weeks |
| Methicillin-resistant staphylococci in the presence of a prosthetic device | Vancomycin, 30 mg/kg daily (maximum 2 g/day unless serum levels are monitored) divided q6h or q12h IV; plus rifampin, 300 mg q8h PO for 6 weeks; plus gentamicin, 1 mg/kg (maximum 80 mg) q8h IV/IM for the first 2 weeks |
| Methicillin-susceptible staphylococci in the presence of a prosthetic device | Nafcillin or oxacillin, 2 g q4h IV for 6 weeks; plus gentamicin, 1 mg/kg (maximum 80 mg) q8h IV/IM for the first 2 weeks; plus rifampin, 300 mg q8h PO for 6 weeks |
| HACEK organisms | Ampicillin, 2 g q4h IV for 4 weeks |
| | Ceftriaxone, 1 g q12h IV; plus gentamicin, 1.7 mg/kg q8h IV for 4 weeks |
| Enterobacteriaceae | Ceftriaxone, 2 g q12h IV |
| | Imipenem, 0.5 g q6h IV |
| | Aztreonam, 2 g q8h IV; plus gentamicin, 1.7 mg/kg q8h IV for 4-6 weeks |
| *Pseudomonas aeruginosa* | Piperacillin, 3 g q4h IV |
| | Ceftazidime, 2 g q8h IV |
| | Imipenem, 0.5 g q6h IV |
| | Aztreonam, 2 g q6h IV; plus tobramycin, 1.7 mg/kg q8h IV for 6 weeks |

Modified from Bisno AL, et al: *Antimicrobial treatment of infective endocarditis due to viridans streptococci, enterococci and staphylococci, JAMA* 261:1471, 1989, and Baldassarre JS, Kaye J. In Kaye D, editor: *Principles and overview of antibiotic therapy in infective endocarditis,* ed 2, New York, 1992, Raven Press.
*MIC,* Minimal inhibitory concentration.
*HACEK, Haemophilus aphrophilus, Haemophilus paraphrophilus, Actinobacillus actinomycetemcomitans, Cardiobacterium hominis,* and *Kingella Kingae.*

endocarditis occurs in most patients without an obvious predisposing event.

The oropharynx is a frequent portal of entry for organisms gaining access into the bloodstream. Blood cultures are positive in 18% to 85% of patients after a dental extraction. Other dental procedures that may result in a transient bacteremia include periodontal operations such as gingivectomy, root canal surgery, and dental cleaning. The frequency of bacteremia correlates with the severity of gingival infection and the extent of tissue trauma. The organisms isolated reflect the normal mouth flora. Viridans streptococci are isolated most frequently. The streptococci are sensitive to penicillin unless the patient is receiving prophylactic penicillin for rheumatic fever or given antibiotic prophylaxis as early as 1 to 2 days before a procedure. Thus prophylaxis should begin just prior to a procedure so that serum levels of the antibiotic are adequate at the time of anticipated bacteremia. Maintenance of good oral hygiene, however, decreases the amount of gum disease, which is a key determinant of the frequency of a transient bacteremia following any dental manipulation.

Diagnostic procedures involving the gastrointestinal tract are another source of transient bacteremias. Positive blood cultures are found in 4% of patients having fiberoptic gastrointestinal endoscopy, 5% of patients having flexible sigmoidoscopy, 11% of patients having a barium enema, and 5% of patients undergoing colonoscopy. The predominant organisms isolated with these procedures are enterococci, a frequent cause of endocarditis, and gram-negative bacilli, organisms rarely involved in native valve endocarditis.

Transient bacteremia and infective endocarditis can also occur following urinary tract, obstetric, and gynecologic procedures. The urinary tract is the portal of entry in 20% to 50% of patients with enterococcal endocarditis.

Prevention of endocarditis requires a knowledge of both the events likely to produce bacteremia as well as the patient with predisposing cardiac lesions. Unfortunately, half the patients with endocarditis have no recognized underlying heart disease, making antibiotic prophylaxis impossible for this group. Patients with mitral valve prolapse–click murmur syndrome have been reported to be at increased risk of endocarditis. Prophylaxis in all patients with mitral valve prolapse would be difficult because of its high incidence (5% to 6% of the American population). One approach is to prescribe prophylaxis only for patients with associated mitral insufficiency and not for those who have only a systolic click and are undergoing procedures associated with endocarditis.

Patients with a previous episode of endocarditis and those with prosthetic or bioprosthetic heart valves should also receive prophylaxis for predisposing events. Since infection of a prosthesis is often difficult to eradicate and carries a high mortality, antibiotic prophylaxis is recommended both for the usual predisposing events and for additional procedures associated with a transient bacteremia with a lower risk of infection, such as upper gastrointestinal tract endoscopy, barium enema, and colonoscopy.

Antibiotic prophylaxis is not indicated for patients at risk for endocarditis undergoing cardiac catheterization, pacemaker insertion, or peritoneal dialysis. Effective use of prophylactic antibiotics requires that adequate drug levels be present at the time of the event posing the risk of transient bacteremia. To accomplish this goal, the antimicrobial drug should be given initially just before the procedure and continued for 6 hours. For dental procedures and other procedures involving the airway the antibiotic selected should be directed against viridans streptococci. Genitourinary manipulation and gastrointestinal, gynecologic, and obstetric procedures require that the antibiotic prophylaxis be directed against enterococci. Antibiotics should be adequate for penicillinase-producing staphylococci in a predisposed person having incision and drainage of an abscess. A urine culture should

**Table 17-3.** Antibiotic prophylactic regimens for adults undergoing dental, oral, or upper respiratory tract procedures*

| Drug | Initial dose | Route | Regimen |
|---|---|---|---|
| Amoxicillin | 3 g | PO | 1 hr before, then 1.5 g 6 hr later |
| Ampicillin | 2 g | IV or IM | 30 min before, then ampicillin, 1 g IV or IM, or amoxicillin, 1.5 g PO, 6 hr later |
| Ampicillin plus gentamicin† | 2 g<br>1.5 mg/kg (max 80 mg) | IV or IM<br>IV or IM | 30 min before, then amoxicillin, 1.5 g PO 6 hr later; or repeat parenteral drugs 8 hr later |
| Erythromycin ethylsuccinate‡ *or* | 1600 mg | PO | 2 hr before, then half the dose 6 hr later |
| Erythromycin stearate‡ | 1 g | PO | |
| Clindamycin‡ | 300 mg | PO | 1 hr before, then 150 mg 6 hr later |
| Vancomycin†‡ | 1 g | IV | Administer over 1 hr and perform procedure immediately when finished |

*Parenteral regimens are recommended for patients with prosthetic or biosynthetic heart valves.
†May be preferred for patients in highest-risk groups, although data to support this practice are not available.
‡If patient is allergic to penicillin or receiving continuous oral penicillin.

**Table 17-4.** Endocarditis prophylaxis for adults undergoing genitourinary, gastrointestinal, or gynecologic procedures*

| Drug | Initial dose | Route | Regimen |
|---|---|---|---|
| Ampicillin plus gentamicin | 2 g<br>1.5 mg/kg (to a maximum of 80 mg) | IV or IM | 30 min before, then repeat 8 hr later; or amoxicillin 1.5 g 6 hr later |
| Vancomycin plus gentamicin† | 1 g<br>1.5 mg/kg (to a maximum of 80 mg) | IV<br>IV or IM | 1 hr before, then repeat 8 hr later |
| Amoxicillin‡ | 3 g | PO | 1 hr before, then 1.5 g 6 hr later |

*Parenteral regimens are recommended for patients with prosthetic or biosynthetic heart valves.
†If allergic to penicillin.
‡Alternative for low-risk patient.

**Table 17-5.** Endocarditis prophylaxis for incision and drainage of skin abscesses caused by coagulase-positive staphylococci*

| Drug | Initial dose | Route | Regimen |
|---|---|---|---|
| Nafcillin or oxacillin | 2 g | IV | ½ to 1 hour before procedure, then 2 g IV q4h |
| Dicloxacillin | 500 mg | PO | 1 hr before procedure, then 500 mg q6h |
| Cefazolin† | 1 g | IM | 1 hour before procedure, then 1 g IV or IM q8h |
| Vancomycin*† | 1 g | IV | Over 30 min; start infusion 1 hr before procedure, then 1 g q12h IV |

Modified from Dajani AS et al: *JAMA* 264:2919, 1990.
*Route and duration of therapy depend on the severity of the infection and whether the predisposed person is at high risk (e.g., prosthetic heart valve). Results of Gram stains and cultures should also guide antibiotic selection.
†If patient is allergic to penicillin.

be obtained before a genitourinary procedure so that any infection can be identified and treated before the instrumentation.

Antibiotic regimens for prophylaxis are listed in Tables 17-3, 17-4, and 17-5. The recommendations for use in the United States are derived from the guidelines proposed by an advisory committee to the American Heart Association. Amoxicillin has replaced penicillin for prophylaxis in patients undergoing dental or upper respiratory tract surgical procedures. Patients who have recently received penicillin or who are allergic to penicillin should receive oral erythromycin or clindamycin for dental procedures. For gastrointestinal, genitourinary, and gynecologic procedures parenteral ampicillin and gentamicin are recommended. Those patients with a penicillin allergy should receive parenteral vancomycin plus gentamicin. Since parenteral regimens are often difficult for outpatients, amoxicillin may be substituted in low-risk patients. Since the recommendations for endocarditis prophylaxis are empirical, clinical judgment must be used in selecting which patients should receive antibiotic prophylaxis for various procedures that might cause a transient bacteremia.

## BIBLIOGRAPHY


Arnett EN, Roberts WC: Valve ring abscess in active infective endocarditis: frequency, location, and clues to clinical diagnosis from the study of 95 necropsy patients, *Circulation* 54:140, 1976.

Baddour LM, Bisno AL: Infective endocarditis complicating mitral valve prolapse, *Rev Infect Dis* 8:54, 1986.

Bisno AL et al: Treatment of infective endocarditis due to viridans streptococci, *Circulation* 63:730A, 1981.

Calderwood SB et al: Risk factors for the development of prosthetic valve endocarditis, *Circulation* 72:31, 1985.

Dajani AS et al: Prevention of bacterial endocarditis, *JAMA* 264:2919, 1990.

Dinubile MJ et al: Cardiac conduction abnormalities complicating native valve active infective endocarditis, *Am J Cardiol* 58:1213, 1986.

Durack DT: Experimental bacterial endocarditis, *J Pathol* 115:81, 1975.

Durack DT: Prevention of infective endocarditis, *N Engl J Med* 332:38, 1995.

Ellner JJ et al: Infective endocarditis caused by slow-growing, fastidious, gram-negative bacteria, *Medicine* 58:145, 1979.

Everett ED, Hirschmann JV: Transient bacteremia and endocarditis prophylaxis. A review, *Medicine* 56:61, 1977.

Johnson JD et al: Splenic abscess complicating infectious endocarditis, *Arch Intern Med* 143:906, 1983.

Mansur AJ et al: The complications of infective endocarditis: a reappraisal in the 1980s, *Arch Intern Med* 152:2428, 1992.

McKinsey DS, Ratts TE, Bisno AL: Underlying cardiac lesions in adults with infective endocarditis: the changing spectrum, *Am J Med* 82:681, 1987.

Pelletier LL, Petersdorf RG: Infective endocarditis: a review of 125 cases in 1963-1972, *Medicine* 56:287, 1977.

Rice LB et al: Enterococcal endocarditis: a comparison of prosthetic and native valve disease, *Rev Infect Dis* 13:1, 1991.

Scully BE, Spriggs D, Neu HC: Streptococcus agalactiae (group B) endocarditis. A description of twelve cases and review of the literature, *Infection* 15:21/169, 1987.

Sussman JI et al: Viridans streptococcal endocarditis: clinical microbiological and echocardiographic correlations, *J Infect Dis* 154:597, 1986.

Tunkel AR, Kaye D: Endocarditis with negative blood cultures, *N Engl J Med* 326:1215, 1992.

van der Meer JTM et al: Epidemiology of bacterial endocarditis in the Netherlands. I. Patient characteristics, *Arch Intern Med* 152:1863, 1992.

van der Meer JTM et al: Epidemiology of bacterial endocarditis in the Netherlands. II. Antecendent procedures and use of prophylaxis, *Arch Intern Med* 152:1869, 1992.
Von Reyn CF et al: Infective endocarditis: an analysis based on strict case definitions, *Ann Intern Med* 94:505, 1981.
Washington JA II: The role of the microbiology laboratory in the diagnosis and antimicrobial treatment of infective endocarditis, *Mayo Clin Proc* 57:22, 1982.
Weisse AB: Febrile drug addicts, *Am J Med* 94:274, 1993.
Wilson WR et al: Short-term therapy for streptococcal infective endocarditis, *JAMA* 245:360, 1981.

CHAPTER

# 18A Peripheral Vascular Disease

**Jay D. Coffman**

## OBSTRUCTIVE ARTERIAL DISEASE

### Epidemiology and etiology

Patients with obstructive arterial disease complain of pain, tightness of muscles, fatigue, or weakness of the legs on walking. Symptoms are relieved by rest within a few minutes. This symptom is termed *intermittent claudication,* which means to limp intermittently.

Most patients have arteriosclerotic obstructive arterial disease. About 2.1% of males and 1.6% of females have symptoms suggesting intermittent claudication. The prevalence is markedly increased in diabetic patients. The incidence is two times greater in smokers than in nonsmokers and increases with the intensity of the habit. The ratio of men to women is about 3:1. Females lag behind males by about 10 years in development of the disease.

### Pathophysiology

The symptoms are usually caused by obstructive arterial disease due to arteriosclerosis. The obstructed or stenosed large or medium size artery limits blood flow to the active muscle. A decreased perfusion pressure distal to the lesion falls further with the vasodilatation of exercise, and the muscle contraction may actually stop blood flow. Diabetic patients may have more severe and progressive arteriosclerosis obliterans than others. The distribution of the disease is different in that diabetic individuals have less aortoiliac disease, a similar incidence of superficial femoral disease, and a greater involvement of the vessels between the knees and ankles. There is not an increased amount of disease in the foot vessels in diabetics. Except for a thickened capillary baseline membrane that is more permeable to large molecules, a small vessel lesion has not been demonstrated. Medial calcification of blood vessels is common in diabetic patients, but these noncompressible vessels usually cause no symptoms. In diabetic patients who develop ulcers of the foot in the presence of normal pulses, the lesions are probably secondary to repetitive trauma unnoticed in the face of peripheral neuropathy.

Other risk factors for arteriosclerotic occlusive disease are tobacco smoking, hypertension, and hyperlipoproteinemias.

### History

The patient's muscle symptoms occur after walking a remarkably constant distance except they are aggravated by walking on inclines or when heavy bundles are carried. The location of the discomfort sometimes helps define the vessel affected; however, calf claudication may occur with the disease at any vascular level, since these muscles are most involved in walking. Low back or buttock claudication suggests aortoiliac disease, thigh pain indicates iliac or common femoral artery disease, and foot symptoms point to diseased vessels at or below the popliteal artery. The most common lesion is an obstruction or stenosis of the superficial femoral artery in the adductor canal, and it causes calf claudication.

In addition to intermittent claudication, the other symptoms of obstructive arterial disease of the limbs are rest pain, numbness, and paresthesia. When these occur, the circulation is severely compromised, since even the small nutritional requirements of the skin are not being met. These symptoms usually occur only in feet; rest symptoms in muscles are rare.

### Physical examination

Most patients with only intermittent claudication have normal appearing limbs. There may be global atrophy of the lower limbs in patients with aortoiliac disease. Hair may be sparse on the lower limbs and absent on the toes. Observation of the limbs in the dependent position may reveal dependent rubor, which is a purplish red discoloration of cool feet seen in patients with rest symptoms. Ulcers and small areas of gangrene may be present usually on the toes.

All pulses are palpated and graded as normal, decreased, or absent. Auscultation for bruits over the femoral arteries and abdominal aorta is performed. A systolic bruit indicates an arterial lesion proximal to the point of auscultation, and if accompanied by a decreased pulse it is a hemodynamically significant obstruction. A diastolic component to the bruit indicates poor collateral blood flow.

The collateral circulation to the affected limbs can be evaluated by a simple office test. With the patient supine, elevation of the limbs at a 45-degree angle should not produce pallor. If the feet become pale, the collateral circulation is not fully compensatory. The patient is then asked to assume a sitting position with the limbs dependent. The feet should flush immediately and the veins of the dorsal foot fill within 20 seconds. If the flushing and venous filling times exceed 30 seconds, the collateral circulation is borderline.

### Laboratory studies and diagnostic procedures

In the few patients in whom the diagnosis cannot be made by physical examination, the most valuable test is the measurement of ankle systolic blood pressure via Doppler methods. This pressure should be equal to or greater than the arm pressure.

Arteriography or magnetic resonance arteriography defines the anatomy of the diseased vascular tree but yields

**Table 18A-1.** Differential diagnosis of leg pain with exercise

| | Sex | Age | Frequency | Cause | Pulses |
|---|---|---|---|---|---|
| Arteriosclerosis obliterans | M > F | Seventh decade | Very common | Occluded or stenosed large or medium size arteries; lower extremity involvement | Abnormal |
| Neurogenic | M = F | Sixth-seventh decade | Common | Spinal cord compression or ischemia | Normal |
| Thromboangiitis obliterans | M >> F | Third-fourth decade | Rare | Vasculitis of medium to small arteries; upper and lower extremity involvement | Abnormal; loss of ulnar pulse |
| Adventitial cysts | M > F | Fourth decade | Rare | Unknown | Usually normal |
| Popliteal artery entrapment syndrome | M > F | Third-fourth decade | Rare | Abnormal origin of muscles | Usually normal |
| Venous claudication | M = F | Any age | Rare | Iliofemoral thrombophlebitis | Normal |
| McArdle syndrome | M = F | Any age | Rare | Deficient muscle phosphorylases | Normal |
| Shin splints | M = F | Any age | Common | Swollen anterior tibial muscle | Normal |

little hemodynamic information. It is useful only if surgery is being considered and is rarely needed as a diagnostic test.

## Differential diagnosis

In over 90% of patients arteriosclerosis obliterans is the cause of intermittent claudication. There are other vascular and nonvascular etiologies (Table 18A-1). Neurogenic claudication may be secondary to a prolapsed intervertebral disk, stenosis of the canal, or hypertrophic bony ridging in the intervertebral canal.

Thromboangiitis obliterans (Buerger disease) is a rare cause of intermittent claudication. The etiology is unknown. Small and medium size arteries and veins are affected by an inflammatory reaction; thrombosis in blood vessels may contain sterile microabscesses and multinucleated cells. There are characteristic areas of normal blood vessel between involved segments. The typical patient is a man 20 to 40 years of age, and almost all patients are smokers. Patients usually present with ischemic symptoms or signs in the feet or intermittent claudication. Vasospasm and migratory superficial thrombophlebitis may occur in up to 40% of patients.

Other rarer causes of claudication include adventitial cysts of the popliteal artery, an abnormal origin of the muscle head from the gastrocnemius or plantaris muscle causing popliteal compression, McArdle syndrome, and venous claudication.

### Clinical course

Several studies have shown that 60% to 90% of patients with intermittent claudication due to arteriosclerosis remain stable or improve over a 5- to 9-year period. Patients with diabetes mellitus usually have progressive disease; their amputation rate is four times greater than that in patients with obstructive arterial disease without diabetes. Acute ischemic events occur in 25% of patients over 4 to 7 years. The amputation rate is about 0.8% to 1% per year but is much higher in diabetics and smokers. Obstructive arterial disease is a marker for shortened survival. Most of these patients die a decade earlier of coronary artery disease and/or diabetes.

## Management

Most patients with intermittent claudication should be treated conservatively. The immediate success rate of graft bypass surgery of the superficial femoral artery is 80% to 90% percent, and the 5-year graft patency rate is 70% in the best vascular centers. Balloon angioplasty of the superficial femoral artery is less successful. Patency rates are much lower in angioplasty of, or grafts to, vessels distal to the popliteal artery and somewhat higher in the aortoiliac area. In ordinary practices the 5-year superficial femoral artery bypass graft patency rate may be only about 50%. In Maryland it was found that the use of balloon angioplasty increased 24-fold and peripheral bypass surgery doubled, but the rate of lower extremity amputation did not change over 11 years. Therefore patients should not be referred for surgery or balloon angioplasty unless the symptoms are interfering with their occupation or lifestyle or there are symptoms and signs of ischemia at rest.

General measures include advice to quit smoking and referral to a cessation program if needed. Following bypass grafting or endarterectomy, the number of vascular or graft occlusions in patients who continue to smoke is much greater than in those who quit smoking. A graded exercise regimen may help improve walking distance. Most patients are fearful of losing a limb and do not express it; it can be explained that should progression occur, surgical bypass grafting can be considered. Patients are instructed to keep their feet warm, clean, and dry; toenails should always be cut straight across. Extremes of temperature should be avoided, since ischemic tissue burns at lower temperatures and is more susceptible to frostbite. Cuts or severe bruises on the limbs and feet should be reported to the physician immediately. Obesity and carrying bundles shortens the walking distance before symptoms, since the muscles receive only enough blood flow for a certain amount of work.

Most vascular specialists consider vasodilator drugs not to be of value. They may enhance stealing blood from ischemic areas. Pentoxifylline purportedly increases blood flow by a decrease in blood viscosity and has been reported to produce a small increase in walking distance. The recommended dosage is 400 mg three times a day with nausea and dyspepsia as side effects. Long-term anticoagulation is without value. Fibrinolytic agents may be beneficial in acute occlusions but have no role in chronic disease.

The treatment of thromboangiitis obliterans is similar to that for arteriosclerosis obliterans except sympathectomy may be helpful in cases with severe vasospasm and smoking must be stopped.

### Sources of arterial emboli

Myocardial infarction with mural thrombi
Atrial fibrillation
- Mitral valve disease (mostly mitral stenosis)
- Thyrotoxicosis
- Hypertensive heart disease
- Ischemic heart disease

Cardiomyopathies
Prosthetic heart valves
Chronic congestive heart failure
Endocarditis
Left ventricular aneurysm
Left atrial myxoma
Sick sinus syndrome
Paradoxical embolus from venous thrombosis
Aneurysms of large blood vessels
Atheromatous ulcers of large blood vessels

## ARTERIAL EMBOLI AND ACUTE THROMBOSIS

### Epidemiology and etiology

Typically in this disorder the patient calls the physician because of the sudden onset of severe leg pain that is usually secondary to abrupt interruption of the arterial supply by an embolus or acute thrombosis of a diseased blood vessel. In the differential diagnosis an embolus is unlikely if a source cannot be found, and an acute thrombosis is likely if other evidence of chronic obstructive arterial disease is present. The most common sources of arterial emboli are from mural thrombi in the left side of the heart with myocardial infarction and from valvular thrombi in patients with atrial fibrillation and mitral valve disease (see the box at right). Paradoxical emboli originate from venous thromboses, travel to the right side of the heart, and reach the peripheral circulation through the foramen ovale.

Emboli may also occur from thrombi in aneurysms or from atheromatous ulcers in any proximal vessel. Atheromatous emboli are often caused by catheterization procedures. Acute thrombosis of an artery usually occurs in a patient with stenosed blood vessels due to arteriosclerosis obliterans.

### Pathophysiology

The clinical picture relates to the acute loss of blood supply to the distal extremity. The symptoms and signs are due to the lack of oxygen and the accumulation of toxic metabolites in the limb. In patients with atheromatous emboli small vessels in skin and muscle are occluded by cholesterol crystals and atheromatous debris.

### History

In 50% of patients embolism or acute thrombosis of large or medium size arteries produces the sudden onset of severe pain in the extremity. The remaining patients complain of a more insidious onset of pain over several hours. Paresthesias and numbness are present in the majority of patients; muscular weakness or paralysis occurs in one of five cases. The pain is usually unrelenting. However, in patients with acute thrombosis of previously diseased arteries, collateral vessels may already be well developed and the symptoms may abate. Questions about the possible etiologies (e.g., heart disease, peripheral vascular disease, smoking, rhythm disturbances) are appropriate.

### Physical examination

Emboli usually lodge at bifurcations of arteries, and therefore the most common sites are the superficial femoral artery–deep femoral artery junction, the aorta at the origin of the iliac arteries, and the popliteal artery above the trifurcation of medium arteries to the calf. Distal to the embolus the extremity is cold, pale, and pulseless, and the veins are collapsed. The muscles may be tender. These manifestations are usually sharply demarcated at some distance distal to the embolus, e.g., the lower third of the thigh in femoral artery embolus.

Small atheromatous emboli produce a typical clinical picture. One or more digits may be cyanotic (blue toe syndrome), petechiae or ecchymoses may be apparent on the distal limb and foot, livedo reticularis is often present, and elevated reddened plaques may appear on the skin. The muscles are usually tender and the extremities cool, but pulses are often present and normal. If collateral circulation is inadequate, hemorrhagic blebs and gangrene may form.

In acute thrombosis of an artery the clues to diagnosis are an absence of pulses in the affected extremity, a history of intermittent claudication, and the absence of a source of emboli.

### Laboratory studies and diagnostic procedures

The clinical picture of acute embolism or thrombosis is usually typical, and special tests are not needed. Devices that detect extremity pulsations show no pulsations. Ankle systolic pressure measured with a Doppler technique is absent (no arterial sounds detected) or very low. In microemboli a source may not be apparent. Atheromatous blood vessels may need to be sought by arteriography and aneurysms by ultrasound studies. In difficult diagnostic cases skin or muscle biopsy shows cholesterol crystals. In acute thrombosis arteriography shows the diseased blood vessels and the site of thrombosis.

### Prognosis

The prognosis for acute arterial embolism patients depends heavily on their underlying disease and the high incidence of recurrent emboli. The mortality in most series is more than 20% because of these factors. The prognosis for a given limb depends on the vessel size, patient age, and ischemic time before operation. Larger vessel emboli (aortoiliac) require surgery or gangrene ensues. Smaller vessels may be managed with watchful waiting.

### Management

A vascular surgeon begins to follow the patient as soon as possible. Anticoagulation with heparin is started to prevent thrombus formation and recurrent embolization. Thrombolytic therapy with streptokinase or urokinase may be used before anticoagulation and is successful in about one third of patients. The affected extremity is placed in the dependent position and the body and limb kept warm. Heat should not be applied directly to the extremity, since ischemic tissues burn at lower temperatures than normal tissue. Adequate analgesia must be given, since the pain is often intense. If conservative therapy does not improve the color and temperature of the extremity or the pain in 1 to 4 hours, and if the patient is stable, embolectomy is indicated. Following embolectomy, anticoagulation must be reinstituted.

Treatment of an acute occlusion of an artery narrowed by arteriosclerosis can be conservative with bed rest, anticoagulation, and analgesics. If the limb improves, no further therapy is necessary. If rest pain continues, vascular surgery may be necessary. If thrombolytic therapy is used and successfully dissolves the thrombus, the stenosed vessel must be dilated by angioplasty or bypassed to prevent recurrence.

The treatment of atheromatous emboli is often unsatisfactory. Anticoagulation with heparin or administration of antiplatelet agents has been advocated. Warfarin is usually avoided, since it has been implicated as a cause of the emboli.

## ERYTHROMELALGIA

### Epidemiology and etiology

The erythromelalgia patient complains of burning pain associated with a bright red color of the feet and, less commonly, the hands on exposure to warmth. The etiology is unknown. It may occur idiopathically or be associated with hypertension, thrombocythemia, lupus erythematosus, or myeloproliferative diseases. Both sexes are affected with no special age incidence.

### Pathophysiology

There is evidently a hypersensitivity of the skin to heat, since symptoms occur with the arterial circulation occluded. Attacks are induced by stimuli that produce vasodilatation or vascular engorgement. In erythromelalgia associated with a high platelet count the symptoms may be caused by prostaglandins or thromboxane, since aspirin relieves the attacks.

### History

Attacks of burning pain in circumscribed areas of the whole hand or foot or an entire extremity occur following exposure to local heat, a warm environment, standing, exercise, or dependency of the extremity. The pain may be mild to disabling; it often occurs in bed at night. The involved foot may be red and hot with profuse sweating. Patients should be asked about symptoms of lupus erythematosus.

### Physical examination

During an attack the affected areas are warm, red, and very sensitive. Arterial pulsations are normal. Between attacks the extremities are normal. Trophic changes usually are absent, but cyanosis and even necrosis of the toes or fingers may occur in thrombocythemia.

### Laboratory studies and diagnostic procedures

Attacks can be produced by exposure to water 32° to 36° C; dependency of the limb or venous engorgement may help produce attacks. It is important to do platelet and white blood cell counts.

### Differential diagnosis

Peripheral neuropathies can usually be diagnosed by the presence of neurologic findings. The dependent rubor and pain of arteriosclerosis obliterans is associated with a cold, pulseless foot.

### Management

Attacks may be relieved by elevating the extremity and cooling. Aspirin relieves symptoms in patients with thrombocythemia. Several treatments have been claimed to relieve symptoms in individual cases, but the treatment is generally unsatisfactory, and large doses of sedatives may be necessary. Patients may become totally disabled by the pain.

## RAYNAUD'S PHENOMENON

### Epidemiology and etiology

Raynaud's phenomenon includes episodic, bilateral ischemic attacks of the digits induced by cold or emotional stimuli. If no underlying cause can be found, the phenomenon is considered primary Raynaud's phenomenon. The primary syndrome occurs more frequently in females and is much more common than the secondary causes of the phenomenon. It may be present in as many as 16% of young women in cool climates. The onset of attacks is usually between puberty and 40 years of age. Raynaud's phenomenon may be secondary to a number of underlying causes, most of which involve ischemia or trauma to the digital tissue or its nerve or vascular supply (see the box below).

### Pathophysiology

Evidence points to a local fault in the digital vessels, causing them to be abnormally reactive to cold; this local problem can be aggravated by a normal amount of reflex sympathetic nerve activity. The initial pallor of the attacks is due to digital artery vasoconstriction; this may be followed by cyanosis due to slow blood flow. When the vessels reopen, a reactive hyperemia occurs, imparting a bright red color to the digits. During the first phase numbness is usual; the patient often describes the part as dead. Pain is more common in the reactive hyperemic stage.

### History

In Raynaud's phenomenon the patient may have only sharply demarcated blanching or cyanosis, or all three color changes, during attacks (Fig. 18A-1). At first only one or two fingers may be affected, but later all fingers of both hands are involved. Episodes may last minutes to hours; they may terminate spontaneously or by warming the digits. The hands are affected alone in the majority of cases, the hands and feet next in frequency, and only the feet in some patients.

### Physical examination

Between attacks the digits appear normal in the primary form. Arterial pulses are normal. Trophic changes appear in progressive cases with the development of sclerodactyly. This is characterized by thin, tapering, contracted fingers with smooth, tight skin. Recurrent painful digital infections, blisters, and small areas of gangrene may occur (Fig. 18A-2). In patients showing these trophic changes, scleroderma may be present, although positive tests or other symptoms or signs may not appear until many years later. Patients with obstructive arterial diseases have an absence of pulses in the afflicted extremity. The attacks in patients with other secondary causes have no distinguishing features.

### Laboratory studies and diagnostic procedures

Important laboratory tests include the white blood cell count, hemoglobin, erythrocyte sedimentation rate, protein electrophoresis, urinalysis, complement levels, and tests for antinuclear antibodies and rheumatoid factor. In some cases cold agglutinins and cryoproteins are sought. The capillaries of the finger nail fold can be examined under a microscope. In scleroderma, mixed connective tissue disease, and dermatomyositis there are enlarged, deformed capillary loops surrounded by avascular areas, and hemorrhages may be present. The capillaries are normal in the primary syndrome.

## Differential diagnosis

Raynaud's phenomenon is often diagnosed from the history of well-demarcated color changes of the digits on exposure to cold, since attacks are difficult to induce in the physician's office. The diagnosis of primary Raynaud's

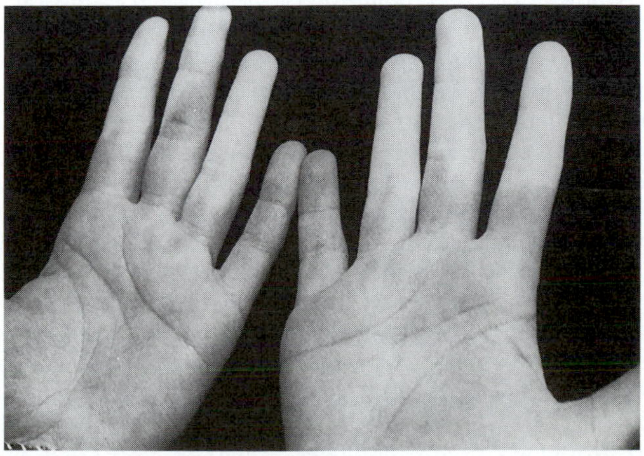

**Fig. 18A-1.** Well-demarcated pallor of the finger occurring during episodes of cold exposure in a young woman with primary Raynaud's phenomenon. (From Coffman JD. *Raynaud's phenomenon,* New York, 1989, Oxford University Press.)

### Secondary causes of Raynaud's phenomenon

- Connective tissue diseases
  - Scleroderma
  - Lupus erythematosus
  - Polymyositis
  - Rheumatoid arthritis
  - Sjögren's syndrome
- Obstructive arterial disease
  - Arteriosclerosis obliterans
  - Thromboangiitis obliterans
  - Arterial emboli
- Traumatic vasospastic disease
  - Chain saw workers
  - Pneumatic hammer workers
  - Pianists
  - Typists
  - Butchers
- Drugs
  - β-Receptor blockers
  - Ergot preparations
  - Methysergide
  - Clonidine
  - Bleomycin, vincristine
  - Bromocriptine
  - Cyclosporine
- Blood dyscrasias
  - Cryoglobulinemia, cryofibrinogenemia
  - Cold hemagglutinins
- Neurogenic causes
  - Thoracic outlet syndrome
  - Carpal tunnel syndrome
  - Poliomyelitis
  - Syringomyelia
  - Reflex sympathetic dystrophy
- Miscellaneous
  - Vasculitis including hepatitis B antigenemia
  - Myxedema
  - Polyvinylchloride exposure

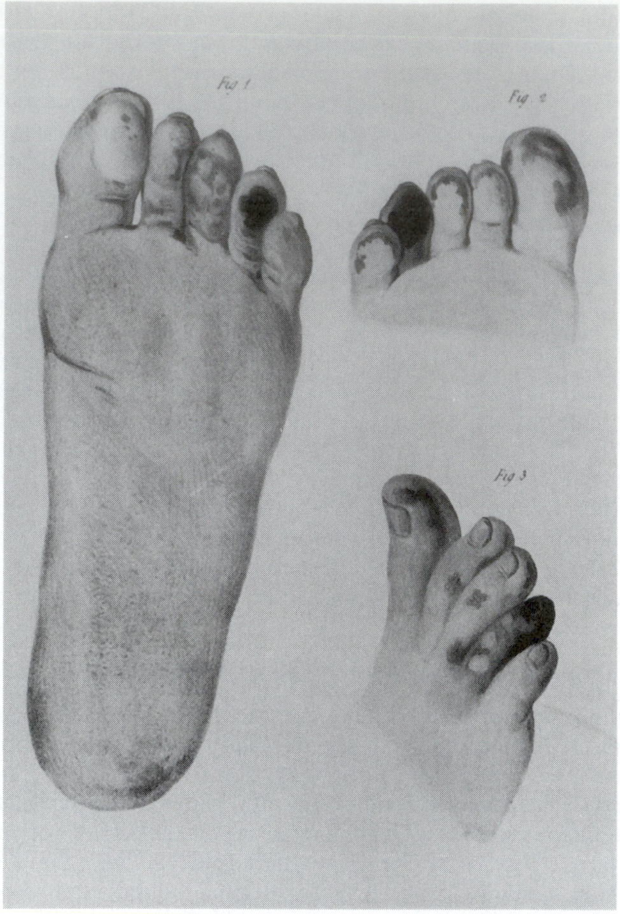

**Fig. 18A-2.** Plate from *de L'Asphyxie Locale et de la Gangrène Symétrique.* Maurice Raynaud, Paris, 1862. (Courtesy of the Boston Medical Library.)

phenomenon depends on exclusion of all secondary causes. A careful history and physical examination eliminates the drug- or work-related cases and elicits symptoms and signs of connective tissue diseases or occlusive arterial disease.

The thoracic outlet and carpal tunnel maneuvers should be performed. The thoracic outlet maneuvers involve three positions: (1) hyperabduction of the arm; (2) extension of the neck while turning the head toward the suspected extremity and holding a deep breath (Adson maneuver); and (3) pulling the shoulders back and down. The radial pulse is palpated, and auscultation is performed over the infraclavicular and supraclavicular spaces in each position. Symptoms or pallor must be produced in the hands, since many patients who do not have symptoms of the syndromes decrease or obliterate their radial pulse and develop a bruit over the subclavian artery.

Patients who present with an unevenly blue-red discoloration of the digits that can extend to the wrists and ankles have acrocyanosis. The etiology is unknown but is probably a vasospastic disturbance of the cutaneous arterioles due to cold hypersensitivity. Acrocyanosis has no special age or sex incidence; it may be associated with various endocrine diseases. The blue discoloration appears in cool environments; the hands usually sweat profusely and are persistently cool. The hands and/or feet are symmetrically involved. The digits may swell and mild hypesthesia may be present, but trophic changes do not occur. Acrocyanosis can be distinguished from Raynaud's phenomenon by the persistent nature of the discoloration in the former entity.

### Prognosis

In primary Raynaud's syndrome about one sixth of the patients improve or even recover, about one third progress, and the rest remain stable. The progressive form with sclerodactyly, recurring infection, or local gangrene can become a disabling, painful disease, but distal digital loss occurs in fewer than 1%. The prognosis for secondary Raynaud's phenomenon depends on the underlying cause.

## Management

In most patients with primary Raynaud's phenomenon reassurance that the prognosis is benign and an explanation of the attacks is the only treatment necessary. The body and extremities must be kept warm to prevent reflex sympathetic vasoconstriction. Loose-fitting warm clothing should be worn. Tobacco smoking is discouraged because it causes cutaneous vasoconstriction, which aggravates the underlying disease.

If these measures fail to allow the patient to engage in usual activities, drug therapy may be tried; it is palliative in approximately two thirds of patients. Nifedipine, a calcium channel blocker, decreases the frequency, severity, and duration of vasospastic attacks and is the most effective treatment. However, some patients cannot tolerate the side effects of headache, anxiety, nausea, edema, and reflex tachycardia. The usual dosage is 10 to 20 mg three times daily, but the extended action tablets (30 to 90 mg) given once daily are probably as effective and have fewer side effects. Another calcium channel blocker, diltiazem, can be used in dosages of 30 to 120 mg three times daily, but it is less effective than nifedipine. Side effects include headaches, dizziness, nausea, ankle edema, and constipation.

Reserpine, in oral dosages of 0.125 to 0.5 mg daily, has had widespread use and does increase finger capillary blood flow. Nausea, lethargy, and symptoms of postural hypotension may occur. Reserpine should never be given to a patient with any indication of previous or current depression. Guanethidine, in dosages of 10 to 50 mg daily, has also been effective and can be used in patients with depression. Diarrhea, lethargy, and orthostatic hypotension are its main side effects. Prazosin, 3 to 6 mg daily, may also be tried; side effects include dizziness, headaches, drowsiness, palpations, and nausea.

Although lumbar sympathectomy has successfully alleviated Raynaud's phenomenon involving the feet, cervicodorsal sympathectomy for the finger symptoms is not recommended. Symptoms usually return within 6 to 24 months after upper extremity sympathectomy.

If there are secondary causes of Raynaud's phenomenon, the treatment is that of the underlying disease. Similar drug therapy outlined above can be tried in the connective tissue diseases or traumatic vasospastic disease. In the latter disease avoidance of the trauma alleviates but does not always cure the vasospastic component. With drug-induced Raynaud's phenomenon the offending drug is withdrawn.

# LIVEDO RETICULARIS

## Epidemiology and etiology

In livedo reticularis the patient complains of a painless, reddish blue mottling of the skin of the extremities or rarely on the trunk of the body on exposure to cool environments or during emotional upsets. The etiology is unknown in the idiopathic cases. Livedo reticularis can accompany other vasospastic diseases, Raynaud's phenomenon, and acrocyanosis. However, it may also be a clue to a systemic disease such as obstructive arterial diseases, connective tissue disease, hypertension, drug reactions (amantadine), hyperviscosity states, endocrine disorders, infections, and neurogenic diseases. It is an important diagnostic feature of atheromatous microembolization to extremities and also of Sneddon syndrome, in which young women with livedo reticularis develop strokes or transient ischemic attacks.

## Pathophysiology

The blanched areas of skin are believed secondary to vasospasm of the small perpendicular arterioles that perforate the skin from the subcutaneous tissue. The bluish periphery around the blanched area is caused by deoxygenated blood in the surrounding horizontally arranged venous plexuses. This gives the characteristic reticular fishnet or lacelike pattern on the skin.

## History

Almost all patients with the idiopathic type are asymptomatic. The reticular pattern in some patients even persists on warming the extremities. Rare patients develop cutaneous ulcerations in the winter, or even the summer, but these patients may actually have an underlying vasculitis.

## Physical examination

The only physical finding in idiopathic cases is the reddish blue reticular pattern of the skin.

## Laboratory studies and diagnostic procedures

There are no laboratory or diagnostic studies helpful in the diagnosis of the idiopathic disease. The appropriate laboratory tests for the other cases are listed under these diseases.

## Management

In the idiopathic syndrome no treatment is necessary. It is a benign condition, and the patient is usually seeking reassurance from a physician. In those who cannot tolerate the appearance of the livedo, it can be blocked with low doses of reserpine or other sympathetic blocking agents. In the rare patients with ulcerations, no treatment has proved satisfactory.

# THROMBOPHLEBITIS

## Epidemiology and etiology

If a patient presents with unilateral, painful swelling of an extremity, acute in onset, the diagnosis is usually thrombophlebitis, although other diagnoses must be considered (Table 18A-2). The diagnosis and management of thrombophlebitis is presented in Chapter 119.

**Table 18A-2.** Differential diagnosis of the swollen limb

| | Pain | Inflammatory signs | Varicose veins | Noninvasive venous studies | Clues to diagnosis |
|---|---|---|---|---|---|
| Thrombophlebitis | + | + | ± | + | Acute onset of swelling |
| Lymphedema | Usually absent | 0 | 0 | Negative | Gradual onset of swelling |
| Postphlebitic syndrome | + | ± | + | Negative | Stasis pigmentation, subcutaneous tissue induration |
| Ruptured popliteal synovial membrane | + | + | 0 | Negative | Fluid in the knee joint, history of arthritis |
| Ruptured calf | + | + | 0 | Negative | Ecchymoses around ankle, tender knot in muscle, sudden onset during exercise—may feel a pop |
| Myositis ossificans | + | + | 0 | Negative | Indurated area in thigh with localized swelling; positive bone scan |

## POSTPHLEBITIC SYNDROME AND VARICOSE VEINS

### Epidemiology and etiology

The postphlebitic syndrome is a chronically swollen limb often with stasis dermatitis, subcutaneous tissue induration, and ulcerations. It can appear soon after phlebitis or 10 to 20 years later and is due to incompetent superficial or deep veins.

Varicose veins are distended, tortuous veins with incompetent valves that may appear following phlebitis or pregnancy or with no apparent instigating cause.

### Pathophysiology

High venous pressure in the limb due to incompetent venous valves leads to capillary leakage of fluid and red blood cells. The tissue reacts to the hemoglobin from red blood cells with inflammation and fibrosis. A brown pigmentation occurs from the inflammatory reaction and deposition of hemoglobin. Ulceration is probably the result of stasis of blood with ensuing hypoxia of the tissue.

Varicosities are due to incompetent venous valves as a result of high venous pressure distending and stretching the veins or to destruction of the valves from thrombophlebitis. For the pathophysiology of ulcers see Chapter 18B.

### History

Patients with the postphlebitic syndrome have a chronically swollen extremity. Often medical care is not sought until very advanced disease with ulcers is present because of the absence of pain. Aching pain in the leg may occur after long periods of standing. The entire extremity is usually involved, but only the calf may be affected.

Most patients with varicose veins have no symptoms, whereas others complain of fatigue or aching in the lower part of the leg or swelling at the end of the day.

### Physical examination

In the postphlebitic syndrome varicose veins are usually present. The edema is pitting but later may become indurated. An itchy, inflamed, scaly rash above or below the medial malleolus is followed by brown pigmentation of the area and finally ulceration. Within this area an incompetent perforating vein can often be palpated as a fluctuant bulge. The ulcers are often painless and show good granulation tissue.

Varicose veins can be seen as dilated, tortuous, sacculated superficial veins.

### Laboratory studies and diagnostic procedures

The clinical picture of the postphlebitic syndrome almost always is diagnostic. When the diagnosis is in doubt, a venogram shows the involved leg to contain an excessive number of veins often with valve destruction and a feathery appearance of the lining of some veins indicating previous phlebitis.

The incompetent valves of varicose veins can be demonstrated by applying a tourniquet on an elevated extremity so that the superficial veins are empty. The patient then stands; release of the tourniquet allows the vein distally to enlarge quickly if incompetent valves are present. If two tourniquets are applied, filling of the saphenous vein between the tourniquets delineates incompetent communicating (perforating) veins.

### Differential diagnosis

The postphlebitic syndrome should not be confused with lymphedema. Patients with lymphedema do not usually have varicose veins, stasis pigmentation, or ulcers. Venograms or lymphangiograms are rarely necessary in the differential diagnosis.

### Management

Postphlebitic syndrome is difficult to treat and requires patient compliance. Heavy-gauge elastic support (30 mm Hg or greater), sometimes with a pad over the perforating vein, must be worn when the patient is ambulatory. Patients must usually sleep with the foot of the bed elevated above heart level to keep edema to a minimum. Ulcers are treated by debridement, antibiotics if infection is present, and pressure dressings or gelatin boots. Rarely the entire fibrosed area must be removed surgically with ligation of the perforating veins and skin grafting.

Uncomplicated varicose veins respond well to heavy-gauge elastic stockings. This prevents symptoms, edema, and further enlargement of the veins. Panty girdles or garters are never worn. Ligation and stripping of veins has decreased in popularity, since the veins may be needed in the future for arterial bypass.

## LYMPHEDEMA

### Epidemiology and etiology

Lymphedema is a chronically swollen, painless limb. It may be hereditary or secondary to destruction of lymphatics by recurrent infections or filariasis, invasion of lymph vessels or nodes by malignancies, or surgical removal or radiation fibrosis of lymph nodes. Primary (idiopathic) lymphedema predominantly affects females. It may be present at birth (congenital), appear at or near puberty (praecox), or occur after age 35 (tarda). Milroy disease is familial and congenital edema of the legs.

### Pathophysiology

The chronic swelling of the limb is due to aplasia, hypoplasia, or varicosities of the lymphatic vessels that drain the tissue fluid. Subcutaneous fibrosis of the edematous tissue gradually occurs.

### History

The swelling in lymphedema is usually gradual in onset and asymptomatic. Some patients do complain of a heaviness and pain. Patients should be questioned about a family history of leg swelling, episodes of cellulitis, radiation therapy, or surgery, and travel to areas where filariasis is common. Recurrent lymphangitis can lead to lymphedema, and extremities inflicted with lymphedema are very susceptible to recurrent episodes of cellulitis. Each attack leaves more residual edema.

### Physical examination

Lymphedema first involves the distal extremity or the entire limb and is soft, pitting, and reversible. Later the edema becomes indurated and nonpitting, the skin thickens and resists wrinkling, and hair follicles become prominent dimples. The lower extremities are involved most often, and approximately 50% of patients have bilateral swelling. Secondary lymphedema usually involves only one extremity. The skin finally becomes coarse, thick, folded, and hard; the extremely disfigured extremities have been aptly termed elephantiasis.

### Laboratory studies and diagnostic procedures

Lymphangiography and venography may confirm the diagnosis but are usually not necessary.

### Differential diagnosis

Painless, chronic swelling of an extremity without varicosities, stasis dermatitis, and collateral veins are diagnostic of lymphedema. In lipodystrophy the subcutaneous tissue of the legs feels nodular; lymphangiography is necessary to demonstrate the normal lymphatics displaced by lipomatous masses.

### Prognosis

Primary lymphedema usually progresses to a chronically swollen limb or limbs, but some patients maintain their state of initial presentation for many years.

### Management

With lymphedema it is important to attempt to keep the involved extremities as free from edema as possible to prevent subcutaneous fibrosis and skin thickening as well as recurrent episodes of lymphangitis. Heavy surgical elastic support garments (30 to 50 mm Hg) covering the entire involved area with graded pressure from distal to proximal extremity must be worn whenever ambulatory. The patient should sleep with the involved extremity above heart level. A low-sodium diet may be instituted and occasional doses of diuretics may help, but continuous therapy has not proved of value. In late, disfiguring cases surgical removal of the subcutaneous tissue has been performed, but it is itself a very disfiguring operation.

## LYMPHANGITIS

### Epidemiology and etiology

In most cases of infection of the lymphatic vessels the agent is the hemolytic streptococcus or the coagulase-positive staphylococcus. Although a portal of entry for the bacteria is not always apparent, fungal infections of the toes are commonly present. Venous or ischemic ulcers and traumatic lesions are also common sources.

### Pathophysiology

The bacterial infection spreads along lymphatics with an inflammatory response often spreading to surrounding tissues (cellulitis).

### History

Patients often show systemic symptoms of infection: fever, shaking chills, headache, general malaise, nausea, and vomiting.

### Physical examination

Red streaks appear, following the pathways of lymphatic vessels, and proximal lymph nodes are often enlarged and tender. The limb may be swollen, and there may be diffuse redness, increased temperature, and tenderness indicative of cellulitis.

### Laboratory studies and diagnostic procedures

The clinical picture is usually typical. Leukocytosis with a left shift in polymorphonuclear cells may be present. Culture of any open lesion may yield the inciting organism.

### Differential diagnosis

Occasionally the differential diagnosis from acute phlebitis, especially in a postphlebitic limb, is difficult, and noninvasive tests for phlebitis must be performed, such as duplex venous ultrasonography and impedance plethysmography.

### Management

Systemic antibiotics to cover the common inciting agents are administered in high doses intravenously until culture reports are obtained. Debridement or drainage of any focus of origin is also very important. Bed rest and extremity elevation may hasten healing by decreasing edema. In recurrent cases, especially with underlying lymphedema, a prophylactic antibiotic, usually penicillin, is administered on a long-term basis.

## BIBLIOGRAPHY

Babb RR et al: Prophylaxis of recurrent lymphangitis complicating lymphedema, *JAMA* 195:871, 1966.

Barnes RW et al: The fallibility of the clinical diagnosis of venous thrombosis, *JAMA* 234:605, 1975.

Coffman JD: Intermittent claudication and rest pain: physiological concepts and therapeutic approaches, *Prog Cardiovasc Dis* 22:53, 1979.

Coffman JD: Principles of conservative treatment of occlusive arterial disease. In Spittell JA Jr, editor: *Clinical vascular disease,* Philadelphia, 1983, Davis.

Coffman JD: Clinical forum: atheroembolism after cardiac surgery, *J Vasc Med Biol* 1:37, 1989.

Coffman JD: *Raynaud's phenomenon,* New York, 1989, Oxford University Press.

Coffman JD: Cutaneous changes in peripheral vascular disease. In Fitzpatrick TB et al, editors: *Dermatology in general medicine,* New York, 1993, ed 4, McGraw-Hill.

Freund U, Romanoff H, Floman Y: Mortality rate following lower limb arterial embolectomy: causative factors, *Surgery* 77:201, 1975.

Goodman RM et al: Buerger's disease in Israel, *Am J Med* 39:601, 1965.

Kinmonth JB: *The lymphatics: diseases, lymphography, and surgery,* Baltimore, 1972, Williams & Wilkins.

Kurzrock R, Cohen PR: Erythromelalgia: review of clinical characteristics and pathophysiology, *Am J Med* 91:416, 1991.

Lensing AW et al: Detection of deep vein thrombosis by real-time B-mode ultrasonography, *N Engl J Med* 340:342, 1989.

Lewis T, Landis EM: Observations upon the vascular mechanism in acrocyanosis, *Heart* 15:229, 1930.

Midge M, Hughes LE: The long-term sequelae of deep vein thrombosis, *Br J Surg* 65:692, 1978.

Tolins SH: Treatment of varicose veins: an update, *Am J Surg* 145:248, 1983.

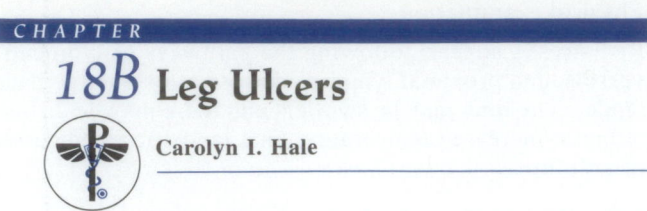

CHAPTER

# 18B Leg Ulcers

Carolyn I. Hale

## EPIDEMIOLOGY/ETIOLOGY

There are many causes of leg ulcers (see box at right). Venous insufficiency accounts for 80% to 90%, arterial insufficiency for 5%, and a mixture of arterial and venous accounts for another 5%. Approximately 2% of ulcers are caused by diabetes and only 1% of ulcers will be caused by one of the many diseases listed in the box. Ulcers are costly to treat, cause loss of work time, and tend to be chronic and recurrent. Median duration of ulceration was 9 months, and 20% had not healed in over 2 years. The great majority of patients have recurrence.

## PATHOPHYSIOLOGY

Venous ulcers, also known as varicose ulcers, venous hypertension ulcers, venous stasis ulcers, or postphlebitic ulcers are caused by the common mechanism of too much hydrostatic pressure in the superficial venous system of the leg. At least 80% of the time this is caused by incompetent valves in deep veins. In the leg, venous blood is returned to the heart via the deep venous system and the superficial venous system. The superficial system, consisting of the short and greater saphenous veins and their tributaries, is emptied into the deep system via perforating veins. Directional flow is maintained by a series of one-way valves. Flow is maintained by the pump action of the calf muscle or elevation of the leg above the level of the heart. Alteration in this system by a previous deep venous thrombosis is the most common predecessor of leg ulcers, although frequently there is no clinical history of thrombosis. Incompetent superficial veins leading to varicose veins account for less than 20% of leg ulcers. This group can be surgically cured and should be identified. Trauma to the leg and rare congenital fistulas can cause arteriovenous fistulas, which also result in venous hypertension.

Basically, an increased venous pressure results in increased pressure in the capillary bed, transudation of fluid and protein into the interstitial space, and altered delivery of oxygen and nutrients to the skin and subcutaneous tissues resulting in ulceration of the overlying tissue. Current theories of the pathophysiology are more complex than this. In 1982, Browse and Burnand suggested that increased back pressure into the capillaries distended endothelial gaps, allowing for leaky capillaries. Fibrin then forms around the capillaries and impedes oxygen diffusion. These findings of pericapillary fibrin cuffs have been confirmed with immunologic staining. It is also known that fibrinolysis is abnormal in this group of patients, but the clinical importance of this is unknown. More recent evidence supports a trapped leukocyte theory. With decreased perfusion pressure, white cells become trapped in the capillaries and release proteolytic enzymes and superoxide radicals that cause endothelial damage. This damage may result in leaky capillaries and fibrin deposition, as well as blockage of local capillary filling and resultant ischemia.

Arterial ulcers are primarily a result of arteriosclerosis obliterans of the lower extremity as previously described. Although this accounts for only 5% to 10% of all leg ulcers, by the age of 80, over 90% of patients have an arterial component. In other words, a venous ulcer at age 50 will become a mixed venous and arterial ulcer by the time the patient reaches 80 and treatment will need to be changed to address the arterial component. Risk factors are diabetes mellitus, smoking, hyperlipidemia, hypertension, and early menopause in women.

Diabetes mellitus results in ulceration from atherosclerosis, peripheral neuropathy, and less commonly necrobiosis lipoidica, diabetic dermopathy, and bacterial and fungal infections. Hyperemia and capillary hypertension, loss of autoregulation and neurogenic regulation, disturbed endothelial function, and abnormal rheology also play a part in the abnormal microcirculation of diabetic patients.

The pathophysiology of other leg ulcers varies with the disease. A few of these are mentioned briefly. Rheumatoid arthritis is associated with ulcers both from vasculitis and from immobility of the leg with resultant inadequate venous return. In sickle cell anemia there is an incidence of ulcers of 25% to 75%, probably from the abnormal rheologic properties of the red blood cells resulting in an ulcer that resembles venous ulcers. Recurrent hemorrhages and infections also play a role. Other hematologic diseases also share common factors with venous ulcers. Polycythemia vera results in increased viscosity, as do various dysproteinemias.

Pyoderma gangrenosum most likely represents a small vessel vasculitis, although not all cases show vasculitis. It may be associated with ulcerative colitis, rheumatoid arthritis, leukemias, regional enteritis, or may occur without any underlying disease.

Drugs may cause ulcers by a number of mechanisms. Hydroxyurea may cause ulcerative lichen planus or a livedo vasculitis-like picture. Some drugs, such as corticosteroids, alter wound healing, although low antiinflammatory products (e.g., cortisone acetate and prednisone in oral doses under 10 mg daily) have no appreciable effect on wound healing. Coumarin necrosis is a rare disease caused by an imbalance in the anticoagulant and procoagulant factors. Inhibition of production of protein C and protein S in hereditary deficiency states or rarely acquired deficiencies associated with disseminated intravascular coagulation, multiple myeloma, and the lupus anticoagulant may disproportionately balance the coagulation system toward thrombosis in early coumarin treatment. (see Chapter 55).

Antibodies to phospholipids cause recurrent thrombosis with a vasculitic-appearing ulcer. These antibodies are manifested by false positive VDRL, a lupus anticoagulant, or anticardiolipin antibodies, and may be associated with lupus and lupus-like diseases and livedo vasculitis and may cause their effects through interactions with protein C or protein S. It has been proposed that they may promote thrombosis by binding to endothelial cells and impairing prostacyclin release or damaging platelet adhesiveness.

The clinical features of leg ulcers are frequently

nonspecific, although several characteristics can help identify the most common types of ulcers (Table 18B-1).

Extensive laboratory testing is not necessary except in unusual ulcers. Generally a complete blood count, glucose, sedimentation rate, albumin, protein, and thyroid screen are sufficient. If a vasculitis is suspected an antinuclear antibody, rheumatoid factor, syphilis serology, cold agglutinins, cryoglobulins, serum protein electrophoresis, protein C and S levels, and anticardiolipin antibodies may be evaluated.

Bacteriologic cultures of the wound are not necessary and are frequently misleading as most wounds are colonized. If there is clinical evidence of cellulitis, a culture should be taken to direct antibiotic therapy. A tissue biopsy is the most accurate method and is necessary if deep fungal or acid-fast organisms are suspected by the clinician.

Biopsies of a leg ulcer should be undertaken with caution. Frequently the biopsy site will not heal, and the patient is left with another ulcer. However, if an ulcer does

## Differential diagnosis of leg ulcers

**Vascular**
- Arterial
  - Arteriosclerosis
  - Thromboangiitis obliterans
  - Cholesterol emboli
  - Hypertension
  - Arteriovenous malformation
- Venous
  - Superficial varicosities
  - Deep venous thrombosis
  - Incompetent perforators
- Lymphatics—elephantiasis nostra

**Vasculitis**
- Small vessel
  - Hypersensitivity vasculitis (leukocytoclastic vasculitis)
  - Lupus erythematosus
  - Rheumatoid arthritis
  - Scleroderma
  - Livedo vasculitis (atrophie blanche)
  - Pyoderma gangrenosa
  - Antiphospholipid antibodies (anticardiolipin or lupus anticoagulant)
- Medium and large vessel
  - Polyarteritis nodosa
  - Nodular vasculitis

**Hematologic**
- Sickle cell anemia
- Spherocytosis
- Thalassemia
- Polycythemia rubra vera
- Leukemia
- Dysproteinemias
  - Cryoglobulinemia
  - Cold agglutinin disease
  - Macroglobulinemia
- Deficiencies of coagulation inhibitors
  - Protein C and S deficiency

**Infectious**
- Fungus
  - Blastomycosis
  - Coccidiomycosis
  - Histoplasmosis
  - Sporotrichosis
- Bacterial
  - Furuncle
  - Ecthyma
  - Ecthyma gangrenosum
  - Septic emboli
  - Pseudomonas
  - Mycobacterial (typical and atypical)
- Protozoal
  - Leishmaniasis

**Metabolic**
- Diabetes
  - Necrobiosis lipoidica diabeticorum
- Gout
- Gaucher's disease
- Prolidase deficiency
- Calcinosis cutis
- Localized bullous pemphigoid

**Tumors**
- Basal cell carcinoma
- Squamous cell carcinoma
- Melanoma
- Kaposi's sarcoma
- Metastatic tumors
- Lymphoproliferative
- Cutaneous T cell lymphoma (mycoses fungoides)

**Trauma**
- Insect bites
- Pressure
- Cold Injury (frostbite, pernio)
- Radiation dermatitis
- Burns
- Factitial

**Neuropathic**
- Diabetic trophic ulcers
- Tabes dorsalis
- Sy ringomyelia

**Drug**
- Halogens
- Methotrexate
- Coumarin necrosis
- Ergotism
- Hydroxyurea

**Panniculitis**
- Webber Christian disease
- Pancreatic fat necrosis
- Alpha 1 antitrypsinase deficiency

**Table 18B-1.** Physical examination

| | Venous | Arterial | Diabetic | Vasculitic |
|---|---|---|---|---|
| **Location** | Medial malleolus, gaitor area. | Toes, heels, bony prominences of foot, lateral malleolus, rarely over medial malleolus. | Same as arterial trophic ulcers on pressure points on the plantar foot, especially metatarsal heads. | Pretibial and dorsum of foot but may be anywhere and frequently is also on other areas. |
| **Appearance** | Irregularly shaped, surrounded by brown pigmentation with edema or sometimes fibrotic, hard skin (lipodermatosclerosis). Ulcer base has granulation tissue and exudate, and the borders may be hyperkeratotic. | Punched out ulcer with round well-demarcated borders and pale or white ulcer bed. Sometimes covered with dry eschar. Surrounding skin cool atrophic and hairless. | Punched out, often surrounded by hyperkeratotic borders. Purulent drainage may indicate osteomyelitis. | Palpable purpura, hemorrhagic vesicle, typically small and multiple, with black, gray, or yellow base and minimal or no granulation tissue. May have thin undermined border. Surrounding skin shows reticulated vascular pattern. |
| **Pain** | Increases with leg dependency, decreases with elevation. | Frequently very painful. Decreases with leg dependency, increases with exercise and leg elevation. | Painless but associated with paresthesia, anesthesia, inconstant, mostly at night. | Extremely painful. |
| **Vascular examination** | Ankle/brachial index greater than 0.9. Pulses present. Plethysmography or doppler studies show abnormal venous system. | Ankle/brachial index less than 0.9. Pulses decreased. Abnormal pallor of leg with elevation, and subsequent rubor with dependency. Delayed venous filling. | Mixed. Usually associated with arterial disease. | Normal. |
| **History** | Edema, trauma, rapid onset. Thrombophlebitis 20% varicosities. | Arteriosclerosis, claudication. Usually >45 yr. Slow progression. | Diabetes mellitus. Peripheral neuropathy. | Association with other systemic disease. Rapid onset. |
| **Treatment** | Leg elevation, compression by elastic bandages or stockings, 30 mm Hg, moist wound dressings. Grafts. | Vascular surgical consultation. No compression. Moist wound dressings. Pentoxyphylline? | Control diabetes. Careful wound care, early intervention for infections. Vascular surgical consult. | Control underlying disease. Nonadherent dressings. Oral steroids, ASA, bed rest. |

## Managed Care Guide
## Flowchart for the management of leg ulcers.

**HISTORY**

Evaluate nutrition, underlying diseases, diabetes, CHF, vasculitis, connective tissue disease, history of deep venous thrombosis, smoking

↓

**PHYSICAL EXAMINATION**

Document size, location, borders, color, surrounding skin, edema, pain

↓

**LABORATORY EVALUATION**

CBC, ESR, glucose, protein, ANA, RF, RPR

*If indicated:* cold agglutinins, cryoglobulins, SPEP, protein C levels, cultures

↓

**DOPPLER INDEX**

(ankle/brachial systolic blood pressure)

**Arterial** (less than .9)
- Nonrestrictive bandaging
- Pain and infection control
- Stop smoking
- Refer for vascular surgical consult
- Pentoxifylline or ASA
- Elevate head of bed
- **Debridement** →

**Venous** (greater than .9)

Superficial
- **Compression**
- Sclerotherapy or stripping

Deep
- **Compression**
- Elevation
- Exercise
- **Debridement** →

**DEBRIDEMENT**

**Superficial slough**
- Hydrocolloids
- Alginates
- Wet dressings
- Whirlpool
- Paste bandages

**Eschar**
- Surgical
- Enzymatic
- Whirlpool

↓

**COMPLICATING FACTORS**

**Stasis dermatitis**
- Topical steroids
- Compression
- Bandages, hydrocolloid or paste

**Cellulitis**
- Antibiotics
  - Systemic
  - Topical

**Contact dermatitis**
- Patch test
- Avoidance of allergen
- Topical steroids

↙ ↘

**GRANULATION TISSUE FORMING**

Moist wound healing and compression →

**NO GRANULATION TISSUE**
- Change dressing
- Reassess
- Biopsy ulcer margin
- Consultation

**SLOW OR NO HEALING**
- Prepare ulcer bed for grafting
- Pinch grafts, split thickness grafts
- Cultured autologous keratinocytes →

**HEALED**
- Protect ulcer site
- **Compression**
- Follow-up frequently to check legs and support stockings

Adapted from Terence Ryan.

not heal for 4 months on adequate therapy, a biopsy from the ulcer edge should be taken.

Vascular studies are needed when pulses are nonpalpable. An ankle/brachial pressure index should be measured in all patients. Venous studies are indicated if needed to confirm the diagnosis of venous ulcers or in the case that superficial varicose veins are the cause. In this case, surgical intervention can prevent recurrent disease and compression stockings will not be needed.

## MANAGEMENT

Although there are a number of causes of leg ulcers the most common cause is venous insufficiency. Compression therapy is the most important treatment for these ulcers. Moist wound dressings, growth factors, and grafting, although beneficial in treatment of venous ulcers, pale in comparison to the use of adequate compression of the leg. Arterial ulcers, however, should *not* be compressed for fear of further arterial compromise. Treatment of this condition is discussed in Chapter 18A. Once an ulcer is healed continued care will be needed to prevent recurrences (see Managed Care Guide on p. 331).

## BIBLIOGRAPHY

Burnand KG et al: Pericapillary fibrin deposition in the ulcer bearing skin of the lower limb, the cause of lipodermatosclerosis and venous ulceration, *Br Med J* 285:1071, 1982.

Callam MJ, Harper DR, Dale JJ et al: Chronic ulcer of the leg: clinical history, *Br Med J* 294:1389, 1987.

Coleridge-Smith PD et al: Causes of venous ulceration: a new hypothesis, *Br Med J* 296:1726, 1988.

Flynn MD, Tooke JE: Aetiology of Diabetic Foot Ulceration: A role for the microcirculation? *Diabetic Medicine* 8:320, 1992.

Harahap M et al: Leg ulcers, *Clinics in dermatology* 1990; 8, number 3/4.

Phillips TJ et al: Leg ulcers, *J Am Acad Dermatol* 25:965, 1991.

Renfro L, Moy J, Sanchez M: Cutaneous ulcers caused by drugs, *Wound* 1990; 2(6):236-246.

Ryan TJ: Current management of leg ulcers, *Drugs* 30:461, 1985.

Young JR: Differential diagnosis of leg ulcers, *Cardiovascular Clin* 13:171, 1983.

# II DERMATOLOGY

CHAPTER

## 19 Diagnosis and Examination Techniques

Frank Parker
James C. Shaw

### AN APPROACH TO DIAGNOSING SKIN DISEASE

Dermatology is a visual specialty. The patient's skin condition is apparent and readily observed by the physician. Because there are hundreds of dermatoses, a logical process of elimination is needed to narrow the possibilities, first to a specific group of diseases and finally to one condition, when initially examining a patient with a skin disease. Such a diagnostic approach is based on specific morphologic description of the skin lesions along with an appropriate history and laboratory tests. This systems analysis approach to diagnosis involves three steps. First, the primary and secondary skin lesions are identified. Second the examiner places the patient in one of several major diagnostic groups of diseases. Many skin conditions are found in each of the groups, but all the diseases in a given group tend to manifest the same primary and secondary lesions. The third step involves selecting the one disease the patient has from the other conditions in the group. This step is accomplished by looking for specific features such as location and distribution of skin lesions, unusual shapes or arrangements of the lesions (annular, serpiginous, dermatomal), color, and surface characteristics (appearance of scales, verrucous or vegetative changes).

#### Step 1: Description of primary and secondary skin lesions

Primary skin lesions are uncomplicated lesions that represent the initial cutaneous pathologic changes uninfluenced by secondary alterations such as infection, trauma, or therapy. Secondary skin lesions are changes that occur as a result of progression of the disease, scratching, or infection of the primary lesion. At times primary changes also can occur as secondary manifestations (i.e., pustules may appear as primary lesions of folliculitis or as secondary lesions when pruritic primary lesions are scratched and infected). The challenge is to recognize a primary skin lesion as the initial change characteristic of a disease.

The terminology used to describe primary and secondary skin lesions is the basic language of dermatology, the means by which skin diseases are accurately described (Table 19-1). Each descriptive term is not only a short account of what is seen on the surface of the skin, but also implies specific information about pathologic processes within the skin.

#### Step 2: Assignment of spectrum of primary and secondary lesions to a major group of skin diseases

Each disease within a given group shares the same primary and secondary skin lesions. Because some diseases have overlapping traits, they may be assigned to more than one group. An arbitrary grouping of common skin diseases listed in Table 19-2 according to their dominant skin lesion is used in this section to facilitate discussion.

#### Step 3: Narrowing the possibilities within a given group to the exact diagnosis

Several factors are important in identifying the specific skin condition within each group. The distribution of the skin lesions is important because many conditions have typical patterns or often affect specific regions. For example, psoriasis commonly affects extensor surfaces and atopic eczema involves flexor areas of extremities. Photoreactions are confined to the sun-exposed areas of the body. Involvement of the palms and soles is seen in erythema multiforme, secondary syphilis, psoriasis, and eczema. Contact dermatitis presents with unusual patterns corresponding to areas where the offending material contacts the skin.

A second important clue in differentiating diseases within a given group is the shape of individual lesions and the arrangement of lesions in relation to one another. For example the lesions of lichen planus characteristically are angular papules, whereas pityriasis rosea presents as oval, raised patches. A linear arrangement of lesions is typical of contact with an exogenous substance brushing across the skin or a cutaneous nevus. "Zosteriform" refers to lesions arranged along the cutaneous distribution of a spinal nerve in a bandlike, unilateral configuration (e.g., herpes zoster, dermatomal hemangiomas in Sturge-Weber syndrome) (see Plate 16). Annular lesions are circular with normal skin in the center. Annular macules are observed in drug eruptions, secondary syphilis, and lupus erythematosus. Scaling annular lesions suggest dermatophytosis (see Plate 17). Iris lesions are a special annular lesion in which a papule or vesicle evolves into the center-target or bullseye lesion typical of erythema multiforme (see Plate 18). Urticaria polycyclic patterns evolve when numerous annular lesions enlarge and run together (hives). Serpiginous (snakelike patterns) are seen in creeping eruption (see Plate 19). Herpetiform refers to the grouping of lesions seen in herpes simplex or dermatitis herpetiformis (see Plate 5).

Other physical features are important in diagnosing skin diseases. Dry, lichenified lesions (see Plate 10) suggest a chronic state of a disease, whereas wet, oozing, macerated lesions (see Plate 15) suggest acute reactions. Nodular lesions that are soft, fluctuant, and tender suggest an abscess, whereas firm nodules are likely to be a benign or malignant tumor (see Plate 1). Redness caused by dilation of superficial blood vessels blanches with pressure, whereas erythema caused by extravasated blood, as occurs in petechiae and purpura, does not blanch (see Plate 20). Hues of blue and black indicate melanin pigment. The deeper the melanin pigmentation deposition in the skin, the bluer the color (see Plate 21).

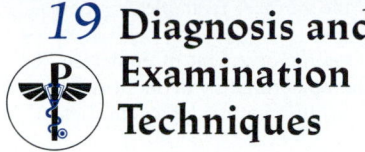

**Table 19-1.** Primary and secondary skin lesions

| Lesion | Description |
|---|---|
| **Primary skin lesions** | |
| Macule | Circumscribed change in skin color without elevation or depression of the surface. Example: erythema, purpura, cafe au lait, vitiligo (see Plate 1). |
| Papule | A solid elevated area no more than 10 mm in diameter. Implies pathologic involvement of epidermis (especially if there is scaling or disturbance of the normal surface of the epidermis) or dermis (usually epidermal surface is normal but redness is present). Example: warts, molluscum contagiosum, lichen planus (see Plate 2). |
| Nodule | Similar to a papule but larger (1 cm or larger in diameter) with visible elevation of the skin. It may represent a pathologic process in the epidermis, in which case it may be associated with scale, erosion, and loss of skin markings or dermis, where it may be fluctuant (if it is a cyst) or firm (if it is a skin cancer or granulomatous infiltrate). Example: cyst, basal cell carcinoma (see Plate 21). |
| Plaque | Evolves from a confluence of papules leading to a flat-topped, circumscribed elevation. Example: psoriasis, urticaria, mycosis, fungoides (see Plate 3). |
| Wheal | Special type of plaque. A slight elevation caused by movement of fluid out of blood vessels. Example: hives (see Plate 4). |
| Vesicles and Bullae | Circumscribed, elevation lesion with cavities containing free fluids that flow out if the lesion is pricked. Vesicles are less than 10 mm in diameter. Bullae are greater than 1 cm in diameter. Vesicles and bullae may evolve within the epidermis (see Plates 5 and 6), in which case the fluid is usually clear serous. The lesions may be flaccid and easily break (i.e., very thin roof), or they may evolve at the dermal-epidermal junction, in which case the lesions are tense, may contain hemorrhagic fluid, and are less likely to rupture (thick roof). Umbilicated vesicles suggest viral induced lesions (herpes simplex and zoster). Example: pemphigus, pemphigoid, porphyria cutanea tarda. |
| Pustule | A vesicle containing purulent exudate. Example: acne, folliculitis (see Plate 7). |
| Scale | Desiccated thin plates of cornified epidermal cells that result from altered keratinization. Scale occurs when the epidermis is perturbed and involved scale assumes different appearances that can be useful in diagnosis, including fine, thin squames seen in eczema or exfoliative dermatitis; thick, silvery scales typical of psoriasis (see Plate 8). |
| Atrophy | Loss of tissue with depression of the surface of the skin. Atrophy may involve the epidermis with fine wrinkling and redness (stria) or the dermis with whitish depression (scleroderma) (see Plate 9). |
| Telangiectasis | Persistent dilation of individual vessels in the skin, usually associated with alterations in the connective tissue of dermis. Example: connective tissue diseases, radiation skin damage (see Plate 7). |
| **Secondary skin lesions** | |
| Lichenification | Dry, leathery thickening of the skin with exaggerated skin markings. Thickening of the epidermis resulting from repeated rubbing and scratching of the skin in chronic dermatitis. Example: Atopic dermatitis, neurodermatitis (see Plate 10). |
| Fissures | Erosion and breaks in the skin of varying depths and causes. Fissures are linear cracks in the skin, usually through the epidermis. Example: chronic eczema, perléche. Erosions are wide, shallow defects in the skin (see Plate 11). |
| Ulcer | Deep loss of skin into the dermis and even into the subcutaneous tissue. Example: Venous and arterial ulcers (see Plate 12). |
| Scar | An area of replacement fibrosis of the dermis or subcutaneous tissues. Scars vary in appearance and may be depressed or raised. Example: Keloids may appear as nodules (see Plate 13). |
| Crusts | Dried exudate of serum, blood, sebum, or purulent material on the skin surface after vesicles; bullae break down to release their contents (see Plate 14). |
| Oozing | Loss of stratum corneum or breakdown of small vesicles with serum covering the skin surface. Example: acute dermatitis (see Plate 15). |

## The dermatologic history

Although the clinical examination is vital in diagnosing skin disease, the history is also important and certain specific information should be determined if possible:

- *Onset*: Where precisely on the body did the condition begin? What did it look like? What are associated symptoms?
- *Course:* How did the disease progress and change? What has been done to treat the condition (by the patient or by physicians)? What is the relationship to vacations, seasons, the environment? Has the condition been continuous or intermittent?
- *Past Medical History:* Does the patient have other cutaneous diseases? Is there a history of atopy, endocrine conditions, skin, or other malignancies or autoimmune diseases?
- *Family History:* Is there a history of atopic diseases and allergies, psoriasis, or other inherited conditions in family members?
- *Work and Hobbies:* What work or hobbies of the patient may expose them to contactants?
- *Topical and Systemic Medications and Materials Used:* Because drug reactions are so common (both to topical and systemic medications—prescribed and over the counter), the physician should always be

**Table 19-2.** Major groups of skin diseases

| Skin disease | Dominant skin lesions |
|---|---|
| Dermatitis or Eczemas | Erythema papules, vesicles, lichenification, oozing, crusts. Example: Contact dermatitis, atopic eczema, nummular eczema, stasis eczema. |
| Papulosquamous Skin Diseases | Unique papules, plaques, and scales. Example: Psoriasis, pityriasis rosea, lichen planus. |
| Pustular Skin Diseases | Papules and pustules. Example: Acne, rosacea, folliculitis. |
| Nodular Skin Diseases | Epidermal and dermal nodules. Example: Benign skin tumors and malignant skin tumors. |
| Vesiculobullous Skin Diseases | Vesicles and bullae. Example: Infectious—impetigo, herpes; immunologic—pemphigus and pemphigoid; mechanical—epidermolysis bullosa. |
| Pigmentary Alterations of the Skin | Hyperpigmented and hypopigmented macules. Example: Vitiligo, Addison's disease, albinism, melasma. |
| Maculopapular Eruptions | Macules and papules. Example: Childhood exanthems, drug eruptions, purpuric lesions. |
| Special Erythematous Reactions of the Skin | Macules and plaques. Example: Urticaria, dermatographism, insect bites. |
| Ulcerative Skin Lesions | Example: Pyoderma gangrenosum, ulcers due to vascular diseases, infectious ulcers. |

alert to this possibility. What medications does the patient apply, especially with rubber gloves? Does the patient use topical steroids? Are other cosmetics, anti-itch products, and other topical medications used? What medications are used in every orifice (i.e., eyedrops, eardrops, suppositories, oral). Even vitamins, cough medications, and birth control pills may cause skin reactions.

The chapters in this section deal with the major disease groups (e.g., dermatitis, papulosquamous, pustular). Not every skin group listed in Table 19-2 is identified as a separate chapter; some chapters are listed based on etiologic factors (e.g., infectious diseases of the skin, common reaction patterns [hives, erythema multiforme], and photoreaction). Nevertheless, it should be possible for the physician to "place" a patient presenting with a common skin condition into the appropriate chapter and further to arrive at a precise diagnosis if the steps in the preceding systematic clinical approach are followed.

In this section, skin conditions are discussed in association with internal diseases and in pediatric, geriatric, and black patients. Finally, a chapter on the general principles of dermatologic therapy is included to help the clinicians treat the common disorders.

## EXAMINATION TECHNIQUES

Inspection of the skin is the most valuable step in dermatologic diagnosis. The use of selected tests can be helpful in confirming or excluding suspected diagnoses. These include the potassium hydroxide examination, Gram's stain, Tzanck smear, selected cultures, and skin biopsy for histologic examination. An understanding of when and how to perform these ancillary tests is essential in making the dermatologic diagnosis (Table 19-3).

### Examination of the skin

Assessment of the morphologic characteristics of most skin diseases requires bright light and magnification. A total body examination is frequently essential to determine the extent of involvement, severity, and any characteristic distribution pattern (see the box on p. 336).

***Distribution.*** Certain diseases have characteristic distributions that are pathognomonic even if the primary lesions are not characteristic (e.g., herpes zoster in a dermatomal distribution and photo-related skin eruptions on the sun exposed areas—central face, extensor arms, and dorsal hands).

***Palpation.*** Palpation of skin lesions helps to assess the level of involvement of the pathologic process. Whereas macules feel like normal skin, palpable lesions may reflect epidermal, dermal, or subcutaneous involvement. A rough surface or scaling indicates an abnormality in the epidermis; a smoother surface usually implies that the pathology is in the dermis or deeper. The firmness of a lesion also can help in the diagnosis: a firm, dermal nodule suggests a dermatofibroma, whereas a rubbery dermal nodule of the same color and size would be more consistent with a neurofibroma.

### Potassium examination

Possibly the most valuable ancillary test in dermatologic diagnosis is the potassium hydroxide (KOH) examination of skin scrapings, which can rapidly confirm or exclude the diagnosis of tineas (dermatophyte fungi), candidiasis, scabies, or tinea versicolor. The rationale for KOH is that the stratum corneum consists of adherent keratinized layers of cells, which optically prevent microscopic visualization. KOH helps dissolve the keratin and allows for separation of the aggregates of stratum corneum cells, but does not disrupt the cell walls of fungi. Perform the following steps to ensure a successful test:

1. Adequate sample of skin must be obtained. This usually requires the use of a scalpel blade; scraping with a glass slide frequently is inadequate. In annular scaly lesions, scraping from the peripheral scale gives the highest yield.

**Table 19-3.** Ancillary tests in dermatology: when to use them

| Test | Indications | Precautions |
|---|---|---|
| Potassium hydroxide (KOH) | Fungal infections of skin or mucosa<br>Tinea versicolor: short, plump hyphae and spores (see Fig. 19-1)<br>Scabies; look for a linear burrow<br>Any red, scaly dermatosis where diagnosis is uncertain | Large depth of field on microscope<br>Never need greater than 40X lens<br>Debris can look like fungal hyphae<br>Scabies: scan at low power (2X or 4X) |
| Gram's stain | Bacterial folliculitis (Gram + cocci in clumps)<br>Pustular eruption (sterile if psoriasis, drug reaction)<br>Candida when there are pustules (Gram +) | |
| Tzanck smear | To confirm or rule out herpesvirus infection:<br>herpes simplex<br>herpes zoster<br>varicella<br>Confirms molluscum bodies in maternal from molluscum lesions | Frequently much cellular debris: PMNS, lymphocytes |
| Cultures | Bacterial infections<br>Nasal staphylococcal carrier state<br>Fungal disease: nail, scalp<br>Herpes simplex- + in 48-72 hours<br>Cytomegalovirus infection | Negative result does not exclude infection<br>Positive bacterial culture may not be the primary cause of the disease (i.e., leg ulcers, mouth ulcers, crusted lesions) |
| Wood's light examination | Fungal infections (tinea capitis from *Microsporum* species fluoresces green)<br>Inguinal dermatitis (erythrasma fluoresces coral red) | Not confirmatory<br>Negative test does not rule out disease |
| Skin biopsy | Any atypical dermatosis where a specific diagnosis will influence treatment<br>If malignancy is in the differential diagnosis<br>If histologic confirmation is desirable by patient, epidermiologists, treating physicians<br>Atypical presentations of common disorders<br>Skin lesions in immunocompromised patients | Consultation by dermatologist may be more cost effective if no biopsy required<br>Many dermatoses do not have pathognomonic histologic findings<br>Sampling errors may hinder making a correct diagnosis<br>Pathology report without diagnostic possibilities (i.e., descriptive only) may not help in making the diagnosis |

*PMNS,* polymorphonucleocytes.

**The dermatologic physical examination (examine entire integument)**

Look and list the primary and secondary lesions observed.

| | |
|---|---|
| Location of skin lesions | Localized, generalized, symmetrically distributed. |
| Unusual configurations | Annular, segmental, dermatomal. |
| Examine mucous membranes, hair, nails | Many skin diseases affect these structures. |

2. The stratum corneum must be dissolved sufficiently. This usually requires a combination of KOH, heat, and mechanical disruption. A 10% to 20% KOH solution is best, and 5% dimethyl sulfoxide (DMSO) can be added to help with the penetration of the KOH. This combination is commercially available from Dermatologic Lab and Supply, Inc. (Council Bluffs, IA). Heating by exposing the bottom of the slide to a flame is necessary to disrupt the keratinized cells, and gentle pressure on the cover slip helps in this process.
3. The microscope must have the appropriate optical settings. The ten power (10×) objective is the best to use when looking for fungal hyphae. The four power (4×) is best for looking for the larger scabetic mites. In both cases, the visualization is optimal with a large depth of field made by closing down the iris or by lowering the condenser lens. The 40 power (40×) lens can be used to confirm findings, but should not be used to search for fungi. The oil immersion (100×) lens is not necessary in the KOH examination and can hinder the chances of finding hyphae.
4. The examiner must build a level of confidence in recognizing fungal hyphae and nonpathologic debris and artifact (e.g., "mosaic" pattern from the trapping of air between the keratinocyte cell walls). Fungal elements can appear different on the different locations of the body; *Candida* organisms have a different appearance from dermatophyte fungi; many nonpathologic structures such as hair, fibers from clothing, and dust can mimic the appearance of fungi. Fig. 19-1 demonstrates an example of common positive findings on a KOH examination.

***Gram's stain.*** Gram's stain is valuable in the diagnosis of some skin infections and occasionally in the diagnosis of candidiasis. When the material to be tested is exudative

A

B

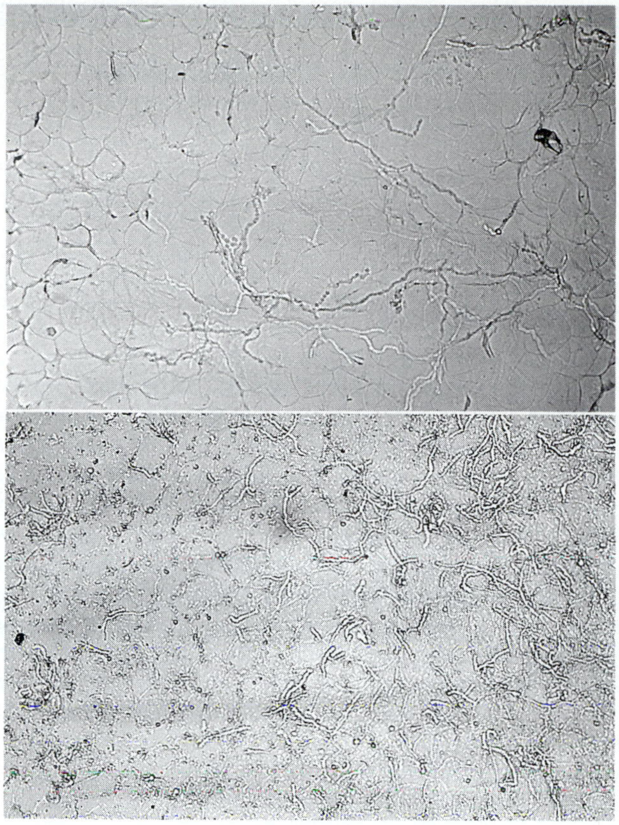

**Fig. 19-1. A,** KOH examination (dermatophyte). Note 10× microscopic picture of branching birefractile hyphae, and size of adjacent keratinocytes **B,** KOH examination (tinea versicolor). Note shorter nonbranching hyphae.

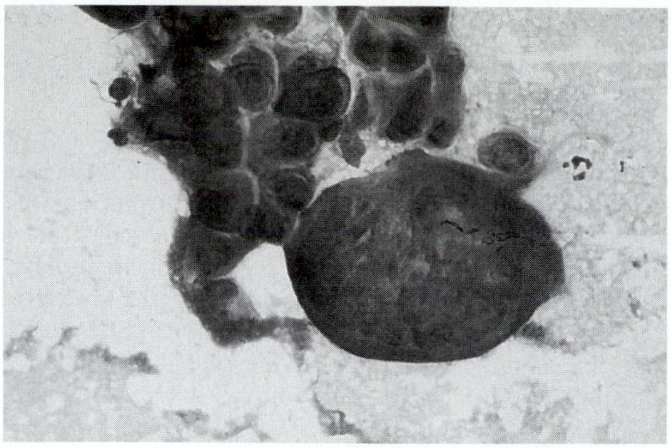

**Fig. 19-2.** Tzanck smear. Note large multinucleated keratinocyte, pathognomonic of all herpes viral infections. Note also neutrophil for size comparison.

or from a pustule, a Gram's stain is indicated. A staphylococcal infection frequently can be identified or excluded with the use of a Gram's stain. *Candida* species are gram positive, and the Gram's stain can be a helpful tool when a candidal infection presents with pustules.

***Tzanck smear.*** The Tzanck smear is the most rapid way to identify herpesvirus infection, including herpes simplex, varicella and herpes zoster. Any dark nuclear stain is acceptable. A 5% methylene blue solution is inexpensive and effective, but Wright's or Giemsa stain also works well.

**Preparation.** The material used in a Tzanck test is the underside of a vesicle roof plus the base of the vesicle. The material is smeared on a glass slide and allowed to dry. It is then fixed by warming under a flame or exposing to absolute alcohol. The stain is applied for several seconds and gently rinsed off with water. A simple method utilizes a slide jar containing the 5% methylene blue solution. The fixed slide is dipped into the jar and then rinsed. The staining is immediate, and the solution remains in the jar for future use. The slide is air dried, a drop of oil is applied, and a cover slip may be placed over the oil because the oil immersion lens is not necessary. Oil on the slide is essential for good optical results.

**Interpretation.** The pathognomonic finding in a Tzanck smear is the presence of multinucleated keratinocytes. Although these cells are large, the term *giant cell* is misleading because that term also is used to describe histiocytes in tissue. The keratinocytes become fused in herpesvirus infections and appear as large cells with multiple nuclei (Fig. 19-2). Neutrophils and mononuclear cells, which frequently also are present on a Tzanck smear, are much smaller than the multinuclear keratinocytes. Low power should be used first to scan the slide to find clumps of larger cells. Higher power can then be used to confirm the cellular findings.

***Cultures.*** In certain cases of suspected bacterial, fungal, or viral infections of the skin, cultures are necessary to make the diagnosis. In most cases, however, a culture is used to confirm a diagnosis that was made by KOH, Gram stain, or Tzanck smear. Fungal culture is most valuable in cases of tinea capitis and nail infections, both of which are difficult to diagnosis by inspection and KOH examination. Bacterial culture can help in any atypical pustular eruption. Culture of the anterior nares is useful to diagnose a staphylococcal carrier state. A herpesvirus culture can help differentiate herpes simplex, which grows in 48 hours, from varicella-zoster, which requires up to 4 weeks to grow. Cultures from tissue specimens obtained by biopsy are indicated when deep fungi, atypical mycobacteria, or other deep bacterial involvement is suspected.

***Wood's light examination.*** The use of a Wood's light (ultraviolet light, 360nm) helps diagnose certain fungal and bacterial infections and helps delineate some disorders of pigmentation. Tinea capitis caused by some *Microsporum* species fluoresces blue-green under a Wood's light, and erythrasma, the intertriginous infection with *Corynebacterium minutissimum* can fluoresce a coral-red color. Although fluorescence suggests certain diagnoses, the presence or absence of fluorescence is not confirmatory.

***Skin biopsy.*** The skin biopsy is an invaluable diagnostic tool when performed in appropriate settings. The punch biopsy is the most common form of skin biopsy, with punches ranging from 2 to 8 mm in diameter. Most skin diseases are best sampled by this diagnostic method because the epidermis, dermis, and subcutaneous fat are present in one sample. If the skin lesion is raised above the skin's surface, a shave biopsy of superficial skin can be used; in cases in which deep tissue or a larger sample is needed, an incisional or excisional biopsy is indicated.

**Indications.** There are no absolute indications for performing a skin biopsy because nonspecific histologic findings frequently do not allow confirmation of a particular diagnosis and because management of the patient may not be affected by a histologic diagnosis. In cases where consultation by a dermatologist may obviate the need for biopsy, considerations pertaining to cost effectiveness may be important. Despite these uncertainties, some general principles apply when considering performing a skin biopsy (see Table 19-1).

**Procedure.** In most cases the required materials include a local anesthetic, a biopsy punch or scalpel, and a means of achieving hemostasis. Healing occurs rapidly following closure with sutures, but it is usually adequate when the wound is allowed to heal by granulation. Hemostatic products include ferric subsulfate (Monsel's solution), aluminum chloride, silver nitrate, and Gelfoam packing.

**Interpretation.** Dermatopathology is a subspecialty of its own. Because of the complexity of skin pathology, a skin biopsy in the primary care setting may not always provide an answer to a dermatologic problem. The following factors determine the quality of the information from a biopsy:

1. Whether the suspected disease has characteristic pathologic findings. Many skin diseases have nonspecific histologic changes, and skin biopsies may be noncontributory (e.g., atopic dermatitis, urticaria, drug eruptions, viral exanthems).
2. Sample location. Generally, a biopsy from the center of an involved area of skin disease has the best chance of demonstrating any characteristic pathologic findings. Occasionally, as in the case of some bullous diseases, a sample from the periphery of the lesion shows the characteristic changes.
3. Sample size or depth. A sample that is not large enough or deep enough may not demonstrate the pathologic changes (e.g., punch biopsy of erythema nodosum).
4. Pathologist. The person who interprets the skin biopsy must be an expert in the histopathology of the skin. Dermatopathologists are the best trained in this field, although general pathologists and dermatologists receive training in skin pathology and may interpret skin biopsy material. Ideally, a pathology report from a skin biopsy either confirms a specific diagnosis, or, if a diagnosis is nonspecific (descriptive only), it discusses differential diagnoses and possibly suggests further diagnostic procedures if indicated.

## BIBLIOGRAPHY

Habif TP: Dermatologic surgical procedures. In Habif TP, editor: *Clinical Dermatology,* ed 2, St Louis, 1990, Mosby.

Sams WM Jr: Diagnostic procedures. In Sams WM, Lynch PJ, editors: *Principles and practice of dermatology,* New York, 1990, Churchill Livingstone.

CHAPTER

# 20 General Dermatologic Therapy

James C. Shaw

## WOUND HEALING

The most important principle of wound healing is adequate hydration. Dehydration of epithelium inhibits migration of epithelial cells and retards the healing process. In contrast moist epithelium migrates over granulation tissue for faster healing. The previously accepted concept of "wet to dry dressings" for healing wounds or ulcers has been modified because this process increases drying of the skin surface. Instead, adequate occlusion to provide a level of humidity that prevents drying results in the most rapid and complete healing. Occlusive dressings can be designed at home or in the office with the use of antibacterial ointments covered with an occlusive film or gauze dressing, or they can be purchased as prepackaged dressings (e.g., DuoDerm, Vigilon, OpSite) (see Chapter 6). Although these products are expensive, they can be helpful in the healing of large ulcers, abrasions, and burns.

## TOPICAL CORTICOSTEROIDS

### The vehicle: cream vs. ointment

An important concept in successful treatment of skin disease is the composition of the vehicle containing the corticosteroid. Creams and lotions are composed of a combination of oil and water. The higher the ratio of oil to water, the thicker the preparation. The presence of water in the vehicle may contribute to skin drying through evaporation. Vehicles containing water also must contain preservatives to prevent contamination with bacteria and fungi. This need occasionally presents problems related to allergic contact dermatitis to preservatives such as quaternium 15 and imidazolidinyl urea. Ointments are composed of only an oil product such as petrolatum and therefore require no preservatives. In general patients tolerate creams and lotions better than ointments, but ointments have some inherent occlusive properties that may enhance the penetration of steroids. Creams and lotions tend to be more effective in intertriginous or moist areas because of their drying properties. Ointments are used preferably on dry skin because of their occlusive properties that retard drying.

### Side effects

Corticosteroids applied topically are generally safe when used for a short time. Chronic use can result in side effects if the steroid is stronger than the lowest potency preparations (hydrocortisone). The main side effect seen with chronic use of potent steroids is skin atrophy resulting in a thinned dermis with prevalent telangiectasis and increased friability. These changes can lead to the development of striae. When potent steroids are used on the face, a rosacea-like papular and pustular dermatitis can occur referred to as steroid-induced rosacea.

### Use of potent steroids

Gradations of potency within the numerous steroid products are available. In general, potency correlates with fluorinated or chlorinated steroids (Table 20-1). Group I (most potent) steroids should be considered in the most recalcitrant dermatoses as short-term treatment only. These steroids, in general, should never be used on the face. Group II through V levels of potency can be used on open areas of the skin for up to several months without concern but should be avoided in intertriginous areas. The weakest groups, VI and VII, are generally safe on the face and in intertriginous areas. Any prolonged use of corticosteroids on the skin can increase chances of developing superinfection with a dermatophyte fungus.

### Occlusion

Steroids have increased effectiveness when they are occluded. The use of an ointment provides some natural occlusion, but additional occlusion can be provided with the use of a plastic or other synthetic dressing such as DuoDerm. Even simple tape increases the penetration of the steroid. Although occlusion increases effectiveness, it also increases the chances of side effects.

### Intralesional steroids

On occasion when a recalcitrant dermatosis is of limited size, the use of intralesional steroids can be helpful. Either

**Table 20-1.** Topical corticosteroids

| Group | Brand name | % | Generic name | Preparation |
|---|---|---|---|---|
| I | Ternovate cream, ointment, scalp application | 0.05 | Clobetasol propionate | 15, 45 g<br>25 ml |
| | Diprolene cream, ointment, lotion | 0.05 | Betamethasone dipropionate | 15, 45 g<br>30, 60 ml |
| | Psorcon cream, ointment | 0.05 | Diflorasone acetate | 15, 30, 60 g |
| | Ultravate cream, ointment | 0.05 | Halobetasol dipropionate | 15, 45 g |
| II | Alphatrex ointment | 0.05 | Betameth. dipropionate | 15, 45 g |
| | Cyclocort ointment | 0.1 | Amcinonide | 15-45 g |
| | Diprosone ointment | 0.05 | Betameth. dipropionate | 15, 45 g |
| | Fluonex cream | 0.05 | Fluocinonide | 15, 30 g |
| | Florone ointment | 0.05 | Diflorisone acetate | 15, 30, 60 g |
| | Halog cream, ointment solution | 0.1 | Halcinonide | 15-240 g<br>20, 60 ml |
| | Lidex gel, cream, ointment, solution | 0.05 | Fluocinonide | 15, 30, 60 g<br>15-120 ml |
| | Maxiflor ointment | 0.05 | Diflorasone diacetate | 15-60 g |
| | Maxivate cream, ointment | 0.05 | Betameth. dipropionate | 15, 45 g |
| | Topicort cream, ointment, gel | 0.25 | Desoximetasone | 15, 60, 120 g |
| III | Alphatrex cream, lotion | 0.05 | Betameth. dipropionate | 15, 45 g |
| | Aristocort cream, ointment | 0.5 | Triamcinolone acetonide | 15, 240 g |
| | Aristocort A | | | |
| | Benisone gel | .025 | Betameth. benzoate | 15, 60 g |
| | Betatrex ointment | 0.1 | Betameth. valerate | 15, 45 g |
| | Cutivate cream, ointment | .005 | Fluticasone propionate | 15, 45 g |
| | Diprosone cream | 0.05 | Betameth. dipropionate | 15, 45 g |
| | Elocon ointment | 0.1 | Mometasone furoate | 15, 45 g |
| | Florone cream | 0.05 | Diflorasone diacetate | 15, 30, 60 g |
| | Kenalog cream, ointment | 0.5 | Triamcin. acetonide | 20 g |
| | Maxiflor cream | 0.05 | Diflorasone diacetate | 15-60 g |
| | Trymex cream | 0.5 | Triamcin. acetonide | 15 g |
| | Uticort gel, ointment | .025 | Betameth. benzoate | 15, 60 g |
| | Valisone ointment | 0.1 | Betameth. valerate | 15, 45 g |
| IV | Aristocort ointment | 0.1 | Triamcin. acetonide | 15-240 g |
| | Benisone ointment | .025 | Betameth. benzoate | 15, 60 g |
| | Cordan ointment | 0.05 | Flurandrenolide | 15-225 g |
| | Cyclocort cream | 0.1 | Amcinonide | 15-60 g |
| | Elocon cream, lotion | 0.1 | Mometasone furoate | 15-60 g |
| | Fluonide ointment | .025 | Fluocinolone acetonide | 60 g |
| | Halog cream, ointment | .025 | Halcinonide | 15-240 g |
| | Kenalog ointment | 0.1 | Triamcin. acetonide | 15-2520 g |
| | Synalar ointment | .025 | Fluocinolone acetonide | 15-425 g |
| | Topicort LP cream | 0.05 | Desoximetasone | 15, 60 g |

*Continued.*

**Table 20-1.** Topical corticosteroids—cont'd

| Group | Brand name | % | Generic name | Preparation |
|---|---|---|---|---|
| V | Aclovate cream, ointment | 0.05 | Aclometasone diprop. | 15, 45, 60 g |
| | Aristocort cream | 0.1 | Triamcin. acetonide | 15-1520 g |
| | Benisone cream | .025 | Betameth. benzoate | 15, 60 g |
| | Beta-Val cream | 0.1 | Betameth. valerate | 15, 45 g |
| | Betatrex cream, lotion | 0.1 | Betameth. valerate | 15-60 g |
| | Cloderm cream | 0.1 | Clocortolone pivalate | 15, 45 g |
| | Cordran cream, lotion | 0.05 | Flurandrenolide | 15-225 g |
| | Cordran ointment | .025 | | 30-225 g |
| | Desowen ointment | 0.05 | Desonide | 15, 60 g |
| | Fluonide cream | .025 | Fluocinolone acetonide | 15, 60 g |
| | Kenalog lotion | 0.1 | Triamcin. acetonide | 15, 60 g |
| | cream | 0.1 | | 15-240 g |
| | ointment | .025 | | 15-240 g |
| | Locoid cream | 0.1 | Hydrocortisone butyrate | 15-60 g |
| | ointment | 0.1 | | 15-60 g |
| | Synalar cream | .025 | Fluocinolone acetonide | 15-425 g |
| | Synemol cream | .025 | Fluocinolone acetonide | 15-60 g |
| | Tridesilon ointment | 0.05 | Desonide | 15, 60 g |
| | Trymex cream, | 0.1 | Triamcin. acetonide | 15-480 g |
| | ointment | .025 | | 15, 80 g |
| | Uticort cream, lotion | .025 | Betameth. benzoate | 15, 60 g |
| | Valisone cream, lotion | 0.1 | Betameth. valerate | 15-430 g |
| | Westcort cream, ointment | 0.2 | Hydrocortisone | 15-120 g |
| VI | Aristocort cream | .025 | Triamcin. acetonide | 15-240 g |
| | Desowen cream | 0.05 | Desonide | 15, 60 g |
| | Fluonid cream, lotion | 0.01 | Fluocinolone acetonide | 15-60 g |
| | Kenalog cream, lotion | .025 | Triamcin. acetonide | 15-240 g |
| | Locorten cream | 0.03 | Flumethasone pivalate | 15, 60 g |
| | Synalar cream | 0.01 | Fluocinolone acetonide | 15-425 g |
| | solution | | | 20, 60 ml |
| | Tridesilon cream | 0.05 | Desonide | 15, 60 g |
| | Trymex cream | .025 | Triamcin. acetonide | 15-480 g |
| | Valisone cream | 0.01 | Betameth. valerate | 15, 60 g |
| VII | Celestone cream | 0.2 | Betameth. valerate | 15 g |
| | Decaderm gel | 0.1 | Dexamethasone | 15, 30 g |
| | Hytone cream, ointment, lotion | 1.0 | Hydrocortisone | 1, 4 oz |
| | Hytone cream, ointment, lotion | 2.5 | | 1, 4 oz |
| | Lacticare HC lotion | 1.0 | Hydrocortisone | 4 oz |
| | | 2.5 | | 2 oz |
| | Medrol cream | 0.25 | Methylprednisolone | 7.5-45 g |
| | Nutracort cream, | 1.0 | Hydrocortisone | 30, 60 g |
| | lotion | | | 4 oz |
| | Oxylone cream | .025 | Fluoromethalone | 15-120 g |
| | Synacort cream | 1.0 | Hydrocortisone | 15-60 g |
| | | 2.5 | | 30 g |
| | Texacort solution | 2.5 | Hydrocortisone | 15-60 g |

Modified from Habif TP: *Clinical dermatology,* ed 2, St Louis, 1990, Mosby.

betamethasone (Celestone) 6 mg/ml or triamcinolone acetonide (Kenalog) 5 mg/ml can be used judiciously in plaques of psoriasis, prurigo nodules, inflamed cysts, and in localized patches of alopecia areata. Skin atrophy is a significant risk whenever intralesional steroids are used.

## COMPRESSES AND SOAKS

### Indications

Wet compresses are helpful in reducing itching and in drying areas of inflamed skin with serous oozing. The main goals of wet dressings are to cool the skin temperature, debride necrotic tissue, and dry out the skin through evaporation. Soaks are used to hydrate dry skin. A 10 to 15 minute soak in warm plain water hydrates dry skin before application of emollients.

### Procedure

Generally, plain water can be used for wet dressings, but occasionally aluminum acetate (Burow's solution and others) aids in the drying of the skin. The compresses should not be occlusive and should allow for evaporation. A thin fabric is wetted and applied to the affected skin for 5 to 10 minutes and repeated for 30 minutes. This protocol can be followed two or three times a day until the skin has achieved the desired dryness.

**Emollients**

1. Emollients containing mineral oil
   A. Lotions
      - Complex 15
      - Keri
      - Lubriderm
      - Neutrogena moisture
      - Nivea
      - Nutraderm
      - Purpose
   B. Creams
      - Eucerine
      - Formula 405
      - Keri
      - Lubriderm
      - Nivea
      - Nutraderm
      - Moisturel
2. Emollients containing glycerine
   - Corn huskers lotion
   - Curel skin lotion
   - Neutrogena Norwegian formula emulsion
   - Shepard's dry skin care
   - Wibi lotion
3. Ointments
   - Aquaphor
   - Vaseline petroleum jelly
   - Petrolatum (generic)
   - Plastibase
   - Moisturel
   - Wondra
   - Acid mantle
   - Unibase
4. Emollients containing lactic acid
   - Lac-Hydrin 5%
   - Lac-Hydrin 12% (Rx)
   - Lacticare lotion 5%
5. Emollients containing urea
   - Aqua care cream 5%, 10%
   - Carmol 10 lotion 10%
   - Carmol 20 cream 20%
   - Nutraplus cream, lotion 10%

Modified from Habif TC: *Clinical dermatology,* ed 2, St Louis, 1990, Mosby.

## EMOLLIENTS

The goal of emollient use is to provide a barrier to evaporation and to deliver some oil content to the skin. Emollients can be pure ointments (Vaseline), which deliver an oil product to the stratum corneum and which provide the greatest protection against evaporation (see the box above). Creams represent a combination of oil product plus water and are thinner and therefore easier to apply. Because of the water content, some evaporation takes place. In the most severe cases of dry skin, creams may not provide an adequate protective barrier. Lotions are the thinnest of the emollients because of a higher water content and a lower oil content. These preparations are effective in the mildest forms of dryness, but tend to be ineffective in severe xerosis.

Emollients are best applied after the skin has been exposed to water through a shower, bath, or soak. Even dry skin absorbs some moisture through gentle bathing, especially if soap is avoided. Emollients can then be applied immediately after the bath or shower to protect the hydrated skin from evaporation.

Emollients contain petrolatum, mineral oil, or glycerin. The addition of urea or lactic acid promotes hydration and removal of excess keratin in the skin and can be helpful in the treatment of dry skin (see the box above).

## TAR

Tar compounds are distilled from organic substances that include coal, wood, and shale. Tar products act primarily as (1) antipruritic agents, (2) antiproliferative agents due to their inhibition of DNA synthesis, and (3) photosensitizing agents used in combination with ultraviolet light, midrange sunbeam spectrum (UVB) therapy in psoriasis.

Products containing tar are most useful in the treatment of psoriasis, seborrheic dermatitis, and pruritic, localized forms of dermatitis such as atopic dermatitis and nummular dermatitis (Table 20-2).

## ANTIHISTAMINES

Antihistamines are valuable in the treatment of numerous skin problems. The main use is for the treatment of histamine-mediated dermatosis such as urticaria, as well as for the general treatment of pruritus (Table 20-3).

The new nonsedating $H_1$ blockers have some place in dermatologic therapy, but they tend to be less potent in their $H_1$ blocking capabilities than the sedating types of antihistamines and therefore have limitations. The use of doxepin, the tricyclic antidepressant and $H_1$ blocking antihistamine, has been valuable in some severely pruritic dermatoses because of the potent $H_1$ blocking effect of this drug. Doses ranging from 25 to 100 ml a day occasionally are used in recalcitrant cases of urticaria and other severe itching dermatoses. Sedation is a potential limiting side effect. The doses of antihistamines need to be reduced in older patients because of their increased susceptibility to sedation. In children a paradoxical effect with antihistamines occasionally results in hyperactivity and hyperalertness.

## ANTIBIOTICS

### Topical antibiotics

Numerous topical antibiotics are available for the treatment of acne and minor bacterial skin problems (Table 20-4).

***Topical antibiotic ointments.*** Several topical antibiotic ointment preparations are available for use in minor

**Table 20-2.** Some common tar preparations

| Preparation | Brand name | Concentration* | Packaging | Use |
|---|---|---|---|---|
| Shampoos | DHS tar | 0.5% coal tar | 8 oz, 16 oz | daily |
| | Ionil-T | 0.85% coal tar | 4-32 oz | daily |
| | Ionil-T plus | 1% coal tar | 120-240 ml | daily |
| | T/Gel | 0.5% coal tar | 4-16 oz | daily |
| | T/Gel extra strength | 1.0% coal tar | 16 oz | daily |
| | Pentrax | 4.3% coal tar | 4 oz | daily |
| | Polytar | 0.5% coal tar | 180-3840 ml | daily |
| | Zetar | 1% whole coal tar | 180 ml | daily |
| Bath oils† | Balnetar | 2.5% coal tar | 240 ml | q.d. to q.wk. |
| | Doak oil | 2% coal tar | 240 ml | q.d. to q.wk. |
| | Polytar bath | 5% coal tar equivalent | 240 ml | q.d. to q.wk. |
| | T/Derm tar emollient | 1.2% coal tar | 4 oz | q.d. to q.wk. |
| Creams | Fototar | 2% coal tar | 85 g, 1 lb jar | daily |
| | Tegrin | 5% crude coal tar extract | 2 oz, 4 oz | daily |
| Gels | Estar | 5% coal tar | 90 g | daily |
| | P&S plus | 1.6% crude coal tar | 105 g | daily |
| | Psorigel | 1.5% coal tar equivalent | 120 g | daily |
| | Aquatar | 2.5% coal tar | 90 g | daily |

*Concentration expressed in coal tar equivalents when possible. On package, stated % may be higher.
†Bath oil directions: add to bath water, soak for 10 to 20 minutes, pat dry.

**Table 20-3.** $H_1$ antihistamines

| Class | Generic name | Brand name | Dose (adult) | How supplied |
|---|---|---|---|---|
| Alkylamines | Chlorpheniramine | Chlortrimeton, others | po: 4 mg q4-6h<br>parenteral: 10-20 mg single | tablets: 4, 8, 12 mg<br>time release: 8, 12 mg<br>syrup, liq.: 1 mg/5 ml, 2 mg/5 ml<br>injection: 10 mg/ml, 100 mg/ml |
| | Brompheniramine maleate | various | po: 4 mg q4-6h<br>parenteral: 5-20 mg | tablets: 4, 8, 12 mg<br>elixir: 2 mg |
| | Triprolidine | Actidil, others | po: 2.5 mg q4-6h | tablets: 2.5 mg<br>syrup: 1.25 mg/5 ml |
| Ethanolamines | Diphrenhydramine | Benadryl, others | po: 25-50 mg q4-6h<br>parenteral: 50-100 mg IV or deep IM | 25 mg, 50 mg<br>syrup: 12.5 mg/5 ml |
| | Clemastine | Tavist | po: 1.34 mg b.i.d.-2.68 mg t.i.d. | tab: 1.34, 2.68 mg<br>syrup: 0.67 mg/ml |
| Ethylenediamines | Pyrilamine | Triaminic | po: 25-50 mg t.i.d.-q.i.d. | tablets: 25 mg |
| | Tripelennamine | PBZ | po: 25-50 mg q4-6h | tab: 25, 50, 100 (SR) mg<br>elixir: 37.5 mg/5 ml |
| Phenothiazines | Promethazine | Phenergan, others | po: 25-50 mg<br>IM: 25-50 mg | tablets: 12.5, 25<br>syrup: 6.25, 25 mg/5 ml<br>injection: 25, 50 mg/ml |
| | Trimeprazine | Temaril | po: 2.5 mg q.i.d.<br>sustained: 5mg q12h | tablets: 2.5 mg<br>sust. release: 5 mg<br>syrup: 2.5 mg/5 ml |
| | Methdilazine | Tacaryl | po: 8 mg b.i.d.-q.i.d. | tablets: 8 mg<br>syrup: 4 mg/5 ml |
| Piperazines | Hydyroxyzine HCL pamoate | Atarax, Vistaril | po: 25-200 mg/day<br>IM: 25-100 mg | tablets: 25, 50, 100 mg<br>oral suspension (Vistaril): 25 mg/5 ml |
| Piperidines | Cyproheptadine | Periactin | po: 4-20 mg/day | tab: 4 mg, syrup 2 mg/5 ml |
| | Azatadine | Optimine | po: 1-2 mg b.i.d. | tablets: 1 mg |
| Tricyclic antidepressants | Doxepin | Sinequan<br>Adapin, others | po: 10-25 mg q6-8h or up to 150 mg single daily dose | capsules: 10, 25, 50, 75, 100, 150 mg<br>oral concentrate: 10 mg/ml |
| Miscellaneous non-sedating | Terfenadine | Seldane | po: 60 mg b.i.d. | tablets: 60 mg |
| | Astemazole | Hismanal | po: 10 mg/day | tablets: 10 mg |
| | Loratadine | Claritin | po: 10 mg/day | tablets: 10 mg |

**Table 20-4.** Topical antibiotics

| Generic name | Brand name | Preparation |
|---|---|---|
| Bacitracin | same | 15, 30, 120 g |
| Chloramphenicol | Chloromycetin cr | 30 g |
| Clioquinol (iodochlorhydroxyquin) | Vioform cr, lo, oint | 15, 30 g |
| | Vioform/hydrocort | 15, 30 g |
| Clindamycin phosphate (1%)* | Cleocin-T soln, gel | 60 g |
| Erythromycin 2%* | Ery-cette pledgets | box of 60 |
| | Em-gel | 30 g |
| | Akne-Mycin oint | 25 g |
| | A/T/S alcohol sol | 60 ml |
| | Eryderm alcohol sol | 60 ml |
| | Erymax alcohol sol | 2 oz, 4 oz |
| | T-Stat alcohol sol | 60 ml |
| | Staticin (1.5%) alcohol sol | 60 ml |
| Erythromycin 3% and Benzoyl peroxide 5% | Benzamycin gel | 23.3 g |
| Gentamycin | Garamycin cr, oint | 15 g |
| Gramicidin & hydrocortisone | Cortisporin oint | 15 g |
| Iodoquinol & HC | Vytone | 30 g |
| Meclocycline* | Meclan cream | 20, 45 g |
| Mefenide acetate | Sulfamylon cream | 60, 120, 480 g |
| Metronidazole† | Metrogel | 30 g |
| Mupirocin 2% | Bactroban oint | 15, 30 g |
| Neomycin | multiple | 7.5-60 g |
| Nitrofurazone | Furacin cream | 30 g |
| Polymyxin/bacitracin | Polysporin (many) | 15, 30 g |
| Polymyxin/bacitracin/neomycin | Neosporin | 15, 30 g |
| | Mycitracin | 15, 30 g |
| Povidone-iodine | Betadine oint | 30 g |
| Silver sulfadiazine | Silvadene cr | 20-1000 g |
| Sulfacetamide sodium† | Sulfacet-R lotion | 30 g |
| | Novacet lotion | 30 g |
| | Sebizon lotion | 85 g |
| Tetracycline HCl* | Achromycin oint | 15, 30 g |
| | Topicycline alcohol sol | 70 ml |

Application: Infections-multiple times daily. Acne-once or twice daily.
Modified from Habif TP: *Clinical dermatology,* ed 2, St Louis, 1990, Mosby.
*Best for acne vulgaris.
†Best for acne rosacea.

wounds (see Table 20-4). Patients can develop allergic contact dermatitis to topical application of neomycin and bacitracin. A newer topical antibiotic, mupirocin (Bactroban ointment) is effective against infections with gram-positive cocci. This antibiotic is especially useful in patients who are carriers of *Staphylococcus aureus* in the nares, and it is effective in mild cases of impetigo.

***Antiseptic cleansers.*** The main antiseptic cleansers include povidone iodine (Betadine), hexachlorophene (pHisoHex), and chlorhexadine (Hibiclens). These effective antibacterial cleaners are useful as adjunctive therapy in superficial skin infections.

***Oral antibiotics.*** Numerous oral antibiotics are available and effective in the treatment of skin infections. A complete discussion of antibiotic choices is found in Chapter 64. In the treatment of acne, the most commonly used oral antibiotics are tetracycline and erythromycin. These antibiotics are inexpensive and generally well tolerated and effective. Effective alternatives, albeit more expensive, include doxycycline and minocycline.

## ANTIFUNGAL THERAPY

*Topical treatment* is effective when involvement is limited to the epidermal or mucosal surface only. With deeper involvement (hair follicles or nails), systemic therapy must be considered. Topical antifungal agents may have activity against *Candida* species only, dermatophytes only, or both (Table 20-5). Application should be once or twice a day until the infection has cleared.

## SYSTEMIC ANTIFUNGAL THERAPY

### Griseofulvin

Griseofulvin has been available since the 1950s to treat dermatophyte fungal infections. It is fungistatic in all dermatophyte fungal infections, but has no activity against *Candida albicans* or *Pityrosporum* species (tinea versicolor). Side effects of griseofulvin can include gastrointestinal upset, headache, and interaction with coumadin anticoagulants to reduce the anticoagulation effect. Griseofulvin is available in microsized 250 to 500 mg once or twice a day, and ultra microsized formulations, 125 to 250 mg once or twice a day. The duration of treatment depends on site of involvement; skin infection such as

**Table 20-5.** Topical antifungal agents

| Generic name | Brand name | Activity | Packaging | Use |
|---|---|---|---|---|
| Amphotericin B | Fungizone | candida (C) | 20 g cream<br>30 ml lotion<br>20 g ointment | twice a day |
| Benzoic acid, salicylic acid | Whitfield's ointment, Antinea ointment otc* | dermatophytes (D) | 1 oz | once or twice a day |
| Ciclopirox | Loprox | C, D | 15, 30, 90 g cream<br>30 ml lotion | twice a day |
| Clotrimazole | Lotrimin AF otc*<br>Mycelex | C, D | 1, 2 oz<br>15, 30, 45, 90 g cream<br>10, 30 ml lotion<br>10 mg troches | every 3-4 hr |
| Econozole | Spectazole | C, D | 15, 30, 85 g cream | twice a day |
| Haloprogin | Halotex | C, D | 15, 30 g cream<br>10, 30 ml lotion | twice a day |
| Ketoconazole | Nizoral | C, D | 15, 30, 60 g cream | twice a day |
| Miconazole | Monostat-derm<br>Micatin otc* | C, D | 15, 30, 85 g cream<br>30, 60 ml lotion<br>15 g cream | twice a day |
| Naftifine | Naftin | C, D | 15, 30, 60 g cream<br>20, 40 g gel | twice a day |
| Nystatin | Mycostatin | C only | 15, 30 g cream<br>15, 30 g ointment<br>60 ml suspension | twice a day<br><br>4 times a day (oral) |
| Oxiconazole | Oxistat | C, D | 15, 30 g cream | twice a day |
| Sulconazole | Exelderm | C, D | 15, 30, 60 g cream<br>30 ml solution | twice a day |
| Terbinafine | Lamisil | D only | 15, 30 g cream | twice a day |
| Tolnaftate | Tinactin otc* | D only | 15 g cream<br>10 ml solution | twice a day |
| Undecylenic acid | Desenex otc* | D only | 30 g ointment<br>45 ml spray<br>42.5 g foam | once or twice a day |

*Over the counter.

tinea cruris responds in 2 to 4 weeks, whereas toenail infection requires 6 to 18 months of treatment.

### Ketoconazole

Ketoconazole is a water-soluble imidazole antifungal drug with activity against dermatophyte fungi, *Candida* species, *Pityrosporum* species (tinea versicolor), and others. Doses of 200 to 400 ml a day are used for most dermatologic fungal infections. The primary precaution with the use of ketoconazole is hepatotoxicity, which occurs in approximately 1 in 10,000 patients. Fatalities have occurred when therapy was continued. Other potential side effects include gastrointestinal upset and decreased libido because of a mild androgen antagonist effect. Gastric acidity facilitates oral absorption and therefore antacids and $H_2$ blockers should not be taken concomitantly.

*Newer Antifungal Medications:* Fluconazole and itraconazole are triazole antifungal agents designed for oral use. These antifungal medications have a broad spectrum of activity that includes most fungal infections found in dermatology. Recent studies have suggested that intermittent dosing (e.g., 100 mg twice a week) may be effective in the treatment of tinea and onychomycosis. Both drugs have the potential for hepatotoxicity.

## ANTIVIRAL THERAPY

### Acyclovir

Acyclovir (Zovirax) is currently the primary antiviral agent used in dermatologic therapy. This medication is effective against herpesvirus infections, including herpes simplex and herpes zoster. The antiviral activity of acyclovir requires activation by the viral enzyme thymidine kinase. Because of this requirement, acyclovir has little toxicity to human cells and therefore has relatively few systemic side effects. The specific treatment recommendations for herpes simplex and herpes zoster are discussed in Chapters 26 and 68.

## PROCEDURAL DERMATOLOGY

### Skin biopsy

Skin biopsy can be essential to making a correct dermatologic diagnosis, and all clinicians should know how to perform this procedure. See Chapter 19 for a detailed description of the skin biopsy.

### Liquid nitrogen cryosurgery

***Indications.*** The correct use of cryosurgery requires confidence in the diagnosis. This treatment should be avoided if the diagnosis is questionable. Liquid nitrogen is

### Liquid nitrogen cryotherapy

The use of liquid nitrogen cryotherapy to treat melanocytic nevi is contraindicated.

effective in treating small, superficial lesions. The best result occurs in a lesion of epidermal origin such as a verruca, seborrheic keratosis, or actinic keratosis because liquid nitrogen causes a separation of the epidermis from the dermis. Small lesions with a dermal component such as acrochordons also may respond to this treatment. Larger dermal lesions and skin malignancies can be treated with liquid nitrogen but require special temperature monitoring techniques to maximize the response and minimize complications. Liquid nitrogen should never be used to treat melanocytic nevi because of the possibility of misdiagnosing what is actually a malignant melanoma (see the box above).

***Procedure.*** Liquid nitrogen (boiling point, -196° C) is commercially available and requires storage in an industrial container. It may be applied by cotton applicator or spray. Cotton applicators generally need to be tailored to a size slightly smaller than the lesion. Q-tip applicators usually do not hold enough liquid to be effective. Rectal/vaginal swabs can be shaped into a point, or cotton can be rolled onto a pointed applicator stick to the desired size. Repeated application of the liquid-soaked cotton, avoiding dripping, achieves the desired amount of freezing.

**Warts.** The amount of freezing required to adequately treat the lesion depends on the size and location. Flat warts and small warts on thin skin require the least amount of freezing. Large and deep warts such as plantar/palmar warts require a relatively more aggressive treatment. Repeated freezing-thawing produces more tissue damage. Although the treatment is painful, local anesthetic is usually not required except in large lesions on the palms, soles, and fingers.

**Seborrheic keratoses.** These epidermal growths tend to be more superficial than warts and therefore require less freeze time than large warts.

**Actinic keratoses.** The time required to treat actinic keratoses with liquid nitrogen depends on the amount of keratinized surface and on the depth of involvement. These lesions generally require less freeze time than warts. If there is concern about squamous cell carcinoma, cryosurgery should be avoided.

***Complications.*** Blister formation is common after cryosurgery. Pain may be severe in the 48 hours after treatment. The use of cryosurgery is limited in dark-skinned people because of the high frequency of healing with hypopigmentation. Infection rarely occurs after cryosurgery, and dressing changes are not required. In general, scarring is usually minimal but is more common on the face. Cryotherapy in children and elderly patients should be performed with caution because of these patients' increased susceptibility to blister formation and scarring.

### Skin tag removal

Acrochordons are treated by a variety of methods depending on the size of the lesions. The smallest lesions can be treated with liquid nitrogen. Larger lesions are best treated by removal with a scalpel or scissors. The need for local anesthesia depends on the size of the lesion, but most can be removed without anesthesia as long as the cutting of each lesion is swift. If hemostasis requires the use of heat or electrocautery, local anesthesia is indicated.

### Cyst removal

Surgical excision of small cysts can be uncomplicated. Large lesions on the face or scalp require the same surgical precautions, as do deeper excisions of malignancies. In a noninflamed cyst, failure to remove the entire cyst wall can result in its recurrence. Small cysts are best excised after local anesthesia by means of an elliptical or punch incision to gain access to the cyst, and removal of the entire cyst wall is achieved with blunt and sharp dissection. Closure can require both dermal and surface suturing.

## BIBLIOGRAPHY

Arndt KA: *Manual of dermatologic therapeutics,* ed 5, Boston, 1992, Little Brown.
Habif TP: *Clinical dermatology,* ed 2, St Louis, 1990, Mosby.

CHAPTER

# 21 Common Skin Disorders

**James C. Shaw**
**Margaret Hewitt Robertson**
**Frank Parker**

## DERMATITIS AND ECZEMA

The words *eczema* and *dermatitis* frequently are used synonymously. Literally, dermatitis means inflammation of the skin; eczema means "bubbling or boiling over." Both terms usually refer to a group of diseases that have similar clinical characteristics. Included in this group are atopic dermatitis, contact dermatitis, stasis dermatitis, xerotic dermatitis, dyshidrotic dermatitis, nummular dermatitis, and lichen simplex chronicus (Table 21-1).

Although the etiology of each disease in this group may be different, the symptoms and primary and secondary lesions are similar. The characteristic symptom in patients with eczema is pruritus. If pruritus is absent, a diagnosis of eczema should be questioned. The common clinical findings usually include erythema, papules, microvesicles, and excoriation in the acute stages and lichenification in chronic forms. The principles of therapy are also similar.

### Atopic dermatitis

Atopic dermatitis is a chronic skin disease characterized by pruritus, erythema, skin inflammation and lichenifica-

**Table 21-1.** Differential diagnosis of dermatitis

| Diagnosis | History | Physical examination | Laboratory | Management |
|---|---|---|---|---|
| Atopic dermatitis | Onset by age 5<br>Family history atopy<br>Pruritus<br>Exacerbating factors<br>Coexistent hay fever, asthma | Flexural dist.<br>Lichenification<br>Papules, erythema<br>Pustules if secondary *Staphylococcus* | Routine: none<br>Consider:<br>culture/pustule<br>IgE | Topical corticosteroids<br>Control environment<br>Antihistamines<br>Emollients |
| Contact dermatitis | | | | |
| Irritant type | Predisposing history of atopy<br>Frequent water exposure<br>Solvents<br>Job description | Hands commonly<br>Erythema, scale, fissuring | None | Topical steroid ointments<br>Protect from wet exposures<br>Gloves<br>Emollients |
| Allergic type | Rapid onset<br>Pruritus<br>Exposures:<br>plants<br>cosmetics | Erythema, vesicles, oozing<br>Location corresponds to exposure | None | Wet to dry dressings<br>Topical or systemic corticosteroids<br>Identify and avoid allergen |
| Stasis dermatitis | Gradual onset<br>Distal legs<br>Previous history<br>Varicosities, leg trauma, etc | Erythema<br>Pigmentation<br>Edema<br>Fibrosis | None | Acute: steroid ointments<br>Long term: compression, leg elevation, emollient ointments |
| Xerotic dermatitis | Winter<br>Low humidity<br>Frequent baths<br>Soap use<br>Pretibial common | Patchy, erythema, scale<br>Extensor areas<br>Spares folds | None | Decrease soap and water exposure<br>Liberal use of thick emollients, especially after bath<br>Steroids short-term prn |
| Dyshidrosis | Pruritic papules and vesicles on hands<br>Recurrent | Papules and small vesicles on hands | None<br>exclude fungus with KOH<br>exclude allergen | Systemic or topical steroids<br>Antibiotics |
| Nummular dermatitis | Gradual onset<br>Pruritic<br>Frequent history<br>Exposure to drying | Round patches<br>Erythema<br>Scaling occasional<br>Oozing occasional | None<br>KOH to exclude fungus | Steroid ointments<br>Tar cream, gel<br>Ultraviolet light |

tion typically distributed in flexural areas, plus a personal or family history of asthma, hay fever, or eczema. The term *atopy* refers to the triad of dermatitis, asthma, and hay fever.

***Epidemiology/etiology.*** Atopy (atopic dermatitis, asthma, or hay fever) is present in 8% to 25% of populations. Atopic dermatitis is present in all races and geographic locations, but appears to be a higher incidence in urban areas and developed countries. Although the trait runs in families, the precise genetics have not been fully elucidated. A family history of respiratory atopy can be obtained in almost 50% of patients with atopic dermatitis.

***Pathophysiology.*** The pathogenesis of atopic dermatitis is not entirely understood. Atopy is characterized immunologically by high concentrations of serum IgE, a high incidence of IgE-mediated responses by skin test to common inhaled antigens, decreased numbers of immunoregulatory T cells, defective antibody-dependent cellular cytotoxicity and reduced cell-mediated immunity.

Criteria for making the diagnosis of atopic dermatitis have been proposed (see box at right). Three major criteria plus three minor criteria should be present to confirm the diagnosis.

***History.*** A suggestive history includes onset of a dermatitis at an early age (most patients have manifestations of atopic dermatitis by age 5 years), pruritus, the existence of exacerbating factors, and a positive family history of atopy.

***Examination.*** Papules, erythema, excoriations, and lichenification are the hallmarks of atopic dermatitis. In adults flexural areas such as the neck, antecubital fossae, and popliteal fossae are most commonly involved (see Plate 10). The face, wrists, and forearms also are common sites of involvement. In severe cases any area of the body can be involved. Infants usually present with pruritic patches of erythema and papules that can be present more centrally on the face, chest, and extensor extremities. The presence of pustules may represent colonization or

### Guidelines for the diagnosis of atopic dermatitis

Must have three or more basic features:
- Pruritus
- Typical morphology and distribution:
  - Flexural lichenification or linearity in adults
  - Facial and extensor involvement in infants and children
- Chronic or chronically relapsing dermatitis
- Personal or family history of atopy (asthma, allergic rhinitis, atopic dermatitis)

Plus three or more minor features:
- Xerosis
- Ichthyosis/palmar hyperlinearity/keratosis pilaris
- Immediate (type I) skin test reactivity
- Elevated serum IgE
- Early age of onset
- Tendency toward cutaneous infections (esp. *S. aureus* and herpes simplex)/impaired cell-mediated immunity
- Tendency toward nonspecific hand or foot dermatitis
- Nipple eczema
- Cheilitis
- Recurrent conjunctivitis
- Dennie-Morgan infraorbital fold
- Keratoconus
- Anterior subcapsular cataracts
- Orbital darkening
- Facial pallor/facial erythema
- Pityriasis alba
- Anterior neck folds
- Itch when sweating
- Intolerance to wool and lipid solvents
- Perifollicular accentuation
- Food intolerance
- Course influenced by environmental/emotional factors
- White dermographism/delayed blanch

From Hanifin JM, Rajka G: *Acta Derm Venereol* Suppl (Stockholm) 92:44-47, 1980.

secondary infection with *Staphylococcus aureus*. Other physical findings that support the diagnosis include xerosis, the infraorbital skin fold (Dennie-Morgan line), periorbital darkening, hyperlinear palms, keratosis pilaris, and nipple dermatitis.

***Management.*** The treatment of atopic dermatitis centers around three principles: (1) treatment of inflamed skin, (2) control of itching, and (3) control of exacerbating factors. The first two usually require pharmacologic treatment, whereas control of exacerbating factors is usually nonpharmacologic.

Topical corticosteroids are the primary modality to treat inflamed skin. For mild disease, a low potency corticosteroid cream is effective. For more severe disease a medium potency corticosteroid cream or ointment may be needed. Secondary infection requires oral antibiotics. Acute flares can sometimes be aborted by a short course of systemic corticosteroids (i.e., prednisone 40 to 60 mg/day for 3 to 4 days, then 20 to 30 mg/day for 3 to 4 days). The most severe cases require combinations of treatments that can include systemic corticosteroids and ultraviolet light therapy.

Antihistamines usually are helpful to control pruritus. Considerable trial and error may be required to identify the best antihistamine for the individual patient. The nonsedating $H_1$ blockers (terfenadine [Seldane], astemizole [Hismanal]) are of limited value in most cases, but can be tried in patients with mild disease. Frequently some sedation is desirable, especially at night. Commonly used $H_1$ blockers include diphenhydramine, hydroxyzine, and cyproheptadine. Doxepin is a potent $H_1$ blocker with sedating properties; its use can be helpful in severe cases. Tepid baths to hydrate and cool the skin can also relieve itching temporarily.

An important aspect of successful treatment of atopic dermatitis is the use of emollients. When used frequently and liberally, emollients can prevent drying of the skin, which is effective in the control of pruritus.

## Contact dermatitis

Contact dermatitis refers to any dermatitis caused by external substances that come in contact with the skin directly. It can occur either by the direct irritating effects of the substance (irritant contact dermatitis), or by the development of a hypersensitivity to the offending substance (allergic contact dermatitis). The dermatitis can be acute, subacute, or chronic.

### Irritant contact dermatitis

Irritant contact dermatitis, which is more common than allergic contact dermatitis, occurs when a chemical disrupts the normal epidermal barrier and causes an inflammatory response. Most irritant substances are used on a daily basis and are found in most living and work environments. They are generally low-grade irritants that require repeated exposure to produce a dermatitis (soapy water, cleansers, rubbing alcohol). Some irritants are highly caustic, producing severe dermatitis after minimal exposure (bleach, strong acids, alkalis). Although anyone can develop irritant contact dermatitis, those with compromised skin (atopic dermatitis, dry skin) are at a higher risk.

***Examination.*** Mild irritants produce erythema, chapped skin, dryness, and fissuring. Pruritus is usually mild to moderate. The hands are the usual site for irritant contact dermatitis (see Plate 11), but the face, especially the eyelids, may be affected. Severe cases can present with edema, serous oozing, and tenderness. Potent irritants cause painful bullae within hours of exposure.

***Management.*** The goals of treatment of irritant contact dermatitis are to restore a normal epidermal barrier and then protect it from the irritating substance. Reduced exposure to soap and water, use of emollient creams or ointments, and use of gloves in hand dermatitis may control a chronic irritant contact dermatitis. In more severe cases, corticosteroid ointments under occlusion may be necessary to treat the acute phase. Systemic corticosteroids, although potentially helpful in reducing acute inflammation, have no place in the treatment of chronic irritant contact dermatitis unless corrective measures are taken to avoid the offending contactants.

### Allergic contact dermatitis

Allergic contact dermatitis occurs when a delayed (type IV) hypersensitivity to a substance develops. This can occur after one exposure or after years of repeated exposure to an antigen. The antigen, usually of low molecular weight, binds to epidermal proteins and is presented to T lymphocytes in the dermis. Further immunologic processing of the antigen takes place in lymph nodes where sensitized T lymphocytes are produced. The allergic dermatitis occurs when the sensitized lymphocytes encounter the antigen in the skin and release inflammatory mediators. The sensitization phase takes 10 to 14 days, but dermatitis may be seen in a sensitized individual within 12 to 48 hours after reexposure.

The most common sensitizer in the United States is the oleoresin of the Rhus family of plants (poison oak, poison ivy, poison sumac). Many substances are capable of sensitizing individuals and causing allergic contact dermatitis. Some common examples include nickel in jewelry, fragrances, preservatives in topical preparations, components in rubber, and chemicals in shoes.

#### History

The patient with allergic contact dermatitis usually complains of intense itching in the area of exposure, followed by the development of a pruritic rash. The exposure can antedate the dermatitis by 2 weeks if it is the result of a primary sensitization. Frequently an exact date of exposure is difficult to identify. In chronic cases, the dermatitis may have been present for months or years.

#### Examination

Clinical findings include erythema, edema, papules, vesicles, and serous oozing in the involved areas. One often sees a sharply outlined configuration corresponding to the area of skin exposure. In Rhus dermatitis linear streaks of dermatitis frequently correspond to areas of contact with the plant resin (see Plate 22). The extent of the dermatitis reflects the source of exposure (e.g., cosmetics on the face, nickel where jewelry is worn, rubber where elastic bands contact the skin, and points of shoe contact on the feet).

***Management.*** Treatment of the acute phase of allergic contact dermatitis depends on the severity of the dermatitis. Wet to dry compresses with water or aluminum acetate (Burow's solution) help dry the vesicular phase (see Chapter 20). Topical corticosteroids are helpful after the skin is dry enough to retain the topical preparation. Soothing lotions such as calamine lotion can provide some relief. In severe cases systemic corticosteroids and antihistamines may be required. Usually the elimination of the offending antigen is curative, but in persistent cases the correct identification of the antigen may require patch testing. Referral to a dermatologist for possible patch testing is especially useful when multiple potential exposures exist such as in certain work environments.

### Stasis dermatitis

Stasis dermatitis occurs on the legs as a result of chronic venous insufficiency. Incompetent venous valves, inadequate tissue support, and postural hydrostatic pressure contribute to the development of venous stasis. The dermatologic changes are secondary to the effects of extravasated blood, which induces a mild inflammatory response in the dermis and subcutaneous fat, plus the low grade tissue ischemia associated with stasis at the capillary level. Superimposed allergic contact dermatitis or recurrent infections are frequently the predominant finding in patients with stasis dermatitis.

***History.*** Symptoms are mild in most cases of stasis dermatitis. There may be a sense of fullness or dull aching in the legs. The patient usually reports a gradual increase in pigmentation and redness.

***Examination.*** In early stasis dermatitis there is mottled pigmentation and slight erythema (see Plate 12). There may be evidence of varicosities, ankle edema, and mild tenderness to deep palpation. Pulses are usually normal. In chronic cases, fibrosis may be the predominant finding, resulting in a woody, hard, sclerotic lower leg.

***Differential diagnosis.*** See box below.

***Management.*** The main emphasis in the management of stasis dermatitis is to counteract the effects of gravity and posture on venous pressure (see Chapter 18). Leg elevation and compression with stockings are the most effective treatment. In mild cases, support hose alone may be sufficient. In more severe cases, daily leg elevation above the level of the head for varying amounts of time may be necessary. Exercise on a regular basis also helps to reduce venous pressure and edema.

The inflammatory component of stasis dermatitis is treated with low or medium potency topical corticosteroids. An ointment base avoids exposure to preservatives, which can cause allergic contact dermatitis.

### Nummular dermatitis

Nummular dermatitis is a chronic pruritic skin eruption consisting of circular, raised patches of erythematous scaly skin. The etiology is not known, although xerosis and emotional stress have been implicated. Adults tend to be affected more than children.

***History.*** Patients usually report patches of itchy skin that gradually enlarge in size and increase in number.

#### Differential diagnosis of stasis dermatitis

Diabetic dermopathy
Allergic contact dermatitis
Cellulitis
Pigmented purpura (Schamberg's disease)

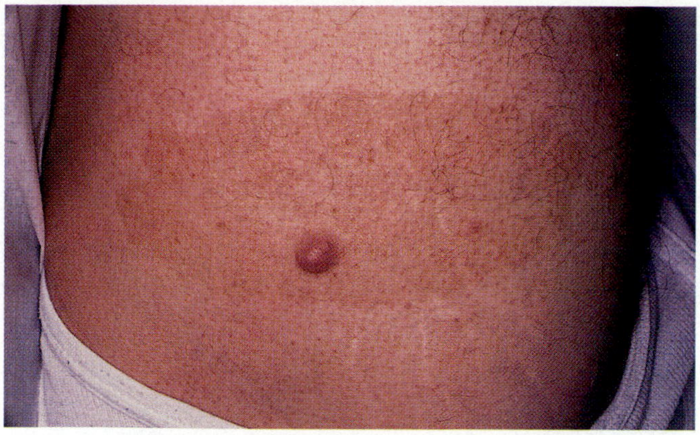

**Plate 1.** Macule (café au lait spot) plus a nodule (neurofibroma).

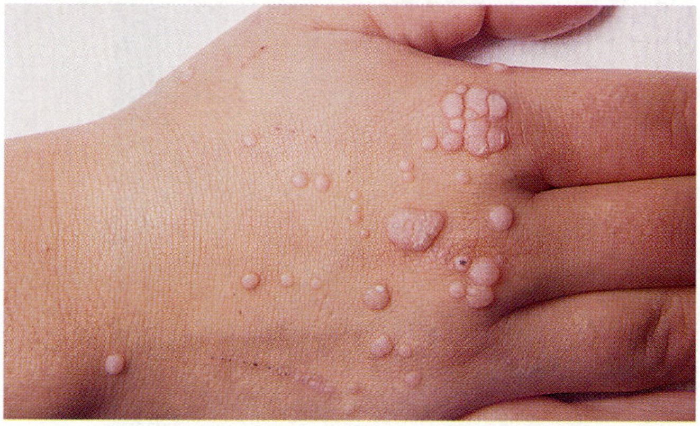

**Plate 2.** Papules (verrucae). Note verrucous surface.

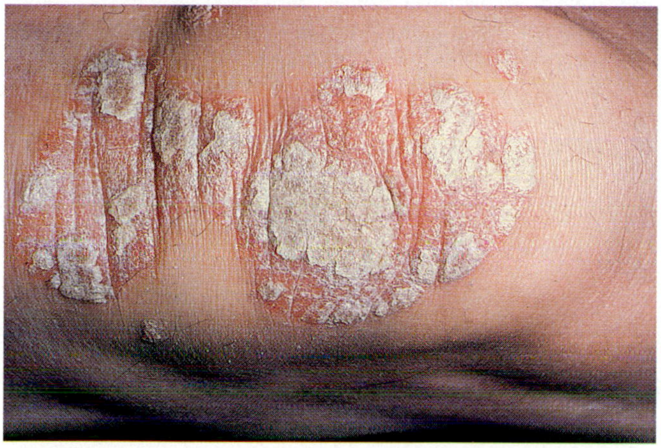

**Plate 3.** Plaques (psoriasis). Note special physical characteristic of scale (silvery, micaceous). Typical location: extensor surfaces (knee).

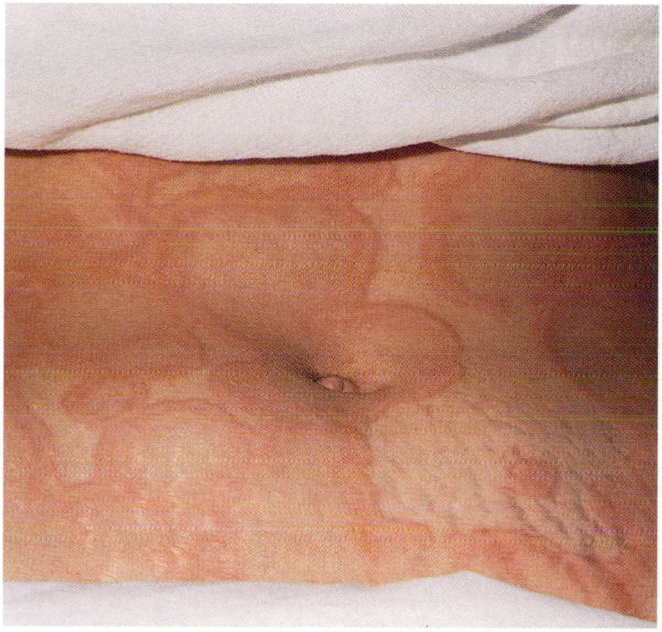

**Plate 4.** Wheal (urticaria). Note central clearing, giving annular configuration.

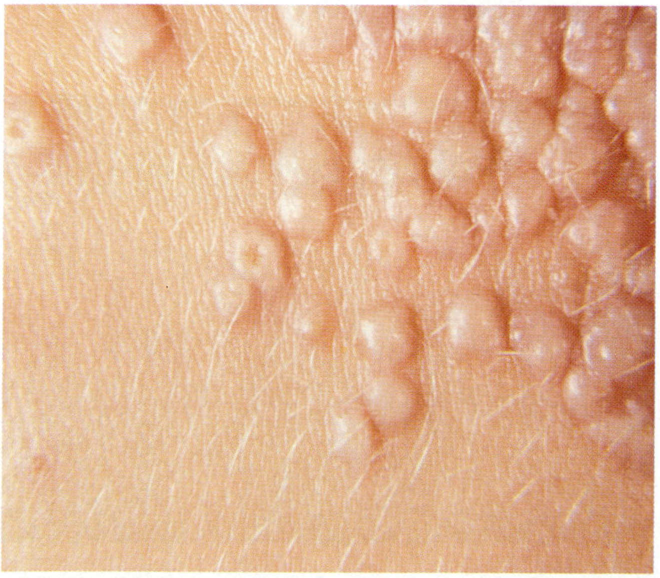

**Plate 5.** Vesicles (herpes simplex). Note umbilication characteristic of viral infection and herpetiform grouping.

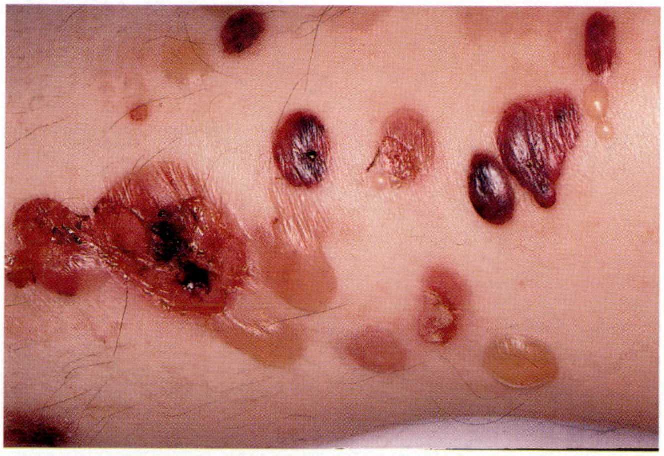

**Plate 6.** Bullae (bullous pemphigoid). Note hemorrhagic nature suggesting subepidermal process.

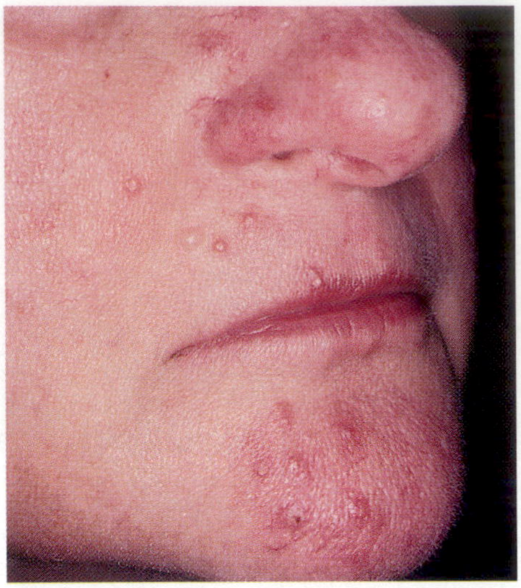

**Plate 7.** Pustules (rosacea). Note also the presence of telangiectasia.

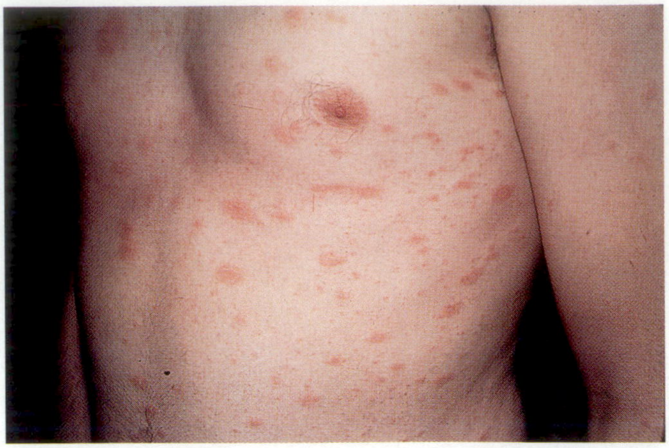

**Plate 8.** Scale (pityriasis rosea). Shows example of how unique scaling (collarette of fine scale within several lesions), distribution and shape of lesions (oval lesions with long axis paralleling natural skin cleavage lines); and color (salmon-pink) help in diagnosing skin disease.

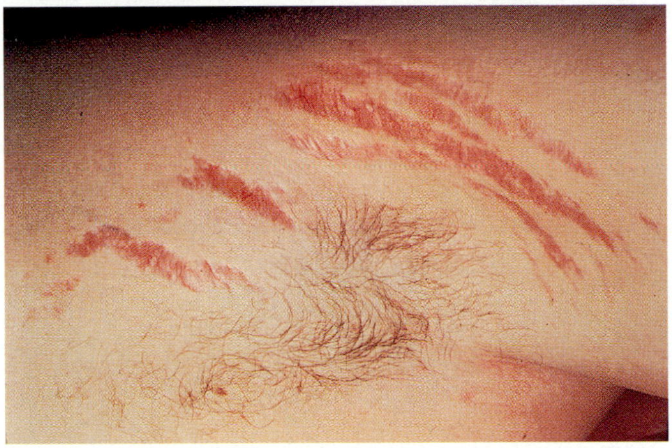

**Plate 9.** Atrophy (striae). Thinning of both the epidermis and dermis contribute to the development of striae.

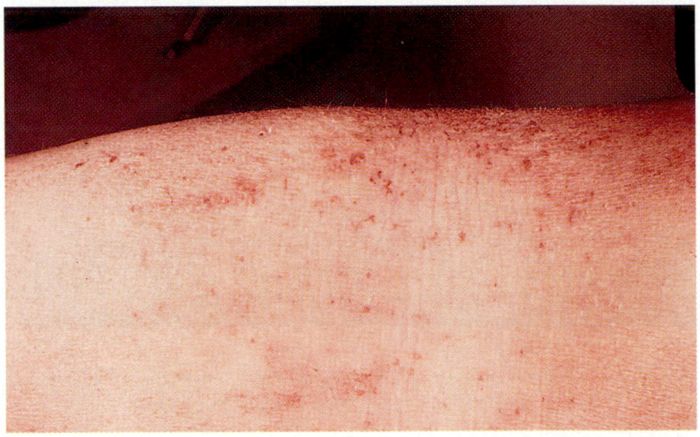

**Plate 10.** Lichenification (atopic dermatitis). Note erythema and pinpoint excoriations in antecubital fossa (typical location for atopic dermatitis—flexural).

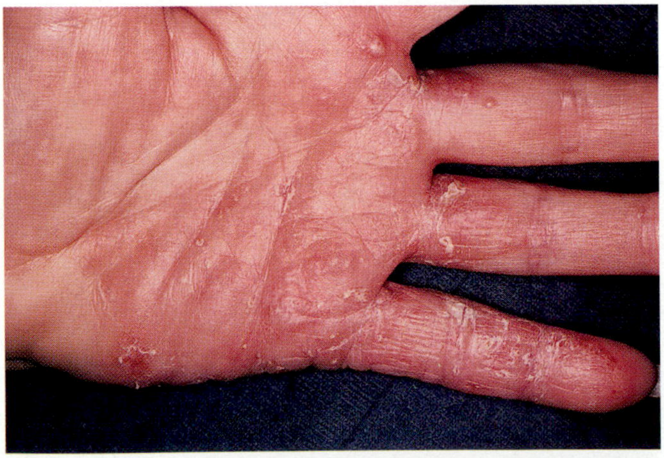

**Plate 11.** Fissures (chronic irritant hand dermatitis). Note superficial fissures in folds along with erythema, lichenification, scaling, and vesicles.

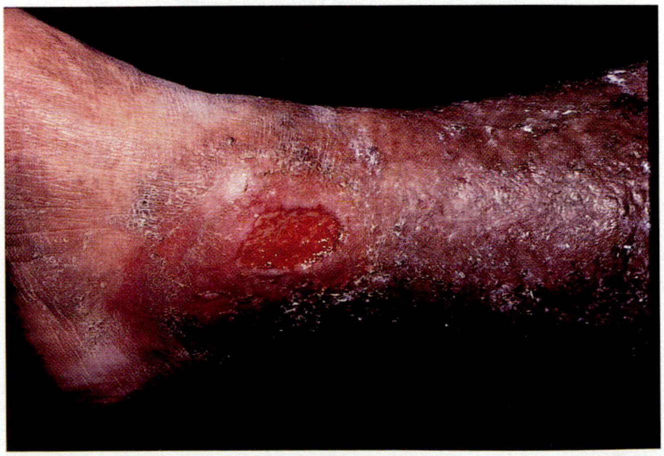

**Plate 12.** Ulcer (stasis dermatitis with ulcer). Note moist ulcer base and typical location near lateral malleolus plus associated dermatitis and stasis pigmentation.

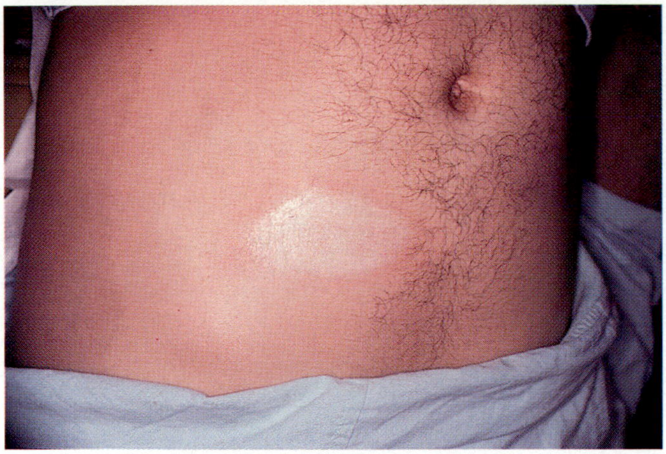

**Plate 13.** Scarring process (morphea). Note ivory white color due to deposition of collagen and loss of hair appendages.

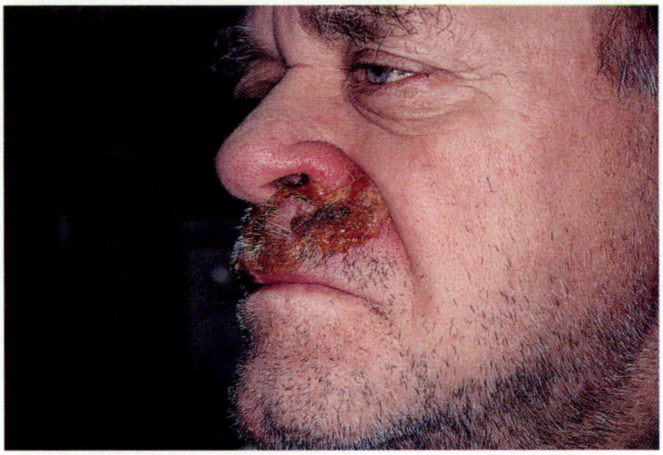

**Plate 14.** Crusts (impetigo). Note both hemorrhagic and honey-colored crust.

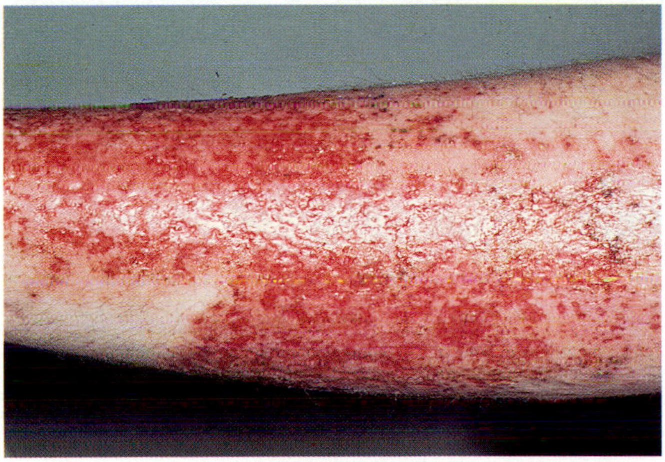

**Plate 15.** Oozing (acute dermatitis). Note multiple erosions with oozing wet glistening surface.

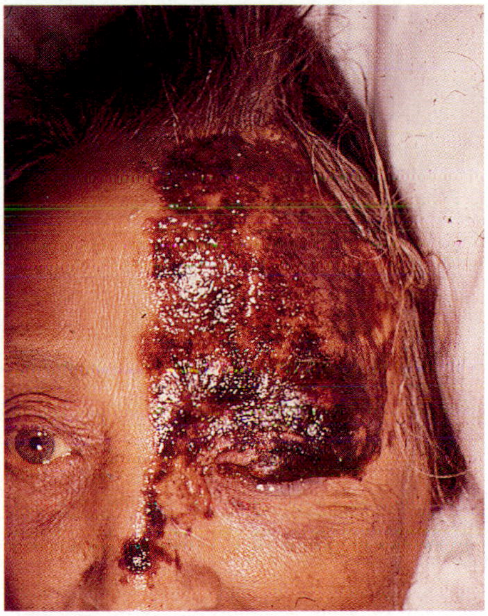

**Plate 16.** Zosteriform lesions (herpes zoster). Note hemorrhagic vesicular involvement of left VI cranial nerve.

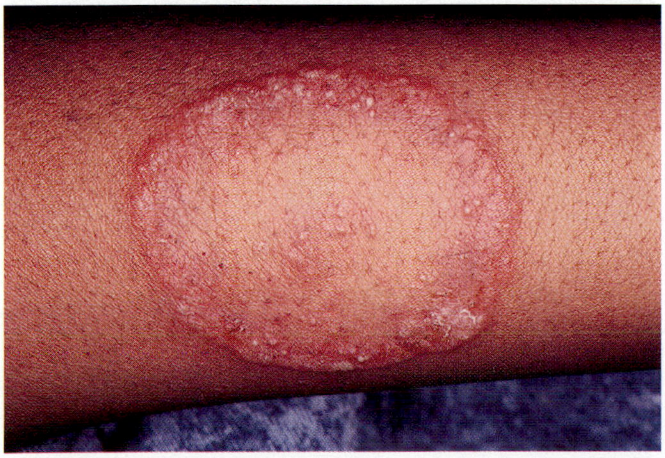

**Plate 17.** Annular lesion (tinea corporis). Note raised erythematous scaling border and central clearing.

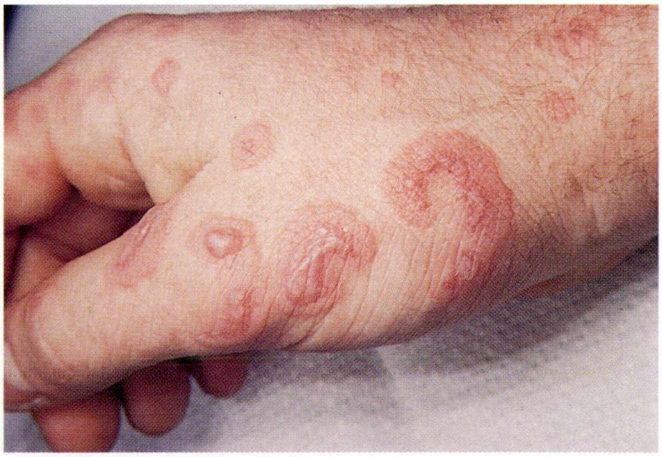

**Plate 18.** Iris and arcuate lesions (erythema multiforme). Note erythematous lesions with multiform configurations—target, arcuate, and vesicles.

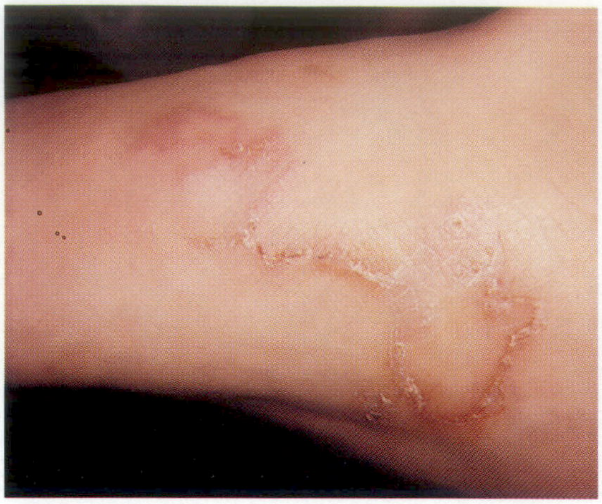

**Plate 19.** Serpiginous lesion (cutaneous larva migrans, creeping eruption). Note snakelike tract of ankylostoma or strongyloides larvae infection of the skin.

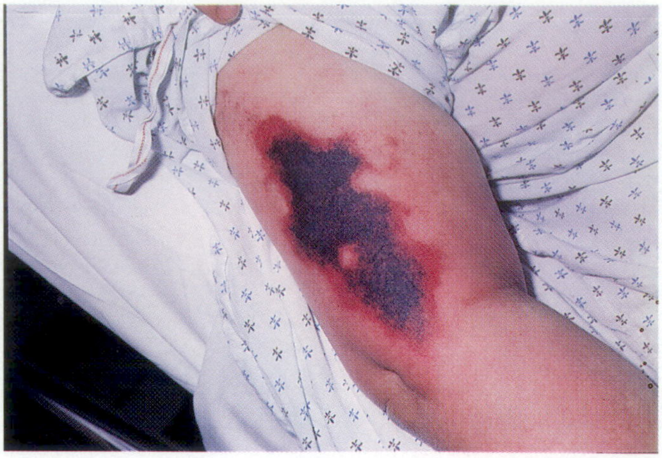

**Plate 20.** Purpuric lesion (purpura fulminans). Note stellate purpuric lesion with surrounding erythema characteristic of disseminated intravascular coagulation secondary to sepsis (e.g., meningococcemia).

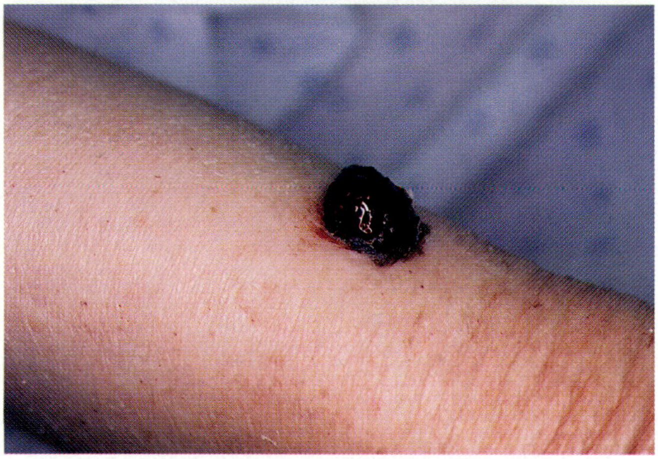

**Plate 21.** Melanin pigment (melanoma). Note variations of hues of color (black and blue) reflecting depth of melanin within the skin.

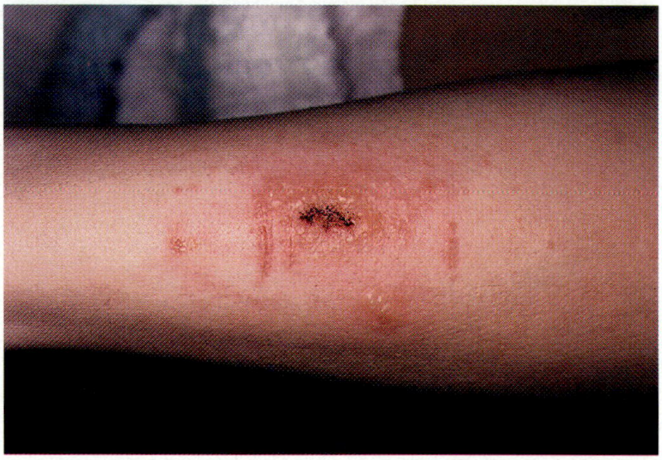

**Plate 22.** Allergic contact dermatitis (poison oak, acute vesicular reaction, and linear features). Dark central pigmentation is oxidized oleoresin.

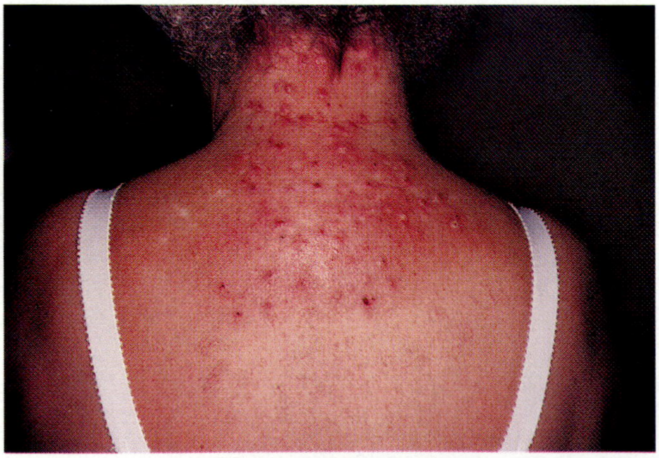

**Plate 23.** Lichen simplex chronicus and prurigo nodules. Note lichenification and excoriated papules that involve only an area on the back that can be reached.

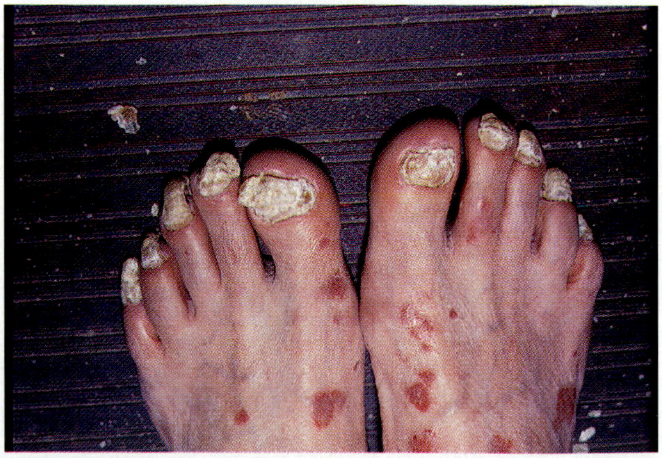

**Plate 24.** Psoriatic nail changes. Note nail dystrophy and accumulation of yellow subungual debris resembling onychomycosis, plus associated cutaneous psoriatic lesions.

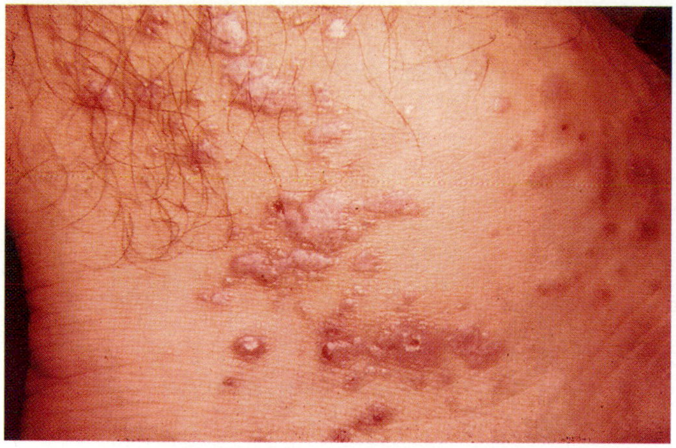

**Plate 25.** Lichen planus. Note polygonal purple, flat, shiny topped papules in typical area (ankles).

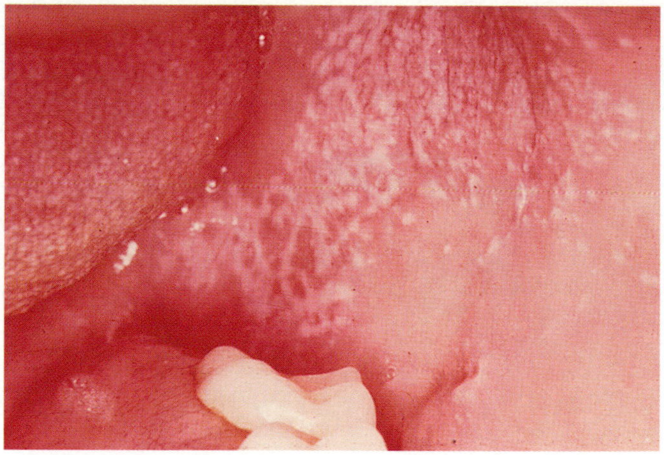

**Plate 26.** Oral lichen planus. Note lacy white streaks on buccal mucosa.

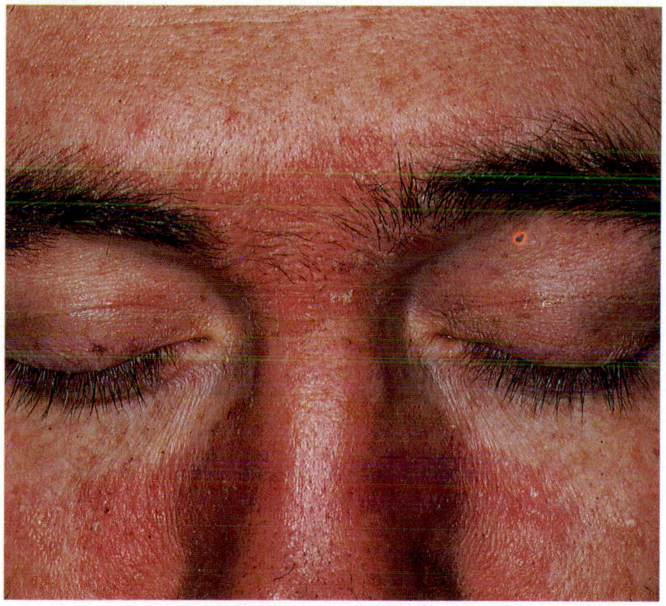

**Plate 27.** Seborrheic dermatitis. (From Habif TP: *Clinical dermatology,* ed 2, St. Louis, 1990, Mosby.)

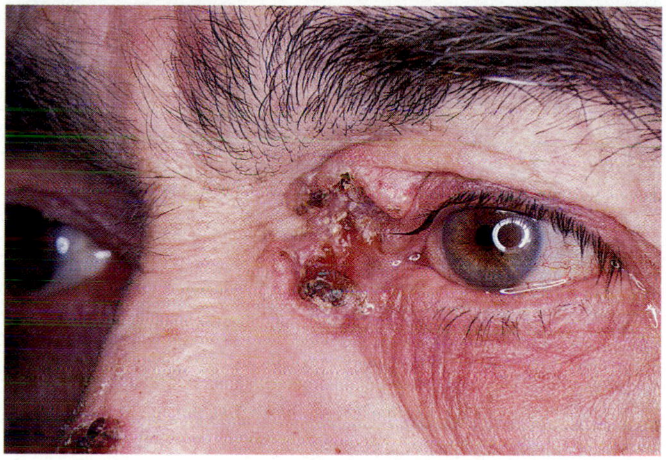

**Plate 28.** Basal cell carcinoma. Note rolled translucent border and central ulceration in typical facial location.

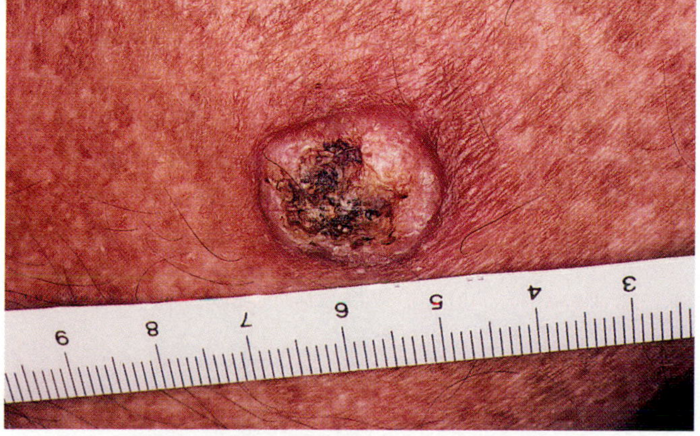

**Plate 29.** Squamous cell carcinoma. Nodular hyperkeratotic lesion with central erosion.

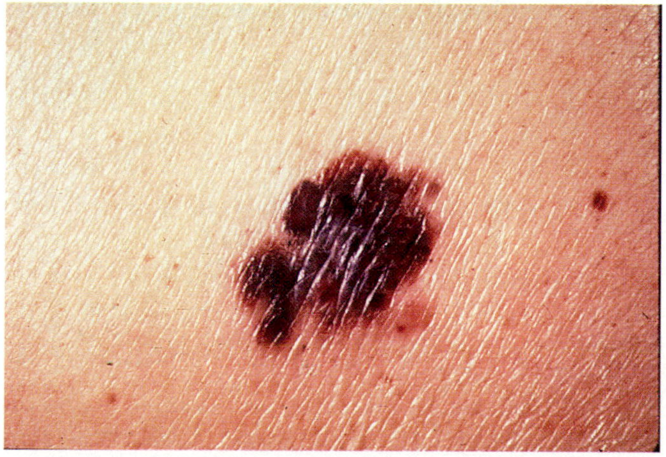

**Plate 30.** Malignant melanoma. Observe the ABCDs in this lesion: Asymmetry, irregular Border, variegate Color, and size (Diameter >6 mm).

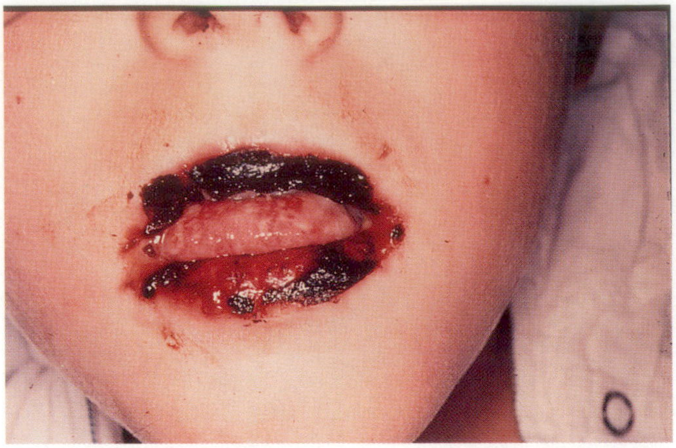

**Plate 31.** Stevens-Johnson syndrome (severe form of erythema multiforme with mucous membrane involvement). Note hemorrhagic erosive crusting of the lips and tongue.

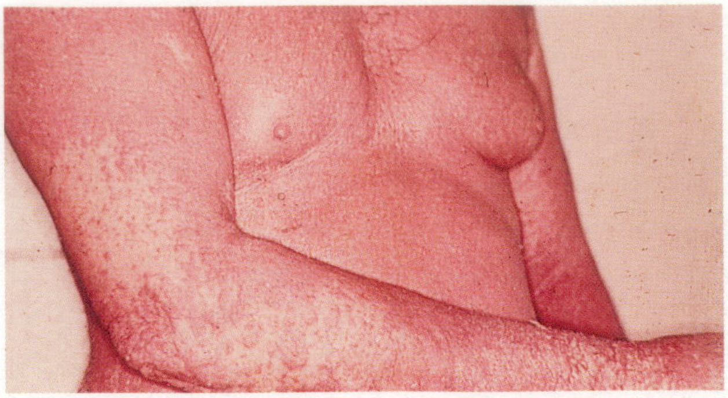

**Plate 32.** Morbilliform drug eruption. Note widespread involvement.

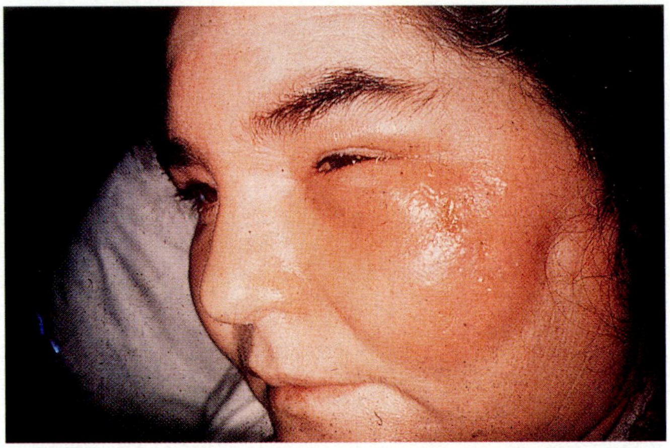

**Plate 33.** Erysipelas. Note bright erythematous sharply demarcated plaque usually associated with fever and pain.

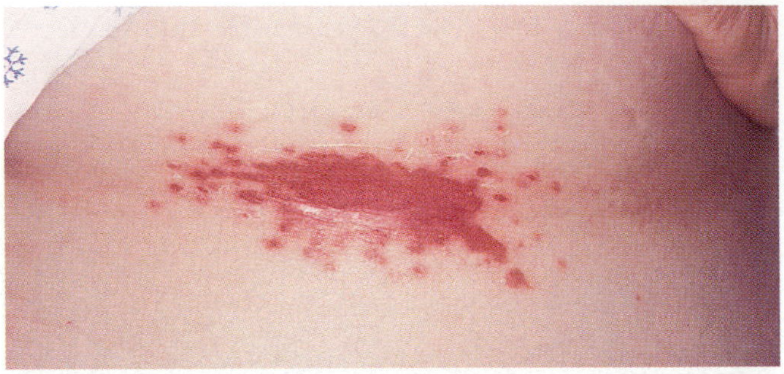

**Plate 34.** Candidiasis. Note erythematous erosive dermatitis with satellite pustules. Location: inframammary.

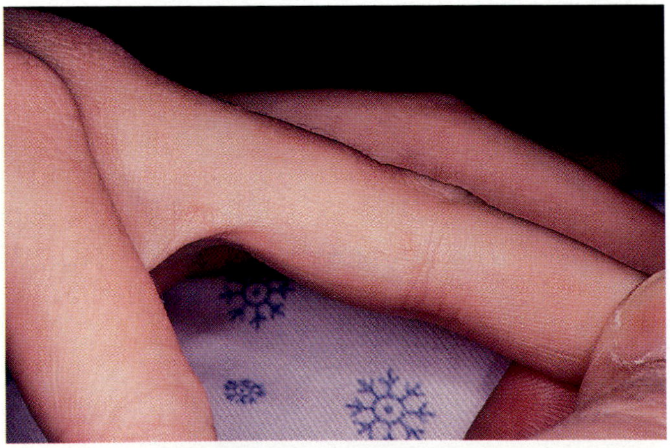

**Plate 35.** Scabies burrow. Note subtle raised linear lesion on the lateral aspect of the finger.

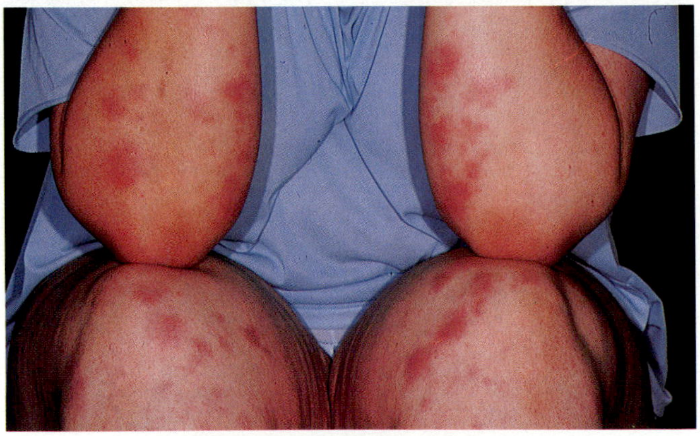

**Plate 36.** Erythema nodosum. (From Habif TP: *Clinical dermatology,* ed 2, St. Louis, 1990, Mosby.)

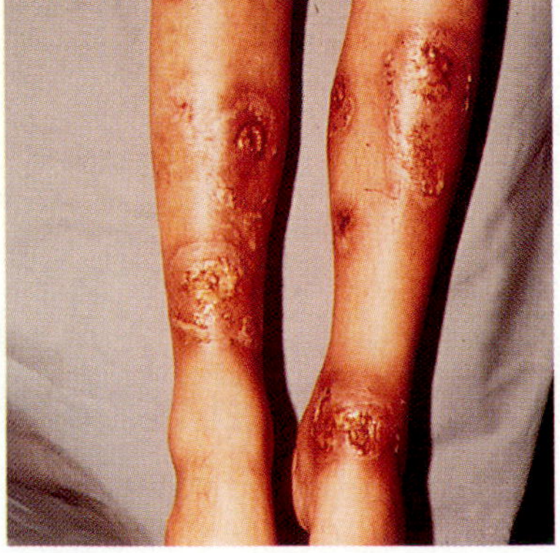

**Plate 37.** Pyoderma gangrenosum. Note ragged ulcerations with surrounding erythema.

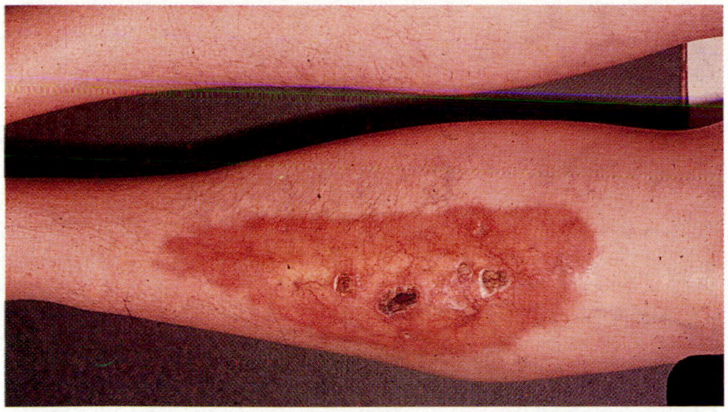

**Plate 38.** Necrobiosis lipoidica diabeticorum. Note red-brown atrophic plaque with telangiectasia.

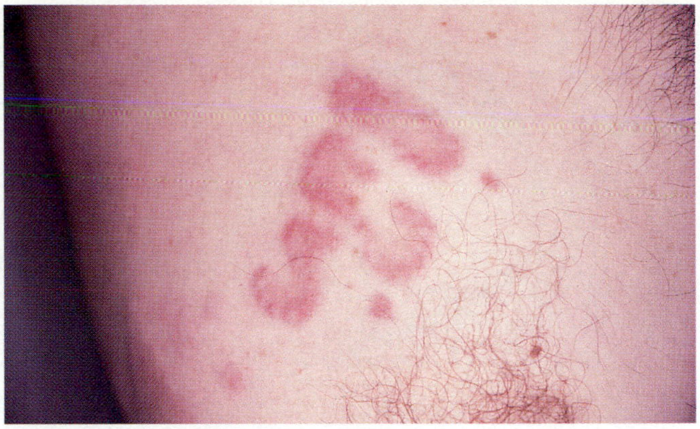

**Plate 39.** Granuloma annulare. Note erythematous plaques of confluent papules arranged in an annular shape.

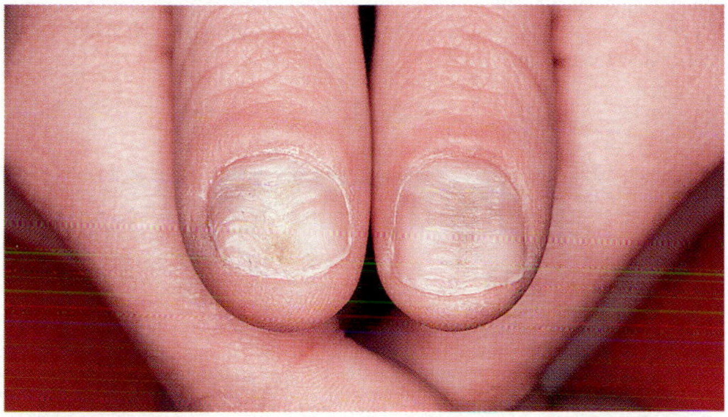

**Plate 40.** Habit tic deformity. Note the pathognomonic horizontal ridges.

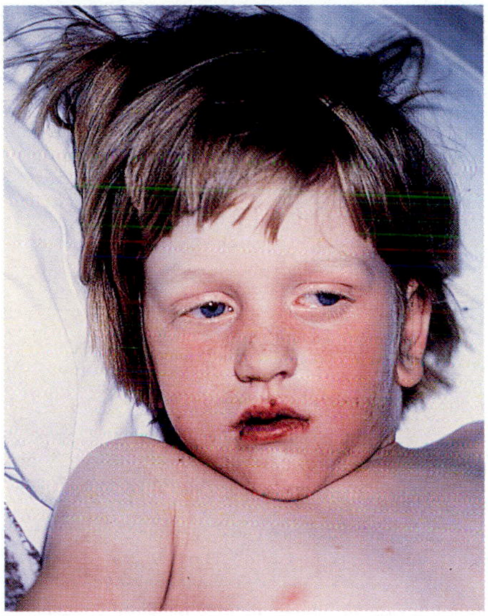

**Plate 41.** Kawasaki's disease—facial erythema, conjunctivitis, and involvement of the lips.

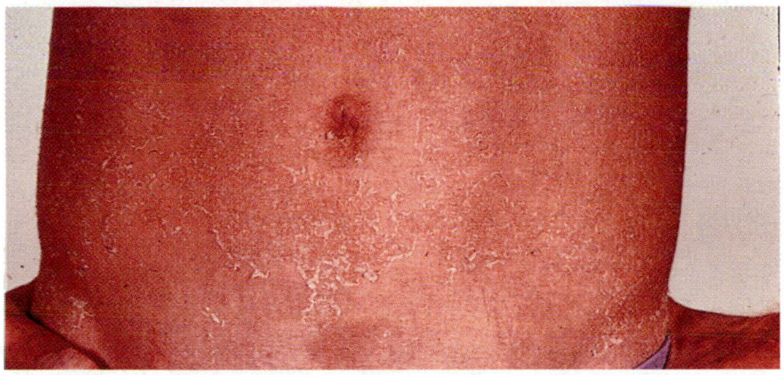

**Plate 42.** Scarlet fever—widespread branny scaling desquamation.

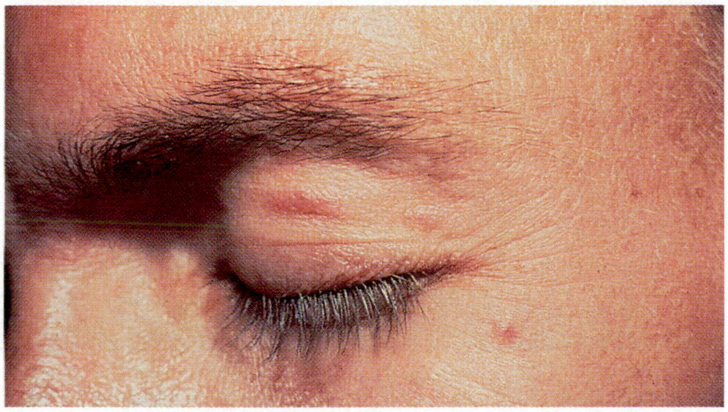

**Plate 43.** Kaposi's sarcoma (early lesion). Note erythematous violaceous plaque on eyelid.

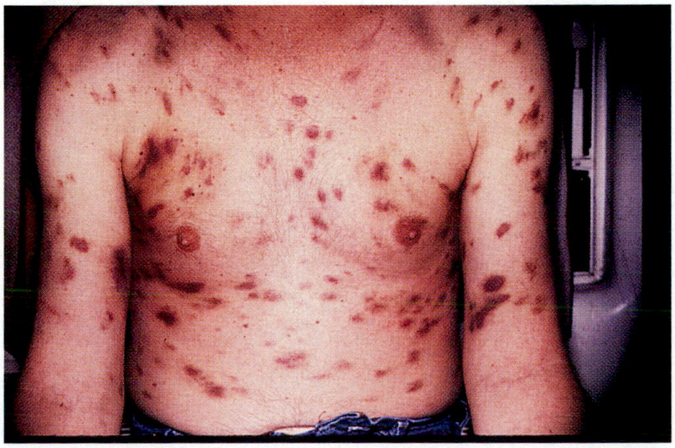

**Plate 44.** Kaposi's sarcoma (more advanced lesions). Note widespread hemorrhagic plaques and nodules.

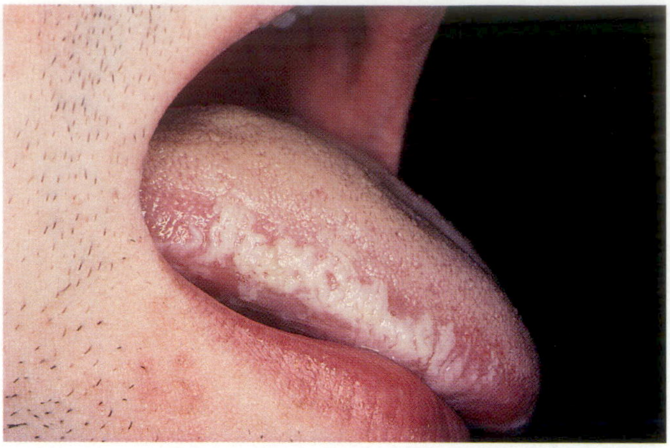

**Plate 45.** Oral hairy leukoplakia. Note white verrucoid plaques on the lateral aspect of the tongue.

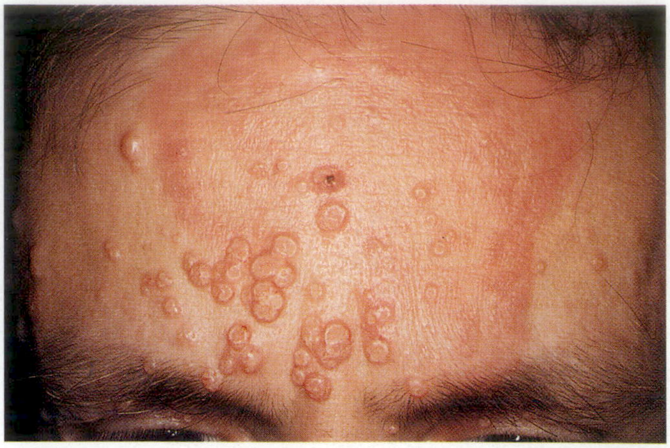

**Plate 46.** Molluscum contagiosum (may appear in atypical manner in HIV positive patients). Note large size varicoid appearance and central keratin plugging.

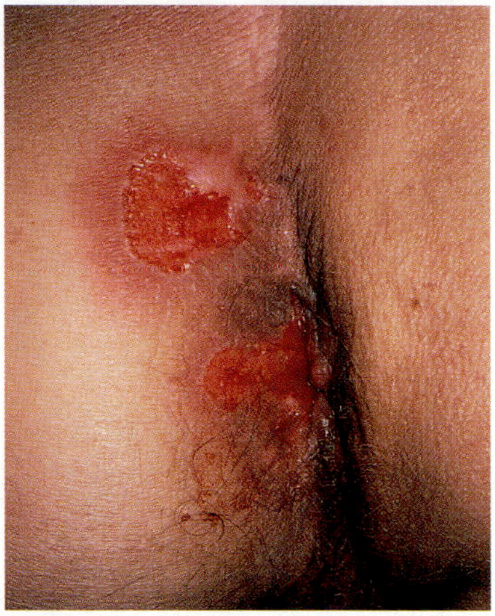

**Plate 47.** Atypical herpes simplex in HIV positive patients. Note deep erosive lesions that are often chronic.

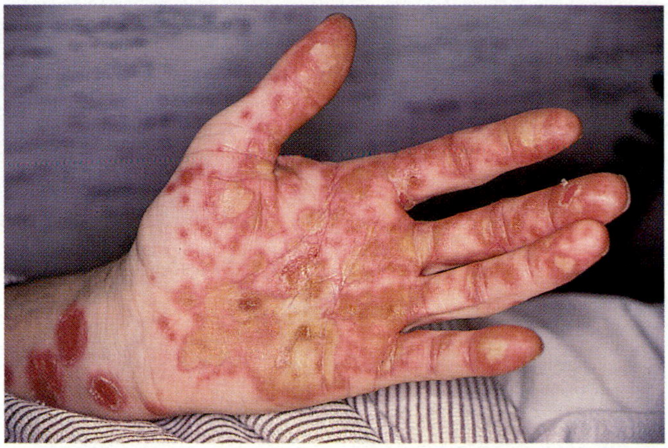

**Plate 48.** Reiter's syndrome (keratoderma blenorrhagicum). Note erythematous and pustular plaques on the palm.

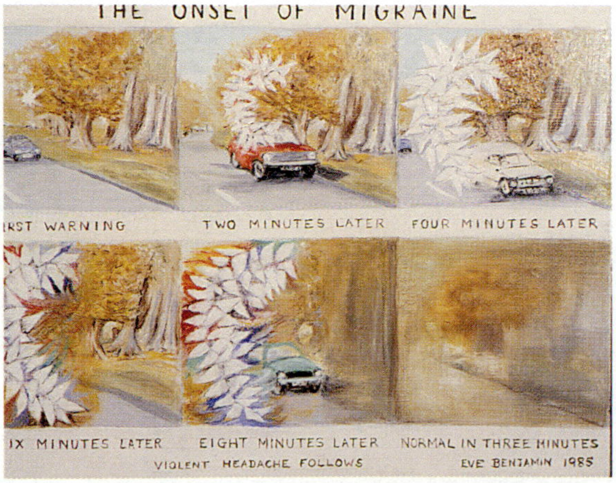


**Plate 49.** Patient artistically depicts visual distortions and scintillating scotoma during aura of migraine headache that may relate temporally with spreading cerebral hypoperfusion. (Courtesy British Migraine Association and Boehringer-Ingelheimer, LTD.)

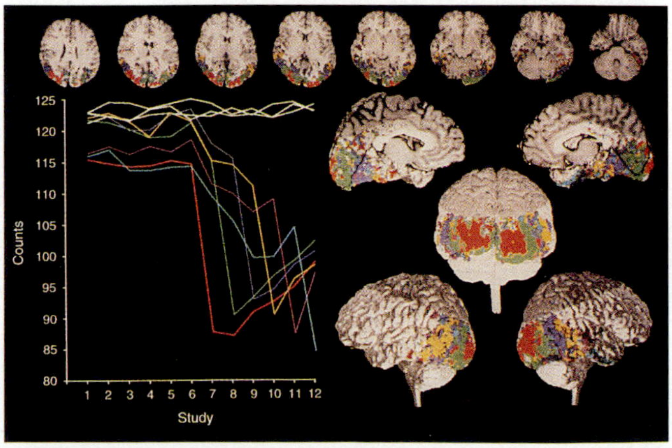


**Plate 50.** Spreading cerebral hypoperfusion demonstrated by cerebral blood-flow measurement using intracarotid Xenon-133 technique. Patient spontaneously developed migraine during procedure. (From Woods RP et al: *N Engl J Med* 331(25):1689, 1992.)

Individual lesions tend to remain fixed for the duration of the disease process. A history of increased water exposure such as frequent showers, swimming, and hot tubs is often reported.

***Examination.*** Round patches of erythema, scaling, and occasional crust or exudation are suggestive of nummular dermatitis. The term *nummular* means coin shaped. The distribution is usually extensor areas of extremities, the back, and buttocks. The differential diagnosis includes psoriasis and tinea corporus. A potassium hydroxide (KOH) examination of any scaly lesions is indicated.

***Management.*** The elimination of exacerbating factors is essential in long-term management. To reduce acute inflammation, potent topical corticosteroids under occlusive dressings or intralesional corticosteroid injections (triamcinolone 5 mg/ml or betamethasone 6 mg/ml) may be necessary. The use of emollients throughout the day and especially after water exposure or bathing is essential. In severe cases systemic steroids, antihistamines, topical tar preparations (see Chapter 20), and ultraviolet light treatments can be used.

### Lichen simplex chronicus and prurigo nodularis

Lichen simplex chronicus refers to thickened skin that develops as a result of chronic scratching. Pruritus is always present in the areas of scratching, but frequently the primary cause for the itching cannot be identified.

***Examination.*** In lichen simplex chronicus there is thickened skin with erythema and accentuation of skin lines (lichenification). Usually there is only one area of involvement. Common sites include extremities, posterior neck, buttocks, vulva, scrotum, and anal area. Prurigo nodularis is characterized by a few to multiple nodules, 0.5 to 1.0 cm in size, scattered over the upper back, arms, and thighs. Areas that are not convenient to reach, such as the central back and posterior thighs, tend to be spared (see Plate 23).

***Management.*** The treatment of lichen simplex chronicus consists of breaking the itch-scratch cycle. Therapy with potent corticosteroids under occlusion may be successful. Intralesional corticosteroid injections and cryotherapy with liquid nitrogen may be required in nodular cases, although the treatment of prurigo nodularis is frequently unsuccessful. Ultraviolet light therapy, antihistamines, and antidepressants can be helpful; but persistence over years is common.

## PAPULOSQUAMOUS SKIN DISEASES

Unique scales are the common feature of papulosquamous skin diseases. The term *squamous* refers to scaling that represents thick stratum corneum and thus implies an abnormal keratinization process. In addition to unusual scales, lesions are characterized by sharply demarcated, red to violaceous papules and plaques that result from thickening of the epidermis and/or underlying dermal inflammation. The sharp delineation of the lesions in this group of diseases helps distinguish them from scaling lesions of eczematous diseases where the borders are usually indistinct (with two exceptions—nummular eczema and seborrheic dermatitis).

The papulosquamous disorders have diverse etiologies and include psoriasis, Reiter's syndrome, pityriasis rosea, lichen planus, pityriasis rubra pilaris, secondary syphilis, mycosis fungoides, and ichthyosiform eruptions. Also included in the differential diagnosis are seborrheic dermatitis, tinea corporis, and discoid lupus erythematosus.

### Psoriasis

***Epidemiology/etiology.*** The exact cause of psoriasis is unknown, but it appears to be a multifactorial disease, with one third of patients genetically predisposed to the condition. The prevalence in the general population is 2% and the condition may begin at any age. Some investigators have proposed two forms of psoriasis. Type I is hereditary (autosomal dominant with 60% penetration), has an age of onset about 20 years of age, and a tendency to follow an irregular course and become generalized; 85% of those with this form are HLA Cw6. Type II is sporadic, has a peak incidence of 60 years old, and is associated with HLA Cw6 in 15% of patients. The precipitating factors responsible for unmasking the genetic predisposition include streptococcal infections, overuse of ethanol, psychologic stress, certain medications (beta blockers, lithium), and trauma to the skin (inducing the Koebner phenomenon, where new skin lesions evolve in areas of injury to the skin).

***Pathophysiology.*** The epidermis is thickened and keratinization is disturbed, leading to the accumulation of parakeratotic stratum corneum (nuclei retained in the corneum), in association with dilated dermal capillaries and neutrophils that extravasate to accumulate within the epidermis. One well-established end result is an acceleration of the epidermal cell cycle whereby cell turnover is increased and transit time for the basal layer to the stratum corneum is decreased from the normal 28 days to 3 to 4 days. This alteration in cell turnover leads to thickened epidermis (causing raised papules and plaques) and defective keratinization and accumulation of stratum corneum (silvery scales).

***History.*** The onset and course of the disease are highly variable. It usually begins gradually, confined to a few areas, but it can be explosive in onset. One cause of the latter presentation is a preceding streptococcal throat infection leading in 2 to 3 weeks to multiple small guttate lesions generalized over the body. Once the disease appears, it follows an irregular chronic unpredictable course. It may remain localized to a few areas or may cause intermittent or continuous generalized lesions.

Itching is usually not a problem in psoriasis but may be severe in individual patients. A family history for psoriasis is elicited in one third of patients, 50% of those with type I psoriasis have an affected parent.

***Physical examination.*** The lesions are erythematous papules and plaques surrounded by thick, silvery scales that resemble mica (micaceous) and that are not easily removed and often accumulate in the patient's clothing or bed (see Plate 3). When the scales are traumatically removed, multiple small bleeding sites appear (Auspitz's sign). In intertriginous areas, maceration and moisture prevent dry scales from accumulating, but the lesions remain red and sharply defined.

Lesions usually are distributed symmetrically over areas of body prominence such as elbows and knees. They also frequently occur on the trunk, scalp and intergluteal cleft and umbilicus. The latter three areas are frequently overlooked by both the patient and physician, but are important diagnostic findings, especially in patients with associated psoriatic arthritis and limited skin disease where the nature of the arthritis becomes apparent if the skin lesions are recognized. Another helpful diagnostic feature is the Koebner phenomenon in which intense trauma to the skin induces new skin lesions; scratches or surgical incisions elicit linear papulosquamous lesions. Such isomorphic lesions also can be induced on the palms of patients whose hands are exposed to friction.

Nail involvement may include stippling or pitting of the nail plate or yellow or red-brown coloring ("oil-staining") of onycholytic patches with accumulation of yellow debris under nails (see Plate 24). Swelling, redness, and scaling of the paronychial margins occur often; associated arthritis of the distal interphalangeal joints may be found.

***Differential diagnosis.*** See Table 21-2.

***Laboratory studies/diagnostic procedure.*** A skin biopsy can substantiate the diagnosis but is seldom necessary because the clinical features of psoriasis are so distinctive. No serologic or other diagnostic tests are available.

***Management.*** The chronic course of psoriasis and the lack of cure can be discouraging but a "nothing can be done" attitude need not be adopted. The patient can be assured that there are several approaches to the control of the disease. Avoidance of aggravating factors such as the excessive use of alcohol, trauma to the skin, emotional stress, and certain drugs should be discussed. No specific dietary manipulations play a role in treating psoriasis. Support groups are of great psychologic help.

The goal of therapy is to decrease epidermal proliferation and underlying dermal inflammation. To achieve remission, topical therapy should be used first if possible. Systemic therapy is applied if topical treatment fails. If the psoriasis is limited to a few plaques, topical therapy is indicated. If it is widespread, ultraviolet light treatment should be considered. If this treatment fails systemic therapy is the final step.

**Table 21-2.** Differential diagnosis of psoriasis

| Disease | Clinical features | Cause | Diagnosis |
|---|---|---|---|
| Tinea and onycholysis | Scaling annular to round patches and onycholysis and crumbling nails. | Dermatophyte infections | KOH. |
| Seborrheic dermatitis | Diffuse lesions with greasy scales on scale behind ears, nasolabial folds, and presternally. | Possibly overgrowth pityrosporum | Skin biopsy may help. |
| Secondary syphilis | Guttate or small scaling plaques over trunk, like pityriasis rosea, but involves palms and soles. | Spirochete | Positive test for syphilis RPR. |
| Cutaneous T-cell lymphoma | Flat to thick plaques with variable scaling, which may be identical to psoriasis anywhere on body. May be erythrodermic-Sézary syndrome. | T-cell lymphoma | Skin biopsy Sézary cells in circulation. T-cell gene rearrangement studies. |
| Reiter's syndrome | Identical skin changes as psoriasis with pustular lesions on palms and soles (keratoderma blennorrhagicum) balanitis circinata; arthritis nail involvement. Mucous membrane changes not seen in psoriasis. | Unknown, but triggered by certain infectious agents | Clinical features, arthritis, conjunctivitis, urethritis. |
| Pityriasis rubra pilaris | Diffuse salmon-colored papulosquamous lesion areas, normal skin in midst, involved skin—"island sparing," keratoderma palm. Keratotic papules on dorsum of fingers. | Unknown | Clinical features, skin biopsy. |
| Pityriasis lichenoides et varioliformis acuta | Red, purpuric, vesicular lesions evolve into scaling macular and papular lesions that scar. Lesions occur over entire body. | Unknown | Clinical features, skin biopsy. |

Three types of topical therapy are available:

1. Topical steroids, usually with intermediate and strong potency are administered once or twice a day
2. Topical tars or anthralin preparation, often used once a day in combination with topical steroids
3. Ultraviolet light, either midrange sunbeam spectrum (UVB) with tar or long wave (UVA) with oral psoralens (PUVA).

Two systemic types of therapy are available, but because of significant side effects, they should be reserved for severe widespread disease that is unresponsive to topical measures: antimetabolites and antimitotic agents including methotrexate or azothioprine, hydroxyurea and cyclosporine. The most commonly used drug is methotrexate in low doses (10 to 25 mg/week), usually given on a weekly basis. Methotrexate is especially useful in patients with severe arthritis. Because these agents can affect bone marrow and the liver, monitoring of blood counts and liver function tests must be performed regularly, together with intermittent liver biopsies (in the case of methotrexate based on accumulative doses). Etretinate, a retinoid, is useful in pustular and erythrodermic forms of psoriasis. Careful monitoring of blood counts, plasma triglycerides, and liver function is required; and avoidance of pregnancy is mandatory; etretinate should probably not be used in women of childbearing age. In severe cases, etretinate can be used in combination with PUVA. About 50% of patients who are refractory to PUVA alone improve when retinoid is added.

***Special patients and issues.*** Guttate psoriasis in the young patient should initiate a search for streptococcal pharyngitis. The patient often is asymptomatic after a day or two of throat soreness. Antibiotic therapy and eradication of the streptococcus may induce a remission of the psoriasis. Only moderately potent steroids, tar, and UVB light should be used in children. Oral agents and PUVA treatment should be avoided if possible in young patients with psoriasis. Pregnancy has a variable effect on psoriasis. Topical steroids and UVB are the best approaches. Avoidance of tar, anthralin, PUVA, or systemic agents is prudent. Special precautions are not necessary for the surgical patient except to warn the patient and surgeon that they may experience the Koebner phenomenon in the surgical scar. Psoriasis does not increase the risk of any skin infection. A patient who has widespread disease that covers at least 40% to 50% of the body and that is resistant to topical therapy should be referred to a dermatologist.

### Reiter's syndrome

Reiter's syndrome can be readily confused with psoriasis because the skin lesions of the two disorders are indistinguishable clinically and histologically. In Reiter's disease, pustular and keratotic papules and plaques commonly occur on the palms and soles (keratoderma blennorrhagicum) and scaling, red patches are found encircling the glans penis and within the groin (balanitis circinata). Other features of Reiter's syndrome may include a seronegative, asymmetric arthritis that may involve the sacroiliac joints as well as uveitis, conjunctivitis, and mucous membrane lesions. The presence of asymptomatic erosions on the tongue and buccal mucosa, urethritis, and occasionally diarrhea distinguish Reiter's syndrome from psoriasis.

### Pityriasis rosea

***Epidemiology/etiology.*** Pityriasis rosea is a self-limited papulosquamous eruption that occurs in young adults. A possible viral etiology has been suggested because of the increased incidence in the winter months and because patients report a history of a preceding upper respiratory infection.

***Physical examination.*** Oval or round, tan-, ink-, or salmon-colored, scaling papules and plaques appear rapidly over the trunk, neck, upper arms, and thighs. Several features of this papulosquamous condition are unique. First, the generalized eruption is preceded by a single lesion, termed the *herald patch* that is commonly misdiagnosed as tinea corporis. The herald patch can occur anywhere, but often appears on the neck or lower trunk and precedes the general rash by several days to a week. Second, the oval patches have an unusual fine, white scale located near the border of the plaques, forming a collarette. Third, the lesions follow skin cleavage lines, with the long axis paralleling these lines in a Christmas tree pattern (see Plate 8).

***Differential diagnosis.*** Tinea corporis and guttate psoriasis must be considered in the differential diagnosis, and two other possibilities always should be ruled out: drug eruption and secondary syphilis. If the rash persists beyond 3 months or generalizes to involve the extremities and face, a drug reaction should be considered (e.g., gold compounds, barbiturates, captopril, clonidine). Serologic tests for syphilis should be obtained if the rash involves the palms and soles and if fever, coryza, or mucous membrane erosions (mucous patches) are present.

***Management.*** Treatment may not be necessary, although topical corticosteroids and antihistamines relieve itching and decrease erythema. Ultraviolet light (UVB) given as three to five treatments to give a mild erythema reaction often clears the rash.

### Lichen planus

***Epidemiology/etiology and pathogenesis.*** Lichen planus is a chronic, pruritic, papulosquamous disease with a wide range of clinical manifestations. The cause of lichen planus is not known, but immune factors may play a role because lichen planuslike eruptions occur in patients undergoing bone marrow transplantation who are experiencing graft vs. host reactions, and certain drug reactions cause widespread lichen planuslike skin reactions.

***Physical examination.*** Lichen planus, a pruritic inflammatory condition of the skin, is included in the papulosquamous group of diseases because the primary lesion is a unique papule with an unusual surface configuration. The papules are flat topped (planus) and polygonal in configuration (i.e., the sides conform to normal fine skin folds and creases) and have a lilac or purple hue (see Plate 25). They may have visible scales on their surface, but more characteristic are subtle, fine, white reticulated lines

(Wickham's striae) surmounting the shiny flat tops of the papules (resembling lichen). Wickham's striae become more apparent under a hand lens after the application of a drop of mineral oil on the surface of the papules. The Koebner phenomenon is seen; thus linear streaks of papules at the sites of skin trauma may be noted.

Although skin lesions can occur anywhere on the body, typical locations are symmetrically distributed papules on the ankles, flexural wrists, mouth, and genitalia. Although the condition is extremely pruritic, one seldom sees excoriations or erosions induced by scratching. Mucous membranes are commonly involved, the lesions appearing most often as asymptomatic white streaks in a reticulate pattern on the buccal mucosa, tongue, gums or lips (see Plate 26). At times blisters and erosions are superimposed on the mucous membrane areas (erosive lichen planus) causing severe discomfort. Lichen planus, on the male genitalia, may appear as violaceous annular lesions and may rarely assume annular and polycyclic forms on the trunk and extremities. Rarely, the lesions may be hyperkeratotic, confined to the hair (follicular), or appear as scarring alopecia.

***Differential diagnosis.*** See Table 21-3.

***Management.*** Treatment is nonspecific and not always successful. For localized patches topical steroids of the moderate to potent forms may be useful in suppressing the itching and inflammation. If the disease is widespread, a 4- to 6-week course of oral corticosteroids may reverse the course (40 to 60 mg/day) with tapering. Erosive oral lichen planus is particularly difficult to control, but at times intralesional steroid injections are helpful. Patients with widespread lichen planus and/or erosive painful oral lichen planus should be referred for dermatologic consultation.

### Seborrheic dermatitis

***Etiology.*** The cause of seborrheic dermatitis is not known; but overgrowth of a normally occurring yeast, *Pityrosporum ovale,* may play some role. The disorder is also possibly genetically determined although its mode of inheritance is not clear.

***Pathophysiology.*** This is an inflammatory scaling reaction that occurs in seborrheic areas of the skin (areas where large numbers of sebaceous glands are found, e.g., scalp, ears, head, and chest). The term *dandruff* is often used to describe seborrheic dermatitis in the scalp.

***History.*** In adults, the process can involve only the scalp or may also cause an erythematous, greasy scaling rash in the nasolabial folds, eyebrows, beard area, external ears, and presternal areas. Blepharitis is also a manifestation. At times stress may cause exacerbation of the condition. Seborrhea is often one of the earliest cutaneous signs of human immunodeficiency virus (HIV) infection.

***Physical examination and clinical features.*** Ill-defined, erythematous patches with greasy yellow scales are typical of seborrheic dermatitis. They may or may not be pruritic. The location of the lesions is often the most important factor in diagnosing this condition; locations include scalp, retroauricular, external ears, eyebrows, nasolabial folds, presternal, and, at times, axillae and groin (see Plate 27).

Seborrhea is often the first sign of HIV infection and is often extensive and difficult to control. For reasons that are not clear, seborrheic dermatitis is common and often severe in patients with chronic neurologic conditions such as Parkinson's disease. Most patients with severe acne have some degree of seborrheic dermatitis, manifested at least by dandruff. At times it is difficult to distinguish seborrhea from psoriasis; some patients appear to have both conditions.

***Differential diagnosis.*** The differential diagnoses include psoriasis, Reiter's disease, atopic eczema (especially in youngsters), and histiocytosis X (again in youngsters). In histiocytosis X an erythematous scaling rash is seen on the scalp, around the ears, and on flexural surfaces. However, petechiae, purpura, and ulcerations occur in histiocytosis X (Letterer-Siwe disease) and not in seborrheic dermatitis.

Although skin biopsy pathology will clearly diagnose histiocytosis X and at times psoriasis, the pathologic changes in seborrheic dermatitis are not distinctive enough to differentiate it from atopic or some of the other eczematous processes.

**Table 21-3.** Differential diagnoses of lichen planus-like skin condition

| Condition | Clinical feature | Etiology | Diagnosis |
|---|---|---|---|
| Discoid LE | Atrophic red patches with follicular plugging | Autoimmune | Skin biopsy for H&E DIF examination |
| Drug-induced lichen planus-like eruption | Skin biopsy same as lichen planus, except at times more eosinophiles in infiltrate | Medications: Thiazide, gold, Quinidine, antimalarials | History |
| Graft versus host | Identical clinical picture, but in patient in clinical situation where graft versus host reaction can occur | Immunologic reaction | Skin biopsy identical to lichen planus. |
| Candidiasis and/or mouth cancer | Oral lichen planus can be white and eroded | Infection—*Candida,* r/o cancer | Swab and KOH of lesion to rule out cancer |

***Management.*** Shampoos containing tar, sulfur, salicylic acid, or selenium, if used daily on a prolonged basis, often control scalp seborrhea and face lesions (when the shampoo is applied to these areas as well). Hydrocortisone cream 1% to 2.5% applied once or twice a day controls seborrhea lesions on the ears and face, and more potent topical steroids in solution form (fluocinolone 0.01%) are useful in controlling scalp lesions when medicated shampoos do not provide complete clearing. Ketoconazole 2% cream and shampoo are alternatives to the topical steroids.

## ACNE AND ACNEIFORM ERUPTIONS

### Acne

Acne is a multifactorial inflammatory disorder of the pilosebaceous units over the face, chest, and back areas where the greatest concentrations of these skin appendages are found. It is the most common cause of pustular reactions of the skin.

***Etiology.*** Several factors play a role as individuals enter puberty: (1) androgenic stimulation of the sebaceous glands and increased serum production; (2) abnormal keratinization in the pilosebaceous canal with obstruction to sebum flow (comedones); and (3) proliferation of anaerobic bacteria, *Propionibacterium acnes,* which lead to rupture of the pilosebaceous unit, extravasation of sebum, and bacteria into the dermis, resulting in inflammatory papules, pustules, and cysts.

***Pathophysiology.*** Weak and strong androgens stimulate the pilosebaceous units at the time of puberty to enlarge and produce large amounts of sebum (an oily substance composed in part of large quantities of triglycerides, diglycerides, and monoglycerides). The vast majority of patients secrete normal amounts of androgens from the ovaries, testes, and adrenal glands; but in occasional instances an underlying endocrine problem may cause acne (polycystic ovarian syndrome, adrenal hyperplasia, adrenal or ovarian tumors). At the same time the increased sebum production is seen, the keratinization process in the pilosebaceous canal is disrupted with impaction and obstruction of the outflow of sebum (comedo formation — open blackheads and closed whiteheads). The wall of the closed comedo may rupture, spilling the follicular contents into the dermis. This leads to the development of inflammatory papules, pustules, and large cysts because under the influence of increased sebum production large numbers of *P. acnes* proliferate (sebum is the substrate for the *P. acnes*), and these bacteria are chemotactic, bringing in neutrophils, which cause the inflammatory response. Stress may accentuate acne. Dietary factors seem to play little or no role in the pathogenesis.

***History.*** The comedones, papules, and pustules that evolve on the face, chest, and back early in puberty occur at the usual time of onset; but acne can occur in patients in their second and third decade. In women, cosmetics with oily bases may aggravate acne. A history of irregular menses and/or hirsutism should lead to an evaluation of possible endocrine disorder. Potent topical or large doses of corticosteroids can also induce an acneiform eruption.

***Physical examination and clinical features.*** The hallmarks of acne, open and closed comedones (dome-shaped black and white papules) erythematous papules, pustules, and deep nodulocystic fluctuant lesions may be seen in varying combination over the face, neck, chest, and back.

The residual of these lesions may also be present: scarring varying from discrete pits to large atrophic depressed or hypertrophic fibrotic areas.

Other variants of acne include the following:

- *Nodulocystic acne* (severe nodular acne) with large fluctuant painful nodules.
- *Acne fulminans:* A rare, acute, severe variety of acne with widespread nodulocystic lesions that contain large quantities of necrotic material that may break down leaving eroded areas over the face and back accompanied by systemic findings of fever, leukocytosis, and arthralgias.
- *Acne due to drugs:* Several medications, including androgens, corticosteroids, and medications with halogens (iodides, bromides, anticonvulsants and lithium), may lead to acne or exacerbate preexisting acne.
- *Gram-negative folliculitis:* May be superimposed on and mimic acne in patients being treated for acne with oral antibiotics or isotretinoin (Accutane). There is overgrowth of gram-negative bacteria in the follicles with sudden flare-up of previously controlled acne as manifested by inflammatory pustules and fluctuant nodules.
- *Perioral dermatitis:* Most often a variant of acne but may be caused by using potent fluorinated topical steroids; a localized condition around the mouth with inflammatory papules, pustules, and scaling macules.

***Differential diagnosis.*** Rosacea may be confused with acne but the presence of telangiectases and lack of comedones should help distinguish this condition. *Flat warts* on the face also should be in the differential diagnosis, but the lack of pustules and comedones help identify warts. Bacterial folliculitis can be diagnosed by Gram stain and cultures of the pustules. Occasionally, acne is confused with adenoma sebaceum (angiofibroma), which consists of fleshy, red papules over the central face associated with tuberous sclerosis.

***Management.*** The principles of therapy involve reversing the etiologic factors that induce the acne lesions: decreased sebaceous activity, decreased *P. acnes* population, and decreased follicular occlusion and inflammation.

1. *Topical Therapy*
   a. Vitamin A acid (all trans-retinoic acid-tretinoin Retin A) is a potent comedolytic agent available as a gel, cream, or lotion in varying concentrations. It is applied to the affected areas once a day beginning with the weakest preparations to avoid its two major side effects, skin irritation and scaling. Although vitamin A acid is used mainly for comedonal acne, it is also beneficial in inflammatory acne.
   b. Benzoyl peroxide, an effective antibacterial agent, as well as a comedolytic agent, is most useful to

treat inflammatory acne. It is available in a lotion base over the counter and in a gel base in 2.5%, 5%, and 10% concentrations as prescription items. Irritation may follow the use of benzoyl peroxide and allergic sensitization may occur. The preparation is usually applied once a day. At times it may be useful to use both vitamin A acid and benzoyl peroxide (inflammatory and comedonal acne).

c. Salicylic acid, sulfur, and resorcinol are agents used alone and in combination that act as mild irritants that have comedolytic properties. One preparation, Sulfacet R, is useful because it is a tinted liquid that can replace the use of make-up.

d. Topical antibiotics including erythromycin and clindamycin are effective in decreasing the *P. acnes* skin population. These preparations in solution, lotion, and gel are used twice a day, often in conjunction with vitamin A acid and/or benzoyl peroxide. Topical antibiotics are not quite as effective as systemic antibiotics, but they do alleviate the many side effects of oral antibiotics.

2. *Systemic Therapy*

a. Antibiotics, particularly tetracycline and erythromycin, are effective in controlling papulopustular and mild nodulocystic acne. Erythromycin is probably just as effective as tetracycline and has the advantage of being effective when taken with food (whereas tetracycline must be ingested 1 hour before or after meals). The usual initial dose for these antibiotics is 500 to 1000 mg/day in divided doses. Minocycline is an effective treatment when the acne does not respond to tetracycline or erythromycin in a dose of 100 to 200 mg/day, although its high cost is a drawback. Perioral dermatitis responds to tetracycline, usually requiring 250 mg twice a day for 6 to 8 weeks.

b. Oral retinoids, 13-cis retinoic acid (Accutane), is a useful therapy in severe nodular acne that is unresponsive to other treatment regimens. The medication produces remarkable clearing in 95% of such patients, but it also provides persistent remissions in 85% of patients. The drug, usually given in doses of 0.5 to 1.0 mg/kg per day for 3 to 4 months, has many side effects characteristic of chronic hypervitaminosis A, including cheilitis, xerosis, epistaxis, eye irritation, myalgias, and bony hyperkeratosis. Accutane is a potent teratogen and is contraindicated during pregnancy. Dose-related elevations in serum triglycerides and night blindness also occur. Because of these potential problems, the medication should be given by those familiar with the use of this drug with frequent monitoring of complete blood count (CBC), serum chemistries (occasionally one sees liver function test abnormalities), and fasting blood lipids. Women of childbearing age must be on birth control measures (both birth control pills and barrier methods) and be monitored for pregnancy before and during treatment.

With appropriate treatment it is possible to control acne but not cure it. Acne may not subside for many years. The goal is to control acne while it is active.

Psychologic ramifications of acne may be important given its cosmetic effects. The physician should be sensitive to the patient's concerns.

## Rosacea

Rosacea is a chronic inflammatory disorder of the blood vessels and pilosebaceous units of the face that occurs most often in middle-aged adults.

***Pathophysiology.*** The cause of this condition is not understood. Some studies suggested a role for the follicular mite *Demodex*. Other aggravating factors that have been incriminated but not well proven include ingestion of foods that cause vasodilation and blushing (hot liquids, caffeine-containing beverages, alcohol, spicy foods, stress, and sunlight).

***History.*** Middle-aged adults are primarily affected. Erythema develops first, followed by telangiectasia, associated with increasing blushing and flushing over the central face and at times neck and chest. Papules and pustules develop and may eventuate in rhinophyma (hypertrophy of the nose). Eye symptoms of burning, itching, and irritation may also occur.

***Physical examination.*** Typically papules and pustules are superimposed on a ruddy complexion and telangiectases most pronounced over the central face. Flushing is an important symptom, often precipitated by heat, hot foods, alcohol, and caffeine-containing beverages. Sebaceous and fibrous enlargement of the nose (rhinophyma) may eventually ensue. Comedones are not present. In severe cases the pustular component may lead to cystic and granulomatous nodules. Ten percent of patients may have ocular complications, including blepharitis, conjunctivitis, chronic chalazion, and keratitis that may impair vision.

***Laboratory studies.*** The diagnosis is based on clinical findings. Laboratory findings are not helpful and skin biopsy is seldom required.

***Differential diagnosis.*** Rosacea may be confused with acne vulgaris, but the former is found in older individuals, lacks comedones, and is accompanied by blushing and telangiectasis. Lupus erythematosus, photodermatitis, and seborrhea may be confused with the vascular element of rosacea, but none of these have pustules. The blushing component of rosacea might cause one to consider the carcinoid syndrome.

***Management.*** Systemic therapy: Low-dose tetracycline or erythromycin, 250 to 1000 mg/day, controls the papules and pustules, but the erythema and telangiectasis are resistant to therapy. The use of antibiotics must be continued lifelong, and some patients require tetracycline 250 mg two to three times a week to suppress the condition.

Topical therapy: Topical metronidazole (Metrogel), 0.75% twice a day, often can control the condition without oral antibiotics. At times both tetracycline and topical metronidazole are needed. Topical sulfur-containing materials (Sulfacet-R) are also useful. Topical steroids should be avoided, especially fluorinated potent steroids, as they may exacerbate the problem and indeed can induce an acnelike eruption.

Although rosacea cannot be prevented, the vascular flushing can be minimized by avoiding sunlight, hot foods, alcohol, and spicy foods. Rhinophyma can be treated with removal of the excess sebaceous and collagenous material with scalpel, electrosurgery, or laser technique. Telangiectasis can be treated with tunable dye laser.

*Indications for consultation.* Patients with severe rosacea that is unresponsive to the usual forms of therapy should be referred to a dermatologist, and ocular symptoms should be evaluated by an ophthalmologist.

## SKIN CANCER

### Basal cell carcinoma

*Epidemiology/etiology.* Basal cell carcinoma (BCC) arising from the basal cell layer of the epidermis is the most common type of human cancer. Estimates of new cases of BCC exceed 400,000 per year in the United States, affecting primarily fair-skinned whites. Chronic exposure to ultraviolet light is thought to be the main factor leading to the development of BCC.

*Physical examination.* The three main variants of BCC are based on the clinical appearance. Nodular BCC, (see Plate 28) the most common, usually develops as a papule and enlarges slowly into a nodule. The lesion is raised, pearly, or translucent in color, with telangiectasias. Ulceration or surface crusting is common. Small lesions tend to be circular in shape, large lesions are more irregular. The most common sites are the sun-exposed areas of the head and neck. Rarely, a BCC can contain melanin and resemble a malignant melanoma. Sclerosing BCC appears as a patch of indurated scarlike change, whitish in color, usually without telangiectasias or ulceration. This variant enlarges horizontally into plaques. Superficial BCC refers to a variant that resembles a dermatitis. In this variant, a patch of erythema with slight scale and friability gradually enlarges over years. A slightly raised advancing border usually surrounds the lesion. The tumor process remains at the base of the epidermis for months to years before larger nodular growth develops (Fig. 21-1).

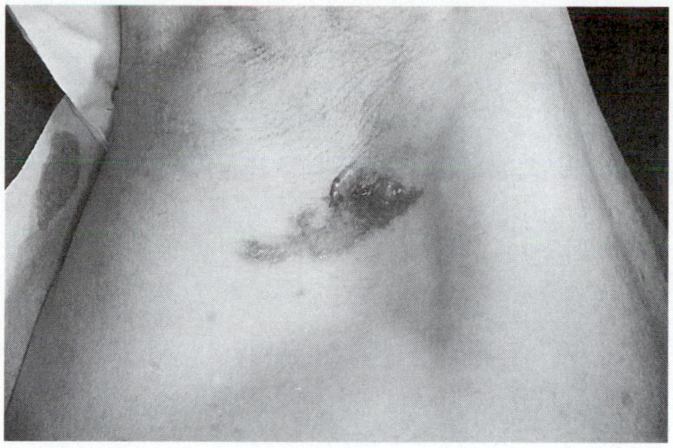

**Fig. 21-1.** Superficial basal cell carcinoma. Note erythematous patch with slightly raised border. This lesion has developed a nodular component at the superior portion.

*Laboratory evaluation.* Diagnosis is confirmed by biopsy. Histologic findings include basophilic cellular collections at the base of the epidermis and in the dermis. There are several histologic variants of BCC, and many benign skin tumors resembling BCC histologically.

*Management.* Prevention. Sun protection beginning in childhood is the best preventive measure. Adults and children should be educated about the damaging effects of excessive sun exposure, the early use of sun screens (minimum SPF 15), and protective clothing. Treatment. Modalities for treating BCC include curettage surgery, excision, radiation, and Mohs' surgery (see later). The choice of treatment depends on the location, size, histologic type, and history of previous treatment. For small lesions, simple excision is usually curative. Large tumors, and those on the central face and around the ears, have a higher treatment failure rate. For these types of BCC, the use of Mohs' surgery may be indicated. Mohs' surgery is a specialized procedure that utilizes excision with frozen section control of all margins by means of quadrant mapping of the specimen. Radiation may be indicated in patients who cannot tolerate excisional surgery or for lesions in difficult anatomic sites.

### Squamous cell carcinoma

*Epidemiology/etiology.* Squamous cell carcinoma (SCC) arises from squamous cells in the epithelium on sun-damaged skin of fair-skinned whites. Ultraviolet light is considered the strongest causal factor, but chemical carcinogens and papilloma viruses may play a role in the development of some forms of SCC of the skin. Human papillomavirus 5 and 16 have both been associated with the development of certain types of cutaneous SCC.

*Physical examination.* Several clinical presentations are considered within the disease spectrum of SCC (Fig. 21-2). Actinic keratoses (solar keratoses) are considered precursors to SCC. They begin as areas of rough or thickened skin, usually with some erythema, and slowly evolve into raised hyperkeratotic plaques or nodules. They are always found on sun-damaged skin. Histologically, actinic keratoses have atypical epidermal growth that is limited to the lower portion of the epidermis. Bowen's disease (SCC in situ) usually presents as a patch of erythematous or brown-red discoloration, slightly raised, with sharp borders. Sun-damaged and sun-protected skin can develop this variant of SCC, which demonstrates atypical epidermal growth throughout the entire thickness of the epidermis, but no invasion into the dermis. Both actinic keratoses and SCC in situ have the potential to evolve into invasive SCC. Keratoacanthoma is a type of SCC that, in the past, has been called self-healing or benign. It develops rapidly as a dome-shaped nodule that can grow to 1 or 2 cm within 8 weeks. Histologic examination usually shows characteristic features but occasionally keratoacanthoma is indistinguishable from

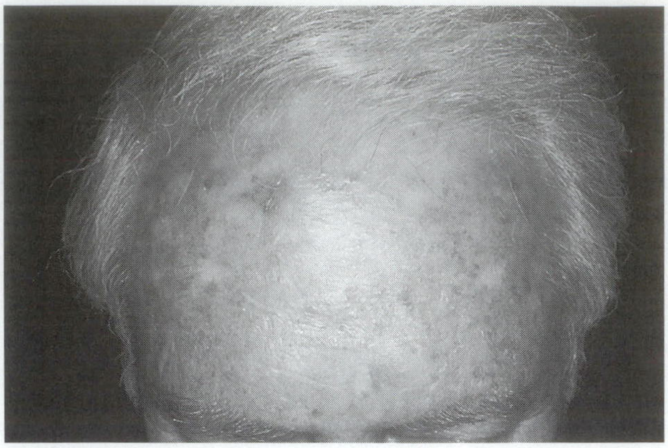

**Fig. 21-2.** Actinic keratoses. Note hyperkeratotic erythematous plaques on the sun-damaged skin of the forehead.

invasive SCC. Although the literature suggests that keratoacanthomas can resolve spontaneously, there have been reports of metastasis, and many authors now regard keratoacanthomas as a variant of SCC. SCC arising de novo without a precursor lesion usually starts with a patch of hyperkeratosis with erythema, which grows slowly into a nodular tumor or a cutaneous horn (see Plate 29).

*Laboratory evaluation.* Skin biopsy frequently is required to confirm the diagnosis. Other tests are not useful.

*Management.* The treatment of choice for SCC is surgical excision. Actinic keratoses can be treated with cryotherapy using liquid nitrogen. Topical chemotherapy with 5-fluorouracil is occasionally used when numerous actinic keratoses are present. Keratoacanthomas are treated with excision or intralesional injection with 5-FU or methotrexate. Systemic retinoids have been used in cases of multiple keratoacanthomas. Squamous cell carcinomas in the setting of immunosuppression require aggressive treatment because of their rapid growth patterns.

## Melanoma

*Epidemiology/etiology.* The worldwide incidence of melanoma is increasing. It is predicted that by the year 2000, 1 of 75 to 90 persons will develop melanoma during their lifetime. Although the incidence is increasing, the death rate from cutaneous melanoma can be reduced by early detection and treatment.

Melanoma primarily affects whites, although it occurs rarely in darker pigmented populations. Epidemiologic data suggest that sun exposure, especially severe sunburns during childhood, may predispose to the development of melanoma in later life. As with other skin cancers, those with the fairest skin (red hair, blue eyes, freckles, always burn in the sun) have the highest incidence.

The cell of origin is the melanocyte, located along the basal layer of skin, and mucous membranes. Genetic factors play a role in familial cases of melanoma, although the role of genetics is not understood in sporadic cases.

*Physical examination.* Several common characteristics of melanoma are the basis for the "ABCDs" of melanoma recognition. **A**symmetry is a common feature of melanoma, whereas most benign tumors tend to be symmetric. **B**order irregularity, although not pathognomonic for melanoma, is a typical finding. **C**olor variegation is an important diagnostic feature of melanoma. Black, blue, and red hues are commonly present in a melanoma. Colors of the brown spectrum (tan to dark brown) are characteristic of benign lesions (nevi, seborrheic keratoses) and are rarely part of a melanoma unless it arises from a preexisting nevus of that color. The **D**iameter of melanoma tends to enlarge with time, whereas benign lesions remain stable. Lesions that enlarge significantly over 1 to 3 months should be evaluated. Bleeding and ulceration may be present in larger lesions. When examining patients with melanoma, examination of the mucous membranes and lymph nodes should be included.

*Clinical variants.* Historically, melanoma has been classified into variants based on appearance, histology, and biologic course. Although there is increasing evidence that the separations may not have prognostic significance, many authors continue to use the terms. Superficial spreading melanoma is the most common type of melanoma (see Plate 30). It is found mostly on the upper back, and in women, on the legs. The horizontal growth pattern results in irregular shapes. Considerable color variation can be seen. Nodular melanoma is a raised lesion found anywhere on the body. It can be black, reddish, or flesh colored. The early vertical growth pattern results in the clinical nodule. Acral-lentiginous melanoma occurs on the palms, soles, finger tips and nails, and mucous membranes. The lesions are usually flat but become nodular if left undiagnosed and untreated. Metastatic spread is common at the time of diagnosis. Lentigo maligna refers to a melanoma in situ that develops on sun-damaged skin of elderly patients. An enlarging pigmented patch on the face is the most common presentation. The process can remain in situ for many years before evolving into melanoma.

*Laboratory evaluation.* Expert pathologic interpretation is critical to the management of patients with melanoma. The implications of a missed diagnosis are obvious. The prognosis is based on the measured thickness of the tumor in millimeters (Breslow level) more than any other histologic finding (Table 21-4). Ideally, the lesion should be excised entirely for diagnosis. Incisional biopsies may be performed for diagnosis when complete excision is not feasible. Shave biopsy should be avoided and freezing or burning of pigmented lesions is contraindicated with the sole exception of seborrheic keratoses. In cases of biopsy-proven melanoma, it may be worthwhile to perform a lymph node drainage scan before excision in order to direct a possible lymph node dissection.

*Management.* The management of a patient with stage I melanoma (local disease only) depends on the type of melanoma and the size and thickness of the lesion. Recent studies have revised the concept of "deep and wide

**Table 21-4.** Survival rates in malignant melanoma

| Tumor thickness (mm) | % Survival | | |
|---|---|---|---|
| | 5 years* | 8 years† | 10 years* |
| 0.0 to 0.76 mm | 99% | 93.2% | 98% |
| 0.76 to 1.69 mm | 94% | 85.6% | 89% |
| 1.7 to 3.60 mm | 81% | 59.8% | 67% |
| greater than 3.60 mm | 49% | 33.3% | 43% |

*Modified from Rigel DS, Friedman RJ: In Sams WM, Lynch PJ: *Principles and practice of dermatology*, New York, 1990, Churchill Livingstone.
†Modified from Clark WH Jr et al: *J Natl Cancer Inst* 81:1893-1904, 1989.

excisions for all melanomas.'' It is now thought that melanomas of a depth of less than 1 mm Breslow thickness can be excised with margins of 1 cm of normal skin. The optimal size of resection for thicker melanomas is not known, and wider resections continue to be performed until this question is answered. The benefit of an elective lymph node dissection is also not established. For melanomas less than 1 mm thick, lymph node dissection is not needed, and for those greater than 4 mm thick, lymph node dissection does not prolong life. In lesions between 1 and 4 mm thick, it may be useful to perform a lymph node dissection, especially if a single drainage pathway can be identified. Follow-up is every 6 to 12 months for thin melanomas (less than 1 mm thick) and every 3 to 4 months for thicker lesions during the first 5 years, with gradual extention up to 10- to 12-month intervals. Patients need lifelong follow-up because metastatic spread can become evident after 10 years. The management of *stage II (lymph node involvement)* and *stage III (systemic involvement)* melanoma is beyond the scope of this section. Most treatments are designed for palliation or temporary remission.

## DISORDERS OF PIGMENTATION

### Abnormalities of pigmentation

Hyperpigmentation and hypopigmentation occur when a variety of things go wrong, including (1) changes in the number of melanocytes, (2) alterations in melanin synthesis, and (3) changes in hormonal balance. These alterations can be either congenital or genetic conditions or acquired diseases.

### Disorders of hyperpigmentation

Generalized hyperpigmentation is usually caused by systemic conditions including endocrine, metabolic, and nutritional conditions. Addison's disease causes diffuse hyperpigmentation with accentuation in scars, palmar and plantar creases, and mucous membrane pigmented patches. Secretion of cortisol from the adrenal glands suppresses melanocyte-stimulating hormone (MSH) and adrenocorticotrophic hormone (ACTH) release from the pituitary. Lack of cortisol with loss of adrenal gland function allows uninhibited release of MSH-stimulating melanocyte pigmentary synthesis. Glucocorticosteroid replacement slowly reverses the hyperpigmentation.

ACTH- and MSH-secreting tumors cause similar Addisonian pigmentation. Pregnancy and oral estrogen stimulate pigmentation of the nipples, areolae, and genitalia, as well as localized patches in the sun-exposed areas on the face (melasma or mask of pregnancy).

Several metabolic diseases (porphyria, cutanea tarda, advanced liver disease, hemochromatosis, and chronic renal failure) and nutritional diseases (kwashiorkor, pellagra, inflammatory bowel disease, and malabsorption) cause hyperpigmentation. Hemochromatosis gives an unusual bronze hyperpigmentation. Certain drugs also cause hyperpigmentation, including bleomycin, fluorouracil, and busulfan.

Several genetic and acquired conditions cause these pigmented lesions:

1. Lentigo: Flat brown to black spots, 2 to 3 mm in diameter on the trunk and proximal extremities, due to an increase in melanocytes at the dermal-epidermal junction. They do not hyperpigment with UV light exposure.
2. Freckles: Tan macules in sun-exposed areas that darken with sun exposure. They are the result of increased melanin synthesis within a normal number of melanocytes.
3. Solar lentigo: Brown flat lesions on sun-exposed areas due to increased numbers of melanocytes. These lesions increase in numbers in individuals over 40.
4. Multiple lentigines syndrome: Including LEOPARD and LAMB syndromes. LEOPARD syndrome includes multiple (L)entigines; (E)CG changes; (O)cular hypertelorism; (P)ulmonary stenosis; (A)bnormalities of genitalia; (R)etardation of growth; and (D)eafness. LAMB syndrome includes multiple (L)entigines (A)trial myxomas, (M)ucocutaneous myxomas, and (B)lue nevi.
5. Various nevi including Mongolian spots (blue-black pigmentation in sacrogluteal region present at birth); *nevus spilus* (light brown patch with speckled dark, brown macules within).
6. Miscellaneous localized pigmented lesions in inherited conditions:
   a. Café au lait macules in neurofibromatosis.
   b. Brown to black macules on the lips and buccal mucosa in Peutz-Jeghers syndrome. Associated polyposis of the large and small intestine are a prominent part of this condition.
   c. Incontinentia pigmenti: A disease in which streaks and whorls of hyperpigmentation occur on the extremities and sides of trunk in females (X-linked dominant disorder) associated with ophthalmologic, bony, and central nervous system (CNS) abnormalities.
7. Post inflammatory hyperpigmentation: Many inflammatory skin conditions result in hyperpigmentation, especially in dark-skinned individuals. Common conditions leaving persistent pigmentation include stasis dermatitis, lichen planus, discoid lupus erythematosus, lichen simplex chronicus, and fixed drug reactions.

***Management.*** Replacing cortisone in Addison's disease will result in slow resolution of the hyperpigmentation. Melasma may be improved using creams containing hydroquinone creams, 3% to 4%, applied twice a day in

**Table 21-5.** Oculocutaneous albinism

| Type | Tyrosine activity | Clinical | Additional findings |
|---|---|---|---|
| Tyrosinase negative | None<br>Hair incubated with tyrosine = no pigment. | Totally devoid of pigment.<br>White hair, skin; ridges pink. | Severe photophobia, nystagmus. |
| Tyrosinase positive | Some tyrosinase activity but decreased activity.<br>Hair incubated tyrosine = small amount pigment. | Some red-yellow color to hair with age.<br>Freckles, nevi lightly pigmented. | Photophobia improves with time. |
| Yellow mutant | Makes some pheomelanin.<br>Hair incubated with cysteine = pheomelanin. | Yellow-red hair.<br>Some freckles. | Severe photophobia, nystagmus; improves with age. |
| Hermansky-Pudlak | Tyrosinase | Pale skin, yellow-red hair.<br>Freckles and pigmented nevi with age. | Hemorrhagic diathesis due to platelet defect.<br>Easy bruising, epistaxis.<br>Pulmonary insufficiency due to accumulation of ceroid.<br>Severe photophobia, nystagmus. |

conjunction with avoidance of sun and the use of sunscreen. Hydroquinone suppresses pigmentation by interfering with tyrosinase activity.

Tretinoin (Retin-A) creams may decrease epidermal hyperpigmentation associated with sun damage. Generally 0.05% retinoid cream should be used initially at night three times a week, slowly increasing its use and concentration.

### Disorders of hypopigmentation

Generalized loss of pigment is usually the result of oculocutaneous albinism due to a variety of conditions in which melanin pigmentation is defective. These conditions include tyrosinase negative, tyrosinase positive, yellow mutant, and Hermansky-Pudlak syndrome (Table 21-5). These conditions are characterized by depigmented skin, light hair color, nystagmus, and poor visual acuity.

### Localized hypopigmentation

Vitiligo is a condition in which melanocytes are destroyed, possibly on an immunologic basis, resulting in symmetric or segmental white macules, usually over bony prominences. Spontaneous repigmentation occurs in some patients. Vitiligo may be seen in association with the autoimmune conditions including Hashimoto's thyroiditis, diabetes mellitus, pernicious anemia, and Addison's disease.

Piebaldism or white forelock consists of depigmentation due to an absence of melanocytes over the forehead and frontal scalp, chest, mid arms, and thighs.

Waardenburg's syndrome is an inherited defect of neural crest-derived elements consisting of poliosis (white forelock), deafness, broad nasal root, epicanthic eyefolds, and heterochromia of the irides.

Tuberous sclerosis. One of the earliest signs of this phakomatosis is hypopigmented macules present at birth. Typically, these macules are "ash leaf" in shape but may be polygonal. Wood's lamp examination of skin accentuates these areas of depigmentation.

Chemically induced depigmentation. Exposure to rubber products, germicidal agents, and industrial cleaning solution can cause irregular depigmented areas simulating vitiligo. These chemicals contain phenols and hydroquinones that destroy melanocytes.

### Treatment of hypopigmentation conditions

Vitiligo is difficult to treat. Sunscreens are necessary to prevent burning. PUVA therapy has had limited success. Patients should be referred to a dermatologist for PUVA therapy. Chemically induced depigmentation also may benefit from PUVA therapy. If the vitiligo is extensive, depigmentation of the remaining normally pigmented skin may be a reasonable option. This procedure should also be supervised by a dermatologist.

## COMMON REACTION PATTERNS

### Urticaria

***Epidemiology/etiology.*** Urticaria (hives) occurs at any age without preference to genetic population, age, or sex. Up to 20% of the population is affected at some time with urticaria. The majority of cases are acute and self-limited. A few persist beyond 6 weeks and are termed *chronic urticaria.* Multiple causative factors are associated with urticaria and are discussed in the box at right.

***Pathophysiology.*** Urticaria occurs when cutaneous mast cells and basophils release histamine and other inflammatory mediators into the dermis. This reaction causes vasodilation and leakage of fluid from small cutaneous blood vessels, resulting in the pruritic raised lesions observed clinically. Although numerous factors can trigger the release of the inflammatory mediators, the process involves a common biochemical pathway of enzyme activation caused by an increased production of cyclic GMP within the cell. This activation can be induced by immunologic and nonimmunologic mechanisms.

Immunologically induced urticaria is most commonly a type 1 IgE-mediated process in which circulating antigens bind with IgE receptors at the cell membrane and trigger the enzyme-activated degranulation. Less commonly, immune complexes cause urticaria through the activation

### Common causes of urticaria

**Foods**
Nuts, strawberries, fish, shellfish, eggs, chocolate, tomatoes

**Food additives**
Benzoates, dyes (Tartrazine), sweeteners (Aspartame), salicylates

**Drugs**
Penicillin, sulfonamides, aspirin, opiates, polymyxin, quinine

**Infections**
Hepatitis A, B, and C, mononucleosis, Coxsackie virus, dental abscesses, sinusitis, fungal infections, intestinal parasites

**Internal disease**
Connective tissue disease, other autoimmune disease, malignancies

**Physical urticarias**
Dermographism, cold, heat, water, vibration, pressure, exercise, ultraviolet light

**Miscellaneous**
Pregnancy, hormones, mastocytosis, contact urticaria, hereditary angioedema

of complement. In non-immunologically–induced urticaria, the same enzymatic cellular response is induced by certain pharmacologic or physical stimuli such as morphine, strawberries, and vibration.

Histamine is the most important chemical mediator of urticaria. Histamine in the dermis produces endothelial cell contraction and increased vascular permeability, which allows for the transudation of fluid into tissue spaces. Clinically this results in vasodilation, erythema and wheal formation (triple response of Lewis). Prostaglandins and beta-adrenergic agents inhibit histamine release by increasing cyclic adenosine monophosphate AMP within the cell. Drugs that inhibit prostaglandins, such as aspirin, can trigger urticaria by their influence on histamine release alone. The pruritus associated with urticaria is also thought to be caused by histamine, although the precise mechanism is unknown.

***History.*** The diagnosis of urticaria is usually evident after a brief history and examination (see box above right). Patients frequently identify their problem as hives and seek medical care for purposes of treatment. The history of pruritic wheals lasting up to several hours is typical. The pruritus can be intense. A history of a swollen tongue or lips and epigastric discomfort can imply gastrointestinal involvement, and the presence of wheezing or pharyngeal swelling suggests an anaphylactoid reaction.

***Examination.*** Urticaria are characterized by sharply demarcated raised areas of erythema with variable size and shape. Ranging in size from 0.5 cm papules to 20 cm plaques, the hives can be circular, annular, or serpiginous in shape (see Plate 4). Central clearing is common. Any area of the body can be involved. Once the diagnosis of urticaria is made, a more complete examination may be needed to identify possible causes. Evidence of infection and signs of internal disease may help determine a reason for the hypersensitivity.

### History in patients with urticaria

**Pattern of development**
Time of day
Acute or chronic pattern
Associated activities (physical urticaria)

**Food history**
Processed foods (food additives)
Other prepared foods (restaurants)
Snacks, candies, diet drinks

**Medications**
Aspirin
Over-the-counter products
Medications taken occasionally

**Environment**
Home (improvement when away from home?)
Work (improvement when away from work?)

**General health**
Underlying chronic illness
Autoimmune diseases
Malignancy
Occult infection (dental, sinus, genitourinary)

***Management.*** If a cause can be identified and eliminated, pharmacologic treatment of the urticaria may not be required. Frequently the cause cannot be identified, and management consists of controlling the development of new lesions and reducing symptoms. Antihistamines control the majority of patients with acute and chronic urticaria. Antihistamines competitively block histamine receptors, but do not prevent the release of the inflammatory mediators. Therefore they are most effective when administered continuously as a preventive therapy. Combinations of antihistamines may be necessary to suppress the development of urticaria. The $H_1$ blockers diphenhydramine and hydroxyzine are commonly used in doses ranging from 25 to 100 mg every 8 hours as tolerated by sedation. The nonsedating $H_1$ blockers can be useful during the day in patients who are intolerant of the sedation (see Table 20-3 on p. 342). The tricyclic antidepressant doxepin is a potent $H_1$ blocker, which can be used in difficult cases. Because of sedation, doxepin is best administered at night. The addition of $H_2$ blockers (cimetedine, ranitidine) may be tried in recalcitrant cases of urticaria, although the evidence for the usage of $H_2$ blockers is inconclusive.

In cases of chronic urticaria, an ongoing search for the cause will sometimes identify the antigen. Although many cases ultimately resolve spontaneously without a proven cause, a systematic elimination of some ingested substances can be helpful (see the box below).

## Erythema multiforme

Erythema multiforme is an acute self-limited disease of skin and mucous membranes that consists of characteristic clinical lesions and histopathology. The severity of erythema multiforme is variable, ranging from mild cases with few lesions to a widespread vesiculobullous form (Stevens-Johnson syndrome). Infections and medications are the most common causes of erythema multiforme (see the box below right).

***Pathophysiology.*** An immunologic mechanism of disease has been postulated as the cause of erythema multiforme. This theory is supported by the frequent association with the administration of medications and with some infections. Immune complexes have been identified within and around the microvasculature of involved skin, and recent studies utilizing the polymerase chain reaction have identified herpesvirus DNA in association with these immune complexes.

### Urticaria elimination list

**Dietary**

- Beer, alcohol
- Chocolate
- Eggs
- Fish, shellfish
- Milk
- Nuts (including peanuts)
- Citrus fruits
- Strawberries
- Cinnamon
- Peas, beans
- Pork
- Cola
- Diet drinks
- Artificial sweeteners
- Tonic water (quinine)

**Medications**

- Aspirin
- Vitamins
- Laxatives
- Lozenges
- Mouthwashes
- Eyedrops

**Miscellaneous**

- Candies
- Cigarettes
- Toothpaste
- Perfume and perfumed soaps
- Cosmetics
- Chewing gum

***History.*** Patients usually report a rapid onset of lesions that may follow a short prodrome of malaise. The hands and feet are commonly involved in early stages. Mouth tenderness is common if there is mucosal involvement. A detailed history of recent illnesses, medications, and infections, including a past history of herpetic infection, is essential to identifying the cause.

***Physical examination.*** The classic lesions of erythema multiforme are raised circular erythematous lesions 0.5 to 3 cm in diameter. Central epidermal pallor with surrounding erythema produces the "target" or "iris" lesions (see Plate 18). The central dusky gray pallor is caused by epidermal necrosis and can be mistaken for pustule formation. Vesicles develop when the necrotic epidermis separates from the dermis. Mucosal lesions erode easily, presenting as shallow ulcerations (see Chapter 29). Although the distribution of erythema multiforme can be widespread, the distal extremities including palms and plantar surfaces are most commonly involved.

***Laboratory evaluation.*** A biopsy of a lesion of erythema multiforme shows findings of a lymphocytic infiltrate at the dermal-epidermal junction, with a characteristic vacuolization of epidermal cells and necrotic keratinocytes within the epidermis. Blood studies may show a slight leukocytosis and elevation of the erythrocyte sedimentation rate; however, no consistent laboratory abnormalities are associated with erythema multiforme.

***Management.*** Erythema multiforme is usually self-limited without treatment. Identification and treatment of any underlying illness may prevent recurrent episodes. Because of the frequent association with herpes simplex virus infection, some authors have recommended the empiric use of oral acyclovir in suppressive doses to treat cases of chronic recurrent erythema multiforme. Analgesics may be necessary in some cases. The use of systemic

### Etiology of erythema multiforme

- Infections
  - Herpes simplex
  - Epstein-Barr virus
  - Streptococcal
  - Mycoplasmal pneumonia
  - Syphilis
- Immunizations
  - Hepatitis B vaccine
  - Immunotherapy (allergy shots)
- Drugs (see the box on p. 361)
- Malignancy
- Radiation therapy
- Connective tissue disease
- Hormonal
  - Pregnancy
  - Menstruation

corticosteroids is controversial, but may be helpful early on in the disease.

### Stevens-Johnson syndrome

A widespread vesiculobullous form of erythema multiforme with involvement of mucosal surfaces is called Stevens-Johnson syndrome. The two diseases are variations of the same pathophysiologic mechanism. Why some patients develop Stevens-Johnson syndrome while others develop milder cases of erythema multiforme is not known but may reflect the quantity of antigen exposure or individual differences in immunologic response.

*Etiology.* The potential causes of both erythema multiforme and Stevens-Johnson syndrome are similar (see box below). Radiation therapy, and particularly cranial radiation therapy, in association with the administration of antiseizure medications, appears to be associated with an increased incidence of erythema multiforme and Stevens-Johnson syndrome (Fig. 21-3). Some authors have recommended avoiding the use of prophylactic phenytoin in patients receiving cranial irradiation.

*History.* A rapid onset of skin and mucosal lesions associated with variable symptoms of malaise and fever is typical in Stevens-Johnson syndrome. Pain or burning in the conjunctiva and mouth is a common early symptom that may at first suggest an infectious etiology until more skin involvement is apparent. A detailed history of underlying diseases and exposure to medications is essential.

#### Drugs commonly associated with erythema multiforme, Stevens-Johnson syndrome, and toxic epidermal necrolysis

**Sulfonamides**
Trimethoprim/sulfamethoxazole
Dapsone

**Anticonvulsants**
Diphenylhydantoin (Dilantin)
Carbamazepine (Tegritol)

**Nonsteroidal antiinflammatory drugs**
Oxyphenbutazone
Phenylbutazone
Piroxicam (Feldene)

**Barbiturates**

**Allopurinol**

**Other Antibiotics**
Penicillins
Tetracyclines
Erythromycin
Cephalosporins

**Salicylates**

**Furosemide**

*Physical examination.* The extensive distribution and severity of the lesions distinguish Stevens-Johnson syndrome from erythema multiforme. Erosive changes on the lips, mouth, conjunctiva, anogenital area, and ears are typical (see Plate 31). Intact vesicles and bullae are uncommon in these areas. Cutaneous lesions may involve the entire skin surface. Individual lesions may be characteristic circular lesions of erythema multiforme, but it is more common to find large confluent areas of dusky erythematous skin, with occasional flaccid vesicles, bullae, and erosions. The lesions are usually tender to touch.

*Differential diagnosis.* Stevens-Johnson syndrome should be differentiated from staphylococcal scalded skin syndrome, vesicular viral exanthems such as varicella, Kawasaki disease, toxic shock syndrome, and paraneoplastic pemphigus. The classic circular "target" or "iris" lesions and the erosive changes on the mucous membranes should confirm a correct diagnosis.

*Management.* The treatment of Stevens-Johnson syndrome is primarily supportive. Control of pain and treatment of secondary infection may require narcotic analgesics and antibiotics. Patients with large areas of denuded skin need fluid and electolyte managment. Liquid diet or intravenous nutrition may be required when mouth lesions prevent oral intake. Eroded areas of skin should be cleansed gently and kept covered with occlusive compresses to prevent drying. Keep mucosal lesions moist by frequent use of antibacterial ointments or protective agents.

The use of systemic corticosteroids is controversial. Some studies have demonstrated delayed healing and higher incidence of complications when steroids are used. Studies have not shown a clear benefit from the use of corticosteroids; however, many physicians routinely use them in cases of Stevens-Johnson syndrome and some believe there may be a positive response.

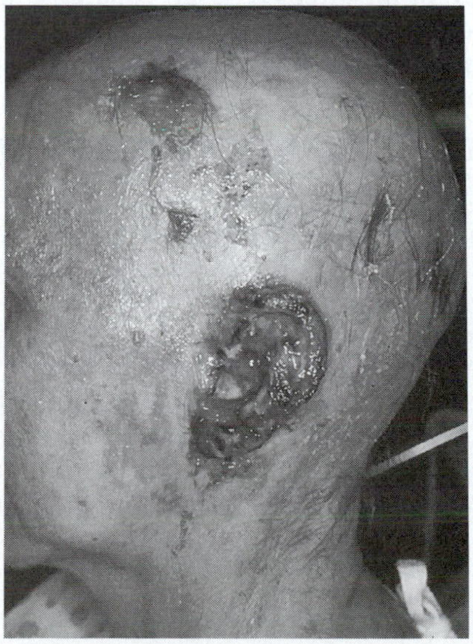

**Fig. 21-3.** Stevens-Johnson syndrome in a patient receiving diphenhydantoin (Dilantin) and x-ray irradiation therapy to the head and neck.

### Toxic epidermal necrolysis (TEN)

Historically, the term *toxic epidermal necrolysis* has been confusing. The main area of confusion has been the use of the term *scalded skin syndrome* to mean toxic epidermal necrolysis. There are many similarities between TEN and Stevens-Johnson syndrome, and many consider the two to be variations of the same disease.

***History.*** The prodrome in TEN is similar to that of Stevens-Johnson syndrome, with 2 or 3 days of fever and malaise. The history of a new drug taken within 1 to 3 weeks before the onset of the illness is strong evidence of a causal relationship.

***Physical examination.*** Extensive epidermal sloughing, along with severe mucosal changes, are characteristic of TEN. The mucosal changes, which are present in over 90% of cases, frequently precede the skin involvement. The percentage of skin surface involvement can range from 40% to 100%. The full-thickness epidermal detachment leaves painful areas of denuded dermis. Primary target lesions also can be seen occasionally.

***Complications.*** Complications are responsible for the mortality rate in TEN that ranges between 25% and 70%. Sepsis is the main cause of death. Gastrointestinal hemorrhage, hypovolemia, and pulmonary edema also have contributed to mortality. Ocular complications include conjunctival scarring, corneal ulceration, and photophobia. Cutaneous complications include alopecia, loss of nails, pigmentary changes, and hypertrophic scarring with contractures.

***Management.*** A burn center provides the best environment for the treatment of TEN. The skills and materials needed to treat TEN are similar to those used in burn care, including xenografts, temperature control, and nutritional management. Treatment consists of supportive measures that are designed to prevent complications and allow healing of all of the affected tissue. A successful approach requires the help of the surgical team, the intensivist or internist, the ophthalmologist, the physical therapist, and an expert nursing staff.

## PHOTOREACTIONS AND PHOTOSENSITIVITY REACTIONS

Photoreactions of the skin most commonly appear after exposure to the sun. They can occur on sunny days, on cloudy days, through window glass, and even from artificial sources of light such as tanning booths. In addition to sun exposure, a second factor usually is responsible for producing a photoreaction. This second factor includes diseases such as porphyria cutanea tarda, oral medications such as griseofulvin, and topical agents such as sunscreens. When a photoreaction is suspected in a patient, this second factor must be found to make an accurate diagnosis.

### "Sunburn"

***Epidemiology/etiology.*** Sunburn is caused by UVB radiation (290 to 320 nm). It also can be caused by UVA irradiation (320 to 400 nm), but the exposure required to induce erythema is much greater.

***Pathophysiology.*** Ultraviolet B erythema has an onset 2 to 6 hours after irradiation. It peaks at 24 to 36 hours. Tanning occurs when ultraviolet light stimulates synthesis of new melanin. This melanin is transferred from melanocytes in the basal cell layer of the upper dermis to keratinocytes. Melanin effectively absorbs ultraviolet B irradiation, providing protection against further damage. Melanogenesis becomes visible 2 to 3 days after UVB exposure.

***Management.*** Sunburn damage is permanent. Patients can be soothed by pain medications such as Tylenol, aspirin, and nonsteroidal antiinflammatories. Moderate-strength topical cortisones in an ointment base can help reduce any discomfort. For severe sunburn, oral prednisone in a dose of 20 to 60 mg daily can reduce the swelling and the pain. Most important, the patient should avoid heat and further solar exposure, even through window glass.

### Photosensitive disorders

***History.*** A careful history is paramount in diagnosing photosensitive disorders. Frequently, a diagnosis can be made by history alone. The following questions can help guide the physician to a correct diagnosis.

1. Can the first photosensitive episode be described in detail?
2. What was the duration of solar exposure required to elicit the reaction? Phototoxic reactions to drugs such as triamterene with hydrochlorothiazide (Dyazide) often occur with minimal exposure, whereas polymorphous light eruption sometimes appears only with extreme exposure such as during a tropical vacation.
3. Does the reaction occur through window glass? Since UVA light penetrates window glass, the action spectrum can be surmised by answering this question. Photoallergic and phototoxic drug reactions usually are caused by UVA light.
4. Was the photoreaction immediate or delayed after solar exposure? Solar urticaria occurs immediately with sun exposure. Polymorphous light eruption is delayed by 4 to 8 hours.
5. What were the cutaneous symptoms? Burning is common with phototoxic drug eruptions. Itching occurs with photoallergic drug eruptions and polymorphous light eruption.
6. What were the systemic symptoms? Systemic symptoms are rare with photodermatitis. Coincidental symptoms not directly related to sun exposure may occur in some diseases such as systemic lupus erythematosus.
7. What topical products were being used? Special emphasis should be made to look for sunscreen use and sunscreens in cosmetic products.
8. What systemic medications were being ingested? See the box on p. 363 for a list of photosensitizing medications.

9. Is there a family history for photosensitivity? Polymorphous light eruption, porphyria cutanea tarda, and systemic lupus erythematosus may have some genetic predisposition.

*Physical examination.* In photodermatitis, the reaction is usually, but not always, limited to sun-exposed areas. These areas typically include the face, the "V" area of the neck and upper chest, dorsal arms, legs, and feet. The spared areas are equally important to the diagnosis. They include the eyelids, upper lip, postauricular area, submen tal area, flexor surfaces of the arms, and finger webs. These areas are typically protected from sun exposure. Because radiation can penetrate clothing, clothing is not always protective. However, sharp clothing cut-off points of the erythema aid in diagnosis.

### Laboratory studies and diagnostic procedures

The answer to the question, "Is a patient photosensitive?" can often be found by determining a patient's minimal erythema dose (MED). The MED is the minimal amount of radiation necessary to induce erythema. For UVB, the average MED in whites is 40 mJ. For UVA, the average MED is 40 J. So thus UVB is 1000 times more effective in producing erythema than UVA. A low MED signifies that the patient gets erythema from an abnormally small amount of radiation. A biopsy can be useful in diagnosing some types of photosensitivity such as polymorphous light eruption, photoallergic eruptions, and some forms of porphyria. If a photoallergic reaction is suspected, photopatch testing can delineate the etiologic chemical. Small amounts of common topical photosensitizers are applied to a patient in duplicate. One side is irradiated to try to elicit a photosensitive reaction at the site of the offending chemical.

*Differential diagnosis.* The most common causes of photosensitivity include polymorphous light eruption, phototoxic reaction, photoallergic reactions, solar urticaria, polymorphous light eruption and systemic lupus erythematosus (Table 21-6).

### Polymorphous light eruption

*Epidemiology/etiology.* Polymorphous light eruption occurs in approximately 10% of the young adult population. It occurs primarily with springtime sunlight exposure and patients tend to become "hardened" as the season progresses. That is, they become less sensitive to sunlight as summer proceeds. Not uncommonly, onset occurs after an unusually intense sun exposure such as a vacation to a tropical climate.

*Pathophysiology.* The pathophysiology of polymorphous light eruption is not clear. Typically, the patient's history is negative for any medications that can cause the photoallergic or phototoxic reactions. Some patients are more sensitive to ultraviolet B light, whereas other patients react to ultraviolet A light. Occasionally, the lesions can be reproduced in the laboratory setting by exposing a focal area of skin repeatedly to the patient's MED.

*History.* The history is the most consistent diagnostic clue. Typically, the patient is a young adult experiencing early springtime solar exposure or extreme exposure. Onset occurs 4 hours to 2 days after the last exposure and lasts up to 7 days after an exposure is discontinued.

*Physical examination.* The lesions appear as papules and papulovesicles. Occasionally, dermal plaques can occur (it does not involve all sun-exposed areas of skin but is typically confined to those areas).

*Laboratory studies.* A biopsy usually shows a superficial and deep mononuclear cell infiltrate. Serologic studies such as an ANA, anti-Ro, and Anti-La antibodies are typically negative.

*Differential diagnosis.* When polymorphous light eruption presents as dermal infiltrates, it can mimic a cutaneous lymphoma. Occasionally, the papules are confluent and appear more eczematous, making the rash appear similar to a photocontact allergy.

*Management.* The rash clears in most patients with topical or systemic corticosteroid use. Nonpharmacologic management of polymorphous light eruption can occur by gradually increasing the patient's exposure to sunlight. Hardening may occur with tanning, and the patient usually will become less sensitive. Beta-carotene, antimalarials, UVB, and PUVA therapy also have been utilized.

### Drug-induced photosensitivity (photoallergic vs. phototoxic)

Drug-induced photosensitivity occurs when photons induce an applied or ingested drug to become a photosensitizer. The most common types of photosensitive drug eruptions are phototoxic and photoallergic. A phototoxic reaction is associated with direct cellular changes induced by the phototoxin. A photoallergic reaction occurs via the immune response.

An example of a phototoxic reaction is the sunburn response that can occur to griseofulvin. Phototoxic reactions can occur with first exposure to the medication. They typically mimic a sunburn reaction.

Phototoxic reactions also can occur to topical substances such as fragrances. Photoallergic reactions most commonly have eczematous morphology. Sunlight has

#### Agents causing phototoxic and photoallergic reactions

*Phototoxic Drugs:* Amiodarone, benoxaprofen, chlorothiazides, demethylchlortetracycline, doxycycline, furosemide, griseofulvin, hydrochlorothiazide, nalidixic acid, naproxen, oxytetracycline, phenothiazine, piroxicam, sulfonamides, tetracycline, thiazides

*Photoallergic Drugs and Chemicals:* Chlorpromazine, promethazine, sulfanilamide

Sunscreens: PABA, Benzophenones, Cinnamates

Fragrances: Musk Ambrette, 6-methylcoumarin

**Table 21-6.** Photosensitivity: differential considerations

| | History | Morphology and physical examination | Laboratory | Management |
|---|---|---|---|---|
| PML | 26-year-old woman: onset with extreme sun exposure; delayed onset 6-8 hours postexposure, lasts 7-10 days; pruritic | Papules, vesicles, or plaques; distribution includes face, neck, dorsal arms | Biopsy: superficial and deep mononuclear cell infiltrate | Topical corticosteroids, oral corticosteroids, B-carotene, PUVA, Trisoralen, antimalarial |
| Solar urticaria | Hives appear immediately with sun exposure, last 1-4 hours; pruritic | Uriticaria appearing in sun-exposed areas | MED testing with UVA and UVB may reproduce lesions; biopsy: superficial perivascular mononuclear cell infiltrates | Antihistamines, UVB/UVA hardening, PUVA, oral corticosteroids |
| Phototoxic | Sunburn appears after minimal exposure; patient may have used new oral medications | Sunburn erythema with sharp cutoffs at nonexposed areas | | Discontinue offending agent; oral corticosteroids; PUVA if becomes chronic |
| Photoallergic | Itchy dermatitis with sun exposure; patient may have used new topical product or oral medication | Eczematous dermatitis; may spread somewhat into non–sun-exposed areas | Reduced MED to UVA; biopsy: spongiosis in epidermis; superficial and deep mononuclear cell infiltrate | Same as above; topical corticosteroids |
| PCT | Estrogen or alcohol intake; history of skin fragility or blisters on hands | Vesicles and bullae on dorsal hands that heal with scarring and milia; mottled hypopigmentation of face; hyperpigmentation of the periorbital area | Biopsy: subepidermal bullae; increased uroporphyrin I and 7-carboxyl porphyrin III in urine; increased isocoproporphyrin in feces | Phlebotomy—500 ml/week until clinical clearing occurs |
| SLE | Sunburn persists days or weeks with no further exposure; rash in butterfly distribution across nose; drugs associated with lupus-like syndrome | Long-lasting sunburn reaction; plaques in butterfly distribution of smaller area | Biopsy: positive ANA; positive Ro antigen; dif–band of fluorescent material at dermal epidermal junction | Chloroquine 125 to 250 mg twice weekly |

*PML,* Polymorphous light eruption; *PCT,* porphyria cutanea tarda; *SLE,* systemic lupus erythematosus; *MED,* minimum erythema dose.

**Managed Care Guide**
**Indications for referral to a dermatologist**

**Specific**

| | |
|---|---|
| Atypical pigmented lesions | • Referral may prevent surgical procedure.<br>• If melanoma suspected, excisional Bx indicated. |
| Blistering diseases | • Wide range of diagnostic evaluations frequently required.<br>• Severe involvement requires multidisciplinary approach. |
| Pigmented skin (African-American, etc.) | • Risk of permanent pigmentary alteration is significant. |
| Acne vulgaris—severe or scarring | • Aggressive therapy necessary to prevent scarring. |
| Any systematically ill patient with undiagnosed dermatosis | • Several diseases have characteristic skin findings. (e.g., toxic shock syndrome, Kawasaki disease, ecthyma gangrenosum, Stevens-Johnson syndrome, others.) |

**General**

| | |
|---|---|
| • If diagnosis uncertain<br>• If treatment is ineffective<br>• If disease severity is high<br>• If expensive or highly toxic medications are indicated. | Referral may be cost effective |

caused the drug to become an allergen, which triggers a delayed contact dermatitis. The most common cause of photocontact dermatitis today is sunscreens. It is important to know the active ingredient of sunscreens because switching brands may not be helpful if the same active ingredient is present.

Fragrances also cause some photocontact allergies. Many cosmetic products contain sunscreens and fragrances without obvious labeling. Phototoxic and photoallergic reactions are most often due to UVA light (see box on p. 363). UVA light occurs with natural sunlight and tanning booths and is transmitted through window glass.

## BIBLIOGRAPHY

Aslanzadeh J et al: Detection of HSV-specific DNA in biopsy tissue of patients with erythema multiforme by polymerase chain reaction, *Br J Dermatol* 126:19-23, 1992.

Avakian R et al: Toxic epidermal necrolysis: a review, *J Am Acad Dermatol* 25:69-79, 1991.

Basruji-Garin S et al: Clinical classification of cases of toxic epidermal necrolysis, Stevens-Johnson syndrome, and erythema multiforme, *Arch Dermatol* 129:92-96, 1993.

Bell WF: *Cutaneous photobiology,* Oxford, England, 1985, Oxford University Press.

Caputo R, Ackerman AB, Sison-Torre EQ, editors: *Pediatric dermatology and dermatopathology,* vol 2, Philadelphia, 1993, Lea & Febiger.

Clark RAF, Nicol N, Adinoff AD: Atopic dermatitis. In Sams WM Jr, Lynch PJ, editors: *Principle and practice of dermatology,* New York, 1990, Churchill Livingstone.

Cookson WOCM et al: Maternal inheritance of atopic IgE responsiveness on chromosome 11q, *Lancet* 340:381-384, 1992.

Cooper KD et al: Immunoregulation in atopic dermatitis: functional analysis of T-B cell interactions and the enumeration of Fc receptor-bearing T cells, *J Invest Dermatol* 80:139-145, 1983.

Darragh TM et al: Identification of herpes simplex virus DNA in lesions of erythema multiforme by the polymerase chain reaction, *J Am Acad Dermatol* 24:23-26, 1991.

Delattre JY, Safai B, Posner JB: Erythema multiforme and Stevens-Johnson syndrome in patients receiving cranial irradiation and phenytoin, *Neurology* 38:194-196, 1988.

Fisher AA: *Contact dermatitis,* ed 3, Philadelphia, 1986, Lea & Febiger.

Fitzpatrick TB: *Sunlight and man,* Tokyo, Japan, 1972, University of Tokyo Press.

Hanifin JM: Atopic dermatitis, *J Am Acad Dermatol* 6:1-13, 1982.

Hanifin JM, Rajka G: Diagnostic features of atopic dermatitis, *Acta Derm Venereol* Suppl (Stockholm) 92:44-47, 1980.

Harbor LC, Bickers DR: *Photosensitivity diseases: principles of diagnosis and treatment,* Philadelphia, 1981, WB Saunders.

Kuster W et al: A family study of atopic dermatitis: clinical and genetic characteristics of 188 patients and 2151 family members, *Arch Dermatol Res* 282:98-102, 1990.

Lever WF, Schaumberg-Lever G: *Histopathology of the skin,* Philadelphia, 1990, JB Lippincott.

Lookingbill DP, Marks JG Jr: *Principles of dermatology,* Philadelphia, 1986, WB Saunders.

Magnus IA: *Dermatologic photobiology,* Oxford, 1976, Blackwell.

Maize JC, Ackerman AB, editors: *Pigmented lesions of the skin,* Philadelphia, 1987, Lea & Febiger.

Mathews KP: Urticaria and angioedema, *J Allergy Clin Immunol* 72:1-13, 1983.

National Institutes of Health (NIH): Diagnosis and treatment of early melanoma. NIH consensus development conference, Consensus statement, October, 1992.

Orkin M, Maibach HI, Dahl MV: *Dermatology,* Norwalk, Conn, 1991, Appleton & Lange Publishers.

Roujeau JC et al: Toxic epidermal necrolysis (Lyell syndrome), *J Am Acad Dermatol* 23:1039-1058, 1990.

Soter NA, Baden HP: *Pathophysiology of dermatologic diseases,* New York, 1991, McGraw-Hill.

CHAPTER

# 22 Drug Reactions

**Frank Parker**

Mucocutaneous reactions to drugs, especially urticaria and morbilliform rashes (generalized confluent erythematous macules and papules), are common. Because drug reactions can cause skin reactions that mimic virtually all forms of skin conditions, the clinician must always consider these possibilities in the differential diagnosis of all skin disease.

## EPIDEMIOLOGY-ETIOLOGY

Drug rashes account for 2% of skin reactions in the hospital setting. In the physician's office, drug rashes may be common, ubiquitous, and easily overlooked and misdiagnosed.

## PATHOPHYSIOLOGY

The mechanism of cutaneous drug reaction is not understood in most instances but a few facts are known. Only

## Drug reactions

**Drug categories most commonly causing skin rash**

Antibiotics
Anticoagulants
Antihypertensive drugs
Psychotropic agents
Rheumatoid agents: nonsteroidal antiinflammatory drugs, gold, allopurinol, penicillamine
Blood products

**Specific drugs commonly causing skin rash**

Amoxicillin/ampicillin
Penicillins
Trimethoprim-sulfamethoxazole
Blood products
Benzodiazepines
Allopurinol
Furosemide

**Table 22-1.** Categorization of drug reaction patterns and their incidence

| Pattern | Incidence (%) |
|---|---|
| Morbilliform (see Plate 32) | 46 |
| Urticarial (see Plate 4) | 23 |
| Fixed drug eruption | 10 |
| Erythema multiforme (see Plate 18) | 5 |
| Other reactions | 16 |
| Acneiform | |
| Alopecia | |
| Bullous | |
| Eczematous and exfoliative | |
| Lichen planus–like | |
| Lupus-like | |
| Photo reaction | |
| Pruritus | |
| Toxic epidermal necrolysis | |
| Vasculitis | |

10% of drug reactions have a clearly identified immunologic basis. Low molecular weight drugs or their metabolites usually combine with a carrier protein to form an antigen. Less commonly high molecular weight drugs (insulin) are a complete antigen and specific antibodies form to initiate the reaction. Factors such as the route of exposure to the drug and its subsequent metabolism influence the likelihood of a reaction (severe reactions occur with intravenous or intramuscular routes). Specific mechanisms of immunologically mediated drug reaction can be due to immediate hypersensitivity (IgE mediated), cytotoxic antibody reactions, circulating immune complexes, and delayed hypersensitivity. The mechanisms of nonimmunologic-mediated drug reactions include toxic overdose, idiosyncratic, drug interactions, and pharmacologic side effects.

## HISTORY

The onset of a drug rash (especially morbilliform and urticarial reactions) is usually 3 to 10 days after the initiation of the drug (1 or 2 days if patient was previously exposed to drug or to a chemically similar drug). Also of importance in the history is prior experience with the drug and cross-reaction to a chemically related drug (i.e., sulfonamides, sulfonylureas, and thiazides may cross react). A history of over-the-counter or illicit recreational drugs also should be determined. When multiple drugs are being used, carefully noting the dates of administration and doses of each drug may be useful. Knowledge of which drugs are most likely to cause a rash is also crucial (see the box above).

## PHYSICAL EXAMINATION

The variety of cutaneous reactions to drugs is vast, but morbilliform and urticarial reactions are the most common. Table 22-1 categorizes and lists the wide variety of drug reaction patterns. Some examples of various types of skin reactions and the drugs that may cause these are noted in Table 22-2.

Morbilliform eruptions are the most common of all drug rashes (see Plate 32). These eruptions often begin on the trunk and evolve onto the extremities. Pruritus is common and mild fever can occur. Both usually begin within the first 2 weeks after a variety of drugs are taken and clear within 2 to 3 weeks after the drug is withdrawn. Urticarial reactions (see Plate 4) are IgE mediated hypersensitivity responses caused most often by aspirin, penicillin, and blood products.

## LABORATORY STUDIES/DIAGNOSTIC PROCEDURES

No laboratory tests can diagnose a drug eruption or identify a specific drug. Skin biopsy can help to identify the specific clinical form of the skin rash, but not whether a drug is the etiology. The presence of a peripheral eosinophilia and eosinophiles seen in the skin biopsy is sometimes seen and increases the suspicion of a drug-related reaction. Skin tests for penicillin are only of use for predicting immediate hypersensitivity reactions such as hives and anaphylaxis. Rechallenging with the suspected drug is potentially dangerous.

## DIFFERENTIAL DIAGNOSIS

It is often difficult to distinguish drug reactions from viral exanthems, scarlet fever, Kawasaki disease, and exfoliative erythroderma (see Chapter 26). Viral exanthems are associated with enanthems, fever, and other viral symptoms. Exfoliative erythroderma also can be due to drugs, psoriasis, eczema, or cutaneous T-cell lymphoma.

## MANAGEMENT

Discontinuing the offending drug will clear the skin rash. When the patient is on multiple drugs, a drug should be withdrawn or switched when possible. Symptomatic therapy includes antihistamines, occasionally systemic steroids, and application of topical steroids. Most cutaneous drug reactions remit within 2 to 3 weeks after the drug

**Table 22-2.** Some specific drugs and clinical associations

| Specific drugs | Possible rash |
|---|---|
| Halogens | Bromide iodide—acne, vegetative granulomas |
| | Fluoride—perioral dermatitis |
| Hydantoins | Morbilliform, erythema multiforme, toxic epidermal necrolysis (TEN) |
| | Purpura, fever, lymphadenopathy |
| | Gingival hyperplasia |
| | Lupus erythematosus–like syndrome |
| Tetracycline | Phototoxicity and photoonycholysis |
| | Fixed drug reaction |
| Thiazide and sulfonamides | Urticaria and morbilliform |
| | Erythema multiforme |
| | Vasculitis |
| | Photosensitivity |
| Trimethoprim-sulfa | Urticaria, TEN, exanthem in 60% AIDS patients |
| Nonsteroidal antiinflammatory drugs | TEN and erythema multiforme |
| | Photosensitivity |
| | Vasculitis |
| Cancer chemotherapeutic agents | Stomatitis, alopecia |
| | Onychodystrophy |
| | Radiation recall reaction—drugs recreate inflammation and erythema in previous skin radiation exposure sites—adriamycin, hydroxyurea, methotrexate, cyclophosphamide, vinblastine, and vincristine |

is stopped. Some drug reactions are serious, such as anaphylaxis, toxic epidermal necrolysis, vasculitis, erythema multiforme, and exfoliative erythroderma and take a longer period to resolve (see Chapter 21).

## ACUTE ALLERGIC REACTIONS—ANAPHYLAXIS

Acute anaphylaxis is a clinical syndrome characterized by the sudden onset of itching, erythema, and urticarial lesions. When severe, there may be upper airway obstruction (laryngeal edema), wheezing, difficulty swallowing, abdominal discomfort, cramps, diarrhea, hypotension, and shock. Most of these reactions occur soon after exposure to drugs, foods, or following insect stings. The term *anaphylaxis* is generally applied to reactions mediated by IgE. When no IgE-mediated mechanism can be demonstrated, the term *anaphylactoid reaction* is used. Some anaphylactoid reactions are due to other antigen-antibody combinations; reactions that do not involve antibodies at all may depend on the release of mediators from mast cells. See Chapter 112 for management of anaphylaxis.

### Acute reactions to drugs

In the past, horse serum given for the treatment of diphtheria, tetanus, and pneumonia was the most common cause of anaphylaxis. Penicillin is now the most common cause. Fatal reactions occur perhaps twice in every 100,000 injections. Acute nonfatal reactions may occur as often as 1 per 1000 injections, but because penicillin is used so often, reactions to it are the most common allergic drug reaction. Severe anaphylactic reactions are associated with specific IgE, and patients will have positive skin reactions to penicillin or its derivatives. Delayed reactions such as rashes are more common and are usually not associated with skin reactivity. Even though it has been shown that most patients who give a history of penicillin reaction years before have a negative skin test and can be given penicillin without adverse effect, it is wiser to avoid penicillin and its analogs unless there is a serious infection that will not respond to another antibiotic. Skin testing should be done then, with penicillin, its breakdown products, and penicilloyl-polylysine. These reagents are not commercially available and testing should be done in the hospital by an expert. If the skin test is negtive, one can cautiously give penicillin or its analogs. If the skin test is positive, an even more cautious program of desensitization should be carried out. Skin tests with most other drugs are unreliable in predicting allergic reactions. It is safer to avoid drugs even if the diagnosis is only presumptive as long as alternatives exist. One is often faced with accepting only a presumptive diagnosis because most reactions occur in patients who are receiving several drugs at one time.

Reactions to intravenous contrast media are usually anaphylactoid and may depend on nonimmunologic activation of complement and histamine release. Patients with a history of such reactions should be managed without further intravenous contrast studies if possible. When another study is essential, reactions can be decreased by pretreatment with corticosteroids, diphenhydramine, and ephedrine.

### Acute reactions to foods

Although many foods can cause acute allergic reactions, 95% of reactions are due to a few foods: eggs, crustaceans (lobster, shrimp, crab), mollusks (clams, oysters, etc.), fish, peanuts, nuts, and seeds. When the history is clear-cut, skin testing is unnecessary and in fact can be dangerous if not done with caution. Skin tests are usually strikingly positive to the food causing the reaction. However, positive skin reactions can occur with foods that the patient tolerates with impunity. Extracts of fruits and vegetables are unstable. The patient can be tested by rubbing the freshly cut surface to a skin scratch. Such techniques can help identify celery as the cause of symptoms, for example, after eating a tuna fish salad sandwich. When a reaction occurs after eating sausage, it can be shown that wheal and erythema are produced not only by the sausage, but also by buckwheat, one of its ingredients. Allergy to foods can begin in adolescence or adulthood despite a history of eating the food with impunity for years.

It is often difficult for patients to avoid exposure to the small amounts of a food allergen that can be unexpectedly present. A ham sandwich may have been cut with a knife previously used to cut a peanut butter sandwich; a hamburger can be grilled on the surface on which an egg has been fried; or a disbelieving hostess may allow small amounts of oyster or nuts in the stuffing. Some exquisitely sensitive patients learn to eat only food prepared at home and may have to carry epinephrine syringes and antihistaminics to use if inadvertently exposed. Immunotherapy has not been shown to be helpful in preventing acute allergic reactions to foods.

### Treatment of the acute reactions

The immediate treatment is the same for both anaphylactic and anaphylactoid reactions. Epinephrine 0.2 to 0.5 mg (0.2 to 0.5 ml of 1/1000 solution) should be given subcutaneously unless the patient is in shock, in which case 1 or 2 ml of 1/2000 aqueous can be given intravenously. Diphenhydramine (Benadryl) 20 to 50 mg can be given subcutaneously to lessen the chance of a delayed reaction or a recurrence. If there is respiratory difficulty or shock, three times this dose should be given (see Chapter 4G for management of bee sting allergy).

If hypotension persists, intravenous saline may be necessary to replace the fluid loss resulting from capillary permeability. If respiratory difficulty is present, then oxygen and intravenous aminophylline should be given. Tracheostomy may be indicated if there is laryngeal edema.

## BIBLIOGRAPHY

Bork K: *Cutaneous side effects of drugs,* Philadelphia, 1988, WB Saunders.

CHAPTER

# 23 Infectious Diseases of the Skin

Bert G. Tavelli

## BACTERIAL INFECTIONS

### Impetigo

Impetigo is characterized by erythematous macules that evolve into vesicopustules, which quickly rupture to form the hallmark honey-colored crusts, usually on exposed skin of the face and extremities. Caused by *Staphylococcus aureus* or *Streptococcus pyogenes,* it is typically seen in children, in whom it is highly contagious. Lesions may burn or itch, but constitutional symptoms are usually absent. Other forms of impetigo include a rare bullous type, mediated by toxins produced by group II *S. aureus* (Fig. 23-1) (which in its most severe form results in staphylococcal scalded skin syndrome) and impetiginized eczema, in which honey-colored crusts and pustules representing staphylococcal or streptococcal superinfection develop on dermatitic skin (see Plate 14).

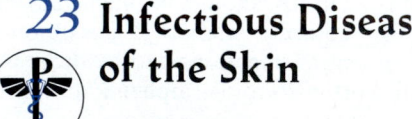

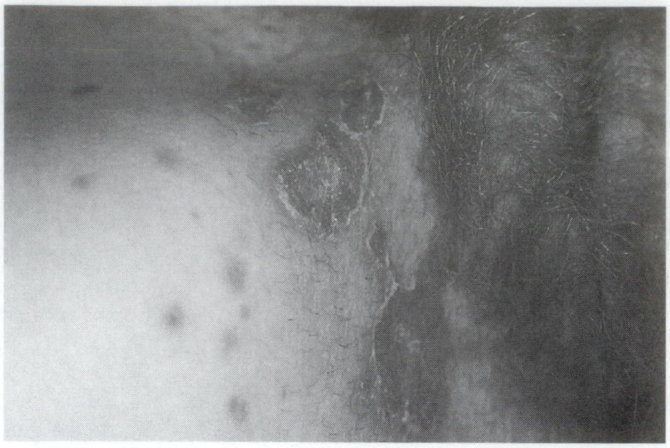

**Fig. 23-1.** Staphylococcal bullous impetigo. Note resolving circular blisters in typical location.

***Management.*** Small areas of superficial involvement respond to local cleansing with antibiotic soaps and topical treatment with mupiricin (Bactroban) ointment, but widespread and bullous lesions are best treated systemically with a penicillinase-resistant antibiotic. In penicillin-allergic patients, clindamycin or erythromycin may be substituted. Impetigo tends to heal without scarring, but certain nephritogenic strains of streptococci can lead to post streptococcal glomerulonephritis.

### Erysipelas and cellulitis

Both erysipelas and cellulitis are caused by rapidly spreading infection with streptococcal, or less commonly, staphylococcal organisms. In erysipelas, more superficial skin and lymphatics are affected, resulting in raised, red, warm plaques with sharply demarcated borders and a brawny (orange-peel) appearance. The face is most commonly affected, and vesicles and bullae also may be seen (see Plate 33). In cellulitis, deeper tissues and subcutaneous fat are involved, most often on the lower extremities, and the plaques are less well marginated or distinct. Local dermatitis, tinea pedis, and stasis ulcers predispose to infection. Both erysipelas and cellulitis can be associated with fever, chills, local pain, lymphangitis, regional lymphadenopathy, and systemic toxicity with tachycardia and hypotension. Tissue culture is usually unnecessary, but blood cultures should be obtained with extensive infection or marked toxicity.

***Management.*** Treatment consists of systemic antibiotic therapy and support. Penicillin is usually adequate, but erythromycin, clindamycin, or cephalosporins may be used. Attention should be given to predisposing conditions

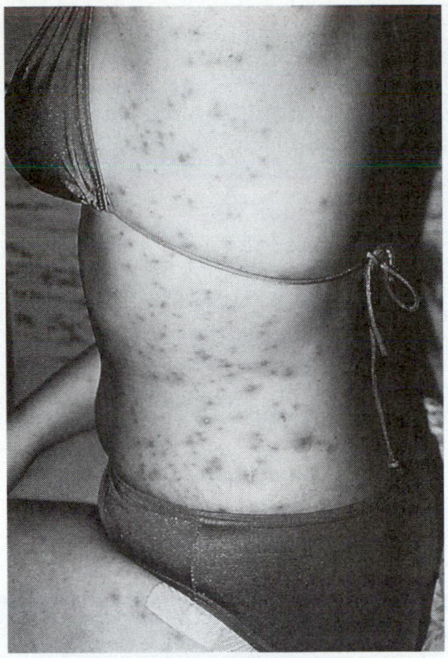

**Fig. 23-2.** Hot tub folliculitis. Note discrete pustules on an erythematous base distributed on the trunk.

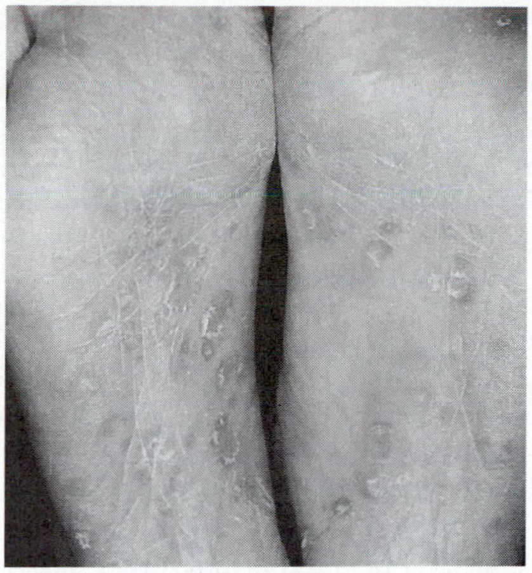

**Fig. 23-3.** Secondary syphilis. Note the papulosquamous red-brown lesions on the plantar surface.

to prevent recurrences, and prophylactic antibiotics in susceptible individuals help prevent chronic lymphedema.

### Necrotizing fasciitis

In some cases, a combination of anaerobic and aerobic bacteria, including staphylococci and streptococci, causes infection of the subcutaneous tissues called necrotizing fasciitis. Usually induced by trauma or extension of an antecedent infection, it rapidly spreads to cause bright red, edematous, tender plaques, associated with superficial gangrene, and marked systemic symptoms. This serious, often fatal infection, requires hospitalization, surgical exploration, and broad-spectrum antibiotics.

### Ecthyma

Ecthyma is caused by streptococcal and staphylococcal infection, often in patients with poor hygiene or at sites of trauma, especially of the lower extremities. Multiple, discrete vesicopustules quickly enlarge and rupture to form superficial purulent ulcers with overlying necrotic crust. Lesions often scar and spread if untreated, but respond quickly to appropriate systemic antibiotics.

### Erythrasma

Erythrasma is a superficial skin infection occurring in skin folds and toe webs, caused by the diphtheroid *Corynebacterium minutissimum.* Asymptomatic flat, dry, brown patches develop, which resemble tinea but can be distinguished by negative potassium hydroxide (KOH) examination and bright coral red fluorescence under Wood's light examination. Topical or systemic treatment with erythromycin is rapidly effective.

### Folliculitis, furuncles, and carbuncles

Folliculitis occurs around hair follicles, caused by occlusion of the ostium with accompanying superficial inflammation and infection. Precipitating factors include trauma, chronic friction, occlusive clothing and chemicals, and excessive sweating. With deeper involvement an inflammatory nodule, or furuncle, is formed, and multiple furuncles can coalesce to form a carbuncle, usually on the posterior neck. *S. aureus* is the cause in most cases. Treatment should begin by addressing underlying causes, including diabetes mellitus. Simple folliculitis can be treated with antibacterial soaps such as Hibiclens, along with topical antibiotics. Moist heat and incision and drainage are used for larger lesions. Recurrent folliculitis or furuncles with surrounding cellulitis respond to systemic antibiotics.

A unique form of folliculitis, so-called "hot tub folliculitis," results from exposure to inadequately disinfected pools or spas contaminated by *Pseudomonas aeruginosa.* One to 2 days after exposure, pinpoint follicular pustules surrounded by bright red macules appear (Fig. 23-2), which resolve without treatment. Systemic infection is rare, but treatment with oral ciprofloxacin may be warranted, including widespread or highly symptomatic infection, and in health care workers.

***Syphilis.*** Syphilis, still common in certain sectors of the population, is an independent risk factor for human immunodeficiency virus (HIV) disease. The primary care practitioner must be vigilant and familiar with its many facets.

Acquired syphilis evolves through three main stages. Primary syphilis is characterized by a painless ulcer (chancre) arising at the inoculation site after an incubation period of 3 weeks (range 10 to 90 days). Because most cases are sexually acquired, any persistent anogenital lesion should be suspected. Regional adenopathy is common, and untreated lesions last 2 to 8 weeks. Additional diagnostic considerations include herpes simplex, chancroid, granuloma inguinale, trauma, and other infections. Dark field microscopy establishes the diagnosis; serologic tests are positive about 75% of the time.

Secondary syphilis begins about 6 weeks (or up to 6 months) after initial contact, most commonly as a widespread, papulosquamous eruption with constitutional symptoms and general lymphadenopathy. Involvement of palms and soles is highly suggestive (Fig. 23-3), as are fissured papules in intertrigious areas, macerated, flat anogenital lesions (condyloma lata), patchy alopecia, and eroded mucous membrane patches. Drug reactions, exanthems, and pityriasis rosea must be considered; but diagnosis can be established by serologic tests, which are nearly always positive.

After a variable latency period, about one third of untreated patients progress to tertiary syphilis, with gummatous skin and bone lesions, cardiovascular disease (aortitis), and neurologic manifestations.

***Diagnosis.*** Dark field microscopy of chancres is best performed at a sexually transmitted disease clinic. The venereal disease reference laboratory (VDRL) or rapid plasma reagin (RPR) tests are used to diagnose secondary or latent syphilis and to quantitatively assess response to therapy. The same test performed by the same laboratory is essential for accurate follow-up results. If positive, initial VDRL or RPR tests should be confirmed by a more specific test, such as fluorescent treponemal antibody absorption (FTA-Abs). All patients with syphilis should be tested for HIV, and contact tracing should be initiated through the local health department.

***Treatment.*** Benzathine penicillin G, 2.4 million units intramuscularly as a single dose, is the treatment for primary, secondary, or early (< 1 year) latent syphilis. Penicillin-allergic patients can use either doxycycline, 100 mg orally twice a day, for 2 weeks, or tetracycline or erythromycin, 500 mg orally four times a day for 2 weeks. Treatment of late latent or tertiary syphilis is best accomplished with benzathine penicillin G, 2.4 million intramuscularly in 3 weekly injections (see Chapter 65 for further details on sexually transmitted diseases).

## SUPERFICIAL FUNGAL INFECTIONS

Superficial fungal infections are divided into two broad categories: dermatophytoses and cutaneous candidiasis. Although dermatomycoses are among the most common infectious diseases in humans, their many clinical variations and their close resemblance to other skin diseases may cause them to be difficult to recognize. A careful skin scraping and accurate KOH examination, along with confirmative cultures when necessary, are essential to ensure proper diagnosis and effective treatment. Infections are caused by the genera *Trichophyton, Epidermophyton,* and *Microsporum;* but the exact species involved is of secondary importance. These mycoses, referred to collectively as dermatophytosis, ringworm, or tinea, are classified according to their location of infection.

### Tinea pedis

Tinea pedis, or athlete's foot, is the most common dermatophytosis. It can present acutely as a blistering eruption with vesicles, pustules, fissures, and marked inflammation. Lesions may burn or itch fiercely, and secondary bacterial infection is frequent (Fig. 23-4). A more common chronic form presents either as maceration and fissuring in toe webs, or as dry, reddish scaly patches around the foot, often in a "moccasin" distribution (Fig. 23-5). Chronic, noninflammatory types may be difficult to treat and frequently lead to development of nail involvement (onychomycosis). Differential diagnosis includes bacterial infections, candidiasis, acute or chronic eczematous conditions, psoriasis, and keratodermas. Topical treatment is usually sufficient for localized involvement, but highly inflamed, widespread, or resistant infection requires systemic treatment for 6 to 8 months (see Management).

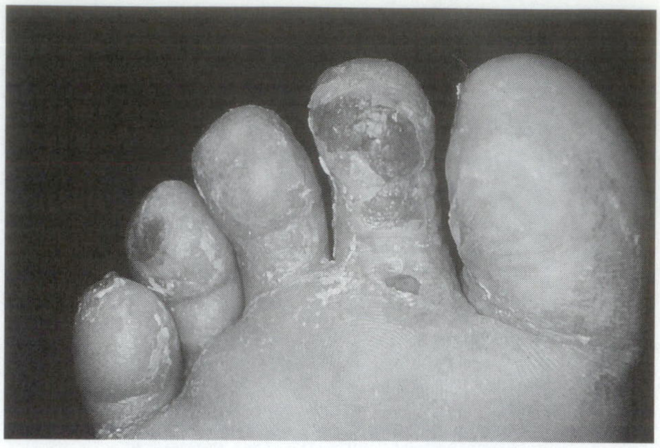

**Fig. 23-4.** Tinea pedis, vesicular inflammatory type. Note small vesicles and erosions.

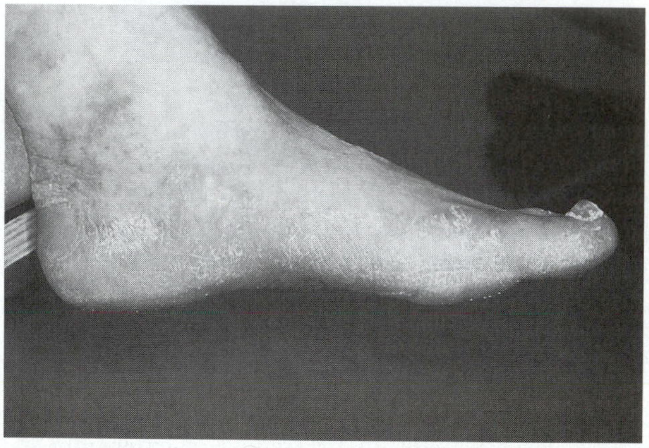

**Fig. 23-5.** Tinea pedis, chronic form. Note the moccasin distribution of scaling and slight erythema.

### Tinea manuum

Like tinea pedis, tinea of the hand can be eczematous, vesicular, and pruritic; but it is much more likely to be mildly red, dry, and scaly. Any combination of hand and/or foot involvement can be seen, most commonly as "two-foot, one hand disease." Treatment approaches are similar to those for tinea pedis.

### Tinea cruris

Tinea involvement of the groin area (jock itch) is characterized by raised, red, scaling, occasionally vesicular plaques, which can expand to involve the thigh, pubic, and perianal skin. Candidiasis, psoriasis, and erythrasma must be considered in the differential diagnosis, although unlike candidiasis, the penis and scrotum are generally spared. Topical treatment for 3 to 4 weeks is effective for most cases, along with attempts to minimize the chafing and excess moisture that precipitate infection.

### Tinea corporis

Fungal involvement of the trunk and extremities most often begins as one or more slightly raised, reddish, scaly patches, which slowly enlarge while clearing centrally (see Plate 17). These annular lesions represent classic "ringworm," but tinea corporis also may be vesiculopustular, eczematous, or nodular. Furthermore, all annular lesions are not ringworm: Sarcoidosis, granuloma annulare, urticaria, and gyrate erythema, to name a few, can present as annular lesions. Psoriasis, contact dermatitis, tinea versicolor, and pityriasis rosea are additional diagnostic considerations.

Superficial, localized infection is usually cured with topical treatment applied twice a day for 2 to 4 weeks. Deeper or more inflamed areas require systemic treatment.

### Tinea facei

Often difficult to diagnose, tinea facei may be present as raised annular plaques, or subtle, indistinct and slightly scaly patches. It may be mistaken for polymorphous light eruption, lupus erythematosus, seborrheic dermatitis, or allergic contact dermatitis, and generally responds to twice a day topical treatment for 2 to 4 weeks.

### Tinea capitis

Scalp ringworm occurs most often in urban children but is also seen in adults. It can present as one or more scaly plaques with short stalks of broken hair ("gray patch" type), or more commonly as smooth, alopecic plaques with pinpoint hair stubs, broken off at scalp level ("black dot" type). Occasionally, lesions are highly inflamed, resulting in an indurated, tender, boggy mass exuding pus called a kerion. Toxic symptoms and adenopathy may be present, and scarring alopecia can result if not treated. These lesions are often misdiagnosed as bacterial infections.

Treatment with systemic antifungals for 4 to 6 weeks is required, along with aggressive local care and consideration of concomitant treatment with prednisone to minimize inflammation and scarring.

### Onychomycosis

Tinea of the fingernails and toenails usually occurs as an extension of adjacent skin involvement. It takes the form of thickened, yellowish, disfigured nails with either proximal or distal nail plate separation (onycholysis) and occasional involvement of adjacent nail folds (paronychia). Onychomycosis must be distinguished from similar infection caused by candidiasis, as well as psoriasis, lichen planus, and contact dermatitis (such as from nail products). Management generally has been unsatisfactory, even with systemic agents, due to prolonged treatment times and high relapse rate. Newer topical and systemic agents promise increased efficacy and shorter treatment periods.

***Management.*** Numerous topical agents are available for treating superficial fungal infections (see Table 20-5 on p. 344). The imidazoles provide broad-spectrum coverage against dermatophytes and *Candida,* and several, including econazole and sulconazole, are also effective against some gram-positive bacteria. Topical steroids blunt local host defenses, may exacerbate infection, and lead to atrophy in occluded skin areas. They have little, if any, place in the treatment of superficial fungal infections.

Griseofulvin is safe and well tolerated as a systemic agent. The ultramicrosize form is generally used, in doses of 250 to 500 mg/day in adults, taken once or twice a day. For tinea infections of the nails, 500 to 750 mg/day is usually effective. It should be taken with food that enhances absorption and minimizes side effects, most commonly gastrointestinal disturbances and headaches. Griseofulvin use has declined with increased development of resistant infections and the advent of newer agents.

The imidazole agent ketoconazole is more effective than griseofulvin, and unlike griseofulvin it is useful against *Candida albicans.* Its widespread use is limited by occasional severe hepatotoxicity.

The newer triazoles, fluconazole and itraconazole, appear to be superior to other agents against dermatophytes, with possibly fewer side effects and the promise of shorter treatment times. Itraconozole accumulates within keratinized tissue and may be especially effective in onychomycosis. Terbinafine, an allylamine, may be useful in resistant infections as it is the first oral fungicidal agent. These newer agents have little use in dermatomycoses; much more study is needed to better define their indications, side effects, drug interactions, and dosage schedules.

### Candidiasis

Cutaneous candidiasis is usually caused by *C. albicans,* and may be associated with underlying conditions such as diabetes mellitus, immunosuppression, or use of systemic antibiotics. Moisture, heat, and maceration greatly predispose to infection, which preferentially involves skin folds of the axillae, groin, breasts, and corners of the mouth (perlèche). Infection is characterized by burning, beefy red erythema with scale and adjacent ("satellite") pustules (see Plate 34).

Candidal involvement of the nail unit can present acutely with pain, redness, and swelling of nail folds (paronychia) or as a chronic form mimicking dermatophyte infection. It greatly favors those exposed to constant wet work, such as health care workers.

***Management.*** KOH examination and cultures, including bacterial, are necessary for a rational approach to treatment. Most superficial infections respond to twice daily topical applications of nystatin or an imidazole cream, along with attention to any predisposing conditions. Severe, resistant, or paronychial infections require systemic treatment with ketoconazole or a newer triazole agent.

## DEEP FUNGAL INFECTIONS

### Sporotrichosis

Sporotrichosis is caused by traumatic inoculation of the organism *Sporothrix schenckii,* most commonly on the distal arm or hand. It is often seen in gardeners or others exposed to thorny bushes, straw, or sphagnum peat moss. It can present as a localized ulcer or nodule, or more classically, an ulcerated papule followed by a chain of painless nodules along lymphatics. Systemic involvement is minimal in immunocompetent hosts. The differential diagnosis includes atypical mycobacterial infection, other deep fungal infections, sarcoidosis, or halogenoderma. Treatment is usually with saturated solution of potassium iodide or systemic imidazole or triazole.

### Blastomycosis

Although the portal of entry for *Blastomyces dermatitidis* is the lung, it often first presents on the skin as an ulcerated nodule, quickly becoming an enlarged, verrucous granuloma. It may be skin limited and mimic other granulomatous disease, but usually includes lung or other organ involvement. It is best diagnosed by tissue culture, and best treated with amphotericin B.

### Histoplasmosis

In most patients histoplasmosis is a self-limited pulmonary infection caused by the saprophytic fungus *Histoplasma capsulatum.* Occasionally, the disease disseminates and ulcerated granulomas develop on skin and mucous membranes. This complication occurs with increased frequency in immunocompromised patients, especially those with acquired immune deficiency syndrome (AIDS). Amphotericin B is the treatment of choice in most of the situations.

### Coccidioidomycosis

Coccidioidomycosis, caused by *Coccidioides immitis,* is primarily a pulmonary disease. In a small percentage of patients, however, it disseminates and forms granulomatous nodules, which coalesce to form ulcerated, verrucous plaques, usually on the head and neck. Disease is best diagnosed serologically. Management of disseminated infection is quite difficult.

## VIRAL INFECTIONS

### Human papillomavirus infection

Long considered benign and uninteresting, infection with human papillomavirus (HPV) has gained considerable importance, emerging as the second most common sexually transmitted disease in the United States and linked to development of genitourinary tract carcinomas. To date more than 60 specific subtypes of HPV have been identified. Although many of these subtypes have been loosely associated with a particular body region, for most purposes these associations are not clinically relevant.

***Common warts.*** Common warts (verrucae vulgares) are quite polymorphous on skin. They begin tiny and smooth, but progress over weeks to months to become typical, raised, keratotic, and often cauliflower-like papules. Common warts occur most often on the extremities but can be found anywhere on the skin in persons of all ages (see Plate 2).

Planar, or flat warts, occur primarily on the face, hands, and pretibial surfaces as tiny, slightly raised, flesh-colored papules. They can be numerous and refractory to treatment.

Palmar and plantar warts present as thick, endophytic papules or plaques, often multiple, which may be exquisitely painful when located over pressure points. These warts may be distinguished from a callous, which they resemble, by the appearance of tiny black dots or bleeding points after paring (Fig. 23-6).

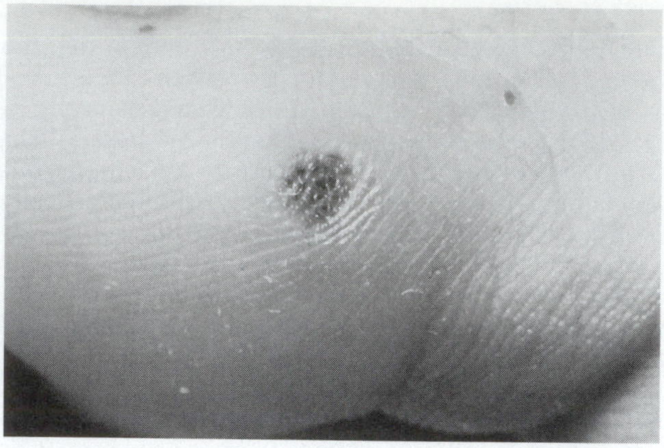

**Fig. 23-6.** Plantar wart (verruca). Note the pinpoint thromboses after the lesion is pared.

***Genital warts.*** An enlarging body of evidence has documented the explosive rise in incidence of genital HPV infection and its recognition as a sexually transmitted disease. Most important though, is the association of certain HPV types, including 16, 18, and 31, with the development of intraepithelial neoplasia of the uterine cervix. Recognition of genital HPV infection by the primary care practitioners has become vital.

Genital warts, or condyloma accuminata, present as single or multiple papillary or fingerlike proliferations which may coalesce to form large, moist, cauliflower-like tumors on mucosal or nonmucosal skin (Fig. 23-7). Presence on the vulva is an important indicator of vaginal or cervical involvement. Subclinical infection is common and can be identified by application of gauze soaked with 4% acetic acid for 10 minutes, which causes inapparent lesions to show up as pinpoint, white macules or papules. The technique is limited by frequent false-positive results.

Bowenoid papulosis is a clinicopathologic variant of HPV infection, in which multiple, smooth, slightly raised papules, ranging from flesh colored to reddish brown, develop on genital skin. Although clinically benign, these lesions show squamous cell carinoma in situ on biopsy and are usually caused by HPV 16, one of the oncogenic subtypes. Their presence in an affected female, or female sexual partner of an affected male, warrants referral to a gynecologist.

***Management.*** Because many warts regress spontaneously, some patients, especially children, may not require treatment. For common warts, topical application of keratolytics, such as salicylic acid (Occlusal), or salicylic and lactic acid in flexible collodion (Duofilm), is useful when applied directly to the wart at bedtime followed by paring of the dead skin the next morning. Cryotherapy with liquid nitrogen for 10 to 20 seconds is also effective.

Flat warts often respond to cryotherapy, but subsequent pigment alteration occurs easily, especially on the face of darker-skinned individuals. Patients also should be advised to avoid shaving or scrubbing affected areas.

Palmar and plantar warts can be refractory, and aggressive treatment with keratolytics and liquid nitrogen is the usual initial approach. Surgical excision and laser ablation are treatments of last resort.

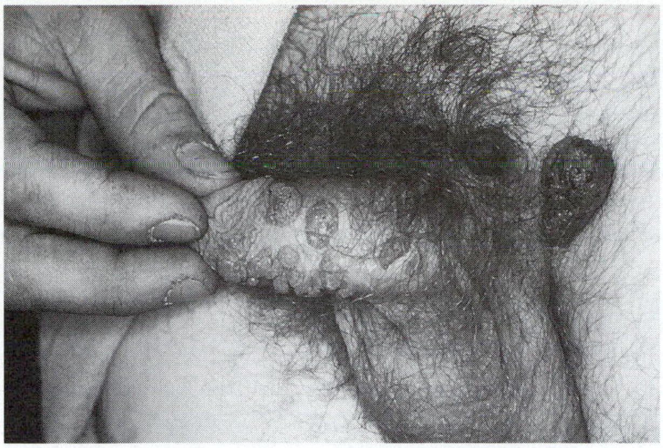

**Fig. 23-7.** Condylomata. Verrucoid pigmented lesions on the penis.

Moist genital lesions respond to topical treatment with 25% to 40% podophyllin, applied weekly until lesions resolve. Treated areas are washed after 3 to 6 hours as tolerated. Podophyllin is toxic and can be a severe irritant and thus should not be dispensed. An additional agent, podophylotoxin (Condylox), is available by prescription for home use by the patient. It is less irritating than podophyllin and is useful in some cases. Liquid nitrogen, and occasionally electrodesiccation, may be necessary for resistant warts.

Referral to a dermatologist should be considered for additional treatment modalities, and for evaluation of persistent lesions, especially of the mouth, genital and periungual areas, where occult squamous cell carcinoma is a concern.

### Herpesvirus infections

***Herpes simplex.*** Herpes simplex virus (HSV) (see Plate 5) infection is an acute, self-limited eruption that is characterized by groups of small vesicles on an erythematous base. After infection by direct inoculation from another individual, the virus replicates within the skin where it involves the sensory nerves. The viral capsid is subsequently transported to the nerve root ganglion where it remains latent, with the potential for reactivation and reinfection at any time. The HSV-1 or HSV-2 subtypes can involve nearly any mucocutaneous or visceral site.

***Oral-facial infection.*** Gingivostomatitis and pharyngitis are the most frequent primary HSV-1 infections, occurring primarily in children. Lesions develop anywhere in the mouth, on the lips, or face. Numerous rapidly evolving vesicles rupture to form painful, necrotic ulcers, associated with fever, malaise, anorexia, and cervical adenopathy. Infection lasts 1 to 3 weeks and heals without scarring. Recurrences present most frequently as herpes labialis (fever blisters, cold sores) where prodromal stinging or burning is quickly followed by one or more typical painful vesicles, usually located on the lips. Viral shedding lasts until the lesions have crusted over, approximately 5 to 7 days. Fever and ultraviolet light may precipitate the recurrences.

***Genital infection.*** Primary genital herpes, usually caused by HSV-2, is characterized by bilaterally distributed groups of vesicles. The infection may also involve the cervix and urethra, with accompanying fever, headache, and malaise. Local symptoms include pain, itching, dysuria, and tender inguinal adenopathy. Viral shedding may persist for 10 to 12 days or more, and the complete course lasts 3 to 4 weeks. Patients with clinical or serologic evidence of prior HSV infection of either type may have a milder illness than those with true primary infections.

Recurrences vary considerably in severity and duration, and asymptomatic viral shedding is not uncommon. Prodromal tingling or burning commonly precedes the eruption, which is unilateral, and usually without adenopathy. Lesions can be painful, but the course is milder than primary disease and lasts 7 to 10 days. Recurrence rates also vary greatly, but most patients will experience at least one within the first 12 months, and average three to four recurrences per year. Patients should be reassured that recurrences tend to become milder and less frequent over time.

***Herpetic whitlow.*** HSV infection of the finger is characterized by redness, swelling, and painful vesicles or pustules resembling bacterial infection. Systemic symptoms and localized adenopathy accompany primary infection, but recurrences are infrequent.

***Herpetic eye infection.*** Herpetic eye infection presents with pain, conjunctivitis, photophobia, and characteristic dendritic corneal ulcers. Both HSV-1 and HSV-2, and to a lesser extent varicella-zoster virus, can cause infection, which can result in blindness. Topical steroids may worsen infection. Patients with herpetic eye infection should be referred emergently to an ophthalmologist.

***Eczema herpeticum.*** Eczema herpeticum occurs in patients with an underlying skin problem, such as atopic dermatitis or Darier's disease, which cause altered skin integrity and thereby allow widespread superinfection with HSV. Diffuse vesiculopustular, eroded, and crusted lesions are accompanied by fever, pain, and adenopathy. Referral to a dermatologist should be considered.

***Postherpetic erythema multiforme.*** Recurrent HSV infection may be followed by development of oral or targetoid acral lesions of erythema multiforme. These lesions occur as a hypersensitivity reaction and respond to suppressive treatment with acyclovir (see Management).

**Laboratory evaluation.** Most HSV infections can be diagnosed by the clinical presentation. When in doubt the quickest and least expensive confirmatory test is the Tzanck smear (see Chapter 19). Like all diagnostic tests for herpesvirus infections, the greatest yield is from intact vesicles or fresh erosions.

Viral culture for HSV confirms the diagnosis, with results usually reported within 48 to 72 hours in most cases. Unfortunately, recent evidence suggests that culture for HSV is not as sensitive as once thought. The more sensitive polymerase chain reaction assay for HSV, from lesional tissue, is not routinely available to clinicians.

When a more timely diagnosis is needed in a symptomatic patient, direct fluorescent antibody tests can be rapid and highly sensitive.

Serologic tests are unreliable in documenting acute HSV infection, but can help demonstrate the presence of a previous infection and are useful in identifying asymptomatic infection in patients undergoing immunosuppressive regimens who should receive prophylactic acyclovir.

**Management.** Most acute primary oral-facial or genital HSV infections can be safely treated with acyclovir, 200 mg orally five times a day for 5 to 10 days. Significant improvement in the rate of healing and the resolution of symptoms can be achieved, especially if initiated early, but treatment has no effect on the development of recurrences.

The benefits of oral acyclovir for acute recurrent disease are less dramatic, but long-term daily therapy to suppress frequent recurrences is safe and effective. Initial doses of 200 mg three times a day to 400 mg twice a day can be tapered as tolerated, with periodic drug holidays to reassess the need to continue. Long-term suppressive therapy does not eliminate ganglionic latency, and reactivation occurs when treatment is stopped.

Topical acyclovir ointment has minimal effect on typical primary or recurrent HSV infection, but has been used adjunctively for chronic disease. Intravenous acyclovir is generally reserved for immunocompromised patients and those with central nervous system (CNS) involvement, but it can be used in severely ill patients with first-episode HSV infection. Other adjunctive therapies include analgesics, sitz baths and Burow's compresses, and topical xylocaine ointment or viscous xylocaine mouthwash.

**Prevention.** Condoms are partially effective in preventing spread to a sexual partner, but abstinence is suggested until complete healing and reepithelialization occurs. Sunscreen agents to block ultraviolet-activated recurrent labial HSV are useful.

***Herpes zoster.*** Herpes zoster (shingles) (see Plate 16) is an acute vesicular eruption caused by reactivation of latent virus from a previous varicella infection. Reactivation can occur at any time and may be triggered by illness, immunosuppression, debilitation, and advancing age. The eruption is unilateral and follows the dermatome of the affected ganglion, although involvement of adjacent dermatomes is common.

**History.** A prodrome of 1 to 4 days or more is common. It consists of tingling, itch, or pain and tenderness, and often is accompanied by systemic symptoms. The pain can be severe, suggesting acute myocardial infarction or acute abdomen in thoracic or lumbar dermatomes. *Physical examination.* Following the prodrome, an eruption develops consisting of several or multiple groups of vesicles on an erythematous base. Vesicles umbilicate, become purulent, rupture and ulcerate, and over 10 to 14 days progress to crusting and complete healing.

Infection may involve motor neurons as well, usually of the same dermatome, and can lead to nerve palsies, weakness, and urinary retention. Zoster in the ophthalmic distribution can lead to severe ocular complications. Dissemination of infection also can occur, primarily in immunocompromised individuals and those with certain underlying malignancies.

The most common sequelae of zoster is postherpetic neuralgia, in which pain in the involved region may persist for months or rarely years. It occurs in 10% to 15% of patients and is more common in those over 60 years of age. Scarring may be seen, especially after severe infection.

**Laboratory evaluation.** Most cases can be diagnosed clinically, but as with HSV infections, Tzanck smears can be a rapid and reliable diagnostic tool (see Chapter 19). Fluorescent antibody tests and tissue culture can provide confirmatory evidence of infection.

**Management.** Pain control is the mainstay of treatment in zoster and should include narcotic analgesics when indicated. In younger and middle-aged patients, who tend to have milder disease courses, pain control and attention to possible secondary infection may be all that is necessary.

Acyclovir attenuates the course and symptoms of herpes zoster. For optimal effect therapy must be initiated early at a usual adult dose of 800 mg taken orally five times a day. It is still considered safe at these doses, but gastrointestinal intolerance is greater, CNS effects such as confusion and lethargy can occur, and the patient should be well hydrated. In patients with reduced renal function, lower doses are required.

Unfortunately, acyclovir has no effect on subsequent pain. Concurrent treatment with prednisone has traditionally been given to lessen the pain and duration of postherpetic neuralgia and is typically reserved for persons over age 55. The usual adult dose is 60 mg/day for 7 days tapered over 2 to 3 weeks. Its use is controversial, however, and must be weighed against known risks and side effects.

***Molluscum contagiosum.*** Molluscum contagiosum (see Chapter 65) is a benign papular eruption, caused by a poxvirus, which is often sexually transmitted in adults. It is characterized by multiple, small, dome-shaped, flesh-colored papules with distinctive central umbilication from which caseous material can be expressed. After an average incubation period of 2 to 3 months, lesions develop primarily on face, trunk, and extremities in children, and on thighs, abdomen, buttocks, and genital areas in adults. The mode of transmission can be sexual, nonsexual, or by fomites. Autoinoculation is also possible, causing linear lesions and distant spread.

Diagnosis is usually clinical, but molluscum contagiosum can be mistaken for many lesions, including warts, nevi, adnexal tumors, and keratoacanthomas. If necessary, the diagnosis can be confirmed by histopathology. Giant or widespread lesions should alert the practitioner to possible immunodeficiency (see Chapter 68).

Without treatment, the lesions can persist for months or for years, but they respond to cryotherapy, light curettage, or any sufficiently destructive or irritating technique. Treatment, which can cause scarring, must be weighed against the benign and self-limited nature of the infection.

### Mycobacterial infections of the skin

***Atypical mycobacteria.*** See Chapter 114 for discussion.

***Tuberculosis and leprosy.*** See Chapter 24 for discussion.

## INFESTATIONS

### Pediculosis

Three forms of lice infest humans: head lice (pediculosis capitis), body lice (pediculosis corporis) and pubic or "crab" lice (*Phthirus pubis*). All are obligate blood-sucking ectoparasites, which produce eggs (nits) that attach firmly to the base of the human's hair shafts or to clothing.

*Head lice* infestation occurs only on scalp hair, particularly the nape of the neck, where intense pruritus may lead to secondary excoriations and furunculosis. Adult lice can be found moving about the scalp, but diagnosis is made more easily by identifying nits. Head lice infestation is rarely seen in blacks.

*Body lice* are similar in appearance, but unlike head lice can be vectors for systemic diseases, such as typhus. Females lay eggs in clothing along seams, where lice reside, emerging to feed on the skin of the back, shoulders, and waist. Transmission occurs by contact with infested skin, clothing, or bedding. Widespread pruritic dermatitis can result, along with excoriations and secondary infection from scratching.

*Pubic lice* are usually contracted from sexual intercourse, but clothing or linen are possible sources. Pubic lice are shorter and rounder than head or body lice, appearing as small yellowish or gray spots. In addition to the genital area, skin, hair of the face, eyelashes, trunk, and axillae can be involved (see Chapter 65.)

***Management.*** Control of all types of louse infestation includes attention to affected clothing, bed sheets, towels, combs and brushes, and measures to limit spread to others. Hot water laundering, dry cleaning, and use of a disinfectant (e.g., Lysol) for combs and brushes are effective measures, as is isolation of fomites for 1 to 2 weeks.

Treatment of head lice in adults is best accomplished with 1% gamma benzene hexachloride shampoo Kwell (lindane) applied to hair for 10 minutes and then thoroughly washed off, or 1% primethrin (Nix), applied as a cream rinse after shampooing, left on for 10 minutes, and then rinsed. Nonprescription products containing pyrethrins and piperonyl butoxide (Rid) are also quite effective. All of the treatments probably should be repeated in 1 week, and nits should be dislodged with tweezers or a fine-toothed comb.

Body and pubic lice are treated by application of 1% gamma benzene hexachloride (Kwell) lotion or shampoo for not more than 8 to 10 hours, then completely washed off. Over-the-counter regimens (pyrethrin with piperonyl butoxide) are also effective.

Close contacts should be treated in all types of pediculosis. Gamma benzene hexachloride can be neurotoxic and should be avoided in patients with widespread dermatitis, pregnant or nursing women, and children less than 3 years of age.

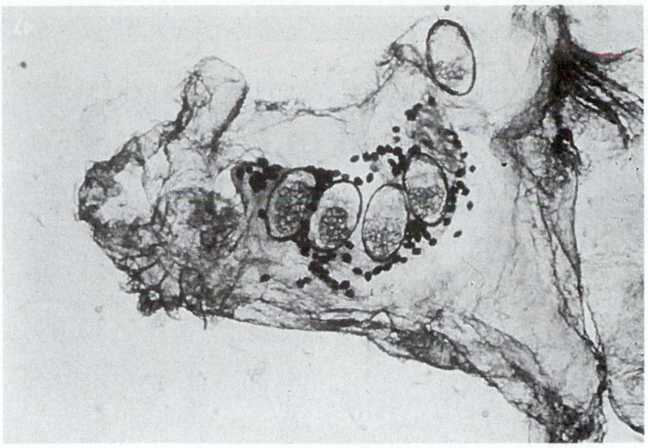

**Fig. 23-8.** Scabies. KOH preparation demonstrating scabetic mites and eggs.

*Scabies* (see Chapter 65 and Plate 35). Scabies is caused by infestation with the itch mite *Sarcoptes scabiei,* resulting in intensely pruritic vesicles, faint red papules, or short linear burrows (see Plate 35). Sites of predilection include finger webs, wrists, axillae, and penis, with sparing above the neck except in infants. Keratotic, crusted scabies (Norwegian scabies) is a variant seen mostly in the debilitated or immunosuppressed patient, in which widespread, crusted lesions teeming with mites are not accompanied by pruritus.

Because the differential diagnosis for scabies includes nearly all pruritic dermatoses, a slide prepared from scrapings of multiple suspected lesions should be prepared to demonstrate mites or ova (Fig. 23-8). Treatment of the nonpregnant adult is usually with 1% lindane (Kwell) lotion applied from the neck down (requires about 1 oz), washed off after 8 to 10 hours, and repeated once only in 5 days. Limiting the prescribed amount helps prevent CNS toxicity and overuse dermatitis. Alternative regimens include 5% precipitated sulfur in petrolatum applied daily for 3 days and repeated in 1 week, or 5% permethrin cream, applied for 6 to 8 hours. As with pediculosis, infested clothing and bedding and close contacts should be treated simultaneously. Patients should be reminded that posttreatment hypersensitivity and pruritis can persist for several weeks. Topical triamcinolone 0.1% cream can be considered to help alleviate the itch.

## BIBLIOGRAPHY

Beutner KR: Rational use of acyclovir in the treatment of mucocutaneous herpes simplex virus and varicella zoster virus infections, *Semin Dermatol* 11:256, 1992.

Buntin DM et al: Sexually transmitted diseases: viruses and ectoparasites, *J Am Acad Dermatol* 25:527, 1991.

Centers for Disease Control and Prevention (CDC): *Sexually transmitted disease treatment guidelines,* 1993, Atlanta.

Roseeuw D, De Doncker P: New approaches in the treatment of onychomycosis, *J Am Acad Dermatol* 29(1):S45, 1993.

Smith EB: Topical antifungal drugs in the treatment of tinea pedis, tinea cruris, and tinea corporis, *J Am Acad Dermatol* 28(5 Pt 1):S24, 1993.

Stiller MJ, Sangueza OP, Shupack JL: Systemic drugs in the treatment of dermatophytoses, *Int J Dermatol* 32(1):16, 1993.

CHAPTER

# 24A Miscellaneous Diseases of the Skin

**Denise Ann Burke**
**John McVey Burket**

## ERYTHEMA NODOSUM

***Epidemiology/etiology.*** Erythema nodosum is a hypersensitivity reaction to an underlying disease process, although it also can occur spontaneously. The box below lists underlying disease entities. Although both males and females can be affected, during the reproductive years women are more often involved than men.

***Pathophysiology.*** Although the actual mechanism is unknown, it is believed to be an immunologic reaction to antigenic stimuli.

***History and physical examination.*** Clinically, the lesions are tender, red, warm, subcutaneous nodules that are more prevalent over the anterior legs; however, they also can be seen in any area that has subcutaneous fat (see Plate 36). The individual lesions tend to resolve spontaneously after about 3 to 6 weeks, but new lesions can continue to develop.

***Laboratory.*** Histopathologic examination demonstrates a septal panniculitis without vasculitis. Laboratory tests should be obtained to rule out underlying disease processes.

***Differential diagnosis.*** See the box at right for differential diagnosis of erythema nodosum.

### Underlying disease processes with erythema nodosum

**Infectious**
***Bacterial***
Brucellosis
*Campylobacter*
Cat scratch disease
Leptospirosis
Salmonella
Streptococcal
Syphilis
Tularemia
*Yersinia enterocolitica*

***Mycobacterium***
Tuberculosis

**Fungal**
Blastomycosis
Coccidioidomycosis
Dermatophytes
Histoplasmosis

**Virus**
Coxsackie virus/enterovirus
Herpes simplex
Infectious mononucleosis
Paravaccinia

***Chlamydia***
Lymphogranuloma venereum
Psittacosis

**Protozoan**
Toxoplasmosis

**Medications**
Antibiotics
Barbiturates
Bromides
Immunizations/vaccinations
Iodides
Oral contraceptives*
Phenacetin
Salicylates
Sulfonamides

**Inflammatory bowel disease†**
Crohn's disease
Ulcerative colitis

**Malignant disease**
Lymphoma or leukemia
Postradiation therapy

**Behçet's disease**

**Sarcoidosis**

**Inhalants (industrial chemicals) and ingestants**

**Foreign tissue**
Blood transfusion
Grafts
Pregnancy
Transplantations

**Damaged tissue**
Chronic abscesses
Hamartomas
Hematomas

**Collagen vascular disease**

*In the United States, these are the most common causes.
†Correlates with disease activity but not duration.

*Management.* The treatment of the underlying process is essential. Supportive care includes bed rest, leg elevation, wet compresses, and support stockings. Medical treatment includes nonsteroidal antiinflammatory drugs, systemic steroids (when stopped, lesions may recur), potassium iodide (400 to 900 mg/day).

## PYODERMA GANGRENOSUM

Pyoderma gangrenosum is an idiopathic inflammatory pustular/ulcerative reaction that is often mistaken for an infectious process.

*Epidemiology/etiology.* The etiology of pyoderma gangrenosum is unknown, but is thought to be immunologic. Bacteria may be cultured from the lesions, but this is thought to be a result of secondary infection.

Approximately 50% of pyoderma gangrenosum cases are associated with an underlying disease process (see box at top right). The highest association is with intestinal and rheumatologic inflammatory conditions.

*Pathophysiology.* Although the exact mechanism is unknown, it is thought to be an immunologic process. The large number of diseases that can be associated with pyoderma gangrenosum contributes to the confusion regarding the development of the lesions. Neutrophils appear to have a major role in the disease process.

*History and physical examination.* Clinical lesions begin as an erythematous papule, pustule, or plaque that enlarges, ulcerates, and eventually scars (see Plate 37). The ulcer's border is undermined and violaceous, with a distal erythematous rim. Pathergy (lesions occurring at sites of skin trauma) is common. The lesions are painful. Although any body area may be involved including mucous membranes, the lower extremities are the most common sites.

*Laboratory.* Skin biopsies, although not entirely diagnostic, frequently demonstrate abnormalities that are suggestive of pyoderma gangrenosum and help rule out infectious causes. Laboratory studies to rule out underlying disease processes may be necessary.

*Differential diagnosis.* See the box at bottom right.

### Differential diagnosis of erythema nodosum

- Contusion
- Arthropod bite
- Superficial thrombophlebitis (large vein in center of lesion)
- Erythema induratum (septal panniculitis with vasculitis)
- Erythema nodosum leprosum (leukocytosis vasculitis in dermis and subcutaneous tissue)
- Benign cutaneous polyarteritis nodosum (medium-sized vessel)

### Diseases associated with pyoderma gangrenosum

- Inflammatory bowel disease
  - Ulcerative colitis
  - Crohn's disease
- Rheumatoid arthritis
- Leukemia
  - AML
  - CML
  - ALL
- Lymphoma
  - Hodgkin's
  - Non-Hodgkin's
- Adenocarcinoma-prostate, colon
- Behçet's disease
- Carcinoid
- Chronic active hepatitis
- Congenital dysfibrinogenemia
- Diabetes mellitus
- Diverticulitis
- Gastric and duodenal ulcers
- Myelofibrosis
- Myeloma
- Osteomyelosclerosis
- Paraproteinemias (especially IgA)
- Paroxysmal nocturnal hemoglobin
- Polycythemia
- Primary thrombocytopenia
- Red cell aplasia
- Sarcoid
- Systemic lupus erythematosus
- Takayasu arthritis (Japan)
- Wegener's granulomatosis

### Differential diagnosis of pyoderma gangrenosum

- Arthropod bite
- Halogenoderma
- Panniculitis
- Atypical mycobacterium
- Behçet's disease
- Brown recluse spider
- Carbuncle
- Chronic herpes in the immunocompromised
- Clostridial infection
- Coumadin or heparin necrosis
- Deep mycosis
- Ecthyma gangrenosum
- Factitial
- Necrotizing vasculitis
- Postoperative gangrene
- Pyoderma vegetans
- Systemic lupus erythematosus
- Stasis ulcer
- Syphilitic gumma
- Tropical ulcer
- Ulcerated necrobiosis lipoidica
- Wegener's granulomatosis

### Management of pyoderma gangrenosum

**Local**

Whirlpool, tub bath
Local measures to keep ulcer clean and free of secondary infection
Biologic dressings
Compression
Topical antibiotics
Debridement
Wet-dry dressings
Elevation
Bedrest
Hyperbaric oxygen
Intralesional steroids
(Triamcinolone 3-5 mg/ml)

**Systemic**

Prednisone (40 to 200 mg/day)*
Dapsone (start 25 to 50 mg/day) or 100 to 500 mg/day with steroids
Sulfasalazine (4 to 6 g qd; decrease to .5-1 g qd after response) alternative to dapsone
Minocycline HCl (100 mg qd)
Cytotoxic agents†
- Azathioprine
- Cyclosporin A
- Cyclophosphamide
- Chlorambucil
- 6-Mercaptopurine
- Melphalan
- Cytosine arabinoside
- Daunorubicin

*Most common systemic therapies
†Usually used for underlying disease processes but seems to help some cases of pyoderma gangrenosum, even if the underlying process is quiescent.

*Management.* The treatment of choice is to treat the underlying disease process. When this is not possible, however, the box above lists some alternatives.

## NONINFECTIOUS GRANULOMATOUS DISEASES (TABLE 24A-1)

### Necrobiosis lipoidica (diabeticorum)

*Epidemiology/etiology.* Necrobiosis lipoidica is an idiopathic inflammatory skin disease frequently associated with diabetes mellitus. The disease is more frequent in women and usually develops over the anterior lower legs. Sixty percent to 75% of patients with necrobiosis lipoidica have either diabetes or an abnormal glucose tolerance curve, but the mechanism of the relationship is unknown.

*Pathophysiology.* Although the etiology is unknown, some insulin-dependent diabetics with necrobiosis lipoidica have increased alpha II macroglobulin, factor VIII-related antigen, and fibronectin. Circulating immune complexes may have a pathogenic role in the vascular occlusive changes seen in the lesions of necrobiosis lipoidica. Deposits of immunoglobulins and complement in the vessel walls and fibrinogen in the necrobiotic areas suggest an immune complex reaction.

*History and physical examination.* The patient, usually a diabetic and often a woman, develops dusky red papule(s) on the lower anterior leg(s). In time the lesions become sclerodermoid in their appearance, enlarging and becoming yellow-brown in coloration. The lesions appear atrophic yet are indurated to palpation and often have a yellow coloration in the center with telangiectases coursing through the lesions associated with an erythematous border (see Plate 38). While most commonly involving the pretibial areas, the lesions may appear on forearms, trunk, face, scalp, palms, and soles. Occasionally the plaques ulcerate.

*Laboratory.* Elevation of blood glucose and/or an abnormal glucose tolerance curve are common findings. Biopsy demonstrates thinning of the epidermis and a dermal infiltrate consisting of histiocytes arranged in a palisaded pattern, lymphocytes, and plasma cells. Collagen degeneration is a common finding.

*Differential diagnosis.* Erythema nodosum commonly occurs on the pretibial area but is distinguished clinically by extreme tenderness of the lesions. Histopathologically, the picture is that of a septal panniculitis, not a palisaded granuloma.

Nodular vasculitis (erythema induratum) may occur on the lower legs, but is usually lateral or posterior rather than anteriorly placed. Histologically, arteritis is in the subcutis associated with a lobular panniculitis.

*Management.* Intralesional corticosteroid (2.5 mg triamcinolone/ml) has been a mainstay of treatment but may not be appropriate with severely atrophic lesions, although it could be used at the peripheral border to prevent further spread. Occasionally, intralesional steroids may induce ulceration.

### Granuloma annulare

Granuloma annulare is a granulomatous response in the skin that frequently presents with annular erythematous papules and plaques.

*Epidemiology/etiology.* The cause of granuloma annulare is unknown. The female/male ratio is 2:1. Of the patients with localized granuloma annulare, 70% are less than 30 years of age, and more than 40% are less than 15 years of age.

*History and physical examination.* Most patients present with a rapid onset of asymptomatic or slightly pruritic lesions, which are usually an annular configuration of confluent papules (see Plate 39). At times they may form plaques and nodules. They tend to be located around joints, especially the elbows, wrists, and ankles. The lesions may be generalized, especially in older patients.

*Laboratory.* Histologically, palisaded granulomas (collections of histiocytes) are found in the dermis, along with

**Table 24A-1.** Noninfectious granulomatous diseases

| Disease | Etiology | Histology | History | Physical examination | Laboratory | Differential diagnosis | Management |
|---|---|---|---|---|---|---|---|
| Gout | Hyperuricemia | Deposition of urate giving palisaded granuloma | Monoarticular arthritis | Inflamed nodules ear helix and around joints | Hyperuricemia and increase in ESR | Darwinian tubercle of ear<br>Rheumatoid arthritis | Colchicine, allopurinol |
| Lichen nitidus | Unknown | Circumscribed collection of histiocytes and lymphocytes engorging single dermal papilla | Sudden onset of mild or no pruritus | Myriads of pinpoint to pinhead size papules, penis, arms, and abdomen | No changes | Lichen planus | ? Combination of psoralen and ultraviolet A for widespread involvement |
| Lichen striatus | Unknown | Histiocytes in papillary dermis with focal vacuolar interface dermatitis | Sudden onset of linear rash in a child | Unilateral linear papules on extremities and sides of neck | No changes | Linear psoriasis<br>Linear lichen planus<br>Linear epithelial nevus | Observation for spontaneous resolution |
| Rheumatoid nodules | Rheumatoid arthritis<br>Lupus erythematosus<br>Rheumatic fever | Deposition of fibrin surrounded by palisaded granuloma | Arthralgias, fever | Subcutaneous nodules near joints | Increase in ESR<br>Positive autoantibody | Gout<br>Granuloma annulare | Dependent on etiology |
| Rosacea | Basically unknown<br>? spicy food<br>? mental stress | Tuberculoid granuloma with telangiectases | Middle age eruption in central aspect of face, papular | Telangiectases, erythematous papules nose and cheeks | No changes | Lupus erythematosus<br>Acne vulgaris<br>Seborrhea | Tetracycline, topical metronidazole |
| Ruptured follicular cyst(s) | Extrusion of keratin from follicular cyst into dermis | Keratin fragments surrounded by foreign body granuloma | Dermal nodule that became inflamed | Dermal nodule face, scalp, neck or trunk with associated erythema | No changes | Pillar cyst<br>Boil<br>Lipoma | Compresses, antibiotics<br>Incision and drainage<br>Excision |

*ESR*, Erythrocyte sedimentation rate.

**Table 24A-2.** Cutaneous tuberculosis

| Type | Clinical | Differential diagnosis | Pathology | Treatment |
|---|---|---|---|---|
| Direct inoculation (exogenous source) | Nonsensitized: red, painless, papule develops enlarging to a plaque that may ulcerate.<br>Sensitized: warty lesion | Squamous cell cancer<br>Atypical mycobacterium<br>Syphilis<br>Deep fungal<br>Warts<br>Cat scratch disease | Epithelioid tubercles<br>Central caseation necrosis*<br>Lymphohistiocytic infiltrate<br>Epidermal hyperplasia<br>(+)AFB | Isoniazid (5mg/kg/d or m q day) + rifampin (10-20 mg/kg/d max. 600 mg) for 9-12 months |
| Endogenous contiguous (scrofuloderma) | Red nodules develop over infected viscera | Deep fungal<br>Tertiary syphilis<br>Lymphogranuloma venereum<br>Nodular cystic acne<br>Hidradenitis suppurativa | Tuberculoid granuloma† caseation necrosis central abscess formation<br>(+)AFB | Same |
| Autoimmune (tuberculosis cutis orificialis) | Small firm nodules that ulcerate.<br>Spread from an infected site.<br>Usually poor health. Mucosa may be involved. | Syphilis<br>Chancroid<br>Lymphogranuloma vencreum<br>Herpes simplex virus<br>Aphthous stomatitis<br>Invasive cancer | Same | |
| Hematogenous spread lupus vulgaris | Brown or red papules, central face or ears. May scale and ulcerate<br>Heal with scarring | Disseminated lupus erythematosus<br>Secondary syphilis<br>Acne vulgaris<br>Rosacea<br>Tinea corporis<br>Leprosy<br>Sarcoid<br>Deep fungal | Tuberculoid granuloma upper dermis<br>Thinned epidermis<br>AFB (−) | Isoniazid + rifampin + ethambutol (15 mg/kd/d) OR Streptomycin (15 mg/kg/d max 1g or 500-750 over age 40)<br>OR pyrazinamide<br>Pyridoxin should be given with isoniazid (15-50 mg) |
| Acute miliary tuberculosis of the skin | Papules, nodules, plaques may have necrosis. Infants and children | Many and varied | Dermal tubercle formation caseation necrosis ulceration<br>(+)AFB | |

*Caseation necrosis: Pink, granular material in the center of tubercle. The cellular outlines are lost.

†Tuberculoid granuloma: "Well-circumscribed collection of epithelioid histiocytes surrounded by a dense cuff of lymphocytes"[1]

a perivascular lymphocytic infiltrate. They are similar to those seen in necrobiosis lipoidica except that the abnormalities in granuloma annulare are more limited, concentric, contain mucin and do not contain plasma cells.

***Differential diagnosis.*** Histopathology is often the only way to differentiate diseases such as sarcoidosis, lichen planus, necrobiosis lipoidica, and papular mucinosis from granuloma annulare.

***Management.*** Many cases, especially in children, resolve spontaneously. Limited and persistent lesions may be treated with topical steroids with or without occlusion or with intralesional steroid (2.5 mg triamcinolone/ml). Persisting *generalized* granuloma annulare often may be cleared with PUVA (8-methoxypsoralen combined with ultraviolet A).

### Sarcoidosis

***Epidemiology/etiology.*** Sarcoidosis is a systemic disease of undetermined etiology. It can involve the skin, lungs, lymph nodes, bones, myocardium, central nervous system, kidneys, spleen, liver, eyes, and parotid glands (see Chapter 116).

***Pathophysiology.*** The pathogenesis of sarcoidosis is unknown. Cell-mediated immunity, as demonstrated by intradermal tests for delayed hypersensitivity, is impaired. The cause of this "anergy" is unknown. Immediate IgE-mediated hypersensitivity is not impaired.

***History and physical examination.*** An acute form of sarcoidosis consists of erythema nodosum, hilar adenopathy, fever, migrating polyarthritis and acute iritis. Granulomatous sarcoidal skin lesions are absent in this form of the disease, and spontaneous resolution usually occurs.

Skin lesions are present in approximately one third of cases. This more chronic form presents with symptoms that depend on the organ system(s) involved. Parotid gland enlargement associated with uveitis (Heerfordt's syndrome, uveoparotid fever) may be seen. Lung involvement along with lymphadenopathy is common. Papules may be noted especially around eyelids, or violaceous smooth and shiny plaques may be seen on the acral areas of the body (lupus pernio), as well as psoriasiform, verrucous, and subcutaneous lesions.

***Laboratory.*** Histopathologically, no matter the location, the characteristic changes are those of a "naked tubercle," that is, a group, sheet, or clump of epithelioid histiocytes surrounded or admixed with few lymphocytes. Laboratory abnormalities include increased erythrocyte sedimentation rate, hypercalcemia, and elevated angiotensin-converting enzyme (ACE). Radiologic examination frequently shows hilar adenopathy and punched out lesions of the bones of distal phalanges.

***Differential diagnosis.*** The skin lesions must be differentiated from granuloma annulare, lichens planus, leprosy, and papular mucinosis. The best way to differentiate among these lesions is biopsy.

***Management.*** When internal organ systems are involved systemic corticosteroids are indicated. If skin lesions are the only manifestation, topical or intralesional steroids are effective.

## INFECTIOUS GRANULOMATOUS DISEASES

### Syphilis

Late secondary and tertiary stages of syphilis demonstrate tuberculoid granulomas on histology. Their infiltrate is notable for abundant plasma cells. This disease process is covered in greater detail in Chapter 65.

### Cutaneous tuberculosis

***Epidemiology/etiology.*** Tuberculosis is a chronic granulomatous disease caused by *Mycobacterium tuberculosis.* It generally affects the lungs, but extrapulmonary involvement can also rarely occur including the skin. *M. tuberculosis* is generally transmitted by airborne droplets; however, contact with broken skin of an infected individual may transmit the organism. Dissemination occurs hematogenously.

***Laboratory, history, physical, management.*** See Table 24A-2.

## BIBLIOGRAPHY


Ackerman AB: *Histologic diagnosis of inflammatory skin diseases,* Philadelphia, 1978, Lea and Febiger.

Bartelsmeyer JA, Roy P: Erythema nodosum, estrogens, and pregnancy, *Clin Obstet Gynecol* 33(4):777, 1990.

Callen JP: Pyoderma gangrenosum and related disorders, *Med Clin North Am* 73(5):1247, 1989.

Demis DJ, editor: *Clinical dermatology,* Philadelphia, 1992, JB Lippincott.

Fitzpatrick TB et al, editors: *Dermatology in general medicine,* New York, 1987, McGraw-Hill.

Gelber RH: Hansen's disease, *West J Med,* 158:583, 1993.

Lever W, Schaumburg-Lever, G: *Histopathology of the skin,* Philadelphia, 1990, JB Lippincott.

Petzelbauer P, Wolff K, Tappeiner G: Necrobiosis lipoidica: treatment with corticosteroids, *Br J Dermatol* 126:542, 1992.

Ullman S, Dahl MZ: Necrobiosis lipoidica: an immunofluorescence study, *Arch Dermatol* 113:1671, 1977.

Wilson J et al, editors: *Harrison's principles of internal medicine,* New York, 1991, McGraw-Hill.


CHAPTER

# 24B Vesiculobullous Diseases of the Skin

Lynne H. Morrison

The blistering diseases discussed here are those that are immunologically mediated. These diseases are uncommon.

## BULLOUS PEMPHIGOID

### Epidemiology/etiology

Bullous pemphigoid (BP) is an acquired bullous disease of the elderly. It is characterized histologically by subepidermal blisters and immunopathologically by deposition of autoantibodies and complement along the basement membrane zone. Most patients also have circulating autoantibodies directed against the epithelial basement membrane zone.

The true incidence of BP is unknown but according to estimates there is one case per 100,000 annually. The vast majority of BP patients are over 60 years old at the time of presentation. In general, men and women are equally affected, there is no racial or geographic predilection, and there is no known HLA association.

### Pathophysiology

BP is considered an autoimmune disease mediated by autoantibodies directed against an antigen (the bullous pemphigoid antigen) in the basement membrane zone of stratified squamous epithelia.

Current evidence suggests the following hypothesis for subepidermal blister formation in BP:

1. Initiating event: Immunologic recognition or alteration of the bullous pemphigoid antigen causes production of various classes of antibasement membrane zone antibodies, with the IgG class predominating.
2. Attachment: The autoantibodies attach to the pemphigoid antigen(s) in the basement membrane zone.
3. Complement activation: Complement is activated, which generates the anaphylatoxins C3a and C5a.
4. Inflammatory response: The complement activation results in massive cell degranulation and release of multiple cytokines, histamine, and proteolytic enzymes. Injury to the basement membrane zone is thought to be mediated by these enzymes and eventually produces dermal-epidermal separation.

### History and physical examination

Most patients with BP present with a pruritic eruption. The degree of pruritus varies from nearly nonexistent to intense. A few patients have prolonged pruritus that precedes the clinical of bullous lesions.

Most patients with BP are not systemically ill, although elderly patients with extensive blistering can become debilitated. Most large series have concluded that there is no increased incidence of malignancy in BP patients compared with age and sex-matched controls.

### Physical examination

Frequently the earliest manifestation of BP includes erythematous macules, papules, and urticarial plaques that may have a serpiginous configuration. Subsequently, tense bullae arise on these erythematous lesions as well as on normal skin. These tense bullae make up the most characteristic clinical feature of BP. The blisters may be filled with clear fluid or may be hemorrhagic; when they rupture they leave denuded areas that become encrusted. The erosions tend to not spread peripherally and generally heal without scarring.

### Laboratory studies/diagnostic procedures

Biopsies submitted for routine histology and for direct immunofluorescence studies are essential in BP and other immunologically-mediated blistering diseases.

The most characteristic histologic finding is subepidermal separation with a mixed inflammatory infiltrate containing lymphocytes and eosinophils. Biopsies for immunofluorescence studies show linear deposition of IgG and $C_3$ along the basement membrane zone. These biopsies are best taken from the edge of an urticarial lesion or

**Table 24B-1.** Differential diagnosis of bullous pemphigoid

| Disease | History | Physical | Laboratory | Management |
|---|---|---|---|---|
| Bullous pemphigoid (BP) | Elderly population; intense pruritus; tense bullae; hives common | Widespread bullae; urticarial lesions; distribution not diagnostic | Skin biopsy; DIF linear IgG along basememt membrane | Systemic oral corticosteroids; occasionally azathioprine or cyclophosphamide |
| Cicatricial pemphigoid | Elderly; mucous membranes and conjunctivae | Erosive blisters on mucous membranes and conjunctivae; skin lesions in 20% | Skin biopsy; DIF | Corticosteroids; tetracyclines |
| Herpes gestationis | Pregnancy; intense pruritus; hives and blisters | Urticaria; vesicles and bullae | Skin biopsy; DIF | Resolves after delivery; may require systemic corticosteroids |
| Epidermolysis bullosa acquisita (EBA) | Adult onset; skin fragility and blisters, extensor areas; pruritus | Bullae and vesicles; erosions; healed areas with scars and milia | Skin Bx, DIF similar to BP; differentiation requires split skin DIF | Corticosteroids; immunosuppressive agents; difficult to treat |
| Dermatitis herpetiformis (DH) | Intense pruritus; extensor areas; gastrointestinal symp. occasionally | Grouped (herpetiforme) vesicles; elbows, knees, back, buttocks | Skin biopsy; DIF; gastrointestinal if diarrhea | Dapsone; gluten-free diet |
| Linear IgA bullous dermatosis | Pruritus; any age; vesicles and bullae | May be similar to DH or BP | Skin biopsy; DIF | Corticosteroids; immunosuppressive agents |

*DIF,* Direct immunofluorescence.

**Table 24B-2.** Differential diagnosis of pemphigus vulgaris

| Disease | History | Physical | Laboratory | Management |
|---|---|---|---|---|
| Pemphigus vulgaris | Widespread erosions; oral lesions | Oral and cutaneous bullae and erosions | Skin biopsy; DIF; indirect IF. | Systemic corticosteroids; immunosuppressive agents; gold |
| Bullous pemphigoid | Elderly; intense pruritus; blisters | Bullae widespread; urticaria common | Skin biopsy; DIF | Corticosteroids |
| Cicatricial pemphigoid | Elderly; mucous membranes and conjunctivae | Bullae, erosions, and scarring on mucous membranes and conjunctivae | Skin biopsy; DIF | Systemic corticosteroids; tetracyclines |
| Erythema multiforme (oral) | Oral mucosal lesions; painful | Oral erosions; may have target lesions on skin | Skin biopsy occ. helpful; DIF to exclude pemphigus | Supportive; eliminate or treat underlying cause (see Chapter 21) |
| Erosive lichen planus | Oral mucosal and tongue lesions | Erosions; white lacy mucosal changes | Skin biopsy helpful; DIF to exclude pemphigus | Topical and systemic steroids; retinoids; cyclosporin |

*DIF,* Direct immunofluorescence.

**Table 24B-3.** Differential diagnosis of pemphigus foliaceus

| Disease | History | Physical | Laboratory | Management |
|---|---|---|---|---|
| Pemphigus foliaceus | Widespread crusted erosions; adult onset | Crusted plaques | Skin biopsy; DIF | Systemic corticosteroids |
| Impetigo | Crusted lesions; face; children | Crusted plaques; honey crusts; serous oozing | Culture | Antibiotics |

*DIF,* Direct immunofluorescence.

**Table 24B-4.** Differential diagnosis of paraneoplastic pemphigus

| Disease | History | Physical | Laboratory | Management |
|---|---|---|---|---|
| Paraneoplastic pemphigus | Erosions; mucous membranes; associated malignancy | Oral and cutaneous erosions | Skin biopsy; DIF | Treat malignancy; systemic corticosteroids; immunosuppressive agents |
| Erythema multiforme (major Stevens-Johnson syndrome) | Mouth, conjunctivae, ears, and widespread; Hx drug, viral infection | Erosions on mucous membranes; target lesions on skin | Skin biopsy | Supportive; treat or eliminate underlying cause |

*DIF,* Direct immunofluorescence.

normal skin immediately adjacent to a blister. Biopsies taken from blistering skin commonly give negative results. Other routine lab abnormalities have not been associated with BP.

### Differential diagnosis

See Table 24B-1.

### Management

Systemic therapy with systemic corticosteroid is the mainstay of therapy. The majority of patients can be controlled with 40 to 80 mg of prednisone daily. In general, mild disease usually responds to lower doses of prednisone than does moderate or severe disease. Once the disease is under control the goal of therapy is to taper the prednisone and eventually maintain the patient on alternate-day therapy to minimize long-term steroid side effects.

Patients who fail to respond to corticosteroids may require the addition of azathioprine or cyclophosphamide. Dapsone or sulfapyridine are alternative steroid sparing agents.

## PEMPHIGUS

### Epidemiology/etiology

The term *pemphigus* refers to a group of chronic blistering skin diseases (Tables 24B-2, 24B-3, and 24B-4) in which autoantibodies are directed against keratinocytes resulting in loss of epidermal cell-to-cell adhesion—a process called acantholysis. In all types of pemphigus, IgG autoantibodies are bound in a characteristic pattern around the cell membrane of affected cells and are also found in patients' serum. Pemphigus is divided into subgroups:

*pemphigus vulgaris* (PV), with suprabasilar acantholysis; *pemphigus foliaceus* (PF), with acantholysis in the superficial layers of the epidermis; and *paraneoplastic pemphigus,* which shows suprabasilar acantholysis as well as histologic features of erythema multiforme and is seen in association with underlying neoplasms.

PV is the most common form of the disease and generally occurs during the fourth to sixth decades of life. It occurs worldwide with an annual incidence of about 0.1 to 0.5 per 100,000 population and is more common in the Jewish population. There is an increased incidence of HLA-DR4, HLA-DR6, and HLA-DR10 haplotypes.

### Pathophysiology

Each major form of pemphigus is characterized by specific autoantibodies directed against epithelial structural proteins. In PV and PF the antigens are found only in stratified squamous epithelia, whereas in paraneoplastic pemphigus the antigens are found in all types of epithelia.

The mechanism of acantholysis is not certain but some data suggest that binding of the autoantibody may induce release of proteolytic enzymes. Antibodies alone in the absence of complement can induce acantholysis although complement may augment the process. Other mechanisms, including the direct effect of the IgG autoantibodies on desmosomal integrity and cell adhesion, may also be important in the pathogenesis of this disease.

### History and physical examination

Most patients with PV present with oral lesions. Typically these are painful and irregularly bordered erosions that extend peripherally and heal slowly. Other mucous membranes may be involved but less commonly than the oral mucosa.

Cutaneous lesions usually appear as flaccid bullae with a predilection for the scalp, face, upper trunk, axillae, and groin. The lesions may develop on normal skin or on erythematous base. They rupture easily to produce painful erosions that extend at the edges. When disease activity increases, large areas of a patient's skin can become denuded, resembling a burn patient's, with marked susceptibility to secondary infection and fluid and electrolyte imbalance. The lesions seen in all groups of pemphigus are restricted to stratified squamous epithelium; internal organs are not affected.

PF usually presents with scaling, crusted lesions on the upper trunk and face. The primary lesions are flaccid, fragile bullae that rupture to produce shallow erosions with subsequent scaling and crusting.

Paraneoplastic pemphigus is a recently described variant in which all patients to date have had a recognized or occult neoplasm, most often non-Hodgkin's lymphomas or hematologic malignancies. Patients most consistently have painful oral erosions and shin lesions that resemble erythema multiforme.

### Laboratory studies/diagnostic procedures

Skin biopsies for routine histopathology and for immunofluorescence are essential. PV histopathologically shows suprabasilar intraepidermal blister formation with acantholysis. In PF, the intraepidermal split is higher up on the plane of the epidermis, often within the granular layer just below the stratum corneum. The remainder of the epidermis stays attached to the basement membrane zone. Paraneoplastic pemphigus characteristically shows a combination of suprabasilar acantholysis similar to PV and keratinocyte necrosis, which resembles erythema multiforme.

Skin biopsies processed for direct immunofluorescence in all three types of pemphigus show deposition of IgG autoantibodies and complement within the intercellular spaces of the epithelium.

### Management

The mainstay of therapy for both PV and PF is corticosteroids, usually in the form of oral prednisone. The goal of therapy is to control the disease at the lowest possible dose of prednisone. When the disease is severe, achieving control in a hospital setting is appropriate. For severe disease higher doses of prednisone, generally 80 mg a day or greater, is necessary to get the disease under control. Once the disease is under control, the prednisone is tapered, if possible, to an alternate-day regimen. The goal is to control the disease at the lowest possible alternate-day dose of prednisone. Half the cases of PV need immunosuppressive medications in addition to prednisone for control. These include azathioprine, cyclophosphamide, and gold.

## DERMATITIS HERPETIFORMIS

### Epidemiology/etiology

Dermatitis herpetiformis (DH) is a severely pruritic papulovesicular eruption characterized by recurrent exacerbations and remissions. DH usually has an onset between the second and fourth decades. The male/female ratio is 3:2. The prevalence of DH in the United States is unknown; however, the prevalence in Utah has been estimated at 15:100,000. Patients with DH have an associated gluten-sensitive enteropathy that is most often asymptomatic. As in patients with isolated gluten-sensitive enteropathy, there is an increased frequency of the HLA-B8 antigen, which is noted in 80% to 90% of DH patients. The frequency in the normal population is 20% to 30%. There is also an increased frequency of HLA-DR3 and HLA-DQW2 haplotypes.

### Pathophysiology

The association of a gluten-sensitive enteropathy, presence of granular IgA in the skin, and strong HLA associations suggest that these three factors are important in pathogenesis. Gluten may act as an antigen, inducing an abnormal mucosal permeability with subsequent production of IgA either locally in the gut mucosa or systemically. This IgA could then bind to the skin as either a cross-reacting antibody or possibly an immune complex. Gluten has been proposed as the dietary antigen important in producing the disease. A strict gluten-free diet controls both the cutaneous and gastrointestinal manifestations. An alternative hypothesis is that a gluten-induced intestinal defect may allow passage of other dietary antigens that then could incite production of IgA that subsequently bind to the skin.

### History and physical examination

Patients with DH typically have severe pruritus, often described as stinging or burning. The onset of pruritus commonly precedes the eruption by several hours. The typical primary lesion of DH is a tense subepidermal vesicle. Patients typically excoriate the primary lesions quickly so that when they are examined only secondary changes of excoriations and crusts are apparent. Typically, the sites of involvement are extensor surfaces including elbows, knees, sacrum, upper back and shoulders, and posterior neck. Mucous membranes are characteristically spared.

### Laboratory studies/diagnostic procedures

The diagnosis is most reliably established by direct immunofluorescence biopsies taken from perilesional skin. Histologically DH shows a subepidermal blister with infiltration of neutrophils in the papillary tips. Perilesional skin biopsies processed for direct immunofluorescence studies show pathognomonic findings of granular deposition of IgA in papillary tips and along the dermal-epidermal junction. Indirect immunofluorescence studies typically are negative. Antiendomesial antibodies have been found in a number of these patients and tend to correlate with severity of underlying gastrointestinal abnormality. An iron deficiency anemia or folate deficiency anemia resulting from malabsorption may be noted in some patients.

### Differential diagnosis

The diseases most likely to be confused with DH are linear IgA bullous dermatosis and BP. Linear IgA bullous dermatosis generally occurs after puberty and presents with heterogenous clinical features. Some cases are indistinguishable clinically from true DH. Unlike DH, however, mucous membranes are affected in up to 50% of patients with linear IgA bullous dermatosis. Pruritus is not as consistent a feature of linear IgA bullous dermatosis as in patients with DH. The disease tends to have exacerbations and remissions similar to DH; spontaneous resolution is noted in approximately one third of the cases. There is no known association between linear IgA bullous dermatosis and gluten-sensitive enteropathy.

### Management

There are two approaches to therapy for patients with DH. One is adherence to a strict gluten-free diet and the other is medical therapy, usually with dapsone. Most patients can completely control their cutaneous disease with dapsone, 100 mg/day. Dapsone does not alter any morphologic changes noted in the intestine or change gastrointestinal symptoms, but it does control cutaneous manifestations of DH quite well. Hemolytic anemia and methemoglobinemia are expected consequences of dapsone therapy and require laboratory monitoring.

Patients following a strict gluten-free diet may be able to significantly reduce the dose of dapsone needed to control the disease or may control the eruption entirely by diet alone. This corrects the abnormality of the small bowel and results in a decrease or loss of cutaneous deposits of IgA. Adherence to this diet is difficult and requires support from a dietician as well as family members. The clinical benefits of a strict gluten-free diet may not be seen for up to 2 years.

CHAPTER

# 25 Hair, Scalp, and Nail Diseases

Phoebe Rich
Janet L. Roberts

## ALOPECIA

The term *alopecia* means hair loss or baldness and requires a qualifying adjective to specify a given pathology. Hair loss is a common complaint, often confusing to both the patient and the treating physician. It can be emotionally devastating to some people.

### Hair physiology

Understanding hair growth cycles is essential to diagnosing hair disorders. The hair shaft is keratin protein produced by hair matrix cells. These cells, located at the base of each follicle and nourished by the underlying dermal papilla, divide every 12 hours, which makes them very vulnerable to physical insult. Individual hair follicles have predictable cycles of growth and rest. The active growth phase is the anagen phase and may last from several months to several years. The length of the growth phase is genetically determined, varies with different hair follicles in different parts of the body, and determines the length to which a person's hair will grow. At the end of the anagen phase, an unknown signal causes the hair follicle to undergo a brief transition or catagen phase, lasting only 2 to 3 weeks. After the catagen phase, the hair follicle enters a relatively long resting or telogen phase lasting 2 to 3 months. During this time a new anagen hair is forming beneath the resting hair. As it grows, it pushes out the telogen hair, which is shed. Normally about 90% of scalp hair is in anagen phase. Approximately 100 scalp hairs are shed daily and are minimally observed by an individual.

#### History in patients with hair loss

- Type of hair loss:
  - Shedding: Increased loss of hairs coming out by the roots
  - Breakage: Increased loss because of hair shafts breaking above the root level
  - Thinning: Having less hair to cover the head
- Duration
- Extent of hair loss
- Distribution of hair loss
- Family history of hair loss
- Associated skin or nail abnormalities
- Chronic illness
- Surgical history
- Nutritional history
- Medication history
- Women: hirsutism, hormonal status
- Cosmetic processing

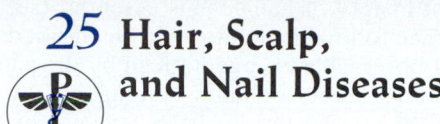

### History of hair loss

A careful patient history of hair loss is essential (see the box on p. 385). The following points must be clarified: (1) whether the first observable change noticed by the patient is shedding (increased loss of hairs coming out by the roots), breakage (increased loss of hairs because of hair shaft fracture above the root level), or thinning (having less hair to cover the head); (2) duration, extent, and distribution of hair loss; (3) family history of hair loss; (4) associated abnormalities of nails and skin; (5) specifics of chronic or acute illnesses, surgeries, nutrition, and medications; (6) in females, hormonal status and hirsutism; and (7) cosmetic processing.

### Physical examination

The successful and appropriate management of hair disorders depends on accurate diagnosis, which requires a systematic evaluation of the patient. The hair and scalp over the entire head must be examined carefully in a strong light. Check for excessive hair (hirsutism) or lack of hair in remote areas and note any associated lesions of skin, mucous membranes, and nails. Note the extent and pattern of hair growth on the scalp and body and any evidence of scalp disease, such as erythema, scaling, crusting, pustules, atrophy, telangiectasias, and presence or absence of follicular orifices. Note any discrete nodules or growths, either superficial or deep, which may suggest malignancy, either primary or metastatic to the scalp. Short hairs, whether blunt (broken off or cut) or tapered (regrowing or miniaturizing hairs) are more easily visualized when viewed against a card of a contrasting color—white for pigmented hairs and black for gray or white hairs.

### Laboratory findings

Microscopic examination of the hair is indicated in patients with breakage problems such as tinea capitis, hair shaft abnormalities, or cosmetic breakage.

In preparing hairs to evaluate for fungus, pluck a few short or broken hairs and cover with potassium hydroxide (KOH) for 15 to 20 minutes. This procedure dissolves the hair keratin and allows for visualization of the fungal elements under high dry magnification. When preparing a hair mount to look for suspected hair shaft abnormalities, the goal is clear visualization of the hair shafts without optical distortion; so place segments of hairs on the slide and cover with a drop or two of Permount (available from most laboratory supply companies).

## TYPES OF ALOPECIAS

Diseases resulting in alopecia are classified as scarring or nonscarring to facilitate making the correct diagnosis (Table 25-1). The nonscarring classification can be divided further into those conditions in which the hair is lost because of hair shaft breakage, hair shedding with the roots attached, and hair thinning with little to no discernible breakage or shedding.

### Scarring alopecias

***Tinea capitis.*** For etiology/epidemiology and management, see Chapter 23.

**History/physical examination.** Tinea capitis may present either as hair breakage, accompanied by minor scaling, or as tender, boggy patches of alopecia (kerion). Symptoms range from none, to pruitus, pain, and tenderness.

**Management.** Usually systemic antifungal agents are required to treat tinea capitis. Combined use of systemic antifungal therapy and systemic corticosteroids are necessary to treat kerions (see Chapter 23).

***Discoid lupus erythematosus.*** For etiology/epidemiology, pathophysiology, and management, see Chapter 81.

**Physical examination.** Discoid lupus erythematosus presents as patches of hair loss with scarring throughout the affected area, hyperpigmentation and hypopigmentation, telangiectasias, and follicular hyperkeratosis.

*Differential diagnosis.* See Table 25-1.

*Management.* Therapy of inflammatory scarring alopecias may include topical, intralesional or oral corticosteroids, topical or oral antibiotics, topical or oral antifungal medications, and in selected, severe cases, antimalarial drugs or dapsone (see Table 25-1).

### Nonscarring alopecias

***Shedding because of breaking hair shafts.*** Structural hair shaft abnormalities can be acquired or congenital. Acquired forms are from breakage due to improper or too frequent use of chemicals for permanent waving, straightening, dying, or bleaching. As a result "weathering" and breakage of the distal hair ends ("split-ends") may occur, as is frequently seen in whites, or breakage of hair shafts proximal to the scalp at weakened fracture points as is seen in black patients. Cessation of the offending cosmetic processing usually results in normal regrowth.

*Congenital* hair shaft abnormalities may be associated with structural weakness and result in hair that is fragile and breaks easily. The major groups include fractures, irregularities, or twisting and coiling of the hair shafts. They may be seen as an isolated finding or be associated with abnormalities of nails, teeth, and sweat glands. A full discussion of these disorders is beyond the scope of this chapter (see bibliography). Microscopic examination of the hair under light magnification is usually sufficient for diagnosis by a sophisticated observer.

**Trichotillomania.** Trichotillomania is an abnormal compulsion to pull out one's own hair (Fig. 25-1).

***Etiology/epidemiology.*** There are two types of trichotillomania. The first, which occurs in those less than 6 years, is usually self-limited, and is more common in boys. The second type begins in those over 6 years and females are affected ten times more often than males. This type has a chronic course. Scalp hair pulling predominates, but any site may be affected.

***History.*** Although the cause is pulling of one's hair, frequently the patient does not admit to pulling and parents are not aware of the habit.

***Physical examination.*** Clinically, trichotillomania presents as irregular, bizarre shapes of hair loss with stubble of different lengths, distorted hair tips from manipulation, and often retained bits of hair at scalp level, which appear as black dots.

***Laboratory evaluation.*** In those patients who deny pulling their hair, a biopsy may be necessary. Pathognomonic histologic findings called trichomalacia (pigmented frag-

**Table 25-1.** Differential diagnosis of alopecias

| Disease | History | Physical | Laboratory | Management |
|---|---|---|---|---|
| **Scarring alopecias** | | | | |
| Congenital (aplasia cutis) | Present at birth | Alopecia<br>Ulceration occasionally | None | Plastic surgery |
| Tinea capitis with inflammation (kerion) | Pruritic, scaly patches<br>Pain and tenderness | Alopecia, scales<br>Boggy patches<br>Pustules | KOH positive<br>Fungal culture | Oral antifungals |
| Bacterial folliculitis | Pruritic pustules | Pustules, papules<br>Some alopecia | Gram stain<br>Bacterial culture | Antibiotics |
| Discoid lupus erythematosus | Pruritus occasionally<br>Lesions other than scalp common | Erythema<br>Scaly thick plaques<br>Pigmentation | Skin biopsy<br>DIF occasionally | Topical steroids<br>Intralesional steroids<br>Antimalarial agents |
| Lichen planopilaris | Pruritus occasionally | Alopecia<br>Peripheral erythema<br>Follicular accentuation | Skin biopsy | Topical steroids<br>Intralesional steroids |
| Folliculitis decalvans | Rare<br>Asymptomatic alopecia, inflammation | Patchy alopecia<br>Follicular erythema at periphery | Skin biopsy | No effective Rx |
| Neoplasm | Asymptomatic alopecia | Evidence of tumor on the scalp | Skin biopsy | Treat tumor |
| Trauma | Hx of traction, excessive hair treatments | Distribution where traction is most severe | None | Eliminate trauma |
| **Nonscarring alopecia** | | | | |
| ***Breakage of hairs*** | | | | |
| Cosmetic treatment | Hx frequent or excessive hair Rx | Broken hairs | None | Eliminate trauma |
| Tinea capitis | Pruritic scaly patches | Erythema, scales | KOH positive<br>Fungal culture | Oral antifungals |
| Structural hair shaft disease | Unmanageable hair<br>Childhood onset usual | Kinky hair<br>Broken hairs | Microscopic hair examination | No effective Rx |
| Trichotillomania (hair pulling) | Children<br>Frequently no history | Hair loss in irregular, bizarre pattern | Skin biopsy in difficult to diagnose cases | Counseling<br>Behavior modification<br>Clomipramine |
| Anagen arrest | Hx chemotherapy<br>Hx radiation Rx<br>Rapid fallout | Widespread shedding | None | Self correcting |
| ***Shedding by roots*** | | | | |
| Telogen effluvium (telogen arrest) | See the box on p. 388<br>Occurs 3 months after physical insult | Diffuse alopecia or thinning | Hair pull >5-10 hairs<br>Forced hair pull analysis for anagen: telogen ratio | Reassurance<br>Correct any identified causes<br>Eliminate offending drug |
| Alopecia areata | Asymptomatic patches of alopecia | Round patches<br>Noninflammatory<br>May be diffuse | Skin biopsy in difficult cases | Topical steroids<br>Intralesional steroids<br>Induce contact dermatitis (DNCB)<br>Ultraviolet therapy |
| ***Thinning without increased shedding*** | | | | |
| Androgenetic alopecia (male pattern balding) | Gradual thinning | Men: temporal and vertex<br>Women: thinning over crown area | None usually<br>Skin biopsy occasionally<br>Rule out other causes | Topical minoxidil<br>Hair transplant |

*DIF,* Direct immunofluorescence; *DNCB,* dinitrochlorobenzene.

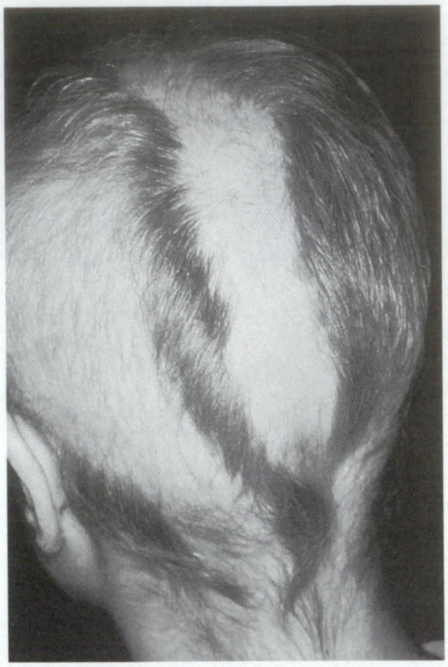

**Fig. 25-1.** Trichotillomania. Note large area of incomplete hair loss.

## Causes of telogen effluvium

Severe acute and chronic illnesses
Childbirth
Surgery with general anesthesia
High fevers
Rapid weight loss
Dietary: protein deficiency, iron deficiency, excessive vitamin A
Hypothyroid, hyperthyroid
Severe psychologic insult
Drugs (see the box below)

## Drugs that may cause telogen effluvium

Anticoagulants
  coumarin, heparin
Nonsteroidal antiinflammatory drugs (including ASA)
Tricyclic antidepressants
Beta-adrenergic blockers (oral, ophthalmic)
  propranolol, metoprolol
$H_2$ antagonists
  cimetidine, ranitidine, famotidine
Antikeratinizing
  vitamin A toxicity, isotretinoin, etretinate
Heavy metals
  lithium, arsenic, lead, gold
Gout medications
  allopurinol, probenecid, colchicine
Hormones
  oral contraceptives, progesterone, clomiphene, anabolic steroids
Antihyperlipemic drugs
  clofibrate, lovastatin, niacin

ments of hair shafts within follicles) confirm the diagnosis.

***Management.*** Treatment is difficult. Behavior modification training is sometimes helpful as may be newer medications used for treating obsessive-compulsive disorders such as chlomipramine and fluoxetine.

**Anagen arrest.** Anagen arrest refers to alopecia in patients receiving systemic chemotherapy or local irradiation. The insult to the matrix cells is severe enough to cause temporary cessation of mitosis of matrix cells in anagen phase, with a resultant breakage of the hair shafts below scalp level. Hairs are shed 2 to 3 weeks after treatment. Because about 90% of scalp hairs are in anagen phase at any given time, the resultant hair loss can be almost complete. Chemotherapy is generally not scarring so that hair regrowth begins when treatments are stopped. Attempts at prevention include ice-filled "chemo-caps" to reduce circulation to the scalp during therapy.

*Shedding with roots attached.* See Table 25-1.

**Telogen arrest (effluvium)**

***Pathophysiology.*** Telogen arrest is caused by insults to the growing hairs sufficient to cause a greater than usual number of anagen hairs to cycle prematurely into the resting or telogen phase. After 30 to 90 days in telogen phase, the hairs are shed. Daily hair counts exceed 100 a day. Acute and chronic causes exist (see the box at top right), and many drugs can cause this form of shedding (see the box at bottom right).

***History.*** (See the box on p. 385).

***Management.*** Treatment includes identification and elimination of any offending causes. It is usually self-limited and reversible.

**Alopecia areata.** Translated literally, alopecia areata means patchy hair loss. However, the disease can be extensive resulting in loss of hair over the entire scalp and face (alopecia totalis), or over the entire body (alopecia universalis).

***Etiology/epidemiology.*** Alopecia areata, a common cause of hair loss, can occur at any age. The peak incidence is between 20 and 50 years, and sex distribution is equal.

***Pathophysiology.*** Alopecia areata is thought to be autoimmune in nature. The precise mechanism is not known.

***History.*** The most common presentation is the sudden appearance of asymptomatic, round patches of complete hair loss, usually limited to the scalp, although any hair may be affected. In the most severe cases, rapid hair loss with extensive total scalp hair shedding can be seen (Fig. 25-2).

***Physical examination.*** Round patches of smooth alopecia with no inflammation are the usual finding. "Exclamation-point" hairs (short broken off hairs) may be present around the perimeter of the patches. Loss may be either limited to an occasional inconspicuous spot or total or universal.

***Laboratory evaluation.*** Usually laboratory evaluation is not required. In atypical cases, a skin biopsy can be helpful. In rare cases there are coexistent autoimmune

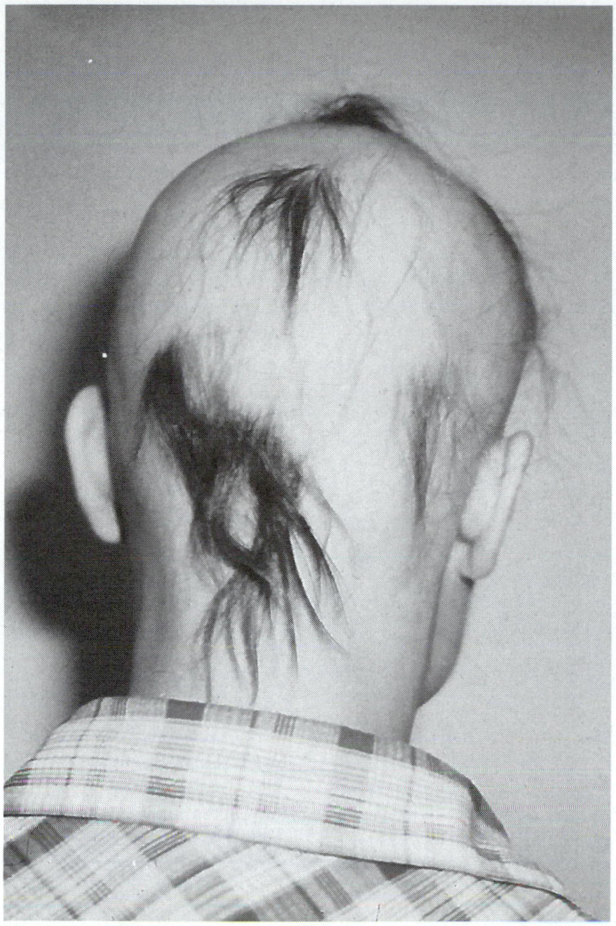

**Fig. 25-2.** Alopecia areata (alopecia totalis). Note completely smooth scalp where hair has fallen out.

associations including thyroid disease, vitiligo, diabetes mellitus, Addison's disease, pernicious anemia, and connective tissue disease. Laboratory evaluation to exclude these diseases should be based on suggestive history.

***Differential diagnosis.*** Tinea capitis and scarring alopecias such as folliculitis decalvans should be considered.

***Disease course.*** In general the disease is more extensive and chronic in childhood, with a poorer prognosis for spontaneous, permanent regrowth. The vast majority of adults with alopecia areata experience the intermittent occurrence of asymptomatic bare patches with spontaneous regrowth.

***Management.*** No treatments are predictably effective, especially in extensive hair loss. Treatments include immune suppressants, such as ultraviolet light, potent topical corticosteroids (Chapter 20), intralesional corticosteroids (betamethasone, 6 mg/ml, or triamcinolone, 3 to 10 mg/ml monthly), and rarely oral corticosteroids. Immune stimulation through irritant or allergenic compounds (dinitrochlorobenzene, anthralin) applied to the affected areas, and direct hair growth stimulation with topical minoxidil also can be effective. In cases of extensive hair loss, a well-styled wig is sometimes the best alternative. Oral corticosteroids should be used for limited periods of time, 3 to 6 months maximum. Intralesional corticosteroids are injected in small increments into the bare patches with a dosage totalling no more than 20 to 30 mg/month over the long term.

#### *Androgenetic alopecia*

**Etiology/epidemiology.** Androgenetic alopecia, or male pattern balding, affects up to about 50% of men. Androgenetic alopecia can be present in as many as 37% of postmenopausal women. Asians appear to be less susceptible than whites or blacks. The genetic predisposition appears to be multifactorial rather than of a single maternal gene as was previously thought.

**Pathophysiology.** The metabolism of androgens within hair follicles and a genetic predisposition are the requirements for the development of androgenetic alopecia. The activity of the enzyme 5-alpha-reductase in the scalp, which converts testosterone to dihydrotestosterone (DHT), appears to play a role in the process of hair miniaturization. Serum levels of circulating androgens are not elevated in most cases. In both men and women there is a progressive shortening of the anagen phase, which leads to smaller, finer hairs with each succeeding cycle.

**History.** Gradual thinning of the scalp hair is typical. A history suggestive of masculinization requires evaluation for possible systemic androgen excess.

**Physical examination.** In men the usual pattern is temporal recession, and thinning on the vertex with gradual progression to total balding of the frontal and vertex scalp. In women the thinning is more diffuse over the crown and usually spares the frontal scalp line and temporal areas. In both men and women, the parietal and occipital scalp are not involved.

**Laboratory evaluation.** In men the diagnosis is usually apparent. In women occasionally there can be uncertainty. In these cases, certain laboratory tests to exclude causes of telogen effluvium (see the box at top left) plus a scalp biopsy can be helpful.

**Management.** The only treatments currently available are the topical use of minoxidil and surgical hair transplantation. Ongoing research in the use of androgen antagonists will possibly result in an effective treatment.

## NAIL DISEASES

Nail disorders (Table 25-2) are common complaints among patients. The physician treating nail disorders must have a thorough understanding of the anatomy of the nail and its growth pattern.

### Anatomy and terminology

The nail plate is that portion of the nail unit commonly referred to as the nail. It is surrounded by folds on three sides: the two lateral nail folds and the proximal nail fold. The nail folds are collectively the paronychium. The area beneath the free edge of the nail, the hyponychium, is contiguous with the volar skin of the digit. The nail bed lies beneath the nail plate and contains the blood vessels and nerves. The nail matrix is the root of the nail, and its distal portion is visible on some nails as the half-moon shaped structure called the lunula.

### Nail growth and kinetics

Nails grow at a rate of approx 0.1 mm/day, which means it takes about 4 to 6 months to regenerate a fingernail and

**Table 25-2.** Differential diagnosis of nail disorders

| Condition | PE/history | Laboratory | Management |
|---|---|---|---|
| Onychomycosis | Hyperkeratosis of nail bed, yellow-brown discoloration, onycholysis. Usually chronic. | KOH positive<br>Culture positive | Systemic or topical antifungal therapy |
| Paronychia, acute | Red, warm, tender nail. Often follows injury to nail fold. | Positive bacterial culture, usually *Staphylococcus* | Systemic antibiotic |
| Paronychia, chronic | Boggy, swollen, red, inflamed nail folds. Usually occurs in people who have wet work jobs. | Pus is KOH positive and culture positive for *C. albicans* | Anticandida therapy, topical or systemic |
| Psoriasis | Usually associated with cutaneous psoriasis. Pitting, onycholysis, splinter hemorrhages, nail bed hyperkeratosis. | KOH negative | Topical or intralesional steroids |
| Lichen planus | Pitting and ridging early. Can eventuate in scarring and pterygium formation. | KOH negative | Systemic, topical, or intralesional steroids |
| Melanoma | Pigmented band in the nail that widens or darkens. | Biopsy nail bed or matrix depending on site of pigment | Wide excision |
| SCC | Hyperkeratosis, onycholysis. | Biopsy lesion | Excision, sometimes Mohs' surgery |
| Habit tic | Usually thumbs, horizontal parallel lines on nail plate. History of manipulating nail folds. | KOH negative | Explain cause to patient; occasionally wrapping nail |
| Mucous cyst | Occurs on proximal nail fold, and over DIP joint. | Mucin expressed from punctured lesion | Excision, repeated liquid $N_2$, intralesional cortisone |

8 to 12 months to replace a toenail. The nail matrix is the germinative portion of the nail and is responsible for the formation of the nail plate. Damage to the matrix usually results in an abnormal nail plate, which may result in a permanent nail dystrophy such as a split nail. Conversely, an injury to the nail plate or nail bed will usually allow for regrowth of a normal nail.

## Infectious nail diseases

***Onychomycosis (fungal nail infection).*** Onychomycosis includes tinea unguium caused by dermatophyte fungi, candidiasis of the nail, caused by *Candida albicans,* and infections caused by other yeast and nondermatophyte fungi. Fungal infections of the nails are common worldwide without racial predilection. Some persons may have genetic predisposition to the development of chronic tinea unguium. Other factors that may increase the development of onychomycosis are humidity, heat, trauma, diabetes mellitus, and underlying tinea pedis.

**Tinea unguium.** An infection of the nail, tinea unguium is caused by a dermatophyte fungus. Tinea ungium is the most common nail disorder and is frequently overdiagnosed. Nonfungal nail conditions such as psoriasis can be indistinguishable from onychomycosis; therefore it is important not to rely on clinical inspection alone to diagnose fungal infections of the nail. A potassium hydroxide (KOH) preparation or fungal culture should be performed to substantiate the diagnosis.

***Physical examination.*** The various subtypes of tinea unguium are based on their pattern of involvement of the nail unit.

1. Superficial white onychomycosis (Fig. 25-3) is characterized by white discoloration on the surface of the patient's nail, which can be easily scraped away with a blade. It occurs only on the patient's toenails and is easily treated with any of the topical antifungal medications. The causative organism is *Trichophyton mentagrophytes* in most of the cases.
2. Distal subungual onychomycosis is so named because the site of invasion is the distal nail bed and progression is distal to proximal. Nail bed hyperkeratosis and yellow brown discoloration is usually present, with eventual crumbling and disintegration of the nail plate. The most common dermatophytes are *T. rubrum* and *T. mentagrophytes,* although others also can be seen. Distal subungual onychomycosis of the toenails is usually associated with tinea pedis (Fig. 25-4). When it occurs in fingernails it is often associated with scaling of the palm of the affected hand and both feet. The organism on the hands is usually *T. rubrum.*
3. Proximal subungual onychomycosis is quite rare in people with intact immune systems. It occurs when the organisms invade the nail plate proximally from the proximal nail fold and involves the ventral nail plate. The clinical presentation is that of white or yellow discoloration on the inferior surface of the nail plate extending out from the proximal nail fold. The causative organisms of this rare form are *T. rubrum, T. mentagrophytes, T. schoenleinii, and T. tonsurans.*

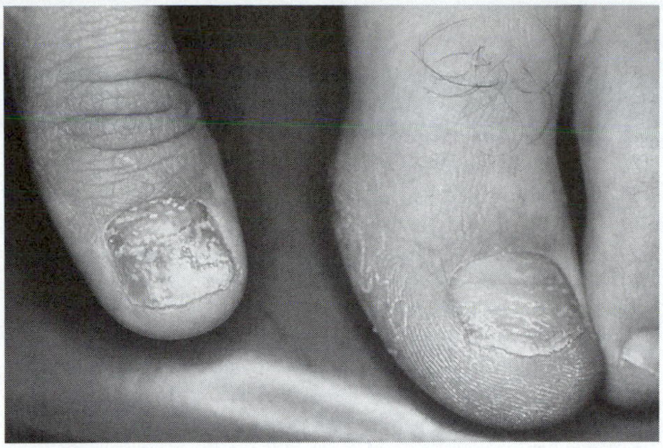

**Fig. 25-3.** Superficial white onychomycosis.

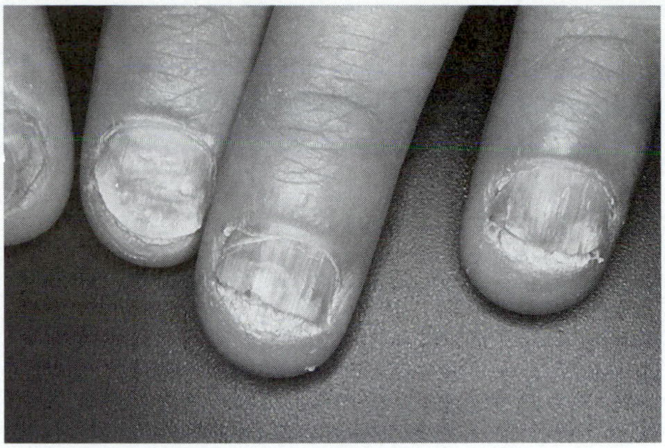

**Fig. 25-4.** Distal subungual onychomycosis.

***Differential diagnosis.*** Psoriasis is the most common nail disorder that can be mistaken for tinea unguium. Usually other signs of psoriasis are present on the body. In uncertain cases, confirmation by KOH examination of nail debris and fungal culture for identification are required.

**Candida onychomycosis.** This organism is caused by *C. albicans,* is unusual and occurs in people with chronic mucocutaneous candidiasis or acquired immune deficiency syndrome (AIDS). Normally *Candida* does not easily invade the nail plate, although it can invade the nail folds (see Chronic Paronychia). The yeast enters the nail distally and can invade the nail plate in those lacking an intact immune system.

**Onychomycosis from molds.** This form is rarely isolated from the nails and their role in the pathogenesis of onychomycosis is still controversial. The most common mold isolated from diseased nails is *Scopulariopsis brevicaulis.*

***Management.*** Treatment of onychomycosis must be tailored to the type of infection and individual patient needs. Because onychomycosis is frequently overdiagnosed, it is important to demonstrate fungus by KOH preparation or culture before initiating systemic antifungal therapy. Except in the case of white superficial onychomycosis, topical antifungal therapy is rarely curative. The treatment of distal subungual onychomycosis, the most common clinical subtype, requires systemic therapy, usually griseofulvin, for the length of time it takes the nail to regrow (see Chapter 20). One to 2 years of treatment are usually required, especially in elderly patients. A case can be made for not treating asymptomatic toenail fungus in patients who are over 50 years old because the nails grow so slowly and fungus is so prevalent in toenails of the elderly. The relapse rate in toenails is as high as 40% to 50% at 1 year after treatment. In cases of griseofulvin resistance, ketoconazole, 200 mg/day, can be used. Due to the potential for hepatotoxicity with ketoconazole, however, the risk/benefit ratio must be carefully weighed, and laboratory monitoring of liver function is essential. Studies are being conducted on newer systemic antifungals such as terbenifine, itraconazole, and fluconazole using creative dosing schedules, which may shorten the time of treatment and minimize the side effects in the treatment of onychomycosis. At the present time, none of these drugs have FDA approval for the treatment of onychomycosis.

**Paronychia.** Paronychia is defined by infection or inflammation of the nail folds. It can be acute or chronic based on the pathogenesis and organism.

***Acute paronychia.*** Acute paronychia results from a bacterial infection of the nail folds. It usually follows some kind of trauma to the nail folds such as overaggressive manicuring or injury. The most common bacterial agents in acute paronychia are *Staphylococcus aureus* and *Pseudomonas* species. Treatment is similar to that of other bacterial infections of the skin and includes draining and administering a systemic antibiotic.

***Chronic paronychia.*** Chronic paronychia causes swollen, red, tender, boggy nail folds. It occurs most frequently in people with wet work jobs or those whose hands are exposed to solvents and chemicals. The first occurrence is separation of the cuticle and nail folds from the nail plate, followed by the formation of a potential space for various microbes to invade, especially *C. albicans.*

***Management.*** Treatment includes drying the area and applying anticandidal agents. In cases of severe inflammation, topical or intralesional steroids can be used. It is important to educate the patient about excessive water and chemical exposure.

## Dermatologic diseases that affect the nails

***Psoriasis.*** Psoriasis occurs in 2% to 3% of the population and between 10% and 50% of psoriatics have nail involvement (see Chapter 20).

**Physical examination.** Psoriasis of the nails can have a variety of clinical manifestation depending on the site of the involved nail unit. Nail pitting (in the nail plate) is due to involvement of the matrix; onycholysis, subungual hyperkeratosis, and yellow discoloration ("oil drop sign") are due to involvement of the nail bed. Psoriasis of the nail is often indistinguishable clinically from fungal infection of the nail (see Plate 24). Clinical inspection of other areas of the body that are psoriasis prone (elbows, knees, scalp, gluteal cleft) and negative KOH examination and fungus culture can provide clues to the diagnosis of psoriasis of the nails. Approximately 5% of psoriatic patients have psoriasis limited to the nails, a situation that poses a great diagnostic challenge.

**Management.** Treatment of psoriasis can be challenging and at times frustrating. Often as cutaneous

**Table 25-3.** Nail signs of systemic disease

| Nail sign | Nail appearance | Systemic disease |
|---|---|---|
| Clubbing | Increased unguophalangeal angle | Cardiopulmonary and gastrointestinal disorders |
| Half and half nail | Proximal half is brown, distal half is white | Renal failure |
| Nail fold telangiectases | Dilated vessels in proximal nail fold and cuticle | Dermatomyositis and systemic lupus erythematosus |
| Splinter hemorrhages | Longitudinal brown streaks under the nail | Trauma is the most common cause but also may be seen in subacute bacterial endocarditis |
| Mees' lines | Transverse white lines | Arsenic poisoning |
| Muehrcke's lines | Double white transverse lines | Chronic hypoalbuminemia |
| Koilonychia | Thin everted distal edge | Anemia, Plummer-Vinson syndrome |
| Azure lunula | Blue lunula | Hepatolenticular degeneration (Wilson's disease) |
| Terry's nails | Milky white nails with prominent onychodermal band | Cirrhosis, chronic congestive heart failure |
| Plummer's nails | Onycholysis | Thyrotoxicosis |

psoriasis clears, the nails will clear as well. Topical steroids may be helpful in some mild cases; however, results are usually disappointing in severe psoriatic involvement of the nails. Intralesional steroids (triamcinolone 3 mg/ml) to the nail matrix are generally more helpful, although not always welcomed by the patient. Psoralen plus ultraviolet A (PUVA) and grenz ray are sometimes beneficial in severe cases. A dermatologist should be consulted for these treatments.

***Lichen planus.*** Lichen planus is a relatively uncommon disorder that can affect the skin and/or nails (see Chapter 21). When it occurs in the nails, it can rapidly destroy the nail matrix, leading to onychorrhexis (longitudinal ridges) and eventual destruction of the nail plate. The end stage of lichen planus of the nails is destruction of the matrix so that portions of the nail fail to grow. The resultant defect is called a pterygium and is characterized by areas of the nail where the proximal nail fold adheres to the nail bed where the nail is absent.

**Management.** Potent topical corticosteroids can be tried, but systemic steroids are sometimes necessary for the treatment of rapidly destructive lichen planus of the nails.

## Neoplastic nail conditions

***Malignant melanoma.*** Malignant melanoma of the nail unit is rare, accounting for only 1% to 4% of melanomas. Although 20% of these are amelanotic, containing little or no pigment, most start as a solitary longitudinal pigmented band in the nail. The band usually widens and darkens over time and frequently there is leaching of pigment into the proximal nail fold (Hutchinson's sign). The most commonly involved nails are the great toe and thumb. Over 25% of patients give a history of prior trauma to the digit, which in some cases causes delay in seeking medical attention. There are many benign causes of longitudinal pigmented bands in the nail ranging from hematoma and certain medications to a normal occurrence in blacks; but any solitary pigmented band that widens, darkens, or otherwise alters the nail plate needs further evaluation. The onus is on the physician to be certain that a pigmented band or spot on the nail is not a melanoma.

**Management.** Early detection and wide surgical excision are essential. When there is doubt about the diagnosis, referral to a dermatologist and biopsy of nail bed, nail matrix, or surrounding tissue are indicated. Once the diagnosis of malignant melanoma is confirmed, referral to an oncologic surgeon experienced in the management of malignant melanoma is mandatory (see Chapter 21).

Other cutaneous neoplasms occasionally are seen in the nail unit. Both basal cell carcinoma and squamous cell carcinoma occur rarely in the nail bed. A benign painful tumor that is often seen in a subungual location is a glomus tumor, an encapsulated tumor of the arteriovenous anastomosis in the nail bed. These tumors may be seen beneath the nail as a red or blue discoloration, but the main distinguishing feature is pain, which may be spontaneous or associated with cold. A benign bony growth called an exostosis can occur subungually, usually beneath the toenail, and often after trauma to the digit.

### *Other common nail disorders*

**Habit tic disorder.** Habit tic disorder (see Plate 40) is a common disorder self-induced and characterized by horizontal parallel ridges in the nail plate. It results from frequent repetitive manipulation of the cuticle and nail fold overlying the matrix. The thumb is the most commonly involved digit. Once the cause of the problem is explained to the patient, the cure is simply a matter of leaving the nail alone.

**Digital mucous cyst.** Mucous cysts are the most common tumor of the digit and usually occur on the dorsal surface of the finger between the nail folds and the distal interphalangeal joint. They are not a true cyst because they lack a cystic lining but are more accurately called focal mucinosis.

***Nail changes in systemic disease.*** Some nail findings provide helpful clues for the diagnosis of systemic disorders. A few nail signs are specific for underlying medical problems. Nail fold telangiectases are associated with connective tissue disorders such as systemic lupus erythematosus and dermatomyositis. Clubbing is associated with pulmonary and gastrointestinal disorders. Other much less specific nail signs such as splinter hemorrhages may be seen in subacute bacterial endocarditis but are commonly seen in trauma (Table 25-3).

## BIBLIOGRAPHY

Baden HP: *Diseases of the hair and nails,* ed 1, Chicago, 1987, Mosby.

Baran R, Dawber RPR: *Diseases of the nails,* Oxford, England 1984, Blackwell Scientific Publication.

Fitzpatrick TB, Eisen EZ, editors: *Dermatology in general medicine,* ed 3, New York, 1987, McGraw-Hill.

Hordinski MK: *Alopecia areata,* Monograph, Kalamazoo, Mich, 1988, Upjohn.

Maibach HI: *Seminars in dermatology,* vol 10, Philadelphia, 1991, WB Saunders.

Moschella SL, Hurley HJ, editors: *Dermatology,* ed 2, vol 2, Philadelphia, WB Saunders.

Olsen EA, editor: *Disorders of hair growth, diagnosis and treatment,* ed 1, New York, 1993, McGraw-Hill.

Orfanos CE, Happle R, editors: *Hair and hair diseases,* ed 1, Berlin, 1990, Springer-Verlag.

Roberts JL: Androgenetic alopecia: treatment results with topical minoxidil, *J Am Acad Dermatol,* 16:705, 1987.

Samman PD, Fenton DA, editors: *The nails in disease,* ed 4, Chicago, 1986, Year Book.

Scher RK, Daniel CR: *Nails: therapy, diagnosis, surgery,* Philadelphia, 1990, WB Saunders Co.

Zaias N: *The nail in health and disease,* ed 2, Norwalk Ct, 1990, Appleton and Lange.

CHAPTER

# 26 Common Exanthems

**Elizabeth Gardner Stratte**

Historically, childhood exanthems were classified on a numerical basis, with the first disease being measles, second disease scarlet fever, third disease rubella, fourth disease "Duke's disease" (now believed to be exanthemata of coxsackie-ECHO group or variants of rubella, rubeola or scarlet fever), fifth disease erythema infectiosum, and sixth disease roseola infantum. Today, childhood exanthems are known to be caused by 50 viral and several bacterial and rickettsial infections (Table 26-1).

The diagnosis and treatment of patients presenting with fever and skin rash is discussed in Chapter 62.

## MEASLES (RUBEOLA)

### Etiology/epidemiology

A paramyxovirus, measles is an RNA virus. There has been a 95% decline in incidence since the vaccine licensure in 1963.

In the 1970s and 1980s new epidemics of measles occurred on college campuses and in urban areas. Fifty percent of cases occurred in children less than 5 years of age. People likely to get measles included unimmunized preschoolers, adolescents aged 15 to 19 years, and certain ethnic groups. Hispanic preschool-aged children are 12 times more likely to contract measles than white children.

Causes of this reemergence included low immunization rates (especially before the trivalent measles-mumps-rubella [MMR] vaccine) and vaccination before 1967 with the "killed" inactivated measles virus vaccine. There was a 5% immunization failure even when properly performed. Outbreaks in school-aged children with documented immunization led to reconsideration of immunization policies and a program of revaccination.

### History and physical examination

Measles occurs in typical, modified, and atypical forms depending on the age and immunity of the patient.

Typical measles is seen in unimmunized or partially immunized preschoolers, adolescents, and young adults. The incubation period is 7 to 12 days with a prodrome lasting 2 to 4 days including high fever, coryza, cough, and conjunctivitis. Koplik's spots are pathognomonic, occur during the prodrome, and last for 2 days after the rash begins. They appear as tiny white or blue-gray specks on an erythematous base on the buccal mucosa adjacent to the molars. The exanthem begins behind the ears and at the scalp margins and rapidly spreads down the torso within 3 days. Lesions begin as discrete erythematous papules that become confluent. The eruption is nonpruritic, lasts 4 to 7 days, and fades with a branny desquamation. Fever resolves on the second or third day of rash. Patients are contagious from 4 days before until 3 days after the onset of the rash. Complications include pneumonia, diarrhea, pharyngitis, otitis media, and, less frequently, myocarditis and encephalitis. The mortality rate from measles is <0.1% and highest in infants less than 12 months. Immunocompromised patients are at risk of developing severe complications, such as giant cell pneumonia and measles encephalopathy.

Modified measles occurs in partially immune hosts, typically young infants with partial protection through maternal antibody at the time of infection or immunization, immunized individuals with partial vaccine failure, or patients who received IgG during prodrome. Patients have an abbreviated, milder form of rubeola. The incubation period is longer, the prodrome is shorter, and the rash less severe. After a prodrome of 2 to 3 days, a red-brown exanthem appears, which is nonconfluent and fades in 5 to 6 days with desquamation.

Atypical measles occurs in individuals who received the killed vaccine, which has been available since 1967. Patients with atypical measles have no immunity to one of the viral surface glycoproteins, F protein (necessary to prevent the spread of infection), but do produce hemagglutinin antibody, which causes hypersensitivity to the wild virus, producing the unusual disease. Two days after the abrupt onset of high fever, myalgias, and cough, a rash appears, beginning on the extremities and spreading centrally. It may be confined to an acral location and have associated peripheral edema. The morphology is papular, papulovesicular, and often hemorrhagic. Koplik's spots are usually absent.

Symptoms usually are more severe than in typical measles and can persist for months. A lobular or segmental pneumonia is virtually always present and pleural effusions are common. Associated findings include hepatosplenomegaly, hyperesthesia or dysesthesia, weakness, leukopenia, and lymphopenia. Measles infection in preg-

**Table 26-1.** Exanthems

| Disease | Age | Prodrome | Skin morphology | Distribution | Other findings | Diagnosis |
|---|---|---|---|---|---|---|
| Measles | Infants<br>Young Adults | Fever, URI, conjunctivitis | Erythematous macules—papules become confluent<br>Nonpruritic | Face first<br>Moves down over entire body | Koplik's spots, cough, photophobia, adenopathy | Clinical; acute/conval hemagglutinin serology |
| Rubella | Adolescents<br>Young adults | Fever, malaise, cough | Rose pink macules and papules<br>Not confluent | Face first<br>Moves downward | Forschheimer spots<br>Postauricular adenopathy<br>Headache | Rubella hemagglutinin inhib or comp fix titers acute/conval |
| Erythema Infectiosum (Fifth Disease) (Parvovirus B19) | 5-15 yr | None or mild fever<br>Malaise | Slapped red cheeks<br>Reticulate erythema or maculopapular<br>Not pruritic | Face—red cheeks<br>Arm/legs reticulate | Rash waxes-wanes several weeks<br>Arthritis; aplastic anemia | IgM Antibody |
| Roseola Exanthem HHV 6 | 6 mo-3 yr | High fever 3-5 days<br>Then rash | Rose-pink, maculopapular<br>Appears after fever resolves | Neck, trunk with little involvement of face<br>Lasts only hours to few days | Cervical and postauricular adenopathy<br>Humanherpes virus-6 may cause neonatal hepatitis | Clinical |
| Varicella Chicken Pox | 1-14 yr | Fever, malaise | Vesicles (often umbilicated) or red base<br>Very pruritic | Generalized involvement<br>Lesions leave scars | Oral lesions<br>Pneumonia in older patients | Tzanck viral culture |
| Enterovirus (Coxsackie, ECHO) | Children | Fever, URI | Variable—maculopapular, petechial, vesicular | Generalized or acral (hand-foot-mouth) | Fever, myocarditis, meningitis, pleurodynia, mouth ulcers | Clinical, viral culture |
| Adenovirus | 5 mo-5 yr | Fever, URI | Maculopapular, morbilliform, rubelliform, petechial, roseola-like | Generalized | Fever, URI, conjunctivitis | Viral culture<br>Acute/conval titer |
| Epstein-Barr (Inf. Mononucleosis) | Children<br>Adolescents | Fever, sore throat | Maculopapular, morbilliform, urticarial, erythema multiforme-like | Trunk<br>Extremities | Cervical adenopathy<br>Hepatosplenomegaly | Mono spot<br>Acute/conval<br>EB Nuclear<br>Ag Titers |
| Kawasaki Disease | 6 mo-6 yr | Fever, eye irritation | Papular, morbilliform, scarletiniform<br>Commonly desquamates as clears | Generalized with palm, sole and perineal accentuation | Conjunctivitis cheilitis, glossitis, adenopathy, peripheral edema, coronary artery abnormalities | Clinical |
| Staph Scalded Skin (Staphy Toxin) | Neonates, infants | | Sudden onset, tender, red rash that exfoliates leaving raw surfaces<br>Nikolsky's sign | Generalized | Fever, conjunctivitis | Culture of coagulase + staph from systemic site<br>Not skin |

| | | | | | | |
|---|---|---|---|---|---|---|
| Scarlet Fever (Beta Strep Toxin) | School age | Fever, sore throat, malaise, headache | Diffuse, erythema with "sandpaper" texture<br>Exfoliative as rash clears | Generalized, circum oral pallor<br>Pastia's lines | Pharyngitis, palate perlèche, abdominal pain, strawberry tongue | Throat culture<br>$\uparrow$ ASO titer |
| Staph Scarlet Fever (Exfoliative Toxin) | School age | | Tender, red, erythroderma with sandpaper quality<br>Doesn't desquamate | | No pharyngitis | Negative throat culture<br>No ASO $\uparrow$ |
| Meningococcemia | <2 years | Malaise, fever, URI | Papules, petechiae, large areas of purpura, purpura-fulminans | Trunk extremities, soles,palms | High fever, meningismus, shock | Blood culture, spinal tap |
| Rocky Mt. Fever (Ricketsii) | Any age | Fever, malaise | Maculopapular, petechial rash | Acral areas first; trunk later | CNS, pulmonary, and cardiac involvement | Serology Weil-Felix test |

*URI*, Upper respiratory infection.

nancy can result in a threefold increase in maternal mortality and pneumonia is the most likely cause of death. Although there is an increase in preterm delivery, the virus is not a teratogen. There is a low rate of transmission to the neonate, but severe disease results in a 30% to 33% mortality rate. Death is usually due to pneumonia.

### Laboratory evaluation

If the diagnosis is in question, the acute and convalescent titers exhibit a fourfold rise in hemagglutination inhibition antibodies. Extremely high antibody titers are characteristic of atypical measles caused by the killed virus vaccine.

### Differential diagnosis

Drug hypersensitivity syndromes, viral exanthems, and meningococcemia should be considered.

### Management

No specific treatment is available. Oral vitamin A is necessary for epithelial cell integrity and plays a role in immune modulation. In a randomized double blind trial in 1990, the group treated with 400,000 IU vitamin A recovered more rapidly from pneumonia and diarrhea, experienced less croup, spent fewer days in the hospital, and had fewer deaths than the placebo group. Other studies have also shown vitamin A to decrease morbidity and mortality in children hospitalized with measles.

Current recommendations are to treat patients 6 months to 2 years of age with vitamin A who are hospitalized and those patients older than 6 months of age who have risk factors and are not already receiving vitamin A. Patients with risk factors include those with immunodeficiency (human immunodeficiency virus [HIV], congenital immunodeficiency, and immunosuppressive therapy), those with ophthalmologic evidence of vitamin A deficiency, those with impaired intestinal absorption (cystic fibrosis or biliary obstruction), those with moderate to severe malnutrition (i.e., eating disorders), and recent immigrants from areas with high mortality rates from measles. The treatment regimen is a single dose of 200,000 IU by mouth for children older than 12 months, and 100,000 IU for children 6 to 12 months. This dose should be repeated in 24 hours and at 4 weeks for patients with ophthalmologic findings. Vitamin A is a teratogen and should not be given to pregnant women.

### Immunization

The current vaccine is the Moraten vaccine, developed by attenuation of the Edmonston strain in 1968. The trivalent MMR (measles, mumps, and rubella) has been in use since 1971 (see Chapter 3 for recommendations and contraindications).

## RUBELLA

### Etiology

Rubella is a mild illness associated with an exanthem, but severe fetal malformations occur if infection occurs in the first half of pregnancy. Rubella is an RNA virus with hemagglutinin and complement fixing antigens.

### History and physical examination

After an incubation period of 15 to 21 days, a prodrome of malaise, cough, fever up to 40° C, headache, and eye pain occur. The exanthem begins on the face and progresses to involve the trunk and extremities, and then the entire body in 1 to 3 days. It is light in color and less confluent than measles with discrete rose pink macules and 1 to 4 mm papules. It fades as it progresses and is absent on the face when it is prominent on the trunk. There may be a final flaky desquamation. The enanthem of pinpoint rose-colored and petechial macules (Forschheimer spots) is present on the soft palate in 20% of patients during the prodrome or first few days of the exanthem. Adenopathy, both suboccipital and posterior auricular, is present. Arthritis and arthralgias occur with increasing age. Fingers and wrists are most commonly involved, and massive effusions may occur and last for 10 to 14 days.

Twenty-five percent to 50% of patients are asymptomatic. Most common in the spring, rubella is highly contagious, with 100% infected in close living conditions. It is spread by respiratory droplets, and during viremia the virus can be recovered from the pharynx, skin, urine, and feces. Infants with congenital infection shed large amounts of the virus for up to 1 year and are potential sources of infection.

### Congenital rubella syndrome

Fetal infection with rubella may result in sensoral deafness, heart disease, and cataracts. One major malformation may be present in 50% of fetuses if infected in the first 1 to 3 months of pregnancy, 5% if infected after the fourth month, and rare if infected after the second trimester. There is also an increased risk of abortion, stillbirth, prematurity, and growth retardation. Sensorineural deafness is the most common malformation and may be unilateral or bilateral. Cardiac lesions are present in 50% of infants infected in the first 2 months. Patent ductus arteriosus is the most common cardiac anomaly. Fifty percent of infants have bilateral cataracts, usually with associated retinopathy. Encephalopathy, mental retardation, diabetes mellitus, and thyroid disorders also have been reported.

Prenatal management includes evaluation and counseling of any pregnant women infected with rubella even though they may have been immunized. Fetal vein sampling for viral culture and RNA probes has been used for antenatal confirmation of infection in the fetus. Administration of immunoglobulin for postexposure prophylaxis during early pregnancy is not recommended because it does not prevent the congenital rubella syndrome. There have been a few reports of seropositive women with infants who develop congenital rubella after maternal reinfection, suggesting that vaccine-induced immunity is not adequate to prevent reinfection.

### Laboratory evaluation

A fourfold rise in acute and convalescent hemagglutinin inhibition or complement fixation IgG titers is diagnostic. For the diagnosis of infection during pregnancy, IgM levels are detected by enzyme-linked immunosorbent assay (ELISA) for 4 weeks after the appearance of the rash.

### Management

There is no specific therapy for rubella. The arthritis responds to aspirin. The rubella vaccine is a live attenuated virus. Current immunization recommendations are to give the rubella vaccine as the trivalent MMR at 15 months of age (see Chapter 3). Women should be tested at child-bearing age and be vaccinated if not immune once pregnancy has been ruled out.

## ERYTHEMA INFECTIOSUM (FIFTH DISEASE)

### Epidemiology/etiology

Human parvovirus B19 is the cause of erythema infectiosum. It is also the cause of aplastic anemia in patients with hemoglobinopathy, chronic anemia in immunodeficient patients, and rarely, intrauterine infection with resultant hydrops or fetal death. Fifth disease is most common in school-aged children 5 to 15 years. Transmission is by respiratory secretions.

### History and physical examination

The incubation period for fifth disease is 4 to 14 days. Sometimes there is a prodrome of low grade fever, malaise, and headache. A fiery red rash appears on the cheeks (slapped cheeks) as macular erythema or raised plaques. One to 4 days later a more generalized rash develops, beginning as discrete erythematous macules and papules but gradually evolving into a distinctive lacy, reticular pattern most prominent on the extremities. This eruption waxes and wanes for several weeks, exacerbated by temperature changes, exercise, sunlight, and emotional factors. Patients typically feel well; but headache, fever, sore throat, and coryza occur in 5% to 15% of children. Adults typically develop gastrointestinal upset and arthritis, with severe pain, stiffness, and swelling of the hands, feet, and knees.

### Laboratory evaluation

Diagnostic tests for B19 are available only at the Centers for Disease Control (CDC) through state health departments. IgM antibody is present at the time the rash begins and declines by 1 to 2 months. B19 DNA by nucleic acid hybridization is the most sensitive test of detection. Fetal infection can sometimes be diagnosed by combining ultrasound with alpha fetoprotein levels.

### Management

A specific antiviral treatment or vaccine for erythema infectiosum is not available. Arthritis responds to aspirin or nonsteroidal antiinflammatory drugs. Hematologic complications have been successfully treated with IV gamma globulin. Isolation is not necessary because once the rash appears virus is no longer being shed.

## ROSEOLA (EXANTHEM SUBITUM)

### Etiology and epidemiology

Humanherpes virus-6, a double-stranded DNA virus, is the etiologic agent. The epidemiology is unique. All cases occur between 6 months and 3 years, with most occurring before age 1 year; the peak prevalence is at 7 to 9 months. This prevalence rate is probably due to a decline of maternal antibodies by 4 to 5 months and widespread exposure to the virus. HHV-6 has been documented in the salivary glands of many asymptomatic carriers, which led to the hypothesis that viral shedding from the saliva in healthy, previously infected individuals is a ubiquitous source of infection.

### History and physical examination

The incubation period is 15 days. A sudden onset of fever, as high as 40° C, lasts 3 to 5 days, followed by defervescence and appearance of the rash.

Children do not appear sick, although reddening of the conjunctivae, puffy eyelids, mouth lesions, and upper respiratory symptoms have been described. Patients are often drowsy during the day and irritable at night. The rash may coincide with the decrease in fever or follow it by 1 to 2 days. Small rose-pink macules and maculopapules, often with a halo of pale skin, appear on the neck and trunk, with only minimal lesions on the face or proximal extremities. The eruption may last only a few hours or 1 to 2 days. Children may have an exanthem of pinpoint pink elevations on the uvula and soft palate. Occipital, cervical, and postauricular adenopathy occur. Postoccipital adenopathy is common. Rare complications include febrile seizures, bulging fontanelle, encephalitis, and thrombocytopenia purpura.

Recent reports include HHV-6 as the cause of neonatal hepatitis, fatal hemophagocytic syndrome, and a mononucleosis syndrome in adults.

### Laboratory evaluation

Diagnosis is by clinical presentation. Tests for IgM and IgG specific for HHV-6 are not yet available. Demonstration of HHV-6 by electron microscopy (EM), DNA hybridization or polymerase chain reaction (PCR) does not indicate acute infection as it apparently can persist as a lifelong latent infection.

### Management

There is no specific therapy and no need to isolate patients due to its ubiquitous nature.

## VARICELLA

### Epidemiology

In the United States, 3 to 4 million cases occur each year, with 4500 hospitalizations for complications including secondary bacterial infections, Reye's syndrome associated with salicylate use, acute cerebellar ataxia, meningoencephalitis, and pneumonia. Half of the cases of varicella occur before age 5 years, and epidemics have a peak incidence in the late winter and spring. Varicella is acquired by aerosolized droplet spread from close contacts who are infected and uncommonly from direct contact with individuals who have active herpes zoster.

### History and physical examination

After an incubation period of 20 to 21 days, patients develop a low-grade fever and malaise. Red macules develop into papules and ultimately into crops of numerous small, discrete vesicles with 1 to 2 mm of surrounding erythema (Figure 26-1). Lesions progress eventually to pustular and finally crusted lesions. The eruption begins on the scalp, face, and trunk and spreads to the extremities over several days. Crops continue to appear for 3 to 5 days, often with significant pruritus. Mucous membrane involvement may include ulcers on the palate, pharynx, tonsillar pillars, conjunctivae, and genital areas. Large blisters may develop, which may be superinfected. Children receiving steroids, especially for underlying malignancy, and children with congenital or acquired immunodeficiency may develop extensive eruptions, with scarring sequelae, severe symptoms, and varicella pneumonia. Chronic and recurrent varicella infection has been described in children with HIV infection.

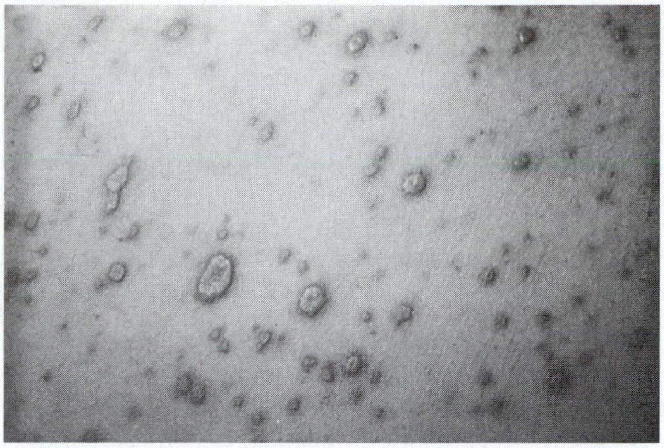

**Fig. 26-1.** Varicella. Note umbilicated papules and vesicles with surrounding erythema.

Varicella is a more severe illness in adults. There is often a prolonged fever, malaise, arthralgias and pneumonia. The pneumonia presents as an interstitial, micromodular, or lobar distribution. It may be associated with cyanosis, dyspnea, or hemophysis and become overwhelming.

Congenital and neonatal varicella occur occasionally. Multiple congenital anomalies may result from maternal infection in the first or second trimester. The risk of varicella for an infant when the mother contracts the illness within 2 weeks of delivery is 25%. This infection in the neonatal period (onset of varicella within 5 to 10 days of delivery) carries a mortality of 30%.

### Laboratory evaluation

The clinical presentation is diagnostic in most cases. Tzanck stains of scrapings from intact vesicles, and viral culture aid in the diagnosis (see Chapter 19).

### Management

Most children with varicella require only supportive treatment consisting of acetominophen for fever, antihistamines for sedation and itching, and local skin care for comfort. Topical antipruritic lotions (Calamine, Sarna) can be soothing. Aspirin is contraindicated in varicella because of the possible relationship to the development of Reye's syndrome.

Patients with varicella pneumonia should be kept in strict isolation, well-segregated from patients receiving steroids or having HIV or other illnesses that compromise the immune system.

Acyclovir is indicated for use in older patients (adolescents and adults) and in immunocompromised patients with varicella. In patients with intact immune systems, oral acyclovir given in high doses during the incubation period and early stages of the disease can reduce the severity of the illness. Usually 200 mg/kg with a maximum dose of 800 mg given every 3 to 4 hours in the early phases is recommended. Since acyclovir is only effective in preventing viral replication, early treatment is essential. Once lesions develop in the skin, viral replication has already taken place, and further use of acyclovir may not be of any benefit. Oral acyclovir also should be considered in patients with chronic skin or pulmonary disease, patients receiving long-term salicylate therapy, and children receiving oral or inhaled corticosteroids.

Intravenous acyclovir is indicated in immunocompromised patients with varicella. A dose of 10 mg/kg every 8 hours for up to 10 days is usual for those patients with normal renal function.

Varicella-zoster immune globulin (VZIG) provides passive immunity after exposure and is indicated in selected groups of patients including pregnant women, immunocompromised patients, and adults.

A varicella vaccine has recently been licensed in the United States.

## ENTEROVIRUS

### Epidemiology

Coxsackie, echo, and poliovirus are now grouped as one genus of picornavirus. This group is the most common cause of summertime infections, causing up to two thirds of viral infections. More than 30 types can cause exanthems. The most notable dermatologic disease in this group is hand-foot-and-mouth disease, which is discussed later.

### History

The presentation of the viral illness is variable and age dependent. The prodrome is usually absent or brief and is followed by variable systemic signs and symptoms including fever, URI symptoms, meningeal signs, conjunctivitis, vomiting, and diarrhea.

### Physical examination

Multiple types of skin eruptions are associated with enterovirus infection. These include rubelliform, morbilliform, scarlatiniform, vesicular, urticarial, petichial, and pustular eruptions. Rare forms include vasculitis, purpura, a zosterlike eruption, a dermatomyositis-like eruption associated with X-linked agammaglobulinemia, and a parvovirus B19-like eruption.

Hand-foot-and-mouth disease is typically caused by coxsackie A16, but other coxsackie serotypes and enterovirus 71 can mimic the clinical picture. The illness is common in the late summer or fall. After a short incubation period of 4 to 6 days, a prodrome of low grade fever, anorexia, malaise, and sore throat are followed by the typical enanthem. In the mouth small vesicles rapidly erode forming sharply marginated ulcers measuring a few millimeters to 2 cm wide on the buccal mucosa and tongue; they also may be on the palate, uvula, and anterior tonsillar pillars. An exanthem of 3- to 7-mm gray-white angulated or round vesicles appear on the dorsum of the hands and feet and also on the palms, soles, and diaper area in young infants. Occasionally a generalized maculopapular or vesicular rash may be present. Eruptions may be asymptomatic, painful, or pruritic. The spread of infection is restricted by enteric precautions.

### Laboratory evaluation

Viral culture is occasionally helpful. Cultures can be obtained from stool, pharynx, urine, and cerebrospinal fluid (CSF). Due to the multitude of viral etiologies, acute and convalescent serologies are impractical.

### Management

Supportive measures, restricted activity, and rest are recommended. Specific antiviral treatment is not available.

## ADENOVIRUS

Adenovirus is a common cause of fever and upper respiratory infection in children 6 months to 5 years of age. Exanthems occur in only 2% to 8% of illnesses, but the number of infections make this a frequent cause of winter and spring eruptions. Exanthems are maculopapular, morbilliform, rubelliform, and petechial. Systemic symptoms include conjunctivitis, rhinitis, pharyngitis, adenopathy, and pneumonia. Viral culture and acute and convalescent titers confirm the diagnosis. Treatment is not useful for these infections.

## EPSTEIN-BARR VIRUS

### Epidemiology

Epstein-Barr virus (EBV) is the etiologic agent of several diseases including infectious mononucleosis, oral hairy leukoplakia, and hepatitis. EBV causes exanthematous skin eruptions in two settings: (1) young children with acute EBV infection and (2) adolescents and adults with EBV infection (mononucleosis) who receive antibiotics. Infective mononucleosis syndromes are described in Chapter 67.

### Physical examination

Thirty percent of young children with acute EBV infection develop maculopapular, petechial, papulovesicular, scarlatiniform, urticarial, or erythema multiforme-like eruptions. Eruptions are often accompanied by facial and peripheral edema. The presentations of fever, rhinorrhea, adenopathy, and hepatosplenomegaly are variable. Diagnosis of suspected infection is with serologic assays. The monospot test is usually negative before 4 years of age. Acute and convalescent titers to Epstein-Barr nuclear antigen confirms an acute infection. Lymphocytosis is seen in 70% of patients and atypical lymphocytes may be present.

Older children and adolescents with mononucleosis given antibiotics develop erythematous and copper-colored macules and papules, which begin on the trunk and spread to involve the entire body, often becoming coalescent predominantly on the extensor surfaces. The eruption persists for 3 to 4 days before fading. Although ampicillin is the usual culprit, the reaction is not a penicillin allergy. The monospot test is positive in these patients.

## KAWASAKI DISEASE

### Epidemiology

Kawasaki disease is an acute multisystem illness of unknown cause. It was first described in Japan in 1967. The median age at presentation is 2 years with 80% of patients younger than 5 years. Kawasaki disease has occurred in community and nationwide epidemics (see Plate 41).

### History/physical examination

Criteria for diagnosis include (1) fever greater than 39.4° C for at least 5 days; (2) bilateral conjunctival injection; (3) erythema of the pharynx with fissured lips and a "strawberry" tongue; (4) acute nonpurulent cervical lymphadenopathy; (5) polymorphous exanthem; and (6) at least one of the following: erythema of the palms and soles, edema of the palms and soles, desquamation of the tips of the fingers or around the nails. The exanthem is typically a truncal eruption with variable morphologies including morbilliform, urticarial, scarlatiniform, or erythema multiforme-like lesions with annular targetoid lesions.

Recent advances in the diagnosis include the realization that a scarlatiniform perineal eruption is a frequent early finding (occurs in 67%). This eruption appears in the first week, 90% of patients within the first 6 days, often as early as the first day of fever and the median time to presentation is 3 days. Confluent, sometimes tender, macular to plaque-type erythema involves part or all of the perineal region. There is no maceration, vesiculation, pustulation, or sparing of the groin folds, suggesting that an erythrogenic toxin is present such as in staphylococcal scalded skin syndrome, toxic shock syndrome, or scarlet fever. This eruption rapidly progresses to peeling. Present in 67% of 58 patients reported, it is more common than oropharyngeal changes.

Kawasaki disease can result in coronary abnormalities in 15% to 20% of patients, effecting long-term morbidity and mortality. Coronary complications include aneurysms, coronary thrombosis or stenosis, angina pectoris, and ultimately myocardial infarction.

### Management

A single dose of intravenous gamma globulin 2000 mg/kg is useful in preventing complications of coronary vascular involvement. Complications of treatment include disseminated intravascular coagulation and serum sickness. Aspirin is given 80 to 100 mg/kg per day in four divided doses for 2 weeks, followed by 3 to 5 mg/kg per day for 6 to 8 weeks. Echocardiograms are followed for 2 months and then each year thereafter.

## STAPHYLOCOCCAL SCALED SKIN SYNDROME

### Epidemiology/etiology

Staphylococcal scaled skin syndrome (SSSS) is a dermatitis caused by an exfoliative toxin elaborated by coagulase positive group II staphylococci, usually phage type 55 or 71. This disease is seen predominantly in children under the age of 10 years. Eighty-five percent of children over the age of 10 years have a specific antistaphylococcal antibody and are able to metabolize and prevent the spread of the toxin. The syndrome is potentially life-threatening and includes a spectrum of severity from limited disease to extensive cutaneous disease.

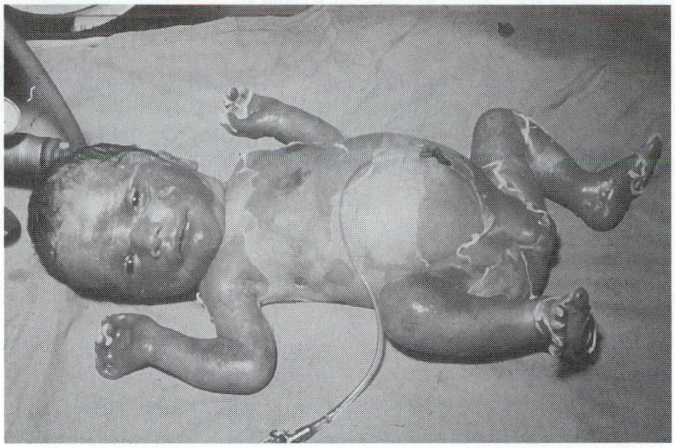

**Fig. 26-2.** Staphylococcal scalded skin syndrome. Note widespread desquamation.

### History/physical examination

Initially a prodrome of malaise, fever, irritability, and generalized tender erythroderma is seen. The eruption spreads from the periorificial, axillae, and other intertriginous areas over the entire body, sparing the hairy parts. Next crusts around the mouth and eyes are noted. Within a few days the upper layer of the skin becomes wrinkled and with light stroking easily rubs off like wet tissue paper (Nikolsky's sign), leaving a moist underlying surface (Fig. 26-2). Shortly thereafter the patient develops flaccid bullae and eventually exfoliation of the skin. Children treated promptly do very well and the skin heals in 10 to 14 days without scarring if the course is uncomplicated.

### Laboratory evaluation

Diagnosis of SSSS is confirmed by isolation of coagulase-positive *Staphylococcus aureus.* The exfoliative toxin is produced by infection from a primary focus, usually in the nose or around the eyes, but also from wound infections or bacteremia. The organism also may be isolated from the conjunctivae, ala nasi, nasopharynx, umbilicus, urinary tract, or stool. The blisters are sterile. For differentiation of SSSS from toxic epidermal necrolysis, a skin biopsy may be necessary. In SSSS the separation occurs in the epidermis; in drug-induced toxic epidermal necrolysis the cleavage is below the dermal-epidermal junction.

### Management

Prompt initiation of antistaphylococcal antibiotics will eradicate the source of infection and halt the production of the exfoliative toxin. In severe SSSS intravenous antibiotics are indicated, but in milder cases oral antibiotics suffice. Appropriate attention must be given to fluid and electrolyte management due to the disruption of the barrier function. In the late stages bland ointments or lubricating lotions may be helpful. Topical antibiotics are unnecessary.

# SCARLET FEVER (SCARLATINA)

## Etiology

Scarlet fever, one of the most common childhood exanthems, is streptococcal pharyngitis accompanied by a cutaneous eruption. It is caused by an erythrogenic toxin produced by group A beta-hemolytic streptococci with either pharyngitis or a cutaneous infection as the primary infection. The scarlet fever exanthem occurs only after previous sensitization to streptococcal exotoxins.

## History/physical examination

After an incubation period of 2 to 5 days, children develop fever, headache, vomiting, malaise, and sore throat. The mucous membranes of the tonsils, pharynx, tongue, and palate are bright red and may have petechiae. Initially the tongue has a heavy coating, and after a few days the edematous papillae protrude through the coating producing a "white strawberry" tongue. In 4 to 5 days the coating peels off leaving a glistening "red strawberry" tongue.

In the first 1 to 2 days an erythematous punctate rash appears on the trunk and then becomes rapidly generalized within 3 to 4 days. The punctate lesions give the skin a fine sandpaper-like appearance. The face is flushed and circumoral pallor is present. The eruption is more intense in areas such as the axillae, antecubital, popliteal, and inguinal regions with Pastia's lines. Transverse areas of hyperpigmentation with a petechial character due to capillary fragility occur in the skin folds. If the eruption is severe, minute vesicular lesions may appear on the abdomen, hands, and feet. In scarlatina, a mild form of scarlet fever, the rash may be faintly erythematous and localized to the trunk. The eruption may be brought out more strongly when the patient is warm or overheated in blankets. The exanthem lasts for 4 or 5 days and as it fades, it leaves a fine branny scale (see Plate 42) that may appear as large exfoliative lamellar scales on the hands, palms, soles, fingertips, elbows, and feet.

## Differential diagnosis

*S. aureus* may cause a scarlet feverlike disease caused by an exfoliative exotoxin produced by staphylococci of bacteriophage group II. It is characterized by an erythematous, tender, sandpaper-like eruption. This disorder is differentiated from streptococcal scarlet fever by the absence of pharyngitis, negative bacterial cultures, and the absence of elevated antistreptolysin titers. Staphylococcal scarlet fever typically does not desquamate. Early complications include otitis media, bronchopneumonia, mastoiditis, septicemia, and osteomyelitis.

## Laboratory evaluation

The diagnosis is based on the clinical presentation, the isolation of group A streptococci from the pharynx, and a rising antistreptolysin-O titer.

## Management

The prognosis for adequately treated streptococcal infection is excellent due to the continued susceptibility of the organism to penicillin. Oral or intramuscular penicillin is the treatment of choice for streptococcal scarlet fever (Penicillin V 25-50 mg/kg per day, divided 6 to 8 hours for 10 days, or benzathine penicillin 25,000 U/kg intramuscularly as a single dose).

# ROCKY MOUNTAIN SPOTTED FEVER

## Epidemiology/etiology

*Rickettsia rickettsii* transmitted by the bite of a wood tick causes this acute febrile illness with a maculopapular eruption. Initially confined primarily to the Rocky Mountain states, the disease is also endemic in the eastern United States and cases have been reported from all parts of the United States.

In the western United States, men are infected by the bite of the wood tick *Dermacentor andersoni.* In the eastern states, women and children are more commonly infected from the bite of the dog tick *Dermacentor variabilis.*

## History/physical examination

After an incubation period of 5 to 7 days, the child develops fever and headache. On the third or fourth day of illness, the rash begins on the flexor areas of the wrists and ankles. Within 2 days the rash spreads to the back, chest, and abdomen and becomes generalized. The face, palms, and soles may be involved; and conjunctivitis, and periorbital and peripheral edema may be present. Initially the macules are erythematous and later become purpuric. The severity and extent of the eruption correlate with the severity of the disease. Disseminated intravascular coagulopathy or purpura fulminans, myocarditis, heart failure, delirium, and seizures may occur in extreme cases.

## Diagnosis and management

Diagnosis can be confirmed by the second or third week of infection by the Weil-Felix agglutination test with OX-19 and OX-2 strains and by the complement fixation tests. The pathogenic organisms cannot be cultured routinely. During the acute stages of the illness, clinical presentation and a history of exposure to a tick bite are important. When in doubt, a rapid diagnosis can be obtained by skin biopsy. Treatment is with tetracycline and in the more severely ill, chloramphenicol may be utilized.

# III Ear, Nose, and Throat

CHAPTER

## 27 Common Problems of the Ear

**Michael D. Seidman**
**George T. Simpson II**
**Mumtaz J. Khan**

Many disorders routinely encountered by primary care physicians may affect the ear, and it is paramount that they possess a comprehensive understanding of a number of otologic problems. There must be a basic understanding of the anatomy (Fig. 27-1) and physiology of the ear. Additionally, the primary care physician must be able to examine and evaluate disorders of the ear, know routine management for common otologic diseases, and know when to refer to an otolaryngologist.

### FOREIGN BODIES

Foreign bodies in the external auditory canal are a common problem, particularly in children. The foreign bodies include peanuts, plastic beads, pins, paper, and pencil erasers, virtually anything that can be placed in the canal. Insects may become trapped in the canal and produce irritating symptoms. Unless the ear canal is traumatized, these foreign bodies may be asymptomatic. When retained for some time, however, infection may develop and produce edema and inflammation of the canal wall itself, as well as purulent and foul-smelling discharge. The true etiology of the problem may be obscured.

The first step in evaluation and treatment of a foreign body in the ear is a complete examination of the head and neck, including the opposite ear and the nose to rule out the presence of multiple foreign bodies. In the absence of a clear history of foreign body placement, a foreign body may not be suspected or detected on the initial examination because of severe inflammation and swelling that can sometimes mimic that of acute or chronic mastoiditis. In this situation, an otolaryngology consultation should be arranged.

Removal should never be attempted by the patient or the family, because it will usually be unsuccessful and may exacerbate the problem and create additional problems. Removal requires complete cooperation by the patient or immobilization to prevent movement of the patient's body and head. Sometimes, particularly in young children, immobilization will require brief general anesthesia. When a live insect is trapped in the ear canal, it may be killed by filling the canal with mineral oil or alcohol.

The basic principle of removal is to apply pressure behind the object so as to pull it from the canal. Instruments such as clamps or alligator forceps should not be used routinely, as they may push the foreign body further into the canal and may traumatize both the canal and the tympanic membrane. Small soft objects that are not occluding the canal may be removed using syringe irrigation in a manner similar to that for removing wax. The water should be at body temperature (lukewarm) to avoid inducing pain or caloric response with vertigo and nausea. Water irrigation should not be used with hygroscopic foreign bodies such as beans or other vegetable material as they will swell with the absorption of water and make removal more difficult.

Small instruments such as wax or wire-loop curet or a blunt hook can be used to remove objects. The curet or blunt hook is passed through the canal until it is beside the

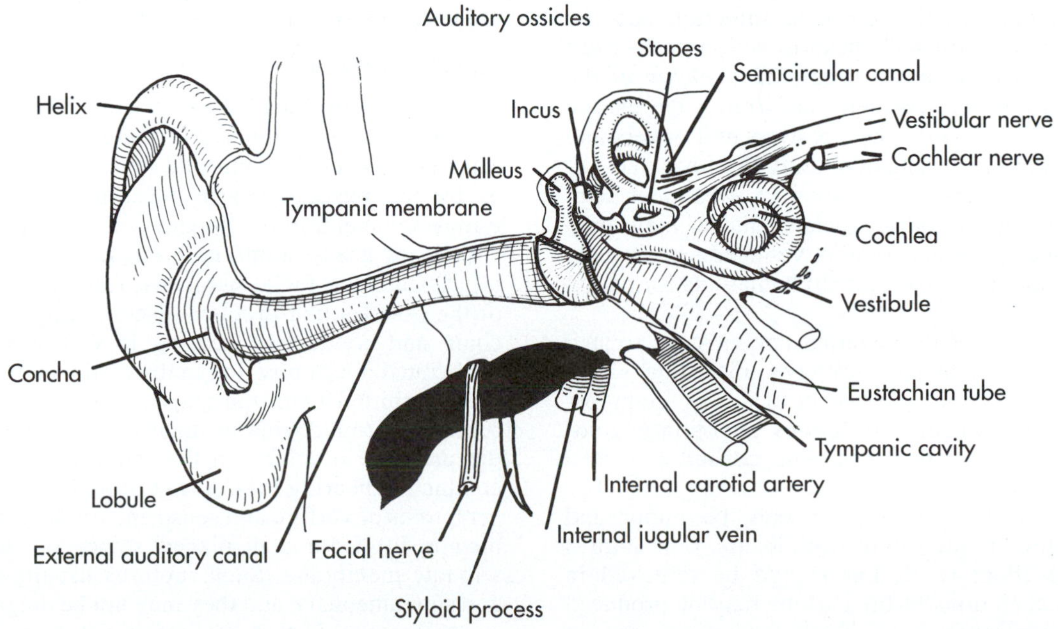


**Fig. 27-1.** Anatomy of the external, middle, and internal ear.

foreign body, and then it is used to pull the object from the canal. As removal is most easily accomplished under direct vision through a binocular operating microscope, an otolaryngologist should be consulted if difficulty is encountered. If the foreign body is near the tympanic membrane, one should consider obtaining an audiogram first to be sure that hearing is not already compromised. If the foreign body has perforated the tympanic membrane, the patient should be seen by an otolaryngologist.

If there has been no gross contamination and there are no signs of inflammation or infection of the middle ear, medication is not usually necessary. An obvious infection should be treated in the manner outlined later (see Otologic Infections). In the presence of lacerations of either the canal or the tympanic membrane, the ear canal should be kept dry to allow healing as will be discussed later. This means preventing water from entering the ear canal while showering, bathing, and hair washing. Cotton balls coated with petroleum jelly may be placed in the external meatus to prevent the entry of water.

Any object in the ear canal that bleeds on manipulation should be suspected of being a mucosal polyp from the middle ear. These polyps occur in the presence of chronic middle ear infections. Their removal should not be attempted, as they may be attached to the facial nerve or ossicles of the middle ear. An otolaryngologist must be consulted for this condition.

## EAR TRAUMA

### External ear trauma

Trauma to the external ear may produce superficial abrasions, contusions, hematomas, lacerations, or partial or complete avulsion. Superficial abrasions are managed as elsewhere in the body. The ear must be inspected for other signs of injury.

Contusions may occur in the postauricular muscles and the muscles of mastication, such as the temporalis. Hematomas may occur when the perichondrium is torn. The accumulation of blood between the perichondrium and the cartilage will produce avascular necrosis and provide an excellent site for soft-tissue infection and abscess formation. If untreated, these infections can result in a loss of portions of the cartilaginous skeleton of the ear resulting in a severe cosmetic deformity: the classic "cauliflower ear" seen in some wrestlers and boxers and in others who engage in physical activities that may result from blunt ear trauma. Temporary treatment with petroleum jelly or collodion-soaked gauze may help to compress the swelling. Protective headgear is now available and should be worn to avert hematoma formation during athletic events.

Large hematomas of the external ear must be treated immediately by incision and drainage, including saline irrigation to remove clots, placement of drains, compression dressings, and systemic antibiotics. An otolaryngologist should be contacted for urgent consultation and surgery if necessary.

Lacerations of the external ear may be minor and require only a few simple sutures for closure. Fine sutures produce an excellent result but should be removed in several days. Lacerations of the earlobe may be produced when earrings are torn away. Such lacerations can be repaired using simple sutures with an excellent result. If not closed primarily, they will require a more complex plastic repair at a later date. Small lacerations extending through skin and cartilage are closed, with care taken to avoid penetration of the cartilage by sutures passing through the skin. This complication may lead to infection of the cartilage. More extensive lacerations and avulsions require the skills of an otolaryngologist.

The external ear canal is occasionally lacerated by a fingernail, cotton-tipped swab, hairpin, or other instrument. These lacerations do not usually cause a significant problem, and they do not require repair. Antibiotic drops may be indicated if a laceration involves more than one half of the external canal, and with larger lacerations, the risk for stenosis increases significantly. Placement of an otowick and application of antibiotic drops may be necessary. Water must be kept out of the ear. It must be determined, however, that the tympanic membrane is intact and that hearing function is normal. The physician must also remember that a laceration of the external canal skin may be associated with a fracture of the temporal bone. If the patient has been struck on the ear, such a fracture becomes more likely.

Trauma may produce injury to the tympanic membranes, including perforations or tears of the membrane. Such injuries may be produced by blows to the outer ear, and barotrauma of an explosive nature may produce a tear in the tympanic membrane. Foreign bodies in the external canal also can cause injury to the tympanic membrane. Most tympanic membrane perforations or tears will rapidly heal spontaneously without intervention. Unless the tympanic membrane is grossly contaminated by dirty water, antibiotics are not usually necessary, although they may be used as a precautionary measure. Occasionally, a small paper patch can be placed over the perforation or laceration by an otolaryngologist to speed the rate of healing. It is most important that the examining physician assess and document the hearing status and other functions of the middle and inner ear at the time of the initial examination. An audiogram should be obtained. If any question remains regarding healing of the injury, an otolaryngology consult must be sought.

### Middle ear trauma

Middle ear injuries result when physical forces are transmitted to structures within the tympanic space. Such injuries may result from loud noises or pressure injuries, or by the introduction of foreign objects through the tympanic membrane. Injuries also may result from significant head trauma with basilar skull fracture. Such injuries include facial paralysis, fracture, and dislocation of the ossicles that produce discontinuity of the ossicular chain and conductive hearing loss. The stapes may be subluxated out of position in the oval window. Forces may be transmitted from the stapes through the cochlea and rupture the round window membrane. Ossicular injury and the presence of blood in the middle ear space result in conductive hearing loss. A leak of perilymph may produce symptoms of vertigo and sensorineural hearing loss, which may result from a displaced stapes or ruptured round window membrane. Such ruptures usually close quickly and spontaneously, and they may not be diagnosed as often as they occur. If they persist, a fistula may result with persistent symptoms and a gradual deterioration of hearing. Perilymph fistulas are considered an otolaryngologic emergency.

### Inner ear trauma

Structures of the inner ear may be injured by sudden forces associated with acceleration, deceleration, or sudden blows to the head. Hydraulic forces transmitted by the ossicles may cause ruptures between the fluid cavities within the labyrinth, disruption or tearing of labyrinthine structures, and bleeding within the labyrinth. Symptoms may vary from hearing loss to dizziness, vertigo, and disequilibrium. These symptoms may be profound, immediate, and incapacitating. They may be irreversible. Significant inner ear injuries usually involve both the vestibular and cochlear systems.

Injuries to the inner ear may be associated with fractures of the temporal bone in the base of the skull. Another form of inner ear trauma is the labyrinthine concussion. Vertigo, hearing loss, and tinnitus constitute the syndrome of the labyrinthine concussion. The most common symptom is positional vertigo, with a brief attack of vertigo and nystagmus being brought on by a change in head position. The syndrome is similar to that of benign paroxysmal positional vertigo. The prognosis for this type of vertigo is quite good, with spontaneous remission usually occurring in 6 months, but occasionally not until more than 2 years after the injury.

In evaluating trauma of the ear, computed tomagraphic scanning (CT) for bony detail is quite helpful.

Function of the ear after trauma must be evaluated by means of audiologic testing. In the presence of any significant likelihood of major injury or significant sequelae, consultation with an otolaryngologist is mandatory and should be obtained on an urgent basis.

## HEARING IMPAIRMENT

Hearing is one of the primary special senses. Impairment of the sense of hearing not only compromises communication, it may result in inappropriate responses to environmental dangers and may induce a sense of isolation that has profound emotional effects.

Probably 10% to 15% of people have some degree of hearing impairment. This estimate means that in the United States, approximately 30 million persons experience some degree of hearing difficulty. Surprisingly hearing loss is frequently overlooked as a major problem despite its common occurrence.

It is important that primary care physicians understand hearing impairment and its socioeconomic ramifications. They have an important responsibility for identifying hearing impairment and obtaining appropriate consultation and remedies for the problem. A normal audiogram has been depicted in Fig. 27-2.

### Causes of hearing loss

Hearing impairment implies a defect in the appropriate identification of acoustic information in the external environment. It may involve any portion of the transducer mechanism of the ear. That is, hearing impairment may result from a defect in the mechanical conduction of sound from the external environment, in sensorineural coding, in transmission of signals to the central nervous system (CNS), or from a mixture of these defects.

***Conductive hearing loss.*** Conductive hearing losses are characterized by mechanical defects or a relative inefficiency in the mechanical portion of the auditory system (Fig. 27-3). Any or all anatomic portions of the external or middle ear may be involved.

**External ear.** In the external ear, any problem or condition that prevents sound energy from reaching the middle ear will result in a hearing loss. The most common condition that produces a hearing loss is occlusion of the external ear canal by cerumen. A buildup of cerumen gradually occludes the canal. Most frequently, cerumen becomes impacted in the ear canal through misguided attempts by the individual to clean the ear canal using a fingertip or a cotton-tipped applicator. Rather than migrating externally, the cerumen is pushed more medially in the canal, eventually occluding it. In this situation, hearing may be restored by removing the cerumen from the canal.

Infection of the soft tissues of the external ear canal produces a conductive hearing loss by closing the canal with edema and retained secretions. Effective management requires removal of all secretions and use of medical therapy.

Overgrowth of the bony wall of the external ear canal may occur. This overgrowth may be the result of contact with cold water while swimming and may be seen in long distance swimmers, surfers, and some scuba divers. The bony knobs may close the ear canal and contribute to retention of the cerumen, fluid, and local inflammation. In addition, occlusion may produce a conductive hearing loss. This condition is called external canal bony exostosis. Exostoses do not require treatment when they are small. When they become large and symptomatic, however, they must be removed surgically by an otolaryngologist.

Rare conditions that produce a conductive hearing loss through occlusion in the external ear canal include tumors and congenital atresias of the canal. Occasionally, multiple recurrent external canal infections can produce a fibrotic or cicatricial stenosis of the canal that requires surgical treatment.

**Tympanic membrane.** When movement of the tympanic membrane is impaired, a mild to moderate mechanical or conductive hearing loss results. Impaired mobility may result from middle ear infection with a buildup of fluid or effusion. A perforation following infection or trauma will impair the mobility and the mechanical efficiency of the tympanic membrane. The mechanical efficiency of the tympanic membrane may be compromised by scar tissue formation within the tympanic membrane and the deposition of calcium, a condition called tympanosclerosis, or by a healed perforation with hypermobility of the membrane at the site of healing. Eustachian tube dysfunction, barotrauma, or barotitis (middle ear inflammation associated with diving injuries or flying) results in negative middle ear pressure and impairs mobility of the tympanic membrane.

**Middle ear.** Many conditions in addition to those involving the tympanic membrane (e.g., middle ear effusion, otitis media, barotitis, tympanosclerosis) affect structures of the middle ear and result in a conductive hearing loss. One such condition is otosclerosis, a bony fusion of the stapes, which reduces the motion of the

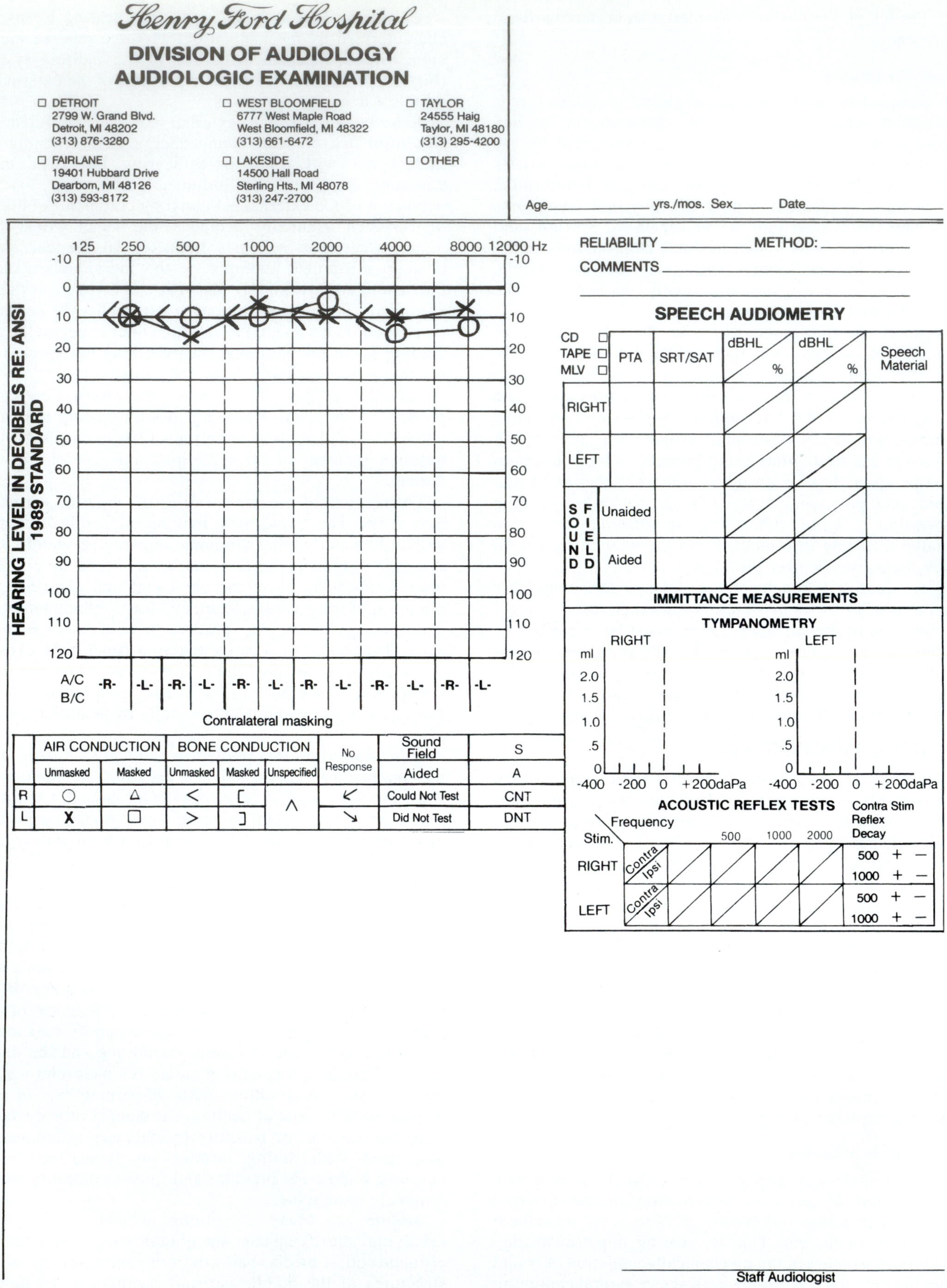


**Fig. 27-2.** Normal audiogram. Pure tone audiograms are graphic representations of the thresholds of perception for tones of various frequencies. Loudness of the tone is measured in decibels (dB) and the frequency or pitch of the tone in hertz (Hz) or cycles per second.

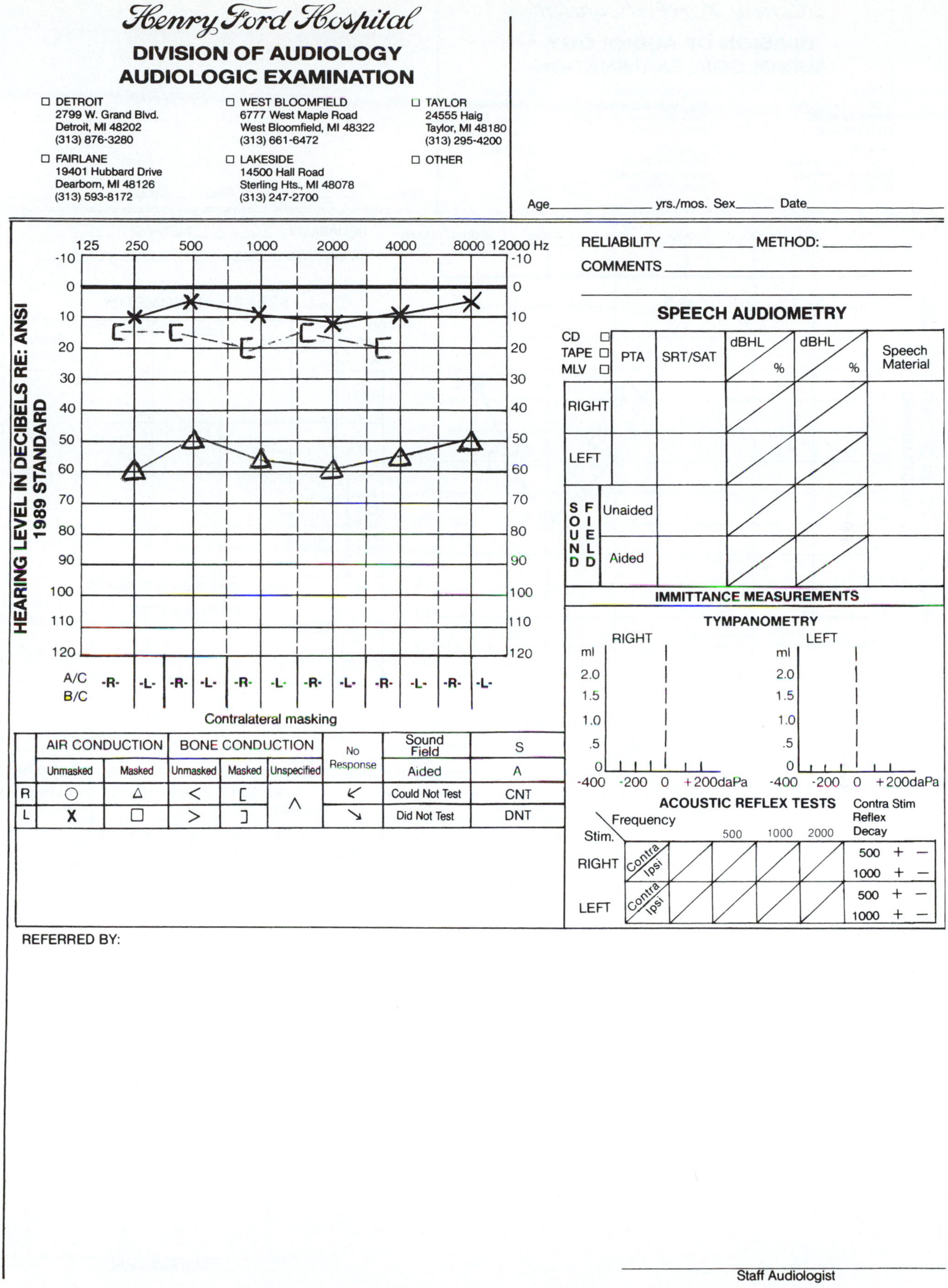


**Fig. 27-3.** Audiogram illustrating moderate conductive hearing loss characterized by air-bone gap in the right ear.

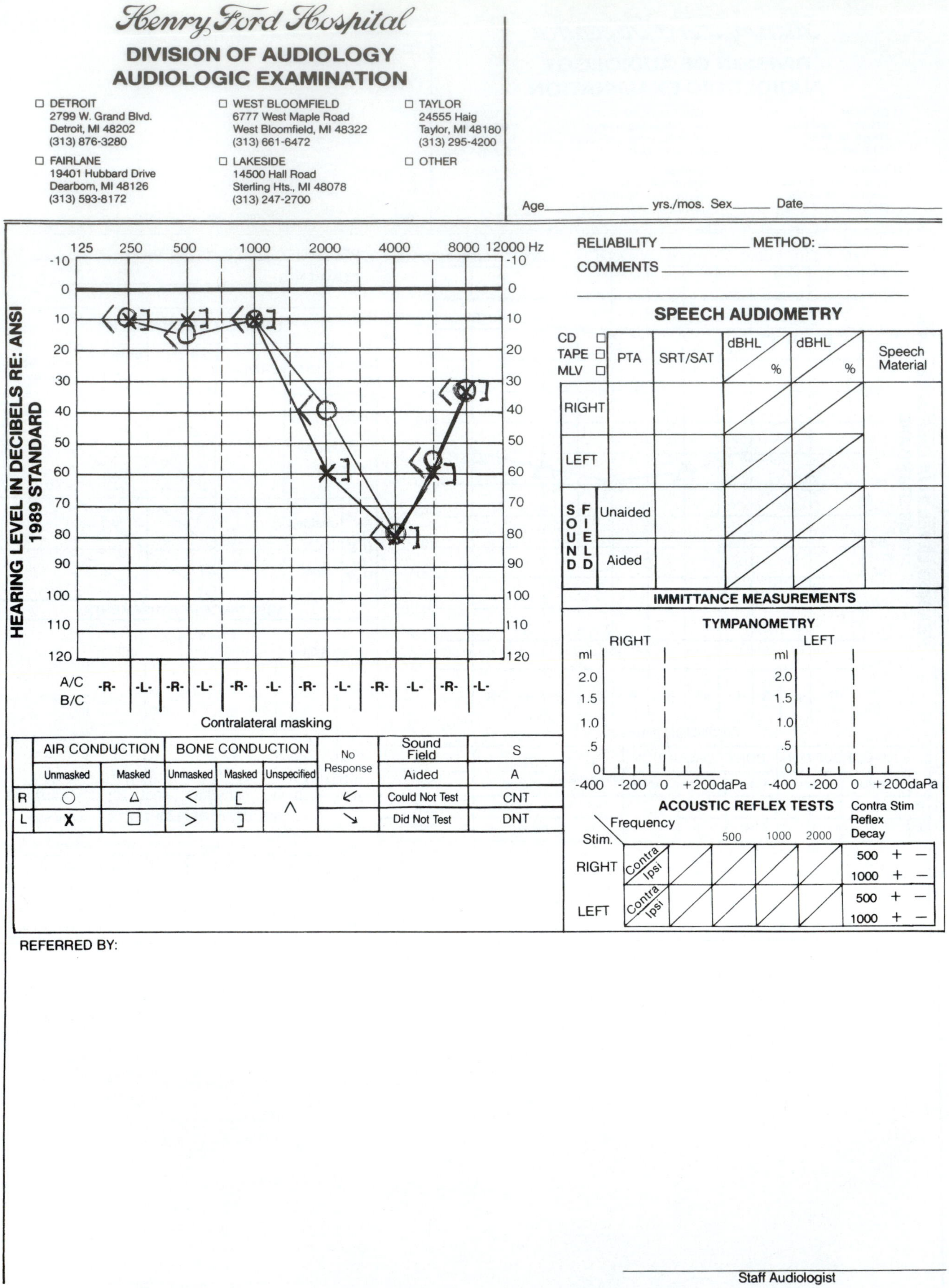


**Fig. 27-4.** Audiogram of bilateral noise-induced sensorineural hearing loss. Typically, it is a high frequency hearing loss, with normal audition at lower frequencies.

ossicle, resulting in hearing loss. It is inherited in an autosomal dominant pattern with variable penetrance. Otosclerosis occurs (but frequently is not detected) in 10% of the population and is treatable with surgery. Ossicular discontinuity, fracture, or subluxation may result from trauma and interfere with the mechanical efficiency of the middle ear sound conduction mechanism. Congenital malformations also may produce conductive hearing loss. Another condition that affects the conduction of sound in the middle ear is the presence of a cholesteatoma (keratoma). This condition is a collection of normal squamous epithelium occurring within a sac or forming a ball within the middle ear space. Cholesteatomas usually follow a perforation or retraction pocket in the tympanic membrane. The ball of squamous epithelium gradually enlarges over time and through a combination of direct pressure and enzymatic resorbtion can cause the destruction of the ossicles and erosion of structures within the inner ear or cranial cavity. If there is communication with the outside, chronic infection and drainage may occur and induce otitis media or disseminated infection with grave sequelae. The degree of destruction may not be appreciated initially, as the collection of squamous cells may become a mechanical transmission device to the inner ear, even when extensive destruction has already occurred.

Mechanical (conductive) hearing loss frequently can be improved or eliminated safely by surgery. Underlying disease must be treated. If surgery is not possible or desired, hearing aids may significantly improve hearing.

***Sensorineural hearing loss.*** Disorders within the cochlea, the auditory nerve and its connections in the brainstem, produce hearing loss that is classified as sensorineural. Sensorineural hearing losses are divided into those involving the cochlea and those involving the retrocochlear region (the eighth cranial nerve and central pathways).

Several disorders within the cochlea produce hearing loss. A common and increasingly recognized form of hearing loss is that induced by noise trauma (Fig. 27-4). This trauma can be explosive noise, but, most commonly, it is prolonged exposure to excessive levels of noise above 85 decibels (dB). Mechanical stress on structures of the inner ear may produce temporary injury and, if prolonged, result in a permanent injury and increasing hearing loss. The most easily damaged structures are the hair cells in the organ of Corti, which is attached to the basilar membrane in the basal turn of the cochlea. As hair cells in this region of the cochlea are involved in the perception of high-frequency sounds, the initial hearing loss is in the area of 4000 hertz, but will gradually progress to involve higher and lower frequencies. Temporary hearing loss from loud noise exposure is called a temporary threshold shift. Such a hearing loss typically improves over 24 to 72 hours. Repeated or persistent noise exposures produce an irreversible hearing loss.

The next most common form of sensorineural hearing loss after traumatic noise exposure is presbycusis. This hearing loss of aging represents gradual degeneration of structures within the cochlea and to some degree, of central neural connections. Some degeneration of the mechanical portion of hearing also may be present. Typically, the hearing loss is most severe in the highest frequencies and is less in lower frequencies (Fig. 27-5). It is gradually progressive. Presbycusis may have a hereditary component involving sensitivity to a variety of factors that produce degeneration.

Sensorineural hearing loss may result from viral or bacterial infections of cochlear structures. Such hearing loss is usually rapidly progressive and frequently total. Similar hearing loss results from labyrinthitis of any etiology, but is usually associated with vestibular symptoms (vertigo and disequilibrium). Syphilitic (luetic) involvement of the labyrinth produces a fluctuating hearing loss and disequilibrium. Symptoms gradually progress, and hearing deteriorates without treatment.

Meniere's disease may be present in patients who experience fluctuating hearing loss. It comprises the syndrome of fluctuating sensorineural hearing loss, tinnitus, pressure symptoms in the ear, and vertigo. The ultimate etiology is unknown, but the pathology involves the buildup of intralabyrinthine pressure, which is called endolymphatic hydrops. The increased pressure distends structures of the labyrinth in an episodic fashion. The episodes are associated with a sudden onset of cochlear and vestibular symptoms. Several therapies have been tried with varying success: the use of salt-restricted diet and vasodilator agents, including nicotinic acid, histamine, 5% carbon dioxide inhalations, diuretic agents, and diazepam. The symptoms may be associated with periods of increased stress. Symptoms wax and wane and may be absent for months to years and then return. Occasionally, profound hearing loss and loss of vestibular function may result. The majority of patients benefit from diuretics and salt restriction. Approximately 15% to 20% fail medical management and several surgical options are available.

While usually associated with conductive hearing losses, otosclerosis also may produce intralabyrinthine symptoms, particularly tinnitus and sensorineural hearing loss, for reasons that are not well understood. Surgery in otosclerosis, while improving hearing, may not affect the other symptoms. Medical treatment with sodium fluoride occasionally leads to stabilization of hearing.

Fistulas involving leakage of perilymphatic fluid from the middle ear or mixing of perilymphatic fluid with endolymphatic fluid may be associated with marked sudden hearing loss. The symptoms do not usually persist, but occasionally may be present for varying periods of time and occur in an episodic fashion. Fistulas are usually associated with physical activity or sudden barotrauma; they may follow external trauma to the ear and head. Bed rest with the head elevated must be begun immediately. An otolaryngologist should be consulted immediately. Surgical correction is occasionally required.

Ototoxic effects of medication are of increasing importance and must be understood by a primary care physician. The most commonly encountered ototoxic drug effect is produced by salicylates. Symptoms include tinnitus, hearing loss, dizziness, and disequilibrium. The hearing loss involves all frequencies. Symptoms rapidly disappear after the cessation of medication. Other drugs producing ototoxic effects include ethacrynic acid and furosemide. Quinine-related antimalarial compounds produce a progressive irreversible hearing loss, sometimes of delayed onset. Malarial infections, however, may produce

*Henry Ford Hospital*

## DIVISION OF AUDIOLOGY
## AUDIOLOGIC EXAMINATION

☐ DETROIT
2799 W. Grand Blvd.
Detroit, MI 48202
(313) 876-3280

☐ FAIRLANE
19401 Hubbard Drive
Dearborn, MI 48126
(313) 593-8172

☐ WEST BLOOMFIELD
6777 West Maple Road
West Bloomfield, MI 48322
(313) 661-6472

☐ LAKESIDE
14500 Hall Road
Sterling Hts., MI 48078
(313) 247-2700

☐ TAYLOR
24555 Haig
Taylor, MI 48180
(313) 295-4200

☐ OTHER

Age_____ yrs./mos. Sex_____ Date_____

RELIABILITY _____ METHOD: _____

COMMENTS _____

### SPEECH AUDIOMETRY

| CD ☐ TAPE ☐ MLV ☐ | PTA | SRT/SAT | dBHL / % | dBHL / % | Speech Material |
|---|---|---|---|---|---|
| RIGHT | | | | | |
| LEFT | | | | | |
| SOUND FIELD — Unaided | | | | | |
| SOUND FIELD — Aided | | | | | |

**IMMITTANCE MEASUREMENTS**

**TYMPANOMETRY**

| RIGHT | LEFT |
|---|---|
| ml 2.0 1.5 1.0 .5 0   -400 -200 0 +200daPa | ml 2.0 1.5 1.0 .5 0   -400 -200 0 +200daPa |

**ACOUSTIC REFLEX TESTS**    Contra Stim Reflex Decay

| Stim. Frequency | | 500 | 1000 | 2000 | |
|---|---|---|---|---|---|
| RIGHT  Contra/Ipsi | | | | | 500 + — |
| | | | | | 1000 + — |
| LEFT  Contra/Ipsi | | | | | 500 + — |
| | | | | | 1000 + — |

HEARING LEVEL IN DECIBELS RE: ANSI 1989 STANDARD

125  250  500  1000  2000  4000  8000  12000 Hz

A/C -R- -L- -R- -L- -R- -L- -R- -L- -R- -L- -R- -L-
B/C

Contralateral masking

| | AIR CONDUCTION | | BONE CONDUCTION | | | No Response | Sound Field | S |
|---|---|---|---|---|---|---|---|---|
| | Unmasked | Masked | Unmasked | Masked | Unspecified | | Aided | A |
| R | ○ | △ | < | [ | ∧ | ↙ | Could Not Test | CNT |
| L | X | □ | > | ] | | ↘ | Did Not Test | DNT |

REFERRED BY:

Staff Audiologist

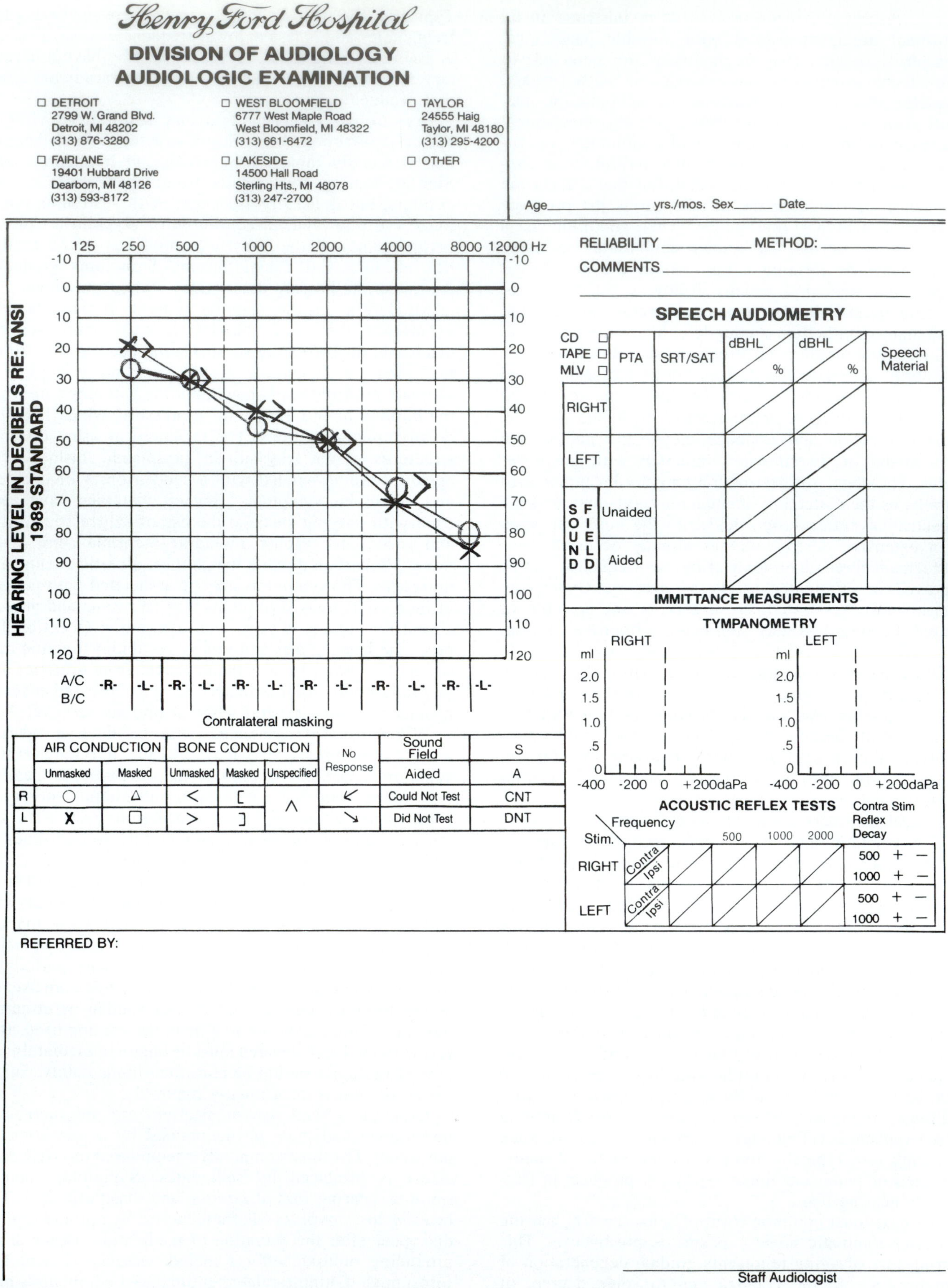

**Fig. 27-5.** Audiogram of mid- to high-frequency sensorineural hearing loss consistent with presbycusis. The hearing loss is most severe at the highest frequencies and is less at lower frequencies.

permanent sensorineural hearing loss if the labyrinth has been infected. Quinine and its analogs may cause fetal injury and congenital deafness. Nitrogen mustard and *cis*-platinum, as used in chemotherapy, also can produce significant hearing loss.

Clinically, the most significant agents producing ototoxicity are the aminoglycosides, all of which produce varying degrees of auditory and vestibular damage. Streptomycin and gentamicin have their greatest effects on the vestibular end organ; kanamycin, tobramycin, and neomycin cause more damage to the cochlear end organ. Patients receiving aminoglycosides rarely complain of vertigo but experience unsteadiness of gait, particularly in darkness. A sensorineural hearing loss is produced, beginning in the high frequencies and progressing to a flat, moderately severe loss across all frequencies. Serial audiograms must be obtained on any patient receiving a prolonged course of these agents. Aminoglycosides produce their effects by damaging the hair cells of the inner ear. Unlike other common antibiotics, aminoglycosides are concentrated in both the perilymph and endolymph so that the hair cells are exposed to high concentrations. The ototoxicity of aminoglycosides does not correlate well with serum drug levels. If the total dose is limited to less than 2 g, however, and the duration of therapy is less than 10 days, the incidence of ototoxicity is low. Because these drugs are eliminated almost exclusively by the kidneys, they must be used with caution in renal failure.

Several congenital disorders may produce a sensorineural hearing loss. When they are not identified at an early age, the acquisition of language skills is severely impaired. Many individuals have been misdiagnosed as having mental retardation when their only problem was impaired hearing. Such events have profound and devastating lifelong consequences for education and quality of life. For this reason, hearing screening should begin at a young age, and full audiologic testing should be used when any child appears to have a significant problem in interacting appropriately with the environment.

Currently, the only effective treatment for sensorineural hearing loss is the use of amplification devices. Research studies have been designed to regenerate cochlear hair cells, and avian models have had some success. All cases of suspected hearing loss should be evaluated by an otolaryngologist.

**Retrocochlear hearing loss.** When the site of the hearing disorder involves the auditory nerve, brain stem, or CNS, it is defined as a retrocochlear hearing loss. Common causes of retrocochlear hearing loss include CNS sequelae of infection or cerebrovascular injury such as a stroke, intracranial bleed, or concussion. Other CNS disorders include demyelinating and other degenerative diseases or neoplasms. A common site of retrocochlear pathology involves the eighth cranial nerve, either within the internal auditory canal or within the posterior fossa in the cerebellar pontine angle near the brainstem. Tumors here are rare but must not be overlooked. Within the auditory canal or near its opening, the most common neoplasm is the vestibular schwannoma, a benign tumor arising in the perineurium of the cochleovestibular nerve. Occasionally, congenital keratomas may occur in this area. Other benign tumors are meningiomas. Primary intracranial malignancies or metastases may produce similar symptoms. Vestibular schwannoma and the cerebellar pontine angle tumors have an insidious onset and thus may be encountered in a primary care practice. Early symptoms may include tinnitus, hearing loss, and disequilibrium.

**Mixed hearing loss.** A mixed hearing loss is present when a conductive hearing impairment occurs simultaneously with sensorineural hearing loss. A mixed or combined hearing loss may follow injury involving structures of the external, middle, and inner ears. Infection may produce acute and chronic changes in the structure of the ear, including acute inflammation and nerve injury, as well as tympanosclerosis. Congenital disorders may involve structures in any or all parts of the ear. A mixed hearing loss may produce variable and confusing signs on physical examination and requires more specialized testing for proper identification.

## DIAGNOSIS OF HEARING LOSS

The diagnosis of hearing loss requires a suspicion of its presence, either by the patient or the examining physician. In moderate to severe hearing loss, it is obvious to everyone that communication is impaired and a hearing loss is likely. In mild degrees of hearing loss, however, a high index of suspicion is necessary. The patient may not be aware of the gradual onset of the loss and may utilize the psychologic defense of denial to avoid facing the realities of aging and altered body image. Because of the socially isolating effects of impaired communication, what may initially appear to be depression or even irrational behavior may actually be the result of hearing loss. Severe or profound hearing loss of long duration prevents proper self-assessment of accurate pronunciation and may result in slurred speech, which can be misinterpreted as resulting from other pathology (Table 27-1).

Family members may become frustrated and angry with the person who has the hearing impairment if the nature of the problem is not recognized. Communication problems may be attributed to antisocial tendencies or impaired mental status. For all of these reasons, awareness of the possibility of hearing impairment and suspicion of its presence are essential if the primary care physician is to adequately aid the patient.

Sudden sensorineural hearing loss is a relatively rare entity that accounts for varying degrees of hearing impairment. The etiology is elusive, but anecdotal information may suggest that vascular, viral, or autoimmune causes are the most common. Treatment is controversial and medicines that have been tried include vasodilators, anticoagulants, steroids, and hypaque. Treatment is much more likely to be efficacious if instituted early in the course (i.e., within 24 hours and preferably earlier).

With a thorough examination of the ear, the primary care physician usually can recognize the presence of a hearing loss even if it is not possible to diagnose the problem more accurately. The physician may desire to have the patient undergo an audiologic evaluation. In most cases of hearing loss, a consultation from an otolaryngologist is essential. During this consultation a complete audiogram may be obtained and appropriate selection of therapy will be arranged.

The primary care physician must understand the process involved in audiologic testing to interpret a report directly from the audiologist or an otolaryngologic consultation.

**Table 27-1.** Relations between hearing threshold level and probable handicap

| Hearing threshold | Probable handicap* |
|---|---|
| <40 dB | Has difficulty hearing faint or distant speech; needs favorable seating, and may benefit from lip reading instruction. May also benefit from a hearing aid. |
| 40-55 dB | Understands conversational speech at a distance of 3 to 5 feet; needs hearing aid, lip reading, favorable seating, and speech correction. |
| 55-70 dB | Conversation must be loud to be understood, and there is great difficulty in group and classroom discussion; needs all of above plus language therapy and maybe special class for the hard-of-hearing. |
| 70-90 dB | May hear a loud voice about 1 foot from the ear, may identify environmental noises, may distinguish vowels but not consonants. A child who needs special education for the deaf with emphasis on speech, auditory training, and language may enter regular classes at a later time. |
| >90 dB | May hear loud sounds; does not rely on hearing as a primary channel for communication; needs special class or school for the deaf; some of these children enter regular high schools. |

*Assumes all medical or surgical treatment has been applied. If the hearing loss is detected in childhood, special education may be required.

## TINNITUS

Tinnitus is noise heard by the patient in the absence of any external stimulation. Recent estimates suggest that approximately 40 million Americans are affected by tinnitus. Rarely, the sound can be heard by the examiner. Subjective tinnitus is that heard by the patient alone, and objective tinnitus is that which can be heard by both the patient and the examiner.

### Objective tinnitus

Objective tinnitus can be heard when the examiner places a stethoscope (with the bell removed) in the patient's external auditory canal or places the bell around the ear on the neck. A blowing sound that coincides with inspiration and expiration can result from an abnormally patent (patulous) eustachian tube. The history may indicate this type of tinnitus because of the association with respiration. This type of tinnitus most frequently follows rapid weight loss or may occur during a debilitating illness.

Sharp clicking sounds that occur in bursts and last for several seconds or minutes may be produced by tetanic contractions of the muscles of the soft palate or the tensor tympani muscle. This phenomenon is known as palatal myoclonus. Occasionally, the palatal contractions can be observed by the examiner when the tinnitus is audible. Disturbances in the vascular blood flow produce a pulsatile sound that is synchronous with the heartbeat. Aneurysms, vascular neoplasms, and arteriovenous malformations may produce this type of tinnitus. A venous hum produced by turbulence within the internal jugular vein can produce a "whooshing" or continuous machinelike sound synchronized with the pulse. The examiner may eliminate the sound by occluding the distal jugular vein while avoiding obstructing arterial flow. Carotid bruits may also manifest as pulsatile tinnitus. Radiologic studies with contrast may reveal an enlarged jugular bulb or carotid vascular disease. Ligation of the internal jugular vein may be curative in some patients.

Recent studies have shown that highly sensitive recording techniques can detect the sound produced by the normal motion of cochlear hair cells. This sound represents mechanical effects produced by the stiffening of the basilar membrane within the cochlea and are called otoacoustic emissions. Although these sounds are found in patients with normal hearing without any symptoms, they may produce subjective tinnitus.

### Subjective tinnitus

Subjective tinnitus is a sound in the ears or head that is heard by the patient alone. Tinnitus may be produced by lesions or conditions within the external ear canal, tympanic membrane, middle ear structures, cochlea, auditory nerve, brainstem, and cerebral cortex. Patients may describe the noise as an ill-defined buzzing, ringing, whistling, or hissing or may identify a specific noise associated with insect or motor sounds. This description can be diagnostically valuable. Meniere's syndrome produces a low-pitched continuous tinnitus similar to an ocean roar and frequently becomes very loud immediately preceding an acute attack of vertigo. It may then disappear after the attack. In otosclerosis, tinnitus is usually low pitched and continuous, but occasionally it can be intermittent. Cerumen, foreign bodies, or loose hairs in the external ear canal may rub against the tympanic membrane and produce a variety of sounds. Noise or physical trauma, including acoustic trauma from an explosion, produces a high-pitched tinnitus that usually subsides after a few hours, although occasionally it can persist if permanent hearing loss has occurred. Continuous bilateral high-pitched tinnitus frequently accompanies hearing loss from chronic noise exposure, presbycusis, and ototoxic chemicals or drugs. A continuous, unilateral, high-pitched tinnitus may be the first symptom of a vestibular schwannoma and may precede loss of hearing or distortion of hearing by several years.

Cochlear and retrocochlear lesions producing tinnitus are usually associated with sensorineural hearing loss or distortion of sounds. The perceived pitch of the tinnitus frequently corresponds to the frequency of greatest hearing impairment. CNS lesions producing tinnitus may not be associated with hearing loss, but are almost always associated with other neurologic signs and symptoms.

Although some patients with tinnitus do not have associated hearing loss, this finding may represent limitations in testing equipment that typically does not measure hearing beyond 8000 hertz.

Many drugs produce tinnitus without associated hearing loss. Such drugs commonly in use include salicylates,

**Table 27-2.** External ear infection

| | Etiology | Clinical findings | Common microbiologic agents | Management |
|---|---|---|---|---|
| Bacterial | | | | |
| Diffuse otitis externa | Swimming; trauma; metabolic disorders (diabetes) | Severe otalgia; tragal tenderness; diffuse inflammation of ear canal | *Pseudomonas*; *Staphylococcus aureus*; *Streptococcus*; *Escherichia coli* | Aural cleansing; topical antibiotic; Burow's solution |
| Localized otitis externa | Furuncles | Otalgia; otorrhea; localized tenderness; furuncle in outer third of ear canal | *Staphylococcus* | Aural cleansing; topical antibiotic; Burow's solution oral anti-*Staphylococcus* |
| Malignant otitis externa | Diabetes; immunosuppression | Diffuse external otitis; necrotizing granulation tissue; facial nerve paralysis | *Pseudomonas* | Systemic antibiotic; necrotic tissue debridement |
| Viral | Unknown | Otalgia; vesicles on ear canal; facial nerve paralysis | Herpes zoster (Ramsay Hunt syndrome); varicella; measles | Analgesics |
| Fungal | Diabetes; tropical climate | Pruritis; minimal otalgia; black, white, or yellow spores | *Aspergillus; Candida* | Aural cleansing; Burow's solution |

indomethacin, quinidine, propranolol, levodopa, carbamazepine, aminophylline, and caffeine. The exact anatomic site where tinnitus is produced by the actions of these drugs in unknown, but the drugs probably have both peripheral and central effects.

The treatment of tinnitus may be frustrating. All efforts should be made to diagnose any associated conditions that may be treated. Several medications taken systemically may suppress tinnitus temporarily, but treatment requires high doses that may be near the toxic range. No drugs are available to "cure" tinnitus; however studies have suggested that amitryptyline and alprazolam may reduce the severity of tinnitus in some patients. These medications are typically reserved for individuals with severe tinnitus, as they may have significant side effects. Ambient or environmental noise is most helpful in suppressing tinnitus. Wide-band, or white, noise suppresses tinnitus, not only while the noise is present but for some time after its cessation. Maintaining background noise from a radio or television set or from a device generating the sound of the ocean or falling rain may be helpful, particularly before sleep. A hearing aid may not only improve hearing, but also suppress tinnitus. Tinnitus masking devices worn by the patient are helpful in some cases. These devices are similar to hearing aids, but they produce a lower level of continuous white noise for tinnitus suppression. The most important single measure in helping a patient with tinnitus is the reassurance of the physician that there is no underlying condition. Proper evaluation and tests are necessary and can readily be obtained. Consultation with an otolaryngologist is often indicated.

## OTOLOGIC INFECTIONS

Ear infections and their sequelae are relatively common problems in all age groups and represent one of the largest categories of illness in the pediatric population. Effective treatment depends on the specific anatomic structures involved, the agents responsible for infection, and appropriate treatment strategies. Ear infections may involve structures of the external ear, the tympanic and mastoid cavities, or even the labyrinth and temporal bone. Infectious agents may be viral, bacterial, or fungal. Effective treatment is based on these considerations.

### External ear infections

External ear infections involve the skin lining, the external auditory ear canal, and the periosteum of the bone immediately beneath the skin. After cleansing the ear canal, the diagnosis is established by the presence of characteristic diffuse inflammation of the ear canal skin, with or without involvement of the tympanic membrane. Edema is not uncommon and frequently moist otorrhea is present. If the tympanic membrane cannot be seen or otitis media cannot be ruled out, treatment must be directed at both external and middle ear infection. Use of a systemic agent is required (see Middle Ear Infection). Absorbent wicks (otowicks) that expand in the external auditory canal are often used when the edema is severe (Table 27-2).

In the presence of infection, the ear must be kept dry. No swimming is allowed, and care must be taken while bathing or hair washing to keep water out of the ear. The external meatus can be temporarily occluded with a cotton ball coated with petroleum jelly. All secretions and debris must be removed at least once or twice a week until the infection resolves. Specific treatments are directed at the infecting organisms (most commonly *Pseudomonas aeruginosa*) and inflammatory effects. Cortisporin otic suspension or colymycin will usually eradicate the infection. Three to four drops in the ear four times a day for 7 to 10 days is the typical course. Other commonly used medications include vasocidin, cetapred, volsol, domboro, garamicin, and boric acid with alcohol.

***Viral infections.*** Viral infections of the external ear are rare. They include varicella, measles, and occasionally herpes virus. Unless secondary bacterial infections develop, treatment is essentially supportive and specific only for symptoms (e.g., pain). In the presence of weeping lesions or edema, astringent agents such as Burow's solution are applied liberally every 4 hours in drops or soaks. Use of steroids is controversial. Symptoms of herpes zoster oticus (Ramsay-Hunt syndrome) include severe otalgia, facial paralysis or paresis, decreased lacrimation on the involved side, loss of taste of the anterior two thirds of the tongue, and vesicles on the external ear canal and on the posterior surface of the auricle. The likelihood of good facial function after Ramsay-Hunt syndrome is 40%. Treatment with acyclovir and occasionally steroids has been advocated but is controversial. Occasionally, surgical decompres sion of the facial nerve is necessary to preserve nerve viability and function. Symptomatic treatment for pain and provision of artificial tears are required pending the resolution of symptoms. Any patient with facial nerve paresis or paralysis should be seen in an urgent consultation with an otolaryngologist, who will evaluate the viability of the nerve and determine whether decompression is required.

***Bacterial infections.*** The most common pathogen involved in an external ear infection is *P. aeruginosa.* Its frequency of involvement, however, may represent opportunistic contamination within the environment in a moist ear. Other bacterial agents include *S. aureus* and *Streptococcus* species. Occasionally, enteric organisms may be present. External ear infections are painful. The pathognomonic sign of external ear infection is pain with manipulation of the auricle. Analgesia must be adequate. Codeine (appropriate for age and weight) may be required. In general, analgesic ear drops are not effective, because inflamed tissue resists local anesthetic agents.

All moist infected ears should be swabbed to obtain specimens for culture and sensitivity determinations. As discussed previously, all foreign materials, debris, and secretions must be removed.

In general the most effective antibiotic agents are those applied topically, but occasionally systemic agents may be required. Some of the most effective topical antibiotic agents currently available are mixtures: neomycin and bacitracin or polymyxin with hydrocortisone. As neomycin is ototoxic, some have suggested that it should not be used with a coexistent perforation; however, most otolaryngologists have used this medication for many years without difficulty. Steroid compounds are included in topical medications to decrease inflammation. A small percentage of patients have an idiosyncratic sensitivity to neomycin and, in its presence, will develop erythema, swelling, and pain at the site of application. If these or other severe external ear symptoms develop or persist for more than 1 or 2 weeks after starting the medication, it should be discontinued and another medication substituted.

Alternative medications for treatment of otitis externa include vasocidin, cetapred, domboro, chloramphenicol otic solution, acetic acid solutions with or without hydrocortisone, and aluminum subacetate (Burow's) solution. These agents have either a bacteriostatic effect or the ability to reduce the pH of the external canal, thus restoring an acid pH to the milieu of the canal skin. In addition some of the medications listed have a mildly astringent effect that aids in drying the skin and decreasing edema.

All medications are given in a dosage of three to four drops, three to four times per day. If Burow's solution is used alone, it should be applied every 2 to 3 hours for the first 48 hours. Acetic acid, in the form of white vinegar, may be used alone, remembering that it will be painful if it enters the middle ear. All medications are instilled into the ear canal with the ear up to allow the medication to contact all portions of the ear canal. The patient should keep the head turned to the side or lie on the side with the treated ear up for 2 to 5 minutes after instillation. Then the medication is allowed to run out by turning the head the opposite way.

In rare instances external ear infections may extend to involve external ear structures and surrounding tissue. Systemic antibiotics are then necessary. Unless culture and sensitivity reports suggest other treatment, penicillinase-resistant penicillin (dicloxacillin orally or oxacillin or cephalosporins parenterally) is usually best. Occasionally, hospitalization is necessary. In this circumstance, applying continuous Burow's solution soaks to the affected area is soothing and helps reduce inflammation, swelling, and pain.

One type of external ear infection that may have lethal consequences and must be recognized by the physician is necrotizing otitis externa (malignant otitis externa). This soft tissue infection, which more commonly occurs in elderly, diabetic, or immunocompromised patients, is typically caused by *Pseudomonas* (or *Pseudomonas* mixed with other organisms). It may begin with an indolent course, minimal symptoms including otorrhea and inflammation, and may lull the patient and physician into a false sense of security. This initially benign-appearing course progresses relentlessly, if untreated, to invasion and necrosis of contiguous soft tissue structures, including the auricle, scalp, and parotid gland. Further extension occurs to structures of the middle and inner ear with eventual extension to the brain. A facial nerve paralysis may be an early and ominous presenting sign. Diagnosis requires a high index of suspicion and the demonstration of granulation tissue. Effective treatment involves a prolonged course of systemic antibiotics and aggressive debridement of necrotic tissue and drainage to prevent further progression. Without treatment, the disease is uniformly fatal, but with aggressive treatment the majority of patients survive.

***Fungal infections.*** Fungal infections of the external ear frequently elicit pruritus. Black, white, or yellow spores may be seen. Contact sensitivity reactions to the fungus may be present. Pain is usually minimal.

Mild fungal infections are best treated by general aural hygiene, which includes removal of all cerumen and debris. A dry ear with a normal mildly acidic pH is restored

**Table 27-3.** Middle ear infection

| | Etiology | Clinical findings | Common microbiologic agents | Management |
|---|---|---|---|---|
| Acute suppurative otitis media | Bacterial contamination with possible eustachian tube dysfunction | Bulging or retracted TM*; air-fluid level; pulsatile discharge | *H. influenzae*; *S. pneumoniae*; *Mycoplasma*; Grp. A strep.; *C. diphtheria*; gram-negative bacilli; parainfluenza virus; RSV† | Aural cleansing; oral antibiotic; analgesia |
| Acute and serous otitis media | Eustachian tube dysfunction; barotrauma; nasopharyngeal tumor | Thickened, retracted TM; gray or amber fluid in middle ear; impaired mobility of TM; conductive hearing loss | Rare | Nasal decongestant autoinflation exercises |
| Chronic suppurative otitis media | Bacterial contamination | Mucopurulent otorrhea; perforated TM; conductive hearing loss; cholesteatoma | Mixed aerobic and anaerobic flora: *S. aureus*; *E. coli*; *Pseudomonas*; *B. fragilis* | Aural cleansing; topical antibiotic; surgical management |

*Tympanic membrane.
†Respiratory syncytial virus.

with Burow's solution, volsol, domboro or boric acid, and alcohol irrigations two to four times a day. Persistent mycoses may benefit from a brief course of tincture of cresylate, three to four drops twice a day for 1 to 2 weeks. This agent should not be used if the eardrum is perforated. Clotrimazol, 1% lotion, in a similar dosage also may be effective. If systemic mycotic allergy is present and associated with local inflammatory changes in the external ear, immunotherapy with desensitization injections can produce dramatic relief of symptoms.

## Middle ear infections (Table 27-3)

***Bullous myringitis.*** In bullous myringitis small blebs or blisters are present on the tympanic membrane. An extremely painful condition, bullous myringitis was once thought to be caused by a *Mycoplasma* infection, but it is now known to be caused by a bacterial middle ear infection. Treatment is both supportive and antibacterial. Medications commonly used to alleviate pain include acetaminophen (Tylenol), ibuprofen, and possibly codeine. Erythromycin, penicillin, or amoxicillin in a dosage of 30 to 50 mg/kg per day is given. Resolution or rupture of the bulla should not be induced unless the pain is severe; in that case lancing of the bulla promptly alleviates the pain.

***Acute suppurative otitis media.*** Acute middle ear infections are one of the most common problems seen by the pediatrician or family physician. Infections typically develop as a result of bacterial contamination through the eustachian tube in the presence of preexisting inflammation in the middle ear. This inflammation results from eustachian tube dysfunction. In the presence of eustachian tube dysfunction, oxygen is absorbed from the air in the middle ear space. A negative partial pressure results, which induces an inflammatory response. This response in turn produces a sterile transudate within the middle ear, which may evolve into an exudative process. Concurrent or subsequent contamination of the middle ear from infective nasopharyngeal contents may occur by aspiration or insufflation during nose-blowing or crying. In infancy it may be produced by the flow of milk or other liquids into the eustachian tube while the infant is lying supine with a bottle propped in his mouth to induce sleep. The major bacterial pathogens in acute suppurative otitis media include *Streptococcus pneumoniae, Moraxella catarrhalis, Haemophilus influenzae,* and group A *S. pyogenes. Staphylococcus aureus, Mycoplasma pneumoniae, Corynebacterium diphtheriae,* and gram-negative bacilli are less frequent causes. The most frequent viruses producing otitis media are the parainfluenza viruses, respiratory syncytial virus, adenoviruses, and coxsackie viruses.

Nontypable *H. influenzae* (nonencapsulated) strains constitute the majority of middle ear isolates. These strains are not associated with invasive or disseminated infections and are responsible for a small, but significant, proportion of middle ear infections in older children and adults. This frequency appears to be increasing. The resistance of *H. influenzae* type B to amoxicillin is increasing and averages approximately 30% in the United States. The drug of choice, as recommended by the American Academy of Otolaryngology, is amoxicillin. Augmentin, cefaclor, Biaxin, or Lorabid are more appropriate to treat *H. influenzae* that is resistant to amoxicillin.

**Diagnosis.** Examination and confirmation of otitis media are best accomplished using a pneumatic otoscope. When fluid is present in the middle ear space, mobility of the tympanic membrane is reduced. Additional signs include a bulging inflamed tympanic membrane or a severely retracted tympanic membrane. Bubbles or an air-fluid level can be seen on occasion. If a perforation of the membrane is present, a pulsatile discharge may be seen, which usually is in the anteroinferior segment of the membrane. It must be remembered that while otalgia will be present, pain or tenderness is not present on manipulating the auricle. Pain is intensified by the insufflation of air with the pneumatic otoscope.

Tympanometry is an objective test in which the mobility of the tympanic membrane is assessed by means of a signal reflected from it while the pressure against the eardrum is continuously changed. The test can be performed by an audiologist, a technician, a nurse, or a physician with only brief training. Although there is some margin for artifact and error, it is less than 10%. There are several commonly seen tympanograms, including type A (normal), type B (flat consistent with middle ear effusion), and type C (retracted, consistent with negative middle ear pressure). Other less commonly seen tympanograms such as type $A_d$ is consistent with a disarticulated ossicular chain leading to hypermobility of the tympanic membrane (Fig. 27-6). This test has a higher reliability in identifying the presence of middle ear fluid than that possessed by many physicians who examine ears infrequently. It can be helpful in supporting a clinical diagnosis.

In most cases, tympanocentesis or myringotomy is not indicated in the diagnosis of otitis media. These procedures involve the removal of secretions from the middle ear to allow bacteriologic studies. These studies are necessary for diagnosis and treatment only in rare circumstances. Almost all cases of otitis media respond quickly to proper management and may even resolve spontaneously. Almost all bacteria implicated in middle ear infections are sensitive to commonly available antibiotics. For these reasons, the risk associated with myringotomy cannot be justified in the usual patient. These procedures should be performed only in rare situations and then only by someone with extensive experience, usually an otolaryngologist, using the proper equipment, including a binocular operating microscope.

The clinical situations in which tympanocentesis or myringotomy can be helpful are in middle ear infections in neonates, immunocompromised or immunosuppressed and leukemic patients, patients who do not respond to adequate doses of antibiotics, or patients who have developed a complication such as meningitis. Here, tympanocentesis may offer specific identification of the etiologic organism and thereby promote an effective choice of antibiotic.

**Therapy.** Antibiotics are the most effective single therapeutic measure in all cases of acute otitis media. Depending on allergic history and the patient's age, any of several antibiotics can be used. Amoxicillin, 20 to 40 mg/kg per day in divided doses by mouth for 10 days, will effectively manage most infections in all age groups. The usual dosage in older children and adults is 250 to 500 mg every 8 hours. If there is a high local prevalence of amoxicillin resistance, amoxicillin plus clavulanate (Augmentin), potassium cefaclor, clarithromycin (Biaxin), or loracarbef (Lorabid) should be substituted.

Another effective medication is the combination of trimethoprim, 8 mg/kg and sulfamethoxazole 40 mg/kg in two divided doses per day. This combination covers most pathogens implicated in otitis media, including *H. influenzae.* Some physicians have recommended avoidance of this medication because of the potential for aplastic anemia. When examining antibiotic choices from an economic perspective, the most economical choice would typically be amoxicillin and the least cost-effective today is cefaclor.

All medications are given for at least 10 days. Some recent studies and clinical experience indicate that a longer course of antibiotic treatment may satisfactorily resolve otitis media and prevent the occurrence of chronic middle ear effusions (serous otitis media), thus possibly reducing the need for myringotomy and pressure equalizing tubes.

Satisfactory analgesia usually can be provided with acetaminophen or ibuprofen supplemented by low doses of codeine as necessary. Codeine should be avoided in very young children, and aspirin is typically avoided because of the potential for Reye's syndrome. Antihistamines and decongestants are usually of no help in acute otitis media except for relieving associated coryza symptoms. Antihistamines may actually impair middle ear clearance by interfering with mucociliary flow through the eustachian tube, but this theory is controversial.

Each patient should be evaluated in 2 weeks. If an effusion persists beyond 4 weeks, the patient is treated for chronic serous otitis media/chronic middle ear effusion, which is described later.

Repeated episodes of acute bacterial otitis media with clearing of middle ear effusions between each attack usually can be managed by the use of a chronic low-dose prophylactic of amoxicillin. Alternatives to antibiotic therapy exist. If acute bacterial otitis media develops in a patient on prophylactic therapy, a myringotomy and insertion of a ventilation tube may be indicated to restore middle ear ventilation and function.

If the tympanic membrane is perforated and drainage is present, this drainage can be cultured for guidance in treatment. Most perforations heal spontaneously. If perforation persists longer than 3 months, the patient should be referred to an otolaryngologist for consultation and treatment.

***Acute mastoiditis.*** Virtually all cases of bacterial otitis media have an associated medical mastoiditis. It is an infection of the soft tissue surrounding the air spaces in the mastoid bone. As this air cell system is confluent with the middle ear space, medical mastoiditis is treated concurrently with therapy for otitis media. No roentgenograms are indicated or necessary, but if taken they almost always reveal clouding of the mastoid air cell system when otitis media is present.

Surgical mastoiditis is an osteitis and periostitis (occasionally associated with thrombophlebitis of the horizontal and sigmoid venous sinuses) that follows acute otitis media. Surgical mastoiditis can be diagnosed clinically by the marked swelling, pitting edema, erythema, and percussion tenderness of the skin over the mastoid bone. Occasionally, edema and displacement of the posterosuperior external canal wall may occlude the canal. The swelling produces an anterior and inferior displacement of the auricle. Facial nerve paresis or paralysis may be present and typically signifies the need for more aggressive management. A fever in the range of

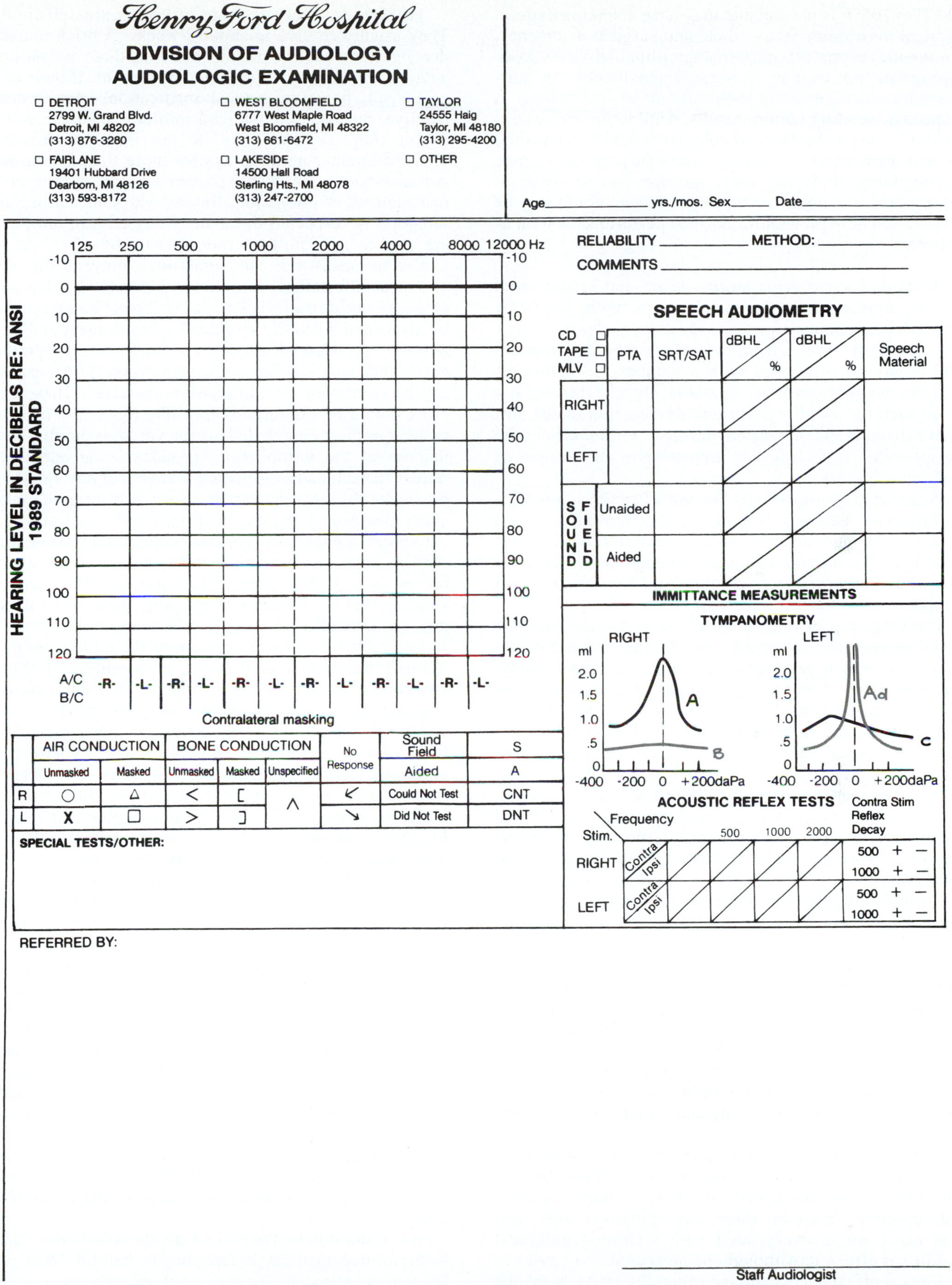

Henry Ford Hospital

DIVISION OF AUDIOLOGY

AUDIOLOGIC EXAMINATION

☐ DETROIT
2799 W. Grand Blvd.
Detroit, MI 48202
(313) 876-3280

☐ WEST BLOOMFIELD
6777 West Maple Road
West Bloomfield, MI 48322
(313) 661-6472

☐ TAYLOR
24555 Haig
Taylor, MI 48180
(313) 295-4200

☐ FAIRLANE
19401 Hubbard Drive
Dearborn, MI 48126
(313) 593-8172

☐ LAKESIDE
14500 Hall Road
Sterling Hts., MI 48078
(313) 247-2700

☐ OTHER

Age________ yrs./mos. Sex_____ Date__________

HEARING LEVEL IN DECIBELS RE: ANSI 1989 STANDARD

125 250 500 1000 2000 4000 8000 12000 Hz

-10 0 10 20 30 40 50 60 70 80 90 100 110 120

A/C B/C -R- -L- -R- -L- -R- -L- -R- -L- -R- -L- -R- -L-

Contralateral masking

| | AIR CONDUCTION | | BONE CONDUCTION | | | No Response | Sound Field | S |
|---|---|---|---|---|---|---|---|---|
| | Unmasked | Masked | Unmasked | Masked | Unspecified | | Aided | A |
| R | ○ | △ | < | [ | ∧ | ↙ | Could Not Test | CNT |
| L | X | ☐ | > | ] | | ↘ | Did Not Test | DNT |

SPECIAL TESTS/OTHER:

REFERRED BY:

RELIABILITY __________ METHOD: __________

COMMENTS __________

SPEECH AUDIOMETRY

| CD ☐ TAPE ☐ MLV ☐ | | PTA | SRT/SAT | dBHL / % | dBHL / % | Speech Material |
|---|---|---|---|---|---|---|
| RIGHT | | | | | | |
| LEFT | | | | | | |
| SOUND FIELD | Unaided | | | | | |
| | Aided | | | | | |

IMMITTANCE MEASUREMENTS

TYMPANOMETRY

RIGHT: ml 2.0 1.5 1.0 .5 0; -400 -200 0 +200daPa; A, B

LEFT: ml 2.0 1.5 1.0 .5 0; -400 -200 0 +200daPa; Ad, C

ACOUSTIC REFLEX TESTS

| Stim. \ Frequency | | 500 | 1000 | 2000 | Contra Stim Reflex Decay |
|---|---|---|---|---|---|
| RIGHT | Contra / Ipsi | | | | 500 + − ; 1000 + − |
| LEFT | Contra / Ipsi | | | | 500 + − ; 1000 + − |

Staff Audiologist

**Fig. 27-6.** Tympanometry. Several commonly seen tympanograms include: Type A—normal; Type B—flat, consistent with middle ear effusion; Type C—retracted, consistent with negative middle ear pressure; and Type $A_d$—consistent with disarticulated ossicular chain.

104°F to 105°F is present and may have a spiking pattern. Surgical mastoiditis is a medical and surgical emergency. Intravenous cephalosporins or ampicillin, in divided doses appropriate for weight, is begun immediately. An antistaphylococcal antibiotic should be given if *S. aureus* is suspected, pending culture results. Antibiotics are continued for 21 days. An otolaryngologist should be consulted on an urgent basis, as in most cases surgery (to include myringotomy, mastoidectomy, incision and drainage of any abscess, and debridement of devitalized bone) may be necessary. These procedures must be performed as soon as possible.

***Acute and serous otitis media.*** Acute and serous otitis media (middle ear effusion) develops with persistent negative intratympanic pressure (as discussed previously). This condition results from eustachian tube dysfunction, which may be associated with a number of conditions, including upper respiratory infection, chronic rhinosinusitis of bacterial or allergic origin, dysfunction of the soft palate (from clefts or surgical defects), and masses in the nasopharynx from adenoid hypertrophy or benign or malignant tumors.

When an effusion persists beyond a few days or weeks, its character changes from a serous transudate to an increasingly mucoid, protein-laden exudate with an increasingly gluelike consistency. Although their role is not clear, bacteria are present in approximately one third of persistent effusions.

The diagnosis of middle ear effusion is established on examination. The tympanic membrane is classically thickened, with a gray or amber fluid seen in the middle ear. Sometimes a fluid meniscus, air bubbles, or bluish fluid may appear behind the tympanic membrane. Mobility of the membrane is always impaired. The membrane is frequently retracted by negative pressure and, if this condition is prolonged, retraction of the pars flaccida area may lead to the formation of a cholesteatoma (keratoma).

Tympanometry is helpful in supporting the clinical impression of serous otitis media, especially in young children. Hearing may be evaluated by tuning forks and audiograms.

Chronic middle ear effusions represent a special problem in young children, as effusions are most common in the early years, when significant speech development occurs. Several recent studies have shown that persistent effusions and mild conductive hearing losses are associated with prolonged impairment of language acquisition skills and that these deficits may last for years. The patient's speech is less well developed than in peers of a similar age. Therefore if medical management does not resolve middle ear effusions within 3 to 4 months, surgical intervention with myringotomy and possibly tubes should be considered.

Chronic middle ear effusions in adults may be secondary to the presence of a nasopharyngeal tumor (poorly differentiated squamous cell carcinoma is most frequent). This diagnosis must be suspected, actively sought, and then ruled out in every adult with a chronic unilateral middle ear effusion. Although the most common causes of middle ear effusions in adults are allergies, eustachian tube dysfunction for other reasons, and barotrauma, the possibility of nasopharyngeal tumor must not be ignored.

**Therapy.** In general, acute effusions are self-limited. They usually resolve in about 2 weeks. A brief course of decongestants such as pseudoephedrine three or four times a day or topical nasal spray may be helpful. If their use is prolonged, however, topical medications may promote reactive mucosal edema and prolong eustachian tube dysfunction. Typically, we do not recommend use of over-the-counter nasal sprays for more than 2 to 4 days. Antihistamines are of no proven benefit, except in the management of coryza or allergic symptoms. If bacterial infection is suspected or cannot be ruled out, antibiotics are used as in acute bacterial otitis media.

Certain measures can sometimes prevent the more severe manifestations in patients prone to develop acute effusions during air travel or diving. Young patients should be awakened when the airplane begins descent and given a bottle or other drink, or chewing gum to promote eustachian tube opening with deglutition. Older patients can be instructed in autoinflation exercises. These exercises should be mastered before the flight. The ingestion of alcohol must be avoided, as the vascular dilation in the mucosa of the nasopharynx produce some edema and impair eustachian tube opening. Patients of any age should be awake during the descent to actively promote eustachian tube activity by chewing, swallowing, or practicing autoinflation exercises. Topical decongestant medications such as nose sprays work rapidly and should be applied before short flights or just before descent. They are used similarly before diving. Use for more than 2 to 4 days is not recommended.

Reestablishing proper aeration of the middle ear is the ultimate therapeutic goal in the management of chronic effusion. Effective therapy depends on establishing, if possible, the cause of eustachian tube dysfunction. Likely causes include chronic rhinosinusitis of bacterial or allergic origin, palatal dysfunction, and hypertrophied adenoid tissue or nasopharyngeal tumors. In infants irritation may be produced by milk or other fluid persisting in the nasopharynx while the infant is supine with a bottle. Fluids may produce local irritation and may actually flow into the eustachian tube and carry bacteria along.

In older children and adults, autoinflation exercises may be helpful. These exercises include blowing the nose forcefully while the mouth and nares are kept closed. A hand held nasal balloon "toy" that children enjoy using can be quickly constructed with a soft, flexible plastic tube such as a disposable medicine dropper. The tip of the bulb is removed with scissors and the balloon or a rubber finger cot is secured over the opposite end with rubber bands. The tube is then placed in one nostril while the other is pinched closed, and the balloon is inflated through the nose. This procedure is repeated several times on both sides. Swallowing and motion of the palate (enhanced by the patient producing a "gunk" sound) while simultaneously maintaining balloon pressure or blowing the nose may open the eustachian tube. Once the patient has mastered such exercises, they should be repeated four to ten times a day.

When autoinflation exercises are unsuccessful or cannot be performed, medical therapy may be helpful. Most cases of chronic effusion resolve spontaneously over several weeks. Although antihistamines and decongestants have been widely used, their efficacy is not supported in clinical studies. Antihistamines and decongestants, however, may be efficacious in the allergic patient. In other cases, these medications may inhibit resolution of the effusion by producing more viscid secretions. Recent evidence indicates that a 7- to 10-day course of tapered steroids also may markedly reduce allergic effusions.

A chronic, low-grade, "steady-state" infectious process may be involved in one third of chronic effusion as is shown by the finding of bacteria in the chronic effusion fluids and the response of effusions to antibiotic treatment. The initial therapy for chronic effusions persisting beyond 3 to 4 weeks should be the same, as in the case of acute otitis media. Effective medications include amoxicillin, amoxicillin plus clavalanate potassium (Augmentin), cefaclor, trimethoprim/sulfamethoxazole, erythromycin, clarithromycin (Biaxin) and loracarbef (Lorabid) over a 14- to 21-day course and then if necessary may be given once nightly at bedtime for 4 to 6 weeks. The effusions frequently resolve with this treatment, which may implicate chronic low-grade bacterial infections in chronic effusions.

If the effusion persists more than 10 to 12 weeks despite adequate medical therapy and autoinflation exercises, an otolaryngologist should be consulted. This recommendation is also true when multiple recurrent episodes of effusion are present, especially if complicated by acute otitis media. In these situations, myringotomy and insertion of ventilation tubes may be considered. This treatment is especially important whenever any conductive hearing loss is present. The ventilation tube allows equalization of middle ear pressure. Conductive hearing loss secondary to the effusion and impaired tympanic membrane mobility usually is markedly improved immediately after surgery.

Chronic effusions may produce tympanic atelectasis when the membrane touches the medial wall of the middle ear space. Retraction pockets may form in the tympanic membrane, and a thick adhesive effusion with chronic inflammation and mucosal hypertrophy may impair its function. Myringotomy and the insertion of ventilation tubes are essential to prevent further progression of these problems. Ventilation tubes will reverse these conditions and help to prevent chronic hearing loss, cholesteatoma formation, and chronic suppurative otitis media.

In occasional patients with adenoidal hypertrophy, the adenoidal tissue may occlude the eustachian tube orifices. Chronically infected adenoid tissue also may produce local edema that interferes with tubal function and, with lymphatic drainage from the middle ear, thereby contribute to recurrent ear infections. In such instances, adenoidectomy may be helpful in resolving the effusion and recurrent infection problem.

***Chronic suppurative otitis media.*** Chronic suppurative otitis media always involves a tympanic membrane perforation or defect with chronic purulent otorrhea and middle ear inflammation. A mild to moderate conductive hearing loss is present. In general the condition is otherwise asymptomatic unless it progresses to involvement of the inner ear and produces sensorineural hearing loss, vertigo, and disequilibrium or facial nerve palsy. Cholesteatoma (keratoma) is the presence of normal squamous epithelium within the middle ear and may occur from retraction of the pars flaccida of the tympanic membrane with chronic negative pressure, with a sac being formed and gradually enlarging to enclose the trapped dead cells of desquamated skin. Alternatively, squamous epithelial tissue may migrate through a perforation of the tympanic membrane and slowly extend to form a large mass within the middle ear. The dead desquamated skin cells form an ideal medium for bacterial growth. The enlarging keratoma or cholesteatoma causes local destruction of bone and the ossicles and may progressively erode into the cranial cavity or inner ear, producing associated symptoms of meningitis and labyrinthitis. Epidural abscesses also may occur. In fact the ear and paranasal sinuses are the most common site from which epidural abscesses arise.

Chronic suppurative otitis media is characterized by a more complex bacteriology than simple otitis media. Cultures frequently reveal a mixed flora of aerobic and anaerobic organisms. The aerobic pathogens commonly found include *Escherichia coli, S. aureus, Proteus mirabilis, Pseudomonas aeruginosa,* and diphtheroid bacilli. The most commonly encountered anaerobes include *Bacteroides fragilis, Bacteroides melaninogenicus,* and *Peptococcus magnus.*

The diagnosis is established by examination and requires removal of secretions, crusts, and debris from the external canal and from against the tympanic membrane. Mucopurulent otorrhea is usually seen, and secretions may have a foul odor. After cleansing, the tympanic membrane is examined as previously described. A defect usually is seen in the superior, posterior, or inferior portion of the tympanic membrane. Mucopurulent fluid may be seen draining through the defect. The middle ear mucosa has a markedly inflamed appearance.

The initial treatment for chronic suppurative otitis media is medical. Topical antibiotics as described for external ear infections are helpful.

In general, chronic suppurative otitis media should be followed up or evaluated by an otolaryngologist who also should direct therapy. Surgery may be required for closure of a tympanic membrane defect or for exploration of the ear and mastoidectomy to eradicate chronic sources of infections such as necrotic bone and cholesteatoma. The goal is to create a safe ear. A secondary but important consideration is improvement of hearing.

### Inner ear infections (Table 27-4)

***Acute labyrinthitis.*** Labyrinthitis is an inflammation of structures of the inner ear. It is caused by invasion of microorganisms or irritation of the inner ear by the passage of toxic products from middle ear infections.

**Viral labyrinthitis.** Many viruses may produce a labyrinthitis, but the most common is the mumps virus. If labyrinthitis occurs, the infection may produce a sudden unilateral inflammation of the cochlea with severe and total sensorineural hearing loss. Vertigo is uncommon with mumps, but it may occur. There is no specific treatment for viral labyrinthitis. If the hearing loss is limited to one ear, no specific further measures are required. Bilateral hearing losses are unusual, but, when present and persistent, amplification is required. Although some advocate the use of systemic corticosteroid therapy to diminish inner ear destruction from viral infection, there is no clear evidence to support its efficacy.

**Table 27-4.** Inner ear infection

| Labyrinthitis | Etiology | Clinical findings | Common microbiologic agents | Management |
|---|---|---|---|---|
| Viral | Middle ear infection<br>Meningitis | Unilateral inflammation of cochlea; sensorineural hearing loss; vertigo | Mumps | Symptomatic |
| Bacterial | Acute or chronic otitis media<br>Meningitis | Severe vertigo; nausea; vomiting; hearing loss | Agents causing acute and chronic otitis media | Myringotomy; Intravenous antibotic; mastoidectomy |
| Vascular | Occlusion of anteroinferior cerebellar artery or labyrinthine artery | Severe vertigo; hearing loss | Vascular insult | Symptomatic; possibly antiplatelet medications |

It should be noted that viral labyrinthitis involves damage to both the cochlea and vestibular system. This condition is permanent and needs to be differentiated from the transient vertigo that occurs in vestibular neuronitis.

**Bacterial labyrinthitis.** Bacterial labyrinthitis may represent a complication of acute or chronic otitis media, or of meningitis. Typical symptoms include severe vertigo associated with nausea and emesis and hearing loss.

Labyrinthitis complicating acute otitis media requires more aggressive therapy than oral antibiotics. An otolaryngology consultation must be obtained on an urgent basis. Treatment requires myringotomy and intravenous administration of appropriate antibiotics as determined by culture, sensitivity, and Gram stain studies of the middle ear exudate. These tests must be performed immediately and before the the institution of the intravenous medication.

If chronic suppurative otitis media is associated with a sudden development of labyrinthitis, effective therapy requires surgical debridement of the diseased tissue by mastoidectomy in addition to the appropriate use of intravenous antibiotics as determined by a culture and Gram stain.

## VERTIGO

Vertigo is the cardinal symptom of a disturbance of the vestibular system. The word refers to any hallucination of movement, whether a sensation of spinning, tilting, swaying, or falling. The pathology may exist anywhere in the vestibular pathway, from the vestibular end organs to the highest cerebral representation of the vestibular system in the temporal lobe. Thus the major priority in the management of the vertiginous patient is anatomic localization. This section stresses the importance of careful history taking and methodical physical examination as the first step toward unraveling the cause of vertigo. Only with information acquired in this manner can the physician select the most useful investigative tests from the large number currently available.

Normal equilibrium requires accurate information from not only the vestibular system, but also sensory input from the proprioceptive, visual, and cerebellar systems. Thus although disequilibrium is often associated with vertigo, many disorders of balance may occur in the absence of vertigo. For instance, a lesion of the dorsal columns, which relay proprioceptive sensation, may cause marked disequilibrium, but will not be associated with vertigo. Vertigo is the result of a conflict between the input to the brain from the vestibular system and from other systems concerned with the maintenance of normal balance.

The vestibular system may be divided anatomically into two parts—peripheral and central. The peripheral system comprises the vestibular end organs (semicircular canals, utricle, saccule, and endolymphatic sac) and their first-order neuronal supply (afferent fibers, Scarpa's ganglia, and the centrally connected fibers). The central system is formed by the vestibular nuclei and their central projections. As will be seen, there are important practical differences between lesions of these two divisions of the vestibular system with which the examining physician must be thoroughly familiar.

### History

The importance of obtaining an accurate history from the vertiginous patient cannot be overemphasized. Many patients have considerable difficulty in describing their symptoms, and such descriptions are often charged with emotion. Taking of a careful and methodical history is tantamount in developing a clinical plan to diagnose and treat the problem efficiently.

***Otologic history.*** The date and circumstances of onset should always be ascertained, as well as the frequency, severity, and duration of attacks. Peripheral lesions cause the greatest systemic upset because they are often associated with pallor, sweating, nausea, and vomiting. Episodic vertigo lasting a few seconds and associated with position changes is typically associated with benign positional vertigo. Vertigo lasting between 30 minutes to 12 hours commonly is seen in Ménière's disease, whereas that lasting several days suggests vestibular neuronitis or labyrinthitis (Table 27-5).

Vertigo of psychogenic origin may have been present for several years. Factors that precipitate or aggravate attacks should be determined. For instance, is the vertigo associated with a particular position or movement? It also is helpful to know what the patient does to alleviate symptoms.

**Table 27-5.** Typical duration of vertigo in some common clinical conditions

| Condition | Duration of vertigo |
|---|---|
| Benign positional vertigo | Few seconds |
| Ménière's disease | 30 minutes to 12 hours |
| Vestibular neuronitis | 2 to 3 days |
| Labyrinthitis | 3 to 10 days |
| Psychogenic | Several years |

**Table 27-6.** Usual hearing status in some syndromes associated with vertigo

| Hearing loss usual | Hearing loss unusual |
|---|---|
| Ménière's disease | Vestibular neuronitis |
| Labyrinthitis | Multiple sclerosis |
| Cholesteatomatous ear disease | Vertebrobasilar ischemia |
| Labyrinthine membrane rupture | Benign positional vertigo |
| Ototoxicity | Basilar migraine |
| Vestibular schwannoma | |

In view of the close anatomic relationship between the hearing and vestibular systems, it is not surprising that vertigo may be associated with auditory symptoms. Such symptoms often provide valuable information about the localization of a lesion within the vestibular system (Table 27-6).

It is important to the patient whether he or she has noticed any hearing loss. Even the most subtle impairment of hearing, particularly if unilateral, is of the utmost importance, as it may be the presenting feature of vestibular schwannoma. Tinnitus may accompany vertigo and may sometimes change character before or during a vertiginous episode. Other derangements of hearing such as diplacusis (hearing the same pitch differently in each ear) or paracusis (distortion) are useful because they tend to suggest cochlear pathology. Symptoms suggestive of suppurative ear disease (e.g., earache, discharge.) should be inquired about. An expanding cholesteatoma (a collection of keratinizing squamous epithelium) may erode the bony labyrinth and cause a fistula in the semicircular canal.

Ototoxicity as a cause of vertigo is likely to be determined only by direct questioning. It should be remembered that the vestibulotoxic effects of some drugs may not become apparent until several weeks after administration.

Labyrinthine membrane rupture (rupture of the oval or round windows) is an often unrecognized cause of vertigo that is eminently treatable. It should be suspected in patients whose symptoms occur after head injury, barotrauma (flying or diving), or unusual physical exertion. Patients presenting in this manner should be referred without delay to an otolaryngologist.

An otologic history would be incomplete without a consideration of previous otologic surgical procedures (e.g., mastoidectomy, stapedectomy) that may have a direct bearing on a patient's symptoms.

***General history.*** Assessment of the vertiginous patient demands evaluation of those other systems that are integrally related with the vestibular system. Patients should be questioned about certain symptoms that may suggest disease within the central nervous or cardiovascular systems. For instance loss of consciousness during an episode of vertigo is strongly suggestive of a nervous system lesion. It is important, however, not to confuse double vision with the disordered visual sensations that are a feature of vertigo. Numbness or weakness in the arms or legs, and difficulty with swallowing or speech are all suggestive of disease within the CNS. Syncopal attacks associated with vertigo may be of cardiogenic origin, and such patients need cardiologic evaluation.

Disorders of equilibrium are not uncommonly a manifestation of an underlying stress phenomenon. Marital or employment difficulties are the usual culprits that may be uncovered by sympathetic questioning.

The old adage that "for every mistake made by not knowing, ten are made by not looking" can be aptly applied to the examination of the vertiginous patient. Particular attention must be paid to the otologic, neurologic, and cardiovascular systems, as the underlying disorder frequently resides in one of these areas.

### Otologic examination

The primary physician should be able to perform a basic examination of the auditory and vestibular systems. The examination is initiated by looking at the pinna. It is inspected for stigmata of previous surgery (such as postauricular incision scars) or, in injured patients, for ecchymosis or hematoma (Battle's sign). The ear canal is examined by gently retracting the pinna upward and backward and gently introducing an otoscope. Cerumen may be removed with a wax hook or by syringing gently. Do not aim the irrigation device directly at the tympanic membrane, as perforation can occur. The tympanic membrane needs to be inspected in its entirety. Signs of an effusion are sought, and the mobility of the membrane is tested with the pneumatic otoscope. A deliberate attempt should be made to scrutinize the uppermost portion of the tympanic membrane (Shrapnell's membrane, or pars flaccida), as cholesteatomas are frequently located in this region. A cholesteatoma may cause a fistula into the lateral semicircular canal; when this occurs increasing the pressure in the external canal (e.g., by tragal pressure or with a pneumatic otoscope) may induce vertigo (a positive fistula sign). Patients with this clinical presentation require urgent referral to an otolaryngologist.

***Deafness.*** It is mandatory to test hearing in the vertiginous patient. Each ear should be tested separately while masking (placing a sound into the nontest ear) the opposite ear. The patient is asked to repeat phonetically balanced words (e.g., *send, thick, daybreak*). As a rough guide, the patient should not miss more than one word in ten. If he or she does, referral to an otolaryngologist should be arranged.

Tuning fork tests (Weber and Rinne) should never be omitted (Table 27-7). They are simple to perform and can

**Table 27-7.** Types of hearing loss associated with vertigo

| Site of lesion | Example | Type of deafness | Tuning fork tests |
|---|---|---|---|
| Middle ear | Cholesteatoma | Conductive | Rinne negative Weber to affected ear |
| Cochlea | Ménière's disease | Sensorineural | Rinne positive Weber to better cochlea |
| Eighth nerve | Vestibular schwannoma | Sensorineural | Rinne positive Weber to better cochlea |

help differentiate between normal hearing and conductive and sensorineural hearing loss.

Weber's test is performed by placing a vibrating tuning fork at the center of a patient's forehead. If the patient has a unilateral conductive hearing loss, the sound localizes to that ear because the better ear is being masked, or "distracted," by the ambient noise. Alternatively, if the patient has a unilateral sensorineural hearing loss, the sound localizes to the opposite ear, which has a better cochlear reserve. A patient who senses the sound in the midline may have normal hearing or bilateral hearing loss (either conductive or sensorineural) of equal severity.

The Rinne test compares the patient's hearing by air and bone conduction. In normal circumstances, sounds are better perceived by air conduction. A vibrating tuning fork is placed on the patient's mastoid process; the examiner should be sure that the patient is hearing it in the test ear. Then the tuning fork is placed opposite the patient's ear canal, and the patient is asked in which position the sound was heard clearest and longest. In patients with normal hearing or with sensorineural hearing loss, the sound is heard better by air conduction (a positive Rinne test). In conductive hearing loss, bone conduction is heard better than air conduction (a negative Rinne response).

***Nystagmus.*** Nystagmus and ataxia are the most objective signs of vertigo. Nystagmus refers to involuntary, repetitive movements of the eye and may be spontaneous or induced. A wide variety of disordered patterns of eye movement have been described; only those forms of nystagmus commonly encountered in clinical practice are described.

**Peripheral nystagmus.** Disease of the labyrinth or of its central connections may cause a jerky or "sawtooth" nystagmus. This term describes a situation in which the eyes move slowly in one direction (the vestibular component) and rapidly return to a midline position (the central component). By convention, the direction of a nystagmus is the direction of the fast component or the central component. Knowledge of the features of this type of vertigo are of the utmost importance (Table 27-8).

To assess spontaneous nystagmus, the patient should sit opposite the examiner in a well-illuminated room. Vestibular nystagmus is enhanced by loss of optic fixation and may be achieved by having the patient use a Frensel lens. These glasses have +20 diopter lenses, which prevent the patient from focusing and have the advantage of giving the observer a clear view of ocular movements. A simple hand lens may be helpful if Frensel lenses are not available. While holding a finger at least 18 inches from the patient, the examiner asks the patient to follow it through an arc within 30 degrees of the primary position. Only sustained nystagmus within this range should be considered pathologic. Outside the range of 30 degrees, nystagmus is a finding in normal subjects and is associated with loss of binocular vision.

**Table 27-8.** General characteristics of peripheral and central nystagmus

| Peripheral nystagmus | Central nystagmus |
|---|---|
| Conjugate | Dysconjugate |
| Unidirectional | Multidirectional |
| Never vertical | May be vertical |
| Temporary | May be permanent |
| Associated with vertigo | May not be vertigo |
| Enhanced by loss of visual fixation | Unaffected by loss of visual fixation |

**Central nystagmus.** The essential features of central nystagmus are shown in Table 27-8 and should be carefully contrasted with those of peripheral nystagmus. Multidirectional or vertical nystagmus is a sinister finding indicating brainstem pathology. Nystagmus that is present only in the abducting eye when the adducting eye is weak is indicative of internuclear ophthalmoplegia. This finding strongly suggests a diagnosis of multiple sclerosis. Nystagmus occurring in the absence of vertigo is most likely due to a central lesion.

**Positional nystagmus.** If there is no spontaneous nystagmus, it may be possible to induce it by the Dix-Hallpike maneuver. While the subject sits on a couch or examination table, the head is rapidly lowered to below the horizontal and turned to either side. It is advisable to check the mobility of the cervical spine before performing this maneuver. In labyrinthine disorders, nystagmus is induced after a latent period of a few seconds, when the affected ear is undermost, and has all the hallmarks of a peripheral nystagmus. Further, the nystagmus is fatigable, as it diminishes in severity each time the test is repeated. In positional nystagmus due to central pathology, the nystagmus may be vertical or multidirectional, is not fatigable, and may not be associated with vertigo.

***Examination of the neurologic and cardiovascular systems.*** Every patient with vertigo requires a full physical examination. Blood pressure should be determined in both arms and in the lying and standing positions. The neck should be auscultated carefully for bruits and for evidence of a subclavian steal syndrome.

In the neurologic examination, all the cranial nerves should be tested, signs of cerebellar dysfunction should be

**Table 27-9.** Outline of neurologic examination

| Cranial nerve | Test |
|---|---|
| I | Sense of smell |
| II | Fundi, visual acuity, visual fields, light reflexes |
| III, IV, VI | Eye movements; check for spontaneous nystagmus (may need Frensel's lenses) |
| V | Corneal reflexes; facial sensation |
| VII | Check for palsy or spasm |
| | Test sensation on posterior wall of ear canal |
| VIII | Hearing and vestibular testing |
| IX | Tonsilar sensation |
| X | Gag reflex, soft palate movements, vocal cord movements |
| XI | Sternomastoid and trapezius contractions |
| XII | Tongue movements |
| Test of equilibrium | Romberg |
| | Gait |
| Cerebellar tests | Evaluate for dysmetria (past pointing), dysdiadochokinesia (inability to perform successive movements), rebound and gait (usually wide based) |

sought, and the peripheral nervous system should be evaluated, with particular reference to the maintenance of posture and gait (Table 27-9).

**Caloric testing.** This test is performed with the patient lying supine on an examination couch with the head raised 30 degrees (in this position, the lateral semicircular canals are in the vertical plane). Each ear is irrigated with cold and warm water. Cold water causes nystagmus to the opposite side, whereas warm water results in nystagmus to the same side as the irrigated ear (hence the mnemonic *COWS: cold, opposite, warm, same*). Impaired responsiveness of a labyrinth to caloric stimuli and assessment of the involved side can be evaluated by this test.

**Other investigations.** Certain basic investigations (e.g., complete blood count [CBC], sedimentation rate, glucose tolerance testing, blood urea nitrogen [BUN], thyroid function) should be performed as indicated by the primary care physician. It is important to consider neurosyphilis as a cause of vertigo; in suspected cases a fluorescent *Treponema* antibody absorption test should be obtained (VDRL misses congenital syphilis in about 50% of cases). Examination of the CSF may be valuable in multiple sclerosis (it may show elevated levels of IgG or oligoclonal bands, which are suggestive but not pathognomonic of the diagnosis).

The radiologic investigations should be appropriate to the nature of the suspected underlying pathology. When a lesion of the internal auditory canal is suspected, an auditory brainstem response is typically obtained. This test is accurate in 96% of the cases and has a false-negative rate of approximately 1% to 2%. It is considered an excellent screening test to evaluate for tumors on the cochleovestibular nerve. In either case, magnetic resonance imaging (MRI) with gadolinium may reveal subtle pathology in exquisite detail and currently is the procedure of choice. In patients who cannot undergo MRI, CT with dye enhancement may be necessary.

### Clinical conditions associated with vertigo (Table 27-10)

***Ménière's disease.*** Ménière's disease consists of four main symptoms: vertigo, hearing loss, tinnitus, and fullness. Classically, all of these symptoms must be present for the correct diagnosis to be made. Ménière's has been further subclassified into cochlear Ménière's and vestibular Ménière's to differentiate patients who have only cochlear symptoms from those with only vestibular symptoms. The symptoms are generally attributed to distention of the membranous labyrinth (endolymphatic hydrops). The vertigo may be violent and is usually associated with nausea and vomiting. It rarely lasts less than half an hour and uncommonly persists for more than 12 hours. The deafness in Ménière's disease is of a fluctuating sensorineural type, most marked initially in the low tones, and is accompanied by loudness recruitment. Eventually hearing loss may be permanent. Every patient with suspected Ménière's disease should be evaluated by an otolaryngologist early in the course of the disease.

The treatment of Ménière's disease is controversial. In the natural history of the disease, spontaneous remission occurs in 50% to 60% of cases. It is thus difficult to evaluate the true efficacy of any treatment modality in these circumstances. Reassurance, after full evaluation, is all that is necessary for many patients. Salt-restricted diets and triamterene (Dyazide) may be beneficial. The most commonly used vestibular suppressants are the antihistamines such as meclizine hydrochloride (Antivert) and cyclizine hydrochloride (Marezine). Diazepam is a valuable adjunct to treatment in the acute attack as well as in patients in whom anxiety is a prominent factor. These drugs should be used for a limited period only. Surgical therapy is indicated when symptoms are disruptive to a patient's life and persist despite appropriate medical therapy. The procedure undertaken depends on the level of hearing and whether the disease is unilateral or bilateral. Some procedures are aimed at decompressing the labyrinth (endolymphatic sac surgery, cochleosacculotomy) and aim at the preservation of hearing. Total destruction of the labyrinth (i.e., labyrinthectomy) is an effective procedure in an ear with total or near total sensorineural hearing loss. Vestibular nerve section has the advantage of treating vertigo while preserving cochlear function.

***Vestibular neuronitis.*** The cause of vestibular neuronitis is uncertain, but some evidence implicates a viral or vascular etiology. The symptoms, severe vertigo with nausea and vomiting, usually last for 2 to 3 days. An important feature of the condition is the absence of cochlear symptoms or signs. After the acute episode subsides, the patient may experience minor episodes of disequilibrium over the ensuing months to years. The condition is self-limiting, and symptomatic initial treatment with vestibular suppressants followed by vestibular rehabilitation with vestibular exercises is all that is typically required.

***Multiple sclerosis.*** The diagnosis of multiple sclerosis may be difficult, and suspected cases should be referred to a neurologist. A plaque of demyelination in the brainstem

**Table 27-10.** Clinical conditions associated with vertigo

| | Etiology and contributing factors | Clinical findings | Diagnosis | Management |
|---|---|---|---|---|
| Ménière's disease<br>Cochlear Ménière's<br>Vestibular Ménière's | Idiopathic; distention of membranous labyrinth (endolymphatic hydrops) | Vertigo; fluctuating sensorineural hearing loss; roaring tinnitus; fullness in ear | Clinical; audiologic and vestibular testing | Reassurance; salt restricted diet; triamterene diazepam; vestibular suppressants; surgical therapy |
| Vestibular neuronitis | Viral or vascular (?) | Severe vertigo; nausea; vomiting; (absence of cochlear signs) | Clinical | Symptomatic-vestibular sedatives; vestibular exercises |
| Multiple sclerosis | Demyelinating plaque in brainstem | Central nystagmus; internuclear ophthalmoplegia | MRI | Symptomatic |
| Benign positional vertigo (Cupulolithiasis) | Deposits of otoconia on cupula; following head injury; positional changes | Vertigo; (no auditory symptoms) | Clinical; positional testing | Cawthorne exercises; particle repositioning maneuver; singular neurectomy<br>Posterior semicircular canal occlusion |
| Vertebrobasilar ischemia | Episodic ischemia of brainstem due to vasospasm, hemodynamic factors or platelet aggregation | Vertigo; tinnitus; signs of brainstem ischemia<br>Subclavian steal syndrome | | Neurologic and cardiovascular management |
| Vestibular schwannoma (Acoustic neuroma) | Benign neoplasm | Mild vertigo; sensorineural hearing loss with poor speech discrimination; involvement of cranial nerves; increased intracranial pressure | MRI | Surgical |

may cause an acute vertiginous episode. The patients are commonly young, healthy adults with no previous neurologic history. The accompanying nystagmus, which may persist after the vertigo has abated, is of a central type. The finding of nystagmus in the abducting eye, with weakness in the adducting eye (internuclear ophthalmoplegia), strongly suggests the diagnosis. Auditory brainstem response may show changes in the auditory system that are not detectable by conventional testing. MRI may demonstrate pathognomonic plaques within the brain and spinal cord.

***Benign positional vertigo (cupulolithiasis).*** Patients with cupulolithiasis complain of vertigo when they adopt particular positions (e.g., turning in bed, bending, stooping). It commonly occurs after head injury. It may be due to release of otoconia from a disrupted utricle into the endolymph. Otoconia then become deposited on the cupula of the posterior semicircular canal, making it unduly sensitive to head movement. It is important to distinguish this condition from postural hypotension in which there are no auditory symptoms and the vertigo lasts only a few seconds.

Positional testing is extremely useful in differentiating those cases caused by end-organ pathology (usually the posterior semicircular canal or utricle) and those due to brainstem pathology. The diagnosis of this condition clearly depends on the correct interpretation of the observed nystagmus. Treatment used to be avoidance of provocative positions; however, current recommendations strongly suggest vestibular habituation exercises known as Cawthorne exercises. These exercises are a program of progressive movements of the head, neck, and upper body that provoke vertigo initially, but over time attenuate the symptoms in approximately 90% of patients. Another conservative possibility includes a maneuver to reposition the otoconia, as described by Epley and more recently by Parnes. Of the 10% that fail conservative management, singular neurectomy (section of the posterior ampullary nerve that innervates the posterior semicircular canal) or surgical occlusion of the posterior semicircular canal may be beneficial. Referral to an otolaryngologist is indicated if patients do not improve significantly after 1 month of exercises.

***Vertebrobasilar ischemia.*** Vertebrobasilar ischemia (VBI) due to episodic ischemia of the brainstem is caused by a circulatory disturbance in the distribution of the vertebrobasilar artery and is a form of transient ischemic attack. Such episodes may be due to hemodynamic factors, vasospasm, or platelet aggregation. Vertigo and tinnitus are the outstanding symptoms; but must be accompanied by symptoms or signs of brainstem ischemia such as diplopia, homonymous hemianopia, facial dysesthesias, dysarthria, or ipsilateral ataxia. Exercising an arm may rarely induce ischemia of the vertebrobasilar system (subclavian steal syndrome). Patients with these transient ischemic attacks should be referred for neurologic and cardiovascular assessment.

## Etiology of facial paralysis

- Infection
  - Bacterial
    - Otitis media
    - Mastoiditis
    - Chronic suppurative otitis media (especially with cholesteatoma)
    - Meningitis
    - "Malignant otitis media"
  - Viral
    - Infectious mononucleosis
    - Herpes zoster
    - Varicella
    - Rubella
    - Mumps
  - Mycobacterial
    - Tuberculous meningitis
    - Leprosy
  - Miscellaneous
    - Syphilis
    - Malaria
- Trauma
  - Temporal bone fracture
  - Facial lacerations
  - Surgical
- Neoplasm
  - Malignant
    - Squamous cell carcinoma
    - Basal cell and adenocystic tumors
    - Leukemia
    - Parotid neoplasms
    - Metastatic tumors
  - Benign
    - Vestibular schwannoma
    - Congenital cholesteatoma
    - Facial nerve neuroma
- Immunologic
  - Guillain-Barré syndrome
  - Reaction to tetanus antiserum
  - Periarteritis nodosa
- Metabolic
  - Pregnancy
  - Hypothyroidism
  - Diabetes mellitus

***Vestibular schwannoma (acoustic neuroma).*** A benign neoplasm, vestibular schwannoma, behaves capriciously. Its presentation may vary from the most subtle audiovestibular disturbance to raised intracranial pressure constituting a medical emergency. The vertigo caused by these neoplasms is usually mild or completely absent. There is commonly an accompanying unilateral sensorineural hearing loss with tone decay and poor speech discrimination. Caloric stimulation may show a canal weakness on the affected side. Involvement of the fifth cranial nerve may be inferred from an impaired corneal reflex or by a disturbance of facial sensation. Large tumors may cause a sixth nerve palsy, lower motor neuron, facial paralysis, ipsilateral cerebellar deficits, and ultimately, raised intracranial pressure and papilledema.

Prognosis is directly related to tumor size, which in turn depends on early diagnosis. Thus patients with even minimal audiovestibular dysfunction, particularly unilateral, should always be referred for otolaryngologic evaluation.

***Facial paralysis.*** Facial paralysis is a symptom of an underlying disease. The physician must localize the site of nerve injury, assess its severity, establish its nature, and, if possible, treat the underlying causes (see box at left).

## LOCALIZATION OF THE SITE OF FACIAL NERVE INJURY

The ability to localize the site of facial nerve injury follows directly from a knowledge of the nerve's anatomy (Fig. 27-7).

Simple tests (topognostic tests) have been devised to evaluate the various branches of the facial nerve. Interpretation of results may be performed best by an otolaryngologist. These tests are not always routinely performed but may include tests to determine lacrimation (Schirmer's test), salivation (electrogustometry), and certain audiologic tests including stapedial reflex testing.

### Clinical examination

The diagnosis of facial paralysis rarely presents any difficulty. However, because there are so many causes of facial paralysis, thorough history taking and physical examination are essential (see box on p. 424).

### Examination of the eye

The single most important structure that may be affected by facial paralysis is the eye; without appropriate care blindness may result.

Several measures are available to temporarily or permanently protect the cornea, and they can be performed either by an otolaryngologist or by an ophthalmologist. Eyedrops, protective eyeglasses, and moisture chambers may be sufficient in milder cases. In some patients, the eyelids may need to be taped together. (Care is required to ensure that the tape does not touch the cornea.) Surgical procedures such as tarsorrhaphy or the implantation of a palpebral spring or gold weight are needed if paralysis is permanent or likely to be prolonged. It is prudent to enlist the help of an ophthalmologist early in the course of a facial paralysis.

### Idiopathic facial paralysis (Bell's palsy)

Although the etiology of Bell's palsy is an enigma, considerable recent support has grown for the viral inflammatory immune concept based on serologic findings in patients with Bell's palsy and the isolation of herpes simplex type I virus from the epineurium of biopsy specimens. Immunofluoroscopic complement fixation studies have shown that immune complexes found in the chorda tympani are of viral origin.

The vascular theory for Bell's palsy also has proponents. This theory suggests that edema of the nerve (possibly initiated by vasospasm or viral infection) causes further ischemia of the nerve within its narrow, unyielding, bony canal.

Treatment of Bell's palsy is controversial and should consider the natural history of the condition. Spontaneous recovery of full function can be expected in 80% of

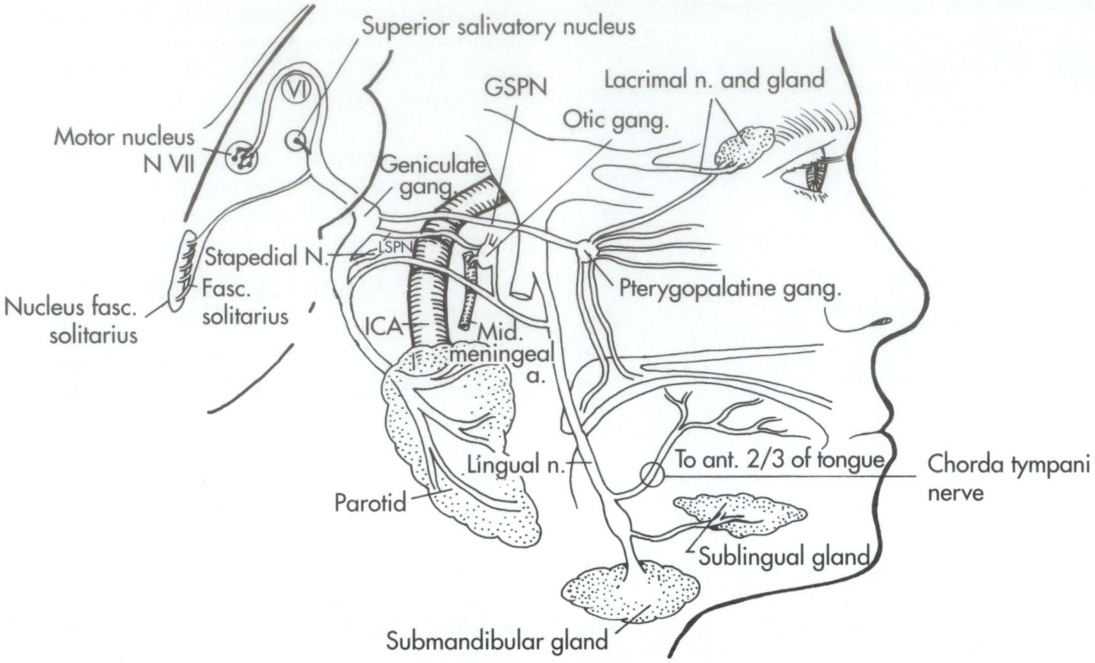


**Fig. 27-7.** Facial nerve anatomy.

## Diagnostic workup in facial paralysis

Examination
- Otolaryngologic and neurologic evaluation
- Photographic records of facial movements
- General physical examination

Topognostic studies
- Schirmer's test, stapedial reflex testing, taste testing

Electrophysiologic studies
- Nerve excitability testing, electromyography, electroneuronography

Audiology
- Pure tone audiometry and impedance tests, electronystagmography

Radiology
- MRI and CT scanning as indicated

Hematology
- CBC, sedimentation rate, other investigations (glucose tolerance, thyroid function tests) as indicated

patients; 10% have mild sequelae. The remainder, about 10% or less, have severe sequelae and poor return of facial function. Steroid therapy is a time-honored choice in Bell's palsy, although statistical evidence supporting its value is lacking. A dose of 1 mg/kg per day of prednisone has been recommended. As in herpes zoster oticus, steroids can be considered. Surgical decompression of the nerve has a limited place in the management of Bell's palsy. Overall, decompression is not routinely performed.

### Suppurative ear disease

***Acute suppurative otitis media.*** The widespread use of antibiotics in acute otitis media has considerably lessened the frequency of facial paralysis as a complication of otitis media. When facial paralysis occurs in otitis media, the nerve is usually dehiscent (incompletely covered by bone), and its sheath becomes involved in the inflammatory process. The paralysis is due to a neuropraxia. Treatment requires the judicious use of antibiotics, myringotomy, and culture of the middle ear aspirate. In acute mastoiditis, a cortical mastoidectomy should be performed. A formal exploration of the nerve is generally not indicated.

***Chronic suppurative otitis media.*** Facial paralysis complicated by chronic ear disease is most often the result of an expanding cholesteatoma, which may exert direct pressure on the nerve. It may also occur in noncholesteatomatous ear disease as a result of a low-grade osteitis involving the nerve sheath. The prognosis for return of facial nerve function depends on the degree of nerve degeneration. Timely surgical intervention may avert permanent facial paralysis, hence the need for early referral to an otolaryngologist.

### Temporal bone fracture

The most frequent temporal bone fracture (about 90% of cases) occurs in the long axis (i.e., longitudinal fractures). Fortunately, the facial nerve is involved in only about 10%. Fractures in the transverse axis of the temporal bone occur less often (about 10% of cases), but about half are complicated by facial paralysis. The time of onset of the facial paralysis is of prime importance. If the onset immediately follows the injury, severe injury to the nerve is likely to occur; if it occurs several hours or days after the injury, nerve continuity is assured and the prognosis for spontaneous recovery is good. Basilar skull fractures usually are managed primarily by a neurosurgeon, and the decision to explore the facial nerve is made in consultation with an otolaryngologist. The decision is clearly influenced by the patient's general condition, the time of onset of the paralysis (immediate or delayed), and the presence or absence of degeneration as evidenced by electrophysiologic testing.

### Herpes zoster oticus (Ramsay Hunt syndrome)

The Ramsey Hunt syndrome comprises a triad of clinical findings: vesication of the auricle, facial nerve paralysis, and audiovestibular disturbances. In many cases, vesicular eruption may be seen in the areas of distribution of the cervical, trigeminal, glossopharyngeal, or vagus nerves—hence the term *cephalic herpes zoster.* The value of steroids in this condition is unproven, but it is common practice to administer them. Acyclovir also has been advocated. There are a plethora of other etiologies in facial nerve paralysis, and the reader is referred to any general otolaryngology text for more details.

## BIBLIOGRAPHY

### General Texts on Otolaryngology


Bluestone CD, Stool S, editors: *Pediatric otolaryngology,* Philadelphia, 1983, WB Saunders.

English GM, editor: *Otolaryngology,* Hagerstown, Md, 1976, Harper & Row.

Goodhill V, editor: *Ear diseases, deafness and dizziness,* Hagerstown, Md, 1979, Harper & Row.

Paparella MM, Shumrick DA, editors: *Otolaryngology,* 2nd ed, Philadelphia, 1980, WB Saunders.

Sade J: *Secretory otitis media and its sequellae,* New York, 1979, Churchill Livingstone.


### Vertigo


Epley JM: The canalith repositioning procedure for treatment of benign positional vertigo, *Otolaryngol Head Neck Surg* 107:399-404, 1992.

Gibson WPR: The functional and physical examination of the vestibular system. In Ballantyne J, Groves J, editors: *Scott Brown's diseases of the ear, nose and throat,* ed 4, vol 2, London, 1979, Butterworth.

Parnes LS, Price-Jones RG: Particle repositioning maneuver for benign paroxysmal positional vertigo, *Ann Otol Rhino Laryngol* 102(5):325-331, 1993.

Schuknecht HF: Cupulolithiasis, *Arch Otolaryngol* 90:765, 1969.


### Facial Paralysis


Esslen E: *The acute facial palsies: investigations on the localization and pathogenesis of meatolabyrinthine facial palsies,* New York, 1977, Springer-Verlag.

Fisch U, Felix H: On the pathogenesis of Bell's palsy, *Acta Otolaryngol* (Stockholm) 95:532, 1983.

Graham MD, House WF, editors: *Disorders of the facial nerve,* New York, 1981, Raven Press.

May M: Facial nerve disorders, *Am J Otolaryngol* 4:77, 1982.


CHAPTER

# 28 The Nose and Paranasal Sinuses


**Samuel A. Mickelson**
**Michael S. Benninger**


The nose and paranasal sinuses provide for the diverse functions of respiration, conditioning and purifying inspired air, and olfaction. Although healthy individuals are not necessarily conscious of these functions, they may be significant sources of discomfort and lifestyle interruption when dysfunctional. In fact, nasal sinus–related disorders are the most common reason that patients now visit physicians in the United States. This chapter concerns the more common disorders affecting these sites and suggests approaches to management of patients with nasal and sinus disorders.

## MEDICAL HISTORY

### Symptoms and their significance

Many disorders affecting the nose and paranasal sinuses can be diagnosed by history and physical examination alone. Most laboratory testing is confirmatory only. It is important to obtain a thorough history and have an understanding of the various symptoms and their significance. The major symptoms related to the nose are nasal obstruction (congestion), drainage, facial pain or headache, epistaxis, and change in smell or taste.

### Nasal obstruction

Nasal obstruction (congestion or stuffy nose) can be caused by a deflected nasal septum, enlargement of turbinates, or polyps or mass lesions within the nose. Nasal obstruction is the most common symptom, since turbinate hypertrophy can result from many disorders. It is important to assess whether the nasal obstruction is unilateral, bilateral, or alternating in sides and determine if it is constant or intermittent. If unilateral, a fixed anatomic problem such as a deviated septum, polyp, or mass lesion is likely. Any intermittent or alternating obstruction must relate to variations in the turbinate size. When bilateral, the obstruction is due to a bilateral process such as polyps or allergy, or from a complex deflection of the septum.

### Nasal drainage and postnasal drip

Drainage from the nose is one of the most helpful symptoms in determining the nature of the disorder. It is important to determine if rhinorrhea is unilateral or bilateral, clear or discolored, and watery, mucoid, or tenacious. Unilateral drainage represents a localized process such as unilateral sinusitis or cerebrospinal fluid (CSF) leak, whereas bilateral drainage is due to a more systemic or general process. Clear drainage suggests a diagnosis of vasomotor, nonallergic, or allergic rhinitis, whereas thick and discolored (yellow, green, or brown) drainage suggests bacterial or viral infection. The sensation of postnasal drainage is influenced more by the thickness of the drainage than the quantity. Though many patients complain that swallowing large amounts of drainage causes nausea, it is unclear if they are causally related. A sense of mucus in the throat, hoarseness, and chronic throat clearing are rarely, if ever, caused by sinus drainage since the normal swallowing mechanism clears the mucus without laryngeal contact. The exceptions are during an allergic or viral episode where both nasal sinus and laryngeal inflammation occur simultaneously.

### Facial pain and headache

Facial pain and headache are not useful symptoms in differentiating disorders because of the multiple different disorders that can cause pain. These include many of the nasal and sinus disorders, tension headache, migraine headache, myofacial pain syndrome, temporomandibular joint syndrome, tic douloureux, and dental caries. Pain overlying the sinuses is not necessarily due to pathology in the underlying sinus. When pain is related to nasal or sinus pathology, it is usually due to ostial obstruction or mucous membrane contact with referred pain to other areas of the face. Severe facial pain associated with swelling over the sinuses and purulent drainage is generally related to sinusitis. Many patients with allergic or nonallergic rhinitis complain of intermittent facial pressure or headache associated with changes in the weather, humidity, or other environmental factors. Malignant tumors are to be considered in patients with persistent unilateral facial pain without purulent rhinorrhea.

### Epistaxis

Epistaxis is a nonspecific symptom that may accompany almost any pathology in the nose, nasopharynx, or paranasal sinuses. The most common cause of bleeding is from breaks in the prominent capillary vessels along the anterior septum (Kiesselbach's plexus or Little's area). This occurs frequently with local trauma such as frequent nose blowing, sneezing, or digitally caused trauma. Once bleeding occurs, it may spontaneously recur if the scab becomes dislodged. Patients with a septal deviation may bleed along the deflected portion of the septum, which becomes dry and excoriated. Blood mixed with purulent drainage generally suggests acute sinusitis. Blood will exit anteriorly if the head is leaned forward and posteriorly if the head is straight or leaned backward. Tumors are rare causes of nasal bleeding.

### Changes in olfaction

Anosmia is the complete loss of olfaction, and hyposmia is a decrease in the sense of smell. Parosmia and dysosmia are conditions resulting in an altered sense of smell. Cacosmia, the sensation of unpleasant smell, can occur with acute sinusitis, when recovering from anosmia after influenza or head trauma, or with the use of tetracycline or streptomycin. Phantosmia is the hallucination of smells and can be seen in schizophrenia and temporal lobe seizures.

Anosmia or hyposmia can occur in any condition that affects nasal air flow to the region of the cribriform plate bilaterally. Therefore an alteration in smell thresholds is common in patients with nasal polyps or severe chronic sinusitis, whereas unilateral anosmia usually goes unnoticed. Anosmia without nasal obstruction is most frequently caused by viral upper respiratory tract infections or severe head trauma. Certain industrial chemicals such as formaldehyde can also lead to anosmia. Lead poisoning, vitamin A deficiency, tobacco use, and radiation therapy have been associated with hyposmia or anosmia. Hyposmia occurring in hypogonadal females or during pregnancy is relieved with hormonal treatments or the completion of pregnancy. Rarely an anterior cranial fossa meningioma can cause slowly progressive anosmia. Other rare causes of anosmia include diabetes, hypothyroidism, pernicious anemia, and amphetamine toxicity.

Congenital or genetic causes of anosmia include Turner syndrome, pseudohypoparathyroidism, and congenital hypogonadotrophic eunuchoidism. A decreased sense of smell frequently occurs with increasing age (presbyosmia).

In patients with anosmia but a normal nasal examination, a thorough history and directed laboratory and radiologic tests usually determine the etiology. Treatment of the loss of olfaction should be directed at the cause. Postviral anosmia often spontaneously resolves. Use of oral zinc supplements has recently been advocated for persistent anosmia but benefit has not been proved. Patient counseling is of utmost importance with regard to use of smoke detectors in the home, avoidance of excessive perfumes or colognes, control of bodily odors, and attention to expiration dates on food products.

### Allergic symptoms

Characteristic symptoms of seasonal allergic rhinitis include sneezing, nasal or ocular pruritus, bilateral clear watery or mucoid nasal drainage, and nasal congestion. Patients also complain of pruritus of the upper palate and ears, and dry, scratchy and erythematous conjunctiva. These symptoms are associated with elevations of specific pollen counts. Springtime allergies typically relate to tree pollens, midsummer symptoms to grasses, and fall symptoms to weed pollens.

Dust and mold perennial allergies are less distinct because nasal congestion and clear drainage frequently occur without sneezing and pruritus. Patients with dust or mite allergies are more symptomatic in the morning and with exposure to upholstered furniture, mattresses, pillows, and carpeting. Mold allergies vary significantly through the year depending on the particular mold sensitivities.

### Tobacco, medications, and chemical exposures

Tobacco smoke is an irritant causing congestion of the turbinates, destruction of cilia, and alteration in the mucus-secreting cells of the nasal mucosa. Smokers have increased symptoms of nasal congestion and thick postnasal drainage and may be predisposed to sinusitis.

A variety of medications can also affect the nose. After just a few days of using topical phenylephrine or oxymetazoline, there is rebound swelling of the turbinates (rhinitis medicamentosa) in which the nose becomes chronically congested. Treatment is the discontinuation of the offending agents. Diuretics cause thicker and more tenacious secretions. Turbinate hypertrophy is caused by many drugs, including β-blockers, reserpine, and exogenous estrogens. Though most medication effects are temporary, long-term use of these drugs can have irreversible effects on the nose.

Many chemicals used in industry cause mucosal edema and increased mucoid secretion from the turbinates. Use of intranasal cocaine can cause large septal perforations with resultant bleeding and crusting from the edges. Wood dust and asbestos exposure can also have irritant effects on the nose with secondary congestion of the turbinates.

### Systemic disorders and their effects

Systemic conditions can affect the nose either directly or indirectly. Rhinitis of pregnancy, due to elevated estrogen levels, causes turbinate engorgement and resolves at the end of pregnancy. When severe it can be treated with an oral decongestant.

Sarcoidosis and Wegener's granulomatosis can affect the nose and are covered in more detail later.

## EXAMINATION AND DIAGNOSTIC STUDIES

### Physical examination

The nasal examination is important in the diagnostic workup of any nasal or sinus disorder because most pathologic conditions can be visualized without special studies (see Managed Care Guide). Otolaryngologists typically examine the nose before and after use of a topical decongestant to allow a better view of the nasal cavity. Anterior rhinoscopy with a nasal speculum and headlight allows delineation of the septum, the inferior and middle turbinates, and portions of the nasopharynx and may allow a limited view into the middle meatus. Posterior rhinoscopy with a tongue blade, nasopharyngeal mirror, and headlight allow examination of the posterior choana, nasopharynx, eustachian tubes, and posterior edges of the septum and inferior turbinates. Though examination of the anterior nares with an otoscope is easy, the view is limited to the first 2 or 3 cm of the nose. If this technique is to be used, the nose should at least be decongested first with a topical decongestant.

Flexible and rigid nasal endoscopes have recently been reintroduced for use in the nose in the office setting. The procedure is done after application of a topical decongestant and anesthetic agent. Nasal endoscopy is a sensitive way to evaluate the nose for gross or subtle changes associated with sinusitis. The scope can frequently identify small polyps, erythema, and purulent drainage coming from sinus ostia that would not be visible by routine anterior or posterior rhinoscopy. The maxillary sinuses can also be examined with the endoscope via a sinus puncture, which can assist in the diagnosis of sinus malignancies. Due to the high cost of the instrumentation, nasal endoscopy should not be used for the routine examination of the nose.

Transillumination is a simple technique whereby, in a darkened room, a bright light is applied to the frontal or maxillary sinuses. Transillumination will occur in a sinus with normal or slightly thickened mucosa, whereas the light will not be transmitted in an opacified or fluid-filled sinus. Transillumination can be used instead of a radiograph before treating acute sinusitis.

### Laboratory studies

Nasal and nasopharyngeal cultures are generally not useful because pathologic bacteria (*Staphylococcus aureus, Streptococcus pneumoniae, Haemophilus influenzae,* and *Moraxella catarrhalis*) are present in both normal and sinusitis patients. Cultures from a sinus tap or from an endoscopic guided culture through the sinus ostia are more precise.

Nasal smears are simple and inexpensive studies that can help differentiate sinusitis from allergic or nonallergic rhinitis by determining the type of white blood cells present. A predominance of eosinophils suggests allergic rhinitis, whereas predominance of leukocytes suggests an infection.

Serum immunoglobulin levels can be helpful in the diagnosis of allergic rhinitis (elevated IgE level). Immunoglobulin G subclass studies are performed when an immune deficiency is suspected as a cause for persistent sinusitis. The patient's immunologic response to a pneumococcal vaccine will confirm or eliminate a functional immune deficiency. A complete blood count is useful to help differentiate bacterial sinusitis (elevated neutrophil count) from viral rhinitis (elevated lymphocyte count).

### Radiographic tests

Routine sinus films are useful to help confirm a suspicion of sinusitis and to follow disease resolution following a course of treatment. They are sensitive for air-fluid levels (Fig. 28-1) in the maxillary or frontal sinuses and for moderate to severe mucosal thickening or complete opacification in the maxillary sinuses (Fig. 28-2). However, their ability to identify mild ethmoid, sphenoid, maxillary, or frontal mucosal thickening is severely limited.

Computed tomography is the most useful of all radiographic studies for the paranasal sinuses. Axial and coronal views give detailed information about the osseous and soft tissues of the nose and paranasal sinuses as well as the region of the osteomeatal complex. While some centers perform screening computed tomography (CT) scans at a fee comparable to routine sinus films, they should rarely be ordered by primary care physicians, since their major roles are in assessing patients refractory to medical therapy, evaluating the extent of disease, and preoperative planning.

Magnetic resonance imaging (MRI) is very accurate in determining the extent of sinusitis and tumors. However, at this time cost and availability preclude it from use in the routine management of sinus disease.

### Allergy testing

Allergy testing is useful in patients who have significant symptoms related to seasonal or perennial allergic rhinitis. RAST testing is a serum test that determines the amount of IgG-mediated immunoglobulin against a specific allergen or allergen group. Prick or scratch skin testing

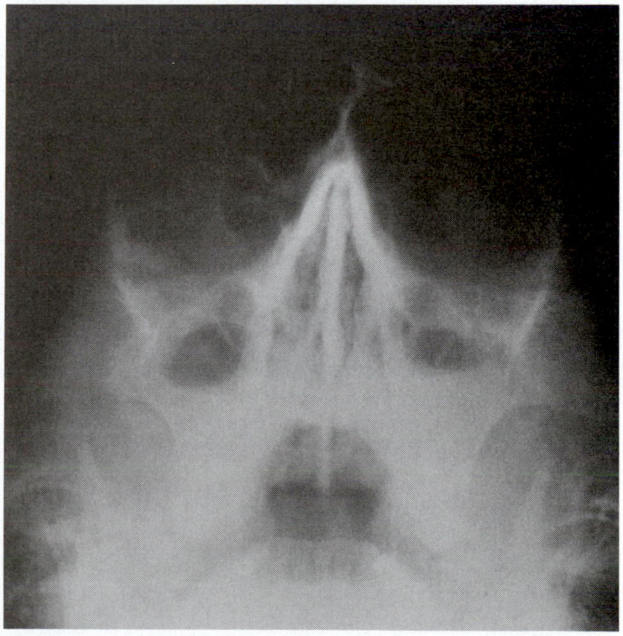

**Fig. 28-1.** Waters' view of maxillary sinus with air-fluid level.

**Managed Care Guide**
**Algorithm describing the treatment of a patient with rhinorrhea**

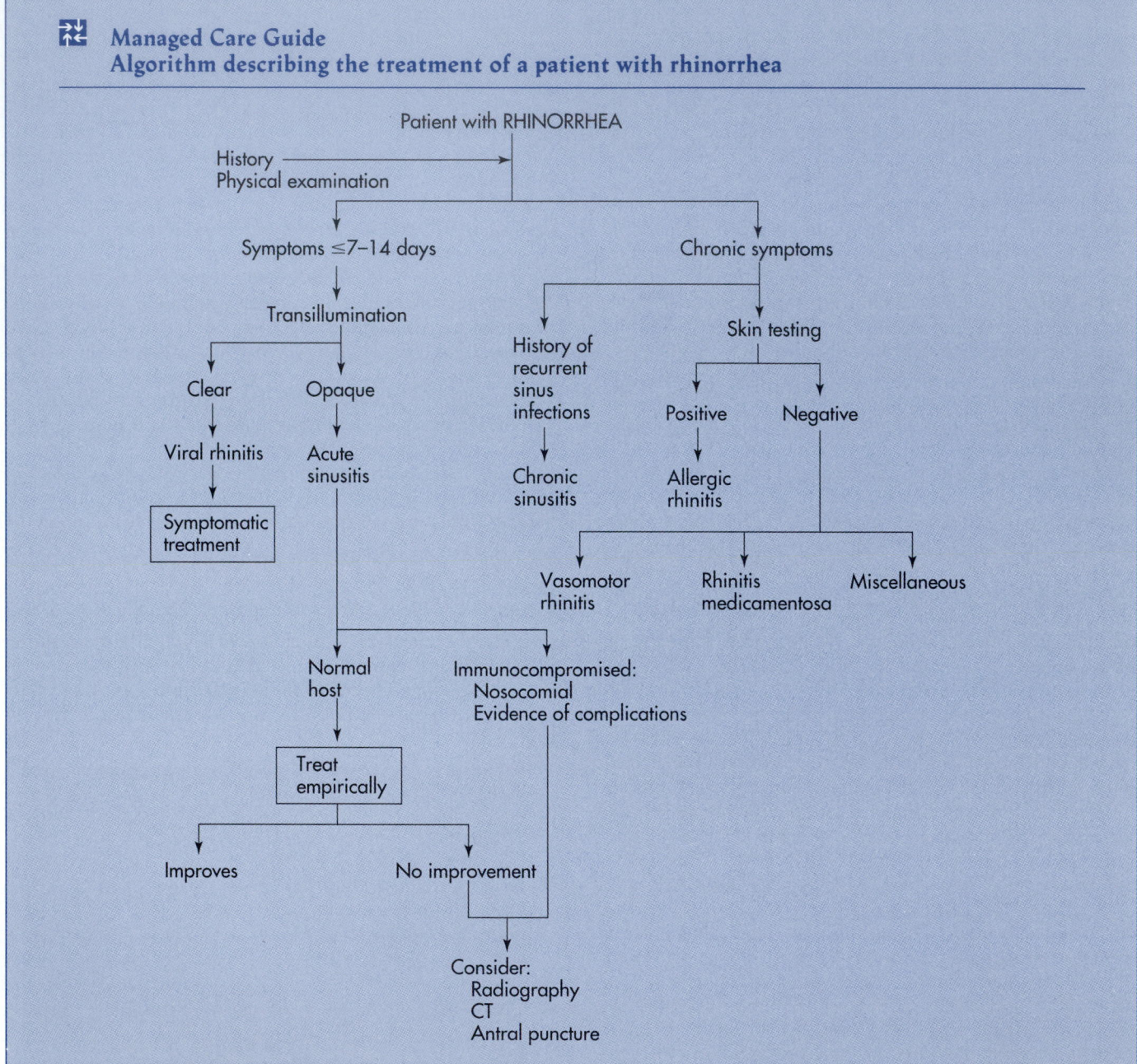

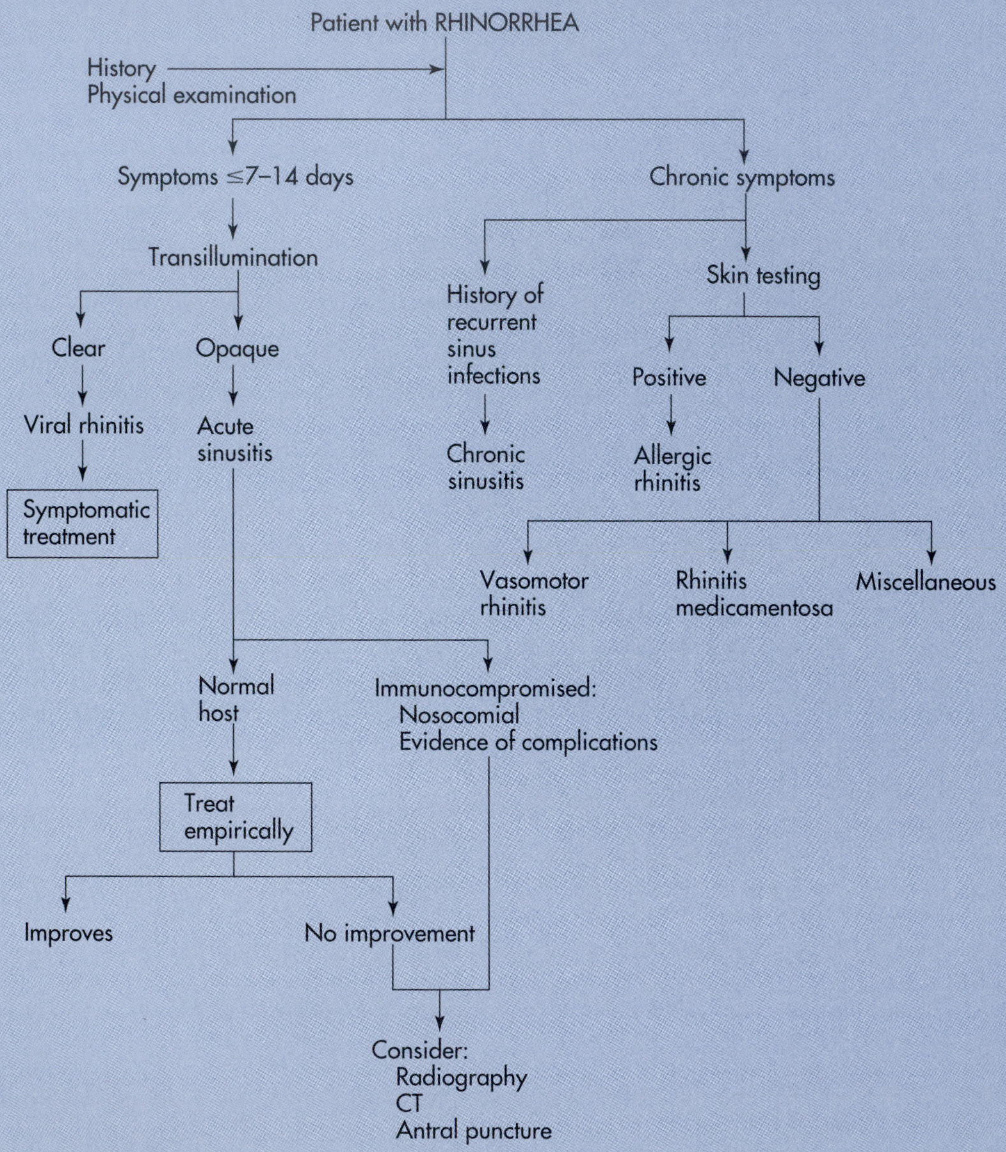

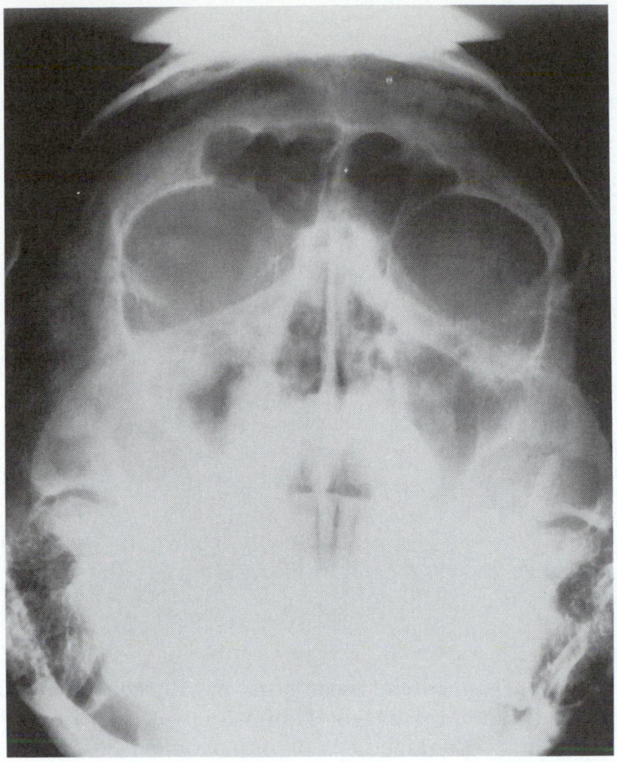

**Fig. 28-2.** Waters' view of maxillary sinus with mucosal thickening.

measures the clinical responses to inoculation with various allergens and is mediated by release of histamine and other chemicals. Intradermal testing is more sensitive than prick tests, yet poses a higher risk of anaphylaxis and is performed if prick testing is negative or not diagnostic.

## EVALUATION OF COMMON DISORDERS

### The common cold

The common cold is an acute viral rhinosinusitis with inflammation of all mucosa of the nose and paranasal sinuses. Generalized symptoms include malaise, fatigue, low-grade fever, chills, and sore throat. The nasal symptoms include nasal obstruction, anterior and posterior clear rhinorrhea, diffuse pressure over the paranasal sinuses, and occasionally plugged ears associated with eustachian tube dysfunction. On the second or third day of infection an increase of neutrophils in the nasal secretions may cause the drainage to be more discolored, but within 1 to 2 days the drainage becomes clear again. The white blood cell count may be slightly elevated, with a predominance of lymphocytes or atypical lymphocytes. Sinus radiographs are normal or show mild mucosal thickening.

### Management

Management is supportive with antipyretics, analgesics, and oral decongestants; hydration and saline nasal sprays aid in mucus clearance. Though a topical decongestant is helpful for the symptoms, one needs to be cautious about the potential for rebound effects from excessive use. Antihistamines decrease nasal drainage but should be avoided when purulent sinusitis is suspected, since they thicken the mucus blanket and slow down mucociliary transport. Symptoms usually resolve in 5 to 8 days without other treatment.

### Epistaxis

The etiologies of epistaxis include both local and systemic factors. Local causes are most common in children and are usually associated with nose picking, excessive blowing, sneezing, or rubbing. Bleeding frequently occurs with the common cold, acute sinusitis, or allergic rhinitis. Recurrent bleeding may occur if a scab forms at the bleeding site and becomes dislodged. Though tumors are rare causes of epistaxis, they should be included in the differential diagnosis, especially with profuse bleeding in adolescent males (juvenile nasopharyngeal angiofibroma) or in adults without other known etiologies. In adults, bleeding tends to be more profuse and may be from the posterior nasal cavity. Systemic causes of epistaxis include acquired coagulopathies, hereditary blood dyscrasias, and the use of aspirin, coumadin, or heparin. Patients with hypertension are not more likely to have a nosebleed, though elevated blood pressure can result in more profuse bleeding and makes it more difficult to control. Antihypertensive agents should be administered to hypertensive patients with epistaxis.

The most common site of bleeding is from Kiesselbach's plexus (Fig. 28-3) on the anterior septum. Posterior epistaxis is less common but can be a serious problem in adults. A posterior bleed is defined as bleeding far enough posterior that the site of bleeding cannot be seen by anterior rhinoscopy.

Evaluation of epistaxis is primarily by physical examination. Anterior rhinoscopy with a nasal speculum and Fraser suction (to remove clots and fresh blood) are usually sufficient to identify the site of bleeding. Areas with prominent vessels or scabs should be examined with caution because manipulation may start up active bleeding. Sinus radiographs should be done only when tumors are suspected as the cause of bleeding. When a severe posterior bleed cannot be controlled by packing, carotid artery angiography may help to delineate the source of bleeding.

The management of epistaxis depends on the site of bleeding, the severity, and the etiology. Patients with coagulopathies should have the nose packed with dissolvable packing materials (Oxycel cotton or Gelfoam), since any localized trauma such as pack removal will cause bleeding from multiple sites in addition to the original site. Attempts should be made to correct the coagulopathy.

Conservative measures can be helpful in all patients. These include improving the humidity of inspired air, moisturizing the nose with saline sprays 6 to 10 times a day, and applying antibiotic ointments to reduce scabbing and speed healing of the excoriated areas. Long-term care with an unscented water-base lotion twice a day along with saline sprays usually prevents recurrences.

Recurrent bleeding along the anterior septum is best treated conservatively. When these measures fail, application of silver nitrate or electrocautery can be helpful. This should be performed after application of a topical decongestant and anesthetic agent (4% cocaine or 1% tetracaine). Silver nitrate cautery should be performed

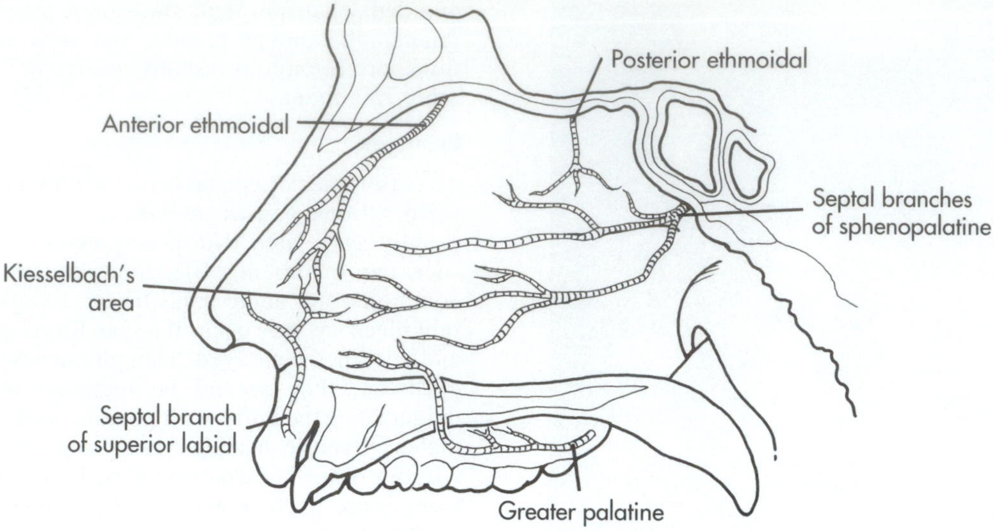


**Fig. 28-3.** Kiesselbach's plexus on the anterior septum derives blood supply from the superior labial, descending palatine, and sphenopalatine arteries.

from the periphery toward the site of bleeding. When done in the opposite direction, there is a risk of precipitating active bleeding that may be difficult to control. A cotton-tip applicator helps remove excessive silver nitrate from the rest of the nose.

Active bleeding from the anterior nasal cavity is best treated with an anterior nasal pack left in place for 2 to 5 days. Vaseline gauze packing impregnated with an antibiotic ointment can be layered in the nose to apply pressure to the bleeding site. Other packing materials include commercially available balloons and Merosel sponge packs. Oral antibiotics should be given to help prevent excessive bacterial growth in the packing and subsequent bacterial sinusitis. A posterior pack is indicated for more posterior bleeding that fails to respond to anterior packing. Posterior packs may be fashioned from gauze materials, Foley catheters, or commercially available balloon packs. Patients with posterior packs are usually admitted to the hospital and given supplemental oxygen, since significant hypoxemia can occur.

Alternative methods of controlling severe posterior bleeds include arterial ligation of the internal maxillary or ethmoidal vessels and occasionally even ligation of the external carotid artery. Arteriography with embolization has also been used for posterior bleeds. Posterior bleeding may be severe enough to require ICU monitoring and multiple transfusions to maintain normal hemodynamics.

### Trauma

Due to their position on the face, the nasal bones are the most frequently fractured bones of the facial skeleton. There is frequently epistaxis associated with fractures from intranasal mucosal tears. Most nasal fractures can be diagnosed by palpation of the bony nasal skeleton finding pinpoint tenderness along with displacement of the nasal bones. Nondisplaced and small fractures at the tip of the nasal bones are more difficult to palpate. Lateral radiographs can confirm a displaced fracture but should be used with caution, since normal suture lines can look like nondisplaced fractures.

Initial management is supportive with head elevation and cold compresses to diminish swelling. Epistaxis usually stops spontaneously or with a topical decongestant spray. Nondisplaced fractures require no active treatment. Nasal fractures are repaired for either functional (nasal obstruction) or cosmetic reasons. Reduction of the nasal fracture is generally done 4 to 8 days after injury. This allows the soft tissue swelling to diminish, allowing for a better reduction of the displaced nasal bones. A comparison to the preinjury state in a recent photograph will help assess the need for reduction. Although management of the fracture is not emergent, it is important to examine and palpate the nasal septum at the time of the initial evaluation to be sure there is no widening and softening that would be suggestive of a septal hematoma. Untreated septal hematomas cause disruption of the blood supply to the septum and can lead to a subsequent saddle nose deformity. When a septal hematoma is suspected, an emergency consultation with an otolaryngologist is in order. All other fractures may be assessed 3 to 4 days after injury, allowing for a better assessment of subtle deformities. Nondisplaced fractures do not require further evaluation.

### Acute sinusitis

Acute sinusitis represents an acute bacterial infection involving the mucosal surfaces of the paranasal sinuses and nasal cavity. It usually occurs following an upper respiratory tract infection. Less common causes include swimming in contaminated water, nasal foreign bodies, and spread from dental infections. Indwelling nasotracheal and nasogastric tubes also predispose to acute sinusitis. When of dental origin, the causative tooth is usually the first or second maxillary molar whose roots extend toward the floor of the maxillary sinus.

Acute sinusitis typically presents with unilateral or bilateral nasal obstruction, purulent rhinorrhea, facial pain, and pressure overlying the paranasal sinuses. There is exacerbation of pain with bending over or straining, and the maxillary teeth may be tender. In contrast to the clear

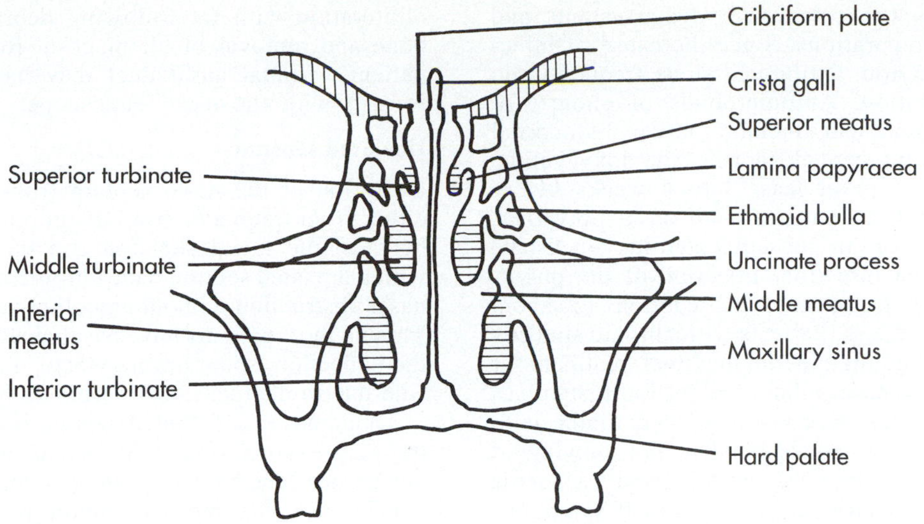


**Fig. 28-4.** Coronal view of nasal cavity, turbinates, and meati and their association with the paranasal sinuses.

secretions of viral infections, the secretions in acute sinusitis are purulent.

The diagnosis can be made by history, along with a physical examination finding tenderness over the paranasal sinuses, congestion of the turbinates, and purulent drainage in the nose, nasopharynx, or posterior oral pharynx. After decongesting with a topical agent, purulent drainage may be seen in the middle meatus and a nasal endoscope may help in identifying swelling, erythema, and purulence coming out of sinus ostia. Transillumination of the sinuses usually shows a decrease in light transmission of the involved sinus. Radiographic studies are generally needed only to support a questionable history or physical examination. Routine sinus films show mucosal thickening or an air-fluid level in the sinuses. Acute bacterial sinusitis is caused by *S. pneumoniae, H. influenzae,* and *M. catarrhalis.*

Acute sinusitis is usually treated empirically without cultures with a 10- to 14-day course of an appropriate antimicrobial agent, saline nasal sprays, oral decongestants, and analgesic agents. Topical decongestants should be used for 2 to 3 days only and then switched to oral agents to prevent potential rebound. Antihistamines should be avoided unless there is also a history of allergic rhinitis. Good first-line agents are amoxicillin, erythromycin plus a sulfonamide, and amoxicillin with clavulanate. Alternatives include cefuroxime, cefprozil, cefpodoxime, doxycycline, and trimethoprim with sulfamethoxazole. Though there is evidence of increasing β-lactamase activity in bacterial pathogens, antibiotics that cover these organisms are generally used as second-line drugs due to their increased cost and potential side effects. When acute sinusitis is from a dental source, the causative tooth should be treated with root canal or drainage of periapical abscess.

Sinus irrigation is indicated when there is severe pain and the maxillary sinus is not draining. The sinus tap obtains a culture and clears the purulent material from the sinus, giving significant symptomatic relief. Surgery is indicated when there is spread of infection to adjacent areas. External ethmoidectomy is used for ethmoiditis with periorbital abscess and frontal sinus trephination for frontal sinusitis with spread to the intracranial cavity. Endoscopic sinus surgery may benefit patients who have sinusitis that recurs more often than three times per year.

The goals of treatment are not only the resolution of symptoms but also the elimination of mucosal thickening that could narrow the ostiomeatal complex and predispose to recurrent or persistent infection. Since sinus radiographs and computed tomography are not routinely performed at the completion of treatment, it would seem prudent to treat the patient for 5 to 7 days after resolution of symptoms. The patient should be referred for otolaryngology evaluation in cases of recurrent infections greater than two to three per year, severe infection that fails to respond to antibiotics, or persistent infection despite a few courses of antibiotics.

## Chronic sinusitis

Chronic sinusitis represents a persistent low-grade infection involving the paranasal sinuses with persistent mucosal thickening. Pansinusitis or multifocal sinusitis is usually due to nasal polyposis or dysfunction of mucociliary transport (Fig. 28-4), whereas more localized infection is due to ostial obstruction. Patients present with persistent low-grade infection with intermittent acute exacerbations more typical of acute sinusitis. The chronic symptoms are persistent nasal obstruction associated with chronic nasal drainage. The drainage is usually discolored, thick, and copious in the morning, slowly clearing by afternoon. Anosmia is not uncommon, and nasal obstruction is also worse in the morning. Facial pain and sinus headaches may occur daily or only with exacerbations of acute sinusitis.

The diagnosis of chronic sinusitis is made by the classic symptoms associated with radiographic findings of mucosal thickening on routine films or sinus CT scans. Allergy testing is helpful, since perennial allergic rhinitis can mimic sinusitis symptoms. Chronic sinusitis is a polymicrobial disease with cultures usually growing multiple pathogens. The most common pathogens are *M. catarrhalis, H. influenzae, S. pneumoniae, S. aureus,* and a variety of anaerobes.

Chronic sinusitis is treated with decongestants and intranasal steroid preparations. Since the cause of infection is ostial obstruction, antibiotics alone frequently do not result in resolution. Antimicrobials of choice for empiric primary treatment include antistaphylococcal penicillin, clindamycin, cephalosporins, and doxycycline. Treatment should be for at least 3 to 4 weeks before surgery is considered. In patients with nasal polyposis, administration of oral or intramuscular steroids can also be helpful in controlling infection. Injection of the polyps with steroids must be done with caution to avoid complications of blindness. Patients with chronic sinusitis and allergic rhinitis should undergo maximal treatment for the allergies to reduce nasal inflammation. Antihistamines should be avoided unless there is an allergic diathesis to avoid thickening of the mucus blanket and slowing of mucociliary transport. Patients with chronic sinusitis should be referred for surgical intervention if symptoms persist despite 1 to 2 months of treatment with intranasal steroids, decongestants, and a trial of antibiotics. Surgery is directed at relieving the obstruction at the sinus ostia.

Chronic infection in the maxillary, anterior ethmoid, and frontal sinuses can be caused by ostiomeatal complex obstruction. Endoscopic sinus surgery can frequently relieve this obstruction, allowing the return of normal function of the sinuses and resolution of the chronic infection (Fig. 28-5). Older surgical options included the nasal antral window, which creates a new opening into the maxillary sinus under the inferior turbinate. This procedure improves aeration of the maxillary sinus but is limited because of a high incidence of closure over time. The Caldwell-Luc procedure involves a sublabial approach to the maxillary sinuses with removal of all mucosa. This procedure is generally reserved for patients with irreversibly damaged, nonfunctioning mucosa. Surgery on the frontal sinuses is indicated for mucoceles or chronic osteomyelitis (Pott's puffy tumor) in which the infectious process has eroded through the anterior or posterior walls of the sinus. Treatment of these patients includes systemic antibiotics plus frontal sinus obliteration with fat following debridement of infected bone and removal of all mucosa. Reconstruction of the patient's frontal nasal duct may have merit when performed with the nasal endoscope.

## Deviated septum

Deviation of the nasal septum from the midline occurs either from trauma or from disproportionate growth rates between the facial skeleton and nasal septum. Patients with a deviated septum have chronic unilateral or bilateral nasal obstruction without any other significant symptoms. Though most patients have nasal obstruction on the side of the deflection, some have a worse airway on the opposite side due to compensatory turbinate hypertrophy.

Diagnosis of a deviated septum is made by history and physical examination. Even small anterior cartilaginous deflections tend to cause worse symptoms than posterior deflections. The more common posterior septal spurs rarely cause significant nasal obstruction. Septal deflections may predispose to recurrent sinusitis due to focal ostial edema, increased turbulence of airflow, or bacterial deposition.

Correction of a septal deformity is a minor elective surgical procedure that is performed under local anesthesia with sedation in the ambulatory setting. In patients who have external nasal deformities, a rhinoplasty may be performed in conjunction with septoplasty to improve both the functional and cosmetic problems. Occasionally a functional rhinoplasty is necessary along with the septoplasty to correct a severe septal deflection.

## Turbinate hypertrophy

The nasal turbinates may enlarge for a variety of reasons, including allergic rhinitis, nonallergic rhinitis, septal deflection, exposure to tobacco smoke, irritants and pollutants, and use of certain drugs (Fig. 28-6). Prescription drugs that cause turbinate hypertrophy include β-blockers, reserpine, and hormones such as estrogen. Frequent cocaine use may cause turbinate congestion similar to the rebound effect associated with overuse of

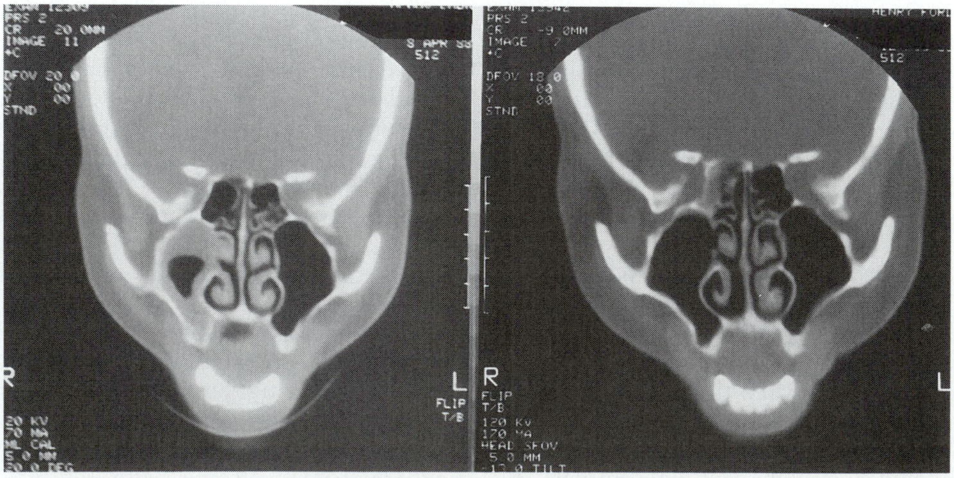


**Fig. 28-5.** Coronal CT of patient before (*left*) and after (*right*) endoscopic anterior ethmoidectomy and enlargement of the maxillary ostium. Maxillary mucosal thickening has resolved following surgery.

topical decongestants. Compensatory turbinate hypertrophy frequently occurs on the side opposite a septal deviation. Aeration of the middle turbinates (concha bullosa) occurs in 10% of adults and, when large enough, can lead to significant nasal obstruction.

The diagnosis of turbinate dysfunction is based on a history of chronic nasal obstruction associated with examination findings of turbinate hypertrophy. Reexamination after a topical decongestant can help differentiate enlargement due to osseous or soft tissue changes. Patients with turbinate hypertrophy that fails to respond to decongestants, antihistamines, or intranasal steroids may be candidates for surgical reduction. A variety of surgical techniques have been used to reduce turbinate size. Cautery of the inferior turbinates causes scarring in the submucosa and limits edema from allergic and nonallergic rhinitis. Lateral turbinate fracture is commonly performed with septoplasty to displace the turbinates away from the septum. Submucosal resection of the turbinate bone with preservation of the mucosa is useful when the bone is the primary cause of enlargement. Turbinoplasty involves removal of a portion of the turbinate bone and mucosa and leads to a greater reduction than submucous resection. Total resection of the inferior turbinates is rarely performed due to the risk of atrophic rhinitis and ozena (foul smelling mucus accumulating underneath large crusts).

## Nasal vestibulitis

Nasal vestibulitis is a common problem caused by *S. aureus* infection around a hair follicle in the nasal vestibule. The infection is associated with excessive nose blowing or picking. Management is directed at limiting digitally induced nasal trauma, application of an antistaphylococcal antibiotic ointment (mupirocin) to help prevent scabbing around hair follicles, and use of an antistaphylococcal oral antibiotic. Patients with diabetes, immune deficiency, or progressive infection despite antibiotics should be placed on intravenous antibiotics due to the potential of spread to the cavernous sinus.

## Nasal polyposis

Nasal polyps represent an inflammatory disorder of the nose and paranasal sinuses of unknown etiology. They usually originate from sinus mucosa and protrude through the ostia, appearing as gray translucent pedunculated masses above or below the middle turbinate. Although patients with allergic rhinitis have an incidence of nasal polyps similar to that of the general population, those with nasal polyps have a 30% incidence of allergy. The growth and persistence of nasal polyps may be exacerbated by inflammatory reactions and release of histamine and other mediators of inflammation. Solitary nasal polyps may be caused by acute or chronic sinusitis, and diffuse nasal polyposis may cause secondary sinusitis. Antral choanal polyps originate from the maxillary sinus and may fill the nasal cavity and nasopharynx and hang into the oral pharynx.

Symptoms of nasal polyps include nasal obstruction, hyposmia or anosmia, and symptoms associated with secondary infection. The diagnosis is made by anterior rhinoscopy or nasal endoscopy after nasal decongestion. Nasal endoscopy allows detection of smaller polyps that may not be visible without magnification. A biopsy should be taken from unilateral or solitary polyps to rule out a benign or malignant tumor. Isolated asymptomatic polyps or retention cysts occurring in the floor or roof of the maxillary sinuses do not require any treatment or evaluation. These lesions should be biopsied only if symptomatic or suspicious for malignancy.

The management of nasal polyps is directed at the control of symptoms. When secondary sinusitis occurs, broad-spectrum antibiotic therapy is beneficial. When polyps produce nasal obstruction or anosmia, topical steroid sprays may reduce the size of the polyps and improve the airway. Large obstructive polyps may require oral steroids, intramuscular steroid injections, or injection of steroid suspensions into the polyps. When medical management fails to adequately control the symptoms, surgical intervention is warranted.

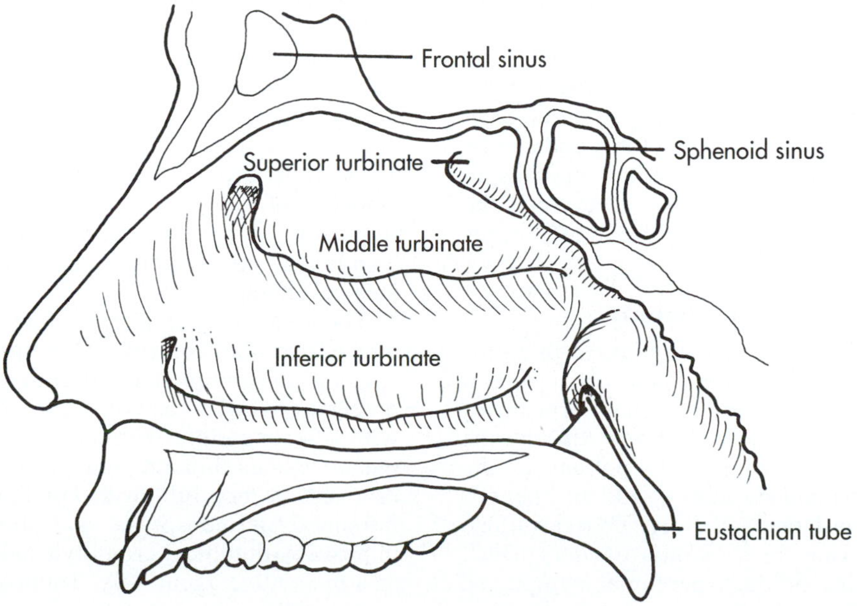


**Fig. 28-6.** View of the lateral nasal wall.

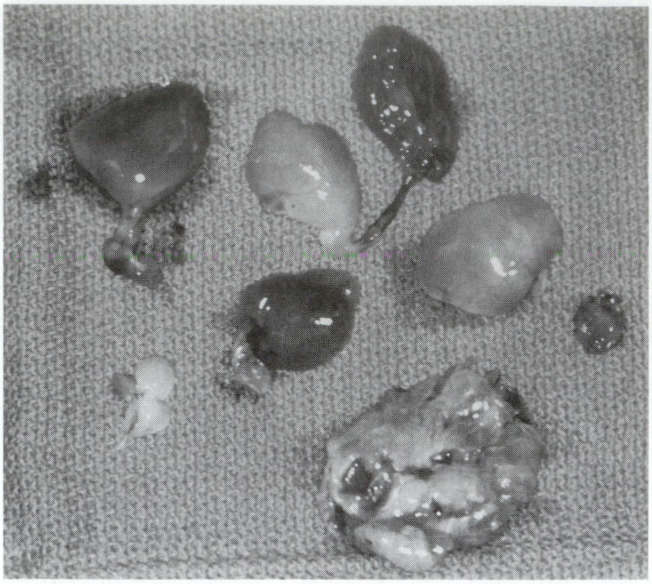

**Fig. 28-7.** Multiple nasal polyps removed from nose and paranasal sinuses.

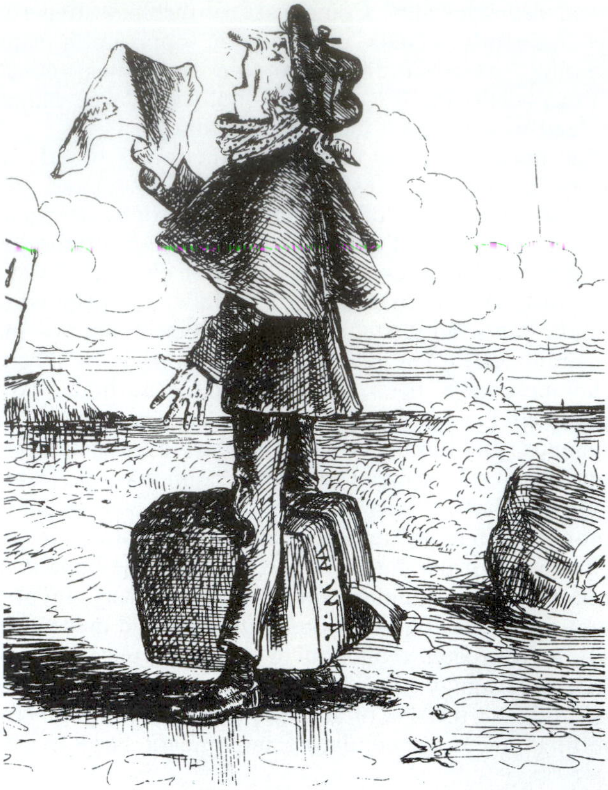

**Fig. 28-8.** Severe pollen allergy as depicted in 1905. (Courtesy Boston Medical Library.)

Nasal polypectomy alone can improve the nasal airway but rarely relieves sinusitis or anosmia, since it fails to open the sinuses, which are the source of polyp growth. Office polypectomy is generally used for diagnosis or for limited or solitary lesions. Sinus surgery with an endoscope or an open approach is used to remove polyps along with enlargement of sinus ostia and removal of the origins of the polyps (Fig. 28-7). This can improve the efficacy of topical steroids and can be beneficial in long-term management of the disorder. Antral choanal polyps are removed by direct visualization of the maxillary sinus through an endoscope or through a Caldwell-Luc approach.

The triad of nasal polyps, asthma, and aspirin sensitivity (Sampters triad) is a particularly difficult combination to treat. Chronic sinusitis from polyp growth and ostial obstruction may cause exacerbation of the asthma. Though surgical intervention is generally not curative, it can be very beneficial for the nasal symptoms and can be helpful in controlling wheezing in selected patients in whom the sinusitis is an exacerbating factor for the asthma. Asthma has been reported to improve after sinus surgery in 40% to 98% of patients.

## Allergic, nonallergic, and vasomotor rhinitis

Allergic rhinitis typically includes symptoms of intermittent nasal obstruction, clear rhinorrhea or postnasal drainage, frequent sneezing, watery eyes, and pruritus of the nose, eyes, and palate (Fig. 28-8). In North America the seasonal allergies are triggered by tree pollens in the spring, grasses in midsummer, and weeds in the fall (typically August 15 until the first frost). Allergies also occur in response to exposure to animal danders. Dust, mite, and mold allergies produce perennial symptoms, with less pruritus and sneezing than seasonal allergies. Dust or mite allergy is worse in the morning from exposure to upholstered furniture, pillows, and mattresses, which have high mite populations. The diagnosis is confirmed with serologic (RAST), epidermal (prick or scratch), or intradermal skin testing. Nasal smears frequently demonstrate an increase in eosinophils in nasal secretions, and serologic testing shows an increase in IgE levels.

Nonallergic rhinitis has symptoms similar to perennial allergic rhinitis but fails to show responses on allergy skin testing. Vasomotor rhinitis is a form of nonallergic rhinitis with exacerbation of symptoms from changes in temperature and humidity, exposure to hot or cold foods, anxiety, or the ingestion of vasoactive substances in foods or drinks. Nonallergic rhinitis with eosinophilia (NARE) is an entity of chronic rhinitis and nasal eosinophilia without evidence of atopy. Nasal polyps have been found more frequently in patients with NARE than in the general population, but symptoms may be more recalcitrant to medical therapy.

The treatment of allergic and nonallergic rhinitis is directed at the control of symptoms. Allergic rhinitis responds to combined oral decongestant and antihistamine preparations, whereas nonallergic rhinitis is better treated with a decongestant without antihistamine. For tenacious mucus, mucus thinners and expectorants such as guafenesin can be helpful. Both conditions may benefit from intranasal steroid sprays, and allergic rhinitis may also improve with topical cromolyn sodium. Cromolyn is used as a preventive agent only. Traditional antihistamines are useful in the primary treatment of allergic rhinitis. When excessive sedation occurs despite use of a reduced dose

**Table 28-1.** Granulomatous diseases affecting the nose

| Disease | Symptoms | Diagnosis | Treatment |
|---|---|---|---|
| Sarcoidosis | Nasal obstruction | 1-3 mm septal nodules, noncaseating granulomas on biopsy | Systemic steroids |
| Wegener granulomatosis | Nasal obstruction, bloody drainage | Septal ulcers and turbinate hypertrophy; vasculitis, acute and chronic inflammation on biopsy; elevated antinuclear cytoplasmic antibody and sedimentation rate | Systemic steroids, cyclophosphamide, methotrexate; oral trimethoprim and sulfamethoxazole |
| Syphilis | Foul smelling drainage and gummatous mass, chondritis, osteitis, saddle nose deformity | Positive FTA-ABS test and VDRL, treponeme on smear | Long course of penicillin |
| Tuberculosis | Beefy red mucosa with ulcerations and exudate, granulomas on septum | Positive PPD, *Myobacterium* spp. on smear, caseating granulomas on biopsy | Isoniazid, rifampin, streptomycin, and ethambutol |
| Rhinoscleroma | Painless submucosal plaques causing airway obstruction | Biopsy and culture grow *Klebsiella* rhinoscleromatous | High dose ampicillin |
| Lethal midline granuloma | Rapidly progressive septal ulceration and perforation | Biopsy similar to lymphoepithelioma | Radiation therapy |
| Leprosy | Red granular ulcers, septal perforations with crusting, bleeding, and atrophic rhinitis | Biopsy and culture show *Mycobacterium leprae* | Dapsone and other sulphone antibiotics, saline and mineral oil sprays for atrophic rhinitis |

*FTA-ABS*, Fluorescent treponemal antibody absorption; *PPD*, purified protein derivative.

(pediatric dosage), the nonsedating antihistamine preparations should be considered.

When medications fail to adequately control allergic rhinitis, hyposensitization can be beneficial in symptom control. While hyposensitization is most effective for seasonal allergic rhinitis, avoidance of causative allergens is important for all patients. Surgical reduction of the turbinates is used only for patients with severe symptoms despite maximal medical therapy.

## MANAGEMENT OF UNCOMMON DISORDERS

### Benign and malignant tumors

These are discussed in Chapter 32.

### Granulomatous disorders

The granulomatous disorders represent systemic diseases with local manifestations. Referral to an otolaryngologist is indicated for nasal symptoms occurring in any patient with a known systemic granulomatous disease. The most common symptoms are persistent nasal obstruction, crusting and bleeding, and secondary sinusitis. Examination may show small nodular areas involving the nasal mucosa, diffuse thickening of the septal and turbinate mucosa, and septal ulceration, granulation tissue, or perforation. The granulomatous diseases that affect the nose, their presenting symptoms, diagnostic criteria, and treatments are listed in Table 28-1.

### Mycotic infections

Mycotic infections are rare, occurring almost exclusively in diabetic or immunocompromised patients in either an invasive or superficial form. The invasive form is a rapidly progressive and destructive infection that causes necrosis of facial soft tissues and the nose. If not contained, infection spreads to the orbit and intracranial cavity, leading to rapid death. Presenting symptoms are severe facial pain, bloody discharge, fever, and facial swelling. A gray or black nonsensate avascular area of nasal mucosa or facial skin is due to fungal vascular invasion with secondary avascular necrosis. Treatment is with aggressive and repeated debridement of avascular tissue along with systemic antifungal agents. *Mucor* and *Aspergillus* are the most common fungi to cause the invasive form.

The superficial form is most likely from aspergillosis but can also be caused by histoplasmosis, blastomycosis, cryptococcosis, rhinosporidiosis, mucormycosis, and sporotrichosis. These infections are most common in hot and humid climates, presenting in an indolent manner or occurring along with chronic bacterial sinusitis due to overgrowth of fungi in retained secretions. Recommended treatment is to surgically open the sinus and remove the infected material. Systemic antifungal treatment is not necessary.

## BIBLIOGRAPHY

Axelsson A, Brorson JE: The correlation between bacteriologic findings in the nose and maxillary sinus in acute maxillary sinusitis, *Laryngoscope* 83:2003, 1973.

Benninger MS: Rhinitis, sinusitis, and their relationship to allergies, *Am J Rhinol* 6(2):37, 1992.

Benninger MS, Mickelson SA, Yaremchuk K: Functional endoscopic sinus surgery: morbidity and early results, *Henry Ford Hosp Med J* 38(1):5, 1990.

English GM: Nasal polypectomy and sinus surgery in patients with asthma and aspirin idiosyncrasy, *Laryngoscope* 96:374, 1986.

Fairbanks DNF: *Pocket guide to antimicrobial therapy in otolaryngology—head and neck surgery,* ed 7, Alexandria, VA, 1993, American Academy of Otolaryngology—Head & Neck Surgery Foundation.

Leopold DA: Physiology of olfaction. In Cummings CW et al, editors: *Otolaryngology—head and neck surgery,* vol 1, ed 2, St Louis, 1993, Mosby.

Rosnagle RS, Yanagisawa E, Smith HW: Specific vessel ligation for epistaxis: survey of 60 cases, *Laryngoscope* 83:517, 1973.

Weiss NS: Relation of high blood pressure to headache, epistaxis, and selected other symptoms: the United States health examination survey of adults, *N Engl J Med* 287(13):632, 1972.

CHAPTER

# 29 Oral Cavity and Salivary Gland Disease

**Vanessa Gayl Schweitzer**

This chapter highlights the most common benign disorders of the oral cavity and salivary glands, concentrating on the cardinal manifestations of the disease processes, the generalist's guide to essential diagnostic tests and procedures, medical/surgical treatments, and indications for hospitalization and consultations with subspecialties.

In general, diseases of the oral cavity and salivary glands may require combined assessment by internal medicine subspecialties (infectious disease, hematology/oncology, rheumatology), as well as dermatology, genetics, dentistry, oral and maxillofacial surgery, and otolaryngology. Clearly, the management of tumors of the head and neck requires prompt referral for diagnosis and treatment planning to the otolaryngologist or head and neck surgical oncologist, in conjunction with evaluation by a head and neck tumor board, to precisely classify the tumor cell type, tumor stage, and treatment modality for a particular neoplasm (e.g., surgery, external beam/interstitial radiation therapy, chemotherapy, immunotherapy, photodynamic therapy). Note that neoplastic oral cavity and salivary gland diseases are discussed in Chapter 32.

## PHYSICAL EXAMINATION

The correct assessment of head and neck problems requires an orderly examination with bright coaxial light (head mirror or fiberoptic headlight), two or more tongue blades, single or double gloves, laryngeal mirrors of different sizes, topical anesthetic (e.g., 10% oral lidocaine, 1% tetracaine oral spray, 14% benzocaine spray), and removal of dentures and dental appliances.

Inspection of the **oral cavity** includes the following structures: buccal and palatal mucosa, anterior tongue, orifices of Stensen's and Wharton's ducts, upper and lower buccogingival sulci, soft palate, anterior and posterior tonsillar pillars, palatine (faucial) and base of tongue (lingual), tonsils, retromolar trigone, floor of mouth, alveolar ridges, and teeth. Note that excessive pressure on the tongue by tongue depressors or forced tongue protrusion can result in gagging and altered tonsil size with a false assessment of tonsil hypertrophy. Anatomically the **oropharynx** comprises the faucial arch (soft palate, uvula, and tonsillar pillars), tonsils, tonsillar fossa, base of tongue, and the posterior pharyngeal wall (to the level of the hyoid bone). Inspection of the three pairs of major salivary glands includes the parotids, the submandibular glands, and the sublingual glands, in conjunction with the cervical region for regional lymph node evaluation.

## ORAL CAVITY

### Normal variations

***Torus palatinus and mandibularis.*** These represent innocuous exostoses that appear as bony, occasionally lobulated, hard growths at the midline of the hard palate **(torus palatinus)** (Fig. 29-2) or on the lingual surface of the lower mandibular alveolus **(torus mandibularis)** (Fig. 29-3). They have been associated with ice chewing. Surgical removal may be necessary for the wearing of dentures and dental appliances, or if the mucosa is chronically traumatized by mechanical or thermal substances. The differential diagnosis for midline soft or firm palatal lesions should include multiple neoplasms such as ectopic pleomorphic adenoma, adenoid cystic carcinoma, and malignant salivary gland tumors, with diagnostic biopsy.

***Ankyloglossia (tongue-tie).*** Ankyloglossia is a short frenulum linguae, which inhibits tongue protrusion.

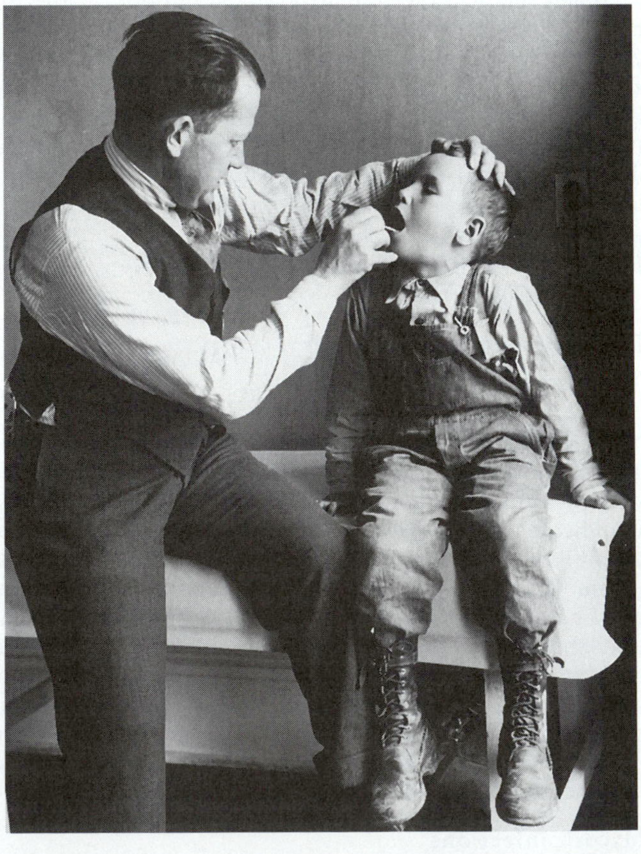

**Fig. 29-1.** Doctor examining boy's throat, Reedsville, West Virginia. (From the Library of Congress.)

Speech defects are rarely attributable to tongue-tie. However, surgical division with or without Z-plasty can be performed for release of the shortened frenulum.

## Mechanical injury

Lesions and abrasions of the oral cavity mucosa are caused by sharp objects. These localized areas of ulceration are frequently surrounded by a white membrane that may become secondarily infected and require treatment. Hyperkeratosis, a thickening of the stratum corneum, accounts for 70% of all white oral lesions (male/female ratio is 2:1), it is most common in the fifth to sixth decades, located in the mandibular mucosa, cheek, and lip. Dentures and self-induced cheek biting are notorious for causing a diffuse, erythematous plaque over the maxillary alveolar ridges along the occlusal plane. Cheek or tongue trauma may follow accidental biting of an anesthetized lower lip or tongue following a regional or local analgesic dental injection. Orthodontic appliances, and more commonly dentures, are also responsible for traumatic oral ulcerations clearly related to appliance location. Chronic trauma can cause a well-defined ulcer with a white keratotic halo.

## Vascular disorders

***Hemangioma.*** Hemangiomas often arise at birth, enlarging with growth until puberty, when spontaneous regression usually occurs. Hemangiomas appear as small, erythematous soft masses usually on the lip, gingiva, or tongue, but may form purplish red plaquelike areas over the buccal mucosa (Fig. 29-4). Steroids and/or sclerosing agents may be injected locally or via angiographic embolization techniques in symptomatic lesions to hasten regression. Surgical removal may be necessary for enlarging hemangiomas causing respiratory obstruction or functional deformity, either via conventional surgical excision or laser surgery (with a $CO_2$, KTP, Nd:YAG, or copper vapor laser).

***Ranula.*** Ranula is a small, painless mucocele on the floor of mouth that forms when the ducts of the sublingual gland or several minor salivary glands become obstructed. Ranula presents as a large, soft, compressible mass, usually blue and occasionally with the profunda vein stretched across the surface. Histologically it demonstrates a thin-walled retention cyst. Occasionally the ranula may penetrate the muscular diaphragm of the floor of the mouth and appear in the neck in a submental region as a plunging ranula. Treatment of the simple ranula is marsupialization. A plunging ranula may require removal by a combined transoral and transcervical approach (Fig. 29-5).

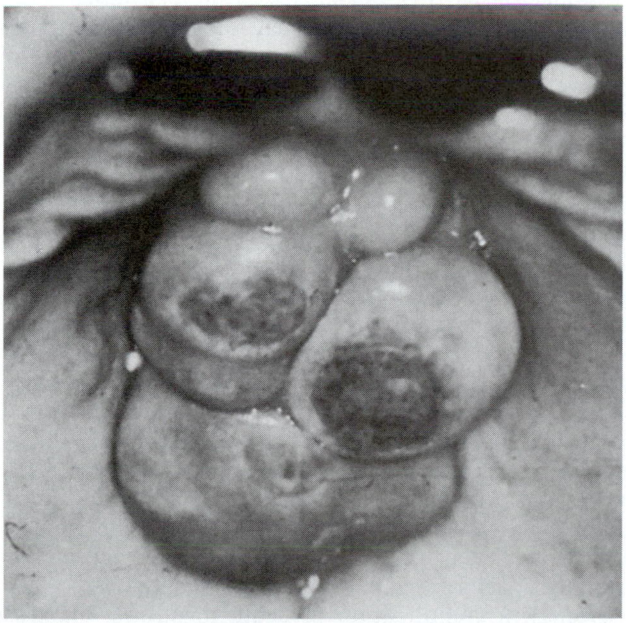

**Fig. 29-2. Torus palatinus.** Bony hard single or lobulated midline swelling that may be traumatized by hot foods or interfere with denture wearing. Differential diagnosis includes fissural cyst, adenoid cystic carcinoma, and ectopic pleomorphic adenoma.

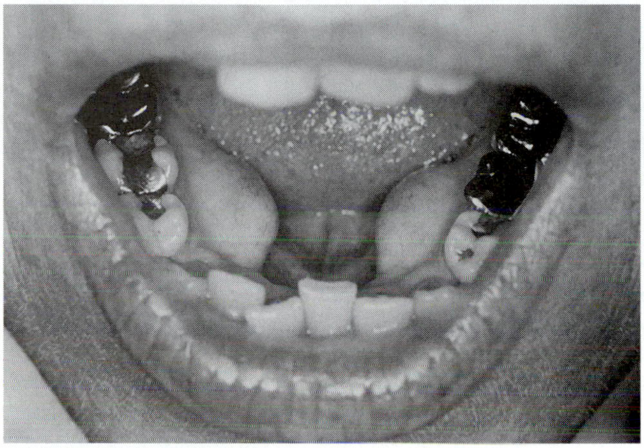

**Fig. 29-3. Torus mandibularis.** Bony hard lobulated swellings rimming the lingual surface of the lower alveolar ridge of the mandible opposite the premolars. Suspected etiology is chronic ice chewing. Less common than torus palatinus.

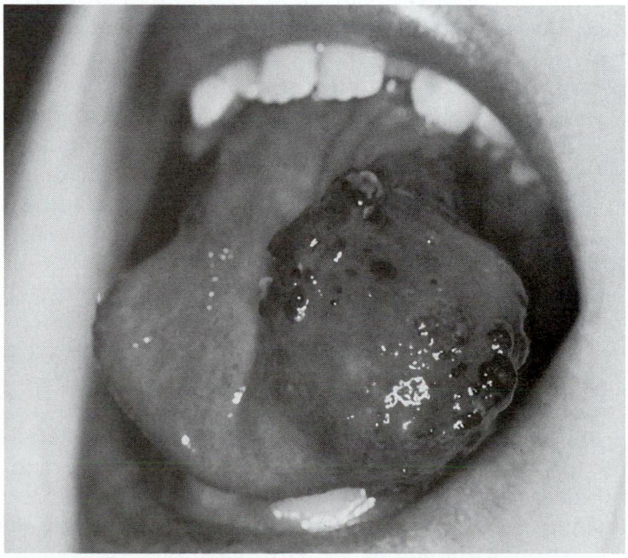

**Fig. 29-4.** Hemangiomas may form purplish to red elevated masses involving the lips, gingiva, and tongue, occasionally contributing to dysphagia, dysarthria, and respiratory obstruction.

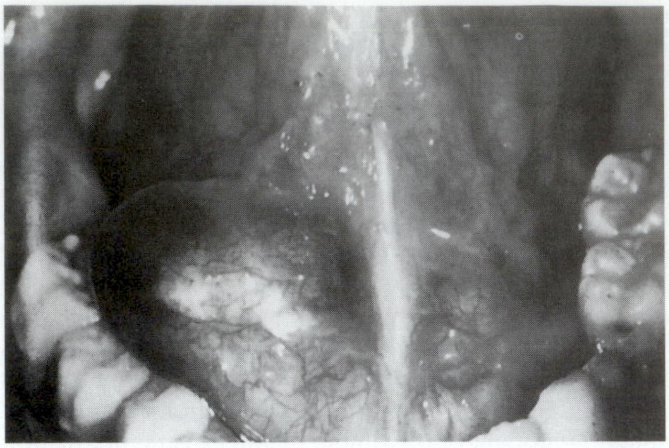

**Fig. 29-5. Ranula.** Mucocele present in the floor of mouth or undersurface of tongue, with occasional extension into the soft tissues of the neck and mouth (plunging ranula).

## Managed Care Guide Tonsillectomy

The *absolute* indications for tonsillectomy include the following:

1. Biopsy for malignancy
2. Recurrent streptococcal infections in a patient with rheumatic fever or febrile convulsions with poor compliance for antibiotic therapy
3. Tonsillar hypertrophy producing respiratory obstruction, dysphagia, or cor pulmonale
4. Diphtheria carrier.

The *relative* indications for tonsillectomy include the following:

1. Recurrent tonsillitis (e.g., three episodes per year for 3 years, or five episodes per year for 2 years, or seven episodes per year)
2. Pyrexia with febrile seizures
3. Cervical lymphadenopathy
4. Tonsillar and pharyngeal exudate
5. Sleep apnea syndrome characterized by snoring or restless sleep with apneic episodes, enuresis, daytime hypersomnolence
6. Peritonsillar abscess
7. Orthodontic complications producing tongue thrust, class II malocclusion with overbite, and midfacial underdevelopment

## Inflammatory diseases

The following are the most common oropharyngeal and deep neck space infections of the head and neck requiring immediate clinical diagnosis and usually medical and/or surgical consultation by a subspecialist.

***Adenotonsillitis/pharyngitis.*** Acute adeno tonsillitis/pharyngitis is characterized by sore throat, dysphagia, odynophagia, pyrexia, and tender anterior cervical tonsillar and digastric lymphadenopathy. Tonsillar appearance demonstrates diffuse or punctate purulent exudate, hypertrophic swelling, occasional halitosis, edema of the palate, and hyperemia of the oropharyngeal mucosa. Severe pain lasting more than a few days (in the absence of cough or hoarseness), fever, marked erythema, pharyngeal exudate, tender cervical lymphadenopathy and recent exposure to streptococcal infection are factors suggesting infection with *Streptococcus pyogenes* (β-hemolytic group A). In high-risk populations both rapid strep tests and conventional throat cultures with vigorous swabbing of tonsil crypts and infected pharynx are recommended to decrease the risk of false negative throat swab analyses. Although *S. pyogenes* is the most important treatable pathogen responsible for acute adenotonsillitis and pharyngitis, culture studies show variability in organisms depending on the patient's age and disease chronicity, including *S. viridans, Staphylococcus aureus, Haemophilus influenzae, Branhamella catarrhalis,* as well as adenovirus and Epstein-Barr viral infections. Differential diagnosis includes diphtheria, scarlet fever, Vincent's angina, infectious mononucleosis, tularemia, cytomegalovirus, toxoplasmosis, pemphigus, and malignancy. The drug of choice for acute adenotonsillitis/pharyngitis is penicillin (or clindamycin for strep eradication in penicillin failures due to β-lactamase–producing organisms). Alternative drug therapies include cefalexin, cefadroxil, and erythromycin, as well as oral sialogogues and oral or topical pain medication. Although the peak for most infections is from 6 months to 4 years of age, a secondary peak occurs in the late teenage and early adult population (see box).

The *absolute* indications for adenoidectomy are adenoid hypertrophy causing respiratory obstruction or cor pulmonale, and recurrent adenoiditis in a patient with rheumatic fever. *Relative* indications for adenoidectomy are adenoid hypertrophy causing eustachian tube obstruction with recurrent otitis media, adenoid hypertrophy causing nasal obstruction or sinusitis, and concomitant adenoidectomy with choanal atresia surgery. In particular, conspicuous persistent **unilateral tonsillar hypertrophy** in the absence of a history of acute inflammation requires bilateral tonsillectomy for a histologic diagnosis of a malignancy, such as lymphosarcoma or lymphoma, versus a chronic inflammatory condition. Of note, (simulated) unilateral tonsillar enlargement is secondary to medial displacement of the tonsil due to a parapharyngeal swelling or mass effect (internal carotid artery aneurysm, deep lobe parotid tumor, chemodectoma, neurofibroma, lymphadenopathy, parapharyngeal space abscess). Referral to an otolaryngologist is indicated, with concomitant contrast computed tomography (CT) or magnetic resonance imaging (MRI) before needle-aspiration biopsy.

Safe antibiotics for the treatment of acute tonsillitis in pregnancy include cephalosporins, erythromycins (except estolate preparations), penicillins, and aztreonam. Drugs considered unsafe or contraindicated for therapy during pregnancy include aminoglycosides, chloramphenicol and sulfonamides near and at term, tetracyclines, erythromycin estolate, clarithromycin, and ciprofloxacin.

*Quinsy,* a complication of acute tonsillitis, manifests symptoms of severe dysphagia, referred otalgia, malaise, fever, tender digastric and cervical lymphadenopathy with acute tonsillitis and medial displacement of the tonsil to the midline due to peritonsillar abscess formation. Quinsy is rare in children, usually unilateral, and more common in patients with recurrent tonsillitis. Treatment requires subspecialty management with needle aspiration or local incision and drainage, culture and sensitivity tests for aerobes and anaerobes, and occasionally intravenous antibiotics and hydration (high-dose penicillin at 24 million U daily) until the acute fever, compromising edema, and severe dysphagia have resolved enough to allow oral antibiotic therapy for a total of 14 days. Elective surgical tonsillectomy should be performed for severe, acute solitary or recurrent peritonsillar abscesses. Bleeding quinsy is a potentially serious sign of the erosion of peritonsillar pus into the tonsillar or internal carotid artery. It requires immediate surgical evaluation. Additional complications of acute tonsillitis include lateral pharyngeal abscess, septicemia, pneumonia, and airway obstruction.

The specialty referral for evaluation of adenotonsillectomy should be with an otolaryngologist. In cases of blood dyscrasias, history of malignant hyperthermia, maxillofacial deformity, congenital cleft palate, or velopharyngeal insufficiency additional evaluation by a hematologist, anesthesiologist, pediatric or adult oral maxillofacial surgeon, and speech therapist may be needed.

### Drug-induced diseases

The following otolaryngologic manifestations of drug-related side effects have been documented:

1. Dilantin produces a gingival hypertrophy that is painless.
2. Tetracycline causes a gray, brown, or yellow staining of the deciduous teeth of a fetus, if consumed by the mother during the last half of pregnancy, and if consumed by the child during the newborn period. Tetracycline should not be given to nursing mothers or children through the age of 8 due to the effects on enamel formation.
3. Several chemotherapeutic agents cause ulceration and necrosis of the oral mucosa, drug-induced mucositis, or secondary leukopenia.
4. Antibiotics may precipitate allergic reactions, such as Stevens-Johnson syndrome and hairy tongue, a black discoloration with or without elongation of the tongue papillae, reflecting an overgrowth of pigment-producing bacteria.

### Metabolic disorders

***Scurvy.*** Vitamin C (ascorbic acid) is required for the maintenance of the intracellular milieu of all mesenchymal cell derivatives. Vitamin C deficiency is characterized by gingivitis and bleeding gums, hemorrhages, skeletal abnormalities, poor wound healing, a proclivity toward infections, and "corkscrew" deformities of body hair.

***Ariboflavinosis.*** Vitamin $B_2$ is necessary for tissue oxygenation. Riboflavin (vitamin $B_2$) deficiency is characterized by atrophic glossitis, angular cheilitis, and gingivostomatitis.

***Pellagra.*** Niacin (vitamin $B_3$) is essential for tissue oxygenation. Deficiency of vitamin $B_3$ is characterized by a red, beefy tongue with occasional ulcerations and patchy loss of papillae.

***Iron deficiency.*** The classic manifestations of iron-deficiency anemia include a smooth and red tongue with loss of the papillae, angular cheilosis, and ashen-gray oral mucosa (Plummer-Vinson syndrome).

***Hypothyroidism.*** Hypothyroidism in the neonatal period causes cretinism with characteristic macroglossia. Hypothyroidism in adolescence may also cause altered bone maturation and subsequent malocclusion.

***Acromegaly.*** Acromegaly, secondary to increased growth hormone production, is characterized by macroglossia and wide spacing of the teeth.

***Diabetes mellitus.*** Diabetes mellitus is characterized by an increased propensity to oral mucosal infections by opportunistic organisms, such as *Candida albicans.* Oral manifestations are thrush, periapical and periodontal inflammation, and caries.

***Amyloidosis.*** The prominent oral feature of amyloidosis is macroglossia with yellow nodules apparent along the lateral and dorsal surfaces of the tongue and gingiva. The primary form is idiopathic; the secondary variety may be in association with other disease processes, such as tuberculosis, leprosy, syphilis, multiple myeloma, and macroglobulinemia. Histologically amyloidosis demonstrates positive metachromatic crystal violet staining and green birefringence with Congo red staining of amyloid tissue deposits.

***Pernicious anemia.*** Vitamin $B_{12}$ deficiency is characterized by a shiny smooth and red tongue, pale yellow-gray oral mucosa and lips, loss of the tongue papillae, and increased susceptibility to oral ulcerations (Möller-Hunter glossitis).

***Menopause.*** Oral manifestations of menopause are typically diffuse gingivostomatitis (dry, burning sensation), diffuse erythema, shininess, senile atrophy of mucosa, and occasional fissuring in the mucobuccal fold.

### Hematologic disorders

***Plummer-Vinson (Patterson-Kelly) syndrome.*** Plummer-Vinson syndrome is characterized by an iron-deficiency hypochromic anemia with acute atrophic glossitis, angular cheilitis, spoon nails, esophageal webbing, and a propensity to carcinomas of the postcricoid region, most commonly in women.

***Polycythemia vera.*** Polycythemia vera is a malignant involvement of bone marrow or hypoxemia characterized by a reddish purple discoloration of the tongue, purplish tinged mucosa, with easy traumatization of the oral mucosa.

***Thalassemia.*** Mediterranean thalassemia demonstrates pallor and cyanosis of the oral mucosa.

***Sickle cell anemia.*** Patients with sickle cell anemia manifest a stepladder alignment of the trabeculae of the interdental septum and a pale yellow discoloration of the oral mucosa.

*Severe leukopenia.* Severe leukopenia, a condition commonly following administration of chemotherapeutic drugs, is characterized by necrotic sloughing of the oral mucosa with underlying ulceration in the absence of any inflammatory response.

*Acute leukemia.* The first manifestations of acute leukemia are often hyperplastic gingivitis, with ulceration, hemorrhages, and occasional necrosis of the gingiva.

### Pigmentation changes of the oral cavity

Systemic disease processes as well as chemical toxicities may manifest as pigmentary changes of the skin, nail beds, and oral mucosa. The following pigmentary changes have been clearly described:

1. Melanosis (physiologic pigmentation)
2. Peutz-Jeghers syndrome—brown (melanin)
3. Bismuth toxicity—black
4. Arsenic toxicity—black
5. Lead poisoning—blue-gray
6. Mercury poisoning—gray or violet
7. Silver poisoning—violet, blue, or gray
8. Addison's disease—brown
9. Hemochromatosis—bronze
10. Xanthomatous diseases—yellow to gray

### Mucocutaneous disorders

*Recurrent aphthous stomatitis (RAS).* Recurrent aphthous stomatitis (RAS) is a common entity of unknown etiology affecting 20% to 50% of the general population, characterized by recurring aphthous ulcers, typically starting in childhood or adolescence. The ulcer typically is small, round, or ovoid with a circumscribed margin, erythematous halo, and a yellow or gray floor, lasting from 1 to 4 weeks before healing. The macules are usually preceded by a prodrome of burning or pain, commonly occur in crops of one or more, and usually are found on the tongue and buccal mucosa. Positive family history is found in one third of patients with an increased frequency of HLA-A2, A11, B12, and DR2, supporting a genetic basis for susceptibility. A minority (10% to 20%) of patients with RAS have an underlying low serum iron or ferritin level, a deficiency of folate, or vitamin $B_{12}$; 3% of RAS patients have celiac disease. Other predisposing factors include stress and trauma, cessation of smoking, menses, and food allergy. There is no evidence that RAS is a classic autoimmune disease. About 20% of the population complain of occasional aphthae, with a higher prevalence in the higher socioeconomic classes, and a tendency for resolution with increasing age. The three main clinical types of RAS are minor aphthous ulcers (80%), major aphthous ulcers (10%), and herpetiform ulcers (10%).

Minor aphthous (Mikulicz's) ulcers are usually 2 to 4 mm in diameter and are found mainly on the nonkeratinized mobile mucosa of the lips, cheeks, floor of mouth, sulci, and ventrum of the tongue; they are uncommon on the gingiva, palate, or dorsum of the tongue. Usually one to six ulcers appear at a time, healing within 7 to 10 days and recurring at variable intervals. Minor ulcers are usually round or ovoid but are often more linear when in the buccal sulcus, a common site. The ulcer is usually yellowish but becomes grayish as epithelialization proceeds and at the same time pain abates. The ulcers heal with little or no evidence of scarring and occur mainly in the 10- to 40-year age group.

Major aphthous (Sutton's) ulcers, previously known as periadenitis mucosa necrotica recurrans, have an age of onset in childhood or adolescence. They are larger than Mikulicz's ulcers, often more than 1 cm in diameter, lasting up to a month in duration, and more frequently recur, with a propensity for the anterior tonsillar pillar. They form on any area of the oral cavity, including the dorsum of the tongue and palate. Major ulcerations are extremely painful, round or ovoid with inflammatory halo, and may heal with scarring.

Herpetiform ulceration (HU) has an age of onset in young adulthood and is extremely painful, usually tiny but coalescent. HU begins with vesiculation and passes rapidly into multiple, minute, pinhead-sized discrete ulcers at any oral site. They increase in size and coalesce to leave large ragged ulcers that heal in 10 days or longer. HU is found in the slightly older adult female population. There is no evidence of involvement of herpes simplex virus.

The treatment for recurrent aphthous stomatitis, in addition to correction of underlying predisposing factors such as vitamin deficiencies, includes (1) oral saline mouthbaths and 0.2% aqueous chlorhexadine gluconate mouthwash, (2) topical tetracycline mouthwash, (3) topical corticosteroids (hydrocortisone pellets or triamcinolone acetonide in carboxymethylcellulose), and (4) systemic corticosteroids or immunosuppressants for HU.

*Erythema multiforme.* Erythema multiforme is a mucocutaneous syndrome characterized by oral and genital ulcerations in conjunction with target skin lesions (see Chapter 21). The lesions are described as bullae surrounded by an area of edema, which itself is surrounded by inflammation. The oral bullae frequently burst early, resulting in an area of ulceration surrounded by edema and inflammation. Typically, the labial mucosa is covered by a serosanguineous exudate that leads to virtually pathognomonic bloody crusting and swollen lips. The mucosal lesions begin as erythematous areas, which vesiculate and form bullae that break down to irregular, large painful erosions with extensive surrounding erythema with or without associated skin lesions. Diagnosis is usually clinical, although biopsy may be required. Immunostaining of oral mucosal lesions demonstrates a pattern of immunofluorescence in the vessel walls of the lamina propria.

Erythema multiforme is a condition that may be caused by immune diseases such as systemic lupus erythematosus, infections (herpes simplex or mycoplasma), or drugs (penicillin, barbiturates, or salicylates). Stevens-Johnson syndrome is a virulent hemorrhagic variety of erythema multiforme, typically occurring in children, with a mortality of 5% to 15%. Treatment is supportive with oral hygiene and in severe cases systemic corticosteroids, levamisole, or azathioprine.

*Pemphigus.* Pemphigus is an oculomucocutaneous syndrome characterized in the most severe form, pemphigus vulgaris, by flaccid bullous lesions throughout the oral cavity, especially the buccal mucosa, palate, and gingiva. Serrated, defined, bright red erosions with gray-white remnants of ruptured blebs are produced. Patients typically present with multiple large painful irregular and persistent erosions that must be differentiated clinically from other erosive lesions such as pemphigoid and superficial mucoceles. Histologically the bullae are intraepithelial, manifesting epithelial intercellular antibody on direct and indirect immunofluorescent staining. Pemphigus bullae manifest the Nikolsky sign (i.e., firm pressure on top of the intact bullae results in extension of the edges). Generalized systemic toxicity accompanies the oral cutaneous lesions in 80% of patients, ultimately ending in death if left untreated. In pemphigus vegetans the bullae are succeeded by verrucous granulations, particularly on the oral commissure, and hyperplastic masses on the tongue may give rise to a cerebriform appearance. Treatment of pemphigus includes steroids and antimetabolites (dapsone).

***Pemphigoid.*** Bullous pemphigoid is an oculomucocutaneous syndrome in which the oral lesions are rarely seen. Mucous membrane pemphigoid involves the oral cavity in one third of cases, but the vesicular lesions develop much more slowly than with pemphigus. Tumorous membrane pemphigoid produces a desquamative gingivitis. The bullae are subepidermal, with absence of acantholysis, and are more tense (i.e., rupture less easily) than in pemphigoid. Linear deposits of IgG and complement 3 at the epithelial basement membrane zone on immunofluorescent staining of oral biopsy specimens are typical. Circulating basement membrane antibodies are not present.

Immunostaining of oral mucosal vesiculobullous disorders with direct and indirect immunofluorescence of biopsy specimens, indirect immunofluorescence of serology, evaluation of oral mucosal deposits for immunoglobulins and complement pattern of immunofluorescence, and the presence of autoantibodies may help differentiate the following disorders: pemphigus, mucous membrane pemphigoid, bullous pemphigoid, dermatitis herpetiformis, linear IgA disease, erythema multiforme, lichen planus, discoid lupus erythematosus, angina bullosae hemorrhagica, and superficial mucoceles.

### Miscellaneous disorders

***Chronic pharyngitis.*** Chronic pharyngitis is generalized hyperemia of the pharyngeal mucous membrane with an orange to red discoloration of lymphoid tissue on the posterior oropharyngeal wall. A persistent feeling of scratchy throat is secondary to several factors, including nicotine exposure, postnasal drainage, allergy, occupational and environmental inhalants, use of tartar control toothpaste or irritating mouthwashes, and chronic mouth breathing.

This is a common syndrome in primary care practice. Treatment is focused on relieving potential causative factors, saline gargles, and reassurance.

***Geographic tongue (glossitis migricans).*** Geographic tongue is a benign glossitis characterized by loss of the filiform (non–taste bud) papillae in a circumscribed fashion, occurring with varying duration. Vitamin B complex may be effective; however, reassurance is the most basic treatment.

***Angioneurotic edema.*** Angioneurotic edema is an inflammatory condition characterized by extravasation of colloid into the soft tissues with formation of mucosal edema and bullae. Typically involving the lips, oral mucosa, and tongue, the process may extend into the larynx and trachea and cause respiratory insufficiency (Fig. 29-6). Agents associated with angioneurotic edema include certain foods (shellfish), antibiotics (penicillin), antihypertensive drugs (ACE inhibitors: captopril, lisinopril, enalapril, fosinopril sodium, benazepril hydrochloride), and insect bites.

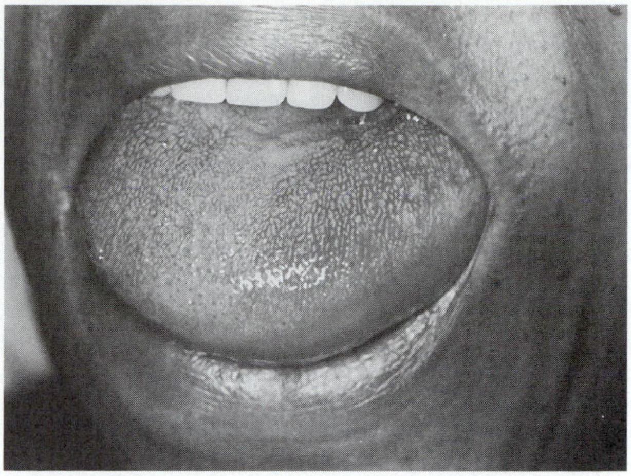

**Fig. 29-6.** Angioneurotic edema following antihypertensive drug therapy with ACE inhibitors may produce diffuse mucosal edema involving the lips, tongue, and oral mucosa.

***Macroglossia.*** Macroglossia, or large tongue, is associated with a variety of conditions including hemangioma, myxedema, acromegaly, amyloidosis, Pierre Robin syndrome, tertiary syphilis, von Gierke's disease, actinomycosis, and Down syndrome.

***Black hairy tongue.*** Black hairy tongue is usually a harmless, black-brown staining with hypertrophy of the filiform papillae, possibly caused by tobacco use, fungi *(Aspergillus niger),* or prolonged antibiotic therapy. Treatment includes scraping and toothbrush cleansing with a baking soda–based toothpaste and Peridex or hydrogen peroxide mouthwash.

### Benign oral conditions associated with distant malignancy

***Acanthosis nigricans.*** Acanthosis nigricans is characterized by wartlike eruptions on the tongue, lips, and buccal mucosa, with brown-black epidermal hyperplasia of the skin and thickened perlèche of the angles of the mouth.

***Oral pigmentation.*** Pigmentation of the oral mucosa is normal in dark skinned populations, but in whites, diffuse light brown oral pigmentation is associated with ectopic adrenocorticotropic hormone production. Biopsy can differentiate a black or bluish black mucosal pigmentation from a benign dental amalgam tattoo.

### Precancerous conditions

***Leukoplakia with dyskeratosis.*** Leukoplakia is a clinical morphologic term for a white patch. The histologic description is dyskeratosis, which is an abnormal orientation in development of epithelial cells with hyperchromatism, altered polarity, increase in nuclear size, and prominence of the nucleoli. There is a tendency for malignant transformation in 4% to 6% of leukoplakia cases and 13% of dysplasia cases. Leukoplakia reportedly accounts for approximately 13% of all white patch lesions, which are usually found in men (male/female ratio is 3:2), and is most common in the fifth to sixth decades; 80% of patients are smokers and 30% have histories of alcohol abuse. The most commonly affected sites are the cheeks, lips, and lower gingiva (see Chapter 32 for Managed Care Guide for oral cancer screening). Tendency for malignant transformation is most common along the floor of mouth, lips, and tongue. Chronic nicotine, betel nut, snuff, oral tobacco, and alcohol use predisposes one to malignant transformation and possible diffuse field cancerization of the mucosa of the oral cavity. Biopsy is mandatory for confirmation of malignant transformation. Analysis for tumor cell markers may be helpful in the genetically predisposed population of patients at risk for multiple upper aerodigestive tract malignancies.

***Erythroplakia.*** Erythroplakia is a descriptive clinical term for a velvety, red mucosal plaque. The lesion may become carcinoma in situ or frank invasive carcinoma and therefore should be referred to an otolaryngologist for biopsy.

***Candidiasis.*** *Candida albicans,* an oral commensal fungus, resides on the posterior dorsum of the tongue. Infections are usually the result of xerostomia, local disturbances in salivary flora due to broad-spectrum antibiotics, pregnancy, diabetes, immunosuppression, AIDS, malnutrition, or underlying malignancy. There are several types of intraoral candidiasis, each with different signs, age of predilection, and predisposing factors. Thrush, or acute pseudomembranous candidiasis, produces soft creamy patches resembling mild curds, which are easily wiped away with gauze, leaving areas of erythema. Thrush is present in both healthy neonates and adults, as well as in patients with xerostomia, chronic antibiotic or corticosteroid use, and T cell immunosuppression. Chronic mucocutaneous candidiasis syndromes are rare; several are familial, associated with autoimmune defects such as hypoparathyroidism and hypoadrenocorticism, and present in the first decade of life. Chronic oral candidiasis produces tough, adherent white patches with a premalignant potential, indistinguishable from clinical leukoplakia except by biopsy. Denture-induced chronic atrophic candidiasis occurs usually beneath the complete upper denture, commonly in the middle aged or elderly, and is characterized by erythema limited to the denture-bearing area and stomatitis predisposing to angular cheilitis. Median rhomboid glossitis (central papillary atrophy of the tongue) produces a nonmalignant red, depapillated rhomboidal area in the center of the dorsum of the tongue, anterior to the sulcus terminalis. It is commonly associated with candidiasis, smoking, and denture wearing. Histologically it shows irregular, pseudoepitheliomatous epithelial hyperplasia.

Diagnosis of *Candida albicans* is by periodic acid–Schiff (PAS) purple staining of blastophores and pseudohyphae. Biopsy is indicated for suspected leukoplakia. Treatment consists of topical antifungals (nystatin or mycostatin mouthwash, suppositories, oral pellets), systemic antifungals (ketoconazole, flucytosine, and fluconazole), and denture cleaning. Barium swallow and/or flexible esophagoscopy may be necessary for suspected esophageal candidiasis.

Also see Chapter 68 for specific manifestations of HIV infection.

### Benign tumors

In general, all oral cavity lesions should be documented clinically by size and descriptive appearance in conjunction with photographic documentation if available with referral to a surgical subspecialist for definitive biopsy and excision.

***Fibroma.*** Fibroma is a circumscribed, firm, smooth, painless mesenchymal lesion, variable in size and either pedunculated or sessile. It contains dense connective tissue with a normal epithelial covering.

***Neurofibroma.*** A single neurofibroma is a hamartoma, usually firm and pedunculated, found anywhere in the oral cavity but with a predilection for the tongue and palate. von Recklinghausen's disease is an autosomal dominant neurocutaneous disorder characterized by multiple neurofibromas, particularly on the tongue, gingiva, and labial mucosa. Neurofibromas in facial soft tissues interfere with lip excursion, mastication, and the nasal airway.

## SALIVARY GLANDS

An outline of nonneoplastic salivary gland disorders is shown in the box at right.

### Diseases

***Sialoadenitis.*** Acute sialoadenitis refers to acute inflammation of a salivary gland that causes erythema, pain, tenderness, swelling, and purulent discharge from the affected duct, presumably due to stasis of the saliva with increased viscosity, allowing for the growth of pathogens, particularly *Staphylococcus aureus* and other gram-positive bacteria, as well as *Pseudomonas, Enterobacter, Klebsiella, Enterococci, Proteus,* and *Candida* species. Predisposing conditions include dehydration and debilitation, trauma, radiation therapy, and chemotherapy. If untreated, increasing induration and pitting of the skin with involvement of the masseteric and submandibular spacial planes may require salivary gland incision and drainage. Treatment consists of rehydration, warm compresses, oral cavity irrigations, sialogogues, and treatment with antistaphylococcal antibiotics. The initial drug of choice for treatment of acute suppurative parotitis or sialoadenitis is amoxicillin plus clavulinic acid with alternative choices including clindamycin, cefoxitin, vancomycin plus metronidazole, and antistaphylococcal penicillins for a minimal duration of 10 days or until the entire acute process has resolved.

Chronic recurrent sialoadenitis is characterized by recurrent, painful enlargement of the gland, usually aggravated by eating and caused by decreased salivary flow, stasis, and alteration in salivary composition. Treatment consists of usually conservative measures (sialogogues, heat and massage, hydration, antibiotic treatment if needed), with sialadenectomy reserved for refractory cases.

***Parotid abscess.*** Parotid abscess is the progression of the acute parotitis into a stage of suppuration with multiloculated areas of pustulence associated with pitting edema of the skin and occasionally trismus. Treatment is the same as for acute parotitis with hospitalization, a surgical incision (located parallel to the facial nerve) and drainage procedure, and intravenous antibiotics.

***Viral parotitis (mumps).*** Viral parotitis, a common viral infection of children between the ages of 4 and 10 years, has an incubation period of 14 to 21 days and a duration of 7 to 10 days characterized by unilateral or bilateral painful swelling of the parotid glands, malaise, and trismus, with other occasional systemic symptoms of orchitis, pancreatitis, encephalitis, meningitis, and cochleitis. Diagnosis is confirmed by measuring antibodies to the S and V mumps antigen (greater than 1:192 is diagnostic). The condition is self-limiting.

***Recurrent parotitis.*** Recurrent parotitis is the result of congenital or acquired sialectasias or at times may be attributed to calculi or strictures (ductal and stomal). Dilatation of the salivary ducts with stasis of secretions in the absence of infections results in recurrent parotitis. Treatment is conservative and usually effective, with surgery reserved for symptomatic patients that fail to respond to medical treatment.

***Sialolithiasis.*** Sialolithiasis primarily affects the submandibular glands (80% of cases) with calculi often composed of hydroxyapatite. Calculi develop more commonly in the Wharton duct because the saliva produced by the submandibular gland is more viscid than that of other glands. Radiopaque stones develop in 40% of cases, most frequently among men of middle age. Symptoms are characterized by fluctuating pain and swelling that are worse at mealtime. Stones occasionally can be removed transorally provided that they are easily palpable within the mouth and if they lie within 1 to 2 cm of the orifice. Punctum dilators are used to dilate the duct after the mucosa is anesthetized and a stitch is placed distal to the stone to prevent its displacement posteriorly by the probe. The danger of transoral removal of a posteriorly situated stone is inadvertent injury to the lingual nerve. Stones positioned close to the hilum of the gland are best removed via an open transcervical approach.

Sialosis refers to bilateral recurrent salivary gland swelling characterized histologically by acinar cell hypertrophy, striated duct atrophy, and interstitial edema. Several causes have been identified including nutritional disorders (vitamin deficiency, malnutrition, bulimia), endocrine (diabetes, hypothyroidism), metabolic disorders (obesity, malabsorption, cirrhosis, anemia), inflammatory disorders (Sjögren's syndrome), and drugs (thiourea). Treatment involves avoiding the causative factors if possible.

***Ptyalism.*** Ptyalism, or hypersalivation, is caused by a number of inflammatory, endocrine, neuropsychiatric, and

### Nonneoplastic salivary gland disorders

**Inflammatory diseases**

***Acute***

- Mumps
- Acute suppurative sialoadenitis
- Allergy
- Drug induced
  - Iodine
  - Mercury
  - Bismuth
  - Arsenic
  - Starch

***Chronic***

*Obstructive*

- Calculi
- Stricture—ductal and stomal (cheek biting)
- Sialoadenitis
- Sialectasia

*Nonobstructive*

- Postmumps sialoadenitis (sialectasia, childhood, and adulthood)
- Nonspecific sialoadenitis
- Specific sialoadenitis (tuberculosis, actinomycosis)
- Benign lymphoepithelial disease (sialectasias)
- Allergy
- Drug related (mercury, iron, copper, thiourea)
- Autoimmune (Sjögren's syndrome)

**Metabolic and endocrine diseases**

- Benign hypertrophy
  - Hypothyroidism
  - Diabetes
  - Alcoholism and cirrhosis
  - Endocrinopathies
- Benign atrophy
  - Fatty (replacement)
  - Fibrous (replacement)
- Menopausal hypertrophy
- Nutritional
  - Vitamin deficiency
  - Malnutrition hypertrophy
  - Bulimia hypertrophy
- Gouty parotitis

**Trauma (internal or external)**

- Contusion
- Laceration
- Penetrating
- Pneumoperitonitis

**Congenital diseases**

- Dermoid cysts
- First cleft
  - Type 1
  - Type 2
- Branchial pouch

**Cysts (acquired)**

- Obstructive (stricture, calculus)
- Traumatic
- Glassblower's
- Parasitic
- Infectious (HIV)

drug-related conditions. Ptyalism is best managed by the elimination of the underlying condition with surgical treatment to either eliminate or divert saliva flow. Elimination of saliva can be achieved by bilateral divisions of the chorda tympani and Jacobson nerves via an endaural tympanotomy approach, but this is seldom long-term. Alernatively, sialadenectomy or ductal ligation eliminates saliva production but only from the resected gland. Salivary diversion may be accomplished by bilateral transposition of Wharton's or Stensen's ducts into the tonsillar fossa and is effective for children with cerebral palsy.

Causes of hypersalivation include inflammatory conditions (stomatitis, rabies), endocrinopathies (pregnancy, Graves' disease), neuropsychiatric disorders (epilepsy, cerebral palsy, hysteria), and drugs (mercury, iodine, pilocarpine).

***Xerostomia.*** Xerostomia, or dry mouth, is caused by several local and systemic diseases producing a distressing sensation of diminished taste, difficulty with deglutition, burning sensation, and the promotion of dental caries. Treatment involves managing the underlying condition and supplying the patient with artificial saliva. Guafenesin is occasionally helpful in decreasing salivary viscosity. Differential diagnosis of xerostomia includes local causes (irradiation, chronic sialoadenitis, surgical interruption of the chorda tympani nerve, sialadenectomy), and systemic causes (Sjögren's syndrome, Mikulicz's disease, sarcoidosis, lymphoma, dehydration, debilitation, menopause, mental stress, opiate derivatives, anticholinergics, nicotine, atropine, acute and chronic renal failure, infection, graft-versus-host rejection, and anemia).

***Sjögren's syndrome.*** Sjögren's syndrome is an autoimmune disorder characterized by keratoconjunctivitis sicca, xerostomia, abnormal taste, intermittent unilateral or bilateral salivary gland enlargement, and a dry tongue with atrophy of the papillae. It is also associated with connective tissue disorders such as rheumatoid arthritis, systemic lupus erythematosus, and polyarteritis nodosa and most commonly occurs in menopausal women. About 10% of patients go on to develop pseudolymphoma and rarely Waldenström's macroglobulinemia. Diagnosis of Sjögren's syndrome is confirmed by minor salivary gland biopsy of the lip, nasal septum, or hard palate in conjunction with laboratory testing (rheumatoid factor, antinuclear factor, protein electrophoresis, autoantibodies). Histopathologic findings demonstrate lymphocytic infiltrates, acinar atrophy, and ductal epithelial hyperplasia and metaplasia. Treatment is supportive for the xerostomia and xerophthalmos.

### Benign tumors

The most common benign tumors of the salivary glands are pleomorphic adenoma, monomorphic adenoma, Warthin's tumor, and oncocytoma (Table 29-1 and the box at right). In general, the diagnosis and therapeutic management of benign tumors warrant otolaryngologic intervention. The minimal diagnostic and therapeutic procedure for benign parotid tumors is superficial parotidectomy with preservation of the facial nerve.

**Classification of epithelial salivary gland tumors according to Batsakis**

Mixed tumor (pleomorphic adenoma)
Papillary cystadenolymphoma (Warthin's tumor)
Oncocytosis—oncocytoma
Monomorphic adenomas
  Basal cell adenoma
  Glycogen-rich adenoma and clear cell adenoma
  Others
Sebaceous adenoma
Sebaceous lymphadenoma
Papillary ductal adenoma
Benign lymphoepithelial lesion

**Table 29-1.** Histologic classification of salivary tumors

| Tumor | Incidence (%) |
|---|---|
| **Benign** | |
| Pleomorphic adenoma | 46 |
| Warthin's tumor | 6.6 |
| Oncocytoma | 0.7 |
| Monomorphic adenoma | 0.2 |
| **Malignant** | |
| Mucoepidermoid adenoma | 16 |
| Adenoid cystic carcinoma | 10 |
| Adenocarcinoma | 8 |
| Malignant mixed tumor | 6 |
| Acinic cell carcinoma | 3 |
| Squamous cell carcinoma | 2 |
| Others | 1.5 |
| TOTAL | 100 |

From Lee KJ, editor: *Textbook of otolaryngology—head and neck surgery,* Norwalk, CT, 1989, Appleton and Lange.

## BIBLIOGRAPHY

Batsakis JD: *Tumors of head and neck,* ed 2, Baltimore, 1979, Williams & Wilkins.
Becker W, editor: *Atlas of ear, nose and throat diseases,* Philadelphia, 1984, WB Saunders.
Bull TR, editor: *Color atlas of ENT diagnosis,* ed 2, London, 1987, Wolfe Medical Publications.
Cummings CC, editor: *Otolaryngology—head and neck surgery,* vol 2, ed 2, St Louis, 1993, Mosby.
English GM: *Otolaryngology,* vols 3-5, Philadelphia, 1993, JB Lippincott.
Fairbanks DNF: *Pocket guide to antimicrobial therapy in otolaryngology—head and neck surgery,* ed 6, Alexandria, Va, 1991, American Academy of Otolaryngology—Head and Neck Surgery Foundations.
Johns ME, Harris AE: *Salivary gland tumors: therapy based on clinical pathologic diagnoses,* Washington, DC, 1985, American Academy of Otolaryngology—Head and Neck Surgery Foundations.
Lee KJ, editor: *Textbook of otolaryngology—head and neck surgery,* New York, 1989, Elsevier.

Levin LS, Johns ME: Lesions of the oral mucous membranes, *Otolaryngol Clin North Am* 19:87, 1986.
Lynch MA, Brightmore VJ, Greenberg MS: *Burkett's oral medicine: diagnosis and treatment,* ed 8, Philadelphia, 1984, JB Lippincott.
Pindborg JJ: *Atlas of diseases of the oral mucosa,* Philadelphia, 1980, WB Saunders.

CHAPTER

# 30 The Larynx and Upper Airway

Michael S. Benninger

The larynx is at the crossroads of the respiratory and digestive tracts. Phylogenetically, its primary function is to protect the lungs from aspiration. A secondary function is for respiration and the most recent function is the development of voice. Many disorders of the larynx and surrounding structures can interfere with airway patency, swallowing, or satisfactory voice production.

## IMPLICATIONS OF ANATOMY AND PHYSIOLOGY WITH VOICE PATHOLOGY

Certain pathologic voice processes can alter pitch, loudness, and breathiness. Anything that increases the mass of the vocal fold tends to decrease pitch. This effect can be seen in the masculinization of the voice, as occurs in women smokers; edema of the vocal folds from vocal overuse; or mucopolysaccharide accumulation in masculinization, which occurs in hypothyroidism. Similarly, vocal nodules, polyps, or tumors tend to cause decreased pitch and increase breathiness as the vocal folds are not allowed to come together. Hyperfunctional voice disorders, in which the vocal folds tend to be tensed at a level greater than would occur with normal speaking or singing, result in a higher pitch. Chronic pulmonary disease, which tends to not provide for adequate subglottic pressure, tends to result in lowering of the voice. The small larynges of a boy have the characteristics of a girl and, therefore, his pitch would tend to be in the same range, which accounts for the lovely soprano voices of the boy choirs. As the mass of the vocal folds increase, both due to size and hormonal changes, masculinization occurs.

## HISTORY

The focus of the history of diseases of the upper airway depends largely on the age of the patient. Because airway dysfunction in small children is often due to developmental causes such as laryngomalacia, congenital disorders, or anatomic abnormalities, the history is more directed at difficulties with breathing or feeding. A patient in middle childhood tends to have fewer problems with airway or eating; rather, more problems may be associated with voice quality or development. Vocal nodules account for a majority of voice problems in these age groups. Tonsil and adenoid hypertrophy not only cause chronic upper airway obstruction or may be associated with recurrent infections, they may also result in changes in resonance. Voice problems in an older adult smoker may precipitate a concern about a laryngeal carcinoma.

A thorough history should include an assessment of the time of onset of the problem, whether it is progressive, what types of behaviors improve or worsen the disorder, and whether the patient had previous treatment with or without success. Voice dysfunction of long duration without progression is less alarming than a recent rapidly progressive problem. It should be determined whether the problem is worse in the morning (which might suggest gastroesophageal reflux) or worse at night (which may suggest vocal overuse). Symptoms of cough might result in a thorough pulmonary evaluation, whereas hemoptysis might lead to a quick referral to an otolaryngologist to rule out laryngeal cancer. A complete medical history is needed because dysfunctions of the cardiopulmonary, digestive, endocrine, neurologic, and musculoskeletal systems can result in airway and voice disorders.

Once a worrisome process has been ruled out, the most important factor guiding treatment of voice disorders is the patient's need and desire to initiate treatment for voice improvement. Voice dysfunction in a 75-year-old retired sedentary individual would likely require much less aggressive management than in a 35-year-old singer or radio broadcaster.

### Laryngeal voice evaluation

The simplest way to evaluate laryngeal function is by listening. From the baby's cry to the final sigh of life, the voice portrays human emotion, thought, and creativity. A trained listener will find that many laryngeal disorders can be suspected by listening carefully to the quality of voice. Although the "hot potato" voice of a child with epiglottitis is well recognized by most pediatricians and family practitioners, subtle alterations in cry are rarely used in assessment of a neonate, infant, or small child. Most textbooks of pediatric medicine fail to describe how changes in cry and voice may be the signs of disease. In adults, careful assessment by listening to the voice, often while obtaining a history, can give major clues to the pathologic processes. A high-pitched voice in comparison to others of the same sex and age is suggestive of a functional dysphonia caused by inappropriate utilization of the laryngeal intrinsic or extrinsic musculature. A breathy voice may suggest a mass lesion, such as a polyp, or a neurologic disorder such as a vocal fold paralysis or myasthenia gravis. A harsh or raspy voice may suggest vocal fold swelling, such as might occur from chronic abuse or smoking. A tape recorder can be used to determine whether vocal modification and hygiene have improved the voice quality. A clinician who takes the time to carefully listen to all patients' voices will become much more experienced in evaluating whether a pathologic process is present.

### Physical examination

Although the natural inclination is to wish to first visualize the larynx when voice dysfunction is present, the clinician should remember that often a thorough physical examination is indicated to exclude a nonlaryngeal etiology for the voice disorder. An ear examination may reveal a hearing disorder, which may cause the patient to speak at loud levels with subsequent voice strain. The nose, oral cavity, and oropharynx should be viewed to rule out sources of difficulty with resonation. The neck and thyroid should be palpated for masses. A pulmonary assessment will determine the presence of problems that may affect the breath "support" of the voice. A neurologic assessment may expose disorders such as myasthenia gravis, amyotrophic lateral sclerosis, or multiple sclerosis, which may present with a change in voice. A musculoskeletal disorder can result in difficulties with appropriate posture needed for efficient voice production. These examinations may guide the clinician toward ancillary tests such as a chest radiograph or thyroid function test.

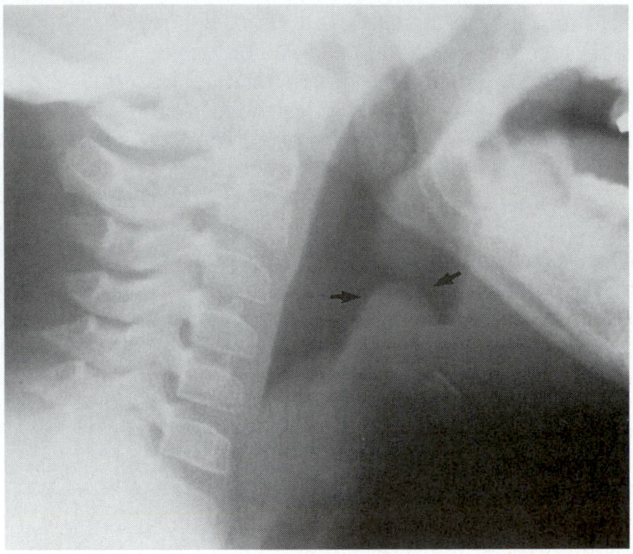

**Fig. 30-1.** Acute supraglottitis. Lateral soft tissue radiograph of neck showing swollen epiglottis (*arrows*), the "thumbprint sign." A normal epiglottis projects a narrow shadow.

Once a general medical condition has been ruled out, and if the dysphonia (abnormal voice) persists, then visualization of the larynx becomes necessary. Although some skilled primary care or emergency room physicians have experience with indirect laryngoscopy, a referral to an otolaryngologist usually is necessary.

The simplest and most cost-effective means of visualization is with reflected light from a head mirror (allowing binocular vision) and a laryngeal mirror. In some patients, where mirror indirect laryngoscopy is difficult, or where a more specific evaluation or video documentation is indicated, indirect flexible nasopharyngolaryngoscopy may be recommended. This simple, safe test is performed during the office visit with minimal discomfort to the patient and is invaluable in visualizing the larynx of small children or infants. The recent development of videostroboscopy allows for a direct assessment of vocal fold vibration, which is too rapid to be seen by the naked eye. The stroboscope pulses light at the vocal fold in a fashion that allows for an image of the vocal fold wave form and can be used to help define disorders of vibration such as scarring, swelling, or masses. It is also useful in voice training, patient education, and assessment of treatment response.

***Ancillary tests.*** Many ancillary tests are used to evaluate voice function. These are primarily used to assess pitch, airflow, harshness or breathiness, or range. A discussion of the specific tests are beyond the scope of this chapter, but the two most important factors needed for laryngologic assessment are the ability to visualize the larynx and a trained ear that can detect subtle voice changes.

A 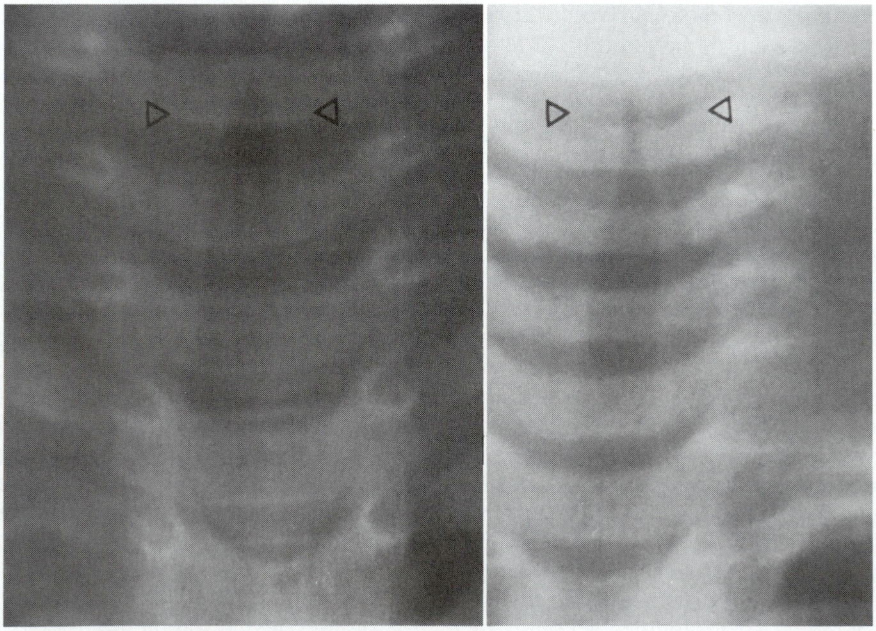 B

**Fig. 30-2.** Acute laryngotracheobronchitis (croup). **A,** Normal anteroposterior soft tissue radiograph of larynx. **B,** Croup. The "steeple sign" (*arrows*) is produced by sublglottic edema, which is soft tissue swelling beneath the vocal cords.

Radiographic imaging rarely plays an important role in the evaluation of the upper airway. Plain radiographs can identify adenoid hypertrophy, are occasionally used to verify epiglottitis by revealing a swollen epiglottis usually described as a "thumbprint" (Fig. 30-1), and are invaluable in assessing subglottic stenosis in an infant and small child because they will show a "steeple sign" (Fig. 30-2). Furthermore, plain radiographs are valuable in assessing potential foreign bodies, although they may be misleading if the foreign body is radiolucent. Computed tomography (CT) scans and magnetic resonance imaging (MRI) are primarily helpful to evaluate mass lesions. MRI with gadolinium can help determine whether a vascular lesion such as hemangioma is present. Usually, however, with mass lesions of the larynx or upper tracheobronchial tree, a biopsy is necessary; therefore radiographic imaging is used only when additional information is required.

Ancillary tests that often may be valuable to evaluate the upper airway tend to be related to specific disorders. Pulmonary function testing with spirometry help identify upper airway rather than lower airway obstruction. Thyroid tests can be performed if hypothyroidism or hyperthyroidism is suspected. A Tensilon test determines whether myasthenia gravis is the etiology for the voice disorder. If directed testing and clinical evaluation do not reveal the source of dysphonia, a functional voice disorder is usually present; that is, the patient is either consciously or unconsciously using the voice improperly. Sometimes, however, subtle changes can occur or the patient may be compensating for an early neuromuscular disorder. In such cases, laryngeal electromyography has proved to be effective in helping to make diagnoses.

## OVERUSE, MISUSE, AND ABUSIVE DISORDERS OF VOICE

Most disorders of voice are related to either overuse or misuse where the individual is not aware of appropriate voice utilization techniques or abusive causes of voice dysfunction. This is best seen in people who use their voice for a living, such as professional speakers or singers. Chronic overuse or misuse may become habitual, and the patients may not be able to reverse their voice behaviors without speech therapy evaluation and treatment.

### Acute laryngitis

Laryngitis by definition means laryngeal inflammation. Although the most common cause is an acute upper respiratory tract infection with secondary inflammatory effects, acute laryngitis can be caused by excessive voice overuse or misuse, exposure to toxic chemicals, allergic laryngitis, or general environmental irritants such as dust, smoke, or dryness. In the acute setting the patient tends to notice a rapid change in voice and may at times actually become aphonic (complete loss of voice) either due to the direct effect of the inflammation or from compensating for discomfort. Fortunately, in the typical setting, acute laryngitis resolves spontaneously and requires no further treatment other than reassurance. In the individual who uses the voice occupationally or avocationally, however, a short period of dysphonia and worse, aphonia, may be a significant detriment. In these individuals, a laryngologic examination is indicated. If gross erythema is present (Fig. 30-3) and there is a potential risk for a vocal hemorrhage, a short period of voice rest is recommended. If there is mild or moderate edema with minimal increased vascularity, however, then relative voice rest is recommended. If the patient has a critical voice need within the next few days, a short course of systemic steroids can be initiated, which frequently will decrease the edema sufficiently to allow for more normal vocalization. Inhaled steroids are generally not recommended, as they provide little short-term benefit and risk side effects due to drying.

Chronic laryngitis is more commonly associated with smoking or prolonged or excessive voice utilization. In such cases, a neoplastic process should be ruled out. Absolute voice rest is not indicated because if the patient does not change behavior, the voice problems tend to be recurrent. Voice moderation, modification, and a course of speech therapy is usually helpful. Smoking cessation programs are always advocated.

### Reinke's space edema

Reinke's space lies just deep to the mucosa. In this space loose connective tissue is present and early edematous changes can frequently occur. Reinke's space edema (Fig. 30-4) can be caused by either the acute or chronic etiologies mentioned under acute and chronic laryngitis. As fluid accumulates in Reinke's space, the voice tends to lower in pitch, there is difficulty with the upper portions of the voice range, and a gravelly or harsh sound may occur. Reinke's space edema is usually reversible with voice moderation and modification. Persistent Reinke's space edema, however, may be a sign of underlying disease such as hypothyroidism and should be investigated. Furthermore, a more chronic infiltration of Reinke's space occurs in smokers and is a prelude to diffuse laryngeal polyposis, which often is not reversible even with smoking cessation.

### Vocal fold nodules

Vocal nodules are small swellings seen at the junction of the anterior one third and middle one third of the vocal folds in the area of the maximal vibratory ex-

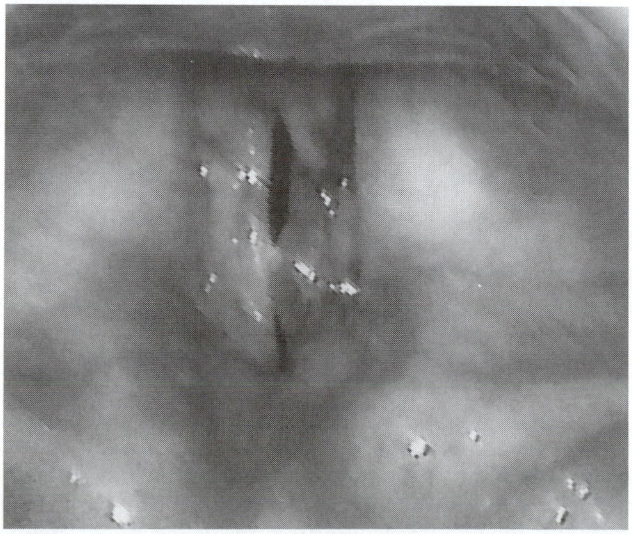

**Fig. 30-3.** Acute laryngitis with edema and increased vascularity.

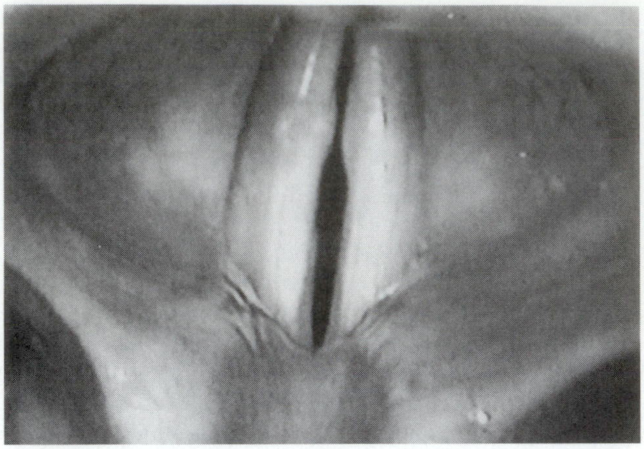

**Fig. 30-4.** Reinke's space edema. Note fullness on free margin of vocal fold.

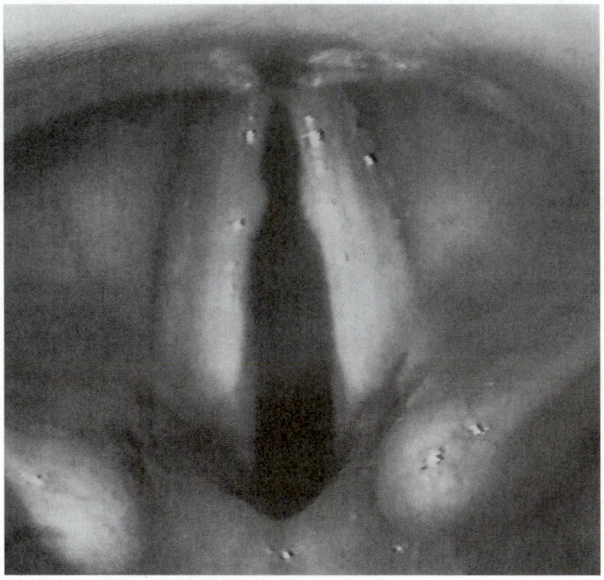

**Fig. 30-5.** Vocal nodules.

cursion (Fig. 30-5). Vocal nodules are one of the most common causes of voice dysfunction. In general, nodules are caused by chronic overuse, misuse, or abuse and result in a breathy, somewhat harsh voice with slight decreases in pitch. Vocal nodules frequently are seen in professional or performing vocalists, particularly those without previous voice training.

Vocal nodules are also common in children. A review of a large series of voice dysfunction in children reported that as many as 17% of school-aged children have some voice derangement at any given time. A majority of these children have vocal nodules. The peak incidence of nodules in children usually begins at about age 5, correlating with school attendance and ending just before puberty. They are more common in boys than in girls. Because nodules are so common in young children, the diagnosis is often made without visualization of the larynx. Clinicians should be cautioned against assuming a diagnosis of vocal nodules without further assessment. If persistent dysphonia occurs in a child, laryngeal evaluation is indicated. The mother, child, and referring physician can then be reassured, and a decision regarding treatment can be made.

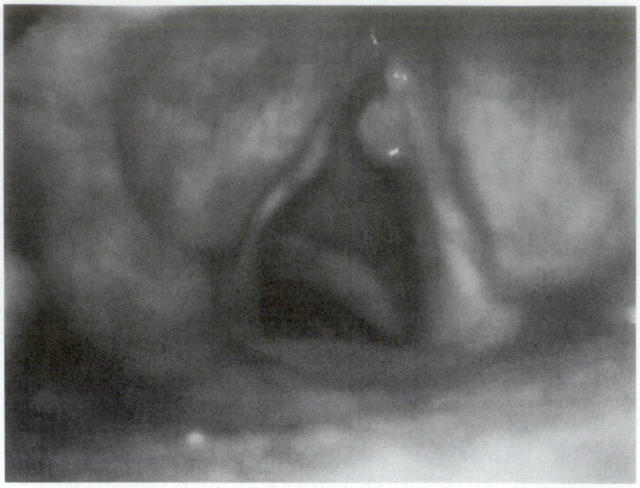

**Fig. 30-6.** Pedunculated unilateral vocal polyp.

Fortunately, vocal nodules are reversible with voice modification in most individuals although the aid of a skilled speech-language pathologist is frequently necessary. It is the unusual patient who requires surgery for vocal nodules, and if voice behaviors are not modified, the nodules will likely recur. Parents are told to gently remind the child when the child uses the voice inappropriately, but to remember that this problem is common in children. It will likely resolve without any intervention at the time of puberty and rarely, if ever, results in any permanent voice changes. Excessive, overbearing parents who demand strict modification for a young child may be more detrimental than persistent nodules. Most children are moderately compliant with voice instructions and gradual resolution is usually seen.

### Vocal polyps

Unlike vocal nodules, vocal polyps (Fig. 30-6) tend to be unilateral, may be diffuse or pedunculated, and usually do not resolve with voice therapy. Although the etiology of polyps is not clearly known, they are frequently associated with an episode of significant voice overuse such as screaming or with an acute viral upper respiratory tract infection. It is postulated, therefore, that bleeding occurs into the vocal fold, and gradual consolidation results in a vocal polyp. In general the voice of an individual with a vocal polyp is much more breathy and harsh than that of the person with simple vocal nodules. Occasionally, the polyp can be quite pedunculated and can lie intermittently in the subglottic area where minimal voice change is present, or it may protrude directly between the vocal fold where significant dysphonia or even aphonia is heard. Therefore the patient may give a history of having a normal voice or complete loss of voice in a single sentence. Occasionally, vocal polyps may be quite hyperemic and erythematous and may bleed slightly with excessive voice use.

Treatment for a unilateral vocal polyp is surgical excision. Excision is curative and can diagnose the rare neoplasm that might be present. Voice therapy is sometimes used both preoperatively and postoperatively, which may prevent recurrence.

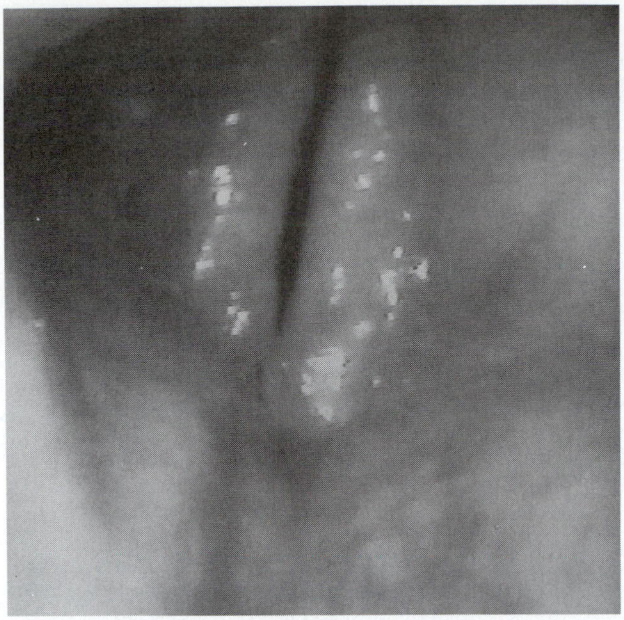

**Fig. 30-7.** Diffuse polypoid changes of the vocal folds secondary to smoking.

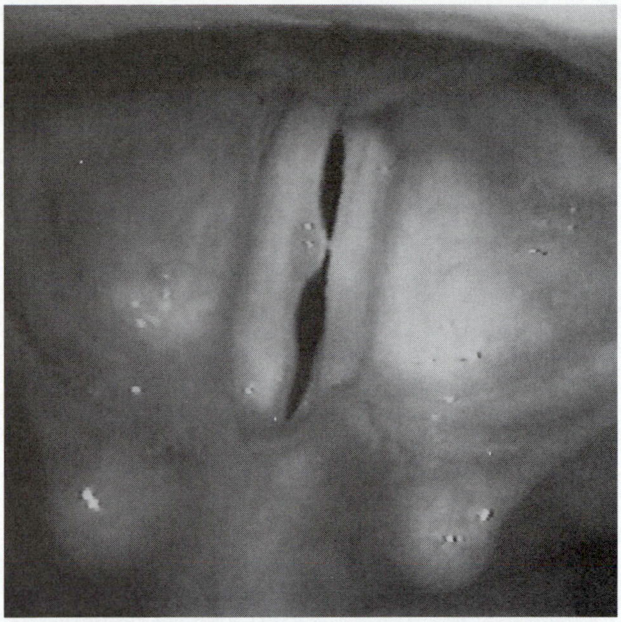

**Fig. 30-8.** Vocal fold mucous retention cyst.

Diffuse vocal polyps (Fig. 30-7) are generally bilateral and are seen primarily in individuals with long histories of smoking or airborne chemical exposure. With chronic diffuse polyposis, smoking cessation may not result in resolution. Significantly decreased pitch due to increased vocal fold mass effect and masculinization are the typical symptoms, although breathiness and harshness also are common. The treatment of diffuse vocal polyps is removal of the smoking irritant; if this approach does not resolve the problem, the thickened mucopolysaccharide deposits in Reinke's space can be removed microsurgically.

### Vocal fold cysts

In comparison to nodules and polyps, vocal fold cysts are uncommon. Epidermoid cysts are more common, accounting for two thirds of vocal cysts; mucous retention cysts (Fig. 30-8) account for one third. Occasionally, vocal cysts can be confused for a vocal nodule or polyp, particularly if a secondary contact nodule is noted on the opposite vocal fold. Cysts are also treated surgically because medical therapy generally does not result in resolution. Because these cysts are usually submucosal, a biopsy may be indicated to rule out a neoplasm.

### Vocal fold granulomas

Vocal fold granulomas occur either secondary to aggressive voice use or to intubation trauma. Granulomas usually are found on the vocal processes of arytenoids in the posterior aspect of the larynx (Fig. 30-9). Chronic esophageal reflux irritating the posterior larynx may be an additional precipitating factor. The treatment of contact granulomas depends on etiology. Granulomas that occur after intubation are treated by excision. In granulomas caused by aggressive speaking, excision along with voice therapy is recommended. As gastroesophageal reflux is common in the general population and may play a role in the development or persistence of vocal granulomas, an antireflux regimen or antireflux medication is usually recommended for all patients with vocal fold granulomas.

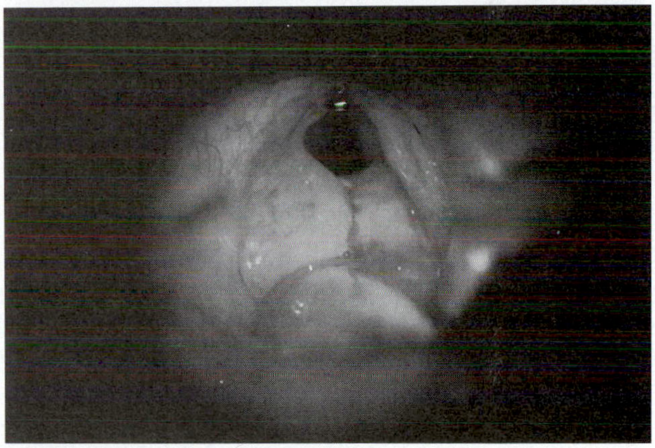

**Fig. 30-9.** Postintubation contact granulomatas on the vocal processes of the arytenoid cartilages.

## ALLERGIC LARYNGITIS

Allergic laryngitis is generally seen only in association with generalized upper airway allergic reactivity. Patients with acute allergic nasal flare-ups occasionally complain of simultaneous changes in voice. Specific treatment of the allergic disease usually improves the laryngeal dysfunction. However, the treatment of allergies with medications such as antihistamines frequently results in a drying effect of the larynx, which may actually worsen the voice. Therefore newer generation, nonsedating $H_1$ antihistamines are preferred in individuals with allergic rhinitis, as the drying effects of these antihistamines are substantially less. The addition of a mucolytic agent, such as iodinated glycol or guaifenesin, and increased hydration generally alleviate some of the difficult drying side effects of these medications.

**Table 30-1.** Medical causes of voice disorders

| Disorder | Symptoms | Differential diagnosis | Testing | Management |
|---|---|---|---|---|
| **Endocrine** | | | | |
| Hypothyroidism | Mild hoarseness (early), decreased pitch, loss of range, loss of fine control | Overuse/Misuse | Thyroid function tests | Thyroid hormone |
| Sex hormone | | | | |
| Premenstrual syndrome | Loss of range<br>Mild raspiness | | Characteristic history is diagnostic | Supportive, conservation<br>Speech evaluation |
| Pregnancy | Decreased pitch, voice fatigue third trimester | | | Voice instruction |
| Diabetes | Voice changes late in disease | Rule out other causes of dysphonia | | Voice instruction |
| **Neurologic disorders** | | | | |
| Vocal fold paralysis | Breathiness<br>Loss of volume | Vocal fold masses<br>Viral upper respiratory infection | Otolaryngology assessment after 2 weeks of hoarseness | Treat underlying cause<br>Surgery |
| Multiple sclerosis | Hoarseness<br>Difficulty swallowing | Other neurologic disorders | MRI, Lumbar puncture | Voice therapy, supportive |
| Amyotrophic lateral sclerosis | Progressive loss of voice<br>Difficulty swallowing | Vocal fold paralysis | | Supportive voice, swallowing instruction |
| Myasthenia gravis | Increased breathiness with use | | Tensilon test | Voice improves with treatment |

## REFLUX LARYNGITIS

One of the most common causes of changes in voice in an adult population is gastroesophageal reflux. Stomach acid reflux can irritate the posterior larynx and can play a role in contact granulomas. More commonly, reflux results in chronic laryngeal irritation. The classic complaints are a voice that is worse in the morning and improves throughout the day, a chronic sense of a foreign body or globus sensation in the throat that requires frequent throat clearing, or voice changes in association with dyspepsia. Frequently, these patients have been told that the source of their voice disorder is nasal or sinus. In actuality, except for the rare individual with allergic laryngitis or acute purulent rhinosinusitis, nasal sinus symptoms do not result in laryngeal complaints. Rather, it is the laryngeal irritation that results in the sense of thick mucus accumulation on the vocal folds and a desire to frequently clear the throat. In patients with such complaints, a trial of an antireflux regimen, hydration, and avoidance of throat clearing is often found to resolve the problem. In the absence of any worrisome symptoms such as hemoptysis or pain and particularly in a nonsmoker, a conservative antireflux trial is indicated before otolaryngologic referral.

Studies utilizing 24-hour pH monitoring have shown a significant association between upper airway disorders and reflux. Sixty percent of patients with chronic laryngitis, 58% of patients with globus, 45% of patients with dysphagia, and 52% of patients with undiagnosed etiology for chronic cough have significant gastroesophageal reflux. Failure of general antireflux measures may require $H_2$-antihistamine therapy (often in higher doses than used for peptic ulcer disease) or the hydrogen-potassium ATP=ase inhibitor, omeprazole.

Reflux is also common in the neonate and infant. Reflux has been implicated in sudden infant death syndrome. Frequently, chronic reflux in such children may result in a change in voice or cry. Because laryngeal disorders in this age group may be significant, a change in voice in a neonate or infant, even if reflux is the probable cause, should prompt a referral to an otolaryngologist.

## ENDOCRINE DYSFUNCTION AND VOICE

### Thyroid disorders

The vocal folds are sensitive to minor changes in body fluid accumulation, the mechanism by which most endocrine disorders affect voice. The most common endocrine source of significant or persistent voice dysfunction is hypothyroidism (Table 30-1). In the acute setting or in early hypothyroidism, small amounts of Reinke's space edema can occur. In the chronic hypothyroid state, myxedematous changes with mucopolysaccharide accumulation can result in a more significant and more chronic change in voice. Because the incidence of hypothyroid disease resulting in changes in voice is much less common than other causes, screening thyroid tests by primary care clinicians or generalists is generally not indicated unless there is other evidence of a hypothyroid state. Hyperthyroidism rarely affects voice until global neuromuscular changes occur.

### Sex hormone dysfunction

The most frequent changes in voice that occur in relationship to sex hormones are usually not due to sexual hormone dysfunction but, rather, normal changes in hormone concentration (see Table 30-1). The most obvious is the masculinization of voice that occurs in puberty in the young man. This change is best exemplified by the voices of boys, which change during puberty to the normal adult male voice. Similarly, women's voices tend to masculinize somewhat after menopause, although the degree is variable. The normal menstrual cycle affects voice in some women. Particularly during the premenstrual syndrome, changes in estrogen and progesterone concentration can result in a small amount of reversible Reinke's space edema. This edema, in combination with the generalized effects of premenstrual syndrome, including abdominal cramping, headaches, fatigue and irritability, can affect voice quality. For the average nonprofessional speaking or singing woman, these changes probably have minimal effect, although they may be important to those who use their voices for a living. In rare circumstances where significant voice changes occur, gynecologic and endocrinologic assessment and perhaps even hormonal treatment may be indicated.

Pregnancy also can result in substantive changes in voice. General fatigue; the expanding uterus, which decreases total lung capacity; and musculoskeletal difficulties, particularly low-back pain can all affect voice support. The nasal congestion and engorgement that frequently accompany pregnancy also can result in some changes in resonation. With proper voice instruction and counseling, most women can still function well up to delivery, even if they have significant voice demands.

### Diabetes

Patients with diabetes, particularly those who are insulin dependent, may notice gradual changes in voice (see Table 30-1). This change tends to correspond to the severity of disease and is likely secondary to microvascular disease or progressive neuropathies that affect the fine-tuning of voice control. It is important to reassure patients that this is not related to a more serious process once that possibility has been eliminated.

## NEUROLOGIC DISORDERS

Many progressive neurologic diseases can result in changes in swallowing and voice function. In certain circumstances, the subtle changes that prompt referral to an otolaryngologist may be the first sign of the disease; however, with progression, these are rarely the only symptoms.

### Vocal fold paralysis

An evaluation of the etiology of unilateral vocal fold paralysis reveals multiple potential causes. Historically, thyroid disease and surgery had been the major etiology but with improvements with diagnosis, technique, and nonsurgical therapy, this cause is less common. More often, nonlaryngeal malignancies or treatment of such cancers, primarily upper lobe pulmonary or mediastinal tumors, have become the most common cause of unilateral paralysis. Nerve injury from surgery for thyroid disease, cervical decompressions, and lung disease are important causes. Many patients develop paralyses of undetermined etiology. Intubation trauma can result in paralysis either by subluxation of the cricoarytenoid joint and subsequent fixation or by subluxing the joint over the recurrent laryngeal nerve, resulting in a neurogenic paralysis. Patients with unilateral vocal fold paralyses tend to present with breathiness, which often improves as they accommodate with the other vocal fold (see Table 30-1). It is important to determine the etiology and to rule out a neoplastic source. Treatment is primarily directed at improvement of voice and the prevention of aspiration.

Bilateral vocal fold paralysis is much less common. In the adult population the etiologies tend to be similar to those of unilateral paralysis, although occasionally, rheumatoid arthritis can result in bilateral vocal fold immobility secondary to cricoarytenoid joint fixation. In the neonate, bilateral paralysis is frequently due to Arnold-Chiari malformation and is an urgent life-threatening situation requiring immediate intubation after birth. In the older child, bilateral vocal fold paralysis tends to be iatrogenic, usually secondary to neck or chest surgery, with injury to the recurrent laryngeal nerves. The principles of treatment of bilateral paralysis are based around airway management initially and frequently require intubation and subsequent tracheotomy. Fortunately, after secondary procedures such as arytenoidectomy, most patients can eventually be decannulated, although such treatment may result in worsening of voice.

### Multiple sclerosis

Beyond the classic Charcot's triad of scanning speech, nystagmus, and vertigo, patients with multiple sclerosis may have dysfunction of pharyngeal or laryngeal musculature. More than 50% of patients with progressive multiple sclerosis eventually have some voice complaints (see Table 30-1). Some patients also develop dysphagia and changes with coordination of swallowing. These symptoms tend to be mild in comparison to the general disease and therefore usually do not require intervention.

### Myasthenia gravis

Myasthenia gravis selectively affects muscles innervated by the cranial nerves. Although the eye muscles are the most visible, other cranially nerve innervated muscles, such as those of the larynx and pharynx, can be affected by this disorder (see Table 30-1). Patients complain of gradual loss of voice with use, which recovers after relatively short periods of voice rest. The voice change may be the presenting sign of the disease. With treatment, complete return of pharyngeal or laryngeal function occurs.

### Amyotrophic lateral sclerosis

Although most patients eventually develop a voice disorder with amyotrophic lateral sclerosis (ALS), usually the general progression has more significant effects and the voice changes do not generally require treatment (see Table 30-1). However, swallowing dysfunction due to pharyngeal muscular involvement can have a substantial effect on patients, resulting in incoordination with swallowing and predisposing to aspiration. In the later stages of the disease, many of these patients require tracheotomy and tube feedings. Conservative treatment with voice and swallowing education and instruction may allow patients to function for prolonged periods of time without tracheotomy or tube feedings.

## BENIGN AND MALIGNANT TUMORS OF THE LARYNX

The most common benign tumors of the larynx originate from tissues of the larynx. Hemangiomas are the most common laryngeal tumor of infants and small children. They are generally not present at birth, become apparent within the first year of life, and are often associated with external facial or neck hemangiomas. Gradual regression is the rule; therefore airway management is the most important treatment consideration. Occasionally, with progressive large hemangiomas, systemic steroid therapy may be indicated. Complete regression occurs in most laryngeal hemangiomas except for large hemangiomas or those that occur with significant facial and skin involvement. Such patients have substantial improvement, but complete regression may not occur. In the older child and adult, arterial venous malformations occur (Fig. 30-10). They are much smaller and do not regress spontaneously. Because they can be confused for malignant tumors such as melanomas, otolaryngologic evaluation is indicated.

The other benign tumors of the larynx are related to minor salivary glands (benign mixed tumors), neurologic tumors such as granular cell neoplasms or neurofibromas, or musculoskeletal derivation such as chondromas, which tend to involve the cricoid cartilage. Such tumors usually present with voice change voice and foreign body sensation and perhaps progressive airway difficulties. Treatment is based on appropriate diagnosis and biopsy; most are amenable to surgical excision.

### Respiratory papillomatosis

Respiratory papillomas are the most common benign neoplasms of the upper airway (Fig. 30-11). They occur in two separate distributions based on age. The initial distribution tends to occur in young children and is frequently called juvenile papillomatosis. A strong association with a viral etiology due to human papilloma virus has been made. There is an increased incidence of juvenile papillomatosis of the upper airway and the larynx in children vaginally delivered from mothers with vaginal venereal warts, although some association also has been found with papilloma of the penis in fathers. The papillomas themselves are wartlike growths that usually involve the larynx, but can involve other areas of the upper airway. In the juvenile form, they tend to be progressive, with gradual hoarseness and occasionally upper airway obstruction. Recurrent surgical procedures are frequently necessary to treat the presenting symptoms and to prevent progression. In rare circumstances, progression can occur into the tracheobronchial tree, particularly after tracheal procedures; therefore tracheotomy should be avoided. Carbon dioxide laser excision is the treatment of choice, although interferon or photodynamic therapy may be considered in severe cases.

The second distribution of papilloma occurs after puberty or in young adults. It is much more indolent than the juvenile form, is often solitary, and rarely presents with airway obstructive symptoms. The principal complaint is usually a change in voice. Simple excision and the use of carbon dioxide laser are frequently curative.

### Malignant neoplasms

Squamous cell carcinoma (Fig. 30-12) is the most common malignant neoplasm of the upper airway. Smoking is the predominant predisposing factor; these tumors are rarely found in nonsmokers. In the pharynx, alcohol also has

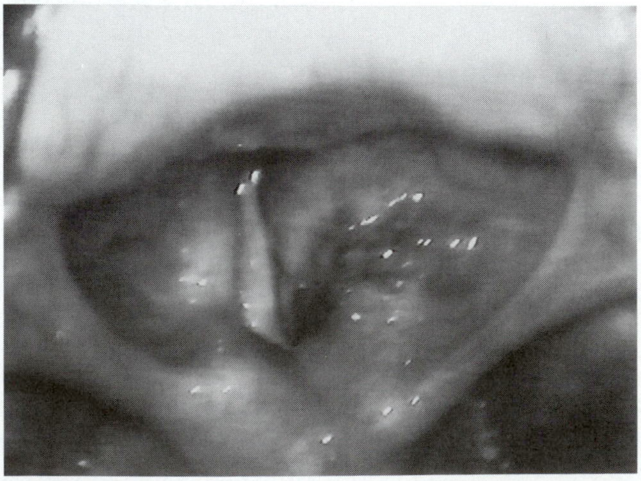

**Fig. 30-10.** Large arterial-venous malformation of supraglottitis and false vocal fold.

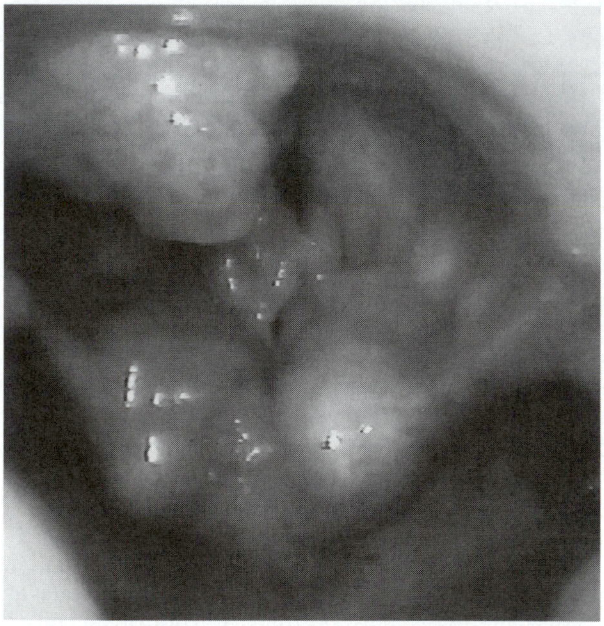

**Fig. 30-11.** Diffuse laryngeal papillomatosis involving vocal folds and epiglottis.

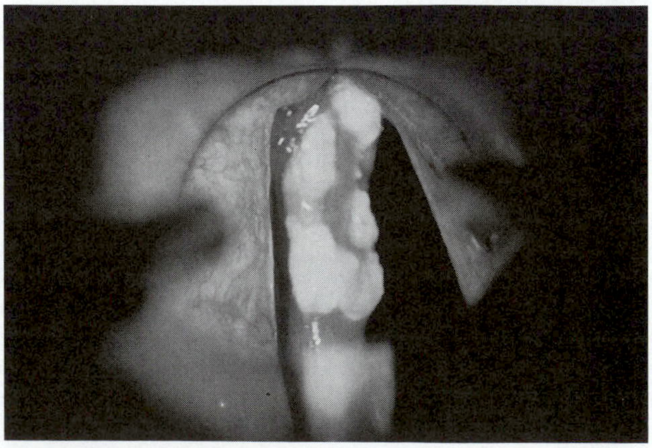

**Fig. 30-12.** Squamous cell carcinoma of the larynx.

been associated, and combined tobacco and alcohol exposure has more than an additive effect. Symptoms that might suggest squamous cell cancer rather than a benign pharyngeal or laryngeal process include progressive voice changes, dysphagia (difficulty swallowing) or odynophagia (painful swallowing), hemoptysis, or referred otalgia. Otalgia is caused by innervation of the ear from the ninth and tenth cranial nerves. A foul odor may be present, particularly in patients with tumor necrosis.

Carcinomas of the true vocal folds tend to present early due to voice changes. However, cancer of the supraglottic larynx, posterior pharyngeal wall or hypopharynx, and the piriform sinuses tend to present late with advanced disease, neck metastases, and poor prognosis.

Treatment of pharyngeal and laryngeal squamous cell cancers is primarily surgery, radiation therapy, or combined modality radiation and surgical treatment. Recently, chemotherapy has been utilized in multicenter studies; however, efficacy has not yet been proven on the basis of long-term mortality rates. This area, however, is dynamic, and combined radiation and chemotherapy may allow for survival rates equivalent to those for surgical treatment while providing for organ preservation.

## ACUTE AIRWAY EMERGENCIES

Most disorders of the pharynx and larynx are gradually progressive, result in subtle disorders that are frequently reversible, and do not result in any potential life-threatening problems. However, as the larynx and upper airway are the conduit to the lungs, certain diseases and disorders can result in rapid, progressive, and life-threatening airway obstruction. The most common sign of upper airway obstruction is noisy breathing (stridor). Stridor is always a sign of upper airway obstruction and appropriate evaluation is always indicated. It is not necessarily a sign of impending respiratory compromise and arrest. Inspiratory stridor, which is mild, may allow time for a more selective evaluation. It is usually due to disorders of the larynx, either in the supraglottis or glottis. Severe inspiratory stridor can occur in the face of an absence of expiratory stridor. The increased negative pressure of the thorax, which occurs during inspiration, can result in a Bernoulli effect and rapid closing of the airway on inspiration despite relatively normal expiration. Biphasic stridor (during both inspiration and expiration) can occur at other levels of the laryngotracheal tree such as the subglottis or trachea, or when severe laryngeal obstruction has occurred. Expiratory stridor without inspiratory stridor is suggestive of a nonlaryngeal site of obstruction such as in the bronchi. Difficulty breathing also can be caused by disorders of the oral cavity or oropharynx. Infectious swelling of the floor of the mouth in Ludwig's angina can force the tongue posteriorly into the pharynx. Angioneurotic edema with tongue base involvement and swelling has become more prevalent with the recent association to ACE inhibitors. Stridor in association with other signs of airway obstruction such as upright posturing, sternal or supraclavicular retractions, pallor, or cyanosis is an acute emergency that must be managed immediately.

### Croup (acute laryngotracheobronchitis)

Croup is a common condition that affects infants and small children, usually under the age of 2 or 3 years. It is more frequent in winter months and in northern climates. Croup is caused by viruses, particularly, parainfluenza and respiratory syncytial infections, with rare cases caused by bacteria (staphylococci). Typically, the child will have a prodrome of an acute upper respiratory tractlike infection, which lasts for 2 to 3 days, and classically parents are awakened at night with a child who has a barking cough and noisy breathing (Table 30-2). Generally, these children are in no distress, although in rare circumstances the obstruction can progress to a degree that requires airway management.

The pathophysiology of croup is due to viral inflammation of the upper trachea and cricoid region. The supraglottic larynx usually is not involved, although some vocal fold swelling occurs. Swelling, particularly of the cricoid, which is the only complete ring of the upper tracheobronchial tree and has the smallest diameter in the airway of infants and small children, results in airway obstruction. Treatment of croup is generally conservative. Parents often can manage the child at home with close observation, humidification, and decreased temperature. Frequently, parents report that once the child was brought outside into the cold air and placed in the car, the noisy breathing and cough subsided. If conservative methods do not result in alleviation of the symptoms, or if there is evidence of progressive airway obstruction, then the child should be seen urgently. A croup tent of high humidity, a lower temperature environment, and intravenous hydration are sufficient treatment in the health care setting. Some have advocated the use of systemic steroids or racemic epinephrine, although these drugs remain controversial. In rare circumstances, the airway obstruction progresses so that intubation and intensive care unit management are necessary. If a child develops recurrent episodes of croup, a laryngeal examination is indicated to rule out other potential causes such as anatomic abnormalities or mass lesions, and bronchoscopy may be recommended.

**Table 30-2.** Airway obstruction

| Disorder | Symptoms | Differential diagnosis | Evaluation | Treatment |
|---|---|---|---|---|
| Acute laryngobronchitis (Croup) | Barking cough and noisy breathing | Epiglottis<br>Foreign body | Rule out airway compromise | Humidification<br>Cool air |
| Epiglottitis | Rapid airway obstruction<br>Drooling | Croup<br>Foreign body | Avoid examination (may precipitate airway crisis) | Immediate otolaryngology referral for airway management<br>Antibiotics |

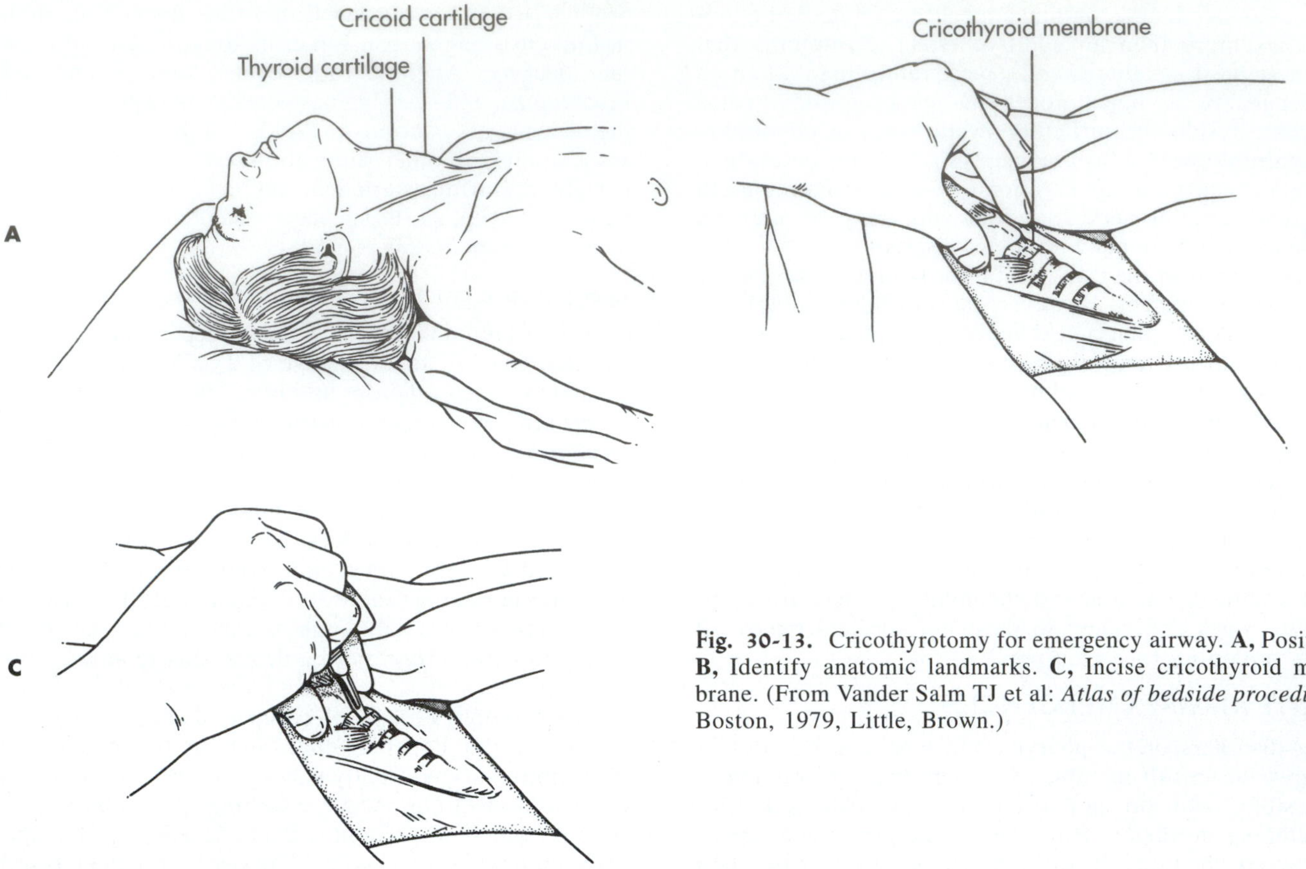


**Fig. 30-13.** Cricothyrotomy for emergency airway. **A,** Position. **B,** Identify anatomic landmarks. **C,** Incise cricothyroid membrane. (From Vander Salm TJ et al: *Atlas of bedside procedures,* Boston, 1979, Little, Brown.)

## Epiglottitis (supraglottitis)

Unlike croup, supraglottitis is an immediate life-threatening disease. Although supraglottitis can occur in any age group, even into adulthood, it is most common in young children between the ages of 3 and 5 years. The etiology of supraglottitis in more than 90% of children is primarily secondary to bacterial infection and inflammation caused by *Haemophilus influenzae type B.* A direct correlation with *H. influenzae* in the adult population is much less common. The incidence is decreasing with the use of *H. influenzae* vaccinations. Because of the looser connective tissue and multiple glands that occur on the lingual surface of the epiglottis in comparison to the laryngeal surface, swelling in this location results in downward directing of the epiglottitis obstructing the laryngeal introitus. Unlike croup, the prodrome tends to last hours rather than days, and the airway obstruction comes on quite rapidly (Table 30-2). Frequently, these children are brought into the Emergency Room in a seated position with their heads thrust forward. They drool as attempts at swallowing worsen their obstruction and appear toxic and frightened, but they are rarely crying, as this also exacerbates the airway blockage. With supraglottitis, complete airway obstruction is imminent in all children. Attempts at visualization of the posterior pharynx should be avoided because the use of tongue blades for visualization may precipitate obstruction. A lateral neck radiograph may show obvious signs of epiglottic edema with a positive "thumb sign" (Fig. 30-2). Radiographic studies in the Emergency Room should be avoided, as they can cause unnecessary delay in the management of the airway obstruction. Because intubation is difficult in these patients, attempts at intubation in the Emergency Room should be avoided unless the child has completely obstructed or unless vital signs and blood gasses suggest imminent respiratory arrest. Suspicion of acute supraglottitis requires controlled observation of the epiglottis and larynx in an operating room setting with an otolaryngologist and anesthesiologist, followed by controlled intubation or tracheostomy.

Once the anesthesiologist and otolaryngologist are present, they accompany the child to the operating room where observation of the larynx via laryngoscopy is achieved. With supraglottitis, a cherry red, boggy, markedly swollen epiglottis is seen, and the child is intubated. Although tracheotomy had been used in the past, recent information suggests that intubation in controlled settings is satisfactory. Attempts at obtaining blood cultures or bloodwork should not be undertaken before airway management is secured. Once the airway is secured, blood cultures should be obtained and empiric systemic antibiotic treatment for *H. influenzae,* such as with a third-generation cephalosporin, should be begun until blood cultures reveal the causative organism. Blood cultures are more frequently positive than direct cultures of the epiglottis.

The tracheotomy tube should be secured, and if necessary, the child should be sedated in an intensive care unit setting. With treatment, resolution usually occurs rapidly, and thus the child can be extubated within 3 days. Before extubation, the larynx and the epiglottis should be visualized by an otolaryngologist to ensure that the epiglottic edema has subsided. The role of steroids is controversial; however, many clinicians empirically use systemic steroids to allow for more rapid resolution.

### Laryngeal trauma

Acute laryngeal trauma rarely occurs independently; it usually is associated with trauma of the head and neck. Exceptions are clothesline type injuries, which occur while riding off-road motorcycles and snowmobiles; attempted strangulation or suicide; direct blows to the neck; or occasionally a motor vehicle accident in which the neck strikes the steering wheel. Bruising or hematomas of the neck should prompt the clinician to suspect laryngeal injury. In the face of global head and neck trauma, laryngeal injury is often overlooked, particularly in the presence of neurologic injury. Furthermore, airway obstruction resulting from laryngeal trauma may not occur until the edema forms sometime after the acute injury. If laryngeal trauma is suspected, a direct laryngeal examination is indicated because acute airway obstruction may occur and because immediate airway management will be necessary.

### Emergency tracheotomy, cricothyrotomy

Fortunately, most episodes of acute upper airway obstruction can be managed with intubation. In unusual circumstances, either because of other injuries, atypical anatomy, or pharyngeal bleeding, intubation may not be possible. Emergency airway access may then become necessary. A simple method of gaining time is to pass large-bore angiocatheter needles through the cricothyroid membrane, allowing for some passage of air. Use of a flexible nasopharyngolaryngoscope to guide intubation may be helpful.

Because most generalists and primary care clinicians have never had to perform immediate airway management other than intubation, possible tracheotomy or cricothyrotomy is intimidating. In unusual circumstances, however, the generalist may be the only trained physician present—particularly generalists who also staff Emergency Rooms—and may be forced to attempt airway control. Emergency tracheotomy is a somewhat difficult procedure and usually requires the expertise of a specially trained otolaryngologist, trauma surgeon, or emergency medicine physician. Cricothyrotomy, however, is easier to perform. The cricothyroid membrane is easy to palpate, except in individuals with very large necks. Because this area has minimal vascularization and lies above the thyroid gland, bleeding is generally not significant. Once the cricothyroid membrane is palpated, a scalpel can be used to stab into the trachea, and an immediate gush of air should be heard (Fig. 30-13). A hemostat can be used to dilate the stab wound and an endotracheal tube can be inserted. Once established, a cricothyrotomy should usually be converted to a formal tracheotomy within 24 hours to prevent subglottic stenosis. In individuals with traumatic airway obstruction or when airway management is necessary before adequate assessment of the cervical spine can be made, cricothyrotomy rather than endotracheal intubation should be performed because manipulation of the neck can result in significant neurologic sequelae.

## FOREIGN BODIES

Foreign bodies of the upper aerodigestive tract can occur in any age group, but are more common in toddlers and small children. In adults with dentures, lack of sensation through the denture may result in swallowing large boluses of food or bones, resulting in the presence of a foreign body, especially fish bones. In toddlers and small children, esophageal foreign bodies tend to be coins and laryngotracheobronchial foreign bodies tend to be pieces of food, particularly nuts and hot dogs.

Fortunately, most upper aerodigestive tract foreign bodies are esophageal, and the child usually presents with difficulty swallowing. Older children may be able to tell parents whether they have swallowed something such as a coin. Frequently, the mother will state that "the child was playing with a coin (or other object) and when I turned around I could no longer find it." Later, the child may develop difficulty with swallowing. With tracheobronchial foreign bodies, a more typical history is one of choking while eating, with subsequent noisy breathing or even obstruction. Occasionally, there may be a history of choking a few days previously, and the child presents with signs of a pneumonia or pneumonitis. All circumstances in which a foreign body is suspected should be evaluated. The diagnosis of a foreign body is made based primarily on adequate suspicion by the primary care physician.

Lateral neck radiographs and anteroposterior and lateral chest radiographs will identify radiopaque foreign bodies (Fig. 30-14). Radiolucent foreign bodies, particularly of the bronchial tree, may be suspected by lobar hyperinflation and a shift of the thorax to the noninvolved side. The later is due to ball-valving caused by the foreign body with retention of inspired air and prevention of expired air. Lobar collapse also may be a sign of a foreign body. Fishbones may be seen through adequate visualization of the pharynx and tongue depression. Even in the presence of normal radiographs or pharyngeal examination, suspicion for foreign bodies should prompt referral to an otolaryngologist for definitive assessment. If a suspected laryngeal foreign body is present that partially occludes the laryngeal airway, and the child is breathing and able to maintain satisfactory oxygenation, attempts at removal or Heimlich maneuver should be avoided to ensure that airway obstruction is not precipitated by shifting of the foreign body. A flexible nasopharyngolaryngoscope is an invaluable tool to observe foreign bodies of the larynx, piriform sinus, and pharynx. Because the cricopharyngeus muscle is a common site for foreign body obstruction in the esophagus, foreign bodies in this location can occasionally be visualized from above.

An upper aerodigestive tract foreign body prompts removal. Occasionally, removal can be accomplished with long, curved forcep and mirror laryngopharyngoscopy or indirect flexible laryngopharyngoscopy. Most commonly, particularly in small children, removal in an operating room setting is required. Meat tenderizers have been used for esophageal bolus foreign bodies, but may result in esophageal perforation. Attempts at removal of esophageal foreign bodies with Fogerty catheters may convert an esophageal foreign body into a laryngeal foreign body. These methods should be avoided.

A

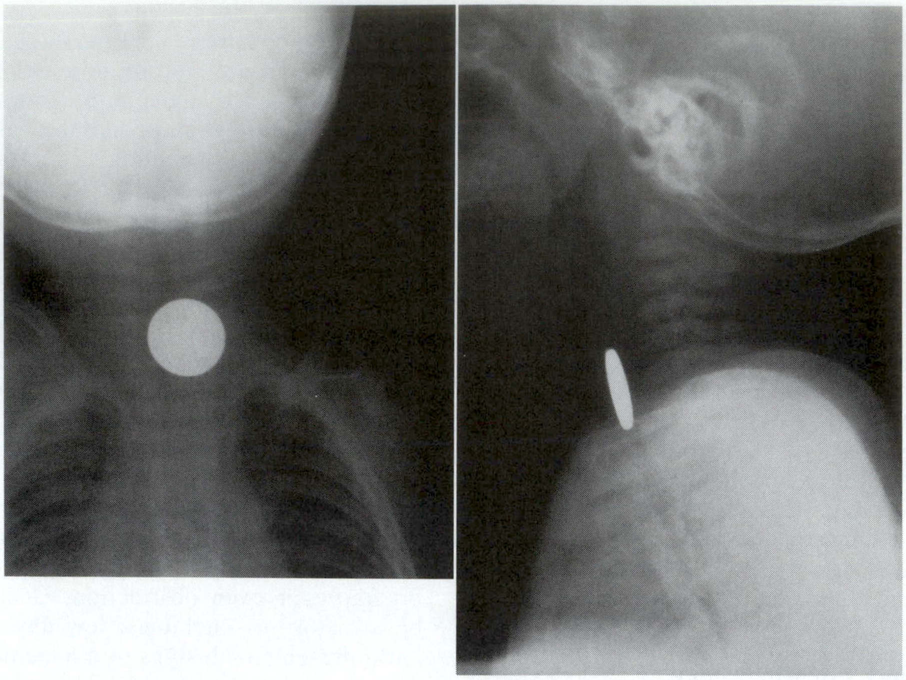

B

**Fig. 30-14.** **A,** A coin in the hypopharynx above the cricopharyngeus muscle. **B,** Lateral view of the neck reveals the usual position of a coin lying above the cricopharyngeus muscle and behind the larynx.

## COUGH

Although chronic cough is explained in detail in other chapters, a discussion of the potential otolaryngologic etiologies of cough is necessary for a complete differential diagnosis. The most common cause of cough related to the upper airways is an acute viral illness and associated laryngeal or pharyngeal inflammation. These problems tend to be self-limited, and no specific intervention except cough suppression is needed. Prolonged paroxysmal chronic cough may be secondary to vocal fold paralysis or paresis and aspiration, or changes in upper airway sensation such as occurs with superior laryngeal nerve paralysis. A diagnosis is easily made with laryngoscopy. Nighttime paroxysmal cough is frequently caused by nighttime gastroesophageal reflux, which may be silent without symptoms of heartburn. Night sweats may be another occult sign of gastroesophageal reflux. The recumbent position, which occurs with sleep, predisposes to gastroesophageal reflux, which can cause laryngeal irritation and paroxysms of cough. Patients often awake claiming difficulty with catching breath, and a short period of laryngospasm may occur. Appropriate antireflux regimens are sufficient to alleviate gastroesophageal reflux-related cough.

Many cough receptors are present within the head and neck region. Cough commonly occurs while removing cerumen from an ear. On rare occasions, hair within the ear can cause cough. Sinuses also have cough receptors, and in the face of acute sinusitis, cough may be initiated without laryngeal or bronchopulmonary inflammation. In a patient with otherwise unknown etiologies for their cough after thorough pulmonary workup, laryngeal examination is indicated, and, if negative, a trial of an antireflux regimen is appropriate.

Chronic cough in children has been well studied. In the absence of an obvious etiology after a thorough medical workup, the source of the cough, if related to the head and neck, varies depending on the child's age. In infants and small children, congenital anomalies of the larynx such as laryngeal cysts, webs, stenoses, or clefts are occasionally discovered, although gastroesophageal reflux is a major etiology. In the child between 18 months and 6 years, sinusitis and cough variant asthma are the most common sources of chronic, previously undetermined cough. Both cough variant asthma and psychogenic cough are more likely associated with chronic cough, lasting for more than 4 weeks in the older child, preadolescent, or teenager.

## BIBLIOGRAPHY


Boucher RM, Hendrix RA: The otolaryngologic manifestation of multiple sclerosis, *Ear Nose Throat J* 70:224, 1991.

Gillen J, Benninger M: The changing etiology of unilateral vocal fold immobility, *Laryngoscope* (In press).

Hirano M: Phonosurgical anatomy of the larynx. In Ford C, Bless D, editors: *Phonosurgery: assessment and surgical management of voice disorders,* New York, 1991, Raven Press.

Holinger LD, Sanders AD: Chronic cough in infants and children: an update, *Laryngoscope* 101:596, 1991.

Johnson A, Jacobson B, Benninger M: Management of voice disorders, *Henry Ford Hosp Med J* 38;44, 1990.

Koufman JA: The otolaryngologic manifestations of gastroesophageal reflux disease (GERD): a clinical investigation of 225 patients using ambulatory 24-hour pH monitoring and an experimental investigation of the role of acid and pepsin in the development of laryngeal injury, *Laryngoscope* 101 (Supp 53):1, 1991.

VonLeden H: Vocal nodules in children, *Ear Nose Throat J* 64:473, 1985.

CHAPTER

# 31 Evaluation of Neck Masses

David W. Stepnick

Although relatively nondescript from its external appearance, the neck is a complex anatomic subunit that serves as a conduit for major blood vessels, the trachea, esophagus, and spinal cord, as well as a variety of motor, sensory, and autonomic nerves passing between the head and the torso. Palpation begins to reveal its complexity. It contains the larynx and various glandular structures, including endocrine glands (the thyroid and parathyroid glands) and salivary glands. It is richly supplied with lymphatics, with approximately 200 lymph nodes, the thoracic duct, and minor lymphatic channels within the neck. Given the variety of structures that are located in this relatively small space, it is no surprise that the differential diagnosis of a neck mass is extensive. As such, the clinician should be familiar with all of the various possibilities to best establish a diagnosis.

Palpable masses greater than 1 cm are considered to be abnormal in adults; masses greater than 1.5 cm in children 6 months to 12 years of age are abnormal. Ptotic submandibular glands are often palpable, especially in elderly patients, and must be distinguished from an abnormal neck mass; intraoral-extraoral bimanual examination is usually sufficient to make this differentiation. The hyoid bone or laryngeal framework can likewise be mistaken for a mass. However, careful bimanual palpation better defines the identity and anatomic relationships of these structures. The carotid bulb is occasionally erroneously identified as an abnormal mass. Palpation reveals pulsation in the normal carotid bulb, although pulsatile masses in this region sometimes represent a carotid body tumor or a pseudoaneurysm.

For the purposes of this discussion, the neck is defined as the region from the base of the skull to the thoracic inlet. It includes the submandibular glands and the tail of the parotid. It likewise includes the cervical vertebrae and spinal cord, although a discussion of masses related to these structures is excluded from this chapter. The differential diagnosis of a neck mass is markedly age dependent. Many lesions commonly found in the pediatric age group are rarely, if ever, seen in the adult population (and vice versa). The most common etiologies of a neck mass in a child are inflammatory processes and masses related to congenital or developmental anomalies. Inflammation remains a frequent cause of neck masses in the adult population, although neoplastic processes become a much more common cause of a neck mass than in children. History and physical examination (as well as the age of a patient) can usually narrow the differential diagnosis substantially so that only a few ancillary diagnostic tests are necessary to make a definitive diagnosis.

Since lymphadenopathy is usually the result of infection or neoplasia, knowledge of the lymphatic drainage pathways of the head and neck helps the clinician focus on the potential site of primary pathology. Neck lymph nodes are anatomically divided into six regions (Fig. 31-1). Group I nodes are found in the submandibular area. Group II, III, and IV lymph nodes are those in the upper, middle, and lower jugular regions, respectively. Group V lymph nodes are found in the posterior triangle, and group VI lymph nodes are those in the paratracheal (midline) region. Adenopathy in region I often results from lower lip, anterior tongue, or submandibular gland pathology. Adenopathy in region II may result from oral cavity or nasopharyngeal pathology. Midjugular adenopathy can be seen with oral cavity, laryngeal, hypopharyngeal, or thyroid lesions; the latter three of these areas also drains to level IV. Esophageal lesions most typically affect level IV (as well as other nodes outside the neck). Pathology in the nasopharynx may be reflected by enlargement of level V nodes. None of these lymphatic channels is entirely predictable.

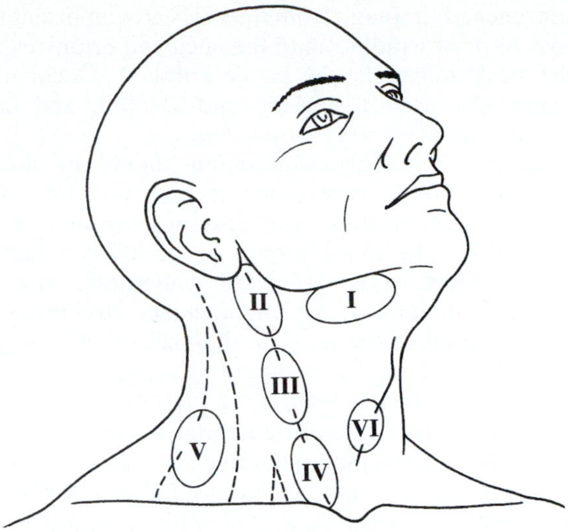


**Fig. 31-1.** The six regions in which neck lymph nodes are found. Group I nodes are found in the submandibular area. Groups II, III, and IV lymph nodes are found in the upper, middle, and lower jugular regions, respectively. Group V lymph nodes are found in the posterior triangle. Group VI lymph nodes are found in the paratracheal (midline) region.

Normal nodes are typically small, have the same consistency as surrounding tissue, and are not palpable. Frequently lymph nodes, especially those which are nontender, can be palpated only by bimanually placing the gloved finger within the mouth and the contralateral hand externally on the neck. Although a node with hard consistency suggests malignancy, the diagnosis of an abnormal neck mass is usually based upon size alone.

## EVALUATION OF A NECK MASS

As with any medical condition, establishment of a diagnosis in a patient with a neck mass begins with a complete history and physical examination. The patient's age is important because inflammatory and congenital causes of neck masses are more likely etiologies in children. Additionally, the speed with which the mass has grown, the presence of associated signs or symptoms in the head and neck region, the race and sex of the patient, and the presence of drainage from the mass are important facts. History of prior irradiation to the neck and prior treatment of the neck mass should be determined. Occupational exposure, the use of tobacco and alcohol, and family history are likewise very important.

A general physical examination should be done in addition to a complete head and neck examination, which includes visualization of the nasopharynx and indirect laryngoscopy. The mass should be carefully examined, noting location, size, firmness, tenderness, effect on overlying skin, and effect on adjacent structures. The specific location of the mass in the neck is often of great help in formulating a differential diagnosis. Thyroid lesions, submandibular lesions, and tail of parotid lesions arise in typical locations. In a similar manner, congenital lesions such as branchial apparatus anomalies, thyroglossal duct cysts, and ranulae are found in characteristic regions. When a mass is suspected to be an enlarged lymph node due to malignant neoplasia, it is important to consider the normal lymphatic drainage pathways in the neck (described previously) such that the most likely primary sites of origin can be examined with special care. Many lesions (e.g., lesions of the soft palate, base of tongue, and supraglottic larynx) have bilateral lymphatic drainage, which can result in early bilateral neck involvement. When a lesion is felt to be malignant, size and attachment of the node to surrounding structures are helpful in determining treatment options and to some degree prognosis. Fixation may indicate invasion into surrounding structures.

Based on the suspected diagnosis, a variety of blood studies may be useful. Complete blood count with differential and a blood chemistry panel are routinely obtained in patients suspected of having a malignant neoplasm. Liver enzymes and alkaline phosphatase are useful in screening for distant metastases. Thyroid function tests are done when a thyroid nodule is identified. Serum calcitonin may be elevated in patients who have medullary carcinoma of the thyroid and is also a useful tool for identifying recurrence.

Chest x-ray (PA and lateral) is important to screen for pulmonary metastases or second primary lesions in patients with head and neck malignancy. If malignancy, deep neck infection, or certain congenital anomalies are suspected and additional information is needed, an axial computed tomography (CT) scan of the neck with contrast seems to provide the most information for the cost. It is especially useful in patients in whom the physical exam is questionable or difficult because of patient anatomy. Modern CT scanning can identify nodes not palpable by the skilled examiner, especially in patients with short, thick necks. Although the test is rarely useful in making a definitive diagnosis, the exact location of the neck mass, its relationship to surrounding structures, and in some cases the primary tumor can readily be seen. CT scanning can show if a lesion involves other structures by pushing or by direct invasion. CT is *not* necessary for every patient with a neck mass; if the primary care physician is unsure about its usefulness in a particular patient, it can always be ordered (if appropriate) by the surgeon to whom the patient is referred.

Radionucleotide scans are useful in the workup of certain neck masses. It is appropriate to obtain a thyroid scan when a thyroid nodule is identified. The presence of multiple nodules in the thyroid suggests benign multinodular goiter. Solitary hot nodules are more likely than cold nodules to be benign. For salivary neoplasms positive technetium scans can help to differentiate oncocytomas and Warthin tumors (which appear hot) from pleomorphic adenomas (which are cold); however, this test is not routinely ordered. Bone scans are useful for identifying sites of osseous metastases but should be obtained only if metastases are likely. Liver and spleen scans are used by some physicians in patients whose screening liver enzyme profile is abnormal to exclude distant metastases to these organs.

Definitive diagnosis of a neck mass is made by tissue biopsy. Fine-needle biopsy or open excisional biopsies are the techniques of choice. Fine-needle aspiration (FNA) biopsy is done with a 22-gauge needle and, with proper training, can easily be done in the office. Many centers provide cytologic diagnosis within minutes or hours. Its primary advantages are that it is relatively easy to do, is of low morbidity, does not seed intervening tissues, and aids in treatment planning. Sometimes a diagnosis can be established without a formal incision. A disadvantage to this procedure is that false negatives and rarely false positives may occur; inconclusive or nondiagnostic results may be obtained. In these cases a definitive diagnosis can be made by excisional biopsy, which should be done following completion of the diagnostic workup. With biopsy-proven malignancy at the primary site, the clinician can treat clinically positive neck disease as such without the need for formal biopsy of the neck mass. Incisional biopsy of a neck mass should be used only if a mass is not surgically resectable.

## TREATMENT

Options for treatment of a neck mass vary considerably based upon the specific lesion being treated; details are included in the following sections. Most neck masses, other than those of inflammatory etiology (and specific benign lesions, e.g., lipomas), should be evaluated by a specialist for confirmation of diagnosis and definitive treatment.

Viral infections are treated with hydration and general supportive care. Persistent adenopathy is frequently seen following viral infections, especially mononucleosis. In general, bacterial infections are treated with penicillin, amoxicillin, or a first-generation cephalosporin. Antistaphylococcal antibiotics should be used if infection is related to the skin, salivary glands, or a congenital anomaly. Inflammatory cervical adenopathy of bacterial origin should respond quickly to antibiotics, and the clinician should see a steady decrease in size of the lymph nodes until they are no longer palpable. Appropriate intravenous antibiotics and referral for incision and drainage are appropriate if suppuration occurs. Associated upper respiratory tract infection helps lower the index of suspicion that a neoplasm may be responsible for the adenopathy, but sometimes definitive conclusions can be reached only via lymph node biopsy. Unexplained persistent adenopathy should be evaluated cytogically by fine-needle biopsy or referred to a surgeon to determine if open biopsy is necessary. Children often have multiple, small palpable lymph nodes present for long periods. Biopsy should be considered if adenopathy is in the posterior triangle, if a lymph node remains larger than 3 cm in diameter after antibiotic treatment, or when a solitary, persistent, enlarged node is found.

In general, congenital lesions and benign neoplasms are excised surgically, sometimes after appropriate antibiotic therapy if these lesions have developed infection. The treatment of neck masses resulting from systemic diseases is aimed at the underlying pathology.

Malignant neoplasms are treated based on the primary site, stage, and cell type by surgery, radiotherapy, and/or chemotherapy. The specific combination of modalities depends on the lesion in question, discussion of which is beyond the scope of this chapter. Regionally metastatic squamous cell carcinoma to the neck with an unknown primary is aggressively treated with radiation therapy delivered to the potential primary head and neck sites and neck. Treatment of locoregional unresectable or distant metastatic disease is considered to be palliative. Radiation therapy, chemotherapy, or a combination of the two may be used.

## INFLAMMATORY MASSES (Table 31-1)

### Cervical adenitis and deep neck infections

Painful swelling of the lymph glands of the neck (cervical adenitis) is commonly seen and usually results from regional viral or bacterial infection. Lymph node size can vary dramatically and tenderness may only be elicited upon palpation. Lymph nodes act as a modulators of the inflammatory response in the immunocompetent host. Lymphadenitis clinically is mirrored by the histopathologic finding of reactive hyperplasia, a nonspecific immune response to an antigenic stimulus. Changes in node architecture and the cell populations result from specific antigenic stimulation. The presence of multinucleated giant cells, granulomas, or certain organisms can sometimes point toward the specific etiology.

Bacterial odontogenic infections together with bacterial or viral tonsillar and pharyngeal infections are the most common causes of cervical adenitis. Less commonly, fungal and acid-fast organisms may be responsible for cervical adenitis. Typically, most of these infections are minor and self-limited and respond to antibiotic therapy. Suppuration may occur when antibiotic therapy is not instituted, when the spectrum of bacterial coverage is inadequate, or when sufficient bacteriocidal effects have not occurred. Once suppuration has been identified, referral to an otolaryngologist–head and neck surgeon is appropriate. The clinician must be vigilant, since morbidity increases and deep neck infections may subsequently result.

A variety of potential spaces exist in the neck that can fill with fluid, blood, or purulent material. These spaces are bounded by dense layers of cervical fascia between which abscess formation may occur and spread along the planes with little resistance. Although described as separate spaces, interconnections exist between them, allowing potential spread of infection.

Peritonsillar abscess is the most common variety of these potential space infections. In this disease, purulence develops between the tonsillar capsule and the superior constrictor muscles. Trismus is one of the hallmarks that helps to differentiate between acute tonsillitis with peritonsillar cellulitis and a true peritonsillar abscess. Incision and drainage with appropriate antibiotic treatment is considered the treatment of choice. Some physicians advocate simple aspiration of the purulent material followed by antibiotics and close follow-up. Hydration is important and sometimes results in the need for hospital admission.

A deep neck infection is one that occurs deep to the level of the platysma. The largest two potential spaces that can become infected are the retropharyngeal space and the parapharyngeal space. Deep neck infections can be life threatening because of the potential for extension into the chest. Other potential complications include airway obstruction, jugular vein thrombosis, and the production of septic emboli. Recognition of these potential complications and early, aggressive treatment with antibiotics and surgical drainage can help decrease potential morbidity. Deep neck infections are commonly caused by *Staphylococcus aureus,* penicillinase-producing organisms, and anaerobes. Deep neck infection should be suspected if intravenous antibiotic therapy does not result in significant improvement of a patient over approximately 3 to 5 days.

The *retropharyngeal* compartment lies between the posterior pharyngeal wall and the alar fascia (found immediately anterior to the prevertebral fascia). It extends from the base of the skull to the level of the tracheal bifurcation. Deep neck infections of the retropharyngeal space (retropharyngeal abscess) almost always involve the pediatric age group. Aspiration of abscess contents may occur if the retropharyngeal abscess ruptures into the pharynx. Careful endotracheal intubation in the Trendelenburg position immediately followed by incision and drainage is the treatment of choice.

The *parapharyngeal* space has been described as an inverted pyramid with its apex at the hyoid bone and its base at the skull base. It is bounded medially by the lateral pharyngeal wall and laterally by the mandible, internal pterygoid muscles, and parotid gland. Anteriorly it is bounded by the pterygomandibular raphe and posteriorly by the prevertebral and visceral layers of fascia and the carotid sheath. Like retropharyngeal abscesses, parapharyngeal infections may not present as a discrete neck mass, especially in early stages. However, as the abscess increases in size, it becomes apparent as a tender, warm, often erythematous swelling of the neck. Fluctuance is not typically found.

Cervical adenitis presumed to be secondary to bacterial odontogenic or pharyngotonsillar origin without evidence of deep neck infection is usually treated on an outpatient basis with oral antibiotics and general supportive care. A 10-day course of antibiotics such as penicillin, amoxicillin, or a first-generation cephalosporin is a good idea. Antistaphylococcal antibiotics are especially important if the primary site of infection is related to the skin, salivary glands, or congenital anomaly (discussed later). As signs of systemic toxicity increase and in younger children treatment with intravenous antibiotics (after appropriate cultures have been obtained) should be considered. Penicillinase-producing organisms, staphylococci, and anaerobes should be adequately covered by the antibiotic chosen. Once culture and sensitivity results are available, appropriate changes in the patient's antibiotic coverage should be made. If a deep neck abscess is diagnosed, appropriate antibiotic therapy and specialist referral for

**Table 31-1.** Differential diagnosis of nonneoplastic inflammatory etiologies of a neck mass

| Etiology | Patient characteristics, signs, symptoms | Testing strategies and findings | Treatment |
|---|---|---|---|
| Adenopathy secondary to peritonsillar abscess | Sore throat<br>Dysphagia<br>Odynophagia<br>Malaise<br>Fever<br>Drooling<br>"Hot potato" voice<br>Trismus<br>Deviation of uvula<br>Bulging of palate<br>Fluctuance in peritonsillar region | Needle aspiration of peritonsillar space | Incision and drainage<br>Antibiotics<br>Hydration |
| Retropharyngeal abscess | Neck mass often not discrete<br>Usually in pediatric age group<br>Fever<br>Malaise<br>Dysphagia | Lateral neck x-ray<br>Axial CT | Incision and drainage (after careful endotracheal intubation) in the OR<br>Antibiotics |
| Parapharyngeal abscess | Spiking fever<br>Rigors<br>Malaise<br>Trismus<br>Dysphagia<br>Odynophagia<br>Aphasia<br>Drooling<br>Torticollis<br>Neck rigidity and pain<br>Paresthesias | Leukocytosis<br>Anemia<br>CT scan w/contrast | IV Antibiotics<br>Hydration<br>Incision and drainage |
| Salivary gland infections | Gland enlargement and tenderness<br>↑ Pain w/eating<br>Mucopurulent discharge from duct (if suppuration)<br>Patients often elderly, dehydrated | X-ray for sialolith<br>CT, if abscess suspected<br>(Radionucleide scanning)<br>(Sialogram) | Hydration<br>Bland diet<br>Analgesics<br>Bed rest<br>Antistaph antibiotics<br>Warm compresses<br>Gentle massage<br>Surgical incision and drainage, if suppuration<br>Gland excision for chronic/recurrent sialoadenitis or sialolithiasis |
| Jugular vein thrombus | Neck swollen, diffuse, usually tender<br>Often H/O indwelling catheter (IJ or subclavian)<br>If *suppurative* thrombophlebitis:<br>Overlying erythema<br>↑ Tenderness<br>Malaise<br>Fever | CT w/contrast or duplex Doppler ultrasound<br>(Angiography) | Broad-spectrum antibiotics<br>Hydration<br>Supportive care<br>Anticoagulants controversial<br>Vein ligation if septic emboli |
| Mononucleosis | Mild and nonspecific URI<br>80% have triad:<br>Sore throat<br>Fever<br>Lymphadenopathy<br>Fatigue sometimes marked<br>Exudative adenotonsillitis<br>Yellowish white<br>Confluent | CBC w/differential<br>Atypical lymphocytes<br>Monospot<br>Heterophile antibodies<br>↑ Serum liver enzymes | Supportive care:<br>Hydration<br>Bed rest<br>(?) Antibiotics<br>Steroids for prolonged or severe cases<br>Endotracheal intubation or tonsillectomy if airway compromised |

**Table 31-1.** Differential diagnosis of nonneoplastic inflammatory etiologies of a neck mass—cont'd

| Etiology | Patient characteristics, signs, symptoms | Testing strategies and findings | Treatment |
|---|---|---|---|
| | Adenopathy<br>Usually bilateral<br>Commonly posterior triangle<br>Tender<br>Can grow to impressive sizes<br>Palatal petechiae<br>Nonallergic rash to ampicillin<br>Hepatosplenomegaly | | |
| CMV | Mild URI sxs<br>Similar to EBV, but less severe<br>*No* exudative pharyngitis | Negative heterophile antibody<br>Serologic test for CMV (+) | Supportive care |
| Tuberculosis | Nodes usually painless<br>Usually nonerythematous<br>Usually enlarging<br>Multiple (66%)<br>Posterior (70%)<br>Overlying skin indurated and slightly brown<br>Sinus tracts may open in skin | Smear or pathologic exam of node or drainage<br>Culture | Systemic antituberculosis medication |
| Atypical mycobacterium | Unilateral cervical lymphadenitis, most commonly submandibular<br>Skin erythematous<br>Usually nontender<br>Usually not warm<br>Changes in color from red to lilac pink<br>Minimal systemic findings<br>Not associated w/pulmonary disease | PPD negative or weakly positive | Surgical excision of infected nodes without antimicrobial chemotherapy |
| AIDS | Opportunistic infections<br>Hairy leukoplakia<br>Kaposi's sarcoma<br>Candidiasis<br>Verrucae<br>Giant aphthous stomatitis | ELISA<br>Western blot<br>Helper/suppressor T cell ratios | Treatment of underlying disease<br>Biopsy of nodes if neoplasm suspected |
| Toxoplasmosis | Common cold sxs<br>Asymptomatic or mildly tender posterior triangle adenopathy<br>Nodes usually confined to one side<br>May fluctuate in size<br>Do not suppurate or develop fistulae | Fluorescent antibody test<br>Compliment fixation test<br>Hemagglutination<br>Sabin-Feldman dye test | Sulfonamides<br>Pyrimethamine |
| Actinomyces | Neck mass: not true lymphadenitis<br>Blue<br>Rubbery<br>Nontender<br>Central loculation<br>Discharge of water material | Curettage and culture | High dose penicillin G IV 4-6 weeks followed by 12 months of oral penicillin |
| Cat-scratch disease | Mild clinical symptoms<br>Regional lymphadenopathy | Serologic test for *Rochalimaea henseale* | Supportive care |
| Syphilis | Cervical adenopathy | FTA-ABS | Penicillin |
| Tularemia | (See text) | | |
| Brucellosis | (See text) | | |
| Leptospirosis | (See text) | | |

Patient characteristics in parentheses are less commonly seen; those testing strategies in parentheses are unnecessary in many patients.
*H/O*, history of; *IJ*, internal jugular; *URI*, upper respiratory tract infection; *sxs*, symptoms; *CBC*, complete blood count; *PPD*, purified protein derivative; *ELISA*, enzyme-linked immunosorbent assay; *FTA-ABS*, fluorescent treponemal antibody absorption.

incision and drainage are considered to be the standards of care.

### Salivary gland infections

Inflammation of the parotid gland (the tail of which extends into the neck) or the submandibular gland may occur as a result of ductal obstruction by inspissated secretions or a salivary gland calculus. Continued stasis can result in infection; the usual causative organism is *S. aureus.* A variety of other etiologies may be responsible for salivary gland inflammation, including viral infections (e.g., mumps) and systemic disease (e.g., Sjögren's disease). Occasionally, patients with a normal ductal system and normal salivary flow develop chronic recurrent infections of the salivary glands.

Acute, nonobstructive suppurative parotitis occurs more commonly in elderly, dehydrated patients. Often these patients are taking diuretics, barbiturates, antihistamines, parasympatholytics, or other medications. Postsurgical patients who have not been kept adequately hydrated are at higher risk.

Radiographic studies may be useful in securing additional information related to the disease. Sialoliths are occasionally seen on x-ray. CT scanning is helpful in establishing the diagnosis of a parotid abscess or deep lobe neoplasm. Radionucleotide scanning and sialograms are not routinely used but have specific indications and are popular in some centers. Cultures obtained from expressed saliva should be obtained, when possible. Development of an abscess may occur and is an indication for surgical referral for incision and drainage. Recurrent sialoadenitis or sialolithiasis is likewise an indication for patient referral.

### Jugular vein thrombophlebitis

Internal jugular vein thrombosis presents as a diffuse swelling of the neck in the region of the internal jugular vein. This entity may also result as an unusual sequela from pharyngeal infection or from indwelling venous catheterization. Treatment of *suppurative* jugular vein thrombosis is with broad-spectrum intravenous antibiotics (ensuring adequate anaerobic coverage), hydration, and supportive care.

### Mononucleosis

The Epstein-Barr virus (EBV) is the etiologic agent responsible for the clinical disease known as mononucleosis. EBV is a small DNA virus of the herpes group. It enters the body via the upper aerodigestive tract and infects the lymphocytes. Clinical disease, especially in children, may be mild and nonspecific and may resemble any other viral upper respiratory tract infection. Although lymphadenopathy usually resolves in a period of several weeks, it can persist for months or even years.

Peripheral blood smear of patients with mononucleosis reveals atypical lymphocytes, but this finding is not pathognomonic and can be found in cytomegalovirus (CMV) infection, toxoplasmosis, mumps, roseola, rubella, and viral hepatitis. Early in the course of the disease monospot testing may be negative. Although heterophile antibodies are often negative when the patient is first seen, they become positive in 90% of adult patients; antibodies are absent in 50% of children less than 10 years of age. In those patients in whom heterophile antibodies remain negative, the etiologic agent may have been another virus causing a similar clinical presentation. Occasionally a patient who has been given ampicillin develops a rash, which seems to indicate worsening of the disease. This nonallergic rash has been said to be a hallmark of mononucleosis. Serum liver enzymes are usually elevated and hepatomegaly or splenomegaly is often seen.

Bacterial superinfection commonly occurs, and many clinicians provide patients with prophylactic antibiotics. Otherwise, treatment is generally supportive, encouraging hydration and bed rest. In some cases systemic steroids may be given if symptoms are particularly severe or do not respond to supportive care after about 5 days.

### Cytomegalovirus

CMV is a herpesvirus that most commonly causes infection in early childhood or young adulthood. Infections are usually subclinical, consisting of mild upper respiratory tract symptoms. Although very similar to EBV infections, CMV usually produces fewer symptoms, runs a more favorable course, does not cause exudative pharyngitis, and does not produce a positive heterophile antibody test. Serologic testing for CMV reveals that peak titers occur 3 to 7 weeks after the onset of symptoms. Treatment is supportive, and very few patients develop complications.

### Tuberculous lymphadenitis

Tuberculosis is centuries old yet remains a leading cause of death among infectious diseases. Although the number of cases in the United States (26,283 in 1991) is relatively small, there are 8 million new cases of tuberculosis per year worldwide with 2.9 million deaths as a result of the disease. There had been a gradual decline in the incidence of tuberculosis until approximately 1985, but the incidence has gradually increased since that time with more cases of resistant tuberculosis reported. *Mycobacterium tuberculosis* is transmitted via droplets that enter the lungs, are consumed by alveolar macrophages, and then multiply intracellularly. It spreads through the blood and lymphatics. About 12% to 23% of cases involve extrapulmonary sites, including lymph nodes, bone, meninges, and the gastrointestinal tract. As many as 80% of patients with tuberculosis exhibit cervical lymphadenopathy.

Since the overall incidence of tuberculosis appears to be increasing, tuberculous adenitis (scrofula) can be expected to occur more frequently. Scrofula is more commonly seen in middle age persons, immigrants, and persons on steroid therapy; 60% of the these lack a primary focus of tuberculosis.

Occasionally diagnosis is made by a lack of responsiveness to conventional antibacterial antibiotics. However, bacterial infections sometimes coexist, and an apparent response may sometimes be seen. Multiple recurrences of an abscess or continued drainage from a wound following incision and drainage of an abscess should cause the clinician to think of tuberculosis infection. Although cervical tuberculous adenitis in the absence of active pulmonary disease is typically not contagious, drainage from infected lymph nodes teems with viable and very communicable bacteria.

Diagnosis is made by finding acid-fast organisms on smear or pathologic examination of the lymph node. Culture can definitively implicate the organism (*M. tuberculosis*), although growth takes many weeks. In the absence of anergy, skin testing should be positive. Systemic chemotherapy with antituberculous medications is the treatment of choice with special attention directed to the increasing incidence of resistant strains of *M. tuberculosis*.

### Atypical mycobacteria

Approximately 90% of extrapulmonary mycobacterial lymphadenopathy is found in cervical lymph nodes. The most common organisms are *M. tuberculosis, M. bovis,* and atypical mycobacteria. *M. bovis* was so named because of its presence in herds of cattle with subsequent human infection caused by drinking infected milk. However, with the development of pasteurization and the destruction of infected herds, it has all but disappeared in North America. Atypical mycobacteria infection has become much more common, especially in children, over the past 40 years: most cases of tuberculous adenitis occurring in children are a result of atypical mycobacteria. Since the treatment is different for *M. tuberculosis* and atypical mycobacterial infections, bacteriologic identification must be made.

The natural history of the disease is that infected nodes slowly increase in size with few other associated symptoms. Spontaneous regression is seen in about two thirds of these patients; the remaining ones can form open, draining wounds. Unlike tuberculous lymphadenitis, surgical treatment is aimed at excision of the infected node often with no subsequent antimicrobial chemotherapy. Since atypical mycobacterial organisms respond poorly to antituberculous agents, residual disease left after incision and drainage often results in a chronic draining sinus tract. Therefore complete excision of these nodes is warranted.

### Acquired immune deficiency syndrome

About 40% to 70% of acquired immune deficiency syndrome (AIDS) patients have signs or symptoms referable to the head and neck region. Lymphadenopathy in AIDS patients can be directly a result of nodal HIV infection, other opportunistic infections, or neoplasia, particularly Kaposi's sarcoma. Although lymph node biopsy can suggest that a patient is infected with HIV, it is not done to establish the diagnosis. When neoplastic processes associated with AIDS (such as lymphoma) are considered in the differential diagnosis of a neck mass, biopsy is done to exclude these other etiologies (see Chapter 68).

### Toxoplasmosis

It is estimated that the protozoan *Toxoplasma gondii* has infected 40% of the population of the United States. Despite this high level of infection, however, only 10% to 20% of those infected manifest clinical disease. This obligate intracellular parasite has as its definitive host the domestic cat. Infection is spread by cat feces; the infectious oocyst can be transported by cockroaches, flies, and earthworms.

Typically, symptoms resemble that of the common cold. Lymphadenopathy usually resolves spontaneously but can persist for months or years. Systemic infection may be heralded by a nonpruritic maculopapular rash that spares the palms, soles, and scalp. The rash usually persists for 3 or 4 days. The disease may progress to involve the myocardium and meninges.

Only months or years after the onset of infection is skin testing of value and, given the frequency of *Toxoplasma* infection, its value is limited. No treatment is indicated for asymptomatic disease. Sulfonamides and pyrimethamine are used in treatment of systemic toxoplasmosis.

### Actinomyces

Actinomyces are gram-positive bacteria previously thought to be fungi because of their morphologic resemblance to fungal hyphae. These organisms cause chronic, suppurative infection with multiple draining sinuses. Typical infections are of periodontal origin and follow dental manipulation or trauma. True lymphadenitis usually does not occur, but a neck mass that contains these organisms may develop. Characteristic discharge of a watery material containing small yellow sulfur granules is seen. Definitive diagnosis is made by curettage and culture. The treatment of choice is high-dose penicillin G given intravenously for 4 to 6 weeks followed by oral penicillin given for up to 12 months longer.

### Cat-scratch disease

Cat-scratch disease, first described in 1950, is characterized by self-limited regional lymphadenopathy that occurs after the bite or scratch of a cat. Most reported patients are males under the age of 20. The disease occurs more frequently in the fall and winter. Greater than 90% of patients have a history of contact with cats, many having been scratched by one. Recent studies suggest that *Rochalimaea henseale* or a closely related organism plays an etiologic role in the development of cat-scratch disease. The serologic test for this organism may be useful in establishing the diagnosis.

Although only mild clinical symptoms are usually associated with this disease, occasional cases of a severe, protracted illness associated with encephalitis have been reported. At present, no specific treatment other than supportive care is recommended. Strategies for prevention of infection are important in control of the disease.

### Syphilis

Enlarging cervical adenopathy may be the first sign of syphilis, although this is not typically the initial presenting complaint of *Treponema pallidum* infection. Serologic testing (e.g., FTA-ABS) may be used to confirm syphilitic infection. Penicillin is the antibiotic of choice for treatment, the dosage and duration of which are based on the duration of infection and the presence or absence of neurosyphilis.

### Other bacterial infections

Several mononucleosis-like illnesses can result from other bacterial infections. Tularemia is caused by *Francisella tularensis* and occurs after inoculation through an infected tick bite or direct contact with infected rabbits. The most common presentation is that of a primary lesion associated with tender regional adenopathy. Alternately, regional adenopathy may be present without a primary lesion, or may be present in conjunction with exudative pharyngitis of oropharyngeal tularemia. Streptomycin is the drug of choice.

Brucellosis is caused by contact with livestock infected with bacteria of the genus *Brucella.* Characteristically, patients have headache, fever, chills, myalgias, hepatosplenomegaly, and lymphadenopathy. Treatment is with rest and supportive care; tetracycline appears to hasten recovery.

When associated central nervous system symptoms are present, the clinician should consider leptospirosis. Agglutination titers confirm the diagnosis.

## CONGENITAL ANOMALIES (Table 31-2)

### Thyroglossal duct cyst

Thyroglossal duct cysts are the most common of the congenital anomalies of the neck. The development of the thyroid gland begins in the embryo as an epithelial-lined tube that arises in the floor of the pharynx at what later becomes the foramen cecum of the base of the tongue. During embryologic development the thyroglossal duct descends through the neck (through or adjacent to the hyoid bone) and ends in the midline of the neck at the median lobe or pyramidal lobe of the thyroid gland. Normally the thyroglossal duct persists for about 6 weeks before complete obliteration. The anomaly occurs when failure of complete obliteration of the duct occurs and a cyst develops anywhere along its course. The anomaly may be a complete fistula tract, cyst(s), or aberrant thyroid tissue found in the midline of the neck.

The cyst or fistula is often asymptomatic, but recurrent inflammation and infection can cause cyst enlargement and prompt a patient to seek medical care. Retraction of the cyst upon protrusion of the tongue is the pathognomonic sign associated with these lesions. Histopathologically they are lined with squamous, respiratory, or transitional epithelium. Subepithelial islands of thyroid tissue in mucous glands are often present, and the tract contains mucoid or mucopurulent material.

Since most of these lesions become infected, complete surgical excision is indicated. Incision and drainage and temporary treatment with antibiotics are used in the face of acute suppuration. It is now well accepted that surgical excision must include excision of the entire potential sinus tract up to the base of the tongue, including removal of the midportion of the hyoid. Recurrence is usually related to incomplete surgical excision.

Thyroglossal duct carcinoma is a very rare disorder in which patients present with a firm midline mass in the neck or base of tongue. Treatment is wide local excision and prognosis is generally good.

### Branchial apparatus anomalies

Remnants of the embryologic branchial arch system are among the most frequent causes of congenital lateral neck anomalies. These anomalies may present as a draining fistula or as a painless or infected mass. They are often asymptomatic and may be completely hidden until inflammation or infection occurs. There is no sex predominance and they are rarely bilateral.

Histopathologically, cysts or fistula tracts are lined with stratified squamous epithelium and contain keratin, hair follicles, and glandular structures. Respiratory epithelium may also be seen, as are lymphoid aggregates in the walls. The course of the tract can be predicted based upon normal branchial apparatus development. Recurrence following excision is usually caused by persistent epithelial remnants left deep to the skin's surface.

Since branchial anomalies characteristically are prone to recurrent infection, the treatment of choice is to control the acute infection with oral antibiotics and then to refer the patient for excision of the cyst and fistula tract. Temporary incision and drainage may be necessary before undertaking definitive surgical excision in the presence of acute inflammation with abscess formation. Other treatment approaches have been used, including the injection of sclerosing solutions and radiation therapy, but these are not curative, have other deleterious effects, and are not advocated.

Carcinoma arising in these branchial cleft anomalies has been reported. Very specific criteria are necessary before making the diagnosis, and they are beyond the scope of this discussion.

### Cystic hygroma

Cystic hygromas or lymphangiomas are endothelial-lined, soft, multiloculated cystic masses that are believed to be the result of abnormal development of the jugular lymphatics. When cystic hygromas are large, they can exert pressure on surrounding structures: airway compromise can occur. Frequently cystic hygromas transilluminate in contradistinction to lipomas, which do not.

A variety of treatment modalities have been described, including the injection of sclerosing solutions, eletrocoagulation, and other techniques, all with limited success. Surgery is usually indicated only in cases of functional impairment, recurrent infection, and very severe cosmetic deformity. Cystic hygromas are rarely removed in their entirety, but fortunately recurrence rates are low.

### Hemangioma

Hemangiomas are the most common tumor of infancy and are reported as the most common salivary gland neoplasm in children. Most are diagnosed by the age of 6 months and rapidly proliferate throughout the first year of life. During this proliferative phase these lesions can grow quite large, and complications such as airway obstruction and high-output cardiac failure may occur. These lesions are to be distinguished from vascular malformations (capillary, arteriovenous, venous, and lymphatic), which typically are present at birth, exhibit a normal rate of endothelial turnover, and grow slowly as the child grows. Gradual spontaneous resolution of true hemangiomas occurs after the proliferative phase and may last until the child reaches the teenage years. In the absence of impending complications, surgical treatment is best avoided, although a variety of issues must be dealt with by appropriate specialists including the child's psychosocial well-being. If no regression is seen by age 5 or if symptoms develop, surgical excision may be indicated.

### Dermoid cysts and teratomas

Dermoid cysts are smooth midline masses not attached to the larynx or the hyoid bone that usually have a doughy consistency. They are most commonly found in the second decade of life. They may be found in the nose as well as deep in the floor of the mouth. Cyst walls are composed

**Table 31-2.** Differential diagnosis of congenital anomalies presenting as a neck mass

| Anomaly | Patient characteristics, signs, symptoms | Testing strategies and findings | Treatment |
|---|---|---|---|
| Thyroglossal duct cyst | Most patients <30 years<br>Midline mass<br>Usually inferior to hyoid<br>Soft<br>Retraction of cyst upon protrusion of tongue is pathognomonic | | Surgical excision<br>Antibiotics, if infected |
| Branchial apparatus anomalies | Usually present in childhood<br>Usually diagnosed by age 30<br>Mass<br>Along anterior border of SCM<br>Between ear canal and clavicle<br>Smooth<br>Fluctuant<br>Nontender<br>Ill-defined margins<br>Varies in size (associated with URIs) | Needle aspiration results in decompression<br>Thin or mucopurulent fluid | Surgical excision |
| Cystic hygroma | Multiloculated cystic masses<br>90% diagnosed before age 2<br>Often enlarge during URIs<br>(Airway compromise)<br>Transilluminate | CT scan<br>May have visible cysts<br>(Aspiration→clear yellow fluid) | Excision *if*<br>Functional impairment<br>Recurrent infection<br>Severe cosmetic deformity |
| Hemangioma | Most diagnosed by age 6 months<br>Proliferate during first year<br>(Airway obstruction)<br>(High-output cardiac failure) | CT scan | Surgical excision *if*<br>No regression by age 5<br>Impending complications |
| Dermoid cysts | Midline masses<br>Smooth<br>Not attached to larynx or hyoid<br>Doughy consistency<br>Commonly found in 20s | | Surgical excision |
| Teratomas | Mass<br>Irregular<br>Firm<br>Lateral | | Surgical excision |
| Laryngoceles | Very soft, compressible mass<br>↑ Size with Valsalva's maneuver<br>Laryngeal component | | Surgical excision<br>(Antibiotics if infection) |
| Ranula | Soft, compressible mass<br>Associated with sublingual gland | CT scan<br>(Salivary amylase) | Surgical excision |

*SCM*, Sternocleidomastoid muscle; *URI*, upper respiratory tract infection.

of squamous epithelium with epidermal appendages. The treatment of choice is surgical excision.

Teratomas are believed to result from errors of fusion of embryonal structures that have developed from pleuripotential cells. They are derived from all three germ layers. Teratomas of the neck are characteristically irregular, firm, lateral lesions. They are treated by surgical excision.

## Laryngocele

A laryngocele, as its name implies, arises as an air-filled mucosa-lined cyst from the larynx. When confined to the larynx, it is referred to as an internal laryngocele. Extension through the thyrohyoid membrane to the neck results in an external laryngocele. This lesion manifests as a very soft compressible neck mass that increases in size with the Valsalva maneuver. It may become infected, requiring antimicrobial therapy. The treatment of choice for laryngoceles is surgical excision.

## Ranula

Ranulas are not true neoplasms, but rather cysts that result from extravasation of saliva from the sublingual gland. Both those confined to the oral cavity and cervical, or plunging, ranulas have been described. Plunging ranulas are located below the level of the mylohyoid muscle and present as a soft, compressible swelling in the upper part of the neck. The cyst is lined with connective tissue rather than true epithelium and therefore is actually a pseudocyst. The pathogenesis of these lesions is poorly understood.

Ranulas may increase or decrease in size. Although infection can occur, ranulas typically do not present as an infected mass. Diagnosis is usually fairly evident based on its compressibility and characteristic location. Specific diagnostic tests are not available; levels of amylase and the protein content of saliva have been used for diagnostic purposes by some physicians. Sialography of the submandibular gland gives no additional information, since the submandibular gland is not involved in the pathophysiology of this lesion. Injection of water-soluble contrast material into the cyst can show the interrelationship between the cyst and sublingual gland and/or the oral portion of the ranula, but this is minimally useful clinically.

A variety of therapies have been advocated including injection of the cavity with a sclerosing agent and marsupialization of the cyst. However, it is becoming more clear that the treatment of choice is excision of the sublingual gland in its entirety without the need for an extensive neck dissection.

## NEOPLASMS

### Neoplastic masses in adults

Neoplasms, both benign and malignant, are frequent causes of a neck mass in the adult population. See Chapter 32 for a complete discussion of these lesions.

### Neoplastic masses in children

Most benign tumors seen in the pediatric age group are congenital and have been previously described. Benign lesions of the salivary glands as well as a variety of other benign masses also develop in children, including lipomas, myomas, fibromas, and fibrous dysplasia. Malignant lesions fairly unique to this age group may also be seen.

***Benign salivary lesions.*** The most frequent benign salivary gland neoplasms in children are hemangiomas. Less frequently benign mixed tumors, vascular proliferative tumors, and a host of others may be encountered. Treatment is generally by surgical excision, preserving the facial nerve.

#### *Malignant neck masses in children*

**Salivary gland tumors.** Salivary gland neoplasms are uncommon in children and, when present, are frequently malignant. The most common malignant salivary gland neoplasm in a child is mucoepidermoid carcinoma. A variety of other tumors are found, including acinous cell carcinoma, undifferentiated carcinoma, adenocarcinoma, carcinoma ex pleomorphic adenoma, undifferentiated sarcoma, adenoid cystic carcinoma, squamous cell carcinoma, rhabdomyosarcoma, and ganglioneuroblastoma.

**Sarcoma.** The most common solid tumor found in the head and neck region in children between the ages of 1 and 4 is a rhabdomyosarcoma. This lesion is most commonly found in the orbit. Other common sites include the ear, nose, nasopharynx, maxilla, oral cavity, pharynx, and larynx. Cervical adenopathy may result from metastatic rhabdomyosarcoma. Diagnosis is made by biopsy of the affected site(s). Treatment includes a combination of surgery, irradiation, and chemotherapy.

**Hodgkin's disease and non-Hodgkin's lymphoma.** Both of these entities may be seen in children, as in their adult counterpart. Presentation and workup are similar to those for the adult patient with the same disease process. The role of surgery is limited to biopsy.

**Neuroblastoma.** Neuroblastoma usually arises from the adrenal medulla but may also arise from neural crest tissue along the sympathetic chain and the cranial ganglia. Although it is one of the most common neoplasms in children, only 5% arise primarily in the neck. Metastases may occur in the neck. Workup should include a urine screen for catecholamines and a bone scan and skeletal survey to rule out bony metastases. Treatment is with radiation therapy.

**Fibrosarcomas and neurofibrosarcomas.** These lesions are rare in children. The mandible is the most frequent site of involvement. These lesions tend to recur after excision, although metastatic disease is rare.

**Malignant thyroid disease.** A solitary nodule in a child has a much higher risk of being a malignant lesion, although typically these have an excellent prognosis. Treatment is by exploration, biopsy, and surgical excision.

**Carcinoma.** Perhaps the most frequent carcinoma to be seen in the childhood age group is that of carcinoma of the nasopharynx. Frequently this lesion initially presents as a neck mass since the primary is often silent. Since the primary site is frequently unresectable, radiation therapy is the treatment of choice.

## MISCELLANEOUS DISORDERS

### Lipomas and epidermal inclusion cysts

Lipomas, benign fatty tumors found just beneath the skin, are soft, slowly growing, usually nondiscrete masses. They are asymptomatic and characteristically found in the posterior triangle when in the neck. Although CT scan is not recommended for helping establish the correct diagnosis, they are of fat or air density radiographically. When found in the characteristic location and when the mass has all of the hallmarks of a lipoma, biopsy or excision is not mandatory. Epidermal inclusion cysts are similarly soft and inseparable from the overlying skin. Fluctuance may help distinguish between the two, but often differentiation is difficult. Epidermal inclusions contain keratin and sebaceous debris and are prone to infection and rupture, unlike lipomas. Because of the tendency to become infected, simple excision is advocated. Simple excision of a lipoma is the treatment of choice if the lesion produces a significant cosmetic deformity or if the diagnosis is in question.

### Sarcoidosis

The adenopathy associated with sarcoidosis is typically nontender and rubbery to palpation. Workup should include chest x-ray, pulmonary function testing, and serum angiotensin-converting enzyme levels. Lymph node biopsy reveals noncaseating granulomas. Patients are treated for the systemic manifestations of this disease (see Chapter 116).

CHAPTER

# 32 Head and Neck Oncology

Dennis H. Kraus
David G. Pfister

The head and neck contain a variety of tissues and organs. Accordingly, a broad spectrum of malignant lesions can occur in this region. Carcinomas, lymphomas, sarcomas, and melanomas arise in the head and neck; salivary gland, thyroid, ocular, and brain tumors are all technically head and neck malignancies. When nonmelanoma skin cancers are excluded, approximately 80,000 such cancers are diagnosed in the United States each year.

Most commonly, however, the term *head and neck cancer* (HNC) refers to squamous cell carcinoma arising from the surface epithelium of the upper aerodigestive tract, including the oral cavity, pharynx, larynx, and nasal cavity/paranasal sinuses (see the box below). When so defined, approximately 45,000 new cases of HNC are diagnosed each year, or 4% to 5% of all newly diagnosed invasive cancers. Squamous cell carcinoma or one of its variants is the histologic type in 95% of these cases. HNC comprises a heterogeneous group of neoplasms, with important site-specific differences in etiology, clinical presentation, staging, prognosis, treatment, and survival. Unless otherwise specified, HNC here refers to cancers of this location and histology. Despite their heterogeneity, certain general principles of management can be identified, and these are stressed. Carcinomas of the salivary glands and thyroid are also briefly reviewed.

### Primary sites of HNC

- Oral cavity
  - Lip
  - Buccal mucosa
  - Floor of mouth
  - Alveolar ridge (lower, upper)
  - Retromolar trigone
  - Hard palate
  - Tongue
- Pharynx
  - Oropharynx
    - Base of tongue
    - Tonsil
    - Lateral wall
    - Posterior pharyngeal wall
    - Inferior surface of soft palate, uvula
  - Hypopharynx
    - Pyriform sinus
    - Posterior pharyngeal wall
    - Postcricoid
  - Nasopharynx
- Larynx
  - Supraglottis
    - False vocal cords
    - Epiglottis
    - Arytenoids
  - Glottis
    - True vocal cords
  - Subglottis
- Nose and paranasal sinuses
  - Maxillary sinus
  - Sphenoid sinus
  - Ethmoid sinus
  - Nasal cavity

## EPIDEMIOLOGY AND RISK FACTORS

The incidence of HNC has shown a minimal increase over the last 30 years. Patients with HNC are predominantly male (3:1), and have a median age of approximately 60 years. An increasing proportion are women, reflecting increased tobacco use in this population. The oral cavity and the larynx are the two most common primary sites. Marginal improvements in survival have occurred over the last 30 years.

HNC is associated with several etiologic factors, especially tobacco and alcohol use. Inhaled tobacco smoke is probably the most important. It affects most sites, although the association is strongest for laryngeal cancer. The risk increases with the number of cigarettes smoked each day. In individuals who stop smoking, it takes over a decade for their risk of HNC to approach that of a nonsmoker. Other tobacco products besides cigarettes, including cigar, pipe, and smokeless tobacco, are associated with a significant increase in HNC. The recent popularity of smokeless tobacco in adolescents and young adults has been associated with increases in oral cavity (especially buccal mucosa) and oropharyngeal cancers. Alcohol consumption is a major risk factor for HNC, especially of the oral cavity, oropharynx, and hypopharynx. As with tobacco, the subsequent incidence of cancer is dose related. When tobacco and alcohol are both used by a patient, the two risk factors appear to be synergistic.

Nasopharynx cancer is especially prevalent in the Far East, where the incidence is 20 to 25 times higher than it is in Western countries. The increased risk is diminished but still present in American descendants of Chinese origin. The exact roles played by genetic and environmental factors, however, remain controversial. The Epstein-Barr virus (EBV) has received great scrutiny as a potential etiologic agent. Patients with nasopharyngeal carcinoma have a greater elevation in their EBV viral capsid titers compared with control patients without the disease, and the level of these titers correlates with the tumor burden present. The EBV genome can be demonstrated in nasopharyngeal cancer tissue. Human papillomavirus has also been considered as an etiologic agent for the development of squamous cell carcinoma throughout the upper aerodigestive tract.

## PATHOPHYSIOLOGY

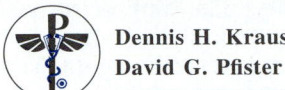

Certain lesions, although not frankly invasive carcinoma, are important to recognize as precursors of squamous cell carcinoma. Since a different histologic diagnosis can dramatically affect prognosis and treatment, direct interaction with the pathologist under these circumstances is crucial. Leukoplakia clinically appears as a white patch, which reflects epithelial thickening. It can be distinguished from a candidal infection in that the leukoplakia placque cannot be removed with direct contact. Leukoplakia most commonly occurs on the buccal mucosa, dorsal tongue, and alveolar ridges. Most of these lesions are not associated with significant cellular atypia and spontaneously regress about 25% of the time; longitudinal follow-up of patients with leukoplakia documents a low incidence of malignant transformation (5% to 10%). Erythroplasia, on the other hand, is an ominous mucosal change. Clinically, it appears as a velvety red patch, most commonly affecting the floor of mouth, ventral tongue, soft palate, and tonsil. This lesion is associated with a high rate of severe dysplasia or in situ/invasive carcinoma at biopsy (80% to 90%). The risk of malignant conversion over time is also significant. As such, erythroplasia always requires biopsy.

Verrucous carcinoma is a low-grade variant of squamous cell carcinoma, most commonly found in the oral cavity and larynx. Clinically it resembles a wart and has an indolent growth pattern. Biopsies of the lesion reveal no invasive cancer. Verrucous carcinoma can be locally aggressive. True verrucous carcinomas rarely develop lymph node metastases.

In the nasopharynx and nasal cavity/paranasal sinuses, the frequency of squamous cell carcinoma is slightly less than other sites (80% to 85%). The incidence of the different types of epidermoid carcinoma of the nasopharynx shows marked geographic variation. Well-differentiated squamous cell carcinoma (World Health Organization [WHO] I), which is more common in North America, occurs in older patients and is more closely linked to traditional carcinogens of the upper respiratory tract, with less association with EBV. Poorly differentiated carcinomas (WHO types II and III), including those with heavy lymphocytic infiltration (so-called lymphoepithelioma), occur in younger patients, with major endemic areas in Asia and the Mediterranean.

## CLINICAL PRESENTATION AND NATURAL HISTORY

HNC is best described as a local and regional disease. In the majority of patients, symptoms and signs related to the primary tumor or its spread to regional (neck) lymph nodes are the primary manifestations of the disease. Asymptomatic cervical adenopathy may be the presenting complaint. An isolated neck mass in an adult should be considered cancer until proven otherwise. Spread of disease to regional lymphatics generally occurs in a predictable manner. For example, tumors of the oral cavity most commonly involve the submandibular and upper jugular nodes; tumors of the larynx, hypopharynx, and oropharynx involve the upper and middle jugular nodes; and nasopharynx cancer affects the retropharyngeal, jugulodigastric, and spinal accessory nodes. The frequency of lymph node metastases at presentation is related to the amount of capillary lymphatics draining the primary site. Sites with a rich supply of capillary lymphatics (e.g., nasopharynx and hypopharynx) commonly present with enlarged lymph nodes, relative to sites with few lymphatic channels (e.g., glottic larynx and paranasal sinuses). The size of the lesion, its grade, and the depth of tumor invasion are also important in predicting the frequency of lymph node involvement. Large, high-grade, and deeply infiltrating tumors are all more likely to have involved lymph nodes.

Tumors most commonly present as a mass or ulcer. Since much of the mucosal surface is not immediately accessible, symptoms are often ignored, leading to a delay in diagnosis. Symptoms that fail to respond to conservative treatment (i.e., antibiotics) in 4 weeks necessitate evaluation by a trained otolaryngologist–head and neck specialist. The symptoms and signs associated with these lesions vary with the primary site (Table 32-1) and are best understood in the context of the anatomy of the area.

Distant metastases are uncommon at presentation in HNC, occurring in less than 10% of patients. Ultimately 20% to 30% of patients manifest distant spread of the disease. Autopsy studies suggest that distant metastases are more frequent, but clinically do not manifest themselves, since the local and regional aspects of the disease are more prominent. The risk of distant metastases increases with involvement of neck nodes. The most common sites of distant spread are lung, liver, bone, and skin. Hypercalcemia occurs in 3% to 5% of cases and generally reflects recurrent or advanced disease.

Given the central roles tobacco and alcohol abuse play in the development of HNC, other problems stemming from their excessive use are associated with these tumors. It has been estimated that 50% to 60% of patients with HNC show significant signs of malnutrition. Many patients with HNC have comorbid ailments that complicate their management, including alcoholic liver disease and cirrhosis, chronic obstructive pulmonary disease, and vascular disease. Second primary cancers are increasingly appreciated in these patients, arising in other head and neck sites, lung, and esophagus. The expressions *field defect, field cancerization,* and *condemned mucosa* have all been used to describe this phenomenon. The risk has been estimated at 3% to 5% each year, although it is much higher in patients who continue to smoke and drink. Ultimately, 10% to 40% of patients develop a second primary cancer.

**Table 32-1.** Clinical presentation of HNC

| Primary site | Clinical presentations |
|---|---|
| Oral cavity | Pain, mouth ulcers, poorly fitting dentures, premalignant lesions, change in speech, foul mouth odor, trismus |
| Oropharynx | Sore throat, neck mass, ear pain, dysphagia, change in speech, trismus |
| Hypopharynx | Sore throat, ear pain, dysphagia, odynophagia, neck mass, hoarseness, foreign body sensation |
| Nasopharynx | Neck mass, hearing loss, otitis media, diplopia, epistaxis, nasal stuffiness, cranial neuropathies (esp. VI) |
| Supraglottic larynx | Odynophagia, sore throat, ear pain, neck mass, hemoptysis, cough, hoarseness, stridor |
| Glottic larynx | Hoarseness, sore throat, dysphagia, dyspnea |
| Paranasal sinuses | Sinusitis, toothache, loose teeth, ill-fitting dentures, epistaxis, proptosis, cheek swelling, hypoesthesia, pain |

## ROUTINE SCREENING

All smokers and users of smokeless tobacco products should have routine screening examinations of the oral cavity (see Managed Care Guides).

## DIAGNOSTIC EVALUATION AND STAGING

A careful history documenting symptoms, potential risk factors, and other comorbid medical problems is important. The percent of total body weight lost in the last 6 months and the patient's performance status as defined by a well-recognized scale quantitates disease impact and symptom severity. Physical examination is central to the appropriate evaluation of these patients. A thorough inspection of the head and neck is essential. Palpation of the parotid, submandibular, and thyroid glands is essential. Although the name of specific nodal groups can be used, a leveling system is now applied at many centers, and has proven to be clinically reproducible (Fig. 32-1). Level I refers to lymph nodes in the submental region and submandibular triangle; levels II, III, and IV refer to the upper, middle, and lower thirds of the internal jugular chain, respectively; level V refers to those nodes in the spinal accessory and transverse cervical chains. Many oral cancers involve the ventral surface of the tongue, and this area needs to be carefully assessed. At certain sites, such as the floor of the mouth and the base of the tongue, visual inspection alone either misses or underestimates the size of a lesion, and palpation or bimanual examination allows a better assessment. The nasopharynx warrants careful scrutiny. Visualization is facilitated by the use of mirrors and rigid and flexible scopes. Flexible scopes are especially useful in patients who continue to have a hyperactive gag reflex after adequate local anesthesia. Assessment of vocal cord mobility and facial nerve function is vital.

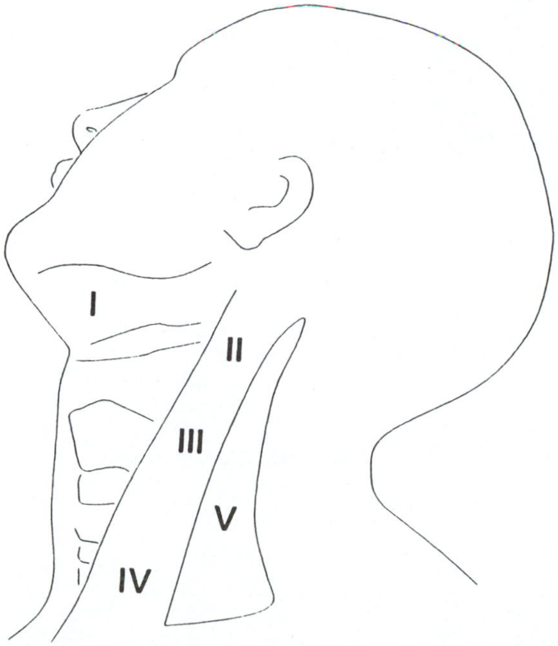


**Fig. 32-1.** *Level I,* lymph nodes in submental region and submandibular triangle; *levels II, III, IV,* lymph nodes in the upper, middle, and lower thirds of the internal jugular chain; *level V,* lymph nodes in the spinal accessory and transverse cervical chains.

Medical imaging with computed axial tomography (CAT) and magnetic resonance imaging (MRI) scans has increasingly been utilized in the evaluation of these patients. A barium swallow may be useful, especially in patients complaining of dysphagia. CAT scan has the advantage of lower cost, faster scanning time, and decreased motion artifact. MRI scan has the advantage of better differentiation of soft tissues and may be the preferable study at certain sites (e.g., nasopharynx and base of tongue). Routinely obtaining both studies is unnecessary; they should be ordered by the otolaryngologist–head and neck surgeon only when appropriate.

Because of the low frequency of distant metastases at presentation, an extensive search for distant metastatic disease is not routinely indicated. A chest x-ray is important, as much to document a possible synchronous lung primary or chronic lung disease in this smoking population as to demonstrate metastatic disease. Liver function abnormalities commonly reflect alcohol abuse or some other nonmalignant process. Formal imaging of the liver and bones is necessary only if appropriate biochemical abnormalities or symptoms are present. A complete blood count may suggest nutritional deficiency or chronic blood loss. Pulmonary function tests and electrocardiogram (ECG) are incorporated into preoperative assessment and may necessitate additional management.

Endoscopy under anesthesia is especially useful in patients with tumors of the larynx and pharynx. The routine use of so-called triple endoscopy (laryngoscopy, esophagoscopy, and bronchoscopy) in the evaluation of these patients is controversial. Proponents emphasize the 5% or higher incidence of synchronous primary cancers that affect prognosis and management. Triple endoscopy is appropriate in two groups: patients at high risk for multiple primaries with clinical evidence of diffuse mucosal abnormalities and patients who have cervical adenopathy without an identifiable primary site.

As with all malignancies, histologic proof is obtained from the primary site. When the primary is occult, histologic confirmation of a suspicious neck node is required. Initially, fine-needle aspiration is preferred instead of an open biopsy.The procedure is well tolerated and accurate (especially for squamous cell carcinoma), with no significant risk of seeding the needle tract. Multiple endoscopies should be performed to exclude an occult primary arising in the nasopharynx, base of tongue, tonsil, or pyriform sinus. If the needle biopsy is noncontributory, an excisional biopsy is indicated and the incision should be placed so it can be encompassed within the customary neck dissection incision. Preoperative counseling of the patient facilitates immediate performance of the neck dissection when malignancy is confirmed at frozen section. When followed long term, the minority of these patients (30%) have their primary tumor identified. It is interesting that the patients in whom the primary site is found generally do worse than those in whom it remains occult (30% versus 60% long-term survival, respectively).

The goal of this evaluation is to appropriately stage the cancer. This process allows one to better define prognosis and management and facilitates uniform reporting of treatment results. The staging system used with HNC is the TNM system, which was recently revised and agreed upon

## Managed Care Guide
## Oral cancer screening form

Date__________ Male____ Female____
Provider #_______ Location/Site______

A. *Risk Factors*

| | | | |
|---|---|---|---|
| 1. Do you smoke cigarettes now?............. | no ___ | yes ___ | pks/day ______ yrs ___ |
| 2. Did you ever smoke cigarettes? ............ | no ___ | yes ___ | pks/day ______ yrs ___ |
| 3. Do you use cigar/pipe/snuff/chewing tobacco? | no ___ | yes ___ | which? ______________ |
| 4. Do you drink alcohol now? .................... | no ___ | yes ___ | |
| 5. If no, did you ever drink alcohol? .......... | no ___ | yes ___ | when quit? ___________ |

B. *Symptoms* (as answered by the patient)

| | | | ≥ 2 weeks' duration? no | yes | unknown |
|---|---|---|---|---|---|
| 1. Do you have any soreness or pain in | | | | | |
| throat .................... | no ___ | yes ___ | ___ | ___ | ___ |
| mouth .................. | no ___ | yes ___ | ___ | ___ | ___ |
| ear ......................... | no ___ | yes ___ | ___ | ___ | ___ |
| jaw ....................... | no ___ | yes ___ | ___ | ___ | ___ |
| neck ..................... | no ___ | yes ___ | ___ | ___ | ___ |
| teeth ..................... | no ___ | yes ___ | ___ | ___ | ___ |
| on swallowing ........... | no ___ | yes ___ | ___ | ___ | ___ |
| 2. Has your voice changed? ............. | no ___ | yes ___ | ___ | ___ | ___ |
| 3. Is your voice hoarse? ................... | no ___ | yes ___ | ___ | ___ | ___ |
| 4. Have you felt any masses or lumps? ......... | no ___ | yes ___ | ___ | ___ | ___ |
| 5. Have you had trouble swallowing? .......... | no ___ | yes ___ | ___ | ___ | ___ |
| 6. Have you had trouble chewing? .............. | no ___ | yes ___ | ___ | ___ | ___ |
| 7. Have you lost >10 lb in the past 2 months? | no ___ | yes ___ | how much? __________ | | |
| 8. Have you coughed up blood? ..................... | no ___ | yes ___ | when? ______________ | | |

C. *Physical Examination*

| | | |
|---|---|---|
| Shortness of breath .......... | no ___ | yes ___ |
| Hoarseness ....................... | no ___ | yes ___ |
| Nose: blood in nares ......... | no ___ | yes ___ |
| Oral cavity: | | |
| caries ....................... | no ___ | yes ___ |
| blood in mouth ......... | no ___ | yes ___ |
| edentulous ............... | no ___ | yes ___ |
| white patches ........... | no ___ | yes ___ |
| red patches ............... | no ___ | yes ___ |
| bleeding areas .......... | no ___ | yes ___ |
| tenderness ................ | no ___ | yes ___ |
| mucosal lesion .......... | no ___ | yes ___ |
| Neck: | | |
| pain ............... | no ___ | yes ___ |
| masses ........... | no ___ | yes ___ |
| nodes .............. | no ___ | yes ___ |

Locate positive findings below:

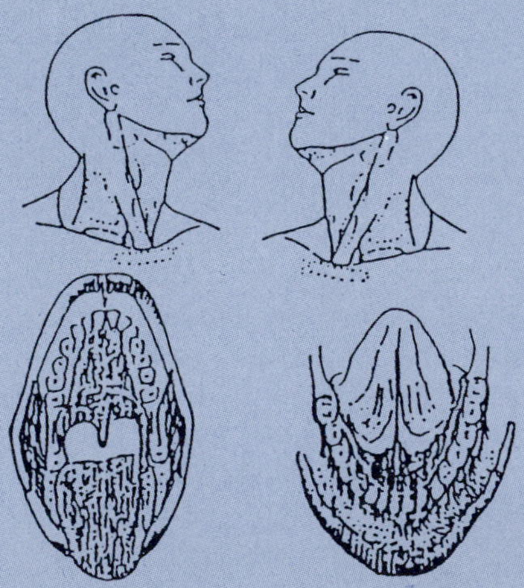

D. Were the above signs and symptoms the reason for this visit? no ___ yes ___

E. *Conclusion* (check one):
Normal ___ Abnormal, cancer not suspected ___ Abnormal, suspicious for cancer ___

F. *Action* (check one):
None required ___ Refer for followup because of: Screening exam ___ Other ___ Exam not done ___ Reason __________

Signature ____________________

From Prout MN, et al: J Cancer Educ 7:139, 1992.

## Managed Care Guide
### Criteria for a positive head and neck cancer screen

The following criteria and recommended actions have been established for "abnormal, suspicious for cancer sign and/or symptom" found at the time of primary screen.

| Criteria | Recommended action |
|---|---|
| Simple leukoplakia: white patch that does not scrape off | Careful oral examination<br>Elective referral to ENT |
| Complex leukoplakia: mixed white and red patches | Immediate referral to ENT |
| Erythroplakia: red velvety patches | Immediate referral to ENT |
| Mucosal lesion with gross appearance of cancer | Immediate referral to ENT |
| Hoarseness or voice change persistent throughout the day for 2 weeks | Immediate referral to ENT |
| Mucosal lesion of uncertain type in high-risk anatomic area: floor of mouth, ventrolateral tongue | Immediate referral to ENT |

From Prout MN et al: *J Cancer Educ* 7:139, 1992.

## TNM system of cancer staging

**Tumor (T)—varies with primary site**

*Examples*

Oropharynx/oral cavity

$T_1$ Tumor ≤2 cm in greatest dimension

$T_2$ Tumor >2 cm but ≤4 cm in greatest dimension

$T_3$ Tumor >4 cm in greatest dimension

$T_4$ Tumor with massive invasion of adjacent structures

Supraglottic larynx

$T_1$ Tumor limited to one subsite of supraglottis with normal vocal cord mobility

$T_2$ Tumor invades more than one subsite of supraglottis or glottis, with normal vocal cord mobility

$T_3$ Tumor limited to larynx with vocal cord fixation and/or invades postcricoid area, medial wall of pyriform sinus, or preepiglottic tissues

$T_4$ Tumor invades through thyroid cartilage and/or extends to other tissues beyond the larynx

**Lymph node (N)—same for all primary sites**

$N_0$ No regional lymph node metastasis

$N_1$ Metastasis in a single ipsilateral lymph node, ≤3 cm in greatest dimension

$N_2$ $N_{2a}$: Metastasis in a single ipsilateral lymph node, >3 cm but ≤6 cm in greatest dimension

$N_{2b}$: Metastasis in multiple ipsilateral lymph nodes, none >6 cm in greatest dimension

$N_{2c}$: Metastasis in bilateral or contralateral lymph nodes, none >6 cm in greatest dimension

$N_3$ Metastasis in a lymph node >6 cm in greatest dimension

**Distant metastasis (M)—same for all primary sites**

$M_0$ No distant metastasis

$M_1$ Distant metastasis

**TNM stage**

| | $N_0$ | $N_1$ | $N_2$ | $N_3$ |
|---|---|---|---|---|
| $T_1$ | Stage I | | | |
| $T_2$ | Stage II | | | |
| $T_3$ | Stage III | | | Stage IV |
| $T_4$ | | | | |

by the American Joint Committee on Cancer and the International Union Against Cancer (see the box at left). The T stage depends on the site, size, and extent of invasion at the primary site. Tumors of the oral cavity and oropharynx use the same criteria; other sites are different. The N stage is defined by the number, size, and location relative to the primary lesion of the regional lymph nodes. The M stage refers to the presence or absence of distant metastases. The N and M formulations are the same for all primary sites. The respective T, N, and M stages are then combined to create four stages. Stage I is the best prognostic group; stage IV is the worst prognostic group. Clinical staging (excluding information obtained at surgery) is the type most commonly used, since clinical decisions are typically based on this information.

## PRINCIPLES OF MANAGEMENT

Patients with HNC present a challenge on many levels. Ongoing tobacco and alcohol abuse are common, as are other medical comorbidities. Their disease and its treatment can cause dysfunction and disfigurement. Optimal treatment and rehabilitation of these patients therefore requires close interdisciplinary cooperation not only among the treating surgical, radiation, and medical oncologists, but also among other health professionals, including dentists and prosthodontists, speech and swallowing therapists, audiologists, nutritionists, occupational and physical therapists, and psychiatrists. Plans for rehabilitating patients should start before treatment.

Control of disease at the primary site and in the neck is the primary goal. Historically, surgery and radiation therapy have been the principal treatment modalities. Chemotherapy's role is best established in the palliative setting but is being actively investigated in combination with surgery and radiation, with important implications for the development of function preserving therapy and the treatment of patients with unresectable disease. In general, treatment is determined by the TNM stage at presentation (Table 32-2), although there are site-specific variations. Management of the primary site and that of the neck are related but also present separate concerns. Treatment plans should consider both survival and quality of life.

For limited disease ($T_1$-$T_2$, $N_0$-$N_1$, $M_0$) single-modality treatment with surgery or radiation is associated with

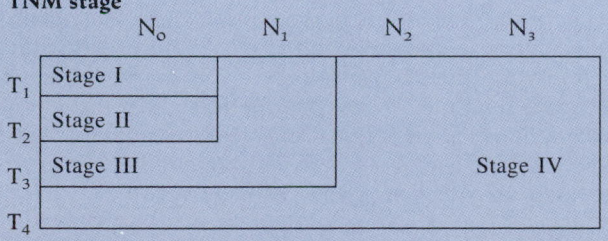

**Table 32-2.** Head and neck cancer treatment

| Disease category | Stage | Standard therapy | Cure rate |
|---|---|---|---|
| Limited | I, II, III ($T_1/T_2$, $N_0/N_1$, $M_0$) | Surgery or RT | 60%-90% |
| Advanced | III, IV ($T_3/T_4$, $N_2/N_3$, $M_0$) | Surgery and RT* | 10%-60% |
| Metastatic | IV ($M_1$) | Chemotherapy; other palliative treatment | Rare |
| Recurrent | Variable | Surgery and/or RT if feasible | Selected patients salvaged |
| | | Chemotherapy; other palliative treatment | Rare |

*RT or chemotherapy/RT if the cancer is unresectable. Chemotherapy/RT with surgery reserved for salvage in patients with advanced larynx cancer.
*RT*, Radiation therapy.

equivalent results (60% to 90% cure rate). The decision as to which modality depends on a variety of factors, including primary site, patient age and general health, local expertise, functional concerns, and patient preference. Patients with an $N_0$ stage can have their necks treated electively depending on the risk of occult nodal disease. This estimate is based on T stage, primary site, differentiation of the tumor, evidence of vascular and lymphatic invasion, and depth of invasion of the primary tumor. If the estimated risk of neck failure is greater than 15%, elective neck staging or treatment is advisable. Obviously, the results of treatment with one modality may require the immediate addition of the other. A positive margin after resection or the finding at neck dissection of multiple positive lymph nodes or extracapsular extension necessitates postoperative radiation therapy; a persistent or growing mass after radiation therapy requires resection.

Patients with bulky, advanced resectable disease ($T_3$-$T_4$, $N_2$-$N_3$, $M_0$) require treatment with a combination of surgery and radiation, since this approach has improved local and regional disease control compared to unimodality therapy. The expected cure rate in this group is 10% to 60%. Because of the poor survival, chemotherapy has been studied in combination with standard local and regional treatment in the hope of improving tumor control. This approach remains investigational. In patients with unresectable disease radiation therapy alone has historically been the standard treatment. The integration of chemotherapy with radiation appears to improve response rates and potentially survival and is an active area of study.

If a patient has recurrent disease after primary treatment, attempts are made to salvage the patient with surgery and/or radiation, depending on previous therapy. If a patient previously received definitive radiation therapy, the options of receiving further radiation are limited. Patients undergoing salvage therapy are at higher risk for disease recurrence compared to similarly staged, untreated patients. Patients with recurrent disease that is not amenable to further surgery or radiation and patients with distant metastatic disease ($M_1$) at presentation or recurrence are treated with palliative chemotherapy.

Five-year survival rates are generally reported for HNC. However, most relapses occur within the first 2 years after treatment. Involved regional lymph nodes reduce the anticipated cure rate within each T stage by approximately 50%. Anticipated survival rates depend on the stage and primary site. For example, hypopharynx primaries have a worse prognosis, stage for stage, than do larynx primaries, even though the structures are immediately adjacent to each other.

The treatment of patients with an occult primary and metastatic squamous cell carcinoma in a cervical node depends on the clinical presentation. Patients with an $N_1$ neck diagnosis can be treated with primary radiation or a neck dissection with equivalent local control. Patients with an $N_2$ or $N_3$ neck diagnosis probably require treatment with neck dissection and radiation therapy. Patients with advanced neck disease have a worse prognosis. Elective irradiation of the potential primary mucosal sites should sterilize the low-bulk disease. However, radiation to the mucosal surfaces will increase the morbidity of treatment in the form of xerostomia and potentially complicate subsequent salvage therapy if necessary.

## Surgery

Certain advantages are associated with surgical treatment of HNC. The treatment time is shorter, and surgery is limited to those tissues at greatest risk of tumor invasion. The immediate and long-term sequelae of radiation are avoided. Pathologic information found at surgery is useful in predicting prognosis and in planning postoperative treatment with radiation.

An adequate surgical procedure requires margins free from tumor. In more advanced lesions this may necessitate a procedure associated with significant functional or cosmetic morbidity. In patients with larynx and pharynx tumors a total laryngectomy may be required. Tumors of the oral cavity and oropharynx may require a composite resection, with removal of part of the mandible and en bloc resection of the primary tumor and regional lymph nodes. Patients with extensive oropharynx tumors often require total laryngectomy, not to remove the primary tumor but to prevent the sequelae of chronic aspiration. Patients with advanced paranasal sinus tumors may require a radical maxillectomy, which occasionally includes orbital exenteration.

There are function-preserving procedures that adhere to sound surgical oncologic principles. Supraglottic laryngectomy and hemilaryngectomy are examples that spare laryngeal function. Successful application of these procedures requires both surgical expertise and careful patient selection. The use of a variety of skin and bone grafts can optimize the functional and cosmetic results. A prosthodontist can customize obturators and other prostheses that facilitate speech and swallowing.

Certain features of a tumor indicate that it is unresectable. The distinction between it being technically unresectable and unresectable for medical reasons is an important one. Contraindications for resection include massive skull base involvement, prevertebral fascia invasion, carotid artery encasement, and skin infiltration. CAT and MRI can be helpful in assessing some of these issues.

The traditional radical neck dissection involves removal of the cervical lymphatic tissues, the sternocleidomastoid muscle, the internal jugular vein, and the eleventh cranial nerve. The procedure can be associated with pain, shoulder weakness, and paresthesia. Because of these potential morbidities, a variety of modified and selective procedures that preserve function have evolved. The clinical decision to use one of these modified or selective techniques requires careful patient selection.

## Radiation therapy

Compared with surgery, radiation is associated with certain advantages. In some instances (e.g., early larynx cancer) the functional results are better. When elective therapy to high-risk lymph nodes is indicated, this treatment can easily be incorporated into patient management. This option is especially relevant in patients who are at risk for bilateral neck node involvement. There is rarely immediate treatment-related mortality.

The ability of radiation therapy to control local and regional disease as a single modality is inversely related to tumor bulk. The probability of tumor control is dose dependent. Large total doses are required to sterilize squamous cell carcinoma. The dose and portals of treatment depend on the primary site and goals of therapy. When single-modality, definitive radiation is used, doses of 6500 to 7000 cGy are necessary. This is generally administered daily over 6 to 7 weeks with a daily fraction size of 180 to 200 cGy. These are optimally delivered either by a megavoltage linear accelerator or $^{60}$Co unit. Careful attention must be paid to the dose received by the spinal cord, since its radiation tolerance is considerably lower.

Radiation therapy can be combined with surgery via either preoperative or postoperative dosing. The customary preoperative dose is 5000 cGy; the difficulty of subsequent surgery and the frequency of serious postoperative complications increase when the radiation dose exceeds this level. The postoperative dose to the primary site and neck are influenced by the findings at surgery and range from 5000 to 7000 cGy depending on factors such as surgical margins and the presence of residual gross disease. Postoperative radiation is currently the more commonly used approach. The local and regional control rate appears to be higher with postoperative treatment, although no survival advantage has been proven. Radiation therapy generally starts 2 to 4 weeks after resection, at which time the wounds are satisfactorily healed.

Adverse effects of radiation in the head and neck can occur both early and late. Mucositis and edema lead to dysphagia, hoarseness, and otitis media. These toxicities are generally managed with conservative measures and resolve with time. Occasionally, temporary placement of a feeding tube, tracheostomy, or myringotomy with pressure-equalizing tubes may be necessary. Fibrosis and induration of irradiated tissues develop to a variable extent. Xerostomia and loss of taste occur during treatment and are related to salivary gland dysfunction. The long-term return of function is variable, in part dependent on dose and portals. Because of the reduction of saliva, dental caries and periodontal disease can be considerable. Dental evaluation before radiation therapy, with extraction of damaged teeth, optimization of oral hygiene, and fluoride treatments, is essential and can prevent long-term complications. Lhermitte's sign, which is characterized by shocklike sensations in the spine, arms, and legs with neck flexion, occurs when the spinal cord is irradiated and is self-limiting. Varying degrees of thyroid dysfunction may develop, and thyroid function tests should be closely monitored in those patients undergoing surgery and radiation to the neck, larynx, or pharynx. Two serious late complications are myelopathy due to overdosing of the cervical spinal cord and osteoradionecrosis of the mandible.

Several techniques aimed at improving the therapeutic index of radiation therapy are under active clinical evaluation and investigation. Radiation implants (brachytherapy) are placed within the tumor bed. The implant can either be permanent (e.g., $^{125}$I) or temporary via afterloading catheters (e.g., $^{192}$Ir). These can be used either alone or in combination with external beam treatment. Their use is associated with excellent local control in selected tumors of the oropharynx (base of tongue) and oral cavity. Hyperfractionated radiation (using more than one fraction per day) has yielded encouraging results in patients with advanced tumors.

## Chemotherapy

By itself, chemotherapy is not curative in HNC. A number of chemotherapy agents cause a major shrinkage of tumor in 20% to 40% of HNC patients. Combinations including the drug cisplatin are generally felt to have the highest response rates. The exact response rate depends on the tumor bulk and previous treatment. Large, previously treated tumors have the lowest response rates.

Historically the prime role of chemotherapy has been in the palliation of patients who have largely exhausted surgical and radiation treatment options or in patients with distant metastatic disease. Under these circumstances the gold standard drug is methotrexate. In general, the treatment is well tolerated, but possible toxicities include mucositis, myelosuppression, hepatotoxicity, nephrotoxicity, and fatigue. Cisplatin is considered to be as active but is associated with more toxicity and greater difficulty of administration. Toxicities include nausea and vomiting, myelosuppression, nephrotoxicity, neurotoxicity, and ototoxity. Unfortunately, the median duration of response with these agents remains short and the median overall survival poor. In hopes of improving these results, a variety of combination chemotherapy regimens have been compared to treatment with a single agent (in most cases methotrexate). These trials have revealed no improvement in survival.

The response rates in patients with previous untreated HNC are higher than in those with recurrent or metastatic disease. Indeed, cisplatin-based combination chemotherapy yields response proportions in the 60% to 90%

range, with complete responses in 20% to 60% of patients. Despite these high response rates, neither induction chemotherapy, adjuvant chemotherapy, nor some combination thereof integrated with standard surgery and radiation has improved survival in these patients compared to results with surgery and radiation alone.

The use of chemotherapy in a treatment scheme that does not improve survival may still be useful, if the functional result of such treatment is superior to that after standard surgery and radiation therapy. Since radiation is most effective when the tumor burden is small, another potential role of chemotherapy would be to decrease the tumor bulk before definitive therapy. A recent randomized trial has tested this approach in advanced cancer of the larynx. Patients with stage III and IV larynx cancer were randomized to one of two treatment arms: standard total laryngectomy and postoperative radiation versus induction chemotherapy followed by definitive radiation, with total laryngectomy reserved for chemotherapy nonresponse or relapse. The survival in both treatment arms was equivalent, and over 60% of surviving patients in the chemotherapy/radiation arm had their larynx preserved.

The use of chemotherapy concomitantly with radiation has been a new area of intense investigation. The emphasis has been on choosing chemotherapy agents that have independent activity in HNC but can also serve as radiation enhancers or sensitizers. Randomized trials suggest this approach yields a higher response rate and improves local control compared with radiation alone. Local mucocutaneous toxicity is generally increased. The potential utility of concomitant chemotherapy and radiation may be a significant part of a function preservation treatment approach and is currently often applied to patients with unresectable disease.

## PREVENTION

Since tobacco and alcohol use are the primary risk factors for HNC, any prevention program must focus on the cessation or modification of these behaviors. Tobacco cessation is most successful when a counseling program is combined with the use of a tapering nicotine patch. Even in patients who stop smoking and consuming alcohol, however, the risk for second malignancy persists for years. Accumulating evidence suggest the retinoids may be important in the prevention of epithelial carcinogenesis. A recent randomized study evaluated the utility in this regard of 13-*cis* retinoic acid (50 to 100 mg/m$^2$/day orally) versus placebo in patients who were disease free after primary treatment for HNC. There was no difference in the number or pattern of relapses or the overall survival in the two groups of patients, but there was a significantly decreased rate of second primary tumors in the treatment arm. Toxicities associated with the 13-*cis* retinoic acid included skin dryness, cheilitis, hypertriglyceridemia, and conjunctivitis. Approximately 20% of patients did not complete treatment because of toxic effects. Less toxic schedules and less toxic substances (β-carotene and vitamin E) are currently being investigated.

## SPECIFIC SITES

### Salivary glands

Cancer of the major and minor salivary glands is uncommon, accounting for about 7% of head and neck malignancies. They arise from the three paired major salivary glands (parotid, submandibular, sublingual) and the approximately 700 minor salivary glands that are distributed throughout the upper aerodigestive tract. There may be an association with previous low-dose radiation exposure, such as that used for acne or lymphoid hypertrophy. There appears to be an association between salivary gland tumors and patients with a history of breast cancer, cancer of the male genital tract, HNC, and skin cancer.

A variety of benign and malignant histologic changes occur in the salivary glands. Approximately 80% of all salivary gland tumors arise in the parotid, 10% to 15% in the submandibular gland, and the remainder in the sublingual and minor salivary glands. The odds of a salivary gland neoplasm being malignant are inversely related to the size of the gland. It is estimated that 20% to 30% of parotid, 40% to 60% of submandibular, and the majority of sublingual and minor salivary gland tumors are malignant. The distinction between benign and malignant tumors can be difficult. The parotid is a potential site for regional and distant metastases, particularly for skin cancer arising on the face.

Salivary gland tumors grow by direct extension and infiltration and generally present as a painless swelling. Rapid growth and facial nerve involvement are both associated with a malignant histology and a poor prognosis. The clinical aggressiveness of the tumors varies with size, histology, and grade. The incidence of clinical and subclinical neck node metastases is lower than with HNC. Distant metastases are uncommon. The risk of distant failure is highest for adenoid cystic tumors, the lung being the most common site.

The use of fine-needle aspiration in the management of salivary neoplasms is controversial. The information does not change therapy in most cases, but it may be useful in treatment planning under certain circumstances (e.g., unresectable tumors). Excisional biopsy should be discouraged, since it only complicates subsequent definitive therapy. CAT or MRI may provide additional useful information. These modalities distinguish between intrinsic and extrinsic glandular masses, extraglandular extension, and the presence of occult metastatic cervical disease. Sialograms were more commonly used in the past but have been replaced by these newer technologies.

Surgery is the treatment of choice for salivary gland neoplasms. Enucleation of salivary gland tumors leads to local recurrence, even with benign tumors, and should be avoided. Excision of the superficial or deep lobe of the parotid gland with facial nerve preservation is performed depending on the tumor's location. The entire gland is removed in submandibular and sublingual tumors. Elective neck dissections are generally not performed, although there may be a role for sampling of the adjacent lymph nodes based on histology and size. Depending on the location and extent of the parotid tumors, resections may include part of the temporal bone, mandible or zygoma, and the facial nerve. There has been success with placement of an immediate nerve graft when the facial nerve must be resected. Management of the eye, including a moisture chamber at night and the use of artificial preparations for replacement of tears, is mandatory to prevent exposure keratopathy, which can accompany facial paralysis. Postoperative radiation is generally indicated for tumors that are high grade, large, deeply invasive, with positive or close margins or positive nodes. Doses are similar to those used with HNC. Primary radiation is generally limited to patients with unresectable tumors. Neutron beam therapy is under investigation in this regard. There is no standard role for chemotherapy in the management of salivary gland tumors.

Parotid tumors tend to have a better survival than other sites. Adenoid cystic cancers often have indolent growth, even when distant metastases are present. Ten-year survival statistics are a more accurate estimate of treatment results for many of these tumors due to the potentially long natural histories.

## Thyroid

Cancer of the thyroid accounts for approximately 12,000 new cases per year and 1000 deaths. There is an increased incidence in female versus males, and they are more common in the white population. Prognosis is improved in women and in patients who develop their disease at a younger age. Exposure to radiation therapy places patients at an increased risk for development of thyroid cancer. Approximately 10% of medullary carcinomas of the thyroid are inherited as an autosomal dominant gene. Medullary thyroid cancer is associated with the multiple endocrine neoplasia syndromes.

Thyroid neoplasms represent an array of benign and malignant processes. The most common thyroid mass represents either multinodular goiter or benign follicular adenomas. The well-differentiated thyroid carcinomas—papillary and follicular adenocarcinomas—represent nearly 90% of all thyroid malignancies. Papillary adenocarcinoma (50% to 60%) is nearly twice as common as follicular adenocarcinoma (25% to 35%). The high-grade variants include medullary (5%) and undifferentiated/anaplastic (5%) carcinomas.

Thyroid malignancies most commonly present as a painless thyroid mass. Cervical lymphadenopathy is consistent with lymph node metastases. Unlike HNC, cervical metastases do not adversely affect long-term survival; distant metastases, however, are associated with reduced long-term survival. Hoarseness may represent recurrent laryngeal nerve paralysis. (See Chapter 34 for diagnosis and management.)

## BIBLIOGRAPHY


Deiter M, et al: Modern management of cervical scrofula, *Head Neck* 11:60, 1989.

de Visscher JGAM, van der Wal KGH, de Vogel PL: The plunging ranula: pathogenesis, diagnosis, and management, *J Craniomaxillofac Surg* 17:182, 1989.

Dillon WP, Harnsberger RH: The impact of radiologic imaging on staging of cancer of the head and neck, *Semin Oncol* 18(2):64, 1991.

Friedman M, et al: Nodal size of metastatic squamous cell carcinoma of the neck, *Laryngoscope* 103:854, 1993.

Jacobs C: The internist in the management of head and neck cancer, *Ann Intern Med* 113:771, 1990.

Johns ME, Goldsmith MM: Incidence, diagnosis, and classification of salivary gland tumors, *Oncology* 3(2):47, 1989.

Johns ME, Goldsmith MM: Current management of salivary gland tumors, *Oncology* 3(3):85, 1989.

Lindberg RD: Distribution of cervical lymph node metastases from squamous cell carcinoma of the upper respiratory and digestive tracts, *Cancer* 29:1446, 1972.

Lucente FE: Impact of the acquired immunodeficiency syndrome epidemic on the practice of laryngology, *Ann Otolol Rhinol Laryngol* 102:(suppl 161), 1993.

McGuirt WF: Panendoscopy as a screening examination for simultaneous primary tumors in head and neck cancer: a prospective sequential study and review, *Laryngoscope* 92:569, 1982.

Million RR, Cassisi NJ, editors: *Management of head and neck cancer: a multidisciplinary approach,* Philadelphia, 1984, JB Lippincott.

Mulliken JB, Glowacki J: Hemangioma and vascular malformations in infants and children: a classification based on endothelial characteristics, *Plast Reconstr Surg* 69:412, 198.

Pfister DG et al: Current status of larynx preservation with combined modality therapy, *Oncology* 6:33, 1992.

Rice DH, Spiro RH, editors: *Current concepts in head and neck cancer,* Atlanta, 1989, The American Cancer Society.

Schantz SP et al: Cancer of the head and neck. In DeVita VT, Hellman S, Rosenberg SA, editors: *Cancer principles and practice of oncology,* ed 4, Philadelphia, 1993, JB Lippincott.

Silverman S, editor: *Oral cancer,* Atlanta, 1990, The American Cancer Society.

Thawley SE, Panje WR, editors: *Comprehensive management of head and neck tumors,* Philadelphia, 1987, WB Saunders.

Witterick IJ, et al: Nonpalpable occult and metastatic papillary thyroid carcinoma, *Laryngoscope* 103:149, 1993.

Work WP: Hemangiomas of the head and neck, *Ann Otol Rhinol Laryngol* 87:633, 1978.

Zangwill KM, et al: Cat scratch disease in Connecticut: epidemiology, risk factors, and evaluation of a new diagnostic test, *N Engl J Med* 329:8, 1993.

# IV ENDOCRINE, DIABETES, AND METABOLISM

CHAPTER

# 33 Diabetes Mellitus

**Stuart R. Chipkin**
**Peter A. Gottlieb**
**David D. Bogorad**
**Frank Parker**

The term *diabetes mellitus* refers to a common clinical syndrome of hyperglycemia that arises from many different causes. Subpopulations of patients with diabetes have had specific genes and biochemical abnormalities linked to their hyperglycemia. For example, an abnormality of glucokinase, a critical gene within the pancreatic β-cell glucose-sensing pathway, appears to identify patients at risk for maturity-onset diabetes of the young (MODY). As further advances refine our understanding of diabetes, treatment strategies will change. For the foreseeable future, glycemic control remains the most effective therapy.

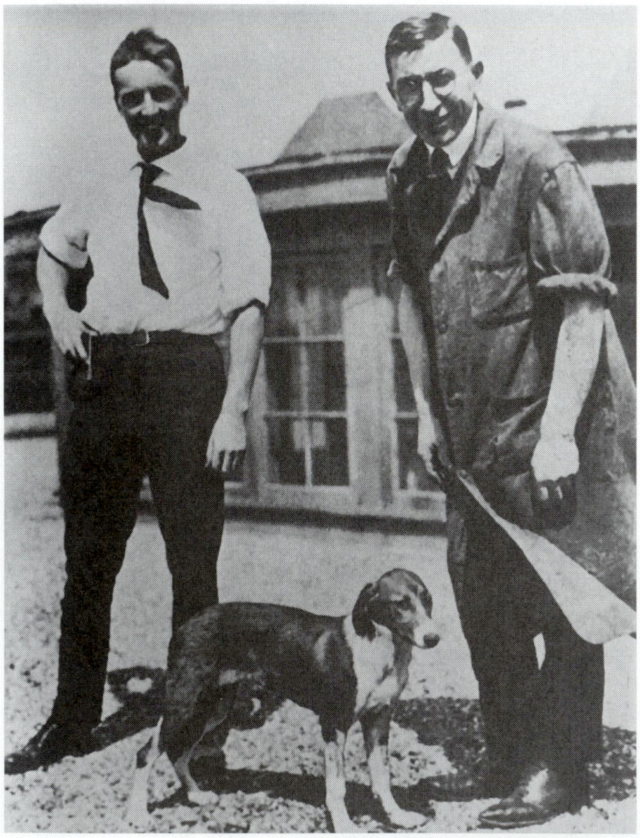

**Fig. 33-1.** Frederick Banting and Charles H. Best standing beside Marge, the pancreatectomized beagle in whom they demonstrated that exogenous insulin could reverse diabetes mellitus and sustain life (1921). (Courtesy of Mrs. Charles H. Best.)

The discovery of insulin at the beginning of this century was predicted to end diabetes as a health problem (Fig. 33-1). However, as we close this century, diabetes and its complications continue to be major causes of morbidity and mortality throughout the world. At present diabetes mellitus affects nearly 14 million people in the United States. Yearly costs of diabetes care are estimated to be over $90 billion, almost half of which reflects direct health care costs, whereas the remainder is for indirect costs such as disability and lost productivity. If costs are divided by the number of patients, the average yearly medical care cost per person with diabetes is three times greater for diabetics ($9493) than for nondiabetics ($2604). The majority of this amount is spent on managing, rather than preventing, the late complications of the disease. A strategy that utilizes resources early to prevent future complications is critical to the successful treatment of diabetes.

Unlike some major health problems such as cardiovascular disease, the frequency of diabetes is increasing in the United States and around the world. The incidence of type I, or insulin-dependent diabetes mellitus (IDDM), is on the rise in many westernized societies for unknown reasons. As certain groups within our society increase, such as people of color and the elderly, the incidence of type II, or non–insulin-dependent diabetes mellitus (NIDDM), can also be expected to rise dramatically (Table 33-1).

## EPIDEMIOLOGY

Although the discovery of insulin markedly reduced the acute mortality of diabetes, chronic complications of diabetes continue to be a leading cause of morbidity and mortality in America (Table 33-2). Diabetes accounts for 8% of all legal blindness in the United States. It is the leading cause of end-stage renal disease, which is of particular concern to African-American and Hispanic diabetic patients, who appear to be at 3 to 6 times the risk for this complication. As a result of both peripheral vascular disease and peripheral polyneuropathy, diabetes is the leading cause of nontraumatic amputation of the lower extremities. Patients with diabetes are at least 1.5 to 2 times more likely than nondiabetic patients to develop cardiovascular disease independent of other known risk factors.

One of the most disconcerting statistics regarding diabetes is the number of undiagnosed cases. Epidemio-

**Table 33-1.** Age-standardized rates of diabetes by race or ethnicity

| Race or ethnicity | Prevalence (%) | Rate relative to whites |
|---|---|---|
| White | 6.2 | 1.0 |
| Cuban | 9.3 | 1.5 |
| African-American | 10.2 | 1.6 |
| Mexican | 13.0 | 2.1 |
| Puerto Rican | 13.4 | 2.2 |
| Japanese-American | 13.9 | 2.2 |
| Pimas (Native American) | 27.5 | 4.4 |

logic surveys continue to estimate that 50% of all people with diabetes, even those who report being under a physician's care, are undiagnosed. A major goal for primary care physicians and health care providers needs to be the accurate diagnosis and initiation of therapy for all patients with diabetes mellitus.

## CLASSIFICATION OF DIABETES

### Insulin-dependent (type I) and non-insulin-dependent (type II) diabetes mellitus

Diabetes mellitus is classified into different types based on etiology and duration of hyperglycemia. Due to the typical age of onset, type I (IDDM) has previously been referred to as juvenile-onset diabetes. However, this term is inaccurate since older patients (over 20 years) can present with classic IDDM. The previously used term *adult-onset diabetes* has also been replaced by NIDDM, since a subset of these patients may develop hyperglycemia during their teenage years (MODY).

Table 33-3 lists some of the differences between type I and type II diabetes mellitus. The importance of understanding the difference between insulin requiring and insulin dependent is not merely semantic. For example, a young obese patient with adequate insulin reserves, arbitrarily given a diagnosis of IDDM because he is treated with insulin, might never be given oral agents even after diet and exercise result in significant weight loss and improved glucose homeostasis. Conversely, an older insulin-dependent patient undergoing general surgery and incorrectly thought to have NIDDM might have insulin doses held due to "normal" blood sugar values, and the condition could potentially deteriorate to ketoacidosis.

### Impaired glucose tolerance

Patients with impaired glucose tolerance (IGT) have plasma glucose levels that are higher than normal but not diagnostic for diabetes. Diagnostic criteria based on an oral glucose tolerance test are (1) fasting glucose less than 140 mg/dl, (2) 2-hour glucose between 140 and 200 mg/dl, and (3) intervening glucose level over 200 mg/dl. Many of these individuals go on to develop NIDDM. Estimates range from a low of 11% after 3 years to a high of 25% at 5 years. Race and ethnicity may increase the risk for NIDDM significantly; 90% of Pima Indians with IGT develop diabetes after 10 years. Other factors that may predict progression to diabetes are glucose concentrations and obesity. Identifying and counseling these patients is important because initiating a diet and exercise program at this stage of disease may prevent or delay the onset of NIDDM and additionally reduce the increased risk that IGT patients have for cardiovascular disease.

### Secondary diabetes

Many conditions can lead to the development of hyperglycemia by interfering with pancreatic insulin secretion or peripheral insulin action (see the boxes on p. 478). Thiazide diuretics, β-blockers, and nicotinic acid are commonly prescribed agents that can significantly raise blood sugars. Hyperglycemia typically improves after stopping any of these medications. Overproduction of counterinsulin hormones such as cortisol, epinephrine, growth hormone, and glucagon can also cause hyperglycemia. Last, conditions that result in the destruction of the insulin-producing β-cells of the pancreas can lead to secondary diabetes.

**Table 33-2.** Frequency and yearly cost of diabetic complications in the United States

| Complication | Frequency | Cost |
|---|---|---|
| Retinopathy | 95% after 20 years<br>2%-6% with blindness | 2000 new cases = $100 million in disability and lost productivity |
| Nephropathy | 34% of IDDM and 19% of NIDDM by 15 years | >10,000 new cases of ESRD = >$300 million in health care costs alone |
| Cardiovascular disease | 1.5-2 times more frequent | 80,000 deaths per year |
| Extremity amputation | >50% of nontraumatic amputations | 30,000 amputations per year<br>$750 million in disability and other costs |

*ESRD*, End-stage renal disease.

**Table 33-3.** Comparison of type I and type II diabetes

| Characteristic | IDDM | NIDDM |
|---|---|---|
| Synonyms | Type I, juvenile onset (formerly) | Type II, adult onset (formerly) |
| Age at onset | Usually <25 years | Usually >40 years |
| Body mass | Lean | Obese (80%-90% of cases) |
| Insulin levels | None, low | Low, normal, or high |
| Glucose at presentation | 300-500 mg/dl | 300-1000 mg/dl |
| Clinical onset | Sudden; 1-3 weeks of acute illness | Gradual; weeks to months |
| Acid/base disturbance | Ketoacidosis | None, or mild lactic acidosis ± rare ketones |
| Genetics | Majority sporadic; only 10% familial; 30%-50% concordance in monozygotic twins | Frequently familial; 100% concordance in monozygotic twins |
| Associated with autoimmune disease | Yes | No |

## Secondary forms of diabetes

**Drug induced**

See the box below.

**Endocrine diseases**

Acromegaly
Aldosteronism
Glucocorticoid excess (Cushing's syndrome; iatrogenic)
Pheochromocytoma
Thyrotoxicosis
Somatostatinoma/hypothalamic disorders
Insulin receptor abnormalities (lipodystrophy; virilization; acanthosis nigricans)

**Other diseases**

Amyloidosis
Cystic fibrosis
Hemochromatosis
Pancreatitis
Pancreatic cancer
Malnutrition
Congenital disorders such as Klinefelter's syndrome, Turner's syndrome, optic atrophy diabetes mellitus, Laurence-Moon-Biedl syndrome, Down syndrome

## Drugs associated with abnormalities in glucose tolerance

**Agents that elevate blood sugar**

***Hormones***

Glucocorticoids
Estrogens
Thyroid hormone ($T_4$ and/or $T_3$)
Catecholamines

***Antihypertensives***

Diuretics—thiazides, furosemide
β-Blockers—propranolol, atenolol
Prazosin
Clonidine

***Other drugs***

Streptozocin
Nicotinic acid (niacin)
Isoniazid
Lithium
Phenytoin
Indomethacin
Tricyclic antidepressants
Phenothiazines

**Drugs that lower blood sugar**

Pentamidine
Ethanol
Choloroquine, hydroxycholoroquine
Quinidine, quinine
Terbutaline, β-agonists
Ritodrine

### Gestational diabetes

Gestational diabetes occurs in previously nondiabetic women who typically develop hyperglycemia during the second half of pregnancy but who become normoglycemic after birth. Similar to patients with IGT, between 30% and 50% of patients with gestational diabetes eventually develop NIDDM within their lifetimes.

### Other statistical categories

Two other groups of patients with glucose abnormalities have been identified. *Previous abnormality of glucose intolerance* is reserved for those patients who have had documented hyperglycemia in the past but whose glucose profiles now appear normal. This category is important because individuals who are now normoglycemic should not be mislabeled as diabetic for insurance and employment purposes. *Potential abnormality of glucose intolerance* is used to classify patients whose risk of diabetes is greater than that of the general population, such as first-degree relatives of people with diabetes.

## PATHOPHYSIOLOGY

Hyperglycemia occurs either when circulating levels of insulin are low or when cellular sensitivity to insulin is impaired. Without insulin to stimulate glucose transport into cells, blood glucose concentrations increase and symptoms of diabetes develop.

### IDDM

In IDDM autoimmune destruction of the pancreatic β-cells results in a severe and eventual total depletion of insulin. Although this autoimmune process appears to be mediated by T lymphocytes, the key target antigens that initiate the β-cell attack and the environmental and possibly viral host factors that perpetuate this destructive process are not yet known. Antibody reactivity to pancreatic islet cells, glutamic acid decarboxylase (GAD), and insulin can be used to identify patients with an immune predisposition to develop IDDM. Determining the human lymphocyte antigen (HLA) status and the degree of loss of first-phase insulin secretion in response to intravenous glucose can further refine the potential for diabetes up to 90% in first-degree relatives of diabetic individuals. Intervention trials utilizing insulin, nicotinamide, and other immunomodulatory agents with the goal of arresting the progression of prediabetes are currently being undertaken throughout the world.

Ultimately, the end result of this β-cell destructive process is the absolute lack of insulin. The absence of insulin produces abnormalities in biochemical pathways of carbohydrate, protein, and lipid metabolism. As circulating insulin levels decrease, glycogen storage is inhibited, glycogen breakdown is enhanced, gluconeogenesis is increased, and blood glucose levels begin to rise. Diminished insulin concentrations decrease protein synthesis and can lead to amino aciduria. Continued low levels of insulin decrease lipogenesis, increase lipolysis, and result in release of free fatty acids into the circulation.

Diabetic ketoacidosis (DKA) begins to develop when excess free fatty acids taken up by the liver are preferentially shunted toward the formation of acetone and acetoacetate and consequently β-hydroxybutyrate. As the concentration of ketone bodies increases, the serum buffering capacity is exceeded and metabolic acidosis occurs. Hyperglycemia induces an osmotic diuresis that eventually leads to dehydration and volume depletion as the kidneys' ability to compensate for elevated glucose levels is exceeded. DKA as a presenting manifestation of IDDM is usually precipitated by a mild underlying stress state, such as a viral infection.

### NIDDM

NIDDM occurs because of a resistance to, rather than an absence of, insulin. It remains unclear whether the primary defect for any given patient is impaired insulin secretion by the β-cell or diminished peripheral sensitivity to circulating insulin. Final disease expression appears to require both the presence of an insulin-resistant state and insufficient β-cell function.

Although the structure of insulin, its receptor, and cellular glucose transport proteins appears to be normal in most individuals, intracellular signals distal to the insulin receptor appear to be abnormal in NIDDM. An absence of first-phase insulin secretion in response to an intravenous glucose load is one of the earliest abnormalities that can be detected. However, basal and postprandial circulating insulin levels are elevated in people predisposed to NIDDM. Both hepatic sensitivity and skeletal sensitivity to insulin have been shown to be impaired in patients with NIDDM. Decreased hepatic sensitivity to insulin results in increased gluconeogenesis. Increasing levels of insulin become required to suppress hepatic production of glucose and overcome skeletal muscle resistance to glucose uptake. These defects combine to stimulate insulin release from the β-cell and so increase circulating levels of insulin before any abnormality of serum glucose is detectable.

Obesity itself appears to promote a hyperinsulinemic state. Weight loss can reverse this effect and so decrease serum insulin concentrations. Since not all obese patients develop hyperglycemia, it has been theorized that individuals whose β-cells cannot continue to maintain a hyperinsulinemic state over time are those who will eventually go on to develop diabetes.

NIDDM patients have sufficient insulin to inhibit ketone formation and thus do not typically develop ketoacidosis. This may be due to the relatively smaller amounts of insulin generally needed to stimulate lipid uptake as compared with glucose transport (Fig. 33-2). Thus these patients often present with very high glucose concentrations (600 to 1200 mg/dl), which produce a hyperosmolar state without ketoacidosis. Under conditions of severe stress (e.g., sepsis) when counterinsulin hormones such as cortisol and epinephrine are released in excess, the physiologic effect of insulin may be further reduced to the point where ketone production does occur.

Other pathways of lipid metabolism are also differentially affected by type II diabetes. NIDDM patients appear to have resistance to the effects of insulin on enzymes responsible for triglyceride metabolism, resulting in elevated triglycerides and very low–density lipoprotein (VLDL). In association with increased triglyceride levels, patients with NIDDM also have decreased high-density lipoprotein (HDL) cholesterol levels.

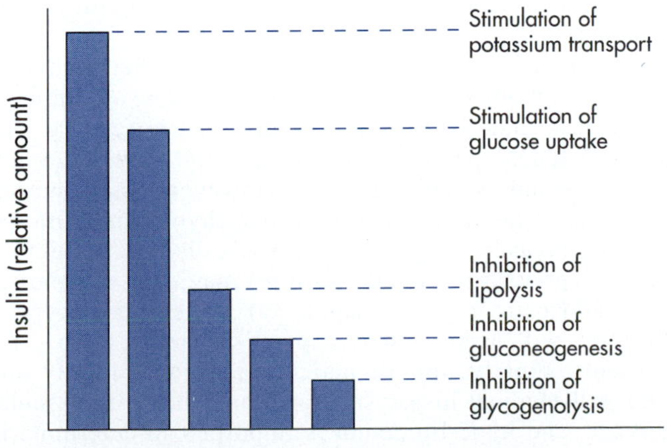


**Fig. 33-2.** Relative sensitivities of various metabolic processes. (From Besser GM, Bodansky HJ, Cudworth AG: *Clinical diabetes—an illustrated text,* New York, 1988, Gower Medical Publishing.)

### Complications of diabetes mellitus

Several mechanisms are now under investigation as causes of the complications of diabetes mellitus. One theory is based on glucose's ability to attach to proteins independent of any enzyme reaction. The rate of protein glycosylation increases as the glucose concentration rises. Glycosylated proteins, referred to as advanced glycation endproducts (AGEs), appear to have altered metabolic characteristics. The increase in AGEs in vascular and neural tissues may be responsible for many of the abnormalities observed in diabetes, such as impaired release of the vasodilator nitric oxide.

Other proposed etiologies of diabetic complications focus on changes in cellular biochemical reactions. The protein that transports myoinositol across cell membranes can also transport glucose. As blood sugars rise, there is increased competition between myoinositol and glucose, resulting in abnormally low cellular myoinositol content. Changes in intracellular myoinositol pools could have significant effects on further downstream signals, such as protein kinase C, diacylglycerol, and intracellular calcium.

Another intracellular abnormality thought to play a role in diabetic complications is the intracellular accumulation of sorbitol. In addition to glycogen synthesis or glycolysis, glucose can be metabolized to fructose and sorbitol intracellularly (the polyol pathway). The accumulation of sorbitol due to hyperglycemia has been linked with abnormalities of nerve conduction. Decreasing sorbitol production by inhibiting the enzyme aldose reductase has been postulated to be beneficial to diabetic patients. Although therapeutic trials with aldose reductase inhibitors have been disappointing, most of these were conducted after the onset of neuropathy. Trials are currently being conducted to evaluate the role of these drugs as preventive therapy for diabetic neuropathy.

Atherosclerosis is the leading cause of death among people with diabetes mellitus. Whereas hyperglycemia has been found to be an independent risk factor for heart disease, the precise mechanism by which glucose predisposes to atherosclerosis is not well understood. Increases in glucose and free fatty acids can damage endothelial cells, resulting in inhibition of fibrinolysis, formation of local thrombus, release of vasoconstrictor prostaglandins, and oxidation of low-density lipoproteins (LDLs). Diabetes can also increase platelet adhesiveness and aggregation via thromboxane and platelet-derived growth factor (PDGF). Hyperglycemia-related production of AGEs may enhance binding of LDL to collagen within arterials walls and may inhibit vasodilatory and antiproliferative effects of nitrous oxide.

Other factors besides glucose may contribute to the increased risk for vascular disease associated with diabetes. Peroxidized LDL, which is preferentially taken up by macrophages and may be more atherogenic, appears to be increased in diabetics. In addition, glycosylated LDL may also be taken up preferentially by macrophage scavenger receptors. HDLs tend to be lower in poorly controlled diabetics and may result in decreased reverse cholesterol transport. Lipoprotein lipase, which metabolizes chylomicrons and VLDLs, is inhibited in insulin-resistant states such as diabetes (see Chapter 7).

## HISTORY

### Initial interview

Although the hallmark symptoms of diabetes mellitus are polyphagia, polydipsia, and polyuria, many individuals with NIDDM have a gradual onset of frequent urination that prevents recognition of symptoms. Many attribute their polyuria to their polydipsia and don't seek medical attention. Nocturia is a particularly helpful indicator of polyuria and the onset of significant hyperglycemia; most patients remember how many times they get up during the night. The association of thirst or dry mouth with frequent nocturia is more consistent with elevated nighttime blood sugars than with benign prostatic hyperplasia or other urogenital conditions. Weight loss despite increased food intake is also very suggestive of diabetes, although it should be noted that hyperthyroid patients may have the same complaint. Conversely, individuals with NIDDM may relate a recent history of weight gain that is sufficient to increase insulin resistance and impair its action.

Patients often complain of excessive fatigue, stiffness particularly in the shoulders and upper back, itching, numbness and tingling in the hands and feet, and cramping of the upper and lower leg. Visual changes such as transient blurriness are very suggestive of fluctuating hyperglycemia. Patients may give a history of having had several pairs of glasses made without perceiving any improvement in visual acuity. Although increased blurred vision suggests worsening glucose control, visual acuity does not immediately return with correction of blood sugars. If individuals are not instructed that their vision can remain blurred for weeks after proper glucose control is established, they may perceive their diabetic regimen as ineffective. By the time objects disrupting vision (floaters) or actual visual loss is reported, diabetic retinopathy may be already far advanced. Thus history is not an adequate tool for detecting early retinopathy.

At the initial interview certain factors may help determine the type, severity, and length of disease. A relatively short (2 to 3 weeks) duration of symptoms precipitated by an acute viral illness often suggests a presentation of IDDM. This does not imply that viral infections cause the onset of hyperglycemia but rather that the stress of these infections unmasks inadequate insulin reserves due to β-cell destruction. In contrast, patients with NIDDM are generally not able to pinpoint when their symptoms began, reflecting the insidiousness of the disorder. In-depth questioning regarding weight changes and nocturia often suggests a history of at least 2 months. Careful review of the patient's medications can be quite rewarding, since removal of a diabetogenic agent ameliorates hyperglycemia (see the box on p. 478).

One reason that patients with IDDM tend to present with a shorter duration of symptoms is the presence of ketoacidosis in addition to hyperglycemia. Although individuals can tolerate moderately elevated blood glucose for long periods, very few can ignore the symptoms of metabolic acidosis. The absolute lack of insulin in type I diabetes shortens the period of unrecognized disease, but the severity of illness at presentation is often greater and requires rapid diagnosis and intervention to prevent excess morbidity and mortality.

When first evaluating a patient, the reason for the current presentation must also be addressed. Symptoms such as heat intolerance, tremor, change in hand or foot size, localized truncal weight gain and episodes of tachycardia with sweating and headache may raise questions concerning secondary forms of diabetes such as hyperthyroidism, acromegaly, Cushing's syndrome, and pheochromocytoma (see the box on p. 478). Although type II diabetes may have existed subclinically for an extended period, extremely high sugars or rapid onset of symptoms in a patient without ketosis suggests an additional underlying process that may have acutely worsened insulin resistance. Production of stress hormones that decrease insulin sensitivity occurs in infection, myocardial infarction, malignancy, and inflammatory diseases. In addition to common infections such as pneumonia, cellulitis, and pyelonephritis, hyperglycemia can also be precipitated by sinusitis, osteomyelitis, meningitis, gynecologic infections, dental infections, and any kind of abscess.

To better assess the onset of diabetes and/or to help document increased cardiovascular risk from impaired glucose tolerance, previous measurements of blood glucose should be reviewed. A history of mildly elevated blood sugars during surgery or during a prior hospitalization suggests a more prolonged period of glucose intolerance and thus an increased risk for atherosclerosis, peripheral neuropathy, and other complications. Gestational diabetes or the history of macrosomia (birth weight over 9 lb), spontaneous abortions, or stillbirth might suggest a previous period of insulin resistance in female patients.

Family history regarding incidence of diabetes, thyroid disease, and other endocrinopathies should be ascertained. Since less than 10% of type I diabetes is familial, the average IDDM patient will typically not know any other family members with diabetes. However, other autoimmune diseases (e.g., Hashimoto's thyroiditis, Graves' disease, myasthenia gravis, Addison's disease, pernicious anemia, premature gonadal failure) may exist in families of IDDM patients (see Chapter 39). Patients with type II diabetes will usually have a positive family history for diabetes. Finally, for all patients additional family and personal medical history of hypertension, cardiovascular disease, and hyperlipidemia is important to determine in order to prevent premature atherosclerotic disease.

In addition to hyperglycemia, problems related to hypoglycemia should be assessed in patients using oral hypoglycemic agents or insulin. These symptoms include those associated with increased catecholamine secretion (sweating, tremor, palpitations, anxiety, hunger) and those associated with central nervous system dysfunction (headache, dizziness, blurry vision, confusion, decreased fine motor skills, abnormal behavior, seizures, loss of consciousness). Patients with tinnitus often report an increase in intensity when hypoglycemic.

Patients with tightly controlled diabetes sometimes do not experience the adrenergic symptoms of hypoglycemia; occasionally confusion or unconsciousness is the only symptom. This phenomenon, called *hypoglycemia unawareness,* is of great concern and precludes patients from being treated with intensive insulin therapy. Treatment with β-blockers may iatrogenically produce hypoglycemic unawareness.

Several factors may contribute to the change in perception and reaction to hypoglycemia. In IDDM patients the loss of counterregulatory hormone secretion in response to hypoglycemia, particularly glucagon and epinephrine, is found after several years of diabetes. Second, the glucose concentration at which patients perceive symptoms can also change. Tightly controlled patients tend to experience symptoms at lower blood sugar levels, leaving less leeway between onset of symptoms and loss of consciousness. Last, the loss of sympathoadrenal responses may be due, in part, to autonomic neuropathy.

Nocturnal hypoglycemia is a common event that frequently goes unrecognized and therefore unreported by patients. In the Diabetes Control and Complications Trial (DCCT) intensively controlled patients were more likely to have hypoglycemic episodes at night than at other times. A history of violent nightmares, vivid and bizarre dreams, night sweats, and/or a headache upon awakening in the morning provide suggestive evidence of these events. However, patients do not always wake up to experience these symptoms and may only report a sense of not sleeping well or not feeling well rested in the morning. Nocturnal hypoglycemic events are not trivial; they may induce seizures or coma and require hospitalization.

Hypoglycemic episodes, which used to be considered a minor annoyance and an indication of tight control, are now recognized to be potentially dangerous and avoidable by using blood glucose self-monitoring. By determining time of day, time since last meal, time since last exercise, and peak of pharmacologic activity, the cause of many hypoglycemic episodes can be explained and treatments or schedules can be adjusted to prevent their recurrence. Judicious placement of snacks and deliberate timing of exercise can dramatically reduce the frequency of hypoglycemic events.

Sudden increases in the frequency of hypoglycemic episodes in an otherwise stable patient deserve further evaluation. Hypothyroidism, adrenal insufficiency, or decline in renal function can present as hypoglycemia or markedly increased insulin sensitivity and are more likely to occur in IDDM patients. Correlation of hypoglycemia with initiation of certain medications (see the box on p. 478) may identify a reversible cause of hypoglycemia. Common clinical agents that lower blood sugars include aerosolized pentamidine and excess alcohol. Any malabsorptive syndrome in which nutrients are not absorbed but still are able to stimulate insulin release can cause hypoglycemia.

### Follow-up visits

At routine follow-up appointments, just as at initial visits, signs and symptoms of hyperglycemia and hypoglycemia should always be elicited. Poor glucose control is suggested by weight loss, whereas weight gain may suggest poor dietary habits or overinsulinization.

For patients with home blood glucose monitors, follow-up visits should include a review of blood sugar records. Log books or other methods of summarizing data can also be reviewed in between visits by mail, telephone, or facsimile. Many meters have memory chips that allow dates, times of day, and glucose values to be downloaded into microcomputers where software can analyze blood glucose patterns. Pictorial representation of blood glucose data can be very effective in motivating patients to achieve better glycemic control.

In addition to routine questions regarding symptoms of potential diabetic complications, it is important to inspect the patient's feet regularly, especially if any neuropathy has been found. It is not uncommon for patients to be unaware of significant pathology, including cellulitis, ulcers, osteomyelitis, and Charcot joints.

## PHYSICAL EXAMINATION

Diabetes has the ability to affect every portion of the physical examination from eyes to feet. Findings on physical examination may vary substantially depending on when in the course of the disease it is conducted. At the time of diagnosis, for example, patients may have documented weight loss and decreased blood pressure (from hypovolemia), whereas in an office setting weight gain and hypertension are more common.

Vital signs provide great insight into volume status, underlying cardiovascular risk, and possible autonomic neuropathy. Patients should have orthostatic vital signs checked yearly and in all acute hospitalizations. Orthostasis may affect decisions regarding hypertensive therapy, advice regarding dizziness prevention, and severity of volume depletion. Resting tachycardia can also represent loss of cardiac parasympathetic function secondary to autonomic neuropathy.

Patients with diabetes should have their weight recorded at each visit. Body weight can be used as a simple but important piece of feedback and goal orientation for patients. However, expectations concerning body weight need to be properly communicated. People with IDDM need to understand the importance of maintaining body weight as part of overall health. Adolescents may intentionally worsen glucose control as a means of losing weight. NIDDM patients may become less compliant if too much emphasis is placed on being overweight. Individuals may become frustrated as they gain weight in response to initial therapy from volume restoration, and reverse their overall metabolic state from catabolic to anabolic. A more effective approach is to explain that an initial weight gain frequently occurs, but that part of the long-term approach is to establish a healthy diet that can slowly and effectively result in weight loss.

Type I patients with diabetes of greater than 5 years' duration should have a yearly dilated funduscopic examination. Since the time of disease onset is less clear in type II patients, yearly examinations are recommended from the time of diagnosis. The ability to detect abnormalities varies with experience and should be conducted by an ophthalmologist when needed. Dilatation with a mydriatic preparation should be preceded by evaluation for risk of open-angle glaucoma. In addition to retinal abnormalities, people with diabetes are at an increased risk for cataract formation.

Although there are few physical findings in the neck and chest that are unique to diabetes, these portions of the examination are of great importance in documenting complications and concomitant illness. Carotid bruits can be an indicator of atherosclerotic complications. The increased risk of autoimmune thyroid disease in patients with IDDM may be manifested as goiter. Findings on cardiac and pulmonary examination are important indicators of impaired myocardial contractility. Although congestive heart failure most often reflects atherosclerotic disease, it may also be a manifestation of a diabetic cardiomyopathy, which is thought to be due to microvascular abnormalities. Electrocardiographic (ECG) recording can document the lack of appropriate heart rate changes with the Valsalva maneuver or reduced respiratory beat-to-beat variation commonly seen in diabetic autonomic neuropathy. Consultation and further testing may be needed to confirm accurately the presence of the disorder. In addition, diabetes seems to predispose patients to silent ischemia and perhaps to an increased incidence of silent myocardial infarctions, which may be noted on the ECG.

The examination of the abdomen can be misleading in diabetes. Patients in DKA often have tenderness that can mimic an acute abdomen. However, since these signs resolve upon treatment of DKA, patients should not be referred for exploratory laparotomy until the ketoacidosis is fully treated. In long-standing hyperglycemia, fatty infiltration of the liver can produce hepatomegaly that improves with glucose control.

Examinations of the reproductive system can reveal consequences and causes of hyperglycemia. In women recurrent yeast infections accompany untreated or poorly controlled diabetes mellitus. In addition, gynecologic pathology such as pelvic inflammatory disease can cause sudden changes in glycemic control. In men with impotence multifactorial causes usually are found; a genitourinary examination is necessary to assess the causes (see Chapter 140). Absence of bulbocavernosis and anal wink reflexes can suggest diabetic neuropathy.

**Table 33-4.** Diabetes and the skin

| Skin change | Clinical | Incidence/pathogenesis | Treatment |
|---|---|---|---|
| Gangrene and skin ulcers | Necrotic toes, feet; punched out leg ulcers | Atherosclerotic peripheral vascular disease and small vessel disease; extremely common in diabetes | If localized arterial obstruction, bypass surgery; diabetic control minimizes hypercholesterolemia |
| Necrobiosis lipoidica diabeticorum | Red, yellow, atrophic areas with telangiectasis; usually lower legs but can be on arms; may ulcerate | 0.3% of diabetics; may precede onset of diabetes; most seen in severe long-standing disease | Topical or intralesional steroids |
| Diabetic dermatopathy | Brown, small atrophic areas on pretibial areas | Not specific for diabetes; seen in 50% diabetics | None |
| Bullous diabeticorum | Small to large tense, noninflammatory blisters usually on lower extremities | Often due to mild trauma | Prevent secondary infection<br>Soaks<br>Diabetic control |
| Cutaneous infections | Impetigo, tinea infections, candida infections, paronychia | Common in diabetes | Specific therapy for each infection |
| Pruritus | Itching without primary skin lesions; may be localized to genital areas or generalized | Not specific for diabetes, but may be seen | Antihistamines, emollients |
| Neurotropic ulcers, malperforans | Painless deep ulceration on pressure areas of foot with hyperkeratosis around edges | Due to peripheral neuropathy and anesthesia with repeated trauma | Prevent secondary infection; protect weight-bearing areas |
| Acanthosis nigricans | Pigmented, velvety areas in body folds | Associated with insulin antibodies | None |
| Lipoatrophy, localized | Localized adipose tissue atrophy | | None |
| Lipoatrophy, generalized (Lawrence-Seip syndrome) | Subcutaneous atrophy and generalized loss of fat; acanthosis nigricans, hirsutism, hepatosplenomegaly | Insulin-resistant diabetes | None |
| Scleroderma adultorum | Nonpitting edema of face and upper trunk; often follows respiratory infection | May be seen in association with diabetes | May resolve slowly with time |
| Xanthomas | Small yellow/eruptive papules (eruptive xanthomas) on the extensor surfaces of extremities and trunk | Lack of insulin prevents clearance of chylomicrons and VLDL lipoproteins (hypertriglyceridemia) | Insulin and diet reverse lesions |

## THE SKIN IN DIABETES MELLITUS

Cutaneous changes associated with diabetes mellitus are outlined in Table 33-4.

Necrobiosis lipoidica diabeticorum (NLD) is perhaps the most distinctive, although relatively unusual, skin sign suggestive of diabetes. Single or multiple atrophic, waxy yellow patches with an erythematous border and telangiectasis coursing through the center are usually seen on the pretibial area. In 15% to 20% of cases these lesions precede overt chemical diabetes. Occasionally the lesions ulcerate and are very difficult to heal. Topical or intralesional steroids may slow the progression of early lesions but require caution, since these lead to skin atrophy in themselves and can cause ulceration.

Recurrent cutaneous or mucous membrane candidal infections (paronychia, nail infection, thrush) should always initiate a search for diabetes. Unexplained pruritus should also alert the physician to the possibility of diabetes (along with liver or renal disease or an underlying lymphoma).

For patients with diabetes, examination of the extremities represents a tremendous source of information and a major opportunity to significantly reduce the risk for amputation. Diabetes is the leading cause of nontraumatic amputation; it is estimated that 50% of these amputations could be prevented by early detection (see the box below). As part of their routine examination, patients with diabetes should be instructed to remove their socks or stockings and have a direct and thorough examination of their lower extremities. Symptoms cannot be relied upon, since patients with neuropathy may not perceive any abnormal sensations. Direct visualization between the toes and of the plantar surface identifies early evidence of skin breakdown, cellulitis, and ulcerations. Dry skin and loss of hair over the lower leg and foot are evidence of both decreased neural innervation and vascular supply. Loss of the Achilles reflex and change in perception of vibration, temperature, and pinprick further document the presence of neuropathy. Assessment of posterior tibial and dorsalis pedis pulses provides evaluation of arterial vascular supply. In patients with long-standing diabetes, decreased sensation can also occur in upper extremities. In patients with upper extremity neuropathy consideration may need to be given to the risks of fingerstick blood glucose monitoring. Upper extremities can also be afflicted with Dupuytren's contractures.

### Examination of the diabetic foot

Remove socks/stockings at each visit
Visual examination
- Skin dryness
- Presence of hair over lower legs and toes
- Breaks in skin, especially between toes
- Formation and location of calluses
- Presence of edema

Vascular
- Check pulses
- Capillary filling

Neurologic
- Achilles reflexes
- Vibration
- Pinprick

## LABORATORY STUDIES

The diagnosis of diabetes mellitus ultimately rests on the presence of hyperglycemia as defined by The National Diabetes Data Group (see the box below). Two fasting blood sugars over 140 mg/dl provide equally as accurate a diagnosis of diabetes as an emergency room visit value of 850 mg/dl. Oral glucose tolerance testing (OGTT) is in practice not needed to make the diagnosis of overt diabetes but can be very useful in selecting those with a predisposition to develop NIDDM. Fasting values between 120 and 140 mg/dl are most likely to be evidence of impaired glucose tolerance and potentially represent a critical time when changes in diet and exercise can have the greatest impact on insulin sensitivity.

The glycosylated hemoglobin is an invaluable tool in assessing the level of diabetes control that a patient has been able to achieve. The test is based on the fact that the nonenzymatic attachment of glucose to hemoglobin is determined by ambient circulating glucose concentrations.

### Diagnosis of diabetes

**In nonpregnant adults**

A random plasma glucose level of 200 mg/dl or greater plus classic signs and symptoms of diabetes mellitus, including polyuria, polydipsia, polyphagia, and weight loss

OR

A fasting plasma glucose level of 140 mg/dl or greater on at least two occasions

OR

A fasting plasma glucose level less than 140 mg/dl *plus* sustained elevated plasma glucose levels during at least two oral glucose tolerance tests; the 2-hour sample and one other between 0 and 2 hours after the 75 g glucose dose should be 200 mg/dl or greater

**In children**

A random plasma glucose level of 200 mg/dl or greater plus classic signs and symptoms of diabetes mellitus, including polyuria, polydipsia, polyphagia, and weight loss

OR

A fasting plasma glucose level of 140 mg/dl on two occasions and sustained elevated plasma glucose levels during at least two oral glucose tolerance tests; both the 2-hour sample and one other between 0 and 2 hours after the glucose dose (1.75 g/kg ideal body weight up to 75 g) should be 200 mg/dl or greater

**In pregnant women**

After an oral glucose load of 100 g; gestational diabetes may be diagnosed if two plasma glucose values (in mg/dl) are ≥ the following:

| Fasting | 1 hour | 2 hours | 3 hours |
|---|---|---|---|
| 105 | 190 | 165 | 145 |

**Table 33-5.** Laboratory tests recommended for diabetic patients

| Test | Frequency |
|---|---|
| Glycosylated hemoglobin or hemoglobin $A_{1c}$ | Every 3 months |
| Fructosamine (for pregnant patients) | Every 3 weeks |
| Urine dipstick for glucose protein, blood | Every 3 months |
| 24-hour urine collection for microalbumin, protein, creatinine clearance (need serum creatinine) | Yearly (beginning after 5 years in IDDM) if:<br>Dipstick is positive<br>Hypersensitive<br>Increase in BUN/creatinine |
| Electrolytes, BUN, creatinine | Yearly |
| Lipid profile | As per NCEP (see Chapter 40) |
| TSH and thyroid antibodies | At initial visit and then as indicated by antibody tests and physical exam |
| ECG | At initial visit |
| Dilated funduscopic exam | Yearly |

*BUN*, Blood urea nitrogen; *NCEP*, National Cholesterol Education Program; *TSH*, thyroid-stimulating hormone.

The percentage of glycosylated hemoglobin is highly correlated with mean blood glucose values for the preceding 2 months and thus serves as an accurate benchmark of overall glycemic control. It is reported as either a total glycosylated hemoglobin, in which all subfractions of hemoglobin are pooled, or as the hemoglobin $A_{1c}$, which is the predominant glycosylated fraction.

The American Diabetes Association (ADA) currently recommends that the glycosylated hemoglobin or hemoglobin $A_{1c}$ assay be performed four times a year in diabetic patients (Table 33-5). More frequent determinations following changes in treatment strategies can provide additional positive feedback to patients. The value of testing glycosylated hemoglobin is diminished if it is done too frequently (less than 2 months apart) or if multiple therapeutic changes have not allowed a steady state to be achieved. Other assays have been developed to detect glycosylated proteins with shorter serum half-lives than hemoglobin, such as fructosamine ($t_{1/2}$ = 2 to 3 weeks), but their utility is limited to special situations such as pregnancy, where more frequent assessments are necessary to obtain tighter diabetes control.

The hemoglobin $A_{1c}$ assay can serve as an unbiased means of determining glycemic control and confirming home blood glucose records. For diabetic patients without home blood glucose meters, these tests are a far more accurate determinant of glycemic control than office-drawn fasting or random blood glucoses. Although the home blood glucose record is critical in serving as the basis for the adjustments in medication regimens, studies have shown it to be less reliable than the hemogloblobin $A_{1c}$ in determining overall glycemic control. Selective omission of high test results and fabrication of blood glucose data to please health care providers are unfortunately common and can lead to inaccurate assessments of diabetes control.

Routine office testing of urine by dipstick can provide information on metabolic control and renal function. Morning urine glucose levels can provide insight into approximate circulating concentrations from the previous night. The detection of urinary ketones can be useful in assessing the patient's level of insulinization. Strongly positive ketones in the morning as opposed to the mildly positive test seen in overnight starvation, or ketones noted during the course of the day without concurrent illness, suggest significant undertreatment of hyperglycemia or omission of insulin doses. The presence of protein (more than 300 mg/24 hours) or blood can be an indication of diabetic nephropathy. Several dipsticks can detect evidence of leukocytes, which indicate risk for urinary tract infections.

Early detection of nephropathy is critical to preventing deterioration to end-stage renal disease. Although yearly blood urea nitrogen (BUN) and creatinine values are currently recommended, these parameters only become elevated after significant kidney damage has occurred. Small quantities of albumin (30 to 300 mg) in a 24-hour urine collection serve as an accurate marker of early nephropathy. Although these amounts cannot be detected by routine urine dipsticks, dipstick immunoassay tests for microalbuminuria have recently become available and can be used for screening random urine specimens. This test should be done yearly on all type I patients with greater than 5 years of diabetes. Those with positive microalbuminuria dipstick tests should then undergo either a timed overnight or 24-hour urine collection for albumin, protein and creatinine clearance to further evaluate renal function. Indications for type II patients have not been determined but probably should include those patients with high blood pressure or a positive family history of hypertensive or renal disease.

Fasting lipid profiles are an important indicator of cardiovascular risk in patients with diabetes mellitus. Hypertriglyceridemia, which is predictive of coronary artery disease in diabetics, is the most common lipid abnormality among these patients. In poorly controlled diabetes, increased triglyceride concentrations reflect decreased metabolism of chylomicrons and VLDL. Impaired insulin action results in decreased stimulation of lipoprotein lipase, which is the rate-limiting enzyme in hydrolysis of triglyceride-rich particles.

Rather than begin therapy with a cholesterol-lowering agent, the first step in managing lipid abnormalities in diabetic patients is to obtain maximal glycemic control. However, hyperlipidemia should not be ignored indefinitely merely because near normal glucose levels have not been achieved. Once glucose control has been optimized, lipids should be assessed even if glucose levels are still elevated, and efforts should then focus on reducing serum cholesterol and triglycerides. Not all cholesterol-lowering medications are useful when diabetes is present. Diabetic patients with impaired gastrointestinal motility frequently cannot tolerate resins. In addition, niacin can worsen glucose intolerance and is probably best used in patients treated with insulin rather than oral hypoglycemic agents. Gemfibrozil may be preferred for patients with high triglycerides and low HDL, whereas 3-hydroxy-3-methylglutaryl coenzyme A (HMG CoA) reductase inhibitors may benefit those with predominantly elevated LDL. All adults with diabetes should have an ECG performed at their initial visit.

Thyroid-stimulating hormone (TSH) should be periodically measured in high-risk diabetic patients. Patients with IDDM are at 2% to 7% increased risk for autoimmune thyroid disease. The presence of antithyroid antibodies can further identify patients who would benefit from yearly TSH measurements. The rate of thyroid dysfunction in the elderly, who also are prone to NIDDM, can approach 5% of the general population.

## DIABETIC COMPLICATIONS

### Retinopathy

Diabetic retinopathy causes about 10% of cases of new blindness in the United States each year and is second only to age-related macular degeneration as a cause of permanent blindness. The risk of diabetic retinopathy increases with the duration of the disease. After 10 years, 27% of insulin-dependent diabetics have retinopathy. After 30 years, the prevalence rises to over 90%, and about 30% of these patients have proliferative changes. The prevalence of diabetic retinopathy in noninsulin-dependent diabetics is lower. The DCCT has shown that rigorous control of blood sugar delays the onset of microvascular complications in the retina.

Renal disease as manifest by proteinuria, elevated blood urea nitrogen (BUN) and creatinine is highly correlated with the presence of retinopathy. In patients with nephropathy, there is a good correlation between the presence of systemic hypertension and retinopathy. In diabetic women who begin pregnancy with no retinopathy, the risk of developing background changes is about 10%. Those who already have background diabetic retinopathy at the start of pregnancy may show progression, and about 4% will develop proliferative changes.

Diabetic retinopathy can be divided into background, preproliferative, and proliferative categories. Microaneurysms are the first ophthalmoscopically detectable change in diabetic retinopathy. Dot, blot, and splinter hemorrhages and venous engorgement follow (Fig. 33-3). Macular edema, secondary to diffuse capillary leakage, is a visually significant complication. If sufficient leakage occurs, lipid will accumulate in the retina, either in a scattered fashion, or in a ring formation around a group of leaking microaneurysms.

In the preproliferative stage, areas of capillary nonperfusion will be seen on fluorescein angiography. On ophthalmoscopic examination increasing retinal hemorrhages, microaneurysms, and cotton-wool spots can be seen. Finally, intraretinal microvascular abnormalities (IRMA) are characteristic of preproliferative retinopathy. IRMA are focal areas of dilated capillaries that may function as collateral channels in areas of capillary drop-out. Ophthalmoscopically, they can be difficult to distinguish from surface neovascularization, but the difference is clear on fluorescein angiography. These preproliferative changes are risk factors for the development of proliferative retinopathy, which can arise on the disc or elsewhere.

As the neovascular vessels proliferate, fibrous connective tissue elements accompany them. The fibrotic tissue can grow into the vitreous cavity or across the surface of the retina. Subsequent contraction of the connective tissue elements can lead to the development of a traction retinal detachment. Additionally, the fragile new vessels can tear easily, causing a vitreous hemorrhage.

The Diabetic Retinopathy Study proved that argon laser panretinal photocoagulation significantly decreases the likelihood that eyes with proliferative retinopathy will progress to severe visual loss. Other controlled studies proved the effectiveness of argon laser photocoagulation in decreasing or stabilizing diabetic macular edema and the value of vitrectomy in managing the severe complications of diabetic retinopathy.

Neovascularization of the iris (rubeosis) is usually seen only in eyes with proliferative retinopathy. Iris neovascularization causes progressive closure of the angle, leading to the development of neovascular glaucoma. Once established, this form of glaucoma is difficult to treat, but in the early phases panretinal photocoagulation can cause regression of the iris vessels and stabilization of any areas of angle closure.

The corneal epithelium is not as adherent to the underlying stroma in patients with diabetes. This condition contributes to delayed healing in the event of a corneal abrasion, and a much greater likelihood of recurrent corneal epithelial erosions after minor corneal trauma. Other ocular findings in patients with diabetes include a twofold to fourfold greater risk of cataract than in the general population; an increased propensity to acute ischemic and nonischemic optic neuropathy; and pupil-sparing third, fourth, and sixth cranial nerve palsies.

Because treatments for diabetic maculopathy and proliferative retinopathy are most effective when initiated early, it is incumbent on the generalist to obtain ophthalmic consultation on patients with diabetes who complain of decreasing vision and/or demonstrate any retinal vascular abnormalities. Yearly dilated funduscopic examinations are therefore critical in preventing diabetes-related blindness. In patients with IDDM, these annual examinations should begin 5 years after the onset of diabetes.

### Nephropathy

The earliest pathologic evidence of diabetic nephropathy appears to be thickening of the glomerular basement membrane. An increase in the mesangium and subintimal thickening of both afferent and efferent arterioles can also be detected at this stage. The deposition of macromolecules such as albumin and other large proteins may

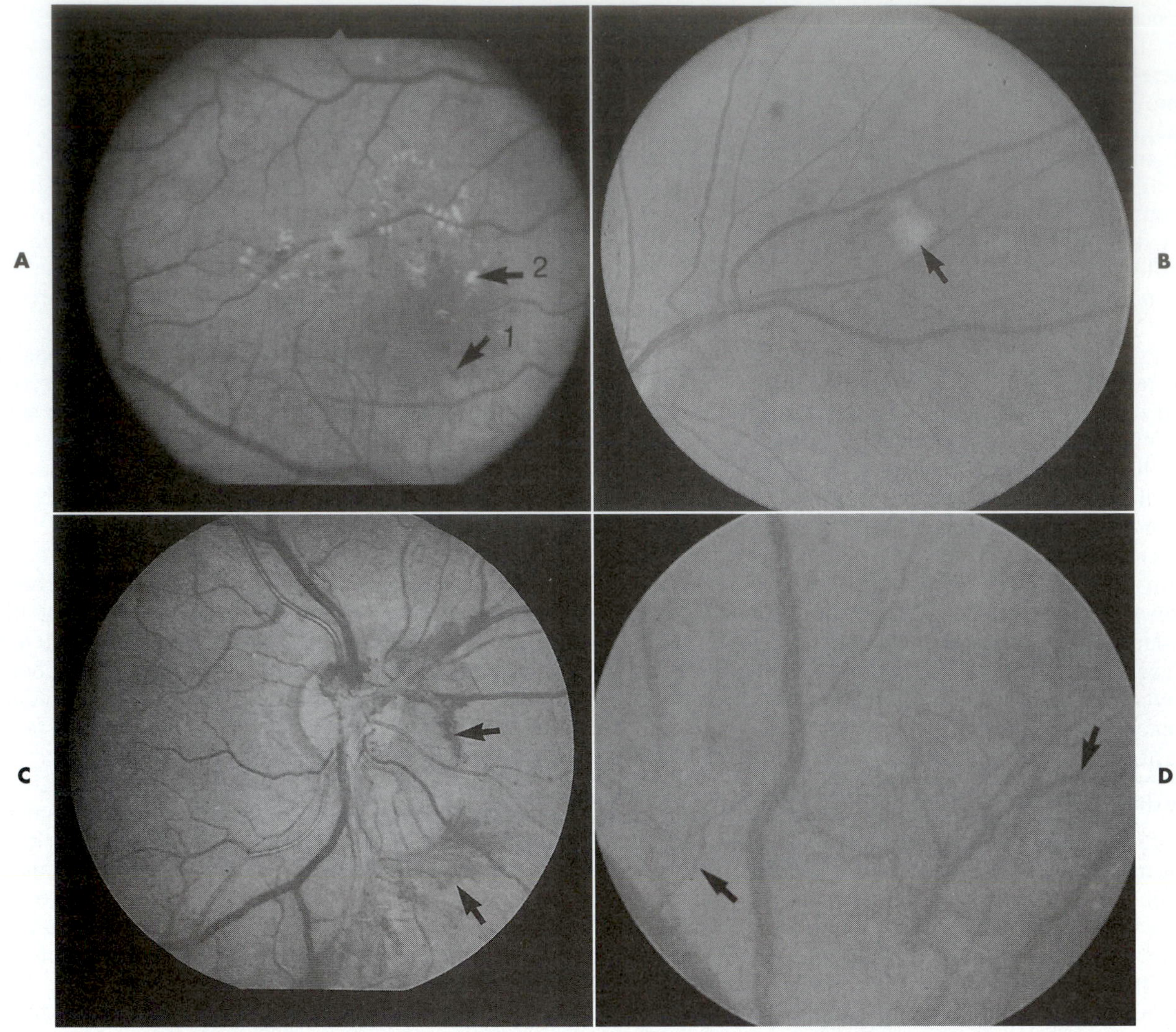


**Fig. 33-3.** **A,** Early background retinopathy showing scattered microaneurysms *(1)* and hard exudates *(2)*. **B,** Background retinopathy in a diabetic patient showing a cotton-wool spot in the center of the field *(arrow)*. These are areas of retinal infarction and evidence of deteriortation in the retinal microcirculation. **C,** Proliferative retinopathy. Fronds of new vessels emerging from the disk and elsewhere. **D,** Neovascular tissue before visible leakage or hemorrhage has occurred. (From Bloom A, Ireland J, Watkins P: The eye. In Bloom A, Ireland J editors: *Color atlas of diabetes,* ed 2, St Louis, 1992, Mosby.)

contribute to the observed thickening and fibrosis seen in the glomerular wall and mesangium. Eventually large accumulations of PAS-positive material are observed (the nodules of Kimmelstiel and Wilson), which denote the development of more advanced diabetic renal disease.

The metabolic consequences of hyperglycemia reduce glomerular filtration of macromolecules and increase intraglomerular pressure. Glomerular hyperperfusion is believed to occur in response to several stimuli, including renal hypoxia. The first clinically detectable abnormality of early or incipient nephropathy appears to be microalbuminuria. This is defined as between 30 and 300 mg of albumin in a 24-hour urine collection. Several studies have correlated the presence of microalbuminuria with the later development of overt diabetic nephropathy. This later stage of disease is typically marked by proteinuria (>300 mg albumin/24 hours), which progresses to nephrotic-range proteinuria, and then to reduced renal function. Incipient nephropathy can be detected as early as 5 years after the diagnosis of diabetes in type I patients, but it generally takes up to 20 years for full-blown expression of nephropathy leading to end-stage renal disease to be seen in the 30% of diabetic patients who develop this complication. It should also be noted that the risk of coronary artery disease is markedly increased in patients with overt diabetic nephropathy.

Current treatments for nephropathy consist of improved glycemic management, exquisite control of hypertension, and reduced dietary protein intake. Improved glycemic control in the DCCT was associated with a decrease in risk of proteinuria. Aggressive control of hypertension in diabetic patients is increasingly recognized as an important strategy to prevent renal complications. Angiotensin converting enzyme (ACE) inhibitors appear to be the agents of choice for treatment of hypertension associated with diabetic nephropathy and perhaps even for microalbuminuria without hypertension. These agents reduce glomerular hyperperfusion independent of their effect on systemic hypertension and have been correlated with amelioration of clinical markers of diabetic nephropathy, including microalbuminuria (less than 300 mg/24 hours; reagent strip negative) and proteinuria (more than 300 mg/24 hours; reagent strip positive). Because glycosylated proteins may be particularly damaging to the mesangium, inhibitors of glycosylation and even aldose reductase inhibitors are being evaluated for their potential role in preventing nephropathy.

### Neuropathy

The three principal types of diabetic neuropathy are mononeuropathy, peripheral polyneuropathy, and autonomic neuropathy. Mononeuropathies and radiculopathies affect either large nerves or nerve roots. These neuropathies are frequently noted at the presentation of diabetes but may also be present after years of treatment. Vascular disease of small arterioles (vasa nervorum) plays an important role in the development of this condition. Both motor and sensory components of the nerve are affected, resulting in weakness, hyperesthesia or hypoesthesia, and pain. Mononeuropathy can be so painful that patients cannot tolerate the touch of their bedsheets on the affected part. Diabetes can also cause the severe pain of a radiculopathy, typically of the chest or abdomen, often mimicking herpes zoster or even an acute surgical abdomen. Major peripheral nerves such as the femoral and obturator are often affected. Although any cranial nerves can be involved in diabetes, the third, fourth, and sixth nerves are most commonly affected. Unlike most diabetic complications, which appear to be more progressive, mononeuropathies develop rapidly but generally resolve within 3 to 12 months.

The differential diagnosis for mononeuropathies includes degenerative disc disease, nerve entrapment syndromes, (e.g., carpal tunnel syndrome), herpes zoster, Graves' disease, and other metabolic conditions. Electromyography (EMG) can often help to distinguish the cause of symptoms and confirm the clinical diagnosis of diabetic neuropathy. CT scan or magnetic resonance imaging (MRI) of the brain should be considered for patients with cranial neuropathies to rule out other causes of oculomotor defects.

Peripheral polyneuropathy, the most common type found in diabetics, and autonomic neuropathy are most likely caused by metabolic consequences of hyperglycemia. The DCCT also demonstrated that lowering of mean blood glucose values over many years reduced the risk for peripheral and autonomic nerve dysfunction. (See Chapter 103 for further discussion of diabetic peripheral neuropathy, diabetic truncal radiculopathy, and diabetic amyotrophy.)

The autonomic nervous system is not exempt from the deleterious effects of prolonged hyperglycemia. Autonomic neuropathy is typically found after many years of diabetes and can affect both the parasympathetic and sympathetic fibers, causing a spectrum of problems for the diabetic patient. It may manifest as impotence, gastroparesis (early satiety, nausea, vomiting), diabetic diarrhea, urinary retention, and cardiac abnormalities such as palpitations, resting tachycardia, or orthostatic hypotension. Diagnosis is often clinical, but the loss of R-R variation and heart rate changes in response to the Valsalva maneuver on ECG monitoring can document its presence. Direct testing of the affected organ systems, such as gastric emptying studies and assessment of urinary bladder capacity, can further confirm clinical suspicion. Treatment is symptomatic and consists of promotility agents such as metoclopramide, erythromycin, and cisapride for gastroparesis; tetracycline or loperamide for diabetic diarrhea (some clinicians have found clonidine to be useful); frequent voiding and cholinergic agents (bethanecol) for urinary retention; and papaverine injections, mechanical devices, or prosthetic implants for impotence.

## DIFFERENTIAL DIAGNOSIS

It is important to consider a differential diagnosis of presenting symptoms and underlying causes of diabetes mellitus rather than hyperglycemia itself. Other causes of polydipsia (diabetes insipidus, medication side effect, psychogenic), polyuria (hypercalcemia, medications, renal wasting, urologic conditions), blurred vision (myopia), weakness/fatigue (hypothyroidism, hyperthyroidism, anemia, adrenal insufficiency, depression), and pruritus (allergy, renal failure) should be considered.

Recognizing underlying etiologies of diabetes mellitus can provide options for the most appropriate therapeutic approach. Identifying secondary causes of diabetes, including glucocorticoid excess, hyperthyroidism, acromegaly, and pheochromocytoma, offers an opportunity to reverse the hyperglycemic state and reestablish normal glucose tolerance. IDDM and NIDDM should be properly differentiated; the terms are often incorrectly used based on insulin use rather than on insulin dependence. The IDDM patient depends on insulin to prevent ketoacid formation and cannot be considered for oral hypoglycemic therapy. The NIDDM patient may use insulin to maintain glucose control but does not depend on it and may be evaluated for oral agents if diet and exercise restore insulin sensitivity.

## MANAGEMENT

### Diabetic ketoacidosis

Although the diagnosis of DKA is still considered a medical emergency, improved treatment has greatly reduced the mortality of this condition. Patients generally present with nausea, vomiting, abdominal pain, and lightheadedness as their main complaints. Physical examination reveals signs of dehydration such as hypotension, dry mouth, and diminished skin turgor. Kussmaul respirations (fast, deep breaths) can frequently be noted, and the breath may reveal the sweet fruity smell of acetone. Abdominal pain suggesting an acute abdomen is often seen but may solely be due to ketoacidosis and usually resolves with its effective treatment.

Laboratory examination demonstrates hyperglycemia between 300 and 600 mg/dl, with serum ketones generally greater than a 1:8 dilution. BUN and creatinine are frequently elevated due to dehydration. Although hyperkalemia or normokalemia may initially be noted on electrolyte examination, total body potassium is decreased and hypokalemia is nearly always found in DKA after initial treatment is begun. Given the intensive management required for DKA (insulin drips, frequent fingerstick blood glucose and electrolyte determinations, assessment of volume status), admission to the intensive care unit should be the rule for nearly all patients when possible. Arterial blood gas measurements may not be required in all patients with DKA but can help in assessing the severity of acidosis and determining if other acid-base disturbances or causes of metabolic acidosis are complicating the acute presentation. Low bicarbonate levels occur due to the acidotic state and should be used in place of serum ketones to follow efficacy of therapy. Hypophosphatemia, hypomagnesemia, elevated amylase, and white blood cell counts between 10,000 and 30,000 can all be found in typical cases of DKA. White blood cell counts greater than 30,000 are more likely to be associated with infection than with stress.

Initial treatment for DKA is fluid replacement with normal saline to expand the intravascular space, followed by half normal saline with potassium chloride or phosphate to replace the rest of the fluid deficit. Treatment of hypokalemia should always precede the administration of insulin to prevent the development of severe potassium deficiency.

Insulinization should begin with boluses of 5 to 20 U of insulin intravenously, followed by the institution of an insulin drip at 1 to 15 U per hour. Frequent fingerstick blood glucose assessments, initially taken every hour, should determine the amount of insulin given to gradually lower the blood sugar toward normal. The insulin drip should not be stopped until the serum bicarbonate has normalized, which usually takes between 12 and 24 hours to achieve. If blood glucose values of approximately 200 mg/dl are reached before normalization of the bicarbonate has occurred, then dextrose should be added to the half normal saline to avoid inducing hypoglycemia by continued insulin administration.

Monitoring the serum electrolytes every 4 hours can further confirm the success of insulin treatment and guide the replacement of potassium. Overlapping the last few hours of the insulin drip with the first dose of subcutaneous insulin can prevent the reemergence of DKA at this last critical point in the care of these metabolically unstable patients.

### Hyperosmolar hyperglycemic nonketotic states

Hyperosmolar hyperglycemic nonketotic state (HHNK) is the result of inadequate insulin coupled with some degree of renal and cerebral impairment, which allows the development of severe hyperglycemia without significant ketosis or acidosis. Older NIDDM patients, whether treated with oral hypoglycemic agents or insulin are susceptible to the development of HHNK. This syndrome most often presents with hyperglycemia (blood glucose 500 to 1500 mg/dl) and dehydration. The presentation of patients in coma from HHNK has become less common, since individuals are usually brought to medical attention earlier than in the past. Physical examination reveals severe dehydration (5 to 10 L) but none of the other manifestations that characterize DKA, such as abdominal pain. Underlying causes for the development of HHNK should be sought as discussed previously.

Despite serum hyperosmolarity, treatment should still begin with normal saline to expand the intravascular space; normal saline is relatively hypo-osmolar compared with the hyperosmolar serum in HHNK. Conversion to half normal saline with potassium should be determined by serum osmolarity, normalization of blood pressure, and establishment of urine output. Fluid treatment alone greatly reduces the blood glucose in HHNK patients. Smaller, judicious doses of insulin (5 to 10 U bolus or 1 to 5 U/hour drip) should be utilized to lower the blood glucose rather than the higher doses recommended for DKA. Overly rapid correction of fluid deficits and hyperglycemia is not indicated for HHNK patients; it may even worsen coexisting conditions such as congestive heart failure and coronary artery disease and also exacerbate the potential risk of cerebral edema.

## Outpatient management

As the major cause of death for patients with diabetes has changed from the acute problems of ketoacidosis to the chronic complications of cardiovascular disease, the focus of treatment has shifted from inpatient therapy to outpatient prevention. The goals of therapy must be determined for each individual with diabetes in the context of that person's lifestyle, work, family, and social situation. The cost in both monetary and human terms must be constantly and repeatedly weighed against the need for better metabolic control. Tight control of the diabetic patient implies the goal of near normalization of not only glycemia but also of blood pressure and serum lipids (Table 33-6). Other factors requiring careful attention include urinary albumin excretion, choice of antihypertensive agent, and prevention of blindness and amputation.

The results of the DCCT have confirmed that maximizing control of blood sugars in IDDM significantly reduces risk for microvascular complications over time (see below). The most effective means of normalizing blood sugars have consistently been diet, exercise, and medication. For IDDM patients, diet and exercise are used to maintain weight and promote growth and development during childhood, puberty, and adolescence. For NIDDM

**Table 33-6.** Control of diabetes-related complications in the 1990s

| Index | Excellent | Fair | Poor |
|---|---|---|---|
| Fasting glucose | ~115 | ~140 | >200 |
| Postprandial glucose | ~160 | ~200 | >235 |
| Hemoglobin $A_{1c}$ | 6 | 8 | >10 |
| Blood pressure | 130/80 | 150/88 | >150/90 |
| LDL cholesterol | <130 (<100 if CAD) | 130-159 | >160 |
| Triglyceride | <200 | 200-300 | >400 |
| HDL cholesterol | | | <35 |

*CAD*, Coronary artery disease.

patients, diet therapy has focused on decreased caloric intake and weight reduction. Recent recommendations have placed greater emphasis on reducing the percentage of calories from fat compared with carbohydrate restriction. Low-protein diets, when adhered to, most likely are of benefit to patients with nephropathy.

A prerequisite to satisfactory management of the diabetic patient is an ongoing frank and open discussion between the clinician and patient regarding the specific goals of therapy. Although the DCCT convincingly showed that a large group of intensively treated IDDM patients had a reduction in risk for diabetic complications, the implementation of these findings on an individual basis can be problematic. It seems reasonable to assume that improved glycemic control in all diabetics is likely to decrease rates of microvascular complications, since the same mechanisms are largely responsible for these complications in both IDDM and NIDDM. Analysis of the retinopathy data implies that almost any improvement in glucose control improves risk. However, since risk for development of microvascular complications cannot be predicted, it is not clear whether intensive therapy will benefit all patients. In addition, the risks of intensive therapy may significantly outweigh the benefits for some patients. The consequences of severe hypoglycemia and weight gain may be far greater for NIDDM patients (especially those with atherosclerosis) than they were for the young, otherwise healthy IDDM participants in the DCCT. In deciding the appropriateness of intensive therapy, assessment should be made of the extent and impact of the proposed lifestyle changes, as well as the risk for hypoglycemia and weight gain. Physicians need to determine whether the resources exist in their practice and/or community to meet the demands of intensive therapy. Only after lengthy discussions can patients make an informed choice about the optimal approach to the management of their particular case of diabetes mellitus. Whereas some may decide that intensive therapy is not worth the necessary changes, others may opt to try to minimize their chance of developing potentially devastating diabetes-related complications.

### Diet

Without proper nutrition therapy, it is nearly impossible to maximize glucose control and minimize complications. In composing a healthy diet, one must consider number as well as distribution of calories. The diet is best designed and implemented by a registered dietitian. Nutrition guidelines differ depending on age, size, physical activity, and level of comprehension. Total daily caloric requirements for adults range from 10 kcal/lb (22 kcal/kg) for sedentary individuals to 16 kcal/lb (35 kcal/kg) for very active people. Adolescent needs tend to be on the higher end of the range (13-15 kcal/lb for females and 15-18 kcal/lb for males). Young patients require sufficient calories and protein to ensure growth and development.

General guidelines for caloric composition established by the ADA closely follow recommendations by the American Heart Association. Previously recommended high-fat–low-carbohydrate diets were found to be associated with very high rates of coronary artery disease and have been replaced with diets high in complex carbohydrates and low in fat. About 55% to 60% of total calories should come from carbohydrates; high-fiber, unrefined forms are preferred. Fat content should be reduced to less than 30% of total calories unless hypertriglyceridemia results. Polyunsaturated fats should comprise 6% to 8% of total calories, and saturated fats should be less than 10% with monounsaturated fats making up the remainder. Cholesterol intake should be less than 300 mg/day. Reduced protein intake is recommended for diabetic patients, since Americans typically eat twice the amount needed and since excess protein may be detrimental to glomerular function. The goal is to decrease protein to 12% to 20% of total calories, which is equivalent to approximately 0.8 g/kg body weight for adults. Use of water-soluble fiber (up to 40 g/day) may increase insulin sensitivity and decrease postprandial glucose levels by delaying intestinal absorption. Reduced intake of sodium (≤3000 mg/day) and alcohol is also advised.

Distribution of calories over the course of the day will be different for people using insulin compared to other people with diabetes. Patients taking insulin must ensure that the timing of their meals takes into account the peak of previously administered insulin. Missed or delayed meals, which may have little impact on diet-controlled diabetic patients, can precipitate serious hypoglycemic reactions in those taking insulin. Although patients using short-acting insulin may need snacks at specific times during the day, NIDDM patients not taking insulin do not need snacks added to their regimen.

A critical role of nutrition planning for obese diabetic patients is weight loss. For the approximately 80% of people with NIDDM who are obese, relatively small amounts of weight loss can markedly improve insulin sensitivity and glucose control. Since achieving and maintaining weight loss is extremely difficult, unrealistic demands for weight loss should not be imposed on patients because inability to comply will ultimately induce frustration, depression, and further eating. Reduction of 500 kcal per day is sufficient to allow loss of 1 lb per week. Sustained effort with 10 to 15 lb of weight reduction over 3 to 4 months can significantly improve hemoglobin $A_{1c}$ values and lipid profiles.

Patients are more likely to lose weight if they feel supported by a team of health care professionals and if they perceive a tangible, immediate benefit from weight loss. Positive comments from doctors, nurses, and dietitians for every pound lost can be a positive reinforcing experience. NIDDM patients who lose sufficient weight to decrease insulin requirements to 20 U per day with appropriate glucose control may be considered for a trial on oral agents. Similarly, patients taking oral agents who lose weight may be able to control their diabetes with diet therapy alone. Losing weight is best accomplished by a combination of diet and exercise; either approach alone is usually unsuccessful.

Weight loss must be placed in the context of the patient's family and culture. Many patients do not perceive themselves as having weight problems despite being obese by medical standards. Traditional family roles may impede changing eating patterns if patients feel they cannot eat differently or prepare separate meals from their family. Recommending foods that are not a part of the patient's culture or not readily available in nearby stores almost ensures noncompliance. Several ethnic groups associate weight loss with illness and poverty; families and others may pressure patients to maintain heavier body size. In some groups heavier women are perceived as more beautiful and as a reflection of their husband's prosperity; weight loss for them will be negatively reinforced by family and friends.

A large part of implementing successful nutrition therapy is communication and education. Inquiries as to what patients want to weigh or think is a healthy weight will help define goals that are acceptable to everyone. Modifying ethnic recipes so that they can still be used will encourage acceptance by patient and family. Emphasis can be placed on incorporating dietary changes into family eating habits so that the children may have less chance of developing diabetes. Family members should be encouraged to attend group or individual nutrition counseling sessions. Communicating with the primary food shopper and the primary cook (not always the same person) can be critical to finding an ally within the family. In some families a specific person (parent or grandparent) makes all health care decisions about its members and needs to be consulted before any therapy can be started. Identifying support groups who can help reinforce weight loss can offset community stereotypes. Community resources, such as religious and other non-profit organizations (including the ADA and Juvenile Diabetes Foundation), can be used to promote health within the community. In addition, most states have Centers for Disease Control and Prevention–funded Diabetes Control Projects through the state departments of public health, which are valuable resources to patients and providers.

While general guidelines are helpful in planning diets, advice to individual patients should be tailored to specific behaviors and patterns. Admonitions such as "watch your diet" and "eat fewer sweets" do not provide means of affecting change. Suggestions about controlling portion size, avoiding snacks (especially while watching television), using diet soft drinks, choosing broiling over frying, drinking 1% or skim milk instead of whole milk helps patients to successfully implement healthy alternative behaviors. Patients with limited knowledge may benefit from primarily emphasizing survival skills, and those with better understanding can learn to read labels effectively and count calories. Food exchanges are a strict way of monitoring food intake but can be very difficult to maintain on a long-term basis.

### Exercise

Exercise provides several benefits to patients with diabetes. Even light exercise requires patients to get out of the house (and kitchen), to make their health a priority, and to gain a sense of control. In addition to reduction of other cardiovascular risk factors such as blood pressure and LDL cholesterol, exercise increases insulin sensitivity by increasing uptake of glucose by muscle.

Exercise programs should be carefully initiated and advanced. Adults should have a risk assessment for underlying coronary artery disease. Risk for arrhythmias should also be evaluated. Exercise sessions ideally should involve 5 to 10 minutes of warm-up, 20 to 30 minutes of actual physical activity, and 15 to 20 minutes of cool-down. The intensity of physical activity should be slowly increased over several weeks until 75% of maximum pulse rate response is obtained. Symptoms of shortness of breath, nausea, sweating, and palpitations should be carefully evaluated in exercising diabetic patients.

Fingerstick blood glucoses should be checked before and at the conclusion of exercise periods. For patients taking insulin or oral agents, exercise should preferably be performed after meals or snacks. Prolonged strenuous exercise (over 1 hour) usually requires additional carbohydrate (bread or fruit) exchanges to prevent hypoglycemic reactions. If blood glucose levels are low at the end of exercise, oral glucose or glucose-containing fluids should be taken and a repeat fingerstick checked 1 hour later. High blood glucose levels at the end of exercise may reflect counterinsulin hormone effects, which can dissipate over a short time or be due to underinsulinization. A fingerstick glucose 2 hours after exercise helps to distinguish between these different states and also reveals the direction the blood glucose is moving in. The prolonged duration of skeletal muscle glucose uptake can result in hypoglycemia many hours (8 to 16) after the actual exercise has occurred.

Other problems associated with exercise in diabetic patients are ophthalmologic and orthopedic. Retinal hemorrhages can occur in patients with underlying retinopathy if intraocular pressures increase while straining. Patients with neuropathy need to be particularly careful to avoid exercise-related injuries to their extremities. Inability to adequately feel pain during exercise can result in callus and blister formation, skin breakdown, and musculoskeletal injury including fracture. Diabetic athletes need to check their feet very carefully after any exercise session that involves running, jumping, or twisting.

### Blood glucose self-monitoring

The ability of patients to determine their own glucose concentration has been one of the most significant advancements in diabetes care since the discovery of insulin. Instead of having to rely on inaccurate perceived symptoms or extrapolations of urine levels, patients get immediate, reliable, accurate estimates of their diabetic control from capillary blood glucose values. Whether using oral agents or insulin, patients can use blood glucose self-monitoring to identify incipient hypoglycemia and early hyperglycemia. Modifications can be made to existing diet, exercise, and pharmacologic regimens in response to the pattern of high and low glucose levels identified by fingerstick glucose records. In addition, acute increases in fingerstick blood glucose values can help identify infections and other stress states early on.

Patients with diabetes should be encouraged to record their glucose levels in a logbook that is reviewed by the physician. Entries in the logbook should include date, time, medication administered and comments that may include hypoglycemic symptoms, specific foods eaten (or meals missed), and exercise sessions. Physicians should evaluate the logbook for times of day of hypoglycemic events and highest blood glucose values. Patients quickly become frustrated with monitoring glucose if physicians do not take an interest in these logs and review them carefully. Observing trends can indicate where the most advantageous adjustments in nutrition, exercise, or insulin therapy lie (Table 33-7).

**Table 33-7.** Adjustments for diabetes therapy

| Observation | Response |
|---|---|
| Increased fasting glucose | Increase nighttime intermediate-acting insulin |
| Increased prelunch glucose | Short-acting insulin before breakfast |
| Increased late afternoon blood glucose | Increase morning intermediate-acting insulin |
| Increased blood glucose before bedtime | Short-acting insulin before supper |
| Decreased blood glucose morning after exercise | Snack following exercise before bedtime |
| Decreased fasting blood glucose with high predinner values | Shift calories from dinner to snack before bedtime |

**Table 33-8.** Sulfonylureas

| Name | Duration | Dosage | Metabolism/excretion |
|---|---|---|---|
| **First generation** | | | |
| Tolbutamide (Orinase) | 6-12 hr | 500-3000 mg | Liver |
| Tolazamide (Tolinase) | 12-24 hr | 100-1000 mg | Liver |
| Chloropropamide (Diabenese) | 36+ hr | 100-750 mg | Liver/kidney |
| Acetohexamide (Dymelor) | 12-38 hr | 250-1500 mg | Liver/kidney |
| **Second generation** | | | |
| Glyburide (Diabeta, Micronase) | 24 hr | 1.25-30 mg | Liver/kidney |
| Glipizide (Glucotrol) | 24 hr | 5-40 mg | Liver/kidney |

Self-monitoring has advanced from color matching estimates to wipe systems using a reflectance meter to no-wipe meters with memory chips that can download data into a microcomputer and provide graphic analysis by day or time. The plethora of meters on the market can be confusing to patients. A certified diabetes educator frequently has extensive experience with several meters and can provide insight into pros and cons of specific meters. Individual features of meters that should be considered by each patient include overall meter size, text display size, button size, ease of pushing buttons, means of communication (choice of languages, graphic images, spoken words for blind patients), and maintenance requirements. Future proposed technologies include measuring glucose from skin capillaries indirectly without having to prick fingers.

## Oral hypoglycemic agents

Oral hypoglycemic agents should be used only for patients with type II diabetes after diet and exercise have proved to be ineffective in controlling blood sugar. Sulfonylureas have been the only oral medications approved in the United States for the treatment of diabetes mellitus (Table 33-8). These compounds primarily act by stimulating insulin release by the β-cell. Additionally, they may also increase the number of insulin receptors on hepatocytes and improve glucose uptake by skeletal muscle and adipose tissue. Almost 80% of type II patients initially respond to these agents, but the secondary failure rate reaches approximately 25%.

Hypoglycemia is the principal severe side effect of sulfonylureas. Since hypoglycemia due to these agents lasts significantly longer than that associated with insulin, hospitalization or monitored observation is typically required. Sulfonylureas are also teratogenic and should not be used in pregnant diabetic women.

Sulfonylureas have been divided into older (first-generation) and newer (second-generation) agents. The increased potency of the second-generation agents is mostly compensated by lower dosing ranges. These agents do have slightly fewer side effects (e.g., alcohol-induced flushing) and may be less likely to produce hyponatremia from drug-induced syndrome of inappropriate antidiuretic hormone (SIADH) because of an increase in free water clearance. If one sulfonylurea drug fails to control blood glucose, there is usually no significant benefit in trying another agent other than to prove to a reluctant patient that insulin is the treatment of last resort.

The value of sulfonylureas was questioned in a 1970 report from the University Group Diabetes Program (UGDP), which documented an increase in cardiovascular deaths in diabetic patients treated with tolbutamide compared with those treated with insulin. The data have been intensively scrutinized and questions have been raised regarding differences in cardiovascular risk factors and degree of glucose control between the two groups. Other studies have not demonstrated similar findings, and no studies have been conducted with second-generation agents. Although some debate still exists, oral sulfonylurea agents have generally been and continue to be considered safe and effective treatment in appropriate NIDDM patients.

Biguanides are a class of oral hypoglycemic agents that lower blood glucose by a different mechanism than that of sulfonylureas. These drugs decrease intestinal absorption of glucose, reduce hepatic glucose production, increase muscle and adipose glucose uptake, and suppress appetite. Although biguanides improve glycemic control as well as sulfonylureas in new-onset NIDDM, they are most often employed as adjunctive therapy when sulfonylureas fail. Production of lactate is the most serious side effect of these medications. Phenformin is no longer used because of the high risk for fatal lactic acidosis. Metformin has been reported to be equally as effective as phenformin at reducing hyperglycemia with less risk for lactate production. Metabolic states that reduce clearance of lactate, such as impaired renal or hepatic function, are contraindications to the use of biguanides. Limitation of the maximum dosage to 2.5 g/day also greatly reduces the incidence of lactic acidosis. Metformin, which has recently become available in the United States, also causes transient gastrointestinal complaints in up to 20% of patients.

### Insulin

***Preparations and characteristics.*** Although insulin is a single hormone, as a drug, it is available from three major sources (beef, pork, and synthetic human) and in three major classes (short, intermediate, and long acting). Previously, use of impure animal insulins was associated with development of insulin antibodies, local and occasionally systemic allergic responses, and lipoatrophy (subcutaneous atrophy). The frequency of these side effects decreased significantly with the introduction of purified pork insulin, which is produced by removing the noninsulin impurities from porcine pancreatic homogenates. The term *human insulin,* unlike beef and pork insulin, does not refer to its source but rather to the final product, which has an amino acid sequence identical to that made by the human pancreas. Human insulin can be made either by modifying porcine insulin, which differs by only three amino acids, or by using recombinant technology to infect bacteria with human insulin–producing genetic sequences. There is little difference in the frequency of side effects just listed when comparing human and purified pork insulins. There is also relatively little difference in the cost of human versus purified pork insulin. There is no benefit to switching patients who have been well maintained on purified pork insulin. Human insulin appears to have slightly shorter peaks and durations of action than purified pork insulin. Table 33-9 lists the major types of human insulins, their peaks of action, and their duration. Lys-Pro insulin, if it becomes available, may represent an ultrashort-acting insulin that can be administered just before a meal for the caloric intake of that meal.

**Table 33-9.** Insulin preparations commonly used to treat diabetic patients

| Type of insulin | Peak of action | Duration of action |
|---|---|---|
| **Short acting** | | |
| Lys-Pro insulin* | 1-2 hr | 3-5 hr |
| Human regular | 1.5-3 hr | 4-6 hr |
| Semilente | 1.5-3 hr | 4-6 hr |
| Pork regular | 2-4 hr | 6-8 hr |
| **Intermediate acting** | | |
| Human NPH | 6-10 hr | 12-16 hr |
| Human Lente | 6-10 hr | 12-18 hr |
| Pork NPH | 8-12 hr | 14-20 hr |
| **Long acting** | | |
| Human Ultralente | 10-16 hr | 16-24 hr |

*Not currently available in the United States.

Once a patient's glucose levels have been stabilized on a particular type of insulin, it is important to continue that type of insulin. This is particularly critical to remember when writing prescriptions. Although many pharmacies stock only human insulin, others may stock both human and animal types and can use their discretion to dispense any type of insulin unless an exact source is specified on a prescription.

In general, patients requiring more than one insulin type at the same time can combine NPH and regular insulins in the same syringe for simultaneous administration. Similarly, the Lente insulins can be mixed in the same syringe. An increasing number of premixed insulin preparations are becoming available to patients with diabetes mellitus. Since many patients respond well to a ratio of two thirds intermediate-acting to one third short-acting insulin (see further), a mixture of 70% NPH and 30% regular insulin (70/30 insulin) has been made available. In this type of preparation, 30 U of 70/30 is equivalent to 21 U NPH and 9 U regular. Other mixtures, including 80/20 and 90/10, are projected to follow. Although premixed insulin can be an added convenience, patients should not be forced to change their activities or diet merely to fit this ratio of intermediate- to short-acting insulin.

***Initiation of therapy.*** Patients with diabetes mellitus are generally started on insulin for one of four reasons: (1) following inpatient admission for ketoacidosis; (2) after failure of diet, exercise, and sulfonylurea drugs to control blood glucose in NIDDM; (3) as part of insulin pump treatment; and (4) after diet fails to control blood glucose in a patient with gestational diabetes. An optimal starting dosage of insulin must aim to prevent recurrent hyperglycemia and prolonged hospitalization without precipitating hypoglycemia. Issues that require careful consideration are the number of shots and the types of insulin to be used. Whereas IDDM patients are usually started on insulin in the hospital after ketoacidosis, NIDDM patients may be started on insulin in the hospital at the time of diagnosis or in the outpatient setting after having failed sulfonylurea therapy.

In IDDM the goal of insulin dosing is to replace physiologic levels previously maintained by intact β-cells. It is important to remember that amounts of insulin required to treat acidosis are greater than daily requirements to maintain normoglycemia. However, as normal pH is restored, dosages of insulin used over a 24-hour period may reflect total daily dose requirements. IDDM patients will, in general, need at least two shots of insulin per day to ensure that some circulating insulin is present over 24 hours. One approach has been to total the amount of short-acting (regular or Semilente) insulin needed to maintain blood glucose control for a 24-hour period and to use two thirds of that as the next day's morning dose, the remaining third being given in the evening. Morning and evening doses are also divided so that two thirds is given as intermediate-acting (NPH or Lente) insulin and one third is given as short acting (regular or Lente). For example, if a patient recovering from ketoacidosis needed 63 U of regular insulin to maintain a glucose level in a range between 150 and 200 mg/dl, 42 U would be given in the morning and 21 U would be allocated for the evening. The morning dose would comprise 28 U NPH and 14 U regular; the evening dose would be 14 U NPH and 7 U regular.

The above approach may work very well for healthy patients who eat consistent meals at regular intervals. It may only serve as an initial approximation for other patients with varying behaviors and activities. Assessing glycemic patterns from blood glucose self-monitoring logbooks usually provides clues as to what changes would be most effective.

Occasionally type II patients are started on insulin in the hospital after being hospitalized for severe hyperglycemic states. For these patients insulin therapy supplements pancreatic production and is used to overcome cellular resistance. Some patients may need extra daytime insulin to maximize caloric intake, and others may need nighttime insulin to adequately suppress hepatic glucose production; some may need both. Since daily pancreatic output of insulin is equivalent to approximately 20 to 25 U, most type II patients can be conservatively started on 18 to 20 U intermediate-acting insulin per day. Another approach is to begin with intermediate-acting insulin in a two thirds morning/one third nighttime ratio and add short-acting insulin as indicated by fingerstick glucose patterns.

When beginning inpatient insulin therapy, preprandial fingerstick glucose levels can be used to determine coverage with short-acting insulin. However, a single sliding scale for all times of day is frequently inappropriate because of overlap between peaks of short- and intermediate-acting insulins. In general, it is best to attempt to achieve tight insulin control as an outpatient, when the patient is eating, exercising, and performing his or her normal activities. It is important not to increase insulin too aggressively, since this can subsequently precipitate a severe hypoglycemic reaction that will serve only to frustrate the patient and may even lead to incorrectly labeling the patient as brittle. Increasing insulin dosages by 10% typically provides safe but significant additional coverage.

Major changes in insulin regimens should not be made daily. Each modification affects glucose beyond the duration of action of the insulin preparation used; 2 to 3 days are needed before a new steady state is reached. As with too large increases in dosage, too frequent adjustments in insulin can also lead to bouts of hypoglycemia and hyperglycemia resulting in patient frustration.

Most patients with NIDDM are started on insulin after failing oral agent therapy. The need to change from oral agents to insulin therapy in type II patients is a common part of diabetes management after 12 to 15 years. Patients who have received nutrition and exercise counseling and are taking maximum doses of oral agents but who continue to have fingerstick glucose or glycosylated hemoglobin levels out of their target range should be considered for insulin therapy. The target range needs to be individualized for each patient based on expected benefits of glucose control, consequences of adverse events such as hypoglycemia, and willingness/ability to comply with a prescribed regimen. For a 46-year-old patient without other medical problems, the target range for preprandial glucose may be 120 mg/dl; measured values of 180 mg/dl or glycosylated hemoglobin two points over the upper limit of normal would thus be an indication for insulin. Conversely, the target range may be much higher for a 75-year-old patient with underlying coronary artery disease because of the risk of a hypoglycemia-induced myocardial infarction. For such a patient, a glucose level of 220 mg/dl on maximum oral agents may be tolerated in light of these other considerations. Whereas the need to begin insulin may be obvious in some patients, it may be unclear in others depending on age, family resources, financial resources, visual acuity, learning abilities, underlying medical conditions, and nutrition behaviors. As noted above, the target range for each individual needs to be clarified through extensive ongoing discussions. Consultation with an endocrinologist can be helpful in these more ambiguous cases because it provides support for the decision of the primary physician and reinforces the importance of the action to the patient. Endocrinologists also have resources available to facilitate the learning and transition to insulin therapy.

Initiating insulin therapy involves motivation, education, and training. Many patients believe that beginning insulin reflects poor compliance or indicates a marked worsening of their diabetes. In addition, they mistakenly attribute a causal relationship between the coincident onset of complications and the initiation of insulin (e.g., "I saw what happened to my friend after he went on insulin; he lost a leg"). Primary physicians need to emphasize the goal of glucose control and educate patients that insulin is one of the tools that is used to achieve this goal. In that way, insulin can be viewed as a therapy for patients who can still have complications prevented.

Starting insulin therapy in NIDDM patients in the outpatient setting has become increasingly common in recent years. The principal requirements for successfully completing this transition include reliable fingerstick monitoring at multiple times of day, consistent (often daily) follow-up (usually by phone), and the ability to implement change within 1 or 2 days. The effectiveness of acute insulin adjustments depends on the accuracy of the reported fingerstick values. Values must also be obtained from different times of day to understand the glycemic pattern (see above). Frequent follow-up is necessary to ensure that blood glucose does not remain too high or too low and place the patient at risk for hospitalization. Admission for severe hyperglycemia can also be prevented if patients have the ability to change dosages or supplement with short-acting insulin. Although some of these functions can be carried out by family members or visiting nurses, lines of communication and guidelines for contact must be clearly established.

The importance of the diabetes educator and/or diabetes nurse cannot be overemphasized in any discussion of instituting insulin therapy in diabetic patients. Valuable time for both the patient and health care professional can be saved if proper techniques are learned for the care and handling of insulin, mixing insulin preparations together, choosing injection sites, and injecting correctly into those areas. Also, periodic review of these basics of diabetes care in even the most experienced diabetic patients can be of great benefit in attaining the goal of better blood glucose management.

## Special cases

***Adolescents.*** Within the spectrum of patients with diabetes mellitus, certain groups require special consideration. Adolescence, with its rebellion against authority and emphasis on peer acceptance, is nearly antithetical to the realities of self-care for diabetes mellitus. Teens with IDDM, resentful of having to take insulin, watch their diet, and check fingersticks, may become noncompliant and set the stage for future complications. These patients may present with frequent hospitalization for mild ketoacidosis or hypoglycemia. Others adjust their insulin to intentionally worsen glycosuria to avoid weight gain and present with extremely elevated glycosylated hemoglobins despite recommendations to increase insulin doses. Admonition by well-meaning parents who may have previously been very involved in glucose monitoring and insulin administration frequently alienates the adolescent further. Extreme problems, including eating disorders and use of illegal drugs, alternate with episodes of unexplained hypoglycemia and severe hyperglycemia. Many of these patients are mistakenly labeled brittle without appreciation of the underlying problems. A delicate balance must be struck between providing emotional support for adolescents with diabetes and encouraging them to accept responsibility for their own health care. Opportunities to interact with other adolescent diabetics will diminish the sense of being different from others. Diabetic summer camps or retreats create a peer network that can provide support and stability through these tumultuous years.

***Elderly patients.*** Older patients with diabetes need to be carefully evaluated for the impact of complications and for the risks versus benefits of tight control. Morbidity from complications can assume different forms in older patients. For example, cataracts are more common than proliferative retinopathy. Neuropathy, in addition to increasing risk for foot ulcers, also increases the likelihood of falling. Falls are also more common in diabetics with impaired vision and orthostasis. The increased probability of atherosclerosis in older patients increases their potential risk for significant cardiovascular events in response to a severe hypoglycemic episode. It is important to emphasize that cardiovascular or other major diseases are the contraindication for intensive therapy and not age per se. Regimens that avoid extremes of hyperglycemia and hypoglycemia may be a reasonable goal for many older diabetic patients with coexisting medical problems. A single injection of a long-acting insulin (e.g., Ultralente) can be used for this purpose in those NIDDM patients requiring insulin to control their diabetes.

***Pregnant patients.*** The etiologies and complications of the pregnant diabetic patient depend on whether she has had preexisting diabetes and becomes pregnant, or develops hyperglycemia after becoming pregnant. Preexisting poorly controlled diabetes affects pregnancy by increasing the risk of fetal malformations and fetal demise (see the box at right). It should be noted, however, that near normalization of blood glucose in women with IDDM, especially during the first 8 to 12 weeks of gestation, has been shown to reduce the risks of major congenital defects to nearly that of healthy women. In addition, diabetic women can have significant worsening of proliferative retinopathy during pregnancy. Even though retinal changes can reverse after delivery, some changes remain and can lead to decreased vision.

### Maternal/fetal complications of diabetes during pregnancy

**Developmental malformations**
CNS defects
Macrosomia, organomegaly
Cardiac abnormalities
Renal anomalies
Situs inversus

**Perinatal morbidity/mortality**
Stillbirth
Asphyxia
Respiratory distress
Increased blood volume, hyperviscosity
Congestive heart failure
Hypocalcemia
Hypomagnesemia
Hypoglycemia
Hyperbilirubinemia

Women of childbearing age with diabetes should consult with an endocrinologist regarding the benefits of tight glucose control before attempting conception. Motivation is usually high in these patients, and most are willing to take three shots per day and check fingersticks four or more times per day. After conception insulin dosage requirements frequently lessen, and hypoglycemic episodes occur more often as insulin sensitivity increases. Target blood glucose concentrations are as follows:

1. Fasting: 60 to 90 mg/dl (3.3 to 5 mmol/L)
2. Preprandial: 60 to 105 mg/dl (3.3 to 5.8 mmol/L)
3. 2 hours postprandial: 90 to 120 mg/dl (5 to 6.7 mmol/L)

Glycosylated albumin or fructosamine levels, which reflect the average blood glucose over the preceding 2 to 3 weeks, can be used to assess glycemic control and effectiveness of therapy. During the second half of pregnancy expected increases in insulin resistance and dosage requirements need to be discussed with patients to avoid frustration from increases in blood glucose despite maintenance of diet and physical activity. However, insulin sensitivity quickly returns to baseline after birth, and careful attention must be paid to prevent severe postpartum hypoglycemia.

The woman with gestational diabetes becomes temporarily glucose intolerant during the second half of pregnancy as a result of insulin resistance. Gestational diabetes very rarely happens during the first half of pregnancy, since insulin sensitivity is increased during that time. In fact, blood glucose values are lower in pregnant women because the hormonal environment of early pregnancy increases insulin sensitivity and because large amounts of glucose are transported across the placenta. Normal fasting glucose levels in nondiabetic pregnant women can be as low as 50 mg/dl. During the second half of pregnancy insulin sensitivity is reduced because of further changes in the hormonal environment; human placental lactogen (hPL), which is similar in structure to growth hormone, is thought to play a significant role. Although most women are able to compensate with an increase in insulin production and secretion, those who cannot compensate develop gestational diabetes.

All women should be screened with a 50-g glucose load between 24 and 28 weeks of pregnancy. Those women with a 2-hour glucose value greater than 140 mg/dl should undergo a 100-g, 3-hour glucose tolerance test. The diagnosis of gestational diabetes is made if two values are abnormal (see the box on p. 483). Using this definition the frequency of gestational diabetes in the United States is approximately 3%. Decisions about treatment must be made quickly in these women to normalize glucose levels and reduce risk for complications. Independent of treatment options, these patients need to be taught blood glucose self-monitoring, the risks of hyperglycemia and hypoglycemia, and risks for future development of type II diabetes. During pregnancy, consultation with a registered dietitian can frequently improve blood glucose values. Patients should not try to lose weight or severely restrict calories, since starvation-induced ketosis may adversely affect fetal CNS development. If glucose values continue to be outside of the desired range, insulin therapy must be initiated, since oral agents are contraindicated during pregnancy. Glycosylated albumin or fructosamine levels can be used to determine average glucose control for the preceding 2 to 3 weeks. Persistent maternal hyperglycemia causes the fetal pancreas to overproduce and oversecrete insulin, which may explain the frequently observed macrosomia. At birth persistent neonatal hyperinsulinemia can induce severe hypoglycemia in the newborn.

Although sensitivity to insulin is rapidly restored in most women after childbirth, it is extremely important to follow up with postpartum patients to make sure that their blood glucose level does not remain elevated. The insulin resistance of the second half of pregnancy can unmask a latent type II patient who requires continued treatment.

The development of gestational diabetes identifies a population of patients at risk for developing type II. Although the etiology of the impaired insulin secretion and diminished insulin sensitivity is different for gestational diabetes, the inability to adequately compensate and the resulting hyperglycemia are final common pathophysiologic pathways. Follow-up studies have reported that 30% to 50% of women with gestational diabetes develop NIDDM within 10 years. Primary care physicians should counsel patients with a history of gestational diabetes about the risk for NIDDM and initiate a diet and exercise program as early as possible. Current studies are evaluating the feasibility of preventing NIDDM with this approach in high-risk patients.

***Changing circadian rhythms.*** Controlling blood glucoses in diabetic patients who do not work typical 9 AM to 5 PM hours can be extremely difficult. Insulin peaks and durations must be balanced against changing meal times and circadian rhythms and are often best handled by endocrinologists. The use of Ultralente insulin, in either single or split doses with doses of regular insulin to cover meals, can be a very flexible and successful approach to patients with this lifestyle. Alternatively, the use of insulin pump therapy, which is imitated by the Ultralente/regular regimen, can also be considered. These approaches can be very satisfying to those individuals looking for more flexibility with improved glucose control or to those who have failed more conventional insulin regimens.

## COMMENTARY/CONTROVERSY

### Intensive therapy—DCCT

The value of maintaining glucose concentrations as close to the normal range as possible has been emphasized by the recently concluded DCCT. This 9-year study enrolled over 1400 type I patients who were randomized to either conventional or intensive insulin therapy. Intensive therapy was achieved using an insulin pump or at least three subcutaneous injections per day. Intensive therapy patients monitored their fingersticks at least four times per day. The trial evaluated patients who had no evidence of complications and those who had early manifestations of retinopathy or nephropathy. Intensive therapy patients achieved lower average blood glucose levels (approximately 155 mg/dl) compared with the conventional therapy (approximately 230 mg/dl) as well as lower glycosylated hemoglobin values (7.1% vs. 9.2%). Retinopathy in the intensive therapy group was lowered by 76%, and the risk for albuminuria was decreased by nearly 50% (Fig. 33-4). Neuropathy was also decreased in the intensive therapy group. The lack of difference in car-

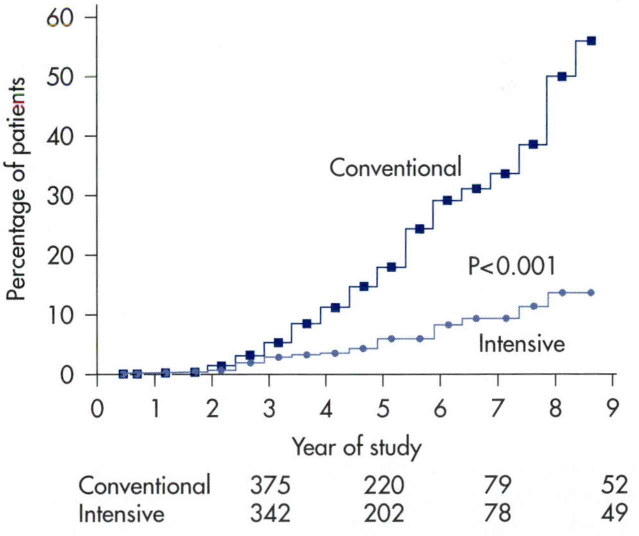


**Fig. 33-4.** Cumulative incidence of a sustained change in retinopathy in patients with IDDM receiving intensive or conventional therapy. A sustained change in the severity of retinopathy was defined as a change observed by fundus photography of at least three steps from base line that was sustained for at least 6 months. In the primary-prevention cohort, intensive therapy reduced the adjusted mean risk of the onset of retinopathy by 76% during course of study, as compared with conventional therapy (P <0.001). Numbers of patients in each therapy group evaluated at years 3, 5, 7, and 9 are shown below graphs. Similar results obtained in patients with mild baseline retinopathy and for development of microalbuminuria. (Massachusetts Medical Society: *N Eng J Med* 329:977, 1993.)

diovascular events between the two groups may have been obscured by the relatively young average age (27) and otherwise good health of the participants.

Adverse effects of intensive insulin therapy included hypoglycemia and weight gain. Patients in the intensive therapy group were three times more likely to have a severe hypoglycemic event requiring assistance from another individual. Intensive therapy patients were also more likely to become over 120% of their ideal body weight.

The results of the DCCT provide strong support for recommending tight control in type I patients. Intensive therapy is not recommended with end stage renal disease or blindness because of the inability to reverse these complications. In addition, intensive therapy is not currently being recommended for children below age 13. Patients with established vascular disease are most likely not good candidates for intensive therapy, since severe hypoglycemia could induce catecholamine release and precipitate myocardial infarction.

For patients with NIDDM the risks of hypoglycemia may exceed the benefit of near normal blood glucose. Since the mechanisms by which excess glucose contributes to diabetic complications are similar in IDDM and NIDDM, it would be expected that improved glycemic control would benefit both groups. However, if NIDDM patients who tend to be older and at risk for coronary disease are subjected to the threefold increased risk of severe hypoglycemia observed in DCCT, the price of tight control could be increased morbidity and possibly mortality. Future studies on NIDDM patients will need to assess the risk versus benefit of intensive therapy. Currently, it seems reasonable for those NIDDM patients expressing interest in intensive therapy to undergo careful evaluation for atherosclerosis. Support from a diabetes team specializing in intensive therapy is also highly recommended.

### Combination therapy with an oral agent and insulin

The use of oral hypoglycemic agents in combination with insulin was proposed in an effort to maximize control and minimize insulin dosing. Several regimens have been proposed, including daytime insulin with nighttime oral agents, and nighttime insulin with daytime oral agents. Long-acting and intermediate-acting insulins have been suggested for increasing basal insulin concentrations, and short-acting insulin has been used near meal times. Initial predictions that these alternatives would induce severe hypoglycemic episodes have not been fulfilled. However, these regimens have not been found to substantially improve overall glucose control, even though they have lowered the dosage of insulin needed to achieve it. Certain patients may respond well to combination regimens, but no predictive factors for success have been consistently identified. Proposed trials using oral agents with insulin are best discussed in consultation with an endocrinologist.

### Hypertension in the patient with diabetes

Hypertension occurs in nearly 50% of patients with diabetes. In type I a family history of hypertension and renal dysfunction are risk factors for elevated blood pressure. Abnormalities in cell membrane sodium pumps, which have been linked to the presence of hypertension, are more common in IDDM patients with hypertension. In type II patients epidemiologic studies have demonstrated a strong association between hypertension, diabetes, obesity, and lipid abnormalities. Insulin resistance and the resulting hyperinsulinemia have been postulated to contribute significantly to the development of these abnormalities (see Chapter 7). Although evidence exists for a role in diabetes, obesity, and hypertriglyceridemia, the contribution of insulin resistance to hypertension is less clear.

The treatment of high blood pressure in the patient with diabetes helps to prevent microvascular and macrovascular disease. Untreated hypertension is associated with increased risk for renal and retinal complications of diabetes. Conversely albumin excretion, which serves as a marker of glomerular function, is improved in diabetic patients with treated hypertension. In studies of atherosclerosis, the risk for heart disease in patients with both hypertension and diabetes is more than additive. The benefit of hypertension treatment on cardiovascular risk is well established.

There is considerable debate as to which pharmacologic agent represents optimal first line therapy. Recommendations by the Joint National Commission have stressed the proven benefits of thiazide and β-blocker drugs on cardiovascular risk reduction. Other experts feel these recommendations do not take into account the absence of diabetic patients in most of these studies, the untoward effects of these drugs on increased blood sugar and VLDL levels, and the increased potential for impotence. In addition, there are now considerable data on the benefit of ACE inhibitors in preserving renal function in patients with diabetes. Reduction in urinary protein and microalbumin excretion and prolongation of the time to dialysis appear to be greater for patients taking ACE inhibitors. Unfortunately, there have been extremely few long-term studies comparing ACE inhibitors with other agents. In short-term studies some (e.g., diltiazem) but not all calcium blockers have been shown to be beneficial in reducing both blood pressure and albumin excretion.

Studies with ACE inhibitors have demonstrated an ability to decrease albumin excretion independent of blood pressure reduction. Beneficial effects of these drugs have also been observed in nonhypertensive diabetic patients. It is important to note that benefits can be demonstrated in the range of 20 to 300 mg protein/24 hours before routine urinalysis tests become positive for protein. Microalbuminuria appears to be a strong predictor of progression to end-stage renal disease. These studies have raised the question as to whether diabetic patients with normal blood pressure should be started on some form of therapy to maximize renal function. Before this question can be answered, further studies need to determine the clinical stage at which intervention produces maximum preservation. For example, recent studies have suggested a greater benefit in macroalbuminuric compared with microalbuminuric patients. In addition, further work needs to identify dosing parameters for normotensive patients, since blood pressure remains largely unchanged.

Although no standard recommendations for pharmacologic therapy to minimize diabetic nephropathy exist, the encouraging results with ACE inhibitors should suggest their use in proteinuric or hypertensive diabetic patients.

> **Necessary tools for good diabetes care**
>
> **Medications**
>
> Oral agents
> Insulin
> Insulin syringes (1/3ml [30 U], 1/2ml [50 U], 1ml [100 U]) or pen.
>
> **For blood glucose self-monitoring**
>
> Blood glucose meter
> Test strips
> Alcohol pads
> Cotton balls
> Lancet device and lancets
> Logbook
> Software for downloading and analysis of data
>
> **For hypoglycemia**
>
> Glucose tablets, glucose gel, cake frosting, juice, or soft candy
> Glucagon, injectable, for some
>
> **For illness**
>
> Urine strips to test for ketones
> Short-acting insulin (regular, semilente)

The case for utilizing them in normotensive diabetic patients with elevated levels of microalbuminuria is less clear. Reasonable factors to consider in making the decision to begin therapy in these patients include current renal function as assessed by 24-hour urine collection, total amount of albumin excretion, concomitant medical conditions, and parental history of hypertension (which may increase the risk of nephropathy). Consultation with either an endocrinologist or nephrologist may be of benefit in this situation.

## WHAT PATIENTS NEED AT HOME

The patient with diabetes mellitus has to have both diagnostic and therapeutic agents available at home to provide optimal self-care. The box at right lists many of the items that should be considered before the diabetic patient walks out the door. All patients need to have educational information concerning diet and exercise. Those who monitor their fingerstick blood glucose will need items to clean their fingertips and prick their fingers before they can place a drop of blood on the proper strip that can be read by the appropriate meter. All patients need to have some agent available to them in case of hypoglycemia. If hypoglycemia unawareness is a significant problem, a family member or close friend needs to be taught how to administer glucagon intramuscularly.

Patients with diabetes need to be able to diagnose and respond to illnesses quickly if they are to prevent visits to the emergency room and inpatient admissions. All type I patients should keep urine strips for testing ketones available to detect ketonuria early on. Health care providers need to react quickly and aggressively when ketonuria is documented. Some patients may be able to manage illnesses at home with frequent physician input, oral rehydration, multiple injections of short-acting insulin, frequent fingerstick and urine monitoring. However, a large proportion of patients are best seen immediately in the office or the hospital emergency department. The availability of short-acting insulin, even if it is not part of their normal regimen, can frequently be helpful to patients with glucose levels getting progressively out of control.

To ensure proper administration of insulin, proper size syringes and alcohol wipes need to be provided to patients. Patients accustomed to 50 U per syringe (0.5 ml) may become confused if 100 U syringes are suddenly prescribed. It is also important to calculate how long the prescription of insulin will last. The vast majority of insulin comes as 100 U/ml with 10 ml per vial. Thus one vial of insulin for a patient on 60 U NPH in the morning and 30 U in the evening will last only about 11 days (1000 U/vial divided by 90 units/day equals 11 days/vial). Such a patient would be better off receiving three vials per monthly prescription.

## CONSULTATION

Primary care physicians provide the majority of health care to patients with diabetes mellitus and thus have an ideal opportunity to coordinate health care and prevent long-term complications of this chronic disease. Consultations are beneficial for specific services and addressing complicated questions. Specific services can include ophthalmologic evaluation, podiatric examination, and diabetes teaching. Diabetes teaching should not be prescribed only at the time of diagnosis. Distinct educational messages are necessary as patients change from oral agents to insulin, begin intensive insulin therapy, lose recognition of typical hypoglycemic symptoms, and develop complications of diabetes. Certified diabetes educators are specially trained in areas of diabetes patient education and are a particularly valuable resource for patients. Specific programs that have achieved recognition by the ADA have an established curriculum and interdisciplinary representation to address patient needs on multiple levels. Endocrinologists often lead these programs and can provide additional education to patients. Pregnant patients with diabetes need intensive insulin therapy, preferably before conception, and would benefit from evaluation by an endocrinologist.

In the early phase of their condition patients with diabetes require education and decisions about optimal therapy. If questions exist concerning benefits of one versus multiple daily injections, alternative regimens and types of insulins, or appropriateness of intensive insulin therapy, an endocrinologist should be consulted. Intensive insulin therapy cannot be accomplished by a single health provider and should be implemented by a team of diabetes health professionals led by an endocrinologist.

As diabetes progresses, changes in symptoms and frequency of hypoglycemia may occur that can benefit from consultation. In addition, decisions regarding insulin therapy in type II patients and modifications to existing insulin regimens may be assisted by an endocrinologist. Portions of the physical examination (funduscopic examination) and specialized treatments (foot care) not within the expertise of the primary physician may be evaluated and followed by ophthalmologists, endocrinologists, and podiatrists. This phase represents a particularly important opportunity for prevention of complications by complete assessment of cardiovascular risk, ophthalmologic status, neuropathic changes, and nephropathic markers.

As chronic complications occur, the focus of consultations changes from prevention to minimizing damage. Yearly visits to an ophthalmologist evaluate the need for photocoagulation therapy. Consultation with nephrologists are needed as serum creatinine rises (over 2.5 mg/dl) and plans for dialysis become necessary. The question of whether new pain symptoms are being caused by neuropathy may be answered by either an endocrinologist or a neurologist. Neurologic consultation may be particularly beneficial for patients with pain unrelieved by standard therapy. Patients with atherosclerosis may benefit from cardiology consultation. During this phase an endocrinology consultation may help adjust insulin doses to minimize hypoglycemia, reevaluate the target range for blood glucose control, and maximize prevention of other complications.

## CONCLUSION

Diabetes mellitus has come to serve as a model for approach and delivery of health care. It is a major public health problem that requires increased public awareness and, for NIDDM, necessitates testing to uncover those who remain undiagnosed and those who are at high risk. With proper education patients can manage diabetes to a large degree on their own. Optimum management involves increasing awareness of healthy nutrition and exercise behaviors, as well as compliance with medication. Diabetes is a condition that is best treated by a multidisciplinary team of health care professionals who work together to prevent complications. Careful attention to present blood glucose values helps reduce risks for retinal, renal, and neurologic complications. State of the art diabetes care is aimed at care of the entire patient, modification of lifestyle and environment, and prevention of complications.

Over the next several years agents that help prevent complications will be tested and introduced. New types of therapies that improve blood glucose control will also become available. Means of identifying those at risk for the disease will ultimately be helpful in delaying or preventing its onset.

## BIBLIOGRAPHY


Barss VA: Diabetes and pregnancy, *Med Clin North Am* 73:685, 1989.

Besser GM, Bodansky HJ, Cudworth AG: *Clinical diabetes—an illustrated text,* New York, 1988, Gower Medical Publishing.

DCCT Group: Effect of intensive treatment of diabetes on the development and progression of long-term complications in IDDM, *N Engl J Med* 329:977, 1993.

Department of Health and Human Services: *The prevention and treatment of complications of diabetes mellitus: a guide for primary care practitioners,* Centers for Disease Control, 1991.

Dyck PJ et al: Nerve glucose, fructose, sorbitol, myoinositol and fiber degeneration and regeneration in diabetic neuropathy, *N Engl J Med* 3199:542, 1988.

Frank RN: On the pathogenesis of diabetic retinopathy: a 1990 update, *Ophthalmology* 98:586, 1991.

Franz MJ et al: Technical review: nutrition principles for the management of diabetes and related complications, *Diabetes Care* 17 (5):490, 1994.

Horton ES: Exercise and diabetes mellitus, *Med Clin North Am* 72:1301, 1988.

Javanovic-Peterson L, editor: *Medical management of pregnancy complicated by diabetes,* Alexandria, Va, 1993, American Diabetes Association.

Lebovitz HE, editor: *Physician's guide to non-insulin-dependent (type II) diabetes: diagnosis and treatment,* ed 2, Alexandria, Va, 1988, American Diabetes Association.

Lewis EJ et al: The effect of angiotensin converting enzyme inhibition on diabetic nephropathy, *N Engl J Med* 329:1456, 1993.

Max MB et al: Effects of desipramine, amitriptyline, and fluoxetine on pain in diabetes neuropathy, *N Engl J Med* 326(19):1250, 1992.

Morley JE, Kaiser FE: Unique aspects of diabetes mellitus in the elderly, *Clin Geriatr Med* 6:693, 1990.

Selby JV et al: The natural history and epidemiology of diabetic nephropathy: implications for prevention and control, *JAMA* 263: 1954, 1990.

Williams G: Management of NIDDM, *Lancet* 343:95, 1994.


CHAPTER

# 34 Thyroid Gland Disorders


**Alan P. Farwell**
**Susana A. Ebner**


Clinical disorders of the thyroid gland are the most common endocrinopathies. As such, it is essential for the primary care physician to recognize the clinical features of the various forms of thyroid dysfunction. In addition, subclinical thyroid disease has become a recognized clinical entity due to recent advances in the measurement of hormone concentrations in blood that allow the identification of clinically euthyroid patients who may develop thyroid dysfunction. Thus the clinician must posses an understanding of the fundamentals of thyroid hormone economy, the laboratory evaluation of thyroid function, and the availability of thyroid imaging techniques to appropriately manage these patients.

## NORMAL THYROID HORMONE ECONOMY

### Regulation

Synthesis and secretion of thyroid hormone is under the control of the anterior pituitary hormone, thyrotropin (TSH). TSH secretion increases when serum thyroid hormone concentrations fall and decreases when they rise, in a classic negative feedback system. TSH is also under the regulation of the hypothalamic hormone, thyrotropin-releasing hormone (TRH). The negative feedback of thyroid hormone is targeted mainly at the pituitary level but probably affects TRH release from the hypothalamus as well. In addition, input from higher cortical centers affects TRH secretion.

Under the influence of TSH the thyroid gland synthesizes and releases thyroid hormone. Thyroxine ($T_4$) is the principal secretory product of the thyroid gland, comprising about 90% of the secreted hormone under normal conditions. $T_4$ is also the most abundant thyroid hormone in serum, with a normal circulating level between 4.5 and 11.0 μg/dl. Although some effects of thyroid hormone are attributed specifically to $T_4$, for the most part $T_4$ functions as a hormone precursor that is metabolized in peripheral tissues to a more active form.

### Metabolic pathways

The major pathway of metabolism of $T_4$ is by sequential monodeiodination. Removal of the 5′-, or outer ring, iodine is the activating metabolic pathway, leading to the formation of the metabolically active form of thyroid hormone, 3,5,3′-triiodothyronine ($T_3$). Removal of the inner ring, or 5-, iodine is an inactivating pathway, producing the metabolically inactive hormone, 3,3′,5′-triiodothyronine (reverse $T_3$, or $rT_3$). Under normal conditions about 41% of $T_4$ is converted to $T_3$, about 38% is converted to $rT_3$, and about 21% is metabolized via other pathways, such as conjugation in the liver and excretion in the bile.

$T_3$ is the metabolically active thyroid hormone and exerts its actions via binding to chromatin-bound nuclear receptors and regulating gene transcription in responsive tissues. Only about 10% of circulating $T_3$ is secreted directly by the thyroid gland, whereas more than 80% is derived from conversion of $T_4$ in peripheral tissues, primarily in the liver. Thus factors that affect peripheral $T_4$ to $T_3$ conversion have significant effects on circulating $T_3$ levels. Peripheral $T_4$ to $T_3$ conversion is catalyzed by type I 5′-deiodinase, which is found primarily in the liver. Serum levels of $T_3$ are about 100-fold less than those of $T_4$, with a normal circulating range between 60 and 180 ng/dl. Like $T_4$, $T_3$ is metabolized by deiodination, forming diiodothyronine, and by conjugation in the liver.

### Serum-binding proteins

Both $T_4$ and $T_3$ circulate in the serum bound to several proteins that are synthesized in the liver. Thyronine-binding globulin (TBG) is the major serum-binding protein and binds about 80% of the serum thyroid hormones. The affinity of $T_4$ for TBG is about tenfold greater than that of $T_3$ and is part of the reason that circulating $T_4$ levels are higher than $T_3$ levels. Other serum-binding proteins include transthyretin, which binds about 15% of $T_4$ but little if any $T_3$, and albumin, which has a low affinity but a very large capacity for binding $T_4$ and $T_3$. Overall, 99.97% of circulating $T_4$ and 99.7% of circulating $T_3$ is bound to plasma proteins.

### Free hormone concept

Essential to the understanding of the regulation of thyroid function is the free hormone concept, i.e., only the unbound hormone has any metabolic activity. Laboratory measurements of serum total $T_4$ and $T_3$ measure both bound and unbound hormone. Thus, because of the high degree of binding of $T_4$ and $T_3$ to the serum-binding proteins, changes in either the concentrations of these proteins or the binding affinity of thyroid hormone to the serum-binding proteins would have major effects on the total serum hormone levels. However, since the pituitary responds to and regulates the circulating free hormone levels, minimal changes in the free hormone concentrations and thus overall thyroid function are seen.

The gold standard for the direct measurement of free $T_4$ concentrations is equilibrium dialysis. However, this technique requires expertise and is time consuming. The free $T_4$ index (FTI) is the most widely available test of free $T_4$ concentrations and is determined by multiplying the total $T_4$ concentration by the thyroid hormone binding ratio (THBR), also known as the $T_3$ or $T_4$ resin uptake. The THBR is an inverse estimate of serum TBG concentrations and is expressed as a percent. Hence the THBR is reduced if the capacity of serum-binding proteins is high and is increased when serum-binding proteins have diminished ability to bind hormone. Other methods to directly measure free thyroid hormone levels besides equilibrium dialysis are also available but are more expensive than the FTI and may be no more accurate.

### Sensitive TSH assays

Serum determinations of TSH have been available since 1965. The first assays were single antibody radioimmunoassays and remained the standard for 20 years. These assays were useful only for diagnosing primary hypothyroidism, since a lower limit to the normal range could not be reliably measured. The first sensitive TSH assay was developed in 1985, utilizing a dual antibody approach. Application of this method resulted in the expansion of the assay detection limit below the normal range. Thus any assay of this type is referred to as a sensitive TSH assay. The main utility of the sensitive TSH assay is to differentiate between normal and thyrotoxic patients, who should exhibit suppressed TSH values. Currently, commercially available TSH assays have a limit of detection of 0.05 mU/L or lower and a typical normal range of 0.5 to 4.6 mU/L.

With the advent of the sensitive TSH assay came the realization that abnormal TSH values, especially subnormal values, were very common. Abnormal TSH values have been reported in over 15% of hospitalized patients, with more than 60% of these patients having no intrinsic thyroid dysfunction on follow-up testing after recovery from illness. In addition, 20% to 30% of patients over the age of 60 have subnormal TSH values. The vast majority of these abnormal TSH values are associated with normal FTI determinations, giving rise to the syndromes of *subclinical thyroid disease* (discussed below).

Despite these pitfalls, the following conclusions can be made regarding sensitive TSH assays: (1) normal TSH values are both sensitive and specific to identify normal patients; (2) subnormal and suppressed TSH values are sensitive but not specific to identify thyrotoxic patients; (3) abnormal TSH values require additional biochemical and clinical evaluation before a diagnosis of thyroid dysfunction can be made.

## HYPOTHYROIDISM

Hypothyroidism is the most common disorder of thyroid function. Worldwide, hypothyroidism is most often the result of iodine deficiency. In the United States, where iodine is sufficient, autoimmune processes account for the majority of cases. Failure of the thyroid to produce sufficient thyroid hormone is the most common cause of hypothyroidism and is referred to as *primary hypothyroidism* (see the box on p. 500.). *Central hypothyroidism*

### Causes of hypothyroidism

**Primary hypothyroidism**

*Chronic autoimmune thyroiditis*
- Goitrous (Hashimoto's)
- Atrophic

*Therapy for hypothyroidism*
- $^{131}$I therapy
- Thyroidectomy
- Use of antithyroid drugs

*Congenital abnormalities*
- Thyroid agenesis or dysgenesis
- Biosynthetic defects in hormone synthesis

*Other*
- Iodine deficiency
- Thyroidectomy for benign or malignant conditions
- Head and neck irradiation

**Secondary hypothyroidism**

Hypopituitarism
Isolated TSH deficiency

**Tertiary hypothyroidism**

Hypothalamic dysfunction
Isolated TRH deficiency

**Generalized thyroid hormone resistance**

**Transient hypothyroidism**

Postpartum thyroiditis
Silent (painless) thyroiditis
Subacute thyroiditis

### Symptoms of hypothyroidism

**Common (seen in >50% of patients)**

Weakness
Fatigue
Lethargy
Decreased energy
Cold intolerance
Dry skin
Decreased sweating
Hair loss
Inability to concentrate
Memory loss
Constipation
Weight gain
Dyspnea
Peripheral paresthesias

**Less common (seen in <50% of patients)**

Depression
Anorexia
Muscle cramps
Musculoskeletal pain
Arthralgias
Infertility
Menorrhagia and anovulation
Carpal tunnel syndrome
Decreased hearing

occurs much less often and results from diminished thyroidal stimulation by TSH due to pituitary failure *(secondary hypothyroidism)* or hypothalamic failure *(tertiary hypothyroidism)*.

Chronic autoimmune thyroiditis accounts for about 60% of the cases of hypothyroidism in the United States and is further subdivided into goitrous *(Hashimoto's thyroiditis)* and atrophic forms. As with other autoimmune diseases, females are affected much more frequently than males. Chronic autoimmune thyroiditis is characterized by the presence of thyroid antibodies. These antibodies are present in about 7% of the population. The prevalence of newly diagnosed overt hypothyroidism ranges from two to six cases per 1000 women, and the prevalence of established cases is in the range of 20 to 40 per 1000 women.

Hypothyroidism resulting from the treatment for hyperthyroidism is the second most common cause and accounts for about 30% of cases. Secondary and tertiary hypothyroidism comprise less than 5% of cases. *Congenital hypothyroidism* occurs in about 1 in 4000 live births and is the major preventable cause of mental retardation in the world today. Untreated congenital hypothyroidism results in multiple developmental abnormalities known as cretinism. Diagnosis is made primarily through newborn thyroid function screening. Early institution of thyroid hormone replacement therapy results in normal IQ values in treated infants. A rare but increasingly recognized cause of hypothyroidism is *generalized thyroid hormone resistance*. Serum thyroid hormone concentrations are elevated but unable to exert any action due to genetic defects in the nuclear receptors for thyroid hormone.

*Transient hypothyroidism* is, by definition, the only reversible form of hypothyroidism. *Postpartum thyroiditis,* occurring 1 to 6 months after delivery, approaches an incidence of 20% in some series. A hypothyroid phase occurs in more than 60% of individuals and may last up to 1 year. Permanent hypothyroidism occurs in 20% to 30% of those affected.

## Clinical manifestations

Regardless of the etiology, the clinical features of hypothyroidism are similar (see the boxes above and at right). The onset of symptoms is usually insidious; thus hypothyroidism may be present for years before it is diagnosed. Despite the fact that every organ system can be involved, most of the symptoms and signs of hypothyroidism are nonspecific. Indeed, in one series a diagnosis of hypothyroidism was established in under 4% of ambulatory patients with symptoms potentially attributable to the disease. In addition, symptoms do not always correlate with the severity of the hypothyroidism and may be lacking altogether in individuals with overt biochemical evidence of the disease. Weakness, lethargy, constipation, dry skin, and hair loss are common nonspecific symptoms. Characteristic clinical features of hypothyroidism include cold intolerance, facial puffiness, deepening of the voice, and carpal tunnel syndrome (Fig. 34-1).

Some presentations are age specific, such as delayed growth in the child, menorrhagia in premenopausal women, and dementia in the elderly. The clinical picture

## Signs of hypothyroidism

**Common (seen in >50% of patients)**

*Physical examination*
- Coarse skin
- Cold skin
- Pallor of skin
- Coarse hair
- Periorbital edema
- Hoarse voice
- Goiter
- Nonpitting edema (myxedema)
- Delayed relaxation of reflexes

*Laboratory Values*
- Pericardial effusion
- Pleural effusion
- Hyponatremia
- Hypercholesterolemia
- Normochromic, normocytic anemia
- Elevated CPK (MM variant)
- Decreased basal metabolic rate

**Less common (seen in <50% of patients)**

*Physical Examination*
- Slow speech
- Sleep apnea
- Joint effusions
- Hypothermia
- Hypertension, especially diastolic
- Hypoventilation
- Macroglossia
- Myopathy
- Cardiomegaly

*Laboratory Values*
- Sinus bradycardia
- Flattened T waves
- Prolonged QT interval
- Low amplitude QRS complexes
- Coagulopathy
- Elevated lactic dehydrogenase
- Elevated transaminases
- Hyperprolactinemia

*CPK*, Creatine phosphokinase.

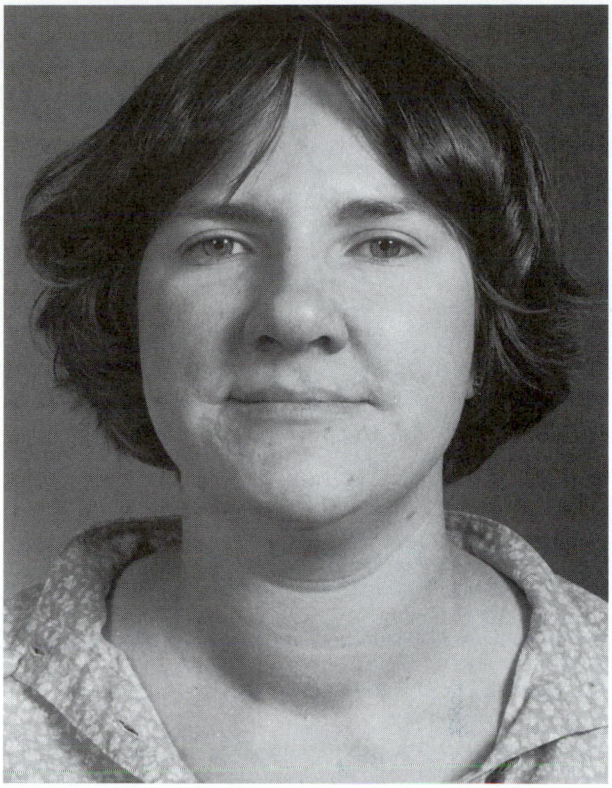

**Fig. 34-1.** Thirty-year-old patient with Hashimoto's thyroiditis and hypothyroidism. Presenting complaint was thyroid enlargement. $T_4 = 4.5$ µg/dl, TSH = 84 µU/ml. Note puffiness of face and visible goiter.

of florid myxedema includes dull, expressionless facies, slow movements, periorbital puffiness, sparse, coarse hair, macroglossia, and cool, pale, coarse skin (Figs. 34-2 and 34-3). The most characteristic clinical finding in hypothyroidism is the delayed relaxation phase of deep tendon reflexes. This is most commonly seen with the Achilles reflex. Small pericardial and pleural effusions are common and occasionally may be massive. Hypothyroid-related pericardial effusions typically do not cause tamponade and nearly always resolve with $T_4$ therapy.

Sinus bradycardia and flattened T waves are characteristic electrocardiographic (ECG) findings in hypothyroidism. Hypercholesterolemia occurs in 95% of patients due to impaired clearance of low-density lipoprotein (LDL) and very low–density lipoprotein (VLDL) particles. Dilutional hyponatremia is common due to impaired water excretion. Increased free water retention also produces increased diastolic blood pressure. Elevated creatine

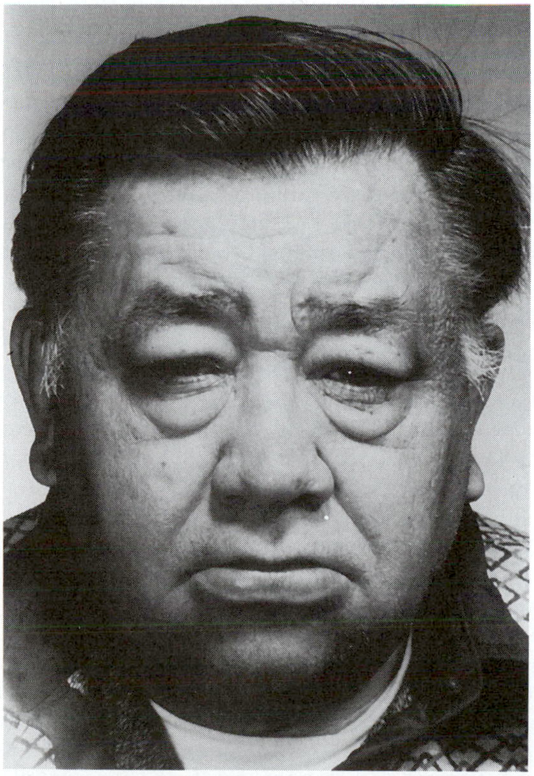

**Fig. 34-2.** Advanced hypothyroidism. Note dulled expression, facial puffiness, and periorbital edema.

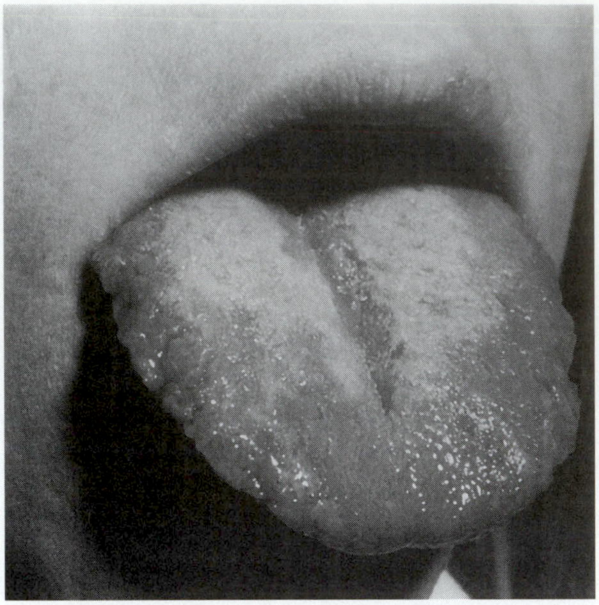

**Fig. 34-3.** Macroglossia of hypothyroidism.

**Table 34-1.** Factors that may obscure the diagnosis of hypothyroidism

| | Increased total $T_4$ by increased TBG binding | Decreased total $T_4$ by decreased TBG binding |
|---|---|---|
| **Drugs** | | |
| | Estrogens | Glucocorticoids |
| | Methadone | Androgens |
| | Clofibrate | L-Asparaginase |
| | 5-Fluorouracil | Salicylates |
| | Heroin | Mefenic acid |
| | Tamoxifen | Antiseizure medications (phenytoin, carbamazepine) |
| | | Furosemide |
| **Systemic factors** | | |
| | Liver disease | Inherited |
| | Porphyria | Acute illness |
| | HIV infection | |
| | Inherited | |

phosphokinase (CPK) concentrations (MM variant), occasionally over 1000 U/L, are often seen due to impaired clearance and may raise the possibility of a myocardial infarction until fractionation is performed. A normochromic, normocytic anemia is frequently found.

### Diagnosis

The hallmark of hypothyroidism is the presence of decreased serum concentrations of thyroid hormone. The most frequently measured thyroid hormone is total $T_4$. The measurement of serum $T_3$ concentrations has a low sensitivity in the laboratory evaluation of hypothyroidism and is almost never indicated. $T_3$ values can be normal in up to one third of patients with the disease and are commonly depressed in euthyroid patients with nonthyroidal illness. Since alterations in serum hormone binding capacity can alter total $T_4$ concentrations and obscure the diagnosis of hypothyroidism (Table 34-1), an estimation of free $T_4$ concentrations by the FTI method is often valuable.

Serum TSH concentrations are almost always elevated, since 95% of hypothyroid patients have primary thyroid failure. Indeed, increased serum TSH concentrations are the most sensitive indicator of the failing thyroid. However, modest elevations of TSH (usually under 15 mU/L) in the presence of normal FTI values *(subclinical hypothyroidism)* do not necessarily progress to overt hypothyroidism. At present there is no consensus on the indications for treatment in healthy individuals with subclinical hypothyroidism (see further).

The vast majority of cases of hypothyroidism can be diagnosed based upon clinical findings and the serum FTI and TSH concentrations. Thyroid antibodies help to provide an etiology for the hypothyroidism and identify a population with subclinical hypothyroidism that has a high risk of progression to overt disease. These antibodies are directed against the thyroid proteins thyroglobulin and thyroid peroxidase (TPO, formerly microsomal protein). Radioisotope scanning is almost never indicated unless used either to document congenital thyroid abnormalities or to evaluate a nodular goiter (see further).

## Differential diagnosis

Changes in serum TBG concentrations can have marked effects on serum $T_4$ values and may obscure the diagnosis of hypothyroidism (see Table 34-1). Factors that either decrease TBG concentrations or interfere with binding to TBG can result in low $T_4$ values in the hypothyroid range. Drugs such as dilantin and salicylates are the most common cause of low serum $T_4$ levels in euthyroid ambulatory individuals. FTI values are often low as well, but a normal serum TSH value in the absence of signs or symptoms of pituitary or hypothalamic failure confirms the diagnosis of drug effect in most cases. Conversely, factors that increase TBG concentrations can result in $T_4$ values in the normal range in the hypothyroid patient.

Abnormal thyroid function tests are often seen in patients with nonthyroidal illness. Mild to moderate elevations of serum TSH concentrations have been reported in up to 20% of hospitalized patients. In one large series fewer than 10% of hospitalized patients with elevated serum TSH values less than 20 mU/L and only 50% of those with serum TSH values over 20 mU/L were subsequently diagnosed with hypothyroidism. An elevated TSH in a patient recovering from severe nonthyroidal illness is likely an adaptive and not a pathologic response. Retesting thyroid functions 2 to 3 months after complete recovery from an acute illness usually distinguishes nonthyroid illness from hypothyroidism.

### Treatment

Synthetic preparations of levothyroxine sodium (L-$T_4$) are the drugs of choice for thyroid hormone replacement therapy. Desiccated thyroid preparations contain both $T_4$ and $T_3$ and have highly variable biologic activity, making these preparations much less desirable. Synthetic combi-

**Table 34-2.** $T_4$ replacement therapy in hypothyroidism

| Age/condition | Initial dosage | Incremental period |
|---|---|---|
| <60 years | 0.05-0.1 mg/day | Every 4-6 weeks |
| >60 years | 0.025-0.05 mg/day | Every 4-6 weeks |
| Preexisting cardiac disease | 0.0125-0.025 mg/day | Every 6-8 weeks |

nations of L-$T_4$ and L-$T_3$ are expensive relative to L-$T_4$ alone and are unnecessary except in special circumstances. Even though the hormonal content of the various brands of synthetic L-$T_4$ is reliably standardized, the deviation of a specific dose can vary between manufacturers. Thus, although brands appear to be interchangeable, clinical experience suggests that it is best to stay with a single brand for an individual patient.

The average replacement dosage of L-$T_4$ in a 68-kg woman is 0.112 mg (112 μg) per day. Institution of therapy in healthy individuals under the age of 60 can begin at dosages of 0.05 to 0.1 mg (50 to 100 μg) per day (Table 34-2). Because of the prolonged half-life of $T_4$ (7 days), new steady-state concentrations of $T_4$ are not achieved until 4 to 6 weeks after a change in dosage. Thus measurement of serum TSH values should not be performed any earlier than this time frame. Reevaluation after a daily dose of 0.1 mg is achieved is reasonable. The goal of L-$T_4$ replacement therapy is to achieve a TSH value in the normal range, since overreplacement of L-$T_4$ suppressing TSH values to the subnormal range has been shown to have a deleterious effect on bone density (see further). Once a normal serum TSH value is achieved, monitoring replacement therapy by determining serum TSH concentrations at 6- to 12-month intervals is appropriate.

Certain drugs can interfere with the absorption of L-$T_4$ in the gut. These include sucralfate, cholestyramine, iron supplements, and certain antacids. Thus L-$T_4$ administration should be spaced as far apart as possible from these medications. Higher L-$T_4$ doses may be necessary in patients who are taking drugs that accelerate the metabolism of $T_4$, such as anticonvulsants and rifampin.

In individuals over the age of 60, institution of therapy at a lower daily dosage (0.025 mg) of L-$T_4$ is indicated to avoid exacerbation of cardiac disease. The dosage can be increased at a rate of 0.025 mg per day every 4 to 6 weeks, with reevaluation after a total daily dose of 0.075 mg is achieved. For individuals with preexisting cardiac disease an initial dosage of 0.0125 mg with increases of 0.0125 to 0.025 mg per day every 6 to 8 weeks is indicated.

Daily doses of L-$T_4$ may be interrupted periodically because of intercurrent medical or surgical illnesses that prohibit taking anything by mouth. A lapse of several days of hormone replacement usually has no metabolic consequences. However, if more prolonged interruption is necessary, L-$T_4$ may be given parenterally at a dosage 25% to 50% less than the daily oral requirements.

## Special considerations

***Myxedema coma.*** Myxedema coma is a rare syndrome that represents the extreme expression of severe, long-standing hypothyroidism. It is a medical emergency, and even with early diagnosis and treatment the mortality can be as high as 60%. Myxedema coma occurs most often in the elderly during the winter months. Common precipitating factors include pulmonary infections, cerebrovascular accidents, and congestive heart failure. The clinical course of lethargy proceeding to stupor and then coma is often hastened by drugs, especially sedatives, narcotics, antidepressants, and tranquilizers. Indeed, many cases of myxedema coma have occurred in hypothyroid patients who have been hospitalized for other medical problems.

Cardinal features of myxedema coma are (1) hypothermia, which can be profound, (2) respiratory depression, and (3) unconsciousness. Other clinical features include bradycardia, macroglossia, delayed reflexes and dry, rough skin. Dilutional hyponatremia is common and may be severe. Elevated CPK and lactate dehydrogenase (LDH) concentrations, acidosis, and anemia are common findings. Lumbar puncture reveals increased opening pressure and high protein content. Hypothyroidism is confirmed by measuring serum FTI and TSH values. Ultimately, however, myxedema coma is a clinical diagnosis.

The mainstay of therapy is supportive care, with ventilatory support, rewarming, correction of hyponatremia, and treatment of the precipitating incident. Because of a 5% to 10% incidence of coexisting decreased adrenal reserve in patients with myxedema coma, intravenous steroids are indicated before initiating $T_4$ therapy. Parenteral administration of thyroid hormone is necessary due to uncertain absorption through the gut. Until recently only L-$T_4$ was available for intravenous use. With both L-$T_4$ and L-$T_3$ now available, a reasonable approach is an initial intravenous loading dose of 200 to 300 μg L-$T_4$ with a second dose of 100 μg given 24 hours later. Simultaneously, with the initial dose of L-$T_4$, some clinicians recommend adding L-$T_3$ at a dosage of 10 μg intravenously every 8 hours until the patient is stable and conscious. The dose of thyroid hormone should be adjusted on the basis of hemodynamic stability, the presence of coexisting cardiac disease, and the degree of electrolyte imbalance.

***Subclinical hypothyroidism.*** Subclinical hypothyroidism is defined as mild elevations of serum TSH in conjunction with normal serum thyroid hormone concentrations and lack of any overt clinical manifestations of hypothyroidism. The prevalence of subclinical hypothyroidism ranges from 10% to 20%, depending on the population, and is most frequently observed in the elderly. The presence of thyroid antibodies in these patients identifies a subset of patients who are at high risk of progressing to overt hypothyroidism. Potential benefits of instituting L-$T_4$ therapy in patients with subclinical hypothyroidism include prevention of overt hypothyroidism, improvement in mild metabolic and physiologic abnormalities, and improvement in symptoms not originally attributed to thyroid dysfunction. Although there is currently no consensus for the management of patients with subclinical hypothyroidism, treatment is reasonable in the following situations: (1) presence of thyroid antibodies, (2) presence of a goiter (to decrease the size of the goiter or to prevent further growth), (3) prior therapy for hyperthyroidism, (4) during pregnancy (see further), (5) presence of hypercholesterolemia, and (6) recent onset hypertension. Therapy is probably not indicated in patients with negative thyroid antibodies or in the recovery phase of nonthyroidal illness. Instead, these patients should be followed with periodic determination of serum TSH concentrations.

***Thyroid hormone replacement and osteoporosis.*** Thyroid hormone has a direct effect on bone resorption and has been shown in several studies to decrease bone density in women taking thyroid hormone for many years. When analyzed carefully, a significant decrease in bone density has been demonstrated in women taking suppressive doses of L-$T_4$ that result in undetectable TSH values, with the hip affected to a greater degree than the spine. This is mainly seen in those individuals requiring suppressive therapy after surgery for thyroid cancer. However, increased fracture rates have not been demonstrated in patients taking L-$T_4$. Women on replacement therapy with normal serum TSH concentrations show no changes in bone mineral density as compared to age-matched women not on L-$T_4$ therapy. Thus, as stated above, the goal of replacement therapy in patients with hypothyroidism should be to achieve a serum TSH in the normal range.

***Thyroid hormone replacement in pregnancy.*** In general, L-$T_4$ replacement requirements increase during pregnancy. This is primarily due to an estrogen-dependent increase in serum TBG concentrations that occurs during the first trimester. In addition, gastrointestinal absorption of L-$T_4$ may be decreased during pregnancy. Approximately 80% of hypothyroid patients need an increase in their replacement dosage during pregnancy, with an average increase equivalent to about 45% of the basal dosage. In addition, pregnancy may unmask hypothyroidism in patients with decreased thyroid reserve, such as those residing in areas of iodine deficiency or in those with euthyroid chronic autoimmune thyroiditis. Thus all patients receiving thyroid hormone replacement who become pregnant should have a serum TSH determination at or near the end of their first trimester. Similarly, evaluation of thyroid function during pregnancy in normal patients is indicated in those patients at high risk for hypothyroidism, such as those residing in areas of iodine deficiency or with a family history of thyroid or other autoimmune disease.

## THYROTOXICOSIS

Thyrotoxicosis is a condition caused by elevated concentrations of the circulating free thyroid hormones $T_4$ and $T_3$. Various disorders of different etiologies can result in this syndrome. The term *hyperthyroidism* is restricted to those conditions in which thyroid hormones are overproduced due to hyperfunction, rather than thyroid inflammation or destruction or thyroid hormone administration.

### Etiology

For practical purposes hyperthyroidism can be classified according to the 24-hour radioactive iodine uptake (RAIU) (see the boxes at right). An elevated RAIU indicates that the etiology of the elevated serum thyroid hormones is a hyperfunctioning thyroid gland. Graves disease is the most common cause of high RAIU thyrotoxicosis. It accounts for 60% to 90% of the cases, depending upon age and geographic region. Toxic nodular and multinodular goiter follows in frequency, accounting for 10% to 40% of the cases and is more common in older patients. A low RAIU is seen in destructive thyroiditides and in thyrotoxicosis resulting from exogenous thyroid hormone. Low RAIU thyrotoxicosis caused by subacute and painless thyroiditis represents about 5% to 20% of all cases. Other causes of thyrotoxicosis are much less common.

#### Causes of high RAIU thyrotoxicosis

- Graves disease
- Toxic multinodular goiter
- Solitary hot nodule
- TSH-secreting pituitary tumor
- Molar pregnancy
- Choriocarcinoma

#### Causes of low RAIU thyrotoxicosis

- Subacute thyroiditis
- Sporadic silent thyroiditis
- Postpartum lymphocytic thyroiditis
- Radiation-induced thyroiditis
- Iodine-induced thyrotoxicosis
- Thyrotoxicosis factitia
- Metastatic thyroid cancer
- Struma ovarii

### Clinical manifestations

Thyroid hormone excess affects multiple organ systems. Although the resulting signs or symptoms in thyrotoxicosis can be nonspecific, their combination usually creates a characteristic clinical picture. Age, presence of other underlying disturbances, and rapidity of onset of the disease can modify both the type and severity of the clinical presentation. Symptoms of thyrotoxicosis may start slowly or precipitously and may range from subtle to florid.

Typical patient complaints include nervousness, irritability, hyperactivity, insomnia, hand tremor, excessive sweating, and palpitations. Most of these symptoms are due to increased sympathetic tone. Weight loss, despite an increased appetite, and heat intolerance are common due to increased energy production and utilization. Pruritus results from increased blood flow to the skin. Proximal muscle weakness is often manifested as difficulty climbing stairs or standing up. Increased gut motility results in hyperdefecation and occasionally in malabsorption or diarrhea. Hyperthyroidism may exacerbate angina pectoris. Oligomenorrhea in women and decreased libido and impotence in men is described.

Less often patients develop nausea, vomiting, and dysphagia. Dyspnea on exertion, due to increased oxygen consumption and respiratory muscle weakness, can be seen. Rarely tracheal compression from a large goiter can cause dyspnea. Periodic paralysis is rare and is seen

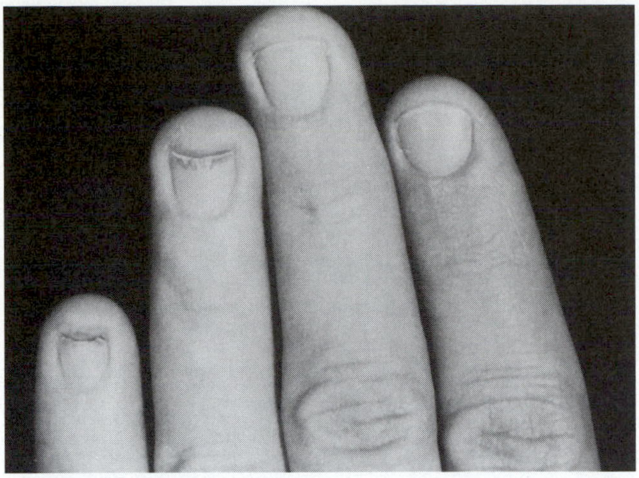

**Fig. 34-4.** Onycholysis involving the ring finger in a patient with Graves' disease.

usually in Asian males usually in association with low serum potassium levels.

The thyroid gland is diffusely enlarged in most patients with Graves' disease. Typically both thyroid lobes are symmetrically enlarged, firm, and nontender. The gland may be particularly firm in those thyroids with coexistent Hashimoto's thyroiditis. In patients with a multinodular goiter the thyroid gland is often asymmetric, irregular, and bumpy. A unilateral nodule, usually larger than 3 cm, is found in a solitary toxic adenoma. A tender thyroid raises the possibility of subacute thyroiditis. A normal or nonpalpable thyroid gland points toward a diagnosis of thyrotoxicosis factitia (see further) or painless thyroiditis, although goiter may rarely be absent in Graves' disease. Hyperthryoidism without goiter is more common in the elderly. Because of increased blood supply to the thyroid, a systolic bruit and a thrill can be found in Graves' disease.

Cardiac findings are the result of both direct thyroid hormone effects on the cardiovascular system and indirect effects through the increased metabolism and oxygen consumption. Sinus tachycardia, elevated systolic blood pressure, and widened pulse pressure are common. A systolic ejection flow murmur may be present. Although sinus tachycardia is the most common rhythm in thyrotoxicosis, other arrhythmias, especially atrial fibrillation, occur in 10% to 25% of patients. Atrial fibrillation is more common in older patients and may be the presenting feature of thyrotoxicosis. In these patients the presence of left atrial enlargement is the rule. Arterial embolism occurs in about 10% of patients with atrial fibrillation.

The skin is often warm, moist, and smooth. Onycholysis, or separation of the nail from the nailbed, is often seen in thyrotoxicosis (Fig. 34-4). Acropachy and clubbing are associated with Graves' disease. Hair texture is fine and alopecia may occur. Hyperpigmentation of the skin may be observed. Vitiligo is associated with Graves' disease.

Distal fine tremor, brisk deep tendon reflexes, and proximal muscle weakness are common neurologic findings. Ophthalmopathy associated with thyrotoxicosis is classified as noninfiltrative or infiltrative. *Noninfiltrative ophthalmopathy* is associated with thyrotoxicosis of any origin. It is characterized by upper lid retraction, which results in lid lag and stare (Fig. 34-5). *Infiltrative ophthalmopathy* is specifically associated with Graves' disease and is discussed later.

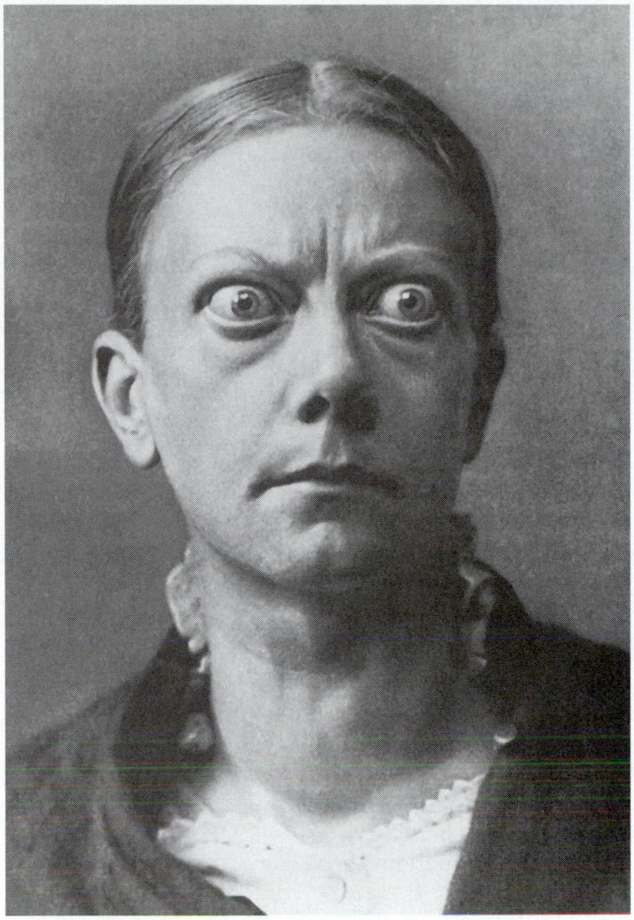

**Fig. 34-5.** Classic appearance of Graves' disease with advanced hyperthyroidism. (From Bramwell B: *Atlas of clinical medicine*, Edinburgh, 1892, University Press.)

## Diagnosis

Elevated serum concentrations of thyroid hormones and suppressed serum TSH concentrations are the hallmarks of thyrotoxicosis. Both total and free thyroid hormone concentrations are elevated, although isolated increases of either $T_4$ or $T_3$ may also occur.

An increase in serum $T_4$ binding protein concentrations or capacity, as seen during pregnancy and estrogen replacement therapy, can result in an increase of total $T_4$ concentrations into the thyrotoxic range. Therefore estimation of free $T_4$ concentrations by the FTI is helpful to clarify the diagnosis in these situations. Disorders that are associated with elevated total $T_4$ concentrations, but normal free $T_4$ concentrations, are collectively known as the euthyroid hyperthyroxinemia syndrome (see the box on p. 506). In these patients serum $T_3$ and TSH concentrations are normal.

$T_4$ toxicosis is described in hyperthyroid patients with concomitant diseases, usually hospitalized patients, in

### Disorders associated with elevated serum $T_4$ concentrations: euthyroid hyperthyroxinemia syndrome

*Increased thyroid hormone binding*
- Abnormal TBG concentrations
- Physiologic: pregnancy, neonatal
- Nonthyroidal illness: acute hepatitis, acute intermittent porphyria
- Drugs: estrogens, heroin, methadone, clofibrate, 5-fluorouracil
- Familial dysalbuminemic hyperthyroxinemia

*Thyroid hormone resistance*
*Drugs: amiodarone, iopanoic acid, propranolol*
*Thyroid hormone autoantibodies*
*Acute nonthyroidal illness*
*Acute psychosis*

whom $T_3$ conversion in peripheral tissues is inhibited because of nonthyroidal illness or drugs. Upon the patient's recovery from the acute illness, serum $T_3$ levels may rise up to the hyperthyroid range. Similarly, hyperthyroid patients who received iodinated preparations, for example those used for radiologic studies, may also develop $T_4$ toxicosis.

Occasionally patients may have increased serum $T_3$ levels and normal $T_4$ levels. Hyperthyroidism due to $T_3$ alone is referred to as $T_3$ toxicosis. This disorder is more frequent in areas of iodine deficiency, in patients with solitary nodules, and in early or relapsing Graves' disease.

Serum TSH determination by a sensitive TSH radioimmunoassay (limit of detection <0.05 mU/L) is a very accurate indicator of thyrotoxicosis. Serum TSH levels should be low or undetectable. Indeed, with the rare exception of a TSH-secreting pituitary tumor, a serum TSH concentration in the normal range rules out the diagnosis of hyperthyroidism. These new sensitive TSH assays have replaced the thyrotropin-releasing hormone stimulation test as a tool in the diagnosis of hyperthyroidism.

Thyroid antibody titers (antithyroglobulin and anti-TPO) are elevated in up to 70% of patients with Graves' disease. Their measurement is not routinely necessary but many times is helpful in establishing the diagnosis, especially in the absence of ophthalmopathy.

TSH receptor antibodies can be commercially measured as thyroid-stimulating (TSI) or thyroid-binding inhibitor (TBII) immunoglobulins. TSI is more sensitive than TBII, but both are very specific. Nevertheless, their measurement is costly and is not routinely recommended. Measurement of TSH receptor antibodies in pregnant women is helpful in predicting the risk of developing neonatal Graves' disease (see further). TSI measurements can occasionally be useful in the diagnosis of euthyroid Graves' disease and in the differential diagnosis of Graves' disease from other hyperthyroid disorders.

Normochromic normocytic anemia and mild neutropenia with lymphocytosis are sometimes found in Graves disease. Liver enzymes (alanine aminotransferase [ALT], aspartate aminotransferase [AST]) may be minimally increased. Mild elevations of serum calcium levels are seen in up to 20% of thyrotoxic patients. This is due to increased bone resorption by thyroid hormones, and resolves with the treatment of hyperthyroidism. Bone and liver alkaline phosphatase fractions may also be elevated. Serum cholesterol levels may be decreased.

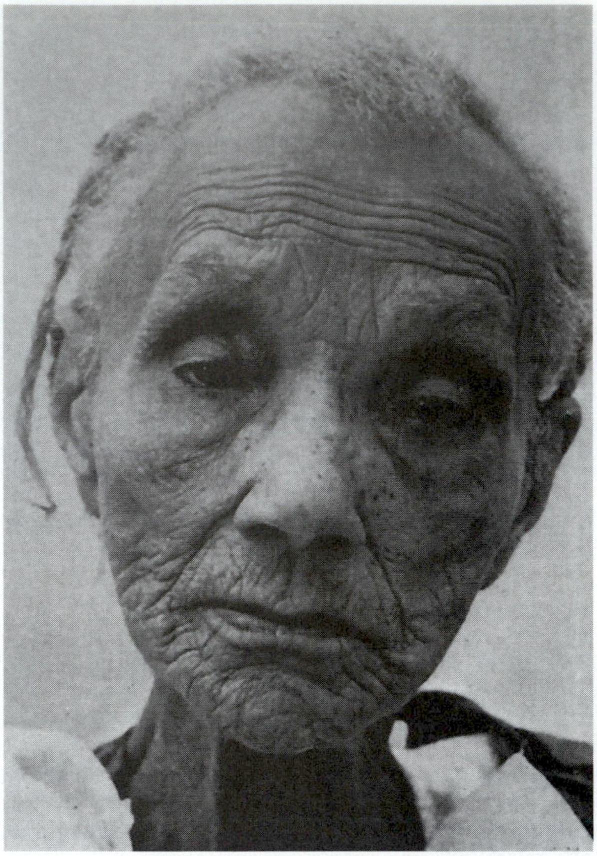

**Fig. 34-6.** Apathetic hyperthyroidism in an older patient. (From Thomas FB et al: *Ann Intern Med* 72:679, 1970.)

As mentioned previously, the 24-hour RAIU separates thyrotoxicosis into two categories. When the diagnosis of Graves' disease is clinically obvious, RAIU determination is not necessary. However, RAIU is a useful tool in the differential diagnosis of thyrotoxicosis in unclear cases. Whereas RAIU distinguishes etiology based on iodine uptake, thyroid radionuclide imaging can distinguish different forms of goiter. A thyroid scan should be requested when the thyroid gland appears to be nodular on physical examination to establish the diagnosis of toxic nodular or multinodular goiter. In addition, a thyroid scan may be ordered in a patient with Graves' disease when a thyroid nodule is felt so as to rule out a coexistent cold nodule.

## Differential diagnosis

When the clinical picture is classic with a diffuse goiter and ophthalmopathy, the diagnosis of Graves' disease is straightforward. The absence of ophthalmopathy or the presence of subtle hyperthyroid symptoms may obscure the diagnosis. This is particularly true in the elderly (Fig. 34-6). Certain psychiatric diseases, such as anxiety and bipolar disorder, can mimic thyrotoxicosis. Conversely,

### Autoimmune diseases associated with Graves' disease

Hashimoto's thyroiditis
Vitiligo
Pernicious anemia
Insulin-dependent diabetes mellitus
Adrenal insufficiency
Myasthenia gravis
Idiopathic thrombocytopenic purpura
Sjögren's syndrome
Systemic lupus erythematosus

thyrotoxicosis can be manifest as a psychiatric disorder or can expose a previously unrecognized one.

History, physical examination, and determination of serum FTI, $T_3$, and TSH concentrations usually provide enough information to make the diagnosis. RAIU is helpful in borderline patients or in those with atypical or few clinical manifestations. High $T_3/T_4$ ratios (greater than 20) are suggestive of Graves' disease. In contrast, inflammatory thyroiditis or exogenous L-$T_4$ administration is characterized by a low $T_3/T_4$ ratio, usually less than 15. TSH receptor antibody determinations and radionuclide imaging studies can be helpful but should be reserved for unusual cases (see above). An elevated sedimentation rate is associated with subacute thyroiditis. Serum thyroglobulin concentration, which is elevated in most forms of thyrotoxicosis, is low or suppressed in thyrotoxicosis factitia.

## Graves' disease

Graves' disease, or toxic diffuse goiter, is an autoimmune disorder characterized by thyrotoxicosis, diffuse goiter, and antibodies directed against the TSH receptor. This is a relatively common disorder, with an incidence of 0.02% to 0.4% in the United States. Endemic areas of iodine deficiency have a lower incidence of autoimmune thyroid disease. As with most types of thyroid dysfunction, women are affected more than men, with a ratio of 5 to 7:1. Graves' disease is more common between the ages of 20 and 50 but can occur at any age. HLA B8 and DR3 haplotypes are associated with Graves' disease in the white population. The disease is commonly associated with other autoimmune disorders (see the box above).

***Pathogenesis.*** Hyperthyroidism results from the stimulation of TSH receptors on thyroid cells by TSH receptor antibodies. The TSH receptor antibody is believed to stimulate the generation of cyclic adenosine monophosphate in the thyroid, resulting in the increased synthesis and release of the thyroid hormones. Proposed hypotheses regarding the abnormal generation of thyroid-stimulating antibody include (1) a primary defect on antigen-specific suppressor T-cells that results in unregulated helper T-cell function and therefore abnormal antibody synthesis, (2) direct helper T-cell activation by thyroid follicular cells expressing HLA class II antigens, and (3) cross-reactivity between bacterial or parasitic antigens and the TSH receptor, provoking the generation of autoantibodies.

The abnormal function of the immune system found in patients with this disease is strongly linked to a genetic predisposition. However, the specific genes involved have not been identified. Concurrence rates for Graves' disease are approximately 50% for monozygotic twins and 5% for dizygotic twins. This lack of complete concordance suggests that environmental factors, including infectious agents such as *Yersinia enterocolitica* or retrovirus, and stressful events, either physical or psychologic, may be involved.

***Specific clinical manifestations.*** The general manifestations of thyrotoxicosis have already been described. Specific findings in Graves' disease include infiltrative ophthalmopathy, pretibial myxedema, and acropachy.

**Graves' ophthalmopathy.** The infiltrative ophthalmopathy associated with Graves' disease is considered an autoimmune-mediated inflammation of the periorbital connective tissue and extraocular muscle. This disorder is clinically evident with various degrees of severity in about 50% of patients with Graves' disease but is present on radiologic studies, such as ultrasound and CT scan, in almost all patients. The majority of patients have mild or moderate disease. Euthyroid Graves' disease refers to patients with ophthalmopathy who have not developed hyperthyroidism. Ophthalmopathy precedes the diagnosis of hyperthyroidism in 15% of patients, whereas 5% of patients remain euthyroid indefinitely. Ophthalmopathy coincides with the diagnosis of hyperthyroidism in about 40% of patients and develops after the diagnosis and treatment of hyperthyroidism in the remaining patients.

Although there is good evidence that this disorder is autoimmune in origin, the target antigen in the orbital tissue has not yet been identified. Thyroid and orbital tissue, such as the eye muscle, may share antigens toward which autoantibodies react. Smoking and radioactive iodine therapy appear to be risk factors for the development or worsening of Graves' ophthalmopathy.

Patients with Graves' ophthalmopathy may complain of retroocular pressure, photophobia, lacrimation, and blurred vision. Muscle inflammation and fibrosis can result in ophthalmoplegia and diplopia. Optic nerve damage due to increased intraocular pressure can lead to decreased vision and blindness.

On physical examination the most obvious sign is proptosis. Although usually bilateral, it can affect only one eye. Conjunctival injection and periorbital and eye lid edema may also be present. The combination of proptosis and lid retraction may lead to corneal exposure and ulceration.

The diagnosis of ophthalmopathy is based on the findings just described. Proptosis is measured with a Hertel exophthalmometer. A reading of 20 to 22 mm is suggestive and more than 24 mm is diagnostic of exophthalmos. Similarly, an asymmetric reading of more than 2 mm is abnormal. Orbital ultrasound, CT, or MRI will show the thickened eye muscle and increased orbital content. These radiologic studies are not routinely ordered to assess the ophthalmopathy, but they may be occasionally useful in the differential diagnosis of exophthalmos, especially if the patient is euthyroid. Unilateral exoph-

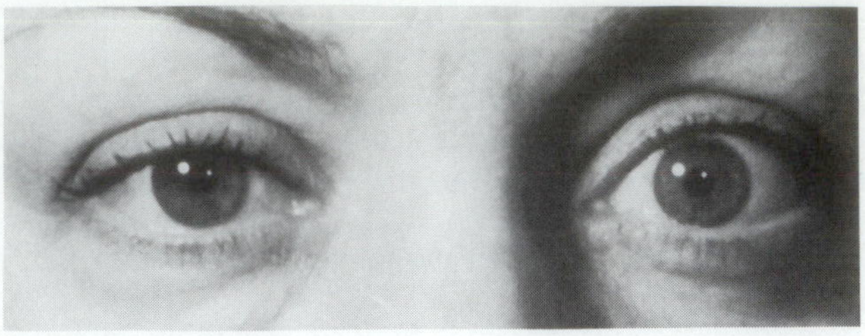

**Fig. 34-7.** Unilateral *(left)* lid retraction in a patient with hyperthyroidism.

thalmos should be evaluated by imaging studies even in patients with documented Graves' disease so as to exclude other causes of orbital pathology (Fig. 34-7).

Treatment of Graves' ophthalmopathy should be performed in conjunction with an ophthalmologist. Conversion to euthyroidism, preferably with antithyroid drugs, is first required. Radioactive iodine treatment should be avoided in patients with clinically significant ophthalmopathy due to potential worsening of the eye disease after treatment, although the frequency with which this occurs is controversial. If the eye disease is mild, local, nonspecific measures should be prescribed for symptom relief and to protect the eye from corneal exposure, including lubricants, dark colored glasses, and adhesive taping of eyelids.

Systemic treatments with immunosuppressive drugs (high-dose steroids or cytotoxic agents) are reserved for severe cases with active and progressive inflammation. Orbital radiation is also used in severe disease. Similar results are obtained with both treatments. When systemic treatment is ineffective or contraindicated, surgical orbital decompression may be beneficial. In patients with severe diplopia, surgical release of the fibrosed extraocular muscle is indicated. Lid retraction that persists after the patient is rendered euthyroid can be corrected with Müller myotomy.

**Pretibial myxedema.** This is an uncommon autoimmune disorder associated with Graves' disease in fewer than 5% of patients. It is characterized by localized dermal accumulation of mucopolysaccharides, most commonly over the tibial surface. It may present as a diffuse nonpitting lesion of the anterior lower leg or as a sharply circumscribed lesion Fig. 34-8. An elephantiasis form is rare. The lesions are usually asymptomatic. Rarely, they may cause pain or ulcerate. Topical occlusive treatment with potent fluorinated steroids has been reported to be successful.

**Thyroid acropachy.** Thyroid acropachy is the rarest manifestation of Graves' disease. It is characterized by subperiosteal new bone formation, predominately of the digits, associated with clubbing of the fingers and localized soft tissue swelling. There is no effective treatment for acropachy.

***Treatment.*** The course of hyperthyroidism in Graves' disease is characterized by cycles of relapse and remission of variable duration, although an unremitting course or a single episode of the disease is also possible. There is no available treatment aimed at the cause of Graves' disease, namely antibodies to the TSH receptor, thus there is no true cure for this disorder. Instead, treatment is aimed at decreasing circulating thyroid hormone levels either by inhibiting thyroid hormone production or by destroying thyroid tissue. There are three major ways of achieving these goals: (1) antithyroid drugs, (2) radioactive iodine, and (3) surgery. The goal of treatment with antithyroid drugs is to alter the natural history of the disease and to induce a remission of the hyperthyroidism. Radioactive iodine and surgery seek to alter the natural history of the disease by decreasing the amount of thyroid tissue available to respond to stimulation by TSH receptor antibodies.

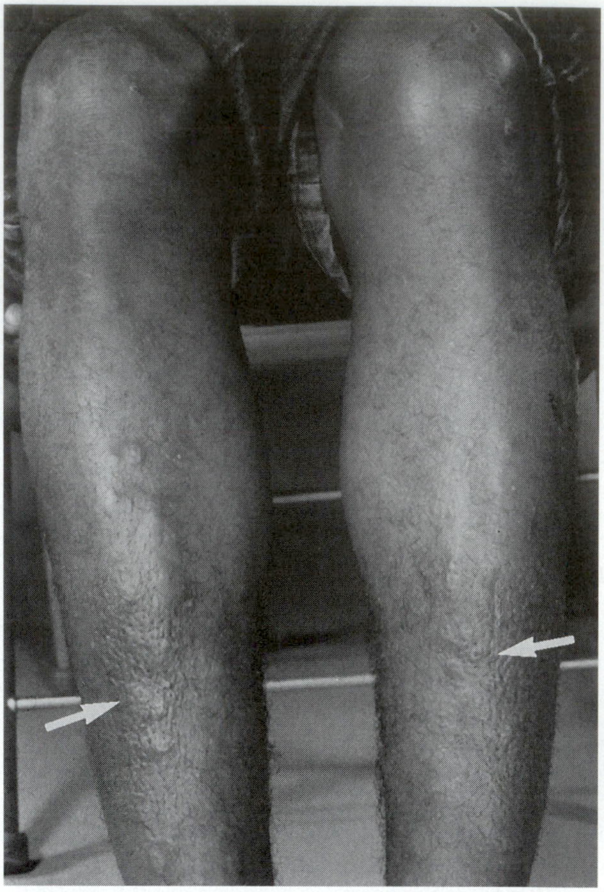

**Fig. 34-8.** Pretibial myxedema (*arrows*) in a patient with Graves' disease.

**Antithyroid drugs.** Antithyroid drugs (ATDs) belong to a group of compounds known as thionamides. They act by inhibiting thyroid peroxidase and therefore block iodine organification and thyroid hormone synthesis. In addition, they exhibit extrathyroidal actions that may be beneficial (Table 34-3). The two available antithyroid drugs in United States are propylthiouracil (PTU) and methimazole (Tapazole). Both are effective in controlling hyperthyroidism. In most cases the choice between the two drugs is up to the physician's individual experience and preference. PTU is recommended for use during pregnancy because its transplacental passage is much less than that of methimazole (see further). PTU is also transmitted into breast milk to a lesser degree than is methimazole and has the additional benefit of inhibiting $T_4$ to $T_3$ conversion.

**Table 34-3.** Characteristics of antithyroid drugs

| Characteristic | PTU | Methimazole |
|---|---|---|
| Intrathyroidal effects | Inhibition of iodination and iodotyrosine coupling | Inhibition of iodination and iodotyrosine coupling |
| Extrathyroidal effects | Possible immunomodulation<br>Inhibition of $T_4$ to $T_3$ conversion | Possible immunomodulation<br>No effect on $T_4$ to $T_3$ conversion |
| Serum half-life | 75 min | 4-6 hr |
| Transplacental passage | Low | High |
| Breast milk levels | Low | High |
| Usual daily dosage | 100-300 mg | 10-30 mg |
| Dose frequency | bid-tid | qd |
| Agranulocytosis | Not dose related | Dose related |

allowing for a more rapid fall in serum $T_3$ concentrations than methimazole and thus a more rapid improvement in symptoms. However, in practice this effect of PTU is important only in the most severely toxic individuals.

The usual starting dosage of methimazole is 20 to 40 mg daily as a single dose; for PTU it is 100 to 150 mg three times daily. Higher dosages may be required for the severely toxic patient, as well as those with very large goiters. After treatment is initiated, patients should be examined and thyroid function tests (FTI and serum $T_3$ levels) monitored every 4 to 6 weeks. Once euthyroidism is achieved, usually within 12 weeks, the dosage of the antithyroid drug can be decreased. Maintenance dosages are usually 5 to 10 mg daily for methimazole and 50 to 200 mg daily for PTU. Thereafter, follow-up visits every 3 months are reasonable.

Remission rates after a treatment course with ATDs vary from 10% to 90% 1 year after stopping the drug, with a mean of about 50%. Longer durations of therapy have been associated with higher remission rates. We recommend that therapy be administered for 1 to 2 years. Remission rates have been lower in recent years compared with those initially described in the 1950s and 1960s. Increased dietary iodine has been implicated in the latter, less favorable, rates. Factors associated with higher chances of remission after discontinuation of antithyroid treatment include negative TPO (antimicrosomal) antibody titers, HLA DR3 negative haplotype, milder thyrotoxicosis at presentation, and reduction in goiter size. Duration and modes of treatment may also influence remission (see further). Among those patients who experience remission, about 25% ultimately become hypothyroid, probably due to concurrent Hashimoto's thyroiditis.

Relapse of Graves' disease after discontinuation of ATDs usually occurs within the first few months. In that case a repeat course of ATDs may be indicated; however, ablation therapy should be considered. Patients who remain in remission should be reevaluated for a relapse every 3 to 6 months or with the recurrence of symptoms.

Concomitant use of L-$T_4$ therapy along with ATDs, primarily methimazole, has been reported to increase rates of remission in Japan. However, this may represent differences in the patient population as well as the iodine intake in Japan. As yet, combination therapy has not been confirmed as an effective therapy in the United States and thus cannot be recommended.

The most serious side effect of ATDs is agranulocytosis, which usually but not always occurs within the first 3 months of treatment. The incidence of agranulocytosis is the same for both PTU and methimazole (0.1% to 0.5%). There is some evidence that methimazole-induced agranulocytosis is dose related and is rarely seen at dosages under 30 mg daily. Patients should be instructed to discontinue the medication and to contact the physician in case of fever or sore throat. Any patient taking ATDs who develops a fever or a sore throat should have an urgent WBC count and differential performed, and the ATD should not be resumed until the results of the WBC count are obtained. Since ATD-related agranulocytosis occurs rapidly, routine monitoring of CBCs is not recommended. It is useful to check a pretreatment CBC, since WBCs are often depressed by Graves' disease itself.

Minor side effects, such as rash and urticaria, are relatively more common (1% to 5%). If acceptable to the patient, the medication can be safely continued and an antihistaminic may be added. Otherwise, one can replace one ATD for the other, but cross-reactivity for both minor and major side effects has been reported.

**Radioactive iodine treatment.** Radioactive iodine (RAI) in the form of $^{131}I$ is taken up by the thyroid gland and produces destruction of thyroid follicular cells. Use of RAI is recommended by many physicians, especially in the elderly. RAI is generally avoided in children and is contraindicated during pregnancy and breastfeeding.

The dosage of $^{131}I$ to be administered is usually in the range of 5 to 10 mCi, with the dosage calculation based on thyroid size and 24-hour RAIU. Administration of ATDs before radioiodine treatment is recommended to decrease thyroid hormone storage and prevent transient worsening of symptoms of hyperthyroidism or development of thyrotoxic storm. About 75% of patients are rendered euthyroid after one dose of radioiodine. The rest of the patients require a second and rarely a third dose. Normalization of thyroid function including normalization of serum TSH usually takes 1 to 2 months but may be delayed for up to a year. Permanent hypothyroidism is the major complication of radioactive iodine treatment. Hypothyroidism eventually develops in about 80% of the patients; therefore, lifelong follow-up is warranted. Extensive studies involving over 5000 patients for up to 40 years have revealed no increase in the incidence of any malignancy after the RAI treatment for hypothyroidism.

**Surgery.** Subtotal thyroidectomy is reserved for the following conditions: (1) patients with large goiters, (2) children who are allergic to ATDs, (3) pregnant women (usually in the second trimester) who are allergic to ATDs, and (4) patients who prefer surgery over ATDs or RAI. Preparation of the patient before undergoing surgery involves depletion of the gland of thyroid hormone with ATDs and decreasing the vascularity of the gland with iodide administration (1 to 3 drops of SSKI daily for 10 days). β-Adrenergic blockers alone have been used in some cases.

The two most common complications from subtotal thyroidectomy are hoarseness due to recurrent laryngeal nerve damage and hypoparathyroidism. Complication rates in the hands of an experienced thyroid surgeon are low (less than 1%). Hyperthyroidism recurs in about 5% of patients, and hypothyroidism develops in up to 60% of patients. RAI should be considered for surgically treated patients who relapse.

**Adjuvant therapy.** Iodide inhibits synthesis and release of thyroid hormones, but its effect is transient. Iodide, in the form of Lugol solution or SSKI (8 drops every 6 hours), is used in the treatment of thyroid storm and for preparation of patients for surgery. Iodinated contrast agents (e.g., iopanoic acid [Telepaque], 1 g/day) have the additional advantage of inhibiting peripheral $T_4$ to $T_3$ conversion and may be used in the management of thyrotoxic crisis.

β-Adrenergic blockers and calcium channel blockers are useful drugs in the symptomatic treatment of hyperthyroidism and are quite effective in decreasing heart rate. Propranolol, 20 to 40 mg four times daily, or atenolol, 100 to 200 mg daily, is the usual starting dosage. Propranolol and esmolol can be given intravenously if needed. Diltiazem can be used for heart rate control if β-blockers are contraindicated. These drugs should be discontinued once the patient is euthyroid.

### Toxic multinodular goiter

Typically, toxic multinodular goiter presents in older patients who have long-standing asymptomatic goiters. Administration of iodine-containing preparations, such as radiographic contrast media, amiodarone, or cough medicines, can precipitate hyperthyroidism in these patients. The onset of hyperthyroidism is more gradual and symptoms are usually milder than those of Graves' disease. Weight loss, atrial fibrillation, and depression are common presentations.

Physical examination usually reveals a large and firm goiter. Discrete nodules may be palpable. Lid lag can be observed, but infiltrative ophthalmopathy is absent. Borderline serum $T_4$ and $T_3$ levels and suppressed serum TSH concentrations are frequent. Thyroid scan is characterized by multiple functioning areas with suppression of other portions of the gland. Substernal thyroid extension may be detected. RAIU is usually elevated but may be normal.

Once hyperthyroidism occurs, it follows an unremitting course; therefore definitive treatment by ablation therapy is recommended. RAI is the treatment of choice in the elderly, and large doses of $^{131}$I are usually required. Surgical removal of the thyroid is advised in patients with large, compressive goiters. Subtotal thyroidectomy is commonly performed in these cases. Antithyroid drugs are given to render the patient euthyroid before radioiodine treatment or surgery to avoid the precipitation of cardiac arrhythmias or thyrotoxic crisis in an unprepared patient.

### Autonomously functioning thyroid nodules (AFTNs)

In this condition hyperthyroidism is associated with a single thyroid nodule that functions independently of the normal thyroid regulatory axis. About 75% of patients with functioning nodules are euthyroid at diagnosis, 20% are overtly hyperthyroid, and 5% are borderline thyrotoxic. AFTNs are more frequent in Europe than in the United States and account for 5% of all solitary nodules. In patients with euthyroid AFTNs, factors that increase the likelihood of developing thyrotoxicosis include (1) nodule size 3 cm or larger, (2) older age, and (3) serum $T_3$ levels in the upper normal range. Overall, about 20% to 25% of functioning nodules become thyrotoxic.

A laboratory picture of $T_3$ toxicosis can be observed, since nodules secrete relatively more $T_3$ than $T_4$. Radionuclide thyroid imaging with either $^{123}$I or $^{99m}$Tc shows a concentration of radioisotope in a single area corresponding to the nodule. There is partial or complete suppression of the rest of the thyroid gland.

In thyrotoxic patients treatment options and considerations are similar to those discussed for a toxic multinodular goiter. For those patients who are asymptomatic, observation and periodic thyroid function monitoring are reasonable, especially if the patient is young and healthy. In older patients and in those with preexisting medical conditions, such as cardiovascular disease, ablation treatment may be indicated.

### Thyroiditis

***Subacute thyroiditis.*** Subacute thyroiditis is a self-limiting inflammation of the thyroid, probably due to a viral infection of the gland. Leakage of large quantities of stored thyroid hormones results in transient thyrotoxicosis. This is followed by a hypothyroid phase that resolves, usually within 6 months.

A prodromal upper respiratory tract illness is common. Typical symptoms include pain in the thyroid area with radiation to the ears or jaw, malaise, and low-grade fever. A mild thyrotoxic picture may be present. On physical examination a tender enlarged thyroid is characteristic. Acute hemorrhage into a thyroid nodule can also cause a painful thyroid. In addition to elevated serum thyroid hormone concentrations and suppressed serum TSH values, an elevated erythrocyte sedimentation rate and a low RAIU confirms the diagnosis.

Treatment is aimed at the relief of symptoms. Aspirin is very effective for mild to moderate thyroid pain. Steroid administration may be necessary for treatment of severe thyroid pain.

***Postpartum and painless thyroiditis.*** These are immune-mediated disorders of the thyroid gland. Postpartum thyroiditis occurs in up to 20% of women, usually within the first 4 months. Painless thyroiditis can affect either sex and is much less common.

Similar to subacute thyroiditis, these disorders are classically characterized by a thyrotoxic phase, followed by a hypothyroid phase and restoration to euthyroidism within 1 year. However, in many cases patients may have only a thyrotoxic or a hypothyroid phase. Relapse of postpartum thyroiditis after subsequent pregnancies has been observed. In addition to the evaluation just mentioned, measurement of the serum thyroglobulin concentration is helpful to differentiate thyroiditis (high serum thyroglobulin concentrations) from surreptitious thyroid hormone administration (low serum thyroglobulin concentrations). Control of the thyrotoxic symptoms can be achieved with β-adrenergic blockers for the duration of these self-limiting disorders.

### Rare causes of thyrotoxicosis

*TSH-induced hyperthyroidism* results from both tumoral and nontumoral TSH hypersecretion from the pituitary. In a hyperthyroid patient the finding of normal or high serum TSH concentrations in conjunction with elevated serum $T_4$ levels is the most distinctive feature of this disorder. Pituitary TSH-secreting tumors are usually large and identifiable on MRI scan of the sellar region and require surgical excision. Octreotide, a long-acting somatostatin analogue, has been successfully used as adjunctive therapy in these patients. Nontumoral pituitary TSH hypersecretion is due to selective pituitary thyroid hormone resistance.

*Trophoblastic tumors,* either *hydatidiform moles* or *choriocarcinomas,* secrete human chorionic gonadotrophin (HCG), which has weak TSH-like biologic activity. Very high concentrations of serum HCG, such as those detected in patients with these tumors, can result in hyperthyroidism. Therapy is aimed at either surgical removal of the tumor or appropriate chemotherapy.

*Differentiated thyroid carcinoma,* particularly if metastatic, is a rare cause of thyrotoxicosis. A whole-body $^{131}I$ scan shows functioning thyroidal and extrathyroidal areas. High-dose radioiodine ablation treatment is warranted in these situations.

*Thyrotoxicosis factitia* results from the ingestion of large doses of thyroid hormone. The self-administration of thyroid hormones is often surreptitious. Occasionally accidental ingestions can occur, especially in children. Thyrotoxicosis may be clinically evident, but the thyroid gland is not enlarged. A low RAIU and a low serum thyroglobulin concentration are characteristic findings. Depending on the thyroid preparation ingested, either or both serum $T_4$ and $T_3$ concentrations are elevated.

*Struma ovarii* is a benign ovarian tumor that contains ectopic thyroid tissue. Very rarely this tumor produces enough thyroid hormone to cause thyrotoxicosis. Surgical removal of the tumor treats the thyrotoxicosis.

### Special considerations

***Hyperthyroidism in pregnancy.*** Thyrotoxicosis occurs in about 0.2% of pregnancies and is most frequently caused by Graves' disease. Physiologic changes that occur in pregnancy result in clinical features that resemble those of hyperthyroidism (i.e., increased heart rate, palpitations, heat intolerance, diaphoresis). Signs that are more specific to thyrotoxicosis include lid lag, tremor, and diffuse goiter. Weight gain during pregnancy may be inappropriately low.

High serum total $T_4$ and $T_3$ concentrations and low serum THBR values are characteristic findings in normal pregnancy and may obscure the diagnosis of thyrotoxicosis. As in the nonpregnant patient, thyrotoxicosis is confirmed biochemically with an elevated FTI, an elevated total $T_3$, and a suppressed TSH. Mild hyperthyroidism may be seen in association with hyperemesis gravidarum. This is due to thyroidal stimulation from elevated serum HCG concentrations and rarely requires the institution of antithyroid therapy. The hyperthyroidism resolves as serum HCG concentrations fall.

RAIU and radioisotope imaging studies are contraindicated in the pregnant patient. ATDs are the treatment of choice. PTU is preferred over methimazole because of lower transplacental passage. PTU dosage should be minimized to keep serum FTI in the upper half of the normal range. As pregnancy progresses, Graves' disease often improves. Indeed, it is not uncommon for patients to require daily PTU dosages of less than 100 mg or to be off all ATDs by the end of pregnancy. Therefore PTU dosage should be reduced and maternal thyroid function should be frequently monitored to decrease chances of fetal hypothyroidism. Relapse or worsening of Graves' disease is common after delivery, and patients should be monitored closely.

If the pregnant woman is allergic to thionamides, subtotal thyroidectomy in the second trimester is recommended. As indicated above, RAI therapy is contraindicated because it can cause fetal hypothyroidism. Similarly, iodide administration is associated with fetal goiter and hypothyroidism and should be avoided. Since ATDs are transferred in small amounts to breast milk, the infant's thyroid function should be frequently monitored if nursing is desired.

Transplacental passage of maternal thyroid-stimulating antibodies may result in fetal hyperthyroidism. The diagnosis is based on increased fetal heart rate and hyperactivity. In this situation increased doses of antithyroid drugs may be advised and methimazole may be preferable.

Neonatal Graves' disease is a transient disorder caused by transplacental passage of maternal thyroid-stimulating immunoglobulins. This disorder occurs in 2% of the infants born to mothers with Graves' disease. Very high values of TSI (over 500% of controls) measured in the mother during the third trimester of pregnancy should alert the physician to the possibility of fetal and neonatal hyperthyroidism.

***Thyroid storm.*** Thyroid storm is an uncommon but life-threatening complication of thyrotoxicosis in which a severe form of the disease is usually precipitated by an intercurrent medical problem. It occurs in untreated or partially treated thyrotoxic patients. Precipitating factors associated with thyrotoxic crisis include infections, stress, trauma, thyroidal or non-thyroidal surgery, diabetic ketoacidosis, labor, heart disease, and RAI treatment (especially if there was no pretreatment with ATDs).

Clinical features are similar to those of thyrotoxicosis, but more exaggerated. Cardinal features include fever (temperature usually over 38.5° C) and tachycardia out of proportion to the fever. Nausea, vomiting, diarrhea, agitation, and confusion are frequent presentations. Coma and death may ensue in up to 20% of patients. Thyroid function abnormalities are similar to those found in uncomplicated hyperthyroidism. Therefore thyroid storm is primarily a clinical diagnosis.

Treatment includes supportive measures such as intravenous fluids, antipyretics, cooling blankets, and sedation. Antithyroid drugs are given in large doses. PTU is preferred over methimazole due to its additional advantage of impairing peripheral conversion of $T_4$ to $T_3$. Recommended initial dose for PTU is 200 to 300 mg every 6 hours. PTU and methimazole can be administered by nasogastric tube or rectally if necessary. Neither of these preparations is available for parenteral administration.

Iodides, orally or intravenously, may be used only after antithyroid drugs have been administered. The radiographic contrast dye iopanoic acid (Telepaque), 1 g daily, is used to block thyroid hormone release and to inhibit $T_4$ to $T_3$ conversion. β-Adrenergic blockers, such as propranolol (oral or IV) and esmolol (IV) are given for heart rate control. Calcium channel blockers may also be used to control tachyarrhythmias. High-dose dexamethasone (0.5 to 1 mg every 6 hours IV) is recommended both as supportive therapy and as an inhibitor of $T_4$ and $T_3$ conversion. Finally, treatment of the underlying precipitating illness (e.g., antibiotics, insulin) is essential.

***Subclinical hyperthyroidism.*** Subclinical hyperthyroidism is defined as TSH values in the subnormal or suppressed range, normal circulating thyroid hormone levels and no specific signs of thyrotoxicosis. The prevalence of subnormal TSH concentrations varies depending on the patient population sample, ranging from 4% in an ambulatory setting to 30% in a hospitalized setting. The prevalence of subclinical hyperthyroidism ranges from 0.1% to 5%. The box below lists other conditions that are associated with low serum TSH values. The majority of the patients with subclinical hyperthyroidism are receiving exogenous thyroid hormone therapy. Endogenous subclinical hyperthyroidism is commonly associated with an autonomous nodular or multinodular goiter and, to a lesser degree, with early Graves' disease, thyroiditis, or an iodine load.

The slight increases in thyroid hormone production or intake that translate in the low serum TSH values seen in subclinical hyperthyroidism have been reported to have adverse effects on both the skeletal and the cardiovascular systems. As noted above, a significant reduction in bone mineral density has been reported in several studies in patients taking suppressive doses of L-$T_4$. Adverse cardiac effects include arrhythmias, such as atrial fibrillation, and worsening of angina. Up to 10% of patients presenting with atrial fibrillation have suppressed serum TSH values, with up to 40% of these patients fitting the definition of subclinical hyperthyroidism.

Management of subclinical hyperthyroidism in patients receiving L-$T_4$ replacement therapy is straightforward. The dosage should be titrated to maintain a serum TSH value within the normal range. In patients taking suppressive doses of L-$T_4$ for goiter reduction or thyroid cancer, the administered dosage should be the lowest necessary to keep serum TSH concentrations in the target level.

Treatment of endogenous subclinical hyperthyroidism should be considered based upon the individual situation. Factors such as age, preexisting medical conditions (i.e., coronary artery disease, osteoporosis, hypertension, arrhythmias), and the likelihood of becoming overtly hyperthyroid should be taken into account. A trial of ATDs to normalize the TSH is reasonable to determine if symptoms possibly related to subclinical hyperthyroidism may improve. RAI therapy may be the best option in patients with a multinodular goiter.

### Causes of suppressed TSH

- Thyrotoxicosis
- L-$T_4$ therapy
- Pituitary or hypothalamic hypothyroidism
- Glucocorticoids
- Dopamine and dopamine agonists
- Recovery from thyrotoxicosis
- Acute and chronic nonthyroidal illness
- Caloric restriction
- Acute psychosis
- Surgical stress

## THYROID NODULES

Nodular thyroid disease is the most common endocrinopathy. The prevalence of clinically apparent nodules is 4% to 7% in the United States, with the frequency increasing throughout adult life. When ultrasound and autopsy data are included, the prevalence of thyroid nodules approaches 50% by age 60. As with other forms of thyroid disease, nodules are more frequent in women. Nodules have been estimated to develop at a rate of 0.1% per year. In individuals exposed to ionizing radiation, the rate of nodule development is 20-fold higher. Although the presence of a nodule raises the question of a malignancy, only 8% to 10% of patients with thyroid nodules have thyroid cancer. There are about 12,000 new cases of thyroid cancer diagnosed annually, with about 1000 deaths from the disease per year. However, many more people have clinically silent thyroid cancer: up to 35% of thyroids removed at autopsy or at surgery harbor a small (under 1 cm) papillary cancer.

The mechanism underlying nodule growth and development remains unknown. Thyroid cancer is more frequent in patients exposed to ionizing radiation. Patients may have received radiation treatments for acne, tonsillitis, enlarged thymus, or cheloid scars, or may have been exposed to nuclear fallout (i.e., Chernobyl and Three Mile Island). Nodules in general are more frequent in these patients, as are multiple nodules in a single patient. In addition, nodules are more frequent in individuals residing in regions of endemic iodine deficiency.

### History and physical examination

Nodules that occur at the extremes of age are more likely to be malignant. Rapid growth and symptoms of local invasion (i.e., vocal cord paralysis, dysphagia) are poor prognostic signs, but few patients present with these symptoms. The most common presentation is that of a nodule discovered incidentally during a physical examination performed for other reasons. Once the nodule is discovered, the patient should be asked about symptoms of hyperthyroidism, exposure to radiation, and family history of medullary or papillary thyroid cancer or familial polyposis (Gardner's syndrome).

Physical examination should reveal nodules larger than 1 cm unless they lie deep in the neck. The physical characteristics may give clues as to the malignant potential of the nodule. However, a hard, firm nodule can be seen in Hashimoto thyroiditis and a cystic papillary carcinoma may be soft and mobile. Cancers are more often found in patients with solitary nodules, although when examined by ultrasound or at surgery multiple nodules are found in up to two thirds of thyroid cancer patients. Most thyroid cancers metastasize locally, so the presence of suspicious lymph nodes in the cervical and supraclavicular regions should be noted.

## Differential diagnosis

The vast majority (over 90%) of thyroid nodules are benign lesions (Table 34-4). The most common benign nodule is the colloid, or adenomatous, nodule, followed by follicular adenomas. Thyroiditis is unusual in a solitary nodule but common in a multinodular gland. Of the malignant nodules, papillary cancer is most common, followed by follicular and then anaplastic carcinoma. Medullary carcinoma occurs most often over the age of 40, with about 20% of cases being associated with the familial multiple endocrine neoplasia type IIA (MEN IIA) (see Chapter 39). Cysts make up 15% to 25% of all nodules and include simple cysts, hemorrhagic adenomas, parathyroid cysts, and necrotic papillary cancers. Rare causes of a solitary thyroid nodule include metastatic carcinoma and *Pneumocystis carinii* infection in the HIV-infected patient.

## Laboratory evaluation

In the absence of signs of hyperthyroidism, thyroid function tests are usually normal. Serum TSH measurement is often the only test needed. Management principles are outlined in the Managed Care Guide. If medullary carcinoma is suspected, serum calcitonin should be measured and a pentagastrin stimulation test considered.

***Radioisotope imaging studies.*** The function of the thyroid nodule can be addressed through the use of radionuclide imaging with either iodine or technetium isotopes. Since the incidence of malignancy in a functioning adenoma is under 1%, radioisotope scans can be useful in the identification of those patients who will benefit the most by a biopsy of the nodule, such as those with a hypofunctioning nodule. Bilateral symmetric cold nodules are most often seen in medullary thyroid cancer. In addition, radioisotope scanning identifies those patients whose nodules are most likely to decrease in size with thyroid hormone suppression therapy (see further). Fig. 34-9 shows $^{123}$I scans of two asymptomatic patients presenting with a 2.5-cm solitary nodule in the right lobe of the thyroid. The patient in Fig. 34-9, A, has a hypofunctioning (cold) nodule, as shown by the absence of radionuclide uptake in the region of the nodule. This patient was referred for biopsy of the nodule. The patient in Fig. 34-9, B, has a functioning nodule that is concentrating almost all of the radionuclide. Patient B was

**Table 34-4.** Differential diagnosis of thyroid nodules

| Type | Incidence (%) |
|---|---|
| **Benign nodules** | 83-92 |
| Colloid (adenomatous) | 42-77 |
| Follicular adenomas | 15-40 |
| Thyroiditis | <5 |
| Nonthyroid | <5 |
| Congenital abnormalities | <1 |
| Other | <1 |
| **Malignant nodules** | 8-17 |
| Papillary | 50-70 |
| Follicular | 10-15 |
| Anaplastic | 5-10 |
| Medullary | 5-10 |
| Lymphoma | 1-5 |
| Metastatic | <5 |
| **Thyroid** | 15-25 |
| Benign | 85 |
| Malignant | 15 |

### Managed Care Guide
### Evaluation of thyroid nodules

1. Evaluation of thyroid nodules with a full array of diagnostic techniques is costly.
2. If the diagnosis of a nodule or diffuse goiter is uncertain, the most cost-effective approach is to have another clinician assess the findings.
3. A discrete, firm, irregular mass associated with suspicious lymphadenopathy is strongly suggestive of malignancy.
4. Thyroid dysfunction implies a background of diffuse and almost always benign disease.
5. Approximately 90% of uninodular thyroid disease proves to be cold on isotopic screening. The 10% of nodules that are hot do not usually require evaluation for malignancy. Clinical follow-up is indicated to detect the rare malignant hot nodule.
6. Isotopic scanning may be 3 to 5 times as expensive as fine needle aspiration (FNA). By performing FNA biopsy first, isotopic scans may be reduced by 50%, saving both time and money
7. Thyroid ultrasounds are not employed in early diagnostic assesment of thyroid nodules because of poor diagnostic discrimination between benign and malignant processes. They may be utilized, however, to accurately guide FNA biopsy and to delineate small or posterior masses.
8. Controversy currently exists over whether to perform isotopic scans on all patients before biopsy to identify cold nodules at greater cost and inconvenience or whether to perform FNA biopsy first and run the risk of indeterminate or false negative biopsy results. Community standards and consultation with an endocrinologist provide the best guide at this time.

Adapted from Clinical Guidelines and Algorithms, Harvard Community Health Plan

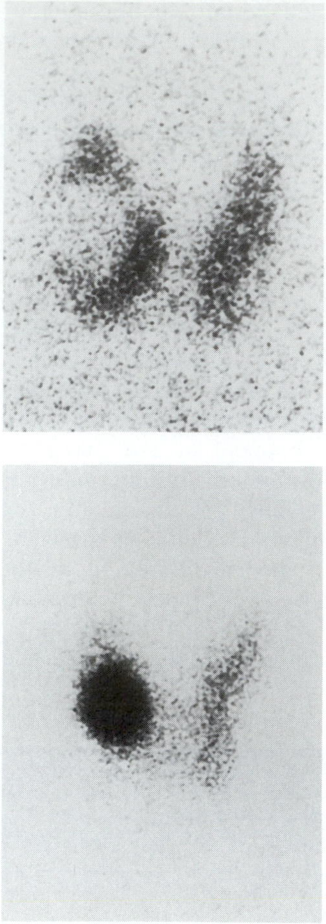

A

B

**Fig. 34-9.** Radionuclide thyroid imaging in the evaluation of the solitary thyroid nodule. Two patients had a solitary 2.5 cm nodule in the right lobe of the thyroid. Thyroid imaging with $^{123}I$ was obtained. **A,** Hypofunctioning nodule, with decreased uptake in the region of the palpable nodule. Uptake in the rest of the gland is homogeneous. This patient was referred for FNA of the nodule. **B,** Functioning nodule, with partial suppression of the remaining thyroid tissue. This patient was placed on L-$T_4$ suppression and a suppression scan was obtained.

placed on thyroid hormone in an attempt to suppress and shrink the nodule.

***Ultrasound.*** Ultrasound rarely adds more to the evaluation of the thyroid nodule over and above the physical examination and a radioisotope scan. Ultrasound can readily diagnose a cyst; however, cysts show up as cold nodules on scans and thus are referred for biopsy, where the diagnosis is made. Ultrasound is most useful in documenting the size of the nodule and assessing the effect of thyroid hormone on shrinking benign nodules. However, physical examination with an experienced physician is adequate in the majority of cases.

***Fine-needle aspiration biopsy.*** Fine-needle aspiration (FNA) biopsy of nodules is a safe and accurate method to diagnose the presence of a thyroid malignancy. Indeed, many clinicians choose FNA as the initial test for the evaluation of a thyroid nodule. Recent studies suggest that FNA is the most cost-effective initial approach and is

**Table 34-5.** Cytologic categories in fine-needle aspiration biopsy of the thyroid

| Cytologic diagnosis | Frequency (%)* |
|---|---|
| Benign | 70.3 |
| Malignant | 3.6 |
| Suspicious | 10.1 |
| Nondiagnostic | 16.3 |

*Average of eight published series.

being increasingly adopted by physicians. Essential to the accuracy of the FNA is the presence of a cytopathologist skilled in the interpretation of the results. Four cytologic results are possible: (1) benign (negative), (2) malignant (positive), (3) suspicious (indeterminate), and (4) nondiagnostic (inadequate). Benign conditions identified by FNA include colloid goiter, cysts, and thyroiditis. Benign FNA smears are obtained in the vast majority of patients (Table 34-5). Positive FNA smears include papillary, medullary, and anaplastic primary thyroid cancer, metastatic cancer, and lymphoma. Since the diagnosis of follicular carcinoma requires the documentation of vascular or capsular invasion, the finding of follicular cells on FNA may indicate either a benign or malignant neoplasm and thus falls into the suspicious category. Nondiagnostic FNA smears often occur in the setting of vascular or cystic lesions or when performed by less experienced physicians. Repeat FNA yields a satisfactory smear in up to 50% of cases. FNA is very accurate, with a false positive rate of 2.9% and a false negative rate of 5.2%, representing the average in seven published series.

## Management

Surgery is indicated for patients with FNA smears in the malignant category. The management of those patients with suspicious FNA results depends on the sequence of procedures performed. If radioisotope imaging is performed first, only those patients with a hypofunctioning nodule will be referred for FNA; thus all suspicious FNA results would be referred for surgery. If FNA is the initial procedure, patients with suspicious FNA smears are referred for radioisotope scanning, after which those with hypofunctioning nodules are referred for surgery (see Managed Care Guide).

***Thyroid cancer.*** The extent of surgery for thyroid cancer is controversial and recommendations vary significantly. Factors affecting surgery include the size of the lesion, pathology, and experience of the surgeon. Lobectomies are performed less frequently since the publication of data demonstrating cancer foci in the opposite lobe in up to 35% of patients. A near total thyroidectomy is thought by many to be appropriate for most lesions and affords less risk of either vocal cord paralysis or hypoparathyroidism compared to total thyroidectomy.

Total body $^{131}I$ scanning should be performed 6 to 8 weeks after near total thyroidectomy surgery to identify metastatic disease. This is done when the patient is hypothyroid (TSH over 50 mU/L); thus the patient should not be started on L-$T_4$ therapy postoperatively. To minimize the time the patient is hypothyroid, L-$T_3$ (Cytomel, 50 to 75 μg per day) may be administered for 3 to 4 weeks after surgery, then discontinued for 2 weeks. Depending on the residual uptake or the presence of metastatic disease, an ablative dose of $^{131}$I ranging from 30 to 150 mCi is administered and a repeat total body scan is obtained 1 week later. The precise amount of $^{131}$I needed to treat residual tissue and metastases is also controversial. Foci of metastatic disease outside the neck should be imaged by CT or MRI to follow the progression or regression of the disease without having to rely on hypothyroid radionuclide scanning.

Suppressive therapy with L-$T_4$ is indicated in all patients after treatment for thyroid cancer. The goal of therapy is to keep serum TSH levels in the subnormal range. Follow-up evaluation every 6 months is reasonable, along with determination of serum thyroglobulin concentrations. A rise in serum thyroglobulin concentration is often the first indication of recurrent disease. Repeat hypothyroid scanning should be performed 1 year after the initial surgery and patients retreated if residual uptake is found. If no uptake is seen on the 1-year scan, a final scan can be obtained 3 to 5 years after surgery as long as thyroglobulin measurements remain stable.

Prognosis in patients with thyroid cancer depends on the pathology and size of the tumor and is generally worse in the elderly. Over all, the vast majority of patients with thyroid cancer will not die of their disease. Papillary cancer is the least aggressive tumor, metastasizes locally, and has a 10-year survival rate greater than 90%. Lymph node metastasis at the time of diagnosis does little to alter the prognosis. Follicular cancer is more aggressive and can metastasize via the bloodstream. Still, prognosis is fair and long-term survival is common. Anaplastic cancer is the exception, since it is highly malignant with survival usually less than 6 months.

***Benign nodules.*** Two options are available for the patient diagnosed with a benign nodule: observation or suppressive L-$T_4$ therapy. The rationale behind L-$T_4$ therapy is that the benign nodule will either stop growing or decrease in size after TSH stimulation to the thyroid gland is turned off. The success rate of such therapy ranges from 0% to 68% in different studies.

Identification of those patients who are most likely to benefit from thyroid hormone therapy can be achieved through measurement of the serum TSH concentration and radioisotope scanning. Suppression therapy has no value if thyroid nodule autonomy exists, as evidenced by a subnormal TSH value. Functioning nodules are the most likely to respond to suppression therapy. However, once TSH concentrations are suppressed, a repeat radioisotope scan (suppression scan) should be obtained. If significant uptake persists on a suppression scan, the nodule is autonomous and L-$T_4$ therapy should be discontinued. Suppression therapy needs to be considered carefully in older patients or those with coronary artery disease. Hypofunctioning nodules are much less likely to respond to suppression therapy. However, a 6-month trial of L-$T_4$ suppression is reasonable. L-$T_4$ therapy should be continued for as long as the nodule is decreasing in size. Once the size of a nodule remains stable for 6 to 12 months, therapy should be discontinued and the nodule observed for recurrent growth. Any nodule that grows during suppression therapy requires repeat biopsy and/or surgical excision.

## SCREENING FOR THYROID DISEASE

Screening for thyroid disease would appear to be beneficial due to the subtle and nonspecific nature of the symptoms of thyroid dysfunction and the fact that thyroid disorders are eminently treatable. In a large study in Wickham, England, about 4.6% of the women were found to have overt thyroid dysfunction. However, over 80% of these patients had been previously diagnosed and the prevalence of new cases was under 0.5%. No new cases of thyroid dysfunction were discovered in men in this study. Thus screening of a general community for thyroid disease has a very low yield and is not recommended.

Case-finding, or identifying disease in patients who seek medical attention for unrelated reasons, may be beneficial in the diagnosis and treatment of thyroid disease. Certain patient subpopulations that do have a higher incidence of thyroid dysfunction can be identified. Included in this group are women over the age of 40, elderly individuals of both sexes, and patients with preexisting autoimmune diseases, hypercholesterolemia, atrial fibrillation, or carpal tunnel syndrome. For these individuals a single screening test is acceptable. The FTI, total $T_4$, or the sensitive TSH may be used. Although the sensitive TSH assay tends to be more expensive, the specificity of a normal TSH value in ruling out thyroid disease is close to 100%.

Case-finding for thyroid disease is not helpful in patients admitted to an acute care medical or psychiatric ward. Abnormal test results are common and rarely indicate previously unrecognized thyroid dysfunction. In these patients thyroid function testing should be reserved for those individuals in whom the clinical suspicion of thyroid disease is high. Both the FTI and a sensitive TSH value are often required to make a diagnosis in these cases. Similarly, case-finding for thyroid disease is not recommended in individuals less than 40 years of age.

In all cases when an abnormal result is obtained, the diagnosis should be confirmed with other tests of thyroid function as well as a directed clinical evaluation. Therapy should not be instituted on the basis of a single abnormal thyroid function test.

## BIBLIOGRAPHY


Braverman LE, Utiger RD, editors: *The thyroid,* ed 6, Philadelphia, 1991, JB Lippincott.

Cooper DS: Subclinical hypothyroidism. In Mazzaferri E, editor: *Advances in endocrinology and metabolism,* St. Louis, 1991, Mosby.

Fisher DA: Management of congenital hypothyroidism, *J Clin Endocrinol Metab* 72:523, 1991.

Gharib H, Goellner JR: Fine-needle aspiration biopsy of the thyroid: an appraisal, *Ann Intern Med* 118:282, 1993.

Helfand M, Crapo L: Screening for thyroid disease, *Ann Intern Med* 112:840, 1990.

Kaplan MM: Assessment of thyroid function during pregnancy, *Thyroid* 2:57, 1992.

Mazzaferri EL: Management of a solitary thyroid nodule, *N Engl J Med* 328:553, 1993.

Nicoloff JT, Spencer CA: Clinical review 12: the use and misuse of the sensitive thyrotropin assays, *J Clin Endocrinol Metab* 71:553, 1990.

Robuschi G et al: Hypothyroidism in the elderly, *Endocrine Rev* 8:142, 1987.

Ross DR: Subclinical thyrotoxicosis. In Mazzaferri E, editor: *Advances in endocrinology and metabolism,* St. Louis, 1991, Mosby.

Singer P et al: American Thyroid Association standards of care for patients with thyroid dysfunction, *JAMA,* 1995.

Singer PA et al: Treatment guidelines for patients with hyperthyroidism and hypothyroidism, *JAMA* 273:808, 1995.

Tunbridge WMG et al: The spectrum of thyroid disease in a community: the Wickham survey, *Clin Endocrinol* 7:481, 1977.

CHAPTER

# 35 Adrenal Gland Disorders

**Melanie J. Brunt**
**James C. Melby**

## ADRENAL ANATOMY AND PHYSIOLOGY

In the adrenal cortex, which constitutes 80% of the total adrenal weight, three zones are responsible for corticosteroid synthesis. The outermost layer, the zona glomerulosa, synthesizes aldosterone, which is the predominant mineralocorticoid, responsible for sodium retention and potassium excretion. The middle and inner layers, the zona fasciculata and the zona reticularis, produce glucocorticoids (principally cortisol) and the sex steroids and their precursor, dehydroepiandrosterone (DHEA). Cortisol functions to promote protein and lipid catabolism and gluconeogenesis. Catecholamines are synthesized in the adrenal medulla, and they are regulated via the autonomic nervous system.

All corticosteroids are derived from cholesterol, which is found in abundance in the adrenal cortex. Regulatory systems for cortisol and aldosterone are outlined in Fig. 35-1. Cortisol is subject to negative feedback regulation via the hypothalamic-pituitary axis (HPA). The majority of the daily cortisol production of 15 to 25 mg is produced between 5 and 9 AM. Metabolic stress such as sepsis or myocardial infarction can raise production levels to 250 mg per day. Aldosterone is regulated via the renin-angiotensin feedback loop, through which low renal perfusion pressure stimulates increased aldosterone production. Extracellular potassium concentration also affects aldosterone secretion, and the HPA plays a small role as well, regulating about 15% of aldosterone production via adrenocorticotropic hormone (ACTH) stimulation.

## ADRENOCORTICAL HYPOFUNCTION

### Pathophysiology

Adrenocortical hypofunction can occur due to primary destruction of the adrenal cortex, with consequent loss of production of all of the corticosteroid hormones. It may also be secondary, due to diminished ACTH production by the pituitary. In the latter disorder only glucocorticoid and androgen production are affected. Mineralocorticoid production remains largely intact because ACTH plays only a small role in aldosterone regulation. Angiotensin II and potassium are the principal factors affecting aldosterone production, and the renin–angiotensin II–aldosterone regulatory axis is independent of regulation by the pituitary. In both disorders the clinical consequences relate to loss of cortisol, a hormone essential for survival, are paramount. Cortisol is essential for the maintenance of vascular tone and cardiovascular output due to its positive inotropic effects; thus hypotension may be present in either disorder. Hypoglycemia also occurs due to the loss of the permissive effects of cortisol on glycogenolysis and gluconeogenesis. Hypercalcemia may be present due to the loss of cortisol inhibition of intestinal absorption and renal reabsorption of calcium. Hyponatremia can also occur. In primary adrenal insufficiency this is due to loss of the sodium-retentive properties of aldosterone. In secondary insufficiency it can occur despite normal aldosterone levels due to (1) decreased cortisol-mediated renal free water clearance and (2) compensatory elevations of arginine vasopressin.

Hyperpigmentation is seen only in primary adrenal insufficiency and is due to increased secretion of β-lipotropin, a component of the precursor peptide that also contains ACTH. Also in primary insufficiency the loss of aldosterone, the principal regulator of potassium excretion in the body, can result in potentially life-threatening hyperkalemia. Increased sodium excretion in the absence of aldosterone can result in profound volume depletion.

### History and physical findings

Adrenal insufficiency often fails to be diagnosed because the clinical presentation can be quite nonspecific. Key clinical features include weakness, fatigue, anorexia, nausea/vomiting, weight loss, and symptoms of volume depletion. The box on p. 518 lists the predominant clinical features of primary adrenal insufficiency, or Addison's disease, which is the most common type. Skin changes in this disease include diffuse hyperpigmentation with accentuation in palmar folds, scars, and oral mucosa, longitudinal pigmented bands under nails, vitiligo in up to 15% of patients, and decreased pubic and axillary hair in females. Associated problems include weakness, fatigue, nausea, and vomiting, and a craving for salt. It may be associated with other endocrine insufficiencies, such as hypothyroidism and hypoparathyroidism, pernicious anemia, thyroiditis, and alopecia areata. Treatment is to replace adrenal hormones. Secondary adrenal insufficiency most commonly occurs in the setting of panhypopituitarism; thus most patients have clinical signs and symptoms suggestive of secondary hypothyroidism and hypogonadism in addition to evidence of cortisol deficiency (see Chapter 36). Rarely secondary adrenal insufficiency is due to isolated ACTH deficiency. In this disorder symptoms and signs of cortisol deficiency such as hypotension, hyponatremia, malaise, and fatigue are present without concomitant evidence of secondary thyroid and gonadal failure.

The following cases illustrate the difficulty in making a diagnosis of adrenal insufficiency:

**CASE 1** A 50-year-old U.S. citizen living overseas in a tropical climate developed malaise, weakness, intermittent abdominal pain, and diarrhea a few months after a brief febrile illness. Physicians prescribed antibiotics without effect.

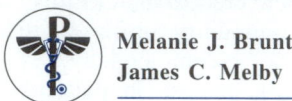

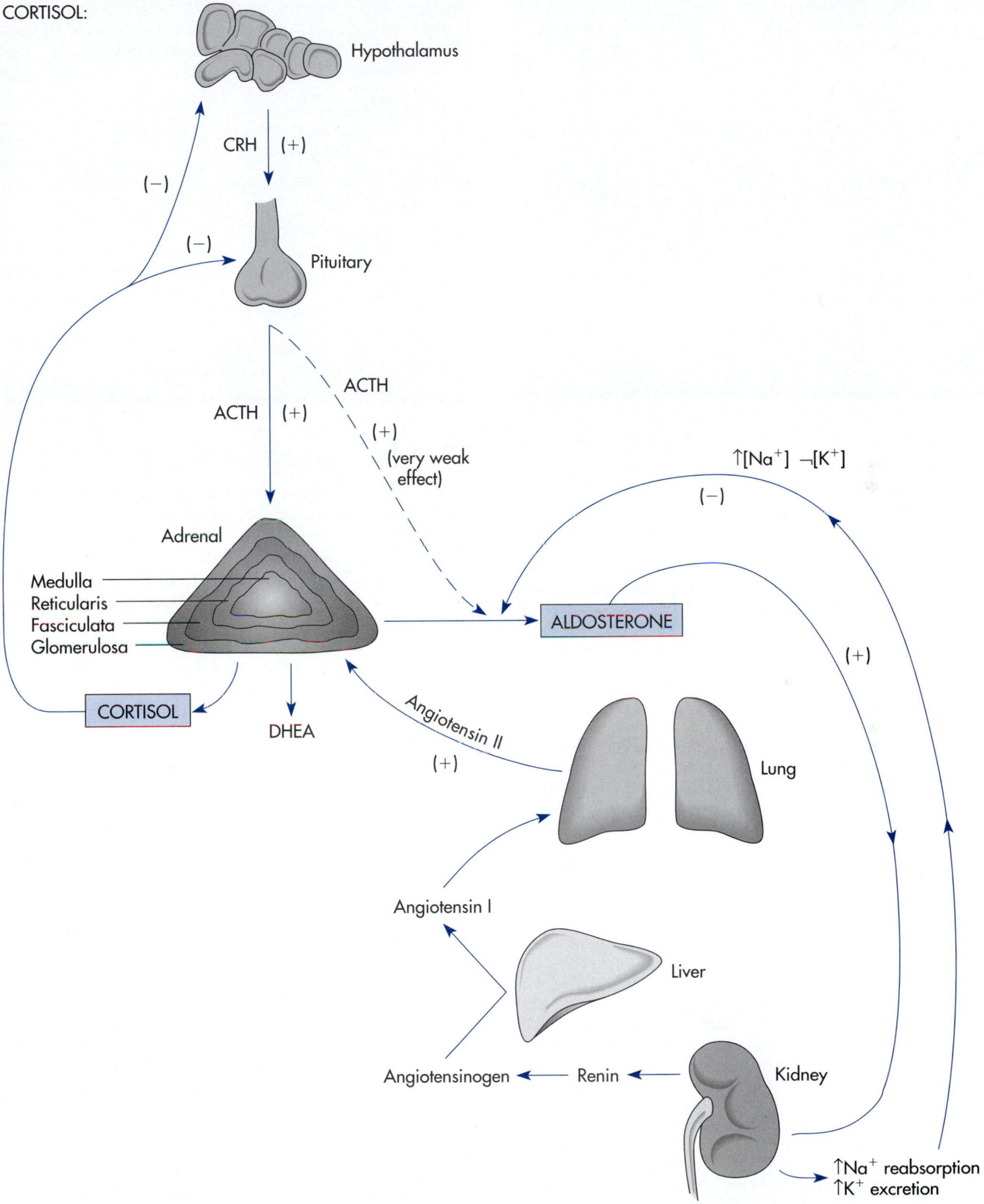


**Fig. 35-1.** Regulatory systems for cortisol and aldosterone. *CRH,* Corticotropin-releasing hormone; *ACTH,* adrenocorticotropic hormone; *DHEA,* dihydroepiandrosterone.

### Frequency of clinical features of primary adrenal insufficiency

**Symptoms**

Weakness and fatigue (100%)
Anorexia (100%)
Nausea and diarrhea (56%)

**Signs**

Weight loss (100%)
Hyperpigmentation (97%)
Hypotension (91%)
Vitiligo (rare)

**Laboratory findings**

Hyponatremia (90%)
Hyperkalemia (66%)
Hypoglycemia (40%)
Hypercalcemia (6%)

### Causes of adrenal insufficiency

**Primary**

Autoimmune/idiopathic (70%)
Tuberculosis (20%)
Other (10%)
Fungal infections
Adrenal hemorrhage
Congenital adrenal hyperplasia
Sarcoidosis
Amyloidosis
HIV/AIDS
Adrenoleukodystrophy
Metastatic disease

**Secondary**

Iatrogenic (following exogenous glucocorticoids) (common)
Isolated ACTH deficiency (uncommon)
Hypothalamic/pituitary lesions (uncommon)

During a visit to the United States he saw his internist, who referred him to a gastroenterologist. Several radiographic studies were performed, no diagnosis was found, and he was treated symptomatically. The patient continued to experience the same symptoms and became depressed, for which he pursued counseling. Upon his permanent return to the United States over a year later, he sought further counseling and was started on a tricyclic antidepressant. A few weeks thereafter he experienced two falls, the second of which was associated with a loss of consciousness. He was brought to an emergency ward, where laboratory data revealed a sodium level of 110 mEq/L. Hyperpigmentation in sun-exposed areas was noted; the patient attributed this to frequent sun exposure. A workup revealed low cortisol levels with absent response to synthetic ACTH injection. A purified protein derivative (PPD) test was positive, and calcification was noted in the area of the right adrenal gland on computed tomographic (CT) scan of the abdomen. All symptoms resolved promptly with glucocorticoid replacement.

**CASE 2** A 35-year-old non–English-speaking immigrant from the Caribbean had a medical history remarkable only for a motor vehicle accident involving a brief loss of consciousness 5 years previously. He was brought to an emergency ward on many occasions over a 3-year period by family members due to confusional episodes associated with violent behavior, recurrent fevers, weight loss, and malaise. The patient was admitted to the hospital from the emergency ward on several occasions. On some of these admissions infections were documented, including streptococcal pharyngitis, pneumococcal pneumonia, and urinary tract infection; on other occasions extensive sepsis evaluations were unrevealing. His mental status remained abnormal but no explanation was found. Electrolytes were consistently within normal limits, though potassium was usually ≥4.5 mEq/L, sodium ≤140 mEq/L, and blood glucose 60 to 70 mg/dl. A blood glucose level of 29 mg/dl finally prompted evaluation of the adrenal axis, and poor response to synthetic ACTH injection was documented.

In both cases primary adrenal insufficiency was finally diagnosed, but the delay led to significant morbidity.

## Etiology and differential diagnosis

***Primary adrenal insufficiency.*** Idiopathic Addison's disease is the predominant cause of primary adrenal insufficiency (see the box above). This is thought in most cases to be an autoimmune disorder of the adrenal cortex characterized by lymphocytic infiltration on histologic examination. The prevalence of antiadrenal antibodies in patients with idiopathic Addison's disease is 70%; therefore the absence of antibodies does not rule out the diagnosis. Nearly half of Addison's disease patients develop associated endocrine disorders with organ-specific antibodies, such as pernicious anemia, gonadal failure, insulin-dependent diabetes mellitus, hypoparathyroidism, vitiligo, or thyroid disorders (see Chapter 39).

Tuberculosis once accounted for over 75% of all cases of Addison's disease. Although it is now less common, the emergence of resistant strains of tuberculosis among HIV-infected persons and increased immigration from countries with high prevalences of tuberculosis may lead to a resurgence of this type of Addison's disease. Features of tuberculous adrenal insufficiency include adrenal enlargement in the early stages (within the first 5 years) followed by adrenal atrophy with calcification. Absence of these features does not rule out tuberculosis as a cause; thus skin testing for tuberculosis should be a standard part of the evaluation of patients with Addison's disease.

Metastatic disease frequently involves the adrenal gland. Cancer of the lung and breast are the two types of malignancies that most commonly metastasize to the adrenals. In 35% of patients with metastatic lung or breast cancer adrenal metastases are found. Despite this high frequency, adrenal insufficiency can be documented biochemically in only about 20% of these patients. This is presumed to reflect the fact that over 90% of the adrenal gland must be destroyed to produce insufficiency. All patients with bilateral adrenal metastatic disease should be tested with short-acting ACTH (Cortrosyn) to rule out insufficiency.

**Table 35-1.** Glucocorticoid characteristics

| Medication | $t_{1/2}$ | Dosages | | Potencies | |
|---|---|---|---|---|---|
| | | Replacement* | Stress† | GC‡ | MC§ |
| Hydrocortisone (cortisol) (Cortef, Solu-Cortef) | 8-12 hr | 20 mg | 200 mg | 1 | 1 |
| Prednisone | 12-36 hr | 5 mg | 50 mg | 4 | 0.25 |
| Methylprednisolone (Solu-Medrol) | 12-36 hr | 4 mg | 40 mg | 5 | 0.25 |
| Dexamethasone (Decadron) | 36-72 hr | 0.75 mg | 7.5 mg | 25 | 0 |
| Fludrocortisone (Florinef) | 12-20 hr | 0.05-2 mg | Increase dietary sodium | 10 | 125 |

*Refers to the dosage required to replace the 24-hour cortisol production of nonstressed adrenal glands.
†Refers to the dosage required to replace the 24-hour cortisol production of the adrenals in situations of severe metabolic stress.
‡Refers to the glococorticoid potency of the medication as compared to cortisol (note the 1,4,5,25 rule may be a helpful way to recall relative potencies).
§Refers to the mineralocorticoid potency of the medication as compared to cortisol.

Acquired immune deficiency syndrome (AIDS) can cause primary adrenal insufficiency. The etiology is usually infection with cytomegalovirus (CMV), *Cryptococcus,* tuberculosis or atypical *Mycobacterium,* or use of medications (e.g., ketoconazole). Although most HIV patients with evidence of adrenal infiltration by one of these organisms do not have adrenal insufficiency because there is sufficient adrenal function preserved, about 20% of patients with HIV have been found in some series to have a subnormal response to ACTH consistent with adrenal insufficiency.

***Secondary adrenal insufficiency.*** Secondary adrenal insufficiency can be related to panhypopituitarism, isolated ACTH loss, or exogenous glucocorticoid suppression of the HPA (see the box at left). Panhypopituitarism is discussed in detail in Chapter 36. Pituitary tumor, infiltration, and infarction are common etiologies. Cases have been reported in the literature of isolated ACTH loss due to selective failure of pituitary ACTH-producing cells. The etiology is unknown in most cases, but an association with other autoimmune endocrinopathies, the postpartum occurrence in some patients, and the measurement of serum antipituitary antibodies have suggested an autoimmune etiology. Exogenous suppression of the HPA during glucocorticoid or ACTH therapy for nonendocrine disorders is common. This can occur up to 12 months after treatment of at least 3 weeks' duration with pharmacologic dosages of these medications. A pharmacologic dosage is defined as any dosage exceeding the 24-hour adrenal replacement dosage (Table 35-1). Although most cases of adrenal suppression follow prolonged use of oral or parenteral glucocorticoids, cases of adrenal suppression following the use of high dosages of inhaled or topical glucocorticoids have been reported as well. In general, the likelihood of suppression increases with dosage and duration of therapy and with use of longer acting agents. However, it is impossible to predict the exact dosage or duration of glucocorticoid use that will produce HPA suppression in an individual patient. Clinically some patients undergoing a taper from prolonged use of glucocorticoids can experience the glucocorticoid withdrawal syndrome, which includes fatigue, weakness, arthralgias, anorexia, nausea, abdominal pain, skin desquamation, and dizziness. This clinical syndrome may or may not be associated with evidence of endogenous adrenal suppression upon testing. In some cases testing is completely normal, suggesting that this syndrome may reflect physiologic and/or psychologic dependence on high doses of glucocorticoids.

### Laboratory studies and diagnostic procedures

As shown in the box at far left, hyperkalemia occurs in 66%, hyponatremia in 90%, and hypoglycemia in 40% of cases. However, as illustrated by Case 2, they can be mild and easily missed. Dynamic endocrine testing is necessary to establish a diagnosis, since random cortisol levels are usually not helpful. Indications for such testing, in addition to electrolyte abnormalities, may include repeated episodes of syncope or hypotension, significant weight loss, unexplained fevers, or fever disproportionate to the type of infection. The Managed Care Guide is an algorithm of the diagnostic evaluation.

***Rapid ACTH test.*** The rapid ACTH stimulation test is highly accurate in establishing or excluding adrenal insufficiency. The test measures only adrenal response to injected ACTH and does not test for endogenous ACTH or corticotropin-releasing hormone (CRH) deficiency. However, the adrenal atrophy that occurs with chronic endogenous ACTH or CRH deficiency often results in poor adrenal response to injected ACTH. Correlation has been demonstrated between rapid ACTH testing results and results of direct testing at higher levels, so the test can be used to assess all levels of adrenal dysfunction. A bolus intravenous injection of 250 μg of synthetic α-1,24 ACTH (Cortrosyn) is administered. Plasma cortisol levels are measured at 0 and 30 to 60 minutes. A 30- to 60-minute plasma cortisol level of greater than 18 to 20 μg/dl excludes the diagnosis of primary adrenal insufficiency and usually excludes chronic secondary adrenal insufficiency as well. However, in acute secondary adrenal insufficiency, cortisol response to Cortrosyn may be normal.

***Plasma ACTH level.*** When the rapid ACTH stimulation test yields abnormal results, a plasma ACTH level differentiates between primary adrenal insufficiency and insufficiency at a higher level. Patients with primary

## Managed Care Guide
## Algorithm for adrenal insufficiency

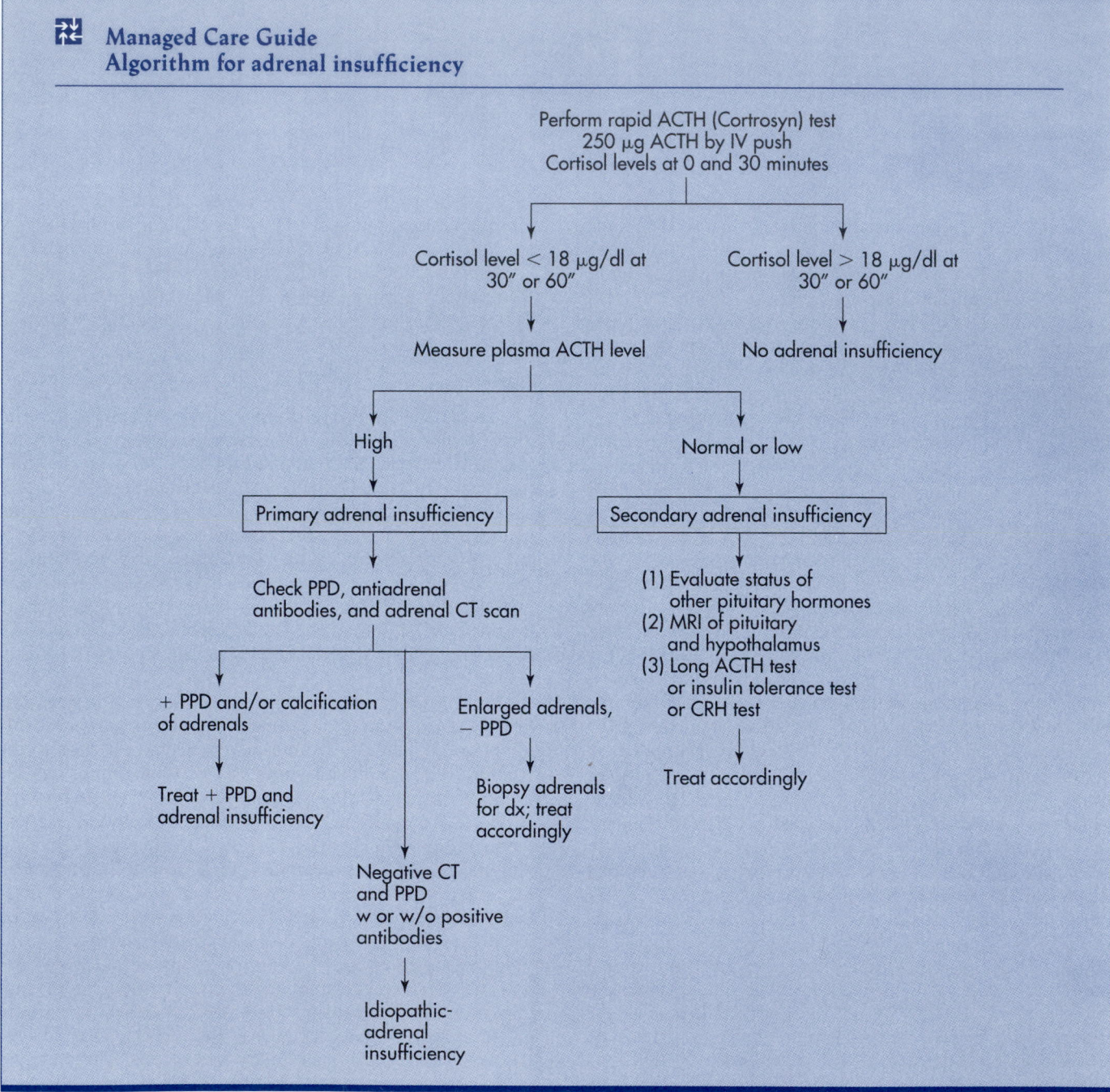

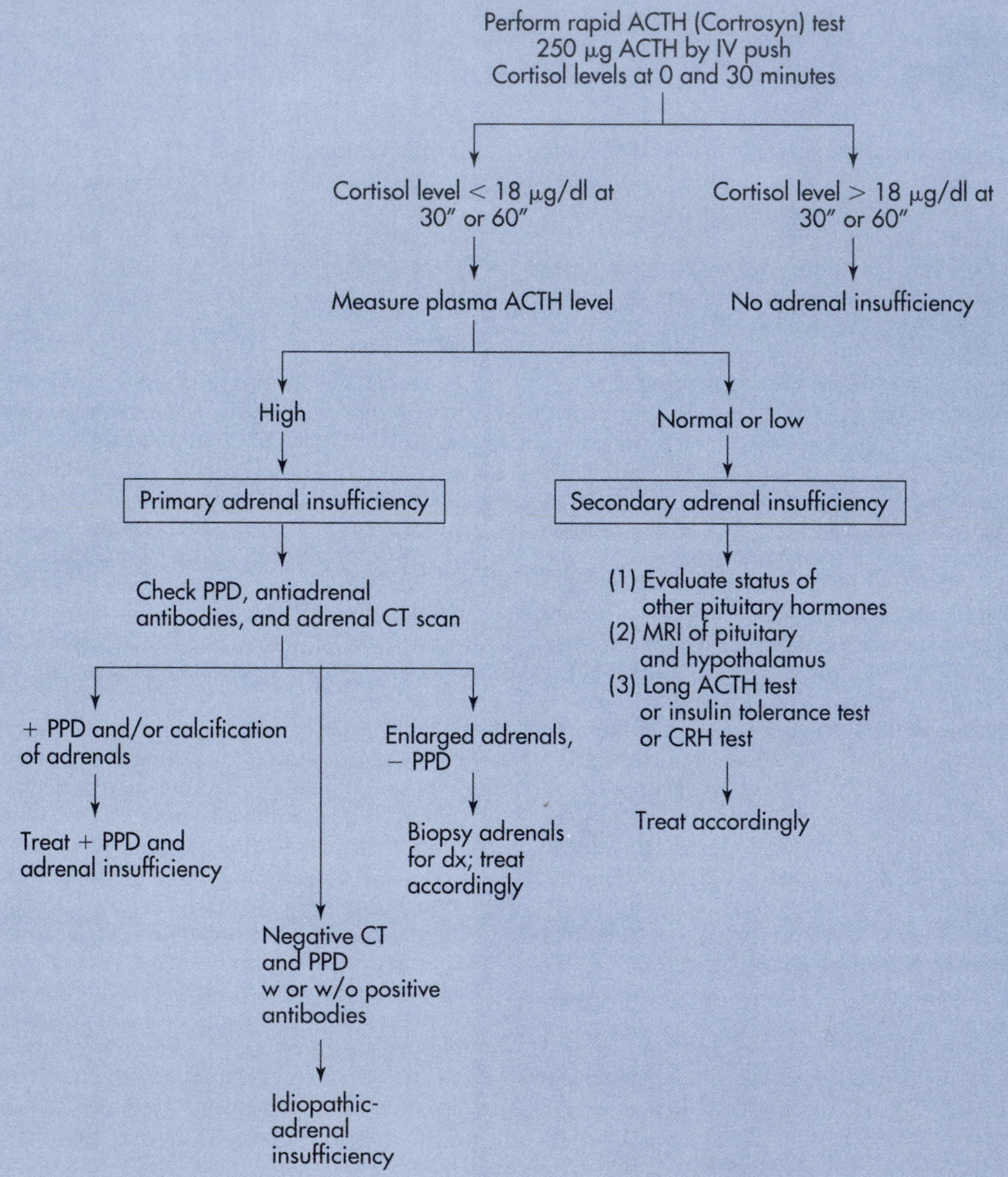
Perform rapid ACTH (Cortrosyn) test
250 μg ACTH by IV push
Cortisol levels at 0 and 30 minutes
Cortisol level < 18 μg/dl at 30″ or 60″
Cortisol level > 18 μg/dl at 30″ or 60″
Measure plasma ACTH level
No adrenal insufficiency
High
Normal or low
Primary adrenal insufficiency
Secondary adrenal insufficiency
Check PPD, antiadrenal antibodies, and adrenal CT scan
(1) Evaluate status of other pituitary hormones
(2) MRI of pituitary and hypothalamus
(3) Long ACTH test or insulin tolerance test or CRH test
Treat accordingly
+ PPD and/or calcification of adrenals
Treat + PPD and adrenal insufficiency
Enlarged adrenals, − PPD
Biopsy adrenals for dx; treat accordingly
Negative CT and PPD w or w/o positive antibodies
Idiopathic-adrenal insufficiency

failure have elevated ACTH levels, whereas patients with secondary failure have normal or low levels. Careful attention must be paid to specimen collection, since falsely low results can occur. This test should be reserved until after abnormal rapid ACTH (Cortrosyn) test results are documented.

***Other tests.*** These tests are usually reserved for endocrine/metabolic units and are not essential for diagnosis if the combined cortisol and ACTH test results establish the level of dysfunction. A long ACTH test involves the administration of 500 µg/dl Cortrosyn as a continuous infusion over 48 hours, with measurement of urinary free cortisol and serum cortisol levels. An insulin tolerance test involves the administration of insulin to invoke hypoglycemia, which is a stimulus to pituitary ACTH secretion. Endogenous ACTH levels are measured as hypoglycemia occurs. This test requires close supervision by experienced personnel. The metyrapone test uses the drug metyrapone to block the final step in cortisol synthesis, thus stimulating an ACTH response to a temporary decrease in cortisol production. A CRH test is sometimes used as well, with measurement of ACTH and cortisol response. This injectable CRH has an ovine source and is similar to endogenous CRH, the hypothalamic releasing factor for cortisol.

Those who are confirmed to have secondary adrenal insufficiency may require additional testing to rule out secondary thyroid or gonadal failure.

***Radiologic imaging.*** If a biochemical diagnosis of primary adrenal insufficiency is established, CT scan imaging of the adrenal glands may be helpful in distinguishing etiology. Normal adrenal glands are often not visualized on CT scan. In idiopathic adrenal insufficiency the atrophic adrenal glands are also not visualized and therefore may not be distinguishable as different from normal. However, infiltrative disorders such as metastatic disease, sarcoidosis, and tuberculosis may cause adrenal enlargement in the early stages of disease. Later adrenal calcification may be seen. If antiadrenal antibodies are negative and calcification is present in the area of the adrenal glands, the presumed etiology is tuberculosis. Patients who have neither adrenal calcification nor positive tuberculin skin testing must be presumed to have idiopathic Addison's disease regardless of antibody status. There is no role for adrenal CT scan in patients who have biochemical evidence of secondary adrenal insufficiency.

For patients who appear to have secondary adrenal insufficiency on biochemical testing, MRI of the brain with views of the pituitary is necessary to rule out a midline CNS lesion. High-resolution CT scanning with contrast may in some cases be adequate to image the pituitary and hypothalamus, but in most centers MRI is now the diagnostic study of choice.

### Treatment

The emergency treatment of acute adrenal crisis is outlined in the box at right. Empiric treatment for adrenal crisis should be considered in all severely ill patients with shock refractory to volume expansion or pressor agents. Factors that would argue strongly for such treatment include risk factors for adrenal insufficiency such as anticoagulant therapy, bleeding diathesis, disseminated intravascular coagulation, disseminated tuberculosis, acquired immune deficiency syndrome, sepsis, or a history of glucocorticoid therapy within the previous 12 months. Treatment is not likely to benefit patients whose refractory hypotension is clearly related to cardiogenic shock. Treatment should be continued until results of the diagnostic evaluation are available. The dosage of glucocorticoid can be tapered at a rate appropriate to the clinical condition of the patient. In patients who are clearly improving clinically, the dosage can be tapered by 50% daily, with a change to oral maintenance therapy within several days.

#### Management of acute adrenal insufficiency

Draw blood for measurement of cortisol and ACTH.
Infuse sufficient normal saline with 5% dextrose to restore normotension.
Administer 2 mg dexamethasone IV immediately (which will not interfere with further testing).
Give 250 µg Cortrosyn (ACTH) IV and measure 30-minute cortisol level.
Begin IV hydrocortisone as a continuous infusion to total 200 mg in 24 hours; or doses can be given in bolus form, 50 mg every 6 hours.
Investigate underlying etiology of adrenal insufficiency with plain film of abdomen to rule out adrenal calcification, tuberculosis testing, and evaluation of thyroid and gonadal status.
Chronic oral replacement therapy can begin as soon as the patient is medically stable and able to take medication orally.

Maintenance therapy for adrenal insufficiency consists of daily oral glucocorticoid, most commonly hydrocortisone or prednisone, plus the mineralocorticoid fludrocortisone in primary adrenal insufficiency (see Table 35-1). For primary adrenal insufficiency, hydrocortisone may be a better choice than prednisone because of its higher mineralocorticoid activity. Thus, for some patients taking hydrocortisone, mineralocorticoid replacement with fludrocortisone may not be necessary. Prednisone is less expensive than hydrocortisone but often requires the concurrent use of fludrocortisone for mineralocorticoid replacement. The need for mineralocorticoid therapy can be monitored via electrolytes and postural blood pressure measurements. Plasma renin activity levels can also be used, since they are elevated if mineralocorticoid replacement is insufficient. Patients should be given the minimum amount of glucocorticoid and mineralocorticoid required to prevent symptoms and maintain normal electrolyte and blood pressure status. Care must be taken to ensure that the patient is indeed on the minimum required dosage, since even small excesses of glucocorticoid therapy can cause osteoporosis and metabolic complications such as hyperglycemia (see the discussion on iatrogenic Cushing's syndrome in this chapter). Excess mineralocorticoid therapy can cause hypertension and hypokalemia.

## Principles of glucocorticoid use and withdrawal

Use the smallest dosage of glucocorticoid for the shortest time possible.
Use shorter acting agents (prednisone, cortisol) given as early in the day as possible and avoid twice daily administration.
Use alternate day therapy when possible (if underlying condition is responsive to this regimen).
Educate the patient as to the appropriate response to major medical stress for 1 year following exogenous glucocorticoid replacement.
To begin to taper, change to the shortest acting agent administered once daily early in the day.
Taper dosage further and switch to alternate day therapy as tolerated by the underlying disease.

In secondary or tertiary adrenal insufficiency, only glucocorticoid replacement is required, unless any concurrent deficiencies of the other pituitary hormones are present.

Patients with adrenal insufficiency should wear some form of easily visible identification stating their diagnosis and therapy. They also must be instructed to increase their medication dosage if any significant illness occurs. Medication should be doubled for illnesses associated with vomiting and/or diarrhea. For milder febrile illnesses dosages should be increased somewhat less. Major medical stresses such as trauma or a surgical procedure require parenteral therapy. For surgery 100 mg of hydrocortisone should be given 8 hours preoperatively and repeated at 1 hour preoperatively. Hydrocortisone should also be added as a continuous infusion to the intravenous fluids at 5 mg/hour during the surgical procedure. A total of 150 to 200 mg should be given in the first 24 hours, with tapering of dosage by 50% per day assuming continued uneventful recovery.

### Management of glucocorticoid withdrawal

Sudden cessation of therapy following at least 3 weeks of supraphysiologic doses of glucocorticoids can precipitate acute adrenal insufficiency (see Table 35-1). Guidelines to prevent adrenal crisis during withdrawal from therapy are outlined in the box above. Changing therapy to shorter acting agents and using alternate day therapy are features that allow HPA axis recovery. The rate of taper of a pharmacologic glucocorticoid dosage depends primarily on the underlying nonendocrine disorder for which the medication is being used. As noted, there may be significant adrenal suppression for up to 1 year after discontinuation of steroids. Major stresses, including surgery, require stress dose steroid therapy (see above and Chapter 5). If patients have symptoms of adrenal insufficiency on withdrawal of steroids, it may be reasonable to perform a Cortrosyn stimulation test to assess adrenal responsiveness.

## ADRENOCORTICAL HYPERFUNCTION (CUSHING'S SYNDROME)

### Pathophysiology

Cushing's syndrome is a constellation of symptoms, signs, and biochemical abnormalities that result from prolonged exposure to excess levels of glucocorticoids. The principal glucocorticoid, cortisol, has primarily catabolic effects in most tissues. Collagen production is impaired, which reduces the tensile strength of dermal structures, including blood vessels, resulting in spontaneous ecchymoses, purple striae, and poor wound healing. Cortisol excess can also result in diffuse fine body hair growth, known as lanugo hair. Muscle wasting and weakness occur due to generalized protein catabolism. Catabolic effects on bone are also seen, since cortisol decreases intestinal calcium absorption, which in turn results in increased bone reabsorption and hypercalciuria, progressing to osteoporosis. Hyperglycemia results from the direct antiinsulin effect of cortisol and a cortisol-mediated increase in hepatic gluconeogenesis and glycogenolysis. Impaired immune and inflammatory response is seen due to a variety of immunologic effects, including impairment of polymorphonuclear cell phagocytosis, depletion of T lymphocytes, monocytes, and eosinophils, and decreased antibody formation. Cell-mediated immune response, vascular permeability, and histamine release are also impaired. The clinical result is an increased susceptibility to bacterial and fungal infections, most commonly with opportunistic organisms such as *Pneumocystis carinii, Aspergillus, Nocardia,* and *Cryptococcus.* Hypertension is also seen due to the permissive effect of cortisol on catecholamine activity and its positive inotropic effects on the heart. The increased catecholamine also has lipolytic effects, as does excess cortisol. This appears to affect adipocytes differentially. In the extremities fat wasting occurs, while fat deposition is increased centrally in the face, neck, and trunk, resulting in the typical Cushing's features of centripetal obesity, moon facies, and buffalo hump.

Clinical manifestations of androgen or mineralocorticoid excess may also be present, depending on the etiology of the syndrome. In the ACTH-dependent forms of Cushing's syndrome, in which excess pituitary or ectopic ACTH production is the primary pathologic feature, signs of androgen excess occur due to stimulation of adrenal production of both classes of hormone by the excess ACTH. Androgen excess is clinically apparent only in women, resulting in coarse terminal hair growth in androgen-sensitive areas, such as the face, chest, and upper back. Acne, oligomenorrhea, temporal balding, and deepening of the voice may also occur. In the ACTH-independent forms of Cushing's syndrome primary overproduction of cortisol results in suppression of ACTH production, which in turn reduces adrenal androgen production, so that features of androgen excess do not occur.

Cushing's syndrome is also associated with accelerated atherosclerosis. In the years before effective treatment evolved, patients with Cushing's syndrome commonly experienced early death from myocardial infarction or stroke. Vascular endothelial cell damage and elevated serum lipid levels due to cortisol excess are thought to be the pathogenic factors.

**Table 35-2.** Cushing's syndrome: etiology and differential diagnosis

| Type | Frequency | Unique features |
|---|---|---|
| Iatrogenic | Common | Absence of signs of androgen excess due to suppression of adrenal androgen production |
| Pituitary (Cushing's disease) | 60% | Signs of androgen excess present; pituitary tumor; suppresses with high-dose dexamethasone testing |
| Adrenal neoplasms | 30% | |
| Adenoma | ~30% | Absence of signs of androgen excess; no suppression with high-dose dexamethasone testing |
| Carcinoma | Rare | May or may not have features of androgen excess; 50% metastatic at diagnosis; no suppression on testing |
| Bilateral nodular hyperplasia | Uncommon | Features of androgen excess present; suppression with high-dose dexamethasone testing; may be Cushing's disease without visible pituitary lesion |
| Ectopic ACTH syndrome | 10% | Most common tumors associated with this are small cell carcinoma of lung, pancreatic carcinoma, bronchial adenoma, thymoma; features of androgen excess may be present; lack of suppression to high-dose dexamethasone |
| Alcoholic pseudo-Cushing's syndrome | Common | Endogenous cortisol overproduction; hypogonadism also present due to direct gonadotoxic effects of alcohol |

### Clinical features of Cushing's syndrome

**Nonspecific features**

Generalized obesity
Hypertension
Abnormal glucose tolerance
Amenorrhea or impotence
Hirsutism

**Specific features**

Central obesity
Ecchymoses
Pigmented striae (>1 cm)
Osteopenia
Muscle weakness
Spontaneous hypokalemia
Erythrocytosis

**Features unique to iatrogenic Cushing's syndrome**

Aseptic necrosis of femoral and humeral heads
Glaucoma
Cataracts
Benign intracranial hypertension
Pancreatitis

Endogenous (noniatrogenic) Cushing's syndrome is a serious disorder with a 5-year mortality of 50% if left untreated. The majority of deaths are due to infection, cardiovascular disease, and suicide.

## History and physical findings

Many of the features of Cushing's syndrome are seen with high frequency in the general population, as shown in the box above. In particular, the triad of obesity, hypertension, and glucose intolerance or diabetes is commonly encountered in an outpatient general medical practice. Alternately, among patients with documented Cushing's syndrome, the presentation is often nonspecific, and typical clinical features may be absent. For example, among patients with pituitary Cushing's syndrome the prevalence of symptoms is obesity 79%, hypertension 77%, easy bruisability 77%, hirsutism 64%, proximal muscle weakness 48%, psychiatric disturbances 48%, abnormal glucose tolerance 39%, clinical diabetes 13%, and hypokalemia 24%. Psychiatric symptoms most frequently include affective changes (mania, depression) but may also present as toxic psychoses, often with paranoia. Symptoms are typically dose-related, although they occasionally follow use of low-dose steroids. Onset is usually within 5 days of starting glucocorticoid therapy, often in the setting of prior psychiatric problems. Resolution is typically within 1 week of discontinuation of glucocorticoids.

Rapid or subacute onset of obesity, hypertension, or other features of Cushing's syndrome is one clue that there is an underlying pathologic process that merits investigation.

## Etiology/differential diagnosis

The differential diagnosis for Cushing's syndrome and the features unique to each type of the syndrome are outlined in Table 35-2.

*Iatrogenic Cushing's syndrome.* This is the most common type seen clinically. Any prolonged use of glucocorticoid at dosages above replacement (see Table 35-1) can result in the adverse metabolic effects and/or clinical features of Cushing's syndrome. Osteoporosis can be a serious problem, with an incidence of 30% to 50% among those treated chronically with glucocorticoids. Reductions in trabecular bone density have been measured after as little as 8 mg of prednisone daily for 4 months. At prednisone dosages of over 10 mg daily for at least 2 months, an increased prevalence of infection is seen. Atherosclerotic disease may also be increased. Several pathologic features of iatrogenic Cushing's syndrome are unique to exogenous glucocorticoid use and are not seen in other types of the syndrome. These include aseptic necrosis of the femoral or humeral heads (which can occasionally occur even with short-term steroid therapy), glaucoma, cataracts, benign intracranial hypertension, and pancreatitis. Signs of androgen excess are not a feature, since exogenous glucocorticoids cause HPA suppression, resulting in decreased ACTH-mediated adrenal androgen production.

*Pituitary Cushing's syndrome (Cushing's disease).* Pituitary Cushing's syndrome accounts for approximately 60% of cases of endogenous hypercortisolism. This is due to an ACTH-secreting pituitary adenoma. These adenomas are often small, resulting in sella turcica enlargement in only 10% of cases. Signs of androgen excess are often present in this disorder due to ACTH-mediated adrenal overproduction of androgen precursors. The HPA appears to be intact but has an abnormally high set point of ACTH feedback regulation. Thus circulating cortisol production can be suppressed with high-dose dexamethasone testing but not with low-dose or overnight testing.

*Ectopic ACTH syndrome.* Ectopic ACTH syndrome accounts for about 10% of endogenous hypercortisolism. The source of ectopic ACTH production is a thoracic tumor in 79% of patients. The most common thoracic tumors are small-cell carcinoma of the lung, bronchial carcinoid, and thymoma. Extrathoracic tumors such as pancreatic carcinoma can also produce ACTH. Both bronchial carcinoid and thymoma are usually benign tumors with a clinical course typical of Cushing's syndrome. The malignant tumors resulting in this syndrome often have a poor prognosis, and patients seldom live long enough to manifest the typical Cushing's stigmata. Metabolic features, such as severe hypokalemia, may predominate. Hyperpigmentation, leg edema, and weight loss may also be predominant features. These tumors are autonomously functioning; thus cortisol and ACTH production are not suppressed following the administration of high doses of the glucocorticoid dexamethasone. Symptomatic treatment may improve quality of life or prolong life and should be pursued.

*Adrenal neoplasms.* Adrenal tumors account for about 30% of cases of endogenous Cushing's syndrome. The majority of these are benign adenomas, which are autonomously functioning and secrete primarily cortisol. Excess cortisol suppresses pituitary production of ACTH; thus, clinically, signs of cortisol excess without androgen excess predominate. These tumors are autonomous and do not decrease cortisol production in response to dexamethasone.

Bilateral nodular adrenal hyperplasia is a poorly understood entity. It is characterized by autonomous cortisol overproduction, but production can be suppressed with high doses of dexamethasone. This may represent a variant of Cushing's disease in which a pituitary adenoma is not visible, since ACTH levels are often elevated.

Adrenal carcinomas are rare, accounting for only 0.2% of cancer deaths in the United States per year. The mean age of presentation is 46 years, with a female/male ratio of 2.5:1. In those cases with hormonal overproduction the majority present with clinical features of Cushing's syndrome. In one series 30% presented with pure glucocorticoid excess, 27% had combined glucocorticoid and androgen excess, 8% had androgen excess alone, 2% had mineralocorticoid excess, 1% had estrogen excess, and the remainder had no hormone overproduction. At diagnosis 50% had regional or distant metastases. Median survival was 21 months.

*Alcoholic pseudo-Cushing's syndrome.* Chronic alcoholism may have many of the stigmata of Cushing's syndrome. Cortisol dynamics are abnormal and cortisol overproduction can be documented. Following abstinence the cortisol dynamics usually return to normal within 3 to 7 days.

### Diagnostic tests

An algorithm that outlines a diagnostic approach to Cushing's syndrome is outlined in Fig. 35-2. The initial step is to perform a screening test to confirm the presence of Cushing's syndrome.

*Hormonal tests.* The overnight dexamethasone (dex) suppression test is the most widely used screen for this disorder. It involves the oral administration of 1 mg of dexamethasone at 11 PM with measurement of plasma cortisol at 8 AM the following day. The normal cortisol response is suppression to less than 5 mg/dl. Obesity, stress, psychiatric disease (especially depression), and medications that increase hepatic metabolism of cortisol and dexamethasone, such as antiseizure medications, estrogen, and rifampin, can falsely elevate the results of this test. If any of these conditions are present, the overnight dexa test should not be performed, and either of the following two tests should be used as the initial screening maneuver (these tests are also used to confirm the diagnosis when the overnight dexa test is positive): (1) the 24-hour urinary free cortisol test is a measurement of unbound, biologically available cortisol; (2) the low-dose dexamethasone suppression test is done by administering 0.5 mg of dexamethasone orally every 6 hours for 2 days. A serum cortisol measured at 8 AM after 48 hours of dexamethasone administration should be suppressed to less than 5 mg/dl. The serum cortisol at 48 hours is easier to perform and appears to have similar diagnostic accuracy to the previously used 24-hour urinary 17-hydroxycorticosteroid levels (measured during the second day of the test).

If Cushing's syndrome is confirmed by one of these tests, further testing is pursued to differentiate among the types of the syndrome. The high-dose dexamethasone suppression test in conjunction with an ACTH level is the first step. The classic high-dose dexa test involves oral administration of 2 mg dexamethasone four times daily for 2 days. Urinary metabolites are measured during day 2. An adequate substitute that obviates the need for urine collection appears to be the administration of a single 8-mg dose of dexamethasone given at 11 PM following a baseline 8 AM cortisol measurement (this is also referred to as a high-dose dexa test). The cortisol is then repeated the following morning. Lack of suppression of the cortisol level, in conjunction with an undetectable to low ACTH

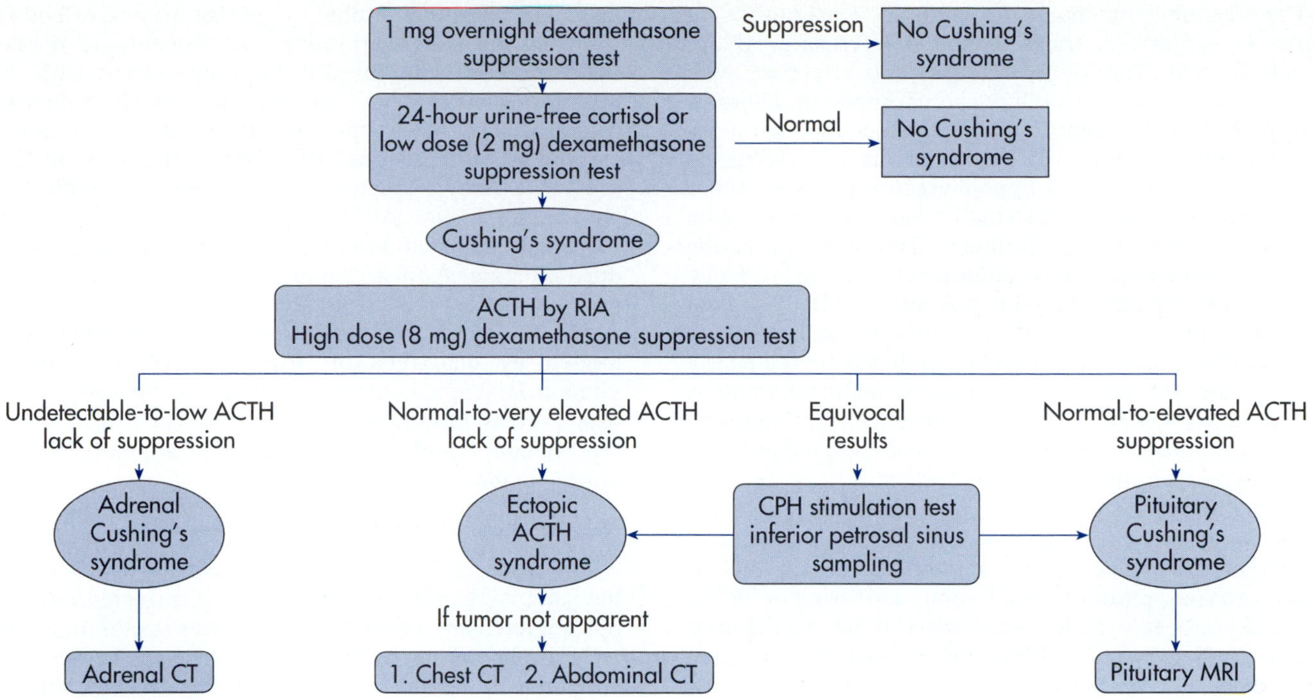


**Fig. 35-2.** Diagnostic algorithm for Cushing's syndrome. (From Kaye, TB, Crapo L: *Ann Intern Med* 112:434, 1990.)

level, is diagnostic of adrenal Cushing's syndrome. Suppression to 50% or less of the baseline cortisol level with normal to elevated ACTH is diagnostic of pituitary Cushing's syndrome. Lack of suppression of cortisol in conjunction with a normal to elevated ACTH suggests the ectoptic ACTH syndrome. If results are equivocal, further testing by use of the CRH stimulation test or inferior petrosal sinus sampling must be performed.

The CRH test involves the administration of a single injection of 100 μg ovine CRH with measurement of ACTH and cortisol before injection and at 15, 30, 60, 90, and 120 minutes following injection. In pituitary Cushing's syndrome an exaggerated increase in plasma ACTH and cortisol levels is seen, whereas in the ectopic and adrenal forms ACTH and cortisol levels remain flat. Although this test can be used instead of the high-dose dexa test to differentiate among the causes of Cushing's syndrome, it is more expensive and therefore may be best suited to problematic cases in which the high-dose dexa test with radiographic studies has failed to distinguish between ectopic and pituitary Cushing's syndrome.

Inferior petrosal sinus sampling is another diagnostic maneuver reserved for this purpose. ACTH levels are measured from blood drawn directly from the petrosal sinuses, which receive the venous drainage from the pituitary. A central/peripheral ACTH ratio of 2:1 or greater indicates a pituitary source of ACTH hypersecretion. A ratio of 1.5:1 or less supports an ectopic cause. If a pituitary source is evident from petrosal sinus sampling, levels may also help to indicate whether it is located on the right or left side of the pituitary.

***Radiologic studies.*** These are performed after localization of the site of excess cortisol production. It is critical that imaging studies be deferred until hormonal studies have been completed, since incidental adrenal or pituitary adenomas are common, occurring in 1% to 8% of normal individuals. If hormonal studies indicate an adrenal source of cortisol overproduction, abdominal CT scanning is performed. CT scanning of the adrenal has a sensitivity of 100%, detecting virtually all adrenal tumors over 1.5 cm in diameter. MRI offers no advantage over CT scan in this setting. Adrenal scintigraphy with $^{131}I$ β-iodomethylnorcholesterol may be helpful in localizing adenomas not seen by CT scan.

If hormonal studies indicate that cortisol overproduction is localized to the pituitary, MRI has higher sensitivity for pituitary imaging than CT scan and should be the diagnostic study of choice. When gadolinium contrast is used, sensitivity of pituitary MRI is approximately 80%.

### Treatment

The treatment of iatrogenic Cushing's syndrome once it has occurred, is to taper the dosage of glucocorticoid as tolerated by the underlying disease. Some of the metabolic effects of excess glucocorticoid use, such as the loss of bone mass, are not reversible. Thus prevention by minimizing dosage and duration of glucocorticoid therapy is critical. Principles of glucocorticoid use and withdrawal are outlined in the box on p. 522. Use of the shortest acting preparation for the shortest time possible is a key feature. Additionally, to minimize bone loss, calcium and vitamin D supplementation should be given to those in whom glucocorticoid use is expected to exceed 1 month. Calcium intake from all sources should total at least 1000 mg per day, and vitamin D, 400 IU per day, should also be administered. For women who are estrogen deficient due to menopause, other disorders, or the effects of the glucocorticoid therapy, estrogen therapy should be strongly considered.

The treatment of choice for pituitary Cushing's syndrome is surgery. A transsphenoidal microsurgical approach is used. The surgery is safe and effective, with tumor localization and removal occurring in approximately 90% of patients without subsequent pituitary hypofunction in most. If no adenoma is visible at operation, total or partial hypophysectomy is sometimes recommended, because very small tumors can be found on careful sectioning of the pituitary. Tumor lateralization with inferior petrosal sinus sampling can be used to guide hemihypophysectomy if no tumor is seen on MRI. Surgical cure rates are high, and surgical morbidity and mortality are low. The success of this technique has rendered nearly obsolete the use of subtotal bilateral adrenalectomy, a procedure associated with high recurrence rates and with Nelson's syndrome, which consists of hyperpigmentation due to excess pituitary ACTH secretion.

Irradiation is also used for pituitary Cushing's syndrome, most often for patients who fail transsphenoidal surgery or for patients with very mild disease. Conventional external pituitary irradiation delivering 4500 to 5000 rad has been used for many years. It may be the most successful therapy for children, but response to it is often inadequate and can be delayed for as long as 6 months. Proton beam therapy is more effective than conventional therapy, since it delivers more irradiation to the pituitary. However, it is available at only a few medical centers. Stereotactic external $\gamma$-irradiation, or the gamma knife, is another promising treatment, but it is expensive and currently available at only a few sites in the United States. Irradiation is associated with a much higher incidence of subsequent pituitary hypofunction than microsurgery, occurring in up to 20% following proton beam therapy.

For Cushing's syndrome due to adrenal adenoma surgical resection is the treatment of choice and is usually curative. Surgery may have to be delayed for a few months while medical adrenolytic agents (see below) are administered to avoid problems with poor wound healing or with metabolic derangement. Surgical resection after medical preparation is also used for adrenal carcinoma, even if metastases are documented preoperatively. If metastatic disease is present, postoperative medical therapy is usually necessary on an indefinite basis to control symptoms and metabolic manifestations. Similarly, the hypercortisolism of ectopic ACTH syndrome is usually controlled with medical therapy, even if the ACTH-secreting malignancy confers a poor prognosis. Medical therapy can substantially improve the quality of life in terminally ill patients by ameliorating the myopathy, hypokalemia, and catabolism of Cushing's syndrome.

Options for medical therapy of Cushing's syndrome include mitotane, an adrenolytic agent that directly lowers corticosteroid production. The starting dosage is 2 to 6 g per day, and 4 to 6 months of therapy may be required before a clinical effect is seen. Side effects may include gastrointestinal disturbances, lethargy, somnolence, and dizziness. Aminoglutethamide is a more rapidly acting adrenolytic agent that blocks the conversion of cholesterol to pregnenolone, a cortisol precursor. This is extremely effective for the rapid reduction of cortisol overproduction. Metyrapone, another effective drug sometimes used in conjunction with aminoglutethamide, is an adrenocortical enzyme (11-$\beta$-hydroxylase) inhibitor that interferes with cortisol synthesis. Trilostane (Modrenal), ketoconazole, and suramin are other drugs that may be effective in lowering cortisol overproduction. Physiologic doses of hydrocortisone must usually be administered with these drugs to avoid adrenal insufficiency. In Cushing's syndrome caused by ectopic ACTH production or adrenal carcinoma, mifepristone (RU 486) is effective. In Cushing's disease cyproheptadine, an antiseratoninergic agent, has been shown to induce clinical and biochemical remission in a small number of patients. Bromocriptine, a dopaminergic agonist, has also produced temporary remission in Cushing's disease.

Finally, alcoholic pseudo-Cushing's syndrome is best treated by detoxification from alcohol. Calcium and vitamin D supplementation should also be considered as osteoporosis prophylaxis in all alcoholics, and estrogen replacement should be considered in amenorrheic alcoholic women.

## MINERALOCORTICOIDS

Aldosterone is the major mineralocorticoid produced by the adrenal gland. Its production is affected primarily by angiotensin II and extracellular potassium, with ACTH playing a small role as well (see Fig. 35-1). Angiotensin II, the predominant factor controlling aldosterone secretion, is in turn responsive to renin, which is secreted by the renal juxtaglomerular apparatus in response to low renal perfusion pressure and low extracellular sodium concentration. Renin stimulates hepatic conversion of angiotensinogen to angiotensin I, which is in turn converted in the lungs to angiotensin II. Stimulation of this axis results in increased aldosterone production, resulting in distal tubular sodium retention and in renal potassium excretion. Aldosterone is metabolized in the liver to tetrahydroaldosterone, which in turn undergoes renal metabolism to aldosterone-18-glucuronide; both of these metabolites can be measured to screen for aldosterone excess. Disorders of aldosterone may result from excess production, as in primary hyperaldosteronism, or inadequate production, as in hypoaldosteronism.

### Primary hyperaldosteronism

***Pathophysiology.*** Estimates of the incidence of primary hyperaldosteronism in the hypertensive population of the United States vary from 0.05% to 2%. Excess mineralocorticoid results in hypokalemia, metabolic alkalosis, and sodium retention. Sodium retention in turn leads to volume expansion and hypertension. Hypokalemia and sodium retention occur because aldosterone acts on the cortical collecting tubules within the kidney to retain sodium and increase potassium excretion. The mechanism is increased aldosterone-mediated synthesis of sodium-potassium-ATPase, which in turn increases the activity of the sodium-potassium pump that draws sodium into the tubular cells and secretes potassium into the lumen. Excess secretion of hydrogen ion into the tubular lumen, resulting in metabolic alkalosis, occurs in the renal medullary collecting tubules under aldosterone's influence as well. Renin and angiotensin II levels are both suppressed due to primary overproduction of aldosterone.

***History and physical findings.*** This disorder presents between the third and fifth decades and is more common in women. The hypertension is clinically indistinguishable from essential hypertension in most cases, since most patients with this disorder are asymptomatic. When symptoms occur, the most commonly reported are headache, easy fatigability, and weakness. The most consistent and overt biochemical manifestation is hypokalemia, which results from renal potassium wastage. More than 50% of hypertensive patients with spontaneous hypokalemia are found to have primary aldosteronism; thus hypokalemia in the absence of diuretic therapy should prompt testing for aldosterone excess, even if the hypokalemia is mild (3.4 to 3.5 mEq/L). It should also be suspected in patients who become severely hypokalemic with the administration of diuretics and who remain so after diuretics are stopped. The hypokalemia causes no symptoms in a substantial proportion of patients. In others, nocturnal polyuria and polydypsia and neuromuscular manifestations such as weakness, paresthesias, intermittent paralysis, and frank tetany can occur. The degree of hypokalemia is related in part to sodium intake. Sodium restriction leads to potassium retention, whereas sodium excess promotes further renal potassium wastage. An additional biochemical feature is abnormal glucose tolerance with insulinopenia, which is demonstrable in over 50% of patients.

***Etiology and differential diagnosis.*** The causes of primary hyperaldosteronism and their frequencies are illustrated in the box below. An aldosterone-producing adenoma (APA) of the adrenal, also known as Conn's syndrome, is the most common cause. These adenomas are usually unilateral, more commonly on the left, and less than 2 cm in size. Although they secrete primarily aldosterone, they may produce some cortisol as well. Aldosterone excess is more pronounced than in other forms of primary hyperaldosteronism. Although plasma renin is completely suppressed by the excess aldosterone, synthesis of aldosterone is only partly autonomous, in that plasma levels still exhibit a circadian rhythm that parallels the plasma cortisol and ACTH levels. Idiopathic hyperaldosteronism (IHA) is due to bilateral nodular hyperplasia of the adrenal cortex. The histologically normal but hypertrophic adrenal glands found in this condition are thought to result from stimulation by an abnormal secretagogue or an amplifier of angiotensin II that has yet to be identified. Suppression of plasma renin may be only partial in this condition, and there is no parallel between cortisol and aldosterone levels. Rarely, primary hyperaldosteronism is due to production of aldosterone by an adrenal carcinoma. Another unusual etiology is glucocorticoid-suppressible hyperaldosteronism, a rare hereditary autosomal dominant trait in which there is ACTH-mediated hypersecretion of aldosterone and little or no regulation of aldosterone by angiotensin II.

Clinical distinctions among these entities are few, and testing must be performed to identify an etiology.

### Frequency of primary aldosteronism

APA (65%)
IHA (34%)
Aldosterone-producing carcinoma (<1%)
Glucocorticoid-suppressible hyperaldosteronism (<1%)

*APA,* Aldosterone-producing adenoma; *IHA,* idiopathic hyperaldosteronism.
Adapted from Melby JC: Clinical review 1: Endocrine hypertension, *J Clin Endo Metab* 69:697, 1989.

***Diagnostic tests.*** Screening for primary hyperaldosteronism can be performed in the outpatient setting. The box below outlines the appropriate screening tests and results. Patients must be off diuretics for at least 4 weeks, spironolactone for at least 6 weeks, and β-blockers for at least 1 week before screening. Hypertension can be controlled with prazosin during this time if diastolic blood pressures exceed 110 mm. Patients should be instructed to consume a normal sodium diet (which approximates 100 to 150 mEq NaCl per day) in the few days before testing. This can usually be accomplished by discontinuing any attempt at sodium restriction but avoiding overtly salty foods. A 24-hour urine collection for aldosterone (or tetrahydroaldosterone) can then be performed. Some authors advocate the captopril test as an initial screening maneuver. This involves the administration of 25 to 50 mg of captopril, an angiotensin-converting enzyme inhibitor that decreases renin-moderated aldosterone secretion in normal subjects. Plasma renin and aldosterone levels are measured 60 to 120 minutes later. This test is more costly, however, and is best reserved for situations in which 24-hour urine results are ambiguous. If screening test results are abnormal, the findings should be confirmed with a renin-aldosterone stimulation test (posture test). Starting at 7:30 AM the patient remains recumbent for 30 minutes. Plasma renin and aldosterone levels are drawn at 8 AM. The patient then remains upright for 4 hours, and the levels are repeated. Persistently suppressed plasma renin levels in conjunction with high 24-hour urinary aldosterone secretion confirm the diagnosis. An alternative to the posture test is the saline infusion test, in which plasma aldosterone is measured after administration of 2 L of saline over 4 hours.

Once a diagnosis of primary hyperaldosteronism is established, the cause must be determined (Fig. 35-3). The renin-aldosterone stimulation test (posture test) results can

### Laboratory features of tests confirming the diagnosis of primary hyperaldosteronism

Stimulated renin-aldosterone test (posture test)
  Suppressed upright renin (<1 ng/ml/hour)
  Plasma aldosterone (supine) at 8 AM (>15 ng/dl)
24-hour urinary aldosterone excretion
24-hour urinary aldosterone
  Normal salt diet (6-25 μg/hr, or 17-69 nmol/24 hr)
  High salt diet (0-6 μg/hr, or 0-17 nmol/24 hr)
  Low salt diet (17-44 μg/hr, or 47-122 nmol/24 hr)
24-hour urinary tetrahydroaldosterone (<65 μg/24 hr)
Saline infusion test—plasma aldosterone (>10 ng/dl)
Captopril test—plasma aldosterone (>15 ng/dl)

Adapted from Melby JC: Clinical review 1: Endocrine hypertension, *J Clin Endo Metab* 69:697, 1989.

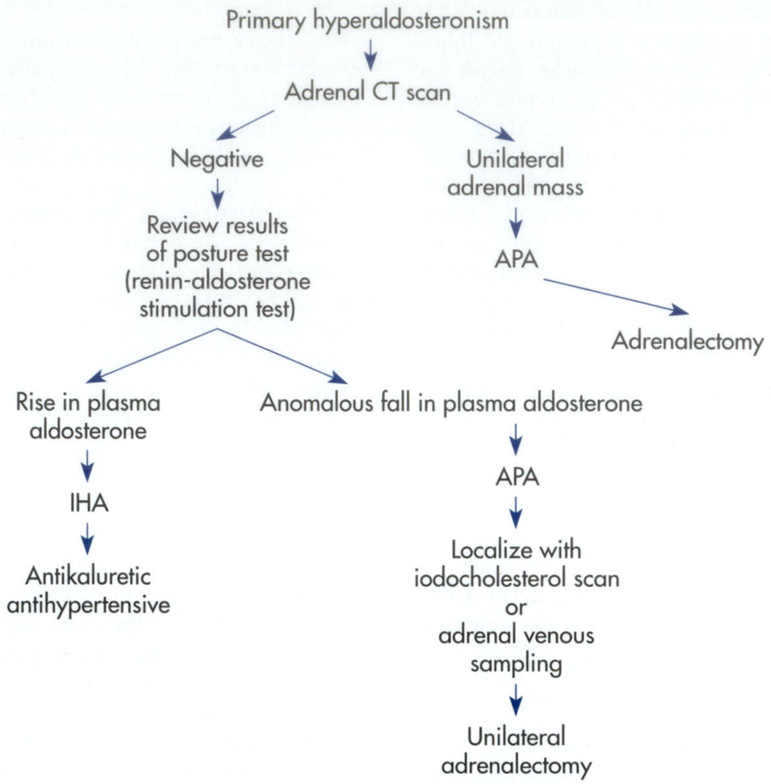


**Fig. 35-3.** Diagnostic approach to primary hyperaldosteronism. (Modified from Melby JC: *J Clin Endocrinol Metab* 69:697,1989.)

be helpful in differentiating IHA from APA in 90% of cases of confirmed primary hyperaldosteronism. Whereas patients with APA have a decline in aldosterone levels at 4 hours, patients with IHA experience a rise in levels.

Because of the small size of most adenomas, adrenal CT scan accuracy is only 65% to 75%. MRI appears to offer no advantage. A promising radiologic maneuver is adrenal scanning with iodocholesterol (NP-59). Patients are pretreated with dexamethasone to suppress normal adrenal functioning, and radioisotope is administered. Imaging is deferred for 5 days, since adrenal uptake and concentration of the isotope are maximal at that time. APA is manifested as lateralization of isotope to one adrenal gland. Accuracy may be as high as 90%, but false negative results have been reported, so this test has not supplanted adrenal venous sampling.

Bilateral adrenal venous sampling continues to be the most accurate test. Normal adrenal venous aldosterone concentration is from 100 to 400 ng/dl. In APA the ipsilateral adrenal venous aldosterone concentration is usually 1000 to 10,000 ng/dl, and the ratio of ipsilateral to contralateral aldosterone levels is usually greater than 10:1. Correct placement of the catheter in the adrenal vein is essential and can be verified by administration of ACTH with subsequent bilateral cortisol measurements. An aldosterone ratio greater than 10:1 in the presence of a symmetric ACTH-induced cortisol response is diagnostic of APA.

***Treatment.*** Surgery is the treatment of choice once APA is identified. Hypokalemia resolves permanently following surgery in all patients, but hypertension may persist. One year after surgery 70% of patients are normotensive, whereas only 50% remain so at 5 years. With IHA fewer than 30% of patients are cured by surgery, so this approach, which invariably results in permanent adrenal insufficiency, is not indicated. Potassium-sparing diuretics are quite effective in IHA. Normokalemia is restored with either amiloride or spironolactone, although additional antihypertensives may be required to control blood pressure. ACE inhibitors can also be quite effective for the control of hypokalemia and hypertension.

### Secondary hyperaldosteronism

This term describes renin-mediated aldosterone excess. This can occur in edematous states such as congestive heart failure (CHF) or cirrhosis, in which intravascular volume depletion stimulates the renin-angiotensin axis. It also can occur in association with hypertension, in disorders such as renal artery stenosis, malignant hypertension, and juxtaglomerular cell tumor. The box at right outlines the causes of secondary hyperaldosteronism. Hypokalemia may not be a prominent feature. Other unusual causes of secondary hyperaldosteronism include Bartter's syndrome. In this disorder chloride absorption is impaired in the ascending limb of the loop of Henle. Impaired chloride reabsorption in turn increases distal tubular delivery of sodium, resulting in increased sodium exchange for potassium in the distal tubule, with loss of potassium. This disorder can be mimicked by diuretic abuse or by chronic self-induced vomiting. Surreptitious vomiting can be recognized from a low urinary chloride level, and diuretics can be detected by a urine screen. Excess ingestion of true licorice, which contains sub-

### Causes of secondary hyperaldosteronism

**Secondary hyperaldosteronism with edema**
Nephrotic syndrome
Hepatic cirrhosis
Congestive heart failure
Severe malabsorption

**Secondary hyperaldosteronism with hypertension**
Renovascular hypertension
Malignant hypertension
Primary hyperreninism (juxtaglomerular cell tumor)

**Secondary hyperaldosteronism without hypertension or edema**
Bartter's syndrome

**Secondary hyperaldosteronism—miscellaneous**
Diuretics
Vasodilators (except prazosin)
Chronic self-induced vomiting
Excess licorice ingestion

### Causes of hypoaldosteronism

**Hyporeninemic hypoaldosteronism**
Diabetes mellitus
Hypertensive nephrosclerosis
β-Adrenergic blocking agents
Chronic volume expansion

**Hyperreninemic hypoaldosteronism**
Aldosterone enzyme defect
Heparin
Lead poisoning
ACE inhibitor
Severe illness

**Pseudohypoaldosteronism**
Chronic interstitial nephritis
Systemic lupus erythematosus
Amyloidosis
Primary mineralocorticoid resistance
Spironolactone

stances that have mineralocorticoid-like effects, can also cause a metabolic picture that mimics endogenous aldosterone excess.

### Disorders of mineralocorticoid deficiency

***Pathophysiology.*** In hypoaldosteronism there is a decrease in aldosterone-mediated synthesis of sodium-potassium ATPase in renal tubular cells, thus the activity of the renal tubular sodium-potassium pump is diminished. Hyperkalemia and sodium wasting are the result. The hyperkalemia can be severe, causing arrhythmias and even sudden death. The sodium wasting is more modest. Although decreased effective blood volume, mild hyponatremia, and postural hypotension may be present, there is often no clinical evidence of volume depletion. Metabolic acidosis may also be present due to decreased aldosterone-mediated renal tubular secretion of hydrogen ion.

***Etiology and clinical findings.*** The box at right outlines the etiologies of this syndrome, which can occur at several levels of the renin-angiotensin axis. Hyporeninemic hypoaldosteronism, also known as type IV renal tubular acidosis, is the most common of these disorders, usually presenting as unexplained hyperkalemia in a patient with diabetes, hypertension, and mild renal insufficiency, occurring spontaneously or with use of ACE inhibitors or administration of a potassium load. The production of renin by the renal juxtaglomerular apparatus is permanently diminished or absent, presumably due to local tissue damage.

Hyperreninemic hypoaldosteronism is seen when renin production by the kidney is intact and the defect is either in the action of angiotensin II or in aldosterone biosynthesis. The mechanism of action of the ACE inhibitors is to interfere with angiotensin II synthesis. Heparin and lead, on the other hand, induce hypoaldosteronism by interfering with aldosterone synthesis at the level of the adrenal gland.

Pseudohypoaldosteronism is characterized by renal resistance to aldosterone, despite high aldosterone and renin levels. The pharmacologic antagonist spironolactone has this effect by interfering with the effect of aldosterone at the receptor level. Less commonly it is caused by a renal resistance to aldosterone seen in association with interstitial nephritis, systemic lupus erythematosus, or amyloidosis.

***Diagnosis and treatment.*** In most cases the clinical setting points to the diagnosis. The level of the defect can be confirmed, however, with the previously described renin-aldosterone stimulation test. Low stimulated renin and aldosterone levels point to a diagnosis of hyporeninemic hypoaldosteronism. Treatment consists of avoidance of potassium loads or inciting pharmacologic agents such as ACE inhibitors or potassium-sparing diuretics. A low-potassium diet with liberalization of sodium intake, potassium-wasting diuretics, or fludrocortisone 100 to 500 μg (0.01 to 0.05 mg) per day may be necessary in some patients. High stimulated renin and low aldosterone levels point to a defect at the level of the adrenal, and high stimulated renin and aldosterone levels point to end-organ refractoriness to aldosterone's effects. Treatment options are the same for these disorders as for hyporeninemic hypoaldosteronism, although treatment of pseudohypoaldosteronism may not be as effective due to renal insensitivity.

## ADRENAL MEDULLA

The adrenal medulla has a different embryologic origin from the adrenal cortex, being composed of chromaffin tissue derived from neural crest ectoderm. Its location next to the adrenal cortex appears to be critical to the synthesis of its major catecholamine—epinephrine. The enzyme critical to epinephrine formation is inducible by high levels of glucocorticoids, delivered from the cortex to the medulla by a rich blood supply. The adrenal medulla is the source of all epinephrine, whereas norepinephrine is produced by extraadrenal chromaffin cells.

## Pheochromocytoma

Pheochromocytoma is the most important disease of the adrenal medulla. It is a tumor of the chromaffin cells that is an uncommon but serious cause of hypertension, with an incidence of 0.1% to 0.4% among hypertensive patients. About 90% of pheochromocytomas are found in the adrenal medulla, and 10% are extraadrenal. In general, once spread occurs to outside the chromaffin tissue, the tumor is considered malignant. This occurs in fewer than 10% of the cases. Intraadrenal tumors are usually unilateral. In the 10% of the cases in which adrenal pheochromocytoma is bilateral, patients often are found to have polyglandular multiple endocrine neoplasia (MEN) type II. Most extraadrenal pheochromocytomas are intraabdominal and can be found anywhere along the sympathetic ganglion chain, which is also composed of chromaffin tissue.

***Pathophysiology.*** Excess production of catecholamines has a variety of physiologic effects. Catecholamines stimulate renal sodium retention by a direct tubular effect, by increased renin secretion, and by reduced intrarenal hydrostatic pressure. Shunting of blood toward the heart, increased cardiac inotropy, and increased peripheral resistance due to vasoconstriction are also consequences of catecholamine excess. Metabolic effects include hyperglycemia, hyperlipidemia, hypokalemia, and increased tissue oxygen consumption. Most of these effects occur due to increased β-receptor–mediated stimulation of adenyl cyclase in cell membranes, which results in increased conversion of ATP to cAMP. Hyperglycemia occurs due to catecholamine-mediated increases in glycogenolysis and gluconeogenesis. Catecholamines also diffusely inhibit gut motility.

***History and physical findings.*** Most patients have persistently elevated blood pressure with superimposed paroxysms of severe hypertension. Despite the hypertension, patients are usually orthostatic due to volume contraction. A minority of patients are normotensive between paroxysmal hypertensive episodes. Episodes are accompanied by headache, sweating, palpitations, anxiety, tremulousness, and nervousness lasting from 15 to 30 minutes. The symptom triad of headache, palpitations, and diaphoresis in association with hypertension has been found to have a high specificity (93.8%) and sensitivity (90.9%) for the diagnosis in hypertensive patients. The absence of hypertension in conjunction with this triad of symptoms excludes pheochromocytoma with a certainty of 99.9%. Other symptoms of pheochromocytoma may include dizziness, constipation, weight loss, flushing, and psychiatric symptoms. Laboratory findings may include hyperglycemia, hyperlipidemia, and hypokalemia.

***Diagnosis.*** Excess production of epinephrine and/or norepinephrine is best determined by measurement of their excreted metabolites. Normal urinary values for catecholamines are listed in Table 35-3. Care must be taken in determining who to screen for this disorder. Because of its low prevalence among hypertensives, even a highly specific screening test results in a significant numbers of false positives. Therefore screening should be performed only in those in whom clinical suspicion is truly high. In particular, it should be reserved for those with hypertension and the above-mentioned symptom triad of headache, palpitations, and sweating, or for those with a personal or family history of disorders suggestive of the MEN syndromes (see Chapter 39).

**Table 35-3.** Normal catecholamine values

| | Range |
|---|---|
| **Urine** | |
| Metanephrine | <1.3mg/24hr |
| VMA | 2-7mg/24hr |
| Epinephrine | 0-34 μg/24hr |
| Norepinephrine | 550 μg/24hr |
| **Plasma** | |
| Norepinephrine | 60-400 pg/ml |
| Epinephrine | 10-55 pg/ml |
| Dopamine | <100 pg/ml |

From Melby JC: Clinical review 1: Endocrine hypertension, *J Clin Endo Metab* 69:697, 1989.

The 24-hour urine collection must be performed carefully. Chlorpromazine, the benzodiazepines, α-methyldopa, and the β-blockers should be eliminated 2 weeks before testing. Ethanol, amphetamines, quinidine, theophylline, tetracycline, reserpine, clofibrate, and disulfiram can also interfere with the test results by raising or lowering catecholamine levels. If antihypertensive agents must be continued, diuretics or vasodilators such as hydralazine and minoxidil cause minimal interference. Levels of metanephrines, vanillylmandelic acid (VMA), and catecholamines should be measured. False negative rates for the metanephrine measurement have been estimated to be 4% to 21%. False negative rates for VMA are also high, up to 58% in one series. Prior VMA assays were subject to false positive results from dietary vanillin and phenolic acids, but this is less of a problem with contemporary assays. Total or fractionated urinary catecholamines using the high-performance liquid chromatography (HPLC) method may be the most sensitive and specific urinary test, with twofold elevations in over 95% of patients with pheochromocytoma. Urinary free norepinephrine was 100% sensitive and 98% specific for pheochromocytoma in one series. Mildly elevated values of all the catecholamine metabolites are common among hypertensives; only very high values are consistent with a diagnosis of pheochromocytoma. Plasma catecholamine measurements can also be used and may be as reliable as urinary measurements, but can be artifically elevated by stress, volume depletion, activity, anoxia, smoking, and medications; thus they must be performed under idealized conditions at complete bed rest. A clonidine suppression test can also be used when the diagnosis is uncertain and plasma norepinephrine levels are only modestly elevated (500 to 1000 pg/ml). Clonidine, 0.3 mg, is given and plasma norepinephrine levels are measured 3 hours later. Virtually all patients with essential hypertension suppress norepinephrine levels to

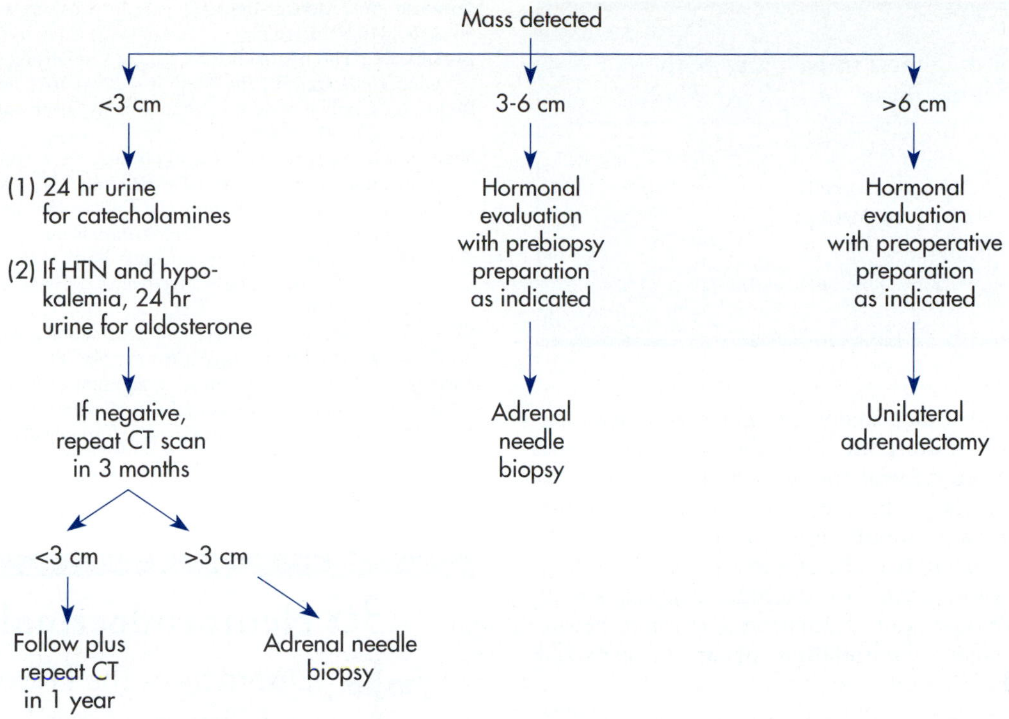


**Fig. 35-4.** Diagnostic approach to incidental adrenal mass. (Data from Ross NS, Aron DC: *N Engl J Med* 323:1401, 1990.)

below 500 pg/ml, whereas patients with pheochromocytoma do not.

Localization of pheochromocytoma after biochemical confirmation may be performed with adrenal CT scan or MRI. The latter may be superior in the detection of small tumors. Extraadrenal pheochromocytomas are harder to localize and may require $^{131}$I metaiodobenzylguanidine (MIBG) scanning. This isotope is specific for catecholamine-producing tissue and detects up to 95% of benign and 40% of malignant pheochromocytomas. Those who are found to have bilateral adrenal tumors should be screened for other manifestations of the MEN syndromes.

***Treatment.*** Surgical removal is the treatment of choice in most cases of benign and malignant pheochromocytoma. Medical treatment must be instituted at least a week before surgery to avoid intraoperative hypertensive crisis. Phenoxybenzamine is the drug of choice, starting at 10 mg twice daily and increasing as tolerated to 0.5 to 1 mg/kg/day until near normotension and control of symptoms are achieved. Prazosin may also be effective preoperatively; however, it does not control intraoperative hypertension well, so phenoxybenzamine must be used intraoperatively. Prazosin is started slowly at 1 mg three times a day to avoid postural hypotension and increased to 2 to 5 mg three times a day. After α-blockade has been achieved, β-blockers can be added if needed to control tachycardia, arrhythmias, or angina. β-blockers should never be administered before α-blockade because they can precipitate hypertensive crisis due to unopposed α-receptor stimulation. Calcium channel blockers have also been used successfully preoperatively and intraoperatively. During surgery volume expansion with blood or plasma is advocated to keep blood pressure normal, since intravascular volume contraction is the usual finding in untreated pheochromocytoma.

The same medications are used to manage the symptoms of malignant pheochromocytoma when complete surgical resection is not possible. An additional agent, α-methylparatyrosine, a catecholamine synthesis inhibitor, actually lowers serum catecholamine levels and can also be effective for these patients.

## INCIDENTAL ADRENAL MASS

The ability of abdominal CT scan or MRI performed for unrelated reasons to detect adrenal masses as small as 0.5 cm has resulted in a diagnostic dilemma. The prevalence of such incidentally discovered masses is 1% to 4% depending on the series. These small adrenal tumors are not new, having been previously reported at autopsy in 1.9% to 8.7% of patients without known endocrinopathy; what is new is our ability to detect them during life.

### Evaluation criteria

Once these lesions are detected, it must be decided whether a diagnostic evaluation is indicated (Fig. 35-4). Features that determine the need for evaluation include the size of the lesion and the coexistence of symptoms or disorders suggestive of hormonal overproduction. Although adrenal carcinoma is rare, lesions over 6 cm in size are significantly more likely to be adrenal carcinoma and

**Prevalence of diagnosis in patients with incidental adrenal mass***

Pheochromocytoma 6500
Aldosterone-producing adenoma 7000
Glucocorticoid-producing adenoma 35
Adrenal carcinoma 58

*Per 100,000 patients. Data from Ross NS, Aron DC: *N Engl J Med* 323:1401, 1990.

should be removed. Since many adrenal carcinomas are hormonally active, lesions this size should be evaluated biochemically before referral for surgery. Lesions of 3 to 6 cm are most likely to be metastatic disease from an unknown primary and should initiate an evaluation. If hormonal studies are unrevealing, adrenal needle biopsy may be necessary to make or exclude a diagnosis of malignancy. Hormonal studies must be performed before needle biopsy, since manipulation of an unsuspected pheochromocytoma is quite dangerous.

Lesions of less than 3 cm can be approached more conservatively. In the absence of a clinical picture suggestive of hormonal excess, a rational approach has been advocated in which screening is performed only for those disorders of highest prevalence. The box above illustrates the estimated prevalence of these disorders among patients with an incidentally discovered mass. These estimates assume that (1) all patients with these disorders have an adrenal mass, and (2) the population prevalence of incidental adrenal mass is 2%. For pheochromocytoma the absence of symptoms and of hypertension yields a negative predictive value of over 99% in patients with an adrenal mass. However, given the severity of pheochromocytomas and the fact that the likelihood of this tumor is substantially increased solely by the existence of a mass, screening is recommended for all patients with an incidental adrenal mass. For APA, screening should be limited only to persons who have hypertension and hypokalemia in addition to the adrenal mass. The absence of hypokalemia has been reported to have a negative predictive value of 95% in the diagnosis of APA in hypertensive persons with an adrenal mass. Routine screening for Cushing's syndrome in asymptomatic patients with adrenal mass is not indicated.

### Monitoring

Those who do not meet the criteria for further investigation should be followed clinically, with repeat CT scan or MRI in 3 months. Tumors evidencing growth to over 3 cm at 3 months should be surgically removed. Small lesions of less than 3 cm that are stable in size for 1 year in asymptomatic patients can be monitored infrequently.

## BIBLIOGRAPHY


Flack MR et al: Urinary free cortisol in the high dose dexamethasone suppression test for differential diagnosis of the Cushing syndrome, *Ann Intern Med* 116:211, 1992.

Greenspoon SK, Bilezikian JP: HIV disease and the endocrine system, *N Engl J Med* 327:1360, 1992.

Jeffcoate W: Alcohol-induced pseudo Cushing's syndrome, *Lancet* 341(8846):676, 1993.

Loriaux DL: The treatment of Cushing's syndrome and adrenal cancer, *Endocrinol Metab Clin North Am* 20(4):767, 1991.

Melby JC: Clinical review 1: Endocrine hypertension, *J Clin Endocrinol Metab* 69:697, 1989.

Nieman LK, Loriaux DL: Corticotrophin releasing hormone: clinical applications (review), *Ann Rev Med* 40:331, 1989.

Oelkers W, Diederich S, Bahr V: Diagnosis and therapy surveillance in Addison's disease, *J Clin Endocrinol Metab* 75:259, 1992.

Ross NS, Aron DC: Current concepts: hormonal evaluation of the patient with an incidentally discovered adrenal mass, *N Engl J Med* 323:1401, 1990.

Sheps SG et al: Recent developments in the diagnosis and treatment of pheochromocytoma, *Mayo Clin Proc* 65:88, 1990.

Snow K et al: BW: Biochemical evaluation of adrenal dysfunction: the laboratory perspective, *Mayo Clin Proc* 67(11):1055, 1992.

Young WF et al: Primary aldosteronism: diagnosis and treatment, *Mayo Clin Proc* 65:96, 1990.


CHAPTER

# 36 Neuroendocrinology

## Disorders of the Hypothalamus and Pituitary Gland

**Robert E. Burr**

Diseases of the hypothalamus, pituitary, and pineal gland are uncommon, occurring at an incidence of only a few per 100,000 individuals per year. Due to the rarity of these conditions and the rapidly advancing concepts of their management, endocrine consultation is usually indicated.

The hypothalamus and the pituitary are part of a complex physiologic (neuroendocrine) system that provides neural and hormonal regulation for a wide variety of physiologic functions (see the box at right). These glands, like all endocrine organs, do not function in isolation. They are part of classic feedback loop systems in which their responses to signals from the structures and tissues are regulated to maintain a stable level of activity. The hypothalamus and pituitary also respond to physiologic states, including, for example, core and skin temperature and plasma osmolarity as well as to an internal circadian clock that imparts a daily pattern to the rates of hypothalamic activity and endocrine secretion.

The most notable characteristic of these two structures is the extraordinary range of physiologic processes regulated by them and, consequently, the great range of clinical presentations for which their disorders can be responsible (see the box at far right).

## CLINICAL ANATOMY AND PHYSIOLOGY

The hypothalamus and pituitary are small organs located deep at the base of the brain closely invested by bone and neural and vascular structures (Fig. 36-1).

The opinions expressed in this chapter are the personal views of the author. They should not be construed as representing official policy of the Department of the Army or the Department of Defense.

## Major hormones of the pituitary gland

- Adrenocorticotropic hormone (ACTH)
  - Regulation:
    - Circadian
    - Stress
    - Cortisol level
  - Hypothalamic releasing factors:
    - Corticotropin-releasing hormone (CRH)
    - Vasopressin
  - Function:
    - Stimulates adrenal synthesis and release of cortisol
- Thyroid-stimulating hormone (TSH)
  - Regulation:
    - Thyroid hormone levels
  - Hypothalamic releasing factor:
    - Thyrotropin-releasing hormone (TRH)
  - Function:
    - Stimulates thyroid synthesis and release of thyroxine
- Follicle-stimulating hormone (FSH)
  - Regulation:
    - Sex steroid level
    - Inhibin
  - Hypothalamic releasing factor:
    - Gonadotropin-releasing hormone (GnRH)
  - Function:
    - Female: stimulates maturation of ovarian follicle
    - Male: stimulates maturation of seminal epithelium
- Luteinizing hormone (LH)
  - Regulation:
    - Sex steroid level
  - Hypothalamic releasing factor:
    - Gonadotropin-releasing hormone (GnRH)
  - Function:
    - Female: stimulates release of oocyte from ovarian follicle and development of corpus luteum
    - Male: testosterone synthesis and release by Leydig cells
- Growth hormone (GH)
  - Regulation:
    - Circadian
    - Stress
    - Fasting
    - Somatomedin C
  - Hypothalamic releasing factors:
    - Somatostatin
    - GH-releasing hormone (GHRH)
  - Function:
    - Stimulates somatomedin C production in hepatocytes
- Prolactin (PRL)
  - Regulation:
    - Estrogen
    - Breast stimulus
    - Stress
  - Hypothalamic releasing factor:
    - Dopamine (inhibits)
  - Function:
    - Stimulates milk synthesis and release

The hypothalamus controls eating and drinking behavior by regulating thirst and appetite. It controls thermal balance by efferent innervation of peripheral skin vasculature and thermoregulatory sweat glands. It controls heart rate and blood pressure through autonomic efferents. The hypothalamus directly secretes two neurohormones that influence peripheral structures: vasopressin (also called antidiuretic hormone, or ADH) and oxytocin. Finally, the hypothalamus secretes neurotransmitters and peptide neurohormones into the pituitary portal blood to regulate the secretion of the six major hormones of the pituitary gland.

## Clinical presentations of hypothalamic and pituitary disease

- Pituitary hormone excess
  - Gigantism and acromegaly
  - Cushing syndrome
  - Hyperthyroidism
  - Amenorrhea
  - Galactorrhea
  - Impotence
  - Infertility
  - Precocious male puberty
- Hypopituitarism
  - Hypothyroidism
  - Adrenal insufficiency
  - Short stature/growth failure
  - Amenorrhea
  - Impotence
  - Infertility
  - Delayed puberty
  - Diabetes insipidus
- Hypothalamic disease
  - Hypothalamic obesity
  - Frohlich syndrome (adiposogenital dystrophy)
  - Central hypothermia (Shapiro syndrome)
  - Central hyperthermia
  - Recurrent hyperthermia paroxysms
  - Diencephalic epilepsy
  - Diencephalic syndrome
- Local effects of pituitary and parasellar masses
  - Visual field defects
  - Diplopia and oculomotor palsies
  - Cavernous sinus thrombosis
  - Temporal lobe epilepsy
  - Cerebrospinal fluid rhinorrhea
  - Hydrocephalus

The pituitary gland is composed of heterogeneous endocrine cells attached during embryonic development to the anterior surface of the infundibular stalk. The major hormones of the pituitary gland are growth hormone (GH), prolactin (PRL), thyroid-stimulating hormone (TSH), adrenocorticotropic hormone (ACTH), follicle-stimulating hormone (FSH), and luteinizing hormone (LH).

The regulatory control of the hypothalamus over the pituitary gland is made possible by two portal vascular plexuses. Both of the portal systems have their first capillary network in close proximity to the neurosecretory cells and their second capillary network in the substance of the pituitary gland itself. For a summary of the relationship of the various hypothalamic regulators to pituitary secretion, the reader should refer to the box at left.

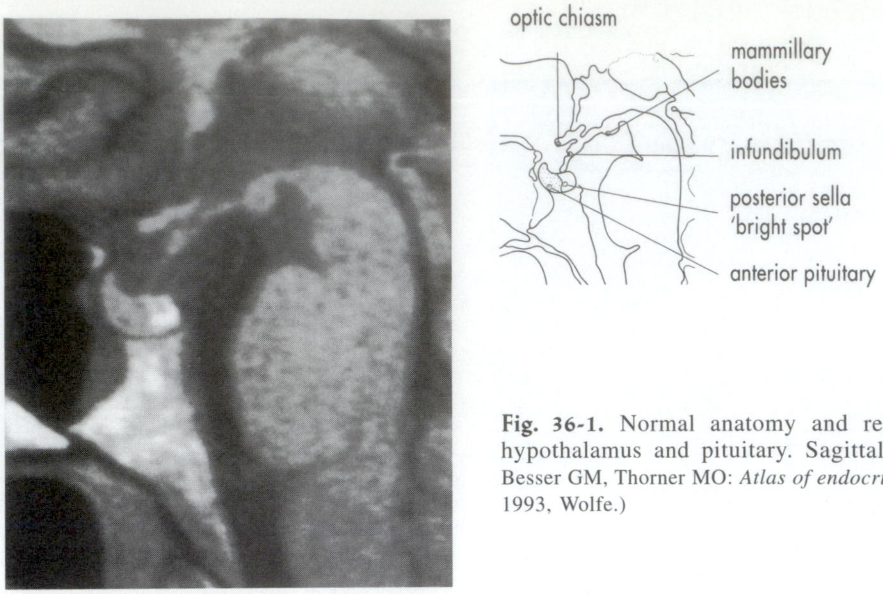


**Fig. 36-1.** Normal anatomy and relationships of the hypothalamus and pituitary. Sagittal view, left. (From Besser GM, Thorner MO: *Atlas of endocrine imaging,* London, 1993, Wolfe.)

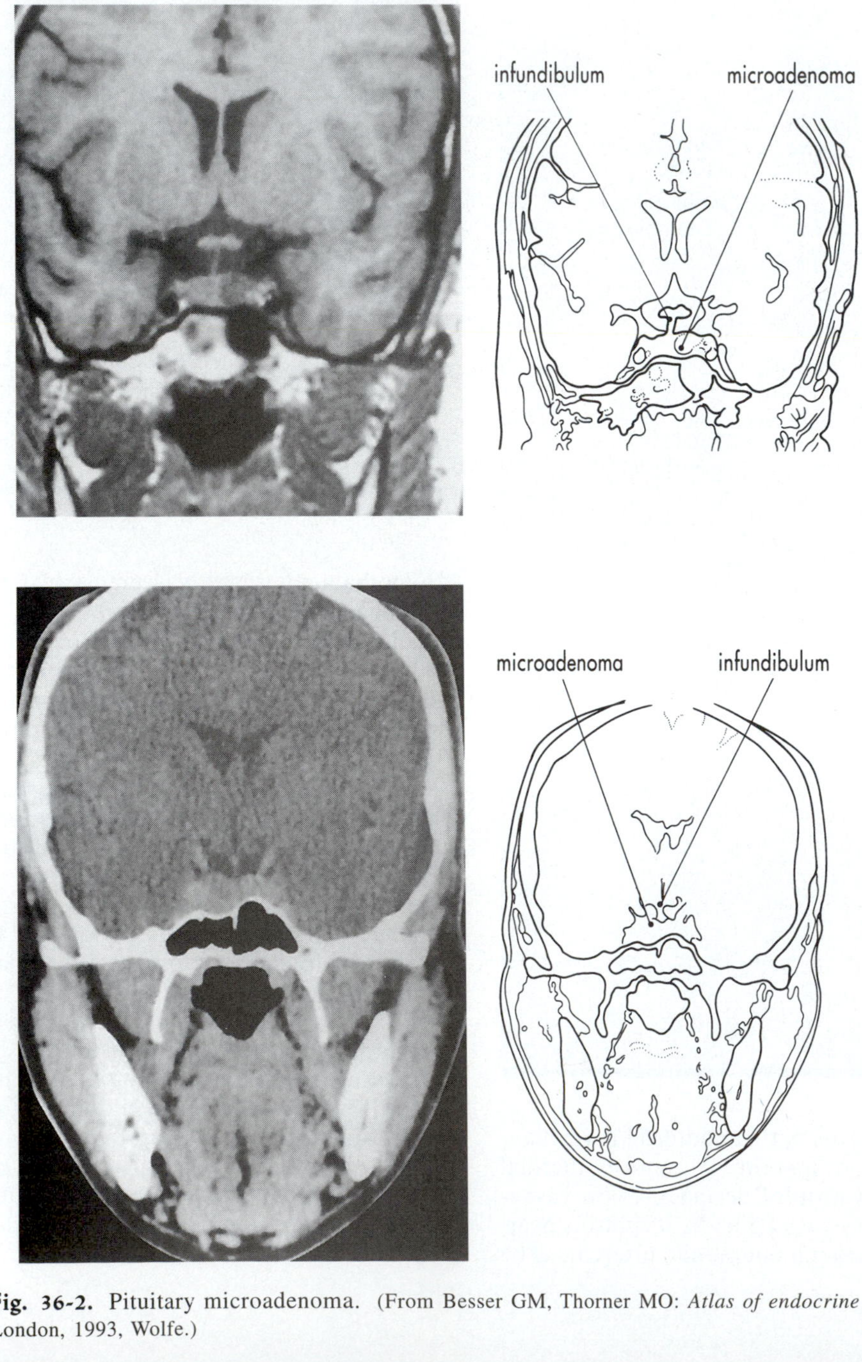


**Fig. 36-2.** Pituitary microadenoma. (From Besser GM, Thorner MO: *Atlas of endocrine imaging,* London, 1993, Wolfe.)

## PITUITARY AND HYPOTHALAMIC TUMORS

### Etiology and presentation

Pituitary tumors are the most common (about 15%) of all intracranial neoplasms. They can arise from any of the cells of the pituitary gland. Most clinically evident pituitary tumors (65%) retain the capacity to secrete pituitary hormones or hormone fragments, which produce a clinical syndrome of hormone excess. A few secrete multiple hormones; growth hormone and prolactin are the most frequent combination (7%). A portion of the pituitary tumors classified as silent produce measurable amounts of α-subunit hormone fragments, which can be used as a tumor marker. Silent tumors can be discovered because of mass effect or incidentally during CNS radiologic studies. Extrapituitary paraneoplastic syndromes can mimic pituitary tumors by the production of hypothalamic releasing hormones that stimulate pituitary secretion of the pituitary hormone itself.

Pituitary adenomas are classified as either microadenomas (under 10 mm in diameter) (Fig. 36-2) or macroadenomas (greater than or equal to 10 mm diameter) (Fig. 36-3). At presentation microadenomas have not usually affected extrasellar structures and are more susceptible to therapy than macroadenomas, which frequently grow beyond the confines of the sella. Enlargement of pituitary adenomas is either by expansion of a well-demarcated tumor or by local invasion. Invasive tumors are more difficult to cure and can cause death by invasion of local vital structures.

Many of the symptoms and signs of pituitary and parasellar tumors result from expansion and compromise of local structures. Tumor expansion superiorly can compress or invade the optic chiasm and produce visual field disturbances. The classic pattern is bilateral temporal field loss (homonymous hemianopsia). Precise visual field measurements are an important part of the assessment and

A

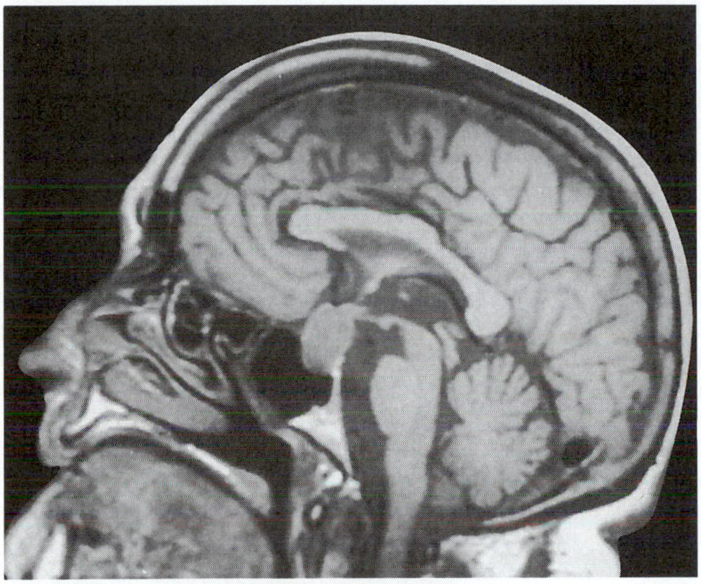

**Fig. 36-3.** Pituitary macroadenoma. **A,** Sagittal view: MRI and schematic. **B,** Coronal view, MRI. (From Besser GM, Thorner MO: *Atlas of endocrine imaging,* London, 1993, Wolfe.)

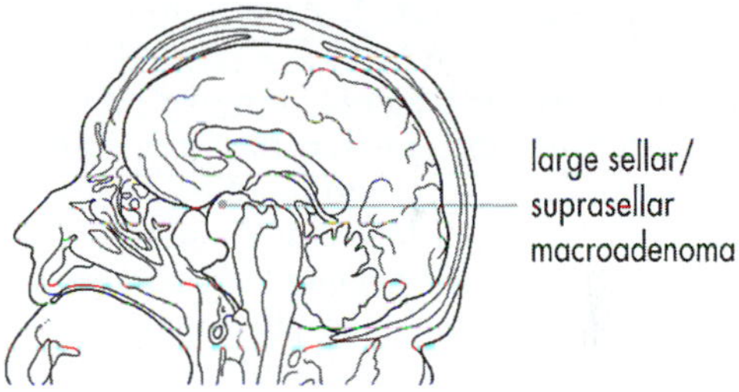


B

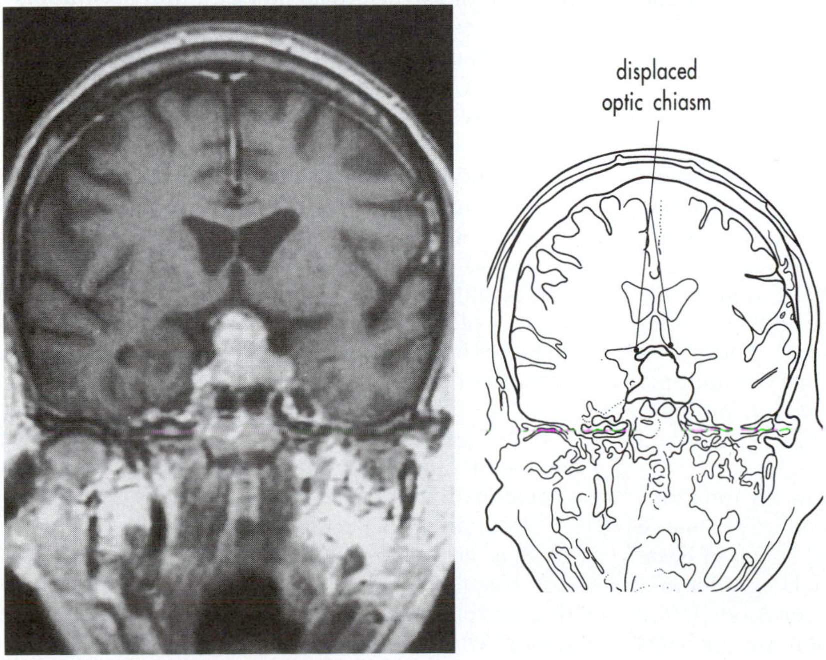

surveillance of pituitary and parasellar tumors. Encroachment on the hypothalamus can cause disturbance of the function of hypothalamic nuclei and interrupt cerebrospinal fluid (CSF) flow from the third ventricle by pressure on the walls of the sylvian aqueduct causing hydrocephalus, which is manifested as ataxia and decrements in cognitive function. Hypothalamic dysfunction is expressed by alterations in body weight, body water, thermoregulation, or other autonomic symptoms including pulse and blood pressure.

Tumor expansion laterally into the cavernous sinus has several consequences. First, if the tumor affects the intravascular portion of any of the three oculomotor nerves, diplopia develops. Second, if the tumor invades the parasellar vascular structures, it makes surgical cure less likely and increases the risk of intraoperative hemorrhage. Third, the tumor mass can cause thrombotic occlusion of the cavernous sinus. Lateral expansion beyond the cavernous sinus can impinge on the medial surface of the temporal lobes, causing temporal lobe epilepsy. Tumor expansion inferiorly, through the roof of the sphenoid sinus, manifests as CSF rhinorrhea.

In addition to pituitary tumors, neoplastic masses in the pituitary and parasellar region include teratomas, gliomas, meningiomas, pineal cell tumors, lymphoma, and leukemia. Nonneoplastic masses are common in the parasellar area, including arteriovenous (AV) malformations, aneurysms, cysts, and granulomas (primary or infectious).

Hypothalamic tumors are similar to those of the rest of the central nervous system. Dysgerminomas arising in the pineal gland frequently extend anteriorly to involve the hypothalamus. Hypothalamic tumors produce clinical disease by destroying nuclei that regulate autonomic functions or pituitary secretion and by destroying axonal tracts that pass through the hypothalamus.

Craniopharyngioma is a benign cystic suprasellar tumor considered to be a remnant of pharyngeal ectoderm from the embryonic union of the hypothalamus and pituitary. Craniopharyngiomas expand superiorly and compress the infundibulum, causing diabetes insipidus and hypopituitarism. Suprasellar calcification in a plain x-ray of the skull is characteristic of craniopharyngioma.

## Evaluation

The clinical evaluation of pituitary and parasellar tumors should include (1) evaluation of suspected endocrine dysfunction, (2) evaluation of pituitary and hypothalamic function, and (3) visualization of the hypothalamus and pituitary.

Specific endocrine syndromes should have appropriate evaluations for that syndrome (e.g., acromegaly, Cushing syndrome, hyperprolactinemia). In addition, family history and review of systems can point toward the multiple endocrine neoplasia syndrome type I in which pituitary tumors are associated with hyperparathyroidism and pancreatic islet cell tumors (see Chapter 39).

Baseline clinical assessment of other pituitary functions should be done for anyone with an adenoma larger than 6 mm. This evaluation should include measurement of basal levels of somatomedin C (as a measure of GH production), PRL, and thyroid, gonadal, and adrenal function. If the patient has polyuric symptoms, evaluation for diabetes insipidus should be done (see further). If the baseline measurements suggest abnormal pituitary function, then formal studies to characterize the degree of abnormal function should be performed.

Neuroophthalmologic evaluation is important to detect subtle visual abnormalities and to establish a baseline to assess visual symptoms that appear subsequently.

Magnetic resonance imaging (MRI) with gadolinium enhancement is the imaging technique of choice for pituitary and parasellar masses. Contrast-enhanced computed tomography (CT) scans, the second choice for visualizing the pituitary, can have specific advantages. For example, calcified lesions without mass effect (e.g., sarcoid and tuberculous granulomas) are seen only on CT.

If a parasellar mass is suspected to represent a vascular lesion such as aneurysm or AV malformation, angiography (including MRI angiography) is required to clarify the diagnosis and define the extent and anatomy of the lesion.

## Management

The management of a pituitary or parasellar mass depends on the specific etiology and the anticipated course of the lesion. The management of pituitary adenomas that cause a specific endocrine syndrome is discussed elsewhere.

Microadenomas found incidentally on radiologic examination of the cranium (pituitary "incidentalomas") require endocrinologic evaluation. The initial laboratory examination should depend on clinical findings, but might include evaluation of somatomedin C, PRL, urine free cortisol, TSH, and total thyroxine. If the microadenoma is not causing any systemic or local symptoms and is not interfering with pituitary function, it can be followed with periodic endocrine and radiologic evaluation. Initial reassessments should be done at intervals of several months. If no progression occurs after 2 or 3 years of regular observation, the interval between evaluations can be increased to 1 or 2 years.

Surgical resection should be considered for pituitary adenomas that cause local symptoms or endocrine dysfunction or are macroadenomas. Pituitary microadenomas usually can be approached transsphenoidally, which avoids many of the difficulties associated with intracranial surgery. Circumstances that favor the intracranial approach over the transsphenoidal are hyperostosis of the sphenoid sinus, significant suprasellar extension, and uncertainty about the nature of the intrasellar mass.

Radiation therapy is not used as primary therapy for pituitary adenomas. It is an adjunct to surgical therapy and is used to treat residual or recurrent tumor. Supervoltage teletherapy is the most commonly used modality. Stereotactic $\gamma$-radiation or beams of $\alpha$-particles or protons are effective but available only in a few centers. The effect of radiation therapy is slow to appear, often taking 5 to 10 years for full effect. Hypopituitarism is a common (90%) result of pituitary radiation therapy. Hypothalamic infarcts are another late complication of pituitary irradiation due to accelerated atherosclerosis.

Depending on the tissue type, up to 95% of microadenomas are cured surgically. Macroadenomas are cured less frequently (under 50%). Patients require postoperative surveillance for hypopituitarism and for recurrence of tumor. After pituitary resection, hypopituitarism should be assumed and appropriate adrenal and thyroid replacement therapy provided. After recovery from surgery, pituitary function can be assessed electively and endocrine replacement therapy discontinued if pituitary function is normal. Surveillance for recurrence should include clinical examination, measurement of hormonal markers, pituitary function, and radiologic assessment. The frequency of surveillance depends on the size and tissue type of the tumor and degree of surgical resection of the pituitary. Surveillance should be continued for at least 5 years in individuals who have not received and at least 10 years in patients who have received radiation therapy.

Craniopharyngiomas are treated surgically but are cured only about 50% of the time. Management of persistent craniopharyngioma is difficult. Diabetes insipidus and hypopituitarism are common complications of craniopharyngioma.

Other nonpituitary parasellar lesions are managed as appropriate to the specific diagnosis. Masses usually require a tissue diagnosis unless they are clearly associated with another already diagnosed illness.

## HYPOPITUITARISM

### Etiology

In addition to pituitary and hypothalamic tumors, hypopituitarism is caused by a number of other processes (see the box at right).

Head injuries, particularly in patients with basilar skull fractures, can cause hypothalamic or pituitary injury. Traumatic section at the proximal infundibulum where it passes through the diaphragma sella can interrupt the vascular communication between the hypothalamus and pituitary, causing hypopituitarism. Interruption of the neurohypophysis can cause diabetes insipidus.

Infections such as cytomegalovirus (CMV) and HIV are becoming a more important cause of hypothalamic dysfunction and hypopituitarism.

Metastasis to the hypothalamus and pituitary occurs in about 3% of patients with carcinoma. The neurohypophysis is particularly susceptible, probably because of the direct systemic arterial blood supply. Consequently, diabetes insipidus is the most common endocrine expression of metastasis to this area.

Pituitary infarction and hemorrhage occur spontaneously in pituitary tumors, during postpartum hemorrhage (Sheehan syndrome), during anticoagulant therapy, or from increased intracranial pressure. Hemorrhagic infarction of the pituitary can cause either permanent or temporary hypopituitarism.

Hypopituitarism can result from surgical hypophysectomy, pituitary stalk transsection, or radiation therapy. Radiation therapy given for any reason to the base of the brain usually induces gradual pituitary failure.

Neuroendocrine dysfunction can result from a wide variety of hereditary and congenital developmental disorders. These conditions usually present in childhood or at puberty.

Autoimmune (lymphocytic) hypophysitis, a rare disorder of women during or after pregnancy, is due to the destructive lymphocytic infiltration of the pituitary and neurohypophysis.

Functional disorders of the hypothalamus and pituitary are mediated by effects of higher brain centers. Hypothalamic amenorrhea is probably the most common neuroendocrine disorder and is caused by the effects of various stresses on menstrual cycling. Depression influences the adrenal axis and can present chemically like Cushing syndrome. In functional disorders the neuroendocrine system is intact and will resume normal function when the external stressors are removed.

### Etiology of hypothalamic and pituitary disease

- Pituitary adenomas
  - Prolactin (25%)
  - Growth hormone (15%)
  - Corticotropin (10%)
  - Gonadotropin (5%)
  - Thyrotropin (1%)
  - Prolactin and growth hormone (7%)
  - Silent (35%)
- Parasellar masses
  - Craniopharyngioma
  - Meningioma
  - Lymphoma/leukemia
  - Arteriovenous malformation
  - Internal carotid artery aneurysm
- Hypothalamic tumors
  - Glioma
  - Astrocytoma
  - Ganglioneuroma
  - Ependymoma
  - Pineal dysgerminoma
  - Third ventricular cyst
- Head injury
- Metastases
- Infectious and infiltrative diseases
  - Meningitis
  - Encephalitis
  - Tuberculosis
  - Sarcoidosis
  - Histiocytosis X (Hand-Schüller-Christian disease)
  - Syphilis
  - HIV/AIDS
- Pituitary infarction and hemorrhage
  - Intrapartum (Sheehan syndrome)
  - Pituitary apoplexy
- Surgical hypophysectomy
- Radiation therapy
- Hereditary and developmental disorders
- Autoimmune (lymphocytic) hypophysitis
- Functional disorders

### Clinical presentation and evaluation

Hypopituitarism presents clinically as the loss of one or more pituitary hormones. In children the usual manifestation is growth failure, which can occur with deficiency of GH, TSH, or ACTH. The other major manifestations are fasting hypoglycemia, delayed puberty, and diabetes insipidus.

In adults with hypopituitarism, hypogonadism is the most common presentation. It can be due to primary loss of hypothalamic releasing hormone, to interruption of the vascular connection between the hypothalamus and pituitary, or to hyperprolactinemia. Moderate hyperprolactinemia (PRL under 200 μg/l) with hypopituitarism suggests hypothalamic disease as the cause of the pituitary dysfunction. Hypogonadism presents as delayed puberty, primary or secondary amenorrhea, or impotence. Hypopituitarism can also present as hypothyroidism or adrenal insufficiency. The syndrome of panhypopituitarism (complete loss of pituitary function) includes asthenia, pallor, weight loss, hypogonadism, and sexual hair loss. The symptoms of hypopituitarism can be subtle, and it can be present for many years before diagnosis.

Laboratory evaluation of patients with suspected hypopituitarism should include an assessment of the secretion of each of the major pituitary hormones. Depending on age and sex, baseline measurements of PRL, TSH, thyroxine ($T_4$), tri-iodothyronine resin uptake ($T_3RU$), cortisol, LH, FSH, and either estrogen or testosterone should be obtained. In addition, dynamic assessment of pituitary response to stress should be done using insulin tolerance testing and pituitary response to releasing hormones.

All patients with hypopituitarism must have a careful radiologic evaluation with MRI or CT to look for structural causes.

### Management

The management of hypopituitarism includes both appropriate hormone replacement and the treatment of causative lesions. This section considers only hormone replacement.

Four endocrine functions require replacement therapy: GH in children and adrenal, thyroid, and gonadal function in children and adults. Oral glucocorticoids are used to treat adrenal insufficiency (see Chapter 35). Mineralocorticoids are usually not required for adrenal replacement therapy in hypopituitarism. There are no objective tests to regulate the replacement glucocorticoid dosage. Myalgias, arthralgia, and nocturia are clinical symptoms of inadequate glucocorticoid replacement.

Since TSH production cannot be used to evaluate the appropriateness of the thyroxine dosage, it must be regulated using clinical response and serum thyroxine concentrations.

Hypogonadism can be treated either with replacement gonadal steroids or with gonadotropic hormones, depending on the patient's interest in fertility. Maintenance of normal gonadal steroid levels is important for both men and women. Hormonal therapy to establish fertility should be managed by specialists skilled in reproductive endocrinology.

## DIABETES INSIPIDUS

Diabetes insipidus (DI) is due either to a failure of the neurohypophysis to produce adequate amounts of antidiuretic hormone (ADH) or by the inability of the kidney to respond to ADH. Reduced ADH secretion is called central DI. Failure of the kidney to respond to ADH is called nephrogenic DI.

ADH increases reabsorption of water in the distal nephron, resulting in more concentrated urine. The maximum concentration that can be achieved depends on the osmolarity of the renal medullary interstitium. ADH secretion is normally stimulated by increases in plasma osmolarity and by reductions in plasma volume.

Central DI can be caused by any process that damages the ADH-synthesizing hypothalamic nuclei or their axons. A significant number of cases (30%) are idiopathic. Central DI can be partial or complete depending on the degree of loss of ADH secretion. Complete DI requires loss of at least 85% of the ADH-secreting neurons.

Nephrogenic DI is caused by conditions that interfere with the ability of the distal nephron to respond to ADH. Reversible causes of nephrogenic DI include hypokalemia, hypercalcemia, and drugs (lithium, demeclocycline, streptozocin, foscarnet). Amyloidosis and sickle cell disease can cause irreversible nephrogenic DI. Nephrogenic DI can be inherited as an X-linked familial trait.

### Clinical manifestations and evaluation

Polyuria is the principal manifestation of DI. Large daily urine volumes of up to 15 L are common. Most conditions causing DI do not affect the hypothalamus directly, and consequently most DI patients have normal thirst responses and can fully compensate for the increased urine production by increased water drinking. If the condition causing DI also affects hypothalamic thirst-regulating centers, patients become hypernatremic. Polyuria and DI can be masked by adrenal insufficiency; occasionally DI first appears with the initiation of glucocorticoid replacement treatment in hypopituitarism.

After acute injury to the neurohypophysis, a three-component disturbance of ADH secretion often occurs. In the first few hours after the injury, ADH release is inhibited, causing a brief period of polyuria. In the next 24 to 48 hours unregulated ADH release occurs, causing a period of reduced water excretion and a considerable risk of water intoxication. If irreversible injury to the neurohypophysis has occurred, then permanent DI develops. Since the course of any individual patient is unpredictable, management of water balance must be individualized.

The diagnosis of DI depends on showing that polyuria is due to an inability to concentrate urine and then determining whether that is due to absent ADH or insensitivity to ADH. In addition to DI, polyuria can be due to excessive water drinking (primary polydipsia), osmotic diuresis due to glucose, mannitol, or glycerol. A history of recent head injury, neurosurgery, or symptoms of parasellar disease should lead to radiologic and functional evaluation of the hypothalamus and pituitary.

If no etiology of polyuria is found on initial evaluation and plasma osmolarity is normal or low, then a formal dehydration test can be done to complete the diagnostic process. The dehydration test measures the neurohypophyseal and renal response to water deprivation and the response of the kidney to exogenous ADH. Dehydration tests are conducted under close medical supervision both to protect the patient with true DI and to ensure that patients do not drink during the test. Baseline measurements of body weight, ADH, plasma sodium, plasma and urine osmolarity, and hourly urine volume are obtained while the patient has *ad lib* access to water. The patient then ceases any water consumption while body weight, plasma ADH and osmolarity, and urine osmolarity are measured hourly. When urine osmolarity has stabilized (less than a 30 mOsm change in 1 hour) or significant dehydration has occurred (loss of 3% to 5% of body weight), 5 U of exogenous ADH are administered and the change in urine osmolarity is measured. ADH deficiency is present when exogenous ADH increases urine osmolarity by 10% or more. Exogenous ADH in complete central DI increases urine osmolarity by at least 50%. There is little change in nephrogenic DI.

### Management

DI due to drugs or electrolyte disorders is managed by correction of the underlying disorder.

#### Commonly used preparations for replacement therapy in hypothalamic and pituitary disease

**Adrenal**

*Cortisone acetate:* 12-20 mg/m$^2$ per day (usually divided and given two-thirds in the AM and one-third in the PM)
*Hydrocortisone:* 12-18 mg/m$^2$ per day (usually divided and given two-thirds in the AM and one-third in the PM)
*Prednisone:* 4 mg/m$^2$ per day (usually single AM dose, but may be divided two-thirds in the AM and one-third in the PM)
*Dexamethasone:* 0.5-0.75 mg/m$^2$ per day (single daily dose)
Emergency glucocorticoid replacement
*Hydrocortisone:* 100 mg IV

**Thyroid**

*Thyroxine*
Adults: 100-150 μg per day
Children: 25-100 μg per day
(single daily dose)

**Testosterone**

*Testosterone enanthate or cypionate:* 150-200 mg IM every 2 weeks or 300 mg IM every 3 weeks

**Estrogen Replacement**

*Conjugated estrogen:* 0.3-1.25 mg orally per day
*Estrone:* 0.75-1.5 mg orally per day
*Ethinyl estradiol:* 0.02-0.05 mg per day
*Estradiol transdermal:* 0.05 or 0.10 mg patch applied twice weekly
*Estradiol valerate:* 1-2 mg orally daily

**Progestogen**

*Medroxyprogesterone acetate:* 5-10 mg orally per day in the last 10-14 days of the induced menstrual cycle

**Vasopressin**

*Vasopressin:* 5-10 units SC 3-4 times per day
*Vaspressin tannate in oil:* 1-5 units IM when previous dose has worn off (every 1-3 days)
*Lysine vasopressin:* 1-4 nasal sprays 3-4 times per day as needed to control symptoms
*Desmopressin for insufflation:* 0.1-0.4 ml insufflated intranasally per day as needed to control symptoms; total daily dose may be divided into up to 3 doses
*Desmopressin for injection:* 0.5-1.0 ml SC or IV per day as 1 or 2 doses

The goal of management in DI is reduction of polyuria to manageable levels without causing water intoxication. ADH-sensitive patients (central DI) can receive ADH or ADH analogues (see the box at left). The most commonly used preparation is desmopressin, an ADH analogue with a prolonged half-life. Desmopressin therapy is initiated in stepwise fashion. After a nightly dose to control nocturia is established, a larger morning dose or two divided doses are used during the daytime. Desmopressin is usually taken intranasally using an insufflator but can also be administered intravaginally and is available in a parenteral form. Two alternative ADH formulations are available for managing chronic DI: pitressin tannate in oil (PTO) and lysine vasopressin. Pitressin tannate in oil is given intramuscularly and has a prolonged duration of action, up to 48 hours. The duration of action for any given dose depends on how well the PTO is resuspended and can vary substantially. PTO doses are administered only after polyuria returns, marking the disappearance of the previous dose. Lysine vasopressin is a relatively short-acting nasal spray that is used by patients as needed to control polyuria. Water intoxication is a risk with any of the ADH preparations, especially with PTO because of its long duration of action. Because patients who have DI often have developed habitual polydipsia to compensate for polyuria, the initiation of ADH therapy must allow time for water consumption to return to normal.

For DI that occurs in the setting of intracranial surgery or head trauma, parenteral aqueous ADH can be used to control polyuria. To minimize the risk of water intoxication, it should be administered in response to hyposthenuria or polyuria, not on a fixed schedule.

Patients with partial central DI or nephrogenic DI can get relief of polyuria either by reductions in distal nephron urine delivery or by the use of drugs that enhance the action of ADH. Thiazide diuretics reduce renal water excretion independent of any action of ADH and can be of considerable benefit in nephrogenic DI, particularly when combined with sodium restriction. Both chlorpropamide and clofibrate enhance the action of ADH and have been effective in controlling polyuria in some patients with partial central DI.

## RELATED CONDITIONS

### Empty sella syndrome

Occasionally radiologic study of the hypothalamus and pituitary demonstrate downward displacement and flattening of the pituitary gland. The sella itself may be enlarged. Usually the finding is incidental or associated with neurologic symptoms that have no endocrine component. When no endocrine disease is present, empty sella is thought to result from herniation of the suprasellar cistern through an incompetent diaphragma sella, which allows the transmission of CSF pulsations into the sellar space, remodeling the structures of the sella.

Although empty sella and abnormal pituitary function can be coincidentally associated, in some individuals pituitary disease may lead to empty sella. Both ectopic pituitary (congenital failure of the pituitary to associate with the neurohypophysis) and acquired loss of pituitary tissue (infarct or hemorrhage) can cause radiologic empty sella.

Empty sella has no significance independent of any conditions with which it is associated. It requires no management or workup in asymptomatic patients.

### Pineal gland disorders

The pineal gland is a neuroendocrine structure at the caudal aspect of the third ventricle, which secretes melatonin in response to sympathetic stimulation as a result of input from both the retina and the hypothalamic nuclei. Consequently, the activity of the pineal responds to both circadian and light-dark cycles. Pineal secretion of melatonin is greatest during darkness and sleep.

Clinical disorders due to abnormal secretion of melatonin have not been described. Tumors of the pineal are the primary clinical problem. Three types of tumors occur: germinoma, pinealoma, and glioma; most tumors of the pineal region are germinomas. The clinical management of germinoma differs significantly from the management of the other two tumor types.

The principal manifestations of pineal tumors are due to impingement on local structures. Hydrocephalus results from obstruction at the sylvian aqueduct and presents as subtle changes in mental status, papilledema, and non-ataxic gait disturbance. Oculomotor disturbances result from interference with the dorsal midbrain structures and hydrocephalus. Paralysis of upward gaze (Parinaud syndrome) is seen frequently in pineal tumors and is associated with lack of ocular convergence and fixed mydriatic pupils. Extension of tumor to the hypothalamus causes disturbances of hypothalamic and endocrine function, manifested as hypopituitarism or disturbances in thermoregulation or body weight. Pineal germinomas commonly secrete human chorionic gonadotropin (HCG) and can occasionally cause precocious puberty in males. Otherwise, pineal tumors produce hypogonadism or delayed puberty.

Radiologic evaluation of the pineal region with MRI or CT is the first step in the evaluation of a patient suspected of having a pinealoma. If a pineal region tumor is demonstrated, HCG should be measured in blood and CSF. HCG, particularly in the CSF, is diagnostic for a germinoma.

Pineal tumors are managed by resection, if possible, and ventriculoatrial shunting to relieve hydrocephalus. Germinomas are particularly sensitive to radiation therapy and have been cured using this modality alone.

### Other hypothalamic disorders

Hypothalamic obesity is the result of lesions in the vicinity of the medial hypothalamus, which houses the hypothalamic nuclei concerned with satiety. Unless it is associated with other evidence of hypothalamic disease, the obesity that develops is indistinguishable from common exogenous obesity. Frohlich syndrome (adiposogenital dystrophy) is the combination of obesity with pubertal delay and occasionally DI. It is usually due to craniopharyngioma, but a number of other hypothalamic tumors have been reported to cause this syndrome.

Central hypothermia, in which body temperature falls inappropriately, results from lesions in the posterior hypothalamus. The disorder may be periodic in association with agenesis of the corpus callosum (Shapiro syndrome).

Central hyperthermia is usually an acute disorder resulting from injury to the anterior hypothalamus caused by trauma or intracranial hemorrhage. Recurrent hyperthermic paroxysms, presumably of hypothalamic origin but of unknown cause, have been described.

Diencephalic epilepsy is characterized by paroxysms of autonomic hyperactivity manifested by sweating, hypertension, flushing, shivering, and pupillary mydriasis. Despite the name, electroencephalographic investigations have not demonstrated an epileptic mechanism. This syndrome is associated with tumors of the third ventricle.

The diencephalic syndrome is seen in children. It is manifested by poor feeding, failure to thrive, delayed psychomotor development, and visual impairment. It is usually due to gliomas of the anterior hypothalamus.

## GROWTH HORMONE DISORDERS

Growth hormone (GH, somatotropin) is the principal hormonal regulator of somatic growth. It produces its effects principally by stimulating hepatic production of somatomedin C (SmC, insulin-like growth factor [IGF] I) and through direct actions on target tissues. The effects of GH include stimulating growth of skin, muscle, visceral tissues, bone, and cartilage. GH also induces insulin resistance and lipolysis.

GH secretion is regulated by the net effect of growth hormone–releasing hormone (GHRH) and somatostatin (growth hormone–release inhibiting hormone, GHRIH), both products of the hypothalamus. GH participates in a feedback loop; its secretion is inhibited by SmC. However, GH secretion is also affected by factors outside the feedback loop. It is increased by acute stress, hypoglycemia, exercise, and fasting. It is reduced by obesity, hyperglycemia and chronic emotional deprivation.

### GH excess

*Gigantism* is a rare condition of children caused by excess GH secretion. Its true incidence is not known but is thought to be much less than one case per million people per year. In adults, *acromegaly* is estimated to have an annual incidence of three cases per million, which sustains a prevalence of about 50 per million. About 5% of acromegalic tumors occur as part of the multiple endocrine neoplasia (MEN) syndrome type I (Wermer syndrome). About 50% of patients with MEN type I have pituitary tumors; about 25% of those pituitary tumors cause acromegaly (see Chapter 39).

Excessive GH secretion is almost always (99%) caused by a pituitary tumor. Other reported sources include carcinoid or pancreatic islet cell tumors and hypothalamic gangliocytomas.

***Clinical manifestations.*** Symptoms of patients with GH excess can be caused by systemic effects of GH, local effect of the tumor, or both. Symptoms develop insidiously and usually progress for years before the patient or an observer becomes aware of the change in appearance. Common presenting complaints due to systemic effects of GH include inappropriate skeletal growth with increased height and arm and leg length in children, and change in ring, glove, or shoe size in adults. Adults also have cortical thickening of the flat bones of the cranium and mandible,

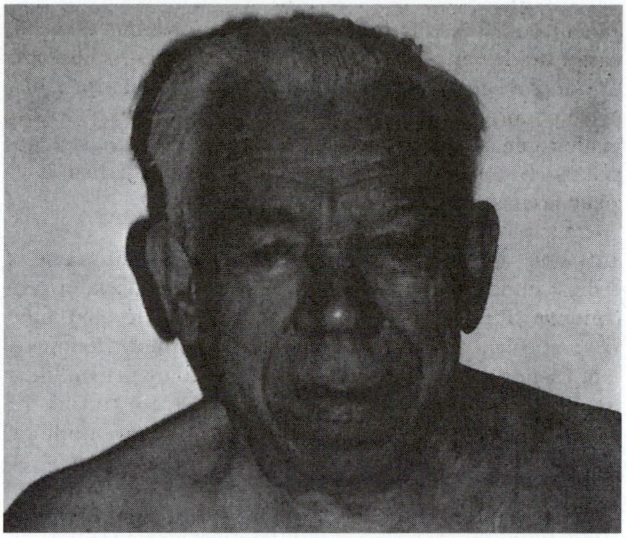

**Fig. 36-4.** Patient with acromegaly.

leading to increased hat size and prognathism of the mandible. Additional common features include excessive sweating, joint pain, muscle weakness, carpal tunnel and other neural entrapment syndromes, and skin tags (Fig. 36-4). Symptoms due to pituitary tumor include headache, abnormal visual field, and impaired secretion of other pituitary hormones. Small pituitary tumors producing PRL can cause hypogonadal symptoms (impotence, amenorrhea) and galactorrhea.

On physical examination the patient with acromegaly has thickened skin with prominent nasolabial folds and thick lips. Hyperhidrosis is common and correlated with disease activity. The voice is deep from laryngeal enlargement. The teeth are widely spaced. The cheeks may seem hollow due to growth of the zygomatic arch and loss of subcutaneous fat. The supraorbital ridge is prominent. The ribs elongate and cause a barrel chest. The joints enlarge due to soft tissue growth and eventually develop significant degenerative arthritis. The patient may have visual field loss or diplopia due to compression of the optic chiasm or oculomotor nerves.

Hypertension occurs in 20% of patients and glucose intolerance or diabetes in 50%. Nephrolithiasis occurs in 10% from increased intestinal calcium absorption and hypercalciuria. Muscular weakness occurs and can be due to a primary myopathy, motor nerve compression by soft tissue, skeletal hypertrophy, or spinal stenosis. Colon polyps and carcinoma occur at an increased rate.

Some of the most useful tools in the evaluation of acromegaly are photographs of the patient in past years. They often provide the clearest demonstration of a change in appearance. Since some individuals can have a normal physiognomy that resembles acromegaly, a demonstration of no change over a number of years can be reassuring.

***Clinical evaluation.*** The diagnosis of acromegaly requires demonstration of the effects of abnormal GH secretion. Random measurements of GH are not helpful in evaluating GH status because GH is secreted in discrete bursts at irregular intervals. Measuring SmC concentration is a useful screening test for the rate of GH secretion, since its concentration varies little during the day.

The diagnosis of acromegaly is confirmed by the failure of a glucose tolerance test to suppress GH below 5 ng/ml at 1 or 2 hours, a consistent clinical examination, and an elevated SmC level. However, a fall in GH below 5 ng/dl does not exclude acromegaly. If testing results are unclear, consultation with an endocrinologist is indicated.

The only way to exclude ectopic secretion of GHRH is to measure GHRH levels in plasma, which is now available in some endocrine reference and academic laboratories. GHRH measurement may be important for patients with no radiologic evidence of pituitary tumor.

Once acromegaly is confirmed, a complete evaluation of pituitary function is required to determine if any other pituitary hormones are being secreted in excess (e.g., PRL) and if there has been any compromise of pituitary function. The usual assessment includes thyroid function tests—a high-sensitivity TSH, an insulin tolerance test for pituitary-adrenal reserve, PRL concentration, and gonadal function. Heel pad thickness is a measure of disease activity and can be used to monitor effectiveness of therapy.

A radiologic evaluation of the pituitary is required. MRI is the preferred technique because of its ability to distinguish vascular and neural structures. High-resolution CT can be used with contrast enhancement. If MRI or CT fails to demonstrate a pituitary tumor in an otherwise clear-cut case of acromegaly, a careful radiologic evaluation of the hypothalamus and the lungs and viscera for GHRH-secreting tumors is required.

Patients with acromegaly need a formal neuroophthalmologic evaluation of their visual fields to assist in planning and monitoring therapy.

***Clinical course and complications.*** Without treatment acromegaly is a progressive condition associated with a considerable premature mortality (two to five times greater than expected). The most common cause of death in men with acromegaly is cardiovascular disease due to hypertension and/or GH-induced hypertrophic cardiomyopathy. Cerebrovascular disease is the most common cause of death in acromegalic women. Respiratory disease is increased in both men and women, including sleep apnea and obstructive airway disease. The excess mortality of acromegaly is clearly reduced by treatment. Therapy ameliorates both direct causes such as cardiomyopathy and indirect causes such as diabetes mellitus and hypertension.

Occasional patients show clear physical evidence of acromegaly and a history consistent with a period of active disease in the past, but without any evidence of current GH oversecretion (fugitive acromegaly). These individuals may have developed a remission of acromegaly through spontaneous infarction of a pituitary tumor. Alternatively, acromegaly without evidence of GH oversecretion can be mediated by insulin or IGF II.

***Management.*** Patients with acromegaly require long-term endocrine management for three reasons: surveillance for recurrence of disease, control of persistent pathologic production of GH, and surveillance for appearance of pituitary failure consequent to therapy. The goal of management of acromegaly is cure of the disease by removal or ablation of the pituitary tumor with preservation of normal pituitary function. This goal unfortunately is achieved infrequently. Cure is determined clinically by the normalization of GH secretion measurements and SmC levels. Skeletal changes of acromegaly are permanent and will not regress.

The primary mode of therapy is neurosurgical resection of the pituitary tumor via the transsphenoidal route. The cure rate by surgery depends primarily on two factors: the initial size of the tumor and the experience of the surgeon. In experienced hands transsphenoidal resection of microadenomas (under 10 mm) results in cure about 75% of the time; macroadenomas (10 mm or larger) are cured about 35% of the time. Neurosurgeons experienced in transsphenoidal pituitary surgery have lower perioperative morbidity and higher rates of surgical cure than surgeons with less experience.

Postoperatively, patients need to be closely followed to assess pituitary function and GH secretion. If abnormal GH secretion persists or reappears after surgery, radiation therapy directed to the pituitary is indicated. Conventional supervoltage radiation therapy is most frequently used, but yttrium implants, α-particle beam, proton beam, and focused γ-radiation (γ-knife) techniques have also been used. The effect of radiation therapy is gradual, reducing residual GH secretion over several years. Pituitary radiation also gradually reduces other pituitary functions, and most patients have hypopituitarism within 10 years.

In cases where surgical cure is not achieved, medical therapies are available to control symptoms while awaiting the effects of radiation. Two drugs are the mainstays of therapy: octreotide and bromocriptine.

Octreotide is a polypeptide analogue of somatostatin with a sufficiently long half-life to be effective by intermittent injection. A typical dosage is 100 μg subcutaneously every 8 hours, although this needs to be individualized. Octreotide satisfactorily reduces GH secretion in about 90% of patients with residual disease. Octreotide has been used preoperatively to reduce tumor size before transsphenoidal resection. Since postsurgical acromegaly is frequently chronic, the duration of octreotide therapy may be many years. The adverse effects of octreotide include decreased gastrointestinal motility, injection site pain, gallbladder bile stasis, and cholelithiasis. Octreotide also inhibits insulin release and has occasionally increased hyperglycemia in acromegalic patients with diabetes. Intranasal and oral octreotide preparations are currently under clinical investigation.

Bromocriptine is another drug that supresses GH secretion. It is less effective than the octreotide but has the advantages of oral efficacy and lower cost. Bromocriptine is effective in reducing GH secretion and acromegalic symptoms in about 80% of patients. A typical dosage is 20 to 30 mg per day in three or four divided doses. The principal adverse effect is nausea, which can be moderated by starting with a small dosage (1.25 or 2.5 mg daily) that gradually increases every few days to tolerance or until symptom control is achieved.

Bromocriptine and octreotide may have synergistic effects on acromegaly. Patients whose disorder is controlled with neither drug alone may benefit from simultaneous treatment with both.

### GH deficiency

GH deficiency is clinically apparent only in children, but the exact incidence is unknown. Complete GH deficiency probably occurs on the order of 1 per 10,000 children. Partial GH deficiency is probably more common, but in the absence of exact criteria for diagnosis, estimates of its prevalence vary substantially. About 10% of children with severe short stature (height below the 1st percentile) and slow growth velocity have GH deficiency. The most common cause of GH deficiency in children is idiopathic isolated GH deficiency that appears to be due to inadequate production of GHRH. Hypothalamic and pituitary function in these children is otherwise normal. Organic disease of the hypothalamus or pituitary accounts for almost all the remainder of cases.

GH deficiency occurs in adults either as a continuation of childhood GH deficiency or as an acquired condition. The most common cause of adult GH deficiency appears to be an idiopathic age-related decline in GH secretion. Problems associated with the manifestations of GH deficiency in adults are depression, osteopenia, reduced lean body mass, and reduced exercise capacity. Osteopenia is a particular problem in adults with GH deficiency since childhood.

In general, the findings of severe short stature (more than 3 S.D. below corrected height for age), inappropriate documented slowing of growth, and truncal obesity suggest GH deficiency, although other endocrinologic and metabolic causes of short stature should be evaluated. GH replacement therapy, now available through recombinant technology, is effective for children with documented GH deficiency and open epiphyses. At this time GH replacement therapy is not indicated for normal children to enhance adult stature or for athletes to increase muscle mass. The reader should consult a pediatric or endocrinology text for further discussion of GH deficiency.

## HYPERPROLACTINEMIA

Prolactin (PRL) is a pituitary hormone whose principal action is to stimulate the synthesis and release of breast milk. It is secreted by specific prolactinotropic pituitary cells. Its synthesis and secretion are stimulated by estrogen in pregnancy and are sustained after delivery by nipple stimulation during suckling. PRL also inhibits the synthesis and secretion of gonadotropin. These two functions are synergistic and appear to provide a physiologic means of inhibiting ovarian function during the period a mother is nursing an infant.

PRL secretion is under tonic inhibition by hypothalamic dopamine. In contrast to the other pituitary hormones, PRL levels rise if the hypothalamic-pituitary connection is disrupted. PRL levels vary in a circadian fashion and are highest during sleep. Exercise, breast stimulation, and other acute stresses can induce PRL secretion.

PRL concentrations vary with age, reproductive status, and gender. Women during the reproductive years have the highest normal PRL levels, about 20 μg/L. PRL levels increase during pregnancy to about six or seven times the preconception level and remain elevated for several months after delivery if breastfeeding is established. PRL levels in men, prepubertal children, and postmenopausal women are about 10 μg/L.

## Etiology

Elevated levels of PRL are relatively common (see the box below). Hyperprolactinemia occurs in about one sixth of all cases of amenorrhea and about 5% of cases of male impotence. Although the exact incidence of PRL-secreting pituitary tumors (prolactinoma, PRLoma) is not known, they are responsible for substantially less than half of hyperprolactinemia cases. Prolactinomas are more likely in individuals with higher PRL concentrations. PRL concentrations over 250 μg/L, except in pregnancy, are almost always due to prolactinomas. Secondary hyperprolactinemia is not autonomous and returns to normal with correction of the underlying condition. The PRL elevation in most secondary hyperprolactinemia is usually less than 100 μg/L.

Prolactinomas are the most common form of pituitary adenoma. About 30% of all pituitary adenomas secrete enough PRL to cause hyperprolactinemia; about 25% of those secrete both PRL and GH. Prolactinomas are the third most common tumor encountered in MEN type I, after parathyroid hyperplasia and gastrinoma.

A substantial number of patients with symptomatic hyperprolactinemia do not have a clinically identifiable cause. Autopsy studies have shown that about 25% of asymptomatic individuals harbor pituitary microadenomas; 70% of these clinically silent microadenomas contain PRL. Therefore it is likely that a number of hyperprolactinemic individuals have PRL-secreting pituitary microadenomas too small to be detected by current radiologic techniques.

Dopamine antagonists block the inhibition of PRL secretion. Primary hypothyroidism causes increased secretion of hypothalamic TRH, which causes PRL secretion. Chronic renal failure is associated with reduced PRL removal and increased PRL secretion. Hyperprolactinemia is common in the polycystic ovary syndrome (about 30%), probably due to tonic estrogen stimulation of the pituitary. PRL levels are increased just after a seizure.

Conditions that interrupt dopamine delivery from the hypothalamus to the pituitary are rare causes of hyperprolactinemia. Examples include primary hypothalamic granulomas, hypothalamic tumors, lesions that compress the infundibular stalk, and pituitary stalk section. Any activation of the breast reflex are also stimulates PRL secretion, including nursing, herpes zoster of the chest wall, and scars from burns or thoracotomy.

Hyperprolactinemia may also be artifactual due either to the stress of venipuncture or sampling too close to sleep or immediately after meals (see further).

### Etiology of hyperprolactinemia

- Prolactinoma
  - Microadenoma
  - Macroadenoma
- Idiopathic hyperprolactinemia
- Pituitary stalk section
- Hypothyroidism
- Dopamine antagonist drugs
  - Phenothiazines
  - Metoclopramide
  - Haloperidol
- Pregnancy and lactation
- Reflex stimulation
  - Nipple stimulation
  - Chest wall scars
  - Postherpetic chest wall pain
  - Breast implants
- Chronic renal failure
- Stress
- Seizures

## Clinical manifestations

Suppression of gonadal function is the major clinical presentation of hyperprolactinemia. At nonreproductive ages hyperprolactinemia is clinically silent. The mechanism of PRL action seems to include suppression of hypothalamic release of GnRH, pituitary secretion of LH/FSH, and direct gonadal inhibition. Hyperprolactinemia induces galactorrhea in both males and females if the other hormonal requirements (insulin, estrogen, and GH) are met. Men with hyperprolactinemia also have gonadal dysfunction, which presents as infertility and/or impotence. Women with prolonged hyperprolactinemic hypogonadism have increased risk of osteoporosis. Hyperprolactinemic women occasionally develop hirsutism with elevated levels of adrenal androgens, presumably due to a direct effect of the PRL on the adrenal gland. In addition to amenorrhea, hyperprolactinemia can cause additional symptoms of hypogonadism such as vaginal dryness and dyspareunia.

If galactorrhea is present with amenorrhea, hyperprolactinemia is found about 75% of the time and prolactinoma about 40% of the time. Galactorrhea may abate late in the course of hyperprolactinemia because progressive gonadal dysfunction can reduce gonadal steroids below the concentrations needed to support milk synthesis and secretion.

Because abnormalities in the menstrual cycle serve so effectively as an early sign of hyperprolactinemia, women of reproductive age rarely present with large pituitary tumors. In contrast, men and postmenopausal women are more likely to present with symptoms due the pituitary tumor itself. Pituitary tumors cause headache, diplopia, ophthalmoplegia, and visual field disturbances. Occasionally prolactinomas produce symptoms of pituitary apoplexy.

GH is cosecreted with PRL in about 7% of pituitary tumors. Patients with hyperprolactinemia may also have evidence of acromegaly.

## Laboratory evaluation

PRL measurement should be done at least 2 hours after awakening (to avoid the sleep-induced PRL rise), preprandially, and with a minimum of distress. The levels obtained should be interpreted using gender, age, and reproductive status. Patients with minimal elevations should have serial measurements to determine if the level is truly elevated. There are no useful provocative or suppressive tests to determine the etiology of hyperprolactinemia or to detect the presence of a prolactinoma.

Patients with hyperprolactinemia need thyroid function testing to rule out primary hypothyroidism. If no secondary etiology of hyperprolactinemia is found or there is clinical suspicion of a pituitary lesion, the pituitary and hypothalamus should be visualized in a search for a prolactinoma or other lesion. MRI with gadolinium enhancement is the preferred technique; CT with contrast enhancement can also be used. Patients with pituitary tumor should have complete workup.

It is important to remember that hyperprolactinemia in association with a pituitary tumor can be caused either by a prolactinoma or by the tumor interrupting dopamine delivery to the pituitary. In the latter case, hypogonadism can result from hypopituitarism as well as from hyperprolactinemia.

## Management

The goals of management of hyperprolactinemia are to maintain normal gonadal function and to prevent any complications related to a prolactinoma. Impaired gonadal function, particularly in women, is a strong indication for pharmacologic treatment of hyperprolactinemia because of the risk of osteoporosis and other clinical consequences of hypogonadism.

Patients with either idiopathic hyperprolactinemia or those who have frank prolactinoma require long-term surveillance and management.

Patients with no evidence of gonadal dysfunction and no evidence of prolactinoma do not require treatment. However, because the hyperprolactinemia may progress, these patients should be periodically reevaluated for evidence of gonadal dysfunction, pituitary tumor, or hypopituitarism. If there is any possibility that hyperprolactinemia is responsible for a reproductive complaint, then a trial of medical therapy is warranted.

Prolactinoma can be treated medically with excellent results. Dopamine agonist drugs effectively reduce PRL secretion and reduce tumor size for the great majority of patients. Surgery and radiation therapy do have a role in the management of some patients with prolactinoma, but only after failure of medical therapy.

Bromocriptine is the most frequently used dopamine agonist drug. PRL levels fall immediately after bromocriptine administration and remain suppressed for 8 to 24 hours after a dose. Bromocriptine also reduces symptoms, such as visual disturbances, caused by local effects of prolactinoma. PRL suppression increases with the duration of therapy, and normal levels are achieved eventually in most patients. Those with very high levels of PRL or large tumors may not achieve normal levels of PRL, but significant falls in PRL should be anticipated. Most patients relapse after bromocriptine withdrawal, so bromocriptine therapy should be assumed to be lifelong. If a trial of bromocriptine withdrawal is attempted, PRL levels should be followed closely and bromocriptine should be resumed if PRL levels rise. Pergolide is an effective alternative drug.

Surgical resection of prolactinoma is indicated if the tumor does not respond to medical therapy or medical therapy is otherwise impossible through patient choice or drug intolerance. Surgery is not indicated for microadenoma and is not needed as a routine adjunct to medical therapy. Prolactinomas are resected usually via the transsphenoidal route. As with all surgery for pituitary tumors, outcome depends on tumor size and the experience of the surgeon. Recurrence of prolactinoma after surgery is common, even in patients whose PRL levels normalize. The exact recurrence rates are not known, but rates increase in proportion to the duration of follow-up. Rates as high as 50% for microadenomas (less than 10 mm) and 90% for macroadenomas have been reported. The conditions of patients who are undergoing surgical therapy must be followed for several years for recurrence of hyperprolactinemia.

Supervoltage radiation therapy has been used both alone and in conjunction with both medical and surgical therapy to treat prolactinomas. Currently it is considered as an adjunctive therapy after surgical resection of prolactinomas that respond poorly to dopamine agonist medication.

### Pregnancy in hyperprolactinemic women

Dopamine agonist therapy in hyperprolactinemic women usually restores normal gonadal function and fertility. Pregnancy is frequently an important goal of therapy. Since estrogen levels rise and dopamine agonist drugs are discontinued during pregnancy, there has been concern that prolactinoma is aggravated by pregnancy. However, the accumulated experience with pregnancy in women with medically controlled hyperprolactinemia has been reassuring in this respect. Women with idiopathic hyperprolactinemia have no significant risk of tumor appearance during pregnancy. Women with microadenomas have a small (about 1%) risk of tumor enlargement. Women with macroadenomas have a moderate risk of tumor enlargement (about 15%).

If prolactinoma enlargement occurs during pregnancy, resumption of dopamine agonist therapy almost always induces tumor regression and resolution of symptoms. There is no evidence that administration of bromocriptine to control hyperprolactinemia during pregnancy is associated with any increase in perinatal morbidity or teratology.

## BIBLIOGRAPHY

Bjerre P: The empty sella syndrome: a reappraisal of etiology and pathogenesis, *Acta Neurol Scand Suppl* 130:1, 1990.

Blackwell RE: Hyperprolactinemia: evaluation and management, *Endocrinol Metab Clin North Am* 21:105, 1992.

Chong BW, Newton JH: Hypothalamic and pituitary pathology, *Radiol Clin North Am* 31:1147, 1993.

Frohman L: Clinical Review 22: Therapeutic options in acromegaly, *J Clin Endocrinol Metab* 72:1175, 1991.

Klibanski A, Zervas NT: Diagnosis and management of hormone secreting pituitary adenomas, *N Engl J Med* 324:822, 1991.

Lamberts SWJ, Hofland LJ, de Herder WW et al: Octreotide and related somatostatin analogs in the diagnosis and treatment of pituitary disease and somatostatin receptor scintigraphy, *Frontiers Neuroendocrinol*, 14:27, 1993.

Melmed S: Acromegaly, *N Engl J Med* 322:966, 1990.

Molitch MM, Russell EJ: The pituitary incidentaloma, *Ann Intern Med* 112:925, 1990.

CHAPTER

# 37 Evaluation and Treatment of Disorders in Calcium, Phosphorus, and Magnesium Metabolism

**Michael F. Holick**

## CALCIUM METABOLISM

Calcium is an important mediator of cell signaling, neurotransmission, and a variety of intracellular biochemical activities. In addition, calcium is the major building block that provides structural integrity to the skeleton. Therefore it is no wonder that the body requires that the circulating concentrations of calcium be tightly regulated. The three hormones responsible for maintaining the blood calcium in the normal range are vitamin D (1,25-dihydroxyvitamin D [1,25$(OH)_2$D]), parathyroid hormone (PTH), and calcitonin. A variety of factors and disease states can alter calcium metabolism, leading to either hypocalcemic or hypercalcemic disorders.

There are approximately 1000 g of calcium in the adult human body. About 99% of the calcium is found in the skeleton and approximately 1% is freely disassociable from the skeleton. The normal blood calcium range is 8.4 to 10.4 mg/dl. Approximately 40% of the blood calcium is protein bound, 50% is in the ionized form, and an additional 10% is complexed to citrate and phosphate ions. At a physiologic pH of 7.4, 1 g of albumin binds 0.8 mg/dl of calcium; therefore the total serum calcium concentrations need to be corrected when circulating albumin levels are abnormal. For example, at pH 7.4 if the total calcium is 7 mg/dl with an albumin of 2 g/dl, then the corrected calcium is $(4\ \text{g/dl} - 2\ \text{g/dl}) \times 0.8\ \text{mg/dl} + 7\ \text{mg/dl} = 8.6$ mg/dl. When the pH is below 7.4, less calcium is bound to albumin; thus a higher fraction is in the ionized form. When pH is above 7.4, the reverse is true. Calcium concentrations are usually reported in mg/dl and can be converted to molar units by dividing the calcium concentrations in mg/dl by 4.

Magnesium is the most abundant intracellular divalent cation and plays an important role in a number of enzymatic reactions and neuromuscular excitability. Since 1% of the total body magnesium is contained in the extracellular compartment, its concentration in the plasma does not provide a reliable index of either total body or soft tissue magnesium content. There is an integral relationship between magnesium and calcium in the body (see magnesium section later).

There is an abundance of phosphorus in the diet, mostly as phosphoproteins. Approximately 85% of the body's phosphorus is present in the skeleton and the other 15% resides in the extracellular fluids and soft tissues. Because our diet has a high phosphorus content, including meats and soft drinks, hypophosphatemia becomes a medical concern only when there is either a phosphate leak in the kidney, malnutrition, or secondary hyperparathyroidism (see phosphate section later).

The three principal hormones that regulate calcium and phosphorus metabolism are PTH, calcitonin, and vitamin D. PTH is a polypeptide that is secreted from the parathyroid glands in response to a decrease in serum ionized calcium concentrations. It acts on calcium and phosphorus metabolism by (1) increasing tubular reabsorption of calcium in the proximal and distal convoluted tubules in the kidney, (2) decreasing tubular reabsorption of phosphate, thereby causing increased loss of phosphate into the urine, (3) mobilizing stem cells to become osteoclasts to liberate calcium and phosphate from the bone, and (4) stimulating the production of 1,25$(OH)_2$D in the kidney, which in turn increases the efficiency of intestinal calcium and phosphate absorption. The precise physiologic function of calcitonin is unknown. Calcitonin interacts with its receptors on mature osteoclasts and decreases osteoclastic function thereby decreasing mobilization of calcium and phosphate from bone.

Vitamin D can be obtained either from exposure to sunlight (vitamin $D_3$) or from dietary sources (vitamin $D_2$ or vitamin $D_3$), including fortified foods such as milk, some cereals, some breads, fatty fish such as salmon and mackerel, and cod liver oil. Vitamin D is biologically inactive and requires successive hydroxylations first in the liver to 25-hydroxyvitamin D (25[OH]D) and then in the kidney to 1,25$(OH)_2$D. 25(OH)D is the major circulating form of vitamin D, and its measurement in the blood is useful to the clinician as an indicator of the vitamin D status of a patient. 1,25$(OH)_2$D is the biologically active form of vitamin D that is responsible for increasing the efficiency of intestinal absorption of calcium. In addition, 1,25$(OH)_2$D mobilizes stem cells to become osteoclasts, which in turn mobilize calcium and phosphorus stores from the bone. Measurement of 1,25$(OH)_2$D has value in patients with hypocalcemia and hypercalcemia disorders when there is suspicion that there is an acquired or inherited disorder in the metabolism of 25(OH)D to 1,25$(OH)_2D_3$ or that there is an abnormal or deficient response to 1,25$(OH)_2$D.

PTH and 1,25$(OH)_2D_3$, when produced in excess, cause hypercalcemia by either directly or indirectly increasing the efficiency of intestinal calcium absorption and by mobilizing calcium stores from bone. Excess production of PTH causes hypercalcemia and hypophosphatemia, whereas excess vitamin D or 1,25$(OH)_2$D can cause hypercalcemia and hyperphosphatemia (although most often the serum phosphate is in the high normal range). A deficiency or defect in the recognition of PTH or vitamin D or an abnormality in the synthesis of 1,25$(OH)_2$D can result in hypocalcemia. A PTH deficiency leads to hypocalcemia and hyperphosphatemia, whereas vitamin D deficiency causes hypocalcemia and hypophosphatemia. Although calcitonin is not absolutely necessary for maintaining calcium homeostasis, when provided in pharmacologic concentrations from an exogenous or endogenous source it transiently lowers blood calcium levels.

### Hypercalcemia

***Epidemiology and etiology.*** Most often hypercalcemia is picked up on a routine blood laboratory evaluation.

Although there are a large number of possible causes for hypercalcemia (Table 37-1), approximately 90% of hypercalcemic patients suffer from either a malignancy or primary hyperparathyroidism. Primary hyperparathyroidism is a relatively common endocrine disorder with estimates of incidence as high as 1 in 500. Primary hyperparathyroidism occurs at all ages but is most frequent in the sixth decade of life, affecting women more often than men by a ratio of 3 to 2. The hallmark of primary hyperparathyroidism is hypercalcemia associated with inappropriately normal or overtly elevated levels of PTH. The disease is most often benign, and 85% of cases are caused by a solitary adenoma. Approximately 15% of patients have a pathologic process characterized by hyperplasia of all four parathyroid glands. Hyperplasia may occur sporadically, but more likely the multiglandular disease is associated with multiple endocrine neoplasia (MEN) type I or II (see Chapter 39). Very rarely primary hyperparathyroidism is caused by parathyroid carcinoma, occurring in fewer than 1% of patients. With the exception of the presentation of a kidney stone in about 20% of patients with hypercalcemia, there are very few symptoms associated with primary hyperparathyroidism, especially when it is detected early. The hypercalcemia is often mild, no more than 1.5 mg/dl above the upper limit of normal (less than 12 mg/dl). Patients who suffer with malignancy are often more ill and manifest the classic signs and symptoms of hypercalcemia. Usually the malignancy is easily detected; however, sometimes an occult malignancy can be the cause.

***Pathophysiology.*** There are three principal causes for hypercalcemia (i.e., PTH, vitamin D, and malignancy related) and several other less common causes (see Table 37-1). PTH and 1,25$(OH)_2$D are the major regulators of calcium metabolism; excess production of these hormones can lead to hypercalcemia. A third hormone that affects calcium metabolism only during malignancy is parathyroid hormone related peptide (PTHrP). As the name implies, the first part of the structure of PTHrP is very

**Table 37-1.** Causes of hypercalcemia

| | PTH | PTHrP | 25(OH)D | 1,25$(OH)_2$D |
|---|---|---|---|---|
| **Parathyroid gland related** | | | | |
| Primary hyperparathyroidism | ↑ | nl or ↓ | nl | nl or ↑ |
| Adenoma (~85%) | ↑ | nl or ↓ | nl | nl or ↑ |
| Hyperplasia (~15%) | ↑ | nl or ↓ | nl | nl or ↑ |
| Carcinoma (<1%) | ↑ | nl or ↓ | nl | nl or ↑ |
| Multiple endocrine neoplasia (hyperplasia) | ↑ | nl or ↓ | nl | nl or ↑ |
| Familial hypocalciuric hypercalcemia | ↑ | nl or ↓ | nl | — |
| Tertiary hyperparathyroidism | ↑ | nl or ↓ | nl | nl or ↓ |
| Severe secondary hyperparathyroidism | ↑↑ | nl or ↓ | nl | ↓ |
| **Malignancy related** | | | | |
| Bone involvement (breast, multiple myeloma, lymphoma) | ↓ | nl or ↓ | nl | ↓ |
| Humoral hypercalcemia (lung, esophagus, cervix, vulva, head, neck, skin, renal, breast, and ovarian carcinomas) | ↓ | ↑↑ | nl | ↓ |
| **Vitamin D related** | | | | |
| Vitamin D intoxication | ↓ | nl | ↑↑↑ | nl, ↓ or ↑ |
| Granulomatous disorders (e.g., sarcoidosis, tuberculosis) | ↓ | nl | nl or ↓ | ↑↑ |
| Williams syndrome | — | — | nl | ↑ |
| **Drug related** | | | | |
| Lithium | ↑ | — | nl | — |
| Thiazides | nl or ↓ | — | nl or ↑ | nl |
| 1,25$(OH)_2D_3$, 1α-OH-$D_3$, calcipotriene, dihydrotachysterol | ↓ | — | nl or ↑ for DHT | ↑ Calcipotriene, nl |
| Androgens (breast cancer therapy) | ↓ | — | nl | — |
| Estrogens and antiestrogens | ↓ | — | nl | — |
| Vitamin A | ↓ | — | nl | — |
| Aluminum intoxication | ↓ or ↑ | — | nl | nl |
| Aminophylline | ↓ | — | nl | — |
| **Miscellaneous** | | | | |
| Immobilization | ↓ | — | nl | ↓ |
| Milk alkali syndrome | ↓ | — | nl | ↓ |
| Hypophosphatasia | ↓ | — | nl | — |
| Acute and chronic renal failure | ↑ | — | nl | ↓ |
| Hyperthyroidism | ↓ | — | nl | ↓ |

*PTH*, Parathyroid hormone; *PTHrP*, parathyroid hormone related peptide; *nl*, normal; ↑, elevated; ↓, decreased; *DHT*, dihydrotachysterol.

similar to PTH (9 of the first 20 amino acids in the *N*-terminal part of PTHrP are identical to those in PTH). When produced in large amounts by the tumor during malignancy, it can act like PTH on bone to mobilize calcium stores. It is estimated that greater than 50% of all hypercalcemia associated with malignancy is due to the abnormal production of PTHrP (especially carcinomas of the head, neck, breast, kidney, lung, ovary, and bladder). The other 50% of tumors that cause humoral hypercalcemia produce other osteoclast activating factors (OAFs) such as interleukin I, prostaglandins, and other cytokines. Activated macrophages in chronic granulomatous diseases and activated lymphocytes in some lymphomas can produce hypercalcemia by an unregulated extrarenal metabolism of 25(OH)D to $1,25(OH)_2D$.

The availability of highly sensitive and specific assays for these calciotropic hormones allows ready identification of the underlying etiology of most hypercalcemic disorders. The etiology of hypercalcemia does affect prognosis. The interval between detection of hypercalcemia associated with malignancy and death is often less than 6 months. As shown in Table 37-1, although several cancers are associated with hypercalcemia, the majority are squamous cell carcinomas of the lung and kidney.

Patients with chronic granulomatous disorders often have hypercalciuria and may have hypercalcemia. For example, in sarcoidosis approximately 50% of patients are hypercalciuric and about 10% are hypercalcemic. The cause for the abnormality in calcium metabolism is due to the unregulated synthesis of $1,25(OH)_2D$ by the granulomatous tissue. Besides treating the underlying disorder, control of the hypercalcemia can often be achieved by inhibiting the extrarenal metabolism of 25(OH)D to $1,25(OH)_2D$ by either high-dose glucocorticoids or the cytochrome P-450 inhibitor ketoconazole. In addition, limiting vitamin D intake and decreasing exposure to sunlight decreases the amount of substrate, thus limiting the extrarenal production of $1,25(OH)_2D$. However, the patient should not be made intentionally vitamin D deficient, since that would cause osteomalacia.

The rare inherited disorder familial hypocalciuric hypercalcemia (FHH) is due to a defect in the calcium sensor in the parathyroid glands, which causes a set point defect and an inappropriate secretion of PTH, resulting in hypercalcemia and hypocalciuria due to increased tubular reabsorption of calcium by PTH. Hypercalcemia may be detected in the first decade of life, whereas hypercalcemia due to primary hyperparathyroidism and MEN syndromes is usually not observed then. The serum PTH values may be elevated in FHH, but they are usually normal or lower for the same degree of calcium elevation when compared to patients with primary hyperparathyroidism. It is difficult to make the diagnosis based on 24-hour urinary calcium excretion because the excretion depends on the glomerular filtration rate. These patients are usually identified because of asymptomatic hypercalcemia. The parathyroid glands demonstrate mild hyperplasia. Partial parathyroidectomy is not recommended because the remaining parathyroid tissue continues to secrete excessive amounts of PTH.

Vitamin D intoxication is a rare cause of hypercalcemia. The most likely settings are ingestion of foods inadvertently overfortified with vitamin D or incorrect prescribing or ingestion by patients (often elderly) who may take 50,000 IU of vitamin D daily instead of biweekly or monthly. Excessive exposure to sunlight does not produce vitamin D intoxication. However, the use of active vitamin D compounds for treating illnesses such as renal osteodystrophy and osteoporosis with oral calcitriol ($1,25[OH]_2D_3$) or dihydrotachysterol, and psoriasis with topical calcipotriene (Dovonex), can cause hypercalcemia.

It is estimated that about 1% of the calcium stores in bone can be mobilized during each month of strict bed rest. Immobilization of adults often causes hypercalciuria. Hypercalcemia is seen only when there is an underlying cause for a high bone turnover such as Paget disease, early or subclinical malignancy-associated hypercalcemia, hyperthyroidism, hyperparathyroidism, secondary hyperparathyroidism associated with renal failure, and in patients with spinal cord injury and paraplegia or quadriplegia; patients can mobilize up to 50% of the calcium from their skeleton within 6 months.

Thiazide diuretics, in combination with hyperparathyroidism, can exacerbate hypercalcemia due to the increased tubular reabsorption of calcium. Vitamin A intoxication is a rare cause of hypercalcemia, as is the hypercalcemia associated with renal failure that is often considered to be due to aluminum intoxication. Lithium carbonate in dosages of 900 to 1500 mg/day causes hypercalcemia in about 5% of patients taking this drug and may be associated with increased PTH levels.

Milk alkali syndrome, which was much more common several decades ago, is caused by excessive ingestion of calcium and absorbable antacids. It causes hypercalcemia in conjunction with some degree of renal failure.

***History.*** It is often difficult to make the diagnosis of hypercalcemia simply based on symptoms unless the patient has a history of kidney stones. The symptoms are often very subtle and limited to the patient or family member reporting increased fatigability, increased sleep requirement, and a change in the ability to concentrate. In more severe cases of hypercalcemia, symptoms may gradually progress to depression, confusion, and even coma. A history of kidney stones (either calcium oxalate or calcium phosphate) or a reduction in height due to spinal compression fractures may be the first presenting symptoms. Gastrointestinal symptoms are often prominent with constipation, anorexia, nausea, and vomiting. Pancreatitis and peptic ulcer disease are unusual but have been associated with hypercalcemia. Polyuria and polydipsia are often present but subtle. Chondrocalcinosis and pseudogout may be the first symptoms of hyperparathyroidism. Hypercalcemia increases the rate of cardiac repolarization, thus shortening the QT interval on the electrocardiogram (ECG). Bradycardia and first-degree atrioventricular (AV) block as well as arrhythmias may occur. Hypercalcemic patients who take digitalis may have an increased sensitivity to the drug. Patients should be asked if they take lithium, thiazide diuretics, excessive quantities of either vitamin A or vitamin D, aminophylline, aluminum-containing antacids, androgens, estrogens, or antiestrogens, since all have been associated with hypercalcemia.

Because of the non–life-threatening and often subtle symptoms associated with mild hypercalcemia, it is not unusual to see an elderly patient complaining of mild confusion, constipation, and fatigue. Thus it is only after a routine blood laboratory evaluation that hypercalcemia is identified.

*Physical examination.* The physical examination is not particularly helpful in the diagnosis of hypercalcemia. Clinical signs are not usually seen until the corrected total calcium is above 12 mg/dl and are more prominent when the total calcium is above 14 mg/dl. Muscle atrophy and proximal muscle weakness may be associated with symptoms of increased fatigue. However, patients with long-standing hyperparathyroidism can have a substantial reduction in their height due to multiple spinal compression fractures. Generalized or local bone pain due to osteitis fibrosa cystica may also be present. Muscle weakness, fatigue, depression, and mental status change in the setting of malignancy or other chronic illnesses could be caused by hypercalcemia. Calcifications in the cornea (band keratopathy) can sometimes be seen in severe chronic hypercalcemia. About 15% to 20% of patients with hyperparathyroidism may suffer from a kidney stone. Soft tissue calcifications are rarely observed in primary hyperparathyroidism because the elevated serum calcium is associated with a low or normal serum phosphorus; thus the Ca × phosphate product is not elevated. However, in situations where there is chronically elevated levels of both calcium and phosphorus (e.g., severe renal failure with secondary hyperparathyroidism and hyperphosphatemia), soft tissue calcifications especially along the tendons and ligaments and ends of digits can be found.

*Laboratory studies and diagnostic procedures.* The most cost-effective way of determining the etiology of hypercalcemia is to obtain at least two fasting serum calcium, phosphorus, and albumin determinations. The reason for a second analysis is that there may be a laboratory error or inadvertent hemoconcentration during blood collection or elevation in serum proteins, particularly albumin. Although fasting does not significantly affect serum calcium or albumin, it is more difficult to evaluate the serum phosphorus level in a nonfasting state. Dietary sources of phosphorus will transiently increase phosphorus levels and a glucose load will decrease serum phosphorus. There is little advantage to obtaining an ionized calcium because of its cost.

*Differential diagnosis.* If hypercalcemia is confirmed with two calcium and albumin levels (preferably in a fasting state), then a determination of intact PTH will differentiate between primary hyperparathyroidism and other causes. Other clinical cues, such as a low or low normal fasting phosphorus level in a patient in the fifth or sixth decade of life, suggest hyperparathyroidism. Because the PTH immunoradiometric assay (IRMA) is so specific (the C-terminal, N-terminal and midmolecule PTH assays are used less frequently because they often give false positive results in hypercalcemia of malignancy caused by PTHrP), an elevation in the circulating PTH levels in association with hypercalcemia essentially makes the diagnosis of some abnormality in the parathyroid glands. There is no need to do an extensive evaluation for other etiologies. All other hypercalcemic disorders, with the exception of FHH and chronic renal failure, will have either suppressed or undetectable levels of intact PTH when the serum calcium is elevated. If a malignancy is found associated with hypercalcemia, it is likely that the two are related and that there is no particular need to measure a PTHrP, which just adds cost to the evaluation. In addition, PTHrP is of no prognostic value. Thus the PTHrP assay is not routinely used for known malignancies. If there is a concern about an occult malignancy, it may be reasonable to measure IRMA PTHrP blood levels, since 50% of occult malignancies in hypercalcemic patients are associated with increased circulating levels of PTHrP. Disorders in extrarenal synthesis of $1,25(OH)_2D$ can be detected by measuring circulating levels of $1,25(OH)_2D$ in conjunction with hypercalcemia. Chronic granulomatous disorders (e.g., sarcoidosis) or lymphoma should be suspected in hypercalcemic patients with low or undetectable PTH levels and high normal or elevated $1,25(OH)_2D$. Since the extrarenal $1\alpha$-hydroxylase is sensitive to prednisone, a course of prednisone (40 mg/day) with an associated drop in serum calcium often makes the diagnosis of a chronic granulomatous disease. To rule out vitamin D intoxication, a markedly elevated 25(OH)D that is at least two times above the upper limit of normal (over 100 ng/ml) is usually necessary.

*Management.* Hypercalcemia is caused by an increase in (1) the mobilization of calcium from the bone, (2) intestinal calcium absorption, and (3) tubular reabsorption of calcium. Thus when the cause is in part due to an increase in intestinal calcium absorption such as patients with hyperparathyroidism, vitamin D intoxication, chronic granulomatous disorders, or lymphoma, patients can benefit by decreasing their dietary calcium intake to 600 to 800 mg a day and increasing their hydration. For patients with mild hypercalcemia (under 12 mg/dl) and no clinical manifestations, this often suffices until a cause is determined. Patients with a moderate elevation (12 to 14 mg/dl), with or without symptoms, usually benefit from treatment because the patients are often dehydrated, leading to a decrease in the glomerular filtration rate (GFR) and the renal clearance of sodium and calcium. Patients with severe hypercalcemia (over 14 mg/dl) usually require immediate therapeutic intervention (Table 37-2).

Hydration with isotonic saline is an important first step in correcting the extracellular fluid deficit. Hydration can usually be achieved by continuous infusion of 3 to 4 L of 0.9% sodium chloride over 24 to 48 hours. This usually results in increased urinary excretion of calcium (100 to 300 mg/dl) and a lowering of the serum calcium by about 1.5 to 2 mg/day. Hydration alone will not return the serum calcium to normal in moderate or severe hypercalcemia. When treating elderly patients with compromised cardiac or renal function in the hospital, fluid inputs and outputs need to be documented. A loop diuretic can help prevent fluid overload.

After hydration has been achieved, a loop diuretic can be used to inhibit tubular reabsorption of sodium and calcium. Usually small doses of furosemide (10 to 20 mg) or ethacrynic acid (50 to 100 mg) will be of benefit.

**Table 37-2.** Management of hypercalcemia

| Therapy | Dosage | Onset | Side effects |
|---|---|---|---|
| **Hydration and diuresis** | | | |
| Hydration | 3-4 L saline/24 hr | Rapid | Congestive heart failure |
| Furosemide | 10-40 mg IV | Rapid | Hypokalemia |
| Ethacrynic acid | 50-100 mg IV | Rapid | |
| **Inhibition of calcium mobilization from skeleton** | | | |
| Calcitonin | 4-8 U/kg SQ, IM, or IV 6-12 hr | 2-6 hr | Nausea, rapid tolerance (1-2 weeks) |
| Etidronate | 7.5 mg/kg IV 2-4 hr | 1-2 days | |
| Pamidronate | 30-90 mg IV 2-4 hr | 1-2 days | Transient fever |
| Plicamycin (Mithracin) | 15-25 μg/kg IV 4-6 hr | 12-24 hr | Thrombocytopenia, neutropenia, nausea, nephrotoxicity, hepatic toxicity |
| Gallium nitrate | 200 mg/m$^2$ IV 24 hr | 3-5 days | Nephrotoxicity, hypophosphatemia |
| Phosphate | 250-350 mg PO qid; 1-1.5 g IV 6-8 hr | Rapid | Soft tissue calcification can cause rapid decline in serum calcium |
| **Decreased intestinal calcium absorption** | | | |
| Hydrocortisone | 100-200 mg/day | 2-3 days | Cushing's syndrome |
| Prednisone | 40-80 mg/day | 2-3 days | Cushing's syndrome |
| Decrease dietary calcium intake to 600-800 mg/day | | | |
| **Miscellaneous** | | | |
| Dialysis | | | |
| Mobilization | | | |

Excessive use of loop diuretics causes dehydration and electrolyte abnormalities, including hypokalemia and hypomagnesemia. Only in life-threatening situations is aggressive hydration with up to 6 L of isotonic saline along with a loop diuretic such as furosemide, 50 to 100 mg every 1 to 2 hours, warranted. Urinary excretion of calcium of up to 1000 mg/day and a decrease of about 3 to 4 mg/dl of serum calcium can be achieved.

Bisphosphonates, in particular intravenous pamidronate or etidronate, have been of great value in inhibiting bone calcium mobilization due to hypercalcemia of malignancy. Daily infusion of 30 to 90 mg of pamidronate for 3 days or 7.5 mg/kg of etidronate over 2 to 4 hours for 3 days causes the calcium to decrease within 2 days and reach a nadir after 7 days. Intravenous etidronate is as well tolerated and safe as pamidronate. Some patients (about 20%) receiving pamidronate develop a transient fever that is usually controlled with acetaminophen. Mild, usually asymptomatic, hypercalcemia lasting for several days to several weeks may develop when using a bisphosphonate. Oral etidronate therapy has not been found to be useful for treating hypercalcemia of malignancy.

Calcitonin is very effective in rapidly lowering hypercalcemia associated with increased bone calcium mobilization. The dosage of calcitonin is 4 to 8 U/kg, given either intravenously, subcutaneously, or intramuscularly every 6 to 8 hours. The serum calcium will begin to decrease within 2 hours. However, tachyphylaxis often occurs, and therefore this drug is only of value for a few days to a few weeks. This drug is especially useful in life-threatening hypercalcemia while waiting for the more sustained effects from intravenous etidronate or pamidronate or other calcium-lowering drugs such as plicamycin and gallium nitrate. Calcitonin therapy may be associated with transient nausea, cramping, abdominal pain, and flushing.

Plicamycin (Mithracin) is a cytotoxic drug that inhibits bone resorption. It has lost favor with the advent of intravenous bisphosphonate therapy because of associated toxicities. The usual dosage of 15 to 25 μg/kg intravenously over 4 to 6 hours causes the serum calcium to decrease within 12 to 24 hours. The serum calcium usually reaches a nadir by 48 to 72 hours. If hypercalcemia recurs, treatment with 10 to 15 μg/kg twice a week often returns the serum calcium to normal. Toxicity is usually associated with the frequency of treatment and total dosage; side effects include thrombocytopenia, hepatocellular necrosis leading to transient increases in transaminases, decreased levels of clotting factors resulting in bleeding, azotemia, proteinuria, and hypocalcemia. Because of the toxicities, plicamycin is of limited value in treating chronic hypercalcemia. Its major benefit is in the rapid control of severe symptomatic hypercalcemia.

Gallium nitrate also inhibits bone resorption. A 5-day infusion of 200 mg/m$^2$/day normalizes calcium in about 75% of patients. However, because of its relatively slow onset and associated nephrotoxicity and severe hypophosphatemia, this therapy has been of limited value.

Other therapies include glucocorticoids, which increase urinary calcium excretion and decrease intestinal calcium absorption when given in a dosage of 40 to 200 mg of prednisone daily in divided doses, or 200 to 300 mg of hydrocortisone or its equivalent intravenously for 3 to 5 days. Glucocorticoids are very effective in treating hypercalcemia from vitamin D intoxication as well as hypercalcemia from extrarenal production of $1,25(OH)_2D$ associated with chronic granulomatous disorders and some lymphomas. They have been less effective in patients with hypercalcemia of malignancy and primary hyperparathyroidism.

Phosphate therapy is effective for treating chronic hypercalcemia and acute hypercalcemia. However, it is important not to increase the blood levels of phosphate so as to cause a high calcium/phosphate product that will increase risk of nephrocalcinosis and soft tissue calcification. The usual treatment is 1 to 1.5 g of phosphate daily for several days, given in four divided doses to minimize chances of developing hyperphosphatemia. Intravenous phosphate is one of the most effective treatments for treating severe hypercalcemia; however, because of its associated toxicity (nephrocalcinosis and hypocalcemia), it is rarely used except in the most severe hypercalcemic patients with cardiac or renal failure. A dosage of 1500 mg of phosphate intravenously over 6 to 8 hours leads to a prompt and precipitous decrease in serum calcium by as much as 3 to 6 mg/dl in patients with initially normal serum inorganic phosphate concentrations. Since the serum calcium concentrations can rapidly drop, it is important to monitor the serum calcium frequently to prevent potentially fatal hypocalcemia.

Thus there are several therapies for treating hypercalcemia. Mild hypercalcemia can usually be treated by decreasing dietary intake of calcium and by hydration. In a hospital setting intravenous isotonic saline with a loop diuretic is reasonable. However, more severe hypercalcemia (over 14 mg/dl) often requires rapid correction. Calcitonin acts rapidly (within hours) and is usually very effective with minimal side effects. At the same time aggressive hydration and sodium and calcium diuresis should be instituted. The bisphosphonates have become the standard treatment for chronic management of hypercalcemia. Because of the associated side effects with phosphate, gallium nitrate, and plicamycin, these agents are less often used.

Patients over the age of 50 with mild hypercalcemia and documented hyperparathyroidism who do not have a history of radiopaque kidney stones, nephrocalcinosis, generalized bone pain, or multiple nontraumatic fractures and have normal renal function and bone mass can be followed with careful monitoring. Patients under age 50 should have surgery, given the high likelihood of osteoporosis and the long surveillance that would be required. Guidelines recommended for surgery in patients with asymptomatic hyperparathyroidism include (1) elevated serum calcium of more than 1 to 1.6 mg/dl above the upper limit of normal of the laboratory, (2) history of a life-threatening hypercalcemia, such as an episode induced by dehydration and recurring illness (3) the presence of kidney stones, (4) a recent reduction in creatinine clearance by greater than 30% compared to aged-matched controls, (5) elevation of 24-hour urine calcium excretion above 400 mg or a urinary Ca/Cr of over 0.35, and (6) reduction in bone mass more than 2 S.D. below the normal by one of several noninvasive methods for measuring bone mass. In patients who do not want immediate surgery, it is advisable to follow bone density measurements regularly. If documented demineralization is found, the potential positive impact of surgery can be stressed more. Also, some post-menopausal women who decline surgery may benefit from estrogen therapy, which may decrease bone turnover.

## Hypocalcemia

***Epidemiology and etiology.*** Hypocalcemia is not often encountered in an outpatient setting because it is corrected physiologically by an increase in the secretion of PTH and the production of $1,25(OH)_2D$, which mobilize calcium stores from bone and increase the efficiency of intestinal calcium absorption. However, a defect in the production or recognition of PTH or $1,25(OH)_2D_3$ or a chronic deficiency of vitamin D can precipitate hypocalcemia. Chronic hypocalcemia is caused by vitamin D deficiency, chronic renal failure, hereditary and acquired hypoparathyroidism, pseudohypoparathyroidism, hereditary disorders in vitamin D metabolism and vitamin D resistance, and hypomagnesemia (Table 37-3).

There are occasions when total serum concentrations of calcium do not reflect the free ionized calcium available to cells. Up to 50% of patients in an intensive care setting are reported to have calcium concentrations below 8.5 mg/dl; however, fewer than 10% have a reduction in ionized calcium. Patients who are critically ill may have transient hypocalcemia in association with burns, severe sepsis, acute renal failure, and extensive transfusions with citrated blood. Acidosis will increase ionized calcium concentrations, whereas alkalosis will decrease ionized calcium concentrations due to decreases and increases in the binding of calcium to albumin, respectively. In many chronic illnesses substantial reductions in serum albumin concentrations are often seen, and this may lower total serum calcium concentrations while the ionized calcium concentration remains normal. At pH 7.4, hypoalbuminemia can be corrected by adding 0.8 mg/dl to the total serum calcium for every 1 g/dl by which serum albumin is lower than 4 g/dl (see previous discussion). Medications such as heparin, glucagon, and protamine may cause transient hypocalcemia. Also, patients with acute pancreatitis have varying degrees of hypocalcemia that usually resolves with the resolution of the acute inflammatory process.

***Pathophysiology.*** The calcium sensor in the parathyroid glands is exquisitely sensitive to small changes in serum ionized calcium concentrations. A small decrease in $Ca^{++}$ results in an increase in the synthesis and secretion of PTH. If a defect in either the synthesis or recognition of PTH is present, hypocalcemia can occur. Idiopathic hypoparathyroidism is manifested by hypocalcemia with a low or absent PTH level. It most often occurs as part of an autoimmune syndrome (see Chapter 39). Congenital aplasia of the parathyroid glands is rare and usually is in conjunction with a defective development of the thymus (DiGeorge syndrome). Surgical hypoparathyroidism can be transient or permanent following neck surgery for thyroid disease due to inadvertent removal of or damage to the parathyroid glands or their vascular supply. The most common form of transient or permanent hypoparathyroidism occurs after surgical correction for primary hyperparathyroidism. Calcium levels decrease for several

**Table 37-3** Causes of hypocalcemia

| Disorder | PTH | 25(OH)D | 1,25$(OH)_2$D |
|---|---|---|---|
| **PTH deficiency** | | | |
| Hereditary (idiopathic) | ↓ | nl | nl or ↓ |
| Postsurgical | ↓ | nl | nl or ↓ |
| Hypomagnesemia | ↓ | nl | nl or ↓ |
| Di George syndrome | ↓ | nl | — |
| Neonatal hypocalcemia | ↓ | nl or ↓ | — |
| **Vitamin D deficiency** | | | |
| Malabsorption syndromes | ↑ | ↓↓ | ↓, nl, or ↑ |
| Liver disease | ↑ | ↓↓ | ↓, nl, or ↑ |
| Lack in diet | ↑ | ↓↓ | ↓, nl, or ↑ |
| Sunscreen use | ↑ | ↓↓ | ↓, nl, or ↑ |
| Lack of exposure to sunlight | ↑ | ↓↓ | ↓, nl, or ↑ |
| Antiseizure medications | ↑ | ↓↓ | ↓, nl, or ↑ |
| **PTH resistance** | | | |
| Pseudohypoparathyroidism | ↑ | nl | nl or ↓ |
| Hypomagnesemia | ↓ | nl | — |
| **1,25$(OH)_2$D insufficiency** | | | |
| Chronic renal failure | ↑ | nl | ↓ |
| Hyperphosphatemia | ↑ | nl | ↓ |
| Vitamin D–dependent rickets type I | ↑ | nl | ↓ |
| Oncogenic osteomalacia | ↑ | nl | ↓ |
| X-linked hypophosphatemic rickets | ↑ | nl | nl or ↓ |
| **1,25$(OH)_2$D resistance** | | | |
| Vitamin D–dependent rickets type II | ↑ | ↓ or nl | ↑↑ |
| **Miscellaneous** | | | |
| Acute pancreatitis | ↑ | nl | — |
| Citrated blood transfusion | ↑ | nl | — |
| Osteoblastic metastases | ↑ | nl | — |
| Acute rhabdomyolysis | ↑ | nl | — |
| Acute renal failure | ↑ | nl | — |
| Hungry bone syndrome after parathyroidectomy | nl or ↓ | nl | — |
| Foscarnet | ↑ | nl | — |
| Radiographic dyes containing EDTA | — | nl | — |

*nl*, Normal; ↓, decreased; ↑, increased; *EDTA*, ethylenediamenetetraacetic acid.

reasons. In patients with an autonomous parathyroid adenoma the chronic hypercalcemia suppresses the normal parathyroid tissue. Chronic hyperparathyroidism also results in osteitis fibrosa cystica, which causes a calcium deficit in the skeleton. Immediately after removal of the adenoma, PTH levels precipitously drop, resulting in hypocalcemia. The remaining suppressed parathyroid glands usually begin secreting PTH, and correction of the hypocalcemia is seen within days. However, hypocalcemia can persist for days to several weeks as the calcium-deficient "hungry bones" begin to remineralize.

Hypomagnesemia below 1 mg/dl is often associated with hypocalcemia. Low magnesium impairs both the release and responsiveness of PTH. Correcting the hypomagnesemia results in an increase in PTH levels and a normalization of serum calcium. Other syndromes associated with a defective production of PTH are listed in Table 37-3.

Hypocalcemia, in association with elevated PTH levels, is most commonly seen in patients with chronic renal failure, vitamin D deficiency, abnormalities in the recognition or metabolism of vitamin D, PTH resistant syndromes, and other miscellaneous causes (see Table 37-3).

In chronic renal failure there is a decrease in the clearance of phosphate, causing hyperphosphatemia, which leads to a decreased production of 1,25$(OH)_2$D and a decrease in the efficiency of intestinal calcium absorption. This results in increased PTH levels, which mobilizes calcium stores from the bone to satisfy the body's calcium requirement. Thus maintaining normal serum phosphate concentrations in the early stages of chronic renal failure ameliorates the secondary hyperparathyroidism that results from mild to moderate renal failure. When the GFR is below about 30% normal, the reserved capacity to produce 1,25$(OH)_2$D is so compromised that, even with a normal serum phosphate, PTH levels rise because of hypocalcemia. Thus, initially, careful management of patients before dialysis with restriction of dietary phosphate and the use of phosphate-binding antacids is of great value (see hyperphosphatemia section). Later calcium supplementation (800 to 1000 mg/day) along with calcitriol (0.25 to 0.5 μg once or twice a day) will maintain serum calcium in the normal range and prevent secondary hyperparathyroidism. Secondary hyperparathyroidism should be avoided because of its devastating consequences to the skeleton causing renal osteodystrophy.

Since it is often assumed that vitamin D deficiency causes hypocalcemia, when the routine blood workup reveals a normal calcium, the diagnosis of vitamin D deficiency is dismissed. However, in the early stages of vitamin D insufficiency the transient hypocalcemia is quickly corrected by secondary hyperparathyroidism. Thus patients with vitamin D insufficiency and early vitamin D deficiency initially have low normal serum calciums with low normal fasting serum phosphorus, an elevated PTH level, and a normal or even elevated $1,25(OH)_2D$ level. If vitamin D deficiency persists, hypocalcemia and hypophosphatemia with low 25(OH)D (under 10 ng/ml) and elevated PTH levels are often seen. Any reduction in the production of $1,25(OH)_2D$ by the kidney can lead to hypocalcemia and secondary hyperparathyroidism. Vitamin D–dependent rickets type I is an inherited disorder of the renal 25(OH)D-1α-hydroxylase leading to low or undetectable levels of $1,25(OH)_2D$. In oncogenic osteomalacia usually a benign tumor secretes a substance that inhibits 1α-hydroxylation of 25(OH)D and causes phosphaturia, resulting in low blood levels of $1,25(OH)_2D$ and phosphorus and painful bones. Patients with vitamin D–dependent rickets type II have markedly elevated levels of $1,25(OH)_2D$ because of a vitamin D receptor defect. This rare disorder is often associated with alopecia totalis.

Vitamin D deficiency is being recognized as a common problem for the elderly, who are less likely to be outdoors where sunlight can stimulate vitamin $D_3$ production in the skin. In addition, aging and sunscreen use substantially diminish the synthesis of vitamin $D_3$ in the skin. Although aging does not decrease the intestinal absorption of vitamin D, intestinal malabsorption syndromes that affect the small intestine (especially the duodenum and jejunum) can markedly reduce the absorption of vitamin D. Similarly, patients with chronic severe parenchymal and cholestatic liver disease often have vitamin D deficiency due to the associated malabsorption syndrome as well as a decreased hepatic capacity to convert vitamin D to 25(OH)D. Patients with seizure disorders who are institutionalized and are not obtaining an adequate source of vitamin D either from the diet or exposure to sunlight are more prone to developing vitamin D deficiency (25[OH]D under 10 ng/ml) and the associated bone disease (rickets or osteomalacia). This is most often seen when patients take more than one antiseizure medication, e.g., phenytoin and phenobarbital. This deficiency state is usually easily corrected by increasing the vitamin D intake to 800 to 1000 IU daily or increasing exposure to sunlight.

Pseudohypoparathyroidism is a hereditary disorder that is associated with elevated PTH levels, hypocalcemia, and hyperphosphatemia. Features such as short stature, round face, skeletal abnormalities (brachydactyly) and heterotrophic calcifications are associated with Albright hereditary osteodystrophy. A defective renal response to PTH can be demonstrated by measuring the urinary output of cyclic AMP in response to PTH administration. Other causes of hypocalcemia include acute pancreatitis, multiple citrated blood transfusions, osteoblastic metastases, and hyperphosphatemia associated with extensive tissue or cell damage such as acute rhabdomyolysis. Usually in these acute and chronic situations the secondary hyperparathyroidism is unable to compensate for the hypocalcemic stimulus, and hypocalcemia ensues.

*History.* A gradual lowering of the serum calcium or a corrected calcium of more than 8 mg/dl often will not cause any symptoms. However, precipitous drops in the serum calcium by 2 to 3 mg/dl observed after surgery for a parathyroid adenoma or after aggressive therapy to treat hypercalcemia can cause neuromuscular irritability, sensations of numbness, and tingling involving fingertips, toes, and the circumoral region (see the box below). When the corrected calcium is below about 7 mg/dl, patients often complain of carpopedal spasms.

*Physical examination.* Increased neuromuscular irritability can be demonstrated by eliciting a positive Chvostek sign by gently tapping the facial nerve just anterior to the ear, resulting in the twitching of the circumoral muscles. Trousseau sign is a carpal spasm elicited by inflation of a blood pressure cuff to 20 mm Hg above the patient's systolic blood pressure for 3 to 5 minutes. Flexion of the wrist and metacarpophalangeal joints, extension of the interphalangeal joints, and adduction of the digits reflect the heightened irritability of the nerves to ischemia in the region below the cuff. Whereas approximately 10% of normal individuals demonstrate a slight positive Chvostek sign, a positive Trousseau sign is rarely seen in the absence of significant hypocalcemia. In more severe hypocalcemia muscle cramps of the legs and feet progress to spontaneous carpopedal spasm (tetany), laryngeal spasm or bronchospasm, seizures of all types, and respiratory arrest. Mental changes include irritability, psychosis, and depression. The QT interval on the ECG is prolonged, and arrhythmias can occur.

Patients with longstanding hypocalcemia due to idiopathic hypoparathyroidism or pseudohypoparathyroidism may have calcification of the basal ganglia and extrapyramidal neurologic symptoms. Subcapsular cataracts and abnormal dentition are also common in these patients.

*Laboratory studies and diagnostic procedures.* The diagnosis of hypocalcemia is most easily made when the serum

**Signs and symptoms associated with hypocalcemia**

Chvostek's sign
Trousseau's sign
Neuromuscular irritability
Paresthesias
Tetany
Laryngospasm
Bronchospasm
Seizures

calcium is below the normal range (usually 8.5 mg/dl) with a normal serum albumin. When hypoalbuminemia exists and the correction for the hypoalbuminemia does not correct the serum calcium, then hypocalcemia is also diagnosed. A low serum PTH associated with hypocalcemia is most likely caused by either idiopathic hypoparathyroidism, surgically induced hypoparathyroidism, or hypomagnesemia (see Table 37-3). An elevated PTH associated with hypocalcemia is due either to a primary defect in the recognition of PTH or secondary hyperparathyroidism. The most common cause of hypocalcemia associated with elevated PTH is secondary hyperparathyroidism due to vitamin D deficiency. A low serum 25(OH)D (usually less than 10 mg/ml) with or without hypophosphatemia and secondary hyperparathyroidism is diagnostic. Measurement of $1,25(OH)_2D$ is of little value in evaluating vitamin D deficiency because it can be low, normal, or elevated depending on the degree and duration of the deficiency except in acquired and inherited disorders of vitamin D metabolism such as chronic renal failure, vitamin D–dependent rickets type I, and oncogenic osteomalacia, where low circulating levels of $1,25(OH)_2D$ with secondary hyperparathyroidism and hypocalcemia are usually seen.

***Differential diagnosis.*** Care must be taken to ensure true hypocalcemia is present. Chronic hypocalcemia can usually be associated with the absence of PTH or its ineffectiveness, the absence of vitamin D, or a defect in vitamin D metabolism or in the recognition of $1,25(OH)_2D$ by its target tissues. Since hypoparathyroidism, pseudohypoparathyroidism, and vitamin D–dependent rickets types I and II are typically lifelong illnesses, the recent onset of hypocalcemia in an adult is usually due to renal failure, small intestinal malabsorption disorders, vitamin D deficiency, magnesium deficiency, or an acquired defect in the metabolism of vitamin D.

Hypomagnesemia can cause neuromuscular irritability and paresthesias similar to hypocalcemia, and this should be ruled out whether hypocalcemia is present or not. Hypocalcemia can also be precipitated by the aggressive treatment of medications intended to reverse hypercalcemia such as plicamycin, bisphosphonates, calcitonin, and oral or parenteral phosphate. Radiographic dyes that contain the calcium chelater EDTA, citrated blood, and the phosphorus-containing drug foscarnet (trisodium phosphonoformate) that is used to treat opportunistic infections in AIDS patients can cause reductions in total and ionized serum calcium concentrations.

***Management.*** Management approaches for hypocalcemia depend in part on the severity of the hypocalcemia, the acuteness of onset, and the symptoms. For acute symptomatic hypocalcemia the intravenous administration of calcium salts such as calcium gluconate (90 mg elemental calcium/10 ml ampule) is recommended. Calcium chloride (272 mg elemental calcium/10 ml ampule) should be used with caution because it causes irritation of the veins. Initially 1 or 2 ampules of calcium gluconate diluted in 50 to 100 ml of 5% dextrose (180 mg elemental calcium) should be infused over 5 to 10 minutes. This procedure should be repeated as necessary to control symptomatic and potentially life-threatening hypocalcemia. Persistent or less severe hypocalcemia can be managed by administration of more dilute calcium solutions over a longer period. Infusion of 15 mg/kg of elemental calcium over 4 to 6 hours will raise the serum calcium by 2 to 3 mg/dl (0.5 to 0.75 mmol/L). For example, to initiate therapy in a 60-kg patient with a calcium level of 4.5 mg/dl, 10 ampules of calcium gluconate (900 mg $Ca^{++}$) in 1 L of 5% dextrose infused at a rate of 50 ml/hour will provide approximately 45 mg of elemental calcium per hour. The rate of infusion can be regulated based on the serum calcium and symptoms. Hypomagnesemic patients who have concomitant hypocalcemia require magnesium supplementation before the hypocalcemia can resolve (see hypomagnesemia section).

Patients with vitamin D deficiency and no associated intestinal malabsorption syndrome can be given 50,000 IU of vitamin $D_2$ twice a week for 1 to 2 months. Once the 25(OH)D levels have returned to normal (optimally 25 to 45 ng/ml), the patient usually remains vitamin D sufficient if provided a multivitamin containing 400 IU of vitamin D. There is no need for concern about potential vitamin D intoxication for a patient who may drink a quart of milk containing 400 IU of vitamin D, take a multivitamin containing 400 IU of vitamin D, and be exposed to sunlight. Vitamin D intoxication is usually seen when patients ingest over 5000 IU of vitamin D daily. Patients with small intestinal malabsorption syndromes can obtain their vitamin D from exposure to sunlight (suberythemal doses on hands, arms, and face two or three times a week; in northern latitudes little vitamin D is produced in the skin in the winter), artificial ultraviolet B radiation, or intramuscular injections of 50,000 to 100,000 IU of vitamin $D_2$. Patients on total parenteral nutrition (TPN) usually get their vitamin D from the multivitamin preparation that is added to their TPN solution. Patients with a partial malabsorption syndrome may benefit from increased doses of vitamin D either with 50,000 units of vitamin D or using the liquid vitamin D (8000 IU/ml) and titrating their dose to maintain their serum 25(OH)D level in the midnormal range (about 25 to 35 ng/ml).

Patients with severe liver disease and malabsorption may benefit from calcidiol ($25[OH]D_3$) therapy. One capsule (20 or 50 μg of $25[OH]D_3$) per day is helpful in treating vitamin D deficiency associated with severe hepatic dysfunction.

Hypocalcemia associated with hypoparathyroidism, pseudohypoparathyroidism, renal failure, and acquired and inherited disorders of vitamin D metabolism and recognition have benefited greatly with the oral or intravenous use of calcitriol ($1,25[OH]_2D_3$). Calcium supplementation of 800 to 1000 mg along with calcitriol of 0.25 μg twice a day is often adequate to increase the efficiency of intestinal calcium absorption to restore serum calcium into the normal range. However, sometimes a dosage as high as 0.5 to 1 μg twice a day is required. Intravenous calcitriol after dialysis has gained favor because of the drug's effect on reversing hypocalcemia and possibly having a direct inhibitory effect on the parathyroid glands. Caution should be exercised when using calcium in combination with calcitriol because hypercalcemia can occur. Therefore this therapy requires frequent serum calcium determinations until a stable dosage of calcium and calcitriol is established. This problem is especially important in treating surgically induced hypoparathyroidism, since the hypocalcemia is transient. Initially, more calcium and calcitriol are needed to satisfy the hungry bone syndrome. However, once normal parathyroid function is restored and the hungry bone is satisfied, calcitriol therapy can often be stopped. Dihydrotachysterol, which is a pseudo-1α-hydroxy analogue that mimics the actions of $1,25(OH)_2D$, has lost favor because of its long half-life in the circulation and potential toxicity.

## PHOSPHORUS METABOLISM

An adult body contains approximately 600 g of phosphorus; 85% is present in the crystalline structure of the skeleton, and the other 15% is found in extracellular fluids. Most of the phosphorus in the circulation is in the form of inorganic phosphate ions $(PO_4)^{-3}$, and in soft tissues the phosphorus is found as phosphate esters such as ATP. Only about 10% of the inorganic phosphorus is bound to protein. In addition to age, sex, and pH, the serum phosphorus concentration is affected by diet, thus making a nonfasting level difficult to interpret. For example, after a meal, the increase in insulin enhances cellular phosphorus uptake, thereby decreasing serum phosphorus levels. Serum phosphorus levels are higher in children and in women after the menopause. There is a circadian variation in phosphorus concentration even during a 24-hour fast; the nadir occurs between 9 AM and noon followed by an increase to a plateau in the afternoon and another small peak after midnight. Alkalosis and acidosis cause a decrease and increase in serum phosphorus, respectively.

Phosphorus is efficiently absorbed by the small intestine. Although most phosphorus absorption is passive, $1,25(OH)_2D$ increases phosphorus absorption in the duodenum, jejunum, and ileum. A low phosphorus intake increases the efficiency of intestinal absorption to 80% to 90%. Up to 70% of phosphorus in foods with a high phosphorus content, such as dairy products, meats, and eggs, can be absorbed. Thus hypophosphatemia due to deficient intestinal absorption is unusual except when nonabsorbable antacids like aluminum hydroxide are consumed.

The major control of phosphorus balance is exerted by the kidney. About 90% of the phosphorus in the circulation is filtered through the glomerulus and is largely absorbed in the proximal tubule, so only 10% to 15% of the filtered load is normally excreted. Urinary excretion of phosphorus reflects dietary intake. Although proximal reabsorption of phosphorus depends on parallel sodium reabsorption in the proximal tubule, sodium reabsorption in the distal convoluted tubule is independent of phosphorus. Therefore volume expansion and decreased sodium reabsorption increase phosphorus clearance.

### Hypophosphatemia

***Pathophysiology.*** Hypophosphatemia can be caused by decreased intestinal absorption of phosphorus, increased losses of phosphate in the urine, and a shift of phosphorus from extracellular to intracellular compartments (see the box at right). Increased renal secretion of phosphorus occurs in states of excess PTH such as primary hyperparathyroidism, vitamin D deficiency, vitamin D–resistant and vitamin D–dependent rickets, as well as hyperglycemic states and oncogenic osteomalacia. Serum phosphorus is low in vitamin D deficiency, due not only to the secondary hyperparathyroidism but also because of a decrease in efficiency of intestinal phosphorus absorption. In X-linked hypophosphatemic rickets and oncogenic osteomalacia there is a severe renal leak of phosphorus into the urine. In hyperglycemic states associated with polyuria and acidosis, inorganic phosphorus is lost in the urine in excessive amounts. Ketoacidosis enhances intracellular organic phosphorus degradation, thereby releasing large amounts of inorganic phosphorus into the plasma that is cleared into the urine. In a ketotic patient the serum phosphorus is often normal because of the continuous shift of phosphorus from intracellular to extracellular pools. However, when the ketoacidosis is corrected, hypophosphatemia often becomes manifest because of the return of phosphorus into the intracellular compartment. Rarely, hypophosphatemia is a paraneoplastic syndrome, most often associated with benign bone tumors but occasionally with small cell lung or prostate cancers.

Alcohol abuse is the most common cause of severe hypophosphatemia. Alcoholics usually have a low dietary phosphorus intake, and the use of calcium- or aluminum-containing antacids and vomiting contribute further. Ethanol also enhances urinary inorganic phosphorus excretion, and marked phosphaturia often occurs during episodes of alcoholic ketoacidosis. Intense hyperventilation for prolonged periods may depress serum phosphorus levels due to the associated alkalosis. Advanced leukemia with blast crisis (leukocyte counts usually above 100,000) has been associated with severe hypophosphatemia; the likely cause is rapid uptake of phosphate into rapidly dividing cells.

#### Causes for hypophosphatemia

- Decreased intestinal phosphate absorption
  - Vitamin D deficiency
  - Vitamin D–dependent rickets types I and II
  - Malabsorption
  - Antacid abuse
  - Alcohol abuse
  - Intracellular shift of phosphorus to extracellular compartment
  - Ketoacidosis
- Increased renal phosphate excretion
  - Hyperparathyroidism
  - Vitamin D deficiency
  - Vitamin D–dependent rickets types I and II
  - X-linked hypophosphatemic rickets
  - Oncogenic osteomalacia
  - Hyperglycemic states
  - Alcohol abuse
- Other
  - Respiratory alkalosis
  - Blast crisis in leukemia
  - Starvation

### Clinical signs and symptoms of severe hypophosphatemia

| | |
|---|---|
| Encephalopathy | Bone pain |
| Seizures | Rickets/osteomalacia |
| Muscle weakness | Cardiomyopathy |
| Rhabdomyolysis | Red cell dysfunction |

***History and physical examination.*** Mild hypophosphatemia is usually not associated with any clinical symptoms. However, severe hypophosphatemia can cause a variety of clinical symptoms compatible with metabolic encephalopathy, as outlined in the box above. Patients may appear irritable and apprehensive and complain of muscle weakness, numbness, and paresthesias. In the most severe form they appear severely confused or are obtunded and suffer from seizures and coma. Diffuse slowing of the EEG can be observed.

Since phosphorus is essential for muscle action through the high-energy bonds (ATP and creatine phosphate), patients with severe hypophosphatemia may suffer from muscle weaknesses, myalgia, and myopathy. Patients with preexisting phosphate deficiency who develop acute hypophosphatemia may develop rhabdomyolysis. Chronic hypophosphatemia causes rickets in children and osteomalacia in adults. Patients with oncogenic osteomalacia with chronic low phosphorus levels often complain of severe bone pain, especially of their long bones. Severe hypophosphatemia has also been associated with cardiomyopathy characterized by a low cardiac output.

***Management.*** Mild hypophosphatemia usually corrects when the underlying cause is addressed. Oral phosphate replacement is sufficient if serum phosphorus is greater than 1 mg/dl and the patient is without symptoms. Milk is an excellent source of phosphorus, containing 1 g of inorganic phosphorus per quart. Neutraphos tablets, which contain 250 mg of inorganic phosphate per tablet as a sodium or potassium salt, can provide up to 3 g a day (3 tablets of Neutraphos every 6 hours). The serum phosphorus level rises by as much as 1.5 mg/dl within 1 to 2 hours after ingestion of 1000 mg of phosphorus.

Severe hypophosphatemia with serum levels lower than 0.5 mg/dl may require as much as 3 g of phosphorus per day over several days to replete the body stores. In patients with severe symptomatic hypophosphatemia who are unable to eat, intravenous phosphorus can be given—up to 1 g in 1 L of fluid over 8 to 12 hours. Some caution is necessary because of the potential for developing associated hypocalcemia and soft tissue calcification. A 15- to 30-ml phosphosoda enema solution composed of buffered sodium phosphate three to four times a day is also useful in correcting severe hypophosphatemia in patients who are unable to take oral phosphorus.

## Hyperphosphatemia

***Pathophysiology.*** Hyperphosphatemia of clinical significance occurs in renal failure and hypoparathyroid states (see the box above). In renal failure the loss of glomerular and tubular function results in impaired phosphorus excretion. Increasing the serum phosphorus level causes a decreased renal production of $1,25(OH)_2D_3$, often producing hypocalcemia. In the absence of renal failure a defect in the renal excretion of phosphorus may be found in pseudohypoparathyroidism and tumor calcinosis. The bisphosphonate etidronate increases renal phosphorus reabsorption and can cause hyperphosphatemia. Vitamin D intoxication either due to excessive ingestion of vitamin D or one of its metabolites or analogues can cause hyperphosphatemia along with hypercalcemia. Severe hyperthermia, crush injuries, nontraumatic rhabdomyolysis, and cytotoxic therapy of hematologic malignancy such as acute lymphoblastic leukemia are also associated with hyperphosphatemia.

### Causes of hyperphosphatemia

Decreased renal phosphate excretion
- Acute renal failure
- Chronic renal failure
- Hypoparathyroidism
- Tumor calcinosis
- Bisphosphonates
- Hypoparathyroid states
- Idiopathic hypoparathyroidism
- Pseudohypoparathyroidism

Other
- Vitamin D intoxication
- Metabolic and respiratory acidosis
- Crush injuries
- Rhabdomyolysis
- Cytotoxic therapy

***History and physical examination.*** When there is a rapid elevation in serum phosphorus levels, the associated hypocalcemia can cause symptoms such as neuromuscular irritability and tetany (see the hypocalcemia section). Chronic hyperphosphatemia in association with a normal calcium can cause nephrocalcinosis and soft tissue calcifications.

***Management.*** The goal is to treat the underlying disorder and return the serum phosphorus to the normal range. Because most foods have a high phosphorus content, it is often very difficult to limit dietary phosphorus intake. However, the goal is to decrease dietary phosphorus to approximately 600 to 1000 mg per day with modest protein restriction. Aluminum hydroxide and aluminum carbonate bind phosphorus in the intestine; therefore 30 to 60 ml of gel or 1 to 4 tablets with each meal help decrease phosphorus absorption. This has been of particular value to patients with renal failure. However, concern about aluminum toxicity causing encephalopathy, osteomalacia, proximal myopathy, and anemia are of concern. Therefore it is now recommended that calcium salts be used in place of aluminum salts as the first line of phosphate binders. Initially 1 g of calcium carbonate with each meal can be gradually increased to 8 to 12 g of calcium carbonate a day; this can be associated with constipation. If the hyperphosphatemia is due to vitamin D intoxication, calcium salts are contraindicated because they will induce severe hypercalcemia.

## MAGNESIUM METABOLISM

Magnesium is the most abundant intracellular divalent cation. It is an essential cofactor for a variety of enzymatic reactions related to the transfer of high-energy phosphate groups from ATP. The maintenance of serum magnesium results from the intestinal absorption of magnesium and the conservation magnesium in the kidney. Approximately 30% of dietary magnesium is absorbed in the small intestine. However, when dietary magnesium is very low or in excess, there is an increase and decrease in the efficiency of magnesium absorption, respectively. It does not appear that either $1{,}25(OH)_2D$ or PTH regulates magnesium absorption in any significant manner. Approximately 96% of magnesium is absorbed along the nephron and about 4% is excreted into the urine.

Approximately 30% of magnesium in the serum is protein bound and 55% is ionized; the remaining 15% is complexed. Similar to calcium, magnesium is bound principally to albumin. Ionized magnesium is the fraction that is important for physiologic processes, including neuromuscular transmission and cardiovascular tone. The serum concentration of magnesium is closely maintained within a narrow range of approximately 1.7 to 2.6 mg/dl. There are no significant differences in magnesium concentration between men and women or with respect to age. Prolonged standing or hemolysis of a blood specimen can lead to a spurious increase in serum magnesium concentrations.

### Hypomagnesemia

***Pathophysiology.*** Magnesium deficiency is a common problem in clinical medicine. It has been estimated that 10% of patients admitted to city hospitals are hypomagnesemic and as many as 65% of the patients in an intensive care unit may be hypomagnesemic. The principal causes of hypomagnesemia are renal or gastrointestinal losses and a decrease in intestinal magnesium absorption. Reduced renal tubular reabsorption of magnesium is the most common cause of hypomagnesemia. Renal magnesium reabsorption is proportional to tubular fluid flow as well as to sodium and calcium excretion. Thus chronic parenteral fluid therapy, especially with saline, and volume expansion states such as primary hyperaldosteronism may result in hypomagnesemia. Hypercalcemia and hypercalciuria decrease renal magnesium reabsorption and contribute to the hypomagnesemia observed in hypercalcemic states. Osmotic diuresesis in diabetes mellitus is one of the more common causes of hypomagnesemia.

The magnesium content of upper intestinal tract fluids is about 1 mEq/L; thus vomiting and nasal gastric suctioning can contribute to magnesium depletion. Similarly, magnesium content in diarrheal fluids can be as high as 15 mEq/L; therefore magnesium depletion is common in acute and chronic diarrhea, Crohn's disease, ileitis, ulcerative colitis, and intestinal and biliary fistulas. Malabsorption syndromes may also be a contributing factor for magnesium depletion. Hypomagnesemia occurs in 30% of severe alcoholics and 80% of those with delirium tremens. The fall in magnesium levels within the first 24 to 48 hours of alcohol cessation is presumably due to intracellular shifts of magnesium following hydration. Drugs associated with renal wasting of magnesium include diuretics (especially loop diuretics, although renal magnesium loss occurs with thiazides), aminoglycosides, cisplatin, cyclosporin, and amphotericin B (see the box above).

#### Causes of hypomagnesemia

Increased renal excretion
- Volume expansion
- Hypercalcemia
- Osmotic diuresis

Increased intestinal losses
- Vomiting
- Nasogastric suctioning
- Malabsorption syndromes
- Ileitis
- Colitis
- Intestinal and biliary fistula
- Ketoacidosis with treatment
- Acute and chronic diarrhea

Drugs
- Diuretics
- Aminoglycosides
- Cisplatin
- Cyclosporin A
- Amphotericin B
- Ethanol

***History and physical examination.*** Neuromuscular hyperexcitability similar to that caused by hypocalcemia is often the presenting complaint in hypomagnesemia. Many of the signs and symptoms of hypomagnesemia are similar to those of hypocalcemia, including muscle weakness, prolonged PR and QT intervals, and cardiac arrhythmias. Chvostek's and Trousseau's signs may be present and the patient may complain of spontaneous carpopedal spasm.

Since magnesium is required for the secretion of parathyroid hormone and the function of parathyroid hormone in the bone, hypomagnesemia can cause hypocalcemia, with its associated symptoms and signs.

***Laboratory studies and management.*** Serum magnesium levels less than 1.5 mEq/L usually indicate magnesium deficiency. Treatment of hypomagnesemia should first be directed at the underlying cause. For a mild deficiency oral magnesium replacement is satisfactory. Diarrhea is the most common side effect. When a patient's magnesium level is less than 1.0 mEq/L, this suggests that there is a significant depletion of total body magnesium stores. The total body magnesium deficit can be as high as 400 mEq. Under these circumstances parenteral magnesium administration is usually indicated. Administration of 2 g magnesium sulfate (16.2 mEq magnesium) can be given intravenously up to 48 mEq over 24 hours.

**Causes of hypermagnesemia**

Renal failure with magnesium-containing antacid
Ketoacidosis without treatment
Familial hypocalciuric hypercalcemia
Volume depletion
Lithium

Alternatively, a 50% solution can be given every 8 hours intramuscularly; but these injections can be painful. Patients with severe hypomagnesemia with seizures or acute arrhythmias may be given 8 to 16 mEq magnesium as an intravenous injection over 5 to 10 minutes, followed by 48 mEq per day.

It should be noted that the restoration of a normal serum magnesium concentration does not indicate repletion of magnesium stores. Therapy should be continued for 3 to 7 days. Once magnesium replacement has been achieved, dietary magnesium is adequate to satisfy the body's requirement. However, patients who have magnesium loss from the intestine or kidney may require continued oral magnesium supplementation of a daily dosage of 300 mg of elemental magnesium given in divided doses. The major side effect is diarrhea. Patients who suffer from renal failure should be monitored carefully to prevent hypermagnesemia.

### Hypermagnesemia

***Pathophysiology and laboratory studies.*** Hypermagnesemia is most often caused by renal failure and can be worsened by the use of magnesium-containing antacids. Elevated magnesium levels encountered in patients with ketoacidosis are often a reflection of dehydration. These patients frequently have a magnesium deficiency. Modest elevations in serum magnesium may be seen in familial hypocalciuric hypercalcemia, lithium ingestion, and during volume depletion (see the box above).

***History and physical examination.*** Neuromuscular symptoms are the most common complaint in patients with magnesium intoxication. Deep tendon reflexes are often absent when magnesium concentrations reach 4 to 7 mEq/L. Depressed respiration and apnea due to paralysis of voluntary musculature may be seen in severe magnesium intoxication. Magnesium concentration greater than 5 mEq/L causes a prolonged PR interval as well as increased QRS duration and QT interval. Complete heart block and cardiac arrest may occur at concentrations greater than 15 mEq/L. Hypermagnesemia causes a suppression of PTH secretion and therefore can be associated with hypocalcemia.

***Management.*** Patients with renal failure who are taking magnesium antacids should be carefully monitored. If hypermagnesemia is present and the patient's antacid contains magnesium, a different antacid such as calcium carbonate should be used. Patients with severe magnesium intoxication require intravenous calcium. Calcium will antagonize the toxic effects of magnesium. The usual dosage is infusion of 100 to 200 mg of elemental calcium over 5 to 10 minutes. The antagonistic effect of calcium is short lived. Patients whose severe magnesium intoxication causes cardiovascular, neuromuscular, and CNS symptoms may require peritoneal dialysis or hemodialysis against a low-dialysis magnesium bath.

## BIBLIOGRAPHY

Attie MF: Treatment of hypercalcemia, *Endocrinol Metab Clin North Am* 18:807, 1990.

Burtis WJ et al: Immunochemical characterization of circulating parathyroid hormone related protein in patients with humoral hypercalcemia, *N Engl J Med* 322:1106, 1990.

Desai TK, Carlson RW, Geheb MA: Prevalence and clinical implications of hypocalcemia in acutely ill patients in a medical intensive care setting, *Am J Med* 84:209, 1988.

Dunlay R et al: Calcitriol in prolonged hypocalcemia due to tumor lysis syndrome, *Ann Intern Med* 110:162, 1989.

Favus MJ, editor: Primer on the metabolic bone diseases and disorders of mineral metabolism, ed 2, New York, 1993, Raven Press.

Holick MF, Krane S, Potts JR Jr: Calcium, phosphorus, and bone metabolism: calcium-regulating hormones. In Isselbacher KJ et al, *Harrison's principles of internal medicine,* ed 13, New York, 1994, McGraw-Hill.

Jacobus CH et al: Hypovitaminosis D associated with drinking milk, *N Engl J Med* 326:1173, 1992.

Pollak MR et al: Mutations in the human $Ca^{2+}$-sensing receptor gene cause familial hypocalciuric hypercalcemia and neonatal severe hyperparathyroidism, *Cell* 75:1297, 1993.

Potts JT Jr: Diseases of the parathyroid gland and other hyper- and hypocalcemic disorders. In Isselbacher KJ et al, editors: *Harrison's principles of internal medicine,* ed 13, New York, 1994, McGraw-Hill.

Ryzen E et al: Parenteral magnesium tolerance testing in the evaluation of magnesium deficiency, *Magnesium* 4:137, 1985.

Shane E: Medical management of asymptomatic primary hyperparathyroidism, *J Bone Miner Res* 6(suppl 2):S131, 1991.

CHAPTER

# 38 Metabolic Bone Disease

**Daniel T. Baran**

## OSTEOPOROSIS

Osteoporosis, which has been linked to inadequate calcium intake and estrogen deficiency as well as to other factors, is an important health problem in the United States. It is estimated that 15 to 20 million women over 45 have osteoporosis. The condition is manifested by a decrease in bone substance and strength. The resulting diminution of bone tissue is expressed as a reduced bone mineral density; the organic matrix (collagen) and mineral component (hydroxyapatite crystal) of bone are affected.

### Epidemiology and etiology

In recent years individuals in our society have become increasingly aware of the contribution of dietary calcium to their health. Several consumer-directed periodicals have discussed the potential benefits of calcium in the prevention of age-related bone loss. However, many American women continue to ingest inadequate amounts of calcium. The median daily calcium intake of American women over age 50 is 475 mg/day, far less than the recommended 800 mg/day. The ultimate consequences of this dietary inadequacy are unclear.

Recent studies have demonstrated that vertebral trabecular bone density appears to reach its peak mass near the end of the second decade, and vertebral bone mass begins to decline during the third decade. Increased calcium intake has been reported to positively affect vertebral bone mass in 25- to 35-year-old women and to prevent vertebral bone loss in 35-year-old women. Increasing calcium intake in the immediate postmenopausal period does not appear to affect the rapid bone loss that occurs during early menopause. Although calcium alone does not prevent this rapid bone loss, which is a result of estrogen deficiency, it does modify the bone response to estrogen. Whereas 0.3 mg per day of conjugated estrogen does not prevent vertebral bone loss, the combination of this much estrogen with calcium does. It has been suggested that calcium may function in an enabling mode in perimenopausal women, permitting the skeleton to respond to hormonal cues, in this case estrogen. In contrast, solely increasing the calcium intake of women between ages 60 and 70 appears to prevent bone loss in the spine, femur, and radius in some studies. Other studies have found that calcium supplementation (1) slows but does not prevent bone loss or (2) has no effect on bone loss in postmenopausal women. Similarly, fracture rates are not clearly related to dietary calcium intake. Epidemiologic data suggest that adequate calcium intake is associated with decreased hip fractures, but a recent study reports that increasing calcium intake does not prevent vertebral fractures. The putative beneficial effects of increased calcium intake on bone mass and fracture rates are supported by studies demonstrating that thiazide diuretics, which decrease calcium excretion and improve calcium balance, decrease the rates of bone loss and hip fracture. As with the conflicting reports on the benefits of calcium intake, not all studies show a beneficial effect of thiazides on hip fracture.

These conflicting studies regarding the value of increased calcium intake on bone mass and fracture rates in postmenopausal women may be confounded by differences in vitamin D intake and levels of the subjects in the various studies. Estimates of the dietary requirement of vitamin D for the elderly vary from 200 to 800 IU daily. Actual dietary vitamin D intake is only about 100 IU in the elderly. Studies have reported low circulating levels of 1,25-dihydroxyvitamin $D_3$ (1,25[OH]$_2$$D_3$) in women with postmenopausal osteoporosis and low levels of 25-hydroxyvitamin $D_3$ (25[OH]$D_3$) in patients with hip fractures. Treatment of postmenopausal women with 1,25(OH)$_2$$D_3$ has had variable effects on bone mass, but the vitamin in combination with calcium does appear to reduce fracture rates.

The role of exercise and the type of exercise that is important for maintenance and accrual of bone mass are unknown. It is agreed that immobilization is detrimental to bone. Bone mass is lost rapidly in quadriplegics, and U.S. astronauts in Space Lab lost bone mass at the rate of 1% a month. Therefore working against gravity seems to be important to maintain bone mass. However, it is not clear that exercise intervention results in a definite increase in bone mass. Although cross-sectional studies suggest that those who exercise have greater bone mass than sedentary individuals, prospective studies indicate that exercise is associated with minimal gains in bone mass in premenopausal and postmenopausal women. It seems clear that exercise in itself does not result in the hoped-for dramatic increments in bone mass, and the increases that do occur may be modulated by dietary factors. Exercise is important, however, in preserving muscle tone and balance in the elderly, and is therefore important in preventing falls.

It is estimated that there are 250,000 hip fractures each year in the United States. Most individuals with hip fractures are hospitalized. Approximately 50% of those who were ambulatory before hip fracture are unable to walk independently afterwards. Ultimately half become totally functionally dependent. About 20% of women sustaining a hip fracture die within 6 months of the event.

The risk of fracturing a bone is related to the strength of the bone and the force applied to it. Since only 1% of falls in the elderly result in hip fracture, the mechanics of falling are thought to be important determinants of fracture, with protective devices decreasing fracture incidence. It has been estimated that density accounts for approximately 75% of bone strength. Each standard deviation decrease in femoral neck density increases the age-adjusted risk of hip fracture 2.6 times. Women with bone density in the lowest quantile have an 8.5-fold greater risk of hip fracture than those in the highest quantile. It is interesting that calcaneal density is nearly as good a predictor of hip fractures as is hip density.

### Pathophysiology

Peak bone mass is attained in the third to fourth decade, and bone loss begins before menopause. Loss of ovarian function, either because of menopause or oophorectomy, is associated with an increase in the rate of bone loss for the ensuing 3 to 4 years. The premenopausal woman with low bone mass is at greatest risk for the development of osteoporosis during the postmenopausal years.

***Type I vs. type II osteoporosis.*** Age-related osteoporosis has been classified into type I and type II. Type I, or postmenopausal, osteoporosis is defined as affecting women within 15 to 20 years of menopause. The main clinical manifestation of type I osteoporosis is vertebral fracture. Estrogen deficiency is thought to underlie this form of osteoporosis, rendering the skeleton more sensitive to parathyroid hormone (PTH), resulting in increased calcium resorption from bone. This in turn decreases PTH secretion, 1,25(OH)$_2$$D_3$ production, and calcium absorption. Type II, or senile, osteoporosis is seen in both men and women over the age of 75 and is manifested mainly by hip and vertebral fractures. Decreased bone formation along with decreased ability of the kidney to produce 1,25(OH)$_2$$D_3$ underlies this type of osteoporosis. The vitamin D deficiency results in decreased calcium absorption, which increases the PTH level and therefore bone resorption. In both types of osteoporosis bone mass decreases because bone resorption exceeds bone formation. Although estrogen deficiency and decreased renal capacity to synthesize $1,25(OH)_2D_3$ affect all elderly women, 70% never develop clinical osteoporosis.

Estrogen replacement therapy (ERT) has a positive effect on bone mass in postmenopausal women regardless of age. Estrogen treatment either increases bone mass or retards the rate of bone loss. Estrogen treatment in combination with progesterone may have a synergistic effect on bone mass. The beneficial effects of ERT on bone mass appear to reduce the risk of vertebral, hip, and other fractures in postmenopausal women. The mechanism of estrogen's effect on bone mass appears to be inhibition of bone resorption with continued bone formation before restoration of coupling. However, recent studies in rat models suggest that estrogen also stimulates bone formation. In addition to its direct effects on bone cells, estrogen treatment in oophorectomized women appears to preserve the intestinal responsiveness to vitamin D. Thus ERT may modulate the effects of vitamin D on calcium absorption, perhaps explaining the synergistic effect of estrogen and calcium on bone mass.

Glucocorticoid excess, either intrinsic or iatrogenic, causes osteoporosis. The glucocorticoids inhibit intestinal calcium absorption and bone formation. Bone resorption is often increased to compensate for the decreased intestinal calcium absorption with cortical and trabecular bone adversely affected. Osteoporosis therapy requires treatment of glucocorticoid overproduction or reduction of steroid dosage to the lowest effective level, preferably every other day.

### History

Women are more likely to develop osteoporosis than men because of a lower peak bone mass and greater rate of bone loss, especially after menopause. White and Asian women are at greatest risk, whereas African-Americans are relatively protected because of greater peak bone mass. A family history of osteoporosis (particularly in a mother), a petite body habitus, cigarette smoking, a sedentary lifestyle, low dietary calcium intake, and an early menopause are additional risk factors for low bone mass. Steroid treatment in doses greater than 5 mg of prednisone or 25 mg of hydrocortisone daily for prolonged periods (over 6 months) contributes to bone loss by increasing bone resorption and decreasing bone formation. Treatment with suppressive doses of thyroxine, e.g., in patients with goiter or after irradiation for thyroid cancer or other causes of hyperthyroidism, also decreases bone mass, particularly in the hip because of activation of osteoclasts and enhanced bone resorption. Prolonged heparin therapy leads to osteoporosis. Hypercalciuria resulting from either increased intestinal calcium absorption or decreased renal calcium reabsorption is a risk factor for low bone mass and may present as kidney stones (see the box at right). It is important to emphasize that these traditional osteoporosis risk factors explain only a small percentage of the individual differences in developing osteoporosis. Therefore an individual without these risk factors still has a reasonable likelihood of developing osteoporosis, which argues for a population-based approach to prevention, including adequate calcium and vitamin D intake and physical exercise. Recent evidence suggests that the expression of the vitamin D receptor is a strong prediction of osteoporosis. Future studies will need to confirm this observation, and, if confirmed, determine the utility of screening vitamin D receptor types and potential therapeutic interventions.

Loss of height and pain may indicate multiple vertebral compression fractures. It is important to realize that even markedly osteoporotic patients without fractures are typically asymptomatic. In patients with bone pain in the absence of fractures, causes other than osteoporosis should be sought.

#### Risk factors for development of osteoporosis

Female
White or Asian heritage
Osteoporosis in mother
Petite body habitus
Sedentary
Cigarette smoker
Low dietary calcium intake (<800 mg/day)
Early menopause (natural or surgical)
Hypercalciuria
Steroid therapy
Treatment with TSH-suppressive doses of thyroxine

*TSH*, Thyroid-stimulating hormone.

### Physical examination

Body habitus and height should be assessed. Multiple vertebral compression fractures result in a dowager's hump and may progress to the point where the rib cage rests upon the pelvis, impairing breathing and appetite. Weight loss may suggest either a malignancy or hyperthyroidism as the etiology of the osteoprosis. In contrast, centripetal obesity, peripheral wasting, easy bruising, and altered fat deposition suggest excessive levels of circulating steroids. In the young man or woman, absence of sexual development suggests hypogonadism.

### Laboratory studies and diagnostic procedures

Routine x-rays of the hips and spine are needed to rule out fractures in the patient with pain and to detect osteoporosis. However, a 30% loss of bone mineral is required before a radiologist can make the diagnosis of osteoporosis on routine x-rays. Before fracture, characteristic features of the osteoporotic spine include codfish vertebrae, accentuation of the vertebral endplates, and accentuation of the vertical trabecular pattern in the vertebral bodies. Progression of the disease results in central or anterior compression fractures (Fig. 38-1). The presence of a posterior compression fracture or a nontraumatic fracture above the fifth thoracic vertebra should alert the physician to the possibility of malignancy metastatic to bone. Accentuation of the trabecular pattern in the femoral neck has been used as an assessment of osteoporotic risk but is at best semiquantitative.

The recent advances in our understanding of osteoporosis and its treatment have been made possible by the development of noninvasive techniques to quantitate bone mass in the spine and hip regions. The newest technique, dual-energy x-ray absorptiometry (DXA), is rapid (10

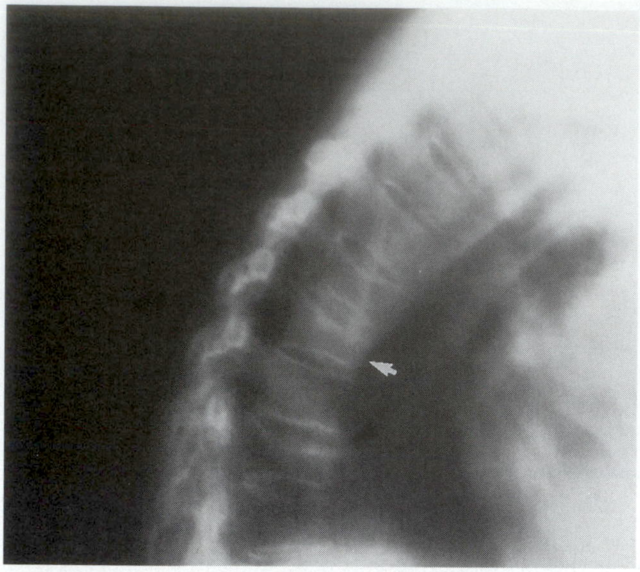

**Fig. 38-1.** Lateral thoracic spine x-ray of a woman with osteoporosis. The arrows indicate vertebrae that are compressed centrally and anteriorly. The x-ray also shows "codfish" vertebrae, the appearance of oval disc spaces.

minutes for each area scanned), reproducible (a coefficient of variation of less than 1%), and exposes the patient to minimal radiation (1.5 mrem) (Fig. 38-2). The advantage of this technique is that it quantitates bone mass in the regions of greatest interest to the physician caring for the osteoporotic patient (the hip and spine). Disadvantages of this technique are its poor images when compared to routine x-rays, and its cost (about $100,000) which has limited its availability. The latest development in the field has involved the improvement in x-ray quality while retaining the ability to quantitate bone mass (Fig. 38-3). The newest equipment generates nearly x-ray quality images, but this has been realized at the expense of greater radiation exposure (about 30 mrem per scan). Although this amount of radiation is negligible (the average chest x-ray exposes the patient to 60 mrem), it might limit the number of serial examinations obtained to assess therapeutic efficacy.

Both single photon absorptiometry of the radius and ulna and ultrasound of the calcaneus have been used to assess osteoporotic risk. Although measurement of bone mass at these sites has been shown to be an excellent predictor of fracture in women, these techniques often fail to diagnose the individual woman at risk. Thus despite their low cost, ease of operation, and suitability for screening procedures, they are not substitutes for quantitation of axial bone mass.

Markers of bone metabolism are currently being evaluated as predictors of bone loss and of response to therapy. These markers reflect osteoblastic (serum levels of alkaline phosphatase, osteocalcin, and the carboxy terminal fragment of type I procollagen) and osteoclastic (serum tartrate–resistant acid phosphatase, and urinary hydroxyproline and collagen crosslinks excretion) activity. Studies suggest that increased levels of serum osteocalcin and urinary hydroxyproline predict those osteoporotic women most likely to respond to calcitonin therapy with an increase in bone density.

Evaluation of patients with osteoporosis should include serum calcium, phosphorus, alkaline phosphatase levels, and a complete blood count. Depending on the results of this evaluation and the clinical presentation, it may be appropriate to perform either serum or urine protein electrophoresis, thyroid function tests, and parathyroid hormone and serum cortisol level assessments. These routine laboratory parameters, when obtained in normal women and women with idiopathic osteoporosis, cannot predict the affected woman but are obtained to rule out secondary causes of the disease. The combination of urinary calcium and hydroxyproline, serum alkaline phosphatase, and determination of body fat mass is said to identify fast bone losers in the perimenopausal period. Theoretically these women are at greatest risk for the future development of osteoporosis.

## Differential diagnosis

Idiopathic osteoporosis accounts for 90% to 95% of cases of osteoporosis that are seen by the general practitioner. As mentioned above, treatment with glucocorticoids or thyroid-stimulating hormone (TSH)–suppressive doses of thyroid hormone may contribute to increased bone loss. Additional causes of osteoporosis include malignancy, Cushing's disease, thyrotoxicosis, hyperparathyroidism, multiple myeloma, and hypogonadism (see the box below). Treatment of Cushing's disease and thyrotoxicosis reverses bone loss. Hyperparathyroidism is associated with cortical bone loss (femur and radius) and with preservation of trabecular bone (spine). Osteoporosis is an indication for surgical therapy of hyperparathyroidism in the otherwise asymptomatic patient. Hypogonadism is a cause of osteoporosis in the young patient. Ovarian and testicular failure increase bone resorption and decrease bone formation, resulting in decreased bone mass.

Osteomalacia is a defect in mineralization and may present with decreased bone density. Because milk in the United States is fortified with vitamin D, osteomalacia is less common in this country than in Europe. However, in the elderly who do not drink milk and lack sun exposure, osteomalacia may contribute to the high incidence of hip fracture. Osteomalacia is diagnosed by measuring serum levels of 25(OH)D, an indication of stores of vitamin D.

### Differential diagnosis of osteoporosis

Malignancy
Multiple myeloma
Cushing disease
Thyrotoxicosis
Hyperparathyroidism
Excess glucocorticoid treatment
TSH-suppressive doses of thyroxine
Hypogonadism
Osteomalacia

*TSH,* Thyroid-stimulating hormone.

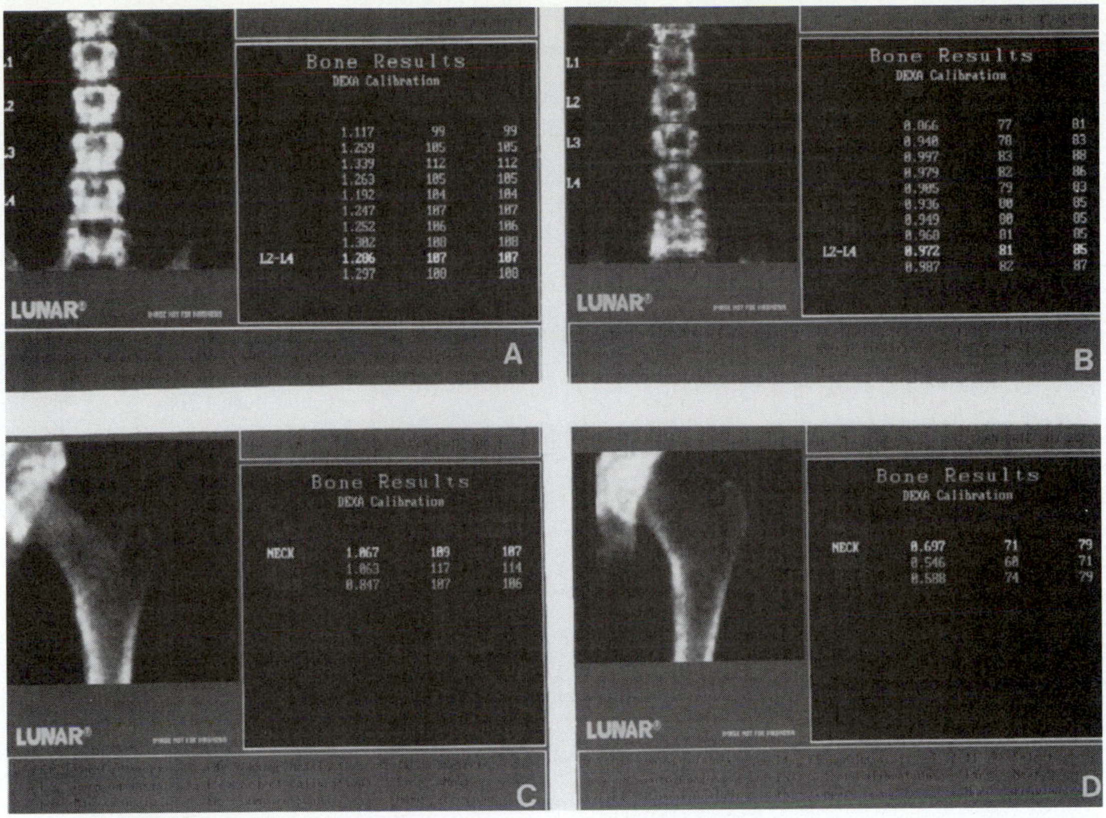


**Fig. 38-2.** Dual energy x-ray absorptiometry of the spine and femur of a normal and an osteoporotic patient. *A*, Normal spine; *B*, osteoporotic spine; *C*, normal femur; *D*, osteoporotic femur. (Courtesy Lunar Corp, Madison, Wis.)

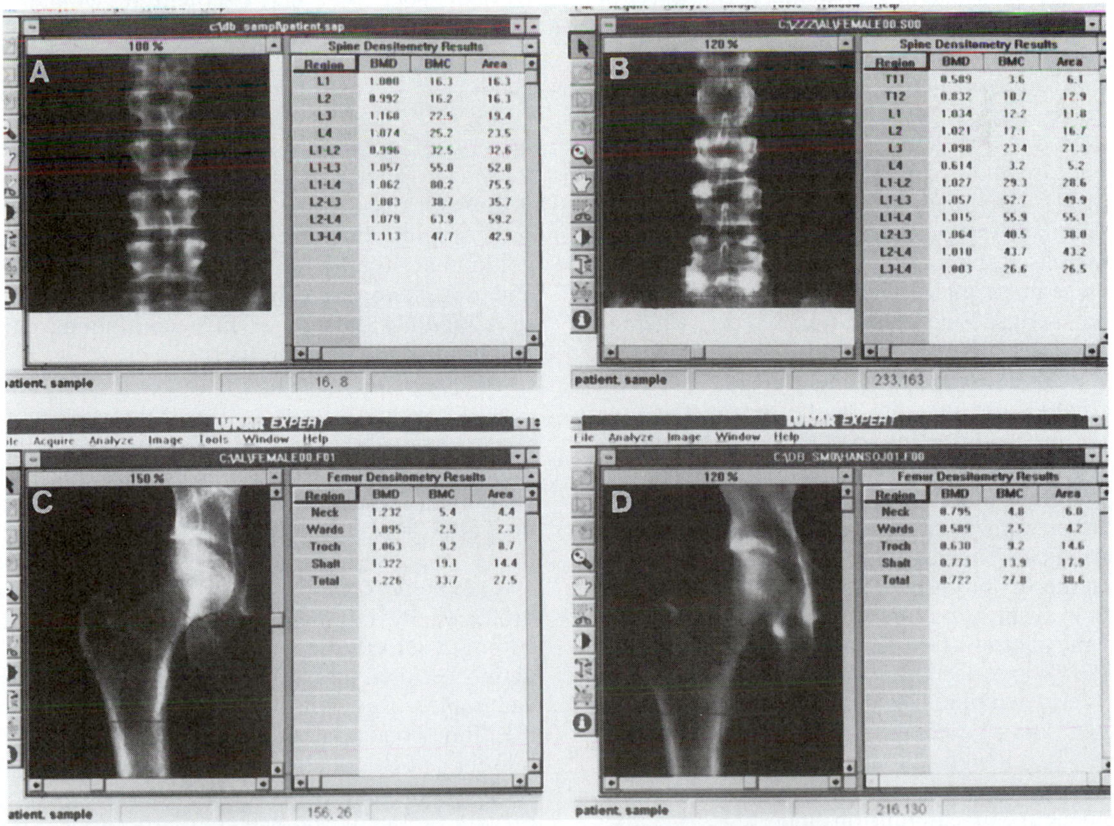


**Fig. 38-3.** Dual energy x-ray absorptiometry of the spine and femur of a normal and an osteoporotic patient with the Lunar Corporation Expert system. Views are nearly x-ray quality. *A*, Normal spine; *B*, osteoporotic spine; *C*, normal femur; *D*, osteoporotic femur. (Courtesy Lunar Corp, Madison, Wis.)

**Table 38-1.** Pharmacologic management of osteoporosis

| Medication | Starting dose | Maintenance dose | Dosage schedule | Retail cost/mo | Common or serious side effects | Comments |
|---|---|---|---|---|---|---|
| Calcium | 1 g PO | 1 g PO | qd | $5-10 | Upset stomach, constipation | |
| Estrogen* | | | | | | |
| Calcitonin | 50 units SC or 100 units SC | 50 units SC | qd (50), qod (100) | $150-200 | Nausea (10%) Vomiting and/or diarrhea (<15%) Facial flush (25%) | Nasal form currently being tested |
| Etidronate | 400 mg | 400 mg | qd × 14 days, then 2½ months; calcium (1 g qd) | $20-25 | Upset stomach (mild) | Etidronate is the only bisphosphonate currently available in the U.S. but is not FDA approved for osteoporosis; calcium and food interfere with absorption |
| $1,25(OH)_2D_3$ | 0.25 μg | 0.25 μg | bid | $45-50 | Hypercalciuria, kidney stones, hypercalcemia | Serum and urine calcium monitoring necessary at least every other month |

*See Chapter 148 for estrogen replacement doses.

## Pharmacologic management

A summary of the pharmacologic treatment options for osteoporosis is found in Table 38-1.

***Calcium.*** Retrospective, cross-sectional, and prospective studies have demonstrated that increased calcium intake is associated with increased bone mass in premenopausal women. In our own prospective randomized intervention trial bone mass of the lumbar spine was measured at 6-month intervals for 3 years in a group of women who increased their calcium intake and in a group whose intake was unchanged. The latter group of women lost 3% of their spinal bone mass after 3 years, whereas those whose dietary calcium increased had no change in their vertebral bone density during the 3 years. The study suggests that increasing calcium intake during the premenopausal period would allow women to enter menopause with a greater bone density.

Increasing calcium intake in the immediate postmenopausal period does not appear to affect the rapid bone loss that occurs during early menopause. In contrast, increasing the calcium intake of 60-year-old women by 500 mg per day appears to prevent bone loss in the spine, femur, and radius. The combination of calcium (1.2 g per day) with vitamin $D_3$ (800 IU per day) has been reported to prevent fractures in elderly women. The number of hip fractures was 43% lower and the total number of nonvertebral fractures was 32% lower among women treated with vitamin $D_3$ and calcium than among those who received placebo. The benefits of calcium on bone mass are also supported by epidemiologic data, which suggest that a lifetime of adequate calcium intake decreases fracture risk.

***Estrogen.*** ERT prevents bone loss by inhibiting bone resorption, thus reducing the risk of fracture. It is usually recommended for perimenopausal women to prevent further bone loss. Although clinical characteristics alone cannot predict the women at risk of osteoporosis, candidates for estrogen treatment include women undergoing early menopause and petite women with a family history of osteoporosis, particularly in their mother. Estrogen treatment also prevents bone loss in older postmenopausal women. For women with an intact uterus, progesterone should be given with the estrogen to prevent continuous stimulation of the endometrium. The estrogen and progesterone may be administered cyclically, resulting in a monthly period, or in a continuous daily fashion, resulting in an atrophic uterus.

Although the majority of studies to date have employed oral estrogens, transdermal estrogen treatment also prevents loss of bone mass in the hip and spine and is an effective alternate route of administration in women not wishing to take oral medications. See Chapter 148 for details of hormone therapy.

***Calcitonin.*** Calcitonin is a 32–amino acid polypeptide produced by the parafollicular C cells of the thyroid. Biologic activity depends on a 7–amino acid ring at the amino terminal end of the peptide. In naturally occurring calcitonins this ring structure is accomplished by a dilsulfide bond. Calcitonin is the most potent endogenous inhibitor of osteoclastic bone resorption. The presence of receptors for calcitonin in the central nervous system may explain the analgesic effects of the drug. Like estrogen, calcitonin is approved by the Food and Drug Administration for the treatment of osteoporosis. It has been demonstrated that the response to calcitonin is determined in part by the activity of the skeletal osteoclasts and osteoblasts. Patients were defined as having either high-turnover osteoporosis (HTOP) or normal-turnover osteoporosis (NTOP) based upon serum osteocalcin levels, urinary hydroxyproline excretion, and skeletal tracer kinetics. Women with HTOP responded to calcitonin with a 20% increase in vertebral bone density during the year study. Those with NTOP had no increase in bone mass. Neither group exhibited an increase in hip density. The skeletal response in the HTOP patients correlated with a reduction in osteocalcin and hydroxyproline levels, indicating a decrease in bone turnover.

Calcitonin has been administered both subcutaneously and intranasally to perimenopausal women. Both routes of administration prevented bone loss in these women (similar to the effect of estrogens). Because of the concerns regarding prolonged estrogen use in postmenopausal women, calcitonin may become an alternative treatment to prevent bone loss in perimenopausal women. Unfortunately, at present only the subcutaneous form of the hormone is available in the United States.

The major effects of calcitonin are gastrointestinal (nausea, vomiting, diarrhea) and vascular (facial flushing, tingling). Urinary frequency, pain at the injection site, and a copper penny taste in the mouth have also been described. The type of calcitonin, the route of administration, and the amount of information provided to the patients contribute to the frequency of side effects.

***Bisphosphonates.*** Bisphosphonates are compounds possessing a strong affinity for the hydroxyapatite crystal. The bisphosphonates can inhibit crystal formation as well as bone resorption. This inhibition of bone resorption is thought to result from a direct effect on osteoclasts. The bisphosphonates are incorporated in the crystal structure, and during osteoclastic bone resorption the diphosphonate enters the osteoclast and subsequently inhibits its function.

The compounds have a low rate of intestinal absorption (approximately 1% to 3% of the ingested dose is absorbed). Both food and calcium interfere with absorption. The absorbed compound either goes to bone or is excreted in the urine. The half-life of the compound in the circulation is brief (minutes), whereas the half-life in bone is long and depends on the turnover of the skeleton. These characteristics of the compounds explain their low toxicity, the restriction of their effects on the skeleton, and the duration of those effects (allowing for discontinuous treatment).

Several recent papers have demonstrated the efficacy of bisphosphonates in the treatment and prevention of osteoporosis. The compounds are administered cyclically with calcium. Treatment with etidronate appears to increase bone mass, decrease fracture rate, and reduce the loss of height that accompanies vertebral fractures. The bisphosphonates also prevent the bone loss that occurs shortly after menopause. During a 6-month trial tiludronate was administered to half of the subjects. During the second 6-month period all subjects received placebo. Tiludronate prevented bone loss; the control subjects had a significant 2.1% decrease in lumbar bone density.

The low cost of these compounds, their ease of administration, and their lack of side effects make bisphosphonates an attractive option for patients. At present, they are not yet approved by the Food and Drug Administration for the treatment of osteoporosis.

***1,25-Dihydroxyvitamin $D_3$.*** Vitamin D is biologically inactive. To attain full biologic activity, it must be hydroxylated (a hydroxy group) at the 25 position in the liver, and then at the 1 position in the renal tubule cells. As a result, diseases of the liver and kidney can adversely affect the metabolism of vitamin D. 1,25(OH)D hydroxyvitamin D increases intestinal calcium absorption, enhances renal tubular calcium reabsorption, stimulates osteoblast synthesis of osteocalcin but decreases osteoblast synthesis of collagen, and augments bone resorption. Because of decreased calcium absorption and reduced circulating levels of $1,25(OH)_2D_3$ in patients with postmenopausal osteoporosis, the hormone has been employed in the treatment of disease.

The major difficulty with the use of $1,25(OH)_2D_3$ in the treatment of postmenopausal osteoporosis is the narrow window between therapeutic efficacy and side effects, e.g., hypercalciuria and hypercalcemia. This was demonstrated in a recent study which showed that $1,25(OH)_2D_3$ increased calcium absorption and bone density of the spine and radius. It also decreased fracture rate from 333 in 1000 patient years in the controls to 250 in 1000 years in the treated patients. However, hypercalciuria occurred in all subjects, and hypercalcemia occurred in 89% of the treated subjects. In a subsequent study the dosage was adjusted to maintain the serum calcium less than 11 mg/dl. In this 2-year prospective study of patients with prior vertebral fractures, $1,25(OH)_2D_3$ increased spine density by 2% compared to a 3% loss in the controls. There were no differences in vertebral fracture rates during the study, and urine calcium increased from 144 mg per day to 256 mg per day, although there were no changes in renal function. The hormone, at a dosage of 0.5 μg per day has been reported to decrease fracture rate after 2 years of therapy. In contrast, in a double-blind randomized 2-year trial no significant differences between control and treated groups were noted in spine density or fracture rate at a dosage of 0.43 μg per day despite twofold increments in urine calcium. A recent prospective, randomized but not blinded study of 622 women with previous vertebral fractures reported that controls ingesting calcium alone had a threefold increased fracture rate compared to those on calcitriol.

Thus, although calcium absorption does decrease with age, there is suggestive but not conclusive evidence that $1,25(OH)_2D_3$ may be an effective long-term treatment for osteoporosis; however, the significant risk of hypercalciuria and hypercalcemia requires close monitoring.

***Fluoride.*** The agents used to treat osteoporosis (calcium, estrogen, calcitonin, bisphosphonates, $1,25[OH]_2D_3$) are inhibitors of bone resorption. Fluoride has been shown to be a stimulator of bone formation. Unfortunately, in prospective randomized trials fluoride has been shown to increase bone mass but not to reduce fracture rate. It has been suggested that fluoride is incorporated into bone as fluorapatite, which is more brittle than the normal hydroxyapatite crystal. Therefore, although bone mass is increased, bone strength is not improved. At present the use of fluoride in the treatment of osteoporosis is not recommended.

***Special cases.*** Steroid treatment and TSH-suppressive doses of thyroid hormone decrease bone mass. In prospective randomized studies both calcitonin and bisphosphonates have been shown to prevent the decreases in bone mass that occurred in patients receiving between 15 and 17 mg of prednisone daily. Estrogen therapy also appears to prevent steroid-induced bone loss, but prospective randomized studies have not yet been completed. Any postmenopausal patient who will be on long-term supraphysiologic steroid therapy should also be treated with agents that prevent bone loss. The dosages of calcitonin, bisphosphonates, and estrogen used to treat individuals taking steroids are identical to those used for postmenopausal osteoporosis.

To date, the studies evaluating prevention of thyroid hormone–induced bone loss have all been conducted in animals. Bisphosphonates, but not calcitonin, prevent the bone loss resulting from TSH-suppressive doses of thyroid hormone. Bisphosphonates have been shown to prevent thyroid hormone–induced changes in markers of bone resorption in humans, so it is presumed that the clinical studies currently being conducted will demonstrate preservation of bone mass as well.

## PAGET'S DISEASE

Paget's disease (Fig. 38-4) is characterized by increased bone resorption mediated by osteoclasts that contain more nuclei than normal. There is also an increase in bone formation resulting in a high turnover state. The collagen produced by the osteoblasts is not laid down in the typical linear fashion, but rather in a disorganized, woven fashion; this characteristic is not specific for Paget's disease but is characteristic of any high turnover state.

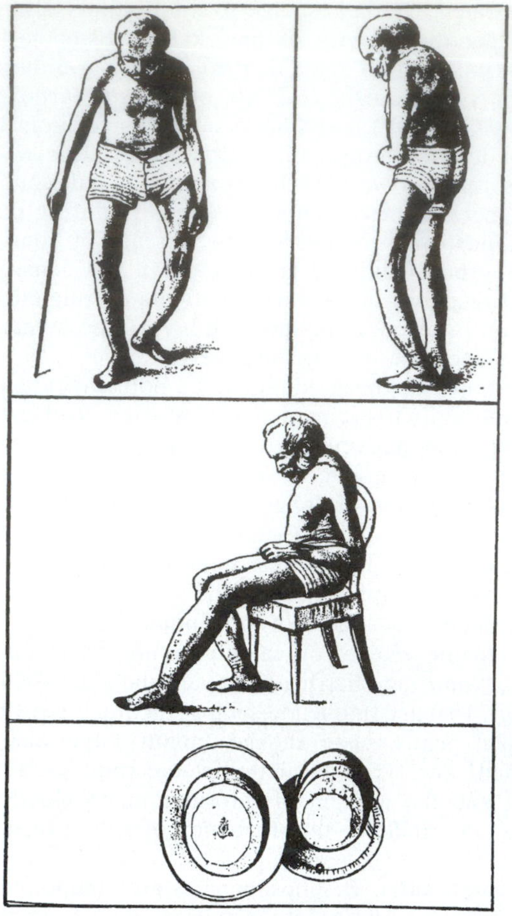

**Fig. 38-4.** Chronic inflammation of the bones (osteitis deformans). Three figures from sketches of the patient (case 1) taken six months before death. The same patient's cap worn in 1844 and hat worn in 1867. (Read by Sir James Paget before the Royal Medical Chirurgical Society of London, November 14, 1876.)

### Epidemiology and etiology

Paget's disease occurs in nearly equal frequency in men and women. It is present in 0.1% to 1% of elderly hospitalized patients in the United States, with a frequency of nearly 3% in some outpatient studies of subjects over 55. It is said to be more common in northern climates.

The etiology of the disease remains controversial. Viral inclusion bodies have been described in the cytoplasm and nuclei of osteoclasts at sites of pagetic involvement but not in the osteoclasts in normal bone from the same subject. It is not clear if these viral particles are causative agents or are secondary phenomena in abnormal osteoclasts. Genetic analyses of some kindreds are consistent with an autosomal dominant mode of inheritance. However, other studies found a low incidence of Paget's disease in twin pairs, suggesting that genetic transmission is less likely. A high percentage (6% to 8%) of people over age 55 in Lancashire, England, have x-rays consistent with Paget's disease. In some communities the high prevalence has been linked to the occurrence of canine distemper, suggesting it may be the putative virus that is responsible for the osteoclastic abnormalities.

### Pathophysiology

As a result of the high turnover state, bone formation occurs in a haphazard fashion, resulting in a woven bone appearance. Although the affected bone may be larger than normal bone, pagetic bone is weaker and more susceptible to fracture. The bones most commonly affected, in order of decreasing frequency are sacrum, spine, femur, skull, sternum, and pelvis. Involvement of the tibia and humerus is less common, but the disease may occur at any skeletal site and may involve one (monostotic) or many (polystotic) bones. Less than 1% of patients with Paget's disease develop osteogenic sarcoma, which usually manifests itself as a lytic lesion on x-ray. Cancerous degeneration usually manifests itself by increasing pain and/or a rapidly increasing serum alkaline phosphatase.

Pagetic bone is highly vascular; this is said to be responsible for the increased warmth of the skin over the affected bones. In patients who have extensive, poorly controlled disease the increased vascularity of the involved bone may contribute to high-output cardiac failure. The greater vascularity makes surgery on the affected bone technically more difficult and may also pose hemorrhagic problems in patients who fracture a pagetic bone.

Pain at the involved site(s) is a common manifestation of Paget's disease. Some studies suggest that prostaglandins may be the responsible pain mediators. Pain may also be a manifestation of neural impingement, spinal stenosis, or degenerative arthritis. The latter is a common occurrence if the disease affects both the pelvis and the proximal femur. If the pain is the result of an accompanying degenerative arthritis, treatment of Paget's disease alone will not relieve symptoms. A common manifestation of Paget's disease of the skull is deafness, resulting from either neural impingement or involvement of the bones of the middle ear.

Hypercalciuria and hypercalcemia can occur in immobilized patients with Paget's disease. The lack of weight bearing decreases bone formation but does not affect bone resorption. The calcium released from bone cannot be reused and is released into the circulation and excreted. Hypercalcemia in patients with Paget's disease who are not immobilized suggests the presence of another problem responsible for the hypercalcemia, such as hyperparathyroidism (see Chapter 37).

### History

The majority of patients with Paget's disease are asymptomatic, and the disease is diagnosed by the radiologist because x-rays are obtained for some other problem. Because pagetic bone becomes larger, changes in hat size may occur in patients with skull involvement. Headache is also a common complaint of patients with Paget's disease of the skull. Bowing deformities of the weight-bearing bones (femur and tibia) reflect the weakness of pagetic bone.

### Physical examination

Neurologic evaluation should be focused on the sites involved (e.g., skull involvement, cranial nerves; lumbar spine involvement, nerves of the lower extremity). Warmth at an affected site suggests active Paget's disease.

### Laboratory studies and diagnostic procedures

Markers of bone metabolism are used to assess the activity of the disease. Most studies to date have employed measurement of serum alkaline phosphatase and/or urinary hydroxyproline. Because of the ease of obtaining blood samples, the serum alkaline phosphatase is a more convenient parameter to follow. Although alkaline phosphatase is produced by osteoblasts, increased alkaline phosphatase may also reflect liver disease, ectopic pregnancy, a healing fracture, or any osteoblastic process in bone. Alkaline phosphatase from bone can be distinguished by either heat fractionating the total alkaline phosphatase or obtaining a radioimmunoassay specific for bone alkaline phosphatase. Urinary hydroxyproline can be affected by gelatin in the diet. Recent studies have also used serum tartrate–resistant acid phosphatase and urinary collagen crosslink excretion to assess disease actively, but there is less experience with these tests.

The extent of disease activity (the number of bones in which disease is active) is best determined by a radionuclide bone scan, which can differentiate between active and quiescent Paget's disease. X-rays should be obtained of positive areas on bone scan. Symptoms originating in an area of quiescent disease suggest an arthritic etiology and do not respond to treatment specific for Paget's disease. Skull involvement is an indication for audiologic evaluation.

## Differential diagnosis

Since Paget's disease is characterized by increased bone resorption with resultant increased bone formation, the stages of the disease involve (1) increased resorption, (2) resorption plus formation, or (3) a sclerotic quiescent phase. The x-ray appearance is virtually diagnostic of the disease. Any osteoblastic process such as metastatic prostate cancer may resemble Paget's disease on x-ray and should be suspected in any male patient with Paget's disease. Acid phosphatase, which is often employed as a marker for prostate cancer, is produced by bone cells and may be evaluated in active Paget's disease. Since metastatic osteoblastic prostate malignancy is in the differential diagnosis, increases in serum acid phosphatase should be further evaluated by assessment of the prostatic fraction of acid phosphatase and prostate specific antigen.

## Management

There is no clear-cut indication as to when to institute therapy. Indications for treatment include increasing severity of symptoms and an alkaline phosphatase greater than three times normal. Active skull disease is usually an indication for therapy because of the likelihood of auditory impairment. Sudden neurologic impairment (e.g., weakness in an extremity), if linked to pagetic disease in a vertebra, may be an indication for surgical intervention since the response to pharmacologic therapy may not be observed for weeks.

***Calcitonin.*** Calcitonin is a potent inhibitor of bone resorption. Since bone resorption and bone formation are coupled, inhibition of resorption ultimately inhibits formation, resulting in decreased urinary hydroxyproline excretion and decreased serum alkaline phosphatase. Although the drug is also used to treat hypercalcemia of malignancy, it does not cause hypercalcemia in patients with Paget's disease or osteoporosis.

The usual dose of calcitonin is 100 IU subcutaneously three times a week. This is similar to the regimen used for treating high-turnover osteoporosis. Some physicians prefer to initiate therapy with daily injections of 100 IU calcitonin, but this regimen has not been shown to dramatically improve response. Between 95% and 100% of patients with Paget's disease respond to calcitonin within 6 months with a 50% decrease in serum alkaline phosphatase. Persistence of symptoms despite decreased disease activity suggests an arthritic component. Therapy is usually discontinued after 6 months and the activity of the disease followed. Return of symptoms and/or an increasing alkaline phosphatase are indications for another 6-month course of calcitonin treatment. Over time some patients become refractory to calcitonin because of either development of antibodies or down-regulation of the calcitonin receptor.

***Bisphosphonates.*** Bisphosphonates are effective in 85% to 100% of patients with Paget's disease. The bisphosphonate currently used in the United States is etidronate disodium. The usual dosage is 400 mg a day (approximately 5 mg/kg body weight). At higher doses (10 and

20 mg/kg body weight) the drug may cause osteomalacia. Both food and calcium interfere with etidronate disodium absorption, so it should be given on an empty stomach. The drug also causes phosphaturia and may result in mild hypophosphatemia, but in the patient on a normal diet this is usually of no clinical significance. Nevertheless, serum phosphorus should be measured along with serum alkaline phosphatase at 3-month intervals. By 6 months there is usually a 50% decrease in serum alkaline phosphatase activity. Although the drug's primary effect is to inhibit bone resorption, inhibition of bone formation can also occur. To prevent osteomalacia, even at doses of 400 mg/day, the drug should be administered for 6 months followed by a 6-month treatment-free period. If the alkaline phosphatase begins to rise or if symptoms recur, the drug may be administered for additional 6-month treatment periods.

Pamidronate is currently available in the United States as an intravenous therapy for hypercalcemia of malignancy. It, and a number of diphosphonates like it, are second and third generations of the drug. They possess greater inhibitory effects on bone resorption than etidronate and fewer effects on bone formation. The intravenous form has been used as a single infusion in the treatment of Paget's disease, producing sustained inhibition of bone resorption. It is relatively free from severe side effects and should soon replace plicamycin as the intravenous therapy for Paget's disease.

***Plicamycin.*** Plicamycin was formerly called mithramycin. It is a cytotoxic antibiotic that is a potent inhibitor of bone resorption. It is administered intravenously over 4 hours at a dosage of 10 μg/kg body weight. Side effects include liver and bone marrow toxicity. Liver function tests, complete blood count, platelet count, and prothrombin time should be obtained before administering the drug. Response to therapy may be observed within hours, especially in patients with very active disease. Because of side effects, the use of the drug should be considered only in the patient who is symptomatic and has failed treatment with etidronate and the calcitonins. It is anticipated that intravenous pamidronate will eventually replace plicamycin for the patient who requires rapid decrease in disease activity.

***Nonsteroidal antiinflammatory agents.*** Nonsteroidal antiinflammatory agents do not specifically treat Paget's disease. They are especially helpful in patients who have secondary arthritic involvement.

## BIBLIOGRAPHY


Baran D et al: Dietary modification with dairy products for preventing vertebral bone loss in premenopausal women: a 3-year prospective study, *J Clin Endocrinol Metab* 70:264, 1989.

Chapuy MC et al: Vitamin $D_3$ and calcium to prevent hip fracture in elderly women, *N Engl J Med* 327:1637, 1992.

Civitelli R et al: Bone turnover in postmenopausal osteoporosis: effect of calcitonin treatment, *J Clin Invest* 82:1268, 1988.

Dawson Hughes B et al: A controlled trial of the effect of calcium supplementation on bone density in postmenopausal women, *N Engl J Med* 323:878, 1990.

Favus MJ, editor: *Primer on the metabolic bone diseases and disorders of mineral metabolism,* ed 2, New York, 1993, Raven Press.

Johnston CC Jr, Slemenda CW, Melton JL: Clinical use of densitometry, *N Engl J Med* 324:1105, 1991.

Naessen T et al: Hormone replacement therapy and the risk for first hip fracture, *Ann Intern Med* 113:95, 1990.

Recker RR: Current therapy for osteoporosis, *J Clin Endocrinol Metab* 76:14, 1993.

Thiebaud D et al: A single infusion of the bisphosphonate AHPrBP (APD) as treatment of Paget's disease of bone, *Am J Med* 85:207, 1988.

Tilyard MW et al: Treatment of postmenopausal osteoporosis with calcitriol or calcium, *N Engl J Med* 326:357, 1991.

Watt NB et al: Intermittent cyclical etidronate treatment of postmenopausal osteoporosis, *N Engl J Med* 323:73, 1990.


CHAPTER

# 39 Endocrine Syndromes

**Robert E. Burr**

This chapter reviews syndromes that do not represent abnormalities of a particular endocrine axis. These include multiglandular syndromes involving several endocrine systems simultaneously, such as the multiple endocrine neoplasia and autoimmune mediated polyglandular failure and paraneoplastic syndromes due to inappropriate hormone secretion by neoplastic tissue.

## MULTIPLE ENDOCRINE NEOPLASIA

The multiple endocrine neoplasia (MEN) syndromes are familial diseases inherited in an autosomal dominant pattern. MEN type I (Wermer's syndrome) includes hyperparathyroidism, pancreatic islet cell tumors, and pituitary adenomas. MEN type II (Sipple's syndrome) is more variable in its manifestations but always includes medullary thyroid carcinoma and can have, in differing degrees, pheochromocytoma, mucosal neuromas, and hyperparathyroidism.

Because of the high likelihood that affected members of a kindred will develop disease, prospective screening is an important component of the management of kindreds. Screening and genetic counseling of kindreds with one of the MEN syndromes allow individuals at low risk to be excluded from lifelong medical screening and stimulate individuals at high risk to be monitored more closely for early signs of disease. The techniques for genetic screening are generally available at referral centers offering medical genetic services and genetic counseling.

### MEN type I

***Epidemiology and etiology.*** MEN type I is expressed as an autosomal dominant with high penetrance. The probability that the offspring of an individual with MEN I will inherit the MEN I allele, located on chromosome 11, is 50%. Almost all members of a family who inherit the genetic predisposition for MEN I will develop some component of the disease.

---

The opinions expressed in this editorial are the personal views of the author. They do not represent official policy of the Department of the Army or the Department of Defense.

***Clinical manifestations and diagnosis.*** The likelihood of expressing one of the components of the syndrome increases with age. Parathyroid hyperplasia usually appears in the third or fourth decade of life. About 50% of affected individuals will have clinical disease by the age of 40.

The three common manifestations of MEN I are parathyroid hyperplasia, pancreatic islet cell tumors, and pituitary adenomas. Hyperparathyroidism occurs in practically all MEN I patients and is usually the first endocrinologic abnormality to appear. Islet cell tumors occur in about 70% to 80% and pituitary adenomas occur in about 50% of MEN I patients. In addition to the classic elements of the MEN I triad, about 50% of patients have nonfunctioning bilateral adrenal hyperplasia and some kindreds have a high incidence of lipomas.

The islet cell tumors can secrete more than one hormone and, consequently, can cause more than one endocrine syndrome (Table 39-1). Pancreatic polypeptide is the most common tumor product and, although it does not produce symptoms, its excessive secretion is a useful marker for the presence of pancreatic tumor. Gastrinomas are the most common clinical islet cell tumor (65% of MEN I patients) and cause the Zollinger-Ellison syndrome, which is characterized by severe hypersecretion of gastric acid and intractable gastroduodenal ulceration. Gastrointestinal complications of hypergastrinemia have been the most significant cause of death and disability in individuals with MEN I. MEN I accounts for about one third of gastrinomas; the other two thirds are sporadic. Insulin-secreting islet cell tumors (insulinomas) are the second most common form (35%) of islet cell tumor in MEN I. The principal manifestation of insulinoma is fasting hypoglycemia, which usually presents as syncope or seizures. Islet cell tumors of MEN I can also secrete a variety of other hormones (see Table 39-1), including glucagon, vasoactive intestinal polypeptide (VIP), somatostatin, and growth hormone–releasing hormone or corticotropin-releasing hormone.

The pituitary adenomas associated with MEN I demonstrate the same endocrinologic spectrum as sporadic adenomas (see Chapter 36). The most common type is prolactinoma, which is the third most common endocrine manifestation of MEN I after hyperparathyroidism and gastrinoma. Acromegaly and Cushing's syndrome are also caused by pituitary adenomas in MEN I but can also be due to production of the releasing hormones by an islet cell tumor.

Patients with islet cell tumors, particularly gastrinomas, are at risk for MEN I (about 22% of individuals with gastrinomas and about 4% of individuals with insulinomas). Consequently, such patients should be evaluated for hyperparathyroidism (see Chapter 37) and pituitary adenoma, and if possible their first-degree relatives should be screened for hyperparathyroidism with serum calcium.

Among patients with hyperparathyroidism those who are at increased risk for MEN I are relatively young (under 50), have recurrent disease, have suggestive family histories (e.g., ulcers, nephrolithiasis), or have parathyroid hyperplasia. Further testing for other endocrine abnormalities depends on symptoms and signs. In patients with hyperparathyroidism, gastrin measurements must be deferred until hypercalcemia has been resolved because hypercalcemia will artifactually elevate gastrin levels.

Patients with pituitary adenomas have a 5% risk of MEN I. If these patients also have hypercalcemia, MEN I should be suspected.

***Prospective screening in MEN kindreds.*** Family members of a MEN I patient are at high risk for disease; each has a 50% probability of inheriting the disease allele and manifesting disease. Early detection of disease by endocrine screening tests can reduce morbidity and mortality and is a standard part of the management of MEN I kindreds. In some cases, carriers of the MEN I allele can be identified by genetic analysis.

Individuals at risk for MEN I should have periodic prospective screening (see the box on p. 568) for the

**Table 39-1.** Pancreatic tumors of MEN I

| Tumor | Hormone | Clinical manifestations |
|---|---|---|
| Gastrinoma | Gastrin | Severe peptic ulceration<br>Diarrhea<br>Gastric mucosal hypertrophy |
| Insulinoma | Insulin | Fasting hypoglycemia<br>Syncope<br>Seizures |
| Glucagonoma | Glucagon | Hyperglycemia<br>Necrolytic migratory erythema<br>Anemia<br>Venous thrombosis |
| VIPoma | Vasoactive intestinal peptide | Secretory diarrhea<br>Hypokalemia<br>Metabolic acidosis |
| Somatostatinoma | Somatostatin | Hyperglycemia<br>Cholelithiasis<br>Diarrhea with steatorrhea<br>Anemia |
| | Growth hormone–releasing hormone | Acromegaly (see Chapter 36) |
| | Corticotropin-releasing hormone | Cushing's syndrome (see Chapter 35) |

### Suggested prospective screening for asymptomatic individuals at risk for MEN I

- Symptoms
  - Hypercalcemia
  - Nephrolithiasis
  - Peptic ulcer disease or hyperacidity
  - Diarrhea
  - Hypoglycemia
  - Menstrual disorder
  - Galactorrhea
  - Pituitary insufficiency
  - Visual field disturbance
  - Acromegaly
  - Cushing's syndrome
- Signs
  - Acromegaly
  - Lipomas
  - Cushing's syndrome
- Laboratory evaluation
  - Serum calcium
  - Parathyroid hormone, if elevated calcium
  - Prolactin as clinically indicated
  - Somatomedin C as clinically indicated
  - Fasting blood glucose as clinically indicated
  - Fasting insulin as clinically indicated
- Test meal for gastrin and pancreatic polypeptide
- Pituitary imaging at 4- to 6-year intervals
- Equivocal results should lead to specific focused evaluation

endocrine tumors that comprise it. Since frank endocrine disease can develop even in childhood, the screening should begin before the age of 10. Screening should be repeated at intervals, no less frequently than every 3 years if results are unequivocally normal, and yearly if a trend to abnormality or equivocal test results are obtained. In addition to clinical and laboratory screening, many experts suggest pituitary imaging by magnetic resonance imaging (MRI) or computed tomography (CT) at 4- to 6-year intervals to detect silent microadenomas.

About 90% to 95% of individuals with the disease allele have abnormal screening results by the age of 40 years. However, the risk of developing disease is lifelong; individuals have presented with their first manifestations as late as the eighth decade. Consequently, screening should be continued indefinitely in an individual who is known to have inherited the disease allele.

***Management.*** Islet cell tumors have been the principal cause of morbidity and mortality in MEN I due either to gastrointestinal hemorrhage in Zollinger-Ellison syndrome, hepatic failure due to hepatic metastases, or intractable hypoglycemia in insulinoma.

The islet cell tumors in MEN I are multicentric, having been found both in the body of the pancreas and in the duodenum, and frequently recur after pancreatic resection. Hepatic metastases are common and, even with prospective screening, are often present at diagnosis. Despite this, surgery or other tumor-directed therapy can reduce tumor burden and hormone production sufficiently to remit symptoms in many patients. Since the growth of islet cell tumors is slow and morbidity from the tumor mass can take many years to develop, asymptomatic individuals with hepatic metastases are usually not treated. A variety of techniques are available to manage patients with symptomatic tumor mass or endocrine manifestations unresponsive to medical control. These include surgical debulking, embolization of tumor via the hepatic artery, chemotherapy, and, more recently, liver transplantation.

If surgical management of MEN I–associated gastrinoma is not possible or is unsuccessful, pharmacologic control of gastric hypersecretion is effective in controlling symptoms in many patients. The $H^+$-$K^+$ pump inhibitor omeprazole reduces gastric hyperacidity very effectively. $H_2$-receptor antagonists (e.g., cimetidine, ranitidine) can also be used, although large doses may be required. If inhibiting acid secretion does not control symptoms, then the somatostatin analogue, octreotide, can be tried as a gastrin secretion–inhibiting adjunct.

Insulinoma is treated initially by pancreatic resection or adenectomy using localization techniques to identify active insulin-secreting adenomas. If surgical therapy is unsuccessful, other techniques are available to ameliorate hypoglycemia. These include diazoxide (5 to 15 mg/kg/day) to inhibit insulin secretion, glucocorticoids to increase insulin resistance, glucagon by subcutaneous infusion, and antitumor therapy by embolization or chemotherapy. Octreotide may be helpful in insulinoma but must be used with great caution because it also inhibits glucose counterregulatory hormones and consequently can aggravate hypoglycemia. Intractable insulin-induced hypoglycemia may require chronic parenteral glucose administration.

Glucagonoma, uncontrolled by resection, can be effectively treated with octreotide. The characteristic rash of glucagonoma, necrolytic erythema migrans, also appears to respond to octreotide.

Octreotide is very effective for the control of diarrheal syndromes associated with islet cell tumors. Life-threatening acute exacerbations of diarrhea (diarrheal crisis) can occur due to sudden release of peptides from islet cell tumors. Octreotide in large doses (1000 to 1500 µg per day) rapidly controls the dehydration and electrolyte imbalance associated with these occurrences. Octreotide should be considered prophylactically before procedures (resection, embolization) that may release diarrheogenic hormones.

Parathyroid hyperplasia is managed by total parathyroidectomy and by autotransplantation of one or two glands to the forearm where later resection, if hyperparathyroidism occurs, can be easily accomplished (see Chapter 37).

Pituitary tumors in MEN I are managed according to their clinical presentation (see Chapter 36).

## MEN type II

***Epidemiology and etiology.*** The penetrance of the MEN II inherited trait is very high and virtually all individuals who have the inherited trait will develop disease. The three clinical subtypes are familial medullary carcinoma of the thyroid (FMCT), multiple endocrine neoplasia IIA (MEN IIA), and multiple endocrine neoplasia IIB (MEN IIB). MCT is common to all three subtypes and is the hallmark of the MEN II syndromes, although 75% of MCT cases are not familial. FMCT is not associated with other endocrine neoplasia but is included because of its close genetic relationship to MEN IIA. MEN IIA is the most common (65%) of the three and, in addition to MCT, includes pheochromocytomas (50% of affected individuals) and parathyroid hyperplasia (20%). The components of MEN IIB besides MCT are pheochromocytoma, marfanoid habitus, and submucosal neuromas. The neuromas appear in the lips and tongue, in the conjunctiva and cornea (where they may be seen by ophthalmoscope or slit lamp), and in the gastrointestinal tract, where they can cause dysmotility and obstruction. Parathyroid hyperplasia is not associated with MEN IIB.

The alleles responsible for the MEN II syndromes are found on chromosome 10. In some kindreds with FMCT and MEN IIA specific mutation of the *ret* protooncogene has been found. In these kindreds it is possible to detect the presence of the mutation early in life and identify those members of the kindred at risk.

***Clinical manifestations and diagnosis.*** Medullary carcinoma of the thyroid is common to all of the MEN II syndromes and is the principal cause of morbidity and mortality. Virtually all members of an MEN II kindred develop MCT.

In MEN II diffuse C cell hyperplasia appears early in life, and abnormal calcitonin secretion usually precedes frank tumor formation. This phenomenon is used to identify individuals at risk for MCT. Whereas MCT in FMCT and MEN IIA appears in the third or fourth decade of life, MCT in MEN IIB is much more aggressive and develops much earlier. This difference in the behavior of MCT is the most important difference between the two syndromes. MCT is usually multicentric and usually has metastasized by the time clinically appreciable abnormalities in the thyroid gland develop (see Chapter 34).

Individuals with MEN IIA have a high incidence (about 50%) of multicentric bilateral intraadrenal pheochromocytomas. Like the changes in the thyroid C cells adrenal medullary cells in individuals with MEN IIA exhibit diffuse hyperplasia that precedes the appearance of pheochromocytomas. Periodic urinary or plasma catecholamine measurements combined with adrenal imaging techniques are used to detect early pheochromocytoma. Pheochromocytoma usually (90%) develops after C cell hyperplasia but can be the first manifestation of MEN IIA. MEN IIA–associated pheochromocytomas secrete relatively high levels of epinephrine (see Chapter 35). Early detection by screening has reduced the incidence of clinically apparent pheochromocytoma in MEN IIA.

Hyperparathyroidism due to parathyroid hyperplasia occurs in 10% to 20% of individuals with MEN IIA. It is usually mild and occurs late in the evolution of the syndrome. Early total thyroidectomy to prevent or treat MCT seems to have substantially reduced the incidence of this component of MEN IIA.

Most individuals with MEN IIB have a marfanoid habitus but do not develop the aortic ring dilatation and ocular lens dislocations characteristic of Marfan syndrome. Ganglioneuromatosis of the gastrointestinal tract is a common feature of MEN IIB and frequently causes significant complaints.

***Screening of MEN II kindreds.*** Screening of members of MEN II kindreds reduces the morbidity and mortality associated with MCT by permitting prophylactic thyroidectomy in individuals who have inherited the MEN II allele. Screening is accomplished either by genetic diagnosis as early as possible in life or by serial biochemical screening. Genetic diagnosis offers the advantage of detecting affected individuals before pathologic changes have occurred and excluding members of the kindred who have not inherited the MEN allele from serial testing. In kindreds with FMCT or MEN IIA with a defined mutation of the *ret* protooncogene, specific genetic testing for the mutation detects affected individuals with certainty. For members of kindreds who have not had genetic markers for the MEN II allele defined, serial endocrine testing for C cell hyperplasia and adrenal medullary hyperplasia is necessary. Testing for C cell hyperplasia in a patient from a kindred with FMCT or MEN IIA should begin in the first year of life; in MEN IIB it should begin in the first month.

Screening is done by examining the calcitonin secretory response to calcium or pentagastrin infusion. Tests producing abnormal or equivocal results should be repeated within 3 months. Two abnormal responses are an indication for total thyroidectomy.

Surveillance for pheochromocytoma should be done annually beginning before the age of 10 years. Screening should include both catecholamine measurement and adrenal imaging. Elevation of catecholamines or the development of an adrenal mass is an indication for adrenalectomy.

Although prophylactic thyroidectomy has reduced the incidence of hyperparathyroidism in MEN IIA, these patients should have periodic surveillance using serum calcium and parathyroid hormone concentrations.

***Management.*** The key to management of MEN II is the identification of individuals who have inherited the MEN II allele by genetic or endocrine screening and the prevention of MCT by prophylactic total thyroidectomy with exploration of the neck and mediastinum. No other modality is effective for preventing MCT. Total thyroidectomy seems also to reduce the incidence of hyperparathyroidism in individuals with MEN IIA.

Pheochromocytoma is also managed surgically by removal of the affected adrenal glands. Since the pheochromocytomas associated with MEN IIB are rarely malignant and adrenalectomy causes significant long-term morbidity, prophylactic adrenalectomy is not recommended.

## PARANEOPLASTIC HORMONE SYNDROMES

The principal paraneoplastic hormone syndromes (Table 39-2) include hypercalcemia of malignancy (see Chapter 37), ectopic Cushing's syndrome (see Chapter 35), hyponatremia due to the inappropriate ADH syndrome, non–insulin-mediated hypoglycemia, gynecomastia, and oncogenic hypophosphatemia (see Chapter 37).

### Syndrome of inappropriate antidiuretic hormone

Syndrome of inappropriate antidiuretic hormone (SIADH) is due to the release of vasopressin or vasopressin-like

**Table 39-2.** Principal paraneoplastic endocrine syndromes

| Syndrome | Manifestations | Hormone | Underlying conditions |
|---|---|---|---|
| Humoral hypercalcemia of malignancy | Lethargy<br>Coma<br>Anorexia<br>Constipation<br>Polyuria<br>Muscle weakness | PTH-related peptide | Squamous cell carcinoma (lung, head and neck, cervix)<br>Renal and ovarian adenocarcinoma<br>T cell leukemia |
| | | Cytokines | Multiple myeloma |
| Hypercalcemia due to bone metastases | Hypercalcemia (see above)<br>Bone pain<br>Pathologic fractures | Various tumor products | Breast cancer |
| Ectopic Cushing's syndrome | Muscle wasting and weakness<br>Hypokalemia<br>Hyperpigmentation<br>Psychiatric disturbance | ACTH<br>ACTH precursors | Small cell carcinoma of the lung<br>Carcinoid tumors<br>Carcinoma of the pancreas, thymus, and other sites<br>Pheochromocytoma<br>Medullary thyroid carcinoma |
| SIADH | Hyponatremia | Vasopressin | Small cell carcinoma of the lung<br>Cancer of the prostate and adrenal cortex<br>Hodgkin's lymphoma |
| Tumor-associated hypoglycemia | Fasting hypoglycemia | Insulin-like growth factors (probable) | Mesenchymal tumors<br>Hepatoma |
| Oncogenic hypophosphatemia | Muscle weakness<br>Osteomalacia | ? | Mesenchymal tumors<br>Primary bone tumors<br>Prostatic carcinoma<br>Small cell carcinoma of the lung |
| Erythrocytosis | Polycythemia | Erythropoietin | Renal cell carcinoma<br>Hepatoma<br>Cerebellar hemangioma |
| Gynecomastia | | HCG | Testicular carcinoma |
| Hyperthyroidism | Goiter<br>Tremor<br>Tachycardia<br>Weight loss | HCG | Choriocarcinoma |
| Renin-mediated hypertension | Hypertension | Renin<br>Prorenin | Renal juxtaglomerular cell tumors<br>Carcinoma of pancreas, ovary, lung |

*PTH*, Parathyroid hormone; *ACTH*, adrenocorticotropic hormone; *HCG*, human chorionic gonadotropin.

peptides in the absence of osmotic or volume mediated stimuli. Classic SIADH is associated with three general categories of disorders: neoplasms (notably bronchogenic carcinoma), primary pulmonary disorders (e.g., severe pneumonia) and central nervous system disorders (e.g., encephalitis, tumor, cerebrovascular accident). SIADH is being increasingly recognized as a complication of AIDS and seems to be caused by several different mechanisms. SIADH may also be a component of exertional hyponatremia, which occurs during prolonged exertion in the heat. SIADH and hyponatremia can also be found in postoperative patients and as a side effect of various drugs (see the box at left on p. 571).

SIADH is the most common cause of hyponatremia in hospitalized patients. The actual symptoms manifested by a particular patient depend on the rate and magnitude of the depression of sodium concentration. The symptoms can range from none to seizures, hypothermia, and coma. In postoperative patients, particularly women of reproductive age and children, hyponatremia due to SIADH is a cause of serious morbidity.

Morbidity and mortality related to hyponatremia are due to edema and infarction of the cerebral hemispheres and brainstem. The risk of encephalopathy is related to the rate of development and degree of hyponatremia. Too rapid correction of hyponatremia also presents a risk to the CNS: the osmotic demyelination syndrome.

The key consideration in the diagnosis of SIADH is proving that hyponatremia is due to inappropriate release of vasopressin. Consequently the diagnosis of SIADH depends on excluding all states that produce appropriate physiologic increases in vasopressin (see the box at right on p. 571).

Laboratory findings in SIADH include hyponatremia, a urine osmolality that is inappropriately concentrated compared with a simultaneously measured serum osmolality, urine sodium over 20 mEq/L, hypouricemia, and low BUN. The low serum uric acid and BUN and the elevated urine sodium are helpful discriminators of SIADH from mild volume contraction, in which uric acid and BUN are high and urine sodium is usually less than 15 mEq/L.

### Causes of SIADH

- Neoplasms
  - Small-cell carcinoma of the lung
  - Leukemia/lymphoma
  - Pancreatic carcinoma
  - Prostate carcinoma
  - Thymoma
  - Uterine carcinoma
- Pulmonary disease
  - Acute respiratory failure/pneumonia
  - Advanced tuberculosis
  - Lung abscess/empyema
- Central nervous system disorders
  - CNS infection
  - Mass lesions
  - Intracranial hemorrhage
  - Acute intermittent porphyria
  - Acute head injury
  - Hydrocephalus
  - Acute psychosis
  - Alcohol withdrawal
- Drugs
  - Bromocriptine
  - Carbamazepine
  - Chlorpropamide
  - Clofibrate
  - Colchicine
  - Cyclophosphamide
  - Fluoxetine
  - Narcotics
  - Nicotine
  - Phenothiazines
  - Tricyclic antidepressants
  - Vinblastine
  - Vincristine
- Other causes
  - AIDS
  - Postoperative state/trauma
  - Exercise-heat stress (exertional hyponatremia)
  - Psychosis
  - Alcohol withdrawal

### Diagnosis of SIADH

All the following criteria are required:

1. Hyponatremia (<135 mEq/L) and hypoosmolarity (<275 mosm/kg)
2. Normal plasma and extracellular fluid volume
3. Relative urine hyperosmolarity (>100 mosm/kg)
4. Urinary sodium concentration >20 mEq/L
5. No other cause of hyponatremia
   a. Normal adrenal and thyroid function
   b. Normal renal function
   c. No congestive heart failure
   d. No portal hypertension or cirrhosis
   e. No drug therapy that may cause hyponatremia

The treatment of SIADH depends on the severity of the hyponatremia. The goal of treatment is to relieve symptoms related to hyponatremia and sustain the serum sodium above 125 mEq/L. If the hyponatremia is asymptomatic, water restriction is an effective initial treatment. Water restriction should be titrated by the response of the serum sodium. Daily water intakes between 500 and 1500 ml are usually sufficient to maintain the serum sodium above 125 mEq/L. If water restriction does not reduce urine sodium concentration despite weight loss, then renal sodium wasting, rather than SIADH, should be considered. Water restriction is difficult to maintain over the long term and usually must be supplemented with other techniques to control hyponatremia.

Symptomatic hyponatremia (lethargy, anorexia, headache, seizures, coma) is an unstable and potentially lethal metabolic state requiring urgent correction. Water restriction alone is not an appropriate therapy in this circumstance. The goal of therapy is to raise serum sodium concentration by 1 mEq per hour until symptoms are controlled. (NOTE: The osmotic demyelination syndrome can be almost entirely avoided by restricting the rate of correction of hyponatremia to less than 2 mEq/L per hour with cumulative change no greater than 12 mEq/L in 24 hours or 18 mEq/L in 48 hours.) Treatment options include normal saline (with or without loop diuretics) and hypertonic saline. The choice between normal and hypertonic saline depends in large part on the urine osmolality. If the urine is more concentrated than normal saline (308 mEq/L), then normal saline administration will cause serum sodium to decrease. Decreasing urine osmolality by use of loop diuretics may allow use of normal saline. However, hypertonic saline is a very effective alternative means of raising serum sodium concentrations. Treatment is continued until symptoms resolve or sodium concentration reaches 125 mEq/L. In patients for whom saline loading may carry a risk of congestive heart failure, diuretic therapy can be used to avoid circulatory overload.

Patients with SIADH can be maintained by water restriction alone if that is sufficient to prevent symptomatic hyponatremia at a level of water intake that is acceptable. Patients who cannot accomplish sufficient water restriction to prevent hyponatremia need some type of additional therapeutic agent. Loop diuretics (e.g., furosemide), which increase free water clearance in combination with a liberal salt intake, are typically the first line of therapy. Demeclocycline inhibits the action of ADH in the renal tubule. The usual dose is 600 to 1200 mg per day in 2 to 4 divided doses. Phototoxic reactions are the principal adverse effect, and patients must be cautioned about the risks of sun exposure while taking demeclocycline. Urea in doses of 30 to 60 g per day produces an osmotic diuresis that has been able to control hyponatremia in some patients.

Patients with nonneoplastic conditions causing SIADH should periodically suspend therapy to see if the SIADH has resolved.

### Non-insulin-mediated hypoglycemia

Hypoglycemia not due to excess insulin production is associated with tumors of mesenchymal origin and primary hepatic carcinomas. Some adrenal and gastrointestinal tumors also manifest this syndrome. The hypoglycemia appears to be caused by insulin-like growth factors secreted by the tumors. Patients present with symptomatic fasting hypoglycemia either with a seizure or syncopal episode.

Management of the hypoglycemia by removal of the inciting tumor is not possible in the majority of cases. No single medical approach has been satisfactory. High-carbohydrate feedings every 3 to 4 hours around the clock, nocturnal infusions of 10% dextrose, and supraphysiologic doses of glucocorticoids to induce insulin resistance have all been used to manage the hypoglycemia.

## CARCINOID TUMORS AND THE CARCINOID SYNDROME

### Carcinoid tumors

Carcinoid tumors are neoplasms that arise from a distinct category of enterochromaffin cells that comprise the dispersed neuroendocrine system. These cells are widely distributed throughout the body, and consequently carcinoids have been reported from many anatomic locations. Carcinoid tumors are relatively common, usually benign in behavior, and are usually discovered incidentally.

Most carcinoid tumors are hormonally silent and produce no systemic symptoms. However, the enterochromaffin cells that give rise to carcinoid tumors normally secrete a wide variety of hormones and other bioactive substances and thus have the potential to produce a number of syndromes. In addition to the typical carcinoid syndrome, carcinoid tumors can produce Cushing's syndrome, acromegaly, SIADH, oncogenic osteomalacia, watery diarrhea with hypokalemia, and hypergastrinemia.

Carcinoid tumors occur most commonly in the appendix (about 65%) and are usually found incidentally during appendectomy. Carcinoid tumors in the proximal appendix are even occasionally the cause of appendicitis. Appendiceal carcinoids almost never metastasize or cause the carcinoid syndrome. The next most common site is the small bowel, particularly the jejunum and ileum (about 15%), where carcinoids are frequently multicentric. The lung is the site of about 10% of carcinoid tumors; the remainder appear in other gastrointestinal sites, the ovary, testis, or pancreas.

Carcinoid tumors are usually indolent and produce significant morbidity or mortality only after many years. They may present with symptoms related to the tumor itself. In the gastrointestinal tract the most common symptoms are intermittent obstruction or bleeding. Carcinoid tumors can cause a fibrotic reaction in the underlying mesentery, which can cause dysmotility and ulceration. Carcinoid tumors in the biliary tree or ampulla (particularly associated with neuroectodermal dysplasia syndromes such as neurofibromatosis) can cause obstructive jaundice or portal hypertension. In the lung, carcinoid tumors produce cough, bronchial obstruction, and hemoptysis. Carcinoid tumors in other locations are usually asymptomatic until a large tumor mass develops or metastases appear.

### The carcinoid syndrome

The carcinoid syndrome is a characteristic group of systemic symptoms produced by some carcinoid tumors. The principal manifestation of the syndrome is paroxysmal facial and truncal flushing lasting 1 to 2 minutes with a sense of cutaneous warmth but without sweating. Diarrhea, which may be severe, is also common. Occasional patients may develop wheezing or cough associated with the flushing. After considerable time patients with uncontrolled carcinoid syndrome may develop (1) a characteristic facies with a permanent plethora and telangiectasia or (2) endocardial fibrosis, which leads to valvular dysfunction and heart failure.

The carcinoid syndrome requires the introduction of tumor products into the systemic circulation. For tumors located outside the gastrointestinal tract (lung, gonad) the carcinoid syndrome can appear early, before metastasis. However, because the liver effectively removes carcinoid tumor products, gastrointestinal carcinoid tumors are usually clinically silent until metastases have developed in liver or other extraintestinal tissues.

The principal mediators of the carcinoid syndrome differ somewhat depending on the location of the tumor. Serotonin is the best characterized tumor product and probably is the primary mediator of endocardial fibrosis and diarrhea. The flushing is due to peptides and, particularly in gastric carcinoids, histamine. Some carcinoids produce primarily 5-hydroxytryptophan, which is converted to serotonin after release.

### Diagnosis

Because clinically significant carcinoids are uncommon and indolent, the symptoms that are finally recognized as due to a carcinoid tumor often have been present for years. The diagnosis should be considered in individuals with flushing spells or persistent diarrhea or other unexplained gastrointestinal complaints. Carcinoid tumors should be included in the differential diagnosis of most syndromes of hormone excess.

Since either serotonin or 5-hydroxytryptophan appears to be produced consistently in the carcinoid syndrome, diagnosis is based on the demonstration of high levels of 5-hydroxyindoleacetic acid (5-HIAA), a metabolite of both, in a 24-hour urine collection. Many substances can interfere with the interpretation of 5-HIAA levels, and specific protocols should be followed to ensure accuracy. 5-HIAA levels greater than 25 mg/24 hours in a patient with clear symptoms and signs of the carcinoid syndrome are diagnostic. Less elevated levels (6 to 25 mg/24 hours) may be due to artifact, carcinoid syndrome, mastocytosis, or primary intestinal disease (most notably gluten enteropathy). If the elevation persists, then a radiologic investigation of the chest and abdomen is indicated. If the patient has flushing spells, mast cell disorders should be considered. Provocative testing with epinephrine can be used to distinguish between flushing due to carcinoid, which can be evoked by epinephrine, and flushing due to mastocytosis, which is usually moderated by epinephrine.

Carcinoid tumors are treated, when possible, by surgical removal. Small tumors, particularly in extraintestinal sites, are often cured by resection. Many intestinal carcinoids have metastasized at the time of diagnosis, but local resection of tumor and regional lymph nodes has produced apparent cure of symptomatic individuals in some cases.

Patients with unresectable carcinoid tumor and the carcinoid syndrome can be treated medically. Octreotide is the mainstay of therapy and controls diarrhea and flushing in most cases. Flushing associated with gastric carcinoids is, at least in part, due to their release of histamine. Combination therapy with $H_1$ and $H_2$ blockers can help control this symptom and any associated bronchospasm and wheezing. Serotonin antagonists (cyproheptadine, methysergide) have been effective in controlling diarrhea in carcinoid syndrome. However, they do not seem to ameliorate the endocardial fibrosis or reduce the later requirement for cardiac valve replacement. Bronchial carcinoids appear to be sensitive to glucocorticoids, which can be used to control carcinoid symptoms for patients with these tumors.

Embolization, antitumor chemotherapy, and resection of large tumor masses have all been used with benefit in the control of carcinoid syndrome unresponsive to medical therapy. Recent reports suggest the combination of interferon $\alpha$-2 and octreotide is particularly effective in controlling carcinoid syndrome.

## AUTOIMMUNE POLYGLANDULAR SYNDROMES

Most cases of autoimmune mediated endocrine disease occur sporadically and affect only one endocrine tissue. However, the two well-defined syndromes in which multiple endocrine tissues are affected are autoimmune polyglandular syndrome type I and type II (see the box below). Both these syndromes have a high incidence of spontaneous adrenal insufficiency. Recognition of either syndrome in an individual or kindred allows prospective surveillance for adrenal or other endocrine gland dysfunction.

### Components of the autoimmune polyglandular syndromes

**Autoimmune polyglandular syndrome type I**

Major
- Mucocutaneous candidiasis
- Hypoparathyroidism
- Adrenal insufficiency

Minor
- Alopecia
- Malabsorption
- Autoimmune chronic active hepatitis
- Hypogonadism
- Pernicious anemia
- Thyroid disease (Graves' disease or primary hypothyroidism)

**Autoimmune polyglandular syndrome type II**

Major
- Thyroid disease (Graves' disease or primary hypothyroidism)
- Insulin-dependent diabetes mellitus
- Adrenal insufficiency
- Hypogonadism
- Myasthenia gravis
- Gluten-induced enteropathy

Minor
- Vitiligo
- Alopecia
- Serositis
- Parkinson's disease
- Pernicious anemia

### Autoimmune polyglandular syndrome type I

Autoimmune polyglandular syndrome type I (APS I) has three principal components: mucocutaneous candidiasis, hypoparathyroidism, and adrenal insufficiency. Chronic candidiasis and primary hypoparathyroidism typically develop in the first or second decade of life. Adrenal insufficiency usually appears after hypoparathyroidism but has been known to precede it. The majority of individuals with APS I eventually acquire all three deficiency diseases but some only develop one or two. APS I is familial and is inherited in an autosomal recessive pattern, affecting siblings but not the immediately preceding or following generations. About 10% of individuals developing idiopathic hypoparathyroidism before the age of 20 have this syndrome and later develop adrenal insufficiency.

Individuals with APS I are prone to develop certain other autoimmune diseases that are considered minor components of APS I: alopecia, malabsorption, autoimmune chronic active hepatitis, hypogonadism, pernicious anemia, and hyperthyroidism or hypothyroidism.

The diagnosis of APS I depends on the appearance of chronic candidiasis and hypoparathyroidism or adrenal insufficiency in a sibship. The appearance of any two major or minor components in a single individual is suggestive of the syndrome and should lead to the evaluation of the patient's siblings. Not all members of a sibship with APS I manifest the complete syndrome. There are no useful markers currently to distinguish those members of a sibship at risk from those who have not inherited the propensity to autoimmune disease. Since adrenal insufficiency may appear late in life, it is prudent to periodically evaluate each member of an APS I sibship. The evaluation should screen adrenal, parathyroid, thyroid, and liver function, and vitamin $B_{12}$ concentration. Antiadrenal and antiparathyroid antibodies should be measured, since they have considerable predictive value for the development of adrenal and parathyroid failure.

All members of a sibship with APS I should be counseled about the risk of late-appearing autoimmune disease, particularly the risk of adrenal insufficiency and about the need for periodic examination.

### Autoimmune polyglandular syndrome type II

Autoimmune polyglandular syndrome type II (APS II) is more common than APS I. It is an inherited condition and appears to be an autosomal dominant with variable penetrance. It is associated with specific HLA antigens, which allows the possibility of detecting kindred members who have inherited the susceptibility to APS II.

The major autoimmune diseases of APS II are thyroid disease (Graves' disease or primary hypothyroidism), insulin-dependent diabetes mellitus, adrenal insufficiency, hypogonadism, myasthenia gravis, and gluten-induced enteropathy. Individuals with APS II can have just one or any combination of these conditions. Kindreds with APS II usually do not exhibit any particular pattern of diseases in their affected members. Rather, it is the susceptibility to disease that is inherited. A number of other autoimmune diseases are encountered in kindreds with APS II. In many cases the association is reported in only one or two instances; however, certain conditions occur at distinctly higher incidence in APS II than in the general population, such as vitiligo, alopecia, serositis, Parkinson's disease, and pernicious anemia.

Individuals with the inherited susceptibility to APS II have about a 50% chance of developing one of the major associated diseases. Individuals who have developed one APS-associated disease have a 50% chance of developing another.

The diagnosis of APS II can be made upon the appearance of a characteristic autoimmune disease in a member of a known kindred or in an individual with two or more APS II-associated autoimmune diseases. Individuals with an APS II-associated disease should be screened periodically for the appearance of additional autoimmune disease. Screening should include a clinical examination looking for evidence of APS II-associated disease and tests of thyroid and adrenal function, vitamin $B_{12}$ concentration, and organ-specific autoantibodies. Screening examinations should be done at 3-year intervals in individuals with no evidence of new autoimmune disease, but more frequently for those with elevated levels of specific antibodies. Because the risk of disease does not diminish with age, screening should be continued throughout life.

Because of the dominant pattern of inheritance, screening and counseling should be offered to all first-degree relatives of patients with APS II. In some kindreds HLA typing can pinpoint with considerable confidence the members at risk for autoimmune disease and so permit a more focused surveillance program for the family, freeing those members with little risk from lifelong concern and repeated medical evaluation. For those family members at risk who have no specific complaints or evidence of autoimmune disease, measurement of thyroid function, glucose tolerance, and antiadrenal antibodies every 2 or 3 years is sufficient.

APS II should be seriously considered in an individual with one characteristic autoimmune disease and a suggestive family history. If APS II is suspected, the patient should be screened for the presence of other APS II-associated autoimmune disease. Where available, organ-specific antibodies to target tissues (e.g., thyroid, gonads, adrenal and islet cell) should be measured. Glucose tolerance, vitamin $B_{12}$ concentration, and thyroid and adrenal function should be measured. First-degree relatives should be screened. In the absence of specific symptoms or signs, screening relatives for thyroid disease and postprandial hyperglycemia has the highest likelihood of detecting silent autoimmune endocrinopathy and confirming the diagnosis of APS II. If confirmed in a kindred, then additional screening for early autoimmune disease becomes appropriate.

The management of an individual with APS II includes appropriate replacement therapy and periodic surveillance for the appearance of new autoimmune disease.

## BIBLIOGRAPHY


Davila DG, et al: Bronchial carcinoid tumors, *Mayo Clin Proc* 68:795, 1993.

Kovacs L, Robertson GL: Syndrome of inappropriate antidiuresis, *Endocrinol Metab Clin North Am* 21:859, 1992.

Marshall JB, Bodnarchuk G: Carcinoid tumors of the gut. Our experience over three decades and a review of the literature, *J Clin Gastroenterol* 16:123, 1993.

Raue F, Frank-Raue K, Grauer A: Multiple endocrine neoplasia type 2: clinical features and screening, *Endocrinol Metab Clin North Am* 23:137, 1994.

Riley RJ: Autoimmune polyglandular syndromes, *Horm Res* 38 (Suppl 2):9, 1992.

Skogseid B, Rastad J, Oberg K: Multiple endocrine neoplasia type 1: clinical features and screening, *Endocrinol Metab Clin North Am* 23:1, 1994.

Sterns RH: The management of symptomatic hyponatremia, *Semin Nephrol* 10:503, 1990.


CHAPTER

# 40 Lipid Disorders

**Stuart R. Chipkin**

## EPIDEMIOLOGY AND ETIOLOGY

Over the past 50 years the focus in the field of lipid metabolism has changed from biochemical reactions to clinical marker to modifiable risk factor. Observational and migration studies have documented the association between cholesterol and atherosclerosis using endpoints ranging from autopsy to myocardial infarction to angiographic coronary disease (see Chapter 7). After recognizing cholesterol as a risk factor, intervention studies have been subsequently conducted to prove that lowering cholesterol improves risk. Basic science research has provided understanding of the cellular abnormalities that help define the relationship between lipids and vascular plaque formation. Public awareness programs (e.g., National Cholesterol Education Program) have helped to change behavior throughout the United States. This approach covering epidemiology, intervention trials, and public health has become a model for primary prevention of chronic disease.

Significant advances have been made in the understanding and treatment of lipid abnormalities. Lipid testing currently allows simple screening for identification of patients at risk. In the future, profiles of proteins that coordinate lipoprotein reactions may serve as more precise markers of risk. Changes in diet are easier to integrate into daily living than they once were, although diets high in saturated fat and cholesterol still are widespread among certain cultural groups. Similarly, routine exercise has become a common part of many people's lives, although this phenomenon decreases with socioeconomic status and age. Pharmacologic alternatives now exist that allow effective treatment of hyperlipidemic states, although not all patient populations have been fully studied. Unfortunately, there are still large numbers of patients who remain undiagnosed and at high risk for development of atherosclerosis.

The majority of lipid disorders faced by the primary physician in the United States are the result of an imbalance between physiologic pathways and behavior. Cellular mechanisms maximize the availability of cholesterol to cells for use as a component of membranes and as a precursor for bile acids, sex hormones, and adrenal steroid synthesis. The two principal sources for the body's cholesterol are the liver (where it is synthesized) and the intestines (where it is absorbed). Dietary intake thus can greatly influence total body cholesterol.

Human biochemical pathways originally developed in an environment of low-fat diets and high physical activity. Over centuries, in Western societies, dietary fat has increased substantially and physical activity has decreased. As excess of dietary fat and cholesterol exceeds cellular capacity, lipid concentrations increase in the vascular space and eventually within the vascular wall, contributing to the development of atherosclerosis.

## PATHOPHYSIOLOGY

Clinical abnormalities of cholesterol and lipid metabolism have their basis in the balance between synthesis, absorption, transport, uptake, and excretion of lipids. Cholesterol enters the circulation from either intestinal absorption or hepatic synthesis. The cholesterol absorbed from the intestinal tract comes from two origins: dietary cholesterol (250 to 500 mg per day in most Americans) or bile (600 to 1000 mg per day). Animal products are the exclusive source of dietary cholesterol; fruits and vegetables contain none. Although biliary cholesterol is excreted into the intestines, bile is still a significant source of cholesterol absorption because 50% is reabsorbed. This reabsorption process probably developed in response to an environment in which metabolic demand for cholesterol was greater than dietary intake. As dietary intake of cholesterol greatly increased, an enhanced ability to absorb cholesterol increased serum levels.

Cholesterol also enters the circulation after being synthesized from 3-hydroxy-3-methylglutaryl coenzyme A (HMG CoA), principally within hepatic cells. The enzyme that converts HMG CoA to mevalonic acid, HMG CoA reductase, determines the rate of cholesterol synthesis. Inhibition of this enzyme decreases cholesterol synthesis. Cholesterol synthesized in the liver may be converted into bile acids, which facilitate intestinal fat absorption, excreted into the intestines via the bile, or released directly into the circulation.

Since lipids are not water soluble, they are transported in the circulation within particles possessing hydrophobic centers and hydrophilic peripheries. The peripheries of these lipoprotein particles contain free cholesterol and phospholipids, which are polar, and apoproteins (or apolipoproteins), which serve to stabilize the particle, enhance membrane transport, and serve as ligands for specific receptors. The relative contribution of lipid and protein changes the density of these particles and creates distinct categories (Fig. 40-1).

### Lipoprotein particles and pathways

Cholesterol and triglyceride pathways involve transportation of lipoproteins from a point of synthesis to target tissues and their return transport to a site of reabsorption and degradation. Since the source of dietary lipid is external, the pathway beginning with intestinal absorption of cholesterol and triglycerides is termed exogenous (Fig. 40-2). Dietary fat is principally transported from intestine to liver within chylomicron particles. After ingestion of a meal containing fat, bile acid micelles containing intestinal lipids stimulate epithelial cells of the small intestine to synthesize chylomicrons. Chylomicrons are the largest lipoprotein particle but, because of their high lipid content, they are also the least dense. Following transport through mesenteric lymph to the thoracic duct, chylomicrons enter the bloodstream. Triglycerides are released from chylomicrons after exposure to lipoprotein lipase. This enzyme is synthesized in adipose tissue, muscle, breast, and lung cells and is located along capillary endothelial cell surfaces. Depending on the tissue, the liberated free fatty acids are used for fuel (muscle), storage (fat), or synthesis of other compounds (breast and liver). The residual particles containing a small amount of triglyceride are termed chylomicron remnants. Impaired stimulation of lipoprotein lipase in diabetes mellitus explains the high level of triglycerides found with hyperglycemia. Lipoprotein lipase deficiency occurs as an autosomal recessive deficiency and produces severe hypertriglyceridemia.

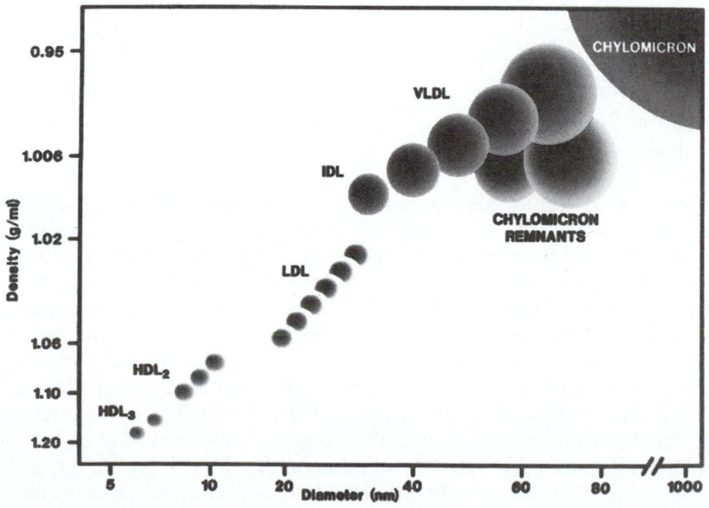


**Fig. 40-1.** Distribution of lipoproteins along a density continuum.

The pathway of lipid transport that originates in the liver is referred to as endogenous. Lipids synthesized in the liver are transported to peripheral tissues via very low–density lipoprotein (VLDL) (see Fig. 40-2). Similar to chylomicrons, these particles have triglyceride released after exposure to lipoprotein lipase. The residual particles, intermediate-density lipoprotein (IDL), are taken up by the liver via the low-density lipoprotein (LDL) receptor. VLDL particles can also be metabolized directly to LDL via the enzyme hepatic triglyceride lipase.

Seventy percent of the total plasma cholesterol is transported within LDL particles to the liver (75%) and

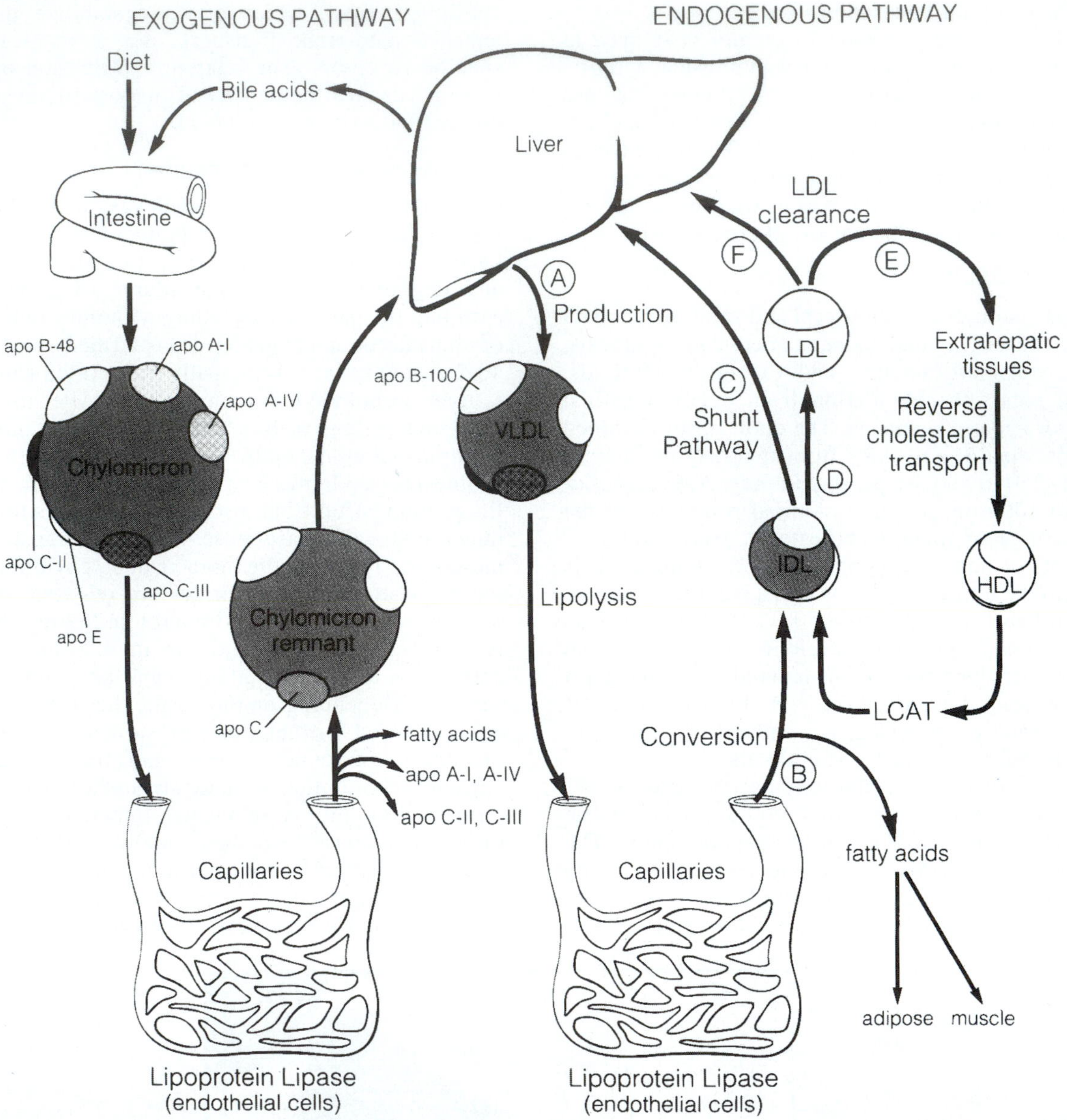


**Fig. 40-2.** Pathways of Lipid Metabolism: The exogenous pathway *(left)* describes the absorption of metabolism of fats ingested from dietary sources. Absorbed fats form chylomicrons, which move from lymph into the bloodstream where insulin activates lipoprotein lipase to release fatty acids for use by muscle or fat. The endogenous pathway *(right)* depicts formation of lipoproteins within the liver followed by metabolism in other parts of the body and return to the liver. After hepatic synthesis of VLDL with apo C,E and B-100, lipoprotein lipase is stimulated in the same fashion as the exogenous pathway. The remnant IDL is either taken up by the liver through apo E receptors or is further metabolized to LDL. LDL circulates through the periphery and is taken up at the liver by the LDL receptor. Although there is essentially no feedback mechanism within the exogenous pathway, the endogenous pathway can exert feedback inhibition through the receptors on the cell service. In the reverse transport pathway, free cholesterol is taken up by nascent HDL in peripheral tissues and transferred to apo E-containing lipoproteins which can then be taken up by apo E receptors in the liver. Direct hepatic uptake of HDL may also exist.

other peripheral tissues. LDL particles encompass a wide array of subtypes. Small, dense LDL particles, which are found more often in males and in patients with diabetes, appear to be more atherogenic.

Many of the mechanisms by which LDL increases risk for atherosclerosis occur beneath the arterial wall. After traversing the intima, LDL can be oxidized by endothelial and smooth muscle cells. Oxidized LDL results in accumulation of circulating monocytes, which take up the modified LDL via alternative scavenger receptors. Upon uptake of oxidized LDL, these monocytes become lipid-filled macrophages that can further oxidize LDL. Continued excess oxidized LDL appears to inhibit macrophage motility and locally derived relaxing factors. As foam cells develop from the lipid-filled macrophages, the first visible lesion in atherosclerosis, the fatty streak, appears.

The return of cholesterol from peripheral tissues to the liver involves high-density lipoprotein (HDL) and is referred to as reverse transport (see Fig. 40-2). HDL contain relatively little lipid and much protein and thus are the smallest and densest lipoprotein particle (see Fig. 40-1). HDL has been found in several studies to correlate inversely with coronary artery disease (see Chapter 7). Of the subclasses of HDL that have been identified, some studies suggest that $HDL_2$ correlates best with protection against coronary artery disease. However, total HDL is currently the most relevant clinical measure. HDL particles, which are initially made in a nascent form in the liver, take up and transport free cholesterol from the periphery to the liver. In addition to the potential protective effect of this reverse cholesterol transport from periphery to liver, HDL may be beneficial because of its ability to inhibit binding of LDL to matrix proteins, oxidation of LDL, and receptor uptake of oxidized LDL.

Lipoprotein (a), or Lp(a), is a particle intermediate in density between HDL and LDL that correlates strongly with risk for atherosclerosis. It is composed of apoprotein B and a glycoprotein, apo (a), which has strong homology to plasminogen. Levels of Lp(a) do not appear to vary with age, sex, total cholesterol, or triglyceride and change little with dietary or pharmacologic therapy.

## Cellular metabolism of lipoproteins

LDLs are taken up by receptors that recognize specific apoproteins. Activation by apoproteins means that LDL receptors may take up many lipoproteins, including IDL and VLDL. For this reason the LDL receptor is also referred to as the apo-B,E receptor. After internalization, the receptor cycles back to the surface and the LDL is broken down. The free cholesterol released from LDL metabolism is used for cellular demands (formation of cell membranes or steroids) or is stored as cholesterol ester.

The number of LDL receptors at the cell surface helps to regulate the amount of intracellular cholesterol. Synthesis of receptors is increased when the amount of cholesterol within the cell is decreased (Table 40-1). In the converse situation an increase in intracellular cholesterol results in decreased cell membrane receptors and prevents further uptake of cholesterol-rich LDL particles. This mechanism, while maintaining intracellular cholesterol, allows the concentration of cholesterol in the vascular space to increase. Although this mechanism may have had no adverse consequences for individuals on a low-cholesterol diet, it may be maladaptive to a Western style diet high in cholesterol and saturated fat.

Two other mechanisms within the cell also serve to maintain concentrations of intracellular cholesterol. A negative feedback from rising intracellular cholesterol causes inhibition of HMG CoA reductase, the rate-limiting step of cholesterol synthesis. In addition, intracellular cholesterol levels can be modified by the enzyme acyl CoA: cholesterol acyltransferase (ACAT), which converts cholesterol to a cholesteryl ester storage form. The result of all these mechanisms is that, when the amount of cholesterol within the body increases, cellular concentrations remain stable while vascular concentrations rise.

Abnormalities in the LDL (apo-B,E) receptor have been identified and associated with hyperlipidemic states and premature coronary artery disease. Mutations have been identified at several sites of receptor synthesis and processing. Familial hypercholesterolemia is a disease resulting from a defect in LDL receptors (Table 40-2).

## Apoproteins

Generally located on the outer hydrophilic portion of lipoproteins, apoproteins serve important roles by stabilizing lipoprotein structure, enhancing membrane trans-

**Table 40-1.** Effect of intracellular cholesterol on receptor synthesis

| | LDL receptor synthesis | HMG CoA reductase activity | ACAT activity |
|---|---|---|---|
| ↓ Intracellular cholesterol | ↑ | ↑ | ↓ |
| ↑ Intracellular cholesterol | ↓ | ↓ | ↑ |

*LDL*, Low-density lipoprotein; *HMA CoA*, 3-hydroxy-3-methylglutaryl coenzyme A; *ACAT*, acyl CoA: cholesterol acyltransferase.

**Table 40-2.** Inherited defects in lipid metabolism

| | Inheritance pattern | Prevalence | Major abnormality |
|---|---|---|---|
| Familial combined hyperlipidemia | Autosomal dominant | 10-15% of all MIs under age 60 | ↑ LDL and VLDL |
| Familial hypertriglyceridemia | Autosomal dominant | 5% of all MIs under age 60 | ↑ VLDL |
| Familial hypercholesterolemia | Autosomal dominant | 5% of all MIs under age 60 | ↑ LDL |
| Tangier disease | Autosomal recessive | | ↓ HDL |

*MI*, Myocardial infarction; *LDL*, low-density lipoprotein; *VLDL*, very-low-density lipoprotein; *HDL*, high-density lipoprotein.

port, acting as receptor ligands, and serving as cofactors for enzymes. They are typically classified into four groups: apo B, A, C, and E. Apoproteins B-48 and B-100 are large proteins located in triglyceride-rich lipoproteins. Apo B-100 is used in the production of VLDL and binds to the LDL receptor. Decreased amounts of apo B result in low triglyceride levels and occasionally deficiencies in vitamins E and A. Genetic excess of apo B-100 is the underlying cause of familial combined hyperlipidemia, found in 10% to 15% of patients with myocardial infarction before age 60 (see Table 40-2). Apoprotein A activates the enzyme that esterifies cholesterol and transfers it to HDL, suggesting an important role in reverse cholesterol transport. Abnormal apo A occurs in Tangier disease and results in hypertriglyceridemia and low HDL (under 5 mg/dl). Cholesterol esters become deposited in the reticuloendothelial system, giving rise to the characteristic orange tonsils, lymphodenopathy, and hepatosplenomegaly. Apoprotein C is required for activation of lipoprotein lipase, which hydrolyzes triglycerides from chylomicrons and VLDL. Abnormalities of apo C-II produce extremely high levels of serum triglyceride and abdominal pain with pancreatitis. Apoprotein E is located on nearly all lipoproteins except LDL and acts as a ligand for LDL and apo E receptors. By stimulating these membrane-bound receptors, apo E plays an important role in cellular uptake of cholesterol. Each parent contributes one of three isoforms of apo E with varying affinity for the apo E receptor; apo E-4 has the greatest and apo E-2 has the least. Homozygotes for apo E-2 have elevated VLDL and IDL, tuberoeruptive xanthomas, VLDL/triglyceride ratio greater than 0.3, and are at risk for premature coronary artery disease.

### Lipid abnormalities

Serum lipid levels become abnormal, as described above, when lipids available to cells exceed metabolic demands. In the most general sense cholesterol or triglyceride levels become elevated if too much lipid enters the vascular space or too little is metabolized or excreted. As points of entry into the bloodstream, both intestine and liver are potential causes of hypercholesterolemia. Impaired degradation of cholesterol can occur because of alterations in reverse transport, receptor number, or receptor signaling via apoproteins (see above).

Increased entry of cholesterol into the bloodstream can be caused by primary or secondary defects. Primary causes of hypercholesterolemia include diet and genetic abnormalities (see below and Table 40-2). Although total cholesterol and LDL levels increase in men and women from Western societies between ages 20 and 60, many believe that the increased production and decreased clearance are due to changes in diet and exercise behaviors.

Major dietary sources of cholesterol are meat, eggs, and animal fats (which include milk products). Increased dietary cholesterol raises LDL levels, which decrease cellular LDL receptor levels, which further decreases uptake of both LDL and VLDL. Reduction in LDL receptors is also thought to occur in response to intake of foods rich in saturated fatty acids such as coconut oil, butterfat, palm oil, and cocoa butter. Excess caloric intake does not always increase serum cholesterol, since those who exercise and eat high-calorie diets do not demonstrate hypercholesterolemia. Obese individuals overproduce VLDL (containing apo B) and have diminished levels of HDL.

Increased serum triglyceride levels are usually the result of excessive dietary intake. Increased VLDL and triglyceride levels are also found in familial hypertriglyceridemia, an autosomal dominant abnormality found in 5% of patients younger than age 60 with myocardial infarction. Patients with familial combined hyperlipidemia have both elevated VLDL and LDL.

### Secondary causes of hypercholesterolemia

Abnormal lipid profiles can also occur secondary to disorders of hormone balance, liver, and kidney. The reversibility of the lipid abnormalities is directly related to the reversibility of the underlying condition. Hypothyroidism causes hypercholesterolemia and hypertriglyceridemia, although the increased risk for myocardial infarction is unclear. Patients with type II diabetes mellitus or poorly controlled type I diabetes have hypertriglyceridemia. Increased triglyceride synthesis is stimulated by increased glucose and fatty acid concentrations. Decreased hydrolysis of triglycerides occurs because of impaired insulin-stimulated lipoprotein lipase activity. Although hypertriglyceridemia is a strong predictor of cardiovascular disease in diabetic patients, this may reflect glucose control, since triglycerides frequently normalize with intensive therapy. These patients also tend to have decreased HDL levels, even after correction for obesity. Estrogen increases HDL and lowers total cholesterol; progesterone tends to decrease HDL; anabolic steroids appear to increase LDL (see Chapter 7).

Obstructive liver disease produces hypercholesterolemia by blocking the only pathway of cholesterol excretion. Similarly, impaired secretion of bile and bile acids feeds back to the hepatocyte and downregulates LDL receptors, causing increased serum cholesterol levels.

The nephrotic syndrome can cause abnormalities in cholesterol and triglyceride. Hypoalbuminemia stimulates lipoprotein synthesis and increases LDL. Impaired metabolism of VLDL has been observed and hypertriglyceridemia has been reported. As renal failure develops, lipoprotein lipase activity is progressively impaired and triglyceride levels become the predominant lipid abnormality.

## HISTORY AND PHYSICAL EXAMINATION

The majority of lipid abnormalities are not associated with specific symptoms or signs. However, portions of the history and physical can be very helpful in identifying high-risk patients and those with very specific lipid abnormalities. Symptoms of pancreatitis or abdominal pain can be due to hypertriglyceridemia. A diet history can detect excess lipid intake and provide insight into simple but effective changes to reduce dietary lipid. Cultural factors may determine methods of food preparation and increase exposure to saturated fat. Simple questions that can provide important clues are: "How many meatless meals do you have per week?" "How often do you use oil to prepare food?" "How many eggs per week do you eat?" Patient histories can also provide clues to underlying secondary causes of hyperlipidemia, including diabetes, hypothyroidism, and renal or hepatic failure.

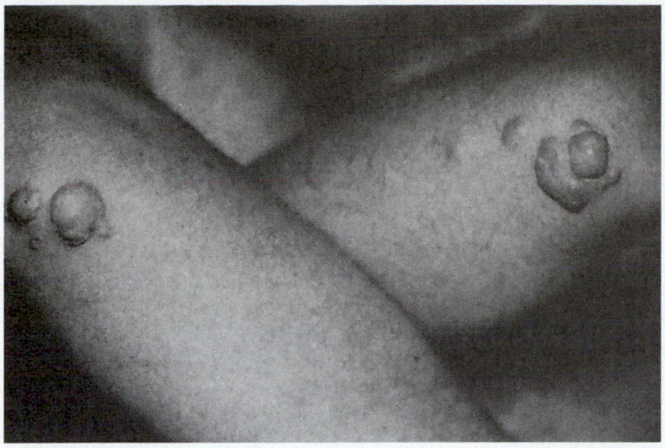

**Fig. 40-3.** Tuberoeruptive xanthomas. Pictured are the firm, yellowish nodules that typically appear on the elbows, knees, buttocks, and palms.

Although not very sensitive for general hyperlipidemic abnormalities, physical findings can be quite specific for certain hyperlipidemic states. Corneal arcus and extensor xanthomas are strongly indicative of familial hypercholesterolemia caused by abnormal LDL receptors. Tuberoeruptive xanthomas (elbows, knees, buttocks, and palms) are seen in apo E abnormalities and familial hypertriglyceridemia (Fig. 40-3). Orange tonsils are virtually pathognomonic for Tangier disease.

## TESTING

Diagnosis of lipid abnormalities currently depends on measurement of cholesterol and triglyceride fractions of specific lipoproteins. Although this minimizes the contribution of specific apoproteins, use of lipoprotein measurement throughout research trials and ease of testing have established these substances as the standard for assessing cardiovascular risk. In the future specific apoproteins may become the preferred measure for deciding on need for therapeutic intervention (see Chapter 7).

Currently the National Cholesterol Education Program recommends that every adult over the age of 20 have total and HDL cholesterol measured. Most experts agree that patients do not have to be fasting for the measurement of total and HDL cholesterol to be accurate. For those patients with a total cholesterol over 200 mg/dl and an HDL less than 35, a full lipid profile should be analyzed to determine the relative contribution of LDL, HDL, and VLDL. If the patient has a cholesterol over 200 and either known cardiovascular disease or more than two risk factors for atherosclerosis (see the box at right), a full lipid profile is also appropriate. In addition, a total cholesterol greater than 240 mg/dl is sufficient to warrant a complete lipid profile.

Children who have a positive family history of premature heart disease may have a genetic hyperlipidemic condition. Early identification of these children may stimulate initiation of dietary modifications that reduce fat and cholesterol intake. Exercise programs can also be established at an early age. Consensus on pharmacologic treatment of pediatric patients is less well defined than that on adults. Cholesterol-lowering medications have not been studied in children, and their use could be harmful.

### Risk factors for coronary heart disease

**Positive**

Age ≥ 45 for men
≥ 55 for women (or premature menopause without estrogen therapy)
Family history of premature coronary heart disease
Smoking
Hypertension
HDL cholesterol ≤ 35 mg/dl
Diabetes

**Negative**

HDL cholesterol ≥ 60 mg/dl

**Table 40-3.** Range of cholesterol values

| | Desirable | Borderline | High risk |
|---|---|---|---|
| **Without known vascular disease** | | | |
| Total cholesterol | <200 | 200-239 | ≥240 |
| LDL cholesterol | <130 | 130-159 | ≥160 |
| HDL cholesterol | ≥35 | | <35 |
| **With known vascular disease** | | | |
| LDL cholesterol | ≤100 | | >100 |

Modified from *JAMA* 269 (23):3015, 1993.

Lipid profiles typically consist of measured concentrations of total cholesterol, HDL and triglycerides, and calculated VLDL and LDL levels. Since triglyceride levels rapidly rise and fall after eating, accurate measurements of circulating triglycerides can be obtained only in the fasting state. Patients should fast for 9 to 12 hours before having a lipid profile drawn. If triglycerides exceed 400, VLDL cannot be estimated and lipoproteins must be measured following centrifugation. If triglycerides are less than 400, the normal 1:5 ratio of VLDL to triglycerides can be used; the VLDL value is calculated by dividing the triglyceride value by five. By using the estimated VLDL and the measured concentrations of total cholesterol and HDL, the LDL level can be calculated by rearranging the equation:

$$\text{Total cholesterol} = \text{HDL} + \text{LDL} + \text{VLDL}$$

into

$$\text{LDL} = \text{Total cholesterol} - \text{HDL} - (\text{Triglycerides}/5)$$

Previously, normal cholesterol concentrations, which were based on the means of apparently healthy individuals, were thought to be desirable. The concept of desirable values for serum lipids has undergone significant change from a statistical definition to an epidemiologic definition based on increased risk for cardiovascular disease. Current guidelines have been established (Table 40-3).

Initiation of cholesterol-lowering therapy depends on lipid concentrations, past cardiac history, and risk for

**Table 40-4.** LDL thresholds for further workup

| Patient characteristics | LDL threshold | Goal |
|---|---|---|
| **For diet therapy** | | |
| No CHD and 1 risk | ≥160 | <160 |
| No CHD and ≥2 risks | ≥130 | <130 |
| Known CHD | >100 | ≤100 |
| **For drug therapy** | | |
| No CHD and 1 risk | ≥190 | <160 |
| No CHD and ≥2 risks | ≥160 | <130 |
| Known CHD | ≥130 | ≤100 |

Modified from *JAMA* 269 (23):3015, 1993.
*CHD*, Coronary heart disease.

atherosclerosis. The goal for patients without known atherosclerosis is to prevent the occurrence of vascular events (primary prevention). Individuals with borderline LDL values and only one risk factor can be instructed on diet and exercise and can be reevaluated yearly. However, the combination of borderline LDL values and two risk factors is an indication for further workup of secondary causes and an active program to decrease serum cholesterol levels.

The goal for patients with already documented clinical atherosclerosis is to prevent further vascular events (secondary prevention). Any patient in this category with an LDL over 100 mg/dl should have further evaluation and receive specific, individualized recommendations. A summary of thresholds for further workup is provided in Table 40-4.

## THERAPY

### Diet

All therapeutic strategies aimed at reversing hyperlipidemia center around reducing dietary intake of saturated fats and cholesterol. The average intake of cholesterol in the United States remains high at 435 mg per day for men and 304 mg per day for women. Saturated fats are not essential to normal human physiology, and their consumption increases total and LDL cholesterol. Polyunsaturated fats, such as omega-3 and omega-6 fatty acids, are necessary for synthesis of cell membranes and prostaglandins and tend to lower total cholesterol. Monounsaturated fats may also have a beneficial effect on lipid concentrations. Sources of each of these nutritional classes are provided in the box at right. Avoidance of animal meat (especially organ meats), whole dairy products, and eggs significantly reduces cholesterol and saturated fat intake.

The method of food preparation can significantly affect the total amount of unsaturated fat in any menu item. Home recipes that rely on frying, particularly with lard or animal fat, can dramatically increase the saturated fat content of any diet. Commercially prepared foods using palm and coconut oils can also have a very detrimental influence on lipid profiles because of the high content of saturated fat (Table 40-5).

Recommendations for modifying diets have been endorsed by the National Cholesterol Education Program (NCEP) as well as the American Heart Association, the American Diabetes Association, and the American Dietetic Association. The initial approach, termed step-one diet, is to lower dietary intake of cholesterol to less than 300 mg per day with total fat representing less than 30% of total calories and saturated fat being less than 10% of total calories (see the Managed Care Guide). Implementing a step-one diet can frequently be attained with relatively simple modifications in composition and method of preparation (Table 40-6). Those patients who have difficulty incorporating the diet into daily living should receive nutrition counseling from a registered dietician. If the step-one diet is not effective at lowering total and LDL cholesterol into the target range (under 240 total and under 160 LDL if there are no risk factors; under 200 total and under 130 LDL if there are more than two risk factors), a more rigorous diet is recommended. The step-two diet restricts dietary intake of cholesterol to less than 200 mg per day and saturated fat to less than 7% of total calories (see the Managed Care Guide).

Motivating patients to change ingrained dietary behaviors is extremely difficult. Although most people plan their daily menus from a relatively small total number of stock recipes, food items and methods of preparation are strongly influenced by underlying factors such as culture and family traditions. In addition, older patients may feel unable to learn new recipes or approaches to menu planning. Specific, simple and practical suggestions can help to slowly change a diet from one that is high in saturated fats and cholesterol to one that provides enjoyable eating and good nutrition without cardiovascular risk (see Table 40-6). Involving the family member who shops and the one who cooks (not necessarily the same) can be critical to achieving compliance. Identifying restaurants in the community that include low-cholesterol and low-fat items on their menus minimizes difficulties faced by patients when they dine out.

### Sources of dietary fatty acids

**Cholesterol**
Egg yolks
Organ meats: liver, sweetbreads, brain
Animal meats: beef, pork, lamb
Butter

**Saturated fatty acids**
Animal fat: beef, pork
Whole dairy products: milk, cream, ice cream, cheese
Palm oil
Coconut oil

**Polyunsaturated fatty acids**
Safflower oil
Sunflower oil
Soybean oil
Corn oil

**Monounsaturated fatty acids**
Olive oil
Canola oil

**Table 40-5.** Saturated fat levels in commercial oils and shortenings

| | Percent saturated fat* | Percent monounsaturated fat | Percent polyunsaturated fat |
|---|---|---|---|
| Coconut oil | 86 | 6 | 2 |
| Palm oil | 49 | 37 | 9 |
| Vegetable shortening | 31 | 51 | 14 |
| Stick margarine† | 19 | 45-60 | 18-32 |
| Soft tub margarine† | 18 | 36-47 | 44 |
| Peanut oil | 17 | 46 | 32 |
| Olive oil | 13 | 74 | 8 |
| Corn oil | 13 | 24 | 59 |
| Sunflower oil | 10 | 20 | 66 |
| Safflower oil | 9 | 12 | 75 |
| Canola oil | 7 | 55 | 33 |

*Percent of total fat.
†Percents vary depending on type of oil used to make margarine.

## Managed Care Guide
## American Heart Association recommended diet

**Step 1***
***Composition***

Limit intakes of total fat to 30%, saturated and polyunsaturated fatty acids to 10%, and monounsaturated fatty acids to 15% of total calories; limit dietary cholesterol to 300 mg/day.

***General description***

Limit to no more than 7 oz/day

Include only chicken and turkey with skin removed, and use lean cuts of fish, veal, beef, pork, or lamb.

Restrict eggs to two per week, including those used in cooking.

Restrict milk products to 1% fat milk, ice milk, sherbert, low-fat frozen yogurt, low-fat cheese, and low-fat cottage cheese.

Avoid hard fats; use only vegetable oils, olive oil, or margarines.

All vegetables and fruits are allowed except for coconut.

Bread, cereals, pasta, potatoes, and rice are allowed except when made with eggs; limit starchy foods to prevent weight gain.

Avoid whole-milk products, marbled meats, fish eggs, organ meats, bakery goods made with hard fats and eggs, and rich desserts.

***Dietary cholesterol goals (mg/d)***

<300

***Dietary fat goals (% of total calories)***

30

**Step 2**
***Composition***

Stricter reduction of meat consumption, use of less fat and cheese (typically instituted with the help of a nutritionist).

***Dietary cholesterol goals (mg/d)***

200-250

***Dietary fat goals (% of total calories)***

25

**Step 3**
***Composition***

Derive calories mostly from cereals, legumes, fruits, and vegetables. Use meat as condiment, eat only low cholesterol cheeses. Reserve consumption of meat, chocolate, candy, coconut for special occasions.

***Dietary cholesterol goals (mg/d)***

100-150

***Dietary fat goals (% of total calories)***

20

*Modified from Grundy SM: Disorders of lipids and lipoproteins. In Stein JH: *Internal medicine,* St. Louis, 1994, Mosby.

**Table 40-6.** Food substitutes to cut cholesterol intake

| Instead of: | Substitute: |
|---|---|
| Processed meats | Poultry substitutes (e.g., turkey franks) |
| Beef | Chicken (no skin) or fish |
| Whole milk | Low-fat (1%-2%) or skim milk |
| Ice cream | Low-fat yogurt, sherbet, or sorbet |
| Butter | Margarine (from unsaturated oil) |
| Natural cheeses (including cream cheese and sour cream) | Low-fat cheeses (<2-6 g fat per ounce) |
| Egg-containing breads | Whole-grain breads |
| Commercial baked goods | Homemade baked goods (using margarine and other low-fat substitutes) |
| Eggs | Egg substitutes or egg whites (2 whites = 1 whole egg in recipes) |
| Lard, palm oil | Unsaturated vegetable oils (corn, safflower, sesame, sunflower, canola, olive) |
| Egg noodles | Rice or pasta |

Lipid profiles should be checked at 4 to 6 weeks and again after 3 months while patients are on either the step-one or step-two diets to determine the effectiveness of these dietary modifications. Compliance with step-one diet can be expected to reduce cholesterol levels by 30 to 40 mg/dl; step-two diet typically decreases cholesterol an additional 15 mg/dl. Diet therapy should be maintained for 6 to 12 months before deciding whether pharmacologic therapy is warranted, unless LDL cholesterol is over 220 mg/dl or the patient has documented coronary heart disease. For a large percentage of patients, adoption of these dietary changes is sufficient to bring total and LDL cholesterol concentrations into the target range.

Aerobic exercise is an important adjuvant to dietary modifications aimed at lowering cholesterol. Exercise lowers total and LDL cholesterol and increases HDL cholesterol. Physical activity is also an important component of weight reduction, which independently decreases serum cholesterol levels. Exercise also lowers triglycerides, blood pressure, and glucose concentrations.

After diet improvements and exercise participation have been maximized, pharmacologic therapy may be necessary to further reduce risk from cholesterol and lipid abnormalities. The available medicines have increased substantially over the past 10 years. As basic mechanisms of lipid metabolism continue to be identified, targeted agents will undoubtedly be developed. Choosing the most appropriate agent depends on several considerations, including expected action, documented benefit, side effect profile, drug interactions, prescribing frequency, and cost (Table 40-7).

## Medications

*Bile acid sequestrants* act in the intestines to bind cholesterol-containing bile acids and prevent reabsorption, thereby promoting excretion of cholesterol. Years of experience with these agents have demonstrated their effectiveness and benefit for reducing risk for coronary heart disease. Treatment with either of the available resins, cholestyramine and colestipol, can typically decrease LDL concentrations by 15% to 25%. The Lipid Research Clinics-Coronary Primary Prevention Trial (LRC-CPPT) documented a 14% decrease in total cholesterol and a 21% decrease in LDL with a 19% risk reduction in nonfatal myocardial infarctions and cardiac deaths. These drugs are very well suited for patients with isolated elevations of LDL cholesterol. Side effects that may affect compliance include gastrointestinal symptoms of constipation, bloating, nausea, and flatulence. These problems tend to increase with dosage and can sometimes be avoided by increasing dietary fiber and using stool softeners. Because they are unable to bind charged particles, these agents can also prevent absorption of other drugs, including digoxin, warfarin, thiazides, β-blockers and thyroxine; patients taking these other medications are usually advised to take them either 1 hour before or 4 to 6 hours after taking the resin. Absorption of fat-soluble vitamins (A, D, E, and K) can also be impaired with high dosages of these drugs. A significant problem can result if these drugs are used in patients with baseline hypertriglyceridemia. The blocked reabsorption of bile acids appears to cause increased hepatic synthesis of VLDL triglyceride and can precipitate pancreatitis. Bile acid sequestrants must be taken two to three times per day in dosages ranging from 4 g (approximately 1 tablespoon) twice daily to 8 g three times per day for cholestyramine, and 5 g (approximately 1 tablespoon) twice daily to 10 g three times a day for colestipol.

*Nicotinic acid* is a B vitamin at physiologic dosages but a cholesterol-lowering drug at pharmacologic doses. It appears to inhibit VLDL secretion and, as a result, its subsequent metabolism to LDL. In addition to reductions in serum cholesterol (15% to 25%) and triglyceride (20% to 50%) levels, increased concentrations of HDL (10% to 20%) are typical. Nicotinic acid was documented to be effective in secondary prevention by reducing recurrent myocardial infarctions in patients with established coronary disease. Although effective, 40% to 50% of patients taking nicotinic acid discontinue the drug because of side effects. Flushing is a major side effect that can be ameliorated by slow dosage adjustments and pretreatment with aspirin; the problem usually decreases over time. Itching and skin rashes also occur commonly. Gastrointestinal side effects, including epigastric discomfort and nausea, can be reduced by taking the medication with meals or in an enteric-coated form. Peptic ulcer or chronic bowel diseases can be exacerbated by nicotinic acid. Nicotinic acid worsens insulin sensitivity and glucose

**Table 40-7.** Agents that influence lipid metabolism

| Drug class | Dosage | Frequency | Average effect | Side effects | Prevention trials | Monthly cost (awp)* |
|---|---|---|---|---|---|---|
| **Resins** | | | | | | |
| Cholestyramine | 4-8 g | bid-tid | 5%-19% ↓ TC | GI symptoms, multiple drug interactions, ↓ absorption of vitamins A, D, E, and K | LRC-CPPT | \$22-\$68 |
| Colestipol | 5-10 g | bid-tid | 20%-25% ↓LDL | | | \$45-\$75 |
| **Nicotinic acid** | 100 mg to 1 g | tid<br>Long acting, bid (max 9 g/d) | 10%-20% ↓ TC<br>15%-25% ↓ LDL<br>40% ↓ VLDL<br>10%-20% ↑ HDL | Flushing, pruritus, rash, GI symptoms, ↑ LFTs, ↑ glucose, ↑ uric acid | CDP | Generic: \$3-\$30 |
| **HMG-CoA reductase inhibitors** | | | | ↑ LFTs, GI symptoms, myopathy (↑ CPK) | | |
| Lovastatin | 20-40 mg | qd-bid (max 80 mg/d) | 17%-29% ↓ TC<br>29%-39% ↓ LDL | | | \$60-\$216 |
| Simvastatin | 20-40 mg | qd-bid (max 40 mg/d) | 27%-33% ↓ TC<br>37%-40% ↓ LDL | | | \$98-\$150 |
| Pravastatin | 10-40 mg | qd-bid (max 40 mg/d) | 16%-25% ↓ TC<br>22%-34% ↓ LDL | | | \$57-\$110 |
| Fluvastatin | 20-40 mg | qd-bid (max 40 mg/d) | 16%-20% ↓ TC<br>18%-25% ↓ LDL | | | \$34-\$38 |
| **Fibric acid derivatives** | | | | Myopathy (↑ CPK), ↑ LFTs, gallstones, GI symptoms | Helsinki Heart | |
| Gemfibrozil | 600 mg | bid | 10% ↓ TC<br>10-15% ↓ LDL<br>10-25% ↑ HDL<br>40% ↓ TG | | | \$33 |

*TC*, Total cholesterol; *GI*, gastrointestinal; *LRC-CPPT*, Lipid Research Clinics-Coronary Primary Prevention Trial; *LFTs*, liver function tests; *CDP*, Coronary Drug Project; *CPK*, creatine phosphokinase; *TG*, triglyceride.
**awp*, Average wholesale price; range provided is for minimum and maximum dosages.

tolerance and is therefore usually avoided in patients with impaired glucose tolerance or diabetes mellitus. It has also been reported to increase hepatic transaminases and uric acid levels and to precipitate arrhythmias in patients with established coronary disease. Fulminant hepatitis has been reported with use of sustained-release preparations of nicotinic acid. Nicotinic acid can be started at doses as low as 100 mg three times a day and increased up to 3 g three times per day. While increasing doses of nicotinic acid, patients should have periodic determinations for glucose, uric acid, and liver function.

Clinical use of *HMG-CoA reductase inhibitors* has been largely based on reduction of risk for coronary heart disease and improvement in coronary artery diameter. A recent secondary prevention trial using simvastatin in 4444 patients over 5 years found a 34% decrease in major coronary events, a 42% decrease in coronary deaths, and a 30% decrease in death from all causes. By inhibiting the rate-limiting step in cellular synthesis of cholesterol, these drugs decrease intracellular cholesterol concentrations and thereby increase LDL receptor number at the cell surface. An increase in hepatic LDL receptor number increases uptake of LDL, VLDL, and IDL. The decrease in intracellular cholesterol may also diminish hepatic production of lipoproteins. Reductase inhibitors have been shown to reduce total cholesterol by 17% to 34% and LDL by 22% to 40%. A small beneficial effect on HDL and triglyceride concentrations is frequently observed. These drugs are well tolerated by most patients. Myopathy, the most common side effect, can present as (1) weakness, tenderness, aches, and cramps, (2) elevations in creatine kinase, or (3) rhabdomyolysis with very high creatine kinase levels, myoglobinuria, and acute tubular necrosis. The risk for rhabdomyolysis is increased in patients with hepatic disease or those taking cyclosporine, nicotinic acid, or fibric acid derivatives (e.g., gemfibrozil). Other side effects include gastrointestinal upset and diarrhea, and elevations in liver enzymes. Since the significance of minor, intermittent rises in liver function tests is not known, reductase inhibitors can be continued as long as liver enzymes continue to be monitored and do not increase. Sleep disturbances have also been reported with these medications. The ability of some of these drugs to cross the blood-brain barrier has been suggested to play a role in causing insomnia but has not been well-documented. Initial concerns regarding cataract formation have not been proven for humans, thus slit-lamp examinations are no longer required. Dosing depends on the specific reductase inhibitor used but is usually either once or twice daily. Some agents are better absorbed with food and appear to be more active at night compared with daytime; these agents are best taken with dinner. To monitor patients for hepatic side effects, it is reasonable to check liver function tests 6 and 12 weeks after initiation of therapy, every 3 months for the remainder of the first year, and twice per year thereafter. Persistent elevation of liver function tests (more than three times the upper limit of normal) or symptomatic elevation of either liver function tests or creatine phosphokinase (CPK) is an indication for cessation of therapy.

*Gemfibrozil* is a fibric acid derivative that significantly lowers triglycerides by inhibiting hepatic VLDL synthesis and may additionally increase lipoprotein lipase activity. Associated with the 40% decrease in triglycerides is a 10% to 25% increase in HDL. A 10% to 15% decrease in LDL cholesterol can also be expected. In the Helsinki Heart Study, which involved 4081 Finnish men between ages 40 and 55, gemfibrozil therapy was associated with a 34% reduction in documented coronary events. Major side effects include gallstones (2% to 4%), myopathy, and gastrointestinal upset. Problems related to myopathy are similar to those related to reductase inhibitors, and the risk is significantly increased when both drugs are used together. Thus the combination should be avoided or, if necessary, monitored closely in conjunction with a specialist. Uncommon side effects include potentiation of warfarin, leukopenia, impotence, weight gain, and increases in hepatic enzymes. Gemfibrozil is typically prescribed as 600 mg twice daily taken before breakfast and dinner. Lower doses may be beneficial in patients with renal insufficiency. Higher doses have not been shown to be beneficial. As with reductase inhibitors, patients taking gemfibrozil should have CPK and liver function tests checked periodically (see above).

Other fibric acid derivatives do not appear to be as beneficial as gemfibrozil. Clofibrate therapy was not associated with a decrease in repeat myocardial infarctions in the Coronary Drug Project. Although clofibrate did decrease primary myocardial infarctions in a study by the World Health Organization, overall mortality was unchanged, raising the question of drug-related increases in noncardiac mortality.

*Probucol* has only mild cholesterol-lowering properties (approximately 15%) and has not been tested in any large clinical trials. In addition, it has been reported to lower HDLl levels. Side effects include prolongation of the QT interval and gastrointestinal disturbances such as diarrhea, flatulence, abdominal pain, and nausea. Side effects may resolve slowly, since the drug is stored in adipose tissue. Due to the effect on QT prolongation, probucol is contraindicated in patients with known arrhythmias or those taking other drugs that might prolong QT intervals. The usual dosage is 500 mg twice daily. Although probucol is not frequently used, its ability to prevent oxidation of LDL has made it a very useful agent to study underlying mechanisms of atherosclerosis in animal and basic science protocols. Ultimately drugs like probucol may become important therapeutic agents for preventing heart disease because of their antioxidant properties rather than their effects on serum lipids.

## STRATEGIES

A complete lipid profile often reveals a characteristic distribution of lipoprotein particles that suggests which drugs may be of particular value (Table 40-8). A predominant elevation in triglyceride concentrations (seen in type I) responds well to fibric acid derivatives. Very high triglycerides with elevated cholesterol (type V) can be similarly treated but also respond to nicotinic acid. Increased VLDL (type IV) presents with relatively greater increases in triglycerides compared with cholesterol. Use of a fibric acid derivative can markedly improve the lipid profile of these patients. Lipoprotein electrophoresis that exhibits an increased amount of β-VLDL particles produces significant elevations in both cholesterol and triglycerides. Both nicotinic acid and gemfibrozil can be very effective in treating these patients. Patients with

**Table 40-8.** Specific drugs for lipoprotein abnormalities

| Abnormality | Phenotype | Typical cholesterol | Typical triglyceride | Suggested drugs |
|---|---|---|---|---|
| Increased chylomicrons | Types I and V | Type I: 320<br>Type V: 700 | Type I: 4000<br>Type V: 5000 | Fibric acid derivatives<br>Nicotinic acid |
| Increased VLDL | Type IV | 220 | 400 | Fibric acid derivatives<br>Nicotinic acid |
| Increased β VLDL | Type III | 500 | 700 | Nicotinic acid<br>Fibric acid derivatives |
| Increased LDL<br>Normal triglycerides | Type IIa | 370 | 100 | Resins<br>Reductase inhibitors<br>Nicotinic acid |
| Increased LDL<br>Increased triglycerides | Type IIb | 350 | 400 | Resins<br>Fibric acid derivatives<br>Nicotinic acid<br>Reductase inhibitors |
| Decreased HDL | — | — | — | Fibric acid derivatives<br>Nicotinic acid |

**Table 40-9.** Secondary hyperlipoproteinemias causing xanthomas

| Disease | Types of xanthomas | Etiology |
|---|---|---|
| Diabetes | Tendinous xanthelasma tuberous eruptive<br>1+, 4+ | Lack of lipoprotein lipase (insulin dependent enzyme) that clears chylomicrons and VLDL. |
| Pancreatitis | 4+ | Lack of insulin and lipoprotein lipase. |
| Myxedema | 2+, 2+, 1+, 3+ | Lipoprotein lipase deficiency. ↑ cholesterol—LDL in blood—less conversion bile salts. |
| Cholestatic liver disease | 2+, 2+, 1+ | Abnormal cholesterol-rich LP (lipoprotein X) formed. |

increased LDL fractions can be divided into those with normal triglycerides (type IIa) and those with elevated triglycerides (type IIb). Type IIa patients are very good candidates for resins. For those unable to tolerate resins, reductase inhibitors and nicotinic acid are excellent therapeutic choices. Type IIb patients can also be treated with resins as long as the triglycerides do not exceed 300 mg/dl. Both fibric acid derivatives and reductase inhibitors are good choices for these patients. Nicotinic acid is also very effective. Medical therapy for patients with isolated low HDL is controversial. When indicated because of other risk factors, fibric acid derivatives or nicotinic acid represents optimal therapy.

## XANTHOMATOSIS

Xanthomas are caused by a variety of metabolic derangements in lipoprotein metabolism. In addition to diagnosing the xanthoma, the clinician should determine if the skin lesion is related to lipoprotein abnormalities caused by an underlying disease (secondary hyperlipoproteinemia) or to a primary inherited defect in lipoprotein metabolism (primary hyperlipoproteinemia). Table 40-9 and the box on p. 586 outline these conditions.

### Primary hyperlipoproteinemia

There are various forms of xanthomas. All xanthomas represent accumulations of macrophage-foam cells, containing large quantities of lipid (especially cholesterol). *Tendinous xanthomas* arise in tendons and ligaments (e.g., Achilles tendons, tendons of the dorsum of the hands, elbows and knees) and appear as smooth, asymptomatic, skin colored nodules. Their movement is linked to movement of the tendon. They invariably occur in relation to hyperlipoproteinemia and atherosclerotic cardiovascular disease. *Planar xanthomas* appear as yellow, soft, macular or plaque-like lesions, usually around the eyelids (xanthelasma). Up to 50% of patients with these xanthomas have hyperlipoproteinemia and cardiovascular disease. *Tuberous xanthomas* are yellow to red nodules over the extensor surfaces of the body and on the palms. Hyperlipoproteinemia and atherosclerotic cardiovascular disease are usually seen with these xanthomas (see Fig. 40-3). *Eruptive xanthomas* appear as small yellow cutaneous papules suddenly erupting over weeks to months on the extensor surfaces of the extremities, buttocks, and trunk. Hyperlipoproteinemia (hyperlipidemic serum) is always found and is seen in association with lipemia retinalis.

The clinical form of xanthoma found in each patient cannot be used precisely to diagnose the specific underlying disease process because both primary and secondary disease processes give rise to the same forms of xanthomas. As a generalization, however, tendinous xanthomas, particularly in association with xanthelasma and arcus senilis, suggest an underlying LDL hyperlipoproteinemia as well as obstructive liver disease and diabetes. Eruptive xanthomas occur when chylomicrons and VLDL are elevated due to the lack of clearance of such lipoproteins as seen in diabetes, pancreatitis and Type I, IV and V

### Primary hyperlipoproteinemia (genetic LP abnormalities)

I. Triglyceride Removal Defects—Lipoprotein Lipase Deficiency
Type I (Hyperlipoproteinemia)—Lack of chylomicron clearing.
Type IV—Lack of VLDL clearing.
Type V—Lack of chylomicron and VLDL clearance.
All associated with eruptive xanthomas, lipedemic sera, lipemia retinalis, and pancreatitis. Occasionally seen in tendinous and xanthelasma lesions. Atherosclerosis seen in Type IV and V.

II. Excessive TG Production—Increase in VLDL production.
Type IV—Lipoproteinemia or endogenous lipidemia. Associated with mild diabetes and obesity. Lipoproteinemia accentuated by carbohydrate and alcohol ingestion. Eruptive xanthoma and planar xanthomas seen. High incidence of atherosclerotic disease seen.

III. Remnant Lipoprotein Accumulation—Broad Beta Disease. Increase in remnant lipoproteins due to genetic alteration in apoprotein E.
Tuberous and tuberoeruptive xanthomas common. May see tendinous lesions as well. Cardiovascular atherosclerotic disease common.

IV. Defective Low Density LP Removal.
Familial hypercholesterolemia Type II disease due to a dominantly inherited deficiency in LDL receptors.

primary hyperlipoproteinemias. Tuberous xanthomas are typically seen in broad beta or type III disease associated with increase in remnant lipoproteins.

***Treatment.*** Xanthomas are usually a sign of significant atherosclerotic cardiovascular disease and primary genetic or secondary diseases. Therapy will depend, therefore, on the underlying cause. Secondary conditions, if treated appropriately (i.e., insulin for diabetes, thyroid replacement for hypothyroidism), will normalize the hyperlipoproteinemia and the xanthomas resolve. Primary hyperlipoproteinemias should be treated first with appropriate dietary manipulation, and if these do not normalize the hyperlipidemia, drugs are employed.

## BIBLIOGRAPHY


Abramowicz M: Choice of cholesterol-lowering drugs, *Med Lett Drugs Ther* 33:1, 1991.

Brown BG et al: Lipid lowering and plaque regression: new insights into prevention of plaque disruption and clinical events in coronary disease, *Clin Prog Series U Wash* 87:1781, 1993.

Brown MS, Goldstein JL: How LDL receptors influence cholesterol and atherosclerosis, *Sci Am* 251:2, 1984.

Brown WV: Review of clinical trials: proving the lipid hypothesis, *Eur Heart J* 11(suppl H):15, 1990.

Chait A, Brunzell JD: Acquired hyperlipidemia (secondary dyslipoproteinemias), *Endocrinol Metab Clin North Am* 19(2):261, 1990.

Ginsberg HN: Lipoprotein physiology and its relationship to atherogenesis, *Endocrinol Metab Clin North Am* 19(2):211, 1990.

Grundy SM et al: Summary of the second report of the NCEP expert panel on detection, evaluation, and treatment of high blood cholesterol in adults, *JAMA* 269(23):3015, 1993.

Havel RJ: Lowering cholesterol, 1988 rationale, mechanisms, and means, *J Clin Invest* 81:1653, 1988.

Henkin Y et al: Niacin revisited: clinical observations on an important but underutilized drug, *Am J Med* 91:239, 1991.

Howard BV, Howard WJ: Dyslipidemia in non-insulin–dependent diabetes mellitus, *Endocrinol Rev* 15(3):263, 1994.

Howard BV: Lipoprotein metabolism in diabetes mellitus, *J Lipid Res* 18:613, 1987.

Jones PH: A clinical overview of dyslipidemias: treatment strategies, *Am J Med* 93:187, 1992.

Rader DJ, Hoeg JM, Brewster HB Jr: Quantitation of plasma apolipoproteins in the primary and secondary prevention of coronary artery disease, *Ann Intern Med* 120(12):1012, 1994.

Rossouw JE, Rifkind BM: Does lowering serum cholesterol levels lower coronary heart disease risk? *Endocrinol Metab Clin North Am* 9(2):279, 1990.

Steinberg D, Witztum JL: Lipoproteins and atherogenesis, *JAMA* 264(23):3047, 1990.

Walden CC, Hegele RA: Apolipoprotein E in hyperlipidemia, *Ann Intern Med* 120(12):1026, 1994.

# V GASTROINTESTINAL DISEASE

CHAPTER

## 41 Esophagus

Robert Burakoff

### REFLUX ESOPHAGITIS

The term *reflux esophagitis* refers to a pathologic process resulting from gastric acid in frequent contact with the esophageal mucosa. Reflux esophagitis is the most common disease affecting the esophagus. The resting lower esophageal sphincter (LES) pressure is mainly responsible for preventing reflux of gastric contents from reaching the esophageal mucosa. When resting LES pressure decreases, reflux of acid occurs. Whether the decrease of the LES pressure is a result of reflux or precedes it is still unknown. It is known that several factors contribute to reflux, however, and these include transient LES relaxations, a low or hypotensive LES, and anatomic disruption of the sphincter associated with hiatus hernia. All three mechanisms do not occur in all patients. In addition, it has been demonstrated that individuals with reflux clear acid more slowly from the esophagus than do normal individuals.

#### Substances that affect lower esophageal sphincter pressure

**Increase**

Protein meal
Coffee*
Urecholine (bethanechol)
Metoclopramide
Antacids
α-Adrenergic agents
β-Adrenergic agents

**Decrease**

Alcohol
Chocolate
Essence of peppermint
Smoking
Fatty foods
β-Adrenergic agents
Estrogen and progesterone
Caffeine*
Calcium blocking agents
Diazepam
Barbiturates

*Note that coffee contains a protein that increases LES pressure; caffeine, however, decreases LES pressure.

#### Clinical symptoms

The most common symptom of reflux is *heartburn,* a burning sensation in the chest usually after meals or when lying down or bending over. Specific foods may provoke heartburn, and we now know that some of these foods (e.g., chocolate) may even decrease the LES pressure and thereby promote gastroesophageal reflux (see the box at left). If reflux is severe, the patient may experience a bitter or sour taste in the mouth or a mouthful of fluid (waterbrash). Relief of these symptoms with antacids helps confirm the presence of heartburn.

*Odynophagia,* or pain on swallowing, is usually seen only when reflux is severe and occurs with long-standing reflux particularly in the presence of severe esophagitis or ulceration of the esophagus.

*Dysphagia* is a sensation of food sticking in the esophagus. This symptom may result from esophagitis and is described as food sticking but only transiently, whereas with an organic stricture the dysphagia persists despite repeated swallowing.

The association of night sweats and esophageal reflux has been noted in many patients. The degree of sweating experienced is usually modest, and only rarely does a patient mention it spontaneously. The history of night sweats is a clue to the presence of a gastroesophageal reflux, which may also be causing chest pain, asthma, or chronic cough, and not necessarily causing heartburn.

#### Differential diagnosis

Though symptoms of gastroesophageal reflux disease (GERD) are quite characteristic, patients who have concomitant chest pain with features of angina pectoris should undergo electrocardiogram (ECG) and exercise stress test before evaluation for GERD. Although many tests can help establish if reflux esophagitis is present, no single test provides the diagnosis in all patients. What is a practical approach to the patient thought to have reflux esophagitis? If a patient has symptoms of single heartburn without dysphagia, clearly the best approach is no tests at all, but rather a therapeutic trial (see the Managed Care Guide). If a patient's symptoms do not improve with antacids and diet, tests are in order. A few questions may help decide which tests are appropriate.

First, is reflux present? The simplest test, which is also the least sensitive, is a barium swallow, often the first test ordered. A barium swallow determines if a stricture is present but unfortunately demonstrates reflux in only about 25% of patients and usually indicates those with severe reflux. The most sensitive test for reflux is the use of a pH probe during esophageal manometry. The usual pH of the esophagus is greater than 4. With a pH probe electrode positioned in the esophagus, reflux can be determined by a fall in pH, which can be documented in approximately 85% of patients. At the same time, the resting LES pressure can be determined with an esophageal manometry catheter. These pressure-sensing catheters determine the resting LES pressure compared to the stomach pressure (usually greater than 10 mm Hg above gastric pressure in normal individuals) as well as the peristaltic activity of the body of the esophagus. About 85% of patients with reflux have decreased LES pressure.

Once reflux has been demonstrated, the second question that must be answered is what has reflux done to the

## Managed Care Guide
### Algorithm describing the treatment of a patient with heartburn

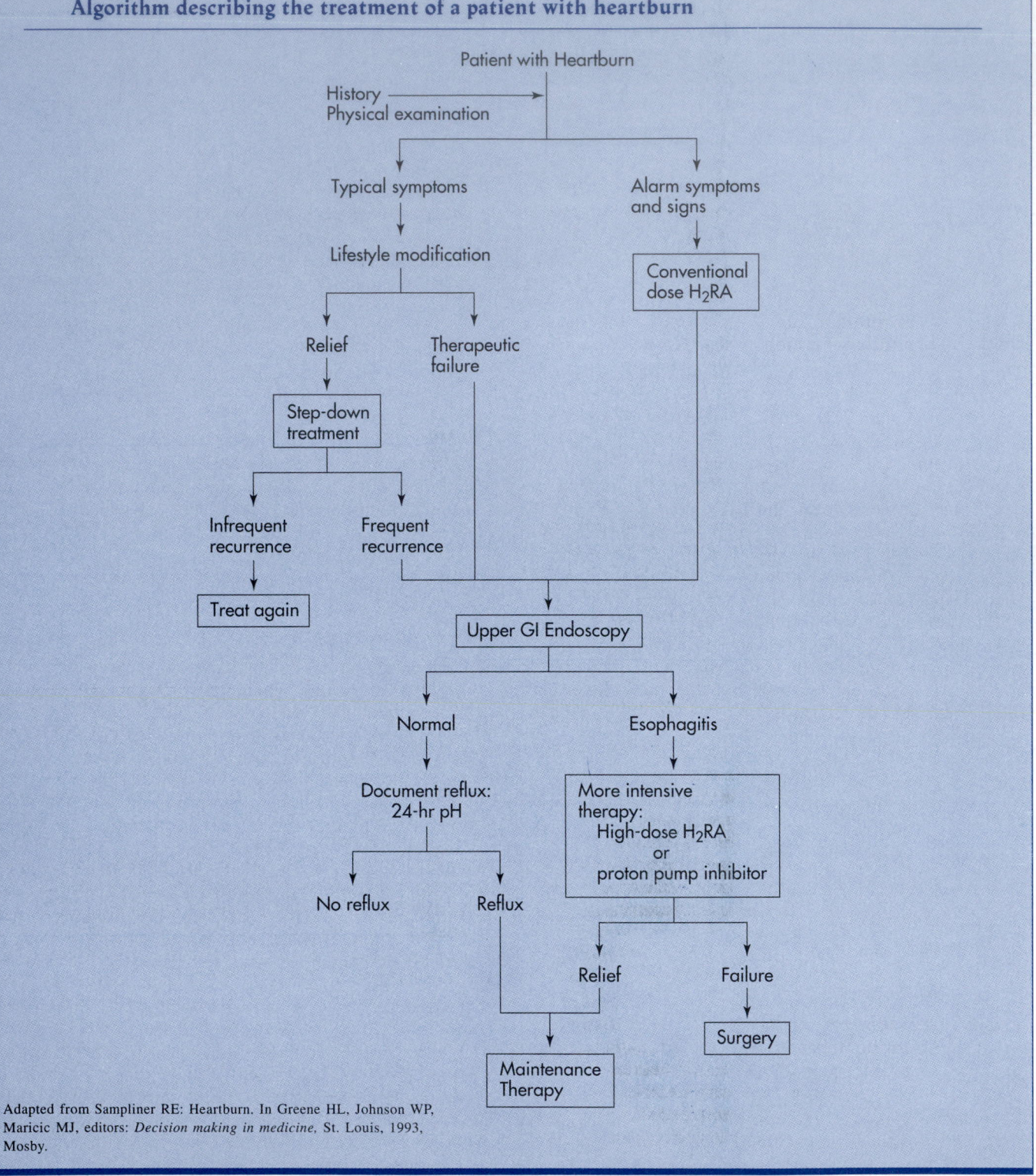

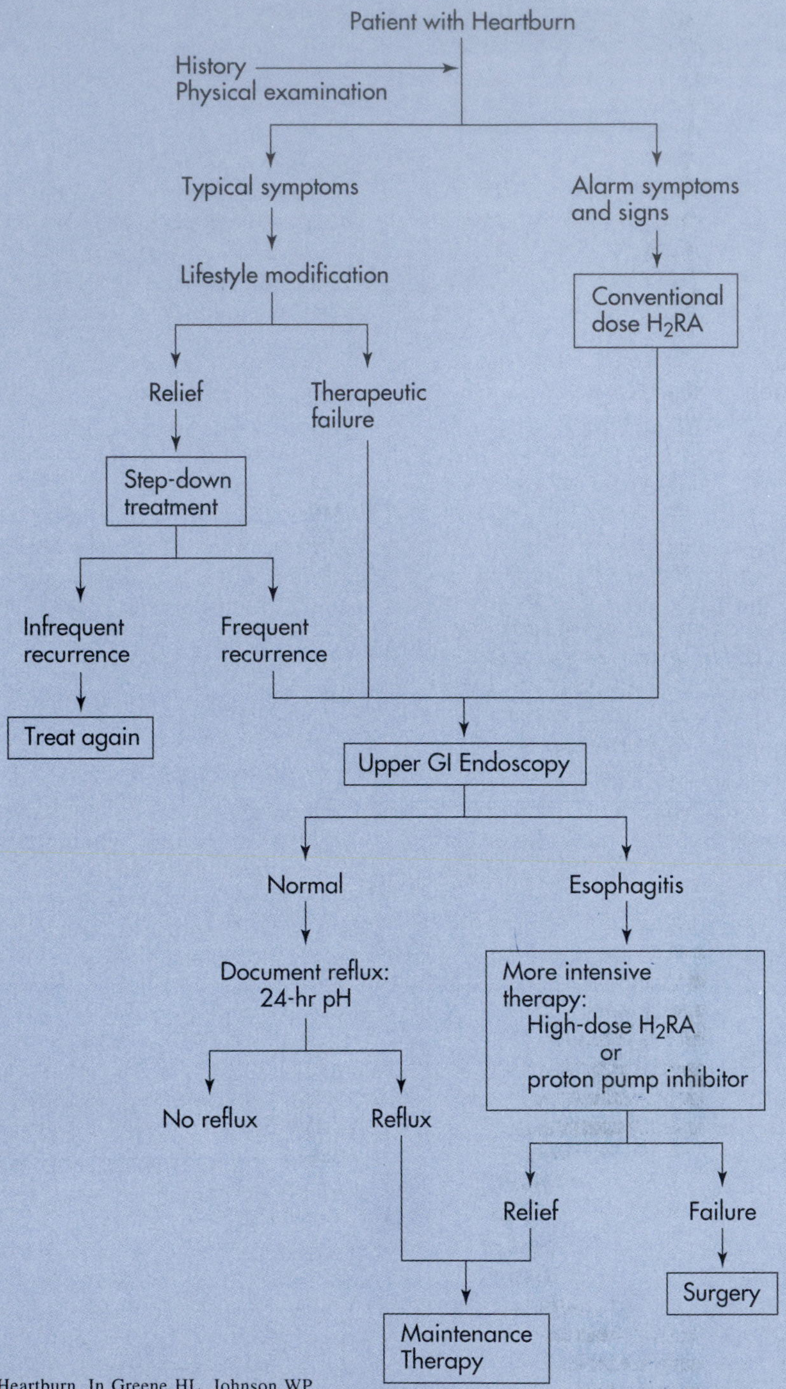


Adapted from Sampliner RE: Heartburn. In Greene HL, Johnson WP, Maricic MJ, editors: *Decision making in medicine*, St. Louis, 1993, Mosby.

esophageal mucosa? This is best determined by endoscopy and biopsy. Finally, are the symptoms due to heartburn? This question may be answered by performing the esophageal acid infusion, or Bernstein, test, which is performed by placing a tube in the esophagus and dripping in 0.1 hydrogen chloride. If the symptoms are reproduced and then disappear or lessen with normal saline, heartburn is confirmed. If the Bernstein test is negative and histologic evidence for esophagitis is lacking, then a 24-hour ambulatory pH recording is indicated to confirm whether the patient has prolonged acid reflux or if the patient's symptoms are temporally correlated with acid reflux. Thus no single test answers all the questions, and the decision to perform a particular test depends on the specific question one desires to answer (Fig. 41-1).

### Complications

*Esophageal stricture* occurs with severe reflux esophagitis and results from the inflammatory process extending into the submucosa. The stricture usually occurs at the distal

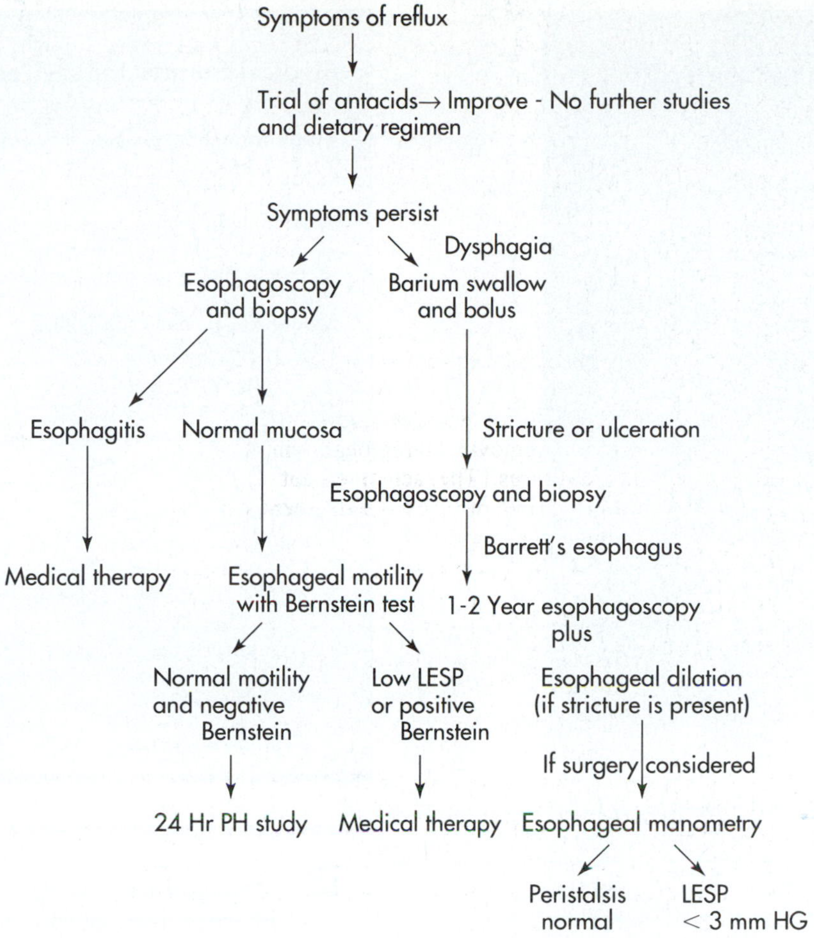


**Fig. 41-1.** Approach to the patient with reflux esophagitis.

esophagus and is most often smooth, in contrast to an irregular stricture from carcinoma. The presenting symptom is dysphagia, which is usually progressive and related to the size of the food bolus swallowed. Patients complain initially of dysphagia with solids but not liquids. With a tight stricture, swallowing of liquids may become impaired. A barium swallow (Fig. 41-2) with a marshmallow or bread bolus helps determine the diameter of the stricture. If a stricture is demonstrated, endoscopy and biopsy are mandatory to help rule out esophageal carcinoma. The medical treatment of esophageal strictures, in addition to a basic antireflux regimen (see below), is dilatation with mercury-filled rubber bougies or dilators. Dilatation is performed until a No. 45 French dilator passes easily. This is equivalent to approximately a 15-mm diameter and allows patients to swallow a typical, well-chewed meal. Esophageal dilatation is successful in most patients and thereby avoids the need for surgery. Those patients who require repeated dilatations or whose strictures are long and tortuous usually require surgery.

*Esophageal ulceration* and *hemorrhage* from esophagitis are uncommon, and if they do not respond promptly to medical management surgery is indicated. Esophageal ulcer is usually diagnosed with a barium swallow and most often presents with worsening of reflux symptoms to a more continuous pain pattern rather than episodic heartburn. The diagnosis of hemorrhage secondary to esophagitis can be confirmed only by esophagoscopy.

A significant complication of reflux esophagitis, but one that fortunately is uncommon, is the development of Barrett esophagus, or columnar dysplasia of the esophagus. In some patients with chronic reflux esophagitis a portion of the squamous epithelium is replaced with columnar epithelium. The importance of this syndrome is the predilection for developing esophageal adenocarcinoma, which in one large series was 10%. It is recommended that endoscopy with biopsy be performed yearly in patients with Barrett's esophagus if low-grade dysplasia is present and every 2 years if it is absent.

Gastroesophageal reflux should be considered in the differential diagnosis of *adult onset asthma.* A causal relationship has been demonstrated in some patients with improvement of pulmonary function tests and symptoms after treatment of gastroesophageal reflux.

## Medical therapy

The primary goal of medical therapy is to keep gastric acid away from the squamous epithelium of the esophagus (see

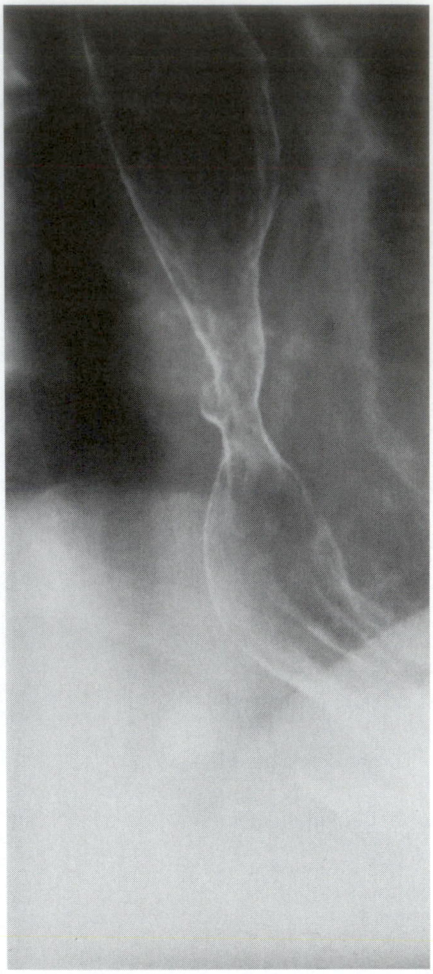

**Fig. 41-2.** Barium swallow demonstrating esophagitis with a hiatus hernia stricture and ulceration.

## Medical therapy for gastroesophageal reflux

**Mild: normal esophageal mucosa**

1. Antireflux regimen: avoid substances that decrease LESP
2. Aluminum hydroxide/magnesium hydroxide antacids: 30 cc after each meal and at bedtime; avoid in renal failure: use aluminum hydroxide only

**Moderate: erosive esophagitis**

1. Antireflux regimen
2. Elevate head of bed
3. $H_2$ receptor antagonist bid × 12 weeks: cimetidine, 400 mg bid; ranitidine, 150 mg bid; famotidine, 20 mg bid; nizatidine, 150 mg bid

**Severe**

1. Antireflux regimen
2. Elevate head of bed
3. **Either** $H_2$ receptor antagonist bid at double Rx × 12 weeks
   **Or** Omeprazole 20 mg qhs × 8 weeks: cimetidine, 800 mg bid; ranitidine, 300 mg bid; famotidine, 40 mg bid; nizatidine, 300 mg bid

*LESP,* Lower esophageal sphincter pressure.

## Managed Care Guide
## Efficacy and cost in treatment of GERD*

| Drug | Dosage | Healed (8 weeks) | AWP cost (8 weeks) |
|---|---|---|---|
| Tagamet (Cimetidine) | 800 mg BID | 30%-50% | ‡$291.94† |
| Zantac (Ranitidine) | 150 mg BID<br>150 mg QID§ | 30%-50% | ‡$178.57<br>‡$357.14 |
| Pepcid (Famotidine) | 20 mg BID<br>40 mg BID§ | 30%-50% | ‡$160.85<br>‡$321.70 |
| Axid (Nizatidine) | 150 mg BID | 30%-50% | ‡$161.65 |
| Prilosec (Omeprazole) | 20 mg QD | 75%-85% (4 weeks) | ‡$103.81 (4 weeks) |
| Propulsid (Cisapride) | 10 mg QID | — | ‡$72.00 (30 days) |

Courtesy of PCS Clinical Management Systems.
*Patients with erosive esophagitis may require up to 12 weeks of treatment.
†Cimetidine has recently become available generically at a cost of about 45% less than Tagamet.
‡Drug is less expensive than price listed due to volume discounts.
§Patient with erosive esophagitis may require higher doses of Zantac or Pepcid.

the box at right). A rational plan to avoid reflux involves three concepts. First, to prevent reflux, the head of the bed can be elevated at bedtime, and lying down after meals is to be avoided. In addition, eating is avoided up to 3 hours before bedtime to avoid the acid load produced in response to a meal. Second, an attempt is made to neutralize gastric acidity with antacids or histamine$_2$ ($H_2$) receptor antagonists (cimetidine, ranitidine, famotidine and nizatidine). The patient ingests 30 ml of an aluminum hydroxide–magnesium hydroxide antacid after meals and at bedtime. Patients are instructed to avoid calcium-containing antacids, since calcium stimulates acid production (via gastrin). The patient is instructed to take antacids at any other time symptoms occur. If antacids are required more than six times daily, resulting in diarrhea, an $H_2$ receptor antagonist should be used. $H_2$ receptor antagonists significantly reduce gastric acid secretion for greater than 6 hours and therefore are required only twice each day. $H_2$ receptor antagonists do not increase LES strength (see the Managed Care Guide).

For patients who have demonstrated moderate to severe esophagitis on esophagoscopy, the use of omeprazole (Losec) is indicated. Omeprazole, a proton pump inhibitor, in a dose of 20 mg per day results in much greater acid suppression than with $H_2$ receptor antagonists. In several studies omeprazole has been shown to be superior to $H_2$ receptor antagonists in healing severe esophagitis and will heal almost 90% of patients over a 12-week period. However, at this time omeprazole has not been approved by the FDA for long-term use.

Gaviscon has weak antacid properties but also produces a foam (alginic acid) that coats the esophagus and floats on top of the gastric contents. Studies have demonstrated a decrease in reflux symptoms when Gaviscon is taken after meals and at bedtime.

The third and final goal in treating reflux is to increase LES pressure in circumstances where the patient continues to have nocturnal reflux in the presence of an $H_2$ receptor antagonist. Metoclopramide, approved in the United States for diabetic gastroparesis, is a potent dopamine inhibitor that increases LES pressure for at least 2 hours and increases gastric emptying. Metoclopramide is usually given as adjunctive therapy with $H_2$ blockers at a dosage of 10 mg before meals and at bedtime. However, approximately 25% to 50% of patients experience restlessness, tremors, parkinsonism, and tardive dyskinesia. Cisapride, a new prokinetic agent released in 1993 in the United States does not have the CNS side effects of metoclopramide and has similar therapeutic effects at a dosage of 10 mg taken 10 minutes before meals and at bedtime. The typical patient with reflux should be advised to avoid foods and drinks that affect LES pressure (see the box on p. 587). The majority of patients respond to the simple three-pronged regimen of elevating the head of the bed, controlled diet, and postprandial antacids.

## ACHALASIA

### Definition and pathophysiology

Achalasia, or cardiospasm, is a diffuse motor disorder of the esophagus characterized by *incomplete* relaxation of the LES and loss of peristaltic activity in the body of the esophagus. These abnormalities result in a functional obstruction of the lower esophagus and dilatation of the body of the esophagus. The etiology is unknown, but a consistent pathologic finding is a significant decrease or absence of ganglion cells in the Auerbach plexus of the esophagus.

### Clinical presentation

This relatively rare disease has a prevalence of approximately 1 in 100,000 per year. Achalasia rarely appears in members of the same family, and onset of symptoms often occurs between the ages of 20 and 40, though the disease can begin at any age, including infancy.

The typical patient presents with dysphagia for *solids* and *liquids,* which is often of several years' duration. In addition, the patient regurgitates retained material from the esophagus usually after lying down or with exercise. Heartburn is rarely a complaint. Further questioning may reveal that the dysphagia worsens with stress or eating rapidly. The more sophisticated patient learns to avoid these symptoms by purposefully regurgitating before dinner to empty the esophagus. As the disease progresses and the esophagus dilates further, episodes of aspiration and bronchopneumonia occur. Odynophagia, or chest pain with swallowing, is seen at the beginning of the illness, but as the esophagus continues to dilate this symptom tends to disappear. If the chest pain continues, the patient may have a variant called vigorous achalasia.

### Diagnosis

The physical examination is rarely if ever helpful in making the diagnosis of achalasia except for the presence of halitosis and weight loss. With long-standing achalasia a presumptive diagnosis can occasionally be made from a chest x-ray showing retained material in the esophagus, sometimes diagnosed as a mediastinal mass on the right side, and by the absence of air in the stomach. The simplest method for diagnosis is a barium swallow (Fig. 41-3). The barium swallow is performed in the supine position to demonstrate the loss of peristalsis, which always involves the lower two thirds of the esophagus. The esophagus is usually quite dilated, and there may be an air-fluid level secondary to retained secretions. The classic finding at the lower end of the esophagus is the gradual tapering to a pointed bird's beak. This results from incomplete relaxation of the hypertonic sphincter.

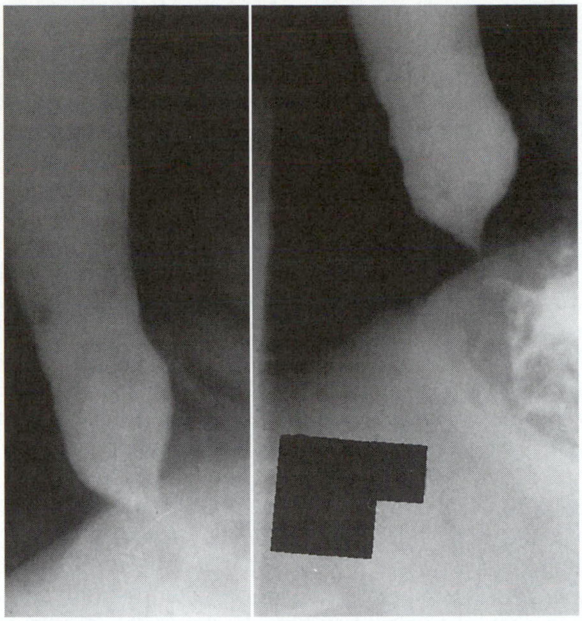

**Fig. 41-3.** Barium swallow demonstrating the classic findings in achalasia, a dilated esophagus *(left)* that terminates at the gastroesophageal junction in a beaklike narrowing *(right).*

The differential diagnosis of these radiologic findings includes a stricture from reflux esophagitis and secondary achalasia from carcinoma involving the fundus of the stomach or the distal esophagus. The tumors one must include in the differential diagnosis are adenocarcinomas of the stomach, pancreas, and lung. Secondary achalasia typically occurs in patients over age 60 with symptoms for less than 1 year.

A radiologic clue to the diagnosis of secondary achalasia is the asymmetric narrowing of the distal esophagus. Esophagogastroscopy can rule out a stricture or tumor, since the endoscope can be passed into the stomach in the presence of achalasia, whereas with a peptic stricture or cancer it cannot. Moreover, in reflux esophagitis the esophagus appears erythematous and friable. During endoscopy careful examination and biopsy of the fundus of the stomach must be performed to rule out adenocarcinoma causing secondary achalasia.

Confirmation of the presumptive diagnosis of primary achalasia requires esophageal manometry, which characteristically shows a lower esophageal sphincter pressure that is high (greater than 30 to 40 mm Hg above gastric pressure), and with a swallow the lower esophageal sphincter pressure never relaxes to gastric baseline pressure. In the body of the esophagus usually all contractions are simultaneous or nonperistaltic. Unfortunately, secondary achalasia gives the same esophageal manometry tracing.

### Treatment

At present no medical or surgical therapy of achalasia can effectively restore normal esophageal function. Therefore the goal of either medical or surgical therapy is to weaken the lower esophageal sphincter to allow solids and liquids to empty by gravity.

Medical therapy is accomplished by pneumatic (balloon) dilatation of the LES. Under fluoroscopic guidance a firm balloon is distended to a predetermined diameter (usually 3 to 3.5 cm) in the area of the LES, thus tearing some of the muscle fibers. Success is obtained in approximately 75% of the patients with one or two dilatations and is determined by more rapid emptying of barium on x-ray and the patient's ability to eat without dysphagia. The major complication of balloon dilatation is a tear into the mediastinum. Fortunately this is rare, occurring in fewer than 5% of patients; it can usually be treated by nonsurgical means with nasogastric suction and antibiotics.

Calcium channel blocking agents, which are potent smooth muscle relaxants, have been tried in patients with achalasia. In one study nifedipine (20 mg) given sublingually before meals resulted in a significant decrease in the LES pressure and a marked decrease in dysphagia. In a placebo-controlled trial neither oral verapamil (160 mg) nor nifedipine (20 mg) consistently alleviated the symptoms from achalasia, but in selected patients either nifedipine or verapamil was beneficial.

In conclusion, pneumatic (balloon) dilatation is still the most definitive medical therapy for treating achalasia. Calcium channel blocking agents certainly should be tried if pneumatic dilatation cannot be performed and before surgery is undertaken.

If medical therapy is unsuccessful, a surgical myotomy (Heller's procedure) can be performed. This operation entails making an incision through the circular muscle down to the mucosa over the entire length of the LES. At least 80% of patients with this procedure have good results. The major problem following surgical myotomy is severe reflux esophagitis, which occurs in 5% to 25% of patients, depending on the experience of the surgeon.

## SMOOTH MUSCLE SPASTIC DISORDERS

### Diffuse esophageal spasm

The term *diffuse esophageal spasm* is frequently misunderstood, since an exact definition has never been agreed on. A good working definition includes the following criteria: (1) symptoms of chest pain and dysphagia, (2) barium swallow that reveals spontaneous, nonperistaltic contractions (so-called tertiary contractions), and (3) esophageal manometry that demonstrates repetitive, simultaneous contractions for at least 50% of the esophagus. Using these strict criteria the prevalence of diffuse esophageal spasm is far less common than achalasia. The etiology is unknown, and consistent pathologic findings have not been documented.

The diagnosis of diffuse esophageal spasm is usually entertained after a patient has undergone complete evaluation for coronary heart disease, often including coronary angiography. The physician should consider the diagnosis of diffuse esophageal spasm *before* coronary heart disease if the patient complains of sharp retrosternal chest pain that occurs while eating solids or liquids. Sometimes the pain occurs at night, awakening the patient from sleep. In addition, patients often complain of dysphagia for solids and liquids, but it is usually intermittent and not progressive, as seen in achalasia.

The presumptive diagnosis is based on the clinical symptoms discussed above and confirmed with a barium swallow and esophageal manometry. On barium swallow, particularly in the lower two thirds of the esophagus, spontaneous random contractions are seen, variously described as corkscrew esophagus, tertiary contractions, and spastic pseudodiverticulosis. Narrowing of the distal esophagus is not seen. However, the clinician should be aware that many patients *without* diffuse esophageal spasm occasionally demonstrate a spontaneous or tertiary contraction on barium swallow.

The diagnosis is confirmed by esophageal manometry, which reveals an LES that relaxes normally after a swallow. The resting LES pressure may also be higher than normal (greater than 30 mm Hg). In the lower two thirds of the esophagus there are spontaneous, high-amplitude, often repetitive contractions after a swallow.

### Nutcracker esophagus

Another motor abnormality of the smooth muscle portion of the esophagus has been termed *nutcracker esophagus* and is characterized by chest pain and dysphagia. Typically this motor disorder is seen more commonly in women at a mean age of 40. The disorder is more common than diffuse esophageal spasm and is diagnosed by esophageal manometry characterized by high-amplitude *peristaltic* contractions in the lower two thirds of the esophagus.

Many patients with noncardiac chest pain secondary to a smooth muscle spastic disorder of the esophagus have a normal esophageal resting manometry or no pain during the stationary manometry. Therefore to increase the diagnostic yield, provocative testing is recommended (Fig. 41-4). Edrophonium chloride (Tensilon) given intravenously can provoke the patient's typical chest pain and does not affect the coronary arteries. Similarly, esophageal balloon distention may produce a positive response. For patients who continue to have noncardiac chest pain with normal manometry and negative provocative testing, 24-hour ambulatory motility manometry has recently become available.

### Treatment of smooth muscle spastic disorders

There is no definitive medical therapy for diffuse esophageal spasm or nutcracker esophagus. The goal of therapy is to relieve the pain and dysphagia, particularly at the time of eating. Traditional therapy has been the use of smooth muscle relaxants, employing agents such as nitrites—either sublingual nitroglycerin or longer-acting nitrites such as isosorbide dinitrate (Isordil). The success of treatment with these agents is variable and unpredictable.

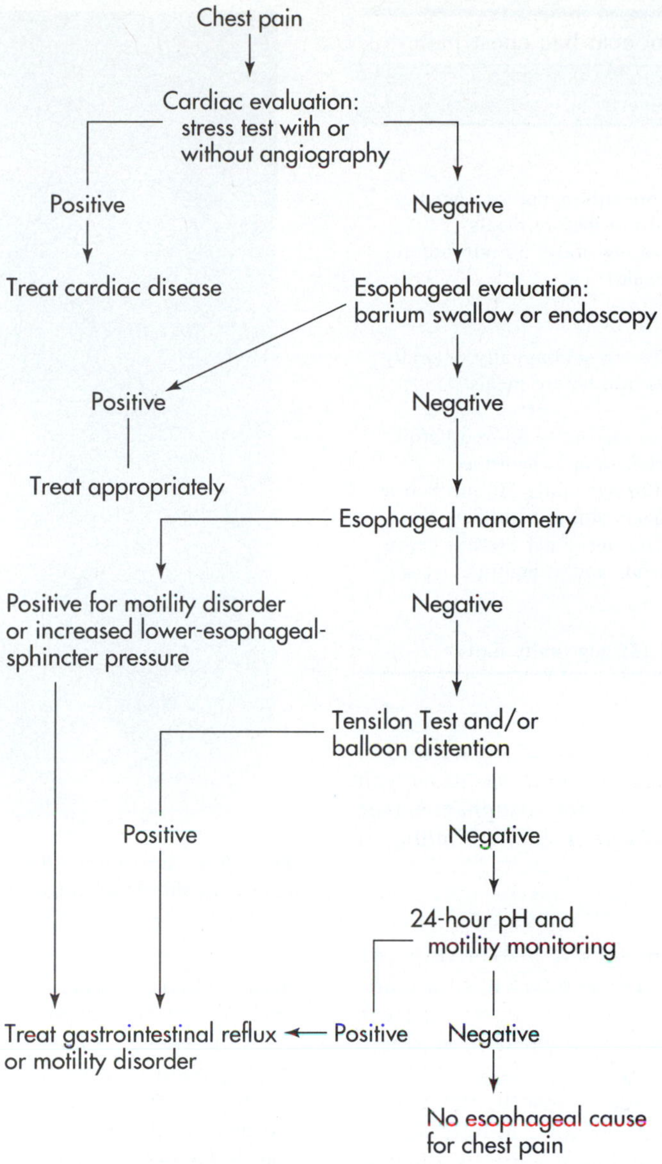


**Fig. 41-4.** Diagnosis of noncardiac chest pain.

Recent studies have noted improvement in symptoms and a decrease in the amplitude of contractions on esophageal manometry with the calcium channel blocking agents nifedipine and diltiazem. Antidepressant therapy (e.g., trazodone hydrochloride) has been used successfully in spastic esophageal motor disorders (Table 41-1). The rationale for antidepressants is that one is treating an irritable esophagus syndrome.

## NONCARDIAC CHEST PAIN

It is estimated that there are approximately 50,000 new cases of noncardiac chest pain each year, based on estimates from the percentage of normal coronary angiograms each year in the United States. In patients with atypical chest pain and no evidence for heart disease (i.e., by ECG and stress testing), one must consider an esophageal cause for the pain. Most frequently patients with noncardiac chest pain are women between the ages of 30 and 60. The etiology of the pain is most commonly reflux of acid or less commonly an esophageal motility disorder. Diagnosis is made by following the algorithm in Fig. 41-4. If the etiology of pain is determined to be reflux of acid, then an aggressive antireflux regimen should be initiated, usually with omeprazole (Prilosec), 20 mg once or twice a day. If this is a motility disorder, then one of the therapies outlined in Table 41-1 should be prescribed.

## CANCER OF THE ESOPHAGUS

The most common tumor involving the esophagus, unfortunately, is a malignant one. Epidermoid or squamous carcinoma is most frequently diagnosed, followed by adenocarcinoma. The adenocarcinoma rarely arises from

**Table 41-1.** Treatment for noncardiac chest pain

| Drug | Dosage |
|---|---|
| **Nitrates** | |
| Nitroglycerin | 0.4 mg sublingually as needed 30 min before meals |
| Isosorbide or dinitrate | 10-20 mg orally 30 min before meals |
| **Calcium channel blockers** | |
| Nifedipine | 10-20 mg sublingually or orally 30 min before meals or 10-20 mg orally 30 min before meals and at bedtime |
| Diltiazem | 90-120 mg orally 30 min before meals and at bedtime |
| Verapamil | 80-160 mg orally 30 min before meals and at bedtime |
| **Sedatives/tranquilizers** | |
| Trazodone (for example) | 100-150 mg orally daily |

the esophageal mucosa but usually is present as a result of extension from the stomach. Adenocarcinoma may result from a malignant change in a Barrett esophagus (see above). Benign tumors are usually an incidental finding of little importance.

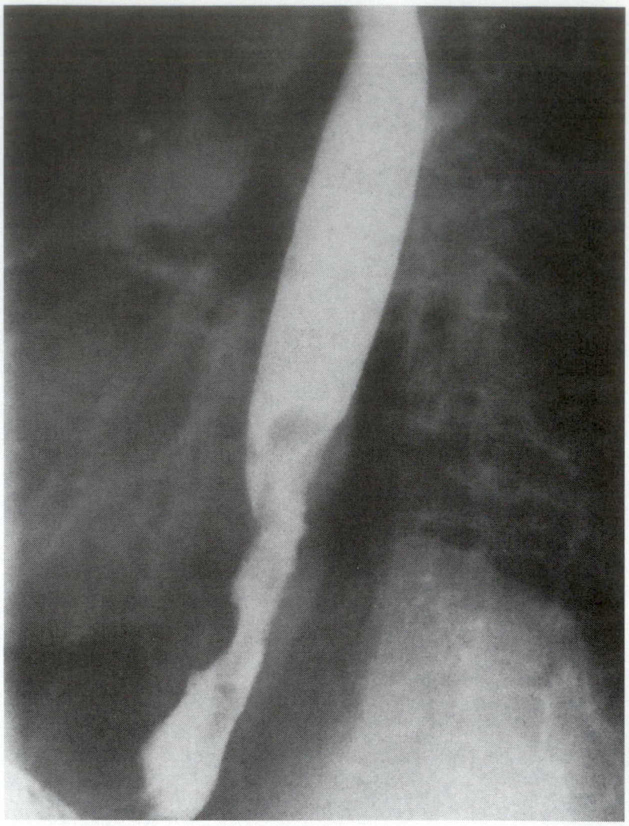

**Fig. 41-5.** Barium swallow demonstrating the classic findings in cancer of the distal third of the esophagus.

## Squamous carcinoma

Fortunately, cancer of the esophagus is a relatively rare tumor in the United States, occurring in two to four white persons per 100,000 and as many as 15 African-American men per 100,000. The incidence is highest in northern China, with 130 cases per 100,000.

It is unclear why the incidence is low in the United States, although it is known that certain etiologic factors contribute and have been associated with esophageal cancer. Alcohol and smoking have been associated with an increase of cancer of the esophagus, as have lye ingestion and radiation exposure. In addition, long-term stasis, as occurs in achalasia, has been associated with increased incidence of esophageal cancer. Patients invariably develop progressive dysphagia for solids, then liquids. By the time of presentation the majority of patients have unresectable disease. Any patient over the age of 40 who has progressive dysphagia of less than 6 months' duration must be given the presumptive diagnosis of esophageal cancer. In addition, many patients have anorexia and weight loss by the time they see their physician. The physical examination is usually not helpful unless supraclavicular lymph node enlargement or hepatomegaly is found, findings that obviously indicate metastatic disease. Other less common presenting symptoms include hoarseness secondary to involvement of the recurrent laryngeal nerve, coughing secondary to aspiration or caused by a tracheoesophageal fistula, and rarely hematemesis (5%).

The presumptive diagnosis can be made by a barium swallow (Fig. 41-5) showing mucosal irregularity and a tumor encroaching on the lumen. The greatest difficulty arises when the tumor causes a smooth narrowing, thereby making differentiation from a benign stricture difficult.

Definitive diagnosis is made by esophagoscopy with biopsy combined with brush cytology in 95% of cases. It is important to know if the tumor is confined to the esophagus alone. Computed tomography (CT) of the chest has been useful in determining the actual extent of the carcinoma in the esophagus as well as the extent of spread into the mediastinum. Most recently endoscopic ultrasonography has been demonstrated to be the most reliable diagnostic technique for staging esophageal cancer.

Irrespective of the type of therapy, the 5-year survival of all patients with esophageal cancer is approximately 5% to 15%. Surgery is the treatment of choice for cancer of the lower third of the esophagus and irradiation for the middle and upper thirds. Before surgery is considered the extent of disease should be ascertained. If there is liver or supraclavicular node involvement, surgery is not performed except for palliation. One form of palliative treatment of esophageal cancer is esophageal dilatation with rubber bougies before and during radiation therapy. This treatment has allowed this unfortunate group of patients to continue eating. Studies are underway to determine if preoperative irradiation combined with surgery improves survival.

## Adenocarcinoma of the esophagus

Adenocarcinoma arising from the mucous glands of the esophagus is extremely rare, but adenocarcinoma arising in columnar epithelium (Barrett's esophagus) is becoming

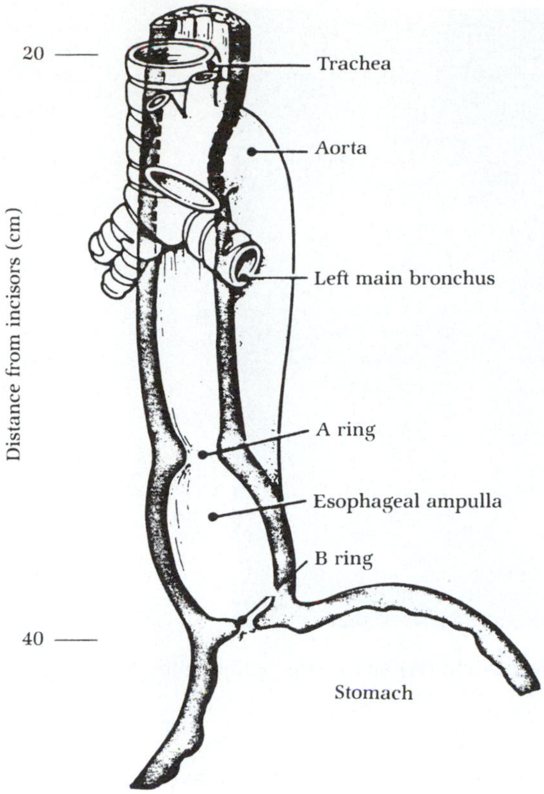


**Fig. 41-6.** The esophagus, demonstrating its relation to the trachea and aorta. (From Spechler S, Burakoff R: The esophagus. In Wilkins R, Levinsky N [editors]: *Medicine: essentials of clinical practice,* ed 3, Boston, 1983, Little, Brown.)

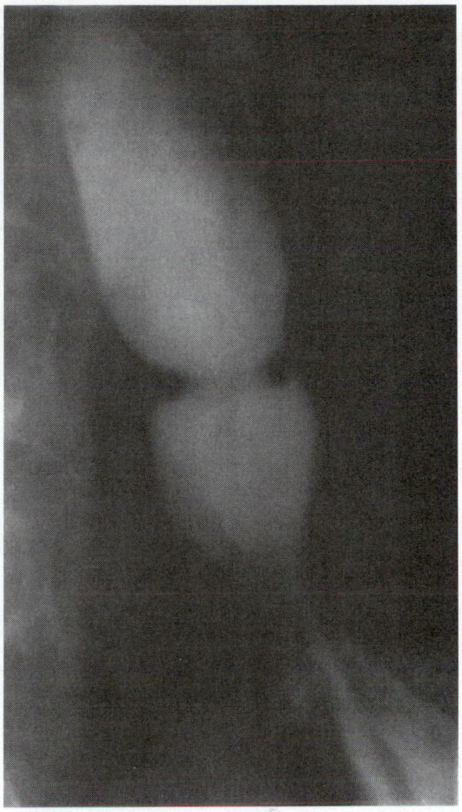

**Fig. 41-7.** Barium swallow demonstrating a lower esophageal *(B)* ring at the gastroesophageal junction.

more common. As discussed above, columnar epithelium results from reflux esophagitis. It is now appreciated that approximately 10% of patients with a biopsy-proved Barrett esophagus develop adenocarcinoma. These patients present with a history of heartburn, then dysphagia. Diagnosis is made by endoscopic biopsy and brush cytology. Radiation therapy is ineffective. Surgery is the treatment of choice, but the 5-year survival is only approximately 5%.

## ESOPHAGEAL RING

The lower esophageal ring, also called the Schatzki or B ring, marks the junction of the esophageal and gastric mucosa (Fig. 41-6). It is composed of squamous epithelium superiorly and gastric epithelium inferiorly. It is the most common clinical entity among the rings and webs, often resulting in clinical symptoms. A patient without heartburn who reports that solid food, invariably meat or bread, gets stuck intermittently in the lower end of the chest probably has a lower esophageal ring. It is still unknown if lower esophageal rings are congenital or acquired. Patients may develop the condition in their 20s or have an initial indication in the fifth to seventh decades.

The diagnosis is made by a barium swallow (Fig. 41-7). During the examination the lower end of the esophagus must be distended and adequately filled or a ring may be missed. In addition, a bolus is swallowed during the barium swallow, which demonstrates hold-up at the gastroesophageal junction. The ring appears as a symmetric indentation at the gastroesophageal junction and is usually less than 5 mm thick. If the ring is thicker, an esophageal stricture must be considered. To rule out carcinoma or stricture, esophagoscopy should be performed. Treatment is accomplished with mercury-filled bougies; simple passage of a No. 50 French bougie dilates the ring in most cases and relieves of symptoms.

## DIVERTICULA

Esophageal diverticula are of three types and represent outpouchings of one or more layers of the esophagus. *Zenker's diverticulum* occurs above the upper esophageal sphincter (cricopharyngeus) and may be associated with incoordination of the pharynx and cricopharyngeus (Fig. 41-8, *A*). The patient presents with intermittent dysphagia, but as the pouch enlarges symptoms progress to aspiration of liquids and regurgitation of food into the mouth. Diagnosis is made by barium swallow. This type of diverticulum usually requires no therapy.

*Epiphrenic diverticulum* occurs just above the lower esophageal sphincter and has been associated with failure of the lower esophageal sphincter to relax and increased amplitude of contractions of the esophagus. Patients present with symptoms of dysphagia and may regurgitate large amounts of fluid when recumbent as a result of fluid accumulating within the diverticulum. Diagnosis is made by barium swallow demonstrating a barium-filled sac in the distal esophagus (Fig. 41-8, *B*). Esophageal manometry is performed to rule out an associated motility disorder. Surgery is necessary only if clinical symptoms are significant.

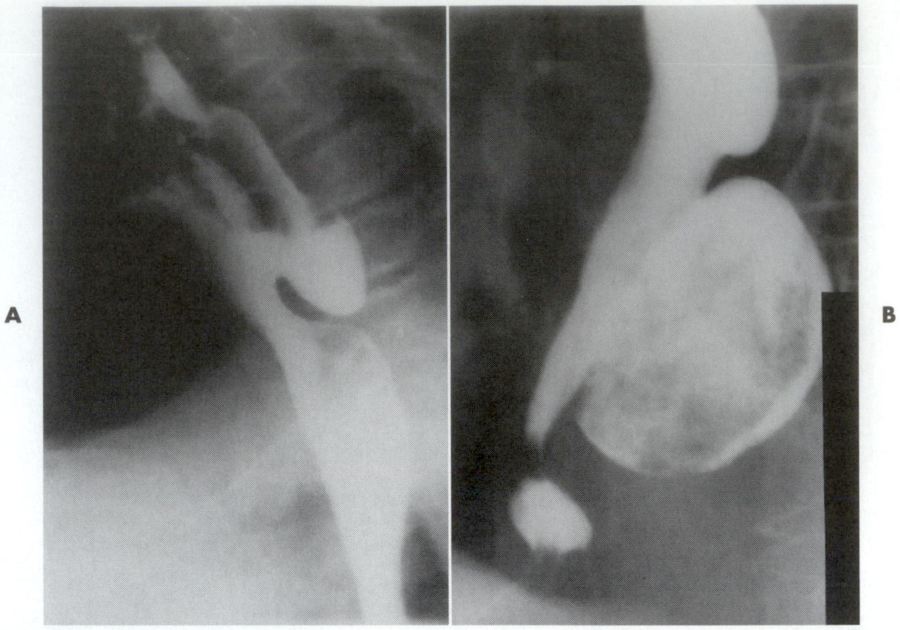

**Fig. 41-8.** Barium swallow demonstrating Zenker's diverticulum (**A**) and a large epiphrenic diverticulum of the distal esophagus (**B**).

## SYSTEMIC DISEASE INVOLVING THE ESOPHAGUS

There are several diseases that can secondarily involve the esophagus (e.g., diabetes mellitus, alcoholism with neuropathy, amyloidosis), but none demonstrates a consistent, characteristic abnormality. Collagen vascular disease can also involve the esophagus, resulting in varying degrees of aperistalsis of the esophagus. Invariably these abnormalities are associated with the Raynaud phenomenon, which has been associated with aperistalsis of the esophagus. Fortunately, except for scleroderma, these other diseases result in insignificant functional impairment of the esophagus.

In scleroderma patients have clinical problems resulting from two abnormalities of the esophagus: (1) aperistalsis of the lower two thirds and (2) incompetence of the LES. The presence of both of these defects results in severe reflux esophagitis. The abnormalities result from atrophy of the smooth muscle of the esophagus as well as an abnormality of the nervous control of the lower esophageal sphincter.

Patients have symptoms of heartburn and dysphagia for solids. On physical examination there is usually evidence of Raynaud's phenomenon. With time heartburn may lessen, and the dysphagia worsens as a stricture develops. The presumptive diagnosis is made on the basis of the patient's history and a physical examination. A barium swallow demonstrates aperistalsis from the aortic arch to the end of the esophagus as well as reflux of barium. With progression of the disease a stricture is seen. The diagnosis can be confirmed by esophageal manometry, which demonstrates aperistalsis of the lower two thirds of the esophagus and a decreased resting LES pressure. All patients should undergo esophagoscopy at some point in their illness to evaluate the severity of the esophagitis and to be sure that a Barrett esophagus is not present.

There is no specific treatment for scleroderma involving the esophagus except to recommend the most effective measures for controlling reflux. These include elevating the head of the bed, avoiding foods that decrease LES pressure, and $H_2$ receptor antagonist therapy. It has been shown that $H_2$ receptor antagonists and omeprazole decrease the reflux symptoms as well as the severity of the esophagitis seen endoscopically.

If a stricture develops, dilatation with rubber bougie is usually successful. As a result of the poor peristalsis in the body of the esophagus, surgery is avoided if possible. If the reflux esophagitis cannot be treated successfully medically, a Belsey repair or partial fundoplication has been attempted with some success.

## DISEASES OF THE HYPOPHARYNX AND PROXIMAL ESOPHAGUS

In addition to systemic diseases involving the smooth muscle portion of the esophagus, several diseases, primarily neurologic, affect the hypopharynx, upper esophageal sphincter, and striated portion of the esophagus. Patients who have difficulty in initiating swallowing may have cerebrovascular accidents, amyotrophic lateral sclerosis, multiple sclerosis, poliomyelitis, diphtheria, or tetanus. Patients recovering from cerebrovascular accidents can benefit from evaluation by a speech therapist who can recommend swallowing exercises to improve deglutition. Patients with dysphagia for liquids and solids involving the upper esophagus may have amyloidosis, dermatomyositis-polymyositis, myasthenia gravis, myotonia dystrophia, myxedema, oculopharyngeal muscular dystrophy, or thyrotoxicosis.

Involvement of the striated muscle is diagnosed by barium swallow and cineradiography and is confirmed by demonstrating aperistalsis in the upper third of the esophagus by esophageal manometry. The dysphagia may be alleviated by treating the systemic disease.

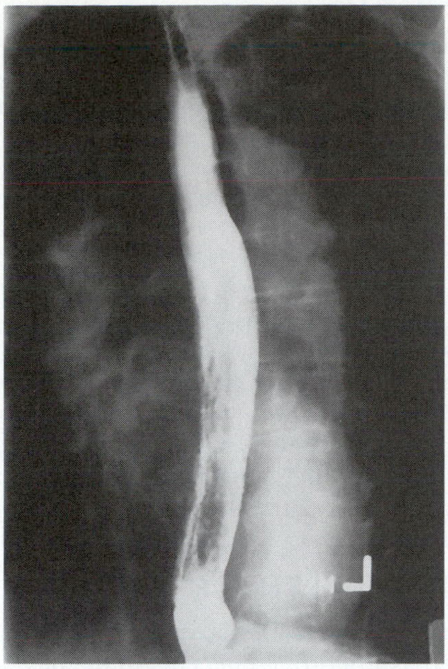

**Fig. 41-9.** Barium swallow demonstrating the mucosal ulcerations of monilial esophagitis.

## INFECTIONS OF THE ESOPHAGUS

The incidence of infectious diseases of the esophagus has increased largely as a result of the dramatic increase in acquired immune deficiency syndrome (AIDS). In caring for patients with AIDS one must always be on the lookout for various infectious organisms that can affect the esophagus, especially moniliasis, herpes simplex (HSV 1), and cytomegalovirus (CMV).

### Moniliasis *(Candida)*

Candidiasis is also seen with increased frequency in patients with neoplastic diseases, diabetes mellitus, chronic renal failure, and other conditions where there is immune incompetence. Patients develop severe odynophagia as well as dysphagia. If the moniliasis is severe, the patient may also experience hematemesis. On physical examination the physician may discover oropharyngeal moniliasis (thrush).

Barium swallow (Fig. 41-9) may demonstrate ulceration of the esophageal mucosa, but the diagnosis is best confirmed by esophagoscopy. Brushings of the mucosal ulcerations demonstrate yeast forms, and biopsy of the ulceration and staining with silver methenamine demonstrate the mycelia.

In the immune competent patient treatment is usually successful with nystatin oral suspension, 250,000 units every 2 hours for 1 week total. A total dose of up to 12 million units a day may be necessary. In the immunocompromised patient excellent results have now been achieved with fluconazole (Diflucan), an antifungal agent administered in dosages of 50 to 200 mg once a day orally.

### Herpes simplex and cytomegalovirus

As in patients with candidal esophagitis, patients with these infections usually complain of odynophagia. Diagnosis can be made only by esophagoscopy and biopsy of the esophageal mucosal lesion with the appropriate staining and culture of the tissue. Successful treatment can be accomplished with acyclovir (Zovirax) for HSV 1 and gancyclovir for CMV.

## MISCELLANEOUS DISORDERS

### Mallory-Weiss syndrome

Mallory-Weiss syndrome comprises a mucosal tear at the gastroesophageal junction resulting from vomiting. With the advent of flexible upper endoscopy it is now appreciated that the Mallory-Weiss syndrome is found in 15% of patients who have hematemesis. The classic description is one of forceful retching followed by vomiting of blood; as many as 25% of patients vomit blood with the initial vomitus.

Diagnosis is made by upper endoscopy, and the tear is usually seen on the gastric side of the gastroesophageal junction. Treatment consists of observation, since nearly all episodes stop spontaneously. Intravenous vasopressin can be used if bleeding continues. The area can be electrocoagulated if bleeding does not stop spontaneously. Surgery is rarely required.

### Foreign bodies

Most commonly foreign bodies are a result of poorly chewed, hastily swallowed food, especially bread and meat. Food impaction usually occurs in the edentulous elderly or very young. Animal bones and other objects, including pins and coins, pass through the gastrointestinal tract more than 90% of the time.

Patients describe ingestion of the food or object and complain of acute chest pain and salivation. A plain film of the chest or neck usually visualizes the object. If not, a barium swallow is performed to determine the location of the obstruction.

A nonobstructing foreign body that has not caused a perforation within 24 hours usually passes into the stomach. If the object or food is impacted or fails to pass, it is removed with a snare by flexible upper endoscopy. Often a lower esophageal ring is found when food impaction occurs. After removal of the material, the ring can be dilated with a mercury-filled rubber bougie.

## BIBLIOGRAPHY

Achem SR, Kolts BE: Current medical therapy for esophageal motility disorders, *Am J Med* 92(5A):98S, 1992.

Burakoff R: Noncardiac chest pain, *Emerg Med* 22(3):49, 1990.

Connolly GM et al: Oesophageal symptoms, their causes, treatment and prognosis in patients with acquired immunodeficiency syndrome, *Gut* 30:1033, 1989.

Fellows IW, Ogilvie AL, Atkinson M: Pneumatic dilatation in achalasia, *Gut* 24:1020, 1983.

Fulp SR, Richter JE: Esophageal chest pain, *Am Fam Physician* 40(3):101, 1989.

Gelfand MD: Gastroesophageal reflux disease, *Med Clin North Am* 75(4):923, 1991.

Hirsch MS, Schooley RT: Treatment of herpesvirus infections, *N Engl J Med* 309:963, 1983.

Janssens JP, Vantrappen G: Irritable esophagus, *Am J Med* 92 (5A):27S, 1992.

Leen CL et al: Once-weekly fluconazole to prevent recurrence of oropharyngeal candidiasis in patients with AIDS and AIDS-related complex: a double-blind placebo-controlled study, *J Infect* 21:55, 1990.

Meyers JO: Prevention and treatment of cytomegalovirus infections, *Ann Rev Med* 42:179, 1991.

Rex DK: Gastroesophageal reflux disease in adults: pathophysiology, diagnosis and management, *J Fam Pract* 35(6):673-681, 1992.
Reynolds WA: Are night sweats a sign of esophageal reflux? *J Clin Gastroenterol* 11(5):590, 1989.
Sutherland JE: Gastroesophageal reflux disease. When antacids aren't enough, *Postgrad Med* 89(7):45, 1991.
Tio TL, Cohen P, Coene PP: Endosonography and computed tomography of esophageal carcinoma, *Gastroenterology* 96:1478, 1989.
Triadafilopoulos G et al: Medical treatment of esophageal achalasia: double blind crossover study with oral nifedipine, verapamil and placebo, *Dig Dis Sci* 36(3):260, 1991.
Zamost BJ et al: Esophagitis in scleroderma: prevalence and risk factors, *Gastroenterology* 92:421, 1987.

CHAPTER

# 42 Gastric and Duodenal Ulcers

W. Paul McKinney
Mark Feldman

Gastric and duodenal ulcers are defects in the mucosa of the stomach or duodenum that penetrate to or through the level of the muscularis mucosa (Fig. 42-2). This depth of penetration distinguishes ulcers from the more superficial gastric and duodenal erosions. Although nearly 100% of patients with benign gastric and duodenal ulcers secrete both acid and pepsin (hence the term *peptic ulcer*), recent insights into the origin of ulcers of the upper gastrointestinal tract have revealed other important factors that play a role in their etiology.

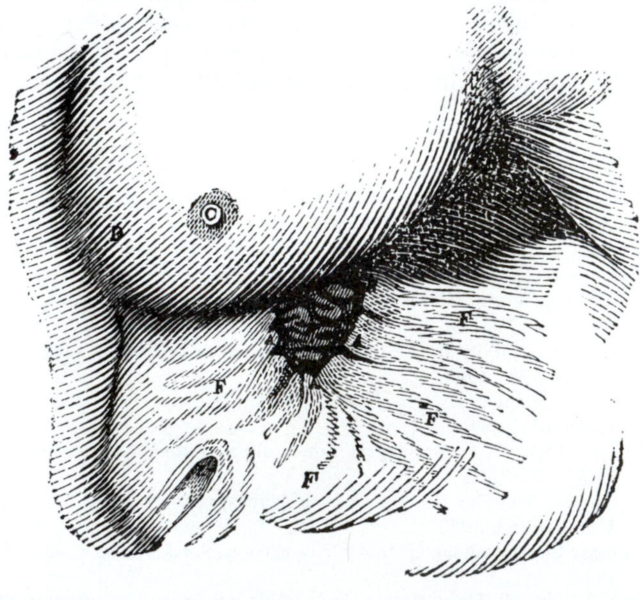

**Fig. 42-1.** Drawing by William Beaumont, M.D., of his famous patient, Alexis St. Martin, representing the appearance of the open gastrocutaneous fistula. With this fistula, Beaumont was able to demonstrate the digestive capabilities of the gastric secretions. (Courtesy of the Boston Medical Library.)

## EPIDEMIOLOGY

The lifetime risk of peptic ulcer disease is 5% to 10%, with an annual prevalence rate of 1.8%. About 350,000 new cases are diagnosed each year in the United States. There is no difference between men and women in the incidence of gastric ulcer, but men are twice as likely as women to develop a duodenal ulcer. The incidence of both gastric and duodenal ulcer increases with age.

A variety of conditions are risk factors for ulcer disease, including cigarette smoking, use of aspirin and other analgesics, dependent personality type, blood group O, and *Helicobacter pylori* infection. Neither alcohol use nor specific dietary factors, including caffeine, have been clearly linked to ulcer disease. Ulcers are more common in patients with chronic obstructive pulmonary disease, cirrhosis, renal failure, and renal transplantation. Less definite associations have been noted for hyperparathyroidism, coronary artery disease, and polycythemia vera.

## ETIOLOGY AND PATHOGENESIS

Gastric hydrochloric acid and pepsin have traditionally been viewed as important elements in the development of ulcer disease. About 30% to 40% of patients with duodenal ulcer have above average rates of acid secretion. Three mechanisms for elevated acid secretion have been described or proposed: (1) gastrin hypersecretion with hypergastrinemia (e.g., Zollinger-Ellison syndrome), (2) elevated histamine production with hyperhistaminemia (systemic mastocytosis, basophilic leukemia), and (3)

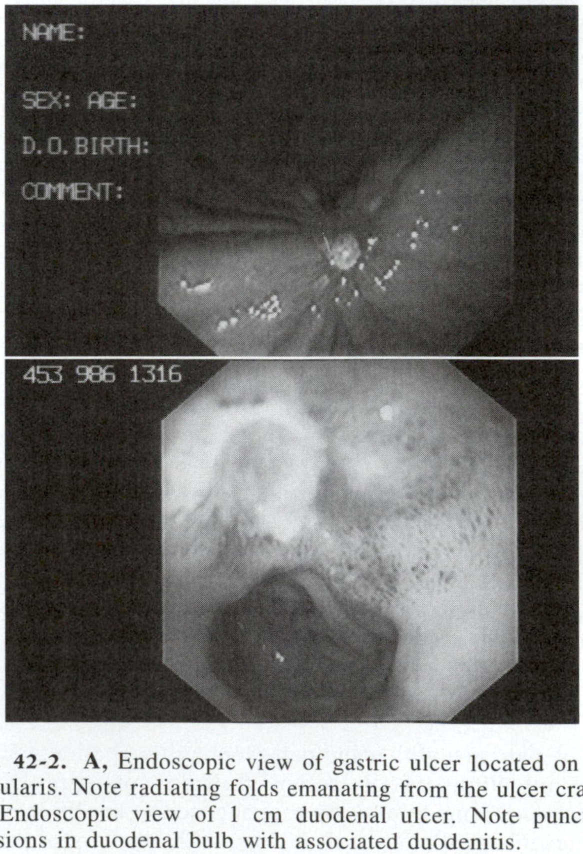


A

B

**Fig. 42-2.** **A,** Endoscopic view of gastric ulcer located on the angularis. Note radiating folds emanating from the ulcer crater. **B,** Endoscopic view of 1 cm duodenal ulcer. Note punctate erosions in duodenal bulb with associated duodenitis.

increased neuronal release of acetylcholine (vagal hyperfunction). The remaining 60% to 70% of patients with duodenal ulcer and almost all patients with gastric ulcer have normal (or even low, in the case of gastric ulcer) rates of acid production. In such individuals a breakdown in local defense mechanisms plays a pathogenetic role. The various factors maintaining mucosal defense include surface mucus and bicarbonate, which form a thin alkaline gel coating mucosal cells, mucosal blood flow, and regular cell renewal, each of which may be enhanced by endogenous prostaglandins. Additional pathogenetic factors that may contribute to the development of ulcer disease include genetics, stress, and a variety of exogenous factors, including infectious agents, as described below.

Ulcers are more common in an identical twin of an affected individual than in a fraternal twin, suggesting a genetic predisposition. Certain genetic disorders may be responsible for peptic ulcer disease in a minority of cases, with multiple endocrine neoplasia type I (MEN I) being the most common example (see Zollinger-Ellison syndrome below and also Chapter 39).

The exact role of psychologic stressors in the development of ulcer disease has not yet been determined. However, some studies suggest that emotional distress may contribute to increased acid production and may be linked to the formation of ulcers in some patients. Although earlier studies suggested that duodenal ulcer patients have excessively dependent personalities, more recent studies indicate that there is no specific ulcer personality.

A variety of external factors may play a role in certain persons. Cigarette smoking is about two times more frequent among ulcer patients than unaffected persons, although the mechanism for ulcer formation is uncertain and probably multifactorial. The risk of ulcer disease is proportional to the number of cigarettes smoked per day. Aspirin and several nonsalicylate nonsteroidal antiinflammatory drugs (NSAIDs) reduce mucosal prostaglandin synthesis and consequently interfere with multiple factors important in maintaining the integrity of mucosal defense barriers, including mucus and bicarbonate secretion. Although some studies support a pathogenetic role in ulcer disease for corticosteroids, especially prednisone, several studies refute an independent role for steroids in the genesis of ulcers; corticosteroids may worsen mucosal injury caused by NSAIDs, however.

Though a host of infectious agents, including viruses (herpes simplex virus 1, cytomegalovirus) and fungi *(Candida albicans)* have been detected in ulcer disease in certain settings, infection with the bacterium *H. pylori* has received the greatest attention. More than 90% of persons with duodenal ulcers and up to 80% of those with gastric ulcers are infected with *H. pylori.* However, the correlation of infection with ulcer disease is far from 1:1; about half of asymptomatic persons over the age of 60 also show evidence of infection. A pathogenic role of the organism in gastritis is supported by the finding that administration of viable bacteria to either animals or human volunteers results in gastritis (but not ulcers). Moreover, eradication of infection with antimicrobial drugs is coupled with resolution of gastritis. Recent evidence supports the hypothesis that infection with *H. pylori* may be responsible for the development of ulcer disease in certain individuals. The rate of duodenal and gastric ulcer recurrence in persons infected with *H. pylori* is substantially lower if infection can be eradicated (Fig. 42-3). Thus *H. pylori*–related gastritis is an important risk factor for ulcer disease.

## PATIENT HISTORY: NONULCER DYSPEPSIA VS. TYPICAL ULCER SYMPTOMS

Classic ulcer pain is a burning or gnawing sensation located in the epigastrium, relieved by food or antacids. However, this pain location is not specific for ulcer disease, and the characterization of pain is a highly insensitive indicator of ulcer disease. The episodic nature of the pain, tending to cluster and last for minutes, with pain episodes separated by long symptom-free periods, is a better predictor of the presence of an ulcer. Pain recurrences, sometimes with a seasonal pattern in the fall or spring, are very typical. In contrast, dyspepsia (indigestion) is a vague constellation of symptoms, including nausea, vomiting, anorexia, an unpleasant sense of satiety, bloating, and poorly defined pain. It may be impossible to distinguish ulcer pain from nonulcer dyspepsia on the basis of the history alone.

## PHYSICAL EXAMINATION

No elements of the physical examination are useful in discriminating uncomplicated ulcer disease from other organic or functional disorders of the gastrointestinal tract. Epigastric tenderness, for example, may be present with ulcer disease as well as with cholecystitis, pancreatitis, nonulcer dyspepsia, and a variety of other disorders.

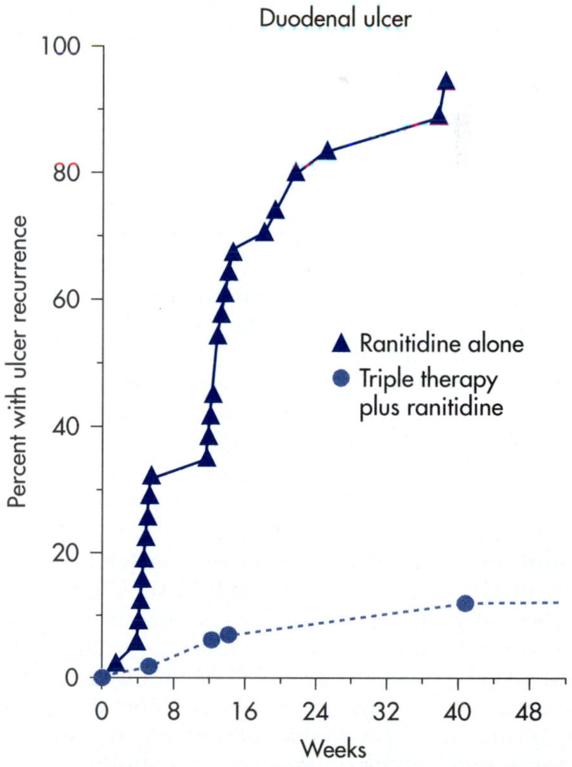


**Fig. 42-3.** One-year recurrence of duodenal ulcers following successful healing with ranitidine alone or ranitidine plus bismuth subsalicylate, metronidazole, and tetracycline. (From Graham DY et al: *Scand J Gastroenterol* 28:939, 1993.)

However, certain findings may suggest the presence of well-known complications of ulcer disease. For example, a succussion splash implies gastric outlet obstruction; a positive fecal occult blood test or coffee ground–like nasogastric aspirate may be present with bleeding; and abdominal rigidity is typical of free perforation of an ulcer.

## LABORATORY STUDIES AND DIAGNOSTIC PROCEDURES

Routine laboratory tests are usually normal in ulcer disease, unless either fluid and electrolyte depletion associated with vomiting or anemia due to bleeding is present.

The standard upper gastrointestinal radiographic series (upper GI) has historically been the procedure of choice for confirming the diagnosis of ulcer disease and has been improved upon with the use of double contrast techniques. However, it involves radiation exposure, a major concern for pregnant patients, and has only 70% to 80% of the accuracy of upper GI endoscopy. Diagnostic accuracy is reduced even further for lesions of the fundus and cardia of the stomach, giant duodenal ulcers, ulcers embedded in duodenal deformities, marginal ulcers at the site of gastrojejunostomy, and superficial mucosal lesions.

Generally viewed as the standard for diagnosis of ulcer disease, upper GI endoscopy allows visualization of ulcers (see Fig. 42-2), directed biopsy of lesions suspected of being cancerous, and bacteriologic analysis for *H. pylori.* It is currently recommended for *all* newly diagnosed gastric ulcers for the purpose of excluding malignancy. Its major drawback is the attendant cost (approximately two or more times that of the x-ray) and the additional preparation required, including intravenous sedation and its associated side effects (e.g., respiratory depression, pulmonary aspiration). There is a small (0.03% to 0.1%) risk of gastrointestinal perforation with endoscopy as well.

A number of tests for diagnosing *H. pylori* infection are available. Serologic antibody tests (enzyme-linked immunosorbent assay, or ELISA) are available but are expensive and do not readily distinguish active from past or successfully treated infection. Breath tests based on metabolism of radiolabeled urea by urease, which is plentiful in *H. pylori,* are being developed. If endoscopic biopsy material is obtained from the stomach, it can be stained and examined microscopically for *H. pylori* (Fig. 42-4) or added to a gel containing urea and phenol red, a pH indicator that turns pink if bacterial urease is present. Alternatively, the biopsy can be cultured for *H. pylori,* although this is tedious. The optimal approach to diagnose *H. pylori* infection is yet to be determined.

In some ulcer patients Zollinger-Ellison syndrome with or without MEN I may be suspected. In such individuals, fasting serum gastrin levels should be measured (see the box above). A high fasting gastrin level (over 200 pg/ml), if confirmed on repeat testing, should be followed by basal and peak acid output measurements. A markedly elevated fasting gastrin level (more than 600 pg/ml) together with high basal acid output (more than 15 mmol/hr; 60% or more of peak acid output) indicates the presence of Zollinger-Ellison syndrome. In persons with mild elevations in serum gastrin levels (200 to 600 pg/ml) and a high basal acid output, serum gastrin should be measured serially following intravenous secretin injection. Increases in gastrin exceeding 200 pg/ml within 10 minutes following secretin injection are diagnostic of Zollinger-Ellison syndrome and should lead to a search for the islet cell tumor, which is usually located in the pancreas or duodenum.

**Clinical situations in which measurement of serum gastrin levels is indicated due to suspicion of Zollinger-Ellison syndrome**

Family history of peptic ulcer
Ulcer associated with hypercalcemia or other manifestations of MEN I
Multifocal peptic ulcer
Peptic ulceration of postbulbar duodenum or jejunum
Peptic ulceration associated with diarrhea*
Chronic unexplained diarrhea*
Enlarged gastric folds on upper GI radiograph
Before surgery for "intractable" ulcer
Recurrent ulcer after ulcer surgery

From Schiller LR. In Wyngaarden JB, Smith LH, Bennet JC, editors: *Cecil textbook of medicine,* ed 19, Philadelphia, 1992, WB Saunders.

*Not due to antacid ingestion.

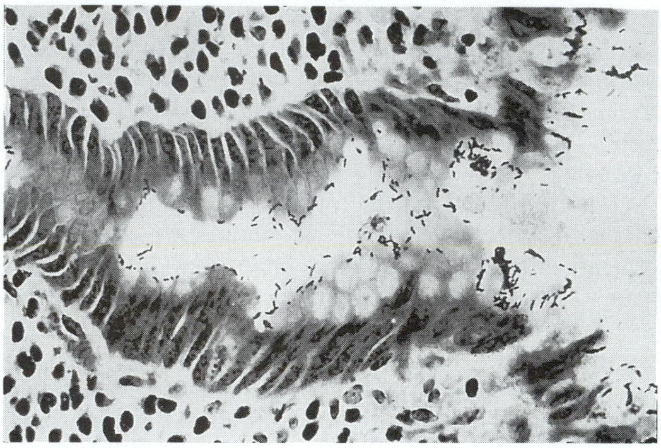

**Fig. 42-4.** Warthin-Starry stain of *H. pylori.* Dark rod-shaped organisms are in proximity to but do not invade gastric mucosa. An associated chronic active gastritis is present.

## DIFFERENTIAL DIAGNOSIS

The differential diagnosis of ulcer disease can be problematic because a wide variety of thoracic and upper abdominal disorders may cause similar pain, including nonulcer dyspepsia, cholecystitis, pancreatitis, irritable bowel syndrome, esophagitis, gastric malignancy, and myocardial ischemia. Other diseases to be considered include hypertrophic gastritis, syphilis, Crohn's disease, giardiasis, strongyloidiasis, and duodenal polyps or webs. The lack of response of pain to food or antacids and the presence of severe pain or rebound tenderness may help suggest a diagnosis other than uncomplicated ulcer

**Table 42-1.** Comparative costs of standard courses of pharmacologic therapy for duodenal ulcer

| Agent | Dosage | Cost of initial treatment* |
|---|---|---|
| **Antacids** | The only preparation shown to be effective in randomized trials conducted in the U.S. is Mylanta II: 30 ml 1 hr + 3 hr pc + hs; equivalent therapeutic efficacy of other preparations with equal acid neutralizing effects has not been proven | Varies widely depending on preparation and dose; cost for Mylanta II 30 ml 1 hr and 3 hr pc and hs is \$93.24 |
| **$H_2$ Antagonists** | | |
| Cimetidine | 400 mg bid or 800 mg qhs | \$67.54 |
| Rantidine | 150 mg bid or 300 mg qhs | \$77.10 |
| Famotidine | 20 mg bid or 40 mg qhs | \$74.85 |
| Nizatidine | 150 mg bid or 300 mg qhs | \$75.70 |
| **Omeprazole** | 20 mg q AM | \$100.18 |
| **Sucralfate** | 1 g qid or 2 g bid | \$73.16 |

*Average wholesale price, assuming four weeks of therapy, as of November 1993.

disease. In situations where weight loss, anemia, or exacerbation of pain with eating are present, the diagnosis of gastric cancer should be excluded.

If mild or vague symptoms of dyspepsia and no indicators of more serious disease or complicated ulcer disease are present, one should consider empiric therapy with ulcer-type dosages of $H_2$ blockers or antacids for about 2 weeks (see Table 42-1 for daily dosages). If antacids are chosen initially and intolerance develops, the patient can be switched to $H_2$ blockers. If symptoms persist or progress during the therapeutic trial period or recur later, then a definitive study should be performed. A schematic approach to this common clinical scenario is found in Fig. 42-5. The decision of whether to approach the diagnosis using radiographic or endoscopic techniques depends on the local situation, including costs, facilities, and experience of the personnel involved (see the Managed Care Guide).

## MANAGEMENT

The goals of ulcer therapy are to relieve pain, promote healing, and prevent complications and recurrence. Several approaches to treatment may be considered.

### Nonpharmacologic

There is no evidence that diet alteration is helpful in promotion of ulcer healing. Consumption of milk, a traditional home remedy for ulcers, transiently buffers acid, but its calcium and protein content also stimulate gastric acid production. Although very spicy foods may lead to pyrosis or dyspepsia, they are not ulcerogenic and do not inhibit healing. Thus a balanced diet, adjusted to caloric needs, is appropriate. Elimination of bedtime and between-meal snacks and of excessive alcohol intake is warranted as well.

Smoking cessation should be strongly encouraged, since cigarette smoking is the major lifestyle factor that increases the risk of ulcer disease, impairs healing, reduces the time between recurrences, and increases overall morbidity and mortality due to ulcers. If the patient is willing to try to stop smoking and to set a quit date, educational materials, referral to support groups, appropriate use of nicotine gum or patches, and early follow-up to ensure continuing abstinence may be helpful in achieving this goal (see Chapter 124).

Although difficult to quantitate, stress is probably a risk factor for peptic ulcer disease. The use of emotional support and relaxation techniques to assist in stress reduction may be of value, though unproven, for persons who are unable to cope with stressful life events. Anxiolytic and antidepressant drugs are warranted only to treat debilitating anxiety or clinical depression.

### Psychosocial/family approach

As noted above, family support in coping with stress is of uncertain value in reducing symptoms or increasing the rate of ulcer healing. However, the family may play a strong supportive role in ensuring continued abstinence from cigarettes and excessive alcohol use and in ensuring compliance with the prescribed medical regimens.

One point should be repeatedly stressed to the patient: disappearance of ulcer symptoms during pharmacologic therapy (see below) does not imply complete healing of the ulcer. Although symptoms may well abate after 1 week, about 6 weeks of therapy are essential to healing the large majority of ulcers.

### Pharmacologic therapy

The usual dosing and costs of the major agents used in ulcer therapy are found in Table 42-1.

***Antacids.*** Antacids were the mainstay of ulcer therapy for decades before the development of antisecretory drugs. The acid-neutralizing capacity of antacids varies widely depending on the preparation. Their main drawback is the requirement for frequent use (e.g., 1 and 3 hours after meals and at bedtime), which may lead to poor compliance. Most preparations contain magnesium hydroxide, which tends to induce diarrhea; aluminum hydroxide, which tends to constipate; or both compounds. With the exception of these side effects and the potential for

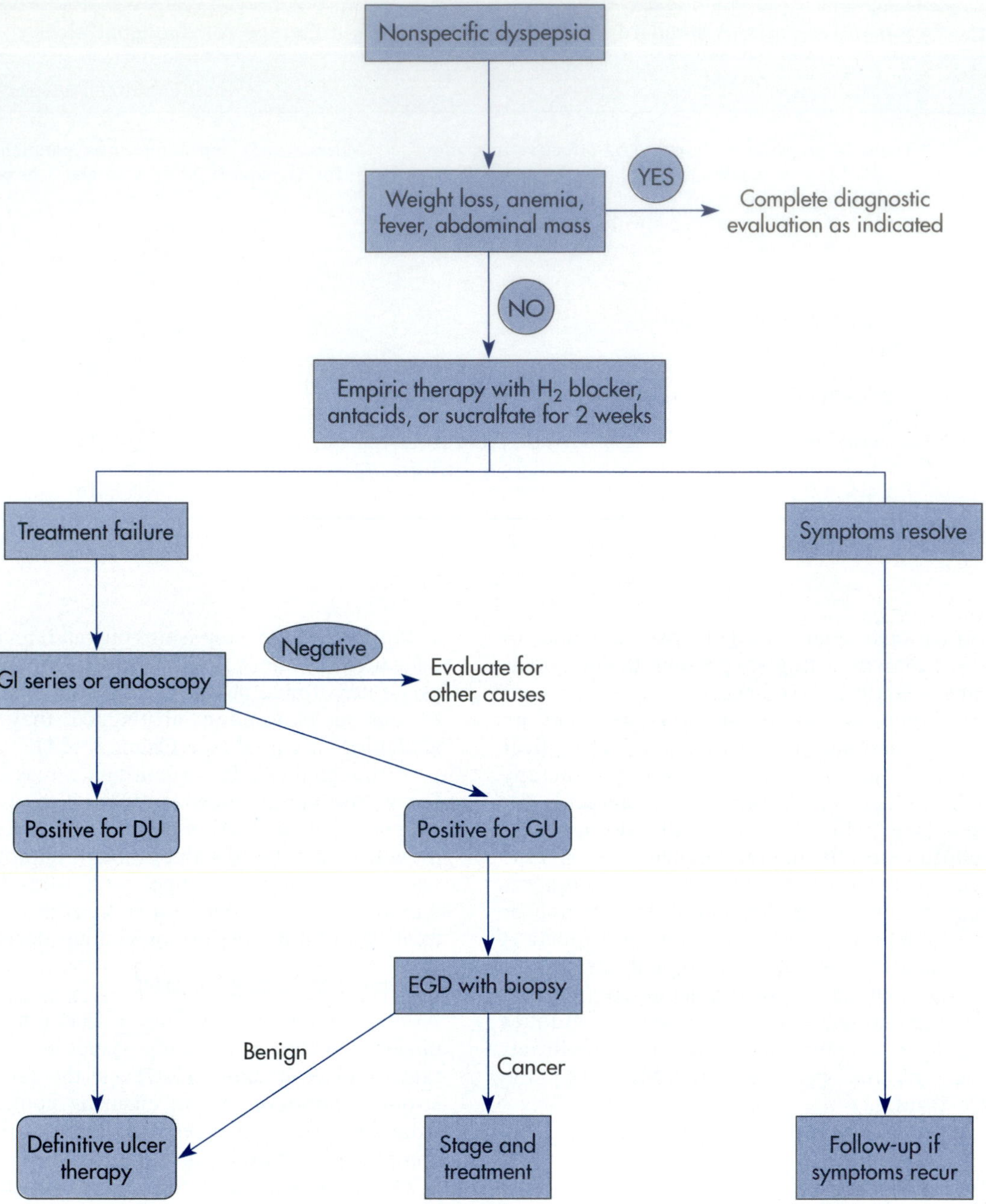


**Fig. 42-5.** Suggested approach to the empiric therapy of nonulcer dyspepsia.

aluminum and magnesium toxicity in the setting of renal failure, antacids are well tolerated.

Calcium-containing antacids should be avoided, due to the rebound in acid secretion induced by calcium products and the risk of hypercalcemia and resultant renal injury. The addition of simethicone has no proven benefit in symptom reduction. Even though their over-the-counter availability increases access to their use, some insurance plans may not reimburse patients for nonprescription drugs such as antacids.

***$H_2$ receptor antagonists.*** $H_2$ receptors involved in gastric acid secretion are blocked by specific antagonists, which reduce basal and food-stimulated acid secretion. They facilitate healing and prevent recurrences of both gastric and duodenal ulcers. There are no important differences in clinical efficacy among the four currently available $H_2$ blockers (cimetidine, ranitidine, famotidine, and nizatidine), with over 80% of ulcers healed after 6 to 8 weeks of therapy.

$H_2$ blockers are very well tolerated. Central nervous system symptoms, especially headache and confusion, are uncommon and seen most often in persons with hepatic or renal dysfunction. Due to inhibition of the hepatic cytochrome P-450 system, cimetidine may lead to elevated levels of concurrently administered drugs that are metabo-

**Managed Care Guide**
**Endoscopy in the evaluation of dyspepsia**

1. Reserving the use of diagnostic esophagogastroduodenoscopy for those patients with symptoms despite 6 to 8 weeks of therapy provides a strategy for cost reduction while maintaining prudent patient care.
2. Those patients who have no response to therapy after 7 to 10 days, those who develop complications of peptic disease, those who show signs of a severe systemic illness, and those with symptom recurrence should require diagnostic evaluation earlier in their course of illness.
3. Adoption of this recommendation must be modified in the light of each patient's clinical presentation, including patients at high risk or with multisystem problems.

From the Clinical Practice Guidelines, Clinical Efficacy Assessment Project (CEAP) of the American College of Physicians, 1994

lized by these enzymes, notably warfarin, theophylline, and phenytoin, with resultant toxicity. These interactions occur less often with the other $H_2$ blockers.

***Proton pump inhibitors.*** Substituted benzimidazoles, of which the prototype is omeprazole, are potent inhibitors of parietal cell hydrogen-potassium adenosine triphosphatase (ATPase), the proton pump mediating secretion of hydrogen ions. In single daily doses of 20 mg, omeprazole is slightly more effective than $H_2$ blockers in producing duodenal ulcer healing but is more expensive (see Table 42-1). Therefore its use in ulcer disease should be reserved for special circumstances, such as in refractory ulcers or in Zollinger-Ellison syndrome, in which cases higher than customary dosages may be required (e.g., 40 mg per day in the former and 60 to 80 mg per day in the latter). Omeprazole is not yet approved for gastric ulcer healing, nor is it approved for chronic maintenance therapy.

***Sucralfate.*** Sucralfate, the aluminum hydroxide salt of sucrose modified by sulfate groups, promotes ulcer healing by an uncertain mechanism, possibly by forming a viscous, acid-resistant gel over the ulcer. For duodenal ulcer a dosage of 1 g four times a day or 2 g twice a day is effective. Sucralfate is probably also effective for therapy of gastric ulcer, although it is not approved for this use by the FDA.

Sucralfate is not appreciably absorbed and therefore has no systemic effects. However, it may be bound by either food or antacids and itself may bind other drugs (e.g., digoxin, ciprofloxacin, phenytoin), reducing their absorption if administered at the same time as the other drug. It is also a large pill and may be more difficult for some patients to swallow.

***Antimicrobial agents.*** A number of regimens employing combinations of antibiotic agents have been tested for their ability to eradicate *H. pylori,* to enhance ulcer healing rates, and most important to reduce ulcer recurrences. We favor their use in patients with duodenal and gastric ulcer as opposed to maintenance therapy with $H_2$ blockers, since the former is much cheaper (Table 42-2). Most regimens employ bismuth subsalicylate, metronidazole, and either tetracycline or amoxicillin, in combination with an $H_2$ receptor antagonist such as ranitidine, for about 2 weeks of total therapy.

Graham and associates reported success using a regimen including ranitidine 300 mg daily, tetracycline 500 mg four times a day, metronidazole 250 mg three times a day, and bismuth subsalicylate 262 mg five or eight times a day for 2 weeks. Duodenal ulcer patients treated with the antibiotic plus $H_2$ blocker regimen had an ulcer recurrence

**Table 42-2.** Comparative costs of pharmacologic regimens used to prevent duodenal ulcer recurrence

| Agent | Dosage | Cost of prophylactic regimen in first year |
|---|---|---|
| **Combination therapy for *H. pylori* eradication** | | |
| Tetracycline | 500 mg qid × 2 weeks | $2.80 |
| Metronidazole | 500 mg tid × 2 weeks | $1.68 |
| Bismuth subsalicylate | 525 mg qid × 2 weeks | $11.20 |
| Ranitidine | 300 mg/d × 2 weeks | $38.36 |
| TOTAL COST | | $54.04 |
| **$H_2$ Antagonists** | | |
| Cimetidine | 400 mg qhs × 1 year | $514.65 |
| Ranitidine | 150 mg qhs × 1 year | $580.35 |
| Famotidine | 20 mg qhs × 1 year | $525.60 |
| Nizatidine | 150 mg qhs × 1 year | $507.35 |
| **Sucralfate** | 1 g bid × 1 year | $474.50 |
| **Antacids** | Wide variation depending on preparation; usually given bid | Varies depending on preparation; cost for Mylanta II 30 ml bid: $347.48 |

rate of 12%, compared to a 95% recurrence rate among those given $H_2$ blockers alone (see Fig. 42-3). Hentschel and associates used ranitidine 300 mg daily, amoxicillin 750 mg three times a day, plus metronidazole 500 mg three times a day for 12 days, with similarly excellent results. The predominant side effect observed among antibiotic-treated subjects has been diarrhea, although dyspepsia and rash may also occur. Several other regimens have been evaluated, including omeprazole plus either amoxicillin or clarithromycin. As shown in Table 42-2, $H_2$ receptor antagonists, sucralfate, and low-dosage antacid can also prevent duodenal ulcer relapses, but these regimens given continuously are relatively expensive.

*Misoprostol.* Analogues of E-type prostaglandins reduce gastric acid secretion by decreasing cyclic adenosine monophosphate production in parietal cells. Although their efficacy in healing ulcers is similar to that of $H_2$ blockers, their use may lead to diarrhea and premature labor. The only prostaglandin commercially available currently is misoprostol, which is approved in a dosage of 200 μg four times a day for prevention of NSAID-induced gastric ulcers in patients at high risk and not for acute ulcer healing.

Reduction in dosage or, ideally, elimination of drugs inhibiting prostaglandin synthesis, namely aspirin and NSAIDs, is advised, especially for gastric ulcer patients. Use of nonacetylated salicylates such as salsalate and choline magnesium trisalicylate as antiinflammatory agents appears to be associated with a low risk of ulcer development. Also, use of an alternative analgesic such as acetaminophen may be considered, if appropriate. When these options are not possible and an NSAID must be given, it should be used in the lowest possible dosage and misoprostol cotherapy should be considered, especially if the patient has a prior ulcer history.

*Anticholinergics.* Anticholinergic agents, such as atropine and propantheline, reduce basal acid and pepsin secretion by blocking muscarinic receptors in the stomach, but they also nonspecifically block muscarinic receptors elsewhere, producing drowsiness, blurred vision, and urinary retention. They have no role in primary therapy for ulcer disease.

## Special cases

Special considerations should be made for patients during *pregnancy.* If diagnostic confirmation of ulcer disease is required, endoscopic procedures are preferred to a radiographic approach based on concern for the safety of the fetus. Given similar theoretical concerns for potential fetal injury, ulcer therapy during pregnancy should employ nonabsorbed medications, (e.g. antacids, sucralfate) rather than systemically absorbed agents.

For persons receiving *multiple drug regimens* the potential for drug interactions, especially with certain $H_2$ blockers, should be considered. Cimetidine, the prototypical agent of this class, acts to increase serum concentrations of a wide variety of drugs, including warfarin, theophylline, phenytoin, carbamazepine, lidocaine, quinidine, and procainamide. Newer $H_2$ blockers, such as famotidine and nizatidine, appear to have little or no drug interaction potential.

Reduced dosages of $H_2$ blockers should be used in the *elderly* and in persons with *renal insufficiency.* The potential of these agents for causing altered mental status in older persons should always be borne in mind.

## Indications for hospitalization and surgery

Almost one third of patients with ulcer disease experience one of the three primary complications of the disorder: bleeding, perforation, and obstruction. Such problems may present before ulcer disease is diagnosed, since about one third of ulcer patients have no symptoms before their first complication. The frequency of complications has not changed dramatically since $H_2$ receptor antagonists become available.

*Hemorrhage.* Bleeding is the most common ulcer complication, affecting about 15% of persons with either gastric or duodenal ulcer. The likelihood of bleeding is not related to duration of disease. The mortality associated with a bleeding episode is 5% to 10% and has not changed in several decades. Use of NSAIDs is an important risk factor for hemorrhage.

Hemorrhage from ulcers usually causes melena, with or without hematemesis. In acute blood loss the hematocrit does not reflect the severity of bleeding. In this circumstance a systolic blood pressure of under 100 mm Hg and a heart rate over 100 beats/min; or an orthostatic rise in pulse and/or fall in blood pressure are more sensitive indicators of hemorrhage.

Actively bleeding ulcers or those with a visibly bleeding vessel may be treated endoscopically using bipolar or multipolar electrodes, heater probe, and laser or by injection of alcohol, epinephrine, or other agents into the base. The most cost-effective endoscopic modality for stopping active bleeding, preventing rebleeding, and for reducing the need for transfusion or surgery has not been established.

Continued bleeding from an ulcer or recurrent major bleeding in the hospital is an indication for surgery. Emergency surgery effectively stops bleeding in 90% to 95% of cases. For patients who do not require surgery for bleeding, an $H_2$ blocker or omeprazole should be given for at least 8 weeks to complete ulcer healing. There is a 30% to 50% chance of rebleeding over the subsequent 5 years after cessation of medical therapy, and therefore maintenance therapy with a nocturnal dose of an $H_2$ receptor antagonist is recommended. Whether eradication of *H. pylori* will reduce rebleeding is uncertain at present, although there is increasing evidence to suggest this.

*Perforation.* Free perforation (rupture of the ulcer into the peritoneal cavity) occurs in about 8% of persons with duodenal ulcer and 3% of those with gastric ulcer. It is more common in the elderly, in men, and in users of NSAIDs. Mortality due to perforation is about 10%. The pain of perforation is usually sudden, severe, and constant. Marked abdominal tenderness, boardlike rigidity, hypotension, and tachycardia usually occur. Upright abdominal films or chest films indicate free intraperitoneal air in about 75% of cases. A duodenal ulcer may also perforate into the lesser sac, causing back pain rather than peritoneal signs. Penetration of the ulcer into a solid organ such as the pancreas may occur, as may fistulization from the duodenum to the common bile duct or from the stomach to the duodenum or colon.

Emergency laparotomy is the preferred treatment for perforation, with closure of the perforation using a portion of omentum and postoperative administration of broad-spectrum antibiotics. Occasionally vagotomy is performed for perforated duodenal ulcer during the procedure. In gastric ulcer resection or biopsy is sometimes performed to exclude cancer, depending on the appearance of the ulcer, the condition of the patient, and the time elapsed since perforation. $H_2$ receptor antagonists or omeprazole should always be prescribed subsequently for at least 8 weeks to facilitate healing, followed by nocturnal $H_2$ blockers for maintenance therapy, unless vagotomy or other acid-reducing procedure has been performed. The effect of *H. pylori* eradication in patients with perforated ulcer is unclear.

***Obstruction.*** Gastric outlet obstruction occurs in almost 5% of ulcer patients. It is more common in pyloric channel ulcers. Mortality from obstructive complications is 7% to 26%, depending on age of the patient and presence of associated diseases. Symptoms of obstruction include nausea, vomiting, epigastric fullness, early satiety, weight loss, and epigastric pain. The physical examination may show signs of volume depletion and reveal a succussion splash. The saline load test may be performed to aid diagnosis. The finding of more than 400 ml of gastric fluid 30 minutes after instilling 750 ml of isotonic saline into an empty stomach strongly supports the diagnosis. Therapy of gastric outlet obstruction has three goals: decompression, replacement of lost fluid and electrolytes, and nutritional support. The first goal is accomplished by continued nasogastric suction for 72 hours, the second by administration of intravenous normal saline with 10 to 20 mEq of potassium per liter, and the third by intravenous calories. Intravenous $H_2$ blocker therapy is also employed. Half of the patients with obstruction improve with such medical management. Failure of the obstruction to resolve in 3 to 7 days indicates surgery may be needed. However, endoscopic balloon dilatation together with $H_2$ blockers is an alternative to surgical intervention, although the long-term outcome following combined endoscopic and medical therapy is not clear at present, nor is the role of *H. pylori* eradication.

### Primary care management vs. referral

Primary care practitioners should be capable of diagnosing and managing uncomplicated ulcer disease. If endoscopy with or without biopsy is required for diagnosis or if malignancy is a consideration, a gastroenterologist should be consulted. If active gastrointestinal bleeding occurs, consult an endoscopist immediately; surgical staff should be alerted. In the case of suspected obstruction, a GI consultant should be asked to assist with patient diagnosis and management, and a surgeon should be advised that assistance may be needed. If perforation of an ulcer occurs, a surgeon should be consulted at once.

## BIBLIOGRAPHY


Cryer B, Feldman M: Smoking and peptic ulcer disease: mechanisms of gastroduodenal mucosal injury in humans, *J Smoking Related Disorders* 5:9, 1994.

Feldman M, Burton ME: Histamine$_2$-receptor antagonists: standard therapy for acid-peptic diseases, *N Engl J Med* 323:1672 (Part I); 323:1749 (Part II), 1990.

Goldschmiedt M, Peterson WL: The role of *Helicobacter pylori* in peptic ulcer disease, *Semin Gastrointest Dis* 4(1):13, 1993.

Graham DY et al: Effect of treatment of *Helicobacter pylori* infection on the long-term recurrence of gastric or duodenal ulcer, *Ann Intern Med* 116:705, 1992.

Graham DY et al: Treatment of *Helicobacter pylori* reduces the rate of rebleeding in peptic ulcer disease, *Scand J Gastroenterol* 28:939, 1993.

Hentschel E et al: Effect of ranitidine and amoxicillin plus metronidazole on the eradication of *Helicobacter pylori* and the recurrence of duodenal ulcer, *N Engl J Med* 328:308, 1993.

Kurata JH: Epidemiology: peptic ulcer risk factors, *Semin Gastrointest Dis* 4(1):2, 1993.

Maton PN: Omeprazole, *N Engl J Med* 324:965, 1991.

Peterson WL, Lee E, Feldman M: Relationship between *Campylobacter pylori* and gastritis in healthy humans after administration of placebo or indomethacin, *Gastroenterology* 95:1185, 1988.

Seymour NE: Surgical therapy of peptic ulcer disease, *Semin Gastrointest Dis* 4(1):39, 1993.

Soll AH: Gastric, duodenal, and stress ulcer. In Sleisenger MH, Fordtran JS, editors: *Gastrointestinal disease: pathophysiology/diagnosis/management,* ed 5, Philadelphia, 1993, WB Saunders.

Van Dam J, Wolfe MM: The Zollinger-Ellison syndrome, *Semin Gastrointest Dis* 4(1):47-59, 1993.

Walker P, Feldman M: Psychosomatic aspects of peptic ulcer disease: a multifactorial model of stress, *Gastroenterol Int* 5:33, 1992.

Walt RP: Misoprostol for the treatment of peptic ulcer and anti-inflammatory drug-induced gastroduodenal ulceration, *N Engl J Med* 327:1575, 1992.


CHAPTER

# 43 Biliary Tract Disease


**Michael S. Karasik**
**Nezam H. Afdhal**


The major function of the gallbladder is the interprandial storage and concentration of hepatic bile, which consists of cholesterol, bile salts, and phospholipids. Postprandially, fat in the duodenum results in the release of the hormone cholecystokinin, which in turn triggers contraction of the gallbladder with ejection of concentrated gallbladder bile through the cystic duct and then the ampulla of Vater into the duodenum. The gallbladder is lined by simple absorptive columnar mucosa whose major functions are the absorption of water and the secretion of mucin glycoprotein and hydrogen ions. The majority of disorders of the gallbladder relate to an inability to maintain cholesterol solubility, resulting in gallstones and their complications.

## CHOLELITHIASIS

### Epidemiology

Because the greatest risk factor for the development of gallstones is increasing age, the incidence of gallstones is on the rise. In the United States, over 20 million people have gallstones, and approximately 1 million new cases

**Table 43-1.** Pathophysiology of cholesterol gallstone formation in high-risk patients

| High-risk groups | Cholesterol supersaturation of bile | Nucleation | Gallbladder stasis |
|---|---|---|---|
| Female | + | + | + |
| Pregnancy | ++ | + | ++ |
| Ileal disease (i.e., Crohn's disease) | +++ | ? | ? |
| Obesity | +++ | + | + |
| Rapid weight loss | ++ | ++ | ++ |
| Spinal cord injury | + | + | +++ |
| New World Indians (i.e., Pima) | +++ | + | + |
| Diabetes mellitus | + | + | +++ |
| Cholesterol-lowering fibric acid agents: Clofibrate, Gemfibrozil, Bezafibrate | ++ | + | ? |
| Somatostatin-analog: Octreotide | ++ | + | +++ |

are diagnosed annually. According to the National Institutes of Health, nearly 600,000 cholecystectomies were performed in 1991, with an estimated health care cost of over $5 billion. Although gallstones can be classified into cholesterol stones and pigmented stones, each with distinct mechanisms of pathogenesis, the vast majority (>75%) of gallstones in Western countries are primarily composed of cholesterol.

## Pathogenesis

***Cholesterol gallstones.*** Three simultaneous defects are necessary for cholesterol gallstone formation: (1) secretion of a cholesterol-supersaturated bile by the liver; (2) nucleation of cholesterol monohydrate crystals from gallbladder bile; and (3) gallbladder stasis with an adequate residence time of crystals within the gallbladder so that they can grow to a size that prevents them from being expelled from the biliary tract. The majority of patients have all three defects, but in certain clinical situations one particular factor may predominate. Table 43-1 lists groups of individuals at increased risk of developing cholesterol gallstones and illustrates which pathophysiologic factors are predominantly responsible.

The identification and recognition of the pathophysiologic mechanism of gallstone formation in high-risk groups has led to attempts at prophylaxis. Ursodeoxycholic acid, an orally administered, naturally occurring, hydrophilic bile acid, completely prevented gallstone formation in a group of obese patients rapidly undergoing weight loss (>20 kg/16 weeks); in comparison, there was an incidence of 25% in similar patients receiving placebo. Studies of antinucleating agents such as nonsteroidal antiinflammatory drugs (NSAIDs) to prevent mucin hypersecretion and promotility agents such as cholecystokinin in patients receiving total parenteral nutrition (TPN) are ongoing; these drugs have great potential.

***Pigmented stones.*** Pigmented stones make up approximately 20% to 25% of cases of cholelithiasis in Western industrialized nations. Pigmented stones are more common in the elderly, in patients after cholecystectomy, and in those who reside in the Orient. Although the two types of pigment stones, brown and black, are primarily composed of calcium bilirubinate, they occur in very different clinical settings. Black stones are formed in the gallbladder and are more common in patients with chronic hemolysis, cirrhosis, or alcoholism and in those receiving TPN. Black stones have an irregular surface, are usually small and hard, and consist of fully cross-linked calcium bilirubinate. Brown stones are usually formed within the bile ducts; consist of calcium bilirubinate, mucin, and cholesterol; and are often soft and friable. Brown stones are more common in the Orient, particularly in patients with cholangiohepatitis, a condition associated with infection by *Clonorchis sinensis,* a liver fluke (Fig. 43-1). In the United States, brown stones usually occur in patients

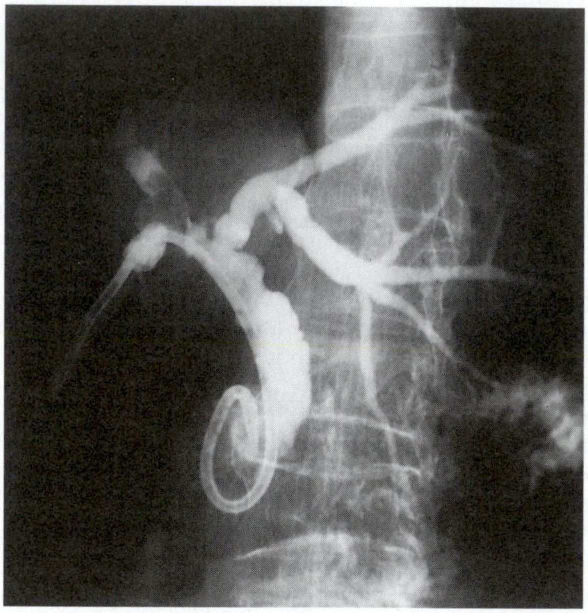

**Fig. 43-1.** A percutaneous transhepatic cholangiogram has been performed after the placement of a stent across a large obstructing stone. The stone is seen in the right hepatic duct, obstructing the entire right hepatic system in this Chinese immigrant with Oriental cholangiohepatitis.

A

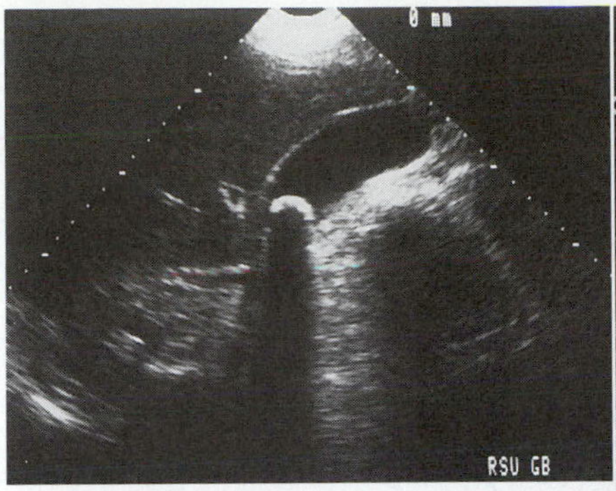


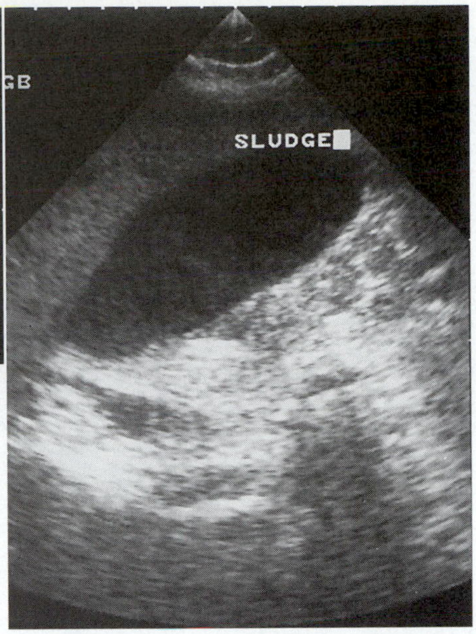


B

**Fig. 43-2.** **A,** An ultrasound demonstration of the gallbladder, longitudinal section. A gallstone is visualized. Notice the characteristic shadowing from the base of the stone. **B,** Longitudinal ultrasound scan demonstrating sludge within the gallbladder. Unlike stones, sludge casts no acoustic shadow.

after cholecystectomy in which bile may be chronically infected with microorganisms that are able to deconjugate bilirubin, such as *Escherichia coli.*

***Biliary sludge.*** Biliary sludge is most often identified by ultrasound examination of the gallbladder as echogenic material that layers out in the dependent portion of the gallbladder and is composed of a mixture of mucin, cholesterol crystals, and calcium bilirubinate granules (Fig. 43-2). Previously assumed to be a completely benign, incidental finding usually associated with conditions of impaired gallbladder emptying (i.e., TPN, pregnancy), it is now recognized that 30% of patients with sludge develop gallstones and that biliary sludge can result in complications of gallstone disease, such as pancreatitis and cholangitis. In a study of 23 patients on TPN, sludge developed in 30% by 3 weeks, in 50% by 4 weeks, and in 100% after more than 6 weeks. Stones formed in almost half (43%) of patients who developed sludge. Half of these patients developed complications necessitating cholecystectomy after a mean of 43 days.

The natural history of biliary sludge formed during pregnancy has also been evaluated. Although biliary sludge formed during pregnancy disappears in the majority (60%) of patients after delivery, postpartum ultrasound examinations have demonstrated the persistence of sludge in 20% of patients and the formation of gallstones in the remaining 20%. Biliary sludge is sometimes present in patients with idiopathic pancreatitis, and cholecystectomy in these individuals may be associated with a significant reduction in the incidence of recurrent acute pancreatitis. Therefore biliary sludge should be considered part of the clinically relevant spectrum of gallstone disease.

## Natural history of gallstones

Gallstones are usually asymptomatic within the gallbladder. However, they may transiently obstruct the cystic duct, producing "biliary colic," or with more significant obstruction produce cholecystitis and its complications. Stones small enough to pass into the common bile duct may then obstruct there. The most common site of obstruction in these cases is at the ampulla; obstruction at this point may be associated with the development of cholangitis or gallstone pancreatitis. Since none of the treatments for any of these conditions is without risk, a knowledge of their natural history and the treatment options is essential (Fig. 43-3).

***Asymptomatic gallstones.*** Even as recently as a decade ago, it was fairly common practice in many medical centers to perform a cholecystectomy when gallstones were found, regardless of whether the patient had symptomatic cholelithiasis. This was especially true for patients with diabetes, a condition felt to increase the risk of complications of cholecystitis and cholangitis.

In the past 10 years, however, a thorough evaluation of the natural history of asymptomatic gallstones has altered this approach. It is now known that with rare exceptions cholecystectomy is not required for the majority of patients with asymptomatic cholelithiasis. Patients with asymptomatic gallbladder stones have up to a 2% to 3% risk of developing biliary pain each year for the first 10 years after the diagnosis of stones. After 10 years the risk decreases to less than 1% annually. Postmortem studies have demonstrated that of known gallstone patients, the cause of death is related to gallstone disease in fewer than 3%. In general, therefore, surgical treatment for gallstones is recommended only for patients with symptomatic disease.

***Symptomatic gallstones.*** In patients whose conditions become symptomatic, the most common presentation is that of biliary colic. Biliary colic is not colicky in nature. It is usually steady, intense, and located in the right upper quadrant, although the pain may be referred to the right shoulder or scapular region, the midepigastrium, or elsewhere in the chest or abdomen. Peptic symptoms, belching, bloating, fatty food intolerance, and chronic pain should not be confused with biliary colic. There are no associated laboratory abnormalities. In 60% of cases the acute attack resolves spontaneously. Recurrent attacks of pain may occur in up to 70% of patients weeks to years after the initial episode. Biliary complications, such as

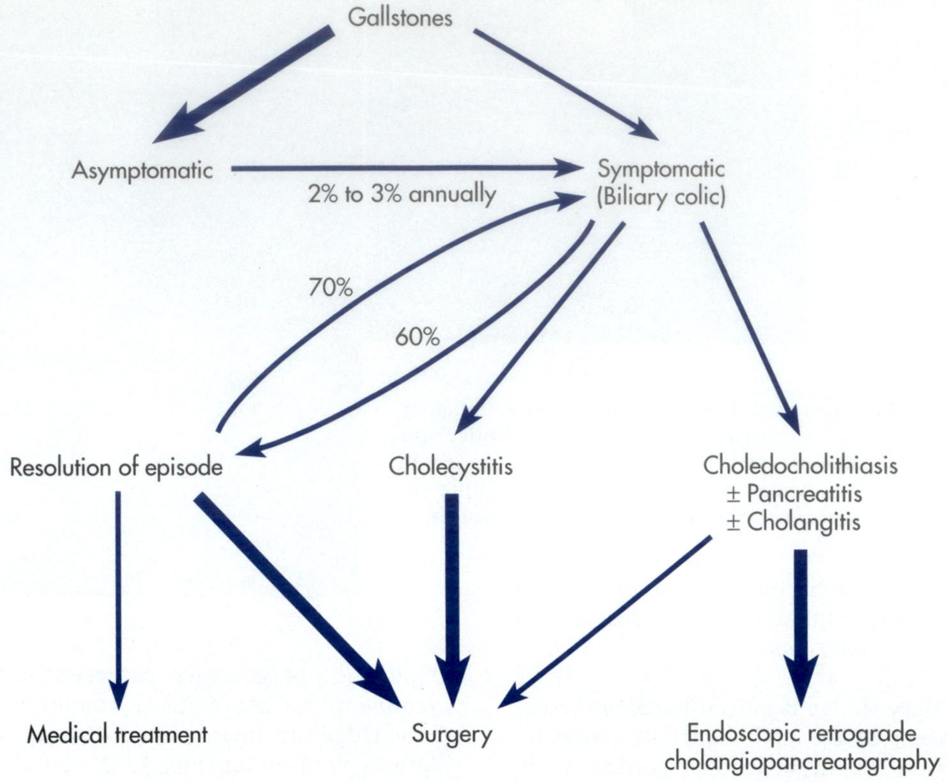


**Fig. 43-3.** The natural history and management of gallstones.

acute cholecystitis, cholangitis, and gallstone pancreatitis, occur in 10% to 20% of patients with symptomatic gallstones. For these reasons, treatment, usually cholecystectomy, is often advised for patients with symptomatic gallstones.

## Differential diagnosis

Although pain in the right upper quadrant should always raise suspicion for gallstone-related disease, it is by no means pathognomonic for these conditions. Acute hepatitis is commonly associated with pain in this location. Pain in this case results from acute hepatic inflammation stretching the liver capsule. The liver edge is often tender. Characteristically, transaminase levels in viral or toxin-mediated hepatitis are elevated at least 5 to 10 times normal compared with less than 2 times normal in cholecystitis and normal values with biliary colic. However, using the symptom and laboratory complex to differentiate between alcoholic hepatitis and acute cholecystitis can sometimes be more difficult. Although alcoholic hepatitis is usually associated with characteristic hepatic enzyme elevations, both conditions generally produce low levels of transaminases, and both may be associated with fever and leukocytosis. Taking a thorough history is essential. Although classically producing mid-epigastric pain, peptic ulcer disease may also present with pain in the right upper quadrant. Unlike pain of biliary origin, however, peptic symptoms often improve or resolve with antacid therapy. Rarely, appendicitis, colitis, or terminal ileitis may also present with right upper quadrant pain.

Atypical presentations of biliary tract disease may occur as well. Pain may rarely occur in the right lower quadrant, left upper quadrant, or even the chest, where it may occasionally be confused with angina pectoris.

## Management

In general, treatment of gallstone disease is directed at alleviating symptoms and preventing complications. New advances in medical and surgical options for symptomatic gallstone disease have occurred in the past decade. Whereas surgery can permanently resolve disease associated with gallbladder stones of any size, number, and makeup, medical therapy can be used only in specific situations and there is a significant risk of recurrence after discontinuation of therapy. Still, medical therapy is occasionally recommended in certain patients, particularly those with extremely high surgical risk.

***Surgical management.*** Surgery has historically been the mainstay of treatment for symptomatic gallstone disease. Cholecystectomy is generally a very safe procedure with an overall mortality rate of 0.1% to 0.3%. It relieves the characteristic biliary type of pain in approximately 90% of patients and prevents future recurrences. In addition, cholecystectomy is also responsible for the incidental discovery and removal of early gallbladder cancers.

Before 1987, cholecystectomy was performed only as an open procedure through one of several possible laparotomy incisions. Based on a review of 12 studies by Ransahoff and Gracie, the operative mortality rates for elective open cholecystectomy in men are estimated at

**Table 43-2.** Factors favoring laparoscopic cholecystectomy over open cholecystectomy

| Factors | Laparoscopic | Open |
|---|---|---|
| Duration of hospital stay | 1 day | 4-5 days |
| Time to convalescence | 7-14 days | 20-40 days |
| Postoperative pain | Minimal | Significant through convalescence |
| Postoperative ileus | Uncommon | Common |
| Cosmetic result | Several small scars (<2 cm) | Laparotomy scar (>8 cm) |
| Relative cost to patient | Significantly reduced by shorter hospital stay and earlier return to work | Significantly more expensive |

0.11% for those under age 30, 0.24% for those aged 31 to 40, 0.54% for those aged 41 to 50, 1.22% for those aged 51 to 60, 2.73% for those aged 61 to 70, 6.15% for those aged 71 to 80, and 13.84% for those aged 81 to 90. Women are apparently more tolerant of this operation; mortality rates in women are approximately half those in men at all age groups. Elective ("late") surgery, performed 6 to 8 weeks after an episode of biliary colic or uncomplicated acute cholecystitis, had formerly been preferred over earlier surgery because it had been felt that actively inflamed tissues complicated surgery and increased the risk of secondary complications. A number of prospective randomized controlled trials, however, have demonstrated early surgery to be associated with lower morbidity and mortality rates.

Although open cholecystectomy is a relatively safe and simple operation, laparoscopic cholecystectomy, first performed in 1987, has superceded the open procedure in popularity over the past few years. In the United States, 75% of all cholecystectomies are being performed laparoscopically. When performed by a surgeon experienced with the technique, laparoscopic cholecystectomy offers most patients a number of advantages over an open procedure without producing any apparent increase in the morbidity or mortality rates (Table 43-2). The exact morbidity rates are as yet unclear because the procedure is relatively new and the experience of surgeons performing it is variable. One disadvantage includes a limited ability to evaluate the common bile duct for stones, and early data have demonstrated a slightly increased incidence of biliary duct injuries compared with those in conventional cholecystectomy.

Conversion from a laparoscopic to an open approach is necessary in approximately 5% of cases because of difficulty in identifying anatomy, excessive bleeding, or complications during the operation. Open cholecystectomy is still the preferred route in patients with peritonitis, sepsis, severe acute pancreatitis, and end-stage cirrhosis.

Initially it was felt that laparoscopic cholecystectomy would reduce the cost of gallstone disease to both the patient and society. A recent study, however, has demonstrated that although each patient's unit cost has decreased, annual total cholecystectomy costs are rising because of an increase in the number of laparoscopic operations being performed.

**Postcholecystectomy syndrome.** After cholecystectomy, fewer than 5% of patients have recurrent or persistent abdominal pain months to years later. However, persistence or early recurrence of pain may imply that the initial diagnosis of gallbladder-related pathology causing the pain was incorrect. Biliary sources of postcholecystectomy pain include retained common bile duct stones, postsurgical bile duct strictures, and sphincter of Oddi dysfunction.

Albeit controversial, sphincter of Oddi dysfunction after cholecystectomy appears to be more common in women and may result in typical biliary pain months to years after surgery. Elevated pressures (>40 mm Hg) within the sphincter of Oddi have been recorded manometrically and are believed to result in intermittant biliary obstruction at the level of the sphincter of Oddi. In addition to their pain, affected patients may demonstrate the following findings: (1) a dilated common bile duct; (2) delayed emptying (>45 minutes) of contrast material from the duct after endoscopic retrograde cholangiography; and (3) hepatic enzyme elevations (usually low grade), especially during "attacks" of pain. It is unclear how or why cholecystectomy might affect sphincter of Oddi function; however, approximately 95% of patients with at least two of the three listed findings appear to respond to sphincterotomy with resolution of biliary type pain.

***Medical management.*** The nonsurgical approaches to gallstone disease are bile acid dissolution therapy and fragmentation of stones with extracorporeal shock-wave lithotripsy (ESWL). These approaches offer the benefit of potentially avoiding surgery in patients at high risk of significant morbidity and mortality from cholecystectomy. However, nonsurgical measures have a number of important disadvantages, the most notable being extremely high recurrence rates after discontinuation of therapy. At present, fewer than 10% of patients with symptomatic gallstones should be considered suitable for nonsurgical therapy of gallstones.

**Bile acid dissolution therapy.** Oral dissolution therapy should be considered for patients with suspected cholesterol gallstones and high surgical risk. Oral dissolution agents include ursodeoxycholic acid (UDCA) and chenodeoxycholic acid (CDCA). Although both work by reducing cholesterol secretion into bile and enhancing cholesterol solubilization, UDCA also inhibits cholesterol crystal nucleation. However, these agents have no effect on calcium bilirubinate stones. Thus candidates for therapy should have noncalcified (cholesterol) gallstones. In addition, an oral cholecystogram should reveal a functioning gallbladder, demonstrating the ability of these agents to reach the gallbladder lumen. Treatment with UDCA is more expensive than that with CDCA; however, CDCA may be associated with diarrhea and hepatotoxicity in a significant number of patients. Combination therapy with both agents reduces the cost and diminishes side effects without substantially affecting dissolution rates. The ideal patient for oral dissolution is not obese and has small (<1 cm), floating stones. Success rates in such patients are as high as 70% total dissolution at 1 year. Biliary colic is alleviated in the majority of patients, even those who do not have complete dissolution. Gallstone recurrence is about 10% per year over the first 5 years, and the role of maintenance therapy is unclear. Gallstones, when they recur, are often small and once again symptomatic.

**Contact dissolution.** Direct instillation into the gallbladder of powerful cholesterol-solubilizing solvents, such as methyltertbutyl ether (MTBE) and ethyl propionate (EP), has been associated with almost 100% dissolution of cholesterol gallstones. The major drawbacks of this therapy are the need to directly catheterize the gallbladder either by a radiologically placed percutaneous catheter or a nasogallbladder tube placed during endoscopic retrograde cholangiopancreatography (ERCP). MTBE is more toxic and volatile than EP and can cause damage to the duodenal mucosa with drowsiness and hemolysis when systemically absorbed. The use of automated pump systems have decreased operator and patient contact with the solvents, have decreased spillage of solvent out of the gallbladder, and can result in complete dissolution of large stones in hours. If delivery systems can be further perfected, this therapy may have benefit in critically ill patients unable to withstand surgery.

**Extracorporeal shock wave lithotripsy.** ESWL is similar to that used for fragmentation of renal calculi. Shock waves are produced by lithotriptors and delivered to the gallbladder using ultrasonic guidance. Oral bile acid therapy is begun simultaneously, both because the resulting stone fragments are more amenable to dissolution therapy and because such therapy promotes bile acid flow for enhanced clearance of stone fragments. ESWL has had variable success, depending on the aggressiveness of the operator and the pain threshold of the patient. Experience in the United States demonstrated 50% stone clearance as compared with greater than 90% from West Germany. Successful lithotripsy is more likely to occur when stones are radiolucent, solitary, and <2 cm in size. Normal gallbladder motility is required for fragment passage. Although the addition of ESWL to dissolution therapy for large stones is theoretically better than either alone, the ESWL has its risk profile. Through the process of fragmentation, larger stones become smaller and may more easily pass into the cystic and common bile ducts, where they may cause acute obstruction. In the 6 months after ESWL, at least one study demonstrated severe biliary pain in 1.5%, acute cholecystititis in 1.0%, and acute pancreatitis in 1.5% of patients. Another problem is the high costs of lithotriptors that have made access prohibitive for many centers. Combined with its variable success rates and side-effect profile, ESWL has not gained the acceptance it was initially expected to achieve.

### Complications

***Acute cholecystitis.*** Acute inflammation of the gallbladder and adjacent peritoneum usually occurs as a result of a stone impaction within the cystic duct. Affected individuals have a history of biliary colic. The pain associated with cholecystitis is similar in location to colic but is usually more severe and persistent, lasting at least 6 hours. In the absence of complications such as gangrene or perforation, fevers are usually low grade and rigors uncommon. The right upper quadrant is very tender, and localized rebound may be present. On examination the patient cannot take a deep breath while the physician's hand is palpating the right upper quadrant because of increased pain as the gallbladder descends to touch the hand (Murphy's sign). Bilirubin levels may be elevated, but jaundice is rare. Transaminase levels are rarely greater than 3 times normal. Leukocytosis with band forms is common. Radiologic imaging is recommended to confirm the diagnosis and to rule out complications such as gallbladder perforation or gangrenous cholecystitis. Ultrasound usually demonstrates stones, gallbladder distention, wall thickening, and localized edema but is often nondiagnostic. Cholescintigraphy, using $^{99m}$Tc-hepatic iminodiacetic acid (HIDA) analogues, is more sensitive than ultrasound for uncomplicated cholecystitis, characteristically demonstrating nonvisualization of the gallbladder in patients with acute cholecystitis. In most cases, however, ultrasound is usually recommended before HIDA scanning because of its added sensitivity in evaluating the anatomy adjacent to the gallbladder. Although most patients with acute cholecystitis respond to conservative management, surgery is recommended because of the high recurrence rate and significant incidence of complications. In patients with a prohibitively high acute surgical risk, a drainage tube can be placed by radiologic guidance into the gallbladder (percutaneous cholecystostomy) during the acute period.

Complications of acute cholecystitis include gangrenous cholecystitis, emphysematous cholecystitis, and gallbladder perforation. Although their presentation is usually associated with a higher incidence of fevers, rigors, and peritoneal signs, they may not appear different from uncomplicated cholecystitis and thus may not be suspected before surgery. These complications have a significantly increased incidence of morbidity and mortality that necessitate emergency surgery. Gangrenous cholecystitis implies necrosis of the gallbladder wall. The diagnosis is suggested during cholescintigraphy by visualization of a rim of increased radioactivity around the gallbladder and within the adjacent hepatic parenchyma. Diabetic persons and the elderly appear to be at increased risk of developing emphysematous cholecystitis, a severe form of acute cholecystitis that is associated with gas-forming organisms, particularly *Clostridium perfringens*. Emphysematous cholecystitis is suggested by the findings of gas bubbles within the gallbladder wall or lumen on plain film and by irregular, indistinct shadowing from the gallbladder on ultrasound (Fig. 43-4). It has been suggested that all diabetic persons with symptoms of acute cholecystitis should have a plain film of the abdomen to search for emphysema. Gangrenous and emphysematous cholecystitis greatly increase the risk of gallbladder perforation.

Other complications of calculous cholecystitis include gallstone ileus, which is gallstone obstruction of the distal small bowel that usually occurs as a result of erosion of a gallstone through the gallbladder wall into the duodenal bulb. The most common site of bowel obstruction is the

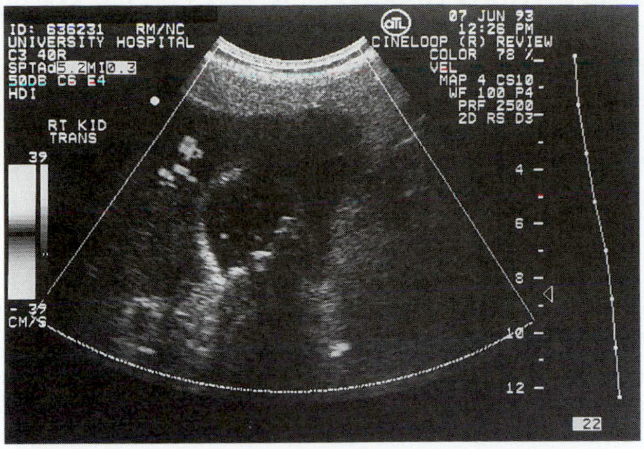


**Fig. 43-4.** Ultrasound demonstration of air within the lumen of the gallbladder and adjacent hepatic parenchyma is seen in this diabetic patient with emphysematous cholecystitis.

ileocecal valve. Bouveret's syndrome occurs when the stone obstructs the duodenal bulb, producing gastric outlet obstruction. Another rare complication of cholecystitis is Mirizzi's syndrome, in which bile duct obstruction occurs secondary to stone impaction within the cystic duct when the impacted stone and its secondary inflammatory mass impinge on the lumen of the adjacent bile duct.

***Choledocholithiasis.*** Stones within the bile duct usually originate in the gallbladder but may arise de novo (see section on brown pigment stones). Up to 15% of patients with cholelithiasis develop choledocholithiasis. Although it is occasionally asymptomatic, the characteristic presentation is jaundice and cholestatic biochemical serum studies. Bilirubin levels rise in proportion to the degree of obstruction, are primarily the direct (conjugated) form, and may be elevated 20 to 30 times normal values. Alkaline phosphatase levels are usually 3 to 6 times normal but may be only mildly elevated. In contrast to the generally benign course in most patients with incidentally found gallbladder stones, 25% to 50% of patients with bile duct stones may develop serious complications of obstruction, (i.e., cholangitis and gallstone pancreatitis); therefore bile duct stones should always be removed.

Radiologic identification of biliary tract stones is not as sensitive as for gallstones. Ultrasound examinations demonstrate stones within the bile duct in 20% of cases but have an 80% sensitivity for demonstrating bile duct dilatation, a marker for extrahepatic obstruction. Bile duct dilatation occurs in virtually all cases of chronic obstruction (i.e., malignancy) but may take up to 2 weeks to develop in some patients with acute obstruction from stones. Thus a patient with acute obstruction who initially had nondilated ducts on ultrasound, may benefit from repeating the examination 2 weeks later. Cholangiography is the most sensitive test for identification of dilatation, stones, and other causes of obstruction. Cholangiography can be performed by the gastroenterologist (ERCP), the radiologist (percutaneous transhepatic cholangiography [PTC]), or the surgeon during surgery. Both of the former techniques have very high success rates, can be performed in elective and emergency situations, and can obviate the need for surgery. ERCP is successful in obtaining a cholangiogram in over 90% of cases and is generally preferred by most patients and physicians because it is more comfortable for the patient and allows for therapeutic intervention during the same session.

Endoscopic stone removal is performed by making a small cut in the ampulla, a sphincterotomy, to enlarge this opening to the bile duct. A basket or balloon can then be introduced into the bile duct through the ERCP scope to clear the duct of stones. In the hands of an experienced endoscopist, this procedure has an 85% to 90% success rate, with complications such as pancreatitis, perforation, and bleeding occurring in 2% to 5%. The most common complication, pancreatitis, occurs in approximately 2% of cases and is usually mild.

PTC is successful in demonstrating the bile ducts in over 95% of cases when the intrahepatic ducts are dilated but significantly less when they are not. Stones can be removed by choledocholithotomy, but several weeks are required to form a dilated tract across the liver and into the bile duct through which the stone can be removed or manipulated.

***Cholangitis.*** The biliary tree is normally an open, sterile system that when obstructed behaves as a closed system. Regardless of the cause of obstruction, impaired biliary excretion into the intestine results in jaundice and the spilling of conjugated bilirubin into the urine. When bacteria are introduced into the system, as occurs often with stones and occasionally with malignancy, the resulting closed system behaves like an abscess. In addition to jaundice, the patient develops significant inflammation of the bile duct, often with *abdominal pain,* intermittent *fevers* and rigors, and *jaundice.* These three form the classic symptom triad of cholangitis, referred to as Charcot's triad. Although obstructive cholangitis is frequently referred to as *pus under pressure,* frank pus (suppuration) is not usually seen within the bile duct. The term *suppurative cholangitis,* however, is used to refer to severe cholangitis, regardless of the presence or absence of pus. This condition is an emergency, requiring emergency ductal decompression. Reynold's pentad, which adds hypotension and altered mental status to the signs of Charcot's triad, is considered pathognomonic for suppurative cholangitis. Clinical findings suspicious for suppurative cholangitis include fever >104° F, hypotension, abdominal rebound, leukocytosis >20,000/mm$^3$, and bilirubin >9 mg/dl. A mortality rate of 40% has been associated with suppurative cholangitis as compared with 10% in the less toxic cases.

The intermittent fevers and rigors seen with cholangitis are presumed to result from bacteremia. Although the bile in 90% of affected individuals contains many different microbes, blood cultures are positive in 40% of patients and usually for only one strain of organism. The most common organisms are *Escherichia coli* (60%), *Klebsiella pneumoniae* (30% to 40%), *Bacteroides fragilis* (5% to 10%), and *Enterococcus faecalis* (5% to 10%). Initial antibiotic therapy is usually broad based and empiric to cover these organisms. Antibiotic coverage should also be widened to include *Pseudomonas aeruginosa,* if the patient has recently had an ERCP, since scope contamination by *P. aeruginosa* has been reported. Although all patients should receive antibiotic and intravenous fluids, the mainstay of treatment is biliary decompression. This can be achieved by ERCP with sphincterotomy or stone extraction, by stenting (placing a drainage tube across the site of obstruction via the endoscope), by PTC, or by surgery. Either ERCP or PTC should be used initially. Even when the condition cannot be cured (i.e., by removal of stones), these treatments may allow for long-term palliation of an otherwise moribund patient.

*Gallstone pancreatitis.* Overall, approximately 40% of cases of acute pancreatitis are related to choledocholithiasis. Surgical series have demonstrated stones within the biliary tree in up to 75% of patients during the initial presentation of presumed gallstone pancreatitis but in as few as a third of such patients if evaluated after their pancreatitis has improved. The mechanism of pancreatic injury may be that of elevated pressure within the pancreatic duct as a result of more distal obstruction from stones and secondary inflammation.

The physician should suspect "gallstone" pancreatitis when a patient with acute, often recurrent pancreatitis has a present or past history of gallstones or common bile duct stones, especially when there are no other known risk factors for pancreatitis. Although patients classically complain of epigastric pain radiating to the back with nausea, vomiting, and anorexia, the symptoms and physical findings may be difficult to differentiate from those of acute cholecystitis. In fact, acute cholecystitis occurs concomitantly with gallstone pancreatitis 5% of the time. In light of this statistic, it is recommended that serum amylase levels be measured in all patients with presumed cholecystitis. Elevation of alkaline phosphatase or bilirubin levels at the onset of an attack of pancreatitis is often a clue to gallstone pancreatitis but may also occur secondary to compression of the intrapancreatic portion of the common bile duct as it passes through an inflamed pancreas.

The diagnosis of gallstone pancreatitis is confirmed by cholangiography, usually by ERCP. Until recently, however, the optimal timing for ERCP and possible sphincterotomy was controversial. Two randomized controlled trials have compared early (within 24 to 72 hours of admission) vs. late ERCP with or without papillotomy for pancreatitis presumed secondary to choledocholithiasis. These studies clearly demonstrated a reduction in complications, including biliary sepsis and death, when ERCP was performed early in patients with moderate-to-severe pancreatitis. One of these studies showed a similar effect for mild pancreatitis as well. When performed within 72 hours of admission in patients with severe pancreatitis, early intervention with ERCP also significantly reduced the length of hospitalization.

Based on these results, the present recommendation is ERCP with possible sphincterotomy performed within 48 hours of the onset of moderate to severe pancreatitis presumed secondary to choledocholithiasis. The treatment of mild pancreatitis is primarily one of supportive care. Affected patients require aggressive fluid resuscitation because of sequestration of fluids into the inflamed retroperitoneum and their inability to eat. Conservative management alone in patients with mild pancreatitis is associated with a success rate of approximately 80%.

## ACALCULOUS DISEASES OF THE GALLBLADDER

### Acute acalculous cholecystitis

Overall, approximately 5% to 15% of patients with acute cholecystitis have acalculous disease, but it has been estimated to be as high as 87% and 50%, respectively, in patients with acute cholecystitis in the postoperative period and in children. Most patients are older (>55), and gender does not affect the incidence. This condition is most often seen in the intensive care unit in patients with multiorgan system failure, trauma (especially after major surgery), burns, and sepsis. Although in most patients the pathogenesis is unclear and is likely multifactorial in origin, the process is believed to be one of secondary infection in a functionally obstructed gallbladder. Rarely, primary infections of the gallbladder with *Salmonella* and *Candida* organisms and cytomegalovirus (CMV) may cause this condition in patients with severe immunosuppression.

Regardless of the etiology, however, the clinical scenario is similar to that of acute calculous cholecystitis. Patients may become bacteremic and septic if the condition is not treated promptly. Delays in diagnosis or treatment have led to a high incidence of complications such as gangrene, empyema, and perforation before surgery. The mortality rate has been reported to be at least twice as high in acalculous cholecystitis as in calculous disease because of the high incidence of comorbid conditions and the delay in diagnosis.

The timely diagnosis of acute acalculous cholecystitis requires an awareness of this entity and suspicion on the part of the physician. Laboratory findings are similar to those seen in acute calculous cholecystitis; most patients demonstrate leukocytosis and mild elevations in the alkaline phosphatase, bilirubin, and transaminase levels. HIDA scanning confirms the diagnosis, and ultrasound may detect complications. Optimal treatment is emergency cholecystectomy, but a percutaneous cholecystostomy is alternative therapy in patients with extraordinarily high surgical risks.

### Hyperplastic cholecytoses

These conditions represent abnormalities of the gallbladder wall of unclear etiology. They are usually clinically silent but may be associated with symptoms of cholelithiasis that respond to cholecystectomy. These conditions may be associated with the formation of nodules. When large in size they may present as a fundal "polyp" on gallbladder ultrasound or oral cholecystogram. The most common forms of hyperplastic cholecytoses are cholesterolosis and adenomyomatosis. Gallbladder cholesterolosis, or cholesterosis, is a condition whereby there is deposition of triglycerides and cholesterol within the gallbladder wall. These yellowish deposits lying within a mildly inflamed, reddened background have given rise to the term *strawberry gallbladder.* The deposits may form small polypoid projections that can break off and serve as seeds for gallstone formation. Gallstones are seen in 10% to 15% of patients with cholesterolosis, but this condition is present in a minority of all patients with gallstones. Adenomyomatosis, or adenomyosis, implies hyperplasia of the gallbladder mucosa and muscularis. Gallbladder wall thickening can increase to 3 to 5 times that of normal gallbladders. This condition is associated with intramural diverticula, crypts, or sinus tracts (Rokitansky-Aschoff sinuses) that may be seen on ultrasound of the gallbladder, and it may present as localized, segmental, or diffuse disease. The localized disease may produce a nodule that is sometimes referred to as an *adenomyoma.* The adenomyoma is a pseudotumor and has no potential for neoplasia. The segmental form produces a constricting ring or septum in the fundus or body, and the diffuse form produces generalized thickening of the gallbladder wall. Hyalocalcinosis, also referred to as the *porcelain gallbladder* because of its egg-shell appearance on plain film, ultrasound, or CT scan, has been associated with a 22% chance of developing gallbladder cancer. Prophylactic cholecystectomy is generally recommended in these cases.

### Gallbladder neoplasia

Gallbladder cancer is the fifth most frequent digestive tract cancer. Epidemiologic studies have demonstrated an association between gallbladder cancer and the presence of gallstones. The risk associated with stones larger than 3 cm is estimated to be 9 times that of 1-cm stones. Certain ethnic groups, in particular North American and Mexican Indians, have increased risk over the general population. The risk is also increased in patients with the porcelain gallbladder and when there are anomalous connections between biliary and pancreatic ducts.

Primary gallbladder cancers are usually adenocarcinomas and are felt to arise in adenomatous polyps. Polyp size appears to be an important risk factor for the presence of carcinoma. In a study by Kozuka and associates of gallbladder neoplasia in 1605 gallbladders removed by cholecystectomy, all benign adenomas were <12 mm in diameter, whereas those with carcinomatous foci were >12 mm. Most invasive carcinomas were >30 mm in diameter. The prognosis associated with gallbladder cancer is uniformly poor when the process has extended beyond the gallbladder wall, with 5-year survival rates of less than 5%. Although distant metastasis of the tumors occurs late, aggressive local extension of the disease along the biliary tract and into the liver is seen very early. This, in combination with late diagnosis, accounts for the poor survival. In general, curative surgery occurs only when an adenoma is found incidentally during routine cholecystectomy for other indications. Because of the aggressive nature of this disease, its poor outcome, and the inability to radiologically differentiate early gallbladder cancers arising in a polyp from benign polyps or pseudotumors (as may occur in the hypertrophic cholecystoses), cholecystectomy should be performed when ultrasound or CT scanning demonstrates a focal, irregular thickening of the gallbladder wall or a polyp. Prophylactic cholecystectomy should be considered in patients with porcelain gallbladders and perhaps in young North American Indians with very large gallstones. Chemotherapeutic trials for gallbladder cancer have demonstrated no benefit. The use of external beam radiation therapy and/or local radiotherapy using implantable iridium ($^{192}$Ir) wires for patients with localized disease and pain or jaundice is being evaluated.

## BILIARY TRACT DISEASES

### Primary sclerosing cholangitis

Primary sclerosing cholangitis (PSC), an uncommon autoimmune condition, is primarily seen in young men in association with inflammatory bowel disease (IBD), particularly ulcerative colitis, but has also been associated with a number of other autoimmune syndromes. Although 50% to 75% of patients have ulcerative colitis, the incidence of PSC in patients with IBD is 1% to 4%. The pathology is one of idiopathic fibrosis and inflammation of the extrahepatic or intrahepatic biliary ducts, resulting in stricturing and obstruction within these systems. Depending on the degree of progression of PSC, the condition may be completely asymptomatic and without laboratory abnormalities, have symptomatic and laboratory-demonstrated cholestasis, or have signs and symptoms of end-stage cirrhosis. Although more advanced cases are more likely to demonstrate cholestasis with alkaline phosphatase levels as high as 10 times normal, they may also be only minimally elevated in advanced disease. PSC is the most common cause of elevated alkaline phosphatase levels in patients with IBD. Patients with IBD and elevated levels of alkaline phosphatase should be evaluated for the possibility of PSC. No diagnostic serum studies exist. Diagnosis usually requires cholangiography. Cystic dilatations arising between strictures have given rise to the classic cholangiographic appearance of "beads on a string" (Fig. 43-5). These strictures are usually not amenable to dilatation or

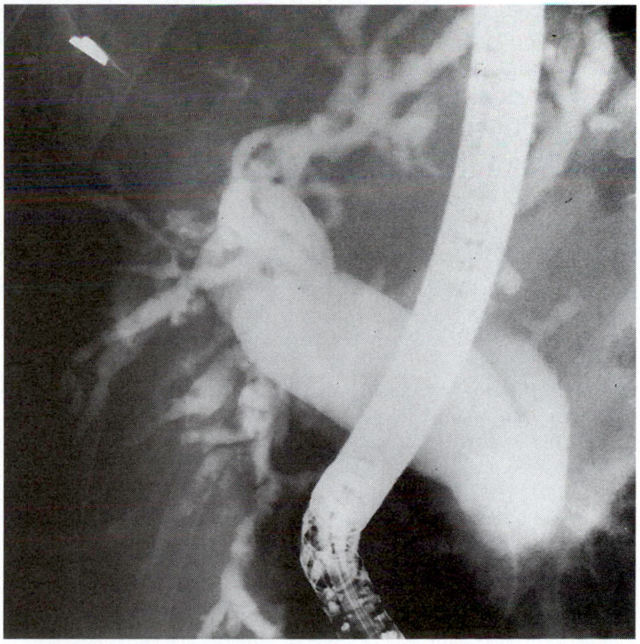

**Fig. 43-5.** An ERCP in a patient with acquired immune deficiency syndrome demonstrates severe sclerosing cholangitis. This patient has severe intrahepatic and extrahepatic disease. His intrahepatic ducts demonstrate dilatation of small ductal segments between areas of stricturing, producing the characteristic appearance of "beads on a string." In addition, there is significant dilatation of the common bile duct resulting from papillary stenosis.

long-term bypass. However, the diagnosis may be made only on liver biopsy, when the primary site of duct involvement is the smallest ductules, "pericholangitis." Numerous experimental protocols using antiinflammatory and antimetabolic agents have been tried without success. Ursodeoxycholic acid and methotrexate appear to have some promise. Liver transplant is indicated for patients with secondary cirrhosis uncomplicated by cholangiocarcinoma, which is a complication of PSC that occurs in up to 10% of patients.

### Secondary sclerosing cholangitis

A cholangiographic appearance similar to that of PSC may occur in some patients as a result of prior biliary surgery, chronic choledocholithiasis, cholangiocarcinoma, and in patients with the acquired immune deficiency syndrome (AIDS).

### AIDS-sclerosing cholangitis or AIDS cholangiopathy

AIDS-sclerosing cholangitis was named because its cholangiographic appearance is very similar to that of PSC. This condition is uncommon, but its prevalence appears to be increasing with physician awareness. It appears to occur during the last stage of AIDS, when T-helper ($CD_4$) cell counts are less than 50/mm$^3$. The condition is most likely a result of opportunistic infection and secondary chronic inflammation within the duct. *Cryptosporidium,* other protozoa, and CMV infections of the duct are most commonly seen. Although most patients with this process have a slow and relatively asymptomatic course, patients may present with severe abdominal pain, anorexia, and symptoms of chronic cholestasis. Bilirubin levels greater than 5 mg/dl are unusual; however, alkaline phosphatase levels in symptomatic patients may be as high as 20 to 30 times normal. Although the incidence of secondary biliary fibrosis has not been evaluated by liver biopsy, clinically apparent cirrhosis has not been seen in our experience. The mortality rate is high in these patients but usually from other complications of AIDS.

## BIBLIOGRAPHY

Afdhal NH, Smith BF: Pathogenesis of cholesterol gallstones, *Viewpoints Digest Dis* 22:13, 1990.

Barkun ANG, Ponchon T: Extracorporeal biliary lithotripsy, *Ann Intern Med* 112:126, 1990.

Fan S-T et al: Early treatment of acute biliary pancreatitis by endoscopic papillotomy, *N Engl J Med* 328:228, 1993.

Geenan JE et al: The efficacy of endoscopic sphincterotomy after cholecystectomy in patients with sphincter-of-Oddi dysfunction, *N Engl J Med* 320:82, 1989.

Johnson LB: The importance of early diagnosis of acute acalculous cholecystitis, *Surg Gynecol Obstet* 164(3):197, 1987.

Kozuka S, Tsubone M, Yasui I et al: Relationship of adenocarcinoma to carcinoma of the gallbladder, *Cancer* 50:22, 1982.

Lee SP, Nicholls JF, Park HZ: Biliary sludge as a cause of acute pancreatitis, *N Engl J Med* 326:589, 1992.

Messing B et al: Does total parenteral nutrition induce gallbladder sludge formation and lithiasis? *Gastroenterology* 84:1012, 1983.

Neoptolemos JP et al: Controlled trial of urgent endoscopic retrograde cholangiopancreatography and endoscopic sphincterotomy versus conservative treatment for acute pancreatitis due to gallstones, *Lancet* 2:979, 1988.

Ransahoff DF, Gracie WA: Treatment of gallstones, *Ann Intern Med* 119:606, 1993.

CHAPTER

# 44 Liver

Raymond S. Koff

## GENERAL DIAGNOSIS

Accurate clinical diagnosis and optimal management of patients with liver disease are common concerns of primary care physicians. Since screening tests for liver disease are now widely used, primary care physicians deal increasingly with asymptomatic patients whose laboratory findings of early liver disease require accurate approaches to avoid costly diagnostic or management errors. Even the approach to jaundice, a venerable feature of hepatobiliary disease, has undergone dramatic changes in the past few years. The introduction of serologic tests for viral hepatitis, noninvasive imaging with ultrasonography and computed tomography (CT), and increased sophistication in the use of invasive procedures have altered and expedited clinical assessment.

### Unconjugated hyperbilirubinemias

Disorders associated with overproduction of bilirubin and impaired hepatic uptake and conjugation of bilirubin in the absence of intrinsic liver disease are the unconjugated hyperbilirubinemias. They are suspected in the jaundiced patient whose urine is normal colored and whose tests for urinary bilirubin are negative. Unconjugated hyperbilirubinemia stemming from overproduction of bilirubin may result from hemolysis, ineffective erythropoiesis, or the breakdown of large hematomas. When evidence of hemolysis or hematoma resorption is absent and the patient seems generally healthy, impaired bilirubin uptake and conjugation resulting from Gilbert syndrome are the suspected causes of unconjugated hyperbilirubinemia. In this disorder other liver tests are usually normal, a family history of unconjugated hyperbilirubinemia may be present, and fasting for 2 or more days may raise the serum bilirubin to levels that trigger recognition of jaundice. Reassurance that a serious or progressive disorder is not present is all that is necessary. Patients with Gilbert syndrome should carry identification indicating that they have this disorder.

### Cholestatic syndromes

Diminution in the flow of hepatic bile into the duodenum is known as cholestasis. Cholestatic syndromes are settings in which impaired bile flow is responsible for a set of typical clinical and laboratory features. Jaundice, dark urine, and light-colored stools are often quite striking. Pruritus, presumably related to serum retention and sequestration in the skin of ill-defined pruritogenic bile salts, is a feature of the cholestatic syndromes. Cholestasis may result from parenchymal liver disease, intrahepatic disorders affecting the smaller bile ducts, or extrahepatic biliary obstruction. Regardless of the cause, it is accompanied by elevation of serum bilirubin, bile acids, cholesterol, and alkaline phosphatase. Serum aminotransferase levels are usually only mildly elevated and serum albumin is at near-normal levels. Malabsorption of fat-soluble vitamins may result from inadequate bile salt micelle formation and leads to hypoprothrombinemia that is responsive to parenteral administration of vitamin K. If cholestasis is prolonged, vitamin D deficiency may result in osteomalacia.

Drug-induced liver injury, alcoholic hepatitis, and acute viral hepatitis top the list of likely causes of intrahepatic cholestasis. Primary biliary cirrhosis, postoperative intrahepatic cholestasis, gram-negative or gram-positive septicemia, Hodgkin disease, recurrent jaundice of pregnancy, and recurrent benign familial cholestasis may also be considered. Because patients with parenchymal liver diseases do not require surgical intervention and may carry an excessive surgical risk, it is critical to distinguish them from patients with extrahepatic bile duct obstruction who may require surgery. In addition to the clinical and laboratory manifestations of cholestasis, patients with extrahepatic cholestasis are at risk for ascending cholangitis with fever, chills, and right upper quadrant pain. Another complication of extrahepatic biliary obstruction is secondary biliary cirrhosis, which develops after many months or more commonly after years of unrelieved obstruction.

When extrahepatic cholestasis seems likely, the procedure of choice is ultrasonographic examination of the biliary tree to detect dilatation of ducts, the presence of gallstones, and the level of anatomic obstruction. Ductal dilatation may be found in as many as 90% of patients with extrahepatic obstruction of 2 or more weeks' duration. In patients with obstruction of shorter duration, the ducts may not be sufficiently enlarged for ultrasonographic detection of dilatation.

If evidence of obstruction is present on ultrasonography, invasive techniques are required for further evaluation. Two techniques are available in most medical centers: percutaneous transhepatic skinny-needle cholangiography and endoscopic retrograde cannulation of the common bile duct and pancreatic ducts. The former procedure is undertaken in patients with evidence of obstruction on ultrasonography; the latter may be preferred for patients in whom extrahepatic obstruction is the likely diagnosis despite an unrevealing ultrasonography, and for patients suspected of having distal obstruction or ampullary or pancreatic disease. If ultrasonography and cholangiographic techniques indicate the absence of extrahepatic cholestasis, needle biopsy of the liver may provide a specific diagnosis of intrinsic liver disease.

## ACUTE HEPATITIS

### Acute viral hepatitis

Primary care physicians need to know about viral hepatitis because it is commonly encountered in the office and clinic; over 500,000 new infections occur annually in the United States. The major objectives in managing viral hepatitis are supportive care of the symptomatic patient and interruption of hepatitis transmission by patient education and, where available, by immunoprophylaxis.

***Prevalence*** A large number of viruses, including cytomegalovirus, Epstein-Barr virus, and herpesvirus, may be associated with features of hepatitis, but the majority of cases of acute viral hepatitis seen in clinical practice in the United States result from hepatitis A virus (HAV), hepatitis B virus (HBV), and hepatitis C virus (HCV). Among reported sporadic cases of viral hepatitis in adults, about half represent HBV infections, one third are due to HCV, and the remainder are attributed to HAV. A very small proportion of reported HBV infections actually may be coinfections with the hepatitis D virus (HDV), a defective virus requiring the simultaneous presence of HBV for its expression. Although rare in the United States, infections resulting from hepatitis E virus (HEV) are common in developing nations. Although HAV, HBV, and HCV have all been implicated in contact transmission of hepatitis in the United States, common-source or community outbreaks in this country are most commonly traced to HAV infection, posttransfusion hepatitis largely results from HCV infection, and hepatitis among health-care workers has classically been related to HBV or HCV infection.

In addition to acute infections, HBV, HDV, and HCV are associated with a carrier state. Carrier frequencies far exceed the annual incidence of new cases of hepatitis B and hepatitis C. In contrast, HAV infections do not lead to persistent infection or a carrier state. Persistent infection by HBV, HDV, and HCV may be associated with chronic hepatitis and cirrhosis and its complications. In the case of HBV and HCV infections, an increased risk of primary hepatocellular carcinoma, the most prevalent nondermatologic malignancy in the world, has been demonstrated.

#### *Etiology and epidemiology*

**Hepatitis A virus.** Hepatitis A virus, a 27-nm RNA-containing picornavirus, has been propagated in a number of human and nonhuman tissue culture systems. Only one human serotype of HAV has been recognized. Infection with HAV leads to the formation of a specific antibody: anti-HAV. In acute-phase sera the anti-HAV belongs to the immunoglobulin M (IgM) class, whereas in convalescent sera immunoglobulin G (IgG) anti-HAV predominates. Anti-HAV confers prolonged, probably lifelong, immunity to reinfection. The incubation period of HAV infection is about 30 days; viremia is short-lived and occurs during the late incubation period and early acute phase of the illness. Fecal shedding of HAV is more prolonged, beginning during the second half of the incubation period and persisting for several days after the onset of symptoms or jaundice. Peak fecal HAV shedding and the period of maximal communicability occur at the onset of illness in the majority of affected patients. Fecal-oral spread is the predominant mode of HAV transmission (Table 44-1). HAV outbreaks have been recognized in day care centers for preschool children, in neonatal intensive care units, in institutions for the mentally retarded, and among homosexual men. Contaminated water and foods, such as raw or inadequately cooked clams, oysters, and mussels, have been implicated in common-source epidemics. Parenteral transmission of HAV appears to be rare because of the brief period of viremia. Maternal-neonatal HAV transmission is not an established epidemiologic entity. A prolonged fecal carrier state is not known in HAV infections.

**Hepatitis E virus.** Hepatitis E virus, a 32-nm RNA agent believed to belong to the caliciviruses or possibly the $\alpha$-like supergroup of RNA viruses, is responsible for large

**Table 44-1.** Characteristic routes of viral hepatitis transmission

| Mode | HAV | HEV | HBV | HDV | HCV |
|---|---|---|---|---|---|
| Percutaneous | | | | | |
| Inoculation | +/– | – | +++ | +++ | +++ |
| Transfusion | – | – | + | + | ++ |
| Permucosal | | | | | |
| Sexual | + | – | +++ | ++ | + |
| Fecal-oral | +++ | +++ | – | – | – |
| Maternal-neonatal | – | – | +++ | + | +/– |

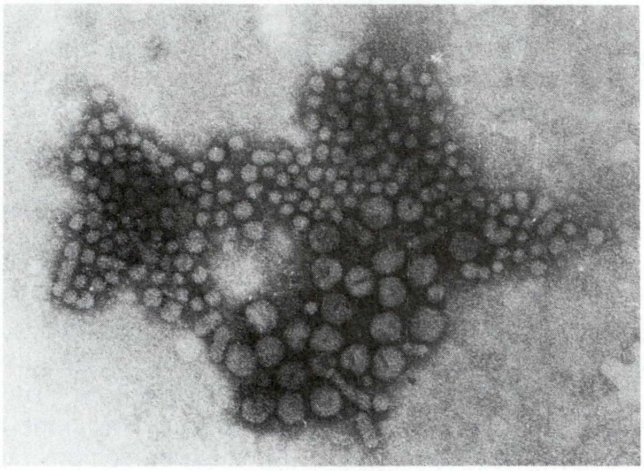

**Fig. 44-1.** Hepatitis B virus. The small particles are composed of hepatitis B surface antigen. The large particles are intact viruses. (Original magnification ×130,000.)

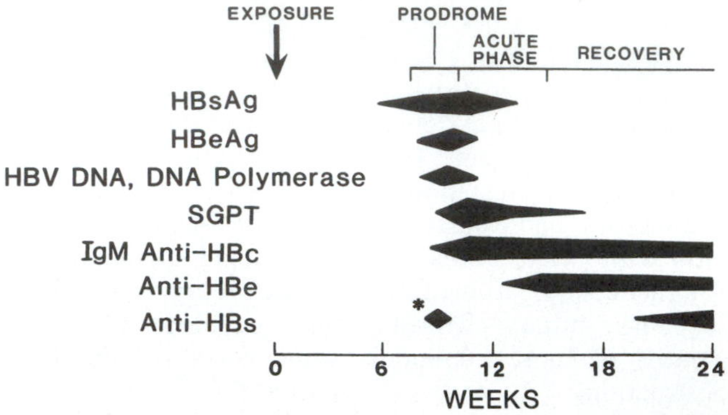


**Fig. 44-2.** The sequence of serologic events in acute hepatitis B is shown here. The asterisk before the anti-HBs shown during the prodrome marks the observation that although anti-HBs may be present early in the infection it is not usually detected as a freely circulating antibody until the recovery phase.

water-borne outbreaks of hepatitis in developing nations; it is the most common cause of sporadic hepatitis in young adults in the third world. Pregnant women who acquire this infection appear to be at very high risk for fulminant hepatitis. The only cases reported in the United States were imported in travelers or visitors from endemic regions. The incubation period is about 6 weeks with a range of 2 to 9 weeks. Immunofluorescent assays for anti-HEV, enzyme-linked immunosorbent assays (ELISA), and Western blot techniques for serologic identification are under development. Neither persistent HEV infection nor chronic liver disease resulting from HEV have been recognized.

**Hepatitis B virus.** A 42-nm, DNA-containing virus, hepatitis B virus appears to belong to a group of closely related viruses that infects humans, woodchucks, ground and tree squirrels, the Pekin duck, and the grey heron. Although HBV DNA has been inefficiently propagated in cell culture, cloning in bacteria and yeast has permitted expression of HBV antigens. The surface of HBV contains a specific antigenic material, the hepatitis B surface antigen (HBsAg), which is also found in excess of the intact virus in the form of smaller 22-nm spheres and tubular particles in the circulation of HBV-infected individuals (Fig. 44-1). HBV DNA, DNA polymerase, and two other antigenic materials, the hepatitis B core antigen (HBcAg) and the hepatitis B e antigen (HBeAg) have been identified in the core of the virus. HBsAg is the first serologic marker of HBV to appear in the infected individual and precedes elevation of the serum ALT (SGPT), as shown in Fig. 44-2. HBeAg appears a few days to a week or so later but disappears well before HBsAg. Antibody to HBcAg (anti-HBc) appears in sera after HBsAg and HBeAg become detectable and persists for a variable but prolonged period. HBeAg is detected only in HBsAg-positive sera and is a marker of infectivity since it is highly correlated with the number of circulating infective HBV particles and concentration of HBV DNA. Antibody to HBeAg (anti-HBe) becomes detectable as HBeAg declines in titer. An HBV variant in which HBeAg is not expressed but viral replication occurs nonetheless has been described more often outside the United States. Antibody to HBsAg (anti-HBs) is the last serologic marker of HBV to appear, usually showing up in the late convalescent phase, and persisting for prolonged periods. This antibody, which may be present well before it is detected in serum (see Fig. 44-2), is neutralizing, and highly correlated with immunity to reinfection. In some patients HBsAg may no longer be detectable during the acute phase of infection and anti-HBs may not have appeared yet. In this circumstance, IgM anti-HBc is present and may be accompanied by anti-HBe.

HBV infection is self-limited in 90% to 95% of adults, but in neonates, infants, and young children persistent infection is far more common. Persistent infection is characterized by the prolonged presence of HBsAg and anti-HBc with little or no detectable anti-HBs. HBsAg carriers who are also HBV DNA and HBeAg positive may transmit infection. Some carriers are asymptomatic; others have chronic hepatitis. The prevalence of the carrier state varies widely from area to area, but in the United States 0.2% to 0.5% of the general population are HBsAg positive. Among Asian-Americans, Pacific islanders, native Alaskans, injection-drug users, homosexual men, and immunosuppressed populations, the carrier rate may exceed 5%.

The long incubation period of HBV infection, averaging from 60 to 90 days, is responsible for the efficiency of bloodborne spread. It is accompanied by viremia, which begins late in the incubation and persists for several weeks to months or, in the case of individuals destined to become carriers, years. Although screening of blood donors for HBsAg has dramatically reduced the frequency of transfusion-associated HBV infection, transfusion of blood products that cannot be sterilized, injection drug use, and accidental needlesticks or splashing accidents in unvaccinated health-care workers remain important sources of HBV transmission. Permucosal transfer of HBV plays an even more important role in the epidemiology of this disease. HBV has been identified in semen, menstrual blood, and saliva, and transmission from acutely infected patients and HBsAg carriers has been established by follow-up study of their sexual contacts. Permucosal transfer during parturition is responsible for maternal-neonatal spread. Women who are HBsAg carriers, particularly those who are HBeAg positive, and women with acute disease in the third trimester may infect their infants. Since infection early in life often results in persistent infection, maternal-neonatal spread serves to perpetuate HBV infection in successive generations. Neither food nor water has been implicated in the spread of HBV.

**Hepatitis D virus.** Individuals with acute or persistent HBV infection appear to be at risk of coinfection or superinfection with HDV, a 36-nm defective agent. This HBsAg-enveloped RNA virus requires the helper functions of HBV for its expression, and during the course of HDV infection HBV replication is temporarily suppressed. The incubation period of HDV infection is 3 to 7 weeks. Acute HDV infection can be recognized by the appearance of IgM anti-HDV, HDV antigen, and HDV RNA in serum. HDV is believed to be spread percutaneously, in a manner similar to HBV, and in the United States injection drug users appear to be at highest risk. HDV coinfection with HBV leads to either a self-limited hepatitis or fulminant disease. HDV superinfection of HBsAg carriers may lead to acute self-limited hepatitis, fulminant hepatitis, or rapidly progressive chronic hepatitis.

**Hepatitis C virus.** The genome of hepatitis C virus, a lipid-enveloped 55-nm RNA virus distantly related to the pestiviruses and flaviviruses, has been sequenced and a number of recombinant antigens have been identified and used in assays for antibodies in serum. Current second- and third-generation assays employ multiple structural and nonstructural antigens and have good sensitivity and specificity. Unfortunately none of the recognized antibodies have been shown to be neutralizing. Available evidence indicates that there are several strains of HCV. Polymerase chain reaction (PCR) amplification to detect HCV RNA in serum permits the identification of viremic patients, but remains an investigational tool. Viremic patients may have acute infection, may be asymptomatic carriers, or may have chronic liver disease. Although HCV usually has an incubation period of about 7 to 10 weeks, the range is extremely wide. HCV has been identified in serum during the late incubation period, the acute phase of illness, and for prolonged periods after convalescence, even in some patients who appear to resolve their hepatitis. Nearly all patients in whom HCV infection leads to chronic hepatitis remain viremic. HCV RNA has been identified in lymphocytes; HCV may be present in low concentrations in some body fluids.

HCV is a bloodborne pathogen spread predominantly by percutaneous transmission. Injection drug use and transfusion are known risk factors. However, the introduction of surrogate tests and anti-HCV screening of blood donors has dramatically reduced the frequency of transfusion-associated HCV infection. Sexual transmission occurs but is less common than in the case of HBV. Maternal-neonatal spread appears to be uncommon unless the mother is also HIV positive or has high titers of HCV RNA.

***Clinical presentation and natural history.*** The spectrum of illness in acute viral hepatitis is broad. Regardless of the responsible virus, many patients have no recognized clinical illness. In such infections, the presence of viral hepatitis may be signaled by recognition of biochemical abnormalities or serologic markers of recent infection. If biochemical abnormalities are transient or absent only serologic evaluation may provide evidence of infection. The overwhelming majority of individuals with silent viral hepatitis are never seen by health-care providers; symptomatic viral hepatitis with or without jaundice is that form most commonly seen by the physician.

Patients with anicteric illness may have transient gastrointestinal or upper respiratory symptoms suggestive of a nonspecific viral infection, short-lived anorexia and fatigue, and a day or two of fever. The decision to seek medical aid is often delayed and then canceled as the illness wanes. In contrast, viral hepatitis with jaundice has a longer, more striking clinical presentation, although it too is usually a self-limited disease. The illness typically begins with a prodrome lasting a few days to a few weeks. Among the characteristic features are malaise, anorexia, nausea and vomiting, fatigue, influenza-like symptoms, diarrhea, arthralgias, right upper quadrant abdominal discomfort, low-grade fever, and distaste for or actual aversion to cigarettes and their smoke. In patients with HAV infection the prodrome tends to begin abruptly, and respiratory symptoms, such as pharyngitis, cough, coryza, and fever (usually 37.5° to 38.5° C) are often more prominent than in other hepatitis virus infections. In HBV and HCV infection the prodrome may have a more insidious onset and a prolonged duration. In about 5% to 10% of patients with HBV infection a syndrome resembling serum sickness may be the earliest manifestation of hepatitis. In affected patients arthralgias are accompanied by objective evidence of polyarthritis simulating an acute rheumatoid arthritis. Urticaria, maculopapular eruptions, angioneurotic edema, and rarely hematuria may be present. The joint and nonarticular manifestations of serum sickness last from a few days to a few weeks. The syndrome subsides and disappears with the development of jaundice or, if the illness is anicteric, with the

**Table 44-2.** Natural history of viral hepatitis

| Outcome or sequela | HAV | HEV | HBV | HDV | HCV |
|---|---|---|---|---|---|
| | Estimated frequency (%) | | | | |
| Complete recovery | >99 | >99 | 90-95 | 95 | 10-40 |
| Fulminant hepatitis | <0.1 | <1-10* | 1 | 1-2 | <1 |
| Persistent infection (carrier state) | 0 | 0 | 5-10† | 1-5 | 50-90 |
| Chronic hepatitis | 0 | 0 | 1-3 | 1-5 | 20-70 |
| Proportion with progression to cirrhosis | 0 | 0 | 33 | 33-50 | 10-20 |
| Hepatocellular carcinoma | 0 | 0 | 5-40 | 5-40‡ | (?)20§ |

*Among pregnant women with HEV infection, case fatality rates may exceed 10%.
†Carrier rates of 50% or greater may follow HBV infection in neonates and infants.
‡HDV infection may promote the development of carcinoma in HBV-infected chronic hepatitis/cirrhosis patients.
§The relative risk of hepatocellular carcinoma in chronic hepatitis/cirrhosis resulting from HCV may be similar to that in HBV-associated disease.

development of laboratory evidence of hepatitis. Chronic joint disease is not seen. Deposition of immune complexes of HBsAg–anti-HBs and/or HBeAg–anti-HBe in the joints, skin, small blood vessels, and kidneys appears to be responsible for this syndrome. A similar syndrome has been reported infrequently in HCV infection.

Jaundice is usually preceded by the appearance of dark brown urine, a lighter stool color, and in some patients mild pruritus. Prodromal symptoms subside as the jaundice increases. However, in patients with severe variants prodromal symptoms may persist. Hepatic enlargement with mild tenderness is typical in the jaundiced patient, and a palpable spleen is present in about 20%. In most cases jaundice is maximal during the second week after onset and then disappears during the next 2 to 8 weeks, marking clinical recovery in the majority of instances. Symptomatic improvement occurs concomitantly with the resolution of the biochemical abnormalities.

The natural history of acute viral hepatitis remains incompletely defined (Table 44-2). HAV infection, whether silent or symptomatic with or without jaundice, is rarely fatal (fatalities are seen in about 2% of patients over 40 years old) and is not associated with the development of either persistent infection (carrier state) or chronic hepatitis. In symptomatic HBV infection with jaundice the case fatality rate approaches 1% and is adversely influenced by the following: increasing age, debility, the coexistence of malignancy, and coinfection or superinfection with HDV.

Persistent infection and chronic hepatitis appear to be common sequelae of HBV, HBV/HDV, and HCV infections. Chronic hepatitis, as determined by persistent aminotransferase elevations for more than 6 to 12 months, has been found in many persistently infected patients and may lead to both cirrhosis and hepatocellular carcinoma, which in turn lead to premature mortality.

***Laboratory studies.*** During the prodrome and early acute phase of the illness there may be normal or low-normal leukocyte counts, or leukopenia. A relative lymphocytosis and atypical lymphocytes may be prominent. Leukocytosis is unusual and suggests the presence of a severe clinical variant (fulminant hepatitis or bridging necrosis) or other disease unrelated to viral hepatitis. Anemia is not a typical feature, although mild hemolysis is rarely observed.

Serum aminotransferase elevations are detected during the prodrome and rise progressively. Alanine aminotransferase levels are usually higher than those of aspartate aminotransferase. In anicteric hepatitis alanine aminotransferase elevations may be the only biochemical abnormality detected; however, minimal increases in serum bilirubin often accompany the serum enzyme elevations. In icteric patients peak serum bilirubin levels are usually reached in the second week of the acute illness and vary between 5 and 20 mg/dl. Serum alkaline phosphatase levels are either normal or mildly increased. Serum albumin is usually normal or slightly decreased, whereas serum globulins may be mildly elevated. The prothrombin time is normal or prolonged, usually to within a few seconds over the control values.

Serologic studies to define the responsible etiologic agent are undertaken during the acute phase of illness and, if necessary, during convalescence (Table 44-3).

Identification of anti-HAV of the IgM class in acute-phase sera is diagnostic for acute HAV infection. The presence of anti-HAV of the IgG class indicates that prior HAV infection has occurred and that the present episode is not hepatitis A. The presence of HBsAg or, if HBsAg is absent, IgM anti-HBc in acute-phase sera is indicative of HBV infection. The development of anti-HBs in late convalescent-phase sera is also indicative of HBV infection or immunization to HBsAg (see Prevention). The diagnosis of HDV infection is only considered in HBsAg-positive individuals. Diagnosis of acute HCV infection requires detection of anti-HCV or HCV RNA.

### *Clinical variants*

**Fulminant hepatitis.** Fulminant hepatitis, the most dreaded variant of viral hepatitis, is seen almost exclusively in patients with symptomatic hepatitis with jaundice, and is characterized histopathologically by massive hepatic necrosis or extensive bridging necrosis (see below). HBV infections (with or without HDV infection), HBV infection by the mutant virus that does not express HBeAg, HEV infection in pregnant women, and, to a lesser extent, HAV and HCV infections are the major causes. Fulminant hepatitis is manifested by signs of hepatic encephalopathy accompanied by profound prolongation of the prothrombin time. Diminution of liver size is a characteristic feature and gastrointestinal bleeding and

**Table 44-3.** Serologic diagnosis of viral hepatitis

| Agent | Acute phase | Convalescence |
|---|---|---|
| HAV | Presence of IgM anti-HAV | Development of IgG anti-HAV |
| HEV | Presence of IgM anti-HEV and/or HEV RNA | Loss of HEV RNA; development of IgG anti-HEV |
| HBV | Presence of HBsAg and/or IgM anti-HBc | Loss of HBsAg; development of anti-HBs and IgG anti-HBc |
| HDV | Presence of HDV RNA or HDV antigen or IgM anti-HDV in HBsAg-positive patient | Loss of HDV RNA or antigen; development of IgG anti-HDV or loss of anti-HDV |
| HCV | Presence or development of anti-HCV; presence of HCV RNA | Loss of HCV RNA |

ascites are common complications. The course in 65% to 95% of patients is rapidly downhill with death occurring in 1 to 4 weeks of onset. Sepsis, cerebral edema, respiratory and renal failure, and refractory hypotension punctuate the course and contribute to the mortality. Hypoglycemia is observed in about 5% of patients. Survivors have no evidence of chronic liver disease.

**Bridging necrosis.** Bridging necrosis is a variant of viral hepatitis in which confluent bands of hepatic necrosis span contiguous central veins, portal tracts, or the zones between central veins and portal tracts. This lesion has been identified in all etiologic forms of viral hepatitis but occurs more often in HBV infections. The presenting features, clinical course, and natural history are usually identical to those of typical viral hepatitis, and the presence of this lesion is not recognized. In probably fewer than 5% of affected individuals, the course of the illness is quite different. Jaundice persists beyond the second week and serum bilirubin levels may exceed 20 mg/dl. Malaise, fatigue, nausea, vomiting, and anorexia persist and evidence of fluid retention may become prominent. The prothrombin time may be prolonged, reaching levels seen in fulminant hepatitis. In these patients, although the evolution of the illness is slower, the course may be identical to that of fulminant hepatitis, with death resulting from hepatic failure complicated by sepsis and bleeding.

**Cholestatic hepatitis.** An uncommon variant of viral hepatitis, cholestatic hepatitis is characterized by clinical features of severe intrahepatic cholestasis. HAV infection appears to be responsible for most instances. Deep jaundice with serum bilirubin levels as high as 30 mg/dl and severe pruritus may persist for many weeks, although other symptoms of hepatitis are less prominent. Serum aminotransferase levels are elevated early in the course but may decline with time, while serum alkaline phosphatase levels may remain elevated by twofold to sixfold. Although the course is prolonged, the prognosis is excellent, with full recovery anticipated. If the diagnosis of viral hepatitis cannot be confirmed by serologic studies, further studies are necessary to avoid confusion with other causes of intrahepatic or extrahepatic cholestasis.

**Relapsing hepatitis.** Several weeks to a few months after clinical recovery from acute hepatitis, recurrent symptoms and liver test abnormalities may be detected in relapsing hepatitis. HAV appears to be the most common virus associated with this variant. During the relapse, IgM anti-HAV remains positive and fecal shedding of HAV may recur. Despite the prolonged course, full recovery is invariable and chronic hepatitis is not seen.

***Indications for consultation and hospitalization.*** Most patients with uncomplicated viral hepatitis are managed at home by the primary care physician without need for a specialist. Consultation with a specialist is necessary for those patients with severe clinical variants, e.g., fulminant hepatitis; the aid of an experienced gastroenterologist-hepatologist may expedite management. Referral may also be reasonable when cholestatic hepatitis is suspected because further diagnostic evaluation requiring special skills, including performance of liver biopsy, may be warranted if early confirmation cannot be obtained.

For typical viral hepatitis, hospitalization is restricted to those few individuals suffering dehydration as a result of persistent vomiting. Parenteral fluids are given until resumption of adequate oral caloric intake. Hospitalization is also indicated for those patients with fulminant hepatitis or a progressively worsening course suggestive of bridging necrosis evolving into fulminant disease. Patients with cholestatic hepatitis and others with uncertain diagnoses after a period of observation and evaluation may require brief hospitalization for invasive studies (e.g., percutaneous liver biopsy performed by a gastroenterologist-hepatologist).

***Management of typical viral hepatitis.*** The treatment of uncomplicated disease is supportive. No specific drug therapy is currently available. The goals of management are to provide adequate nutrition; to reduce discomfort and distressing symptoms; to avoid exposure to known or suspected hepatotoxic drugs; and to interrupt, where possible, transmission of infection (see Prevention). Careful monitoring of the course is necessary to identify clinical variants and initiate required therapeutic maneuvers if the course deteriorates. A clear discussion of the illness, its typical course, and reassurance about the generally self-limited nature of the disorder may reduce anxiety and prevent psychogenic disability.

Adequate caloric intake of a balanced diet may require multiple small meals. Because anorexia and nausea usually worsen during the day, breakfasts are often best tolerated and the bulk of calories may be consumed in the morning. Although it is often said that fatty foods are poorly tolerated, self-selection of foods is usually highly satisfactory and no foods need be restricted on medical grounds. High-protein diets have no important influence on recovery rates.

Malaise, fatigue, and abdominal discomfort may be reduced by restriction of physical activity. The degree of restriction is best determined by the patient. Enforced bed rest has no value in management, but if fatigue is excessive bed rest for a few days may be desired. Mild physical exercise is generally well tolerated, but excessive exercise in a poorly conditioned individual or even in a physically active one may exacerbate symptoms and is best avoided. Restrictions in physical activity are progressively lifted as symptoms diminish, the sense of well-being improves, and biochemical studies reflect waning of the hepatitis. Complete resumption of normal activities should not be hampered by the persistence of minor aminotransferase elevations during convalescence.

All nonessential medications are discontinued since their metabolism may be altered in the patient with unstable liver disease. However, oral contraceptive use may be continued during the illness; such use does not adversely influence the course. Alcohol ingestion is prohibited until the convalescent phase, when social use may be resumed without harm. Corticosteroid therapy has no benefit and is potentially harmful. Treating severe nausea and vomiting with drugs remains unsatisfactory. For patients who cannot retain oral fluids or food, hospitalization is required. Intravenous glucose with supplemental potassium, sodium, thiamine, and vitamin B complex is used to restore body water, provide calories, and maintain electrolyte balance. Intravenous amino acids have no proven therapeutic value in this setting.

Monitoring the course of hepatitis requires weekly or biweekly visits to the practitioner's office or clinic, supplemented by telephone contact. At each visit symptoms and physical findings are reviewed and serum bilirubin, alanine aminotransferase and the prothrombin time are measured. Progressive prolongation of the prothrombin time necessitates further evaluation for the presence of severe disease. Once it is clear that the clinical illness is over, further monitoring at 3 months to determine whether HBsAg has cleared, in the case of hepatitis B, and that aminotransferase levels are once again normal seems reasonable. Persistent abnormalities are rechecked at 6 months and, if present, require further evaluation for chronic hepatitis.

### *Management of clinical variants*

**Fulminant hepatitis and bridging necrosis.** Patients with fulminant hepatitis and bridging necrosis should be hospitalized as soon as their illness is identified by significant worsening of the clinical course or the development of encephalopathy and striking hypoprothrombinemia. Management should be undertaken in centers with liver transplantation programs. Survival rates, which had been 10% to 35% for fulminant hepatitis, are now 65% to 70% if liver transplantation is promptly performed before the development of irreversible brain injury.

**Cholestatic hepatitis.** No specific therapy is available. Pruritus may respond to oral administration of the anion-exchange resin cholestyramine or to treatment with ursodeoxycholic acid.

***Screening.*** Screening for prior infection by HAV or HEV, as detected by the presence of IgG antibodies, has limited value at present. Screening of blood donors for HBsAg has been a requirement for federally-licensed blood banks for nearly two decades. Screening for evidence of past HBV infection, as determined by the presence of anti-HBc or anti-HBs, is cost-effective before vaccination in health-care workers who are repeatedly exposed to blood or blood derivatives during their medical or dental careers and in whom high rates of HBV infection are likely. Screening of health-care workers just beginning their careers (e.g., nursing, medical, and dental students), is unlikely to be cost-effective. To interrupt maternal-neonatal transmission of HBV, all pregnant women should be tested for HBsAg. Neonates born to HBsAg-positive women are candidates for immunoprophylaxis (see Prevention). Screening of blood donors for anti-HCV and for serum alanine aminotransferase elevations has detected some HCV carriers and some individuals with chronic hepatitis C; exclusion of these donors has reduced the risk of posttransfusion hepatitis C by over 80%.

### *Management of HBsAg and HCV carriers*

**HBsAg carriers.** Two major issues to consider when managing HBsAg carriers are their health status and the risk of their transmitting the HBV infection to susceptible contacts. Counseling of the carrier and the family is necessary to avoid maladaptive anxiety reactions, depression, and social isolation responses associated with stigmatization of the carrier as someone with inordinately high personal health risks and high risks of infectivity. It should be emphasized that the HBsAg carrier state is not invariably lifelong and that HBsAg may be cleared with time. Effective chemotherapy or immunologic measures to clear HBV infection in carriers without active liver disease are not yet available. Fortunately the majority of carriers have normal serum aminotransferase levels, and liver biopsy in these carriers infrequently reveals chronic hepatitis or cirrhosis. Immune complex-mediated extrahepatic disorders, such as necrotizing vasculitis and glomerulonephritis, have been described in HBsAg carriers, but limited data suggest that these disorders develop in 1% or fewer of the patients.

The infectivity of HBsAg carriers appears to diminish with time. Active immunization with the hepatitis B vaccine protects susceptible contacts of infective carriers and neonates of carrier women but has no value if administered to HBV carriers. Health-care workers who are HBsAg carriers may continue to be employed provided that personal hygiene is adequate and evidence of HBV transmission to patients is absent.

**HCV carriers.** The guidelines for managing HCV carriers without recognized liver disease should probably be similar to those described for HBsAg carriers, since HBV and HCV infections share so many clinical and epidemiologic features. However, the HCV carrier state is poorly understood and many questions remain unanswered. For example, it is not yet known whether viremia and infectivity diminish with time or whether there is a risk of the delayed development of chronic liver disease in HCV carriers.

#### *Prevention*

**Hepatitis A virus infection.** Because fecal shedding of HAV is usually greatest during the prodrome when clinical recognition of hepatitis is difficult, strict isolation precautions have little value. Two forms of immunoprophylaxis are available: administration of immunoglobulin or hepatitis A virus vaccine. Immunoglobulin may be given, in a dosage of 0.02 ml/kg of body weight, to household and other close personal contacts of the index patient within 2 weeks of exposure. Protective efficacy rates approach 90%, and the duration of protection is about 2 to 3 months. Casual contact in the workplace, office, or school classroom is not an indication for immunoglobulin prophylaxis.

Immunoglobulin has been used in the control of common-source outbreaks, outbreaks in institutions for the mentally retarded, and outbreaks in day care centers for preschool children. Preexposure immunoprophylaxis with inactivated HAV vaccine replaces preexposure immunoglobulin administration in many of these settings, as well as in the following high-risk populations: travelers to endemic regions, military and peacekeeping personnel, sewage workers, caretakers of children, food handlers, and health-care workers. Protective efficacy rates for HAV vaccines in the preexposure setting should approach 100% and the duration of protection may exceed 10 years before booster doses are necessary. Transient pain at the injection site is the major adverse effect of HAV vaccine.

**Hepatitis E virus infection.** Neither passive immunoprophylaxis nor active immunization is available.

**Hepatitis B virus infection.** Passive immunoprophylaxis with hepatitis B immunoglobulin (HBIG) and active immunization with hepatitis B virus vaccine (recombinant yeast-derived HBsAg subunit vaccine) have emerged as mainstays in the prevention of HBV transmission (see the box at right). Administration of HBIG, containing large amounts of anti-HBs, is indicated for postexposure prophylaxis in three major settings: (1) after accidental inoculation, ingestion, or splashing onto mucous membranes or conjunctive of HBV-positive blood or secretions in nonvaccinated individuals, (2) for the sexual contacts of the acutely infected patient, and (3) concurrently with HBV vaccine, for the neonate of HBsAg-positive mothers. In the first two settings HBIG in an intramuscular dosage of 0.04 to 0.07 ml/kg is given as early as possible, and if the individual is susceptible when tested for anti-HBs before HBIG injection, it is repeated 1 month later. For the neonate at risk HBIG should be given in a dosage of 0.5 ml shortly after birth (within hours) and HBV vaccine administered in a three- or four-dose schedule beginning within the first week of life. Combined passive-active immunization in these circumstances can prevent 95% of maternal-neonatal infections.

Active immunization is the measure of choice for preexposure prophylaxis against HBV infection. Protective efficacy rates are about 90% to 95%. The recombinant yeast–derived HBsAg preparations are administered intramuscularly, into the deltoid only or in infants into the anterolateral muscle of the thigh. In the three-dose schedule, after the initial injection a second injection is given at 1 month and a third 6 months after the first. In the four-dose schedule the third dose is given 2 months after the first, and the fourth is given 12 months after the first. The four-dose schedule may provide more rapid protection in some individuals. The recombinant vaccines induce seroprotective levels of anti-HBs in over 95% of recipients. Booster doses are recommended only in dialysis patients whose antibody levels may fall below the seroprotective threshold. Excepting transient soreness at the injection site in 10% to 15% of the recipients and fever of less than 24-hours' duration in fewer than 3%, no important adverse reactions have been attributed to the vaccine.

### Indications for immunoprophylaxis of HBV infection

**Preexposure immunoprophylaxis with HBV vaccine**

Neonates/infants of HBsAg-negative women
Selected high-risk adolescents
Catch-up vaccination of early adolescents
High-risk adult populations
- Health care workers
- Homosexual men
- Heterosexuals with multiple partners, sexually transmitted diseases
- Injection drug users
- Hemophiliacs, thalassemics
- Developmentally disadvantaged individuals in institutions
- Hemodialysis patients
- Prisoners
- Pacific islanders
- Alaskan natives

**Postexposure immunoprophylaxis with HBV vaccine**

Sexual and household contacts of newly identified HBV carriers

**Postexposure immunoprophylaxis with HBIG and HBV vaccine**

Accidental tissue penetration/mucous membrane contamination in nonvaccinated individual
Sexual contact of acutely infected individual*
Neonate of HBsAg-positive woman

* The role of HBV vaccine in this setting is unsettled; it may be most useful if the index patient develops persistent infection and exposure is repeated.

Indications for HBV vaccine are shown in the box above. Universal immunization of all infants in the United States should result in control of HBV infection and, eventually, disease eradication. Catch-up vaccination of adolescents (age about 11 years) should accelerate eradication.

**Hepatitis D virus infection.** Active immunization against HBV is the only current method of preventing HDV infection.

**Hepatitis C virus infection.** Although immunoglobulin preparations may contain anti-HCV, a neutralizing antibody has not been identified, and evidence of efficacy in the prevention of HCV infection is largely absent. Prospects for an HCV vaccine have seemed dim because of absence of evidence of homologous immunity and because of the multiple genotypes of HCV observed. However, a prototype recombinant vaccine providing partial protection in chimpanzees appears promising in early studies.

### Drug-induced hepatitis

Drug-associated liver disease may simulate acute viral hepatitis and its variants or extrahepatic bile duct obstruction. It may also induce chronic liver disease, including chronic hepatitis, cirrhosis, granulomatous disease, and even malignant disorders of the liver.

*History.* The broad spectrum of pathologic lesions produced by drug hepatotoxicity requires the practitioner to document all drug exposures in any patient with abnormal liver tests or jaundice. The history is incomplete until all medications, prescribed and over-the-counter, are enumerated. Because some patients consume medications prescribed for other household members, thorough questioning may be necessary to obtain an accurate history. Although most drug-induced hepatotoxicity occurs within the first few months after the responsible drug is taken, in some poorly understood instances hepatic injury does not become manifest until several months of drug use have elapsed. Rarely, drug-induced injury may be seen after a year or more of drug use.

Liver disease induced by drugs is occasionally accompanied by extrahepatic clinical manifestations that can cause confusion with other forms of liver disease. For example, the presence of rash, arthralgias, and fever may be seen in liver injury resulting from sensitizing drugs as well as in viral hepatitis. However, the absence of extrahepatic features does not exclude drug-induced hepatotoxicity. Similarly, although the presence of eosinophilia is suggestive of drug sensitivity, it is not an invariable finding and its absence is characteristic of some forms of drug hepatotoxicity.

*Diagnosis and management.* The diagnosis of drug-induced hepatotoxicity is confounded by the recognition that hundreds of drugs have been implicated, and confirmation of drug-induced liver disease may be exceedingly difficult. Furthermore, hepatotoxicity may be recognized in only a minute fraction of patients exposed to the offending drug, and newly approved drugs may not have been used with sufficient frequency to identify their hepatotoxic potential; thus recognition may be hindered until widespread use. Practitioners must become familiar with the hepatotoxicity of commonly prescribed drugs and maintain a high index of suspicion when dealing with less well-known agents. If liver injury is recognized, all nonessential drugs are discontinued. Although consistent with drug-induced disease, improvement is not necessarily diagnostic and further evaluation for other causes of liver disease is necessary. Drug rechallenge may provide more convincing evidence; however, since rechallenge has led to life-threatening liver disease in some situations, it requires informed consent and should not be undertaken unless the drug is essential and cannot be substituted. It should be emphasized that drug rechallenge is rarely required for the patient's care. Suspected drug-induced liver injury should be reported to the pharmaceutical manufacturer and to the Food and Drug Administration on their adverse-reaction forms.

*Follow-up.* After discontinuation of the suspected drug the liver tests should be sequentially measured to ascertain that improvement in laboratory studies occurs concomitantly with clinical improvement. In many instances clinical and biochemical improvement are seen within a few days of drug discontinuation. However, for some drugs liver injury progresses nonetheless and peaks at variable times thereafter. Unfortunately, in a small proportion of patients with drug-induced hepatitis fulminant disease ensues. Progression of disease for more than a few days after drug discontinuation requires reassessment to make sure that other hepatic disorders have not been missed. Referral to a gastroenterologist-hepatologist at this time is appropriate.

A distinction between clinically important drug-induced liver disease and transient minor aminotransferase elevations in the asymptomatic patient is worth drawing. A number of drugs, including those in many different therapeutic classes, may produce minor increases in serum enzyme levels in as many as 15% of individuals during the first several weeks of treatment. This phenomenon, in which enzyme levels may be either slightly increased or as much as two or three times the upper limits of normal, appears to reflect an adaptive process, since levels usually return to normal despite continuation of the drug. There is no convincing evidence that symptomatic drug hepatotoxicity is a sequel to this adaptive change. If the patient is asymptomatic at the time the abnormality is found, the drug may be continued, provided it is still needed, enzyme levels are sequentially measured and do not exceed three times the upper limit of normal, and the patient fails to develop symptoms suggestive of hepatotoxicity. The drug must be immediately discontinued if the enzyme levels are higher than a threefold increase, if the drug is no longer needed, if the patient cannot be monitored, or if on monitoring, the enzymes continue to rise or symptoms develop.

### Alcoholic hepatitis

Although it may be considered as simply another form of drug-induced liver disease, the extraordinary prevalence of alcoholism and alcohol-induced liver injury in our society and the contribution of alcoholic hepatitis to the morbidity and mortality of cirrhosis mandate that it receive special attention in this text. Furthermore, the management of the patient with alcoholic hepatitis presents issues for the practitioner that are distinctly different from those concerned with viral or drug-induced hepatitis.

*Prevalence and pathophysiology.* Alcoholic liver disease is one of the most common causes of liver disease in the United States, and alcoholic hepatitis, both a precursor of and accompaniment of alcoholic cirrhosis, is responsible for a large proportion of hospital admissions for alcohol-related liver disease, including many of those directly related to cirrhosis and its complications. In contrast to alcoholic fatty liver, which is a universal feature of excessive alcohol consumption, alcoholic hepatitis is seen in only about 10% to 20% of heavy imbibers. The bulk of men with recognized alcoholic hepatitis have consumed over 70g of alcohol daily for more than 10 years. In women the threshold appears to be as low as 35 to 40 g for the same period. Since the prevalence of alcoholism has increased in recent years among young people and women, the prevalence of alcoholic hepatitis has also increased in these groups.

The pathogenesis of alcoholic hepatitis remains ill defined. Direct ethanol toxicity, mediated by acetaldehyde and acetaldehyde adducts, may play a role in the initiation of liver injury but perpetuation of alcoholic liver disease may be linked to cell-mediated immune mechanisms. The role of malnutrition or nutrient deficiency as a contributing factor remains to be established.

***Natural history and clinical presentation.*** Early in the development of alcoholic hepatitis recognition of liver disease is difficult because most patients are asymptomatic and do not seek medical attention. Denial of excessive alcohol ingestion is common, and family members may be unaware of the patient's alcohol dependence. Minor abnormalities of liver chemistries (e.g., aspartate aminotransferase elevations with normal alanine aminotransferase levels) may provide the sole clue to the presence of liver disease. In many patients persistence of clinically silent alcoholic hepatitis or exacerbations consequent to binge drinking are accompanied by nonspecific complaints or symptoms suggestive of extrahepatic organ involvement such as pancreatitis or erosive gastritis. Workup of these manifestations may reveal incidental evidence of hepatic disease and thereby lead to consideration of alcoholic hepatitis as a likely diagnosis. In other patients the diagnosis of alcoholic liver disease is preceded by complaints that suggest prodromal manifestations of viral hepatitis. Such presenting complaints include anorexia, nausea, vomiting, abdominal pain, malaise, fever, and weight loss. Jaundice may be striking, particularly in patients who have had repeated bouts of alcoholic hepatitis superimposed on alcoholic cirrhosis. In jaundiced patients the clinical picture may resemble that of extrahepatic bile duct obstruction. There is a broad spectrum of severity, and case fatality rates of 2% to 10% are commonly reported. Hepatomegaly with or without mild tenderness is a characteristic feature of alcoholic hepatitis. Spider angiomas are common, and ascites may be present in as many as 25% of patients without cirrhosis. When cirrhosis is present, the frequency of ascites in alcoholic hepatitis may exceed 80%.

After alcohol ingestion is discontinued, most patients with alcoholic hepatitis recover over a period of weeks to months. If cirrhosis has not yet developed and abstinence is maintained, the lesion is reversible and the prognosis is good; however, in some patients the disease is rapidly progressive over a period of weeks and ultimately leads to death from hepatic failure despite alcohol withdrawal. This pattern may be seen in patients without underlying cirrhosis but is most commonly encountered in alcoholic hepatitis superimposed on alcoholic cirrhosis. In a minor proportion of patients with alcoholic hepatitis, markers of HCV infection may be present. The precise contribution of HCV infection to the pathogenesis of alcoholic liver disease remains to be determined.

***Complications and clinical variants.*** The major complication of alcoholic hepatitis is the development of alcoholic cirrhosis. Even in the absence of cirrhosis, evidence of portal hypertension may be recognized. Ascites, splenomegaly, and esophagogastric varices may reflect elevation of portal venous pressure because of the combined effects of perivenular fibrosis, venoocclusive disease, hepatic inflammation, hepatic triglyceride accumulation, and increased hepatocyte water content. The management of portal hypertension and its manifestations in alcoholic hepatitis is identical to that for portal hypertension in the cirrhotic patient. However, to the extent that the underlying lesions are reversible (e.g., hepatic inflammation), portal pressure falls with abstinence, and resolution of clinical manifestations of portal hypertension abates in alcoholic hepatitis.

The most troublesome variant of alcoholic hepatitis is that which simulates extrahepatic biliary tract obstruction. The presence of jaundice (with or without pruritus), fever, leukocytosis, and liver tests compatible with cholestasis is suggestive of ascending cholangitis. Painless and unrecognized pancreatitis leading to compression of the common bile duct may be responsible for a minority of such instances. In an even smaller number of patients choledocholithiasis resulting from either pigment stones or incidental cholesterol gallstones may be responsible. In most patients evaluation with ultrasonography fails to disclose bile duct dilatation, and invasive cholangiography confirms the absence of an obstructing anatomic lesion. Evidence of cholestasis subsides with resolution of alcoholic hepatitis. The precise mechanism responsible for cholestasis in these patients remains to be established.

***Laboratory studies.*** Hematologic abnormalities are common. Anemia is present in about two thirds of cases and reflects folate deficiency, alcohol-induced marrow depression, iron deficiency secondary to gastrointestinal bleeding as a result of alcoholic gastritis, or hemolysis. Even in the absence of folate deficiency the mean corpuscular volume of the red cell may be strikingly increased. Leukopenia is not uncommon (about 10% to 20% of cases), and leukocytosis is seen in about 40%. A leukemoid reaction is seen in fewer than 5%. Thrombocytopenia may be present in about 10% to 15%. The serum bilirubin is elevated, but the range of values may be extreme, and levels exceeding 30 mg/dl are found in about 10%. In about 80% to 90%, the serum aspartate aminotransferase level is at least twice as high as the alanine aminotransferase, which is often normal or only trivially elevated. Peak levels of aspartate aminotransferase exceed 300 IU in fewer than 10% of cases. The serum alkaline phosphatase is usually elevated, often to levels of two or three times the upper limit of normal. Threefold or greater increases may be seen in patients with cholestasis. Serum albumin levels may be depressed and globulins elevated. Occasionally, exceedingly high globulin levels may be found because of striking increases in IgG and IgA levels. The prothrombin time is prolonged in patients with severe disease.

***Indications for consultation and hospitalization.*** The major indication for consultation is consideration of liver biopsy. Liver biopsy is useful in confirming the diagnosis and in determining the reversibility of the liver lesion. Consultation is also necessary when the clinical picture suggests extrahepatic bile duct obstruction. Hospitalization is necessary for symptomatic patients who have fever, persistent vomiting, or signs of hepatic failure (e.g., hepatic encephalopathy). Home management is particularly difficult because cessation of alcohol ingestion can rarely be assured and failure to improve may indicate either continuing alcoholism or a severe course. Consultation with an alcoholism treatment program may be initiated during hospitalization or on an ambulatory basis.

*Management.* Treatment of alcoholic hepatitis is difficult. Specific drug therapy is not available. However, the mortality of severe alcoholic hepatitis, manifested by spontaneous hepatic encephalopathy or a calculated discriminant function based on the serum bilirubin and prothrombin time, can be reduced by treatment with corticosteroids. The efficacy of corticosteroid treatment is strikingly reduced in patients with acute gastrointestinal bleeding. Colchicine and insulin-glucagon infusions have been used in clinical trials of patients with severe disease, but convincing evidence of efficacy is not available, and the latter regimen may be hazardous. The major objectives of management are to ensure alcohol withdrawal, provide supportive care during the symptomatic illness, and offer prolonged counseling and intensive medical supervision supporting continued abstinence.

## CHRONIC LIVER DISEASE (CHRONIC HEPATITIS AND CIRRHOSIS)

### Non-alcoholic disease

***Chronic viral hepatitis.*** The term *chronic hepatitis* or *chronic viral hepatitis* includes a spectrum of histopathologic lesions, previously known as chronic persistent, chronic lobular, and chronic active hepatitis. Intensive study and prolonged follow-up of affected patients indicate that the distinctions between these lesions are arbitrary, difficult to draw, and of limited clinical utility. Hence the term chronic hepatitis has gained favor and is used here. Chronic viral hepatitis refers to a virus-induced necroinflammatory disorder persisting for more than 6 months. It is characterized histopathologically by the presence of hepatocyte necrosis, a dense mononuclear and plasma cell infiltration of the portal triads variably spilling into the adjacent parenchyma, with or without fibrosis. In most cases the necrosis is irregularly distributed among periportal hepatocytes. In others contiguous necrosis of hepatocytes results in bridging necrosis similar to that seen in severe viral hepatitis. Progression of fibrosis with distortion of the normal hepatic architecture and the development of cirrhosis is seen in some patients. Additionally patients with chronic viral hepatitis, particularly those with cirrhosis, are at risk for the development of hepatocellular carcinoma.

**Prevalence and etiology.** Chronic viral hepatitis is the major cause of nonalcoholic chronic hepatitis in the United States. Persistent HBV, HBV and HDV, and HCV infections are established precursors of chronic viral hepatitis. No more than 5% of adult patients with acute HBV infection are at risk for the development of chronic hepatitis B. However, 20% to 70% of patients with HCV infection develop chronic hepatitis C. Limited serologic studies suggest that approximately 40% of the chronic viral hepatitis cases in the United States are attributable to HCV infection, about 25% to HBV infection, and about 5% to HBV and HDV infection. The remainder have been attributed to unknown agents, but the etiology in these cases remains obscure until more sensitive tests for HCV and HBV are available.

**Clinical presentation and natural history.** Many patients with chronic viral hepatitis are asymptomatic and may never come to medical attention. Others are asymptomatic for long periods, but the development of end-stage disease, including complications of cirrhosis, may be the earliest clinical manifestation of the disease. In a small proportion mild to moderately severe fatigue and anorexia prompt medical attention, and in a small number of patients mild jaundice leads to evaluation. Some patients may be identified on follow-up after acute viral hepatitis; in these individuals serum aminotransferase levels remain elevated or fluctuate in and out of the normal range for prolonged periods. Multiphasic health screening tests demonstrating elevation of serum aminotransferases or positive tests for HBsAg or anti-HCV may be the sole abnormalities pointing to the presence of chronic viral hepatitis. Other patients are identified through screening of blood donors.

Recurrent episodes of acute hepatitis-like illness are infrequent but appear to be more common in chronic hepatitis B than in chronic hepatitis C. Such exacerbations, often termed HBeAg seroconversion flares, may be seen when replication of HBV is reduced either spontaneously or during treatment. In general, disease activity diminishes after transition to a low or nonreplicative state in which HBeAg and HBV DNA are absent. Other exacerbations have been attributed to HBV reactivation from a quiescent state to active replication in which HBeAg and HBV DNA are again detectable and may lead to further disease progression. Although chronic viral hepatitis might remain stable and clinically unchanged over many years, the disease may be slowly progressive. In a small proportion of patients the disease is rapidly progressive and evidence of hepatic failure or cirrhosis is manifest within a 5-year period. As many as 50% of patients with chronic hepatitis B may develop cirrhosis; 10% to 20% of those with chronic hepatitis C develop cirrhosis.

**Laboratory studies.** Serum aminotransferase levels are variably elevated between nearly normal and values greater than several thousand units. Peak serum alanine aminotransferase levels are usually increased less than tenfold. Aspartate aminotransferase levels are equal to or lower than the alanine aminotransferase levels. Hyperbilirubinemia is also variable; in many patients normal levels are found, but levels exceeding 20 mg/dl may be seen in severe cases. Mild to moderate increases in serum alkaline phosphatase levels may be found. Hypoalbuminemia and prolongation of the prothrombin time are found in severe disease. In patients with chronic hepatitis B tests for HBsAg are positive, and in those with biochemically active disease HBeAg and HBV DNA are usually detected. In a small proportion of patients with HBsAg-positive chronic hepatitis positive tests for HDV infection indicate the contribution of this agent to the disease process. Positive tests for anti-HCV, combined with aminotransferase elevations, are typical in chronic hepatitis C.

**Diagnosis.** Criteria for the diagnosis of chronic viral hepatitis include laboratory documentation of liver disease for 6 or more months. Persistent or fluctuating serum alanine aminotransferase levels may be sufficient. Liver biopsy may be undertaken toward the end of this period, regardless of whether the patient has symptoms, to confirm the diagnosis and exclude other treatable disorders and to assess the severity of the lesion and its progression. Although a single biopsy that confirms the absence of severe disease or evidence of cirrhosis may seem reassuring to patient and physician, progression may still occur. Nonprogression, based on multiple liver biopsies obtained over several years, supports the notion that the prognosis is good but cannot predict future nonprogression. These considerations should be discussed with the patient.

### Management

***Indications for consultation.*** Consultation is necessary for liver biopsy (an outpatient procedure in most medical centers), for patients with clinical or biochemical evidence of deterioration, and for initiation of antiviral therapy.

***Drug therapy.*** Treatment with injections of 5 million units (daily) or 10 million units (three times weekly) of interferon alfa-2b, for 16 weeks, is indicated for patients with compensated chronic hepatitis B, in whom HBeAg and HBV DNA are present and serum aminotransferase levels are elevated. Patients with decompensated disease, manifested by hypoalbuminemia, jaundice, hypoprothrombinemia, gastrointestinal bleeding, ascites, or encephalopathy, should not be treated except by experienced investigators following a defined protocol. Treatment of compensated chronic hepatitis B has resulted in inhibition of HBV replication and biochemical evidence of a reduction in hepatocyte necrosis and inflammation in 40% to 50% of the cases. Furthermore, this virologic and biochemical response appears to be prolonged and associated with improvement in histologic evidence of hepatic injury. Adverse reactions are common and include a flulike syndrome, bone marrow suppression, and depression. Patients must be monitored frequently, and dose reductions may be necessary in as many as 25% of treated patients. Whether treatment reduces the risk of progression to cirrhosis or hepatocellular carcinoma remains uncertain, but this seems likely, particularly in those patients in whom even HBsAg disappears on follow-up. Unfortunately, interferon treatment of patients with HBV and HDV chronic hepatitis has produced few sustained responses.

Treatment of patients with compensated chronic hepatitis C with 3 million units, three times weekly for 6 months, of interferon alfa-2b produces a biochemical response (i.e., normalization of serum alanine aminotransferase levels in about 50%); however, relapses are common on cessation of treatment and durable remissions occur in no more than 20% of treated patients, some of whom may lose viremia. Whether the progression of chronic hepatitis to cirrhosis and hepatocellular carcinoma is interrupted by effective therapy for chronic hepatitis C remains uncertain. Long-term follow-up studies are needed.

***Liver transplantation.*** In patients with life-threatening, far-advanced chronic hepatitis B in whom HBV replication is active, liver transplantation is not curative. In fact, because HBV may replicate in extrahepatic sites, the grafted liver is likely to be infected and the course of the disease may be markedly accelerated and severe, leading to liver failure and recurrent transplantation. In many medical centers transplantation is not an available option for patients with active HBV infection. Preliminary studies of long-term immunotherapy with hepatitis B immune globulin suggest a reduced risk of graft infection. In contrast, although HCV infection may recur when transplantation is undertaken in the patient with end-stage chronic hepatitis C, clinically important injury of the graft is uncommon.

***Autoimmune chronic hepatitis.*** Autoimmune chronic hepatitis is a chronic (persisting for more than 6 months), progressive, inflammatory disease of the liver of unknown etiology, predominantly affecting young women, and frequently associated with hypergammaglobulinemia. Left untreated it is associated with a high mortality. A number of markers of autoimmunity and extrahepatic autoimmune manifestations may be present, suggesting an immunologically mediated disorder; a response to immunosuppressive therapy also is characteristic.

**Etiology and classification.** Although some similarities to systemic lupus erythematosus have been observed, and the term *lupoid hepatitis* was once applied, the diseases are separate and readily distinguished in most instances. Autoimmune hepatitis may take a variety of serologic forms, based on the presence of different autoantibodies. The best known is classic autoimmune hepatitis, also known as type I autoimmune hepatitis, a disease found predominantly in women and associated with antinuclear and antismooth muscle (antiactin) antibodies. Evidence of genetic susceptibility is available: an association with HLA-A1-B8-DR3 haplotypes has been found.

**Clinical presentation and natural history.** Autoimmune chronic hepatitis may present with jaundice and fatigue accompanied by extrahepatic manifestations of systemic disease. Abdominal pain, severe acne, arthralgias or polyarthritis, amenorrhea, pleuritic pain, diarrhea, and fever may be prominent. In the absence of jaundice these features may fail to raise the suspicion of underlying liver disease unless hepatomegaly or splenomegaly is detected. In the fully expressed disorder jaundice is present in as many as 80% of patients, hepatomegaly is found in a similar percentage, and the spleen is enlarged in about 50%. Spider angiomas may be present, and signs of portal hypertension (e.g., ascites) may develop. Postnecrotic cirrhosis and its complications (e.g., gastrointestinal bleeding from esophageal varices) may be presenting features or sequelae.

The course of the disease is variable. Inactive phases may occur in as many as 20% of untreated patients, and the lesion may resolve before the development of cirrhosis. However, in most patients the disease, if untreated, is associated with high morbidity and mortality, particularly within the first few years after diagnosis. Approximately one third of patients succumb to hepatic failure within 5 years, and about three fourths have died at the end of 10 years if untreated.

**Laboratory studies and diagnosis.** In contrast to patients with chronic viral hepatitis, those with autoimmune chronic hepatitis may have immune-mediated anemia, leukopenia, and thrombocytopenia. However, hypersplenism may be responsible for hematologic abnormalities in both viral and autoimmune chronic hepatitis.

Elevations of gamma globulin and IgG levels are common in autoimmune disease. High titers of antinuclear and antismooth muscle antibodies are typical, and positive tests for the LE cell factor are commonly found. Liver biopsy reveals the lesions of chronic hepatitis with or without cirrhosis.

**Differential diagnosis.** Although it probably represents fewer than 10% of all cases of chronic hepatitis, drug-induced chronic hepatitis may closely simulate autoimmune chronic hepatitis. Markers of autoimmunity may be found and immune-mediated hematologic abnormalities may be present. In general, implicated drugs are those causing an acute hepatitis-like illness, women are at highest risk, and regression usually occurs after cessation of the offending drug. Isoniazid, α-methyldopa, nitrofurantoin, and phenytoin, are a few of those drugs in which a relationship to chronic hepatitis has been postulated. Chronic viral hepatitis must be considered, as can other disorders that may masquerade as autoimmune chronic hepatitis—Wilson's disease and α 1-antitrypsin deficiency. Iron overload may be considered, although the serum transaminases tend to be lower in this disorder.

**Management.** The treatment of choice for autoimmune chronic hepatitis is corticosteroids with or without azathioprine. A number of trials have indicated that corticosteroid treatment prolongs life but may not reduce the risk of progression to cirrhosis and the development of portal hypertension. Enthusiasm for corticosteroid therapy is tempered by recognition of important side effects in many patients, and prednisone-azathioprine regimens require frequent white cell and platelet counts to monitor for azathioprine toxicity.

Therapy may be initiated either with high-dose prednisone (60 mg) daily, moderate-dose prednisone (30 mg) daily with 50 mg of azathioprine, or a maintenance dosage of 10 to 20 mg prednisone with or without azathioprine. The high-dose and moderate-dose prednisone regimens are tapered to maintenance levels (10 to 20 mg) over a 4-week period. Symptomatic improvement on these regimens is expected within 3 months and biochemical remission within 6 months. Histologic remission may be delayed for 1 to 2 years. Treatment should be continued for 1 to 2 years before an attempt is made to discontinue therapy. Relapse may be expected in one half to two thirds of those who respond on withdrawal of immunosuppressive treatment. Repeated courses of treatment may also be associated with a relapse rate of 50%. Limited data suggest that, after induction of remission with prednisone and azathioprine, prednisone may be discontinued and azathioprine alone may maintain remission. Pulse prednisone is ineffective for autoimmune hepatitis in relapse. Promising small series and case reports suggest a possible role for cyclosporine as immunosuppressive therapy. Liver transplantation has been successful for patients with end-stage liver disease resulting from autoimmune hepatitis. Recurrence is rare.

## Cirrhosis

Cirrhosis implies irreversible chronic injury to the liver in which diffuse disorganization of the lobular architecture results from the combined effects of connective tissue proliferation and nodular regeneration of surviving hepatocytes. Hepatic necrosis and inflammation appear to be responsible for collapse and collagenization (fibrosis) of the reticulin framework of hepatocyte cords. Total liver cell mass is reduced and chronic inflammation is an associated feature. Distortion of the microcirculation of the liver and collagen deposition in the space of Disse lead to impaired sinusoidal transport and reduced extraction of protein-bound substrates, as well as increased resistance to blood flow. Portal venous hypertension, intrahepatic anastomotic channels between inflow and outflow veins, and extrahepatic collaterals between the portal and systemic veins are sequelae of the cirrhotic process. Cirrhosis is one of the 10 leading causes of death for both sexes in the United States and is an important cause of mortality throughout the world.

***Alcoholic cirrhosis.*** Although a variety of disorders are associated with cirrhosis, alcoholic cirrhosis is the predominant cause, accounting for at least 40% of cirrhosis deaths in the United States.

**Clinical presentation and natural history.** Alcoholic cirrhosis may be clinically latent and discovered incidentally at laparotomy, during evaluation of unrelated illness, or as a consequence of the development of complications, such as portal hypertension. Asymptomatic phases of cirrhosis may be detected during the workup of impotence, infertility, hepatosplenomegaly, or minimal abnormalities of liver biochemical tests. Evaluation of clinically apparent alcoholic hepatitis may lead to identification of underlying cirrhosis. Since alcoholic cirrhosis is usually not detected until after 10 or more years of excessive alcohol ingestion, children and adolescents are unaffected. The incidence of the disease peaks in midlife, and affected men exceed affected women by about 2:1. Presenting features may include jaundice, particularly in patients with acute alcoholic hepatitis and those with advanced disease and markedly reduced liver cell mass. The jaundice is associated with nonspecific complaints such as nausea, vomiting, anorexia, fatigue, weight loss, low-grade fever, and decreased libido. In a variable proportion of patients evidence of portal hypertension, hepatic encephalopathy, or abnormalities of hemostasis may be presenting clinical features.

The liver is enlarged, with a rounded edge and a firm consistency. However, in advanced disease hepatomegaly may be less prominent and the liver edge may be grossly irregular, a result of macroscopic nodular regeneration. Splenomegaly is common, and venous collaterals in the abdominal walls may be striking. Spider angiomas, palmar erythema, evidence of muscle wasting, and an emaciated appearance accompanied by parotid gland enlargement are commonly found. Gynecomastia and testicular atrophy are frequent findings.

The course of alcoholic cirrhosis is highly variable and appears to depend on the stage and activity of the disease at the time of diagnosis, the subsequent alcohol consumption of the patient, and the occurrence of complications, which in themselves are life-threatening. Variceal bleeding because of portal hypertension, progressive hepatic encephalopathy, intercurrent bacterial infections, and hepatocellular carcinoma are the major causes of death. Life expectancy is reduced in alcoholic cirrhotic patients.

Five-year survival rates vary between 25% and 60%.

**Laboratory studies and diagnosis.** Hematologic abnormalities are similar to those found in alcoholic hepatitis, and liver chemistries may reflect the presence of alcoholic hepatitis superimposed on alcoholic cirrhosis. In patients without evidence of acute alcoholic hepatitis the spectrum of biochemical abnormalities is wide. In patients who have abstained for prolonged periods, results of liver tests may be completely normal despite established cirrhosis. In most patients, and particularly in those who continue to imbibe, mild elevations of serum bilirubin, serum aspartate aminotransferase, and serum alkaline phosphatase are found. As liver cell mass diminishes with progression of the disease, prolongation of the prothrombin time resulting from reduced synthesis of prothrombin precursor proteins, impaired conversion of the inactive protein to the active molecule, and consumption coagulopathy may be recognized. In severe cases and in malnourished patients hypoalbuminemia is common. Serum globulins and the gamma globulin fraction may be mildly to moderately elevated. Hyponatremia, hypokalemia, and low blood urea nitrogen levels are characteristic. However, cirrhosis may be complicated by the development of progressive azotemia, the hepatorenal syndrome (see Ascites).

The clinical diagnosis of alcoholic cirrhosis is based on recognition of the characteristic clinical features, physical findings, and laboratory studies in the alcoholic patient. Since alcoholic hepatitis, a reversible disorder, may simulate alcoholic cirrhosis, an irreversible one, and because both may be present, liver biopsy is a useful confirmatory procedure. Histologic examination helps define the stage of the disease and exclude other disorders that may affect the alcoholic patient (e.g., iron overload disease).

**Complications and indications for consultation and hospitalization.** Complications of alcoholic cirrhosis are identical to those seen in nonalcoholic cirrhosis and are presented in detail in a later section. Such complications as variceal bleeding, infection, nonresponsive ascites, and progressive hepatic failure are indications for consultation and should prompt hospitalization. Surgical procedures for a patient with alcoholic cirrhosis often are associated with excessive operative morbidity-mortality and should be avoided or delayed unless failure to operate is life-threatening.

**Management of uncomplicated alcoholic cirrhosis.** No specific therapy is known to reverse alcoholic cirrhosis or halt the progression of the disease in a patient who continues to consume alcohol. Complete abstinence is the major goal of management, since compliance with such a regimen may lead to clinical improvement, biochemical resolution, and reduction in the rate of loss of hepatic mass. Although a balanced and nutritious diet containing greater than 2000 kcal and 1 g protein per kilogram of body weight is prescribed, except for patients with hepatic encephalopathy, it should be emphasized that dietary treatment has limited value in the patient who continues to drink. Thiamine and multivitamins may be given as well as supplemental folic acid, magnesium, and pyridoxine or pyridoxal phosphate.

Because occult sepsis is common, careful evaluation for bacterial infection may be warranted even in the absence of high fever or shaking chills. Patients with cirrhosis, including those with nonalcoholic disease, should be cautioned about the high risk of *Vibrio* septicemia resulting from ingestion of raw or undercooked mollusks. On each visit to the physician's office or outpatient clinic, evidence of early encephalopathy, fluid retention, and gastrointestinal bleeding should be sought. Successful long-term management of the patient with alcoholic cirrhosis requires that the practitioner be sympathetic and supportive but also firm in stressing a program of abstinence. Referral to a formal alcohol withdrawal program may be useful. Counseling of the patient's family and employer may facilitate adherence to such a program. Psychotropic drugs such as hypnotics, sedatives, and tranquilizers are best avoided, since their administration is potentially hazardous in this setting. Disulfiram has induced fatal fulminant hepatitis in a number of patients; it should not be used.

***Primary biliary cirrhosis.*** Primary biliary cirrhosis is a chronic, progressive inflammatory disease of the liver characterized by destruction of the intrahepatic bile ducts and the eventual development of cirrhosis. In contrast to secondary biliary cirrhosis, a complication of prolonged anatomic obstruction of the extrahepatic biliary tree, the extrahepatic biliary tree is normal in patients with primary biliary cirrhosis.

**Etiology and prevalence.** Although the cause of primary biliary cirrhosis is unknown, an autoimmune mechanism may be involved; cytotoxic T-lymphocytes infiltrate and attack the bile duct epithelium, granulomas surround injured bile ducts, circulating antibodies against mitochondria are present in nearly all patients, immune complexes may be found in the circulation, and other autoimmune disorders are seen in 10% to 15% of patients. Although triggering events such as urinary tract infections have been postulated, firm evidence of a role for bacterial or viral infection in the pathogenesis of primary biliary cirrhosis remains absent. A disorder resembling primary biliary cirrhosis has been described in a handful of patients after exposure to chlorpromazine, tolbutamide, methyltestosterone, and oral contraceptive agents.

The disease largely affects women between the ages of 35 and 65, but the age range is wide and onset in the third and eighth decades of life has been described. Fewer than 15% of patients are men. Based on studies in England, the prevalence has been estimated to be 50 per million population. Familial cases of primary biliary cirrhosis are documented, and some family members may have the antimitochondrial antibody characteristic of the disease, but no association with HLA types has been recognized.

**Clinical presentation and natural history.** As many as 15% of affected patients are asymptomatic at the time of diagnosis. These patients are usually identified as a result of evaluation of unexplained hepatomegaly, or by the discovery of elevated serum alkaline phosphatase or, more rarely, serum aminotransferase levels during routine evaluation. Such patients may remain asymptomatic for decades although the liver lesion may progress silently. In most cases pruritus with or without fatigue is the earliest symptom, followed months to years later by jaundice, xanthomas, and the clinical picture of prolonged and slowly progressive intrahepatic cholestasis. Weight loss, right upper quadrant abdominal pain, anorexia, nausea and vomiting, and increased skin pigmentation are described in 5% to 15% of patients. The CREST syndrome (calcinosis, Raynaud's phenomenon, esophageal hypomotility, sclerodactyly, and telangiectasia), and Sjögren's syndrome, or renal tubular acidosis, may be present. Although variceal bleeding, ascites, and hepatic failure are terminal features of disease progression, in a small proportion of patients these are presenting features. Bone thinning secondary to osteomalacia and osteoporosis may lead to vertebral collapse.

Hepatomegaly is present in about 50% to 75% of patients at the time of diagnosis and splenomegaly in 10% to 50%. Hyperpigmentation and xanthomas are present in about 10% to 30% of cases at diagnosis, but the frequency of physical abnormalities increases with time.

The rate of progression of the disease is highly variable. In asymptomatic patients life expectancy may be minimally reduced. In symptomatic cases, average survival appears to vary between 6 and 12 years, but the range is wide. Jaundice, weight loss, ascites, bridging fibrosis, and cirrhosis on presentation are correlated with a poor prognosis.

**Laboratory studies and diagnosis.** Isolated elevation of serum alkaline phosphatase of liver origin, exceeding twice the upper limits of normal with or without mild increases in serum aminotransferase levels, is an early feature. Mild elevations of serum bilirubin and hypercholesterolemia are present in about half of asymptomatic patients and may become more prominent with time. Elevated serum IgM levels may be found in about 50% of patients. In patients with cholestasis malabsorption of vitamin K, secondary to impaired bile salt excretion, leads to prolongation of the prothrombin time. Antimitochondrial antibodies are found in 95% of cases, and the titer exceeds 1:500 in about half. The antibodies are directed against an inner mitochondrial antigen, termed M2, which comprises components of the pyruvate dehydrogenase complex. Antimitochrondrial antibodies also are found in some patients with autoimmune chronic hepatitis, but low titers are characteristic.

The diagnosis can be confirmed by liver biopsy, which demonstrates destruction of portal triad bile ducts; these ducts are surrounded by mononuclear and plasma cells resembling lymphoid follicles, with or without granulomas and piecemeal necrosis. Portal fibrosis, bridging fibrosis, and cirrhosis may be present. Cholestasis is prominent in most specimens and may be accompanied by increased hepatic copper concentrations. Patients with a suggestive liver biopsy but absent antimitochondrial antibodies may require endoscopic retrograde cholangiography to exclude secondary biliary cirrhosis. It is not necessary in patients with antimitochondrial antibodies and a biopsy compatible with primary biliary cirrhosis.

**Indications for consultation and hospitalization.** Consultation is necessary for liver biopsy or cholangiography, and for patients with progressive disease manifested by hepatic failure or complications of cirrhosis. In the latter circumstances, referral to a liver transplantation center may be necessary.

**Management.** Specific therapy is not yet available. Neither corticosteroids nor azathioprine is effective, and the former may enhance bone thinning and the frequency of vertebral collapse. D-penicillamine, the antiinflammatory copper-chelating agent, has limited efficacy if any and such a high frequency of serious side effects that it cannot be recommended. Colchicine, which also has antiinflammatory and antifibrotic properties, has been used but evidence of efficacy is minimal. Ursodeoxycholic acid, in a dosage of 13 to 15 mg/kg, has improved biochemical tests and pruritus and is well tolerated by most patients. It has not had a major effect on the histologic lesion, but it does appear to delay the development of hepatic failure and improve survival. It has gained widespread favor and appears to be the current treatment of choice. Methotrexate has been used in some centers and is reported to improve liver tests, relieve pruritus, and improve histology. Large-scale controlled clinical trials are not yet available, and pulmonary fibrosis may complicate treatment. Use of methotrexate should probably be limited to those centers observing research protocols.

Supportive, symptomatic therapy includes parenteral administration of vitamins D, A, and K and oral vitamin E and calcium supplements. Pruritus often responds to ursodeoxycholic acid. For patients not treated with this bile acid, pruritus may be controlled by administration of cholestyramine, the bile salt sequestrant, in a dosage of 4 g with each meal. Rifampin, plasmapheresis, or ultraviolet light may lessen pruritus in patients not responding to ursodeoxycholic acid or cholestyramine but is reserved for those with extreme symptoms.

For patients with intractable pruritus, jaundice, and evidence of early hepatic failure, prolonged survival and a return to full activities of daily living have resulted from hepatic transplantation. Posttransplantation recurrence of disease has been reported, but differentiation from chronic rejection has obscured its frequency.

***Wilson's disease.*** Wilson's disease is a rare, autosomal recessive disorder of copper metabolism that affects children and young adults and leads to chronic hepatitis and cirrhosis. If untreated it inevitably leads to progressive and fatal liver and central nervous system damage.

**Etiology and prevalence.** The gene for Wilson's disease has been localized to the long arm of chromsome 13. The prevalence of the homozygous disease state is about 1:30,000; the prevalence of the heterozygous carrier state is 1:90. Defective biliary excretion of copper from the hepatocyte is the defect that leads to the accumulation of toxic amounts of copper in the liver and subsequently in the brain, cornea, lens, and kidney.

**Clinical presentation and natural history.** Liver involvement, resembling acute viral hepatitis or fulminant hepatitis often complicated by hemolytic anemia and chronic hepatitis with or without cirrhosis (or cryptogenic cirrhosis), is the usual presenting manifestation of affected children and young adolescents. In adults neurologic or psychiatric features may be more prominent, and liver disease may be inapparent although it is invariably present. Parkinson-like tremors, dysphagia, dysarthria, and dystonia are commonly seen. Emotional liability, adolescent adjustment problems, depression, and psychosis are well-known findings. Golden-brown Kayser-Fleischer rings, a result of the deposition of copper in

Descemet membrane of the cornea, are usually demonstrable by slit lamp examination in patients with CNS involvement.

**Laboratory studies and diagnosis.** Liver chemistries are usually abnormal but nonspecific, reflecting variable degrees of hepatocyte necrosis, fatty infiltration, and inflammation. Reduced serum levels of ceruloplasmin, the copper-binding glycoprotein, are found in 95% of patients, but in children with symptomatic liver disease only 85% have low ceruloplasmin levels. Hypouricemia, hypophosphatemia, uricosuria, aminoaciduria, and phosphaturia may be present. Diagnosis requires a high index of suspicion as well as documentation of low serum ceruloplasmin levels, increased urine copper, and increased hepatic copper concentrations in specimens obtained by biopsy.

**Management.** If Wilson's disease is suspected, the patient should be referred to a specialist familiar with the disease. Screening of family members may permit detection of asymptomatic Wilson's disease. Both the propositus and identified asymptomatic individuals require treatment. Treatment is designed to reduce copper stores by lifelong administration of the copper-chelating agents D-penicillamine or triethylene tetramine. Oral zinc salts and avoidance of high copper–containing foods may be useful adjunctive maneuvers. Successful decoppering prevents disease when begun early, improves liver and neurologic symptoms, and prolongs survival.

***Iron-overload diseases.*** The accumulation of excessive amounts of iron in the liver and extrahepatic tissues may be a consequence of a genetic disorder or a complication of chronic hemolysis, transfusion therapy, porphyria cutanea tarda, alcoholic cirrhosis, portacaval anastomosis, or dietary iron overload. Hepatic fibrosis, cirrhosis, complications of portal hypertension, and an increased risk of hepatocellular carcinoma are sequelae of the progressive liver disease in untreated patients and may be accompanied by diabetes, dilated cardiomyopathy, hypogonadism, hyperpigmentation, and arthropathy. This section focuses upon the genetic disorder only.

**Etiology and prevalence.** Genetic iron overload is transmitted as an autosomal recessive disease. The responsible gene has been localized to the short arm of chromosome 6, probably between the HLA A and B loci; the prevalence of the homozygous state may be as high as 1:400 and the heterozygous state may have a prevalence of 1:12. The linkage with HLA haplotype is useful in screening siblings, since the presence of the same haplotype as in the proband confirms the presence of the homozygous genetic iron overload disorder. The pathogenesis of genetic iron overload remains controversial. Although enhanced intestinal iron absorption appears to be the major defect, impaired regulation of iron metabolism in the mononuclear phagocytic system, enhanced iron uptake by the liver, and decreased biliary excretion of iron also may play a role.

**Clinical presentation and natural history.** Although iron accumulation begins early in life, tissue injury is not usually seen until the fourth decade, and clinical manifestations of iron toxicity may not be seen for another 10 to 20 years. The disorder is about 10 times more common in men than women and usually begins earlier. Early symptoms include weakness and weight loss. Hepatomegaly, splenomegaly, and signs of cirrhosis and portal hypertension may be found. The development of hepatocellular carcinoma is the most devastating complication of liver involvement. Diabetes mellitus is present in approximately 65% of the cases and retinopathy, renal involvement, and neuropathy may complicate the course. Loss of libido, impotence, and testicular atrophy in men and secondary amenorrhea and early menopause in women may be seen. Patients with iron overload disease appear to be at increased risk of *Listeria, Yersinia,* and pathogenic *Vibrio* infections.

**Laboratory studies and diagnosis.** Liver biochemical tests may be normal, except for slight increases in serum aminotransferase levels commonly found. Elevations usually do not exceed three times the upper limits of normal. Diagnosis requires demonstration of increased serum iron levels and decreased transferrin levels, yielding a transferrin saturation usually in excess of 60%, elevated serum ferritin levels (often above 1000 mg/L), and quantitative evidence of increased hepatic iron concentration.

**Management.** Patients with suspected iron overload disease should be referred to a specialist for definitive diagnosis (liver biopsy with quantitative hepatic iron determinations) and initiation of iron depletion by phlebotomy. Subsequent management can be undertaken by the primary care physician. Phlebotomies are undertaken weekly or biweekly and continued at that rate until the hemoglobin falls because of mild iron deficiency anemia. Transferrin saturation may decline precipitously just before the decrease in hemoglobin levels. Maintenance of iron balance thereafter may require occasional phlebotomy. Siblings of the propositus should be screened by HLA haplotyping or sequential measurement of iron parameters. If iron overload is identified, it is necessary that phlebotomy therapy be initiated, since effective iron depletion prevents all clinical manifestations. Treatment of patients with clinical iron overload disease may reverse cardiac dysfunction, hepatomegaly, glucose intolerance, and hyperpigmentation but not hypogonadism, arthropathy, cirrhosis, and the risk of hepatocellular carcinoma.

## COMPLICATIONS OF CIRRHOSIS

Regardless of the etiology of cirrhosis, the complications are often life-threatening in themselves and may contribute to the reduced life expectancy of the patient. The primary care physician must be familiar with these complications, recognize them early on, and plan a course of appropriate management. Early consultation with an experienced gastroenterologist-hepatologist may be helpful, since management of the major complications of cirrhosis is difficult and the efficacy and safety of many therapeutic measures remain controversial. Furthermore, early referral for consideration for hepatic transplantation is recommended for most patients with cirrhosis, except those with alcoholic cirrhosis who have continued to drink.

### Esophagogastric varices

***Pathophysiology.*** Portal hypertension secondary to cirrhosis leads to the development of extensive collateral channels between the left gastric and azygos veins. These channels are usually most prominent in the lower third of the esophagus and fundus of the stomach. Esophagogastric varices, as well as varices in the small or large bowel and retroperitoneal space, may be asymptomatic for prolonged periods. However, when the varices are large and associated with marked elevations of portal pressure, spontaneous hemorrhage may result. Although many affected patients have ascites, no specific precipitants of bleeding from esophagogastric varices are recognized. Hence the occurrence and onset of hemorrhage are unpredictable. Impaired hemostasis may contribute importantly to the initiation or perpetuation of variceal bleeding in some patients. Thrombocytopenia in cirrhosis may reflect hypersplenism secondary to congestive splenomegaly resulting from portal hypertension, disseminated intravascular consumptive coagulation, or, in the alcoholic cirrhotic patient, folate deficiency or alcohol-induced bone marrow depression. Prolongation of the prothrombin time in cirrhosis may be multifactorial (see Alcoholic cirrhosis) and may also contribute to persistent bleeding.

***History and diagnosis.*** Hematemesis and melena are the cardinal manifestations of bleeding esophagogastric varices. Because patients with cirrhosis may bleed from other lesions, such as erosive gastritis, peptic ulcer disease, and Mallory-Weiss tears, endoscopic visualization of the bleeding site is essential as soon as hemodynamic stabilization is achieved. Prompt admission to the hospital and early consultation with a skilled endoscopist are required. Even in large medical centers with considerable experience in its management hemorrhage from esophagogastric varices is associated with a mortality of 30% to 50%. Recurrent bleeding occurs in 30% to 70% of survivors. The 5-year survival rate after variceal hemorrhage varies between 5% and 20%.

***Management.*** Optimal treatment of bleeding varices remains controversial. Transfusion of whole blood and, if necessary, fresh frozen plasma and platelet concentrates may restore circulating blood volume and improve the clotting mechanism. In some patients these measures may be sufficient to control bleeding. If bleeding persists esophagogastric tamponade with the triple-lumen, double-balloon tube has its advocates; however, morbidity and mortality as a result of tamponade complications have dampened enthusiasm for this mechanical approach. Intravenous administration of aqueous vasopressin through a peripheral vein may provide temporary control of hemorrhage, although the efficacy of vasopressin's vasoconstrictive effects is limited. The combination of vasopressin and nitroglycerin (intravenous, sublingual, or transdermal administration) may be more effective than vasopressin alone. In some medical centers embolization of the left gastric vein and its branching collaterals has been achieved during transhepatic portal vein catheterization. Although this technique may halt bleeding, recurrent hemorrhage is commonplace as new collaterals develop or the embolized vessels recanalize.

In recent years endoscopic injection of varices with sclerosing agents has gained favor in the management of bleeding varices. Although technically difficult when hemorrhage is active, sclerotherapy has been used both in the acutely bleeding patient and after cessation of bleeding. Repeated injections are necessary over a period of weeks to months in an attempt to obliterate all varices. Sclerotherapy appears to be superior to medical management in interrupting active bleeding, preventing recurrent bleeding, and improving survival rates.

Complications such as esophageal perforation, ulceration, stricture formation, and pneumonia and renal adverse effects have been recognized in as many as 40% of treated patients. In terms of survival and preservation of liver function endoscopic sclerotherapy also appears to be equivalent or superior to surgical construction of a portacaval anastomosis or selective splenorenal shunt. Although the surgical procedures dramatically reduce the risk of variceal bleeding, they carry an excessive operative mortality when performed as emergency treatment for active bleeding; they also have little influence on overall survival, since a reduction in deaths resulting from bleeding is more than matched by increased mortality resulting from hepatic failure. In recent studies endoscopic ligation of varices with elastic rings (banding) appears to be superior to sclerotherapy with fewer recurrences of bleeding, fewer complications, and better survival rates.

Another approach to the management of bleeding varices is the construction of a transjugular intrahepatic portal-systemic shunt (TIPS) by an interventional radiologist. This approach may be most appropriate for the liver transplantation candidate in whom bleeding cannot be controlled by other techniques and immediate transplantation is not possible.

Prophylactic pharmacologic therapy with propranolol, the nonselective β-blocking agent, has been reported to moderately reduce the risk of the first episode of variceal bleeding in cirrhotic patients and to lower the mortality associated with bleeding. Unfortunately, some patients do not have a satisfactory reduction in portal hypertension, while others are not suitable candidates for β-blockade because of contraindications or side effects. Selective β-blockers are not as effective. Early studies suggest that the combination of a vasodilator with propranolol will enhance the efficacy of prophylaxis. Both propranolol or sclerotherapy prevent recurrent bleeding, but neither appears to prolong survival.

### Hepatic encephalopathy

Hepatic encephalopathy is a neuropsychiatric syndrome that may develop insidiously or abruptly and may be transient, recurrent, or persistent in a cirrhotic patient. A major complication of surgical portacaval and splenorenal anastomosis, hepatic encephalopathy also occurs, in the absence of surgical intervention, in patients with spontaneous portal-systemic shunting and in cirrhotic patients with end-stage hepatic failure whose functional hepatic mass is reduced.

***Pathophysiology.*** The pathogenesis of hepatic encephalopathy remains uncertain. Both the liver's reduced ability to detoxify nitrogenous metabolites and impaired clearance of nonnitrogenous materials have long been postulated to play roles. Elevated CNS and peripheral blood levels of ammonia, methanethiol, false neurotransmitter amines, aromatic amino acids, and short-chain fatty acids have been implicated individually or through synergistic action. The progressive neural inhibition characteristic of hepatic encephalopathy suggested a GABA-mediated effect (GABA is the major inhibitory neurotransmitter in mammalian brain) and benzodiazepine receptor ligands have been identified in patients with hepatic encephalopathy. Since benzodiazepine receptors were shown to be a component of the GABA–chloride channel complex in neural tissues, and benzodiazepines produce neuroinhibition through this GABA link, these observations have stimulated considerable new research into the mechanism of encephalopathy and the development of agents that might reverse the disorder at the neural level.

Most episodes of hepatic encephalopathy are, in fact, precipitated by exogenous factors (Table 44-4). Correction of these precipitants leads to reversal of the encephalopathy. The major inciting factors are gastrointestinal bleeding; excessive protein ingestion; treatment with sedatives, hypnotics, opiates, or tranquilizers; azotemia; infection; hypokalemia; and metabolic alkalosis. Excessive diuresis, surgical anesthesia, hypoxemia, and constipation are also established precipitants.

***History and diagnosis.*** The earliest phases of hepatic encephalopathy are subtle personality changes that may be difficult to recognize. Episodic slowing of speech and alertness may follow and sleep patterns may be reversed. Confusion, slurred speech, and gait disturbances mark a deeper stage. Asterixis, the flapping tremor, is usually present as is constructional apraxia. Trail-making (number connection) tests are useful in quantitating the degree of impairment in early stages but have little value in the full-blown syndrome, of which coma is the end stage. Electroencephalography reveals evidence of slowing of wave frequency typical of metabolic encephalopathy. In some patients muscle rigidity, pyramidal tract signs, and seizures are prominent features. In patients with long-standing hepatic encephalopathy the clinical presentation may be that of psychosis, choreoathetosis, dementia, or myelopathy. The diagnosis of hepatic encephalopathy is a clinical one based on the presence of the characteristic clinical picture in a patient with advanced liver disease. Elevated arterial ammonia levels may be found, but their sensitivity and specificity are sufficiently low to limit their value. Because other disorders (e.g., subdural hematoma and meningitis), may resemble hepatic encephalopathy, further evaluation with lumbar puncture and CT may be necessary.

In its early phases and in acute episodes with an identifiable precipitant, the syndrome is completely reversible and the brain is histologically normal. In persistent hepatic encephalopathy reversibility is less likely and glial hyperplasia and neuronal loss may be observed in the cortex, cerebellum, and basal ganglia.

***Management.*** Therapy is initiated at the first sign of encephalopathy before coma supervenes. Hospitalization is usually required if encephalopathy is more than mild. Identification of precipitating factors and, where possible, their elimination or correction are the first steps of treatment. Concurrently, control of encephalopathy is sought by reducing nitrogenous materials, and supportive therapy is initiated to maintain vital functions. Restricting dietary protein to near zero levels while maintaining caloric balance through increased oral intake of carbohydrate and fat may sufficiently control mild encephalopathy. Consultation with experienced dieticians often helps achieve compliance with this regimen. Cathartics and enemas also may be used to remove protein or blood from the gut. If clinical improvement results from protein restriction alone, dietary protein may be restarted at levels of 20 g daily and increased in 10 g increments every few days as tolerated. In general, vegetable protein is better

**Table 44-4.** Precipitants of hepatic encephalopathy in cirrhosis

| Precipitating factor | Example |
|---|---|
| Drug administration | Antianxiety agents (particularly benzodiazepines) |
| | Sedatives-hypnotics |
| | Analgesics |
| Electrolyte and acid-base abnormalities | Hypokalemia |
| | Metabolic alkalosis |
| | Severe hyponatremia |
| | Azotemia |
| Hypovolemia | Overzealous diuresis |
| | Dehydration |
| Increased gastrointestinal intraluminal nitrogenous materials | Gastrointestinal bleeding |
| | Excessive dietary protein |
| | Azotemia |
| | Constipation |
| Miscellaneous catabolic states | Infection |
| | Surgical anesthesia |
| | Portacaval, splenorenal, or other portal-systemic shunting |
| | Superimposed acute hepatic injury |
| | Hypoxemia |

tolerated than animal protein at equivalent intake levels. However, patient acceptance of a vegetarian diet is often poor, and compliance in the ambulatory setting may be difficult. For patients who fail to respond to protein restriction or for those with recurring encephalopathy despite protein intake well below the recommended daily requirement of 0.8 g/kg adjunctive therapy is indicated. One approach is the parenteral administration of amino acid preparations rich in branched-chain amino acids and low in aromatic amino acids. High cost and uncertain efficacy limit enthusiasm for their use.

Control of encephalopathy may be achieved in more than 80% of patients by oral administration of lactulose, a synthetic nonabsorbable disaccharide that lowers the pH in the lumen of the colon, traps ammonia as ammonium ions, favors the bacterial assimilation of ammonia, and reduces the concentration of short-chain fatty acids in the colon. It is given in a dosage of 15 to 30 ml by mouth or nasogastric tube three or four times daily, with adjustments of dosage determined by improvement in encephalopathy, usually occurring within 2 to 3 days. In general, lactulose must be given in doses sufficient to produce two or three soft stools each day with a fecal pH of less than 6.0. Overdoses of lactulose may induce severe diarrhea with crampy abdominal distress, bloating, and electrolyte disturbances. Rectal instillation of lactulose may also be effective but is less suitable for ambulatory patients than is oral administration. If lactulose fails, neomycin may be used in dosages of 0.5 g every 6 hours with or without continued lactulose. Neomycin therapy is associated with a small risk of ototoxicity and nephrotoxicity and should be reserved for lactulose-intolerant patients. Metronidazole may be as effective as neomycin but experience with this agent is still limited and comparisons with lactulose are not yet available. Prolonged administration of lactulose may permit resumption of near normal protein intake without recurrence of encephalopathy. Clinical assessment of mental status, asterixis, constructional ability, handwriting, and trail-making tests should be employed on follow-up of treated patients at each office visit.

Other approaches to the treatment of encephalopathy are under study. These include the oral administration of sodium benzoate, a drug that has been used in managing the ammonia toxicity seen in urea cycle disorders, and administration of benzodiazepine receptor antagonists. At present these treatments must be considered experimental. Liver transplantation should be considered among the therapeutic options for patients with progressive or recurrent encephalopathy.

## Ascites

Ascites, the accumulation of fluid in the abdominal cavity, is a cardinal feature of advanced liver disease but may also be seen in peritoneal tuberculosis, nephrotic syndrome, congestive heart failure, and neoplastic diseases. Although ascites may be a complication of cirrhosis or extensive liver disease without cirrhosis, the pathophysiologic mechanisms are believed to be similar.

***Pathophysiology.*** In patients with advanced liver disease excessive retention of sodium and water leading to ascites and edema formation appears to result from the combined effects of portal hypertension, increased hepatic lymph production, hypoalbuminemia, splanchnic venous pooling, and peripheral arterial vasodilatation consequent to release of vasodilator factors and arteriovenous shunting (see the box above). The precise mechanisms and the sequence in which they occur remain controversial. One hypothesis indicates that systemic vasodilatation is the key phenomenon. It leads to arterial underfilling, enhanced sympathetic efferent discharge, release of arginine-vasopressin through nonosmotic baroreceptor mechanisms, and activation of the renin-angiotensin-aldosterone system.

The increased sympathetic tone, angiotensin II activity, and decreased renal perfusion pressure result in increased proximal sodium and water reabsorption. Avid distal renal tubular sodium reabsorption results from decreased distal sodium delivery as well as from the decreased glomerular filtration rate secondary to renal vasoconstriction. Resistance to the distal renal tubular effect of atrial natriuretic factor and impaired escape from aldosterone's sodium-retaining action are also postulated to play a role. Impaired free water clearance resulting in part from excessive arginine-vasopressin levels is characteristic.

### Mechanisms responsible for ascites formation

**Initiating factors**

Portal hypertension/splanchnic venous pooling
Increased hepatic lymph flow with accumulation in peritoneal space
Hypoalbuminemia/decreased colloid osmotic pressure
Peripheral arteriolar dilatation resulting from vasodilator factors and arteriovenous shunting

**Secondary factors**

Decreased "effective" central blood volume
Enhanced sympathetic efferent discharge
Nonosmotic release of arginine-vasopressin
Activation of renin-angiotensin-aldosterone
Resistance to atrial natriuretic factor
Impaired escape from aldosterone-induced sodium retention

**Consequences**

Avid distal renal tubular sodium reabsorption
Increased proximal renal sodium reabsorption
Impaired free water clearance

***History and diagnosis.*** Ascites may not be recognized by the patient. In those instances in which increasing abdominal girth is noted by the patient, the onset is usually insidious and few symptoms may be present. When extensive, ascites may lead to respiratory compromise, umbilical hernia formation and rupture, an impaired sense of well-being, and early satiety resulting in reduced calorie intake. Spontaneous bacterial peritonitis is rarely seen in the cirrhotic patient without ascites; it is usually a complication of ascites and should be considered in every cirrhotic patient with ascites. When clinical examination at the bedside is equivocal, ascites may be detected by abdominal ultrasonography. Diagnostic paracentesis with removal of 50 to 100 ml of fluid is necessary in all patients

**Fig. 44-3.** Ancient Chinese drawing of traditional method of treatment of ascites. Note centrifugal obesity, respiratory distress of the patient, and the "appropriate concern" of the members of the family. (Courtesy C. Michael Bliss, M.D.)

with new-onset ascites and in those with long-standing ascites in whom fever, abdominal pain, azotemia, or hepatic encephalopathy may indicate the presence of a complicating disorder. In uncomplicated ascites secondary to cirrhosis, the serum-ascites albumin gradient is nearly always 1.1 g/dl or more. The ascitic fluid total protein is less useful in classifying ascites. Cell counts in uncomplicated ascites are usually less than 400 leukocytes/mm$^3$ per cubic millimeter and of these fewer than 25% are polymorphonuclear leukocytes. The presence of more than 250 polymorphonuclears strongly suggests bacterial infection. In spontaneous bacterial peritonitis the serum-ascitic albumin gradient is unchanged, the cell count is elevated, polymorphonuclear leukocytes predominate, and the ascitic fluid lactic acid dehydrogenase (LDH) may be increased. Bacterial culture of the fluid is mandatory.

***Management.*** In the stable patient with cirrhosis and uncomplicated ascites, management may be initiated in the office. A key element in therapy is restriction of dietary sodium to no more than 0.5 to 2.0 g daily. Consultation with a dietitian is necessary to achieve compliance, which is often difficult and requires an exceedingly conscientious approach. In patients with severe dilutional hyponatremia (serum sodium below 125 mEq/L), fluid intake should be limited to no more than 1500 ml per day. If weight reduction, diminution in abdominal girth, and diuresis are not achieved within a few days after dietary sodium restriction, diuretic agents are added to the therapeutic regimen. Spironolactone, in a single oral dose of 100 mg daily, is the initial drug of choice. If no response is observed after 3 to 5 days of therapy, the dosage is increased in increments of 100 to 200 mg daily every 4 to 5 days, until a maximal dosage of 600 mg is achieved. If weight still remains unchanged, the dosage is reduced to 100 to 200 mg daily and oral administration of furosemide, 40 mg daily, is added. If necessary, furosemide may be increased every 2 to 3 days in 40 mg increments until a maximal dosage of 160 mg is achieved. The goal of diuretic treatment in the patient with ascites without peripheral edema is a loss of no more than 0.4 kg of body weight daily. In patients with extensive edema, the latter serving as a reserve for plasma volume, no limit on daily weight loss is needed until edema disappears. It is essential that throughout the treatment period serum electrolytes and renal function be regularly monitored. Diuretic-induced hypovolemia, hypokalemia or hyperkalemia, hyponatremia, hyperchloremic metabolic acidosis, azotemia, or encephalopathy may require temporary cessation of therapy and, if severe, corrective measures.

Large-volume paracentesis with removal of 4 to 6 L of fluid appears to be as safe and effective as diuretic therapy and considerably more rapid in achieving a therapeutic effect. For patients with tense ascites and respiratory embarrassment or imminent rupture of an umbilical hernia (Fig. 44-3), and for those who are refractory to diuretic therapy, it is the treatment of choice. In some, but not all, medical centers in which ascites is treated by multiple large-volume paracenteses, intravenous colloid infusion with albumin or dextran is used to prevent volume depletion. The clinical importance of colloid replacement in this setting remains unsettled.

For the rare patient who fails to respond to the regimens outlined above, a surgically implanted peritoneovenous shunting device may produce a temporary diuresis. However, the combination of limited efficacy and multiple complications has so diminished enthusiasm for this procedure that it is rarely performed. The presence of spontaneous bacterial peritonitis is an absolute contraindication to shunt placement; spontaneous bacterial peritonitis may also be responsible for failure to respond to diuretics. If spontaneous bacterial peritonitis is suspected,

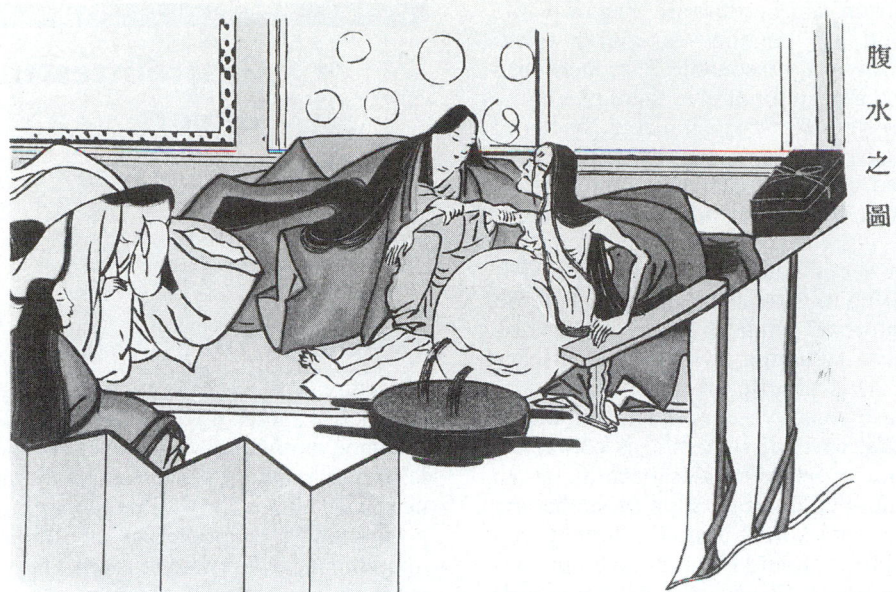

parenteral broad-spectrum antibiotics are begun while cultures of ascitic fluid are pending. Use of a third-generation cephalosporin is a reasonable approach until sensitivity tests dictate the need for altered therapy. For the patient who has recovered from spontaneous bacterial peritonitis, a high recurrence rate can be anticipated; recurrences are reduced by prophylactic antibiotic treatment with norfloxacin or triple oral nonabsorbable antibiotic regimens.

Another cause of or accompaniment to treatment failure, almost invariably seen in patients treated for ascites in the hospital, is the hepatorenal syndrome, characterized by oliguria and progressive azotemia, with a low urinary sodium concentration. This almost invariably fatal syndrome, linked to intense renal vasoconstriction-induced hypoperfusion with renal cortical ischemia, is characterized by a marked diminution in glomerular filtration rate in the absence of structural renal disease. Supportive therapy for this form of oliguric renal failure is similar to that used in other forms; management should be undertaken in consultation with the nephrologist. Liver transplantation may be required for patients with refractory hepatorenal syndrome or with recurrent ascites resistant to therapy.

## BIBLIOGRAPHY

Basile AS, Jones EA, Scolnick P: The pathogenesis and treatment of hepatic encephalopathy: evidence for the involvement of benzodiazepine receptor ligands, *Pharmacol Rev* 43:27, 1991.

de Franchis R et al: The natural history of asymptomatic hepatitis B surface antigen carriers, *Ann Intern Med* 118:191, 1993.

Edwards CQ, Kushner JP: Screening for hemochromatosis, *N Engl J Med* 328:1616, 1993.

Gines A et al: Incidence, predictive factors, and prognosis of the hepatorenal syndrome in cirrhosis with ascites, *Gastroenterology* 105:229, 1993.

Imperiale TF, McCullough AJ: Do corticosteroids reduce mortality from alcoholic hepatitis? A meta-analysis of the randomized trials, *Ann Intern Med* 113:299, 1990.

Koff RS: Viral hepatitis. In Schiff L, Schiff E, editors: *Diseases of the liver,* Philadelphia, 1993, JB Lippincott.

Krawczynski K: Hepatitis E, *Hepatology* 17:932, 1993.

Maddrey WC, Combes B: Therapeutic concepts of the management of idiopathic autoimmune chronic hepatitis, *Semin Liver Dis* 11:248, 1991.

Niederberger M, Schrier RW: Pathogenesis of sodium and water retention in liver disease, *Prog Liver Dis* 10:329, 1992.

Resnick RH, Koff R: Hepatitis C–related hepatocellular carcinoma, *Arch Intern Med* 153:1672, 1993.

Runyon BA et al: The serum-ascites albumin gradient is superior to the exudate-transudate concept in the differential diagnosis of ascites, *Ann Intern Med* 117:215, 1992.

Stiegmann GV et al: Endoscopic sclerotherapy as compared with endoscopic ligation for bleeding esophageal varices, *N Engl J Med* 326:1527, 1992.

Wong DKH et al: Effect of alpha-interferon treatment in patients with hepatitis B e antigen–positive chronic hepatitis B. A meta-analysis, *Ann Intern Med* 119:312, 1993.

CHAPTER

# 45 Gastrointestinal and Liver Tumors

Paul C. Schroy III

## TUMORS OF THE STOMACH

A variety of benign and malignant tumors can arise in the stomach (Table 45-1). Adenocarcinoma is the most common malignant neoplasm, followed by lymphoma and leiomyosarcoma. Leiomyoma is the most common benign neoplasm but is rarely clinically significant. Benign gastric polyps tend to be more relevant clinically but are relatively uncommon. Carcinoid tumors may also arise in the stomach. In general, these tumors are detected during radiographic or endoscopic evaluation of patients with nonspecific gastrointestinal complaints such as epigastric pain, nausea, vomiting, and bleeding. Progressive weight loss and the presence of a palpable mass are more ominous signs suggestive of malignancy. Because these tumors share similar radiographic appearances with each other as well as with benign diseases, particularly gastric ulcer, endoscopy with biopsy and brush cytology is the diagnostic modality of choice. Management varies considerably depending on tumor type and, in the case of malignancy, tumor stage.

### Gastric cancer

Gastric cancer is one of the most common cancers worldwide, even though both the incidence and death rate from gastric cancer have declined dramatically worldwide over the past 50 years. In the United States gastric cancer currently ranks eighth among causes of cancer-related death, accounting for more than 14,000 deaths per year. Overall 5-year survival is in the range of 12% to 14%.

***Epidemiology.*** Gastric cancer rates vary considerably. Japan, Russia, China, Iceland, Scandinavia, and parts of Latin America exhibit the highest rates, whereas India, parts of Africa (Uganda), and the United States have the lowest. In the United States the annual incidence of gastric cancer is approximately 9.6 cases per 100,000 population. In general, migrants tend to acquire a cancer risk similar to that of their host country, thus suggesting a strong role for environmental factors in the etiology of this disease.

***Etiology.*** The etiology of gastric cancer is obscure. Epidemiologic data provide strong evidence that that environmental factors, particularly diet, play a dominant role. Diets rich in complex carbohydrates (e.g., fava beans), salt, pickled or smoked foods, and dried fish have all been linked with an increased risk of gastric cancer. Conversely, diets rich in fresh fruits and vegetables have a negative association. Dietary nitrates have also been implicated on the basis of both epidemiologic evidence and rodent models of gastric carcinogenesis. It has been postulated that dietary nitrates may be reduced by bacteria

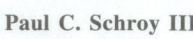

**Table 45-1.** Most common gastrointestinal and liver tumors

| Site | Benign | Malignant |
|---|---|---|
| Stomach | Leiomyoma<br>Hyperplastic polyp<br>Adenomatous polyp<br>Hamartomatous polyp | Adenocarcinoma<br>Primary lymphoma<br>Leiomyosarcoma<br>Carcinoid |
| Small bowel | Adenomatous polyp<br>Leiomyoma<br>Lipoma | Adenocarcinoma<br>Primary lymphoma<br>Carcinoid<br>Leiomyosarcoma |
| Large bowel | Adenomatous polyp<br>Hyperplastic polyp<br>Juvenile polyp<br>Pseudopolyp<br>Lipoma | Adenocarcinoma |
| Liver | Hemangioma<br>Adenoma<br>Focal nodular hyperplasia | Hepatocellular carcinoma<br>Cholangiocarcinoma |

into nitrites, which then combine with secondary amines in food, drugs, or pesticides to form carcinogenic nitrosamines.

Genetic factors also appear to play a role in the etiology of gastric cancer. Gastric cancer is one of the malignancies found in families with the cancer family syndrome. Gastric cancer has also been reported in patients with familial polyposis coli. Familial clustering has also been observed in the absence of these well-defined genetic syndromes. As with colon cancer, family members have a twofold to threefold increased risk of developing gastric cancer with one affected first-degree relative. It is interesting that familial risk is more strongly associated with the diffuse histopathologic type of gastric cancer than the intestinal type.

***Predisposing conditions.*** A variety of conditions have been associated with an increased risk of gastric cancer. Chronic atrophic gastritis with intestinal metaplasia and achlorhydria is found in the majority of patients with gastric cancer, but its etiologic role is unclear, since fewer than 10% of patients with this condition ultimately develop gastric cancer. Both pernicious anemia and adenomatous polyps, which are also associated with chronic atrophic gastritis, reduced gastric acidity, and intestinal metaplasia, are well-recognized predisposing conditions. Prior gastric surgery for peptic ulcer disease, particularly partial gastrectomy with Billroth II anastomosis, is associated with an increased risk of cancer in the gastric remnant 15 to 20 years after the initial surgery. Other premalignant conditions include Ménétrier's disease and common variable immunodeficiency syndrome. Recent epidemiologic data support an association between chronic *Helicobacter pylori* infection and gastric cancer. Surveillance with periodic endoscopic examinations has been recommended for many of these conditions, but strict guidelines have not been established.

The relationship between chronic gastric ulcer and gastric cancer is controversial. Most authorities currently agree that gastric ulcer does not predispose to gastric cancer. However, since gastric cancers may present as an ulcer, histologic and cytologic assessment is recommended for all gastric ulcers, regardless of their radiographic or endoscopic appearance. Follow-up endoscopy after 8 to 12 weeks of appropriate medical therapy is also indicated, since a small but significant number of malignant ulcers can demonstrate healing by radiographic criteria alone.

***Histopathology.*** Gastric cancers can arise in any region of the stomach. Over the past three decades there has been a proximal shift in distribution, with fewer cancers arising in the distal stomach and a greater number in the fundus, cardia, and gastroesophageal junction. Gastric cancers are also more likely to arise along the lesser curvature than the greater curvature.

Gastric cancers can assume a myriad of gross morphologic configurations. *Early gastric cancers* (i.e., tumors confined to the mucosa or submucosa regardless of lymph node status) may appear as a subtle polypoid protrusion, superficial plaque, mucosal discoloration, depression, or ulceration. More advanced cancers commonly present as polypoid or fungating masses with superficial ulceration; less commonly superficial spreading or infiltrating (linitis plastica) forms are encountered. Histologically the vast majority of malignant neoplasms of the stomach are adenocarcinomas. These can be subdivided into *diffuse* and *intestinal* types according to Lauren's classification system, or *infiltrative* and *expanding* types according Ming's classification system. The intestinal or expanding type tends to predominate in high-risk populations and is more common in men and older patients, associated with a relatively better prognosis, and preceded by a prolonged precancerous state. In contrast, the diffuse or infiltrative type predominates in women and younger patients, carries a poorer prognosis, and is not preceded by a known precancerous lesion.

***Clinical features.*** Although early gastric cancers may be diagnosed by routine endoscopy and biopsy, 90% of patients with gastric cancer seek medical help only when the cancer has progressed to a more advanced stage. Persistent abdominal pain, often mild and vague, associated with weight loss is the most common presentation. Weight loss is due to anorexia in 25% of patients and early satiety in 10%. Although occult gastrointestinal blood loss is quite common, gross hematemesis is rare. About half of the patients have a palpable epigastric mass. Jaundice, ascites, a periumbilical metastatic nodule (a Sister Mary Joseph node, named after a nun who noted that, when a palpable mass beneath the umbilicus was present, death was near), a Virchow node (left supraclavicular), and a firm mass palpable on rectal examination in the anterior cul de sac (Bloomer shelf) all suggest widespread metastases and a poor prognosis.

***Diagnosis.*** In high-risk countries such as Japan, mass screening of asymptomatic individuals with endoscopy, double-contrast radiography, and cytology have been successful in detecting a high percentage of early gastric

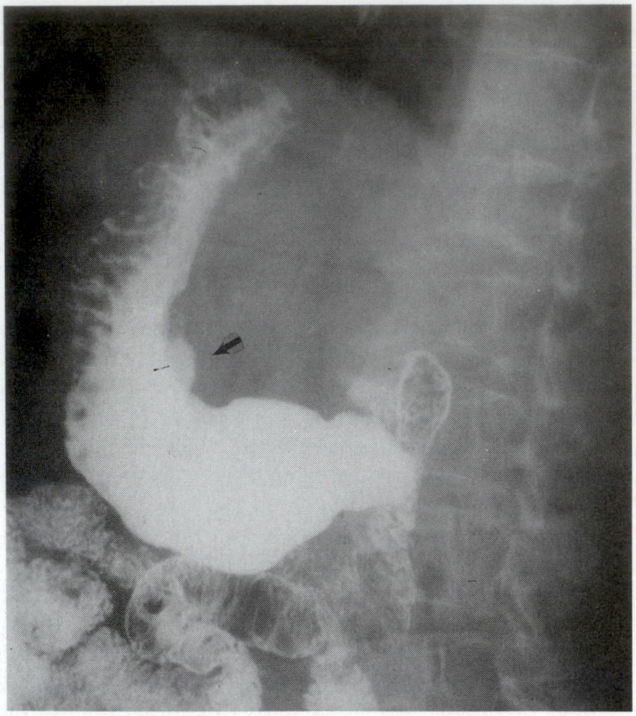

**Fig. 45-1.** The appearance of a gastric ulcer on an upper gastrointestinal series. Note that the ulcer *(arrow)* is within a mass.

cancers. Unfortunately, mass screening cannot be justified in the United States because of the relatively low incidence. Physicians must therefore rely on a high degree of suspicion when evaluating patients with vague nonspecific gastrointestinal complaints, particularly older patients with new dyspeptic symptoms or high-risk patients. Upper gastrointestinal (UGI) radiography and endoscopy are the principal diagnostic modalities. UGI radiography is widely used as an initial diagnostic test for symptomatic patients. Air-contrast studies afford greater accuracy, particularly for early mucosal abnormalities. Abnormal findings such as a mass with or without ulceration (Fig. 45-1), enlarged gastric folds, and lack of distensibility (leather bottle appearance) require endoscopic follow-up and tissue confirmation. Endoscopy is also warranted in patients with equivocal radiographic findings, as well as in those with suspicious clinical presentations but negative x-ray results. At endoscopy multiple biopsies and brush cytology should be obtained of any mass lesion, ulceration, area of discoloration, unexplained mucosal depression, or prominent fold(s). Repeat endoscopy with tissue sampling may be necessary if histologic or cytologic assessment is nondiagnostic.

Once the diagnosis is established, an extent of disease evaluation is warranted to optimize treatment planning and determine prognosis. Endoscopic ultrasound provides an accurate assessment of depth of tumor invasion into the bowel wall and may give useful information regarding perigastric lymph nodes. Computerized tomography (CT) provides an accurate assessment of regional and retroperitoneal lymph node involvement, direct extension into contiguous organs, liver metastases, and ascites. Paracentesis with cytologic examination should be performed if ascites is present. Laparoscopy may also be useful in the evaluation of patients with unexplained ascites and negative or equivocal CT scans. Enlarged peripheral lymph nodes (e.g., Virchow's node) require biopsy. Additional studies such as abdominal ultrasound, radionuclide scanning, magnetic resonance imaging (MRI), and angiography may be useful in select cases.

***Treatment.*** Surgical resection is the only potentially curative treatment for gastric cancer. All patients should be considered for surgery unless there is evidence of widespread metastatic disease, the patient is a poor surgical candidate, the primary tumor is clearly unresectable, or total gastrectomy is required with only palliative intent. Curative resection requires wide excision of the primary tumor and en bloc removal of regional lymph nodes and contiguous structures. The actual extent of resection is determined at the time of surgery and depends on a number of factors, most notably tumor size, location, and lymph node status. A palliative resection should be considered in patients with incurable disease to diminish the risk of complications, such as bleeding, perforation, or gastric outlet obstruction. Chemotherapy should be considered for patients with surgically incurable disease. Combination regimens comprising the most active single agents, such as 5-fluorouracil, doxorubicin plus mitomycin C, or cisplatin, have yielded the best response rates but have had little impact on long-term survival. Radiotherapy has been used primarily as a palliative approach to specific tumor-related problems, such as bleeding, obstruction and pain secondary to local extension, liver infiltration, and bone metastases.

***Follow-up.*** The postoperative management of patients with gastric cancer is largely dependent on the status of the disease after resection. Patients with residual or inoperable disease should be considered for radiation or chemotherapy. Those without evidence of disease should be closely monitored for signs or symptoms of recurrence. Since 85% occur within the first 2 years, patients should be evaluated at frequent intervals during this period. Follow-up should include a careful history, physical examination, and routine laboratory tests (complete blood count and liver profile) every 3 to 6 months for the first 2 years and every 6 to 12 months thereafter. In addition, a CT scan of the abdomen, chest radiograph, and UGI endoscopy with biopsy of the anastomosis should be obtained 6 to 12 months after surgery, and then yearly. Suspicious findings warrant aggressive diagnostic evaluation and tissue confirmation.

***Prognosis.*** Prognosis depends largely on tumor stage at the time of diagnosis. The tumor, node, metastasis (TNM) classification system is currently the most widely used staging system (Table 45-2). Based on this system, 5-year survival rates range from 85% to 90% for stage I disease to 3% for stage IV. Unfortunately, overall survival is only 12% to 14%, indicating that most patients present with advanced, incurable disease.

## Gastric polyps

Gastric polyps are uncommon, occurring in less than 2% of autopsy surveys. Because of their rarity, epidemiologic

**Table 45-2.** Gastric cancer: 5-year survival by stage of disease at time of diagnosis

| Stage | TNM | | Description | 5-year survival (%) |
|---|---|---|---|---|
| I | $T_1\ N_0\ M_0$ | T1 | Tumor limited to mucosa or submucosa | 85-90 |
| | | N0 | No lymph node metastases | |
| | | M0 | No distant metastases | |
| II | $T_{2\text{-}3}\ N_0\ M_0$ | T2 | Tumor involves muscularis, does not penetrate serosa | 52-55 |
| | | T3 | Tumor penetrates serosa, does not involve contiguous structures | 45-47 |
| III | $T_{1\text{-}3}\ N_{1\text{-}3}\ M_0$ | N1 | Involvement of perigastric nodes within 3 cm of tumor | 17-20 |
| | | N2 | Involvement of regional nodes more than 3 cm from tumor, resectable | 5-10 |
| | | N3 | Other intraabdominal and nonremovable nodes involved by tumor | |
| IV | $T_4\ N_{1\text{-}3}\ M_0$ | T4 | Tumor invades contiguous structures (includes unresectable tumors) | 3 |
| | $T_{1\text{-}4}\ N_{0\text{-}3}\ M_1$ | M1 | Distant metastases present | |

and etiologic data are scant. They are almost always asymptomatic and usually discovered incidentally at endoscopic or radiologic examination. Patients may complain of vague epigastric pain unrelated to eating, bloating, belching, or nausea. Occult gastrointestinal bleeding and iron-deficiency anemia may also occur, but hematemesis is rare. Pedunculated polyps located near the pylorus may occasionally present with symptoms of intermittent gastric outlet obstruction due to prolapse.

*Hyperplastic* polyps are the most frequent histologic type, accounting for 75% to 90% of all benign gastric epithelial polyps. These polyps are also referred to as regenerative or inflammatory polyps, since they comprise a proliferation of normal gastric mucosal elements without evidence of atypia and inflammatory cells. Often small (under 2 cm) and solitary, they exhibit no predilection for site, occurring with equal frequency in the proximal and distal stomach. A diffuse hyperplastic polyposis may be seen in up to one third of patients and may represent a form of Ménétrier's disease. Hyperplastic polyps may be associated with chronic *H. pylori* infection and active gastritis. Malignant transformation is rare but has been reported.

*Adenomatous* polyps are far less common, accounting for 10% to 20% of benign gastric epithelial polyps. Unlike hyperplastic polyps, adenomatous polyps are true neoplastic lesions that carry a significant risk of malignant transformation, particularly over 2 cm. Histologically villous, tubulovillous, or, rarely, tubular patterns of growth may be observed with varying degrees of cellular atypia (dysplasia). These lesions typically present as large (over 2 cm), solitary lesions in the gastric antrum. They may coexist with gastric adenocarcinoma and are not uncommon in pernicious anemia.

*Hamartomatous* polyps are rare. These occur either sporadically or as part of a polyposis syndrome. They are usually small (under 5 mm) and multiple. Because of a predilection for the proximal stomach, they are sometimes referred to as fundic gland polyps. Histologically they resemble normal fundic mucosa with cystic gland dilatation of the upper half of the gland. Hamartomatous polyps are nonneoplastic and have no malignant potential.

Gastric polyps are frequently encountered in patients with inherited polyposis syndromes. Hamartomatous polyps of the stomach have been described in familial adenomatous polyposis coli and Gardner's syndrome, Peutz-Jeghers syndrome, Cronkhite-Canada syndrome, and Cowden's disease. Adenomatous gastric polyps are also found in persons with familial adenomatous polyposis coli and Gardner's syndrome.

The management of gastric polyps largely depends on clinicopathologic considerations. All polypoid gastric lesions require biopsy to establish a histologic diagnosis. All symptomatic polyps should be removed either endoscopically or surgically. Asymptomatic hyperplastic polyps, if small and adequately biopsied, do not need to be removed. The same is true for hamartomatous polyps. Adenomatous polyps should be completely excised because of their premalignant nature. Surgical resection is indicated for any polyp containing malignant tissue, adenomatous polyps not amenable to complete endoscopic removal, and polyps with nondiagnostic histology. Patients with adenomatous gastric polyps require annual endoscopic surveillance because of the risk of developing new polyps or cancer. Surveillance is not recommended for patients with only hyperplastic or hamartomatous polyps.

### Gastric lymphoma

Primary gastric lymphoma accounts for 1% to 5% of all gastric malignancies and is anatomically the most common extranodal type of non-Hodgkin's lymphoma. The stomach is also commonly involved in patients with disseminated disease arising elsewhere. Grossly, gastric lymphoma is often indistinguishable from gastric adenocarcinoma, presenting as an infiltrating submucosal lesion, ulcerated mass, or polypoid lesion. Histologically most are of the diffuse large cell (histiocytic) type. Symptoms are nonspecific and include abdominal pain, nausea, vomiting, anorexia, weight loss, and bleeding.

The diagnosis of gastric lymphoma should be considered in any person found to have diffuse mucosal hypertrophy with irregular thickening of the rugal folds or an ulcerated or polypoid mass at endoscopy or upper gastrointestinal series. Endoscopic biopsies and brush cytology should be obtained to establish the diagnosis but may be nondiagnostic due to the submucosal location of the tumor. Newer modalities such as endoscopic ultrasound and fine-needle aspiration may be useful in difficult cases. In many cases laparotomy may be required to confirm the diagnosis. CT of the abdomen and chest and a bone marrow aspiration/biopsy provide additional staging information.

The treatment of gastric lymphomas, albeit controver-

**Table 45-3.** Ann Arbor classification of gastric lymphomas

| Stage | Extent of disease |
|---|---|
| IE | Disease limited to stomach |
| IIE | Extention to abdominal nodes |
| IIIE | Involvement of stomach, abdominal nodes, and nodes above the diaphragm |
| IV | Disseminated |

*E*, Extranodal site.

sial, largely depends on the stage of disease. Among the many staging systems that have been proposed, the Ann Arbor classification (Table 45-3) is the most suitable and widely used. Surgery is the mainstay of treatment for stage IE disease (*E* refers to extranodal) and may be curative. Complete resection of all gross tumor with pathologic confirmation of negative margins rather than total gastrectomy is the most widely accepted approach. Postoperative radiation and/or chemotherapy may further improve outcome. Optimal treatment for Stage IIE is unclear but often includes combination chemotherapy, either alone or in combination with surgery or radiation. Stage IIIE or IVE should be treated with combination chemotherapy. Surgery should be considered, regardless of the stage, if there is uncertainty regarding the diagnosis, or if there is bulky transmural involvement so as to prevent treatment-induced hemorrhage or perforation. The overall 5-year survival in patients with gastric lymphoma is approximately 40% to 45%.

### Stromal tumors

*Leiomyomas* are the most common benign tumor of the stomach, occurring in up to 50% of persons over the age of 50. The vast majority are small (under 2 cm) and clinically silent. Larger lesions may ulcerate the overlying mucosa and produce bleeding or abdominal pain. These tumors arise from the smooth muscle layer of the stomach and therefore appear as intramural filling defects with or without superficial ulceration on upper gastrointestinal series or submucosal masses endoscopically. Endoscopic biopsies are frequently nondiagnostic, unless the lesion is ulcerated. Local surgical excision is the treatment of choice for symptomatic lesions.

*Leiomyosarcomas* account for approximately 1% of gastric malignancies. These tumors are sometimes difficult to distinguish from benign leiomyomas, unless there is evidence of local extension or distant metastasis. Like leiomyomas, gastrointestinal bleeding and abdominal pain are the most common presenting symptoms. The presence of a palpable abdominal mass and weight loss are highly suggestive of malignancy. Surgical resection is the treatment of choice, but unfortunately two thirds of patients have extragastric spread at the time of initial laparotomy. Neither radiotherapy nor chemotherapy has demonstrated significant efficacy. Five-year survival rates are in the range of 25% to 50%.

### Gastric carcinoids

Carcinoid tumors of the stomach are rare. Although the pathogenesis of gastric carcinoids is not well understood, hypergastrinemia appears to be a predisposing condition, since there is an increased frequency of such tumors in patients with pernicious anemia, atrophic gastritis with achlorhydria, and Zollinger-Ellison syndrome. Most gastric carcinoids are small and asymptomatic. Grossly they may resemble an ordinary ulcer, polyp, or tumor mass; occasionally multiple lesions are present. Histologically it is often difficult to distinguish between benign and malignant tumors, unless metastases are present. Gastric carcinoids are of foregut origin and may secrete a variety of hormones, including 5-hydroxytryptophan, ACTH, or 5-hydroxytryptamine (serotonin). Hence patients may present with clinical manifestations of the carcinoid syndrome or Cushing's syndrome, but both are rare in the absence of liver metastases. An elevation in 24-hour urinary levels of 5-hydroxyindoleacetic acid (5-HIAA) confirms the diagnosis in such patients. Decisions regarding management are contingent upon size and histology. Complete endoscopic or surgical excision is the treatment of choice for small (under 1 cm) incidentally discovered lesions. Larger lesions tend to exhibit more aggressive biologic behavior and warrant wide surgical resection with lymph node dissection. Management of metastatic disease and the carcinoid syndrome is discussed below under Small Bowel Carcinoid Tumors.

## TUMORS OF THE SMALL BOWEL

Primary tumors of the small bowel are uncommon by comparison with other sites in the gastrointestinal tract. The relative paucity of small bowel tumors is particularly intriguing when one considers that the small bowel accounts for 75% of the length of the gastrointestinal tract and more than 90% of its mucosal surface area. Neutral or alkaline luminal pH, rapid transit, the liquid nature of the luminal contents, a paucity of anaerobic bacteria, and the presence of detoxifying enzymes (e.g., benzopyrene hydroxylase) capable of nullifying the effects of putative carcinogens have all been implicated as plausible explanations for this phenomenom. Despite their rarity, small bowel tumors should be considered in the differential diagnosis of patients with symptoms suggestive of intermittent partial small bowel obstruction or unexplained occult gastrointestinal blood loss. The most common types of benign and malignant small bowel tumors are listed in Table 45-1.

### Epidemiology

The epidemiology of benign small bowel tumors is not well defined because most are asymptomatic and not evident clinically. Conversely, accurate epidemiologic data for malignant small bowel tumors are available due to their progressive and ultimately symptomatic nature. Overall, tumors of the small bowel account for approximately 1% of all gastrointestinal malignancies. In 1992 there were approximately 3400 new cases and 950 deaths from malignant small bowel tumors in the United States. Incidence figures suggest a slight male predominance, with an overall incidence of less than 1 case per 100,000 population. Malignant small bowel tumors tend to be more common in developed countries, with the exception of immunoproliferative small intestine disease (IPSID) (also known as $\alpha$-chain disease), Mediterranean lymphoma, and diffuse primary small intestine lymphoma, which predominates in impoverished geographic regions.

## Etiology

The etiology of most small bowel tumors is poorly understood. Although causative factors undoubtedly vary with histologic type, common factors must exist, since patients with celiac sprue are predisposed to both adenocarcinoma and lymphoma of the small bowel. As in the colon, small bowel adenocarcinomas probably arise from preexisting benign adenomas, but the molecular mechanisms responsible for malignant transformation are unknown. Microbial colonization appears to be an important etiologic factor in the IPSID form of primary small bowel lymphoma based on its epidemiology and the observation that the disease is reversible if treated with tetracycline at the early prelymphomatous stage. Impairment of the normal mechanical or immunologic barriers resulting in increased mucosal penetration of deleterious pathogens and/or antigens has also been implicated in the etiology of small bowel tumors in patients with Crohn's disease and celiac sprue.

## Predisposing conditions

A number of mostly rare conditions appear to be associated with an increased risk of malignant small bowel tumors. Celiac sprue, Crohn's disease, familial adenomatous polyposis coli/Gardner's syndrome, neurofibromatosis, and various reconstructive procedures involving the ileum such as an ileal conduit, ileocystoplasty, and ileostomy have all been associated with an increased risk of small bowel adenocarcinomas. Celiac sprue, IPSID, nodular lymphoid hyperplasia, and the acquired immunodeficiency syndrome (AIDS) predispose to small bowel lymphomas. With the exception of familial adenomatous polyposis coli, periodic surveillance is generally not recommended for these conditions.

## Histopathology and differential diagnosis

***Benign tumors.*** Adenomas, leiomyomas, and lipomas are the most common benign tumors of the small bowel. *Adenomas* arise from the epithelial elements and can display tubular, tubulovillous, or villous growth patterns. Although the natural history of small bowel adenomas is not well defined, available evidence would suggest that they probably have a similar malignant potential to colorectal adenomas. Most are small and may be sessile or pedunculated. Both sporadic adenomas and those associated with familial polyposis syndromes have a predilection for the proximal small intestine, particularly in the periampullary region of the duodenum. Periampullary adenomas, particularly of the villous type, are associated with a high risk of invasive adenocarcinoma.

*Leiomyomas* and *lipomas* form from smooth muscle and fatty tissue, respectively. It is unknown if they can degenerate into malignant forms, but if this occurs it must be very rare. Other benign tumors are curiosities.

***Malignant tumors.*** *Adenocarcinomas* are the most common malignant tumors of the small bowel. Most of these malignancies originate in the proximal small bowel, from the second part of the duodenum to about 20 to 30 cm distant to the ligament of Treitz. Structurally they may be flat, stenosing, infiltrating, ulcerating, or polypoid lesions. Histologic appearance is similar to that of colorectal adenocarcinomas.

*Lymphomas* of the small bowel can be divided into three general types. First, in the Western world primary small bowel lymphomas usually present as localized tumors in the jejunum or, most commonly, the ileum. Virtually all are of the non-Hodgkin's type and are usually staged according to the Rappaport classification system. Most are of B cell origin, except for those associated with long-standing celiac sprue, which are of T cell origin. Second, in the Middle East and other developing countries diffuse IPSID-related lymphomas predominate. These lymphomas arise from IgA-secreting B cells in the lamina propria. During the early stages of the disease an $\alpha$–heavy chain paraproteinemia may be detectable, hence the name $\alpha$-chain disease. Malabsorption is common. Third, secondary lymphomas, which originate elsewhere and spread to the small intestine, are the most common type of small bowel lymphoma.

Like benign leiomyomas, *leiomyosarcomas* arise from smooth muscle cells. Early stage tumors may be difficult to distinguish from leiomyomas. More advanced tumors tend to be less differentiated and easier to diagnose histologically.

*Carcinoids* belong to the neuroendocrine or amine precursor uptake and decarboxylation (APUD) family of tumors. Although carcinoids can occur anywhere in the gut, the small bowel, particularly the ileum, is the most common site of malignant tumors. These tumors arise in the epithelial compartment, presumably from specialized hormone-producing cells derived from the neural crest. Carcinoid tumors are capable of producing a variety of biologically active substances. Depending on the site of origin, these may include serotonin, gastrin, histamine, somatostatin, pituitary hormones, catecholamines, kinins, or prostaglandins, to name only a few. Foregut carcinoids (duodenum and jejunum) tend to produce a wide range of humoral mediators, whereas midgut carcinoids (ileum) produce mainly serotonin and substance P or other tachykinins. In general, localized tumors are rarely associated with the carcinoid syndrome, since they secrete only small amounts of hormone(s), which are rapidly inactivated by the liver. The carcinoid syndrome is much more frequently associated with bulky metastatic disease involving the liver. Histologically, it is often difficult to distinguish benign from malignant tumors. Localized tumors less than 1 cm are generally regarded as benign and those greater than 2 cm as malignant.

## Clinical features

Benign tumors are often asymptomatic and clinically insignificant. Fluctuating abdominal pain due to intermittent partial small bowel obstruction is the most frequent presenting manifestation of symptomatic lesions. Obstruction is often due to intussusception. Of note are benign small bowel tumors, particularly lipomas, the most common cause of intussusception in adults. Occult gastrointestinal bleeding may also be seen, but frank hematemesis or rectal bleeding is rare.

Because of their progressive nature, malignant tumors eventually become symptomatic and ultimately fatal unless detected early. Abdominal pain is the most common presenting symptom and may be colicky or more constant. Occult gastrointestinal blood loss is also common, but frank bleeding is rare except in the case of leiomyosarcomas. Weight loss occurs in up to 50% of patients and

**Table 45-4.** Clinical manifestations of the carcinoid syndrome

| Organ | Manifestation |
|---|---|
| Skin | Flushing |
| | Telangiectasia |
| | Cyanosis |
| | Pellagra |
| Gastrointestinal tract | Diarrhea |
| | Cramping |
| Heart | Valvular lesions |
| Respiratory tract | Wheezing |
| Kidney | Peripheral edema |
| Joints | Arthritis |

may be secondary to malabsorption, particularly in the case of diffuse lymphomas of the α-chain or Mediterranean type. Perforation is rare but may be seen with lymphomas or leiomyosarcomas. Jaundice is a common presenting feature of malignant periampullary tumors. The constellation of flushing, diarrhea, abdominal pain, and valvular heart disease typify the carcinoid syndrome, but other manifestations may also be present (Table 45-4). Foregut carcinoids may also cause symptoms of hypoglycemia, gastric hypersecretion, or Cushing's syndrome.

## Diagnosis

Historically barium contrast radiography has been the principal modality for the preoperative detection of small bowel tumors. The routine small bowel follow-through after oral ingestion of barium is useful in assessing the terminal ileum but less sensitive than enteroclysis (small bowel enema) in assessing other parts of the small bowel. Since enteroclysis requires duodenal intubation, it is reasonable to obtain a routine small bowel study with compression views of the terminal ileum as the initial diagnostic study in patients with suspected small bowel tumors. If this examination is negative or inconclusive, enteroclysis should be performed.

Endoscopic approaches are also useful in the diagnosis of small bowel tumors. In addition to direct visualization, endoscopy provides a means of obtaining tissue for histologic evaluation of abnormal findings. Endoscopy is the procedure of choice in patients with occult gastrointestinal blood loss. Otherwise asymptomatic patients, however, should first undergo colonoscopy to exclude the presence of a colonic neoplasm. Evaluation of the UGI tract is indicated if the colonoscopy is negative or if the condition suggests UGI disease. UGI endoscopy should also be performed to further evaluate abnormal radiographic findings. Standard forward-viewing gastroduodenoscopes permit direct visualization of the proximal gastrointestinal tract down to the level of the second and sometimes third part of the duodenum, including the ampulla of Vater. Push enteroscopy with either a pediatric or adult colonoscope permits visualization beyond the ligament of Treitz into the proximal jejunum. Retrograde ileoscopy during colonoscopy permits visualization of the terminal ileum. Until recently the jejunum and proximal ileum could be evaluated only intraoperatively. However, fiberoptic enteroscopes that potentially obviate the need for laparotomy have been developed. These so-called Sonde enteroscopes are passed nasally and advanced by peristalsis. Unfortunately these instruments are difficult to maneuver and, because of their small diameter, lack a biopsy channel. Moreover, Sonde enteroscopy should not be performed in cases of partial or complete obstruction because of the prolonged time required for passage and impaired visualization due to excessive secretions. Finally, side-viewing endoscopes are useful in evaluating the periampullary region and performing endoscopic retrograde cholangiopancreatography in patients with evidence of extrahepatic biliary tract obstruction.

Other potentially useful diagnostic modalities include CT, particularly for preoperative staging of malignant tumors and, in select cases, arteriography.

Urinary 5-HIAA, a metabolite of serotonin, should be measured in patients with clinical features suggestive of carcinoid syndrome. Levels greater than 10 mg per 24 hours confirm the diagnosis in most cases. Serotonin-containing foods and drugs (e.g., phenothiazines) that elevate serotonin levels can give false positive results and should be withheld during testing. Malabsorption and chronic intestinal obstruction can also cause modest elevations in urinary 5-HIAA levels. Plasma or platelet serotonin levels can also be measured, but these tests are not widely available.

## Treatment and prognosis

***Benign tumors.*** Adenomas of the small bowel should be treated because of their premalignant status. Appropriate therapy depends on a number of factors, including location, size, shape (sessile or pedunculated), and histologic type (tubular or villous). Duodenal adenomas, with the exception of periampullary lesions, are usually amenable to endoscopic removal or ablation. Although some periampullary adenomas can also be treated endoscopically, surgical resection is preferred for most because of their sessile shape, villous histology, and propensity for malignant transformation. Local resection is considered adequate for completely benign tumors; more radical resection (i.e., pancreaticoduodenectomy [Whipple procedure]) is indicated for adenomas containing carcinoma. Unlike for colorectal adenomas, long-term surveillance is not indicated for sporadic adenomas unless there is the concern of incomplete removal. Surveillance is recommended for patients with familial polyposis coli or Gardner's syndrome. Although strict guidelines have not been adopted, it is reasonable to perform a UGI endoscopy before prophylactic colectomy at age 30 and every 5 years thereafter.

Limited resection is adequate treatment for other benign tumors of the small bowel. Observation alone may be sufficient for asymptomatic tumors discovered incidentally at endoscopy, assuming biopsies confirm benign histology.

***Malignant tumors.*** Surgical resection is the only potentially curative treatment for adenocarcinomas of the small bowel. Palliative resection or bypass should be considered if curative resection is not feasible. Palliative procedures should also be considered to control bleeding or relieve obstruction. Unfortunately, neither chemotherapy nor radiation therapy is effective in the treatment of advanced disease. Overall 5-year survival is only 10% to 20% even after "curative" resection.

Optimal treatment of primary small bowel lymphomas depends on extent of involvement and stage. Surgical resection is indicated for localized lymphomas confined to the bowel wall (stage IE) or involving contiguous nodes only (stage IIE). The role of adjuvant radiation therapy or chemotherapy following curative resection is controversial. Resection should also be considered for more advanced segmental disease in hope of both reducing tumor burden and obviating the risk of bleeding or perforation induced by radiation therapy or chemotherapy. Radiation therapy, alone or in combination with chemotherapy, is the treatment of choice for patients with diffuse unresectable small bowel disease. Disseminated disease is usually treated with radiation therapy plus combination chemotherapy. Five-year survival rates range from 40% to 47% for resectable disease to less than 25% for unresectable disease. For unclear reasons patients with preexisting celiac sprue have a worse prognosis, stage for stage, than those without underlying small bowel disease.

*Carcinoid* tumors of the small bowel should be resected because of their potential to invade and metastasize. Tumors less than 1 cm are usually benign and can be cured with a limited surgical resection. Larger tumors, particularly those greater than 2 cm, require more radical surgical resection. Surgical debulking, hepatic artery embolization with materials such as Gelfoam, hepatic artery ligation, and hepatic dearterialization procedures have been advocated for patients with metastatic disease in hope of minimizing symptoms of the carcinoid syndrome. Synthetic analogues of somatostatin, including octreotide and ondansetron, have demonstrated impressive efficacy in controlling both the clinical features and biochemical abnormalties of the carcinoid syndrome. Tumor regression has also been observed with long-term octreotide therapy. Combination chemotherapy with 5-fluorouracil plus streptozocin has demonstrated response rates of about 40% but has little impact on overall survival. Although overall 5-year survival is only around 54%, prolonged survival is not uncommon, even in the setting of metastatic disease.

Surgical resection is the treatment of choice for leiomyosarcoma. Chemotherapy with doxorubicin-containing regimens and radiation therapy both have a role in the management of unresectable disease. Surgery has also been advocated in the treatment of solitary liver or lung metastases. Overall 5-year survival rates of 20% to 50% have been reported.

## TUMORS OF THE LARGE BOWEL

Colorectal tumors are commonly encountered in the evaluation of both symptomatic and asymptomatic individuals. Polyps are the most common benign tumors and may be classified as neoplastic (adenomatous polyps), nonneoplastic (e.g., hyperplastic polyps), or submucosal (e.g., lipomas). Adenomatous polyps (adenomas) are premalignant precursors of most colorectal cancers; in contrast, nonneoplastic polyps have little or no malignant potential. Adenocarcinomas are by far the most common malignant tumors. Lymphomas, carcinoids, sarcomas, and a variety of extremely rare malignant tumors may also occur in the large bowel. This discussion focuses primarily on adenocarcinoma of the large bowel, commonly referred to as colorectal cancer, and its precursor, the adenomatous polyp.

### Epidemiology

Worldwide incidence and mortality of colorectal cancer vary considerably. With the notable exception of Japan, industrialized countries are at greatest risk. High rates are found in North America, Western Europe, and New Zealand, whereas lower rates are found in Eastern Europe, most South American countries, Asia, and Africa. Incidence rates have been increasing worldwide over the past several decades. In the United States incidence rates appear to be stable but remain in excess of 40 cases per 100,000 persons. In 1994 alone there were approximately 149,000 new cases and 56,000 deaths—figures second only to lung cancer. Americans of average risk have approximately a 5% chance of developing colorectal cancer during their lifetime. Age is an important determinant of risk. Although extremely uncommon in individuals below the age 35 (except with rare predisposing genetic syndromes), the incidence of colorectal cancer increases steadily with age, particularly after age 50. Cancers of the colon affect men and women at similar rates, whereas cancers of the rectum are more common in men. Overall 5-year survival rates have improved significantly in recent years, presumably due to improved therapy and early detection, and are currently in the range of 54% to 57%. Low-income minority groups, particularly African-American males, tend to have lower survival rates even after adjustment for tumor stage.

The epidemiology of colorectal adenomas is similar to that of colorectal cancer. In general, the prevalence of colorectal adenomas in a given country parallels the prevalence of colorectal cancer. Age is an important determinant of prevalence in high-risk countries. In the United States autopsy studies suggest an overall prevalence of 50%, ranging from around 30% at age 50 to 55% at age 80. Unlike colorectal cancer, adenomas are more common in men.

### Etiology

The etiology of colorectal adenomas and subsequent colorectal cancer is unknown but seems related to both environmental and genetic factors. The importance of environmental factors is supported both by the wide geographic variation in incidence rates and studies of migrant populations. Diet has been strongly implicated as the major environmental factor by which to explain these epidemiologic associations. In general, populations with a relatively high prevalence of colorectal adenomas and cancer consume high-calorie, high-fat diets. Conversely, populations at low risk consume diets rich in fruits, vegetables and crude fiber. A variety of mechanisms have been proposed by which to explain these associations. It has been suggested that increased fat intake results in (1) increased luminal concentrations of secondary and deconjugated bile acids, which have been shown to have tumor-promoting activity in experimental models of colorectal cancer; (2) increased deleterious lipid peroxidation radicals generated from fat metabolism; (3) increased incorporation of fatty acids in cell membranes; (4)

increased synthesis of prostaglandins, which can stimulate cell proliferation; (5) alterations in gut bacteria; and (6) an increase in available calories. Conversely, high-fiber diets might have a dilutional effect on luminal carcinogens and/or facilitate transit time, thereby reducing the time of mucosal exposure to noxious substances; alter the gut flora such that it is capable of detoxifying potential carcinogens; and/or decrease fecal pH, causing deionization of potentially harmful free fatty acids and bile acids. Although these associations have been documented by both epidemiologic studies and experimental models, it remains unknown whether dietary alterations can reduce the risk of colorectal cancer.

Genetic factors also appear to be of considerable importance in the etiology of colorectal adenomas and cancers. There are well-established hereditary polyposis and nonpolyposis colorectal cancer syndromes, most of which exhibit an autosomal dominant mode of inheritance. Together these syndromes account for approximately 6% of new cases of colorectal cancer annually. Genetic factors have also been implicated in many sporadic cases. It has long been recognized that first-degree relatives (parents, children, siblings) of individuals with colorectal cancer are at increased risk. Moreover, recent data from pedigree studies of a large kindred of affected individuals suggest an autosomal dominant mode of inheritance for most sporadic colorectal adenomas and cancers.

Elucidation of the molecular genetics of colorectal cancer has provided additional evidence for the role of genetic factors. The gene responsible for familial adenomatous polyposis and Gardner's syndrome, referred to as the *APC* (adenomatous polyposis coli) gene on chromosome 5, has been identified and cloned. Alterations in a number of other genes, including the *ras* protooncogene on chromosome 2, the *MCC* (mutated in colon cancer) gene on chromosome 5, the *p53* tumor suppressor gene on chromosome 17, and the *DCC* (deleted in colon cancer) gene on chromosome 18 have also been identified in a variable percentage of familial and sporadic colorectal cancers and adenomas.

### Predisposing conditions for colorectal cancer

Personal history
- Colorectal adenomas
- Colorectal cancer
- Breast, ovarian, endometrial cancer

Inherited adenomatous polyposis
- Familial adenomatous polyposis
- Gardner's syndrome
- Turcot syndrome

Hereditary nonpolyposis colorectal cancer
- Lynch I (site-specific)
- Lynch II (family cancer syndrome)

Family history
- Colorectal adenomas
- Colorectal cancer

Inflammatory bowel disease

Inherited nonadenomatous polyposis
- Generalized juvenile polyposis
- Peutz-Jeghers syndrome

## Predisposing conditions

A number of conditions have been associated with an increased risk of colorectal cancer (see the box above). Recognition of these high-risk groups has important implications with respect to screening.

***Personal history of colorectal adenomas/cancer.*** It is widely accepted that, with rare exception, virtually all colorectal cancers arise from adenomas. Evidence supporting the adenoma-carcinoma sequence is derived from epidemiologic, morphologic, biologic, clinical, and therapeutic data. Patients with a history of adenomatous polyps have at 50% risk of developing a metachronous adenoma and a 5% to 8% risk of developing a cancer within 15 years of follow-up. The risk of developing a metachronous cancer in patients with a history of colorectal cancer is less well defined but is probably in the range of 5%.

***Inherited adenomatous polyposis syndromes.*** The inherited adenomatous polyposis syndromes include familial adenomatous polyposis coli (FAP), Gardner's syndrome, and Turcot syndrome. FAP is a rare autosomal dominant condition characterized by the presence of 100 or more colorectal adenomas. The disease is caused by mutations of the *APC* gene on chromosome 5. The polyps are not present at birth but appear during the second or third decade of life. If left untreated, the risk of colorectal cancer is 100% by age 40. There is also an increased incidence of gastric and small bowel polyps. The duodenal papilla and periampullary region have a particular propensity for adenomatous and occasionally carcinomatous change.

Gardner's syndrome is distinguished from FAP by the presence of extraintestinal manifestations, including desmoids, osteoma, benign soft tissue tumors (e.g., lipomas), dental abnormalities, and congenital hypertrophy of the retinal pigment epithelium. There is also an increased incidence of CNS, thyroid, adrenal, and liver (hepatoblastoma) cancers. Otherwise, the syndrome is identical to FAP.

Turcot syndrome is an extremely rare autosomal dominant disease characterized by CNS tumors and colorectal adenomatous polyposis. Extraintestinal manifestations of Gardner's syndrome may also be seen. Colorectal cancer risk is similar to that of FAP.

***Hereditary nonpolyposis colorectal cancer syndromes.*** Two types of familial nonpolyposis colorectal cancer syndromes have been identified. Lynch syndrome I, or hereditary site-specific colorectal cancer, is an autosomal dominant condition with high penetrance characterized by early onset colorectal cancer (average age 44 years) in the absence of polyposis, a predominance of tumors proximal to the splenic flexure (approximately 70%), and an excess of both synchronous and metachronous colorectal cancers. Lynch syndrome II, or cancer family syndrome, is a closely related condition that includes all of the features of Lynch syndrome I but is also characterized by early onset of cancers of other sites, including the endometrium, ovaries, stomach, and brain. Torre's syndrome, a rare familial condition characterized by multiple sebaceous gland tumors and colorectal cancer, is a subtype of Lynch syndrome II. Although the absence of multiple polyps is a prerequisite for the diagnosis, the colorectal cancers in both syndromes arise from preexisting adenomas.

***Family history of colorectal adenomas/cancer.*** It has long been recognized that a family history of colorectal cancer increases an individual's risk of colorectal cancer. Results of several epidemiologic surveys indicate that individuals with a single first-degree affected relative have a twofold to threefold increased lifetime risk of developing colorectal cancer compared to the average person in the general population. Individuals with two first-degree affected relatives have an even greater risk. The same is true for individuals with a family history of colorectal adenomas.

***Inflammatory bowel disease.*** Patients with both chronic idiopathic ulcerative colitis and Crohn's disease have an increased risk of colorectal cancer. The actual degree of risk, however, is debatable. For ulcerative colitis the duration of disease and extent of involvement are important determinants of risk. Patients with pancolitis of greater than 7 years' duration or left-sided colitis of 15 years' duration are at increased risk. Duration of disease also appears to be a factor in patients with Crohn's disease. Unlike most colorectal cancers that arise from adenomas, cancers associated with inflammatory bowel disease tend to arise in flat mucosa and therefore are more difficult to detect at an early stage. Dysplasia, the presence of DNA aneuploidy, and mutations of the *p53* tumor suppressor gene are early markers of neoplastic transformation.

***Inherited nonadenomatous polyposis syndromes.*** Generalized juvenile polyposis and Peutz-Jeghers syndrome are both associated with an increased risk of colorectal cancer. Generalized juvenile polyposis is an autosomal dominant condition characterized by the presence of numerous juvenile polyps of the colon. Juvenile polyps are nonneoplastic hamartomas composed of a fibrovascular stoma, cystic epithelial glandular structures, and a conspicuous inflammatory component. The increased risk, albeit small, of colorectal cancer is related to the presence of adenomatous epithelium in some juvenile polyps. Single juvenile polyps are not associated with an increased risk of colorectal cancer.

Peutz-Jeghers is another autosomal dominant hereditary disease characterized by hamartomatous polyposis of both the small and large bowel and mucocutaneous pigmentation. A small percentage of affected individuals develop colorectal cancer at a young age, presumably related to the occasional presence of adenomatous epithelium within the hamartomas.

***Miscellaneous conditions.*** Women with a history of breast, ovarian, or endometrial cancer are at increased risk of colorectal cancer, as are patients with a history of abdominal or pelvic irradiation. Additional risk factors include the presence of a ureterosigmoidostomy, *Streptococcus bovis* bacteremia and endocarditis, *Schistosoma japonicum* infections of the colon, and Bloom syndrome, which is a rare genetic disease characterized by dwarfism, characteristic facies, and a photosensitive telangiectatic erythema of the face. The association between cholecystectomy and colorectal neoplasia appears to be relatively weak.

## Histopathology and differential diagnosis

***Adenomatous polyps.*** Adenomatous polyps are benign glandular neoplasms. They are classified as tubular, villous, or tubullovillous. Clinicopathologic studies suggest a strong correlation between the extent of villous component and adenoma size. Based on endoscopic surveys, approximately 80% of adenomas are tubular, 10% to 15% tubulovillous, and 3% to 5% villous. The distribution of adenomas is similar to that of colorectal cancers, with approximately two thirds of adenomas occurring in the left colon and rectum (Fig. 45-2).

All adenomas display some degree of dysplasia, which is defined on the basis of cytologic atypia and architectural abnormality. According to the World Health Organization classification system, the terms *low-grade* and *high-grade* are used to describe the degree of dysplasia. Low-grade dysplasia incorporates the categories of mild and moderate dysplasia, whereas high-grade dysplasia incorporates the categories of severe dysplasia and carcinoma in situ. Adenomas with mild dysplasia exhibit few of the pathologic criteria of malignancy; those with severe dysplasia have most of the cytologic and structural characteristics of cancer, but the glands themselves are not invasive. Adenomas containing invasive cancer are referred to as malignant polyps. It is estimated that fewer than 5% of adenomas undergo malignant transformation. The likelihood of finding invasive cancer in an adenoma increases with size (larger than 2 cm), villous component, and presence of high-grade dysplasia. Multiplicity and age may also be determinants.

In addition to adenomas, other types of benign polyps arise in the colon and rectum. The most common of these is the *hyperplastic polyp.* Hyperplastic polyps tend to be small (under 5 mm) and have a predilection for the rectum and sigmoid colon. Depending on the method of study, hyperplastic polyps may be found in up to 80% of individuals. Like adenomas, their frequency increases with age. It is important to note that hyperplastic polyps are nonneoplastic and have no malignant potential. Although subtle differences have been described in terms of gross appearance, it is nearly impossible to distinguish

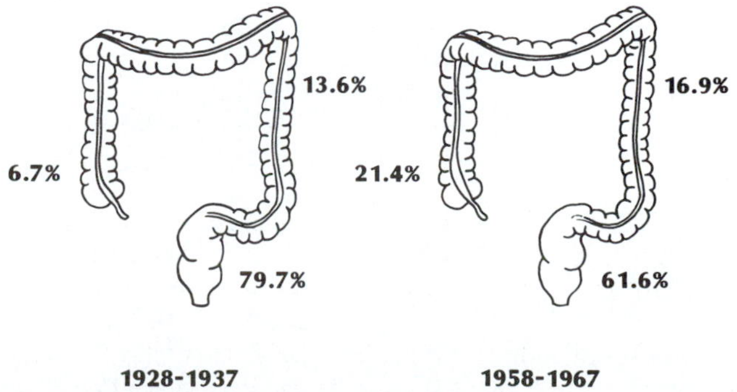


**Fig. 45-2.** Proximal shift of colorectal cancer; distribution of primary sites.

these lesions from small adenomas endoscopically.

*Juvenile polyps* are nonneoplastic hamartomas with a characteristic histology. They are the most common polyps of childhood. Bleeding and rectal prolapse are the most common clinical manifestations. Many will infarct and pass spontaneously. Unlike generalized juvenile polyposis, isolated juvenile polyps have no malignant potential.

*Pseudopolyps* are nonneoplastic polypoid remnants seen in long-standing inflammatory bowel disease. Usually multiple lesions are found throughout the involved area of colon, and they frequently have a friable, inflamed appearance. Although these pseudopolyps are not themselves neoplastic, the entire colon of a patient with inflammatory bowel disease is at risk of developing a malignancy.

*Lipomas* originate within the wall of the colon, but as they enlarge they frequently become polypoid. They may be found anywhere in the colon but are usually seen near the ileocecal valve. The surface is smooth and red and may have a yellow tinge reflecting the fat content. Usually these tumors are asymptomatic and do not require removal.

*Leiomyomas* and *lymphoid polyps* are very unusual. When seen, they are smooth, sessile, and firmly attached to the wall. They rarely cause symptoms.

*Carcinoid tumors* of the colon are almost always benign. They are usually seen as small yellow nodules in the rectum. No treatment is needed unless they enlarge.

***Adenocarcinomas.*** Colorectal cancers may present as exophytic, ulcerative, infiltrating, or annular lesions. With the exception of the cecum where exophytic, polypoid lesions predominate, there is no correlation between site and configuration. The anatomic distribution of colorectal cancers has shifted proximally in recent years (see Fig. 45-2). Currently approximately 30% of cancers arise in the rectum, 25% in the sigmoid, 6% in the descending colon, 11% in the transverse colon, 9% in the ascending colon, and 13% in the cecum. Histologic grades for colorectal adenocarcinomas include well differentiated, moderately differentiated, poorly differentiated, and undifferentiated or anaplastic, depending on the degree of cytologic atypia and glandularity. Mucinous or signet-cell carcinomas are variants of undifferentiated tumors.

Metastatic pathways usually involve lymphatic invasion with spread to mesenteric lymph nodes first, then hematogenous spread via the portal system to the liver. Ultimately, spread occurs via the systemic circulation to the lungs and other parts of the body. Rarely, tumors in the rectal region metastasize directly to the lungs, presumably via hemorrhoidal veins that connect directly to the systemic circulation.

Occasionally, other types of colorectal tumors are encountered. Malignant tumors of the anorectal junction are *squamous cell* or *cloacogenic* carcinomas. These metastasize via lymphatics to groin nodes before spreading systemically. These tumors are rare, comprising only about 1% of colorectal tumors. Other primary malignant tumors are extraordinarily rare. *Lymphomas, leiomyosarcomas,* and *liposarcomas* have all been reported but are curiosities.

Direct invasion of the colon from adjacent malignancy (ovary or prostate) or metastases to the colon from distant sites (breast, lung, stomach, and melanoma) may occur late in the course of the disease but rarely presents a diagnostic problem.

## Staging and prognosis

Since Dukes' original staging system for rectal cancers in 1932, several modifications have been made in an attempt to incorporate additional prognostic information. The Astler-Coller system and the TNM system (proposed by the American Joint Committee on Cancer and International Union Against Cancer) are currently the most widely used and are applicable to both colon and rectal cancers (Table 45-5). Both are defined on the basis of depth of mural invasion and lymph node status. Prognosis, as defined by 5-year survival rates, is closely correlated with tumor stage at diagnosis, and ranges from over 80% for Dukes' A (stage I) tumors to 3% for Dukes' D (stage IV) tumors.

Poorly differentiated histology, mucin production,

**Table 45-5.** Staging classifications and prognosis of colorectal cancer

| Dukes' | Astler-Coller | AJCC/UICC | Description | 5-year survival (%) |
|---|---|---|---|---|
| A | | | Penetration into bowel wall | >80 |
| | A | T1 } Stage I | Submucosa | |
| | B1 | T2 } | Muscularis | |
| B | B2 | T3 } Stage II<br>T4 } | Penetration through bowel wall ± involvement of adjacent organs | 60 |
| C | | | Lymph node involvement | 20 |
| | C1 | | Without penetration of bowel wall | |
| | C2 | Stage III | With penetration of bowel wall | |
| | | N1 | 1-3 nodes | |
| | | N2 | >4 nodes | |
| | | N3 | Any node along a major vascular trunk | |
| D | D | Stage IV<br>M1 | Any T, any N, distant metastases present | 3 |

*AJCC*, American Joint Committee on Cancer; *UICC*, International Union Against Cancer.

abnormal DNA content (aneuploidy), perforation, tumor invasion of adjacent organs, venous involvement, and a preoperative elevation in the plasma carcinoembryonic antigen (CEA) titer (over 5 ng/nl) are also correlated with a poor prognosis. Unlike most other carcinomas or sarcomas, prognosis is not influenced by tumor size.

### Clinical features

***Adenomas.*** Adenomatous polyps usually are asymptomatic. Intermittent bleeding, which is usually occult, is the most common manifestation. Occasionally visible scant bleeding occurs, either mixed in the stool or on its surface; massive bleeding is rare. Patients may complain of a change in bowel habits, but this is unusual. Rarely profuse watery diarrhea, resulting in dehydration and electrolyte abnormalities, is associated with large villous adenomas of the distal colon and rectum. Patients may also complain of vague discomfort; more severe pain is very uncommon and may be attributable to intussusception. Rectal prolapse of polyps has also been described.

***Cancers.*** The clinical manifestations of colorectal cancers tend to vary with anatomic location. Cancers of the right colon most commonly present with occult bleeding and iron deficiency anemia. Obstruction is unusual because of the voluminous and distensible nature of the cecum. On occasion a mass may be palpated in the right lower quadrant. Since stool becomes more concentrated as it passes through the transverse and descending colon, cancers of these sites cause crampy abdominal pain, obstruction, or less commonly even perforation. Cancers of the transverse colon may also present with occult bleeding but more often obstruction. Cancers of the left colon and sigmoid commonly produce rectal bleeding or symptoms related to partial bowel obstruction, such as crampy abdominal pain, change in bowel habits, and/or changes in stool size and consistency. Cancers of the rectum characteristically produce increased stool frequency, changes in stool caliber or consistency, small amounts of bright red bleeding, rectal urgency, tenesmus, and incontinence. Advanced tumors may also produce perianal pain, hematuria, urinary frequency, or vaginal fistula due to local invasion. Cancers of any site may perforate, resulting in signs and symptoms of a localized abscess or peritonitis.

Anorexia and weight loss are common systemic symptoms. Their presence is not specific for colorectal cancers, and patients may have far-advanced colon cancers without these findings. When present, however, especially in the older age group, colon cancer must be a prime diagnostic possibility. Signs and symptoms of metastatic disease vary according to the site of involvement.

### Diagnosis

A variety of diagnostic modalities may be used to detect and diagnose colorectal neoplasms. The three main indications for diagnostic evaluation include (1) symptoms of obstruction, bleeding or locally invasive disease, (2) a positive test for occult blood, and (3) screening of asymptomatic patients.

***Evaluation of symptomatic patients.*** Colonoscopy is the most widely used diagnostic modality for symptomatic patients, since it permits direct visualization of the entire large bowel in 90% to 95% of patients, as well as a means of obtaining tissue for histologic evaluation of suspicious lesions or removing polyps. Depending on the nature of the symptoms or other mitigating circumstances, a sigmoidoscopy and/or barium enema may also be obtained. If a lesion is found by sigmoidoscopy or barium enema, a colonoscopy should be performed to ascertain the nature of the lesion, obtain tissue for histologic evaluation, and determine whether synchronous lesions are present elsewhere in the bowel. A colonoscopy should also be performed in patients with persistent symptoms and negative sigmoidoscopy or barium studies. If the entire bowel is not well visualized due to an obstructing lesion, technical difficulties, or poor patient tolerance, a double-contrast barium enema should be obtained.

***Evaluation of a positive fecal occult blood test.*** The likelihood of finding a neoplastic lesion in patients with a positive fecal occult blood test increases with age. Approximately 50% of patients with a positive fecal occult blood test have either an adenoma (38%) or cancer (12%). Available data support the use of colonoscopy as the diagnostic procedure of choice in evaluating a positive fecal occult blood test. Double-contrast barium enemas are nearly as sensitive for lesions over 2 cm, but demonstrate much lower sensitivity for lesions smaller than 1 cm. Moreover, colonoscopy is still indicated to obtain tissue or remove polyps if a lesion is detected by barium enema.

***Evaluation of asymptomatic patients (screening).*** Although the survival rates from colorectal cancer have improved significantly in recent years, more than 40% of patients still die from their disease. Like many other cancers, prognosis is closely correlated with stage of disease at the time of diagnosis. Despite improvements in diagnostic capability, nearly 40% of patients have local or regional spread of their tumors, and another 20% have metastatic disease. This is largely because most patients remain entirely asymptomatic until their tumors reach an advanced stage. Survival is inversely correlated with duration of symptoms (Fig. 45-3). Together these observations provide a strong rationale for secondary prevention through screening programs aimed at detecting localized, presymptomatic cancers. By identifying and removing colorectal adenomas, screening also has the potential to reduce the incidence of colorectal cancer.

Proponents of colorectal cancer screening widely agree that case finding rather than mass screening is the most appropriate approach for early detection. Case finding refers to the performance of screening individuals at increased risk for the disease of interest. High-risk groups have been identified for colorectal cancer. Patients in whom age (over 50) is the only risk factor are considered to be of average risk; those belonging to high-risk groups are listed in Table 45-5.

The digital rectal examination, fecal occult blood test, and sigmoidoscopy have been advocated as screening tests for average risk individuals. The importance of the digital rectal examination has diminished as a result of the proximal shift of colorectal cancer but is still recom-

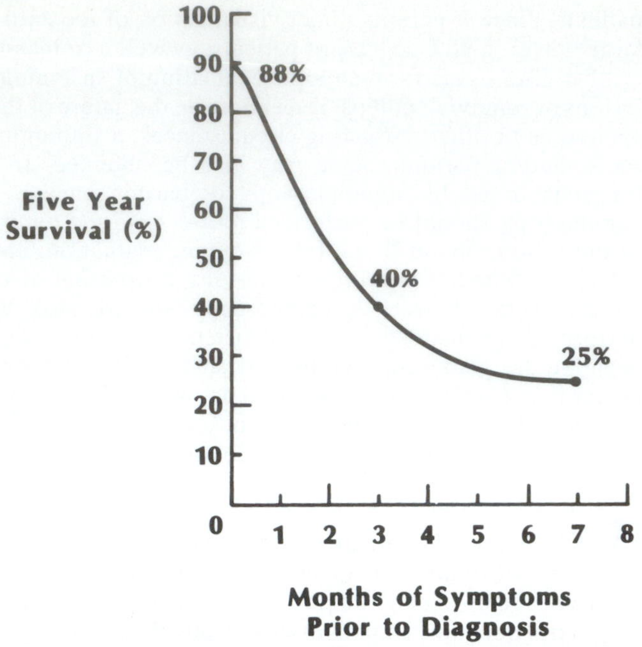


**Fig. 45-3.** Survival rate related to duration of symptoms.

mended by most on a yearly basis. It is estimated that fewer than 10% of cancers are now detectable by this approach.

It has long been recognized that occult bleeding is an early sign of colorectal cancers. The fecal occult blood test is based on the phenolic oxidation of guaiac to a blue compound by the peroxidase-like activity of hemoglobin. Available data suggest that, with the exception of meat, diet has little effect on standard guaiac slide tests. Iron and laxatives have unpredictable effects on both positives and negatives, but in general iron should not be held responsible for a positive test. Vitamin C can inhibit the reaction, resulting in a false negative test. Hydration with water before adding the reagent increases sensitivity but also decreases specificity, due to an increase in the number of false positives. Controlled trials of asymptomatic patients suggest that fecal occult blood testing may enhance detection of early stage (Dukes' A and B) cancers. Although it is safe to assume that earlier detection translates into improved 5-year survival rates, it remains unproven whether this approach improves overall mortality. However, a recent randomized trial involving over 46,000 participants demonstrated a 33% reduction in mortality with annual testing. On the negative side, fecal occult blood testing is associated with false negative rates of over 50% for cancers and over 80% for adenomas, largely because not all neoplasms bleed or bleed only intermittently. Moreover, false positives result in unnecessary tests with their attendant risks and costs.

The other major screening test for average risk individuals is sigmoidoscopy. The rationale for sigmoidoscopy is that it permits direct visualization of that region of the large bowel most likely to harbor either an adenoma or cancer. Several types of sigmoidoscopes are available, including the 25-cm rigid scope, the 35- or 60-cm flexible fiberoptic scope, and the 40- to 60-cm flexible videoscopes. Flexible instruments have two to three times greater yield than the rigid scopes and have demonstrated much better patient tolerance. The 60-cm flexible scope is associated with a higher diagnostic yield than the 35-cm scope but also with greater patient discomfort; a higher degree of technical proficiency is also required. Although the effectiveness of sigmoidoscopy in screening has not been well studied, available data from uncontrolled trials using rigid sigmoidoscopy suggest that sigmoidoscopy is effective in detecting early stage lesions, improving survival, and reducing the incidence of colorectal cancers through the identification and removal of polyps. Recent case-control studies have provided strong evidence that sigmoidoscopy is effective in reducing mortality from cancers arising within reach of the scope.

Based on these data, the American Cancer Society has recommended that asymptomatic men and women at average risk should be offered digital rectal examinations and stool blood tests annually beginning at age 50, with flexible sigmoidoscopy every 3 to 5 years also beginning at age 50. Patients found to have a positive stool test or a biopsy-proven adenoma by sigmoidoscopy should undergo colonoscopy to rule out the possibility of a synchronous adenoma or cancer. Up to 50% of patients with adenomas detected by sigmoidoscopy have a proximal adenoma. Although controversial, colonoscopy is not recommended for patients with only a hyperplastic polyp found by sigmoidoscopy.

Screening strategies for high-risk groups are outlined in Table 45-6. Colonoscopy is the preferred diagnostic modality for all such patients, with the exception of individuals at risk for FAP or Gardner's syndrome in whom sigmoidoscopy should be performed every 6 to 12 months, beginning in adolescents who are *APC* gene positive by blood testing. Guidelines for individuals who are *APC* gene negative are not well established, but some authorities recommend colonoscopy every 3 to 5 years beginning at age 40. Individuals at risk for hereditary nonpolyposis colorectal cancer should undergo colonoscopy every 2 years beginning at age 25 and then yearly after age 35. Individuals with one or two first-degree relatives with colorectal cancer should undergo colonoscopy every 3 to 5 years beginning approximately 5 years before the age of diagnosis for the youngest affected relative. Patients with long-standing ulcerative colitis should undergo colonoscopy with biopsy for dysplasia beginning at 8 years after age of onset for pancolitis and at 15 years for distal disease. Recommendations for surveillance of patients with a history of colorectal cancer or adenoma(s) are discussed below.

## Treatment

***Adenomas.*** Endoscopic polypectomy is the treatment of choice for all colorectal adenomas, regardless of whether they are symptomatic or discovered incidentally. Since histologic evaluation is the only reliable means of distinguishing adenomas from nonneoplastic polyps, particularly for diminutive (less than 5 mm) lesions, endoscopic removal or ablation is recommended for all colorectal polyps. The major risks of endoscopic polypectomy are bleeding and perforation. If a polyp cannot be removed endoscopically, surgical resection should be considered after careful assessment of the patient's operative risk versus the risk of malignancy. Periodic endoscopic assess-

**Table 45-6.** Colorectal cancer screening strategies for high-risk groups

| Risk group | Strategy |
|---|---|
| Prior colorectal cancer | Colonoscopy at 1 yr; thereafter every 3 yr |
| Prior colorectal adenoma | Colonoscopy every 3 yr |
| FAP/GS | |
| *APC* gene positive | Sigmoidoscopy every 6-12 mo beginning at adolescence |
| *APC* gene negative | Colonoscopy every 3-5 yr beginning at age 40 |
| HNPCC | Colonoscopy every 2 yr beginning at age 25 until age 35; yearly thereafter |
| Family history 1 or 2 FDR | Colonoscopy every 3-5 yr beginning at least 5 yr before age of youngest affected relative |
| Ulcerative colitis | Colonoscopy every 1-2 yr after 8 yrs of pancolitis or after 15 yr of distal colitis |

*FAP*, Familial adenomatous polyposis; *GS*, Gardner's syndrome; *APC*, adenomatous polyposis coli; *HNPCC*, hereditary nonpolyposis colorectal cancer; *FDR*, first-degree relative.

ment and piecemeal removal every 6 months to 1 year is a reasonable alternative in poor surgical candidates. Laser ablation is also an option in such patients.

The treatment of malignant polyps (i.e., adenomas containing invasive cancer) depends on polyp morphology and histology. Endoscopic polypectomy is considered curative for pedunculated polyps provided that (1) the stalk is tumor free, (2) there is no lymphatic or vascular invasion, (3) the cancer is well or moderately differentiated, and (4) there is no residual or recurrent tumor at the polypectomy site on follow-up examination. If all of these criteria are not met, surgical resection is warranted. Surgical resection is recommended for all patients with malignant sessile polyps provided they are of acceptable operative risk.

***Cancer.*** Surgical resection is the only potentially curative treatment for colorectal cancer. Curative resection requires wide excision of the primary tumor and en bloc removal of draining lymph nodes, lymphatics, and contiguous structures. The actual extent of resection varies according to anatomic location. The introduction of stapling devices has been an important advance in that it has shortened operative time, reduced the incidence of anastomotic leaks and infection, and reduced the need for colostomy in patients with low-lying rectal cancers. Although an abdominoperitoneal resection with colostomy is often recommended for rectal tumors not amenable to low anterior resection with primary anastomosis, alternate sphincter-sparing approaches, including local excision, irradiation, electrofulguration, or a combination thereof, may be curative in select patients. A more limited palliative resection is recommended for patients with metastatic disease at the time of diagnosis.

An emerging body of evidence supports the use of adjuvant therapy following curative resection. Combined modality treatment with chemotherapy (5-fluorouracil alone or in combination with levamisole) and postoperative radiation has been shown to reduce local recurrence rates and improve disease-free survival and overall survival in patients with Dukes' B2 and C rectal cancers. Combination chemotherapy with 5-fluorouracil and levamisole has also been shown to improve disease-free survival and overall survival in patients with Dukes' C cancers arising above the pelvic-peritoneal reflection; its efficacy in the treatment of Dukes' B2 tumors remains unproven. The regimen of 5-fluorouracil plus leucovorin is also effective.

Chemotherapy is the treatment of choice in patients with metastatic disease. Since this approach is rarely curative, efficacy is generally defined in terms of initial response rates (i.e., tumor shrinkage) and improved 5-year survival. 5-Fluorouracil is the most active single agent, with response rates in the range of 20%. Combination regimens, with the exception of 5-fluorouracil plus leucovorin, however, have exhibited superior activity in preliminary trials and are currently the regimens of choice outside the setting of a protocol. Intraarterial hepatic infusion of 5-fluorouracil or floxuridine has demonstrated superior efficacy in the treatment of hepatic disease but has had little impact on survival and is associated with significant toxicity. Radiation therapy has a palliative role in the management of advanced or recurrent pelvic disease, particularly in patients with pain unresponsive to chemotherapy.

Aggressive surgical intervention may be warranted in the case of isolated hepatic or pulmonary metastases in an otherwise healthy patient. Although the cure rate is not high, many case reports document the value of attempting tumor removal in this otherwise 100% fatal situation.

### Follow-up

***Adenomas.*** Periodic surveillance colonoscopy is warranted in patients with a history of colorectal adenomas because of the risk of metachronous adenomas and cancer. Based on recent data from the National Polyp Study, an interval of at least 3 years has been recommended for repeat colonoscopy after removal of all adenomas. Patients with malignant polyps or large sessile adenomas and those in whom all identified polyps have not been removed may require more frequent examinations.

***Cancer.*** Close surveillance is also indicated for patients with colorectal cancer following curative resection. A reasonable follow-up program includes office visits every 3 months for the first 3 years and then every 6 months, with a carcinoembryonic antigen (CEA) determination every visit and a complete blood count (CBC) and liver profile every 6 months. An annual CT scan of the abdomen and pelvis and a chest x-ray should also be obtained for the first 5 years. Colonoscopy should also be performed at 1 year to detect anastomotic recurrences, and every 3 years thereafter to detect metachronous adenomas or cancer. Patients in whom a complete preoperative colonoscopy or double-contrast barium enema could not be performed because of obstructing tumors should undergo a postoperative examination at 3 to 6 months.

The detection of a rising CEA level after stable low levels necessitates thorough evaluation. Some oncologists and surgeons even suggest exploratory second-look laparotomy in an attempt to find a localized recurrence. Unfortunately, most patients with rising CEA values have substantial spread and cure is not possible.

## TUMORS OF THE LIVER

Tumors of the liver are frequently encountered in clinical practice. Depending on geographic location, the majority of such tumors may be either primary liver tumors or metastatic tumors. Primary liver tumors may be benign or malignant and may arise from hepatic parenchymal tissue, the biliary tree, or vascular structures (see Table 45-1). Hepatocellular carcinomas (hepatomas) and cholangiocarcinomas are the most common malignant tumors; hemangiomas are the most common benign tumors. All other types of benign or malignant primary tumors are rare.

### Epidemiology

The incidence of hepatocellular carcinoma varies considerably worldwide, ranging from only 1% to 2% of malignant tumors found at autopsy in North and South America and Europe, to 20% to 30% in parts of Africa and Asia. Hepatocellular carcinoma is up to four times more common in men than women. The peak incidence occurs in the fifth or sixth decades of life in low-risk countries but one to two decades earlier in high-risk areas.

Unlike hepatocellular carcinoma, the incidence of cholangiocarcinoma is dispersed more evenly throughout the world. Peak incidence is in the sixth decade of life, and there is no male predominance.

Hemangiomas are the most common benign tumors, found in approximately 5% based on all autopsies. The epidemiology of other types of benign tumors is essentially unknown.

### Etiology

Between 30% and 70% of patients with hepatocellular carcinoma have underlying cirrhosis. The risk of hepatocellular carcinoma varies with the type of cirrhosis. Cirrhosis due to hemochromatosis has the highest risk; up to 22% of such patients develop hepatocellular carcinoma even if treated with phlebotomy. Hepatocellular carcinoma also occurs in approximately 2% to 3% of patients with alcoholic cirrhosis and 10% of patients with postnecrotic cirrhosis associated with chronic hepatitis B infection. Other forms of chronic liver disease, such as chronic hepatitis C infection, $\alpha_1$-antitrypsin deficiency, and tyrosinemia, are also predisposing conditions. In parts of Asia chronic parasitic infection with *Clonorchis sinensis* is associated with the development of cholangiocarcinoma.

Epidemiologic studies have established a close association between hepatocellular carcinoma and chronic hepatitis B (HBV). In high-risk areas 90% to 95% of patients with hepatocellular carcinoma have serologic evidence of active or remote infection. Approximately 60% to 70% have evidence of chronic hepatitis and/or cirrhosis at presentation. Integration of HBV-DNA into the host genome appears to be an inciting event. Chronicity of infection and vertical transmission predispose to HBV-DNA integration and hence hepatocellular carcinoma.

Environmental carcinogens have also been implicated in the etiology of hepatocellular carcinoma. Mycotoxins derived from saprophytic fungi, particularly aflatoxin B1, are potent hepatocarcinogens and are believed to contribute to the increased incidence of hepatocellular carcinoma in high-risk areas such as Africa and China. Long-term use of androgenic steroids is also associated with an increased risk of hepatocellular carcinoma. Vinyl chloride and the contrast agent Thorotrast are associated with angiosarcomas of the liver. Oral contraceptives and pregnancy have both been associated with liver cell adenomas and focal nodular hyperplasia. Rare cases of malignant transformation of liver cell adenomas into hepatocellular carcinomas have been reported.

### Histopathology and differential diagnosis

***Benign tumors.*** *Hemangiomas* are the most common benign tumors of the liver. They are typically solitary and small but may be multiple or large. Most are subcapsular and have a predilection for the right lobe of the liver. Two forms commonly occur in the liver: (1) the cavernous hemangioma, which is the more common and due to dilatation of existing blood vessels, and (2) the true hemangioma, which results from a proliferation of embryonic vascular tissue.

*Liver cell adenomas* are rare benign tumors associated with oral contraceptive therapy and pregnancy. They are usually large with a smooth appearance and soft consistency. They occur with equal frequency throughout the liver and are usually visible at the surface. The histologic differentiation of a liver cell adenoma from a well-differentiated liver cell carcinoma can be quite difficult.

*Focal nodular hyperplasias* are also rare benign tumors associated with oral contraceptive use and pregnancy. They are usually solitary, often less than 5 cm in diameter, and occur in either lobe of the liver. Like adenomas, these lesions occur with equal frequency throughout the liver and are usually located peripherally. Unlike adenomas, they are nonneoplastic hamartomas. Focal nodular hyperplasias are often pedunculated and highly vascular.

***Malignant tumors.*** *Hepatocellular carcinomas* account for 80% to 90% of primary liver cancers. Grossly, hepatocellular carcinomas may exhibit a nodular pattern characterized by the presence of small multiple nodules throughout the liver or a massive tumor that often totally replaces one lobe. A diffuse fibrolamellar type has also been described, which occurs primarily in younger, noncirrhotic patients and carries a better prognosis. Histologically it is sometimes difficult to distinguish benign from malignant tumors, and even normal parenchymal cells in the case of well-differentiated tumors.

*Cholangiocarcinomas* are glandular malignancies that arise from bile duct epithelium. Although these tumors may be found coincidentally within hepatocellular carcinomas, cholangiocarcinomas are generally not associated with underlying cirrhosis.

*Angiosarcomas* are rare hepatic malignancies that arise from vascular elements. *Hepatoblastomas* are rare tumors seen primarily in infants and young children. Unlike other types of liver cancer, these tumors tend to be unifocal, resectable, and highly curable.

In the United States the incidence of clinically significant metastatic disease is at least 20 times greater than that of primary malignancies. The liver is the most frequent site of bloodborne metastases, which occur in about 30% of all cancers, including half of those from stomach, breast, and lung, and tumors arising in the portal vein drainage system.

## Clinical features

***Benign tumors.*** Most benign tumors of the liver are asymptomatic. Vague right upper quandrant pain or discomfort is often the major complaint in symptomatic patients. Severe right upper quadrant pain with hypotension suggests spontaneous rupture, which can be fatal. Physical examination is often normal but may reveal a palpable mass, hepatomegaly, or, in the case of large hemangiomas, a vascular hum. Thrombocytopenia due to platelet adherence has been reported in patients with large hemangiomas.

***Malignant tumors.*** The onset of symptoms in patients with hepatocellular carcinoma may be insidious or sudden. In general, symptomatic patients have advanced, incurable tumors. Abdominal pain is the most common presenting feature. The pain may be characterized as a dull localized ache due to stretching of the liver capsule or sudden and severe due to spontaneous rupture. Patients may also complain of diffuse pain due to rapidly accumulating ascites. Weakness, anorexia, and weight loss are also frequent. Early satiety may occur due to liver enlargement or ascites. Occasionally, patients present with manifestations of Budd-Chiari syndrome due to hepatic vein thrombosis or variceal hemorrhage due to portal vein thrombosis. Tender hepatomegaly, often with a palpable mass, ascites, and in some cases a bruit are the most common physical findings. Overt jaundice is often a very late finding except in patients with cholangiocarcinomas.

A variety of paraneoplastic syndromes have been described in patients with hepatocellular carcinoma. Hypercalcemia, erythrocytosis, hypoglycemia, hyperlipidemia, sexual precocity or feminization, coagulapathy due to dysfibrogenemia, hyperthyroidism, and pseudoporphyria have all been reported.

## Diagnosis

Accurate diagnosis of hepatic tumors relies on clinical suspicion, radiologic imaging, serologic testing for tumor markers, and in most cases tissue confirmation. The vast majority of benign or malignant tumors present as space-occupying lesions easily detectable by a variety of imaging modalities (Figs. 45-4 and 45-5). Ultrasonography is the most widely employed imaging modality because it is readily available, reliable, inexpensive, noninvasive, and avoids the potential risks of radiation. CT and MRI are useful modalities for confirming the findings at ultrasound, helping to distinguish benign from malignant tumors, and assessing extent of disease. Dynamic CT scanning (CT angiography) and MRI may be particularly useful in detecting small tumors and in evaluating invasion of vascular structures. Hepatic arteriography is also useful for characterizing vascular status of small lesions, determining operability, and defining anatomy in potentially resectable tumors.

Hepatic isotope scans have limited utility in the detection of many primary hepatic tumors. Technetium-labeled red blood scans are most useful in the diagnosis of hemangiomas but otherwise lack both sensitivity and specificity, particularly in the setting of cirrhosis. Dynamic CT scanning using a bolus injection is also helpful in distinguishing hemangiomas from other hepatic tumors. Occasionally gallium scans have proven useful, since this tracer preferentially accumulates in some hepatocellular carcinomas but not in normal liver nor cirrhosis. Gallium does, however, accumulate in liver abscesses and granulomas.

Most patients with hepatocellular carcinoma at some

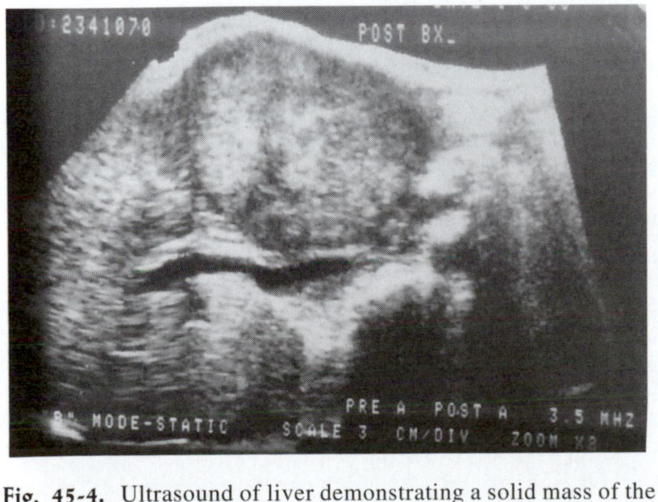


**Fig. 45-4.** Ultrasound of liver demonstrating a solid mass of the left lobe with area of central necrosis. Mass proved to be a hepatocellular carcinoma.

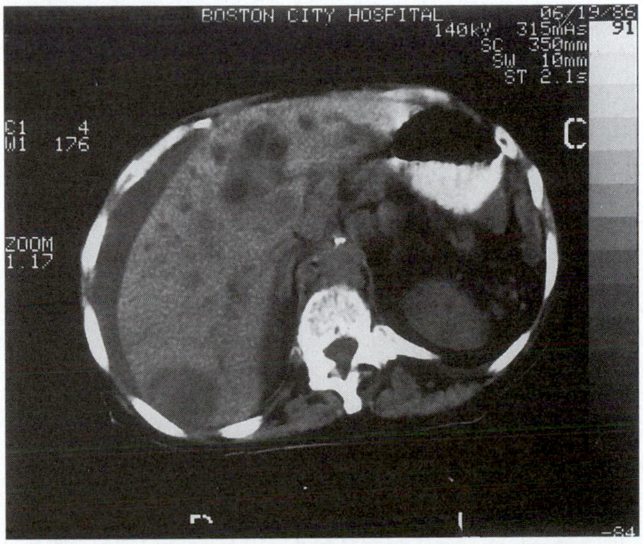


**Fig. 45-5.** CT scan of metastatic carcinoma of the liver with ascites. Note the multiple filling defects.

time have elevated serum levels of α-fetoprotein; levels greater than 500 ng/ml are diagnostic. Lower levels are less specific, since they may also be seen in the setting of hepatitis or active cirrhosis. High-risk patients, particularly those with chronic HBV infection or hemochromatosis, should have annual α-fetoprotein determinations and ultrasound studies in hope of detecting early, potentially curable tumors. Measurement of serum CEA levels is another useful tumor marker in the diagnosis of metastatic disease, particularly for primary cancers of the gastrointestinal tract, breast, or lung.

Liver biopsy is often necessary to confirm the diagnosis of most liver tumors. Although a blind percutaneous biopsy may suffice in patients with large tumor masses, ultrasound or CT-guided biopsies have a much higher yield. Laparoscopy with directed liver biopsy is an even more accurate method for establishing the diagnosis. Caution is warranted in patients with localized tumors, since skin metastases at the biopsy site have been reported.

## Treatment

***Benign tumors.*** Most benign tumors are asymptomatic and do not require treatment. Both adenomas and focal nodular hyperplasias are known to regress in patients taking oral contraceptives once the drugs are discontinued. Surgical resection may be indicated in rare patients with intractable pain or in whom there is a strong fear of rupture. Corticosteroids are effective in the treatment of thrombocytopenia associated with large hemangiomas.

***Malignant tumors.*** Surgical resection is the only proven effective treatment for hepatocellular carcinoma or cholangiocarcinoma. Unfortunately, relatively few patients have localized, potentially curable disease. Even in the rare event that an early, resectable lesion is detected, the presence of cirrhosis often precludes aggressive surgical intervention. Careful preoperative assessment, including an extent of disease workup as well as an assessment of hepatic functional reserve in patients with known or suspected cirrhosis, is essential. Because of major advances in surgical technique and perioperative care, resections as extensive as a trisegmentectomy have an acceptable operative mortality in carefully selected patients. Palliative surgery is generally not recommended except in patients with obstructive jaundice.

The treatment of advanced primary malignancies of the liver is rarely successful. The role of liver transplantation for patients with disease confined to the liver is still under investigation, but results thus far are less than impressive, with the notable exception of young patients with the fibrolamellar variant of hepatocellular carcinoma. Chemotherapy delivered either systemically or by hepatic artery infusion is commonly used but rarely effective. Of the many agents studied, doxorubicin (adriamycin) appears to be the most active agent currently available. Radiation therapy has no role because of its lack of efficacy and risk of radiation hepatitis. Embolization, alone or in combination with chemotherapy, and hepatic artery ligation have had limited success as palliative approaches but very little impact on survival. There is a growing body of evidence suggesting that percutaneous injection of alcohol directly into tumor deposits under ultrasound guidance may be the most efficacious approach to patients with unresectable disease. There are also data to suggest that this approach may be as effective as surgery in many resectable tumors.

The management of patients with metastatic liver disease varies according to the site of origin. In general, chemotherapy is the most commonly employed therapeutic intervention. Embolization and hepatic artery ligation have been used for palliation in select patients. Surgical resection has also been advocated in patients with very limited involvement.

## Prognosis

The overall prognosis for patients with malignant tumors of the liver is poor. Although cure rates as high as 30% have been reported after surgical resection, the median survival without resection is in the range of 4 to 6 months.

## BIBLIOGRAPHY

American Cancer Society National Conference on Colorectal Cancer, *Cancer* 70 (suppl):1205, 1992.

DiBisceglie AM, moderator: NIH conference on hepatocellular carcinoma, *Ann Intern Med* 108:390, 1988.

Kvols LK et al: Treatment of the carcinoid syndrome: evaluation of a long-acting somatostatin analogue, *N Engl J Med* 315:663, 1986.

Lance P: Tumors and other neoplastic disease in the small bowel. In Yamada T, editor: *Textbook of gastroenterology,* vol 2, Philadelphia, 1991, JB Lippincott.

List AF et al: Non-Hodgkin's lymphoma of the gastrointestinal tract: an analysis of clinical and pathologic features affecting outcome, *J Clin Oncol* 6:1125, 1988.

Mandel JS et al: Reducing mortality from colorectal cancer by screening for fecal occult blood, *N Engl J Med* 328:1365, 1993.

Schein PS, Sherlock P, editors: Gastric cancer, *Semin Oncol* 12:2, 1985.

Schroy PC: Gastric cancer. In Bayless TM, editor: *Current therapy in gastroenterology and liver disease*-3, Philadelphia, 1990, BC Decker.

Schroy PC, Hesketh PJ: Colorectal cancer: adjuvant therapy. In Bayless TM, editor: *Current therapy in gastroenterology and liver disease,* ed 4, Philadelphia, 1994, BC Decker.

Selby JV et al: A case-control study of screening sigmoidoscopy and mortality from colorectal cancer, *N Engl J Med* 326:653, 1993.

Vogelstein B et al: Genetic alterations during colorectal tumor development, *N Engl J Med* 319:525, 1988.

Winawer SJ et al: Colorectal cancer screening, *J Natl Cancer Inst* 83:243, 1991.

Winawer SJ et al: Randomized comparison of surveillance intervals after colonoscopic removal of newly diagnosed adenomatous polyps, *N Engl J Med* 328:901, 1993.

CHAPTER

# 46 Diseases of the Pancreas

Norton J. Greenberger

## ACUTE PANCREATITIS

### Epidemiology/etiology

The incidence of pancreatitis varies in different countries and depends on etiologic factors (e.g., alcohol, gallstones), metabolic factors, and drugs (see the box at right). In the United States acute pancreatitis is related to alcohol ingestion more commonly than to gallstones, whereas in England the opposite is true. Pancreatitis is classified as acute or chronic. An attack is defined as acute if the patient becomes asymptomatic after recovery, whereas with chronic pancreatitis the patient has persistent pain or insufficient exocrine or endocrine pancreatic function. Epidemiologic data of autopsy surveys indicate in the United States the overall prevalence of acute pancreatitis is approximately 0.5%; the annual death rate is an estimated 1.5 per 100,000, or approximately 4000 cases per year.

### Pathophysiology

There are many causative factors in the pathogenesis of acute pancreatitis, but the mechanism by which the conditions trigger pancreatic inflammation have not been clearly elucidated. The final common pathway in the pathogenesis of acute pancreatitis is thought to be autodigestion by activated enzymes. The autodigestion theory postulates that proteolytic enzymes (e.g., trypsinogen, chymotrypsinogen, proelastase, phospholipase) are activated within the pancreas rather than the intestinal lumen. A variety of factors (such as endotoxins, exotoxins, viral infections, ischemia, noxae, and direct trauma) are believed to activate these proenzymes. Activated enzymes are then believed to digest cellular membranes and cause proteolysis, edema, interstitial hemorrhage, vascular damage, coagulation necrosis, fat necrosis, and parenchymal cell necrosis. In addition, activation of bradykinin peptides and vasoactive substances (e.g., histamine) are believed to produce vasodilatation, increased vascular permeability, and edema. There is thus a cascade of events culminating in the development of acute necrotizing pancreatitis.

The second theory proposed to account for the development of acute pancreatitis concerns inappropriate release of pancreatic lysosomal hydrolases, which causes inappropriate activation of zymogens and autodigestion. Several factors ordinarily protect the pancreatic acinar cell: (1) zymogens and lysosomal hydrolases are packaged in intracellular organelles; (2) pancreatic tissue and juice contain inhibitors of pancreatic trypsin; and (3) plasma

#### Causes of acute pancreatitis

**Common**

Alcoholism
Gallstones
Postoperative (abdominal, coronary bypass)
Drugs
Post-ERCP
Abdominal trauma
Hypercalcemia (drugs, TPN)
Hypertriglyceridemia

**Less common**

Vasculitis (SLE)
Thrombotic thrombocytopenic purpura
Refeeding after fasting (anorexia nervosa)
Periampullary duodenal diverticulum
Pancreas divisum
Cancer of the pancreas
End-stage renal disease

*ERCP,* Endoscopic retrograde cholangiopancreatography; *TPN,* total parenteral nutrition; *SLE,* systemic lupus erythematosus.

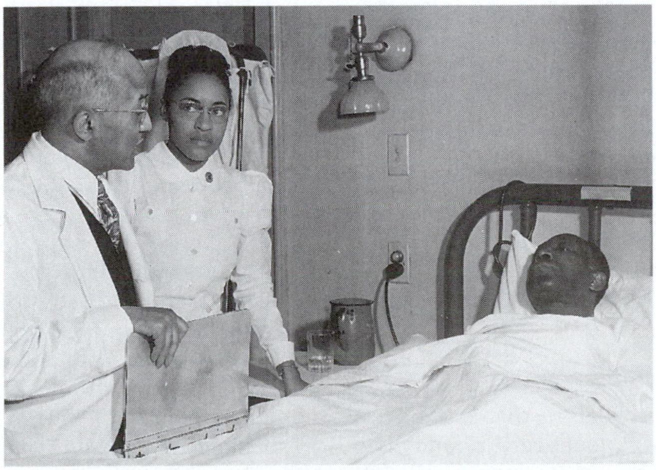

**Fig. 46-1.** Bedside consultation. (From the Collections of the Library of Congress.)

## Drugs causing acute pancreatitis

**Definite**
Thiazides
Furosemides
Sulfonamides
Estrogens
Azathioprine/6-MP
ACE inhibitors
DDI
Valproic acid
Pentamidine
L-Asparaginase

**Probable**
Ethacrynic acid
Acetaminophen
5-Aminosalicylic analogues
Codeine

*ACE,* Angiotensin converting enzyme; *6-MP,* 6-mercaptopurine.

contains antiproteases (e.g., $\alpha_1$-antitrypsin, $\alpha_2$-macroglobulin).

The two most common causes of acute pancreatitis are alcohol ingestion and gallstones. Alcoholic pancreatitis develops in susceptible persons after heavy ethanol ingestion for many years. Chronic alcoholism may produce proteinaceous plugs in the small pancreatic ducts, causing atrophy of pancreatic parenchyma drained by the obstructed duct. Thus in first episodes of alcohol-associated acute pancreatitis approximately 50% of patients already have evidence of chronic pancreatic disease. Patients with gallstone pancreatitis frequently have gallstones in their feces that are not obvious. Certain clinical features should suggest the diagnosis of gallstone-associated pancreatitis. Drugs have also been implicated as a cause of acute pancreatitis (see the box above).

### History

Abdominal pain is the cardinal symptom of acute pancreatitis. This pain may vary from a mild and tolerable discomfort to severe, constant, and incapacitating distress. Characteristically the pain, which is steady and boring, is located in the epigastrium and periumbilical region, and often radiates to the back as well as to the chest, flanks, and lower abdomen. It is important to note that pancreatic pain frequently is more intense when the patient is supine and that patients often obtain relief by sitting with the trunk flexed and knees drawn up. Nausea, vomiting, and abdominal distention from gastric and intestinal hypomotility and chemical peritonitis also are frequent complaints.

### Physical examination

Physical examination typically reveals a distressed and anxious patient. Low-grade fever, tachycardia, and hypotension are fairly common. Shock is not unusual and may result from several factors, including (1) hypovolemia secondary to exudation of blood and plasma proteins in the retroperitoneal space (i.e., a retroperitoneal burn); (2) increased formation and release of kinin peptides, which cause vasodilatation and increased vascular permeability; (3) impairment of myocardial contractility by kinins and other poorly characterized peptides; and (4) systemic effects of proteolytic and lipolytic enzymes released into the circulation. Jaundice occurs in approximately 10% of patients and usually is caused by edema of the head of the pancreas with compression of the intrapancreatic portion of the common bile duct. Abdominal tenderness and muscle rigidity are present to a variable degree, but when compared with the intense pain these signs may be unimpressive. Bowel sounds usually are diminished or absent. A pancreatic pseudocyst may be palpable in the upper abdomen. A faint blue discoloration around the umbilicus (Cullen's sign) may occur as a result of hemoperitoneum, and a blue, red, purple, or green-blue discoloration of the flanks (Turner's sign) reflects tissue catabolism of hemoglobin. The last two findings, which are uncommon, indicate the presence of severe necrotizing pancreatitis. Approximately 10% to 20% of patients develop pulmonary findings, which include atelectasis, basilar rales, mediastinal abscesses, and pleural effusion, the last most frequently left sided. Erythematous skin nodules, which mimic erythema nodosum, may occur; such lesions are caused by subcutaneous fat necrosis.

The physical findings indicating the presence of severe disease include hypotension, tachycardia greater than 130 beats/min, altered sensorium, abnormal physical examination of the lungs, and Cullen's and Turner's signs.

### Laboratory studies and diagnostic procedures

The diagnosis of acute pancreatitis usually is established by the presence of an increased serum amylase exceeding two times the upper limit of normal values. There appears to be no definite correlation between the severity of pancreatitis and the degree of serum amylase elevation. In acute pancreatitis the serum amylase usually is elevated within 24 hours and remains so for 1 to 3 days. Levels return to normal values within 3 to 5 days unless there is extensive pancreatic necrosis, incomplete ductal obstruction, or pseudocyst formation. Approximately 75% of patients with acute pancreatitis have an elevated serum amylase. Normal values, however, may occur if (1) there is a delay of 2 to 5 days in obtaining appropriate blood samples; (2) the underlying disorder is chronic pancreatitis with an acute exacerbation rather than acute pancreatitis; and (3) hypertriglyceridemia is present. Serum lipase levels are increased in approximately 70% to 85% of patients, and lipase may now be the single best enzyme to measure for the diagnosis of acute pancreatitis. If both serum amylase and serum lipase levels are determined, one test is abnormal in approximately 80% to 85% of patients with acute pancreatitis.

The serum amylase is often elevated in other conditions (see the box on p. 653) in part because the enzyme is found in many organs in addition to the pancreas (salivary glands, liver, small intestine, kidney, fallopian tubes), and can be produced by various tumors (carcinoma of the lung, esophagus, breast, and ovary). No blood test is reliable for the diagnosis of acute pancreatitis in patients with renal failure. The serum amylase can become elevated when the

### Causes of hyperamylasemia

**Pancreatic disease**

Acute pancreatitis
Pancreatic pseudocyst
Pancreatic trauma
Pancreatic carcinoma

**Nonpancreatic disease**

Renal insufficiency
Salivary gland lesions*
Tumor (lung, esophagus,* ovary, breast)
Diabetic ketoacidosis*
Burns
Pregnancy
Renal transplantation
Drugs (morphine, codeine)
Pregnancy
Macroamylasemia

**Other abdominal disorders**

Biliary tract disease (cholecystitis, choledocholithiasis)
Perforated peptic ulcer
Intestinal obstruction or infarction
Postoperative hyperamylasemia
Peritonitis
Ruptured ectopic pregnancy

*Salivary isoamylase elevated and not pancreatic isoamylase.

creatinine clearance is less than 50 ml/min. In such patients the serum amylase is usually less than 500 IU/L in the absence of other objective evidence of pancreatitis. A serum amylase may be spuriously normal in certain conditions (e.g., hypertriglyceridemia). In this setting values for urine amylase and serum lipase are often abnormal, thus supporting the diagnosis of acute pancreatitis. Imaging procedures such as ultrasound and computed tomography (CT) scan are helpful in further confirming the diagnosis of acute pancreatitis (Fig. 46-2). Imaging techniques show a diffusely enlarged pancreas in 70% to 90% of patients during an acute attack of pancreatitis. In patients with clinical findings suggesting the presence of a *severe* attack of pancreatitis (see the box above right), CT scan is indicated and often provides important information. In this regard a contrast-enhanced CT scan provides the best means to visualize the pancreas and is very accurate in diagnosing pancreatitis and detecting its local complications. Over 90% of CT scans performed within 72 hours of admission are abnormal in patients with acute pancreatitis. Identification of pancreatic and peripancreatic necrosis by dynamic CT scanning is useful in distinguishing between mild and severe pancreatitis. Areas of the pancreas not enhanced by contrast are thought to be necrotic, and the extent of pancreatic necrosis does correlate with the severity of the disease. The vast majority of patients with acute pancreatitis do not require a CT scan. Rather, this should be reserved for patients with more than three Ranson prognostic signs, one or more major factors, or evidence of one or more systems undergoing organ failure.

### Assessing the severity of acute pancreatitis

**Prognostic signs in acute pancreatitis (modified Ranson)**
***At admission or diagnosis***

Age > 55 years
WBC > 16,000
Blood glucose > 200 mg/dl
Serum LDH > 350 IU/L
AST > 250 IU/L

***During initial 48 hours***

↓ Hct > 10% with hydration or Hct ≤ 30%
↑ BUN > 5 mg/dl
Serum calcium < 8 mg/dl
Arterial $Po_2$ < 60 mm Hg
Fluid sequestration > 5000 ml

*Interpretation:* ↑ mortality with three or more signs

**Major factors adversely influencing survival in acute pancreatitis**

Hypotension
Need for massive fluid and colloid replacement
Respiratory failure
Hypocalcemia
Chocolate brown (hemorrhagic) peritoneal fluid

*Interpretation:* If three or more factors present, mortality can be as high as 50%

**Banks' clinical criteria for grading the severity of pancreatitis**

Cardiac: Shock, tachycardia > 130 beats/min
Pulmonary: Arterial $Po_2$ < 60 mm Hg; acute respiratory distress syndrome
Renal: Azotemia, urine output < 50 ml/hr with hydration
Metabolic: ↓ Serum albumin, ↓ serum calcium
Hematologic: ↓ Hct > 10% with hydration
Neurologic: Confusion, obtundation
Abdominal: Hemorrhagic peritoneal fluid, tense ascites.

*Interpretation:* One or more signs indicate severe disease

*WBC,* White blood cell count; *LDH,* lactate dehydrogenase; *AST,* aspartate aminotransaminase; *Hct,* hematocrit; *BUN,* blood urea nitrogen.

Other routine studies in patients with acute pancreatitis include chest x-ray, electrocardiogram (ECG), arterial blood gases and routine serum chemistries. Careful attention is given to the white blood cell count, blood glucose, liver tests, blood urea nitrogen (BUN), serum calcium, serum albumin, and arterial $Po_2$, which are also of prognostic value (see the box above).

## Differential diagnosis

Any severe acute pain in the abdomen or back should suggest acute pancreatitis. The diagnosis usually is considered when a patient with a reason to have developed pancreatitis presents with severe and constant abdominal pain, nausea, emesis, fever, tachycardia, and abnormal findings on abdominal examination. Laboratory studies frequently reveal leukocytosis, abnormal x-rays of the

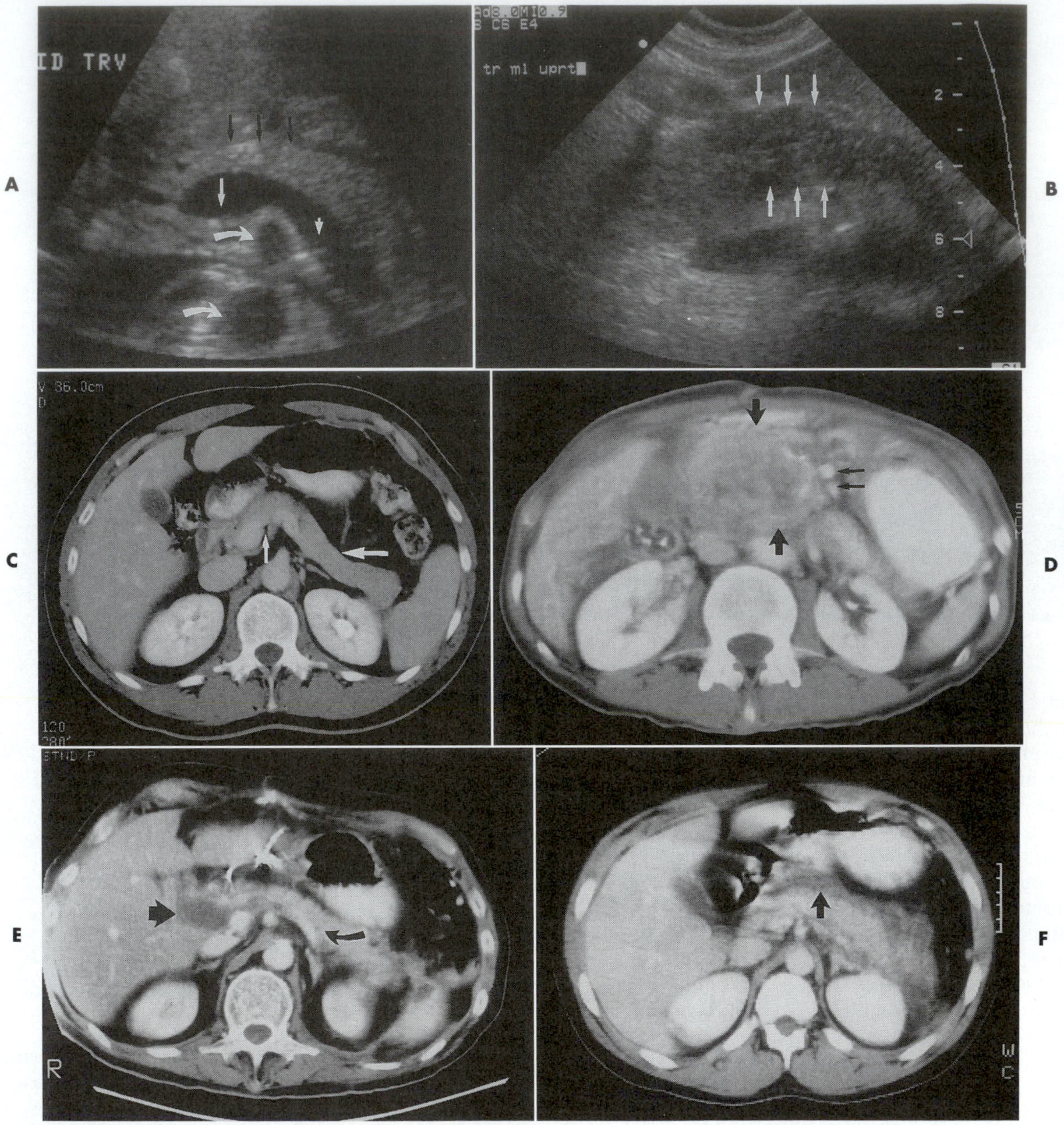


**Fig. 46-2.** Normal pancreas and pancreatitis. **A,** Normal pancreas *(black arrow)* and normal landmarks. Portal vein *(large white arrow),* splenic vein *(small white arrow),* superior mesenteric artery *(top curved white arrow),* and aorta *(linear curved white arrow).* **B,** Ultrasound demonstrating an enlarged pancreas outlined by arrows in acute pancreatitis. **C,** Dynamic (contrast-enhanced) CT scan showing a normal pancreas *(white arrows).* **D,** CT scan showing a necrotic pancreas *(broad black arrows)* impinging on the superior mesenteric artery and vein *(horizontal thin arrows).* **E,** Dynamic CT in acute pancreatitis showing viable pancreas *(curved arrow)* and necrotic pancreas *(straight arrow).* **F,** CT scan in acute pancreatitis showing enlarged pancreas and peripancreatic fluid collection *(arrow).*

**Table 46-1.** Diagnosis of acute pancreatitis

| Criterion | Definite | Probable | Possible |
|---|---|---|---|
| 1. Causal factor identified | X | X | X |
| 2. Compatible physical examination | X | X | X |
| 3. Nonspecific indications of an inflammatory response (i.e., fever, tachycardia, ↑WBC) | X | X | ±* |
| 4. Biochemical confirmatory tests<br>Serum amylase ↑3 × normal or ><br>Serum lipase ↑2 × normal or ><br>Urine amylase ↑<br>Other reasons for elevated serum amylase excluded | X† | — | — |
| 5. Imaging procedures<br>Ultrasound<br>CT scan | X† | — | — |

*All three are not present.
†If no. 1-3 and either no. 4 or 5 are positive, a definite diagnosis of acute pancreatitis is established.

### Differential diagnosis of acute pancreatitis

Acute appendicitis
Acute cholecystitis
Perforated viscus, especially peptic ulcer
Alcohol hepatitis
Mesenteric vascular occlusion
Connective tissue disorders with vasculitis (SLE, polyarteritis nodosa) and related disorders (TTP, Henoch's purpura, Schönlein purpura)
Renal colic
Dissecting aortic aneurysm
Gynecologic problems (pelvic inflammatory disease, ectopic pregnancy, mittelschmerz, ruptured ovarian cyst)
Medical problems that can cause acute abdominal pain (pneumonia, myocardial infarction, diabetic ketoacidosis, sickle cell anemia, porphyria)

*SLE,* Systemic lupus erythematosus; *TTP,* thrombotic thrombocytopenic purpura.

abdomen, hyperglycemia, hypocalcemia, raised BUN levels, and decreased serum albumin values. The diagnosis usually is confirmed by finding an elevated serum amylase or serum lipase. Obviously, not all of these features need be present for the diagnosis to be established. It is convenient to consider the diagnosis of acute pancreatitis in terms of definite, probable, and possible pancreatitis. The criteria for these diagnostic categories are summarized in Table 46-1.

The differential diagnosis of acute pancreatitis is summarized in the box above. Acute appendicitis must be considered in all patients with acute abdominal pain. Localization of pain to the right lower quadrant, low-grade fever, and moderate leukocytosis point to the diagnosis of acute appendicitis. It may be quite difficult to distinguish between acute cholecystitis and acute pancreatitis, since an increased serum amylase may be found in both disorders. That the pain of biliary tract origin is more right sided and gradual in onset and the fact that ileus usually is absent are helpful clues pointing toward a diagnosis of acute cholecystitis. A perforated duodenal ulcer is usually diagnosed by the presence of free intraperitoneal air, which is present in over 75% of patients. Alcoholic hepatitis should be considered in patients with a history of excessive alcohol ingestion, hepatomegaly, and elevated values for mean corpuscular volume (MCV), serum aspartate aminotransferase (AST; formerly SGOT), an AST:ALT (alanine aminotransferase; formerly SGPT) ratio greater than 3:1, and gamma glutamyl transpeptidase (GGTP). The diagnosis of intestinal obstruction caused by mechanical factors should be entertained with a history of colicky abdominal pain, compatible findings on physical examination of the abdomen, and x-rays of the abdomen showing characteristic changes of mechanical obstruction. Acute mesenteric vascular occlusion should be considered in elderly debilitated patients with a history of weight loss, postprandial abdominal pain, and an abdominal bruit who present with brisk leukocytosis, abdominal distention, and bloody diarrhea. Arteriography in such patients frequently shows evidence of vascular occlusion in two or more major arteries. It is important to remember that serum amylase levels are increased in approximately 25% of patients. In patients with systemic lupus erythematosus (SLE) or polyarteritis nodosa it may be quite difficult to differentiate between the abdominal pain caused by vasculitis and gut ischemia with or without infarction, and that caused by pancreatitis per se.

Diabetic ketoacidosis often is accompanied by abdominal pain, leukocytosis, and elevated serum amylase levels, thus simulating acute pancreatitis. However, the serum amylase frequently is of salivary and not of pancreatic origin. Metabolic acidosis per se can result in elevated serum amylase levels (especially salivary isoamylase). However, the serum lipase level is not elevated in diabetic ketoacidosis and with an imaging procedure is useful in excluding a diagnosis of acute pancreatitis. Renal colic usually is associated with an abnormal urinalysis and sonogram and often with an abnormal intravenous pyelogram. All patients with acute abdominal pain must have a chest film examination to exclude acute pneumonia, which can mimic a surgical abdomen. A constellation of the

## Complications of acute pancreatitis

**Local**

- Pancreatic phlegmon
- Pancreatic pseudocyst
  - Pain
  - Rupture with/without hemorrhage
  - Hemorrhage
  - Infection
- Pancreatic ascites
  - Disruption of main pancreatic duct
  - Leaking pseudocyst
- Pancreatic abscess
- Involvement of contiguous organs by necrotizing pancreatitis
  - Massive intraperitoneal hemorrhage
  - Thrombosis of blood vessels
  - Bowel infarction
- Obstructive jaundice

**Systemic**

- Pulmonary
  - Atelectasis
  - Pneumonitis
  - Pleural effusion
  - Mediastinal abscess
  - Adult respiratory distress syndrome
- Cardiovascular
  - Hypotension
    - Hypovolemia
    - Sepsis
  - Sudden death
  - Nonspecific ST-T changes in ECG simulating myocardial infarction
  - Pericardial effusion
- Hematologic
  - Disseminated intravascular coagulation (DIC)
- Gastrointestinal hemorrhage
  - Peptic ulcer disease
  - Erosive gastritis
  - Hemorrhagic pancreatic necrosis with erosion into major blood vessels
  - Portal vein thrombosis; variceal hemorrhage
- Renal
  - Oliguria } usually caused by hypovolemia
  - Azotemia }
  - Renal artery and/or renal vein thrombosis
- Metabolic
  - Hyperglycemia
  - Hypertriglyceridemia
  - Hypocalcemia
- Central nervous system
  - Psychosis
  - Fat emboli
  - Encephalopathy
- Fat necrosis
  - Subcutaneous tissues/erythematous nodules
  - Bone
  - Other organs (mediastinum, pleura, nervous system)
- Miscellaneous
  - Sudden blindness (Purtscher's retinopathy)

*Adapted from Greenberger NJ et al: *The medical book of lists: a primer of differential diagnosis in internal medicine,* ed 3, St Louis, 1990, Mosby.

following clinical features should suggest the diagnosis of gallstone-associated acute pancreatitis: (1) age over 50 years; (2) female; (3) serum amylase over 1000 U; (4) serum AST over 100 U; and (5) serum bilirubin over 2 mg/dl. If all five features are present, there is an 85% probability the diagnosis is gallstone pancreatitis.

Although the vast majority of patients with acute pancreatitis recover without major complication, 5% to 10% develop *severe* pancreatitis. Accordingly, it is important to identify factors that increase the likelihood of a fatal outcome in patients with acute pancreatitis. Several schemes to assess the severity of pancreatitis have been proposed, and these are summarized in the box on p. 653. Note that the major factors are identified in all three classifications. Patients with severe acute pancreatitis need to be hospitalized in intensive care units, and consultations with a surgeon and gastroenterologist are indicated.

### Management of acute pancreatitis

As indicated above, in most patients with acute pancreatitis (85% to 90%) the disease is self-limited and subsides spontaneously, usually within 3 to 5 days after treatment is initiated. Medical treatment is aimed at reducing pancreatic secretion and, in essence, putting the pancreas at rest. Conventional measures include (1) analgesics for pain; (2) intravenous fluids and colloids to maintain normal intravascular volume and correct electrolyte abnormalities; (3) no oral alimentation; and (4) nasogastric suction. However, since nasogastric suction offers no clear-cut advantages in the treatment of mild to moderately severe acute pancreatitis, its use should be considered elective rather than mandatory. The patient with mild to moderate pancreatitis usually requires treatment with intravenous fluids, remaining NPO, and possibly nasogastric suction for 3 to 5 days. A clear liquid diet frequently is started on the fifth day and a regular diet by the seventh day.

No drugs have been demonstrated to improve the course of mild, moderate, or severe pancreatitis. The list includes anticholinergic drugs (which are contraindicated), antibiotics (except for infected pancreatic necrosis and other proven infection), somatostatin analogues such as octreotide, $H_2$ receptor antagonists, and calcitonin.

The patient with fulminant pancreatitis requires intensive therapy. This usually includes large amounts of intravenous fluids, treatment of cardiovascular collapse and respiratory insufficiency, and treatment of hypocalcemia. Removal of toxic pancreatic exudate from the peritoneal cavity may alter the course of the disease, although controlled trials of peritoneal lavage have not established that this procedure is effective. In patients with failure in one or more organ systems (see the box at left), intensive supportive therapy, preferably in an ICU, is indicated. Such patients with severe acute pancreatitis usually require parenteral nutrition. Consultation with a surgeon or gastroenterologist should be obtained.

In patients acutely ill with severe pancreatitis and major risk factors, the presence of pancreatic abscess or infected phlegmon needs to be excluded. This is usually accomplished by CT-guided biopsy, aspiration of pancreatic tissue, and preparation of appropriate cultures. Infected pancreatic necrosis should be removed by debridement; this should be done surgically because it is difficult to evacuate solid infected material by percutaneous catheter drainage. The optimum treatment of patients with severe pancreatitis and *sterile* pancreatic necrosis is controversial. If such patients develop organ failure or have acute physiologic and chronic health evaluation (APACHE II; a scale used to assess severity of illness) scores greater than 13, surgical debridement is reasonable because the mortality in this setting can be as high as 40%. The complications of acute pancreatitis are summarized in the box on p. 656.

## PSEUDOCYST OF THE PANCREAS

Pseudocysts of the pancreas are collections of tissue, fluid, debris, pancreatic enzymes, and blood that develop over a period of 1 to 4 weeks after the onset of acute pancreatitis. In contrast to true cysts, pseudocysts do not have an epithelial lining and the walls consist of necrotic, granulation, and fibrous tissue. Disruption of the pancreatic ductal system is common. It should be noted that transient edema and fluid collections within the pancreas may give rise to epigastric pain, a palpable abdominal mass, and distortion or displacement of the upper gastrointestinal tract on barium study, thus mimicking a pancreatic pseudocyst. The use of ultrasonography and CT scanning should permit differentiation between an edematous and inflamed pancreas and an actual pseudocyst.

### Etiology

Pseudocysts are preceded by pancreatitis in approximately 90% of cases. In several reports the incidence of acute and chronic alcoholism in patients with pseudocysts has ranged from 88% to 93%. Gallbladder disease was identified in approximately 5% and trauma in approximately 10% of cases; rarely are there other etiologic factors.

### Clinical features

Pseudocysts develop in 10% to 15% of patients with acute pancreatitis. Pseudocysts are solitary lesions in more than 90% of patients and multiple in less than 10%. Approximately 90% of pseudocysts are located in the body or tail of the pancreas and 10% in the head. Abdominal pain is a cardinal symptom and is present in more than 90% of patients. Nausea and vomiting, anorexia, and weight loss are common symptoms, whereas diarrhea and fever are relatively infrequent. A palpable mass, often tender and usually in the midabdomen or left upper quadrant, is present in approximately 50% of patients. However, on the basis of physical examination alone it is difficult to differentiate between an edematous, inflamed pancreas (which can give rise to a palpable mass) and a pseudocyst. Ascites is present in approximately 20% and jaundice in 10% of patients.

Several laboratory tests are important in the evaluation of patients with pseudocysts. Serum amylase is raised in approximately 75% of patients. The white blood cell count is 12,000/mm$^3$ or higher in approximately half of the patients, the blood sugar is elevated in one third, and the hemoglobin level is under 10 g/dl in approximately one fourth of the patients. Chest x-ray evidence of pulmonary and/or pleural disease is found in approximately 25% of such patients. The serum bilirubin is elevated to values greater than 2 mg/dl in approximately 10% of patients, usually as a result of compression of the intrapancreatic portion of the common bile duct. Ultrasound, CT scan, and

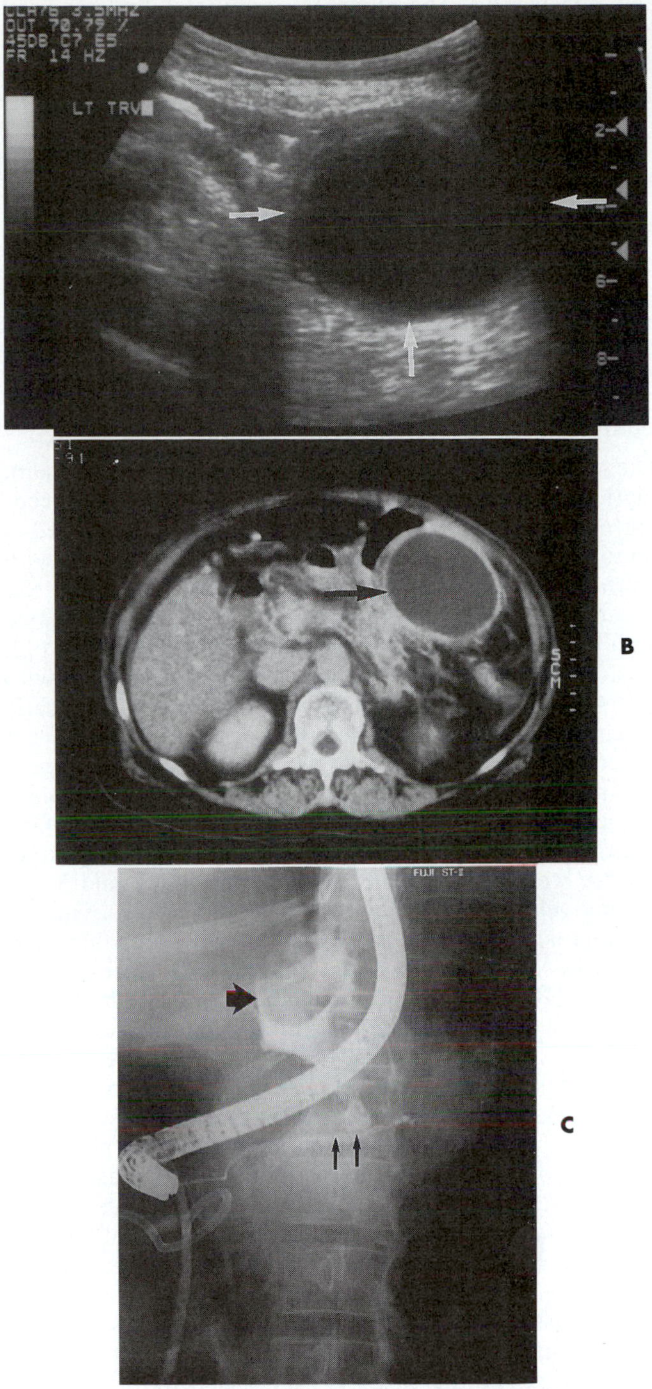

A

B

C

**Fig. 46-3.** Pseudocyst of the pancreas. **A,** Ultrasound showing a large pancreatic pseudocyst *(white arrow).* **B,** CT scan showing a well-encapsulated pseudocyst *(arrow).* **C,** ERCP showing a disrupted pancreatic duct *(vertical arrows)* communicating directly with a pancreatic pseudocyst *(horizontal arrow).*

endoscopic retrograde cholangiopancreatography (ERCP) findings in pancreatic pseudocyst are shown in Fig. 46-3.

### Differential diagnosis

The diagnosis of pseudocyst often is difficult, however, because the clinical features, physical examination, and conventional radiologic evaluations are both insensitive and nonspecific. The symptoms, physical findings, and laboratory and radiographic studies have been summarized previously. An ultrasound or CT scan should be obtained to confirm the diagnosis. The differential diagnosis of pancreatic cysts includes (1) pseudocysts; (2) retention cysts; (3) neoplasms such as cystadenoma and cystadenocarcinoma; (4) congenital causes; and (5) desmoids.

In studies utilizing serial ultrasound or CT scan, pseudocysts resolved in 25% to 40% of patients. However, pseudocysts that are greater than 5 cm and present for longer than 6 weeks infrequently disappear. Persistent pseudocysts can be treated by CT-guided percutaneous drainage (if the location is favorable) or by surgical or endoscopic cystogastrostomy or cystoenterostomy.

### Course of the disease and complications

The major complications of pseudocyst include pain, rupture with and without bleeding, gastrointestinal bleeding, abscess, and pancreatic ascites. The most dreaded is rupture with hemorrhage, which is associated with mortality rates of 50% to 60%. Pancreatic abscess can occur (1) because of communication of the pseudocyst with the colon; (2) after inadequate surgical drainage of a pseudocyst; (3) after needling a pseudocyst; and (4) with infected severe pancreatic necrosis. In addition, pancreatic abscess is much more common in patients with severe pancreatitis. In a representative series, pancreatic abscess occurred in 28 of 330 patients with pancreatitis. The cause of pancreatitis in these cases of pancreatic abscess most commonly was surgery; alcoholism and biliary tract disease were the etiologic insult in only 6.6% and 3.0%, respectively. In patients with lethal pancreatitis, evidence of pancreatic abscess is found at autopsy in more than 90% of cases. The incidence of pancreatic abscess rises appreciably with an increasing number of risk factors present in a given case, being less than 3% with fewer than three risk factors and greater than 50% with five or more risk factors. Characteristic signs of pancreatic abscess are the development of fever, tachycardia, leukocytosis, toxicity, and rapid deterioration after an initial period of stabilization. Serial CT scans may provide additional evidence to support a diagnosis of infected pseudocyst and/or pancreatic abscess, but the absence of telltale gas on a CT scan does not exclude a diagnosis of pancreatic abscess.

Pancreatic ascites occurs because of one of two factors: (1) disruption of the main pancreatic duct or (2) a leaking pseudocyst. The diagnosis is established by the triad of findings of (1) persistently increased serum amylase; (2) elevated ascitic fluid amylase; and (3) increased ascitic fluid protein concentration (over 3 g/dl). Patients frequently require surgery.

### Management

If the patient is stable and serial ultrasound examinations show that the pseudocyst is decreasing in size, observation only is indicated. However, patients with an expanding pseudocyst or those complicated by rupture, hemorrhage, or abscess should undergo operation. Elective cyst drainage usually is indicated if pseudocysts persist for longer than 6 weeks. ERCP may be important in this setting in that a leaking pancreatic duct can be identified and treated by stenting (see Fig. 46-3). The long-acting somatostatin analogue octreotide, which inhibits pancreatic secretion, is also useful in this setting.

## CHRONIC PANCREATITIS

### Epidemiology and etiology

Chronic pancreatitis is usually characterized by recurring or persistent abdominal pain with or without steatorrhea or diabetes. Morphologically, chronic pancreatitis is characterized by irregular sclerosis with destruction and permanent loss of pancreatic parenchyma that may be focal, segmental, or diffuse and variable dilatation of the pancreatic ducts.

Chronic pancreatitis may present as episodes of acute inflammation superimposed upon a previously injured pancreas or as chronic damage with persistent pain or malabsorption. The box below lists the causes of both chronic pancreatitis and pancreatic exocrine insufficiency. Patients with chronic pancreatic damage of mild to moderate severity usually come to medical attention because of chronic abdominal pain. Often the only abnormal laboratory test at this stage of the disease is a test of pancreatic exocrine function such as the secretin test or bentiromide (Chymex) test. Patients with extensive chronic pancreatic damage frequently present with diarrhea, steatorrhea, and weight loss; these patients have pancreatic exocrine insufficiency. Because of the enormous reserve capacity of the pancreas, malabsorption is a late manifestation of chronic pancreatitis resulting only when more than 90% of the exocrine pancreas is destroyed.

#### Causes of chronic pancreatitis and pancreatic exocrine insufficiency

**Chronic pancreatitis**

Chronic alcoholism*
Etiologic factor unknown (idiopathic)*
Hereditary pancreatitis
Hemochromatosis
Radiation injury
Trauma
Sicca syndrome

**Cystic fibrosis***

**Following surgery**

Gastric surgery (subtotal gastrectomy, antrectomy, vagotomy, and pyloroplasty)
Whipple procedure
≥ 95% pancreatic resection for chronic pancreatitis

**Neoplasms**

Adenocarcinoma of the pancreas*
Islet cell tumors (gastrinoma, VIPoma)
Duodenal adenocarcinoma obstruction of pancreatic duct

**Severe protein-calorie malnutrition**

*VIP,* Vasoactive intestinal polypeptide.
*Most common.

**Recurrent bouts of acute pancreatitis without an obvious cause**

- Biliary microlithiasis (most common; 60% to 75% of cases)
- Occult disease of biliary tree, pancreatic duct system, ampulla of Vater
- Hypertriglyceridemia
- Pancreas divisum
- Hereditary pancreatitis
- Drugs

In the United States alcohol is by far the most common cause of clinically apparent pancreatic exocrine insufficiency, whereas cystic fibrosis accounts for the majority of cases in children. Approximately 85% of patients with cystic fibrosis have impairment of pancreatic exocrine function. With improvement in the treatment of their pulmonary problems, an increasing number of patients with cystic fibrosis are reaching adulthood, at which time their pancreatic exocrine insufficiency can become clinically relevant. In adult patients 20 to 40 years of age with exocrine pancreatic insufficiency without obvious cause, the diagnosis of cystic fibrosis should be excluded. In adult patients over age 40 with pancreatic insufficiency without obvious cause, pancreatic cancer needs to be excluded (see the box above). It is important to note that in up to 25% of adults in the United States with chronic pancreatitis, the disorder is idiopathic.

### Pathophysiology

The pancreas has an enormous reserve capacity for the digestion of nutrients. Studies by DiMagno and his associates clearly demonstrated that there is an inverse relationship between intraduodenal and intrajejunal levels of lipase and development of steatorrhea. Similarly, there is also an inverse relationship between intraluminal trypsin and chymotrypsin levels and the development of azotorrhea (increased nitrogen in the stool) and creatorrhea (undigested muscle fibers in the stool). The data of DiMagno et al. indicate that steatorrhea, azotorrhea, and creatorrhea are late manifestations of pancreatic exocrine insufficiency and develop when the capacity of the exocrine pancreas to secrete these enzymes is less than 10% of normal values. Thus patients may have evidence of exocrine dysfunction, that is, an impaired response to intravenously injected secretin or secretin plus cholecystokinin or an abnormal pancreatic ductal system demonstrated by ERCP but without any obvious impairment in digestive function.

Many patients with chronic pancreatitis have persistent abdominal pain as the major manifestation of their disease. The mechanism of pain in chronic pancreatitis has not been clearly elucidated, but there are several postulated mechanisms. These include (1) persistence of pseudocysts with perifocal inflammation; (2) dilatation of the pancreatic duct due to elevated ductal pressures; (3) continued pancreatic parenchymal inflammatory processes; (4) pressure of an enlarged or inflamed gland on retroperitoneal structures; and (5) infiltration or entrapment of sensory nerves. Pseudocysts can be important in the pathogenesis of pancreatic pain as evidenced by the repeated observation that up to 50% of patients with chronic pancreatitis and pain have obtained pain relief by simple drainage of pseudocysts. Therefore it is important that, in all patients with chronic pancreatic pain, imaging studies (preferably a CT scan) are performed to exclude the possibility of an underlying pseudocyst. An abnormal pancreatic ductal system is frequently documented in patients with chronic pancreatitis. However, there is no consistent relationship between the severity of pain due to chronic pancreatitis and the presence of strictured or dilated ducts. However, some patients with pancreatic pain and stenotic ducts may obtain relief when the pancreatic ductal system is stented.

Studies in experimental animals and in humans have supported the concept of an enteropancreatic axis. This theory postulates that, after initiation of intraluminal digestions by pancreatic enzymes, increased levels of proteases in the duodenal and jejunal lumen act in a feedback manner to decrease release of cholecystokinin from the small bowel mucosa, which in turn results in decreased stimulation of the pancreas. The concept has led to the use of pharmacologic doses of pancreatic enzymes, rich in protease content, in the treatment of persistent pain in patients with chronic pancreatitis (see p. 661).

### History

Although patients with chronic pancreatitis may have symptoms identical to those found in patients with acute pancreatitis, it is important to note that patients with chronic pancreatitis often complain of persistent or recurring pain. Although many patients may have severe epigastric pain that radiates through to the back, the pain pattern often is atypical. The pain may be maximal in the right upper or left upper quadrant, in the back, or diffuse throughout the abdomen; it may even be referred to the anterior chest or flank. Characteristically the pain is severe, persistent, deep seated, unresponsive to antacids or food ingestion, and increased by alcohol ingestion or heavy meals (especially foods rich in fat). Often the pain is so severe as to require the frequent use of narcotics. Nausea, vomiting, and abdominal distention are seen less frequently and usually are secondary to the pain and use of medications (especially narcotics), which decrease gastric and intestinal motility.

Weight loss, diarrhea, and steatorrhea frequently are present. However, clinically apparent deficiencies of fat-soluble vitamins are noted less frequently than in patients with steatorrhea secondary to small bowel disease. The stool characteristically has an oily appearance and may cling to the sides of the toilet bowl, requiring several flushes of the toilet.

### Physical examination

The physical findings in patients with chronic pancreatitis and/or pancreatic exocrine insufficiency usually are not impressive. Indeed, the disparity between the severity of the abdominal pain and the paucity of physical findings is remarkable. Abdominal tenderness and mild fever may be seen, especially in those with episodes of acute superimposed on chronic pancreatitis. Weight loss may be profound. Jaundice may be noted in 10% to 20% of

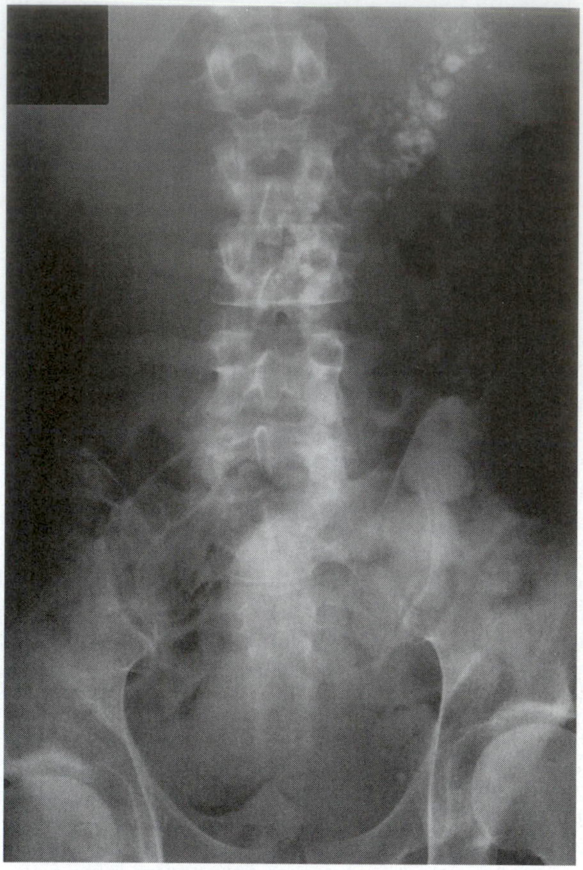

**Fig. 46-4.** Calcification in the pancreas.

patients from obstruction of the common bile duct secondary to edema or fibrosis of the duct above or in the head of the pancreas. Ascites and a palpable abdominal mass (pseudocyst) may be noted in 2% to 5% of patients. Patients with severe malabsorption often show evidence of malnutrition with cachexia, muscle wasting, edema, and stigmata of vitamin deficiencies.

### Laboratory studies and diagnostic procedures

Several studies can be used to evaluate pancreatic exocrine function, but many of these are not widely available. Direct tests of pancreatic secretory capacity include the secretin test or the secretin plus cholecystokinin test. These tests are usually available only in academic health centers. A practical and useful test of pancreatic secretory function is the bentiromide (Chymex) test. This test is based on administering a tripeptide (benzoyl-tyrosyl-para-aminobenzoic acid) with the tyrosyl-para-aminobenzoic acid linkage being specifically susceptible to chymotrypsin action. If there is pancreatic exocrine insufficiency and decreased intraluminal amounts of chymotrypsin, the para-aminobenzoic acid is not split off, absorbed, and excreted in the urine. If less than 50% of the available para-aminobenzoic acid is recovered in the urine, the test is definitely abnormal and should prompt further investigative studies. A reliable test to document evidence of intraluminal maldigestion is to examine stools for evidence of fatty acid crystal and undigested muscle fibers (creatorrhea). The finding of more than five muscle fibers in the stool provides strong evidence of impaired intraluminal digestion. Although a very specific test, this test is rather insensitive in that positivity requires that more than 95% of the exocrine pancreas has been destroyed.

Several diagnostic procedures are available to image the pancreas. The simplest test is the plain film of the abdomen; if this shows evidence of pancreatic calcification, it establishes the diagnosis of chronic pancreatitis (Fig. 46-4). Ultrasound studies may reveal evidence of pancreatic calcification (before it is evident on the plain film), enlargement of the pancreas, or irregularities in the pancreas. The CT scan is the diagnostic procedure of choice to evaluate the pancreas in patients with suspected chronic pancreatitis. In addition to showing evidence of calcification, it may show evidence of duct dilatation, focal enlargement, fluid collections, biliary ductal dilatation, alterations of peripancreatic fat, or fascia. A normal-appearing pancreas appears in only 10% of the patients with chronic pancreatitis. ERCP often shows varying degrees of ductular dilatation and may show marked dilatation of areas of stenosis as well.

## Diagnosis of pancreatic exocrine insufficiency

Identify etiology of pancreatic insufficiency (e.g., alcoholism, pancreatic cancer)
Steatorrhea
Pancreatic calcification } The classic diagnostic triad
Diabetes mellitus
Undigested muscle fibers in stool (creatorrhea)
Tests of pancreatic exocrine function; frequently necessary since diagnostic triad found in approximately 20% of patients
- Secretin-CCK test
- Chymex (bentiromide) test

↓ Absorption vitamin $B_{12}$ (part II Schilling test)
Normal tests of mucosal function (D-xylose, small bowel biopsy)
Response to pancreatic enzyme replacement therapy
- Gain in weight
- Amelioration of diarrhea/steatorrhea

There may be a poor correlation between pancreatic function tests and ERCP findings

*CCK,* Cholecystokinin.

### Differential diagnosis

The criteria for the diagnosis of pancreatic exocrine insufficiency are summarized in the box at left. To begin with, the etiology of pancreatic insufficiency must be identified. In adults past age 40 and especially past age 60 who present with evidence of pancreatic malabsorption (steatorrhea, creatorrhea) the diagnosis of pancreatic cancer must be excluded. The classic diagnostic triad for pancreatic exocrine insufficiency comprises steatorrhea, pancreatic calcification, and diabetes mellitus. The presence of these three findings obviates the needs to carry out additional tests of pancreatic secretory capacity. Unfortunately, only one fourth of the patients with pancreatic exocrine insufficiency manifest the diagnostic triad. Therefore it is often necessary to carry out additional studies (i.e., qualitative examination of the stool and Chymex test, as already discussed). Absorption of vitamin $B_{12}$ with the part II Schilling test is often done, since over 40% of patients with pancreatic exocrine insufficiency have impaired absorption of vitamin $B_{12}$. In patients with malabsorption, as evidenced by the presence of steatorrhea, it is also necessary to confirm that tests of mucosal function are normal. These include a normal D-xylose test, normal small bowel x-rays, and a normal small bowel biopsy. An important parameter that confirms the presence of malabsorption due to pancreatic exocrine insufficiency is a positive response to pancreatic enzyme replacement therapy. Such a positive response is characterized by gain in weight and amelioration of diarrhea, steatorrhea, and creatorrhea.

In patients with chronic pancreatitis manifested only by chronic abdominal pain, it is important to exclude other painful conditions and to confirm that patients are not surreptitiously using alcohol. If available, the secretin test is useful in establishing the diagnosis of chronic pancreatitis, since patients with pain due to chronic pancreatitis almost invariably have a peak bicarbonate concentration under 80 mEq/L.

The differential diagnosis of pain in chronic pancreatitis should include all of the following: (1) pseudocysts; (2) peptic ulcer disease; (3) cholelithiasis; (4) pancreatic cancer; (5) biliary tract obstruction; (6) pancreatic stones; and (7) narcotic addiction. The latter is an important issue and can usually be diagnosed by taking a careful history and trying to wean the patient off narcotics under clonidine cover. This usually requires hospitalization and administration of clonidine (usually as a patch, but at least in a dosage of 5 μg/kg). Because the drug may cause hypotension, it should be done in a hospital setting where the narcotic dosage can be reduced 20% to 25% per day.

## Management and course of the disease

The Managed Care Guide on p. 662 provides an algorithm for approaching the management of patients with pancreatogenous steatorrhea. It is usual to start with pancreatic enzymes that have both potent lipase and protease content and to take a minimum of 12 capsules per day, four with meals. If treatment with 12 capsules per day is not effective, this can be increased to 16, or even up to 24 capsules per day. If diarrhea or steatorrhea persists, the fat content in the diet should be reduced. If there are still problems with persistent steatorrhea or diarrhea, either bicarbonate or an $H_2$ receptor blocker can be added. The evidence that $H_2$ receptor blockers bring about additional improvement in this setting is still somewhat controversial.

The management of pain in chronic pancreatitis requires an understanding of the natural history of this problem. A classic study by Ammann evaluated 245 patients with chronic pancreatitis and persistent pain for a median period of 10 years. In this group alcohol was the etiologic factor in 173 patients, 58 had idiopathic chronic pancreatitis, and 14 had various rare disorders. Irrespective of medical or surgical therapy, 85% of the patients obtained lasting pain relief within 4.5 years. In many patients pain relief was accompanied by further pancreatic dysfunction and the development of malabsorption. It is imperative to be sure that the use of alcohol is discontinued in all patients with chronic pancreatitis, and especially those with persistent pain. This simple expedient will result in pain relief in approximately 50% of patients with chronic pancreatitis.

Because there is evidence supporting the concept of an enteropancreatic axis, a trial of high-dose pancreatic enzyme therapy should be considered in all patients who have pain due to chronic pancreatitis. This should include pancreatic enzyme therapy (18 to 24 capsules per day), and the capsules should not be the enteric coated, slow release type of enzyme preparation. The patients most likely to respond to pancreatic enzyme replacement therapy are females with idiopathic pancreatitis, in whom a response rate of about 75% may be seen. By contrast, the response rate is much less in males (20% to 25%), male alcoholics (12% to 15%), and males and females with severe chronic pancreatitis (25%). The Managed Care Guide on p. 663 is the algorithm for assessment and management of pain in chronic pancreatitis. It should be emphasized that, in all patients with chronic pancreatitis and persistent pain, it is important to exclude the presence of the pseudocyst since drainage of the pseudocyst often results in amelioration of pain. Finally, risk of narcotic addiction in such patients is high, and the pain in such patients should be controlled by using nonnarcotic analgesics. Drugs such as Darvon plus Tylenol combinations or nonsteroidals such as ketorolac, taken orally, are often effective. A regular schedule of Extra Strength Tylenol (1 g every 8 hours) is also effective. Patients who have been alcoholic should be cautioned about using even small doses of alcohol if they are taking 3 g of Tylenol per day.

The complications of chronic pancreatitis are summarized in the box above. Certain complications merit special mention. The first is pancreatogenous ascites, which can develop either as a result of a leaking pseudocyst or a disrupted pancreatic duct. The second is common bile duct

### Complications of chronic pancreatitis and pancreatic exocrine insufficiency

Pancreatic ascites
Chronic pain
Narcotic addiction
Steatorrhea and diarrhea
Diabetes mellitus
Cobalamin malabsorption
Ascites
Common bile duct obstruction
Biliary cirrhosis
Splenic vein thrombosis
Portal hypertension
Nondiabetic retinopathy
Pancreatic cancer

**Managed Care Guide**
**Management of pancreatogenous steatorrhea**

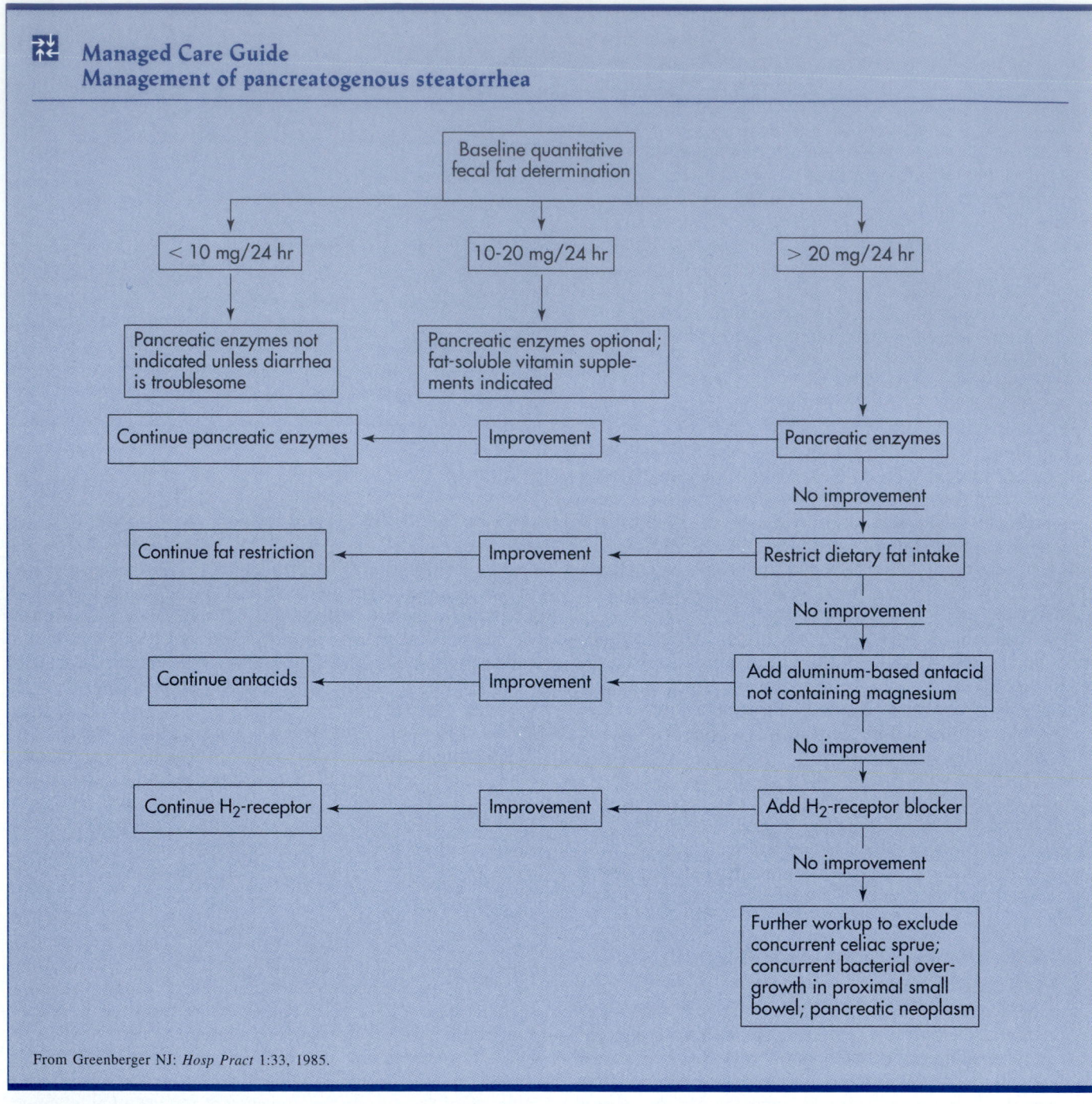

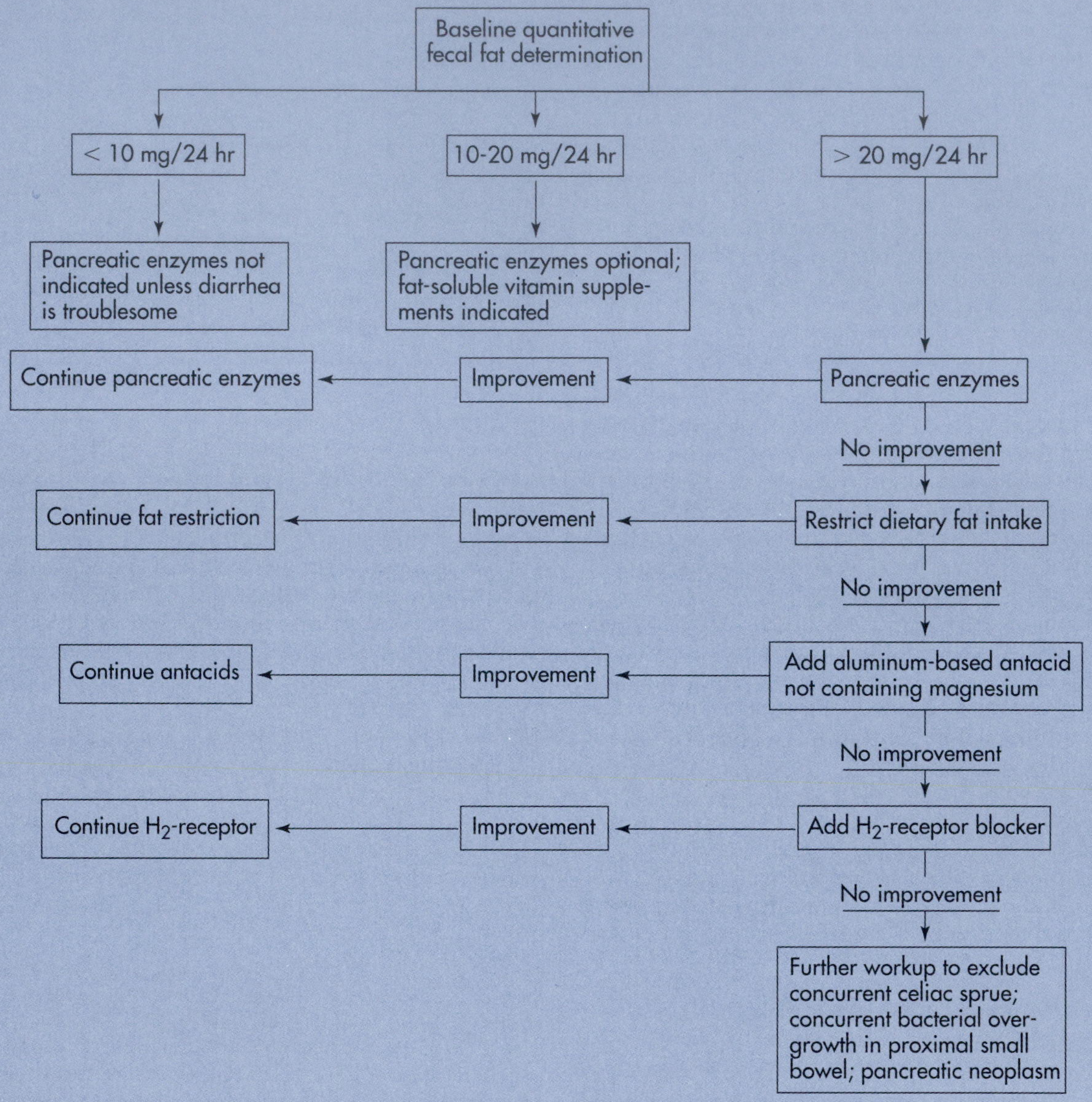


From Greenberger NJ: *Hosp Pract* 1:33, 1985.

obstruction with obstructive-type tests of liver function and the development of secondary biliary cirrhosis. Accordingly, in all patients with chronic pancreatitis who have persistent and sustained elevation of the serum alkaline phosphatase to values greater than two times normal for more than 2 months, studies should be undertaken to evaluate the presence of extrahepatic biliary tract obstruction. This usually means the performance of an ERCP. If this shows evidence of a stricture, then a liver biopsy should be performed. If this shows evidence of a secondary biliary cirrhosis, then decompression of the biliary tract obstruction should be undertaken.

## PANCREATIC CANCER

### Epidemiology

Carcinoma of the pancreas, one of the most dreaded of all tumors, strikes adults in all age groups; the peak age of risk is about 60 years. The overall incidence has risen 300% over the past 30 years, and pancreatic cancer now ranks as the fourth most common tumor behind lung, colorectal, and breast cancer. The disease attacks men twice as frequently as women.

Only a few risk factors have been clearly identified as predisposing to the development of pancreatic cancer. These include cigarette smoking, diabetes, and chronic

### Managed Care Guide
### Management of chronic pancreatic pain

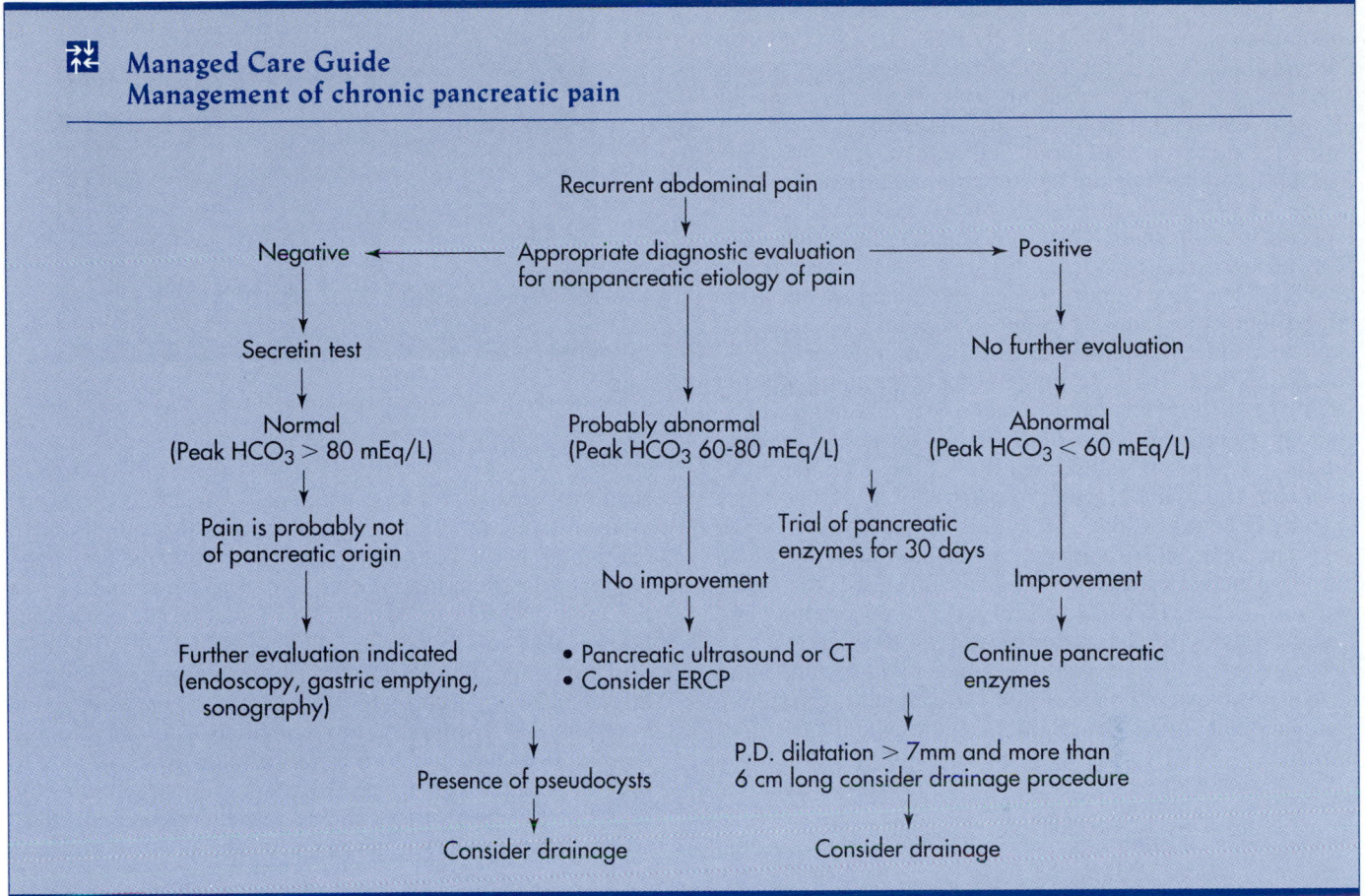

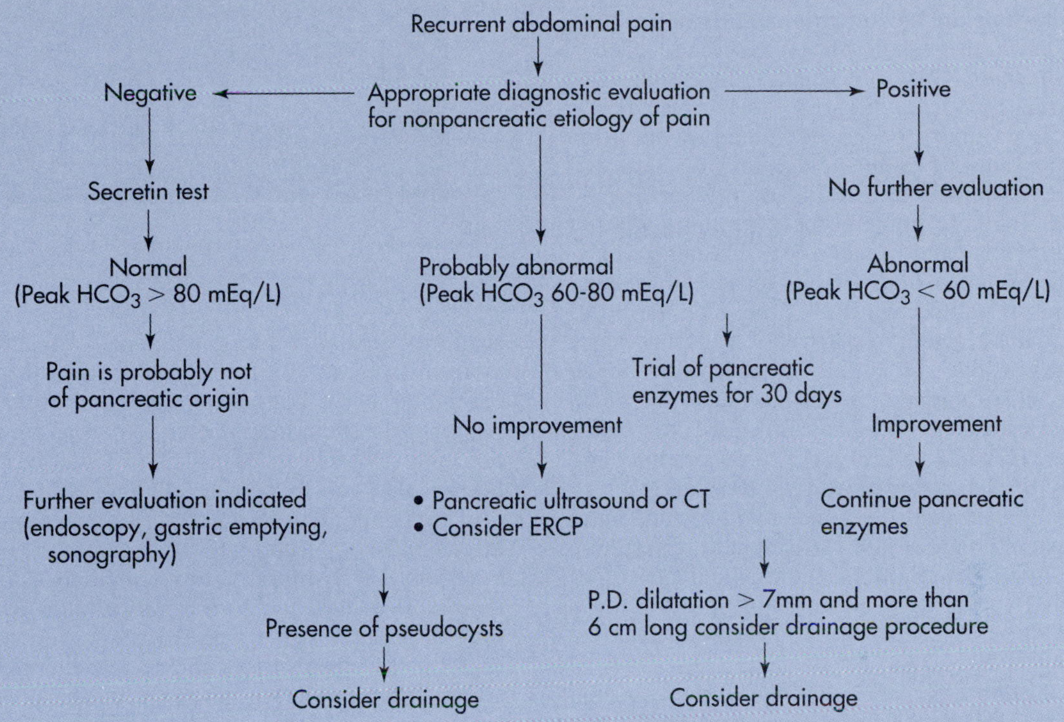


pancreatitis. However, the vast majority of patients with this tumor have none of these risk factors. This inability to identify subgroups at risk for the disease is one of the major problems limiting the development of screening techniques for early detection.

### Pathophysiology

The clinical presentation of pancreatic carcinoma, at least initially, can be quite variable, and these features are summarized in the box at right. The most common presentation, which is that of new onset, obscure and unrelenting abdominal pain, is due to an enlarging mass in the pancreas causing pressure on retroperitoneal structures and the stomach and duodenum. Presentation with diarrhea and malabsorption can be a consequence of a localized obstruction of the main pancreatic duct and head of the pancreas, resulting in pancreatic exocrine insufficiency and steatorrhea with diarrhea. Accordingly, the new onset of an irritable bowel–type syndrome in any patient past 50 with no prior history of such a disorder should always raise the question of pancreatic cancer. Pancreatic cancers located at the head of the pancreas often cause obstruction of the common bile duct resulting in new onset of jaundice with obstructive features. Approximately 40% of patients with pancreatic carcinoma have an abnormal blood glucose level detected within 2 years before diagnosis. Accordingly, in any patient past age 50 who develops signs of unexplained carbohydrate intolerance, especially if this is accompanied by abdominal pain or weight loss, the diagnosis of pancreatic carcinoma should be excluded.

### Clinical presentations of pancreatic carcinoma

New onset of persistent abdominal pain without an obvious cause
Onset of diarrhea (irritable bowel–type symptoms) without obvious cause in an adult over 50 years of age
Unexplained weight loss
Onset of diabetes without obvious risk factors (see text)
Onset of obstructive-type jaundice in adults over 50 years of age
Onset of depression without obvious cause
Onset of malabsorption with stigmata of pancreatic exocrine insufficiency in adults over 50 years of age
Metastatic adenocarcinoma with primary of unknown origin
Malignant ascites
Recurrent thrombophlebitis
Onset of symptoms of gastric outlet obstruction (nausea, postprandial distention)

### History

Persistent abdominal pain, weight loss, and unremitting jaundice are the outstanding symptoms of pancreatic carcinoma. As noted above, the site of the lesion, however, greatly influences the character and time of onset of symptoms. Obscure abdominal pain is one of the most difficult of all symptoms to evaluate. Clues to a pancreatic origin include a persistent gnawing, boring upper abdominal discomfort referred through to the back. This upper abdominal pain may have no particular exacerbating or relieving factors. If there is already some mechanical compromise to gastric emptying, the patient may complain of vague abdominal distress and fullness made worse by eating. Cancer in the body or tail of the pancreas frequently produces more severe pain, and its unrelenting nature should raise the suspicion of pancreatic cancer, especially if the pain is worse when lying supine and relieved by sitting forward. Although painless jaundice is touted as a presentation of pancreatic cancer, more often the patient complains of vague abdominal distress that may be difficult to characterize. In adults over age 50 presenting with irritable bowel–type symptoms without any prior such history, and especially if this is accompanied by weight loss, the diagnosis of pancreatic cancer should be kept in mind. Similarly, the new onset of malabsorption with stigmata of pancreatic exocrine insufficiency in adults past age 50 without an obvious reason to have pancreatic insufficiency should also raise the question of pancreatic cancer. Patients with anaplastic carcinoma of the pancreas have a lesion that grows rapidly and spreads quickly to distant locations, and this can result in evidence of malignant ascites or metastatic carcinoma at the time of presentation. Finally, patients with obstructive type jaundice often complain of intense and persistent pruritus.

### Physical examination

Pertinent physical findings in the patient with suspected pancreatic cancer include the following: (1) jaundice; (2) excoriations or scratching that may reflect pruritus; (3) evidence of recent weight loss; (4) Virchow supraclavicular adenopathy; (5) hepatomegaly, especially with the palpable left lobe of the liver; (6) a palpable gallbladder (Courvoisier's sign), which occurs in approximately one fourth to one third of patients; (7) palpable periumbilical (Sister Mary Joseph) lymph nodes; (8) splenomegaly, which may be due to splenic vein thrombosis because of invasion of the splenic artery and vein by the tumor; and (9) new detection of a left upper quadrant bruit, again due to invasion of the splenic artery and/or vein (this occurs in approximately 25% of patients with carcinoma of the body and tail of the pancreas).

### Laboratory studies and diagnostic procedures

Routine studies to obtain in patients suspected of harboring a pancreatic cancer include CBC, chemistry profile, and chest film. Chemistry profile may provide an initial clue to the presence of metastatic disease by the presence of a disproportionately elevated serum alkaline phosphatase. In patients with classic obstructive jaundice the serum aminotransferases, if elevated, are less than 400 IU. The serum alkaline phosphatase may be 2 to 10 times normal, and markers for viral hepatitis should be negative. Key tests to confirm suspected pancreatic cancer include ultrasound, CT scan, ERCP, CT-guided biopsy of a pancreatic mass lesion, and arteriography if surgery is contemplated (Fig. 46-5).

For a patient with obstructive-type jaundice the ultrasound study is an important initial consideration. The presence of dilated intrahepatic ducts points to a mechanical, obstructive process, where the absence of dilated ducts points to the diagnosis of intrahepatic cholestasis. CT scan, especially contrast-enhanced (dynamic) scan, is abnormal in approximately 90% of the patients with carcinoma of the pancreas, and especially so if the lesion is more than 2 cm in diameter. When an obvious lesion is detected by CT scanning, a CT-guided percutaneous biopsy may establish the diagnosis. ERCP may also provide important diagnostic information as well as affording an opportunity to decompress the obstructed bile duct. If CT scanning shows evidence of potentially resectable disease, an arteriogram should be performed to provide a road map for the surgeon and to exclude the presence of sheathing of the pancreaticoduodenal artery and/or splenic vein thrombosis which, if present, preclude a curative resection.

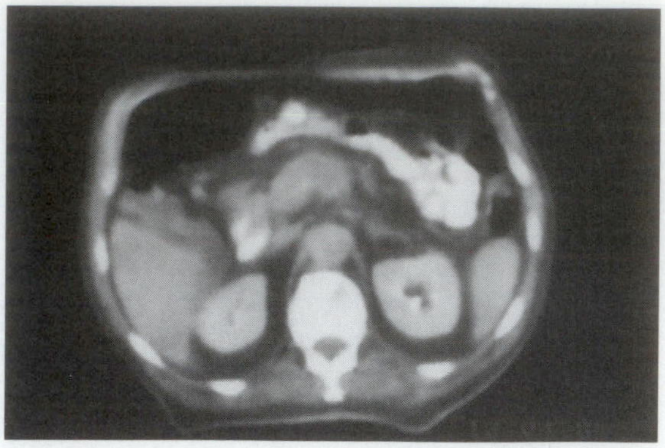

**Fig. 46-5.** CT scan demonstrating a mass in the pancreas.

## Differential diagnosis

For any patient presenting with new onset of persistent abdominal pain, jaundice with obstructive-type liver tests, new onset of diarrhea and malabsorption, the diagnosis of pancreatic carcinoma must be considered. In patients past age 60 with jaundice and obstructive-type liver tests, the differential diagnosis in 80% of cases lies between pancreatic cancer and choledocholithiasis with viral hepatitis, posttransfusion hepatitis, drug-induced jaundice, and alcoholic liver disease comprising the remainder. Therefore, if there is no history suggesting any of the latter four disorders, an imaging procedure should be carried out to determine whether the biliary ducts are dilated and, if so, further studies are indicated. Choledocholithiasis is rarely painless. Carcinoma of the ampulla of Vater can mimic many of the features of carcinoma of the pancreas but has a much better prognosis. This condition is diagnosed by ERCP, which reveals a tumor protruding into the duodenal lumen. CT-guided percutaneous biopsy of the pancreas is an effective means of establishing the diagnosis and provides positive results in approximately 85% of cases. For pancreatic duct adenocarcinomas, ERCP has a sensitivity of approximately 90% and a similar specificity. Arteriography has a sensitivity of approximately 65%, and a specificity of 90% at vessel sheathing and/or splenic vein thrombosis is demonstrated.

## Management

For patients with a lesion demonstrable by CT scan that measures less than 3 cm and in whom arteriography shows no evidence of vessel involvement or metastases, exploration with intent to carry out a Whipple procedure is recommended. If the operative findings confirm a lesion that is 3 cm or less in size with no adenopathy and no extension, a Whipple procedure results in a 2-year survival of up to 40%. The resectability rate in patients with pancreatic carcinoma is approximately 20%, owing to the presence of small metastases at presentation not detectable by CT scanning. The 5-year survival rate is still a dismal 5% or less in cases of nonresectable lesions. For patients with obstructive jaundice and evidence of metastases or nonresectability, it is reasonable to attempt stenting of the common bile duct to relieve both the symptoms and sequelae of high-grade extrahepatic obstruction. If a carcinoma of the head of the pancreas is causing gastric outlet obstruction, then it is reasonable to explore the patient and carry out a gastric bypass procedure as well as a cholecystojejunostomy. It should be emphasized that these procedures are palliative and will not affect the patient's long-term survival. Only 10% of patients with pancreatic cancer survive 1 year. There is no effective chemotherapy or radiation therapy for carcinoma of the pancreas. Approximately 15% of patients will respond briefly to chemotherapy. The addition of radiotherapy to chemotherapy results in an increased survival of only 1 to 2 months.

***Glucagonoma syndrome.*** Tumors of the pancreatic alpha cells result in high levels of circulating glucagon. This syndrome is associated with angular cheilitis, glossitis, and necrolytic migratory erythema—intertriginous, red, scaling, arcuate, erosive lesions in the body folds. The lesions are often confused with candidiasis. Skin biopsy is often diagnostic of the condition. Diabetes, anemia, and weight loss are commonly seen. Removal of the tumor results in healing of the cutaneous lesions.

## BIBLIOGRAPHY


Ammann RW et al: Course and outcome of chronic pancreatitis: longitudinal study of mixed medical-surgical series of 245 patients, *Gastroenterology* 86:820, 1984.

Balthazar EJ: Acute pancreatitis: prognostic value of CT, *Radiology* 156:767, 1985.

Banks PB: Acute pancreatitis: identification of high risk patients and aggressive treatment, *Gastrointest Dis Today* 2(1):2, 1993.

Campbell DR, Greenberger NJ: Management of pain in chronic pancreatitis. In Burn GR, Bank S, editors: *Disorders of the pancreas,* New York, 1992, McGraw-Hill.

DiMagno EP, Go VLW, Summerskill WH: Relations between pancreatic enzyme outputs and malabsorption in severe pancreatic insufficiency, *N Engl J Med* 288:813, 1973.

Eckfeldt JH, Lentherman JH, Levitt MD: High prevalence of hyperamylasemia in patients with acidosis, *Ann Intern Med* 104:362, 1986.

Karimgani I et al: Prognostic factors in sterile pancreatic necrosis, *Gastroenterology* 103:1636, 1992.

Lowenfels AB et al: Pancreatitis and the risk of pancreatic cancer, *N Engl J Med* 328:1433, 1993.

O'Malley VP et al: Pancreatic pseudocysts: cause, therapy, and results, *Am J Surg* 150:680, 1985.

Ranson JHC: Risk factors in acute pancreatitis, *Hosp Pract* 20:69, 1985.

Toskes PP: Bentiromide as a test of exocrine pancreatic function in adult patients and pancreatic exocrine insufficiency, *Gastroenterology* 85:565, 1983.


CHAPTER

# 47 Acute Abdomen


**Erwin F. Hirsch**
**Desmond H. Birkett**
**Joseph T. Ferrucci**


Patients with acute abdominal pain continue to challenge physicians and surgeons despite the sophisticated diagnostic and therapeutic armamentarium of modern medicine. The syndrome of the acute abdomen requires prompt investigation to establish a diagnosis and appropriate therapy. Delay in the implementation of appropriate treatment is usually associated with increased mortality and morbidity.

## HISTORY

Patients with an acute abdomen characteristically complain of abdominal pain, vomiting, change in bowel habits, or a combination of these symptoms. Most of these patients also demonstrate signs or have symptoms of significant systemic disease (e.g., tachycardia, tachypnea, fever, hypotension). Accurate and early diagnosis requires a careful overall evaluation of the patient and a review of symptoms.

### Pain

Abdominal pain is mediated through the autonomic nervous system and the intercostal nerves. The intraperitoneal organs and visceral peritoneum derive their nerve supply from the autonomic system. The parietal peritoneum is innervated by the intercostal nerves, which arise from the fifth to the eleventh spinal cord segments, and the diaphragm is innervated by the phrenic nerve.

The single most important component in the evaluation of patients is a careful medical history that focuses on the type, duration, location, and radiation of the abdominal pain. The characteristics of abdominal pain and its location provide a clue in many instances to its etiology and to the diagnosis. Crampy, colicky abdominal pain is the result of constrictive spasms of a hollow viscus. When longer free intervals occur between bouts of pain, gastrointestinal obstruction usually is located in the distal small bowel or the colon. Conversely, short free intervals between painful episodes that are usually accompanied by vomiting are characteristic of obstruction in the proximal portion of the small bowel or stomach. Steady abdominal pain usually is associated with nonobstructive conditions such as penetrating duodenal ulcers, pancreatitis, dissecting aortic aneurysm, pelvic inflammatory disease, or a perforated viscus complicated by the formation of abscess and/or generalized peritonitis.

The location and radiation of abdominal pain are important indicators of the abdominal organs involved. Pain in the right lower quadrant at MacBurney point, 3 to 5 cm below the umbilicus and 3 to 5 cm to the right of the midline, for example, characterizes acute appendicitis; tenderness in the right upper quadrant over the liver, called

*Murphy's sign,* suggests acute cholecystitis. Diaphragmatic irritation and the presence of shoulder pain in the recumbent position is usually caused by free blood in the peritoneal cavity resulting from a ruptured ectopic pregnancy or from an injury to the spleen.

### Vomiting

Vomiting is a common symptom in patients with an acute abdomen. It is usually associated with constant or colicky pain. A careful history regarding the frequency of vomiting, its relation to pain, and the characteristics and volume of the vomitus provides concrete leads to the eventual diagnosis.

Frequent vomiting of bilious fluid, associated with pain, is usually produced by upper abdominal pathology (acute cholecystitis, pancreatitis), whereas clear vomitus that occurs soon after the ingestion of liquids may indicate an upper gastrointestinal site of obstruction (pyloric obstruction, carcinoma of the stomach). Delays of 2 to 6 hours between pain and the onset of vomiting are characteristic of small bowel obstruction, whereas large bowel obstruction may be present without any history of vomiting at all. In elderly patients abdominal distress, nausea, and vomiting may be produced by fecal impaction, which can mimic the signs and symptoms of an acute abdomen.

Generalized or localized peritonitis may be produced by a ruptured viscus, ischemia, inflammation of a retroperitoneal hematoma, shock, or an unassociated major systemic illness. The peritonitis itself may cause a dynamic ileus, which is manifested in many instances by vomiting, with or without a history of abdominal pain. The absence of vomiting, however, does not exclude a major intraabdominal catastrophe such as a perforated duodenal ulcer, ruptured acute appendicitis, or major intraabdominal hemorrhage.

### Bowel function and habits

A detailed history that describes the patient's bowel habits (stool and gas) must be obtained to the extent possible given the condition of the patient. The absence of bowel movements but the passage of gas per rectum should not be worrisome. The total absence of stool and gas, however, usually indicates significant intraabdominal pathology. Diarrhea may be associated with regional inflammatory changes within the peritoneal cavity such as acute appendicitis, pelvic abscess, pelvic inflammatory disease, and inflammatory disease of the bowel. Nevertheless, a significant number of non-surgical gastrointestinal syndromes are also characterized by abdominal pain and diarrhea. These syndromes have to be kept in the differential diagnosis when diarrhea is frequent and there is no history that supports a surgical condition. A history of hematochezia, melena, or documented occult blood in the stool must be sought.

The effects of an acute abdomen on body temperature, pulse, blood pressure, and state of hydration may be influenced by preexistent illness. Therefore a good review of systems must be obtained to reveal any history of diabetes, renal disease, jaundice, or dehydration. Pulmonary infiltrates, pneumonia, anemia, and cardiac problems may complicate medical and surgical management. The patient must be maintained in a hemodynamically stable condition, since patients with an acute abdomen often require immediate surgical therapy. Hemodynamic instability associated with an intraabdominal crisis is usually the result of acute intravascular blood loss such as hemorrhage from a ruptured spleen, a ruptured aorta, or an ectopic pregnancy. Hemorrhage in these conditions is often life threatening. A milder form of hemodynamic instability results from loss of functional extracellular fluid, which may result from an adynamic ileus, intestinal obstruction, pancreatitis, and generalized or localized peritonitis with subsequent loss of intravascular volume. The latter is the most common etiology for the hemodynamic and metabolic instability of these patients.

## PHYSICAL EXAMINATION

Following a careful history, examination of the abdomen includes inspection, auscultation, percussion, palpation, rectal examination, and evaluation of the abdominal wall for the presence or absence of hernia. During inspection of the abdomen the presence of distention, scars, masses, or abnormal circulatory patterns are carefully noted. With normal breathing patterns the upward and downward exertion of the diaphragm results in abdominal motion during inspiration and expiration. When these normal movements are absent and a pure intracostal breathing pattern is noted, significant peritoneal pathology is often present.

### Auscultation

Perhaps the most significant component of the abdominal examination is auscultation. The presence, absence, or characteristics of bowel sounds determine in many instances whether there will be an operative or a nonoperative intervention. Hyperactive bowel sounds followed by rushes and periods of silence accompanied by colicky pain are characteristic of intestinal obstruction. Hyperactive bowel signs are usually associated with mild forms of peritonitis or other forms of ileus. The absence of bowel sounds, however, indicates total peristaltic paralysis associated with an acute inflammatory process, intraabdominal hemorrhage, a major surgical or nonsurgical retroperitoneal process, or a major systemic disease.

### Percussion

Percussion of the abdomen is extremely valuable to establish whether distention is caused by air or fluid.

### Palpation

Palpation should be gentle and initiated away from the site of pain to have the maximum cooperation possible from the patient. The presence of cutaneous hyperesthesia is usually a sign of intraabdominal pathology. The abdominal wall is carefully palpated in the inguinal, umbilical, and femoral areas. The presence or absence of abnormal masses as well as the size of the intraabdominal organs are carefully noted. Inflammatory changes in the peritoneal cavity are manifested by a variety of signs depending on the magnitude of the process. Voluntary or involuntary guarding may be present. Rigidity, or the presence of rebound tenderness, and referred rebound tenderness may be present.

No abdominal examination is complete without rectal and vaginal examinations. The presence of masses, tenderness, and fluid collections is carefully noted and evaluated in reference to the patient's total complaints. Fecal impaction may be noted to cause severe pain and abdominal distention, vomiting, and distress in chronically ill or elderly patients.

Although the symptoms and signs characteristic of the acute abdomen syndrome are present in most patients, they may be absent in many elderly individuals. Fever, pain, and tenderness may be less evident. The lack of these early signs and symptoms often delays elderly patients from seeking medical attention. Their lack may also give the physician a false sense of security. It is imperative that minimum signs of abdominal discomfort in elderly patients be fully evaluated and closely monitored by repeated clinical examination and laboratory studies to avoid missing a life-threatening process.

## LABORATORY AND RADIOGRAPHIC STUDIES

Laboratory and radiographic procedures can be of significant help in the evaluation, initial management, and definitive therapy of the patient with an acute abdomen. However, overemphasis on the utilization of these studies to pursue a definitive diagnosis may delay definitive therapy, with a resultant increase in mortality and morbidity.

The complete blood count (CBC) is a useful laboratory aid. Unfortunately, however, it does not establish a diagnosis. Its value is primarily to establish the relative proportions of the hemogram (e.g., anemia, leukocytosis, dehydration). A CBC without a differential may be of little value at times when decisions need to be made as to observation or operation. As an example, when patients present with right lower quadrant pain, a normal white blood cell count, and a normal differential, they may be observed despite clinical findings suggestive of acute appendicitis, whereas other patients with similar signs and symptoms and leukocytosis with a shift to the left may be operated on more urgently. Serum electrolytes and blood gas analyses, which are indicated in many instances for evaluation of the patient, do not usually provide the physician with clear diagnostic clues of an acute abdomen. They provide indispensable data, however, in the evaluation of the metabolic and biochemical status of a patient before a major surgical procedure. The leukocytic response of elderly patients may be minimal, and intraabdominal infection in these patients may be suggested only by a slight shift to the left in the differential count.

Urinalysis is a simple laboratory test that is mandatory in all patients evaluated for abdominal pain. Nearly all pathologic syndromes involving the urinary tract can mimic signs of the acute abdomen. Many of these conditions (e.g., pyelonephritis, cystitis, urinary tract infections, nephrosis, nephritis) can be diagnosed or first suspected by this examination.

The serum amylase assay is a reliable test to diagnose acute pancreatitis. However, elevated serum amylase in the presence of a clinical syndrome that is not consistent with this disease raises the question of a different diagnosis. Serum amylase levels can be elevated by a number of major intraabdominal processes.

Of all the liver function tests, there are some that have a direct bearing on the diagnosis and management of a patient with an acute abdomen. These are the prothrombin time, partial thromboplastin time, thrombin time, serum alkaline phosphatase, and serum bilirubin. The thrombin time and partial thromboplastin time are essential screening tests to assess the patient's coagulation status, particularly if surgical therapy is contemplated. An elevated serum bilirubin level in itself is not diagnostic of an acute abdomen; however, a significant elevation associated with chills and fever supports a diagnosis of cholangitis, which requires prompt therapy.

Appropriately ordered radiographs interpreted by radiologists or physicians knowledgeable of the patient's history and physical findings can be of immense help in establishing a secure diagnosis in patients presenting with an acute abdomen.

An upright chest film is mandatory in all patients with an acute abdomen. This film is ideal for demonstrating the presence of free air under the right or left diaphragmatic domes as well as for demonstrating pulmonary, pleural, and cardiac pathology (Fig. 47-1).

The most commonly ordered of all abdominal films (supine and upright views), if properly interpreted, can be of invaluable help. The supine film under normal conditions characterizes the position and size of the normal

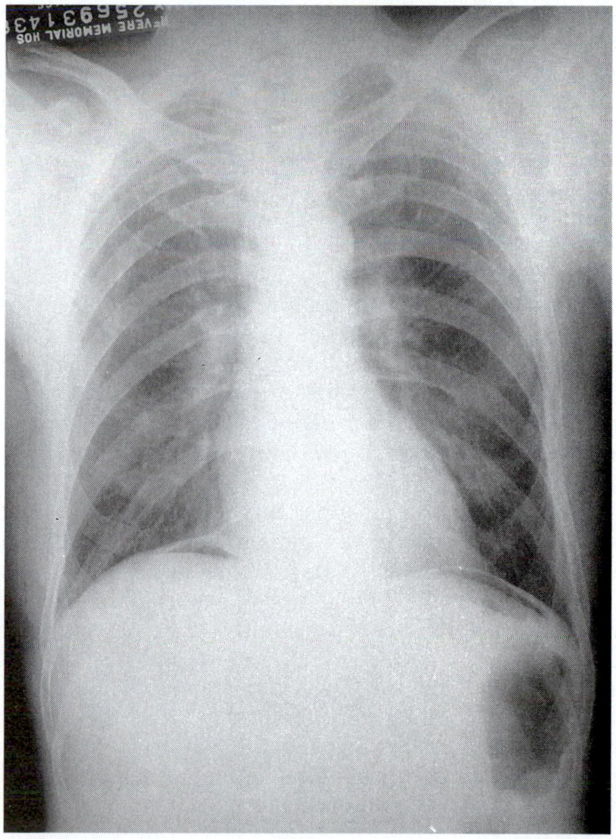

**Fig. 47-1.** Posteroanterior upright chest x-ray reveals free air under the domes of the right and left diaphragm in a patient with a perforated duodenal ulcer.

intraperitoneal organs and establishes the normal or pathologic characteristics of intraluminal gas patterns. A careful evaluation may indicate the presence or absence of psoas shadows, air in the retroperitoneal space, and radiopaque calculi in the ureter and kidneys. The upright film of the abdomen is also essential for the evaluation of the acute abdomen. It can demonstrate the presence of free air in the peritoneal cavity, pathologic air-fluid levels in the small and large bowel, and air-fluid collections representing abscess cavities. If properly carried out, films of the abdomen can also show displacement of certain interperitoneal organs as a result of a mass effect from other organs (e.g., the downward midline displacement of the splenic flexure of the colon as a result of an enlarged spleen). In certain instances plain film studies can be complemented by an intravenous pyelogram if suspicion of urinary tract or retroperitoneal process exists or by a barium enema when an obstructive lesion of the colon is suspected.

Diagnostic ultrasound is extremely helpful in the evaluation of patients with an acute intraabdominal process. It provides an accurate delineation of the biliary tree, both intrahepatic and extrahepatic, as well as the presence or absence of gallstones, liver tumors, pancreatic enlargement, and renal obstruction or pathology. Furthermore, diagnostic ultrasound is essential in the evaluation of gynecologic conditions unless there are life-threatening or otherwise clear indicators for surgical intervention. A pelvic ultrasound is essential in the workup of women being evaluated for acute lower abdominal pain.

The usefulness of computed tomography (CT) in the diagnostic workup of a patient with an intraabdominal catastrophe is reserved for complicated clinical presentations such as the possibility of a slowly leaking aortic abdominal aneurysm, perforated diverticulitis or appendicitis, intraabdominal abscess, ischemic bowel disease, and gynecologic masses.

Both ultrasound and CT are now widely available. They sometimes lead to specific diagnosis and often disclose entities and the extent of disease anticipated clinically. Both are noninvasive and require minimal patient preparation. The optimal sequence of imaging is plain film, ultrasound (biliary, renal, ob-gyn), and CT if needed (aorta, pancreas, bowel). Most of the information required for the diagnosis and the decision to operate or not operate can easily be obtained by the modalities previously explained.

Angiographic studies in patients with signs of an acute abdomen are reserved for patients in whom ischemic lesions of the gastrointestinal tract are suspected or when the source of gastrointestinal bleeding must be established. The studies are carried out promptly while other resuscitative procedures are performed. Angiographic studies can determine the presence or absence of occlusive or nonocclusive mesenteric ischemia as well as the location and size of the occlusive process. Furthermore, vasodilatory therapy or control of intraabdominal hemorrhage by embolization can be achieved during angiography.

## THERAPY

The therapeutic approach to a patient with an acute abdomen should stress resuscitation, stabilization, diagnosis, and definitive therapy. If not seen by a surgeon initially, a surgical consult is obtained early so that appropriate therapeutic decisions can be promptly carried out. Most acute intraabdominal syndromes are characterized by a hypovolemic state (anemia or dehydration), and intravenous fluids are essential in the early stages of management. Insertion of a nasogastric tube is both diagnostic and therapeutic. Gastrointestinal decompression is essential for the patient's comfort, the improvement of pulmonary function, and the removal of nonfunctional gas and fluid. The volume and characteristics of the fluid, as described above under Vomiting, may help to establish a definitive diagnosis. If it is not possible to pass a nasogastric tube in a patient with acute upper abdominal pain, the diagnosis of a gastric volvulus should be considered. A lateral radiograph of the chest reveals elevation of the left diaphragm and a characteristic double gastric air bubble.

The quality and quantity of the urine reveal renal function, the presence or absence of urinary tract sepsis, and the patient's cardiovascular status. Therefore a Foley catheter is inserted in these patients to allow evaluation of renal function as well as the adequacy of resuscitation.

The use of antibiotics for these conditions is described below.

## BILIARY DISEASE

Biliary disease is one of the most common pathologic problems in a patient presenting with an acute upper abdominal process, particularly when confined to the right upper quadrant. It can present at any age; however, it is more common in middle-aged and elderly patients. The pain caused by biliary disease may present with or without evidence of peritoneal inflammation. The known presence of gallstones in a patient with an acute abdomen, particularly an acute upper abdominal process, is not necessarily an indication of biliary disease, since silent or symptom-free gallstones are common in elderly patients.

### Acute cholecystitis

Acute cholecystitis presents as an acute upper abdominal inflammatory process. The patient may first complain of vague upper abdominal pain either in the epigastrium or confined to the right upper quadrant. The pain may be referred through to the right shoulder blade. The patient is anorectic. He or she may complain of vomiting and exhibit manifestations of a generalized systemic illness. The inflammatory process produced by acute cholecystitis causes the patient to experience an increase of pain on movement or coughing.

On examination the patient looks unwell and has a fever, tachycardia, and normal blood pressure. The abdomen moves poorly with respiration, and bowel sounds are reduced but not absent unless the gallbladder has perforated resulting in a generalized peritonitis. On palpation of the abdomen there is tenderness, guarding, and rebound or percussion tenderness confined to the right upper quadrant. In some instances the inflammatory mass of omentum, colon, and small bowel surrounding the gallbladder may be felt when palpating the abdomen

A

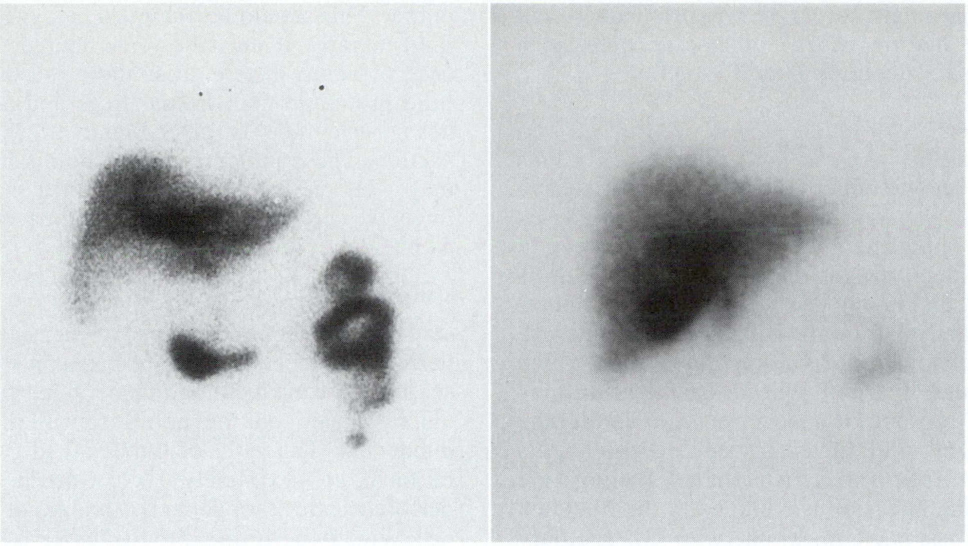

B

**Fig. 47-2.** **A,** Normal HIDA scan demonstrating a normal biliary tract. **B,** Nonvisualization of the gallbladder in a HIDA scan performed on a patient with a blocked cystic duct and acute cholecystitis.

gently. The patient may exhibit a positive Murphy's sign, which is indicated by an increase in pain when a hand is placed gently on the right upper quadrant and held stationary while the patient takes a deep breath. The contracting diaphragm moves the liver down and compresses the inflammatory mass against the palpating hand.

Initial clinical examination may be followed by a sonogram of the right upper quadrant. In addition to gallstones, thickening of the gallbladder wall and pericholecystic fluid are readily seen findings in many cases of acute cholecystitis.

In the majority of cases of acute cholecystitis the diagnosis can be established firmly on clinical grounds from a history and physical examination with no need for further ancillary tests. In a few patients, however, the diagnosis may not be clear from the history and physical examination. The first investigation performed should be KUB (kidney, ureter, bladder) and upright radiographic studies of the abdomen to look for radiopaque stones in the region of the neck of the gallbladder that do not move with a change of position of the patient, suggesting a blocked cystic duct. The performance of an HIDA scan that demonstrates good visualization of the biliary tree with flow of nuclide into the intestine but no filling of the gallbladder after 1.5 hours indicates possible blockage of the cystic duct, suggesting acute cholecystitis (Fig. 47-2). There is a small but definite false positive rate (approximately 5%) with the HIDA test, particularly in patients who have been starved for a number of days.

Early treatment for a person with acute cholecystitis includes intravenous fluids for hydration, passage of a nasogastric tube to decompress the stomach, antibiotic coverage with ampicillin, and surgical consultation.

### Biliary colic

A patient presenting with biliary colic has severe epigastric pain that comes on rather suddenly, gradually builds to a peak intensity, and lasts from several hours to a maximum of 12 to 18 hours. The pain is steady and is located in the epigastrium; it does not move to the back. It may be accompanied by vomiting. The pain is not made worse by movement, and the patient often moves around to try to get relief. A careful history may elicit similar but less pronounced episodes of pain. On examination the patient is afebrile, is reluctant to stay still, and has a normal pulse rate and normal blood pressure. On abdominal examination there is no evidence of tenderness, guarding, or rebound tenderness, and the bowel sounds are normal. Blood tests are entirely within normal limits.

Treatment includes analgesia for the relief of pain followed by an elective workup for biliary disease when the pain has stopped. A cholecystectomy is frequently indicated once biliary tract cholelithiasis is diagnosed.

### Acute hydrops of the gallbladder

Patients with acute hydrops present with epigastric and right upper quadrant pain that is moderately severe and has been present for many hours. The patient is not systemically ill, but the pain is made worse by movement and there may be intermittent vomiting. The patient is afebrile. On abdominal examination the abdomen moves well, and bowel sounds are normal. On palpation there is usually mild tenderness in the right upper quadrant with a palpable globular mass under the right costal margin that is the distended gallbladder. Diagnosis is usually made on clinical grounds; however, a KUB and upright x-ray examination, sonogram, and an HIDA are of diagnostic value. These patients may develop acute cholecystitis if the hydrops does not resolve spontaneously or if it is not treated operatively. The initial treatment comprises intravenous fluids, placement of a nasogastric tube, and analgesics. If the hydrops does not resolve quickly, a semiemergent cholecystectomy is performed.

### Ascending cholangitis

Ascending cholangitis presents in a rather insidious manner. It occurs most commonly in patients who have choledochal calculi causing obstruction. The cholangitis then arises from infected bile as a closed infection occupies the bile duct system. In mild cases the bile is markedly infected, and in more severe cases the bile ducts may become filled with frank pus. Patients present with pain in the upper abdomen or right upper quadrant, which may be accompanied by vomiting. On examination they are febrile, are mildly icteric, and have tachycardia and hypotension. Patients with severe ascending cholangitis present in severe septic shock. Abdominal findings are minimal because the infection is confined to the bile duct system. The diagnosis is a clinical one with few ancillary investigations that help in establishing the diagnosis in the immediate situation. Ultrasound may demonstrate dilated bile ducts, and blood workup shows elevated white blood cell count, bilirubin, enzymes, and alkaline phosphatase levels. A routine examination of the patient's urine demonstrates the presence of bile.

The patient has immediate blood samples taken for culture, intravenous fluids for resuscitation, and placement of a nasogastric tube. Antibiotic therapy is started immediately. By and large these patients respond poorly to noninterventional therapy. In experienced hands the patients can be managed by endoscopic retrograde cholangiopancreatography (ERCP), papillotomy, and drainage of the biliary tree. Surgical drainage and cholecystectomy remain the standards of care.

### Acute pancreatitis

The most common causes of acute pancreatitis are alcohol abuse and gallstones. It may therefore be possible to elicit a history of recent heavy alcohol ingestion and, particularly in alcoholics, repeated attacks of pancreatitis.

Patients with acute pancreatitis present with evidence of an acute upper abdominal process. They complain of epigastric pain that goes through to the back accompanied by vomiting. On examination the patient is in severe pain and is afebrile with tachycardia. In severe cases of acute pancreatitis the patient may be hypotensive with evidence of dehydration. Abdominal examination may range from reduced or absent bowel sounds with mild epigastric tenderness and guarding to a silent abdomen with generalized severe tenderness and guarding with rebound tenderness.

Patients require blood tests for full blood count, electrolytes, calcium, amylase, and blood gases. The serum amylase level may be only slightly elevated, if at all, in patients who have had repeated episodes of pancreatitis and have evidence of pancreatic insufficiency. This is because there is insufficient acinar tissue left to cause a high serum amylase level. In this group of patients the diagnosis often must be based on the history and clinical grounds.

Immediate treatment is directed to resuscitation and establishment of a normal blood pressure and normal urine output. This should be achieved by aggressive intravenous fluid therapy. It must be remembered that, in the severe case of acute pancreatitis, there is marked secretion of fluid in and around the pancreas and retroperitoneum. A nasogastric tube is placed and attached to continuous suction. These patients require admission to hospital and may well require management in a medical or surgical intensive care unit. CT can detect local complications such as phelgmon and abscess formation.

## PERFORATED PEPTIC ULCER

One of the complications of peptic ulcer disease is perforation, occurring more often in the spring and fall seasons. The most common ulcer to perforate is a duodenal ulcer situated on the anterior wall of the bulb of the duodenum. The ratio of duodenal to gastric ulcer perforation is approximately 10:1. Gastric ulcers most often perforate into the general abdominal cavity, but they occasionally perforate into the lesser sac, which makes the diagnosis harder. The perforation sets up a chemical peritonitis initially caused by bile and sterile intragastric contents. A bacterial peritonitis then develops on top of the chemical peritonitis after 8 to 12 hours, depending on the degree of contamination.

Patients presenting with a perforated peptic ulcer often give a typical history of the sudden onset of epigastric pain. The onset of the pain is so sudden that the patient can almost document the exact time the ulcer perforated. By the time of admission to hospital the patient is complaining of generalized abdominal pain. He or she is often mildly diaphoretic and may not give a history of peptic ulcer disease. In a significant number of patients perforation is the initial presentation of peptic ulcer disease.

On examination, these patients are afebrile, are mildly diaphoretic, have mild tachycardia, and are normotensive. The abdomen is rigid with generalized tenderness, guarding, and rebound tenderness. The abdomen may show signs of true boardlike rigidity. Bowel sounds are absent, and there is loss of liver dullness to percussion because of the free air in the peritoneal cavity.

In a patient suspected of having a perforated peptic ulcer on clinical grounds, the first step is to obtain an erect abdominal x-ray with particular reference to the diaphragm, looking for intraperitoneal air under the diaphragm (see Fig. 47-1). A posteroanterior chest film often reveals free air under the diaphragm, although a separate film centered on the diaphragm is sometimes required. In 20% to 30% of patients with a perforated ulcer there is no free intraperitoneal air visible under the diaphragm on an erect abdominal x-ray. In rare patients who have perforated a gastric ulcer into the lesser sac, the only abnormality on x-ray is that of air outlining the lesser sac. In those patients who are highly suspected of having perforation but no evidence of air under the diaphragm, the diagnosis may be confirmed by an upper gastrointestinal series using Gastrografin that has been either swallowed or put down a nasogastric tube. Extravasation of the contrast medium usually indicates a perforation.

The CBC, electrolyte, and blood urea nitrogen (BUN) on these patients is usually within normal limits, particularly if the patient is admitted to the hospital within 12 hours of perforation. Leukocytosis may appear after 12 hours, and dehydration may produce a high hematocrit and elevated BUN. The treatment of a patient with a perforation must include intravenous fluids for the correction of dehydration, the passage of a nasogastric tube which is then placed on continuous suction, and admission to a surgical service for operation.

### Leaking peptic ulcer

A few patients present with a leak from a duodenal ulcer. The perforation is not overt; it does not produce a generalized peritonitis and free air under the diaphragm. The leakage does soil the right upper quadrant, however, and the intestinal contaminants run down the right paracolic gutter. These patients may present with a right-sided peritonitis, which can appear similar to appendicitis. On giving a careful history, however, the patients describe a relatively sudden episode of epigastric pain rather than the classic picture of appendicitis.

Patients with a severe acute exacerbation of duodenal ulcer disease occasionally appear on initial presentation to have an acute abdomen; however, when carefully examined they have severe pain and mild tenderness in the right upper quadrant but no evidence of peritonitis. Bowel sounds are active in these patients, and there is no rebound or referred rebound tenderness.

## INFLAMMATORY BOWEL DISEASES

### Appendicitis

Appendicitis is one of the more common surgical emergencies and tends to present in young people. However, appendicitis cannot be completely ruled out because of age in any patient.

Patients with appendicitis typically complain of periumbilical pain, anorexia, nausea, and vomiting. Although they often present a history of vomiting, it is rarely severe or continuous. As the inflammatory process extends beyond the visceral peritoneum of the appendix and involves the parietal peritoneum in the right lower quadrant, the pain appears to move from the periumbilical region into the right lower quadrant. In those patients in whom the appendix lies in the right paracolic gutter, the pain may localize higher and more laterally than the usual position in the right lower quadrant. As the process continues, the patient feels generally unwell and complains of increasing pain on movement.

On examination the patient is usually febrile, lies quietly, and has fetor oris. On abdominal examination there is reduced movement, tenderness in the right lower quadrant with accompanying guarding and rebound, or percussion tenderness. The bowel sounds are usually present but may be reduced. If the patient has progressed to the stage of a frank perforation and has generalized peritonitis, he or she presents with generalized tenderness, guarding, and rebound tenderness. Rectal examination is an important part of assessing the patient with appendicitis, and if the appendix is in the more classic position, hanging over the pelvic brim, there will be tenderness to examination on the right side.

The diagnosis is usually based on clinical findings and rarely requires ancillary investigations. A white blood cell count shows leukocytosis, and the electrolytes are usually normal. Only in rare cases is it necessary to proceed further with investigation. In these situations the most useful investigation is ultrasound of the right lower quadrant. Acute appendicitis is diagnosed when the appendix is seen to be greater than 8 mm in diameter and appears noncompressible with the ultrasound probe. An appendicolith is easily documented with ultrasound as an echogenic focus. Disorders simulating appendicitis such as abscess or ovarian cyst can be readily differentiated. Barium enema may show an absence of filling of the appendix. Although the latter may show a pericecal mass indentation, it is not a sign of appendicitis, but it may be supportive of the clinical diagnosis.

The complete filling of the appendix to its tip with barium essentially rules out appendicitis.

As previously noted, in complicated or late cases CT may also show the calcified appendicolith and an appendiceal abscess.

Treatment is admission to hospital, administration of intravenous fluids, and preparation for appendectomy. It is not necessary to place a nasogastric tube unless there is generalized peritonitis in association with appendicitis.

### Mesenteric adenitis

In children and adolescents mesenteric adenitis—the enlargement of lymph nodes of the small bowel mesentery—presents with a clinical picture that is often indistinguishable from that of appendicitis. This condition is part of a generalized viral infection in which the patient gives a history of a recent sore throat and associated viral symptoms. On examination there is lymph node enlargement in the neck, axillae, and groin. On abdominal examination there is tenderness and guarding in the right lower quadrant.

When the diagnosis is established with extreme confidence, an operation is not necessary. In a significant number of patients, however, the diagnosis is not clear cut, and in these patients it is very reasonable to perform an appendectomy to ensure that appendicitis is not missed and at the same time to remove the possibility of appendicitis in the future. The associated morbidity and complications of appendicitis are low, particularly when the appendectomy is performed in young people early in the course of the disease.

### Acute Crohn's disease of the ileum

In young people a condition of acute regional ileitis (Crohn's disease) may present as an acute abdominal emergency. Patients give a history of abdominal pain that starts in the center of the abdomen and moves to the right lower quadrant. The pain tends to be intermittent and colicky. There is usually a history of recent weight loss and diarrhea. On examination the patient has a low-grade fever and tachycardia, and on abdominal examination the bowel sounds are increased, suggesting a partial small bowel obstruction. There are tenderness and guarding in the right lower quadrant. In patients suspected of having acute ileitis, a barium enema, to look for reflux of barium into the terminal ileum, may make the diagnosis. These individuals require admission to hospital, intravenous fluid administration, and observation. It may not be possible to distinguish this entity from appendicitis, and the majority of patients are explored for the diagnosis of appendicitis.

## Diverticulitis

Diverticulosis is an acquired condition that is rarely seen in persons less than 40 years of age. It starts in the sigmoid colon and extends proximally. The incidence of diverticulosis increases with aging and is an asymptomatic condition. On occasion, however, sigmoid diverticula become inflamed and cause diverticulitis. The complications of diverticulitis are obstruction, perforation, and abscess formation.

Patients present with a history of lower abdominal pain that moves to the left lower quadrant and is accompanied by general malaise, fever, anorexia, sometimes vomiting, constipation, and the absence of passing flatus. On examination the patient has a fever and tachycardia and is normotensive. He or she appears to be in discomfort, particularly on moving, and on abdominal examination has some mild distention with tenderness and guarding confined to the left lower quadrant. On gentle palpation a mass effect may be discernible. Bowel sounds are reduced. On rectal examination there is tenderness on the left side of the pelvis, and a mass may be palpable.

The diagnosis is based mainly on clinical findings, and the workup includes a CBC and electrolytes, especially when the patient is vomiting significantly. KUB and upright x-ray studies of the abdomen may show no more than nonspecific small bowel and large bowel distention, suggesting a partial paralytic ileus.

Diverticulitis may rarely result in large bowel obstruction with the patient having marked abdominal distention associated with vomiting. On abdominal x-rays a classic picture of a large bowel obstruction with a large dilated colon proximal to the sigmoid region is usually present (Fig. 47-3). Edema, inflammation, and swelling in an adynamic segment of sigmoid colon produce the obstruction.

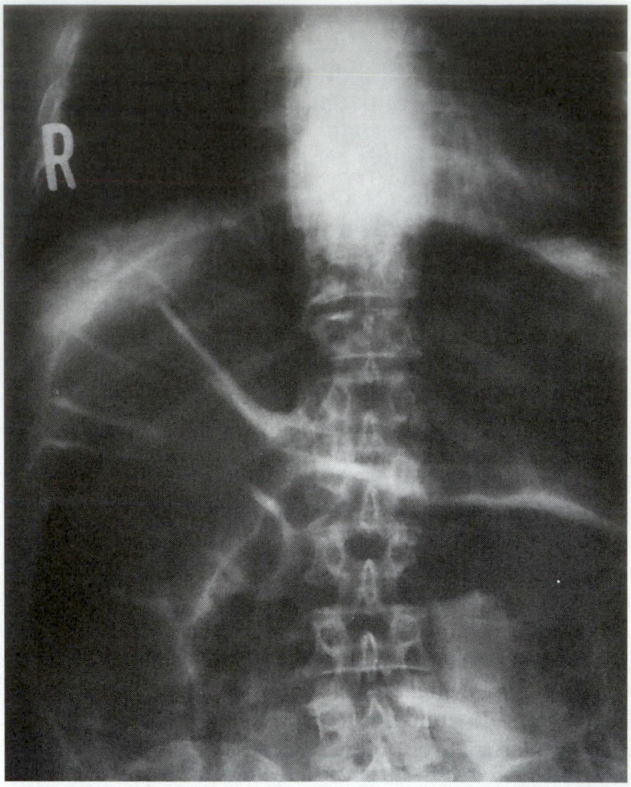


**Fig. 47-3.** Large dilated colon proximal to diverticulitis of the sigmoid colon which has produced obstruction.

Patients with colonic obstruction due to diverticulitis are treated with fluid resuscitation, a nasogastric tube, and intravenous fluids. The large bowel obstruction usually subsides as the inflammatory component of the diverticulitis resolves.

Diverticular abscess is another complication of diverticulitis. These patients usually give a history of 4 to 5 days of abdominal pain and illness that has been localized in the left lower quadrant. On examination they have a fever, tachycardia, dehydration, and normal blood pressure. On abdominal examination there is a marked and well-defined tender mass in the left lower quadrant which can usually be palpated rectally as well. When observed long enough, the patient shows signs of an abscess with spiking fever. These patients need to be treated with a nasogastric tube, intravenous fluids, and antibiotics before laparotomy for drainage of the abscess and resection of the diverticular segment. CT with rectally administered contrast is an excellent diagnostic modality to confirm the presence of characteristic pericaloric abscess formation.

On occasion the diverticular abscess associated with diverticulitis does not remain localized and may rupture into the generalized peritoneal cavity. These patients give a long history of illness and abdominal pain. When seen by the physician they are usually febrile with tachycardia, hypotension, and significant dehydration. Immediate treatment is nasogastric suction, intravenous fluid resuscitation, and antibiotics. Definitive treatment is laparotomy and colon resection.

The most serious complication of diverticulitis is a free perforation with fecal peritonitis. These patients initially have an abscess surrounding the diverticulitis. This ruptures into the peritoneal cavity and results in a free communication between the sigmoid colon and the peritoneal cavity. The patients are extremely ill with fever, tachycardia, and hypotension, and have evidence of severe sepsis. On examination the abdomen is distended. The bowel sounds are absent, and there is a loss of liver dullness because of free air in the peritoneal cavity. Laboratory studies include a complete blood count, electrolytes, and an x-ray study of the abdomen. It is often not possible to perform an upright x-ray examination because of the general state of the patient. In these circumstances a lateral decubitus x-ray view is obtained, to look for free intraperitoneal air. The treatment is vigorous intravenous resuscitation, antibiotic administration, and placement of a nasogastric tube in preparation for a laparotomy. This complication carries a high mortality.

Diverticulitis and its complications tend to occur in elderly patients. One of the main reasons for high morbidity and mortality in this group of patients is the problem of associated diseases, particularly those involving the cardiac, respiratory, and renal systems. These associated diseases should be looked for carefully and may have to be treated along with resuscitative measures and surgical treatment of the acute abdomen.

### Mesenteric ischemia

Ischemia in any part of the body causes significant pain, and the bowel is no exception. There are two types of mesenteric ischemia: (1) occlusive varieties result from an embolus or a thrombus that forms on an atheromatous plaque and (2) nonocclusive, or low flow, mesenteric ischemia, which presents as a result of associated conditions that critically reduce mesenteric flow in an elderly patient with a vascular system that is already compromised. When mesenteric ischemia appears to be secondary to an embolus, the possibility of atrial fibrillation or another cardiac problem such as a mural thrombus associated with a recent myocardial infarction is sought. In the nonocclusive group there may well be a precipitating factor (e.g., marked dehydration). This variety of mesenteric ischemia also has a high incidence in those patients undergoing digoxin therapy.

Mesenteric ischemia is most difficult to diagnose when severe abdominal pain starts initially without any signs of an acute abdomen. These patients develop abdominal signs later, bowel sounds are usually absent or reduced, generalized tenderness and guarding may be present, and hypotension may occur. On workup the patients have an elevated white blood cell count and dehydration, which increases the hematocrit and BUN. There may be an elevated amylase level of bowel origin, and blood gases often show marked, resistant metabolic acidosis. Treatment includes prompt rehydration and an immediate mesenteric arteriogram in the early or mild cases, to look for evidence of an occlusion that may be corrected operatively or evidence of marked vascular spasm suggesting a low flow state. Patients with occlusive disease are prepared for operative correction, and those with a low flow state are perfused with papaverine for 6 hours through a catheter placed in the superior mesenteric artery. This is followed by laparotomy. Those patients who have evidence of severe mesenteric ischemia probably benefit more from immediate laparotomy with resection of dead gut and correction of an occlusion if one is found. In patients who have evidence of a low flow state, laparotomy must be performed to be certain there is no infarcted or severely compromised bowel. A subsequent arteriogram may be performed after laparotomy to continue perfusion with vasodilator agents.

The mortality associated with this condition is extremely high, mainly because by the time the diagnosis can be made, there is extensive necrosis of the small and sometimes the large bowel; the best results are in those patients who are treated early. Elderly patients who present with severe abdominal pain and no evidence of abdominal findings should be considered for an early arteriogram to confirm or exclude the diagnosis because these are the patients who have the lower rates of mortality and morbidity.

## BOWEL OBSTRUCTION

The Greek word for obstruction is *ileus.* Patients may present with a mechanical ileus or a paralytic ileus. The most common cause of paralytic ileus is abdominal surgery; however, in the emergency room it is most commonly caused by an associated intraabdominal process, usually a mechanical ileus, which is called a small or large bowel mechanical obstruction.

### Small bowel obstruction

Small bowel obstruction is a common cause of an acute abdomen in patients presenting to an emergency room. The patient complains of colicky midabdominal pain lasting one to several days. The pain lasts for a few seconds and subsides only to return again a few minutes later. This is accompanied by vomiting and abdominal distention, although with small bowel obstruction the distention is not always marked, particularly when the obstruction is high. In late cases there may be constipation and lack of passing flatus. If the patient gives a history of previous intraabdominal operations, it may help to make the diagnosis of the small bowel obstruction.

The pathophysiology of small bowel obstruction explains some of the signs and symptoms experienced by patients. The small bowel contracts to overcome the obstruction and subsequently dilates proximal to the obstruction. As it becomes dilated, the two-way mechanism of absorption and secretion in the bowel is compromised. Although absorption is inhibited, secretion into the intestinal lumen continues. This results in very significant fluid loss and dehydration in these patients. Dehydration is not a manifestation of their vomiting. In patients who have had obstruction for a long time, the colicky abdominal pain may be less intense and less frequent because of the impaired function of the dilated bowel.

Strangulated or incarcerated inguinal hernia is the most common cause of small bowel obstruction. Other causes are strangulated femoral hernia, small bowel adhesions, congenital bands, small bowel carcinomas, internal hernia, and limited segments of mesenteric ischemia.

On examination the patient may be noted to complain of intermittent abdominal pain. There may be striking evidence of marked dehydration with loss of skin turgor, a dry tongue, and occasionally sunken eyes. The pulse rate is usually increased, and blood pressure is normal unless there is marked evidence of bowel ischemia from either strangulation of a loop or mesenteric ischemia. Abdominal distention varies with the level of obstruction. The umbilicus and both groins are carefully examined to look for inguinal and femoral hernias. It should be noted that an inguinal or femoral hernia can be hidden in an obese person with a large, pendulous abdomen. The apron must be retracted and the inguinal regions examined thoroughly. Adhesions may belie abdominal scars and may be the cause of obstruction. Bowel sounds are usually increased with evidence of high-pitched sounds and rushes. Although mild direct tenderness may be present, guarding and rebound tenderness are not unless the patient truly has ischemic bowel impairment.

The laboratory investigation necessary to make the diagnosis of small bowel obstruction consists of KUB and upright abdominal x-rays to look for evidence of distended small bowel. Often a typical stepladder appearance of the small bowel on the flat plate and multiple air-fluid levels in loops of small bowel on the upright film are the radiologic hallmarks of small bowel obstruction (Fig. 47-4). Occasionally evidence of a further specific entity

A 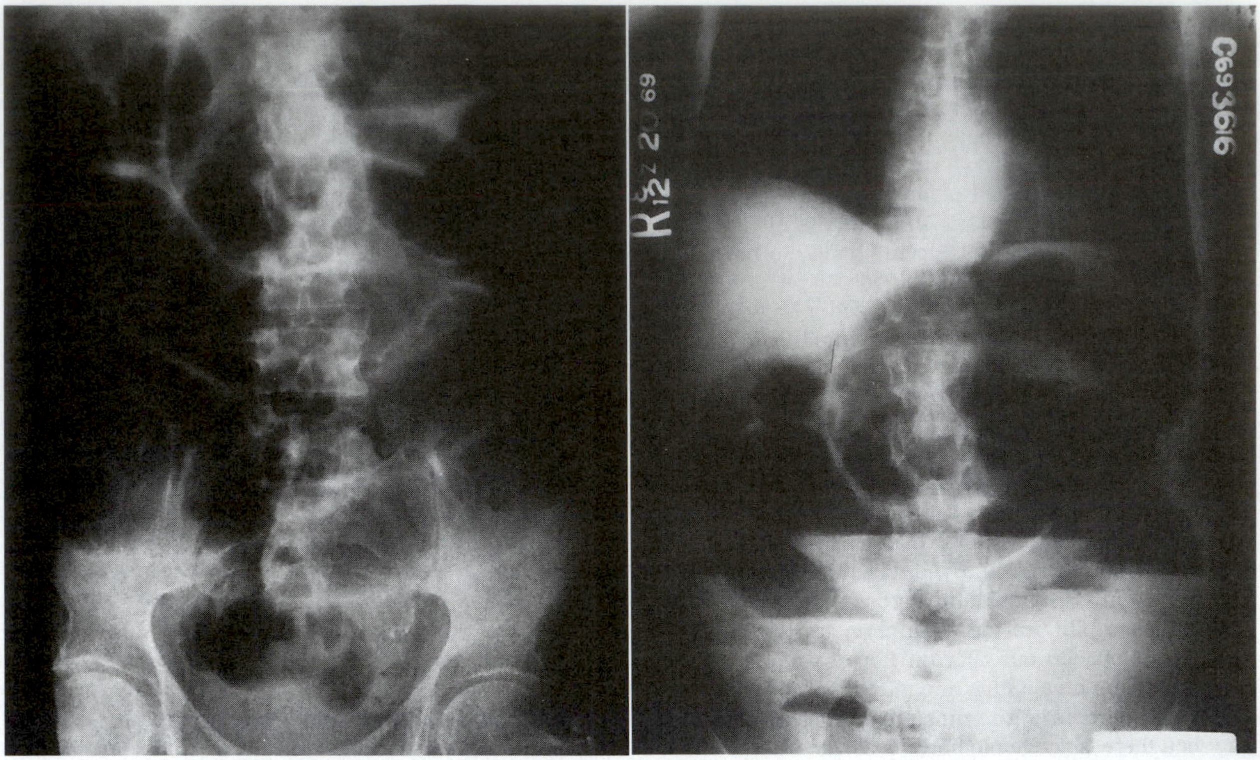 B

**Fig. 47-4. A,** Multiple loops of distended small bowel noted on abdominal flat plate, producing a stepladder appearance. **B,** Multiple air fluid levels on an upright film of the abdomen are produced by small bowel obstruction.

such as gallstone ileus, ingested foreign body, or frank bowel infarction may be seen. In problem cases oral contrast material for small bowel follow-through may show an area of partial obstruction more clearly. A CBC and electrolyte assays help with the estimation of dehydration and guide fluid replacement therapy.

Nasogastric suction is started immediately, and intravenous fluids are administered to correct the dehydration and to establish an adequate urinary output. Once the patient is resuscitated, a laparotomy is performed to relieve the obstruction.

## Large bowel obstruction

Elderly patients with large bowel obstruction commonly present to hospital emergency rooms. This problem is rarely seen in patients below the age of 50. Patients with large bowel obstruction complain of gradual and then marked abdominal distention associated with pain in the lower abdomen. The pain is colicky in nature and is less frequent and less intense than the pain caused by small bowel obstruction. There is a history of constipation and a lack of passing flatus for a number of days before admission. In severe and prolonged cases of large bowel obstruction there may be vomiting that results from superimposed small bowel obstruction. Dehydration does not become as prominent a feature of large bowel obstruction as it is with small bowel obstruction, unless small bowel obstruction is superimposed on the large bowel obstruction.

The most common cause of large bowel obstruction is carcinoma of the sigmoid colon. An inquiry is made, therefore, into the patient's history for recent change in bowel habits, with or without the passage of blood per rectum. In elderly patients, particularly in institutionalized ones who have had previous episodes of intermittent abdominal pain and distention, the possibility of a sigmoid volvulus must be entertained. Although colonic obstruction may be caused by clinical diverticulitis, it is not usually as severe as the obstruction associated with carcinoma.

Patients with large bowel obstruction are usually afebrile unless there is an associated diverticulitis. They may have tachycardia and may rarely be hypotensive and dehydrated. On examination there is marked distention of the abdomen, particularly in the flanks and across the upper abdomen, due to distensibility of the ascending, transverse, and descending colon. On auscultation bowel sounds tend to be normal, and on manual examination there is usually no abdominal tenderness or guarding. Tenderness is usually present when there is nonviable bowel, as occurs in patients with volvulus of the sigmoid colon that has strangulated or in patients who have marked distention of the small bowel and evidence of impending cecal rupture. In this situation the tenderness is in the right lower quadrant. On occasion the cecum in fact ruptures, resulting in free intraperitoneal air and cecal distention, seen on abdominal x-ray studies. The viability of the sigmoid should be considered in patients with a sigmoid volvulus in whom there is tenderness over the large sigmoid loop. Rectal examination is an important part of assessing a patient with large bowel obstruction. Obstructing rectal carcinomas may be palpated, as may masses on

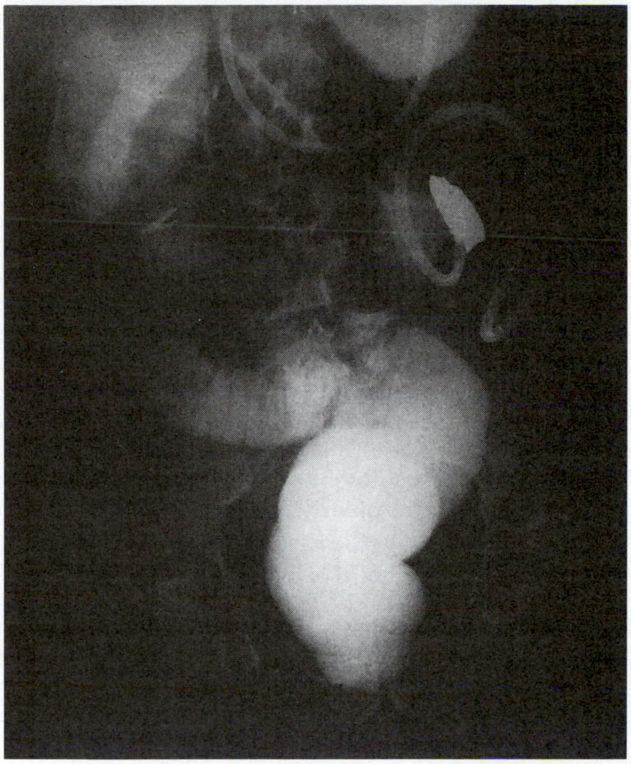

**Fig. 47-5.** Distended colon noted on abdominal flat plate in patient with large bowel obstruction produced by sigmoid volvulus.

the left side of the pelvis caused by carcinoma or diverticulitis.

KUB and upright x-rays of the abdomen are the most important investigations for confirming the diagnosis of large bowel obstruction. In such cases the distended large bowel extends down to the level of the colonic obstruction. The size of the cecum is noted. When the cecum reaches 14 cm in diameter, it must be assumed to be at or near the point of perforation. Air is looked for under the diaphragm to rule out a sigmoid or cecal perforation. When a volvulus of the sigmoid is present, the distended sigmoid assumes the appearance of a large coffee bean arising from the pelvis (Fig. 47-5). To distinguish large bowel obstruction from large bowel ileus, the patient is placed in a prone position and an abdominal x-ray obtained, which often reveals air filling the rectum in patients with ileus. In most cases of suspected large bowel obstruction a barium enema is performed to document the presence and nature of the lesion preoperatively.

Treatment of a patient with large bowel obstruction requires admission to hospital and placement of an intravenous line and a nasogastric tube. Because the colon is mainly an organ for fluid absorption, the dehydration that accompanies small bowel obstruction is not usually as marked as with obstruction of the large bowel. The patient with a volvulus of the sigmoid is admitted to hospital for surgical consultation and an urgent attempt to reduce the volvulus with sigmoidoscopy. If this is not satisfactory, the patient requires an emergency laparotomy.

## GYNECOLOGIC DISEASE

Not all acute abdominal processes are due to disease of the gastrointestinal tract in the female patient. Gynecologic causes for an acute abdomen must be considered.

### Salpingitis

Salpingitis is an inflammatory process of the fallopian tubes and is invariably bilateral. The patient gives a history of constant lower abdominal pain that, because of the bilateral nature of the disease, is situated in the suprapubic region and extends out into both sides of the lower abdomen. It is accompanied by a vaginal discharge, and the patient gives a history of recent sexual intercourse.

On examination the patient is febrile with tachycardia and normal blood pressure. No distention is seen on examination of the abdomen. Bowel sounds may be normal or reduced, depending on the degree of paralytic ileus associated with the inflammatory condition in the pelvis. On palpation there is tenderness above the pubic symphysis that extends into the right and left sides of the lower abdomen. In severe cases this tenderness is marked and may be accompanied by guarding. On vaginal examination there is a discharge arising from the os of the cervix, and the adnexa are swollen and tender.

Investigations show an elevated leukocyte count and positive vaginal cultures for bacteria. The treatment is antibiotic therapy, which in mild cases can be given on an outpatient basis. The patient is followed by a consulting gynecologist.

Tuboovarian abscess may form in severe cases. This abscess may be palpated on vaginal examination as well as on abdominal examination in some cases. Occasionally these abscesses rupture, causing severe prostration and the signs and symptoms of generalized peritonitis. Ultrasound of the lower abdomen accurately reveals the presence of a tuboovarian abscess. Such patients require intravenous fluids, antibiotics, and operative drainage.

### Mittelschmerz

Mittelschmerz is sometimes confused with appendicitis, especially if an inadequate medical history is taken. Mittelschmerz is due to peritoneal irritation associated with ovulatory bleeding. Symptoms occur exactly in the middle of the menstrual cycle. The patient presents with pain that has arisen initially in the right lower quadrant and remains there. This pain is unlike that of appendicitis, which starts in the periumbilical region and migrates later to the right lower quadrant. The patients are not anorectic and may in fact be hungry when questioned. Vomiting may occur in severe cases. On examination the patients may have a low-grade fever resulting from blood in the peritoneal cavity. The abdomen is often tender in the right lower quadrant; this is usually mild, and there is rarely any guarding. There is often tenderness on rectal and pelvic examination but no other abnormalities. These patients have a normal white blood cell count occasionally accompanied by a significant fall in the hematocrit level.

### Ovarian torsion

Ovarian torsion occurs more commonly in young women than in old women. The pain arises from ischemia of the ovary as a result of obstruction of the blood supply by the torsion. As a result the pain comes on rather quickly and is often severe; it may be referred to the low back. The patient often gives a history of minimal nausea and sometimes vomiting.

On examination the patient is usually afebrile but may have tachycardia caused by the pain. There is tenderness and guarding in the right or left lower quadrant depending on which ovary is twisted. On rectal and pelvic examination there is usually tenderness, and sometimes a mass can be palpated on the involved side.

Ultrasound may show some evidence that would support torsion of the ovary; however, it may be necessary to admit the patient for laparoscopy to confirm or rule out the diagnosis.

### Ectopic pregnancy

An ectopic pregnancy in the fallopian tube may present as an acute abdominal emergency when the tube ruptures into the peritoneal cavity. The patient presents with sudden lower abdominal pain which, when the patient is lying down, may also be associated with shoulder tip pain due to irritation of the diaphragm by blood.

The patient gives a history of sexual intercourse and a missed menstrual period. The condition of the patient at the time of presentation is directly related to the amount of blood loss from the ruptured fallopian tube. In severe cases of blood loss the patient may have fainted or she may have tachycardia and be hypotensive at the time of presentation at hospital. On examination there is tenderness and guarding in the lower abdomen. The tenderness may also be generalized because of the presence of blood in the peritoneal cavity. Mild cases may present with pain and with little sign of blood loss, and in these patients pelvic ultrasonography may be helpful in making the diagnosis. All patients are admitted to hospital for operation. Those who have severe signs of hemodynamic instability require resuscitation with intravenous fluids and blood replacement. Patients suspected of having an ectopic pregnancy require pregnancy testing, ultrasound, and possible admission to hospital for observation. This is a life-threatening condition, and so patients must be managed expeditiously.

## DISEASES THAT MIMIC AN ACUTE ABDOMEN

### Renal colic

Patients presenting with renal colic typically have severe pain in either flank that radiates down to either lower quadrant. As the stone causes an obstruction, there may be pain in the posterior flank caused by the dilated kidney and acute hydronephrosis. When the stone is in the lower ureter there may be referred pain to the labia or scrotum. The pain is constant and severe and often causes the patient to roll around in an effort to seek relief. Although this is not an intraperitoneal process, it may well result in abdominal signs that range from mild abdominal tenderness on one side of the abdomen or the other to mild abdominal distention and reduction; bowel sounds are occasionally absent. There is rarely any evidence of guarding. To support the diagnosis there may or may not be a history of hematuria.

Urinalysis reveals blood cells on microscopic examination. Should a patient be suspected of having renal colic, renal ultrasound or intravenous pylography is performed to demonstrate either hydronephrosis, hydroureter, or delayed excretion on the side of the stone. A scout film may well show the presence of the stone initially in the line of the ureter.

### Pleurisy

Chest infections resulting in pleuritic pain on many occasions give clinicians the impression that a process is ongoing in the abdominal cavity, particularly when it is on the right side. The most likely false diagnosis is that of acute cholecystitis. On careful examination, however, there are often symptoms referable to the lungs. The patient may have pleuritic pain made worse by taking a deep breath. Occasionally contraction of the upper abdominal musculature to splint the rib cage is mistaken for intraabdominal pathology. A false Murphy sign may be present because of the pleuritic pain causing the patient to catch his breath. If there is any doubt as to whether the Murphy sign is positive, the patient is asked to take a deep breath in the absence of palpation of the upper abdomen. X-ray studies are an essential part of the workup and diagnosis of the patient with possible pleurisy; however, such studies may not confirm the diagnosis, particularly in the presence of viral conditions.

## BIBLIOGRAPHY

Beal J: The acute abdomen. In *Textbook of surgery,* Philadelphia, 1981, Saunders.

Dunphy SE: Acute abdomen. In *Current surgical diagnosis and treatment,* ed 5, Los Altos, Calif, 1981, Lange.

Schwartz S, Storeer E: Manifestations of gastrointestinal disease. In *Principles of surgery,* New York, 1969, McGraw-Hill.

CHAPTER

# 48 Hernia

**Leon G. Josephs**

No disease of the human body, belonging to the province of the surgeon requires in its treatment a better combination of accurate, anatomical knowledge with surgical skill then Hernia in all its varieties.

**Sir Astley Paston Cooper, 1804**

*Stedman's Medical Dictionary* defines hernia as "the protrusion of a part or structure through the tissues normally containing it." For a hernia to occur, two factors must be present: (1) a defect in the wall of tissue between two cavities and (2) a pressure differential between the cavities. In the process of protruding into another cavity the herniating structure becomes enveloped by the lining of its own surroundings in addition to the lining of its neighbor. This fused structure is known as the hernia sac. If the sac and its contents are easily returned to the original cavity the hernia is described as reducible. An incarcerated or irreducible hernia is one that cannot be returned. If the blood supply to a herniated structure becomes obstructed, it is called a strangulated hernia. This is a surgical emergency that, without intervention, will result in tissue ischemia and necrosis.

It is estimated that 5% to 10% of the population has a hernia in some form or another. In 1991 there were 750,000 hernias repaired in the United States, the most common type being groin hernias. Groin hernias are further classified as indirect inguinal (50% of the total number), direct inguinal (25%), and femoral (6%). Ventral hernias are any herniation of the anterior abdominal wall other than the groin and represent only 14% of all hernias. They include epigastric (5%), incisional (5%), umbilical (3%), and spigelian (<1%). Other less common hernias include lumbar, obturator, diaphragmatic, and parastomal.

The history of hernia surgery dates back to ancient times, with mention in an Egyptian papyrus in 1550 BC. At that time treatment included applying constricting bandages to the offending area and a change of diet. In 25 AD the Greek encyclopedist Celsus documented the first surgical repair of an inguinal hernia. The principles of hernia repair changed little as the practice of surgery passed from the barber-surgeons of the Dark Ages to the anatomists of the Renaissance. The era of contemporary surgical repair of groin hernias began in 1884, when Edoardo Bassini (1844-1924) performed the first modern groin herniorrhaphy in Italy. Since Bassini the basic theory of hernia repair has remained constant with added adaptations by surgeons such as McVay, Lichtenstein, and Shouldice. With the advent of laparoscopic surgery new techniques of hernia repair are being implemented.

Perhaps the most important recent revolution in hernia surgery is not technical but economical, with the procedure being performed in an outpatient setting. During the decade of the 1980s same-day surgical centers grew so that 70% of the 680,000 groin hernias repaired in 1991 were done on an ambulatory basis. As a result, the primary care physician has taken on a greater role in the preoperative and postoperative care of the patient.

In all types of hernia one must determine if the hernia is due to an abnormal increase in intraabdominal pressure. It is therefore important to elicit a careful review of systems, especially urinary, pulmonary, and gastrointestinal.

In older men an accurate voiding history and prostate examination looking for enlargement or nodules should be done. If it is determined that the patient has some degree of bladder outlet obstruction, the proper referral to a urologist should be sought. Repairing a hernia in the presence of urinary obstruction is associated with a high rate of recurrence.

Chronic cough due to chronic obstructive pulmonary disease (COPD) should also be evaluated. It is important to optimize pulmonary function to decrease recurrence rates. The degree of pulmonary dysfunction plays a critical role in the repair of large hernias, which may have lost the right of domain to the abdominal cavity. If the abdominal viscera are placed back into a space that is not large enough, the upward pressure on the diaphragm greatly reduces the patient's capacity to breathe.

Finally, a complete gastrointestinal history must be obtained. Any new onset of change in bowel habits, stool consistency, or heme-positive stools must be investigated before elective repair of a hernia. In addition, the first symptom of ascites may be the onset of a hernia.

## GROIN HERNIA

In its simplest anatomic form the groin consists of two layers, superficial and deep, that are mirror images of one another. The superficial layer consists of skin, abdominal wall fat, Scarpa fascia, and external oblique aponeurosis and muscle. The deep layer begins after the spermatic cord and inguinal canal with the aponeurosis and muscle of the internal oblique and transversus. It continues with the transversalis fascia, below which lies preperitoneal fat and finally the peritoneum. A hernia in this area is thus a failure of these layers to contain the enclosed abdominal viscera.

An indirect inguinal hernia is a herniation through the internal inguinal ring that extends along the spermatic cord through the inguinal canal. If the process continues for a long time the sac can reach the scrotum. A direct inguinal hernia is a weakness of the floor of the inguinal canal in the area of Hesselbach's triangle. The borders of the triangle are classically defined as the inguinal ligament inferiorly, the inferior epigastric vessels laterally, and the rectus muscle medially. Traditionally an indirect hernia is defined as a hernia lateral to the inferior epigastric vessels, where a direct hernia occurs medial to the vessels within the triangle. A femoral hernia is a protrusion beneath the inguinal ligament into the femoral canal medial to the femoral vein (Fig. 48-1).

The etiology of groin hernias is multifactorial. Congenital, biologic, and environmental influences have all been implicated. The most important event in the etiology of groin hernias is considered to be human evolution to the standing position. When we assumed an upright posture, the groin became a vulnerable spot for herniation. Thus the musculature of the groin area developed two protective mechanisms to prevent herniation: (1) a shutter mechanism, where the internal oblique and transversus abdominis muscles contract toward the inguinal ligament, strengthening the posterior wall of the canal, and (2) a closure or sphincter mechanism, where contraction of the transversus abdominis muscle causes the cranial or caudal displacement of the transversalis fascia narrowing the deep inguinal ring.

The primary cause of an indirect hernia is congenital. The herniation occurs through a patent vaginal process that is left behind after the descent of the testicle. In women the vaginal process is present in the canal of Nuck. Since autopsy studies have shown more patent processes then hernias, it is believed that this alone cannot be responsible for indirect hernias in the adult. Hence indirect herniation is due to a congenitally present patent vaginal process plus a breakdown of the sphincter protective mechanism through various environmental conditions such as local trauma, increased intraabdominal pressure, and weakening of the muscles.

Direct inguinal herniation can also be attributed to several causes. If the tranversus abdominis and internal oblique musculature attach with a high arching inferior border, the shutter mechanism is faulty, predisposing to herniation. This congenital abnormality doesn't explain the increase in direct herniation in later life. As in indirect herniation, environmental factors that increase intraabdominal pressure play an important role. Peacock found

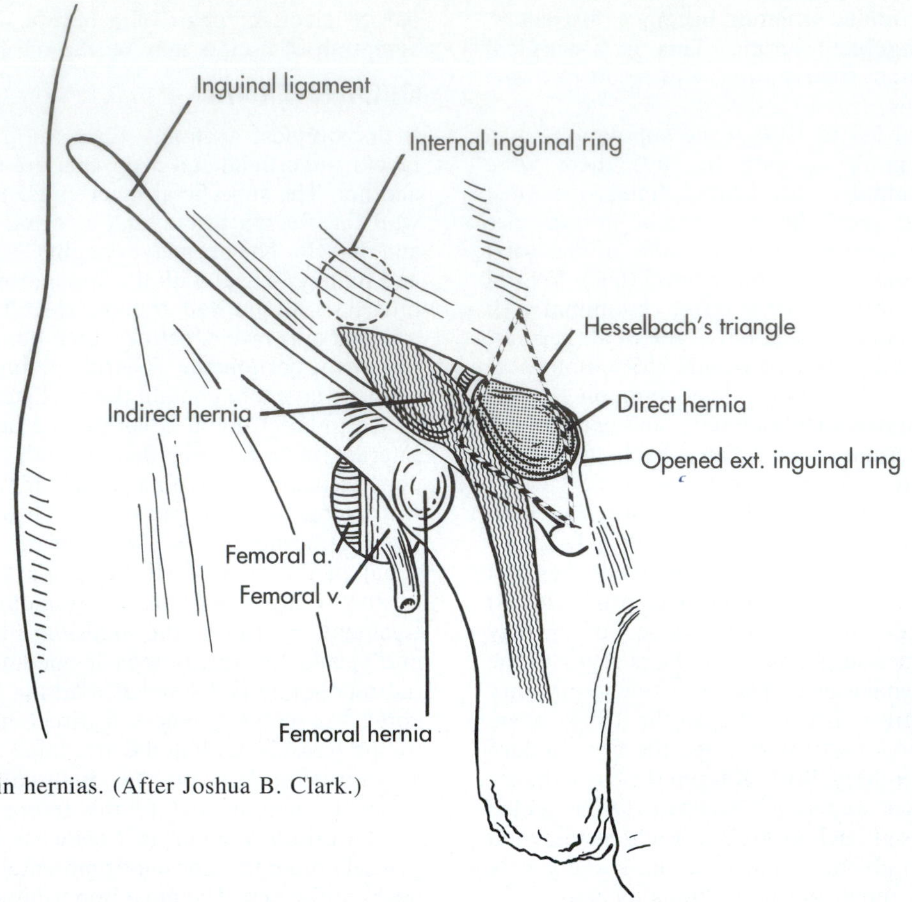


**Fig. 48.1** Groin hernias. (After Joshua B. Clark.)

that patients with hernias have an abnormality of collagen metabolism in the inguinal area. In addition, factors that influence collagen synthesis, such as malnutrition, lead to weakening of the abdominal musculature.

A femoral hernia is thought to be caused by a breakdown in the shutter mechanism and an enlargement of the femoral canal. Women have larger femoral canals, and therefore femoral hernias are more common in women then in men. Several factors contributing to the widened canal include the size of the female pelvis, the smaller size of the iliopsoas muscle, and the chronic engorgement of the femoral vein during pregnancy.

Of the 700,000 groin hernias repaired each year, 7% to 14% are for recurrence. The literature estimates that indirect and direct hernias both have about a 10% recurrence rate, whereas a recurrent hernia has a further recurrence rate of 35%. It is generally recognized that, if a hernia recurs before 2 years, it is regarded as an error in technique or judgment. Improper choice of operation, overlooking an indirect component to a direct hernia, and technical difficulty are common reasons for an early recurrence. After 2 years failures are generally attributed to weakening of tissues secondary to collagen metabolism.

The examination for groin hernias begins with a visible inspection of the groin and the external genitalia. With the patient standing the spermatic cord is palpated bilaterally for any localized swelling in the scrotal contents. When palpating the inguinal canal the physician must examine three areas. The examiner's finger follows the path of the spermatic cord and invaginates the scrotal skin. The first area to inspect is the external inguinal ring and the fascia of the external oblique. Following the spermatic cord up the canal the posterior wall is inspected for weakness. Finally the invaginated finger palpates the internal ring. After feeling the internal ring, the finger is removed slightly and the patient is asked to cough or strain, increasing intraabdominal pressure. A hernia is present if the examiner feels the sac tapping against the finger. Other positive findings include a rush of peritoneal fluid under the examining finger, reproduction of the patient's pain, or a bulge through a weakened posterior wall. In females the examination is confined to palpation of the groin and femoral area with the patient straining. Any noticeable swelling is a positive finding.

When a patient complains of groin pain and swelling, it is important to determine whether the hernia is undergoing an acute event such as incarceration or strangulation or if it is a long-standing problem that can be dealt with electively. This differentiation requires both a careful history from the patient about reducibility of the sac and the ability to reduce the hernia on physical examination. Differential diagnoses, including inguinal or femoral adenopathy, ectopic testis, hydrocele, psoas abscess, and saphenous varix, must be considered (Fig. 48-2).

Although many techniques have evolved over the years, the basic concept remains reenforcement of the two defense mechanisms already in place: strengthen the posterior wall and narrow the internal inguinal ring. In indirect herniorrhaphy the hernia sac must be dissected free and reduced whereas in femoral hernias the femoral canal is narrowed. The repair is made either by using the

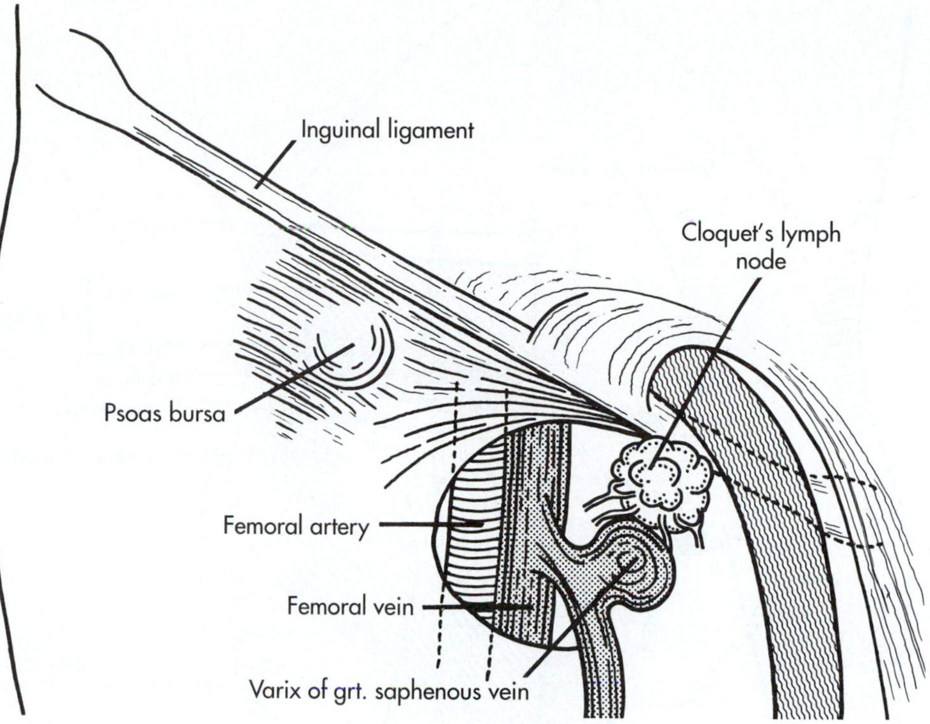


**Fig. 48-2.** Femoral masses that may be confused with hernias. (After Joshua B. Clark.)

tissue already present or by utilizing synthetic materials to reconstruct the posterior wall, a so-called tension-free repair. With the advent of laparoscopic surgery a new technique utilizing these basic concepts has been added. Proponents point out the shorter postoperative recovery time and its value for recurrent hernias and bilateral repairs. Opponents state that laparoscopic hernia repair is more costly and the recurrence rates are unknown.

Minimal wound discomfort can continue postoperatively for several days; if it continues longer or is unrelieved by oral analgesics a reason must be sought. Early postoperative wound infections may present as a continued painful incision, erythema, and swelling. Severe postoperative pain may be secondary to a nerve entrapment, which may require reoperation. Slight erythema and bruising of the skin extending into the scrotum is normal postoperatively. If the hernia had a large scrotal component, swelling of the scrotum can be relieved by scrotal support and ice packs. Any increasing pain or testicular tenderness should be evaluated by the surgeon to rule out ischemia.

After a standard groin herniorrhaphy the patient is generally allowed to go back to normal activities after 1 to 2 weeks and should wait 4 to 6 weeks before heavy work or contact sports. With laparoscopic repairs the data are not yet in, but it is my practice to allow patients to begin heavy activity as soon as they feel fit, generally 2 to 3 days postoperatively.

Late postoperative complications, though uncommon, are distressing to both patient and physician. As mentioned previously, recurrence is seen in approximately 10% of first-time hernia repairs and 35% of recurrent herniorrhaphies. With a recurrence the patient generally complains of the same symptoms as with the primary defect, and the physical findings are similar. In repairing a recurrent hernia different types of techniques should be offered; it is here that laparoscopic repair may find its niche.

Other complications of herniorrhaphy include a reactive hydrocele, which is a result of incomplete excision of the hernia sac in the scrotum. This problem usually resolves without intervention; however, it can be treated with sterile aspiration. Ilioinguinal or femoral neuroma can be caused by nerve entrapment or regeneration of a cut nerve. In a neuroma the patient generally presents with unresolving postoperative pain. Treatment can include local nerve blocks; however, they generally resolve on their own. If persistent, wound exploration and excision may be necessary.

Testicular atrophy is an uncommon complication of primary hernia repair but is more prevalent in surgery for recurrent hernia. If the vascular pedicle of the testicle is injured during an extensive cord dissection, venous outflow is compromised, leading to ischemia and eventually testicular atrophy. The testicle can generally stay in place as a natural prosthesis unless pain control is an issue. The patient should be assured that both fertility and potency will not be affected if the other testicle is functional.

## VENTRAL HERNIA

All other hernias of the anterior abdominal wall besides groin hernias are termed ventral hernias. The following sections define these hernias and how to recognize and treat them (Fig. 48-3).

### Epigastric hernia

An epigastric hernia occurs in the midline between the umbilicus and xiphoid process of the sternum. A defect in the decussation of the fibers of the linea alba allows a

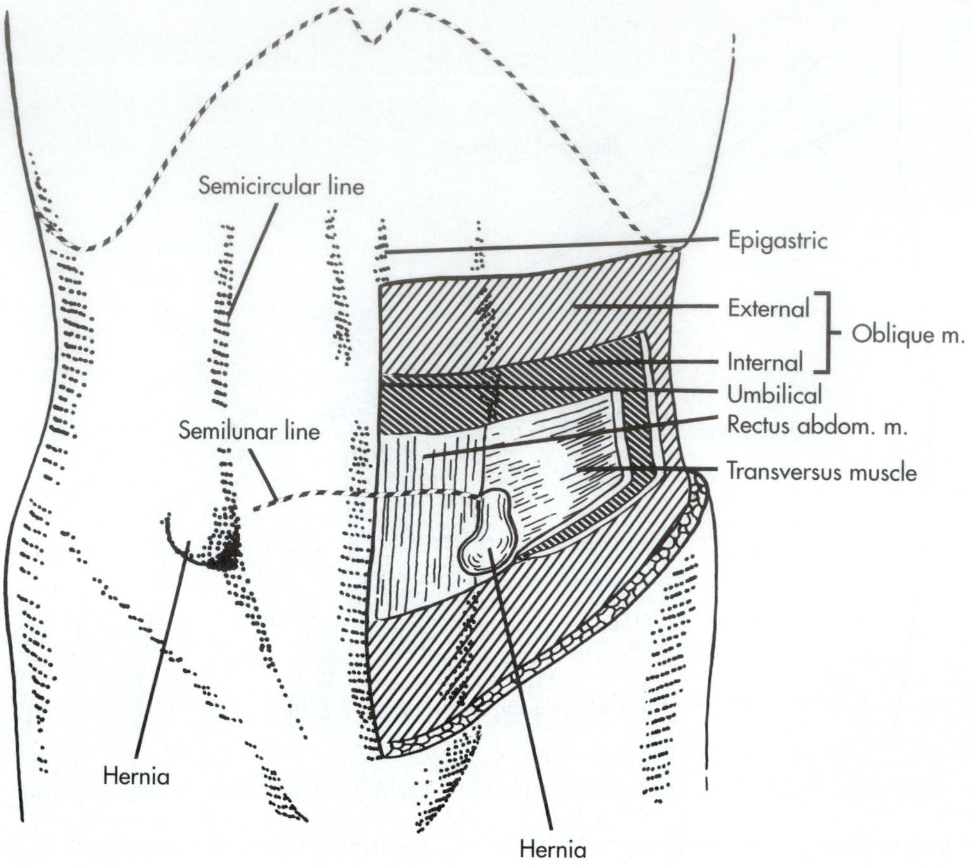


**Fig. 48-3.** Spigelian hernia protrudes through the abdominal wall at the semilunar line. (After Joshua B. Clark.)

protrusion of the contents below. It is three times more common in men than women, and the age of peak occurrence is between 20 and 50. About 20% of epigastric hernias are multiple. The most common manifestation is herniation of preperitoneal fat, but herniation of omentum or bowel can occur.

Epigastric hernias are usually asymptomatic. A small bump or swelling may be found in the midline, which increases with exertion or straining. The smaller ones can be very painful because of the irritation of the preperitoneal fat through a small defect. Large hernias can incarcerate and, if they contain bowel, may cause obstruction.

Repair of ventral hernias is recommended due to the possibility of incarceration. Smaller hernias can be repaired using local anesthesia. The hernia sac is dissected free of surrounding tissues and reduced. The defect is then closed. Postoperative recovery time is minimal, especially for small defects.

## Umbilical hernia

An umbilical hernia is a congenital defect caused by a patent umbilical ring left after the umbilical vessels are obliterated. It is a normal occurrence in 20% of all newborn infants, greater in males and African-Americans. In the pediatric population umbilical hernias are observed until the age of 2; if they persist after age 2, it is suggested that they be repaired.

In adults all umbilical hernias should be repaired because of the propensity to incarcerate, obstruct, and possibly strangulate. New hernias in adulthood should be investigated for all the previously stated causes of increased intraabdominal pressure. In umbilical hernias it is especially important to look for other stigmata of liver disease, since a new umbilical hernia is often the first sign of ascites.

The repair follows the same principles common to all hernia surgery. The sac is dissected free of the surrounding tissues and reduced, and the defect in the umbilical ring is then closed. The umbilicus itself is left in place during the procedure. Postoperatively the patient should experience minimal discomfort and be back to normal activities in 1 to 2 weeks.

## Incisional hernia

An incisional hernia is a herniation through a surgical incision and is the one true iatrogenic hernia. The incidence is reported to be between 2% and 11% of all patients undergoing abdominal operations. The interval between the original procedure and the development of an incisional hernia is variable. There is a 2:1 female to male predominance in incisional hernias.

The factors responsible for incisional herniation can be placed into two groups: those which surgeons can control and those which they can not. Controllable factors include technical aspects such as choice of incision, suture choices, and surgical techniques. Uncontrollable factors include the age of the patient, general debility, steroid use, nutritional status, and postoperative wound infection.

One manifestation of an incisional hernia is a swelling or bulge at the incision site that may be painful. As in all hernias, examination is best when the patient strains to increase intraabdominal pressure. A patient with an incarcerated incisional hernia may also present with signs and symptoms of a bowel obstruction.

Before repair of an incisional hernia an explanation for the first breakdown should be explored. Nutritional status should be reviewed: overweight patients should reduce their weight and malnourished patients should increase nutritional intake. Pulmonary function should be optimized to reduce intraabdominal pressure increases resulting from coughing or dyspnea. Skin hygiene with cleansing agents should be undertaken to decrease the incidence of wound infection.

The repair of an incisional hernia can be a formidable task. In large defects with incarcerated bowel, multiple adhesions must be taken down before repair of the fascia can be done. Depending on the size of the defect and the preference of the surgeon, synthetic material, such as polypropylene mesh, may be used to repair the hernia. Postoperative recovery then depends on the extent of the procedure and what was done for the repair.

### Spigelian hernia

A spigelian hernia, also known as a lateral ventral hernia, is a protrusion through the spigelian fascia that, by definition, is the area of the transversus abdominis aponeurosis lateral to the edge of the rectus sheath but medial to the transition of the transversus abdominis muscle to its aponeurotic tendon. This lateral border is also known as the spigelian line. A spigelian hernia can occur anywhere in the spigelian fascia, but its most common origin is just below the umbilicus in the region of the semilunar line of Douglas; it is here that the spigelian fascia is widest and weakest. Lower spigelian hernias can be confused with an inguinal hernia, the difference being that a direct inguinal hernia occurs below the transversus abdominis aponeurotic arch, and a spigelian hernia protrudes through it (see Fig. 48-3).

Spigelian hernia is seen most in older patients, particularly in women, in whom a predisposing factor may be recent weight loss. Spigelian hernias are more common on the right side. Coincidentally, groin hernias must also be searched for. The presenting symptom is often pain in the area of the spigelian fascia. If the physician is unable to diagnose the herniation on physical examination, computed tomography (CT) scan or ultrasound may be helpful in patients in whom the diagnosis is strongly suspected. Repair is recommended, since incarceration occurs in 25% of the cases. The procedure involves reducing the hernia sac and its contents and then repairing the fascial defect. The defect is generally small, so prosthetic material is usually not necessary. Results of surgery are excellent and the recurrence rates are very low.

## MISCELLANEOUS HERNIAS

### Lumbar hernia

There are two potential spaces for herniation in the lumbar area. The more common of the two is the superior lumbar triangle, where the Dolee or Grynfeltt type occurs. The herniation is below the twelfth rib through the quadratus lumborum muscle mass. The inferior lumbar hernia occurs through the Petit space, which is bounded by the iliac crest inferiorly, latissimus dorsi posteriorly, and external oblique anteriorly. The hernia generally contains preperitoneal fat; rarely bowel or omentum is present. When one is evaluating any mass or bulge in the lumbar area, a hernia must be kept in mind. CT scan or ultrasound may be helpful in making the diagnosis. Repair generally requires synthetic mesh due to the size and position of the defect.

### Obturator hernia

An obturator hernia is a rare herniation through the obturator foramen internally. It usually is seen in elderly women and presents as an acute bowel obstruction without any prior surgical history. Referred pain along the distribution of the obturator nerve (Howship-Romberg

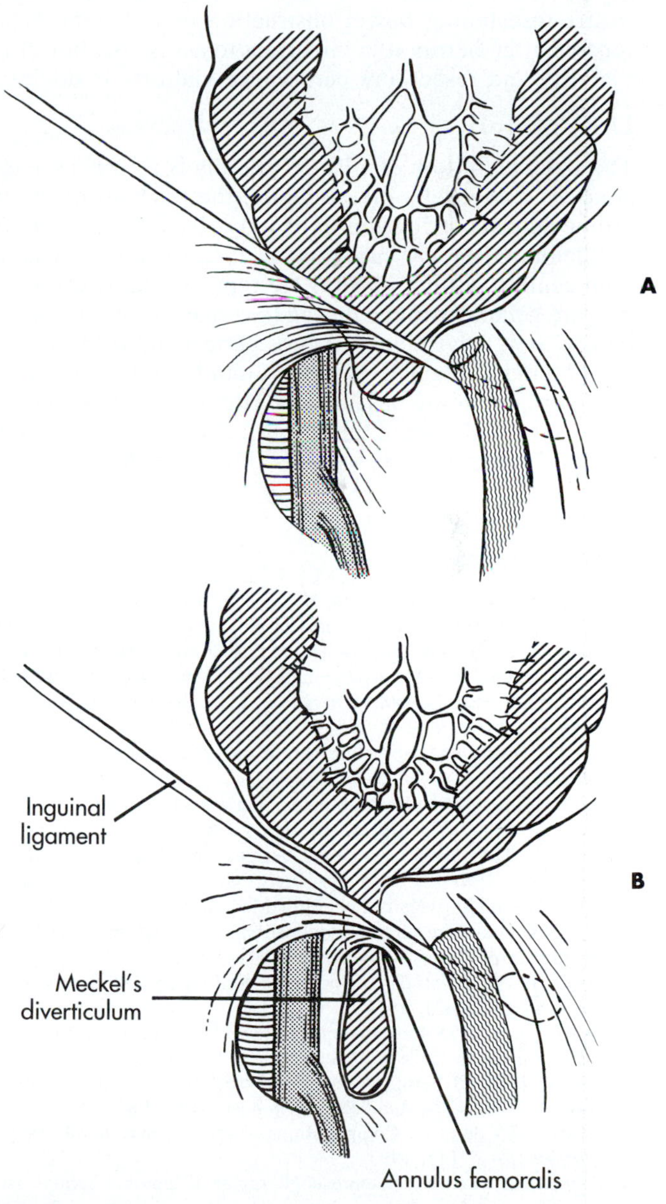


**Fig. 48-4.** Special hernias. **A,** Richter's hernia. **B,** Littre's hernia.

sign) may be present. Another clue is bowel gas below the superior pubic ramus on abdominal radiographs. The hernia sac may be palpable on vaginal examination. Reduction and repair are generally done by exploratory laparotomy, but if the diagnosis is highly suspected preoperatively, a retroperitoneal approach can be used.

### Richter's hernia

Richter's hernia occurs when only part of the circumference of a loop of bowel protrudes through a hernial orifice. Although any part of the small or large bowel may protrude, the terminal ileum is the most common. Usually the antemesenteric border protrudes into the sac and the mesenteric portion remains in the abdomen. Richter's hernias are most common in the groin and umbilicus, but they have also been described in incisional, obturator, and lumbar hernias (Fig. 48-4, *A*).

Clinical presentation runs the gamut from being asymptomatic masses discovered on physical examination to life-threatening bowel obstruction or ischemia. When repairing the hernia it is important to assess the bowel for viability and resect any part whose viability is doubtful.

### Littre's hernia

The strict definition of a Littre's hernia is a hernia sac that contains a Meckel's diverticulum, the remnant of the vitelline duct occurring approximately 30 cm from the terminal ileum. Of the 50 case reports of Littre's hernias in the 20th century, all hernia sites are represented. Littre's hernias are generally found during the repair of another sort of hernia. It is advisable that in a patient older than 30 an asymptomatic Meckel's diverticulum be left alone. In the younger population or if the diverticulum is symptomatic, it is resected. Repair of the hernia defect is then done in the standard fashion for its location (Fig. 48-4, *B*).

## BIBLIOGRAPHY

Activity and recurrent hernia, *Br Med J* 2:3, 1977 (editorial).

Altschule MD: Hernia as the presenting complaint in patients with cirrhosis of the liver and ascites, *N Engl J Med* 224:351, 1941.

Cannon DJ, Reed RC: Metastatic emphysema, *Ann Surg* 195:270, 1981.

Chapman CB, Small AM, Roundtree LG: Decompensative portal cirrhosis, *JAMA* 97:237, 1931.

Deitch EA, Engel JM: Spigelian hernia: an ultrasonic diagnosis, *Arch Surg* 115:93, 1980.

Engeset J, Youngson GG: Ambulatory peritoneal dialysis and hernial complications, *Surg Clin North Am* 64:385, 1984.

Gaston EA: The repair of inguinal hernias. In *Annual of the Boston University School of Medicine Division of Surgery,* vol 1, Boston, 1981, Boston University School of Medicine.

Gomella LG et al: The surgical implications of herniation of the urinary bladder, *Arch Surg* 120:964, 1985.

Harrison JH: Resection of the spermatic cord in inguinal hernia repair, *Am J Surg* 121:631, 1971.

Haug JN, Seeger R: *Socioeconomic factbook for surgery 1982,* Chicago, 1982, American College of Surgeons.

Lewin JR: Femoral hernia with upward extension into the abdominal wall: CT diagnosis, *Am J Roentgenol* 136:206, 1981.

MacFadyen BV Jr et al: Complications of laparoscopic herniorrhaphy, *Surg Endosc* 7:155, 1993.

McKernan JB, Laws HL: Laparoscopic repair of inguinal hernias using a totally extraperitoneal prosthetic approach, *Surg Endosc* 7:26, 1993.

Myers R, Zollinger R: Gastrointestinal symptoms and inguinal hernia, *N Engl J Med* 227:660, 1941.

Ray B et al: Massive inguinal scrotal herniation, *J Urol* 118:330, 1977.

Smedberg SGG et al: Herniography in athletes with groin pain, *Am J Surg* 149:378, 1985.

Spangen L: Spigelian hernia, *Surg Clin North Am* 64:351, 1984.

CHAPTER

# 49 Infectious and Inflammatory Diseases of the Intestines

J. Thomas LaMont

Inflammation and infection of the intestine are commonly encountered diseases, seen in about 10% to 15% of patients examined in medical practice. On a worldwide basis infectious diarrheas are second only to cardiovascular diseases as a cause of death. The evaluation and treatment of these common disorders can be initiated by the generalist in the office; only a minority of patients require specialized consultation. The cornerstone in diagnosing intestinal infection and inflammation is a meticulous history of the present illness, with particular attention to duration and frequency of symptoms. The differential diagnosis should be constructed to include not only the more likely possibilities but also those entities which can be verified by specific laboratory testing.

## INFECTIOUS DIARRHEA

### Office diagnosis of infectious diarrhea

The diagnosis of infectious diarrhea of viral or bacterial etiology is aided considerably by a careful history of the time course of the illness and exposure to possible sources of these pathogens (Table 49-1). Viral gastroenteritis and toxin-mediated food poisoning are brief illnesses with short incubation periods, as is traveler's diarrhea. Bacterial dysenteries are generally longer in duration, more severe, and accompanied by more serious signs and symptoms of enteritis including bloody diarrhea, fever, prostration, and weight loss. Familiarity with the basic patterns of these dysenteries allows a tentative diagnosis to be made at the time of the initial visit.

A simple algorithm can be used to diagnose most patients with infectious diarrhea encountered in office practice (Fig. 49-1). Acute diarrhea of less than 1 week's duration is highly suggestive of infectious diarrhea. The physician should inquire about antibiotic exposure, recent travel, exposure to infected persons, and homosexual contacts. Patients with bloody diarrhea, fever, chills, and dehydration are likely to have bacterial or amebic dysentery, whereas watery diarrhea with only mild cramps suggests viral infection.

As shown in Table 49-2 and the box on p. 683, infectious diarrheas can be categorized according to the agent involved (viral, bacterial, parasitic), the mode of acquisition (food poisoning, traveler's diarrhea), and the

**Table 49-1.** Clinical features of common infectious diarrheas

| Class / Typical agent | Incubation period | Duration of illness | Epidemiology |
|---|---|---|---|
| Viral gastroenteritis: Norwalk agent | 1-2 d | 1-2 d | Family and school outbreaks usually in winter and summer |
| Food poisoning: *Staphylococcus aureus* | 4-8 hr | 12-24 hr | Point source outbreaks common |
| Bacterial dysentery: *Shigella sonnei* | 1-2 d | 3-7 d | Contaminated food, water |
| Enteric fever: *Salmonella typhosa* | 3-10 d | 3-6 wk (untreated) | Contaminated food or water, often via an asymptomatic carrier |
| Traveler's diarrhea: *Escherichia coli* | 4-6 d | 2-4 d after arrival in epidemic area | Common in Mexico, Latin America, Far East; usually transmitted via cooked food, tap water, salad |
| Antibiotic-associated pseudomembranous colitis: *Clostridium difficile* | 1-3 d | 3-10 d | Usually acquired in hospital during or following antibiotic therapy |

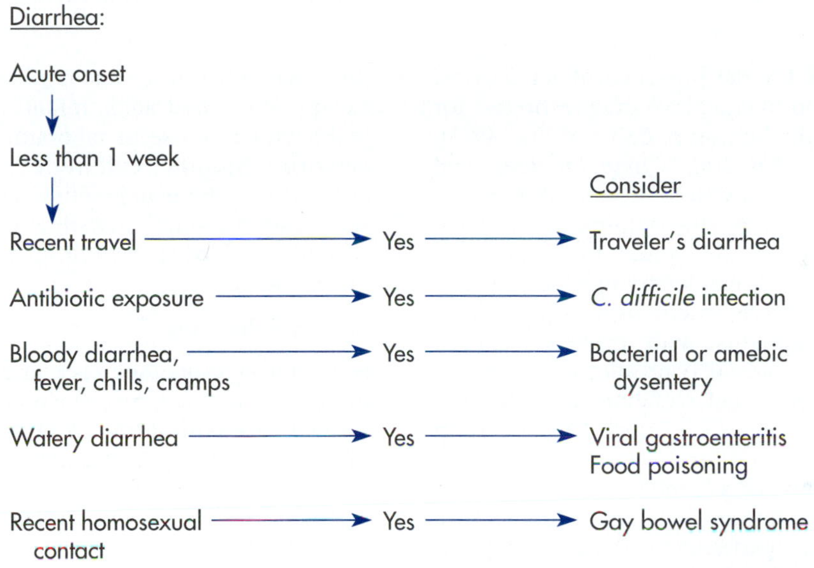


**Fig. 49-1.** Diagnostic algorithm for infectious diarrhea: history.

pathophysiologic mechanism (ingestion of preformed toxin, epithelial invasion). The salient clinical features of the most common infectious diarrheas encountered in practice are described below.

A brief physical examination of the abdomen may provide additional diagnostic information. Tenderness in both lower quadrants suggests infectious colitis (*Shigella, Campylobacter, Entamoeba histolytica*), whereas middle or upper abdominal tenderness suggests *Salmonella* or *Campylobacter* infection or viral gastroenteritis. In some elderly patients *Clostridium difficile* infection may cause an ileus with only minimal diarrhea, abdominal distention, and reduced bowel sounds. Rectal examination provides the opportunity to examine the stool for blood or mucus and to test for the presence of occult blood. Significant abdominal tenderness, rebound, and rigidity are signs of severe disease and are indications for hospital admission and prompt surgical consultation.

Following a careful history the physician should obtain a fresh stool specimen for bacterial culture, parasite

### Incidence of leukocytes in infectious diarrheas

**Usually (50% or more)**
*Shigella* dysentery
*Campylobacter* dysentery
Amebic colitis
Enterohemorrhagic or enteroinvasive *Escherichia coli*

**Sometimes (30% to 50%)**
*Yersinia enterocolitica*
*Clostridium difficile*
*Salmonella* gastroenteritis
*Giardia lamblia*

**Rarely (<5%)**
Viral gastroenteritis
Acute food poisoning
Enterotoxigenic *E. coli;* enteric or typhoid fever

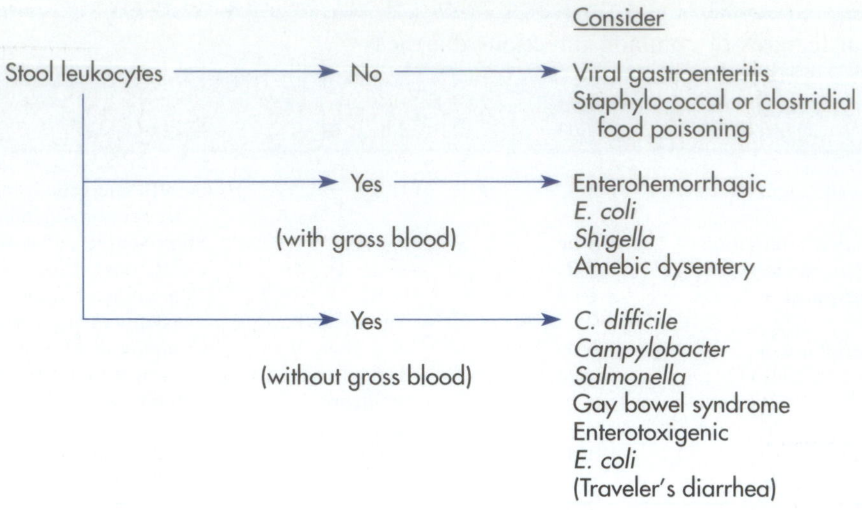


**Fig. 49-2.** Diagnostic algorithm for infectious diarrhea: stool leukocyte examination.

examination, and to test for the presence of leukocytes, which is a convenient and inexpensive diagnostic test for infectious diarrhea (see the box on p. 683 and Fig. 49-2). Invasive pathogens like *Shigella, Campylobacter,* and enterohemorrhagic or enteroinvasive strains of *Escherichia coli* produce a leukocyte-containing diarrhea, whereas viral gastroenteritis and some toxin-mediated diarrheas are usually not accompanied by fecal leukocytes. However, stool leukocytes are absent in 40% to 50% of stool specimens from patients with proven bacterial enteritis. Stool leukocytes are also present in idiopathic inflammatory bowel disease and ischemic enteritis, but these conditions can generally be excluded by a careful history.

Flexible sigmoidoscopy or colonoscopy can provide useful diagnostic information in selected patients with acute infectious diarrhea, particularly those with pseudomembranous colitis, amebic dysentery, ischemic colitis, or gay bowel syndrome. Advanced radiologic tests including barium enema, abdominal computed tomography (CT) scan, and ultrasound are seldom necessary in the evaluation of acute infections.

### Viral gastroenteritis

The major pathogens of viral gastroenteritis are the Norwalk agent and *Rotavirus,* which account for approximately 30% to 40% of gastrointestinal infections worldwide. Outbreaks of *Rotavirus* diarrhea occur more commonly during the winter and summer months, particularly among children from 6 to 24 months of age. Viral gastroenteritis in older children and adults caused by the Norwalk agent is one of the commonest causes for work absenteeism in our society, at a cost of many millions of dollars annually. Transmission is by the fecal-oral route, and the incubation period is approximately 1 to 2 days. Symptoms of viral gastroenteritis are mild and brief, usually lasting 24 to 48 hours. The illness can be quite debilitating in some patients, with vomiting, frequent loose watery stools, diffuse myalgias, chills, and occasionally fever. Because Norwalk agent and *Rotavirus* are highly infectious, family outbreaks are quite common, with preschool-age children frequently affected. The disease is self-limited and rarely requires special treatment except in dehydrated infants. The absence of fecal leukocytes is a useful laboratory finding in viral gastroenteritis. Specific culture or serologic tests are not currently available in practice. Transient lactase deficiency secondary to small intestine villous damage can cause secondary diarrhea lasting up to several weeks after the initial attack.

### Bacterial diarrheas

Bacterial enteropathogens can cause diarrhea by at least three well-defined mechanisms: (1) secretion of a preformed exotoxin during storage of food, (2) colonization of the intestinal tract without mucosal invasion but with release of enterotoxin, and (3) invasion of the intestinal epithelium with or without enterotoxin production (see Table 49-2).

Food poisoning refers to infectious diarrhea of various etiologies acquired by eating contaminated food. Outbreaks of food poisoning are typically more common in warm weather, when food is stored at higher temperatures that allow bacterial multiplication and release of protein exotoxins. These organisms or their toxins are then ingested; they then cause an acute illness within a few hours.

***Staphylococcus aureus.*** Food poisoning caused by *Staphylococcus aureus* is attributed to ingestion of a preformed enterotoxin produced by certain strains of staphylococci, typically carried by a food handler with an *S. aureus* infection on the hand. The onset of staphylococcal food poisoning occurs abruptly 4 to 8 hours after ingestion of the contaminated food. The cardinal manifestations of nausea, vomiting, abdominal colic, profuse watery diarrhea, and prostration rarely last more than 24 hours. Occasional patients become dehydrated and require intravenous fluid replacement.

The diagnosis of *S. aureus* food poisoning is based on the short incubation period and duration of symptoms, the almost universal presence of vomiting, the absence of fever, and the occurrence of the same illness in other patients who shared the food. A definitive diagnosis can be

**Table 49-2.** Classification of infectious diarrheas

| Mechanism | Bacterial pathogen | Source of pathogen |
|---|---|---|
| Ingestion of preformed exotoxin | *Staphylococcus aureus* | Custard, pudding, potato salad, mayonnaise |
| | *Bacillus cereus* | Rice |
| Colonization of bowel with enterotoxin production | *Vibrio cholerae* | Fecal contamination of food or water |
| | *Escherichia coli* (enterotoxigenic strains) | |
| | *Clostridium perfringens* | Meat |
| Epithelial invasion | *Salmonella* sp. | Eggs and poultry |
| | *Shigella* sp. | Various |
| | *Campylobacter fetus* | Various |
| | *Yersinia enterocolitica* | Milk, meat |
| | *V. parahaemolyticus* | Fresh or cooked seafood |
| | *E. coli* (enteroinvasive strains) | Various |

made only if the contaminated food is shown to contain large numbers of enterotoxin-producing staphylococci; this, however, is impractical in most instances. Antibiotic treatment is not indicated for this short-term disease, since bacterial proliferation in the host does not occur.

***Clostridium perfringens.*** *Clostridium perfringens* is nearly ubiquitous in the environment and can be routinely isolated from human and animal feces, air, water, and soil. *C. perfringens* type A is primarily responsible for food poisoning in humans. The usual vectors are meat and poultry, which are often contaminated with heat-resistant *C. perfringens.* When food is cooked more than 24 hours before eating and left to cool or stand at room temperature, the organism may multiply to form an infectious inoculum. When the food is served cold or with only brief rewarming, sufficient numbers of organisms are present to produce an exotoxin in the small intestine. Symptoms may occur simultaneously in several individuals who ate the same meal 6 to 24 hours after ingestion. Diarrhea and cramping abdominal pain lasting for 12 to 24 hours are the typical symptoms. Nausea may be present, but vomiting is distinctly rare. As with staphylococcal food poisoning, no specific therapy is required. Isolation of *C. perfringes* from the stool is not diagnostic, since this organism is part of the normal fecal flora.

***Bacillus cereus.*** *Bacillus cereus,* an organism increasingly implicated as a cause of food poisoning, is ubiquitous in soil and frequently present in raw, dried, and processed foods. The organism is able to produce two distinct enterotoxins, one very similar to the heat-labile *E. coli* enterotoxin that causes watery diarrhea and one similar to the enterotoxin of *S. aureus* that produces emesis. *B. cereus* food poisoning is usually associated with rice dishes that have initially been boiled, which the spores of *B. cereus* can withstand, and then left to simmer or kept warm in steam heaters for prolonged periods during which the pathogen multiplies and produces toxins.

***Shigella species.*** Shigellosis, an acute self-limited enteric infection, is one of the most common causes of bacillary dysentery. The most important isolates are *S. dysenteriae, S. flexneri, S. boydii,* and *S. sonnei.* In the United States *S. sonnei* accounts for three fourths of stool isolates, with *S. flexneri* found in the majority of remaining cases.

Shigellosis is encountered worldwide, particularly in areas of poor hygiene and overcrowding. Outbreaks in the United States tend to be sporadic, but minor epidemics from a single food source or in custodial institutions or day care centers have been described. The mode of spread is predominantly fecal-oral, with infected food handlers posing the major health hazard. A distinguishing feature of this pathogen is the small number of organisms required to constitute an infective dose. Controlled studies in volunteers have demonstrated clinical disease after ingestion of several hundred organisms. *Shigella* causes disease primarily by invasion of and multiplication within the colonic epithelium, which induces an acute colitis. Certain strains of *Shigella* release an enterotoxin that causes a profuse watery diarrhea in the early stages of the disease.

After an incubation period of 24 to 48 hours the onset of diarrhea is heralded by abdominal pain, tenderness, and cramping. The diarrhea is liquid and greenish with strands of mucus, blood, and leukocytes; 20% to 30% of patients may pass gross blood (hematochezia). The entire colon may be involved, and the sigmoidoscopic appearance in severe cases may mimic ulcerative colitis with mucosal hyperemia, friability, and ulceration. Diagnosis depends on isolation of the organism from stool culture or rectal swabs.

In general, *Shigella* dysentery is a self-limited disease; fever abates within approximately 4 days and diarrhea and abdominal cramping subside in a week. Stool cultures commonly remain positive for several days or weeks after the clinical illness has subsided. In severe childhood infections bacteremia and hemolytic-uremic syndrome have been reported.

***Salmonella species.*** *Salmonella* is one of the major diarrheal pathogens of the world, with 20,000 to 30,000 cases reported annually in the United States. Since most diarrheal infectious diseases are underreported, the actual figure is likely to be much higher. *Salmonella* is divided into three species: *S. typhi,* the causative agent of classic typhoid fever, *S. choleraesuis,* and *S. enteritidis,* which is subdivided into many serotypes. *Salmonella* species, particularly *S. enteritidis* and *S. choleraesuis,* can be cultured from a variety of nonhuman hosts, including poultry, rats, reptiles, wild birds, and flies.

The main animal reservoirs for human disease are poultry and livestock. Supermarket chicken and eggs are often contaminated with *Salmonella* species, which are present in the intestinal tracts of commercially raised animals. It is estimated that 85% of community-acquired salmonellosis in the United States is related to ingestion of contaminated food, whereas 15% arises from person-to-person spread. The seasonal incidence of salmonellosis peaks in the summer and autumn. In contrast to *Shigella* species, where small inocula can cause disease, infection with *Salmonella* requires ingestion of 10,000 to 100 million organisms and less in patients with low gastric acidity.

*Salmonella* infection produces two forms of illness: (1) gastroenteritis similar to other bacterial dysenteries and (2) enteric fever. When the infecting organism is *S. typhi,* the resultant illness is typhoid fever; other species of *Salmonella* produce a similar illness called *paratyphoid fever.*

**Enteric fever.** In enteric fever the organism multiplies in the small intestine and invades the epithelium but produces minimal inflammation and cell destruction. The organisms then gain access to the bloodstream via the intestinal lymphatics, and a short-lived primary bacteremia ensues 24 to 72 hours after inoculation. This primary bacteremia is transient and terminated by phagocytosis of the organisms by the cells of the reticuloendothelial system. The organisms survive intracellularly and continue to multiply, giving rise to a second, more prolonged bacteremia accompanied by fever, headache, abdominal pain and myalgias that can last days to weeks, the so-called enteric fever. During this phase of continuous bacteremia all organs are exposed to viable organisms, and abscess formation occasionally occurs. Patients with sickle cell disease, aortic aneurysms, cancer, hemolytic anemia, and valvular heart disease are more prone to develop prolonged bacteremia and tissue abscesses. For unknown reasons the gallbladder is almost universally infected during this period, and organisms multiply to a higher titer in bile, usually without the production of cholecystitis. Stool cultures become positive secondary to the shedding of a large number of organisms into the bile during the third to fourth week of the disease.

Chronic carriage of *Salmonella* after enteric fever provides a human reservoir for this organism. Approximately 50% of patients continue to shed organisms in the stool at 6 weeks, and 5% to 10% continue to excrete up to the third month. A chronic carrier is defined as an individual with positive stool culture 1 year after initial infection, usually from continuous gallbladder shedding.

**Gastroenteritis:** *Salmonella* gastroenteritis is caused primarily by serotypes of *S. enteritidis,* including *S. typhimurium, S. heidelberg, S. newport,* and *S. agona.* This disease shows seasonal variation, with the highest incidence reported during July through November, and is usually connected with infection from poultry products—chicken, turkey, duck, and particularly eggs. Apparently domestic birds harbor *Salmonella* in their intestines without developing symptoms. Poultry from avian carriers becomes contaminated during evisceration and packing. Thus adequate cooking of poultry and poultry products is important in disease prevention. The high incidence of *Salmonella* in raw poultry and eggs makes food handlers particularly susceptible to infection.

Onset of clinical symptoms occurs 8 to 48 hours after ingestion of organisms, reflecting the time required for multiplication and invasion of the epithelium. Nausea and vomiting are prominent and are initially followed by colicky abdominal pain and diarrhea frequently mixed with mucus and blood. The course of the disease is 2 to 5 days followed by a gradual reduction of symptoms. The carrier state is significantly less frequent following gastroenteritis than enteric fever, with only 15% of stool cultures positive at 4 weeks. Antimicrobial therapy has not been shown to clearly improve the course of gastroenteritis and may prolong the carrier state (Fig. 49-3). In previously healthy hosts the illness is usually mild, but patients with sickle cell disease and other chronic debilitating conditions may develop bacteremia and abscess formation after a bout of *Salmonella* gastroenteritis.

***Escherichia coli.*** Diarrhea-producing strains of *E. coli* can be classified into five groups based on the mechanisms of diarrhea: enterotoxigenic, enteropathogenic, enteroadherent, enteroinvasive, and enterohemorrhagic. These groups produce different clinical syndromes that vary considerably in their clinical features, geographic incidence, and host susceptibility (Table 49-3). Specific strains of *E. coli* are diagnosed by serotyping the flagellar and somatic antigens. In clinical practice the results of specific typing on stool samples are not available for at least several days, by which time patients have often recovered. An important application of serotyping is in the study of *E. coli* epidemics. For example, a large outbreak of enterohemorrhagic *E. coli* was reported recently as the

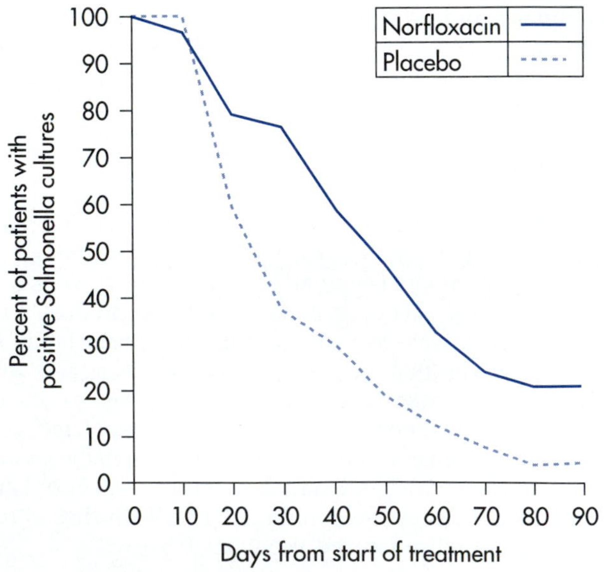


**Fig. 49-3.** Effect of antibiotic therapy in prolonging the carrier state in acute *Salmonella* gastroenteritis. (From Wiström J et al: *Ann Intern Med* 17:207, 1992.)

cause of fatal dysentery in children following ingestion of undercooked hamburgers from a fast food chain.

Enterotoxigenic *E. coli* (ETEC) organisms adhere to the small bowel mucosa and produce diarrhea by release of several toxins. LT, or heat-labile toxin, resembles cholera toxin and produces a watery diarrhea by triggering fluid secretion in the intestine. ST, or heat-stable toxin, is a peptide that stimulates intestinal guanylate cyclase, causing fluid secretion.

ETEC is a major cause of diarrhea in travelers from industrialized societies who are visiting developing or third world countries, and in infants and children in these countries. The usual mode of transmission is via contaminated food or water. ETEC produces a mild illness lasting 2 to 4 days characterized by abdominal cramps, low-grade fever, diarrhea, and passage of watery stool. Anorexia and vomiting may occur early in the illness.

Enteropathogenic *E. coli* (EPEC) organisms are an occasional cause of profuse watery diarrhea in infants in the United States and Europe. These strains possess as a virulence factor the ability to adhere to intestinal epithelial cells, a property lacking in nonpathogenic *E. coli*. As with ETEC, diarrhea associated with EPEC is usually self-limited, except in infants where massive dehydration may occur.

Enteroadherent strains of *E. coli* (EAEC) are seldom encountered in clinical practice, and the mechanism for diarrhea is still not clear. These strains adhere to liver cells in culture, a feature that distinguishes them from other pathogenic strains. Infected individuals develop a mild nonbloody diarrhea.

The enteroinvasive and enterohemorrhagic forms of *E. coli* involve the colon primarily and produce a clinical picture of acute dysentery with abdominal cramps, fever, and watery or bloody diarrhea containing leukocytes. Enteroinvasive *E. coli* (EIEC) may cause traveler's diarrhea or foodborne outbreaks of dysentery. The main pathogenic feature is invasion of and proliferation within enterocytes, a feature that also characterizes *Shigella* species. Patients infected with EIEC complain of fever, malaise, anorexia, cramps, and watery diarrhea with passage of mucus or blood that contains leukocytes. The diarrhea is short-lived, and complications are very rare except in malnourished infants.

The most serious form of *E. coli* diarrhea is caused by infection with enterohemorrhagic *E. coli* (EHEC). As the name suggests, this strain produces a hemorrhagic infection of the colon that can be fatal. The 0157:H7 strain of *E. coli* was first identified as the cause of hemorrhagic colitis following ingestion of contaminated hamburger. Outbreaks are now reported with increasing frequency, particularly from the Pacific Northwest region of the United States, but sporadic cases are diagnosed in all areas. *E. coli* 0157:H7 produces two toxins that inhibit protein synthesis within intestinal cells, but their role in hemorrhagic colitis is obscure.

As with all types of dysentery, a wide range of symptoms follows infection with EHEC. In a typical case 12 to 24 hours of abdominal cramps and watery diarrhea are followed by fever and bloody stools. Severe infection, particularly in children and the elderly, may be complicated by hemolytic-uremic syndrome or thrombotic thrombocytopenic purpura, which carries a fatality rate of 25%. Severe cases of EHEC infection are often accompanied by white blood cell counts in excess of $20,000/mm^3$, dehydration, and azotemia.

The enteroinvasive strains of *E. coli* (EIEC) are rarely implicated in the United States as a cause of traveler's diarrhea or food poisoning. In developing countries EIEC has been associated with bloody diarrhea in children. The clinical features of EIEC are fever, malaise, anorexia, crampy lower abdominal pain, and watery diarrhea, with spontaneous recovery within 2 to 4 days of onset. Although not well studied, antibiotics may reduce the duration of illness as in shigellosis (see the box on p. 688).

***Campylobacter* species.** Infection with *Campylobacter jejuni* and *C. coli* accounts for about 20% of cases of bacillary dysentery in our society. *Helicobacter pylori* (formerly *Campylobacter pylori*) is unrelated to these diarrheal pathogens and causes chronic gastritis (see Chapter 2). *Campylobacter* resembles *Salmonella* in its mode of transmission to humans from eggs and poultry. In addition, sick pets and other domestic animals may harbor *Campylobacter* as a pathogen and may serve as reservoirs of human disease. *Campylobacter* is a common cause of traveler's diarrhea, especially in subtropical areas where it is spread by ingestion of contaminated food and water. The pathogenesis of *Campylobacter* colitis involves invasion of the mucosa and toxin production, as in shigellosis.

Typically, *C. jejuni* and *C. coli* produce a moderate to severe dysentery with diarrhea, bleeding, fever, and

**Table 49-3.** Mechanisms of diarrhea in *E. coli*

| E. coli strains | Illness | Typical illness |
|---|---|---|
| Enterotoxigenic (ETEC) | Watery diarrhea, 2-4 d duration | Travelers to developing countries, infants in those countries |
| Enteropathogenic (EPEC) | Mild, watery diarrhea | Rare cause of sporadic diarrhea in the United States |
| Enteroadherent (EAEC) | Mild diarrhea without blood or leukocytes | Unclear; may cause outbreaks of food poisoning |
| Enteroinvasive (EIEC) | Dysentery like that in *Shigella* infections, but milder | Food poisoning outbreaks in developing countries; rare in the United States |
| Enterohemorrhagic (EHEC) | Hemorrhagic colitis occasionally with hemolytic-uremic syndrome | Epidemics related to ingestion of meat and dairy products; infants and elderly most severely affected |

## Effectiveness of antibiotic therapy for bacterial diarrheas

**Antibiotics effective**

*Salmonella* enteric fever (esp *S. typhosa*)
*Shigella* dysentery
*C. difficile*
*Yersinia* septicemia
Traveler's diarrhea, severe or with bloody stools
*Campylobacter* dysentery or sepsis

**Antibiotics possibly effective**

Enteroinvasive *E. coli*
Enteropathogenic *E. coli*
*Campylobacter* enteritis

**Antibiotics probably not effective**

Enterohemorrhagic *E. coli*
*Salmonella* gastroenteritis
*Yersinia* enteritis without septicemia
Acute food poisoning (*S. aureus, B. cereus*)

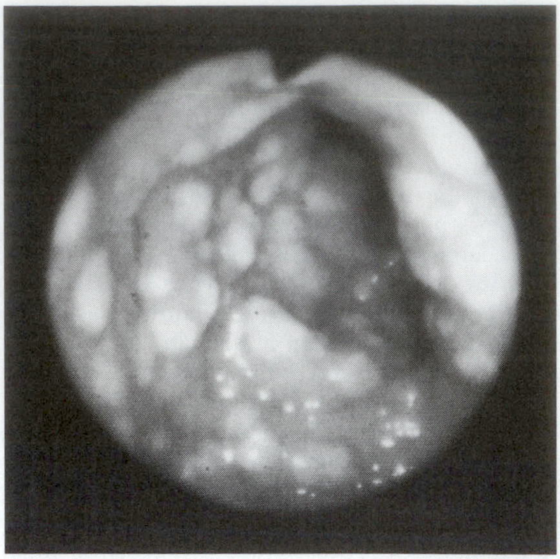

**Fig. 49-4.** Proctoscopic appearance of pseudomembranes in the rectum. The white raised plaques scattered over the mucosa are typical of acute pseudomembranous colitis secondary to *C. difficile* infection. (From Triadafilopoulos G, LaMont JT: Pseudomembranous colitis. In Walker WA et al, editors: *Pediatric gastrointestinal disease,* vol 1, Philadelphia, 1991, BC Decker.)

abdominal pain. The latter may be so severe as to mimic acute appendicitis or other causes of an acute abdomen. In patients with bloody diarrhea, proctosigmoidoscopy may reveal evidence of acute proctocolitis resembling *Shigella* colitis. Indeed, prolonged or relapsing *Campylobacter* infection may mimic idiopathic ulcerative colitis. Rarely, *Campylobacter* colitis can lead to perforation or hemolytic-uremic syndrome. An association between Guillain-Barré syndrome and preceding *Campylobacter* diarrhea has also been reported recently.

***Clostridium difficile.*** *C. difficile,* the pathogen responsible for antibiotic-associated colitis and diarrhea, is now considered one of the most common causes of nosocomial infections in this country. The organism is a gram-positive anaerobe that exists in spore form in hospital rooms and soil and that cannot colonize the bowel except when the normal colonic microflora is altered by antibiotics. Once it has colonized, *C. difficile* releases two toxins that are implicated in pathogenesis: toxin A, an enterotoxin, and toxin B, a cytotoxin.

*C. difficile* infections for the most part are hospital acquired; although outpatient cases do occur, they account for fewer than 1% of total cases. Patients in hospital are often exposed to the two conditions necessary to develop disease: (1) antibiotic therapy and (2) spores of *C. difficile.* These spores are nearly ubiquitous in the hospital and persist for months or even years on commodes, toilets, soiled bed linen, bed rails, call buttons, and hospital floors. Hospital personnel, although not themselves infected or colonized, often carry *C. difficile* on their hands, rings, or stethoscopes and may carry the organism from patient to patient.

Risk factors known to be associated with acquisition of *C. difficile* infection include recent exposure to an antibiotic in the hospital, occupying a hospital room with an infected roommate, exposure to rectal thermometers, sigmoidoscopy or enema, and treatment in an intensive care unit. According to a recent hospital study, approximately one patient in five acquires *C. difficile* infection after admission, and of these a third develop diarrhea or colitis. Most culture-positive patients remain asymptomatic and probably serve as a reservoir for infection of other patients. At the time of discharge a considerable number of patients are still culture positive for *C. difficile* and presumably carry the organism home or to chronic care facilities.

*C. difficile* causes a very wide spectrum of disease, ranging from the asymptomatic carrier state to life-threatening colitis with toxic megacolon and perforation. In a typical case diarrhea starts during the administration of antibiotics or within a few days of stopping antibiotics. The most frequently implicated antibiotics are ampicillin, amoxicillin, cephalosporins, and clindamycin, but nearly all antibiotics (including metronidazole) have been implicated in this condition. Diarrhea is usually watery or mushy. It may occasionally be blood tinged, but frank rectal bleeding is rare and should suggest another diagnosis. Lower abdominal cramps, distention, and low-grade fever are not uncommon. The presence of persistent or worsening fever, abdominal pain, and distention may indicate severe disease with impending megacolon or perforation. Elevation of the white blood cell count above 20,000, hypoalbuminemia, ascites, and metabolic acidosis indicate severe colitis.

Diagnosis of *C. difficile* infection is based on demonstration of the cytotoxin in stools with either the cytotoxin assay or one of the recently developed immunoassays for toxins A and B. Culture of the organism is considered too sensitive for routine clinical use, since up to 20% of inpatients treated with antibiotics become transient carriers without diarrhea or other symptoms and do not require treatment. Diagnosis can be easily confirmed by bedside sigmoidoscopy without bowel preparation; it confirms the

**Table 49-4.** Treatment of viral and bacterial diarrheas

| Infection | Treatment | Comment |
|---|---|---|
| *S. aureus* or *B. cereus* food poisoning | None required | Duration of illness <24 hr |
| Viral gastroenteritis | Rehydration for infants<br>Loperamide | Transient lactose intolerance common in children |
| *Shigella* dysentery | Quinolone antibiotic or TMP/SMX | Antibiotic resistance common in strains from subtropical areas |
| *Salmonella* enteric fever | Select antibiotic on basis of drug sensitivity | Chronic carriers may require prolonged therapy, especially *S. typhosa* |
| *Salmonella* gastroenteritis without sepsis | Antibiotics not recommended | Antibiotic therapy prolongs the carrier state |
| Traveler's diarrhea | Quinolone antibiotic or TMP/SMX | Mild diarrhea may be treated with antidiarrheals, without antibiotic |
| Hemorrhagic colitis (EHEC) | Antibiotics not effective | |
| *Campylobacter* colitis | Quinolones may reduce duration of diarrhea if started early | Quinolone resistance increasing |
| *C. difficile* colitis | Metronidazole or vancomycin | 20% relapse rate |

*TMP/SMX*, Trimethoprim/sulfamethoxazole.

presence of pseudomembranes, visible as yellow or white raised plaques studding the rectal mucosa (Fig. 49-4). The great frequency of this infection in hospitals and its variety of manifestations make diagnosis of *C. difficile* a challenge.

***Treatment of bacterial diarrheas.*** Oral rehydration with clear liquids, chicken broth, or Gatorade is the mainstay of therapy for patients with mild viral or bacterial diarrhea. Intravenous hydration may be required in the presence of severe diarrhea or abdominal pain. Most authorities caution against the use of antidiarrheal agents such as diphenoxylate, codeine, and paregoric on the grounds that these drugs interfere with the flushing effect of diarrhea on removing organisms and their toxins. However, bismuth subsalicylate suspensions (Pepto-Bismol), 2 tablespoonsful four times daily, or kaopectate in the same dosage is useful in controlling diarrhea, nausea, and other symptoms in mild infectious enteritis.

The main controversy regarding therapy relates to the effectiveness of antibiotics for bacterial dysentery. Confusion arises because some, but not all, bacterial infections of the bowel have been shown to respond to antibiotic therapy. Moreover, the specific diagnosis of the offending organism is usually not available for 3 or 4 days or longer after stool samples are submitted to the laboratory, by which time the patient is usually better. As shown in Table 49-4 and the box on p. 688, antibiotic therapy has clearly been shown to benefit patients with *Salmonella* enteric fever, shigellosis, traveler's diarrhea, and *C. difficile* infection. *Campylobacter* septicemia is benefited by antibiotics, but the benefit of antibiotics in uncomplicated *Campylobacter* enteritis is not proven.

Another problem in antibiotic treatment of enteric infections is the rapid acquisition of antibiotic resistance by *Shigella, Salmonella,* and *Campylobacter* species. Currently many strains of *Shigella* isolated in developing countries are resistant to ampicillin, tetracycline, and trimethoprim/sulfamethoxazole. The quinolone antibiotics (norfloxacin and ciprofloxacin) are still effective against a wide range of diarrheal pathogens, including *E. coli, Shigella, Salmonella,* and *Yersinia.* Ciprofloxacin at a dosage of 500 mg twice a day is very effective against nearly all isolates of these pathogens, including *S. typhosa.* A second-line antibiotic is trimethoprim/sulfamethoxazole, but many strains of *Shigella* and other pathogens acquired in developing countries are resistant to this organism.

The asymptomatic carrier state is quite common after recovery from most forms of bacterial dysentery. Stool cultures are positive for *Salmonella* species in approximately 5% of placebo-treated patients at 90 days versus 20% of those receiving norfloxacin (see Fig. 49-3). Fecal shedding of enteric pathogens is quite common after clinical recovery, does not necessarily indicate relapse, and usually does not require therapy.

A practical therapeutic approach is to avoid antibiotics in patients with mild gastroenteritis or acute food poisoning (predominantly vomiting). For patients with moderate or severe diarrhea, fever, tachycardia, chills, rectal bleeding, or abdominal pain empiric broad-spectrum antibiotic coverage can be initiated with ciprofloxacin, 500 mg twice daily, or trimethoprim/sulfamethoxazole, 160 mg/800 mg twice daily. Antibiotics can be stopped or changed when stool culture results are available. *C. difficile* can be treated with metronidazole, 250 mg four times a day for 10 days, or alternatively with oral vancomycin, 125 mg four times a day for 10 days. The response to therapy is rapid, with many patients reporting disappearance of symptoms within 3 to 5 days. As shown in Fig. 49-5, 125 mg vancomycin four times a day is just as effective as 500 mg four times a day. Because of its lower cost, metronidazole is the drug of first choice. Relapse of *C. difficile* colitis occurs in 15% to 20% of patients following successful initial therapy and should be treated with a second course of metronidazole or vanco-

**Geographic incidence of traveler's diarrhea**

**High Risk (20% to 50%)**
Indian subcontinent
Southeast Asia
Africa
Mexico
Developing countries in Latin America and Middle East

**Intermediate Risk (10% to 20%)**
Eastern Europe
Former Soviet Republics
Caribbean countries
China
Mediterranean European countries

**Low Risk (less than 10%)**
Canada, United States
Japan
Australia, New Zealand
Developed areas of Latin America and Caribbean

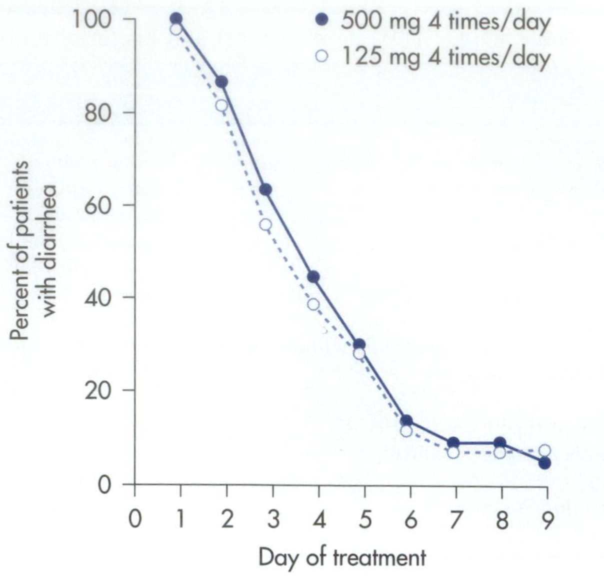


**Fig. 49-5.** Response to treatment of pseusdomembranous colitis with 125 mg qid vs 500 mg qid of vancomycin. The lower dose is equally effective and results in considerable cost saving for the patient. (From Fekety R et al: *Am J Med* 86:15, 1989.)

mycin. Multiple relapses occur in some patients and may respond to tapering doses of either agent for 1 to 2 months, in combination with cholestyramine, 4 g four times a day to bind toxins in the lumen.

***Traveler's diarrhea.*** Traveler's diarrhea commonly disrupts the vacations of millions of travelers, primarily those visiting countries where sanitation and public hygiene measures are not well developed. The incidence of traveler's diarrhea varies considerably with the destination (see the box above) and with the duration of the sojourn. Younger tourists are more likely than older adults to develop diarrhea, probably because their travel budget requires that they eat in lower quality restaurants or from street vendors. However, one study reported that traveler's diarrhea occurred in 50% of gastroenterologists attending a conference in Mexico City. Risk factors for traveler's diarrhea include drinking tap water and using ice, eating uncooked vegetables, especially salad, and eating raw or undercooked shellfish or seafood. In urban areas food rather than water is the most likely source of traveler's diarrhea.

The pathogens isolated from patients with traveler's diarrhea vary with the country visited and the timing and techniques of the stool culture. The commonest pathogen isolated from United States visitors to Mexico is enterotoxigenic *E. coli* (ETEC), an organism prevalent in water supplies. ETEC is found in 26% to 72% of tourists to Mexico with diarrhea and is common in Asia and Africa. Approximately 15% to 20% of tourists develop *Shigella* infection. Pathogens found in traveler's diarrhea are *Salmonella, Campylobacter* species, *Amoeba, Giardia, Cryptosporidium,* and *Rotavirus.*

The clinical features of traveler's diarrhea depend on the pathogen involved. ETEC produces a mild 2- to 4-day illness with acute watery diarrhea and mild nausea and abdominal cramps without vomiting. Usually the patient is confined to bed for a day or 2, but a change in itinerary is not required. In some travelers, especially those remaining in rural areas for longer than 2 weeks, protracted diarrhea for 6 to 10 weeks may be secondary to disaccharidase deficiency.

Avoidance of food from street vendors, tap water, and raw food decreases the risk of traveler's diarrhea. Washed citrus fruits, carbonated drinks, and dried foods are usually safe. Most authorities do not recommend prophylactic antibiotics because of the risk of side effects and the development of antibiotic resistance in *Shigella* and other pathogens. Prophylactic antibiotics (e.g., trimethoprim/sulfamethoxazole, 160/800 mg twice a day) are recommended for high-risk patients, including those with AIDS, inflammatory bowel disease, diabetes mellitus, severe heart disease, and those taking $H_2$ blockers or omeprazole. Healthy travelers should be given two medicines to carry on their journey: loperamide or a similar antidiarrheal agent and a broad-spectrum antibiotic effective against enteric organisms, such as ciprofloxacin. In the event of mild diarrhea during or after the trip the traveler should be advised to avoid milk, alcohol, and spicy foods and to take loperamide to reduce the frequency of diarrhea. If the traveler experiences diarrhea with blood, more than 10 watery stools in a 24-hour period, or cramps with fever, then ciprofloxacin, 500 mg twice a day, should be taken for 3 days. An alternative regimen is trimethoprim/sulfamethoxazole, 160/800 mg for 3 days. Oral hydration with bottled water or soft drinks is also encouraged. If dysentery symptoms persist for more than 3 or 4 days, then medical consultation is recommended to exclude parasites or other conditions and to ensure rehydration.

## Parasitic infestations causing diarrhea

The diagnosis of parasitic infestation requires proper stool examination by an experienced parasitologist. In this age of international travel, many parasitic infections are acquired abroad and become symptomatic after the patient returns home. A careful travel history and a high index of suspicion are critical to the diagnosis of parasitic disease.

***Giardia lamblia.*** The organism is distributed worldwide, with the vast majority of infestations being asymptomatic. *Giardia* is a common cause of diarrhea among travelers, with certain areas posing exceptionally high risks. In the past, attack rates of up to 30% have been reported in travelers to St. Petersburg. In the United States *Giardia* infestations are acquired from contaminated water supplies. Individuals with hypogammaglobulinemia, particularly selective immunoglobulin A deficiency, are at highest risk.

The major symptom of giardiasis is diarrhea, which may be acute, intermittent, or chronic, often accompanied by dull cramping pain, anorexia, nausea, and flatulence. A less common but important presentation is steatorrhea and progressive weight loss. The mechanism of diarrhea and malabsorption in giardiasis is not clearly established. Patients with immunoglobulin deficiency syndromes frequently have flat or clublike villi on small bowel biopsy with a marked decrease in the number of plasma cells in the lamina propria. Diagnosis of giardiasis can be made by examination of a duodenal aspirate for the characteristic organisms. The cysts or trophozoites can also be found in stool, but up to 50% of confirmed cases having a negative fecal examination.

Treatment with quinacrine in an oral dosage of 100 mg three times a day for 7 days is effective in 90% to 95% of patients. Metronidazole at a dosage of 250 mg three times a day for 7 days is also highly effective. For individuals with immunoglobulin deficiency a prolonged course of metronidazole has been shown to restore the normal villous architecture and reverse the malabsorption syndrome.

**Amebiasis.** Of the seven species of ameba known to parasitize the human intestinal tract, only *Entamoeba histolytica* is pathogenic. Infection with this organism occurs on a worldwide basis but is much higher in tropical areas in which poor sanitary conditions prevail. Clinical symptoms of amebiasis are more frequent in endemic areas, in military servicepersons returning from duty in the Far East, and in migrant laborers from Mexico, but the disease may also occur in individuals who have not traveled outside the United States.

Humans are the principal host and reservoir for this organism, and infection takes place by ingestion of cysts from contaminated water or food sources. Spread is predominantly by the fecal-oral route, although venereal transmission does occur and is a significant hazard among the homosexual population.

The most commonly encountered clinical variant of this disease is the *asymptomatic cyst passer.* In these asymptomatic patients *E. histolytica* exists as a commensal in the lumen of the large intestine. Once the ameba is encysted and passed into the environment, it is relatively resistant and can survive up to 10 days. The invasive motile trophozoite *E. histolytica* cannot survive in the environment and plays no role in fecal-oral spread of disease. Occasionally an asymptomatic cyst passer develops acute invasive amebiasis, and current recommendations are that all symptomatic cyst passers (except in highly endemic areas) be treated, since they are the reservoir of the disease and pose an infective risk to others.

*Symptomatic intestinal amebiasis* produces a wide variety of symptoms. Some individuals present with a chronic disease characterized by intermittent bouts of diarrhea, abdominal pain, and weight loss. The diarrhea usually contains blood and mucus, and tender hepatomegaly and pain over the cecum and ascending colon may be present. Other individuals present with an acute dysenteric illness with fever, abdominal pain, tenesmus, and bloody diarrhea. A critical concern is to distinguish amebiasis from ulcerative or Crohn's colitis, since mistaken treatment with corticosteroids can accelerate amebic colitis and foster systemic invasion. Sigmoidoscopy usually reveals discrete rectosigmoid ulcers with normal intervening mucosa. The indirect hemagglutination test is quite sensitive in detecting invasive amebic disease, including hepatic abscess and colonic mucosal invasion, but remains positive for an extended period after treatment of the disease. Metronidazole, 750 mg three times a day for 5 to 10 days, is effective therapy for active intestinal infection with *E. histolytica* (see Chapter 6).

### Gay bowel syndrome: anorectal infections in homosexual men

Acute and chronic infections of the rectum, anus, and intestine in homosexual men are collectively referred to as gay bowel syndrome (Table 49-5). Two forms of gay bowel syndrome are described: acute proctitis and gastroenteritis. The classic sexually transmitted pathogens such as *Neisseria gonorrhoeae, Treponema pallidium,* herpes simplex virus, condylomata accuminata, *Chlamydia trachomatis,* and chancroid have all been identified in anorectal lesions in acute proctitis. Venereal transmission of enteric pathogens such as *Shigella, Salmonella, Entamoeba histolytica, Giardia lamblia,* and *Campylobacter jejuni* may produce a picture of acute bacillary dysentery.

The clinical features of acute proctitis in homosexuals are nonspecific and mimic idiopathic inflammatory bowel disease. The most common presenting symptoms include discharge, rectal pain, tenesmus, hematochezia, and diarrhea. Likewise, the sigmoidoscopic appearance of the rectal mucosa is nonspecific and includes mucosal erythema, granularity, friability, and frank ulceration. A specific infectious agent usually cannot be identified on the basis of clinical symptoms or sigmoidoscopic appearance. Before the institution of therapy, cultures must be obtained for the variety of organisms expected in this setting. Rectal swabs should be cultured for *N. gonorrhoeae* and *C. trachomatis,* and viral cultures should be sent to a reference laboratory for herpes simplex virus isolation. Routine bacterial stool cultures and examination for *E. histolytica* are also obtained. After identification of specific pathogens, therapy is directed toward each of the organisms identified; broad-spectrum, empiric therapy is to be avoided. The clinical features of common anorectal infections are summarized in Table 49-5. The additional difficulties of treating immunocompromised individuals suffering from AIDS are discussed in Chapter 68.

**Table 49-5.** Clinical features of gay bowel syndrome

| Disease | Signs and symptoms | Diagnosis | Treatment |
|---|---|---|---|
| Anorectal gonorrhea | Creamy rectal discharge, constipation, pain | Culture of *Neisseria* on selective medium | Procaine penicillin, 4.8 million U IM, plus 1 g probenecid orally<br>or<br>Spectinomycin, 2 g IM |
| Herpes simplex infection | Extreme rectal pain and tenderness, bloody discharge; discrete on sigmoidoscopy | Viral isolation from stool, discharge, or acute and convalescent sera | Acyclovir, 5 mg/kg IV q8h |
| Anorectal syphilis | Mild or no symptoms | Darkfield examination of ulcer, serologic testing | Benzathine penicillin, 2.4 million U IM (single dose)<br>or<br>Tetracycline, 500 mg qid for 15 days |
| Amebiasis | Diarrhea with mucus or blood; diffuse proctitis with scattered ulcers at sigmoidoscopy | Motile trophozoites or cysts in stool, serologic studies | Metronidazole, 750 mg qid for 10 days |
| Lymphogranuloma venereum | Diarrhea, discharge; diffuse proctitis at sigmoidoscopy | Granulomas in rectal biopsy or stool | Tetracycline, 500 mg PO qid for 2-3 weeks |

**Table 49-6.** Diagnostic features of chronic inflammatory bowel disease

| Parameter | Ulcerative colitis | Crohn's disease |
|---|---|---|
| Organ involved | Colon alone | Colon and small bowel (60%); small bowel alone (30%); colon alone (10%) |
| Symptoms | Bloody diarrhea, pain, weight loss | Diarrhea, rarely bloody; abdominal pain or mass; fever; nausea, vomiting |
| Distribution | Continuous involvement; may involve rectum alone or rectum plus varying amounts of proximal colon | Segmental involvement, right-sided colitis |
| Rectal involvement | 100% | 50% |
| Intestinal complications | Megacolon, colon cancer, stricture | Enteric and perianal fistula; obstruction from strictures; malabsorption if ileum involved or removed |

## CHRONIC INFLAMMATORY BOWEL DISEASE

Chronic inflammatory bowel disease is a general term applied to ulcerative colitis and Crohn's disease, disorders of unknown etiology characterized clinically by chronic relapsing diarrhea, bleeding, and abdominal pain and pathologically by inflammation of the colon and small intestine. Although these two diseases share some epidemiologic and clinical similarities, they can be distinguished on the basis of diagnostic, pathologic, and clinical criteria. The major differences are that ulcerative colitis involves the mucosa and submucosa of the colon, whereas Crohn's disease is characterized by transmural inflammation of both small and large bowel and is usually accompanied by granuloma formation. Despite well-defined diagnostic criteria (Table 49-6), some patients with chronic inflammatory bowel diseases have features of both diseases and cannot be definitely assigned to either group.

### Ulcerative colitis

Ulcerative colitis or proctocolitis is a chronic inflammatory disease affecting primarily the mucosa and submucosa of the rectum and colon. Although a number of etiologic theories have been advanced, the cause of ulcerative colitis is unknown. The most likely mechanism involves a type of autoimmune process whereby an initial insult (e.g., bacterial or viral enteritis) triggers the activation of intestinal T lymphocytes and macrophages, which continue to evoke a chronic inflammatory response. Genetic factors are also involved, since approximately 15% to 20% of patients have a blood relative with either ulcerative colitis or Crohn's disease.

Most cases occur between the ages of 15 and 25, with a small secondary peak in incidence between ages 55 and 65. Ulcerative colitis is more common in whites, women, urban dwellers, upper socioeconomic groups, and Jews. The disease is rare in developing countries and in immigrants to the United States from developing countries.

***Clinical features.*** The major symptoms are rectal bleeding and diarrhea with the daily passage of up to 15 movements of blood and mucus associated with tenesmus.

Diarrhea at night is particularly common and argues against irritable bowel syndrome or osmotic diarrhea secondary to lactose intolerance or dietary indiscretion. Symptoms of fatigue, anorexia, and weight loss are common. Fever is frequent, and abdominal pain may be present but is less common than in Crohn's colitis. Surprisingly, constipation occurs in about 10% of patients with proctosigmoiditis, although some of these individuals complain of frequent, rectal discharges of blood and mucus without actual stool.

Five percent or less of patients with ulcerative colitis have a fulminant course, with toxic megacolon, perforation, or massive hemorrhage, and may require emergency colectomy during their first attack. One of the hallmarks of ulcerative colitis is the spontaneous waxing and waning of symptoms with long periods of complete remission; a few have continuous distress. Up to 10% of patients may be symptom free for years after the first episode. Occasionally the onset of illness is insidious or heralded by extracolonic manifestations such as arthritis or iritis. Long-term complications of ulcerative colitis include inflammatory stricture and colon cancer. The risk of colonic cancer is increased significantly in patients with pancolitis for more than 10 years and increases steadily with time.

The initial diagnosis of ulcerative colitis is a process of exclusion. The most important conditions to exclude are bacterial and amebic infections of the bowel, since these are responsive to specific therapy and may become much worse if the patient is mistakenly treated with corticosteroids. Thus stool cultures are done for bacterial pathogens and are examined carefully for evidence of *Giardia* or amebae. *C. difficile* infection may coexist with ulcerative colitis and should be excluded, especially in patients recently exposed to antibiotics. Patients with AIDS may develop cytomegalovirus colitis, which is easily confused with chronic inflammatory bowel disease.

The major diagnostic tests for ulcerative colitis are *sigmoidoscopy* (or *colonoscopy*) and *barium enema.* Sigmoidoscopy reveals a friable, reddened, edematous mucosa that bleeds easily when touched. Granularity and small ulcerations are common. Biopsy of the rectum reveals typical changes of inflammation, ulceration, and crypt abscesses. A normal barium enema is seen early in the course of ulcerative colitis in a small percentage of patients. The earliest abnormalities detected on barium enema are spiculation and ulceration of the mucosa. Contraction or foreshortening of the colon develops later with loss of haustration (Fig. 49-6), deeper ulcers, pseudopolyp formation, and strictures.

The differential diagnosis includes Crohn's disease (see below), ischemic colitis in patients more than 50 years old, bacterial and amebic dysentery, and antibiotic colitis. In younger patients with bloody diarrhea one must exclude familial polyposis. Crohn's colitis is differentiated by its propensity to spare the rectum, the presence of small bowel involvement in many patients, and the tendency to form fistulas. Ischemic colitis is a disease of the elderly that causes acute bloody diarrhea and abdominal pain, usually with sparing of the rectum. Infectious diarrheas are excluded by appropriate bacteriologic studies or, in the case of acute amebic colitis, by demonstration of mobile trophozoites or cysts in the stool.

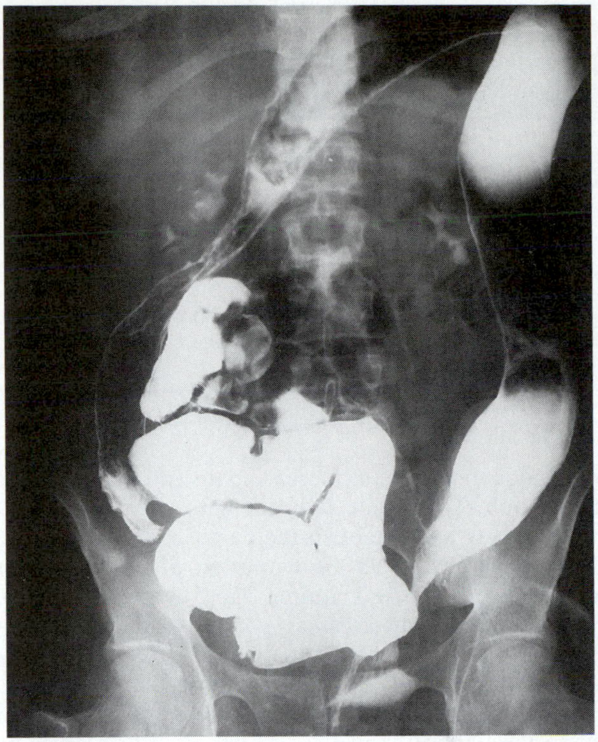

**Fig. 49-6.** Barium enema in a patient with long-standing ulcerative colitis showing loss of haustral markings in the left and transverse colon and considerable shortening of the colon.

***Indication for consultation*** Consultation with a gastroenterologist is recommended at initial diagnosis for colonoscopy and for guidance regarding drug therapy. Failure of medical therapy, recurrent bleeding, extracolonic manifestations, and possible surgical management are also appropriate indications for consultation. Colonoscopic surveillance for colon cancer is recommended every 3 years, beginning 10 years after the initial diagnosis for ulcerative colitis.

***Management.*** Management of ulcerative colitis has as its main goal returning the patient to a normal level of function in society. Success in treating this disease requires that the physician educate patients and help them accept the fact that they have a lifelong illness. A useful analogy is diabetes mellitus, a chronic disease that when controlled with diet, drugs, and insulin allows a normal and productive life. Failure by the physician to gently lead the patient to optimistically accept the reality of a lifelong condition will reduce the effectiveness of subsequent therapeutic maneuvers.

Some patients (and their families) with ulcerative colitis are convinced that a "proper" or "strict" diet will control the disease. Unfortunately, this expectation is not matched by any convincing research data to support specific long-term diet recommendations. During flares of disease patients should avoid roughage and fiber (salad, cereals, fruits, nuts). Elemental liquid formula diets are recommended when patients are unable to tolerate solid food because of strictures or inflammatory masses. Otherwise, patients are advised to eat a regular diet and to

**Table 49-7.** Drug therapy for inflammatory bowel disease

| Drug | Mechanism | Indication | Typical dosage |
|---|---|---|---|
| Sulfasalazine | Active agent, 5-aminosalicylate | Maintenance of remission | 1 g tid or qid |
| 4-Aminosalicylate, 5-aminosalicylate | Antiinflammatory agent | Mild ulcerative colitis or proctitis | 2-3 g/d |
| Hydrocortisone retention enemas | Reduction of inflammation in rectum and left colon | Mild left-sided colitis or proctitis | 125-mg enemas at bedtime |
| Prednisone | Systemic antiinflammatory and immunosuppressive effect | Induction of remission in moderate or severe disease | 40-60 mg/d |
| Azathioprine; 6-mercaptopurine | Immunosuppressive | Maintenance therapy after failure of sulfasalazine | 50 mg/d |

avoid foods that seem to increase pain and diarrhea. Most patients quickly become familiar with their own dietary idiosyncrasies and establish their own diet.

The role of stress in the evolution of chronic inflammatory bowel disease requires careful attention by the physician. Although stress is not the primary cause of ulcerative colitis or Crohn's disease, life stresses may trigger flares of disease and increase the psychologic burden of illness. The sources of stress may be obscure, both to the patient as well as to the attending physician, and only skillful interviewing may bring it to light.

Most patients with ulcerative colitis have intermittent symptoms or mild continuous symptoms that generally respond well to medical treatment. The mainstays of drug therapy are sulfasalazine (Azulfidine) and corticosteroids, both of which are aimed at reducing colonic inflammation (Table 49-7). Corticosteroids are best used to control acute flares of disease, whereas sulfasalazine and 5-aminosalicylate preparations are designed as maintenance therapy. Sulfasalazine at a dosage of 2 to 4 g per day decreases the frequency of attacks of ulcerative colitis and reduces symptoms of colitis. Newer forms of this drug containing only the salicylate moiety have recently been introduced. These include oral and enema preparations of 5-aminosalicylate and 4-aminosalicylate, which offer the theoretic advantage of avoiding side effects related to the sulfa portion but are much more expensive than sulfasalazine. Up to 10% of patients taking sulfasalazine experience nausea, vomiting, headache, skin rash, and hemolytic anemia. Corticosteroids are reserved for more severe episodes of disease, especially those not responsive to other therapeutic measures. Severely ill patients may require hospitalization to allow parenteral nutrition, bowel rest, and corticosteroids. Patients with ulcerative proctitis or left-sided colitis may respond to enemas containing corticosteroids, thereby avoiding systemic side effects.

## Crohn's disease

Crohn's disease differs from ulcerative colitis in its tendency to involve the small intestine and colon in a segmental fashion (skip areas) and the frequency of recurrence after surgical resection (see Table 49-6). Although the terminal ileum and right colon are most commonly involved, any area of the gastrointestinal tract from mouth to anus may be affected. Three patterns of involvement in Crohn's disease have been recognized: isolated small bowel involvement, ileocolitis, and involvement of the colon alone—Crohn's colitis or granulomatous colitis. In all locations the transmural inflammatory lesion causes thickening of the bowel secondary to edema and fibrosis and narrowing of the lumen. Noncaseating granulomas in the submucosa occur in most resected specimens of Crohn's disease bowel.

***Crohn's disease of the small intestine.*** Crohn's disease of the small intestine usually affects the distal ileum but rarely ever the duodenum or stomach. The typical features are chronic right lower quadrant abdominal pain, fever, diarrhea, and weight loss. Significant rectal bleeding is quite rare, in contrast to ulcerative colitis. In children or teenagers the presenting complaint may be failure to thrive, growth retardation, or obscure fever without diarrhea. The patient may also present with a clinical picture resembling acute appendicitis. Partial small bowel obstruction secondary to stricture is also a common mode of presentation.

Diagnosis of ileal Crohn's disease is based on the clinical history and a small bowel barium study demonstrating narrowing and distortion of the terminal ileum with or without skip areas (i.e., areas of inflammation separated by various lengths of uninvolved bowel). In long-standing disease one can see sinus tracts, enteric fistulas, and inflammatory masses caused by walled-off perforations. These radiologic features may also occur in patients with lymphoma, ischemic disease, tuberculosis, and carcinoid tumor.

***Crohn's ileocolitis and colitis.*** In the typical patient with Crohn's ileocolitis the disease involves the terminal ileum, cecum, and ascending colon in continuity. These patients typically complain of nonbloody diarrhea, right-sided abdominal pain, a mass, fever, weight loss, and perianal problems such as fistula or hemorrhoids. Sigmoidoscopy is often negative, an important differential point with ulcerative colitis in which sigmoidoscopy is almost always positive. Rectal biopsy through the sigmoidoscope or colonoscopic biopsies may show noncaseating granuloma. Barium enema reveals cobblestoning, asymmetric involvement or skip areas, and longitudinal ulcers. Small intestinal involvement may be diagnosed on barium enema if sufficient barium refluxes through the ileocecal valve to adequately fill the terminal ileum. In about 25% of patients with Crohn's colitis the entire colon including the rectum

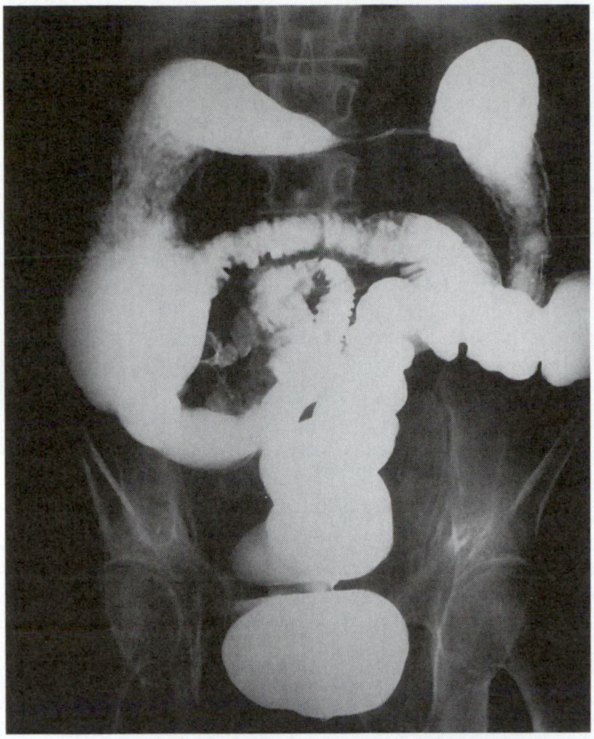

**Fig. 49-7.** Barium enema of Crohn's colitis with stricture formation in the transverse colon.

is involved, whereas in others a right colonic or segmental distribution is noted (Fig. 49-7). In contrast to ulcerative colitis, Crohn's colitis is a more indolent disease. Patients may often complain initially of perianal fistula or abscess, low-grade diarrhea without blood, or extracolonic manifestations such as erythema nodosum or arthritis. Intermittent right-sided abdominal pain and weight loss are typical. Megacolon or severe acute colitis with bloody diarrhea and fever are distinctly unusual.

***Treatment of Crohn's disease.*** The treatment of Crohn's disease is similar to that described for ulcerative colitis (see Table 49-7) and depends on disease severity, presentation, and complications. Although the efficacy of sulfasalazine in Crohn's disease has not been established, a trial of therapy is warranted in mild cases. Symptoms of intestinal obstruction are treated with continuous nasogastric suction and intravenous fluids. Cachexia secondary to extensive bowel disease or obstruction may respond to hyperalimentation. Corticosteroid therapy is required if the patient does not respond to conservative therapy; however, corticosteroids are contraindicated in patients suspected of having intraabdominal abscess. In the acutely ill patient with moderate or severe symptoms, oral or parenteral corticosteroids may be replaced by the equivalent oral dosage, which is slowly reduced over a period of months. Long-term immunosuppressive maintenance therapy with low-dosage azathioprine or 6-mercaptopurine is effective in some patients. Surgery is indicated in the acutely ill patient with persistent obstruction, enteric fistula, perforation, massive hemorrhage, or suspected abscess. Unfortunately, the clinical recurrence rate following surgery for small intestinal Crohn's disease is virtually 100% at 5 years. Despite the complications of this disease and the inevitable recurrence following surgery, patients with Crohn's disease are able to lead normal lives most of the time and total life span is not substantially reduced.

## ISCHEMIC COLITIS

Ischemic colitis usually results from reduced blood flow to the colon (low flow state) even though the major arteries and arterioles of the colon and rectum are patent. This may be caused by cardiac disease, sepsis, or shock of any cause. Less commonly it is caused by arterial or venous occlusion, embolus or thrombosis of the inferior mesenteric artery, volvulus and intussusception, aortic dissection, and inadvertent surgical ligation. Rarely, amyloidosis, vasculitis, and colon cancer are associated with arterial occlusion. The typical patient is between the ages of 50 and 90, but younger patients are being reported with increasing frequency.

### Clinical features

The sudden onset of crampy, left-sided lower abdominal pain and bloody diarrhea in an elderly patient with known vascular disease suggests ischemic colitis. In fulminant cases the patient presents in shock with bloody diarrhea, fever, tachycardia, and severe abdominal pain accompanied by rebound tenderness and rigidity. If the rectum or rectosigmoid is involved, sigmoidoscopy reveals submucosal hemorrhages protruding into the lumen. These same submucosal hemorrhages are visualized radiologically as "thumbprints" on a plain film of the abdomen or barium enema. In some cases air is seen in the wall of the bowel, indicating transmural necrosis or impending perforation. Because most patients with ischemic colitis do not have occlusion of a major artery, mesenteric angiography is seldom helpful in the acute situation and is not recommended.

### Treatment

Mild ischemic colitis can be treated conservatively with nasogastric suction, bowel rest, and antibiotics. Surgery is indicated for patients with signs of localized or diffuse peritonitis or those with fulminant disease, characterized by high white blood cell count or metabolic acidosis. Bloody diarrhea with active disease persisting beyond 2 weeks indicates a poor prognosis. It is important to obtain a barium enema several months after an episode of ischemic colitis to rule out the development of stricture, which may require surgical excision.

## DIVERTICULOSIS AND DIVERTICULITIS

Diverticula of the colon are saclike herniations of the mucosa through the muscularis (Fig. 49-8). These outpouchings are composed of mucosa and serosa and follow the course of a nutrient artery within the muscularis of the bowel wall. Diverticula occur most commonly in the sigmoid colon and decrease in frequency in the proximal colon. The incidence ranges between 20% and 50% in Western populations over age 50 and increases with age. Thickening of the muscle coat of the colon in areas involved with diverticulosis suggests that diverticula are caused by the increased force of colonic muscle contractions. The rarity of colonic diverticula in underdeveloped nations in contrast to Western countries has led to the unproven theory that diverticula result from the highly refined Western diet, which is relatively deficient in dietary fiber or roughage. Such diets result in decreased fecal bulk, narrowing of the colon, and an increase in intraluminal pressure to move the smaller fecal mass.

Colonic diverticula are asymptomatic in 70% of patients and are found incidentally on a barium enema performed for other reasons. About 30% of patients develop complications of inflammation, both acute and chronic, and hemorrhage. Because diverticulosis is quite common in older patients, one must use caution in attributing pain or bleeding to the diverticula unless other conditions, especially a colonic neoplasm, have been excluded.

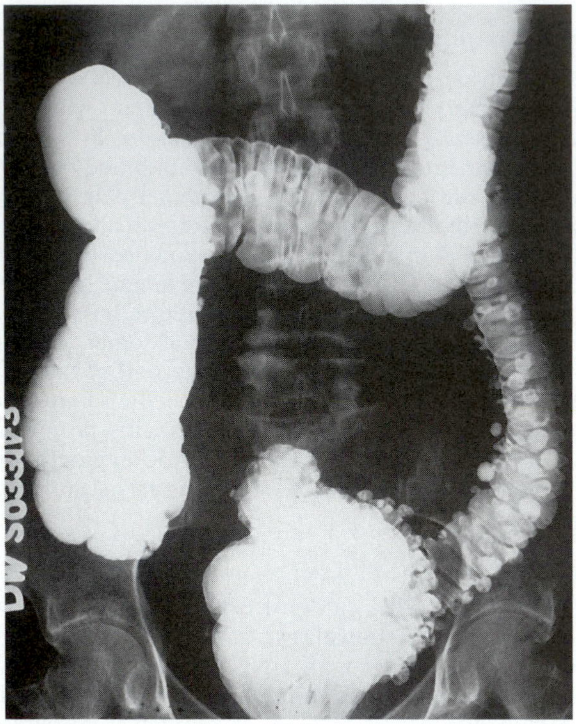

**Fig. 49-8.** Barium enema appearance of colonic diverticulosis in an asymptomatic patient. Note the larger number in the left colon versus the right.

## Diverticulitis

Inflammation in or around the diverticular sac is related to retention of undigested food residues and bacteria, which may form a hard mass called a fecalith. This compromises the blood supply to the thin-walled sac and renders it susceptible to invasion by colonic bacteria. The inflammatory process may vary from a small intramural or pericolic abscess to generalized peritonitis. Some attacks are accompanied by minimal symptoms and seem to heal spontaneously. Most perforations of the diverticular sac are minor and result in inflammation of the sac and its serosal surface. Diverticulitis occurs more often in men than in women and three times as often in the left colon than in the right colon (see Fig. 49-8). This suggests that diverticulitis may be related to the higher intraluminal pressures and the more solid fecal material in the sigmoid and descending colon.

Acute diverticulitis is a disease of variable severity characterized by lower abdominal pain made worse by

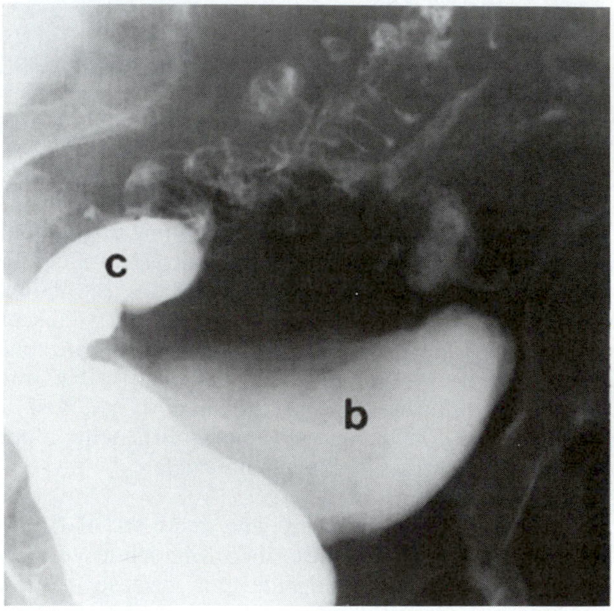


**Fig. 49-9.** Barium enema of colovesical fistula following acute diverticulitis. Barium fills the urinary bladder *(b)* from a fistula from the sigmoid colon *(c)*.

**Table 49-8.** Complications of colonic diverticulosis

| Complication | Pathophysiology | Typical clinical manifestations |
|---|---|---|
| Acute diverticulitis | Microperforation of diverticulum with localized peritonitis | Pain and tenderness in left lower quadrant, fever, constipation |
| Fistula formation | Following acute diverticulitis, a passage forms between the colon and urinary bladder (colovesical fistula), adjacent loop of bowel (enteroenteric fistula), or vagina (rectovaginal fistula) | Urinary tract infection, fever, abdominal, pain, mass, passage of air or stool through vagina |
| Obstruction | Fibrous stricture following acute diverticulitis | Crampy lower abdominal pain, altered bowel habit |
| Hemorrhage | Erosion of artery within diverticular sac | Painless hematochezia |

defecation and signs of peritoneal irritation: muscle spasm, guarding rebound tenderness, fever, and leukocytosis (Table 49-8). Inflammation around the colon often results in some degree of constipation. Rectal bleeding, usually microscopic, is noted in 25% of cases, but massive bleeding is rare in the presence of acute diverticulitis. Complications include free perforation, which results in acute peritonitis, sepsis, and shock, particularly in the elderly. The perforation may be walled off by adherent omentum or neighboring structures such as the bladder or small bowel. Abscesses or fistulas arise as the inflammatory mass tracks into other organs. Severe pericolitis causes a dense fibrous reaction or stricture around the bowel, which can be associated with colonic obstruction and on barium enema may mimic a colon cancer. Sometimes surgical removal is indicated to rule out malignancy or alleviate obstructive symptoms. Repeated attacks may result in fistulas between the colon and neighboring organs, especially the bladder (Fig. 49-9) and vagina.

Differential diagnosis in milder cases is principally that of a neoplasm in the area of the diverticulosis. Sigmoidoscopy may show an acutely inflamed mucosa over an apparent extrinsic mass; passing the instrument through the contracted lumen is usually impossible. During acute diverticulitis barium enema may be dangerous, since the contrast material under pressure may rupture an inflamed diverticulum and cause a free perforation. Abdominal ultrasound or CT scan is useful in diagnosing peridiverticular inflammatory masses or abscess. The examination is best deferred until after adequate treatment and healing of the diverticulitis. The radiologic findings of diverticulitis are leakage of barium from a diverticular sac, stricture formation, and the presence of a pericolic inflammatory mass. Often the distortion caused by inflammation cannot be differentiated from cancer, in which case colonoscopy or laparotomy is required.

Treatment in mild cases consists of bed rest, stool softeners, liquid diet, and a broad-spectrum antibiotic. Hospitalized patients with acute peritoneal signs, suspected abscess, or perforation require intravenous broad-spectrum antibiotics. Surgical intervention may be necessary to drain abscesses or to resect an obstructing inflammatory mass. The usual procedure is to perform a diverting colostomy with resection of the involved colon; reanastomosis is then performed at a second operation. Repeated attacks of diverticulitis in the same area of the left colon generally require surgical resection.

### Painful diverticular disease without diverticulitis

Some patients develop colicky recurrent left lower quadrant pain without clinical or pathologic evidence of acute diverticulitis. They complain of alternating constipation and diarrhea, and the pain may be relieved by defecation or the passage of flatus. Examination during a bout of pain reveals tenderness over the sigmoid colon, but signs of peritoneal inflammation such as rebound tenderness, muscle guarding, fever, and leukocytosis are absent. Barium enema shows typical diverticula without evidence of inflammation or stricture, plus a sawtooth irregularity of the lumen reflecting associated muscle spasm. The pain is severe enough in some cases to warrant observation in hospital and restriction of food, but some patients can be treated at home with oral antibiotics and a low-residue diet. After initial improvement the patient is started on a high-residue diet or given a bulk laxative such as hemicellulose, unprocessed bran, or psyllium extract. Surgical excision is usually not indicated unless full-blown acute diverticulitis or its complications occur.

### Hemorrhage from diverticula

Hemorrhage is a rare complication that occurs in elderly patients, usually in the absence of signs or symptoms of diverticulitis. The pathogenesis is presumably erosion of a vessel within the diverticular sac, often in the right colon. The degree of bleeding is often mild and self-limited, although in some patients massive, life-threatening hemorrhage occurs. In some patients with severe hemorrhage urgent colonoscopy after cleansing the colon of blood may help establish the diagnosis. Surgery is required in only a small fraction of cases for persistent bleeding, since most bleeding stops spontaneously.

## BIBLIOGRAPHY

Guerrant RL, Bobak DA: Bacterial and protozoal gastroenteritis, *N Engl J Med* 325:327, 1991.

Kelly CP, LaMont JT: Treatment of *Clostridium difficile* diarrhea and colitis. In Wolfe M, editor: *Gastrointestinal pharmacology,* Philadelphia, 1993, WB Saunders.

Keusch GT: Antimicrobial therapy for enteric infections and typhoid fever: state of the art, *Rev Infect Dis* 10(suppl 1):S199, 1988.

Levine MM: *Escherichia coli* that cause diarrhea: enterotoxigenic, enteropathogenic, enteroinvasive, enterohemorrhagic, enteroadherent, *J Infect Dis* 155:377, 1987.

Murphy GS, et al: Ciprofloxacin and loperamide in the treatment of bacillary dysentery, *Ann Intern Med* 118:582, 1993.

Peppercorn MA: Advances in drug therapy for inflammatory bowel disease, *Ann Intern Med* 112:50, 1990.

Pithie AD, Wood MJ: Treatment of typhoid fever and infectious diarrhea with ciprofloxacin, *J Antimicrob Chemother* 26(suppl F):47, 1990.

Podolsky DK: Inflammatory bowel disease, *N Engl J Med* 325:928, 1008, 1991.

Pothoulakis C, LaMont JT. *Clostridium difficile* colitis and diarrhea, *Gastroenterol Clin North Am* 22(3):623, 1993.

Thompson WG, Patel DG: Clinical picture of diverticular disease of the colon, *Clin Gastroenterol* 15:903, 1986.

CHAPTER

# 50 Functional Gastrointestinal Disease

**Richard I. Rothstein**

Functional gastrointestinal diseases are those disorders consisting of varying combinations of chronic or recurrent symptoms with no identifiable physiologic, biochemical, infectious, anatomic, or structural cause. These disorders comprise a large percentage of primary care patient visits and account for about 40% of visits to gastroenterologists.

A recent survey of a random sample of individuals in the United States revealed that 69% reported having at least one of 20 defined functional gastrointestinal symptoms during the previous 3 months. With significant overlap, symptoms were attributed to four major regions: esophagus (42%), gastroduodenum (26%), bowel (44%), and anorectum (26%). In general, symptom reporting declined with increasing age, and low socioeconomic status was associated with increased symptom reporting. The rate of physician visits and work or school absenteeism was increased for those having a functional gastrointestinal disorder.

The functional gastrointestinal disorders encompass those related to the esophagus (globus, rumination, atypical chest pain), gastroduodenum (nonulcer dyspepsia, aerophagia), bowel (irritable bowel syndrome, chronic constipation, painless diarrhea, bloating/excessive gas, chronic abdominal pain), pancreaticobiliary tree (pancreaticobiliary dyskinesia), and anorectum (proctalgia fugax, levator syndrome) (see the box below). The unifying pathophysiology for functional gastrointestinal disorders is thought to be a primary disorder of gut motility. With no specific gold standard to assist in identification, the functional disorders require that comprehensive and careful histories be taken, along with physical examinations and judicious use of laboratory studies. Increased effort in establishing diagnostic criteria for functional disorders based on epidemiologic and clinical research has resulted in enhanced diagnostic certainty and the ability to make a positive diagnosis rather than a diagnosis of exclusion.

The functional gastrointestinal diseases share similar biopsychosocial models and a close relationship of psychophysiologic effect. Stress, anxiety, depression and heightened emotional states affect symptom production and response (Fig. 50-1). The seeking of medical attention for functional symptoms may be prompted by increased frequency or severity of symptoms, reduced coping mechanisms or concomitant illness, or fear of serious illness. Individuals with functional complaints who seek medical attention for their symptoms have significant psychiatric disorders more frequently diagnosed, when compared to individuals with functional disorders who do not seek medical attention. Psychologic factors influence the decision to seek health care, and examining the motivation for an office visit is a key step in the evaluation and management of this group of disorders.

This chapter examines the functional gastrointestinal disorders, with a focus on irritable bowel syndrome as representative of this group and a review of related syndromes and their differential diagnoses.

## Functional gastrointestinal disorders

Esophagus: globus, rumination, atypical chest pain
Gastroduodenum: nonulcer dyspepsia, aerophagia
Colon/small bowel: irritable bowel syndrome, chronic pain, chronic constipation
Pancreaticobiliary tract: pancreaticobiliary dyskinesia, pancreatitis
Anorectum: proctalgia fugax, levator syndrome

## IRRITABLE BOWEL SYNDROME

The term *irritable bowel syndrome* is used by some to connote all the functional gastrointestinal disorders, from globus to proctalgia fugax, and has gained the reputation of being a wastebasket diagnosis for complaints not attributable to organic disease. The shared similarities of the various functional syndromes in pathophysiology and presentation have suggested the concept of the irritable gut or irritable person syndrome, with symptoms arising principally from global physiologic changes that accompany emotional tension.

Irritable bowel syndrome (IBS) is defined as a functional gastrointestinal disorder attributed to the intestine and includes chronic or recurrent abdominal pain, altered bowel habit (consistency, frequency, feeling of incomplete evacuation), abdominal bloating and feeling of excessive intestinal gas, and mucus with the stools. These symptoms, continuous or intermittent, should be present for at least 3 months. The diagnostic symptom criteria for IBS as outlined by an international working party are found in the box on p. 699.

### Epidemiology and etiology

The syndrome of IBS occurs in 15% to 20% of adults. There is a predominance among women in the United States (nearly 2:1) but a reported predominance among men in other parts of the world, such as in India. In the

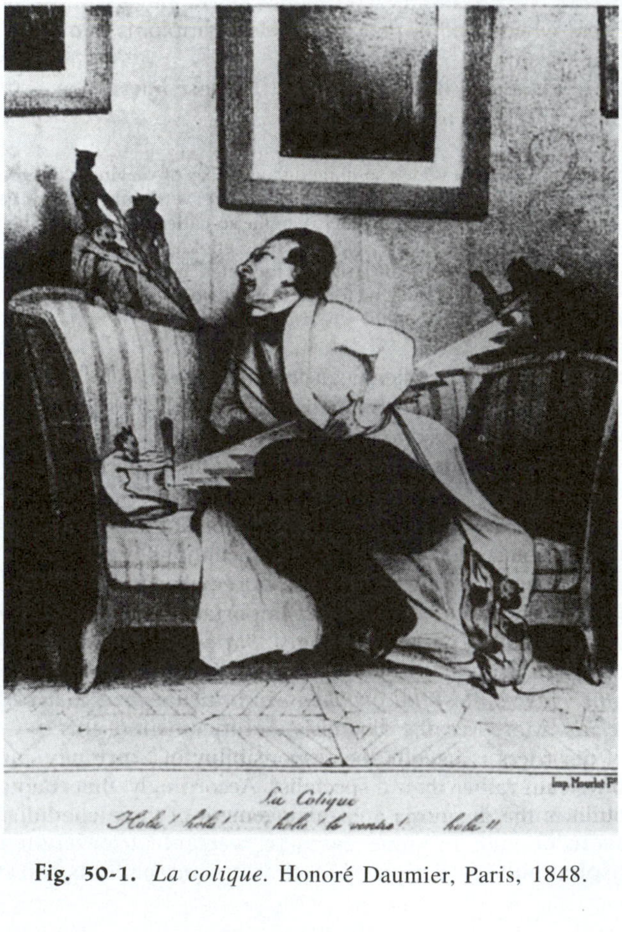


Fig. 50-1. *La colique.* Honoré Daumier, Paris, 1848.

United States no reported difference exists between different racial subgroups. Symptoms usually begin in young adulthood and persist in the majority throughout life, although in an intermittent fashion. The childhood gastrointestinal disorder of recurrent abdominal pain may be equivalent in symptoms and pathophysiology to IBS, and about one third of affected children have irritable bowel syndrome in adulthood.

Of note, less than half of the *people* with irritable bowel symptoms seek medical attention for their symptoms, becoming *patients* with IBS when they do so. The overall prevalence of IBS in a population remains stable, although there is a dynamic shifting, with some individuals becoming asymptomatic while others develop symptoms or experience a recurrence.

## Pathophysiology

The frequent location of pain in the lower abdomen, the relief of pain by defecation, and the passage of scybala (pelletlike stools) implicate irritability of the distal colon as a principal mechanism of the disorder. Sigmoid contractions are paradoxically increased in IBS patients with symptoms of constipation, effecting increased segmentation and decreased propulsive movement, with resultant scybala and distention. Segmental contractions may be decreased in diarrhea-prone patients, with more rapid intestinal transit time. Abdominal pain in IBS most likely arises from areas of intestinal distention occurring proximal to areas of spasm.

Altered myoelectrical activity of the colon, with a higher proportion of slow waves in the frequency range of 2 to 4 cycles per minute, has been reported for patients with IBS. The specificity of this marker has been questioned, since it is also found to occur in psychoneurotic patients who have no bowel symptoms. Small intestinal transit has been documented to be more rapid in diarrhea-prone IBS patients, whereas it is prolonged in those complaining of constipation or abdominal pain or distention.

An altered sensation of visceral pain may occur in IBS, with a lowered threshold for gut distention. Balloon distention of the lower bowel provokes pain in patients with IBS at volumes that do not usually cause symptoms in controls. Patients with IBS frequently complain of bloating and increased gas; however, studies have shown that IBS patients have abdominal symptoms with the same or lower colonic gas volumes as nonsymptomatic controls. Balloon distention at various sites along the large or small bowel during colonoscopy or during the passage of a small bowel tube resulted in the exact reproduction of right upper quadrant pain in a group of patients initially thought to have gallbladder symptoms by their clinicians. All patients had negative screening tests for gallbladder disease. This possibly explains the return or persistence of symptoms in those patients who undergo cholecystectomy for right upper quadrant pain suspected to be biliary in origin, who may have had a silent gallstone but noisy gut.

The pathophysiology of IBS involves the enteric nervous system, visceral smooth muscle, and neurohumoral control of gut function. Symptoms arise as the lower gut participates in the whole organism response to emotional arousal, as part of the fight or flight emergency reactions. Release of neurotransmitters and interchange of information from the central nervous system to the enteric nervous system modulate the activity of the bowel and its irritability.

Measured alterations in bowel motility in response to stimuli such as eating, stressful interviews, and acute psychologic or physical stress have been documented. Measurement of sigmoid motility during hypnosis, using an indwelling transrectal manometric catheter, has provided information about brain-gut emotional relationships, with the ability to isolate an emotion (hostility, anger, sadness) and its related manometric pattern.

The prevalence of psychologic symptoms and psychoneurotic personality traits in *patients* with IBS is higher than in non-IBS controls and, it is important to note, higher than in those with IBS who do not seek medical care. Depression, somatization, and frequency of consulting a physician for minor complaints of all kinds (learned illness behavior) is found more frequently in patients than nonpatients with IBS. These psychologic factors relate to the health care–seeking behavior in patients with IBS and not to the illness itself. Patients presenting to primary care practices may demonstrate less somatization than those referred to gastroenterologists, although mood disturbances are commonly present in IBS patients visiting primary care settings.

The total dependency needs of the patient need to be recognized, including attitude toward illness and the sick role. Several recent surveys of IBS patients and matched controls have shown that childhood physical, emotional, and sexual abuse occurred more commonly in IBS patients, and abuse was not confined to women. Childhood sexual abuse was associated with findings of depression, increased medical visits, and multiple somatic complaints in the IBS patients.

### Rome criteria for IBS

Continuous or recurrent symptoms for at least 3 months of:
- Abdominal pain, relieved by defecation or associated with changes of frequency or consistency of stool
- An irregular pattern of defecation at least 25% of the time, with two or more of the following:
  - Altered stool frequency
  - Altered stool form (scybala or loose and watery)
  - Altered stool passage (straining, urgency, feeling of incomplete evacuation)
  - Passage of mucus, usually with bloating or feeling of abdominal distention

From Drossman DA et al: *Gastroenterol Int* 3:159, 1990.

## Clinical presentation and physical examination

A wide range of symptoms prompts the division of IBS into symptom-predominant subtypes, although it may be best considered as a single entity with variable manifestations. Patients who offer one of the predominant IBS symptoms (pain, constipation, diarrhea) as their chief complaint are found most of the time to have all three symptoms following rigorous history taking and inspection of the stools. Dyspepsia, without organic explanation, is found in the majority of patients with IBS, and symptoms of esophageal dysfunction are found in 50%. The noncolonic gastrointestinal symptoms of nausea, vomiting, dysphagia, and early satiety were found more often in a group of patients with IBS than in matched controls. In two studies in which the IBS patients and age-matched controls were 90% to 100% female and middle aged, anxiety, fatiguability, hostile feelings, sadness, and sleep disturbances were reported to occur more often in the IBS group, as were palpitations, hand tremor, and fear of serious disease. Bladder dysfunction symptoms (nocturia, frequency and urgency of micturition, and feeling of incomplete bladder emptying) were more commonly present in the IBS patients, as were the symptoms of back pain, an unpleasant taste in the mouth, constant feelings of tiredness, and dyspareunia. This range of symptom reporting represents global physiologic responses and heightened emotional arousal.

The usual patient with IBS has had at least months of symptoms, and many relate a lifelong history of altered bowel habits and abdominal distress. New onset of IBS symptoms in an elderly patient should prompt a thorough examination for organic etiology, although prevalence of functional symptoms may be level throughout all age groups.

Patients may describe the initial passage of a formed bowel movement, possibly following straining, with a sense of incomplete evacuation. Subsequent need to defecate results in several looser bowel movements, which may be described as diarrhea. Other patients may relate the passage of pelletlike stools and a changing frequency of bowel habits. Alteration in consistency, color, and shape may be reported by those with IBS, who often may go to great lengths to observe and document their eliminations (with daily output diaries and photographs on occasion!). Patients may have long periods of normal stool habits and no abdominal symptoms, only to develop sudden recurrence of symptoms.

Crampy lower abdominal pain, usually on the left, is often mentioned by IBS patients and may be worsened or precipitated by eating (gastrocolic reflex); it is relieved, perhaps only transiently, by passage of flatus or stool. Some patients complain of bloating and of being full of gas with variable increases in eructation or passage of flatus, although most do not have demonstrable changes in abdominal girth. Occasional patients have proptosis of the abdomen caused by contraction of the diaphragm and lumbar muscles, pushing the abdominal contents forward.

Female patients may relate exacerbations of all their IBS symptoms to phases of their menstrual cycle, with exacerbation of diarrhea being common during menstrual or premenstrual phases. About half of IBS patients may describe episodes of fecal or mucus incontinence, and many complain of stool urgency. Sleep disturbance is commonly reported and may relate to exacerbation of symptoms.

A history of rectal bleeding, weight loss, fever, and nocturnal diarrhea or pain awakening the patient from sleep would not be expected in IBS and should prompt investigation for other cause. Although it is possible to develop bleeding from hemorrhoids or an anal fissure from straining due to constipation, bleeding per se is not part of IBS and should always be fully investigated.

### IBS features

**Key features**

Abdominal pain; relief with defecation
Irregular bowel habits with alternating diarrhea and constipation
Feeling of incomplete bowel evacuation
Passage of mucus
Bloating with abdominal distention
Absence of weight loss
Absence of rectal bleeding
Left lower abdominal tenderness to palpation

**Common associated features**

Dyspepsia, nausea, heartburn, dysphagia
Fatiguability, sleep disturbances, sadness, anxiety
Fear of serious disease
Bladder dysfunction symptoms, back pain
Multiple abdominal surgical procedures

The physical examination in patients with IBS is usually normal, with the exception that a fullness and tenderness may be found during palpation of the left lower quadrant, relating to sigmoid colon spasm and distention. This finding is not specific for IBS, since it may be present in diverticular disease.

The digital rectal examination is quite valuable to perform to determine stool character, since patients whose chief complaint was diarrhea may be found to have formed, hard scybalous stool in the rectal vault; an empty rectum can be found in constipated patients. A careful bimanual pelvic examination should be done for female patients with lower abdominopelvic pain to check for a possible gynecologic cause of symptoms (see the box above).

### Laboratory studies and diagnostic procedures

The range of symptoms of IBS encompasses those found in the organic diseases that form its differential diagnosis. Abdominal pain and altered bowel habit are common symptoms in a variety of gastrointestinal illnesses, and a review of the disorders that produce symptoms of IBS should always be undertaken. When diarrhea is a predominant symptom, stool samples should be analyzed for fecal leukocytes and ova and parasites, to check on possible infectious or inflammatory colitis. Depending on the specific clinical situation, a stool culture for enteric pathogens and assay for *Clostridium difficile* toxin may be sent. The stool *Giardia* antigen immunoassay may be performed, requires only one sample, and has excellent sensitivity and specificity.

In most situations performance of flexible sigmoidoscopy is a necessary diagnostic test, as is stool analysis for occult blood. Biopsy of the bowel mucosa to check for microscopic or collagenous colitis or possible mast cell disease might be considered. Young patients with infrequent symptoms and good response to initial treatments do not need endoscopic examination of the lower bowel. Those with diarrhea or who do not improve with initial treatment should undergo this procedure. Reproduction of the patient's usual abdominal pain during air insufflation of the sigmoid and its reduction with removal of the air and endoscope is commonly found in IBS patients undergoing sigmoidoscopy. Any patient with rectal bleeding needs lower gastrointestinal endoscopy, since hematochezia is not part of IBS and its source needs to be determined.

Lactose intolerance should be considered, since it may result in altered bowel habit, bloating and excess intestinal gas and can be easily identified by the lactose hydrogen breath test or lactose tolerance test. An inexpensive lactose tolerance test involves asking the patient to drink a quart of milk at one sitting and record the ensuing gut symptoms, if any. This usually works better to identify lactose-related symptoms than the dairy-free diets sometimes recommended.

A complete blood cell count is recommended to check for anemia or inflammation. Tests for thyroid disease, carcinoid, or other systemic disease are usually not indicated unless specific clinical indicators are present in the history or physical examination.

Depending on the clinical situation, barium enema studies or colonoscopy may be undertaken to look at the proximal colon and ileocecal region. Localized pain and other features may dictate ultrasound study of gallbladder, liver, and pancreas, computed tomography (CT) scanning of these organs, or imaging the colon, as in suspected diverticulitis. Small bowel radiography may be needed in patients with periumbilical pain and other symptoms possibly related to Crohn's disease. Some patients with constipation, especially those with laxative abuse or dependency, benefit from study of colonic transit, and those who complain of fecal incontinence may be studied with anorectal manometry. Dyspeptic patients may require upper gastrointestinal radiography or endoscopy.

Patients with unexplained diarrhea who have been extensively evaluated and are without obvious cause should have a stool sample alkalinized to check for the presence of phenolphthalein from surreptitious laxative abuse. This can be done from a small stool smear upon which are added a few drops of sodium hydroxide, with a resultant red color change in the presence of the laxative. Laxative abuse was found to be the cause in about one third of patients who came to a tertiary medical center for chronic diarrhea.

At the present time the minimal workup for IBS should include the history and physical examination of the stools, complete blood count, and in most cases performance of flexible sigmoidoscopy. Tests for lactose intolerance should be considered. Other possible tests should be reserved for specific clinical indicators, based on patient age, or performed at a later time if subsequent clinical information suggests alternative etiologies (see the box at right).

### Laboratory and diagnostic tests

**Initial**

History: check for positive IBS features
Physical examination: include digital rectal examination
Complete blood count, stool guaiac
Flexible sigmoidoscopy: needed for most patients
Rule out lactose malabsorption

**Subsequent or symptom directed**

Stool analysis for leukocytes, ova, and parasites
Stool for *Giardia* antigen, *C. difficile* toxin
Gastrointestinal radiography or ultrasound
Upper and lower gastrointestinal endoscopy
Blood studies for thyroid disease, other metabolic disorders
Colonic transit marker study, anorectal manometry
Alkalinization of the stool: check for laxative abuse

## Differential diagnosis

The symptoms of IBS are not specific for it. Abdominal distress with altered bowel habits may result from many conditions affecting the gastrointestinal tract, and careful consideration of these entities is necessary.

Complaint of diarrhea should prompt a search for lactose intolerance, an extremely common condition that can result in loosening of bowels, increased bowel frequency, increased intestinal gas and passage of flatus, and feeling of bloating. The amount of lactose load affects resultant symptoms, and patients should be encouraged to look for a relationship of dietary intake to gut symptoms. Overall prevalence of lactose intolerance ranges from about 6% in white Americans, to 75% to 90% in groups of Native Americans, African-Americans, and those of Asian background. There is no relationship between lactose intolerance and IBS, and since both occur with a significant frequency, they will occur concomitantly in some individuals. Tests for lactase deficiency should be done as indicated above, and if confirmed, most patients will be easily managed with the use of lactase supplements with little need to alter dairy intake. Other individuals may need to reduce the total intake of lactose-containing foods.

The conditions of giardiasis, sprue, Crohn's disease, bacterial overgrowth and other small bowel disorders should be considered and appropriately searched for if strongly suspected. Food intolerance, different from true food allergy, has been reported to cause abdominal pain and diarrhea in patients who are often atopic. Food diaries, to record intake and symptoms, may assist in discovering food relationships. The history taking should include an inquiry into possible sorbitol ingestion from sugarless gums, candies, or soft drinks, since a large number of adults have sorbitol intolerance due to excessive intake and may experience abdominal pain, cramping, bloating, and altered bowel habits.

Abdominal symptoms arising from peptic ulcer disease or gallbladder disease are not generally accompanied by altered bowel habit and should not usually be confused with IBS. Upper gastrointestinal radiography or abdominal ultrasound should be reserved for those patients whose clinical picture is not clear.

Inflammatory bowel disease, and less commonly infectious colitis, may give rise to symptoms simulating IBS and require consideration. The common feature of hematochezia in ulcerative colitis separates it from IBS, which lacks rectal bleeding. Collagenous colitis, microscopic colitis, and eosinophilic gastroenteritis are unusual disorders with features overlapping those of IBS, with chronic diarrhea and abdominal discomfort predominating. Symptoms of diarrhea, abdominal pain, urinary frequency, headache, flushing, hives, and dermatographia are seen in some individuals with mast cell mediated disease, and increased numbers of mast cells may be found in colonic or terminal ileal mucosal biopsies. Lower abdominal pain may arise from pelvic processes, such as ovarian cysts, pelvic inflammatory disease, or endometriosis and can be searched for with pelvic examination, ultrasound, or CT scan.

Constipation may result from anatomic obstruction, such as bowel malignancy, or as a result of medication side effect or myochotic sigmoid spasm in diverticulosis. It may be part of idiopathic pseudoobstruction, Hirschsprung's disease, or a sequela of laxative abuse. Sigmoidoscopy allows screening for luminally obstructing processes, the presence of diverticulosis, or melanosis coli (resulting from laxative abuse). Since the pathophysiology of colonic diverticulosis involves sigmoid spasm and segmentation, some patients with diverticulosis have symptoms similar to those of IBS patients, and the two disorders may coexist. The majority of patients with diverticulosis are asymptomatic. Patients with constipation and abdominal symptoms dating to infancy should be considered for anorectal manometry to determine the presence of reflex internal sphincter relaxation, which is lacking in Hirschsprung's disease.

With similarity of symptoms possible from IBS and those disorders in its differential diagnosis, an important issue is to avoid extensive, expensive, repetitive, or hazardous workups in approaching an IBS diagnosis as a diagnosis of exclusion. Several investigators, using a strict definition for IBS and following a limited workup, offer evidence of the possibility of making a positive diagnosis, with excellent reliability. Positive historical features reliably favoring the functional diagnosis of IBS include pain eased by a bowel movement, looser stools and more frequent bowel movements at onset of pain and abdominal distention, scybala, diarrhea alternating with constipation, passage of mucus, and absence of weight loss. A normal screening complete blood count and flexible sigmoidoscopy add to diagnostic certainty. With confidence in diagnosis, treatment should be instituted for the IBS. Rectal bleeding, fever, anemia, evidence of malnutrition, and other atypical features in presentation or laboratory findings are not part of the IBS and should prompt investigation into elements of its differential diagnosis. An overview of the differential diagnosis is presented in Table 50-1.

**Table 50-1.** Differential diagnosis

| Condition | Evaluation |
|---|---|
| Lactose intolerance | Tests of lactase deficiency |
| Giardiasis | Stool O&P, *Giardia* antigen |
| Sprue, other mucosal diseases | Malabsorptive tests, small bowel biopsy |
| Crohn's disease | Small bowel radiography |
| Bacterial overgrowth | Lactulose hydrogen breath test |
| Food intolerance | Food diaries and avoidance |
| Sorbitol intolerance | Dietary elimination |
| Hyperthyroidism | Thyroid function tests |
| Peptic ulcer disease | Upper GI radiography or endoscopy |
| Gallbladder disease | Abdominal ultrasound, ERCP |
| Inflammatory bowel disease | Endoscopy, mucosal biopsy, barium enema |
| Infectious colitis | Stool O&P, culture, *C. difficile* toxin |
| Mast cell disease | Rectal biopsy |
| Painful diverticulosis | Flexible sigmoidoscopy |
| Diverticulitis | Abdominal CT scan |
| Laxative abuse | Alkalinize stool for phenolphthalein |
| Abdominal angina | Doppler ultrasound to check vascular flow |
| Gynecologic disorders | Pelvic exam, ultrasound, CT scan |
| Bowel neoplasia | Flexible endoscopy, barium radiography |
| Hirschsprung's disease | Anorectal manometry, rectal biopsy |
| Intestinal pseudoobstruction | Colonic transit marker studies |

*O&P*, Ova & parasites; *GI*, gastrointestinal; *ERCP*, endoscopic retrograde cholangiopancreatography.

## Management

An important feature of caring for patients with IBS is the clinician-patient relationship. A willingness to provide ongoing longitudinal care, with appropriate consultation as indicated, is prerequisite for successful management. Many patients shop around in a search for explanation of their symptoms and might be shunted around a primary provider, since multiple specialists do extensive medical investigations or invasive surgery.

The initial encounters should provide adequate time for exploration of symptoms and explanation of gastrointestinal function and dysfunction. Some patients are able to correlate the onset or recurrence of symptoms with critical or stressful life events. Many IBS patients demonstrate excessive somatic focusing and more health-related fears, a common feature of patients in referral practices. They complain of more nongastrointestinal symptoms and more frequently utilize health care services than their IBS counterparts who tolerate their symptoms without consulting a physician. This illness behavior may be, in part, based on familial factors, with learning of a sick role, having reinforcement for symptoms, or even due to physical or sexual abuse. A significant minority of patients meet the criteria for a psychiatric illness such as depression, anxiety, somatoform disorder or posttraumatic stress disorder, and this should be recognized and managed. IBS patients in primary care practices may demonstrate less chronic somatization than those seen in referral gastroenterology practices, although mood disorders are common in IBS patients attending primary care sites.

It is most important to establish a positive diagnosis of IBS, beginning with the first encounter, if it appears to be the reason for the patient's symptoms. Confidence on the part of the clinician minimizes the frequent desire for more testing "to be sure no other hidden disease" exists to explain the symptoms. Scheduling return visits demonstrates an ongoing interest, and follow-up encounters enable the assessment of changes in clinical features and response to treatment measures. As the clinical course progresses, less frequent and shorter appointments are needed as the patient responds to treatment and gains an understanding of the disease.

The impact of irritable bowel symptoms on the quality of an individual's life is often underrecognized or not explored to the extent needed by the patient. In a group of patients, two thirds of whom were female with a mean age of 45 and mean duration of symptoms of 7 years, the reported areas of quality-of-life impact were those affecting activities and schedules, diet and nutrition, lack of social support and interpersonal relationships, and mood changes. Patients were concerned about not being taken seriously, being told "it's in your head," undergoing many tests without adequate explanation, and a perceived lack of physician concern for their symptoms. Many of these issues are easily avoided by giving adequate time to patient education and empathic listening. Failure to attend to these issues contributes to doctor shopping and using alternative health care venues.

Management of IBS may involve dietary, pharmacologic, and psychologic intervention (see the box at right). The intermittent nature of IBS directs intervention to symptomatic relapses and to strategies for management of its chronic forms. There is a marked placebo response rate in patients with IBS, and many interventions appear successful, at least initially. Patients need to be reassured of the benign nature of the disorder, that it waxes and wanes, has an excellent prognosis, and is not related to colon cancer. Although most patients respond to reassurance and supportive therapy, along with symptom-specific medical treatment, some patients are quite challenging and require frequent telephone or office contact. The dependency issues in these patients are related to their more commonly found psychopathology, especially neuroticism and hypochondriasis. When psychiatric disease is identified in IBS patients, appropriate referral for treatment is indicated.

Specific dietary recommendations involve lactose avoidance for those IBS patients who also have lactase deficiency, or they may use lactase supplements when eating foods containing dairy products. Yogurt and aged cheeses may be better tolerated, since lactose is diminished by the microbial action in those products. Specific foods that trigger symptoms should be avoided. For some patients with either constipation or diarrhea, bulking the stools with fiber may be helpful and is accomplished with increased bran in the diet. A significant number of patients are intolerant of too much added bran, developing bloating and increased intestinal gas. The fiber supplements of hydrophilic colloid (psyllium, methylcellulose) may be better tolerated by some individuals and can be ingested as liquids, tablets, or even as cookies. Patients with constipation and those taking fiber supplements should be encouraged to drink at least 2 quarts of fluid each day. Bland or restrictive diets do not generally benefit the IBS patient and may be harmful if done long term.

Although it has been documented that patients with an initial complaint of constipation, diarrhea, or abdominal pain have all three identified following careful questioning and physical examination, it is helpful in initiating medication therapy to focus the drug intervention at the chief complaint. Patients with abdominal cramps or spastic abdominal pain may obtain benefit from anticholinergic agents, which function to diminish sigmoid contractility and decrease intestinal distention occurring proximally. L-Hyoscyamine and dicyclomine are frequently prescribed agents for this effect, and patients need to be aware of the side effects of dry mouth, dizziness, and possible blurred vision. Anticholinergics coupled with minor tranquilizers (phenobarbital, chlordiazepoxide) may be of benefit for patients with anxiety, although controlled trials to demonstrate clinical efficacy are lacking. The natural antispasmodic peppermint oil may be of benefit, and its encapsulation, in the form available in Europe, allows dissolution distal to the stomach to avoid the possible side effect of pyrosis, caused by its lowering of esophageal sphincter tone if released at a higher level. Tricyclic antidepressants can manage symptoms of abdominal pain, perhaps because of their anticholinergic effect as well as their central effects.

Diarrhea may be controlled with diphenoxylate or loperamide, the latter being particularly useful when there is also fecal incontinence. Some patients benefit from stool bulking to solidify their looser stools; calcium supplements are potentially useful, as are cholestyramine and cholestipol. Although diarrhea may not be fully controlled

## Management of IBS

Key is ongoing supportive physician-patient relationship. Therapy is directed to the initial predominant symptom.

**Abdominal pain**

Anticholinergics: L-Hyoscyamine, 0.125 mg tablets po 20 minutes ac and qhs; dicyclomine, 20 mg po qid
Anticholinergics/anxiolytics: Clidinium bromide, 2.5 mg, with chlordiazepoxide, 5 mg 20 minutes ac and qhs; hyoscyamine, atropine, scopolamine with phenobarbital, 16.2 mg tid to qid
Tricyclic antidepressants: Amitriptyline, 50 - 100 mg po qhs
Behavioral therapy, psychotherapy, hypnotherapy

**Diarrhea**

Antidiarrheals: loperamide, 2 mg bid to qid prn; diphenoxylate, 2.5 mg, with atropine, 0.025 mg qid prn
Fiber: Bran, psyllium seed husk, methylcellulose qd to tid
Calcium, cholestyramine, cholestipol
Tricyclic antidepressants
Psychotherapy, hypnotherapy, behavioral therapy

**Constipation**

Fiber, fluids, exercise
Occasional stool softeners
Lactulose, colonoscopy prep solution (rarely)

**Gaseousness, Bloat**

Lactase supplement/lactose reduction in lactose intolerance
Food diaries to correlate symptoms and dietary intake
Avoidance of specific offending dietary components
Trial of activated charcoal with meals

with these measures, urgency and frequency may be reduced. Some patients with diarrhea may also benefit from treatment with the tricyclic antidepressants. Long-term use of paregoric or codeine is not recommended.

Constipation in IBS usually responds to bulking agents, increased fluids, and exercise. Stool softeners (dioctyl sodium sulfosuccinate) are of occasional benefit, but patients should be counseled to avoid long-term use of laxatives. Infrequently a patient may require treatment with lactulose or polyethylene glycol and electrolytes (colonoscopy prep solution) to enhance colonic transit. Initial use of enemas may help wean a patient from laxative use.

For patients complaining of intestinal gas or bloating, specific food avoidance (leguminous vegetables, beans) may be of benefit. The yeast-derived enzyme food supplement (Beano), marketed to diminish intestinal gas production, is not likely to offer benefit nor will simethicone products, whose target is gas bubble dissolution in the upper gastrointestinal tract. One intervention that may offer clinical relief is activated charcoal capsules taken with meals, which are able to diminish intestinal fermentation and gas production, although patients should be advised that charcoal will darken their stools.

Psychotherapy, behavioral therapy, and hypnotherapy offer alternative approaches or adjunctively assist in management of the patient suffering from IBS. Compared to continued medical therapy, dynamically oriented short-term psychotherapy is more likely to result in diminished abdominal pain and bowel dysfunction. Patients refractory to at least six different therapeutic regimens over a period of a year or more were recently shown to have significantly improved in symptoms of abdominal pain and bowel irregularity following hypnosis, compared with medically treated controls. Most impressive is that the improvement persisted in long-term follow-up and has also been demonstrated in patients who underwent group hypnotherapy. Behavioral therapies such as biofeedback have met with mixed success and may be considered.

The future management of IBS may include therapies directed at neuroendocrine manipulation (leuprolide, ondansetron) or prokinetic motility stimulation (cisapride), but further clinical evaluation of these agents is needed.

It is clear that for the management of IBS many interventions are possible, and no one management strategy works for all patients. Directing therapy at the initial or chief complaint should effect symptom relief. Searching into what prompted an individual to seek medical attention for his or her symptoms is rewarding and may permit the identification and modification of stressful situations. Patients need to be educated about the relationship of IBS symptoms to diet and stress. Although most patients with IBS can be managed completely in a primary care practice, referral to a gastroenterologist should occur when endoscopic examination is anticipated, when the patient fails to respond to initial therapies, for second opinions, and for periodic follow-up assessments. The primary care physician serves a critical role as health adviser and counselor for the patient with IBS, and the most important tool of management is the ongoing, supportive physician-patient relationship.

## GLOBUS

The sensation of a lump or ball in the throat that occurs independently of the act of swallowing is called globus. Typically this sensation is present all the time and seems to interfere with swallowing and breathing. Often the onset may follow a swallowing event in which the patient believes a food item may have gotten stuck or caused irritation, such as a fishbone or seed. Many individuals with globus sensation relate significant stress or anxiety as a precipitant to symptom onset.

Globus may be a common complaint, experienced by about one third of patients with the IBS, found to be present in 18% of a control group of women in a gynecology clinic, and accounting for 4% of new otolaryngologic clinic appointments. In younger patients globus was three times more prevalent in women than men, but over age 50 the prevalence for globus is equal in men and women.

Although its pathophysiology is not understood, a presumed mechanism for the production of globus sensation is cricopharyngeal spasm, which may occur during heightened emotional arousal. A tense individual may become aware of the previously subconscious act of swallowing, and this increased attention to initiating a swallow coupled with anxiety-related reduction of saliva may result in further tension and spasm. Manometric studies to document increased cricopharyngeal tone have been contradictory. In about one fourth of globus patients abnormal gastroesophageal reflux may be present, although the nature of its association or its relationship to symptoms is not clear.

Globus should be differentiated from true dysphagia, which may be high, with difficulties in initiating a swallow, or may be low with the typical symptom of food or pills lodging substernally in the esophagus. A careful history allows separation of globus from dysphagia, the latter occurring only with swallow attempts (Table 50-2). If high or low dysphagia is suspected, investigation should be directed at identifying an anatomic obstruction or motility disorder. Barium radiography, laryngoscopy,

**Table 50-2.** Comparison of globus and dysphagia

| Findings | Globus sensation | Dysphagia |
|---|---|---|
| Timing | Not related to swallow | With swallowing |
| Location | Upper chest, throat | Neck, esophagus |
| Associated symptoms | Difficulty breathing, anxiety | Regurgitation, weight loss |
| Psychologic stress | Common | Uncommon |
| Barium x-ray endoscopy | Normal | Usually abnormal |

upper gastrointestinal endoscopy, esophageal manometry, and other specialized tests may identify oropharyngeal or cricopharyngeal disorders, esophageal stenosis from ring or stricture, or possible motility disorder. The workup for globus may involve cineradiography to evaluate the swallowing function and to provide reassurance. Since globus sensation has been found to occur in some patients with reflux esophagitis, suspicion of that condition should prompt appropriate investigation and treatment.

Management of the globus sensation relies heavily on adequate explanation of the mechanism of symptom production and reassurance. Some patients with gastroesophageal reflux disease may benefit from acid suppressive or prokinetic agents. Treatment of globus sensation is often difficult and recurrence common. Inquiry into stressful trigger events may prove revealing and supportive therapy rewarding. Some patients benefit from treatment with antidepressants, behavioral therapy, or psychotherapy.

## RUMINATION

Rumination, also called merycism, involves painless regurgitation of swallowed food into the mouth. The regurgitated food is rechewed and reswallowed, and this behavior is not upsetting to the individual. In fact, the regurgitated material is considered to be pleasant tasting. The process is involuntary, usually begins shortly after meals, lasts about a half hour, and decreases as the regurgitant material changes its taste from increased acidity. In contrast to vomiting, rumination is not associated with nausea. In contrast to gastroesophageal reflux disease, patients have no pain. The motility of the esophagus and stomach is normal in ruminators.

The habit has its onset in childhood, with persistence in some individuals into adulthood. Although this behavior is unusual, within certain families it may be fully acceptable, with familial ruminators developing in several generations. Rumination appears to be a learned behavior, and it is only infrequently upsetting to the patient when it results in social embarrassment. It is important to distinguish rumination from vomiting or gastroesophageal reflux disease to avoid unnecessary treatments. Some ruminant patients respond to behavioral therapies.

## ATYPICAL CHEST PAIN

The evaluation of patients with chest pain occurs with regularity in primary care practices and in emergency departments. Diagnosing possible coronary artery disease is the first step in the evaluation of chest pain, and this has involved the performance of about 600,000 coronary arteriograms annually in the United States. With up to one third of these examinations having normal results, about 200,000 new cases of noncardiac chest pain are diagnosed each year. The number is actually higher, since younger patients or those without classic anginal symptoms do not undergo catheterization. Within this group of noncardiac chest pain patients, about one third have an esophageal cause of the pain after investigation, with gastroesophageal reflux disease a more common finding than esophageal dysmotility or spasm. Noncardiac chest pain assumes the exclusion of valvular heart disease or pericarditis, and disorders of the lung or pleura (tumor, pleurisy) and chest wall musculoskeletal origin (costochondritis) are in its differential diagnosis. The term *chest pain of unknown origin* (CPUO) can be used to describe a chest pain syndrome in the absence of discernable cause. The pain is often atypical for classic angina. Patients with CPUO have a high prevalence of anxiety disorders, depression, somatization, and perceived vulnerability to serious heart disease. High levels of neuroticism and poor coping strategies are found in some CPUO patients, with less symptom improvement, more frequent pain episodes, and greater social maladjustment.

Patients with CPUO may have a lower threshold to visceral sensation and interpret normal physiologic events as being uncomfortable. Studies incorporating balloon inflation in the esophagus show that CPUO patients experience chest discomfort at significantly smaller balloon volumes than do asymptomatic volunteers. The pathophysiology of CPUO may parallel that for IBS, with a lowered threshold to visceral stimulation (sensing distention above an area of spasm), induction of abnormal motility during acutely stressful stimulation, a close relationship to emotional arousal, and similar psychometric profiles for personality characteristics. About one third of CPUO patients have panic disorder, with features of tachycardia, sweating, dyspnea, dizziness, hot flashes, nausea, choking, trembling, depersonalization, paresthesias, fear of dying, or fear of going crazy.

The diagnostic investigation for a patient with chest pain involves careful review of the history and physical examination (checking for chest wall tenderness) and performance of an electrocardiogram (ECG) and chest radiograph. Echocardiography may be indicated, and treadmill exercise tolerance testing is important to look for a possible cardiac origin of symptoms. Some patients need referral to cardiologists for assessment and coronary catheterization. The entity of microvascular angina (syndrome X) may be diagnosed during atrially paced coronary catheterization, as may be coronary spasm during ergonovine stimulation. When coronary disease is ruled out as the cause of chest pain, or if the pain is accompanied by esophageal symptoms initially (dysphagia, reflux), esophageal investigation should be performed. Upper gastrointestinal radiography or endoscopy provides information concerning possible gastroesophageal reflux disease, the latter permitting acquisition of esophageal biopsies to check for histologic evidence of reflux esophagitis, even when the endoscopic view is normal. Referral to a gastrointestinal motility laboratory for ambulatory 24-hour pH probe testing allows quantification of esophageal acid exposure and correlation of reflux events to symptoms. Stationary or ambulatory esophageal motility testing may reveal a baseline dysmotility associated with the chest pain (achalasia, diffuse spasm, nutcracker esophagus), and provocative testing with edrophonium or balloon inflation may implicate a probable esophageal cause for symptoms.

The differential diagnosis for CPUO includes the disorders reviewed above along with consideration of possible peptic ulcer disease, biliopancreatic disease, IBS, upper gastrointestinal malignancy, and panic disorder.

Management of patients with CPUO begins with the reassurance that none of the determinable disorders that cause its symptoms has been found. Patients should be educated about the possible mechanisms of pain production and assessed for psychologic disease. Patients should know that the prognosis in CPUO is excellent with no determinable increased risk of mortality. Patients with reflux-type symptoms or evidence of increased esophageal acid exposure may benefit from acid suppression or prokinetic medications. If esophageal motility changes are evident on manometric studies or by clinical suspicion, nitrates, calcium channel blockers, or anticholinergics should be tried. Some patients may respond to low-dosage anxiolytics or to antidepressant therapies. Behavioral therapies may also be of benefit for some patients with CPUO.

## NONULCER DYSPEPSIA

Dyspepsia is a clinical syndrome characterized by symptoms that include epigastric pain, early satiety, belching, bloating, and nausea. Although these symptoms are commonly found in peptic ulcer disease, only about one fourth of dyspeptic patients have mucosal lesions when studied. The remaining patients, if further study fails to reveal an etiology, are considered to have nonulcer (functional) dyspepsia.

The cause of nonulcer dyspepsia (NUD) is unknown, and it is defined by the absence of discernable diseases capable of producing its symptoms, including peptic ulcer disease, esophageal reflux, pancreaticobiliary disease, aerophagia, and IBS. *Essential dyspepsia* has been proposed as an alternative term to represent this syndrome. The prevalence of dyspepsia ranges from 20% to 30%, being about twice as common as peptic ulcer disease.

Several pathophysiologic mechanisms may contribute to the pathogenesis of NUD. Patients with NUD usually have normal gastric acid secretion, and treatment of these patients with acid suppressors has not been universally successful to diminish symptoms. It is not likely that acid secretion plays an important role in NUD pathogenesis. Disorders of upper gastrointestinal tract motility have been implicated in causing functional dyspepsia, and some patients have mild gastroparesis. No differences in circulating gastrointestinal peptide hormones have been found. Some NUD patients have increased amounts of duodenogastric reflux, but that it occurs in asymptomatic healthy controls without accompanying symptoms makes it less likely to be an important cause for most patients.

Studies have variously reported that 30% to 50% of NUD patients have type B chronic antral gastritis, with associated *Helicobacter pylori* infection. It is now known, however, that most people with chronic gastritis and *H. pylori* infection are asymptomatic. It is likely that the infection results in a chronic inflammatory response, but it is not likely that the gastritis causes dyspepsia. Although some studies have indicated that NUD patients are more frequently anxious, depressed, or neurotic when compared to controls, there are no substantial data to support a particular personality profile in functional dyspepsia. Stress and emotional arousal may certainly be related to onset or increased NUD symptom reporting, and a lowered pain threshold may be another contributing factor.

The differential diagnosis for NUD includes peptic ulcer disease, gastric cancer, gastroesophageal reflux disease, biliary tract disease, pancreatic disease, medication side effects, metabolic disorders (diabetes, thyroid disease, electrolyte imbalance), intestinal or coronary ischemia, aerophagia, and IBS. Laboratory studies with complete blood count and screening chemistry profile, upper gastrointestinal radiography and endoscopy, ultrasonography, CT scanning, and endoscopic retrograde cholangiopancreatography (ERCP) may be used in the search for potential causes of the NUD symptom complex.

The management of a patient with dyspepsia begins with a detailed history and physical examination. After considering the conditions in the differential diagnosis, a determination of the need for endoscopic or other investigation should be based on the patient's age and symptom severity. It is reasonable to recommend initial investigation for patients over age 40, for those with chronic symptoms, or when organic disease is suspected (e.g., weight loss, evidence of gastrointestinal bleeding, anemia, jaundice, vomiting, dysphagia). Dyspeptic patients under age 40 with no evidence of organic disease and short duration of symptoms that are generally mild should not need early investigation. Empiric therapy with acid suppressors may be of benefit to relieve symptoms in these individuals, and reassurance and education should be given. If little or no improvement occurs within 2 weeks, then further investigation is warranted. The absence of mucosal disruption by endoscopy or radiography places the dyspeptic patient into the NUD category. Investigation for IBS, gastroesophageal reflux, aerophagia, and biliopancreatic disorders results in these disorders being found in three fourths of the NUD group. The remaining fourth have essential dyspepsia.

Treatment of NUD patients should be individualized, and the broad range of medications employed highlights the uncertainties in pathogenesis and lack of uniform patient response. Agents with potential efficacy include the $H_2$ receptor antagonists (cimetidine, ranitidine, famotidine, nizatidine), proton pump inhibitor (omeprazole), prokinetics (metoclopramide, bethanecol, cisapride), cytoprotectives (sucralfate), and even antibiotics to eradicate *H. pylori* when present. The use of these medications remains empiric, and individual patients may respond to one or another agent. Some patients may benefit from behavioral therapy or psychotherapy, but evidence for their efficacy is lacking. The primary care physician plays the central role in the ongoing management of patients with NUD, referring patients to gastroenterologists when initial therapies are unsuccessful, endoscopy is contemplated, for a second opinion, or for periodic assessment.

## AEROPHAGIA

Aerophagia means excessive air swallowing followed by belching. Normal individuals swallow approximately 2 to 3 ml of air with each swallow, accumulate air in the gastric fundus as a bubble, and intermittently eructate (burp). Following a meal or the ingestion of carbonated beverages, large amounts of gas may be belched from the stomach, and depending upon the norms of a society burping may be socially appropriate and expected or inappropriate and discouraged.

Patients with aerophagia complain of excessive stomach gas and feel bloated after meals. They may have abdominal pain or dyspepsia in addition to distention. Eructating seems to offer relief of symptoms, and the patient complains of constant need to belch, which can be accompanied by some regurgitation. Individuals with aerophagia commonly believe their gas to arise from poor digestion or fermentation. Although these two mechanisms account for production of gas in the colon, gas in the stomach is primarily derived from swallowed air and has a composition similar to that of room air. Anxiety has been shown to increase the frequency of swallowing and may contribute to the excess ingestion of air.

Patients with aerophagia should be observed during the initial visit for repetitive air swallowing, which usually precedes a belch. The mechanism of air intake into the esophagus and stomach, with forced expulsion, can be easily explained by making the person aware of the activity as it happens. Attention during eating often reveals excessive air intake with slurping of some foods or high intake of carbonated drinks.

The symptoms of bloating, abdominal distention, pain, and eructation may be found in other gastrointestinal conditions such as peptic ulcer disease, giardiasis, and IBS. Some of these symptoms may be seen in patients with gastroesophageal reflux, gallbladder disease, and gastroparesis. Bloating, distention, and abdominal pain with increased flatus but not excessive eructation are characteristic of lactose intolerance and some malabsorptive diseases. In selected patients barium radiography, abdominal ultrasound, upper gastrointestinal endoscopy, and tests of lactase deficiency may be indicated. For the majority of patients minimal workup is required, especially if active air swallowing is witnessed during the initial encounter.

Patients with aerophagia should be educated about the origin of their symptoms. Pointing out each air-swallowing event, as it is observed during the office visit, can demonstrate the mechanism and frequency of aerophagia to the patient. An explanation of the mechanism of esophageal speech taught to patients with laryngectomies is often helpful in permitting an understanding of air intake and belching. On occasion the clinician's demonstration of air swallowing and belching can have impressive results. Most important, patients need to have a heightened awareness of the frequency of their maladaptive behavior, and this awareness often reduces the frequency of air swallowing. Simethicone, with an ability to coalesce smaller air bubbles into larger ones, does not reduce total ingested air but does offer significant placebo effect. Again, reassurance and education provide impressive benefit in managing patients with aerophagia.

## PANCREATICOBILIARY DYSKINESIA

Dysfunction of the sphincter of Oddi can give rise to distinct clinical disorders of biliary and pancreatic type. Biliary dyskinesia results in elevated common duct pressure due to heightened sphincteric resistance to bile flow, either from sphincter stenosis, hypertonicity (spasm), or dyssynergic motility. Sphincter stenosis may occur from passage of a stone, with resultant papillitis and fibrosis. Dysfunction of the sphincter from spasm or abnormal contractile activity has been variously termed tachyoddia, sphincterismus, and dyssynergia. Abdominal pain is presumed to develop when elevated bile duct pressure is transmitted to liver ductules. Cholecystectomy removes the capacitor for bile storage, with more direct pressure changes exerted on the proximal biliary tract, and biliary dyskinesia should be considered in the evaluation of the postcholecystectomy syndrome. Sphincter of Oddi dysfunction has also been implicated in the pathophysiology of pancreatitis and pancreatic pain.

Patients with pancreaticobiliary dyskinesia are most often women and are usually seen after cholecystectomy. Other functional gastrointestinal disorders are frequently found in patients with biliary dyskinetic syndromes, including irritable bowel syndrome, esophageal dysmotility, and gastroparesis. An increased reporting of neuropsychiatric complaints and increased somatization scoring on psychometric testing has been found in groups of dyskinetic patients compared to controls, as has been the increased incidence of temporomandibular joint syndrome and a higher likelihood of having undergone hysterectomy.

Most patients with biliary dyskinesia report a recurrence of the same pain that led to their previous gallbladder removal. The pain is usually episodic, located in the epigastrium or right upper abdominal quadrant, and may radiate to the back or flank. The pain in some patients is more chronic, with variations in intensity. Pancreatic dyskinesia may produce chronic or intermittent pancreatic-type pain, epigastric in location with radiation to the back. Initial diagnostic studies to define pancreaticobiliary dyskinesia include screening for elevations in liver function tests or amylase/lipase during or following pain episodes and searching for a dilated common bile duct or pancreatic duct on ultrasound. Referral for ERCP allows definition of ductal anatomy and bile duct drainage time, and some specialists can perform sphincter of Oddi manometry at the time of ERCP to determine ductal pressures and sphincteric function. Diagnosis of pancreaticobiliary dyskinesia is based on the history of classic symptoms, with elevated liver or pancreatic enzymes, dilated biliary or pancreatic ducts, and often delayed ductal drainage at ERCP. Sphincter of Oddi manometry has become a gold standard to demonstrate elevated ductal pressures and dysfunction of sphincter motility. The differential diagnosis includes other disorders of the biliopancreatic ducts such as stones, strictures, and tumors. Patients with postcholecystectomy pain should be reevaluated for possible IBS or peptic diathesis.

Management of pancreaticobiliary dyskinesia has included utilization of pharmacologic agents that lower sphincteric tone (calcium channel blockers, nitrates, anticholinergics). Pancreatic enzyme supplementation may be of benefit for management of pancreatic pain by suppressing pancreatic exocrine secretion and decreasing ductal pressure.

Endoscopic sphincterotomy and surgical sphincteroplasty have been shown to be effective in reducing or alleviating symptoms in selected patients with elevated sphincter of Oddi pressures determined by manometry. Patients with pancreaticobiliary dyskinesia should benefit from the behavioral and supportive therapies found useful in the other functional disorders, and future trials of noninvasive treatment are awaited.

## CHRONIC ABDOMINAL PAIN

Chronic functional abdominal pain is defined as pain persisting at least 6 months for which no defined cause is discernible after extensive review of the history, physical examination, and laboratory testing. The majority of patients with this syndrome are women, and many had chronic abdominal pain as children. The true prevalence is not known, but patients with this disorder are frequent users of the health care system, often for multiple chronic pain syndromes.

Pain is usually reported to be present constantly and not related to positional changes, diet, eating, or defecation. The patient may have fixed beliefs about the cause of the pain that do not correlate with anatomic or physiologic processes. Increased symptom reporting is usually associated with heightened stress and emotional arousal. Many patients with chronic pain have experienced sexual or physical abuse in childhood. Some individuals manifest depression, and there is a high frequency of somatoform disorders.

The physical examination usually elicits pain with palpation of the abdomen but without focality. Patients asked to demonstrate the area of pain with one finger often rub the entire abdomen with the whole hand. Multiple surgical scars are often present. The laboratory evaluation should be directed at symptoms suggestive of particular organ systems, and often patients are extensively studied. It is important to review prior studies and avoid unnecessary repetition.

The differential diagnosis is extensive; however, features of the history and laboratory should guide the appropriate workup (Table 50-3).

Management of patients with chronic pain is best accomplished with a multidisciplinary team approach including the primary physician and referral specialists. Some institutions have a pain clinic with a coordinated program of analgesic, behavioral, psychologic, and medical management. The primary physician should establish an ongoing relationship with the patient and provide reassurance. Goals should be focused on minimizing the impact of the illness on the patient and the patient's family and not on curing the illness. The patient must be an active participant in the treatment process.

Various pharmacologic agents have been used in managing chronic abdominal pain, including opiate analgesics, tricyclic antidepressants, and anxiolytics. Psychologic treatments have encompassed behavioral therapy, psychotherapy, and hypnotherapy. Chemical or surgical nerve destruction has been successful in some patients with intractable chronic abdominal pain, and transcutaneous electrical nerve stimulation (TENS) and acupuncture have helped others. Relaxation training and biofeedback techniques are useful adjuncts in comprehensive multidisciplinary treatment.

**Table 50-3.** Chronic pain differential diagnosis

| Condition | Evaluation |
|---|---|
| Intestinal angina | Doppler ultrasound |
| Crohn's disease | Gastrointestinal radiography, endoscopy |
| Pancreatic disease | ERCP, CT scan |
| Slipping rib syndrome | Trial of nerve block, rib resection |
| Gynecologic disorders | Pelvic exam, ultrasound, CT scan |
| Metabolic disorders | Porphyrin screen, check for diabetes, uremia, Addison's disease |
| Poisoning | Lead, arsenic levels |
| Adhesions | Laparoscopy |
| Muscular hematoma | Ultrasound |
| Superior mesenteric artery syndrome | Upper GI radiography, check for impingement |
| Miscellaneous | Rule out familial Mediterranean fever, sickle cell disease, paroxysmal nocturnal hemoglobinuria, tabes dorsalis |

## CHRONIC CONSTIPATION AND LAXATIVE ABUSE

Chronic constipation is a common disorder that can lead to chronic laxative abuse and resultant colonic dysmotility. Constipation in IBS often alternates with diarrhea and is associated with abdominal pain, whereas chronic functional constipation may be painless and constant. Some patients with lifelong symptoms may defecate once weekly or even less frequently. Individuals with chronic constipation often begin their symptoms in childhood, related to improper toilet training, lack of bathroom privacy, or embarrassment. With suppression of the normal urge to defecate the rectum fills with stool and becomes capacious. Subsequent stool passage may be painful due to hardness or volume of the feces or because of an associated anal fissure or inflamed hemorrhoid. This prompts further stool holding and leads to reduced rectal sensation of the urge to defecate. The capacious rectum affects normal anorectal reflex relaxation of the internal sphincter, requiring ever increasing volumes of rectal contents to trigger this initial defecatory event. Some children and elderly patients may develop encopresis, described as involuntary fecal incontinence occurring as a result of overflow of looser stool past a full rectum. Encopresis in childhood is usually accompanied by behavioral or personality changes and may be secondary to significant family psychopathology. Occasional elderly patients have an associated stercoral ulcer of the rectum.

Constipation in adult patients is usually related to dysfunction of the colon in one of three patterns: pancolonic inertia, sigmoid spasm, or anorectal dysmotility. Pancolonic inertia may result from neuropathic illnesses, medication side effects, or as a result of laxative abuse. Sigmoid spasm is a mechanism for diminished bowel transit in irritable bowel syndrome or diverticulosis, resulting from paradoxical hypermotility of the left colon and excessive segmenting contractions. Anorectal dysfunction may result from rectal distention and diminished rectal sensitivity as described above, or from failed relaxation of the internal sphincter with megacolon in Hirschsprung's disease. Hirschsprung's disease involves congenital absence of ganglion cells in a segment of bowel wall, with resultant chronic segmental contraction and failure of relaxation of the anal sphincter. The colon dilates above the hypertonic segment with ensuing megacolon. The affected segment varies in length and usually produces symptoms in childhood or adolescence, although some individuals with short segment involvement might not show symptoms until adulthood. Treatment involves surgical resection of the aganglionic segment.

The diagnostic evaluation in chronic constipation involves performance of a complete history and physical examination, with attention to signs of possible metabolic or neurologic illness. The digital rectal examination may reveal a fecal impaction in the rectum and gives information about the anal sphincter. Patients with Hirschsprung disease have large amounts of stool in the colon but none palpable with the examining finger, whereas patients with functional constipation but not IBS usually have abundant stool felt in the rectum by digital examination. Performance of anoscopy to search for an anal fissure is important if painful defecation is described by the patient. Flexible sigmoidoscopy permits screening for left-sided colonic lesions associated with obstruction (neoplasia, stricture, myochosis with diverticulosis). Endoscopy also permits the discovery of melanosis coli, a brown pigment found in the colonic wall in patients who chronically ingest anthroquinone laxatives (senna, cascara, aloe). Barium enema examination gives information about form and function of the colon, and plain radiographs are helpful to quantify stool content and distention of bowel loops.

The most important examination in chronically constipated patients may be the marker study of colonic transit. In this study patients ingest a gelatin capsule containing 20 plastic opaque 1-mm rings, and the progress of these markers is documented with plain abdominal films over the subsequent 5 days. During the study individuals need to avoid taking laxatives and should supplement their diets with 30 g of fiber daily, beginning 3 days before swallowing the marker capsule and throughout the duration of radiographic study. The location of the markers at the end of 5 days directs further investigation and management: for pancolonic inertia if the markers are scattered throughout the colon, for sigmoid spasm or obstruction if markers pile up at the left colon, and for possible Hirschsprung disease if markers make it to the rectum but do not exit by the end of the study. If Hirschsprung disease is suspected, anorectal manometry should be performed to investigate sphincter function. Quite often all markers are gone from the intestine by day 5, indicating normal colonic function, and frequently patients attribute an improvement in their symptoms to the use of a high amount of fiber supplements. Fiber then becomes a basis for treatment.

The differential diagnosis for constipation is broad, but the usual chronic nature of functional constipation allows it to be distinguished from metabolic, neurologic, or anatomic causes. Appropriate evaluation screens for these other etiologies.

The management of chronic constipation begins with educating the patient about the physiology of defecation and the pathophysiology of constipation. Bowel retraining should be instituted, with encouragement to visit the toilet after a meal, taking advantage of the gastrocolic reflex, and regular exercise to help stimulate colonic transit. Judicious use initially of laxatives may assist in regularizing the bowel habit, but these agents should not be used long term. Enemas may be of benefit to empty the lower colon initially.

High intake of supplemental fiber (bran, hydrophylic colloid) is safe and effective, and should be accompanied by generous intake of fluids. Dried fruits and fiber-rich fruit juices are excellent adjuncts. Stool softeners or glycerin suppositories are of occasional benefit. Some patients require initial and periodic enemas to help empty the lower bowel, but chronic enema therapy should not be necessary.

Long-term management sometimes involves the use of daily lactulose, a nonabsorbed carbohydrate fermented by colonic bacteria that results in increased stool fluidity and colonic output. A rare patient may require intermittent use of colonoscopic prep solutions (polyethylene glycol with electrolytes) taken in small daily amounts and effecting increased stool output. All treatment regimens need to be individualized, and response depends on duration of symptoms, antecedent laxative abuse, and general activity status of the patient.

## PROCTALGIA FUGAX AND LEVATOR SYNDROME

Proctalgia fugax may be considered a variant of the levator syndrome, and both disorders involve chronic or intermittent anorectal pain. Proctalgia fugax is characterized by fleeting attacks of severe, intense anorectal pain that occurs at irregular intervals with complete absence of symptoms in between episodes. From surveys of healthy adults its prevalence appears to be around 15%, with more women than men experiencing the disorder. The prevalence rates for proctalgia were found to be higher in populations of individuals attending gastroenterology clinics, especially in patients with IBS.

Episodes of proctalgia are found to be precipitated by stress and anxiety. It is not certain whether individuals who do not seek medical attention for this functional disorder would demonstrate the high frequency of psychopathology (anxiety, depression, hypochondriasis) seen in patients with proctalgia who seek medical advice.

The pathogenesis of proctalgia fugax is not understood. Its diagnosis is based on clinical symptoms of fleeting pain, and the absence of demonstrable anorectal disease. Symptoms may be precipitated by defecation and rarely following sexual intercourse. Patients often describe intense anal pain, lasting seconds to minutes, with subsequent total resolution of the pain, and long intervals (months) of complete freedom from symptoms. Most individuals experience only a few episodes of pain per year, but some have symptoms weekly or monthly.

The diagnostic workup should include examination in men of genitalia and prostate and a pelvic examination in women, along with digital examination of anus, coccyx, and rectal musculature. In some affected individuals a tender muscle is palpable. Anoscopy and flexible sigmoidoscopy should be performed to screen for other possible anorectal disease and to provide reassurance.

Treatment for proctalgia fugax is made difficult by its fleeting nature and infrequent occurrence of episodes. Some individuals gain benefit from direct pressure manually applied to the anal area during an attack. Pharmacotherapy with muscle relaxants has been studied but has not been generally helpful. Biofeedback techniques and relaxation training may be of benefit, and supportive psychotherapy is important in the management of proctalgia symptoms.

The levator syndrome is characterized by a dull ache or firm pressure felt higher in the rectum in contrast to the anal location of proctalgia. More women than men experience its discomfort, usually in middle age ranges. In contrast to the fleeting nature of pain in proctalgia fugax, patients with levator syndrome, also called coccygodynia, experience pain for hours to days. The pain is most often constant or rhythmic and may be likened to sitting on a ball or feeling like a ball (or corncob) was inside the rectum. Precipitants include defecation, sexual intercourse, sitting for long periods, and stress or anxiety. The pathophysiology is thought to involve spasm of the pelvic floor muscles.

Digital rectal examination in levator syndrome demonstrates tender rectal muscles. Palpation of the coccyx should be done to reveal possible tenderness or excessive mobility from traumatic injury, suggesting an alternative diagnosis. As for proctalgia, patients with levator syndrome should undergo flexible sigmoidoscopy to screen for other anorectal diseases. Careful pelvic and prostate examinations need to be conducted, and ultrasound or CT scanning of the pelvis may be warranted.

Management of this disorder has included digital puborectalis massage, sitz baths, electrogalvanic stimulation, and biofeedback training utilizing electromyography. Medications possibly helpful in controlling symptoms include muscle relaxants, nonsteroidal antiinflammatories, and calcium channel blockers.

## BIBLIOGRAPHY


Almy TP, Rothstein RI: Irritable bowel syndrome: classification and pathogenesis, *Ann Rev Med* 38:257-65, 1987.

Bradley LA, McDonald JE, Richter JE: Psychophysiological interactions in the esophageal diseases: implications for assessment and treatment, *Semin Gastrointest Dis* 1:5, 1990.

Camilleri M, Prather CM: The irritable bowel syndrome: mechanisms and a practical approach to management, *Ann Intern Med* 116: 1001, 1992.

Drossman DA et al: Identification of subgroups of functional gastrointestinal disorders, *Gastroenterol Int* 3:159, 1990.

Drossman DA, Thompson WG: The irritable bowel syndrome: review and a graduated multicomponent treatment approach, *Ann Intern Med* 116: 1009, 1992.

Lynn RB, Frieman LS: Current concepts: irritable bowel syndrome, *N Engl J Med* 329: 1940, 1993.

Talley NJ, Philips SF: Non-ulcer dyspepsia: potential causes and pathophysiology, *Ann Intern Med* 108:865, 1988.

Thompson WG, Pigeon-Reesor H: The irritable bowel syndrome, *Semin Gastrointest Dis* 1:57, 1990.

Whitehead WE, Crowell MD, Schuster MM: Functional disorders of the anus and rectum, *Semin Gastrointest Dis* 1:74, 1990.

Zighelboim J, Talley NJ: What are functional bowel disorders? *Gastroenterology* 104:1196, 1993.


CHAPTER

# 51 Outpatient Evaluation of Common Anorectal Disorders

David J. Schoetz, Jr.

Anorectal diseases afflict a considerable number of patients in any large outpatient practice. Evaluation of disorders of the anus and rectum should follow the same logical progression used in all other fields of medicine. Comprehensive evaluation of the patient is facilitated by the availability of instrumentation that, in many instances, permits accurate diagnosis at the time of the original outpatient presentation.

## HISTORY

Careful and comprehensive history taking requires diligence, experience, and sympathy on the part of the examiner. A pertinent medical history must be obtained when evaluating patients with anorectal complaints. Preexisting systemic diseases, such as diabetes mellitus, or neurologic disorders, such as multiple sclerosis, may be the primary causal factor in the patient's complaint. Previous abdominal operations and anal procedures should be documented. In women the obstetric history, especially performance of an episiotomy, may be relevant. Medications the patient is currently taking may cause or alter symptoms. Family history, with particular reference to the presence of polypoid disease, inflammatory bowel disease, and carcinoma of the colon, is essential.

Social history includes recent or remote travel and whether any diarrheal illnesses were incurred during that time. Sexual history, when pertinent, must be detailed and frank. The current increase in both homosexual and heterosexual anal intercourse has resulted in an appreciable increase in sexually transmitted anal and rectal diseases. The examiner should not permit personal prejudices to prevent the collection of such valuable information.

A complete review of systems should be obtained when appropriate. Recent weight loss and other constitutional symptoms, such as fevers and chills, are important data. Of particular importance is a urologic and gynecologic history. Information about the presence of recurrent urinary tract infections, recurrent vaginal infections, pneumaturia, and fecaluria should be recorded.

### Bleeding

Bleeding is the most common reason patients are seen for evaluation (see the box on p. 711). Of primary importance is the distinction between bleeding from the anorectal region and bleeding from a more proximal site. Blood from the anorectum is nearly always bright red, often clotted, and is most frequently associated with the act of defecation. When blood is noticed on the toilet paper and occasionally dripping into the toilet bowl, the source is

### Causes of rectal bleeding

**Anorectal region**
Hemorrhoids
Anal fissure
Carcinoma of anus or rectum
Polyps of rectum

**Colon**
Diverticulosis
Angiodysplasia
Carcinoma
Inflammatory bowel disease
Infectious disease
Rare neoplasms, benign and malignant
Ischemic colitis

**Other**
Peptic ulcer disease, gastritis
Meckel's diverticulum
Small bowel neoplasms

usually internal hemorrhoids. Blood that is noticed on the surface of the stool is also associated with hemorrhoids.

When bleeding is accompanied by pain during the act of defecation, the diagnosis is almost always anal fissure. Although ulcerated, thrombosed external hemorrhoids may also produce these symptoms. Bright red blood associated with diarrhea and the passage of mucus or pus per rectum should alert the historian to the presence of an acute inflammatory condition involving the colon or rectum. Dark red blood with or without blood clots, melena, and blood intermixed with the stool indicate that the source of bleeding is above the anus and rectum. After the examiner has excluded the possibility of hemorrhage from the upper gastrointestinal tract, the most common sources of large amounts of rectal bleeding are diverticulosis and angiodysplasia of the colon. The bleeding from angiodysplasia is characteristically intermittent, whereas that of diverticulosis is more often unrelenting. Massive bright red rectal bleeding is seldom caused by lesions within the anus and rectum.

### Pain

Pain arising from the anal canal is usually described as burning, stinging, or stabbing (see the box above). Anal fissure is the most common cause. Characteristically, the pain is increased during the act of defecation. Throbbing pain associated with swelling in the perianal region indicates the presence of either thrombosed hemorrhoids or perianal abscess. Proctalgia fugax is classically described as a deep boring pain in the rectum that frequently awakens the patient from sleep and lasts for variable periods of time; this type of pain is intermittent and has no known organic cause. Advanced carcinoma of the rectum may also cause a deep boring pain in the rectal area, but unlike proctalgia it is constant and indicates extrarectal extension of the carcinoma. Pain in the coccygeal region, also known as coccygodynia, is rarely of anorectal origin. Patients with this disorder complain of pain at the tip of the coccyx that is aggravated by sitting on hard surfaces for long periods.

### Causes of anorectal pain

**Common**
Anal fissure
Hemorrhoids
Abscess, anorectal or pilonidal
Proctalgia fugax
Coccygodynia

**Less common**
Inflammatory conditions
Neoplasms

## PHYSICAL EXAMINATION

Outpatient evaluation of the anus and rectum requires proper equipment for adequate visualization. The examining room should be well lit and supplied with all materials the examiner might need. Trained assistants are essential during the examination to expedite the procedure and to prevent injury. Preparation of the patient before examination should be conducted on an individual basis. In general, the administration of a disposable enema to patients who are to undergo proctosigmoidoscopic examination facilitates the procedure. However, the presence of symptoms of inflammatory bowel disease or proctitis may necessitate foregoing the enema to obviate any mucosal changes that may be induced by the enema solution itself. Similarly, the presence of fissure and other painful conditions of the anal region may prevent administration of an enema. Adequate suction, illumination, probes, biopsy instruments, and electrocautery should be present at the start of the examination.

### Position

Several positions are acceptable for examination of the anorectal region (Figs. 51-1 to 51-3). The left lateral decubitus (Sims) position is convenient and precludes the need for a specialized examination table. In this position the patient lies on the left side with the knees drawn up as far as possible toward the chin. The buttocks should overhang the edge of the examining table to facilitate the examination. Although the Sims position is comfortable for the patient, many believe that performance of proctosigmoidoscopy in this position is difficult. The knee-chest position, with the patient kneeling on the examination table and resting the shoulders and head on the pillow, is appropriate in the absence of an examining table. However, this position is uncomfortable because no support is provided for the chest or thighs. Most examiners agree that any of the commercially available proctoscopy tables enable optimal patient positioning for a complete examination. The position afforded by the table is one that is unfamiliar to many patients and consequently provokes appreciable anxiety in some. With this table the patient is securely supported in the head-down position, and gravity is used to move the abdominal viscera and mucus out of the pelvis. In addition, little air is insufflated, and consequently the examination is usually less painful.

Complete visual examination of the anorectal region may begin before positioning the patient on the table. Rectal prolapse and the mucosal prolapse associated with advanced hemorrhoidal disease are frequently spontaneously reduced in the prone jackknife position. Consequently, if the history suggests either of these diagnostic possibilities, the anus should be examined in the bathroom after the patient has expelled a preparatory enema.

## Inspection

When the patient is on the examining table, the examiner should note the position of the anus and the presence of any scars associated with previous surgery. The patulous anus associated with rectal prolapse and primary incontinence of neuromuscular origin may be appreciated. Thrombosed external hemorrhoids are readily recognized, as are prolapsed internal hemorrhoids and hypertrophied anal papillae. The erythema and swelling associated with perianal suppurative disease may be identified easily. Epidermoid carcinoma of the anus and malignant melanoma must not be excluded from consideration in the visual differential diagnosis of these other common anorectal problems. A single edematous skin tag, commonly seen in the posterior midline, is associated with the presence of anal fissure. Manual traction on the buttocks permits visual identification of a fissure in most patients. The presence of fissures in unusual locations or the presence of multiple fissures should suggest the possibility of inflammatory bowel disease or syphilis.

Dermatologic conditions affecting the perianal region may also be evident by inspection. Circumferential erythema with lichenification and superficial fissuring is commonly seen with pruritus ani. Moist skin eruptions should suggest the presence of eczema or fungal infestations. A dry scaling skin eruption extending up the natal cleft suggests the presence of psoriasis. Vegetative warts are easily recognized as condyloma acuminatum. Less frequently flat, velvety, wartlike growths may indicate condyloma latum, a manifestation of secondary syphilis.

Fistulous openings of various causes may also be appreciated. Pilonidal disease is characterized by single or multiple orifices in the midline of the natal cleft posterior to the anus. Hairs may be extruding from the orifices. External openings in the perianal region may also indicate the presence of a fistula in ano. The site of these external orifices should be documented carefully because the external opening suggests the position of the internal opening of the fistulous tract. Suppurative hidradenitis may also demonstrate multiple fistulous tracts, frequently extending toward the scrotum and out onto the skin of the buttocks. In addition, chronically indurated and edematous skin surrounds these sinuses.

## Palpation

After inspection a gloved finger that is liberally lubricated should be inserted into the anal canal. Patients with acute fissure and perianal abscess may not tolerate even the most gentle digital examination and consequently require general or regional anesthesia for complete evaluation. As the finger negotiates the anal canal, the examiner is able to palpate the intersphincteric groove and the anorectal ring. The tone of the sphincter mechanism can be examined at rest and during voluntary maximal contraction. The prostate gland should be examined for size,

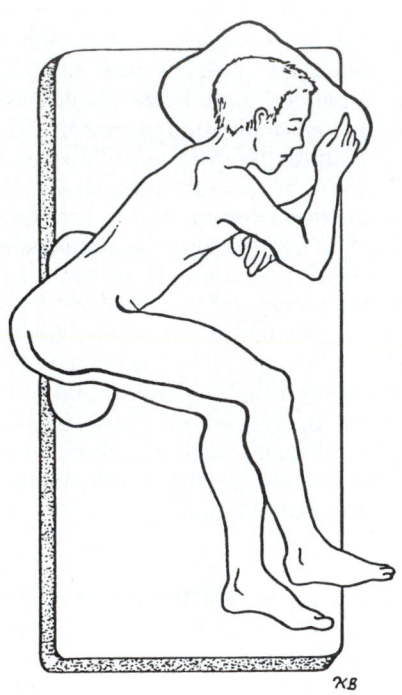

**Fig. 51-1.** Left lateral decubitus (Sims) position.

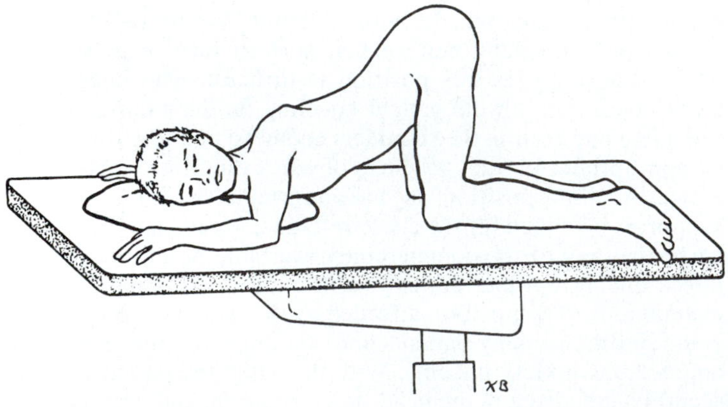

**Fig. 51-2.** Knee-chest position.

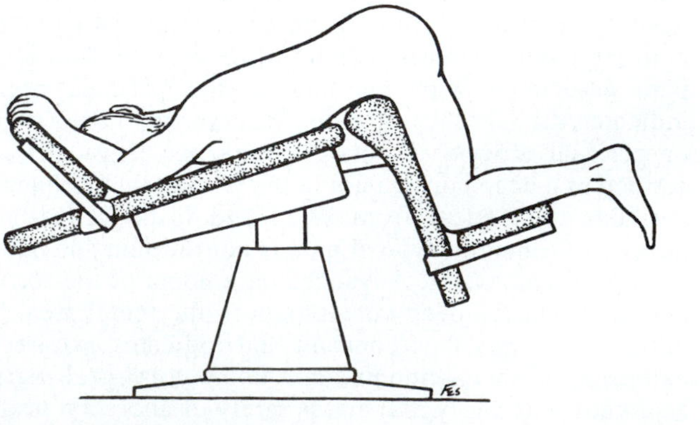

**Fig. 51-3.** Prone jackknife position on special examining table.

consistency, and the presence of masses. Hypertrophied papillae are frequently palpable, as are anal fissures, which are felt as longitudinal grooves in the anal canal. After the finger has passed into the ampullary portion of the rectum, a complete search of all aspects of the lower rectum is made. Particular attention must be directed to the posterior aspect of the rectum because this area is not readily visualized during proctosigmoidoscopy. Meticulous examination is particularly important in the diagnosis of villous adenoma and retrorectal masses. Rectal masses must be described in terms of size, consistency, degree of mobility and infiltration of the pararectal tissues, and presence of ulceration. Pararectal adenopathy associated with carcinoma of the rectum frequently may be suggested by digital examination. Submucosal lesions, such as leiomyoma, should be distinguished from mucosal abnormalities. Concurrently the examiner should be cognizant of the presence of advanced carcinoma of the cervix or ovary in women and of the presence of Blumer's shelf associated with advanced intraabdominal malignancy. When the examining finger is removed, the presence of blood, pus, and mucus should be noted. Any stool adherent to the examining finger should be tested for the presence of occult blood when this examination is appropriate.

## Anoscopy

Many types of anoscopes are commercially available, and each has its major proponents. Different sizes of anoscopes should be available to accommodate all situations (Fig. 51-4). In all instances the anoscope must be well lubricated (Fig. 51-5). After the anoscope has been inserted, the obturator is removed, and a quadrant of the anal canal is inspected.

Mucosal abnormalities, such as ulceration, exudate, polyps, and tumors, should be noted. The dentate line must be examined for the presence of internal orifices of suspected fistulas or abscesses; such areas may be recognized by the appearance of a drop of pus exuding from one of the crypts. Hypertrophied anal papillae and anal polyps may also be seen. Anal fissures should be characterized with regard to the apparent chronicity as indicated by scarring of the edges and the presence of fibers of the internal sphincter muscle at the base of the fissures. Visualization of hemorrhoids is undertaken, and performance of the Valsalva maneuver by the patient accentuates the appearance of internal hemorrhoids.

## Proctosigmoidoscopy

Rigid proctosigmoidoscopy is one of the most misunderstood and underutilized tools in the diagnostic armamentarium of physicians. When properly performed, however, this examination should be painless and free from serious morbidity. Many types of proctosigmoidoscopes are available (Fig. 51-6), and the ultimate choice rests with the examiner. In situations in which large numbers of daily examinations are performed or when insufficient personnel are available to provide adequate cleansing of the instruments between examinations, the advantages of disposable sigmoidoscopes should be considered. Small

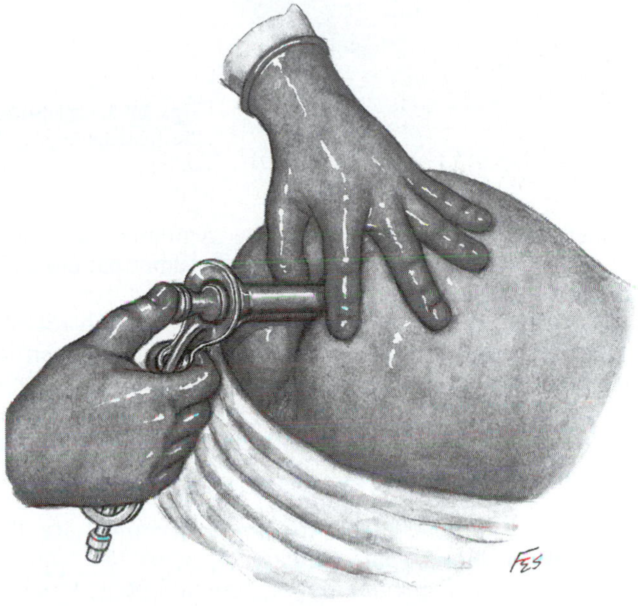

**Fig. 51-5.** Insertion of the anoscope. Pressure is kept on the obturator during insertion. Stabilization is afforded by the left hand to prevent injury if the patient moves.

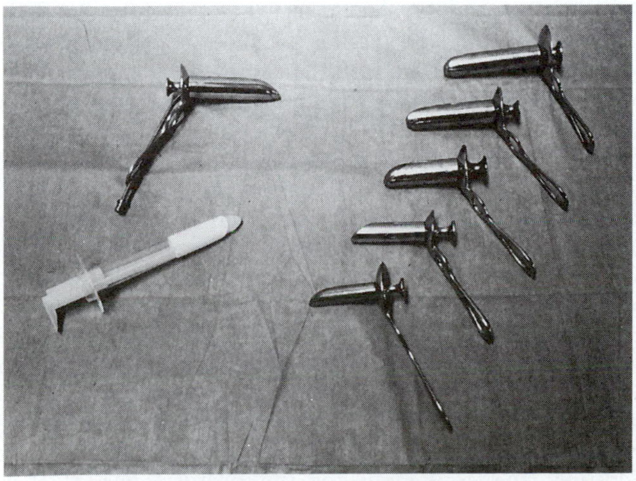

**Fig. 51-4.** Anoscopes.

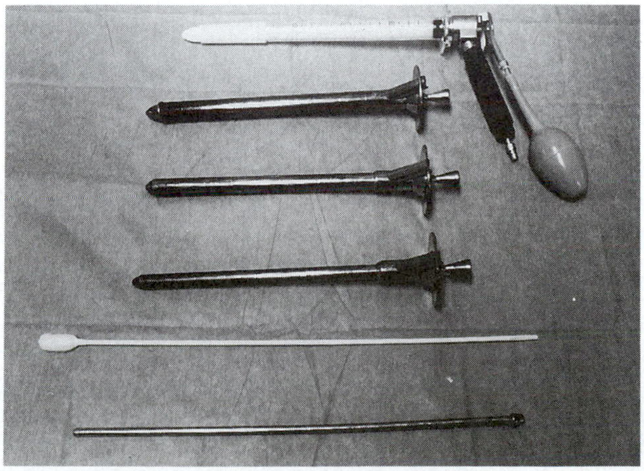

**Fig. 51-6.** Sigmoidoscopes.

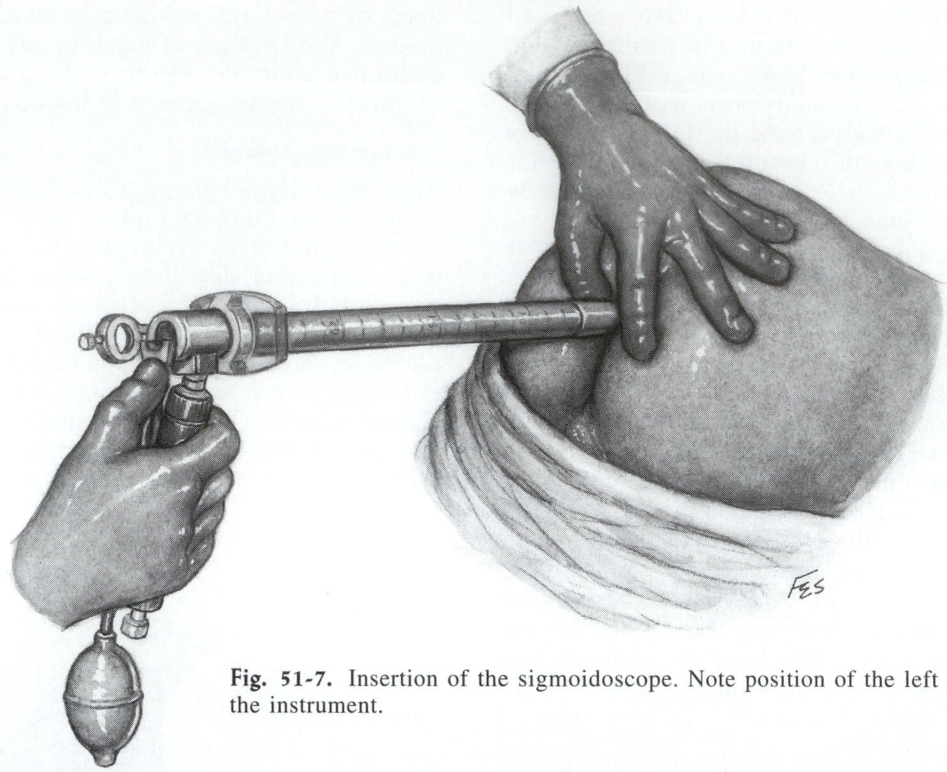


**Fig. 51-7.** Insertion of the sigmoidoscope. Note position of the left hand to stabilize the instrument.

diameter sigmoidoscopes should be available for examination of the pediatric patient and of the adult patient with anal stenosis or stricture within the rectum.

Digital examination dilates the anus and also reveals any potentially obstructing lesions that may alter performance of the examination. The importance of "verbal anesthesia" cannot be underemphasized. After digital examination, the well-lubricated sigmoidoscope is passed into the distal rectum (Fig. 51-7). As soon as the examiner feels the resistance of the sphincter has been overcome, the obturator is removed, and its tip is examined for the presence of blood, pus, mucus, or stool. No further advancement of the sigmoidoscope should be undertaken without direct visualization of the lumen.

Because the rectum in most individuals lies anterior to the sacrum, the sigmoidoscope is directed posteriorly and advanced with the lumen in direct view (Fig. 51-8). As the instrument reaches the rectosigmoid junction, it is common to lose sight of the lumen. Initial redirection to the patient's left and then to the right advances the instrument into the distal sigmoid colon in most patients. Maneuvering at this juncture must be gentle because stretching of the mesentery produces considerable discomfort. Excessive insufflation results in cramping. When the lumen cannot be visualized, the instrument should be withdrawn, and another attempt should be made to negotiate the area. In no instance should the bowel be stretched so tightly that the mucosa blanches. Further attempts at advancement under these circumstances may result in perforation. Residual stool and enema fluid should be suctioned as it is encountered to permit adequate visualization of the lumen. Observation should be made during both insertion and removal of the instrument. Most agree that the average distance the rigid sigmoidoscope can be passed is about 20 cm. Persistent attempts to insert the instrument beyond the limit of the patient's tolerance will be self-defeating because patients are unlikely to return for repeat examinations if their initial sigmoidoscopy has been unduly painful.

Mucosal detail should normally be readily apparent with a fine vascular pattern easily appreciated beneath a thin, healthy rectal mucosa. Edema associated with inflammatory bowel disease results in the loss of vascular pattern. Ulcerations, when present, may be serpiginous and deep, or discrete aphthous ulcerations suggesting Crohn's disease, or superficial and diffuse suggesting ulcerative colitis or proctitis.

Neoplastic disease involving the rectum and distal sigmoid is not infrequently encountered. Polypoid lesions should be characterized with regard to size, consistency, appearance of the surface, and the presence or absence of a pedicle. Carcinoma must be described with regard to ulceration, portion of the circumference involved by the tumor, and degree of fixation. After the lesion has been described accurately, appropriate investigations should be undertaken, and the patient should be referred to a qualified surgeon or gastroenterologist for appropriate biopsy or snare excision and subsequent histologic diagnosis.

Submucosal lesions of the rectum are not rare. Both lipomas and carcinoids are seen as raised yellowish submucosal masses. Both leiomyomas and leiomyosarcomas, however, may more easily be palpated than observed. If diagnostic consideration is being given to the presence of a submucosal tumor of the rectum, consultation for the performance of operative excision should be obtained.

Although the risk of perforation from rigid sigmoidoscopic examination is negligible, the performance of transsigmoidoscopic biopsy and fulguration appreciably increases the risk of both hemorrhage and perforation. In addition, the equipment for the performance of these procedures is highly specialized. The expense required to

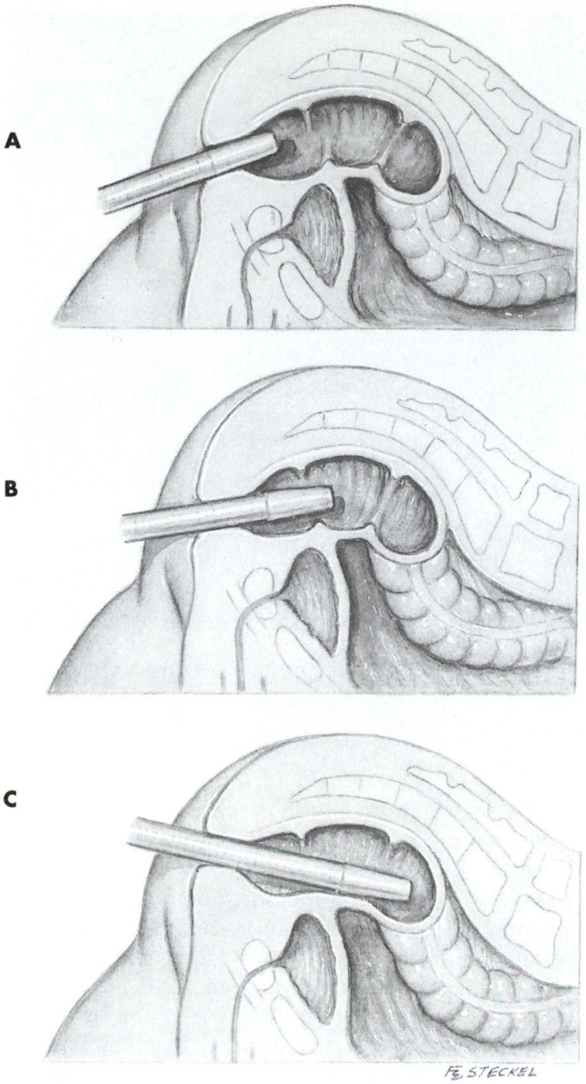


**Fig. 51-8.** Initial direction of the sigmoidoscope is posterior **(A).** As the instrument advances into the rectum, it is more horizontal **(B).** At the rectosigmoid, it is directed anteriorly and toward the patient's right side **(C).**

obtain and maintain such equipment may not be justified for individuals not specifically trained in operative sigmoidoscopy.

Recent advances in fiberoptic technology have resulted in the development of flexible fiberoptic sigmoidoscopes for outpatient use (Fig. 51-9). Most patients can be prepared for this examination with two disposable enemas, and no premedication is required. With the patient in the left lateral decubitus position, the flexible sigmoidoscope can be advanced to the 55 to 60 cm level in at least half of the patients. The superiority of the optics, when combined with the increased length of bowel examined, results in a diagnostic yield of neoplasms approximately three times greater than with the rigid sigmoidoscope. Potential disadvantages to the routine use of flexible sigmoidoscopy include the considerable increase in expense, the degree of sophistication required of the examiner, and the potential risk of explosion during the performance of electrosurgical procedures through the flexible instrument. Nevertheless, flexible sigmoidoscopy

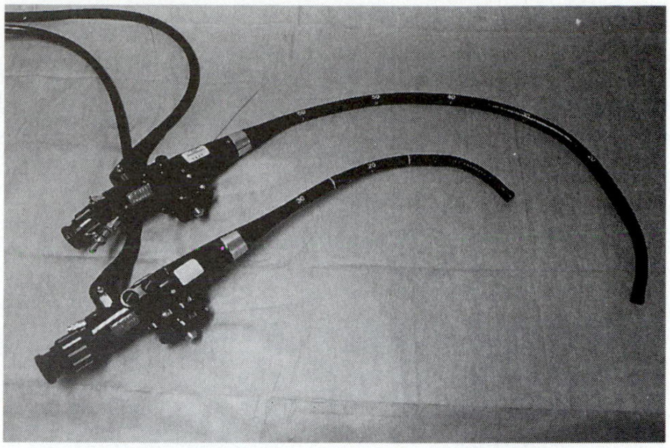

**Fig. 51-9.** Flexible sigmoidoscopes (American Cystoscope Makers, Inc., Stamford, CT). *Top,* Standard 65-cm instrument. *Bottom,* Newer, more easily used 35-cm instrument.

represents an important addition to the diagnostic and therapeutic armamentarium of the physician interested in the diagnosis and treatment of diseases affecting the colon and rectum.

## COMMON ANORECTAL PROBLEMS

### Hemorrhoids

Although hemorrhoids are a common anorectal disorder, they are one of the most misunderstood and overdiagnosed afflictions of the anorectum. At least 5% of the general population experience symptoms of hemorrhoids. The disease may occur at any age, although the incidence appears to increase with age.

The cause of dilated veins in the anal canal is not completely understood. Although hemorrhoids were previously believed to represent varicosities of the hemorrhoidal veins, this theory is now known to be an oversimplification. The relative prevalence of hemorrhoids in the Western world, which has a fiber-deficient diet, suggests that excessive straining during the act of defecation is an important predisposing factor to the development of this disease. Chronic diarrheal states, such as inflammatory bowel disease, may also be associated with hemorrhoids. Heredity may contribute; approximately 10% of patients with hemorrhoids have a family history of hemorrhoidal disease.

Hemorrhoids may be classified as external or internal (Fig. 51-10). External hemorrhoids represent dilated veins of the inferior hemorrhoidal system and are located below the dentate line in the perianal area. Internal hemorrhoids represent dilation of the superior hemorrhoidal venous system and are present in the distal rectum and anal canal. The classification of internal hemorrhoids can be subdivided further into varying degrees. First-degree internal hemorrhoids protrude into the lumen of the anal canal without a subjective sensation of protrusion and are found during examination for complaints of bleeding. Second-degree internal hemorrhoids protrude during the act of defecation but spontaneously reduce after the bowel movement is completed. Third-degree internal hemorrhoids require manual reduction after the termination of bowel action. Fourth-degree internal hemorrhoids are permanently prolapsed and are not reducible despite

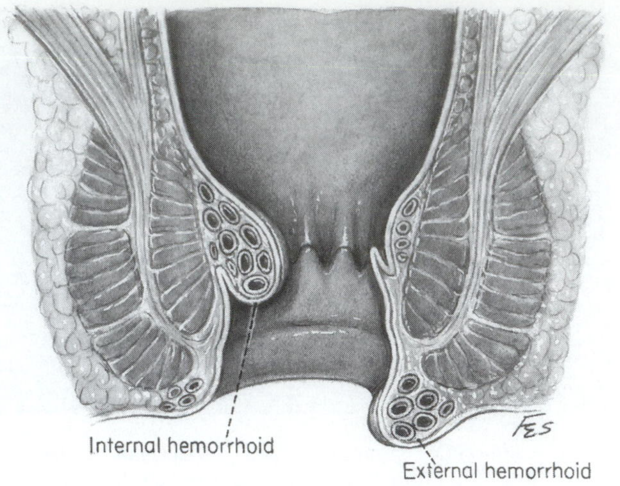


**Fig. 51-10.** Anatomy of internal and external hemorrhoids.

attempts at manual reduction (Fig. 51-11). Mixed hemorrhoids are those in which components of both internal and external hemorrhoids are present in the same individual.

***External hemorrhoids.*** These may be the source of considerable discomfort. Many patients complain of pain in the perianal region after straining maneuvers that result in inflammation and in engorgement of external hemorrhoids. In addition, mucus discharge and difficulties in providing adequate perianal hygiene may result in pruritus.

***Management.*** Treatment for symptomatic external hemorrhoids should be directed at decreasing the necessity for straining at stool. Frequently, modification of toilet habits and particularly discouragement of sitting on the toilet for prolonged periods should be emphasized. Bulk-forming laxatives and a high-fiber diet provide regular and easy evacuation. Control of diarrhea, when possible, also appreciably improves symptoms. Instruction on proper anal hygiene should be provided. Sitz baths, witch hazel, and application of topical hydrocortisone should control pruritus in most individuals. Finally, insertion of creams containing hydrocortisone may be used to diminish inflammation within the anal canal.

External hemorrhoids may also be complicated by the formation of thrombosis. Thrombosed external hemorrhoids present as the abrupt onset of severe perianal pain with a mass. Examination reveals a tender subcutaneous perianal lump that has a characteristic bluish discoloration. Treatment depends on the severity of pain. If the pain is not severe or is resolving, nonoperative treatment is indicated. Bulk-forming agents, mild analgesics, sitz baths, and topical steroids should be prescribed. When the pain is severe, consideration should be given to referral for prompt surgical excision.

***Internal hemorrhoids.*** The most common symptom of internal hemorrhoids is bleeding. Classically, the bleeding is described as bright red blood on the toilet paper and is frequently noticed dripping into the toilet bowl at the time of defecation. Prolapse may occur to varying degrees as previously described. Pain is not a symptom of uncomplicated internal hemorroids, but the occurrence of pain should indicate the presence of a fissure, a thrombosis, or an abscess as an associated condition.

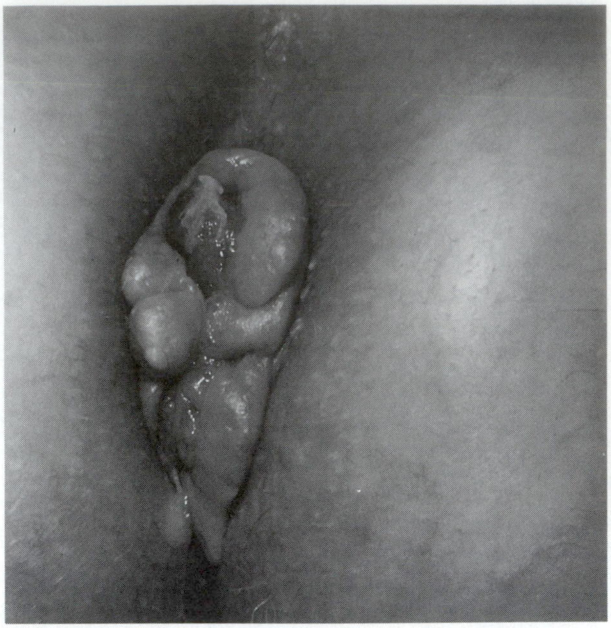

**Fig. 51-11.** Fourth-degree hemorrhoids with thrombosis and ulceration.

The diagnosis of internal hemorrhoids cannot be made by inspection when the hemorrhoids are at an early stage of development. Similarly, digital rectal examination is notoriously inaccurate in the diagnosis of early hemorrhoidal disease. Definitive diagnosis requires the performance of anoscopy. Proctosigmoidoscopy must be performed to exclude the presence of coexistent diseases of the colon and rectum. Similarly, barium enema examination and colonoscopy must be performed when any doubt exists as to the origin of rectal bleeding after initial outpatient evaluation.

***Management.*** When the diagnosis of internal hemorrhoids is secure, treatment may take one of several forms. Medical therapy of hemorrhoids is directed primarily toward the avoidance of straining during defecation. The consumption of a high-fiber diet and sufficient liquid to ensure the passage of a soft, well-formed stool is the mainstay of treatment. Bulk-forming agents and stool softeners may also be used to supplement these dietary maneuvers. Education of patients with regard to the proper methods of ensuring adequate bowel evacuation with a minimum of straining is an important adjunct to medical therapy.

First-degree, second-degree, and some third-degree hemorrhoids may be treated on an outpatient basis by specialized techniques that do not involve formal hemorrhoidectomy. First-degree hemorrhoids may be treated by injection sclerotherapy or infrared coagulation. Second-degree and third-degree hemorrhoids are most often treated by rubber band ligation (Fig. 51-12). This technique uses a device that places a rubber ring around the base of the hemorrhoid within the lower rectum that acts as

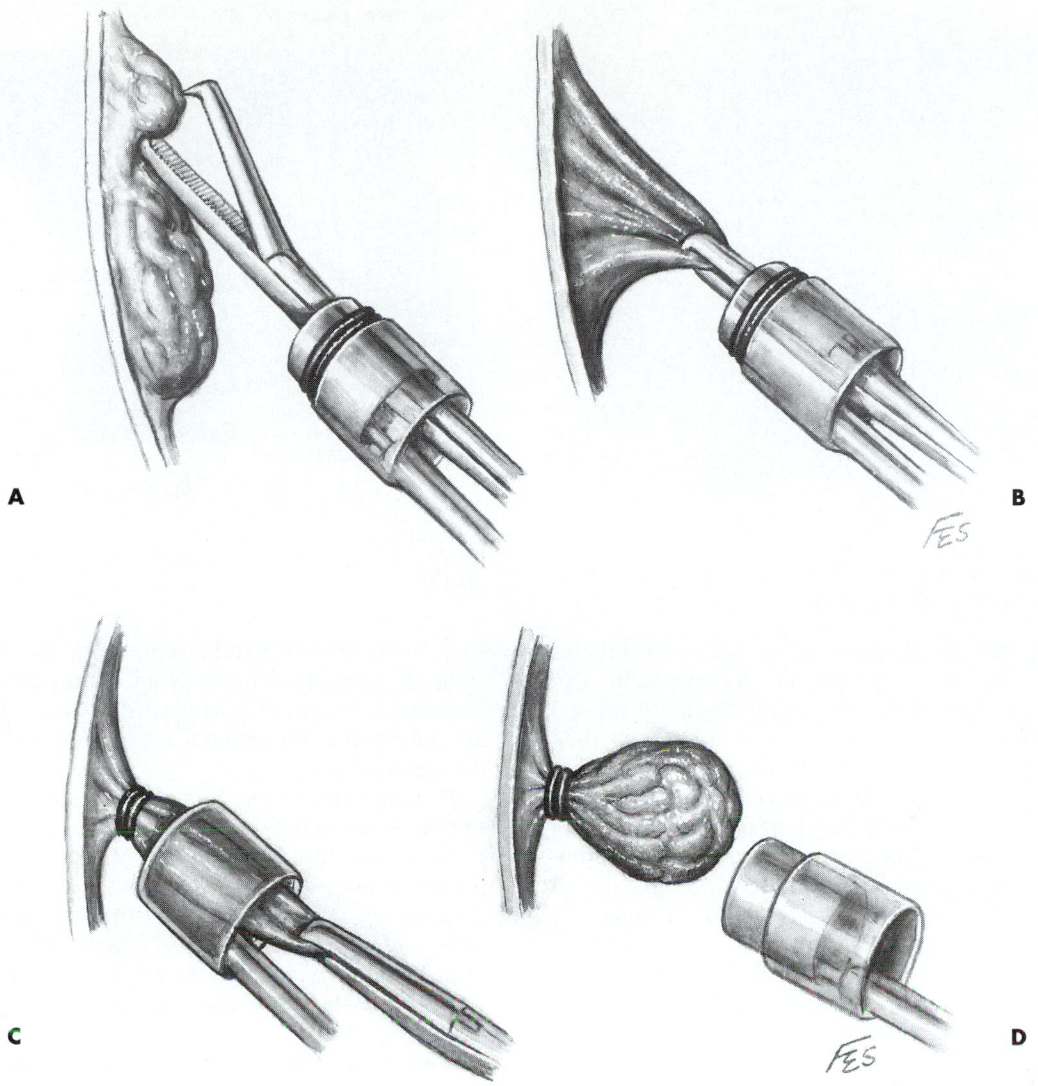


**Fig. 51-12.** Rubber band ligation of hemorrhoids. **A,** Redundant mucosa at the base of the hemorrhoid, within the lower rectum, is grasped. **B,** Excess tissue is drawn into the ligator as long as the procedure is not painful for the patient. **C** and **D,** The instrument is fired.

a tourniquet to strangulate the excess tissue while fixing the mucosa into the muscularis. Other techniques include cryosurgery, direct current coagulation, and laser coagulation. Each of these instruments has some associated cost, which may be prohibitive. More important, all are associated with complications, such as pain and bleeding. These procedures should be performed by individuals thoroughly familiar with the diagnosis, treatment, and management of complications of hemorrhoids. Advanced degrees of internal hemorrhoids or combined internal and external hemorrhoids require formal hemorrhoidectomy.

## Fissure in ano

Anal fissure may be defined as a painful linear ulceration within the anal canal extending from the dentate line to the anal verge. This common condition is extremely painful owing to the somatic innervation of the anus. Although fissure is encountered more often in young adults, it may be seen in infants and children as well as in the elderly. It is generally accepted that the initiating factor in the development of fissure is trauma to the anal canal, which is most often caused by the passage of a hard fecal bolus.

The diagnosis of anal fissure is made by inspection (Fig. 51-13). The classic triad of anal fissure is the presence of a linear ulceration with a sentinel pile at the distal margin and a hypertrophied anal papilla at the proximal margin. The distribution of fissures in the anal canal is in the midline; in men 99% of anal fissures are in the posterior midline, whereas in women 10% of fissures are in an anterior location. The presence of multiple fissures or fissures that are not in typical locations should suggest the presence of secondary factors, including Crohn's disease of the anus, tuberculosis and syphilis of the anus, and anorectal trauma.

The chief complaint of patients with anal fissure is pain during defecation and for a variable period thereafter. Bleeding, although common, is not invariably present. In most instances history alone establishes the diagnosis. Physical examination by simple inspection confirms the presence of a fissure. Digital examination, if possible,

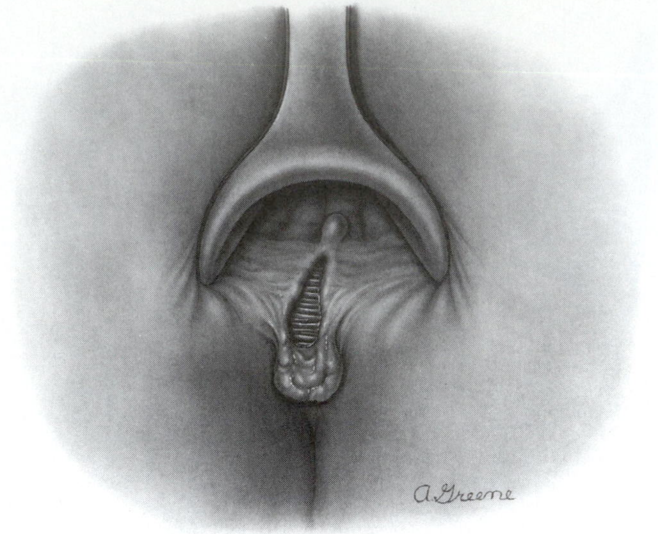


Fig. 51-13. Chronic anal fissure. Note the sentinel pile, indurated ulcer, and hypertrophied papilla.

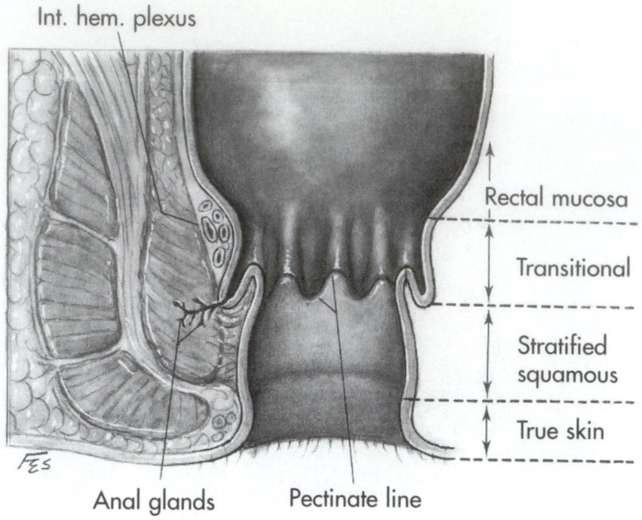


Fig. 51-14. Anatomy of the anal canal. Note position of the anal glands.

reveals variable degrees of spasm of the internal sphincter and tenderness to direct palpation. Examination can sometimes be facilitated by the application of topical anesthetic agents in a gel form. Nevertheless, office endoscopic procedures are frequently impossible because of the degree of the patient's discomfort. In some instances diagnosis must be made under anesthesia. At some point in the patient's course a proctosigmoidoscopic examination must be undertaken to exclude a diagnosis of inflammatory bowel disease. Once again, it must be stressed that fissures in an aberrant position as well as multiple fissures must prompt intensive investigation for the presence of an underlying disease process.

***Management.*** Acute fissures, evidenced by a lack of previous symptoms and the absence of physical signs of chronic fissure, may be treated by nonoperative therapy. The aim of medical therapy is to break the cycle of hard stool, pain, and consequent constipation caused by sphincter spasm and an aversion to bowel movement. Warm baths, bulk-forming agents, and stool softeners are useful. Anesthetic ointments, although helpful in the acute phase of the illness, may be associated with the development of cutaneous sensitivity and dermatitis with prolonged use. Finally, the use of antinflammatory suppositories and ointments has been tried with variable success. The result of these nonoperative maneuvers in the treatment of anal fissure is healing in about half of the patients.

Operative treatment should be recommended for patients in whom a trial of medical management of acute fissure fails and for individuals with uncomplicated chronic fissures. Current opinion favors the performance of internal sphincterotomy as definitive operative treatment.

## Anal suppurative disease

It is now generally accepted that both abscess and fistula in ano share a common cause. Perianal abscess is the acute manifestation of the underlying suppurative disease process, whereas the fistula represents the chronic disease state. A fistula is defined as an abnormal communication between two epithelial surfaces; thus the fistula in ano is an abnormal communication between the anal canal and the perianal skin.

Complete understanding of the anatomy of the anorectal region is essential in the diagnosis and treatment of a patient with abscess or fistula. A critical structure is the pectinate line, which represents the junction of the rectal mucosa with the anoderm. At this level the ducts of the anal glands empty into the crypts (Fig. 51-14). Other important areas are the muscles of the pelvic floor and the relationship between the internal and external anal sphincters.

Current evidence suggests that infection originating within an anal gland is the most common cause of abscess and fistula. Careful anatomic dissections have demonstrated that about two thirds of the anal glands penetrate into the internal sphincteric muscle, and half of these glands penetrate through the internal sphincter into the intersphincteric plane. Obstruction of the ducts of these glands results in formation of an abscess in the intersphincteric plane. The precipitating events resulting in anal gland obstruction may be constipation, diarrhea, or anal trauma. Abscess may complicate fissure in ano. In addition, anal suppuration is a well-recognized complication of surgery of the anal region.

Specific predisposing factors must be excluded. Crohn's disease may primarily involve the anorectum. Active Crohn's disease of the rectum and chronic ulcerative colitis may also predispose to formation of abscess. Various specific anorectal infections, such as tuberculosis, syphilis, and lymphogranuloma venereum, may result in anorectal abscesses. Careful history and examination should exclude the presence of these underlying conditions.

Anorectal abscesses result from extension of the abscess in the intersphincteric plane. The route of extension determines the presentation of the abscess (Fig. 51-15). When the tracking is toward the perianal region in the intersphincteric plane, the presentation is that of a

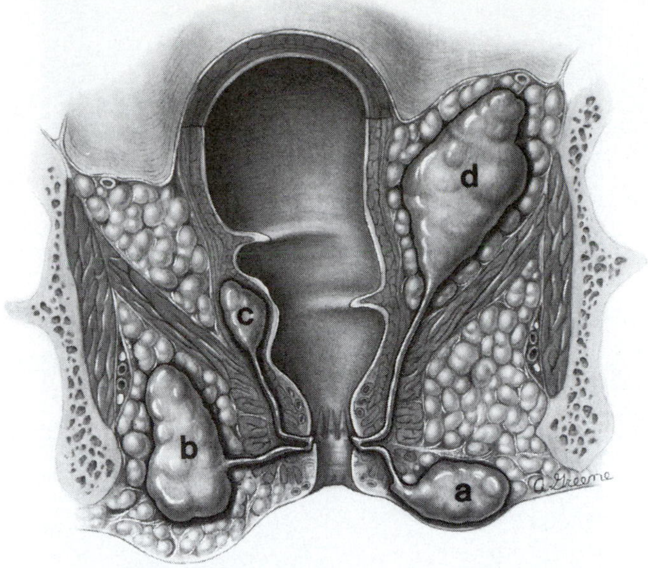


**Fig. 51-15.** Common sites of anorectal abscesses: perianal *(a)*, ischiorectal *(b)*, intersphincteric *(c)*, and supralevator *(d)*.

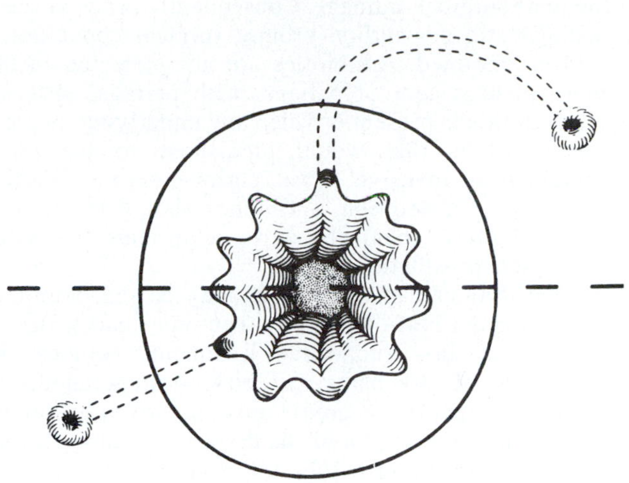


**Fig. 51-16.** Graphic representation of the Goodsall rule.

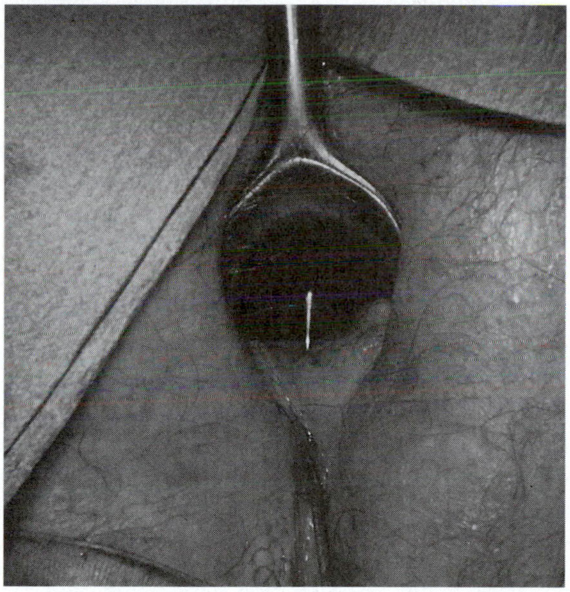

**Fig. 51-17.** Fistula in ano with probe in the fistulous tract.

perianal and perirectal abscess. When the purulence penetrates the external sphincter into the ischiorectal fossa, the presentation is that of an ischiorectal abscess. Both of these abscesses present with the classic findings of perianal swelling with redness, heat, and pain. When the purulence tracks in a superior direction, a supralevator abscess is formed. The purulence may remain in the intersphincteric plane and present without external swelling or induration. In these instances rectal examination reveals exquisite tenderness with fluctuation within the anal canal. With supralevator or postanal space extension, examination under anesthesia may be necessary to establish the diagnosis.

Anoscopy and sigmoidoscopy are usually impossible to carry out in the presence of an acute abscess. These examinations should be performed, however, after definitive therapy has resulted in relief of discomfort. When examination under anesthesia is required to establish the diagnosis, endoscopic procedures should be included as part of the evaluation. Associated underlying conditions as well as the internal openings of the abscess will be identified by these procedures.

Fistula in ano represents the chronic form of anal suppurative disease. Patients with chronic fistulas have complaints of intermittent perianal pain and drainage. A previous history of operative drainage of an anal abscess or of spontaneous drainage is usually elicited. Again, underlying pathologic conditions should be sought before definitive therapy is given.

Diagnosis depends on careful examination of the perianal region. On inspection, an external opening is observed in the perianal skin. The position of the external opening is paramount in determining the position of the internal opening. The Goodsall rule states that, if the external opening is anterior to a horizontal line bisecting the anus, the internal opening will lie in a radial direction within the anal canal (Fig. 51-16). On the other hand, if the external opening is posterior to this line, the internal opening will lie in the posterior midline. Multiple fistulous tracts also indicate a probable origin from the posterior midline with a chronic horseshoe fistula. The farther the external opening is from the anal verge, the more likely it is that a complicated fistulous tract will be found.

After inspection, palpation is undertaken to delineate the fistulous tract. A probe may then be passed from the external opening to demonstrate the course of the fistula (Fig. 51-17). When this procedure is carried out in an outpatient setting, it must be performed carefully to minimize discomfort to the patient and to prevent the formation of false channels. In many instances of chronic fistula, however, the entire fistulous tract may be demonstrated by the judicious passage of a probe.

*Management.* The treatment for perianal suppuration is adequate surgical drainage. Consequently, when abscess is a diagnostic possibility, prompt surgical consultation should be obtained. Antibiotics are not indicated in the primary management of patients with perianal abscess. When cellulitis is present or when any underlying medical condition exists that would predispose to the rapid development of invasive sepsis, perioperative antibiotics are indicated. In addition, antibiotics should be used in patients who have rheumatic or valvular heart disease or intravascular prosthetic devices.

Simple drainage of an abscess may be the definitive therapy in about half of patients. The other half progress to fistula in ano. Supportive treatment includes the frequent use of sitz baths and bulk-forming agents to prevent constipation. Careful postoperative follow-up examination of the region of the crypts indicates whether the drainage procedure will be followed by the formation of a chronic fistula.

The presence of a fistula in ano is an indication for operative intervention. Spontaneous healing is extremely rare. A neglected fistula may result in repeated abscess formation and potential extension of the process into a more complicated fistula. The principles of operative management are beyond the scope of this review, but operation should be performed by surgeons who are well trained in the treatment of fistulas to minimize serious complications related to division of the sphincter muscle.

## Pruritus ani

Itching of the perianal region is an extremely common complaint. Although the potential causes of pruritus are numerous, most often careful evaluation does not uncover any specific cause. Characteristically, perianal itching is episodic and more intense at night. Often a history of mucus seepage and fecal soiling can be obtained.

Careful evaluation of the patient's history for the presence of generalized dermatologic conditions, such as psoriasis, seborrheic dermatitis, eczema, and contact dermatitis, should be sought. The prolonged use of topical agents on the perianal skin may also be associated with the development of allergic dermatitis. Other systemic diseases that may predispose to perianal itching are diabetes and underlying liver disease with jaundice.

After appropriate evaluation of the history, complete examination of the perianal skin, anal canal, and rectum should be performed. The presence of anorectal abnormalities, such as cryptitis, prolapsed hemorrhoids, and large perianal skin tags, should be documented. All of these conditions may predispose the patient to increased mucus soilage and difficulties in cleaning the perianal skin. Rarely, mucus-secreting neoplasms may result in pruritus. In the younger age group consideration should be given to the presence of pinworm infection, and appropriate diagnostic maneuvers should be undertaken.

*Management.* In the absence of specific predisposing conditions treatment consists primarily of careful attention to perianal hygiene. Many patients use soap to cleanse the perianal skin, causing superficial abrasion and a defatting of the keratotic layers with subsequent aggravation of perianal irritation. Careful attention should be given to the avoidance of soap and to the use of moist absorbent cotton for cleansing. The perianal skin should be kept dry. Application of topical hydrocortisone preparations has been demonstrated to be effective in the overall treatment of idiopathic pruritus. In some individuals in whom leakage is a prominent symptom the use of perineal strengthening exercises results in a diminution of fecal soiling and subsequent improvement. Irradiation of the perianal skin and subcutaneous resection of its nerve supply are previously performed practices, and they are mentioned here only to be discouraged. Careful attention to all aspects of perianal hygiene ensures successful control of symptoms in most individuals.

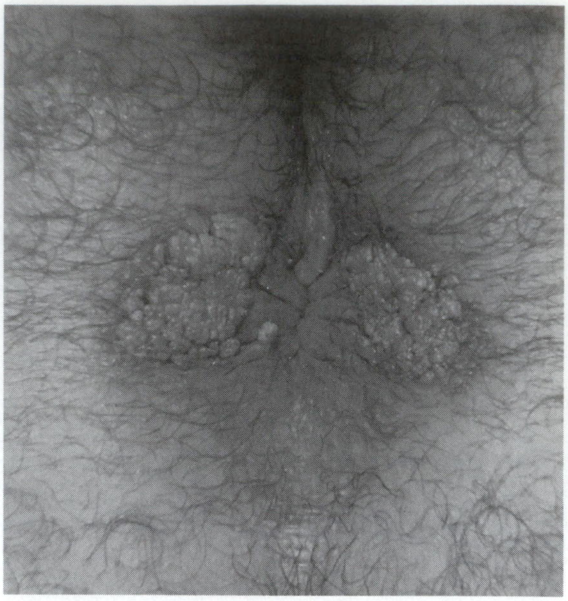

**Fig. 51-18.** Condyloma acuminatum with typical mirror-image plaques of warty tissue around the anus.

## Sexually transmitted diseases of the anorectum

Changing social mores have resulted in a dramatic increase in the number of sexually transmitted diseases affecting the anorectum. Familiarity with these diseases is essential for the outpatient evaluation of anorectal complaints. Prompt recognition and treatment can prevent considerable morbidity and help control the spread of these disorders.

*Condyloma.* Condyloma acuminatum is a disease believed to be caused by a transmissible and autoinoculable papillomavirus. The incubation period is usually from 1 to 6 months but may be considerably longer. Commonly referred to as genital warts, the lesions are found in the perianal and anal canal as well as in other portions of the perineum, vulva, vagina, and penis (Fig. 51-18). The incidence is greatest in male homosexuals. A history of anal intercourse is elicited in 70% to 90% of patients presenting with anal condyloma.

Condyloma may appear as multiple tiny lesions to massive perianal plaques. The surface of the warts is papilliform and may be pink or white. They frequently extend into the anal canal and even into the rectum. Most often the symptoms are irritation with discharge and bleeding. The presence of other sexually transmitted diseases must be determined.

**Management.** Local treatment of condyloma is associated with a 25% to 70% incidence of recurrence. Podophyllin and bichloracetic acid are caustic agents that have demonstrated effectiveness. The former is contraindicated in the presence of warts within the anal canal because of the formation of burns on the contralateral side. Podophyllin, 25% in tincture of benzoin, may be applied on a weekly basis to perianal, perineal, and vulvar warts. Care must be exercised to prevent damage of surrounding normal skin. Various surgical procedures include fulguration, surgical excision, and cryotherapy. Recently immunotherapy has been successfully used. Preparation of vaccine from 5 g of wart tissue with subsequent weekly injections into the deltoid muscle has resulted in improvement in patients with recurrent warts. α-Interferon may be injected at the base of condylomata to stimulate immune-modulated eradication. The reasons for the difficulty in eradicating this disease are numerous. Because the disease is probably sexually transmitted, resumption of sexual activity before the completion of treatment, the acquiring of new sexual partners, and the long incubation period may cause reinfection or delayed recurrence.

***Nonspecific venereal proctitis.*** Nonspecific venereal proctitis, a disease of unknown origin, is associated with nonspecific urethritis in sexual partners. Patients are most often seen because of the onset of anorectal pain and tenesmus with irritation and mucoid discharge. Proctoscopic examination reveals distal proctitis with mucopurulent exudate. Specific culture for *Chlamydia trachomatis* may be undertaken. Tetracycline, 250 mg four times a day for 5 to 10 days, most often results in complete cure. Once again, it is important to differentiate this condition from gonococcal proctitis by appropriate culture techniques. Differentiation from idiopathic ulcerative proctitis and other forms of inflammatory bowel disease requires repeated proctoscopic examination. Biopsy should be obtained in all patients with antibiotic-refractory proctitis.

***Acquired immune deficiency syndrome.*** The acquired immune deficiency syndrome (AIDS) in the homosexual population must be considered when dealing with anorectal diseases. This syndrome is described in Chapter 68.

Practically speaking, the diagnostic approach to the homosexual patient with anorectal pain or discharge should begin with a complete sexual history and detailed examination of the anorectum. The presence of a fissure indicates possible syphilitic lesions, and an exudate from the fissure should be examined with darkfield illumination. If a mucopurulent discharge is present within the distal rectum, appropriate cultures for *Chlamydia* organisms and gonorrhea should be obtained. When neither of these cultures is positive, empiric treatment with tetracycline as previously described should be undertaken, with a presumptive diagnosis of nongonococcal proctitis. When symptoms are not resolved, specific cultures for herpes and cytomegalovirus should be obtained. Multiple potentially infecting organisms may be present in one person, thus complicating both diagnosis and treatment. Fortunately, most acute proctitis in this population is either chlamydial or gonococcal and can be treated effectively by many therapeutic regimens. The implications of active viral proctitis are unknown at present. Current information and speculation on the pathogenesis of AIDS suggest that careful long-term follow-up studies for all individuals identified as having active viral proctitis should be mandatory.

Anorectal diseases in patients with human immunodeficiency virus (HIV) and AIDS is confined almost exclusively to persons practicing anal receptive intercourse. Some form of anorectal disease develops in about one third of these patients during their illness. More than one disease in one patient is the rule rather than the exception. Perianal sepsis is most common, followed by condyloma and herpes simplex. Cytomegalovirus may cause anal ulceration, as may invasive carcinoma and lymphoma. Investigation of HIV-positive patients should, in addition to the basic examination, focus more intently on the skin to exclude Kaposi's sarcoma and on peripheral lymph nodes. Viral and bacterial cultures of lesions should be obtained. An associated diarrhea may be the result of bacterial, fungal, protozoal, or viral causes. It is important to remember that, in patients with AIDS, opportunistic infections are common, such as tuberculosis, histoplasmosis, cryptosporidiosis, and cytomegalovirus as well as the more usual pathogens.

Idiopathic ulceration of the anus in patients with AIDS is a challenge. These lesions are usually deeply burrowing painful ulcers associated with leakage of mucus as a result of diminished sphincter tone. Biopsy is essential to determine the cause. Empiric therapy with topical and oral acyclovir is begun, although this drug is not uniformly successful.

Surgery for anal disease is controversial. Current data suggest that HIV-positive patients without AIDS may have good results from conservative anorectal operations. Patients with established AIDS fail progressively as the degree of immunosuppression progresses. Anal surgery in these patients has a prohibitive morbidity, with failure of healing, fecal incontinence, and progressive sepsis.

## BIBLIOGRAPHY

Beck DE, Wexner SD, editors: *Fundamentals of anorectal surgery,* New York, 1992, McGraw-Hill.

Coller JA: Technique of flexible fiberoptic sigmoidoscopy, *Surg Clin North Am* 60:465, 1980.

Corman ML: *Colon and rectal surgery,* ed 3, Philadelphia, 1993, JB Lippincott.

Fazio VW, editor: *Current therapy in colon and rectal surgery,* Toronto, 1990, BC Decker.

Gordon PH, Nivatvongs S: *Principles and practice of surgery for the colon, rectum, and anus,* St Louis, 1992, Quality Medical Publishing.

# VI Hematology/Oncology

CHAPTER

## 52 Anemias and Other Red Cell Disorders

Liberto Pechet

The term *anemia* translates literally to "lack of blood." We can redefine this term as a reduction in hemoglobin or red blood cells (RBCs) or hematocrit. The common denominator is a decrease in the oxygen supply to peripheral tissues due to a decreased red cell mass. A main concept leading to our ability to understand how to approach anemias is to consider them secondary manifestations of underlying disease processes. Hence, discovering a patient with anemia should automatically lead to a search for its etiology.

The first step in understanding anemias is to develop a logical classification. This entails both a pathophysiologic (i.e., understanding the underlying mechanism) and a morphologic grouping of anemias. The latter is based both on the size of peripheral blood RBCs and the bone marrow appearance of red cell precursors. According to this approach the pathophysiologic mechanism of anemia can be either a failure of the bone marrow to produce enough RBCs or excessive loss or destruction of RBCs due to bleeding or hemolysis. Morphologically, anemias can be classified as macrocytic when the red cells are oversized, normocytic when they are of normal size, and microcytic when they are smaller than normal. The RBC indices are calculated by electronic laboratory cell counters and give an accurate description of cell size at a glance.

The reticulocytes are also helpful since, by representing young anucleated RBCs, they tell us the ability of the bone marrow to compensate for the reduced cell mass, or in other words its ability to respond to anemia. The reticulocyte count is usually increased in hemolytic anemia and in the regenerative phase after bleeding (if the iron stores are sufficient) or following effective therapy for anemia. They are very low or absent whenever the bone marrow fails, such as in aplastic anemia and immediately following chemotherapy. From a clinical point of view anemia produces rather nonspecific symptoms such as shortness of breath, dizziness, weakness, lack of energy, and even congestive heart failure depending on its severity, rapidity of onset, and integrity of the cardiopulmonary system.

### ANEMIAS DUE TO DISORDERED OR DECREASED RED BLOOD CELL PRODUCTION

#### Deficiencies of essential nutrients

Nutritional anemias are caused by a lack of one or more elements essential for the normal maturation of RBCs and, in some cases, of white blood cells (WBCs) and platelets as well. The most common deficiency encountered in clinical practice is that of iron. Its absence results in a defect in the synthesis of heme, leading to a delay in the maturation (hemoglobinization) of the cytoplasm of RBC precursors. Deficiencies of folate and vitamin $B_{12}$ (cobalamin), both of which are necessary for DNA synthesis and normal nuclear maturation, are less common.

***Iron-deficiency anemia.*** Iron deficiency is the most common cause of anemia in the United States. Typical patients include infants on a prolonged milk diet with no other nutrients, multiparous women, and patients with bleeding from a gastrointestinal or gynecologic neoplasm. Because of the potential for serious underlying pathology, the etiology of iron deficiency must be ascertained.

**Iron metabolism.** Iron absorption is finely regulated to meet metabolic needs. Iron is absorbed most effectively within the duodenum and upper portion of the jejunum. Intestinal absorption is sensitive to changes in total RBC mass and not to total body iron stores; this accounts for increased iron absorption in all anemias, independent of iron stores. Under normal circumstances the daily loss of iron is about 1 mg, exactly the amount absorbed through the gastrointestinal tract. A menstruating woman needs to absorb iron at a rate of approximately 2 mg daily because of excess loss in menstrual blood. During pregnancy the need for absorbed iron reaches 2.5 to 3 mg per day to meet the demands of the fetus.

**Etiology.** Dietary deficiency of iron in the United States in found almost exclusively in infants on a prolonged milk diet or in elderly people whose diet is grossly inadequate (Table 52-1). The daily recommended iron intake for infants is 1 mg/kg/day beginning at approximately 3 to 4 months of age. The infant consuming 1 quart of human milk per day receives only 0.4 mg of iron; those consuming cow's milk receive less than 0.1 mg.

Female adolescents with heavy menstrual bleeding occasionally develop iron deficiency despite iron's ready availability in food. About 15% to 20% of menstruating women are deficient in iron. In contrast, iron deficiency as the result of diet is rare among American men. Resection of the proximal intestine or gastroenterostomy, ulcerative colitis, regional enteritis, rapid gastrointestinal motility, and sprue may be associated with iron deficiency due to malabsorption. Iron deficiency may also develop with chronic intravascular hemolysis and urinary iron loss (hemosiderinuria) or with excessive blood donations. Any unexplained iron-deficiency anemia must be investigated for a source of bleeding. In principle an adult man or postmenopausal woman who develops iron deficiency has gastrointestinal or gynecologic bleeding until proven otherwise. The possibility of such bleeding, particularly from age 40 on, obligates the primary care physician to do a thorough gastrointestinal (and in women a gynecologic) workup. One should not treat patients with iron without investigating the cause of the anemia.

**Clinical findings and diagnosis.** The clinical manifestations of iron deficiency depend on whether it has developed over a short or a long period. Iron loss through acute hemorrhage is often a problem of volume loss and may require immediate blood transfusions. Chronic iron deficiency may be clinically subtle. Some of the signs are related to changes in the surface epithelium in various parts of the body. These changes result in glossitis, angular stomatitis, achlorhydria and atrophic gastritis, spooning of nails, and rarely dysphagia. Pica, a craving for unusual substances such as clay, starch, ice or compulsive consumption of one kind of food, is occasionally seen with severe iron deficiency.

The laboratory diagnosis of iron deficiency is based on the characteristics of RBCs and an evaluation of iron stores (Table 52-2). A decreased hemoglobin with hypochromic, microcytic RBCs (Fig. 52-1) is characteristic. The typical serum findings are low serum iron and high transferrin levels, measured as the total iron binding capacity (TIBC). The normal saturation of transferrin, which fluctuates between 30% and 40%, decreases to less than 15% with iron deficiency. A very low serum ferritin level, usually below 12 μg/L, is also characteristic. We recommend the use of ferritin alone, since serum iron and TIBC are frequently affected by chronic inflammatory conditions. Ferritin can also be falsely elevated in acute liver disease, but finding very low or absent ferritin is pathognomonic for iron deficiency. When in doubt, a bone marrow aspirate is obtained to evaluate iron stores. Because thalassemia minor also presents with microcytosis and hypochromia, ancillary laboratory tests may be necessary, such as hemoglobin electrophoresis and determination of hemoglobin $A_2$ (discussed under hemoglobinopathies).

**Table 52-1.** Etiology of iron deficiency

| Cause and source | Pathology |
|---|---|
| **Bleeding** | |
| Gastrointestinal tract | Carcinoma of the stomach or colon |
| | Duodenal and gastric ulcer |
| | Esophageal hiatal hernia |
| | Hemorrhoids |
| | Regional enteritis, ulcerative colitis |
| | Hookworms |
| Gynecologic | Excessive menstrual bleeding |
| | Uterine malignancy |
| Urinary tract | Hemorrhagic cystitis |
| | Prostatic hypertrophy |
| | Prostatic carcinoma with bleeding |
| | Hypernephroma |
| | Excessive anticoagulation and other hemostatic defects |
| | Chronic dialysis |
| | Paroxysmal nocturnal hemoglobinuria |
| | Microangiopathic hemolytic anemia |
| Lung | Idiopathic pulmonary hemosiderosis |
| Systemic | Excessive blood donations |
| | Uncorrected operative blood loss |
| | Factitious self-induced blood-letting |
| **Nutritional deficiency** | |
| Dietary | Infants on prolonged exclusive milk intake |
| | "Tea and biscuits" diet |
| | Multiple pregnancies and lactation with diet poor in iron |
| Malabsorption | Extensive gastrointestinal resection |
| | Specific iron malabsorption (not well documented) |
| | Part of the sprue syndrome |
| | Ulcerative colitis and regional enteritis |
| | Excess intake of antacids, clay, grain |

**Therapy.** While pursuing the etiology of documented iron deficiency, patients can be started on oral iron therapy. The least expensive form of iron is ferrous sulfate, containing 60 mg elemental iron per tablet. To avoid gastrointestinal irritation, it may be advisable to start with one tablet a day and increase the dosage to two to three tablets a day, as tolerated. The hematocrit and reticulocyte count are determined approximately 1 week after initiation of treatment, at which time a mild increase in the reticulocyte count should be seen. If no reticulocytosis is present, one must consider lack of patient compliance, poor absorption, continuous bleeding, or the wrong diagnosis. If iron sulfate is not tolerated, other oral preparations such as ferrous gluconate should be substituted. If oral iron is not tolerated or is poorly absorbed, or

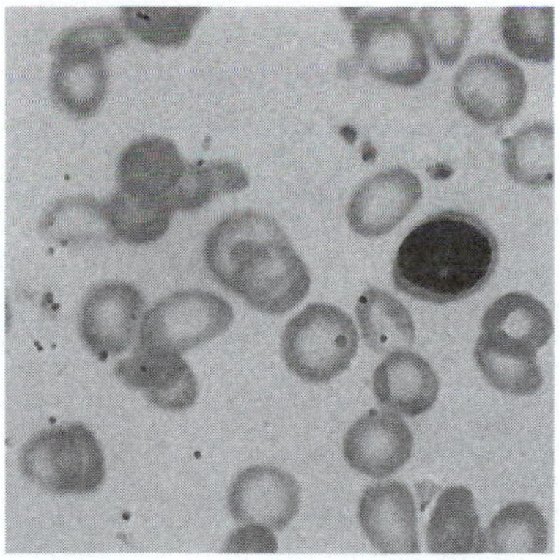

**Fig. 52-1.** Severe iron deficiency.

**Table 52-2.** Relationship between iron stores, laboratory findings, and clinical manifestations with worsening iron deficiency

| Laboratory test | Normal | Early iron deficiency | Mild anemia | Severe anemia |
|---|---|---|---|---|
| Bone marrow iron stores | Normal | Absent | Absent | Absent |
| Serum ferritin | Normal | Reduced | Low | Very low |
| Serum iron | Normal | Reduced | Low | Very low |
| Total iron binding capacitiy (TIBC) | Normal | Increased | High | High |
| TIBC % saturation | 30-40 | 20-30 | <20 | <15 |
| RBC indices | Normal | Normal | Microcytic, hypochromic | Microcytic, hypochromic |

if iron reserves have to be replenished rapidly, parenteral iron therapy may be given. The commonly used preparations are iron dextran complexes for intramuscular or intravenous use containing 50 mg iron per milliliter. The total dose of parenteral iron is calculated from tables supplied by the manufacturer.

***Megaloblastic anemias.*** Megaloblastic anemias (macrocytic anemias) are seen less frequently than iron-deficiency anemias. When they are diagnosed or suspected, a hematologist can be helpful.

**Pathophysiology.** Megaloblastic anemia results from defective nuclear maturation, commonly a consequence of either folic acid or vitamin $B_{12}$ deficiency. The term *pernicious anemia* is used specifically for the deficiency of vitamin $B_{12}$ that results from its malabsorption due to lack of intrinsic factor and not to its malabsorption for other reasons or its absence from the diet. These anemias are grouped together because the term *megaloblastic* refers to specific changes in the morphology of red cell precursors best seen in bone marrow aspirates. Myelodysplastic syndromes may also present with macrocytic red cells and megaloblastic morphology.

Folic acid deficiency may result from an inadequate dietary intake (absolute or relative to needs), lack of absorption, or a block in the conversion of folate to tetrahydrofolate (see the box below). The normal serum folate level ranges between 6 and 21 mg/L. It takes approximately 4 months for anemia to develop in the absence of folate. Nutritional folate deficiency is found predominantly in alcoholics, in persons with special or unusual diets (diets predominant in starches and grain with little animal protein or fresh fruit and vegetables), or in those on prolonged parenteral nutrition administered without folate supplements. Inadequate absorption is seen in association with tropical and nontropical sprue (celiac disease).

Vitamin $B_{12}$ (cobalamin) is actively absorbed in the presence of intrinsic factor, a glycoprotein produced in gastric parietal cells. Large hepatic stores and the slow utilization by the marrow explain the long latent period preceding the development of vitamin $B_{12}$ deficiency after total gastrectomy (up to 6 years) and the long remissions seen in patients with pernicious anemia after cessation of therapy. The most common cause of vitamin $B_{12}$ deficiency is addisonian pernicious anemia caused by the absence of intrinsic factor with associated gastric atrophy. It is seen more often in middle-aged and elderly persons, particularly of northern European descent. African-American women appear to develop it earlier in life. The absence of intrinsic factor may be due to an immune mechanism combined with a genetic predisposition. Vitamin $B_{12}$–deficiency anemia has also been described in vegans and strict vegetarians who do not drink milk. After total and occasionally partial gastrectomy, malabsorption of vitamin $B_{12}$ develops as a result of removal of the source of intrinsic factor. Removal of the distal ileum can also result in vitamin $B_{12}$ deficiency because of the elimination of the site of absorption. Gastrointestinal surgical procedures resulting in a blind intestinal loop can lead to excessive utilization of vitamin $B_{12}$ by overgrowth of bacteria, thereby causing a decrease in the availability of the vitamin for absorption. A similar situation exists with infestation of the fish tapeworm, *Diphyllobothrium latum,* which utilizes available $B_{12}$. Chronic alcoholism can also produce vitamin $B_{12}$ malabsorption in conjunction with chronic gastritis and damage to the parietal cells.

**Clinical findings.** Typical symptoms of chronic anemia develop insidiously in megaloblastic anemias. In pernicious anemia there is usually a yellowish pallor to the skin and oral mucosa. Physical examination occasionally reveals slight enlargement of the spleen. More important, severe vitamin $B_{12}$ deficiency may be accompanied by neurologic complications such as paresthesias, abnormal gait, difficulty with coordination, and mental deterioration. As pernicious anemia progresses, impaired vibratory and position sense and ataxic or spastic gait develop. The neurologic changes reflect involvement of the dorsal and lateral columns of the spinal cord (subacute combined systems disease). These changes are not found with folate deficiency. Because folate administration partially corrects the anemia of vitamin $B_{12}$ deficiency, the neurologic complications of this deficiency may progress when such treatment is inadvertently administered. The possibility of such complications makes the specific differential diagnosis between folate and vitamin $B_{12}$ deficiency mandatory in every case of megaloblastic anemia.

**Diagnosis and therapy.** Megaloblastic anemia should be suspected when blood counts reveal a high mean corpuscular volume (MCV) (usually above 115 $fL^3$) and the following abnormalities are present on the peripheral blood smear: macroovalocytes, severe poikilocytosis, and hypersegmentation of the nuclei of polymorphonuclear leukocytes (mean lobe count 3½ or greater, or nuclei with six nuclear segments). Mild leukopenia and thrombocytopenia are frequently present. The diagnosis is confirmed by finding low serum levels of either vitamin $B_{12}$ (usually

### Causes of folate deficiency

**Decreased availability**
Low dietary folate
Goat's milk anemia
Long-term oral antibiotics

**Decreased absorption**
Tropical sprue
Nontropical sprue
Celiac disease in children

**Increased demand**
Pregnancy
Chronic hemolysis
Chronic hemodialysis
Neoplasm
Exfoliative dermatitis

**Interference with folate metabolism**
Alcohol abuse
Anticonvulsants
Oral contraceptives
Inhibitors of dihydrofolate reductase (methotrexate, pyrimethamine, triamterene, pentamidine, trimethoprim)

less than 100 pg/ml) or serum folate (less than 4 μg/L) and by bone marrow cellular morphology that shows typical megaloblastic maturation. When the serum $B_{12}$ concentration is low, pernicious anemia must be differentiated from malabsorption due to other causes. The Schilling test determines the immediate cause of cobalamin deficiency. Other less specific laboratory findings in megaloblastic anemias are an elevated indirect bilirubin level and a very high serum lactic dehydrogenase level due to intramedullary hemolysis. If dietary folate deficiency is diagnosed, it is necessary to correct the dietary habits that led to it. In addition, administration of 1 mg of folate daily by mouth is recommended. Therapy results in a reticulocytosis reaching a peak within 6 to 8 days followed by a slow rise in hemoglobin. When there is a chronic increased demand for folic acid, as in chronic hemolytic anemias or pregnancy, it is advisable to administer 0.1 to 0.3 mg folic acid daily. If megaloblastic anemia occurs in conjunction with anticonvulsant drugs, they may be continued provided folic acid supplements are administered. For vitamin $B_{12}$ deficiency the vitamin is administered parenterally, except in rare cases of nutritional deficiency. Pernicious anemia is initially treated with 1000 μg of vitamin $B_{12}$ weekly for the first 6 weeks, followed by 1000 μg every 2 to 3 months for maintenance or 100 μg monthly for the rest of the patient's life.

## Decreased red cell production

***Anemia of chronic disease/inflammation.*** The second most common form of anemia (after iron deficiency) seen by the primary care physician is the anemia that accompanies an underlying inflammatory disease, usually chronic inflammation, the anemia of chronic disease. The discovery of a mild to moderate normochromic, normocytic anemia may be secondary to and lead to the diagnosis of any of the diseases listed in the box at right. In some cases no underlying disease is found despite a thorough evaluation. One is left with an uneasy feeling of having missed something. In such cases hematologic consultation is advisable. The anemia of chronic disease usually develops within 1 to 2 months of an illness. There is only a rough correlation between the severity of the underlying disease and that of the anemia, which results from diminished production of red cells. Iron therapy is never indicated in the anemia of chronic disease unless concomitant iron deficiency is documented. A very similar hematologic picture may be seen in patients with malignancies, especially if advanced.

**Diagnosis and therapy.** This anemia is most often normochromic normocytic and occasionally hypochromic microcytic, with a low reticulocyte count, increased reticuloendothelial iron stores, low serum iron, and low TIBC. Serum ferritin is increased, reflecting increased iron stores. When iron deficiency coexists, serum ferritin is usually reduced. In most cases there is no need to treat the anemia of inflammation. Remission of the underlying disease results in rapid amelioration of the anemia.

***Anemia of chronic renal failure.*** Severe anemia is a common complication in patients with end-stage renal disease. Red blood cell morphology is more disturbed than in anemia of inflammation, and burr cells are common (Fig. 52-2). Erythropoietin deficiency is probably the most important factor in this anemia, although uremic toxins may directly inhibit erythropoiesis. Concomitant inflammation may also be a factor. Iron deficiency may occur in patients on chronic hemodialysis as a result of blood loss on the dialysis membrane as well as from bleeding secondary to uremic gastroenteritis and platelet dysfunction. The anemia of chronic renal disease may be ameliorated by the use of erythropoietin administered parenterally. In addition, patients on dialysis are given 1 mg folic acid daily. Iron may be necessary to facilitate erythropoietin's full potential.

***Stem cell defects***

**Aplastic anemia.** Perhaps one of the most disturbing experiences a physician can have is dealing with aplastic anemia, particularly in a previously healthy individual and especially when the anemia develops as the result of exposure to a drug or chemical that could have been

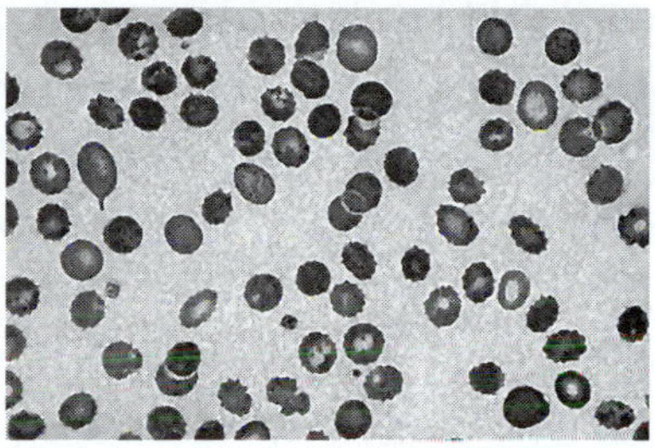

**Fig. 52-2.** Burr cell and basophilic stippling.

### Causes of anemia of chronic disease

**Chronic infection**
Any

**Chronic inflammation**
Connective tissue (immune) disorders
Severe trauma
Myocardial infarction
Burns

**Malignancy**
Carcinomas, sarcomas
Hodgkin's disease
Other lymphomas
Leukemias
Myeloma

**Chronic liver disease with or without alcoholism**

**Chronic renal disease**

**Endocrine disorder**
Hypothyroidism
Hypopituitarism
Hypogonadism
Hyperparathyroidism

avoided. The primary care physician is the first to be consulted, usually concerning hemorrhage or infection. Because of the grim prognosis and difficulty in treatment, a hematologist must be involved in the care of such patients immediately upon discovery or suspicion of the disease. Aplastic anemia is characterized by a progressive reduction of RBCs, granulocytes, and platelets. RBC morphology may be normocytic or macrocytic. The reticulocyte count is less than 1%. The granulocytes and the platelets are decreased but maintain normal morphology. Bone marrow biopsy shows predominantly lymphocytes, plasma cells, and fat cells. Occasionally small islands of hematopoiesis are found. Their persistence denotes a better prognosis with a better chance of bone marrow recovery.

**Pure red cell anemia.** Pure RBC anemia is a rare disorder in which patients present with anemia and the near or total absence of bone marrow erythrocyte precursors. The finding of a very severe anemia, no reticulocytes, and normal WBCs and platelets, should raise the clinician's suspicion for this diagnosis, and a hematologist's help should be obtained.

## ANEMIAS DUE TO INCREASED DESTRUCTION OF MATURE RED CELLS (HEMOLYTIC ANEMIAS)

The term *hemolysis* literally means "destruction of blood." The pathophysiologic abnormality is a shortening of RBC survival, normally 100 to 120 days. Regardless of the primary abnormality leading to hemolysis, the final hemolytic event results from injury to the RBC membrane. Thus any disorder that affects the membrane may result in a shortened red cell survival. The hemolytic anemias are broadly categorized as those resulting from an intrinsic defect of red cells, usually congenital, and those related to an extrinsic defect, usually acquired. They can also be categorized by the site of RBC destruction: in some situations the major site of destruction is in the circulation (intravascular), whereas in others the final hemolytic event takes place extravascularly in macrophages, primarily the spleen (Fig. 52-3). The liver becomes the predominant hemolytic organ in the absence of the spleen. The usual response of the bone marrow to hemolysis is an increase in erythropoiesis up to eightfold, reflected by a very high reticulocyte count. If the bone marrow's ability to respond to hemolysis is limited by another disease, even mild RBC destruction can lead to anemia.

Symptoms due to hemolysis depend on its severity and the rapidity with which anemia develops. Patients may be pale and slightly jaundiced. A history of cholelithiasis and splenomegaly may be found in association with congenital or long-standing hemolysis. The history may reveal similar hereditary forms in the family, and a study of parents or siblings may reveal reticulocytosis, splenomegaly, or both in otherwise compensated, silent cases. In chronic hemolytic syndromes exacerbation of hemolysis may produce a hemolytic crisis with a severe worsening of

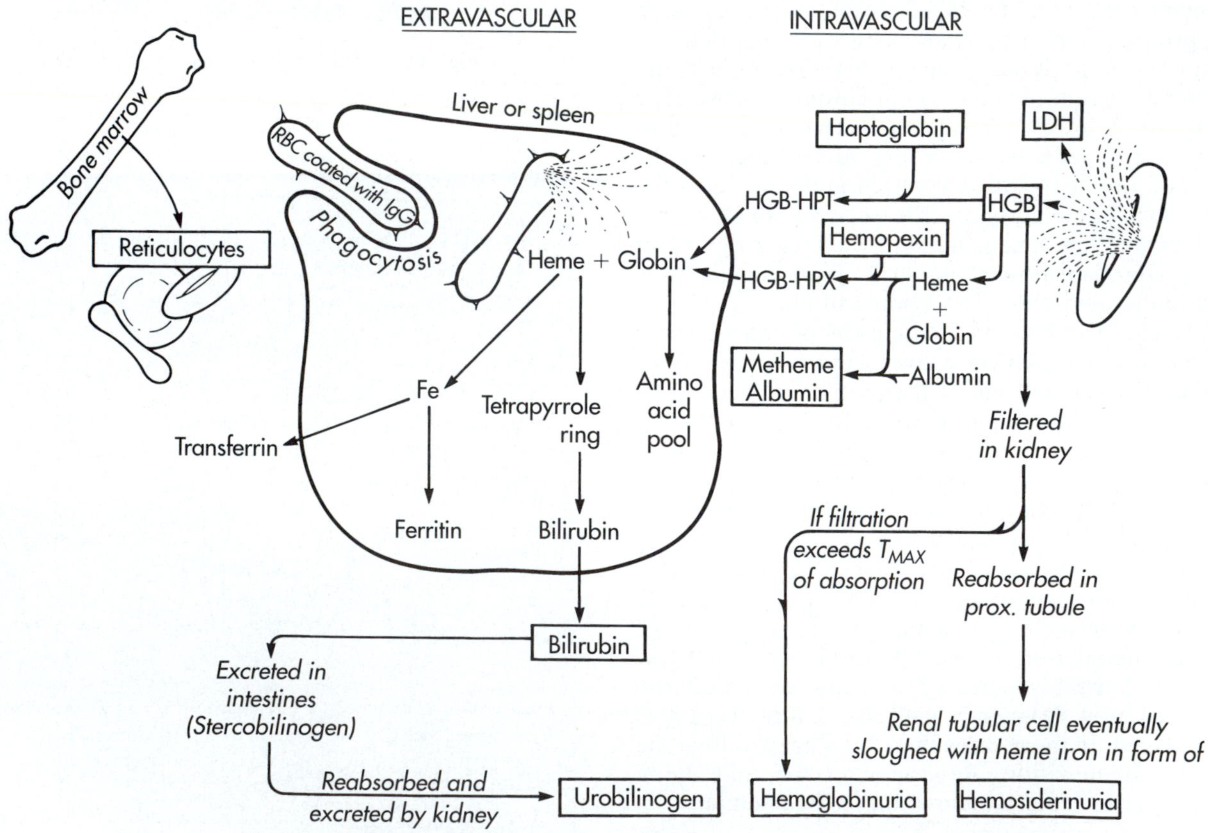


**Fig. 52-3.** Hemoglobin metabolites and other substances resulting from intravascular and extravascular hemolysis. Items enclosed in rectangles indicate assays routinely obtained that reflect hemolysis. These tests are more likely to be positive with intravascular hemolysis than with extravascular hemolysis. *HGB*, Hemoglobin; *HPT*, haptoglobin; *HPX*, hemopexin; *LDH*, lactic dehydrogenase.

the anemia. Hemolysis should be suspected whenever the reticulocyte count is increased without evidence of blood loss. Depending on the cause of the hemolysis, spherocytes or other abnormalities in red cell shape may be present on the peripheral blood smear (Fig. 52-4). Definitive proof of the existence of hemolysis is provided by a shortened red cell survival, although survival studies are infrequently indicated. Unconjugated bilirubin is usually increased in hemolytic states because of the release of hemoglobin breakdown pigments from macrophages. Jaundice becomes clinically detectable when bilirubin levels exceed 4 mg/dl. Decreased plasma haptoglobin (a protein synthesized in the liver that binds free hemoglobin), hemoglobinemia, hemoglobinuria, hemosiderinuria, and an elevated lactic dehydrogenase (LDH) level may be present, particularly in association with intravascular hemolysis (see Fig. 52-3).

### Anemias resulting from extrinsic red cell defects

***Immune hemolysis.*** Immune hemolysis is due to immunologic damage to the erythrocyte membrane, caused by antibodies. Immunoglobulin M–coated RBCs are removed primarily in the liver, whereas those coated with IgG antibodies are preferentially cleared by the spleen. When the RBCs are coated with complement, its complete activation results in severe membrane damage, causing intravascular hemolysis, which may occur in IgM-mediated hemolysis. Drugs have been implicated in approximately 17% of all cases of acquired immune hemolytic anemia (see the box at right). Four mechanisms result in drug-induced hemolytic anemia (Table 52-3).

Autoimmune hemolytic anemias (AIHAs) of the IgG type are the most common form of acquired immune hemolytic anemias. They are estimated to occur in approximately 1 to 2 per 100,000 population, and they account for 70% of cases. Hematologic consultation is often helpful for their diagnosis and therapy. AIHAs can be classified into two major categories: those due to cold-reactive antibodies and those due to warm-reactive antibodies. Cold AIHA, or the cold agglutinin syndrome, is characterized by the presence of IgM autoantibodies, and it commonly accompanies an infection or malignant disease. Sometimes no associated disease is found. The most common infections associated with cold agglutinin AIHA are those caused by *Mycoplasma pneumoniae* and infectious mononucleosis. Clinical manifestations reflect the anemia and vascular disturbances related to cold agglutinins (e.g., acrocyanosis, Raynaud's phenomenon, and gangrene of the extremities), all of which are precipitated by exposure to cold and partially relieved by rewarming of extremities. In warm-reactive AIHA usually induced by IgG autoantibodies, hemolysis is mainly extravascular, with the spleen being the major site of RBC destruction. Warm AIHA may be primary (idiopathic) or secondary to an underlying disease (see the box on p. 728). Physical examination reveals moderate splenomegaly in more than half of the patients, mild to moderate hepatomegaly, occasional lymphadenopathy, and frequent jaundice. There may be a history of passing dark urine.

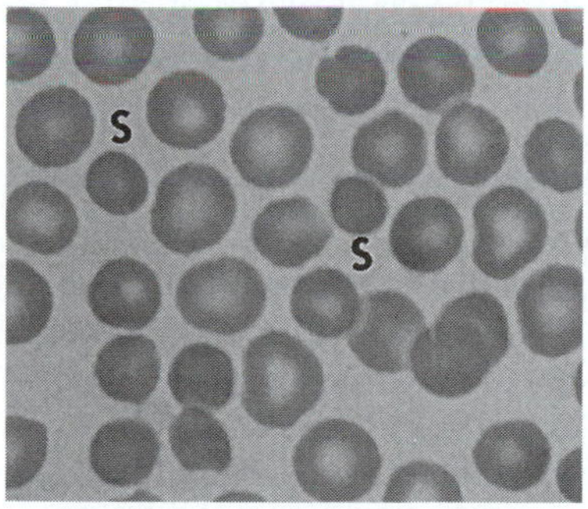


**Fig. 52-4.** Spherocytes (S). Wright's stain. Magnification × 1000.

#### Drugs implicated in immune hemolytic anemia

- Stibophen
- Quinidine
- Quinine
- Para-aminosalicylic acid
- Phenacetin
- Pyramidon
- Penicillin
- Cephalosporins
- Dipyrone
- α-Methyldopa
- Levodopa (L-dopa)
- Mefenamic acid
- Sulfonamides
- Phenothiazides
- Antihistamines
- Barbiturates
- Amphetamines
- Mesantoin
- Methylene blue
- Insecticides

**Table 52-3.** Mechanisms of drug-induced immune hemolytic anemia

| Type | Role of drug | Antibody attachment |
|---|---|---|
| Innocent bystander or immune complex (quinidine) | Induces antibody to drug | Drug antibody absorbed to red cell membrane |
| Hapten (penicillin) | Combines with red cell membrane | Antibody bound to drug–red cell complex |
| Autoantibody (α-methyldopa) | Induces antibody to drug | Binds to Rh antigen on red cell membrane |
| Nonspecific (cephalosporins) | Alters red cell membrane | Plasma proteins absorbed to red cell membrane |

## Disorders frequently associated with warm-antibody AIHA*

**Reticuloendothelial disease**
Chronic lymphocytic leukemia
Hodgkin's disease
Non-Hodgkin's lymphomas
Thymoma
Multiple myeloma
Waldenström macroglobulinemia

**Collagen disease**
Systemic lupus erythematosus
Scleroderma
Rheumatoid arthritis

**Infectious diseases, especially childhood viral syndromes**

**Immunologic diseases**
Hypogammaglobulinemia
Dysglobulinemias
Other immune deficiency syndromes

**Gastrointestinal disease**
Ulcerative colitis

**Benign tumors**
Ovarian dermoid cyst

*Does not include drugs that cause AIHA.

Laboratory studies are essential. Most important, a direct antiglobulin, or Coombs, test is positive in the vast majority of cases of AIHA. The reticulocyte count is invariably increased unless there is concomitant bone marrow depression. The hematocrit may be moderately to severely decreased, and spherocytes are characteristic. In some patients with warm-reacting IgG antibodies nucleated RBCs may be present in the peripheral blood smear. Serum bilirubin is moderately increased (usually 2.5 to 5 mg/dl) and mostly unconjugated. Urine and fecal urobilinogen are elevated as well. When hemolysis is suspected, hematologic consultation can be helpful.

The first step in the evaluation of a patient with AIHA is a thorough search for an underlying disease such as a lymphoma or chronic lymphocytic leukemia. If discovered and treated successfully, the hemolytic anemia may abate. If no underlying cause is found or if the hemolysis is severe enough to necessitate immediate treatment, corticosteroids are administered. Unfortunately, steroids are ineffective in most patients with idiopathic cold agglutinin disease. In chronic high-titer cold agglutinin disease, exposure to cold should be avoided. With warm-reactive AIHA, if no response to prednisone is obtained within 3 weeks, splenectomy should be considered. A trial of intravenous gammaglobulins (1 g/kg once or 0.4 g/kg daily for 3 days) may also be beneficial, but it is expensive. RBC transfusions are occasionally necessary, but this can be a difficult undertaking. In general, patients with AIHA are serologically incompatible with most blood donors' red cells, resulting in difficulty in crossmatching. In patients with cold agglutinin disease the administered RBCs are warmed to body temperature. Finally, plasmapheresis has been tried in the cold agglutinin hemolytic anemias to remove antibodies, but its results may be short lived.

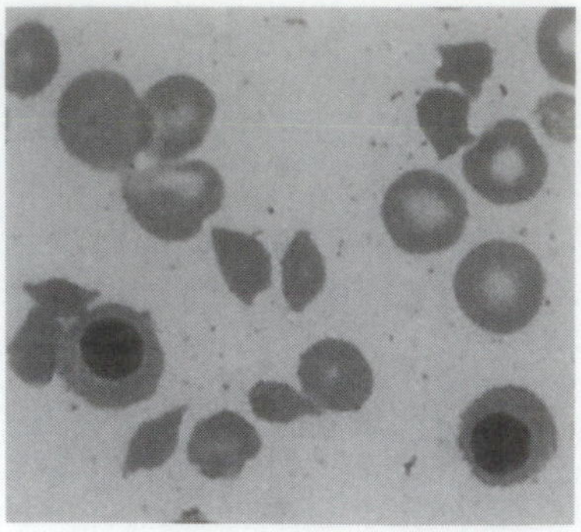

**Fig. 52-5.** Schistocytes and nucleated red cells. Wright's stain. Magnification × 1000.

*Mechanical injuries.* Microangiopathic hemolytic anemia (mechanical red cell destruction) develops when erythrocytes are traumatized in the microcirculation. The hallmark of this type of anemia is finding schistocytes, or fragmented, deformed, helmetlike erythrocytes (Fig. 52-5). These broken nonpliable cells become entrapped and engulfed by macrophages, thus leading to a shortened survival. Disseminated intravascular coagulation (DIC), in which RBCs are sheared on fibrin strands, is a typical cause of microangiopathic hemolytic anemia. In carcinomatosis the red cell shearing is probably the result of direct contact with intraluminal embolic tumor cells. Red cell fragmentation also occurs in thrombotic thrombocytopenic purpura, severe peripheral vascular disease, amyloidosis, immune disorders, malignant hypertension, and eclampsia. Mechanical hemolysis also occurs with severely damaged cardiac valves, as with severe atherosclerotic aortic valvular disease, or after replacement of heart valves with prostheses, the so-called Waring blender syndrome.

### Anemias resulting from intrinsic red cell defects

*Membrane defects*

**Hereditary spherocytosis.** Hereditary spherocytosis (HS) is the most common of the hereditary hemolytic anemias among persons of northern European descent. It is transmitted as an autosomal dominant trait, although sporadic cases have also been described. HS is characterized by the presence of anemia, jaundice, splenomegaly, and spherocytes. There is usually a family history of anemia. The intrinsic membrane defect renders the cells highly susceptible to membrane loss, which probably accounts for their spherocytic shape (see Fig. 52-4). Patients usually become symptomatic before age 10, but mild cases may not be diagnosed until adulthood, and many affected subjects are found only by systematic studies of HS families. Cholelithiasis is prevalent, even in asymptomatic patients. Although the anemia is usually mild to moderate, aplastic crises (temporary decrease in the bone marrow's ability to compensate for hemolysis) may produce severe exacerbations. HS must be distinguished from acquired hemolytic disorders, which can also be accompanied by spherocytosis. The direct antiglobulin test is negative, and the RBCs' osmotic fragility is increased. Splenectomy is the single most important therapeutic intervention in HS. Splenectomy results in a clinical cure, although spherocytes and abnormal osmotic fragility persist because the membrane defect remains.

**Paroxysmal nocturnal hemoglobinuria.** PNH is a rare hemolytic anemia characterized by intravascular hemolysis with hemoglobinuria. PNH is not a hereditary form of hemolytic anemia, but an acquired genetic disorder due to a mutation in a bone marrow hematopoietic cell precursor. It affects all the descendants arising from this mutated clone: RBCs, WBCs, and platelets. Nevertheless, the most obvious and early manifestations are related to hemolysis, since the acquired erythrocyte membrane defect renders them markedly sensitive to complement activation. Patients present with intermittent dark red urine, particularly at morning voiding, a moderate degree of anemia due to chronic hemolysis, leukopenia, and thrombocytopenia. When suspected, PNH should be managed with the help of a hematologist experienced in this condition. The disease progresses over a few years. It may evolve into aplastic anemia or acute leukemia. The diagnosis is based on the Ham acidified serum lysis test. A simple screening test, the sugar-water test, is suggestive of the disease if positive. Occasionally it may be negative and the Ham test may still be positive. Treatment involves intermittent transfusion therapy with washed RBCs (to eliminate complement). Iron is given to replace iron lost in urine as hemosiderin. Surgery is avoided, since these patients are poor surgical risks. Anticoagulation prophylaxis has been recommended for patients with PNH because they are prone to thrombotic events. When thrombotic episodes develop acutely, thrombolytic therapy may be salutary. Finally, bone marrow transplantation may be considered.

***Hemoglobinopathies.*** Two major hemoglobinopathies are considered here: the sickle cell syndromes and the thalassemias. A hematologist must be involved in managing patients who are severely affected (usually homozygotes), so this discussion focuses on the heterozygote condition, which is only mildly symptomatic or asymptomatic. More than 300 types of hemoglobinopathies have been described, most being characterized by single or, rarely, multiple amino acid substitutions in the globin chains, which reduce the solubility of hemoglobin leading to increased RBC intracytoplasmic viscosity, decreased membrane pliability, and shortened RBC survival. The thalassemias, however, are characterized by reduced synthesis of either $\alpha$-chains ($\alpha$-thalassemia) or $\beta$-chains ($\beta$-thalassemia), which results in precipitation of the normal (but excess) $\beta$- or $\alpha$-chains, respectively, and causes membrane ridigity and shortened RBC survival. In both situations the final hemolytic event is precipitated by a change in the properties of the cell membrane. The electrophoretic mobility of hemoglobins with amino acid substitutions is usually abnormal and can be identified by hemoglobin electrophoresis.

**Sickle cell disease.** Homozygous sickle cell anemia is an inherited disease found primarily in people of African ancestry, the gene having originated in two regions of West Africa and providing a possible survival advantage to individuals infected with the malarial parasite. The basic defect in sickle cell disease is replacement of glutamic acid by valine at position 6 of the $\beta$-chain, leading to hemoglobin S (two normal $\alpha$ and two $\beta_s$ chains). Polymerization of deoxyhemoglobin is the ultimate cause of the sickling phenomenon. The end result of sickling is occlusion of precapillary arterioles and infarction of surrounding tissues. Hemolysis occurs because of increased membrane rigidity of the deformed cells.

Patients with sickle cell trait or the heterozygous condition have erythrocytes that contain 20% to 40% hemoglobin S, with most of the remainder being normal adult hemoglobin (hemoglobin $A_1$). Sickle cell trait may be associated with a mild renal tubular defect that results in an inability to concentrate urine, but generally the condition is completely asymptomatic. Rarely, upon exposure to severe hypoxia, the sickling phenomenon can be induced and can lead to symptoms. Sickle cell trait is present in approximately 8% to 10% of African-Americans. Hemoglobin S also occurs in association with other abnormal hemoglobins, such as hemoglobin C and hemoglobin D, or with thalassemia trait. These are called sickle cell variants and produce symptoms of varying severity.

The clinical picture of sickle cell anemia is that of a severe, constant, hemolytic anemia interrupted by vasoocclusive (painful) or aplastic crises. Symptoms first occur during the second half of the first year of life when most fetal hemoglobin has been replaced by hemoglobin S. Patients become progressively more anemic and develop splenomegaly. Eventually splenic function is lost from repeated thromboses (autosplenectomy), which can lead to an increased risk of infections during childhood. Such children should be managed by hematologists with expertise in this condition.

One major problem experienced by patients is pain crisis (vasoocclusive episodes) caused by infarctions that lead to recurrent attacks of pain involving the chest, abdomen, and skeleton. Aplastic crises resulting in acute exacerbation of anemia develop as a result of infections when compensatory RBC production is impaired. This situation can be fatal if the anemia becomes severe. Bone disease develops owing to multiple infarctions and expansion of the bone marrow cavity. Vascular occlusions may cause avascular necrosis of the hip or shoulder. Osteomyelitis caused by *Salmonella* organisms is not an uncommon sequela. The sequence of marrow infarction, necrosis, and the healing process results in new bone formation, which produces characteristic radiographic changes. Cardiomegaly and pulmonary disease develops secondary to anemia and repeated infections and infarctions. The acute chest syndrome is a complication characterized by fever, pleuritic pain, lung infiltrates, and hypoxemia. It is fatal in 2% to 14% of cases due to infection, infarction, or both.

Antibiotics should be immediately instituted in the presence of fever and arterial $Po_2$ should be monitored. The right upper quadrant syndrome manifests as pain, fever, and jaundice. It may be due to acute cholecystitis, extrahepatic biliary tract obstruction, viral hepatitis, or infarction in the liver. Stroke may be another catastrophic complication of sickle cell anemia. If CT scan or MRI examination is considered, one must be careful with the use of contrast dyes, even the newer nonionic contrast agents, unless the hemoglobin is at least 5 g/dl. Hyposthenuria, hematuria, priapism, and the nephrotic syndrome are occasionally encountered. Retinal detachment, blindness, and vitreous hemorrhages are common ocular complications. As a result of complications and repeated crises, not many patients live beyond the third decade.

Hemoglobin electrophoresis demonstrates only a hemoglobin S band in sickle cell anemia, and both hemoglobin $A_1$ and hemoglobin S in sickle cell trait. Hemoglobin F may be slightly elevated. Screening tests are based on rapid sickling of red cells under hypoxic conditions on peripheral smears or on solubility properties that allow distinction between Hb AS, SS, and A. In sickle cell anemia the presence of numerous sickled cells on Wright-stained blood smears is easily seen. Technical advances in amniocentesis have enabled the diagnosis of sickle cell anemia as early as the sixteenth week of gestation. When this is not feasible, fetoscopy and fetal blood sampling are required, although these procedures are associated with an increased risk of fetal loss and occasional false positive or false negative results. Because one out of four offspring has the homozygous disease if both parents have sickle cell trait, genetic counseling of young couples carrying the sickle cell gene can prevent the trauma of caring for a child afflicted with sickle cell anemia.

Treatment of sickle cell anemia is aimed at relieving the painful vasoocclusive crises, treating the secondary effects of the chronic anemia, and if possible correcting the anemia. Treatment also requires supplementation with folic acid (1 mg daily) and prevention of infections with prompt antibiotic treatment or by vaccination (pneumococcal vaccine). The treatment of vasoocclusive crises relies on supporting measures: analgesics, intravenous fluids, and oxygen. With severe and prolonged pain, narcotic analgesics are often necessary. Oxygen is commonly used to diminish hypoxia, but its benefits have not been substantiated. If acidosis is present, sodium bicarbonate is added, usually one ampule (44 mEq) to each liter of 0.45% saline in 5% glucose, but as with oxygen therapy its benefits have not been proven. Partial exchange transfusions may be indicated in situations of prolonged vasoocclusive crises, before elective surgery, for priapism, or during pregnancy. It is advisable to maintain the hematocrit at 25% throughout pregnancy, since sickle cell blood is closest to normal viscosity at this level. At delivery regional or spinal anesthesia should be used and proper oxygenation ensured. Recently efforts to optimize erythropoiesis by administering erythropoietin and to increase fetal hemoglobin with hydroxyurea or butyrate have undergone initially promising trials.

**Hemoglobin C disease.** Hemoglobin C disease is found in approximately 3% of heterozygotes. In West Africa the carrier rate may reach 25%. The homozygous form of hemoglobin C disease has a characteristic picture on peripheral blood smears. The interaction between hemoglobin S trait and hemoglobin C trait is quite common, occurring once in every 833 births to African-Americans. Individuals with hemoglobin SC disease tend to have a variable course, with complications occurring less frequently than with sickle cell anemia but with more symptoms than either trait alone. These patients have been reported to develop thromboembolic complications, retinopathy, and renal papillary necrosis more frequently than patients with sickle cell anemia.

***Thalassemias.*** The thalassemia syndromes are a heterogenous group of inherited disorders resulting from suboptimal synthesis of either the α- or β- globin chains, called, respectively, α- and β-thalassemia. They result from genetic defects at any one of a number of sites in the production of globin. The clinical expression of the thalassemic defect depends on the globin chain involved, the extent of the defect, and the adequacy of compensatory adjustments in the production of other globin chains. The normal globin chains become unbalanced because of a decrease in the affected chains, forming intraerythrocytic inclusions that damage the RBC membrane and lead to hemolysis. For instance, in homozygous β-thalassemia, excess α-chains precipitate on the red cell membrane, forming inclusions called Heinz bodies. These inclusions in turn cause increased red cell rigidity, membrane damage, and subsequent hemolysis. The homozygous thalassemias should be treated in specialized centers.

**β-Thalassemia.** β-Thalassemia major (Cooley's anemia, Mediterranean anemia) is a severe, transfusion-dependent anemia that can be fatal by late childhood or early adolescence. It is found in persons homozygous or doubly heterozygous for a mutation that affects the capacity for synthesis of β-globin subunits of hemoglobin. In the fully manifested case a severe anemia with drastically reduced MCV and mean corpuscular hemoglobin concentration (MCHC) is always found. In β-thalassemia trait (heterozygous β-thalassemia) normal α-chains are synthesized in parallel with decreased (but not absent) β-chains. Patients develop hypochromic, microcytic indices, mild poikilocytosis, and anisocytosis and are often misdiagnosed as having iron-deficiency anemia. In β-thalassemia trait, however, the RBC count is normal or even elevated in relation to the hematocrit, whereas it is decreased in iron-deficiency anemia. The two conditions must be distinguished and a firm diagnosis of β-thalassemia trait established for purposes of genetic counseling and to avoid iron therapy. With thalassemia trait hemoglobin $A_2$ levels average 5.1% (normal upper limit is 3.7%), and in 50% of cases the hemoglobin F levels are mildly elevated to 2% to 5% (the upper normal limit being 2%).

The major problem in β-thalassemia major is the severity of the anemia. Compensatory mechanisms result in extramedullary hematopoiesis with hepatosplenomegaly. Expansion of the bone marrow leads to skeletal abnormalities, secondary thinning of cortices of long bones, and pathologic fractures. Patients require frequent transfusions, which result in hemosiderosis. Elimination of excess iron may be achieved with iron chelators (e.g., deferoxamine B) administered intramuscularly or via continuous intravenous infusion. Such treatment may result in a significant decrease in iron accumulation in tissues and hopefully longer and healthier survival. Bone marrow transplantation or molecular manipulations that would allow insertion of messenger RNA containing normal genetic information for the synthesis of β-chains are in preliminary stages of research.

**α-Thalassemia.** The α-thalassemia syndromes are a group of inherited disorders with decreased synthesis of α-chains. They are especially common in Chinese and Southeast Asians but may also be encountered in people originating from Africa, the Middle East, and the Mediterranean area. In contrast to β-thalassemia, hemoglobins

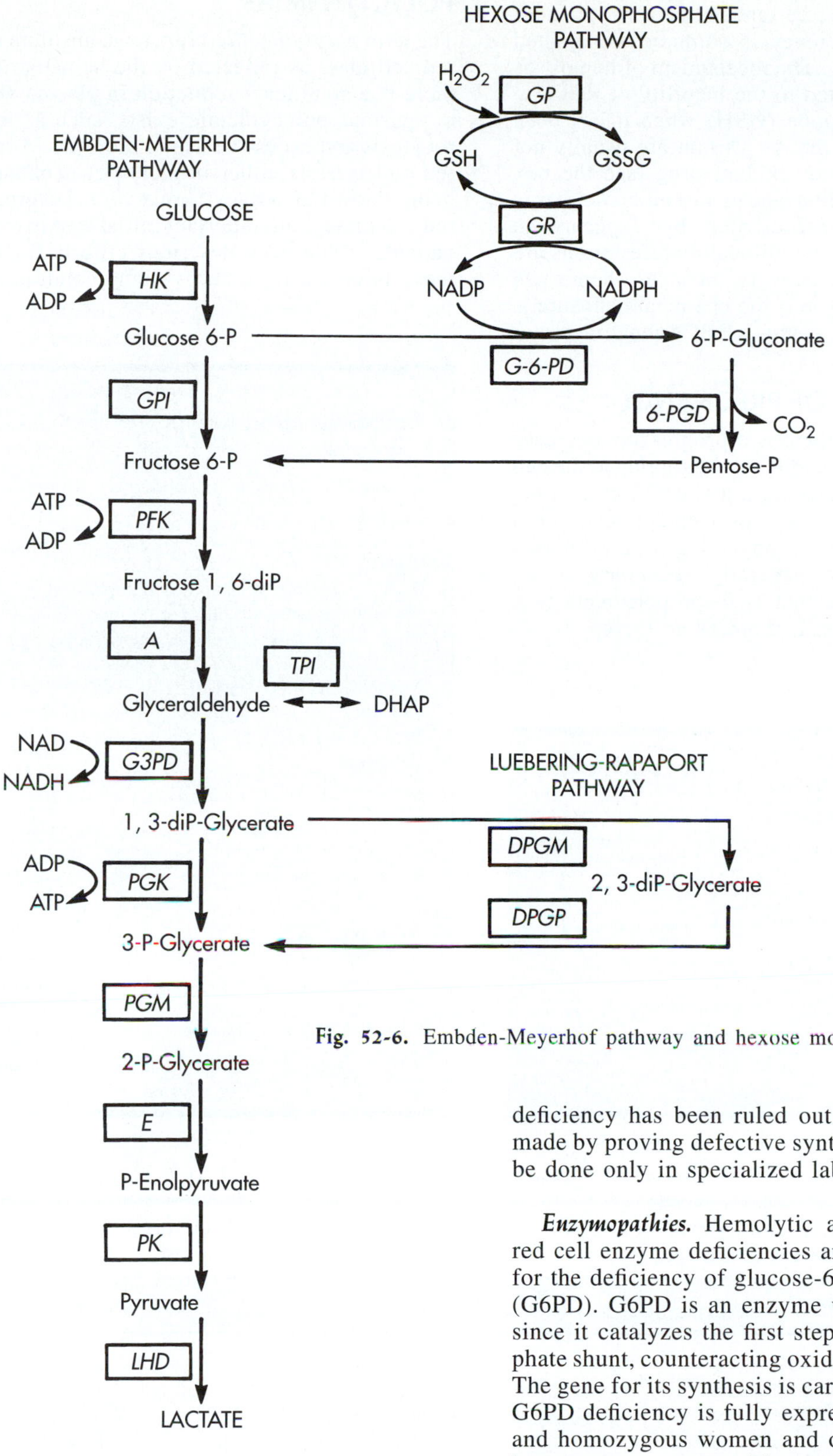


**Fig. 52-6.** Embden-Meyerhof pathway and hexose monophosphate shunt in RBCs.

$A_2$ and F are decreased because of decreased α-chains, which are constituents of both $A_2$ and F hemoglobins. α-Thalassemia trait should be suspected in a patient belonging to the appropriate ethnic group who presents with microcytic, hypochromic anemia, normal or decreased hemoglobins $A_2$ and F, and in whom iron deficiency has been ruled out. A definitive diagnosis is made by proving defective synthesis of α-chains. This can be done only in specialized laboratories.

***Enzymopathies.*** Hemolytic anemias due to hereditary red cell enzyme deficiencies are exceedingly rare except for the deficiency of glucose-6-phosphate dehydrogenase (G6PD). G6PD is an enzyme vital to the RBC integrity, since it catalyzes the first step in the hexose monophosphate shunt, counteracting oxidative processes (Fig. 52-6). The gene for its synthesis is carried on the X chromosome. G6PD deficiency is fully expressed in heterozygous men and homozygous women and only partially expressed in heterozygous women. The enzyme deficiency appears to offer a selective advantage against the malarial parasite. There are two normal variants of the enzyme differing by one amino acid and designated A+ and B+ (+ denotes the presence of the enzyme and − denotes its absence), the former of which is prevalent in people of African ancestry. In the United States the most common deficiency is the A− type: approximately 12% of African-Americans are affected, and 20% of African-American women are heterozygous. Among Mediterranean persons a more severe type of G6PD deficiency is common, designated G6PD Mediterranean or B–. The mechanism of hemolysis in G6PD deficiency is related to the inability of RBCs to regenerate reduced glutathione (GSH) when it has been oxidized. Individuals with the A– variant are usually not anemic unless exposed to an oxidant drug (see the box below), whereas in the Mediterranean variant hemolysis is chronically present and exacerbated by exposure to oxidants. In the A– variety the clinical manifestations are episodic, with complete recovery between hemolytic episodes. This can occur even if the chemical exposure is continued because the new, younger RBCs contain greater amounts of the G6PD.

## DILUTIONAL ANEMIA OF PREGNANCY

During normal pregnancy there is a progressive decrease of hemoglobin, hematocrit, and RBCs beginning at the end of the first trimester and reaching a maximum around the twentieth week, with a slight improvement near term. These changes, referred to as physiologic or dilutional anemia of pregnancy, are generally secondary to an increase in plasma volume that is disproportionate to a mild increase in RBC mass. It requires no therapy.

### Drugs that produce hemolysis of G6PD-deficient RBCs

Sulfonamides
Antimalarials
Nitrofurans (nitrofurantoin)
Analgesics (aspirin, phenacetin)
Diuretics (thiazides, acetazolamide)
Hypoglycemic agents (tolbutamide, chlorpropamide)
Sulfones
Miscellaneous (naphthalene, vitamin K, quinidine, probenicid, isoniazid)

## POLYCYTHEMIAS

The term *polycythemia* refers to an absolute increase in the red cell mass as reflected by the hematocrit. However, if there is a significant reduction in plasma volume, a false or spurious polycythemia exists, such as in stress erythrocytosis and excessive use of diuretics. A true increase in red cell mass is either primary or secondary, the former being known as polycythemia vera. Determination of the red cell mass is an important initial step in evaluating these patients. Table 52-4 describes criteria for distinguishing these three entities. The various conditions resulting in

### Causes of secondary polycythemias

**Appropriate increase in erythropoietin production**
High altitude
Chronic lung disease
Right-to-left cardiovascular shunt
High oxygen affinity hemoglobinopathy
Massive obesity with chronic hypoxia
High concentration of carboxyhemoglobin

**Inappropriate increase in erythropoietin production**
Tumors
Renal carcinoma
Hepatoma
Cerebellar hemangioblastoma
Pheochromocytoma
Carcinomas of the ovary, prostate, lung, breast, adrenal cortex
Uterine fibroid

**Renal abnormalities**
Hydronephrosis
Nephrotic syndrome
Renal cysts
Kidney transplantation

**Benign familial erythrocytosis**

**Table 52-4.** Differential diagnosis of relative erythrocytosis, secondary erythrocytosis, and polycythemia vera

| Examination | Relative erythrocytosis | Secondary erythrocytosis | Polycythemia vera |
|---|---|---|---|
| RBC mass | N | I | I |
| Plasma volume | D | N or I | N or I |
| Granulocytes | N | N | N or I |
| Platelets | N | N | N or I |
| Serum vitamin $B_{12}$ | N | N | I |
| Transcobalamin 1 | N | N | I |
| Serum iron | N | N | Usually D |
| Leukocyte alkaline phosphatase | N | N | N or I |
| Arterial oxygen saturation | N | N or D | N |
| Bone marrow | N | Erythroid hyperplasia | Panhyperplasia |
| Erythropoietin | N | I | N or D |
| Splenomegaly | Absent | Absent | Usually present |

*N,* Normal; *D,* decreased; *I,* increased.

secondary polycythemia are listed in the box on p. 732. In all cases erythropoietin is increased and the primary stimulus for its secretion must be found.

### Polycythemia vera

Polycythemia vera is a chronic myeloproliferative disease. It occurs mostly after the fifth decade and is characterized by an increased production of RBCs with variable increases in granuloycytes and platelets. The red cells are responsive to, but not dependent on, erythropoietin for their maturation. In fact, their precursors may be excessively sensitive to erythropoietin. The disease starts insidiously with fatigue and weakness. When hyperviscosity develops, the patients present with dizziness, headaches, and visual problems. Occasionally the disease is discovered after an episode of acute thrombosis or during investigation of a bleeding tendency. In some cases patients complain of itching, particularly after a warm bath. The typical patient is plethoric with congestion of the oral mucosa and a ruddy complexion. Splenomegaly is present in more than two thirds of patients.

To establish the diagnosis of polycythemia vera, two groups of criteria have been established (see the box below). The diagnosis is considered firmly established if the three major criteria are present or if the first two major criteria plus two minor criteria are documented. Polycythemia vera is a chronic disorder with a median survival of 9 years. The disease transforms into acute nonlymphocytic leukemia in some patients. In most other cases patients become progressively anemic with increasing bone marrow fibrosis and reduction of hematopoietic tissue (i.e., spent polycythemia). Extramedullary hematopoiesis may develop, and the spleen may become enormous. Complete bone marrow failure with severe pancytopenia develops in the final phase of such cases.

Once the diagnosis of polycythemia vera has been established, the red cell mass should be reduced to normal levels. This should best be managed in collaboration with a hematologist. Therapy must be individualized for the stage of disease and for symptoms. Three therapeutic approaches are available: phlebotomy, myelosuppressive agents, and radioactive phosphorus ($^{32}P$). Recent studies suggest that Interferon-$\alpha$ is a promising agent. Elective surgery should not be performed until polycythemia vera has been well controlled because of the high incidence of postoperative thrombotic and hemorrhagic complications.

#### Criteria for the diagnosis of polycythemia vera

**Major criteria**

RBC mass: Male >36 ml/kg
Female >32 ml/kg
Arterial $O_2$ saturation >92%
Splenomegaly

**Minor criteria**

Thrombocytosis >400,000/µl
Leukocytosis >12,000/µl
Leukocyte alkaline phosphatase activity >100 (no fever or infection)
Serum vitamin $B_{12}$ >900 pg/ml or unbound vitamin $B_{12}$ binding capacity >2200 pg/ml
Polycythemia vera is considered present if the patient has all three major criteria or the first two major criteria plus any two minor criteria.

Modified from Wasserman IR: The management of polycythemia vera, *Br J Haematol* 21:371, 1971.

## HEMOCHROMATOSIS

Iron overload refers to total body iron stores in excess of 50 mg/kg. Hemochromatosis denotes a group of clinical disorders characterized by parenchymal tissue damage resulting from progressive accumulation of iron in the body. Chronic inflammation or repeated transfusions lead to excessive trapping of iron by macrophages. When the excess iron lodges in parenchymal cells, the iron leads to fibrosis of the liver and damage to the heart and other organs.

### Primary (idiopathic) hemochromatosis

Primary hemochromatosis, or idiopathic hemochromatosis, results from a somatic gene mutation, creating an inherited disorder of iron metabolism associated with the histocompatibility HLA-A3 gene on chromosome 6. It takes many years of excessive iron accumulation for the disease to become manifest in the homozygous state. That is why the advanced disease is usually seen in middle-aged and elderly persons. This disease is more common in men (10:1). Laboratory diagnosis of the disease is based on the quantitation of body iron stores through blood studies and liver biopsy. Transferrin saturation of greater than 60% in males and 50% in females is suggestive of iron overload. Serum ferritin levels above 300 µg/L in males and 200 µg/L in females indicate increased iron stores in the absence of inflammation or liver disease. Liver biopsy allows actual quantitation of stainable parenchymal iron. If the iron overload is not corrected, death from hepatic or myocardial failure often results. Hepatoma is a late but frequent complication. To treat homozygotes with established iron overload, regular phlebotomy is used to remove iron. The usual practice is to remove a unit of blood (approximately 500 ml, containing 250 mg iron) one to three times a week. After the iron stores have been depleted, the patient may be kept in normal iron balance by lifelong phlebotomies.

### Transfusional hemosiderosis

Transfusional hemosiderosis develops in patients subjected to numerous transfusions, as practiced in patients with various forms of severe chronic anemias. To avoid tissue damage produced by increasing iron deposits, chelation of the metal is recommended, particularly after 100 or more transfusions. Deferoxamine B is most effective when given by continuous infusion, which can now be administered at home through the use of portable infusion pumps.

## BIBLIOGRAPHY

Adams JA et al: Primary polycythemia, essential thrombocythemia, and myelofibrosis—three facets of a single disease process, *Acta Haemat* 79:33, 1988.

Berk PD et al: Therapeutic recommendations in polycythemia vera based on polycythemia vera study group protocols, *Semin Hematol* 23:132, 1986.

Beutler E: Glucose-6-phosphate dehydrogenase: new perspectives, *Blood* 73:1397, 1989.

Brittenham GM: Development of iron-chelating agents for clinical use, *Blood* 80:569, 1992.

Collins PW, Newland AC: Treatment modalities of autoimmune blood disorders, *Semin Hematol* 29:64, 1992.

Cook JD, Skikne BS: Iron deficiency: definition and diagnosis, *J Intern Med* 226:349, 1989.

Dessypris EN: The biology of pure red cell aplasia, *Semin Hematol* 28:275, 1991.

Edwards CQ, Kushner JP: Screening for hemochromatosis, *N Engl J Med* 328:1616, 1993.

Engelfriet CP, Overbeeke MAM, von dem Borne AE G Kr: Autoimmune hemolytic anemia, *Semin Hematol* 29:3, 1992.

Esbach JW: The anemia of chronic renal failure: pathophysiology and the effects of recombinant erythropoietin, *Kidney Int* 35:134, 1989.

Fosburg MT, Nathan DG: Treatment of Cooley's anemia, *Blood* 76:435, 1990.

Frickhofen N et al: Treatment of aplastic anemia with antilymphocyte globulin and methylprednisolone with or without cyclosporine, *N Engl J Med* 324:1297, 1991.

Kark JA et al: Sickle cell trait as a risk factor for sudden death in physical training, *N Engl J Med* 317:781, 1987.

Kazazian HH, Boehm CD: Molecular basis and prenatal diagnosis of beta thalassemia, *Blood* 72:1107, 1988.

Kernan NA et al: Analysis of 462 transplantations from unrelated donor facilitated by the national marrow donor program, *N Engl J Med* 328:593, 1993.

Means RT et al: The erythropoietin receptor in polycythemia vera, *J Clin Invest* 84:1340, 1989.

Miyata T et al: Abnormalities of PIG-A transcripts in granulocytes from patients with paroxysmal nocturnal hemoglobinuria, *N Engl J Med* 330:249, 1994.

Nissen C: The pathophysiology of aplastic anemia, *Semin Hematol* 28:313 1991.

Ohene-Frempong K, Schwartz E: Clinical features of thalassemia, *Pediatr Clin North Am* 27:403, 1980.

Perrine SP et al: A short-term trial of butyrate to stimulate fetal-globin gene expression in the β-globin disorders, *N Engl J Med* 328:81, 1993.

Rodgers GP et al: Augmentation by erythropoietin of the fetal-hemoglobin response to hydroxyurea in sickle cell disease, *N Engl J Med* 328:73, 1993.

Schilling RF: Anemia of chronic disease: a misnomer, *Ann Intern Med* 115:572, 1991.

Silver RT: A new treatment for polycythemia vera: recombinant interferon alfa, *Blood* 76:664, 1990.

Speck B: Allogeneic bone marrow transplantation for severe aplastic anemia, *Semin Hematol* 28:319, 1991.

Vichinsky EP: Comprehensive care in sickle cell disease: its impact on morbidity and mortality, *Semin Hematol* 28:220, 1991.

Wayne AS, Kevy SV, Nathan DG: Transfusion management of sickle cell disease, *Blood* 81:1109, 1993.

Weatherall D.: Bone marrow transplantation for thalassemia and other inherited disorders of hemoglobin, *Blood* 80:1379, 1992.

CHAPTER

# 53 Nonmalignant White Cell Disorders

**Philip A. Lowry**

The primary nonmalignant disorders of leukocytes (white blood cells) encountered in an adult practice represent abnormalities of number. Congenital functional abnormalities are usually manifested in childhood. Acquired functional abnormalities may result from infection such as human immunodeficiency virus (HIV-1), treatment with drugs such as chemotherapy agents and corticosteroids, or as an additional aspect of malignant leukocyte disorders. This chapter describes the normal mechanisms of hematopoiesis and then reviews the various nonmalignant abnormalities of leukocyte subclasses. It concludes with a brief discussion of the role of the newly available myeloid cytokines in the treatment of these disorders.

## NORMAL HEMATOPOIESIS

An understanding of the basic concepts of normal hematopoiesis forms the foundation for approaching the diagnosis and therapy of malignant and nonmalignant blood disorders. Normal hematopoiesis proceeds from a pluripotent hematopoietic stem cell in the bone marrow that is capable of self-renewal and of proliferation and differentiation into all the recognized mature hematologic lineages under the control of the various hematopoietic cytokines (Fig. 53-1). Leukocytes derived from this process can be divided into two general classes: the myelomonocytic and lymphocytic. All leukocytes monitor and react to infection, inflammation, and endogenous tissue damage or degeneration.

Myelomonocytic cells (neutrophils, eosinophils, basophils, and monocytes/macrophages) are capable of phagocytosis of infecting agents or cellular debris and release of inflammatory or chemotactic mediators. These cells have no inherent specificity but react to foreign antigens that have been opsonized by antibody or complement.

Mature segmented neutrophils are released from the marrow and circulate for 6 to 8 hours before migrating to extravascular tissues, where they perform their bactericidal function and persist for only a few days. Less is known about the kinetics of basophils and eosinophils, although they are probably similar. They participate in allergic reactions and in the response to parasitic and fungal infections.

Monocytes have a similar short half-life in the circulation but are longer lived in the extravascular tissues. Monocytes that develop specialized phagocytic function are recognized as macrophages. In addition to phagocytic functions, monocytes/macrophages play a key role in antigen presentation to lymphocytes.

The lymphocytic class of leukocytes synthesizes specialized reactive molecules that interact with foreign antigens forming a specific arm of the immune response. Differentiated B cells are responsible for humoral immu-

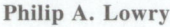

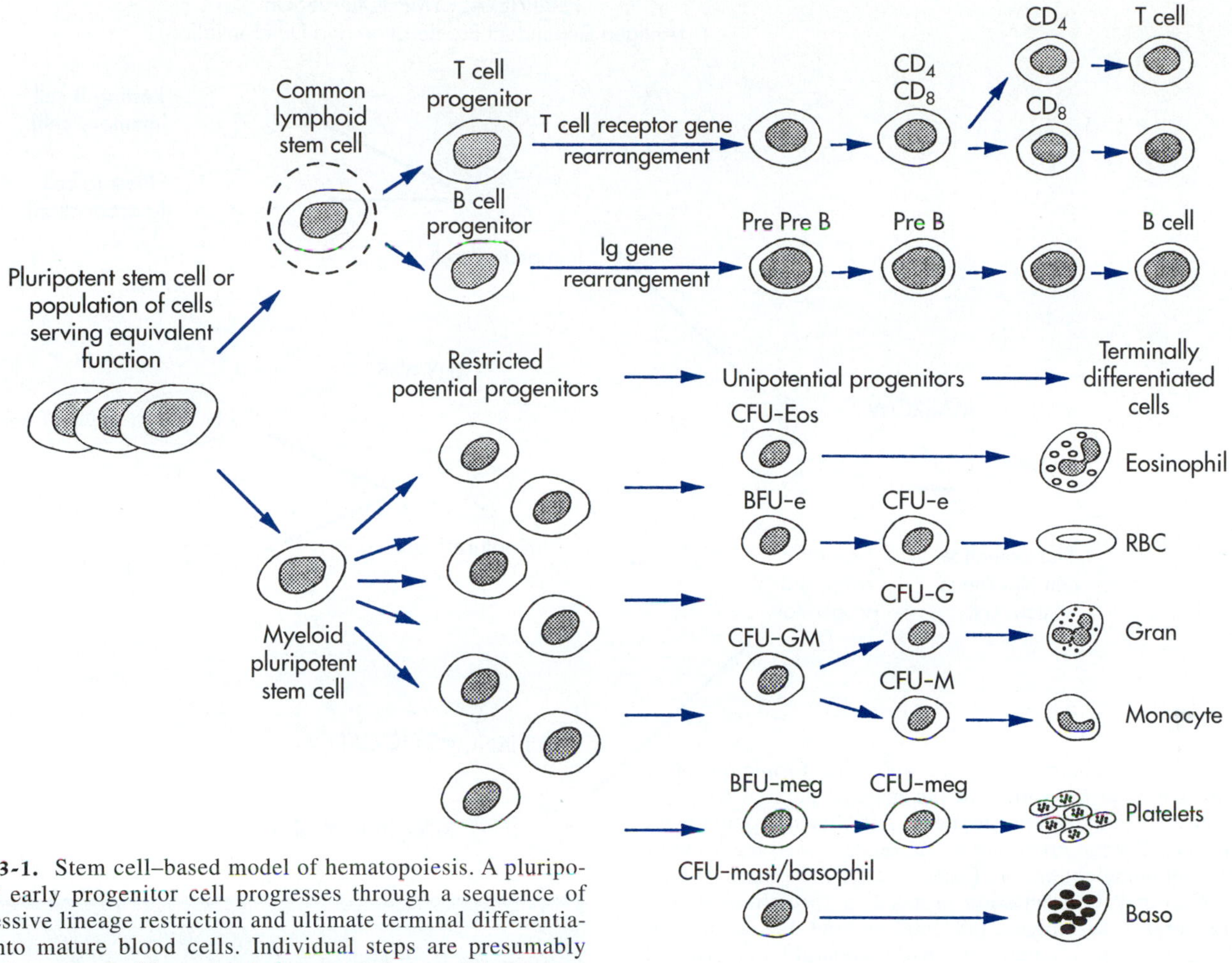


**Fig. 53-1.** Stem cell–based model of hematopoiesis. A pluripotential early progenitor cell progresses through a sequence of progressive lineage restriction and ultimate terminal differentiation into mature blood cells. Individual steps are presumably under the control of hematopoietic growth factors. The various hematologic malignancies may represent an "arrest" at one of these developmental stages.

nity through production of immunoglobulins. They circulate and initiate complement-mediated lysis or opsonized phagocytosis, particularly of bacterial pathogens. T cells control cell-mediated immunity. Differentiated T cells have a surface-bound T cell receptor that is similar to immunoglobulin in its unique structure and specificity for limited antigen interaction. In addition to specific recognition and destruction of endogenous tissues altered by viral infection or neoplastic degeneration, T cells modulate the overall immune response through direct cell-to-cell interaction with B cells and monocytes and the release of lymphokines and inflammatory modulators.

Development of these specialized reactive molecules starts with apparently random rearrangements of multiple genetic loci that are ultimately combined to produce mature immunoglobulin and T cell receptor molecules. After initial development in the marrow, final lymphocyte proliferation and differentiation proceed in specialized tissues capable of antigen presentation to select appropriate clones and of eliminating pathologically autoreactive cells (Fig. 53-2).

## NONMALIGNANT DISORDERS

Since leukocytes are primarily directed to the immune response, abnormalities are most often manifested as susceptibility to infections or inflammation. Qualitative abnormalities are rare, and most are typically congenital and manifest in childhood. Acquired qualitative defects may be seen with HIV-1 infection, treatment with corticosteroid or chemotherapeutic agents, or as complicating features of autoimmune or lymphoproliferative disorders. The box on p. 736 summarizes the evaluation of a patient with suspected immunodeficiency.

Adult practitioners more often encounter problems related to quantitative leukocyte disorders. General depression of leukocyte counts usually reflects an abnormality of production or an increased rate of loss or destruction. Production problems typically reflect abnormalities of the marrow related to inherent abnormalities of the hematopoietic stem cell, acute toxic insults such as those from chemotherapy or irradiation, a metabolic abnormality such as that from a vitamin deficiency, or a malignant or storage disorder that invades or replaces the marrow cavity. These mechanisms affect all of hematopoiesis and therefore rarely manifest as a single lineage deficit but more often as pancytopenia. Unusual disorders may result from specific growth factor abnormalities. These disorders are rare, but those such as cyclic neutropenia and Kostmann's syndrome are now recognized to result from specific deficiencies of granulocyte colony–stimulating factor (G-CSF), a cytokine involved in the direction of terminal granulocyte differentiation and ultimate function. Increased loss or destruction may relate to severe infections,

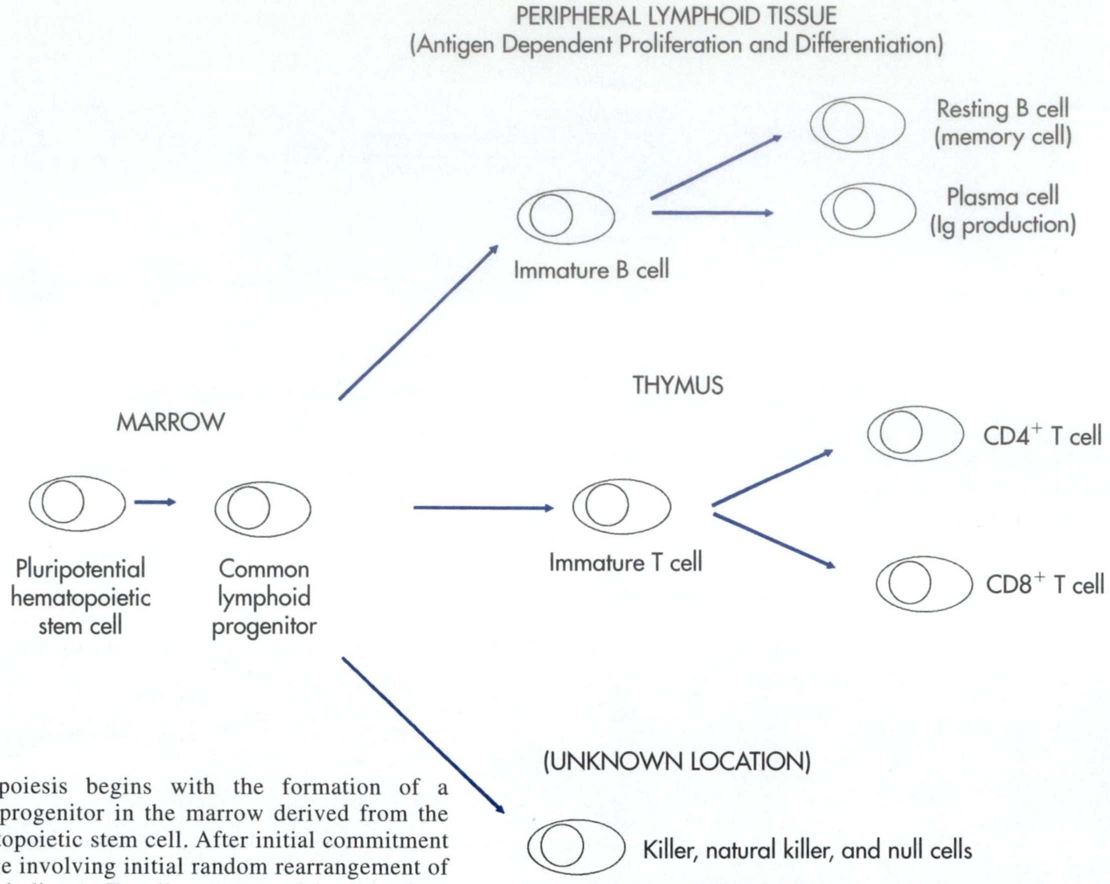


**Fig. 53-2.** Lymphopoiesis begins with the formation of a common lymphoid progenitor in the marrow derived from the pluripotential hematopoietic stem cell. After initial commitment to B or T cell lineage involving initial random rearrangement of loci for immunoglobulin or T cell receptor molecules, final proliferation and differentiation proceed in specialized tissues and are subject to antigen presentation and the control of modulating cells and lymphokines. Killer, natural killer, and null cell subsets are rare, are poorly characterized, and apparently do not undergo antigen-dependent and restricted proliferation and differentiation.

extensive tissue necrosis, splenic hyperfunction, or rarely to autoimmune mechanisms.

Syndromes of cellular excess are most typically due to malignant transformation with autonomous proliferation or are reactive to a specific pathologic state. Tables 53-1 and 53-2 list normal ranges of leukocyte numbers and related evaluations, and the box on p. 737 summarizes the quantitative leukocyte disorders.

## Granulocyte disorders

Qualitative defects in granulocytes are rarely encountered de novo in adult practice. They are associated with recurrent suppurative bacterial infections that may be fatal in childhood or, if persistent to adult life, typically respond to antibiotics. The nitroblue tetrazolium test is a rapid screen.

Neutropenia is seen most often in the context of previous treatment with cytotoxic therapy and in such a situation is usually anticipated and recognized before the onset of major secondary problems. Acute neutropenia can also be seen in certain infectious diseases, particularly bacterial sepsis and a variety of viral syndromes related to increased destruction. Vitamin $B_{12}$ or folate deficiency may also cause neutropenia resulting from abnormal maturation, and it may be seen as the first manifestation of an acquired marrow disorder such as myelodysplasia, aplastic anemia, leukemia, or other malignancy involving the marrow. More chronic forms of neutropenia may be seen as an expression of a congenital disorder (e.g., cyclic neutropenia), in the context of an autoimmune disease (e.g., systemic lupus erythematosus, Felty's syndrome), or as a manifestation of hypersplenism.

Neutropenia, particularly when the absolute neutrophil count is less than 500/µl, constitutes a potential medical emergency requiring prompt evaluation and, in the context of manifestations of infection, immediate intervention to

### Approach to the patient with suspected immunodeficiency

History and physical: Establish frequency and type of infections, signs or symptoms of other congenital problems, signs or symptoms of autoimmune or lymphoproliferative disorder, medications, family history, risk factors for HIV infection.
Complete blood count and differential: Screen for quantitative leukocyte abnormalities.
HIV serology: Screen for acquired immunodeficiency syndrome (AIDS).
Nitroblue tetrazolium test: Screen for phagocytic defect (recurrent pyogenic infections).
Quantitative immunoglobulins: Screen for B cell defect.
*Candida* skin test: Screen for T cell defect.
Hemolytic complement ($CH_{50}$): Screen for complement deficiency.

From Buckley RH: Immunodeficiency diseases, *JAMA* 268:2797, 1992.

**Table 53-1.** Normal total and differential leukocyte counts

| Cell type | Absolute number ($\times 10^9/L$) | Differential percentage (%) |
|---|---|---|
| Total leukocytes | 4.4-11.3 | (100) |
| Neutrophils (total) | 1.8-7.7 | 25-62 |
| Lymphocytes | 1.0-4.8 | 20-52 |
| Monocytes | 0-0.8 | 2-12 |
| Eosinophils | 0-0.45 | 0-9 |
| Basophils | 0-0.2 | 0-4 |

**Table 53-2.** Normal values for selected additional laboratory determinations

| Test | Normal values |
|---|---|
| Serum vitamin $B_{12}$ | 160-1000 pg/ml |
| Serum folate | 6-21 ng/ml |
| Leukocyte alkaline phosphatase | 13-130 (rating score) |
| Serum immunoglobulin G (IgG) | 8-16 mg/ml |
| Serum IgM | 0.5-2 mg/ml |
| Serum IgA | 1.4-4 mg/ml |

Modified from Williams WJ et al, editors: *Hematology,* ed 4, New York, 1990, McGraw Hill.

### Summary of quantitative disorders of leukocytes

**Disorders associated with neutrophilia**

Pyogenic infections
Burns
Tissue necrosis
Myeloproliferative syndromes
Leukemias

**Disorders associated with neutropenia**

Aplastic anemia
Folate or $B_{12}$ deficiency
Marrow infiltrating disorders (including leukemia)
Myelodysplastic syndromes
Rickettsial or viral infections
Alcoholism
Chemotherapy or radiation therapy
Drug reaction

**Disorders associated with lymphocytosis**

Viral infections including infectious mononucleosis
Syphilis
Lymphoma or lymphocytic leukemia
Thyrotoxicosis

**Disorders associated with lymphopenia**

Corticosteroid administration
Hodgkin's disease
Infectious hepatitis
HIV infection

**Disorders associated with eosinophilia**

Allergic or hypersensitivity reactions
Parasitic infections
Solid malignancy
Skin diseases
Loeffler syndrome
Pulmonary eosinophilia
Eosinophilic leukemia
Idiopathic eosinophilia

**Disorder associated with eosinopenia**

Hyperadrenalism or corticosteroid administration

**Disorders associated with monocytosis**

Chronic myelomonocytic leukemia
Systemic lupus
Solid malignancy
Rickettsial infections
Subacute bacterial endocarditis
Acute monocytic leukemia

**Disorders associated with basophilia**

Urticaria pigmentosa
Myeloproliferative disorders

forestall life-threatening complications. A complete history and physical examination should focus on antecedent treatments or conditions. Review of the peripheral blood and marrow smears may identify potential malignant forms or signs of vitamin or cellular deficiency. Additional laboratory studies that may be helpful include antinuclear antibody, rheumatoid factor, serum immune electrophoresis, and determination of folic acid and $B_{12}$ levels. Antineutrophil antibodies are available on an investigational basis but are rarely returned in time to help with acute decision making and may not be sufficiently specific and reliable to help with a diagnostic evaluation.

Although definitive therapy for neutropenia and its underlying causes may require the assistance of a hematologist, several immediate measures may be required and often should be instituted by the primary physician even in advance of hematologic consultation. Potential toxic drugs or other potential contributing factors should be eliminated at the time of diagnosis. Any signs of infection, including fever even without other localizing signs, mandate prompt initiation of broad-spectrum antibiotics. This issue has been recently reviewed by Pizzo in the *New England Journal of Medicine* (see bibliography) and is discussed in detail elsewhere in this text.

Neutrophilia, in contrast, is rarely a medical emergency in and of itself except as a marker of a more serious underlying disorder. Neutrophilia is seen acutely most often as a manifestation of underlying infections, particularly those related to bacterial organisms. It may also be seen in response to acute stress related to burns, major trauma, or organ infarction. In these cases the primary disorder is usually manifestly evident from the history and physical examination. Treatment with drugs such as epinephrine, corticosteroids, and the more recently available recombinant growth factors may also induce neutrophilia. A mild neutrophilia may be seen occasionally as a response to extreme heat or cold exposure or with exercise, convulsions, or severe pain.

Chronic neutrophilia may be seen in the context of

persistent infections or inflammatory conditions or occasionally as a chronic response to untreated malignancies of another organ system. Chronic neutrophilia may complicate therapy with corticosteroids or lithium or may accompany certain endocrinologic disorders such as adrenocorticotropic hormone–producing or glucocorticoid-producing tumors or thyroid storm. Chronic neutrophilia is rare as a congenital abnormality, although it may be seen in association with Down syndrome. In these forms the neutrophilia represents a reactive process, and its treatment is simply the treatment of the primary disorder.

The major differential concern in neutrophilia is to identify a primary myeloproliferative disorder. A definitive evaluation may require bone marrow aspiration and cytogenetics to search for the characteristic Philadelphia chromosome (t9:22 translocation), but a screen of a leukocyte alkaline phosphatase level may provide an initial clue to which of these two diagnoses is operative. Although leukemoid reactions or other reactive causes of neutrophilia are usually associated with an elevated leukocyte alkaline phosphatase level, chronic myelocytic leukemia is typically associated with a very low value.

### Eosinophil disorders

Patients presenting with excess numbers of eosinophils require evaluation of stool for ova and parasites; cultures and evaluation for fungal, mycobacterial, or other chronic bacterial diseases; and evaluation for autoimmune or chronic allergic disorders, all of which may be associated with a reactive eosinophilia. Hypereosinophilia that persists for more than 6 months with the exclusion of reactive forms of eosinophilia suggests a primary hypereosinophilic syndrome.

Hypereosinophilic syndrome most often afflicts white males. Total leukocyte counts may be elevated to the range of 10,000 to 50,000/μl, with 30% to 70% of cells being mature-appearing eosinophils. Hypereosinophilic syndrome is an idiopathic condition with a range of eosinophil morphology from very mature to very immature leukemic-appearing cells.

Chronic eosinophilia from any cause may result in severe cardiac toxicity with restrictive congestive heart failure and mitral valve regurgitation and also may be associated with chronic pulmonary infiltrates or effusions. At one time, primary hypereosinophilia was often fatal when severe and prolonged. More recently the prognosis is dramatically improved with treatment, including corticosteroids, hydroxyurea, and leukopheresis.

### Monocyte disorders

Chronic disorders of monocytes are rare other than as a marker of an underlying malignant disease such as myelodysplasia, a myeloproliferative disorder, or occasionally as a marker of underlying lymphoma. Normally, monocytosis is seen as a manifestation of chronic inflammation or an immune disorder, such as collagen vascular disease, inflammatory bowel disease, or sarcoidosis. It is also seen with chronic infectious states, particularly tuberculosis, subacute bacterial endocarditis, and syphilis. Treatment of monocytosis is directed toward the underlying causative disease.

### Basophilia

Basophilia is similarly a marker for underlying malignant and nonmalignant disease. Basophilia may be seen with allergic or inflammatory conditions or with certain infectious conditions such as viral or a tubercular infection. The underlying cause is usually obvious, and the treatment is directed toward it. Basophilia may also be a marker for the myeloproliferative diseases or for occult carcinoma, and a search for these conditions should be undertaken when no other cause is manifested.

### Lymphocyte disorders

Lymphocytopenia can result from a variety of causes and, although not associated with the explosive infectious susceptibility of neutropenia, may nevertheless be a marker of severe immune compromise. Congenital B cell deficiencies typically result in immunoglobulin defects and recurrent bacterial infections. Congenital T cell deficiencies are not only associated with loss of cell-mediated immunity but, because of the simultaneous loss of helper/suppressor function necessary for B cell proliferation and differentiation, result in the combined immunodeficiency states. These disorders typically present in childhood and are usually fatal at an early age, with the exception of mild B cell disorders that may respond to chronic treatment with antibiotics and immunoglobulins. (For a more detailed discussion of these disorders refer to the Bibliography.)

Lymphopenias or abnormalities of lymphocyte function may also be secondary manifestations of a variety of other autoimmune states and of malignancies such as lymphoma and Hodgkin's disease. Chronic therapy with glucocorticoids or antineoplastic agents may induce functional or numeric abnormalities of lymphocytes as well.

With the recent emergence of AIDS a new category of lymphopenia and lymphocyte dysfunction has developed (see Chapter 68). Screening for HIV infection should be a standard part of the evaluation of a patient presenting with lymphopenia.

Lymphocytosis, as with the other disorders of lymphocyte excess, can be divided into two broad categories: a

## Myeloid cytokines

**Current Uses**

Definite utility: G-CSF for congenital neutropenia
Probable utility: Recovery after marrow transplantation, mobilization of peripheral stem cells for transplant
Possible utility: Prophylactic use in support of dose-intensive chemotherapy without stem cells
No data: Use in established neutropenia after chemotherapy
Adverse effects: Possible acceleration of leukemic transformation in myelodysplastic syndromes and stimulation of solid tumor growth

**Toxicities**

GM-CSF: Fever, bone pain, myalgias, edema/pericarditis, first dose reaction
G-CSF: bone pain, splenomegaly (with prolonged use), neutrophilic dermatitis (rare)

manifestation of a primary hematologic malignancy or a reactive process. Lymphocytosis may be seen with the various mononucleosis syndromes related to Epstein-Barr virus, cytomegalovirus, or toxoplasma infection and may also be seen in the early presentation of HIV-1 infection. Acute lymphocytosis may also be seen with a number of other viral infections or in the context of noninfectious inflammatory processes associated with autoimmune disease or hypersensitivity reactions.

With the increasing use of screening blood counts, patients with chronic lymphocytic leukemia are frequently diagnosed in an asymptomatic and early stage on the basis of an elevated lymphocyte count noted on a routine determination. Although suspicion of such a syndrome usually requires a bone marrow biopsy and hematologic evaluation, it is important for the primary care physician to recognize that the early stage of chronic lymphocytic leukemia may be associated with a relatively normal life span. Even as lymphocyte counts reach very high levels of 1 to 3 million/μl, intervention may not be specifically required, since leukostasis is rare. Patients with chronic lymphocytic leukemia usually develop problems not related to lymphocytosis but rather to associated infectious complications of other cytopenias.

## HEMATOPOIETIC GROWTH FACTORS

A major addition to the therapeutic armamentarium in the treatment of hematologic disorders has been the identification, production, and promulgation of the hematopoietic cytokines, such as erythropoietin, granulocyte macrophage colony–stimulating factor (GM-CSF), and G-CSF.

Although erythropoietin enjoys established applications, the use of the myeloid cytokines has preceded the rigorous scientific justification of their value to patient care. Particularly in the context of the need to control health care costs it is essential that the medical community continue to critically evaluate the efficacy of these new agents and rigorously establish the appropriate contexts for their use. The box on p. 738 summarizes current uses of the myeloid growth factors.

## BIBLIOGRAPHY

Buckley RH: Immunodeficiency diseases, *JAMA* 268:2787, 1992.

Demetri GD: Hematopoietic growth factors: current knowledge, future prospects, *Curr Prob Cancer* 16(4): 1992.

Mazza JJ, editor: *Manual of clinical hematology,* Boston, 1988, Little, Brown.

Pizzo PA: Management of fever in patients with cancer and treatment-induced neutropenia, *N Engl J Med* 328:1323, 1993.

Williams WJ et al, editors: *Hematology,* ed 4, New York, 1990, McGraw-Hill.

Yang KD, Hill HR: Neutrophil function disorders: pathophysiology, prevention, and therapy, *J Pediatr* 119:343, 1991.

CHAPTER

# 54 Hematologic Malignancies

**Philip A. Lowry**

The hematologic malignancies range from indolent disorders to the highly aggressive leukemias and lymphomas whose explosive onset and rapid progression are among the most dramatic in all of medicine. The primary care physician must be particularly concerned with an initial suspicion of hematologic malignancy, more so than with a final diagnosis. A thorough history and physical examination, complete blood count (CBC), and evaluation of the peripheral blood smear often suffice to construct a well-focused differential diagnosis. This chapter focuses on the initial signs of hematologic malignancies and the basics of their diagnosis (see Chapter 53). It also reviews disease-specific treatment decisions and outcomes and summarizes the prognosis of the primary hematologic malignancies and related disorders.

## ABNORMALITIES OF THE HEMOGRAM

Abnormalities of the CBC may signal a hematologic malignancy. Leukemia, lymphomatous involvement of the marrow, myelodysplasia, and myeloproliferative disorders should be included in the differential diagnosis of anemia or other cytopenias. A monotonous, sustained increase in a single cell population without an obvious inciting event, such as infection, suggests a myeloproliferative or leukemic process. Basophilia may be a marker of myeloproliferative disorder. An abnormal CBC should prompt inspection of the peripheral smear with a particular evaluation for abnormal morphology and the presence of blasts signaling acute leukemia. Bone marrow evaluation may be necessary to establish a final diagnosis.

## HISTORY

Involuntary weight loss, fevers, or night sweats may be a presenting symptom with lymphoproliferative disorders, and pruritus may be a clue of Hodgkin's disease. Abdominal distention and discomfort may reflect splenomegaly that accompanies lymphoma or myeloproliferative disorders. Back pain may reflect retroperitoneal adenopathy, direct spinal involvement with lymphoma, or compression fractures resulting from myeloma. Similarly, myeloma can produce lytic skeletal lesions, pathologic fractures, or unusual osteoporosis.

Hematologic malignancies frequently suppress normal bone marrow function, resulting in fatigue secondary to anemia, recurrent infections related to neutrophil or lymphocyte defects, or petechiae or bleeding related to platelet deficiencies. Bleeding may also signal disseminated intravascular coagulation. Myeloproliferative disorders may present with thrombosis.

## LYMPHADENOPATHY AND SPLENOMEGALY

Lymphadenopathy should focus attention on the possibility of an underlying hematologic malignancy. Causes of

## Common causes of lymphadenopathy

- Infections
  - Acute suppurative lymphadenitis
    - *Staphyloccus aureus*
    - *Streptococcus pyogenes*
    - Tuberculosis
  - Viral infections: human immunodeficiency virus (HIV-1), rubella, rubeola, mumps, roseola (predominantly in children), infectious mononucleosis (Epstein-Barr virus, positive or negative), toxoplasmosis
- Immune disorders
  - Systemic lupus erythematosus
  - Rheumatoid arthritis
  - Sjögren's syndrome
    - Benign adenopathy
    - Malignant adenopathy
  - Dermatomyositis
  - Sarcoidosis
  - Serum sickness
  - Hypersensitivity reaction
- Endocrine disorders
  - Hyperthyroidism
  - Adrenocortical insufficiency
- Dermatopathic diseases
- Drug-induced disorders
  - Benign
  - Malignant
- Neoplastic disorders
  - Leukemia
  - Lymphoma
  - Myeloproliferative syndromes
  - Metastatic (see text)
- Miscellaneous disorders
  - Angioimmunoblastic lymphadenopathy
  - Lipid storage disorders
    - Gaucher's disease
    - Niemann-Pick disease
  - Other disorders

## Causes of splenomegaly

- Infections
  - Subacute bacterial endocarditis
  - Brucellosis
  - Infectious mononucleosis, cytomegalovirus
  - Tuberculosis
  - Parasites
    - Malaria
    - Schistosomiasis
    - Kala-azar
    - Other
  - Sepsis
- Immune disorders
  - Systemic lupus erythematosus
  - Sarcoidosis
  - Rheumatoid arthritis (Felty's syndrome)
- Hematologic disorders
  - Hemolytic anemias, acute and chronic
  - Immune thrombocytopenic purpura
  - Lymphomas
  - Leukemias
  - Myeloproliferative diseases
- Metastatic diseases
- Infiltrative splenomegaly
  - Lipid storage disease
  - Amyloidosis
  - Diabetic lipemia
  - True cysts
    - Epithelial
    - Endothelial
    - Dermoids, lymphangiomyomatosis, hydatid
- Vascular congestion
  - Congestive heart failure
  - Portal hypertension secondary to cirrhosis
  - Splenic vein obstruction
  - Budd-Chiari syndrome

lymphadenopathy are summarized in the box above, and a general scheme for its evaluation is presented in the Managed Care Guide. Persistent lymphadenopathy of greater than 2 weeks' duration or lymphadenopathy with pathologic features (firm, hard, or very large lymph nodes in unusual locations unassociated with obvious localized infection) requires prompt diagnostic consideration. It is ***not*** acceptable to pursue multiple empiric antibiotic courses in the vain hope that adenopathy will resolve.

Young patients or others at risk should be screened for HIV infection. Severe or persistent pharyngitis should suggest the possibility of infectious mononucleosis.

Fever, weight loss, or night sweats may be particularly suggestive of lymphoma. Chest tightness, progressive dysphagia or dyspnea, or facial plethora may suggest a primary lung or esophageal process. A change in bowel habits or abdominal discomfort may suggest an occult gastrointestinal malignancy.

Cervical adenopathy in an older, smoking man suggests a primary head and neck cancer and should prompt full ear, nose, and throat evaluation before lymph node biopsy, which can compromise subsequent lymph node dissection. Supraclavicular adenopathy is frequently an indicator of more distant disease in the lung, breast, or abdomen. Axillary adenopathy suggests carcinoma of the breast, lung, skin, lymphoma, and even occasionally prostate.

Inguinal adenopathy can be problematic in that many individuals have long-standing, rubbery nodes that are nonpathologic. Small nodes that are unchanged over a long period and unassociated with focal signs of pelvic disorder may not require further evaluation. Adenopathy of a more suspicious nature should prompt a thorough evaluation of the rectal and perineal regions as well as specific genital examination.

A complete history and physical examination, chest x-ray study, mammogram, or computed tomography (CT) scan of the chest or abdomen as indicated by the location of the adenopathy may provide the diagnosis or suggest additional diagnostic procedures. If a diagnosis is not clear, fine-needle aspiration of a pathologic lymph node may initially suggest a diagnosis, but definitive excisional biopsy is often required. In all cases the least invasive procedure to make a diagnosis should be selected first.

Other than in the occasional young, asthenic individual whose normal-sized spleen is palpable solely because of body habitus, a palapable spleen may suggest an under-

**Managed Care Guide**
**The workup of lymphadenopathy**

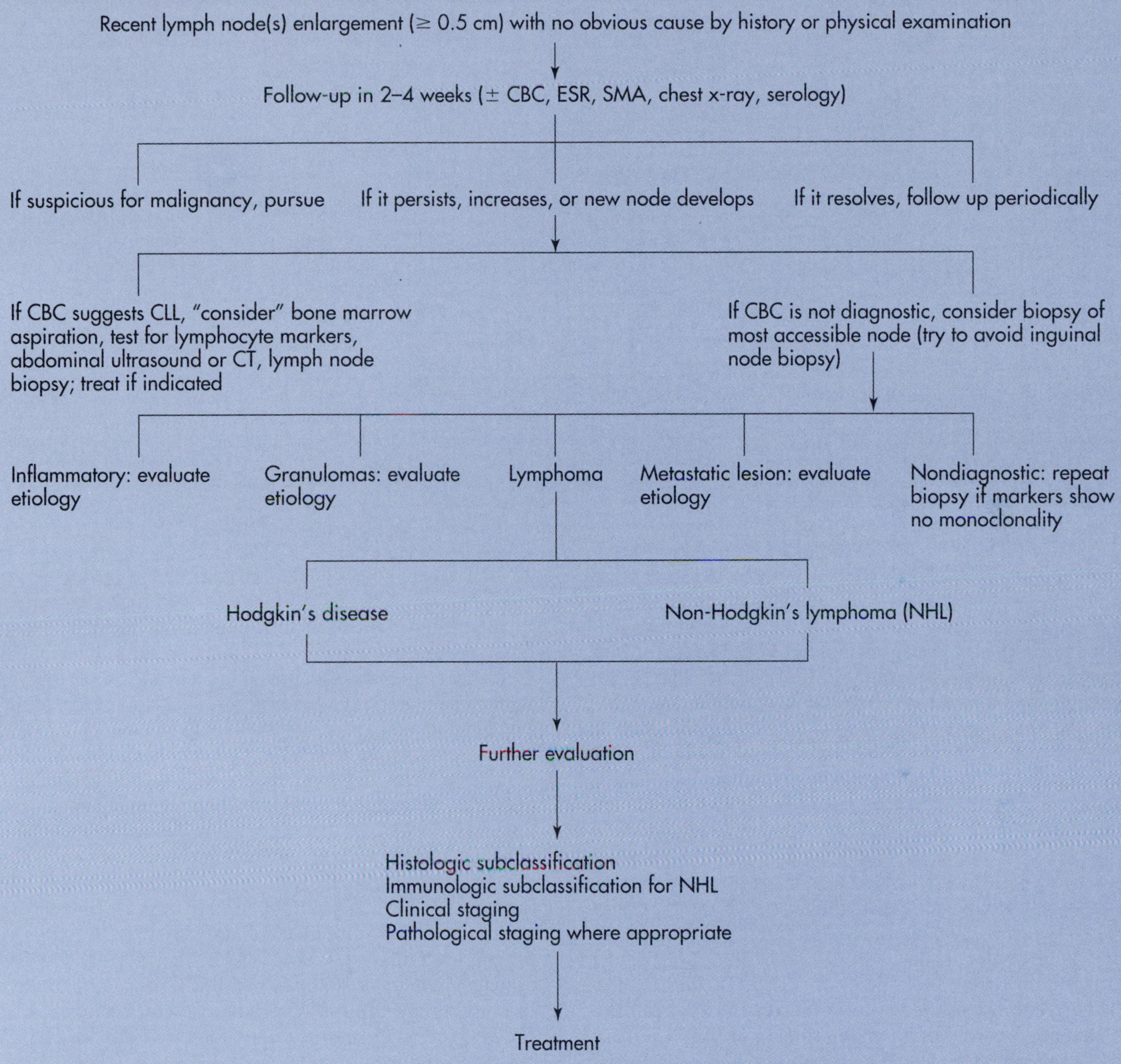
Recent lymph node(s) enlargement (≥ 0.5 cm) with no obvious cause by history or physical examination
Follow-up in 2–4 weeks (± CBC, ESR, SMA, chest x-ray, serology)
If suspicious for malignancy, pursue
If it persists, increases, or new node develops
If it resolves, follow up periodically
If CBC suggests CLL, "consider" bone marrow aspiration, test for lymphocyte markers, abdominal ultrasound or CT, lymph node biopsy; treat if indicated
If CBC is not diagnostic, consider biopsy of most accessible node (try to avoid inguinal node biopsy)
Inflammatory: evaluate etiology
Granulomas: evaluate etiology
Lymphoma
Metastatic lesion: evaluate etiology
Nondiagnostic: repeat biopsy if markers show no monoclonality
Hodgkin's disease
Non-Hodgkin's lymphoma (NHL)
Further evaluation
Histologic subclassification
Immunologic subclassification for NHL
Clinical staging
Pathological staging where appropriate
Treatment

lying hematologic malignancy. Conditions associated with splenomegaly are listed in the box on p. 740. If splenomegaly is mild, there are no other signs or symptoms of hematologic malignancy, and the patient has a condition frequently associated with splenomegaly, observation may suffice.

In other cases the patient should be evaluated for hematologic malignancy. Splenectomy is rarely required as a diagnostic procedure, since bone marrow or lymph node aspiration typically reveals the diagnosis. Splenectomy may be performed as part of the staging workup for early Hodgkin's disease. Immune cytopenias complicating lymphoproliferative disorders, cytopenias resulting from splenic sequestration, and intractable symptoms from massive splenomegaly may require therapeutic splenectomy.

## MYELOPROLIFERATIVE DISORDERS

The myeloproliferative disorders represent an abnormal proliferation of relatively mature cells of the erythrocyte, megakaryocytic and/or myeloid lineage, although the abnormality resides in the earliest stem cell. Although the cells in excess may appear at least superficially normal on morphologic examination, they may be functionally abnormal. The myeloproliferative disorders are usually classified based on the primary cell in excess, although all lineages are affected. Clinical features of these disorders are summarized in Table 54-1.

**Table 54-1.** Clinical features of myeloproliferative disorders

| | Essential thrombocythemia | CML | Polycythemia vera | Myelofibrosis with myeloid metaplasia |
|---|---|---|---|---|
| Symptoms | Hemorrhage, thrombosis | Bone pain, fever/sweats | Hemorrhage, thrombosis, pruritus | Hemorrhage, thrombosis, portal hypertension |
| Splenomegaly | 30%-40% | 95% | 90% | 100% |
| Primary cell in excess | Platelets | Granulocytes | Red blood cells* | (Marrow fibrosis)† |
| LAP | →↑↓ | ↓ | ↑ | ↑ |
| Cytogenetics | Normal | Philadelphia chromosome*,‡ | Normal | Normal |
| Marrow | ↑Megakaryocytes | ↑All lines | ↑All lines | ↑All lines, fibrosis |
| Treatment | Plateletpheresis, anagrelide | Hydroxyurea, allogeneic bone marrow transplantation | Phlebotomy, radioactive phosphorus | Occasionally require splenectomy |
| Progression to acute leukemia | Rare | Most | 1%-2% (13% if treated with radioactive phosphorus) | 6% |

*Platelet defects may induce occult gastrointestinal blood loss, producing an artifactually normal or decreased hematocrit and morphologic changes consistent with iron deficiency.

†Myelofibrosis with myeloid metaplasia (MMM) has as its primary manifestation marrow fibrosis rather than a specific cellular excess. This fibrosis produces a luekoerythroblastic peripheral smear with immature white cells, nucleated red cells, and teardrop red cells. MMM is grouped with the myeloproliferative disorders because it may be an end-stage evolution of the other syndromes as well as a primarily presenting syndrome and probably represents a proliferation of megakaryocytes with release of secondary factors inducing the characteristic fibrosis.

‡Gross chromosomal translocation may occasionally be absent, but genetic rearrangements involving the *bcr* locus on chromosome 22 and c-*abl* locus on chromosome 9 should be detectable on Southern blot analysis.

The primary differential diagnosis in the myeloproliferative disorders is to distinguish reactive proliferations of normal cells. Chronic myelocytic leukemia (CML) must be distinguished from a benign leukemoid reaction. Patients with a leukemoid reaction frequently have a history of infection or another inciting process, lack splenomegaly, and have an elevated leukocyte alkaline phosphatase (LAP) score. Patients with CML, in contrast, have low LAP scores and lack signs or symptoms of a clear inciting event. CML is confirmed by bone marrow examination with identification of a characteristic genetic rearrangement involving the *bcr* locus on chromosome 22 and c-*abl* locus on chromosome 9, producing the abnormal Philadelphia chromosome.

Polycythemia vera must be distinguished from secondary polycythemias related to chronic obstructive pulmonary disease, congenital or another cardiopulmonary disease, inheritance of a hemoglobin with abnormal oxygen affinity, or elevated carboxyhemoglobin levels related to smoking. Neoplasms of the kidneys or liver may rarely produce erythropoietin, autonomously inducing a secondary polycythemia.

The diagnosis of polycythemia vera is based on the determination of an elevated red blood cell mass, exclusion of secondary causes, and the presence of other indicators, including splenomegaly, leukocytosis, or thrombocytosis. Secondary polycythemia may be excluded by history and physical examination, determination of arterial blood gas level, and determination of carboxyhemoglobin where appropriate. Direct determination of circulating erythropoietin levels is becoming a useful adjunctive procedure: erythropoietin levels in secondary polycythemias are elevated, whereas they are depressed in polycythemia vera.

Essential or primary thrombocytosis must be differentiated from thrombocytosis related to inflammation, iron-deficiency anemia, or postsplenectomy thrombocytosis. Reactive thrombocytosis rarely reaches levels greater then $10^6/\mu l$.

Clinical symptoms of the myeloproliferative syndromes may relate to organomegaly or to the qualitative or quantitative cellular changes. Platelet changes may paradoxically produce thrombosis or hemorrhage. Plateletpheresis can be acutely effective, especially in essential thrombocytosis; long-term control requires pharmacologic therapy. Aspirin should generally be avoided in the treatment of thrombocytosis associated with any myeloproliferative disorder, since it may greatly exacerbate the bleeding tendency without preventing thrombosis, except in occasional patients who have severe, recurrent thromboses. Polycythemia increases intravascular viscosity and may also induce thrombosis.

Treatment for the myeloproliferative disorders is usually directed to controlling the cellular excess and is not curative. Simple phlebotomy may suffice for polycythemia vera; hydroxyurea is useful in all the conditions but especially in CML. Survival in essential thrombocytosis and polycythemia vera may be prolonged except in patients with severe thrombotic problems. CML uniformly evolves in time to acute leukemia and therefore is treated with bone marrow transplantation in selected younger patients in whom it may be curative. Myelofibrosis with myeloid metaplasia is more difficult to treat, and survival is typically short.

## MYELODYSPLASTIC SYNDROMES

The terms *myelodysplastic* and *myeloproliferative* are often confused. Although myeloproliferative disorders demonstrate proliferation of morphologically relatively normal-appearing cells, the myelodysplastic syndromes present a different problem of abnormal maturation, with cytopenias rather than cellular excess in the peripheral blood. Like the myeloproliferative disorders the myelodysplastic syndromes originate from the transformation of an early hematopoietic stem cell and typically have effects in multiple cell lineages. Because of the high frequency of acute leukemic evolution, these disorders are often referred to as *preleukemic*.

The median age of patients affected with myelodysplastic syndromes is 60 to 70 years, though younger patients may occasionally present with similar abnormalities, particularly 5 to 10 years after intensive chemotherapy or radiotherapy for other malignant disorders. Presenting signs may be fatigue or weakness related to anemias, bleeding related to thrombocytopenia, and infectious complications related to leukopenia. CBC and differential usually reveal cytopenias. Morphologic changes often include poorly granulated or hyposegmented neutrophils and hypochromic red cells with moderate to marked anisocytosis and poikilocytosis. Because of the maturation abnormalities, developing hematologic cells are incapable of normally completing their maturation sequence and thus accumulate in increased numbers within the marrow. Reflecting the preleukemic nature of this disorder, myeloblasts are increased in number. Chromosome abnormalities are frequent, particularly those involving chromosomes 5, 7, 8, 17, and 21. Survival is generally short, with only rare cures in selected patients who are candidates for bone marrow transplantation. The box at right summarizes the myelodysplastic syndromes.

## CHRONIC LYMPHOCYTIC LEUKEMIA

The malignant cell of chronic lymphocytic leukemia (CLL) is a mature-appearing lymphocyte that is morphologically indistinguishable from its normal counterpart. Patients with CLL can tolerate leukocyte counts exceeding 1 million/μl without leukostasis or other major direct sequelae. Patients ultimately succumb to cytopenias resulting from marrow replacement or more frequently from infectious complications resulting from disordered lymphocyte development or function. In contrast to the acute leukemias and to CML, survival in patients with CLL presenting at a relatively early stage is frequently prolonged and may not be dramatically different than that of age-matched control patients.

Individuals with CLL are typically over 60 years of age and are often discovered coincidentally based on lymphocytosis noted on a routine CBC. They may occasionally present with mild symptoms of peripheral lymphadenopathy, splenomegaly, fatigue related to anemia, or infectious complications. Bone marrow morphology confirms the diagnosis, but additional confirmation can be obtained by finding the expression of the cell surface antigen CD5, which is not expressed on normal B cells.

In the absence of marked cytopenias or other specific complications a simple policy of watchful waiting may be the most effective initial therapy. Once specific therapy is required, the traditional approach is to combine an oral alkylator such as cyclophosphamide or chlorambucil with prednisone in pulse or continuous therapy.

### Myelodysplastic syndromes

**General features**

Myelodysplastic syndromes show abnormal (dysplastic) hematopoietic maturation. Marrow cellularity is *increased*, reflecting ineffective hematopoiesis, but inadequate maturation results in peripheral *cytopenias*.

**Syndromes**

*Refractory anemias:* Refractory anemias typically present in older patients, with anemia being the most prominent feature, although it is accompanied by mild to moderate pancytopenia. These syndromes are subdivided based on the number of blasts and the presence or absence of ringed sideroblasts:

| | % Marrow Blasts | Survival |
|---|---|---|
| Refractory anemia | < 5% | 2-4 years |
| Refractory anemia with ringed sideroblasts* | < 5% | 3-5 years |
| Refractory anemia with excess blasts | 5%-20% | 1-2 years |
| Refractory anemia in transformation | 20%-30% | < 1 year |

*Chronic myelomonocytic leukemia:* CMML presents with splenomegaly, monocytosis, and mild leukocytosis, which may be confused with CML. In contrast to CML, marrow maturation is dysplastic and the Philadelphia chromosome is absent. The clinical course is more similar to the refractory anemias.

*Miscellaneous primary myelodysplasia:* Patients may present with dysplastic marrow maturation but not the specific features of the above syndromes. Cytogenetic abnormalities involving chromosomes 5 or 7 are frequent. Those with a deletion of 5q may show a more indolent course and prolonged survival.

*Secondary myelodysplasia:* Previous exposure to benzene or other toxins or treatment with chemotherapy may induce myelodysplasia.

**Treatment**

Myelodysplastic syndromes and their resulting leukemias tend to be highly resistant to chemotherapy and are best treated with supportive measures using antibiotics and transfusion. Occasionally, young patients may be considered for allogeneic bone marrow transplantation. The role of myeloid growth factors (granulocyte colony–stimulating factor granulocyte macrophage colony–stimulating factor) is undefined with possible stimulation of leukemic progression in others.

**Differential diagnosis**

Hereditary dysplasias (hereditary sideroblastic anemia, Fanconi anemia, Diamond-Blackfan syndrome, Kostmann's syndrome, Shwachmann syndrome); $B_{12}$/Folate deficiency; toxins (drugs, alcohol, chemotherapy); irradiation; renal failure; tuberculosis; autoimmune disease; viral infections (Epstein-Barr virus, parvovirus, HIV); paroxysmal nocturnal hemoglobinuria.

*Ringed sideroblasts are erythroid precursors with a defect in iron metabolism, producing iron-laden mitochondria that ring the nucleus and produce a characteristic appearance on marrow smears stained for iron.

The vast majority of patients with CLL are older and not candidates for allogeneic bone marrow transplantation. Occasionally, a younger patient presenting with this disease should be considered for such therapy, since it offers the potential for cure.

## ACUTE LEUKEMIAS

Acute leukemia is a maturation arrest of an immature hematopoietic progenitor that rapidly proliferates and displaces normal elements within the marrow and peripheral blood. Classification schemes have historically been based on morphologic and immunohistochemical criteria dividing the acute leukemias into lymphoblastic and nonlymphoblastic types. Monoclonal antibodies detecting specific cell surface membrane antigens have provided a more rapid and precise means of separating the various types of acute leukemia. Increasingly, leukemias are being classified on the basis of specific chromosomal or oncogene rearrangement. Classification schemes and treatment outlines for acute lymphoblastic and nonlymphocytic leukemia are summarized in the boxes below.

Acute leukemias can be rapidly fatal because of infections related to granulocytopenia or bleeding related to thrombocytopenia. Occasional individuals presenting with hyperleukocytosis, particularly of immature blasts, may develop leukostasis reactions in the pulmonary or cerebral circulations and require immediate leukopheresis. Patients with acute promyelocytic leukemia or the monocytic variants may present with disseminated intravascular coagulation, necessitating factor transfusion and platelet support in the face of active bleeding. The role of heparin remains controversial in this circumstance. Patients with acute leukemias have high levels of spontaneous cell turnover, which increases after the institution of therapy. The sudden transfer of the intracellular contents to the extracellular space can cause life-threatening elevations of uric acid, potassium, and phosphate. Thus patients with acute leukemia should be routinely treated with intrave-

### Acute lymphoblastic leukemia

**Classification schemes**
***Morphologic classification***

L1: Small regular blasts, fine chromatin (65% of cases; especially children)
L2: Larger blasts, irregular nuclei, increased cytoplasm (30% of cases; especially adults)
L3: Burkitt (5% of cases)

***Immunologic classification***

Null cell (pre-B cell): $CALLA^+$ (CD10), $TdT^+$, $CD19^+$ ± IgH rearrangement (70%)
T cell: $CD2^+$, $TdT^+$, TCR rearrangement (25%)
B cell (Burkitt): Surface $Ig^+$ (5%)

***Genetic classification***

Karyotypic abnormalities in up to 50%
t9:22 (p190 rather than p210): High CR but high relapse
t8:2, t8:14, t8:22 (involving c-*myc* on chromosome 8): Burkitt
Altered ploidy

**Prognostic features**

Poor prognostic features include
- Age < 2 or > 9
- White blood cell count at presentation > $30 \times 10^9$/L
- (?)T cell phenotype with mediastinal mass
- CNS involvement

**Treatment considerations**

Induction with vincristine and prednisone; add anthracycline for poor risk
CNS therapy
Prolonged maintenance therapy
Bone marrow transplantation in first remission for poor risk; second remission for others

### Acute nonlymphocytic leukemia

**Classification schemes**
***Morphologic classification***

M0: Primitive stem cell–like leukemia
M1: Undifferentiated myelogenous leukemia
M2: Acute myelogenous leukemia
M3: Acute promyelocytic leukemia
M4: Acute myelomonocytic leukemia
M5: Acute monocytic leukemia
M6: Erythroleukemia
M7: Megakaryoblastic leukemia

***Immunologic classification***

Morphologic classification schemes are supplemented by determination of leukemia cell expression of surface antigens including CD34 (expressed on stem cell–like leukemias), HLA-DR, CD11 (myelomonocytic cells), CD14 (monocytic cells), glycophorin A (erythroleukemia), and glycoprotein Ia/IIb (megakaryoblastic leukemia).

***Genetic classification***

t9:22—ANLL complicating previous CML
t8:21—M2 (good prognosis)
t15:17—M3 (rearrangement of the retinoic acid receptor)
inv16—M4 with eosinophilia (good prognosis)
del 5, del 7, $5q^-$, $7q^-$—previous myelodysplastic syndrome (poor prognosis)
tri 8, tri 13—(poor prognosis)
t1:3, t3:3—increased platelets (poor prognosis)
t4:11—biphenotypic (features of both ALL and ANLL)

**Prognostic features**

Poor prognostic features include infection at diagnosis; ANLL arising from previous chemotherapy, radiation therapy, or myelodysplasia; older age; cytogenetics (see above); hyperleukocytosis.

**Treatment considerations**

Induction with cytosine arabinoside and daunorubicin followed by intensive consolidation.
Disseminated intravascular coagulation complicating M3 and M5 subtypes.
Radiation and/or leukopheresis occasionally required for hyperleukocytosis.
Bone marrow transplantation for selected patients.

nous fluids and allopurinol in anticipation of rapid application of definitive chemotherapy.

Definitive therapy requires aggressive chemotherapy with antibiotic and transfusion support, which usually requires hospitalization in a tertiary care center. The use of allogeneic bone marrow transplantation may yield long-term disease-free survival rates approaching 50% among appropriately selected patients.

## HODGKIN'S DISEASE

Hodgkin's disease probably represents a more diverse group of disorders then previously recognized. The Reed-Sternberg cell is the putative malignant cell without whose presence it is difficult or impossible to establish a diagnosis of Hodgkin's disease. The precise origin of this cell remains a subject of debate, and it may have different lineage derivation in the different subtypes of Hodgkin's disease.

Hodgkin's disease has a bimodal age distribution, with peaks in the second and third decades and then again in the sixth and seventh decades of life. Typical presentation is with cervical or axillary adenopathy or the detection of a mediastinal mass on chest x-ray film. Patients may develop associated symptoms of fevers, night sweats, weight loss, or pruritus. The diagnosis is established by characteristic lymph node histology. Based on histology, patients are subcategorized as having lymphocyte-predominant, mixed cellularity or lymphocyte-depleted disease. A separate category of Hodgkin's disease is nodular sclerosing Hodgkin's, in which bands of sclerosis divide the lymph node into lobules. Nodular sclerosis has a somewhat better prognosis. The histologic classification is summarized in Table 54-2.

Hodgkin's disease is usually spread by the lymphatic route to contiguous lymphoid groups. Staging is critical, since limited disease may be treated with radiotherapy, but more extensive disease requires systemic chemotherapy. Staging is largely based on physical examination, computed tomography (CT) scans of the chest, abdomen, and pelvis, and bone marrow examination. Lymphangiograms are used less often, and gallium scans are an increasingly useful adjunct. Staging is summarized in the box at right.

Splenectomy was traditionally done in patients with low-stage disease to rule out occult involvement before proceeding to radiotherapy. Although CT scanning has increased the diagnosis of occult abdominal disease, splenectomy may still be required in selected cases. Because of the low incidence of abdominal disease, young women with clinical stage I disease confined to cervical or axillary nodes, especially with lymphocyte-predominant or nodular sclerosing histologies, may not require splenectomy.

Therapy for Hodgkin's disease has been highly successful relative to other hematologic malignancies. For localized disease (stages IA and IIA) radiotherapy is frequently curative. Stage IV disease or the presence of B symptoms, especially in stage III, often requires combination chemotherapy but still has a high rate of response. The treatment of intermediate stages, especially IIB and IIIA, varies depending on the experience of radiotherapists involved in the patient's care. Combination radiation therapy and chemotherapy is associated with an unfortunate increase in late secondary leukemias or solid malignancies and is generally avoided except in the presence of massive disease in the mediastinum. Bone marrow transplantation may be useful in the treatment of relapse.

## NON-HODGKIN'S LYMPHOMA

Non-Hodgkin's lymphomas are predominantly of B cell origin and typically present with lymphadenopathy or an abdominal mass. Non-Hodgkin's lymphomas are classified based on individual cellular histologic characteristics and the general pattern of organization of malignant tissues within the lymph nodes. Details of the classification systems can be found within standard hematology or oncology textbooks, but for general purposes can be thought of as falling into three categories.

The *indolent lymphomas* are composed of relatively small, well-differentiated cells. The most common forms encountered are diffuse small lymphocytic and follicular small cleaved cell lymphoma (well-differentiated lympho-

**Table 54-2.** Histopathologic classification and clinicopathologic correlations of Hodgkin's disease

| Classification | Frequency (%) | B symptoms* (%) |
|---|---|---|
| Lymphocyte predominance | 3-10 | 0 |
| Nodular sclerosis | 20-50 | 35 |
| Mixed cellularity | 25-40 | 43 |
| Lymphocyte depletion | 5-10 | 70 |

*Fever, weight loss, night sweats.

### Staging classification of Hodgkin's disease (modified Ann Arbor)

The classification is labeled A if the patient has none of the three B symptoms (fever, night sweats, or unexplained loss of 10% or more of the body weight) during the 6 months before admission. Presence of these symptoms prompts a B classification.

Stage I: Single lymph node region (I) or a single extralymphatic site ($I_E$)

Stage II: Two or more lymph node regions on the same side of the diaphragm (II) or a localized site of extralymphatic involvement plus one or more node regions on the same side of the diaphragm ($II_E$)

Stage III: Lymph node regions on both sides of the diaphragm (III), which may include the spleen ($III_S$), a single extralymphatic site ($III_E$), or both $III_{SE}$)

Stage IV: Diffuse or disseminated involvement of one or more extralymphatic organs:
- Marrow = M+
- Lung = L+
- Liver = H+
- Pleura = P+
- Bone = O+
- Skin = D+

cytic and nodular poorly differentiated lymphocytic lymphoma in the Rappaport classification scheme). Although slow growing, this group of lymphomas often become evident in an advanced stage. The indolent nature of this class of lymphoma usually results in prolonged survival approaching that of age-matched controls in selected patients. Though responsive to chemotherapy, the indolent lymphomas are rarely curable except with the application of therapy such as allogeneic bone marrow transplantation, which is usually not medically appropriate in this age group.

The *aggressive lymphomas* occupy an intermediate territory composed of larger, more immature cells that usually replace the normal node in a diffuse pattern of growth. Large cell and immunoblastic lymphomas (histiocytic lymphoma in the Rappaport classification) make up this group. Left untreated, the natural history of these lymphomas is more rapid, resulting in death within a short time. This rapid growth, however, renders them highly susceptible to chemotherapy and potential cure in a high proportion of cases.

Finally, the small subset of the *highly aggressive lymphomas* includes diseases such as lymphoblastic lymphoma and Burkitt's lymphoma. They tend to be explosive in onset and their course progresses rapidly to death when left untreated. They have a high predilection toward involvement of the central nervous system or other sanctuary sites. These lymphomas may be so highly responsive to chemotherapy that the rapid lysis of large numbers of tumor cells can cause a tumor lysis syndrome, with excessive levels of phosphate, potassium, and uric acid that may precipitate renal failure, cardiac arrhythmias, and other serious sequelae. Although the highly aggressive lymphomas may respond very well to chemotherapy, their aggressive growth and extensive nature make them more difficult to cure than the intermediate aggressive lymphomas.

Non-Hodgkin's lymphomas are staged in a manner analogous to that of Hodgkin's disease, although the lack of orderly spread and more unitary treatment approaches make staging less useful than in Hodgkin's disease. Newer classification systems based on age, a more general distinction of localized versus advanced disease, extent of extranodal involvement, performance status, and a variety of biologic markers will probably emerge as more useful predictors of prognosis and guides to therapy.

Treatment depends mostly on histologic diagnosis, with consideration given to stage and patient status. For the indolent lymphomas, therapy is usually minimal and is often delayed until necessary to treat symptoms. Judicious use of oral alkylating agents and/or local irradiation may be as efficient as more aggressive chemotherapeutic interventions. Occasionally, a patient who has symptoms at a young age may benefit from aggressive treatment with autologous or allogeneic bone marrow transplantation.

Combination chemotherapy with cyclophosphamide, doxorubicin hydrochloride (Adriamycin), vincristine (Oncovin), and prednisone, collectively known as *CHOP*, remains standard therapy for patients with large cell lymphoma. A recent cooperative group study showed no superiority of more aggressive five- and six-drug regimens. Selected patients may be treated with bone marrow transplantation at relapse.

The preferred treatment for the highly aggressive lymphomas is patterned after that for acute lymphoblastic leukemia. To be successful, it must incorporate therapy directed toward the central nervous system. Though these malignancies may show a dramatic response with marked tumor lysis, long-term survival unfortunately remains poor, particularly in the older patient with advanced disease. Autologous and allogeneic transplantations play an important role in helping appropriately selected patients to achieve long-term disease-free survival.

## MYELOMA AND RELATED PLASMA CELL DISORDERS

Myeloma is a disease of plasma cells, the terminally differentiated immunoglobulin-secreting B cell. The classic presentation of myeloma is that of a monoclonal immunoglobulin spike detectable in the peripheral blood or urine and punched out lytic lesions of the major marrow-containing bones, including the skull, proximal long bones, and axial skeleton; when severe it is associated with hypercalcemia. Plasmacytoma is a histologically similar plasma cell lesion presenting as a soft tissue mass.

Myeloma should be suspected in cases of pathologic fracture, unexplained anemia, unexplained renal failure, unexplained hypercalcemia, and with the detection of a monoclonal protein. Diagnosis is made by serum protein electrophoresis combined with marrow evaluation. Treatment includes chemotherapy and radiotherapy to skeletal lesions. Cure is achievable only with marrow transplantation in selected individuals.

Patients with low levels of monoclonal protein and fewer than 10% plasma cells in the marrow are labeled as having a monoclonal gammopathy of unknown significance. Most such patients are older at diagnosis and more often die of unrelated causes, although the disease in long-term survivors may evolve into frank myeloma. Watchful waiting may be the most appropriate intervention.

## BONE MARROW TRANSPLANTATION

Bone marrow transplantation is an increasingly important therapy used in the treatment of hematologic malignancies whose general features are summarized in the box on p. 747. The two major forms of bone marrow transplantation are *allogeneic* transplantation, in which donor marrow is typically derived from a matched sibling, and *autologous* transplantation, in which the patient's own marrow is harvested in advance and stored in liquid nitrogen until the time of use.

The performance of bone marrow transplantation follows a *preparation* phase in which high doses of chemotherapy with or without concomitant radiation are administered to treat the malignancy and, in the case of allogeneic transplants, suppress host immunity to adequately accept the marrow graft. This is followed by infusion of the marrow graft through a central vein. The cells in the graft can then migrate to the marrow cavity and reestablish hematopoiesis.

Marrow transplantation offers the opportunity to rescue patients who would otherwise succumb to fatal hematologic toxicities of the accelerated chemotherapy doses used in the preparative regimen. Allogeneic transplant further offers the opportunity to replace diseased marrow

### Bone marrow transplantation

**Types**

*Syngeneic:* Donor is an identical twin.

*Allogeneic:* Donor is typically a sibling matched at the A, B, DR loci of the major histocompatibility (HLA) complex.

*Unrelated:* HLA-matched volunteer (unrelated); the results are comparable to standard transplant when done with careful matching in experienced center.

*Autologous:* Marrow is previously harvested from the patient and cryopreserved until the time of use.

*Peripheral stem cell:* Cells derived from blood rather than marrow are used; it is typically autologous.

**Phases**

*Initial evaluation:* Patient is evaluated for ability to tolerate and benefit from transplant.

*Marrow harvest:* Autologous transplant patients have stem cells harvested in advance and cryopreserved.

*Preparative phase:* Patients receive high-dose chemotherapy/radiotherapy to suppress or eradicate malignant cells and, in heterologous transplantation, to suppress recipient immunity sufficiently to receive the donor marrow.

*Transplant:* Previously harvested autologous marrow is thawed, or heterologous marrow is harvested and infused into the patient via a central vein. Cells then "home" to marrow cavities.

*Immediate recovery:* Immediate recovery period is similar in all patients with the possibility of acute pulmonary, hepatic, or cardiac toxicity from the preparative regimen and a period of absolute cytopenias resulting in bleeding or infectious risk.

*Long-term recovery:* Although patients undergoing autologous transplantation typically return to relatively normal with hematologic recovery, heterologous transplant recipients may have additional complications related to graft-versus-host disease and related immune deficiencies.

with normal donor marrow and may create an ongoing immunologic reaction against residual malignant cells that contributes to disease control. An expensive and toxic therapy, the ultimate role of bone marrow transplantation is not yet fully established, but it seems to play a role in the treatment of chronic myelocytic leukemia, high-risk acute leukemia in first remission, relapsed lymphoma, and selected patients with myelodysplasia and myeloma. Allogenic transplantation may also benefit nonmalignant disorders such as aplastic anemia, storage diseases, osteopetrosis, and severe thalassemia.

## BIBLIOGRAPHY

Bloomfield CD, Herzig GP, editors: Advances in the management of adult acute leukemia, *Hematol Oncol Clin North Am* 7(1), 1993.

DeVita VT Jr, Hellman S, Rosenberg SA: *Cancer: principles and practice of oncology,* ed 4, Philadelphia, 1993, JB Lippincott.

Forman SJ, editor: Bone marrow transplantation, *Hematol Oncol Clin North Am* 4(3), 1990.

Jacobs P: Hodgkin's disease and the malignant lymphomas, *Dis Mon* 34:215, 1993.

Mazza JJ, editor: *Manual of clinical hematology,* Boston, 1988, Little, Brown.

Rosenthal DS: Clinical aspects of chronic myeloproliferative diseases, *Am J Med Sci* 304:109, 1992.

Williams WJ et al, editors: *Hematology,* ed 4, New York, 1990, McGraw-Hill.

CHAPTER

# 55A Hemorrhagic and Thrombotic Disorders

**Jack E. Ansell**
**Michael Thane**
**Frank Parker**

Primary care physicians often encounter clinical problems of bleeding or thrombosis. Easy bruising is a common complaint in the office setting. Posttraumatic or postsurgical bleeding in a hospitalized patient may first be seen by the family physician for management. Physicians are commonly faced with an unexpected or unexplained prolonged partial thromboplastin time or bleeding time. Deep venous thrombosis of a lower extremity, although a common medical condition, is notoriously tricky to diagnose, and its treatment may be fraught with complications. Accordingly, primary care physicians must have a working knowledge of the rudiments of hemostatic and thrombotic reactions, associated pathologic conditions, and especially appropriate treatment of disorders that can evolve into life-threatening emergencies. This discussion touches on a wide range of hemorrhagic and thrombotic disorders and their treatment, beginning with a brief overview of coagulation and platelet physiology.

## NORMAL HEMOSTASIS

Normal hemostasis depends on the close interaction of platelets and the coagulation proteins in a normally functioning vascular system. As a consequence of vascular injury, platelets exposed to subendothelial collagen are stimulated to undergo a sequence of reactions leading to primary platelet plug formation. This plug is then reinforced by the activation of coagulation and fibrin formation to form a stable hemostatic plug.

Platelet reactions can be divided into three physiologic processes: *adhesion* to subendothelial collagen; activation, shape change, and *secretion* of a number of substances; and *aggregation* between adjacent activated platelets. Adhesion depends on specific platelet membrane receptors (glycoprotein $I_b$) and on von Willebrand factor, a plasma factor that serves as a bridge between platelets and collagen. Deficiencies of either can lead to platelet dysfunction and bleeding. Platelet secretion depends on a sequence of reactions in the platelet membrane. These include phospholipase C activation, which leads to calcium mobilization in the platelet cytosol, and phospho-

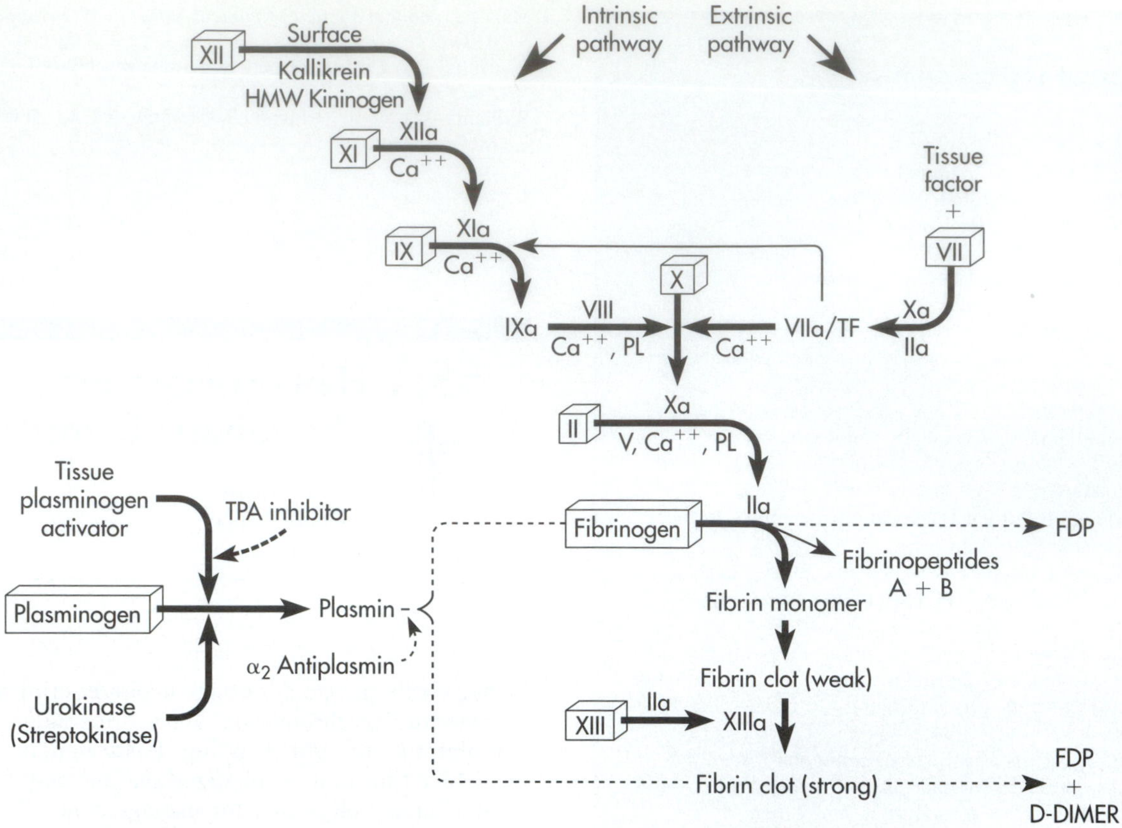


**Fig. 55A-1.** Coagulation cascade. Fibrin clot formation results from the generation of thrombin, which is dependent on the sequential interaction of proenzymes and activated coagulation factors in the intrinsic, extrinsic, and common pathways of coagulation. *HMW*, High molecular weight; *PL*, phospholipid.

**Table 55A-1.** Characteristics of coagulation factors

| Factor | Descriptive name | Source | Approximate half-life (hr) | Function |
|---|---|---|---|---|
| I | Fibrinogen | Liver | 120 | Substrate for fibrin clot (CP) |
| II | Prothrombin | Liver (VKD) | 60 | Serine protease (CP) |
| V | Proaccelerin, labile factor | Liver | 12-36 | Cofactor (CP) |
| VII | Serum prothrombin conversion accelerator, proconvertin | Liver (VKD) | 6 | (?) Serine protease (EP) |
| VIII | Antihemophilic factor or globulin | Endothelial cells and (?) elsewhere | 12 | Cofactor (IP) |
| IX | Plasma thromboplastin component, Christmas factor | Liver (VKD) | 24 | Serine protease (IP) |
| X | Stuart-Prower factor | Liver (VKD) | 36 | Serine protease (CP) |
| XI | Plasma thromboplastin antecedent | (?) Liver | 40-84 | Serine protease (IP) |
| XII | Hageman factor | (?) Liver | 50 | Serine protease contact activation (IP) |
| XIII | Fibrin-stabilizing factor | (?) Liver | 96-180 | Transglutaminase (CP) |
| Prekallikrein | Fletcher factor | (?) Liver | ? | Serine protease contact activation (IP) |
| High–molecular weight kininogen | Fitzgerald factor, Flaujeac or Williams factor | (?) Liver | ? | Cofactor, contact activation (IP) |

*CP*, Common pathway; *VKD*, vitamin K–dependent; *EP*, extrinsic pathway; *IP*, intrinsic pathway.

lipase $A_2$ activation, which leads to release of arachidonic acid through the prostaglandin cascade and formation of thromboxane $A_2$. As a result, platelets secrete a number of endogenous proteins, platelet agonists, and vasoactive factors. This process also exposes the glycoprotein $II_b$-$III_a$ complex on the platelet membrane, which binds fibrinogen and serves as a linking site to bind other platelets and thus complete the process of platelet aggregation.

As the platelets are activated by vascular injury, the coagulation cascade is also initiated, leading to fibrin formation and stabilization of the primary platelet plug. The participants in the coagulation reactions can be functionally grouped and characterized (Table 55A-1) and their sequential interactions illustrated (Fig. 55A-1). A number of serine proteases or proenzymes require activation; cofactors accelerate the enzymatic reactions, and inhibitors limit the reactions. Factors XII and XI in the intrinsic system are activated by contact with damaged endothelial cells. Prekallikrein accelerates the reaction and high–molecular weight kininogen serves as a cofactor. Factor IX in turn is activated by $XI_a$ but can also be activated through the extrinsic system by factor VII-tissue factor. Factor VIII is a cofactor accelerating the activation of factor X by $IX_a$. Factor X can also be activated through the extrinsic system by factor VII and tissue factor. Factor VII is activated by the release or exposure of tissue factor from injured endothelial cells. The common pathway proceeds with activation of factor II (prothrombin), with factor V serving as a cofactor. Factor $II_a$, or thrombin, then cleaves two small peptides from fibrinogen (peptides A and B), and the remaining fibrin monomers polymerize to form long fibrin strands and ultimately a fibrin clot. Factor XIII stabilizes the association of fibrin monomers by introducing covalent disulfide bonds between strands.

There are a number of natural inhibitors in this process serving to limit fibrin formation. These include antithrombin III, heparin cofactor II, protein C and protein S, and tissue factor pathway inhibitor (Fig. 55A-2). Deficiencies of any of these proteins can lead to hypercoagulable or prethrombotic conditions.

Last, fibrin formation is limited by the fibrinolytic system, the principal factor being plasminogen (see Figs. 55A-1 and 55A-2). The primary activator of plasminogen is tissue plasminogen activator (tPA) released from damaged endothelial cells. tPA has its own natural inhibitor, plasminogen activator inhibitor, which can be altered in disease states.

## SCREENING

There are a large number of assays of the functional status of the coagulation and platelet mechanisms, but many are relevant only to the coagulation specialist consulting in the evaluation of complex hemorrhagic or thrombotic disorders. The primary care physician, however, should be

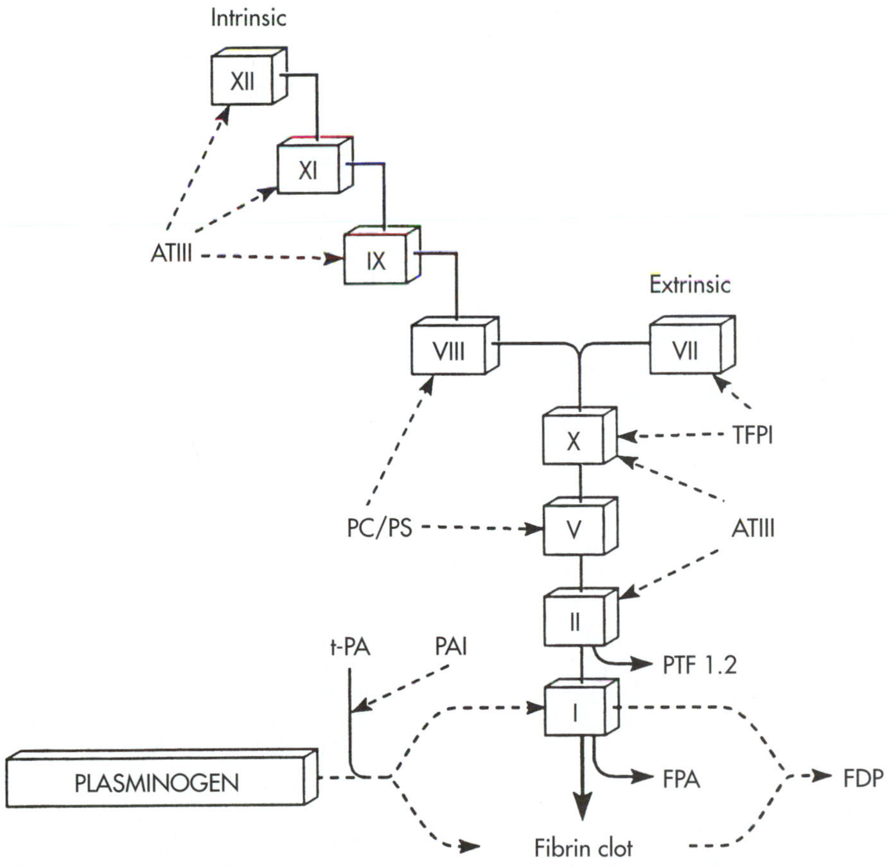


**Fig. 55A-2.** Coagulation cascade illustrating the site of action of coagulation inhibitors and the fibrinolytic system. *ATIII,* Antithrombin III; *PC/PS,* protein C/protein S; *t-PA,* tissue plasminogen activator; *PAI,* plasminogen activator inhibitor; *TFPI,* tissue factor pathway inhibitor; *PTF 1.2,* prothrombin fragment 1.2; *FDP,* fibrin(ogen) degradation products.

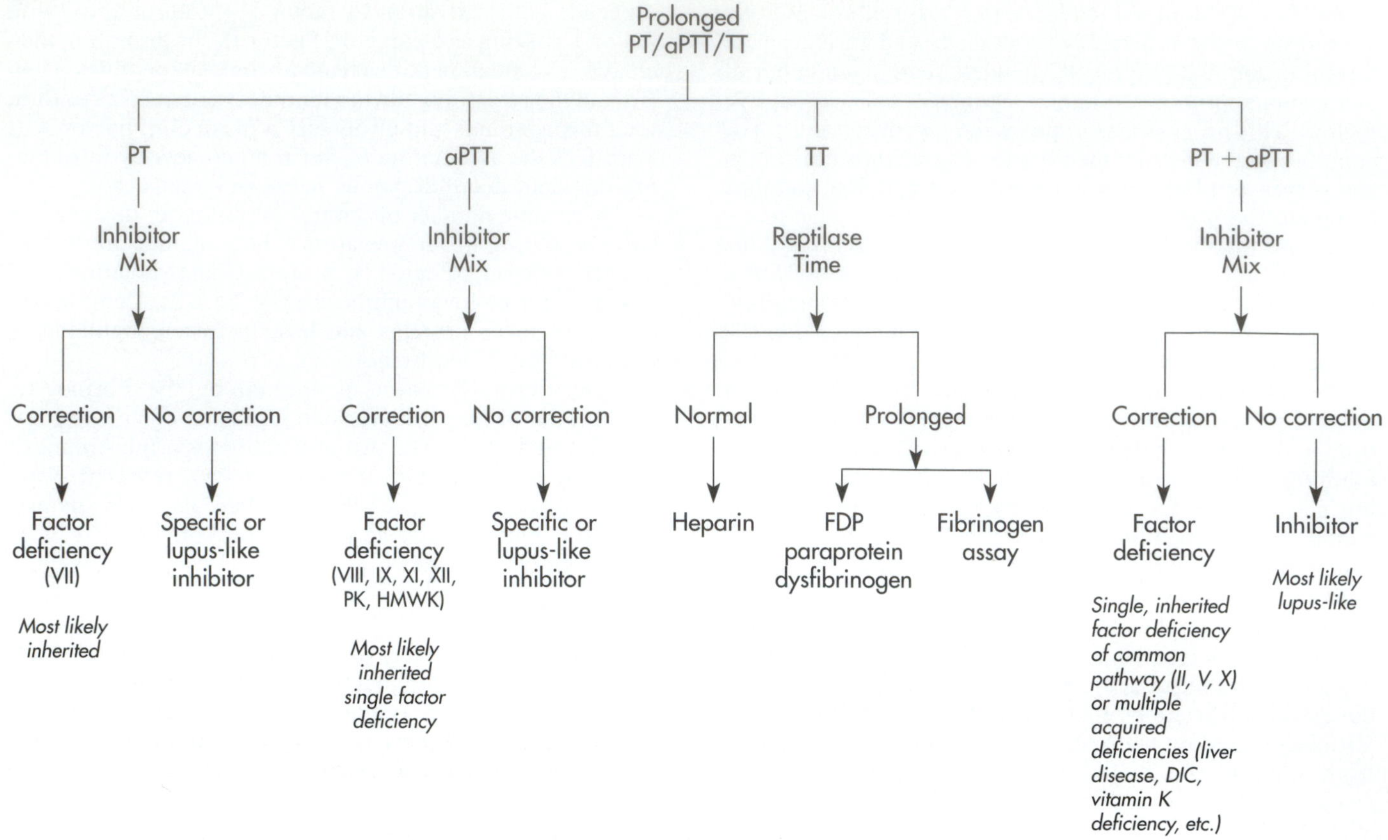


**Fig. 55A-3.** Approach to the evaluation of a prolonged prothrombin time (PT), activated partial thromboplastin time (aPTT), or thrombin time (TT).

familiar with the usual screening tests and the conceptual approach to evaluating hemostatic disorders.

## History and physical examination

The evaluation begins with the clinical history to determine whether a patient truly has a bleeding tendency based on history (if acute bleeding is not currently present), and whether it is congenital or acquired based on data such as family history, male or female occurrence, and childhood bleeding. Clues to a coagulation vs. platelet defect can also be discerned by noting the history of petechiae (platelet defects) or ecchymoses (coagulation defects). None of these historical elements is definitive, but they do help in the overall evaluation. A detailed medication history is imperative, particularly noting aspirin or nonsteroidal antiinflammatory agent use. Physical examination provides limited clues in this evaluation but may help support a platelet or coagulation defect by the presence of petechiae or ecchymoses. Furthermore, the presence of other abnormalities may indicate an underlying systemic illness associated with specific hemorrhagic or thrombotic disorders.

## Laboratory evaluation

The laboratory evaluation can be extensive, but the initial tests almost always include a prothrombin time (PT) and activated partial thromboplastin time (aPTT) for screening of the entire coagulation cascade, and a platelet count and bleeding time to screen for quantitatively and qualitatively normal platelets. The bleeding time has been shown not to be a good preoperative screening test to predict bleeding potential, but it is useful for evaluating known or suspected qualitative platelet defects. The platelet count is obviously useful to detect reduced or increased platelet numbers. Fig. 55A-3 highlights the approach to evaluating an abnormal PT or aPTT and the diagnostic possibilities. A prolongation of either test can be the result of a coagulation factor deficiency or circulating inhibitor (antibody). The distinction between these two possibilities is made by performing a mixing assay with patient and normal plasma and repeating the abnormal test. A correction in the result suggests a factor deficiency, whereas no correction suggests an inhibitor. Factor assays or other tests can then be performed to further distinguish the abnormalities.

Additional assays with which physicians should be familiar include a thrombin time (an indirect measure of fibrinogen) and assays of fibrin(ogen) degradation products (FDP) or D-dimers. A positive FDP assay can result from plasmin lysis of fibrinogen or fibrin, whereas a positive D-dimer indicates plasmin lysis of fibrin, an indicator that thrombin has been generated and has converted fibrinogen to fibrin (i.e., intravascular coagulation).

Clinicians should not feel reticent about seeking consultative help from a coagulation specialist when confronted with a hemorrhagic or thrombotic disorder. Given their usual complexity, these disorders may require extensive laboratory evaluation. Table 55A-2 illustrates some of the more common disorders and how they would alter the usual screening tests just discussed.

**Table 55A-2.** Presumptive diagnosis of common bleeding disorders based on routine screening tests

| Platelet count | Bleeding time | PT | PTT | TT | Miscellaneous | Presumptive problem |
|---|---|---|---|---|---|---|
| ↓ | N-↑ | N | N | N | | Thrombocytopenia |
| N | ↑ | N | N | N | | Platelet function defect or vascular defect |
| N | ↑ | N | ↑ | N | ↓ $VIII_e$, ↓ $VIII_{ag}$, ↓ $VIII_{vWF}$ | von Willebrand disease |
| N | N | ↑ | N | N | | Extrinsic pathway defect (VII) |
| N | N | N | ↑ | N | | Intrinsic pathway defect (VIII, IX, XI, XII, prekallikrein, high–molecular weight kininogen, inhibitor) |
| N | N | ↑ | ↑ | N | | Common pathway or multiple pathway defects excluding fibrinogen |
| N | N | ↑ | ↑ | ↑ | High levels of FDP | Fibrinogen deficiency or dysfunction, vitamin K deficiency, liver disease, primary fibrinolysis |
| ↓ | N-↑ | ↑ | ↑ | ↑ | High levels of FDP | DIC |
| N | N | N | N | N | Positive clot solubility | XIII deficiency |

*N*, Normal; ↓, decreased; ↑, increased; *FDP*, fibrin(ogen) degradation products; *DIC*, disseminated intravascular coagulation.

## HEMORRHAGIC DISORDERS AND THEIR TREATMENT

### Thrombocytopenia

A prolonged bleeding time as a result of thrombocytopenia does not develop until the platelet count reaches the 50,000 to 75,000/µl range (normal 150,000 to 350,000/µl). The risk of significant spontaneous bleeding, however, is not present until the count reaches the 10,000 to 20,000/µl level. Furthermore, the risk of bleeding is somewhat less for the same level of platelet count when the thrombocytopenia is due to peripheral destruction vs. inadequate production of platelets. A bone marrow biopsy is commonly used to distinguish between inadequate production and increased destruction as a cause of the thrombocytopenia.

Inadequate production of platelets may result from a stem cell defect and usually affects all three cell lines, as in the myeloproliferative and myelodysplastic syndromes. Invasion of the marrow by carcinoma, granuloma, or fibrosis also interferes with thrombopoiesis. Cancer chemotherapy is probably the most common cause today for a drug-induced reduction in platelet production, although some other drugs can also interfere, usually in an idiosyncratic fashion. Vitamin $B_{12}$ and folic acid deficiencies are well-known causes of ineffective thrombopoiesis. Platelet transfusions are indicated to treat bleeding in these situations, but prophylactic platelets are not generally recommended unless the platelet count is reduced to the 10,000 to 20,000/µl range. When platelets are transfused, the quantity obtained from a single apheresis donor is used, which is equivalent to the platelets obtained from approximately 6 to 8 random donor units. Alternatively, random donor platelets can be used.

Thrombocytopenia in the setting of a normal bone marrow can be attributed to either immune or nonimmune peripheral destruction, and rarely to excessive dilution. Nonimmune thrombocytopenia is most often encountered with disseminated intravascular coagulation (DIC), where platelets are activated and destroyed when they come in contact with intravascular fibrin or are exposed to thrombin. Treatment is generally directed at the underlying cause of the DIC or at interrupting the consumption process (see discussion of DIC later). Platelets may be given, but their overall effectiveness is questionable unless the DIC is corrected. Severe thrombocytopenia can also occur in the rare disorder of thrombotic thrombocytopenic purpura (TTP), a primary disorder of platelet consumption of unknown etiology. The TTP syndrome consists of thrombocytopenia, microangiopathic hemolytic anemia, often transient neurologic deficits, renal impairment, and fever. TTP, once a highly fatal disorder, is responsive to the simultaneous administration of fresh frozen plasma (FFP) and plasmapheresis. High-dose adrenal corticosteroids may provide some benefit, and aspirin is often given to interfere with platelet activation. In some cases splenectomy may also be of benefit. With these treatments mortality has been reduced considerably, but TTP and DIC are still life-threatening emergencies that require hematologic consultation.

Immunologic thrombocytopenia may be mediated by drug-induced antibodies, isoantibodies, or autoantibodies. Drug-induced antibodies may attach to platelet membranes by an innocent bystander mechanism (immune complex deposition), in response to neoantigen formation by a drug and platelet membrane complex, or by specific membrane receptor targeting induced by a drug. Heparin is the most common cause of drug-induced thrombocytopenia. Heparin-induced thrombocytopenia (HIT) usually occurs after 6 to 8 days of intravenous heparin therapy, although it can occur sooner, especially in previously exposed patients, and it may develop after exposure to subcutaneous therapy or even heparin flushes used to maintain catheter patency. It is thought to be an immune mediated thrombocytopenia. The diagnosis is based on the clinical presentation with other causes being excluded. Heparin-induced platelet aggregation or serotonin release assays may help confirm a diagnosis.

Although platelet counts may be low, bleeding is

unusual. Rather, paradoxical thromboembolism is the most worrisome complication and may be attributable to in vivo heparin-induced platelet aggregation. HIT occurs in about 1% to 5% of patients taking heparin for 5 to 10 days, and heparin-induced thrombosis occurs in only a small fraction of these patients. Cessation of heparin is mandatory, and alternative anticoagulation is initiated with warfarin or a new low–molecular weight heparinoid called danaparoid (Org 10172, Orgaran).

Idiopathic (immune) thrombocytopenic purpura (ITP) is the most common form of immunologic thrombocytopenia. It occurs in acute (often in children) and chronic (in adults) forms. In children 90% or more of cases have an acute onset, often preceded by a viral illness, and resolve on their own over the course of 1 to 3 months. Physical findings are limited to the skin, where petechiae may be seen, especially in the dependent extremities. Splenomegaly is not seen. Specific treatment is often unnecessary, although corticosteroids may be given to boost the count from very low levels until spontaneous recovery occurs. ITP in the adult is most often chronic with an insidious onset of easy bruising or minor bleeding noted over the preceding months. Women are more commonly affected. Bleeding manifestations include petechiae, ecchymoses, menorrhagia, hematuria, melena, epistaxis, and gingival bleeding. The onset is not associated with an antecedent infection. The physical examination is unremarkable. The diagnosis is traditionally based on clinical grounds (i.e., the exclusion of other causes of thrombocytopenia in the setting of peripheral destruction of platelets as determined by a bone marrow biopsy). A platelet antibody assay may be helpful but should not be used as a definitive test. Treatment is more complex than for childhood ITP. Corticosteroids are indicated initially, but definitive responses are uncommon. Splenectomy is generally indicated next in low surgical risk candidates. Other treatment modalities include intravenous γ-globulin, attenuated androgens, immunosuppressive agents, staphylococcal protein A columns, and plasmapheresis. After all therapeutic modalities are exhausted, about 10% of patients continue to have serious thrombocytopenia for which no therapy is effective. Table 55A-3 highlights the differences between the acute and chronic forms of ITP.

Thrombocytopenia resulting from isoantibodies occurs after multiple platelet transfusions, or in a syndrome called posttransfusion purpura caused by transfusion of mismatched platelets. Thrombocytopenia can also occur on a dilutional basis in individuals transfused large volumes of blood over a short interval (e.g., 10 to 20 units of blood over a 24-hour period). Finally, thrombocytopenia can occur as a result of a hyperfunctioning spleen (hypersplenism) in individuals with splenomegaly for a variety of reasons.

### Qualitative platelet disorders

Functional platelet defects produce a long bleeding time in the presence of a normal platelet count and may predispose to bleeding. Inherited disorders are uncommon, the most likely one being von Willebrand disease, which is a defect or deficiency in von Willebrand factor, a component of the factor VIII complex that is important for normal platelet adhesion. Acquired defects are much more common and are usually the result of drugs, aspirin being the major

**Table 55A-3.** Clinical features of the acute and chronic forms of idiopathic thrombocytopenic purpura

| | Acute (predominating in children) | Chronic (predominating in adults) |
|---|---|---|
| Age of onset | 2-6 yr | 20-40 yr |
| Sex predilection | None | 3 females : 1 male |
| Presentation | Sudden | Insidious |
| Preceding illness | Common | Unusual |
| Onset of bleeding | Abrupt | Insidious |
| Serious bleeding | Uncommon | Uncommon |
| Palpable spleen | Rare | Rare |
| Platelet count | <20,000/μl | 20,000-80,000/μl |
| Clinical course | 2-6 wk | Months to years |

**Table 55A-4.** Laboratory findings in disorders of platelet function

| Laboratory test | Thrombasthenia | Storage pool disease | Abnormal release mechanism (aspirin-like) | Bernard-Soulier syndrome (giant platelet) |
|---|---|---|---|---|
| Platelet count | Normal | Normal | Normal | Mild to moderate thrombocytopenia |
| Platelet morphology | Normal | Normal | Normal | Characteristic giant platelets |
| Bleeding time | Prolonged | Prolonged | Prolonged | Prolonged |
| Clot retraction | Deficient | Normal | Normal | Normal |
| Platelet retention in glass bead columns (glass adhesion) | Reduced | Reduced | Reduced | Reduced |
| Platelet aggregation by 5 μm ADP | Absent | Normal | Normal | Normal |
| Platelet aggregation by threshold concentrations of ADP (0.2-1.5 μm) | Absent | Primary wave normal | Primary wave normal | Normal |
| Platelet aggregation by collagen suspensions and 5 μm epinephrine | Absent | Abnormal | Abnormal | Normal |
| Platelet aggregation by ristocetin (1.2-1.5 mg/ml) | Normal | Normal | Normal | Abnormal |
| Storage nucleotide pool | Normal | Diminished | Normal | Normal |

offender. Aspirin and other nonsteroidal antiinflammatory drugs (NSAIDs) impair platelet prostaglandin production and induce a release defect; aspirin-induced impairment is irreversible, whereas NSAID effect is not. Rarely platelet transfusions are needed to correct an aspirin defect in the face of serious bleeding. Uremia also produces a qualitative defect that can sometimes be improved by dialysis or by the infusion of cryoprecipitate or the use of deamino-8-D-arginine vasopressin (DDAVP). Last, myeloproliferative disorders can be associated with a platelet defect resulting from an abnormal stem cell. Table 55A-4 summarizes the laboratory findings one might see in the spectrum of qualitative platelet disorders.

### Acquired coagulation disorders

A discussion of the inherited coagulation disorders is a pediatric topic, but the more common acquired disorders are important to review, since the primary care physician will be called upon to diagnose and treat these problems. The reader is referred to other texts in the bibliography for a more detailed discussion of the congenital factor deficiencies.

***Vitamin K deficiency.*** Vitamin K deficiency is most often seen in seriously ill patients, especially in the postoperative state when patients are poorly nourished and receiving antibiotics. Poor nutrition removes vitamin K from the diet, and antibiotics kill the gut bacteria that produce vitamin K. Vitamin K deficiency produces an initial rise in the prothrombin time because of the rapid decline of factor VII activity, the vitamin K–dependent factor with the shortest metabolic half-life. An elevation of the activated partial thromboplastin time follows as other vitamin K–dependent factors decline (factors IX, X, and II). This condition, which often leads to serious bleeding, is easily reversed by parenteral vitamin $K_1$ therapy (5 to 10 mg intramuscular or subcutaneous). Prophylaxis in patients at risk can easily prevent the condition, but unfortunately vitamin K deficiency often goes unrecognized until bleeding occurs.

***Liver disease.*** Impairment of the synthetic capacity of the liver is one of the most common causes for an acquired hemostatic defect. Hemostatic failure usually reflects the degree of liver failure and is usually subtle in acute liver failure unless the destruction of parenchymal tissue is fulminant. The PT, dependent on the short 6-hour half-life of factor VII, is prognostically helpful. Patients with biliary tract disease and obstructive jaundice may also develop a coagulopathy, but the mechanism in this situation is closely linked to levels of the vitamin K–dependent coagulation factors resulting from impaired absorption of vitamin K.

Hemostatic failure in liver disease involves both the platelet and coagulation phases of clotting. Thrombocytopenia, usually of mild degree when the platelet count is 50,000 to 100,000/μl, is frequently encountered because of hypersplenism that accompanies portal hypertension. Qualitative defects in platelet function, if they occur, are probably not a major factor.

Coagulation is impaired primarily because of decreased factor synthesis, but abnormal factors may be produced, excessive consumption can occur, and fibrinolysis may be enhanced as contributing causes of hemostatic failure. A low fibrinogen, one of the last factors to be reduced, is a poor prognostic sign.

Treatment depends on the severity of the coagulopathy and the presence of bleeding and usually includes FFP. Treatment simply for the purpose of correcting an abnormal PT and aPTT, however, is not recommended, since it takes a large volume of plasma to correct the abnormality, the correction is short lived, and the protein load contained in the plasma may be enough to induce hepatic encephalopathy in a patient who is so predisposed. Platelet transfusions can be given in the face of clinically important bleeding with a very low platelet count, but generally they are ineffective in hypersplenism.

***Disseminated intravascular coagulation.*** Disseminated intravascular coagulation (DIC) is conceptually a simple disorder, yet it is frustratingly complex in its diagnosis and treatment. It often occurs in critically ill patients and is common in the intensive care setting. However, DIC can also occur in relatively well patients, a result of certain underlying diseases such as malignancy. Its onset can be fulminant and rapidly fatal or can be more subtle and gradual. Although its name implies a disorder of intravascular clotting, its clinical expression is often one of a diffuse hemorrhagic disorder.

DIC involves the pathologic activation of coagulation by an underlying disease process that leads to fibrin clot

#### Causes of disseminated intravascular coagulation

Infection
- Gram-negative endotoxemia with hypotension or shock
- Severe gram-positive septicemia
- Rocky Mountain spotted fever
- Viral infections (herpes)
- Malaria (*Plasmodium falciparum*)
- HIV 1 infection

Complications of pregnancy and delivery
- Gram-negative sepsis
- Abruptio placentae
- Amniotic fluid embolism
- Retained dead fetus
- Toxemia

Pediatric disorders—especially in newborns

Malignant disease
- Metastatic carcinoma (prostate, pancreas, lung, stomach, colon, breast)
- Leukemia, especially APL

Liver disease (cirrhosis)

Complications of surgery
- Extracorporeal circulation

Critical tissue damage
- Brain tissue destruction
- Massive trauma
- Heat stroke
- Extensive burns

Miscellaneous
- Hemolytic transfusion reactions
- Vasculitis
- Aneurysms
- Giant hemangioma
- Snakebite

**Table 55A-5.** Laboratory findings in disseminated intravascular coagulation

| Test | Low-grade DIC | Fulminant DIC |
|---|---|---|
| Blood smear (microangiopathic) | ± | + |
| Platelets | Low normal to low | Very low |
| PT | Normal; short | Long |
| PTT | Normal; short | Long |
| TT | Normal; short; long | Long |
| Fibrinogen | Elevated; normal; low normal | Low |
| Fibrin monomers (protamine sulfate, ethanol gelation) | ± | + |
| Fibrin(ogen) degradation products | Mildly elevated | High |

All tests are easily obtainable within a short period of time (e.g., 1 to 2 hours) and constitute a DIC screen.

formation and secondary fibrinolysis, which then cause further consumption of coagulation factors, platelets, and red cells. In the fulminant syndrome bleeding results from factor deficiency (primarily factors I, II, V, VIII, and XIII), thrombocytopenia, excessive fibrinolysis, and high levels of FDP superimposed on a vascular system already damaged by diffuse microvascular thrombi. Bleeding is typically manifested by diffuse superficial hemorrhage in the form of ecchymoses and petechiae as well as oozing from the gingiva, the oral mucosa, or from the gastrointestinal and urinary tracts. Most hemorrhage tends to be from the microvasculature, although major vascular hemorrhage and central nervous system bleeding can occur. The diffuse thrombus formation may result in flat stellate-shaped purpuric necrotic areas, along with hemorrhagic bullae, acral cyanosis and the widespread mucosal bleeding mentioned above.

The pathophysiology of the consumption process depends on the underlying disease process or initiating event. The common mechanism is activation of a pathway of coagulation, usually the tissue factor pathway. The box on p. 753 summarizes those conditions likely to cause a DIC syndrome.

The diagnosis of DIC is complicated by the fact that the clinical manifestations range from no findings to those of an extensive thrombotic or hemorrhagic disease. Bleeding is usually generalized and from the microvasculature. Table 55A-5 highlights those tests commonly used to diagnose DIC. The most important component in the treatment of DIC is correction of the underlying disease. Supportive measures include FFP and platelet transfusions. Recent studies suggest a benefit to infusions of antithrombin III concentrates, but it is too premature to recommend their use. In rare cases low doses of intravenous or subcutaneous heparin may be useful to interrupt the process of consumption by neutralizing activated coagulation factors. This may be most helpful in well-characterized conditions such as acute promyelocytic leukemia associated with a high incidence of DIC. Efficacy of therapy can be monitored by looking for a decrease in FDP, an increase in fibrinogen, or the normalization of the PT and aPTT.

### Factors that enhance the risk of thromboembolism

Acquired risk factors
- Age >40 years
- Prior major surgical procedures
- Prior thromboembolism
- Immobilization
- Stasis (e.g., congestive heart failure, edema)
- Malignancy
- Sepsis
- Stroke
- Obesity
- Inflammatory bowel disease
- Pregnancy
- Estrogen therapy
- Nephrotic syndrome
- Polycythemia rubra vera
- Lupus anticoagulant
- Paroxysmal nocturnal hemoglobinuria

Inherited
- Antithrombin III deficiency
- Protein C deficiency
- Protein S deficiency
- Abnormal factor V
- Dysfibrinogenemia
- Disorders of plasminogen and plasminogen activator

## THROMBOTIC DISORDERS AND THEIR TREATMENT

Modern concepts of thrombogenesis originated in the mid-1800s with Rudolph Virchow, who attributed thrombosis to abnormalities of blood vessels, blood flow, or blood constituents. One can similarly conceptualize the pathophysiology of hypercoagulability in these same terms. In other words not all prethrombotic conditions are necessarily attributable to abnormalities of coagulation, but rather in the majority of cases the defect resides in a vascular or blood flow disturbance. The hemostatic system is involved only in that it is the final common pathway to thrombosis. Consequently the evaluation of an individual suspected of having an increased risk of thrombosis may focus on vascular and flow abnormalities as well as on an assessment of factors intrinsic to the blood, such as a deficiency of coagulation inhibitors. In the search for the etiology of a thrombotic event it is essential to take into account factors known to enhance the risk of thrombosis (see the box above). When a primary disorder of coagulation is the suspected cause, one begins by measuring the activities of the principal inhibitors of coagulation, including antithrombin III, protein C, and protein S. A recently described genetic defect in factor V that makes it resistant to protein C inactivation is a relatively common cause of hypercoagulability that can be detected. Fibrinolytic system disorders can also be investigated. Analysis is best done when the acute thrombotic episode has stabilized and ideally when the patient is not receiving anticoagulants.

## Antithrombotic Therapy

The following discussion focuses on the major antithrombotic agents in clinical use. Discussion of the various thromboembolic syndromes can be found elsewhere in this text.

There are three principal modes of antithrombotic therapy: anticoagulant therapy, antiplatelet therapy, and thrombolytic therapy. Both anticoagulants and antiplatelet agents can be considered prophylactic in the sense that they prevent thrombi from forming de novo (primary prophylaxis) or they prevent the further growth and extension of established thrombi (secondary prophylaxis). These agents do little to reduce the size of the existing thrombus. Thrombolytic agents, however, work more directly by activating the fibrinolytic system and hastening thrombus dissolution. The following discussion focuses on the practical use of the most common antithrombotic agents.

### *Anticoagulants*

**Heparin.** Heparin is a glycosaminoglycan of heterogeneous molecular weight that is commercially derived from porcine intestinal mucosa or bovine lung. First isolated in 1916 at Johns Hopkins by McLean, Howell, and Holt, heparin became available for clinical use several decades later as purification procedures were improved.

Heparin causes its anticoagulant effect through high-affinity binding with circulating antithrombin III (AT III), an antithrombotic regulatory protein that promotes gradual neutralization of several activated coagulation factors. Binding with heparin produces a conformational change of AT III, which greatly accelerates its inactivation of coagulation factors Xa, IXa, and thrombin, thereby causing a rapid anticoagulant effect.

Heparin is given parenterally as a constant intravenous infusion, intermittent intravenous injection, or subcutaneous injection. For hospitalized patients who require rapid anticoagulation, administration by constant intravenous infusion is preferred to permit accurate titration of the heparin dose. To initiate heparin therapy, patients are given a loading dose of approximately 5000 U by intravenous bolus, followed by a constant infusion of approximately 1000 U hourly. Heparin dosing nomograms have recently been shown to provide for a more rapid achievement of therapeutic anticoagulation, and their use is recommended (Table 55A-6). Heparin may also be given by intermittent intravenous bolus at 4-hour intervals, but such therapy has been shown to be less effective than continuous infusions.

When heparin is given intravenously, the intensity of anticoagulation is monitored using the aPTT. The heparin infusion is adjusted to prolong the aPTT to the recommended therapeutic range of 1.5 to 2.5 times the aPTT mean of normal range. Clinicians encounter considerable variability in patients' heparin requirements not only because of differences in aPTT reagent sensitivity to heparin, but also because of differences in heparin clearance and neutralization by heparin-binding proteins. Reagent differences can be overcome by performing in vitro heparin titration curves to determine the correlation of the aPTT with therapeutic heparin concentrations in the range of 0.2 to 0.4 U/ml. The overall variability of response to heparin demands frequent monitoring of the aPTT while treatment with heparin proceeds.

**Table 55A-6.** Guidelines for dosing heparin according to a weight-based nomogram

| aPTT response | Heparin dosage |
|---|---|
| Initial dose | 80 U/kg bolus, then 18 U/kg/hr |
| aPTT <35 sec (<1.2 × control) | 80 U/kg bolus, then ↑ by 4 U/kg/hr |
| aPTT, 35-45 sec (1.2-1.5 × control) | 40 U/kg bolus, then ↑ by 2 U/kg/hr |
| aPTT, 46-70 sec (1.5-2.3 × control) | No change |
| aPTT, 71-90 sec (2.3-3.0 × control) | ↓ infusion rate by 2 U/kg/hr |
| aPTT >90 sec (>3 × control) | Hold × 1 hr, then ↓ rate by 3 U/kg/hr |

From Raschke RA et al: The weight-based heparin dosing nomogram compared with a "standard care" nomogram, *Ann Intern Med* 119:874, 1993.

Bleeding is the most common adverse effect of heparin therapy. The overall risk of important heparin-induced bleeding is approximately 5% and is influenced by anticoagulation intensity, duration of heparin therapy, concomitant use of other drugs, and severity of illness. If major bleeding occurs, heparin anticoagulation may be rapidly reversed with protamine sulfate, given at a ratio of 1 mg per 100 U of estimated heparin reserve (the amount of heparin thought to remain in the body). Heparin-associated thrombocytopenia occurs in approximately 1% to 5% of patients receiving heparin and is occasionally associated with arterial thrombosis and bleeding (see discussion of heparin-induced thrombocytopenia earlier in this chapter). Chronic subcutaneous heparin therapy may cause osteoporosis in a minority of patients, leading to spontaneous fractures. Heparin does not cross the placenta and may be used for thromboembolic treatment during pregnancy.

**Low–molecular weight heparin.** Recently low–molecular weight heparins (LMWHs) have become available in the United States for primary prophylaxis in selected conditions (e.g., total hip and knee replacement). LMWHs are obtained by enzymatic or chemical depolymerization of unfractionated heparin. They have a more uniform distribution by molecular weight and shorter chain length of polysaccharides, with an average molecular weight of 4500 to 6000. LMWHs are advantageous compared to standard heparin in their greater ability to neutralize factor $X_a$. Compared to thrombin, they have less binding to heparin-binding proteins and platelets, a longer half-life, and are more uniformly absorbed from subcutaneous depots. They are safer with regard to bleeding and heparin-induced thrombocytopenia. They can be given subcutaneously once or twice daily depending on the indication and the preparation. Dosages are determined on a fixed or weight basis and do not require monitoring, at least when used for primary prophylaxis. They have only recently been approved for use in the United States, but as clinical trials are completed, indications for their use should increase for both primary and secondary prophylaxis.

**Oral anticoagulants (warfarin).** Because heparin must

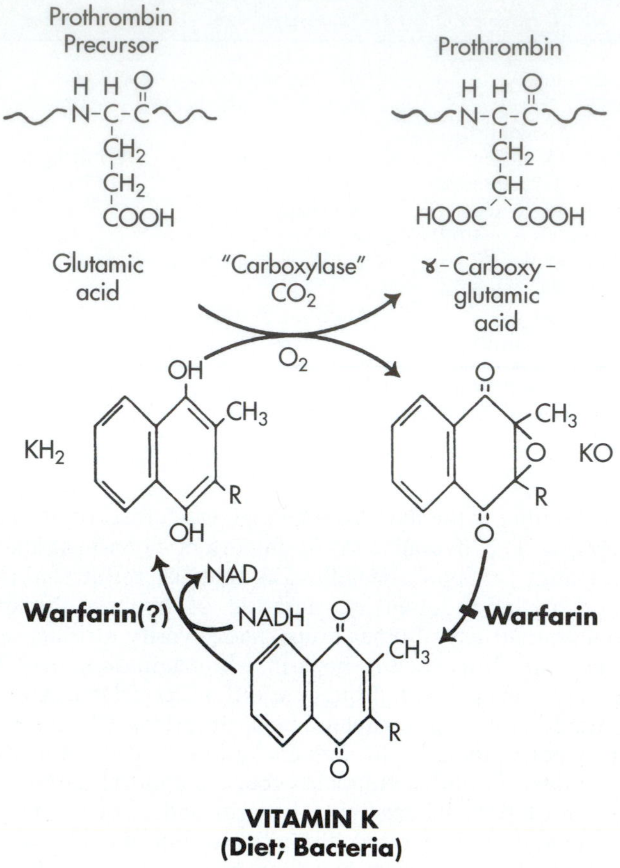


**Fig. 55A-4.** Site of action of warfarin. Warfarin interferes with a reductase enzyme responsible for reducing vitamin K from its oxidized state. The oxidized form accumulates in the blood during warfarin therapy. (Adapted from Corrigan JJ: *Ann NY Acad Sci* 393:366, 1982.)

To convert a prothrombin time ratio to an INR:

$$INR = PT\ ratio^{ISI}$$

Example:

17.9 s = PT ratio
12.2 s = Mean of normal range
2.3 = ISI of thromboplastin

Then:

$17.9 / 12.3 = 1.47$
$1.47^{2.3} = 2.4$ INR

**Fig. 55A-5.** Calculation of the International Normalized Ratio (INR). A comparative rating of prothrombin time ratios. The PT ratio one would have obtained if using the international reference thromboplastin. The International Sensitivity Index (ISI) is a comparative rating of different thromboplastins.

be given parenterally, its use is usually restricted to the hospital setting. Patients requiring intermediate-term or chronic anticoagulation are treated with warfarin, the most widely used oral anticoagulant. Warfarin is a synthetic analogue of dicumarol, originally derived from spoiled sweet clover and identified as the cause of sweet clover disease of cattle by Link and Campbell in 1939. Widespread use of dicumarol as treatment for thromboembolic disorders was aided by the development of the one-stage PT by Quick and co-workers. Today warfarin is the primary oral anticoagulant marketed in the United States, although other synthetic analogues are used worldwide.

Warfarin exerts its anticoagulant effect through competitive interference with vitamin K, which is essential for the normal synthesis of factors II, VII, IX, and X, and the antithrombotic factors protein S and protein C. Vitamin K serves as a cofactor that catalyzes the γ-carboxylation of certain glutamic acid residues on the vitamin K–dependent coagulation factors; the reaction provides critical calcium binding sites essential for full function. By competitive inhibition of microsomal reductases warfarin interferes with the conversion of oxidized vitamin K to its active reduced form, causing an acquired vitamin K deficiency and hepatic production of functionally inactive coagulation factors (Fig. 55A-4). Because the half-lives of the vitamin K–dependent factors vary, the full effect of a given dose of warfarin on the PT is not seen for several days after initiation of therapy. Early prolongation of the PT is due to depletion of factor VII, which has an estimated half-life of 6 to 8 hours.

Conversely, treatment with intravenous vitamin K reverses warfarin-induced anticoagulation via synthesis of new vitamin K–dependent factors within 24 to 48 hours. When necessary, treatment with intravenous FFP gives a rapid (although temporary) reversal of warfarin effect by direct replacement of active vitamin K–dependent factors.

Warfarin therapy is usually initiated with a dosage of 5 to 10 mg daily for the first 2 or 3 days. When heparin anticoagulation precedes warfarin therapy, treatment with warfarin should begin 3 to 5 days before termination of heparin to permit full depletion of vitamin K–dependent factors and achieve a therapeutic PT. Usually both heparin and warfarin can be started at the same time when a patient enters the hospital with a deep venous thrombosis or pulmonary embolism.

The international normalized ratio (INR) is the standard reporting methodology for monitoring warfarin anticoagulation; earlier monitoring methods using the PT alone, PT percentages, or PT ratios are no longer recommended because they fail to correct for differences in reagent sensitivity, and thus PTs from different laboratories are not comparable. The INR provides a method to compare different PTs based on an international standard. It is calculated by raising the laboratories' PT ratio (PT ÷ mean normal range) to the power expressed by the international sensitivity index, a measure of thromboplastin reagent sensitivity (Fig. 55A-5). Two intensity levels of warfarin anticoagulation are currently recommended: less intense warfarin therapy (INR of 2.0 to 3.0) is sufficient for most thromboembolic indications, and more intense warfarin therapy (INR of 2.5 to 3.5) is reserved for mechanical heart valves and failure of less-intensive treatment with warfarin (Table 55A-7). During warfarin treatment the patient's INR must be monitored regularly to ensure the desired intensity of anticoagulation. After initiating therapy the INR is checked at least weekly, adjusting the warfarin dose when necessary. When stable anticoagulation is attained, the frequency of INR testing may be reduced, based on the patient's compliance with medication and follow-up. Compliance can be improved significantly with regular education about warfarin dosing, drug interactions, and potential side effects of warfarin therapy.

Clinicians who observe patients on warfarin anticoagulation encounter many difficulties in maintaining their patients within a desired therapeutic range. Variations in dietary vitamin K, drug interactions with warfarin, and patient compliance all may cause rapid fluctuations in response to a given warfarin dose. Clinicians must be aware of the many potential drug interactions with warfarin and should avoid those medications known to alter warfarin's anticoagulant effect. As a precaution, anticoagulated patients starting a new medication should be monitored with more frequent INR testing to detect any changes in anticoagulant effect induced by the drug. Table 55A-8 lists the different mechanisms of drug interactions with warfarin and selected drugs known to alter the PT.

Bleeding is the most frequent side effect of warfarin therapy. The risk increases with greater intensity of anticoagulation, history of previous bleeding, concurrent use of antiplatelet agents, severe intercurrent illness, and old age. Periodic assessments for bleeding should include a hematocrit, urinalysis, and stool occult blood testing. Bleeding during warfarin anticoagulation may unmask occult pathology, such as lung, colon, uterine, or bladder neoplasia. Clinicians must consider obtaining appropriate diagnostic studies if anticoagulated patients develop hemoptysis, rectal or vaginal bleeding, or hematuria. Warfarin-induced skin necrosis is a rare complication caused by thrombosis of small vessels supplying subcutaneous fat, often associated with occult protein C or protein S deficiency. Warfarin is *contraindicated during pregnancy* because of fetal bleeding and multiple teratogenic effects. Women of childbearing age who require warfarin therapy should be counseled in effective methods of birth control, and a pregnancy test is a prudent precaution for such patients before beginning treatment with warfarin.

**Table 55A-7.** Therapeutic range for oral anticoagulant therapy based on the international normalized ratio

| Indication | Recommended INR |
|---|---|
| Prophylaxis of venous thrombosis<br>Treatment of venous thrombosis<br>Treatment of pulmonary embolism<br>Prevention of systemic embolism<br>Tissue heart valves<br>Acute myocardial infarction<br>Valvular heart disease<br>Atrial fibrillation | 2.0-3.0 |
| Mechanical prosthetic valves<br>Recurrent systemic embolism | 2.5-3.5 |

### *Antiplatelet agents*

**Aspirin.** Aspirin and most other NSAIDs inhibit platelet aggregation by interfering with cyclooxygenase, an enzyme important in the generation of prostaglandins. Aspirin irreversibly inhibits this enzyme, whereas NSAIDs usually cause reversible inhibition of cyclooxygenase. Only small doses of aspirin are needed (less than one 5-grain tablet) to affect most of the platelets in the circulation. This effect persists for the lifetime of those platelets affected (about 10 days). Nonacetylated forms of salicylate (e.g., choline, sodium salicylate) do not have this inhibitory effect. Dipyridamole and sulfinpyrazone, agents used in the past for their supposed antiplatelet effect, have been shown not to have any beneficial effect mediated by antiplatelet activity.

**Table 55A-8.** Drugs that interact with warfarin or alter its effect on hemostasis

| Drug | Mechanism of interaction |
|---|---|
| **Prolongs prothrombin time** | |
| Amiodarone | Decreases clearance |
| Anabolic steroids | Unknown |
| Cephalosporins (second and third generation) | Interferes with vitamin K recycling |
| Cimetidine | Decreases clearance |
| Clofibrate | Unknown |
| Disulfiram | Decreases clearance |
| Erythromycin | Unknown |
| Fluoroquinolones | Displaces binding to albumin |
| Glucagon | Unknown |
| Metronidazole | Decreases clearance |
| Miconazole | Decreases clearance |
| Omeprazole | Decreases clearance |
| Phenytoin | Unknown |
| Piroxicam | Unknown |
| Quinidine | Unknown |
| Phenylbutazone | Decreases clearance |
| Salicylates | Enhances hypoprothrombinemia |
| Sulfinpyrazone | Decreases clearance |
| Tamoxifen | Unknown |
| Trimethoprim/sulfamethoxazole | Decreases clearance |
| Vitamin E | Unknown |
| **Reduces prothrombin time** | |
| Alcohol | Increases clearance |
| Barbiturates | Increases clearance |
| Carbamazepine | Increases clearance |
| Cholestyramine | Decreases absorption |
| Griseofulvin | Increases clearance |
| Nafcillin | Increases clearance |
| Rifampin | Increases clearance |
| Sucralfate | Decreases absorption |
| **Enhances risk of bleeding** | |
| Aspirin | Inhibits platelet function |
| Heparin | Inhibits other coagulation factors |
| Penicillins | Inhibits platelet function |

**Table 55A-9.** Approved indications and suggested dosages for thrombolytic agents

| Thrombolytic agent | Deep venous thrombosis | Pulmonary embolism | Acute myocardial infarction | Occluded catheters/arteries/veins |
|---|---|---|---|---|
| Streptokinase | 250,000 IU × 30 min, then 100,000 IU/hr × 24 hr | 250,000 IU × 30 min, then 100,000 IU/hr × 24 hr | $1.5 \times 10^6$ IU × 20 min | 250,000 IU × 60-120 min |
| Urokinase | 4400 IU/kg × 10 min, then 4400 IU/hr × 24 hr | 4400 IU/kg × 10 min, then 4400 IU/hr × 24 hr | $2 \times 10^6$ IU bolus or $3 \times 10^6$ IU over 90 min | 5000 IU |
| Alteplase (t-PA) | – | 100 mg over 2 hr | 60 mg × 1 hr (6-10 mg as bolus), 20 mg over second hr, 20 mg over third hr | – |
| Anistreplase | – | – | 30 U ($1.25 \times 10^6$ IU streptokinase) bolus | – |

**Ticlopidine.** Ticlopidine is a new antiplatelet agent that mediates its effect by inhibiting platelet aggregation possibly by interfering with the binding of von Willebrand factor and fibrinogen to the platelet membrane. It has a delayed onset of action up to 48 hours after beginning therapy and its effect may persist for several days after cessation of therapy. Ticlopidine has been shown to be an effective platelet inhibitor in a number of conditions, but its use is not recommended because of potentially serious side effects, unless individuals are unable to take aspirin. These side effects include diarrhea, skin rash, and a low incidence of neutropenia.

***Thrombolytic agents.*** The major fibrinolytic or thrombolytic agents currently in use include streptokinase, urokinase, tissue plasminogen activator (t-PA), and anisoylated plasminogen-streptokinase activator complex (APSAC or anistreplase). These agents are most often used in ischemic cardiovascular disease (see Chapter 11). They are also recommended in fulminant pulmonary embolism and some cases of deep venous thrombosis, but because of a high-risk profile they should be used with great care and in those with no risk factors for bleeding. At a minimum, these agents are contraindicated in the setting of active internal bleeding, recent (within 2 months) cerebral vascular event or intracranial/intraspinal surgery, intracranial neoplasm, arteriovenous malformation or aneurysm, severe uncontrolled hypertension, or a known bleeding diathesis. Thrombolytic agents are used for the clearance of thrombi that obstruct indwelling catheters such as those used in cancer patients.

Streptokinase, the least expensive agent, binds to plasminogen, and the streptokinase-plasminogen complex activates other plasminogen molecules to the active enzyme plasmin. Urokinase directly activates plasminogen. Tissue plasminogen activator, which also activates plasminogen directly, has a greater affinity for clot-bound plasminogen than circulating plasminogen and thus is less likely to activate plasminogen in a systemic fashion, leading to hypofibrinogenemia. However, in the dosages needed to be effective, some of this specificity is lost. Through molecular manipulation anistreplase has greater affinity for fibrin than circulating fibrinogen and thus on a theoretical basis is less likely to produce systemic hypofibrinogenemia. It also has a longer half-life than the three other agents.

Thrombolytic therapy does not require close monitoring of coagulation parameters, since a fixed dosage is given in most situations. The major reason to monitor therapy in some cases is to ensure that a lytic state has been achieved; this can easily be determined by a thrombin time that should be at least 3 seconds above baseline value or a fibrinogen level that should be reduced to the 1.5 g/L level. Streptokinase has the problem of being susceptible to neutralization by existing antistreptococcal antibodies as well as producing allergic reactions resulting from these antibodies. It is recommended to coadminister corticosteroids with streptokinase to prevent such reactions, and if a lytic state cannot be achieved, another thrombolytic agent should be used. Table 55A-9 summarizes the recommended dosages of these agents for their currently approved indications.

## BIBLIOGRAPHY

Ansell J: Hypercoagulability: a conceptual and diagnostic approach, *Am Heart J* 114:910, 1987.

Ansell J: Oral anticoagulant therapy: fifty years later, *Arch Intern Med* 153:586, 1993.

Ansell JE, Kumar R, Deykin D: The spectrum of vitamin K deficiency, *JAMA* 238:40, 1977.

Bick RL: Platelet function defects: a clinical review, *Semin Thromb Hemost* 18:167, 1992.

Broze GJ: The role of tissue factor pathway inhibitor in a revised coagulation cascade, *Semin Hematol* 29:159, 1992.

Clouse LH, Comp PC: The regulation of hemostasis: the protein C system, *N Engl J Med* 314:1298, 1986.

Hirsh J: Heparin, *N Engl J Med* 324:1565, 1991.

Hirsh J: Oral anticoagulant drugs, *N Engl J Med* 324:1865, 1991.

Hirsh J, Levine MN: Low molecular weight heparin, *Blood* 79:1, 1992.

Kirkwood TBL: Calibration of reference thromboplastin and standardization of the prothrombin time ratio, *Thromb Haemostast* 49:238, 1983.

Landefeld SC, Beyth RJ: Anticoagulant-related bleeding: clinical epidemiology, prediction, and prevention, *Am J Med* 95:315, 1993.

Levine MN, Hirsh J: Hemorrhagic complications of anticoagulant therapy, *Semin Thromb Hemost* 12:39, 1986.

Plow EF, Ginsberg MH: The molecular basis of platelet function. In Hoffman R et al, editors: *Hematology: basic principles and practice,* New York, 1992, Churchill Livingstone.

Raschke RA et al: The weight-based heparin dosing nomogram compared with a "standard care" nomogram, *Ann Intern Med* 119:874, 1993.
Schmaier AH: Disseminated intravascular coagulation: pathogenesis and management, *J Intens Care Med* 6:209, 1991.

CHAPTER

# 55B Purpuric Skin Conditions

Frank Parker

Purpura is the change in the skin brought about by extravasation of blood (red blood cells) into the dermis and adipose tissue. As such, purpura appears as a purplish-blue discoloration and in distinction to erythema (a red coloration) the discoloration cannot be blanched by pressure. Purpura can be divided into two categories: nonpalpable (macular) and palpable (raised). Nonpalpable purpura is usually the result of bleeding into the skin without inflammation of the cutaneous vessels, whereas palpable purpura is the result of inflammation and damage of the skin vessels, the inflammation causing the elevation of the lesions.

## NONPALPABLE PURPURA

Nonpalpable purpura is due to either a bleeding disorder or alterations in blood vessel fragility; classically this category is primarily divided into thrombocytopenic and nonthrombocytopenic conditions.

### Thrombocytopenic purpura

Thrombocytopenic purpura characteristically appears as petechiae (small purpuric macules) and is caused by a reaction to drugs, hematologic malignancies, viral infections, and autoimmune conditions (idiopathic [ITP] and thrombotic [TTP] thrombocytopenic purpura). In each instance platelet counts below 50,000/mm$^3$ are seen, causing generalized petechiae with pronounced cutaneous bleeding. Mucosal bleeding may also occur so oral and conjunctival petechiae may be seen.

***Pathogenesis.*** A variety of factors cause the thrombocytopenia. Drugs can cause thrombocytopenia on an immunologic basis (the drug becomes a hapten on the platelets with subsequent immunologic attack). Hematologic malignancies decrease platelets by replacing bone marrow. ITP is due to circulating antiplatelet antibodies.

### Nonthrombocytopenic purpura

In the absence of low platelets, nonpalpable purpura can result from a variety of *coagulation disorders* (lack of various clotting factors) or from alterations in *skin fragility* and small vessel competence (see below) caused by a variety of underlying conditions. Purpura resulting from skin fragility changes maybe associated with necrosis of the skin.

***Changes in skin fragility and vessel competence.*** *Senile* or *actinic purpura* is the most common cause of changes in skin fragility and vessel competence is in older patients or in those on prolonged use of either systemic or potent topical steroids where minor trauma causes ecchymosis. The skin itself is often more fragile as aging and steroids decrease the collagen connective tissue supporting the superficial cutaneous vessels. *Hypergammaglobulinemic conditions* can also cause flat petechial lesions on the legs and *Schamberg's disease,* an idiopathic capillaritis that results in mild inflammation and leakage of the capillaries causing petechial and pigmented areas resembling cayenne pepper on the lower legs. When an etiology can be found it is often a reaction to a medication being taken. Other much rarer causes of nonpalpable purpura include *Ehlers Danlos syndrome* (where there is increased blood vessel fragility) and *amyloidosis* where amyloid infiltrates cutaneous blood vessels making them more permeable to minor trauma ("pinch purpura" can be seen when pinching the skin, especially on the eyelids).

Several serious conditions can cause nonpalpable purpura but these may be associated with skin necrosis. These include disseminated intravascular coagulation, antiphospholipid antibody syndrome and Coumadin skin necrosis.

*Antiphospholipid antibody syndrome* is associated with the presence of a mixture of autoantibodies that bind to phospholipids. They are comprised of the lupus anticoagulant and the anticardiolipin antibodies. Such antibodies induce an anticoagulant effect *in vitro* but are associated clinically with arterial and venous thrombosis that can cause livedo reticularis (red to purple reticulate skin pattern usually on the lower extremities and arms), leg ulcers resembling pyoderma gangrenosum, thrombophlebitis, cutaneous infarcts and digital gangrene, and subungual splinter hemorrhages. The condition can be seen with or without systemic lupus erythematosus, Sjögren syndrome, scleroderma and rheumatoid arthritis. Women with repeated idiopathic abortions are often found to have antiphospholipid antibodies. The antiphospholipid syndrome can be diagnosed by special tests. In the case of lupus anticoagulant, the dilute Russell viper venom time is the most sensitive and specific while anticardiolipin antibodies are detected by ELISA test for IgM and IgG.

*Coumadin skin necrosis* is a severe reaction to Coumadin found mostly in young women, 3 to 10 days after initiating these drugs. Petechiae or ecchymotic lesions usually on the lower extremities rapidly become deep, large necrotic areas. Biopsies reveal occlusion of dermal and subcutaneous veins with fibrin. Coumadin skin necrosis has been associated with protein C deficiency.

## PALPABLE PURPURA

Raised or thickened purpuric papules, nodules, or plaques usually represent a necrotizing reaction in blood vessels. Whether clinically the purpuric lesion is a papule, a nodule, or a plaque, and whether it becomes necrotic depends on the size and position of the cutaneous vessels involved in the process (Fig. 55B-1).

***Pathogenesis.*** A variety of clinical settings or conditions may be associated with leukocytoclastic vasculitis, the most common type of vasculitis of the superficial vessels

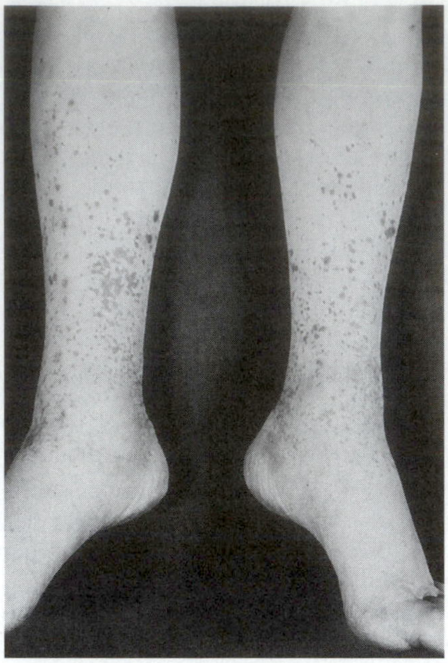

Fig. 55B-1. Palpable purpura (leukocytoclastic vasculitis). Note discrete purpuric papules on the distal extremities.

of the skin: sepsis (bacterial and viral); medications or drugs; collagen vascular diseases (especially rheumatoid arthritis and systemic lupus erythematosus); cryoglobulinemia; malignancies (lymphomas) and Henoch Schönlein purpura. The vasculitis associated with these conditions is an immune complex disease in which antibodies (IgG, IgM, or IgA) are formed to a variety of antigens (e.g., bacteria, drugs, etc.) and the immune complexes lodge within small cutaneous vessel walls activating complement. Some of the complement components are chemotactic, bringing polymorphonuclear leukocytes into the vessel walls. When they release their lysosomal enzymes, the vascular wall inflammation causes perivascular accumulation of red blood cells (RBC) and the clinical picture of raised purpuric papules, nodules, and plaques—so-called palpable purpura. Occasionally leukocytoclastic vasculitis can be associated with systemic signs and symptoms, including fever, glomerulonephritis, neuropathy, GI bleeding, and abdominal pain (Henoch-Schönlein purpura).

Medium-sized vessel vasculitis is seen in polyarteritis nodosa and Wegener granulomatosis while large vessel vasculitis includes giant cell arteritis, Takayasu arteritis, and Buerger's disease.

***Management.*** The treatment of vasculitis depends first on identifying the cause of the vasculitis and eliminating factors that may be causing the condition (e.g., drugs, sepsis). Oral steroids, Cytoxan, and dapsone are all useful in controlling vasculitis.

## BIBLIOGRAPHY

Callen JP: *Cutaneous aspects of internal disease,* Chicago, 1981, Year Book Medical Publishers.

Lookingbill DP, Marks JG Jr: *Principles of dermatology,* Philadelphia, 1986, WB Saunders.

CHAPTER

# 56 Transfusion Therapy in General Practice

Elzbieta B. Griffiths
Irma O. Szymanski

Modern transfusion practice began with the discovery of ABO blood groups by Landsteiner in 1901. Further progress was made possible by development of effective anticoagulant/preservative solutions, discovery of other blood groups, introduction of the antiglobulin (Coombs) test, and modern blood collection and transfusion equipment. During the last decade, the pace of development has been particularly rapid. New advances include the introduction of sensitive methods to detect blood-borne pathogens, preparation of blood components and derivatives of high purity, improved understanding of immunologic effects of blood transfusion, and emphasis on educational efforts to disseminate the new information to physicians.

Although careful screening of blood donors and extensive testing of donated blood have increased the safety of transfusion, adverse effects cannot be totally eliminated. Through the latest technology donated blood is tested for the following disease markers: anti-HIV 1/2 (human immunodeficiency virus), anti-HTLV I/II (human T cell leukemia/lymphoma virus), HBsAg (hepatitis B surface antigen), anti-HBc (hepatitis B core antigen), anti–hepatitis C virus (HCV), alanine aminotransferase (ALT), and syphilis. The chance of acquiring an infectious disease through transfusion is shown in Table 56-1; immunologic complications, their etiology, and their incidence rates are listed in Table 56-2.

## BLOOD COMPONENT THERAPY

Currently blood components rather than whole blood are transfused in most medical centers. Although some surgeons prefer whole blood in the setting of massive hemorrhage, this practice is not recommended because stored whole blood does not contain functional platelets or coagulation factors V and VIII. Furthermore, whole blood has a large quantity of immunogenic material such as leukocytes and platelets. The following blood components are prepared from whole blood by centrifugation: packed red cells, platelets, and plasma. Red cells can be further processed and purified by washing, freezing, or filtering. Platelets, prepared from whole blood (random donor platelet concentrates) or collected by apheresis, can also be purified by filtration. Cryoprecipitate is isolated from thawed fresh frozen plasma (FFP) at 4° C. Plasma derivatives (albumin, immunoglobulin, coagulation factor concentrates, antithrombin III) are prepared commercially. The presence of multiple blood components and derivatives allows for efficient use of scarce blood resources and enables the storage of each component under optimal conditions to maximize viability, function, and availability. It is now possible to transfuse a therapeutic blood component in a small volume, thus decreasing circulatory

**Table 56-1.** Magnitude of the risk of transfusion-associated infections

| Infection | Risk per unit | Comment |
|---|---|---|
| HIV | 1/60,000 to 1/225,000 | Varies regionally |
| HBV | 1/200,000 | |
| HCV | 1/6000 | Chronic hepatitis in 50% of cases |
| HTLV I/II | 1/50,000 | Associated with T cell leukemia and HAM/TSP |
| CMV | Unknown | Some groups of patients at risk |
| Malaria, Chagas disease | Rare in United States | Common in certain parts of the world |
| Babesiosis | Rare | Cases reported in the northeastern United States |
| *Yersinia enterocolitica* | Very rare; 29 cases reported | Bacterium growing at 4° C, producing endotoxin |

From Dodd RY: *N Engl J Med* 327:419, 1992; and Rossi E, Simon T, Moss G: *Principles of transfusion medicine,* Baltimore, 1991, Williams & Wikins.
*HAM/TSP*, HTLV I–associated myelopathy/tropical spastic paraparesis; *CMV*, cytomegalovirus.

**Table 56-2.** Immunologic complications of transfusions

| Type | Etiology | Incidence |
|---|---|---|
| Immediate hemolytic reactions | Antibody-induced destruction of donor red cells | 1/25,000 |
| Delayed hemolytic reactions | Destruction of donor red cells by antibodies appearing after transfusion | 1/2500 |
| Febrile reactions | Reaction of antibodies to donor WBC | 1/200 |
| Transfusion-related acute lung injury (TRALI) | Extensive complement activation usually resulting from antibodies in donor plasma to recipient WBC | 1/10,000 |
| Allergic reactions, mild (urticaria) | Immunization to plasma factors | 1/100 |
| Allergic reactions, moderate with bronchospasm and laryngeal edema | Immunization to plasma factors | 1-2/1000 |
| Anaphylactic reactions | Immunization of IgA-deficient individuals to IgA | 1/150,000 |
| GvHD | Inability of the recipient to reject donor lymphocytes | Not defined |

*WBC*, White blood cells; *GvHD*, graft-vs.-host disease.

overload. Current medical practice requires that patients be informed about the benefits and risks of blood transfusion and that consent be obtained.

## Indications for red cell transfusions

Red cell transfusions are given to increase oxygen-carrying capacity in anemic patients. The most accurate definition of *anemia* is decreased red cell mass. However, the measurement of red cell mass is impractical, and the hematocrit (Hct) or hemoglobin (Hb) level is measured instead. Red cell mass can decrease acutely related to rapid blood loss (e.g., trauma, surgery, and obstetric, gynecologic, or gastrointestinal problems) or accelerated red cell destruction (e.g., autoimmune hemolytic anemia). Anemia can also develop slowly because of chronic bleeding or inadequate red cell production. The guidelines for correcting acute blood loss or chronic anemia are discussed next.

***Acute blood loss.*** Acute blood loss may result in hypovolemia and anemia. Hypovolemia must be corrected promptly, usually with crystalloid infusions. A patient may be considered normovolemic when vital signs, tissue perfusion, and urine output have normalized. Depending on the amount of blood loss and the adequacy of fluid replacement, the Hct decreases and reflects the degree of anemia. If anemia is severe enough, impairment in tissue oxygenation may result, necessitating red cell transfusion. The level of Hct at which this occurs varies according to the patient's health status. It is stated that normal individuals can tolerate an Hct as low as 21% without adverse effects. However, studies involving Jehovah's Witnesses have shown an increased perioperative mortality rate when the preoperative Hct was less than 24%.

***Chronic anemia.*** Some patients tolerate chronic anemia well because of the development of compensatory mechanisms, such as a shift in the oxygen dissociation curve and an increase in cardiac output. Therefore unless the Hct is below 18%, the decision to transfuse should be based on the symptoms present rather than the Hct alone. Patients with cardiovascular, cerebrovascular, or pulmonary disease may not tolerate even mild anemia and might require an Hct of about 30%. Red cell transfusions should not be given if anemia can be corrected with hematinics (Iron [Fe], vitamin $B_{12}$, or folic acid) or erythropoietin (EPO). EPO is approved for treatment of anemia resulting from chronic renal failure and azidothymidine (AZT) treatment of AIDS. In cases in which anemia is caused by chronic blood loss, its etiology should be established and appropriate treatment instituted. Studies have shown that quality of life is improved when the Hct is maintained at a higher level. Since the total number of red cell units transfused to patients receiving chronic transfusion

**Table 56-3.** Composition and relative advantages of different red cell products

| Red blood cell product | Content: plasma (no. lymphocytes/unit) | Relative advantages |
|---|---|---|
| Packed | 50-70 ml (1-2 × $10^9$) | Least expensive, readily available |
| Washed | Minimal (1-2 × $10^8$) | For prevention of allergic and febrile reactions |
| Previously frozen | Minimal (5 × $10^7$) | Same as washed red blood cells for decreasing HLA alloimmunization, prevention of CMV, transmission, and GvHD |
| Filtered (4th-generation filters) | 50-70 ml (<1 × $10^6$) | For prevention of HLA alloimmunization, febrile reactions, and CMV transmission |

*HLA*, Human leukocyte antigen.

**Table 56-4.** Characteristics of platelet concentrates

| Platelet concentrate | Content: volume/no. platelets/no. WBCs | Relative advantages |
|---|---|---|
| Random | 50 ml/5.5 × $10^{10}$/4 × $10^7$ | Least expensive, readily available |
| Apheresis | 300 ml/3 × $10^{11}$/1 × $10^8$ | Decreased disease transmission; can be HLA and HPA matched |

*HPA*, Human platelet antigen.

therapy is similar regardless of the level of Hct maintained, it might be advisable to maintain these patients at an Hct of about 30%.

***Practical aspects of red cell transfusion.*** The relative advantages of various red cell products are listed in Table 56-3. The number of units required for each transfusion depends on the initial and desired Hct. One unit of packed red cells is expected to increase the Hct by 2% to 3% in an average adult, although in some cases this is not seen because of an increase in plasma volume induced by red cell transfusion. The usual infusion rate is 2 to 4 ml/kg/hr. For patients at risk for circulatory overload the rate should not exceed 1 ml/kg/hr. In actively bleeding patients the unit can be administered as rapidly as physically possible. The effectiveness of red cell therapy should be evaluated by measuring the Hct within 24 hours of transfusion and assessing the clinical status of the patient.

## Indications for platelet transfusions

Characteristics of random donor and apheresis platelet concentrates are shown in Table 56-4. Platelets are given prophylactically to prevent bleeding or therapeutically to stop bleeding related to thrombocytopenia or thrombocytopathy. The majority of platelet transfusions are given prophylactically. Traditionally, nonbleeding patients are given platelet transfusions when the platelet count is lower than 20,000/μl. However, this practice has been recently questioned in light of data showing that spontaneous bleeding does not occur unless the platelet count is less than 5,000/μl. Table 56-5 gives guidelines for prophylactic platelet transfusions according to platelet counts and associated conditions. Platelet transfusions are contraindicated in autoimmune thrombocytopenic purpura, thrombotic thrombocytopenic purpura, and posttransfusion purpura except when life-threatening bleeding is present. In these patients the transfused platelets are destroyed rapidly and may aggravate the disease process.

**Table 56-5.** Indications for prophylactic platelet transfusions

| Platelet count/μl | Associated conditions |
|---|---|
| <5,000 | None |
| 5000-10,000 | Fever or minor hemorrhage |
| 10,000-20,000 | Heparin therapy, coagulation disorder |
| <60,000 | Surgery contemplated |
| >100,000 | Bleeding time >15 min and surgery contemplated |

***Practical aspects of platelet transfusions.*** The usual therapeutic dosage of platelets for an adult is a pool of 6 U of random donor platelets or 1 U of apheresis platelets. The response to platelet transfusions should be assessed by measuring the platelet count 1 or 24 hours later. In a stable, adult leukemic patient 1 U of apheresis platelets increases the platelet count by 20,000 to 30,000/μl. Patients alloimmunized to HLA or HPA do not respond to platelet transfusions. HLA- or both HLA- and HPA-matched platelets may be effective in these patients. However, transfusion of HLA-matched platelets is not necessary in nonimmunized patients. To prevent alloimmunization, patients who are candidates for long-term platelet support should receive only leukodepleted blood products.

## Indications for transfusion of plasma and derivatives

***Fresh frozen plasma.*** The characteristics of plasma and its derivatives are shown in Table 56-6. FFP contains all normal plasma constituents such as immunoglobulins, coagulation factors, albumin, and complement components. FFP is indicated for the treatment of acquired or congenital coagulation factor deficiencies other than factor VIII or IX deficiency, when bleeding is present, or when

**Table 56-6.** Characteristics of plasma and derivatives

| Product | Volume | Content | Risk of transmitting infectious disease |
|---|---|---|---|
| FFP | 200-300 ml | All plasma constituents | As in Table 56-2 |
| Cryoprecipitate | 10-25 ml | Factor I (fibrinogen), factor VIII, vWF, factor XIII, fibronectin | As in Table 56-2 |
| Albumin 5% | 250 ml | 96% albumin, 4% globulin | Practically nil |
| Albumin 25% | 50 ml | 96% albumin, 4% globulin | Practically nil |
| Intravenous IgG, 5% | As required | Mainly IgG, some IgM and IgA | Practically nil |
| Factor VIII concentrate, 1000 U | 10 ml | Factor VIII | Practically nil |
| Factor IX complex, 1000 U | 25 ml | Factors IX, II, VII, X | Practically nil |

*vWF,* von Willebrand factor.

surgery is scheduled. The current recommendation is to give FFP only when the prothrombin or partial thromboplastin time is at least 1.5 times the control value. The usual dosage is 10 to 20 ml/kg. FFP is not recommended for blood volume expansion. In the future, units of solvent/detergent-treated, pooled plasma may be available.

***Cryoprecipitate.*** Cryoprecipitate contains plasma proteins that remain insoluble after thawing a unit of FFP at 4° C. One bag of cryoprecipitate contains about 80 IU of factor VIII and vWF, between 100 and 350 mg of fibrinogen, and about 50% of the factor XIII and fibronectin originally present in the unit of FFP. Cryoprecipitate is used to treat congenital or acquired afibrinogenemia, vWF deficiency, and factor XIII deficiency. Disseminated intravascular coagulation (DIC) is an example of acquired fibrinogen deficiency in which cryoprecipitate infusions are helpful. Usually, multiple doses of 10 U pools are required for therapy.

***Albumin.*** Albumin is manufactured from pools of donor plasma and subsequently heat treated to inactivate microorganisms. It is effective as a plasma volume expander and has been commonly used to treat hypovolemia and burn injuries. However, controlled trials in settings of extensive vascular surgery or trauma have shown that patient outcomes are similar regardless of whether albumin or crystalloids are used. In burn patients, albumin infusions are considered beneficial when given 24 hours after the injury. It is generally accepted that albumin should not be used to treat malnutrition.

***Intravenous IgG.*** Intravenous IgG is now commonly used to treat agammaglobulinemia and certain immune disorders, such as autoimmune thrombocytopenic purpura, Kawasaki disease, and some neurologic disorders (acute Guillain-Barré syndrome). The beneficial effects are thought to result from the blockade of the reticuloendothelial system by the infused immunoglobulin, immunomodulation through antiidiotype antibodies, or prevention of binding of the activated complement component C3 to target cells. The usual dosage is 0.4 g/kg/day for 5 days, although smaller doses have also been effective.

***Coagulation factor concentrates.*** Isolation of coagulation factors by immunoabsorption and treatment of the concentrates by heat and solvent/detergent methods to inactivate microorganisms have increased their purity and safety. Although most factor VIII concentrates (e.g., antihemophilic factor [Monoclonal Purified]) contain only the antihemophilic factor, preparations enriched in vWF are also available (Humate-P). Recombinant factor VIII has been in clinical use for some time (e.g., Kogenate) and is safe and effective but also quite expensive.

The prothrombin complex (Profilnine) for treatment of factor IX deficiency actually contains the vitamin K–dependent factors IX, II, VII, and X. Its use has been associated with DIC and thrombotic episodes because of the presence of activated coagulation factors. Purified factor IX concentrates (Alphanine, Mononine) containing less thrombogenic material than the prothrombin complex are now available.

## TRANSFUSION REACTIONS, SYMPTOMS, AND TREATMENT

A transfusion reaction is any adverse event resulting from the infusion of a blood component or derivative. Reactions are immediate if they occur during or within a few hours of transfusion or delayed if they occur within days or weeks after administration of a blood product. Transfusion-induced alloimmunization that might complicate subsequent transfusions and bacterial contamination of blood, a relatively rare event, are not discussed here. The magnitude of the risk of transfusion-associated infections is shown in Table 56-1. All transfusion reactions, when they occur, should be reported to the blood bank for immediate evaluation of their etiology.

### Immediate hemolytic transfusion reactions

Most immediate hemolytic transfusion reactions are due to *clerical errors* resulting in transfusion of ABO-incompatible blood. The *symptoms* often include pain in the vein through which blood is infused, back pain, chest pain, difficulties in breathing, anxiety, chills, and fever. The blood pressure may decrease, shock may ensue, and DIC may develop as a result of complement activation. Patients with severe hemolytic transfusion reactions may sustain transient or permanent renal failure. The death in the early period after a transfusion reaction is due to shock or bleeding. Prompt treatment of these complications is essential for successful outcome.

Treatment must be started *immediately.* The goals in the initial phase are to prevent shock and to maintain urine output. If DIC is present, it is important to provide appropriate blood component replacement therapy. When anemia is present, compatible red cell transfusions should be given. Dialysis should be considered for renal failure.

### Delayed hemolytic transfusion reactions

Delayed hemolytic transfusion reactions occur usually 2 to 14 days after transfusion in a patient previously sensitized to blood group antigens during pregnancy or transfusion. In these patients, antibodies may be undetectable at the time of pretransfusion testing. However, antibody titer rises rapidly after transfusion of red cells that bear the offending antigen. The symptoms are typical: fever, unexplained anemia, and hyperbilirubinemia, but DIC and renal failure are rare. For diagnosis of this problem, blood samples should be sent to the blood bank for transfusion reaction evaluation. Other necessary tests include urine analysis, creatinine, lactase dehydrogenase, haptoglobin, and a DIC screen. Usually no therapy is needed except for compatible red cell transfusions if symptomatic anemia is present.

### Febrile transfusion reactions

Febrile transfusion reactions are considered to be the result of immunization of the recipient to donor white cells. These reactions manifest themselves as fever above the baseline value (increase of at least 2° F), usually associated with chills and slight elevation of blood pressure. The symptoms may occur during or within 2 hours of transfusion. In the case of a febrile reaction the transfusion should be discontinued and blood samples sent to the blood bank to rule out red cell incompatibility. Treatment includes a fever-lowering drug such as acetaminophen. For prevention, leukodepleted products should be used.

### Transfusion-related acute lung injury

Sometimes leukocyte antibodies in donor plasma can initiate a severe reaction called a *transfusion-related acute lung injury.* This syndrome is also called *noncardiogenic pulmonary edema* because of the radiographic appearance of bilateral pulmonary infiltrates in the absence of heart failure. The symptoms, which may occur during or within 6 hours after transfusion, include severe respiratory distress and hypoxemia. Fever and hypotension unresponsive to fluid administration may also occur. Complement activation associated with release of the anaphylatoxin C5a causes an increase in capillary permeability and clumping of leukocytes in the microvasculature of the lung, impeding pulmonary blood flow and oxygenation of red cells. Although this complication is potentially life-threatening, with prompt and vigorous respiratory support, including oxygen administration and mechanical ventilation in the intensive care unit, patients usually recover.

### Allergic reactions

Patients sensitized to donor plasma factors might have mild allergic reactions manifesting as urticaria, whereas more severe reactions may include extensive geographic urticaria, laryngeal edema, bronchospasm, abdominal pain, joint pains, and headaches. When mild reactions occur, the transfusion can be stopped temporarily while the patient is given antihistamines. When symptoms subside, the transfusion can be started again. In the case of more severe reactions the transfusion should not be restarted, and the patient may need corticosteroids and epinephrine. Subsequent reactions can be prevented by giving washed or previously frozen red cells.

### Anaphylactic reactions

Anaphylactic reactions occur within minutes of initiating blood transfusion or immunoglobulin infusion in an IgA-deficient patient who has developed anti-IgA antibodies. The patient becomes flushed, has intense sensation of heat on the skin, feels very anxious, and may develop laryngospasm and shock. Treatment with epinephrine, intravenous fluids, and possibly intravenous corticosteroids is necessary. For future transfusions, blood from IgA-deficient donors should be used. One may also transfuse previously frozen red cells, washed extensively to remove plasma and selected on the basis of low levels of red cell–bound IgA.

### Transfusion-associated GvHD

The symptoms of GvHD, a rare but increasingly recognized complication, occur usually 2 to 14 days after transfusion and include fevers, skin rash, liver failure, diarrhea, and marrow aplasia. The condition is fatal in about 95% of the cases but can be prevented by irradiation of blood products, which inhibits the ability of donor T lymphocytes to undergo blast transformation and engraftment.

### Circulatory overload

Patients with poor cardiac function may not tolerate standard volumes of blood components and may develop circulatory failure with pulmonary edema. Symptoms include dyspnea, pounding headache, and constrictive feeling in the chest. Standard therapy for cardiac decompensation should be initiated, and such patients should receive aliquots of blood at a slow rate.

### Managed Care Guide
### Practice strategies for elective red blood cell transfusion

1. Avoid an empiric, automatic transfusion threshold (for example, hemoglobin <100 g/L [10 g/dL]).
2. Regard elective transfusion with homologous blood as an outcome to be avoided.
3. Plan for the availability of autologous blood when acute blood loss can be predicted (before elective surgery).
4. Administer transfusion on a unit-by-unit basis, according to symptoms. Remember: One unit of blood may be sufficient.
5. Consider erythropoietin therapy to treat the anemia associated with chronic diseases (for example, anemia associated with drug-induced myelosuppression in patients who have the acquired immune deficiency syndrome [AIDS] or anemia associated with chronic renal insufficiency).

Data from *Ann Intern Med* 16:403, 1992.

## ALTERNATIVES TO HOMOLOGOUS TRANSFUSION THERAPY

The risk of disease transmission, alloimmunization, and transfusion reactions can be eliminated by using autologous, rather than homologous, blood. Autologous blood donations should be considered for every patient scheduled for an elective surgery for which blood use is anticipated. Contraindications for predepositing autologous blood include an Hct less than 33%, unstable angina, severe aortic stenosis, and the possibility of existing bacteremia (e.g., osteomyelitis). Intraoperative and postoperative salvage of autologous blood and preoperative hemodilution are also commonly used to reduce homologous blood transfusions.

In some instances patients want to provide their own donors, a procedure known as *directed donation.* Blood banking organizations do not encourage this practice because it does not increase the safety of donated blood.

The usefulness of blood substitutes, such as perfluorocarbons and modified hemoglobin solutions, despite their potential to reduce homologous blood use, has not yet been demonstrated. Therefore modern medical practice still depends on volunteer blood donations.

## BIBLIOGRAPHY


Basta M et al: Mechanism of therapeutic effect of high-dose intravenous immunoglobulin: attenuation of acute, complement-dependent damage in a guinea pig model, *J Clin Invest* 84:1974, 1989.

Beutler E: Platelet transfusions: the 20,000/μL trigger, *Blood* 81:1411, 1993.

Dodd RY: The risk of transfusion-transmitted infection, *N Engl J Med* 327:419, 1992.

Erstad B, Gales B, Rappaport W: The use of albumin in clinical practice, *Arch Intern Med* 151:901, 1991.

Harmening D: *Modern blood banking and transfusion practices,* ed 2, Philadelphia, 1989, FA Davis.

Petz L, Swisher S: *Clinical practice of transfusion medicine,* ed 2, New York, 1989, Churchill Livingstone.

Plasma-Consensus Conference: Fresh frozen plasma: indications and risks, *JAMA* 253:551, 1985.

Red Cell-Consensus Conference: Perioperative red blood cell transfusion, *JAMA* 260:2700, 1988.

Rossi E, Simon T, Moss G: *Principles of transfusion medicine,* Baltimore, 1991, Williams & Wilkins.

Schlichter SJ, Harker LA: Thrombocytopenia: mechanisms and management, *Clin Haematol* 7:523, 1978.

Sultan Y et al: Anti-idiotype suppression of autoantibodies to factor VIII (antihaemophilic factor) by high-dose intravenous gammaglobulin, *Lancet* 2:765, 1984.

Valeri CR et al: Increase in plasma volume after the transfusion of washed erythrocytes, *Surg Gynecol Obstet* 162:30, 1986.

Von dem Borne AEG, Decary F: Nomenclature of platelet-specific antigens, *Transfusion* 30:477, 1990.

Walker RH, editor: *Technical manual,* ed 10, Arlington, Va, 1990, American Association of Blood Banks.

Welch HG, Meehan KR, Goodnough LT: Prudent strategies for elective red blood cell transfusion, *Ann Intern Med* 116:393, 1992.


CHAPTER

# 57A Cardinal Manifestations of Cancer

**Kathryn L. Edmiston**

Cancer is the second leading cause of death in the United States and as such is a concern for most patients seeing their primary care physicians (Table 57A-1). The magnitude of the cancer problem is likely to increase in the coming decades as the U.S. population ages. At the beginning of the 20th century fewer than 10% of Americans were over the age of 55. By 1989 this figure had doubled, and it is expected to increase through the year 2030. The risk of developing cancer increases dramatically with age; more than 65% of all cancer deaths occur in patients over the age of 55. Because patients frequently visit their primary care physician for routine health maintenance or the evaluation of new symptoms, primary care physicians need to have a thorough knowledge of the clinical signs and symptoms associated with cancer and the initial evaluation of the patient who is suspected of having cancer.

## ASYMPTOMATIC PATIENTS

Patients may be diagnosed with cancer before symptoms occur or may come to medical attention because of symptoms resulting from their cancer. For most types of cancer, diagnosis in the early stages of disease before symptoms have occurred is critical. Treatment of early stage lung cancer may be cured, whereas advanced lung cancer is never curable even with aggressive treatment. This creates a particular dilemma for the primary care physician. How can cancer be diagnosed in its earliest and potentially curable stages *before the patient has developed any symptoms?* A thorough risk assessment during a routine visit and the appropriate use of cancer screening tests may lead to the diagnosis of cancer in the asymptomatic patient.

A thorough risk assessment can easily be accomplished during the medical interview. Risk assessment should include a history of habits such as smoking and alcohol use, occupational and other environmental exposures, diet, and family history. Cancers associated with specific risks are shown in Table 57A-2. Once a patient is found to be at risk, what interventions are necessary? First, and most important the patient should be counseled regarding the elimination of cancer-causing behaviors. Patients who smoke should be advised of the increased frequency of lung cancer and other cancers of the aerodigestive tract, as well as the risk of cardiovascular and peripheral vascular disease. It is estimated that 90% of all lung cancers are directly caused by tobacco use. Patients who wish to discontinue smoking should be provided with smoking cessation tools (see Chapter 124).

Early intervention to prevent the development of cancer may be warranted for patients with certain types of risk. For example, patients with familial adenomatous polypo-

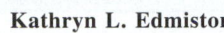

**Table 57A-1.** Estimated incidence and mortality of common cancers in the United States in 1995

| Primary cancer | Incidence | Deaths |
|---|---|---|
| Bronchogenic | 170,000 | 157,400 |
| Breast | 183,000 | 46,300 |
| Colorectal | 138,200 | 55,300 |
| Prostate | 244,000 | 40,400 |
| Head and neck | 39,750 | 12,460 |

**Table 57A-2.** Risk factors associated with common primary cancers

| Primary cancer | Risk factors |
|---|---|
| Bronchogenic carcinoma | Tobacco<br>Asbestos<br>Radiation exposure |
| Breast carcinoma | First-degree relative with breast cancer<br>Prior personal history of breast cancer<br>Nulliparity<br>Early menarche<br>Late menopause |
| Colon carcinoma | High-fat, low-fiber diet<br>Personal history of colonic adenomatous polyps or previously resected colon cancer<br>Inflammatory bowel disease |
| Cervical carcinoma | Multiparity<br>Infection with human papillomavirus |
| Esophageal cancer and head and neck cancer | Tobacco and alcohol use |

sis are almost certain to develop colon cancer by age 50 if left untreated. Prophylactic colectomy is recommended for prevention. Similarly, patients with a strong family history of bilateral, premenopausal breast cancer may wish to consider early mammography or even prophylactic bilateral mastectomy in selected cases.

Finally, careful evaluation of organ systems at risk should be performed during the routine physical examination. Patients with heavy sun exposure or a family history of melanoma should have a thorough skin examination. A thorough inspection and manual examination of the oral cavity in patients with a history of tobacco and alcohol use may detect premalignant lesions or potentially curable invasive carcinomas of the oral cavity. The breasts should be carefully examined, particularly in women over the age of 50 or any woman with a family history of breast cancer.

A number of cancer screening tools such as mammography and sigmoidoscopy are recommended by the American Cancer Society for the early detection of cancer.

## SYMPTOMATIC PATIENTS

Symptoms of cancer may be vague and nonspecific, such as weight loss, fatigue, and malaise. Specific symptoms may occur because of physiologic or mechanical effects of the primary tumor or metastases at distant sites.

Weight loss occurs commonly at the time of diagnosis in many patients with advanced cancer. Although a wide constellation of gastrointestinal symptoms are common in patients with cancer, decreased caloric intake may not be sufficient to explain weight loss. An aggressive search for an undiagnosed cancer is probably not warranted in most patients with unexplained weight loss as their *only* symptom until changes in dietary intake, depression, and stresses at work or in family have been assessed. Patients at high risk for cancer, such as smokers or those with additional symptoms, should undergo further evaluation without delay.

Pain is the most feared symptom resulting from cancer. Pain occurs at some time during the clinical course of most cancer patients and may be a result of the treatment or the underlying malignancy. Although chronic pain affects nearly all patients with advanced cancer it usually can be adequately controlled with medication.

Somatic pain caused by involvement of bone, muscle, or other soft tissues is typically well-localized and described as aching, stabbing, or pressurelike. Pain can frequently be elicited by palpation over the affected site. Weight-bearing and movement may exacerbate the pain caused by bony involvement. Visceral pain varies with the organ affected. Pain from bowel obstruction may be crampy, whereas pain from liver involvement may be sharp and throbbing. Neuropathic pain results from involvement of peripheral or central nervous system pathways by tumor. This type of pain is typically described as a burning, tingling, or unpleasant sensation in a region of neurologic dysfunction. Neuropathic pain may be difficult to treat with analgesics alone.

Trousseau first described superficial migratory thrombophlebitis associated with gastrointestinal malignancies in 1865. Since that time it has been noted that a hypercoagulable state is frequently associated with a diagnosis of cancer. Patients with advanced cancer are clearly at increased risk for the development of deep venous thrombosis (DVT). In 1951 Ackerman suggested that DVT may be the presenting problem of patients with undiagnosed cancer. This continues to be debated. About 70% of patients with DVT have an identifiable risk factor for thrombosis such as bed rest, recent surgery, or varicosities. The risk of occult malignancy in this group is less than 5%. In patients with idiopathic DVT the incidence of undiagnosed cancer is 30% to 35%. Many patients with idiopathic DVT who are concurrently diagnosed with cancer after an extensive screening evaluation (abdominal ultrasonography, abdominal computed tomography [CT], and upper gastrointestinal endoscopy) are found to actually have symptoms of the primary cancer. The appropriate evaluation for patients with idiopathic DVT should be a complete history and physical examination, complete blood count and differential, serum lactase dehydrogenase (LDH), chest x-ray, and evaluation of any additional signs or symptoms consistent with a diagnosis of malignancy.

## PHYSICAL EXAMINATION

### Skin

A thorough inspection of the skin is useful for detecting skin cancer. The incidence of malignant melanoma has increased dramatically over the last six decades. The principal risk factor is sun exposure. The prognosis for patients with deeply invasive primary lesions, regional or distant metastases is grim, so early detection is paramount. Pigmented skin lesions should be examined for size, color, shape, and symmetry. Guidelines for assessing hyperpigmented skin lesions (the ABCD acronym) and the characteristics of suspicious lesions are described in Chapter 21. Patients with suspicious lesions should be promptly referred to a dermatologist or plastic surgeon for excisional biopsy (see Chapter 57B).

### Oral cavity

A careful inspection and manual examination of the oral cavity should be a routine part of the physical examination, particularly in patients over the age of 40 who use tobacco and alcohol. The American Cancer Society estimated that there would be 28,150 new cancers of the oral cavity diagnosed in 1994. Tobacco and alcohol are the principal etiologic factors in these cancers. About 90% of oral cancers occur in regions easily visualized during the routine physical examination. Premalignant lesions such as leukoplakia and erythroplakia may also be detected and treated early. Leukoplakia appears as thick, white hyperkeratotic plaque most commonly on the buccal mucosa, dorsal tongue, and alveolar ridge. Although considered a premalignant lesion, there is a low frequency of transformation to invasive cancer. Erythroplakia appears as an erythematous granular lesion most commonly on the floor of the mouth, ventral tongue, and soft palate. About 60% to 85% of patients with erythroplakia have early invasive squamous cell cancer at biopsy. Patients with the above diagnoses should be advised to stop smoking and drinking alcohol and should continue under routine surveillance. Vitamin A derivatives may help prevent the subsequent development of second primary tumors of the head and neck in patients previously treated for squamous carcinoma of the oral cavity. See Chapter 32 for further information.

### Lymphadenopathy

Inflammatory adenopathy, congenital abnormalities, and neoplasia are all broad categories that need to be considered when evaluating cervical adenopathy. In the pediatric population inflammatory and congenital lesions are the most common cause of neck masses. In young adults the frequency of neoplasia, especially lymphoma, increases but it is still less common than inflammatory adenopathy. In contrast, 50% of patients over the age of 40 with an enlarged asymmetric neck mass are diagnosed with carcinoma or lymphoma (see Chapter 32). If a careful head and neck examination fails to reveal any abnormalities, a fine-needle aspiration biopsy can usually be performed as an outpatient procedure. Special stains may be necessary to determine the precise nature of the abnormality. If the cytology is consistent with a diagnosis of lymphoma, an excisional biopsy may be required for more precise diagnosis.

Axillary adenopathy is a frequently encountered abnormality in clinical practice and most often is due to benign processes. Large, multiple, matted or enlarging lymph nodes should be biopsied. Supraclavicular adenopathy is almost always of pathologic significance and requires further evaluation. Lung cancer is the most common cancer to metastasize to supraclavicular lymph nodes, and a chest x-ray should be obtained promptly. A Virchow node in the left supraclavicular fossa may represent involvement from a gastrointestinal cancer.

### Breast mass

The breast examination is a complex and difficult part of the routine physical examination because of the wide variability in normal anatomy. The breast is a composite of fat and glandular tissue that changes throughout the menstrual cycle. These changes are typically referred to as fibrocystic change and should not be considered abnormal. However, any discrete palpable mass in the breast requires further evaluation. Although mammography is a useful screening test for breast cancer, it should not be used alone in the diagnosis of a palpable breast mass. *A normal mammogram particularly in a young, premenopausal woman does not definitively exclude the diagnosis of cancer.*

The differential diagnosis of a palpable breast mass includes fibroadenoma, benign cyst, and carcinoma. See Chapter 149 for a detailed presentation of breast diseases.

Signs on physical examination that require urgent evaluation are redness, warmth, and tenderness of the breast. There may be a palpable mass in the breast. Although a biopsy is required to confirm the diagnosis, these are signs of inflammatory breast cancer and prompt staging and treatment are indicated.

### Chest

A chest x-ray is the most important diagnostic test in a patient with pulmonary complaints. Pleural effusions may result from inflammatory, cardiovascular, and neoplastic disorders. Thoracentesis obtains fluid that may yield a precise diagnosis. Fluid should be analyzed for LDH and protein content, cell count and differential, culture, pH, and cytology. The characteristics of a malignant pleural effusion are listed in the box below. Malignant pleural effusions occur most commonly in patients with lung and

#### Characteristics of malignant pleural effusions

Appearance
- Bloody or serous

Biochemistry
- $LDH_{pl}/LDH_{ser} > 0.6$
- $TP_{pl}/TP_{ser} > 0.5$
- pH may be $< 7.0$

Cytology
- Malignant cells identified

$LDH_{pl}/LDH_{ser}$, Ratio of lactic acid dehydrogenase in pleural fluid to LDH in serum; $TP_{pl}/TP_{ser}$, ratio of total protein in pleural fluid to total protein in serum.

breast cancer. A chylous effusion with high lipid content occurs most commonly from lymphomatous involvement of lymph nodes in the retroperitoneum and mediastinum.

A solitary pulmonary nodule (SPN) is an opacity seen on chest x-ray measuring less than 4 cm and completely surrounded by lung parenchyma. It is a common incidental finding that requires further evaluation. The purpose of further diagnostic evaluation is to distinguish malignant neoplasms that are potentially curable with surgery from benign lesions and incurable malignant lesions. If the patient has had prior chest x-rays, these should be obtained for comparison to the most recent examination. If the SPN has been present and unchanged over 2 years, it is probably benign and a subsequent chest x-ray should be obtained to ensure stability. If previous chest x-rays are not available, further study is warranted. Fluoroscopy may be useful for clarifying subtle or questionable abnormalities on chest x-ray. For larger lesions or when the fluoroscopy is equivocal, CT scanning is the most useful diagnostic test. Lesions with benign appearing calcifications or CT-detectable fat in a well-circumscribed pulmonary nodule are probably benign and do not require further evaluation. The presence of enlarged mediastinal or hilar lymph nodes or multiple nodules is more likely to occur with malignant disease. See Chapter 120 for a presentation of neoplasms of the lung.

### Abdomen

Unexplained ascites, hepatomegaly, or a palpable abdominal mass may all suggest the presence of an intraabdominal malignancy. Ascites in a middle-aged woman is a common presentation for ovarian cancer. The first step in evaluating such a patient is a pelvic examination to assess the presence of an adnexal mass. Additional studies should include transvaginal ultrasound or an abdominal CT scan to assess the extent of disease and a blood test for CA 125. CA 125 is a marker for ovarian cancer and is elevated in 80% of patients with ovarian cancer.

When the pelvic examination is normal, and for men with unexplained ascites, paracentesis should be performed. Malignant ascites typically is bloody with malignant cells seen on cytologic analysis.

Hepatomegaly can occur as a result of benign infiltrative disease of the liver or involvement of the liver by tumor. Involvement of the liver by metastasis is far more common than the occurrence of primary hepatocellular carcinoma. Lung, colon, and breast cancer frequently metastasize to the liver, and a prior history of these cancers should raise the clinical suspicion of metastatic liver disease in a patient with hepatomegaly. A CT scan provides the most diagnostic information in evaluating hepatomegaly. If lesions consistent with metastatic or primary liver cancer are seen, a biopsy may be required to establish the precise diagnosis (see Chapter 44).

A palpable abdominal mass should be evaluated by a CT scan to determine its origin and relation to normal intraabdominal organs. A tumor mass in the abdomen may be a primary or metastatic focus of disease. Further evaluation and biopsy depend on the location and radiographic appearance of the mass. A mass arising from the large bowel may be further evaluated with colonoscopy (see Chapter 45). Upper gastrointestinal endoscopy may be indicated for upper abdominal masses or those that may be of pancreatic origin. A percutaneous fine-needle biopsy/aspiration under CT or ultrasound guidance is the procedure of choice for diagnosing a renal mass.

Testing for fecal occult blood is recommended as part of the routine physical examination for patients over the age of 40. Those patients who are found to have occult blood in the stool or iron-deficiency anemia may have an occult gastrointestinal malignancy. Further evaluation should be guided by the presence of any associated symptoms (see Chapter 45 for a detailed presentation of GI neoplasms).

### Prostate

Prostate cancer is the most common cancer affecting men in the United States. The American Cancer Society estimated that there would be 244,000 new cases of prostate cancer diagnosed in the United States in 1995. Enlargement of the prostate is part of the normal aging process and often results in symptoms of frequency, urgency, and hesitancy. It is often very difficult to distinguish on clinical criteria alone whether symptoms are due to benign prostatic hypertrophy or cancer. Patients who are symptomatic, even if the digital rectal examination is normal, should probably be evaluated with the following tests.

Patients with prostate cancer may be asymptomatic or have symptoms similar to those in patients with benign disease. Asymptomatic patients may come to attention because of palpable findings on digital rectal examination (DRE) such as diffuse enlargement or focal, well-localized nodules. Any hard area or discrete nodule detected on routine DRE should arouse suspicion for carcinoma. Transrectal ultrasound (TRUS) and determination of the prostate specific antigen (PSA) add significantly to the information obtained during the DRE. The diagnostic workup for prostate cancer is presented in detail in Chapter 138.

### Testis

Testicular cancer is the most common malignancy occurring in young men between ages 20 and 35. The only identifiable risk factor for testicular cancer is cryptorchid testis. There is an 11- to 50-fold increased risk in the undescended testis compared to the frequency in normally located organs. Orchiopexy does not decrease this risk but may allow for earlier diagnosis.

Since the diagnosis of testicular cancer is frequently delayed and often misdiagnosed, young men are now being instructed in testicular self-examination as a means of improving early diagnosis of testicular cancer. The differential diagnosis of a testicular mass is shown in Table 57A-3 and includes acute and chronic epididymitis, varicocele, hydrocele, and inguinal hernia.

Transscrotal ultrasound is a useful diagnostic tool in the evaluation of a testicular mass. Patients who are found to have a solid mass should be referred for inguinal orchiectomy (see Chapter 141).

Human chorionic gonadotropin (hCG) and $\alpha$-fetoprotein (AFP) are serum tumor markers for testicular cancer. hCG is elevated in 40% to 60% of patients with nonseminomatous testicular cancer. Although AFP can be elevated in a variety of benign and malignant conditions, 70% to 90% of patients with advanced nonseminomatous

**Table 57A-3.** Differential diagnosis of a testicular mass

| Diagnosis | Age | Symptoms | Location | Ultrasound |
|---|---|---|---|---|
| Tumor | 20-45 | Painless swelling | Attached to testis | Solid |
| Epididymitis | Any | Acute painful swelling with or without fever | Around testis | — |
| Hydrocele | Any | None | In vaginal sac around testis | Cystic |
| Spermatocele | Middle | Painless swelling | On top of testis | Cystic |
| Varicocele | Young | None; bag of worms | Left > right | Cystic |

testicular cancer have an elevated level. These markers should be checked preoperatively and throughout the course of treatment and follow-up.

## DIAGNOSIS

Symptomatic or asymptomatic patients may have a variety of findings consistent with a diagnosis of cancer. Although patients may be suspected of having cancer based on abnormal physical findings or radiographic studies, a diagnosis of cancer *always* requires a biopsy. A biopsy may confirm the diagnosis of malignancy and may provide important prognostic information. Biopsy material may be obtained in a variety of ways depending on the site.

A fine-needle aspiration biopsy can be accomplished with a minimum of morbidity in the outpatient department. Material is sent to the pathology lab for cytologic evaluation. This is a particularly useful procedure for evaluating palpable masses in the breast and enlarged palpable lymph nodes. Needle aspiration biopsy guided by ultrasound or CT can be used to biopsy abnormalities in a variety of sites including breast, thyroid, and essentially all abdominal and pelvic organs except bowel and bladder. Incisional or excisional biopsy or a more extensive procedure may be necessary to obtain tissue for diagnosis if the fine-needle biopsy is nondiagnostic or if additional material is thought to be necessary for a complete histologic evaluation.

The pathologist plays an essential role in evaluating the patient with a suspected diagnosis of cancer. The patient's age, symptoms, physical findings, suspected diagnosis, and the site of the biopsy should all be communicated to the pathologist before the procedure to be certain that an optimal speciman is obtained, handled, and fixed in a manner that maximizes diagnostic accuracy. The pathologist has a variety of tools that are used to establish a precise diagnosis of cancer. Immunohistochemical markers may help to distinguish a carcinoma from a sarcoma or a lymphoma. Additional special stains may be necessary to reach a precise diagnosis or to identify a primary site when it is not clinically evident.

Once a diagnosis of cancer has been established, further studies may be needed to determine the extent of the disease and the precise stage of the cancer even if the patient is otherwise healthy. All patients should have a complete history and physical examination. Laboratory evaluation should include a complete blood count and differential and blood tests to screen for kidney, liver, and bone disease. Any abnormalities in the history, physical examination, or laboratory studies that may be due to cancer require further diagnostic evaluation. Even if all of the above studies are normal, selected radiographic studies may be required based on the natural history and usual pattern of metastases from the specific primary site. For example, all patients with cancer do not require a head CT unless there are symptoms, abnormalities in the neurologic examination, or if cancer from the patient's primary site frequently involves the brain.

Most solid tumors are staged by the TNM classification. The T stage designates the extent of the primary lesion; N designates the extent of regional lymph node involvement; $M_0$ is the absence of any distant metastases; and $M_1$ indicates the presence of distant metastases. The TNM are then grouped into a stage classification. Stage 1 usually represents early stage disease. Patients with stage 4 disease usually have distant metastases.

Complete staging evaluation is essential for further management. The stage at diagnosis often determines the appropriate treatment modality. Patients with localized disease may require only local therapy such as radiation or surgery, whereas patients with disseminated disease may be considered for systemic therapy. Second, the stage at diagnosis has a major impact on prognosis. Patients with localized disease may be curable, in contrast to most patients with disseminated cancer in whom the disease may be treatable but not curable. Finally, it is essential that patients enrolled in clinical trials be uniformly staged so that the results are generally valid.

### Carcinoma of unknown primary site

Most patients with metastatic cancer have a clinically obvious primary site where the tumor began. However, approximately 5% of patients with metastatic cancer have a clinically occult primary site despite a complete history, physical examination, routine laboratory studies, and a chest x-ray. Myriad extensive diagnostic testing can be undertaken in an attempt to identify the primary site, but this is generally futile because a primary site is not identified. Moreover, specific identification of the primary site usually does not have a major impact on the subsequent outcome. Efforts should be directed at identifying treatable tumors such as the lymphomas, hormonally responsive malignancies such as breast and prostate carcinomas, germ cell tumors, and small cell carcinoma of the lung.

Some situations need special consideration. Poorly differentiated carcinoma or poorly differentiated adenocarcinoma of unknown primary site describes a subset of patients who may have a favorable response rate to cisplatin-based combination chemotherapy. The most favorable responses occur in young patients with a limited number of metastases located in the retroperitoneum or peripheral lymph nodes. About 30% of these patients are disease-free after treatment, and prolonged complete remissions may be achieved.

Adenocarcinoma in an axillary node in an otherwise asymptomatic woman should be treated as an occult breast primary. Immunohistochemical stains for estrogen and progesterone on the biopsy specimen may provide corroborative evidence of a breast primary. Mammography may be useful in identifying an occult breast cancer, but a normal mammogram does not rule out the possibility of a breast primary. Women who have adenocarcinoma of unknown primary only in an axillary lymph node should undergo breast surgery and axillary dissection and receive adjuvant therapy similar to that for patients with stage 2 breast cancer. In contrast to other patients with adenocarcinoma of unknown primary, the prognosis is good with approximately 65% 5-year disease-free survival.

Patients with upper or midcervical lymphadenopathy secondary to squamous cell carcinoma should be evaluated for a head and neck primary. This should include a chest x-ray and endoscopic evaluation of the whole upper aerodigestive tract. If no primary is identified, aggressive combined modality therapy with radiation therapy and neck dissection should be prescribed in the same dosage and fields as in patients with a known head and neck primary. With this approach the 5-year survival is 30% to 50%.

Occult prostate cancer should be searched for in men with osteoblastic metastases involving the axial and appendicular skeleton, since patients with diffuse metastatic prostate cancer are likely to benefit from hormonal therapy. In a male patient with diffuse osteoblastic metastases and adenocarcinoma on biopsy, an elevated serum PSA or immunohistochemical staining of the biopsy specimen for PSA is sufficient to initiate treatment for metastatic prostate carcinoma.

### The multidisciplinary approach

Once the diagnosis of cancer is established, it should be communicated and explained to the patient. It is always helpful to have a family member or significant other present during this discussion. A thorough explanation of the treatment plan, potential complications, and expected outcome is essential.

Although many specialists are frequently involved in caring for the patient with cancer, the primary care physician is a vital part of the multidisciplinary team. Patients often look to their primary provider to help them understand the complicated aspects of their cancer management. Subspecialists also appreciate the unique perspective of the primary care physician for assessing the impact of other chronic diseases on future care. The primary care physician should continue to counsel the patient and family even after the diagnosis of cancer is established.

When the diagnosis of cancer is made, referral to the appropriate subspecialist is often necessary. This may include a medical oncologist, radiation oncologist, and surgical oncologist. Nurses, social workers, physical therapists, enterostomal therapists, occupational therapists, and clergy are also important members of the health-care team.

## FUTURE DIRECTIONS

Clinical research is being done to improve the care of patients with most solid tumors. Patients who are referred to tertiary care cancer centers are often candidates for participation in clinical research trials either through cooperative groups or pharmaceutical companies. Patients should be encouraged to participate in clinical trials to obtain the best possible care for their cancer *and* to help develop new and innovative cancer treatments for the future.

## BIBLIOGRAPHY


Allison JE, Feldman R, Tekawa IS: Hemoccult screening in detecting colorectal neoplasm: sensitivity, specificity and predictive value, *Ann Intern Med* 112(5):328, 1990.

Boring CC, Squires TS, Tong T: Cancer statistics, 1993, *CA Cancer J Clin* 43(1):7, 1993.

Cooper HS, Slemmer JR: Surgical pathology of the colon and rectum, *Semin Oncol* 18(4):367, 1991.

Donegan WL: Evaluation of a palpable breast mass, *N Engl J Med* 327(13):937, 1992.

Hainsworth JD, Greco FA: Poorly differentiated carcinoma and poorly differentiated adenocarcinoma of unknown primary tumor site, *Semin Oncol* 20(3):279, 1993.

Hainsworth JD, Greco FA: Treatment of patients with cancer of an unknown primary site, *N Engl J Med* 329(4):257, 1993.

Harris JR et al: Breast cancer, *N Engl J Med* 327(5):319; (6):390; (7):473, 1992.

Heelan R: Lung cancer imaging: primary diagnosis, staging and local recurrence, *Semin Oncol* 18(2):87, 1991.

King MC, Rowell S, Love S: Inherited breast and ovarian cancer, *JAMA* 269(15):1975, 1993.

Leonard RJ, Nystrom JS: Diagnostic evaluation of patients with carcinoma of unknown primary tumor site, *Semin Oncol* 20(3):244, 1993.

Mcguirt WF: Diagnosis and management of masses in the neck, with special emphasis on metastatic malignant disease, *Oncology* 4(8):85, 1990.

Mettlin C et al: The American Cancer Society National Prostate Cancer Detection Project, *Cancer* 67(12):2949, 1991.

Monreal M et al: Occult cancer in patients with deep venous thrombosis, *Cancer* 67:541, 1991.

Portenoy RK: Cancer pain management, *Semin Oncol* 20 (suppl 1):19, 1993.

Smart CR: Screening for cancer of the aerodigestive tract, *Cancer* 72:1061, 1993.

Swenson SJ et al: An integrated approach to evaluation of the solitary pulmonary nodule, *Mayo Clin Proc* 65:173, 1990.

White CS, Templeton PA, Belani CP: Imaging in lung cancer, *Semin Oncol* 20(2):142, 1993.

CHAPTER

# 57B Cutaneous Signs of Internal Malignancy

James C. Shaw

## SPECIFIC CUTANEOUS SIGNS OF INTERNAL MALIGNANCY

### Cutaneous T-cell lymphoma

Mycosis fungoides (MF) is the common term used to describe cutaneous T-cell lymphoma (CTCL). The term mycosis fungoides, although widely used, is a misnomer since there is no relationship to fungal disease. Clinicians should be familiar with both terms (MF and CTCL).

***Epidemiology/etiology.*** CTCL (MF) is a malignancy of helper T-cells that involves the skin. Men are affected more than women, and blacks twice as much as whites. The disease is usually diagnosed in the fifth and sixth decades although a trend toward earlier diagnosis has been observed recently. The incidence in the United States is twice that observed in England, Wales, Norway, the Netherlands, and Western Australia. The etiology of CTCL is unknown although there is speculation concerning the role of retroviral infection, since an aggressive form of T-cell lymphoma/leukemia similar to late stage MF is associated with the retrovirus HTLV-1, and a new retrovirus, HTLV-5, has been isolated from several patients with CTCL.

***Pathophysiology.*** The precise pathophysiology leading to the development of CTCL is uncertain. One theory is that CTCL begins as a malignancy of helper T-cells, and, because of effective immune host response, is not easily detectable in early stages. The malignancy then becomes more aggressive as host response declines and the total number of malignant cells increases. An alternative theory is that CTCL is the result of chronic antigen stimulation (no antigen has yet been identified); this results in T-lymphocyte proliferation with the potential for transformation into malignant cell lines.

***History.*** CTCL develops slowly in most cases. Patients usually seek medical attention because of asymptomatic or pruritic patches of abnormal-appearing skin. Rarely, CTCL presents with raised tumors noticed by patients. Constitutional symptoms are usually absent but may include fever, night sweats, and weight loss.

***Physical examination.*** There are three clinical stages in CTCL: the *patch stage,* the *plaque stage,* and the *tumor stage* (Fig. 57B-1). The patch stage consists of fixed erythematous patches with slight scaling and wrinkling of the epidermis. They range in size from a few millimeters to 10 to 20 cm in diameter and can be present anywhere on the body. The plaque stage evolves from the patch stage as the lymphocytic infiltrate in the dermis enlarges and the lesions develop a raised component. The plaques can be arcuate or irregular in shape and usually take on a reddish-brown color. The tumor stage represents further evolution from the plaque stage, with raised reddish-brown to violaceous cutaneous tumors with central necrosis and ulceration. All three stages can be present simultaneously, and regional or generalized lymphadenopathy can be present during any of the stages. Occasionally CTCL presents as a generalized exfoliative erythroderma. *Sézary syndrome* is a variant of CTCL presenting as a leukemic phase of the disease. Although this form can be present with any of the stages, it presents more frequently with erythroderma or an exfoliative dermatitis.

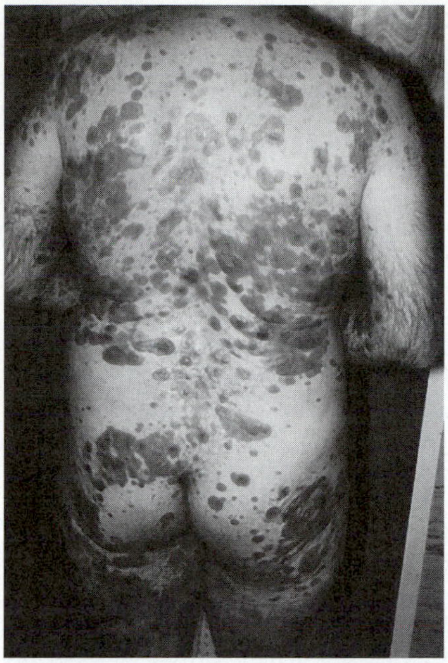

**Fig. 57B-1.** Cutaneous T-cell lymphoma (mycosis fungoides). Note patch, plaque, and tumor stages.

***Differential diagnosis.*** The diagnosis of CTCL can be difficult to make on the basis of clinical appearance, especially in the early phases. Allergic contact dermatitis, other chronic dermatitis, pigmented purpura, psoriasis, and drug eruptions can be in the differential diagnosis of patch stage. Once raised lesions are present, the differential diagnosis includes other cutaneous malignancies, deep fungal infections, granulomatous disease, and deep forms of vasculitis. In all phases of CTCL, diagnosis is made by biopsy.

***Laboratory examination.*** Confirmation of the diagnosis requires histopathologic examination from lesional skin, and in early stages the histologic diagnosis can be difficult to make. The hallmark of CTCL is the presence of a dense accumulation of mature and atypical lymphocytes in the upper dermis. In most cases the lymphocytes are also present within the epidermis (epidermotropism), a feature that may be lost in late tumor stages. Multiple biopsies over time may be necessary to confirm the diagnosis. In addition to routine histopathologic examination, cell surface markers and gene rearrangement studies of the T-cell antigen receptors from sampled lymph node tissue can help make the diagnosis. Laboratory evaluation for evidence of systemic involvement includes routine hematology and chemistry, a Sézary cell count (examination of the buffy coat for atypical lymphocytes called Sézary cells), and imaging studies of liver, spleen, and paraaortic lymph nodes.

*Management.* At the present time CTCL is difficult to cure, and the goal of treatment is a prolonged remission. In many cases, the disease is maintained in a chronic form for many years and patients die of unrelated causes. The decision to treat therefore is not always straightforward. There is literature suggesting that treatment may not prolong life. The treatment of CTCL depends on the level of involvement and frequently requires a team approach using the skills of dermatologists, oncologists, and radiation therapists. Because the therapies available for late stage disease are disappointing, most of the emphasis is on the treatment of patch and plaque stage disease. *Topical nitrogen mustard* has been used in early disease for many years and has been associated with remissions for up to 12 years in approximately 20% of those treated. Contact dermatitis is a common complication, and there is an increased risk of developing skin cancers with continued use. *PUVA (psoralens plus ultra-violet light A)* is also effective in early disease although recurrences usually develop if treatment is stopped. *Total body electron beam* therapy has been the most successful treatment, with total remissions achieved in 80% to 95% of patients with early disease, and disease-free periods of up to four years. Other beneficial treatments include extracorporeal photophoresis, single and multiple drug chemotherapy, and combinations of electron beam plus adjuvant chemotherapy. More studies are necessary to determine whether any treatments increase survival, especially in late stage disease.

### Lymphoma cutis

All types of lymphoma can involve the skin although rarely. The most common presentation is the development of asymptomatic erythematous to violaceous firm nodules that require biopsy for diagnosis. Treatment is systemic treatment of the underlying lymphoma.

### Leukemia cutis

Leukemia can involve the skin with infiltrative nodules and plaques although rarely. Diagnosis is based on histopathologic examination and treatment is directed toward the leukemic process.

### Cutaneous metastasis

Cutaneous metastasis of an underlying malignancy is rare, occurring in approximately 1% to 2% of patients with malignancy. The incidence by tumor classification of cutaneous metastasis reflects the incidence of the underlying malignancy: lung cancer and colon cancer are most common in men, and breast cancer is most common in women. Any area of the body can be involved. The lesions usually develop rapidly and are noticed by patients although they are asymptomatic. Cutaneous metastases usually consist of firm dermal nodules measuring 0.5 cm to 1.5 cm in diameter. The color is erythematous or reddish-brown with occasional violaceous hues (Fig. 57B-2). Diagnosis is made by biopsy and treatment is directed toward the underlying malignancy.

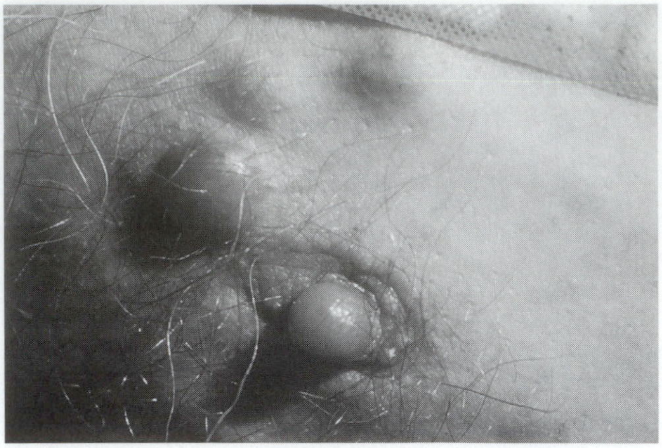

**Fig. 57B-2.** Metastatic carcinoma (bronchogenic carcinoma). Note reddish-brown dermal nodules.

## NONSPECIFIC CUTANEOUS SIGNS OF INTERNAL MALIGNANCY (Table 57B-1)

### Acanthosis nigricans

Acanthosis nigricans is a dermatosis that can occur unrelated to malignancy, but occasionally develops in association with internal malignancy, usually gastric carcinoma or other adenocarcinoma. Clinically acanthosis nigricans consists of hyperpigmented areas of hyperkeratosis that result in plaques or patches of thickened skin with a velvety or slightly verrucous texture. Common sites of involvement are the skin fold areas of the neck, axillae, groin, and antecubital/popliteal fossae. In paraneoplastic acanthosis nigricans, involvement of the dorsal and palmar hands, or other atypical sites are clues to the malignant association.

### Pruritus

Generalized pruritus is associated with several systemic diseases, most notably obstructive liver disease, renal disease, diabetes mellitus, and iron deficiency. The most common malignancies associated with pruritus are lymphomas, polycythemia, and multiple myeloma.

### Sweet's syndrome

Sweet's syndrome (acute febrile neutrophilic dermatosis) may be associated with malignancy in approximately 10% of cases. Hematologic malignancy is most common, usually acute myelogenous leukemia. Clinically, Sweet's syndrome consists of tender, erythematous dermal nodules anywhere on the body, with associated systemic findings of fever, malaise, arthralgias, and neutrophilia. Biopsy of skin lesions shows a neutrophilic dermal infiltrate. Response to treatment with systemic corticosteroids (i.e., prednisone 40 to 60 mg/day) is usually excellent regardless of whether there is an associated malignancy or not. Recurrences are common.

**Table 57B-1.** Cutaneous reactions to internal malignancy

| Disease | History | Physical | Malignancy |
|---|---|---|---|
| Acanthosis nigricans | Thickening of skin on hands and intertriginous areas | Hyperpigmented, velvety hyperkeratotic changes | Gastric carcinoma |
| Acquired hypertrichosis lanuginosa | Increased hair on face or other areas | Fine hypertrichosis; face common | Lymphoma |
| Acquired ichthyosis | Thickening, scaling on palms, soles, or other areas | Hyperkeratotic changes | Lymphoma |
| Bazex's syndrome (hyperkeratosis paraneoplastica) | Thickening of skin on nose, hands, feet | Focal hyperkeratotic plaques | Squamous cell carcinoma in the upper respiratory tract |
| Dermatomyositis | Muscle weakness; photo accentuated dermatitis | Erythema, telangiectasia, atrophy, Gottron's papules, heliotrope rash (eyelids) | Multiple associated malignancies have been reported |
| Erythema gyratum repens | Rare; pruritus, scaling | Characteristic swirls of erythema, scaling | Lung carcinoma |
| Erythroderma | Rapid onset total erythema | Erythema, some scaling | Cutaneous T-cell lymphoma |
| Flushing | Episodic head and neck flushing | Erythema (transient) | Carcinoid |
| Necrolytic migratory erythema (NME) | Periorificial shallow erosions; sore tongue; weight loss | Superficial blisters and erosions, perioral, perineal; glossitis | Glucagonoma |
| Herpes zoster | Pain and blisters; pain may precede lesions by 72 hours | Dermatomal; vesicles, papules, pustules | Any malignancy; immunosuppression |
| Leser-Trélat sign (multiple seborrheic keratoses) | Rapid onset of large numbers of asymptomatic small lesions | Multiple (>100) small to medium seb. keratoses | Breast carcinoma; GI carcinomas |
| Migratory thrombophlebitis | Painful swelling on an extremity; occasionally generalized hypercoagulability | Firm, linear, cordlike lesions involving superficial vessels | Visceral carcinomas, prostate carcinoma |
| Pruritus | Total body pruritus; sometimes worse after shower | No primary skin findings | Multiple malignancies; lymphomas |
| Pyoderma gangrenosum | Enlarging painful ulcers | Pustules, ulcerations; erythematous rolled edge | Leukemia, lymphoma; adenocarcinoma |
| Sweet's syndrome (acute febrile neutrophilic dermatosis) | High fever; malaise, arthralgias; skin rash | Erythematous nodules, plaques; lesions are tender; arthritis | Hematologic; AML most common |
| Urticaria | Pruritic hives | Urticaria | Multiple |

### Glucagonoma syndrome

There is a specific cutaneous finding associated with the α cell pancreatic malignancy, glucagonoma. The skin change, called *necrolytic migratory erythema (NME),* consists of shallow erythematous erosions from superficial blisters, along with some scaling. The most common sites are the perineum and other periorificial areas, distal legs, and sites of trauma. Associated findings include stomatitis and glossitis, anemia, and hyperglycemia with glycosuria. Histopathology of the skin lesions can demonstrate pallor and necrotic cells in the epidermis that are characteristic of NME. The clinical and histologic differential diagnosis includes nutritional deficiencies (zinc, amino acid, thiamine), acrodermatitis enteropathica, and superficial blistering diseases such as bullous impetigo and pemphigus foliaceus. The definitive test is a serum glucagon level that is markedly elevated. The precise mechanism of the skin lesions is not clear, but rapid resolution occurs when the tumor is resected.

## BIBLIOGRAPHY


Braverman IW: Cutaneous T-cell lymphoma, *Curr Probl Dermatol* 3:181, 1991.

Brodland DG, Zitelli JA: Mechanisms of metastasis, *J Am Acad Dermatol* 27:1, 1992.

Habif TP: *Clinical dermatology,* ed 2, St Louis, 1990, Mosby.

Holloway KB, Flowers FP, Ramos-Caro FA: Therapeutic alternatives in cutaneous T-cell lymphoma, *J Am Acad Dermatol* 27:367, 1992.

Poole S, Fenske NA: Cutaneous markers of internal malignancy: I. Malignant involvement of the skin and the genodermatoses, *J Am Acad Dermatol* 28:1, 1993.


CHAPTER

# 57C Benign Tumors of the Skin

**Bert G. Tavelli**

There are dozens of benign proliferations of the skin and its appendages, each with numerous variations. Familiarization with the most common of these helps in deciding when it is best to treat or advise the patient, and when it is best to refer.

## FRECKLES AND LENTIGINES

*Freckles* (ephelides) are small, sun-induced pigmented macules, characterized histologically by increased melanin along the basal layer of the epidermis. Their color varies in relation to sun exposure. *Solar lentigines* are sun-induced macular lesions that are larger than freckles. The even, tan or brown pigmentation is caused by increased melanin along the base of the epidermis. Solar lentigines are also known as "liver spots." *Simple lentigines* are small, symmetric, evenly pigmented macules that are usually darker than freckles or solar lentigines. Often appearing in childhood, they are randomly distributed and not sun-sensitive. Histologically they have increased numbers of normal melanocytes, along with increased melanin pigmentation throughout the epidermis. No treatment is usually needed for these lesions.

## MELANOCYTIC NEVI

Melanocytic nevi are a group of benign proliferations of nevus cells, forming symmetric, well-circumscribed, evenly-pigmented lesions anywhere on the skin.

Acquired melanocytic nevi vary considerably in clinical appearance (Fig. 57C-1). Typical benign nevi present as symmetric, round to oval lesions with distinct, rounded borders. They range in contour from flat (junctional), to slightly raised or papillated (compound), to dome-shaped or pedunculated (intradermal); pigmentation may vary from tan to all shades of brown or black. Many intradermal nevi eventually become flesh-colored, or only slightly pigmented. They tend to enlarge in proportion to body growth, but may do so more rapidly during pregnancy.

Though variations in size, shape, color, and growth characteristics occur within a given individual's nevi, the "ABCDs" provide a rationale for the clinical identification of lesions suggestive of melanoma: **Assymetry** (not round or oval); ***Border*** irregularity (notching or poorly defined); ***Color*** variegation (shades of brown, red, white, black, blue, or combinations of colors); ***D***iameter (greater than 6 mm). An otherwise benign-appearing, pigmented or nonpigmented nevus that changes rapidly in any way can represent melanoma, which is presented in Chapter 21.

Several clinical variants of melanocytic nevi deserve discussion. *Blue nevi* are acquired, usually solitary dark blue or blue gray papules located anywhere on the skin or mucous membranes. They are thought to represent ectopic accumulations of melanocytes in the dermis that reflect

### Managed Care Guide
### Atypical nevi

**Terminology**

The term "dysplastic nevi" is misleading and should be avoided. They are presently classified clinically as "atypical nevi" or "nevi with atypical architecture," and histologically as "nevi with architectural disorder."

**Frequency**

Estimates vary by tenfold, but atypical nevi are common.

**Familial atypical mole and melanoma syndrome**

Familial atypical mole and melanoma syndrome (FAM-M) seems to be well established, and defines families with (1) occurrence of melanoma in one or more first- or second-degree relatives; (2) large numbers of nevi, some of which are atypical; and (3) nevi that show certain histologic features. Individuals with this syndrome have a significantly high risk of developing melanoma. Referral to a dermatologist is required for intensive surveillance and to promote early diagnosis.

**Nonfamilial atypical moles**

The risk of melanoma developing in individuals having nonfamilial atypical nevi is unknown. It is certainly far less than with the familial type, but there may be an increased relative risk compared to the general population. These cases must be individualized and assessed by every criterion available.

**Management**

Lesions that are clinically suggestive of malignant melanoma require biopsy. As with the clinical evaluation where inspection of small portions of the lesion are inadequate for diagnosis, so it is with the histopathologic evaluation. When possible, total excisional biopsy is required. A large incisional wedge biopsy is preferred for lesions that are too large or technically or cosmetically inappropriate for excision. Shave biopsies or punch biopsies are never acceptable. Because of the difficulty in diagnosing melanoma, both clinically and histopathologically, referral to a dermatologist should be considered (see Chapter 21).

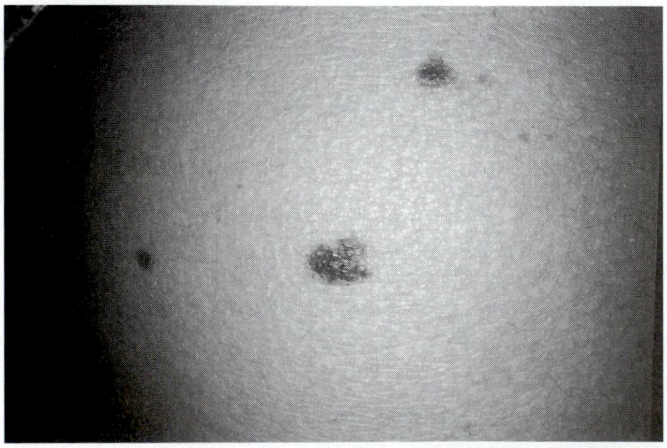

**Fig. 57C-1.** Melanocytic nevus—junctional type.

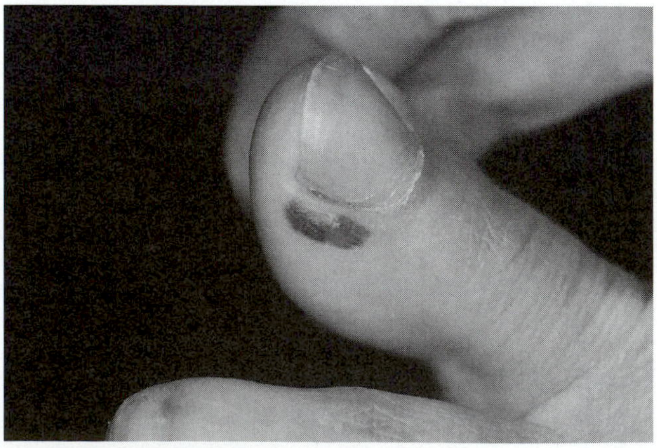

**Fig. 57C-2.** Atypical melanocytic nevus, compound type. Note large size and colors.

light of a blue wavelength because of their density and depth. They are benign, although clinically can resemble melanoma. *Atypical nevi* are a more common but controversial variant that have been difficult to classify and for which there are no strict diagnostic criteria. Previously referred to as "dysplastic nevi," they are generally larger than other acquired nevi, with somewhat indistinct or irregular borders (Fig. 57C-2). Pigmentation varies within lesions from dark brown to tan or flesh-colored, often on a reddish background. They are usually flat but may have a centrally raised portion that can be darker than the surrounding macular area.

Clearly, an individual lesion like this (large, asymmetric or irregular shape, color variation) might be suggestive of melanoma. However, when many such nevi occur on the same person, management becomes more difficult. Additionally, the histology of these lesions has been similarly difficult to define, with no clear cut, reproducible criteria with which to distinguish them from other pigmented lesions.

The main importance of atypical nevi lies in the possible increased risk of development of melanoma, either in an individual lesion, or in patients or families in whom these nevi are seen. These issues have been highly controversial and the field is constantly in flux, making clinical management difficult. A reasonable approach for the primary practitioner, based in part on a recent National Institutes of Health consensus conference, is summarized in the Managed Care Guide.

## CHONDRODERMATITIS NODULARIS

Chondrodermatitis nodularis (Fig. 57C-3) is a painful, pressure-induced papule or nodule occurring primarily along the helical rim of the ear. Lesions are precipitated by focal, often minor trauma, and develop into inflamed, intensely painful papules with central necrosis or ulceration. They may resemble basal cell or squamous cell carcinoma. Treatment with topical or intralesional corticosteroids may be useful, but surgical excision is often necessary.

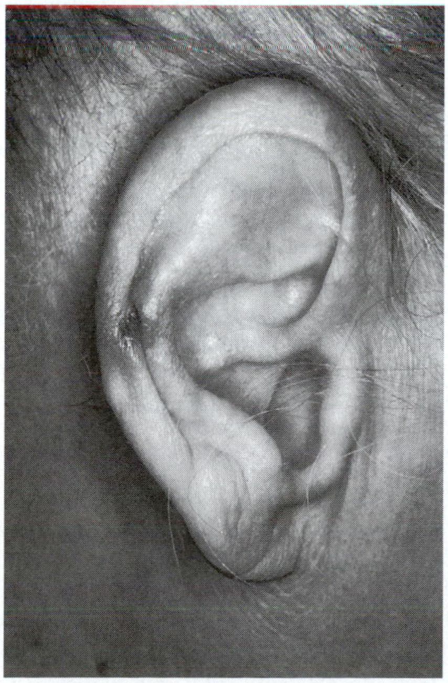

**Fig. 57C-3.** Chondrodermatitis nodularis helicis. Note erythematous eroded nodule on ear helix. These lesions are tender on palpation.

## KELOIDS

Keloids are firm, smooth, often tender proliferations of scar tissue at sites of injury to the skin (Fig. 57C-4). They may be flesh-colored, pink, or hyperpigmented, and occur mostly on the chest, shoulders, back, and earlobes. They are differentiated from a simple hypertrophic scar in that, by definition, they extend beyond the boundaries of the original injury. Keloids can attain a size of many centimeters and are also more common in darker-skinned individuals. Treatment is problematic, since surgery usually results in a larger keloid. A combination of intralesional corticosteroids, pressure dressings, and specialized surgical techniques is useful in some cases.

## SEBORRHEIC KERATOSES

Seborrheic keratoses are symmetric, keratotic papules or plaques that appear stuck on the skin (Fig. 57C-5). They

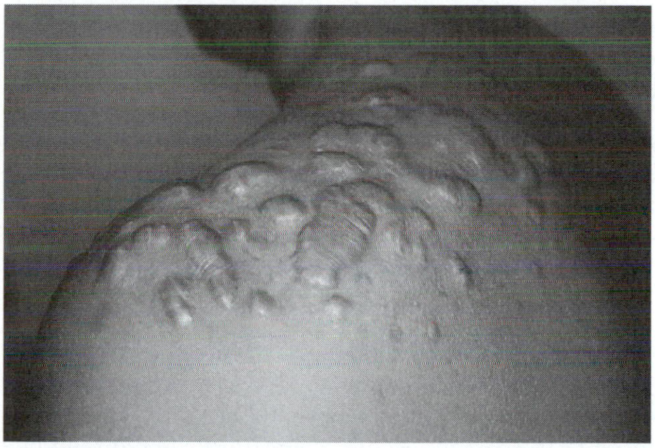

**Fig. 57C-4.** Keloids. Raised, flesh-colored lesions in typical area (shoulder).

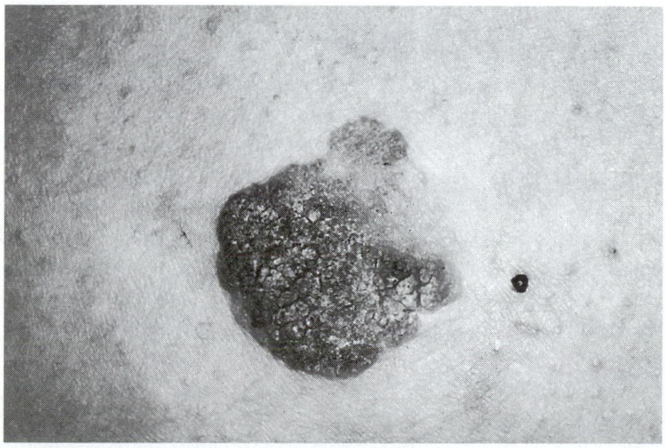

**Fig. 57C-5.** Seborrheic keratosis. Note raised stuck-on appearance.

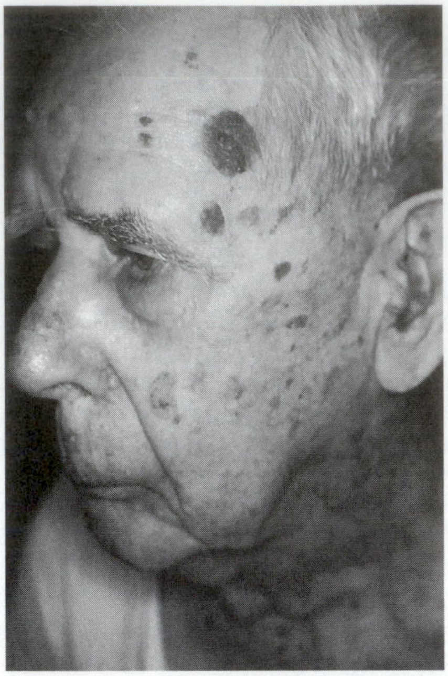

**Fig. 57C-6.** Seborrheic keratoses. Note several waxy hyperkeratotic pigmented lesions of varying size.

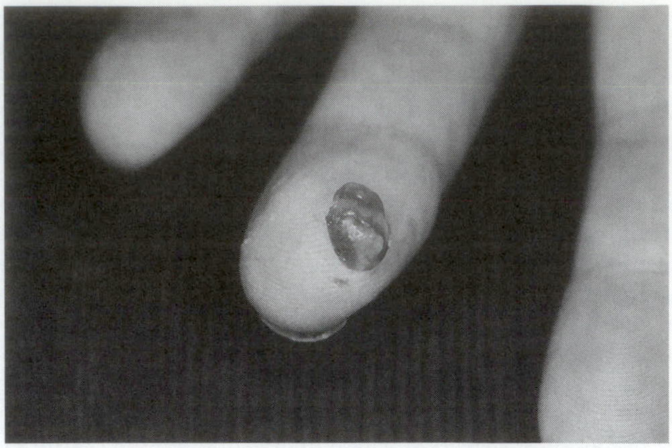

**Fig. 57C-7.** Pyogenic granuloma. Note exuberant granulation tissue.

arise in the fourth or fifth decade, most commonly on the trunk, but can occur anywhere on the skin, including the face (Fig. 57C-6). Seborrheic keratoses range in color from light tan to dark brown or black, and often have a waxy consistency. They can be distinguished from melanoma, which at times they closely resemble, by the presence of multiple, dilated follicular ostia filled with keratin. Biopsy by excision is necessary when the diagnosis is uncertain. If needed, symptomatic lesions can be treated with a light liquid nitrogen spray.

## CALLUSES AND CORNS

Both calluses and corns represent hyperkeratotic, thickened skin arising in response to chronic trauma from pressure or friction. A corn is generally smaller and more focal, occurring over bony pressure points on the sides of the toes or foot. Elimination of the abnormal pressure forces is necessary to allow for healing. Manipulating or changing footware is often successful.

## SEBACEOUS HYPERPLASIA

Sebaceous hyperplasia is the term given to symmetric, raised, 2 to 4 mm papules that appear on the face in middle age. The distinctive yellow color and typical umbilication around a central pore (follicular ostium) help distinguish them from basal cell carcinoma and other epidermal neoplasms. Fordyce's condition is characterized by multiple tiny, yellowish lesions of sebaceous hyperplasia located on mucosal surfaces of the lips and vaginal labia. No treatment is needed for these benign lesions.

## HEMANGIOMAS

Hemangiomas are benign proliferations of blood vessels forming variously sized, soft, red, compressible papules that occur anywhere on skin. The most common type seen in adults is the "cherry hemangioma," which is small, usually less than 3 mm, and difficult to blanch. They are seen primarily on the chest and back, and increase in number with age. No treatment is required, and excision for cosmetic purposes must be weighed against the resultant scar.

## PYOGENIC GRANULOMAS

Pyogenic granulomas (Fig. 57C-7) are reddish-purple, friable, vascular tumors that range in size from several millimeters to greater than a centimeter. They can arise anywhere on the skin, often as a response to local trauma. They bleed profusely when abraded, and are often ulcerated or covered with scale crust. Though at times these lesions involute spontaneously, they usually require surgical excision. Recurrences are common. Occasionally malignant melanoma can resemble a pyogenic granuloma and should be considered in the differential diagnosis.

## LIPOMAS

Lipomas are subcutaneous tumors of adipose tissue, usually located on the trunk and proximal extremities. They are soft, symmetric, and easily movable over deeper structures, and can be confused with various cystic lesions. They may be single or multiple, and any size from 1 to many centimeters in diameter. The term *angiolipoma* is given to a variant that histologically contains multiple small blood vessels, and clinically may be associated with pain. These symptomatic lesions may be surgically excised.

## FOLLICULAR CYSTS

Follicular cysts are dermal tumors containing sebum and keratin debris that are derived from the lining of the hair follicle. They appear as firm, raised, slowly enlarging nodules anywhere on the skin, predominantly on the scalp, face and trunk. They are also termed wens, and erroneously referred to as epidermal, inclusion, or sebaceous cysts. Most lesions are left untreated, though surgical excision may be needed for larger cysts or those in sensitive anatomic sites.

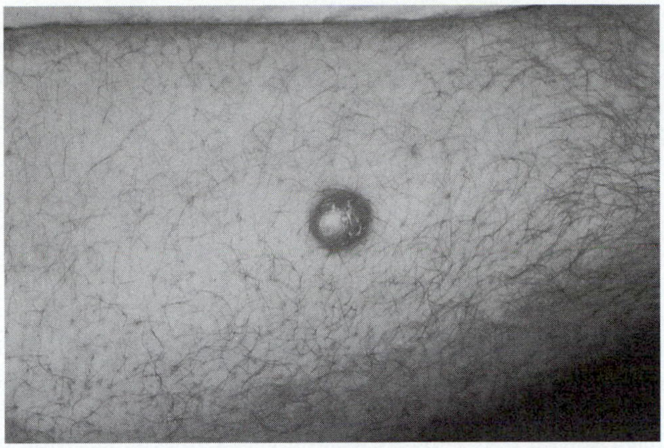

**Fig. 57C-8.** Dermatofibroma. Note reddish-brown nodule with regular margin.

## DERMATOFIBROMAS

Dermatofibromas (Fig. 57C-8) are firm, scarlike, pigmented dermal nodules that occur most frequently on the extremities of women, but can be found anywhere on the skin in either sex. Most present as slowly enlarging, reddish-brown, slightly elevated papules or nodules. Individual lesions can reach a centimeter or more in size, and can be painful. They are not attached to fat or fascia, but are affixed to overlying epidermis. This can be demonstrated by applying lateral pressure to the lesions and looking for a buttonhole-like depression, a technique useful in helping to distinguish them from other pigmented lesions. Dermatofibromas should be referred for evaluation if they are large or rapidly enlarging, irregularly pigmented, bleeding, or painful, so that malignant melanoma, dermatofibrosarcoma protuberans, and other malignant processes can be excluded.

## FIBROUS PAPULE

Fibrous papules (adenoma sebaceum, angiofibroma) are smooth, 1 to 2 mm, grayish to flesh-colored papules that occur almost exclusively on the nose and central face. They are common in middle-aged individuals and are usually solitary, though multiple lesions are sometimes seen and should alert the practitioner to the possibility of tuberous sclerosis. Biopsy is required at times to distinguish them from basal cell carcinoma.

## ACROCHORDONS

Also called skin tags, acrochordons are among the most common of benign skin tumors. They most often involve the axillae, neckline, and groin, where they appear as pinpoint to 5 mm or larger flesh-colored papules. The surface can be smooth or rough, and they are often pedunculated. Acrochordons are most often confused with nevi or seborrheic keratoses. Surgical removal is used for those lesions that interfere with function or become persistently inflamed.

## BIBLIOGRAPHY

Lever WF, Schaumberg-Lever G: *Histopathology of the skin,* ed 7, Philadelphia, 1990, JB Lippincott.

Maize JC, Ackerman AB editors: *Pigmented lesions of the skin,* Philadelphia, 1987, Lea and Febiger.

National Institutes of Health (NIH): *Diagnosis and treatment of early melanoma.* NIH consensus Development Conference, Consensus Statement 10(1):1992.

CHAPTER

# 58 Principles of Cancer Therapy

Diane Savarese

Despite recent advances in basic science and clinical research, cancer remains the second leading cause of death in the United States. Historically, surgical extirpation offered the only possibility of cure, however small. This changed with the introduction of radiation therapy and combination chemotherapy in the twentieth century. The modern approach to cancer therapy usually involves an integrated approach by medical, surgical, and radiation oncologists, nursing, nutrition, social work, and physical therapy.

## SURGICAL MANAGEMENT

Surgery may play a role in the diagnosis, staging, primary therapy, and palliation of malignant disease. The decision to use primary surgical therapy for the treatment of a malignancy depends on the patient, the tumor type, and the extent of disease (stage). Most clinicians use the American Joint Committee on Cancer (AJCC) staging system to classify tumor extent. In general, primary surgical treatment is most appropriate for early stage tumors, whereas more advanced disease implies spread beyond locoregional areas and the inability of even aggressive surgery to cure the patient. In some cases, even in early stage disease, chemotherapy or radiation therapy is preferable for primary treatment (e.g., lymphomas, small cell lung carcinoma), with surgery playing a diagnostic rather than therapeutic role. In other malignancies patients who have disseminated (stage IV) disease may be amenable to surgical intervention for cure (e.g., osteogenic sarcoma, Wilms' tumor). Surgical debulking of large tumor masses in advanced epithelial ovarian cancer enhances the effectiveness of subsequent chemotherapy. Palliation of specific complications from local tumor involvement may also require surgical intervention (e.g., diverting colostomy for bowel obstruction in locally advanced or metastatic colorectal cancer).

## RADIATION THERAPY

Irradiation destroys cancer cells because they, unlike normal cells, cannot repair the cumulative cellular deoxyribonucleic acid (DNA) damage induced by x-rays administered in multiple doses over several days (fractionated radiation therapy). There are two types of radiation therapy in clinical use: external beam and interstitial radiotherapy (brachytherapy). External beam radiation is delivered by a source outside of the patient such as an x-ray generator, cobalt unit, or linear accelerator. Interstitial therapy entails placing the radiation source directly within or adjacent to the tumor itself. Radiation therapy may be delivered with curative intent, resulting in total and permanent eradication of tumor (e.g., early laryngeal or prostate cancer, Hodgkin's disease), or palliatively to relieve symptoms or reduce tumor bulk (e.g., brain metastases, spinal cord compression from epidural metastases, localized pain from bone metastases) (Table 58-1).

There is a direct relationship between the radiation dose administered, tumor cell kill, and the likelihood of complications (Fig. 58-1). In general, the larger the tumor, the higher the dose needed to sterilize the area. Radiotherapy is therefore better able to eradicate small- rather than large-volume tumors. It may also be used with other modalities such as surgery or chemotherapy. Preoperative radiotherapy may be used to reduce tumor volume, making a locally advanced tumor more amenable to surgical removal (e.g., rectal cancer). More commonly, postoperative radiotherapy is used to eradicate gross or microscopic disease left behind at the time of surgery. One example is the use of breast conservation therapy for early stage breast cancers. Treatment with lumpectomy followed by radiation therapy has shown equivalent long-term results when compared with modified radical mastectomy alone. Postoperative radiotherapy is most useful in decreasing locoregional recurrences, but it usually has little effect on overall survival from cancer. Radiation may also be used with chemotherapy to maximize systemic benefit and locoregional control. Specific examples include Hodgkin's disease with bulky mediastinal masses and the addition of chest radiation to chemotherapy for limited stage small cell lung cancer. Low-dose chemotherapy has also been used to sensitize cells to radiation therapy. This approach has been most useful for tumors of the cervix, rectum, pancreas, and head and neck.

**Table 58-1.** Results from palliative radiotherapy

| Reason for irradiation | Likelihood of response/relief of symptoms |
|---|---|
| Brain metastases | 80% |
| Bone metastases | 80%-90% (50% complete) |
| Spinal cord compression | |
| Ambulatory patient | 70%-85% |
| Nonambulatory patient | 16% |
| SVC obstruction | 50%-70% |
| Bronchial obstruction | 25%-60% |

*SVC*, Superior vena cava.

## DRUG TREATMENT

Useful chemotherapy agents include not only classic cytotoxic drugs but also hormones, biologic response modifiers, and other drugs that by themselves have no or limited antitumor activity but that act to modify the activity or toxicity of other drugs or the body's immune system.

### Cytotoxic chemotherapy agents

Cytotoxic chemotherapy agents directly kill tumor cells by interfering with cellular mechanisms such as DNA, ribonucleic acid (RNA), and protein synthesis. The mechanism of action is generally different for different classes of antineoplastic agents (see the box on p. 779). Although some drugs are designed to be selectively more toxic to malignant cells (e.g., 5-fluorouracil [5-FU], methotrexate), all agents are somewhat toxic to normal cells, resulting in side effects.

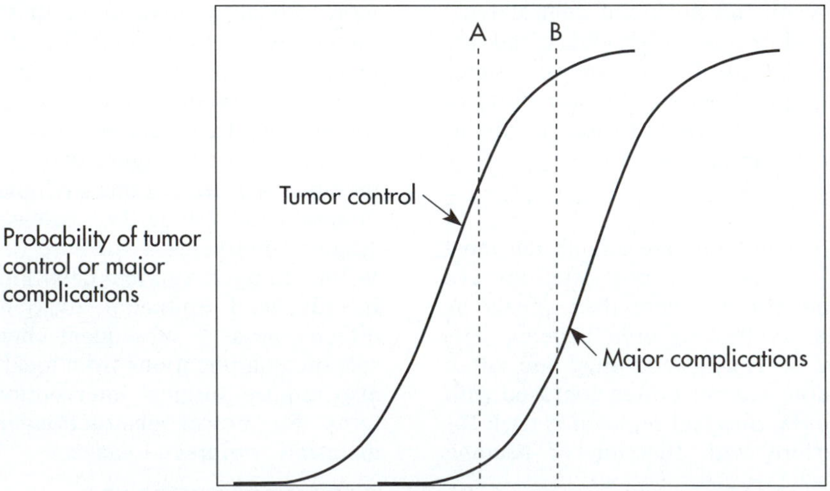


**Fig. 58-1.** Therapeutic index of radiation portrayed as two parallel sigmoid curves indicating the likelihood of tumor control and the likelihood of significant toxicity. *A,* Dose required for tumor control with minimum complications; *B,* dose resulting in maximum tumor control. (Adapted from DeVita VT Jr et al, editors: *Cancer: principles and practice of oncology,* ed 2, Philadelphia, 1993, JB Lippincott.)

The normal tissues most commonly affected by toxicity are those with the highest intrinsic turnover rate: bone marrow, hair follicles, gastrointestinal tract, and skin. Most cytotoxic drugs exhibit a dose-response relationship, in that dose reduction may mitigate toxicity, but it may also compromise the anticipated therapeutic effect. In general, cytotoxic drugs are administered in combination rather than as single agents because simultaneous interference with multiple biochemical pathways may result in more tumor cell kill with a delay in the appearance of drug resistance. To diminish the likelihood of intolerable toxicity, drugs whose adverse effects overlap as little as possible are combined. Commonly prescribed combination therapy regimens for several solid tumors are presented in Table 58-2.

### Classes of cytotoxic chemotherapy drugs

**Antimetabolites**
- Methotrexate
- 5-Fluorouracil (5-FU)
- 6-Mercaptopurine
- 6-Thioguanine (6-TG)
- Deoxycoformycin
- Cytarabine (Ara-C)

**Alkylating Agents**
- Nitrogen mustard
- Melphalan
- Cyclophosphamide
- Ifosfamide
- Chlorambucil
- Busulfan
- Thiotepa

**Nitrosoureas**
- Carmustine (BCNU)
- Lomustine (CCNU)
- Semustine (methyl-CCNU)
- Streptozotocin

**Antitumor Antibiotics**
- Doxorubicin
- Daunorubicin
- Mitoxantrone
- Mitomycin C
- Bleomycin
- Actinomycin D
- Mithramycin

**Vinca Alkaloids**
- Vincristine
- Vinblastine
- Vindesine

**Epidophyllotoxins**
- Etoposide (VP-16)
- Teniposide (VM-26)

**Miscellaneous**
- Cisplatin
- Carboplatin
- Hexamethylmelamine
- Dacarbazine
- Hydroxyurea
- L-Asparaginase
- Procarbazine
- Amsacrine (m-AMSA)

## Hormonal therapy

Steroid hormones are useful for the therapy of tumors whose growth is hormone dependent (Table 58-3). These agents are usually minimally toxic and are used most often for palliation of advanced disease, except for glucocorticoids, which are useful for the primary treatment of hematologic malignancies.

## Biologic response modifiers

These agents include an ever-expanding array of molecules that augment the natural immune-mediated host response to malignant cells. These molecules are normally produced in vivo in response to viral infection and other antigenic stimuli but are synthesized for clinical use by recombinant DNA techniques. Interferons have shown

**Table 58-2.** Commonly used combination chemotherapy regimens

| Disease | Regimen |
|---|---|
| Breast cancer | Cyclophosphamide, methotrexate, 5-FU (CMF) |
| | Cyclophosphamide, doxorubicin (Adriamycin), 5-FU (CAF) |
| Lung cancer | Cisplatin, etoposide |
| Colorectal cancer | 5-FU, leucovorin |
| Lymphoma | |
| Non-Hodgkin's | Cyclophosphamide, doxorubicin, vincristine, prednisone (CHOP) |
| Hodgkin's | Nitrogen mustard, vincristine, procarbazine, prednisone (MOPP) |
| | Doxorubicin, bleomycin, vinblastine, dacarbazine (ABVD) |
| Bladder cancer | Methotrexate, vinblastine, doxorubicin, cisplatin (MVAC) |
| Testicular cancer | Cisplatin, etoposide, bleomycin (PEB) |

**Table 58-3.** Hormone therapy of malignant disease

| Disease | Hormone agent | Mechanism of action |
|---|---|---|
| Breast cancer | Tamoxifen | Antiestrogen |
| | Aminoglutethimide | Steroidogenesis inhibitor |
| Prostate cancer | Leuprolide | LHRH agonist |
| | Flutamide | Antiandrogen |
| Endometrial cancer | Medroxyprogesterone | Progestin |
| Lymphomas | Glucocorticoid | Lymphocytolytic |

*LHRH*, Luteinizing hormone–releasing hormone.

activity in hairy cell leukemia, Kaposi's sarcoma, chronic myelogenous leukemia (CML), and non-Hodgkin's lymphoma. Interleukins, especially IL-2, have demonstrated activity against melanoma and renal cell cancer. Multiple ongoing trials are examining the role of these and other cytokines in the management of malignant disease. Monoclonal antibodies, proteins directed against antigenic molecules on the surface of tumor cells, may be useful in vivo to locate tumor cells, may be used to kill cells directly, or be used as vehicles for toxins and radioisotopes. These molecules and tumor vaccines are being studied.

### Adjuncts to therapy

Some drugs used to treat cancer do not kill tumor cells directly but instead act to enhance the activity of other drugs (e.g., levamisole and leucovorin used with 5-FU in the treatment of colorectal cancer) or to ameliorate chemotherapy-associated toxicity (e.g., leucovorin rescue after high-dose methotrexate). Cytokines, including granulocyte colony–stimulating factor (G-CSF), and granulocyte macrophage colony–stimulating factor (GM-CSF), have also been used to mitigate neutropenia after cytotoxic chemotherapy.

### Indications for systemic chemotherapy

***Primary systemic therapy.*** Primary systemic therapy is the use of chemotherapy as the primary treatment modality with curative intent. Tumors for which chemotherapy alone may be curative include lymphomas, advanced testicular cancer, and small cell lung cancer.

***Palliation of advanced disease.*** Palliation represents the use of chemotherapy to achieve objective tumor shrinkage, subjective improvement in symptoms, and prolongation of life. The first two objectives may be frequently achieved. However, improved survival is difficult to demonstrate for most patients with solid tumors. Unfortunately, response rates are often low (Table 58-4), both the number and severity of side effects increase as performance status declines, and most tumors eventually become resistant to chemotherapy.

***Combined-modality therapy.*** Combined-modality therapy indicates the addition of chemotherapy to radiotherapy and/or surgery to achieve maximal tumor cell kill. Some tumors that are apparently localized at presentation have a high likelihood of systemic relapse despite optimal initial surgery or radiotherapy. Occult micrometastases left behind may provide a nidus for regrowth of tumor at a later time, resulting in clinically evident metastatic disease. *Adjuvant therapy* is systemic chemotherapy administered after primary curative therapy by other means (usually surgery). It may decrease the likelihood of recurrence by eradicating micrometastatic foci. For women with resectable breast cancer a highly significant decrease in the rate of breast cancer recurrence and death has been demonstrated with the use of adjuvant chemotherapy or tamoxifen. Adjuvant treatment with 5-FU and levamisole reduces recurrence rates and mortality in patients with lymph node–positive colon cancer (Dukes' stage C), whereas for rectal cancers, adjuvant treatment with both 5-FU and radiation therapy can decrease recurrence and death rates in patients with Dukes' stage B or C disease.

*Neoadjuvant therapy* refers to the use of chemotherapy with or without radiotherapy before definitive local therapy. This approach is used most often for initially large tumors of the head and neck or locally advanced esophageal tumors in an attempt to increase surgical resectability. Although this approach may enhance local control and surgical resectability of solid tumors, controlled trials have failed to show a survival advantage compared with that of conventional treatment.

**Table 58-4.** Results of combination chemotherapy for initial treatment of stage IV disease

| Tumor type | Overall response rate (%) | Complete response rate (%) | Response duration (mo) | Median survival (mo) |
|---|---|---|---|---|
| Breast | 60-70 | <20 | 12 | 24 |
| Colorectal | 25-35 | <10 | 12-18 | 12-24 |
| NSCLC | 20-40 | <5 | 2-4 | 5-6 |
| Bladder | 30-50 | 10-20 | | 9-18 |
| Head and neck | 50-70 | 15-30 | 3-5 | 5-8 |

*NSCLC*, Non–small cell lung cancer.

***Experimental vs. standard therapy.*** When a widely accepted, standard therapy may not exist, the patient may be asked to participate in a clinical trial. Clinical trials of antineoplastic therapy are no longer restricted to specialized large cancer centers; community physicians are increasingly being asked to participate. Clinical trials fall into phase I, II, and III trials. The goal of phase I studies is to determine the relationship between toxicity and dose. Phase II studies attempt to identify the specific tumor types for which a new treatment may be promising. In general, patients who have failed standard therapy or for whom no standard therapy exists are appropriate for these types of studies. Phase III trials are randomized trials designed to compare standard treatment for a specific tumor or tumor-related condition to a newer alternative treatment to determine whether the new treatment may be more efficacious and/or less toxic. These trials are usually offered to previously untreated patients. Randomized trials with concurrent control groups are necessary to definitively demonstrate the superiority of one treatment over another. The randomization procedure, which may be difficult to understand from the viewpoint of the patient, is necessary in trials of this design to prevent bias introduced by other factors that could cause an investigation or a patient to select one treatment over another.

### Evaluation of the benefit of chemotherapy

***Risk/benefit ratio.*** Choosing optimal cancer therapy is not always easy. Guidelines for new regimens are frequently published, and it may be difficult to recommend a potentially beneficial new program of treatment without much knowledge of the results. Usually a rough estimate of the relative benefit from chemotherapy (likelihood, quality, and duration of response) may be compared with an estimate of the likelihood and severity of the side effects involved in the therapy (risk/benefit ratio). To accurately determine the value of a given response and what constitutes acceptable risk (toxicity), each patient's values and preferences, the impact of the therapy on lifestyle, and the repercussions of therapy on the patient's family must be considered.

***Definition of response status.*** *Objective response* refers to measurable shrinkage of tumor masses as assessed by physical examination or radiologic studies. A complete response (CR) implies eradication of all clinically apparent tumor. This necessitates repeating all studies that showed tumor presence before the start of treatment. CR is not necessarily synonymous with cure. Patients who have a CR may harbor residual tumor cells, and the rapidity of recurrence depends on the number of cells and how quickly they grow. *Cure* implies the persistent eradication of tumor for a proscribed period, the duration of which depends on differences in growth rate and biologic behavior. For example, of the patients destined to relapse after potentially curative treatment of early stage breast cancer, 65% to 85% do so within 2 years; however, the risk of relapse persists for 10 to 20 years. By contrast, over 95% of expected relapses from testicular cancer occur within 2 years of the original treatment, and late relapses are rare. In general, a CR is a necessary prerequisite for long-term survival and cure. Therefore chemotherapy regimens expected to result in CR for potentially curable neoplasms should be administered aggressively, with a fair amount of toxicity accepted.

A partial response (PR) is a decrease of at least 50% in the sum of the products of the perpendicular diameters of all measurable lesions. Treatments that result in a PR may lead to clinical improvement, may not represent a significant decrease in tumor burden, and may not have any meaningful impact on survival. Subjective response is a patient-reported sense of improved well-being after treatment; most subjective responses occur in the setting of objective response. Attempts to quantify this measure of improvement have included the use of quality of life scales, which assess functional status by using indirect measures such as performance status (see the box below), weight, duration of hospitalization, and amount of analgesics, antiemetics, and other supportive measures used by the patient.

***Prognostic factors.*** In general, good performance status and low tumor burden correlate most closely with better survival and higher response rates. More specific prognostic factors may be derived for individual tumors such as breast cancer, which may then be used to identify patients with a higher risk of relapse who may benefit from systemic chemotherapy after definitive local therapy (Table 58-5). Unfortunately, prognostic factors are not perfect for predicting which of these relatively good prognosis patients will eventually relapse.

***High-dose therapy.*** Most cytotoxic drugs display a dose-response relationship with higher doses resulting in greater tumor cell kill and, in theory, better cure rates. The limiting factor in increasing drug dose is toxicity, usually myelotoxicity. Hematopoietic support with bone marrow and/or peripheral blood stem cell transplantation has been used in an attempt to improve cure rates by allowing administration of higher-dose chemotherapy. Unfortunately, for most solid tumors, this approach has not yet been shown to result in greater survival compared with standard-dose chemotherapy and remains experimental.

### Risks and side effects of chemotherapy

All organ systems may be adversely affected by chemotherapy, with a wide variation in severity. In addition to anticipated tissue toxicities to bone marrow, hair, gastrointestinal tract, and skin, other less common toxicities may be characteristic of particular drugs (Table 58-6). The occurrence of toxicity, especially myelotoxicity, after chemotherapy may force dose reduction to where toxicity occurs at a more tolerable level but efficacy is preserved. It may be impossible to achieve this goal in individuals.

Many patients are fearful of chemotherapy, having heard about the bad experiences of a friend or family member. The primary physician may be able to reduce anxiety by realistically defining and quantifying the specific risks involved. Not all potential side effects occur in all patients. When toxicity does occur, it is usually of limited duration and reversible. In the event of severe or persistent adverse effects, doses can be reduced, the treatment stopped, or often alternative drugs substituted.

### Eastern Cooperative Oncology Group (ECOG) performance status scale

0 Normal activity
1 Symptoms of disease, but ambulatory and able to carry out activities of daily living
2 Out of bed more than 50% of the time; occasionally needs assistance
3 In bed more than 50% of the time; needs nursing care
4 Bedridden; may need hospitalization

**Table 58-5.** Prognostic factors for axillary node negative breast cancer

| Prognostic factor | Risk of relapse: Lower | Risk of relapse: Higher |
|---|---|---|
| Tumor size | Small | Large |
| Hormone receptors | Present | Absent |
| Nuclear grade | Low | High |
| Proliferative rate/S phase | Low | High |
| DNA-ploidy | Diploid | Aneuploid |
| HER-2/*neu* oncogene amplification | Absent | Present |
| Cathepsin D overexpression | Absent | Present |

**Table 58-6.** Hematologic and nonhematologic toxicity

| Drug | Bone marrow toxicity | Skin* | | | GI Tract† | | Hepatic |
|---|---|---|---|---|---|---|---|
| | | Necrosis | Rashes | Hair | Mucositis | Nausea and vomiting | |
| Actinomycin D | 3 | 3 | 3 | 3 | 3 | 3 | 0 |
| Amsacrine (AMSA) | 2 | 3 | 0 | 3 | 1 | 1 | 1 |
| Ara-C (cytarabine) | 3 | 0 | 0 | 0 | 2 | 2 | 3 |
| L-Asparaginase | 0 | 0 | 0 | 0 | 0 | 2 | 3 |
| Azathioprine | — | | | | | | 3 |
| Bleomycin | 0 | 0 | 3 | 2 | 3 | 1 | 0 |
| Busulfan | — | 0 | 2 | 0 | 0 | 1 | 1 |
| Carboplatin | 3 | 0 | 1 | 1 | 0 | 1 | 0 |
| Carmustine (BCNU) | 3 | 2 | 2 | 1 | 0 | 3 | 3 |
| Chlorambucil | 2 | 0 | 1 | 0 | 0 | 1 | 1 |
| Cisplatin | 1 | 0** | 0 | 0 | 0 | 3 | 0 |
| Cyclophosphamide | 3 | 0 | 1 | 3 | 1 | 2 | 1 |
| Dacarbazine (DTIC) | 1 | 2 | 0 | 0 | 0 | 3 | 2 |
| Deoxycoformycin | 1 | 0 | 1 | 0 | 0 | 1 | 2 |
| Daunomycin/doxorubicin | 3 | 3 | 3 | 3 | 3 | 3 | 0 |
| Etoposide/teniposide | 2 | 2 | 0 | 1 | 1 | 1 | 2 |
| Fludarabine | 2 | 0 | 2 | 0 | 1 | 2 | 1 |
| Fluorouracil | 1-2 | 1 | 2 | 2 | 3 | 1 | 2 |
| Hexamethylmelamine | 1 | 0 | 0 | 0 | 0 | 1 | 0 |
| Hydroxyurea | 3 | 0 | 1 | 1 | 0 | 1 | 0 |
| Ifosfamide | 2 | | 0 | 3 | 1 | 2 | 1 |
| Lomustine (CCNU) | 3 | 0 | 0 | 0 | 0 | 3 | 3 |
| Melphalan | 3 | 0 | 0 | 0 | 0 | 1 | 1 |
| Mercaptopurine | 2 | 0 | 1 | 0 | 2 | 1 | 3 |
| Methotrexate | 1-2 | 0 | 1 | 1 | 3 | 1 | 3 |
| Mithramycin | 1 | 2 | 2 | 0 | 2 | 3 | 3 |
| Mitomycin C | 1 | 3 | 1 | 0 | 0 | 1 | 0 |
| Mitotane | — | 0 | 1 | 0 | 0 | 2 | 0 |
| Mitoxantrone | 2 | 3 | 0 | 1 | 2 | 2 | 1 |
| Nitrogen mustard | 3 | 3 | 2 | 1 | 1 | 3 | 0 |
| Procarbazine | 2 | 0 | 1 | 0 | 0 | 2 | 0 |
| Streptozocin | 1 | 2 | 0 | 0 | 0 | 3 | 3 |
| Taxol (paclitaxel) | 3 | | 1 | 3 | 2 | 2 | 2 |
| Thioguanine (6-TG) | 2 | 0 | 1 | 0 | 2 | 1 | 2 |
| Thiotepa | | 0 | 0 | 1 | 0 | 0 | 0 |
| Vincristine | 1 | 3 | 0 | 2 | 1 | 1 | 2 |
| Vinblastine | 3 | 3 | 0 | 2 | 2 | 1 | 0 |
| Vindesine | 2 | 3 | 0 | 2 | 1 | 1 | 0 |

*0,* Very mild or very rare; *1,* occasional, usually not severe; *2,* moderately severe; *3,* frequent or severe; *SIADH,* syndrome of inappropriate antidiuretic hormone; *MAO,* monoamine oxidase; *RTA,* renal tubular acidosis; *XRT,* radiation therapy.
*Necrosis if extravasated, or phlebitis; rashes, pruritus, changes in pigmentation; alopecia.
†Stomatitis.
‡Arrhythmias or congestive heart failure.
§Hypersensitivity reactions.
||CNS toxicity.
¶Peripheral neuropathy.
#Toxicity unique to agent.
**High drug concentration infusion.

## Occurrence and management of chemotherapy toxicity by organ site

Postchemotherapy side effects may be acute or short term and generally reversible, or they may be long-term chronic toxicities, which may be reversible. A brief synopsis of selected adverse effects by organ system follows. An extensive discussion of the adverse effects associated with biologic response modifiers is beyond the scope of this text (see Bibliography).

### *Bone marrow*

**Leukocytes.** Myelotoxicity may range from clinically insigificant decreases in the formed elements of the blood to life-threatening cytopenias. The *nadir count* refers to

| Cardiac‡ | Allergic§ | Pulmonary fibrosis | Nephrotic | Neurologic: Central‖ | Neurologic: Peripheral¶ | Other# |
|---|---|---|---|---|---|---|
| 1 | 0 | 0 | 0 | 0 | 0 | Fever, radiation recall |
| 3 | 0 | 0 | 0 | 1 | 0 | Cardiac arrhythmias |
| 0 | 1 | 2 | 0 | 2 | 2 | Fever, conjunctivitis |
| 0 | 2 | 0 | 0 | 2 | 0 | Fever, coagulopathy, pancreatitis |
| 2 | | 1 | 0 | 0 | 0 | — |
| 1 | 1 | 3 | 0 | 1 | 0 | Pericarditis, fever |
| 0 | 0 | 2 | 0 | 0 | 0 | Addisonian syndrome, cataracts |
| 0 | 2 | 0 | 0 | 1 | 1 | Cumulative myelosuppression |
| 0 | 0 | 2 | 2 | 2 | 0 | Prolonged nausea and vomiting |
| 0 | 1 | 1 | 0 | 1 | 0 | |
| 1 | 3 | 0 | 3 | 2 | 3 | Vascular toxicity, prolonged nausea and vomiting |
| 0 | 1 | 2 | 0 | 0 | 0 | Fever, SIADH, cystitis |
| 0 | 0 | 0 | 0 | 1 | 0 | Flulike syndrome |
| 0 | 1 | — | 2 | 1 | 0 | |
| 3 | 1 | 0 | 0 | 0 | 0 | Radiation recall |
| 0 | 2 | 0 | 0 | 1 | 2 | |
| 0 | 1 | 1 | 1 | 3 | 1 | |
| 1 | 1 | 0 | 0 | 2 | 1 | Conjunctivitis |
| 0 | 0 | 0 | 0 | 2 | 2 | |
| 0 | 1 | 0 | 0 | 1 | 0 | |
| 1 | 1 | 0 | 2 | 2 | 1 | Prolonged nausea and vomiting, cystitis, fever |
| 0 | 0 | 1 | 2 | 0 | 0 | Prolonged nausea and vomiting |
| 0 | 1 | 1 | 0 | 0 | 0 | |
| 0 | 0 | 0 | 0 | 0 | 0 | |
| 0 | 1 | 2 | 2 | 2 | 0 | Fever, conjunctivitis |
| 0 | 0 | 0 | 3 | 0 | 0 | Coagulopathy, fever |
| 1 | 0 | 2 | 2 | 0 | 0 | Hemolytic-uremic syndrome |
| 0 | 1 | 0 | 0 | 2 | 0 | Adrenal insufficiency |
| 1 | 0 | 0 | 0 | 0 | 0 | |
| 0 | 0 | 0 | 0 | 1 | 0 | |
| 0 | 2 | 2 | 0 | 2 | 2 | MAO inhibitor |
| 0 | 0 | 0 | 3 | 0 | 0 | Prolonged nausea and vomiting; proximal RTA |
| 3 | 3 | 0 | — | 0 | 0 | Cardiac arrhythmias, fever |
| 0 | 0 | 0 | 0 | 0 | 0 | |
| 0 | 0 | 0 | 0 | 0 | 0 | |
| 1 | 0 | 0 | 0 | 2 | 3 | Hepatotoxic with XRT, SIADH |
| 0 | 0 | 1 | 0 | 0 | 1 | |
| 0 | 0 | 1 | 0 | 2 | 3 | |

the lowest absolute value of the circulating blood cells after chemotherapy. Different chemotherapy drugs result in variable degrees of myelosuppression (see Table 58-6), but it may vary depending on the dose (methotrexate) or schedule of administration (5-FU). The time to the nadir averages 9 to 12 days after chemotherapy. Some agents cause prolonged or delayed granulocyte nadirs (nitrosoureas, chlorambucil, mitomycin C, busulfan, procarbazine). Patients whose neutrophil nadir is under 1000/µl have severe myelotoxicity; fever in the presence of neutropenia (less than 500/µl neutrophils) is a medical emergency.

Prophylactic antibiotics are usually not indicated for patients who are neutropenic from standard dose chemotherapy. While neutropenic, patients should avoid persons who are ill and report fever immediately. When fever does occur, patients must receive parenteral broad-spectrum antibiotics until the neutropenia resolves. Visitors and medical personnel should observe strict handwashing techniques. Unnecessary instrumentation and invasive procedures should be avoided. Granulocyte transfusions are not generally used because of the high risk of complications. Recombinant colony–stimulating factors such as G-CSF and GM-CSF decrease the duration of the neutrophil nadir and the duration of empiric antibiotic use and hospitalization when administered prophylactically during the chemotherapy cycle. They have not been shown to alter the course of febrile neutropenia once it develops. Nevertheless, despite their expense, they are frequently prescribed in this scenario.

**Platelets.** Some agents are relatively less toxic to platelets than to other bone marrow cells (cyclophosphamide, etoposide, vinca alkaloids, mitoxantrone). A platelet decrease to under 50,000/µl represents severe thrombocytopenia, but in general spontaneous bleeding rarely occurs unless platelet counts fall below 5000/µl.

It is important to avoid intramuscular injections, unnecessary instrumentation, and the use of medications (such as aspirin or nonsteroidal antiinflammatory drugs) that could exacerbate a bleeding tendency. Platelet transfusions should be reserved for patients with platelet counts under 5000/µl, patients with significant bleeding, and patients in whom invasive procedures become unavoidable.

**Erythrocytes.** Hypoproliferative anemia secondary to chemotherapy is less common than thrombocytopenia and leukopenia, although cisplatin and the nitrosoureas can cause refractory anemia. Cisplatin may also cause Coombs positive hemolytic anemia. In addition, a syndrome of microangiopathic hemolytic anemia, renal insufficiency, and thrombocytopenia has been described with mitomycin C, generally at cumulative dosages above 50 mg/m$^2$. Transfusion of packed red blood cells is the recommended management. Some studies suggest that administration of erythropoietin may ameliorate chemotherapy-induced hypoproliferative anemia.

In the differential diagnosis for all of these myelotoxicities, one must consider tumor replacement of the marrow, autoimmune destruction, sepsis, and myelosuppression from other drugs. If cytopenias do not resolve within the expected time, it may be appropriate to perform a diagnostic aspiration and/or biopsy of the bone marrow.

***Hair.*** Alopecia usually begins 2 to 3 weeks after the institution of cytotoxic chemotherapy. Not all cytotoxic agents produce the same degree of hair loss (see Table 58-6). Hair usually regrows after the discontinuation of chemotherapy. Although hair loss from the scalp is most noticeable, it may occur from all areas of the body, including eyebrows, axillary, and pubic areas.

Patients should be forewarned of this complication; a wig may be purchased if desired. Scalp hypothermia reportedly decreases the amount of hair loss, but protection depends on the type and dosage of drug. These devices should not be used during leukemia treatment, since circulation of the drug to the scalp may be impaired.

### *Gastrointestinal tract*

**Mucositis.** Mucositis usually presents as a burning or tingling sensation, especially in response to acid foods, and may be followed by erythema, superficial erosions, ulcerations, and sloughing of the mucosa. The oral mucosa is most commonly symptomatic. However, any mucosal area may be involved. Symptoms usually last 3 to 7 days. The worst offenders are bleomycin, doxorubicin, 5-FU, and methotrexate (see Table 58-6).

In the differential diagnosis, herpesvirus and *Candida albicans* mucosal infections should be considered. The patient should avoid dentures and irritating foods and rinse the mouth frequently with a salt or baking soda solution. Oratect gel, "miracle mouthwash" (mixture of viscous lidocaine, Maalox, diphenhydramine elixir, and/or nystatin), and systemic pain medication may help a great deal. In severe cases the patient may require hospitalization for nutrition and fluid support. Fungal or herpetic superinfections should be treated.

**Nausea and vomiting.** Symptoms may range from mild nausea to intractable vomiting. Symptoms usually begin 1 to 6 hours after chemotherapy and last less than 24 hours. Cisplatin, ifosfamide, and nitrosoureas may result in protracted nausea and vomiting up to 72 hours. Psychologic factors can influence vomiting, and anticipatory nausea and vomiting may occur when patients think about treatment or see the treatment facility just before chemotherapy.

The differential diagnosis includes tumor obstruction, ileus, metabolic abnormalities (especially hypercalcemia), and brain metastases. Prophylaxis is important in management. Mildly emetogenic drugs (see Table 58-6) may be accompanied by oral phenothiazines. Moderately emetogenic drugs may require a combination of agents, including lorazepam, phenothiazines, metoclopramide, and steroids. More severely emetogenic drugs such as cisplatin are usually managed with a serotonin antagonist like ordansetron. Other effective agents include barbiturates, haloperidol, and droperidol. Patients with anticipatory nausea and vomiting may benefit from behavioral techniques, hypnosis, or the use of lorazepam.

### *Heart and lungs*

**Cardiac.** Transient dysrhythmias may occur during or shortly after the administration of amsacrine, paclitaxel (Taxol), or doxorubicin. Anthracyclines and amsacrine may lead to a characteristic dose-dependent cardiomyopathy. The differential diagnosis should consider volume overload, intrinsic cardiac disease, cor pulmonale, and malignant pericardial effusion.

To avoid cardiomyopathy, the total doxorubicin dosage should be limited to less than 450 mg/m$^2$. If this is exceeded or if patients have a higher than usual risk of developing cardiomyopathy, serial radionuclide ventriculograms should be followed. If congestive heart failure occurs, it is frequently irreversible but can be managed with diuretics, inotropic agents, and afterload reduction.

**Pulmonary.** Pneumonitis and pulmonary fibrosis may be caused by bleomycin, Ara-C, mitomycin C, nitrosoureas, alkylating agents, procarbazine, and methotrexate. Patients usually present with insidious onset of fever, dyspnea and nonproductive cough. Pulmonary lymphangitic spread of tumor, adult respiratory distress syndrome (ARDS), infection, and other toxins should be considered in the differential diagnosis.

Discontinuation of the offending agent and treatment with corticosteroids may help, although pulmonary fibrosis is frequently irreversible. Although chest x-ray studies and single breath diffusion capacity of the lungs for carbon monoxide (DLCO) are less than perfect screening tests for early bleomycin pulmonary toxicity, they should be done periodically during therapy. Patients should inform anesthesiologists about prior bleomycin exposure, and inspired oxygen concentration should always be less than 30% (lifelong).

***Kidneys.*** Renal insufficiency may be the result of direct tubular damage (cisplatin, streptozotocin), glomerular injury (nitrosoureas), acute tubular necrosis from drug precipitation (high-dose methotrexate), or drug-induced vasculitis (mitomycin C).

**Dosage modification for renal or hepatic dysfunction**

**Renal dysfunction**

Methotrexate
Cisplatin
Deoxycoformycin
Cyclophosphamide
Bleomycin
Mithramycin
Streptozotocin
Mitomycin C

**Hepatic dysfunction**

Amsacrine
Vinca alkaloids
Anthracyclines
Paclitaxel (Taxol)

Differential diagnosis includes prerenal azotemia, diabetic nephropathy, paraprotein-induced renal insufficiency, other drugs, ureteral obstruction or direct kidney invasion by cancer or amyloid, infection, tumor lysis syndrome, and paraneoplastic syndromes.

For cisplatin use prevention is best accomplished by aggressive prechemotherapy hydration with 1 to 2 L of saline over several hours. Alkaline hydration should be used for high-dose methotrexate. The use of concomitant nephrotoxins such as radiologic contrast media or aminoglycosides should be avoided if possible. If renal insufficiency develops, potentially reversible causes should be ruled out and all drugs discontinued if possible. Patients with renal insufficiency may require dose reduction of chemotherapeutic agents whose excretion is predominantly renal (see the box above). Chemotherapy agents excreted by the hepatic route may need dose adjustments in the presence of hepatic insufficiency also.

***Genitals.*** Azoospermia and anovulation develop in the majority of patients treated with alkylating agents. Cisplatin causes temporary infertility in most patients. Reversibility depends on drug dosage, concomitant radiotherapy, and age. Children treated before puberty are most likely to recover normal sexual development and fertility. Adult women older than 25 years are least likely to recover normal fertility after treatment. Many drugs are teratogenic, especially in the first trimester, but pregnancies have been successfully completed in the second or third trimester despite treatment with chemotherapy. There appears to be little if any increase in birth defects in children born of parents who have received prior chemotherapy.

Pretreatment factors may cause anovulation (stress, weight loss, heavy exercise) or azoospermia (Hodgkin's disease). Hypothyroidism, sometimes treatment related, may be a potentially reversible cause of infertility.

Patients should be counseled before therapy. The opportunity for sperm banking should be explored if pretreatment sperm counts are adequate. Unfortunately, oocyte cryopreservation is not routinely available in this country.

Second malignancies, both hematologic and solid tumors, may occur after chemotherapy, particularly when long-term treatment with alkylating agents is combined with radiation therapy. The risk for acute leukemia peaks at about 5 years, whereas that of secondary solid tumors may peak later, at 10 years.

Other side effects may also occur with various chemotherapy drugs. A full enumeration is beyond the scope of this text. They are summarized in Table 58-6.

## APPROACH TO CANCER PAIN

Pain is one of the most frequent and least well-managed aspects of cancer care. Undertreatment of pain is a common problem despite the widespread availability of effective pharmacologic agents and other, nonpharmacologic means of pain control. Barriers to effective pain management are summarized in the box on p. 786.

### Assessment of pain

The initial assessment should focus on identifying the cause of the pain, and should include a detailed history of pain intensity, character, and location. Psychosocial assessment of the patient is important. Physical examination should place emphasis on the area affected by pain and, in particular, the neurologic examination. An appropriate diagnostic workup to determine the cause of pain may be warranted.

### Management of cancer-related pain

Specific antineoplastic therapy should be considered to control cancer-related pain. Surgery for curative excision or palliative debulking has the potential to reduce pain; however, many pathologic processes leading to severe pain are not amenable to surgery. Radiotherapy may be particularly helpful in alleviating the pain of tumor invasion or compression. Alternatively, pharmacologic or neurosurgical/anesthetic approaches may be used to control pain. The World Health Organization (WHO) pain ladder (Fig. 58-2) portrays a rational progression in the doses and types of analgesic drugs for effective pain management. Fig. 58-3 is a flow chart depicting an algorithm for cancer pain management from the initial assessment of pain and its cause to the various treatment modalities, including the WHO analgesic ladder and other pharmacologic and nonpharmacologic modalities.

***Pharmacologic management of cancer pain.*** Nonsteroidal antiinflammatory drugs (NSAIDs) are especially useful in patients with bone pain or inflammatory lesions. They may also provide additive analgesia when combined with opioids. Their usefulness is limited to mild to moderate pain, and there is a ceiling dose above which no further analgesia occurs despite increasing doses. Adverse effects include gastritis, impaired platelet function, and renal insufficiency.

Opioids are the analgesics most used in managing moderate to severe pain. Opioids are classified as full agonists, partial agonists, or mixed agonist/antagonists. Commonly used narcotic agonists include morphine, hydromorphone, codeine, oxycodone, methadone, and fentanyl. These opioids are classified as full agonists because they do not have a ceiling to their analgesic effect, and do not reverse or antagonize the effects of other

### Barriers to effective pain management

**Problems related to health care professionals**

Inadequate knowledge of pain management
Poor assessment of pain
Concern about regulation of controlled substances
Fear of patient addiction
Concern about side effects of analgesics
Concern about patients becoming tolerant to analgesics

**Problems related to patients**

Reluctance to report pain
- Concern about distracting physicians from treatment of underlying disease
- Fear that pain means disease is worse
- Concern about not being a "good" patient

Reluctance to take pain medications
- Fear of addiction or of being thought of as an addict
- Worries about unmanageable side effects
- Concern about becoming tolerant to pain medications

**Problems related to the health care system**

Low priority given to cancer pain treatment
Inadequate reimbursement
- The most appropriate treatment may not be reimbursed or may be too costly for patients and families

Restrictive regulation of controlled substances
Problems of availability of treatment or access to it

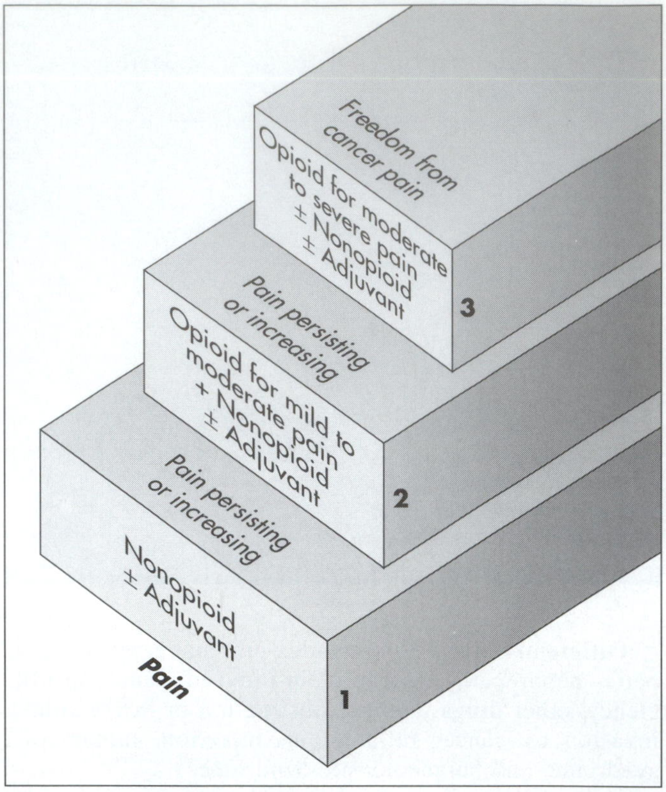


**Fig. 58-2.** The World Health Organization (WHO) three-step analgesic ladder. (Adapted from the World Health Organization.)

opioids within this class. Mixed agonist/antagonists and partial agonists are rarely used in chronic management of cancer pain, since they may reverse opioid effects and can precipitate abstinence syndrome in patients who are physically dependent on opioids.

Adjuvant medications, or co-analgesics, are used to enhance the analgesic efficacy of opioids. Corticosteroids, anticonvulsants such as phenytoin and carbamazepine, antidepressants, bisphosphonates, and antihistamines may all be useful in various settings.

Side effects of opioids are numerous and may result in a failure of opioid treatment, even when managed judiciously. Opioids decrease peristalsis and GI secretions, leading to increased transit time and desiccated feces difficult to pass. A prophylactic bowel regimen should be prescribed to elderly patients, nonambulatory patients, those with intrinsic bowel disease, and to patients receiving concurrent constipating drugs. Unfortunately, tolerance usually does not occur to this side effect. Management may include stool softeners, bulk agents such as psyllium, or mild stimulant laxatives.

Over 50% of patients receiving opioids experience nausea; it is usually multifactorial in etiology, constipation, CNS effects, delayed gastric emptying, and increased vestibular sensitivity may all contribute. Treatment with phenothiazine antiemetics or a prokinetic agent like metoclopramide may be helpful.

Sedation is a property of all opioids. Fortunately, tolerance usually develops within several days. Excess sedation may be managed by administering smaller, more frequent doses of narcotic. Mental status changes including euphoria, dysphoria, and confusion may occur, especially with the initiation of narcotic therapy. Patients receiving long-term opioid therapy usually develop tolerance to the respiratory depression effects of these agents. Occasionally, respiratory depression may occur when sedative effects of opioids are no longer opposed by the stimulatory effects of pain. If rapid reversal of opioid effect resulting from excessive respiratory depression is necessary, repetitive doses of a dilute solution of naloxone should be used.

Tolerance refers to the need to increase doses over time to maintain pain relief. Increasing dose requirements are most consistently correlated with progressive disease. Opioid tolerance and physical dependency are expected with long-term opioid treatment and should not be confused with psychologic dependency (addiction). Patients should be warned not to abruptly discontinue narcotics; when a decrease is warranted, they should be tapered.

***Nonpharmacologic management of cancer pain.*** Nonpharmacologic management may include psychosocial interventions such as relaxation and imagery and anesthetic/neurosurgical approaches. Anesthetic techniques may include nerve blocks and intraspinal or epidural administration of narcotics or local anesthetics. Neurosurgical approaches include peripheral neurectomy, rhizotomy, anterolateral cordotomy, commissural myelotomy, or, rarely, hypophysectomy. A full discussion of nonpharma-

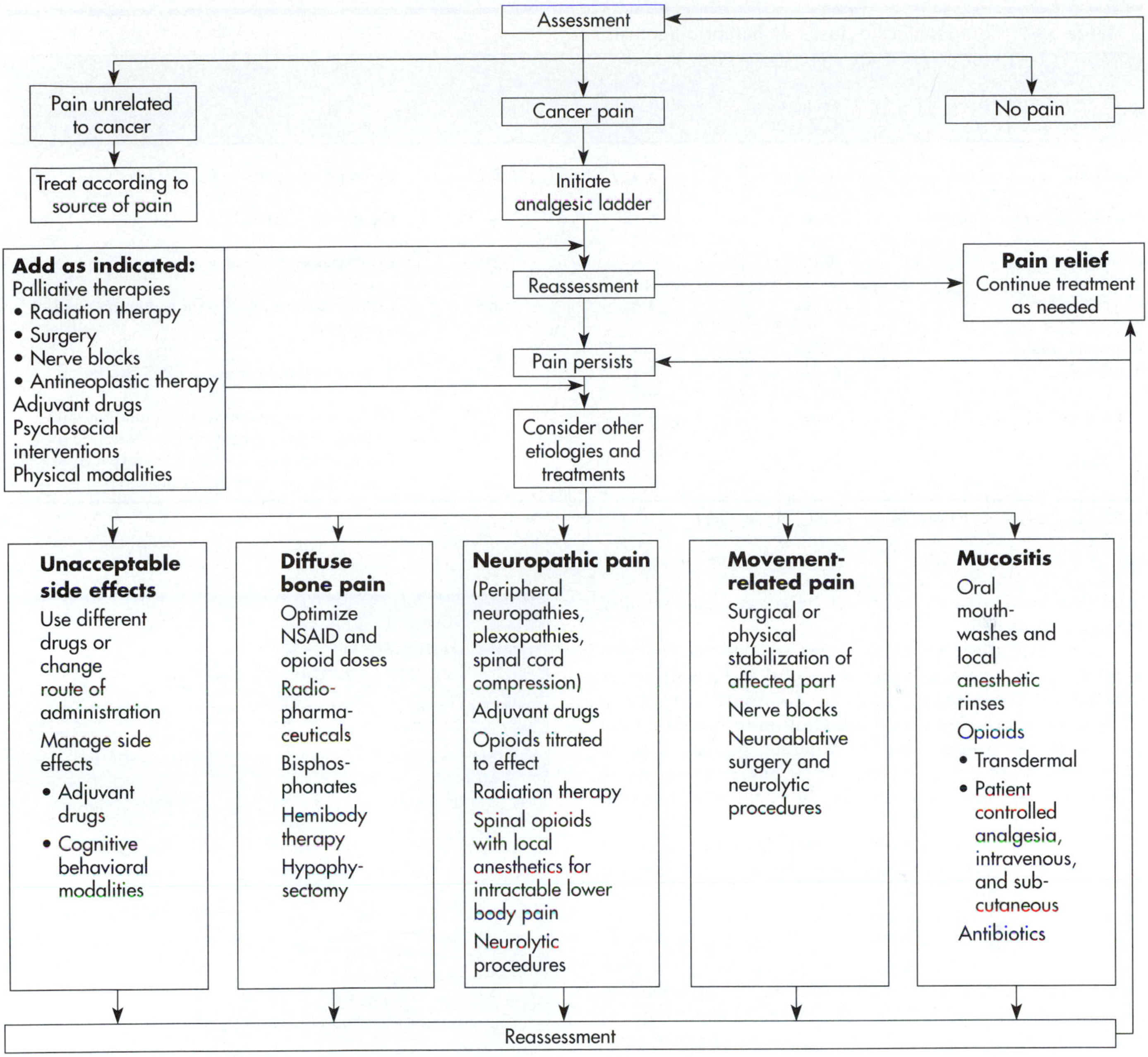


**Fig. 58-3.** Algorithm for pain management in patients with cancer.

cologic modalities available for the management of cancer-related pain is beyond the scope of this text.

It is common clinical practice to initiate opioid therapy with a "weak" opioid such as codeine, oxycodone, or hydrocodone. These agents are most commonly available in fixed combination with acetaminophen or aspirin. In many cases the limiting factor to obtaining adequate analgesia with these agents is ingestion of maximal doses of the co-analgesic. If pain relief is inadequate with these agents, then it is appropriate to switch to a stronger opioid. Some general principles of narcotic management are listed in the box on p. 788. The oral route is usually preferred as it is safe, acceptable to patients, economical, and effective. Morphine is the prototype drug, and is probably the drug of choice in most cancer patients requiring long-term analgesia for chronic pain. Morphine is easy to administer because of the availability of many different dose forms. Immediate release oral morphine has a short half life and therefore must be dosed every 3 to 4 hours (Table 58-7). It is especially useful for "rescue" doses, when breakthrough pain necessitates the use of an opioid with a rapid onset of action. Sustained release oral morphine eliminates the need for frequent dosing of oral morphine; it is dosed every 8 to 12 hours. This dose form requires one day to approach steady state concentrations. Effective pain relief can best be accomplished by anticipation and prevention of pain. Because many patients have persistent or daily pain, it is important to use opioids on a regular schedule rather than as needed. Opioid doses should be adjusted in each patient to achieve acceptable pain relief with a

**Table 58-7.** Equianalgesic doses of narcotic agonists

| Opiate | Equi-analgesic dose (mg) | Usual dosing interval (hr) | Plasma half life (hr) | Comment |
|---|---|---|---|---|
| Morphine | 10 IM<br>30-60* | 3-4 | 2-3 | Standard comparison for opioids |
| Controlled release morphine | 30-60 po<br>5 IV | 8-12<br>2-4 | — | Cannot be crushed |
| Codeine | 200 po | 3-4 | 2-3 | Combination product with acetaminophen or aspirin |
| Oxycodone | 30 po | 3-4 | 2-3 | Combination product with acetaminophen or aspirin |
| Hydromorphone | 7.5 po | 3-4 | 2-3 | |
| Meperidine | 75 IM<br>300 po | 3-4<br>4-6 | 2-3 | Toxic metabolite leads to CNS excitation |
| Methadone | 20 po | 4-6 | 15-30 | Delayed toxicity due to accumulation with chronic dosing causing excessive sedation |
| Fentanyl | 25 μg/hr | 48-72 | — | Patches should be initiated at lowest dose and titrated every 3d as needed |

*1:6 relative potency po: IM changes to 1:3 during chronic dosing.

tolerable level of adverse effects. Dosages may require frequent readjustment.

IM injections are generally to be avoided for management of chronic pain, as they are painful and absorption is unreliable. The subcutaneous or IV route may be a reasonable alternative for administration of opioids if the patient is no longer able to tolerate po, if there is discontinuity of the GI tract, or if more analgesia is required than can realistically be achieved by oral administration.

A transdermal preparation of fentanyl, a potent narcotic that is 90% absorbed through skin, has recently become available. Advantages include convenience and the avoidance of peaks and troughs during continuous dosing. Disadvantages include expense, poor adhesion to hairy or sweaty skin, and the long elimination half life that, although allowing for dosing every 3 days, also results in a slow titration of effect. The transdermal route is therefore not appropriate for management of acute pain.

Cross tolerance is not universal among the various members of the class of narcotic agonists. If one agent is not effective, another may be tried. It is important to be aware of equianalgesic doses.

### Managed Care Guide
### General principles of narcotic analgesic management

1. Start with the lowest doses possible (equivalent to 5 to 10 mg IM morphine)
2. Titrate dose to desired effect OR to intolerable side effects
3. Use the appropriate route of administration
4. Anticipate pain; most patients require around-the-clock dosing plus additional "as needed" rescue doses
5. Know equianalgesic doses; knowledge of relative potency important
6. Use a combination of drugs: addition of co-analgesics (NSAID or adjuvant)
7. Manage side effects judiciously
8. Understand physical dependence and tolerance

*NSAID*, Nonsteroidal antiinflammatory drugs.

## BIBLIOGRAPHY

American Joint Committee on Cancer: *Manual for staging of cancer,* ed 3, Philadelphia, 1988, JB Lippincott.

DeVita VT Jr et al, editors: *Cancer: principles and practice of oncology,* ed 2, Philadelphia, 1993, JB Lippincott.

Early Breast Cancer Trialists' Collaborative Group: Systemic treatment of early breast cancer by hormonal, cytotoxic, or immune therapy, *Lancet* 339:1,71, 1992.

Fisher B et al: Eight year results of a randomized clinical trial comparing total mastectomy and lumpectomy with or without irradiation in the treatment of breast cancer, *N Engl J Med* 320:822, 1989.

Frei E, Canellos GP: Dose: a critical factor in cancer chemotherapy, *Am J Med* 69:585, 1980.

Gabrilove JL et al: Effect of granulocyte colony–stimulating factor on neutropenia and associated morbidity due to chemotherapy for transitional cell carcinoma of the urothelium, *N Engl J Med* 318:1414, 1988.

Hansen RM, Borden EC: Current status of interferons in the treatment of cancer, *Oncology* 6:19, 1992.

Myers SE, Schilsky RL: Prospects for fertility after cancer chemotherapy, *J Clin Oncol* 19:5597, 1992.

NIH Consensus Conference: Adjuvant therapy for patients with colon and rectal cancer, *JAMA* 264:1444, 1990.

Perry MC, editor: *The chemotherapy source book,* Baltimore, 1992, Williams & Wilkins.

Pignon J-P et al: Meta-analysis of thoracic radiotherapy for small-cell lung cancer, *N Engl J Med* 327:1618, 1992.

Spitzer G et al: Autologous bone marrow transplantation in solid tumors, *Curr Opin Oncol* 4(2):272, 1992.

Urba WJ et al: Hodgkin's disease, *N Engl J Med* 326:678, 1993.

Vokes EE, Weichselbaum R: Concomitant chemoradiotherapy: rationale and clinical experience in patients with solid tumors, *J Clin Oncol* 8:911, 1990.

CHAPTER

# 59 Management of Oncologic Emergencies

Ana Maria Lopez

Although patients with cancer are often seen as having chronic and debilitating medical problems, emergent symptom complexes may arise. Oncologic emergencies are predictable complications of malignant primaries, metastases, or their treatments. Cancer-related deaths are the overall second leading cause of mortality among adults in the United States, and patients frequently visit their primary care physician for initial evaluation of a cancer-related sign or symptom. The generalist is responsible for pursuing the signs and symptoms of oncologic emergent or urgent problems, which if unrecognized, could result in preventable morbidity and mortality. When a diagnosis of malignancy is established, oncologic consultation is appropriate, and further investigative studies can be pursued with an oncologist.

## METABOLIC EMERGENCIES

### Hypercalcemia

*Etiology.* Hypercalcemia resulting from malignancy is the leading cause of hypercalcemia in hospital practice. The most common cause of hypercalcemia in the outpatient setting is hyperparathyroidism. An elevation in the calcium level is the most common life-threatening metabolic disorder associated with cancer, affecting 10% to 20% of all patients. At the time of presentation the underlying tumor is known in nearly all cases. Approximately 150 new cases per million people are diagnosed each year, with the highest incidence being in the inpatient population. Once identified, malignant hypercalcemia can often be corrected with the proper interventions, but survival is not significantly prolonged.

Malignancies associated with hypercalcemia may be of solid tumor or hematologic origin. The solid tumors most often associated with hypercalcemia are of squamous cell origin: lung, head, neck, esophageal, and female genital tract. The remainder of solid tumors involved are of breast (20%) and renal cell (8%) origin. Hematologic malignancies resulting in hypercalcemia are multiple myeloma and leukemia (see the box above).

*Pathophysiology.* Abnormalities in the calcium level may be the result of changes in skeletal resorption or in hormonal changes affecting calcium metabolism. Malignant hypercalcemia may result from bone resorption secondary to skeletal invasion or from production of humoral factors, specifically parathyroid-like hormone. Biochemically, high calcium levels are accompanied by low phosphate levels, but unlike primary hyperparathyroidism, parathyroid hormone levels are normal. High levels of a parathyroid hormone–related protein are present in most patients with primary or metastatic cancer–associated hypercalcemia. Humoral factors explain the lack of correlation between the extent of bone metastases and the level of hypercalcemia.

**Malignant etiologies of hypercalcemia**

**Solid tumor**

Lung (squamous cell)
Other squamous cell cancer
- Head
- Neck
- Female genital tract

Breast
Renal cell

**Hematologic**

Multiple myeloma
Leukemia
Lymphoma

Elevated calcium levels impair the kidneys' ability to concentrate urine, resulting in diuresis and further volume depletion; consequently, the patient's hypercalcemia is complicated and worsened by the dehydration.

*Signs and symptoms.* The clinical findings in hypercalcemia have been well documented and range from constipation to obtundation and death. Rapid recognition of this symptom complex may be lifesaving (see the box on p. 790). Symptoms may occur at calcium levels lower than those noted with benign hypercalcemia, perhaps because of the more rapid onset of calcium elevation in malignant hypercalcemia.

*Diagnosis.* Clinical suspicion in recognizing the symptom complex is the first step in making the diagnosis of malignant hypercalcemia. Hypercalcemia is an elevation in unbound, ionized serum calcium concentration. Since serum calcium levels measure total calcium values, a simple calcium level is insufficient to confirm the diagnosis of hypercalcemia. Calcium is normally bound to albumin in the serum. Since many patients with underlying malignancies have low albumin levels because of poor nutrition and depletion of protein stores, a normal calcium level may actually represent hypercalcemia. The calcium level should be corrected on the basis of the albumin level to make the diagnosis of hypercalcemia. The equation for a corrected calcium level follows:

Corrected calcium (mg/dl) = Measured calcium (mg/dl) + 0.8 mg/dl for each gram of measured albumin less than 4.5 g/dl

In addition, changes in acid-base balance influence the albumin-binding capabilities of calcium. If available, the clinician may obtain a direct measurement of the ionized calcium level.

*Treatment.* The goal of treatment is to improve the patient's quality of life by improving mental status and decreasing the need for inpatient days. Hypercalcemia may be reversed by reducing or eliminating tumor burden,

### Symptoms of hypercalcemia

**Nervous system**
Lethargy
Weakness
Decreased deep tendon reflexes
Confusion
Apathy
Agitation
Psychosis
Stupor
Obtundation
Coma
Death

**Gastrointestinal**
Constipation
Obstipation
Ileus
Anorexia
Nausea
Vomiting

**Renal**
Diabetes insipidus–like syndrome
Nocturia

**Cardiac**
Short QT complex
Broad T wave

increasing renal clearance or calcium, and inhibiting osteoclastic bone resorption (Fig. 59-1). When possible, treatment of the underlying malignancy should be aggressively pursued. When resulting from multiple myeloma or lymphoma, malignant hypercalcemia may be controlled with steroids, which begin treatment of the underlying neoplasm. The usual steroid side effects are seen, and a drop in the calcium level is noted in 3 to 5 days. Since most cases of malignant hypercalcemia occur late in the course of the disease, curative options are usually limited.

As discussed earlier, hypercalcemia is often aggravated by dehydration; therefore the cornerstone of therapy is volume replacement with isotonic fluid. Although furosemide can treat the calciuria, it must be used with extreme caution so that it does not increase dehydration. Rehydration alone is effective in 30% of cases but is short lived and confines the patient to a continuous intravenous line. The response to fluids is usually not long lasting, since the underlying process has not been affected. Drug therapy is often required to provide longer control.

Calcitonin is a potent inhibitor of bone resorption; it acts rapidly, often within 12 to 24 hours, and is nontoxic. Patients with a history of organ failure—renal, hepatic, cardiac, and hematopoietic—may use the drug safely, and nearly 80% of patients respond. The usual therapeutic dosage is 4 to 8 U/kg given intramuscularly or intravenously every 12 hours. Calcitonin acts by directly binding to osteoclast receptors and inhibiting bone resorption. Although drug effects last approximately 72 hours, patients may quickly become refractory to the drug, necessitating further interventions.

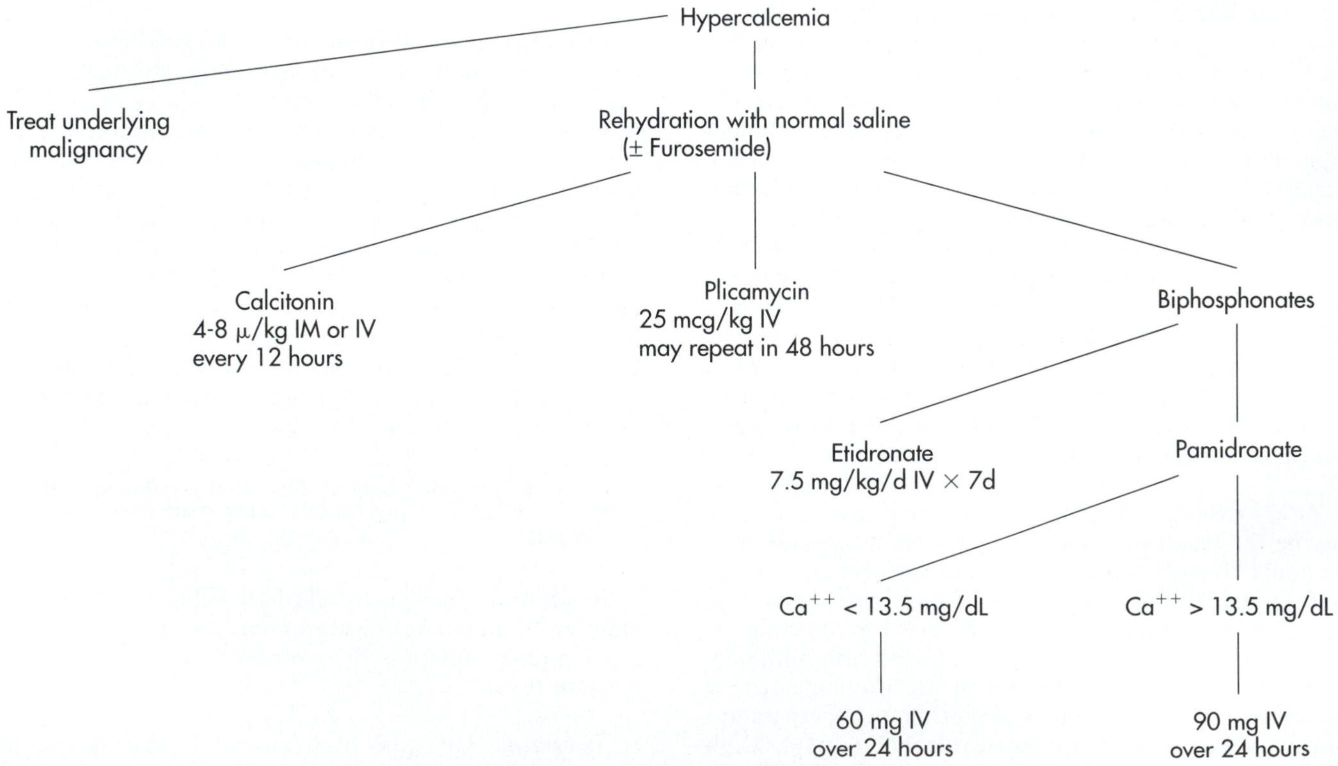


**Fig. 59-1** Therapy for hypercalcemia.

Mithramycin, also known as *plicamycin,* is an antineoplastic antibiotic derived from *Streptomyces plicatus.* Mithramycin possesses direct osteoclast inhibitory effects in addition to potentially blocking the effects of vitamin D and inhibiting parathyroid hormone. The standard dose for mithramycin is 25 μg/kg given intravenously, which usually leads to a decline in serum calcium levels in 6 to 48 hours. If no response is evident in 48 hours, the dose may be repeated. Although a rapid onset of action is seen, hypercalcemia may recur, requiring repeat treatment. Mithramycin has renal, hepatic, and bone marrow toxicities, with the latter resulting primarily in thrombocytopenia.

Biphosphonates and diphosphonates are pyrophosphate analogues that bind to the hydroxyapatite crystals in areas of increased bone turnover to inhibit osteoclastic function directly. Phagocytized bone crystals are toxic to osteoclasts and inhibit further bone resorption. Etidronate was the first drug in this class to be approved for the treatment of hypercalcemia. In a multicenter, double-blind randomized controlled study, its effects were significantly superior to those of hydration alone. The standard dose is 7.5 mg/kg per day given intravenously for up to 7 days. Once calcium homeostasis is restored with the intravenous form, maintenance therapy with etidronate, 20 mg/kg daily given orally, may be effective. Oral use beyond 90 days has not been adequately studied. Etidronate's main side effect is hypocalcemia. Although azotemia may occur, it is preventable in patients with normal renal function by initiating etidronate therapy after fluid replacement has been completed. Pamidronate has recently been approved for use in malignant hypercalcemia at the dosage of 60 mg infused over 24 hours for mild hypercalcemia. For calcium levels greater than 13.5 mg/dl, 90 mg over 24 hours is recommended as a continuous infusion. Maintaining patient hydration and electrolyte balance are important to decrease side effects. Patients may experience a febrile reaction with the first dose, and phlebitis at the intravenous site is not uncommon. New agents in this class are being investigated and may be promising.

## Syndrome of inappropriate antidiuretic hormone

***Etiology.*** Syndrome of inappropriate antidiuretic hormone (SIADH) is a common cause of hyponatremia and affects 1% to 2% of all patients with cancer. A common malignant etiology is small cell lung cancer; however, SIADH is associated with a plethora of benign causes that must be considered before deciding that cancer is responsible. Pulmonary infections such as pneumonia, tuberculosis, and lung abscesses may produce SIADH. Abnormalities in the central nervous system such as a mass lesion, an infection, or a hemorrhage may also result in hyponatremia related to SIADH. Medications such as opiates, thiazides, chlorpropamide, and the chemotherapeutic agents cyclophosphamide and vincristine may also contribute to SIADH.

***Pathophysiology.*** SIADH is thought to result in hyponatremia resulting from sustained endogenous production and release of ADH or ADH-like substances. Malignancy-related SIADH is similarly attributed to the secretion of humoral factors with ADH-like activity by the tumor. Vasopressin, the ADH, acts on the renal tubule to conserve water and results in dilutional hyponatremia. In a typical patient, water retention results in a weight gain of approximately 3 kg or roughly 10% of body water. Increased volume status promotes water and sodium losses despite a low serum sodium level and precludes the formation of edema. Natriuresis produces the characteristically elevated urinary sodium concentration coupled with serum hyponatremia.

***Signs and symptoms.*** Clinical findings in SIADH are related to water intoxication. Initial drops in the serum sodium level cause the patient to complain of nausea, anorexia, fatigue, headache, and myalgia. When the serum sodium level drops below 120 mEq/L, increases in the total body water level result in brain swelling and cause neurologic symptoms to predominate. At this level of hyponatremia an extensive range of nervous system symptoms are evident: mental status changes, confusion, lethargy, pathologic reflexes, papilledema, seizures, focal neurologic signs, coma, and death. Hyponatremia is a medical emergency that, if progressive and untreated, is uniformly fatal (see the box below).

***Diagnosis.*** Diagnostic evaluation of hyponatremia may frequently be prompted by a sudden change in mental status or by the finding of a low serum sodium level (less than 130 mEq/L) on routine chemistry testing. A careful physical examination and history, laboratory evaluation of renal function, and measurement of urinary and serum osmolality and sodium concentration allow the clinician to determine the physiologic appropriateness of the patient's hyponatremia. An elevated urine osmolality (over 120 mOsm/kg) associated with a decreased serum osmolality (280 mOsm) is consistent with a diagnosis of SIADH. A low serum sodium level must be associated with an elevated urinary sodium concentration to confirm the diagnosis of SIADH. A patient with normal renal, adrenal, and thyroid function and with a urinary sodium greater than 20 mEq/L demonstrates natriuresis, which with a

### Symptoms of SIADH

**Early**

Nausea
Anorexia
Fatigue
Headache
Myalgia

**Late**

Mental status changes
Confusion
Lethargy
Pathologic reflexes
Papilledema
Seizures
Focal deficits
Coma
Death

decreased serum sodium level is not a normal physiologic response and is characteristic of SIADH (Table 59-1).

***Treatment.*** After determining the etiology of the hyponatremia and assessing its clinical severity, the course of therapy can be determined. The goal of therapy is to raise the serum sodium concentration and to restore serum osmolality to normal. When possible, attempts to control the underlying malignancy must be made with efforts to restore electrolyte balance. If efforts to control the tumor with chemotherapy are instituted, care must be taken not to further promote hyponatremia with the pretreatment hydration required by some chemotherapeutic regimens. Fluid restriction to 800 to 1000 ml per day may be sufficient in mild cases of hyponatremia to produce volume contraction with an approximate 2- to 3-kg weight loss, reverse sodium wasting, and correction of serum sodium.

**Table 59-1.** Diagnostic criteria of SIADH

| | Serum | Urine |
|---|---|---|
| Osmolality | Low (<280 mOsm/kg) | High (>120 mOsm/kg) |
| Sodium level | Low (<130 mmol/L) | High (>20 mEq/L) |

If the patient is unable to comply with fluid restriction, demeclocycline may be used. Demeclocycline is a tetracycline that restores sodium homeostasis by interfering with the renal tubular effects of vasopressin. As with all tetracycline drugs, hypersensitivity to the sun and decreased gastrointestinal absorption with antacids, milk, and vitamins may occur. Demeclocycline's main side effect is azotemia, which can be monitored with the sodium level. Dosages should be reduced for patients with renal insufficiency. Demeclocycline at a daily dosage of 600 mg may be used in two or four divided doses. To correct severe hyponatremia (less than 120 mEq/L), serum sodium levels must be corrected slowly with normal or hypertonic saline. The latter may be necessary in life-threatening hyponatremia. Sodium replacement needs may be calculated as follows:

Sodium deficit (mEq/L) = 125 mEq/L − (Measured serum sodium [mEq/L] × 0.6 × body weight in kg)

The goal is to correct the serum sodium level to 125 mEq/L at a rate of 0.5 mEq/L per hour or 14 mEq per day to minimize the risk of central nervous system damage in the form of central pontine myelinolysis (CPM). CPM is characterized clinically by dysphagia, facial weakness, flaccid quadriplegia or paraplegia, and eventually coma resulting from demyelination in the pons (Fig. 59-2).

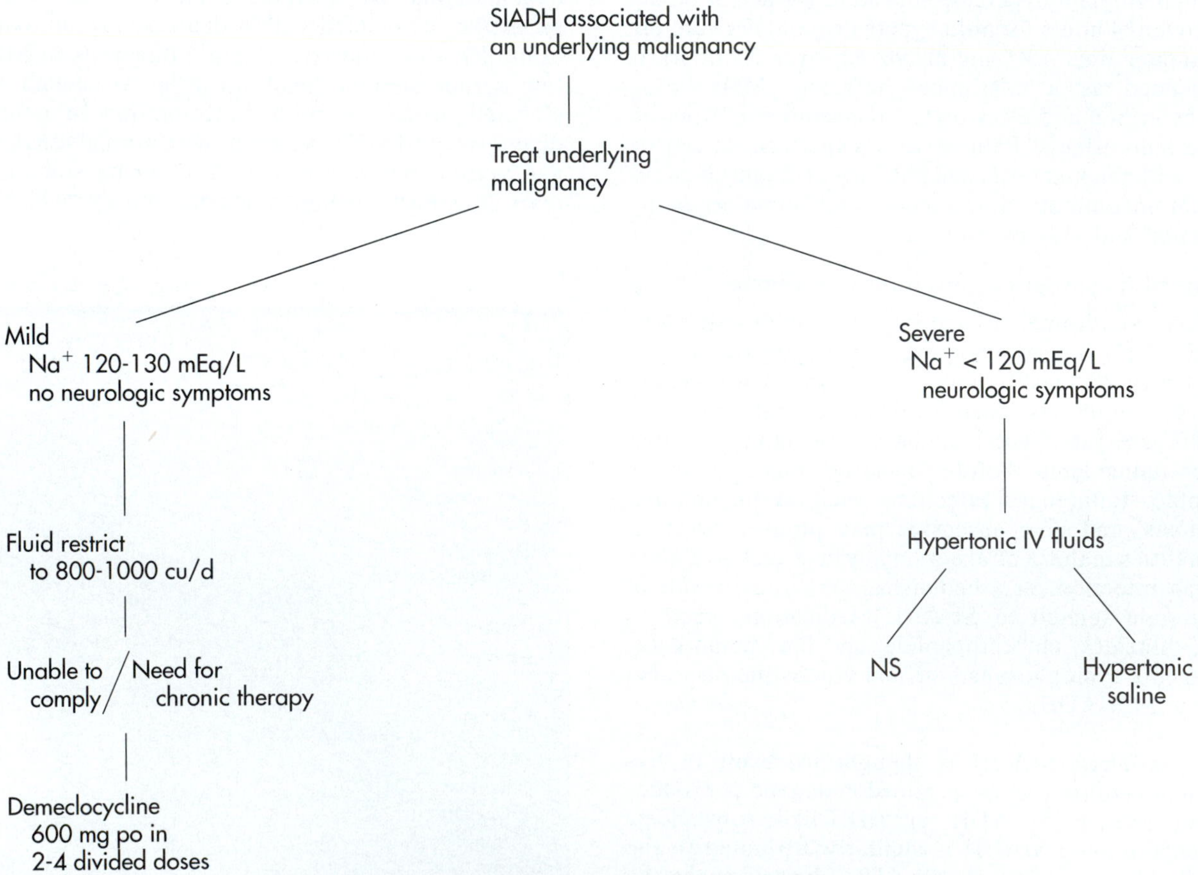


**Fig. 59-2** Treatment of SIADH associated with malignancy.

### Tumor lysis syndrome

*Etiology.* Tumor lysis syndrome can occur in relation to the effects of chemotherapy or rapid tumor growth. Both can result in the rapid release of the products of cytolysis into the systemic circulation, which may lead to irreversible renal compromise and death. Patients with both solid tumors and hematopoietic malignancies are at risk for tumor lysis syndrome, particularly if the tumor is highly proliferative or exquisitely sensitive to therapy (e.g., high-grade lymphoma or acute leukemia).

*Pathophysiology.* Tumor lysis syndrome can occur in relation to the effects of chemotherapy or rapid tumor growth. Patients with both solid tumors and hematopoietic malignancies are at risk for tumor lysis syndrome, particularly if the tumor burden is high or the tumor is in a stage of rapid cell division, in which sensitivity to chemotherapy is increased. The rapid release of the products of cytolysis into the systemic circulation leads to elevations in the levels of uric acid, potassium, and phosphate, all of which may contribute to renal failure. Hyperphosphatemia promotes hypocalcemia. The release of these intracellular metabolites occurs at a rate that exceeds the excretory capacity of the kidneys. Uric acid and phosphorus may precipitate in the renal tubules, impairing renal excretory function and causing further elevations in these metabolites. At particular risk is the patient who is dehydrated or who has baseline renal insufficiency.

*Signs and symptoms.* One of the earliest clinical signs of nephropathy related to uric acid elevation is oliguria. Signs and symptoms of uremia (nausea, vomiting, mental status depression, fluid overload), edema, and congestive heart failure may follow. High phosphate levels contribute to the nephropathy, and acidosis and anuria may develop.

Hyperkalemia and hypocalcemia primarily affect cardiac function. Dysrhythmias such as ventricular tachycardia are evidenced symptomatically and on the electrocardiogram (ECG). If they are not identified and reversed in a timely fashion, sudden death may result. In addition, hypocalcemia may result in complaints of muscle cramps, tetany, and seizures (see the box at right).

*Diagnosis.* When oliguria is reported in the appropriate clinical setting and ultrasound evaluation of the kidneys rules out obstruction as the cause of decreased urine output, tumor lysis syndrome should be considered. Elevated uric acid levels are seen, and electrolyte abnormalities may be noted. Microscopic examination of the urine may reveal the precipitated uric acid crystals and confirm the diagnosis of tumor lysis syndrome; however, their absence does not exclude the diagnosis.

*Treatment.* Since tumor lysis syndrome is a common and predictable complication of certain malignancies, therapeutic intervention is primarily focused on prevention (Fig. 59-3). Hydration and the prophylactic use of allopurinol are the cornerstones of preventive intervention. Normal saline at rates of 100 to 150 ml per hour is usually sufficient to produce a dilute urine. Allopurinol directly impairs the production of uric acid, which causes the intermediary xanthine to accumulate. Allopurinol at oral dosages of 300 to 600 mg per day should be initiated 48 hours before the onset of chemotherapy, and continuation is advised until all risk of tumor lysis is passed. Alkalinization of the urine with an infusion of sodium bicarbonate (100 mEq/L) may prevent uric acid crystals from precipitating in the urine. Monitoring of electrolytes and uric acid levels and renal function allows for early detection of metabolic aberrations. Once oliguria has developed, attempts at diuresis should be made with furosemide or mannitol.

When metabolic aberrations are present and more conservative measures are failing, hemodialysis is often successful in recuperating renal function. Hemodialysis is considered when potassium levels are greater than 6 mEq/L, uric acid levels are greater than 10 mg/dl, or phosphate levels are greater than 10 mg/dl. These interventions have resulted in a significant decline in mortality resulting from tumor lysis.

## CARDIAC EMERGENCIES

### Superior vena caval syndrome

*Etiology.* The etiology of superior vena caval syndrome (SVCS) has changed since Ehrlich's review in 1934 (Table 59-2). At that time, 46% of the cases were associated with malignancies, 36% were due to aortic aneurysms, and 18% were due to infectious or other benign etiologies. Recent reviews have demonstrated that malignant causes account for 97% of the cases of SVCS, with most attributed to lung cancer or lymphoma.

**Table 59-2.** Etiology of SVCS

| | 1934 | 1990 |
|---|---|---|
| Cancer | 46% | 97% |
| Benign causes | 54% | 3% |

**Signs and symptoms of tumor lysis syndrome**

Oliguria
Uremia
  Nausea
  Vomiting
  Mental status depression
Hypervolemia
  Congestive heart failure
  Edema
Hyperkalemia
  Ventricular tachycardia
Hypocalcemia
  Muscle cramps
  Tetany
  Seizures
Hyperphosphatemia
  Worsened nephropathy
Acidosis
Anuria

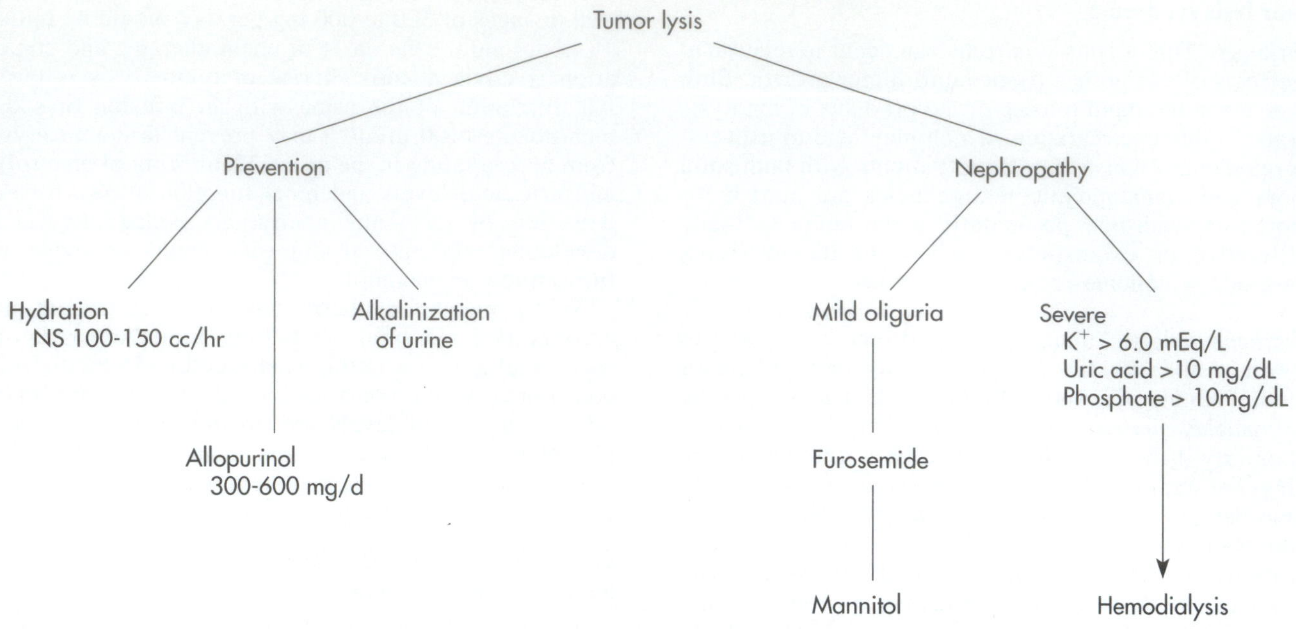


**Fig. 59-3** Treatment of tumor lysis syndrome.

***Pathophysiology.*** The mass effect of a tumor, aneurysm, abscess or other space-occupying lesion may be a partial or complete obstruction of blood flow through the SVC to the right atrium, producing SVCS.

The SVC is sensitive to mass effect because of its thin walls and low pressure. Abnormalities in the nondistensible nearby structures may easily compress the SVC. The obstruction may develop acutely and not allow for the formation of collateral blood flow, leading to a more rapid development of SVCS.

***Signs and symptoms.*** The most dramatic presentation of SVCS is a rapid progressive development of facial and upper body edema. Alternatively, clinical symptoms may develop slowly over the course of several weeks. The patient may complain of headache, nausea, dizziness, vision changes, hoarseness, cough, dysphagia, and syncope. With progression, more severe symptoms develop. Stridor and dyspnea, especially when the patient is supine, are associated with airway obstruction. Increased intracranial pressure and consequent cerebral edema are evidenced by nightmares, stupor, and seizures, but death is rarely attributed to SVCS.

Physical examination is often remarkable for neck vein distention, facial edema, and trunk and upper extremity swelling. Enlarged, dilated, cutaneous vessels in the anterior chest and upper abdomen provide evidence for collateral blood flow. Plethora and tachypnea may also be noted. In later stages, papilledema, lethargy, mental status changes, seizures, and coma may develop (see the box at right).

### Signs and symptoms of SVCS

**Nervous system**
Headaches
Nightmares
Nausea
Dizziness
Vision changes
Papilledema
Lethargy
Mental status changes
Syncope
Seizures
Stupor
Coma
Death

**Respiratory**
Hoarseness
Cough
Dyspnea
Tachypnea
Stridor

**Vascular**
Collateral flow
- Plethora
- Dilated cutaneous vessels

Obstruction
- Neck vein distention
- Facial edema
- Upper extremity and trunk swelling

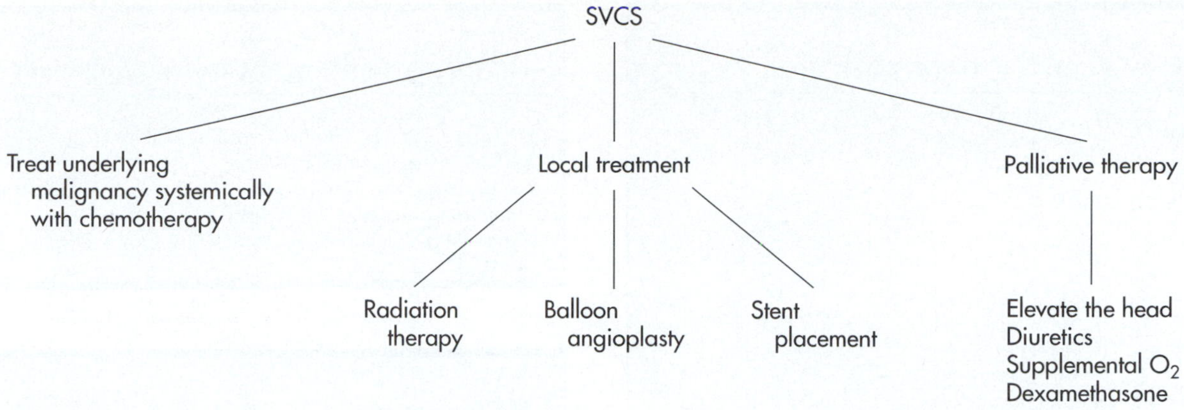


**Fig. 59-4** Treatment of superior vena caval syndrome.

*Diagnosis.* The diagnosis of SVCS is based primarily on the patient's symptoms and the physical examination findings. Chest radiographs may reveal a superior mediastinal mass or hilar adenopathy. Computerized tomography (CT) allows for visualization of the obstruction and evaluation of the extent of the disease.

SVCS usually arises as a subacute oncologic problem and not as a true emergency, since unrelieved obstruction is not life threatening except when tracheal obstruction is also present. In most previously undiagnosed cases, measures to determine the etiology of the mass lesion may be performed and are essential guides to therapy. Radiation therapy induces necrosis; therefore, when initiated before the diagnosis, diagnostic efforts may be impaired.

*Treatment.* Interim therapeutic measures such as elevation of the head, diuretics, and supplemental oxygen may be instituted for symptomatic relief. Dexamethasone may be used in patients with evidence of intracerebral edema. In patients with highly chemosensitive tumors, lymphoma, germ cell carcinoma, and small cell carcinoma of the lung, chemotherapy plays a significant role in treatment; however, in most patients, radiotherapy is the cornerstone of therapy. Balloon angioplasty and stent placement have been used to relieve the obstruction, but experience is limited (Fig. 59-4).

## Cardiac tamponade

*Etiology.* Cardiac tamponade is a life-threatening condition that, when recognized early, is treatable and reversible. Tamponade occurs when fluid accumulates in the pericardial space, not allowing for adequate filling of the atria and ventricles. When caused by a malignant condition, this fluid contains malignant cells.

*Pathophysiology.* The pericardial space normally contains approximately 20 ml of fluid maintained at a very low pressure. Malignant cells bring about changes in oncotic pressures that cause fluid to accumulate. Increased pericardial fluid increases the intrapericardial pressure, which may lead to hemodynamic compromise and collapse. The amount of pericardial fluid does not directly correlate with the intrapericardial pressure. Fluid that accumulates quickly may reach a hemodynamically significant pressure earlier than fluid that accumulates slowly and provides time for the heart to adapt to the hemodynamic changes.

Similar hemodynamics may occur with tumor encasement of the heart and radiation-induced pericarditis with fibrosis. Postradiation pericarditis may occur several years after radiation therapy. Tumors that encase the heart may be of primary or metastatic etiology. Common primary malignancies that encase the pericardium are teratomas, sarcomas, and mesotheliomas. Metastatic disease surrounding the heart is frequently due to spread of breast or lung cancer, lymphoma, or melanoma. Cardiac tamponade may occasionally be the initial presenting sign of a primary or metastatic malignancy (see the box above).

### Differential diagnosis for increased pericardial pressure

- Tumor encasement
  - Primary malignancies
    - Teratoma
    - Sarcoma
    - Mesothelioma
  - Metastatic malignancies
    - Breast
    - Lung
    - Lymphoma
    - Melanoma
- Cardiac tamponade
- Postradiation pericarditis

### Symptoms of cardiac tamponade

**Symptoms**
Nausea
Hiccups
Cough
Hoarseness
Chest pressure
Dyspnea

**Signs**
***Early***
High jugular venous pressure
Tachycardia
Pulsus paradoxus

***Late***
Bradycardia
Low-output heart failure
Shock
Death

### Diagnostic findings of cardiac tamponade

Chest radiograph: Globular cardiac shadow
ECG: Electrical alternans
Echocardiogram: Intrapericardial fluid and collapse of atrial and/or ventricular walls from increased pressure
Swan-Ganz measurement: Equalization of pressures

### Malignant etiologies of DIC

AML (especially M3)
Adenocarcinoma
  Gastrointestinal
  Prostate
  Lung
  Breast

***Signs and symptoms.*** The patient's symptom complex is variable and may range from mild nausea and hiccups to cough, hoarseness, chest pressure, and dyspnea. Physical examination is often notable for tachycardia and high jugular venous pressures. Pulsus paradoxus, the exaggerated decrease in pulse pressure during inspiration, is pathognomonic for tamponade. With frank tamponade bradycardia, low-output failure, shock, and death may occur (see the box above).

***Diagnosis.*** Once the diagnosis of cardiac tamponade is suspected clinically, a definitive evaluation must be pursued. The chest radiograph is often remarkable for a large, globular heart shadow. ECG may reveal sinus tachycardia and low voltage. Electrical alternans with alternating larger and smaller QRS complexes may also be seen. Echocardiogram allows for the visualization of the pericardial fluid and the collapse of the atrial and ventricular walls caused by high intrapericardial pressure. Swan-Ganz pressure measurements characteristically reveal equalization of the right atrial, right ventricular, pulmonary artery, and pulmonary capillary wedge pressures (see the box above).

***Treatment.*** The goal of intervention is to decompress the heart. This may be accomplished with pericardiocentesis. The pericardial fluid may be serous, serosanguineous, or hemorrhagic. It may be distinguished from cardiac chamber blood because of its absence of clot formation and because its hematocrit is lower than that of venous blood. Once it is identified as pericardial fluid, a sample should be sent for culture, sensitivity, and cytologic testing. Potential complications of pericardiocentesis are laceration of the myocardium or coronary artery, hemorrhage, arrhythmia, and cardiac arrest.

If it is caused by a malignant etiology, the fluid reaccumulates without a more definitive intervention. An intrapericardial catheter may be placed in the pericardial space and left to drain until this space is essentially dry. Doxycycline may then be infused in an attempt to fibrose the pericardium and inhibit further fluid accumulation. Repeated doses of doxycycline are often required, and the patient may complain of chest discomfort, palpitations, and fever. Intrapericardial methotrexate has also been used with some success. Sclerosis is often successful but may cause significant discomfort and require narcotic analgesia in some patients. Creation of a pericardial window is reserved for cases that are difficult to control, since thoracotomy is required. Whenever possible, treatment options should address the underlying malignancy (Fig. 59-5).

## HEMATOLOGIC EMERGENCIES

### Disseminated intravascular coagulopathy

***Etiology.*** Disseminated intravascular coagulopathy (DIC) is seen with many disease states, including malignancies (see the box above). After infection and trauma, cancer is the third most common cause of DIC; DIC is the principal coagulopathy encountered in cancer patients. The most common malignant associations are melanoma, acute myelogenous leukemia (AML), especially the M3 promyelocytic subtype (APL), and mucin-producing adenocarcinomas such as those from the gastrointestinal tract, prostate, lung, and breast. Nearly two thirds of those patients with promyelocytic leukemia develop DIC, which is associated with a 32% fatality rate related to hemorrhage.

***Pathophysiology.*** DIC results from general activation of the coagulation system. Investigation into hemostatic abnormalities in this patient subset has revealed the presence of tissue procoagulants in the leukocytes of patients with APL and other forms of AML. Similarly, tumors and necrotic tissue may release procoagulants,

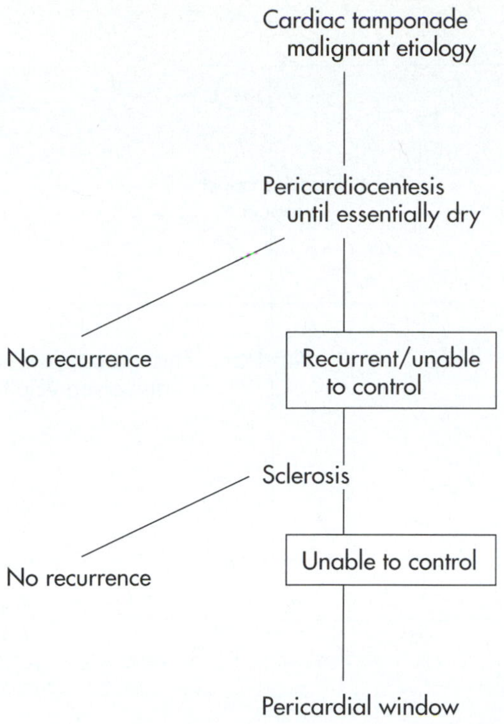


**Fig. 59-5** Management of malignant pericardial effusion producing cardiac tamponade.

which induce the thrombotic phase of DIC. The formation of small thrombi throughout the microvasculature results in the consumption of platelets and coagulation factors associated with the hemorrhagic phase of DIC. In addition, thrombotic events may produce ischemia and subsequent tissue damage.

***Signs and symptoms.*** Patients may have hemorrhagic or thrombotic events, which can range from minor mucosal bleeding to life-threatening visceral bleeding. Any site of trauma such as a venipuncture site or surgical incision may demonstrate poor hemostasis associated with the depletion of coagulation factors and thrombocytopenia. Thrombotic complications are less common than hemorrhagic ones but may be seen if significant blood flow obstruction takes place. Cancer patients may be asymptomatic with the chronic form of DIC.

***Diagnosis.*** DIC is characterized by specific laboratory findings, including a prolonged prothrombin time (PT), partial thromboplastin time (PTT), and thrombin time (TT) accompanied by evidence of clotting factor consumption with low fibrinogen levels, elevated fibrin split products, and thrombocytopenia. Examination of the peripheral smear may reveal schistocytes. In chronic DIC, laboratory abnormalities may be only minimally out of range (see the box above).

***Treatment.*** Once it is recognized, DIC should be urgently addressed to prevent potentially fatal complications (Fig. 59-6). When feasible, control of the underlying malignancy is essential; however, symptom control and subsequent prevention of recurrence often constitute the sole therapeutic option. Blood product support with platelets, packed red cells, cryoprecipitate, and fresh frozen plasma is frequently necessary. The use of heparin is controversial but is generally favored in conditions in which the thrombotic component predominates. Patients with chronic DIC may require long-term heparin therapy.

### Diagnostic characteristics of DIC

| | |
|---|---|
| PT | Increased |
| PTT | Increased |
| TT | Increased |
| Fibrinogen level | Decreased |
| Fibrin split products | Increased |
| Thrombocytopenia | Decreased |

### Migratory thrombophlebitis: Trousseau syndrome

***Etiology.*** Various malignant conditions are thought to be associated with hypercoagulability and thrombosis. It is clinically characterized primarily as a migratory superficial thrombophlebitis, although larger vessels also may be affected. Clinical thromboembolic disease has been estimated to occur in 10% of patients, although postmortem studies often reveal a higher incidence. On occasion a thrombotic event may be the harbinger of an underlying malignancy. The most common malignancies associated with increased thrombotic events are melanoma, lymphoma, leukemia, and carcinoma of the lung or gastrointestinal tract, etiologies similar to those that result in DIC. As in all patients, hypercoagulability is heightened in the postoperative period and with bed rest.

***Pathophysiology.*** The mechanism of migratory thrombophlebitis is not clearly understood and may precede detection of the underlying malignancy by several months. Normal hemostasis may be disrupted mechanically or biochemically by the presence of the tumor. Disseminated clotting may be triggered by the release of procoagulant substances from mucin-producing carcinomas; however, thrombotic complications are usually prevented by intact hepatic and hematopoietic systems. The role of other hypercoagulability risk factors such as advanced age and sedentary lifestyle needs to be considered in evaluating disruptions of the delicate coagulation system balance.

***Signs and symptoms.*** The patient typically comes to the primary care physician with complaints of swollen, erythematous, and tender extremity consistent with deep venous thrombosis or with evidence of superficial thrombophlebitis. Less commonly, symptoms of pulmonary embolus with dyspnea and acute-onset pleuritic chest pain occur and require urgent attention. The hallmark of this syndrome is its recurrent nature, and documentation of

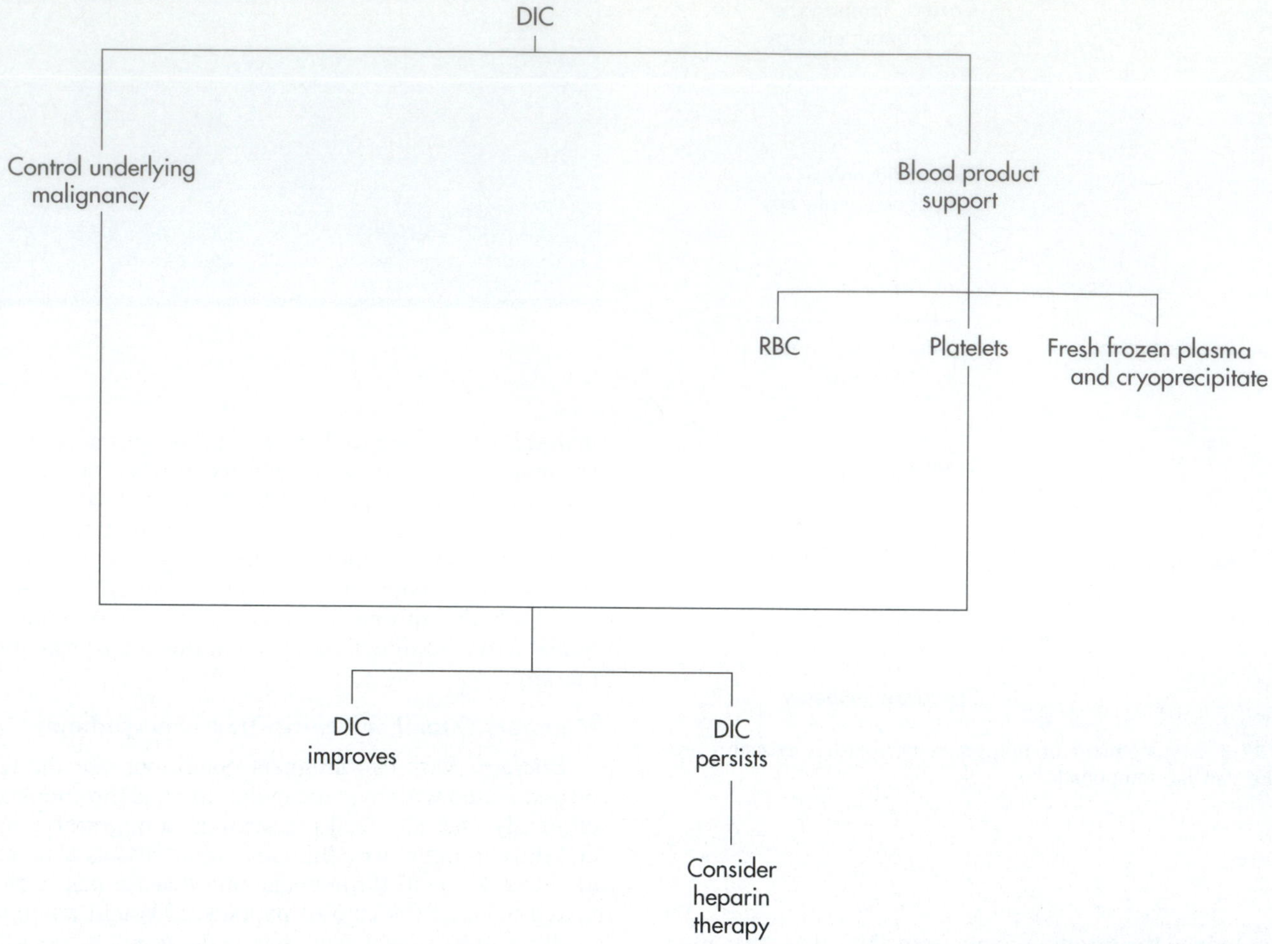


**Fig. 59-6** Therapeutic approach to DIC.

recurrent thromboses is cause to begin a search for common malignancies.

***Diagnosis.*** The usual diagnostic approach to superficial thrombophlebitis, deep venous thrombosis, and pulmonary embolus should be pursued and is not reviewed here. Although the presence of a malignancy may predispose to hypercoagulability, a single thrombotic event does not mandate an extensive search for a malignancy. Recent investigation, however, reveals a higher incidence of subsequent carcinoma in patients who have idiopathic deep venous thrombosis or pulmonary embolism.

***Treatment.*** The therapeutic approach is not particular to cancer patients. The use of heparin quickly followed by oral anticoagulants is standard. Unlike other patients, in whom anticoagulation is continued for 3 to 6 months, hypercoagulable cancer patients require anticoagulation for as long as the malignancy is active, which for many patients is the remainder of their life. For patients who are refractory to anticoagulation or in whom anticoagulation is contraindicated, a Greenfield filter may be surgically placed in the inferior vena cava (see Chapter 2).

## NEUROLOGIC EMERGENCIES

### Cord compression

***Etiology.*** Although back pain is a common complaint for patients coming to primary care physicians, the mangagement of new onset back pain in a patient with a known malignancy should be considered a medical emergency for which the usual approach of rest and observation cannot be pursued. If the new onset of back pain is due to compression of the spinal cord, prompt diagnosis and urgent intervention may prevent serious and permanent neurologic impairments and result in a marked improvement in the patient's quality of life.

Nearly 20% of patients develop neurologic complications related to underlying cancer. Spinal cord or cauda equina compression occurs in 5% to 10% of patients with cancer, affecting approximately 20,000 persons annually. An increased incidence of this oncologic complication appears to be related to the increased survival of patients with cancer (see the box on p. 799).

***Pathophysiology.*** The most common scenario for cord compression is the direct extension of a metastatic lesion from the vertebrae into the epidural space. Although

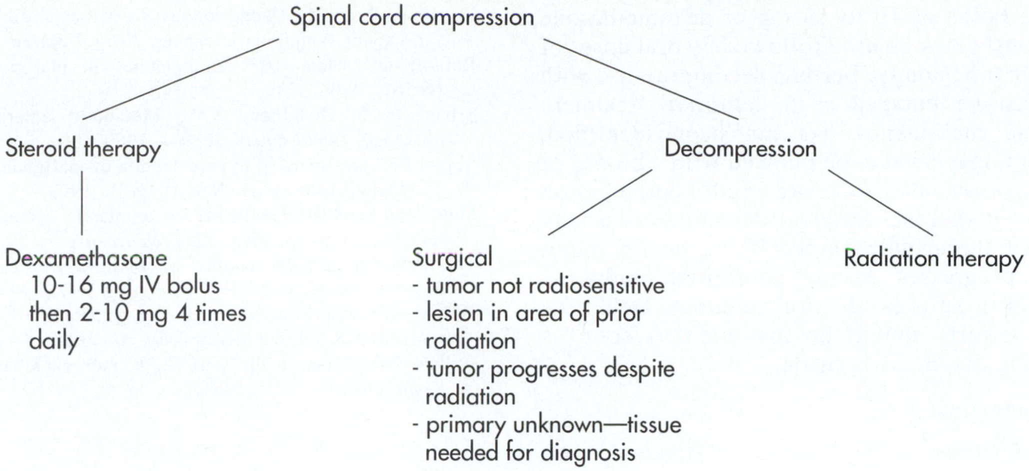


**Fig. 59-7** Management of spinal cord compression.

### Malignant etiologies of cord compression

**Primary malignancy**
Lymphoma
Melanoma
Sarcoma
Multiple myeloma
Renal cell carcinoma

**Metastatic malignancy**
Lung
Breast
Prostate

metastatic lesions are more common, cord compression may be the initial presentation of the tumor. Half of the metastatic lesions are due to lung, breast, or prostate cancer. Other common etiologies are lymphoma, melanoma, sarcoma, multiple myeloma, and renal cell cancer. In children, neuroblastoma, lymphoma, and sarcoma are the usual causes of cord compression.

The site of compression is the thoracic spine, with 70% of the compressions occurring in this area. The lumbar spine is affected 20% of the time, and the cervical spine is the site of the lesion in 10% of cases.

***Signs and symptoms.*** About 95% of patients have new onset back pain. Characteristically, this pain is worse with movement, including involuntary actions such as coughing, and is accompanied by motor and sensory deficits that progressively move upward. In time, autonomic dysfunction may take place, with bladder and bowel incontinence.

In contrast, back pain caused by degenerative joint disease is often improved with recumbancy. It is not associated with progressive neurologic impairment and is most frequent in the cervical or lumbar spine.

Physical examination is remarkable for tenderness to percussion of the involved vertebrae, brisk deep tendon reflexes, and motor and sensory deficits. Sequential neurologic examinations may be used to clinically document the progression of the cord compression.

***Diagnosis.*** Clinical suspicion of cord compression is based on a thorough history and physical examination. In over half of cases the malignant lesion may be visualized on plain radiographs of the spine. Although better visualization of the spinal cord compression may be made with either a spinal myelogram or magnetic resonance imaging (MRI), MRI is noninvasive, has no radiation exposure, and carries no risk of allergic reaction to dye. Intramedullary disease may be visually enhanced with the use of gadolinium.

***Treatment.*** Untreated sensory loss produces progressive anesthesia; motor deficits result in paralysis, and loss of sphincter control takes place. The best prognostic markers regarding the potential effectiveness of treatment are the patient's physical findings and functional status at the time that therapy is instituted. The majority of patients who are ambulatory at the time of diagnosis are ambulatory at the completion of treatment. Approximately 20% of patients who are paraplegic at the onset of treatment are able to ambulate after treatment, but fewer than 10% of patients who begin treatment with paralysis are ambulatory at the end of treatment.

The goal of therapy is to decompress the spinal cord (Fig. 59-7). Steroid therapy should be begun promptly; however, the exact steroid dosage remains controversial.

Traditionally, a bolus of 10 to 16 mg of dexamethasone given intravenously may be used followed by oral doses of 2 to 10 mg four times daily. Further decompression with radiotherapy can be pursued as a definitive treatment measure. If the malignancy has not been identified, diagnostic efforts may need to be pursued with a biopsy of the affected site, especially if the site of cord compression is the only site of disease. Surgical decompression may also be the best therapeutic choice if the lesion is not radiosensitive, progresses despite appropriate radiation doses, or occurs in an area of prior radiation. Definitive decompression efforts should be instituted as soon as possible after the diagnosis is made.

### Intracerebral metastases

***Etiology.*** Metastases to the brain are a frequent complication of bronchogenic carcinoma as well as a number of other adenocarcinomas, lymphoma, and melanoma.

***Pathophysiology.*** As with any other mass lesion within the skull, the mass may produce edema and elevation in the intracranial pressure. Increased pressures produce the symptoms that are described in the next section. Metastatic lesions are often multiple and therefore less amenable to resection.

***Signs and symptoms.*** Patients frequently visit the physician at the urging of family members who express concern regarding changes in mental status or personality. Focal neurologic deficits and new-onset seizures may also be noted. The clinical spectrum of increased intracranial pressure can range from headache and papilledema to loss of consciousness associated with frank herniation.

***Diagnosis.*** The neurologic symptoms described should lead the clinician to obtain a thorough history and to perform a complete physical examination. The diagnosis of intracerebral metastases relies on a thorough evaluation of the symptoms, a thoughtful consideration of the differential diagnoses, and an imaging study to visualize the lesion. The greatest risk of a mass-producing lesion is increased intracranial pressure with potential uncal herniation, which carries a grave prognosis.

***Treatment.*** The initial treatment goal is to decrease the edema caused by the mass. This is accomplished with steroids as described in the management of spinal cord compression. Radiotherapy is the key therapeutic intervention for radiosensitive metastases. Because of their multiple nature, surgical resection of intracerebral metastases is usually not a therapeutic option.

## BIBLIOGRAPHY


Bryne TN: Spinal cord compression from epidural mets, *N Engl J Med* 327:614, 1992.

Helms SR, Carlson, MD: Cardiovascular emergencies, *Semin Oncol* 6:463, 1989.

Kamholtz R, Sze G: Current imaging in spinal metastatic disease, *Semin Oncol* 18:158, 1991.

Paterson AHG et al: Double-blind controlled trial of oral clodronate in patients with bone metastases from breast cancer, *J Clin Oncol* 11:59, 1993.

Prandoni P et al: Deep venous thrombosis and the incidence of subsequent symptomatic cancer, *N Engl J Med* 327:1128, 1992.

Ratnoff OD: Hemostatic emergencies in malignancy, *Semin Oncol* 16:561, 1989.

Silverman P, Distelhorst CW: Metabolic emergencies in clinical oncology, *Semin Oncol* 16:504, 1989.

Singer FR: Treatment of hypercalcemia of malignancy with intravenous etidronate, *Arch Intern Med* 151:471, 1991.

Sundersan N et al: Treatment of neoplastic spinal cord compression: results of a prospective study, *Neurosurgery* 29:645, 1991.

Theriault RL: Hypercalcemia of malignancy: pathophysiology and implications for treatment, *Oncology* 7:47, 1993.

Walpole HT et al: Superior vena cava syndrome treated by percutaneous transluminal balloon angioplasty, *Am Heart J* 115:1303, 1988.

Willson JKV, Masaryk TJ: Neurologic emergencies in the cancer patient, *Semin Oncol* 16:490, 1989.


CHAPTER

# 60 Living with Cancer: Psychosocial Implications

**Debra M. Lundquist**

> Coping with cancer means more than coping with a chronic disease. It is coping with the human predicament. Cancer can be an exhaustible, relentless and resourceful foe.
>
> **A.D. Weisman, 1976-1977**

The very thought of cancer is frightening to most people. The diagnosis of cancer is devastating and affects every aspect of the person's life. It is often the first time one confronts mortality, questioning life and its meaning. To many, cancer implies a death sentence; to others it implies suffering and pain. Despite advances in diagnosis and treatment, cancer remains a fatal disease for a significant number of patients.

Cancer is a heterogenous group of diseases characterized by uncontrolled growth and spread of abnormal cells. Many cancers can be cured if detected and treated promptly. However, if the spread of disease is not controlled or checked, it results in death.

In the United States, cancer is the second leading cause of death and accounts for 23% of all deaths. There were approximately 1.17 million new cases diagnosed in 1993 with 526,000 deaths in the United States. For women ages 35 to 74, cancer is the leading cause of death. Cancer is the second leading cause of death for men in the United States.

In the early 1900s few cancer patients survived. By the 1940s only one patient in four was alive 5 years after diagnosis, and in the 1960s, it was one cancer patient in three. Today, there are 8 million living Americans who have a history of cancer. Half of this group were diagnosed 5 or more years ago and can be considered cured. The remaining 4 million still have evidence of cancer and will sometimes endure years of fighting the disease.

## MEANING OF A CANCER DIAGNOSIS

The diagnosis of cancer elicits a wide range of emotions, including shock, disbelief, numbness, powerlessness, and vulnerability. Concerns about death and the feeling that time is running out are common. For most people, illness is a slight inconvenience of short duration, with rapid recovery and minimal disruption in lifestyle. The person who is diagnosed with cancer finds the diagnosis is only the beginning of many life changes.

Cancer is regarded as a chronic illness that affects every aspect of a person's life. Like most chronic illnesses, cancer is characterized by uncertainty, whether it involves unpredictable disease trajectories, uncertain remissions, or recurrence of disease. According to Weisman, like cancer's ability to spread through the body, it also is able to also spread into the emotional and social domains of an individual, causing disruptions in families and causing one to question the meaning of life. Weisman also identified uncertainty as a major coping problem.

A diagnosis of cancer is considered a catastrophic event that causes physical and psychologic changes to the individual and family. Weisman identified seven major areas of concern for these individuals: health, self-appraisal, work and finances, family and significant relationships, religion, friends and associates, and existential issues. Weisman identified coping with the problems associated with a cancer diagnosis as a major task of the individual and family. He described good coping as an action that consists of the principal parts of hope, trust, quality of survival, and reasonable control of symptoms.

Martocchio compared living with a chronic illness such as cancer to walking along the ocean. Even if one is walking with another person, one may still be alone with his or her thoughts, desires, fears, joys, and suffering. For those individuals who have not developed a relationship with the sea, a walk along the edge of the ocean can be of terrifying intensity at times. Like the ocean, life with cancer has many moods, and there is a constant, changing action.

Martocchio also described four patterns of living and dying that are useful in understanding the uncertainties of living with a life-threatening illness such as cancer. These patterns, which can be influenced by both the natural disease process and the effects of treatment modalities, follow:

1. Peaks and valleys: A time characterized by a series of exacerbations and remissions
2. Descending plateaus: A pattern of steplike losses of functional ability occurring an unpredictable number of times for indeterminate periods
3. Downward slope pattern: A continuous and rapid downhill course
4. Gradual slant pattern: A gradual decline over time

According to Martocchio, there may be combinations of these patterns; they do not have to be isolated from each other. Common to all of these patterns is a high level of uncertainty and a need for continuous monitoring. Of note is the fact that Martocchio does not address those individuals who are cured and also face fears and uncertainty about the future.

In a study done by Weisman and Worden, 120 newly diagnosed cancer patients were interviewed in 4- to 6-week intervals, beginning 10 days after diagnosis. The purpose of the study was to further explore the impact of a cancer diagnosis. This study examined how newly diagnosed cancer patients coped with the existential plight of being diagnosed with a life-threatening illness. *Existential plight* was defined as "a luckless predicament in which one's very existence seems endangered." This study confirmed that newly diagnosed cancer patients are most concerned about dying regardless of their prognosis. These concerns occur most intensely during the first 100 days, the time known as "existential plight."

This finding was supported by a study done by McCorkle and Quint-Benoliel. Their study revealed that newly diagnosed lung cancer patients experienced more health and existential concerns than those newly diagnosed with myocardial infarction. The cancer patients also experienced more mood disturbances than the myocardial infarction group. An interesting finding was that, although symptom distress remained the same for both groups at both time intervals, patients reported being less worried as well as in better spirits than at the first interview. This led to the inference that, as patients understand more about their illness, they may conclude that their situation is not as life threatening as previously thought. Mood disturbances are not uncommon in the newly diagnosed cancer patient. Northouse interviewed women with breast cancer and found the level of mood changes improved over time, although the subjects' levels of distress did not.

## TREATMENT-RELATED CONCERNS

The initiation of treatment for cancer is a time characterized by fear, uncertainty, and feelings of loss of control. Patients realize that treatment is essential to combat the disease. However, fears related to the physical and psychologic aspects of the treatment as well as the impact on the family and financial ramifications can be overwhelming. Concerns about the physical aspects of treatment include potential side effects, changes in body image, and changes in functional status. Psychologic concerns include the fears related to the outcome of treatment, the uncertain future, and the ability of the individual to cope with the treatment. Feelings of uncertainty are paramount. Common questions asked by newly diagnosed patients with cancer include: How will I be affected by the treatment? Will the treatment help me? Will I be cured? and Is it really worth it? Many patients fear being a burden to their family and have concerns about their ability to maintain employment. Concerns about employment and the financial implications predominate, particularly if the individual with cancer is the provider for the family.

The treatment itself is a source of anxiety. Many individuals have misconceptions based on the public perception of cancer and its treatment. It is important to clarify misconceptions before initiating treatment. This knowledge helps the person regain a sense of control in a situation that causes many to feel out of control.

Patients also experience difficulties at the completion of treatment. For many, there is often a sense of ambivalence. Patients are happy at the thought of completing treatment but fear distancing themselves from the health care team. There is also a sense that they are no longer actively fighting the cancer. It is not unusual for some patients to develop behaviors such as hypochondriasis as a means of coping with anxiety about completing treatment. Reassurance about the availability of the health care team is encouraged as is education about symptoms that would need to be reported. Routine checkups and yearly comprehensive examinations help alleviate anxiety. As the duration of time from the completion of treatment increases, patients become more comfortable with the distance that has developed from the health care team.

## CANCER RECURRENCE

Cancer recurrence poses as great a threat as, if not greater than, the initial diagnosis of cancer. Mahon found the time of recurrence of cancer was more upsetting than the initial diagnosis and that people were less hopeful than at the time of initial diagnosis. Fear of recurrence is almost always present whether the prognosis is excellent or poor. A number of psychosocial stressors are experienced at the time of recurrence. For most patients the realization that the focus of treatment shifts from cure to control of disease is extremely stressful and frightening. Many patients perceive that, once treated, cancer is cured and will not recur. Therefore when the recurrence is confirmed, feelings of disbelief, uncertainty, anger, and fear are experienced. Many patients experience feelings of hopelessness and depression and question the benefit of additional treatment if cure is no longer the goal.

Chekryn identified several stressors experienced at the time of recurrence by both patients and spouses (see the box below).

In addition, Mahon identified health and health-related concerns, work and finances, and self-appraisal issues. It is important to assess patients and families who are most vulnerable to the stressors that result from recurrence and provide support and guidance to facilitate adjustment. For many patients and families the opportunity to verbalize feelings of grief, anger, and fear enables them to move forward and make decisions regarding treatment and the future.

## TERMINAL PHASE

The transition from active treatment to supportive care of the dying patient is important in the cancer continuum. Palliative care is the shift in treatment goals from a curative intent to providing relief from suffering. Relief of suffering for the dying patient goes beyond the management of physical symptoms. The emotional, spiritual, and existential concerns must all be addressed.

Martinez and Wagner identified the principles of palliative care, as shown in the box below.

When the decision is made to shift the focus to palliative care, persons experience many responses, often in a cyclic process. Initially, one may experience shock and denial at the realization that no further treatment will stop the cancer's spread. This is followed by varying degrees of denial, bargaining, sadness, anger, and acceptance. Coping patterns in the terminal phase can be predicted by the patient's history of coping with past events.

Many patients choose to die at home with hospice services (if available). Hospice care and death at home give the patient and family a sense of control over their environment at a time when they feel out of control. Remaining at home in familiar surroundings is also comforting for many people. However, this option is not feasible for all dying persons. Some patients may be too acutely ill to be managed at home. Lack of resources to provide adequate care in the home is another barrier.

For patients who choose to die at home, an individualized plan of care must be developed with the involvement of the patient and family. Information regarding the dying process as well as anticipated signs and symptoms of approaching death are important to best prepare the family to care for the dying patient. Anticipation of predictable changes in the patient who is dying can help the patient and family effectively cope. The major processes underlying cancer death include infection, organ failure, extensive carcinomatosis, pulmonary problems, myocardial infarction, and hemorrhage. Common symptoms include dyspnea, pain, altered elimination, and seizures. Assessment and care of the dying patient need to focus on the physical, psychosocial, and spiritual aspects of the individual. The focus shifts to maintaining comfort and managing symptoms to promote a peaceful death with dignity. See Chapter 128 for further discussion of death and dying.

### Chekryn's stressors at time of cancer recurrence

Difficulty with closure related to the expectation of cure or remission
Pervasive feelings of uncertainty
Grief about present and potential losses
Feelings of injustice, anger, and fear
Existential concerns
Concerns related to ability to cope with recurrence
Impact on the marital relationship

From Chekryn J: *Cancer Nurs* 7(6):491, 1984.

### Managed Care Guide
### Principles of palliative care

The goal of treatment is to optimize quality of life.
Death is regarded as a natural process, to be neither hastened nor prolonged.
Diagnostic tests and other invasive procedures are minimized unless the intervention will result in the alleviation of symptoms.
Use of heroic treatment measures is discouraged.
When using narcotic analgesics, the right dosage is the one that provides pain relief without unacceptable side effects.
The patient is the expert on whether pain and symptoms have been adequately relieved.
Patients eat if they are hungry and drink if thirsty; fluids and feeding are not forced.
Care is individualized and based on the goals of the patient and family, as the unit of care.

From Martinez J, Wagner S: Hospice care. In Groenwald S et al, editors: *Cancer nursing: principles and practice,* ed 3, Boston, 1993, Jones & Bartlett.

## SURVIVORSHIP ISSUES

Early detection and intervention using a multimodality treatment approach have significantly increased the number of cancer survivors. Cancer is now considered a chronic, life-threatening illness rather than a terminal illness.

Cancer survivorship can be described as the experience of living through or beyond illness. It is a process that encompasses all phases of survival but is best defined as long-term survival. Historically, cancer survivors were considered cured of their disease 5 years after the completion of treatment. When thinking of cancer survivorship, the term *cure* is not accurate because some persons have cancers that may be controlled for several years. Although these individuals are not cured, they are indeed survivors with a chronic disease. Long-term survivors may experience a variety of problems ranging from minor, short-term difficulties to major psychosocial crises.

The major psychosocial themes identified for cancer survivors include interrelationships between long-term physical effects and psychosocial outcomes, fears of relapse and death, dependence on health care providers, survivor guilt, uncertain sense of longevity, social adaptation dilemmas, and the effects on the family. The ability of a person to cope as a survivor of cancer is influenced by the degree of physical changes experienced relating to treatment. Certainly, fear of recurrence and death are present to some degree regardless of the time since initial diagnosis. This is probably the most common concern for cancer survivors. Dependence on health care providers is often the result of ambivalence that develops as the patient completes treatment. There is a sense of euphoria about completing treatment, which is in conflict with fears experienced relating to the change in intensity and frequency of interactions with health care providers.

Feelings of survivor guilt are common for cancer survivors. These feelings may be experienced on routine follow-up visits when there is interaction between the survivor and others in the waiting room.

A sense of uncertainty regarding the future is experienced by many cancer survivors. Concerns focus on the potential long-term implications after having survived a chronic illness. Many persons identify a greater appreciation of life and the desire to live life in a more meaningful way as positive approaches to this uncertainty.

An additional area of difficulty is the transition from the sick role to the healthy role. This is not always easy for cancer survivors. McCaffrey and co-workers identified the presence of physical disability, negative expectations from the support network, personal concerns about the ability to readjust, and social stigma as social dilemmas encountered by the cancer survivor. These are areas that require exploration and discussion. The ability to discuss these concerns by a member of the health care team may help the individual to look at them in a more objective manner.

Finally, the effects on the family of the survivor need to be considered. There is limited information regarding the effects of long-term psychologic stress on the family. However, this is an area of assessment that must not be minimized. The diagnosis of cancer affects not only the individual but those around him or her. Throughout the diagnostic and treatment phases the family often struggles to respond and support the loved one with cancer. Health care professionals must be sensitive to the needs of families of survivors.

Additional areas of concern for the cancer survivor include financial, employment, and insurance issues. Access to insurance is usually through employment. Unfortunately, some cancer survivors experience discrimination in the workplace. McCaffrey and co-workers identified three categories of employment-related concerns: dismissal, demotion, and reduction or elimination of work-related *benefits;* problems resulting from co-workers' *attitudes* about cancer; and problems arising from attitudes of the *survivor* regarding how he or she should be perceived in the workplace. Federal and state laws were developed to prohibit discrimination against qualified individuals with a history of cancer. Both the Federal Rehabilitation Act of 1973 and the more recent Americans with Disabilities Act prohibit discrimination against cancer survivors in the workplace.

Access to comprehensive insurance continues to be problematic. The availability of adequate insurance is not a guarantee for many people. Unfortunately, there is no state or federally mandated legal right to health insurance, although this may change in the future. Barriers to obtaining insurance include refusal of new applications, waived or excluded preconditions, policy cancellations or reductions, higher premiums, and extended waiting periods. These barriers may also affect the spouse or family member who carries the insurance. Studies have found that 25% to 30% of cancer survivors experience some form of insurance discrimination.

In an effort to protect survivors of cancer, the American Cancer Society published the Cancer Survivor's Bill of Rights. The goal of this document was to call public attention to the needs of the cancer survivor, to enhance cancer care, and to bring greater satisfaction to cancer survivors. Resources are becoming increasingly available to better support cancer survivors, on both the local and national levels. The National Coalition for Cancer Survivorship (NCCS) serves as a resource for those interested in issues of survivorship. The continued development of programs, support networks, and resources is essential to ensure that cancer survivors are treated fairly and maintain their quality of life.

## IMPACT OF CANCER ON THE FAMILY

Cancer is a disease that affects not only the patient, but also the entire family. One in four Americans will be diagnosed with cancer in his or her lifetime, and two of every three families will have at least one member diagnosed with cancer. Some families may have multiple members of more than one generation being treated for cancer at the same time. It is essential that the health care team assess the ability of the family to mobilize itself and its resources in response to the needs of the person with cancer. Acknowledgement of the importance of the family enhances the care of the person experiencing the disease.

Worry about the impact of the illness on loved ones is very real. The diagnosis of cancer places a strain on the entire family, and often the person experiencing the disease expresses feelings of guilt or worry because of what "I'm putting my family through." This concern reinforces the need to include the family in the plan of care.

The major issues affecting the family and their ability

### Issues affecting the family and their coping ability

Emotional strain
Physical demands of care
Uncertainty
Fear
Altered roles and lifestyles
Financial considerations
Comforting the patient
Perceived inadequacy of services
Philosophic and spiritual concerns
Sexuality
Incongruent needs and perceptions

From Woods NF, Lewis FM, Ellison ES: *Cancer Nurs* 12(1):28, 1989.

to cope with a cancer diagnosis were identified by Woods, Lewis, and Ellison (see the box above). Whether the family can respond to these issues is related to disease characteristics such as the patient's age at diagnosis, prognosis, disease severity and progression, the duration of illness, and associated disabilities.

The location of the person in the cancer trajectory is an important point to consider. Giacquinta and Christ identified transition points in the cancer experience (see the box above). Families may remain at a transition point for an extended time or may progress quickly from one point to the next. The movement through these transition points serves as a reminder of the many changes experienced by the family that drain family strength and resources. Compounding this are the uncertainty and fear experienced at each transition point by the person with cancer and the family.

Family members may assume many different roles throughout the cancer experience. They may function in the role of partner, actively participating in decision making with the person with cancer and providing care to the ill family member. A family member fulfills the participant role by taking an active role in care and being included in decisions. However, the ill patient remains responsible for decision making. As an observer the family member does not participate in the care or decision making. It is important to identify who is functioning in the different roles to better care for the patient and family.

In a study of 41 family members of adult cancer patients, Welch identified five specific family needs when a family member has cancer. These are listed in the box above.

Similar concerns of the family were identified by Wright and Dyck. The primary concerns of the family include dealing with symptoms, waiting, fear of the future, and obtaining information. Families of patients who had a recurrence had significantly higher needs. The highest priority of all families regardless of phase of illness was the need to be kept informed about the patient's condition and to be assured that the patient was comfortable.

Research in this field has identified three consistent findings: the family affects the patient's adjustment to cancer, family members do not necessarily share the same

### Transition points in the cancer experience

Diagnosis
Treatment initiation
Treatment completion
Cure
Failure to respond to treatment
Recurrence
Decision to discontinue treatment
Terminal illness
Death

From Giacquinta B: *Am J Nurs* 10:1585, 1977; and from Christ GH: *Health Social Work* 8:57, 1983.

### Specific family needs

Knowing the patient is receiving excellent care
Being informed about cancer and treatment
Participating in patient care
Communicating with the health care team
Participating in a support group

From Welch D: *Cancer Nurs* 4:365, 1981.

concerns about cancer, and family members cope with cancer in individual ways. Regardless of the person's phase of illness, care of the family is critical in caring for the person with cancer. In caring for the family, the needs of the individual with cancer are best met.

## HEALTH CARE TEAM

Use of a multidisciplinary team is essential in helping the patient adapt to the many changes encountered as the result of a cancer diagnosis. Involvement of the team in planning care for the individual facilitates the restoration of physical and emotional well-being as the members focus on the goal of promoting quality of life. In addition to the patient and family, members of the team include physicians, nurses, social workers, clergy, nutritionists, and physical therapists. When appropriate, other members are psychologists, occupational therapists, and other health care providers. Regular team meetings are essential to maximize care and identify potential obstacles of goal attainment.

The goals are individualized to the patient. To formulate realistic goals, a thorough discussion of the treatment plan, potential complications, and expected results is essential. For some the goal is curative, whereas for others it may be palliative. Regardless of the goal, maintaining quality of life underlies all interventions.

In addition to the resources available by the members of the team, knowledge of additional resources available is important in providing care. Community-based resources include support groups, educational groups, and organizations such as the American Cancer Society and the Leukemia Society of America, both of which offer programs and services to persons with cancer. Most major cities and towns have local chapters. Written publications are available from the American Cancer Society and the National Cancer Institute. These materials are written for medical professionals and laypersons; they are free of charge and informative.

## BIBLIOGRAPHY


Chekryn J: Cancer recurrence: personal meaning, communication, and marital adjustment, *Cancer Nurs* 7(6):491, 1984.

Christ GH: A psychosocial assessment framework for cancer patients and their families, *Health Social Work* 8:57, 1983.

Giacquinta B: Helping families face the crisis of cancer, *Am J Nurs* 10:1585, 1977.

Jassak P: Families: an essential element in the care of the patient with cancer, *Oncol Nurs Forum* 19(6):871, 1992.

Mahon SM, Cella DF, Donovan MI: Psychosocial adjustment to recurrent cancer, *Oncol Nurs Forum* 17(3)(suppl):47, 1990.

Martinez J, Wagner S: Hospice care. In Groenwald S et al, editors: *Cancer nursing: principles and practice,* ed 3, Boston, 1993, Jones & Bartlett.

Martocchio BC: Authenticity, belonging, emotional closeness and self-representation, *Oncol Nurs Forum* 14(4):23, 1987.

Martocchio BC: Family coping: helping families help themselves, *Semin Oncol Nurs* 1:292, 1985.

Weisman AD: *Coping with cancer,* New York, 1979, McGraw-Hill.

Weisman AD, Worden JW: The existential plight in cancer: significance of the first 100 days, *Int J Psychiatry Med* 7:1, 1976-77.

Welch D: Planning nursing interventions for family members of adult cancer patients, *Cancer Nurs* 4:365, 1981.

Welch-McCaffrey D et al: Psychosocial dimensions: issues in survivorship. In Groenwald S et al, editors, *Cancer nursing: principles and practice,* ed 2, Boston, 1990, Jones & Bartlett.

Woods NF, Lewis FM, Ellison ES: Living with cancer: family experiences, *Cancer Nurs* 12(1):28, 1989.


CHAPTER

# 61 Cancer Prevention, Screening, and Follow-up

**Linda M. Sutton**

More than a million Americans are diagnosed with cancer every year. Since the 1950s cancer has been the second leading cause of death in the United States, and it was estimated that 526,000 deaths in 1993 would be attributed to cancer. Furthermore, with current trends demonstrating a decline in mortality rates from heart disease, cancer may well be the leading cause of death in the United States by the year 2000. The box above details the five primary sites of malignancy that account for approximately 60% of the estimated annual cancer incidence and nearly 60% of all deaths related to cancer. The primary care physician plays a pivotal role in the reduction of cancer-associated morbidity and mortality through aggressive approaches to prevention and early detection. In addition, anticipated improvement in diagnostic techniques and treatment modalities will result in a greater proportion of patients who survive after a diagnosis of cancer. The future of health care is such that the primary care physician will play a key role in the management and follow-up of successfully treated cancer patients.

### Leading sites of estimated cancer incidence and mortality for 1994

**Incidence**
Prostate
Breast
Lung
Colorectal
Bladder

**Mortality**
Lung
Colorectal
Breast
Prostate
Pancreas

From Boring CC et al: *CA Cancer J Clin* 44(1):7, 1994.

## PREVENTION

The term *prevention* is meant to imply prevention of cancer-related mortality and, where possible, morbidity. Carcinogenesis is a multistep process with long periods of latency for individual steps along the way. There are several levels in the ontogeny of a neoplasm at which specific interventions may prevent subsequent morbidity and mortality. Unfortunately, cancer is not a single target at which preventive strategies can be aimed. Rather, *cancer* is the collective term for many distinct neoplasms with different etiologies, risk factors, and behavioral characteristics. This complicates but does not preclude effective preventive programs.

Until the latter half of this century the preventive armamentarium consisted largely of antineoplastic therapies. Unfortunately this tertiary prevention led to declines in cancer-related morbidity and mortality rates for only a minority of malignancies. Lack of curative therapies for the majority of cancers and a limited knowledge base precluded effective use of other preventive approaches. The explosion of basic science and clinical information over the past few decades has advanced our understanding of the process of carcinogenesis, allowed better identification of high-risk groups, and led to enthusiasm for primary and secondary preventive strategies.

Secondary preventive measures are successful through screening techniques. Screening allows detection of an established neoplasm at a stage that remains amenable to curative therapy. The performance of screening mammography in asymptomatic women is one example of a successful secondary prevention. Mortality from breast cancer has decreased for women over the age of 50 who have undergone recommended screening. However, for many cancers the use of secondary prevention is hampered by the lack of adequately sensitive and specific screening

### Risk factors associated with cancer mortality

Tobacco
Diet
Alcohol
Radiation exposure
  Ultraviolet
  Ionizing
Chemical exposure
  Drugs
  Pollution
  Occupational
Reproductive factors
Infections
Genetic predisposition

tests as well as by the low prevalence of cancers at individual primary sites. Noncompliance by patients and physicians further compromises the efficacy of available screening tests.

Primary preventive methods, on the other hand, seek to interrupt neoplastic development before a malignant growth is established. This can be accomplished through modification of patient characteristics or environmental factors that have been identified through epidemiologic studies as being associated with increased cancer risk. Although risk factors such as age and gender are not amenable to modification, other risk factors, such as tobacco use, are felt to play a causative role in the transformation of a normal host cell to a neoplastic clone. Elimination of such causative factors can have a major impact on cancer incidence and mortality. Alternatively, neoplastic development could be reversed or inhibited through chemoprevention. A number of chemical agents, both naturally occurring and pharmaceutically engineered, inhibit carcinogenesis in experimental systems. Recent clinical trials have suggested that this might be an important part of cancer prevention in the future.

## High-risk groups

Successful preventive interventions require that factors associated with an increased risk of developing cancer can be defined and individuals or groups who possess these high-risk characteristics and behaviors can be identified before the diagnosis of cancer. Furthermore, the identified risk factors must be amenable to modification such that for individual patients the development of a particular cancer is delayed or prevented. It has been estimated that between 75% and 80% of cancers in the United States could be avoided through alterations in behavior. Numerous environmental factors have been identified as having a causative or permissive role in the development of human malignancies (see the box above). Tobacco use and diet are responsible for a large proportion of the cancer-related deaths in the United States. Although other factors are responsible for some definite proportion of overall cancer mortality, their contribution is smaller. Some of these factors, such as pollution and occupational exposures, are not as readily amenable to modification as are those that reflect personal behaviors.

### Tobacco-related cancers

Lung
Oral cavity
Larynx
Esophageal
Pancreas
Kidney
Bladder
Uterine cervix

***Tobacco.*** Tobacco is responsible for more cancer-related deaths than any other single risk factor and accounts for more than 30% of all cancer deaths. The box above underscores the impact of tobacco use on cancer incidence. Clearly, tobacco use is a high-risk behavior, and its elimination would have a profound impact on cancer-related mortality in the United States. For example, the incidence of lung cancer would decline by approximately 90%, with an estimated 25% reduction in overall cancer mortality if smoking alone were completely eradicated. Elimination of other forms of tobacco use would further decrease cancer incidence and mortality. There would be additional health benefits in the form of decreased incidence of cardiovascular and respiratory disease.

***Diet.*** There is a substantial body of evidence supporting the role of diet in the development and inhibition of neoplastic growth. In vitro laboratory studies and animal experiments provide clues to the role that various nutrients might play in human carcinogenesis. As early as the 1940s the permissive role of a high-fat diet in neoplastic development in laboratory animals exposed to carcinogens was demonstrated. However, animal studies must be interpreted with caution and are not always immediately relevant to human biology.

The evidence linking factors in the human diet to neoplastic growth are largely derived from epidemiologic studies conducted at the population level or through specific cohort or case control studies. The interpretation of such epidemiologic data is complicated by numerous factors. Retrospective epidemiologic studies attempting to link nutrient intake to risk of subsequent cancer suffer from recall bias. The recall of nutrient intake by study participants may be unreliable and biased toward the socially correct answer rather than reflective of true behavior. In addition, in the United States approximately one third of the money spent on food annually is for food prepared outside the home. Study participants may not be able to accurately report the composition of these foods. Even if recall of recent nutrient intake is accurate, the culprit in carcinogenesis may well be the intake of foodstuffs many years before a particular study. Confounding variables also complicate the interpretation of epidemiologic data. Many studies may not examine lifestyle differences other than diet, such as physical activity, that could alter the conclusions obtained. Randomized prospective trials, which would provide the strongest evidence of causation between diet and cancer, are prohibitively expensive to conduct and fraught with

**Nutrient categories**

**Macronutrients**
Carbohydrates
Proteins
Fiber
Fat

**Micronutrients**
Vitamins
Minerals
Trace elements

scientific difficulties in controlling or measuring nutrient intake. The compilation of data from many sources forms the basis of the current state of imperfect knowledge regarding the interaction between diet and carcinogenesis.

**Fiber.** The human diet is composed of macronutrients and micronutrients (see the box above). Deficiencies and excesses of these elements within the diet appear to contribute to the development of specific malignancies. The role of fat and fiber intake in carcinogenesis has been the most widely studied. Numerous case control and prospective studies have demonstrated a link between a low-fiber diet and subsequent development of colorectal cancers. It is hypothesized that a high-fiber diet may lower the risk of colon cancer by increasing fecal bulk and diluting the concentration of carcinogens within the colon, thereby limiting the exposure of colonic mucosa to potential mutagens. A high-fiber diet may also modulate the effect of other dietary substances. Countries with very high–fiber diets, such as Finland, have decreased incidences of colon cancer despite high fat intake.

**Fat.** Clinical studies have demonstrated an association between excessive consumption of fat and calories with cancers of the breast, colon, prostate, ovary, endometrium, gallbladder, and most recently lung. Obesity has been associated with cancers of the endometrium, kidney, and pancreas. International epidemiologic studies have identified strong associations between per capita fat intake and age-adjusted rates for specific cancers. The prevalence of breast, colon, and prostate cancers is much higher in the Western world than in countries such as Japan. The diet of the Western world derives approximately 35% to 40% of the calories consumed from fat, whereas the amount of fat consumed in the Japanese diet is more limited. It is interesting that the incidence of breast cancer is rising in Japan as fat consumption has risen from about 10% of the caloric intake in the 1950s to the current 25%. The increased risk of these cancers may not be uniform for all types and amounts of fat consumed. The mechanism by which dietary fat enhances carcinogenesis is unclear. Current research is focused on dissecting out the components of dietary fat that may promote the development of cancer. Dietary fat may enhance the development of colon cancer by increasing the concentration of bile salts within the colon. Bile acids alter the metabolic activity of microbial flora within the colon such that the colonic mucosa is increasingly exposed to weakly carcinogenic bile acid metabolites. Mechanisms of mutagenesis in other malignancies are lacking.

**Vitamins and Minerals.** The number of studies that have investigated the role of vitamins and minerals in carcinogenesis is relatively small. Diets deficient in vitamins A, C, and D have been associated with increased cancer risk. The strongest evidence exists for vitamin A deficiency, which has been implicated in the development of cancers of the lung, breast, oropharynx, stomach, bladder, prostate, and colon. Vitamin A is necessary for normal epithelial tissue growth and development. A deficiency of this important vitamin can increase the susceptibility of normal tissues to mutagens. Squamous tissues deficient in vitamin A exhibit metaplastic differentiation that can be reversed by administration of vitamin A and related compounds. There is evidence to suggest that diets rich in vitamin A and related compounds not only diminish the risk but also protect against the development of certain cancers. A decreased intake of vitamin D has been associated with an increased risk of colon cancer in several recent studies, and diets composed of foods rich in vitamin A, C, and E are associated with decreased cancer incidence. Vitamin C may inhibit the formation of carcinogenic nitrosamines that have been associated with the development of gastric cancer. Nonetheless, the role of vitamins C and E in neoplastic development remains particularly unclear. Although vitamins C and E function as antioxidants, there is little evidence to support any direct role for these vitamins in the inhibition or reversal of neoplastic growth and development.

Among the many minerals required for normal tissue development, calcium and selenium have received the most attention with regard to carcinogenesis. There is laboratory as well as preliminary clinical data to support a role for calcium deficiency in the development of colon cancer. Results of the numerous studies focusing on the role of dietary selenium are contradictory and inconclusive. Data on other micronutrients, such as molybdenum and zinc, are scanty, and further investigations are necessary.

***Alcohol.*** The chronic consumption of alcohol is strongly associated with cancers of the oropharynx, larynx, and esophagus. The risk of these cancers is greatly magnified by concomitant use of alcohol and tobacco. Nonetheless, there is a dose-response relationship between alcohol consumption and the development of oral and esophageal cancers that is independent of concomitant tobacco use. In addition, there is some evidence, although not conclusive, that cancers of the liver, stomach, pancreas, colon, and breast are also associated with increased alcohol consumption. The risk of moderate or occasional alcoholic intake for cancer development is not well established. The mechanism through which alcohol influences carcinogenesis is currently under investigation. Animal studies have failed to identify pure ethanol as a carcinogen. Alcohol may exert its influence through alterations in cellular metabolism and permeability that permit carcinogenic disruption of normal cellular behavior by other chemical substances. Alternatively, alcohol consumption may contribute to malnutrition and increased consumption of other substances associated with enhanced cancer risk.

***Radiation exposure.*** The carcinogenic potential of radiation exposure was appreciated shortly after its discovery as the pioneering scientists who worked with radiation developed skin cancers and leukemias at alarming rates. Radiation comes in a variety of forms and energies. It is an omnipresent risk factor within the environment. Nearly all tissues within the body are susceptible to its carcinogenic effects. Background radiation provides the largest source of exposure for the general population. Light emitted from the sun contains a broad spectrum of radiation energies. The ultraviolet portion of these energies is a major risk factor for the development of basal and squamous cell carcinomas of the skin, as well as melanoma. Ultraviolet radiation is thought to be directly carcinogenic, and risk of subsequent malignancy is directly proportional to received dose. The risk of developing a skin cancer, particularly melanoma, is highest in populations who have the highest exposure by virtue of geographic latitude and skin type. The worldwide incidence of melanoma increases with increasing proximity to the equator. Skin cancers occur most frequently on the areas of the body with the greatest exposure to sunlight. In addition, there are genetically determined differences in susceptibility to ultraviolet radiation. Patients with conditions such as xeroderma pigmentosum are exquisitely sensitive to sunlight-induced skin damage and are at very high risk of developing skin cancer.

Ionizing radiation is also thought to be directly mutagenic. Many of the data regarding the role of ionizing radiation in neoplastic development are derived from studies of individuals exposed to the radiation fallout of the atomic bomb and those receiving medical x-rays for either diagnostic or therapeutic purposes. These populations generally have exposures in excess of 50 Gy and clearly have an increased risk of leukemias and lung and breast cancers. There is also an increased incidence of thyroid and bone cancers within the field of radiation in some studies. Age at the time of exposure appears to be an important ameliorating factor, since the latency period for radiation-induced cancers is often years to decades.

**Table 61-1.** Chemically induced tumors

| Chemical | Tumor site |
|---|---|
| Arsenic | Lung, skin |
| Asbestos | Lung |
| Bis(chloromethyl)ether | Lung |
| Chromium | Lung |
| Nickel | Lung, nasopharynx |
| Betel nut | Oropharynx |
| Isopropyl alcohol | Nasopharynx |
| Cutting oils | Skin |
| Soot, coal tar | Skin |
| Nitrosoamines | Stomach |
| Aflatoxin B1 | Liver |
| Vinyl chloride | Liver, bladder |
| Aromatic amines | Bladder |
| Benzene | Leukemia |
| Radiopharmaceuticals | Liver, bone |

***Chemical exposure.*** The number of chemicals with carcinogenic potential seems to be endless. The daily exposures of individuals to carcinogenic chemicals is difficult to accurately assess given the number and variety of chemicals present in the air, water, and food. Exposures occur within the home as well as through recreational and occupational activities. Certain chemicals have well-documented associations with human neoplasms (Table 61-1). In addition, some medical therapies are also closely linked with increased risk of subsequent cancer. Alkylating agents, such as chlorambucil, cytoxan, and melphalan, were originally developed for use in antineoplastic regimens. These agents are associated with increased risk of subsequent malignancies when used to treat patients with collagen vascular diseases such as rheumatoid arthritis as well as those with cancers. Hormonal therapy with estrogens or androgens has also led to increases in the incidence of particular malignancies. In women the use of exogenous estrogens has been associated with an increased risk of endometrial and breast cancers. Use of diethylstilbestrol (DES) in pregnant women is associated with the development of vaginal clear cell adenocarcinoma in their female offspring. The use of androgens in male athletes has been associated with increased risk of liver cancers. The use of immunosuppressive therapy after organ transplantation is associated with a dramatic increase in the incidence of lymphoma. The potential neoplastic risk of any proposed medical therapy must be clearly understood and weighed carefully against the expected benefit.

***Infections.*** Worldwide infectious agents play an important role in neoplastic development. There are well-documented associations between a number of agents and specific cancers (Table 61-2). The contribution of infectious agents to cancer morbidity and mortality rates within the United States is more limited. Nonetheless, the prevalence of certain infectious agents, particularly herpes simplex II, HBV, and the HIV, mandates heightened public awareness of the role of these agents in neoplastic development.

## Can modification of personal behaviors alter cancer risk?

***Tobacco.*** Numerous clinical trials have demonstrated that physicians are a powerful force in shaping the behavior of patients. Physician-based smoking cessation trials have repeatedly demonstrated that *any* intervention can effectively reduce tobacco use by smoking patients.

**Table 61-2.** Cancers associated with infectious agents

| Infectious agent | Neoplasm |
|---|---|
| Human immunodeficiency virus (HIV) | Lymphoma, Kaposi's sarcoma |
| Human T cell lymphotrophic virus | T cell lymphoma/leukemia |
| Human papillomaviruses | Anogenital carcinoma |
| Herpes simplex virus II | Cervical cancer |
| Epstein-Barr virus | Nasopharyngeal cancer<br>African Burkitt lymphoma |
| Hepatitis B virus (HBV) | Hepatocellular cancer |

Schwartz concluded, after a review of 28 smoking cessation trials, that physician interventions consisting of advice or brief counseling alone resulted in smoking cessation rates of 5% to 10%, whereas more intensive interventions helped 20% to 25% of participants to quit smoking. More intensive smoking cessation programs include specific instructions and prescriptions for pharmacologic measures such as nicotine gum and transdermal patches, extended counseling, or follow-up visits to deal specifically with smoking cessation. The success rates of these interventions may appear disappointingly small. However, if every physician in the United States implemented a smoking cessation program within her or his practice, the public health impact would be enormous. In addition, patients who are unable to eliminate tobacco use completely may benefit from reducing their exposure, since the risk of developing tobacco-related cancers is dose related. Glynn and his colleagues at the National Cancer Institute recommend adopting a simple protocol when counseling individual patients as well as a practice-wide approach to smoking cessation (see the boxes below). See Chapter 124 for further discussion.

***Diet and alcohol.*** Populations with high caloric intakes of fat and low consumption of fiber and certain micronutrients are clearly at increased risk of developing a number of malignancies. How this risk should be interpreted for individual patients is unclear; whether dietary modification for individual patients will alter neoplastic development is controversial; and how diets are modified is also a much debated issue. Kritchevsky, in a review of cancer and diet, emphasized that a high-fiber diet may not be equivalent to a low-fiber diet supplemented with fiber. Vitamin and mineral supplementation may be complicated by unexpected toxicities and may not decrease cancer risk as well as adoption of a diet containing foods rich in these same vitamins and minerals. Several interventional trials designed to address the impact of dietary modifications on neoplastic development and growth are currently under way. These trials are limited by the large number of patients required to achieve statistically reliable results and the long duration between neoplastic incitement and clinically detectable cancer. Several studies have used intermediate markers of neoplastic transformation such as colonic polyp formation and indicators of proliferative activity within target tissues as means of restricting study length. Clinical trials assessing the effect of fiber, calcium, and vitamin supplementation on colonic polyp formation are ongoing. Although colonic polyps are established neoplastic precursors, the import of increased proliferative activity for malignant transformation in other tissues is not clearly established. There is currently a large research effort aimed at the identification and validation of intermediate markers of cancerous growth. An alternative approach is to modify the diet of patients diagnosed with cancer who are at high risk of recurrence or a second primary cancer. The ongoing Women's Intervention Nutrition Study (WINS) addresses the impact of a low-fat diet as an adjuvant to hormonal therapy or chemotherapy for women with early stage breast cancer.

Many authorities feel that the complexity of the human diet, coupled with the many undefined interactions with other factors such as physical activity, precludes firm dietary recommendations for individuals. Other authorities, such as the American Cancer Society and the National Research Council, feel that sufficient data are available on some dietary components to allow for general dietary recommendations. The most recent dietary guidelines promulgated by the American Cancer Society and those of the National Research Council are listed in the boxes below and on p. 810. Specific dietary instructions must be individualized with consideration to comorbid illnesses and conditions. It is notable that most authorities who offer dietary guidelines include limitation of alcoholic intake.

***Radiation and chemical exposure.*** Although exposure to ultraviolet radiation and the consequent risk of skin

### Patient protocol for smoking cessation

Ask about smoking at every opportunity.
Advise all smokers to stop.
Assist patients with stopping by setting a quit date, providing self-help materials, and prescribing nicotine gum if indicated.
Arrange follow-up visits to foster maintenance and prevent relapse.

From Glynn TJ et al: *Semin Oncol* 17(4):391, 1990.

### Office protocol for patient smoking cessation

Select an office smoking-cessation coordinator.
Create a smoke-free office.
Identify all smoking patients.
Develop patient smoking cessation plans.
Provide follow-up support.

From Glynn TJ et al: *Semin Oncol* 17(4):391, 1990.

### Dietary guidelines of the American Cancer Society

Maintain a desirable body weight.
Eat a varied diet.
Include a variety of both vegetables and fruits in the daily diet.
Eat more high-fiber foods, such as whole grain cereals, legumes, vegetables, and fruits.
Cut down on total fat intake.
Limit consumption of alcoholic beverages, if you drink at all.
Limit consumption of salt-cured, smoked, and nitrite-preserved foods.

From Weinhouse S et al: *CA Cancer J Clin* 41(6):334, 1991.

## National Research Council dietary guidelines to prevent cancer

Eat a variety of foods.
Maintain a healthy weight.
Choose a diet low in fat, saturated fat, and cholesterol.
Choose a diet with plenty of vegetables, fruits, and grain products.
Use salt and sodium only in moderation.
If you drink alcoholic beverages, do so in moderation.

From Ashley JM: *Oncology* 7(115):27, 1993.

cancers can be minimized through the use of protective clothing and sunscreens, the largest source of radiation exposure is from the general background. Not only is this exposure difficult to quantify and almost impossible to limit, it is also likely to increase with progressive deterioration of the atmospheric ozone layer. However, exposure to medical and dental radiation, the second largest source of radiation exposure, can be limited. Physicians should demonstrate restraint in the use of diagnostic and therapeutic radiation, particularly in patients who are young, are pregnant, or have benign medical conditions. The cumulative exposure to medical radiation can be monitored by carefully recording within a patient's medical record all diagnostic radiographic studies as well as the total dose and target of any therapeutic radiation administered. The careful recording of radiation exposure as routinely practiced by radiation oncologists might serve as a paradigm for primary care physicians and as a mechanism for monitoring individual exposures.

In a similar fashion, patients who receive treatment with medications such as alkylating agents and hormones, which carry an increased risk of subsequent malignancy, should have the dosage and duration of treatment carefully monitored in the medical record. Prominent labeling of individual charts can facilitate a monitoring program. The risks and benefits of these potentially carcinogenic therapies should be reviewed periodically in any patient who receives treatment for prolonged periods.

The exposure to occupational and industrial carcinogens can be minimized by the use of equipment such as gloves, protective clothing, and masks in appropriate situations. Physicians should encourage the use of such protective gear.

However, often the hazards of chemical substances are unknown or patients are unaware of the specific exposures they have experienced. Recent legislation requiring employers to inform workers of potentially hazardous substances in the workplace may improve patients' cognizance of exposures. This in turn might lead to a better understanding of the role some chemical substances play in carcinogenesis in humans. Discussion of the occupational environment of individual patients and documentation of reported exposures within the medical record may serve several purposes. The patient may not be aware of the risk inherent in agents that are known to have carcinogenic potential and therefore may not adequately use protective equipment. Second, documentation of exposures may allow associations to be identified at a future date.

**Table 61-3.** Selected chemopreventive agents under investigation

| Agent | Mechanism of action |
|---|---|
| 4-HPR | Stimulates differentiation |
| Piroxicam | Is prostaglandin synthesis inhibitor |
| DMFO | Is ornithine decarboxylase inhibitor |
| DHEA, DHEA analogue(s) | Is glucose-6-phosphate dehydrogenase inhibitor |
| 4-HPR–tamoxifen | Stimulates differentiation |
| 4-HPR–selenite–vitamin E | Has various mechanisms |
| β-Carotene | Is antioxidant |
| β-Carotene–vitamin A | Stimulates differentiation, is antioxidant |
| Molybdate | Maintains differentiation |

*DHEA*, Dehydroepiandrosterone; *4-HPR*, all-trans-4-hydroxyphenylthetinamide.
From Kelloff GJ et al: *Semin Oncol* 17(4):438, 1990.

***Infections.*** Alterations in sexual behavior might well lead to diminished risk for cancers associated with sexually transmitted infectious agents such as herpes simplex II and HIV. Patients who engage in unprotected sexual activities with multiple partners are at particularly high risk of becoming infected. Physicians should ask about sexual practices and advise patients of the associated risks of infection and subsequent malignancy. This is particularly important in those patients who have no current evidence of infection with these agents. Patients who do manifest evidence of infection should receive regular follow-up with attention to evaluating the presence of neoplastic processes.

Patients with exposure to bloodborne agents should be encouraged to take appropriate precautions. Individuals with occupational exposures to blood and body fluids should be advised to routinely use protective gear. Intravenous drug users should be discouraged from sharing hypodermic needles. Finally, the HBV vaccine should be offered to all individuals at high risk of exposure to this infectious agent.

### Chemoprevention

Despite the best efforts of physicians and patients, not all malignancies are avoidable through alterations in personal behaviors. The nascent science of chemoprevention offers hope that the development of neoplastic processes can be interrupted and reversed. Although the term *chemoprevention* was coined in the 1970s, the concept of using specific chemical compounds to interfere with neoplastic development and prevent cancer dates back to the earliest days of anticancer research. However, the enhanced understanding of carcinogenesis at the biochemical, molecular, and genetic level that has arisen over the past decade has allowed this concept to become a reality.

There are many chemical compounds that effectively inhibit carcinogenesis. Table 61-3 provides a partial list of compounds under active investigation for application to

### CAUTION: Cancer's warning signals

*C*hange in bowel or bladder habits
*A* sore that does not heal
*U*nusual bleeding or discharge
*T*hickening or lump in breast or elsewhere
*I*ndigestion or difficulty in swallowing
*O*bvious change in wart or mole
*N*agging cough or hoarseness

cancer prevention. Preliminary studies have demonstrated that several agents can decrease the risk of second malignancies in patients diagnosed with cancer. Use of tamoxifen after the diagnosis of breast cancer has led to a decrease in the incidence of second primary breast cancers in the contralateral breast. A randomized, double blind clinical trial of a derivative of vitamin A, 13-*cis*-retinoic acid, has demonstrated the ability to prevent second primary squamous cell carcinomas when administered at high doses to patients successfully treated for squamous cell carcinomas of the head and neck. In addition, vitamin A and related retinoids appear to have some activity in preventing the initial development of head and neck cancers when administered to patients at high risk for these malignancies. Toxicity and compliance have been major problems in chemoprevention trials. Currently there are several ongoing, large cooperative group trials investigating chemoprevention for a variety of malignancies—breast, prostate, colon, and lung. The results of these large clinical trials will not be available for some time. Nonetheless, the results are anxiously awaited and may radically change the management of oncologic processes.

## SCREENING

Early detection of cancers through screening has the potential to reduce cancer-related mortality significantly. It is estimated that successful implementation of screening programs could reduce the mortality of specific cancers by as much as 60%.

### Screening methods

A broad array of methods can be used to enhance early detection of cancers. The spectrum includes public education to heighten awareness of malignancies and increase familiarity with early warning signs (see the box above), as well as risk assessment, health surveys, instruction in self-examination, physician examination, and mass screening. The vast majority of these methods are directly within the purview of the primary care physician. However, the extent of screening activity varies widely among physicians' practices. Those practices with a systematic approach to the preventive services are often the most successful at achieving and maintaining high levels of screening. The components of a successful practice-based implementation of cancer screening are outlined in the box above. For specific recommendations on screening guidelines please refer to Chapter 2 for breast cancer, cervical cancer, colorectal cancer, and prostate cancer; to Chapter 21 for skin cancer; to Chapter 32 for head, neck, and oral cancer; and to Chapter 141 for testicular cancer.

### Implementation of office-based cancer screening

Determine level of current practice screening activity.
Set measurable screening goals.
Develop a comprehensive plan to achieve and maintain goals.
Encourage staff training and active participation in screening activities.
Ensure that office systems, design, and organization facilitate screening.
Develop state-of-the-art skills in early detection and screening techniques.
Develop state-of-the-art counseling and communication skills.
Use reminder systems to ensure that patients at risk are identified, screened, and followed.
Exploit every opportunity to perform screening and prevention.
Minimize cost barriers for patients whenever possible.

## FOLLOW-UP

Cancer is increasingly curable. Approximately 40% to 50% of those diagnosed with cancer survive the disease. Countless others live for extended periods with treatment-responsive disease. These numbers are likely to increase in the future as the anticancer armamentarium expands with new strategies and methods. All of these patients require follow-up to monitor for distant effects of cancer therapy, recurrence of disease, or development of additional primary tumors.

A reasonable follow-up strategy for the most common and/or most treatable malignancies is suggested in Table 61-4. The natural history of the primary cancer determines the frequency and procedures of follow-up. In addition, cancer survivors may be at increased risk of primary cancers in second or third sites and should continue to undergo routine cancer screening. It is important to note that few follow-up strategies have been subjected to the same rigorous analyses that have been required for screening strategies. Nonetheless, early detection of recurrent tumors may allow some patients to be saved with additional treatment. For example, a rising carcinoembryonic antigen (CEA) after resection of a colon cancer might detect local recurrence or isolated hepatic or pulmonary metastases. Some patients with hepatic metastases confined to one lobe or region of the liver can be cured by hepatic resection. Whereas the mean survival for patients with metastatic disease is 24 months, the 5-year survival for patients with isolated hepatic or pulmonary metastases is approximately 30%.

Some investigators question the benefit of periodic follow-up, suggesting that the improved survival associated with detection of occult recurrences may result from lead time and length bias. The increasing use of tumor markers for periodic follow-up has fueled the controversy over what constitutes appropriate follow-up. Many tumor markers are nonspecific and can be elevated by nonma-

**Table 61-4.** Possible strategies for follow-up of selected cancers

| Cancer site | Follow-up frequency | Regimen for each follow-up visit | Additional follow-up |
|---|---|---|---|
| Prostate | Every 3-4 mo × 3 yr; then every 6 mo × 2 yr; then annually | Complete history<br>Physical examination<br>Complete blood count<br>Hepatic transaminases<br>Alkaline phosphatase<br>PSA | |
| Breast | Every 3 mo × 3 yr; then every 6 mo × 2 yr; then annually | Complete history<br>Physical examination<br>Complete blood count<br>Hepatic transaminases<br>Alkaline phosphatase<br>Calcium | Mammography every 12 mo; CXR every 6-12 mo |
| Lung | Every 3 mo × 3 yr; then every 6 mo × 3 yr; then annually | Complete history<br>Physical examination<br>Complete blood count<br>Hepatic transaminases<br>Alkaline phosphatase<br>BUN/creatinine<br>Calcium phosphate<br>CXR | Chest CT with cuts through the liver and adrenals every 6-12 mo |
| Colorectal | Every 3 mo × 2 yr; then every 6 mo × 3 yr; then annually | Complete history<br>Physical examination<br>Complete blood count<br>Hepatic transaminases<br>Alkaline phosphatase<br>CEA (if elevated before surgery)<br>Sigmoidoscopy (if S/P anterior resection of rectal lesion) | CXR annually<br>Colonoscopy (every 3-6 mo after surgery in patients with obstructing lesion)<br>*or*<br>Colonoscopy (at 1 yr after surgery; if negative then every 2-3 yr in patients without an obstructing lesion) |
| Bladder | Every 3 mo × 2 yr; then every 6 mo × 3 yr; then annually | Complete history<br>Physical examination<br>Complete blood count<br>Hepatic transaminases<br>Alkaline phosphatase<br>BUN/creatinine<br>Urinalysis, urine cytology | Cystoscopy and urethral washings with each visit (when organ has been preserved) |
| Uterine cervix | Every 3 mo × 1 yr; then every 4 mo × 1 yr; then every 6 mo × 3 yr; then annually | Complete history<br>Physical examination<br>Complete blood count<br>Hepatic transaminases<br>Alkaline phosphatase<br>BUN/creatinine<br>Urinalysis<br>CXR<br>Colposcopy | Abdominal/pelvic CT every 6-12 mo × 3-5 yr |
| Testicular | Every 1 mo × 1 yr; then every 2 mo × 1 yr; then every 3-6 mo thereafter | Complete history<br>Physical examination<br>Complete blood count<br>Hepatic transaminases<br>Alkaline phosphatase<br>CXR<br>Serum tumor markers (α-fetoprotein, β-subunit of human chorionic gonadotropin) | Abdominal/pelvic CT every 2-3 mo × 1 yr; then every 6 mo |
| Oropharyngeal | Every 1 mo × 1 yr; then every 2-3 mo × 2 yr; then every 6 mo × 2 yr; then annually | Complete history<br>Physical examination | CXR<br>Indirect laryngoscopy<br>Sputum cytology |
| Skin (melanoma) | Every 3 mo × 2 yr; then every 6 mo × 4 yr; then annually | Complete history<br>Physical examination<br>Complete blood count<br>Hepatic transaminases<br>Alkaline phosphatase | |

*BUN*, Blood urea nitrogen; *CXR*, chest x-ray; *CT*, computed tomography; *CEA*, carcinoembryonic antigen.

**Table 61-5.** Tumor-associated antigens with efficacy in follow-up

| Serum tumor marker | Useful in following |
|---|---|
| Prostate-specific antigen | Prostate cancer |
| Carcinoembryonic antigen | Colon cancer |
| CA 125 | Ovarian cancer |
| α-Fetoprotein | Testicular, liver cancer |
| β-Subunit of human chorionic gonadotropin | Testicular cancer |

lignant as well as malignant processes. An elevated CEA after breast cancer can lead to an extensive, costly search for a pathologic etiology. The sensitivity of the CEA assay may exceed the ability to detect recurrent lesions. The resultant fruitless search may leave the alarmed patient and clinician unsatisfied and frustrated. Some tumor markers have well-defined roles in cancer follow-up, as outlined in Table 61-5. Although controversy over appropriate follow-up regimens persists, detection of abnormalities in any follow-up study should prompt a complete diagnostic evaluation and referral when appropriate.

## BIBLIOGRAPHY

Ashley JM: Dietary guidelines for cancer prevention and control, *Oncology* 7(11S):27, 1993.

Boring CC et al: Cancer statistics, 1994, *CA Cancer J Clin* 44(1):7, 1994.

Chu KC, Smart CR, Tarone RE: Analysis of breast cancer mortality and stage-distribution by age for the Health Insurance Plan Study: a randomized trial with breast cancer screening, *J Natl Cancer Inst* 80(14):1125, 1988.

Cullen JW, Greenwald P: Prevention of cancer. In Edelstein BA, Michelson L, editors: *Handbook of prevention,* New York, 1986, Plenum Press.

Eddy DM: Screening for cervical cancer, *Ann Intern Med* 113(3):214; (5):373, 1990.

Fahs MC et al: Cost effectiveness of cervical cancer screening for the elderly, *Ann Intern Med* 117(6):520, 1992.

Garfinkel L: Nutrition and cancer: current status, *CA Cancer J Clin* 41(6):325, 1991.

Gerber GS et al: Disease-specific survival following routine prostate cancer screening by digital rectal examination, *JAMA* 269(1):61, 1993.

Gilbertsen VA: Cancer of the prostate gland, *JAMA* 215(1):81, 1971.

Glynn TJ et al: Cancer prevention through physician intervention, *Semin Oncol* 17(4):391, 1990.

Glynn TJ: Relative effectiveness of physician-initiated smoking cessation programs, *Cancer Bull* 40:359, 1988.

Hong WK et al: Prevention of second primary tumors with isotretinoin in squamous-cell carcinoma of the head and neck, *N Engl J Med* 323(12):795, 1990.

Jenson CB, Shahon DB, Wangensteen OH: Evaluation of annual examinations in the detection of cancer, *JAMA* 174(14):1783, 1960.

Kelloff GJ et al: Progress in applied chemoprevention research, *Semin Oncol* 17(4):438, 1990.

Kritchevsky D: Diet and cancer, *CA Cancer J Clin* 41(6):328, 1991.

Lashner BA, Silverstein MD: Evaluation and therapy of the patient with fecal occult blood loss: a decision analysis, *Am J Gastroenterol* 85(9):1088, 1990.

Littrup PF, Goodman AC, Mettlin CJ: The benefit and cost of prostate cancer early detection, *CA Cancer J Clin* 43(3):134, 1993.

Mandel JS et al: Reducing mortality from colorectal cancer by screening for fecal occult blood, *N Engl J Med* 328(19):1365, 1993.

Mettlin C, Dodd GD: The American Cancer Society guidelines for the cancer-related checkup: an update, *Cancer* 41(5):279, 1991.

Miller AB: Screening for cancer: state of the art and prospects for the future, *World J Surg* 13(1):79, 1989.

Rogers AE, Conner MW: Interrelationships of alcohol and cancer. In Alfin-Slater RB, Kritchevsky D, editors: Human nutrition: a comprehensive treatise, volume 7, New York, 1991, Plenum Press.

Sackett DL, Holland WW: Controversy in the detection of disease, *Lancet* 2(7930):357, 1975.

Schwartz JL: Review and evaluation of smoking cessation methods: the United States and Canada, 1978-1985, *NIH Pub No 87-2940,* Bethesda, MD, 1987, National Cancer Institute.

Smart CR: Screening and early cancer detection, *Semin Oncol* 17(4):456, 1990.

Tomin R, Donegan WL: Screening for recurrent breast cancer: its effectiveness and prognostic value, *J Clin Oncol* 5(1):62, 1987.

Trock B, Lanza E, Greenwald P: Dietary fiber, vegetables, and colon cancer: critical review and meta-analyses of the epidemiologic evidence, *J Natl Cancer Inst* 82(8):650, 1990.

Vargas PA, Alberts DS: Colon cancer: the quest for prevention, *Oncology* 7(11S):33, 1993.

Weinhouse S et al: American Cancer Society guidelines on diet, nutrition, and cancer, *CA Cancer J Clin* 41(6):334, 1991.

Wynder EL, Cohen LA: Nutritional opportunities and limitations in cancer prevention, *Oncology* 7(11S):13, 1993.

CHAPTER

# 62 Fever and Rash

Jennifer S. Daly
Richard H. Glew

Fever has long been recognized by the public as a sign of disease. For physicians, the integument is a large organ system that provides a window into conditions that commonly present with fever. Throughout history rash and fever have often been associated with contagious infectious diseases and may instill fear in the patient as well as in family and neighbors. The presence of a rash often brings the patient to seek medical care and at the same time provides important diagnostic clues to the physician as to the nature of the underlying cause. On occasion the presence of skin lesions permits rapid diagnosis of an easily recognized exanthematous illness, whereas in other instances an etiologic diagnosis is established only after extensive cultures, serologic and immunologic evaluation, other laboratory examinations, or a skin biopsy. Fever and rash occur not only as part of an acute microbial infection, but also may be the presenting signs of a connective tissue disorder, microangiopathic disorders, or related to the immune response to an infectious agent.

## EPIDEMIOLOGY AND ETIOLOGY

The first priority in evaluating a patient with fever and rash is to decide the degree of urgency suggested by the clinical presentation. The practitioner must decide if the patient is likely to be suffering from a benign, self-limited disease requiring no confirmatory tests or therapy, or is critically ill with a potentially fatal illness requiring immediate diagnostic evaluation and prompt therapy. The examiner must decide if the patient is possibly infected with a highly contagious organism and requires isolation precautions.

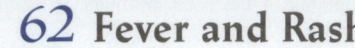

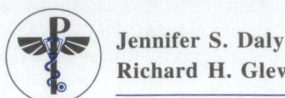

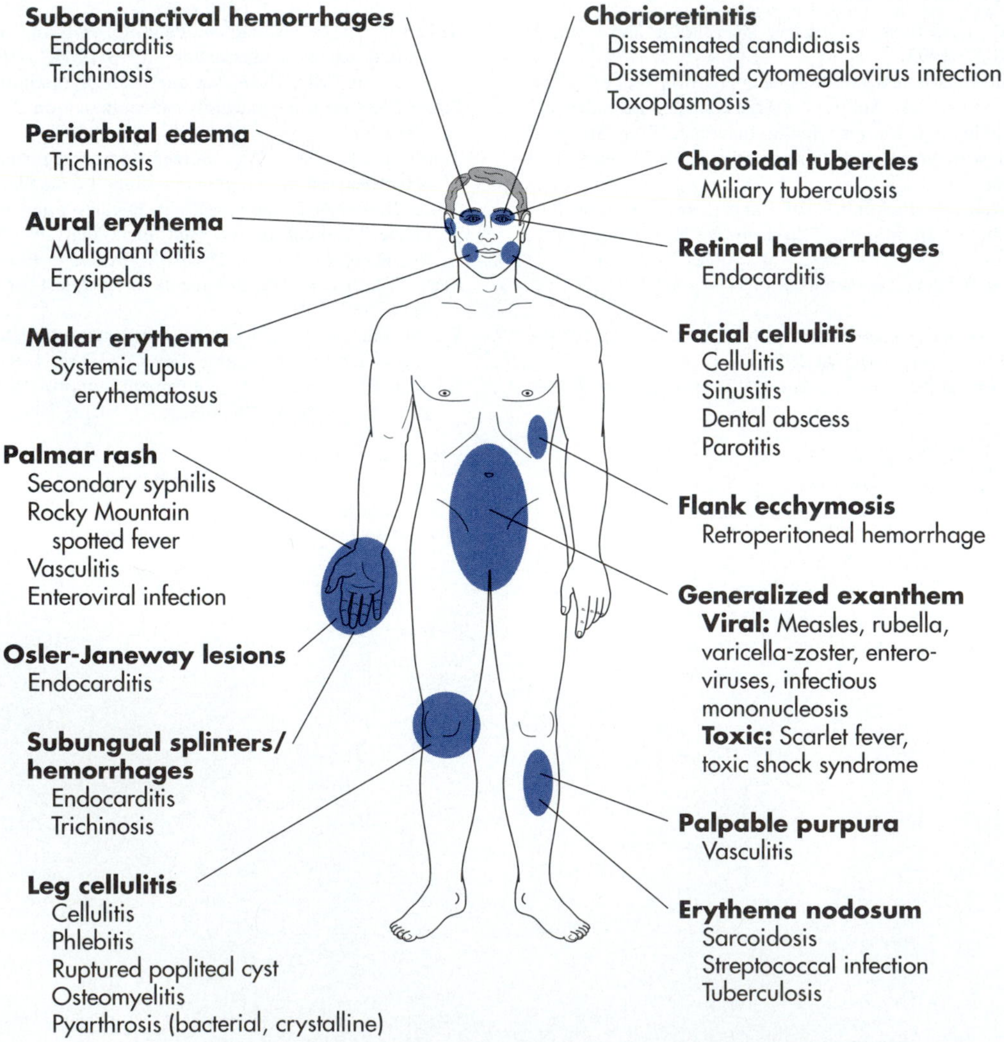


**Fig. 62-1.** Integumentary evidence of disseminated infections.

**Table 62-1.** Febrile illnesses frequently associated with rash

| Disease | Pathogen |
|---|---|
| **Maculopapular eruptions** | |
| ***Classic exanthems of childhood*** | |
| Rubeola (measles) | Rubeola virus |
| Rubella (German measles) | Rubeola virus |
| Exanthema subitum (roseola) | Human herpes virus 6 |
| Scarlet fever | Group A streptococci |
| Erythema infectiosum (fifth disease) | Human parvovirus B19 |
| ***Herpes viruses*** | |
| Mononucleosis syndromes | Epstein-Barr virus (with or without antibiotic administration)<br>Cytomegalovirus |
| ***Enteroviruses*** | |
| Aseptic meningitis | Coxsackieviruses |
| Febrile syndromes | Echoviruses |
| ***Retroviruses*** | |
| Mononucleosis-like illness | HIV-1 (acute infection) |
| ***Bacteria*** | |
| Lyme disease | *Borrelia burgdorferi* |
| Leptospirosis | *Leptospira* species |
| Relapsing fever | *Borrelia* species |
| Syphilis (secondary) | *Treponema pallidum* |
| Typhoid fever | *Salmonella typhi* |
| ***Mycoplasmas*** | |
| Primary atypical pneumonia | *Mycoplasma pneumoniae* |
| ***Rickettsiae*** | |
| Rocky mountain spotted fever | *Rickettsia rickettsii* |
| Endemic murine typhus | *Rickettsia typhi* |
| Epidemic louse-borne typhus | *Rickettsia prowazekii* |
| ***Parasites*** | |
| Mononucleosis/lymphadenopathy | *Toxoplasma gondii* |
| ***Immune-mediated conditions*** | |
| Medication reaction | Many agents, especially sulfa drugs, penicillins, allopurinol, diuretics, dilantin |
| Systemic lupus erythematosus | |
| Adult Still's disease | |
| Dermatomyositis | |
| Acute rheumatic fever (erythema marginata) | |
| Papules, urticaria, and pruritus of pregnancy (PUPP) | |
| Contact dermatitis | |
| **Diffuse erythema** | |
| Scarlet fever | Group A streptococci |
| Toxic shock syndrome | *Staphylococcus aureus* (occasionally group A streptococci) |
| Kawasaki disease, (mucocutaneous lymph node syndrome) | Unknown |
| Staphylococcal scalded skin syndrome | *S. aureus* |
| Medication reaction | See above |
| Toxic epidermal necrolysis | Graft-versus-host disease |

*Continued.*

Finally, the practitioner must decide if the patient's illness is a localized cutaneous process or a manifestation of a systemic disease (Fig. 62-1).

Epidemiologic clues are uncovered via extensive, meticulous, and dogged historical analysis. Physicians should explore the patient's recent or past exposure to infectious diseases and potential allergens or toxins. History should be sought concerning travel to exotic lands and within temperate regions (e.g., coccidioidomycosis via travel to the southwestern United States or Lyme disease via travel to the coastal Northeast); occupations and avocations; sexual practices; use of illicit drugs; dietary habits (e.g., consumption of raw or undercooked meats or fish, unpasteurized milk); pet or animal contacts, including hunting or fishing; and similar illnesses recently in family members or the local community.

## Pathophysiology

A localized or discrete rash can occur secondarily to infections, toxins, inflammatory conditions, or contact allergy. Localized infections of the skin and skin structure often become established via a disruption in normal skin integrity and often involve minor trauma not apparent to the patient at the moment of occurrence or to the physician at the time the infection is diagnosed. Secondary infections occur in areas with a preexisting abnormality or lesion, such as atopic dermatitis, chronic edema (occasionally subtle and commonly related to prior surgery, long-bone fracture, cellulitis, thrombophlebitis, or radiation therapy), peripheral vascular disease, or in patients with obvious penetrating trauma, allergic dermatitis (e.g., poison ivy), burns, or insect bites and stings. Systemic symptoms, such as fever, chills, and malaise, may occur.

**Table 62-1.** Febrile illnesses frequently associated with rash—cont'd

| Disease | Pathogen |
|---|---|
| **Vesiculobullous eruptions** | |
| ***Viruses*** | |
| Chickenpox | Varicella-zoster virus |
| Shingles | Varicella-zoster virus |
| Fever blisters/gingivostomatitis | Herpes simplex virus |
| Eczema herpeticum | Herpes simplex virus |
| Hand, foot, and mouth disease | Coxsackievirus |
| Herpangina | Coxsackievirus |
| Aseptic meningitis | Echoviruses, coxsackievirus |
| ***Rickettsiae*** | |
| Rickettsialpox | *R. akari* |
| ***Immune-mediated conditions*** | |
| Medication reaction (see above; Stevens-Johnson syndrome) | |
| **Pustular** | |
| ***Viruses*** | |
| Febrile syndrome | Coxsackieviruses |
| ***Bacteria*** | |
| Folliculitis | *S. aureus*<br>*Pseudomonas aeruginosa* (hot tubs) |
| Furunculosis | *S. aureus* |
| Dermatitis/arthritis | *Neisseria gonorrhoeae* |
| ***Noninfectious conditions*** | |
| Behçet disease (keratoderma blennorrhagicum) | Unknown |
| **Papulosquamous** | |
| Reiter's syndrome | Triggered by enteritis or urethritis |
| **Purpuric** | |
| ***Bacteria*** | |
| Bacteremia/endocarditis | *S. aureus* |
| Bacteremia/ecthyma gangrenosum | *P. aeruginosa* |
| Tularemia/necrotic eschar | *Francisella tularensis* |
| ***Rickettsiae*** | |
| Rocky mountain spotted fever | *R. rickettsii* |
| Typhus | *R. prowazekii*<br>*R. typhi*<br>*R. tsutsugamushi* |
| ***Postinfectious/autoimmune conditions*** | |
| Allergic (Henoch-Schoenlein) purpura | Poststreptococcal infection |
| Thrombotic thrombocytopenic purpura | Unknown |
| Hemolytic-uremic syndrome | Postenteritis condition (e.g., enterotoxigenic *Escherichia coli*) |
| Leukocytoclastic vasculitis | See text |

Diffuse, generalized rash and fever can be the result of infectious agents or noninfectious processes such as medication allergy, autoimmune disease, neutrophilic dermatoses, toxins, and neoplasia. Idiopathic disorders such as Kawasaki disease are uncommon but may need to be considered if the etiology of the patient's illness evades diagnosis after several days. In both infection-associated and noninfectious cases the rash is often a result of vasculitis, a process characterized pathologically by inflammatory changes and necrosis of blood vessels. Vasculitic lesions may be composed of various inflammatory cells, including neutrophils and lymphocytes, or granulomas. Vessel-based neutrophilic dermatoses include leukocytoclastic vasculitis (hypersensitivity angiitis), Sweet's syndrome (acute febrile neutrophilic dermatosis), pyoderma gangrenosum, pustular vasculitis, familial Mediterranean fever, and erythema nodosum (Table 62-1). Leukocytoclastic vasculitis presents clinically as palpable purpura and is encountered commonly on skin biopsy of vasculitic lesions. Histologically the small blood vessels in the skin exhibit infiltration with neutrophils, including neutrophil debris or dust. Various microorganisms can produce rashes by different pathophysiologic mechanisms. Some agents are bloodborne and multiply in the skin (e.g., herpes viruses), others produce toxins (e.g., *Staphylococcus aureus* and *Streptococcus* species), some evoke an inflammatory response (*Neisseria gonorrhoeae, Salmonella typhi*), and others have a direct effect on blood vessels (e.g., *Rickettsiae*).

## HISTORY

The physician needs to obtain a complete inventory of current or recently consumed medications, chronic illnesses and conditions, significant past illnesses and operations, allergies (both to natural products and medications), exposures to chemicals, and recent changes in the patient's lifestyle or personal habits. Specific areas to address within each part of the history follow.

### Host factors

Review of the patients underlying conditions, illnesses, and treatments can help the physician decide whether the patient is predisposed to infections that are likely to be fulminant or fatal and therefore must be treated urgently, such as (1) gram-negative bacteremia in the patient with malignancy, neutropenia, or alcoholism or (2) staphylococcal bacteremia in the parenteral drug user, dialysis patient, or patient recently hospitalized. Toxic shock syndrome should be considered in a menstruating woman or a patient with recent surgery, including nasal surgery with packing in place. Fulminant bacteremia due to *Streptococcus pyogenes, S. pneumoniae,* or *Neisseria meningitidis,* occasionally occurs in previously healthy patients but should be suspected in a patient who has had a splenectomy, and it should be treated promptly with antibiotics. Additional host factors, such as therapy with immunosuppressive drugs, infection due to human immunodeficiency virus (HIV-1), malignancy, and immunoglobulin deficiency or complement disorder, may lead to unusually severe infection with a common pathogen or infection with organisms that are usually nonpathogenic. Deficiencies of the terminal components of complement (C6, C7, C8) predispose individuals to recurrent meningococcemia and disseminated gonococcal infection.

### Medical history

The patient should be asked about prior illnesses, hospitalizations, surgery, and blood transfusions. Transfusion of blood or blood components can result in hepatitis B, which can present as fever, arthralgia/arthritis, and a diffuse rash (often urticaria). Superficial or deep surgical wounds and seromata may become infected with *S. aureus* and produce toxic shock syndrome without overt local wound infection.

### Family history

The physician should take a complete family history involving parents, grandparents, siblings, and children. A family history of immune deficiency, recurrent infections, or diseases associated with autosplenectomy (such as sickle cell disease and other hemoglobinopathies) may predispose the patient to overwhelming infection, especially with *Streptococcus pneumoniae, Haemophilus influenzae,* and other encapsulated organisms. Hereditary or acquired disorders associated with hemolysis can predispose to unusually severe infection due to *Mycoplasma pneumoniae* or *Salmonella* species. A family history of autoimmune disorders may be a clue suggesting the need for rheumatologic evaluation.

### Personal and social history

A history of travel or residence in areas endemic for fungal pathogens or parasitic diseases, including Lyme disease, or recent exposure to animals or insect vectors can be a clue to etiology. The physician should inquire about recent exposures to febrile illnesses in the family or social/work/school setting. The eating of raw or undercooked meat can predispose to an infectious mononucleosis-like illness such as toxoplasmosis, brucellosis (also may present as arthritis, relapsing fever, or osteomyelitis), or trichinosis (presentation with myalgia, fever, periorbital edema, and splinter hemorrhages subconjunctivally and subungually). Ingestion of unpasteurized milk or cheese may result in toxoplasmosis and brucellosis. Ingestion of raw shellfish by patients with cirrhosis can produce disseminated infection due to *Vibrio vulnificus,* resulting in fever, shock, and hemorrhagic skin lesions. Questions about sexual encounters and practices may reveal likely exposure to gonorrhea, syphilis, or hepatitis B. However, many patients may be reluctant to give an accurate sexual history. If skin lesions suggest sexually transmitted disease (see Chapter 65), the physician should not hesitate to perform appropriate diagnostic tests even if the patient reports no risk factors or behavior. If a sexually transmitted disease is confirmed, the physician should again question the patient firmly but compassionately, since there may be a need for contact tracing.

### Present illness

A careful history of the temporal evolution of symptoms and signs is important. Patients with a diffuse rash and fever may be categorized according to the type of skin lesions, the tempo and sequence of their evolution, and the spectrum and the pace of development of associated signs and symptoms. For example, the patient who presents with fever, rash, and joint pain due to gonococcal septic arthritis commonly relates an antecedent history of several days of polyarthralgias and is noted to have an asymmetric acral distribution of papulopustular skin lesions, occasionally with a history of symptoms suggesting prior or ongoing genital gonorrhea. The patient who presents with a history of fever and rash occurring over weeks to months may be more likely to have an autoimmune disorder or may need the thorough, sequential, and deliberate evaluation undertaken in patients with classic fever of unknown origin (see Chapter 63). The physician must listen to the patient and repeat questions to encourage recall of historical information, to find forgotten or suppressed details, and to gain new insights.

## PHYSICAL EXAMINATION

The physical examination of the febrile patient begins with the skin and mucous membranes, including conjunctivae, oropharynx, and the anogenital region. Externally, primary infections of skin (e.g., cellulitis) may be detected or there may be integumentary evidence of disseminated infection: (1) the petechial-to-purpuric rash of meningococcemia (Fig. 62-2, *A*) or Rocky Mountain spotted fever, (2) embolic lesions (splinter hemorrhages, Osler's nodes or Janeway lesions) of endocarditis (Fig. 62-2, *B*), and (3) palpable purpura or necrotic papules of systemic vasculitis or gonococcemia (Fig. 62-2, *C*). Alternatively, exanthemata may reflect disease resulting from toxins, such as the

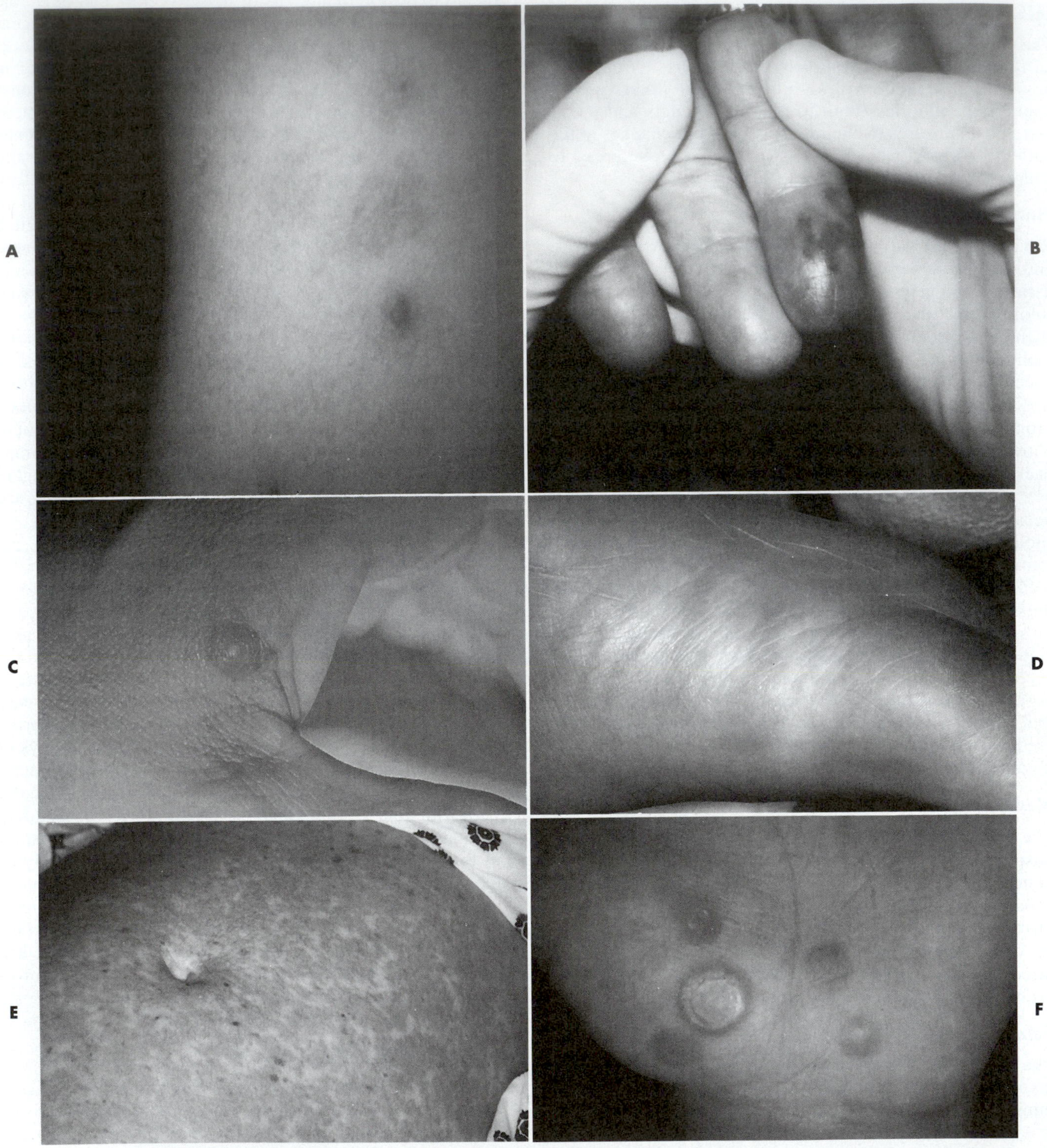


**Fig. 62-2.** **A,** Papular/purpuric lesions (arm) in a patient with meningococcal meningitis; **B,** purpuric lesions (finger) in a patient with *Staphylococcus aureus* endocarditis; **C,** pustular lesion (hand) in a patient with disseminated gonococcemia; **D,** diffuse erythroderma (foot) in a patient with toxic shock syndrome; **E,** maculopapular rash (abdomen) in a patient with primary infection with rubeola (measles); **F,** maculopapular rash (hand) in a patient with secondary syphilis.

sunburnlike erythroderma of scarlet fever and toxic shock syndrome (Fig. 62-2, *D*) or immunologic mechanisms (medication reactions, connective tissue diseases, vasculitis). Although the childhood exanthematous diseases (e.g., rubella, rubeola [Fig. 62-2, *E*]) may produce classic eruptions in children or adults, these can be simulated in adults by infections due to viruses (infectious mononucleosis) and spirochetes (secondary syphilis [Fig. 62-2, *F*]) and manifested in unusual or muted fashion in patients with prior immunization (atypical measles).

Careful examination should be conducted of the chest, heart, and abdomen. Examination of the musculoskeletal system includes a search for local tenderness, warmth, swelling, or erythema, as well as manipulation of all accessible joints for the presence of effusions or restriction of motion. A diligent search must be carried out for localized or generalized lymphadenopathy. Particular attention should be directed to areas highlighted in the history. In the acutely ill, febrile patient examination of the tympanic membranes, mouth, genitalia, rectum, and pelvis and neurologic assessment should not be deferred because one may chance upon clues that will allow diagnosis of the underlying etiology in a patient presenting with fever and rash. In persistently enigmatic cases the patient may need to be examined repeatedly during the day. For example, the rash associated with adult Still's disease is often evanescent and is most obvious during a period of high fever.

## LABORATORY STUDIES

No laboratory test is routine in the evaluation of the patient with fever and rash. The extent and timing of laboratory use are determined by several factors: (1) severity and acuity of the patient's condition, (2) presence of debilitating or compromising underlying diseases, (3) occurrence of symptoms that indicate focused investigation (abscess, drainage, cough, sputum production, pleurisy, or petechial lesions), (4) physical findings that establish a virtually certain diagnosis with little need for laboratory assistance, (5) the likelihood that presumptive antibiotic therapy will be instituted before the diagnosis is confirmed, and (6) the differential diagnosis arrived at by the physician first examining the patient. Because antibiotics may inhibit the growth of bacteria from subsequent blood cultures, at least two blood cultures should be obtained before beginning antibiotic therapy in certain outpatients (e.g., patients with organic valvular heart disease who are about to be given oral antibiotics for a febrile illness and who may be harboring bacterial endocarditis) and in virtually all patients acutely ill enough to warrant parenteral antibiotic therapy. Patients who are producing sputum warrant a sputum culture. It should be recalled that *S. aureus* pneumonia, often complicating influenza, can produce a diffuse erythroderma and toxic shock syndrome, and patients with mycoplasmal pneumonia may present with a nonspecific erythematous macular rash or with erythema multiforme.

A low threshold should be maintained for sampling abnormal collections of fluid (pleural or joint effusions and ascites) for examination and culture. An often troubling question is whether to perform a lumbar puncture. Although headache may occur in many febrile illnesses without direct central nervous system involvement, cerebrospinal fluid should be sampled immediately in patients with fever and rash who have severe headache, altered mental status, or stiff neck. A lumbar puncture should be considered in patients whose sensorium is difficult to interpret, such as infants and the elderly, and in patients with altered mental status and cutaneous manifestations compatible with disseminated bacterial infection even in the absence of fever. Cultures for respiratory viruses (via throat washings/swab or sputum) or enteroviruses (via throat washings/swab or stool) are relatively expensive and only moderately sensitive, thereby proving more useful as an epidemiologic tool than as a guide to management of the individual patient. Skin biopsy may be helpful in establishing the diagnosis either through pathologic examination, culturing of the specimen, or immunologic staining, but it is expensive, and results may not be available for days. Biopsy of skin lesions may be of utility in diagnosing Rocky Mountain spotted fever, since serologic tests usually require several days to provide positive results in rickettsial diseases.

Serologic evaluation is helpful in establishing a diagnosis. Screening tests for collagen vascular diseases include the erythrocyte sedimentation rate, antinuclear antibodies, rheumatoid factor, and complement levels. More specific tests to document rheumatologic disorders are needed in selected cases and are described in Chapter 79.

To document seroconversion for diagnostic confirmation of acute infection both acute and convalescent specimens must be obtained. In many infections the diagnosis can be confirmed only retrospectively, weeks to months after the illness. For example, a late convalescent specimen, obtained 6 to 8 weeks after the illness began, may be the only specimen to display the greater than fourfold increase in antibody titer necessary to confirm a diagnosis of legionellosis or leptospirosis. A cost-effective approach to laboratory diagnosis is to freeze and store an acute phase serum sample, since patients whose clinical course or bacterial cultures make the etiology of their fever and rash clear do not need a battery of expensive serologic tests for uncommon diseases, and the serum can be discarded without testing.

### Special considerations for hospitalized patients with fever and rash

The appearance of fever and rash in a hospitalized patient not recently evaluated for fever merits a fresh, abbreviated history, physical examination, and laboratory evaluation. A review of all medications and recent diagnostic and therapeutic maneuvers may provide information needed to suspect a medication-related rash or postprocedure urinary tract infection. Particular attention should be given to mucous membranes and the optic fundi, and a complete skin examination should be performed. A white blood cell count with differential and two blood cultures, via separate venipuncture sites, should be obtained unless the rash appears typical for a medication-induced etiology (symmetric erythema multiforme) or a clinically diagnosable infection (e.g., herpes zoster). Additional fluids and specimens should be sampled for culture as dictated by the history and physical examination. Abdominal findings may suggest the need for liver chemistries, amylase, or abdominal imaging (such as radiographs, ultrasonography, or computed tomographic [CT] scanning) to diagnose an

**Table 62-2.** Common bacterial skin and soft tissue infections

| Type of lesion/disease | Etiologic agents | Risk factors | Antibiotic treatment | Fever |
|---|---|---|---|---|
| Impetigo | *Staphylococcus aureus*<br>Group A streptococci | Warm climate, young age | Dicloxacillin; topical mupirocin | Rare |
| Folliculitis | *S. aureus* | Chronic nasal carriage of *S. aureus* | Dicloxacillin; erythromycin | Occasional |
| | *Pseudomonas aeruginosa* | Hot tub immersion | Ciprofloxacin | |
| Furunculosis | *S. aureus* | Chronic nasal carriage of *S. aureus* | Dicloxacillin or clindamycin | Occasional |
| Erysipelas | Group A streptococci | Minor trauma | Oxacillin, nafcillin, penicillin G, or ampicillin/sulbactam | Common |
| Cellulitis | *S. aureus*<br>β-Hemolytic streptococci | Chronic edema, minor trauma, tinea pedis, dermatoses | Oxacillin, nafcillin, or first-generation cephalosporin | Common |
| | *Pasteurella multocida* | Cat bite or scratch | Ampicillin or parenteral cephalosporin | |
| | Gram-negative rods | Water exposure | Third-generation cephalosporin | |
| | *Erysipelothrix rhusiopathiae* | Fish handling | Penicillin G | |
| Necrotizing cellulitis | See cellulitis; also frequently mixed anaerobic/aerobic flora | Diabetes, vascular insufficiency, colon cancer | Broad-spectrum agents active against fecal flora and *S. aureus* | Common |
| | *Clostridium* species | | Penicillin G | |

occult abscess that could be responsible for skin lesions due to bacteremia (e.g., ecthyma gangrenosum or purpuric lesions from bacteremia-induced disseminated intravascular coagulation) or for a toxin-mediated rash (diffuse erythroderma).

## DIFFERENTIAL DIAGNOSIS

As an aid to the formulation of a differential diagnosis, the rash should be characterized using standard descriptive terminology. The term *exanthem* designates a skin eruption, whereas *enanthem* refers to a rash involving mucosal surfaces. Exanthematous rashes are commonly characterized by their appearance: diffuse erythroderma, maculopapular, nodular, vesicular-bullous, or petechial-purpuric. Table 62-1 lists potential etiologies for these types of rash. The differential diagnosis of other skin reactions/syndromes such as urticaria, erythema multiforme, and erythema nodosum are described in Chapters 21 and 24.

In establishing a differential diagnosis for a patient with fever and a rash, one should take into consideration the pace of the illness, appearance of the rash, degree of overall clinical acuity, associated symptoms and signs, the host immune system, and whether the process is systemic or localized to the skin and soft tissue. Tables 62-1 and 62-2 outline microorganisms and noninfectious disorders responsible for localized and systemic processes involving the skin. Table 62-3 lists conditions characterized by fever and rash for which antimicrobial treatment is indicated.

## MANAGEMENT

The physician must first decide whether the patient is suffering from a nonfatal condition and can be managed as an outpatient or requires hospitalization for aggressive management of a suspected fulminant, life-threatening infection. If one suspects infection due to meningococcemia, gonococcemia, septic shock due to gram-negative or gram-positive bacteremia, endocarditis, toxic shock syndrome, or Rocky Mountain spotted fever, prompt institution of treatment with appropriate antibiotics (see Table 62-3) is imperative. Potentially treatable viral infections such as disseminated herpes simplex or varicella in an immunocompromised host (treated with acyclovir), or Hantaan viral infection (possibly treatable with ribavirin) in a patient with exposure to rodents must be considered and therapy initiated promptly. For most other viral infections only supportive care is available. In an immunocompromised patient the mere presence of fever, with or without a rash, may dictate empiric treatment, for example, broad-spectrum antibiotics administered to a febrile neutropenic patient. If the patient is pregnant, at either extreme of age, or without adequate family or social support, hospitalization may be necessary. For example, pregnant patients are at greater risk of severe pneumonia as a complication of primary infection due to varicella-zoster (e.g., chickenpox) and may benefit from treatment with acyclovir, although this antiviral agent has not been approved for use during pregnancy. Patients with severe hemolytic uremic syndrome may require hospitalization for management of anemia, renal failure, or hypertension, and those with thrombotic thrombocytopenic purpura may benefit from plasmapheresis. Patients with systemic vasculitis require immunosuppressive therapy, preferably via consultation with a rheumatologist.

Traditionally the presence of fever and rash has signaled the possibility of contagious disease to the lay public and physicians alike. Because the differential

**Table 62-3.** Selected systemic infections for which antimicrobial treatment is indicated

| Disease syndrome | Causative organisms | Type of rash | Empiric treatment |
|---|---|---|---|
| **Bacteria** | | | |
| Bacillary angiomatosis | *Bartonella (Rochalimaea)* species | Nodular, verrucous | Erythromycin |
| Endocarditis | *Streptococcus viridans* group | Petechial, purpuric, nodular; acral | Ampicillin plus gentamicin |
| | *Staphylococcus aureus* | Petechial, purpuric, nodular; acral | Oxacillin, nafcillin, or vancomycin plus gentamicin |
| | Fastidious gram-negative organisms | Petechial, purpuric, nodular; acral | Ampicillin plus gentamicin |
| Gonococcemia | *Neisseria gonorrhoeae* | Petechial, purpuric; acral | Ceftriaxone |
| Lyme disease | *Borrelia burgdorferi* | Erythema chronicum migrans; erythema multiforme | Tetracyclines, ceftriaxone, or penicillin G |
| Leptospirosis | *Leptospira* species | Maculopapular | Penicillin G or tetracyclines |
| Meningococcemia/meningitis | *N. meningitidis* | Petechial, purpuric; acral | Penicillin G or ceftriaxone |
| Rat bite fever | *Streptobacillus moniliformis, Spirillum minor* | Maculopapular, morbilliform, petechial | Penicillin G |
| Relapsing fever | *Borrelia* species | Maculopapular | Tetracyclines or penicillin G |
| Scarlet fever | *S. pyogenes* | Scarlatiniform, maculopapular erythroderma | Penicillin G |
| Septic shock | Gram-negative bacilli, *S. aureus* | Ecthyma gangrenosum (petechial, purpuric) | Broad-spectrum β-lactam agent plus an aminoglycoside |
| Syphilis (secondary) | *Treponema pallidum* | Maculopapular; mucous patches | Penicillin G |
| Toxic shock syndrome | *S. aureus*, group A streptococci | Diffuse erythroderma, mucosal erythema | Oxacillin, nafcillin |
| Tularemia | *Francisella tularensis* | Eschar; maculopapular | Streptomycin plus tetracyclines |
| Typhoid fever | *Salmonella typhi* | Maculopapular, rose spots | Ceftriaxone or quinolones |
| **Rickettsiae** | | | |
| Rickettsialpox | *Rickettsia akari* | Maculopapular, vesicular | Tetracyclines or chloramphenicol |
| Rocky Mountain spotted fever | *R. rickettsii* | Maculopapular, petechial, purpuric; begins peripherally, spreads centrally | Tetracyclines or chloramphenicol |
| Typhus | *R. prowazekii* (louse-borne)<br>*R. typhi* (murine)<br>*R. tsutsugamushi* (scrub) | Maculopapular; begins centrally, spreads peripherally | Tetracyclines or chloramphenicol |
| **Chlamydiae** | | | |
| Pneumonia | *Chlamydia pneumoniae* | Maculopapular, erythema nodosum | Tetracycline or erythromycin |
| Psittacosis | *C. psittaci* | Maculopapular | Tetracycline or erythromycin |
| **Mycoplasmas** | | | |
| Pneumonia, cough | *Mycoplasma pneumoniae* | Maculopapular, vesiculobullous | Macrolides or tetracyclines |
| **Viruses** | | | |
| Oral/genital herpes | Herpes simplex | Vesicular, pustular | Acyclovir |
| Chicken pox, shingles/zoster | Varicella-zoster virus | Vesicular, pustular | Acyclovir |
| Acute HIV-1 (mononucleosis syndrome) | HIV-1 (see Chapter 68) | Maculopapular | ? Antiretroviral agents |

diagnosis of fever and rash includes diseases that require isolation procedures, health care providers must explain carefully the transmissibility and clinical prognosis of illnesses diagnosed or under consideration. The practitioner should discuss whether household members, contacts via school, day care, work, or social activities, or any other friends or family should be notified of the illness. Fears and prejudices should be considered and dealt with by the physician and hospital staff. For an ill child with a specific etiologic diagnosis for fever and rash, there may be questions about return to school or day care.

If the diagnosis is not clear or the patient is not improving, consultation with specialists (e.g., infectious diseases, rheumatology, dermatology) may be indicated. Follow-up should be continued until the patient is well or a definitive diagnosis is made. Serologic tests should be repeated in 2 to 6 weeks as needed, to pursue unresolved diagnostic confusion.

## BIBLIOGRAPHY

Allen ST et al: Toxic shock syndrome associated with the use of latex nasal packing, *Arch Intern Med* 150:2587, 1990.

Bunch TW: Hypersensitivity angiitis and panniculitis. In Kelley WN, editor: *Textbook of internal medicine,* ed 2, Philadelphia, 1992, JB Lippincott.

Chaplain BS, Proesmans W: The hemolytic uremic syndrome of childhood and its variants, *Semin Hematol* 24:148, 1987.

Ellison RT et al: Prevalence of congenital or acquired complement deficiency in patients with sporadic meningococcal disease, *N Engl J Med* 308:913, 1983.

Fauci AS, Haynes BF, Katz P: The spectrum of vasculitis: clinical, pathologic, immunologic, and therapeutic considerations, *Ann Intern Med* 89:660, 1978.

Fitzpatrick TB: Fundamentals of dermatologic diagnosis. In Fitzpatrick TB et al, editors: *Dermatology in general medicine,* ed 2, New York, 1979, McGraw-Hill.

Fox MD, Schwartz RA: Erythema nodosum, *Am Fam Physician* 46:818, 1992.

Glew RH: Fever. In Green HL, editor: *Introduction to clinical medicine,* Philadelphia, 1991, BC Decker.

Gran JT, Andreassen AH: Pneumonia, myocarditis, and reactive arthritis due to *Chlamydia pneumoniae, Scand J Rheumatol* 22:43, 1993.

Huston DP, Bressler RB: Urticaria and angioedema, *Med Clin North Am* 76:805, 1992.

Jordaan HF: Acute febrile neutrophilic dermatosis: a histopathologic study of 37 patients and review of the literature, *Am J Dermatopathol* 11:99, 1989.

Kingston ME, Mackey D: Skin clues in the diagnosis of life-threatening infections, *Rev Infect Dis* 8:1, 1986.

Kurzrock R, Cohen PR, Markowitz A: Clinical manifestations of vasculitis in patients with solid tumors: a case report and review of the literature, *Arch Intern Med* 154:334, 1994.

Patterson R et al: Erythema multiforme and Stevens-Johnson syndrome: descriptive and therapeutic controversy, *Chest* 98:331, 1990.

Weber DJ, Gannon WR, Cohen MS: The acutely ill patient with fever and a rash. In Mandell GL, Douglas RG, Bennett JE, editors: *Principles and practices of infectious diseases,* ed 3, New York, 1990, Churchill Livingstone.

CHAPTER

# 63 Fever of Undetermined Origin

**Howard Libman**
**Cynthia J. Whitener**

Fever is a common presenting problem in primary care practice. Often its cause is determined by the presence of associated localized symptoms, and its course is self-limited. Examples include upper respiratory tract infection manifesting as fever and nasal congestion and acute gastroenteritis presenting with fever and diarrhea. Less frequently fever occurs without localization of symptoms and is persistent. In these instances there is concern about the possibility of occult disease, and decisions regarding the appropriate nature and extent of diagnostic evaluation sometimes become problematic.

In general, fever is caused by infections, neoplastic diseases, and inflammatory disorders. It may also be the result of drug toxicity, granulomatous disease, vascular thrombosis, tissue infarction, and metabolic disorders. It is less commonly related to central nervous system diseases that affect the thermoregulatory center of the hypothalamus directly.

Febrile illnesses of less than 2 weeks' duration are often infectious in etiology, most frequently viral, or secondary to drug toxicity, and a specific diagnosis is sometimes not established. For an immunocompetent patient who does not appear particularly ill and has a normal physical examination, a limited diagnostic evaluation is indicated. Many systemic disorders begin with a prodrome characterized by fever, and observation ultimately leads to localization of the illness.

Fevers lasting longer than 2 weeks are generally associated with localized symptoms or signs that suggest an appropriate diagnostic evaluation. For patients without localized complaints occult bacterial infection is more likely if they are 50 years of age or older, or have diabetes mellitus, a complete blood count characterized by leukocytosis or a leftward shift in the white blood cell count, or an erythrocyte sedimentation rate (ESR) of 30 or above. Consideration should be given to evaluating such patients, as well as ill-appearing individuals, immunocompromised hosts, and those who have a history of valvular heart disease or injectable drug use, in a hospitalized setting.

Fever of undetermined origin (FUO) is defined as a febrile illness of more than 3 weeks' duration in which temperatures exceed 38.3° C on several determinations and with no diagnosis reached after 1 week of intensive evaluation. The purpose of these restrictive criteria is to eliminate most self-limited conditions. The differential diagnosis of FUO includes a wide variety of infections (approximately 30% of cases), neoplastic diseases (30%), inflammatory disorders (15%), and miscellaneous conditions (15% to 20%) (see the box on p. 823). However, because the medical literature describes hospitalized

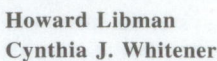

### Differential diagnosis of fever of undetermined origin

**Infections**

***Bacterial***

Dental abscess
Sinusitis/mastoiditis
Endocarditis
Intraabdominal/pelvic abscess
Biliary tract infection
Prostatitis
Septic pelvic vein thrombophlebitis
Osteomyelitis
Prosthetic device infection
Systemic infections
- Tuberculosis
- Atypical mycobacterial infection
- Salmonellosis
- Disseminated gonococcal infection
- Syphilis
- Lyme disease
- Leptospirosis
- Brucellosis

***Viral***

Cytomegalovirus
Epstein-Barr virus
Human immunodeficiency virus

***Chlamydial***

Psittacosis

***Rickettsial***

Q fever
Rocky Mountain spotted fever

***Fungal***

Cryptococcosis
Histoplasmosis

***Parasitic***

Malaria
Amebiasis
Toxoplasmosis
Pneumocystosis

**Neoplasia**

Lymphoma
Leukemia
Renal cell carcinoma
Hepatoma
Metastatic carcinoma
 to bone, liver, or central nervous system
Atrial myxoma
Malignant histiocytosis

**Inflammatory diseases**

Rheumatic fever
Systemic lupus erythematosus
Juvenile rheumatoid arthritis
Mixed connective tissue disease
Vasculitis

**Miscellaneous conditions**

Drug fever
Sarcoidosis
Multiple pulmonary emboli
Regional enteritis
Whipple's disease
Alcoholic hepatitis
Hemolysis
Occult hematoma
Tissue infarction
Metabolic disorders
Familial Mediterranean fever
Thermoregulatory disorders
Factitious fever

patients, it is important to realize that the prevalence of specific diagnoses in an outpatient population with undifferentiated febrile illness may be different.

In a comparison of the two major studies of patients with FUO performed by Petersdorf et al. in 1960 and 1980, tuberculosis, subacute bacterial endocarditis, rheumatic fever, systemic lupus erythematosus (SLE), and familial Mediterranean fever were sharply decreased or absent in the latter series. Conditions that increased in frequency included cytomegalovirus (CMV) infection, osteomyelitis, sinusitis, malignant histiocytosis, juvenile rheumatoid arthritis of the adult (Still's disease), regional enteritis, and occult hematomas.

## PATHOPHYSIOLOGY OF FEVER

Normal body temperatures taken orally in the basal state range between 36° and 37.8° C, with rectal temperatures generally 0.6° higher. Accurate oral temperatures may be difficult to obtain in patients with central nervous system impairment or hyperventilation, and rectal, axillary, or tympanic membrane temperatures are preferred in these settings. Diurnal variation in body temperature is usual in healthy individuals, with the lowest reading in the early morning and the highest in the late afternoon and early evening.

Fever, defined as a sustained abnormally high body temperature, occurs when heat production exceeds heat loss for an extended period. Chills, which may be experienced by the patient at the onset of fever, are characterized physiologically by muscular contraction, cutaneous vasoconstriction, and piloerection. Other commonly associated symptoms include fatigue, sweats, arthralgias, and myalgias. Altered mental status may occur in the chronically ill and the elderly, especially in the context of underlying cardiopulmonary or central nervous system disease. Although fevers above 41° C are uncommon, sustained higher temperatures are frequently associated with neurologic dysfunction and death.

Heat production occurs from energy-producing biologic reactions, and under normal circumstances heat dissipation is accomplished through loss of water vapor during respiration and by insensible cutaneous evaporation. When there is a transient increase in heat production, such as occurs with vigorous exercise, sweating, hyperventilation, and cutaneous vasodilatation provide the means for additional heat loss.

The hypothalamus gland, specifically its thermoregulatory center located anteriorly near the base of the third ventricle, is important in the control of body temperature. This region serves as a thermostat regulating the temperature set point and is susceptible to stimulation by cytokines known as endogenous pyrogens. Endogenous pyrogens are polypeptides released by monocytes and tissue macrophages in response to a variety of stimuli, including exogenous pyrogens (e.g., viruses, bacterial products, endotoxin, yeast, protozoa), cell phagocytosis, immune complexes, and tissue injury. The major types of endogenous pyrogens identified to date include interleukin-1 and cachectin, also known as tumor necrosis factor. Interferons are also thought to be pyrogenic, although their pathophysiologic mechanism is as yet undefined.

Endogenous pyrogens act on the hypothalamus by inducing phospholipases, which make arachidonic acid available for prostaglandin synthesis. Prostaglandin $E_2$, through the generation of cyclic adenosine monophosphate (AMP), serves to increase the thermal set point of the hypothalamus. Aspirin and nonsteroidal antiinflammatory agents such as ibuprofen lower body temperature by inhibiting cyclooxygenase activity, thereby blocking prostaglandin synthesis.

## FEVER PATTERNS

Although fever patterns are generally nonspecific, the following patterns are sometimes useful in differential diagnosis:

1. Intermittent: This pattern is characterized by an exaggeration of normal diurnal variation of temperature. It is most commonly associated with irregular use of antipyretic drugs and with pyogenic abscesses, tuberculosis, and lymphoma.
2. Sustained: This pattern is characterized by little variation in temperature and is often related to significant systemic infections such as bacterial endocarditis and pneumococcal pneumonia.
3. Relapsing: This pattern is characterized by alternating extended periods of fever and normal temperature and frequently occurs with malaria, lymphoma, and some unusual infections.
4. Temperature-pulse disparity: This pattern is characterized by high temperature with a disproportionately slow pulse. It is commonly described with salmonellosis, chlamydial and rickettsial infections, Legionnaire's disease, drug fever, and factitious fever.

It is important to note that febrile response to disease may be attenuated or absent in elderly patients, uremic and diabetic individuals, and persons receiving corticosteroid or antipyretic therapy.

## DIAGNOSTIC EVALUATION

The general diagnostic approach to FUO begins with a careful history and physical examination. Based upon these data and the age and underlying medical condition of the patient, a selective laboratory evaluation is then performed. Initial diagnostic efforts are directed at the early identification of potentially serious illnesses that are amenable to specific treatment.

Common causes of FUO in young adults include CMV infection, lymphoma, SLE, and regional enteritis. In the elderly bacterial endocarditis, tuberculosis, lymphoma, and temporal arteritis should be considered. Atypical presentations of common diseases are more frequent than uncommon conditions. In immunocompromised patients the differential diagnosis is expanded to include opportunistic, as well as common, diseases (Table 63-1).

### History

A careful history of the present illness is essential in focusing the differential diagnosis and determining an appropriate laboratory evaluation of the patient with FUO. An inaccurate or incomplete history may lead to the use of inappropriate diagnostic tests, potentially subjecting the patient to increased morbidity. Attention should be paid to the nature of the onset of symptoms and to any localization of them that occurs over time.

The patient's medical history, including any chronic or immunocompromising disorders, recent hospitalizations or surgeries, and medications, should be elicited. Travel history, exposure to tuberculosis, wild and domestic animal exposure, drug use, work environment, avocations, geographic origins, and HIV risk factors should be reviewed in detail. The patient should be questioned about whether other persons with whom he or she lives or associates have similar symptoms. If the preliminary history is not revealing, it should be reviewed periodically; input from family members and close friends should be solicited.

### Physical examination

A careful physical examination should be performed and repeated at periodic intervals. An assessment should be made as to whether the patient appears acutely or chronically ill, and any fever pattern noted should be described.

The skin may reveal peripheral stigmata of endocarditis, the malar rash of SLE, maculopapular rash of drug eruption, generalized rash of secondary syphilis, or evidence of vasculitis. Lymphadenopathy may indicate the presence of CMV, EBV, or HIV infections, syphilis, or lymphoma. Funduscopic examination may reveal evidence of retinitis secondary to CMV infection or toxoplasmosis or Roth's spots suggestive of bacterial endocarditis. Percussion and transillumination of the sinuses may indicate the presence of sinusitis. Examination of the pharynx may show occult dental infection, pharyngitis or tonsillitis, or manifestations of HIV disease, such as thrush or oral hairy leukoplakia.

The presence of new or changing cardiac murmurs may indicate endocarditis or atrial myxoma. Cardiopulmonary auscultation may also establish the diagnoses of pneumonia, pericarditis, or pleuritis. Palpation of the abdomen may reveal hepatomegaly, splenomegaly, abscess, or mass. Digital rectal examination may suggest the diagnosis of prostatitis or show evidence of occult blood. Bimanual pelvic examination may indicate the presence of pelvic

**Table 63-1.** Differential diagnosis of fever in the immunocompromised host

| Underlying condition | Compromising factor(s) |
|---|---|
| Solid tumor | D, E |
| Acute leukemia | A, D |
| Chronic lymphocytic leukemia | B |
| Lymphoma | C, E |
| Multiple myeloma | B |
| Asplenism | B |
| Organ transplantation | C, D |
| HIV disease | C, D |
| Injection drug use | D, F |
| Corticosteroid therapy | C |

| Compromising factor | Pathogens | Sites of infection |
|---|---|---|
| A. Granulocytopenia | Enteric bacteria<br>*Staphylococcus*<br>*Candida*<br>*Aspergillus* | Skin<br>Oropharynx<br>Esophagus<br>Lungs<br>Perianal region |
| B. Defective humoral immunity | *Pneumococcus*<br>*Haemophilus* | Lungs |
| C. Defective cellular immunity | Tuberculosis<br>Atypical mycobacteria<br>Cytomegalovirus, herpes simples virus, varicella-zoster virus<br>*Listeria*<br>*Nocardia*<br>*Candida*<br>*Cryptococcus*<br>Cytomegalovirus<br>*Pneumocystis*<br>Toxoplasmosis | Depends on pathogen |
| D. Disruption of skin or mucosa | Regional flora | Skin<br>Lungs<br>Gastrointestinal tract<br>Urinary tract |
| E. Anatomic obstruction | Regional flora | Lungs<br>Biliary tract<br>Urinary tract |
| F. Altered consciousness | Pharyngeal flora | Lungs |

inflammatory disease. Musculoskeletal examination may show arthritis, bursitis, or localized bony tenderness suggesting osteomyelitis. Neurologic examination may reveal evidence of meningismus or occult focal deficits indicative of pyogenic central nervous system disease.

## Laboratory evaluation

The initial laboratory evaluation of all patients with an occult febrile illness should consist of a complete blood count with differential count, kidney and liver function tests, blood cultures, syphilis serology, serum protein electrophoresis, skin test for tuberculosis (PPD) with controls, chest radiograph, and urinalysis (see the box on p. 826). An acute phase serum sample should also be obtained. Additional diagnostic testing should be individualized based upon findings from the history and physical examination.

The complete blood count may show lymphocytosis, suggestive of viral infection, leukocytosis or leftward shift of white blood cells, indicative of bacterial infection, or evidence of leukemia. Monocytosis is described with tuberculosis, CMV infection, lymphoma, and metastatic carcinoma. Eosinophilia is often associated with lymphoma, drug fever, and vasculitis. Anemia and thrombocytosis are described with many acute and chronic infections and neoplastic and inflammatory diseases. Thrombocytopenia may indicate the presence of an acute infection or immune-mediated disorder. Liver function test abnormalities may suggest hepatitis or infiltrative disease of the liver or biliary tract disease, both of which are generally associated with a disproportionate increase in serum alkaline phosphatase. The ESR and C-reactive protein, nonspecific markers of acute and chronic diseases, are not sufficiently sensitive or specific to be clinically useful in most instances.

Three sets of blood cultures obtained through separate venopunctures are generally sufficient to diagnose conditions associated with continuous bacteremia such as en-

## Laboratory evaluation of the patient with occult febrile illness

**Initial evaluation**

Complete blood count
Differential white blood cell count
Kidney and liver function tests
Blood cultures
Syphilis serology
Serum protein electrophoresis
Skin test for tuberculosis with controls
Chest radiograph
Urinalysis
Acute phase serum sample

**Additional studies based upon clinical presentation**

Viral hepatitis serologies
Serologies for EBV, CMV, HIV, Lyme disease, toxoplasmosis, or other infectious diseases
Antinuclear antibody
Rheumatoid factor
Antistreptolysin O test

**Radiologic imaging studies**

Sinus radiographs
CT or MRI scan of the head
Echocardiography
Doppler studies of extremities
Ventilation/perfusion lung scan
Upper GI series/barium enema
CT or MRI scan or ultrasound of the abdomen and pelvis
Intravenous pyelogram
Bone radiographs/scan

**Invasive studies**

Skin biopsy
Liver biopsy
Bone marrow biopsy
Lymph node biopsy
Aspiration of abnormal fluid collections
Lumbar puncture
Exploratory laparotomy

docarditis. Infections with intermittent bacteremia, such as pneumonia and visceral abscess, may require repeated blood cultures over time. The microbiology laboratory should be notified if there is suspicion of an atypical or slow-growing organism.

The serum protein electrophoresis may show nonspecific hypergammaglobulinemia or a monoclonal spike characteristic of a plasma cell dyscrasia. The skin test for tuberculosis should be performed with control studies to exclude the possibility of cutaneous anergy. Chest radiograph may reveal hilar adenopathy, diffuse or localized infiltrates, or pleural effusion suggestive of infectious, neoplastic, or connective tissue diseases. Urinalysis may show proteinuria, microscopic hematuria, or evidence of infection.

A positive screening test for syphilis should always be confirmed by specific serology. Hepatitis A, B, and C viral serologies are indicated if there are unexplained liver function test abnormalities. Serologies for EBV, CMV, HIV infection, Lyme disease, toxoplasmosis, and other infectious diseases should be considered in the appropriate clinical settings.

The ANA test and rheumatoid factor are reserved for those situations in which SLE and rheumatoid arthritis are suspected clinically. An antistreptolysin O titer to establish the presence of antecedent streptococcal infection is indicated if rheumatic fever is a diagnostic consideration.

### Radiologic imaging studies

Radiologic imaging studies are useful in establishing specific diagnoses suggested by history, physical examination, and initial laboratory evaluation. Sinus films may indicate the presence of sinusitis, and CT or MRI scans of the head may show occult brain abscesses. Echocardiography may reveal valvular vegetations indicative of endocarditis or atrial myxoma. Doppler studies of the lower extremities or ventilation/perfusion lung scan may suggest the diagnosis of multiple pulmonary emboli.

The diagnosis of inflammatory bowel disease may be supported by findings on upper gastrointestinal series or barium enema. Abdominal/pelvic ultrasound or CT or MRI scan may show biliary tract disease, pelvic inflammatory disease, or occult abscess. An intravenous pyelogram with nephrotomogram or renal ultrasound may be useful in diagnosing renal cell carcinoma or abscess. Plain radiographs or radionuclide scans of the bone may suggest the presence of osteomyelitis. Gallium and indium scan findings are generally nonspecific but sometimes helpful in localizing an occult disease process.

### Invasive studies

Invasive studies and biopsy procedures are reserved for (1) when the initial clinical assessment is suggestive of systemic or localized disease but insufficient to establish a definitive diagnosis, and (2) when there is reasonable likelihood that findings from the procedure will significantly alter clinical management.

Skin biopsy may be useful in establishing the diagnosis of vasculitis or drug toxicity. Lymph node biopsy is indicated if lymphoma or adenitis secondary to disseminated infection such as tuberculosis is suspected. In general, an excisional biopsy is preferred, and the inguinal region should be avoided if possible because of an increased rate of nonspecific findings. Liver biopsy should be considered if there is evidence of chronic hepatitis or infiltrative disease. In the context of pancytopenia, bone marrow biopsy may be useful in establishing the diagnosis of hematologic malignancy or disseminated infection. Abnormal fluid collections involving the pericardial, pleural, abdominal, or joint spaces should be aspirated and sent for cell count, chemistries, culture, and cytology. A lumbar puncture is indicated in the context of meningismus or central nervous system dysfunction. Exploratory laparotomy is reserved for those relatively few instances in which there is compelling evidence of significant undiagnosed intraabdominal disease.

## DIFFERENTIAL DIAGNOSIS

### Infections

Tuberculosis, bacterial endocarditis from slowly growing or difficult-to-grow organisms, biliary tract infection, intraabdominal abscess, septic pelvic vein thrombophlebitis, and viral infections, including CMV, Epstein-Barr virus (EBV), and human immunodeficiency virus (HIV), are frequent causes of FUO.

Abscesses, the most common type of bacterial infection presenting as an FUO, are often localized in the abdomen or pelvis. Renal abscess with obstruction, perinephric abscess, or prostatic abscess in males may not be associated with any abnormalities on urinalysis. Diagnosis of these conditions is generally established with a radiologic imaging study, such as ultrasound, computed tomographic (CT) scan, or magnetic resonance imaging (MRI) scan.

With the widespread use of blood cultures in recent years, intravascular infection is now a relatively infrequent cause of FUO. However, atypical causes of endocarditis (e.g., *Haemophilus* species, fungi) and infections that cause intermittent bacteremia, including salmonellosis, disseminated gonococcal infection, and brucellosis, are still described. Culture-negative endocarditis is suggested by the presence of vegetations on echocardiogram. Diagnosis of other bacteremic infections may require multiple or special blood cultures, aspiration of fluid from affected body sites (e.g., bone marrow, joints), or specific serologic tests.

Other occult bacterial infections that may cause FUO include sinusitis, mastoiditis, and chronic osteomyelitis. Iatrogenic infections should be considered in patients with prosthetic joints, vascular devices, or other implanted synthetic materials.

Tuberculosis, particularly extrapulmonary disease, and atypical mycobacterial infection, especially *Mycobacterium avium* complex in patients with advanced HIV disease, are important causes of FUO. After decades of decreasing prevalence, tuberculosis has increased in frequency in the United States, with urban areas affected disproportionately. Symptoms of extrapulmonary tuberculosis are variable and depend upon the site(s) of involvement. Diagnosis is made by isolation, blood culture, or tissue biopsy. Symptoms of *M. avium* complex infection are generally nonspecific, but there may be evidence of bone marrow or liver involvement on diagnostic evaluation. Diagnosis is most often established by isolator blood culture.

EBV and CMV infections may be prolonged and have few, if any, localizing signs. Generalized lymphadenopathy, splenomegaly, and rash may be present. Diagnosis is made by serology or culture. Primary HIV infection may present in a similar manner, and patients with advanced HIV disease sometimes have persistent fever and constitutional symptoms not attributable to a specific opportunistic infection or neoplasm. Diagnosis of primary HIV infection is established serologically, and fever attributable to advanced HIV disease is determined by the exclusion of other conditions (see Chapter 68).

The chlamydial and rickettsial infections, psittacosis and Q fever, sometimes present with fever and constitutional symptoms. Their diagnosis is often suggested by history of contact with birds or farm animals and can be confirmed serologically. Parasitic infections that may cause FUO include malaria and amebic liver abscess, and toxoplasmosis and pneumocystosis in patients with advanced HIV disease. Diagnosis is made by appropriate serologic and imaging studies. Spirochete diseases, including secondary syphilis, Lyme disease, and leptospirosis, may also present with fever, but the presence of localized symptoms often provides a clue to their etiology. Diagnosis of each condition is made serologically.

### Neoplasms

Lymphoma, leukemia, renal cell carcinoma, hepatoma, and metastatic carcinoma to the bone, liver, or central nervous system are the most frequent neoplastic causes of FUO.

Hodgkin's disease, especially early in its course, may present with fever alone, and lymphadenopathy may be limited to the abdomen or retroperitoneal space. Non-Hodgkin's lymphoma is generally associated with palpable lymphadenopathy, hepatosplenomegaly, or both. Diagnosis of lymphoma is made by excisional biopsy of affected lymph nodes or, less commonly, by bone marrow biopsy. Acute leukemia may present with high-grade fever in conjunction with anemia and leukopenia or leukocytosis. Bone marrow aspiration and biopsy are usually diagnostic. In patients with chronic lymphocytic or granulocytic leukemia, fever often indicates the presence of accompanying infection.

Most solid tumors are not associated with fever in the absence of obstruction or tissue necrosis. Notable exceptions include renal cell carcinoma, which may present with flank pain and hematuria, and hepatoma, which generally occurs in the context of chronic hepatitis B infection. Presumptive diagnosis is most often made by radiologic imaging study. Metastatic gastrointestinal and ovarian tumors to the bone, liver, or central nervous system may also be associated with fever. Atrial myxoma, an infrequent cause of FUO, may be clinically confused with bacterial endocarditis, presenting with fever, changing heart murmurs, and peripheral embolic phenomena. Diagnosis is made by echocardiography.

### Inflammatory diseases

Rheumatic fever, SLE, juvenile rheumatoid arthritis, mixed connective tissue disease, and vasculitis are the most common inflammatory disorders responsible for FUO.

Rheumatic fever generally occurs during childhood or in a young adult with the diagnosis established by specific clinical and laboratory criteria in the context of serologic evidence of recent streptococcal infection. The diagnosis of SLE is also established by specific clinical, laboratory, and serologic findings. Fever associated with SLE may represent a manifestation of the disease or of a complicating infection in the context of immunosuppressive therapy. The diagnosis of rheumatoid arthritis is generally established by the presence of polyarthritis and a positive rheumatoid factor. However, a seronegative variant, Still's disease, which manifests with fever, polyarthritis, generalized lymphadenopathy, organomegaly, and rash, is a diagnosis of exclusion.

Vasculitic conditions, including periarteritis nodosa, Wegener's granulomatosis, and temporal arteritis may also present with fever. Diagnosis is made by angiography and vascular biopsy. Polymyalgia rheumatica is a disease of elderly persons manifested by fever, headache, myalgias, and arthralgias. It may occur with or without temporal arteritis and is often associated with a very high ESR.

### Miscellaneous conditions

Drug fever, sarcoidosis and other granulomatous diseases, multiple pulmonary emboli, regional enteritis, Whipple's disease, alcoholic hepatitis, hemolytic episodes, occult hematomas, metabolic diseases, familial Mediterranean fever, factitious fever, and thermoregulatory disorders constitute the miscellaneous causes of FUO.

*Drug fever.* Drugs are a relatively common cause of fever, and drug fever should be considered in the differential diagnosis of all febrile illnesses. Although fever has been attributed to many different medications, it is commonly associated with a relatively small number of agents (see the box at right). Fever related to drug treatment may also be the result of endotoxin release in response to antibiotic therapy (e.g., Jarisch-Herxheimer reaction) or the lysis of tumor cells following chemotherapy. Self-limited fever is also common following administration of many vaccines.

Drug fever may be low or high grade, sustained or intermittent, and in some instances it is disproportionate to the degree of systemic toxicity. Its onset often immediately follows initial use of a medication but may be delayed weeks, months, or even years. Clinical improvement is generally noted within 24 to 48 hours of discontinuation of the causative agent.

Drug fever may present with rash, hemolysis, bone marrow suppression, or eosinophilia. Certain drugs, especially barbiturates, methyldopa, penicillin, phenytoin, and sulfonamides, have been associated with a serum sickness–like syndrome, manifested by rash, lymphadenopathy, arthritis, nephritis, and edema. An SLE-like syndrome, characterized by fever, arthralgias, and positive antinuclear antibody (ANA) test, has been described with hydralazine, phenytoin, procainamide, and other agents.

#### Agents commonly associated with drug fever

Allopurinol
Amphotericin B
Antihistamines
Antituberculous medications
Atropine
Barbiturates*
Bleomycin
Cephalosporins
Clofibrate
Heparin
Hydralazine†
Meperidine
Methyldopa*
Nifedipine
Nitrofurantoin
Penicillin*
Phenolphthalein
Phenytoin*†
Procainamide†
Quinidine
Sulfonamides*
Thiouracils

*May be associated with serum sickness–like syndrome.
†May be associated with SLE-like syndrome.

*Granulomatous diseases.* Sarcoidosis is a systemic granulomatous disease of unknown etiology. Fever has been described in association with hilar lymphadenopathy, arthritis, or hepatic involvement. Diagnosis is made through biopsy of an affected organ, with the characteristic finding of noncaseating granuloma. Granulomatous hepatitis manifests as fever, hepatomegaly, and increased serum alkaline phosphatase. Diagnosis is made by liver biopsy, with the differential diagnosis including tuberculosis, syphilis, histoplasmosis, lymphoma, sarcoidosis, drug reactions, and other conditions.

*Other disorders.* Multiple pulmonary emboli, generally the result of asymptomatic deep venous thrombosis of the lower extremities, typically present with recurrent respiratory symptoms associated with low-grade fever. Diagnostic evaluation includes Doppler studies of the legs, ventilation/perfusion lung scan, or pulmonary angiography. Myocardial infarction is also sometimes associated with a low-grade fever secondary to tissue necrosis.

Gastrointestinal disorders presenting with fever include regional enteritis and Whipple's disease, which are usually characterized by weight loss, abdominal pain, and malabsorption syndrome. Alcoholic hepatitis may manifest as fever with unexplained abnormalities in liver function tests. Hemolysis attributable to a hematologic disorder, systemic disease, or drug toxicity may present as fever without localizing symptoms, as may occult hematomas secondary to trauma or bleeding dyscrasia. Rarely, FUO is the result of metabolic diseases such as gout, hyperthyroidism, thyroiditis, hyperparathyroidism, and pheochromocytoma.

Familial Mediterranean fever, also known as periodic disease, is an uncommon autosomal recessive disease characterized by periodic fevers associated with atypical chest and abdominal pain in men of Mediterranean background. Arthritis and skin lesions have also been described. Diagnosis is established clinically.

Thermoregulatory disorders caused by hypothalamic dysfunction secondary to encephalitis, stroke, or hemorrhage occur infrequently. Diagnosis is made by CT or MRI scan of the brain. Fever secondary to hypothalamic disease may respond to chlorpromazine therapy.

*Factitious fever.* Factitious fever, most often described in young women and persons with medical training or experience, is a fever that has been artificially produced by the patient. Clinical clues to the diagnosis include the lack of constitutional symptoms and systemic toxicity and the presence of a temperature-pulse disparity. Diagnosis is established by the use of supervised temperatures with

**Table 63-2.** Management of fever

| Intervention | Adult dosage | Comments |
|---|---|---|
| Acetaminophen therapy | 650 mg every 3 to 4 hr | Avoid high dosage in patients with significant hepatic dysfunction |
| Aspirin therapy | 650 mg every 3 to 4 hr | Avoid in children because of association with Reye's syndrome<br>May induce gastritis, platelet dysfunction |
| Ibuprofen* therapy | 200 mg every 6 hr | Appears useful in controlling fever associated with malignancy<br>May induce gastritis, platelet dysfunction |
| Cool compresses or baths | As needed | No advantage to use of alcohol over water |
| Cooling blanket | As needed for hyperpyrexia | Reduce temperature to 39.5°C and then use traditional measures<br>May induce cutaneous vasoconstriction |

From Gartner JC Jr: *Adv Pediatr Infect Dis* 7:6, 1992.
*Other nonsteroidal antiinflammatory agents can be used in equipotent dosages.

thermometers whose results are not easily manipulated. Rarely, fraudulent fever has been described that is the result of self-inoculation of pyogenic substances or the ingestion of foreign material.

## MANAGEMENT

Except for extreme hyperpyrexia, defined as a temperature over 41° C, which can cause central nervous system dysfunction, there is no information to suggest that fever is deleterious in humans. In addition, there is indirect evidence which implies that fever may be beneficial to patients through the activation of specific host defense mechanisms. Indiscriminate treatment of fever could theoretically interfere with immune responsiveness. It could also obscure the natural history of an undiagnosed condition and the response to specific therapy of an identified disease. Despite these concerns, many physicians choose to initiate antipyretic therapy in febrile patients in an effort to alleviate their physical discomfort.

Definite indications for treatment of fever include avoidance of tachycardia in persons with a history of or at increased risk for congestive heart failure, hyperventilation in those with pulmonary decompensation or dehydration, encephalopathy in those with underlying central nervous system disease, and febrile convulsions in predisposed younger children.

Commonly used antipyretic agents include acetaminophen, aspirin, and nonsteroidal antiinflammatory agents such as ibuprofen (Table 63-2). Each appears to be effective when given in adequate dosage. Aspirin is contraindicated for the management of fever related to viral illness in children because of its association with Reye's syndrome. Because intermittent antipyretic therapy usually results in alternating fever, chills, and sweats, continuous therapy is generally preferable.

Alternative methods for fever control include sponging the body with tepid water and the use of cooling blankets, although the latter sometimes induces cutaneous vasoconstriction and shivering. There is no particular advantage to alcohol baths. Extreme hyperpyrexia should be managed by immersing the patient in an ice-water bath until fever is reduced to 39.5° C, followed by traditional measures.

Over 90% of adults with FUO are diagnosed with a specific disorder over time, and with few exceptions blind therapeutic trials should be avoided. Empiric antimicrobial therapy increases the risk of superinfection and drug toxicity. However, antituberculous therapy is indicated for high-risk patients diagnosed with granulomatous disease pending culture results, and the combination of penicillin G and an aminoglycoside is recommended if the working diagnosis is culture-negative endocarditis.

Empiric corticosteroid therapy should be reserved for instances of suspected connective tissue disease; it may mask the clinical symptoms of other disorders without affecting their natural history. A trial of nonsteroidal antiinflammatory agents has been suggested as a means of distinguishing infectious from neoplastic causes of fever in patients with preexisting cancer.

## BIBLIOGRAPHY


Chang JC: Neoplastic fever: a proposal for diagnosis, *Arch Intern Med* 149:1728, 1989.

Dinarello CA et al: New concepts in the pathogenesis of fever, *Rev Infect Dis* 10:168, 1988.

Esposito AL, Gleckman RA: A diagnostic approach to the adult with fever of unknown origin, *Arch Intern Med* 139:575, 1979.

Larson EB, Featherstone HJ, Petersdorf RG: Fever of undetermined origin: diagnosis and follow-up of 105 cases, 1970-1980, *Medicine* 61:269, 1982.

Leibovici L, Cohen O, Wysenbeek AJ: Occult bacterial infection in adults with unexplained fever: validation of a diagnostic index, *Arch Intern Med* 150:1270, 1990.

Lipsky BA, Hirschmann JV: Drug fever, *JAMA* 245:851, 1981.

Mellors JW et al: A simple index to identify occult bacterial infection in adults with acute unexplained fever, *Arch Intern Med* 147:666, 1987.

Musher DM et al: Fever patterns: their lack of clinical significance, *Arch Intern Med* 139:1225, 1979.

Petersdorf RG, Beeson PB: Fever of unexplained origin: report on 100 cases, *Medicine* 40:1, 1961.

Vickery DM, Quinnell RK: Fever of unknown origin: an algorithmic approach, *JAMA* 238:2183, 1977.

CHAPTER

# 64 Guidelines for Antimicrobial Therapy and Prophylaxis

Margaret Durkin

The specifics of the treatment of various infections are dealt with in sections of this text concerned with those infections. This chapter is divided into two sections, the first dealing with general principles of antimicrobial therapy and the second with the characteristics and adverse effects of various drugs and groups of drugs. The latter discussion is synoptic owing to considerations of length. A number of excellent textbooks concerned with antibiotics and antimicrobial agents are available (see Bibliography), and these should be referred to for more detail. Several useful and convenient pocket guides to antimicrobial therapy are also available. These guides are frequently updated and provide ready assistance as to drugs of choice, alternative agents, appropriate dosages, and adverse reactions.

## GENERAL PRINCIPLES

### Mechanisms of action

Antimicrobial agents include naturally occurring compounds produced by plants, synthetic compounds, and substances produced by a variety of fungi and bacteria. Antimicrobial agents used to treat infection have one common characteristic: they have a lethal or inhibitory effect on the infecting agent and an effect on host cells that is of a significantly lesser degree. Antimicrobial agents work by several mechanisms (see the box at right). Some, represented by penicillins, cephalosporins, and vancomycin, interfere with the synthesis of the bacterial cell wall, causing instability of this support structure. This action leads to lysis of the bacterial cell or inhibition of cellular division. Other agents, such as polymyxin and amphotericin B, cause loss of integrity of the cell membrane. A large number of agents affect bacterial protein synthesis, causing inhibition of cell growth (chloramphenicol, tetracycline, macrolides) or lethal errors of translation of genetic information (aminoglycosides). Still other agents, such as sulfonamides and trimethoprim, inhibit microorganisms by interfering with enzymes involved in pathways of cellular metabolism.

Some antimicrobial agents are classified as bacteriostatic, meaning that they inhibit but do not kill microorganisms, whereas some are considered bactericidal in that they have a lethal effect on the microorganism (see the box at right). These designations reflect the concentration of drug required to inhibit the growth of the organism (usually measured as the minimal inhibitory concentration [MIC]) and the concentration that kills the organisms (minimal bactericidal concentration [MBC]). Antibiotics thought of as static may in fact be able to kill a particular organism, but not at concentrations safely obtainable in humans. This classification is somewhat arbitrary, and there are a number of exceptions. For example, penicillins are generally considered bactericidal, but enterococci are inhibited and not killed within the range of achievable in vivo concentrations. Similarly, clindamycin is classified as bacteriostatic but kills many strains of staphylococci. In any case, most bacteriostatic agents are capable of killing bacteria if sufficient concentrations are achieved. The only

### Mechanisms of action of some commonly used antimicrobial agents

**Act on bacterial cell wall**

Penicillins
Cephalosporins
Aztreonam, imipenem
Vancomycin

**Act on microbial cell membrane**

Polymixin
Amphotericin B

**Act on protein synthesis at the level of the ribosome**

Aminoglycosides
Chloramphenicol
Erythromycin, azithromycin, clarithromycin
Clindamycin
Tetracycline
Spectinomycin

**Affect microbial DNA synthesis, replication, or translation**

Sulfonamides
Trimethoprim
Rifampin
Metronidazole
Acyclovir
Flucytosine

### Bactericidal and bacteriostatic antimicrobials

**Bactericidal**

Aminoglycosides
Aztreonam
Imipenem
Cephalosporins
Penicillins
Quinolones
Vancomycin

**Bacteriostatic**

Chloramphenicol
Clindamycin
Macrolides
Sulfonamides
Tetracyclines
Trimethoprim

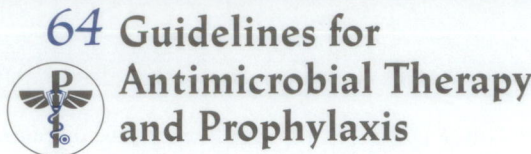

**Table 64-1.** Major mechanism of resistance to antimicrobials

| Antibiotic | Mechanisms of resistance |
|---|---|
| β-Lactams | Inactivation by β-lactamases (both chromosomal and plasmid in origin) |
| | Change in the permeability of the outer membrane |
| | Changes in the penicillin-binding proteins |
| Aminoglycosides | Aminoglycoside-modifying enzymes |
| | Changes in permeability of the inner membrane |
| | Alteration in ribosomal target sites |
| Chloramphenicol | Inactivation by acetyltransferase |
| | Membrane impermeability |
| | Alteration in ribosomal target sites |
| Macrolides | Inactivation by erythromycin esterase |
| | Alteration in ribosomal target sites |
| Clindamycin | Alteration in ribosomal target sites |
| Sulfonamides and trimethoprim | Overproduction of PABA |
| | Membrane impermeability |
| | Structural changes in the enzyme dihydropteroate synthetase and dihydrofolate reductase |
| Tetracyclines | Membrane impermeability |
| | Alteration in binding to target site |
| | Active efflux of tetracycline across the cell membrane |
| Quinolones | Mutations in DNA gyrase leading to decreased affinity for the agents |
| Vancomycin | Membrane impermeability |
| Rifampin | Alteration in DNA-dependent RNA polymerase |

clinical situation in which the significance of a bactericidal versus a bacteriostatic agent is well documented is in endocarditis, in which a bactericidal agent is required for effective therapy. Some infectious disease authorities believe that optimal management of meningitis also requires an agent that is bactericidal for the infecting organism, but this proposal has not been clearly established. In essentially all other bacterial infections appropriate antibiotics appear to be equally effective, regardless of whether they are bactericidal or bacteriostatic. If the physician has multiple antibiotic choices, a cidal drug should usually be chosen over a static antimicrobial.

## Efficacy

The clinical efficacy of an antimicrobial agent is established by clinical use. Measures of antimicrobial susceptibility are extremely valuable in determining the likelihood of efficacy; however, the only definite statement that can be made is that infection caused by an organism that is resistant to a drug in vitro would not be expected to respond to therapy with that drug. Standard measurement of antimicrobial susceptibility is performed by evaluating the inhibition or killing of an organism exposed to varying concentrations of a drug. This testing results in the determination of an MIC and an MBC. Because twofold dilutions of drug usually are employed, this is at best an approximation. Many laboratories use an agar diffusion technique to measure susceptibility, in which paper disks impregnated with standard amounts of antibiotics are placed on agar seeded with the organism to be tested. The antibiotic produces a diffusion gradient in the agar that inhibits growth of organisms such that the size of the zone of inhibition around the paper disk correlates with the susceptibility of the organism. The laboratory reports organisms to be sensitive or resistant (and occasionally intermediate), depending on the size of the zone of inhibition. The availability of newer, more cost-effective technology has led some laboratories to use modifications of the standard dilution techniques of susceptibility testing so that MICs may be reported. All the methods of susceptibility testing are done according to standardized procedures, ensuring reproducibility.

Certain organisms are not routinely tested because of known, uniform susceptibility to agents of choice. Group A β-hemolytic streptococci, for example, have not shown a tendency toward increased resistance to penicillin. Certain other organisms such as pneumococci and meningococci should be screened in at least a limited manner, since isolates resistant to penicillin have been reported. In a similar manner gonococcal resistance to penicillin was initially rare but is currently an increasing problem, and penicillin should never be presumed effective therapy for gonorrhea. Susceptibility tests for some of these organisms are difficult to perform and interpret. Many strains of *Haemophilus influenzae* are resistant to ampicillin. A simple test for production of ampicillin-inactivating β-lactamase is often performed, and if it is positive the organism is considered resistant to ampicillin. A negative β-lactamase test in the case of *H. influenzae* or any other organism, however, does not guarantee susceptibility, since some strains are resistant through mechanisms other than production of an inactivating enzyme.

Since the introduction of antimicrobial agents, some bacteria have been able to evolve in a manner that protects the organism against the action of the antimicrobial agent. Several different mechanisms resulting in bacterial resistance have been identified (Table 64-1). About 95% of *Staphylococcus aureus* strains were initially sensitive to penicillin, but now most *S. aureus* are resistant to the drug because of the production of penicillinase, which inactivates the penicillin. Many hospital-acquired, bacterial pathogens are multiresistant (i.e., resistant to a number of agents to which they might be expected to be susceptible). Resistance patterns of such organisms, primarily gram-negative aerobic bacilli, *S. aureus,* and enterococci vary from species to species, strain to strain, and hospital to hospital. It is important for practitioners who use antibiotics to be aware of the observed resistance patterns at their institution to utilize appropriate empiric therapy for hospital-acquired infection.

Susceptibility testing should guide the use of antimicrobial agents; however, in most cases the clinician must select empiric antimicrobial therapy while awaiting the results of cultures. Empiric therapy is based on the suspected diagnosis (e.g., pneumonia, peritonitis), the common pathogens involved in that diagnosis, and the known or expected pattern of susceptibility of the suspected pathogen(s). Antibiotic therapy may be adjusted on the basis of the results of susceptibility testing.

In most instances an effective antimicrobial agent with the narrowest spectrum of activity against the organism(s) causing the infection should be used. The normal microbial flora of the human body is an established ecosystem that contributes to host protection. This ecosystem is upset by the use of any antibiotic, but the broader the spectrum of activity of the agent(s) the more radical is the effect. For example, in a given clinical situation if penicillin, cefazolin, and ceftriaxone are effective agents for the treatment of an infection, penicillin, which has a narrower spectrum of activity, is preferred. In some situations, such as intraabdominal infection and sepsis due to unknown organisms, broad-spectrum therapy must be used to provide activity against a number of possible pathogens. Therapy may be narrowed when an etiologic agent or agents are identified. The use of a broad-spectrum agent such as ceftriaxone when a narrower spectrum drug would have sufficed may lead to an increased incidence of colonization and superinfection with organisms, such as the yeast *Candida albicans.* In the hospital setting abuse of broad-spectrum agents may lead to the emergence of multiresistant flora.

### Toxicity

An obvious consideration in the selection of an antimicrobial agent is potential toxicity (Table 64-2). An effective agent with the least toxicity should always be selected. For each patient an adequate history regarding allergy to antimicrobial agents should also be elicited. This history should be as detailed as possible. Many patients attribute minor symptoms such as gastrointestinal upset to allergy, when the adverse effect would be better termed an intolerance. Nonspecific rashes are generally less worrisome than urticaria. Although a cephalosporin might be considered an alternative agent for the treatment of some infections in the penicillin-allergic patient, a history of an acute anaphylactic reaction to penicillin would be a contraindication to this substitution. One specific adverse event needs to be factored into every decision to use an antibiotic. *Clostridium difficile* colitis is a complication that has been associated with virtually every antibiotic. Although some antibiotics may have a stronger association with *C. difficile* disease than others, *C. difficile* colitis should always be considered in the differential diagnosis of a patient with diarrhea who either is taking or has taken antibiotics (see Chapter 49).

### Synergy

Occasionally antimicrobial combinations are chosen for synergistic effect. Synergy exists when two antimicrobials are more effective together against a single pathogen than either would be if used individually. Synergy may be necessary to exert a bactericidal effect against organisms such as *Enterococcus* and *Pseudomonas* species. Synergy may also be desired in treating serious infections such as endocarditis. The most accepted example of synergy is the combination of β-lactams and aminoglycosides.

### Cost

A final consideration in the choice of an antimicrobial agent is cost. If one has several agents to choose from, each of which is expected to be equally effective, the least expensive agent is preferred. Obviously, considerations of spectrum and toxicity must be weighed in the selection. An example of this type of cost analysis is the treatment of a community-acquired urinary tract infection with sulfonamide or ampicillin, rather than one of the oral cephalosporins, which are considerably more expensive. In the case of a pregnant patient with a urinary tract infection who is allergic to penicillin or sulfonamide and in whom tetracycline should not be used, however, the more expensive cephalosporin might be the drug of choice.

• • •

In summary, the antimicrobial agent(s) selected should have confirmed activity against the pathogen with the narrowest spectrum, least toxicity, and lowest cost. The availability of a large number of agents makes this a realistic approach in most situations.

The efficacy of antimicrobial therapy is assessed clinically. Depending on the disease being treated, signs and symptoms of infection should resolve in an expected fashion. The typical patient with pneumococcal pneumonia should show signs of improvement within the first 48 hours of therapy. Thus awareness of the natural history of appropriately treated infections is important. Serum levels of antibiotics are occasionally assessed to ensure adequate dosage. The use of antimicrobial agents with potential toxicity requires careful monitoring of pertinent organ function.

### Real or apparent failure of antimicrobial therapy

There are a number of reasons for real or apparent failure of antimicrobial therapy. Correctness of diagnosis and appropriateness of the antibiotic(s) chosen should be reconfirmed. Compliance is a special problem in outpatient therapy. Several studies have documented complete compliance rates of less than 25%. Other factors contributing to clinical failure relating to the drug used are inappropriate dosage, route of administration, or dose interval, poor absorption, inactivation of drug by other drugs used concomitantly, and foci of infection with local environments that affect drug activity. Emergence of drug resistance in the primary pathogen during therapy is relatively unusual: superinfection with a different, resistant organism is a more common cause of what may appear to be treatment failure. Persistent fever in a treated patient may be related to the natural history of the disease, an undrained abscess, phlebitis at the site of intravenous catheters, an infected foreign body, or immunodeficiency.

**Table 64-2.** Adverse effects of antimicrobials

| Frequent | Occasional | Rare |
|---|---|---|
| **Penicillins** | | |
| Rashes, allergic reactions, diarrhea | Hemolytic anemia, drug fever, *C. difficile* colitis | Myoclonus and seizures, interstitial nephritis, hemorrhagic cystitis (methicillin), granulocytopenia, platelet dysfunction, prolonged PT |
| **Cephalosporins** | | |
| Thrombophlebitis with IV use, nausea, diarrhea | Allergic reactions, drug fever, neutropenia, thrombocytopenia, *C. difficile* colitis, prolonged PT (moxalactam) | Positive Coombs' test hemolytic anemia, minimal hepatitis, pneumonitis, interstitial nephritis, disulfiram-like reaction with ETOH, gallstones (ceftriaxone) |
| **Aminoglycosides** | | |
| | Renal toxicity, rash, nausea and vomiting, ototoxicity (auditory and vestibular) | Neuromuscular blockade |
| **Tetracyclines** | | |
| Nausea, vomiting, diarrhea, inhibition of bone growth,* discoloration of teeth,* mucocutaneous candidiasis | Malabsorption, *C. difficile* colitis, photosensitivity, liver damage (with dosages >1 g/day), prolonged PT, vertigo (minocycline) | Allergic reactions, rash, pseudotumor cerebri, diabetes insipidus (demeclocycline) |
| **Macrolides** | | |
| Epigastric pain, nausea, vomiting, diarrhea, thrombophlebitis with IV infusion | Cholestatic hepatitis (erythromycin estolate), reversible ototoxicity with IV infusion | Allergic reactions, rash, *C. difficile* colitis, pancreatitis |
| **Clindamycin** | | |
| Diarrhea, hypersensitivity reactions, rash | Nausea, vomiting, *C. difficile* colitis | Reversible neutropenia |
| **Vancomycin** | | |
| | Thrombophlebitis, hearing loss, nausea, nephrotoxicity (mild), urticaria, rash, upper body redness after rapid IV infusion | Neutropenia, thrombocytopenia |
| **Chloramphenicol** | | |
| | Anemia or leukopenia (reversible), gray syndrome in newborns, nausea, vomiting, diarrhea, mucocutaneous candidiasis | Aplastic anemia, rashes, drug fever, confusion, headache, peripheral neuritis, optic neuritis |
| **Sulfonamides** | | |
| Hypersensitivity reactions (Stevens-Johnson syndrome, rashes, photosensitivity, serum sickness–type reaction), nausea, vomiting | Crystalluria, hemolytic anemia, agranulocytosis | Hepatitis, aplastic anemia, renal tubular necrosis, necrotizing angiitis, pancreatitis, aseptic meningitis, confusion/agitation |
| **Quinolones** | | |
| | Nausea, vomiting, diarrhea, rash, restlessness, lethargy, headache, tremor, mucosal candidiasis | Crystalluria, hematuria, cystitis, *C. difficile* colitis, abnormal LFTs, eosinophilia, neutropenia |

*Occurs primarily in children younger than age 8, or in children whose mothers took tetracycline while pregnant.
*PT*, Prothrombin time; *ETOH*, ethanol; *LFT*, liver function tests.

**Table 64-3.** Available sulfonamides and trimethoprim

| Generic name (trade name) | Adult dosage | Comments |
|---|---|---|
| Trimethoprim/sulfamethoxazole (Bactrim, Septra) | 1 DS tab PO bid<br>8 mg/kg/day, divided q6-12h<br>For PCP, 2 DS tabs PO qid<br>20 mg/kg/day, divided q6-8h | Dosage based on trimethoprim component<br>PO therapy for PCP should be considered only in stable patients without respiratory impairment |
| Trimethoprim (Proloprim, Trimpex) | 100 mg PO q12h or 200 mg PO q24h | May be tolerated in patients with sulfa allergy |
| Sulfisoxazole* (Gantrisin) | 0.5-1 g PO q6h<br>25 mg/kg IV q6h | Used primarily for the treatment of urinary tract infections |
| Sulfamethoxazole* (Gantanol) | 1 g PO q8-12h | Used primarily for the treatment of urinary tract infections |
| Sulfacytine* (Renoquid) | 0.5 g PO load, then 0.25 g PO q6h | |
| Sulfadiazine* (Sulfadyne) | 2-4 g PO load, then 0.5-1 g PO q4-6h | Preferred sulfonamide for the treatment of toxoplasmosis, currently available only through CDC |
| Sulfadoxine† (Fansidar) | 3 tabs PO (d) | Used in the treatment of chloraquine resistant malaria |
| Sulfasalazine (Azulfidine) | 0.5-1 g PO q4-6h | Used in the treatment of ulcerative colitis |

*Short-acting sulfonamides.
†Long-acting sulfonamides.
*PCP, Pneumocystis carinii* pneumonia; *CDC,* Centers for Disease Control and Prevention.

Drug fever may occur with antimicrobial agents and should be considered in patients who continue to have or who redevelop fever during therapy without a demonstrable focus of persistent or new infection. Drug fever may be associated with peripheral blood eosinophilia or rash, but these often are absent.

## SPECIFIC AGENTS

### Sulfonamides and trimethoprim

***Sulfonamides.*** The sulfonamides are bacteriostatic agents that inhibit bacterial growth by interfering with folic acid metabolism, interrupting purine synthesis, and thereby inhibiting DNA synthesis. They are competitive inhibitors of the enzyme dihydrofolic acid synthetase, which catalyzes the conversion of paraaminobenzoic acid (PABA) to dihydrofolic acid. Because mammals can absorb preformed folic acid and therefore are not dependent on this metabolic pathway, bacteria are preferentially affected by this action.

The sulfonamides are active against a wide variety of microorganisms, but the emergence of sulfonamide resistance has limited their utility (Table 64-3). Resistance to the sulfonamides is mediated through the overproduction of PABA (which drives the inhibited metabolic step overcoming competitive inhibition) or through structural changes in the enzyme dihydrofolic acid synthetase (disfavoring the interaction with sulfonamides). Many gram-negative bacilli and cocci are susceptible to sulfonamides; however, the significant prevalence of resistant strains makes empiric use untenable in all but community-acquired *Escherichia coli* urinary tract infection. Drug resistance has limited the use of sulfonamides against many gram-positive cocci, and organisms such as enterococci are always resistant. *Nocardia asteroides* is susceptible to sulfonamides, and these drugs, alone or in combination with others, are standard therapy in infections caused by this organism. The sulfonamides also are active against protozoa such as *Toxoplasma gondii* and malarial parasites.

Sulfonamides are partially metabolized in the liver, with metabolites and unchanged drug excreted in the urine. They vary in their protein binding in serum, with longer acting agents being more highly protein bound than those more rapidly excreted.

The sulfonamides in common use in the United States have a low incidence of side effects (e.g., gastrointestinal upset, dizziness, headache, and fever) compared to some early preparations. Crystalluria and resultant complications of renal damage and urinary tract obstruction also are rare. An important danger of sulfonamides in the newborn is kernicterus. Sulfonamides successfully compete with bilirubin for protein-binding sites in blood, leading to an elevation of free bilirubin levels. For this reason *sulfonamides should never be given to pregnant women during the third trimester.*

Hypersensitivity reactions remain the most important complications of sulfonamide therapy. Systemic reactions, and in particular rashes, are not uncommon. Erythema multiforme, even to the extent of the generalized mucocutaneous involvement of the Stevens-Johnson syndrome, has been clearly associated with sulfonamide therapy. Patients should be specifically questioned as to sulfonamide allergy before use of these drugs.

The oral hypoglycemic agents include sulfonamide derivatives. Drug interaction between sulfonamide antimicrobials and these agents have been reported to cause potentiation of hypoglycemia. Cross-allergy between sulfonamides, oral hypoglycemic agents, and sulfonamide-related diuretics such as furosemide also may occur.

***Trimethoprim.*** Trimethoprim is a pyrimidine derivative that is active against a wide variety of bacteria. The drug inhibits folate and purine metabolism by inhibiting the enzyme dihydrofolic acid reductase, which mediates the step after that inhibited by sulfonamides. The comparable enzyme in humans is more than 10,000 times less susceptible to trimethoprim than the bacterial reductase. Many gram-negative bacilli and gram-positive cocci are susceptible to trimethoprim. Although resistance is easily produced in vitro, it has not yet become a clinical problem.

Trimethoprim was initially available in the United States as a fixed-combination oral preparation with sulfamethoxazole, which, as mentioned above, has similar pharmacologic characteristics. The two agents were combined for a potential synergistic effect, since together they inhibit two sequential steps in a metabolic pathway. Combination therapy reduces the likelihood of the development of resistance to either component of the combination. Trimethoprim is approved for use as a single agent, but the majority of its use occurs in combination with sulfamethoxazole. Trimethoprim-sulfamethoxazole is available in oral and intravenous forms.

Trimethoprim-sulfamethoxazole has been used primarily in the treatment of urinary tract infection. The relatively broad spectrum of activity of the drug against gram-negative bacteria and the convenience of twice daily administration have contributed to a high degree of popularity. Trimethoprim-sulfamethoxazole is well absorbed when taken orally and achieves good tissue levels. High concentrations of trimethoprim-sulfamethoxazole in the prostate make this drug one of the preferred agents in the treatment of prostatitis particularly in men over 50 in whom gram-negative rods are the primary etiologic agents. Single evening doses of trimethoprim-sulfamethoxazole also have been shown to be effective in the prophylaxis of recurrent urinary tract infection.

Trimethoprim-sulfamethoxazole, especially the preparation for intravenous administration, may be used in the treatment of serious infections and bacteremia due to gram-negative bacilli that are resistant to other agents or in patients with allergies to β-lactams. Serious *Salmonella* infections, including typhoid fever, have been treated successfully with trimethoprim-sulfamethoxazole. Trimethoprim-sulfamethoxazole is also effective in the treatment of shigellosis and may be useful in the prevention of traveler's diarrhea (see Chapter 49).

Trimethoprim-sulfamethoxazole is effective against pneumococcus and *Haemophilus influenzae* and can be used to treat chronic bronchitis, otitis media, and other respiratory tract infections. It has become the drug of choice in the treatment of *Pneumocystis carinii* pneumonia. Dosages required are eightfold to tenfold higher than those recommended for other indications. Experience with *P. carinii* pneumonia in the acquired immune deficiency syndrome (AIDS) suggests that these patients have a higher incidence of adverse reactions to trimethoprim-sulfamethoxazole therapy than do other patients. Patients with allergic manifestations to trimethoprim-sulfamethoxazole may tolerate trimethoprim singly or in combination with other agents. Trimethoprim-sulfamethoxazole has been found effective in preventing *P. carinii* and toxoplasmosis in patients with AIDS when taken two to three times per week. Trimethoprim-sulfamethoxazole is also used in selected patients undergoing chemotherapy, primarily for hematologic malignancies, to prevent *P. carinii* pneumonia.

Trimethoprim is excreted as an active drug as well as metabolites in the urine. The dosages of trimethoprim and trimethoprim-sulfamethoxazole must be adjusted in renal failure, and these drugs should be avoided in patients with serious renal functional impairment. Trimethoprim and sulfamethoxazole are removed by hemodialysis.

All the side effects, toxic reactions, and hypersensitivity reactions observed with the sulfonamides also may occur with trimethoprim-sulfamethoxazole, including bone marrow suppression. This effect may be diminished with the administration of folinic acid. Nephrotoxicity also has been associated with trimethoprim-sulfamethoxazole therapy. Trimethoprim and trimethoprim-sulfamethoxazole should be avoided in pregnancy.

### β-Lactam antibiotics

The β-lactam antibiotics include the penicillins, cephalosporins, monobactams, carbapenams, and other groups of compounds currently under development. The prototype of this group, and indeed the first antibiotic in clinical use, is penicillin. Penicillin was discovered as a product of the mold *Penicillium notatum* by Fleming in 1929 and was developed for clinical use by Chain, Florey, and their colleagues at Oxford before and during World War II. Since that time a number of derivatives of penicillin have been and continue to be discovered and produced. The first cephalosporin was discovered by Giuseppe Brotzu in Sardinia in 1946 as a fermentation product of *Cephalosporium acremonium.* Manipulations of the side chains of the cephalosporin nucleus have resulted in dozens of active derivatives. Completely novel β-lactam compounds have been developed and promise even more potential derivatives. The large number of β-lactam agents available and under investigation has resulted from greater sophistication in the manipulation of chemical structures to produce novel compounds with increased potency, expanded antimicrobial activity, and advantageous pharmacologic properties.

The β-lactam antibiotics share a similar mode of action. They interact with a set of enzymes (also called penicillin-binding proteins), which mediate production of the bacterial cell wall glycopeptide. Various agents affect different enzymes or groups of enzymes. The result is impairment of the bacterium's ability to construct the latticelike, giant single molecule of glycopeptide, which is the main structural support of the bacterial cell. The defective cell wall may result in a loss of rigidity of the cell or an inability of the cell to maintain its integrity under the stress of osmotic conditions. The defect may also result in fruitless elongation of a cell into a filament incapable of successful division. Other, more subtle, changes in the integrity of the cell wall may make it more susceptible to enzymes that cause breaks in the glycopeptide. Such enzymes are necessary for new cell formation at the time of cell division. The bacterial cell may also become more susceptible to other environmental factors.

The most important mechanism of bacterial resistance to the β-lactam antibiotics is the production of inactivating enzymes, or β-lactamases. A number of β-lactamases have been identified. Some are genetically coded in plasmids, and others are the product of genes in the bacterial chromosome. Some β-lactamases break the β-lactam ring of some of the β-lactam agents and not others, and some of these enzymes have broad-spectrum effects. Semisynthetic β-lactam antibiotics have been engineered to resist a broad spectrum of β-lactamases. Resistance to β-lactam agents may also be mediated through an impermeability of the surface of the bacterium, which prevents the drugs getting to their sites of action. Resistance to β-lactam antibiotics is a field of increasing investigational interest. New mechanisms are regularly being identified.

The β-lactam antibiotics are a remarkably safe group of drugs. The human organism does not have any metabolic processes similar to bacterial glycopeptide production or maintenance. As a group, compounds containing the β-lactam ring appear to have only one direct toxic effect, and that is neurotoxicity. Penicillin directly placed on the cerebral cortex causes seizures. Similarly, seizures and abnormal myoclonic movements may be seen in patients with renal impairment who are given large doses of penicillin. The neurotoxic potential of other β-lactam antibiotics has not been fully assessed. A number of β-lactam agents have been associated with renal toxicity, acute tubular necrosis, or interstitial nephritis. Nephrotoxicity has been clearly demonstrated with some β-lactams, associated with others, and not yet observed with the use of some.

Penicillin is associated with a relatively high incidence of hypersensitivity reactions. A variety of hypersensitivity reactions have been described, including acute anaphylaxis, angioneurotic edema, erythema multiforme, nondescript rashes, erythema nodosum, and serum sickness syndromes. A significant percentage of patients who have been treated with penicillin give a history of a variety of adverse reactions. It is necessary to take a careful history to determine the risk of β-lactam administration. Many patients describe allergies when in truth the adverse reaction is more accurately an intolerance, such as gastrointestinal distress. Skin test material, although available, is not very reliable (i.e., false negative skin tests may give rise to dangerous confidence). A significant incidence of cross-reactivity between cephalosporins and penicillins has been cited; however, clinical experience suggests that this may be more a case of associated allergies (allergy to multiple allergens rather than cross-reaction). As a rule, treatment with a β-lactam should be avoided in any patient with a history of allergy to any other β-lactam agent, especially if the previous reaction was urticarial or anaphylactic. Imipenem is structurally closer to penicillin than cephalosporins and should be used extremely cautiously in patients with true penicillin allergy. If satisfactory alternative therapy is not available, a drug of a different group (e.g., a cephalosporin in a patient allergic to a penicillin) may be administered with informed consent and provision for emergency treatment of anaphylaxis. The probability of an allergic reaction in a particular setting is difficult to predict, since repeat penicillin therapy in a patient with documented allergy may result either in a life-threatening reaction or no reaction at all. In rare instances desensitization with sequential doses of penicillin may be attempted after obtaining expert consultation.

All the β-lactam antibiotics are excreted in urine. They are cleared by glomerular filtration, and most are actively secreted by the renal tubule. Secretion can be competitively inhibited by drugs such as probenecid. Some of the most recently developed β-lactam agents appear to be excreted primarily by glomerular filtration without significant tubular secretion. All β-lactams require some dosage adjustment for significant renal dysfunction with the exception of nafcillin, cefoperazone, and ceftriaxone, which are hepatically metabolized.

***Penicillin G.*** The earliest preparations of penicillin were mixtures of various forms of the drug and were defined according to units of activity, which are still used to prescribe penicillin. Among the various forms of penicillin, penicillin G had the best clinical characteristics and became the standard. Production of pure, soluble salts of penicillin G capable of forming crystals gave rise to the term *crystalline penicillin G.* The designation *aqueous penicillin G* specifies the soluble salts of the antibiotic. One unit of penicillin is equivalent to 0.6 μg of pure sodium penicillin G.

Although much attention is directed toward broad-spectrum "big gun" antibiotics, penicillin G is still the drug of choice for a number of the most significant infections affecting humans. Among these are infections due to group A β-hemolytic streptococci, *Streptococcus pneumoniae,* other streptococcal species, the meningococci, clostridia, many other anaerobic bacteria, and spirochetes (in particular syphilis). Penicillin can no longer be given empirically for gonococcal infection due to increasing resistance. In certain communities, penicillin cannot be used with confidence for empiric treatment of pneumococcal infection. The vast majority of strains of *S. aureus* have become resistant to the drug, but infection due to penicillin-sensitive *S. aureus* is still best treated with penicillin.

Aqueous penicillin G is available as very soluble sodium or potassium salts. In this form the drug is usually given by intravenous infusion or occasionally, intramuscularly. Intermittent administration is preferred because the drug is relatively unstable in many infusion solutions and may achieve higher tissue levels as a result of high concentration gradients following intermittent dosing. Penicillin G is rapidly excreted, and the half-life of the drug after bolus infusion is approximately 30 minutes. Because of this short half-life, the drug should be administered with an interval between doses of no longer than 4 hours. Usual doses of intravenous penicillin G range from 400,000 U every 4 hours for uncomplicated pneumococcal pneumonia, to 6 to 10 million U per day for anaerobic pleuropulmonary infections, to 2 million U every 2 hours for meningococcal or pneumococcal meningitis.

Penicillin can also be administered intramuscularly in procaine or benzathine form (Table 64-4).

***Penicillin V.*** Penicillin V, or phenoxymethyl penicillin, is an acid-stable, naturally occurring penicillin available as potassium and sodium salts for oral administration. Its gastrointestinal absorption is significantly better than that of penicillin G, and it has become the oral penicillin in general use. Penicillin V is only slightly less active against most gram-positive organisms that are susceptible to penicillin G but is of an order of magnitude less active against gram-negative penicillin-sensitive organisms such as gonococcus and meningococcus. Penicillin V is used for the oral therapy of streptococcal disease, pneumococcal pneumonia, and dental infections of mild severity. It also is used for rheumatic fever prophylaxis and for endocarditis prophylaxis when parenteral therapy is impractical.

***Penicillinase-resistant penicillins.*** This refers to penicillins that are resistant to staphylococcal penicillinase and thus may be used interchangeably with the term *antistaphylococcal penicillin.* These penicillins include methicillin, oxacillin, nafcillin, cloxacillin, dicloxacillin, and several others not in common use. They are active against penicillinase-producing *S. aureus* but are less active than penicillin G against penicillin-susceptible *S. aureus.* The drugs are active against other penicillin-susceptible gram-positive organisms at achievable blood and serum levels but are inactive against gram-negative organisms. As compared to the other penicillins, antistaphylococcal penicillins are inactive against enterococci.

Methicillin was the first penicillinase-resistant penicillin available. It is rapidly excreted in the urine and is only 35% protein bound in serum. It has been associated with a higher incidence of interstitial nephritis than other available penicillins and therefore is now used less frequently. This same adverse effect has been described less frequently with other penicillins. Nafcillin is somewhat more active against susceptible organisms than methicillin but is highly protein bound (87%) in serum. Nafcillin is excreted to a significant extent by the liver and thus requires no dosage adjustment in renal insufficiency. Methicillin is not absorbed after oral ingestion, and nafcillin is only minimally absorbed. Methicillin can be administered by intramuscular injection, but the preferred route is intravenous.

The isoxazolyl penicillins are penicillinase resistant and acid stable. They are semisynthetic penicillins that are better absorbed after oral administration than methicillin and nafcillin. Oxacillin is available for intramuscular, intravenous, and oral administration. The oral form is less well absorbed than other available agents, and the drug is usually given parenterally. It is rapidly excreted by the kidneys. Cloxacillin and dicloxacillin are well absorbed after oral administration and are usually preferred for oral use.

Serious infections due to *S. aureus* are treated with large parenteral doses of the penicillinase-resistant penicillins. Methicillin, nafcillin, and oxacillin are interchangeable for most clinical purposes and are given in dosages of 8 to 12 g per day in adults. In clinical situations such as skin infections, where either *S. aureus* or streptococci may be significant pathogens, one of these agents is usually sufficient. Many hospitals use nafcillin and oxacillin interchangeably for parenteral administration, depending on cost. In some uncommon situations nafcillin is preferable to another of this group because of its somewhat higher intrinsic activity against *S. aureus* (e.g., nafcillin has an added advantage of slightly better penetration into the central nervous system in patients with staphylococcal meningitis).

Oral penicillinase-resistant penicillins are used primarily for skin infections of limited severity. Both cloxacillin and dicloxacillin are well absorbed and well tolerated; however, dicloxacillin gives higher serum levels after identical doses.

The emergence of *S. aureus* resistant to penicillinase-resistant penicillins (often called methicillin-resistant *S. aureus* is an increasing problem worldwide. These organisms are usually found in the hospital environment, although increasing numbers of isolates are coming from community sources, especially from among drug addicts in urban areas. These methicillin-resistant strains of *S. aureus* are frequently resistant to a variety of agents, and alternative agents, such as vancomycin, will have to be used pending susceptibility studies.

***Ampicillin, amoxicillin, and other aminopenicillins.*** Ampicillin was the first semisynthetic, broad-spectrum penicillin derived from 6-aminopenicillanic acid. Since its discovery, a number of derivatives of the compound and related compounds have been developed. Ampicillin and related drugs are active against most bacteria susceptible to penicillin G, and are also active against some *E. coli,* other Enterobacteriaceae, and *H. influenzae.* Unfortunately, resistance to ampicillin is now increasing in these pathogens, and susceptibility cannot be assumed.

Ampicillin and the other aminopenicillins are used in the treatment of upper and lower respiratory tract infections (e.g., otitis media in children and bronchitis in adults, which are usually caused by pneumococci or *H. influenzae*). They are also prescribed for urinary tract infections (most community-acquired *E. coli* remain sensitive) and are used in oral regimens for the treatment of *Salmonella* and *Shigella* infections. Parenteral ampicillin is used in the treatment of bacterial meningitis caused by *Listeria* and for therapy of endocarditis secondary to enterococci. Ampicillin is the preferred therapy for severe enterococcal infection and is commonly used in combination with other agents to cover enterococci in the setting of abdominal or biliary infection. Ampicillin should always be used with an aminoglycoside to produce a bactericidal effect in the setting of enterococcal endocarditis and bacteremia. Intravenous dosages amount to 2 to 6 g per day.

Although ampicillin is available in an oral form that results in adequate levels after ingestion, amoxicillin is frequently the preferred oral equivalent to ampicillin. Amoxicillin gives higher levels than ampicillin after oral administration, and it may provoke less diarrhea and other types of gastrointestinal upset. Compliance may also be better with amoxicillin because of its every 8 hour dosing as opposed to ampicillin's every 6 hour dosing. Amoxicillin has a similar spectrum of activity when compared to ampicillin. It is frequently used in the treatment of otitis media, urinary tract infections, and upper and lower respiratory tract infections.

The adverse reactions observed with ampicillin and related compounds are similar to those observed with other penicillins, as described above. Ampicillin is, however, associated with *ampicillin rash,* a bright red, maculopapular eruption usually occurring sometime after 5 days of therapy. The etiology of this rash is obscure and may not be truly allergic. Although it may resolve despite continued therapy, the possibility of morbidity from allergic mechanisms requires both the discontinuation of the drug and designation of the patient as penicillin allergic. The documentation of ampicillin rash is important, however, because in some instances (e.g., endocarditis, meningitis) the benefits of penicillin therapy may outweigh the

**Table 64-4.** Classification and characteristics of the penicillins

| Generic name | Trade names | Route of administration | Adult dosage*† |
|---|---|---|---|
| **Natural penicillins** | | | |
| Penicillin G | Pentids, Pfizerpen | IV, IM, PO | 0.25-0.5 g q6h PO; 1.2-24 × $10^6$ U/day IV/IM |
| Penicillin G procaine | Wycillin, Duracillin | IM | 0.3-4.8 million U q6-12h |
| Penicillin G benzathine | Bicillin, Permapen | IM | 2.4 million U IM‡ |
| Penicillin V | Pen-Vee K, V-Cillin, Penapar | PO | 0.25-0.5 g q6h |
| **Penicillinase-resistant penicillins** | | | |
| Methicillin | Staphcillin | IV, IM | 1-2 g IV/IM q4-6h |
| Oxacillin | Prostaphlin | IV, IM, PO | 0.5-1 g PO q6h; 0.5-2 g IM/IV q4-6h |
| Nafcillin | Unipen, Nafcil | IV, IM | 0.5-2 g IV/IM q4-6h |
| Cloxacillin | Tegopen, Cloxapen | PO | 0.25-0.5 g q6h |
| Dicloxacillin | Dynapen, Dycill | PO | 0.25-0.5 g q6h |
| **Aminopenicillins** | | | |
| Ampicillin | Polycillin, Omnipen | IV, IM, PO | 0.25-0.5 g PO q6h; 1-2 g IV/IM q6h |
| Amoxicillin | Amoxil, Polymox | PO | 0.25-0.5 g q8h |
| Bacampicillin | Spectrobid | PO | 0.4-0.8 g q12h |
| Hetacillin | Versapen | PO | 0.225-0.45 g q6h |
| Cyclacillin | Cyclapen | PO | 0.25-0.5 g q6h |
| **Carboxypenicillins** | | | |
| Carbenicillin | Geopen | IV, IM, PO | 0.38-0.76 g PO q6h; 5-6.5 g IV/IM q4-6h |
| Ticarcillin | Ticar | IV, IM | 1-3 g IV/IM q4-6h |
| **Ureidopenicillins** | | | |
| Mezlocillin | Mezlin | IV, IM | 3-4 g IV/IM q4-6h |
| Piperacillin | Pipracil | IV | 3-4 g q4-6h |
| **Penicillin plus β-lactamase inhibitors** | | | |
| Amoxicillin/clavulanic acid | Augmentin | PO | 0.25-0.5 g q8h |
| Ampicillin/sulbactam | Unasyn | IV, IM | 1.5-3 g IV/IM q6h |
| Ticarcillin/clavulanic acid | Timentin | IV | 3.1 g q4-6h |
| Piperacillin/tazobactam | Zosyn | IV | 3 g/0.375 g IV q6h |

*All penicillins other than nafcillin and oxacillin require dosage adjustment for creatinine clearance.
†The higher end of the dosage spectrum should be used for severe infections.
‡Newborns (<1 mo of age) require specific dosing, see Mandell et al. and Sanford for dosage recommendations.
§Not FDA approved for pediatric use.
||Indications are generalized for the penicillin subgroup rather than for specific agents unless mentioned by name.

potential risk of a serious allergic reaction. It is noteworthy that virtually all patients who receive ampicillin during active infectious mononucleosis develop the ampicillin rash.

***Antipseudomonal and extended spectrum penicillins.*** Several penicillins, when given in large enough doses, have significant in vivo activity against *P. aeruginosa.* Carbenicillin was the first of these drugs and was developed at a time when *P. aeruginosa* was becoming an increasing problem in the compromised host. Ticarcillin was developed later and is more active than carbenicillin against most strains of *P. aeruginosa.* Both carbenicillin and ticarcillin must be given in large dosages (approximately 5 and 3 g, respectively, every 4 hours) to patients with normal renal function to achieve serum levels adequate for inhibiting most strains of *P. aeruginosa.* Each of these drugs contains 4.7 mEq of sodium per gram, so the sodium load can be substantial (equivalent to 1 L of normal saline per day with carbenicillin). The large dosages and rapid renal clearances of these drugs also result in the delivery of large amounts of nonabsorbable anion to the renal tubule, which may lead to hypokalemia. Carbenicillin, and probably most penicillins in large enough dosages, may also interfere with platelet function.

Mezlocillin and piperacillin are more recently developed antipseudomonal agents. These drugs are active against a variety of gram-negative bacilli including *P. aeruginosa,* although the susceptibility of *P. aeruginosa* may vary among communities. In general, piperacillin is active against a higher percentage of isolates than is mezlocillin. These drugs have essentially replaced carbenicillin and ticarcillin. They are being used as single-drug therapy for intraabdominal infection because of their broad spectrum of activity against aerobic and anaerobic gram-negative organisms and gram-positive cocci, includ-

| Pediatric dosage*†‡ | Indications‖ |
|---|---|
| 6.25-12.5 mg/kg q6h PO;<br>100,000-250,000 U/kg/day IV/IM q2-12h<br>25,000 U/kg q12-24h<br>50,000 U/kg*<br>6.25-12.5 mg/kg q6h | Streptococcal infections including pneumococci, *Actinomyces, Clostridium tetani, C. perfringens, Pasteurella,* oral anaerobes, *Neisseria meningitidis,* syphillis; benzathine penicillin used in prophylaxis of rheumatic fever |
| 25-33 mg/kg IV/IM q4-6h<br>12.5-25 mg/kg PO q6h; 37.5-50 mg/kg IV/IM q6h<br>150 mg/kg/day IV/IM q4-6h<br>12.5-25 mg/kg q6h<br>3.125-6.25 mg/kg q6h | Sensitive *Staphylococcus aureus, Streptococcus pyogenes* (group A streptococci) |
| 12.5-25 mg/kg PO q6h; 25-50 mg/kg IV/IM q6h<br>6.6-13.3 mg/kg q8h<br>12.5-25 mg/kg q12h<br>5.6-11.25 mg/kg q6h<br>12.5-25 mg/kg q6h | Penicillin-sensitive enterococci, other streptococci, *Listeria, Escherichia coli, Proteus,* and *Haemophilus influenzae,* which have tested susceptible to ampicillin |
| 7.5-12.5 mg/kg PO q6h; 24-100 mg/kg IV/IM q4-6h<br>50 mg/kg IV/IM q4-6h | Active against many gram-negative bacilli including some *Pseudomonas* strains, but preferred therapy is usually the other antipseudomonal penicillins |
| 50 mg/kg IV/IM q6h<br>50 mg/kg q4-6h§ | Active against most *P. aeruginosa* strains; also effective against penicillin-sensitive enterococci and other gram-negative bacilli; if used at maximal dosage, active against *Bacteroides fragilis* |
| 20-40 mg/kg/day, given q8h§<br>200 mg/kg/day q4-6h§ | Streptococcal species including enterococci and pneumococci; methicillin-sensitive *S. aureus,* oral and bowel anaerobes, sensitive gram-negative rods such as *E. coli, Klebsiella, Proteus* and *H. influenzae;* piperacillin/tazobactam and ticarcillin/clavulanic acid active against most isolates of *P. aeruginosa* |

ing enterococci. In many hospitals mezlocillin or piperacillin, in combination with an aminoglycoside, is used as empiric therapy for febrile neutropenic patients in which *P. aeruginosa* remains a major concern. These drugs have pharmacokinetic properties similar to those of carbenicillin and ticarcillin, but they have less sodium per gram. All of the antipseudomonal penicillins should be used with an aminoglycoside for synergy if a bactericidal effect against *P. aeruginosa* is desired.

All of the antipseudomonal and extended-spectrum penicillins are rapidly excreted by the normal kidney. Because all are given in large dosages (16 to 30 g per day) any impairment in renal function may lead to accumulation of the drugs. Thus in the presence of renal function impairment the dosages of these drugs should be modified. Mezlocillin and piperacillin are given in dosages of 2 to 4 g every 4 to 6 hours.

***Penicillin/β-lactamase inhibitor combinations.*** One method of broadening the spectrum of the penicillins has been the addition of β-lactamase inhibitors to specific agents (see Table 64-4). These inhibitors function by neutralizing the enzyme produced by the bacteria, which ordinarily would have inactivated the penicillin. The β-lactamase inhibitors have a high affinity for the β-lactamases, and by binding to them prevent the enzyme from binding to the β-lactam ring of the penicillin. Adding a β-lactamase inhibitor does not improve activity against organisms whose method of resistance is other than β-lactamase production.

Three β-lactamase inhibitors are available in combination with agents of the penicillin class: sulbactam, clavulanic acid, and tazobactam. These agents inhibit some β-lactamases but not all. In general, the β-lactamases produced by *S. aureus,* most anaerobes, and some gram-negative bacilli are affected by β-lactamase inhibitors. β-Lactamase inhibitors do not act against the type of β-lactamases (termed class I) produced by *Pseudomonas;* consequently their addition does not extend activity against *P. aeruginosa.* There is at least a theoretical disadvantage in using sulbactam in that it has been shown to induce the production of class I β-lactamases.

Amoxicillin/clavulanic acid was the first available drug in this category. The spectrum of activity of

**Table 64-5.** Classification and characteristics of cephalosporins

| Generic name | Trade name | Route of administration | Adult dosage* normal creatinine clearance† |
|---|---|---|---|
| **First generation** | | | |
| Cefazolin | Ancef, Kefzol | IM, IV | 1-2 g q8h |
| Cephalothin | Keflin, Seflin | IM, IV | 0.5-2 g q4-6h |
| Cephapirin | Cefadyl | IM, IV | 0.5-2 g q4-6h |
| Cephalexin | Keflex | PO | 0.25-0.5g q6h |
| Cephradine | Velosef, Anspor | IV, IM, PO | 0.25-0.5g PO q6h |
| Cefadroxil | Duricef | PO | 0.5 mg q12h or 1 g qd |
| **Second generation** | | | |
| Cefaclor‖ | Ceclor | PO | 0.25-0.5 mg q8h |
| Cefamandole | Mandol | IM, IV | 0.5-2 g q4-6h |
| Cefonicid | Monocid | IM, IV | 1-2 g q24h |
| Cefotetan | Cefotan | IM, IV | 1-3 g q12h |
| Cefoxitan | Mefoxin | IM, IV | 1-2 g q4-8h |
| Cefmetazole | Zefazone | IV | 2 g q6-12h |
| Ceforanide | Precef | IM, IV | 0.5-1 g q12h |
| Cefuroxime | Zinacef, Kefurox | IM, IV | 0.75-1.5 q 6-8h |
| Cefuroxime axetil | Ceftin | PO | 0.125-0.25 g q12h |
| Cefprozil | Cefzil | PO | 500 mg q12h |
| Loracarbef | Lorabid | PO | 200 mg q12-24h |
| **Third generation** | | | |
| Cefoperazone | Cefobid | IV | 2-4 g q6-12h |
| Cefotaxime | Claforan | IV | 1-2 g q8h |
| Ceftriaxone | Rocephin, Nitrocephin | IM, IV | 1-2 g q12-24h |
| Ceftazidime | Fortaz, Tazicef | IM, IV | 1-2 g q8h |
| Ceftizoxime | Ceftizox | IM, IV | 1-2 g q8h |
| Cefsulodin | Cefomonil | IV | 1-1.5 g q6h |
| Cefixime | Suprax | PO | 400 mg qd |
| Cefpodoxime | Vantin | PO | 100-400 mg q12h |
| Ceftibuten# | Cedax | PO | 200 mg q12h |
| Cefetamet# | | PO | 500 mg q12h |
| **Fourth generation** | | | |
| Cefipime# | | IV | 1-2 g q8-12h |

*The higher end of the dosage spectrum should be used for serious infections.
†All cephalosporins other than cefoperazone and ceftriaxone require dosage adjustment for creatinine clearance <50.
‡Newborns (<1 month of age) require specific dosing; see Mandell et al. and Sanford.
§None of the cephalosporins have any activity against enterococci or methicillin-resistant *S. aureus*.
‖Some sources refer to cefaclor as a first-generation cephalosporin.
¶No pediatric dosing available.
#Not as yet FDA approved.

amoxicillin is broadened by the clavulanic acid to include methicillin-sensitive *S. aureus,* β-lactamase–producing *H. influenzae,* most anaerobes, and the majority of *E. coli, Proteus,* and *Klebsiella* species. This agent is well absorbed with excellent tissue penetration. It is commonly used in the treatment of upper and lower respiratory tract infections, including sinusitis and otitis. Ampicillin/clavulanic acid is active against *S. pyogenes,* most *S. aureus,* and *Pasteurella multocida,* which makes it a preferred oral agent for treatment of soft tissue infections resulting from animal bites.

Ampicillin/sulbactam is a parenteral agent with a spectrum of activity similar to that of amoxicillin/clavulanic acid. Ampicillin/sulbactam is used in the treatment of lower respiratory tract infections and complicated intraabdominal and soft tissue infections in patients at risk for infection with gram-negative bacilli.

The addition of clavulanic acid to ticarcillin extends its coverage to include β-lactamase–producing *S. aureus* and additional strains of *Bacteroides, H. influenzae, Morganella, Klebsiella,* and *Proteus.* Ticarcillin/clavulanic acid is used in settings in which broad-spectrum gram-positive and gram-negative coverage is desired.

Piperacillin/tazobactam has coverage comparable to that of ticarcillin/clavulanic acid, with perhaps better gram-negative and pseudomonal coverage as a result of the intrinsic activity of piperacillin as compared to that of ticarcillin.

***Cephalosporins.*** The cephalosporins are a large and growing group of β-lactam antibiotics. The first practical and clinically useful cephalosporin derivative was cephal-

| Dosage in children*†‡ | Comments/Indications§ |
|---|---|
| 8.3-25 mg/kg q6-8h<br>75-160 mg/kg q4-6h<br>10-20 mg/kg q6h<br>6.25-25 mg/kg q6h<br>6.25-12.5 mg/kg q6-12h<br>15 mg/kg q12h | Spectrum of all agents similar; effectiveness against nonenterococcal streptococci and *S. aureus* (methicillin-S) allows their use for PO and parenteral therapy of skin and soft tissue infections; cefazolin is used for surgical prophylaxis; these drugs are alternative agents for treatment of community-acquired urinary tract infections and for therapy of infections caused by susceptible gram-negative rods |
| 6.6 mg/kg q8h<br>50-150 mg/kg/day q4-8h<br>¶<br>20-30 mg/kg q12h<br>80-160 mg/kg/day q6h<br>¶<br>¶<br>50-250 mg/kg/day q6-8h<br>125-250 mg q12h<br>15 mg/kg q12h<br>15-30 mg/kg/day q12h | Cefotetan and cefoxitan have good activity against *B. fragilis* as well as most enteric gram-negative rods; used as prophylaxis for abdominal surgery and to treat intraabdominal infections; remaining agents have a similar spectrum of activity, including effectiveness, against respiratory flora such as *H. influenzae, Branamella,* and pneumococci; widely used in the treatment of otitis, sinusitis, bronchitis, and pneumonia |
| 25-100 mg/kg q12h<br>50-180 mg/kg/day q6h<br>50-100 mg/kg/day q12-24h<br>30-50 mg/kg q8h<br>200 mg/kg/day q6h<br>15-25 mg/kg q6h<br>8 mg/kg qd<br>10 mg/kg/day q12h<br>4 mg/kg q12h<br>¶ | All third-generation cephalosporins have increased activity against gram-negative bacilli, with diminished effectiveness against streptoccocci and *S. aureus;* ceftazidime and cefaperazone have activity against *P. aeruginosa;* ceftazidime, cefotaxime, ceftriaxone, and ceftizoxime achieve therapeutic levels in cerebrospinal fluid; as a result of this broad spectrum of activity, third-generation cephalosporins are frequently used for patients who appear bacteremic or who are seriously ill without a clear focus of infection; ceftriaxone and cefixime are indicated as one-dose therapy for gonococcal infection |
| ¶ | |

othin, which became available in 1964. Currently there are at least 20 different cephalosporins. They tend to be the most confusing group of antibiotics to clinicians because of the similarity of their names and because the different agents have very similar coverage. For example, there are six cephalosporins available for coverage of gram-positive cocci, *E. coli,* and some isolates of *Klebsiella* and *Proteus.* To help make sense of the cephalosporins, they have been roughly organized into first-, second-, and third-generation agents, with this division based primarily on similarity of coverage and order of development. In general, first-generation cephalosporins are the preferred cephalosporins to use against *S. aureus* and most streptococci, whereas the third-generation cephalosporins have the broadest coverage against gram-negative pathogens. The second generation includes agents with coverage against *Bacteroides fragilis,* and the third generation contains the agents with the best central nervous system penetration. Cephalosporins are frequently used for surgical prophylaxis because of their relatively broad spectrum of activity and their comparatively long half-life, which reduces the need for multiple doses. Cephalosporins are universally ineffective against enterococci, methicillin-resistant *S. aureus,* and most coagulase-negative staphylococci. Cephalosporins can be considered as alternative therapy in penicillin-allergic patients, but only with extreme caution. They should be avoided if the allergy is of the immediate hypersensitivity type such as urticaria or anaphylaxis.

Most hospital formularies carry only two or three representative cephalosporins from each generation, so it is usually not necessary to become familiar with every agent available. Table 64-5 lists all the available cephalosporins.

**First-generation cephalosporins.** The first-generation cephalosporins, with cephalothin as the representative drug, are broad-spectrum agents active against most gram-positive cocci and some aerobic gram-negative bacilli. They are relatively stable in the presence of *S. aureus*–produced penicillinase and are almost as effective as methicillin and other penicillinase-resistant drugs in the treatment of serious infections caused by this organism.

In addition to their activity against *S. aureus* and streptococci, the first-generation cephalosporins can be effective against *E. coli* and some *Proteus* and *Klebsiella* species. This gram-negative coverage is variable and limits their empiric use. First-generation cephalosporins are frequently used as surgical prophylaxis for procedures in which the risk of anaerobic and gram-negative infection is low. Cefazolin usually is preferred for prophylactic purposes because of the persistence of serum levels achieved after administration by either intravenous or intramuscular injection.

Adverse reactions observed with first-generation cephalosporins are similar to those observed with β-lactam agents as a whole. Diarrhea, dyspepsia, and rarely pseudomembranous colitis may occur. Allergic reactions, neutropenia, and thrombocytopenia are also occasional side effects. In addition, nephrotoxicity has been described with members of this group. Dosages of the first-generation drugs need only minor to moderate adjustment with diminished renal function.

Several first-generation cephalosporins are available for oral administration. These drugs are similar in antibacterial spectrum to the parenteral first-generation cephalosporins. They vary slightly in activity against particular organisms and in pharmacokinetics after oral administration. Cefaclor is more active against gram-negative organisms, such as *H. influenzae,* than the other oral first-generation agents, but serum levels are somewhat less. Available first-generation cephalosporins are summarized in Table 64-5.

The oral cephalosporins are excreted by the kidney, and high urinary concentrations are achieved. The drugs are useful in the treatment of urinary tract infection, especially those caused by *E. coli* and *Klebsiella,* as well as skin and soft tissue infections. The activity of cefaclor against *H. influenzae* and gram-positive cocci, and its usual three times per day dosing, has made it popular for the treatment of otitis media in children.

**Second-generation cephalosporins.** Cefoxitin and cefamandole were the first second-generation cephalosporins and were marketed in the United States during the late 1970s. Chemically, cefoxitin is actually a cephamycin and is a derivative of a natural product different from the cephalosporins. Officially, however, cefoxitin is grouped among the cephalosporins. Cefuroxime and cefotetan are other second generation agents commonly used in the United States (see Table 64-5).

The second-generation cephalosporins differ from the first-generation agents in their much broader activity against Enterobacteriaceae and other gram-negative pathogens and their lesser potency against susceptible gram-positive cocci. Cefoxitin and cefotetan are highly resistant to a number of β-lactamases, including that produced by *B. fragilis,* and these drugs are active against most strains of this organism. As compared to the first generation, agents including cefaclor, cefuroxime, and cefamandole provide almost complete coverage against *H. influenzae,* including β-lactamase–producing strains. Cefoxitin is active against penicillin-susceptible and penicillin-resistant gonococci.

The second-generation cephalosporins are useful mainly in two capacities. Cefoxitin and cefotetan are used in the prophylaxis and treatment of abdominal infections involving bowel anaerobes and gram-negative organisms. Cefamandole and cefuroxime, because of their activity against *H. influenzae* and pneumococci, are used to treat ear infections in children and lower respiratory tract infection in adults. Second-generation cephalosporins have been replaced by the third-generation cephalosporins in the treatment of meningitis due to their ability to achieve superior cerebrospinal fluid (CSF) drug levels.

Adverse effects seen with the second-generation cephalosporins are basically the same as those of the first generation. Cefamandole is excreted in the bile and has been associated with hypoprothrombinemia reversible with vitamin K (see discussion of moxalactam below). Cefamandole also inhibits alcohol dehydrogenase and may cause a disulfiram-type reaction in patients imbibing alcohol. The second-generation cephalosporins are excreted primarily via the kidneys by filtration and tubular secretion.

All these drugs can be given intramuscularly, with cefuroxime being the best tolerated. Cefoxitin has been reported to interfere with serum and urine creatinine determinations, and cefamandole may give a false positive reaction with certain tests for glucose. Cefuroxime is available in oral form as cefuroxime axetil. This drug has a longer half-life than the oral first-generation cephalosporins and can be administered twice daily. Cefuroxime axetil has a similar spectrum of activity to that of intravenous cefuroxime and is used for similar indications.

**Third-generation cephalosporins and moxalactam.** The third-generation cephalosporins include both true cephalosporins and moxalactam, which is a 1-oxa-β-lactam with oxygen in place of the sulfur atom in the cephem ring. Available third-generation drugs include cefotaxime, moxalactam, cefoperazone, ceftizoxime, ceftriaxone, and ceftazidime. A number of other agents are under investigation or close to release.

The third-generation agents have an extended coverage against gram-negative bacilli as well as increased potency against susceptible organisms compared to the second generation cephalosporins. These drugs are among the most active antibiotics against Enterobacteriaceae. Activity against gram-positive cocci is less than that observed with first- and second-generation drugs. Although some of the third-generation agents have modest activity against staphylococci and streptococci, they are not preferred as therapy for gram-positive infections.

The primary use for third-generation cephalosporins is the treatment of infections caused by gram-negative bacilli resistant to other agents and, in particular, multiresistant organisms. Ceftriaxone, cefotaxime, and ceftizoxime are also recommended agents in the treatment of meningitis, specifically that caused by *H. influenzae* and other susceptible gram-negative bacilli. This efficacy derives from tissue penetration characteristics and very high levels of activity (low MICs). Ceftazidime is effective against most *P. aeruginosa* and achieves excellent CSF levels. For this reason it is used in the empiric treatment of meningitis usually in combination with vancomycin in patients following neurosurgery. Ceftazidime is also used in other clinical situations where coverage of *P. aeruginosa* is desired, such as nosocomial pneumonia and the empiric treatment of the febrile neutropenic patient. As with the antipseudomonal penicillins, combination therapy with an aminoglycoside is usually recommended. Ceftriaxone has the longest half-life of the third-generation cephalosporins and can be given once daily. For that reason it has become a commonly used agent in outpatient intravenous antibiotic therapy. Ceftriaxone is also the preferred agent in the treatment of CNS Lyme disease.

The third-generation cephalosporins appear to share the adverse reactions of the first- and second-generation drugs. Cefoperazone, cefotetan, and moxalactam share a tetrazol substituent with cefamandole, which appears to be responsible for inhibition of alcohol dehydrogenase leading to the potential for a disulfiram-type reaction seen in some patients exposed to alcohol. Moxalactam may cause impaired platelet function and may also affect the production of vitamin K–dependent clotting factors. This latter activity is associated with the above-mentioned methylthiotetrazole side chain. Currently moxalactam is rarely used because of the possibility of increased risk of bleeding. The effects of these very broad-spectrum agents on normal flora may lead to colonization and superinfection with organisms such as enterococci and resistant *P. aeruginosa*.

The third-generation cephalosporins are excreted via renal filtration with little or no active secretion. Most of the drugs are metabolized only to a small extent, if any, in vivo.

#### *Novel β-lactam antibiotics*

**Carbapenams.** A number of β-lactam agents with novel chemical structures have been isolated from fungi and actinomycetes. These compounds differ in structure from penicillins and cephalosporins and have interesting antibacterial activities. The thienamycins (or carbapenems) are β-lactam agents with an extremely broad spectrum of activity. The first carbapenem approved for use in the United States, imipenem, is marketed in combination with an enzyme inhibitor, cilastatin, as Primaxin. The enzyme inhibitor prevents inactivation of the active agent by an enzyme of the renal tubule.

Imipenem/cilastatin has the broadest spectrum of activity of any single antimicrobial agent. It is effective against nonenterococcal streptococci and oral and bowel anaerobes. Imipenem/cilastatin is active against *S. aureus* and enterococci if they are sensitive to methicillin and ampicillin, respectively. This compound is active against a broad array of gram-negative bacilli, including *P. aeruginosa, Acinetobacter,* Enterobacteriaceae and *H. influenzae.*

Clinically, imipenem/cilastatin should be used in patients who are seriously ill, with multiple potential sources of infection. This agent is especially appropriate when concern exists regarding resistant gram-negative bacilli. Imipenem/cilastatin is effective in the treatment of nosocomial pneumonia and intraabdominal infection, although frequently there are more cost-effective appropriate choices available. Imipenem is effective in the empiric treatment of the febrile neutropenic patient. This drug may also be appropriate in complicated, life-threatening soft tissue infections such as synergistic gangrene or necrotizing fasciitis, where potential pathogens range from group A streptococci to mixed anaerobic/aerobic gram-negative bacilli.

Imipenem given with cilastatin has a half-life of 1 hour. About 70% of imipenem is excreted unchanged in the urine, and consequently dosing should be adjusted for renal dysfunction. Imipenem/cilastatin achieves relatively low levels in bile and as a result may not be an optimal drug for the treatment of cholecystitis and cholangitis. It can be given either intravenously or intramuscularly, in dosages ranging from 500 mg every 6 hours to 1 g every 8 hours, depending on the indication. It is not recommended for the treatment of meningitis.

Imipenem/cilastatin is structurally similar to penicillin and should be used with caution in patients with penicillin allergies. High doses of this agent have been associated with seizures, frequently in the setting of unstable renal function. Imipenem/cilastatin can rarely cause nausea, vomiting, leukopenia, and minor transaminase elevation.

**Monobactams.** Monobactams are monocyclic β-lactam agents isolated from assorted soil bacteria. Aztreonam is a synthetic monobactam with a bactericidal effect on aerobic gram-negative bacilli. As seen with the previously described β-lactam agents, aztreonam acts by inhibiting cell wall synthesis. Its structure includes an iminopropyl carbonyl side chain, which resists the activity of β-lactamases, including those produced by *P. aeruginosa*.

Aztreonam has no activity against gram-positive or anaerobic pathogens. It is very effective against most Enterobacteriaceae, *N. meningitidis, N. gonorrhoeae, P. aeruginosa,* and *H. influenzae. Citrobacter, Acinetobacter,* and nonaeruginosal pseudomonal species may be resistant. This agent can be administered either intravenously or intramuscularly, at dosages of 1 to 2 g every 8 hours, with the higher dosage used for coverage of *P. aeruginosa*. Serum half-life in patients with a normal creatinine clearance is 1.5 to 2 hours. Excretion is renal as unmetabolized drug. As with most other β-lactam agents, dosage adjustment is required in renal dysfunction.

Aztreonam administration has been associated with relatively rare reports of rash, nausea, vomiting, diarrhea, and minimal transaminitis. Renal toxicity has been very uncommon, and bleeding disorders and platelet dysfunction have not been reported. Aztreonam may be less likely than cephalosporins to cause type I allergic reactions (urticaria, anaphylaxis) in patients allergic to penicillin. Serious allergic reactions to aztreonam have occurred, however, so this drug should still be used with caution in the penicillin-allergic individual.

The use of aztreonam is limited to infections in which the etiologic pathogen is clearly an aerobic gram-negative bacillus. In situations such as sepsis of unclear etiology, pneumonia, or abdominal infection, it may constitute part of an appropriate regimen that also includes an agent with gram-positive, anaerobic coverage. Aztreonam has been used in penicillin-allergic patients when *P. aeruginosa* infection is suspected, such as in the febrile neutropenic patient. Although aztreonam has a similar bacterial spectrum as the aminoglycosides, it is frequently misused as an aminoglycoside substitute. As discussed in the next section, the current preferred use of aminoglycosides is not for isolated gram-negative coverage but to provide synergy with other agents. Though a β-lactam, aztreonam has not been shown to act synergistically with other β-lactams or vancomycin.

### Aminoglycosides

The aminoglycoside antibiotics are compounds composed of amino sugars and hexoses or aminohexoses joined by glycosidic linkages. Although chemical differences among these drugs are significant, they share basic characteristics of antibacterial activity, pharmacology, and toxicity. The aminoglycosides include streptomycin, neomycin, kanamycin, gentamicin, tobramycin, amikacin, sisomicin, and netilmicin. The -mycins are derived from *Streptomyces* species and the -micins from the fungus *Micromonospora;* amikacin is produced semisynthetically from kanamycin.

The aminoglycosides are active against a variety of bacteria, but because of their relatively small toxic/therapeutic ratio they have been used primarily in the treatment of infections caused by gram-negative bacilli. They are active against most facultative anaerobic and aerobic gram-negative bacilli at clinically achievable serum levels. Their activity against gram-positive organisms is limited at achievable serum levels, and more satisfactory agents are available. The aminoglycosides are used, however, in combination with penicillins in the treatment of streptococcal endocarditis, particularly when due to enterococci. They are also indicated in combination with rifampin and vancomycin in the treatment of prosthetic valve endocarditis caused by coagulase-negative staphylococci. In these situations they act synergistically with the other antibiotics to kill bacteria. The aminoglycosides are bactericidal. They interact with bacterial ribosomes to cause irreversible impairment of protein synthesis leading to cell death. They enter the bacterial cell primarily through oxygen-dependent active transport.

Indications for the use of aminoglycosides have changed over the past decade. Previously aminoglycosides were used as primary agents for the treatment of gram-negative aerobic bacilli. Their limitations are as follows: they may not be active in acidic or anaerobic environments such as abscesses. They achieve minimal levels in sputum and purulent fluids. Their toxicity is significant. Multiple options currently exist for the treatment of gram-negative infections, including the third-generation cephalosporins, imipenem, aztreonam, and parenteral quinolones. Consequently most clinicians choose not to use aminoglycosides in settings where other agents will be effective. Aminoglycosides are reserved for situations that require their unique qualities; primarily when synergy with β-lactams or vancomycin is desired or for unusual pathogens for which limited alternative therapy is available. Several of the aminoglycosides are active against mycobacteria, including amikacin, kanamycin, and streptomycin, which is well established in the treatment of tuberculosis.

Organisms may be resistant to aminoglycosides due to impermeability of the cell wall or a change in the structure of the ribosome, preventing effects on protein synthesis. The production of inactivating enzymes, which attack aminoglycosides at various sites on the molecule, is a more frequent mechanism of resistance. Inactivating enzymes may be carried on bacterial plasmids and may be passed from one organism to another, even across species lines. Six or seven of the inactivating enzymes affect gentamicin and tobramycin, whereas only two affect amikacin, accounting for some of the broader spectrum of the latter drug.

The aminoglycosides are very water soluble and are administered intravenously or intramuscularly. They are not absorbed after oral administration. Neomycin, because of toxicity, is used only topically or orally. Streptomycin and kanamycin are most commonly administered intramuscularly but can also be given intravenously if clinically indicated. Aminoglycosides are excreted via the kidney by glomerular filtration and excretion. Their accumulation in renal failure parallels the creatinine clearance. Half-lives of the drugs in adults with normal renal function range from 2 to 4 hours. Serum levels of the drugs are influenced not only by renal function but also by the age of the patient, clinical status, presence of fever, presence of burns, hematocrit, and various other factors. Thus serum levels in any given patient are not entirely predictable.

The unpredictability of serum levels, the closeness of mean serum levels to MICs, and the potential for toxicity with these drugs (see below) contribute to the value of obtaining serum level determinations. Rapid immunoassays are now generally available. Levels are usually measured 1 hour after (peak) and less than 1 hour before (trough) administration of a dose of the drug. Typically, peak and trough therapeutic levels of streptomycin, kanamycin, and amikacin are 20 to 30 and 5 to 10 μg/ml, respectively. Serum concentrations at peak and trough usually recommended for gentamicin, tobramycin, and netilmicin are 6 to 10 μg/ml and less than 2 μg/ml, respectively. If the particular aminoglycoside is being used in the treatment of a life-threatening infection, the higher end of the spectrum given for peak level is desired. If these drugs are being used for synergy, a lower peak is acceptable. Current theory suggests that an elevated trough is more likely to contribute to drug toxicity than an elevated peak. Also, aminoglycoside activity may be greater at a higher peak concentration. For that reason the administration of a larger aminoglycoside dosage given less frequently is being evaluated. No conclusions regarding the once daily administration of aminoglycosides can be drawn at this time, although most specialists in the area of antimicrobial dosing advocate using a 12-hour interval rather than 8 hours.

Dosing for all the parenteral aminoglycosides must be adjusted for alterations of renal function, or else accumulation of the drugs with dose-dependent toxicity may result. A number of nomograms for dosage have been developed, and each package insert contains a satisfactory nomogram based on serum creatinine and other patient characteristics. Elderly patients, patients with unstable renal function, and those who require prolonged therapy should have serum levels monitored carefully to ensure adequate levels outside the potentially toxic range. The aminoglycosides are removed by hemodialysis and peritoneal dialysis and should be readministered following dialysis. Aminoglycosides may be added to peritoneal dialysis fluid at concentrations near the mean serum level so as to provide persistent, nontoxic concentrations.

Oral preparations of neomycin, kanamycin, and gentamicin have been used as nonabsorbable bowel preparations for prophylaxis in bowel surgery and in immunocompromised patients. Topical neomycin is frequently used for dressing minor wounds and in solutions, and topical gentamicin has been used in the treatment of burns.

The most important toxicities of the aminoglycosides

are the effects on the hair cells of the ear and the tubular epithelial cells of the kidney. All the aminoglycosides have the potential of causing ototoxicity, which may be manifested as either a vestibular or cochlear effect. Although some of the agents are more likely to cause one or the other, all the agents are capable of both. Hearing loss is irreversible and permanent. Vestibular damage is also permanent and can be severely uncomfortable, but the effects are usually ameliorated by compensatory mechanisms after months to years. Renal damage is reversible with the regeneration of new tubular epithelium. The clinical picture is one of acute tubular necrosis with nonoliguric renal failure.

Serum aminoglycoside levels do not always correlate with nephrotoxicity and ototoxicity. Some patients may develop toxic reactions despite documentation of serum levels in the therapeutic range. Toxicity is, however, usually seen in patients with levels above the therapeutic range. The elderly appear to be particularly susceptible to ototoxicity.

Aminoglycosides may cause neuromuscular blockade. This usually occurs in the setting of rapid infusion and can lead to respiratory paralysis. Fortunately, with the usual methods of administration it is a rare occurrence, but the neuromuscular blocking effect may complicate recovery from anesthesia-related paralysis and may be a problem in patients with neuromuscular disorders such as myasthenia gravis and botulism. These drugs should be avoided or used very cautiously in patients with myasthenia. Peripheral and optic neuritis has been described with aminoglycosides but is rare. Hypersensitivity reactions to aminoglycosides are relatively unusual and typically manifest as rash and drug fever.

Table 64-6 is a summary of the characteristics of available aminoglycosides.

***Streptomycin.*** Streptomycin is still useful in the parenteral therapy of tuberculosis but is not recommended as first-line therapy for most patients because of the availability of safer and more easily administered agents. With the resurgence of multidrug-resistant tuberculosis, streptomycin use is making a comeback. It is used both empirically and based on susceptibility testing in patients with suspected or documented drug-resistant tuberculosis (see Chapter 114).

Although most common aerobic bacilli are resistant to it, streptomycin is still the drug of choice for tularemia and plague because of its proven efficacy. It also remains a useful drug in the treatment of brucellosis, usually in combination with tetracycline. Although most of the original studies evaluating synergy between β-lactams and aminoglycosides featured streptomycin, gentamicin is now the commonly used aminoglycoside in addition to penicillin for the treatment of enterococcal or *S. viridans* endocarditis.

Streptomycin is usually administered intramuscularly, but if therapy is to be prolonged or the clinical situation limits the use of this route (e.g., thrombocytopenia), it can be given intravenously. The usual adult dosage is 1 to 2 g per day given as one dose.

***Neomycin and kanamycin.*** Neomycin is no longer available for parenteral use because of its toxicity. It is a frequent component of many topical antibacterial ointments, creams, and irrigating solutions. It is also available in oral preparations for suppression of bowel organisms preparatory to surgery and in the treatment of hepatic encephalopathy. Kanamycin can be used for the treatment of gram-negative bacillary infections caused by susceptible organisms.

***Gentamicin and tobramycin.*** Gentamicin and tobramycin are the primary aminoglycosides used in clinical practice. As described above, these agents are seldom used primarily for their gram-negative activity but are chosen for synergy in the treatment of specific infections. An

**Table 64-6.** Aminoglycoside antibiotics in clinical use

| Agent (trade name) | Route of administration | Usual dosage* | Therapeutic serum levels (μg/ml) Peak† | Therapeutic serum levels (μg/ml) Trough |
|---|---|---|---|---|
| Neomycin | PO, topical | PO 1-3 g/day | — | — |
| Streptomycin | IM‡ | 15 mg/kg q24h | 20-30 | <5 |
| Kanamycin (Kantrex) | PO | 2-8 g/day | — | — |
| | IM | LD 10 mg/kg; 7.5 mg/kg q12 | 20-30 | 5-10 |
| Gentamicin (Garamycin) | IM, IV | LD 2 mg/kg; 3-5 mg/kg/day§‖ divided q8-12h | 4-10 | <2 |
| Tobramycin (Nebcin) | IM, IV | LD 2 mg/kg; 3-5 mg/kg/day§‖ divided q8-12h | 4-10 | <2 |
| Amikacin (Amikin) | IM, IV | LD 10 mg/kg; 7.5 mg/kg q12h‖ | 20-30 | 5-10 |
| Netilmicin (Netromycin) | IM, IV | LD 2.2 mg/kg; 3-5 mg/kg/day§‖ divided q8-12h | 4-10 | 4-10 |

*LD,* Loading dose.
*The dosage given is for adult patients with normal creatinine clearance; all drugs require dosage adjustment with renal dysfunction.
†The higher peak given will be needed for certain organisms such as *P. aeruginosa* or in life-threatening infections.
‡Although only approved for IM use, streptomycin may be given IV in situations that make IM use difficult or impractical.
§The higher dosages should be used for the treatment of serious infections.
‖IM and IV dosages are the same.

aminoglycoside, usually gentamicin or tobramycin, should be used with a β-lactam in all serious (nonurinary tract) infections caused by *P. aeruginosa.* Gentamicin and tobramycin are also useful in the treatment of certain staphylococcal and streptococcal infections. Although controversial, most experts recommend the addition of gentamicin, tobramycin, or amikacin to antipseudomonal β-lactam therapy in the treatment of febrile neutropenic patients.

In most clinical situations gentamicin and tobramycin are virtually interchangeable, although some organisms are resistant to gentamicin but sensitive to tobramycin. Tobramycin has approximately twice the activity as gentamicin on a weight basis against most strains of *P. aeruginosa,* but most isolates of *Serratia* are more sensitive to gentamicin than tobramycin. Clinical and experimental evidence suggests that tobramycin is somewhat less nephrotoxic than gentamicin, but this difference is of questionable clinical significance.

Gentamicin and tobramycin may be administered intravenously or intramuscularly in dosages of 3 to 5 mg/kg per day in two or three divided doses. Doses must be adjusted according to renal function, and serum levels should be monitored.

***Amikacin.*** Amikacin is a derivative of kanamycin with a spectrum of activity that is somewhat broader than gentamicin and tobramycin. This antibiotic was synthesized to resist inactivating enzymes. Strains of gram-negative bacilli resistant to gentamicin and tobramycin and sensitive to amikacin are observed with some frequency in hospitals with large intensive care units, but in other settings the three drugs usually are interchangeable.

Amikacin is given in a dosage of 15 mg/kg per day in two or three divided doses with adjustment made for renal impairment. It can be given intramuscularly or intravenously. The pharmacokinetics of this drug, with peak serum levels to MIC ratios for most susceptible organisms higher than those obtained with gentamicin and tobramycin, may be advantageous in some situations.

***Netilmicin and sisomicin.*** Netilmicin has been released for use in the United States, and sisomicin is available in other parts of the world. These drugs do not differ enough in clinical utility from other available drugs to offer any advantage under present circumstances. Netilmicin may be less likely to cause ototoxicity when compared with the other aminoglycosides, but it is not clear that this difference is clinically significant.

### Tetracyclines

The first tetracycline, chlortetracycline, was introduced in 1948 after it was discovered during efforts to screen for new natural antibiotics. Over the ensuing 20 years a number of other tetracyclines were discovered from natural sources or were produced semisynthetically. The original sources of the tetracyclines are various species of the genus *Streptomyces.* As the name implies, the chemical structure of the tetracyclines contains four fused six-carbon rings. Currently available tetracyclines include chlortetracycline, oxytetracycline, tetracycline, methacycline, demeclocycline, doxycycline, and minocycline.

Chlortetracyclin (Aureomycin) was the first truly broad-spectrum antibacterial antibiotic. The tetracyclines are active against many gram-positive cocci (except for resistance in most strains of enterococci), gram-negative cocci, many enteric gram-negative rods, strains of *Haemophilus* species, anaerobic bacteria, *Mycoplasma, Chlamydia, Rickettsia,* and, to an extent, some protozoa. Resistance to tetracyclines among these groups of organisms is frequent enough that they are drugs of first choice only in infections caused by *Rickettsia, Chlamydia,* and *Mycoplasma.* In other situations, use is avoided while susceptibility testing is pending, except in infections of limited severity or in situations where the susceptibility of the pathogen is already established. Even when susceptibility is ensured, tetracyclines are rarely the drug of choice for commonly encountered bacteria such as streptococcal or staphylococcal species. Susceptibility to tetracycline implies susceptibility to the whole group. Doxycycline and minocycline, however, tend to be more active against susceptible organisms, especially pneumococci, gonococci, and *H. influenzae,* than the other members of the group. An organism resistant to one member of the group should be considered resistant to all the agents in that group.

Tetracyclines exert their antibacterial effect through binding to the 30S ribosomal subunit, thereby preventing protein synthesis. This inhibition of protein synthesis is reversible and nonlethal, and thus the tetracyclines are bacteriostatic agents. Resistance to tetracycline usually is based on the impermeability of the cell membrane to the drug.

The pharmacokinetics of the various tetracyclines vary much more than their antibacterial activity (Table 64-7). Absorption of these drugs after oral administration is significantly impaired by antacids as the drugs complex with cations. Doxycycline and minocycline are well absorbed (more than 90%), whereas chlortetracycline is the least well absorbed (30%) after oral administration. All the tetracyclines are excreted in the urine; however, excretion across the gastrointestinal tract and in the bile may be significant, especially with doxycycline. The dosage of all the tetracyclines, except doxycycline, must be adjusted in the presence of renal impairment. The tetracyclines penetrate most tissue fairly well, cross the placenta (see below), and are present in breast milk.

Tetracyclines inhibit bacterial protein synthesis, and similar effects can be seen in human cells during functional interference with cellular or mitochondrial ribosomes. This becomes clinically apparent in patients with renal insufficiency in whom tetracycline accumulates, causing a catabolic effect on tissue and exacerbation of azotemia. Tetracyclines also may have some intrinsic nephrotoxicity, but mechanisms have not been defined. Doxycycline is the only member of the group not contraindicated by renal insufficiency. A syndrome of acute hepatotoxicity has been described with the tetracyclines when they are given in large intravenous dosages, especially during pregnancy. Liver damage can be as severe as acute hepatic necrosis. Intravenous dosages of less than 2 g tetracycline and recommended dosages of doxycycline appear to be relatively safe, but the drugs should not be used during pregnancy or in patients with any renal function impairment. Tetracyclines bind to teeth and bones, causing discoloration in the former and

**Table 64-7.** Characteristics of available tetracycline antibiotics

| Generic name | Trade name | Dosage* | Half-life | Comments |
|---|---|---|---|---|
| Tetracycline | Achromycin | 250-500 mg q6h† | 8 hr | Least expensive |
| Oxytetracycline | Terramycin | 250-500 mg q6h† | 9 hr | |
| Chlortetracycline | Aureomycin | 250-500 mg q6h† | 6 hr | Poorest GI absorption |
| Demeclocycline | Declomycin | 150-300 mg q6h† | 12 hr | Can cause nephrogenic diabetes insipidus |
| Methacycline | Rondomycin | 150 mg q6h | 14 hr | |
| Doxycycline | Vibramycin | 200 mg, followed by 100 mg q12h | 18 hr | Excreted by the GI tract in the presence of renal failure; preferred agent in renal failure |
| Minocycline | Minocin | 200 mg, followed by 100 mg q12h | 16 hr | Well absorbed when taken orally; may cause vertigo as a side effect; least hepatic metabolism of the tetracyclines; preferred in hepatic dysfunction |

*All agents are available PO or IV; the dosage for both routes is the same.
†Higher dosages, especially >2 g per day, have been associated with fulminant hepatic necrosis.

inhibition of growth in the latter. Tetracyclines should not be used during pregnancy or in children for this reason. Additionally, they can cause increased intracranial pressure in neonates. Tetracyclines may rarely cause skin photosensitivity.

Tetracyclines have a broad effect on the normal flora of the body, and use of these drugs may be associated with mucosal or intertriginous candidiasis, diarrhea, pseudomembranous colitis, and superinfection. Gastric upset and heartburn are not uncommon complaints. As a result of their relatively low pH, tetracyclines can also cause esophageal ulceration when taken orally.

Studies on the use of minocycline to treat meningococcal carriers found that a significant number of patients developed dizziness, vertigo, nausea, and malaise. This particular syndrome has been associated only with this tetracycline. Demeclocycline may cause diabetes insipidus as a peculiar side effect, and this drug is used in the treatment of syndrome of inappropriate antidiuretic hormone (SIADH) production.

The tetracyclines have been supplanted in many clinical situations by other available agents. Although they can be used in the treatment of minor respiratory tract infections such as bronchitis and urinary tract infections, other drugs are usually preferable. Tetracyclines, especially doxycycline, are being used with increasing frequency in the treatment of genital and pelvic infections caused by *Chlamydia trachomatis* and *Mycoplasma*. Doxycycline is active against *C. pneumoniae,* which is an increasingly recognized cause of community-acquired respiratory tract infection. Tetracyclines are drugs of choice for all the rickettsial diseases, brucellosis, myeloidosis, *Vibrio* species, *Chlamydia* infections, mycoplasmal pneumonia, and relapsing fever. In some of these situations chloramphenicol or erythromycin is an alternative agent. Tetracyclines also are used frequently in the treatment of acne as chronic therapy to suppress the skin flora. Minocycline is the preferred agent for this indication and may also act by decreasing the amount of fatty acids on the surface of the skin.

Tetracycline and doxycycline are the two most commonly used tetracyclines in the United States today. The former is adequate for most indications. The latter is preferred in the setting of renal functional impairment. Intramuscular tetracyclines usually are tolerated poorly and give poor serum levels.

## Macrolides

Macrolides are semisynthetic compounds composed of carbon atoms linked in a circular manner, with various side chains. The macrolides are bacteriostatic antibiotics that act by inhibiting protein synthesis at the level of the ribosome. They are able to penetrate well into tissues and achieve intracellular levels that exceed the levels measured in serum. Erythromycin is the oldest and most commonly used macrolide. Spiramycin and kitasamycin are used in other parts of the world but are not approved for use in the United States. Azithromycin and clarithromycin are two recently developed macrolides that have just been approved for clinical use. Table 64-8 is a summary of the macrolide antibiotics.

***Erythromycin.*** Erythromycin was discovered in 1952 as a product of *Streptomyces erythreus.* It has a complex chemical structure with a large lactone ring.

Erythromycin is active against most gram-positive cocci and bacilli, including *Corynebacterium diphtheriae.* It also is active against *N. gonorrhoeae.* It has some activity against *N. meningitidis* and *H. influenzae* but not at a clinically relevant concentration. It is active against *Bordetella pertussis* and *Legionella* species and is the drug of choice in infections caused by these organisms. Erythromycin is effective in the treatment of pneumonia caused by *M. pneumoniae* and is used to treat *C. trachomatis* pneumonia and conjunctivitis in infants. Erythromycin is not very active against strains of genital *Mycoplasma.* Aerobic gram-negative bacilli are resistant to erythromycin, apparently on the basis of impermeability of the cell wall. Most strains of *S. aureus* are sensitive to erythromycin, but resistance is prevalent enough in some areas to require routine susceptibility testing. Pneumococci and other nonenterococcal streptococci are rarely resistant. Most anaerobic bacteria are moderately sensitive, and erythromycin is often used as an alternative to penicillin in allergic patients with a minor oral infection. Erythromycin is also effective against *Campylobacter jejuni* and is an option in the treatment of syphilis in a penicillin-allergic patient. There is a significant failure

**Table 64-8.** Macrolide antibiotics

| Agent (trade name) | Route and dosage | Comments |
|---|---|---|
| Erythromycin | | Half-life of 1.2-2.6 hr |
| Base (Ilotycin, E-Mycin) | 0.333 g PO q8h | Absorption improved if taken on an empty stomach |
| Stearate (Erythrocin) | 0.25-0.5 g PO q6-12h | |
| Ethylsuccinate (Eryped, E.E.S.) | 0.4 g PO q6-12h | |
| Estolate (Ilosone) | 0.25-0.5 g PO q6-12h | Best absorbed; associated with hepatotoxicity in adults |
| Lactobionate (Erythrocin Lactobionate) | 0.25-1 g IV q6h | Intravenous therapy recommended for serious infection caused by *Legionella* sp; high incidence of phlebitis, large volume of diluent needed; reversible ototoxicity has been observed |
| Gluceptate (Ilotycin Gluceptate) | 0.25-1 g IV q6h | |
| Azithromycin (Zithromax) | 0.5 g PO on day 1; 0.25 g PO qd starting day 2 | Complex pharmacokinetics, with half-life variable depending on sampling schedule, can be up to 57 hr as a result of redistribution from tissue; appears not to interact with other liver-metabolized agents; single dose of 1 g approved for the treatment of uncomplicated genital chlamydial infection |
| Clarithromycin (Biaxin) | 0.5 g PO q12h | Less GI toxic than erythromycin; useful in the treatment of *Mycobacterium avium-intracellulare* and other atypical mycobacterial infections |

rate when erythromycin is used to treat syphilis, so careful follow-up is required.

Erythromycin may be administered orally and intravenously. Intramuscular injection is painful. It comes in several oral preparations: erythromycin base and erythromycin stearate, estolate, and ethylsuccinate. The estolate form is the best absorbed but has caused hepatitis and cholestatic jaundice in some patients, especially adults. The ethylsuccinate form is the next best absorbed, followed by the stearate and then the base. Absorption of these preparations is better in the fasting patient. Absorption of all the preparations is probably adequate to treat relatively minor infections caused by organisms that are very sensitive.

Many patients complain about gastric distress and various degrees of nausea after erythromycin ingestion. Two preparations of erythromycin for intravenous administration are available, a lactobionate and a gluceptate. Irritation and thrombophlebitis may complicate intravenous therapy; this, combined with the amount of diluent needed to prepare material for infusion, leads to the need for relatively large infusion volumes. Erythromycin is excreted in the bile and via the intestine. In most cases adjustment of dosage in the presence of renal insufficiency is not necessary.

Erythromycin is remarkably nontoxic. Gastrointestinal distress, as mentioned above, and diarrhea may limit therapy or lead to noncompliance, however. Reversible ototoxicity has been documented in rare instances in association with the administration of large dosages intravenously. Allergic reactions occur but are relatively infrequent. Gastrointestinal intolerance is much more frequent than allergy and should not be confused with documented allergy. Erythromycin may increase theophylline and cyclosporin levels by decreasing hepatic metabolism. There have been reports of dose-related cardiac toxicity, primarily arrhythmias, in individuals taking erythromycin and the nonsedating antihistamines such as astemizole (Hismanal) and terfenadine (Seldane). This has occurred more commonly in patients with baseline cardiac disease.

Erythromycin is the alternate drug of choice for several infections in the penicillin-allergic patient, including group A streptococcal and pneumococcal infection. The drug is an alternative agent for minor skin and periodontal infection, otitis media, rheumatic fever prophylaxis, and in certain circumstances for prophylaxis against endocarditis. It is the drug of choice in the treatment of mycoplasmal pneumonia, pertussis prophylaxis, eradication of *C. diphtheriae* in carriers, and the treatment of infections caused by *L. pneumophila* and other species of *Legionella.* In the latter disease it is usually given parenterally. The nature of other indications, except the treatment of disseminated gonococcal disease in the penicillin-allergic patient, is such that oral administration is usually sufficient. Erythromycin combined with sulfisoxazole is used to treat otitis media in children. Topical erythromycin is used for the treatment and prophylaxis of conjunctivitis.

***Clarithromycin.*** Clarithromycin is a semisynthetic 14-membered ring macrolide that was approved for clinical use in 1991. Only oral preparations are available. It is not degraded by gastric acid, so it may be taken with meals. Clarithromycin has a longer half-life than erythromycin and can be given twice a day. It achieves excellent tissue and intracellular levels. Clarithromycin dosage should be reduced if the creatinine clearance is less than 30.

Clarithromycin is active against those pathogens that are sensitive to erythromycin, including nonenterococcal streptococci, sensitive *S. aureus,* oral anaerobes, *Legionella,* and *Mycoplasma.* Clarithromycin has greater activity than erythromycin against respiratory gram-negative bacteria such as *H. influenzae* and *Moraxella.* It is also active against *Neisseria* species, *Chlamydia,*

*Helicobacter pylori,* and atypical mycobacteria. Clarithromycin has shown promise in the treatment of *M. avium-intracelluare.*

Both clarithromycin and azithromycin appear to cause less gastrointestinal irritation than erythromycin. Transient hearing loss has been reported with both. Clarithromycin does elevate theophylline levels and may have some cardiotoxicity when given with nonsedating antihistamines. Clarithromycin may rarely cause mild to moderate transaminitis, elevated blood urea nitrogen (BUN), elevated prothrombin time, and decreased white blood cell count.

***Azithromycin.*** Azithromycin is a newly developed macrolide that has a nitrogen group added to the 14-member macrolide ring of erythromycin. As compared with that of clarithromycin, the absorption of azithromycin is reduced by the presence of food; consequently this drug should be taken 1 to 2 hours before meals. At present it is available only in oral form, but current trials are evaluating an intravenous form of azithromycin.

Azithromycin achieves very high tissue and intracellular levels in the setting of very low serum levels. Half-life in tissues can be as long as 76 hours, allowing once daily dosing. This drug is primarily excreted unmetabolized by the biliary system, with a small amount excreted in the urine. No data are available regarding the dosing of azithromycin in hepatic or renal failure. Some data suggest that, as compared with erythromycin and clarithromycin, azithromycin may not affect theophylline metabolism, but conclusive studies have not been done. Theophylline levels, as well as levels of any hepatically metabolized agent, should be followed closely in any patient also on a macrolide antibiotic. Azithromycin has not been studied in children younger than age 16 or in pregnant women.

With respect to spectrum of activity, azithromycin appears less active against gram-positive organisms (staphylococci and streptococci) than either erythromycin or clarithromycin. Azithromycin is more active than any of the other macrolides against *H. influenzae.* Azithromycin is also active against *Mycoplasma, Chlamydia,* and *Legionella* species. Clinical trials have shown azithromycin to be effective in the treatment of streptococcal pharyngitis, sinusitis, mild cases of community-acquired pneumonia, and minor soft tissue infections. Its utility may be greatest in the treatment of uncomplicated cervicitis or urethritis caused by *C. trachomatis.* Clinical trials have shown a single 1-g dose of azithromycin to be as effective as a 7-day course of doxycycline for this indication.

Azithromycin is relatively well tolerated, with minimal gastrointestinal side effects when compared to erythromycin. Headache, dizziness, transaminitis, and reduced white cell count have been described.

In summary, the optimal clinical indications for using clarithromycin or azithromycin remain undetermined. Cheaper agents are available for most of the studied indications. There may be some advantage to their use in respiratory infections, where the coverage of *Mycoplasma, Legionella,* and chlamydial pneumonia as well as *H. influenzae* may be desired. There is clearly some benefit to giving individuals with urethritis or cervicitis a directly observed method of therapy with respect to expected compliance. Clarithromycin has definitively improved therapeutic options in the treatment of atypical mycobacteria and appears useful in therapy for *H. pylori.*

### Clindamycin

Clindamycin is a 7-chloro-7-deoxy derivative of the older, naturally occurring antibiotic lincomycin. The derivative has eclipsed the use of the parent compound in the United States. Both agents are classified as lincosamides and inhibit protein synthesis at the level of the ribosome.

Clindamycin is active against most gram-positive cocci, except most strains of enterococci, which are resistant. Clindamycin differs from erythromycin, with which it is often grouped, in its significantly limited potency against aerobic and facultatively anaerobic gram-negative organisms, which are usually sensitive to erythromycin (e.g., *N. gonorrhoeae*) and against *M. pneumoniae.* On the other hand, clindamycin is very active against most gram-negative anaerobes at concentrations similar to those that inhibit aerobic and anaerobic gram-positive cocci. Resistance to clindamycin does occur among usually susceptible organisms, and testing of organisms such as staphylococci and pneumococci is warranted. Enteric and other aerobic gram-negative rods are almost uniformly resistant to clindamycin, *except* for several peculiar organisms, e.g., certain strains of *Flavobacterium.* Some species of *Clostridium* are resistant.

Clindamycin can be administered orally, intravenously, or intramuscularly. Oral preparations are well absorbed and are only slightly affected by eating. Intravenous and intramuscular administrations are well tolerated. Clindamycin penetrates tissues well, except for the central nervous system; it is concentrated in bone and is as much as fortyfold more concentrated in polymorphonuclear leukocytes than in serum. The serum half-life of the drug is about 2½ hours in normal volunteers but may be significantly prolonged in the presence of a number of clinical situations. The drug is excreted to some extent in urine and bile. Dosage adjustment is necessary only with concomitant renal and hepatic dysfunction.

Adverse reactions with clindamycin include hypotension, bronchospasm, rash, and anxiety with too-rapid infusion and occasional allergic reactions. The drug received attention during the early 1970s because of an up to 20% incidence of diarrhea, with or without colitis, associated with its use. It is now clear that most cases of diarrhea and pseudomembranous colitis with clindamycin and a variety of other antibiotics is the result of overgrowth of *C. difficile* in the bowel. This organism is usually clindamycin resistant and produces cytotoxins that damage the bowel epithelium. Abnormal liver function tests and blood dyscrasias have been associated with clindamycin administration.

Clindamycin usually is used in two ways. First, it is a substitute for penicillins in penicillin-allergic patients with infections caused by gram-positive cocci (e.g., group A streptococci and staphylococci). As mentioned above, neither is clindamycin interchangeable with erythromycin nor is the susceptibility of pathogens completely predictable. The other major use of clindamycin, treatment of anaerobic infection, has led to its becoming a major parenteral antibiotic for hospitalized patients. Clindamycin is an alternative agent to penicillin for treatment of anaerobic infections of the respiratory tract (e.g., head and neck abscesses, aspiration pneumonia, and lung abscess). The drug also is useful in those situations when *S. aureus* is of concern as a potential pathogen. Clindamycin is frequently used in the treatment of anaerobic infections arising in the abdomen and pelvis. It is active against both gram-negative and gram-positive anaerobic bacteria. Resistance among *B. fragilis* isolates is still limited in most places. Clindamycin is a useful drug for the treatment of staphylococcal infections. Although it is frequently bactericidal for staphylococci in vitro, treatment failures in endocarditis have been reported. Topical clindamycin is used occasionally in the treatment of acne, but safer therapeutic modalities are available.

### Chloramphenicol

Chloramphenicol was discovered as a product of *Streptomyces venezuelae* during the late 1940s but now is synthesized chemically. The drug inhibits protein synthesis at the ribosome in a reversible fashion and therefore is bacteriostatic for most organisms.

Chloramphenicol is a broad-spectrum agent active against many gram-positive and gram-negative aerobic and anaerobic bacteria. However, resistance to the drug is prevalent among many groups of generally sensitive organisms. The drug can be used in the treatment of infections caused by *S. typhi* and ampicillin-resistant *H. influenzae,* although resistance is becoming increasingly more frequent. *Rickettsia, Chlamydia,* and *Mycoplasma* are sensitive to chloramphenicol. Resistance to chloramphenicol either is based on bacteria becoming impermeable to the drug or as a result of the production of inactivating enzymes. Resistance transfer, mediated through R factors, is important in the epidemiology of resistance to the drug, especially among *Salmonella* and *Shigella* strains.

Chloramphenicol is extremely well absorbed after oral administration and is well tolerated when given intravenously. Paradoxically, absorption from intramuscular sites is relatively poor, and this route should be avoided. Chloramphenicol penetrates tissue well, especially the central nervous system, and therefore is useful in the treatment of infections of the brain and meninges. It also is effective against many intracellular pathogens. The drug is metabolized to various derivatives and conjugates in vivo and is excreted in the urine. Active chloramphenicol does not accumulate in renal failure; the metabolites accumulate, however, although they do not seem to be toxic. Active chloramphenicol is toxic and may accumulate in the presence of immature or otherwise compromised hepatic function. The use of the drug should be avoided in patients with these problems (neonates and patients with severe liver disease).

The toxicity of chloramphenicol is not insignificant, but fortunately serious problems are uncommon. The drug is a dose-related inhibitor of bone marrow, presumably on the basis of interaction with mitochondrial ribosomes; inhibition reverses when the drug is stopped. This reversible effect may result in blockage of iron utilization with increased serum iron levels and anemia, as well as thrombocytopenia and neutropenia. The histologic hallmark of this toxicity is cytoplasmic vacuolation of marrow cell precursors. A more ominous and idiosyncratic non–dose-related toxicity is aplastic anemia with pancytopenia, which occurs in approximately 1 of 100,000 patients receiving the drug. This effect is irreversible and often fatal. Aplastic anemia has been said to occur only when all or part of the therapy has been oral. This statement is clearly not true, since aplastic anemia has been described in patients who have received parenteral therapy alone. Aplastic anemia also has been associated with ophthalmic preparations.

If the drug is used in infants at all, it must be done with extreme caution, and the serum level of the drug should be measured. Prolonged prothrombin times (correctable with vitamin K) and neurotoxicity also have been described with extended administration of chloramphenicol. Chloramphenicol inhibits certain hepatic enzymes and may interact unfavorably with other drugs.

Chloramphenicol remains a drug of choice for typhoid fever, although epidemics of disease caused by chloramphenicol-resistant organisms have been observed. Ampicillin (or amoxicillin), quinolones, and trimethoprim-sulfamethoxazole are alternative agents. Chloramphenicol is as effective as tetracycline in the treatment of rickettsial diseases. Because of its ability to enter the central nervous system in the presence or absence of inflammation, chloramphenicol frequently is used in the treatment of brain abscess and can be used to treat pneumococcal or meningococcal meningitis in the penicillin- and cephalosporin-allergic patient. The drug also penetrates the eye. Chloramphenicol has been used for a variety of other infections, but safer alternative agents are available in most situations.

### Vancomycin

Vancomycin is a chemically complex glycopeptide antibiotic isolated during the mid-1950s from *Streptomyces orientalis.* It is active only against gram-positive bacteria, and it irreversibly inhibits cell wall synthesis by direct interaction with the mucopeptide. Resistance to the drug among gram-positive organisms is unusual, but enterococci are inhibited but not killed at low concentrations. Vancomycin-resistant enterococci are still uncommon but are being isolated with increasing frequency.

Original preparations of vancomycin contained much extraneous material. Preparations are now much purer. Toxicities initially observed with vancomycin use were probably secondary to these impurities. The drug is poorly absorbed after oral administration and there is no intramuscular preparation. The drug is well tolerated when administered intravenously, but too-rapid infusion may cause a histamine-type reaction with flushing, pruritus, rash, and general discomfort, termed red man syndrome. The drug is almost exclusively excreted via glomerular filtration, and the dosage must be carefully adjusted to renal function. Serum levels should be monitored to avoid accumulation. The drug is not removed by hemodialysis. Vancomycin diffuses into the CSF in the presence of meningeal inflammation but achieves low levels, and depending on the clinical situation intrathecal doses may be also needed. Both reversible and irreversible deafness have been associated with excessive serum levels of vancomycin. Nephrotoxicity also is possible, but the full potential for such toxicity has not been clearly established. Allergic reactions are uncommon.

Vancomycin is used primarily as an alternative bactericidal agent in serious infections caused by gram-positive cocci, especially *S. aureus* and *S. epidermidis,* in penicillin-allergic patients, and in particular in endocarditis. Increased use of the drug also has resulted from the increasing prevalence of methicillin-resistant *S. aureus* and *S. epidermidis.* Vancomycin, as a single agent, appears to be highly effective in the treatment of endocarditis due to gram-positive cocci, but to achieve a bactericidal effect against enterococci requires combined therapy with an aminoglycoside. Vancomycin given orally is also effective in the treatment of diarrhea and pseudomembranous colitis caused by toxigenic *C. difficile.* Oral vancomycin is sometimes used as part of a bowel prep to decrease resident flora.

## Spectinomycin

Spectinomycin is a naturally occurring aminoglycoside antibiotic produced by *Streptomyces spectabilis* that is antibacterial through inhibition of protein synthesis. Although the drug has activity against a variety of organisms, it has clinical utility only as alternative treatment of uncomplicated gonorrhea. The drug is available only as a preparation for intramuscular injection. In this form it has the advantage of single-dose therapy for gonorrhea when given in a 2-g dose. The drug is excreted in the urine. The use of this drug in common practice is not associated with significant toxicity, although it may rarely cause dizziness, nausea, headache, or allergic manifestations.

## Metronidazole

Metronidazole is a synthetic antimicrobial agent that has been used in the treatment of protozoal infections, such as amebiasis, trichomoniasis, and giardiasis. The drug is active against anaerobic bacteria, especially gram-negative bacilli and notably penicillin-resistant *B. fragilis.* The drug is not active against microaerophilic, facultative, and aerobic organisms.

Metronidazole is very well absorbed after oral administration and is well tolerated when given intravenously. It penetrates tissues well, including the central nervous system, and is metabolized by the liver.

Seizures, encephalopathy, and peripheral neuropathy have been associated with metronidazole therapy. The drug has been reported to be tumorigenic in animals and mutagenic in bacteria. Although follow-up of treated patients thus far has not revealed an increased incidence of neoplasms, the potential for long-term problems has not been clearly defined. The drug can cause a disulfiram-like reaction when taken with alcohol. Many patients complain of an unpleasant metallic taste while receiving the drug.

Metronidazole is primarily used in the treatment of infections caused by susceptible anaerobes, especially in combination with other antimicrobials for the treatment of intraabdominal and pelvic infections. Its role in respiratory tract infection has not been clearly established. The drug has been shown to be effective in the treatment of endocarditis caused by anaerobic, gram-negative bacilli. Metronidazole also may be valuable in the treatment of brain abscesses due to anaerobic bacteria, since the drug appears to penetrate these lesions well. The drug may have an additional advantage for some therapeutic indications in that oral therapy can be instituted early in the course of therapy. Metronidazole also has been used to treat diarrhea and colitis caused by *C. difficile,* and it appears to be effective therapy for nonspecific vaginitis.

## Rifampin

Rifampin is a derivative of the naturally occurring antibiotic rifamycin B. The compound inhibits RNA synthesis by binding to DNA-dependent RNA polymerase. Rifampin is active against a wide range of microorganisms, including gram-positive and gram-negative bacteria, mycobacteria, *Chlamydia,* and some fungi and viruses (at relatively high concentration). Unfortunately, many organisms quite rapidly acquire resistance to rifampin upon exposure, presumably through changes in the susceptibility of RNA polymerase. This rapid emergence of resistance in vitro and in vivo has limited the use of rifampin to several situations, and it is usually administered with another agent.

A number of toxic effects of rifampin have been described. Some of these toxic effects may be related to effects on mitochondrial RNA synthesis, although mitochondria appear to be relatively impermeable to rifampin. The most important toxicity is hepatotoxicity, which is usually mild but may rarely manifest as overt hepatitis. Hematologic and renal toxicity have been described. Hypersensitivity to the drug may play a role in some of the observed abnormalities. A syndrome of abdominal discomfort after intermittent doses of the drug has been described. Rifampin penetrates tissue extremely well, to the point that its presence in tears may stain soft contact lenses pink, and sweat may have an orange discoloration.

The clinical use of rifampin in the United States has been limited to three situations. Rifampin is a first-line drug in the treatment of tuberculosis and is usually combined with isoniazid and pyrazinamide to prevent emergence of resistance and to facilitate sterilization of sputum. Rifampin is effective for the eradication of meningococci from the pharynx of carriers. It is now the drug of choice for this purpose because of the high prevalence of sulfonamide resistance among meningococci and the prevalence of annoying side effects with minocycline. It is usually given in a regimen of four doses of 300 mg over 2 to 4 days. Rifampin also is used in combination with other agents in the treatment of serious infections caused by *S. aureus* and *S. epidermis,* especially multiresistant strains. Rifampin may be particularly helpful when added to a primary antistaphylococcal regimen when the infection involves prosthetic material.

## Quinolones

The quinolones represent a relatively new and unique group of antimicrobials (Table 64-9). Some of the agents in this group have been available for several years, and clinical experience has led to some consensus regarding their use. New quinolones continue to be developed, and multiple investigational agents with potentially new properties are currently under study. Nalidixic acid was the first quinolone in clinical use, but low serum levels limited its usefulness. Currently ciprofloxacin, ofloxacin, lome-

**Table 64-9.** Quinolone antimicrobials

| Agent (trade name) | Route and dosage | Peak serum levels (μg/ml) | Comments |
|---|---|---|---|
| Ciprofloxacin (Cipro) | 0.5-0.75 g PO q12h; 0.2-0.4 g IV q12h | 0.8-2.8; 0.46 | Renal and hepatic excretion; most active against *M. tuberculosis* |
| Ofloxacin (Floxin) | 0.2-0.4 g PO q12h; 0.2-0.4 g IV q12h | 3.5-5.3; 4-4.5 | Primary renal excretion; best quinolone to use against *Chylamydia* and genital *Mycoplasma* sp. |
| Lomefloxacin (Maxaquin) | 400 mg PO qd | 1.4 | Renal and hepatic excretion; approved for treatment of UTIs and nonstreptococcal bronchitis |
| Norfloxacin (Noroxin) | 400 mg PO bid | 1.4-1.8 | Renal and hepatic excretion; low serum levels limit use to the treatment of UTIs |
| Enoxacin (Penetrex) | 400 mg PO bid or 600 mg PO qd | 2 | Renal and hepatic excretion; approved for the treatment of UTIs and *N. gonorrhoeae* |

*UTI*, Urinary tract infection.

floxacin, norfloxacin, and enoxacin are available in the United States.

Quinolones are bactericidal agents that act by binding to and inhibiting DNA gyrase, resulting in impairment of DNA synthesis and potentially the cleavage of bacterial DNA. Resistance is a significant and increasing problem with quinolones and is caused by mutations in the DNA gyrase that limit the binding of the quinolone. Resistance may also result from the development of impermeability of the outer membrane. Resistance may develop after exposure of particular bacteria to subinhibitory concentrations of quinolone.

As a group, quinolones can be characterized by rapid and excellent absorption when taken orally, with therapeutic levels achieved in almost all tissues and fluids. Quinolones also achieve excellent intracellular levels. In most settings oral therapy is as effective as intravenous. Quinolones chelate with metal cations, resulting in decreased absorption; consequently they should not be taken with magnesium- or aluminum-containing antacids, zinc compounds, or calcium. Quinolone absorption is also impaired when taken with sucralfate or bismuth subsalicylate. Quinolones do cross the blood-brain barrier but do not achieve adequate levels for the treatment of streptococcal or staphylococcal meningitis, and experience in the treatment of gram-negative pathogens in the spinal fluid is minimal. Quinolones are one of the few antimicrobials to achieve good levels in prostatic tissue. The majority of the drugs of this class are excreted via both the renal and hepatic routes. Ofloxacin is the only available quinolone with primarily renal excretion. All quinolones currently approved for use in the United States require some dosage reduction in the presence of renal failure.

Ciprofloxacin and ofloxacin are both available in oral and intravenous formulations and have been studied in patients with serious infections. They have a similar spectrum of coverage, with activity against the Enterobacteriaceae, *H. influenzae, Neisseria* species (including *N. gonorrhoeae*), *Branhamella, Aeromonas* species, and *P. aeruginosa.* Other pseudomonal species may be resistant to the quinolones. *Salmonella, Shigella, E. coli, Campylobacter,* and *Vibrio* species are susceptible to the quinolones, making them ideal agents for the prophylaxis or treatment of traveler's diarrhea. Ciprofloxacin is active against mycobacteria and is being used in the treatment of drug-resistant tuberculosis. In vitro the quinolones show significant activity against *Legionella* species, but clinical trials have not been performed. Ofloxacin is active against *C. trachomatis,* but therapy must continue for 7 to 10 days. Ofloxacin is also the preferred quinolone in the treatment of *M. hominis* and *Ureaplasma* species. Although the quinolones are active against staphylococcal infections, the clinical experience has been variable. Quinolones have proven ineffective against streptococci, including enterococci, and they have no activity against anaerobes. Though the quinolones may be used for the treatment of gonorrhea, they are inactive against syphilis. Lomefloxacin, norfloxacin, and enoxacin have a similar spectrum of activity when compared with ciprofloxacin and ofloxacin, but they have not been approved for the treatment of significant systemic infection.

Adverse events associated with quinolones are limited. Gastrointestinal toxicity, including nausea, diarrhea, and vomiting, is the most commonly reported side effect. As with all other antimicrobials, *C. difficile* colitis can occur during or following therapy with the quinolones. Central nervous system toxicity has been reported; specifically headache, restlessness, confusion, and agitation have been associated with quinolone use. Hypersensitivity reactions such as rash, urticaria and anaphylaxis have occurred rarely in patients taking quinolones. Animal studies have suggested that quinolones can impair cartilage development. For that reason they are contraindicated in pregnant women and children under age 16.

Clinical indications for the use of the quinolones remain under review. They offer unique benefits in treating infections, including the opportunity for oral treatment, which otherwise would require intravenous therapy and efficacy against difficult-to-treat pathogens. However, the emergence of resistance to the quinolones has changed the approach to their use. To preserve their utility, quinolones should be used only for well-delineated indications. All the quinolones are approved for the treatment of urinary tract infections, particularly complicated ones, where infection with *P. aeruginosa* is a concern. Ciprofloxacin, ofloxacin, and lomefloxacin are approved for the treatment of respiratory tract infections caused by gram-negative pathogens, with the corollary that they should never be used when there is a question of anaerobic or streptococcal infection. Quinolones are very helpful in the treatment of respiratory tract infections in patients with cystic fibrosis, where *Pseudomonas* species are common pathogens. As discussed, it is appropriate to use quinolones in the prophylaxis or treatment of traveler's diarrhea. Quinolones have also been used as prophylaxis in immunocompromised patients, where they have been successful in decreasing the absolute number of infections caused by gram-negative pathogens. In other settings, quinolones are best used for therapy in patients who are allergic to penicillins and cephalosporins, or when isolates are resistant to more commonly used antimicrobials. Quinolones should be used with caution in the treatment of staphylococcal infection, preferably in settings where other agents cannot be used.

### Urinary tract antibacterial agents

Urinary tract antibacterials are a group of compounds that provide antibacterial activity in the urine with little or no activity in the serum. The oral agents are sometimes used in the treatment of uncomplicated cystitis but more commonly are selected for the prophylaxis or chronic suppression of urinary tract infection.

Nitrofurantoin is a synthetic compound with a broad spectrum of activity against many bacteria that commonly cause urinary tract infection. The drug is rapidly excreted in the urine and inactivated in tissue. It has no usefulness in patients with impaired renal function, since toxic levels may accumulate despite inactivation, and it is not effectively delivered to its site of action. The drug has been reported to cause acute, subacute, and chronic pneumonitis, which may be severe. This pulmonary toxicity appears to be both idiosyncratic and a result of hypersensitivity to the drug. Nitrofurantoin also can cause significant peripheral neuritis when toxic levels accumulate in the body. Nausea and vomiting are dose-related side effects. The drug comes in two preparations, a crystalline form and a macrocrystalline form. The latter seems to have better gastrointestinal tolerance characteristics.

Nalidixic acid and cinoxacin are synthetic chemotherapeutic agents that achieve antibacterial levels in the urine. These drugs interfere with bacterial DNA synthesis and are active against a variety of enteric gram-negative bacilli. They are relatively nontoxic, although neurotoxicity in adults and increased intracranial pressure in infants have been described. The drugs should be avoided in patients with renal functional impairment and in children.

Methenamine mandelate and hippurate are salts of methenamine, a drug that has been used as a urinary antiseptic for almost 100 years. In acidic urine methenamine is converted to formaldehyde, which is active against bacteria and fungi. Mandelic and hippuric acids in the preparations serve to lower the urine pH and have some antibacterial activity of their own. The usefulness of these agents is limited by the difficulty of lowering the urine pH to 5.0 for maximum activity; additional acidification, usually with ascorbic acid, is often necessary. These drugs are inactive against urea-splitting organisms, since the urine cannot be adequately acidified. Enteric-coated capsules are used to prevent release of formaldehyde in the stomach. These drugs are well tolerated except for occasional gastrointestinal upset and urinary tract irritation from formaldehyde production. They are used for chronic suppression of infection, usually in patients with indwelling catheters.

### Agents used to treat tuberculosis

The treatment of tuberculosis is discussed in sections of the text dealing with infections due to *M. tuberculosis* (see Chapter 114).

### Antifungal agents

Antifungal agents can be grouped into those used systemically to treat severe and deep fungal infections and those used to treat superficial infections. The therapy of fungal infections is discussed in Chapters 25 and 113. Some clinical and pharmacologic aspects of particular agents bear review.

Amphotericin B is the most reliably effective antifungal agent available. It is active against a wide variety of fungi, and resistance to it is rare. The drug binds to sterols in the fungal cell membrane, affecting permeability. Although amphotericin has greater affinity for ergosterol (the primary membrane sterol or fungi) than cholesterol (the primary sterol of animal membranes), much of the toxic effect of the drug in humans is probably due to a mechanism similar to that which produces its antifungal activity.

The most important side effect of amphotericin B is nephrotoxicity, which is predictable and unavoidable. The drug also may suppress the bone marrow. Cardiovascular, neurologic, and hepatic toxicity are rare but have been described. Fever, chills, hypotension, nausea, and vomiting are not uncommon with intravenous administration and make therapy very difficult in some patients. Premedication with steroids, antihistamines, and antiemetics is often tried to avert some of these infusion side effects. Efforts are ongoing to develop a carrier for amphotericin, such as lipids, that would increase the tissue levels of the drug while reducing toxicity. Currently liposomal amphotericin is available only on an investigational basis.

The fate of amphotericin B in the body remains a mystery. It is not excreted in the urine, and no metabolites have been measured. Detectable drug may persist in the serum for weeks to months after cessation of therapy.

Nystatin is a drug closely related to amphotericin B that is too toxic for systemic therapy but is nonabsorbable and is used for topical and oral therapy of mucosal and cutaneous yeast infections. When used topically or orally the drug has virtually no side effects.

Flucytosine (5-fluorocytosine) is an antimetabolite active against many pathogenic yeasts, although primary and acquired resistance to the agent is common. It is converted to 5-fluorouracil in the fungal cell and thereby interferes with nucleic acid synthesis. Flucytosine has synergistic activity with amphotericin B presumably due to increased permeability of the fungal cell. The drug is relatively nontoxic in clinical use; however, its accumulation to toxic levels (more than 100 μg/ml) can lead to bone marrow depression and hepatotoxicity. Because the drug is excreted in the urine, dosages must be adjusted for renal impairment. Many centers that frequently use the drug assay its serum levels routinely.

Clotrimazole and miconazole are imidazole derivatives with activity against a wide variety of fungi. Both are available as topical agents for mucosal and skin infections, and the latter is available as an intravenous preparation for the treatment of severe systemic fungal infections. Parenteral miconazole therapy may be associated with fever, chills, nausea, vomiting, rash, and phlebitis; hyperlipidemia has been associated with the vehicle of administration (castor oil). Parenteral miconazole has a limited role in the therapy of severe fungal infections because of the demonstrated efficacy of amphotericin B and the availability of ketoconazole, fluconazole, and itraconazole.

Ketoconazole is an antifungal oral agent with a broad spectrum of antifungal activity. It appears to interfere with ergosterol synthesis. The drug has been used successfully in the treatment of a variety of fungal infections including candidiasis, coccidioidomycosis, dermatophytoses, and others. Its use has declined due to the development of the newer azole antifungal agents. The drug is well tolerated with a low incidence of gastrointestinal distress. Idiosyncratic hepatotoxicity has been described, and the drug may interfere with human steroid metabolism.

Fluconazole is a triazole antifungal agent that increases the permeability of the fungal cell wall by inhibiting the synthesis of ergosterol, a major cell wall constituent. It is available as both an oral and intravenous formulation. When taken orally, fluconazole has excellent bioavailability. As compared to ketoconazole and itraconazole, it is well absorbed in the setting of achlorhydria or when $H_2$ blockers are also given. Fluconazole achieves high levels in all tissues and fluids, including the prostate and CSF. With a half-life of 25 hours, fluconazole can be given once daily. Fluconazole is partially metabolized in the liver, but significant renal excretion occurs and the dosage should be adjusted in the presence of renal failure.

Fluconazole has very limited toxicity. Nausea and vomiting are the most commonly reported adverse events. Rash, headache, and elevated liver enzymes have also been described. Severe hapatitis in two patients may have been associated with fluconazole use. Rifampin increases the metabolism of fluconazole, resulting in decreased levels. Fluconazole can increase the levels of phenytoin, warfarin, and oral hypoglycemic drugs. Effect on cyclosporin levels appears to be minimal.

Fluconazole is active against *C. albicans* and other candidal species, with the exception of *C. krusei* and *Torulopsis glabrata.* It is also very effective against *Cryptococcus neoformans.* It is not useful for the treatment of *Aspergillus* infections or in the treatment of coccidioidomycosis or histoplasmosis. Fluconazole is approved for the treatment of mucocutaneous candidiasis, preferably in immunocompromised patients in whom topical therapy is less than optimally effective. It is also the drug of choice for maintenance therapy for cryptococcal meningitis. Fluconazole prophylaxis has been shown to decrease the incidence of serious fungal infections in patients after bone marrow transplant, and some clinicians also use it prophylactically in neutropenic patients after chemotherapy. Concern does exist regarding the emergence of resistant fungi as a result of long-term treatment with fluconazole, as well as the potential for an increase in the incidence of *Aspergillus* infection in these populations.

Itraconazole is a newly developed triazole agent that is active against a broad spectrum of fungal pathogens. It is available only as an oral agent. Similar to the other azoles, itraconazole acts by inhibiting the fungal cytochrome P-450 enzyme system, which results in a decrease in the synthesis of ergosterol.

Itraconazole absorption is improved in the presence of food. It appears to accumulate in tissues. As compared with fluconazole, itraconazole does not achieve significant levels in the CSF. It is metabolized in the liver and excreted in the feces and urine. No dosage adjustment is necessary in renal failure, but this drug should be used with caution in the setting of hepatic failure. Drugs that induce hepatic enzymes, such as isoniazid, rifampin, phenobarbital, and phenytoin, may decrease itraconazole levels when given concomitantly. Itraconazole may reduce the metabolism of other hepatically metabolized agents such as cyclosporin, digoxin, and warfarin. Itraconazole has been associated with nausea, diarrhea, rash, headache, dizziness, and elevated liver function tests.

Itraconazole is active against *Histoplasma, Blastomyces, Cryptococcus,* and dermatophytes. At higher levels it is also active against *Candida* species and *Aspergillus.* Currently itraconazole is approved for use in the treatment of blastomycosis, histoplasmosis, paracoccidioidomycosis, and sporotrichosis. Although it has been utilized in the treatment of aspergillosis, the drug of choice for that infection remains amphotericin B.

Griseofulvin is an oral antifungal agent used in the treatment of dermatophyte infection. It appears to interfere with fungal DNA synthesis. The drug is well tolerated but can cause gastrointestinal upset. Headaches, confusion, and fatigue may occur. The drug is usually administered for a prolonged period. It interferes with porphyrin metabolism and should not be used in patients with porphyria. It also has a disulfiram-like effect, and concurrent intake of alcohol should be avoided. The role of griseofulvin in the treatment of fungal skin infections has been and will be further supplanted by more effective topical and systemic agents.

A variety of nonprescription topical agents are marketed for the treatment of dermatophytic infections of the skin, such as athlete's foot, jock itch, and ringworm. Many of these agents contain zinc salts, especially zinc undecylenate, and undecylenic acid; they are mainly useful prophylactically. Topical preparations of tolnaftate, miconazole, clotrimazole, econazole, and ciclopirox are available without prescription and are more effective. Haloprogin is a topical antifungal agent available by prescription that is also effective against dermatophytes. Topical nystatin is ineffective against dermatophytes but is the therapy of choice for minor mucocutaneous candidiasis. The use of ketoconazole in the treatment of trivial skin and mucous membrane infections is inappropriate pending full evaluation of the usefulness of the drug in more serious infections and its long-term toxicity.

### Antiviral agents

A great deal of progress has been made in the development of antiviral chemotherapy, but this field is still in its infancy. Several effective antiviral agents exist for the treatment of specific infections. Some of these drugs have not been completely evaluated and should be reserved for specific indications pending further clinical investigation.

Idoxuridine was among the first specific antiviral agents to be studied. The drug is very toxic when used parenterally, and its use is now limited to one indication: topical therapy in herpes simplex keratitis. The drug is active against DNA viruses and interferes with human as well as viral DNA synthesis.

Vidarabine (adenine arabinoside) is an antiviral agent by virtue of its interference with DNA synthesis. It is active against herpes viruses. It has been shown to be of use in the treatment of herpes simplex encephalitis and in ameliorating systemic herpes zoster infection in immunocompromised patients. Topical vidarabine is of use in the treatment of herpes keratoconjunctivitis. The drug is relatively nontoxic but does cause neurotoxicity and mental disorders and can cause bone marrow suppression. The potential for long-term toxicity has not been clearly established. The parenteral form of the drug is administered by intravenous infusion. Vidarabine has been almost entirely replaced by acyclovir in the treatment of herpes and varicella infections.

Acyclovir is the most commonly utilized antiviral agent, primarily due to its efficacy and safety. It inhibits viral DNA synthesis and thus is active against herpes viruses. Topical and parenteral forms of the drug have been used in the treatment of initial infection in herpes genitalis with reduction of healing time and diminished viral shedding. The drug is much less effective in the treatment of recurrent lesions, but if taken prophylactically in patients with frequent recurrences it has been shown to reduce the incidence of the episodes. Acyclovir is the drug of choice in the treatment of herpes encephalitis. It also has been used successfully in the treatment of herpes simplex and herpes zoster infections in immunocompromised patients. Resistance to acyclovir occurs spontaneously in some herpes simplex isolates, and the emergence of resistance in patients on long-term therapy or prophylaxis with acyclovir has been described.

Acyclovir is excreted in the urine by glomerular filtration and tubular secretion. If given in a high dosage with inadequate hydration, acyclovir can cause renal failure by inducing crystalline nephropathy. Neurotoxicity has been described with the drug, characterized primarily by seizures. Possible long-term adverse reactions to the drug have not been established.

Foscarnet and ganciclovir are two antiviral agents that have been developed primarily for the treatment of cytomegalovirus retinitis in patients with HIV infection. Both agents are effective in the treatment of herpes and varicella infections. Foscarnet has the additional benefit of activity against herpes strains that appear resistant to acyclovir and ganciclovir. The antiviral drugs are discussed more fully in Chapter 68.

## BIBLIOGRAPHY

Bennett WM et al: Drug therapy in renal failure: dosing guidelines for adults. I. Antimicrobial agents, analgesics, *Ann Intern Med* 93:62, 1980.

The choice of antimicrobial drugs. In *The Medical Letter.* Issues published frequently.

Cunha BA, editor: Symposium on antimicrobial therapy, *Med Clin North Am* 66:1, 1982.

Garrod LP, Lambert HP, O'Grady F: *Antibiotics and chemotherapy,* ed 5, New York, 1981, Churchill Livingstone.

Greenwood D, editor: *Antimicrobial chemotherapy,* Philadelphia, 1983, WB Saunders.

*Handbook of antimicrobial therapy,* New Rochelle, NY, 1986, Medical Letter on Drugs and Therapeutics.

Kucers A, Bennett N: *The use of antibiotics,* ed 3, London, 1979, Heinemann.

Mandell GL, Douglas RG, Bennett JE, editors: *Principles and practice of infectious diseases,* ed 3, New York, 1990, Churchill Livingstone.

Ristuccia AM, Cunha BA: *Antimicrobial therapy,* New York, 1984, Raven Press.

Rubenstein E, Federman DD, editors: *Scientific American medicine: infectious disease,* New York, 1978-1994.

Sanford JP: *Guide to antimicrobial therapy,* Dallas, 1994, Antimicrobial Therapy Inc.

Symposium on antimicrobial agents, *Mayo Clin Proc* 66, 1991.

CHAPTER

# 65 Sexually Transmitted Diseases

**Robin R. Ingalls**
**Peter A. Rice**

Many American physicians are aware that sexually transmitted diseases (STDs) are a growing public health problem and that the "traditional" venereal diseases, including syphilis, gonorrhea, chancroid, lymphogranuloma venereum, and granuloma inguinale, account for only a part of STDs in industrialized societies. Whether the measure of the problem is the number of infections and the accompanying physical and psychologic morbidity in individual patients or the resulting complications such as pelvic inflammatory disease, infertility, and perinatal morbidity, most of the problems are caused by microorganisms outside the traditional sphere of venereology. Primary physicians and other health care providers must understand the increased scope of the etiology, epidemiology, prevention, and pathogenesis of STDs if these conditions are to be recognized and managed in individual patients and controlled in populations.

In this chapter genitourinary infections, which are frequently transmitted sexually, are classified according to the patient's presenting complaints. Although this approach serves as a useful initial guide to a differential diagnosis, most of these infections have overlapping modes of presentation, and individual infections may produce several complaints (Fig. 65-1). Hence further evaluation, including physical and laboratory examinations, are almost always necessary to make a specific diagnosis and to formulate a plan for management.

Identification and treatment of sexual partners are essential parts of the management of the patient with STDs. Since many of the infections are not reportable, the physician cannot rely on the partners being contacted by

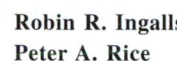

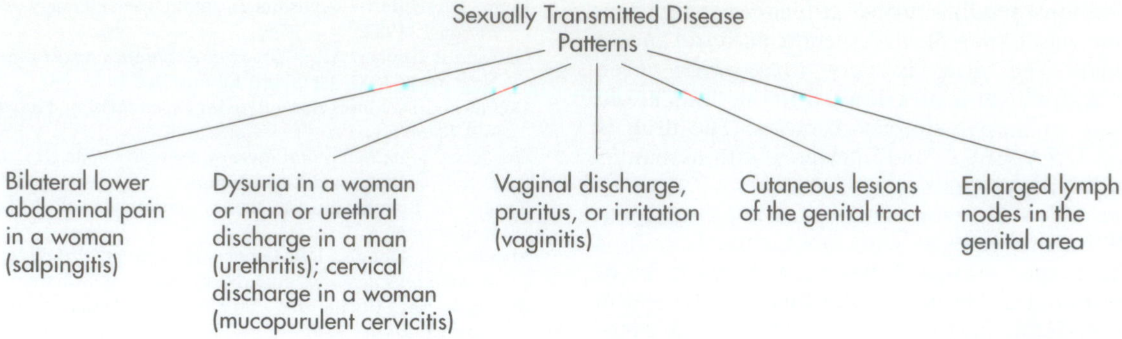


**Fig. 65-1.** Frequent clinical patterns of presentation of sexually transmitted diseases. (Modified from Woo B et al: In Branch WT, editor: *Office practice of medicine,* Philadelphia, 1982, WB Saunders.)

public health authorities, and the need to evaluate the partners must be judiciously emphasized to the patient.

## VAGINITIS

The major causes of infection of the vagina, vulva, cervix, and urinary tract (lower genitourinary tract) in women may have overlapping symptoms such as vulvar irritation, dysuria, and dyspareunia. The most common presenting syndrome in women with a vaginal infection (often sexually acquired) includes a constellation of symptoms: vaginal discharges (often malodorous), vulvar irritation or pruritus, dysuria (often external), and dyspareunia. These symptoms are so common that milder forms may not be perceived as abnormal by the woman, and therefore she may not mention them to her physician until they are elicited during a routine gynecologic examination when the accompanying signs are identified. Because vaginal infections are not reportable in the United States, their incidence can be only crudely estimated. Vaginitis accounts for half of patient visits to private gynecologists, and three forms are categorized as follows: (1) bacterial vaginosis, (2) vaginitis caused by *Candida albicans,* and (3) vaginitis caused by *Trichomonas vaginalis.* These infections account for nearly 30% of visits by women to clinics for STDs.

Vaginal infection appears to be rising in frequency. Although growing public discussion and media attention may have contributed to the apparent increase, much of the rise is probably real. Greater sexual activity among the population as a whole, as well as a higher proportion of people within the ages of peak sexual activity, may be responsible. The extent to which sexual contact contributes to each of the major forms of vaginitis remains uncertain. Trichomoniasis is clearly linked to sexual activity, and a significant proportion of cases of bacterial vaginosis appear to be sexually acquired. Sexual contact, however, is probably a minor contributor to the epidemiology of vulvovaginal candidiasis.

Pharmaceutical advances may also have aided the spread of vaginitis. Systemic antibiotics often disturb the normal composition of genital flora. By widely replacing barrier methods, oral contraceptives have removed an obstacle to sexual acquisition of certain pathogens. Moreover, these compounds may favor the growth of yeasts by directly altering the vaginal milieu.

***Evaluation of the patient's history and symptoms.*** The patient's symptoms are usually the determining factor in decisions about therapy. Asymptomatic carriage of *C. albicans* or *Gardnerella vaginalis* probably does not require treatment. On the other hand, a patient's symptoms may suggest infection where none exists. For example, physiologic vaginal discharge is partially under hormonal control and may increase at ovulation, during pregnancy, or with the use of oral contraceptives. When accompanied by a change in sexual activity, such discharge may arouse fear of infection. Physiologic discharges account for 10% of vaginal complaints presented to private practices. In contrast to infectious vaginitis, these cases are not usually accompanied by vulvar soreness, vaginal malodor, or urinary complaints. In more than 90% of patients, microscopic examination of the discharge reveals less than one polymorphonuclear neutrophil per vaginal epithelial cell.

It is important to note that vaginal odor is often perceived as unpleasant even under normal circumstances. Moreover, the intensity and subjective quality of the odor vary with the menstrual cycle. Nevertheless, odor is a cardinal symptom of bacterial vaginosis even in the absence of vulvovaginal irritation, and a complaint of vaginal odor should always be taken seriously.

Symptoms of urinary frequency and dysuria, including not only external dysuria (burning pain over the vulvar area upon urination) but also internal dysuria (burning pain within the urethra), may be more commonly associ-

**Table 65-1.** Clinical and laboratory features of vaginitis

| Feature | Normal | Bacterial vaginosis | *Candida* | *Trichomonas* |
|---|---|---|---|---|
| Appearance of discharge | White, gray, clear; nonhomogenous | Gray, white; homogenous and frothy | White; adherent plaques; curdy | Gray, creamy; homogenous; frothy (25%) |
| Amount of discharge | Variable | Large | Scant | Large |
| Vulvar irritation | None | Uncommon | Common | Occasional |
| pH of discharge | <4.7* | >4.7 | <4.7* | >4.7 |
| Amine test (fishy odor upon addition of 10% NaOH or KOH to discharge) | Negative | Positive | Negative | Positive |
| Microscopy (saline and 10% NaOH or KOH) and Gram stain | Epithelial cells; rare white blood cells; gram-negative and gram-positive rods | Clue cells†; coccobacilli; absence of gram-positive rods | Leukocytes; yeasts and pseudomycelia | Leukocytes; motile trichomonads; coccobacilli |

Modified from Hansfield HH: *Hosp Prac* 17:99, 1982.
*Except during menses; pH is normal >5.0 when blood is present.
†Clue cells are epithelial cells with a ragged and refractile appearance due to large numbers of adherent bacteria (see Fig. 65-2).
*NaOH,* Sodium hydroxide; *KOH,* potassium hydroxide.

ated with vaginitis, particularly in young women, than infection of the urinary tract without accompanying genital infection.

Patients should also be questioned about their menstrual history, including the date of the previous menstrual period, earlier pregnancies and abortions, methods of contraception, previous vaginal or urinary infections, and a history of STDs or possible exposures. They should also be questioned about their personal hygiene including their douching habits, and their use of sprays and deodorants, tight-fitting undergarments, and tampons. All of these have been implicated as potential predisposing factors in vaginitis. The presence of systemic illnesses, such as diabetes, or the use of drugs such as sulfonamides or corticosteroids may be associated with both infectious and noninfectious vaginitis.

***Physical and laboratory examinations.*** The physical examination of the patient and a microscopic examination of the discharge should be performed at the time the patient is being evaluated to establish, if possible, a specific cause of the vaginitis. During a speculum examination the quantity and quality of the discharge should be noted. This should include the color and consistency of the discharge, the presence or absence of bubbles (frothiness) in the discharge, and the presence of odor. The vaginal walls should be examined for erythema and the vulva for erythema and edema. Laboratory examinations that should be performed in evaluating vaginal secretions in women with vaginitis include (1) pH determination, (2) microscopic examination of a wet mount preparation of the secretions, looking for signs of specific infection (see below) and the presence of polymorphonuclear leukocytes (PMNs), (3) Gram stain of the secretions, and (4) a test for amine liberation using sodium or potassium hydroxide. Special cultures can be performed if the methods outlined above do not provide a specific diagnosis. Although these features of the physical and laboratory examination should adequately predict most cases of vaginitis, it is important to remember that other genitourinary infections, which are sometimes sexually acquired, may coexist with vaginitis. In particular the urethra should be examined for mucopurulent discharge, particularly in women complaining of internal dysuria, and the cervix should be carefully examined for signs of cervicitis or discharge. These findings should prompt additional laboratory investigations; the presence of cervicitis warrants a bimanual pelvic examination.

***Diagnostic considerations.*** The major causes of vaginitis include bacterial vaginosis and vaginitis caused by *C. albicans* and *T. vaginalis.* The major clinical and laboratory features of the three most common forms of vaginitis are summarized in Table 65-1. Other less common etiologies include atrophic vaginitis and in the young nonmenstruating girl vaginitis caused by *Neisseria gonorrhoeae.* The use of irritants in douches, sprays, deodorants, or tampons and tight-fitting undergarments may produce a nonclassifiable vaginitis.

Many of these infections are sexually transmitted, and patients with bacterial vaginosis or trichomoniasis should be screened for clinically inapparent infection with organisms such as *N. gonorrhoeae* or *C. trachomatis,* which may be more important. One study showed that 28% of patients with bacterial vaginosis had another sexually acquired disease. In clinics that treat sexually transmitted diseases gonorrhea is diagnosed 1½ to 2 times more often in women carrying *T. vaginalis.*

### Bacterial vaginosis

Bacterial vaginosis (BV), sometimes termed nonspecific vaginitis and previously known as *Gardenerella*-associated vaginitis, represents nearly half of all cases of vaginitis. Because signs of inflammation in the vagina are either minimal or absent altogether, and because an accompanying polymicrobial etiology is currently assumed, the term *bacterial vaginosis* is now used for this condition.

BV is probably an infection involving certain anaerobic bacteria and possibly *G. vaginalis,* which is almost always present. *G. vaginalis* is fastidious and slow growing, but it can be cultured from over 90% of women who have symptomatic BV, and it has been isolated from up to 30% of asymptomatic women. In university women lacking both signs and symptoms of vaginitis, isolation rates have been as high as nearly 70%. However, good clinical responses in women harboring *G. vaginalis* to antibiotics to which the organism is resistant in vitro suggest that effective treatment is directed principally at other organisms present in the vagina. For example, metronidazole is highly effective in BV with accompanying *G. vaginalis,* but in vitro the organism is resistant to the drug. In fact, some women cured of vaginal symptoms with the drug are still colonized with *G. vaginalis.*

Anaerobic bacteria (*Peptococcus* and *Bacteroides*) are often cultured from vaginas of healthy women but are present in numbers an order of magnitude higher in patients with vaginitis. Vaginal odor, a prominent feature of BV, results from the release of aromatic amines by these bacteria. These amines are produced from bacterial decarboxylases acting upon free amino acids, which may be generated by *G. vaginalis* and which are required for growth of anaerobic bacteria. Thin-layer chromatographic analysis permits the diagnosis of BV with a sensitivity and specificity of nearly 90%, if the percent of diamines present approaches 20% of the concentration of alanine in vaginal fluid. Aromatic amines become volatile at basic pH. An increased odor after coitus may be the result of volatilization of amines subjected to the basic pH of semen. Certain amines irritate the skin, and some organic acid metabolites may damage epithelial cells, thereby producing additional symptoms in patients.

Certain curved gram-negative or gram-variable rods may also accompany BV. These organisms, recently classified under the genus *Mobiluncus,* are motile, curved, fastidious, anaerobic bacilli with a gram-positive type wall that frequently stains gram negative or gram variable. They appear in vaginal smears from about 50% of BV patients and are absent in normal women.

An added characteristic of BV is the usual lack of facultative lactobacilli isolated from the cultures and the dearth of large gram-positive rods, typical of lactobacilli, present in normal Gram-stained vaginal secretions. These secretions also contain few PMNs. One explanation is that anaerobic bacteria may inhibit chemotaxis and phagocytosis of aerobic bacteria by PMNs, resulting in protection of aerobic flora that would otherwise cause an inflammatory response.

***Diagnosis.*** The diagnosis of BV is based on a combination of the patient's symptoms, findings on physical examination, and laboratory tests. No single aspect is pathognomonic of this infection.

About 85% of BV patients notice a slight rise in vaginal discharge and 7% complain of a moderate increase. Significant vulvar irritation and dyspareunia are usually absent. Often the patient notices an odor, particularly during or just after coitus. However, similar odors are often noted by trichomoniasis patients; in fact, none of these findings is highly specific for BV.

Discharge is frequently present at the introitus and visible on the labia minora. Usually the labia and vulva are not erythematous or edematous. A thin, homogenous discharge often adheres to the vaginal walls, which are uninflamed and may appear moist. The appearance of this discharge contrasts with the clumped or floccular, nonadherent quality of normal vaginal discharge. Small bubbles, which contain carbon dioxide generated by bacterial decarboxylase, may be present, as well as a pungent odor. Usually the discharge is white. To determine this, the examiner should remove the discharge with a swab and check it against a white background. The cervix is normal in BV; abnormalities on bimanual examination are highly unusual and should prompt a search for other causes.

In most women with BV the pH of vaginal secretions is abnormally high. To measure vaginal pH, the examiner should collect some of the discharge on the inferior speculum blade, then dip a strip of indicator paper into the sample. The paper should have a range of 4.7 to 7 pH units; normal vaginal pH is about 4.7 or lower, whereas 90% of BV patients have a pH above 4.7. Because menstrual blood and semen also give pH readings above 4.7, the sample should be free from these substances. Successful treatment restores the high pH to normal. The examiner should be aware that elevated vaginal pH is also associated with trichomoniasis. The addition of 10% of potassium or sodium hydroxide to vaginal discharge of a BV patient causes aromatic amines to be volatilized and produces a distinct fishy odor.

Microscopic examination of a wet mount of vaginal discharge may aid the diagnosis of BV. Large rods comprise the normal vaginal flora. In BV clumps of tiny coccobacilli (probably *G. vaginalis*) predominate. Clue cells, epithelial cells with coccobacilli attached, are often present. Frequently the coccobacilli are so numerous that they obscure the structure of the epithelial cells (Fig. 65-2). Clue cells occur in 90% of BV patients, and over 90% of patients with clue cells yield positive cultures for *G. vaginalis.* PMNs are not a prominent feature; their presence in a ratio of more than one PMN per epithelial cell suggests a second inflammatory process of the vagina or cervix. The wet mount of vaginal discharge is, of course, also useful for detecting trichomonads and fungi.

A Gram stain of vaginal discharge may be highly specific for BV diagnosis. Before staining, one prepares the smear by rolling a thin film of secretion over the slide. A normal vaginal smear shows a preponderance of gram-positive rods that are mostly lactobacilli. In contrast, a smear from a BV patient yields no lactobacilli. Instead, gram-negative coccobacilli (presumed *G. vaginalis*) prevail, often accompanied by gram-negative rods, gram-positive cocci, and the previously noted curved rods that stain gram negative or gram variable.

A number of different culture media can be used for *G. vaginalis.* Included among these are Columbia blood agar, Columbia chocolate agar, and peptone-starch-dextrose agar, any of which provides a useful adjunctive means to diagnose BV. However, standard laboratory techniques including examinations of wet mounts and gram-stained smears provide a more practical means to diagnose BV. A reasonable approach to the diagnosis might include looking for a pH above 4.5, identifying the presence of a white adherent discharge, odor after treatment of secretions with potassium or sodium hydroxide, and clue cells.

A

B

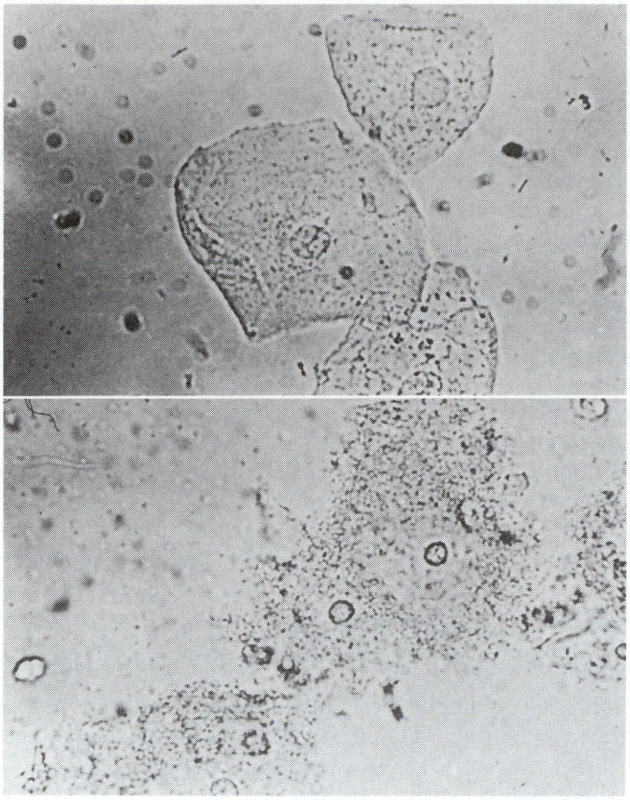

**Fig. 65-2.** Phase contrast photomicrographs of vaginal wet mounts. **A,** Normal wet mount showing clean epithelial cells and flora consisting of large rods. **B,** Wet mount from a woman with bacterial vaginosis (BV) showing clue cells covered with clumps of adherent bacteria. These tiny coccobacilli and curved rods may obscure the structure of epithelial cells in BV. (×400)

The presence of three of these four signs signifies the presence of *G. vaginalis* in 98% of cases.

*G. vaginalis* is recovered from 70% to 90% of male sexual partners of infected women. However, most of these men are asymptomatic, and whether they are treated does not seem to affect rates of recurrent BV among their female partners. *G. vaginalis* also occurs in vaginal secretions of up to 30% of sexually inexperienced women.

***Treatment.*** Many drugs have been used to treat BV, but the discrepancies between in vitro activity and in vivo effectiveness are often sharp. These inconsistencies may stem from several factors, including the complex synergistic microbial etiology of BV and the influence of the vaginal milieu on antimicrobial capacity.

Metronidazole is the most effective treatment for BV. A 7-day oral regimen of 500 mg twice daily cures over 90% of patients. Metronidazole itself is not active against *G. vaginalis* but is active against most of the anaerobic bacteria that participate in the infection. The hydroxy metabolite of metronidazole, however, is toxic to *G. vaginalis.* It is not known whether the efficacy of metronidazole is due to its action against anaerobes, its metabolites activity against *G. vaginalis,* or both. Therapy with metronidazole usually eradicates *G. vaginalis* but some patients, though rendered asymptomatic, still harbor the organism. Regimens of fewer than 7 days, including single-dose regimens effective in treating trichomoniasis, have proven inadequate against BV and should not be used. Metronidazole is not a completely benign drug, and it should be avoided in pregnancy. Its toxicities are further discussed in the section on trichomoniasis. Oral clindamycin, 300 mg twice daily for 7 days, is an alternative regimen for patients unable to take metronidazole. In addition, there is limited experience with intravaginal clindamycin cream 2% (5 g, one full applicator at bedtime for 7 days) and metronidazole gel 0.75% (5 g, one full applicator twice a day for 7 days).

Asymptomatic carriage of *G. vaginalis* is common and most authorities do not recommend treatment, even if accompanied by clue cells on vaginal wet mount as an isolated finding. On the other hand, a woman may deny symptoms but show obvious signs of BV, including excessive vaginal discharge of a chronic nature. In such a case treatment should be considered using the recommendations outlined above. There is no equivalent of BV in the male, and treatment of the male sexual partner has not been shown to be of any benefit to the patient.

### Vulvovaginal candidiasis

A greater understanding of vulvovaginal candidiasis (VVC) has evolved since it was first described years ago; however, several major questions still remain. Conversion of asymptomatic vaginal carriage of yeasts to symptomatic disease and the associated problem of managing women with frequent recurrences are among the most important problems. VVC is second only to BV in frequency of infectious vaginitis and accounts for about one third of cases of infectious vaginitis seen by private gynecologists. Of the yeasts isolated from the vagina, 80% to 95% are *Candida* species, and the remainder are *Torulopsis* species or other yeasts. The therapeutic response for these other yeasts is basically the same as for VVC.

It is uncertain whether sexual transmission plays an important role in VVC, but it is generally not considered an STD. Many patients note the onset of symptomatic VVC during the administration of systemic, broad-spectrum antimicrobials. The condition is probably brought about by changing the normal flora of the vagina. This occurs less frequently following metronidazole therapy, perhaps because metronidazole is less active against lactobacilli than other antibiotics. The association of uncontrolled diabetes and VVC has been reported frequently, and the patient with diabetes may present with recurrent bouts of VVC. In addition, recurrent VVC can be seen in the early stages of human immunodeficiency virus (HIV) infection.

During pregnancy the incidence of VVC is high and progresses during the course of gestation. In addition, recurrences during pregnancy are frequent; nearly half of women with symptomatic disease have a second episode during the same pregnancy. The role of oral contraceptives in predisposing to VVC is still controversial, and in some instances where infection recurs repeatedly changing to lower dosages or sequential oral contraceptives or discontinuation of oral contraceptives altogether has been suggested, although efficacy may be unpredictable.

In addition to the vagina, the rectum may become

colonized with yeasts. Although it has been stated that rectal yeasts may reinoculate the vagina after topical therapy for symptomatic disease has been completed, this notion has not been supported by two controlled treatment studies utilizing vaginal therapy in combination with oral nystatin, which is not absorbed systemically but which does eradicate rectal yeasts. In neither study was cure improved by the addition of nystatin.

***Diagnosis.*** Accurate diagnosis of VVC may be difficult because the clinical features are insufficiently specific. The typical complaint of women with active VVC is prominent vulvar and perivaginal pruritus, which may be aggravated at night or after bathing. Itching may also increase around the beginning of menstruation but decrease during menses.

The labia may appear either pale or erythematous and edematous, as may the vulva. Satellite lesions, pustulopapules extending beyond the main margin of erythema, strongly suggest candidiasis. A curdy, adherent vaginal discharge may occur, but discharge may also be thin or even absent. Odor, if present, tends to be mild. Vaginal pH is usually around 4.5, the same as in normal women. Normal vaginal pH in a woman with vaginitis suggests candidal infection because the pH usually increases in patients with BV or trichomoniasis.

Gram stain and wet mounts reveal fungal elements in 20% to 70% of VVC cases, and cervical cytology detects only about 25% of infections. Therefore negative direct microscopic examination does not rule out active VVC. *In the absence of another specific diagnosis, a symptomatic patient with marked vulvar pruritus and normal vaginal pH might be given a trial of antifungal therapy.*

***Treatment.*** Topical imidazoles are effective treatment for vulvovaginal candidiasis, and many preparations are available. Miconazole (Monistat), clotrimazole (Gyne-Lotrimin, Mycelex-G), butoconazole (Femstat), terconazole (Terazol), and tioconazole (Vagistat) are all effective. Clotrimazole and miconazole are available over the counter. Miconazole can be administered as a 200-mg vaginal tablet at bedtime for 3 consecutive nights or as a 2% cream (5 g) also at bedtime for 7 days. Dosages for the other imidazoles are as follows: clotrimazole, two 100-mg vaginal tablets for 3 nights or 1% cream (5 g) at bedtime for 7 days; butoconazole 2% cream (5 g) at bedtime for 3 days; tioconazole 6.5% vaginal ointment for one dose, 80-mg vaginal tablet at bedtime for 3 days, or 0.4% cream (5 g) at bedtime for 7 days. Single-dose treatment is appropriate for mild to moderate disease, and multiday regimens should be reserved for severe or complicated disease. A single dose of fluconazole, 150 mg, is as effective as 3 days of clotrimazole intravaginally. However, the judicious use of a systemic drug for local disease should be critically evaluated. Currently there is no oral agent approved by the FDA for the treatment of acute VVC.

Treatment of VVC with lactobacillus preparations is popular, but there are no recent data to confirm a beneficial effect of either oral or vaginal administration of lactobacillus preparations. Povidone-iodine preparations are 65% effective, but they should be avoided in pregnancy because absorption might suppress normal fetal thyroid development. Boric acid (600 mg in gelatin capsules, 1 capsule inserted in the vagina nightly for 2 weeks) eradicates *Candida* species within 1 week after therapy in 92% of women, and it is inexpensive.

When samples from VVC patients are recultured 3 to 6 weeks after completion of treatment, 2% to 50% have been recolonized. The regimen used does not affect the recolonization rate. Prevention of recurrent symptomatic infection is the main problem in management of VVC. Eliminating the risk factors mentioned previously in this discussion may benefit some individual cases. Short courses of antifungal therapy administered from the fifth to eleventh days of the menstrual cycle significantly reduce the rate of recurrence, but such retreatments are very expensive.

Patients with recurrent, unexplained episodes of vaginal candidiasis should be evaluated for a predisposing condition such as diabetes mellitus and HIV. Treatment of the male sexual partner is not necessary unless candidal balanitis is present. Patients should be cautioned that many of the creams and suppositories are oil based and may weaken latex condoms and diaphragms.

### Trichomoniasis

Trichomonas infection was diagnosed in just over 10% of women attending STD clinics in 1977. It is the cause of 16% of vaginitis cases seen by private physicians. Approximately 2.5 to 3 million American women acquire the disease yearly. *Trichomonas vaginalis* is a protozoan transmitted by sexual contact, and it can be recovered in at least 30% of the male sexual partners of infected women. The prevalence of infection in men increases markedly to 70% of those who are examined within 48 hours of their contact with an infected woman. As stated earlier, women with trichomoniasis may harbor an additional sexually acquired agent. For example, 8% to 50% of women infected with *T. vaginalis* also have gonorrhea. *T. vaginalis* usually involves the squamous epithelium of the vagina, but not columnar epithelium; hence the endocervix is spared. About 90% of infections also involve the urethra and Skene glands, and examinations of wet mounts of urethral material demonstrate organisms in about half of infected women. Therapeutic regimens that eradicate organisms from the vagina but not from the urethra may permit reinoculation of the vagina. For this reason urinary tract involvement is very important and may account for the poor efficacy of topical therapy for *T. vaginalis*. The vaginal discharge in trichomoniasis contains many PMNs resulting from the inflammatory response to the organism. Proper diagnosis requires a thorough evaluation of symptoms, a physical examination, and appropriate laboratory testing; the diagnosis based only on clinical features is often incomplete.

***Diagnosis.*** Symptoms in infected women occur in ranges from 10% to 50%, whereas 25% of documented infections are asymptomatic. Most infected patients have vaginal discharge and 25% to 50% have pruritus. Mild dysuria is present in about 20% of patients. Exacerbation of symptoms may accompany or immediately follow the menstrual period. Lower abdominal pain may occur, but the examiner must always be aware that such pain may represent coincident pelvic inflammatory disease.

Vulvar involvement is seen in fewer than 20% of patients and the appearance of the labia may vary from normal to erythematous or edematous. Most women exhibit a profuse vaginal discharge which may be gray in most and yellow or green in fewer than 20%. Although it is commonly believed that the discharge in trichomoniasis is often frothy, it is visibly so in only 10% of cases and correctly predicts the disease in 50% to 70% of these. Frothy discharge may also be present in BV. Most of the other common signs associated with vaginitis have no discriminating value in making a diagnosis of trichomoniasis. Erythema of the vaginal walls is present in two thirds of patients, and they may appear granular when more extensive disease is present. Punctate hemorrhages of the cervix, which give a strawberry appearance, are highly specific for *T. vaginalis* infection but are seen in only 2% of cases. Motile trichomonads are seen on wet mounts in only about 70% of infections; therefore a negative examination of the wet mount does not exclude this infection. Epithelial cells in the wet mounts are easily distinguished from those seen in BV because of the sharply defined edges. When more than one PMN per epithelial cell is visualized on the wet mount, an inflammatory process should be suspected and the cervix should be examined because the source of the PMNs cannot otherwise be determined. *Large numbers of PMNs are absent in BV; therefore a patient having a frothy vaginal discharge, an elevated vaginal pH, and a large number of PMNs on examination of the wet mount more likely has T. vaginalis infection than BV. The two diseases may coexist, however, and can be simultaneously treated with metronidazole.*

***Treatment.*** Symptomatic and asymptomatic infection with *T. vaginalis* should be treated. When the likelihood of reinfection has been diminished, either by simultaneous treatment of sexual partners or by isolation of the woman, numerous regimens have been found to be equivalent in their cure rates. A single 2-g dose of metronidazole cures approximately 95% of women and is now the recommended treatment for trichomoniasis. Treatment for 7 days with 500 mg twice daily may improve this cure rate to as high as 98%. It is important that sexual partners be treated as well, and patients should be instructed to avoid sexual intercourse until both partners are cured.

The single 2-g dose of metronidazole has several advantages. These include supervised administration, which is independent of patient compliance, a total dose comprising 38% of the standard regimens, a shorter time during which the patient's anaerobic flora are disturbed, and a shorter period during which the patient should abstain from alcohol. However, effectiveness of the single dose relies more on simultaneous treatment of partners than do the standard regimens.

The majority of strains of *T. vaginalis* are easily killed by metronidazole, although strains with high levels of resistance have been isolated from patients who have been treated repeatedly with metronidazole. Some patients have been cured with high intravenous doses of metronidazole administered for prolonged periods, but this regimen has not been approved by the Food and Drug Administration (FDA).

Metronidazole is absolutely contraindicated during the first trimester of pregnancy, and its safety during the second and third trimesters is not established, although single-dose therapy has been used. Pregnant women who receive standard doses of metronidazole during the first trimester experience a 2.5% incidence of perinatal death and an 11% rate of spontaneous abortion. Although these rates do not exceed those seen in untreated control groups, these observations fail to account for the possibility that other STDs might have similar effects. In one study of 61 women who were treated with metronidazole during pregnancy, none bore children with congenital malformations. However, in another study of pregnant women who received the drug during their first trimester, 3.8% gave birth to babies with developmental abnormalities, a slightly higher rate than that expected in the overall population. Despite the absence of direct evidence of a teratogenic effect of metronidazole in humans, it seems prudent to avoid all unnecessary drugs in pregnancy. Many pregnant women continue to harbor *T. vaginalis* after therapy; hence curative therapy with metronidazole could be delayed.

Among the side effects of metronidazole are a disagreeable or metallic taste and nausea, which is described by up to 10% of patients taking a single 2-g dose. Of patients treated with the 7-day course, 7.5% experience transient neutropenia with peripheral white blood counts of 1000 to 1400 cells/mm$^3$. However, this reaction is always reversible and has never been linked with significant infectious complications.

There is no significant evidence linking metronidazole to oncogenesis in humans. In one extended study of 771 women treated with metronidazole, 24 women developed cancer where 18 to 22 cases would have been expected, but this difference was not statistically significant. Four women acquired lung cancer, a higher than expected proportion, but all four were smokers. Thus the risk of short-term, low-dose treatments appears to be extremely small.

Like disulfiram, metronidazole blocks the hepatic metabolism of ethanol to aldehyde, giving rise to systemic symptoms including nausea and flushing. It is important that patients avoid alcohol during treatment and for an additional 24 hours after completing therapy. Metronidazole also appears to prolong the prothrombin time in patients taking warfarin, probably by competing for binding sites on serum proteins. Patients taking oral anticoagulants should be carefully monitored during metronidazole therapy.

### Atrophic vaginitis

Atrophic vaginitis may induce abnormal vaginal discharge in women who lack estrogen due to either natural menopause or castration by radiation or surgery. When deprived of estrogen, the vaginal epithelium atrophies. Superficial vaginal epithelial cells are lost, leaving only the basal cell layer, which is prone to infection and inflammation even with little or no trauma. This leads to atrophic vaginitis, pruritus of the vulvovaginal area, dyspareunia, and an increased risk of cystitis.

***Diagnosis.*** Abnormal vaginal discharge is often accompanied by vaginal and vulvar burning, soreness, or itching. Dysuria, vague lower abdominal discomfort, and vaginal bleeding may also occur. The vaginal epithelium appears dry and pale pink rather than moist and bluish red, and the skin of the vulvar area is thin and parchmentlike. A urethral caruncle, representing prolapsed urethral epithelium, may be present. Constricting fibrosis may partially occlude the upper part of the vagina.

***Treatment.*** Atrophic vaginitis is treated with local estrogen, which may be given as a cream, although most women find vaginal suppositories more convenient. Topical estrogen treatment thickens the vaginal mucosa, rapidly relieving symptoms within a week of starting therapy. Daily applications of conjugated estrogens (Premarin) or estradiol produce stable serum estrogen levels equivalent to the normal follicular phase levels in ovulating women. After about 1 month of therapy the frequency of application may be decreased to once a week or even once a month to maintain healthy vaginal epithelium and avoid systemic effects of estrogen.

### Gonococcal vaginitis

Because the stratified vaginal epithelium in the normal adult protects against infection by *N. gonorrhoeae,* gonococcal vaginitis is rare except in children and in pregnant and postmenopausal women. Since the vaginal epithelium is altered by pregnancy and may be thin and fragile in postmenopausal women, the gonococcus may cause vaginitis in these cases.

***Diagnosis.*** In any patient with gonococcal vaginitis the physical examination may be exquisitely painful. It reveals an intense inflammation that causes the vaginal canal to be extremely red, swollen, and edematous; there may also be an abundance of pus. Often the urethra and Skene and Bartholin glands are involved. In premenopausal women the gonococcus sometimes involves only the endocervical epithelium without producing salpingitis, in such a case the cervical os contains pus and the cervix may be edematous and soft. Inflamed cervical erosion or small abscesses in nabothian cysts may occur. However, very few adult women with symptoms of vaginitis have a gonococcal etiology. In one study 29 of 478 symptomatic females (4%) had positive *N. gonorrhoeae* cultures, but all were considered to be asymptomatic carriers with vaginitis of a different cause. Pelvic examination of the asymptomatic carrier often reveals no findings at all, or merely an abnormal but scanty discharge. Diagnostic tests for and treatment of gonococcal infection are described in the section on cervicitis.

## URETHRITIS AND CYSTITIS IN WOMEN

Urethritis in women usually produces symptoms of internal dysuria. Urinary symptoms commonly bring the young woman to the physician. Approximately 25% of women attending STD clinics have dysuria as their major complaint. A similar frequency is seen in women seeking care from general practitioners. More than 20% of adult women experience at least one episode of dysuria annually, and it is common in adult women of all ages. Younger women more often seek medical care because of their symptoms. The majority of women with acute dysuria and frequency have infections of the urethra, vagina, or bladder. However, the relative proportion of cases attributable to vaginitis remains uncertain and probably varies depending on the population studied. In one large study a group of younger women who complained of acute dysuria were twice as likely to have vaginitis rather than a bacterial urethritis or cystitis as a cause for their urinary symptoms. In this group vaginitis was more than five times as common as bacterial cystitis or urethritis. Thus, although the presence of dysuria is less common in individual women with vaginitis than in women with urethritis or cystitis, in many populations of young women the prevalence of vaginitis may so exceed the prevalence of urinary tract infection that vaginitis becomes the most common cause of dysuria. It has not been established whether the vaginitis-associated organisms in BV, VVC, or trichomoniasis produce dysuria because they also infect the urethra (producing a urethritis accompanied by internal dysuria in some women) or because they cause sufficient vulvar and labial inflammation that painful urination results from urine passing over these infected areas. Although external dysuria is probably more common, agents associated with vaginitis can be readily cultured from the urethras of women with vaginal discharge and symptoms of dysuria and frequency. This suggests that an actual urethritis may well occur in some women. In women with *T. vaginalis* infection this may be associated with pyuria, or PMNs may be seen on a urethral gram-stained specimen.

Approximately two thirds of women who develop dysuria acutely, who do not have vaginitis, have significant colony counts ($>10^5$ colony-forming units [CFU] per milliliter) in a midstream urine specimen and therefore are diagnosed as having cystitis. The remaining one third of these women have the acute urethral syndrome, namely acute dysuria, and frequency without significant colony counts in the urine.

Women with the acute urethral syndrome can be further subdivided into three groups: (1) those with lower urinary tract infection (bladder and/or urethra) caused by coliforms or *Staphylococcus saprophyticus* ($<10^5$ CFU/ml), (2) those with sterile pyuria, often due to chlamydial or gonococcal infection, and (3) those without pyuria who usually are not infected.

Coliforms and *S. saprophyticus* may infect both the urethra and the bladder. Women having $>10^5$ CFU/ml of these organisms in their urine have cystitis, whereas those with $<10^5$ CFU/ml have the acute urethral syndrome. Both groups have pyuria and may otherwise appear similar clinically. Laboratory tests other than quantitative urine cultures also do not distinguish the two groups. In coliform infection the pathogenesis is presumed to begin with periurethral and vaginal colonization, subsequently spreading upward to the bladder and sometimes to the kidneys. The pathogenesis of *S. saprophyticus* infection is not known precisely, but it is probably similar to coliform infection and may also be spread by sexual transmission.

Primary genital herpes simplex virus (HSV) infection may produce dysuria and can be distinguished from other causes of dysuria by the presence of typical herpetic lesions and adenopathy. These lesions may occasionally appear after the onset of dysuria, making initial diagnosis difficult.

***Diagnosis.*** The pathogens that cause urethritis (*C. trachomatis* and *N. gonorrhoeae*) and urinary pathogens (coliforms and *S. saprophyticus*) warrant consideration after vaginitis has been excluded. Clinical criteria alone do not differentiate these two groups; however, the presence of suprapubic pain, hematuria, or a history of previous urinary tract infection favors coliform or staphylococcal infection. In this group symptoms usually begin abruptly and patients seek medical assistance within 1 to 4 days. The accompaniment of pyuria by hematuria in half of cases suggests coliform infection. If coliforms or staphylococci are present in excess of $10^5$/ml they can be seen on Gram stain of unspun urine. A Gram stain is performed as follows: (1) flood the slide with gentian violet for 5 seconds and rinse thoroughly with cold water; (2) flood the slide with Gram iodine for 5 seconds, and rinse with cold water; (3) flood the slide with 95% alcohol until the blue coloring begins to wash out (about 10 seconds), and rinse with cold water; (4) flood the slide with basic fuchsin or safranin, allow to sit for 15 seconds, and rinse with cold water. Dry the slide completely, either by patting it with a paper towel or by letting it air dry.

When fewer than $10^5$/ml bacteria are present, such as in the acute urethral syndrome, the Gram stain is negative, and preparing a culture is necessary to make a specific diagnosis. In women who have a clinical presentation typical of cystitis but with $10^1$ to $10^4$/ml coliforms grown from a carefully collected specimen, the diagnosis of acute urethral syndrome is probable. Isolation of these lower numbers of bacteria is confirmatory, particularly if PMNs are seen in the urine. Particular care should be taken in securing clean-voided urine specimens from these patients to minimize contamination of the urine with perineal or fecal coliforms. In some patients urethral catheterization or suprapubic aspiration may be the only adequate means of distinguishing coliform infection with low counts from a contaminated specimen. It should be realized, however, that studies suggesting the usefulness of urine colony counts of less than $10^5$/ml in predicting infection were performed in young, acutely dysuric women (mostly university women), that these criteria may not be applicable to other populations of women with acute urinary tract infection, and that almost certainly they are not applicable to women with asymptomatic infection.

Lower urinary tract infection caused by either *C. trachomatis* or *N. gonorrhoeae* usually occurs in young women who may have recently changed sex partners. Women who experience acute dysuria and frequency resulting from chlamydial infection generally do not complain of urgency, hematuria, or suprapubic pain. They have had a gradual onset of symptoms (1 to 3 weeks), and when they are examined they may have mucopurulent cervicitis accompanied by PMNs but no intracellular gram-negative diplococci on examination of a cervical Gram stain. Examination of the urine shows pyuria, but no hematuria and no coliforms on Gram stain of the unspun urine. Women who have gonococcal urethritis and/or cervicitis have a more florid illness, and they may experience suprapubic pain or hematuria, they may have a more abrupt onset of their illness accompanied by pyuria. A Gram stain of cervical material reveals intracellular gram-negative diplococci in about half of women.

If possible, the clinician should obtain specimens from both the urethra and cervix from a woman with sterile pyuria to test for chlamydial infection. A thin, cotton-tipped, or Dacron swab should be used for the former and a small brush supplied with direct immunofluorescent microscopy kits used for the latter. In both cases care should be taken to collect many epithelial cells. For culturing, the specimens are collected into a tissue culture transport medium containing antibiotics. If they cannot be processed within 48 hours, they should be frozen immediately at -60° C and sent to the laboratory on dry ice. Currently cell culture is the most sensitive of the available assays, but polymerase chain reaction (PCR) assays for *Chlamydia* species may be even more sensitive. Detection of *Chlamydia* antigen by direct immunofluoroscopy or enzyme linked immunosorbent assay (ELISA) has proven to be highly specific if performed by qualified laboratory personnel. However, the sensitivities of individual *Chlamydia* antigen detection assays may be unacceptably low, particularly in asymptomatic women. If *Chlamydia* culturing facilities, PCR, or *Chlamydia* antigen detection methods are unavailable, the following findings suggest that *C. trachomatis* is the etiologic agent: sterile pyuria (pyuria associated with neither coliforms nor *S. saprophyticus*), negative gonococcal culture, acute dysuria, frequency, and clinical features typical of chlamydial infection.

The examiner should bear in mind that simultaneous infection with two or more agents may occur. In women without demonstrable pyuria, it has usually been impossible to establish an infectious agent responsible for acute dysuria and frequency.

***Treatment.*** Women with chlamydial infection should receive doxycycline, 100 mg orally twice daily for 7 days, or azithromycin, 1 g orally in a single dose. Because the safety and efficacy of azithromycin have not been established for persons under age 15, it should not be used in that group. Pregnant women should be treated with erythromycin base, 500 mg orally four times a day for 14 days.

Several effective regimens are available for women whose dysuria and frequency arise from coliform or staphylococcal infection of the urethra or bladder. Women with uncomplicated cystitis may be successfully treated by single doses of ampicillin (3.5 g orally), amoxicillin (3 g orally), or trimethoprim-sulfamethoxazole (TMP-SMX) (four single-strength tablets at once, orally). These regimens are as effective as 7 to 10 days of ampicillin, sulfamethoxazole, nitrofurantoin, or TMP-SMX in standard dosages used for urinary tract infections. Single-dose therapy should be restricted to reliable patients who will return for posttreatment cultures and for persistent or recurrent symptoms. It should be avoided in women with urologic abnormalities, symptoms of pyelonephritis, and those who have experienced dysuria and frequency for more than 10 days.

Women with acute urethral syndrome due to coliforms or staphylococci also benefit from antimicrobial treatment, although few regimens have been studied. The similarities of clinical picture and pathogenesis between these patients and those with cystitis suggest that the same regimens will work well in both cases.

Usually the clinician will want to begin treatment without waiting for the etiologic diagnosis. The presence or absence of pyuria affects the choice of therapy. In women with pyuria infection is nearly always present, and thus empiric treatment is reasonable. When clinical, epidemiologic, and laboratory evidence suggests coliform or staphylococcal infection, the appropriate treatment is single-dose or traditional 7 to 10-day therapy with the regimens outlined above for urinary tract infection. When the findings point toward chlamydial infection, doxycycline or azithromycin should be used until culture results are available. If a gonococcal infection is identified, one of several regimens can be used: (1) intramuscular ceftriaxone, 125 mg or 250 mg in a single dose; (2) cefixime, given as a single 400-mg oral dose; (3) ciprofloxacin, 500 mg orally as a single dose; or (4) ofloxacin, 400 mg as a single dose. Women with sterile pyuria should also receive doxycycline.

According to most evidence, women without pyuria do not benefit from antimicrobial therapy. Such patients should receive Pyridium to relieve symptoms and be asked to return in 48 hours in the unlikely event that symptoms persist. If they do, the clinician should conduct another examination and evaluation for pyuria and etiologic agents.

Urethrotomy, urethral dilatation, and other urologic procedures have failed to be useful in treatment of acute urethral syndrome. Since most patients have demonstrable infection, these methods should be avoided. Their role in treating recurring or prolonged dysuria also requires further evaluation.

## URETHRITIS IN MEN

Gonococcal and nongonococcal urethritis (NGU) are the most frequent STDs found in men in developed countries. Significant developments in these diseases over the past decade have included the appearance of penicillinase-producing *N. gonorrhoeae,* the identification of *C. trachomatis* and *Ureaplasma urealyticum* as major etiologic agents of NGU, an improved understanding of the range of illness caused by these pathogens, and the use of new systems of therapy.

Traditionally it has been thought that men with gonococcal infection of the urethra become symptomatic and seek treatment. Although the frequency of asymptomatic infection is low among men seeking care at STD clinics, it has been reported to be as high as 60% in studies that have screened sexually active males or examined contacts of women with symptomatic infections. The true incidence of asymptomatic gonorrhea in men is therefore not known with certainty and varies with the population studied. In the general civilian population, however, the best estimate is that between 2% and 10% of infected men never become symptomatic. These asymptomatic men represent the major reservoir of gonorrhea in the community, and their recognition comes only from aggressive tracing of identified sexual contacts. It is of great epidemiologic importance that physicians and health care providers attempt to judiciously identify contacts of persons they are treating for STDs. The importance of *C. trachomatis* and *U. urealyticum* is unclear. But the asymptomatic urethral carriage of these organisms in men may be an even more important epidemiologic problem than with *N. gonorrhoeae.*

***Evaluation of the patient's history and symptoms.*** The symptoms of urethral infection in men may vary from vague discomfort to dysuria, or urinary frequency without a discharge to frank dysuria accompanied by a thick purulent discharge. The major historical features to be elicited from the patient are (1) recent sexual exposure; (2) an estimate of the incubation period if that is possible (i.e., single sexual contact); (3) a recently acquired and treated STD, since the current event may represent a treatment failure; (4) drug allergies, particularly to penicillin; and (5) identification of sexual contacts. It is possible for urethritis to also occur in association with urinary tract infections, bacterial prostatitis, urethral stricture, phimosis, and secondary to catheterization or other instrumentation of the urethra.

***Physical and laboratory examinations.*** If the patient is not circumcised, the foreskin should be retracted to completely examine the glans. Inability to retract the foreskin may indicate adhesion to the glans or phimosis. Edema of the foreskin may be present as a result of vigorous sexual activity. Hypospadias or displacement of the urethral meatus to the underside of the shaft, however, is common and usually causes no problem. A careful inspection for the presence and characteristics of a urethral discharge should be sought; sometimes this may be seen only as staining of the underwear. Other lesions on the penile shaft and at the base of the shaft and the presence or absence of inguinal lymphadenopathy should also be determined.

If a discharge is not present, the penis should be milked or stripped by applying gentle pressure over the ventral and dorsal surfaces of the base of the penis and moving the fingers toward the meatus to bring forward small amounts of discharge. Gonococcal urethritis classically results in a profuse and purulent discharge, whereas NGU is more often associated with a scant mucoid discharge (Fig. 65-3). A calcium alginate swab or a small spun cotton-tipped swab mounted on wire (not the routine wooden or nylon cotton swab) should be inserted 2 cm into the urethra to obtain a specimen for microscopic examination and culture. If sufficient moist material is obtained, first roll the swab on a glass slide for Gram stain. The remaining sample should then be transferred onto a modified Thayer-Martin plate for culture by rolling the swab in a large Z pattern. Because *N. gonorrhoeae* grows best in relatively anaerobic conditions, culture plates should be incubated in candle jars while awaiting transportation to the laboratory. Cultures can also be mailed to the laboratory, provided they are grown on media specially prepared for this purpose.

A Gram stain should be performed as described in the previous section, and the stained smear should be examined under oil-immersion microscopy for PMNs as well as for gram-negative intracellular diplococci. The examiner should take care to record exactly what is seen on the slide. To avoid counting superimposed cells, an area of the slide consisting of a monolayer of separate cells should be found. The presence of 4 or more PMNs per field

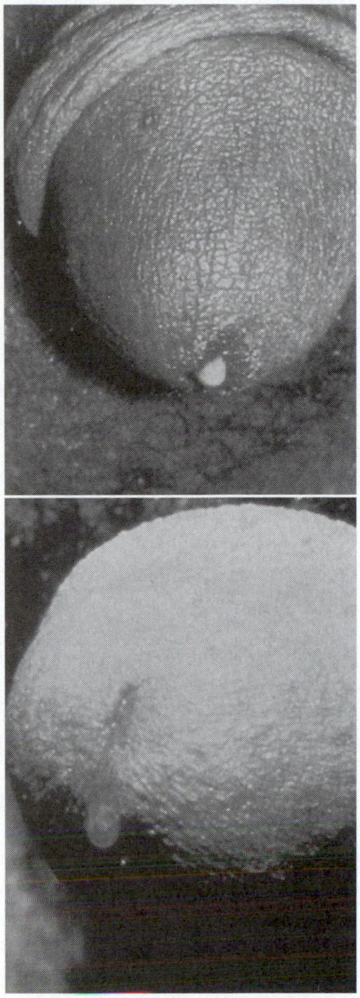


**Fig. 65-3.** Urethritis in men. Gonococcal urethritis classically produces a profuse and purulent discharge **(A)**, whereas nongonococcal urethritis more often results in a scant mucoid discharge **(B)**.

in five 1000× oil-immersion fields indicates an inflammatory discharge. These criteria are analogous to those employed in men without apparent urethral discharge who are undergoing evaluation for signs and symptoms of urethritis.

*If diagnostic facilities for Chlamydia are available and are to be utilized, a second swab should be obtained, with particular attention paid to rolling the swab against the walls of the urethra so as to obtain sloughing cells where the Chlamydia organisms reside intracellularly. Obtaining discharge alone is not sufficient either for C. trachomatis antigen detection assays or for culturing.* Cotton-tipped or Dacron swabs are superior to Calgi-swabs. For culturing, the specimens are collected into a tissue culture transport medium containing antibiotics. If they cannot be processed within 48 hours, they should be frozen immediately at -60° C and sent to the laboratory on dry ice.

The objective diagnosis of urethritis relies on the demonstration of PMNs in the urethral swab or voided urine, preferably first-voided urine. The presence of a visibly clear urethral discharge or even small amounts of mucoid discharge does not always indicate urethritis. The presence of more than 4 PMNs per field in five 1000× oil-immersion fields of the Gram stain warrants a diagnosis of urethritis. When urethritis is suspected but PMNs are not detected on the Gram stain of the urethral swab, the patient should be examined in the morning before his first void. A Gram stain of the urethral swab should be repeated and a first voided urine specimen obtained to examine for the presence of PMNs. To detect PMNs in urine, the first 10 to 15 ml of urine should be collected and spun at 400 *g* (2000 rpm in a standard bench-top centrifuge) for 10 minutes. All but 0.5 ml of the supernatant is decanted, and the sediment is resuspended in the residual urine. Sufficient sediment is placed on a slide to cover approximately 1 cm, and a coverslip is placed over it. The area under the coverslip is examined at a magnification of ×400 (high dry objective), and the number of PMNs in each of five fields is enumerated. Fifteen PMNs in any of 5 random 400× fields of sediment of the first voided urine specimen is abnormal. This markedly enhances the likelihood of reaching a firm diagnosis, and the value of this procedure has been shown repeatedly.

Recently the urinary dipstick leukocyte esterase test (LET) has also been used to predict culture-verified urethral infections with *C. trachomatis* and *N. gonorrhoeae.* Although the sensitivity of this test varies with the status of clinical symptoms and the overall prevalence of infections in the population being tested, the specificity for either of these infections can be greater than 90%.

Unfortunately, some men do have *N. gonorrhoeae* or *C. trachomatis* despite negative urethral Gram stain, urine sediment, or LET.

***Diagnostic considerations.*** The diagnosis of gonorrhea requires demonstration of *N. gonorrhoeae* by Gram stain or culture but not necessarily the presence of urethritis. PCR and *Chlamydia* antigen testing are specific for detection of *Chlamydia,* but there is no simple test to detect *U. urealyticum.* Diagnosis of NGU requires not only exclusion of urethral infection with *N. gonorrhoeae* but also demonstration that urethritis is present, since asymptomatic carriage of the responsible organisms may be common.

### Urethritis caused by *N. gonorrhoeae*

Because *N. gonorrhoeae* preferentially infects columnar and transitional epithelium, the usual manifestation of infection is acute anterior urethritis. Typically an incubation period of 3 to 5 days is followed by rapid onset of dysuria and purulent urethral discharge. Both symptoms are present in over 70% of men with gonococcal urethritis; about 30% complain of discharge only and 2% have dysuria only.

***Diagnosis.*** A fast and reliable way to diagnose gonorrhea in men with symptomatic urethritis is to make a Gram stain of a smear of urethral exudate. Smears with typical gram-negative intracellular diplococci (GNID) located within PMNs are diagnostic for gonorrhea. When compared to culture results, such smears are highly sensitive (83% to 95%) and specific (95% to 99%). In contrast, smears with extracellular gram-negative diplococci or atypical GNID predict positive cultures 15% and 29% of the time, respectively. Therefore if typical GNID are present, culture is optional. In all other cases it is necessary for the diagnosis to be confirmed by culture. Confirmation usually depends on colony morphology, Gram stain, and the oxidase test. Sugar fermentation reactions may be required in some cases where NGU is under consideration.

The sensitivity of cultures in detecting gonorrhea may vary depending on methods used in obtaining samples, on reduced viability during transport, and on inhibition by selective media. Modified Thayer-Martin medium, currently the most widely used selective medium due to its ease of preparation and low cost, contains the antibiotics vancomycin (4 μg/ml), colistin (7.5 μg/ml), nystatin (12.5 μg/ml), and trimethoprim (6.25 μg/ml). Vancomycin may prevent growth of between 0.3% and 30% of gonococcal isolates. Therefore in areas where vancomycin-sensitive gonococci are widespread it may be appropriate to use a nonselective medium such as enriched chocolate agar. Such areas can be identified by periodically growing gonococci on both selective and nonselective media or by monitoring culture results from patients whose urethral smears contain GNID.

***Treatment.*** For the treatment of gonococcal urethritis the Centers for Disease Control and Prevention (CDC) recommend ceftriaxone, 250 mg intramuscularly in a single dose. Newer single-dose oral regimens include cefixime, 400 mg; ciprofloxacin, 500 mg; or ofloxacin, 400 mg. Coinfection with *C. trachomatis* takes place in 15% to 25% of males with gonorrhea, and a treatment for *Chlamydia,* such as doxycycline, 100 mg orally twice a day for 7 days, should be given along with therapy for gonorrhea. Because of their high risk of acquiring infection, even asymptomatic sex partners of gonorrhea patients should be examined and given appropriate treatment.

### Nongonococcal urethritis

NGU includes all urethritis from which *N. gonorrhoeae* is not isolated. In developed countries NGU is at least as prevalent as gonorrhea among men attending STD clinics; among men seen by private physicians and at student health centers NGU may be 3 to 10 times more common. In particular, NGU occurs more frequently than gonorrhea among white heterosexual males of relatively high socioeconomic status. Because of recent decreases in gonorrhea, NGU is also overtaking gonorrhea as the major cause of urethritis in the urban poor.

NGU is a clinical syndrome with many possible etiologies. *C. trachomatis* is isolated from 30% to 50% of patients with NGU compared to 0.5% of men without urethritis. Evidence from cultural studies, animal experimentation, and other sources has demonstrated that *C. trachomatis* is a cause of NGU. Although evidence for its role in NGU is less conclusive, *U. urealyticum* is believed to account for 20% to 25% of NGU. The cause for the remaining 20% to 30% of NGU cases is unknown. HSV, *T. vaginalis,* and *C. albicans* are believed to be infrequent causes of NGU (<5%). *G. vaginalis, Mycoplasma hominis, Corynebacterium genitalum, C. pseudogenitalum,* coliform bacteria, and commensal bacteria of the urethra and perineum have not been causally associated with urethritis.

***Diagnosis.*** The symptoms of NGU are much like those of gonorrhea, but they are less vivid and develop more slowly after a longer incubation period. Dysuria and urethral discharge occur in only about 38% of patients with NGU, as opposed to 78% of gonorrhea patients. Men with NGU are more likely to present with a single symptom than men with gonococcal urethritis. When present, discharge in NGU usually appears only after penile stripping; compared with gonorrhea discharge, it is sparse and appears mucoid rather than purulent.

The practical diagnosis of NGU usually rests on documentation of urethritis (PMNs on Gram stain or in first voided urine, as earlier discussed) and the exclusion of gonococcal infection, since most clinicians do not have access to cultures for *C. trachomatis* or *U. urealyticum.*

***Treatment.*** Although many drugs have been tried against NGU, antibiotics have proved less successful with NGU than with gonorrhea. Currently the therapy of choice is oral doxycycline, 100 mg twice a day for 7 days. Alternative regimens include ofloxacin, 300 mg orally twice a day for 7 days, or erythromycin base, 500 mg orally four times a day for 7 days. Persistent or recurrent NGU occurs within 6 weeks of initiating treatment in up to one third of men. Once the presence of urethritis is established, the patient should be questioned about compliance and sexual contact. The physician should carefully examine the external genitals for skin lesions, inguinal lymphadenopathy, urethral foreign bodies, meatal warts, and epididymitis or testicular abnormalities. If present, urethral exudate should be checked for *T. vaginalis* and fungi. If cultures for *T. vaginalis* are available, they should be performed on exudate and possibly expressed prostatic secretion; cultures for *N. gonorrhoeae* should be done if indicated. Sex partners should also be examined. Most men with persistent or early recurring NGU are culturally negative for both *C. trachomatis* and *U. urealyticum;* however, *C. trachomatis*–positive recurrences sometimes follow intercourse with new or untreated partners.

Frequent recurrences or persistent urethritis that is unresponsive to antibiotics call for microbiologic tests to detect prostatic infection (see Chapter 138). If no pathogen is detected, as is usually the case, the patient should be referred to a urologist. Urethroscopy to detect strictures, foreign bodies, or endourethral lesions may be warranted. Unless major abnormalities are discerned, it is usually better to observe the patient without further therapy than to blindly implement more antimicrobial treatment. There are no known connections between persistent urethritis and either strictures or involuntary infertility.

## EPIDIDYMITIS

Acute epididymitis is characterized by acute pain and swelling of the epididymis. Commonly it is associated with a genitourinary infection (see Chapter 141).

## MUCOPURULENT CERVICITIS

Mucopurulent cervicitis in a woman may be considered the microbiologic equivalent to male urethritis. It is the most common STD syndrome in American women, although it may be difficult to recognize and to distinguish from cervical ectopy (see further). In some instances it can lead to pelvic inflammatory disease. Cervicitis may accompany vaginitis caused by *C. albicans* or *T. vaginalis.* However, in the absence of vaginitis it is usually caused by *N. gonorrhoeae, C. trachomatis,* HSV, or combinations of these microorganisms. In the United States, *C. trachomatis,* overall, is the most common cause of cervicitis and HSV is the least common. In about one third of women the diagnosis cannot be established.

***Evaluation of the patient's history and symptoms.*** Women with acute cervicitis complain primarily of increased vaginal discharge or an associated symptom such as dysuria. As with other conditions in women who complain of lower genitourinary symptoms, a sexual history must be obtained to establish the possibility of an STD and to manage the contact. Leukorrhea from chronic cervicitis sometimes produces a secondary, nonspecific vulvovaginitis, and the women may complain of symptoms associated with this condition as discussed earlier. In some cases infection of the cervix may extend deeply enough to produce symptoms of dyspareunia, lower abdominal pain, or back pain. Women should be asked specifically about these symptoms, since pelvic inflammatory disease, an important complication, warrants consideration in any woman with acute cervicitis.

***Physical and laboratory examinations.*** The diagnosis of mucopurulent cervicitis rests on the demonstration of a mucopurulent discharge (mucopus) from the cervical os, analogous to demonstrating purulent exudate in the male urethra (Fig. 65-4). In women without visible mucopus diagnosis depends on the demonstration of increased numbers of PMNs on a Gram-stained smear of endocervical discharge.

The examiner may check for mucopurulent discharge by swabbing a sample of mucus from the endocervix and observing its color against the background of the white swab. If the mucus is yellow or green, mucopus is present. After noting the results of this swab test, the clinician should roll a thin film of the mucus onto a slide for a Gram stain determination of PMNs. The examiner should then transfer the remaining sample into a modified Thayer-Martin plate for culture, tracing a Z on the plate and making sure all parts of the swab come in contact with the plate. A second cotton-tipped or Dacron swab should be obtained if *Chlamydia* diagnostic facilities are available, paying particular attention to roll the swab against the walls of the endocervix so as to obtain sloughing cells where *chlamydiae* reside intracellularly. Gram stain and culture techniques for *N. gonorrhoeae* and *C. trachomatis* are described further in the sections on urethritis. The mucus smear should be examined microscopically for PMNs and GNID. The criteria for an inflammatory discharge, 4 or more PMNs per field in five 1000× oil-immersion fields, are identical to the criteria employed for men with signs and symptoms of urethritis.

Cervical ectopy that is edematous and friable, bleeding readily when swabbed, is a common sign of mucopurulent cervicitis due to *C. trachomatis.* A bimanual pelvic examination should be performed and the results systematically documented as described in the section dealing with the evaluation of a woman with pelvic inflammatory disease.

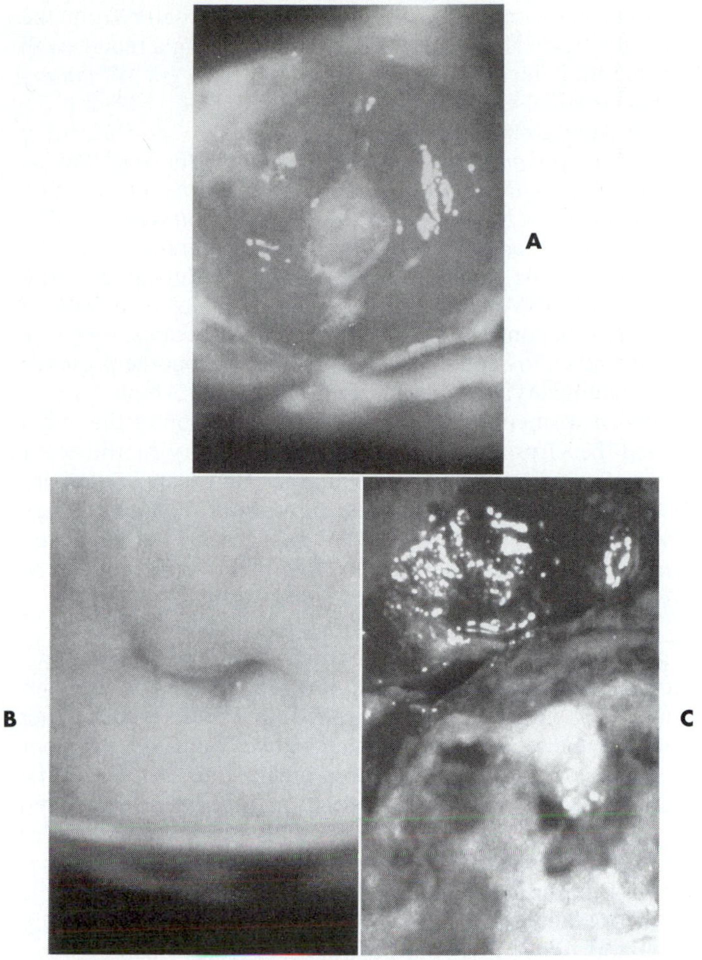


**Fig. 65-4.** Cervicitis. Like gonococcal urethritis in men, gonococcal cervicitis usually produces a mucopurulent discharge from the cervical os (**A**). Chlamydial infection, on the other hand, may be asymptomatic or result in significant cervical edema and discharge (**B** and **C**).

***Diagnosis.*** Studies in STD clinics and student gynecology clinics have shown that *C. trachomatis* infection occurs in about 50% of women with mucopurulent cervicitis by the above criteria and in fewer than 10% of women without it. The diagnosis of gonococcal cervicitis must be made by Gram stain and culture, since only approximately 35% of women with gonococcal cervicitis have a mucopurulent discharge by the above criteria. Culture facilities for *N. gonorrhoeae* are generally available, and a specimen for Gram stain and culture should be collected from the endocervical os of all women with cervicitis after first wiping the cervix clean to remove vaginal flora. The sensitivity of a Gram stain showing intracellular GNID (in comparison with culture) is nearly 50% and the specificity is 100%. The sensitivity of a single endocervical culture for *N. gonorrhoeae* onto a Thayer-Martin plate is about 80% to 90% and can be improved by taking a second specimen for culture, usually from the rectum. Care should be taken to avoid taking a rectal swab containing fecal material, since the yield for *N. gonorrhoeae* will be diminished.

*A diagnosis of HSV infection should be considered if there is inflammation of the exocervix (beyond the os where the red granular appearance of the endocervix, which is lined by thin vascular columnar epithelium, meets the normal squamous epithelium).* Ulcerations of the cervix may be apparent, more commonly during an initial attack of HSV when the virus can be isolated in 80% of women. In contrast, recurrent HSV usually does not cause overt cervicitis and then almost never without the presence of accompanying external genital lesions. About 10% to 20% of women with recurrent HSV infection of the vulva shed the virus from the cervix. If laboratory facilities for isolation of HSV are not available, HSV can be demonstrated by Papanicolaou smear in about 50% of women with HSV cervicitis. In the absence of vaginitis no infectious cause of cervicitis other than *C. trachomatis, N. gonorrhoeae,* and HSV has been identified.

***Cervical ectopy.*** In some women the normal squamous epithelium of the cervix may be replaced by the thinner, more vascular columnar epithelium normally occurring within the endocervical canal. This condition, whether congenital or caused by lacerations of the exocervical os during childbirth or instrumentation, gives the cervix a red granular appearance sometimes called cervical erosion or ectopy. In general, ectopy is asymptomatic or accompanied by minimal amounts of mucoid discharge or friable mucosa that bleeds easily with slight trauma. Occasionally patients may have minor intermenstrual bleeding or a thick, gelatinous discharge. Ordinarily, however, a mucopurulent discharge is absent.

Colposcopy shows that epithelium is intact and not ulcerated. Occasionally a chronic cervicitis with mucopurulent discharge may develop, but cervicitis caused by the aforementioned agents or cervicitis accompanied by vaginitis should be excluded before this diagnosis is made. In chronic cervicitis the cervix appears boggy and inflamed and may resemble carcinoma. Occasionally infection of the cervix may extend deep to cause a low-grade cellulitis with symptoms of dyspareunia, lower abdominal pain, or back pain. Leukorrhea from chronic cervicitis sometimes results in a secondary, nonspecific vulvovaginitis in which many PMNs, but no specific pathogens, are found on the vaginal wet prep. No therapy is required in this situation.

Normally present during early adolescence, ectopy gradually disappears as squamous metaplasia replaces the ectopic columnar epithelium; however, pregnancy or the use of oral contraceptives favors its persistence or reappearance. Traumatic cauterizing procedures are no longer routinely used to eliminate ectopy. The presence of ectopy may render the cervix more susceptible to infection with *N. gonorrhoeae* or *C. trachomatis.*

***Treatment.*** In cases of *C. trachomatis* infection of the endocervix the organism can often be isolated in tissue culture. Newer methods that employ amplification of *Chlamydia* DNA may prove to be more sensitive than culture. If these methods are unavailable and culture for *N. gonorrhoeae* is negative, the clinician should consider doxycycline therapy for nongonococcal mucopurulent cervicitis, as recommended for NGU in men. Oral doses of 100 mg of doxycycline twice daily for 1 week, or azithromycin, 1 g orally in a single dose, are the recommended therapies. Alternative regimens include ofloxacin, 300 mg orally twice a day for 7 days, and erythromycin base, 500 mg orally four times a day for 7 days. Pregnant women should receive erythromycin.

For uncomplicated gonorrhea in women, individual treatment should take into account the sites of infection, patient preference, hypersensitivity, presumed compliance, and cost. The following are suggested regimens for treatment of uncomplicated gonorrhea in adults, including gonococcal mucopurulent cervicitis and gonococcal urethritis in men. It is also recommended that patients receive cotreatment for chlamydial infection with doxycycline or an equivalent regimen, since *C. trachomatis* coexists in up to 45% of cases of gonorrhea.

Many antibiotics are effective for treating gonorrhea, including ceftriaxone, cefixime, ciprofloxacin, and ofloxacin. Ceftriaxone, 250 mg intramuscularly in a single dose, is the standard to which the newer regimens are compared. It is about 95% effective against anogenital gonorrhea and is also successful against pharyngeal infection. Clinical trials have shown that the lower 125-mg dose is as effective as the 250-mg dose. Disadvantages of ceftriaxone include cost and the discomfort of administration. The newer oral regimens can all be given as a single dose in the following strengths: cefixime, 400 mg; ciprofloxacin, 500 mg; ofloxacin, 400 mg. Quinolones are contraindicated in pregnant or nursing women and in persons under the age of 17. In those cases patients should receive 2 g cephalosporin or spectinomycin intramuscularly in a single dose.

It is critical that male sexual partners of infected women be evaluated for gonococcal infections, even if they lack symptoms. Such men should be treated on their initial visit, without waiting for confirmation of the diagnosis of gonorrhea.

Women treated for gonococcal cervicitis should return 3 to 8 days after conclusion of therapy for posttreatment cultures. The clinician must obtain culture specimens from the rectum as well as the cervix, because 20% of treatment failures yield positive cultures from the rectum.

Patients treated for uncomplicated infections do not need to return for further follow-up unless their symptoms persist. However, because the rate of reinfection is high in some studies, rescreening women several months after therapy may be an effective strategy to control infection in certain populations.

## PELVIC INFLAMMATORY DISEASE

Pelvic inflammatory disease (PID) refers to ascending infection of the uterus, fallopian tubes, and broad ligaments, and may include endometritis, salpingitis, tuboovarian abscess, and pelvic peritonitis. Unfortunately, the sequelae of PID can be devastating for women of childbearing years, resulting in tubal infertility, ectopic pregnancy, chronic abdominal pain, and recurrent PID. Although some cases arise from predisposing events such as surgical trauma or obstetrically related events, the majority of cases occur as a result of lower genital tract infections. In these cases microorganisms in the vagina and lower cervix enter and traverse the normally sterile endometrial cavity and initiate an inflammatory reaction in any or all of the aforementioned structures. Spontaneously occurring PID may occur in acute or chronic forms. Chronic PID may develop from chronic infection with *C. trachomatis* or from the use of intrauterine devices (IUDs); tuberculosis is no longer a significant cause of chronic PID in developed countries.

About 1 million cases of PID are recognized each year in the United States. About 25% of those treated for the disease require hospitalization. The direct and indirect costs of the disease and its complications were estimated to exceed $4 billion in 1990; this figure will undoubtedly be pushed higher by the rising costs of tubal microsurgery and in vitro fertilization for women rendered infertile by salpingitis. If the current PID incidence persists, costs are projected to approach $10 billion by the year 2000.

The long-term sequelae of PID were emphasized in a large cohort study from Sweden. Out of 900 women with laparoscopically proven salpingitis, tubal infertility occurred in 11.4% following one episode of PID. Increased age adversely affected reproductive outcome, with a tubal infertility rate of 19% in women ages 25 to 34 years and 9% in women ages 15 to 24 years. Laparoscopic grade of PID also adversely affected outcome, with tubal infertility rates of 30% in the most severe disease. They also found that etopic pregnancy occurred in 4.1% of women with a history of PID, a seven- to tenfold increase over the control women studied. In addition, chronic abdominal pain was noted in 18% of the women in the cohort and was related to the number of episodes of PID.

In the United States the number and rate of ectopic pregnancies have increased over the past two decades. In the National Hospital Discharge Survey conducted by the CDC, the rate of ectopic pregnancy per 1000 reported pregnancies between 1970 and 1989 increased almost fourfold, from 4.5 to 16.1. The case fatality rate for ectopic pregnancy in 1989 was 3.8 deaths per 10,000 ectopic pregnancies, and ectopic pregnancy remains the leading cause of pregnancy-related death during the first trimester. These statistics just begin to describe the morbidity and mortality associated with PID.

Because of the spectrum of disease, clinical diagnosis of PID is imprecise. Up to 12% of women with suspected acute PID have other conditions such as acute appendicitis, endometriosis, ectopic pregnancy, or corpus luteum bleeding at laparoscopy. Another 23% display no laparoscopic abnormalities. Only about 65% of suspected cases have laparoscopic evidence of acute salpingitis. PID probably exists within a clinical continuum ranging from uncomplicated cervicitis to endometritis, salpingitis, parametritis, and pelvic peritonitis. PID encompasses the latter three conditions; laparoscopy or laparotomy is required to distinguish between them. In this discussion PID refers to the clinical syndrome that includes each of these conditions, and the term salpingitis is restricted to cases of visually or histopathologically confirmed inflammation of the fallopian tubes.

The introduction of organisms into the upper tract may be exogenous or endogenous. Sexually acquired agents such as *C. trachomatis* and *N. gonorrhoeae* may migrate upward or be surgically implanted during procedures such as dilatation and curettage or hysterosalpingography. Bacterial species that are part of the indigenous flora of the lower genital tract may also produce PID, particularly when it is recurrent or associated with the use of an IUD. The agents most often implicated in acute PID include those which are primary causes of cervicitis (i.e., *N. gonorrhoeae* and *C. trachomatis* in young, sexually active women) and those which can be regarded as normal components of the vaginal flora (see the box above). In the United States *N. gonorrhoeae* organisms have been isolated from 45% to 80% of women with acute PID. Extension of gonococcal infection from the endocervix to the fallopian tubes occurs in at least 15% of women with gonorrhea, and one prospective study has suggested that half of women who become infected after recent exposure to *N. gonorrhoeae* develop signs of adnexal tenderness that suggest salpingitis. However, there are some complications to this picture. In some patients with positive endocervical cultures for *N. gonorrhoeae* tubal cultures show other organisms that may or may not be accompanied by gonococci. Only about one third to two thirds of women with positive endocervical cultures for *N. gonorrhoeae* have positive peritoneal or tubal cultures for the pathogen. In general, PID is most often associated with gonorrhea in populations having a high incidence of gonorrhea, in developing countries, or in the indigent central city urban population of developed countries. In cases of PID where no STD organisms can be identified, microbiologic studies of specimens from the upper genital tract have resulted in the isolation of other bacterial species, including *Streptococcus, Escherichia coli, H. influenzae,* and anaer-

### Organisms implicated as causative agents in pelvic inflammatory disease

**Cervical pathogens**
*N. gonorrhoeae*
*C. trachomatis*

***Anaerobic bacteria***
*Prevotella* spp.
Peptostreptococci
*Mobiluncus* spp.
*Actinomyces* spp.

**Vaginal flora**
***Facultative bacteria***
Enterobacteriaceae
*H. influenzae*
*G. vaginalis*
*Streptococcus* group B

***Mycoplasma***
*M. hominis*
*U. urealyticum*

From Holmes KK: In Isselbacher KJ et al, editors: *Principles of internal medicine,* ed 13, New York, 1994, McGraw-Hill.

obes (*Bacteroides, Peptococcus,* and *Peptostreptococcus*). Hence PID is considered a polymicrobial disease.

It is extremely difficult to pinpoint the microbial etiology in the individual PID patient because mixed infections are frequent, the fallopian tube is difficult to sample, and the pathogens that usually cause PID require complex techniques for detection. For example, anaerobic and facultative bacteria and genital mycoplasmas have been isolated from the peritoneal fluid or fallopian tubes in a high proportion of PID patients in the United States (especially in those with nongonococcal PID), but in only a small fraction of those in Scandinavian countries. These discrepancies are poorly understood. Also, much of the evidence implicating vaginal organisms in salpingitis is based on cultures obtained by culdocentesis, a procedure in which vaginal flora could contaminate the aspirating needle. However, studies in which cultures were obtained by laparoscopy have also implicated anaerobic and facultative organisms in PID. The bacterial mixtures found have generally resembled the abnormal vaginal flora characteristic of nonspecific vaginitis, except that *B. fragilis,* which is rarely found in the vagina, sometimes is isolated from the peritoneal fluid of women with PID.

In general, first episodes of acute PID are usually caused by *N. gonorrhoeae, C. trachomatis,* or both. Recurrent bouts of acute PID, episodes occurring in IUD users, and cases precipitated by invasive intrauterine diagnostic or therapeutic procedures usually stem from ascending infection caused by *C. trachomatis* or by the endogenous vaginal flora.

### Criteria for establishing a clinical diagnosis of pelvic inflammatory disease

**Minimum criteria**

Lower abdominal pain
Adnexal tenderness
Cervical motion tenderness

**Additional useful criteria**
***Routine***

Oral temperature >38.3° C
Abnormal cervical or vaginal discharge
Elevated ESR and/or C-reactive protein
Cervical infection with *N. gonorrhoeae* or *C. trachomatis*

***Elaborate***

Histopathologic evidence on endometrial biopsy
Tuboovarian abscess on sonography
Laparoscopic abnormalities consistent with PID

Modified from Centers for Disease Control and Prevention: 1993 Sexually transmitted diseases treatment guidelines, *MMWR* 42:77, 1993.

***Evaluation of the patient's history and symptoms.*** A varied symptom complex may be offered by the woman with PID depending on the extent of involvement of the upper genital tract and the associated findings that may occur with infection of the lower genitourinary tract or the rectum. The sequence of events leading to the first episode of PID caused, for example, by *N. gonorrhoeae* and *C. trachomatis* is probably cervicitis, then endometritis, then salpingitis, then peritonitis. A vaginal discharge may be an accompanying symptom as a result of involvement of the cervix; this is associated with dysuria and frequency due to an accompanying urethritis in approximately 20% of cases. It is important to carefully elicit these symptoms, which, though less severe, may be useful in establishing the specific microbiologic cause of PID. Anorectal pain, tenesmus, rectal discharge, and bleeding due to proctitis occurred in 7% of women with PID in one series. Midline abdominal pain due to endometritis is a common complaint, and abnormal menstrual bleeding is present in 35% to 40% of patients. Bilateral low abdominal pain and pelvic pain caused by salpingitis may be present. Typically the patient describes the abdominal pain as dull or aching. In some cases, however, pain may be absent or atypical, and the inflammatory symptoms may be discovered during the course of an unrelated evaluation or procedure such as a tubal ligation. Dyspareunia due to movement of the cervix, particularly with deep penetration, may be a prominent complaint, and the presence of this symptom should be elicited from the patient as a part of the sexual history. The use of oral contraceptives or an IUD should be requested of the patient as these agents affect the likelihood of PID (see further). About 25% of PID patients experience general abdominal pain caused by generalized peritonitis; 5% to 10% have pleuritic right upper quadrant pain caused by perihepatitis.

The pattern in which symptoms evolve is related to the etiology of the disease and varies from one patient to another. The onset of IUD-associated PID is often gradual and may be preceded by a malodorous vaginal discharge typical of nonspecific vaginitis. The onset of gonococcal PID is usually more acute than that of chlamydial PID and often occurs during menses.

***Physical and laboratory examinations.*** The clinical criteria for establishing a diagnosis of PID are listed in the box above. In most women with gonococcal or chlamydial PID a speculum examination reveals evidence of mucopurulent cervicitis. Cervical motion tenderness results from stretching of the adnexal attachments on the side toward which the cervix is pushed. Bimanual examination demonstrates uterine fundal tenderness due to endometritis and abnormal adnexal tenderness due to salpingitis that is usually but not always bilateral. About half the women with acute salpingitis exhibit a palpable adnexal swelling, but evaluation of the adnexae is not completely reliable. Fever is not required for the diagnosis; only about one third of patients with acute salpingitis have an initial temperature above 38° C.

Laboratory findings include elevation of the erythrocyte sedimentation rate (ESR) in 75% of patients with salpingitis and an increase in the peripheral white blood cell count in about 60%. In nearly all patients with laparoscopically confirmed salpingitis vaginal secretions contain more than one PMN per vaginal epithelial cell, as revealed by microscopic examination of a saline wet mount. According to some experts the absence of white blood cells from vaginal fluid rules out the diagnosis of acute PID. Cervical secretions should be cultured and examined microscopically as previously described in the

**Table 65-2.** Special diagnostic studies for consideration in women with lower abdominal pain and/or vaginal bleeding

| Test | Indications | Findings |
|---|---|---|
| Radioimmunoassay for β subunit of hCG | Possible ectopic pregnancy or intrauterine pregnancy | Highly sensitive and positive in low titer by the time of presentation in ectopic pregnancy; positive in high titer in the first trimester of intrauterine pregnancy |
| Culdocentesis | Suspected rupture of ectopic pregnancy | Aspiration of blood from the pelvis that will not clot within a glass syringe |
| Endometrial aspiration biopsy (not desirable if pregnant) | Suspected spontaneous abortion | Chorionic villi obtained from uterus |
| Ultrasonography of the pelvis | Suspected ectopic pregnancy or ovarian cyst | Provides reasonably good sensitivity and specificity for detecting cysts or ectopic pregnancy |
| Laparoscopy | Diagnosis uncertain or response to therapy incomplete | Will confirm or exclude diagnosis of salpingitis; will detect appendicitis, endometriosis, or ectopic pregnancy |

Modified from Woo B et al: In Branch WT, editor: *Office practice of medicine,* Philadelphia, 1982, WB Saunders.

section on cervicitis. To help improve diagnostic accuracy, more elaborate testing has been suggested, including endometrial biopsy and laparoscopy, but both tools have limitations.

***Diagnosis.*** The major diagnostic considerations in the evaluation of a woman suspected of having PID are other causes of pelvic pathology that mimic salpingitis, such as appendicitis and ectopic pregnancy. Table 65-2 indicates a diagnostic approach for women in whom the diagnosis of PID is insecure before performing laparoscopy. However, no finding short of laparoscopy is pathognomonic for salpingitis, and in the United States most physicians are reluctant to perform laparoscopy every time salpingitis is suspected. Laparoscopy confirms salpingitis in 60% of the patients who meet the following criteria: (1) lower abdominal pain of less than 3 weeks' duration; (2) pelvic tenderness on bimanual pelvic examination; and (3) evidence of lower genital tract infection (e.g., white blood cells outnumber all other cells in the vaginal fluid).

The probability of salpingitis increases in the presence of additional findings, including a rectal temperature above 38° C, a palpable adnexal mass, and elevation of the ESR above 15 mm/hour. Laparoscopy reveals salpingitis in 68% of patients with one of these additional findings, in 90% of those with two, and in 96% of those with three or more. Although the combination of all these findings is highly specific, it is quite insensitive; these three additional findings occur in only 17% of patients with laparoscopy-confirmed salpingitis.

In the hands of an experienced physician laparoscopy has a low morbidity and is considered the most specific method for diagnosis of acute salpingitis; ultrasonography is not sufficiently sensitive. Patients with suspected PID who have normal laparoscopy have a better prognosis, with few if any sequelae. For women with lower abdominal pain the primary value of laparoscopy is exclusion of other surgical problems. The most common and serious problems that are apt to be confused with salpingitis are usually unilateral (see the box at right). Therefore unilateral pain or pelvic mass is a strong indication for laparoscopy unless the clinical picture warrants laparotomy instead. Other frequent indications for laparoscopy include absence of lower genital tract infection, a missed menstrual period, and failure to respond to appropriate therapy.

About 5% to 10% of women with acute PID develop symptoms of perihepatitis, including pleuritic upper abdominal pain and tenderness, usually localized to the right upper quadrant. Symptoms of perihepatitis, also called the Fitz-Hugh–Curtis syndrome, appear during or after onset of PID symptoms and may overshadow the lower abdominal symptoms, possibly causing an errone-

### Laparoscopic findings in patients with false positive or false negative clinical diagnosis of pelvic inflammatory disease

**False-positive clinical diagnosis**

Acute appendicitis (24%)
Endometriosis (16%)
Corpus luteum bleeding (12%)
Ectopic pregnancy (11%)
Pelvic adhesions only (7%)
Benign ovarian tumor (7%)
Chronic salpingitis (6%)
Miscellaneous (15%)

**False-negative clinical diagnosis**

Ovarian tumor (20%)
Acute appendicitis (18%)
Ectopic pregnancy (16%)
Chronic salpingitis (6%)
Acute peritonitis (6%)
Endometriosis (5%)
Uterine myoma (5%)
Atypical pelvic pain (6%)
Miscellaneous (6%)

From Jacobson L: *Am J Obstet Gynecol* 138:1007, 1980.

ous diagnosis of cholecystitis. Some studies have shown that in up to 25% of acute salpingitis cases early laparoscopy reveals inflammation ranging from edema and erythema of the liver capsule to exudate with fibrinous adhesions between the visceral and parietal peritoneum. If treatment is delayed, late laparoscopy shows dense violin-string adhesions covering the liver; when tractions is placed on these adhesions, they cause chronic exertional or positional right upper quadrant pain. Although perihepatitis was formerly attributed only to gonococcal PID, it is now known that chlamydial salpingitis, and possibly other types of salpingitis, can also lead to perihepatitis.

Besides right upper quadrant tenderness, physical findings of perihepatitis often include adnexal tenderness and cervicitis, even in patients lacking symptoms suggestive of salpingitis. Liver function tests may be normal or slightly abnormal. Although an oral cholescystogram may indicate gallbladder malfunction, ultrasonography of the right upper quadrant is normal. To summarize, a diagnosis of perihepatitis is warranted in a young woman with mucopurulent cervicitis, pelvic tenderness, and subacute pleuritic right upper quadrant pain with normal ultrasonography of the gallbladder.

Certain clinical manifestations of acute PID correlate with specific etiologic findings. For example, onset of salpingitis is related to menses in women with gonorrhea but not in those without gonorrhea. Gonococcal or chlamydia-associated salpingitis occurs in women who are significantly younger than those with other forms of salpingitis. Chlamydia-associated salpingitis tends to bring on milder symptoms of longer duration and with less fever than the gonococcus-associated disease. Paradoxically, however, patients with chlamydial salpingitis have higher ESR and more severe inflammation, as seen in laparoscopy. It is suspected that chlamydial salpingitis may occur as an indolent subclinical disease that could be a major cause of infertility in women. IUD-associated PID also tends to be indolent; compared to other PID types it is more often linked with adnexal masses but less often with fever.

***Treatment.*** Four principles form the basis for recommendations regarding the treatment of PID. First, the goals of treatment are both short and long term. Second, treatment requires broad-spectrum antibiotic therapy. Third, treatment is usually empiric. And finally, the choice of therapy must be flexible. The physician should at least consider hospitalization for all women with a diagnosis of PID (see the Managed Care Guide).

The 1993 CDC recommendations for treatment of PID are that unhospitalized patients should receive a combined regimen with broad activity, such as cefoxitin, 2 g intramuscularly, plus probenicid, 1 g orally in a single dose, or ceftriaxone, 250 mg intramuscularly followed by doxycycline. An alternative to this is ofloxacin, 400 mg orally twice a day, plus either clindamycin or metronidazole for 14 days. Disadvantages of the ofloxacin regimen are that it is considerably more expensive than the cephalosporin regimen, and patient compliance with a 2-week regimen cannot be guaranteed.

Hospitalized patients should be given antibiotics parenterally. Inpatient regimen A consists of cefoxitin, 2 g intravenously every 6 hours, or cefotetan, 2 g intravenously every 6 hours, plus doxycycline. Regimen B includes high-dose clindamycin, 900 mg intravenously every 8 hours, plus gentamicin. The former regimen is preferred if either *C. trachomatis* or *N. gonorrhoeae* is isolated. These regimens should be continued until at least 48 hours after the patient has improved; a 14-day course of therapy is completed with either doxycycline or clindamycin. Doxycycline is preferred if chlamydial infection is suspected; clindamycin is preferable for treatment of tuboovarian abscess.

In treating PID the most important goal is to prevent the disastrous long-term complications. The physician should begin treatment as soon as the diagnosis is made, and therapy should never be withheld while awaiting the results of cultures for microorganisms.

If a patient is wearing an IUD, the device should be removed. It is uncertain whether it is better to remove the IUD at the beginning of therapy or to wait until the inflammation has resolved, although there are theoretical arguments for each approach. If a woman has one episode of PID while wearing an IUD, she should stop using the device unless no other means of contraception are feasible.

### Managed Care Guide for hospitalization of patients with PID

1. Uncertain diagnosis
2. When surgical emergencies such as appendicitis and ectopic pregnancy must be excluded
3. Suspicion of pelvic abscess
4. Pregnancy
5. Severe illness that precludes outpatient management
6. Inability of the patient to follow or tolerate an outpatient therapy
7. Failure of the patient to respond to outpatient therapy
8. Inability to arrange clinical follow-up 48 to 72 hours after beginning antibiotic treatment

***Management of PID patients.*** Whether or not they are hospitalized, patients being treated for PID should be monitored closely. They should receive a thorough examination on the second or third day of treatment, by which time improvement is usually apparent. Fever, if it was initially present, and abdominal pain and tenderness should all be subsiding. If the patient has not responded to therapy, the diagnosis and need for hospitalization (if the patient is not already in the hospital) should be reconsidered. To resolve any uncertainty, diagnostic laparoscopy should be performed; ultrasonography may also be useful in detecting an inflammatory adnexal mass. If the diagnosis of PID is secure, the physician should consider changing the antimicrobial regimen based on the results of cultures obtained at the time of treatment initiation.

***Follow-up of partners.*** If *N. gonorrhoeae* or *C. trachomatis* is present, the patient's recent male sexual partners should be examined and appropriately treated, even if they are without symptoms. The patient should also be seen about 1 week after the completion of antibiotic therapy, at which time a pelvic examination should be performed to check for residual pelvic abnormalities. In addition, the physician should examine endocervical samples for *N. gonorrhoeae* and *C. trachomatis.*

***PID in teenagers.*** Acute PID occurs almost exclusively in sexually active women. The risk for teenagers of 15 to 16 years of age who are sexually active appears to be several times greater than for women ages 20 to 24. Factors contributing to this higher susceptibility may include a larger number of sex partners, higher frequency of anovulatory cycles, less likelihood of immunity to pathogens, and possibly delay in seeking medical attention. Besides youth, risk factors include a previous history of gonorrhea or salpingitis and IUD use. The relative risk of PID among IUD users compared with women using no contraception varies from 1.4 to 7.3 depending on the study. With a few exceptions studies have shown that, among IUD users, the relative risk of PID was higher in nulliparous women than in parous women. In contrast, use of oral contraceptives appears to decrease the risk of PID.

***Infertility and PID.*** The rate of infertility resulting from salpingitis is related to the patient's age, the etiology of salpingitis, the duration of symptoms before initiation of treatment, the severity of salpingitis as seen by laparoscopy at the time of diagnosis, and the number of previous episodes of salpingitis. The rate of infertility as a result of tubal occlusion among women exposed to a chance of pregnancy is 14% for women ages 15 to 24 and 26% for those ages 25 to 35. The average risk for women of all ages is 11% after one episode of salpingitis, 23% after two episodes, and 54% after three or more episodes. One episode of gonococcal salpingitis carries a risk of 6%, as opposed to 21% for one episode of nongonococcal salpingitis.

Although the rate of infertility due to *C. trachomatis*–associated salpingitis has not been determined, a preliminary analysis of such cases points toward about a 10% rate of tubal occlusion after therapy. Studies in several countries have revealed a strong connection between infertility due to tubal occlusion and the prevalence and titer of antibody to *C. trachomatis.*

***Pelvic pain and PID.*** Persistent or recurrent pelvic pain in a sexually active woman may pose a difficult problem for the clinician. Frequently the clinician responds by administering multiple antibiotics for possible recurrent salpingitis. Various studies have reported that salpingitis has recurred in about 15% to 25% of treated women. The physician must be aware of other diagnostic considerations such as endometriosis, pelvic adhesions from previous salpingitis or surgery, tuboovarian mass, cyst or abscess, myometritis, and chronic ectopic pregnancy. In one study of young women with histories of PID undergoing laparoscopy for persistent or recurrent pelvic pain, the diagnosis of chronic salpingitis was proved wrong in 13 to 23 cases. Conversely, small ovarian cysts were found in 8 of 18 patients whose findings on physical examination had been normal. Thus the establishment of a diagnosis for such patients appears to require pelvic ultrasound examination and radioimmunoassay to detect the β subunit of hCG, followed by laparoscopy. However, numerous studies have reported that about half such patients have normal laparoscopic findings.

There are few clinical features that distinguish between patients with PID and those with normal laparoscopic findings. Patients with positive laparoscopic findings are more likely to have pain that interferes with sleep and that can be reproduced by movement of the cervix. Pain associated with deep penetration during sexual intercourse, as opposed to pain during initial penetration, often signifies intrapelvic disease. A normal ESR is strong evidence against chronic salpingitis; other causes of pain, such as ovarian cyst, chronic ectopic pregnancy, or endometriosis, should be considered. A palapable mass in a patient taking oral contraceptives must be regarded as possibly neoplastic; if the patient both smokes and takes oral contraceptives, mesenteric thrombophlebitis is a possibility.

## GENITAL SKIN LESIONS

Genital skin lesions can be classified as ulcerative or nonulcerative, and they may or may not have an infectious etiology. They may present in patients who are considered likely either by themselves or by their physician to have an STD; however, even when all available tests are used by experienced dermatovenereologists, as many as 40% of ulcerative lesions on the penis, for example, do not yield a specific diagnosis. Genital lesions may be infectious but not sexually transmitted. Numerous lesions are related to trauma. Some are secondary to a dermatologic disorder or a neoplastic process. The box on p. 874 broadly classifies the differential diagnosis, but the ensuing discussion emphasizes sexually transmitted or sexual activity–related causes of genital lesions.

Lymphogranuloma venereum (LGV) and donovanosis (granuloma inguinale) are rare causes of genital infections in the United States. The incidence and etiology of sexually transmitted infectious causes of genital ulceration also vary according to geographic area. There are parts of Asia and Africa where genital ulceration is the usual reason for a patient to attend a clinic, and both syphilis and chancroid are very common. In Western industrial societies urethritis and vaginitis are much more common reasons to visit clinics than is genital ulceration; genital HSV infection is the most common form of ulceration, and chancroid is relatively uncommon. Syphilis has been the second most common form of ulceration in the United States and must always be excluded. Casual sexual encounters during overseas travel, however, may result in the appearance of patients with unusual forms of genital ulceration.

***Evaluation of the patient's history and symptoms.*** Initially the patient should be questioned to discover if trauma is the obvious cause of the genital lesion, particularly if it is an ulcerative lesion. If trauma is implicated, the onset of the lesion should have been noted shortly after the trauma, and the traumatic event should have been noticeably painful at the time. A complete history of sexual activity and uncommon sexual exposure should be requested of the patient. A history of preceding vesicular lesions in a patient with genital erosion, particularly if the lesions are recurrent, suggests HSV infection. Patients who are infected with pediculosis pubis or scabies may complain of a significant pruritic component, and if they have erosions they may be secondary to excoriation.

***Physical and laboratory examinations.*** In the assessment of patients with genital lesions, simple and careful clinical observations are essential in evaluating potential causes and in establishing priorities for the implementation of laboratory methods to assist and confirm the clinical impression. Genital lesions can be broadly subdivided into ulcerative and nonulcerative (Table 65-3). However, it is important to remember that more than one STD may coexist and hence the clinical patterns may be mixed. Although the clinical findings are sometimes diagnostic (e.g., presence of herpetic vesicles) and these together with epidemiologic consideration may help guide initial therapy, many genital ulcerations cannot be diagnosed on examination alone. It is essential to exclude syphilis by appropriate serology in all cases. Darkfield or direct immunofluorescent microscopy should also be performed, by experienced technicians when possible, on lesions that suggest primary (usually ulcerative) or secondary (usually nonulcerative) syphilis.

### Differential diagnosis of genital skin lesions

**Infectious**

***Viral***

*Usually sexually transmitted*

Condylomata acuminata*
Herpes simplex (primary)†
Epstein-Barr virus
Molluscum contagiosum*

*Probably not sexually acquired*

Herpes zoster

***Bacterial***

*Usually sexually transmitted*

Chancroid†
Syphilis*†
Lymphogranuloma venereum†
Donovanosis
Furospirochetal (e.g., human bites)

*Probably not sexually acquired*

Impetigo
Cellulitis
Erythrasma
Folliculitis/carbuncle/abscess
Secondary pyoderma

***Fungal***

*Probably not sexually acquired*

Candidiasis
Deep fungal infection
Tinea cruris
Tinea versicolor

***Parasitic***

*Usually sexually transmitted*

Pediculosis pubis
Scabies

**Noninfectious**

***Traumatic***

*Usually sexually transmitted*

Human bite
Laceration of vagina, anus
Penile venereal edema
Suction edema, purpura, erosions, bullae

*Probably not sexually acquired*

Zipper lacerations
Contact dermatitis
Foreign body/injection of drugs

***Dermatologic disorders***

*Usually sexually transmitted*

Aphthous ulcers
  Simple, severe, Behçet's disease
Balanitis xerotica obliterans
Bullous disorders
  Epidermolysis bullosa
  Erythema multiforme
  Pemphigoid
  Pemphigus vulgaris
Eczematous dermatitis
Epidermal inclusion cyst

*Probably not sexually acquired*

Fixed drug eruption
Hidradenitis, suppurative
Lichen planus
Penile lymphangitis
Pityriasis rosea
Plasma cell balanitis
Psoriasis
Sebaceous cyst
Seborrheic dermatitis

***Neoplastic***

*Usually sexually transmitted*

Malignant melanoma
Squamous cell carcinoma in situ

Modified from Woo B et al: In Branch WT, editor: *Office practice of medicine,* Philadelphia, 1982, WB Saunders.
*Nonulcerative.
†Ulcerative.

**Table 65-3.** Genital ulcers

| Clinical observation | HSV | Syphilis | Chancroid | Lymphogranuloma venereum | Donovanosis |
|---|---|---|---|---|---|
| Incubation period | 2-7 days | 10-90 (avg 21) days | 1-14 (avg 3-5) days | Initial lesion rarely noticed, 1-4 wk (avg 10-14 days) | Unknown, probably 1-12 wk |
| Location of ulcer | Male: glans, prepuce, shaft of penis<br>Female: cervix, vagina, labia | Male: coronal sulcus, glans, shaft of penis, perianal area<br>Female: cervix, vagina | Male: frenulum, prepuce, coronal sulcus, glans, shaft of penis<br>Female: cervix, vagina, fourchette, labia, perianal area | Male: glans, shaft of penis<br>Female: vagina, labia | Male: glans, prepuce, shaft of penis, perianal area<br>Female: labia, fourchette |
| Number of lesions | Multiple, at times confluent, more lesions with first infection than with recurrences | Usually one, multiple not rare | Usually 1 to 3, may be up to 10 | Usually single | Single or multiple |
| Initial appearance of lesion | Vesicle | Papule | Inflamed macule/papule/pustule | Papule/vesicle/pustule | Papule |
| Shape of typical ulcer | Small, grouped, variable border | Round, oval; if irregular, symmetrically so | Irregular ragged, variable size | Discrete | Sharply defined, but irregular |
| Depth of ulcer | Superficial | Superficial cup or saucer shape, elevated edges | Hollow, excavated, undermined | Superficial | Elevated |
| Surface of ulcer | Bright red | Smooth, shiny, glazed, crust | Rough, uneven, grayish | | Clean, friable, beefy granulation, depigmentation |
| Secretion | Moderate, serous | Scanty, serous | Abundant, purulent, and frequently necrotic | Variable | Rare |
| Induration | None | Firm, parchmentlike, movable, circumscribed, does not change shape with pressure | Rarely present, changes shape with pressure, boggy | None | Firm granulation tissue |
| Pain | Often; more pain with initial infection than with recurrences | Rarely | Often | Variable | Rare |
| Inguinal adenopathy | Tender, bilateral in approximately 50% of primary disease | Bilateral, multiple, constant, and painless | Usually single, unilateral, tender, and unilocular; overlying erythema; bilateral involvement can occur; suppuration and rupture of fluctuant nodes in 5-8 days may occur, leaving single large ulcer | Cause of usual presentation; initially firm, tender, discrete, movable, later indolent fixed, matted, occasionally leading to suppuration and fistulas, sign of groove; unilateral (60%) and bilateral (40%) involvement | Rare |
| Constitutional symptoms | Common in primary, less common in recurrences | Rare in primary | Rare | Frequent | Rare |
| Course | Recurrence is the rule; reinfection occurs | Slowly resolves to latency without treatment; relapse and reinfection possible | Frequently progresses to erosive lesions; relapses or reinfections reported | Local lesion heals without scars; systemic disease proceeds | Worsens slowly; deep ulcers occasionally develop |

Modified from Wiesner P et al: Genital ulcers. In Holmes KK, Mardh P-A, editors: *International perspectives in neglected sexually transmitted diseases,* New York, 1983, McGraw-Hill.

**Table 65-4.** Laboratory procedures for diagnosis of sexually acquired genital ulcerative lesions

| Procedure | Specific technique | Specimen | Criteria | Diagnosis |
|---|---|---|---|---|
| Reagin test | RPR-CT (rapid plasma reagin card test) or VDRL test | Serum | Reactive titer | Probable syphilis |
| Direct immunofluorescopy | Fixation<br>Reaction with fluorescein-conjugated specific monoclonal antibody | Exudate from lesion or aspirate of bubo | Yellow-green fluorescence<br>Elementary bodies<br>Spirochetes | LGV<br>Syphilis<br>HSV |
| Dark-field microscopy | Unstained preparation | Exudate from lesion or aspirate of bubo | Motile *Treponema pallidum* | Syphilis |
| Bacteriologic cultures | Chocolate agar enriched with 1% Isovitalex and vancomycin (3 μg/ml) added | Exudate from lesion or aspirate of bubo | Normucoid, yellow-gray, translucent, movable colonies containing pleomorphic clumps of gram-negative bacilli, *Haemophilus ducreyi* | Chancroid |
| Light microscopy | Papanicolaou smear (or other specially stained preparation) | Exudate from lesion | Intranuclear inclusions in multinucleated giant cells | HSV |
| | Gram-stained preparation | Exudate from ulcer or aspirate of bubo | Gram-negative bacilli in chains | Possible chancroid |
| | Wright-Giemsa stain | Crushed tissue from biopsy | Donovan bodies | Donovanosis |
| Basic serology | LGV complement fixation assay | Serum | Reactive titer >1:64 | Probable LGV |
| Tissue culture | *Chylamydia* culture | Exudate or aspirate of bubo | Typical stains and cytopathic effects | LGV |
| | HSV culture | Exudate from lesion | Typical stains and cytopathic effects | HSV |
| Advanced serology | Microimmunofluorescence<br>Serologic typing | Sera, agent | | Research tools |

Modified from Wiesner P et al: In Holmes KK, Mardh P-A, editors: *International perspectives in neglected sexually transmitted diseases,* New York, 1983, McGraw-Hill.
*LGV,* Lymphogranuloma venereum; *HSV,* herpes simplex virus.

To establish specific etiologic diagnoses of genital ulcers, the following tests should be performed. First, the physician should assess the possibility of syphilis by microscopic examination; a Tzanck test should also be carried out to check for HSV infection (see Chapter 19).

In addition, Gram stain or other specific stains may need to be performed on smears of exudates or aspirates, impression smears, or crushed or fixed tissue. These preliminary results may guide the selection of further serologic, viral,and bacteriologic testing.

In general, the clinician should proceed from clinical diagnosis to microscopy, then to more sophisticated laboratory tests. However, with the exceptions of darkfield or direct immunofluoroscopy for syphilis and special stains for donovanosis and HSV infection, direct microscopy is no longer considered reliable for the diagnosis of genital ulcers. Similarly, skin tests are now regarded as inadequate for diagnosis. In determining what techniques should be routinely required, two important considerations are the prevalence of specific conditions and the capabilities of the health services in the community. Table 65-4 briefly summarizes, in order of sophistication, the laboratory procedures used to assess the possibility of sexually acquired ulcerative lesions.

Nonulcerative lesions may also appear on the genital surfaces. Some may be infected but not sexually acquired; others are due to STDs. The most common of these are genital warts, and their appearance is familiar though varied. Condylomata acuminata must be distinguished from warts seen in secondary syphilis, condylomata lata. Often this is only possible with darkfield analysis and serologic testing for syphilis. Again, the two diseases may coexist, so inclusion of one does not always exclude the other. The presence of a smooth rounded papule varying in size from barely visible to 3 to 4 mm in diameter suggests a diagnosis of molluscum contagiosum. Pruritic lesions that are sexually transmitted are usually caused either by scabies or crab lice. Specific diagnostic features, including laboratory investigations, of these diseases are described under each condition.

## Ulcerative genital lesions

The infectious causes of genital ulcers include HSV, *Treponema pallidum, Haemophilus ducreyi,* three specific serotypes of *C. trachomatis,* and *Calymmatobacterium granulomatis.* Clinical features can often help differentiate between these diagnoses (Fig. 65-5). The presence of painful vesiculopustules warrants a clinical diagnosis of herpes, although a reaginic serologic test for syphilis should also be carried out. The diagnosis can be confirmed by isolation of HSV in 90% of such patients and by Papanicolaou smear in about two thirds.

If painful nonvesicular ulcers or inguinal nodes are present, the physician should suspect herpes, chancroid, or LGV. Attempts to demonstrate HSV, *H. ducreyi,* or *C. trachomatis* are indicated. However, culture and cytology for demonstrating HSV are less sensitive at the ulcerative stage than at the vesicular stage. Syphilis should be excluded by darkfield or direct immunofluorescent microscopy and serology; these tests should be repeated 1 to 2 weeks later if negative initially and other diagnoses have not been confirmed. The physician should check for *H. ducreyi* by culturing the lesion or the aspirate of a suppurated node (bubo) and also for *C. trachomatis* by culturing a node aspirate. If there are grounds to suspect syphilis, whether clinical (painless ulcerative lesions) or epidemiologic (recent exposure), then direct immunofluorescent or darkfield microscopy or a rapid reagin test should be performed promptly. If these are negative, two or more microscopic examinations should be done on successive days, and serologic tests should be repeated 1 week and 6 weeks later.

The persistence of chronic, painless genital ulceration warrants a test for syphilis and a culture for *H. ducreyi;* a biopsy is required to exclude donovanosis and carcinoma.

***Genital herpes.*** Genital herpes is caused by HSV, a DNA virus with two serotypes. Type 1 is usually found in oral lesions but also causes 10% to 20% of genital herpes. In contrast, type 2 occurs predominantly in genital infections. The two types can be distinguished by various laboratory techniques, including differing cytopathic effects, neutralization, and immunofluorescence tests.

**Pathophysiology.** The incubation period of primary genital herpes is typically 3 to 5 days; however, the period may be longer or shorter and cannot be determined in some patients. At the onset prodromal burning of the skin appears, usually followed by the appearance of grouped vesicles. These vesicles rupture to form multiple shallow painful ulcers, which may coalesce into one or more larger ulcers (see Fig. 65-5). In men herpetic lesions commonly occur on the glans, prepuce, or shaft of the penis; in women the labia minora and majora and the fourchette are often affected. In 90% of women with primary genital herpes, HSV can be recovered from the cervix, even without clinically apparent lesions. In homosexual men perianal herpetic lesions are quite common, making defecation intensely painful.

Inguinal lymphadenopathy develops in about 50% of primary herpes patients; also common are constitutional symptoms such as malaise, fever, and headache. Acute meningitis may also ensue. In some patients HSV causes a sacral radiculitis, leading to constipation, urinary retention, and perigenital anesthesia. In recurrent genital herpes the ulceration is often somewhat milder, and the associated constitutional symptoms are slight or absent.

**Diagnosis.** At present the most sensitive laboratory method for HSV diagnosis is tissue culture isolation. Recovery of virus is easier from an intact vesicle or early ulcer than from a late ulcer and easier from primary lesions than recurrent ones. The sample should be collected in virus transport medium, held at 4° C, and sent to the laboratory within 12 hours. Although smear tests (immunofluorescence, immunoperoxidase, Papanicolaou) are specific, their sensitivity may be as low as 50%. The serology test demonstrates a fourfold rise in titer of antibodies to HSV as detected by complement fixation or neutralization tests; however, the practical difficulties of collecting acute and convalescent sera from patients, and the delay involved, make this an inferior method of diagnosis.

**Treatment.** Oral acyclovir, 200 mg five times a day for 7 to 10 days, may be administered for initial episodes of genital herpes and will generally halt the development of new lesions, hasten the period of crusting and healing, and shorten the time of viral shedding. For recurrent episodes of genital herpes, treatment is generally not recommended unless it can be instituted during the prodrome or within the first 2 days of onset. For patients with frequent recurrences daily suppressive therapy with acyclovir is effective in reducing the frequency of attacks. Acyclovir administered at a dosage of 400 mg twice a day has been shown to reduce the frequency of herpes recurrences by at least 75% among patients with six or more recurrences a year. Safety has been documented for as long as 5 years. Although acyclovir-resistant strains have been isolated from patients on supressive therapy, these strains have not been associated with treatment failure, at least among immunocompetent patients. Recurrences were not affected immediately after discontinuance of the drugs, although the natural course of recurrent episodes may diminish with time, and patients should be reevaluated after 1 year of

A

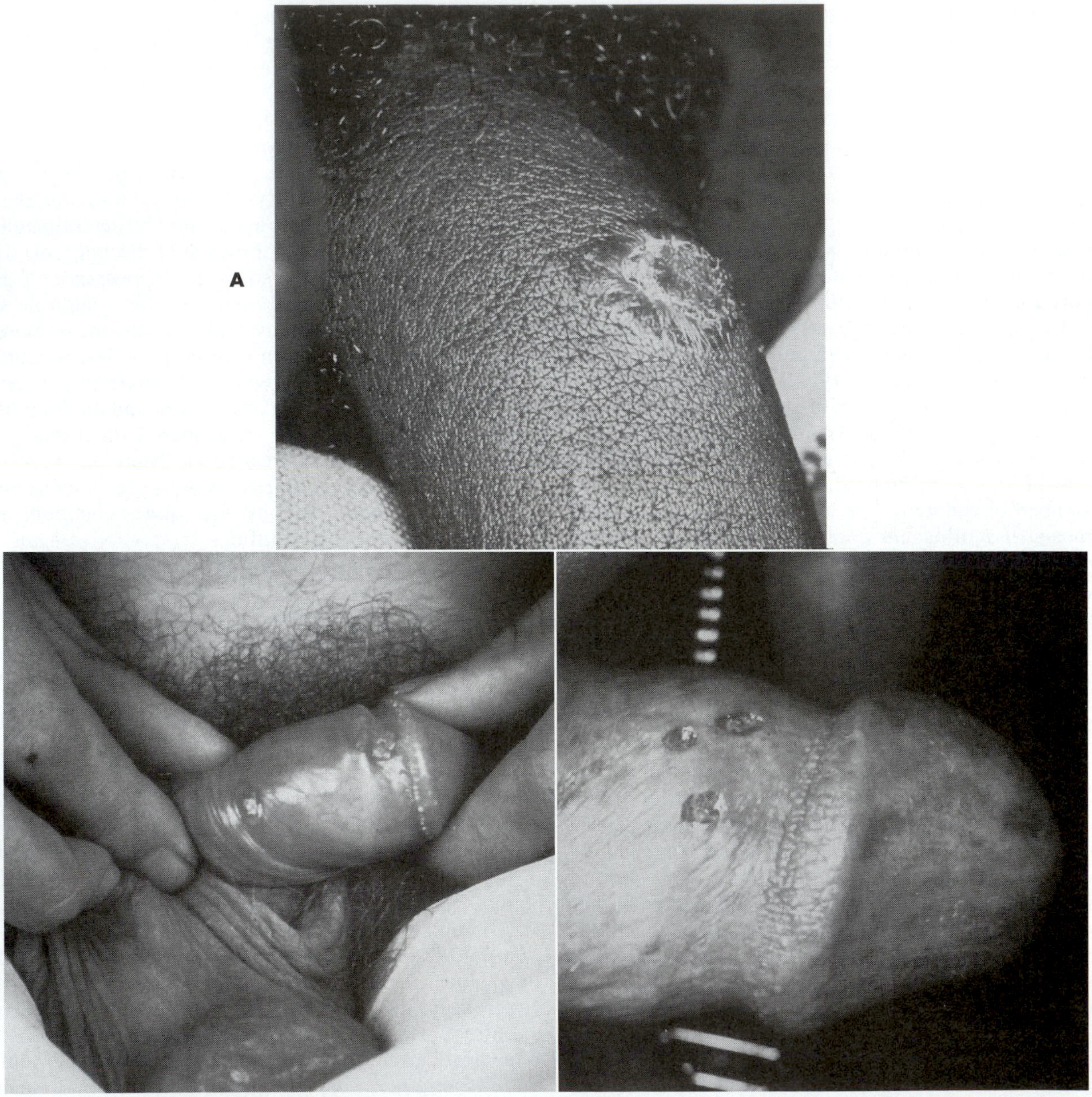

B

C

**Fig. 65-5.** Genital ulcerative lesions in men. Primary syphilis is associated with solitary, round ulcers that are usually superficial with raised edges **(A)**. The chancre associated with chancroid may be multiple, with an irregular shape, rough surface, and undermined edges **(B)**. Herpetic ulcers initially appear as vesicles that evolve into multiple, painful, superficial ulcers **(C)**. (**A** and **C** from Meheus A, Ursi JP: *Sexually transmitted diseases,* Kalamazoo, Mich, 1982, Upjohn.)

suppressive therapy. It should be noted that suppressive therapy does not totally eliminate viral shedding or the potential for transmission.

Local treatment of recurrent genital herpes should be limited to bathing the area as often as possible with warm physiologic saline or tap water, followed by air drying. Women should be urged to sit in a lukewarm bath, spread the labia, and bathe the vulva thoroughly; this cannot be done properly in a shower. When necessary, analgesics should be administered. Local antiseptics are useless, and steroid applications contraindicated. Because secondary infection is rare, there is no place in genital herpes management for systemic antimicrobials unless microbiologic studies have indicated their necessity. Patients with severe cases of primary genital herpes often have viremia and feel miserable and uncomfortable; oral acyclovir therapy or even admission to the hospital for intravenous therapy with acyclovir and supportive treatment may be warranted, especially for women. The physician should be aware that some patients may develop meningitis or sacral radiculitis leading to retention of urine. Because of the pain, catheterization of such patients is difficult and may require a general anesthetic.

Most uncomplicated cases of primary genital herpes heal completely in 7 to 14 days, after which it is safe to resume sexual activity. Since recurrent episodes are usually briefer, the period of abstinence may be correspondingly shorter. The most important aspect of genital herpes management is sympathetic explanation and discussion of the disease. Many patients respond with horror, having heard about herpetic infection of newborns and the association of HSV type 2 with cervical carcinogenesis. The physician should discuss these subjects in a calm and reassuring way so that the patient's knowledge is not limited to articles in the popular press. Patients should be tactfully alerted to the possibility of recurrence and advised to avoid intercourse at these times. Condoms have not been proven to protect against genital herpes. Because of the connection between genital herpes and cervical cancer, women who have had herpes should undergo cervical cytology for premalignant disease once a year indefinitely. The woman's obstetrician must also be informed of her history. If delivery occurs at a time when HSV is being released in the mother's genital tract, there is a 25% to 40% chance that the baby will be infected, possibly with severe or fatal consequences. Therefore under these circumstances many obstetricians perform a cesarean section.

***Syphilis.*** Syphilis is a systemic infectious disease caused by *T. pallidum,* a close-coiled, slender, spiral organism that is motile and multiplies by binary fission every 30 hours. Although too slender to be seen by ordinary light microscopy, it is visible by darkfield or direct immunofluorescent microscopy. It has never been propagated in artificial media or in tissue culture but will grow in rabbit testicle tissue.

**Pathophysiology.** Primary syphilis has an incubation period of between 9 and 90 days and is characterized by an ulcer or chancre at the site of infection (see Fig. 65-5). In men the primary chancre develops at the frenulum, coronal sulcus, urinary meatus, or shaft of the penis. In women primary chancres occur on the labia, at the fourchette, near the clitoris, or sometimes on the cervix. In anoreceptive homosexual men chancres may appear at the anus or in the anal canal, although they may easily escape diagnosis because they are often inconspicuous.

A primary chancre first appears as a papule that soon becomes eroded, forming a well-defined, hardened ulcer with a sloughing or granulating floor. Although slow to heal, the ulcer is painless unless it becomes secondarily infected. Primary chancres are usually single, but about 15% of patients have multiple chancres. Within a week or so of chancre appearance, inguinal lymphadenopathy develops in most patients; this may be unilateral or bilateral. The nodes are discrete, rubbery in consistency, and usually painless.

In secondary syphilis the spirochete disseminates, usually 2 to 8 weeks after the appearance of the chancre. Secondary syphilis has many manifestations including papular cutaneous lesions on the genitals or near the anus that may erode to form shallow ulcers. Mucous patches may appear on the glans penis, the vulva, the vaginal introitus, or the perianal region. Patients with these lesions also have the other signs and symptoms of secondary syphilis, including maculopapules, lymphadenopathy, and constitutional symptoms. Late syphilis or tertiary syphilis is a slowly progressive disease that can affect any organ system in the body, most notably the central nervous system.

**Diagnosis.** The diagnosis of early syphilis is positive if *T. pallidum,* detected by darkfield or direct immunofluorescent microscopy is present in fluid obtained from lesions or in an aspirate from a swollen lymph node. A single negative result is not conclusive and may be due to self-treatment with local antiseptics or antibiotics, or simply to a low concentration of treponemes. A negative first test should be followed by at least two more examinations on successive days; during the interim the patient should simply bathe the lesions with saline or tap water.

To collect specimens for microscopic viewing of *T. pallidum,* clean the ulcer with physiologic saline, abrade its surface with a scarifier, and gently squeeze out the fluid. Collect the fluid on a clean coverslip, which is then inverted onto a glass slide for immediate darkfield microscopy. Do not dilute the sample with saline. If fluorescent microscopy is to be used, smear a drop of the fluid onto a slide, fix with acetone, and send to the microscopist. For patients whose ulcers are healing or who have applied antiseptics, a specimen may be obtained by lymph node puncture. After preparation of the skin, insert a 20-gauge needle into a lymph node and inject up to 1 ml sterile saline. This material is then aspirated and examined for *T. pallidum.*

At the patient's first visit blood should be collected for syphilis serology. This should include a reagin test such as the Venereal Disease Research Laboratory (VDRL) or rapid plasma reagin (RPR) test, as well as a specific test such as the fluorescent treponemal antigen-absorbed (FTA-ABS) test or the microhemagglutination assay (MHA-TP). Reagin tests are reactive in about 75% of patients with primary syphilis and in 100% of those with secondary syphilis; for FTA-ABS the corresponding figures are 80% and 100%, respectively. A rising titer of reagin strongly suggests an early infection. The FTA-ABS is particularly useful in diagnosing early syphilis. Another test, the FTA IgM, may be particularly useful in the diagnosis of early syphilis in patients who have had the disease before (and have a persisting positive FTA-ABS, performed regularly), but false positive reactions can occur. For routine screening where other diagnoses besides syphilis are under consideration, the reagin tests alone should be used first and a positive reagin test confirmed with FTA-ABS.

**Treatment.** The current recommended therapies for syphilis in the nonimmunocompromised patient are given below. Penicillin G is the drug of choice for treatment of all stages of syphilis. The tetracyclines are also effective and can be used in nonpregnant, penicillin-allergic patients. Penicillin is the only therapy with documented efficacy for neurosyphilis. The Jarisch-Herxheimer reaction may occur within the first 24 hours after therapy for syphilis. This reaction consists of an acute febrile illness accompanied by headache and myalgias. Patients should be warned about this acute illness, and antipyretics may be used as needed.

For cure, serum levels of penicillin must reach at least 0.03 μg/ml for a minimum of 7 days. The treatment recommended by the CDC for primary and secondary syphilis, which is 2.4 million U of benzathine penicillin G administered intramuscularly in a single dose, will ensure that these levels are reached. Patients who are allergic to penicillin should be treated with oral doxycycline, 100 mg twice a day, or tetracycline, 500 mg four times a day for 2 weeks. For the pregnant woman there are no proven alternatives to penicillin; it is recommended by the CDC that a pregnant woman with penicillin allergy be treated with penicillin after undergoing desensitization. Erythromycin should not be used because it does not reliably cure an infected fetus.

Some physicians treat secondary syphilis with longer regimens than those recommended above, reasoning that, as the disease progresses, the duration of therapy must increase. Such prolonged regimens may include a second injection of benzathine penicillin G, 2.4 million U administered 1 week after the first. Some physicians prescribe the second dose of benzathine penicillin G for primary syphilis as well.

Patients who have latent syphilis should be evaluated for evidence of tertiary disease. If there is no evidence of neurosyphilis on CSF examination, treatment consists of benzathine penicillin G, 7.2 million U total, administered as three doses of 2.4 million U intramuscularly at 1-week intervals. Patients with neurosyphilis or syphilitic eye disease should be treated with 12 to 24 million U of aqueous penicillin G daily for 10 to 14 days.

**Follow-up.** Response to therapy should be monitored by clinical examination and a quantitative reagin test (VDRL or RPR) at 3 and 6 months after treatment. Patients being treated for neurosyphilis should also have CSF examination repeated every 6 months until it is normal. Successful treatment of seropositive early syphilis reduces the reagin titer. The FTA-ABS test often remains reactive indefinitely and is therefore not useful for follow-up. Persistent or recurrent symptoms or a sustained fourfold rise in the nontreponemal test titer suggests treatment failure or reinfection. Failure of the test to decline by fourfold at 3 months also identifies a patient at risk for treatment failure. In a pregnant woman this titer should reduce at 1 month, and if it has not decreased, she should be retreated. After 1 year all adequately treated patients with seropositive primary syphilis have become seronegative; after 2 years 95% to 100% of patients with secondary syphilis have become seronegative. If, after 2 years, reagin tests have either become negative or stabilized at a low titer, further follow-up is not needed. However, homosexual men and members of other high-risk groups should be urged to undergo serologic testing every 6 months indefinitely. Sexual partners of patients with syphilis of any stage need to be evaluated clinically and serologically.

*Chancroid.* The cause of chancroid is *H. ducreyi,* a short gram-negative rod with rounded ends. In stained clinical specimens it is usually obscured by the presence of other organisms. The organism is fastidious, requiring special enriched media for culture.

**Pathophysiology.** The incubation period of chancroid is between 1 and 5 days. The lesions are papular at first but soon form superficial ulcers that are multiple, ragged, and painful, but not indurated (see Fig. 65-5). The granulation tissue at the ulcer base may be covered with a necrotic exudate and easily bleeds with manipulation. In men they occur at the meatus (where they may cause phimosis or paraphimosis) or on the glans or shaft of the penis. In women ulcers often affect the introitus, labia, and vagina; homosexual men often develop perineal or anal ulceration. Genital and perianal chancroid heals slowly. More than 50% of patients develop regional inguinal lymphadenopathy. Lymph nodes become painful and tender and suppuration may cause a fluctuant inguinal abscess (see Table 65-3).

**Diagnosis.** Culture of *H. ducreyi* is difficult, but special enriched media are available and are successful in up to 80% of cases of clinically diagnosed chancroid. Cultures should be performed whenever these media are available. Material obtained from the patient may be cultured directly onto enriched chocolate agar (1% Isovitalex plus vancomycin, 3 μg/ml, added), which is then incubated in a 5% to 10% $CO_2$ environment at 33° C. Colonies may not appear for a week or longer. In areas where only occasional cases are seen, the results of culture are correspondingly less satisfactory. There is no reliable serologic test for chancroid. The disease prevails in developing countries with limited laboratory facilities, and the diagnosis must usually be based on clinical findings. More reliable diagnostic aids would also be helpful in industrialized countries, where few physicians are familiar with chancroid.

**Treatment.** There are three regimens currently recommended by the CDC for treatment of chancroid. Single-dose therapy can be given with azithromycin, 1 g orally, or ceftriaxone, 250 mg intramuscularly. Erythromycin base, 500 mg orally four times a day for 7 days, is an alternative. Because its safety has not been established, azithromycin should not be administered to pregnant or lactating women. Patients should be reexamined 3 to 7 days after starting therapy. If there is no clinical improvement, the clinician should reconsider the diagnosis or the patient's compliance.

After successful treatment, prolonged follow-up of chancroid is not necessary. However, if nontreponemecidal drugs were used in the treatment, the patient should undergo a final serologic test for syphilis 3 months after the original exposure to infection.

***Lymphogranuloma venereum.*** LGV is a rare disease in the United States caused by *C. trachomatis* serovars $L_1$, $L_2$, and $L_3$, which are immunologically distinct from ocular and other genital strains. The incubation period of LGV is typically less than a week. The initial lesion is a small herpetiform ulcer, usually single but occasionally multiple. Usually transient and inconspicuous, these lesions often escape notice by patient or physician. In particular, the lesions are rarely seen in women; in men they appear on the glans or shaft of the penis.

**Pathophysiology.** The most prominent feature of early LGV is inguinal adenitis, which follows the primary lesion by a few days to several weeks. Both inguinal and femoral lymph nodes may be affected. Large, tender masses of nodes appear, sometimes grooved by the inguinal ligament. Abscesses form, causing fluctuant swellings that can discharge spontaneously. The inflammation is chronic, with much fibrosis. Recovery from lymphadenitis is slow, especially if treatment has not been prompt.

**Diagnosis.** Because LGV patients nearly always present at the stage of inguinal adenopathy, diagnosis of LGV involves distinguishing it from other causes of lymph node enlargement, such as syphilis, herpes, chancroid, bacterial lymphadenitis, and lymphoproliferative disorders. The most commonly used diagnostic test is a complement fixation test, which uses either LGV or psittacosis antigens; a microimmunofluorescence test is somewhat less widely available. In a patient with LGV the complement fixation test becomes positive a week or two after the infection is acquired, usually with a titer of 1:64 or higher. It is usually impractical to demonstrate a rising titer of antibodies, since in clinical practice serology is often limited to a single test.

If chlamydial culture facilities are available, LGV may be conclusively diagnosed by isolation of the agent from pus from buboes. Although the *Chlamydia* antigen detection test that utilizes monoclonal antibody recognizes LGV strains, use of these reagents employing pus from bubos has not been rigorously tested.

**Treatment.** Doxycycline is the preferred regimen, 100 mg by mouth twice a day for 3 weeks. Sulfonamides are also effective for the therapy of LGV; they have the advantage of not masking incubating syphilis. Sulfisoxazole, 500 mg orally four times a day for 21 days, or erythromycin, 500 mg orally four times a day for 3 weeks, is also effective. Patients should have follow-up until symptoms have resolved. If the chosen regimen has not resulted in a good clinical response, it may have to be repeated. The stage of the disease when treatment is begun appears to be the most important predictor of success. Inguinal abscesses should undergo aspiration rather than incision.

***Granuloma inguinale.*** The apparent cause of granuloma inguinale (formerly called donovanosis) is *C. granulomatis,* a gram-negative encapsulated bacillus, best seen in large mononuclear cells from tissue smears. Because this organism is very difficult to culture and has not been thoroughly characterized, the Koch postulates have not been fulfilled.

**Pathophysiology.** Granuloma inguinale is a poorly understood disease; in fact, some researchers have questioned whether the infection is transmitted sexually. Initially painless papules appear on the genitals. These lesions ulcerate and slowly develop into granulation tissue, which spreads over large areas of the genitals. Although inguinal adenitis does not occur, pseudobuboes (subcutaneous granulations in the inguinal region) may appear. In anoreceptive homosexuals granulating lesions develop at the anus and may spread to surrounding areas.

**Diagnosis.** Microscopy of lesion specimens can confirm a clinical diagnosis. The clinician removes from the edge of the lesion a small fragment of granulomatous tissue and smears the undersurface on a glass slide. The specimen is then dried, fixed with methanol, and stained with Wright-Giemsa stain. Microscopic viewing reveals Donovan bodies within large mononuclear tissue cells; these pink, ovoid bodies are surrounded by two capsules and exhibit bipolar staining. This may be the only aid to diagnosis, since culture for *C. granulomatis* is not routinely available and there is no serologic test.

**Treatment.** Doxycycline, 100 mg twice a day, or tetracycline, 500 mg every 6 hours, for 14 days is effective against donovanosis. An alternative is TMP-SMX, 1 double-strength tablet twice a day for 14 days. Patients should be seen for monthly follow-up until all lesions are healed.

### Nonulcerative genital lesions

With the exception of syphilis, the diagnosis of nonulcerative genital lesions is predominantly clinical. However, this clinical diagnosis must be supplemented by biopsy if the diagnosis is unclear or if a premalignant condition is suspected. The problem of biopsy for anogenital warts is difficult. Although the greater proportion are benign, malignancy does undoubtedly develop in some. Therefore warts that fail to respond to treatment or that are in any way atypical should be excised for histopathologic examination. Previous podophyllin therapy may make the histology difficult to interpret.

Pruritic lesions should be evaluated for scabies or crab lice (see further). Some nonulcerative genital or anal lesions are due to STDs. Others are infective but are caused by organisms that are not sexually transmitted. Others are noninfective, but since they enter into the differential diagnosis of STDs, the physician needs to be familiar with them.

***Anogenital warts.*** Human papillomavirus (HPV) is the etiologic agent of genital warts. Infection with HPV has increased tenfold over the past 15 years, making anogenital warts the most commonly diagnosed STD in the United States. Over 60 HPV genotypes have been identified, and at least 20 are associated with anogenital warts, most commonly HPV types 6 and 11. Other HPV genotypes may be found in the anogenital region (e.g., types 16, 18, 31, 33, and 35) and have been associated with genital dysplasia and carcinoma.

HPV has a specific cell tropism and infects the basal layer of squamous or transitional epithelium. As a result of HPV infection, epithelial cells are stimulated to grow, producing hyperplastic proliferation of the epidermis (acanthosis) often associated with increased superficial keratin (hyperkeratosis). The host response to HPV infection is poorly understood, but an intact immune system is clearly important in the control of infection. Patients with immune deficiencies, such as HIV infection or transplant recipients, have much more frequent and severe disease.

**Physical and laboratory examination.** Genital warts often result from intercourse with individuals who already have warts, following an incubation period of 2 to 3 months. On moist surfaces these lesions appear as sessile or pedunculated exophytic lesions, known as condylomata acuminata. Condylomata begin as minute swellings, rapidly growing into fleshy exophytic lesions with pointed surfaces and sometimes fusing into large, irregular masses. In men condylomata often develop on the glans penis, prepuce, coronal sulcus, or within the urethral meatus (see Fig. 65-6). Typical sites in women include the labia, vaginal introitus, and perianal region. Condylomata may also occur internally on the cervix or vagina and should be suspected in women with vulvar warts.

Other clinical manifestations of HPV infection include papular warts, which are usually small, multiple, keratotic, and less papillary. These usually occur on nonmucosal surfaces such as the penile shaft in men or the labia majora in women. More commonly, however, HPV infection is subclinical. Detection in those cases can be accomplished only by soaking the area with 3% to 5% acetic acid for 2 to 5 minutes and examining either directly or under magnification for shiny, aceto-whitened areas. Acetowhitening is not, however, specific for HPV, and false positive tests are common. Colposcopy has been the traditional method of detecting HPV infection in women, but it has recently been advocated for use in male patients as well.

Cytologic and histopathologic examination is helpful in establishing a diagnosis of HPV infection, but its accuracy is difficult to determine because there is no gold standard to which it can be compared. The classic cytologic findings of HPV infection include squamous cells with hyperchromatic nuclei surrounded by a perinuclear clear zone (koilocytes), multinucleated giant cells, acanthosis, and papillomatosis. Newer methods of detecting HPV infection include nucleic acid hybridization techniques, Southern blot analysis, immunohistochemical techniques, and polymerase chain reaction. The accuracy of Papanicolaou smears is variable and depends on the sampling method and the pathologic criteria used. About 10% or more of tissue specimens from women with normal Pap smears may contain HPV DNA as determined by these other methods, but the clinical significance of this viral DNA is unclear.

**Treatment.** HPV infection is treated for a variety of reasons, including cosmetic purposes, symptomatic improvement, reduction of viral transmission, and to prevent the development of neoplasia. There are, however, no current data to prove that treatment affects either the transmission or natural history of the disease. The usual treatment for warts is cytotoxic therapy or ablative therapy. Podophyllin resin, an antimitotic agent, has been used for years as the first-line therapy. A 10% to 25% solution of podophyllin in compound tincture of benzoin is applied to the lesions once or twice a week by a medical professional or trained paramedic, not by the patient. A single application should not exceed 0.5 ml of a 25% solution because of the risk of absorption and ensuing toxic symptoms. Podophyllin should remain in contact with the lesions for 4 hours, or up to 24 hours if there are no adverse reactions, before being washed off. When treating vaginal warts, the physician should make sure that the treated area is dried before removing the speculum. Podofilox 0.5% solution for self-treatment of genital warts is also available. Patients apply the compound daily for 3 days, followed by 4 days of no therapy, and repeat this cycle three more times if necessary. Pregnancy and cervical warts are contraindications to the use of podophyllin and podofilox.

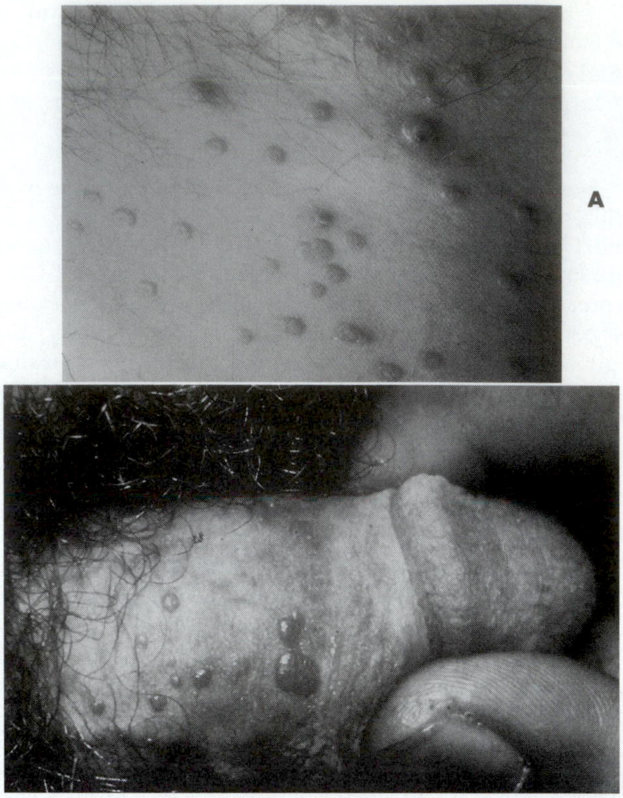

A

B

**Fig. 65-6.** Nonulcerative genital lesions. Molluscum contagiosum of the suprapubic area. Note the flesh-colored papules with central umbilication **(A).** Typical condyloma of penile warts, most often associated with HPV type 6 or 11 **(B).** (**A** from Holmes KK et al, editors: *Sexually transmitted diseases,* New York, 1984, McGraw-Hill. **B** from Bingham JS: *Pocket picture guides: sexually transmitted diseases,* London, 1994, Gower Medical Publishing.)

The CDC currently recommends cryotherapy as first-line management for anogenital warts. Early studies on bichloroacetic and trichloroacetic acid (TCA) cryotherapy are promising. Unlike podophyllin, TCA can be used in pregnant women and for cervical warts. Liquid nitrogen cryotherapy is popular and can be swabbed or sprayed onto a lesion, usually. Each individual lesion is frozen down to its base along with some adjacent epithelium. Unfortunately, the depth of tissue destruction cannot be controlled, and cervical lesions extending into the endocervical canal cannot be reached. Ablative therapy can also be done by specialists with surgical excision, electrocautery/electrodissection, $CO_2$ laser therapy, and the loop electroexcisional procedure. Finally, intralesional interferon appears to be efficacious, although recurrence rates are high and side effects such as a flulike illness have been reported.

It is important that all women with external anogenital warts or contacts of patients with anogenital warts undergo Pap smear. Any evidence of atypical cervical cytology is an indication for colposcopy. Patients with condylomata located at the urethral meatus or perianal area should also undergo urethroscopic or proctoscopic examination, respectively. In the absence of coexisting dysplasia, treatment of subclinical HPV infection as detected by Pap smear, colposcopy, biopsy, acetic acid whitening, or nucleic acid detection is not recommended.

***Genital molluscum contagiosum.*** Genital mulloscum contagiosum is caused by a poxvirus that has not yet been cultured in vitro; thus virologic techniques are not used for diagnosis. Although lesions can occur anywhere on the body, in adults they are particularly common on the genitals. The incubation period lasts from 2 to 8 weeks, after which lesions appear. These are raised, flesh-colored, umbilicated papules, 2 to 5 mm in diameter, each with a central depression containing a white plug made up of degenerate epithelial cells and viral inclusion bodies (see Fig. 65-6). The lesions are found on the penis or scrotum in men, on the labia majora in women, and on the inner thighs and pubic area of both sexes.

The lesions should be lanced and their contents destroyed. The traditional method, opening the lesions with a pointed wooden applicator dipped in liquid phenol, is quite effective, but some physicians prefer to use cautery under local anesthesia. Unless every lesion is destroyed, the disease will recur.

***Scabies.*** Scabies are caused by the itch mite. The adult female, a round-bodied, eight-legged mite measuring 400 µm in length, travels across human skin at the rate of 2.5 cm per minute. The mite chooses a suitable location and burrows into the horney layer to the boundary of the stratum granulosum; remaining there for the rest of its approximately 30-day life. Within hours of burrowing it begins laying huge eggs that develop into adult mites in 10 days. The average infested patient hosts about 11 adult female mites.

The mites tend to settle in specific areas, especially the hands and wrists. Since eruption is partially caused by immature stages of the mite and by sensitization, the distribution of scabietic lesions does not correspond to that of the adult females. In primary infestation itching and eruption occur only after sensitization, which takes several weeks. Itching characteristically occurs at night.

The hands are frequently the first areas infested. Here the lesions, which are often eczematous, appear primarily on the finger webs and the sides of the digits. Lesions often develop on the flexor surfaces of the wrists, as well as on the extensor surfaces of the elbows (where lesions may be nodular but are usually dry and eczematous) and the anterior axillary folds. In women eczematic lesions may develop on the breasts. Papular lesions often occur on the abdomen; frequently arranged in a spokelike pattern around the umbilicus. The penis is typically involved; here the lesions may take the form of nodules, pyoderma, or chancriform changes. The infestation may spread to the crease where the buttocks join the upper part of the thighs, causing impetigenous crusting in this area. In adults the palms, soles, scalp, face, neck, and upper back are usually not involved.

The pathognomonic burrow is a short wavy line, dirty in appearance, which often crosses skin lines. It appears most frequently on the fingerwebs, volar wrists, elbows, and penis. Most infested areas have small, erythematous, often excoriated papules, many of which are larval sites. Secondary eczematization and infection may obscure other features and make diagnosis more difficult. In general, scabies causes polymorphic lesions, although occasionally a patient appears in whom urticaria is the only cutaneous feature.

**Diagnosis.** For diagnosis of scabies it is necessary to obtain a specimen from freshly developed, unexcoriated papules or burrows; these can be located with the aid of a hand lens or head loupe. The clinician places mineral oil on a sterile scalpel blade and allows the oil to trickle onto the lesions. Six or seven vigorous scrapes of the scalpel remove the surface of the burrows or papules, along with the oil. The specimen is placed on a glass slide, covered by a coverslip, and viewed under the microscope. The presence of any stage of the mite, or the more numerous fecal pellets, confirms the diagnosis.

**Treatment.** The two recommended regimens are 5% permethrin cream (Elmite) applied to all areas of the body from the neck down and washed off after 8-14 hours, or 1% lindane (Kwell), 1 oz of lotion or 30 g of cream applied thinly from the neck down and washed off thoroughly after 8 hours. Lindane should not be used following a bath, and it is not recommended for persons with extensive dermatitis, pregnant or lactating women, and children under 2 years of age. An alternative regimen is 10% crotamiton (Eurax) applied to the body for two consecutive nights and washed off 24 hours after the second application. Bedding and clothing should be decontaminated as well, but decontamination of the living areas is not necessary. Pruritus can persist for several weeks; however, some experts recommend retreatment if patients are still symptomatic after 1 week. Sexual and close household contacts should be evaluated and treated if necessary.

***Crab lice.*** Lice are wingless insects that are obligate parasites. Two species parasitize humans: *Pediculus humanus* (which is subdivided into two populations, the head louse and the body louse) and *Phthirus pubis,* the pubic or crab louse, which causes pediculosis pubis. The pubic louse ranges from 0.8 to 1.2 mm in length and is broader than it is long. Powerful claws on the second and third pairs of legs enable the louse to latch onto the pubic hair. From egg to egg, the life cycle of the pubic louse is about 25 days.

The pubic area is the most common site of infestation. Although the lice tend to remain at the initial site of contact, they occasionally spread to the hairs of the thighs and trunk, especially in hairy individuals, and even to the beard and mustache. Involvement of the eyelashes and periphery of the scalp occurs mainly in children and is probably acquired by close contact with an infested mother.

Pruritus, the most common symptom, begins about 30 days after exposure. Brought about by the louse inserting its mouthparts into a cutaneous cavity and sucking blood, the itching may be immunologic in origin, rather than mechanical. Excoriations may lead to pyoderma, which may obscure the organisms. Lymphadenitis and febrile episodes may ensue, although these secondary symptoms are probably less common in developed countries due to early diagnosis and prompt, effective therapy.

**Diagnosis.** Although not common, the maculae ceruleae are characteristic of pubic lice infestation. These asymptomatic, bluish or slate-colored macules appear on the trunk and thighs and fade shortly thereafter. Two likely causes of the macules are hemoglobin breakdown products of the host and secretions from the parasite's salivary gland.

Involvement of areas other than the pubic region may complicate the diagnosis. Any pruritic eruption of a hairy area should be cause for suspicion of crab lice. In some cases examination of other areas such as the axillae may lead more easily to a diagnosis, since the patient may have already eradicated the pubic infestation by self-treatment. Eyelash infestation is especially troublesome to diagnose because seborrheic, infectious or eczematous blepharitis may be simulated; however, careful examination shows that the crusts consist of the parasites.

Pediculosis pubis is rare among STDs in that it can be diagnosed by physical examination alone. The adult lice can be identified with the aid of a magnifying lens, especially after feeding when they become rust colored. Particles of rust-colored excreta may be visible at sites of infestation.

Usually, however, the disease is diagnosed by recognizing the numerous nits or ova, which the parasites attach to the pubic hair with a cementlike secretion. Since the nits are initially affixed to the hair at skin level, and grow out with the hair, the length of the infestation can be estimated by the distance of the nits from the skin surface. Although the nits are visible to the naked eye, they can be confused with kinks and knots in the hair or flakes of seborrheic dermatitis. The diagnosis should be confirmed by plucking the hair and identifying the nit under the microscope.

**Treatment.** All infested sites and adjacent hairy areas should receive medication, particularly the pubic mons and perianal region. In hairy individuals the thighs, trunk, and axillae are frequently infested and should be treated. The most common medication is lindane (Kwell). A typical treatment consists of lindane shampoo lathered into infested areas for 4 minutes, then thoroughly washed off. A single application is usually sufficient; if viable ova persist or new ones appear at the bases of hairs, the patient should receive a treatment a week after the first. An equally effective treatment is 1% permethrin cream rinse (Nix) applied to affected areas and washed off after 10 minutes. Lindane is the least expensive treatment, but permethrin has less potential for toxicity in the event of inappropriate use. Children may be given the shampoo treatment. However, lindane should not be used by pregnant or nursing women. If the eyelashes are infested, occlusive ophthalmic ointment should be applied to the eyelid margins for 10 days to smother lice and nits; lindane and other drugs should never come in contact with the eyes. Although corticosteroids may reduce the pruritus associated with pediculosis, they should be avoided. If used before diagnosis they potentiate the infestation, allowing it to become generalized.

Sexual contacts of pediculosis patients should be treated simultaneously to prevent reinfection; other uninfested household members need not be treated. Once the parasites have been eradicated, the patients and sexual partners should wash and dry all used underwear, pajamas, sheets and pillowcases by machine (hot cycle) or have them dry cleaned.

## Noninfective genital ulceration

***Traumatic ulceration.*** Traumatic ulceration may stem from physical or chemical causes. During intercourse the external genitalia may become abraded or fissured particularly at the frenulum or coronal sulcus in men and at the fourchette in women. The penis may be bitten during fellatio. Injuries from zippers are common, and psychiatric disorders may result in self-mutilation of the genitals. Regardless of origin, the lesions may become secondarily infected, leading to persistent painful ulceration with tender inguinal adenitis.

Chemical ulceration may result from the application by the patient of strong antiseptics to prevent infection. Such ulcerations may be iatrogenic, for example, after cautery or treatment of genital warts with podophyllin. The use of corticosteroid-containing medications on small infective ulcers may enlarge them.

***Behçet's disease.*** This relapsing vasculitis disease is characterized by oral and genital ulceration and uveitis, often with hypopyon. The etiology is unknown. The genital ulcers occur on the penis and scrotum in men, and on the vulva and vagina in women; in both sexes perianal ulceration may develop. The ulcers range from 2 to 20 mm in diameter and may be deep or shallow. Very painful, the ulcers persist for several weeks before healing, often with fibrosis. Relapses often occur.

The prognosis of Behçet's disease may be poor. Although systemic corticosteroids may be somewhat helpful, there is no satisfactory treatment for this condition.

### *Premalignant and malignant disease*

**Erythroplasia of Queyrat.** A premalignant disease of unknown cause, erythroplasia of Queyrat usually affects men over the age of 50. It is characterized by a red plaque appearing on the glans penis or adjacent lining of the prepuce; diagnosis is based on histologic evidence that shows the changes of intraepidermal carcinoma. Symptoms indicating the onset of malignancy include hardening and fixation of the ulcerative lesion and enlargement of the inguinal lymph node.

**Genital cancer.** Cancer of the penis, vulva, or anus usually occurs in individuals over the age of 50. The condition may take the form of an infiltrative lesion or of a raised ulcer with everted edges.

### Noninfective conditions causing nonulcerative genital lesions

***Normal variants.*** Patients having these features may misinterpret them as symptoms of STDs. Fordyce's spots, which appear as clusters of small yellow dots on the vulva or inner lining of the prepuce, are ectopic sebaceous glands. Fibroepithelial polyps, which are common around the anus and vaginal introitus, may be mistaken for warts. Coronal papillae may also be confused with warts; these are hypertrophic papillae with a normal epithelial covering. Lymphocele is a transitory condition in which the lymphatics above the coronal sulcus become blocked, leading to the appearance of a stringlike swelling that can encircle the penis. Edema of the glans penis or prepuce may also occur. Lymphocele may be linked with frequent or prolonged intercourse or masturbation, but the cause is unknown. The condition resolves in 2 to 3 weeks without treatment.

***Dermatoses.*** Balanitis xerotica obliterans, believed to be a genital form of lichen sclerosis et atrophicus, usually affects men between the ages of 30 and 50. White plaques with associated scarring develop on the glans penis and around the urinary meatus, spreading into the terminal urethra for a short distance. In women a similar condition affects the vulva and perianal area. Irritation often ensues, and eventually contraction of fibrous tissue may decrease urinary flow in men and cause dyspareunia in women. This chronic progressive disease in some cases converts to malignancy. No cure is available, although corticosteroid ointments may reduce the amount of scarring. Constriction of the terminal urethra requires regular urethral dilatation.

Lichen planus is a skin disease of unknown cause that may appear on the penis, scrotum, or vulva. The purple flat-topped lesions occur in papular or annular form and usually cause irritation. Similar lesions may emerge on other parts of the body; in some patients silver spots appear inside the mouth. No specific treatment is known, but lichen planus usually resolves spontaneously. Topical corticosteroid medications may alleviate the irritation.

Psoriasis may affect the genitals of both sexes, with papules or silvery scaled plaques appearing on the penis, scrotum, and vulva. Lesions on the glans penis may be similar to the circinate balanitis of Reiter's disease; in fact, the histologic features of psoriasis are much like those of keratoderma blenorrhagica. Psoriasis rarely affects the genitals alone; lesions often appear on the elbows, knees, or scalp, and the nails may be pitted and irregular. A patient with psoriasis should be referred to a dermatologist.

***Benign neoplasms.*** Fibroma, lipoma, hemangioma, and pigmented nevia are among the benign neoplasms. Small sebaceous cysts often occur on the genitals, especially near the median raphe of the penis and scrotum. For many benign neoplasms the exact histologic diagnosis is reached only after excision.

***Malignant neoplasms.*** Intraepidermal carcinoma may appear either alone or associated with condylomata acuminata. Bowen's disease emerges as a raised scaly plaque, Paget's disease as persistent eczema with discharge and crusting. Both disorders can affect the genitals or the perianal area and may persist as intraepidermal carcinomas for years before invasive carcinoma develops.

Squamous cell carcinoma may develop on the penis, vulva, or anus. This condition may be preceded by chronic irritation, condylomata acuminata, and premalignant conditions such as erythroplasia of Queyrat, leukoplakia, Bowen's disease, and Paget's disease. Carcinoma of the penis, usually found in uncircumcised men over age 50, begins as a small, warty plaque or nodule that soon ulcerates and develops into a hard fixed mass, which may fungate. Involvement of inguinal lymph nodes may come later and indicate a poor prognosis. Carcinoma of the vulva, most often occurring in postmenopausal women, may develop from leukoplakia or from preexisting condylomata acuminata. Usually starting on the labia major, it develops into an infiltrated ulcer or proliferative tumor. Lymph nodes become involved at a later stage.

## BIBLIOGRAPHY

Centers for Disease Control and Prevention: 1993 sexually transmitted diseases treatment guidelines, *MMWR* 42:77, 1993.

Holmes KK et al, editors: *Sexually transmitted diseases,* New York, 1984, McGraw-Hill.

Jacobson L: Differential diagnosis of acute pelvic inflammatory disease, *Am J Obstet Gynecol* 138:1007, 1980.

Rice PA, Dale PA: Infections of the genitourinary tract in women: selected aspects. In Stollerman GH et al, editors: *Advances in internal medicine,* Chicago, 1984, Mosby.

Steinberg JL, Cibley LJ, Rice PA: Genital warts: diagnosis, treatment, and counseling for the patient. In Remington JS, Swartz MN, editors: *Current clinical topics in infectious diseases,* Boston, 1993, Blackwell Scientific Publications.

Steinberg JL, Rice PA: Pelvic inflammatory disease. In Carr, Freund, editors: *The medical care of women,* Philadelphia, 1993, WB Saunders.

CHAPTER

# 66 Parasitic and Tropical Diseases, and Advice for Travelers

**Manoj Jain**
**Alfred DeMaria, Jr.**

## PARASITIC AND TROPICAL DISEASES

Parasitic diseases occur worldwide. Tropical diseases are only "tropical" because of climatologic factors affecting vectors and intermediate hosts. Tropical and parasitic diseases can be imported readily into nonendemic areas in an age of rapid air travel and mass migration. An individual acquiring Lassa fever in West Africa may fly to

Paris, then to New York, and on to Kansas City within 24 hours, with the evolution of symptoms and the potential for spread throughout the trip. This may lead to secondary cases in persons who are in transit to dozens of other destinations.

This chapter is designed as an overview for the primary care practitioner to suggest diagnostic possibilities in a limited number of settings. The reader is referred to detailed textbooks of parasitic and/or tropical diseases and geographic medicine for more comprehensive coverage of particular diseases.

Many parasitic diseases are easily diagnosed and treated by well-established routine procedures and management options. The diagnosis and management of other parasitic diseases may be challenging and may require special expertise, uncommon tests, and unusual drugs. The practitioner should be aware of the services provided by the appropriate departments in medical and public health schools and by local public health agencies. The U.S. Centers for Disease Control and Prevention (CDC) provides advice in the diagnosis and management of parasitic diseases and telephone health advice for travelers. It is a source of unreleased and investigational drugs. The CDC also publishes information about parasitic and tropical diseases in the *Morbidity and Mortality Weekly Reports* and its supplements. Periodic supplements review recommendations for health aspects of world travel. Similar services are available through public health ministries and agencies in other countries, as well as from the World Health Organization (WHO).

**Table 66-1.** Parasitic worms that commonly infest or infect the alimentary tract and associated structures

| Parasite | Common name |
|---|---|
| **Roundworms** | |
| *Ascaris lumbricoides* | Large roundworm |
| *Ancylostoma duodenale* | Old World hookworm |
| *Necator americanus* | New World hookworm |
| *Strongyloides stercoralis* | Threadworm |
| *Trichuris trichiura* | Whipworm |
| *Enterobius vermicularis* | Pinworm |
| *Capillaria philippinensis* | |
| **Flatworms** | |
| Tapeworms | |
| *Taenia solium* | Pork tapeworm |
| *Taenia saginata* | Beef tapeworm |
| *Diphyllobothrium latum* | Broad fish tapeworm |
| *Hymenolepis nana* | Dwarf tapeworm |
| *Hymenolepis diminuta* | Rat tapeworm |
| *Dipylidium caninum* | Dog tapeworm |
| Blood flukes | |
| *Schistosoma mansoni* | |
| *Schistosoma japonicum* | |
| *Schistosoma mekongi* | |
| *Schistosoma malayensis* | |
| *Schistosoma haematobium* | |
| *Schistosoma intercalatum* | |
| Intestinal flukes | |
| *Fasciolopsis buski* | |
| *Heterophyes heterophyes* | |
| *Metagonimus yokogawai* | |
| Liver flukes | |
| *Clonorchis sinensis* | Chinese liver fluke |
| *Opisthorchis felineus* | |
| *Opisthorchis viverrini* | |
| *Fasciola hepatica* | Sheep liver fluke |
| *Fasciola gigantica* | |

## Parasites of the alimentary tract

Parasitic worms of the alimentary tract are highly adapted to existence in the human gastrointestinal tract, its vasculature, and the biliary tract. Table 66-1 lists the parasitic worms that commonly infest and infect the alimentary tract and related structures. The successful parasite causes limited morbidity in its host. The vast majority of people infested with the common worm parasites are asymptomatic. In fact, symptoms are usually the result of a larger than usual number of parasites, or a heavy "worm load." Asymptomatic infestation, however, may have chronic effects on the host that are not immediately apparent. Symptomatic bearers of worms usually have nonspecific complaints, except for peculiar clinical syndromes discussed later. Many times alimentary tract worms are discovered incidentally when stool is examined in the course of a diagnostic workup for complaints that may or may not be related to the infestation. Diarrhea caused by the protozoan parasites is discussed later.

The worm or metazoan (multicellular) parasites of the human alimentary tract and associated organs are divided between two phyla: the flatworms or Platyhelminthes and the roundworms or Nematoda. The worms of both major groups have complex life cycles involving varied intermediate and definitive hosts and larval stages.

***Roundworms of the alimentary tract.*** The intestinal nematodes, or roundworms, have a worldwide distribution and infest hundreds of millions of individuals. The human intestinal roundworms include *Strongyloides stercoralis,* the hookworms (*Ancylostoma duodenale* and *Necator americanus*), *Ascaris lumbricoides,* the whipworm *(Trichuris trichiura),* and the pinworm *(Enterobius vermicularis).* Over one billion persons worldwide are estimated to be carriers of *Ascaris;* at least 500 million carry *Trichuris,* and an estimated 42 million in the United States are infested with pinworms. Other worms include *Capillaria philippinensis,* which is an intestinal nematode that causes a severe disease in humans, mostly limited in distribution to parts of the Phillippines, but rarely reported in other parts of the world as well. These worms live in the mucosa of the small bowel and are occasionally invasive. They are acquired by ingesting freshwater fish containing larvae. The intestinal nematodes have host dependence of varying degree. *S. stercoralis* can live and reproduce in soil as a free-living organism. The larvae of hookworms feed in soil but require a host for maturation and reproduction. The larvae of *Ascaris, T. trichiura,* and *E. vermicularis* develop in excreted eggs and hatch when the eggs are ingested by another host.

***Strongyloides stercoralis.*** The life cycle of *S. stercoralis* is summarized in Fig. 66-1. Eggs hatch in the host intestine, giving rise to free-living rhabditiform larvae that are passed in the stool. In warm, moist soil the rhabditiform

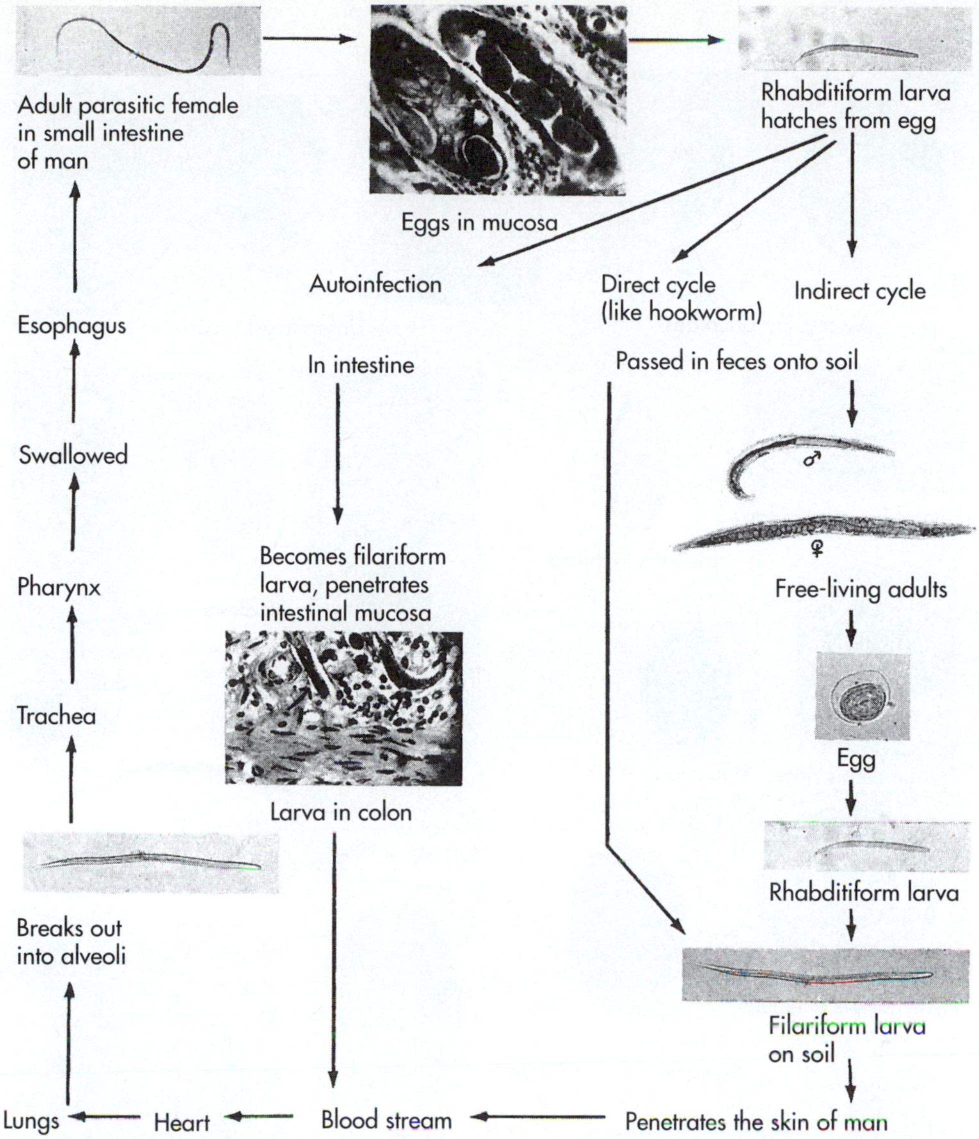


**Fig. 66-1.** Life cycle of *Strongyloides stercoralis.* (From Brown HW, Neva FA: *Basic clinical parasitology,* ed 5, Norwalk, CN, 1983, Appleton-Century-Crofts.)

larvae may go on to mature to free-living adult forms or develop into filariform larvae that are capable of invading human skin. Larvae migrate from the skin to the bloodstream and are carried to the lung where they penetrate the airway, climb the trachea, and are subsequently swallowed. In the proximal small bowel the larvae mature to the adult forms that invade the mucosa. The rhabditiform larvae also may develop into filariform larvae in the gut lumen, leading to autoinfection and maintenance of the disease despite removal of the host from an endemic area. In immunosuppressed and debilitated patients, patients with human immunodeficiency virus (HIV) infection and in patients on corticosteroids, this cycle of autoinfection may lead to a syndrome of hyperinfection with *S. stercoralis.*

Most patients with strongyloidiasis are asymptomatic. A heavy worm load can lead to epigastric pain, weakness, malaise, and watery diarrhea, perhaps due to an absorptive defect. Upper gastrointestinal radiographic studies may show duodenal and jejunal mucosal edema. Ulceration and even intestinal perforation may occur. The hyperinfective syndrome can be an overwhelming systemic disease that is often fatal. Extensive migration of larvae can lead to derangement of multiple organs, abscesses in the liver and other organs, and development of adult worms in the bronchial tree. The diagnosis of strongyloidiasis is made by demonstrating larval forms in the stool (Fig. 66-2) or parasites in duodenal aspirates or biopsies.

**Hookworm.** Hookworm disease is transmitted by passage of eggs in the stool, which hatch in warm, moist soil forming rhabditiform larvae that develop within a few days into filariform larvae. There are no free-living adult forms. Filariform larvae invade the skin and migrate in the same way as the larvae of *S. stercoralis.* The life cycle of the hookworm is summarized in Fig. 66-3. Once the larvae reach the small intestine, they mature to adults that attach to the duodenal and jejunal mucosa and suck blood. An adult *A. duodenale* is capable of sucking up to 0.1 to 0.3

A

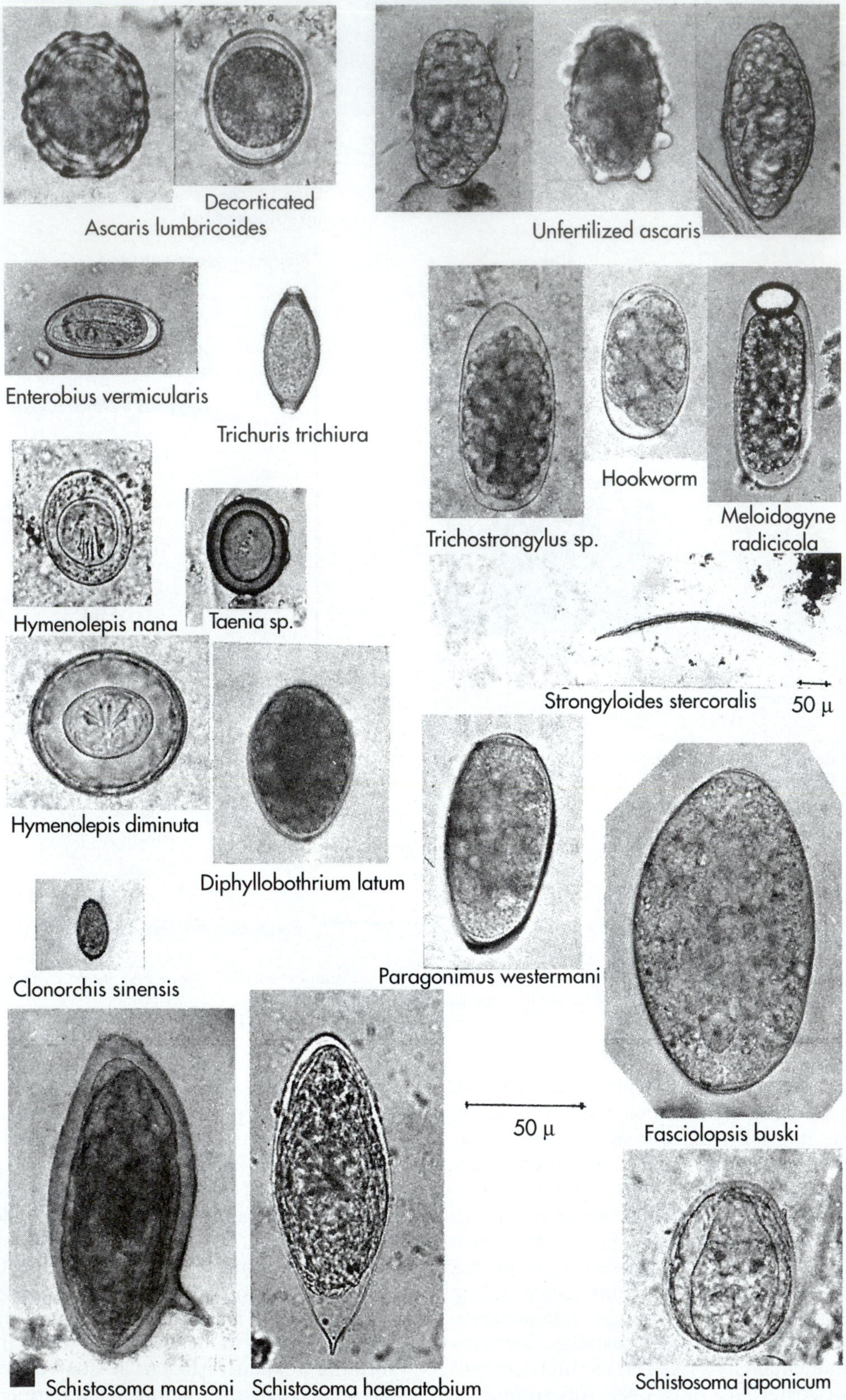


**Fig. 66-2.** Worm eggs (**A**) encountered during microscopic examination of stool and fecal vegetable artifacts (**B**) that may be confused with ova and parasites. (From Brown HW, Neva FA: *Basic clinical parasitology,* ed 6, Norwalk, CT, 1994, Appleton-Century-Crofts.)

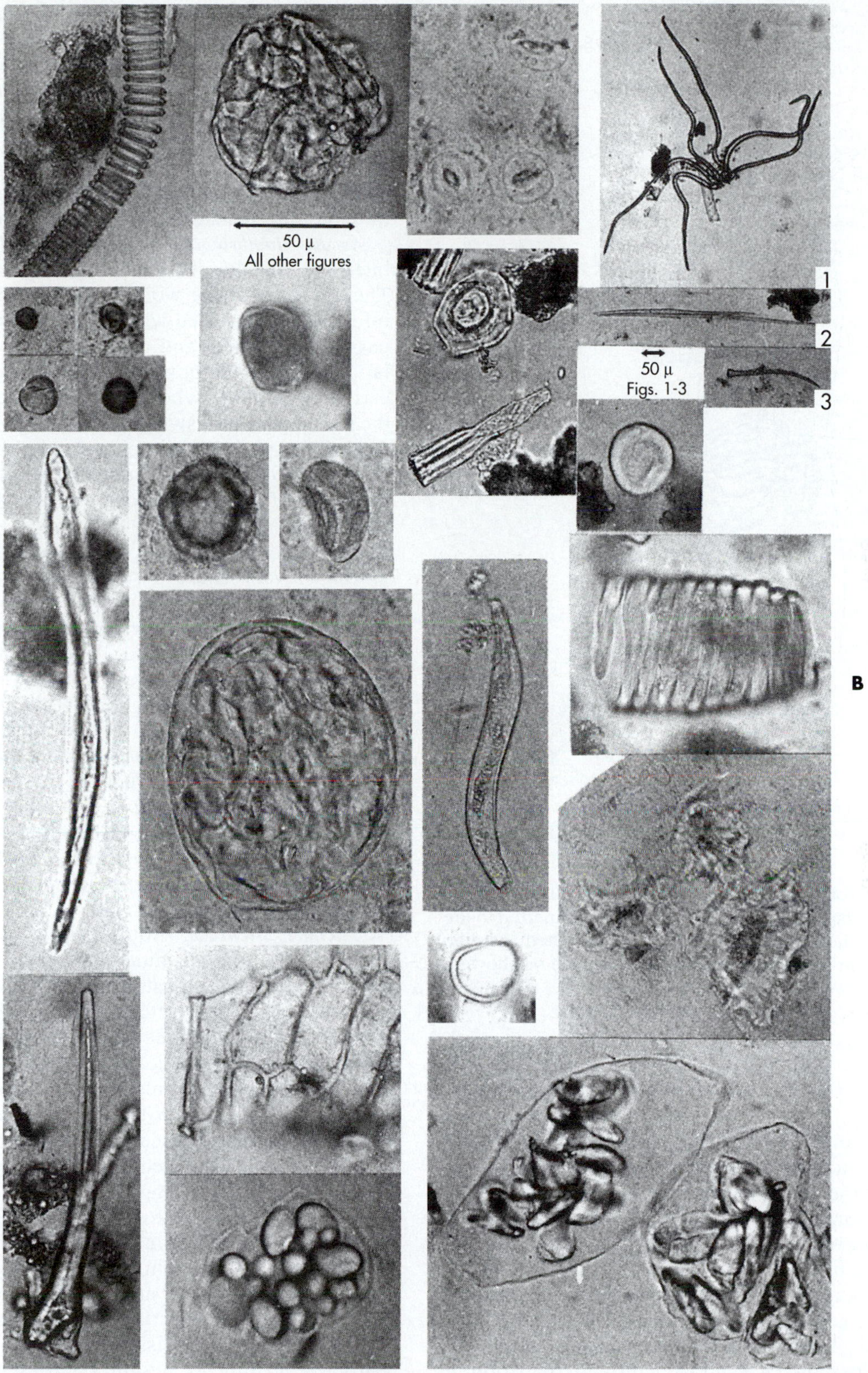


**Fig. 66-2, cont'd.** For legend see opposite page.

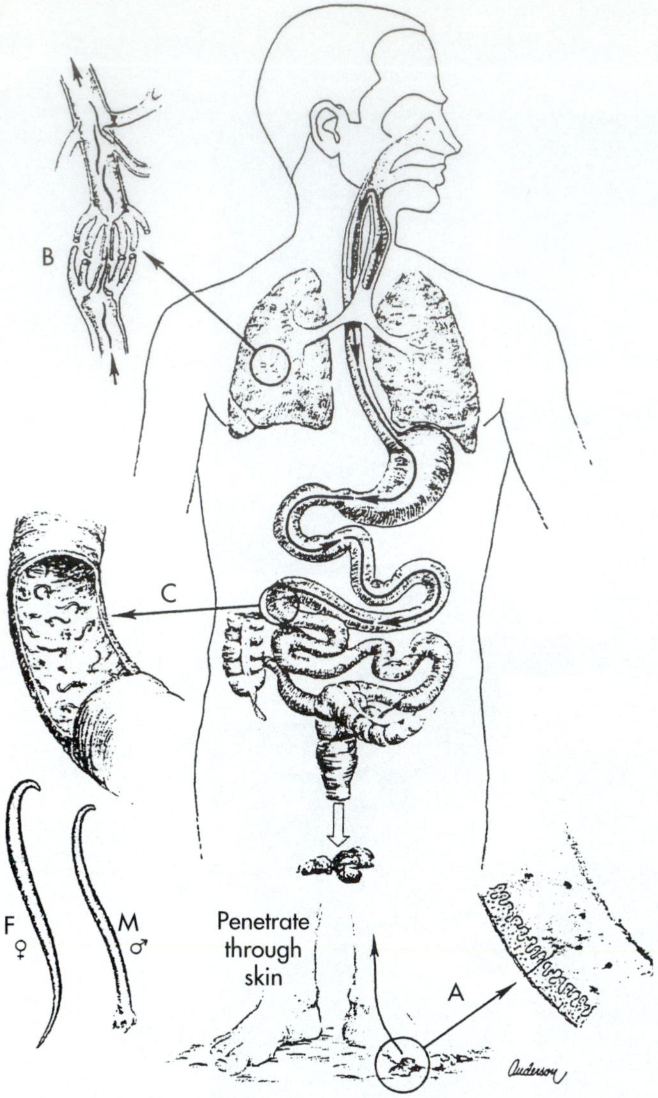


**Fig. 66-3.** Life cycle of the hookworm. Filariform larvae in *(A)* the soil penetrate the skin and are carried in the circulation to the lungs *(B)* where they break out of the capillary bed into the alveolar spaces, are swept up the bronchial tree, are swallowed, and become adult worms *(C)* in the small intestine. (From Beck JW, Davies JE: *Medical parasitology,* ed 3, 1981, Mosby.)

ml of blood per day; *N. americanus* removes somewhat less. The worms produce an anticoagulant that causes blood to ooze around the feeding worm, leading to blood in the stool and more blood loss. Worm load can be in the thousands, and the life span of adult hookworms may be several years. Humans may develop infestation with other species of hookworm that have animals, such as dogs and cats, as primary hosts.

The most important clinical manifestation of hookworm disease is anemia. The degree of anemia is a function of the worm load. This iron deficiency anemia is due to chronic blood loss and is compounded by malnutrition; it may be severe enough to lead to cardiomegaly. Varying degrees of malabsorption are a concomitant of the infestation and further complicate the disease. Children with significant worm loads may experience growth retardation and inanition. Individuals with hookworm disease may also complain of hunger and nondescript abdominal pain. The diagnosis is made by demonstrating the hookworm ova in the stool (see Fig. 66-2). Hookworm should be suspected in any patient with hypochromic, microcytic anemia who is living in a warm climate with direct exposure to moist soil.

The filariform larvae of *S. stercoralis* and the hookworms can cause a localized dermatitis, called ground itch, when they invade the skin. The usual setting is warm, moist soil and bare feet. Likewise, larval migration through tissues may lead to systemic and pulmonary symptomatology. Skin and systemic syndromes produced by migrating nematode larvae are discussed later.

***Ascaris lumbricoides.*** *A. lumbricoides* is the largest intestinal roundworm, reaching lengths of up to 30 cm. The life cycle of the worm is presented in Fig. 66-4. The infestation is acquired when embryonated eggs, which are passed in the stool and mature in soil, are ingested. The larvae hatch in the bowel, invade the bowel wall, and are carried to the lungs where they penetrate the alveoli, climb the trachea, and are swallowed. This migration can lead to marked peripheral eosinophilia and pulmonary infiltrates. The adult worms mature in the small intestinal lumen, and the mature female worm can produce more than 200,000 eggs a day.

The major symptoms of ascariasis are due to the migrating larvae. These systemic symptoms are discussed later in the chapter. Individuals carrying adult worms are usually asymptomatic. Symptoms, when they occur, are related to the worm load. With light to moderate infestation, vague abdominal pain may occur. With heavy infestation, especially in children, the major complication is mechanical obstruction of the intestine caused by the mass of worms. Worms may migrate to aberrant locations causing biliary tract obstruction, pancreatitis, or appendicitis. Occasionally bowel perforation and peritonitis occur. Diagnosis of ascariasis is made by demonstrating fertilized and unfertilized eggs in stool (see Fig. 66-2). Adult worms in the bowel lumen may appear on intestinal radiographic contrast studies.

***Trichuris trichiura.*** Adult *T. trichiura,* the whipworm, attach to the colonic mucosa. Eggs passed in the stool mature in the soil. Ingested eggs hatch in the small bowel, and the larvae pass into the colon where they mature. The larvae do not invade tissue. Most patients with whipworm are asymptomatic. Heavy infestation may lead to dysentery-like symptoms and occasionally hemorrhage and anemia. Rectal prolapse may occur, and the small white worms may be seen attached to the prolapsed mucosa (''coconut cake'' rectum). Diagnosis is made by demonstrating the typical eggs in the stool (see Fig. 66-2).

***Enterobius vermicularis.*** The pinworm, *E. vermicularis,* also inhabits the colon. Adult female worms migrate through the anus at night and deposit eggs on the perianal and perineal skin. The migration causes intense pruritus. The eggs become infective within hours and are resistant to drying. They can disseminate widely, similar to dust particles, leading to autoinfection as well as family and institutional outbreaks (Fig. 66-5). Whole families typically become infested. After ingestion, the eggs hatch in the small bowel and migrate to the colon, where they mature. There is no tissue invasion.

The primary symptoms of pinworm infestation are

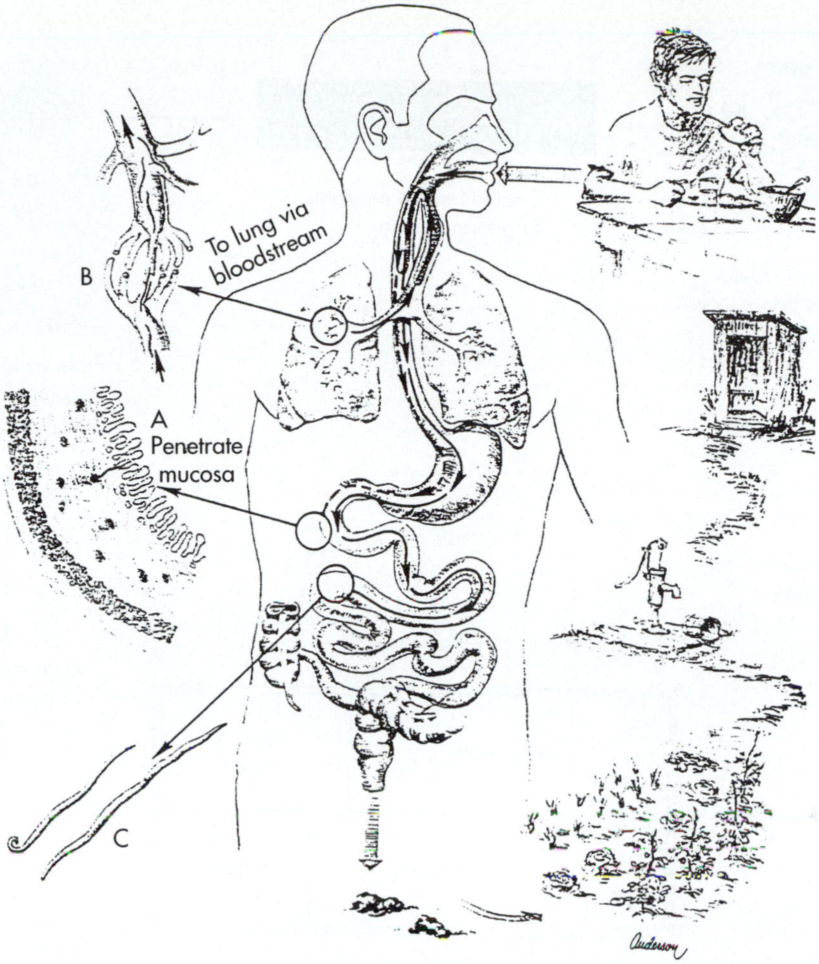


**Fig. 66-4.** Life cycle of *Ascaris lumbricoides.* Infective eggs, ingested in contaminated food and water, hatch in the small intestine where *penetration of the mucosa, (A)* results in invasion of the bloodstream by the larvae, which are carried to the lungs. The larvae, too large to cross the capillary bed, break out into the alveolar spaces, *(B)* are carried up the bronchial tree, are swallowed, and reach the small intestine where they become adult worms, *(C).* (From Beck JW, Davies JE: *Medical parasitology,* ed 3, 1981, Mosby.)

related to the nocturnal migration of the gravid female worms. Moderate to severe perianal pruritus occurs, and excoriation from scratching results. Migration to the vagina may cause vaginitis. The diagnosis may be made by demonstrating eggs or worms in the stool, but it is more easily established by microscopic examination of transparent (Scotch) tape, the adhesive side of which has been pressed to the anus and perianal skin (see Fig. 66-5). The highest yield is obtained during the night or early morning. Adult female worms are captured on the adhesive tape.

The treatment for intestinal nematodes has been made simpler by the availability of mebendazole (Vermox). This agent can be used for all the worms except *S. stercoralis.* Asymptomatic, light infestation with hookworms, without anemia, need not be treated. In the case of mixed infestations, including *Ascaris,* treatment is directed against *Ascaris* first, as inadequate treatment of these worms may result in their aberrant migration. Entire families of patients with pinworm should be treated to prevent recurrence. *S. stercoralis* infestations are treated with thiabendazole. Current recommendations for the treatment of persons with intestinal roundworms are summarized in Table 66-2. Mebendazole is teratogenic in animals and should not be used during pregnancy (albendazole is a related benzimidazole), although the alternative, pyrantel pamoate, has not been established as safe in pregnant women and the fetus.

***Tapeworms.*** The tapeworms, or cestodes, are hermaphroditic flatworms. Adults live in the gut lumen of the definitive host. These worms have no gut and absorb nutrients across their integument. Larval forms encyst in the tissues of intermediate hosts.

Four tapeworms are important human intestinal parasites: *T. saginata* (beef tapeworm), *T. solium* (pork tapeworm), *D. latum* (broad or fish tapeworm), *H. nana* (dwarf tapeworm). The first three are named after the usual food source from which people acquire the parasite. Larval forms, encysted in meat or fish (the cysticercus or plerocercoid, respectively), are ingested and develop into adult forms in the gut lumen. *H. nana* uses the human as both definitive and intermediate host. Cysticerci of this

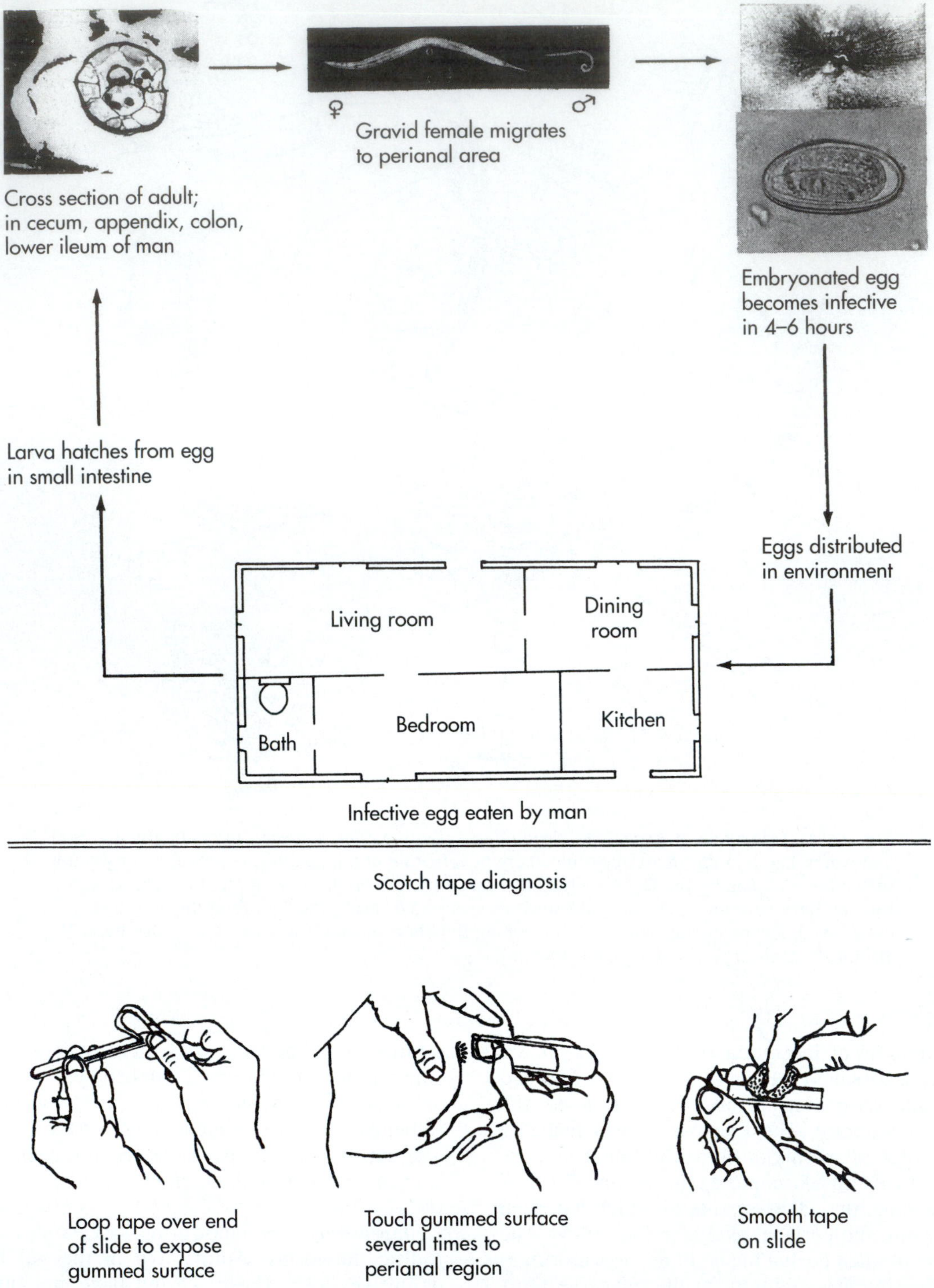


**Fig. 66-5.** Life cycle of *Enterobius vermicularis* and the procedure for the adhesive tape test to reveal migrating worms. (From Brown HW, Neva FA: *Basic clinical parasitology,* ed 5, Norwalk, CT, 1983, Appleton-Century-Crofts.)

**Table 66-2.** Treatment for intestinal roundworms

| Parasite | Drug of choice | Alternative agent | Comment |
|---|---|---|---|
| *S. stercoralis* | Thiabendazole, 25 mg/kg, by mouth, bid for 2 days (maximum dose 3 g/day) | Ivermectin, 200 μg/kg/day, by mouth for 1 to 2 days | Hyperinfection syndrome requires longer therapy or other agents. |
| Hookworms *A. duodenale* *N. americanis* | Mebendazole, 100 mg, by mouth, bid for 3 days | Pyrantel pamoate, 11 mg/kg, by mouth, as a single dose (maximum 1 gram) | Doses are the same for children >2 years old. Pyrantel is considered investigational in the treatment of hookworm. |
| | | Albendazole, 400 mg, by mouth, once | Nutritional support and iron supplements are important. Blood loss may continue after worms are shed. |
| *A. lumbricoides* | Mebendazole, 100 mg, by mouth, bid for 3 days | Pyrantel pamoate, as above<br>Albendazole, 400 mg by mouth, once | Pediatric (>2 years) doses are the same. |
| *T. trichiura* | Mebendazole, 100 mg, by mouth, bid for 3 days | Albendazole, 400 mg, by mouth, once | Heavy infestation may require 3 days of albendazole. Pediatric (>2 years) doses are the same. |
| *E. vermicularis* | Mebendazole, 100 mg, by mouth, one dose; repeat in 2 weeks | Pyrantel pamoate, as above, as one dose; repeat in 2 weeks<br>Albendazole, 400 mg, by mouth, once; repeat in 2 weeks | Family and household contacts should be treated.<br>Pediatric doses are the same. |

species develop in the bowel wall, and larvae are released into the lumen to form more adults. *H. nana* is transmitted through ingestion of ova passed in stool. *T. solium* (Fig. 66-6) also is capable of using humans as its intermediate host. Ova may be ingested with material contaminated with stool from an affected person, or ova may reach the stomach or duodenum by reverse peristalsis. The ova hatch, producing larvae that invade tissue leading to cysticercosis, a disease discussed below in the section dealing with parasites that cause mass lesions in tissue.

Several tapeworms, which are primarily parasites of other animals, are occasionally found in the human gut. Of note are *D. caninum* (dog or cat tapeworm) and *H. diminuta* (rat tapeworm), which infect humans when the intermediate host, the flea, is inadvertently ingested.

Tapeworms are composed of a scolex, or head, that attaches to the intestinal mucosa, and a chain of progressively mature segments (proglottids) that contain the reproductive parts and produce ova. Gravid proglottids and eggs are shed in the stool. These ova may then reinfect in the case of *H. nana* or are ingested by intermediate hosts, hatch, invade, and form tissue cysts. Tapeworms are cosmopolitan parasites. Epidemics of *D. latum* in the United States have been associated with eating certain types of fish from Midwestern lakes. Control measures for tapeworms include adequate cooking of meat and fish, sanitary hygiene practices, and assurance of safe feed for hogs and cattle.

Most patients with tapeworms are asymptomatic. Worms may be harbored in the gut for many years. Symptoms, when they occur, may be related to heavy worm load and are usually nondescript; they include mild abdominal pain, diarrhea, malaise, and occasionally constipation. The motile proglottids of *Taenia* sometime force their way through the anus. *D. latum* can successfully compete with the host for vitamin $B_{12}$ and infestation with this tapeworm can lead to megaloblastic anemia. The ability of *H. nana* to autoinoculate may lead to heavy worm loads and cramping pain, diarrhea, nausea and vomiting, and headache. Intestinal erosions may occur. In children, heavy *H. nana* infestation may be associated with irritability and rarely seizures. These neurologic manifestations have been ascribed to absorption of toxic substances produced by the worms. The diagnosis of tapeworm infestation is made by demonstrating eggs (see Fig. 66-2) or proglottids in the stool.

Praziquantel is the drug of choice for tapeworm disease. The oral dose is 5 to 10 mg/kg in one dose for *T. solium, T. saginata,* and *D. latum* and 25 mg/kg in one dose for *H. nana.* The alternative agent for tapeworms is niclosamide in an adult dose of 2 g once for all the tapeworms except for *H. nana,* which is treated with 2 g as one dose, then 1 g/day for 6 days, as the drug is inactive against the cysticerci in the bowel wall that erupt after 4 days. The pediatric doses of niclosamide are adjusted to 1.0 or 1.5 g.

### *Flukes*

**Schistosomiasis (blood flukes).** Acute schistosomiasis may present as a febrile, systemic process. It occurs 1 to 2 months after exposure to cercariae, at a time corresponding to the onset of egg production by the parasite. It is characterized by fever, weight loss, diarrhea, cough, abdominal pain, and headache. Acute disease may be especially severe with *S. japonicum* infection and is called Katayama fever. Peripheral blood eosinophilia is often of marked degree.

Several trematode worms, or flukes, are capable of infecting humans. The most important human flukes are in the genus *Schistosoma.* More than 200 million people worldwide have schistosomiasis. The predominant species that infect humans are *S. mansoni, S. japonicum, S. mekongi,* and *S. haematobium. S. malayensis* occurs in

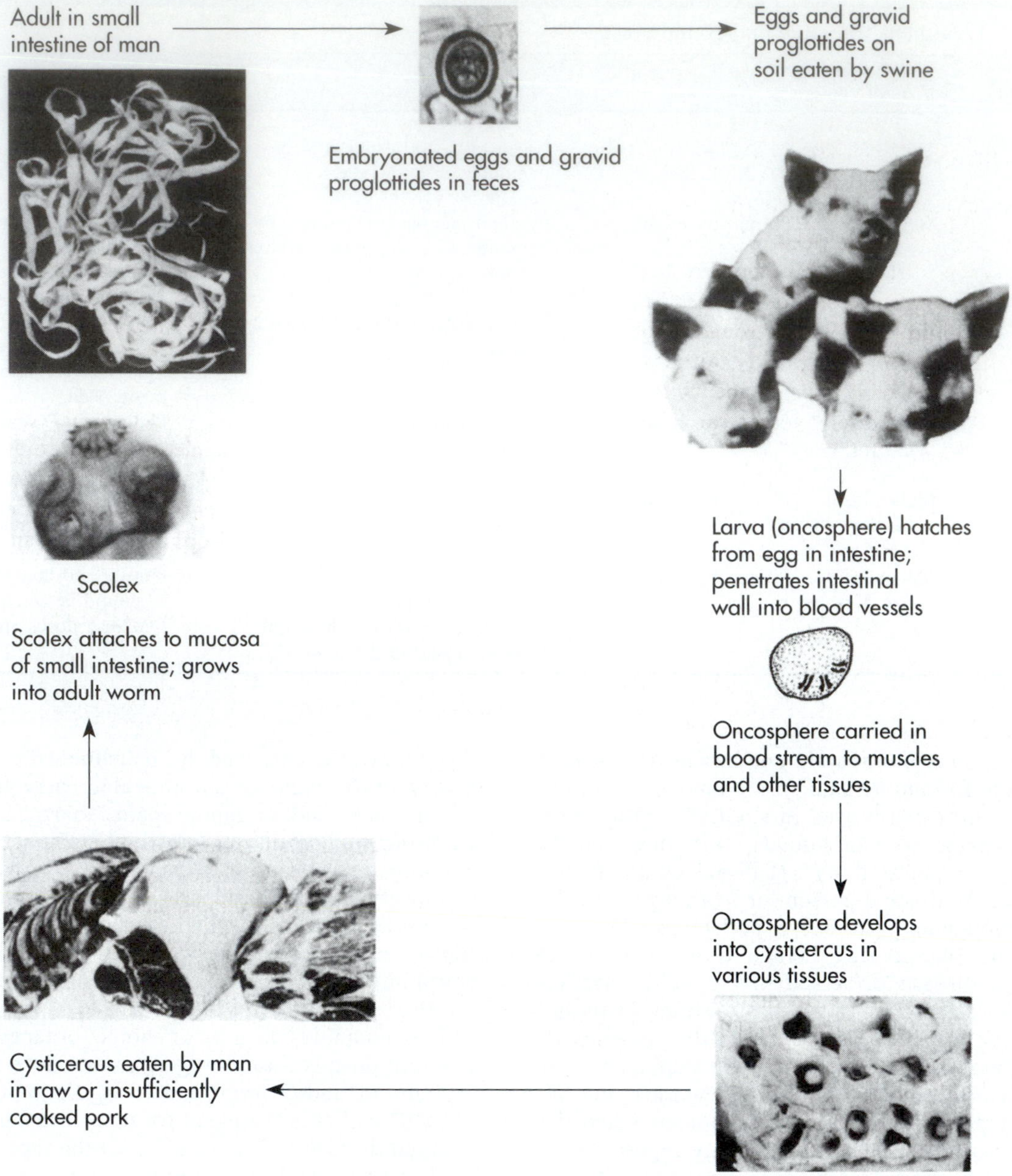
Adult in small intestine of man
Eggs and gravid proglottides on soil eaten by swine
Embryonated eggs and gravid proglottides in feces
Larva (oncosphere) hatches from egg in intestine; penetrates intestinal wall into blood vessels
Oncosphere carried in blood stream to muscles and other tissues
Oncosphere develops into cysticercus in various tissues
Cysticercus eaten by man in raw or insufficiently cooked pork
Scolex
Scolex attaches to mucosa of small intestine; grows into adult worm

**Fig. 66-6.** Life cycle of *Taenia solium.* (From Brown HW, Neva FA: *Basic clinical parasitology,* ed 5, Norwalk, CT, 1983, Appleton-Century-Crofts.)

Southeast Asia and resembles *S. japonicum* and *S. mekongi. S. intercalatum* is closely related to *S. haematobium* and is an increasing problem in Africa.

Schistosomes have complex life cycles (Fig. 66-7), which involve specific snails as intermediate hosts. The disease occurs in many parts of the world. Its distribution depends of the distribution of particular species of snail. The disease is acquired by exposure to fresh water containing the fork-tailed larvae, called cercariae, which are released from the intermediate host. Cercariae are capable of penetrating the skin where they lose their tails and become schistosomulae. Schistosomulae migrate to the lung, then the liver, where they mature to adult forms. The adult forms then join in permanent sexual coupling and migrate to their final intravascular location, the mesenteric veins in the case of *S. mansoni, S. japonicum, S. mekongi,* and *S. malayensis;* the perirectal venules in the case of *S. intercalatum;* and the venous plexus of the urinary bladder in the case of *S. haematobium.* The mating pair of adult worms produce hundreds to thousands of eggs daily over several years. These eggs make their way across the intestinal and bladder mucosae and are excreted. In fresh water the eggs hatch larvae, called miracidia, which invade snails and continue the cycle.

The signs and symptoms of schistosomiasis depend on the worm load. An acute illness usually occurs about 1 month (2 weeks to 2 months) after exposure to the cercariae and correlates with the time of initial egg production. This syndrome is characterized by fever, abdominal pain, diarrhea, and pulmonary complaints associated with marked peripheral blood eosinophilia. *S. japonicum* is the most prodigious egg producer; and the

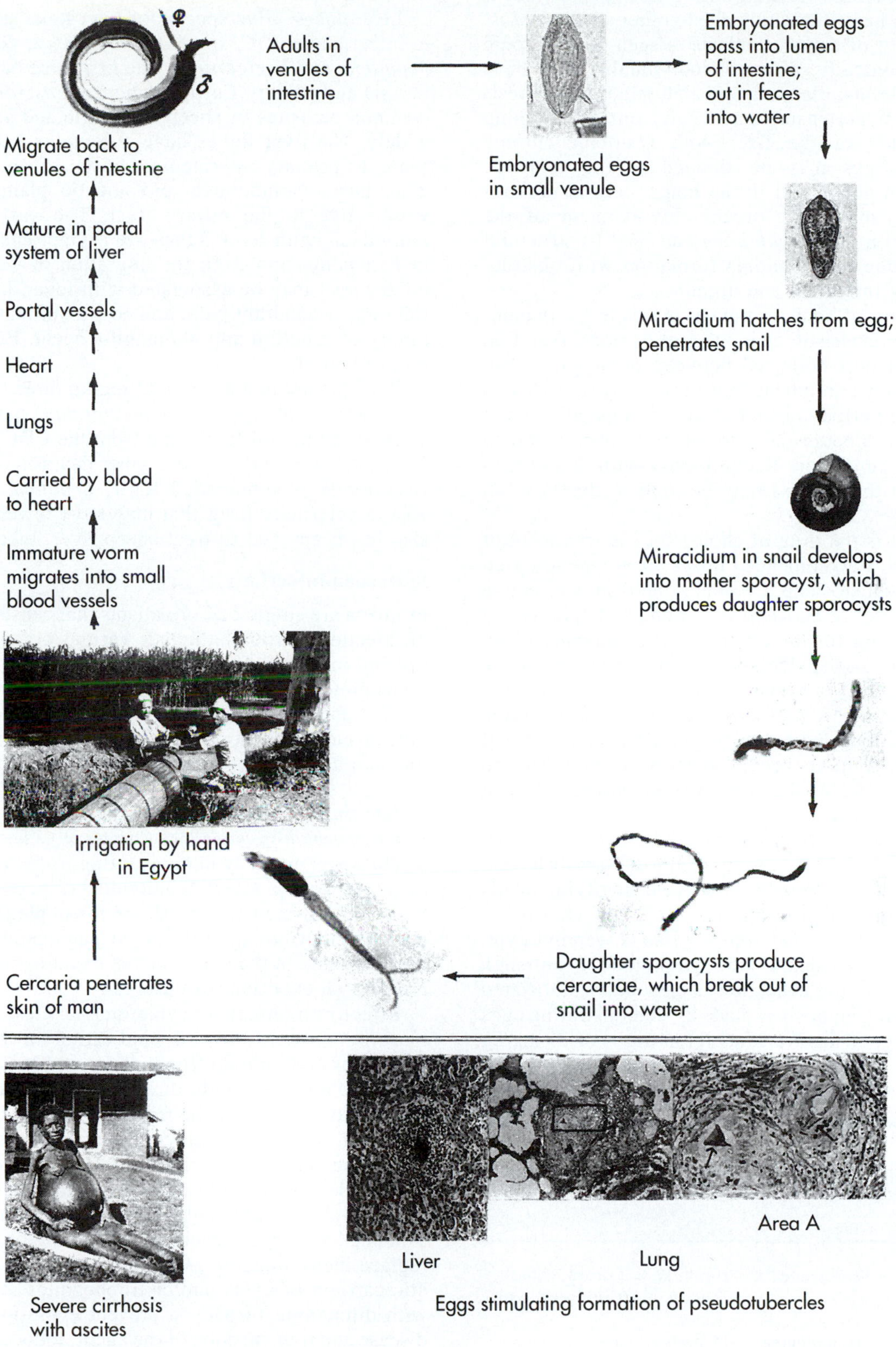
Adults in venules of intestine
Embryonated eggs in small venule
Embryonated eggs pass into lumen of intestine; out in feces into water
Miracidium hatches from egg; penetrates snail
Miracidium in snail develops into mother sporocyst, which produces daughter sporocysts
Daughter sporocysts produce cercariae, which break out of snail into water
Cercaria penetrates skin of man
Irrigation by hand in Egypt
Immature worm migrates into small blood vessels
Carried by blood to heart
Lungs
Heart
Portal vessels
Mature in portal system of liver
Migrate back to venules of intestine
Severe cirrhosis with ascites
Liver
Lung
Area A
Eggs stimulating formation of pseudotubercles

**Fig. 66-7.** Life cycle of *Schistosoma mansoni.* (From Brown HW, Neva FA: *Basic clinical parasitology,* ed 5, Norwalk CT, 1983, Appleton-Century-Crofts.)

syndrome it produces, Katayama fever, usually occurs with the most severe infection due to this species, but it may occur with heavy infection due to other species. Most of the morbidity of schistosomiasis is seen with chronic infection. Chronically affected individuals may have systemic complaints, diarrhea, and abdominal pain. Presinusoidal portal hypertension may result from eggs lodging in the sinusoids of the liver with resultant chronic inflammation. Eggs may be shunted to the systemic circulation with deposition in the lungs, central nervous system (CNS), and other organs. Involvement of the urinary tract with *S. haematobium* can lead to structural abnormalities due to granuloma formation with obstruction, secondary infection, and uremia.

The diagnosis of schistosomiasis is made by demonstrating the characteristic eggs in stool or urine (see Fig. 66-2). Urine is best collected between noon and 2 PM. Because eggs may continue to make their way into excreta for a prolonged period, a count of viable eggs, allowed to hatch in vitro, is a better indicator of live worm load than simple stool examination. Rectal biopsy with demonstration of eggs in the mucosa may be used to diagnose all species.

Praziquantel is the drug of choice for the treatment of schistosomiasis. Recommended doses vary depending on the species of schistosome. Oxamniquine also is effective in the treatment of *S. mansoni* infection. Metriphonate is an alternative drug for the treatment of *S. haematobium.* The latter drugs and advice about their use are available through the CDC. Current recommendations for the treatment of schistosomiasis are summarized in Table 66-3. Many patients with schistosomiasis have a small worm burden and do not require thearpy. The decision to treat should be based on the severity of symptoms, clinical activity, and worm load.

**Intestinal flukes.** The intestinal flukes, *F. buski, H. heterophyes,* and *M. yokogawai,* inhabit the small bowel. These worms have a complex life cycle involving snails and aquatic plants or fish as intermediate hosts. They occur primarily in Asia, but *H. heterophyes* also is seen in Egypt. Most affected individuals are symptomatic, although abdominal pain and diarrhea are occasionally associated with infestation. Diagnosis is made by demonstrating eggs in stool (see Fig. 66-2). Praziquantel in doses of 25 mg/kg three times in 1 day is effective for the treatment of intestinal flukes.

**Table 66-3.** Treatment for schistosomiasis

| Schistosome parasite | Drug | Dose |
|---|---|---|
| *S. mansoni* | Praziquantel | 20 mg/kg × *2 doses*, 4 to 6 hours apart in 1 day, with meals |
| | Oxamniquine | 15 mg/kg, once |
| *S. japonicum*<br>*S. mekongi*<br>*S. malayensis*<br>*S. intercalatum* | Praziquantel | 20 mg/kg × *3 doses*, 4 to 6 hours apart in 1 day, with meals |
| *S. haematobium* | Praziquantel | 20 mg/kg × *2 doses*, 4 to 6 hours apart in 1 day, with meals |

**Liver flukes.** Five species of liver fluke are most likely to infect humans: *C. sinensis, O. felineus, O. viverrini, F. hepaticia,* and *F. gigantica.* The first three occur primarily in Asia and Eastern Europe, whereas *Fasciola* species are common parasites of sheep and cattle and are distributed widely. The liver flukes have a complex life cycle, with snails as primary intermediate hosts; secondary intermediate hosts include fish and aquatic plants. The adult worms live in the biliary tract. The vast majority of individuals with liver flukes are asymptomatic, but early in *F. hepatica* infection the migration of worms into the biliary tract may be associated with fever, hepatomegaly, right upper quadrant pain, and eosinophilia. Occasionally, biliary obstruction and cholangitis occur. Eggs appear in bile and stool.

Praziquantel in a dose of 25 mg/kg three times in 1 day is effective therapy for *Opisthorchis* species and *C. sinensis.* Bithionol (available from the CDC) in a dose of 20 mg/kg twice a day, every other day, for 10 to 15 doses is currently recommended for *F. hepatica.* Triclabendazole, a veterinary drug that may have fewer side effects, also has been used to treat sheep liver flukes.

## Protozoan infections

Protozoa are single cell organisms that cause a wide range of infections. Protozoa invade various organs of the body causing infection of the intestine, blood, or deep tissues. Some protozoa, such as *Pneumocystis carinii, Toxoplasma gondii,* and *Cryptosporidium parvum* have become significant causes of morbidity and mortality among acquired immune deficiency syndrome (AIDS) patients.

### *Intestinal protozoan infections*

***Entamoeba histolytica*** (see Chapter 49). The diagnosis of amebiasis is made by demonstrating trophozoites or cysts in the stool of the affected individual (Fig. 66-8). These are best demonstrated in a fresh stool sample. Several other amoebae that are of little or no pathogenic significance may be found in the stool, so that examination of the stool requires an experienced observer.

Effective treatment of symptomatic intestinal amebiasis must be directed toward eradication of both invasive organisms and luminal trophozoites and cysts. Metronidazole (750 mg, by mouth, three times a day for 10 days) is the drug of choice for the former, followed by iodoquinol (650 mg, by mouth, three times a day for 20 days; exceeding the dose carries the risk of optic neuritis) or diloxanide furoate (500 mg, by mouth, three times a day for 10 days; available only through the CDC) for the latter. Tinidazole, a drug closely related to metronidazole, may replace metronidazole as the drug of choice. Asymptomatic carriers of cysts and/or trophozoites may be treated with diloxanide furoate to prevent evolution of invasive disease and transmission of the agent. Iodoquinol (650 mg, by mouth, three times a day for 20 days) is an alternative to diloxanide, but doses in excess of those recommended have been associated with optic neuritis.

***Giardia lamblia.*** *G. lamblia* is a flagellate protozoan parasite of the intestine that is being increasingly recognized as a cause of diarrhea. The parasite attaches to the epithelium of the proximal small bowel and causes

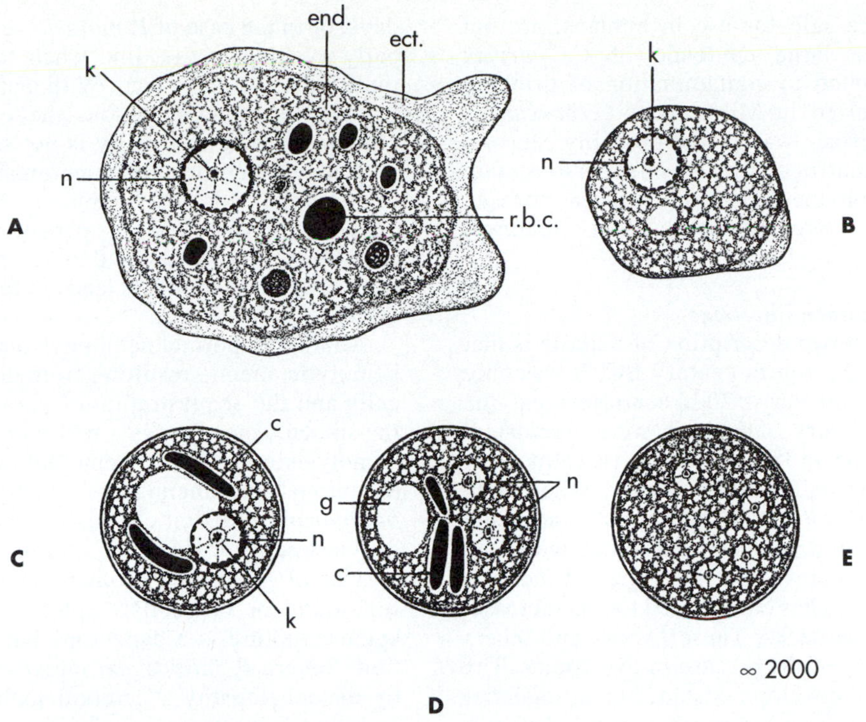


**Fig. 66-8.** *Entamoeba histolytica.* **A,** Trophozoite containing phagocytized red blood cells. **B,** Precystic ameba. **C,** Young cyst. **D,** Binucleate cyst. **E,** Mature cyst (with four nuclei). *c,* Chromatoid bodies; *ect.,* ectoplasm; *end.,* endoplasm; *g,* glycogen acuole; *k,* karyosome; *n,* nucleus; *r.b.c.,* red blood cells. (From Brown HW, Neva FA: *Basic clinical parasitology,* ed 6, Norwalk CT, 1994, Appleton-Century-Crofts.)

abdominal cramps, bloating, and diarrhea. Symptoms may be remittent. Cyst forms passed in the stool transmit the infection.

The natural history of the parasite is poorly elucidated, and several primary animal hosts have been proposed. Most outbreaks of giardiasis have been associated with waterborne transmission, although the fecal-oral route is clearly important in households, family day care, and institutional transmission. Sporadic cases of giardiasis occur throughout the world, and it is a frequent cause of diarrhea in travelers.

The diagnosis of giardiasis depends on demonstrating the trophozoite or cyst in stool or other specimens. If stool is negative, and if the diagnosis is strongly suspected on clinical and epidemiologic grounds, aspiration of duodenal contents or the "string test" may be undertaken. The string test is accomplished by having the patient swallow a commercially available gelatin capsule containing 140 cm of nylon string, the free end of which is secured to the face. The string usually passes to the duodenum and may be gently removed after several hours. Examination of material expressed from the distal end of the string is examined for parasites.

Treatment of giardiasis is with quinacrine (100 mg, by mouth, three times a day for 10 days) or metronidazole (250 to 750 mg, by mouth, three times a day for 5 to 10 days). Metronidazole appears to be safe and effective, but larger than usual doses may be required in some cases. Treatment of asymptomatic as well as symptomatic household contacts may be indicated.

***Blastocystis hominus.*** *B. hominus* is a protozoan parasite first described in the early part of this century. It has been associated with diarrhea for many years, but its role as a cause of diarrheal illness has not been clearly established. Diarrhea with *B. hominus* in the stool in large numbers (>5 per oil immersion field) has been linked epidemiologically with travel and with drinking of untreated water. The drug of choice has not been determined. Metronidazole is usually selected because of its efficacy in other similar infections, and iodoquinol has been used as an alternative.

**Other intestinal protozoan infections.** Recently a newly recognized protozoan parasite has been described in association with outbreaks of diarrhea in widespread parts of the world. This organism is thought to be either a cyanobacterium or a coccidian parasite and has been named *Cyclospora cayetanensis.* The disease has an abrupt onset of watery diarrhea, nausea, and anorexia with a waxing and waning prolonged course of 2 to 12 weeks. Resolution is also abrupt, but may be followed by prolonged fatigue. Organisms have been seen in duodenal aspirates, as well as in stool. The disease tends to occur during warm and wet seasons. Transmission seems to be predominantly waterborne. Sporadic cases may occur in the absence of a recognized outbreak. Successive infections in the same individual have been documented. Treatment options are under investigation, but trimethoprimsulfamethoxazole appears to be promising.

Human infection with protozoal parasites of the gastrointestinal tract of domesticated animals is becoming recognized in widespread parts of the world. In immunocompetent hosts, symptomatic disease related to these parasites appears to be confined to a self-limited episode of gastroenteritis, although asymptomatic carriage of organisms may be prolonged. Severe, intractable diarrhea has been observed in patients with AIDS due to *C. parvum, Isospora belli,* and other protozoa. Effective drugs against these parasites that are safe for use in humans, are not available. Recently, a large epidemic of *C. parvum* infection that was related to contamination of drinking water with cysts occurred in Milwaukee. *C. parvum* is commonly found in surface waters and probably causes a number of sporadic diarrheal illnesses in persons with altered immune function due to underlying disease or age. Vigorous pursuit of more effective water treatment methods is underway.

### *Blood and tissue protozoan infections*

**Malaria.** The first known description of malaria is that of Hippocrates during the fourth century BC. It was only during the late 19th and early 20th centuries that the etiology and natural history of malaria were elucidated. Great strides were made in the control and treatment of malaria during the first half of this century. Whereas in many areas, such as Europe and the United States, the disease has been eradicated, in other areas of the world the parasite is making new gains. The emergence of mosquitoes resistant to pesticides has contributed to this increase, as have sociopolitical setbacks. These factors and others have led to a resurgence of the disease in the tropics. The ability of the parasite to develop resistance to antimalarial drugs has made treatment and prevention more difficult. Thus malaria is an increasing world health problem. The effect of this disease on the health and economy of the world is immeasurable. In the United States most cases of malaria are imported. Failure to diagnose and treat early results in a more than tenfold increase in mortality rate over that observed when the diagnosis is considered at clinical presentation.

Human malaria is caused by four species of the protozoan genus *Plasmodium: P. falciparum, P. vivax, P. ovale,* and *P. malariae.* Disease is transmitted by infection of the sporozoite form through the bite of an anopheline mosquito. Sporozoites invade liver parenchymal cells, and after 2 weeks merozoites are released into the bloodstream. Merozoites invade erythrocytes and the parasite develops into a trophozoite. Trophozoites differentiate in erythrocytes to produce either more merozoites or gametocytes. Merozoites continue the cycle of erythrocyte parasitism.

Male and female gametocytes, taken up by mosquitoes during a blood meal, initiate a phase of sexual reproduction, and development ultimately produces sporozoites. The life cycle of *Plasmodium* is summarized in Fig. 66-9. *P. vivax* and *P. ovale* are capable of latent infection of liver cells, which may give rise to merozoites and therefore clinical disease at times distant from exposure. *P. falciparum* does not have an exoerythrocytic phase. Malaria also may be transmitted by blood transfusion and intravenous injection using contaminated needles.

Clinical signs and symptoms of malaria relate directly to red blood cell parasitism. Erythrocytes parasitized with developing parasites lodge in the microvasculature, causing tissue ischemia with resultant dysfunction and damage. Such tissue ischemia contributes to the dangerous process of cerebral malaria. The malarial paroxysm consists of chills and headache progressing to high fever, severe headache, myalgia, abdominal pain, delirium, nausea, and vomiting. The classic paroxysm of malaria occurs every 2 days, or in the case of *P. malariae* every 3 days, during the early evening at the time when the vectors, anopheline mosquitoes, usually feed. With acute malaria and malaria in the nonimmune person, the classic paroxysm with regular periodicity usually is not seen. Patients are often persistently febrile and symptomatic or have irregularly intermittent fever and symptoms. The paroxysm is associated with the lysis of parasitized erythrocytes with release of merozoites and other parasite products. The release of these products leads to fever and other systemic effects.

Another important pathophysiologic consequence is the hemolytic anemia resulting from destruction of red blood cells and the sequestration of parasitized erythrocytes in the spleen. Anemia may vary from mild to severe. Severe hemolysis may lead to hemoglobinuria and renal failure. Symptoms and anemia are usually most severe with *P. falciparum* infection, as this organism tends to cause the heaviest parasitemia because of its ability to invade erythrocytes of all ages (the other species have a predilection for young or old cells). Splenomegaly is frequent and splenic rupture is a dangerous but uncommon complication. Severe *P. falciparum* infection may be complicated by encephalopathy, "cerebral malaria," due to hypoxia resulting from deep vascular sequestration of parasitized erythrocytes. Nephrotic syndrome occurs only with *P. malariae* infection. This is probably related to the chronic, low grade, subclinical parasitism that occurs with this species. Such subclinical parasitism accounts for the observation that most transfusion-related cases of malaria are caused by *P. malariae.*

The diagnosis of malaria is made by examining stained smears of the peripheral blood. In a patient with unexplained fever, suspicion of malaria should be aroused by a history of residence in an endemic area. Blood smears may show ring forms, trophozoites, schizonts, and gametocytes. Interpretation of smears as to species usually requires expert consultation. Simultaneous infection with more than one species may occur.

The therapy of malaria is complicated by the widespread emergence of chloroquine resistance by *P. falciparum,* the species that causes the most severe disease. Chloroquine had been an effective, relatively inexpensive, and safe therapy for all forms of malaria. *P. falciparum,* probably related to the high levels of parasitemia it achieves, is capable of evolving mechanisms of drug resistance through pressure of natural selection. The widespread use of chloroquine provided this selective pressure. Chloroquine-resistant strains of this species are present, and new treatment strategies have been developed and are under investigation. Unfortunately, *P. falciparum* is becoming more resistant to other agents as well.

Treatment of choice for uncomplicated malaria caused by *P. vivax, P. ovale,* and *P. malariae* is chloroquine phosphate, 1 gram (600 mg base) orally, followed by half this dose at 6 hours and then once a day for 2 days. The equivalent initial pediatric dose would be 10 mg base/kg. Severe illness is treated with intravenous quinidine gluconate (with electrocardiographic [ECG] monitoring) followed by oral therapy if possible. Treatment of *P. vivax* and *P. ovale* must include primaquine phosphate, 15 mg base daily for 14 days or 45 mg base weekly for 8 weeks

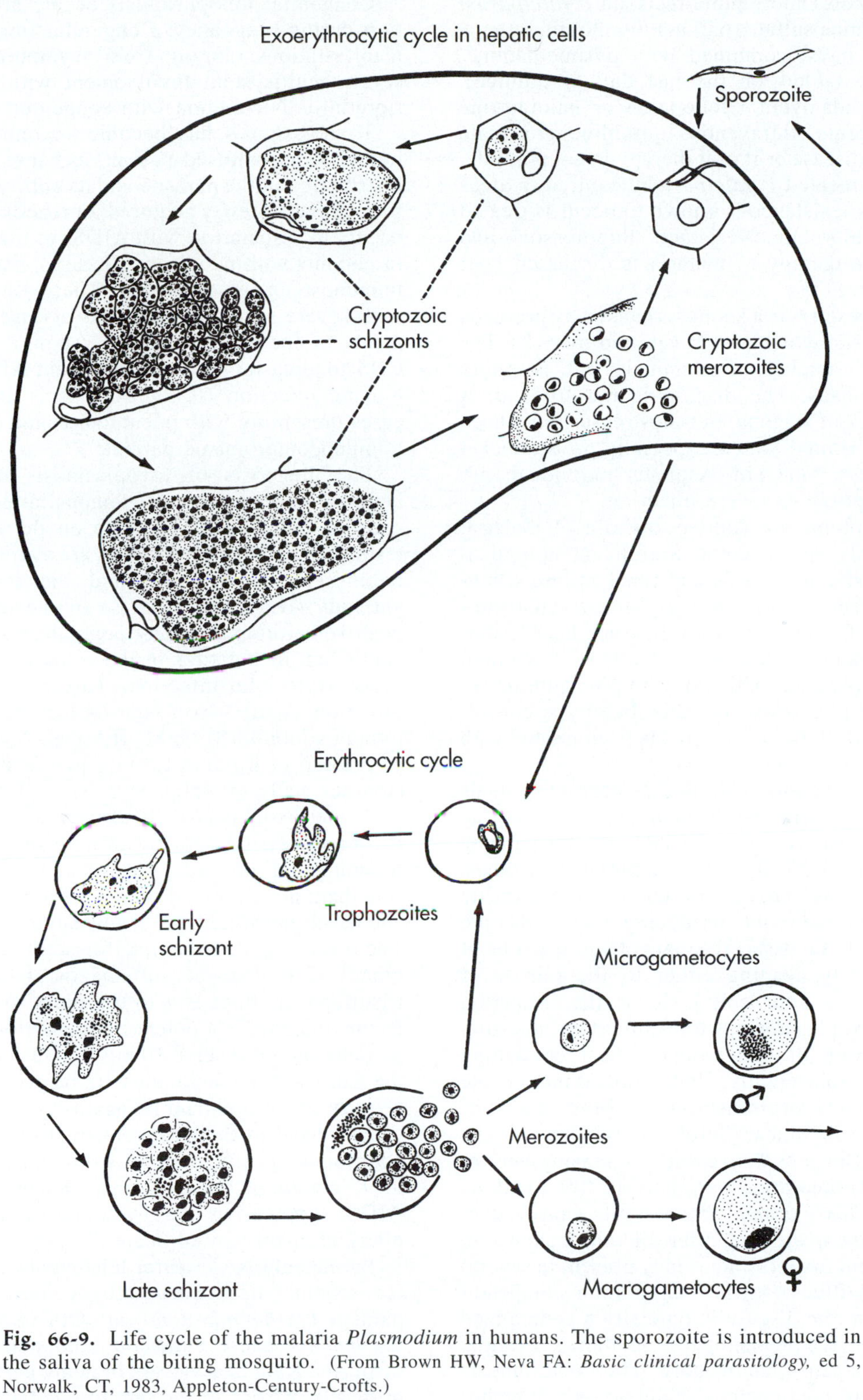


**Fig. 66-9.** Life cycle of the malaria *Plasmodium* in humans. The sporozoite is introduced in the saliva of the biting mosquito. (From Brown HW, Neva FA: *Basic clinical parasitology,* ed 5, Norwalk, CT, 1983, Appleton-Century-Crofts.)

(0.3 mg base/kg/day for 14 days in children) for "radical" cure with elimination of exoerythrocytic forms. Glucose-6-phosphate dehydrogenase deficiency must be ruled out before initiating primaquine therapy, because the drug may precipitate hemolysis. Chloroquine-resistant *P. falciparum* is treated with quinine sulfate (650 mg, by mouth, every 8 hours for 3 to 7 days) combined with pyrimethamine/sulfadoxine (three tablets on the last day of quinine), tetracycline or clindamycin. Mefloquine or halofantrine are alternative agents. Intravenous quinidine gluconate is used for severe disease or if oral therapy is not possible. Suspected or documented *P. falciparum* acquired in areas where chloroquine resistance is known to occur is treated as if it were chloroquine-resistant. Suppressive and chemoprophylactic therapy of malaria is discussed later (see Advice to Travelers).

**Babesiosis.** Babesiosis is a zoonosis caused by protozoa of the genus *Babesia,* which are transmitted by ticks. The parasite infects a number of mammals but is rarely transmitted to humans. The disease is not tropical. It occurs in a number of regions, but most cases have been reported from the United States, especially on Nantucket Island and Martha's Vineyard. Asplenic individuals are particularly susceptible to severe infection.

Signs and symptoms are similar to those of malaria: fever, splenomegaly, and anemia. Significant complications include massive hemolysis and renal failure. Diagnosis is made by demonstrating intraerythrocytic parasites on blood smears. Effective therapy has not been established. Chloroquine may cause symptomatic relief without eradication of the parasites. Clindamycin plus quinine are often used to treat babesiosis, but this therapy is considered investigational. Babesiosis also has been treated with exchange transfusion.

**Toxoplasmosis.** Toxoplasmosis is a disease of animals and people, widely distributed throughout the world. The protozoan *Toxoplasma gondii* is an intracellular parasite capable of invading virtually all mammalian cell types. The definitive host is the cat. In the cat the parasite undergoes sexual reproduction, producing oocysts that are passed in the stool. In tissue the parasite is capable of multiplying asexually, leading either to the release of invasive trophozoites after cell lysis or the formation of tissue cysts. Toxoplasmosis is transmitted by ingestion of oocysts, ingestion of undercooked meat containing tissue cysts, or transplacentally. Undercooked meat is the most common means of transmission. Most cases of toxoplasmosis are subclinical. Serologic evidence of past infection increases in prevalence with increasing age. In some parts of the United States, as many as 70% of adults have antibody to *Toxoplasma.* Tissue cysts cause latent disease that may reactivate long after the initial exposure.

Clinically evident toxoplasmosis may present in several different forms of illness. In normal immunocompetent adults and children, the disease is typically a generalized febrile illness with lymphadenopathy, malaise, myalgia, sore throat, and hepatosplenomegaly. This syndrome is similar to infectious mononucleosis, and atypical lymphocytes may appear in the peripheral blood. Occasionally, a maculopapular rash occurs. The disease also may present predominantly as a localized process involving the CNS, liver, heart, or other organ. Of special importance is ocular toxoplasmosis, which is usually the result of congenital infection, but occasionally is acquired after birth. Characteristic lesions of chorioretinitis may be seen on funduscopic examination. These lesions may remain latent or reactivate with increasing damage to vision.

Congenital toxoplasmosis occurs after primary infection during pregnancy. Congenital infection has protean manifestations ranging from asymptomatic infection to severe multisystem involvement with retardation. Chorioretinitis is common with congenital infection.

Toxoplasmosis has become an important problem in immunocompromised patients because of the ubiquitous distribution of the parasite and its ability to exist in a latent form. Severe, newly acquired, or reactivated latent disease occurs in association with AIDS, in transplant recipients, in patients with neoplastic diseases, and others receiving immunosuppressive therapy. These patients may present with severe systemic illness or disease located predominantly in one organ or organ system, especially the CNS. CNS toxoplasmosis is an important AIDS-related opportunistic infection. Toxoplasmosis is among several diseases presenting with pneumonitis and encephalitis in the immunocompromised patient.

The diagnosis of toxoplasmosis may be made by isolating the parasite or demonstrating it in histologic sections, but usually is made on the basis of serologic testing. Several serologic tests are available, including the Sabin-Feldman dye test and the indirect fluorescent antibody (IFA) test. Because of the high prevalence of positive serology in many populations, the presence of a single significant titer in these tests cannot differentiate acute from old infection. Rising titers imply recent infection. Acute toxoplasmosis may be diagnosed by the immunoglobulin M (IgM)-IFA test. A single titer of 1:80 or greater, or a rising titer on two or more observations, signifies acute infection.

Acute toxoplasmosis is usually self-limited. Treatment is limited to patients with severe disease or those who are immunocompromised. The therapy of choice is pyrimethamine combined with a sulfonamide, sulfadiazine, and trisulfapyrimidines ("triple sulfa") being most active. The dose of pyrimethamine for adults is 25 mg/day for 1 month. The dose of sulfadiazine is 1 to 2 g and of trisulfapyrimidines is 2 to 6 g daily for the same period. Pyrimethamine is a potent bone marrow suppressant, and patients should receive 10 mg folinic acid a day to support the marrow. Folic acid must not be given, as it inhibits the activity of pyrimethamine against *T. gondii.* Steroids are usually used in the treatment of ocular toxoplasmosis in addition to specific therapy, as the inflammatory response to *T. gondii* increases retinal damage. In patients with AIDS, suppressive therapy should be maintained indefinitely after therapy of acute disease.

**Leishmaniasis.** Visceral leishmaniasis, or "kala-azar," is a systemic disease caused by the intracellular protozoan parasite *Leishmania donovani.* Other species of the genus *Leishmania* cause cutaneous and mucocutaneous leishmaniasis. Kala-azar occurs in many parts of the world but primarily in tropical and semitropical regions. The parasite has many animal reservoirs and is transmitted by the bite of sandflies of the genus *Phlebotomus.* The parasites invade reticuloendothelial cells throughout the body, leading to marked proliferation and hyperplasia. Hyperglobulinemia and antigen-antibody complexes further complicate the disease and glomerulonephritis may occur. The onset may be insidious or acute and is associated with high fever. Chills and diarrhea frequently are present. The disease then has a progressive course of prolonged fever, weight loss, organomegaly (which is often of a marked degree), anemia, hypoalbuminemia, and peripheral edema. Visceral leishmaniasis may complicate HIV infection and other causes of immunocompromise.

The diagnosis is made on the basis of typical clinical findings in the right epidemiologic setting or the demonstration of parasites in tissue.

The disease is treated with stibogluconate (antimony) 20 mg/kg per day (up to 800 mg/day) intramuscularly or intravenously for 20 to 28 days. The dose in children is 10 mg/kg per day (up to 600 mg). Stibogluconate resistance has been seen in some areas of the world. Pentamidine and amphotericine B are alternative therapeutic agents when stibogluconate cannot be used or resistance is encountered. The combination of gamma interferon and stibogluconate may be superior to stibogluconate alone. Untreated, symptomatic disease is usually fatal.

**Trypanosomiasis.** Trypanosomes are hemoflagellate protozoans that cause African trypanosomiasis, or sleeping sickness, and American trypanosomiasis, or Chagas' disease. *Trypanosoma brucei gambiense* (West African) and *T. brucei rhodesiense* (East African) are the etiologic agents of sleeping sickness and are transmitted by various strains of the tsetse fly. After the bite of an infected fly, a skin lesion appears at the site. The parasites reproduce in the skin lesion. Dissemination from the initial lesion leads to fever, severe headache, rash, and localized areas of edema. Lymphadenopathy then becomes prominent, especially of the posterior cervical chain. Hepatomegaly and splenomegaly may occur. The disease spreads to the CNS where cerebral damage occurs, leading to the characteristic signs of somnolence, headache, and other neurologic manifestations that eventually lead to continuous sleep. *T. brucei rhodesiense* tends to cause a fulminant disease over months, whereas *T. brucei gambiense* causes a disease that progresses over years. Inapparent infection has been described with the latter.

Diagnosis usually is made by demonstrating parasites in the blood or lymph node aspirates, although serologic tests also are available. Early disease, characterized by a predominance of systemic signs and lymphadenopathy, is treatable with suramin, eflornithine or pentamidine, whereas CNS disease is treated with melarsoprol or eflornithine. These drugs are available through the CDC and should be used only with the guidance of the Parasitic Diseases Division of the CDC.

Chagas' disease is caused by *T. cruzi* and is transmitted through the feces of biting insects of the reduvid group. These insects defecate while taking their blood meal, and parasites in the feces make their way into small wounds, conjunctivae, and mucous membranes. The disease is limited to the Western Hemisphere and has occurred as far north as Texas. Reduvid bugs capable of transmitting *T. cruzi* are found in large parts of North America; therefore the potential for spread of infection in the United States exists wherever small mammals live in close proximity to humans. Transmission of trypanosomiasis by blood transfusion from asymptomatic, chronically infected donors also is a concern.

Among infected individuals, 10% to 30% eventually develop symptomatic disease. The morbidity of American trypanosomiasis is primarily related to chronic infection. In endemic areas, Chagas' disease is a major cause of myocarditis and cardiomyopathy, as well as alimentary tract dysfunction manifested by megaesophagus and megacolon. Acute Chagas' disease is a febrile illness that appears 1 to 2 weeks after exposure to the parasite. It is characterized by systemic toxicity, variable fever, lymphadenopathy, hepatosplenomegaly, and signs of myocarditis. A "chagoma" (a macular, desquamating lesion) may be seen at the site of inoculation. Romaña's sign, unilateral ophthalmia with palpebral edema, may occur. In most cases the acute disease lasts approximately 2 weeks. Acute Chagas' disease in the immunocompromised host can follow a fulminant course. This development has been observed in patients immunosuppressed from cancer chemotherapy. It can be presumed that similar severe disease may occur in patients with immunosuppression due to HIV infection.

The classic means of diagnosing acute Chagas' disease is by xenodiagnosis (i.e., allowing laboratory-bred bugs to bite the patient and examining the bugs for parasites after 1 to 2 months). Parasites also may be demonstrated directly in peripheral smears or by injection of blood into mice. Several serologic tests are available including an enzyme-linked immunosorbent assay (ELISA) that are useful in screening for chronic infection.

Acute Chagas' disease is treatable with two agents, nifurtimox and benznidazole; but the required treatment is prolonged and associated with a high rate of adverse reactions. All cases are not cured. Chronic disease is treated supportively.

## Tissue-invasive roundworms

***Filariasis.*** Filarial infections are caused by a number of tissue-dwelling nematodes. These diseases occur primarily in tropical and semitropical regions and are transmitted by biting insects. The sexually mature filarial worms live in various tissues and produce microfilarial larvae that migrate in blood and tissues. Clinical manifestations of these infections result from the residence of adult forms in tissue, migration of the adult worms, and the release and migration of the larvae. Much of the morbidity results from hypersensitivity to the parasites. Filarial infections are summarized in Table 66-4.

The major filarial infections, due to *Wuchereria bancrofti, Brugia malayi, Loa loa,* and *Onchocerca volvulus,* affect millions of people in endemic areas; but only a small proportion of those affected develop overt clinical disease. The adult worms cause most of the signs and symptoms of these infections, except for *O. volvulus* infection, in which the microfilariae cause eye damage leading to "river blindness." Hypersensitivity reactions to microfilariae cause most of the systemic manifestations of these diseases, and eosinophilia is usually prominent (see later). Several animal filaria have been described in humans, almost all cases of which have been recognized in the United States. Human zoonotic filarial disease is basically the result of the host reaction to parasites that find themselves in an incompatible host.

Diethylcarbamazine is effective against most of the human filariae, but the adult forms of *O. volvulus* are not

**Table 66-4.** Filarial infections in humans

| Agent | Distribution | Vector | Clinical manifestations related to: Residence of adult worms | Clinical manifestations related to: Migration of microfilariae | Diagnostic procedure | Treatment |
|---|---|---|---|---|---|---|
| *Wuchereria bancrofti* | Asia<br>Latin America<br>Pacific islands | Mosquitos | Lymphatic tissue<br>Lymphadenitis<br>Lymphadenopathy<br>Elephantiasis<br>Hydrocele<br>Chyluria | Blood<br>Eosinophilia<br>Allergic reactions<br>Usually nocturnal periodicity | Membrane filtration of blood | Diethylcarbamatine [DEC] PO<br>Day 1: 50 mg, once<br>Day 2: 50 mg, tid<br>Day 3: 100 mg, tid<br>Days 4-21: 2 mg/kg, tid |
| *Brugia malayi*<br>*B. timori* | Southeast Asia<br>India<br>China, Korea<br>Indonesia | Mosquitos | | Some subperiodicity | | |
| *Loa loa* | West Africa<br>Central Africa | Tabanid horseflies (*Chrysops* sp.) | Migratory in subcutaneous tissue<br>Erythematous "Calabar" swellings<br>Visible subconjunctival migration | Blood (Eosinophils)<br>Diurnal periodicity | (At peak microfilaria parasitemia, when periodicity present) | DEC, PO<br>Days 1-3: as above<br>Days 4-21: 3 mg/kg, tid |
| *Mansonella perstans* | Africa<br>South America | Midges | Body cavities<br>Asymptomatic to mild abdominal pain and swellings | Blood<br>Minimal to no symptoms<br>Nonperiodic | | Mebendazole, PO 100 mg, bid for 30 days |
| *M. ozzardi* | South America<br>Central America | Midges | Body cavities<br>Mild systemic symptoms | Blood<br>Nonperiodic | | Ivermectin, PO 150 μg/kg, once |
| *M. streptocerca* | Central Africa<br>West Africa | Midges | Skin | Skin, lymph nodes<br>Dermatitis | Skin biopsy | ? DEC (see above) |
| *Onchocerca volvulus* | Africa<br>Central America<br>South America<br>Yemen | Black flies (*Simulium* sp.) | Soft tissue<br>Subcutaneous nodules | Skin and subcutaneous tissue<br>Rash<br>Keratitis, iritis<br>Blindness | Skin snips (larvae)<br>Biopsy of nodule (adult) | Ivermectin 150 μg/kg once<br>Repeat every 6 to 12 months |

killed and go on to produce more microfilariae unless excised or treated with an effective drug such as ivermectin. Ivermectin has become the drug of choice for the treatment of *O. volvulus.* Diethylcarbamazine can produce an encephalopathy in patients who have a heavy infection with *Loa loa.* Relatively severe allergic reactions can result from the breakdown of killed microfilariae of *L. loa* and *O. volvulus* when diethylcarbamazine is used. Such reactions may require treatment with steroids and antihistamines.

***Trichinosis.*** *Trichinella spiralis* is an intestinal roundworm, the invasive larvae of which encyst in muscle tissue and produce the systemic disease trichinosis. The life cycle of *T. spiralis* is presented in Fig. 66-10. The disease is acquired by ingestion of poorly cooked meat, especially pork, that contains encysted larvae. Outbreaks in the United States also have been associated with bear meat. The ingested larvae become sexually mature in the small intestine, and the adults attach to the mucosa and produce offspring; these larvae invade the gut, migrate to muscle tissue, and encyst. The adult worms are shed in the stool after 2 to 4 weeks. The severity of trichinosis depends on the number of invading larvae and ranges from asymptomatic to fatal.

The disease manifests as an early phase of diarrhea and abdominal pain followed by characteristic periorbital edema, myalgia, fever, sweats, weakness, and eosinophilia. Myocarditis is an important cause of death, and the disease may affect the CNS.

The diagnosis is usually made on clinical grounds, especially when there is a history of ingestion of suspect meat. Subingual sphincter hemorrhages and a low sedimentation rate are hallmarks of the acute illness. Diagnosis is made definitively by biopsy of muscle. Several serologic tests also are available, the simplest and most rapid being the bentonite flocculation test.

Specific therapy for muscle disease is not available. Mebendazole and steroids are usually used in severe disease. Control of this disease depends on adequate cooking of meat (freezing for 3 weeks or more is also effective) and safe food sources for swine.

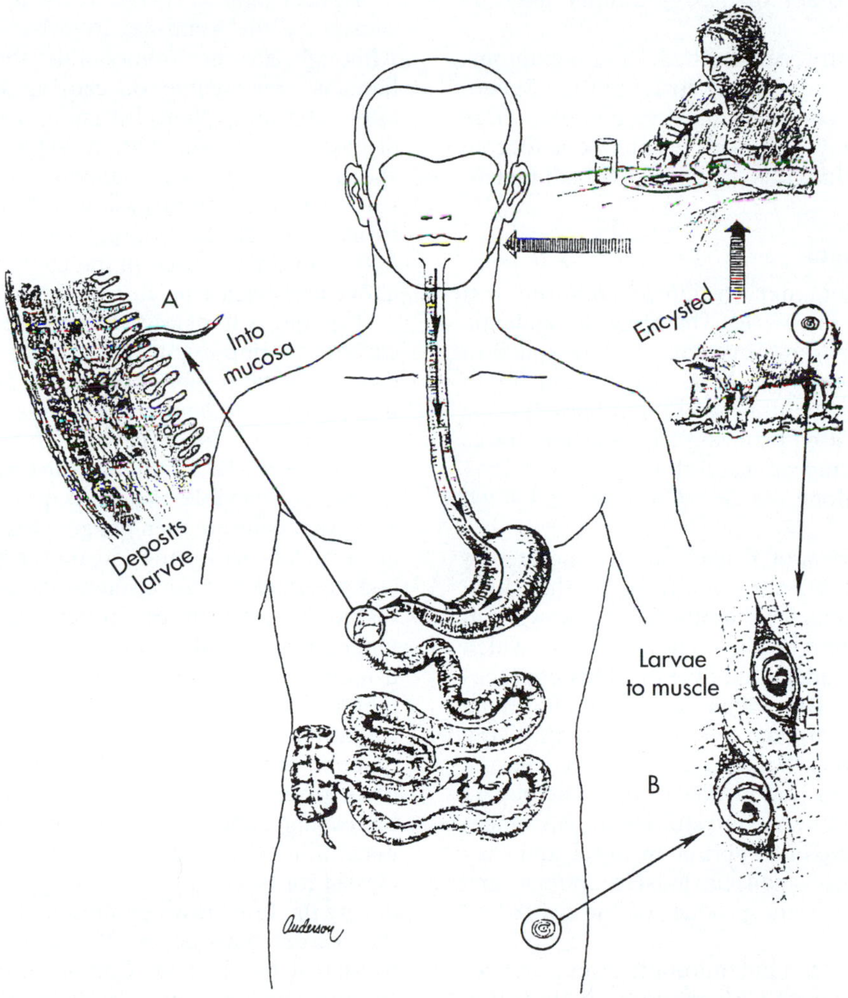


**Fig. 66-10.** Life cycle of *Trichinella spiralis.* Infective larvae, encysted in pork and other meat, when ingested, become adult worms in the small intestine. The female burrows into the mucosa and deposits larvae into lacteals and blood vessels. Circulating larvae eventually penetrate skeletal muscle and become encysted *(A).* In humans these larvae are at a dead end, but in the pig and other animals they become a source of infection *(B).* (From Beck JW, Davies JE: *Medical parasitology,* ed 3, 1981, Mosby.)

***Visceral larva migrans.*** Visceral larva migrans is a systemic disease, usually occurring in children, which is caused by tissue migration of the larvae of nonhuman ascarid parasites of the genus *Toxocara*. The usual host of *T. canis* is the dog and of *T. cati* the cat; *T. leonina* occurs in both. Eggs are shed in the feces of young dogs and cats. Children become infected by ingesting contaminated soil. The eggs hatch in the intestine and larvae invade the bowel and begin a persistent migration through the liver, CNS, muscle, and other organs. This migration may persist for weeks to months to years.

Most patients with visceral larva migrans are asymptomatic but may have pronounced peripheral blood eosinophilia. Symptomatic disease is primarily due to the host response to the parasite and is characterized by fever, cough, bronchospasm, hepatomegaly, and abdominal pain. CNS abnormalities and seizures may predominate. Endophthalmitis also may occur, usually in older children and often without significant systemic signs.

The diagnosis is made by association of the clinical picture with eosinophilia and a history of pica. These larval parasites share A and B blood group antigens with humans and elevated titers of isoagglutinins may be helpful in diagnosis.

The disease is usually self-limited, and symptoms usually resolve despite continued eosinophilia. Severe disease is treated with diethylcarbamazine, 2 mg/kg, three times a day for 7 to 10 days; alternatives are mebendazole or albendazole. Endophthalmitis is treated with adjunctive steroids.

## Enteric bacterial infections

***Vibrio cholerae.*** Cholera due to *Vibrio cholerae* still occurs in many parts of the world. The seventh pandemic caused by the "el tor" strain began in 1961 in southern Asia and has spread to central Asia, Africa, and South America, with occasional outbreaks in southern Europe and the South Pacific. Cases resulting from earlier strains of the organism surviving in natural habitats for long periods have occurred along the Gulf Coast of the United States.

When sufficient numbers of *V. cholerae* are ingested to provide an infective dose, they multiply in the small intestine lumen and adhere to epithelial cells without damaging them. They then produce cholera toxin, which stimulates epithelial cell adenylate cyclase. This produces elevated levels of cyclic adenosine monophosphate (AMP), blocking sodium uptake by the cells and causing massive flux of water, bicarbonate, and chloride into the lumen. The organisms do not invade tissue. The severe watery diarrhea produced by the physiologic derangement resulting from cholera toxin is abrupt in onset and may lead to severe dehydration, nausea, muscle cramps, and shock. The disease state is the product of the water and electrolyte loss.

Diagnosis is based on the epidemiologic circumstances and the severe, watery diarrhea. Microscopic examination of stained stool smears may show a monotonous flora of curved gram-negative rods. Treatment is designed to compensate for the water and electrolyte losses with intravenous fluids. Oral replacement fluid composed of sodium and potassium chloride, glucose, and bicarbonate is used. This solution provides sodium in the presence of glucose. The glucose-linked uptake of sodium by the intestinal epithelium is a system independent of the sodium uptake system blocked by the effect of cholera toxin. Preparations of oral rehydration solution ingredients are available for use in cases of diarrhea of any cause and are the mainstay of supportive treatment of moderate to severe diarrhea. Tetracycline and other antimicrobial agents are used to eradicate organisms.

Some strains of *V. Cholerae* are not of the 01 serotype (which includes the classic and *eltor* strains). These so-called nonagglutinable or non-01 strains occasionally have been implicated in small outbreaks of diarrheal illness and cases of invasive diarrhea similar to shigellosis. In 1992, a non-01 *V. cholerae* of the 0139 serotype caused epidemics of cholera-like illness in Bangladesh and India. *V. cholerae* 0139 produces cholera toxin and causes illness indistinguishable from cholera. It has continued to spread and cause epidemic disease and may be on its way to causing the eighth pandemic of cholera. The management of infection and disease with *V. cholerae* 0139 is the same for *V. cholerae* 01 of both the classic and *eltor* varieties.

***Typhoid fever.*** Typhoid fever is the systemic infection caused by the gram-negative bacillus *Salmonella typhi*. Although all the salmonellae that are pathogenic for humans are capable of causing disseminated infection after gastrointestinal invasion, i.e., enteric fever, such disease is the rule with *S. typhi*. This organism has a special virulence for humans, and people are its only natural hosts. The disease is still a major health problem in parts of the developing world. Approximately 400 to 500 cases are reported in the United States each year, with about half occurring in recent travelers.

Typhoid is transmitted by the fecal-oral route. Chronic carriers are important sources of disease in areas where the disease occurs sporadically. In places where there are many cases and sanitation is poor, sewage contamination of water and foodstuffs is important. The organisms reproduce in the small intestine and, like all the salmonellae, are capable of penetrating the intestinal mucosa. The organisms are then phagocytosed by macrophages, but are resistant to killing, so they reproduce intracellularly and eventually cause bacteremia and disseminated foci of viable bacteria in the reticuloendothelial system. The incubation period from ingestion to clinical disease is usually 1 to 2 weeks; however, it may be as long as 1 month.

Patients with typhoid fever may present with severe toxemia or relatively mild fever and systemic complaints of headache and myalgia. They then go on to develop increasing abdominal pain, constipation, and abdominal distention. Rose spots, the maculopapular rash that is classic for typhoid fever may appear, usually on the trunk, during the full-blown evolution of the disease. Bleeding in the rectum may occur. The disease is characterized by persistent bacteremia. Complications include bowel perforation, hemorrhage, and metastatic foci (e.g., osteomyelitis, meningitis, and pyelonephritis). Most patients have peripheral leukopenia during the disease. Overwhelming disease may lead to hepatic and renal damage. The untreated disease may progress for weeks with increasing fever and debilitation, or it may remit after 2 to 3 weeks (with the possibility of relapse). Some patients (about 3%)

retain a focus of gallbladder infection after acute disease and remain chronic asymptomatic carriers of the organism and potential sources of new infection.

The diagnosis of typhoid fever is made in a patient who has the characteristic signs and symptoms of the illness with a history of possible exposure consistent with the epidemiology of the disease. Blood cultures provide the definitive diagnosis. During the first 1 to 2 weeks of illness, blood cultures are almost always positive. Later these cultures may be negative, but they usually become positive with relapse. Stool and urine cultures are more likely to be positive late in the disease. Serologic tests are available and a fourfold rise in agglutination (Widal test) titer is consistent with disease, although cross-reactions with other salmonellae may occur.

Ciprofloxacin and third-generation cephalosporin antibiotics, such as ceftriaxone and cefoperazone, have become drugs of choice for the treatment of typhoid fever. Although chloramphenicol, trimethoprim-sulfamethoxazole, and ampicillin have remained effective for susceptible strains of *S. typhi,* many multidrug-resistant strains that are resistant to some or all of these agents are being isolated in developing countries. Ciprofloxacin in a dose of 400 mg, intravenously, every 12 hours for 10 to 14 days and orally, 500 mg, twice a day for an additional 7 to 11 days should be effective in most cases. In patients with mild illness who are capable of oral therapy, ciprofloxacin 500 to 750 mg orally twice a day for 14 to 21 days may be used. Neither ciprofloxacin nor any other fluoroquinolone should be given to children or pregnant women because of interference with cartilage formation and possible teratogenic effects. Ceftriaxone may be given in a dose of 2 g intravenously a day and cefoperazone as 2 g intravenously twice a day, both for 14 days. Ampicillin and trimethoprim-sulfamethoxazole, parenterally and orally, are satisfactory and less costly alternatives when the infecting strain is known to be sensitive. Corticosteroid therapy with dexamethasone is beneficial as adjunctive therapy in severe typhoid fever.

Typhoid vaccine affords some protection against acquisition of *S. typhi* infection, but is no substitute for caution (see Advice for Travelers). Parenteral heat-phenol-inactivated vaccine has been available for many years. It is administered in two doses, 4 weeks apart with a booster every 3 years. A more recently developed oral, live-attenuated vaccine of the Ty21a strain of *S. typhi* also has efficacy. The oral vaccine is given with cool liquids, 1 hour before meals, every other day, for four doses.

The best preventive measures for typhoid are good sanitation, good personal hygiene, identification of carriers, and careful follow-up of cases.

## Systemic bacterial diseases (including plague)

Many bacterial diseases have a higher prevalence in tropical regions. Diseases such as cholera, typhoid fever, and meningococcal, staphylococcal, and streptococcal infections are discussed elsewhere in the text. Certain febrile diseases caused by bacteria have particular geographic distributions and are associated with tropical and semitropical areas. The following discussion is limited to bacterial diseases that cause systemic, febrile illness and that are not discussed in sections dealing with particular organ systems.

***Brucellosis.*** Brucellosis is a disease of worldwide distribution, but is especially prevalent along the Mediterranean (where it is known as Mediterranean fever) and in Mexico and South America. The disease is primarily a zoonosis affecting many domestic and wild animals. Four species of gram-negative bacilli of the genus *Brucella* infecting humans have been described: *B. abortus* (usually from a bovine source), *B. melitensis* (goats), *B. suis* (swine), and *B. canis* (dogs). People acquire disease through close exposure to infected animals, meat, and dairy products. Most cases in the United States are related to occupational exposures (e.g., meat packing and farming).

The spectrum of the disease can range from mild inapparent infection, to localized abscess formation, to severe systemic disease. Onset of disease is usually insidious with nonspecific symptoms of fatigue, sweats, chills, myalgia, arthralgia, and headache. Fever ranges from hectic to intermittent to absent. Axillary and cervical lymphadenopathy may occur, and splenomegaly has been observed in about 50% of patients with bacteremia. Fatality is rare with brucellosis, but some patients develop chronic infection with persistent malaise, anorexia, depression, and visceral or skeletal abscesses. The course of brucellosis may be complicated by mycotic aneurysm, encephalitis, meningitis, endocarditis, pneumonia, renal disease, and osteomyelitis.

Diagnosis of brucellosis is made by isolating the organism from blood or tissues or serodiagnosis, usually using agglutination tests. Treatment is with tetracycline for 3 to 4 weeks, combined with streptomycin for severe disease. Relapses after therapy are common.

***Bartonellosis.*** *Bartonella bacilliformis* is a gram-negative bacillus that is the causative agent of bartonellosis, or Oroya fever, and the skin disease verruga peruana. The organism is transmitted from person to person through the bites of sandflies of the genus *Phlebotomus.* The disease occurs naturally in only one part of the world, the Andean mountain valleys of Peru, Ecuador, and Colombia. Asymptomatic carrier rates approach 5% in this area.

The bacilli are capable of invading endothelial cells and erythrocytes. Hemolytic anemia results from destruction of parasitized erythrocytes. The clinical disease is associated with irregular fever, anemia, headache, myalgia, arthralgia, bone pain, and lymphadenopathy. Fatality rates in untreated cases approach 40% and patients with bartonellosis have a peculiar susceptibility to invasive salmonellosis that commonly complicates the disease. Survivors of Oroya fever may go on to develop the cutaneous phase of the disease, verruga peruana, which consists of pathognomonic skin lesions and nodular hemangiomas.

The diagnosis is made on clinical grounds by the association of fever and hemolytic anemia in a person exposed to the endemic area. The organism may be isolated in blood cultures or demonstrated on the surface of erythrocytes on a blood smear. The drug of choice for treatment is chloramphenicol.

***Plague.*** Plague is an ancient disease of enormous historical significance that still warrants fear and concern. The etiologic agent is the gram-negative bacillus, *Yersinia pestis.* Sylvatic plague is a zoonosis of wild rodents that is prevalent in large parts of the world including South America, South and Central Africa, Central Asia, the Near East, and the southwestern United States. The disease is maintained in wild, burrowing rodents as a relatively mild illness. Sylvatic plague may be passed to people by the bite of a flea from an infected wild rodent, and sporadic cases of human plague occur in endemic areas. The great plague epidemics resulted from a domestic cycle of infection involving rats and their fleas. Domestic rats with plague usually die and their fleas go to other rats or people, thereby spreading the epizootic and epidemic.

Plague occurs in several forms in humans. Bubonic plague is usually the result of flea-transmitted infection. The incubation period is 2 to 7 days. Bubonic plague begins as a febrile illness associated with the development of painful, swollen lymph nodes, or buboes. After evolution of the lymphadenitis, a secondary septicemia occurs with severe toxicity, prostration, and shock. Pestis minor is a clinical variant of bubonic plague characterized by the presence of a bubo with less severe systemic signs. Primary septicemic plague without evident localized infection occurs in few cases during epidemics. Approximately 5% of patients with plague develop pneumonia, usually as a preterminal event. Primary pneumonic plague results from person-to-person transmission of plague via droplets or as the result of inhalation of other material contaminated by plague bacilli. Pneumonic plague may be maintained in a cycle of person-to-person transmission.

Patients with plague often develop hemodynamic instability, staggering gait, confusion, and delirium. The course of plague may be complicated by meningitis, pneumonia, and disseminated intravascular coagulation. The fatality rate of untreated bubonic plague is 50% and higher, and pneumonic and primary septicemic plague are almost always fatal.

Diagnosis of plague is made by demonstrating organisms in smears of bubo aspirates, blood, or spinal fluid. It is confirmed by culture.

Treatment must begin before culture results are known, as delays result in failure of clinical cure despite bacteriologic response, and the patient may die of irreversible toxic effects of infection. The drug of choice is streptomycin, and it is often combined with chloramphenicol or tetracycline. Persons closely exposed to wild rodents in plague endemic areas or who have potential laboratory exposure to plague should receive plague vaccine. Case contacts are handled by defleaing, surveillance, quarantine, and chemoprophylaxis.

In the American Southwest, sporadic cases of human plague occur as the result of exposure to prairie dogs, squirrels, chipmunks, and other burrowing rodents. The disease frequently is seen in hunters. Because the plague bacillus is endemic in most of the Southwest United States, it must always be considered in the diagnosis of severe febrile illness or lymphadenopathy in that area, be diagnosed as rapidly as possible, and be treated early. Proper isolation precautions must be taken to prevent spread.

***Tularemia.*** Tularemia is an infection of rodents and rabbits caused by the gram-negative bacillus *Francisella tularensis,* which is transmitted to people by exposure to infected tissues, by inhalation of contaminated material, and by biting arthropods. The disease occurs only in the northern temperate zones.

Tularemia in humans appears as several clinical syndromes that might be confused with plague. Ulceroglandular tularemia is characterized by an ulcerative skin lesion with regional lymphadenitis. Glandular tularemia refers to the presence of bubolike lymphadenitis without a skin lesion. Oculoglandular disease results from conjunctival inoculation and involves the periorbital tissues and lymph nodes of the head and neck. Septicemic tularemia is similar to primary septicemic plague in that localized lymph node or skin involvement may not be apparent. Ingestion tularemia is characterized by gastrointestinal symptoms with or without pharyngitis. Pulmonary tularemia may be primary, but more commonly occurs as a complication of septicemic disease.

Tularemia in the United States occurs primarily as the result of occupational exposure to animal materials (e.g., pelts) or in hunters similarly exposed. Fleas are important vectors. An epidemic of tularemia pneumonia occurred in New England that was related to inhalation of drafts from a chimney containing a dead animal. Tularemia should be suspected in any case of relatively severe systemic disease (especially with skin lesions) or pneumonia in an individual exposed to wild animals.

Diagnosis of tularemia is confirmed by culture or serology. Streptomycin is the drug of choice for therapy.

***Rat-bite fever.*** The term *rat-bite fever* is used to describe two diseases. Rat-bite fevers occur in areas of crowding and poor socioeconomic conditions where close exposure to rats leads to bites or other contacts. One rat-bite disease is caused by the gram-negative rod *Streptobacillus moniliformis* and is called Haverhill fever. The disease is characterized by edema, ulceration, and abscess formation at the rat-bite site, which is associated with intermittent fever paroxysms, a maculopapular to petechial rash, and polyarthritis. The rash frequently involves the palms and soles. Diagnosis is made by the clinical history and the course of the disease, by serologic studies, or by animal inoculation.

The other disease, sodoku, is caused by *Spirillum minus,* a gram-negative organism that is transmitted primarily by rat bite. The disease is characterized by inflammation at the bite site, lymphadenitis, paroxysmal fever, and a dark red, macular rash. Arthritis is absent. The diagnosis is made by darkfield examination of exudates or animal inoculation.

Haverhill fever has been described primarily in the United States, whereas sodoku is the prevalent rat-bite fever in Japan and Asia. A fatality rate of 10% is reported in untreated cases of both diseases. The treatment of choice for both is penicillin, with tetracycline and streptomycin as alternatives.

### Rickettsial diseases

Rickettsiae are obligate, intracellular bacteria that infect a variety of mammals and arthropod vectors. The organisms invade endothelial cells and cause vasculitis. Most diseases caused by rickettsiae can be categorized into two groups: the spotted fevers and the typhus group. Other rickettsial diseases are Q fever, trench fever, and the ehrlichoises.

Among the rickettsial spotted fevers are Rocky Mountain spotted fever (caused by *Rickettsia rickettsii*); boutonneuse fever, South African tick bite fever, and Indian and Kenyan tick typhus (all caused by *R. conorii*); Queensland tick typhus *(R. australis);* and North Asian tick typhus *(R. sibirica).* All of these diseases are transmitted by ticks and have wild rodent and other animal reservoirs.

The spotted fevers are characterized by an acute febrile illness with chills and headache, followed in several days by the eruption of a maculopapular rash often involving the palms and soles. The rash may become petechial to purpuric. A primary ulcerative lesion with an eschar at the site of the tick bite usually occurs with *R. conorii* and *R. sibirica* infections, occasionally in Queensland tick typhus, but never in Rocky Mountain spotted fever. Rocky Mountain spotted fever occurs in North and South America. Boutonneuse fever and the other *R. conorii* infections occur along the Mediterranean Sea and in Africa and India. The geographic distribution of the other rickettsial spotted fevers are indicated by their name.

Rickettsialpox is another member of the spotted fever group and is caused by *R. akari,* which has the house mouse as reservoir and a mite as vector. The course is usually mild. This disease is characterized by a primary papule followed by a febrile illness and a maculopapular rash that becomes vesicular. The primary papule becomes vesicular and then evolves into an eschar. Rickettsialpox has been described primarily in the United States and Russia in urban settings, but sporadic cases from tropical areas also have been reported.

Rocky Mountain spotted fever is the most important of the rickettsial spotted fevers in the United States. The name of the disease derives from where it was first studied. Most cases now occur along the East Coast of the United States, especially in suburban areas of Virginia and Maryland, and places such as Cape Cod. The disease occurs in any area in which the tick vector, usually of the genus *Dermacentor,* is prevalent. The most important preventive measure is avoidance of ticks.

Rocky Mountain spotted fever should be suspected in any patient who has a febrile illness with severe headache that progresses in association with the development of a petechial or purpuric rash. In Rocky Mountain spotted fever, prodromal symptoms usually occur for several days before the rash; whereas in meningococcal disease the rash usually appears shortly after the onset of illness. Obviously the differential diagnosis of these two diseases is critical. Treatment must be prompt in either case.

The typhus group of rickettsial diseases includes epidemic typhus *(R. prowazekii).* Epidemic typhus appears to have humans as its only reservoir, although flying squirrels have been implicated; it is transmitted by the body louse. Epidemic typhus may occur anywhere in the world under situations of deprivation, crowding, and pediculosis. Recurrent typhus, known as Brill-Zinsser disease, may occur many years after initial infection and may appear in immigrants to areas where practitioners are unfamiliar with epidemic typhus. Murine typhus occurs worldwide in domestic cycles involving rats and their fleas. Scrub typhus, which occurs in the South Pacific and Asia, is transmitted by chigger bites from a natural reservoir in small mammals.

Epidemic typhus and murine typhus are characterized by fever, headache, myalgia, and a macular rash. Murine typhus is a milder disease than epidemic typhus, with the fatality rate among untreated cases being 2% in the former and 10% to 40% in the latter. Brill-Zinsser disease is typically milder than primary disease, and the rash may be absent. Scrub typhus is associated with an ulcer that has an eschar at the site of the chigger bite, febrile illness, a maculopapular rash, lymphadenopathy, and often pulmonary signs and symptoms.

*Coxiella burnetii,* a rickettsial organism, is the etiologic agent of Q fever. *C. burnetii* differs from organisms of the genus *Rickettsia* in several ways, including the ability to invade a wider variety of cells and a relative resistance to desiccation and heat. The organism has a number of wild and domestic animal reservoirs and has been found in several varieties of tick. It occurs worldwide. The usual transmission to humans is through the air via dusts contaminated by animal tissues, placental material, and birth fluids. Outbreaks in the United States have been associated with the handling of cattle, abattoirs, and aerosolized material emanating from slaughterhouses. Cases also have occurred in laboratory workers handling the organism.

The disease is characterized by a sudden onset of febrile illness with chills, myalgia, and prominent headache that lasts 1 to 2 weeks and occasionally longer. Multiple areas of pneumonitis may be apparent on chest radiograph, and the patient may complain of nonproductive cough and pleuritic chest pain. Abnormal liver function tests are frequent, but clinical jaundice is unusual. Rash and lymphadenopathy are absent. *C. burnetii* also can cause a chronic syndrome that is essentially Q fever endocarditis. Q fever endocarditis should be suspected in patients with "culture-negative" endocarditis with possible environmental exposure to *C. burnetii* and associated active liver disease.

Trench fever is caused by *Rochalimaea quintana* and is transmitted by lice. The reservoir is human and the disease occurs under conditions of crowding and pediculosis. It is usually a mild systemic febrile illness, frequently with characteristic shin pain. Occasionally, chronic or relapsing infections occur.

*Ehrlichia sennetsu* is the etiologic agent of sennetsu fever. The organism was formerly assigned to the genus *Rickettsia.* The mode of transmission has not been clearly established, but ticks are suspected. Sennetsu fever is a systemic febrile illness associated with lymphadenopathy and hepatosplenomegaly that occurs in Japan and other parts of Asia. In the 1980s, human ehrlichiosis was recognized in the United States. The organism is now identified as *E. chaffeensis,* closely related to the dog pathogen *E. canis.* The vector of human disease has not been established, but canine ehrlichiosis is transmitted by ticks. Human ehrlichiosis is generally a mild, nondescript systemic illness that, in some instances, is associated with macular or petechial rash. Severe illness is complicated by shock and multisystem organ failure and, in some cases, a toxic shocklike syndrome.

**Table 66-5.** Epidemiologic, clinical, and laboratory characteristics of diseases caused by rickettsia

| Disease | Organism | Vector | Reservoir | Occurrence | Rash/eschar | Serology* (Weil-Felix) |
|---|---|---|---|---|---|---|
| *Spotted fever group* | | | | | | |
| Rocky Mountain spotted fever | *R. rickettsii* | Tick | Rodents | North America South America | +/– | OX-19, OX-2 |
| Boutonneuse fever | *R. conorii* | Tick | Rodents | Mediterranean Africa, Southeast Asia | +/+ | OX-19, OX-2 |
| North Asian tick typhus | *R. sibirica* | Tick | Rodents | North Asia | +/+ | OX-19, OX-2 |
| Queensland tick typhus | *R. australis* | Tick | Rodents, marsupials | Australia | +/+ | OX-19, OX-2 |
| Rickettsialpox | *R. akari* | Mite | Mice | Temperate zones | +/+ | 0 |
| *Typhus group* | | | | | | |
| Epidemic typhus | *R. prowazekii* | Louse | Humans | Worldwide | +/– | OX-19, +/–OX-2 |
| Murine typhus | *R typhi* | Flea | Rodents | Worldwide | +/– | OX-19, +/–OX-2 |
| Scrub typhus | *R. tsutsugamushi* | Chigger | Rodents | Asia, South Pacific | +/+ | OX-K |
| *Other* | | | | | | |
| Trench fever | *Rochalimaea quintana* | Louse | Humans | North and South America, Africa, Europe | +/– | 0 |
| Q fever | *Coxiella burnetii* | None | Domesti canimals | Worldwide | –/– | 0 |
| Sennetsu fever | *Ehrlichia sennetsu* | ?Tick | | Asia | –/– | 0 |
| Ehrlichiosis | *E. chaffeensis* | ?Tick | ?Domestic animals | North America | +/– | 0 |

*Specific serologic diagnostic tests are available for each infection.

The diagnosis of rickettsial disease depends on the recognition of acute febrile illness associated with rash. Important diagnostic clues derive from the epidemiology of the diseases, geographic distribution, history of arthropod bites, and animal exposures. The character of the rash, or its absence, and the presence or absence of an eschar also help make the diagnosis.

The Weil-Felix reaction, which is based on the agglutination of three strains of *Proteus vulgaris* (OX-19, OX-2, OX-K) by serum from patients with various rickettsial diseases, is the classic serologic test for infection due to rickettsiae. Agglutinin titers against OX-19 and OX-2 typically rise in all the diseases of the spotted fever group, except rickettsialpox. Agglutinin to OX-19 usually rise in epidemic and murine typhus, whereas the antibody response to OX-2 is variable in these. The OX-K, but not the OX-19 and OX-2, agglutinins are elevated in scrub typhus. None of the agglutinins rise in rickettsialpox or Q fever, and titers may not change in Brill-Zinsser disease.

The Weil-Felix reactions generally have been supplanted by specific serologic tests for confirmation of diagnosis. All of the serologic tests show titer changes late in disease and usually are not useful for acute diagnosis. Serologic tests for various Q fever antigens can help in the diagnosis of Q fever endocarditis. Demonstration of rickettsia in skin biopsies from patients with rashes can be accomplished by direct immunofluorescent staining. In vitro isolation of rickettsiae and in vivo isolation by injection of patient material into laboratory animals are occasionally performed, but the techniques required are available only in special research laboratories, and such isolations are dangerous to laboratory personnel. The differential diagnosis of rickettsial diseases is summarized in Table 66-5.

Tetracycline and chloramphenicol are the drugs of choice for the treatment of rickettsial infections. These drugs are equally effective in the treatment of the spotted fevers and diseases of the typhus group. Tetracycline is usually preferred because of the potential toxicity of chloramphenicol. Response to therapy is prompt, except for Q fever, which is much less responsive, especially in the endocarditis form. Relapses of rickettsial infections may occur after treatment; they are usually related to therapy being initiated early in the course of disease and respond to retreatment. Treatment, however, should not be delayed to avoid relapse. The morbidity and mortality associated with Rocky Mountain spotted fever, typhus, and scrub typhus are substantial in untreated patients.

### Spirochetoses

Spirochetes are the cause of several human diseases. Nonpathogenic spirochetes are ubiquitous members of the normal oral flora. Syphilis is discussed in Chapter 65, and the other diseases caused by spirochetes of the genus *Treponema* are discussed under Skin Lesions. *Leptospira* species and *Borrelia* species are spirochetes that cause systemic, febrile illnesses.

The various serotypes of *Leptospira* causing human infection were previously given individual species names but are now considered varieties of one species, *Leptospira interrogans.* Leptospirosis is a zoonosis that affects many animals worldwide. The disease is present in rural and urban parts of the developing world. Humans acquire leptospirosis by contact with infected animals or their urine, or contaminated water or soil. The organisms are capable of penetrating damaged skin and mucous membranes.

Evidence suggests subclinical infection occurs. The clinical disease is usually biphasic. Mild disease, referred to as "anicteric," manifests as a septicemic phase (characterized by fever, myalgia, headache, malaise, and gastrointestinal complaints lasting several days to 1 week) and an "immune" phase (that may overlap the initial phase and primarily manifests as meningitis, rash, and uveitis). Severe disease—icterohemorrhagic fever, or Weil's disease—compose 10% or fewer clinical leptospirosis infections and is characterized by jaundice, renal functional impairment, and vasculitis with bleeding.

The diagnosis of leptospirosis is made by recognizing the characteristic clinical features, with or without a history of exposure to animals or to water likely to contain animal urine. Leptospires may be isolated in culture using special techniques. Blood cultures may be positive early in the disease, and later the organism may be isolated from cerebrospinal fluid and urine. Serologic tests also are available.

It is unclear whether antibiotics significantly alter the course of leptospirosis. Penicillin or tetracycline may be beneficial if therapy is started early in the course of disease. Doxycycline has been used as a prophylactic agent to prevent leptospirosis in situations in which unavoidable exposure is expected.

Relapsing fever is caused by spirochetes of the genus *Borrelia.* The disease occurs as two epidemiologic types, louse-borne and tick-borne. Although the disease may occur in virtually any area of the world, the epidemic louse-borne infection occurs under socioeconomic conditions associated with the presence of lice and is seen primarily in the higher elevations of Africa and South America. Endemic tick-borne disease occurs in widespread geographic foci (including areas of North America) where ticks and the small animals that serve as the reservoir reside. The clinical disease is related to the cyclic appearance of the spirochetes in the bloodstream.

The organisms, which reappear in the blood after sequestration in tissue, are capable of changing their surface antigens to overcome specific antibody. This results in relapses with fever, chills, myalgia, headache, and cough (lasting 3 to 6 days); about 1 week elapses between episodes. The febrile periods usually end in a crisis. Hepatosplenomegaly; bleeding; and a papular, petechial, or macular rash may occur. Louse-borne infection usually results in one relapse, whereas multiple relapses with higher fever are typical of the tick-borne infection. CNS involvement may present as "aseptic" meningitis.

The diagnosis of relapsing fever is made by demonstrating blood-borne spirochetes during febrile episodes by darkfield examination or on stained smears. Animal inoculation also is used, but serologic tests are of limited value because of the antigenic variability of the organism.

Tetracycline is the drug of choice for treatment, although chloramphenicol, penicillin, and erythromycin also are effective. A Jarisch-Herxheimer reaction (fever, chills, myalgia) typically occurs with therapy. Untreated epidemic disease has a mortality rate of up to 40%, but with treatment the mortality rate is low.

### Arbovirus diseases and hemorrhagic fevers

Several acute viral illnesses are transmitted by arthropod vectors, and the viruses that cause these diseases are often referred to as arboviruses (for arthropod-borne). Approximately 80 to 100 of these viruses infect humans. Diseases occur primarily in tropical and semitropical regions, although some arboviruses cause summer epidemics in the temperate zones. The arboviruses belong to several distinct families of viruses, but all are RNA viruses. Arboviruses cause three disease syndromes—nondescript febrile illnesses, hemorrhagic fevers, and encephalitis—although there is overlap in many cases.

Many arboviruses cause acute, relatively benign, nondescript febrile illnesses often with arthralgia, myalgia, and rash. An example of this group is dengue, or "breakbone fever." This disease is widespread in tropical areas and is transmitted by mosquitoes. Its endemic areas are currently enlarging, especially in the Caribbean and Gulf of Mexico. Dengue has been acquired in Texas. Large parts of the southern United States are at potential risk of dengue activity. The disease is characterized by sudden onset of fever, chills, severe headache, retroorbital pain, conjunctivitis, lymphadenopathy, and severe myalgia and arthralgia. The acute disease lasts about 1 week, often with "saddleback" fever, with a fall and then a rise of daily fever spikes over the week. A diffuse, scarlet fever-type maculopapular rash occurs in the midst of the acute disease. Leukopenia is typical. Recovery is often followed by a prolonged period of depression and fatigue. Similar diseases occur in various parts of the world and are often marked by more severe joint pain with or without rash. These include such exotically named diseases as chikungunya, o'nyong-nyong, Rift Valley fever, and Colorado tick fever. These diseases are transmitted by mosquitoes, ticks, and sandflies.

More severe systemic arbovirus diseases are referred to as hemorrhagic fevers. The classic example is yellow fever, although dengue and chikungunya viruses also cause hemorrhagic fever, especially in Asia. The pathophysiology of hemorrhagic fevers is not well defined and is under intense investigation. Dengue hemorrhagic fever and the "dengue shock syndrome" appear to have an immunologic basis and occur with subsequent episodes of dengue. The hemorrhagic fevers are characterized by leukopenia, thrombocytopenia, ecchymoses, and gross bleeding. In severe cases, shock and death result. Yellow fever is a hemorrhagic fever so named because of the hepatitis and jaundice it produces. It has an important history in the United States, with epidemics occurring as far north as Philadelphia up to 150 to 200 years ago. The conquest of yellow fever contributed to the success of the effort to build the Panama Canal. Nephritis also may occur in patients with yellow fever. Severe yellow fever is associated with profound jaundice, hemorrhage, and hypotension, with a peculiar relative bradycardia. Mortality rates in arbovirus hemorrhagic fevers are approximately 5% to 10%. Other examples are Omsk hemorrhagic fever, Kyasanur Forest disease, and Crimean-Congo fever.

The third disease syndrome associated with arboviruses is encephalitis. The arbovirus encephalitides include eastern equine, western equine, Venezuelan equine, St. Louis, Japanese, California, West Nile, Russian spring-summer, Powassan, and others. These diseases have several animal reservoirs and are transmitted by mosquitoes and ticks. The diseases begin with fever, headache, and systemic viral symptoms; the patients then become somnolent, develop meningeal signs, and may go on to seizures, paralysis, coma, and death. Aseptic meningitis is common. The diseases have a spectrum of severity, and fatality rates range from 50% to 60% for Japanese and eastern equine encephalitis to 5% and less for others, with California encephalitis usually being the least severe. Long-term neurologic sequelae may result, especially in young survivors.

Japanese B encephalitis is transmitted by mosquito throughout large parts of Eastern and Southern Asia. Pigs are important reservoirs of the virus. Whereas mild infections are more common than severe and are associated with myalgia, fever, and headache, severe disease with life-threatening acute illness and neurologic sequelae in survivors also occurs. Incubation period is approximately 1 week. An inactivated vaccine recently was licensed in the United States and is recommended for anyone who will be spending a month or longer in Asia during the warm season, especially if there is to be exposure to rural areas. Three doses of vaccine are given over 1 month, but an accelerated 2-week schedule may be used if necessary. The last dose should be given at least 10 days before travel commences.

Several non-arthropod-borne viruses cause hemorrhagic fevers, often with renal impairment or other systemic and organ-specific complications. These viruses belong to several taxonomic groups and include the Junin and Machupo viruses, which cause Argentine and Bolivian hemorrhagic fever, respectively; the Lassa fever virus, which occurs in West Africa; and the *Hantavirus,* which causes Korean hemorrhagic fever in Asia, nephropathia epidemica in Europe, and *Hantavirus* pulmonary syndrome in the United States. These viruses have rodent reservoirs and are transmitted through exposure to the excreta of infected mice and rats. Mortality rates are high, and Lassa fever is highly communicable. A related virus with a worldwide distribution and the house mouse as a reservoir is lymphocytic choriomeningitis (LCM) virus, which causes a nonspecific, systemic viral syndrome with or without meningoencephalitis. Two additional viruses, the Marburg and Ebola viruses, cause hemorrhagic fever in Africa. The reservoirs and modes of transmission of these viruses are not established. Mortality rates during outbreaks have been high (30% to 70%).

There are no specific therapies for the viral fevers, hemorrhagic fevers, and viral encephalitides. Ribavirin, active against RNA viruses, is being investigated as a specific therapy through several protocols. Serum from survivors of Lassa fever and Ebola virus infection has been used to treat these diseases with some success.

### Ectoparasites

Detailed information about pediculosis, lice, and scabies is presented in Chapter 65.

Chiggers are trombiculid mites, the larvae of which attach to the skin and feed on tissue fluid and necrotic debris. Chiggers occur worldwide in areas of scrub vegetation. They are the vector of scrub typhus in the South Pacific and Asia. The area of chigger skin attachment develops a macular lesion that may evolve into a papular, then vesicular, and then hemorrhagic lesion. Pruritus leads to removal of the parasites by scratching. A systemic reaction may occur in the very young and very old. Chiggers of the skin are treated with a variety of alcoholic solutions and other topical agents such as fingernail polish.

Myiasis is the infestation of the skin with fly larvae or maggots. Maggots may be present in preexisting traumatic lesions and, in fact, have been purposely used for debridement of wounds in the past. Certain species of fly are capable of injecting eggs into undamaged skin causing furuncular myiasis. Several such species occur in South America, North America, and Africa. Furuncular myiasis results in painful, furuncle-like lesions that may be secondarily infected. Furuncular maggots may be removed by means of forceps or by excision. Maggots of colonizing superficial lesions may be treated with chloroform dressings or by pouring ether over the lesions.

Ticks are arachnid parasites that bury their mouth parts in the skin and take a blood meal (see Chapter 4G).

## DISEASE SYNDROMES IN TRAVELERS

### Fever

Fever in a traveler from the tropics is often a cause of anxiety in the traveler and the primary care provider. The traveler may be terrified about an exotic infectious disease acquired overseas. The primary care physician may be anxious about recalling numerous parasite syndromes, shapes, and life cycles learned in medical school.

The differential diagnosis of fever in a returned traveler or an immigrant is extensive, but can be quickly narrowed by a good history, physical examination, and appropriate laboratory data. The box on p. 911 presents the relative risk for several infections, diseases, and injuries for international travelers. Initially, the "nontropical" causes of fever such as community acquired respiratory diseases and urinary tract infection must be ruled out, because they account for over half of fevers among returned travelers. A detailed travel history, food exposure, and animal contact history can narrow the list of diagnoses. A physical examination to look specifically for rash, lymphadenopathy, and hepatosplenomegaly is essential. Distinctive clues in the laboratory findings such as anemia or eosinophilia are extremely helpful. A list of diseases to be considered in the differential diagnosis of febrile illness in travelers and immigrants with some of the clues leading to those diagnoses is provided in the box on p. 911.

The physician must then order specific diagnostic tests unique in the diagnosis of parasitic diseases such as thick and thin blood smears for malaria and examination for ova and parasites in the stool. If the diagnosis is still not evident, often the case, the physician must make a decision to treat empirically and consider consultation with an infectious diseases or a tropical medicine specialist.

***Common causes of fever.*** Common causes of difficult-to-diagnose fever in travelers are malaria, hepatitis, and

### A differential diagnosis of some selected systemic febrile illnesses to consider in returned travelers and immigrants*

**Common**

*Acute respiratory tract infection* (worldwide)
*Gastroenteritis* (worldwide) [foodborne, waterborne, fecal-oral]
Enteric fever, including typhoid (worldwide) [food, water]
*Urinary tract infection* (worldwide) [sexual activity]
Drug reactions [antibiotics, prophylactic agents, other] {rash frequent}
Malaria (tropics, limited areas of temperate zones) [mosquitoes]
Arboviruses (Africa; tropics) [mosquitoes, ticks, mites]
Dengue (Asia, Caribbean, Africa) [mosquitoes]
Viral hepatitis (worldwide)
Hepatitis A (worldwide) [food, fecal-oral]
Hepatitis B (worldwide, esp. Asia, sub-Sahara Africa) [sexual contact] {long incubation period}
Hepatitis C (worldwide) [blood or sexual contact]
Hepatitis E (Asia, North Africa, Mexico, ?others) [food, water]
Tuberculosis (worldwide) [airborne, milk] {long period to symptomatic infection}
*Sexually transmitted diseases* (worldwide) [Sexual contact]

**Less common**

Filariasis (see Table 66-4) (Asia, Africa, South America) [biting insects] {long incubation period, eosinophilia}
*Measles* (developing world) [airborne] {in susceptible individual}
Amebic abscess (worldwide) [food]
Brucellosis (worldwide) [milk, cheese, food, animal contact]
Listeriosis (worldwide) [foodborne] {meningitis}
Leptospirosis (worldwide) [animal contact, open fresh water] {jaundice, meningitis}
Strongyloidiasis (warm and tropical areas) [soil contact] {eosinophilia}
Toxoplasmosis (worldwide) [undercooked meat]

**Rare**

Relapsing fever (western Americas, Asia, northern Africa) [ticks, lice]
*Hemorrhagic fevers* (worldwide) [arthropod and nonarthropod transmitted]
Yellow fever (tropics) [mosquitoes] {hepatitis}
Hemorrhagic fever with renal syndrome (Europe, Asia, ? North America) [rodent urine] {renal impairment}
*Hantavirus* pulmonary syndrome (western North America, ?other) [rodent urine] {respiratory distress syndrome}
Lassa fever (Africa) [Rodent excreta, person to person] {high mortality rate}
Other–chikungunya, Rift Valley, Ebola-Marburg, etc. (various) [insect bites, rodent excreta, aerosols, per son to person] {often severe}
*Rickettsial infections* (see Table 66-5) {Rashes and eschars}
Leishmaniasis, visceral (Middle East, Mediterranean, Africa, Asia, South America) [biting flies] {long incubation period}
Acute schistosomiasis (Africa, Asia, South America, Caribbean) [fresh water]
Chagas' disease (South and Central America) [reduvid bug bites] {often asymptomatic}
African trypanosomiasis (Africa) [Tsetse fly bite] {neurologic syndromes, sleeping sickness}
Bartonellosis (South America) [sandfly bite] {skin nodules}
HIV infection/AIDS (worldwide) [sexual and blood contact]
Trichinosis (worldwide) [undercooked meat] {eosinophilia}
*Plague* (temperate and tropical plains) [animal exposures and fleas] {bubos, pneumonia}
*Tularemia* (worldwide) [animal contact, fleas, aerosols] {ulcers, lymph nodes}
*Anthrax* (worldwide) [animal, animal product contact] {ulcers}
*Lyme disease* (North America, Europe) [tick bites] {arthritis, meningitis, cardiac abnormalities}

*Diagnoses for which particular symptoms are indicative are in *italics*. Exposure to regions of the world that are most likely to be significant to the diagnosis are presented in (parentheses). Vectors, risk behaviors, and sources associated with acquisition are presented in [brackets]. Special clinical characteristics are listed within {braces}.

upper respiratory infection. Other causes of fever include enteric fever, arboviral infection (dengue), and tuberculosis.

Malaria must be suspected in every patient who returns from the tropics without a localized source for fever. Even if the traveler reports compliance with chemoprophylaxis, malaria can occur due to the resistant *Plasmodium falciparum* and possible inadvertent noncompliance. Failure of chemoprophylaxis may occur in the compliant individual. Eighty percent of the malaria cases reported in the United States from 1980 to 1988 were acquired in sub-Sahara Africa. Even with appropriate prophylaxis, *P. vivax* and *P. ovale* can cause relapse months after the traveler returns, with the persistence of the extraerythrocytic (hepatic) stage.

Enteric fever may be due to *Salmonella typhi* or nontyphoidal *Salmonella* species. Typhoid fever and enteric fever must be considered in returning travelers even if immunized, especially if at risk for hypochlorhydria due to age, blockers of gastric acid secretion, or previous surgical procedure. Blood and stool cultures are usually positive.

Arboviruses are capable of causing flulike illness, hemorrhagic fever, or encephalitis. Dengue is a classic example in which the patient presents 1 to 2 weeks after returning with fever, chills, myalgia, arthralgia, and in some instances rash. Recovery is characterized by prolonged fatigue. Hemorrhagic fever caused by viruses such as the Lassa fever virus must be considered in patients with leukopenia, thrombocytopenia, ecchymoses, and gross bleeding. Immediate strict isolation and public health consolation are necessary. Encephalitis due to arboviruses needs to be considered if a history of headache, meningeal signs, and mental status changes present after a nonspecific prodrome.

Fever patterns in general are unreliable guides to diagnosis. Fever-pulse dichotomy may occur in typhoid fever or brucellosis. Relapsing fever presents classically as febrile episodes of 3 days followed by afebrile periods of 6 to 7 days in patients returning from western South America. Dengue fever may have "saddle back" pattern with relapse after 2 to 3 weeks.

***Region traveled.*** Travel history is essential for appropriate differential diagnosis. Activity, length of stay, and site of stay, help include or exclude specific diagnoses. A traveler who has ventured into rural areas, or lived for a prolonged time with native populations, is at a much greater risk of tropical diseases, such as dengue or typhoid fever, than businessmen who go for short visits and stay in western-style hotels. In addition, a disease such as bartonellosis need only be considered in a traveler returning from Peru, Ecuador, or Colombia with possible exposure to sandflies. African trypanosomiasis should be considered in patients who present with fever 2 to 4 weeks after returning from a rural site in East or West Africa with a history of remembered or potential fly bite.

***Onset of fever after return.*** Incubation periods for tropical diseases vary greatly and are important indicators of possible diagnoses. Arboviral infection, spotted fevers, and plague have short incubation periods and occur within 1 or 2 weeks of return from the tropics, whereas malaria, acute schistosomiasis, and leishmaniasis can occur up to 1 month or more after return.

Acute schistosomiasis can present 4 to 6 weeks after return from an endemic area such as Egypt with fever, weight loss, diarrhea, and marked peripheral eosinophilia. Visceral leishmaniasis may present 2 to 4 months or longer after return from endemic areas such as India, with high fever and organomegaly associated with a history of exposure to sandflies.

***Exposures.*** Specific exposure to animals, flies, ticks, foods, or fresh water add a new set of diagnoses to be considered in the febrile patient. The traveler often does not volunteer the information because he or she does not realize its significance. For example, brucellosis usually requires exposure to animals, meat, or dairy products and presents with hectic fevers, myalgia, adenopathy, and positive blood cultures. Plague must be considered in patients with potential exposure to rodents presenting with fever and painful and swollen lymph nodes (buboes) within a week after return from an endemic area.

***Empiric therapy.*** Indiscriminate use of antibiotics should be avoided; however, when patients are critically ill or malaria is suspected, empiric treatment is required. Empiric treatment for malaria should be considered in persons who return from endemic regions, with or without history of prophylaxis, who are systemically ill with no focal signs of infection, even if initial thick or thin blood smears are negative.

Broad-spectrum antibiotics used for empiric therapy of bacterial and rickettsial infections include chloramphenicol and the tetracyclines. Chloramphenicol is often effective for many potentially lethal diseases that are difficult to diagnose on presentation including typhoid fever, brucellosis, relapsing fever, bartonellosis, glanders, melioidosis, anthrax, plague, tularemia, Rocky Mountain spotted fever, epidemic typhus, and scrub typhus.

Of course, fever may not be the only sign of illness. Rash, diarrhea, lymphadenopathy, or respiratory symptoms can point to diagnoses. The differential diagnoses of illness with these findings is presented in the designated sections of this chapter and in other parts of this book under specific organ systems.

Traveler's diarrhea is described in Chapter 49.

## Respiratory infections

Respiratory illness is among the most common causes of morbidity and mortality in the tropics, largely due to crowded living conditions and socioeconomic deprivation. The causes of illness are quite similar to those in the developed countries with additional organisms specific to the tropics. Travelers who acquire respiratory tract pathogens in the tropics may present special diagnostic problems. A list of unusual infections with pulmonary infiltrates that may be encountered in returning international travelers is presented in the box on p. 913.

Several organisms that cause systemic infection may cause pulmonary illness. *S. typhi* frequently causes bronchitis or nonspecific bronchopneumonia. *Yersinia pestis,* the etiologic agent of plague, is infectious through the respiratory route and causes a rapidly progressive pneumonia. If the patient has been exposed to rabbits or slaughtered animals, tularemic pneumonia should be considered. Half of leptospirosis cases have nonspecific pulmonary involvement. Several etiologic agents that cause pneumonia and that are not discussed in other sections of the text are included below.

Meliodosis is an infection caused by the gram-negative bacillus *Pseudomonas pseudomallei.* The organisms live in water and soil and are capable of infecting several animals in addition to people. The disease is uncommon and occurs primarily in Southeast Asia and the Pacific, with sporadic cases occurring in various other areas. It is acquired through close contact with soil and water. The disease is usually pulmonary, although inapparent infection, skin infection, lymphadenitis, septicemia, and visceral abscesses have been encountered. Acute pulmonary disease is characterized by fever, pleuritic chest pain, myalgia, and headache. Consolidation in the upper lobes, often with cavitation, is the typical radiographic finding. Septicemia and metastatic suppurative infection may complicate pneumonia. Chronic pulmonary infection, with recrudescence at a later time, may occur, and the disease may resemble tuberculosis. Diagnosis is made on the basis of Gram stain and culture. Serologic tests also are available. Treatment is with tetracycline, chloramphenicol, or a sulfonamide, alone or in combination depending on susceptibility tests, for 30 to 60 days or longer

**Infections associated with pulmonary infiltrates that may be encountered in returning international travelers**

**Bacterial:**
Tuberculosis
Legionellosis
Q fever
Melioidosis
Tularemia
Glanders
Psittacosis
Plague
Brucellosis
Typhoid
Rickettsiosis

**Fungal:**
Blastomycosis
Coccidioidomycosis
Histoplasmosis

**Viral:**
Measles
Hemmorrhagic fevers
Influenza
Adenovirus

**Parasitic:**
Amebiasis
Toxoplasmosis
Ascariasis
Hookworm
Strongyloidiasis
Filariasis
Paragonimiasis
Schistosomiasis (Katayama fever)
Echinococcosis
Toxocariasis
Trichinosis

Other causes of pneumonia that commonly occur in the United States are not listed, but should always be ruled out because they are common causes of pneumonia worldwide.

depending on the location of infection and chronicity. Ceftazidime also has been used successfully.

Glanders, a disease of horses and other equine animals, has a worldwide distribution and is caused by *Pseudomonas mallei.* It occasionally occurs in humans, causing syndromes simliar to melioidosis. The disease is differentiated from melioidosis by culture. Treatment is usually with streptomycin combined with tetracycline or a sulfonamide.

Psittacosis is a systemic disease caused by *Chlamydia psittaci* that usually presents in humans as a respiratory disease. *C. psittaci* is primarily a pathogen of birds, especially psittacine birds, e.g., parrots and parakeets. People acquire the disease by exposure to sick or well birds that are shedding the organism. The disease is characterized by fever, severe headache, myalgia, lethargy, cough productive of scant sputum, dyspnea, splenomegaly, and occasionally a macular rash similar to the rose spots of typhoid. Chest radiograph may show diffuse, patchy infiltrates or nodular or miliary lesions. The diagnosis is usually made on the basis of clinical signs and symptoms in a patient with a history of avian exposure and is confirmed serologically or, less commonly, by isolating the organism from blood or sputum. Treatment is with tetracycline, to which there is usually a prompt response, although relapses may occur.

*Paragonimus westermani,* the lung fluke, is a trematode that infects the lung. The disease occurs primarily in Asia, especially Korea, although foci of infection are present in other parts of the world. Other species of *Paragonimus* also infect humans. The disease is acquired by ingestion of larvae encysted in the secondary intermediate hosts, freshwater crabs and crayfish. Snails are primary intermediate hosts. Encysted larvae migrate through the intestinal wall and make their way to the lung and other organs. Fibrous cysts form around adult worms in the lung and other tissues. Chronic cough productive of copious sputum and hemoptysis are the usual symptoms. A variety of neurologic symptoms and signs results from cerebral involvement.

Chest radiograph shows small nodular infiltrates or larger lesions that are seen with heavy pulmonary worm loads. The diagnosis is suspected on the basis of residence in an endemic area, productive cough, hemoptysis, eosinophilia, and chest radiographic findings. The diagnosis is confirmed by demonstrating the characteristic operculated eggs in sputum (see Fig. 66-2). Treatment with praziquantel in a dose of 75 mg/kg per day in three divided doses for 2 days is safe and effective. Bithionol is an alternative agent.

Among viral causes of pneumonia, measles-associated pneumonia still accounts for 25% of pneumonia among children in developing countries. Several parasitic diseases can cause primary or associated respiratory illness. Hepatic abscess due to *Entamoeba histolytica* can lead to sympathetic pleural effusion or secondary pneumonitis. Worms can cause pulmonary disease as they migrate through the lung alveoli (ascaris or hookworm) or as they pass through the pulmonary vasculature (schistosomiasis or filariasis) or as they lodge in the lung tissue (paragonimiasis or echinococcosis). Pulmonary infiltrates with eosinophilia are discussed under eosinophilia.

A traveler who presents with a respiratory illness is most likely to be infected with a cosmopolitan organism. Several diagnoses, however, need to be kept in mind. *Mycobacterium tuberculosis* infection is present in 50% to 60% of people in developing countries and is a particular threat to travelers returning from prolonged stays in the tropics. Epidemiologic clues of animal exposure are often essential to reach the diagnosis of Q fever, psittacosis, or tularemia. Workup must include the standard sputum Gram stain and culture, along with acid-fast stain and mycobacterial culture. Blood count with differential count to check for eosinophilia is important. Examination of sputum and stool for ova and parasites may be helpful.

## Eosinophilia

The eosinophilic granulocyte is a cell that participates in hypersensitivity reactions and plays a role in host defenses, particularly against multicellular parasites. Peripheral blood eosinophilia, usually defined as more than

450 eosinophils/mm$^3$, occurs with a number of allergic reactions and disease processes, but on a worldwide basis the most common cause is parasitic infection.

Peripheral blood eosinophilia is associated with helminthic parasites, not single cell protozoa such as *E. histolytica* or *Giardia* species. Tissue-invasive or tissue-dwelling worms or those that have invasive larvae are most commonly associated with eosinophilia. Among the intestinal roundworms, the larval migration stages of *Ascaris,* the hookworms, and *Strongyloides stercoralis* are associated with eosinophilia, whereas pinworm and *Trichuris trichiura,* which do not have invasive larvae, are not. *S. stercoralis,* which has the potential for autoinfection, may cause persistent eosinophilia in affected individuals. High degrees of eosinophilia are seen with trichinosis, and eosinophilia is observed with all forms of filariasis.

Several parasites with nonhuman usual hosts may infect humans and cause tissue infection associated with eosinophilia. These include *Echinococcus granulosus* and *E. multilocularis,* which cause hydatid cysts; *Toxocara* species, which cause visceral larva migrans; and animal hookworms, the invasive larvae of which cause cutaneous larva migrans. The rodent parasite *Angiostrongylus cantonensis* causes the syndrome eosinophilic meningitis with an eosinophilic pleocytosis in the cerebrospinal fluid. *Gnathostoma spinigerum,* a dog and cat nematode, can cause a similar syndrome. Eosinophilic gastritis is associated with the fish-borne, sea mammal ascarid *Anisakis,* and eosinophilic gastroenteritis may be seen with the nematode parasite of rodents, *Angiostrongylus costaricensis.* The early phase of infection with the liver fluke *Fasciola hepatica* is associated with marked eosinophilia, as in infection with the lung fluke *(Paragonimus westermani).* Severe scabies may be associated with eosinophilia.

"Tropical eosinophilia" is a syndrome seen in all parts of the tropics but most commonly in Asia. It is due to unidentified microfilariae. The disease is characterized by dyspnea, cough, wheezing, systemic complaints, and peripheral blood eosinophilia. The diagnosis is usually presumptive and the syndrome is treated with diethylcarbamazine.

The syndrome of "pulmonary infiltrates with eosinophilia" (PIE) is closely related to tropical eosinophilia. PIE is seen in some cases of asthma, polyarteritis nodosa, infections with nematodes that migrate through the lung (*Ascaris, S. stercoralis,* hookworms, trichinosis, etc.) and ectopic migration of *F. hepatica* larvae. When idiopathic and self-limited, the PIE syndrome is referred to as Loeffler's syndrome.

Several noninfectious conditions may be associated with peripheral blood eosinophilia. These conditions, the infections already discussed, and some other infections associated with eosinophilia are listed in the box at right.

Patients with eosinophilia should have a careful history taken for geographic exposure and other contacts that might cause one to suspect helminthic disease. A thorough physical examination may be helpful in distinguishing parasitic from nonparasitic causes. A stool specimen for ova and parasite examination is of obvious importance, and duodenal aspiration for *S. stercoralis* may be required. The blood should be examined for microfilariae depending on the history of travel and residence. A negative history and the absence of evidence of parasitic infection should lead to a more extensive workup for the other causes of eosinophilia. The differential diagnosis indicated by the conditions listed in the box above can serve as a guide to other diagnostic tests and procedures.

## Causes of significant peripheral blood eosinophilia

**Helminthic parasites:**

*Ascaris lumbricoides* (invasive larval stage)
Hookworms (invasive larval stage)
*Strongyloides stercoralis* (initial infection and autoinfection)
Trichinosis
Filariasis
*Echinococcus granulosus* and *E. multilocularis*
*Toxocara* species
Animal hookworms
*Angiostrongylus cantonensis* and *A. costaricensis*
Schistosomiasis
Liver flukes
*Fasciolopsis buski*
Anisakiasis
*Capillaria philippinensis*
*Paragonimus westermani*
"Tropical eosinophilia" (Unidentified microfilariae)

**Other infections/infestations:**

Pulmonary aspergillosis
Severe scabies

**Allergies:**

Asthma
Hay fever
Drug reactions
Atopic dermatitis

**Autoimmune and related disorders:**

Polyarteritis nodosa
Necrotizing vasculitis
Eosinophilic fasciitis
Pemphigus

**Neoplastic diseases:**

Hodgkin's disease
Mycosis fungoides
Chronic myelocytic leukemia
Eosinophilic leukemia
Polycythemia vera
Mucin-secreting adenocarcinomas

**Immunodeficiency states:**

Hyperimmunoglobulin E with recurrent infection
Wiscott-Aldrich syndrome

**Other:**

Addison's disease
Inflammatory bowel disease
Dermatitis herpetiformis
Toxic/chemical syndrome
(Eosinophilic myalgia syndrome-tryptophan, toxic oil syndrome)
"Hypereosinophilic syndrome" (unknown etiology)

## Mass lesions

Several parasites of humans and other animals and a variety of other infectious agents cause diseases that result in mass lesions of the soft tissue and organs.

Extraintestinal amebiasis results when trophozoites of *E. histolytica* invade the bowel wall, are carried in the bloodstream, and settle in tissue. Lesions usually occur in the liver via seeding of the portal blood. Amebic liver abscesses typically occur in the setting of asymptomatic bowel infection, most commonly as single in the right lobe. They are characterized by liquefaction necrosis centrally, with invasive amoebae in the wall of the lesion. Patients may have insidious development of symptoms or abrupt systemic signs. A tender mass may be palpated through the abdominal wall. Rarely, amebic abscesses occur in the brain, lung, or spleen. Liver abscess may be complicated by rupture into the peritoneal cavity and extension into the pleural space, lung, or pericardial sac.

Diagnosis is made on clinical grounds, or the lesion may be demonstrated on radionuclide scan. Needle aspiration of liver abscesses reveals necrotic material that may resemble "anchovy paste." Serologic tests are usually positive in patients with invasive amebiasis.

Amebic liver abscess may be treated with oral metronidazole, 750 mg, three times a day (35 to 50 mg/kg per day in children) for 10 days. Needle aspiration also may have therapeutic benefit in some cases. Diloxanide furoate or iodoquinol are often used in conjunction with metronidazole to ensure eradication of amoebae in the intestinal lumen.

Migrating adults of the filarial worm *L. loa* cause localized areas of inflammation in subcutaneous tissue resulting in characteristic "calabar swellings." *Dracunculus medinensis,* the guinea worm, is a tissue-invasive nematode that causes characteristic serpiginous lesions in the subcutaneous tissue of the lower extremities. Dracunculosis occurs in Africa, the Middle East, and southern Asia. The parasite is acquired by ingesting the intermediate host, copepods (small crustaceans), with drinking water. Larvae penetrate the intestinal wall, mature, and mate in the retroperitoneum. Adult female worms migrate to the lower extremities and may reach lengths of up to 80 cm in the subcutaneous tissue. Motile larvae are released through a blister in the skin. Worms may be removed by incising the skin or by gradual extraction by winding the worm on a stick. Niridazole, thiabendazole, and metronidazole have been used and the result is extrusion of the worm.

Humans are both definitive and intermediate hosts of the pork tapeworm *Taenia solium.* The larvae of *T. solium* invade the intestinal wall and migrate to tissue, where they encyst as cysticerci, causing cysticercosis. Infection may result from ingestion of eggs or by autoinfection from eggs shed by adult tapeworms in the intestine. Cysticerci may be widely distributed in many tissues, but of most significance are lesions in the eye and brain. Cerebral cysticercosis may result in recurrent seizures or increased intracranial pressure secondary to obstruction of cerebrospinal fluid flow. Cysticerci remain viable for several years.

Lesions containing dead *T. solium* cysticerci may calcify and diagnosis may be made by radiographic demonstration of calcified lesions in soft tissue that have a characteristic "puffed rice" appearance or by biopsy of accessible lesions. Computed tomography (CT) of the head is useful in diagnosing cerebral cysticercosis. Surgical resection of lesions, especially in the case of anatomic compromise, is indicated. Praziquantel is useful in treatment of cysticercosis in a dose of 50 mg/kg per day in three divided doses for 15 days. Albendazole is an alternative agent. Steroids are usually used in conjunction with treatment to limit tissue damage.

Hydatid cysts are mass lesions caused by the larvae of the canine tapeworms *Echinococcus granulosus* and *E. multilocularis.* The disease occurs primarily in areas where dogs are used for herding. Humans become intermediate hosts after ingesting eggs with material contaminated by canine feces. Larvae invade the intestinal wall and migrate to tissue where they produce progressively enlarging cysts. Lesions usually occur in the liver and lung and may involve any tissue. Invasion of blood vessels may result in dissemination. Symptoms are related to the mass effect of lesions. Rupture of cysts, either spontaneously or at surgery, may result in anaphylactic reactions and seeding of new lesions. Cysts may calcify and thus be demonstrable radiographically. Eosinophilia may be present. Serologic tests are available, but cross-reactions with other parasites exist. Treatment is limited to careful surgical excision of symptomatic lesions or careful drainage of cysts previously sterilized with formalin or silver nitrate. Albendazole is effective adjunctive therapy for *E. granulosus.*

Actinomycosis is caused by the anaerobic gram-positive filamentous bacterium *Actinomyces israelii* and related species. *Actinomyces* species are normal inhabitants of the human oral cavity. Disease due to these organisms usually manifests as suppurative and/or granulomatous lesions, often in the jaw and occasionally in the thorax, abdomen, or skin. Lesions are firm and slowly spreading, and they develop draining sinuses that may contain macroscopic colonies of the organism with the appearance of "sulfur granules." The diagnosis is suggested by the characteristic lesions and confirmed by culture. Treatment is usually with penicillin for a prolonged period, with tetracycline as an alternative agent.

*Nocardia asteroides* is an aerobic actinomycete that causes pulmonary and disseminated infection. The organism is a ubiquitous saprophyte in soil. Infection of the skin can produce abscesses with draining sinuses. Treatment is with sulfonamides.

Mycetoma is an infection of the skin, subcutaneous tissue, and often bone that is characterized by mass swelling with draining sinuses and extensive tissue destruction. Lesions usually occur in the feet (i.e., Madura foot), but also occur on the legs and hands. The disease is caused by a variety of actinomycetes, e.g., *N. asteroides* and *Streptomyces* species, as well as several fungi, including *Madurella* and *Cephalosporium* species. These organisms are soil saprophytes. The disease occurs in tropical and semitropical areas worldwide. It is acquired through abrasions and puncture wounds. Lesions of the shoulder and back have been described in burden bearers. Treatment depends on the causative agents, but cure with chemotherapy alone is difficult.

Pyomyositis, or tropical pyomyositis, is a bacterial abscess of striated muscle, virtually always due to

*Staphylococcus aureus.* The disease is common in several tropical areas, including Asia, Africa, and the West Indies; it occurs only rarely in temperate areas. Patients present with complaints of fever, chills, and malaise, as well as pain and swelling in the muscle involved, usually in the thigh and buttocks. The pathogenesis of this disease is unclear, as muscle tissue is normally resistant to bacterial infection. One suggestion as to the etiology of pyomyositis is that migrating helminth larvae damage tissue, making it susceptible to bacteria of hematogenous origin or organisms carried by the worm. Treatment involves surgical drainage and antistaphylococcal agents.

### Skin lesions

A new skin lesion in a traveler can be a cause of concern. Among the most common skin disorders for which returned travelers are seen by their primary care provider are secondarily infected insect bites, pyodermas, cutaneous larva migrans, and nonspecific dermatitis. Short-term travelers are unlikely to acquire diseases such as leprosy, yaws, or filariasis. As in other diseases in travelers, the exposure history is crucial in reaching a diagnosis and workup is greatly dependent on suspected diagnoses.

Viral exanthems, purpuric lesions from viral and bacterial infections, rickettsial diseases, syphilis, and fungal infections are all causes of skin lesions in developed countries. Several skin lesions that occur primarily in the tropics or are caused by parasites are discussed here.

Orf is a disease caused by a pox virus of sheep. It is seen in areas where sheep are raised. Lesions usually occur on the hand, but any area of skin may be involved. Lesions may be single or multiple and begin as reddish blue papules that progress to bullous lesions that rupture, leaving ulcers covered by gray-white crusts. The disease is self-limited; significant systemic signs are absent, but it is occasionally associated with a transient maculopapular rash of the trunk. A similar lesion called "milker's nodule" is caused by a bovine pox virus.

Anthrax is a zoonosis of several domesticated animals caused by *Bacillus anthracis.* The disease usually begins as a cutaneous lesion at an inoculation site. The lesion is initially a vesicle and then becomes a painless ulcer covered by a black eschar surrounded by erythema and edema. Patients may go on to develop lymphadenitis and septicemia, and the fatality rate in untreated disease is 5% to 20%. Treatment is with penicillin. Ulcerative lesions with lymphadenopathy also occur with tularemia, bubonic plague, glanders, and rat-bite fever (see earlier discussion).

Several spirochetal diseases are endemic in the tropics and are caused by organisms that are similar to or identical with *Treponema pallidum* of syphilis. Pinta is a disease of the skin alone caused by *T. carateum;* it occurs in Central and South America and is transmitted by close contact and perhaps biting insects. The initial lesion is a papule that enlarges and develops satellite papules. Secondary pinta occurs after 1 to several months. The lesions of secondary pinta, called pintides, and are scaly macular lesions that develop blue pigmentation. The bluish lesions gradually progress to depigmentation and late lesions are white.

Yaws is caused by *T. pertenue* and is usually a childhood disease. It has a widespread distribution in the tropics. This disease involves bone as well as skin. The initial lesion at the inoculation site is a pruritic papilloma, called the "mother yaw." Secondary lesions include scaly macules, papules, and small papillomas. Painful papules occur on the palms and soles. Late lesions are destructive gummas of the skin and bones.

Bejel, or nonvenereal syphilis, usually occurs in children, mostly in the desert regions of Asia and Africa. Initial lesions appear on mucous membranes or in mucocutaneous areas. They are usually papules or condylomas. Later manifestations are similar to those of secondary and late syphilis. All these treponematoses are associated with positive serologic tests for syphilis. Spirochetes are demonstrable in skin lesions at various times, and the diseases can be spread by contact. Treatment is with penicillin or, in the penicillin-allergic patient, tetracycline.

Leprosy, or Hansen's disease, is a chronic infection due to *Mycobacterium leprae,* a bacterium that has not been cultured in artificial media. Currently the disease occurs primarily in tropical and subtropical regions, but sporadic cases occur worldwide. Lesions of the skin and peripheral nerves are the most notable manifestations. Two forms of the disease occur—lepromatous and tuberculoid leprosy—but there is considerable overlap. The lepromatous form is characterized by enormous numbers of organisms in lesions without a significant delayed hypersensitivity response. The tuberculoid form is characterized by more limited lesions, a cellular reaction, and few organisms in tissue.

With all types of leprosy, peripheral nerve involvement leads to varying degrees of denervation. Palpable thickening of superficial nerves is often noted. The skin lesions of tuberculoid leprosy are well demarcated, hypopigmented macules with hypesthesia that tend to develop circular borders. The lesions of lepromatous leprosy may be macules, papules, or nodules. There is also marked thickening of the skin leading to the typical leonine facies and pendulous ear lobes. Skin lesions of leprosy preferentially occur on the coolest portions of the skin: face (especially the cheek, nose, and brow), elbows, knees, buttocks, etc. The midline of the back is usually spared, and in lepromatous leprosy loss of the lateral eyebrows is typical. An immune reaction, erythema nodosum leprosum, occurs in lepromatous leprosy and is characterized by tender, erythematous, subcutaneous nodules associated with fever and lymphadenopathy. "Lucios phenomenon" is seen in lepromatous leprosy, especially in Mexico, and is characterized by angular dermal ulcers secondary to arteritis.

The diagnosis of leprosy is based on clinical appearance and demonstration of acid-fast organisms in skin biopsies. Treatment is with sulfones (e.g., dapsone). Several other drugs are being evaluated for efficacy, especially since the emergence of dapsone resistance. Thalidomide is curiously effective in the treatment of erythema nodosum leprosum.

*Mycobacterium marinum,* a saprophytic water organism, causes a localized skin lesion called "swimming pool granuloma." The lesion is papular to nodular and often ulcerates. The disease occurs sporadically in many parts of the world. It is treated with minocycline or antituberculous agents. Primary cutaneous tuberculosis may result in a similar lesion.

Visceral leishmaniasis has been discussed. Severe, progressive, diffuse leishmaniasis can occur with any form of cutaneous disease and appears to be related to immune compromise. There are several forms of cutaneous leishmaniasis. Old World cutaneous leishmaniasis, or oriental sore, occurs along the Mediterranean Sea, in the Middle East, and in southern Asia; it is caused by *Leishmania tropica.* The protozoan parasites are transmitted by the bite of sandflies of the *Phlebotomus* species. Two types of lesion occur at the site of the bite. In the rural, or moist, type an ulcer forms after a period of weeks to months and is associated with regional lymphadenopathy. In the dry, or urban, form a purple, pruritic nodule forms and breaks down to form an ulcer. These ulcers heal after several months to a year leaving hypopigmented scars.

Three species of *Leishmania* occur in Central and South America. *L. mexicana* causes "chiclero ulcer" in Central America. Ulcers that heal within several months occur on exposed surfaces, usually the hands or face, or forest workers, especially chicle harvesters. *L. peruviana* causes "uta," which occurs at high altitude and is characterized by single or multiple ulcers that heal. The most significant form of American leishmaniasis is caused by *L. brasiliensis.* It is transmitted by sandflies in jungle areas. A primary skin ulcer is followed by disseminated lesions to the mucous membranes. The disease is thus called American mucocutaneous leishmaniasis, or espundia. The mucous membrane lesions can be destructive or hypertrophic leading to deformity of the nose, palate, and larynx, as well as obstruction of the airway. Systemic signs and symptoms of fever, anorexia, and anemia are frequent.

The diagnosis of all forms of cutaneous leishmaniasis is usually made on clinical grounds. It is confirmed by demonstrating organisms in lesions or by culture. Several drugs are used for treatment, stibogluconate being the usual one. Amphotericin B has also been used in cases of severe American mucocutaneous leishmaniasis.

Helminthic parasites of humans and other animals that have skin-invasive larvae can cause dermatitis. Human hookworm larvae may cause a pruritic, edematous, maculopapular rash, usually on the feet, called ground itch. Larvae of cat and dog hookworms of the genus *Ancylostoma* cause a comparable rash called creeping eruption, or cutaneous larva migrans. Similar dermatitis from larvae of *Strongyloides stercoralis* occasionally occurs. Autoinfection with this worm can lead to erythematous and urticarial skin lesions. Pruritus and urticaria may appear at the time of invasion of the skin by the cercariae of *Schistosoma* species. Schistosome dermatitis may result from exposure to nonhuman, especially avian, schistosome larvae after sensitization. This dermatitis is called swimmers' itch.

Systemic fungal infections such as blastomycosis, cryptococcosis, and histoplasmosis occasionally cause skin lesions. African histoplasmosis caused by *Histoplasma duboisii* is primarily a skin disease characterized by granulomas. *Sporotrichum schenckii* is a saprophytic fungus that causes ulcerative skin lesions along lymph channels, usually after contact with rose thorns or sphagnum moss. Chromoblastomycosis is a fungal disease of the skin caused by *Phialophora* species that occurs mostly in the rural tropics; the disease is characterized by spreading cauliflower-like lesions. Rhinosporidiosis is a rare destructive skin and mucous membrane disease of the tropics caused by the fungus *Rhinosporidium seeberi.*

## GENERAL ADVICE

It is important to remind travelers of some basic common sense tips about their travel.

- Plan ahead. If planning travel, ask early about potential health concerns. Immunization is most effective when given at the appropriate time. Information gathering may take time.
- Review general health status regarding underlying conditions and medication requirements that may be affected by foreign destinations (e.g., insulin supply, needles and syringes, transport of medications, allergies, air travel, and pulmonary disease). Persons with conditions that may require emergency care should carry appropriate health status identification. Persons who wear glasses should carry a copy of their prescription.
- Travelers should be counseled as to the risk of bloodborne infection from nonsterile needles, syringes, and transfusions in the developing world.
- The risk of sexually transmitted infections, including HIV and infections caused by antibiotic-resistant organisms, is higher in many other parts of the world than in the United States. Vacationing travelers and lone travelers may be especially vulnerable to unsafe sex. Sexual contact with persons who may be infected should be avoided, and persons choosing to have sexual contact may reduce their risk of acquiring a sexually transmitted disease by always using a latex condom and avoiding anal intercourse.
- Activities should be modified for conditions of heat, humidity, and altitude.
- Adequately chlorinated pools are generally safe for swimming. Salt water is generally safe, but sea water and beaches may be contaminated with human sewage or animal feces. Swimming or wading in freshwater streams, ponds, or lakes may present risk for diseases such as schistosomiasis, leptospirosis, and giardiasis.
- Patients should be reminded that illnesses developing even months after return from a trip may be related to travel, and travel history should be reported to health care providers from whom treatment is sought.
- For diarrhea prevention, see Chapter 49.

## VACCINE RECOMMENDATIONS

Chapter 3 discusses routine and travel-specific immunizations that must be considered for travelers and reviews special considerations for use of vaccines in travelers.

## MALARIA PREVENTION

Malaria is an important problem in many tropical countries and occurs in up to 2% of travelers who visit West Africa without prophylaxis. The only areas considered not to have risk of malaria are the United States, Canada, Europe, and Japan. Risk in other areas varies from country to country, and place to place within countries, as do the recommendations. Specific details about areas of risk are available.

Avoiding contact with arthropods is an important method of preventing malaria; this fact must be emphasized by the health care provider. The best defenses against arthropod bites are avoidance of outdoor activities at dawn, dusk, and evening; use of insect repellent; and appropriate use of screens and bednetting. Such precautions also are helpful against other arthropod-borne diseases such as dengue fever.

Chloroquine-resistant *P. falciparum* has now spread to most areas with malaria. Chloroquine phosphate is still recommended for prevention of malaria for travel to areas where chloroquine-resistant *P. falciparum* has not been reported. The dose is 300 mg base (500 mg salt) once a week beginning 1 to 2 weeks before and continuing for 4 weeks after exposure to an area of low or no risk for chloroquine-resistant malaria. Travelers to areas of where chloroquine-resistant *P. falciparum* malaria has been reported should take mefloquine alone. The adult dose is 228 mg base (250 mg salt) per week starting 1 week before travel and continuing weekly during stay in the area of risk and for 4 weeks after leaving the area. Doxycycline alone is an alternative agent for short-term travelers who cannot take mefloquine; however, doxycycline failure has been well documented. Mefloquine is not approved for pregnant women, and an approved pediatric dose has not been established. Mefloquine is contraindicated in travelers on beta-blockers, those with a history of seizures, or those whose occupation requires fine coordination. Chloroquine alone is an alternative for pregnant women and children, but travelers who take chloroquine alone in areas at risk for chloroquine-resistant *P. falciparum* should be provided with and counseled about pyrimethamine-sulfadoxine (Fansidar) self-treatment for febrile illness occurring when professional medical care is not available. Mefloquine in therapeutic dose is associated with a high frequency of side effects and is not recommended for self-treatment. There are also mefloquine-resistant *P. falciparum* on the Thailand-Myanmar border; hence daily doxycycline is recommended for travelers in this region.

## BIBLIOGRAPHY

American College of Physicians Task Force on Adult Immunization and Infectious Diseases Society of America: *Guide for adult immunization,* ed 2, Philadelphia, 1990, American College of Physicians.

Ash LR, Orihel TC: *Atlas of human parasitology,* ed 3, Chicago, 1990, American Society of Clinical Pathologists Press.

Beck JW, Davies JE: *Medical parasitology,* ed 3, St Louis, 1981, Mosby.

Benenson AS, editor: *Control of communicable diseases in man,* ed 15, Washington DC, 1990, American Public Health Association.

Centers for Disease Control and Prevention: *Health Information for international travel,* Washington DC, yearly, Government Printing Office.

Garcia LS, Bruckner DA: *Diagnostic medical parasitology,* ed 2, Washington DC, 1993, American Society for Microbiology.

Lederberg J, Shope RE, Oaks SC Jr, editors: *Emerging infections. Microbial threats to health in the United States,* Washington DC, 1992, National Academy Press.

Neva FA, Brown HW: *Basic clinical parasitology,* ed 6, Norwalk Conn, 1994, Appleton & Lange.

Strickland GT, editor: *Hunter's tropical medicine,* ed 7, Philadelphia, 1991, WB Saunders.

The Medical Letter: Drugs for parasitic infections, *Med Lett Drugs Ther* 35(911): 111-122, 1993.

Warren KS, Mahmoud AAF, editors: *Tropical and geographical medicine,* ed 2, New York, 1990, McGraw-Hill.

Wilson ME: *A world guide to infections. Disease, distributions, diagnosis,* New York, 1991, Oxford University Press.

CHAPTER

# 67 Infectious Mononucleosis and Mononucleosis-like Disorders

Nelson M. Gantz

A 19-year-old man presenting with malaise, fever, sore throat, and cervical lymphadenopathy should suggest the diagnosis of acute infectious mononucleosis. Supporting this diagnosis is a white blood cell count showing a lymphocytosis with atypical lymphocytes and a positive Monospot test, which measures the presence of heterophile antibodies. In addition to the positive Monospot test, this patient will develop virus-specific antibodies to the Epstein-Barr virus (EBV). In most cases, the diagnosis of EBV infectious mononucleosis is not difficult. Problems occur for the clinician when the clinical findings are not classic and the Monospot test is negative. Several disorders can cause a Monospot-negative, mononucleosis-like illness including cytomegalovirus (CMV), EBV, toxoplasmosis, group A beta-hemolytic streptococci, and human immunodeficiency virus (HIV).

The complaint of chronic fatigue, defined as fatigue present for at least 6 months, accounts for about 20% of visits to primary care physicians. A syndrome characterized by chronic fatigue, recurrent sore throat, arthralgias, myalgias, fever, and cognitive dysfunction has been called the chronic fatigue syndrome. This chapter reviews the epidemiology, clinical manifestations diagnosis, complications, clinical course, and management of acute EBV infectious mononucleosis. The disorders that clinically mimic infectious mononucleosis are reviewed and the chronic fatigue syndrome is discussed.

EBV is one of seven herpes viruses. The other viruses in this group include herpes simplex virus-1, herpes simplex virus-2, varicella-zoster virus, CMV, human herpes virus-6, and human herpes virus-7. EBV is a DNA virus that infects B lymphocytes and nasopharyngeal epithelial cells. The virus does not produce cytopathic changes in the infected cells. In response to EBV infection, numerous antibodies are produced including heterophile antibodies and virus-specific EBV antibodies.

## EPIDEMIOLOGY

Antibodies to EBV are found in persons all over the world, and their prevalence is highest in lower socioeconomic groups. For example, in China by age 5 years, about 95% of persons have EBV antibodies; in contrast in the United

States and Great Britain the seropositive rate for EBV antibodies is about 50% by that age. Acute infectious mononucleosis is diagnosed most frequently in adolescents in higher socioeconomic groups. The incidence of acute infectious mononucleosis is highest in persons 15 to 24 years of age. The symptoms of acute EBV infection depend on the age during which the infection is acquired. Those acquiring an acute EBV infection before age 15 years have usually an asymptomatic infection or a mild "flulike" illness. Persons acquiring EBV infection after age 15 years usually have the typical acute infectious mononucleosis illness with fever, pharyngitis, malaise, and cervical and axillary lymphadenopathy.

## METHODS OF TRANSMISSION

Using special techniques, EBV can be demonstrated in the pharynx of patients with acute infectious mononucleosis for up to 18 months after recovery from an acute illness. The virus also can be identified in throat washings from patients with leukemia or lymphoma, as well as renal transplant recipients. The virus is not highly contagious, and most cases probably are acquired from asymptomatic shedders after close contact. Exchange of saliva with kissing may be responsible for viral transmission; the disease has been called the "kissing disease." The paradox of a high seroprevalence rate and low degree of contagion results because infected persons shed the virus for prolonged periods after an acute illness. Documented cases of intrafamilial transmission are unusual as are clusters of acute infectious mononucleosis. In experimental studies, the usual incubation period is 35 to 50 days in the adult. No precautions are required once an index case is identified. Acute infectious mononucleosis also can spread by a blood transfusion and is a cause for the "postpump perfusion" syndrome; however, most cases of postpump perfusion syndrome are caused by CMV.

## CLINICAL MANIFESTATIONS

Classic acute infectious mononucleosis is an illness characterized by fever, sore throat, malaise, and lymphadenopathy. The clue to the diagnosis is a young adult with a "toxic" appearance with a pharyngitis of more than 3 days' duration with posterior cervical lymphadenopathy. Pharyngeal exudates are often present (50%) and palatal petechiae may be seen. Other complaints include headache, anorexia, myalgias, chills, nausea, and abdominal discomfort. On physical examination, in addition to the lymphadenopathy, fever, pharyngitis, and splenomegaly occur in 50% of patients. Other findings include hepatomegaly, jaundice, periorbital edema, and a rash. The skin rash does not have a characteristic pattern and may be erythematous, maculopapular, or petechial. Interestingly, when a patient with acute infectious mononucleosis is given the antibiotic ampicillin, a nonallergic skin rash occurs in about 90% of patients. A skin rash also occurs in patients with CMV mononucleosis who have been given ampicillin, although less often than in patients with acute EBV infectious mononucleosis. However, this difference is not the way to establish the diagnosis of acute EBV mononucleosis. Table 67-1 lists the symptoms and signs of acute infectious mononucleosis. In addition to posterior cervical adenopathy, patients may have submandibular, anterior cervical, axillary, and inguinal lymphadenopathy.

**Table 67-1.** Clinical features of acute infectious mononucleosis

| Symptoms and signs | Frequency (%) |
|---|---|
| **Symptoms** | |
| Sore throat | 80 |
| Malaise | 60 |
| Headache | 50 |
| Anorexia | 20 |
| Myalgias | 20 |
| Chills | 15 |
| Nausea | 10 |
| Abdominal pain | 10 |
| **Signs** | |
| Lymphadenopathy | 95 |
| Pharyngitis | 85 |
| Fever | 75 |
| Splenomegaly | 50 |
| Periorbital edema | 30 |
| Hepatomegaly | 10 |
| Palatal exanthem | 10 |
| Jaundice | 10 |
| Skin rash | 5 |

Splenomegaly is present in 50% of patients and is usually maximal in size during the second week of illness. Splenic rupture is a rare complication of infectious mononucleosis, and trauma such as contact sports should be avoided during the first few weeks after diagnosis.

## DIAGNOSIS

Laboratory features of acute infectious mononucleosis include the presence of more than 50% lymphocytes with at least 10% atypical lymphocytes. The total white blood cell count is usually in the range of 10,000 to 20,000 cells/mm$^3$. A characteristic laboratory abnormality is the presence of heterophile antibodies. The term *heterophile antibody* refers to an antibody that reacts with an antigen of another species. These antibodies in patients with acute infectious mononucleosis react with sheep or horse red blood cells, but not guinea pig kidney cells. In contrast, heterophile antibodies found in patients with serum sickness react with guinea pig kidney cells. The heterophile antibody is detected in 90% of patients with acute infectious mononucleosis, but may require 3 weeks to become positive.

Most laboratories use the Monospot test to detect heterophile antibodies. The heterophile antibody is an IgM antibody and is not directed against the EB virus. The heterophile antibody usually disappears in most patients by 3 months, but rarely may persist longer. Thus the presence of a positive Monospot test indicates an acute infection. There is no need to follow or repeat the Monospot test because the titer or duration of the heterophile antibody response does not correlate with the clinical course of the illness. Rarely, false-positive Monospot tests occur in patients with varicella, influenza, or lymphoma. The most frequent cause of a false-positive Monospot test is laboratory error.

**Table 67-2.** Antibodies to Epstein-Barr virus

| Antibody | Time of appearance | Persistence | Comments |
|---|---|---|---|
| Viral capsid antigens | | | |
| VCA IgM | At presentation | 2 months | Indicates an acute infection |
| VCA IgG | At presentation | Lifelong | Not helpful for acute diagnosis |
| Early antigens (EA) | | | |
| Anti EA | At presentation | Lifelong | — |
| EBNA | | | |
| Anti EBNA | 1 month after presentation | Lifelong | A positive test on presentation usually indicates past infection. A negative test followed by a positive test 1 month later suggests a recent infection. |

### Complications of acute Epstein-Barr virus infection

**Hematologic**
Hemolytic anemia
Thrombocytopenia
Neutropenia

**Gastrointestinal**
Liver function test abnormalities
Jaundice
Splenic rupture

**Neurologic**
Aseptic meningitis
Guillain-Barré syndrome
Transverse myelitis
Bell palsy
Seizures

**Dermatologic**
Maculopapular rashes

**Cardiac**
Myocarditis

**Other**
Postanginal sepsis

Approximately 80% to 90% of patients with EBV mononucleosis have a positive Monospot test by the third week of illness. In the other 10% to 20% of patients, the diagnosis can be established by obtaining EBV antibody titers. EBV antibodies are listed in Table 67-2. There is usually no need to follow EBV serology by repeating the test because most of the antibody levels persist for life. However, the appearance of antibody to Epstein-Barr nuclear antigen (EBNA) in a patient with a prior negative EBNA antibody test is suggestive of a recent infection. Other laboratory abnormalities include mild liver function test dysfunction, mild thrombocytopenia, positive cold agglutinins, and the presence of cryoglobulins.

## COMPLICATIONS

The majority of patients with an acute EBV infection recover spontaneously in 3 to 4 weeks. Rarely, complications occur (see the box at left). Splenic rupture, especially during the second or third week, can be life-threatening. Thrombocytopenia is common but severe thrombocytopenia with an intracerebral bleed has been reported only rarely. Neurologic complications occur in less than 1% of patients but can dominate the clinical picture. At the time of presentation in patients with central nervous system (CNS) disease, the Monospot test can be negative, and the numbers of atypical lymphocytes are low or absent. Rarely, neurologic complications, splenic rupture, or upper airway obstruction results in death.

## MANAGEMENT

Treatment of acute infectious mononucleosis is mainly supportive. Contact sports should be avoided during the initial 3 weeks of the illness to avoid splenic rupture. Corticosteroids may be useful in patients with impending airway obstruction, severe thrombocytopenia, or hemolytic anemia. A 1- to 2-week course of corticosteroid therapy usually is administered. For normal hosts, acyclovir or other antiviral agents are not appropriate therapies for this disorder; if a throat culture reveals group A-beta hemolytic streptococci, however, then antibiotic therapy should be given.

## DIFFERENTIAL DIAGNOSIS OF MONONUCLEOSIS-LIKE SYNDROMES

Heterophile-negative and EBV-negative infectious mononucleosis can be caused by several disorders. The various disorders are listed in the box on p. 921.

### Cytomegalovirus

In most studies, CMV is the most frequent cause of this syndrome. Patients with CMV are usually older (mean age 28 years) than those with EBV infectious mononucleosis (peak age 17 years). Fever tends to be more prolonged in patients with CMV mononucleosis compared with that seen in patients with EBV infectious mononucleosis. Pharyngitis and lymphadenopathy occur more often in patients with EBV infectious mononucleosis, and are noted in only 20% of patients with CMV infectious mononucleosis. A rash occurs in about one third of patients with CMV mononucleosis. Atypical lymphocytes also can be present. The diagnosis of acute CMV can be established by demonstrating CMV IgM antibodies. However, this test is associated with both false-positive and false-negative

### Mononucleosis-like disorders

EBV
Hepatitis
CMV
HIV
Trichinosis
Malaria
Toxoplasmosis
Lymphogranuloma venereum
Secondary syphilis
Lyme disease
Cat scratch disease
Subacute bacterial endocarditis
*Yersinia enterocolitica*
Brucellosis
Tularemia
*Salmonella* bacteremia
Miliary tuberculosis
Leptospirosis
Systemic lupus erythematosus
Drug-induced mononucleosis syndrome
Juvenile rheumatoid arthritis
Lymphoma
Chronic fatigue syndrome

Modified from Gleckman RA, Czachor JS. In Gleckman RA, Gantz NM, Brown RB, editors: *Infections in outpatient practice: recognition and management,* New York, 1988, Plenum Press.

results. A diagnosis by serology also can be made by showing a fourfold rise in CMV IgG antibody titers.

## Hepatitis

The prodrome of acute viral hepatitis can mimic acute EBV infection, although pharyngitis and lymphadenopathy are absent. Fever, malaise, myalgias, arthralgias, and a rash may occur. Atypical lymphadenopathy may be present. The diagnosis is suggested by the marked elevation in liver function tests. Diagnosis is established by obtaining the serologic tests for the hepatitis viruses.

## Human immunodeficiency virus

HIV can produce a self-limited infectious mononucleosis-like illness 2 to 4 weeks after the virus is acquired. The illness is characterized by fever, sore throat, headache, anorexia, malaise, arthralgias, myalgias, and weight loss. A diffuse erythematous rash may occur. Symmetric lymphadenopathy is common. Laboratory abnormalities most often include leukopenia, lymphopenia, and thrombocytopenia. Atypical lymphocytes also may occur. Detection of HIV antibody by enzyme-linked immunosorbent assay (ELISA) may be negative during the first few weeks of an acute primary infection. HIV seroconversion usually occurs 3 months after the virus is acquired. During the acute primary HIV infection, which mimics EBV infectious mononucleosis, a transient decline in the CD 4 cell count may occur. Determination of serum p24 HIV antigen levels or use of the polymerase chain reaction (PCR) to detect HIV virus may be useful to establish the diagnosis of HIV disease. Otherwise, if there is a suspicion of HIV infection, the HIV antibody test should be repeated over time.

## Trichinosis

Trichinosis is acquired by eating raw or poorly cooked meat containing the viable larvae of *Trichinella spiralis.* The protean manifestations of trichinosis—fever, myalgias, malaise, and rash—may mimic the symptoms of infectious mononucleosis. Pharyngitis and lymphadenopathy are absent. Clues that suggest the diagnosis of trichinosis include diarrhea, periorbital edema, subconjunctival hemorrhages, eosinophilia, and a low or normal erythrocyte sedimentation rate. The diagnosis can be established by demonstrating antibodies 3 weeks after the infection using the bentonite flocculation test. A muscle biopsy is usually unnecessary, but when obtained from a tender muscle reveals the characteristic worm (see Chapter 66).

## Malaria

A history of travel should alert the clinician to the possibility of malaria. Features that suggest acute infectious mononucleosis include fever, chills, fatigue, myalgias, and arthralgias. Pharyngitis and lymphadenopathy are absent (see Chapter 66).

## Toxoplasmosis

Acute toxoplasmosis can mimic EBV or CMV infectious mononucleosis in the normal host. Toxoplasmosis, however, causes less than 1% of mononucleosis syndromes. Clinical features include fever, malaise, myalgias, and sore throat. Cervical lymphadenopathy is a prominent feature. Atypical lymphocytes may be present. The diagnosis of toxoplasmosis is made by demonstrating IgM antibody to *Toxoplasma.* Acute toxoplasmosis in the normal host is a self-limited illness, and specific acute toxoplasmosis therapy is not indicated.

## Lymphogranuloma venereum

Lymphogranuloma venereum (LGV) is caused by a type of *Chlamydia trachomatis* designated as types L1, L2, and L3. The initial stage is characterized by a small, asymptomatic ulcerative lesion. In the secondary stage, lymphadenopathy and prominent constitutional symptoms may mimic infectious mononucleosis. The consititutional symptoms include fever, chills, anorexia, myalgias, and arthralgias. Inguinal lymphadenopathy occurs but enlarged cervical lymph nodes and pharyngitis are lacking. Diagnosis of LGV usually is established by demonstrating an antibody rise to one of the LGV-specific types (see Chapter 65).

## Secondary syphilis

Constitutional symptoms such as fever, malaise, anorexia, pharyngitis, arthralgias, and painless lymphadenopathy occur in patients with secondary syphilis. A macular, maculopapular, and/or pustular rash, especially involving the palms and soles, strongly suggests the diagnosis. A characteristic feature is enlargement of the epitrochlear lymph nodes. Except in patients with HIV disease, the serologic tests for syphilis (RPR, VDRL, and FTA-ABS) are always positive in patients with secondary syphilis and will establish the diagnosis (see Chapter 65).

### Lyme disease

Lyme disease caused by *Borrelia burgdorferi* may resemble infectious mononucleosis in the early stages. Early symptoms include malaise, fatigue, headache, fever, arthralgias, myalgias and sore throat. These constitutional symptoms may occur before and persist after the characteristic rash of erythema chronicum migrans (ECM) disappears. Lymphadenopathy also occurs and is usually regional but may be generalized. The diagnosis of Lyme disease in the presence of the rash of ECM is not difficult. In the absence of the rash, the diagnosis is based on the epidemiologic findings and correlating the clinical features of the illness with the serologic results (see Chapter 87).

### Cat-scratch disease

Cat-scratch disease can resemble acute infectious mononucleosis. The infection is caused by a fastidious gram-negative bacillus identified as *Rochalimaea henselae* or *Afipia felis.* The disease is characterized by a primary lesion, a papule or pustule, which develops 3 to 10 days after a cat scratch. The hallmark of the illness is chronic regional lymphadenopathy, which develops about 2 weeks after the cat scratch. Constitutional symptoms that mimic infectious mononucleosis include fever, fatigue, sore throat, headache, and anorexia. The diagnosis is suggested by the history of localized lymphadenopathy in a patient with cat contact or a scratch. The organism can be identified on a lymph node biopsy. A serologic test also may be helpful in establishing the diagnosis.

### Subacute bacterial endocarditis

The clinical features of subacute bacterial endocarditis (SBE) can mimic several disorders such as malignancy, cerebrovascular accident, rheumatic disease, and infectious mononucleosis. Patients with SBE can present with fever, fatigue, anorexia, myalgias, and arthralgias. Pharyngitis and lymphadenopathy are absent. The diagnosis of SBE is made by obtaining three sets of blood cultures.

### *Yersinia enterocolitica*

*Yersinia* is a gram-negative bacillus that usually causes diarrhea and abdominal pain. The organism also can cause acute pharyngitis with fever not associated with diarrhea. The diagnosis can be established by cultures.

### Brucellosis

Acute brucellosis can mimic infectious mononucleosis. Symptoms include malaise, headache, anorexia, myalgias, arthralgias, and fever. Lymphadenopathy and splenomegaly may occur. Because patients with brucellosis present with nonspecific symptoms a history of an epidemiologic exposure to animals or dairy products is key to suspect the diagnosis. Cases are diagnosed by serology or culture.

### Tularemia

Tularemia is caused by *Francisella tularensis,* a small, gram-negative rod. Most infections are acquired from the bite of an infected animal such as a rabbit. The illness can mimic acute infectious mononucleosis, with patients having fever, chills, malaise, fatigue, and sore throat. On examination, pharyngitis and cervical lymphadenopathy may be present. Although the organism can be identified by culture, most infections are diagnosed serologically.

### Leptospirosis

Leptospirosis is a zoonosis with clinical features that can mimic acute infectious mononucleosis. Fever, headache and myalgias may occur. A rash, lymphadenopathy, and hepatosplenomegaly may be present. Pharyngitis is present in about 20% of patients. A history of exposure to animals such as rats or dogs is an important clue to the diagnosis (see Chapter 66). Most infections are diagnosed serologically.

### Other disorders

Several other disorders, including salmonella bacteremia, miliary tuberculosis, systemic lupus erythematosus, juvenile rheumatoid arthritis, and lymphoma, may at times mimic acute infectious mononucleosis. Drugs such as procainamide, isoniazid, and phenytoin also can be associated with a mononucleosis-like illness.

### Chronic fatigue syndrome

Chronic fatigue syndrome (CFS) is a disorder characterized by fatigue for at least 6 months and a complex or other symptoms. The illness is not new but has attracted increased attention and controversy since the late 1980s. The cause of the syndrome is unknown. In addition to the presence of chronic relapsing fatigue present for at least 6 months, clinical features include low-grade fever, chills, sore throat, lymphadenopathy, myalgias, arthralgias, headache, sleep disturbances, decreased ability to concentrate, and decreased memory.

The diagnosis of CFS is one of exclusion. Laboratory studies are normal; the erythrocyte sedimentation rate is low or normal. Several illnesses can mimic CFS including psychiatric disease such as depression. Efforts must be undertaken to exclude other potential causes of prolonged fatigue. Management of a patient with CFS is based on symptomatic therapy of a patient's complaints. Depression often occurs as a consequence of the disorder, and antidepressants may be helpful. Other effective measures include drugs to improve sleep and therapy for the muscle and joint complaints. The illness is associated with considerable morbidity but no increase in mortality. It is important to advise patients to avoid exotic, untested remedies that may be expensive and even harmful.

## BIBLIOGRAPHY

Bergman MM, Gleckman RA: Heterophile negative infectious mononucleosis-like syndrome, *Postgrad Med* 81:313, 1987.

Cohen JE, Corey GR: Cytomegalovirus infection in the normal host, *Medicine* 64:100, 1985.

Cooper DA et al: Acute AIDS retrovirus infection: definition of a clinical illness associated with seroconversion, *Lancet* 1:537, 1985.

Davidsohn I, Walker PH: The nature of the heterophilic antibodies in infectious mononucleosis, *Am J Clin Pathol* 5:455, 1935.

Evans AS: Infectious mononucleosis and related syndromes, *Am J Med Sci* 276:325, 1978.

Evans ME et al: Tularemia: a 30 year experience with 88 cases, *Medicine* 64:251, 1983.

Gantz NM, Holmes GP: Treatment of patients with chronic fatigue syndrome, *Drugs* 38(6):855, 1989.

Gleckman RA, Czachor JS: Mononucleosis and mononucleosis-like syndromes. In Gleckman RA, Gantz NM, Brown RB, editors: *Infections in outpatient practice: recognition and management,* New York, 1988, Plenum Press.

Holmes GP et al: Chronic fatigue syndrome: a working case definition, *Ann Intern Med* 108:387, 1988.

Klonoff DC: Chronic fatigue syndrome, *Clin Infect Dis* 15:812, 1992.

McCabe RE et al: Clinical spectrum of 107 cases of toxoplasmic lymphadenopathy, *Rev Infect Dis* 9:754, 1987.

Niederman JC et al: Infectious mononucleosis: clinical manifestations in relation to EB virus antibodies, *JAMA* 204:203, 1968.

Schluederberg A et al: Chronic fatigue syndrome research definition and medical outcome assessment, *Ann Intern Med* 117:325, 1992.

Sumaya CV, Ench Y: Epstein-Barr virus infectious mononucleosis in children: I. Clinical and general laboratory findings, *Pediatrics* 75:1003, 1985.

Sumaya CV, Ench Y: Epstein-Barr virus infectious mononucleosis in children: II. Heterophile antibody and viral specific responses, *Pediatrics* 75:1011, 1985.

Tacket CO et al: *Yersinia* enterocolitis pharyngitis, *Ann Intern Med* 99:40, 1983.

CHAPTER

# 68 Primary Care of the HIV-infected Patient

**Eliot W. Godofsky**
**Joel E. Gallant**
**John J. Zurlo**
**James C. Shaw**
**Peter R. Bergethon**

## HUMAN IMMUNODEFICIENCY VIRUS (HIV) AND THE PRIMARY CARE PROVIDER

Before the era of acquired immune deficiency syndrome (AIDS), immunodeficiency disorders were rare, typically congenital diseases. Comparatively little was known about the immune system, its specialized cells, complex web of interactions, and unique chemical messengers, the cytokines. Care of affected patients typically was relegated to specialized physicians at tertiary care centers. With early recognition that profound immune dysfunction defined the nature of AIDS, medical care was provided by the same specialists at the outset. Yet as the epidemic unfolded through the early and middle 1980s, two facts became obvious. First, the numbers of infected patients would quickly outstrip the numbers of available specialists. Second, with both the explosion of scientific information about the immune system and increased familiarity with the clinical course of AIDS patients that ensued, the nonspecialist could play a significant role in management. Since those early days, HIV infection has become an integral part of the practice of a large number of primary care practitioners throughout the country.

HIV disease is a chronic infection with a clinical course measured over years and a finite number of clinical manifestations and complications. As a result, with a thorough knowledge of the differential diagnoses associated with several major symptom complexes (i.e., cough, fever, headache, diarrhea), the primary care provider should easily be able to diagnose and treat the majority of the complications that patients experience.

## CLINICAL PATHOPHYSIOLOGY OF HIV INFECTION

HIV is a retrovirus and possesses the unique ability to convert its own single-stranded RNA to double-stranded DNA for incorporation into the host cell genome. This reaction is catalyzed by the enzyme reverse transcriptase, the major target for all currently licensed anti-HIV drugs. Two types of HIV, HIV-1 and HIV-2, cause immunodeficiency in humans. HIV-1 is the predominant viral species infecting patients in the United States and throughout most of the developed world. HIV-2 is found almost exclusively in western Africa where it is the predominant viral type. Detailed descriptions of HIV structure, life cycle, and molecular pathophysiology can be found in several major AIDS textbooks (see Bibliography). This focuses primarily on clinical aspects of HIV infection.

### Host response to infection

Immediately following infection with HIV, rapid viral replication occurs. High levels of viremia and p24 antigenemia can be measured early in the peripheral circulation. During this period an estimated 50% to 70% of patients develop symptomatic illness termed primary HIV infection. Symptoms include fevers, chills, malaise, diffuse lymphadenopathy, diarrhea, skin rash, headaches, and sore throat. This syndrome typically lasts for 1 to 3 weeks and then resolves. The host's immune system responds as evidenced by the presence of antibodies to specific viral proteins. Viral markers in plasma, notably p24 antigen concentration and viremia, drop precipitously. The T-helper lymphocyte (CD4) count drops transiently during primary HIV infection, sometimes to very low levels. Along with the development of antiviral antibodies, the CD4 count rises, although not completely back to baseline levels.

The initial host immune response to HIV infection is brisk and aggressive. High antibody levels can be measured to virtually all viral proteins. Some antibodies have neutralizing effects on the virus and cytotoxic T cells appear that specifically target virally infected cells. Unfortunately, the immunologic response to HIV is inadequate. It is interesting that in the blood compartment, the initial immune response is clearly adequate to eliminate plasma viremia. In addition the number of circulating lymphocytes estimated to be infected early in the course of infection drops to 1 in 10,000 or fewer. At this point a shift seems to occur in viral activity from the bloodstream to the lymphoid organs. The rate of viral replication within the lymphoid organs increases over time and ultimately spills back over into the blood compartment. With ongoing, high-level viral replication progressive immune system decline occurs, resulting in the clinical manifestations that are now well described.

### Immunologic abnormalities associated with HIV infection

Given that the primary target cell for HIV is the CD4 cell, and given the pivotal role of the CD4 cell in the orchestration of the immune response, it is not surprising to find that virtually all arms of the immune system are damaged during progressive infection. Qualitative and quantitative CD4 cell defects induced by the virus impair overall T-helper cell function. CD4 cells do not proliferate normally when stimulated, nor do they elaborate the necessary messengers (cytokines) to generate the appropriate responses from other arms of the immune system. Cells of the macrophage/monocyte lineage become dysfunctional in antigen presentation. The humoral immune response is impaired and worsens with advancing disease. As a result, patients develop an inadequate antibody response when exposed to new antigens. All of these immune system defects ultimately lead to the host becoming susceptible to a large group of opportunistic pathogens that are common to other cellular immunodeficiency states. Abnormalities in immune surveillance of neoplastic clonal expansion may be one important mechanism by which HIV-infected patients develop non-Hodgkin's lymphoma.

### Human immunodeficiency virus infectivity of various body fluids

**Fluids known to transmit infection**

Blood
Blood products
Semen
Vaginal fluid
Breast milk

**Fluids not known to transmit infection**

Saliva
Tears
Urine
Cerebrospinal fluid
Amniotic fluid

### Cellular targets of HIV infection

In addition to lymphocytes and macrophages, several other cells can be infected by HIV, although the mechanism of attachment and viral entry may differ. In particular, virus has been isolated from several types of cells in the central nervous system (CNS). It is likely that CNS invasion occurs early in the course of infection, at the same time that lymphoid organ seeding is occurring during and after primary HIV infection. Infected macrophages are thought to be responsible for introducing the virus into the CNS. The clinical implications of CNS infection for the host are great, because many patients suffer from CNS manifestations ranging from benign aseptic meningitis to encephalopathy and myelopathy. Infection of gut epithelial cells may be an important etiologic factor in the unexplained diarrhea and weight loss, which are so common in infected patients. Finally, infection of myeloid precursor cells in the bone marrow may be responsible for the neutropenia often observed in late stage disease.

## ACQUISITION AND TRANSMISSION OF HIV

Although HIV has been isolated from a variety of body fluids, the only fluids that have been recognized to transmit disease are blood and blood products, semen, vaginal fluid, and breast milk (see the box above). Other fluids such as saliva and tears, which contain low concentrations of viral particles, as well as cerebrospinal fluid, which has measurably high viral titers, have not been proven to transmit infection. Of course any body fluid can be rendered infectious if contaminated with blood or plasma. The major means of HIV transmission worldwide is by heterosexual intercourse. Other recognized modes of transmission include homosexual sexual activity, sharing of contaminated needles among injection drug users (IDUs), transfusion of infected blood products, and by mother to child transmission, either in utero, during the perinatal period, or by breast-feeding.

### Heterosexual transmission

During vaginal intercourse either partner can infect the other, although male-to-female transmission is more efficient than the reverse. In the case of semen, inflammatory cells, which are commonly found in the seminal secretions, probably represent the major means by which virus is transmitted. Virus then infects macrophages and lymphocytes within the cervix or higher up in the uterine body with subsequent dissemination of infection. For HIV-infected women vaginal secretions also contain cell-associated and cell-free virus, which probably infects macrophages within the male urethra, leading to disseminated infection. The presence of an active sexually transmitted disease (STD) clearly increases the efficiency of transmission. Whether the lesions are ulcerative, such as syphilis and chancroid, or nonulcerative, such as gonorrhea, the common feature among STDs is the preponderance of inflammatory cells which, coming from the infected partner, can increase the infectivity of the fluid or, in the noninfected partner, can increase the number of exposed susceptible targets.

### Homosexual transmission

Among homosexuals anal-receptive intercourse has the highest likelihood of HIV transmission. It was originally believed that small tears in the rectal mucosa provided a portal for viral entry. Most investigators now believe that virus attaches to and infects mucosal epithelial cells from which spread to underlying tissue macrophages leads to widespread dissemination. As with heterosexual transmission, active STDs probably increase the efficiency of transmission.

### Transmission secondary to infected blood products

Within the blood compartment, virus can be isolated in both the cellular compartment (mononuclear cells) and plasma. Infected cells are probably the more important, owing to the absolute number of viral particles that can be detected intracellularly in comparison with plasma. Before universal testing of blood products for HIV in 1985, many patients were infected after having received blood components, including packed red cells, platelets, or fresh-frozen plasma. Patients who received transfusions from donors with later stage HIV infection have tended to progress more quickly than those transfused with blood products from early stage, asymptomatic donors. This reflects the higher viral inoculum transmitted from the blood of patients with late stage disease, or the greater virulence of HIV associated with advanced disease. Patients with hemophilia A and other clotting disorders also have been infected from contaminated blood products pooled from many donors, some of whom were infected with HIV. At the present time all blood products in the United States are tested for HIV antibodies and are considered safe. The chances of HIV transmission from a single unit of transfused blood now is estimated to be 1 in 250,000.

### Injection drug users

The sharing of needles without sterilization between users results in parenteral exposure to HIV-infected blood. The efficiency of transmission is not clear. The use of a syringe/needle contaminated with blood from an individual with late stage HIV infection probably imparts the highest risk of transmission.

### Mother-to-child transmission

An HIV-infected mother can transmit infection in utero, perinatally, or by breast feeding. Taken together, in utero and perinatal transmissions account for the vast majority of mother-to-child infections. In utero transmission occurs transplacentally, most likely during the third trimester. Perinatal transmission probably takes place as the fetus is exposed to infected body fluids while passing through the birth canal. It is uncertain which of the two is the more common means by which infection is transmitted. Infection of an infant from exposure to infected breast milk certainly occurs, but is an uncommon mode of transmission in this country.

### Other modes of transmission

With the exception of a few rare reports, the transmission of HIV by casual contact is extremely unlikely. Family members and close friends who care for sick and dying patients have no appreciable risk of contracting HIV infection provided that they follow standard infection control procedures.

### Transmission in the health care setting

The occupational risk of transmission of HIV to health care workers (HCWs) from infected patients is extremely low but it is nonetheless a source of great concern. Of the reported cases of work-related HIV transmission, percutaneous exposures from HIV-contaminated needlestick injuries have been the most common mode of infection. HCWs also have become infected by mucous membrane or nonintact skin exposure, but these modes of transmission are extremely rare. The risk of seroconversion following a percutaneous exposure to HIV-infected fluid is approximately 0.3%. The seroconversion rates following the other types of exposures mentioned are likely to be much lower. Injuries that likely represent the highest risk of transmission include deep sticks involving hollow bore needles contaminated with freshly drawn blood. Based on animal data suggesting that postexposure prophylaxis with zidovudine may have some role in preventing infection, many hospitals and health care facilities offer the drug to health care workers after a significant occupational exposure. The lack of proven efficacy and the short-term toxicity of the drug, however, have caused many to question the practice.

The risk of transmission of virus from HCW to patient has received a great deal of attention during the past few years. If transmission occurs, it will most likely happen in the setting of an invasive procedure in an operating room. Although the transmission rate cannot be established reliably, it is likely to be several orders of magnitude less than the rate for patient-to-HCW transmission.

## COURSE AND NATURAL HISTORY OF INFECTION

### Course of disease

Following primary HIV infection during which there is a transient fall in the CD4 count, patients typically become asymptomatic (Fig. 68-1). During the early stages of infection, women may experience recurrent *Candida* vaginitis. Perisitent generalized lymphadenopathy (PGL) may also occur during early stage infection. With PGL, lymph nodes in multiple locations—especially the occipital, posterior cervical, and axillary regions—become enlarged, firm, nontender, and unattached to the underlying tissue. Although some patients note a waxing and waning of lymph node size, the adenopathy generally persists for many months. Pulmonary tuberculosis and bacterial pneumonia also occur at all stages, although they are more frequent when the CD4 count falls below 500 cells/mm$^3$. During this "asymptomatic" period the CD4 count remains at or near the normal range (>500 cells/mm$^3$). Over time the CD4 count declines at a rate of approximately 70 to 100 cells per year (10%/year).

With further CD4 count decline, the first symptoms and clinical conditions begin to appear. Symptoms include fatigue, intermittent unexplained fevers, diarrhea, and night sweats. For the first time patients feel ill. By now the CD4 count has typically dropped to between 200 and 500 cells/mm$^3$. Among the early conditions are oropharyngeal candidiasis, cervical neoplasia, and idiopathic thrombocytopenic purpura. Other conditions seen in early stage disease include oral hairy leukoplakia and herpes zoster (shingles), which can be recurrent and involve more than one dermatome during a single outbreak. Kaposi's sarcoma (KS) and B-cell lymphoma are conditions that meet the Centers for Disease Control and Prevention (CDC) surveillance case definition for AIDS during this stage of disease.

At a CD4 count of 200 cells/mm$^3$, patients are at risk to develop *Pneumocystis carinii* pneumonia (PCP), which, until the widespread use of prophylaxis, was the most common opportunistic infection seen in patients with AIDS. With the CD4 count in the 100 to 200 cells/mm$^3$ range, other conditions that may be seen are the early peripheral and central nervous system complications of infection. Once the CD4 count has dropped to between 50 to 100 cells/mm$^3$, patients become susceptible to the remaining AIDS-related conditions including cryptococcal meningitis, cytomegalovirus retinitis, *Toxoplasma* encephalitis, disseminated *Mycobacterium avium*-complex infection, and AIDS wasting syndrome.

As of January 1, 1993 the CDC revised its surveillance case definition for AIDS, which was first proposed in 1986 (see the box on p. 926). Two important changes were made. First the definition of AIDS was expanded to include all

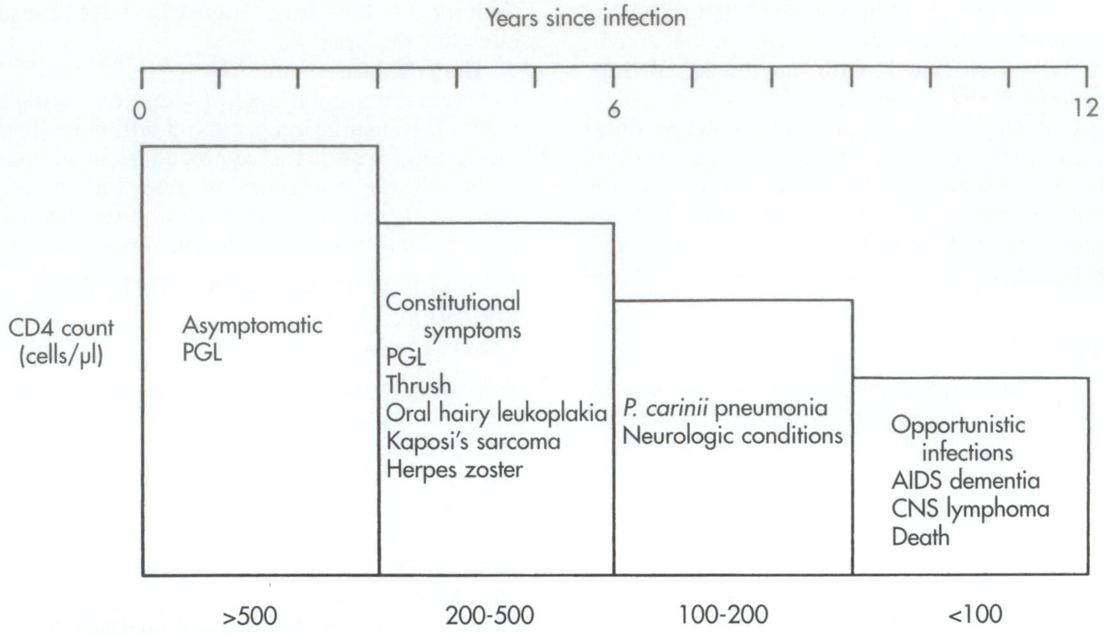


**Fig. 68-1.** The clinical course of HIV infection. The diagram shows the disease progression associated with CD4 count over approximately 12 years. *PGL,* Persistent generalized lymphadenopathy.

## 1993 Expanded surveillance case definition for AIDS

**HIV seropositivity AND CD4 count <200/mm³**
**OR one or more of the following conditions**

Candidiasis, esophageal, bronchial or pulmonary
Cervical cancer, invasive
Coccidioidomycosis, disseminated or extrapulmonary
Cryptococcosis, extrapulmonary
Cryptosporidiosis, chronic intestinal
Cytomegalovirus, retinitis or nonlymphoid
Encephalopathy, HIV-related
Herpes simplex, esophagitis, pneumonitis, or chronic ulcerative
Histoplasmosis, disseminated or extrapulmonary
Isosporiasis, chronic intestinal
Kaposi's sarcoma
Lymphoma, primary CNS, immunoblastic, or Burkitt's
*Mycobacterium avium*-complex or *M. kansasii,* disseminated
*Mycobacterium tuberculosis,* pulmonary or extrapulmonary
*Mycobacterium* species (other), disseminated or extrapulmonary
*Pneumocystis carinii* pneumonia
Pneumonia, recurrent
Progressive multifocal leukoencephalopathy
*Salmonella* septicemia, recurrent
*Toxoplasma* encephalopathy
Wasting, HIV-related

From Centers for Disease Control: *MMWR* RR-17:1-19, 1992.

HIV-infected patients with CD4 counts below 200 cells/mm³, whether or not they have suffered from a recognized complication. Second, pulmonary tuberculosis, recurrent bacterial pneumonia, and invasive cervical cancer in women were added to the list of AIDS-defining conditions.

The preceding account is a stylized description of the typical course of an HIV-infected patient. Unfortunately, there are a great many exceptions to this course of events. For example, symptomatic primary HIV infection is not recognized in 30% to 50% of patients. Also, the rate of decline of CD4 cells varies considerably among individuals. More important, many patients remain completely asymptomatic, even as their CD4 counts drop to low levels. Therefore one cannot reliably predict the CD4 count in an asymptomatic HIV-infected patient. In contrast, the CD4 count is predictably low in symptomatic patients, particularly if they have been diagnosed with a non-KS, AIDS-defining condition. As a result, some of the early staging systems used in HIV infection that were based on symptoms alone inaccurately reflected the true stage of disease in many cases. Similarly, staging systems based on the CD4 count alone are also inaccurate because symptoms influence prognosis. For example if one were to look at two groups of patients with similar CD4 counts, one asymptomatic and one symptomatic (fevers, diarrhea, night sweats, weight loss, thrush), the symptomatic group would progress more rapidly. The revised CDC staging system includes both symptoms and CD4 count (Table 68-1).

### Natural history of infection

HIV infection causes disease that is measurable not in weeks or months but in years. Several studies have examined time course of infection in selected populations. In San Francisco a cohort study of gay men originally begun in the late 1970s to study hepatitis B was adapted to study HIV. Among the cohort, only 2% of patients developed AIDS within 2 years of seroconversion, and 10 years were required for just over 50% of patients to develop AIDS. Interestingly, a small percentage of patients (<5%) have remained symptom-free with normal CD4 counts for more than 15 years.

The natural history of HIV infection also has been

**Table 68-1.** 1993 CDC classification system for HIV infection

| CD4 Count | Clinical categories (A) Asymptomatic, 1° HIV infection or PGL | (B) Symptomatic, not (A) or (C) conditions | (C) AIDS-indicator conditions |
|---|---|---|---|
| (1) >500/$mm^3$ | A1 | B1 | C1 |
| (2) 200-499/$mm^3$ | A2 | B2 | C2 |
| (3) <200/$mm^3$ | A3 | B3 | C3 |

From Centers for Disease Control: *MMWR* RR17:1-19, 1992.

**Table 68-2.** Cumulative AIDS cases according to risk category for adults and adolescents through December 1992

| Exposure category | Cumulative total (%) |
|---|---|
| Homosexual/bisexual men | 142,626 (57) |
| Injection drug use | 57,412 (23) |
| Homosexual/bisexual and injection drug use | 15,899 (6) |
| Coagulation disorder | 2,026 (1) |
| Heterosexual contact | 16,254 (7) |
| Blood component transfusion | 4,980 (2) |
| Other/undetermined | 10,002 (4) |
| TOTAL | 249,199 (100) |

From CDC: HIV/AIDS surveillance report, February 1993, pp 1-23.

**Table 68-3.** Cumulative AIDS cases according to race/ethnicity for adults and adolescents through December 1992

| Race/ethnicity | Cumulative total (%) |
|---|---|
| Caucasian, non-Latino | 131,754 (53) |
| African-American, non-Latino | 73,686 (30) |
| Latino | 41,172 (17) |
| Asian | 1,591 (<1) |
| Native American | 435 (<1) |
| Unknown | 561 (<1) |
| TOTAL | 249,199 (100) |

From CDC: HIV/AIDS surveillance report, February 1993, pp 1-23.

studied for hemophiliacs and transfusion recipients. Hemophiliacs appear to progress less rapidly than gay men, with one study reporting that only 27% had progressed to AIDS by 7 years from the time of seroconversion. The rate of progression to AIDS correlated inversely with age; younger patients, particularly those less than 17 years of age, had a much slower progression than did patients older than 35 years. In contrast, transfusion recipients as a group appear to progress more rapidly than either gay men or hemophiliacs, with approximately 50% of patients developing AIDS by 7 years. Natural history data for HIV-infected injection drug users (IDUs) is limited. Many investigators believe that the prognosis for these patients is generally poor, owing to such factors as the lack of ongoing medical care, noncompliance with treatment plans, poor nutrition, and greater exposure to tuberculosis and other infectious agents.

## EPIDEMIOLOGY OF HIV INFECTION

### United States

The CDC estimates that 1 million people in the United States are infected with HIV, almost all those infections being HIV-1. As of December 1992, 253,448 cases of AIDS had been reported to the CDC. The number of new AIDS cases for 1993 is likely to increase substantially from the previous year due to the changes in the CDC AIDS surveillance case definition discussed earlier. Table 68-2 lists the cumulative AIDS cases according to risk group category for adolescents and adults through December 1992. Homosexual and bisexual men remain the largest risk group followed by IDUs. Hemophiliacs represent a small portion of the whole (1%). Four percent of adults/adolescents with AIDS have been listed as having undetermined risk of infection. This group includes a large number of patients for whom there is incomplete information including patients who are currently under investigation, who died, or who refused interview or were lost to follow-up. As of December 1992, the CDC had identified 584 individuals for whom no identifiable risk could be determined.

Table 68-3 lists the cumulative AIDS cases through December 1992 by race/ethnicity. Although Caucasians represent the largest number of AIDS cases, African-Americans and Latinos make up a disproportionately large number of cases relative to their percentages within the population. Table 68-4 lists the cumulative AIDS cases through December 1992 for women according to both risk group and race/ethnicity. A total of 27,485 female AIDS cases had been reported representing 11% of all adults/adolescents in the United States with AIDS. Although cumulatively most women were infected by injection drug use, the CDC noted that in 1992, for the first time, the number of cases acquired from heterosexual contact exceeded those acquired from injection drug use.

Fig. 68-2 compares the relative percentages between the first and second 100,000 AIDS cases in the United States according to risk group and race/ethnicity. During the early part of the epidemic, the male/female ratio was 10:1, due to the preponderance of cases occurring in homosexual and bisexual men. For the second 100,000 cases the ratio dropped to 7:1, reflecting the higher proportion of heterosexually acquired cases among women. Also notable is the increasing proportion of cases transmitted among injection drug users.

## THE WORLDWIDE PERSPECTIVE

An estimated 100,000 individuals were thought to be infected worldwide in 1980, a number that increased to about 10 million cases by 1992. Of these, approximately 6 million are in Africa alone. Along with African countries, explosive spread has been observed in developing countries in other parts of the world in recent years. India and countries in Southeast Asia have seen an enormous rise in

**Table 68-4.** Cumulative female AIDS cases according to risk category and race/ethnicity for adults and adolescents through December 1992

| Exposure category | Race/ethnicity | | | | | |
|---|---|---|---|---|---|---|
| | Caucasian non-Latino | African-American non-Latino | Latino | Asian | Native American | TOTAL |
| Injection drug use | 2,901 (42) | 7,860 (54) | 2,784 (48) | 19 (13) | 35 (57) | 13,626 (50) |
| Coagulation disorder | 32 (0) | 8 (0) | 3 (0) | — | — | 43 (0) |
| Heterosexual contact | 2,275 (33) | 5,191 (36) | 2,280 (40) | 54 (38) | 15 (25) | 9,835 (36) |
| Blood component transfusion | 1,201 (17) | 419 (3) | 271 (5) | 45 (31) | 5 (8) | 1,944 (7) |
| Other/undetermined | 518 (7) | 1,073 (7) | 407 (7) | 25 (17) | 6 (10) | 2,037 (7) |
| TOTAL | 6,927 | 14,551 | 5,745 | 143 | 61 | 27,485 |

From CDC: HIV/AIDS surveillance report, February 1993, pp 1-23.

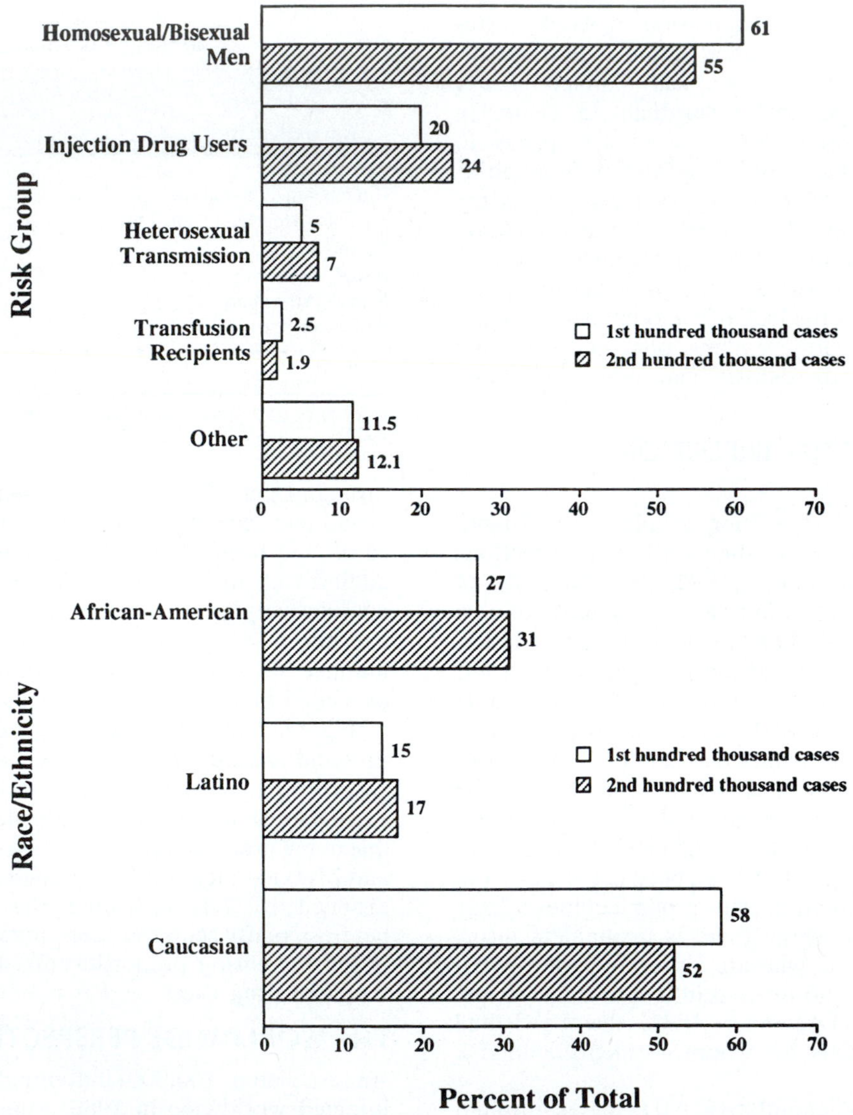


**Fig. 68-2.** The relative proportions of patients with AIDS according to risk group and AIDS/ethnicity comparing the first and second 100,000 cases. The risk group, "Other," consists primarily of homosexual/bisexual men who also are injection drug users along with patients whose risk for infection is uncertain. (From *MMWR* 41:28, 1992.)

the number of AIDS cases during the early 1990s. From a worldwide perspective the major means of spread (~75% of all cases) has been and continues to be sexual intercourse. The male/female ratio is approximately 1.5:1. The World Health Organization estimates that somewhere between 40 million and 110 million individuals will have become infected with HIV by the year 2000.

## AIDS-RELATED MORTALITY

Of the 249,199 adults/adolescents reported to have AIDS in the United States through December 1992, 169,623 (68.1%) had died. The case/fatality ratio for all HIV-infected patients has been estimated to exceed 90%. In the United States in 1992, HIV infection became the leading cause of death for men between the ages of 25 and 44 years and the fourth leading cause of death among women in the same age group. The death rate was three times higher for African-American men than for white men and 12 times higher for African-American women than for white women. Not surprisingly HIV-related death almost always occurs late in the course of disease. Death usually occurs secondary to opportunistic infections, AIDS-related malignancies, or wasting.

## EVALUATION OF THE HIV-INFECTED PATIENT

### Identifying patients at risk

The majority of the approximately 1 million Americans infected with HIV are unaware of their infection, and do not benefit from early intervention. The role of the primary care practitioner in diagnosing HIV disease is of critical importance. During the early years of the AIDS epidemic, surveillance focused on members of "high risk groups" (gay and bisexual men, intravenous drug users, and hemophiliacs); however, that approach is less useful today. A growing number of HIV-infected individuals contract their infection through heterosexual contact or are unaware of their mode of transmission. It has become more accurate therefore to think in terms of *risk behaviors* rather than *risk groups.* As a result, the taking of a thorough history, including nonjudgmental but specific questioning about sexual activity and drug use, has become even more important in identifying patients at risk for HIV infection.

Indications for voluntary testing also include sexually transmitted diseases, pregnancy, and active tuberculosis. Voluntary testing is also recommended for adults hospitalized in facilities where the seroprevalence exceeds 1% or where the AIDS case rate exceeds $1/1,000$ discharges. Finally, HIV testing should be considered in patients with generalized lymphadenopathy; unexplained dementia, aseptic meningitis, or peripheral neuropathy; chronic, unexplained fever, diarrhea, or weight loss; generalized herpes simplex or multidermatomal herpes zoster infection; unexplained cytopenias; B cell lymphoma; or other opportunistic conditions suggestive of defective cell-mediated immunodeficiency.

### Diagnosis

Unfortunately, the diagnosis of HIV disease may still lead to social stigmatization, loss of health insurance, and discrimination in employment and housing. Because of the potential consequences to the patient, informed consent is recommended before HIV testing and is required in most states. In addition HIV testing should be accompanied by pretest and posttest counseling, which should include discussion of the purpose of the test, prognosis and natural history of HIV infection, transmission of HIV and risk reduction, partner notification, and other medical and social issues related to the diagnosis.

The criteria for a positive HIV test are a repeatedly positive enzyme-linked immunosorbent assay (ELISA) followed by a positive Western Blot, usually requiring the presence of p24, gp41, and pg120/160 bands. The accuracy of the test is extremely high. False-negative results are uncommon and usually occur during the window period between infection and seroconversion, a period with a maximum duration of 6 months. False-positive results are extremely rare. Patients with a positive ELISA and a single band on Western Blot are reported as indeterminate. Indeterminate tests may occur in seroconverting patients, patients with advanced HIV disease, patients with HIV-2 infection, and patients with alloantibodies (pregnancy, transfusions, or organ transplantation) or autoantibodies (autoimmune diseases, malignancy). Although patients in low-risk categories with indeterminate tests are unlikely to be infected, repeat tests in 3 and 6 months are usually performed for confirmation. If the indeterminate test is due to seroconversion, it will usually become positive within 1 month.

Other methods to detect HIV infection include viral isolation, polymerase chain reaction (PCR), and p24 antigen assay. Because of the accuracy of the standard HIV test, however, these techniques are rarely necessary. The p24 antigen assay, which is less difficult and expensive than PCR and viral culture, can be helpful in making the diagnosis of the acute retroviral syndrome. Rapid tests for HIV antibodies are available and comparable in accuracy to the ELISA. They are highly sensitive; a negative result is definitive and can be reported in several minutes. Specificity is lower, however, and all positive results must be confirmed with standard tests.

### The initial evaluation

Clinicians evaluating patients with newly diagnosed HIV infection should take a careful history, focusing specifically on common HIV-related symptoms, including fevers, night sweats, weight loss, diarrhea, skin rashes or lesions, oral thrush or ulceration, and changes in neurologic function or mental status. Patients should be questioned about their past medical history, including STDs, chickenpox, hepatitis, bacterial infections, gynecologic problems, and exposure to tuberculosis.

A complete physical examination should be performed, with special attention to the evaluation of lymph nodes, funduscopic examination, examination of the oropharynx and skin, abdominal examination to detect enlargement of the liver or spleen, genital examination for STDs, and neuropsychologic testing to evaluate cognitive function and detect early dementia. Depression is common in HIV-infected patients, and clinicians should be alert to the possibility of this treatable condition. Frequent gynecologic examinations are mandatory in HIV-infected women. Patients who are cachectic or who report significant weight loss require medical evaluation to look for reversible causes.

## Laboratory studies

Several initial laboratory studies are appropriate in patients presenting with HIV infection. Patients who have no documentation of their HIV serology results or who were tested anonymously should have a repeat HIV test. Anemia, leukopenia, and thrombocytopenia are common in HIV-infected individuals and are readily detected with a complete blood count (CBC), which is also used to calculate the total CD4 lymphocyte count. A chemistry panel is important, especially to rule out HIV- or drug-related renal insufficiency and because of the high prevalence of chronic hepatitis B and C infections in HIV-infected populations. A nontreponemal test for syphilis, such as a VDRL or RPR, and a PPD skin test, should be performed at baseline, and repeated yearly.

Serologic testing for prior exposure to *Toxoplasma gondii* using the anti-*Toxoplasma* IgG is useful in determining the need for prophylaxis against toxoplasmic encephalitis. Seropositive patients should receive appropriate prophylaxis after the CD4 count has fallen sufficiently (see p. 957). Seronegative patients should be counseled on preventing infection by avoiding ingestion of undercooked meat, and by using proper precautions when handling cat feces. Seronegative patients should probably be retested when their CD4 count approaches 100/mm$^3$, especially if they are sulfa-intolerant. Although the *Toxoplasma* serology can never be used diagnostically, a seronegative patient with a space-occupying lesion of the CNS is less likely to have toxoplasmosis than a seropositive patient.

Because many patients with HIV-infection continue to engage in high-risk activities and because chronic hepatitis is more common in HIV-infected individuals, prevention of hepatitis B is appropriate for those without evidence of prior infection (negative anti-HBs). Patients with abnormal liver function tests should be tested for hepatitis B surface antigen (HBsAg) and for hepatitis C antibody (anti-HCV). Serologic tests for prior cytomegalovirus (CMV) infection are recommended, as those who are seronegative should receive only CMV-negative blood products. Furthermore, although routine prophylaxis against CMV disease is not currently recommended, it may one day be indicated for seropositive individuals with advanced HIV disease. Serologic tests for herpes simplex virus are not recommended. It has been recommended, however, that anti-varicella IgG be performed in patients who are unable to give a history of chickenpox. This baseline test will help to determine the need for post-exposure prophylaxis with varicella zoster immune globulin (VZIG) in patients who are exposed to chickenpox or shingles. The cryptococcal antigen assay is a sensitive screening test for active cryptococcosis in patients with advanced HIV disease and fever or headache, but it is not useful in the baseline evaluation of the patient.

Routine screening for glucose-6-phosphate dehydrogenase (G-6-PD) deficiency is sometimes recommended, especially in black patients and patients of Mediterranean descent. Several oxidant drugs, such as dapsone, primaquine, and sulfonamides, are commonly used in HIV-infected patients and may lead to hemolysis in G-6-PD-deficient patients.

Because HIV-infected patients are highly susceptible to a variety of pulmonary complications and infections, a baseline chest radiograph may be useful. Injection drug users are especially likely to have radiographic abnormalities that may be mistaken for infiltrates. A radiograph obtained when the patient is asymptomatic may be useful for comparison during the evaluation of respiratory complaints. Furthermore, because anergy is common in HIV-infected patients, the chest radiograph may be helpful in looking for evidence of tuberculosis.

HIV-infected women are at increased risk for several gynecologic problems, including pelvic inflammatory disease and tubo-ovarian abscesses, *Candida* vaginitis, cervical dysplasia, and invasive cervical carcinoma. All HIV-infected women should have a baseline pelvic examination with Pap smear. The use of routine colposcopy is controversial, but the test is indicated in women with abnormal Pap smears or a history of vaginal condylomata. Pap smears should be repeated at least annually in asymptomatic women; more frequent evaluations are recommended in women with abnormalities on Pap smear or with more symptomatic HIV disease.

The single most important test in the evaluation of patients with HIV infection is the CD4 lymphocyte count. The CD4 count is used in staging HIV infection, determining the need for antiretroviral therapy and for prophylaxis of opportunistic infections, assessing the risk of specific HIV-related conditions, and as of 1993, for making and reporting the diagnosis of AIDS. The clinician and patient must be aware of the substantial variation in the results of CD4 counts. Factors affecting the CD4 count include seasonal and diurnal variation, the use of corticosteroids, intercurrent illness, coinfection with HTLV-I, interlaboratory and intralaboratory variation, and variation in the components of the white blood cell count. Because in most laboratories, the absolute CD4 count is determined by multiplying the white blood cell count, the percentage of lymphocytes, and the percentage of CD4 lymphocytes, variation in any one of these components can affect the total CD4 count. Because the CD4 percentage is not subject to variation based on the white blood cell count and lymphocyte count, it may provide a more accurate reflection of the patient's immunologic status when the white blood cell count or lymphocyte count is unusually high. Total CD4 counts of 200 and 500/mm$^3$ generally correspond to CD4 percentages of 14% and 29%, respectively. New technologies are being developed that will allow more direct determination of the absolute CD4 count, eliminating the variability due to the other components of the complete blood count.

In addition to the CD4 count, other surrogate markers are sometimes used for evaluation of HIV infection. These include the p24 antigen, neopterin, beta-2 microglobulin, erythrocyte sedimentation rate (ESR), quantification of plasma viremia, and HIV strain phenotype. Although all correlate with disease progression or activity, they are used primarily in the evaluation of antiretroviral drugs in clinical trials and are less useful in the management of individual patients. Tests designed to quantify viral load are becoming available; however, they are not yet licensed, and the appropriate use of these tests in the management of patients has not been defined.

## Vaccinations

Advancing HIV infection impairs the natural ability to form specific antibodies after infection or immunization.

It is important therefore that vaccinations be given as early in the course of HIV infection as possible. Although its efficacy is not well established in this population, the pneumococcal polysaccharide vaccine is indicated for all HIV-infected patients, because of the high incidence of pneumococcal pneumonia and bacteremia associated with HIV disease. It is given as a single dose, with revaccination after 6 years. It is recommended that the influenza vaccine be given yearly, both to prevent influenza and its potential complications (primarily bacterial pneumonia) and to prevent clinical syndromes that may mimic more serious opportunistic infections. HIV-infected patients who are infected with hepatitis B virus are at greater risk of developing chronic infection and should be offered hepatitis B vaccine if they are at continued risk of infection. Although there is an increased frequency of *Haemophilus influenzae* infections in adults with HIV disease, many are non–type b infections. It is recommended that the *H. influenzae* type-b (Hib) vaccine be "considered" in HIV-infected adults. The efficacy of the vaccine has been more clearly established in children. Recommendations for the tetanus-diphtheria (dT) vaccine and the measles, mumps, and rubella (MMR) vaccine do not differ from those for immunocompetent adults. All other live vaccines are contraindicated, including Bacillus Calmette-Guérin (BCG), oral polio vaccine, oral typhoid vaccine (Ty21a), and yellow fever vaccine. If polio vaccination is indicated for HIV-infected individuals or their household contacts, the enhanced potency inactivated polio vaccine (eIPV) should be used. For international travelers, the inactivated (parenteral) typhoid vaccine can be used in place of the oral vaccine if necessary.

### Charting materials/frequency of office visits and routine labs

Now that patients are identified and treated early in the course of their infection, HIV disease is accurately regarded as a progressive but chronic disorder. As with any such disease, it is important for the primary health care provider to be able to monitor clinical changes and laboratory data in a longitudinal fashion. HIV disease lends itself particularly well to the use of flow charts, which help clinicians keep track of those data, and to observe and respond to changes in their patients' health over time. An example of such a flowchart is shown in Fig. 68-3.

The frequency of evaluation depends in part on the stage of HIV disease. Asymptomatic patients with normal CD4 counts (greater than 600/mm$^3$) can be followed infrequently, repeating CD4 counts every 6 months. Although HIV-related complications are unlikely at this stage, these visits are useful for addressing health care maintenance issues (performance of periodic PPD skin tests, syphilis serologies, and Pap smears, for example), for education about HIV disease and the prevention of transmission, and for building the therapeutic relationship that will become increasingly important as patients progress to more advanced disease. The CDC has recommended that, in patients who are not taking antiretroviral therapy, CD4 counts be repeated every 3 months after the CD4 count falls below 600/mm$^3$. Antiretroviral therapy is currently considered when the CD4 count falls below 500/mm$^3$. Once therapy has been initiated, monitoring of CD4 counts should continue, both to evaluate the response to the antiretroviral agent and to determine the need for opportunistic infection prophylaxis. It is recommended that, in patients with CD4 counts between 200 and 300/mm$^3$, monitoring be performed every 3 months, so that *Pneumocystis* prophylaxis can be initiated when indicated.

There are now good reasons to continue monitoring CD4 counts in patients with advanced HIV disease. As discussed earlier, the risk for a number of opportunistic infections increases after CD4 counts fall below 50 to 100/mm$^3$. Because many of these infections, such as toxoplasmosis, disseminated *Mycobacterium avium* complex, and fungal infections, can be prevented with appropriate prophylactic therapy, CD4 counts continue to provide useful information. Frequent ophthalmologic examinations in patients with very low CD4 counts may lead to early detection and treatment of CMV retinitis. In patients whose CD4 counts are consistently less than 50/mm$^3$, however, there is no reason to continue testing.

It is important to educate patients about the meaning of the CD4 count in the context of the natural history of HIV disease. All too often, HIV-infected individuals place excessive emphasis on minor fluctuations in the CD4 counts, becoming despondent over decreases that are well within the range of normal laboratory variation, or interpreting minor increases as important clinical improvements. This fixation may reflect the attitudes of clinicians and researchers, who are often more comfortable dealing with objective laboratory tests than with the other less quantifiable components that make up a patient's health. Although it is natural for clinicians to be enthusiastic and optimistic when informing a patient of a rising or stable CD4 count, when the count inevitably falls, the patient may respond with pessimism disproportionate to the clinical importance of the test result. The CD4 count is a surrogate marker that provides us with an important but indirect measure of the state of a patient's HIV disease and immunosuppression. The prognostic information it provides is useful, but incomplete. Both patients and clinicians must maintain a holistic approach to HIV disease, which incorporates the CD4 count as only one component of the total picture.

## ANTIRETROVIRAL THERAPY FOR HIV INFECTION

Specific antiretroviral therapy for HIV infection was made available 5 years after the first descriptions of AIDS, and 3 years after the identification of the responsible virus. Such an unprecendented acceleration of the drug approval and availability process in the 1980s has been equally matched by controversy and confusion in the 1990s. Effective use of antiretroviral agents presents a formidable challenge for both patients and physicians. Patients must be sufficiently motivated to follow complicated regimens involving expensive, potentially toxic drugs, that are often recommended when the patient is asymptomatic. Physicians have the equally difficult task of keeping current in a rapidly changing and controversial field that uses surrogate markers of disease progression, lacks conventional sensitivity testing, and uses drugs with significant toxicities and interactions.

| | | | | |
|---|---|---|---|---|
| Name | | Primary Provider | | |
| Patient ID# | | D.O.B. | Phone | |
| Dates | HIV Diagnosis | | AIDS Diagnosis | |
| | 1st visit | | Psychosocial evaluation | |
| Immunizations | Pneumovax (q 6y) | | dT (q 10yr) | |
| | | | | |
| Baseline studies | HBsAg | HBsAB | anti-HCV | Other |
| (dates & results) | Toxo IgG | G6PD | VZV Ab | Other |
| Contacts | | Case Manager | | |
| AIDS Reported? (Initials & Date) | | Visiting Nurse | | |
| Allergies/Drug Reactions | | | | |
| Advance Directives | | | | |

| YEAR | | | | | |
|---|---|---|---|---|---|
| Major diagnoses & clinical events | | | | | |
| Weight/Nutrition | | | | | |
| Clinical stage | | | | | |
| CD4 count<br>as indicated | | | | | |
| Antiretrovirals<br>(drug & start dates) | | | | | |
| PCP prophylaxis<br>(drug & start dates) | | | | | |
| Other major therapy<br>(Ongoing prophylaxis<br>or maintenance) | | | | | |
| Flu vaccine | | | | | |
| RPR<br>yearly if negative | | | | | |
| PPD/controls | | | | | |
| Ophtho. referral<br>CD4<50-100 | | | | | |
| PAP smear | | | | | |

Fig. 68-3. An example of a health maintenance flowchart used in an HIV Clinic.

**Table 68-5.** Potential targets and agents for antiretroviral therapy

| Stage | Agents |
|---|---|
| Viral attachment and penetration | Vaccines<br>HIV antibodies |
| Reverse transcription | Nucleoside analogs (e.g., AZT*)<br>Non-nucleoside RT inhibitors<br>Foscarnet |
| Transcription and translation | Interferons<br>Antisense oligonucleosides<br>Tat antagonists |
| Post-translational processing | Glycosylation inhibitors<br>Protease inhibitors |
| Assembly and budding | Interferons<br>HIV antibodies<br>Cytotoxic lymphocytes |

*AZT, Zidovudine.

## Principles of antiretroviral therapy

Antiretroviral agents can target any number of several steps in the viral replicative cycle that are distinct from mammalian cell processes (Table 68-5). The development of effective antiretroviral compounds has been a relatively difficult process due to the complex nature of HIV infection. Drug development and testing have been streamlined by the availability of rapid and sensitive assay systems to screen large numbers of potential agents, the use of combination phase multicenter trials, and expanded access programs. Unfortunately, both physician and patient must often deal with problems of supply and demand even before sufficient efficacy data are available.

Developing a practical approach to antiretroviral therapy will be reviewed.

## Zidovudine (AZT, Retrovir)

Zidovudine is a nucleoside analog of thymidine that interferes with HIV replication by competitive inhibition of the viral enzyme reverse transcriptase. Zidovudine and related compounds have no effect on previously infected cells. Interim analysis of a 1987 study of 1500 mg/day of zidovudine versus placebo in patients with AIDS or severe AIDS-related complex (ARC) found that patients receiving zidovudine had significantly decreased mortality, fewer opportunistic infections, increased CD4 counts, and weight gain compared with the placebo group. The results of this study led to prompt FDA approval of zidovudine for AIDS patients with a prior episode of *P. carinii* pneumonia or whose CD4 count was below 200/mm$^3$. Subsequent studies found that 500 to 600 mg/day was better tolerated and as efficacious as the higher dose regimens. Current practice is to give zidovudine, 200 mg, every 8 hours. Patients should be seen within 2 weeks of starting therapy to obtain a CBC and evaluate for potential side effects. The CBC should be monitored routinely every 4 weeks for the first 3 months of therapy, and then every 8 to 12 weeks if the counts remain stable. Doses as low as 300 mg/day may be beneficial in some individuals, but should be reserved for patients intolerant to the standard doses.

Determining the optimal time to intervene with antiretroviral therapy has been difficult. Early studies supported "early" intervention with zidovudine in symptomatic and mildly symptomatic patients with CD4 counts from 200 to 500/mm$^3$. While the "rule of 500" rapidly became accepted, important questions remained as only a few studies appeared to demonstrate a survival advantage in patients receiving AZT.

Controversy peaked in the summer of 1993 when preliminary results from the Concorde I study raised questions about the institution of AZT therapy for asymptomatic patients. Investigators found that rates of disease progression did not differ between treatment and placebo groups at 3 years of follow-up. Subgroup analysis showed a trend to benefit from AZT in patients with initial CD4 count above 500/mm$^3$ and a nonsustained benefit with therapy at 12 to 16 months. Although these results did not dispute the efficacy of AZT, they challenged the benefits of early therapy. At the same time, extended follow-up from a cohort of asymptomatic patients treated with AZT versus placebo since 1989 found that progression to AIDS decreased with AZT therapy. The effect lasted for at least 2 years in patients with a baseline CD4 count above 300/mm$^3$ and for 18 months in patients with lower initial counts. Despite the delay in disease progression, early AZT therapy did not prolong survival compared with later treatment. More recent studies have reported similar results, with the duration of AZT benefit related to the patient's immune status when therapy is initiated.

How might the physician interpret these seemingly conflicting results and apply them to clinical practice? On one side, numerous multicenter trials over the last 5 years have substantiated the efficacy of AZT using a variety of laboratory measures and clinical indicators. More recent evidence however, suggests that early therapy with AZT may offer little or no advantages compared to treatment at more advanced stages of HIV infection. Therapy with AZT in patients with CD4 counts above 500/mm$^3$ can slow the decline of CD4 counts without any clinical benefit. Despite misconceptions, many of these findings are not necessarily contradictory as the recurring theme seems to be that benefit from AZT is time-limited in the range of 1 to 2 years. Most of the survival curves converge after 2 to 3 years, despite differences in rates of disease progression. Nonetheless, the ability of AZT to prolong the period during which patients are asymptomatic or minimally symptomatic is an important therapeutic consideration for the HIV-infected patient. Data do not indicate that early therapy with zidovudine is detrimental or has a negative impact on survival. Therefore the benefits of AZT therapy may be greatest if therapy is started when the CD4 count is relatively high. More modest results would be expected in patients with advanced HIV infection. Laboratory demonstration of antiretroviral resistance is consistent with these observations, as drug resistance develops more rapidly in patients with advanced disease. Because viral replication takes place in the lymphatic tissue of asymptomatic HIV-infected individuals with high CD4 counts, antiretroviral therapy may be considered as soon as the diagnosis of HIV infection is made.

Finally, AZT use in pregnant women and their newborns has been shown to decrease the risk of vertical transmission. AZT therapy instituted in the second trimester can reduce maternal transmission of HIV from 25% to 8%. The

U.S. Public Health Service now recommends this treatment in selected women.

Myelosuppression is the major toxicity of AZT (see the box below). The incidence of cytopenias is increased with higher dosages of AZT, advanced disease, lower CD4 counts, low serum levels of $B_{12}$ or folic acid, and baseline anemia or neutropenia. Anemia occurs in approximately 1% of asymptomatic patients, 6% of patients with early symptomatic infection (ARC), and up to 39% of patients with AIDS. Neutropenia occurs in approximately 2% of asymptomatic patients, 4% of patients with early disease, and up to 37% of patients with advanced HIV infection. Recombinant erythropoietin (rEPO) and colony stimulating factors (G-CSF, GM-CSF) lessen or reverse the cytopenias associated with zidovudine administration. Subcutaneous erythropoietin (Procrit, Epogen) given three times a week reduces the transfusion requirement of severely anemic AZT-treated patients with serum erythropoietin levels of less than 500 mU/ml. However, cytokine therapy is inconvenient and extremely expensive, and switching antiretroviral agents is often a more cost-effective approach. Recommended management strategies for common AZT-associated toxicities are outlined in the box at right.

Common subjective side effects of AZT include nausea, headache, myalgias, fatigue, restlessness, flulike symptoms, and abdominal discomfort. These generally occur early in therapy and resolve within 2 months. Other toxicities associated with prolonged AZT therapy include myopathy, cardiomyopathy, transaminase elevation, and bluish discoloration of the nail beds. AZT-associated myositis develops in 1% to 2% of patients during long-term administration. The proximal muscle pain, weakness, and exercise-induced myalgias are accompanied by marked elevations in creatine kinase (CPK) and generally respond to a dose reduction or discontinuation. Some clinicians advocate the routine monitoring of CPK levels at 3-month intervals after 6 to 12 months of AZT therapy. If myositis fails to resolve or worsens several weeks after therapy, primary HIV-related myositis should be considered.

### Didanosine (ddI, Videx)

Didanosine is a nucleoside analog that inhibits the replication of HIV by inhibiting viral reverse transcriptase. The drug was approved by the FDA in 1991 for patients who were intolerant of or "failing" AZT monotherapy. Subsequent studies found that didanosine was more effective than AZT in delaying the development of new op-

---

### Toxicities of currently approved antiretroviral agents

**Zidovudine (AZT)**

Myelosuppression
Myopathy
Headache, insomnia, flulike illness, fevers
Abdominal discomfort
Bluish discoloration of the nail beds
Lactic acidosis (rare)
Hepatomegaly with steatosis (rare)

**Didanosine (ddI)**

Pancreatitis
Peripheral neuropathy
Diarrhea
Hyperamylasemia
Hypertriglyceridemia
Hyperuricemia

**Zalcitabine (ddC)**

Peripheral neuropathy
Pancreatitis
Urticaria
Oral/esophageal ulcers
Cardiomyopathy (rare)

**Stavudine (d4T)**

Peripheral neuropathy

---

### Management of AZT-associated toxicities

**Anemia (hemoglobin $<8$ g/l) - discontinue AZT and:**

Allow bone marrow to recover. Restart AZT at reduced dose (300 mg/day).
Consider supportive blood transfusions. Restart AZT at reduced dose (300 mg/day).
Administer erythropoietin at 50 to 100 µg/kg/day subcutaneously three times each week.
Change to alternate antiretroviral (ddI, ddC, d4T*).

**Neutropenia (neutrophil count $<750$ cell/mm$^3$)- discontinue AZT and:**

Reinitiate at lower dose (300 mg/day) after marrow recovery
Change to alternate antiretroviral (ddI, ddC, d4T).
Administer colony stimulating factor (G-CSF, GM-CSF) starting at 1 to 5 µg/kg/day SQ and titrated in weekly increments up to 10 µg/kg/day to achieve absolute neutrophil count $>750$ cells/mm$^3$. Maintenance dose is usually 0.1 to 1.0 µg/kg/day to achieve an absolute neutrophil count of 750 to 1500 cells/mm$^3$.

**Myositis**

Consider CPK monitoring at 2- to 3-month intervals after 6 months of therapy.
Discontinue AZT for clinical myopathy with significant increase in the CPK level. Over 70% of patients will improve over 6 to 8 weeks.
Continue AZT with modest elevations in CPK in asymptomatic patients.
If symptoms persist or worsen after therapy, consider primary HIV-related myopathy.

**Conditions generally requiring only observation and support:**

Malaise or fatigue
Nausea or vomiting
Abdominal discomfort
Headache
Insomia
Flulike symptoms

*Currently available for compassionate use.

portunistic infections in patients with at least 16 weeks of previous AZT exposure. Additional data suggested that while AZT is the most effective initial therapy, patients with as little as 8 to 16 weeks of prior AZT therapy may benefit from switching to ddI. These studies have prompted some clinicians to change the drug regimen from AZT to ddI much earlier in the patient's clinical course.

Because didanosine is degraded rapidly at an acidic pH, the drug is prepared with a gastric acid buffer that improves bioavailability. ddI is available as a buffered chewable tablet and as a powder for solution in water. Tablets must be taken in pairs to ensure the proper buffering ratio and must be chewed, crushed, or dissolved in cold water to release the buffer before they are swallowed. Current dosage recommendations for the tablet formulation are 200 mg twice a day for patients weighing more than 60 kg and 125 mg twice a day for patients weighing less 60 kg. Doses for the buffered powder are 250 mg twice a day, and 167 mg twice a day, respectively, by weight. Because the bioavailability of both formulations of ddI is decreased when administered with food, the drug should be taken 30 to 60 minutes before a meal and no sooner than 2 hours after the last meal.

The major side effects of ddI are pancreatitis and peripheral neuropathy (see the box on p. 934). Pancreatitis occurs in approximately 7% of patients treated with the lower doses of ddI (400 to 500 mg/day) and ranges from mild abdominal pain with an increased amylase to fatal disease. Some clinicians monitor the serum amylase at 4- to 8-week intervals and reduce the dose if elevations of two to four times normal occur in the absence of clinical pancreatitis. Unfortunately, an elevated serum amylase does not always occur before an episode of pancreatitis, or it may be due to increased salivary amylase production. If a patient on ddI develops abdominal pain, nausea, vomiting, and/or a substantial rise in serum amylase, the medication should be stopped until the diagnosis of pancreatitis can be excluded. Risk factors for the development of pancreatitis include a past history of pancreatitis, alcohol consumption, elevated triglycerides, and advanced HIV infection. Alternative therapy, or at least more frequent monitoring, should be considered in these patients.

Peripheral neuropathy is the major dose-limiting toxicity of ddI, occurring in 13% to 34% of patients on recommended doses. Symptoms include distal numbness, tingling, or burning in the hands and feet that may progress proximally. This condition is more common in patients with a history of peripheral neuropathy or nutritional deficiency, or in those receiving other neurotoxic medications (e.g., isoniazid). Peripheral neuropathy due to ddI generally resolves 2 to 12 weeks after the medication is stopped. In mild cases, the medication has been reintroduced successfully at a lower dose. Diarrhea due to the osmotic effect of the buffer may occur in up to 34% of patients.

### Zalcitabine (ddC, HIVID)

Like AZT and ddI, zalcitabine is a potent inhibitor of reverse transcriptase. A 1992 trial found that combination therapy with AZT and ddC in patients with advanced HIV resulted in greater increases in CD4 cell counts than AZT alone. A subsequent study comparing AZT and ddC in patients with advanced HIV infection and less than 12 weeks of previous AZT, found higher survival rates among patients receiving AZT. On the basis of these studies, the FDA initially approved ddC only in combination with AZT in patients with advanced HIV infection who were failing AZT therapy alone. Subsequent studies have examined the role of ddC monotherapy in patients previously treated with AZT. One large multicentered study found that ddI and ddC are equally effective in slowing disease progression in patients intolerant of or failing AZT. Another study that compared ddC with continued AZT in patients previously treated with 48 weeks or more of AZT found slightly slower rates of decline in weight and CD4 cell count in the ddC group. In 1993, an FDA committee recommended approval of ddC as second-line monotherapy in patients with intolerance or significant clinical deterioration during AZT therapy. Surprisingly, the same committee also recommended withdrawal of the combination approval originally granted by the FDA. Currently, the best studied indication for ddC appears to be as alternate monotherapy based on disease progression and/or the side effect profile of other agents.

Zalcitabine is formulated in tablets of 0.375 and 0.75 mg. The standard dose is 0.75 mg taken every 8 hours and should be reduced by 50% in patients weighing less than 35 kg or with significant impairment of renal function.

Painful sensorimotor peripheral neuropathy is the major dose-limiting toxicity of ddC occurring in approximately 10% of patients on the currently recommended doses (see the box on p. 934). The incidence of this complication is more common in patients with a CD4 count less than 50 cell/mm$^3$. The neuropathy usually responds to cessation of therapy and the judicious use of narcotics or tricyclic antidepressants. In some patients, symptoms of neuropathy may initially progress despite discontinuation of ddC and irreversible cases have been reported. Reinstating therapy after resolution of mild symptoms is possible if a reduced dose is prescribed.

Pancreatitis is relatively uncommon, with ddC therapy occurring in <1% of patients. Oral and esophageal ulcers, cardiomyopathy, urticaria, hyperglycemia, fatigue, and fever have been reported. Intravenous pentamidine, ddI, and stavudine (d4T) should not be given concurrently with ddC. Drugs with the potential to cause peripheral neuropathy (e.g., isoniazid, metronidazole, dapsone, and dilantin) also should be avoided if possible.

### Stavudine (d4T, Zerit)

Stavudine is the most recently approved antiretroviral agent. Like its three predecessors, it is a reverse transcriptase inhibitor. It is readily phosphorylated in cells to its active triphosphate form and displays potent activity against retroviruses in vitro. At this time, no mutations indicative of resistance have been identified; however, they will probably occur with prolonged usage as has been seen with the other drugs in this class.

Early phase I and II clinical studies revealed that a dose of 1 mg/kg/day divided twice daily was the most efficacious best on rates of CD4 response and the development of peripheral neuropathy. Subjects in these studies experienced weight gain, improvement in all parameters of viral expression, and minimal side effects.

Current studies comparing stavudine with zidovudine in patients with CD4 counts of 50 to 500 cells/mm$^3$ are shortly to be completed. The exact role for stavudine is not yet determined. However, based on its efficacy and safety profile it is expected to become one of the first line drugs in the antiviral armamentarium.

The drug is dispensed as capsules in strengths of 15 mg, 20 mg, 30 mg, and 40 mg. The recommended starting dose based on body weight is 40 mg twice daily for patients >60 kg, and 30 mg twice daily for patients <60 kg. Dosage adjustment is necessary for patients with significant impairments in renal function. There are no known problems with absorption and the drug has negligible gastrointestinal side effects.

Stavudine is remarkably free of major side effects apart from peripheral neuropathy. The incidence is approximately 12%, is dose related, and is usually reversible if identified early. Often the drug may be restarted at a lower dose without recurrence of the neuropathy. Apart from mild hepatic dysfunction and some subjective complaints of insomnia, anorexia, and nausea, the drug is generally well tolerated. Care should be taken when other drugs are used that also may cause peripheral neuropathy (isoniazid, metronidazole, ddI, vincristine).

## New therapies

Recent excitement has been generated by the addition of 3TC (lamivudine) to the antiretroviral arsenal. Although ineffective as monotherapy, combination of this inhibitor of reverse transcriptase with AZT has resulted in impressive and sustained (48 to 52 weeks) increases in CD4 counts. Surprisingly, this synergistic effect can be seen in individuals previously treated with long courses of AZT and with falling CD4 counts. Toxicity is minimal with this drug and several phase II/III trials are nearing completion. Nonnucleoside reverse transcriptase inhibitors (e.g., nevaripine, delavridine) interfere with viral enzyme activity without incorporation into DNA. Unfortunately, the rapid emergence of high-level resistance will probably limit the usefulness of these drugs as monotherapy. Preliminary results of combination therapy are more encouraging.

By cleaving precursor viral proteins, HIV protease is a key enzyme in assembly of new viral particles. Protease inhibitors (e.g., saquinavir) are effective at a late stage of infection (after syncytia have started to form), giving these drugs the potential to affect newly and chronically infected cells. A three-drug combination of saquinavir, ddC, and AZT was superior to two-drug combinations in patients with CD4 counts of 50 to 300 in terms of CD4 cell count increases and reduction in viral burden. Despite problems with oral bioavailability, ongoing studies with saquinavir and second-generation protease inhibitors continue to be very encouraging.

Modulation of the immune system to combat HIV infection and its consequences may be accomplished through therapies that use specific cytokines such as interferons, interleukins, and tumor necrosis factor. Treatment with interleukin-2 has been found to augment and prolong increases in CD4 counts in a small number of patients treated with conventional antiretroviral therapy. Particularly promising is the ability of interleukin-12 (IL-12) to boost cell-mediated immune response of peripheral white blood cells in vitro. The potential of IL-12 to increase immune surveillance and CD4 counts with decreased toxicity has promoted intense investigation of this cytokine.

## Combination therapy

Combination therapy directed against HIV offers the following potential advantages: (1) synergistic activity against the virus (2) delay in the development of drug resistance (3) reduced toxicity by using one or more drugs at lower dosages (4) use of agents with different mechanisms of activity against the virus, and (5) activity against different cell types or tissues infected by HIV. A prolonged antiviral effect in vitro may even be obtained when multiple drugs against a single target are used.

Studies on combination therapy have generally been small, early phase trials evaluating regimens of two or more antiretrovirals or an antiretroviral compound combined with a cytokine. A 1992 phase I/II trial of AZT plus ddC in 56 patients with advanced HIV and no prior antiretroviral therapy demonstrated improvement of weight, CD4 cell count, and p24 antigenemia with combination therapy. The results of this trial led to the initial FDA approval of ddC for use in combination with AZT, an indication that has subsequently been withdrawn. Several small studies have suggested that weekly or monthly alternating regimens of antiretrovirals are efficacious and may reduce toxicity compared with monotherapy.

Combination therapy was evaluated recently in a large, multicentered trial in which patients were randomized to receive AZT alone, ddC alone, or the combination. At 1 year of follow-up, there were no differences in overall efficacy between the groups. When stratified by pretreatment CD4 count, however, patients in the 150 to 300/mm$^3$ group who received combination therapy had a statistically significant reduction in AIDS-defining events and improvement in CD4 cell count. Mortality rate was not affected by treatment in any group, and patients in the 50 to 100/mm$^3$ did poorly on all regimens. Although this study suggests a specific patient population that might benefit from combination therapy, the number of clinical end-points used was small and many patients had received more than 18 months of AZT therapy before enrollment.

Future studies are designed to evaluate different antiretroviral regimens in patients stratified by CD4 count and duration of prior therapy. In vivo drug studies strongly support the use of multidrug regimens. The concept is to generate drug pressure that forces the viral enzyme to develop multiple drug-resistant mutations in order to survive. Combination therapy with two or more agents appears more effective in vitro at slowing HIV infection than monotherapy, and is becoming the standard of clinical practice. Patients at early and intermediate stages of infection seem best able to tolerate multidrug regimens. The best combinations, timing of initiation of therapy, and laboratory markers to assess during therapy are not yet determined.

Finally, mention should be made about the potential benefits of acyclovir in combination with AZT therapy. Although acyclovir has little or no direct antiretroviral activity, current evidence suggests that coinfection with herpes virus may enhance HIV replication and accelerate clinical progression. Several large-scale studies have now documented improved survival in patients treated with zidovudine plus acyclovir. The optimum acyclovir dosage for survival benefit appears to be 600 to 800 mg/d. Many practitioners are now adding acyclovir to the treatment regimen of patients with CD4 counts below 200/mm$^3$.

### A practical approach to antiretroviral therapy

The most successful approach to administering antiretroviral therapy has yet to be defined. Most specialists in the field concede that the current group of available agents are generally weak and that better agents and/or more effective combinations are desperately needed.

Overall there is little doubt about the value of treating symptomatic patients with antiretroviral therapy. Whether to initiate drug treatment in asymptomatic patients is a more difficult decision, and rests largely on the belief that new effective drugs will be available in the near future. Multidrug treatment is more likely to reduce viral load and increase CD4 counts than monotherapy and has become the preferred treatment in clinical practice. Patients at early and intermediate stages of HIV infection are best able to tolerate combination therapy, whereas the toxicities are often too problematic for patients with CD4 counts below 50/mm$^3$. The advent of viral load monitoring and better combinations of antiretrovirals will greatly improve future therapy.

## RECOGNIZING AND TREATING COMPLICATIONS OF HIV INFECTION

This section reviews the diagnosis and management of the major complications associated with HIV infection and AIDS that the primary care provider is likely to encounter. Prevention of infectious complications is addressed in the section on prophylaxis.

### Pulmonary infections

***Pneumocystis carinii.*** Although antiretroviral therapy and *Pneumocystis* prophylaxis have reduced the morbidity and mortality due to PCP, it is still one of the most common opportunistic infections in patients with AIDS. *P. carinii* is discussed in this chapter under its traditional category as a protozoan, although recent data suggest that it may in fact be a fungus. Disease most likely occurs as a result of latent infection acquired via the respiratory route early in life.

PCP is usually insidious in onset, with progression of symptoms over weeks or months. The patient typically presents with fever, dyspnea, and a cough, which is often nonproductive. Fatigue and weight loss also may be present. Physical examination may reveal fever and tachypnea, but findings on chest examination are often normal. The chest radiograph typically reveals diffuse, bilateral interstitial or alveolar infiltrates; however, PCP may also present with focal infiltrates, consolidation, cavitary or cystic lesions, pleural effusions, nodular densities, or a normal radiograph. Atypical radiographic features, especially apical infiltrates, have been associated with the use of aerosolized pentamidine for PCP prophylaxis. Spontaneous pneumothorax may occur in association with concurrent or prior PCP and appears to be more common in persons who have received aerosolized pentamidine.

PCP is unusual in patients with a CD4 lymphocyte count less than 200 to 250/mm$^3$. Laboratory abnormalities are nonspecific. Although the serum lactate dehydrogenase (LDH) level is elevated in most patients with PCP, LDH elevations are also seen in other AIDS-related respiratory illnesses. The arterial blood gas may demonstrate hypoxemia, an elevated alveolar-arterial gradient, hypocarbia, or respiratory alkalosis; but a normal arterial blood gas does not exclude PCP. Although oxygen saturation also may be normal, a low oxygen saturation or desaturation with exercise is suggestive of PCP. Other tests used to support the diagnosis of PCP in selected cases include the diffusing capacity for carbon monoxide (DLCO) and Gallium$^{67}$ citrate scintigraphy of the lung. Both are highly sensitive for PCP, but nonspecific. Because of their high sensitivity and negative predictive value, these tests are sometimes useful in the evaluation of patients with normal chest radiographs and arterial blood gases to determine the need for further diagnostic procedures.

Because many other HIV-related conditions can mimic the presentation of PCP and because therapy is prolonged and associated with significant toxicity, empiric treatment should be avoided. The initial diagnostic procedure in patients suspected of having PCP is usually an examination of sputum induced by nebulized hypertonic saline. With proper induction techniques and the use of appropriate stains or monoclonal antibodies, the sensitivity of this test can exceed 90%, approaching that of bronchoscopy.

When examination of an induced sputum specimen is negative, fiberoptic bronchoscopy should be performed. The sensitivity of bronchoalveolar lavage alone ranges from 79% to 98%, and when combined with transbronchial biopsy, the sensitivity of bronchoscopy is between 94% and 100%. Repeat bronchoscopy or open lung biopsy should be considered in patients who have had nondiagnostic bronchoscopy and who are clinically deteriorating.

A growing number of acceptable treatment options are available for patients with PCP. Trimethoprim-sulfamethoxazole (15mg/kg per day of trimethoprim and 75 mg/kg per day of sulfamethoxazole), given orally or intravenously in three to four divided doses for 21 days, is effective in the treatment of *P. carinii* infection and is the drug of choice for initial therapy in most cases. Adverse reactions are common and include fever, rash, leukopenia, neutropenia, and hepatic dysfunction. The traditional alternative to trimethoprim-sulfamethoxazole (TMP-SMX) is daily parenteral pentamidine (4 mg/kg) given intravenously over 1 hour. Pentamidine also is associated with frequent adverse reactions, including renal dysfunction, hypoglycemia, hyperglycemia, hypotension, fever, and neutropenia. Intravenous administration is preferred, as intramuscular administration is painful and associated with sterile abscesses.

The combination of oral trimethoprim (15 to 20 mg/kg a day in 3 to 4 divided doses) and dapsone (100 mg a day) is an alternative to TMP-SMX and appears to be as effective and better tolerated in patients with mild-to-moderate PCP. Toxicities of dapsone include hemolytic anemia in patients with G6PD deficiency and rash, nausea, and methemoglobinemia. Dapsone is ineffective as monotherapy.

A regimen of oral or intravenous clindamycin (1800 to 2400 mg a day) and oral primaquine (15 mg primaquine base a day) is also effective in treating PCP. Side effects include rash, diarrhea, leukopenia, and mild methemoglobinemia. Primaquine should be avoided in G6PD-deficient patients.

Atovaquone is approved for use in patients intolerant to TMP-SMX. Although it is somewhat less effective than

TMP-SMX, it is associated with fewer treatment-limiting adverse reactions. The recommended dose is 750 mg orally three times a day. Absorption of atovaquone is variable, and patients with diarrhea may have inadequate serum levels. Absorption is improved by administering the drug with fatty foods. A new formulation designed to provide better bioavailability is being studied.

Trimetrexate, a folate antagonist, is approved for use in patients with moderate-to-severe PCP who cannot be treated with TMP-SMX. It is given as a daily intravenous infusion of 45 $mg/m^2$ over 60 to 90 minutes. As with atovaquone, it is less effective but better tolerated, than TMP-SMX. Patients taking trimetrexate also should be given folinic acid to minimize bone marrow toxicity. The most common adverse effects are neutropenia, thrombocytopenia, and elevations in serum aminotransferase concentrations.

Adjunctive corticosteroids reduce short-term mortality and respiratory deterioration in patients with moderate-to-severe PCP. Steroids are recommended for patients with PCP with an oxygen pressure ($PO_2$) of less than 70 mm Hg or a $P(A\text{-}a)O_2$ gradient of greater than 35 mm Hg on room air. The recommended regimen is prednisone 40 mg twice a day for 5 days, then 20 mg twice a day for 5 days, followed by 20 mg a day for the remaining 11 days of therapy.

***Toxoplasma gondii.*** *T. gondii,* the most common cause of CNS mass lesions in patients with AIDS, is an uncommon cause of pneumonitis in HIV-infected patients in the United States. Patients with toxoplasmic pneumonitis usually present with dyspnea, nonproductive cough, fever, and diffuse interstitial infiltrates on chest radiograph. Diagnosis is made by demonstration of tachyzoites from respiratory specimens, using hematoxylin and eosin or Giemsa staining. As with toxoplasmic encephalitis, serology is nondiagnostic. Because specific studies of therapy of toxoplasma pneumonia have not been carried out, patients should be treated with regimens recommended for *Toxoplasma* encephalitis.

***Community-acquired pneumonia.*** The association of community-acquired pneumonia with HIV infection was recognized early in the AIDS epidemic. The most common causative organisms are *Streptococcus pneumoniae* and *Haemophilus influenzae.* Intravenous drug users are at greater risk than homosexual men, and individuals who smoke tobacco or other drugs are also at increased risk. Because profound immunosuppression is not required, pyogenic bacterial infections, including pneumonia, may be one of the earliest manifestations of HIV disease and should prompt consideration of HIV testing.

The clinical presentation of bacterial pneumonia is similar in patients with and without HIV infection. The onset of symptoms is more abrupt than with PCP, and the patient is more likely to experience a productive cough and pleuritic chest pain and to have localized findings on chest examination. A relative leukocytosis and left shift are common. Radiographic features typically include localized segmental or lobar consolidation, especially in the case of pneumococcal pneumonia. Radiographic manifestations of *H. influenzae* pneumonia are more variable and include the diffuse bilateral infiltrates characteristic of PCP. Bacterial pneumonia in HIV-infected patients may be associated with a more severe course, a higher incidence of multilobar involvement and bacteremia, a less rapid response to antibiotics, and a higher rate of recurrence.

Patients presenting with clinical and radiographic features of pneumonia should have bacterial cultures of blood and sputum performed. Gram stain of the sputum is helpful in making a presumptive diagnosis, particularly when the sputum is purulent. The diagnosis of concurrent PCP is difficult when purulence is present. Thus when suspected pathogens include both *P. carinii* and pyogenic bacteria, treatment with high-dose TMP-SMX should be considered, as it provides excellent coverage not only against *P. carinii,* but also *S. pneumoniae, H. influenzae, Moraxella catarrhalis,* and *Legionella pneumophila.* When PCP is less likely to occur, as in a patient with a focal infiltrate or a total CD4 count greater than 200/$mm^3$, options for empiric treatment include second-generation cephalosporins or ampicillin-clavulanic acid. When Gram stain or culture is indicative of pneumococcal pneumonia, specific therapy with penicillin or erythromycin is preferred. In patients who fail to respond appropriately to antibiotic therapy or who deteriorate after initial improvement, coinfection with another pathogen, especially *P. carinii,* should be considered.

***Other causes of bacterial pneumonia.*** Nosocomial pneumonia in patients with AIDS is usually caused by gram-negative bacilli, including *Pseudomonas aeruginosa,* or by *S. aureus.* As with other hospitalized patients, risk factors include neutropenia, the use of broad-spectrum antibiotics, and the presence of central venous catheters. Nosocomial pneumonia has a higher morbidity and mortality than community-acquired pneumonia. *Pseudomonas* pneumonia is now a recognized complication of HIV infection, and is not always hospital-acquired or fulminant in presentation.

Other bacterial pathogens reported to cause pneumonia in patients with HIV infection include *Bordetella bronchiseptica, Moraxella catarrhalis,* group B streptococcus, *Mycoplasma pneumoniae, Salmonella typhimurium,* and *Streptomyces* species. Pneumonia due to *L. pneumophila* and *L. micdadei* has been described in patients with HIV infection, causing cavitation in some cases.

*Rhodococcus equi* is a gram-positive, aerobic, nonmotile, non–spore-forming pleomorphic bacillus that causes pulmonary disease in HIV-infected patients. Patients usually present with unilobar, often upper lobe infiltrates that progress over several weeks. Effective antimicrobial agents include erythromycin, vancomycin, clindamycin, chloramphenicol, and TMP-SMX. Prolonged courses of parenteral antibiotics are recommended, and surgical intervention is sometimes necessary for persistent abscesses.

Nocardiosis is unusual in HIV-infected patients, although the actual incidence is unknown, as it is not an indicator disease for AIDS. In most cases, disease occurs in patients CD4 cell counts less than 200/$mm^3$. Patients usually present with an indolent course and nonspecific, constitutional complaints. Pulmonary symptoms such as cough or dyspnea also may be present. The lung is the most common site of disease, although dissemination is common. Radiographic features include nodules, cavities, and diffuse or focal infiltrates. The diagnosis should be suspected when filamentous, beaded, branching, gram-positive, acid-fast rods are seen on Gram stain or modified acid-fast stain of sputum or other respiratory specimens. Sulfonamides are the mainstay of therapy in nocardiosis. Therapy for 6 to 12 months or longer has been recommended.

***Mycobacterium tuberculosis.*** The HIV epidemic has resulted in a worldwide rise in the incidence of tuberculosis. Because *M. tuberculosis* is more virulent than many of the other HIV-associated opportunistic pathogens, it often causes disease at an earlier stage of HIV infection and is frequently the initial manifestation. The incidence is higher in populations with an increased likelihood of prior exposure to *M. tuberculosis,* such as intravenous drug users, blacks, Hispanics, and residents of developing countries.

The natural history of tuberculosis is altered dramatically by HIV infection. In individuals with latent *M. tuberculosis* infection who acquire HIV infection, the risk of reactivation is 2% to 8% per year. HIV-infected persons who acquire new *M. tuberculosis* infection have a high risk of developing primary tuberculosis. The clinical presentation of tuberculosis in HIV-infected patients varies depending on the degree of immunosuppression. Patients with mild to moderate depression of the CD4 count who present with reactivation tuberculosis usually have isolated pulmonary disease with typical radiographic features. In patients who develop tuberculosis at a more advanced stage of HIV infection, however, radiographic findings may be atypical or may mimic those of primary tuberculosis. Cavitary disease is unusual in these patients, and lower lobe infiltrates or miliary patterns occur frequently. Intrathoracic adenopathy, extrapulmonary dissemination, and bacteremia also are more common in patients with advanced HIV disease.

Diagnosis of pulmonary tuberculosis is made by examination of sputum for acid-fast bacilli (AFB), followed by mycobacterial culture. The diagnostic yield of the sputum smear is lower in patients with more advanced HIV disease. The sensitivity of smear and culture may be increased by bronchoalveolar lavage. Because bacteremia occurs in a substantial proportion of patients, blood cultures for AFB should be performed on all patients in whom tuberculosis is suspected. A positive tuberculin skin test with intradermal PPD may provide supportive evidence for a diagnosis of tuberculosis, but a negative skin test should never be used to exclude tuberculosis, as patients may become anergic with progressive depression of cellular immunity.

Patients with AFB on smear or culture of respiratory specimens should be treated for presumed tuberculosis until culture results are obtained. Standard treatment is effective and long-term maintenance therapy or prophylaxis is unnecessary. Rates of treatment failure and relapse do not appear to be higher than in patients without HIV infection. Patients should receive isoniazid 300 mg/day, rifampin 600 mg/day (or 450 mg/day for patients weighing less than 50 kg), pyrazinamide 20 to 30 mg/kg/day, and ethambutol 25 mg/kg/day. The four-drug regimen should be continued for 2 months, and therapy with isoniazid and rifampin should then be continued for a minimum of 9 months, and for at least 6 months after cultures have become negative. Six-month treatment regimens may be equally effective, but have not been adequately studied in HIV-infected patients. Adverse reactions to chemotherapeutic agents occur more frequently than in patients without HIV infection.

Recently, several large outbreaks of multidrug-resistant tuberculosis (MDR-TB) have occurred. These outbreaks involved large numbers of patients, occurred in institutional settings, and were characterized by rapid propagation, high mortality, and rapid progression to death. The isolates were resistant to both isoniazid and rifampin, and in many cases to other drugs as well. Most cases have occurred in HIV-infected patients, presumably because they are more likely to develop tuberculosis soon after infection than are patients without concomitant HIV infection.

Satisfactory therapy for MDR-TB is not currently available. If multidrug resistance is suspected patients should be treated with a standard four-drug regimen consisting of isoniazid, rifampin, pyrazinamide, and ethambutol, plus at least two other agents to which local MDR-TB strains are susceptible. The regimen should be modified when susceptibility tests become available. Because of the poor response to treatment, appropriate isolation procedures must be used to reduce the risk of nosocomial transmission.

***Other mycobacteria.*** *Mycobacterium kansasii* is a cause of serious pulmonary disease in patients with advanced HIV disease. Although only disseminated *M. kansasii* infection is an AIDS-indicator condition, pulmonary disease appears to be considerably more common. The clinical presentation of pulmonary *M. kansasii* disease is similar to that of pulmonary tuberculosis. Radiographic features vary considerably, but diffuse interstitial or apical infiltrates and thin-walled cavities are characteristic. Extrapulmonary disease or dissemination is not uncommon in HIV-infected patients. Treatment with a regimen of isoniazid, rifampin, and ethambutol is usually effective.

Although *Mycobacterium avium* complex (MAC) is a common cause of morbidity in advanced HIV disease, it has only rarely been reported to cause lung disease. Endobronchial lesions containing granulomas also have been reported. Although it may predict dissemination and be an indication for prophylaxis, growth of MAC from respiratory specimens without histopathologic evidence of disease is not an indication for treatment. The same is true for many other nontuberculous mycobacterial species, such as *M. gordonae, M. fortuitum, M. chelonei, M. xenopi, M. haemophilum,* which rarely cause isolated pulmonary disease in HIV-infected patients.

***Fungal infections.*** Although the majority of patients with disease due to *Cryptococcus neoformans* present with meningitis, it also is the most common cause of fungal pneumonia in AIDS patients. The portal of entry of *C. neoformans* is the lung, and clinically silent pulmonary infection is probably more common than overt pneumonitis. Cryptococcal pneumonia may be an indolent or rapidly progressive disease. Patients usually present with fever and nonspecific constitutional symptoms. At least two thirds have respiratory symptoms, such as productive cough, dyspnea, and pleuritic chest pain. The most common radiographic findings are focal or diffuse interstitial infiltrates; but other findings include nodular or miliary infiltrates, alveolar infiltrates, mass lesions, cavitation, pleural effusion, and mediastinal adenopathy. Detection of cryptococcal antigen in the serum is a rapid and highly sensitive screening test for invasive cryptococcal disease such as meningitis, but it may be negative when disease is confined to the lungs. Definitive diagnosis of cryptococcal pneumonia requires culture of *C. neoformans* from respiratory specimens or identification of typical-appearing encapsulated yeast forms in respiratory secretions. Most data about the treatment of cryptococcosis come from studies on patients with meningitis, and amphotericin B or fluconazole is recommended.

The filamentous fungus *Aspergillus* is an uncommon cause of pneumonia in AIDS patients; however, both invasive aspergillosis and obstructing bronchial aspergillosis have been described as a late complication of AIDS. Potential predisposing factors include drug-induced neutropenia, corticosteroid therapy, and marijuana use. Radiographic findings of invasive pulmonary aspergillosis are variable and include upper-lobe cavitation and pleural-based infiltrates or nodules. Diagnosis is made by bronchoalveolar lavage and transthoracic biopsy of lesions. Therapy consists of amphotericin B or itraconazole.

*Histoplasma capsulatum, Coccidioides immitis,* and *Blastomyces dermatitidis* are important causes of pneumonia and disseminated disease in AIDS patients from endemic areas. They are discussed further in the section on endemic mycoses.

***Viral infections.*** Although CMV is an important cause of ocular and gastrointestinal disease in HIV-infected patients, the isolation of CMV from pulmonary secretions usually represents infection without true pneumonitis. Patients in whom both *P. carinii* and CMV are isolated from respiratory specimens do not appear to have a worse prognosis than patients with PCP alone. In the rare cases in which CMV does cause pneumonitis, clinical features are similar to those seen in PCP: nonproductive cough, progressive dyspnea, hypoxemia, and diffuse interstitial infiltrates. The definitive diagnosis of CMV pneumonitis requires a compatible clinical picture, as well as (1) positive cultures for CMV from lung tissue or bronchoalveolar lavage, (2) the presence in pulmonary tissue of typical intranuclear inclusion bodies and CMV antigen or nucleic acid, and (3) the absence of other pathogenic organisms, such as *P. carinii.* Treatment options include ganciclovir or foscarnet.

Varicella pneumonia may complicate both primary varicella zoster virus (VZV) infection or disseminated secondary infection in patients with HIV infection. Patients may present with mild respiratory symptoms or may develop severe hypoxia and respiratory failure. Clinical findings may be minimal, despite markedly abnormal radiographic findings. Patients should be treated with intravenous acyclovir at a dose of 30 mg/kg per day.

### Neurologic complications of HIV infection

The neurologic manifestations of AIDS are protean and cause significant morbidity and mortality. HIV infection affects the central, peripheral, and autonomic nervous systems and causes neuromuscular disease. In addition to the disease caused by primary HIV infection, the nervous system is subjected to a variety of opportunistic infections because of the depressed immune state. Drugs used to treat AIDS are frequently neurotoxic, and their use confounds the complicated clinical picture. One of the most important points to be appreciated is that the clinical picture, natural history, and response to treatment of many neurologic complications of HIV infection are dramatically different from the same diseases occurring in patients without HIV infection.

The stage of HIV disease correlates with a variety of the neurologic syndromes. Most of the neurologic disease occurs against a background of a low-grade chronic meningitis. The typical picture of the abnormal cerebrospinal fluid (CSF) in the otherwise neurologically well HIV-infected patient consists of a mild lymphocytic pleocytosis (5 to 50 cells), a mildly elevated protein level (50 to 100 mg/dl), and normal glucose. HIV can be cultured from 20% of the CSF samples. As the disease progresses, the pleocytosis often decreases, but the CSF protein may vary unpredictably. In general the CSF pattern is not useful in determining the stage of HIV disease, and care must be taken to factor in the underlying chronic changes in the interpretation of an acute syndrome.

The multiple mechanisms leading to nervous system damage are varied and usually poorly understood. The HIV-1–related encephalopathies, myelopathy, myopathy, and peripheral neuropathy are somehow associated with HIV-1 infection of the neural tissues, but the relationships are not yet understood. HIV-1 has a clear predilection for the mesothelial-derived brain elements (blood-derived macrophages, microglial cells, multinucleated giant cells). However, HIV-1 has not been well demonstrated in tissues of neuroectodermal origin (astrocytes, oligodendrocytes, neurons). The neuropathologic changes in HIV-1 infection include widespread myelin pallor, neuronal loss, reactive astrocytic gliosis, and alterations in the neocortical dendritic processes. The widespread damage to the neuroectodermal elements without direct tissue invasion supports the hypothesis that the primary mechanisms for neuronal injury are indirect damage from either HIV-1 proteins or secretory products from infected cells. Research to elucidate this aspect of the neurology of HIV infection is ongoing, and it is hoped this will be clinically fruitful in the near future. In contrast, the destruction of tissue by microbial infection occurring in the presence of a depressed and dysfunctional immune system is reasonably well explicated. The acute and chronic demyelinating polyneuropathies associated with HIV-1 disease are probably secondary to a disordered, rather than depleted, immune system. The mechanism of malignant transformation of B lymphocytes that gives rise to cerebral lymphoma is unknown.

The correct diagnosis of a neurologic syndrome in the HIV patient can be arrived at through a systematic clinical approach that considers the broader context of HIV-1 infection along with the associated systematic diseases and medications. Combining this clinical formulation with judicious use of computed tomography (CT) or magnetic resonance imaging (MRI) imaging of the brain and spinal cord, CSF analysis, nerve conduction testing and electromyography, and selective use of neural and muscle biopsy will frequently lead to the rapid, correct diagnosis.

Often a therapeutic trial with a specific drug may provide a reasonable diagnostic test instead of a tissue diagnosis.

The neurologic complications associated with HIV-1 infection are discussed later.

### *Mass lesions of the CNS*

**Toxoplasmosis.** Encephalitis caused by the obligate intracellular parasite *Toxoplasma gondii* is the most common mass lesion and opportunistic infection of the CNS in adult patients with AIDS. More than 95% of cases in this country are due to reactivation of latent infection in patients with AIDS and advanced immune dysfunction (CD4 count < 100/mm$^3$). In the United States, approximately 10% to 70% of AIDS patients are latently infected (positive *Toxoplasma* IgG), and 25% to 50% of these patients are likely to develop toxoplasmosis. Cats are the definitive host and reservoir for the oocyst form of *T. gondii;* other mammals serve as incidental hosts for the tachyzoites and cyst forms. All three forms are potentially infectious to humans, and transmission may occur by oral and congenital routes. Ingestion of undercooked meat and foods contaminated with oocysts is the most common mechanism. Reactivation of latent organisms encysted within the brain results in the multifocal, necrotic, and inflammatory abscesses characteristic of toxoplasmic encephalitis. The clinical presentation is variable, with headache, altered mentation, seizures, and lethargy the most common symptoms. Fever, focal neurologic deficits, and abnormal level of consciousness are the most common signs. Analysis of the CSF may be entirely normal or may reveal only a mild pleocytosis and elevated protein. Serum and CSF anti-*Toxoplasma* IgG antibodies are positive in greater than 80% of patients. IgM antibodies to *Toxoplasma* are rarely positive, as expected in a reactivated infection. Contrast CT scan typically shows multiple, bilateral, ring-enhancing lesions with edema and/or mass effect and a predilection for the frontal lobes, basal ganglia and corticomedullary junction. Single lesions are seen in approximately 25% of patients and nonenhancing lesions in 5% to 10% of patients. MRI with enhancement is more sensitive than CT (especially if the patient has a nonfocal neurologic examination) and frequently demonstrates lesions not evident on contrast CT.

The diagnosis of toxoplasmosis is usually made presumptively with the appropriate clinical and neuroradiologic presentation, and empiric therapy is indicated. Seronegative patients who have a single lesion on MRI, an atypical clinical presentation, or who are refractory to empiric therapy, are candidates for a stereotactic CT-guided brain biopsy. A clinical and radiographic response to therapy occurs within 2 to 3 weeks in nearly 95% of affected patients. Less than 5% of patients die during the initial episode of infection. Because of the high response rates to empiric therapy, failure to respond to initial therapy generally suggests another diagnosis (usually lymphoma).

Primary therapy for toxoplasmosis consists of pyrimethamine (200 mg loading dose followed by 50 to 75 mg/day), sulfadiazine (4 to 6 g/day in four divided doses), and folinic acid (10 to 50 mg/day). The CBC should be monitored frequently during initial therapy, as pyrimethamine may be associated with bone marrow toxicity. Adjunctive corticosteroids should be considered only in patients with significant edema/mass effect. Anticonvulsants may be indicated to control seizure activity. Nearly 40% of AIDS patients treated with this combination manifest drug toxicity (usually rash or cytopenia) severe enough to warrant discontinuation of drug(s). Therapy with pyrimethamine and clindamycin (600 mg every 6 hours) appears to be equally effective and is associated with less hematologic toxicity and cutaneous eruptions. Primary therapy is continued until a complete or marked clinical and radiographic improvement is achieved (usually 6 to 8 weeks). Because the currently available drugs are unable to eradicate the infection, relapse occurs routinely if therapy is withdrawn. Therefore, life-long suppressive therapy is required using pyrimethamine (50 mg/d) and either sulfadiazine (500 mg po qid) or clindamycin (300 mg po qid). Median survival after diagnosis is approximately 9 months. Prophylaxis in patients at risk for toxoplasmosis is discussed in a later section. Avoidance of cat litter and undercooked meat is recommended for seronegative patients.

**Primary CNS lymphoma.** Primary CNS lymphoma is the second leading cause of CNS mass lesions in patients with AIDS. Affected patients typically have CD4 counts less than 50/mm$^3$. These tumors are high-grade B cell malignancies of the non-Hodgkin's type and almost always contain Epstein-Barr virus DNA sequences integrated into the genome. Focal findings may be absent in up to 50% of patients, and the radiographic appearance is virtually indistinguishable from toxoplasmosis. Lymphoma is more likely (~70%) if a single lesion is present on MRI or located centrally at the corpus callosum. Unfortunately, none of these indicators are completely reliable, and up to 40% of patients with CNS lymphoma have multiple lesions. The diagnosis is usually made presumptively in patients seronegative for toxoplasma with atypical neuroradiology or who are unresponsive to empiric antitoxoplasma therapy. Definitive diagnosis requires brain biopsy. Radiation is standard therapy, with steroids given for edema or increased intracranial pressure. Response rates are poor, with a median survival of less than 6 months.

**Progressive multifocal leukoencephalopathy (PML).** PML is an opportunistic infection caused by a human papovavirus, JC virus. Viral infection of oligodendrocytes causes progressive demyelination. There is no associated brain edema, and patients are rarely obtunded. The clinical course is subacute, with focal neurologic deficits, most commonly aphasia, visual field deficits, sensory loss, and ataxia. MRI is the imaging modality of choice and demonstrates single or multiple nonenhancing white matter lesions situated at the gray-white junction. Characteristic neuroradiology combined with a slowly progressive clinical course is generally sufficient for the diagnosis, although brain biopsy for histologic examination is occasionally needed. Adequate therapy for this infection is not available, and death invariably occurs over weeks to months. Prognosis is somewhat better in those patients with higher T-cell counts.

### *Meningitis*

**Cryptococcal meningitis.** Cryptococcal meningitis is the most common CNS infection in patients with AIDS. *C. neoformans* is an encapsulated yeast of global distribution. Infection occurs through the respiratory route, but meningitis is the most common clinical presentation. Because

*C. neoformans* is a pathogen of relatively low virulence, profound immunosuppression (CD4 lymphocyte counts less than 50 to $100/mm^3$) is required for disease to occur.

The clinical presentation of cryptococcal meningitis is often nonspecific. Patients may present with a prolonged febrile illness with or without headache. Overt signs of meningeal irritation, such as meningismus and photophobia, are present in a minority of patients. Fortunately, the serum cryptococcal antigen test is highly sensitive for invasive cryptococcal disease. Patients with a positive test should undergo lumbar puncture to confirm the diagnosis of meningitis. The CSF cryptococcal antigen and India ink preparation are far more useful than routine CSF studies, although neither is as sensitive as the serum cryptococcal antigen. The CSF white blood cell count is generally low, with a predominance of lymphocytes. The absence of cells in the CSF is not uncommon and is associated with more severe illness. Although protein is often elevated, the CSF glucose is usually normal or only slightly decreased. Culture of *C. neoformans* from CSF is the "gold standard" for the diagnosis of cryptococcal meningitis.

Treatment of choice for cryptococcal meningitis is amphotericin B, with or without 5-flucytosine (5-FC). Traditionally, amphotericin B has been given at doses of 0.7 to 0.8 mg/kg a day for a total dose of 750 to 1000 mg, or until CSF cultures are negative. Fluconazole has been investigated as a possible alternative to amphotericin B and may be an appropriate therapy (at doses of 400 mg/day) for patients with mild disease. However, patients with severe disease, as defined by altered mental status, CSF cryptococcal antigen titers greater than 1:1024, or CSF white blood cell count less than $20/mm^3$, have a higher mortality rate when treated with fluconazole. Because most of the deaths due to cryptococcosis occur early in the course of therapy, an alternate strategy is to treat with amphotericin B for 2 weeks, followed by fluconazole therapy. Studies are being conducted to determine whether the addition of 5-FC provides added benefit.

All patients who complete therapy for cryptococcal meningitis require lifelong suppressive therapy with a triazole agent. Fluconazole (200 mg/day) is currently the most widely used and well-studied agent. The serum cryptococcal antigen test is less useful in diagnosing relapse than first episodes of disease, so that patients with a history of cryptococcal meningitis who develop evidence of recurrent disease require lumbar puncture with CSF fungal culture.

**Aseptic meningitis.** A syndrome of aseptic meningitis may occur in 1% to 2% of individuals after seroconversion representing the initial CNS response to viral invasion. Presenting features include headache, meningismus, cranial neuropathies, and occasionally encephalitis or myelopathy. The illness is self-limited and patients improve over several weeks. CSF analysis shows a mild lymphocytic pleocytosis and elevated protein. A second form of HIV-related aseptic meningitis occurs most commonly during the transition period from asymptomatic to symptomatic HIV infection (CD4 count 200 to $500/mm^3$) and affects up to 60% of patients. Acute symptoms include headache, cranial neuropathies, photophobia, and meningeal signs. The CSF may demonstrate chronic pleocytosis and mild abnormalities of glucose and protein.

**Other meningitides.** For a patient population at increased risk for infection with encapsulated organisms, bacterial meningitis is distinctly uncommon in the setting of HIV infection. The extensive use of prophylactic antibiotics (e.g., TMP/SMX) may be the reason. An exception may be meningitis caused by *Listeria monocytogenes,* which appears to occur with increased frequency in HIV-infected patients. Uncommon causes of meningitis that complicate HIV infection include tuberculosis, syphilis, histoplasmosis, coccidioidomycosis, and lymphomatous meningitis.

***Encephalopathies.*** Diffuse encephalopathies can be divided into (1) those conditions associated with impairment of both cognition and alertness and (2) the AIDS dementia complex (ADC) or HIV encephalopathy, characterized by preserved alertness in the face of impaired cognition, motor function, and behavior. The first group includes metabolic encephalopathies (e.g., drug-induced, hypoxemia-related), the encephalitic form of toxoplasmosis, CMV encephalitis, and herpes encephalitis. CMV encephalitis may be difficult to distinguish from the subacute decline in memory and cognition seen with ADC. Changes in the periventricular white matter may be visualized with enhanced CT or MRI, and hyponatremia from CMV adrenalitis is frequently present. Conventional therapies for CMV (foscarnet, ganciclovir) have not been studied for CMV-related dementia or encephalitis. Rare cases of focal and diffuse encephalitis caused by herpes simplex viruses have been described in AIDS patients. High-dose acyclovir would be the preferred treatment. ADC is the most common CNS complication of HIV infection, affecting the majority of AIDS patients to some degree during their illness. Therefore it is reviewed in greater detail.

**AIDS dementia complex.** Subcortical dementia due to HIV, or ADC, refers to a constellation of disturbances believed to result from HIV infection of the brain. This AIDS-indicator condition is found in all stages of infection. In patients with early stage AIDS, nearly 50% exhibit mild dementia or subclinical cognitive dysfunction on neuropsychologic testing. Approximately 60% of patients have evidence of clinical dementia by the time of death, and 90% of patients dying of AIDS have pathologic correlates of ADC at autopsy. The most common histologic abnormalities include (1) multinucleated encephalitis, (2) diffuse myelin pallor and gliosis, and (3) vacuolar myelopathy (see later). These findings may occur alone or in combination and are believed to be independently related to HIV infection. The correlation between clinical severity and neuropathology is often poor, making the pathogenesis of this syndrome imperfectly defined.

Cognitive impairment, altered motor performance, and abnormal behavior define the clinical triad of ADC. It is useful to divide ADC into progressive stages from subclinical or mild involvement to severe dementia. Early symptoms reflect difficulties in memory and concentration. Patients describe a generalized "slowness" of the thought process. Routine neuropsychologic testing may be essentially normal at this time, although response times on tests of attention (serial 7s) are often delayed. With disease progression, difficulty in managing daily affairs is followed by a more general, and debilitating confusion. Behavioral changes resulting in indifference and apathy

## Diagnostic criteria for AIDS dementia complex

Confirmed HIV seropositivity
History of progressive cognitive/behavioral decline with apathy, memory loss, and slowed mental processing
Neuropsychiatric assessment: deterioration on serial testing in at least two areas, including frontal lobe, motor, speech, and nonverbal memory
Absence of major affective disorder or active substance abuse
Absence of metabolic derangement (i.e., hypoxia, sepsis)
Absence of CNS opportunistic infections or neoplasms
- CT/MRI normal cranial atrophy or white matter rarefaction
- CSF: negative VDRL and cryptococcal antigen

Modified from McArthur JC. In Asbury AK, Mckhann GM, McDonald WI, editors: *Diseases of the central nervous system*, Philadelphia, 1992, WB Saunders.

are frequently misinterpreted as signs of depression. Judgment tends to be retained until the later stages, but a small number of patients may become agitated or overtly manic. On examination, subtle evidence of motor dysfunction can be detected before symptoms are obvious. Motor performance gradually deteriorates, as the patient becomes clumsy, unsteady, and finally too weak to ambulate. Frontal release signs and bowel/bladder incontinence are often present in the late stages of disease. The final phase of ADC is a near-vegetative state characterized by global dementia, mutism, and paraplegia or quadriplegia, although the patient usually remains arousable.

Accurate diagnosis of ADC is particularly important because of the prognostic and legal implications. Evaluation for other potentially reversible causes of dementia should include CSF analysis, VDRL, drug history, and metabolic profile. Neuroradiologic imaging is also useful to rule out other conditions, and to visualize the typical (but not pathognomonic) changes consistent with brain atrophy. Neuropsychological testing emphasizing psychomotor speed, attention, and memory are fairly sensitive for early ADC, and should be monitored serially. The box above outlines the basic criteria for diagnosis of ADC.

Several studies have demonstrated improvement of ADC using standard, as well as high doses (1000 to 1200 mg/day) of AZT. The efficacy of AZT in this setting supports a direct role for HIV in the pathogenesis of ADC. Other nucleoside analogs (ddI, ddC) have not been evaluated sufficiently for this use. Patients with predominant symptoms of depression may respond to small doses of tricyclic antidepressants, and 5 to 10 mg twice a day of methylphenidate (Ritalin) may be useful for mild-to-moderate inattention/apathy. Advanced dementia rarely responds to any intervention, and is associated with poor survival.

**HIV associated myelopathy.** Subacute vacuolar myelopathy is the most common spinal cord syndrome associated with HIV infection and closely resembles the subacute combined spinal cord degeneration of the posterior and lateral columns seen with vitamin $B_{12}$ deficiency. The clinical presentation consists of progressive spastic paraparesis, sensory ataxia, and dementia. This condition is probably a variant form of ADC in which motor abnormalities predominate over cognitive impairment. $B_{12}$ deficiency, spinal cord compression, and HTLV-1 infection should be ruled out. Antiretroviral therapy does not tend to be useful in reversing the myelopathy, although antispasticity agents may be palliative. Rarely, an acute myelopathy (transverse myelitis) may be caused by VZV, CMV, toxoplasmosis, or tuberculosis. Patients have rapid onset of paraparesis, bowel and bladder incontinence, and a distinct sensory level (unlike HIV-associated myelopathy) on examination.

### *Peripheral neuropathies*

**Sensory neuropathy.** A distal symmetric polyneuropathy caused by nerve fiber degeneration develops in as many as 30% of AIDS patients. Patients experience numbness, tingling, burning, and contact hypersensitivity involving the distal lower extremities. Physical examination reveals depressed or absent ankle jerks, loss of vibration sense, and hyperalgesia. The diagnosis is made clinically; electrophysiologic studies or nerve biopsy is rarely needed for confirmation. The differential diagnosis includes entrapment neuropathies, drugs, and $B_{12}$ deficiency. Treatment of this often painful and occasionally debilitating condition is mainly symptomatic. Pain-modifying tricyclic antidepressants (amitripyline, nortriptyline) given at modest doses may be helpful. Patients with severe cases often require narcotic analgesics.

**Inflammatory demyelinating polyneuropathies.** This group of possibly immune-mediated polyneuropathies occurs in association with primary or early HIV infection. The acute form (Guillain-Barré syndrome) presents as an ascending motor paralysis with a mononuclear pleocytosis on CSF analysis. The chronic form develops over several months with a tendency for a relapsing course. Plasmapheresis is the treatment of choice.

**Viral radiculitis.** CMV may cause a necrotizing vasculitis of the lumbosacral nerve roots leading to a cauda equina syndrome. Affected patients have advanced immunosuppression and present with rapidly progressive weakness and numbness of the lower extremities, sphincter paralysis, and areflexia. CSF analysis shows a polymorphonuclear pleocytosis, increased protein, CMV antibodies, and often positive cultures for CMV. Intravenous ganciclovir therapy is effective if started early in the illness.

Up to 10% of HIV-infected patients develop dermatomal herpes zoster. For localized infection, famciclovir (500 mg Tid) or acyclovir (800 mg, 5 times per day) for 7 days may be used to reduce symptoms and risk of dissemination. Disseminated infection, multiple dermatomes, or zoster ophthalmicus requires high-dose intravenous acyclovir (30 mg/kg per day).

**Other neuropathies.** Less common neuropathies described in association with HIV infection include mononeuritis multiplex, toxic neuropathies, entrapment syndromes, and autonomic neuropathy. Mononeuritis multiplex develops over days to weeks to involve several cranial, limb, and truncal nerves in a scattered distribution. The condition may progress into a chronic inflammatory demyelinating polyneuropathy, stabilize, or improve spontaneously. The most common drug-induced neuropathies are related to ddI, ddC, vincristine, dapsone, and isoniazid. Bedridden patients are prone to entrapment neuropathies involving the ulnar and peroneal nerve compartments. Autonomic neuropathies may be present asymptomatically in AIDS patients or manifest as orthostasis, gastrointestinal dysfunction, and urinary incontinence.

### Mental health considerations in HIV-infected patients

In addition to medical management, HIV health care providers must be able to recognize and treat many of the psychiatric complications common in HIV-infected patients. The accurate identification of potentially treatable psychiatric conditions in patients with an ultimately fatal disease can be particularly difficult. HIV-infected patients have an increased lifetime risk of major mental illness, especially major depression.

Persistent signs and/or symptoms of emotional distress in any HIV-infected patient are indications for a thorough psychiatric evaluation including directed history, physical examination, laboratory studies, and cognitive testing. History should focus on any family history of mental illness, substance abuse, present medications, and any previous psychiatric disorders. Laboratory studies to rule out organic etiologies include rapid plasma reagin (RPR), thyroid-stimulating hormone (TSH), folate and $B_{12}$ levels, and CNS imaging in selected patients.

Major depression is the most commonly diagnosed psychiatric disorder in this population. In addition to depressed mood, patients manifest social withdrawal, fatigue, loss of self-esteem, feelings of helplessness, and vegetative features (sleep disturbances, anorexia, weight loss, psychomotor retardation). The incidence of depression appears to increase with advancing HIV infection and declining CD4 counts. Antidepressant therapy can be helpful in more than 75% of patients, with nearly 50% experiencing complete recovery. Useful agents include nortriptyline, desipramine, and fluoxetine. Low doses should be used initially, with slow escalation until a therapeutic response is achieved. Risk assessment for suicidal ideation is an important consideration in any depressed patient.

Anxiety is also common in the HIV-infected population, and providers should attempt to identify specific stressors in the patient's environment. Psychotherapy and the judicious use of anxiolytics may be helpful. Obsessive behavior in the form of fixation with health-related issues is not unusual. Overt psychotic disorders (schizophrenia, mania) may be related to a premorbid condition, medication, or secondary to another psychiatric disorder. Conventional treatment with psychotherapy and antipsychotics is indicated.

Because a high proportion of HIV-infected patients have a history of significant substance abuse, the primary provider often becomes an integral figure in formulating and perpetuating an effective treatment plan. Important components include (1) detoxification and management of withdrawal, (2) continued abstinence (maintenance), and (3) diagnosis and treatment of conditions predisposing to substance abuse. Community programs such as Alcoholics Anonymous, Narcotics Anonymous, and AIDS support groups are excellent resources.

### Oral manifestations

Oral lesions are commonly found in nearly 30% of HIV-infected patients. Except for the higher incidence of Kaposi's sarcoma in gay men, there are few differences in the prevalence of oral lesions based on risk group, geography, or ethnic origin. Diagnosis is usually made clinically and may be confirmed with culture and/or biopsy.

*Neoplasms.* Frequently the first manifestation of AIDS, oral lesions of KS are blue, purple, or red patches or nodules most commonly involving the palate. Ulceration and secondary infection may cause the lesions to become painful. Small lesions respond well to local therapy (intralesional vinblastine, laser excision), but larger lesions may require radiation therapy. Non-Hodgkin's lymphoma of the oral cavity presents as a variety of swellings, nodules, and ulcers. These lesions are often indicative of more widespread disease.

*Fungal infections.* Oropharyngeal candidiasis is a common manifestation of HIV infection. It usually occurs before the development of other opportunistic infections and is predictive of progression to AIDS, independent of the CD4 lymphocyte count. The most common form, pseudomembranous candidiasis, is easily recognized as a removable white plaque on the oral mucosa. Oropharyngeal candidiasis also can present in an erythematous form, with smooth red patches on the palate, buccal mucosa, or tongue; as angular cheilitis, with cracks and fissures at the corners of the mouth; and as candidal leukoplakia, with nonremovable white lesions resembling oral hairy leukoplakia. Although oropharyngeal candidiasis can be diagnosed by potassium hydroxide preparation or fungal culture, the diagnosis is usually made clinically. Therapy with topical antifungal agents, such as clotrimazole oral tablets or nystatin solution, is preferred. Although the azole antifungal drugs are effective, they are expensive and may increase the risk of resistant candidiasis. Rare cases of oral histoplasmosis, cryptococcosis, and aspergillosis have been reported.

*Viral lesions.* Hairy leukoplakia induced by the Epstein-Barr virus is a white lesion involving the lateral surfaces of the tongue. This common lesion is present in 20% of asymptomatic HIV-infected patients, with an increasing incidence as immunosuppression advances. On examination, these adherent lesions may be smooth or corrugated, or may have vertically oriented folds. Hairlike projections may be visualized macroscopically or microscopically. Although recurrences are common, treatment with systemic acyclovir is often effective.

Oral lesions may be caused by other members of the herpes virus family. Intraoral ulcers and recurrent herpes labialis due to HSV-1 and HSV-2 occur with greater frequency and more severity in HIV-infected patients. Symptomatic lesions generally respond to oral acyclovir (200 mg five times a day); higher doses of acyclovir or foscarnet are needed to control the increasing problem of resistance.

*Bacterial infections.* Periodontal disease is the most common bacterial infection of the oral cavity associated with HIV infection. Patients with gingivitis may have the typically mild gumline erythema seen in immunocompetent individuals, or present with a necrotizing ulcerative gingivitis. HIV-periodontitis is a painful condition distinguished by severe soft tissue necrosis and rapid loss of supporting bone and periodontal attachments. A necrotizing stomatitis may occur, with spread to adjoining soft tissue and intraseptal sequestration of alveolar bone. Organisms implicated in the pathogenesis of these conditions include a mixture of aerobic and anaerobic gram-negative bacteria, spirochetes, and yeast. Therapy is difficult and involves debridement of necrotic tissue, irrigation with povidone-iodine/chlorhexidine oral solutions, and antibiotics (e.g., metronidazole).

***Idiopathic/autoimmune lesions.*** Recurrent aphthous ulcers occur with increased frequency and severity in HIV-infected patients. Three lesions have been described: (1) "herpetiform" crops of tiny (1 to 2 mm) ulcers, (2) small (3 to 5 mm) often persistent ulcers, and (3) large (1 to 2 cm) painful ulcers that occur singly or in groups. Before initiating therapy for symptomatic lesions, it is reasonable to culture and/or treat empirically for herpes simplex infection. Treatment options directed at idiopathic lesions include (1) Listerine brand mouthwash, (2) tetracyline suspension, (3) topical steroids, (4) systemic steroids, and possibly (5) thalidomide (under investigation). Viscous lidocaine may be indicated for symptomatic relief in severe cases.

### Gastrointestinal manifestations

***Esophagitis.*** Odynophagia and dysphagia are the primary symptoms related to esophageal involvement in HIV-infected patients. Although *Candida* esophagitis is the most common etiology, other infectious and noninfectious causes are possible. Esophageal candidiasis, which requires a much greater degree of immunosuppression than oropharyngeal candidiasis, is an AIDS-indicator condition according to the CDC case definition. It typically presents with dysphagia, usually in a patient with fewer than 100 CD4 cells and oral thrush. Odynophagia also may be present, but is more common with CMV or herpes esophagitis. Because esophageal candidiasis is so common and easily treatable, diagnosis based on symptoms is appropriate, and an empiric 7- to 14-day course of fluconazole (100 mg/day) or ketoconazole (200 mg/day) should be initiated. Patients who do not respond to therapy should undergo upper endoscopy to rule out CMV, herpes, or aphthous esophagitis. Patients who develop recurrent esophageal candidiasis are candidates for suppressive therapy with daily fluconazole or ketoconazole.

Patients with herpes esophagitis often have concurrent oral ulcers. In contrast to candidiasis, odynophagia, chest pain, and focal pain are characteristic. Endoscopic examination with biopsies is necessary for definitive diagnosis. Oral acyclovir (200 mg five times a day) for 7 to 14 days is effective for mild symptoms, intravenous acyclovir (15 mg/kg per day) is needed for severe cases or to overcome partial viral resistance. Relapses may occur following discontinuation of therapy. The presentation and endoscopic appearance of CMV esophagitis are similar to that of herpes simplex virus. Intravenous ganciclovir or foscarnet given for 2 to 3 weeks is effective. The need for maintenance therapy has not been established.

Noninfectious causes of esophagitis include lymphoma, Kaposi's sarcoma, aphthous ulceration, and pill-induced (ddC, AZT) ulcers. Discontinuing the offending agent improves pill-induced ulcers. Idiopathic ulcers may respond to tapering doses of oral prednisone. Omeprazole and/or a sucralfate slurry are useful adjuvants for symptomatic pain relief.

***Gastric diseases.*** Stomach lesions particular to HIV-infected patients are usually neoplastic or viral processes. Kaposi's sarcoma involving the gastrointestinal tract is common in patients with documented cutaneous disease. The lesions tend to be asymptomatic findings on endoscopy, but bleeding or obstruction may occur. Non-Hodgkin's lymphoma of the gastric antrum may be associated with outlet obstruction and/or bleeding. Although single lesions may occur, extensive abdominal involvement is generally observed. CMV esophagitis is rarely associated with a concurrent gastritis.

***Intestinal disorders.*** Intestinal disease is one of the most common HIV-related manifestations, with 30% to 80% of patients experiencing some form of diarrhea during the course of their illness. The CDC defines AIDS-associated diarrhea as three or more liquid stools per day that persist for longer than 1 month. The incidence of chronic diarrhea correlates with advancing HIV infection and may lead to an AIDS-defining diagnosis. Enteric infection as a cause of diarrhea occurs in 30% to 50% of HIV-infected patients in this country, with a higher prevalence in homosexual men, and in over 90% of patients in developing countries. Patients with diarrhea that is predominantly related to the small bowel present with malabsorption, voluminous stools, dehydration, weight loss, and periumbilical pain. Distinguishing features of large bowel diarrhea include small volume stools, relatively intact absorption, lower quadrant pain, and the presence of white blood cells in the stool.

A recently recommended diagnostic evaluation for AIDS-associated diarrhea is shown in the box on p. 946. A complete evaluation is costly, ranging from several hundred dollars for stool cultures to several thousand dollars if endoscopy is needed. Specific pathogens can be identified in 40% to 60% of cases with the use of stool studies alone, and in 70% to 85% of cases when combined with endoscopy and biopsy. Multiple pathogens are present in up to 30% of cases. Several unidentified pathogens, viruses, and HIV enteropathy are likely responsible for cases with a negative evaluation. Unfortunately, a treatable pathogen is identified in only 30% to 40% of evaluated patients. Clinical features, diagnosis, and management of the most common enteric pathogens will be reviewed.

***Bacterial pathogens.*** Enteric bacterial infections are more common, severe, and prolonged in HIV-infected patients. Diagnosis is usually established by stool culture. *Salmonella* infection is 20 to 100 times more common than in the general population and is associated with a higher incidence of bacteremia and recurrence. Patients present with abdominal pain, high fever, and bloody or nonbloody stools. Antibiotics (e.g., ceftriaxone, ciprofloxicin) are usually required, and oral suppressive therapy may be

### Diagnostic evaluation of patients with AIDS who have diarrhea

Step 1
- Stool cultured for *Salmonella* and *Shigella* species, and *Campylobacter jejuni* at least three times, and assayed for *Clostridium difficile* toxin
- Stool specimens (direct, concentrated, or both) examined for parasites using saline, iodine, trichrome, acid-fast preparations

Step 2
- Gastroduodenoscopy and colonoscopy to inspect tissue and to obtain biopsy specimens and luminal material
- Duodenal biopsy specimens cultured for CMV and mycobacteria
- Colonic biopsy specimens cultured for CMV, adenovirus, mycobacteria, and herpes simplex virus
- Biopsy specimens stained with hematoxylin-eosin for protozoa and viral inclusion cells, with methenamine silver or Giemsa for fungi, and with stains for mycobacteria
- Duodenal fluid specimens examined as above for parasites

Step 3
- Biopsy specimens examined by electron microscopy for *Microsporidia* (duodenal tissue) and adenovirus (colonic tissue)

From Smith PD, et al, *Ann Intern Med* 116(1): 63-77, 1992.

needed after the acute episode. The presentation of *Campylobacter* gastroenteritis is similar. Erythromycin or a quinolone is the preferred therapy. *Shigella* infects the large bowel and presents with abdominal pain, tenesmus, fever, and bloody diarrhea. Treatment is the same as for Salmonella. *Clostridium difficile* may occur in the setting of prior antibiotic therapy. Fever and profuse watery diarrhea are observed. Toxin assays of the stool are highly sensitive. Oral vancomycin or metronidazole may be less effective than in patients without HIV. Nearly 40% of patients with advanced AIDS have disseminated *M. avium* complex infection. The small bowel is commonly involved, resulting in fever, abdominal pain, chronic diarrhea, and malabsorption. Diagnosis requires evidence of invasive disease on small bowel biopsy. Treatment for disseminated disease involves multidrug therapy.

***Protozoan infections.*** Cryptosporidiosis is the AIDS-indicator condition in 2% to 4% of patients and represents 10% to 20% of AIDS-related diarrhea in this country. Persistent large-volume diarrhea, abdominal pain, and malabsorption are typical. Fever is uncommon and symptoms may be intermittent. Diagnosis is made by modified AFB stain or by antibody testing of the stool. Treatment to date has been poor, although paromomycin 500 mg four times a day, appears to be effective in some patients. The small intestinal parasite *Isospora belli* is an uncommon cause of diarrhea in this country. Diagnosis is made by visualization of the characteristic oocyst in Kinyoun-stained specimens. TMP-SMX is effective therapy. *Microsporidia* is an intracellular parasite of the small bowel that is a likely (although controversial) pathogen in patients with AIDS. Diagnosis is made by electron microscopy of a small bowel biopsy specimens. Albendazole (not available in the United States) has been effective in some patients. *Giardia* and *Entamoeba histolytica* are encountered with a low frequency, and the manifestations and response to therapy do not appear affected by HIV infection. Diagnosis is made by ova and parasite examination of the stool or by immunofluorescent antibody (giardiasis). Symptomatic cases can be treated with metronidazole or luminacidal agents.

***Viruses.*** Evidence of disseminated CMV infection is demonstrated at autopsy in 90% of AIDS patients. Colonic manifestations include diarrhea, abdominal pain, and occasionally hemorrhagic ulcers. Colonoscopy shows focal inflammation with hemorrhagic plaques and ulcerations secondary to vasculitis. Therapy with foscarnet or ganciclovir may be of some benefit, but the relapse rate is high. Direct invasion by HIV (HIV enteropathy) may be associated with villous atrophy and malabsorption in the absence of identifiable pathogens.

***Neoplasms.*** Kaposi's sarcoma involves the gastrointestinal tract in 50% of patients with skin disease, and although it is usually asymptomatic, it may cause diarrhea, enteropathy, obstruction, and ulcerations in a small number of cases. Diagnosis is made by endoscopic appearance and biopsy. Gastrointestinal symptoms related to lymphoma include obstruction, perforation, and bleeding. Biopsy is required for diagnosis, and combination chemotherapy is the usual treatment.

***Perirectal and anorectal disorders.*** Diseases involving the rectum are significantly increased in homosexual men. Typical symptoms include pain, discharge, ulceration, and bleeding. Herpes simplex infections and lesions related to human papilloma virus (HPV) infection (warts, squamous cell cancer) are most commonly encountered. Syphilis, gonorrhea, CMV, and chlamydia also may be diagnostic considerations.

***Liver diseases.*** Although seldom the cause of substantial morbidity or mortality, hepatobiliary involvement becomes increasingly common as HIV infection advances. The high incidence of viral hepatitis in patients at risk for HIV infection, the use of potentially hepatotoxic medications, and the liver function test abnormalities seen with systemic illnesses all contribute to the complexity of the problem.

Intrahepatic and extrahepatic causes of biliary tract obstruction have been described in patients with AIDS. Patients generally have right upper quadrant pain, fever, increased serum alkaline phospatase, and jaundice. Acute acalculous cholecystitis, papillary stenosis, and sclerosing cholangitis are the most common syndromes. Infection with *Cryptosporidium, Microsporidium, Candida* species, or CMV may cause any of these conditions. Diagnosis is made by nuclear scan (acalculous cholecystitis) or by endoscopic retrograde cholangiopancreotography (ERCP) (papillary stenosis, cholangitis). Urgent surgery or endoscopic improvement of biliary drainage (sphincterotomy or stent) may be required.

Parenchymal involvement of the liver may be caused by infection, neoplasm, or drug effect. Varying degrees of transaminase elevation can be seen with drug-induced hepatic injury. Implicated medications in HIV-infected patients include sulfonamides, ketoconazole, AZT, isoniazid, and pentamidine. Disseminated tuberculosis and MAC are the most common opportunistic infections affecting the liver. Patients present with fever, hepatomegaly, elevated transaminases, and elevated alkaline phosphatase or g-glutamyl transpeptidase. Diagnosis can be made only by biopsy (see later). Cryptococcosis, histoplasmosis, coccidioidomycosis, CMV, and herpes simplex infection of the liver occur rarely. Lymphoma and Kaposi's sarcoma also can involve the liver.

Serologic evidence of hepatitis B (HBV) infection can be seen in a significant proportion of HIV-infected persons, depending on the specific population studied. Although there appear to be no clinical or biochemical differences in the HIV-infected patients with acute HBV, the risk of becoming a chronic carrier is significantly increased. The impairment of cell-mediated immunity in this population seems to result in a milder chronic HBV infection with less hepatocellular destruction. Unfortunately, hepatitis B viral load and infectivity increase accordingly. Vaccination of seronegative individuals to prevent this complication is able to confer immunity in only 30% to 50% of HIV-infected patients and varies with the CD4 count. Response to interferon therapy is poor. The overall seroprevalence rate of hepatitis C in HIV-positive individuals approximates 7%. The rates are higher among hemophiliacs and intravenous drug users than homosexual males. Progression to chronic hepatitis C infection occurs in more than 50% of infected patients and carries a significant risk of cirrhosis. Treatment with interferon and/or AZT may be effective.

The diagnostic approach to liver disease in HIV-infected patients generally should include the following: (1) viral hepatitis serologies, (2) liver function tests, (3) blood cultures for mycobacterium and fungus, and (4) abdominal imaging. Liver biopsy is usually not indicated, as several studies have shown that the results seldom affect therapy or survival in patients with AIDS. Biopsy may be useful in unexplained cases of fever, hepatomegaly, and abnormal liver function tests or in suspected cases of tuberculosis.

## Nutritional aspects

Malnutrition is common in HIV-infected patients and is frequently associated with anorexia and weight loss. Weight loss may be related transiently to infection, or progressive up to the time of death. Survival in AIDS patients has been found to correlate with serum albumin levels. One study found the median survival to be less than 3 weeks in patients with albumin levels less than 2.5 g/dl. Primary mechanisms of malnutrition include the following: (1) inadequate dietary intake resulting from depression, fatigue, drugs, and systemic infection, as well as conditions affecting the CNS or any part of the gastrointestinal tract; (2) enteropathies from opportunistic infections or HIV leading to malabsorption with nutrient depletion; and (3) hypermetabolism during both symptomatic and asymptomatic phases of HIV infection, which decreases lean body mass even when weight appears stable.

It is important to readily identify nutritional problems, as current evidence suggests early intervention may enhance immune function, prolong survival, and improve quality of life. A comprehensive nutritional assessment should include evaluation of gastrointestinal function, serum albumin level, calculation of calorie intake, estimation of protein/energy requirements, and documentation of the degree of lean body mass loss. Counseling allows specific dietary deficiencies to be addressed, vitamin/mineral supplements prescribed, and high calorie/protein-containing foods to be recommended. Continued and/or severe malnutrition should prompt a more aggressive therapeutic approach.

Treatment of any underlying processes should be optimized if possible. Chronic diarrhea from a variety of etiologies may be reduced with the judicious use of antidiarrheal agents such as loperamide. Oral supplementation with standard preparations (Ensure, Sustecal) are readily available, inexpensive, and often effective. Appetite stimulation with megestrol acetate (Megace) or marinol may increase caloric intake and weight gain in AIDS patients. Total parenteral nutrition (TPN) is most useful for patients with deficient energy intake, as opposed to the metabolic derangements associated with systemic infection. Infectious complications related to the intravenous catheter and the expense associated with TPN are important considerations for this type of therapy. Enteral nutrition by tube is useful in patients with relatively preserved absorptive function, even in the presence of systemic complications. If tolerated, oral feedings should be continued along with enteral supplementation, and the need for tube feeding reevaluated periodically. TPN and enteral nutrition can be managed successfully in both the in-patient and out-patient setting.

## Endocrine manifestations

Diffuse endocrine pathology may occur at any stage of HIV infection and is usually related to neoplasia, opportunistic infections, drugs, or HIV itself. The adrenal gland is the most commonly involved organ, with CMV being the most common pathogen. Less frequent etiologies include mycobacterial infection, toxoplasmosis, cryptococcosis, lymphoma, and Kaposi's sarcoma. Frank adrenal insufficiency is rare, as 90% of the adrenal mass must be destroyed for overt dysfunction to occur. Subclinical defects of cortisol or aldosterone synthesis can be elicited on provocative testing. Routine screening is not recommended unless typical signs and symptoms of insufficiency are present. Mineralocorticoid deficiency may be more common than adrenal insufficiency and may be corrected with replacement therapy (e.g., fludrocortisone).

Some asymptomatic patients have increased T4/T3 due to increased levels of thyroid-binding globulin early in HIV infection. An unusual feature of thyroid function testing in HIV is a "more normal" T3 level than in non-HIV patients with comparable systemic illness. Thyroxine therapy is not indicated unless overt hypothyroidism is present as cachexia may be exacerbated. Clinically silent, nonspecific inflammation of the pancreas with hyperamylasemia can be caused by CMV or malignancy. Hypoglycemia, followed by hyperglycemia, can occur from pentamidine toxicity. Acute pancreatitis from ddI and ddC have been described. Testicular function may be reduced in advanced HIV infection. Spermatogenesis is decreased, hair loss may occur, and some patients report decreased libido. Multifactorial etiologies include CMV, lymphoma, and drugs (e.g., ketoconazole).

### Rheumatologic manifestations

See Chapter 87.

### Cardiac disease

Evidence of cardiac involvement at autopsy is reported in up to 50% of HIV-infected patients, and approximately 6% of patients develop clinically significant cardiac disease. Pericardial effusions are common in HIV infection (23% to 40%), usually asymptomatic, and rarely progress to tamponade. Potential etiologies include hypothyroidism, radiation, CMV, HSV, mycobacteria, fungi, lymphoma, KS, and drugs. Patients are tachycardic and tachypneic, with increased jugular venous pulsations, and a pericardial rub on examination. Evaluation should include an echocardiogram, blood cultures, PPD, and possibly a pericardiocentesis. Mild to moderate asymptomatic effusions can be observed or treated with nonsteroidal antiinflammatory drugs (NSAIDs). Tamponade requires pericardiocentesis and recurrent effusions often necessitate pericardectomy.

Lymphocytic myocarditis is found commonly at autopsy (46%), but only a few patients have ventricular dysfunction. Usually there is nonspecific inflammation suggestive of a viral process (HIV, CMV, coxsackie A and B). Cardiac involvement with toxoplasmosis, cryptococcus, mycobacteria, lymphoma, or KS can occur. Symptomatic patients present with classic clinical signs of congestive heart failure and cardiomegaly on chest film. Biopsy is rarely indicated, and echocardiogram is the best test to assess chamber size and function. Therapy is supportive or directed at the underlying process.

Biventricular dilation resulting in an overt cardiomyopathy may be associated with histologic/serologic evidence of viral myocarditis. Drug toxicity (e.g., adriamycin), autoimmune dysfunction, nutritional deficiency, sepsis, and HIV infection itself also may result in this condition. Patients with symptoms suggestive of congestive heart failure (CHF) should be evaluated with functional cardiac imaging and treated with diuretics, afterload reduction, and digoxin as indicated. Steroid therapy should be considered in selected cases of active myocarditis.

Bacterial endocarditis in HIV-infected patients generally occurs in the setting of injectable drug use. Response to conventional therapy appears to be satisfactory. Lesions of nonbacterial, thrombotic endocarditis with systemic emboli have been described in autopsy series.

### Renal disease

Etiologies of renal disease in AIDS patients include (1) nephrotoxic medications (foscarnet, sulfonamides, amphotericin B), (2) systemic infection and sepsis, (3) vasculitis, (4) injection drug use, and (5) HIV nephropathy (HIVN).

HIVN occurs in up to 10% of infected patients and is strongly associated with a history of injection drug use (50% of cases). Similar to the histologic distribution seen in idiopathic and heroin nephropathy, focal sclerosing glomerulonephritis and mesangial hyperplasia are the most common histologies. Presenting features include (1) azotemia (63%), (2) proteinuria (19%), (3) electrolyte abnormalities (6%), and (4) hematuria (3%). Urine sediment shows increased protein, oval fat bodies, and casts. Absence of hypertension, large kidney size, hypoalbuminemia disproportionate to the proteinuria, and accelerated pace of the disease distinguish HIVN from related disorders. Rapid progression to end-stage renal disease is common, and response to hemodialysis has been poor. Overall survival at 10 months is 50% in affected patients. Patients with AIDS have a much poorer prognosis than those with asymptomatic or symptomatic HIV. Peritoneal dialysis may offer a modest survival advantage.

### Hematologic complications

The hematologic system may be affected during any stage of HIV infection. The peripheral cell lines, bone marrow, and coagulation system may be involved alone, or in combination. Multifactorial etiologies include myelosuppressive drugs (e.g., AZT, ganciclovir), direct suppression by HIV, bone marrow infiltration, infections (e.g., disseminated MAC), neoplasms, and nutritional disorders.

Classic bone marrow findings are not associated with HIV infection. Cellularity is often abnormal, plasma cells and eosinophils tend to be increased, and granulomas may be observed with mycobacterial or fungal infections. Lymphoma, and less often KS, may infiltrate the bone marrow.

Anemia occurs in over 60% of AIDS patients. The usual pattern is a normochromic, normocytic anemia, with increased iron stores, that worsens over time. Macrocytosis is observed with AZT therapy. A clinically silent, Coombs'-positive hemolytic anemia occurs in 20% of AIDS patients with increased gamma globulin. Gastrointestinal bleeding, bone marrow infiltration, and drugs (e.g., AZT, dapsone) should be considered in the differential diagnosis of anemia. Treatment strategies include discontinuation of the offending agents, treatment of underlying processes, and erythropoietin (rEPO) for patients with EPO levels less than 500 mU/ml.

Leukopenia is found in 75% of symptomatic HIV patients and 20% of asymptomatic patients. Drug-induced neutropenia commonly results from AZT, high dose TMP-SMX, ganciclovir, $\alpha$-interferon, and antineoplastic therapy. Granulocyte colony-stimulating factor (G-CSF) is effective in reversing neutropenia from a variety of HIV-related causes.

HIV-induced thrombocytopenia was recognized early in the AIDS epidemic. The mechanism appears to be an autoimmune IgG-mediated peripheral destruction of platelets that occurs early in symptomatic HIV infection (CD4 > 200). Normalization of platelet count often precedes progression to AIDS. Significant hemorrhage is rare. The CBC shows an isolated thrombocytopenia, and increased megakaryocytes are present on bone marrow studies. AZT often reverses the thrombocytopenia early in infection with sustained effects. Fifty percent of patients respond initially to oral prednisone, but the risks of further immunosuppression may outweigh the benefits. Despite an initial response rate of 75%, intravenous immunoglobulin is expensive and associated with a high incidence of relapse. Splenectomy for refractory cases may be considered.

**Table 68-6.** Cutaneous diseases characteristic of HIV infection

| Diagnosis | History | Physical | Laboratory | Differential | Management |
|---|---|---|---|---|---|
| Kaposi's sarcoma | Gradual onset of pigmented or violaceous nodules | Brown to purple nodules anywhere on body; oral lesions common | Confirmation by biopsy | Pyogenic granuloma<br>Bacillary angiomatosis<br>Stasis dermatitis | Small lesions: excision, liq. N2, intralesional vinblastine, vincristine, radiation<br>Widespread: chemotherapy |
| Oral hairy leukoplakia | Asymptomatic tongue lesions | White verrucoid patches on lateral tongue | Usually none<br>R/O *Candida*<br>Consider Bx | Candidiasis | None required<br>May use Retin-A gel 25% podophyllin |
| Bacillary angiomatosis | Skin and mucosal lesions; may have arthritis | Raised, vascular-appearing nodules | Confirmation by biopsy | Kaposi's sarcoma | Erythromycin<br>Rifampin<br>Tetracycline |
| Eosinophilic folliculitis | Pruritic lesions on upper body | Urticarial-like follicular papules on upper body | CD4 <300<br>Elevated IgE<br>Confirmation by biopsy | Bacterial folliculitis<br>Insect bites | Ultraviolet light<br>Fluconazole<br>Topical steroids |
| Large facial molluscum contagiosum | Gradual onset of facial papules; asymptomatic | Hyperkeratotic or smooth papules and plaques | Confirmation by biopsy if uncertain | Verrucae<br>Basal cell carcinoma | Destruction<br>liq. N2<br>curettage<br>excision |

## Neoplastic complications

More than 40% of patients develop neoplastic disease during the course of their illness. KS, non-Hodgkin's lymphoma, and invasive cervical cancer are all AIDS indicator conditions. Kaposi's sarcoma is discussed in detail in the next section on cutaneous manifestations of HIV infection.

***Non-Hodgkin's lymphoma.*** Non-Hodgkin's lymphoma is the AIDS-defining condition in 3% of US cases and occurs in all risk groups. Nearly 25% of all cases occur in the setting of HIV infection. Unlike non HIV-related cases, these lymphomas are intermediate or high-grade neoplasms of the immunoblastic or small noncleaved cell type (Burkitt's or non-Burkitt's) with prominent extranodal involvement. The incidence increases with prolonged survival in HIV. The etiology is unclear, but may be related to polyclonal B cell stimulation and to Epstein-Barr virus coinfection in the case of primary CNS lymphoma.

Classic B symptoms are present in 80% of patients at diagnosis, and many have extranodal disease involving the gastrointestinal tract (4% to 28%), bone marrow (21% to 33%), and liver (9% to 26%). Staging evaluation should include a CT scan, bone marrow biopsy, and lumbar puncture to rule out meningeal disease. As discussed in the section on CNS lesions, non-Hodgkin's lymphoma may be confined to the brain. Factors associated with decreased survival include bone marrow involvement, prior diagnosis of AIDS, Karnofsky score less than 70%, and primary CNS lymphoma.

Therapy is complicated by toxicity, poor bone marrow reserve, and infection. Treatment options range from low-dose combination therapy (e.g., M-BACOD) to high-dose chemotherapy with colony-stimulating factor support (e.g., MACOP-B). Multiagent regimens can achieve a complete response in 30% to 50% of patients depending on the histologic grade of the tumor. Median survival is 4 to 7 months overall and 2 months with immunoblastic lymphoma.

***Anal neoplasia.*** An increased incidence of HPV-associated anal neoplasia is recognized in homosexual men, HIV infection, and chronic immunodeficiency. Screening with routine anoscopy and possible anal Pap smears are recommended for high-risk men. The threshold for biopsy and/or follow-up examinations should be low. Treatment with electrocautery or cryotherapy is effective.

## Cutaneous manifestations of HIV infection

Skin or mucous membrane disease occurs in almost all patients infected with HIV. Some dermatoses are characteristic of HIV infection, whereas others are merely seen in a higher frequency or with atypical features when associated with HIV infection. Examination of the entire skin surface and mucous membranes is essential to making an accurate diagnosis. This section focuses on the most common cutaneous manifestations of HIV infection.

### *Diseases characteristic of HIV infection* (Table 68-6)

**Kaposi's sarcoma**

***Epidemiology/etiology.*** Before the AIDS epidemic was recognized in 1981, KS was observed in three forms: (1) Classic KS seen on the legs of elderly men, (2) African KS seen in a variety of forms in African children and adults, and (3) KS associated with immunosuppressive therapy. The form now called AIDS-associated KS (AIDS-KS) was first seen in the early 1980s in homosexual men who showed other signs of immunosuppression. It was observed to be a rapidly progressive form of KS, frequently with a fatal outcome. AIDS-KS affects mostly men, with a male/female ratio of 106:1 and a mean age of onset of 37 years. In 1989, KS was the AIDS-defining illness in approximately 15% of new cases of AIDS in the United States.

The etiology of KS has recently been related to a novel herpesvirus, consistent with the epidemiology of a sexually transmitted disease. Evidence suggests that factors other than HIV may play a role in the development and growth of AIDS-KS. In recent years, the proportion of patients with AIDS diagnosed with AIDS-KS has declined, possibly reflecting a change in high-risk sexual behaviors and a resultant reduction in transmission of KS as a second sexually transmitted disease distinct from HIV.

***Pathogenesis/pathophysiology.*** The cell of origin in KS is uncertain. Possibilities include vascular endothelial cells, dermal dendrocytes, and vascular smooth muscle cells. KS cells and retrovirus-infected CD4+ T cells produce angiogenic growth factors and cytokines that maintain and promote the growth of KS.

***History.*** Patients usually present with asymptomatic lesions or are diagnosed as part of a complete physical examination.

***Physical examination.*** KS commonly affects the oral cavity, nasal mucosa, genitalia, and feet in addition to the trunk; careful examination of these areas is important. Early lesions (see Plate 43) may start as macular areas of discoloration that enlarge to form papules, nodules, and large plaques. Initially the color may be a red-brown and as the tumor enlarges, a violaceous color becomes more prominent (see Plate 44). Early lesions usually are asymptomatic, but extensive large areas may become ulcerated and painful, and lymphatic involvement can lead to lymphedema. Oral involvement most commonly affects the hard and soft palate.

***Laboratory evaluation.*** Histologic confirmation of KS is indicated, even when the diagnosis appears evident clinically. Patients, oncologists, and epidemiologists frequently need histologic confirmation to direct management. The pathology is usually diagnostic, although there is a wide spectrum of histologic variation.

***Management.*** None of the existing treatments for AIDS-KS are curative, but several treatments for both local and widespread disease effectively reduce the extent of disease and provide palliation. The goals of therapy should be based on the individual needs of the patient and may include correction of cosmetic disfigurement, size reduction of oral lesions to allow normal eating and speaking, and correction of lymphedema, pain, or symptomatic visceral involvement.

***Local therapy.*** Excision, cryotherapy, intralesional chemotherapy and radiation are all effective. *Liquid nitrogen cryotherapy,* although incomplete histologically, results in clinical improvement of small lesions, which lasts up to 6 months. *Intralesional injection* with vinblastine or vincristine provides an acceptable clinical response in more than 60% of patients. Vinblastine, 0.1 mg/cm$^2$ of lesion is used by injecting up to 0.5ml of a 0.2 mg/ml solution. This amount may be increased (up to 0.6 mg/ml) in recalcitrant lesions, but the volume of injected drug should not exceed 0.5 ml/cm$^2$ of lesion, and the maximum amount of drug injected should not exceed 0.2 mg/cm$^2$. Side effects include pain, ulceration, and alopecia. *Radiation therapy* is indicated in large oral lesions or cutaneous plaques not amenable to other treatments. Radiation dermatitis or mucositis is commonly seen after use of this modality. Excision successfully removes small lesions.

***Systemic therapy.*** Interferon alpha used alone or in combination with AZT has resulted in responses of 20% to 40%. Daily therapies include vincristine, vinblastine, etoposide, and bleomycin, all of which are well tolerated, and doxorubicin, which is effective but has a higher incidence of side effects. Careful monitoring for bone marrow suppression is essential. Systemic chemotherapy may be offered to patients with aggressive cutaneous disease, symptomatic visceral disease, pulmonary involvement, or lymphedema. Response rates range from 30% to 70% with active single agents, and from 45% to 88% with combination therapy. Toxicity is problematic and discontinuation almost invariably results in relapse.

**Oral hairy leukoplakia.** Oral hairy leukoplakia (HL) is a lesion that occurs on the tongue and has a high predictive association with HIV infection and the subsequent development of AIDS. It is thought to be caused by infection with Epstein-Barr virus.

***Physical examination.*** HL usually involves the lateral aspects of the tongue. Asymptomatic verrucous white patches that cannot be scraped off are the typical presentation (see Plate 45). The differential diagnosis is candidiasis (thrush) which is similar to HL in appearance but can be diagnosed by potassium hydroxide (KOH) examination of some removable plaque. In uncertain cases, a biopsy demonstrates characteristic features of HL, although on occasion patients can have both candidiasis and HL concomitantly.

***Management.*** Frequently treatment is not required because the lesions are asymptomatic. Successful treatments have been reported with oral acyclovir, single applications of 25% podophyllin, and daily use of topical tretinoin gel (Retin-A gel, 0.01%).

**Bacillary angiomatosis.** Bacillary angiomatosis (BA) is a newly recognized infectious disease first observed in patients with AIDS. Two species of gram-negative organisms, *Rochalimaea quintana* (the agent of trench fever) and *R. henselae* (a newly identified species also thought to be the etiologic agent of cat-scratch disease) have been isolated from skin lesions of BA and are thought to be causative agents of the disease. Epidemiologic evidence suggests that both cat scratches and cat bites are strong risk factors for the development of BA, which also can be seen in immunocompetent hosts.

***Pathophysiology.*** The mechanism of disease in BA is not known. Angiomatous proliferation in skin and viscera is most common but a spectrum of disease including bacteremia with fever, lymphadenitis, and bone lesions also may be present.

***History.*** BA usually develops over several months. Tender skin lesions are the usual presentation. Other symptoms may include fevers, bone pain, focal cutaneous swelling, and abdominal pain.

***Physical examination.*** The typical skin manifestations are raised nodules with a friable or eroded surface and an erythematous base. The lesions can resemble pyogenic granulomas or Kaposi's sarcoma. They are present anywhere on the skin or mucosal surfaces and number from one to hundreds. Less commonly a cellulitic plaque or a subcutaneous mass is the presenting finding.

***Laboratory evaluation.*** A biopsy for histologic confirmation is essential for diagnosis. Characteristic histologic findings are usually evident with light microscopy using routine and special stains. Electron microscopy is occasionally helpful. Culture of the organisms (*R. quintana, R. henselae*) is still an investigational tool.

***Differential diagnosis.*** Kaposi's sarcoma is the main diagnosis that needs to be differentiated from BA.

***Management.*** Erythromycin (2 g/day) or rifampin are effective and can result in complete resolution. Tetracyclines are effective alternative drugs. The appropriate duration of therapy is not established because cases have been reported of relapse in immunodeficient patients after treatment was stopped. Some patients may require indefinite treatment. An immunologic reaction similar to the Jarisch-Herxheimer reaction in syphilis can occur during the first 48 hours of treatment, and pretreatment with antipyretics should be considered. Untreated cases can progress to death.

**HIV-associated eosinophilic folliculitis.** Eosinophilic folliculitis is a characteristic dermatosis of HIV infection. It consists of intensely pruritic urticarial follicular papules on the head and neck, trunk, and proximal extremities. Lesions tend to be individual and can resemble arthropod bites. All patients studied so far have had significant reductions in total CD4 counts (less than 250 to 300 cells/mm$^3$), making the disease a marker of advanced HIV disease. Eosinophilia and elevated levels of IgE may be present.

Diagnosis requires biopsy confirmation. The characteristic histopathologic changes are dense cellular inflammation involving follicular epithelia plus the presence of many eosinophils in the dermis. Staphylococcal folliculitis should be excluded by culture or Gram stain of biopsy material. Treatments include ultraviolet light (UVB) therapy, antihistamines, and topical corticosteroids. Oral ketoconazole has been reported to be successful, although some patients are receiving systemic antifungal treatment at the time they develop eosinophilic folliculitis. Most cases resolve gradually with treatment.

**Molluscum contagiosum.** Mollusca contagiosa are caused by a virus of the poxvirus group and in healthy individuals consist of small dome-shaped papules with a central punctum or umbilication. In persons with HIV infection, the lesions are usually on the face and are frequently large (1 to 2 cm) compared to those in healthy hosts (0.5 cm). The surface may be hyperkeratotic, resembling verrucae, or smooth, resembling basal cell carcinomas (see Plate 46). Usually patients are asymptomatic and the goal of treatment is usually to correct the disfigurement. Cryotherapy or other destructive measures including curettage or excision are effective. Periodic retreatment is usually required and eradication is not possible.

### *Diseases with atypical presentations in HIV disease* (Table 68-7)

**Herpes simplex.** Infection with herpes simplex (type 1 or 2) in HIV-infected individuals usually presents with ulcerative lesions or erosions. Common sites include anogenital, (see Plate 47) oral, and digital areas (Fig. 68-4). Vesicles frequently are absent and Tzanck smears of involved skin or mucosa are frequently negative. Diagnosis is by culture and occasionally by skin biopsy. A hyperkeratotic papular form of chronic HSV infection can be seen in patients with AIDS. Treatment is with acyclovir or, in resistant cases, foscarnet.

**Herpes zoster.** Herpes zoster may be the first sign of HIV infection. It is important to assess HIV risk factors in patients with herpes zoster and to serotest those at risk. Herpes zoster usually presents in its typical form in HIV disease, although severe forms involving more than one dermatome can be seen. Recommended treatments vary and tend to be on the basis of severity. Some routinely use oral acyclovir for 5 days and reserve intravenous treatment for cases of established dissemination. Others recommend prolonged high dose acyclovir as the initial management in HIV patients with herpes zoster to prevent complications with resistant strains.

***Hyperkeratotic herpes zoster.*** In patients with advanced HIV disease, an atypical form of herpes zoster can exists in which persistent hyperkeratotic papules develop in a dermatomal or disseminated distribution (Fig. 68-5). These usually occur after treatment with acyclovir and are thought to be caused by the development of a thymidine kinase-negative strain of the virus that is resistant to acyclovir. The lesions are fixed and tend to be painful. Diagnosis of hyperkeratotic herpes zoster usually requires biopsy confirmation or culture. Treatments include prolonged use of acyclovir or foscarnet. New antiviral agents continue to be studied and may prove to be helpful.

***Scabies.*** In the setting of HIV disease, scabies can present in a hyperkeratotic form similar to the type described in neurologically impaired patients (Norwegian scabies). Hyperkeratotic plaques located anywhere on the body are characteristic of this form of scabies (Fig. 68-6). Pruritus is frequently less than in cases of scabies in healthy individuals. The large amount of mites in the

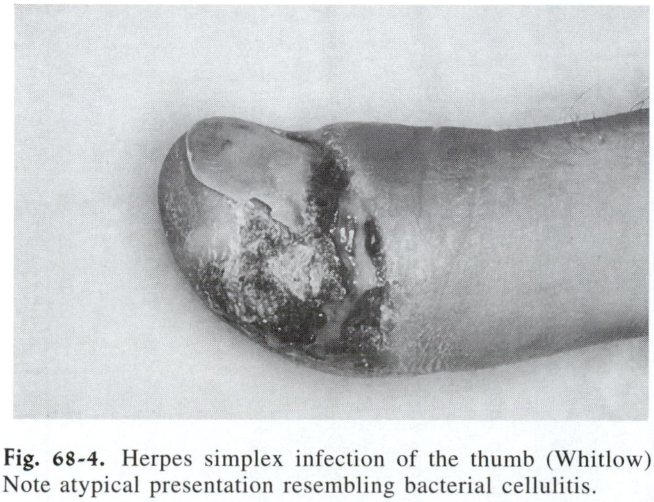

**Fig. 68-4.** Herpes simplex infection of the thumb (Whitlow). Note atypical presentation resembling bacterial cellulitis.

**Table 68-7.** Cutaneous diseases with atypical presentations in HIV infection

| Diagnosis | History | Physical | Laboratory | Differential | Management |
|---|---|---|---|---|---|
| Herpes simplex | Persistent erosive areas or nonhealing ulcer | May see vesicles, erosions, ulcers, or hyperkeratotic papules | Culture + for HSV | Usually characteristic | Acyclovir<br>Foscarnet |
| Herpes zoster | Dermatomal painful vesicles<br>May be widespread | Several dermatomes<br>Persistent hyperkeratotic variant | Tzanck smear + biopsy confirmation | Folliculitis | Acyclovir<br>Foscarnet<br>Famciclovir |
| Scabies | Scaly patches<br>Some pruritus | Hyperkeratotic plaques<br>Anywhere on body | KOH teeming with mites and eggs | Psoriasis<br>Ichthyosis<br>Contact dermatitis | Permethrin 5%<br>Kwell |
| Syphilis | Variable (see Chapter 65) | Papulosquamous chancre<br>Plaques, papules | RPR, VDRL<br>FTA-ABS<br>Biopsy in atypical cases<br>CSF evaluation | Psoriasis<br>Dermatitis<br>Pityriasis rosea | Penicillin (see Chapter 65) |
| Psoriasis and Reiter's disease | Worsening scaling skin lesions<br>Arthritis common | Erythema, scaling, plaques: scalp, genitalia, hands, feet | Confirmation by biopsy in difficult cases | Seborrheic dermatitis<br>Scabies | Topical steroids<br>Emollients<br>Ultraviolet light<br>Etretinate |

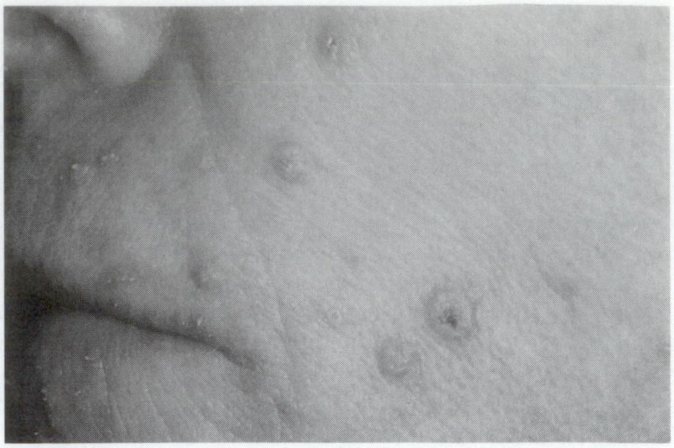

**Fig. 68-5.** Hyperkeratotic herpes zoster. Note papular (nonvesicular) and hyperkeratotic lesions distributed on facial dermatome.

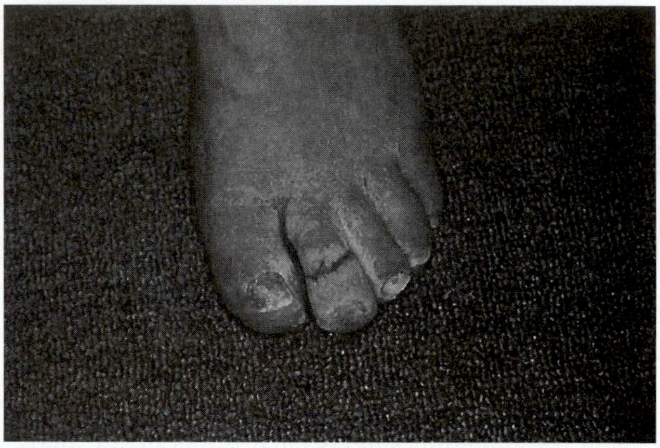

**Fig. 68-6.** Hyperkeratotic scabies in patient with AIDS. Note localized hyperkeratotic patch containing large numbers of mites.

plaques makes these patients able to transmit the disease through fomites such as linens, clothing, and office furniture. Diagnosis is easily made by KOH examination of skin scrapings, which demonstrates numerous mites and eggs. Treatment is usually with applications of gamma benzene hexachloride (Kwell) or permethrin 5% cream (Elimite). Repeated applications may be required. An alternative inexpensive treatment in recurrent cases is with the use of 6% precipitated sulfur in petrolatum for 12 hours, three days in a row, then weekly as needed. Attention to subungual areas is important because these areas can be a source of reinfestation if not adequately treated.

**Psoriasis.** In HIV-infected persons, psoriasis occurs with higher frequency and greater severity than in the general population. The onset may precede or follow the diagnosis of HIV infection and can progress rapidly. Peripheral arthritis occurs commonly in HIV-associated psoriasis. Recent evidence suggests that HIV-associated psoriasis may be part of the disease spectrum of Reiter's syndrome. The clinical presentation of HIV-associated psoriasis includes guttate lesions, papules, plaques, and pustules anywhere on the body including palms and soles. Nail involvement is common.

***Treatment.*** Standard modalities such as topical corticosteroids, tar, and UVB are frequently adequate. The synthetic retinoid etretinate can be tried in recalcitrant cases. Good responses have been reported with AZT alone. Methotrexate has been associated with progression of the underlying HIV disease and most authors do not recommend its use.

**Reiter's syndrome.** Reiter's syndrome is associated with HIV disease and is frequently severe and progressive. It is not known whether this association is directly related to the HIV infection or other factors. Most patients are HLA B27-positive. Characteristic features of Reiter's syndrome include asymmetric large joint oligoarthritis, inflammatory eye disease, and urethritis. The cutaneous lesions of Reiter's syndrome are erythematous, scaly papules and plaques that resemble psoriasis clinically and histologically. When present on the palms and soles, they are called keratoderma blennorrhagica (see Plate 48). On the penis the lesions may be annular and are called circinate balanitis. Nail involvement can be extensive, with hyperkeratotic painful nails and surrounding erythema. Treatment is similar to that for psoriasis. Successful treatment with etretinate has been reported.

### *Diseases with increased frequency in HIV infection* (Table 68-8)

**Seborrheic dermatitis.** HIV-associated seborrheic dermatitis frequently precedes other signs of HIV infection and can be considered a possible marker of HIV infection. The cause is not known but recent evidence implicates overgrowth of the yeast *Pityrosporum* as a causative factor.

***Physical examination.*** Typical signs are patches of erythema with scaling on the sides of the nose, central forehead, and hair-bearing areas of the scalp and beard region. In more severe cases the ears, chest, axillae, and pubic area are involved. Symptoms are usually minimal. Diagnosis can be made by inspection in most cases. Biopsy can be helpful in difficult cases because of characteristic histologic findings in HIV-associated seborrheic dermatitis.

***Management.*** Treatment choices include medicated shampoos containing zinc, tar, selenium sulfide, or ketoconazole, plus topical preparations containing corticosteroids or imidizole antifungal agents. Maintenance therapy is usually required. Oral ketoconazole may be helpful in severe cases.

**Drug reactions.** Reactions to drugs occur frequently in HIV-infected persons including those with profoundly impaired immune status. Reactions are usually in response to antibiotics and are most commonly a morbilliform type of reaction. This occurs most often with the administration of TMP-SMX. The precise immunologic mechanism in this reaction is not known. Some authors recommend a desensitization procedure in patients who develop this reaction to TMP-SMX. Other reactions to drugs seen in HIV disease include urticaria, erythema multiforme, Stevens-Johnson syndrome, and vasculitis.

**Pruritic dermatoses in HIV disease**

Eosinophilic folliculitis
Bacterial folliculitis
Tinea corporis
Tinea versicolor
Granuloma annulare
Insect bite reactions
Hyperkeratotic scabies
Drug reactions
Photosensitivity
Xerosis

**Pruritus.** Many HIV-associated skin diseases present with pruritus. Most patients with pruritus have an identifiable dermatosis (see the box above). Generalized pruritus without skin disease requires a search for an underlying cause.

**CMV infection.** Although CMV infection is seen in all forms of immunosuppression, the prevalence has increased in the setting of HIV disease. While most of the disease manifestations are noncutaneous (retinitis, pneumonitis), the characteristic skin lesions of CMV infection are ulcers in the perioral, perineal skin, and oral mucosa. The diagnosis can be made by viral culture, although biopsy is frequently required to confirm the diagnosis. CMV also has been reported to cause cutaneous vesicles, bullae, and vasculitis. Treatment is with intravenous ganciclovir. Perioraficial ulcers are commonly infected with both CMV and herpes simplex virus; in these combined infections, treatment of the HSV with acyclovir can result in complete responses.

**Fungal infections.** Fungal disease is common in HIV-infected persons. Mucocutaneous fungal infection is usually not life-threatening itself, but cutaneous lesions may be the presenting sign of systemic fungal disease. In these cases a correct dermatologic diagnosis can influence morbidity and mortality.

**Bacterial infections.** Only recently have bacterial infections been appreciated as opportunistic pathogens in the setting of HIV infection. Several clinical presentations already have been discussed including gastroenteritis, pneumonia, skin infection, meningitis, and disseminated infections.

Sinusitis is extremely common in HIV-infected patients. Despite the frequency of sinusitis, relatively little is known about its pathogenesis, microbiologic etiology, or treatment. It appears to be more frequent in patients with late stage disease, at which time it is often recurrent and refractory to therapy. Multiple sinus involvement is the rule, with the maxillary and ethmoid sinuses being those most frequently involved. The best-described bacterial pathogens associated with sinusitis include *S. pneumoniae* and *H. influenzae.* Initial treatment of sinusitis, particularly for patients with an established history of frequent relapses, should include an antibacterial agent with activity against beta-lactamase producing *H. influenzae,* a decongestant combined with guaifenesin, and inhaled nasal steroids. For patients who fail initial antibiotic therapy, substitute antibacterial agents that

**Table 68-8.** Cutaneous diseases with increased frequency in HIV infection

| Diagnosis | History | Physical | Laboratory | Differential | Management |
|---|---|---|---|---|---|
| Seborrheic dermatitis | Flaking in scalp and on face | Erythema, scaling | R/O fungus with KOH examination | Psoriasis<br>Contact dermatitis<br>Impetigo | Selenium, tar shampoo<br>Topical steroids<br>Antifungals occasionally helpful |
| Drug eruptions | Widespread eruption usually<br>Frequent pruritic TMP-SMX history often | Morbilliform rash usually<br>Erythema multiforme | None | Viral exanthem<br>Psoriasis | Supportive<br>Remove drug<br>Desensitize occasionally |
| Pruritus | Pruritus | Variable | Depends on diagnosis | See the box on p. 953 | Depends on diagnosis |
| CMV infection | Periorificial ulcer<br>May have retinitis | Ulcer most common<br>Vesicles, bullae | Culture<br>Biopsy | Herpes simplex<br>Cryptococcus<br>Aphthous ulcer | Treat coexistent HSV<br>Ganciclovir |
| Fungal infections | | | | | |
| Candidiasis | Painful oral, esophageal symptoms | White patches oral mucosa | KOH + biopsy to R/O<br>Oral hairy leukoplakia | Oral hairy leukoplakia | Miconazole troches p.o.<br>Ketoconazole<br>Fluconazole |
| Cryptococcus | CNS symptoms<br>Painful skin nodules | Dome-shaped papules<br>Ulcerations | Confirmation by biopsy<br>Cryptococcal antigen (serum)<br>CNS workup | Molluscum<br>Herpes simplex | Amphotericin B<br>Fluconazole |
| Histoplasmosis | Systemic illness<br>Variable skin symptoms | — | Biopsy confirmation | Folliculitis<br>Dermatitis<br>Aphthous ulcer<br>Vasculitis | Amphotericin B<br>Itraconazole |

should be considered include clindamycin to treat anaerobes, amoxicillin/clavulanate, or a fluoroquinolone to treat *P. aeruginosa.* For patients with truly refractory disease, antral puncture for microbiologic culture may be helpful, although many such patients likely will require surgical drainage.

***Syphilis.*** Transmission and pathogenesis of HIV and *T. pallidum* are intimately intertwined. As an ulcerative STD, the presence of active cutaneous or mucosal syphilitic lesions increases the efficiency of HIV transmission. In turn, the cell-mediated immunodeficiency induced by HIV appears to increase the virulence of *T. pallidum.* Both the frequency of coinfection and the altered clinical course of syphilis in patients with HIV infection have prompted a renewed effort to understand the pathogenesis of syphilis in the immunocompromised patient and to define optimal treatment regimens for the various stages of infection.

Several features about syphilis in HIV-infected patients appear to be unique. First, the course of syphilis may be accelerated in HIV-infected patients. In particular, symptomatic CNS involvement occurs earlier and with greater frequency. Second, treatment for all stages of syphilis may need to be more intensive than what is generally accepted for normal immune hosts. Finally, the standard serologic tests used in the diagnosis may be unreliable. Therefore the primary care provider should maintain a high clinical suspicion for syphilis and a low threshold to biopsy-suspicious lesions.

The clinical presentation of syphilis in the setting of HIV infection is often similar to that observed in noninfected patients. Chancres and maculopapular rashes are common. Unusual nodular or ulcerative lesions have been described less commonly. Ocular infection can result in keratitis, retinitis, and optic neuritis. Patients may occasionally present with sensorineural hearing loss. Symptoms of neurologic disease are variable, ranging from isolated cranial nerve abnormalities to aseptic meningitis to significant behavioral changes.

Diagnosis of syphilis can be made using the standard nontreponemal serologic tests (RPR or VDRL), followed by confirmatory testing utilizing treponemal tests (FTA-ABS). In seronegative patients for whom there is a high clinical suspicion of active syphilis, biopsy of potential lesions should be considered. Various tissue stains for *T. pallidum* can be used to identify the spirochete. CSF sampling is required for all patients, irrespective of disease stage, who have neurologic signs or symptoms, including behavioral changes or visual or auditory symptoms or signs. Sampling also should be performed in any patient with disease of greater than 1 year's duration, a positive RPR for greater than 1 year, or whose RPR or VDRL titer does not fall with standard treatment. It has been suggested that lumbar puncture should be performed on all HIV-infected patients with a positive syphilis serology, although this may be unnecessarily aggressive. The CDC does not advocate this approach.

Penicillin is the agent of choice for the treatment of all forms of syphilis. For disease of less than 1 year's duration, a single intramuscular dose of benzathine penicillin G (2.4 million units) may be adequate, but three doses are often recommended. For the treatment of disease greater than 1 year's duration in the absence of proven or likely CNS involvement, intramuscular benzathine penicillin G (2.4 million units) given weekly for three doses should be used. Treatment of patients with refractory disease or those with proven or suspected neurosyphilis should consist of 10 to 14 days of aqueous intravenous penicillin G (12 to 24 million units/day) or procaine penicillin G (2.4 million units intramuscularly per day) along with probenecid 500 mg four times a day, both for 10 days. Symptoms and quantitative serologic titers should be followed to determine response to treatment.

***Mycobacterium avium complex.*** MAC includes a group of related species that cause serious, disseminated infection in AIDS patients. Disseminated MAC infection occurs almost exclusively in patients with profoundly depressed CD4 counts (typically $<50/mm^3$). With the decline in the frequency of *P. carinii* pneumonia, disseminated MAC infection may now be the most frequent opportunistic complication, occurring in up to 40% of late stage HIV-infected patients.

The organism is ubiquitous in the environment and is easily culturable in soil and water. Patients likely become infected by ingestion or inhalation of the organism. The organism then is engulfed by macrophages. Lacking the capacity to kill the organism, infected macrophages subsequently disseminate the organism widely to lymph nodes in the gastrointestinal tract and abdomen and to the liver, spleen, and bone marrow. Patients typically present with the insidious onset of fevers, night sweats, chills, weight loss, anorexia, and diarrhea. Examination often reveals hepatosplenomegaly but is otherwise nondiagnostic. Commonly associated laboratory abnormalities include anemia and granulocytopenia as a consequence of bone marrow infiltration and elevated liver enzymes (especially alkaline phosphatase). Mycobacterial blood cultures are positive in the majority of cases. The diagnosis also can be made by bone marrow biopsy or by culture and biopsy of other involved organs. Positive cultures from sputum and/or stool specimens may reflect only colonization and have only weak predictive value for the development of disseminated disease. The organism load in tissue is typically overwhelming, in excess of $10^{10}$ organisms/gram of tissue. If patients are untreated the median survival with disseminated MAC infection ranges between 4 and 7 months.

Treatment of disseminated MAC infection has improved greatly with the introduction of the new broad-spectrum, long-acting macrolide antibiotics, clarithromycin, and azithromycin. Both agents have significant activity against MAC and are orally active. The use of either macrolide in combination with one or more additional agent(s) (ethambutol, clofazimine, rifampin, rifabutin, ciprofloxicin, amikacin) improves symptoms and reduces the level of bacteremia in a high proportion of patients. The United States Public Health Service currently recommends clarithromycin plus 1 to 2 additional agents for the treatment of disseminated MAC infection.

***Candidiasis.*** Candidiasis usually presents as oral or oropharyngeal plaques (thrush). Symptoms are variable but usually consist of burning and pain. Examination by KOH preparation or Gram stain of scraped material from the plaques confirms the presence of pseudohyphae and budding yeast. Confirmation is necessary when the differential diagnosis includes oral hairy leukoplakia. Less frequently, candidiasis involves cutaneous surfaces including the palms and soles. Treatment is with imidazole antifungal agents or nystatin. Oral ketoconazole or fluconazole should be considered in severe cases involving the esophagus.

***Tinea.*** Tinea (infection with dermatophyte fungus) does not have a higher prevalence in HIV-infected individuals. The presentation, diagnosis, and treatment are discussed in Chapter 21.

***Cryptococcus.*** A potentially lethal infection usually involving the CNS, cryptococcal infection may present with cutaneous lesions that are characteristic. There are two cutaneous forms. The most common form is the presence of multiple dome-shaped papules on the face that resemble mollusca contagiosa. The other form consists of raised ulcerative lesions anywhere on the body. The diagnosis in both cases is made by skin biopsy that demonstrates the cryptococcal organisms. A diagnosis of cutaneous cryptococcal infection warrants further evaluation for CNS involvement and treatment for systemic disease. Treatment modalities include the use of amphotericin B and fluconazole.

**Endemic mycoses**

***Histoplasma capsulatum.*** *H. capsulatum* is an important cause of pneumonia and disseminated disease in AIDS patients from endemic areas. In the United States, the principal endemic regions are the central and south-central states. Disease occurs as a consequence both of exogenous exposure and reactivation of latent infection.

The presentation is often chronic or subacute, and progressive constitutional symptoms are more common than pulmonary complaints. Isolated pulmonary disease is uncommon in patients with advanced HIV disease; the vast majority of patients present with disseminated disease. Radiographic abnormalities occur in approximately half of patients and typically consist of diffuse infiltrates, which are usually interstitial, but may be reticulonodular or alveolar. Localized infiltrates occur, but are less common. Mediastinal adenopathy and calcification, hallmarks of pulmonary histoplasmosis in patients with normal immune function, are rarely seen in HIV-infected patients with disseminated disease.

A septicemia-like syndrome, with hypotension, coagulopathy, and multiorgan system failure is seen in 10% to 20% of cases. Neurologic manifestations, including encephalopathy, meningitis, and focal brain lesions occur in 5% to 20% of patients. Patients with CNS involvement are less responsive to treatment and have a higher mortality than other patients with disseminated disease.

Histoplasmosis is diagnosed definitively by culture. Diagnostic evaluation should include fungal cultures of blood and bone marrow and of respiratory specimens in those with pulmonary manifestations. Growth of *H. capsulatum* may take many weeks, however, so that a presumptive diagnosis must be made by histopathology or serology. Smears of peripheral blood, bone marrow, respiratory specimens, or tissue stained with periodic acid-Schiff (PAS) or Gomori methenamine silver may demonstrate the typical intracellular yeast forms. Biopsy of skin lesions, which occur in up to 18% of patients, may be especially useful in making a rapid diagnosis of disseminated histoplasmosis. Demonstration of *Histoplasma* polysaccharide antigen (HPA) in serum or urine allows for the presumptive diagnosis of both new infection and relapse. More widely available serologic tests for anti-*H. capsulatum* antibodies, such as immunodiffusion and complement fixation, are less sensitive and specific, but may provide clues to the diagnosis.

Patients with disseminated histoplasmosis should be treated with at least 15 mg/kg of amphotericin B given over 4 to 6 weeks. Itraconazole also show promise for treatment of mild to moderate histoplasmosis. As with many other opportunistic infections in patients with AIDS, *Histoplasma* infection cannot be eradicated, and effective treatment requires lifelong maintenance. Itraconazole (200 mg twice a day) is the most effective of the azole antifungal agents in suppressing histoplasmosis.

***Coccidioides immitis.*** *C. immitis* is a soil fungus, found in the United States, primarily in the deserts of the Southwest. Infection is acquired via inhalation of arthroconidia, and disease usually results from reactivation of latent infection. In patients with AIDS, pulmonary involvement is the most common clinical manifestation, although disseminated or extrapulmonary disease occurs more frequently than in patients without HIV infection. In patients with early stage HIV infection and intact cellular immunity, disease is similar to that seen in patients without HIV infection. In patients with more advanced immunosuppression, however, disease is more severe, and is more often disseminated or extrapulmonary. As with histoplasmosis, patients present with slowly progressive constitutional symptoms, although respiratory symptoms, such as dyspnea, dry or productive cough, and pleuritic chest pain occur more frequently. Radiographic findings often are much more extensive than those seen in patients without HIV infection. Diffuse interstitial or nodular infiltrates are common, although miliary infiltrates, adenopathy, and nodular and cavitary lesions have been described.

Diagnosis should be considered in any HIV-infected patient with pulmonary disease who has spent time in an endemic area. Although serology (tube precipitin or complement fixation) may be helpful, false-negative tests are not uncommon, and the definitive diagnosis is made either by visualization of the coccidioidal spherule on potassium hydroxide mount of sputum or by culture. Patients should be treated with 1 to 2.5 g of amphotericin B, followed by chronic maintenance therapy with oral triazole agents. The limited data available support the use of itraconazole (200 mg twice a day) or fluconazole (400 mg a day) as maintenance therapy.

***Blastomyces dermatitidis.*** Blastomycosis, caused by the dimorphic fungus *B. dermatitidis,* is endemic in the midwestern and south-central United States. In the few cases of blastomycosis reported in patients with AIDS, disease has been either disseminated or limited to the lungs and pleura. In most cases the CD4 count is less than $200/mm^3$ at the time of presentation. Patients with pulmonary blastomycosis present with fever, weight loss, cough, and sometimes pleuritic chest pain and dyspnea. Radiographic abnormalities include focal lobar infiltrates, miliary or diffuse interstitial infiltrates, and bilateral pulmonary nodules. Therapy should be initiated with amphotericin B. After clinical improvement, chronic suppressive therapy with an oral azole compound is required.

**Ophthalmologic complications of HIV infection.** As

many as 80% of HIV-infected patients develop clinically apparent ophthalmic lesions. Most ophthalmologic complications fall into one of three categories: opportunistic infections, microvascular abnormalities, and neoplasms. In addition to these major categories, neuroophthalmologic signs indicative of CNS diseases also may be seen. Other complications that do not fall under these general categories have been described, including retinal vasculitis and closed-angle glaucoma.

***Opportunistic infections.*** CMV retinitis from reactivation of latent virus is one of the most common AIDS-related opportunistic infections in patients with CD4 counts lower than 100/mm$^3$. Symptoms of CMV retinitis can be insidious in onset, developing over several weeks. Patients complain of seeing flashes, spots, "floaters," or visual field defects. CMV retinitis develops unilaterally in most cases, although untreated it inexorably spreads to the unaffected eye. Within the retina, disease can begin either peripherally or centrally. With peripheral disease, retinal involvement may be quite extensive at the time of presentation, because patients may not notice visual symptoms until the central areas become affected.

The primary care provider must always be attentive to the retinal examination in patients with low CD4 counts. CMV retinal lesions appear as areas of fluffy exudate intermixed with hemorrhage ("ketchup and scrambled eggs"). Disease can be recognized readily if the pupils are dilated before the funduscopic examination.

Ganciclovir was the first drug found to have significant anti-CMV activity. Patients are given induction therapy at a dose of 5 mg/kg intravenously every 12 hours. After a 2-week induction period, patients continue the medication at a dose of 2.5 to 5.0 mg/kg a day indefinitely because relapse is invariable once the drug is stopped. An oral form of ganciclovir, taken at a dose of 1 gram three times daily with food, has recently been approved for use following parenteral induction. The principal dose-limiting toxicity of ganciclovir is bone marrow suppression. Granulocytopenia is the most common feature, and sometimes necessitates the use of G-CSF. The other available drug for the treatment of CMV retinitis is foscarnet. Foscarnet can be administered only intravenously. Patients are given induction therapy at a dose of 60 mg/kg every 8 hours, adjusted for renal function, for 2 weeks. Lifelong maintenance therapy at a dose of 90 to 120 mg/kg a day is then instituted. The principal toxicities of foscarnet include renal impairment, electrolyte imbalances, anemia, and seizures.

Ganciclovir and foscarnet may suppress CMV activity only for several months, after which retinitis almost inevitably progresses. Patients with recurrence can be reinduced with the same agent followed by higher dose maintenance therapy, they can be switched to the alternate drug, or they can receive both drugs. Studies are under way to determine the most effective treatment for relapse. Both drugs appear to be equivalent in their anti-CMV activity. Survival for patients diagnosed with CMV retinitis is poor for reasons that are not well understood. Foscarnet may offer a survival advantage over ganciclovir due to specific antiretroviral activity, but is more difficult to tolerate. Patients generally survive for only 4 to 7 months from the time of diagnosis, even if CMV is adequately suppressed. It is likely that the profound immunosuppression that permits expression of CMV also allows other complications to develop, which leads to the death of the patient.

Other opportunistic infections of the retina and choroid are quite uncommon. Toxoplasmic chorioretinitis is surprisingly rare in HIV-infected patients given the frequency of other clinical syndromes caused by the organism in this population. Overall *T. gondii* causes less than 5% of all ocular infections in HIV-infected patients. When it occurs, toxoplasmic chorioretinitis can cause diffuse or localized disease affecting one or both eyes. An inflammatory response is highly variable. Patients should be treated with standard therapy for toxoplasmosis consisting of pyrimethamine with either sulfadiazine or clindamycin. Lifelong maintenance therapy is required to prevent recurrence of disease.

Herpes simplex and herpes zoster have rarely been implicated in causing retinal disease. Their more common ocular manifestations include keratitis and conjunctivitis. Herpes zoster keratitis occurs during outbreaks of disease involving the trigeminal nerve. The diagnosis can be established easily when the characteristic dermatomal zoster rash is seen in the ophthalmic trigeminal distribution. Herpes simplex occasionally causes keratitis in this patient group. For herpes simplex keratitis, treatment with trifluridine ophthalmic solution should be initiated. For both types of herpesvirus infection, treatment with acyclovir may help ameliorate the course of disease and, particularly in the case of herpes simplex virus, prevent recurrence.

***Microvascular abnormalities.*** Cotton-wool spots are perhaps the most frequent ocular abnormality recognized in HIV-infected patients. They have been described most frequently in patients with low CD4 counts but can be seen at any stage of disease. On examination, they appear similar to the cotton-wool spots seen in diabetics. Their presence is a reflection of focal retinal ischemia. Cotton-wool spots are typically asymptomatic and require no treatment. They often resolve spontaneously even as new lesions appear elsewhere in the retina. Microaneurysms and retinal hemorrhages also are seen frequently in HIV-infected patients.

***Neoplasms.*** KS is the most frequent neoplasm to involve the eye. KS lesions typically are observed in the conjunctiva and within the skin of the eyelids. Lesions are violaceous in appearance and can be raised. Beyond the cosmetic defect and the rare impairment in lid function caused by the lesions, KS in this location is otherwise asymptomatic. Localized radiation therapy is effective in reducing the size of lesions while causing little damage to the eye.

## PROPHYLAXIS FOR OPPORTUNISTIC INFECTIONS

The institution of prophylaxis against *Pneumocystis carinii* pneumonia (PCP) has been one of the most important advances in the management of patients with HIV disease. PCP prophylaxis decreases morbidity, prolongs survival, and delays the progression of HIV disease. Its success has led to a search for effective regimens for the prevention of other common HIV-related infections. The issue of prophylaxis becomes especially important in patients with advanced HIV disease, who are at high risk for opportunistic infections, and who may have ceased to benefit from antiretroviral therapy.

The following section focuses on *primary prophylaxis,* or prevention of the first episode of opportunistic disease, and in some cases on *secondary prophylaxis,* or prevention of recurrence of disease. Discussion of maintenance or suppressive therapy given to prevent relapse, also referred to as secondary prophylaxis, is discussed in relation to the particular infection.

### *Pneumocystis carinii*

Although AZT was shown to prolong survival for patients with an initial diagnosis of *P. carinii* pneumonia, the rate of recurrence is high without secondary prophylaxis. *Pneumocystis* prophylaxis not only decreases the incidence of PCP but prolongs survival.

Studies have shown that PCP rarely occurs in patients with CD4 counts greater than 200 to 250/mm$^3$. These studies have provided the basis for the recommendation that *Pneumocystis* prophylaxis be given to all HIV-infected adults with a total CD4 count of less than 200/mm$^3$. Prophylaxis also should be given, regardless of CD4 count, to patients with a history of PCP, or with more than 2 weeks of unexplained fevers or other constitutional symptoms, oral candidiasis, or opportunistic infections that typically occur with CD4 counts less than 200/mm$^3$.

TMP-SMX is the preferred agent for *Pneumocystis* prophylaxis. Although the recommended regimen is one double-strength tablet daily, smaller doses may be equally effective and associated with fewer side effects. In addition to being the most effective drug in preventing PCP, TMP-SMX also appears to protect against toxoplasmic encephalitis and bacterial infections. Adverse reactions occur less frequently with prophylactic doses of TMP-SMX than with the higher doses used for treatment of PCP. A history of non–life-threatening reactions to sulfonamides is not an absolute contraindication to prophylaxis with TMP-SMX.

Oral dapsone is an effective and inexpensive alternative for patients who cannot tolerate TMP-SMX. Toxicities of dapsone include rash, nausea, and methemoglobinemia, and hemolytic anemia in patients with G6PD deficiency. The recommended dose is 100 mg daily, although lower doses (50 mg daily or 100 mg twice weekly) may also be effective. The combination of dapsone and pyrimethamine has shown efficacy in preventing both PCP and toxoplasmosis. A typical regimen would combine dapsone, 50 mg a day, with pyrimethamine, 50 mg a week. Folinic acid is added to pyrimethamine-containing regimens to minimize marrow toxicity.

Aerosolized pentamidine is a less effective alternative for patients who cannot take TMP-SMX. It is well tolerated, although some patients may experience bronchospasm during administration. Bronchospasm usually can be prevented by pretreating with inhaled beta-adrenergic agonists.

### *Toxoplasma gondii*

It is estimated that 20% to 47% of HIV-infected patients with latent *T. gondii* infection will develop cerebral toxoplasmosis at some point in the course of their HIV disease. There is growing evidence that some of the agents effective in PCP prophylaxis also may prevent toxoplasmosis. Because *Toxoplasma* seroprevalence is far less common in the United States than in other parts of the world, the most appropriate strategy is to reserve prophylaxis for patients at highest risk for toxoplasmic encephalitis: anti-*Toxoplasma* IgG seropositive patients with advanced HIV disease.

Multiple studies of PCP prophylaxis have demonstrated a lower incidence of toxoplasmosis in patients given TMP-SMX than in those given aerosolized pentamidine. While neither dapsone nor pyrimethamine appear to be effective as single agents, when used in combination they also reduce the risk of toxoplasmosis.

It is reasonable to consider specific prophylaxis in patients with a positive anti-*Toxoplasma* IgG and a CD4 count less than 100/mm$^3$. In patients already taking TMP-SMX for PCP prophylaxis, no further intervention is necessary. Patients who cannot tolerate TMP-SMX should receive dapsone and pyrimethamine with folinic acid, which also are effective in preventing PCP. The role of other agents such as atovaquone, azithromycin, and clarithromycin in the prevention of toxoplasmosis has not been determined.

### Fungal infections

Although fungal infections are common complications of HIV disease, enthusiasm for routine antifungal prophylaxis has been tempered by lack of data, the high cost of oral antifungal agents, and by the potential for the promotion of resistance.

Mucosal candidiasis is exceedingly common in HIV-infected patients; nevertheless, candidal infections may not be appropriate targets for primary prophylaxis because they respond readily to treatment. Patients who develop frequent recurrences may be candidates for chronic suppressive therapy.

The morbidity, mortality, and cost of therapy for cryptococcal meningitis make it an attractive target for primary prophylaxis. Fluconazole has been shown to decrease the incidence of serious fungal infections, especially cryptococcal meningitis and esophageal candidiasis, in patients with advanced HIV disease. However, fluconazole-resistant candidiasis is a growing problem in this population, and antifungal prophylaxis has not been shown to prolong survival. Routine primary prophylaxis is not currently recommended. When used, it should probably be reserved for patients with CD4 counts less than 50/mm3, as patients with earlier disease are unlikely to develop serious fungal infections, and excessive use of oral antifungal agents may predispose them to azole-resistant fungal infections.

### Mycobacterial infections

Disseminated infection with MAC is the most common opportunistic bacterial infection in patients with AIDS. A late manifestation of HIV disease, it rarely occurs until the CD4 cell count has fallen below 50/mm$^3$. Rifabutin (300 mg a day) was effective in preventing MAC bacteremia in two randomized, placebo-controlled trials in patients with CD4 counts less than 200/mm$^3$. Rifabutin reduced the incidence of MAC bacteremia by 50%, decreased hospitalization, and prolonged the time to fever, fatigue, anemia, alkaline phosphatase elevation, and decline in Karnofsky performance score. The efficacy was most pronounced in patients whose initial CD4 count was less than 75/mm$^3$. Primary prophylaxis with rifabutin is now recommended for patients with CD4 counts less than 50/mm$^3$, or less than 75/mm$^3$in patients with a history of an opportunistic infection. It should not be given as a single drug to patients with active tuberculosis or MAC disease because of the possibility of promoting resistance. Rifabutin is well tolerated, but like rifampin, it induces hepatic microsomal enzymes, causing altered metabolism of oral contraceptives, warfarin, dilantin, methadone, and zidovudine. Patients taking rifabutin should be monitored closely for evidence of drug interactions.

Clarithromycin and azithromycin are effective in treating MAC bacteremia. Clarithromycin (500 mg twice daily) is effective in preventing MAC. However, patients who develop MAC while taking clarithromycin frequently have clarithromycin-resistant isolates, making their infection more difficult to treat. Therefore, this drug should be reserved for patients unable to tolerate rifabutin.

HIV-infected patients with latent *M. tuberculosis* infection are at high risk for the development of reactivation tuberculosis and should be given prophylaxis regardless of age. Candidates for prophylaxis include patients with a PPD reaction of at least 5 mm of induration, a history of a positive PPD, or a recent history of close contact with a person with infectious tuberculosis. The predictive value of anergy testing is poor in HIV-infected patients, and these tests are no longer believed to be helpful in determining the need for prophylaxis.

Isoniazid prophylaxis appears to be as effective in HIV-infected persons as in non-immunosuppressed patients. The CDC recommends that prophylaxis be administered for 12 months, but studies of shorter duration prophylaxis are underway. Isoniazid, 15 mg/kg twice a week, may be substituted for daily therapy in patients whose therapy can be supervised. Pyridoxine, 50 mg a day, is often added to isoniazid therapy to reduce the incidence of peripheral neuropathy. For patients unable to take isoniazid, rifampin may be given for 6 to 12 months.

HIV-infected individuals who are exposed to patients with active MDR-TB should receive high-dose ethambutol, pyrazinamide, and a fluoroquinolone such as ofloxacin or ciprofloxacin. Prophylaxis against MDR-TB in an HIV-infected person should be given for at least 1 year.

### Viral infections

CMV is the most common cause of serious opportunistic viral disease in patients with HIV infection. Patients with CD4 count less than 50/mm$^3$ have a high risk of developing end-organ disease, especially retinitis. The high incidence, significant morbidity, and high cost and toxicity of therapy make CMV disease an appropriate target for prophylaxis. Despite conflicting data in solid-organ transplant recipients, acyclovir does not appear to prevent HIV-associated CMV disease. Oral ganciclovir (1 gm three times daily) decreases the risk of CMV disease in patients with advanced HIV disease who are CMV seropositive. Currently, the drug is licensed only for the maintenance therapy of CMV disease. Although the prospect of CMV prophylaxis is promising, more informaion is needed, especially with respect to the risk of antiviral resistance in patients who have received prophylaxis, before such a practice can be routinely recommended.

Recurrent herpes simplex virus infection is common in HIV-infected patients, and oral acyclovir (600 to 800 mg a day) is effective as secondary prophylaxis. VZV infection is also common in HIV-infected individuals. Because most adults have had primary varicella (chickenpox) during childhood, HIV-infected patients typically develop dermatomal zoster (shingles). Patients at risk for primary varicella should be given varicella-zoster immune globulin (VZIG) after exposure to individuals with active varicella infection. Because VZIG is only protective if given within 4 days of exposure, it may be useful to obtain baseline anti-varicella IgG in patients who cannot recall having chickenpox during childhood. Herpes zoster infection recurs less frequently than herpes simplex virus infection, so secondary prophylaxis is not usually necessary.

### Bacterial infections

HIV-infected patients are at increased risk for bacterial infections with common community-acquired pathogens such as *S. pneumoniae* and *H. influenzae*. Not surprisingly, the use of TMP-SMX for *Pneumocystis* prophylaxis reduces the risk of bacterial infections. The pneumococcal polysaccharide vaccine is also indicated for all HIV-infected adults and should be given as early as possible in the course of HIV infection. The use of a conjugated *H. influenzae* type b vaccine has been suggested, although efficacy data are lacking in adult patients. Although the risk of invasive *H. influenzae* type b infection is increased by HIV infection, the actual number of cases is probably small.

## SPECIAL CONSIDERATIONS IN HIV-INFECTED WOMEN

Rates of new HIV infections in women aged 15 to 44 years have increased faster than any other demographic group in the United States. Over 30,000 U.S. women have been diagnosed with AIDS through 1993, and AIDS has become a leading cause of death in young women. Epidemiologic data collected through the CDC indicate that the female/male ratio of new cases should continue to increase through the 1990s. Also notable is that in women heterosexually acquired HIV-infection is a more common risk factor than intravenous drug abuse. Approximately 75% of HIV-infected women are African American or Hispanic, and a large proportion are poor, uninsured, with inadequate access to health care.

Although HIV infection likely progresses at similar rates in women and men, delays in the recognition of a woman's risk of HIV infection may lead to a relatively late diagnosis. Women infected through heterosexual sex often are unaware of the HIV infection status of their male partners and do not perceive themselves to be at increased risk. This situation is particularly highlighted in the adolescent age group. Although the CDC recommends prenatal HIV testing of women with recognized risk factors, physicians should consider all women who are sexually active to be at risk for HIV. Multiple episodes of vaginal candidiasis or pelvic inflammatory disease, severe genital herpes, cervical dysplasia, and other sexually transmitted diseases should prompt the health care provider to discuss HIV testing. Effective counseling and voluntary testing are essential for the prevention of transmission and the institution of appropriate medical care.

The first HIV-related clinical manifestations in women often involve the reproductive tract. A recent study found that nearly one third of women had an active gynecologic problem at their first HIV clinic visit. The most common of these complications are (1) recurrent vaginal candidiasis, (2) severe genital HSV-2 infection, (3) cervical dysplasia and neoplasia, and (4) recurrent and/or severe pelvic inflammatory disease. Recurrent vaginal candidiasis is the most common initial manifestation of HIV, as well as one of the most frequently encountered opportunistic infections during the course of HIV infection in women. Recurrent or severe *Candida* vaginitis may not be recognized as HIV-related. Perineal herpetic infections may be more severe and persistent with HIV infection. As discussed earlier, women with HIV infection are at increased risk for cervical dysplasia due to human papilloma virus. In general, Pap smears are more often abnormal, cervical dysplasia more severe and extensive, and progression to invasive cancer more common with poor response to conventional therapy. Women with HIV infection should have Pap smears performed at least every 12 months (every 6 months is recommended in women with a previously abnormal Pap smear). Conversely, the presence of a high-grade cervical lesion on routine Pap screening should alert the physician to the possibility of HIV infection. Pelvic inflammatory disease, like many other STDs, is commonly encountered in HIV-infected patients, who may have an increased rate of complications related to pelvic inflammatory disease (e.g., tubo-ovarian abscess) and require surgical intervention more often than HIV-negative women.

The spectrum of AIDS-defining conditions is somewhat different in women than in men. *Candida* esophagitis appears to be a more common AIDS-defining illness in women. Kaposi's sarcoma is unusual in HIV-infected women, but occurs most often in women who acquired HIV through sexual contact with a bisexual man.

Management guidelines for HIV-infected pregnant patients have not been established at this time. When HIV infection is diagnosed during pregnancy, a baseline CD4 count should be obtained as soon as possible. AZT therapy has been offered to women with CD4 counts less than $500/mg^3$. The safety of AZT in pregnancy has not been extensively evaluated, although small, preliminary reports have demonstrated good tolerance and no fetal complications. A multicentered trial has demonstrated the efficacy of AZT in preventing vertical transmission (risk approximately 25% to 30%) of HIV from pregnant women to their offspring. The effect of pregnancy on the natural history of HIV-infection also is unknown. Isolated case reports have suggested that certain opportunistic infections may be more severe during pregnancy.

The social impact of HIV infection in women has yet to be fully appreciated. No longer a problem predominantly of substance abusers, heterosexually acquired HIV infection promises to expand dramatically over the next decade. Many HIV-infected women are mothers, and the implications of their role as primary caregiver for their families are tremendous. By the year 2000, it is expected that millions of children worldwide will be orphaned as a result of the HIV epidemic. Childcare and other family-related concerns may be the driving force behind the need of many women to obtain and comply with medical care. As the numbers continue to increase, the primary care provider needs to assume an integral role in the diagnosis, treatment, and education of women with HIV infection.

## SPECIAL ISSUES IN THE MANAGEMENT OF HIV-INFECTED PATIENTS

Although HIV infection shares many features of other chronic diseases, caring for HIV-infected patients also entails certain unique responsibilities. Frequent discussion of the avoidance of transmission is important. Although laws regarding sexual and drug-use contact notification vary from state to state, primary caregivers often play a role in encouraging or assisting with the disclosure of the patient's HIV status. In many communities practitioners care for patients for whom substance abuse, mental illness, homelessness, child care, lack of medical insurance, and poverty are of more immediate concern than their HIV infection. They must be aware of resources in the community that can assist their patients with these obstacles, so that their medical problems can be addressed. Practitioners may also become involved in issues of employment or housing discrimination, or may have patients who are rejected by their families or friends because of their disease, leaving them without the support that is so crucial as they become increasingly ill. Progress in the understanding and management of HIV disease takes place extremely rapidly, and patients will expect their caregivers to maintain an up-to-date knowledge of the latest advances. Patients may also ask for unapproved or experimental treatment or may take alternative therapies concurrently with or in place of standard drugs. Practitioners must be aware of experimental protocols and make them available to their patients, when appropriate. They also must be familiar with the potential risks and benefits of the alternative therapies being advocated in the community, so that they can counsel their patients about the use of these therapies, and monitor them appropriately if they choose to take them.

As with any chronic disease, practitioners caring for HIV-infected patients will interact frequently with their patients' families and support networks. HIV disease is unique, however, in that in many cases, the patient's spouse, partner, friends, or family members may also be infected. Practitioners must recognize the importance of nontraditional families. Among gay couples, for example, the patient's partner is usually a more appropriate decision maker than the next of kin, if the patient is unable to speak for himself. For this role to be legally recognized, however, the partner must have been designated as the "health care proxy" or "durable power of attorney for health." Patients should be encouraged as early as possible in the course of the disease to make their wishes known to their physician and family regarding their proxy for health care decisions, their wishes regarding terminal care and the aggressiveness with which it should be approached, and the disposition of their property after their death. Whenever possible, their wishes should be formalized with the legal arrangements appropriate to their particular state.

Although issues of death and dying are not unique to HIV care, they play a more prominent role than in many other fields of medicine. At some point in the course of their disease, most patients with HIV infection begin to confront their mortality, and may want to discuss their concerns with their primary care provider. They may ask direct questions about their prognosis and life expectancy, about what to expect as their disease becomes more advanced, or even about suicide or euthanasia. For many patients, these discussions are both informative and comforting. Practitioners who are comfortable discussing death and dying openly can learn more about their patients' fears and misconceptions and about how they wish to be cared for as their disease progresses. Ultimately, the practitioner must help the patient and family acknowledge the inevitability of death and, at some point, the futility of further aggressive intervention. Quality of life issues play an important role in the care of HIV-infected patients and become increasingly important in patients with advanced disease. For example, in some cases the diminishing benefits of continued antiretroviral therapy in patients with CD4 cell counts less than $50/mm^3$ may no longer outweigh the associated adverse reactions, and therapeutic efforts may be better directed toward preventing opportunistic infections. Eventually, the manner of death must be viewed as an important quality of life issue, and assurance that the patient will die without pain or unwanted intervention may become the overriding concern.

## BIBLIOGRAPHY


American Medical Association: *HIV early intervention: physician guidelines,* ed 2, Chicago, 1994, Division of Health Science.

Armstrong D: Treatment of opportunistic fungal infections, *Clin Infect Dis* 16:1, 1993.

Bartlett JG: *The Johns Hopkins Hospital guide to medical care of patients with HIV infection,* Baltimore, 1994, Williams & Wilkins.

Bartlett JG, Feinberg J: Update on management of opportunistic infections in patients with HIV infection, *Infect Dis Clin Pract* 2:233, 1993.

Centers for Disease Control: 1993 Revised classification system for HIV infection and expanded surveillance case definition for AIDS among adolescents and adults, *MMWR* 41 (RR-17):1, 1992.

Coldiron BM, Bergstresser PR: Prevalence and clinical spectrum of skin disease in patients infected with human immunodeficiency virus, *Arch Dermatol* 125:357, 1989.

Corey L, editor: *AIDS problems and prospects,* New York, 1993, WW Norton.

Cotton DJ, Friedland GH, editors: *HIV infection: a primary care approach,* rev ed, Waltham, 1992, Massachusetts Medical Society.

Fauci AS: Multifactorial nature of human immunodeficiency virus disease: implications for therapy, *Science* 262:1011, 1993.

Gallant JE, Moore RD, Chaisson RE: Prophylaxis for opportunistic infections in patients with HIV infection, *Ann Intern Med* 120:932, 1994.

Greenspan D et al: Relation of oral hairy leukoplakia to infection with the human immunodeficiency virus and the risk of developing AIDS, *J Infect Dis* 155:475, 1987.

Hecht FM, Soloway B: *HIV infection: a primary care approach,* Waltham, 1992, Massachusetts Medical Society.

Hoppenjans WB, et al: Prolonged cutaneous herpes zoster in acquired immunodeficiency syndrome, *Arch Dermatol* 126:1048, 1990.

Kaplan MH et al: Dermatologic manifestations of acquired immunodeficiency syndrome (AIDS), *J Am Acad Dermatol* 16:485, 1987.

Koehler JE, et al: Cutaneous vascular lesions and disseminated cat-scratch disease in patients with the acquired immunodeficiency syndrome (AIDS) and AIDS-related complex, *Ann Intern Med* 109:449, 1988.

Koehler JE et al: Isolation of *Rochalimaea* species from cutaneous and osseous lesions of bacillary angiomatosis, *N Engl J Med* 327:1625, 1992.

Levy JA: The transmission of HIV and factors influencing progression to AIDS, *Am J Med* 95:86, 1993.

Masur H: Prevention and treatment of *Pneumocystis* pneumonia, *N Engl J Med* 327:1853, 1992.

Meduri GU, Stein DS: Pulmonary manifestations of acquired immunodeficiency syndrome, *Clin Infect Dis* 14:98, 1992.

Odom RB, Berger TG: *The cutaneous manifestations of AIDS: current concepts,* Kalamazoo, 1990, Upjohn.

Penneys NS: *Skin manifestations of AIDS,* Philadelphia, 1990, JB Lippincott.

Reveille JD, Conant MA, Duvic M: Human immunodeficiency virus-associated psoriasis, psoriatic arthritis, and Reiter's syndrome: a disease continuum? *Arthritis Rheum* 33:1574, 1990.

Sande MA, Volberding PA: *The medical management of AIDS,* ed 3, Philadelphia, 1992, WB Saunders.

Smith PD et al: Gastrointestinal infections in AIDS, *Ann Intern Med* 116(1):63, 1992.

Tappero JW, et al: Kaposi's sarcoma, *J Am Acad Dermatol* 28:371, 1993.

Wormser GP, editor: *AIDS and other manifestations of HIV infection,* ed 2, New York, 1992, Raven Press.

# VIII Musculoskeletal

CHAPTER

## 69 Diagnostic Imaging of Rheumatologic Disorders

**James M. Coumas**
**Brian A. Howard**
**Eric W. Jacobson**

The diagnosis of immune-mediated disease cannot always be made by clinical features alone. Rheumatologic laboratory tests are helpful in establishing the presence of immune-mediated illness and possibly the specific subset of disease. Tests in rheumatology, however, are generally nonspecific and nondiagnostic. Laboratory results must be interpreted in the context of the particular clinical situation. Ordering a routine "battery" of rheumatologic screening tests is neither cost effective nor clinically warranted. Rather, tests should be ordered selectively based on the patient's clinical presentation.

One of the most helpful rheumatologic diagnostic procedures is joint aspiration (arthrocentesis). *Arthrocentesis* is performed for both diagnostic and therapeutic purposes. In general, patients presenting with acute monoarthritis require joint aspiration to ascertain whether the joint is infected. In addition, synovial fluid analysis is an important component of the evaluation of any arthritis of unknown cause. Arthrocentesis also is used for joint injection. Long-acting corticosteroid preparations can be injected directly into joints to relieve arthritic symptoms.

Radiologic studies are another important part of the rheumatologic evaluation. Routine radiographs help distinguish inflammatory from noninflammatory causes of arthritis. Certain radiographic features assist in differentiating various arthritides.

This chapter describes common studies to assist in the evaluation of patients with rheumatic disease. Selective test ordering is emphasized as well as the interpretation of test results.

## RHEUMATOLOGIC LABORATORY TESTS

### Acute phase response

The acute phase response refers to the change in systemic and metabolic factors that occurs in response to inflammatory stimuli such as infection or tissue injury. The most dramatic aspect of the acute phase response is a rapid change in the concentration of certain plasma proteins produced primarily in the liver including increased production of fibrinogen, haptoglobin, C-reactive protein, and serum amyloid A. The erythrocyte sedimentation rate (ESR) and C-reactive protein (CRP) are the two tests used most commonly to assess for the presence of an acute phase response.

***Erythrocyte sedimentation rate.*** Erythrocyte sedimentation depends on the ability of red blood cells to aggregate and form linear clumps (rouleaux). When large amounts of acute phase proteins such as fibrinogen are produced, binding of these proteins to erythrocytes neutralizes the negatively charged, repulsive electrostatic forces and allows the erythrocytes to aggregate and thus sediment more quickly. This forms the basis of the ESR. The more rapidly the red blood cells sediment, the higher the ESR. The normal range for the Westergren method is usually less than 20mm/hour. This range may vary among laboratories.

The ESR tends to be higher in women than in men, probably because of androgens in men, which may lower the ESR. ESRs increase steadily with age, presumably due to increased levels of fibrinogen. They also can be increased in the presence of certain medications such as oral contraceptives and heparin.

The ESR may be falsely lowered by any condition that interferes with the ability of red blood cells to aggregate (see the box on p. 963), including diseases in which (1) erythrocyte shape is abnormal, thus interfering with rouleaux formation (sickle cell disease, hereditary spherocytosis, anisocytosis); (2) hepatic dysfunction is present, which impairs production of acute phase proteins; and (3) fibrinogen is consumed (such as disseminated intravascular coagulation). Drugs such as corticosteroid preparations and high-dose antiinflammatory agents may lower the ESR. Congestive heart failure and diseases associated with an extreme elevation of the white blood cell count (such as chronic lymphocytic leukemia) also may be associated with low ESRs.

The ESR is a nonspecific test; it can be elevated in many conditions associated with inflammation and/or tissue necrosis. The disease states most commonly associated with dramatically elevated (more than 100 mm/hour by Westergren technique) ESRs are malignancy (10%), collagen vascular disease (25%), and infection (50% to 60%). A thorough history, physical examination, and routine laboratory screens usually suggest the correct diagnosis.

***C-reactive protein.*** CRP is one of the acute phase proteins. The properties of CRP include the ability to bind to phosphocholine, to activate the complement cascade, and to interact with polymorphonuclear leukocytes. It tends to rise and fall quickly in response to acute phase stimulation.

The CRP and ESR do not always correlate. CRP is a direct measure of one particular acute phase protein, whereas the ESR reflects multiple processes. The CRP concentration rises and falls rapidly only in response to inflammation or necrosis. Therefore it accurately reflects *acute* changes in clinical status. The ESR tends to rise more slowly and remain elevated for prolonged periods in response to acute phase stimulation. Thus the level of CRP may be more indicative of a patient's clinical status at a single point in time as compared to the ESR.

CRP, like ESR, can be used clinically to assess for underlying inflammation or necrosis. It can also be used to follow the course of a disease and response to treatment. In chronic inflammatory states, CRP levels rarely exceed 6 to 8 mg/dl. Levels greater than this should suggest

### Conditions that falsely lower the erythrocyte sedimentation rate

Abnormal red blood cell shape
- Sickle cell disease
- Hereditary spherocytosis
- Anisocytosis

Hepatic dysfunction

Hypofibrinogenemia
- Hereditary
- Fibrinogen consumption-disseminated intravascular coagulation

Medications
- Corticosteroids
- High-dose antiinflammatory agents

Congestive heart failure

Extreme elevations of white blood cells
- Chronic lymphocytic leukemia

superimposed infection. Interestingly, CRP levels are frequently normal in active systemic lupus erythematosus (SLE). Therefore when CRP levels are elevated, a search for infection should be considered.

## Rheumatoid factor

Rheumatoid factor (RF) is an antibody directed against the Fc portion of human IgG. The classic RF is an IgM antibody; however, all immunoglobulin classes of RF have been described. Only IgM RF is assayed routinely.

Several methods can be used to detect IgM RF. The most common are the latex fixation agglutination assay (LF) and the sensitized sheep red blood cell agglutination assay (SSCA). The LF and SSCA are considered to be positive at a dilution equal to or greater than 1:20.

The importance of RF lies in its incidence and distribution in disease, its association with the course and severity of rheumatoid arthritis (RA), and in its possible pathogenic role in RA. RF is positive in approximately 80% of patients with RA; however, it is nonspecific and is also present in many other diseases (connective tissue diseases, chronic inflammatory diseases, certain malignancies) as well as in up to 5% of the normal population, especially the elderly (see the box above right). It is often present in high titers in mixed essential cryoglobulinemia.

The probability that a patient has RA increases in direct proportion to the titer of RF. Additionally, in patients with RA, high titers of RF correlate with more severe and active joint disease, as well as the presence of rheumatoid nodules, systemic complications, and a poorer prognosis. Titers, however, are not typically helpful in following the course of the disease over time.

It is unclear exactly what role RF plays in the pathogenesis of RA. Possible pathophysiologic roles for RF include (1) enhanced clearance of immune complexes; (2) increased complement fixation; (3) enhanced inflammatory response; and (4) antiviral properties.

The physician should order an RF test when considering a diagnosis of RA. The result must be interpreted in the context of the clinical presentation. A positive result supports the diagnosis of RA if the clinical features are consistent.

### Diseases in which rheumatoid factor is commonly present

**Rheumatic diseases**

Rheumatoid arthritis
Sjögren's syndrome
Systemic lupus erythematosus
Polymyositis/dermatomyositis
Mixed connective tissue disease
Scleroderma

**Infectious diseases**

Subacute bacterial endocarditis
Tuberculosis
Infectious mononucleosis
Hepatitis
Syphilis
Leprosy
Influenza

**Malignancies**

Lymphoma
Multiple myeloma
Waldenstrom's macroglobulinemia
Postradiation or postchemotherapy

**Miscellaneous**

Normal adults, especially the elderly
Sarcoidosis
Chronic pulmonary disease (interstitial fibrosis)
Chronic liver disease (chronic active hepatitis, cirrhosis)
Mixed essential cryoglobulinemia
Hypergammaglobulinemic purpura

## Antinuclear antibodies

Antibodies to various nuclear (or cytoplasmic) antigens are found in the serum of many patients with systemic rheumatic diseases. A search for antinuclear antibodies (ANAs) may be appropriate as a screen for autoimmune disease if the clinical situation suggests that the patient has an autoimmune illness. ANAs cannot only support a diagnosis of autoimmune disease, but also sometimes define a specific subset of disease based on staining patterns and further identification of the specific target antigen.

ANAs are detected by an indirect immunofluorescent assay. Many different tissues or cell lines may be used as a substrate for this assay. If ANAs are present, the pattern and intensity of nuclear staining are documented. ANAs of all immunoglobulin classes will be detected, but IgM and IgA antibodies are detected with less sensitivity than IgG. False-positive tests are common with serum dilutions of less than 1:20; positivity at lower titers is considered a negative result.

ANAs are positive in over 95% of patients with SLE. They are thus an excellent screening test for this disease; however, they are present in many other disease states and therefore are a nonspecific test. ANAs are present in other autoimmune diseases, chronic infections, certain neoplasms, chronic liver disease, pulmonary fibrosis, hypergammaglobulinemia of any cause, multiple sclerosis, as

**Table 69-1.** Drug-induced ANAs: commonly implicated agents

| Category | Drug |
|---|---|
| Cardiovascular/antihypertensives | Procainamide<br>Quinidine<br>β-blockers<br>Hydralazine<br>Methyldopa<br>Captopril |
| Antimicrobial | Isoniazid<br>Sulfonamides<br>Nitrofurantoin |
| Anticonvulsants | Phenytoin<br>Ethosuximide<br>Trimethadione |
| Psychotropics | Chlorpromazine<br>Lithium carbonate |
| Antithyroid | Propylthiouracil<br>Methylthiouracil |
| Miscellaneous | D-penicillamine<br>Oral contraceptives<br>Sulfasalazine |

well as in other illnesses. ANAs can be produced transiently following viral illnesses or burns. They also can be induced by certain drugs, with or without associated clinical symptoms (Table 69-1). Procainamide is the medication most commonly associated with the presence of ANAs; up to 80% of patients taking this medication exhibit ANA. Only about 20% of these patients, however, experience a lupus-like illness. ANAs also are commonly seen in normal people; the incidence increases steadily with age.

Four main staining patterns are observed with ANAs. The type of pattern gives a clue to the etiology of the ANA. One pattern is homogeneous (or diffuse), in which the entire nucleus is fluorescent. It is produced by antibodies to deoxyribonucleoprotein (or the DNA-histone complex). It is nonspecific. In another pattern, termed speckled, the nucleus appears spotted. The speckled pattern occurs with antibodies directed against the extractable nuclear antigens (ENAs), which include Smith (Sm), ribonucleoprotein (RNP), Ro (formerly SS-A), and La (formerly SS-B). Sm is highly specific for SLE but found in only 20% to 30% of cases. RNP is nonspecific but found in high titer in mixed connective tissue disease. Ro and La are strongly associated with Sjögren's syndrome but also are nonspecific. A third pattern is rim or peripheral, a pattern produced by antibodies directed against double-stranded (native) DNA, which is specific for SLE. The outer rim of the nucleus is stained. In the last pattern, nucleolar, the nucleoli are stained. This pattern is most commonly seen in scleroderma (Table 69-2).

The physician should order an ANA when considering the possibility of a connective tissue disease. As with other rheumatologic tests, the result must be interpreted in the context of the particular clinical situation. Typically, the higher the titer, the more significant the finding of a positive ANA. Rim or nucleolar patterns are more specific, and their presence should strongly suggest a diagnosis of SLE or scleroderma, respectively. Speckled and homogeneous patterns are less specific. A positive speckled result can be further evaluated by ordering an ENA panel. Anti–double-stranded DNA and complement levels can provide additional important information when pursuing a workup of a positive ANA.

**Table 69-2.** Common staining patterns of ANAs

| Pattern | Antigen | Disease association |
|---|---|---|
| Homogeneous (diffuse) | Deoxyribonucleoprotein | Nonspecific |
| Speckled | Extractable nuclear antigens (Smith, RNP, Ro, La) among others | Nonspecific |
| Rim (peripheral) | Double-stranded (native) DNA | SLE |
| Nucleolar | Nucleoli | Scleroderma |

### Anti–double-stranded DNA

Anti–double-stranded DNA (aDNA) is found almost exclusively in non–drug-induced SLE. Antibody titers often correlate with clinical disease activity, although changes may precede relapse or remission by several months. The presence of aDNA also correlates with the development of lupus nephritis, in which it probably plays a direct pathogenic role.

### Complement

The complement system comprises a group of distinct glycoproteins involved in the clearance of immune complexes and microorganisms from the circulation, as well as promotion of the inflammatory response. The measurement of complement factors and function identifies the presence of complement-consuming diseases and hereditary complement deficiencies.

A screening test for complement levels is the quantitative $CH_{50}$ photometric assay. The dilution of the patient's serum that will induce 50% lysis of antibody-coated sheep red blood cells is measured. For suspected complement deficiency, $CH_{50}$ will be low. $C_3$ and $C_4$ may be measured directly if specific quantitation is desired.

Complement glycoproteins are acute phase reactants; *elevated* levels may be present in several conditions including many inflammatory diseases. Elevations also have been noted in certain noninflammatory diseases such as diabetes mellitus, obstructive jaundice, and in acute myocardial infarction.

*Decreased* levels of complement factors can result from (1) decreased production; (2) in vivo activation and consumption of complement factors; or (3) in vitro consumption occurring in the test tube (postphlebotomy). The first mechanism is seen in hereditary factor deficiencies and severe liver disease. The second mechanism occurs with classic immune-complex deposition, as well as with other infectious and inflammatory conditions. In vitro activation can be the result of poor specimen handling or the presence of complement activators in the serum. Inflammatory diseases result in normal complement levels when increased production equals in vivo consumption.

Complement levels are measured to assess for immune complex-mediated diseases such as active SLE and vasculitis. When immune complexes are produced, the classic pathway is activated. As complement is consumed, levels decline. Other disease states in which complement levels may be low due to consumption include serum sickness, chronic active hepatitis, subacute bacterial endocarditis, glomerulonephritis, malaria, and mixed essential cryoglobulinemia. In SLE and vasculitis, complement levels may correlate with disease activity. Patients with inherited complement deficiencies also have low levels of complement. Some complement deficiencies (such as $C_4$ deficiency) have been associated with autoimmune diseases, possibly due to the inability to clear immune complexes from the circulation. Deficiencies of factors $C_5$ through $C_9$ predispose to recurrent infections with encapsulated microorganisms (such as *Neisseria* species), presumably due to reduced ability to lyse these organisms.

### Antiphospholipid antibodies

Antibodies to phospholipids are a heterogeneous group of "autoantibodies" that have been associated with thrombotic events. Some of the more common antigens to which these antibodies are produced include cardiolipin, phosphatidylserine, and phosphatidic acid. They are uniformly present in the primary antiphospholipid syndrome, which is characterized by venous and arterial thrombosis, recurrent fetal loss (typically in the second or third trimesters), thrombocytopenia, and Coombs'-positive hemolytic anemia. These antibodies are seen frequently in SLE (20% to 30%) and may be identified in association with use of certain drugs, as well as in other chronic inflammatory and infectious diseases.

Multiple laboratory assays may detect antiphospholipid antibodies. Presence of these antibodies may be indicated by a false-positive Venereal Disease Research Laboratory (VDRL) or prolongation of clotting time as measured by the partial thromboplastin time (PTT) or Russell's viper venom time (RVVT). Antiphospholipid antibodies bind to the prothrombin activation complex (which consists of activated factor X [Xa], factor V, factor II [prothrombin], ionized calcium, and a phospholipid template) and thereby delay the conversion of prothrombin to thrombin. Prolongation of in vitro clotting times is a paradox because the presence of these antibodies predisposes to thrombosis in vivo. Antiphospholipid antibodies also may be detected by an enzyme-linked immunosorbent assay (ELISA), which identifies the specific subclass of immunoglobulin present (IgG, IgA, or IgM). Most pathogenic antiphospholipid antibodies are of the IgG variety.

The clinician should consider screening for the presence of antiphospholipid antibodies when a patient presents with recurrent arterial or venous thrombi, emboli, and/or recurrent second- or third-trimester miscarriages. Screening may be especially important in younger patients presenting with myocardial infarction or cerebrovascular accident in the absence of classic risk factors.

### Antineutrophil cytoplasmic antibodies

Antineutrophil cytoplasmic antibodies (ANCAs) are directed against cytoplasmic antigens (lysosomal enzymes) of neutrophils. ANCAs may be detected using immunofluorescent techniques similar to those used to detect ANAs. Two different granular immunofluorescent patterns are commonly described: one in which the staining is in granules in the *peri*nuclear region of the neutrophil (P-ANCA) and one in which a granular staining is seen more diffusely throughout the *cytoplasm* (C-ANCA). ANCAs are used to screen for the presence of vasculitis. C-ANCAs are strongly associated with Wegener's granulomatosis. P-ANCAs are less specific, but have been described in patients with systemic necrotizing vasculitis associated with glomerulonephritis (such as polyarteritis nodosa [PAN]) and with idiopathic crescentic glomerulonephritis.

### Lyme antibodies

See Infectious Arthritis in Chapter 87.

### HLA-B27

See Chapters 79 and 83.

## ARTHROCENTESIS

Arthrocentesis is a safe and relatively simple procedure in which a needle is introduced into the joint space to remove synovial fluid. It is an essential part of the evaluation of any arthritis of unknown cause and is required to diagnose an infection in the joint. Arthrocentesis also can be used therapeutically, either to fully drain an inflamed joint or to introduce long-acting corticosteroids into the joint.

Joint aspiration requires sound knowledge of the joint anatomy, including the bony and soft tissue landmarks used for joint entry. Strict aseptic technique is crucial to minimize the risk of infection. The physician must practice universal precautions. The procedure is accomplished more easily when the patient is able to relax the muscles surrounding the joint.

Absolute contraindications to performing arthrocentesis include local infection of the overlying skin and severe coagulopathy. If coagulopathy is present and if septic arthritis is suspected, every effort should be made to correct the coagulopathy (with fresh-frozen plasma [FFP] or alternate factors) before joint aspiration. Therapeutic anticoagulation is not an absolute contraindication, though every effort should be made to avoid excessive trauma during the aspiration.

The major complications of arthrocentesis include iatrogenically induced infection and bleeding. Both are extremely rare. The risk of infection after arthrocentesis is less than 1 in 10,000. Correction of prominent coagulopathy before arthrocentesis reduces the risk of excessive hemorrhage.

The knee is one of the most accessible joints for aspiration. Initially, the physician should describe the procedure to the patient, including risks of complications. The entry site should be cleaned with an iodine-based antiseptic solution. After the area dries, it should be wiped once with alcohol. Local anesthesia (subcutaneous lidocaine or topical ethyl chloride) may be applied. With the patient supine and the knee fully extended, the knee joint is entered medially, under the patella (Fig. 69-1). The joint should be fully drained if possible. The needle is then removed and pressure is applied to the site until bleeding has stopped. Finally, the area is cleaned with alcohol and a bandage applied. Other joints that a primary care

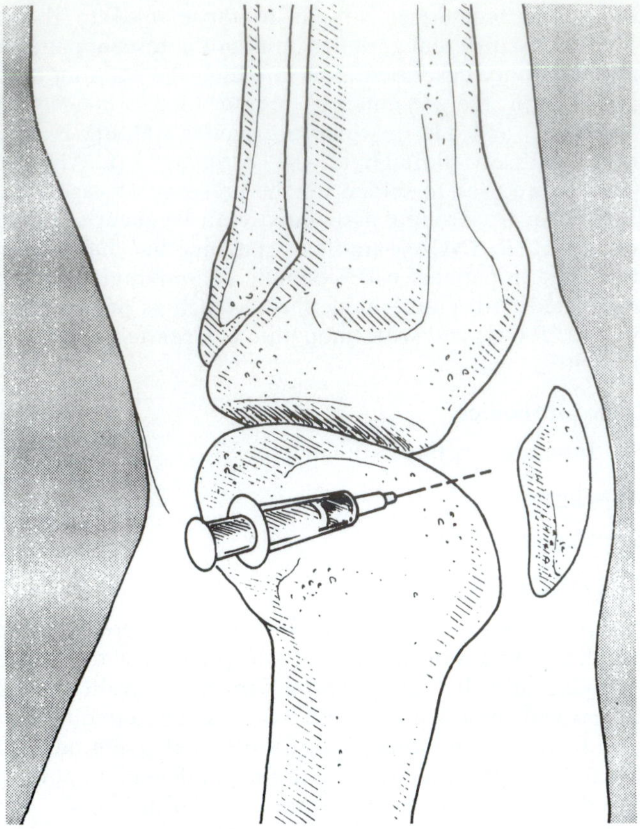

**Fig. 69-1.** Technique for arthrocentesis of the knee: medial approach.

## Common causes of inflammatory arthritis

Rheumatoid arthritis
Spondyloarthropathies
 Psoriatic arthritis
 Reiter's syndrome/reactive arthritis
 Ankylosing spondylitis
 Ulcerative colitis/regional enteritis
Crystal-induced arthritis
 Monosodium urate (gout)
 Calcium pyrophosphate dihydrate (CPPD - "pseudogout")
 Hydroxyapatite
Infectious arthritis
 Bacterial
 Mycobacterial
 Fungal
Connective tissue diseases
 SLE
 Vasculitis
 Scleroderma
 Polymyositis
Hypersensitivity
 Serum sickness

physician may consider aspirating include shoulder, elbow, and ankle (Figs. 69-2 through 69-4).

Once fluid is obtained, synovial fluid analysis is performed to distinguish noninflammatory from inflammatory fluid. Less than 2000 white blood cells (WBC)/mm$^3$ is consistent with noninflammatory fluid (as is seen in osteoarthritis). Greater than 2000 WBC/mm$^3$ indicates inflammatory fluid (see the box above for causes of inflammatory arthritis). In addition to absolute nucleated cell count, synovial fluid is divided into various categories based on the gross appearance, viscosity, WBC differential, and culture results (Table 69-3).

Synovial fluid analysis begins with bedside observation of the fluid. Normal synovial fluid is colorless. Both noninflammatory and mildly inflammatory fluid appear yellow or straw-colored. Septic effusions frequently appear purulent and whitish in color. Hemorrhagic effusions appear red or brown. The clarity of synovial fluids depends on the number and types of cells or particles present. To test clarity, a glass tube filled with synovial fluid is placed in front of black print on a white background. If the print is easily read, the fluid is transparent, indicating normal and noninflammatory fluid. If the print is distinguishable from the background but is not clear, the fluid is translucent, indicating inflammatory effusions. Grossly inflammatory, septic, and hemorrhagic fluids are opaque, preventing any visualization through the tube.

Synovial fluid viscosity, the result of hyaluronic acid content, also can be assessed at the bedside. Degradative enzymes such as hyaluronidase released from inflammatory cells produce a thinner, less viscous fluid. Viscosity can be assessed using the "string sign" while adhering to universal precautions. A drop of fluid is allowed to fall from the end of the needle or syringe, and an estimate is made of the length of the continuous "string" that forms.

**Table 69-3.** Joint fluid characteristics

| | Normal | Group I (noninflammatory) | Group II (inflammatory) | Group III (septic) |
|---|---|---|---|---|
| Color | Clear | Yellow | Yellow or opalescent | Variable, may be purulent |
| Clarity | Transparent | Transparent | Translucent | Opaque |
| Viscosity | Very high | High | Low | Typically low |
| WBC/mm$^3$ | 200 | 200-2000 | 2000-100,000 | >50,000, usually >100,000 |
| PMN (%) | <25 | <25 | >50 | >75 |
| Culture | Negative | Negative | Negative | Usually positive |

*PMN,* Polymorphonuclear leukocytes.

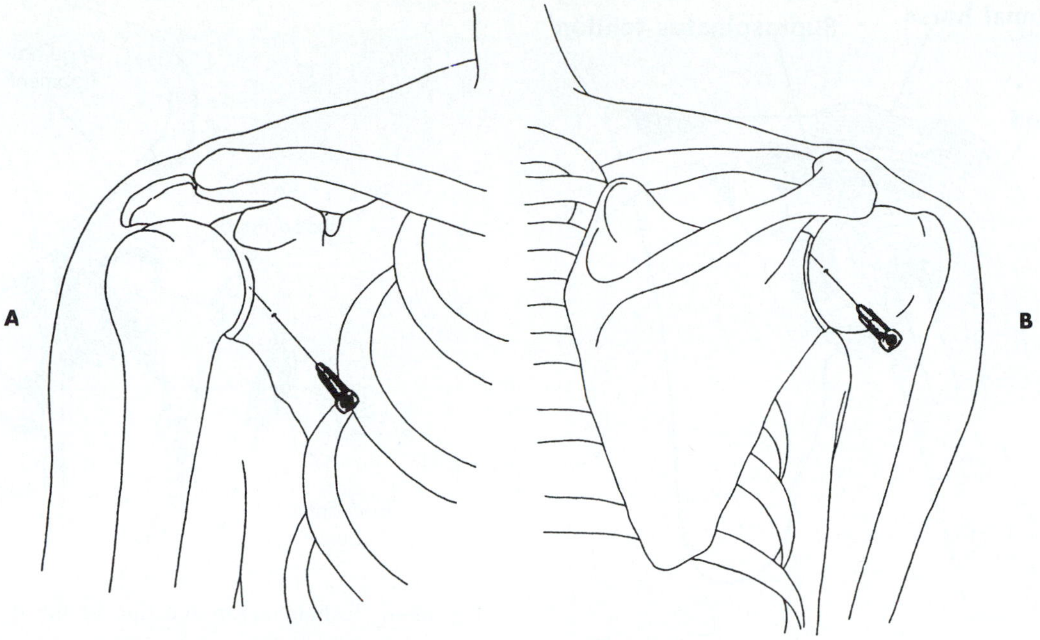


**Fig. 69-2.** Technique for arthrocentesis of the shoulder: anterior and posterior approach.

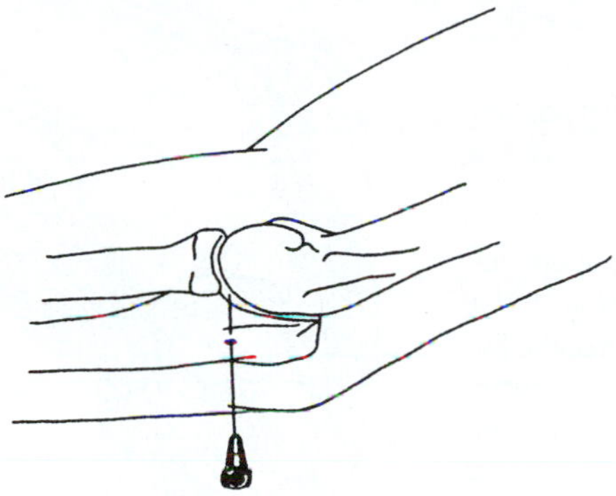

**Fig. 69-3.** Technique for arthrocentesis of the elbow.

Normal fluid typically forms at least a 6 cm continuous "string." Inflammatory fluid will not form a "string." Instead it drops like water dripping from a faucet.

After bedside assessment, the synovial fluid is sent to the laboratory for a cell count and differential, crystal analysis, Gram stain, and culture. Cell counts approaching 100,000 WBC/$mm^3$ suggest septic arthritis and/or a crystal-induced arthritis. Normally, synovial fluid has a predominance of lymphocytes. The percentage of polymorphonuclear leukocytes present increases with inflammatory conditions. In most circumstances, an infected joint has synovial fluid with more than 75% polymorphonuclear cells (see Table 69-3).

All fluid should be assessed for the presence of crystals, specifically monosodium urate and calcium pyrophosphate dihydrate, using a compensated polarized light microscope (see Chapter 82). If the fluid cannot be examined immediately, refrigeration of the fluid helps preserve the crystals.

A Gram stain and culture should be performed on most synovial fluid specimens. Cultures for aerobic and anaerobic bacterial organisms are performed routinely. In certain circumstances, (for example, in *chronic* monoarticular arthritis), fluid may be cultured for the presence of mycobacteria and fungi. If disseminated gonorrhea is suspected, fluid should be plated directly onto chocolate agar or Thayer-Martin media. A positive culture confirms septic arthritis. Other studies on synovial fluid (glucose, protein, complement) usually are not helpful.

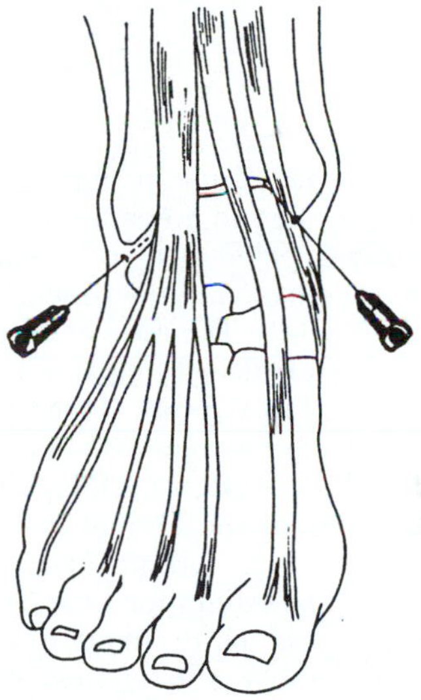

**Fig. 69-4.** Technique for arthrocentesis of the ankle: medial and lateral approach.

Arthrocentesis also is used therapeutically. In septic arthritis, serial joint aspirations are required to remove accumulated inflammatory or purulent fluid. This allows serial monitoring of the total WBC count, Gram stain, and culture to assess response to treatment and provides complete drainage of a "closed space." Inflammatory fluid contains many destructive enzymes that contribute to cartilage and bony degradation. Removal of the fluid may slow this destructive process.

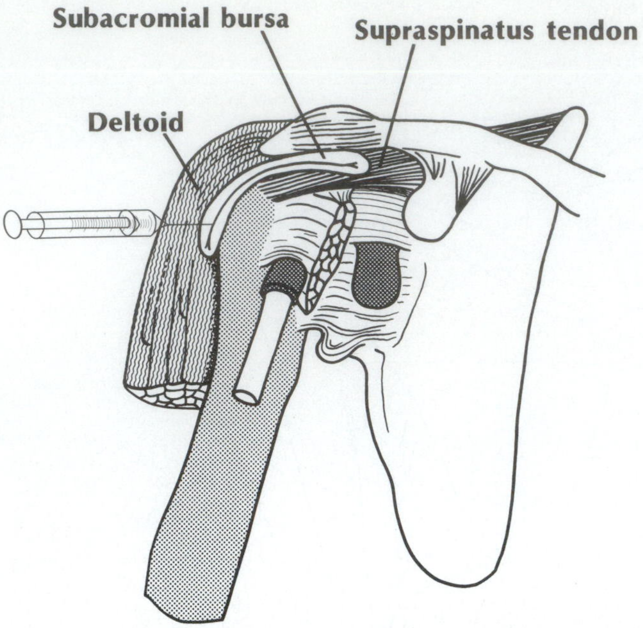


Fig. 69-5. Technique for injection of the subacromial bursa.

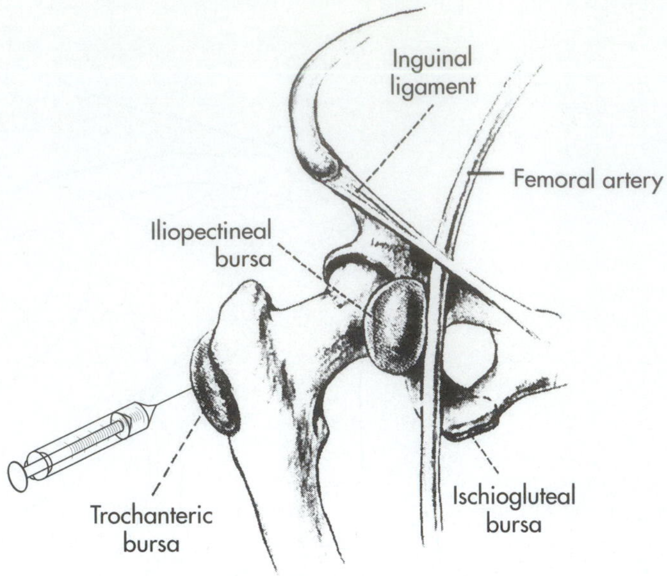


Fig. 69-6. Technique for injection of the trochanteric bursa.

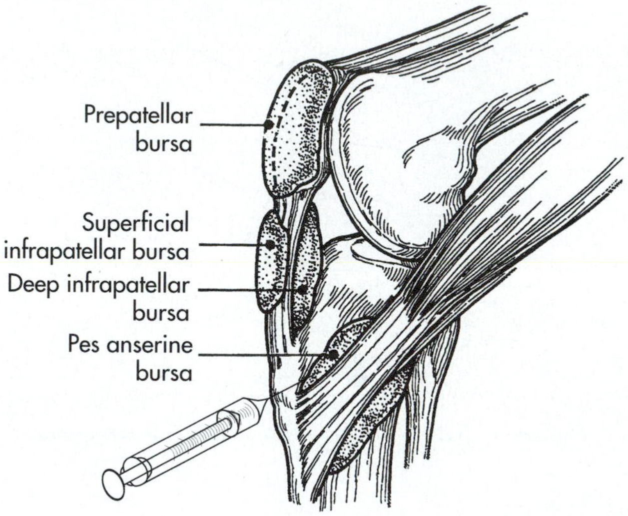


Fig. 69-7. Technique for injection of the anserine bursa.

Arthrocentesis is necessary for intraarticular injection of long-acting corticosteroid preparations. Corticosteroids also are frequently injected into soft tissue sites such as bursae, tendon sheaths, and myofascial trigger points (Figs. 69-5 through 69-7). The dose of corticosteroid used depends on the size of the particular joint or soft tissue site being injected (Table 69-4). Three commonly used corticosteroid preparations are triamcinolone diacetate (e.g., Aristocort Forte, Amcort), methylprednisolone acetate (e.g., Depo-Medrol and Medralone), and triamcinolone hexacetonide (e.g., Aristospan). Triamcinolone hexacetonide has a longer duration of action than the other two preparations. It is more likely to produce tissue atrophy or tendon injury and is thus mainly used for intraarticular injections. A local anesthetic such as lidocaine is frequently mixed with the corticosteroid before injection.

In addition to infection and bleeding, other complications must be considered with injection of a corticosteroid. Lipoatrophy and skin discoloration can occur with any of the steroid preparations, especially when injecting superficial soft tissue areas. Tendon rupture also can occur when injecting tendon sheaths, possibly due to a weakening effect caused by the corticosteroid. A brief postinjection "flare" has been described in up to 1% to 2% of intraarticular injections. This complication generally occurs within the first few hours after the injection. If marked inflammatory symptoms persist for more than 24 hours, the joint or soft tissue region requires reaspiration to rule out infection. Finally, some systemic absorption of the corticosteroid does occur, which may be associated with a transient increase in blood glucose in patients with diabetes.

Repeated injections with corticosteroid preparations into the same joint (or soft tissue region) may accelerate connective tissue degradation. As a rule, an interval of at least 3 to 4 months should be allowed before reinjecting an individual site. If a single site is injected on a regular basis for more than 1 year, an alternate treatment approach should be considered.

## RADIOLOGIC EVALUATION

This section focuses on the radiologic appearance and evaluation of the more common rheumatologic arthropathies. Common applications of alternate imaging modalities with their individual strengths and limitations are included. Despite a diagnostic armamentarium that includes plain film tomography, computed tomography (CT), ultrasound, magnetic resonance imaging (MRI), and nuclear scintigraphy, plain radiographs are still the most cost-effective approach to the diagnosis, evaluation, and

**Table 69-4.** Dose of corticosteroid preparation used in injections

| | Triamcinolone diacetate (Aristocort Forte, Amcort) | Methylprednisolone acetate (Depo-Medrol, Medralone) | Triamcinolone Hexacetonide (Aristospan) |
|---|---|---|---|
| Joint | | 2.5-10 mg | 2-5 mg |
| Small joint of hand/foot | | | |
| Wrist/elbow | | 10-30 mg | 10 mg |
| Knee/ankle/shoulder | | 20-40 mg | 20-40 mg |
| Bursae | 20-40 mg | 20-60 mg | |
| Trigger points | 5-10 mg | | |
| Epicondyles | 5-10 mg | | |

assessment of therapeutic management of inflammatory arthropathies. It is essential that the clinician appreciate the supportive role that roentgenograms and laboratory studies play in evaluating arthritis. They are not intended to supplant a careful history and physical examinations.

Plain film radiographs should provide a survey of the symptomatic region of interest and adjacent articulations. A wide range of valuable information is provided to the clinician and most easily extrapolated from the radiograph if an orderly and sequential approach to plain film interpretation is used. The most common approach involves evaluation of "A"lignment, "B"ony mineralization, joint space or "C"artilage thickness and adjacent "S"oft tissues sequentially, and as such is referred to as the "A B Cs" of radiographic evaluation.

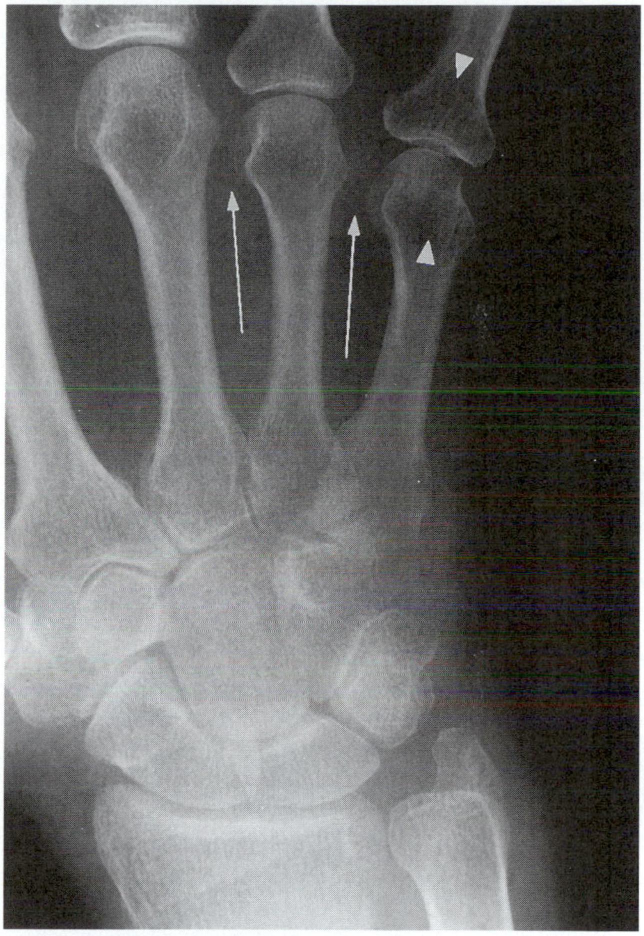

**Fig. 69-8.** Rheumatoid arthritis. Early changes may be confined to juxtaarticular osteopenia *(arrowhead),* periarticular soft tissue swelling *(arrow),* and loss of normal fat fascial planes (i.e., navicular fat stripe) and superficial fat fascial border along ulna styloid.

## Rheumatoid arthritis

Rheumatoid arthritis is a disorder of the synovial lined joints, cartilaginous articulations, bursa, tendon sheaths, and ligamentous and tendinous attachments to bone in addition to abnormalities of the adjacent soft tissues and bone (see Chapter 79). A symmetric polyarticular disease principally involving the appendicular skeleton is seen. Radiographs of the hands and wrists are obtained with posterior/anterior (PA) and Norgaard (semisupinated oblique) views. Common early findings include the following:

1. Soft tissue swelling or periarticular inflammation.
2. Juxtaarticular osteopenia in part attributable to hyperemia with indistinct cortical outline and loss or thinning of the trabecular bone pattern.
3. Symmetric joint space narrowing or cartilage thinning with a predilection for the metacarpophalangeal and proximal interphalangeal joints of the hand. Radiocarpal and midcarpal joint space narrowing is seen in the wrist.
4. Erosions that appear initially as subtle cystic changes are located at the margin of the capsular insertion and the cartilaginous articulation of the joint often referred to as the *bare area.* In the wrist erosion of the ulnar styloid process, distal radioulna articulation, radial styloid, and midscaphoid are common.

Late changes include the following:

1. Subluxation or frank dislocation seen principally at the metacarpophalangeal articulation and interphalangeal articulation of the hand. Subluxation of carpal bones culminate in dorsal or volar intercalated instabilities of the wrist or ulnar translocation. Swan-neck and boutonniere deformities of the digits also may be seen.
2. Progression of juxtaarticular osteoporosis to a generalized or diffuse osteopenia.
3. Ankylosis of the carpal bones.
4. Progression of small erosions to larger erosions.
5. Synovial cyst formation with extension of cyst into the soft tissues.
6. Soft tissue rheumatoid nodules.
7. Superimposed degenerative arthritis.

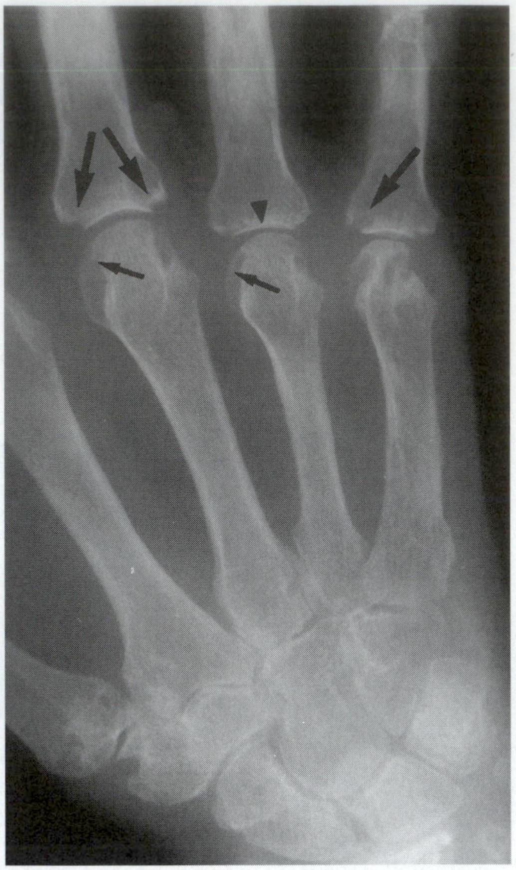

Fig. 69-9. Rheumatoid arthritis. Later changes include symmetric joint space narrowing *(arrowhead)*, loss of subchondral cortical margin *(small arrows)*, and marginal erosions *(large arrows)*.

Analogous changes to those in the hand (Figs. 69-8 and 69-9) occur in the feet in approximately 80% of patients. The knee and hip are the next most commonly involved articulation, with elbow and shoulder not infrequently involved. Principally an appendicular disorder, the axial skeleton shows changes most frequently involving the cervical spine. Approximately 60% to 70% of patients with rheumatoid arthritis develop symptoms related to the cervical spine (Fig. 69-10). Erosions and symmetric narrowing of the apophyseal joints of the cervical spine may culminate in a fibrous ankylosis. Subluxation or "staircasing" at multiple cervical levels is not uncommon. Atlantoaxial instability due to laxity or destruction of the transverse ligament also is seen.

A specific radiographic appearance of rheumatoid arthritis is seen in men with a high level of physical activity and termed *robust rheumatoid arthritis.* This condition is attributable to prominent subchondral cyst formation produced by high intraarticular pressure and intravasation of synovial fluid or granulation tissue through fissures in the articular cartilage with prominent subchondral cyst formation.

Nuclear scintigraphy has been used in the past to evaluate the "activity" of the inflammatory process and assess the success of therapeutic management. More recently, MRI has been used to evaluate the extent of synovial hypertrophy and pannus formation. Ultrasound is especially helpful in the evaluation of juxtaarticular soft tissue masses to exclude a solid mass versus a synovial cyst.

Although routine MRI usually is not necessary, common clinical applications for its use include the exclusion of superimposed infection, abscess formation with or without associated osteomyelitis, or primary neural compromise.

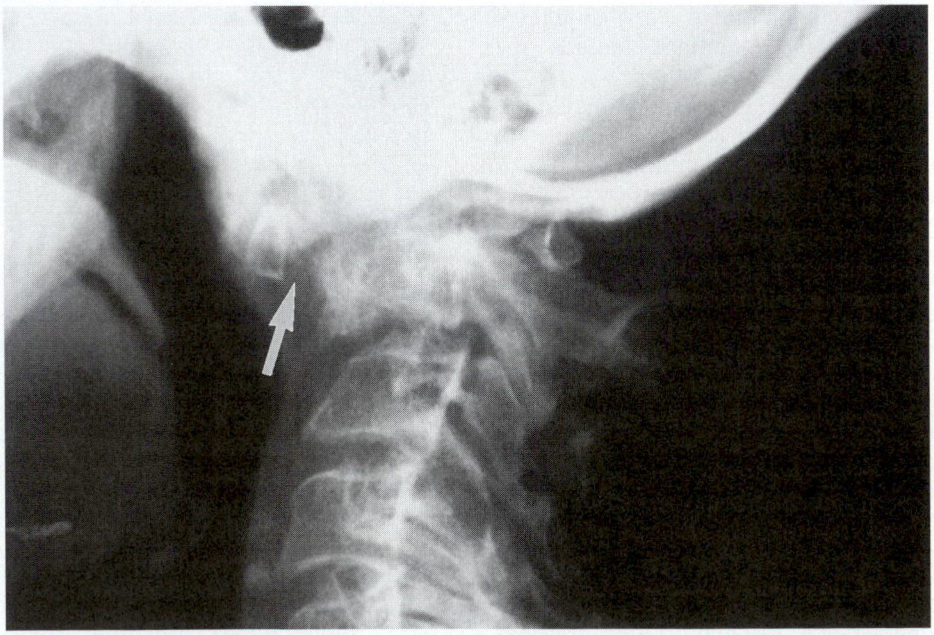

Fig. 69-10. Rheumatoid arthritis of the axial skeleton. Osteopenia, "staircasing" (multilevel subluxation) and erosion/subluxation at the atlantoaxial articulation are common, with widening of the atlanto-dens interval *(white arrow)*.

## Seronegative spondyloarthropathies

***Psoriatic arthritis.*** Psoriatic arthritis may present as a monoarticular or polyarticular disorder with predilection for interphalangeal joints of the hands and feet. (Psoriatic arthritis is presented in Chapter 83 and dermatitis in Chapter 21.) It is a disorder of synovial lined joints with involvement of cartilage, bone, ligamentous and tendinous attachments to bone, and perijuxtaarticular soft tissue changes. Although the frequency of articular disease increases in patients with progressive or severe psoriatic skin manifestations, articular changes may antedate the appearance of any skin disease.

Standard plain film radiographs of the hand and wrist or feet show characteristic radiographic features and distribution of involvement distinct from rheumatoid arthritis. Early hand findings include the following:

1. Normal plain film radiographs.
2. Periarticular or fusiform soft tissue swelling typically confined to a single interphalangeal joint without associated bony changes. This is commonly referred to as a *sausage digit.*
3. Maintenance of normal bone mineralization or subtle juxtaarticular osteopenia that resolves.
4. Asymmetric or unilateral distribution of involvement.

Later radiographic changes include the following:

1. Joint space narrowing involving the distal interphalangeal joint and interphalangeal joints.
2. Bone proliferation—typically adjacent sites of articular erosion or a fluffy irregular, poorly outlined proliferated change at capsular or ligamentous attachment—indicate inflammation at the tendoperiosteum or ligament-periosteum conjunction, which is called *enthesitis.*
3. Periosteal reaction, which presents as a periostitis of the diaphyseal shaft.
4. Tuftal resorption characterized by a loss of the normal sharp cortical outline of the distal tuft and subsequent tapering or "pencilling" of the tuft or digit.
5. Erosions are marginal but may extend subchondrally to produce central erosions or large asymmetric erosions with subsequent "widening of the joint."
6. Bony ankylosis of the joint typically seen in the digits.
7. Subluxation with possible telescoping of bone.

Although the distribution of disease is highly variable, areas of characteristic involvement in the hand and wrist would include the distal interphalangeal (DIP) and interphalangeal (IP) joints (Figs. 69-11 and 69-12). A high incidence of the first metacarpophalangeal joint involvement is noted. The frequency of wrist involvement usually follows that of the hand.

In the foot, forefoot changes parallel those of the hand with bilateral and asymmetric disease. A predilection for the interphalangeal joint of the first digit is noted. In the hindfoot, characteristic bony changes are seen at the retrocalcaneal bursa and proliferative changes at the attachment of the plantar aponeurosis to the calcaneus with associated periostitis of the plantar calcaneus (Fig. 69-13).

Involvement of the axial skeleton occurs with paravertebral ligamentous ossification and progressive nonmarginal osteophyte formation parallel to the disc space and seen principally in the thoracolumbar spine. Cervical spine changes show prominent anterior osteophyte formation with associated discal resorption and subchondral sclerosis.

Erosive changes and findings mimicking rheumatoid arthritis at the atlantoaxial articulation with possible atlantoaxial instability are seen.

Up to 50% of patients with psoriatic arthritis develop radiographic changes at the sacroiliac joints. Reactive sclerosis with associated erosive disease involving the iliac wing aspect of the sacroiliac joint is noted. Although erosive changes are typically confined to the synovial lined aspect of the joint, ligamentous mineralization can occur at the nonsynovial lined portion of the sacroiliac joint.

Differentiating psoriatic arthritis from rheumatoid arthritis on plain film radiographs usually is possible by the distribution of bony involvement. The presence of periostitis, bony ankylosis, tuftal resorption, and enthesitis, coupled with a lack of juxtaarticular demineralization, may be helpful in differentiating features characterizing psoriatic arthritis. Differentiating psoriatic arthritis from other seronegative spondyloarthropathies also may prove difficult.

As in rheumatoid arthritis, the use of alternate modalities is most common in cases of questionable soft tissue injury or infection. MRI excels in the assessment of the

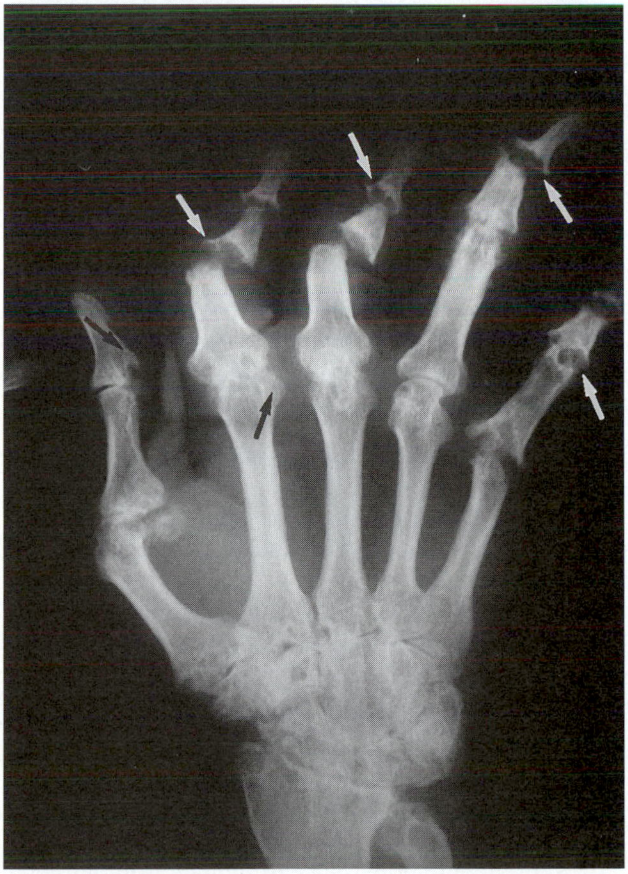

**Fig. 69-11.** Psoriatic arthritis. Erosions involving the distal interphalangeal joint and proximal interphalangeal joint *(white arrow)* with associated periosteal reaction and proliferative change *(small black arrow).* Note "pencil in thimble" configuration.

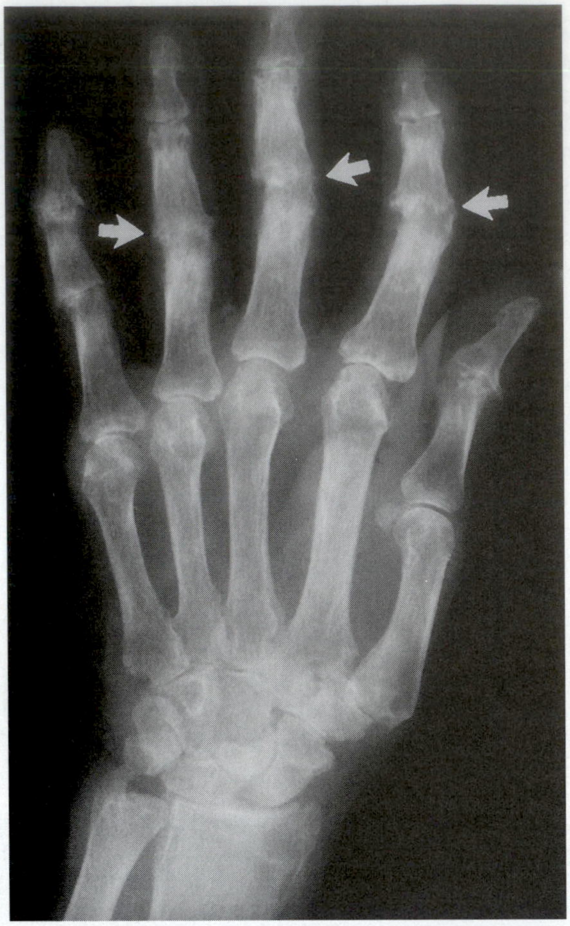

**Fig. 69-12.** Psoriatic arthritis. Bony ankylosis *(white arrow),* maintenance of bone mineralization and localization to target sites (distal interphalangeal and interphalangeal involvement) help differentiate this arthritis from rheumatoid arthritis.

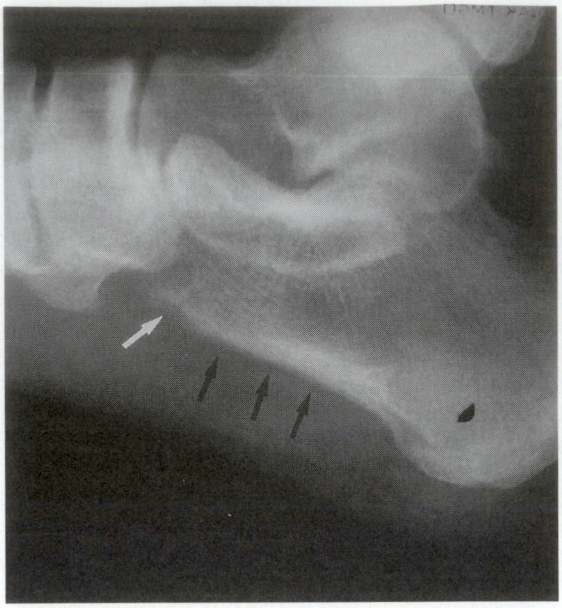

**Fig. 69-13.** Psoriatic arthritis. Periostitis along the plantar calcaneus *(black arrows)* and poorly delineated erosion *(small white arrow)* support the diagnosis.

soft tissue structures about the articulation and the exclusion of underlying abscess formation or associated osteomyelitis.

***Reiter's syndrome.*** Reiter's syndrome consists of the triad urethritis, conjunctivitis, and arthritides. The arthritic component of this seronegative spondyloarthropathy is evaluated with plain film radiographs (see Chapter 83). The joint disease is an asymmetric, monolateral or bilateral polyarticular disorder of synovial lined joints, cartilage, and tendon and ligamentous attachment sites, with a predilection for involvement of the feet (lower extremities).

Early radiographic changes in the metatarsal and interphalangeal joints of the forefoot are the following:

1. Periarticular or fusiform soft tissue swelling with early demineralization. An alternating soft tissue inflammatory process followed by resolution and subsequent normal-appearing plain film radiographs is not uncommon.
2. Symmetric joint space narrowing.
3. Periostitis with or without articular abnormality. The periostitis is often ill defined or "fluffy" in appearance.
4. Bone proliferation at ligamentous and tendinous attachments, which is most evident at the calcaneus, with fluffy poorly delineated mineralization at the plantar aponeurosis attachment and associated calcaneal spurring.
5. Bursal and/or tendon sheath inflammation. A particular predilection for the retrocalcaneal bursa is noted.
6. Erosions are marginal early in the disease process, but ultimately produce uniform joint space narrowing. Narrowing may appear asymmetric at varying intervals in the disease process.

Late radiologic findings include the following:

1. Uniform joint space loss at multiple articulations.
2. Bulky, well-defined periostitis.
3. Subluxation about the metatarsophalangeal joints referred to as a Launois deformity.

The disorder may involve the larger joints of the lower extremities such as the knee and ankle, but tend to spare the hip. Upper extremity involvement is less common and shows a predilection for the proximal interphalangeal joints of the hand. The sacroiliac joints show a bilateral asymmetric involvement confined to the true synovial lined portion of the joint, which parallels the findings of psoriatic arthritis. Changes in the axial skeleton also parallel those of psoriatic arthritis.

Differentiating Reiter's syndrome from the other seronegative spondyloarthropathies can be difficult. Reiter's arthritis typically shows less upper extremity involvement, axial skeleton involvement, and ankylosis than psoriatic arthritis or ankylosing spondylitis. Intraarticular bone production, adjacent sites of bone erosion, and poorly defined "fluffy" periostitis also are hallmarks of Reiter's arthritis (Figs. 69-14 and 69-15). The plantar and retrocalcaneal changes are highly characteristic of Reiter's syndrome. Minimal axial skeleton involvement is helpful

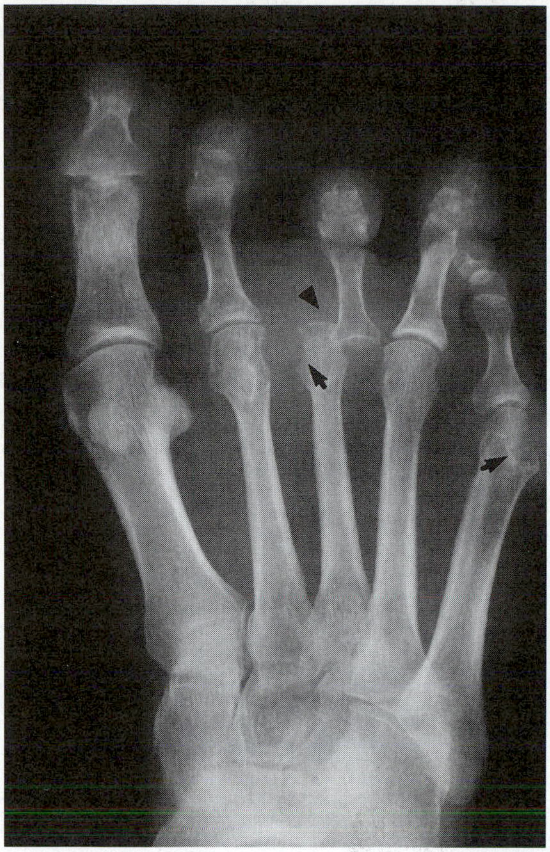

**Fig. 69-14.** Reiter's arthritis. Joint space narrowing, erosions *(black arrow)* and subluxation *(arrowhead)* make differentiating this disorder from other seronegative spondyloarthropathies difficult.

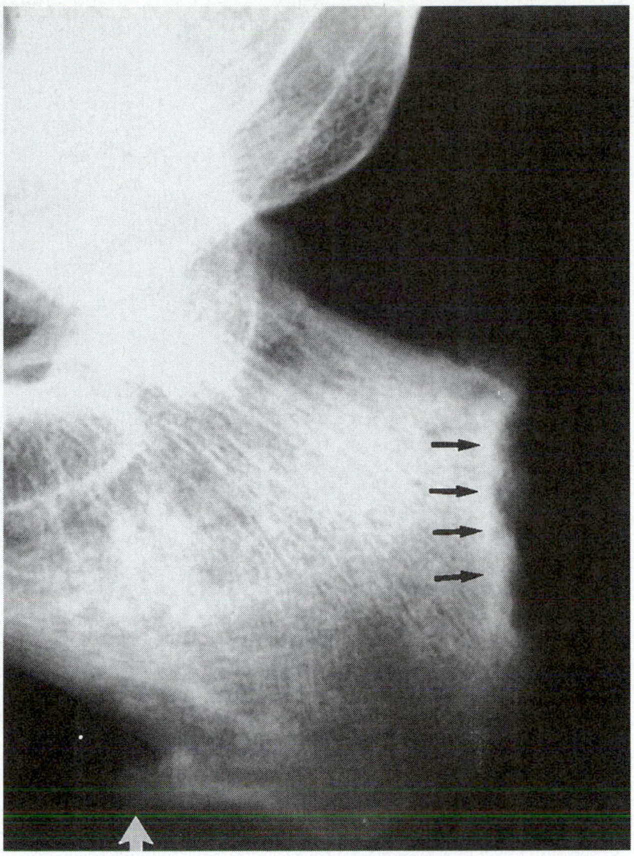

**Fig. 69-15.** Reiters arthritis. Retrocalcaneal bursitis with associated erosions *(black arrows)* and prominent plantar calcaneal spur *(white arrow)* with poor cortical delineation.

in differentiating Reiter's syndrome from ankylosing spondylitis.

Nuclear scintigraphy may help detect subtle proliferative and inflammatory changes, which may not be apparent on plain film radiographs. Early asymmetric, bilateral polyarticular involvement with changes involving both the hindfoot and forefoot are helpful in establishing the early diagnosis of Reiter's syndrome.

***Ankylosing spondylitis.*** Ankylosing spondylitis is an inflammatory joint disorder of the spine and limbs (see Chapter 83). The arthritis begins in the sacroiliac joints and presents radiographically with symmetric erosions and reactive sclerosis and subsequent fusions (Fig. 69-16). Radiologic diagnosis focuses on axial skeleton involvement with sacroiliac joint changes, proliferative enthesopathy, and joint fusions. Early spinal involvement in the thoracolumbar junction with squaring of the vertebral body contours is followed by continuous progression up and down the spine with the formation of symmetric syndesmophytes bridging the vertebral bodies with apophyseal joint ankylosis and ligamentous ossification (Fig. 69-17). End stage spinal changes have a bamboo appearance.

Radiographic findings of ankylosing spondylitis:

1. Bilateral symmetric apparent joint widening with loss of cortical definition of the iliac articular margin.
2. Erosions and reactive sclerosis of the articular surfaces, especially the lower third of the sacroiliac joint.
3. Narrowing and obliteration of the joint with similar changes at the symphysis pubis.
4. Inflammatory resorption of the annulus fibrosus insertion at the corners of the vertebral endplates resulting in the squaring of the vertebral body contours.
5. Bony proliferation at the vertebral corners, which forms delicate vertical bridges of bone that create marginal syndesmophytes best appreciated on oblique views. The continuous undulant contour has a bamboo appearance. Occasionally, destruction of the discovertebral joint occurs and simulates septic discitis.
6. Apophyseal and costovertebral joint ankylosis.
7. Inflammation and erosion at the craniocervical junction may be associated with transverse ligament insufficiency and instability.
8. Hips, heels, and shoulders may be affected with diffuse inflammatory narrowing, erosive destruction, and proliferative "wiskering" periostitis, respectively.
9. The ankylosed spine may fracture with minimal trauma due to the marked rigidity and osteoporosis.
10. The peripheral joints may undergo ankylosis.

Appropriate initial radiographic views to help confirm

A

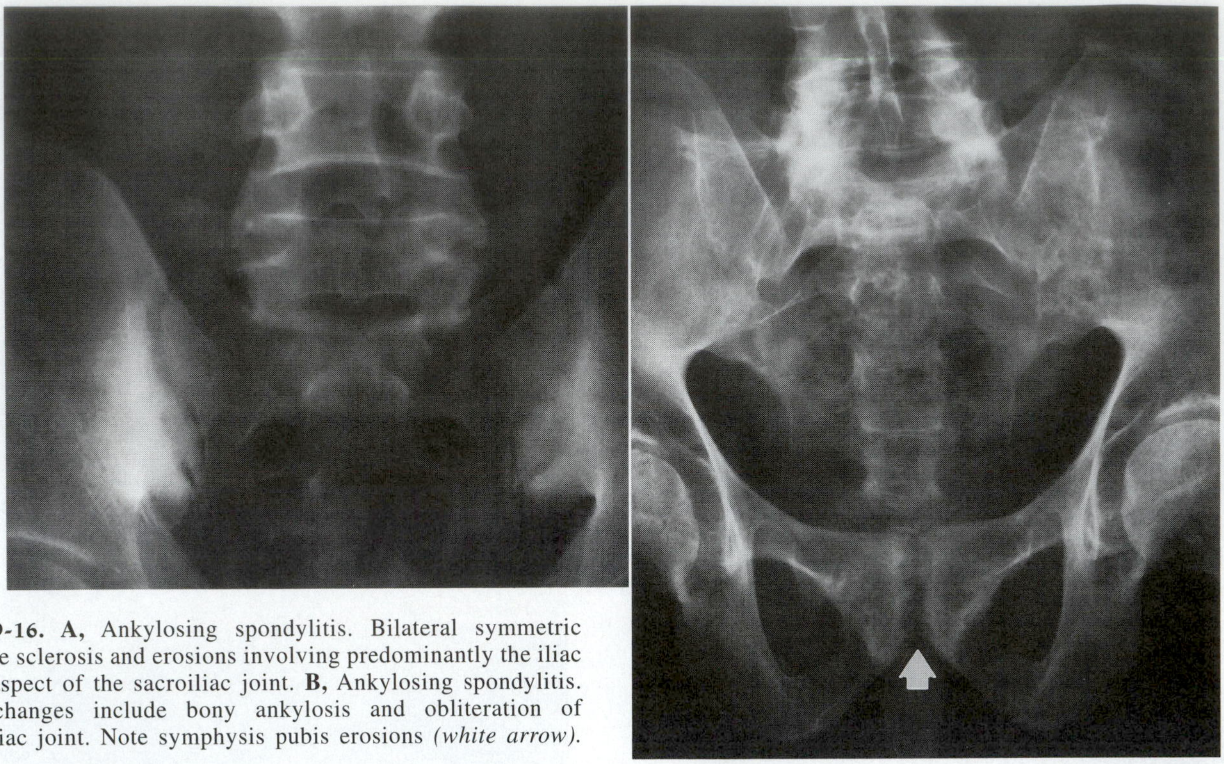

B

**Fig. 69-16.** **A,** Ankylosing spondylitis. Bilateral symmetric reactive sclerosis and erosions involving predominantly the iliac wing aspect of the sacroiliac joint. **B,** Ankylosing spondylitis. Late changes include bony ankylosis and obliteration of sacroiliac joint. Note symphysis pubis erosions *(white arrow).*

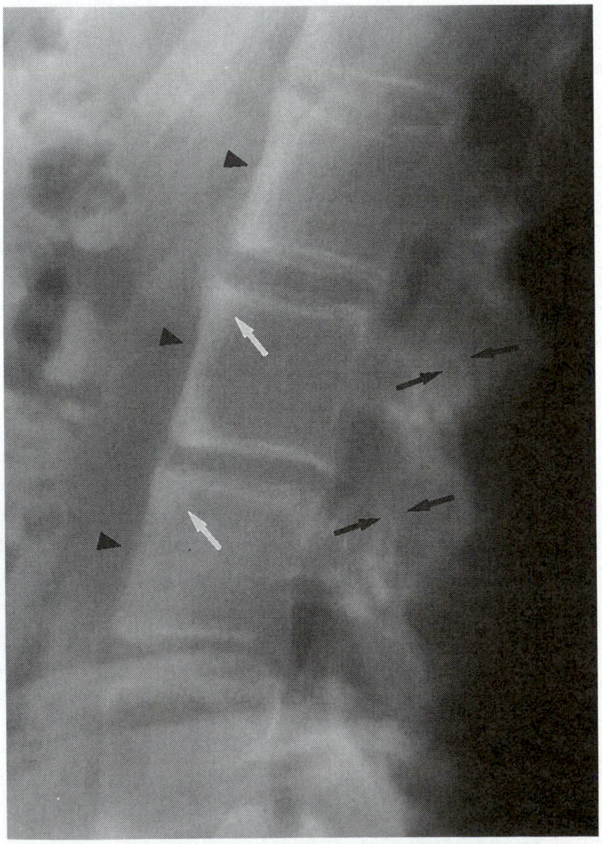

**Fig. 69-17.** Ankylosing spondylitis. Axial skeleton shows squaring of vertebral bodies *(arrowhead),* classic "shiny corners" *(white arrows),* and ankylosis of interarticular facet joints *(black arrows).*

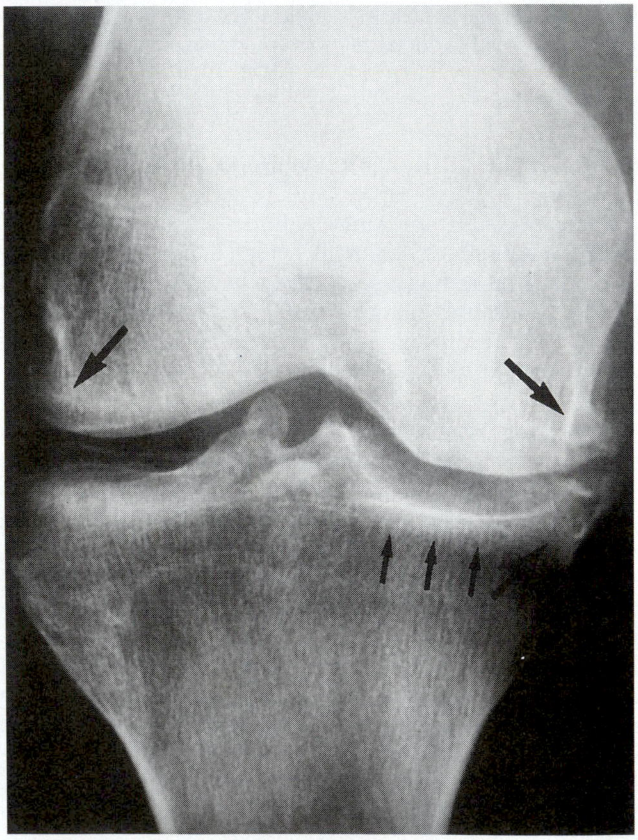

**Fig. 69-18.** Osteoarthritis. Proliferative marginal osteophytes *(black arrow),* narrowing of the medial weight bearing joint space, and subchondral eburnative changes *(small black arrows)* are shown.

the diagnosis of ankylosing spondylitis include anteroposterior and lateral views of the lumbar spine and sacroiliac joint views. CT performed in the axial or preferentially the coronal plane of the sacroiliac joint may demonstrate disease before findings are evident on plain films. MRI has been used to assess associated spinal cord arachnoiditis, spinal canal stenosis, and posttraumatic changes to the spinal cord.

## Osteoarthritis

The term osteoarthritis is typically used interchangeably with degenerative joint disease. Osteoarthritis is characterized by asymmetric joint space narrowing secondary to articular cartilage thinning and associated with subchondral eburnative and cystic changes (Fig. 69-18). Osteoarthritis may occur as a primary process or secondary to another joint insult or destructive joint disease. It is important to determine radiographically whether osteoarthritis is a primary or a secondary process.

In the appendicular skeleton, osteoarthritis is characterized as a proliferative process with predilection for osteophyte formation. There is an asymmetric joint involvement with the absence of erosions, osteopenia, and ankylosis helping to differentiate osteoarthritis from rheumatoid arthritis and the seronegative spondyloarthropathies.

Abnormalities of the synovial lining and adjacent ligamentous and soft tissue structures occur secondarily. A predilection for large weight-bearing joints occur; however, the small distal interphalangeal and interphalangeal joints of the hand are principally involved (Fig. 69-19). In the wrist the trapezial metacarpal and trapezial scaphoid joints are commonly involved. The elbow and shoulder are less commonly involved. If either is the principal abnormality, it is likely that the osteoarthritis is secondary.

Early radiographic changes in the appendicular skeleton include the following:

1. Asymmetric joint space narrowing best shown on weight-bearing or stress films.
2. Subchondral reactive sclerosis or bone formation best seen in the large weight-bearing joints.
3. Subchondral changes of the bone trabecula seen on both sides of the joint space.
4. Effusions that are activity related.
5. No juxtaarticular osteopenia.

Late radiographic findings in the appendicular skeleton include the following:

1. Prominent marginal osteophyte formation.
2. Subchondral cyst formation with a well-delineated margin.
3. Malalignment or angular deformity about weight-bearing joints.

A

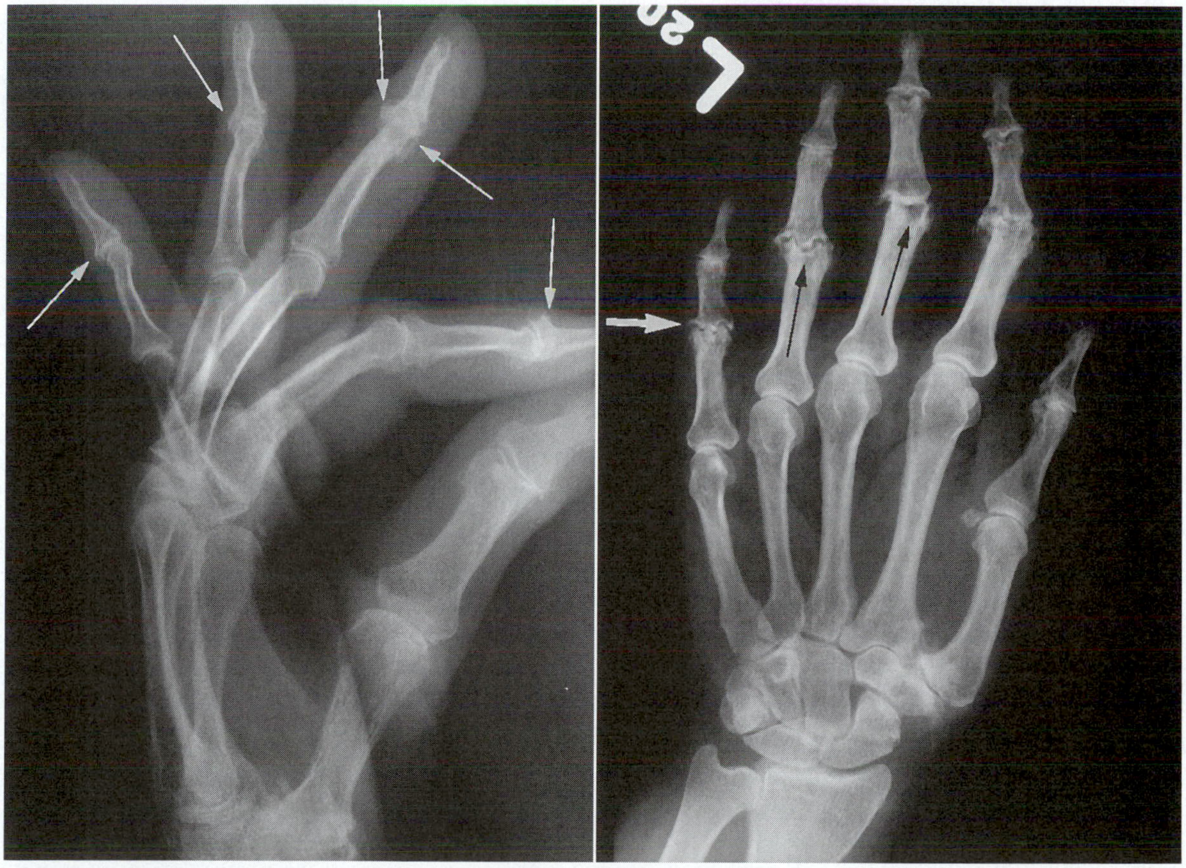

B

**Fig. 69-19.** **A,** Osteoarthritis. Lateral view of the digits show asymmetric extensor and volar proliferative spurs *(arrows)* with associated subchondral eburnative reaction and asymmetric narrowing of the joint space. **B,** Erosive osteoarthritis. Prominent central erosions of the proximal interphalangeal joints *(black arrow)*, gull-wing deformity best shown at fifth posterior interphalangeal joint *(white arrow)*, and subluxation are characteristic radiologic findings.

4. Loose intraarticular bodies (cartilaginous or osseous).
5. Alterations in mechanical stress bearing characterized by cortical and trabecular stress buttressing.
6. Chronic effusions.

In the axial skeleton, osteoarthritis specifically refers to changes at the apophyseal joints. Disk space narrowing or changes of the end-plates resulting from discal resorption are more properly termed intervertebral osteochondrosis. The changes of osteoarthritis at the apophyseal joints parallel those in the appendicular skeleton. In addition to the classic radiographic findings of cartilaginous thinning, marginal proliferation, subchondral eburnation, and cystic changes, capsular and ligamentous laxity occur, which foster subluxation. A pseudospondylolisthesis is produced as the bony vertebral ring remains intact.

Erosive or inflammatory osteoarthritis refers to a specific arthritis seen principally in women and characterized by central erosions of the interphalangeal joints. A predilection for the proximal and distal interphalangeal joints is noted. Marginal proliferative changes characteristic of osteoarthritis in the appendicular skeleton also are present. The central erosion and marginal proliferative changes with associated joint space narrowing have been likened to a sea gull wing and thus termed "gull wing deformity." Late radiographic changes can include angulation about the joint and ankylosis.

## Calcium pyrophosphate dihydrate arthropathy

Calcium pyrophosphate dihydrate (CPPD) crystals are deposited in articular and fibrocartilage, ligament, tendon, capsule, synovium, and synovial fluid (see Chapter 80). Radiologic hallmarks of chondrocalcinosis or abnormal mineralization of hyaline and fibrocartilage is seen. Target areas for chondrocalcinosis include the menisci of the knee, triangular fibrocartilage complex of the wrist, articular cartilage of the hips, and fibrocartilage of the symphysis pubis. Plain film radiograph of the knee (anteroposterior view [AP]), wrist (posteroanterior view [PA]), and pelvis (AP) are the standard radiographs initially ordered to evaluate this disorder.

Although the radiologic findings simulate those of a degenerative process, an atypical pattern of distribution is noted. Chondrocalcinosis of the large weight-bearing joints in addition to smaller non–weight-bearing joints with associated capsular and/or soft tissue mineralization are highly suggestive of a systemic process of calcium crystal deposition arthropathy. Unicompartmental or bicompartmental involvement of the knee with isolated or severe patellofemoral disease is a common radiologic presentation. A characteristic notching (erosion) of the anterior distal femur also is seen frequently (Fig. 69-20). Subtle articular mineralization involving the small joints of the wrist and hand, and mineralization of the triangular fibrocartilage complex, should suggest the diagnosis (Fig. 69-21).

Early radiographic changes include the following:

1. Normal plain film radiograph.
2. Subtle chondrocalcinosis in one or more target areas (knee, wrist, pelvis).
3. Mild symmetric joint space narrowing.
4. Subtle subchondral cyst formation.
5. Effusion.

Later radiographic findings include the following:

1. Prominent chondrocalcinosis.
2. Mineralization of ligaments, tendons, capsule, synovium, and periarticular soft tissues.
3. Prominent symmetric joint space narrowing.
4. Prominent subchondral cyst formation with disproportionately large cysts.
5. Subchondral eburnation.
6. A disproportionately small amount of osteophyte formation for the degree of joint space narrowing and subchondral change.
7. Bilateral weight-bearing and non–weight-bearing joint involvement suggesting a systemic disorder.

The anteroposterior view of the pelvis is radiologically helpful, as early or subtle chondrocalcinosis may be seen in the superolateral articular cartilage of either hip, the synovial lined sacroiliac joints, or at the level of the symphysis pubis.

In the axial skeleton, annular mineralization and discal mineralization are clues that lead to the diagnosis. The radiographic features again mimic those of a degenerative arthritis with the exception of more widespread involvement consistent with a systemic rather than mechanical abnormality. Widespread vacuum phenomenon, multiple levels of discal calcification, and calcification of associated paraspinal ligaments are very characteristic.

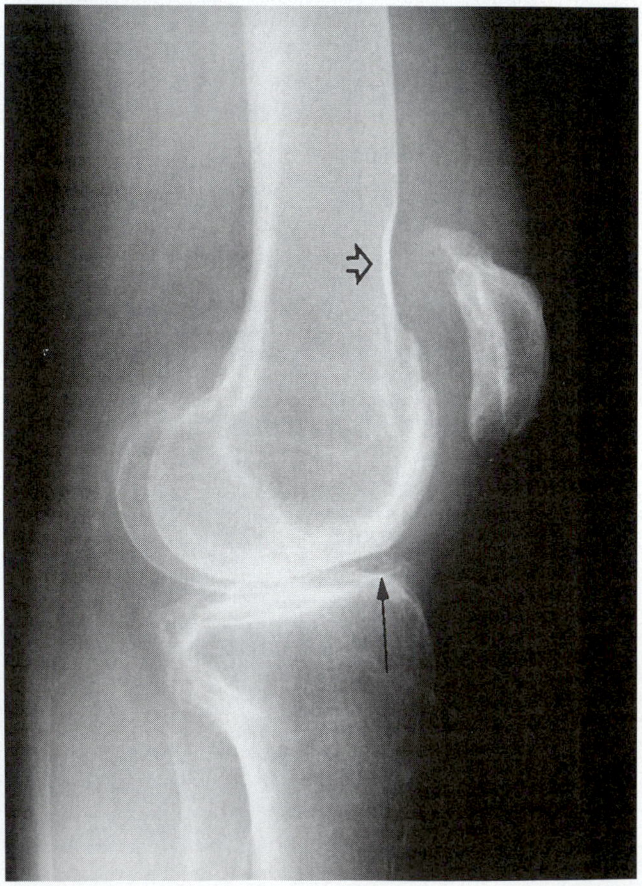

**Fig. 69-20.** Calcium pyrophosphate deposition disease (CPDD). Chondrocalcinosis of the menisci best shown anteriorly *(black arrow)* and characteristic distal femoral cortical notching noted *(black open arrow)*.

Currently, nuclear scintigraphy, MRI, or CT are not helpful in the evaluation of this disorder. The diagnosis is most frequently suggested by the plain film radiographs and corroborated through crystal isolation from joint aspirate.

## Gout

Gout is a crystal deposition arthropathy secondary to deposition of monosodium urate crystals in soft tissues, synovium, cartilage, and joint capsule (see Chapter 82). Osseous and soft tissue changes characterize the radiologic findings of primary gouty arthritis (Fig. 69-22).

Radiographs of initial episodes of gouty arthritis do not show articular abnormality. Juxtaarticular soft tissue swelling is the typical presenting finding. Bony demineralization is not noted. Less than 50% of patients with documented gouty arthritis show osseous change. Radiologic findings of bony change document the chronicity of the disease process, which typically requires more than 5 years for bony changes to occur.

The first metatarsophalangeal joint is the most commonly involved articulation (Fig. 69-23). Beyond the feet, the ankle, knees, hands, and elbows are commonly involved. Bilateral olecranon bursitis is a clinical and radiologic clue to the diagnosis of gouty arthritis.

Tophaceous deposits may occur juxtaarticularly, causing pressure erosion to the underlying bone. Deposits are seen in tendons, ligaments, capsule, and bursa. Extraarticular deposits are seen in the helix of the ear, palm of the hand, sole of the foot, and fingertip.

Involvement of the axial skeleton is uncommon. In rare cases of sacroiliac joint involvement, changes are similar to those in other articulations including large cystic or erosive changes of the true synovial lined joint in an asymmetric unilateral or bilateral pattern of involvement.

Early radiologic findings of gouty arthritis include the following:

1. Normal mineralization.
2. Soft tissue swelling without articular abnormality.
3. Asymmetric monoarticular or polyarticular involvement.

Late radiologic findings include the following:

1. Soft tissue tophi with or without mineralization.
2. Chondrocalcinosis.
3. Osseous erosions with characteristic overhanging bony margin.
4. Geographic sclerotic margination to bony erosion.
5. Intraosseous mineralization.

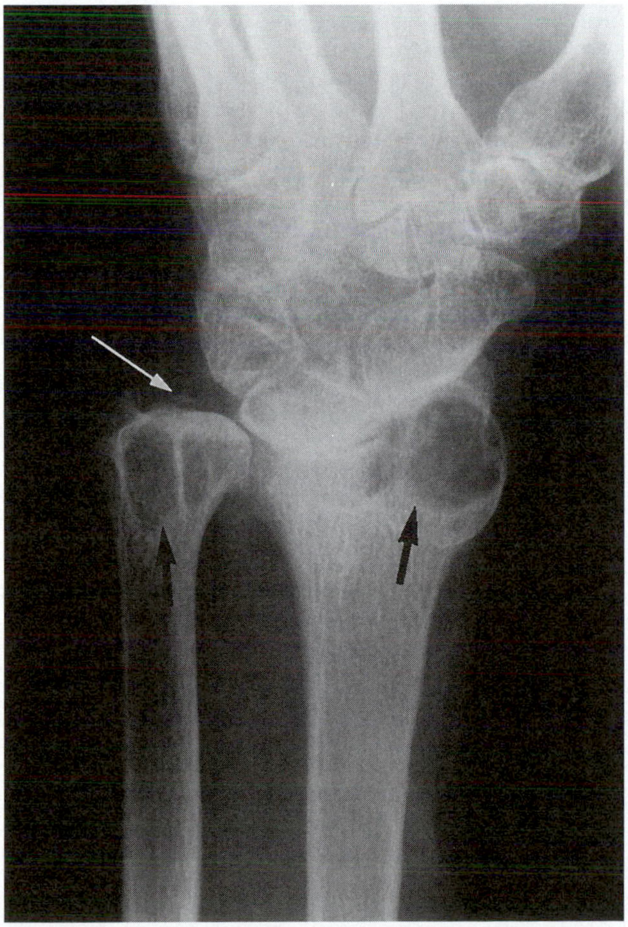

**Fig. 69-21.** Calcium pyrophosphate deposition disease (CPDD). Chondrocalcinosis of the triangular fibrocartilage *(white arrow)* in addition to large subchondral cyst formation *(black arrow).*

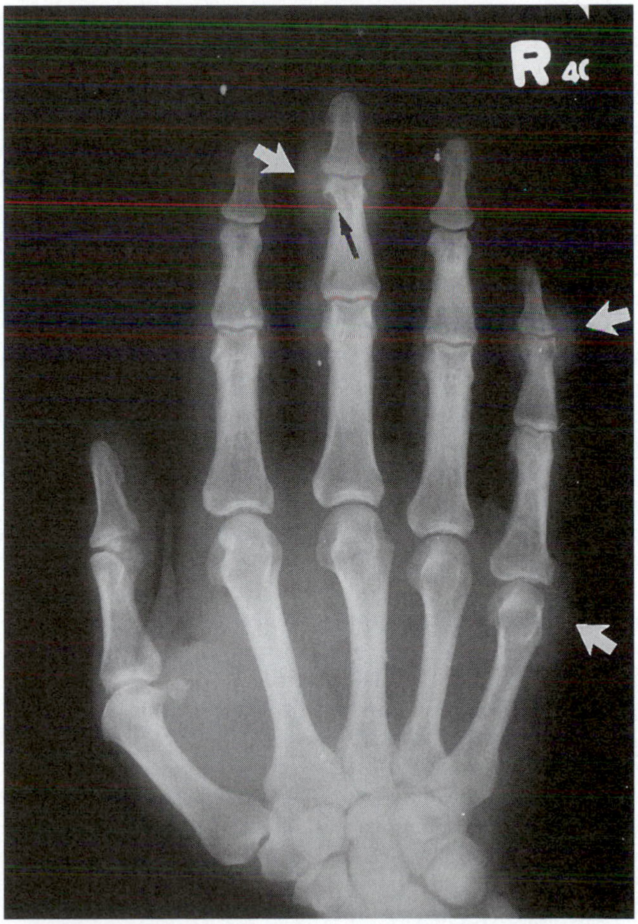


**Fig. 69-22.** Gouty arthritis. Prominent soft tissue tophi *(white arrow)* and associated bony erosion with geographic sclerotic margination *(black arrow).*

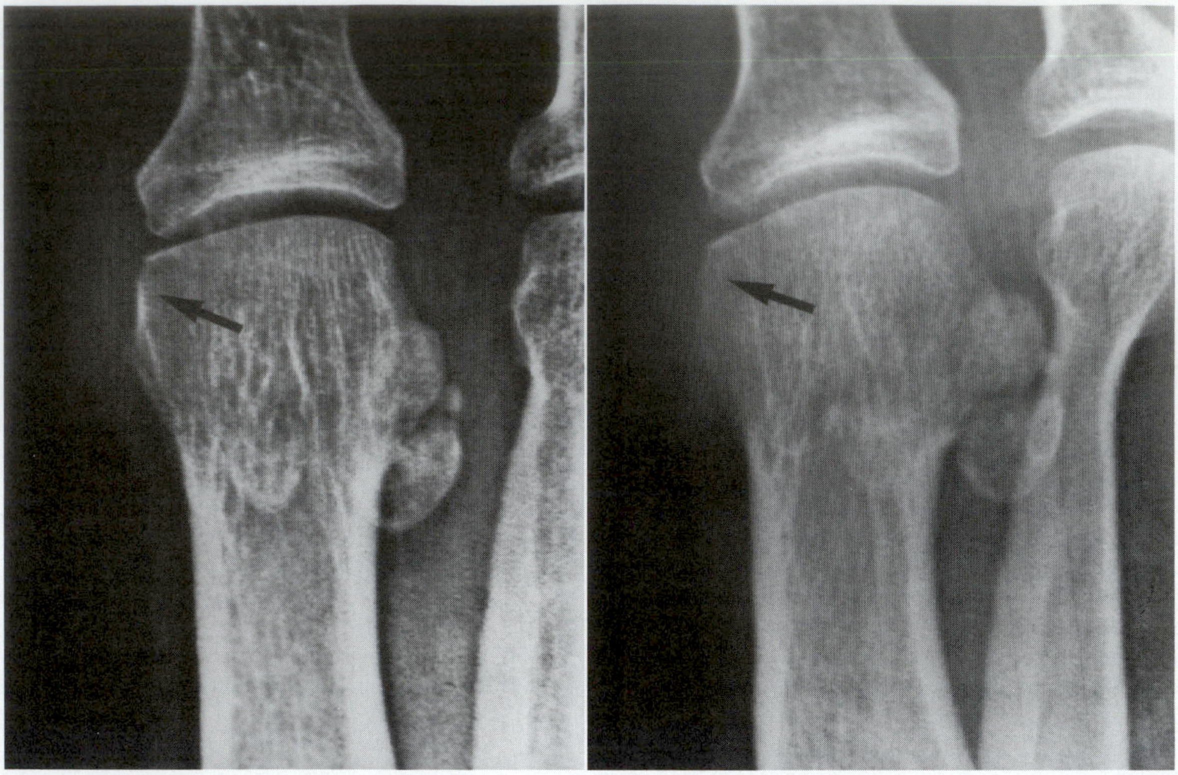


**Fig. 69-23.** **A** and **B,** Gouty arthritis. Progressive erosion of first metatarsal head with loss of subchondral cortical delineation over an 8-month period *(black arrows).*

Gouty arthritis is differentiated from rheumatoid arthritis by the absence in gout of juxtaarticular osteopenia, symmetric joint space loss, and symmetric polyarticular involvement. The distribution of involvement is also different in these two joint diseases.

Differentiating seronegative spondyloarthropathy such as psoriatic arthritis from gout may be more difficult due to the overlap of target sites such as the first metatarsophalangeal joint. Periosteal reaction, progressive bony erosive destruction without associated soft tissue mass or tophus, and ankylosis of an articulation make gouty arthritis less likely. The high predilection of axial skeleton involvement in ankylosing spondylitis and its rare involvement in gouty arthritis help distinguish these two disorders.

Differentiating gout from other crystal deposition arthropathies such as CPPD can be challenging, especially early in the disease process. Joint fluid aspiration and crystal evaluation is most helpful. Radiologic findings of extensive chondrocalcinosis, joint space narrowing, and large subchondral cyst formation without associated soft tissue tophus are helpful in excluding gouty arthritis.

Alternate radiologic imaging modalities do not provide diagnostic or therapeutic advantage in the evaluation of gouty arthritis. The diagnosis is most frequently suggested by plain film radiographs and corroborated by crystal isolation from joint and periarticular sites.

## BIBLIOGRAPHY


Bedell SA, Bush BT: Erythrocyte sedimentation rate—from folklore to facts, *Am J Med* 78:1001, 1985.

Brower AC: *Arthritis in black and white,* Philadelphia, 1988, WB Saunders.

Doherty M et al: *Rheumatology examination and injection techniques,* London, 1992, WB Saunders.

Forrester DM, Brown JC: *The radiology of joint disease,* Philadelphia, 1987, WB Saunders.

Fritzler MJ: Antinuclear antibodies in the investigation of rheumatic diseases, *Bull Rheum Dis* 35:1, 1985.

Gatter RA: *A practical handbook of joint fluid analysis,* Philadelphia, 1984, Lea and Febiger.

Gray RG, Tenenbaum J, Gottlieb NL: Local corticosteroid injection treatment in rheumatic disorders, *Semin Arthritis Rheum* 10:231, 1981.

Harmon LE: Antinuclear antibodies in autoimmune disease—significance and pathogenicity, *Med Clin North Am* 69(3):547, 1985.

Kushner I: C-reactive protein and the acute phase response, *Hosp Practice* 25:13, 1990.

Resnick D, Niwayama G: *Diagnosis of bone and joint disorders,* Philadelphia, 1988, WB Saunders.

Sox HC Jr, Liang MH: The erythrocyte sedimentation rate—guidelines for rational use, *Ann Intern Med* 104:515, 1986.

CHAPTER

# 70 Neck

John H. Bland

The extremely flexible cervical spine is the body's most complicated and mobile articular system; it is designed for mobility at the expense of stability. The seven small, comparatively fragile cervical vertebrae with their extensive ligaments, capsules, tendons, and muscle attachments are poorly designed to protect their contents compared to the skull above and the thorax below. The cervical spine balances a 10- to 15-pound ball, the head, on the lateral masses of the atlas.

Many clinically reported and distinct syndromes arise from abnormalities of the tissues of the cervical spine alone. Even more syndromes arise from distant structures, but they are associated with signs and symptoms referable to the cervical spine, head, shoulders, and upper extremities. These disorders constitute a considerable portion of any physician's practice.

## EPIDEMIOLOGY

More than 10% of the Swedish population recalled having at least three episodes of pain in the neck in a 1984 study. Up to 12% of women and 9% of men experienced neck pain with or without associated arm pain. Seventy percent of adults who visited their doctors for neck pain were well or improving within 1 month. Neck pain is a recurring ubiquitous clinical event, a mild-to-modest transitory nuisance to most of us.

## CLINICALLY RELEVANT ANATOMY

The nucleus pulposus, present at birth, gradually disappears between the age of 12 to 14 years and 35 to 40 years. Little if any nucleus pulposus remains in any of the discs in the cervical spine. Thus persons over age 40 cannot herniate the nucleus pulposus. The uncinate process is a bony development laterally and posterolaterally, which enlarges with increasing age and presents a bulwark that prevents herniation of the intervertebral disks posterolaterally.

From the level of C3-4, the posterior nerve root exits are below the level of the disk. Thus the nerve roots are found regularly with increasing obliqueness from above downward. Clinically, it seems impossible for the disc to compress nerve roots within the spinal canal, because the root exit zone is below the level of the disk.

After age 40 to 45, all dural root sleeves (exit sites) become fibrotic and stiff. All zygapophyseal joints (posterior joints) have menisci capable of proliferation into a pannuslike structure over the surface of the cartilage. This structure has clinical significance.

The anterior nerve root is low in the intervertebral foramen; hence it is unlikely to be subject to compression. The posterior root is well protected from the point of view of any disc herniation; however, the zygapophyseal joints could become enlarged, osteoarthritic, and osteophytic and compress the posterior nerve roots. Any radiculopathy (although radiculopathy itself is rare) is a consequence of the zygapophyseal joint abnormality, not of the uncinate process or the alleged joints of Luschka.

There is a considerable disparity between the anteroposterior diameter and the transverse measurement of the spinal cord as it relates to the internal diameter and transverse diameter of the spinal canal. There are "fat" cords and "thin" cords—seemingly a genetic endowment; the ideal is a thin cord and a capacious spinal canal, a constitutional characteristic.

Preganglionic sympathetic fibers are not present in the cervical spine because they all come from T1, T2, and T3 levels and have their first synapse in one or more of the three cervical sympathetic ganglia. The postganglionic fibers go in three directions: (1) out into the upper extremity, providing all autonomic function to the arm and hand; (2) reentering the intervertebral foramina and the spinal cord and having connections in the vestibular apparatus, the cerebellum, the hypothalamus, and the thalamus, as well as connections to the spinal nerves; and (3) large segments of postganglionic fibers accompany both the vertebral and carotid arteries, following their distribution in the brain with multiple connections.

The anterior portion of the spinal canal is characterized universally by bars of osteophytes at the level of the intervertebral discs, sometimes compressing the cord to varying degrees. The ligamentum flavum is hypertrophic and hyperplastic in most instances, projecting into the posterior spinal canal.

A 30-degree turn of the head normally kinks the ipsilateral vertebral artery. A 45-degree turn kinks both vertebral arteries. In the presence of osteoarthritis, disc disorders, and facet disease, vertebral artery compression is not rare and can become symptomatic.

Physiologically, the cervical spine is characterized by a high degree of motion. Any part of the musculoskeletal system that is put to complete rest will result in an unfortunate series of events culminating in total destruction of a joint within approximately 4 to 6 months. Wherever there is the least motion, there will be the greatest degree of pathophysiologic change in the involved tissues. Because the cervical spine is virtually never completely still, it is especially vulnerable to partial immobilization and at considerable risk by total immobilization. Prolonged immobilization in a cervical collar may result in stiffness, pain, and limited motion. Immobilization, partial or total, should be avoided as much as possible.

## PATIENT HISTORY

Knowing the patient's age and occupation is extremely important. Cervical osteoarthritis with myriad syndromes is a disease of later life. Trauma and "crick" (spasmodic torticollis) occur in younger people. Occupations requiring continued or intermittent hyperflexion, hyperextension, or over-rotation of the cervical spine may produce and prolong symptoms. Details about previous injury are important. Whether the patient wears bifocal glasses may be pertinent because bifocals usually require the patient to extend the occiput, atlas, and axis complex and to flex the lower cervical spine. Inquiry about the type of pillow the patient uses, if any, frequently reveals useful information.

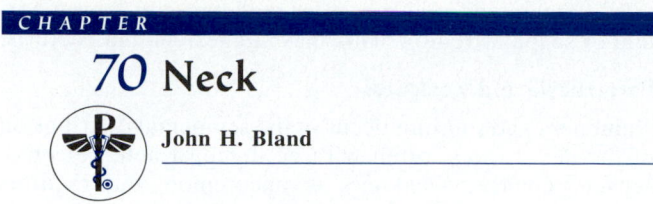

## Physical characteristics

Physical characteristics such as neck length, receding mandible, high arched palate, crooked teeth, and asymmetry of facial bones and muscles should be noted. Information about temporomandibular joint function is important. Investigation of a painful bite, limited jaw opening, or swelling of the temporomandibular joint area may lead to a proper diagnosis.

## Pain characteristics

(See the box for common disorders causing cervical and shoulder pain.) Three phases or periods of the patient's pain history should be investigated during the interview: onset, course, and present status. The location, size, distribution, quality, intensity, severity, and duration of the first pain should be noted. Fig. 70-1 illustrates patterns of reflexly referred pain from visceral and somatic structures. Head pain is common in and characteristic of cervical syndromes.

A lesion at the level of C6-7 may cause neurologic or myalgic pain and real muscular tenderness in the precordial or scapular region. This may suggest angina pectoris.

## Paresthesia and weakness

Numbness and tingling occur in the segmental distribution of the nerve roots, often with no demonstrable objective sensory change. Weakness is uncommon, but requires inquiry. Patients who have trouble balancing their heads

### Common disorders of the cervical spine that cause neck and shoulder pain

- Spasmodic torticollis
- Intervertebral disc protrusion
- Cervical osteoarthritis
- Fibromyalgia syndrome
- Trauma, cervical spine fracture
- Injuries caused by hyperflexion or hyperextension (whiplash)
- Rheumatoid arthritis of cervical spine
- Ankylosing spondylitis of cervical spine
- Infection of cervical spine
- Thoracic outlet syndromes
- Metastatic malignant disease of cervical spine
- Carotid and vertebral artery atherosclerosis

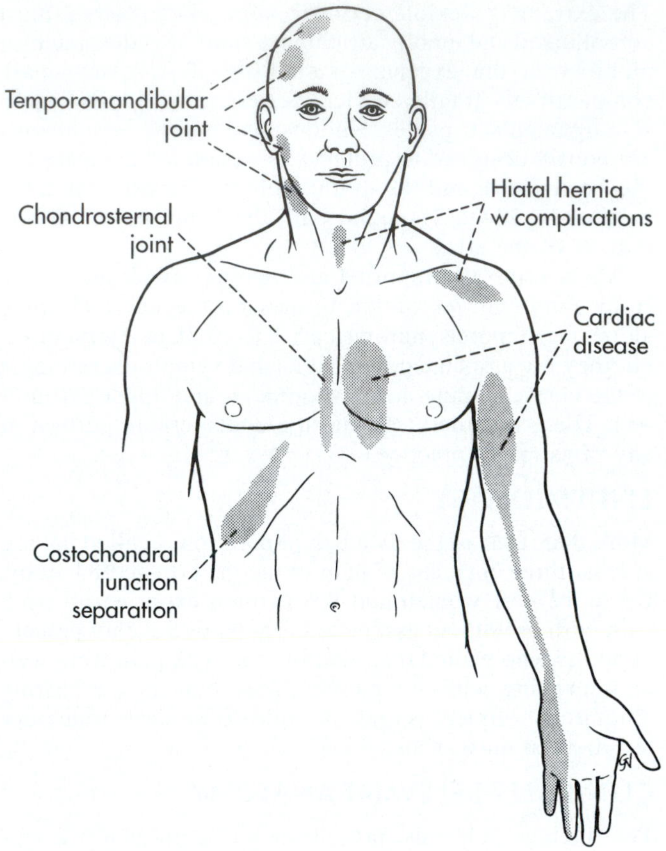


A

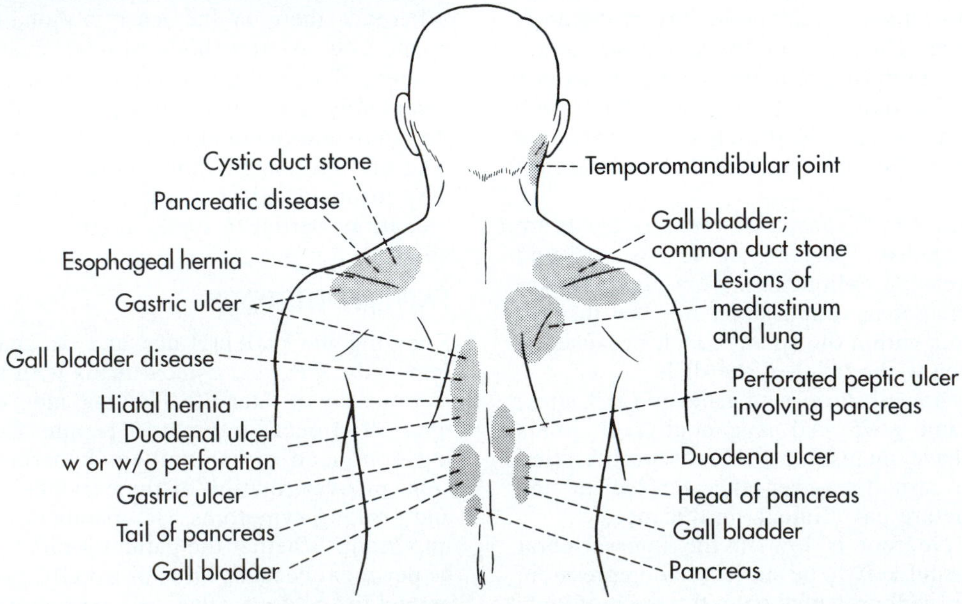


B

**Fig. 70-1. A,** Anterior and posterior referral sites from distant visceral or somatic structures. **B,** Posterior referral sites.

because of muscle weakness have clearly lost power.

## Symptoms

Eye symptoms and signs may occur in cervical syndromes. These signs and symptoms include blurring of vision, frequent change of glasses without improvement, relief of pain by changing neck position, increased tearing, retro-orbital pain, and strange description of eyes "being pulled backward or pushed forward." The etiology of these signs and symptoms is likely the result of irritation of the cervical sympathetic nerve supply to eye structures.

Change in equilibrium occurs because of irritation of sympathetic plexuses surrounding the vertebral arteries or as a result of vascular insufficiency.

Dysphagia is not unusual in cervical syndromes and can be caused by muscle spasm and anterior osteophyte compression of the pharynx and esophagus (Fig. 70-2).

A large group of bizarre symptoms, some of which are unrelated, are explicable in terms of multivalent pathogenetic mechanisms. A patient comment such as "I can't get a deep breath" may be due to C-3–C-5 lesions whose roots innervate the diaphragm and other respiratory muscles. Cardiac palpitation and tachycardia may result from unusual positions or hyperextension of the neck due to irritation of the C4 nerve root supplying the diaphragm and pericardium, or by irritation of the cardiac sympathetic nerve supply. Nausea and vomiting, ill-defined pain, and paresthesia may be caused by cord compression. Drop attacks may be caused by abrupt loss of proprioception, collapse without loss of consciousness, often with the ability to rise and continue with previous activity.

Differentiating psychoneurosis from cervical syndromes is a common problem, usually reflecting the examiner's inexperience with the enormous and complex variety of symptoms and signs explicable as nerve root compression, sympathetic nervous system involvement, cervical cord compression, vascular insufficiency, and diseases and trauma of cervical bone, muscle, and joint.

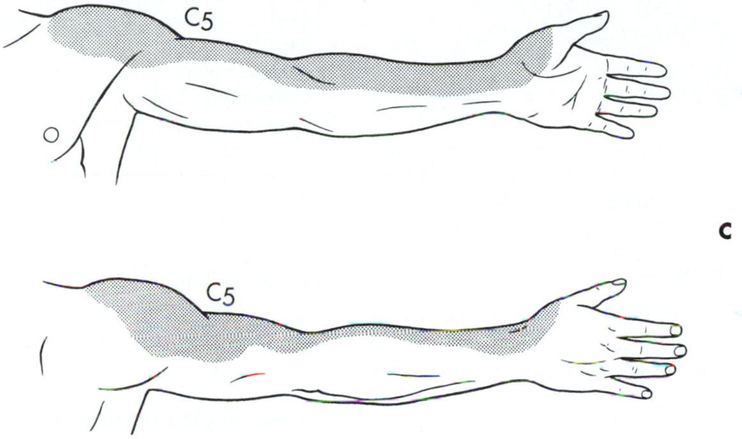


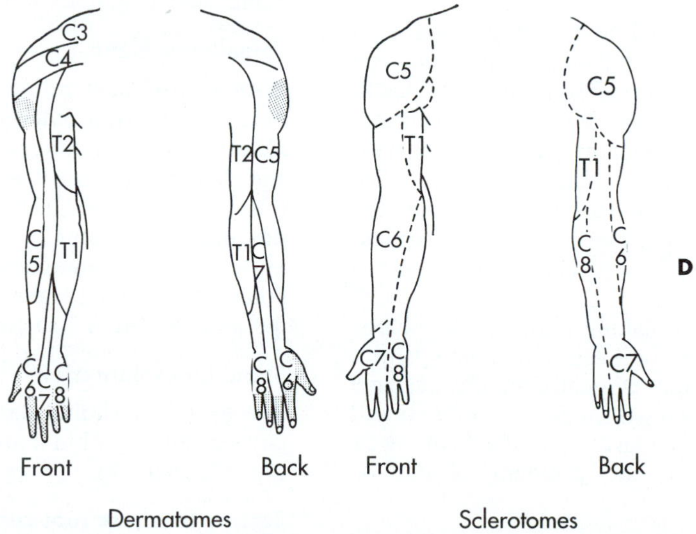


**Fig. 70-1, cont'd. C,** The distribution of all structures of the shoulder derived from the C5 dermatome-myotome-sclerotome. **D,** The distribution of dermatomes and sclerotomes of the upper extremities. (**D** from Lance JW, McLeod JG: *A physiological approach to clinical neurology,* ed 2, Reading, MA, 1975, Butterworth.)

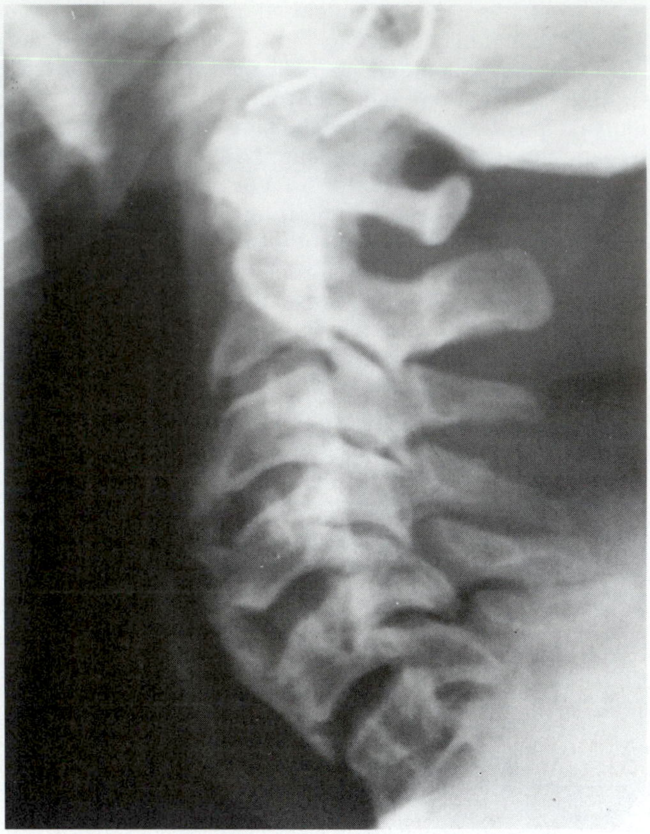

Fig. 70-2. Diffuse idiopathic skeletal hyperostosis. Note the laminar bone at the C3-C4 level has pushed the esophagus forward, stretching the tissues and causing dysphagia.

**Table 70-1.** Neurologic screening tests

| | |
|---|---|
| **Motor function (active and against resistance)** | |
| ***Action*** | ***Nerve(s)*** |
| Rotation of cervical spine | C1,2,3 |
| Shrug | C2,3,4,5 |
| Arm abduction | C5 |
| Forearm flexion, supination | C5,6 |
| Forearm extension | C7 |
| Wrist extension (with elbows extended) | C6 |
| Wrist flexion | C7 |
| Thumb extension | C8 |
| Fifth finger abduction | C8 |
| Interosseal and lumbrical muscle function | T1 |
| **Deep tendon reflexes** | |
| ***Tendon*** | ***Nerve(s)*** |
| Pectoral | C5-T1 |
| Deltoid | C5-6 |
| Biceps | C5-6 |
| Triceps | C7 |
| Brachioradial | C5-6 |
| **Somite areas (light touch, pinprick, and vibration)** | |
| ***Site*** | ***Nerve(s)*** |
| Acromioclavicular joint | C4 |
| Deltoid; lateral arm | C5 |
| Thumb | C6 |
| Middle finger | C7 |
| Fifth finger | C8 |
| Forearm, medial border | T1 |
| Arm, medial border | T2 |

## PHYSICAL EXAMINATION

Most patients with cervical spine syndromes require a complete physical examination in addition to a thorough musculoskeletal examination with appropriate regional focus.

### Posture and movement

The patient should be gowned and sitting upright to determine the range of motion of the cervical spine. The patient's posture should be observed from the front, back, and side while the patient is sitting, standing, and walking. Anatomic details such as scapular height, spinal curves, head tilt, and head position should be noted. The cervicothoracic and thoracolumbar junctions and the sacral area should be examined. The presence of cervical lordosis, kyphosis, and lumbar lordosis should be specifically investigated.

Gait analysis may help in making a diagnosis such as scoliosis, congenital lesions, or even a lumbar spondylolisthesis, which is reflected clinically in the cervical spine. The patient's ability and willingness to move should be observed, looking particularly for head or neck guarding. The acuteness of the problem should be assessed.

### Physical abnormalities

The patient should be observed for any abnormal appearance such as extreme height or shortness, an unusually long or short neck, retracted mandible, crooked teeth, or high palate. These abnormalities, as well as facial asymmetry, abnormal facial development, and asymmetric bone and muscle development suggest congenital anomalies of the cervical spine, particularly the upper third.

### Neurologic examination

Table 70-1 describes clinical neurologic screening tests.

### Spinal movement

With the patient standing, movement of the entire spine in flexion, extension, lateral flexion, and rotation should be observed. Passive ranges of motion should be determined and then an attempt made to actively increase them. All four motions should be tested against resistance to observe the patient's motor power and to determine whether muscle contraction against resistance produces pain. The goal is to produce signs and symptoms that will identify the pain-sensitive structure for a precise diagnosis.

### Shoulder examination

The examiner should determine whether the shoulder or any structures within it are contributing to pain in the neck (see Chapter 71).

### Testing for nerve root compression

The quadrant position is used to alter the size of the intervertebral foramina and determine whether the nerve root can be compressed. Head extension is tested first, so that the inferior facet of the vertebra above glides

**Table 70-2.** Cervical spine diseases with unusual pathogenesis

| Condition | Pathogenic process |
|---|---|
| Ankylosing spondylitis | Inflammation |
| Osteomyelitis | Infection |
| Bursitis in cervical spine | Inflammation |
| Neoplastic lesion (Horner's syndrome) | Neoplastic disease |
| Hyoid bone syndrome | Tendinitis |
| Neck-tongue syndrome | Nerve entrapment |
| Calcific retropharyngeal tendinitis | Tendinitis |
| Ligamentum flavum calcification | Calcific deposits |
| Occipital neuralgia | Neuritis of second cervical spine nerve |
| Simple long neck | Normal anatomic variant; extracervical vertebra |
| Syndrome of third neuron of cervical sympathetic system | Neoplastic or vascular disease, trauma |
| Neck sprain | Trauma (whiplash injury); psychological mechanisms |
| Fibrous dysplasia of the bone (progressive) | Genetic |
| Atlantooccipital and atlantoaxial dislocation | Trauma, infection, inflammation |
| Bilateral facet dislocation below C3 level | Trauma |
| Tennis elbow, carpal tunnel syndrome, rotator cuff lesion | Secondary to cervical osteoarthritis |
| Posterior cervical sympathetic syndrome; Barre-Lieou syndrome | Inflammation; sepsis; neoplasm; psychological and psychiatric mechanisms |
| Psychiatric syndrome of the cervical spine | Mental mechanism (e.g., hysteria) |
| Paget's disease | Unknown; possibly viral origin |
| Vertebral artery syndromes | Osteoarthritis; trauma; atherosclerosis; rheumatoid arthritis |
| Esophageal syndromes | Osteoarthritis; hyperostosis |
| Axial osteomalacia | Metabolic bone disease |
| Osteoporosis | Metabolic bone disease, idiopathic |
| Radiculopathy | Osteoarthritis; various root entrapment diseases |
| Peripheral neuropathy of C1-T1 peripheral nerves | Neuritis (multiple causes) |
| Myelopathy | Osteoarthritis intervertebral discs; trauma; others |
| Vertebrobasilar insufficiency syndromes | Vascular; osteoarthritis; atherosclerosis |
| Thoracic outlet syndrome | Vascular/neuropathic |
| Subclavian steal syndrome | Variety of causes |
| Gout | Monosodium urate crystal deposition |
| Double crush syndrome | Nerve entrapments |
| Postural cervical syndromes | Abnormal posture |
| Levator scapulae muscle syndrome | Specific muscle strain; trauma; postural defects |

posteriorly on the facet of the vertebra below, thereby narrowing the foramina. If this maneuver produces shoulder pain, paresthesia, or numbness, the nerve root is compressed in the foramina. Other maneuvers should not be attempted. If the patient does not experience these symptoms, lateral flexion should be attempted, which closes the foramina toward the side of the flexion and opens it on the opposite side. If this maneuver produces the syndrome, other maneuvers should not be made. If it does not produce the pain or dysesthesia syndrome, full rotation should be added, which maximally closes the foramina on one side and opens it on the opposite side. If active range of motion produces the syndrome, you need not use the quadrant position.

### Head compression test (Spurling test)

Compression of the head, causing force transmission to the cervical spine, may induce pain by narrowing the intervertebral foramina. Upper extremity radicular pain or paraesthesia produced or intensified by this maneuver is indicative of nerve root irritation. Localized, nonradicular pain suggests that soft tissue or joints are the pain-sensitive structures.

The test is performed with the patient sitting. The physician places one hand across the other on the top of the patient's head and gradually increases downward pressure. The patient is instructed to report pain or paresthesia and its distribution. Repeating the test with the patient's head tilted to either side, backward, and then forward, increases the sensitivity of the test.

### Distraction test

This test predicts somewhat the effect of cervical spine traction in relieving pain or paresthesia. Nerve root compression may be relieved, with disappearance of the symptoms and signs, if the intervertebral foramina are opened or the disc spaces extended. Pressure on joint capsules of apophyseal joints is also decreased by distraction. Muscle spasms of any cause may be relieved.

The test is performed with the patient sitting. The physician places the palm of one hand under the patient's chin and the other under the occiput and gradually increases the force of lifting, removing the weight of the skull and distracting the foramina, discs, and joints. This test is continued for 30 to 60 seconds.

### Palpation

The examiner palpates the anterior and posterior cervical triangles for the brachial plexus and examines the site of the subclavian artery. Deep palpation also allows exami-

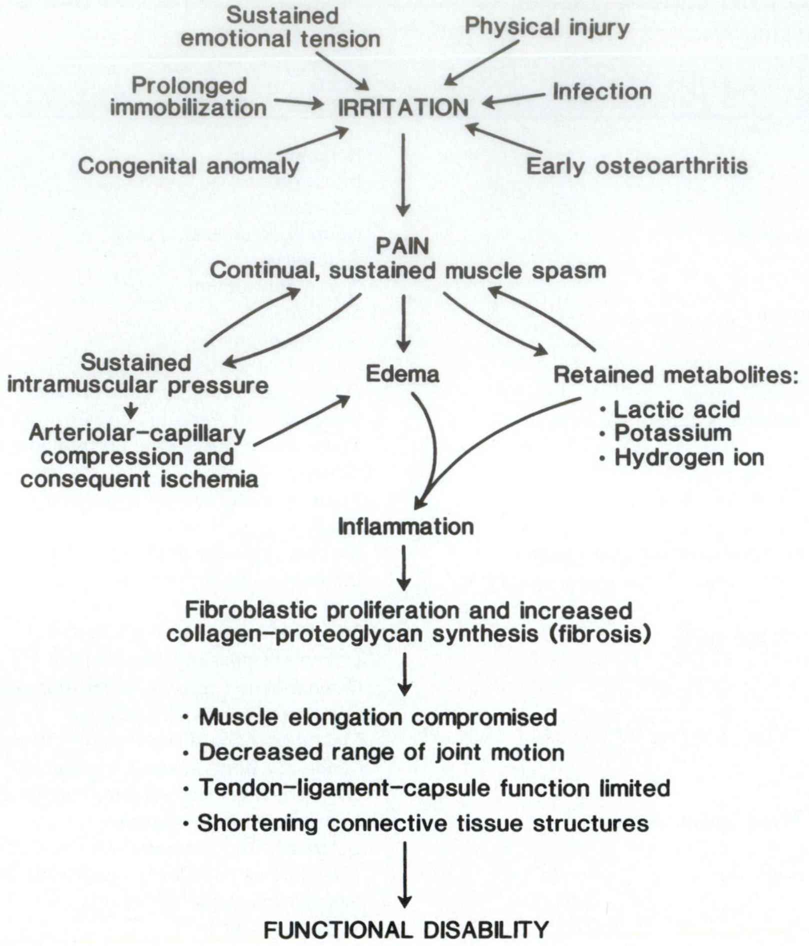


**Fig. 70-3.** Pathophysiologic mechanisms of soft tissue cervical spine syndromes.

nation of the transverse processes of the atlas and axis and sometimes the third vertebra.

In the anterior triangle, the landmarks should be identified. They will help in clinical orientation, such as in the identification of a fractured cervical vertebra. The hyoid bone is at the level of C3. If there are signs and symptoms relating to C3, tenderness may be present at this level. The thyroid cartilage is at the upper level of C4, and the thyroid gland is at the lower level of C5. The first ring of cricoid cartilage is at the level of C6.

### Appearance of the back

The levator muscle of the scapula, the trapezius, rhomboid and scalene muscles, and the superior angle of the scapula should be observed, checking for atrophy, weakness, and neurologic signs. The deltoid, supraspinatus, and infraspinatus muscles should be observed for atrophy. The skin should be examined for thickness, color, scars, temperature, old incisions, and ecchymoses. The carotid arteries are palpated for tenderness. The sternocleidomastoid muscle and its function are examined. Sites of tenderness are marked with a felt pen and correlated, if possible, with the local structures.

Table 70-2 lists cervical spine diseases with unusual pathogenesis. Fig. 70-3 review the pathophysiologic mechanisms of common soft tissue cervical spine syndromes.

## RADIOLOGIC ASSESSMENT

Technologic advances in the past few decades have revolutionized radiology and greatly improved imaging of the cervical spine. Arthrography and diskography are rarely used. Development of low toxicity, water-soluble myelographic contrast has ushered in the era of computed tomography (CT) myelography. Magnetic resonance imaging (MRI) with continuing refinement in software technology and surface coils has added a new dimension of noninvasive evaluation of the cervical spine and spinal cord.

### Plain film radiographic examination

Conventional radiography of the cervical spine includes anteroposterior (AP), AP odontoid, lateral, and right and left oblique views. Two AP views are needed. The AP odontoid through the open mouth demonstrates the entire odontoid process and may also show atlantooccipital or atlantoaxial joints. The second AP view includes the lower cervical spine from C3 to T1.

A lateral cervical spine radiograph should show the base of the skull, seven cervical vertebrae, and the end plate of the first thoracic vertebrae. If shoulders prevent clear imaging of the lower vertebral bodies, a coned-down, or "swimmer's view," of the cervicothoracic junction is obtained. Oblique views illustrate the neural foramina, pedicles, and the superior and inferior articulating facet joints.

The radiographic evaluation of trauma patients must be carefully tailored to prevent further neurologic injury. In a cooperative, neurologically intact patient, AP, AP odontoid, lateral, and right and left oblique views are obtained. Only if these radiographs are normal is it safe to proceed to flexion-extension views.

In severely traumatized patients or those with neurologic deficits, only AP and lateral survey films are obtained without moving the patient. Further cervical spine evaluation of trauma patients is accomplished by CT scan. CT scanning accurately demonstrates fractures and displaced bone fragments that could cause serious neurologic injury by compromising either the spinal canal or neural foramina.

### Magnetic resonance imaging

In radiologic evaluation of the cervical spine, MRI has several advantages over CT scanning. In contrast to CT, no ionizing radiation is involved. MRI has a higher contrast resolution, allowing it to differentiate between soft tissues, both normal and pathologic, with great sensitivity. Unlike CT scanning, bone artifact does not degrade MRI imaging. Multiple imaging planes (e.g., sagittal, axial, coronal, and oblique) are available without repositioning the patient or significantly prolonging the length of the examination, an important advantage in the injured patient. The entire cervical spine is studied in sagittal and coronal images.

MRI study requires a cooperative patient. Disadvantages of MRI include striking motion sensitivity. In addition dense cortical or compact bone has very few hydrogen protons; therefore it is seen as a signal void on MRI with limited spatial resolution. Thus MRI can fail to delineate fractures and poorly defines bone spurs and calcification. MRI is a more expensive imaging method than CT scanning, and patients occasionally are too claustrophobic to endure the study.

## LABORATORY STUDIES/DIAGNOSTIC PROCEDURES

Relatively few laboratory studies are guided by results of historical elicitation and physical examination (e.g., occasional spinal tap, HLA typing, immunoglobulins, rheumatoid factor, antinuclear antibody).

Diagnostic procedures include radiologic evaluation, occasional biopsy or electrodiagnostic studies, and less commonly CT scans, MRI, angiogram, or radionuclide studies. These diagnostic studies as well as chest radiographs and electrocardiograms also help to exclude neck pain from causes such as metastatic disease, referred pain from chest pathology such as Pancoast tumor, pneumonia, and heart disease.

## GENERAL MANAGEMENT

Maintaining optimum overall fitness contributes significantly to the success of management of cervical spine disorders and disease. Management and active treatment of disease, as well as rehabilitation of cervical spine disorders, are strongly linked to the rest of the spine and to the body as a whole.

Patient education is a major contributor to the success of management. Patient education classes about various kinds of arthritis are available through the Arthritis Foundation. Patient handbooks and educational materials also are useful.

Physical therapy modalities are clearly useful in many aspects of cervical spine management. Modalities of physical therapy can be categorized as follows: cryotherapy, the use of physical cold; thermotherapy, both superficial and deep, the use of heat by any method that provides heat; mechanical therapy, the use of massage, whirlpool, and methods that move the tissues about in a variety of ways; and electrotherapy, stimulation of nerve and muscle by electrical current.

Cervical collars play a relatively small role in stabilizing the spine, but they may remind the patient to minimize neck motion. The cervical spine is particularly vulnerable to loss of function when immobilized. The collar may provide comfort and warmth, psychologic benefit, and marginal control of movement.

### Cervical spine pillows

The use of pillows specifically designed for cervical spine disorders is an important part of management. They usually provide comfort and relief of pain and allow for normal sleep.

A frequent complaint in cervical spine patients is night pain. Correction of poor sleeping posture is often successful in alleviating discomfort. Most people sleep on one or more pillows, promoting long flexion of the neck, with subsequent aggravation of or increase in pain due to muscle spasm. Sleeping with no pillow almost always makes symptoms worse. To sleep prone is to keep the neck rotated, strained, and laterally flexed for long periods. When poor sleeping posture results in head and neck pain, the use of a pillow may be helpful.

Cervical pillows vary in size and types, from air pillows blown up to the thickness that raises the head to the most comfortable level, to a tubular-shaped pillow (Cervipillow), to a multipurpose pillow (Wal-Pil-O). Wal-Pil-O provides four combinations of head and neck support, one of which is proper for almost all cervical spine problems. The Wal-Pil-O cradles the head and supports the neck in both side-lying and back-lying postures. It comprises four pillows in all, with soft and medium centers for head and narrow and wide, firmer borders for the neck.

Another pillow, "The Shape of Sleep," features a neck support ridge that fits under the neck and is a physiologic, biomechanically sound model. A bolster-type pillow is available in several different diameters, and pillows with a contour cutout for the head are also obtainable.

### Cervical spine traction

The usefulness and effectiveness of cervical spine traction are well established; it does cause vertebral distraction. This separation allows alteration of the pathologic relationship between the nerve root and compressing disc or between the nerve root and zygapophyseal joints. About 75% to 80% of patients with radicular symptoms receive clear benefit, usually lasting months to years, from optimally applied traction.

Intermittent traction is the best initial application. The clinical problem may be solved that simply. The weight applied ranges from a minimum of 10 pounds to a

A

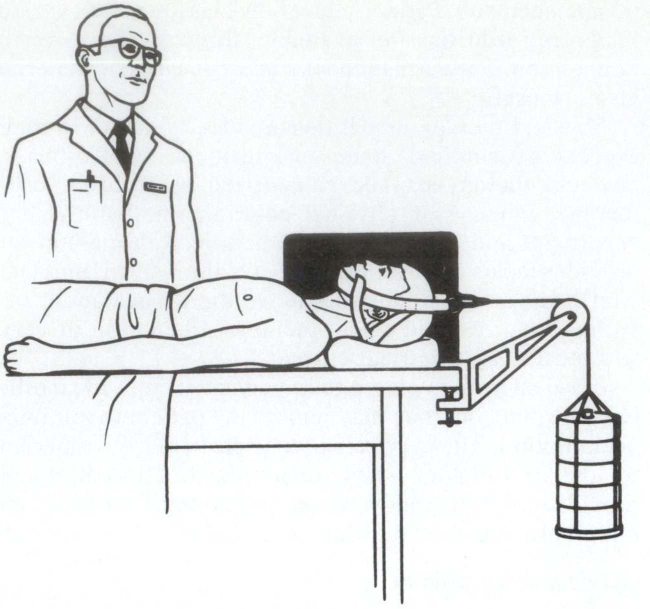

B

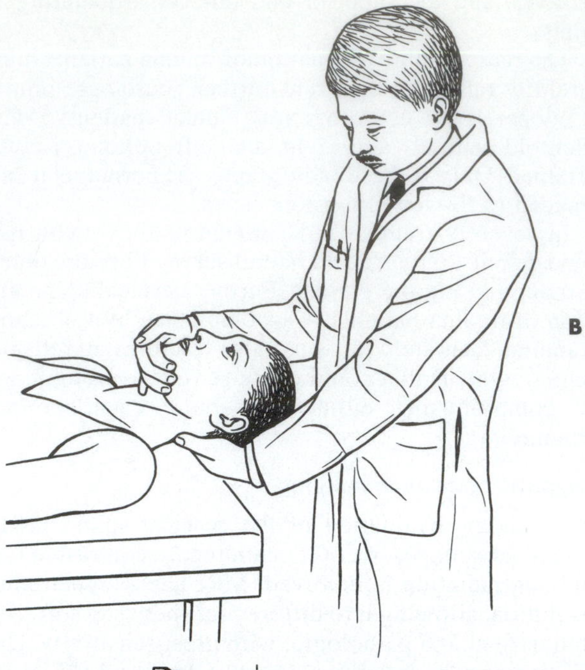

C

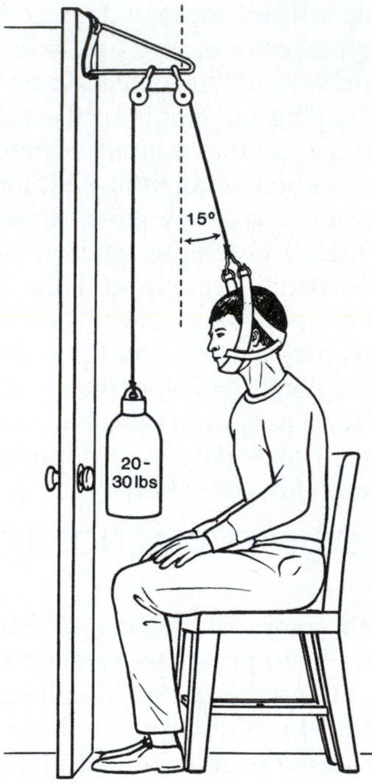


**Fig. 70-4.** **A,** Static cervical traction. **B,** Manual cervical spine traction. **C,** Static home cervical traction.

maximum of 50 pounds (the latter only very rarely) over 15 to 20 minutes. If significant improvement does not occur over 8 to 10 sessions of optimally administered traction, it should be discontinued. If symptoms have clearly worsened, there is little point in continuing traction and the physician should identify precisely why the therapy was not successful.

The amount of weight used in traction is a function of the size of the patient, the presence of neurologic symptoms or signs, the specific lesion for which traction is prescribed, and the patient's general sense of comfort and improvement. The physician is guided by the results of each traction session. With secure improvement, patients may purchase home traction equipment and continue traction under those circumstances until all symptoms resolve. In such cases, the patient should maintain close contact with a medical authority.

Continual traction does not permit the use of as much weight as that permitted in intermittent traction. Increments of weight are added with each traction session, usually beginning with about 10 pounds, depending on the degree of the patient's personally reported progress, or lack of it. Trial-and-error method is the best way to deal with variables such as the distance that the patient sits from the traction pulley, the direction of traction, and the position of the patient during traction. An average level of traction is 15 to 20 pounds for 20 minutes. The patient sits in slight cervical spine flexion facing the door or apparatus, and the angle of the rope is 20 to 30 degrees from vertical. This is a physiologic position (Fig. 70-4, *A*). In general the relief of pain occurs sooner and more completely in patients with radicular symptoms than in those with symptoms arising from the connective tissue structures of the neck itself—ligaments, tendons, muscles, and joints.

Symptoms related to the upper extremities are much more likely to be relieved by traction, whereas symptoms related to the cervical spine connective tissue structures are more likely to respond to other measures. Traction is manipulative therapy, but it is vastly different from adjustments involving rotational and lateral stretches, which pose a greater risk of root irritation.

Cervical traction may be achieved manually. Some authors regard manual traction as preferable because of the immediate sensory feedback to the therapist by the patient and the presumed specificity of treatment (see Fig. 70-4, *B*). In manual traction, one hand is placed under the chin with the other under the occiput, or both hands are placed under the occiput. A longitudinal force is exerted at varying angles of cervical flexion, extension, lateral flexion, and rotation. Degree, direction, and duration of the tractive force are guided by the patient's response, the clinical disorder, and the goal of treatment. Relaxation is urged before initiating traction. The degree to which a patient relaxes can be used as a method of assessing potential response to mechanical traction.

Self-administered or home traction should always be undertaken initially in a teaching session, so that the patient completely understands the procedures and probable perceptions in the process.

Self-traction can be performed with the patient in either supine or sitting position (see Fig. 70-4, *C*). Supine position combines the advantages of increased stability and the possibility of relaxation of muscles.

The angle of traction is between 15 and 35 degrees, depending on the clinical response and the patient's interpretation of its efficacy. The type of head halter used affects the angle of traction provided. The perception of force should be about equal under the occiput and the chin. In most cases slight cervical flexion is preferred because it is the position in which the posterior zygapophyseal joints are separated, the intervertebral foramina are enlarged, and the lateral nerve root canals are released. The application of moist heat before traction is recommended.

Before application of cervical traction, the patient's clinical, historical, and physical data are collected, assessed, and analyzed and the decision for traction made based on these data. Two mechanisms by which cervical spine soft tissues can be damaged and fail are a short duration, high amplitude loading and a long duration, low amplitude loading. The first represents an obvious acute trauma—the classic automobile collision from the rear with "whiplash" injury. The second is a chronic sprain of soft tissues that occurs inconspicuously and gradually, usually with some final event that precipitates a more acute syndrome superimposed on a chronic condition.

### Pharmacologic treatment

Drugs occupy a relatively small place in the management of cervical spine syndromes unless specifically indicated.

### Rest and exercise

Stretching exercises for the cervical spine are used for the same reasons they are used elsewhere in the body: to prevent contracture, to increase range of motion if contracture has occurred, and to maintain biomechanical function of the supporting structures in the cervical spine. Range of motion exercises maintain or increase a limited range of motion. Strengthening exercises are especially important, because the cervical spine is extremely mobile compared to other areas of the body.

## INDICATIONS FOR CONSULTATION

### Neurology

Neurologic consultation is indicated in the following general clinical circumstances:

1. The patient has rheumatoid arthritis of the cervical spine with subluxations associated with definite neurologic symptoms and signs. If the neurologic signs are progressive, the indication becomes urgent.
2. In instances of peripheral neuropathy of unidentified type, entrapment neuropathy at the thoracic outlet, at the elbow, and associated with carpal tunnel syndrome at the wrist; these may be symptoms and signs of cervical myelopathy.
3. Neurosurgical or orthopedic surgical operation is being contemplated for treatment and management of a patient with cervical osteoarthritis—facetectomy, laminectomy, or chondroosteophyte removal.
4. Severe and progressive inflammatory disease of muscle—polymyositis and dermatomyositis.

### Neurosurgery

Neurosurgical consultation may be needed in cervical spine subluxations in rheumatoid arthritis in which surgical stabilization of the spine is required. The following clinical circumstances may require neurosurgical consultation:

1. Rheumatoid arthritis of the cervical spine with subluxations, signs and symptoms of myelopathy, radiculopathy, and peripheral neuropathy.
2. Osteoarthritis of zygapophyseal joints or overproduction of osteophytes in the uncinate processes, or vertebral chondral osteophytes with progressive symptoms and signs identified with it.
3. Cervical spine fractures, particularly fractures in ankylosing spondylitis, rheumatoid arthritis with fracture subluxations or juvenile polyarthritis with soft tissue injury or fracture.
4. Any circumstance of trauma with fracture dislocation or both.

### Orthopedic surgery

The scope of consultative services provided by the orthopedic surgeon and the neurosurgeon overlap.

In general, orthopedic consultation is usually indicated when reconstructive surgery is being considered as in the following:

1. Reconstructive surgery in ankylosing spondylitis, hip, lumbar spine, and cervical spine.
2. Surgical subluxations of the cervical spine in rheumatoid arthritis (various fusions and wiring techniques to stabilize the cervical spine).

## SPECIFIC DISORDERS OF THE CERVICAL SPINE

### Cervical spondylosis (osteoarthritis of the cervical spine)

Osteoarthritis describes all joint involvement in the cervical spine, including all secondary manifestations in vertebrae, tendons, ligaments, capsules, muscles, and hyaline cartilage.

*Genetic factors.* Primary generalized osteoarthritis has strong genetic implications. This disorder is dominant in women and recessive in men. Further hereditary factors occur in ochronosis, calcium pyrophosphate dihydrate (CPPD) crystal disease, gout, and rheumatoid arthritis, all of which may play a role in secondary osteoarthritis. Cervical spine osteoarthritis becomes virtually universal in individuals 50 years of age and older.

Clinical syndromes, symptoms, and signs in osteoarthritis of the cervical spine are conveniently divided into the following five general categories with considerable overlapping: (1) involvement of the joints, intraarticular and extraarticular structures with consequent clinical reflections; (2) nerve rootlets, anterior and posterior nerve roots, principally posterior; (3) compression of the spinal cord, cervical myelopathy; (4) involvement of the vertebral artery by the osteoarthritic process, notably at the atlas-axis-occipital level; and (5) esophageal involvement.

***Joint involvement, intraarticular and extraarticular structures.*** Attacks occur approximately once a year. The patient awakes with severe unilateral pain in the neck; the neck is sometimes fixed by definite deformity; acute torticollis, constant, severe pain, may last 2 to 3 days, with recovery in 7 to 10 days. Pain caused by joint involvement is more likely to arise from the upper cervical spine, whereas pain caused by intervertebral disc osteoarthritis is more likely to arise from the lower cervical spine. These attacks occur roughly from the ages of 35 and 40 to 55 and 60 and gradually become more frequent, depending on the progression of the pathologic events. Pain may be of variable severity and referred to the occipital, retroorbital, and forehead areas. Pain is usually worse in the morning and associated with stiffness, making neck rotation difficult. Moderate to severe unilateral cervical posterior root pain may occur after age 35. It is worse at night, with paresthesias in the hands. Arm pain is at its worst for 2 to 3 weeks, but lasts for 1 to 2 months and subsides gradually. An episode may last about 3 months. When bilateral disc protrusion occurs, pain is present in both upper limbs, and paresthesia occurs in the digits of both hands. Central protrusion may press on the posterior longitudinal ligament and dura mater, becoming adherent, fibrotic, and adhesive and resulting in constant bilateral aching from occiput to scapula. Bilateral disk protrusion occurs mostly in patients 60 years of age or older. Cervical spine motion usually is in only one to three of the six classic movements of the cervical spine; flexion is usually preserved, with limited lateral flexion, extension, and rotation. Painless restriction (painless stiffness) is interpreted as due to osteoarthritis.

Signs of cervical spondylosis include limitation of movement of the cervical spine in all but flexion; tenderness on manual compression of the zygapophyseal joints; and osteoarthritis of zygapophyseal, atlantoaxial, and atlantooccipital joints cause ligamentous contracture.

Radiologic characteristics include zygapophyseal and uncinate processes, and show increased density of bone, varying degrees of chondroosteophytosis, irregular narrowing of joint spaces, and somewhat unusually, pseudocysts. There are no specific laboratory findings. Occasionally, routine radiologic studies are supplemented by CT or MRI.

### Management of cervical spondylosis

- Patient education. The patient is taught the natural history of osteoarthritis of the cervical spine. The majority of patients continue to be functional and effective.
- Exercises. Emphasis should be placed on daily stretching and range of motion exercises. Cervical, thoracic, and lumbar portions of the spine should be included.
- Physical therapy: heat, ultrasound, diathermy, heating pads, infrared lamps, hot wet packs (hydrocollator), hot tub baths, and Hubbard tank.
- Special pillows.
- Analgesic and antiinflammatory drugs, muscle relaxant drugs.
- Special attention to patients with complications of cervical spine osteoarthritis: radiculopathy, peripheral neuropathy, myelopathy, esophageal involvement by osteophytes and vertebral artery compressive syndromes.
- Neurologic, neurosurgical, or orthopedic consultation.
- Traction in selected instances.
- Relaxation techniques two to three times a day, particularly at night.
- Cervical massage.

The prognosis is generally good.

### Neurologic disorders of the cervical spine

The clinical manifestations of nerve root involvement include compression of the posterior root, as well as involvement by viruses such as herpes zoster affecting the dorsal root ganglia. The anterior or motor root is so well protected and anatomically quite low in the intervertebral foramen that it is only very rarely involved; thus most of these syndromes are sensory, involving the posterior nerve root and the dorsal root ganglia.

Sensory changes include perversions of function, pain, paresthesia, anesthesia, hypesthesia, and hyperesthesia, confined to the dermatomes (skin areas supplied by specific cord segments, dorsal roots, or ganglia).

Symptoms of nerve root irritation, termed *radicular,* are increased by motion, coughs, sneezes, strain, nerve root stretching, or any increase in intraspinal pressure. The pain is lancinating in character, intermittent, and rarely constant.

Etiologies for nerve root involvement are osteoarthritis, pachymeningitis, extramedullary tumors, protruded intervertebral discs, extradural abscesses, and a variety of viral disorders and active inflammation (nonspecific, noninfectious granuloma of rheumatoid arthritis). Sometimes muscle spasm alone causes nerve root compression.

Cervical radiculopathy of osteoarthritis may be single or multiple, bilateral, symmetric, or asymmetric; and the magnitude of involvement of each separate root is variable. It also is commonly associated with myelopathy. Clinical syndromes are divided into acute, subacute, and chronic radiculopathies.

***Acute radiculopathy.*** Acute radiculopathy is characterized by an abrupt onset of severe pain and aching in the dermatomal distribution of the cervical root involved. Pain perception is supplied to bone, joints, muscles, and blood vessels, as well as skin; hence the radiation is wide—neck, shoulder, down the arm and forearm, and to the digits. It may extend into the chest anteriorly and posteriorly, especially with C5-7 nerve root involvement. Pain is altered by head or neck position. Scalp, retroorbital, and cervical pains worsen with both active and passive rotation; lateral flexion, extension, and rotation are the most painful. Pain is not worsened by coughing unless there is acute intervertebral disc protrusion. In a few patients, muscular weakness or decreased-to-absent reflexes are seen, reflecting involvement of the motor and sensory root. Atrophy may occur rapidly with fasciculations. Tendon reflexes are diminished or lost.

*Subacute radiculopathy—typical "brachial neuritis."* With this type of radiculopathy, usually more than one root is involved. It is characterized by pain in the neck with associated paresthesias and rather severe muscle spasm. Mild muscle atrophy and hypotonia and muscle weakness are uncommon. Frozen shoulder is a frequent complication, as are tennis elbow and carpal tunnel syndrome.

*Chronic radiculopathy.* This radiculopathy usually follows unaccustomed exercise or work in an awkward position. Symptoms and signs develop insidiously, only partially clearing after an acute attack with lingering pain. Radiologic characteristics include narrowing of intervertebral disc spaces and zygapophyseal joints along with chondro-osteophytes of the uncinate processes. Special studies include electromyography and special radiologic views to identify narrowed intervertebral foramina. Occasionally, an MRI is required.

**Management of radiculopathy**

- Patient education regarding the likely ultimate outcome—usually a good prognosis with optimum management.
- Physical therapy: heat, occasionally cold therapy, one following the other occasionally; gentle stretching and strengthening exercises; range of motion exercises; intermittent soft or hard plastic collar.
- Antiinflammatory drugs, occasional analgesic medication (little or no role for narcotic or potentially addictive drugs).
- Traction judiciously applied with close follow-up; monitor traction according to specific results obtained.
- Cervical spine pillow.
- Massage.
- Occasional lidocaine and corticosteroid injection in areas of pain and spasm.
- Hydrotherapy.

*Cervical myelopathy.* Symptoms are related to ischemia and compression of the spinal cord by osteoarthritic bars, hypertrophied ligamenta flava (posteriorly), cervical disc material anteriorly, and surrounding structures. Clinical symptoms vary greatly.

Disability increases subtly, often preceded by a history of radicular symptoms and recurrent attacks of brachial neuritis. The patient also may experience paresthesias and dysesthesia of hands, weak and clumsy function of hands, weakness in the lower limbs, and vague deep pain in the lower extremities. Numbness and tingling in the tips of the digits occur. The pain is often, but not necessarily, radicular. Gross compromise of touch perception is not usually a feature. However, the patient may have vague impairment of light touch and tactile discrimination, with pin prick sensation diminished to absent. Sensory loss may be one or two dermatomes above the upper segmental level of spinal compression. Vibration sense is impaired or lost below the iliac crest or costal margin. There may be some loss over the digits of the hands. Perception of passive movement in fingers and toes is slightly impaired.

In the case of acute cervical disc protrusion, sudden spinal cord compression may occur associated with severe disabling neck pain and weakness with paresthesias of the upper or of all four extremities. Paresthesias in the soles of the feet are increased by neck flexion.

Onset may be painless and slow. There is difficulty in gait, with upper motor neuron signs affecting both legs. Both hands and feet are paresthetic, with the patient experiencing the sensation of pins and needles from the anterior knees to all toes. Myelography shows protrusions that are often multiple (several sites of compression of the spinal cord). It also shows the occurrence of both chondroosteophyte formation and disc herniation, which is distinguishable only at laminectomy. The posterior longitudinal ligament has adhesions to the dura mater due to proliferative, thick fibroses. Neck flexion causes overstretch and further damage to spinal cord. Pressure on the anterior spinal artery may cause widespread ischemia and cord infarction with paraplegia.

Atrophy of the upper limbs is variable. If upper cervical enlargement is compromised, the supraspinatus and infraspinatus muscles and the deltoid-triceps-biceps-greater pectoral muscles may be involved, as well as the dorsiflexion muscles of the wrists and fingers. If the lower part of the cervical enlargement is involved, most wasting will be in the flexor muscles of the wrist and fingers and in the intrinsic muscles of the hands; wasting is variable. Corticospinal tract involvement is below the level of other involvement if there is coexisting motor radiculopathy. This causes signs of a lower motor neuron region; muscle fasciculation is not conspicuous; spastic weakness of the lower extremity occurs (one leg more than the other); mild generalized wasting as in paraplegia. Muscular wasting and pain may be associated with concomitant osteoarthritis of the lumbar spine.

Tendon reflexes are of great diagnostic importance. A normal jaw jerk with exaggerated tendon reflexes of the upper extremity suggests that the lesion is below the level of the foramen magnum. An exaggerated, diminished, or absent jaw jerk suggests a lesion above the level of the pons.

Tendon reflexes in myelopathy are a function of both upper and lower motor neuron lesions. Compression of the anterior horn cells causes lower motor nerve dysfunction, whereas compression of the corticospinal tract causes upper motor neuron dysfunction. Ultimately, reflexes disappear, but this is preceded by an exaggeration of reflexes, inverted radial reflex, exaggeration of flexor finger jerks, and positive Hoffman and Babinski reflexes. Abdominal reflexes diminish, but are rarely lost; clonus, bowel, and bladder symptoms and signs rarely if ever disappear.

If only the corticospinal tract is involved, symptoms are limited to the lower limbs, with spastic paraplegia and no upper limb symptoms. Rarely, symptoms are motor only, with muscular wasting of the upper limbs and spastic weakness of the lower limbs simulating motor neuron disease. Severe paraplegia or quadriplegia and loss of sphincter control also occur rarely.

Cerebrospinal fluid often shows increased protein content (18 to 125 mg/100ml). Pressure may be elevated and the Queckenstedt test result may be positive. Passive extension of the neck may raise the pressure, indicating partial but not complete block.

Radiologic studies reveal the changes of usual osteoarthritis. Decreased sagittal diameter of the spinal canal in lateral view of plain films also may be noted.

Laboratory data are not usually helpful.

Special studies show narrowing of the sagittal diameter of the spinal canal as measured on standard radiographic film. MRI may be required for precise diagnosis.

**Management of cervical myelopathy**

- Note all features previously discussed with special adaptations for problems of cervical cord compression.
- Surgical therapy is indicated only in unusual circumstances. Extensive laminectomy, foraminotomy, and excision of osteophytes are often unsuccessful.

The natural history of cervical osteoarthritic myelopathy is one of mild disability, and after an initial period of deterioration, a static period may last for several years.

## FRACTURES OF THE CERVICAL SPINE

As a rule of thumb, any patient with a severe head injury should also be evaluated for possible neck injuries. Cervical spine fractures have to be ruled out in any patient who has multiple trauma or is unconscious. Every patient who is seen literally holding his or her head in hands and complaining of neck pain should also be treated as if a fracture were present until proven otherwise. During the initial examination, stabilization of the head and neck is of top priority to prevent further possible spinal cord damage. Patients who have head injuries or are in shock or patients with multiple trauma are frequently combative, requiring restraints. Every emergency room should be equipped with a four poster (rigid cervical collar) or an adjustable cervical collar, which stabilizes the spine until x-rays are obtained.

Fractures of the cervical spine are usually the result of severe trauma inflicted to the head or head and neck. These fractures are usually caused either by an axial load or flexion and rarely result from an extension force acting on the head and neck. Each one of these forces can have a rotatory component that will add to the displacement. The neurologic examination is of the utmost importance in all cervical spine injuries and should be properly documented as soon as the patient arrives at the emergency room. X-rays should include an anteroposterior or a swimmer's view of all the vertebrae including C7. In a swimmer's view, while one arm is abducted to 180°, the other one is pulled down and an x-ray is taken at T1. Frequently oblique views, tomograms, or a CT scan has to be added.

C1 trauma results in the fracture of the posterior arch and/or fracture of the anterior tuberosity that constitute the C1 vertebral body. This injury when not associated with any subluxation or dislocation does not involve any spinal cord damage. The diagnosis can be overlooked if the posterior arch of C1 is not properly visualized. Computed tomographic scans or tomograms are helpful and immediate treatment is immobilization of the spine (Fig. 70-5). Cranial-skeletal traction is preferable until swelling and muscle spasm subside. The neck can then be immobilized in a cervical brace until bony union occurs.

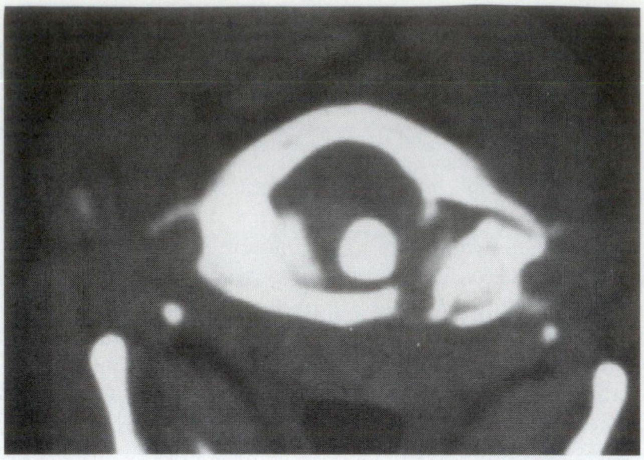

**Fig. 70-5.** CT scan of the C1 vertebra or atlas, showing fracture of the ring structure without compression of the internal neural structures.

## ODONTOID FRACTURES

Fractures of the odontoid have become more frequently recognized, and most of them are reported in relation to motor vehicle accidents. There are different classifications of this fracture. It can be located either high or low on the odontoid process. The fractures that occur in the lower part where the odontoid is essentially part of the C2 vertebral body have a greater incidence of bony union. Fractures that occur at or above the waistline of the odontoid have a high incidence of nonunion. These fractures should be differentiated from a congenital os odontoideum. The latter condition is developmental and indicates failure of union between separate ossification centers. With the exception of the lower type of odontoid fractures, most authors agree that the preferred treatment for these fractures is fusion of C1-C2. The immediate treatment, however, should consist of rigid immobilization in the form of a cervical brace, cranial-skeletal traction, or halo vest, depending on the associated soft tissue injuries. This helps protect against further spinal cord injury.

## HANGMAN'S FRACTURE

Hangman's fracture occurs through the pedicles of C2. This fracture has been associated with capital punishment. In early times the victims died slowly from asphyxiation. To eliminate prolonged suffering, the long drop was employed at hangings for the first time in London in 1784. This resulted in a C2 fracture. The submental knot, applied in judicial hangings, causes a traumatic spondylolisthesis of the axis (C2). This injury can also occur in head-on automobile collisions with the victim's head hitting the windshield, causing extension with fractures of the pars of C2.

When these fractures are associated with severe displacement, the spinal cord is damaged and the patient cannot survive (Fig. 70-6). However, undisplaced fractures are frequently not associated with any neurologic symptoms. Occasionally there is pain along the greater occipital nerve but more often pain in the neck and muscle spasm are the presenting symptoms.

Treatment should be cranial-skeletal traction and then rigid immobilization, usually in a halo vest. Occasionally the traction has to be placed in such a way as to realign minor displacement of the fragments. Surgery is rarely if ever indicated.

A
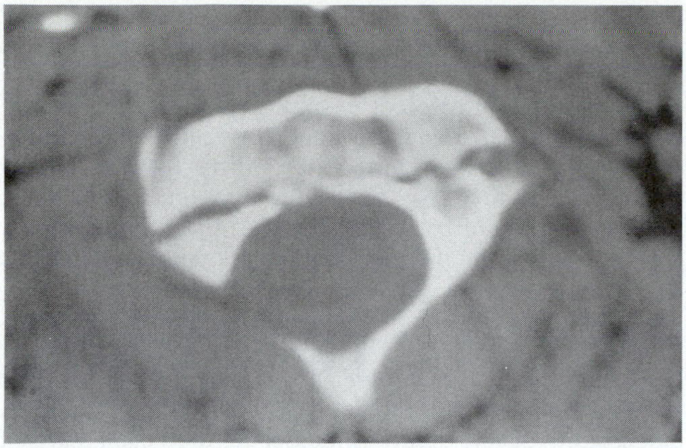

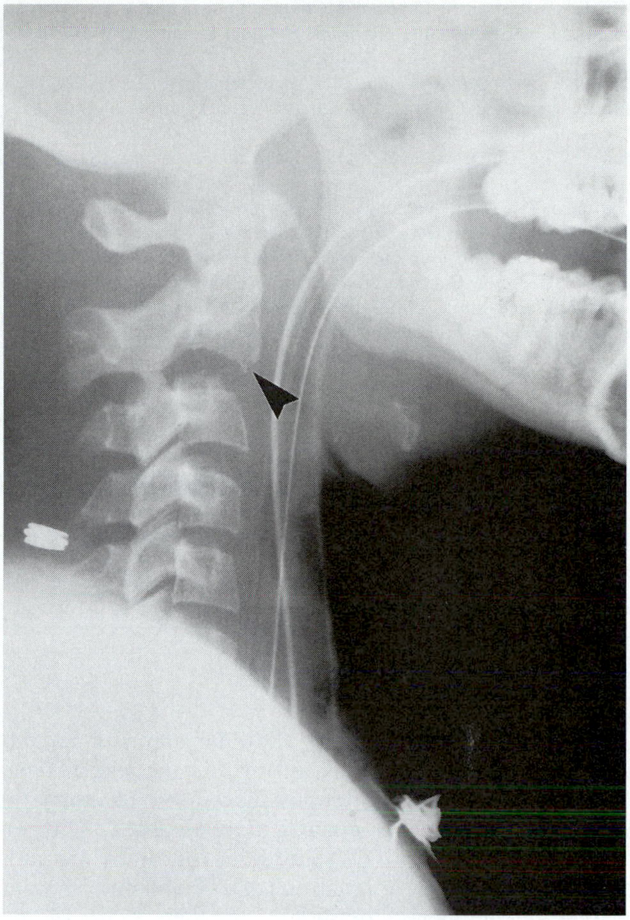
B

**Fig. 70-6.** **A,** CT scan of C2 vertebra or axis, showing a fracture and discontinuity of the ring structure. **B,** Lateral view showing the C2 fracture (*arrow*) complicated by almost total ligamentous disruption between C2 and C3.

## FRACTURES AND DISLOCATION OF C3 TO C7

Injuries to the cervical spine in the area of C3 to C7 can be devastating. They are frequently associated with spinal cord injuries and, depending on the level of paralysis, the extent of the neurologic loss can vary from complete quadriplegia involving paralysis of the upper and lower extremities to high paraplegia with sparing of the upper extremities. The cause for the neurologic deficit is ischemia, bleeding, decreased blood supply, or contusion of the cord followed by swelling and oligemia, which result in necrosis of the spinal cord with complete paralysis below the level of the injury.

The diagnosis is established after careful neurologic evaluation confirmed by x-ray findings.

The first treatment for fractures of the lower cervical spine is immediate immobilization to the fracture in the form of cranial-skeletal traction. It is hoped that this treatment will provide temporary stabilization and alignment of the fracture. The patient may require surgical stabilization of the fracture and, rarely, a decompression laminectomy at a later time.

Surgical stabilization is performed after the patient's general condition has improved to the point that he or she can withstand surgery. Spinal stabilization permits earlier rehabilitation and a reduction in the time the patient must spend at complete bed rest or in a surgical orthosis. Very few patients will require surgical decompression for a cervical spine fracture and surgery does not alter or lessen the neurologic deficit.

Minor, less devastating injuries to the cervical spine include stable fractures without neurologic deficit. An example is the clay shoveler's fracture, which is an avulsion injury of the posterior spinous process.

## ESOPHAGEAL COMPRESSION IN OSTEOARTHRITIS

Osteoarthritis can cause esophageal compression by osteoarthritic chondroosteophytes or by subluxated cervical vertebrae (atlantoaxial subluxation or subaxial subluxation in rheumatoid arthritis).

Dysphagia may manifest as difficulty in initiating the act of swallowing (atlantoaxial subluxation), perception of discomfort or pain during swallowing, and referred pain from esophagus or gastroesophageal junction to the chest.

Evidence of radiologic esophageal compression by anterior chondroosteophytes in osteoarthritis is noted on lateral cervical spine films. Some lesions may be asymptomatic even though they appear grossly compressive. Esophageal compression also can be demonstrated by barium swallow, lateral view of the cervical spine in neutral, flexion and extension positions, and esophagoscopy or gastroscopy if there is any suggestion of ulceration at sites of pressure by chondroosteophytes.

### Management of osteoarthritis

- No treatment is indicated unless the patient has symptoms.
- Apply the many possible therapeutic maneuvers previously listed.
- Surgical removal of anterior osteophytes.

## BIBLIOGRAPHY

Akeson WH, et al: The chemical basis of tissue repair. In Hunter LY, Fink FJ, editors: *Rehabilitation of the injured knee,* St Louis, 1984, Mosby.

Bland JH: *Disorders of the cervical spine: diagnosis and medical management,* ed 2, Philadelphia, 1994, WB Saunders.

Bland JH, Boushey DR: Anatomy and physiology of the cervical spine, *Semin Arthritis Rheum* 20:1, 1990.

Brain WR, Wilkinson M: *Cervical spondylosis,* Philadelphia, 1967, WB Saunders.

British Association of Physical Medicine: Pain in the arm and neck, a multicenter trial of the effects of physical therapy, *Br J Med* 1:253, 1966.
Cailliet R: *Neck and arm pain* ed 3, Philadelphia, 1991, FA Davis.
Hult L: The cervical, thoracic, and lumbar spine syndromes, *Acta Orthop Scand* (Suppl) 17:1, 1956.
Hult L: The Munkfors investigation, *Acta Orthop Scand* (Suppl) 16:1, 1954.
Lawrence JS: Disc degeneration; its frequency and relationship to symptoms, *Ann Rheum Dis* 28:121, 1969.
McKenzie R: *Treat your own neck,* Lower Hutt, New Zealand, 1983.
Shernk HH, editor: Cervical Spine Research Society: *The cervical spine,* ed 2, Philadelphia, 1989, JB Lippincott.
Wilkinson M: *Cervical spondylosis, its early diagnosis and treatment,* Philadelphia, 1971, WB Saunders.

CHAPTER

# 71 Disorders of the Shoulder

John H. Bland

In a general medical practice, shoulder pain is a common complaint in the outpatient setting. As the link between arm and thorax, the shoulder is susceptible to injury that can masquerade as a nonarticular disorder. With the exception of dislocation, shoulder syndromes are more common in the older population (age 40 and on). Shoulder lesions occur more commonly in men than women. Lesions of the cervical spine, nerves, and blood vessels entering the upper extremity and even functional abnormalities of remote structures, diaphragm, and thoracic and abdominal viscera may be perceived symptomatically in the shoulder.

On assumption of erect posture in evolutionary development, primates freed the upper extremity for prehension, sacrificing shoulder joint stability for remarkably increased mobility. No other joint has such extensive, free-ranging mobility. The shoulder joint is strikingly unstable, highly mobile, and continually subject to injury, strain, sprain, and a variety of diseases.

## ANATOMY

Medically, the word *shoulder* means much more than the glenohumeral joint; it includes the intricate and complex mechanism of the entire shoulder girdle, each part of which plays an important role in the coordinated movements of the arm (Fig. 71-1). The term *shoulder joint* is misleading because the shoulder includes three large bones—the humerus, scapula, and clavicle—and four joints—the sternoclavicular, acromioclavicular, scapulothoracic and glenohumeral. Shoulder motion is a summation of movement resulting from synchronous movement of all these joints, no one unit ever moving without the others. The scapula is free floating, suspended by its muscles and having its only connection to the axial skeleton at the sternoclavicular joint. When shoulder movement is started, rhythm and coordinated motion occur as the muscles attached to clavicle, humerus, and scapula increase or decrease in contraction while the scapula seeks its position of greatest stability, the scapular setting phase.

The term *scapulohumeral rhythm* describes events noted on inspection of the normally moving scapula and humerus (Fig. 71-2). Mosely referred to the mechanism of the shoulder girdle as the arm-trunk mechanism. This

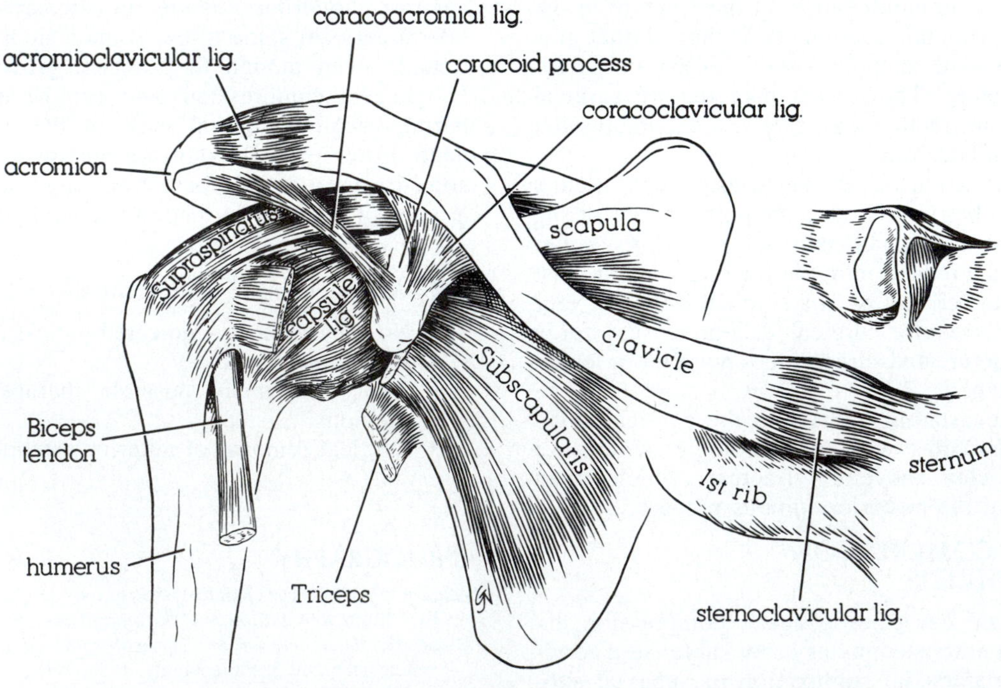


**Fig. 71-1.** Glenohumeral, acromioclavicular, and sternoclavicular joints. The thoracoscapular joint is between the anterior scapular surface and the chest wall.

broad concept allows greater comprehension and interpretation in examination of the shoulder.

The acromion is large and powerful, presumably to stabilize the joint in its function as a non-weightbearing hypermobile, prehensile structure. The acromion functions like the mast of a derrick or crane, providing attachment to the large deltoid muscles. The supraspinatus muscle, relatively small, is used to hold the boom, or the humerus, on the fulcrum, or the glenoid. The clavicle is also like a boom that holds the entire shoulder out away from the body, allowing extensive and remarkable relative hypermobility, adduction, and abduction (Fig. 71-3).

## Muscles

There are three topographic groups of muscles acting on the shoulder: those going from scapula to humerus (scapulohumeral group), those going from trunk to humerus (axiohumeral group), and those going from trunk to scapula.

The scapulohumeral group includes the supraspinatus, infraspinatus, teres minor, subscapularis, deltoid, and teres major. The first four are commonly called the rotator cuff, or the short rotators; the first three insert on the greater tuberosity, and the subscapularis tendon inserts on the lesser tuberosity. The tendons are broad and flat, and about 1 inch in length. It is impossible to dissect the tendons from the capsule; in fact, it is useful to think of the capsule of the glenohumeral joint as being a conjoined tendon containing the insertions of the powerful capsular muscles. The subscapularis and teres major are medial rotators, and the supraspinatus and infraspinatus and the teres minor are lateral rotators. The subscapularis, teres minor, and infraspinatus functional groups depress as well as rotate the head of the humerus (see Figs. 71-1 and 71-4).

The axioscapular group consists mainly of the trapezius, rhomboids, serratus anterior, and levator scapulae. The trapezius rotates the scapula, raising the point of the shoulder and holding the scapula at a certain distance from the vertebral border, important to the setting phase of fixation of the scapula. The serratus anterior and levator scapulae originate on the transverse processes of the cervical vertebrae and upper eight or ten ribs and insert on the vertebral border of the scapula. These muscles are also important for scapular fixation. The rhomboids, antagonists to the trapezius, pull the shoulders backward; they arise from the ligamentum nuchae and the spine of C7 and T1 to T5 and insert on the medial border of the scapula. The trapezius overlies the rhomboids (see Fig. 71-4).

The axiohumeral group consists of the pectoralis major, pectoralis minor, and latissimus dorsi, muscles that connect the humerus to the trunk. The pectoralis major arises from the manubrium and body of the sternum and medial clavicle and inserts into the lateral lip of the bicipital groove of the humerus as well as the capsule. The pectoralis minor arises from the third, fourth, and fifth ribs under the pectoralis major and inserts into the coracoid process. The latissimus dorsi forms the posterior axillary fold and arises from the lower six thoracic vertebrae and

A

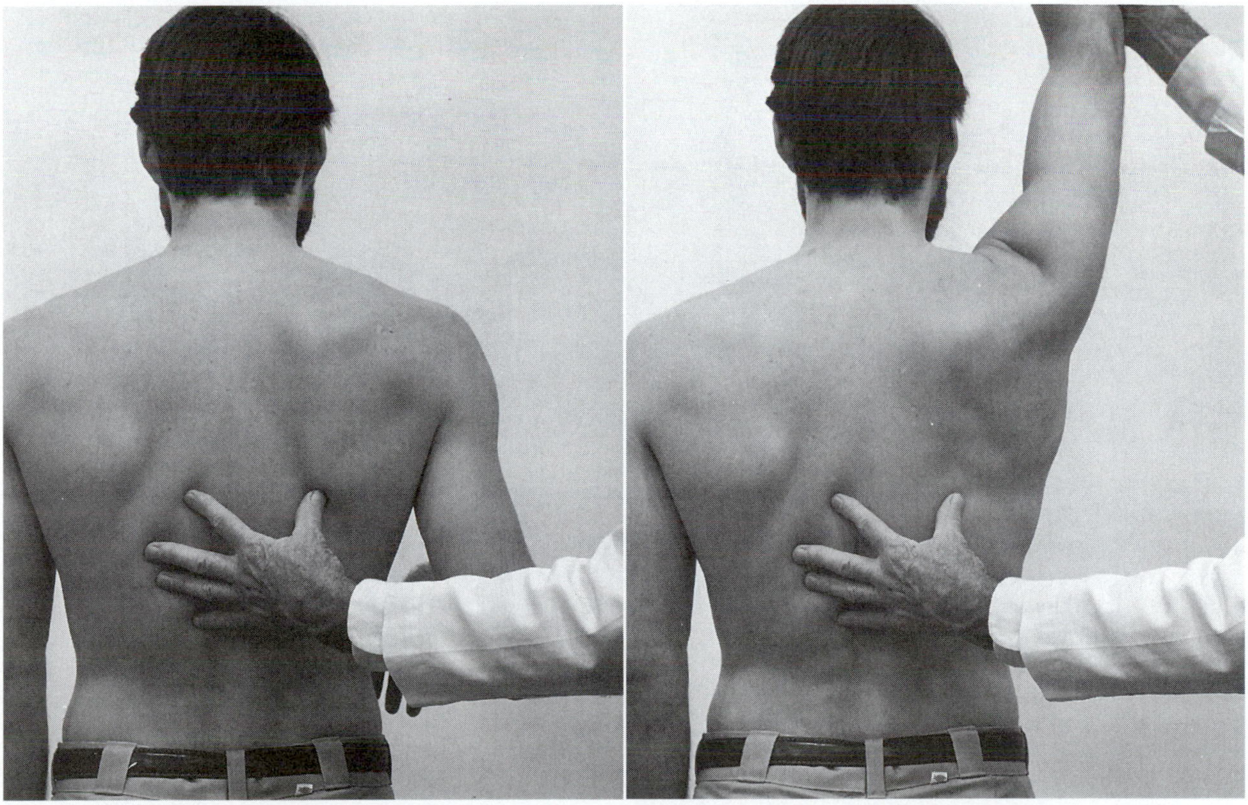

B

**Fig. 71-2. A,** Examiner's thumb is at the inferior angle of the scapula, the bone being somewhat prominent and in slight shrug, with the elbow in flexion. **B,** Scapula has moved anteriorly, upward and laterally on passive abduction, elevation, and hyperabduction. Normal passive scapulohumeral rhythm.

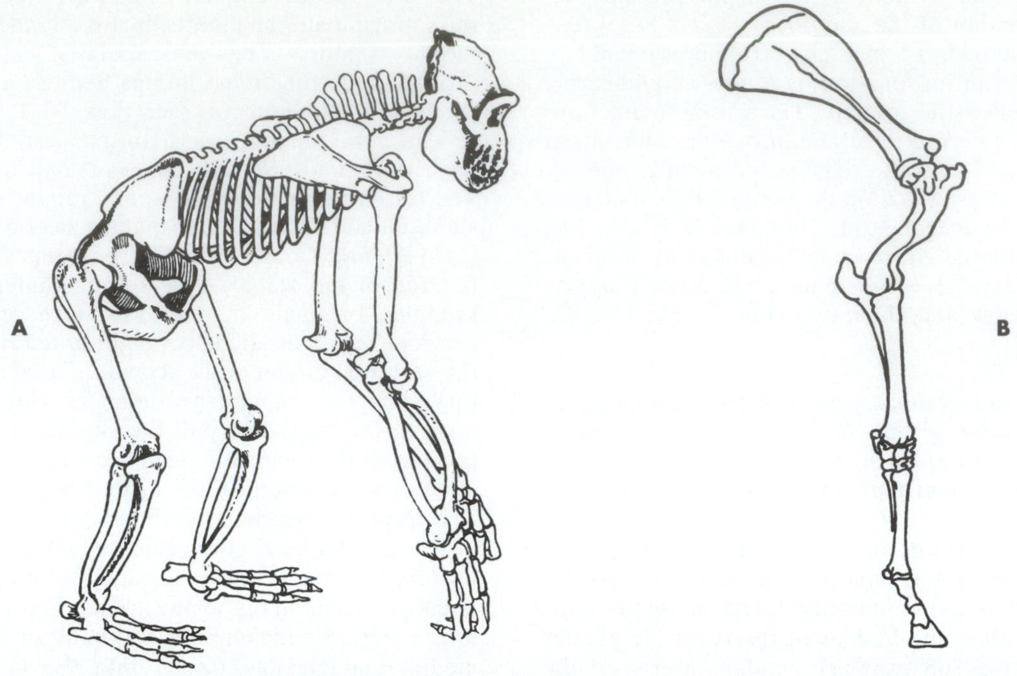


**Fig. 71-3.** **A,** Gorilla shoulder has a massive acromion, a broad scapula, a very large clavicle, a relatively large deltoid muscle, and a small supraspinatus. **B,** Horse shoulder with a long thin scapula positioned on the side of the horse's thorax (rather than posteriorly as in man), no clavicle, a tiny acromion, and a very large supraspinatus muscle that efficiently accelerates the pendulum action of the foreleg. The deltoid is absent. (From Codman EA: *The shoulder: rupture of the supraspinatus tendon and other lesions in or about the subacromial bursa,* Boston, 1934, Thomas Todd.)

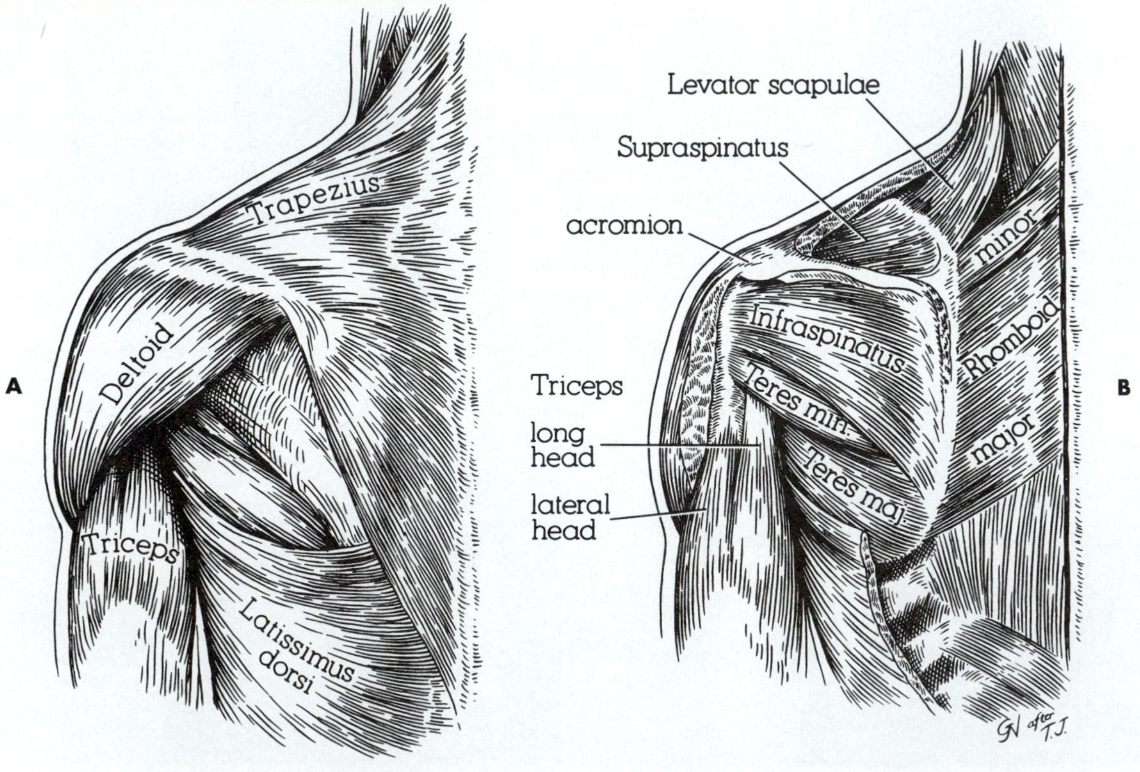


**Fig. 71-4.** **A,** Posterior view of the shoulder. Surface muscles, all groups. **B,** Rotator cuff: subscapularis not shown (medial rotator). Note rhomboids and levator scapula displace the scapula medially toward the midline, while the scapulohumeral group rotates the humerus laterally.

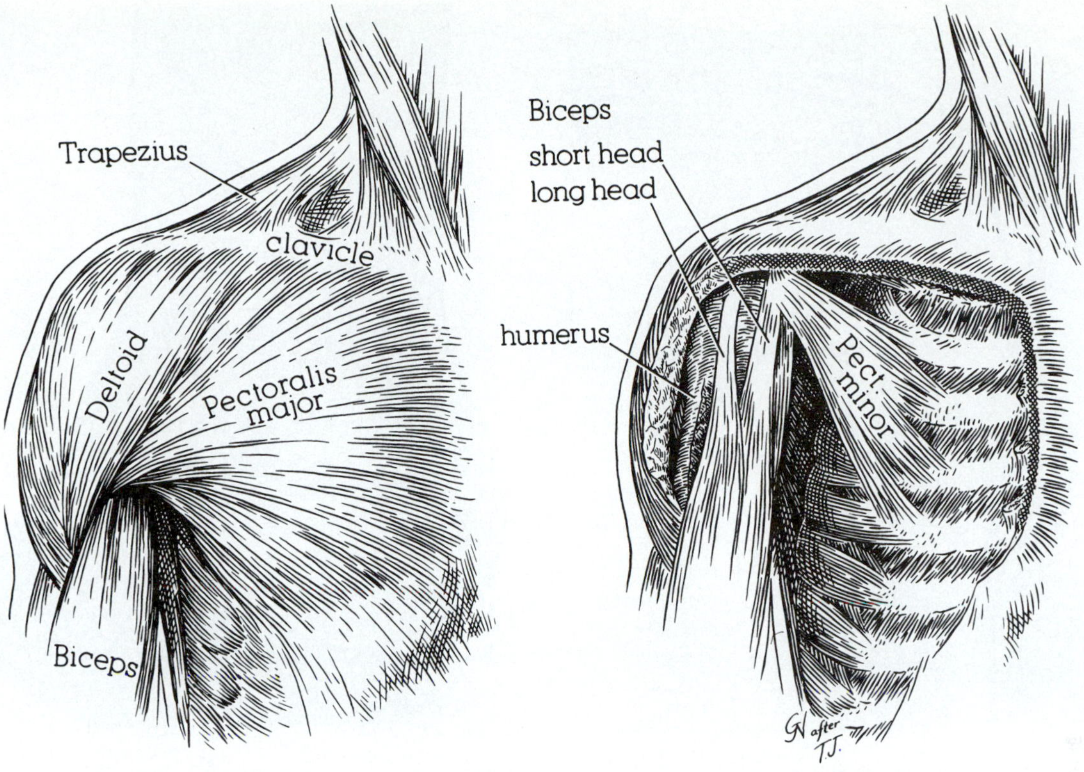


**Fig. 71-5.** Interior view of the shoulder. Surface muscles and deep layer of muscles.

the heavy lumbar fascia and inserts into the floor of the bicipital groove of the humerus (Fig. 71-5).

The biceps and triceps are in a special category, connecting the scapula and the bones of the forearm. If the arm is externally rotated, the bicipital tendon is restored to its original position and can, in fact, abduct the shoulder. The triceps arises by three heads, lateral and medial from the humerus and a long head from the intraglenoid tubercle of the scapula, inserting into the posterior proximal humeral olecranon and the deep fascia on either side of it.

## Bursae

Bursae provide easy gliding movement in areas where there is a great deal of movement but no real need for a complete diarthrodial joint, such as where two muscles cross each other in opposite directions or where tendon or muscle must move on one another without any real articular contact. Synovial sacs, or spaces, are formed allowing smooth gliding movement. The only significant bursa about the shoulder may well be the subacromial bursa, and such designations as subdeltoid bursa, subcoracoid, and supraspinatus bursa describe extensions of the subacromial bursa or the glenohumeral capsule. Some of the subacromial bursal base covers the bicipital grooves; the roof is attached to the underside of the acromion and the coracoacromial ligament. The roof and base are in intimate contact, each lined by a thin synovial membrane. This bursa is an integral and essential component of the shoulder mechanism. The subacromial bursa normally provides a smooth gliding mechanism between the coracoacromial arch above and the rotator cuff tendons below. When bursal surfaces are inflamed, the friction is so painful as to preclude arm abduction or rotation. Adhesive bursitis grossly limits serviceable motion (Fig. 71-6).

## Coracoacromial arch

The coracoacromial ligament is a tough, triangular structure joining the coracoid and the acromion, overhanging the humeral head anteriorly (Fig. 71-7). The combination of the bony acromial roof and this ligamentous arch protects both the rotator cuff tendons and the humeral head from direct trauma. However, the close relationship of the humeral head in abduction reduces the space available for rotator cuff tendons to glide beneath. Chronic impingement and tendon attrition with or without calcific tendinitis may result in a painful arc on abduction. The subacromial bursa may be secondarily inflamed by calcific deposits in the tendon, ultimately rupturing into the bursal sac or rotator cuff. Tendon tears may result in spread of inflammation to the bursa (see Fig. 71-6, *A*).

## Articular capsule

The capsule of the glenohumeral joint has a demonstrated volume twice as large as that of the humeral head, allowing for the unusual mobility as well as some obvious instability. The capsule arises from the glenoid labrum and its surrounding bone and inserts into the upper part of the anatomic neck and into the periosteum of the humeral shaft. It is lined with synovium, which may be reflected along the neck of the humerus, around the periphery of the articular cartilage. Synovial membrane extends into the lining of the biceps tendon sheath, which is an extension of the joint cavity.

Some areas of the fibrous capsule are thickened to ligamentous proportions. The coracohumeral ligament

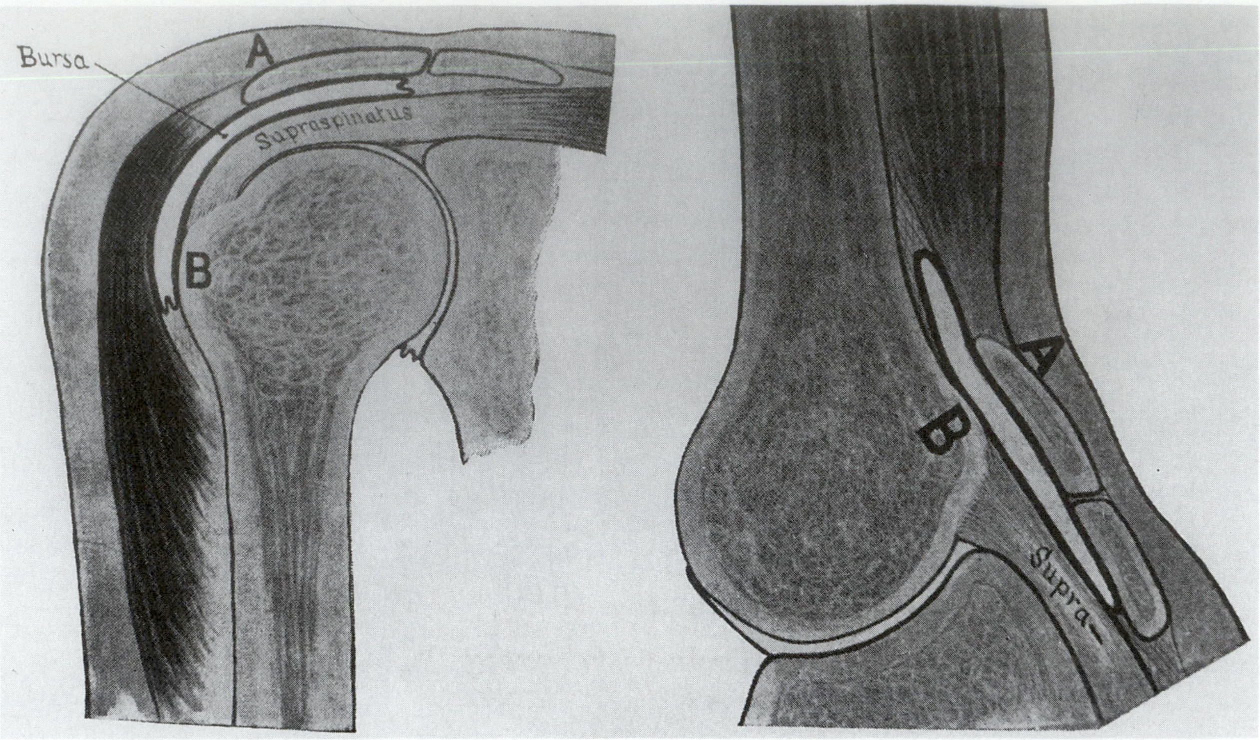


**Fig. 71-6.** (*Left*) Subacromial bursa in normal anatomic position. Supraspinatus insertion. After normal anatomic position: acromion *(A)* and the greater tuberosity and supraspinatus insertion *(B)*. (*Right*) Position of the bursa in extreme abduction; deltoid muscle *(A)* and greater tuberosity of the humerus *(B)*.

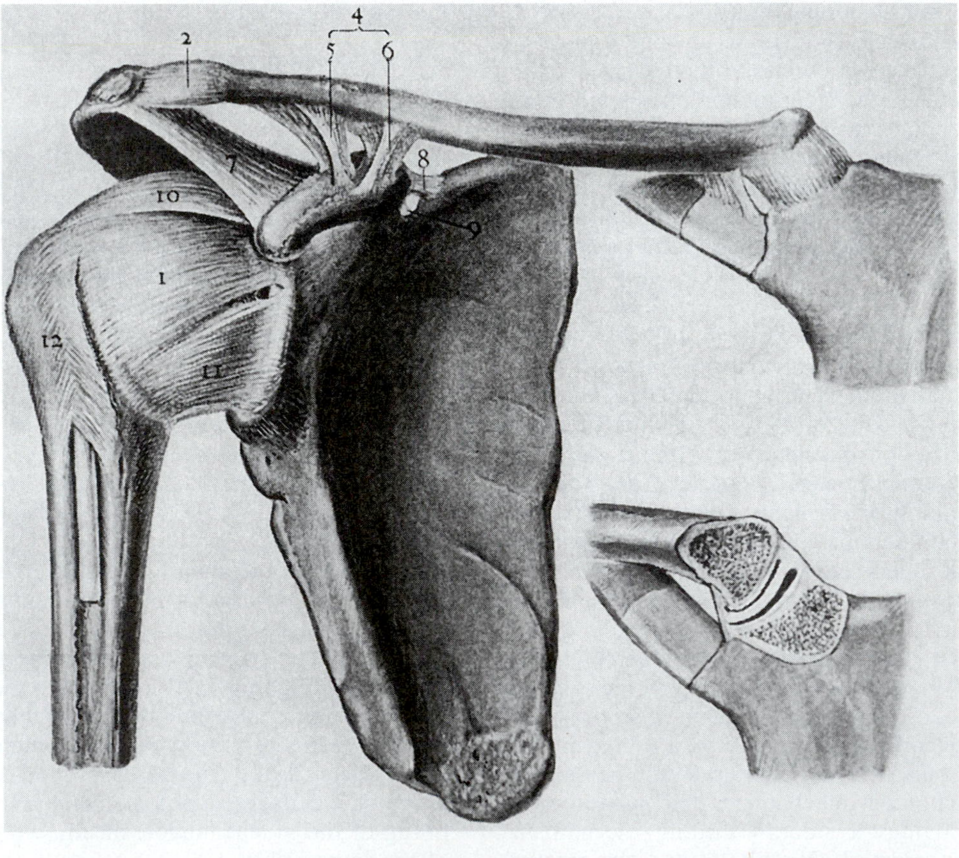


**Fig. 71-7.** Ligaments of the shoulder joint. *1,* Capsule blends with rotator cuff tendon; *2,* acromioclavicular ligament; *4,* coracoclavicular ligament; *5,* trapezoid ligament; *6,* conoid ligament; *7,* coracoacromial ligament or arch; *8, 9,* superior and inferior transverse ligament; *10,* coracohumeral ligament; *11,* glenohumeral ligament; *12,* transverse humeral ligament.

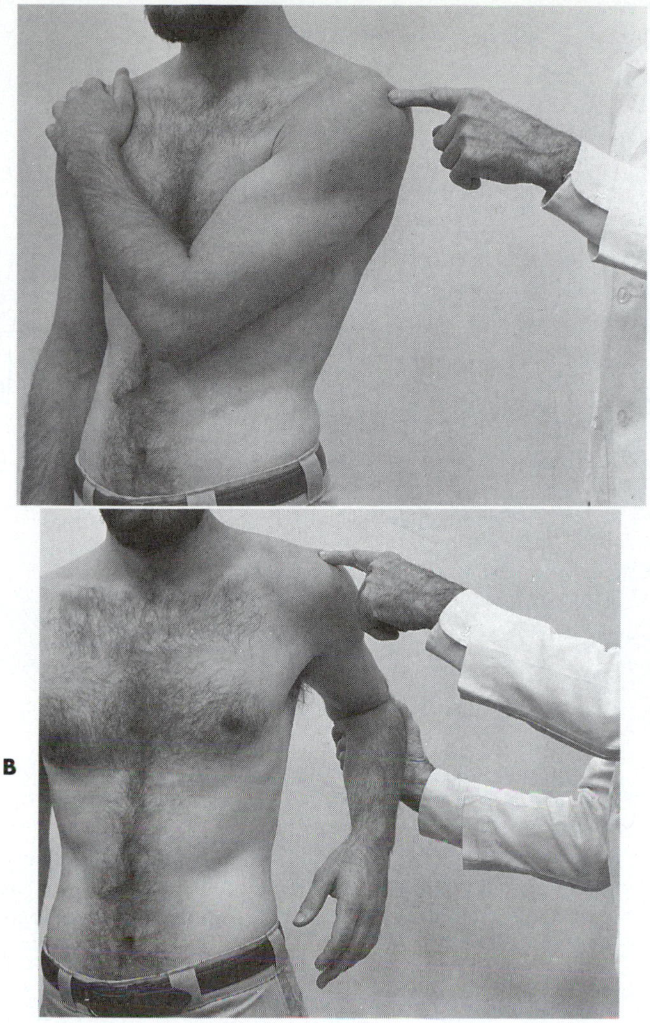


Fig. 71-8. A, Examiner palpates under the shelving edge of the posterior acromion for tenderness of the rotator cuff or swelling and tenderness of the subacromial bursa. B, Anterior aspect is exposed to the examining fingers with the arm in extension or with the hand behind the back in marked medial rotation.

arises from the lateral edge of the coracoid process and extends over the top of the humerus to insert on the greater tuberosity. The capsule thickens anteriorly, forming the superior, inferior, and middle glenohumeral ligaments. These ligaments have quite variable recesses formed between them, sometimes being quite large and redundant. If the fibrous capsule is attached to the neck of the scapula rather than the glenoid, a large anterior pouch appears. The middle glenohumeral ligament is absent or too thin, and anterior dislocations may occur (Fig. 71-8).

### Glenoid fossa

The scapular glenoid fossa, shaped like an upside-down comma, broad below and narrow above, is surrounded by the glenoid labrum, a fibrocartilaginous rim giving stability to the glenohumeral joint. The articular surface of the humeral head is oriented posteriorly, medially, and upward; only a fraction of the surface is in contact with the glenoid surface at any one time. The greater tuberosity directed laterally forms the outer wall of the bicipital groove, and the lesser tuberosity forms the inner wall. New bone formation in and about the bicipital groove may result in damage, fraying, and even rupture of the long head of the biceps tendon.

### Blood supply

There are six major arteries supplying the shoulder: the suprascapular, anterior circumflex humeral, and posterior circumflex humeral are always present; the thoracoacromial, suprahumeral, and subscapular arteries are present less often. There is an area of rather severe undervascularization in the distal part of the supraspinatus tendon, just proximal to its insertion in the greater tuberosity. The infraspinatus and subscapularis tendons may also show hypovascularization but do so much less frequently. This is called the critical zone, and the pathogenetic assumption is that this ischemic area is subject to cellular hypoxia, fiber tears, release of lysozymes with further destruction of tendons, and spread of traumatic inflammation. Such areas have limited repair potential for attritional tears. A further contributing force to tendon damage is the sharp angulation of the rotator cuff tendons over the humeral head, with vessel compression in the tissue of the tendon.

### Nerve supply

Only two sensory nerves supply the shoulder region: the axillary, or circumflex, and the suprascapular. The axillary nerve goes to the anterior surface of the capsule, sending branches into the joint from below. The suprascapular nerve separates from the superior division of the brachial plexus, goes laterally and downward under the trapezius muscle to the upper border of the suprascapular notch, passes under the supraspinatus muscle, and penetrates the infraspinatus fossa, there dividing into terminal branches. The nerve supplies the superior and posterior portion of the joint capsule, most of the tendon sheath, and the acromioclavicular joint. Both nerves supply the coracoclavicular, coracoacromial, coracohumeral, and glenohumeral ligaments. The long thoracic nerve sends a branch to the coracoid process and the acromioclavicular joint. Cartilage and bone are not very pain sensitive, but the tissues of the shoulder can be listed in decreasing degree of pain sensitivity: tendons, bursae, ligaments, synovial tissue, joints, their capsular reinforcements, muscles.

## CLINICAL ANALYSIS

### History

Elicitation of detailed history, is of the utmost importance. Details of the history should include type of onset, location of initial pain, pain behavior from onset, history and nature of injury, type and degree of pain, rapidity of onset, magnitude of disability, spread of symptoms and their precise timing, true appearance of reproducible signs, factors relieving or aggravating it, effect of position, relationship to time of day or night, effect of passive or active movements, and presence or absence of neurologic symptoms or signs.

Attention should be paid to the age of the patient, habitus, occupation, body type, posture, and mental and intellectual status. Emotional tension, complaint threshold, anxiety states, and hysteria affect shoulder complaints.

The following historical points are explored:

1. *Pain location.* Pain is most commonly in the lower

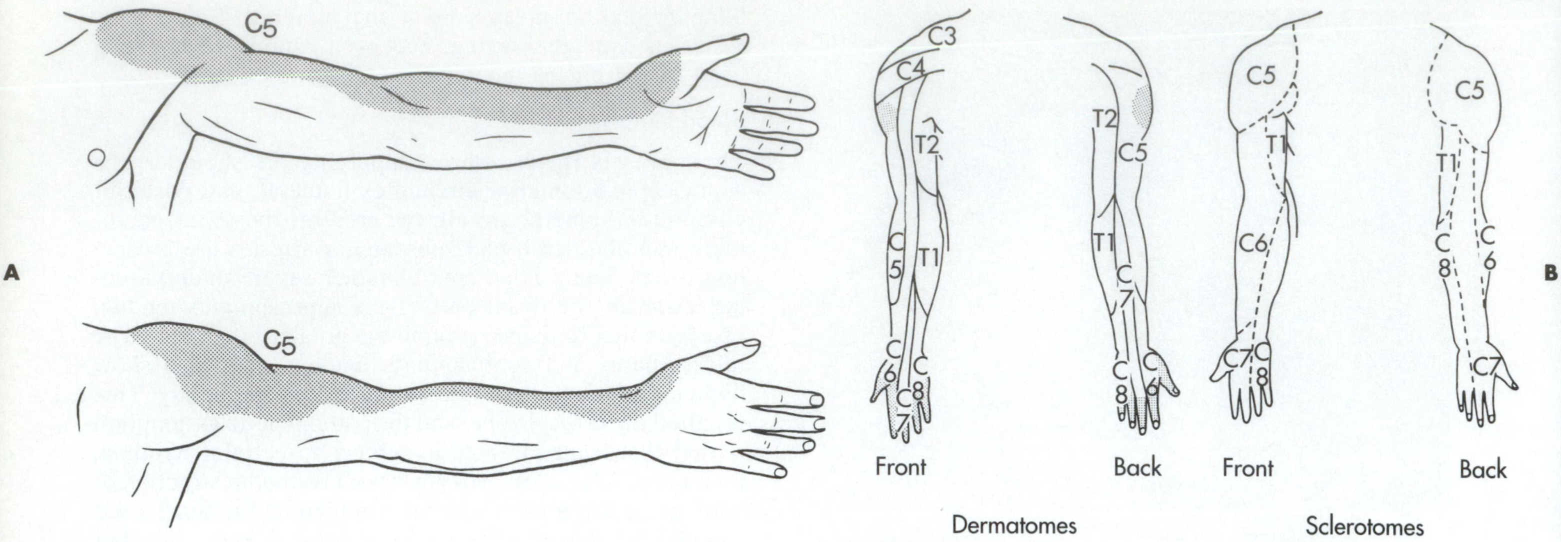


**Fig. 71-9.** C5 sclerotome distribution of pain. (**B,** from Lance JW, McLeod JG: *A physiological approach to clinical neurology,* ed 2, Reading, MA, 1975, Butterworth.)

part of the deltoid area, the referral area for the supraspinatus tendon. Though the lesion may be only millimeters in size, the pain can be great, often involving most of the deltoid area and the proximal arm. Pain at the acromioclavicular joint area means disturbance in and about that joint. Pain in any other part of the arm, shoulder, or neck or in the C5 sclerotome is common to all other possible shoulder lesions (Fig. 71-9).

2. *Duration of symptoms.* Initial symptoms in supraspinatus tendinitis are pain in the deltoid insertion area initiated by abduction, especially active but also on passive abduction. Spread of inflammation to the subacromial bursa is characterized by extension of the pain to the distal arm and into the forearm. Pain involving the forearm as far as the wrist indicates that the process has spread to the capsule and has been present for 3 to 6 months. If the entire arm is painful and there is marked limitation of motion, the inflammation has spread to involve the capsule and synovium, and a frozen shoulder is developing or already present.
3. *Other joint involvement.* This suggests rheumatoid arthritis, gout, or some systemic rheumatic disease.
4. *Preceding injury.* Osteoarthritis rarely involves the shoulder primarily. If preceding injury has occurred, osteoarthritis may gradually develop. Tears in the supraspinatus tendon or capsule and other injuries to the shoulder may appear later, well after the primary injury.
5. *Pattern of pain and its behavior from onset.* The more the arm is involved by pain, the more extensive is the lesion. Tendinitis evolves into subacromial bursitis, which becomes capsulitis and then synovitis.
6. Is it painful to lie on the side of the affected shoulder? If so, it suggests supraspinatus tendinitis or some part of that syndrome.
7. Spontaneous pain without aggravating event? Spontaneous pain indicates an extensive spread, from tendinitis to bursitis and later capsulitis.
8. Head, neck, chest, or upper abdominal pain? These suggest a lesion apart from the shoulder, such as diaphragmatic hernia, cervical spondylosis, or cardiac involvement.

### Physical examination

Inspection should include the head, cervical spine, shoulder, arm, forearm, wrist, and hand, including the area the patient designates as the painful site. Note the effect of gravity (Fig. 71-10).

***Cervical spine.*** The cervical spine should be examined by active flexion, extension, lateral flexion, and rotation to determine if any of these movements causes pain. Second, carry out passive flexion, extension, lateral flexion, and rotation of the cervical spine to determine if these movements produce the characteristic pain. The aim is to determine whether mobile structures—muscles and tendons—are pain sensitive or whether capsules, ligamentous structures, joints, osteophytes, and anterior and posterior longitudinal ligaments are the source of pain.

Ask the patient to flex, extend, laterally flex, and rotate the cervical spine against resistance, the aim being to identify pain-sensitive structures by selective tension. These maneuvers identify lesions of the origin and insertion of muscle.

***Shoulder.*** Inspection anteriorly, laterally and posteriorly of the shoulder is an important aspect of the examination. Comparison with the unaffected side is informative.

Observations of scapulohumeral, claviculohumeral, and arm trunk rhythm may be revealing and often diagnostic. Characteristics to look for are atrophy, loss of muscle tone, fasciculations and fibrillations, and reflex and

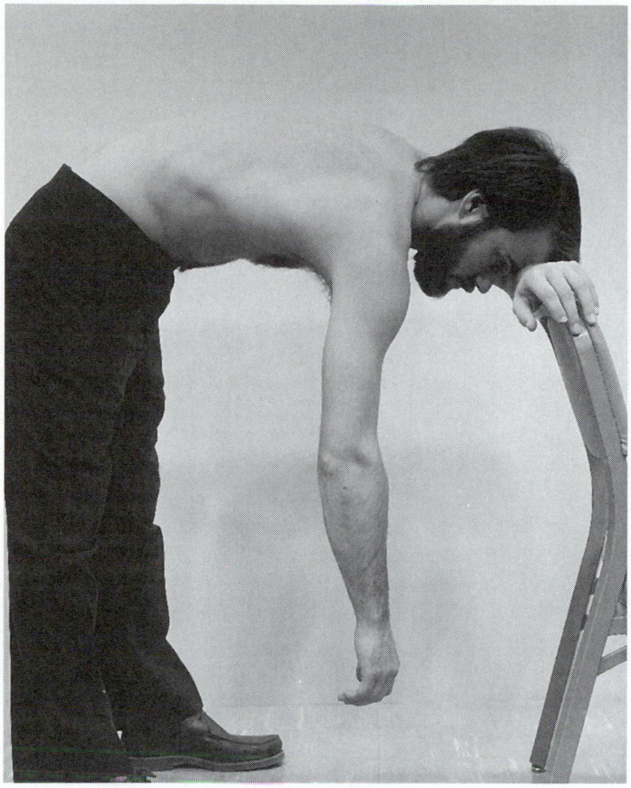

**Fig. 71-10.** Note that the effect of gravity on shoulder (full trunk and hip flexion) separates pain-sensitive structures, relieving pain.

sensory changes. The entire upper limb should be inspected for color change, swelling, skin alteration, and abnormal posturing.

Next a full range of active motion is inspected. Shoulder flexion, extension, adduction, abduction, and medial and lateral rotation are observed anteriorly, posteriorly, and laterally, especially noting the upper trapezius. Note whether or not abduction is accomplished by shrugging, and observe the clavicular movements. Posterior inspection centers on the scapular motion, the scapulohumeral rhythm, the lower angle of the bone moving out or in as it seeks stability. At 45 degrees or so the outward movement accelerates laterally, forward, and upward as the serratus anterior muscle acts. Fig. 71-11 shows normal complete abduction and scapular rotation.

If the glenohumeral or acromioclavicular joint is fixed, the humerus and scapula move as one, and abduction to as much as 60 degrees occurs by the shrugging mechanism (i.e., elevation of the entire shoulder girdle). The lateral view focuses on the deltoid muscle. A look from above with the patient seated is helpful, with occasional inspection in supine and prone positions to see the relaxed musculature and conformation of the shoulders.

The full range of the above motions is noted passively, with the examiner lifting the shoulder and arm through its motions. Full passive motion, gently and slowly done, is common in shoulder problems, even with marked limitation of various active ranges of motion in the presence of muscle and tendon lesions. In tears or ruptures of the rotator cuff active abduction may be impossible or grossly limited, whereas with assisted complete passive motion abduction to 90 degrees can be shown. However, when the support is removed, marked weakness in holding the abduction is noted—the drop-arm sign. By fixing the scapula, glenohumeral restriction in movement is readily shown. Rotation of the humeral head in the glenoid should be shown both in adduction and abduction (to 90 degrees). One must distinguish humeral rotation from pronation and supination of the hand.

Last demonstrate the ranges of motion against resistance to study lesions of the origin and insertion of tendon and ligament.

***Palpation.*** All landmarks are palpated: sternoclavicular and acromioclavicular joints, the coracoid process, the spine of the scapula and clavicle, the acromion about its periphery, the rotator cuff and the muscles of the shoulder joint, adductors, latissimus dorsi, teres major, pectoralis major and minor, and the deltoid. The posterior aspect of the rotator cuff is readily palpable with the arm adducted across the chest, the anterior and upper portions by placing the arm in extension with and without adduction behind the back in medial rotation.

Acromioclavicular lesions are detected by the presence of pain in the superior aspect of the shoulder, by referral to the neck and jaw, plus local joint tenderness, exaggerated by adduction of the arm across the chest.

Crepitus is elicited by placing the palm of the examiner's hand over the top of the patient's shoulder with the other hand rotating the humerus at various angles of adduction, abduction, and rotation. Crepitus is generally indicative of severe rotator cuff disease with secondary osteoarthritis of the glenohumeral joint.

The painful arc is pain production at about 60 degrees abduction with freedom from pain before and after this level, indicating impingement of the greater tuberosity under the acromion, an instance in which there is a supraspinatus tendinitis with or without calcific deposits (Fig. 71-12).

***Special procedures.*** In rotator cuff lesions most muscles about the shoulder develop varying degrees of spasm, itself a source of pain. The pain frequently disappears in full trunk and hip flexion allowing the arm to hang limp, separating by the weight of the arm the inflamed area from the acromion and the coracoacromial arch. The muscles then relax on passive swinging and pendular movements of the arm, so-called pendulum exercises (see Fig. 71-10).

In instances of partial rupture the patient is asked to swing the arm forward and the examiner holds it there, the patient then returning to an erect position with the arm in full abduction, or elevation. Thus the shoulder can be put through a full range of painless motion. Pain in rotator cuff tendinitis may also be relieved by supporting the forearm in flexion, putting the arm at about 30 to 40 degrees abduction, and exerting gentle traction downward. Mosely called this test the depression of the head, and it has diagnostic usefulness.

Lidocaine (Xylocaine) infiltration in the tissues of suspected involvement is often helpful, diagnostically and therapeutically. In rotator cuff tears, with the pain gone, painless movements are possible and a determination of loss of power can be made. With normal movement and power after Xylocaine infiltration the outlook for successful nonsurgical therapy is good.

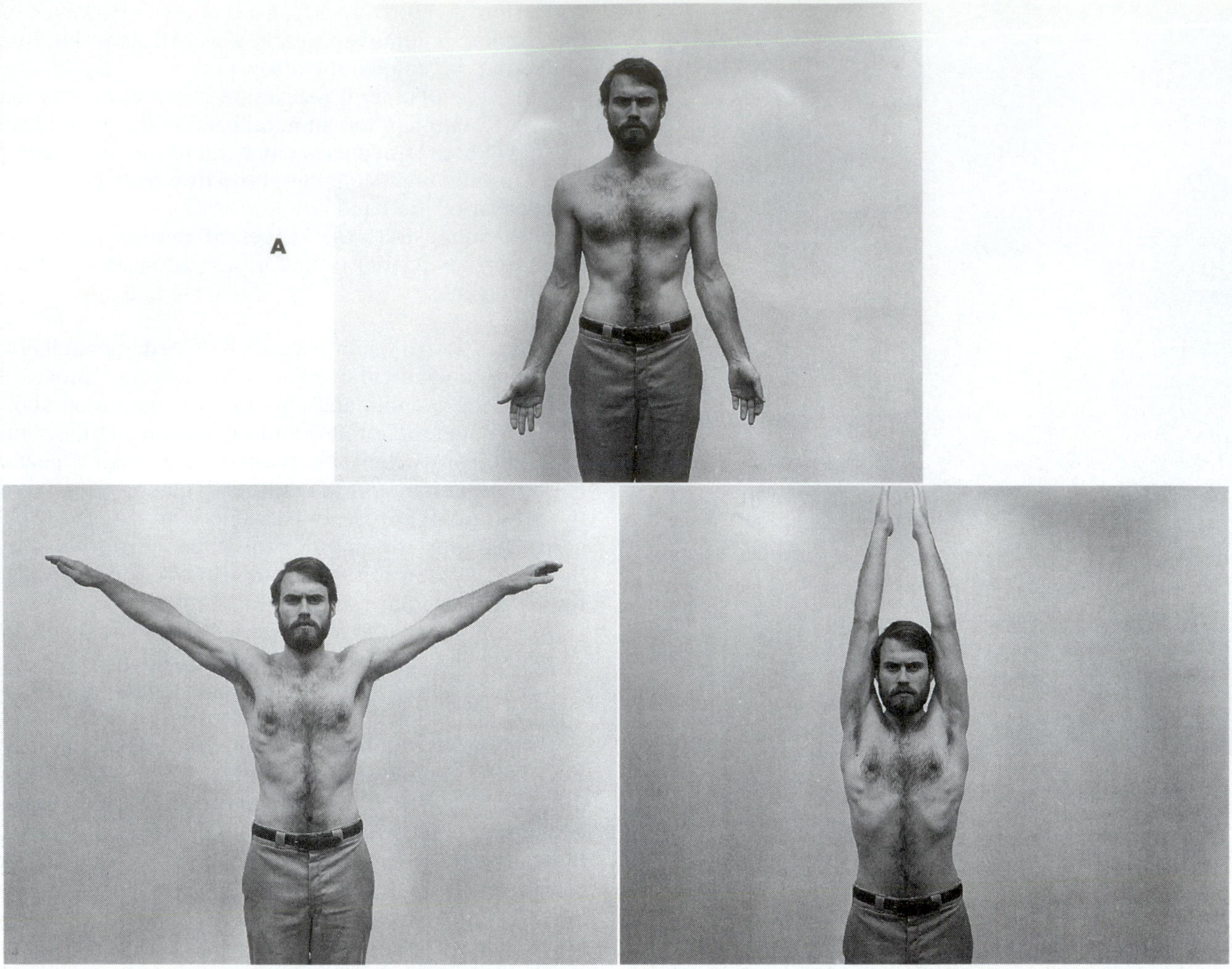

A B C

**Fig. 71-11. A,** Normal anatomic position. **B,** Arms abducted just above 90 degrees until humeri are medially rotated (palms facing down). The next 60 degrees abduction cannot occur. **C,** Note palms facing, scapulae have rotated allowing 60 degrees more; finally the last 30 degrees with distal arm touching the head are achieved by abduction of the humerus across the front of the scapula, the coracoid, and the acromion.

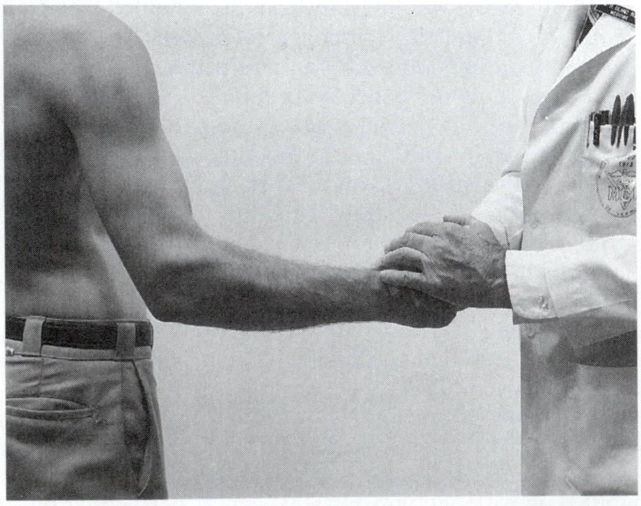

**Fig. 71-12.** Note the right arm abduction to just 30 degrees when pain was felt.

## Systematic clinical plan

A systematic and orderly clinical approach to identification of the pain-sensitive structure generally leads to a precise diagnosis and successful management in the great majority of cases. With the exception of the acromioclavicular joint (derived from the C4 sclerotome embryologically) all structures of the shoulder, which include subacromial bursa, capsule, synovium, glenohumeral joint, periosteum, biceps tendon (long head), and rotator cuff muscles and tendons, are derived entirely or partially from the C5 sclerotome, and thus shoulder pain originating in any structure is perceived only in its distribution (see Fig. 71-9, *A*). Pain arising from structures deep to the deep fascia is referred in a segmental distribution not following the dermatome distribution. The area of pain is always very large, severe, never perceived at the site of the lesion, and always distant. Rhomboid muscle irritation causes severe transient pain over the shoulder region anteriorly and posteriorly following the deep segmental sensory distribution of the fifth cervical root. Irritation of the periosteum of the humerus near the capsule insertion causes diffuse, severe pain over the same segmental area. Thus in disorders of deep structures—muscles, ligaments, capsules, tendons, fascia—broad intrasegmental distribution of pain occurs. Hence, pain caused by shoulder lesions is felt in some part of the C5 sclerotome. Pain may also arise as referred pain from the cervical spine, intrathoracic structures, diaphragm and even intraabdominal structures, as noted later.

Initial approach to the patient is that of a survey of all the segments possibly involved. Pain occurring in the scapular area, the shoulder, or anywhere in the arm indicates a lesion in one of the tissues forming the C5 to T2 sclerotomes (see Fig. 71-9, *B*). Thus a survey of the segments from neck to fingertips tells the examiner whether there is a lesion of tissues in and about the shoulder, a lesion perceived in the shoulder but not arising from shoulder tissues, or pain referred from a distant site, visceral or somatic; hysteria, anxiety state, and psychoneurosis are detectable through clinical inconsistencies. The patient is first asked to actively flex, extend, laterally flex, and rotate the cervical spine; next to shrug the shoulders maximally and actively elevate the scapula (C3 to C4); next the shoulder is taken through a full range of active motion (C5); then the elbow is examined in flexion, against resistance and in extension against resistance to study C5 to C7; next the wrist is examined in resisted extension (C6) and resisted flexion (C7); then the thumb is examined in resisted extension (C8) and resisted adduction (C8); last, the fifth finger is examined in adduction against resistance (T1). The patient is instructed during all these maneuvers to describe pain occurring at any point; weakness, production of paresthesias, and neurologic symptoms are likewise sought.

At the end of these movements the examiner should have a fairly clear idea of whether the tissues of the shoulder are the cause, whether tissues peripheral to that area are involved, or whether the problem is nonorganic or psychogenic. The following 12 movements, systematically done, determine the pain-sensitive structure:

1. *Elevation of the arm.* The arm is abducted to 90 degrees and the patient notes pain in the process. The glenohumeral joint abducts normally to 90 degrees, at which point the greater tuberosity impinges under the coracoid and the coracoacromial arch. The next 60 degrees of elevation are due to scapular rotation, and the last 30 degrees constitute adduction of the humerus across the front of the scapula; the coracoid and acromion processes now point upward instead of forward (see Fig. 71-11). Psychogenic symptoms can be identified in this process, since the degree of elevation minus 60 degrees represents the abduction range at the glenohumeral joint. If marked discrepancy is noted later, psychogenic mechanisms may be invoked.
2. *Passive elevation.* The examiner goes through the same motions as noted in step 1. Pain is noted and the end feel is observed (i.e., whether the movement comes to a hard or soft stop at the extreme of the range, a perception that comes with experience).
3. *Painful arc.* The patient abducts the shoulders. Pain between 60 and 120 degrees indicates impingement between the acromion, the greater tuberosity, and the supraspinatus tendon (Fig. 71-12).
4. *Passive scapulohumeral abduction.* The thumb is placed at the lower angle of the scapula to determine whether it moves. The other hand elevates the arm until the examiner feels the scapula begin to rotate. This occurs normally at 90 degrees (see Fig. 71-2).
5. *Passive lateral rotation.* The patient's elbow is bent at a right angle and the forearm as a lever rotates it outward in the sagittal plane. Normal range is 90 degrees; range, end feel, and pain are noted.
6. *Passive medial rotation.* The examiner rotates the humerus medially, noting how far behind the patient's back the forearm can be placed. Normal range is 90 degrees; restriction and pain are noted.
7. *Resisted abduction.* With the elbow tight against the body, the patient is asked to abduct against resistance by the examiner, who prevents the joint from moving. Resisted abduction examines the deltoid and supraspinatus. Since the deltoid muscle rarely if ever has painful lesions, pain with abduction generally indicates supraspinatus tendinitis (Fig. 71-13, *A*).
8. *Resisted medial rotation.* With the elbow fixed against the body, the patient is asked to rotate medially against resistance, testing pectoralis major, teres major, latissimus dorsi, and subscapular muscles (Fig. 71-13, *B*).
9. *Resisted lateral rotation.* This rotation tests the infraspinatus and teres minor muscles; if lateral rotation results in pain, only the infraspinatus tendon is at fault (Fig. 71-13, *C*).
10. *Resisted adduction.* This adduction tests the thoracohumeral group of muscles (Fig. 71-13, *D*).
11. *Resisted flexion at the elbow.* Resisted flexion tests biceps and brachialis, but if supination against resistance is painful, the lesion is bicipital.
12. *Resisted extension at the elbow.* This extension tests the triceps function (Fig. 71-13, *E*).

**Shoulder range of motion.** The shoulder lends itself well to measurements of range of motion. Clinically useful are extension, 35 degrees from neutral; flexion, 95 to 100 degrees from neutral; adduction, 25 to 30 degrees; abduction, 90 degrees before gross scapular movement; medial and lateral rotation, either from neutral or 90 degrees abduction and 90 degrees both ways. A practical clinical method of recording progress is to observe points that the patient can touch on the body. In the superior plane place the hands behind the head and brace the elbow backward as far as possible; with palms facing and extending maximally vertically over the head, arms touch the sides of the head; in the inferior plane note the dorsum of the hand reaching variably up the back, the buttock, the small of the back, or up between the shoulder blades, all reflecting varying degrees of shoulder mobility (Fig. 71-14).

**Survey of degree of power.** Each muscle or muscle group can be tested for power by having the patient make the

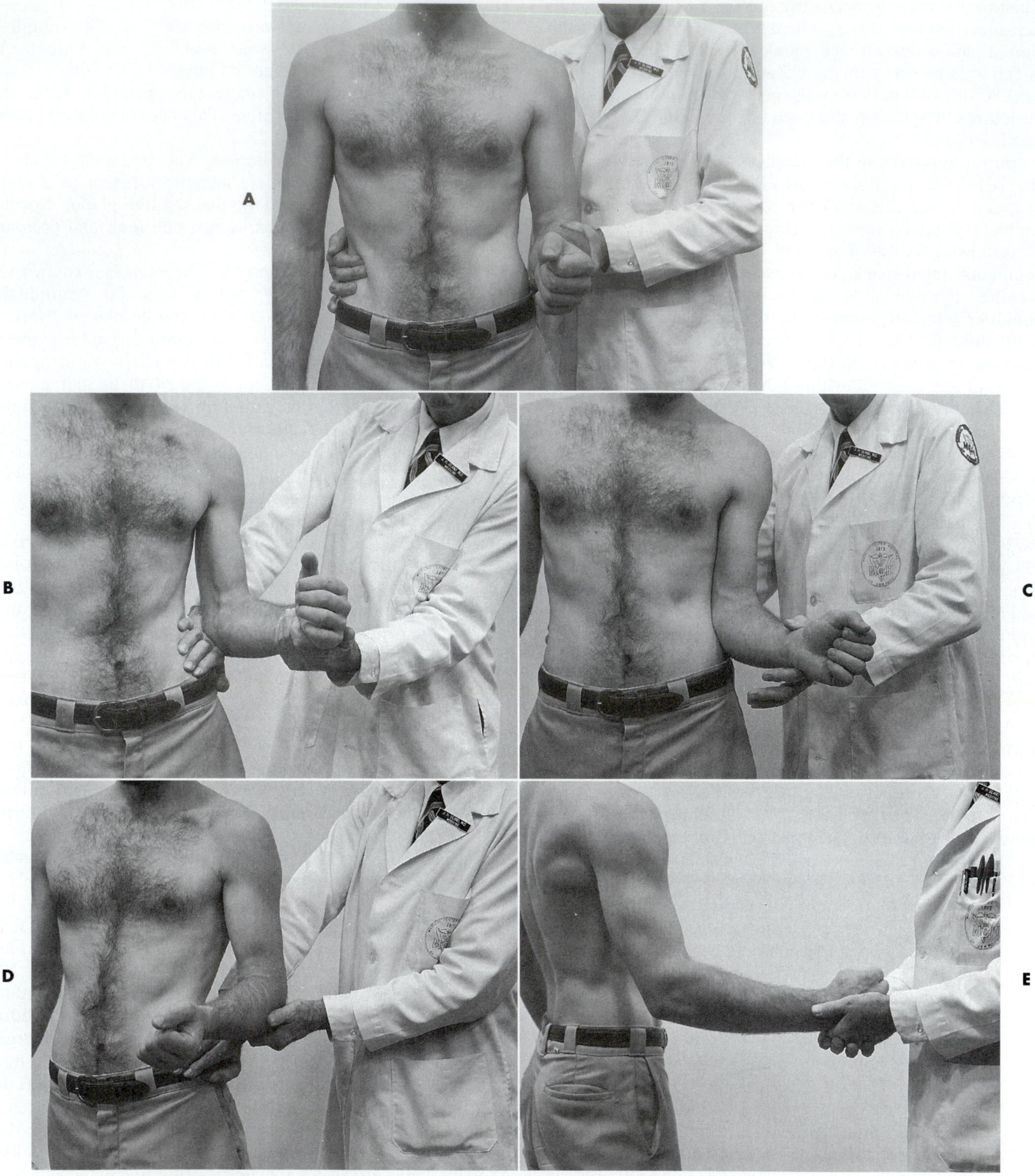


**Fig. 71-13.** **A,** Abduction against resistance; supraspinatus muscle and tendon; **B,** medial rotation against resistance; subscapular muscle and tendon; also pectoralis major, teres major, and latissimus dorsi; **C,** lateral rotation against resistance; infraspinatus and teres minor; **D,** resisted adduction; thoracohumeral muscle group; (*not shown*) flexion against resistance at the elbow; if supination against resistance is painful the lesion is bicipital; **E,** extension against resistance at the elbow; triceps.

A, B

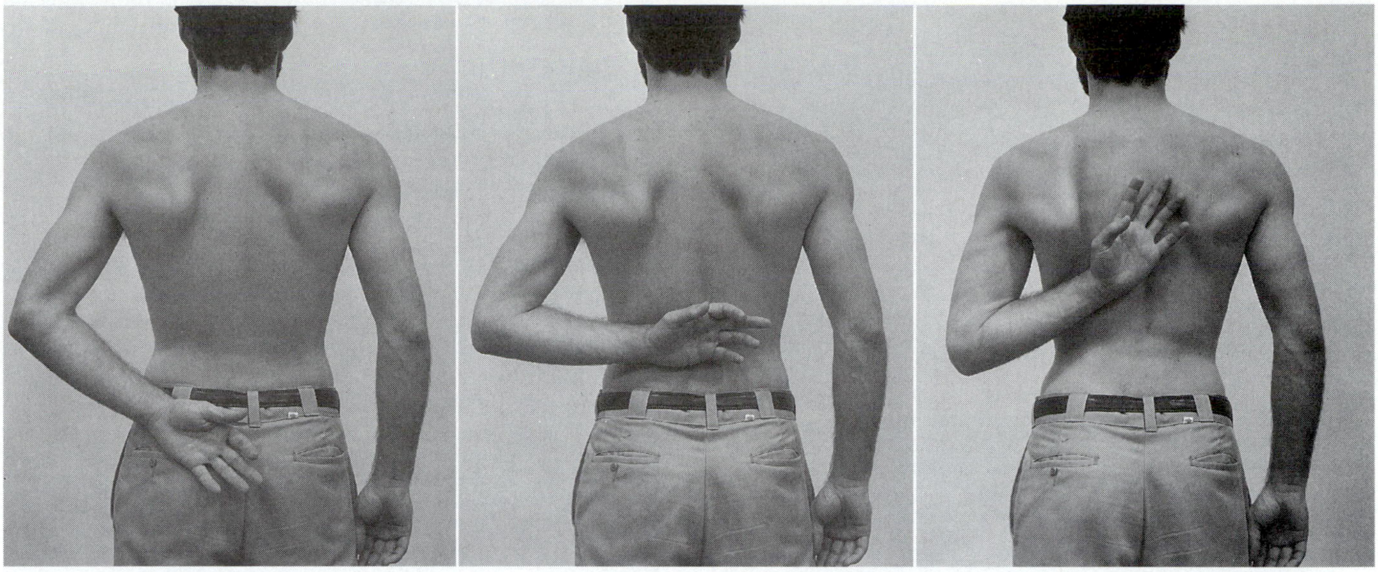

C

**Fig. 71-14.** Parameters of progress. **A,** Hand at buttock only. **B,** Hand can reach to the flank. **C,** Hand can reach to the interscapular area.

appropriate effort against resistance. Weakness may be due to loss or impairment of nerve supply, rupture of tendons, or pain too severe to allow movement.

***Laboratory studies.*** Few laboratory studies are needed in studying the painful shoulder. Erythrocyte sedimentation rate (Westergren), latex fixation, antinuclear antibody, serum calcium, phosphorus, alkaline phosphatase, quantitative immunoglobulins, culture of joint fluids, synovial fluid analysis, and various metabolic and endocrine studies may be helpful in the diagnosis of rheumatoid arthritis, thyroid and parathyroid disease, septic arthritis, and neoplasms involving the shoulder.

***X-ray of the shoulder.*** Most shoulder problems are diagnosed and treated using history and physical examination. For more difficult presentations or cases of tendinitis with persistent disability x-ray study is useful.

**Plain films.** The standard views are anteroposterior (AP) with the beam centered on the coracoid process with both medial and lateral rotation views of the humerus. These views document and locate a calcific deposit in the cuff or in the bursa (Fig. 71-15). Plain films may suggest a full-thickness rotator cuff tear. Note the subluxation of the acromioclavicular joint in Fig. 71-16, *A,* as the patient laterally rotates the arm. The freed humeral head drives the acromion upward. Full-thickness tears may show simply as a narrowing of the acromiohumeral gap. Superior migration of the humeral head is a direct consequence of the loss of supraspinatus function (Fig. 71-16, *B*). The acromioclavicular joint is best studied with the beam passing anteroposteriorly with 30 to 35 degrees angulation upward.

A chest film offers diagnostic clues to the origin of shoulder pain. It may reveal a cervical rib, an old clavicular fracture with malalignment, or an apical lung tumor (Pancoast tumor).

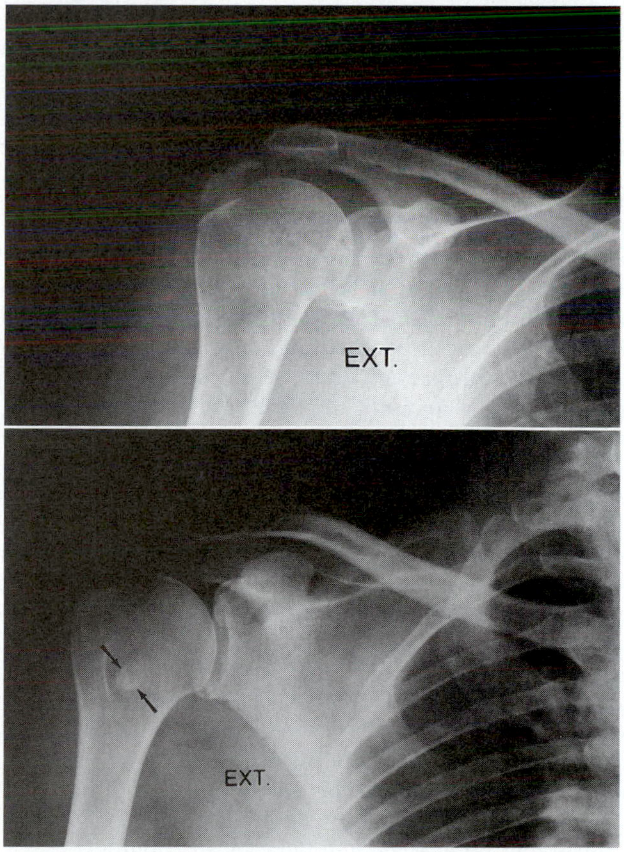


A

B

**Fig. 7-15.** **A,** Calcific tendinitis localized by anteroposterior x-rays. Supraspinatus tendon with extensive calcific deposit. **B,** Subscapularus tendon with calcific deposits; deposit moves across the front of the humeral head on medial rotation.

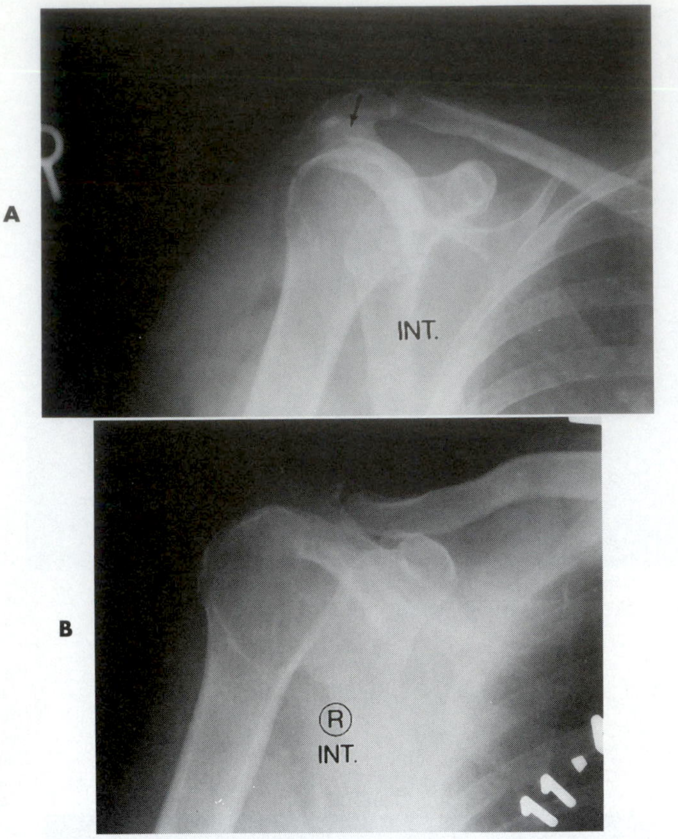


**Fig. 71-16.** **A,** Normal film in lateral rotation. **B,** Two years later the humeral head is elevated. The patient had a full-thickness tear.

### Impingement syndrome

**Clinical characteristics**

Sudden incapacitating or dull ache; painful arc as arm is abducted and elevated forward
Tenderness in anterior edge of acromion and bicipital groove
Instillation of short-acting local anesthetic in subacromial space obliterates symptoms, confirming diagnosis

**X-ray findings**

Normal stage I
Sclerosis, periostitis, cyst formation in stage II; traction osteophyte under surface acromion
Narrowing of acromiohumeral gap, superior subluxation of humeral head in relation to glenoid; erosions of anterior acromion; arthrography shows full-thickness tear and communication between joint space and subacromial bursa

**Treatment**

Stage I: rest, graduated exercise; strictly avoid immobilization (risk of adhesive capsulitis); stretching and strengthening exercises; aspirin or other nonsteroidal antiinflammatory agents
Stage II: all of the above; local injection of anesthetic and corticosteroid (recommend combination of 3 ml 1% lidocaine, 3 ml 0.5% bupivacaine, and 20 mg triamcinolone; (i.e., short-acting anesthetic for diagnosis, long-acting anesthetic for analgesia, and a steroid preparation in depot form)
Stage III: all of the above; anterior acromioplasty

**Contrast study.** Shoulder arthrography demonstrates the shape and capacity of the glenohumeral joint space. It is the only way to distinguish between complete and incomplete tears of the rotator cuff. Complete ruptures can be surgically repaired. Arthrography may be helpful in adhesive capsulitis and recurrent shoulder dislocations. It is not helpful in bicipital rupture.

## THE PAINFUL SHOULDER

Pain syndromes arising from structures in and about the shoulder joint suffer from an unfortunate surfeit of names in textbooks and the published literature, with subsequent confusion of terminology, diagnosis, and treatment. The following syndromes refer to the same basic process: supraspinatus tendinitis, rotator cuff tendinitis, subacromial bursitis, subdeltoid bursitis, painful arc syndrome, calcific tendinitis, calcific bursitis, and impingement syndrome.

Overlapping and usually following these are a group of names also referring to the same process: periarthritis, adhesive capsulitis, frozen shoulder, adhesive bursitis, periarticular adhesions, and check rein shoulder.

The great majority of painful nontraumatic lesions and syndromes about the shoulder are due to tendinitis of the rotator cuff. There are four rotator cuff tendons inserting into the greater and lesser tuberosities. The long head of the biceps tendon passes through the intertubercular groove to insert on the superior rim of the glenoid. The supraspinatus tendon is usually the first and ultimately most involved of the cuff tears. The initial lesion is almost always a localized supraspinatus tendinitis with subsequent extension to other members of the rotator cuff and the subacromial bursa, later extending to the joint capsule and intraarticular and extraarticular structures leading to frozen shoulder. The pathologic process of rotator cuff tendinitis may be a continuum of inflammation, degeneration, and attrition of the rotator cuff by impingement on the anterior edge of the acromial process, the coracocromial ligament, and sometimes the acromioclavicular joint. The wear and attritional tears of the cuff occur on the supraspinatus tendon and may extend into the infraspinatus tendon and the long head of the biceps tendon. See the box above for the stages of impingement. Most cases of rotator cuff tendinitis improve with time, and there is a good case for very conservative management.

Some experts conclude that stiff and painful shoulders all improve irrespective of treatment, whereas others strongly advocate localized steroid injections in all cases of both intracapsular and extracapsular lesions affecting tendons, their sheaths, and bursae.

The term *periarthritis* has become an umbrella term to describe inflammatory syndromes involving all structures about the shoulder. It describes a continuum of pathology with many subsets of sufficient clinical distinction to separate them, culminating in the frozen shoulder. Most physicians with primary interest in shoulder syndromes

### Differential diagnosis of the painful shoulder

**Musculoskeletal syndromes**

Supraspinatus and rotator cuff tendinitis and tenosynovitis
Calcific tendinitis of rotator cuff and biceps tendon
Calcific periarthritis involving multiple sites
Rotator cuff rupture, partial or complete (full thickness)
Bicipital tendinitis and tenosynovitis
Bicipital rupture, long head, partial and complete
Subacromial bursitis (almost always secondary to tendinitis and tenosynovitis)
Capsulitis, adhesive, secondary to tendinitis and bursitis
Frozen shoulder
Myositis, fasciitis, muscle contracture, and adhesions in and around the shoulder
Osteoarthritis, usually secondary, arcromioclavicular, glenohumeral, osteophytic overgrowth in bicipital groove and sternoclavicular joints
Primary septic arthritis (rare)
Scapulothoracic syndromes
- Coracoclavicular disruption
- Fibrositis (fibromyalgia)
- Scapulothoracic grating
- Scraping scapula

**Trauma**

Acromioclavicular separation, partial or complete
Direct capsular injury
Dislocation with secondary trauma to soft bursa
Fractures of scapula, clavicle, and proximal humerus
Nerve injuries
Various injuries: automobile, athletic, vocational

**Systemic disease**

Rheumatoid arthritis or other nonspecific inflammatory arthritis
Septic joint superimposed on rheumatic disease
Metabolic and endocrine disease
- Hyperthyroidism
- Myxedema
- Acromegaly
- Hyperparathyroidism
- Chondroclavicular disease and pseudogout
- Gout

**Reflex sympathetic dystrophy (shoulder-hand syndrome)**

believe that the continuum can and should be interrupted and reversed before it reaches the extreme of this disabling condition.

Inflammation of the supraspinatus or bicipital tendon may spread by contiguity to the tendon sheaths, other tendons, and their sheaths (tenosynovitis), the bursa, capsule, synovium, cartilage, bone, and all immediately surrounding muscles (Fig. 71-17).

The box above lists the differential diagnosis of shoulder pain. Uncomplicated supraspinatus tendinitis and tenosynovitis (with or without extension to other members of the rotator cuff) and bicipital tendinitis and tenosynovitis are associated with the normal range of passive motion. Involvement of the capsule (adhesive capsulitis), the bursa, muscles, and synovium is associated with a

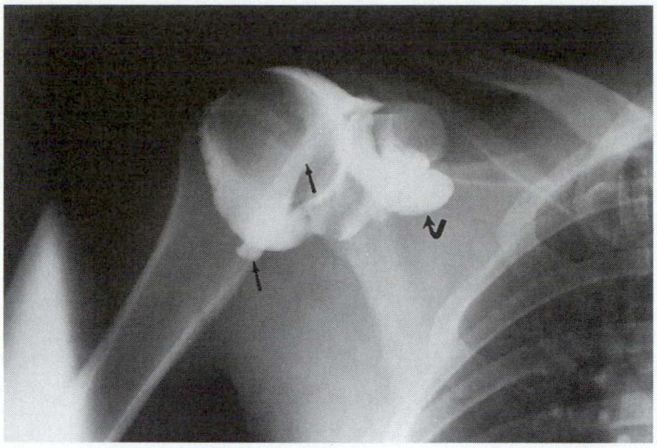

**Fig. 71-17.** Normal study. Note dye in the biceps sheath (*straight arrows*) and in the subscapular recess (*curved arrow*).

limited range of motion. It is important to make this distinction on initial examination.

## SUPRASPINATUS TENDINITIS, TENOSYNOVITIS, AND ROTATOR CUFF LESIONS

The first pathologic event occurs in the supraspinatus tendon where, after the fifth decade, there is almost always thinning, fraying, fissuring, and fibrilliation of the distal tendon in the critical zone of hypovascularity, all arising because of the mechanical disadvantage plus the constant stress on the tissue resulting from humeral impingement against the coracoacromial arch. Traumatic inflammation occurs, possibly also an autoimmune mechanism with antibody produced against denatured collagen and other structural proteins, and spreads to the contiguous tendon sheath, subacromial bursa, and other joint structures.

The patient is usually over 45 years of age with an occupation or leisure activity that entails unusual shoulder stress. The pain is a dull ache in the deltoid insertion area, often over a wider area, even the entire C5 sclerotome, with acute and severe pain on certain movements (abduction to 60 degrees or more, reaching over the head, putting on a coat). There is usually no arm or neck radiation. Night pain is characteristic, and the patient cannot lie on the affected side in bed due to marked increase in pain. He or she often grabs the affected shoulder with the opposite hand, complaining of a catch, or a severe twinge in the shoulder. The shoulder is diffusely tender, especially over the humeral head lateral and posterior to the acromion and over the supraspinatus insertion. More posterior tenderness suggests teres minor and infraspinatus involvement. Pain in resisted medial rotation suggests subscapularis involvement. Weakness and atrophy are uncommon. The anterior and superior aspects of the rotator cuff can be examined by having the patient reach behind the low back.

The posterior aspect of the rotator cuff can be best examined by adducting the arm across the chest. Downward pull on the relaxed arm is painful, owing to tension in the rotator cuff. Adduction and forward-backward swing are without pain. Scapulohumeral rhythm is reversed, with the patient shrugging to rotate the scapula with the least glenohumeral adduction. The pain is much increased by forced abduction against resistance, and there is a painful

## Calcific tendinitis

### Pathophysiology

Most common cause of shoulder pain in young patients
Calcific mass 1 to 1.5 cm in diameter
- Always symptomatic
- Involves overlying subacromial bursa distended with fluid
- Tendinitis and bursitis coexistent

Rotator cuff calcification in 8% asymptomatic population over age 30; ⅓ of calcific deposits cause symptoms; deposits multiple or bilateral about 75% of the time
Hydroxyapatite crystals identified

### Clinical characteristics

Young patient
Severe aching pain 1 to 4 days
All positions painful, unable to sleep
All movement painful
Pain relief if and when deposit inspissates from toothpaste consistency to powder or ruptures along fascial planes into the bursa

### Physical examination

Allows no movement
Palpation in rotator cuff, point maximum tenderness, fullness and swelling
Marked spasm in all shoulder muscles

### X-ray findings

Round or oval deposit between acromion and humeral head may be several cm in length

### Management

Nonsteroidal antiinflammatory drugs
Temporary rest in sling
Local heat or cold, or both serially
Injection of deposit with local anesthetic and steroid, needling the area at same time
With relief of pain, physical therapy, range of motion exercises
If calcific boil does not rupture, operation may be necessary; over 90% of patients recover completely, most of calcification disappears

## Rupture of the rotator cuff

### Pathophysiology

Supraspinatus component most frequently torn, varies from few fibers to massive tears, full thickness of the cuff, even the capsule and floor of overlying bursa, resulting in communication between shoulder joint and subacromial bursa
Rare before age 50, common after age 60 (nearly impossible to rupture tendons in a healthy, young adult)
Occurs at insertion of cuff into bone
Supraspinatus and infraspinatus atrophy in 3 weeks
Shoulder muscles in severe spasm

### Etiology

Degenerative changes
Fraying
Attritional wear
Minor recurrent trauma culminating in loss of collagen fibrillar structure

### Clinical characteristics

Over age 50, often a laborer; abrupt pain in deltoid area; snap following strain or fall
Pain very severe for 6 to 12 hours; cannot continue working if rupture extensive
Abduction mainly affected; patient shrugs to move arm. scapulohumeral rhythm lost; arm can be lifted passively in abduction; power to maintain it gone (drop-arm sign)
Lidocaine infiltration relieves pain; range of motion serviceable if tear incomplete

### X-ray findings

Humeral head high on the glenoid on adduction
Shoulder held in adduction

### Physical examination

Pain relieved by pendulum exercise position (see Fig. 71-10) or downward traction on the arm (depression of the head test)
Extreme tenderness over greater tuberosity

### Management

Complete ruptures recognized early, surgically repaired
Partial ruptures heal surprisingly well, good return of function with conservative management

## Bicipital syndromes

**Anatomy**

Intraarticular: bicipital groove between greater and lesser tuberosities
Extraarticular: lies between subscapularis and supraspinatus tendons in synovial sheath, an extension from the shoulder joint proper

**Four clinical syndromes**

- Tendinitis and tenosynovitis
  - History
    - Chronic pain anterolateral shoulder
    - Pain in trapezius, scalene, deltoid, sometimes extending into arm and forearm
    - No history of acute trauma
    - Pain on repetitive activity overhead
  - Examination
    - Shoulder stiffness, limited movement
    - Extreme tenderness in bicipital groove
    - Audible click when fully abducted and laterally rotated arm slowly brought to side (from tendon being dislocated)
    - Pain caused on resistance against flexed elbow and supinated hand (Yergason sign)
  - Management
    - Rest, heat, gentle exercise, nonsteroidal antiinflammatory drugs
    - Physical therapy
    - Avoidance of excessive tendon use
    - Local steroid/lidocaine injection
- Elongation of bicipital tendon
  - Pathophysiology
    - Related to dislocation from groove
    - Part of attrition wear and tear
  - History
    - Shoulder pain and stiffness
    - Usually an older patient
  - Examination
    - Tenderness in bicipital groove
    - Crepitus on marked rotary movements
    - Laxity long belly of biceps
    - Laxity with elbow flexed at 90 degrees and forearm supinated against resistance
    - Audible click as with tendinitis
  - Management: conservative; operation occasionally
- Tendon dislocation
  - History
    - Painful audible click in external rotation of the shoulder
    - Arm locking in painful condition, relieved by reversing movement, i.e., medial rotation
  - Physical findings:
    - Manual pressure over groove with humerus rotated prevents tendon from dislocating
  - Management: surgery if disability is severe
- Rupture of long head of biceps
  - History
    - Chronic stiffness, shoulder pain
    - May or may not be history of a snap
    - Lump appears with elbow flexion
    - Acute traumatic rupture
    - Abrupt sharp pain, loss of power
  - Examination: lump appears
  - Management
    - Young patient: surgical repair
    - Older patient: usually conservative

arc of 10 to 15 degrees just beyond 60 degrees' abduction (as the tendons and cuff impinge over the coracoaromial arch). Passive range of motion is normal.

X-ray study is usually not helpful, although later calcific densities may be seen, bony flakes, spicules, sclerosis, and osteophytosis of the tuberosities occur, and eburnation and cystic changes follow. Infiltration of the cuff with 1% lidocaine with relief of pain, especially the arc of pain, is both diagnostic and therapeutic (see Figs. 71-15 and 71-16).

Management of rotator cuff tendinitis includes (1) extensive patient education with definition of the problem, prognosis, and reassurance regarding recovery; (2) heat as well as cold intermittently; (3) pendulum exercises (see Fig. 71-10); (4) range of motion exercises; (5) nonsteroidal antiinflammatory drugs; (6) injection of steroid and local anesthetic agents; (7) pain medication; and (8) occasional short course of steroids (e.g., prednisone, 15 mg in the morning and at supper for 5 days reduced by decrements of 5 mg each 5 days to stop). About 90% of patients recover with this therapy.

The boxes on pp. 1006 to 1010 summarize calcific tendinitis, rupture of the rotator cuff, bicipital syndromes (Fig. 71-18), frozen shoulder (Fig. 71-19), acromioclavicular syndromes, reflex sympathetic dystrophy syndrome, neurovascular syndromes, and visceral and somatic lesions.

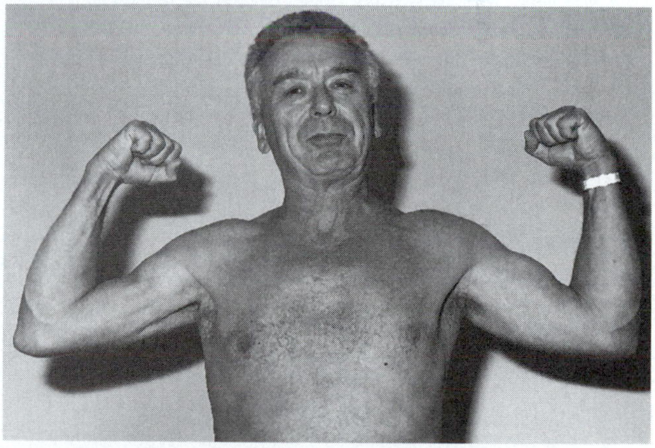

**Fig. 71-18.** Note "lump" in right biceps (*left side of photograph*) compared to the left. The long head of the biceps tendon is completely ruptured.

## LANDMARKS FOR SHOULDER ARTHROCENTESIS AND INTRAARTICULAR INJECTION

The procedure is best accomplished with the patient seated and the shoulder internally rotated. A mark in the skin is made just medial to the head of the humerus and slightly

## Frozen shoulder

### Etiology and pathogenesis

Most likely a reflex sympathetic dystrophy (shoulder-hand syndrome, Sudeck atrophy)

Onset follows prolonged, sustained immobilization of the arm (shoulder sling for trauma, rotator cuff or bicipital tendon lesions, myocardial infarction); immobilization may promote autonomic circulatory impairment, muscle contracture, fibrosis, osteoporosis

### History (clinical features)

Middle-aged people, more common in women than men

Associated with diabetes mellitus

Appears at varying rates and intensity; limitation of motion in one plane to complete fibrous ankylosis with glenohumeral motion compromise, development of pain and restricted motion and duration a few months to several years

Pain severe, worse at night, radiates into the neck and down arms to fingers

### Physical findings

Tender anterior capsule, rotator cuff, and bicipital tendon

Disrupted scapulohumeral rhythm

Markedly restricted passive and active shoulder motion in all planes

Patient may appear systemically ill

### Radiologic and pathologic findings

Osteopenia of humeral head with cystic changes

Narrowing of space between acromion and humeral head

Periarticular soft tissue calcifications on occasion

Markedly thickened, contracted fibrotic capsule, adherent to humeral head with adhesion of long head of biceps tendon in its sheath

Glenohumeral joint space contraction to 0.5 to 3 ml in contrast to normal volume of 30 to 40 ml

### Management

Rest

Physical therapy with graded passive and active exercise program

Nonsteroidal antiinflammatory drugs

Systemic corticosteroids in tapering fashion (i.e., 15 mg prednisone twice a day for 5 days, then taper by 5 mg every 5 days for 4 to 5 weeks, then discontinue)

Injection of periarticular and intraarticular structures with depot corticosteroids and local anesthetic

Manipulation of shoulder under anesthesia

### Prevention

Avoid immobilization

Exercise shoulder to pain limit

## Acromioclavicular syndromes

### Lesions part of differential diagnosis of shoulder pain

Acromioclavicular joint contains meniscus

Minor injuries (without clavicle dislocation) and negative x-ray may be symptomatic due to internal derangement of meniscus

Osteoarthritis, rheumatoid arthritis, direct or indirect trauma may cause pain

Subacromial bursa just below acromioclavicular joint and critical zone of supraspinatus tendon and biceps tendon are in close relationship

Acromioclavicular joint osteoarthritis associated with osteophytes and joint space narrowing (x-ray)

Spread of inflammation from acromioclavicular to contiguous structures accounts for instances of periarthritis

### Clinical characteristics

Pain in superior aspect of shoulder

Sharply localized tenderness at the joint

Pain radiates toward perceived base of neck and in the jaw on the side of the lesion

Motion of throwing a ball overhand produces or exaggerates characteristic pain

Adduction of arm across chest in horizontal plane causes severe pain

### Management (very satisfactory)

Nonsteroidal antiinflammatory drugs

Physical therapy

Surgical repair or resection of outer ½ inch of the clavicle rarely necessary (at no time should this joint be fused).

## Reflex sympathetic dystrophy syndrome

### Synonyms

Causalgia, Sudeck atrophy, traumatic angiospasm, reflex dystrophy of the extremities, postinfarctional sclerodactyly, shoulder-hand syndrome, reflex neurovascular dystrophy, reflex sympathetic dystrophy

### Pathophysiology

Arterial blood: vessels mainly on volar side of arm; lymphatics on dorsal side; venous return aided by pumping through muscle contractions in hand, forearm, and arm derangement of pumping mechanism

- Swelling and limitation of shoulder and hand motion
- Shoulder contraction
- Limitation of wrist movement

### History

May involve wrist, elbow, and other arm tissue, other extremities; most striking usually in hand and shoulder

Painful, stiff shoulder; pain in arm, hand

Hyperesthesia

### Examination

Limitation of shoulder motion (may reach magnitude of frozen shoulder)

Swelling, edema, diffuse tenderness

Painful dystrophy in hand, fingers

Often bilateral; one side can be subtly affected, often later

Incomplete and painful digital flexion

Vasospasm, vasodilatation, vasomotor instability

*Continued.*

### Reflex sympathetic dystrophy syndrome—cont'd.

Trophic skin and nail changes
- Swelling, cyanosis, shiny skin
- Hypertrichosis and hyperhidrosis
- Hypertrophic nails

**Radiologic findings**

Early: subchondral bone erosion (as early as a few days after onset)
Late: diffuse extensive osteoporosis

**Precipitating events**

Myocardial infarction
Painful trauma
Cerebrovascular accident, epilepsy, other CNS disease
Cervical spine disk disease
Painful intrathoracic or upper intraabdominal disorder, Pancoast tumor
Herpes zoster
Calcific tendinitis of shoulder

**Clinical course: three stages**

Rapid or gradual onset painful shoulder; periarthritis of shoulder, arm, hand, finger involvement with redness, duskiness, edema, progressive limitation of movement
Duration: weeks to 6 months
Decreased pain, increased shoulder mobility, decreased hand edema, skin, subcutaneous and muscle tissue atrophy, palmar fascia contractures (simulates Dupuytren contracture); months duration
Dystrophic changes, inelastic skin, cold, cyanotic hands, nail changes, frozen shoulder in adduction, hand and fingers in stiff flexion deformity, muscle atrophy

**Management**

Early mobilization; maximal movement, active and passive
Avoidance of immobilization
Physical therapy: active and passive exercises
Corticosteroids: prednisone, 30 mg per day in divided doses, reducing dose by 5 mg each 5 days, for 5 to 6 weeks
Nonsteroidal antiinflammatory drugs
Analgesics

inferior and just lateral to the coracoid process, both being readily palpable with little practice. Strict sterile skin preparation is accomplished. Of considerable comfort to the patient is to raise a wheal in the skin using a syringe with lidocaine and a 26-gauge needle at the marked spot. A 20- to 22-gauge needle is then directed posteriorly, slightly superiorly, and laterally. Ideally, one should feel the needle enter the joint space. If bone is hit, the physician should pull back and redirect the needle at a slightly different angle. (See Fig. 71-1 for the anatomic structures involved.)

For injection into the subacromial bursa the physician follows the clavicle laterally to palpate the shelving edge of the acromion process, usually readily identified. The needle is directed under the shelving acromion edge. Again, skin anesthesia is advised. The entry into the bursa can usually be perceived.

### Thoracic outlet syndrome

**Anatomy**

Upper extremity neurovascular supply exit arm at root of neck
Clinical syndromes result from compression of brachial plexus, subclavian vein or artery
Medial cord (C8-T1) ulnar distribution (most inferior portion brachial plexus) commonly involved
Sites of neurovascular element compression
- Cervical ribs and fascial connections
- Thoracic rib anomalies
- Compression between scalene muscles
- Rib-clavicle compression
- Compression during hyperabduction or other unusual positions with normal anatomy

**Clinical manifestations**

Rare causes of shoulder pain; diagnosis best made on basis of history and examination

**History**

Paresthesias (numbness, tingling)
Pain
Weakness in shoulder, arm, forearm, hand
Swelling, coldness of extremity
Pain on arising from sleep, related to sleep position

**Examination**

Sensory loss
Muscle atrophy (especially hand) (late finding)
- Hypothenar, interosseus with ulnar involvement
- Abductor pollicis brevis, opponens pollicis with medial nerve involvement
- Fasciculations

Pallor, edema, cyanosis, coldness of involved extremity
Blood pressure discrepancies between arms
Provocative maneuvers (may produce abnormal responses in normal patient)
- Adson: neck extension, chin rotated toward affected side, deep inspiration, pulse obliterates or decreases in intensity, symptoms reproduced (tenses anterior and middle scalene muscles, decreasing interscalene space)
- Costoclavicular: exaggerated military posture (bracing shoulders back and down); pulse intensity decreases
- Pain exacerbation by downward traction on shoulder

**Management**

Conservative measures effective in 80% of cases
- Reassurance
- Patient education
  - Exercise and physical therapy to correct faulty posture and strengthen shoulder girdle musculature
  - Situational change (occupation change, redesign of kitchen or work area)
- Treatment of muscle spasm

Surgery considered only after conservative treatment has failed

A lateral approach to both the shoulder joint and the subacromial bursa can be done, inserting the needle between the acromion process of the scapula and the head of the humerus.

Corticosteroids are commonly mixed with a local

## Visceral and somatic lesions (diaphragmatic disorders) and diseases characterized by referred pain to the shoulder

Pain referred via the phrenic nerve (C3-4 and C4-5) to the supraclavicular region, trapezius, and superior angle of the scapula
Gallbladder and hepatic parenchymal disease: scapular and shoulder top pain associated with epigastric tenderness
Gastric and pancreatic disease: interscapular pain
Perforated hollow viscus via phrenic nerve distribution
Pulmonary infarction: diaphragmatic irritation
Pancoast or apical lung tumor, may have coincident Horner's syndrome
Myocardial ischemia: pain is infraclavicular, ulnar, and at base of the neck
Transverse and descending aortic arch disease: pain, left side of neck and shoulder
Cervical osteoarthritis with neural, muscle, joint, and ligamentous (deep pain) referral pattern at C5 to T1 levels
Pleural disease: diaphragmatic irritation
Peritoneal disease: diaphragmatic irritation
Neoplasms of cervical cord and nerve roots
Neurovascular syndromes (see text)
Objective clinical findings in the shoulder joint are usually absent in referred visceral or somatic disease; Active and passive shoulder motion is not limited, nor does movement produce the patient's pain or other symptoms; an inclusive differential diagnosis is imperative, owing to the complexity and diversity of shoulder disorders

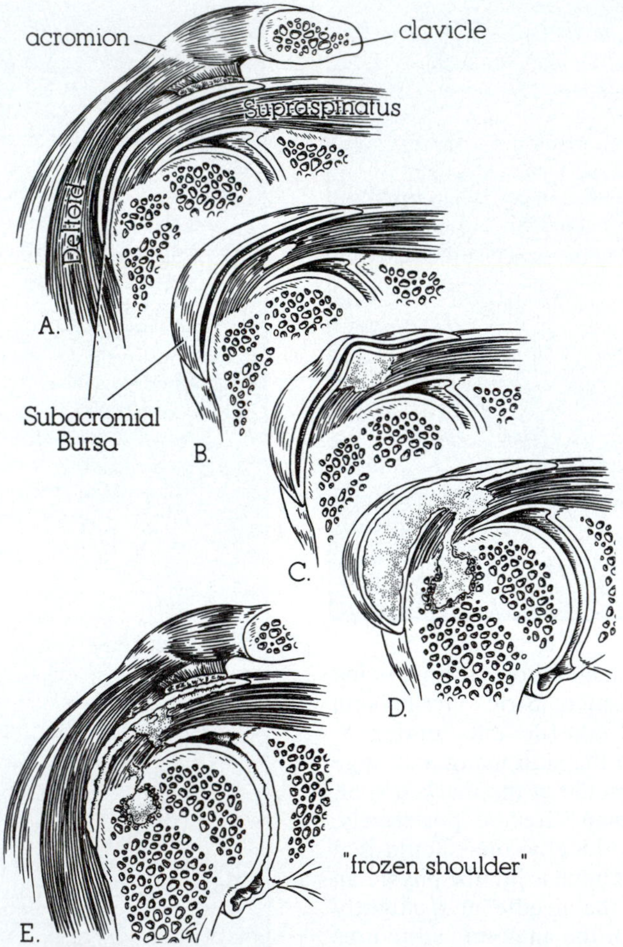


**Fig. 71-19.** Sequence of events terminating in frozen shoulder. **A,** Normal structures of the shoulder. **B,** Supraspinatus tendinitis, sometimes calcific, in the "critical zone." **C,** Spread of inflammation to the tendon sheath and a bulge into the floor of the subacromial bursa. **D,** Rupture into the subacromial bursa and extension of the inflammatory process as an osteitis into the humeral head and greater tuberosity. **E,** Frozen shoulder with involvement of tendons, bursa, capsule, synovium, and muscle with fibrous contracture and markedly diminished volume of the shoulder joint space.

### Possible sequelae of intraarticular and soft tissue corticosteroid injections

**Corticosteroid preparations**

Methylprednisolone acetate (Depo-Medrol) 20, 40, 80 mg/ml
Triamcinolone hexacetonide (Aristospan)20 mg/ml
Betamethasone sodium phosphate and a citrate suspension (Celestone Souluspan) 6 mg/ml
Dexamethasone acetate (Decadron LA) 8 mg/ml
Hydrocortisone acetate (Hydrocortone) 25 mg/ml
Prednisolone tebutate (Hydeltra-T.B.A.) 20 mg/ml

**Possible sequelae to intraarticular and soft tissue injections**

Tendon rupture
Iatrogenic infection (rare)
Deterioration of joints, evidenced radiologically: steroid arthropathy, Charcot-like arthropathy osteonecrosis
Nerve damage
Postinjection flare
Tissue atrophy and fat necrosis
Pancreatitis (rare side effect from systemic absorption)

anesthetic, notably procaine or lidocaine. Package inserts from the major pharmaceutical manufacturers advise against this practice. Most local anesthetics contain preservatives that may result in flocculation of the corticosteroid. Lidocaine for intravenous use does not contain a preservative. A conservative practice is advised. A short- or intermediate-acting steroid preparation such as triamcinolone diacetate or methylprednisolone acetate is recommended for periarticular injections. A long-acting preparation such as triamcinolone hexacetonide may be used for intraarticular injection (see Chapter 69).

There is no consensus regarding the ideal volume and dose of corticosteroid to be injected into joints. The shoulder is a large joint with considerable intrasynovial volume; 2 to 3 ml is advised. The box above lists corticosteroid preparations and sequelae of intraarticular and soft tissue steroid injections.

## BIBLIOGRAPHY

Anderson TE: Rehabilitation of common shoulder injuries in athletes, *J Musculoskel Med* 5(12):15, 1988.

Barth E, Berg E: Practical pointers for common shoulder pain complaints, *J Musculoskel Med* 6(6):38, 1989.

Binder Al et al: Frozen shoulder: a long-term prospective study, *Ann Rheum Dis* 43:361, 1984.

Bland JH, Merrit JA, Boushey DR: The painful shoulder, *Semin Arthritis Rheum* 7:21, 1977.

Bulgen DY et al: Frozen shoulder: prospective clinical study with an evaluation of three treatment regimens, *Ann Rheum Dis* 43:353, 1984.

Chard MD, Hazleman BL: Shoulder disorders in the elderly (a hospital study), *Ann Rheum Dis* 46:684, 1987.

Dacre JE, Beeney N, Scott DL: Injections and physiotherapy for the painful stiff shoulder, *Ann Rheum Dis* 48:322, 1989.

Glousman RE, Jobe FW: How to detect and manage the unstable shoulder, *J Musculoskel Med* 7(3):93, 1989.

Halverson PB et al: Milwaukee shoulder. II. Synovial fluid studies, *Arthritis Rheum* 24:474, 1981.

Hoppenfeld S: *Physical examination of the spine and extremities,* New York, 1976, Appleton-Century-Crofts.

Kleinman KS, Coburn JW: Amyloid syndromes associated with hemodialysis, *Kidney Int* 35:567, 1989.

Kozin F et al: The reflex sympathetic dystrophy syndrome. I. Clinical and histologic studies: response to corticosteroids and articular involvement, *Am J Med* 60:321, 1976.

Kozin F et al: The reflex sympathetic dystrophy syndrome. III. Scintigraphic studies, further evidence for the therapeutic efficacy of systemic corticosteroids and proposed diagnostic criteria, *Am J Med* 70:23, 1981.

Kozin F et al: The reflex sympathetic dystrophy syndrome. II. Roentgenographic and scintigraphic evidence of bilaterality of periarticular accentuation, *Am J Med* 60:332, 1986.

Mavrikakis ME et al: Calcific shoulder periarthritis (tendinitis) in adult onset diabetes mellitus: a controlled study, *Ann Rheum Dis* 48:211, 1989.

McCarty DJ et al: Milwaukee shoulder—association of microspheroids containing hydroxyapatite crystals, active collagenase, neutral protease with rotator cuff defects. I. Clinical aspects, *Arthritis Rheum* 24:464, 1981.

Neer CS II: Anterior acromioplasty for the chronic impingement syndrome, *J Bone Joint Surg* 54A:41, 1972.

Parker RD et al: Frozen shoulder, *Orthopedics* 12:869, 1989.

Warren RF, O'Brien SJ: Shoulder pain in the geriatric patient, *Orthop Rev* 19:129, 248, 1989.

CHAPTER

# 72 Hand

**Joseph M. Lenehan**

A survey published in 1980 entitled "Extremity Disorders, A Survey of their Frequency and Cost in the United States" estimated that one third of all injuries involve the upper extremities. Injuries restrict the patient's activity or require a visit to a physician. This study indicated that there were 16 million injuries annually. These injuries were responsible for 90 million days of restricted activity and 16 million days of work lost per year in the United States. They accounted for 6 million hospital visits and 12 million physician visits per year. The total cost to society was $10 billion. These data indicate that upper extremity, and in particular hand, wounds represent a significant percentage of injuries seen by primary care physicians and emergency room physicians. Hand injuries not only cause significant physical disability; they also produce deformities that are often a source of major psychological trauma (Fig. 72-1).

## ASSESSMENT

In addition to information regarding the patient's age, occupation, dominant hand, previous injury, and general health, a detailed history of the injury is needed. This should include the position of the fingers and hand at the time of injury, the degree of contamination, the type of initial treatment, and the interval between the injury and initial care of it.

An understanding of functional anatomy is important in

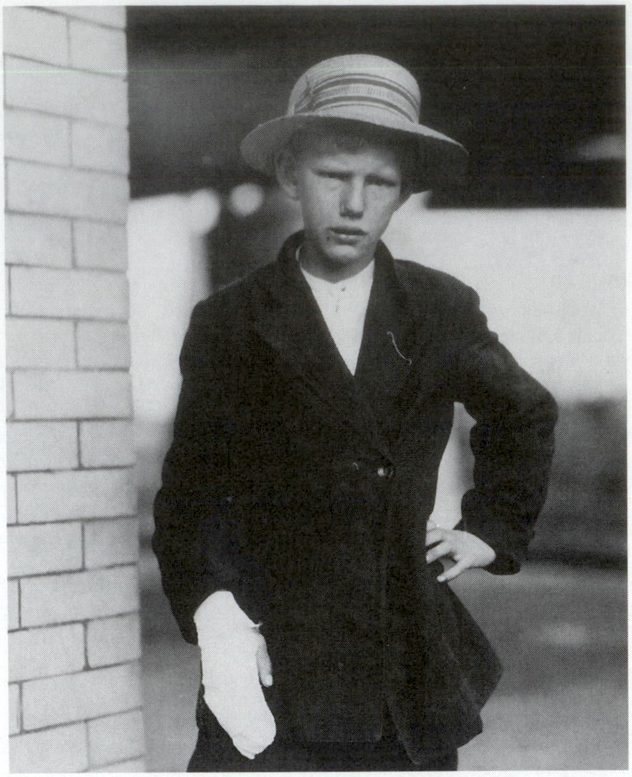

**Fig. 72-1.** Alfred Paggett, a 13-year-old doffer at Shaw Cotton Mills, Weldon, North Carolina, November 1914. (Photograph by Lewis Wick Hine.)

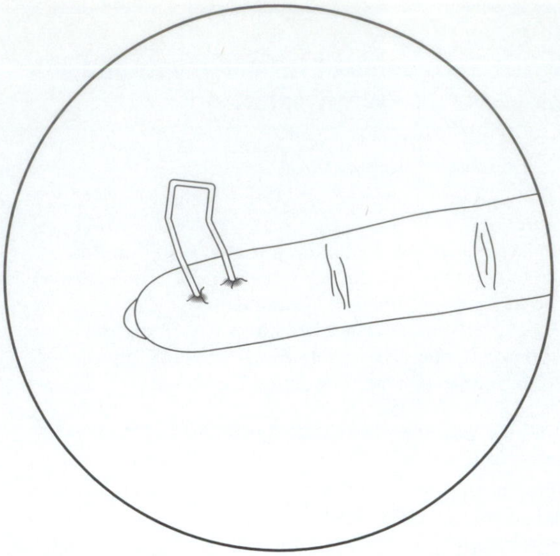

**Fig. 72-2.** The Weber two-point discrimination test is the most sensitive test to detect intact sensation. Normally the two points can be perceived to a distance of <6 mm. Testing should be longitudinally oriented along the radial and ulnar borders of the pulp to test individual proper digital nerve sensation.

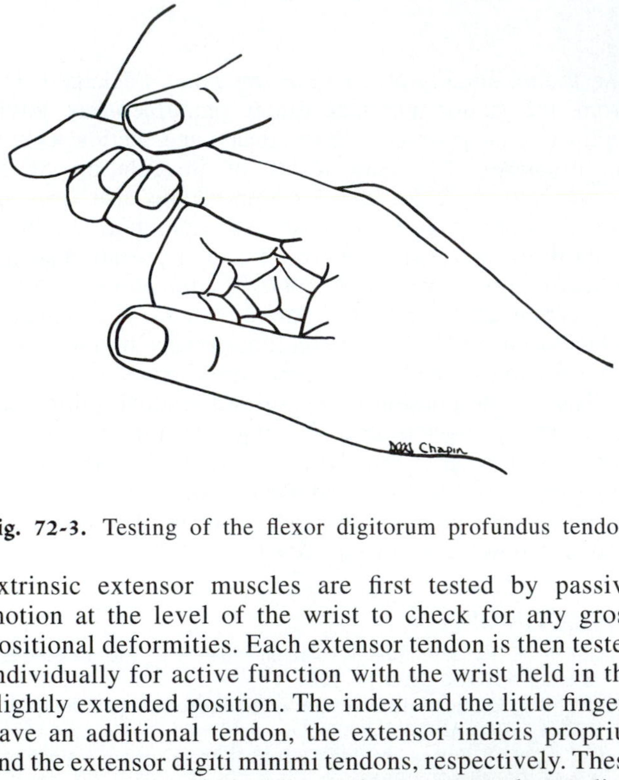

**Fig. 72-3.** Testing of the flexor digitorum profundus tendon.

assessing the injured hand. Physical examination should be performed systematically to assess the skin, musculotendinous units, nerve and vascular supply, and bone and joint function. This is best accomplished by obtaining as much information by inspection as possible before asking the patient to actively move the hand, which may cause discomfort. Any gross positional deformity indicative of tendon or bone injury should be noted. The skin should be inspected for penetrating wounds or gross lacerations. An examination of the sensation in all digits, using the Weber two-point discrimination test, is important in determining median, ulnar, and radial nerve function (Fig. 72-2). The vascular supply should be assessed by inspecting color and capillary filling. Once this information has been obtained, the musculotendinous units and motor function can be assessed.

### Extrinsic muscles

The extrinsic muscles of the hand consist of the digital flexors and extensors; they should be tested individually. The flexor digitorum profundus tendons of the fingers are tested by stabilizing the proximal interphalangeal joint of the fingers and asking the patient to flex the distal interphalangeal joint actively (Fig. 72-3). The flexor digitorum superficialis tendons of the fingers are tested by holding the adjacent fingers in full extension and asking the patient to flex the proximal interphalangeal joint of the involved digit (Fig. 72-4). This effectively prevents the profundus tendon from acting on the digit being tested. The flexor pollicis longus tendon is tested by stabilizing the metacarpophalangeal joint of the thumb and asking the patient to flex the interphalangeal joint (Fig. 72-5). The extrinsic extensor muscles are first tested by passive motion at the level of the wrist to check for any gross positional deformities. Each extensor tendon is then tested individually for active function with the wrist held in the slightly extended position. The index and the little fingers have an additional tendon, the extensor indicis proprius and the extensor digiti minimi tendons, respectively. These can be tested by asking the patient to extend one digit alone while holding the others flexed. The extensor pollicis longus tendon is best tested by asking the patient to hold the hand flat on the table and then extend the thumb (Fig. 72-6). The wrist extensors are tested by active extension against gravity with the fingers fully flexed in a fist with simultaneous palpation of the distal tendons.

### Intrinsic muscles

When testing the intrinsic muscles, a clear understanding of the motor supply from the median and ulnar nerves is

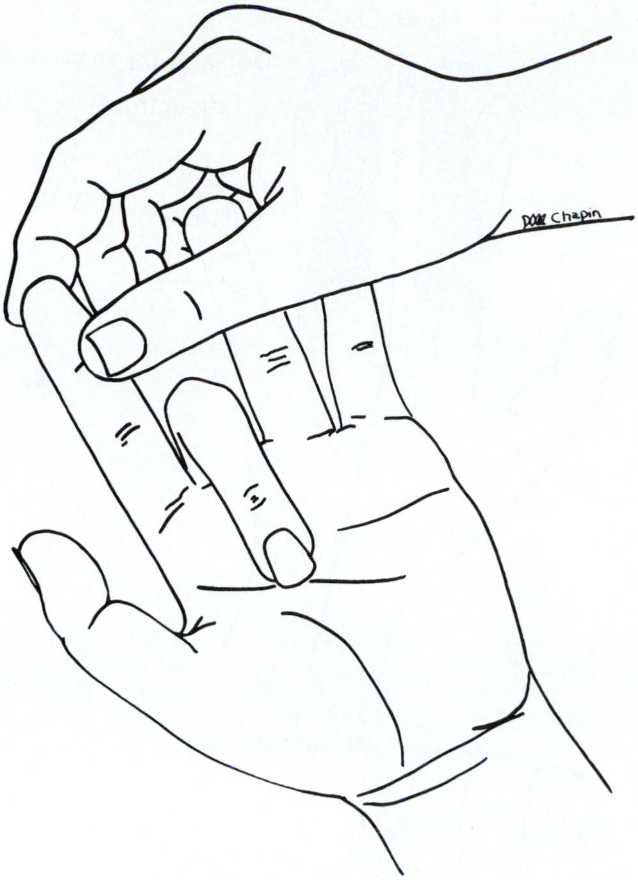

Fig. 72-4. Testing of the flexor superficialis tendon.

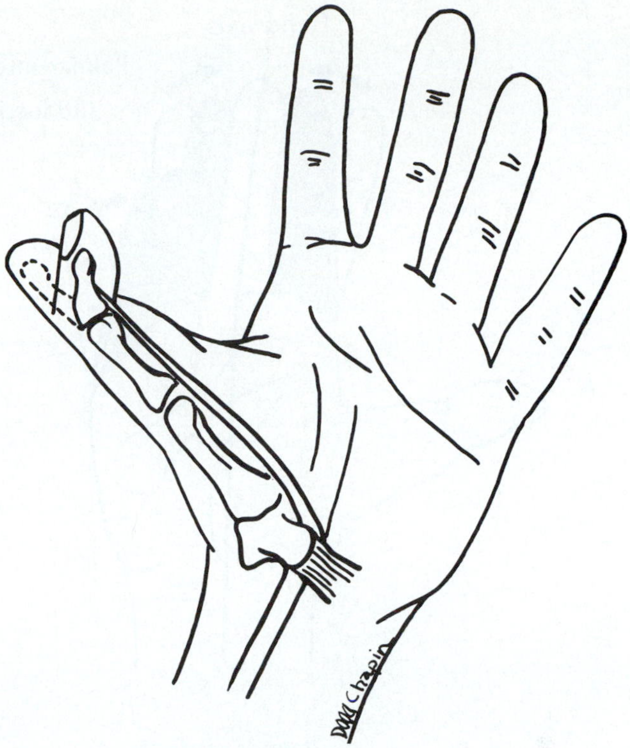

Fig. 72-5. Testing of the flexor pollicis longus tendon.

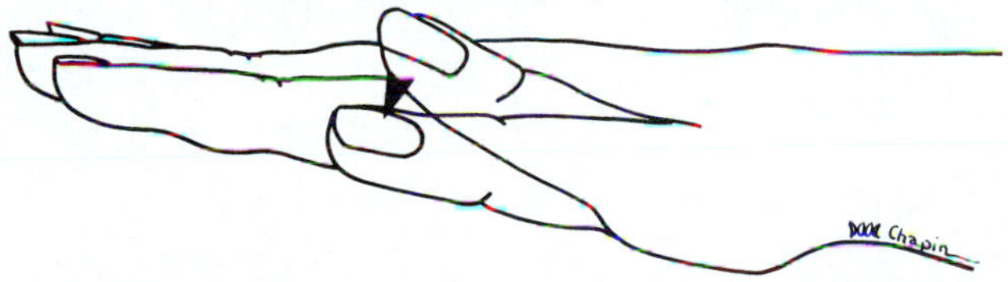

Fig. 72-6. Testing of the extensor pollicis longus tendon.

needed. The median nerve supplies the abductor pollicis brevis, opponens pollicis, and the superficial head of the flexor pollicis brevis muscles, which contribute to opposition of the thumb (Fig. 72-7). The ulnar nerve supplies the interosseous muscles, the deep head of the flexor pollicis brevis muscle, the adductor pollicis muscle, and the hypothenar musculature. The lumbrical muscles to the index and long fingers are supplied by the median nerve, while the lumbrical muscles to the ring and little fingers are supplied by the ulnar nerve. To test for thenar muscle function supplied by the motor branch of the median nerve, the patient must demonstrate opposition of the thumb with the examiner palpating the thenar muscle group. Ulnar nerve motor function is tested by observing the patient's ability to abduct and adduct the fingers and to flex the metacarpophalangeal joints with the interphalangeal joints in the extended position, and by checking the adequacy of the adductor pollicis muscle by assessing the power of a key pinch (Fig. 72-8).

A sensory examination should include a mapping of the areas of diminished sensation that are revealed by light

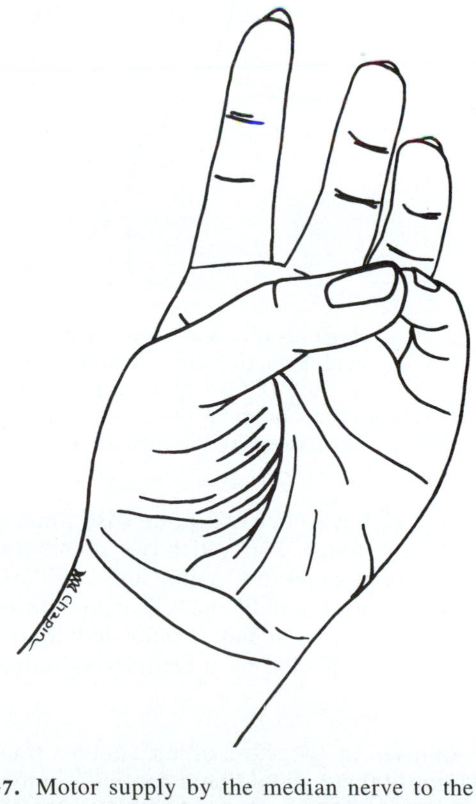

Fig. 72-7. Motor supply by the median nerve to the abductor pollicis brevis, opponens pollicis, and superficial head of the flexor pollicis brevis muscle.

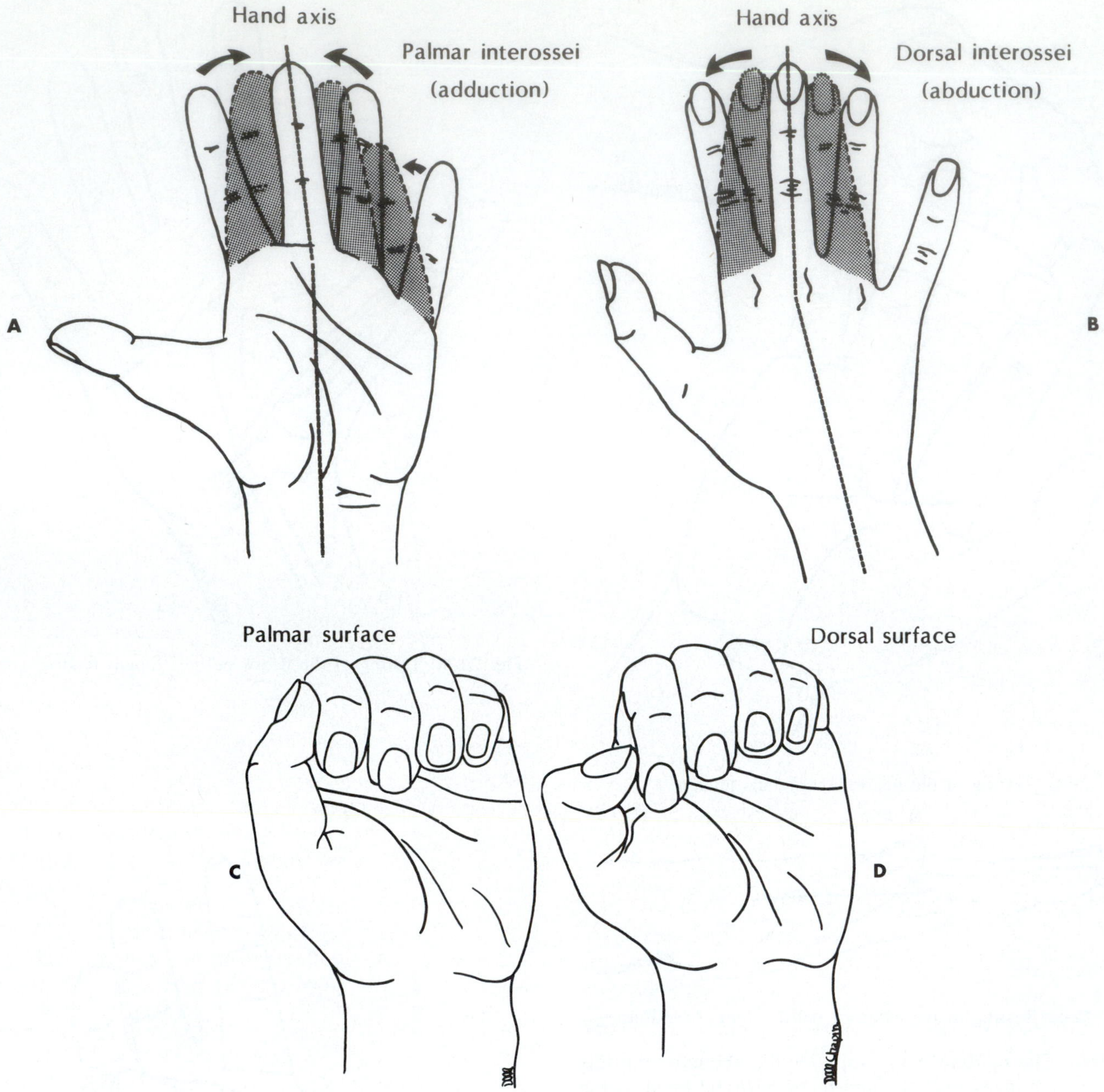


**Fig. 72-8.** Ulnar nerve testing. Weakness of the intrinsic muscle is revealed by adduction **(A)** and abduction **(B)** when there is ulnar nerve injury. When ulnar innervation to the adductor pollicis **(C)** is intact, Froment's test reveals a normal pinch. Injury to the ulnar nerves results in an abnormal pinch **(D),** which can only be performed by using the flexor pollicis longus, innervated by the median nerve.

touch and use of the Weber two-point discrimination test. Normal subjects cannot distinguish two points less than 6 mm apart. Besides assessing pallor and capillary filling, vascular examination should include palpation of pulses and an Allen's test at wrist and, if indicated, digital levels. This may be accompanied by a Doppler examination.

## Injuries

***Acute trauma.*** In the case of an acutely traumatized upper extremity there should be a routine examination of all structures possibly involved. A sterile dressing should be placed on the wound, and the patient should be placed in the supine position with the hand elevated. Bleeding in the hand should be controlled by direct pressure alone. Avoid clamping a bleeding vessel because of its proximity to vital structures such as nerves and tendons. The sterile dressing should be left in place and the extremity assessed distal to the site of injury. A systematic examination can determine whether tendon, vascular, or nerve injuries exist. This is especially true for children, who often become uncooperative once the physician causes pain when examining the injury or exploring the wound.

**Tendons.** Tendon injuries can occur with small, superficial-appearing wounds if the tendon is under

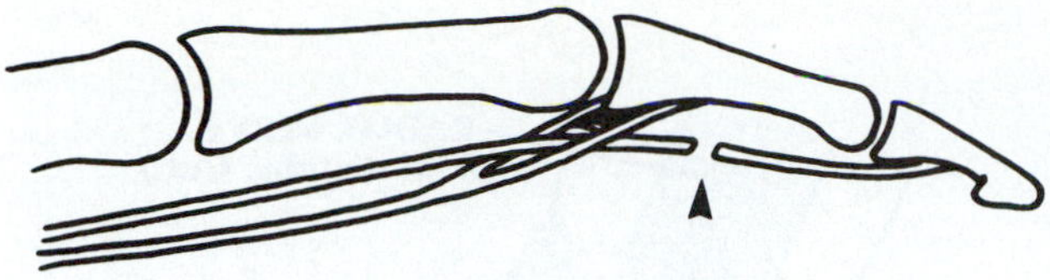

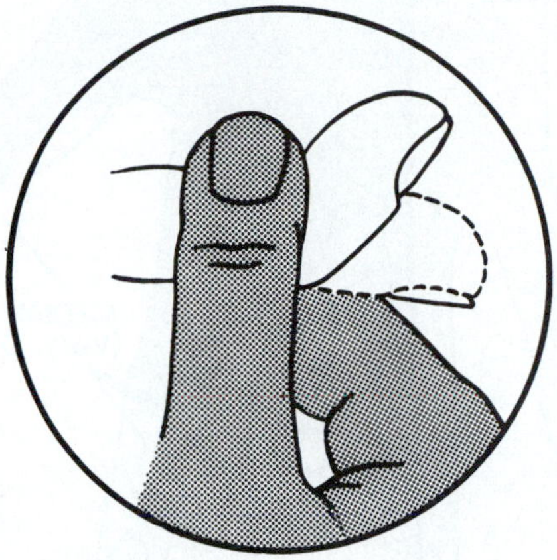

**Fig. 72-9.** Transection of the flexor digitorum profundus tendon distal to the superficialis insertion.

tension at the time of the injury. This is most evident with superficial lacerations over the flexor creases of the fingers or wrist, which often result in significant nerve and tendon injuries.

***Flexor tendons.*** The flexor creases have no subcutaneous fat at the interphalangeal joint level, and a small puncture wound to that area often results in an injury to the flexor sheath. The patient with a partial tendon injury may not have a gross positional deformity but may complain of pain when flexing the finger actively. Testing finger flexion against resistance may elicit pain if there is a partial tendon injury; such testing must be done with caution, however, because it may cause a partial tendon transection to rupture. Critical areas include the flexor digitorum profundus tendon distal to the superficialis tendon insertion and distal to the flexor crease at the proximal interphalangeal joint. The transection of the flexor pollicis longus tendon at the level of the flexor crease at the metacarpophalangeal joint is also a common injury. In examining for flexor tendon injuries, the flexor digitorum superficialis and profundus tendons should be tested independently (see Figs. 72-3 and 72-4). Examination of the flexor pollicis longus tendon requires the demonstration of active flexion at the interphalangeal joint. It is also important to note that a number of patients do not have significant independent flexion at the proximal interphalangeal joint of the little finger. The superficial tendon of the opposite little finger should be tested (Fig. 72-9). A closed rupture of the flexor digitorum profundus tendon can occur. Usually it involves the ring finger in a sports-related grasping injury. If this injury is recognized early, the tendon can be reinserted on the distal phalanx.

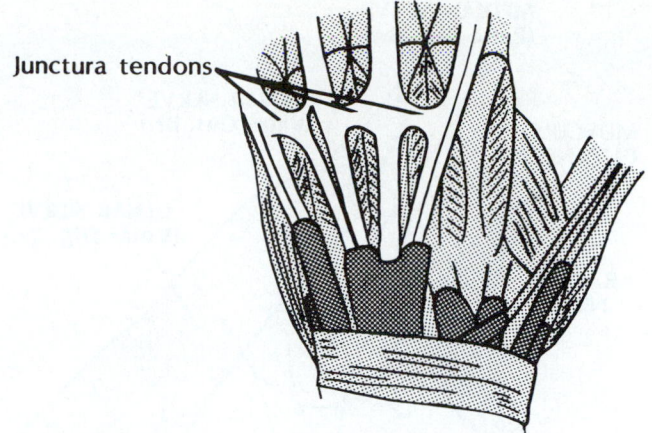

**Fig. 72-10.** Role of the juncturae tendinum.

***Extensor tendons.*** Extensor tendon injuries occur with the fingers fully flexed or extended. Thus all dorsal wounds should be explored for tendon injuries. The fingers should be flexed and then extended so that the tendon can be examined through the full range of its excursion. The two tendons to the index and little fingers, which allow for independent extension of these digits, must be identified. When examining dorsal wounds for possible extensor tendon injuries, it is important to recognize the role of the juncturae tendinum, which are communications between the common digital extensor tendons on the dorsum of the hand (Fig. 72-10). Lacerations over the dorsum of the metacarpophalangeal joint area usually result in a lack of metacarpophalangeal extension, provided the transection is distal to the juncturae tendinum. The interphalangeal joint extension is due to intrinsic muscle function and the metacarpophalangeal joint extension is due to extrinsic tendon function. In the absence of the extrinsic tendons, the interphalangeal joints can be completely extended. Any laceration over the metacarpophalangeal joint should alert the examiner to the possibility of a human bite wound.

**Nerves.** When assessing lacerations of the hand, the physician should understand the anatomic characteristics of the nerves that might be involved (Fig. 72-11). The proper digital nerves on the volar aspect of the thumb are immediately adjacent to the flexor pollicis longus tendon sheath near the metacarpophalangeal joint and are susceptible to injury. The radial and ulnar proper digital nerves at this point are approximately 1 to 1½ cm apart. The dorsal sensory branch of the ulnar nerve and the superficial radial nerve with its multiple branches pass in the subcutaneous tissue over the dorsal ulnar and dorsal radial aspect of the wrists, respectively. They are easily palpated and susceptible to injury by relatively superficial lacerations. On the volar aspect of the fingers the proper digital nerves are volar to the digital arteries. A patient presenting with a volar finger laceration and arterial bleeding is most likely to have a transected digital nerve in addition to the transected artery. A digital sensory examination using a paper clip should be performed to determine two-point discrimination before any anesthesia is instilled. In addition, if regional block anesthesia is performed, motor muscle testing of the intrinsic musculature should be carried out first. Regional nerve blocks

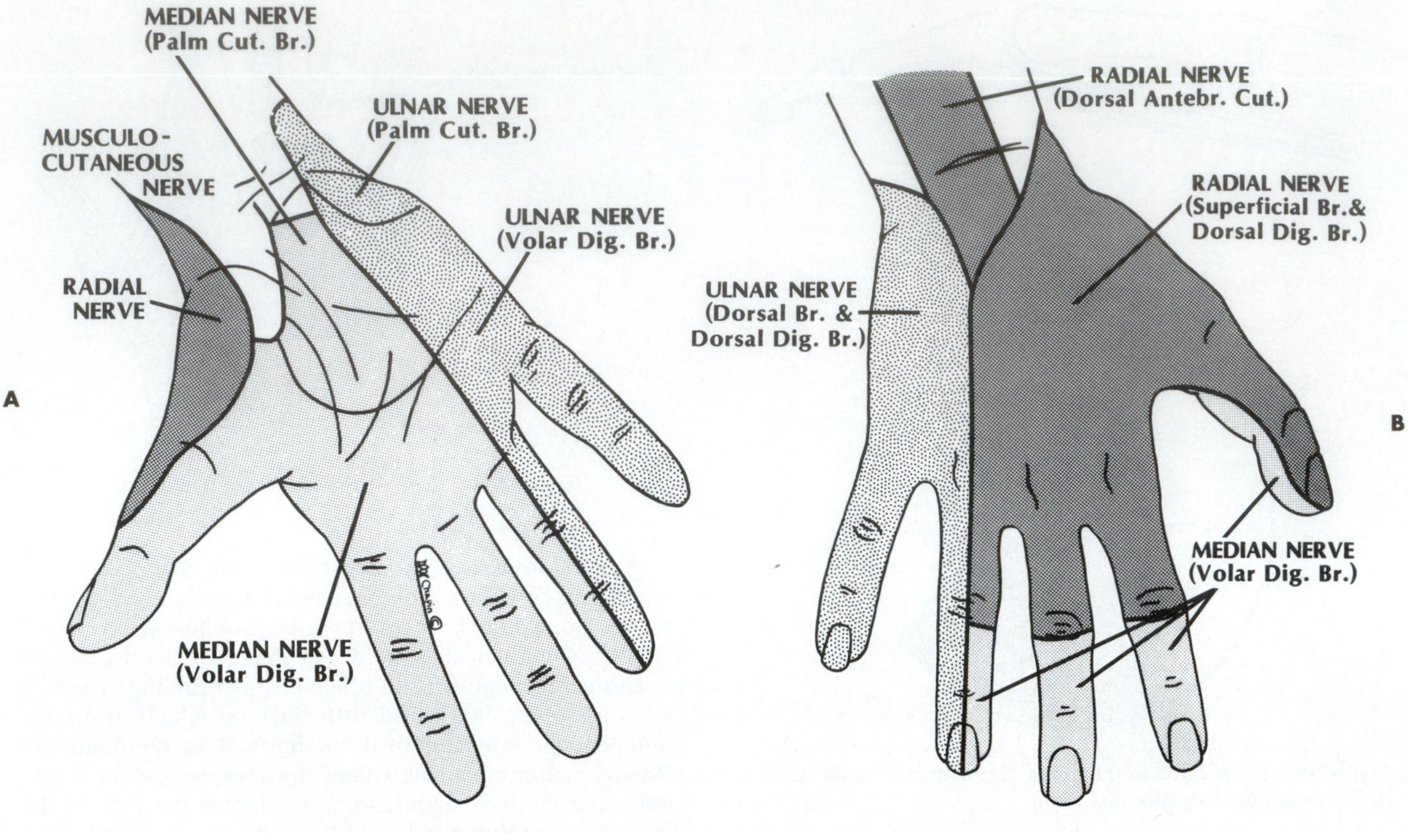


**Fig. 72-11.** Nerves of the hand. **A,** Volar aspect. **B,** Dorsal aspect. *Cut. br.,* Cutaneous branch; *dig. br.,* digital branch; *antebr.,* antebrachial.

include the intermetacarpal block and, at the wrist, the superficial radial nerve, dorsal sensory branch of the ulnar nerve, the median nerve, and the ulnar nerve blocks. With the widely-used techniques of magnification for nerve repairs, it is possible to repair a proper digital nerve at the level of the distal interphalangeal joint. There are different opinions regarding the timing of nerve repair; however, for sharp, clean wounds with nerve injury, primary repair is usually indicated.

**Radiographic examination.** X-ray examination of the hand or finger is needed for most hand injuries and certainly for lacerations resulting from glass; however, wood and nonopaque glass often are not demonstrated on x-ray examination. In addition to searching for foreign bodies, an x-ray should be obtained to assess the hand for fractures, puncture wounds of the bone, dislocations, and ligamentous injuries with small avulsion fragments. Additional x-ray studies are sometimes helpful; they can provide true lateral views of the proximal interphalangeal joint for assessment of intraarticular fractures and/or dislocations, and oblique views of the ring and little metacarpals for assessment of fractures and/or dislocations of the carpal metacarpal joints. Once it has been established that nerve, tendon, joint, or open fractures exist, further exploration of the wound is not indicated. The injury requires surgical exploration and repair in the operating room. Local exploration of the wound only serves to increase the possibility of contamination and may possibly cause a blood clot to be dislodged, resulting in bleeding, which would need to be dealt with on an emergency basis.

### Diagnostic considerations

When dealing with hand injuries it must be remembered that vital structures lie immediately beneath a thin covering of skin, especially over the joint surfaces on the dorsum of the hand and over the flexor creases on the volar aspect of the hand. In open injuries it is important to recognize a partial flexor or extensor tendon laceration, a transection of the flexor digitorum profundus tendon distal to the superficialis insertion (see Fig. 72-9), a transection of the common digital extensor tendon without extension lag resulting from the presence of the tendinous junction (see Fig. 72-10), digital nerve injuries, and crush injuries to the fingertip with subungual hematoma and nail bed injuries.

In closed injuries, long-term morbidity can result from mallet deformity at the distal interphalangeal joint, boutonnière deformity at the proximal interphalangeal joint, collateral ligament injuries at the metacarpophalangeal joint of the fingers and thumb and the proximal interphalangeal joint of the fingers, and rupture of the flexor digitorum profundus tendon from its insertion. Minor hand injuries must be properly splinted to allow uncomplicated wound healing in areas over mobile joint surfaces.

## TREATMENT

### Fractures

Basic orthopedic principles for the treatment of fractures apply to the hand, with the understanding that accurate reduction is required to restore maximal function to small hand bones and joints. Stable fractures usually can be

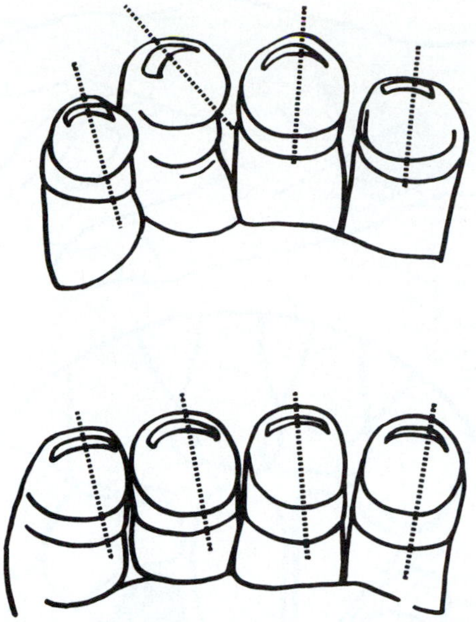

**Fig. 72-12.** Flexed fingertips should be checked for rotational alignment. **A,** Rotational malalignment of fourth finger because of metacarpal or phalangeal fracture. **B,** Normal alignment.

treated by closed reduction and splinting. Unstable and displaced intraarticular fractures often need open reduction with internal fixation. Fractures are classified as either open or closed, an open fracture being one that communicates with the wound.

***Rotational deformities.*** Gross angular or rotational deformity may allow easy recognition of a bone or joint injury. Palpation for tenderness at the injury site can be performed before x-ray examination. Motion or stress examination is usually reserved until adequate radiographic assessment has been accomplished. Proper x-ray examination, often including anterior and true lateral views, must be performed. Careful examination is required to evaluate for rotational deformities. Flexed fingertips normally point toward the scaphoid (Fig. 72-12). Overlapping or malpositioning of the fingertips should be observed in both the flexed and extended positions. In the extended position, rotation is assessed by noting the relationships of the curve of the fingernails with the adjacent fingers and comparing this with the opposite hand.

***X-ray examination of the hand.*** X-rays may be misleading because overlapping structures can obscure a small fragment of bone. In hand injuries small fragments of bone are often attached to a collateral ligament, a volar plate, or a displaced tendon (Fig. 72-13). The fragment may signify a potentially unstable condition that must be treated to avoid deformity. Particular attention should be directed to interarticular fractures. In the case of specific ligamentous injuries, x-rays should be obtained before testing for instability, e.g., the metacarpophalangeal joint of the thumb. Stress testing may displace a previously undisplaced interarticular fracture that could have been treated by immobilization alone.

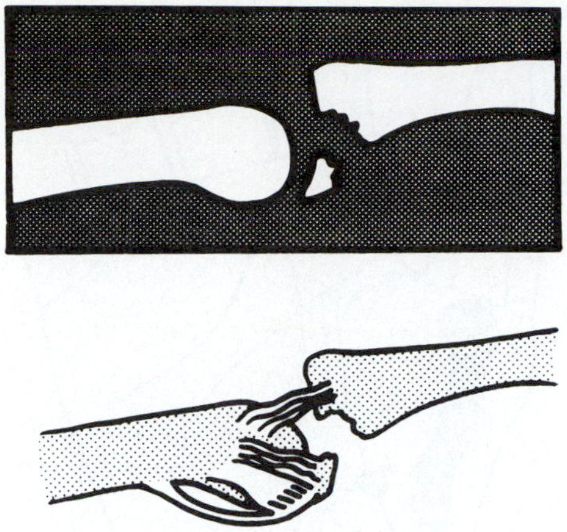

**Fig. 72-13.** Unstable fracture of the proximal interphalangeal joint.

***Fractures of the terminal phalanx.*** Fractures of the terminal phalanx are usually the result of crush injuries and are associated with subungual hematomas and nail bed injuries. In most instances the subungual hematoma should be evacuated; if nail bed injuries exist, the nail should be removed and the laceration of the nail bed repaired with fine absorbable sutures. Adequate repair of the nail bed in soft tissue injuries usually results in a satisfactory reduction of the fracture fragments. Occasionally, with more proximal terminal phalanx fractures, open reduction and internal fixation is indicated. If there is a concomitant flexion deformity at the distal interphalangeal joint, a tendon injury may exist in addition to the fracture.

***Fractures of the middle and proximal phalanx.*** Fractures of the middle and proximal phalanx can be displaced by a number of forces. Because of the extrinsic flexor and extensor tendons' longitudinal pull and the potential for rotational deformities, these fractures must be assessed for both rotational and angulation deformities (see Fig. 72-12). Furthermore, intraarticular fractures at the proximal interphalangeal joint and distal interphalangeal joint may produce fragments involving the articular surface that are potentially unstable (see Fig. 72-13). These fractures can be complicated by subluxation or fracture dislocation; this requires open reduction and internal fixation. Small fractures involving one fourth of the articular surface on the volar lip of the middle phalanx can be associated with late dorsal dislocation. Intraarticular injuries with small fragments, even if not displaced, have a potential for significant morbidity.

***Fractures of the metacarpal.*** Fractures of the metacarpal are usually treated by closed reduction. These must be assessed for overriding with shortening and angulation. Rotational alignment is critical in the assessment and treatment of metacarpal fractures. It can be checked by observing the position of the fingernails and the rotational alignment of the fingertips (see Fig. 72-12). Postreduction rotation should be checked clinically and radiographically. With open injuries and multiple displaced fractures, internal fixation is often recommended.

Bennett's fracture is an oblique intraarticular fracture through the base of the thumb (Fig. 72-14). The metacarpal shaft, the larger segment, is displaced proximally, a result of the pull of the thumb's long abductor tendon. The volar

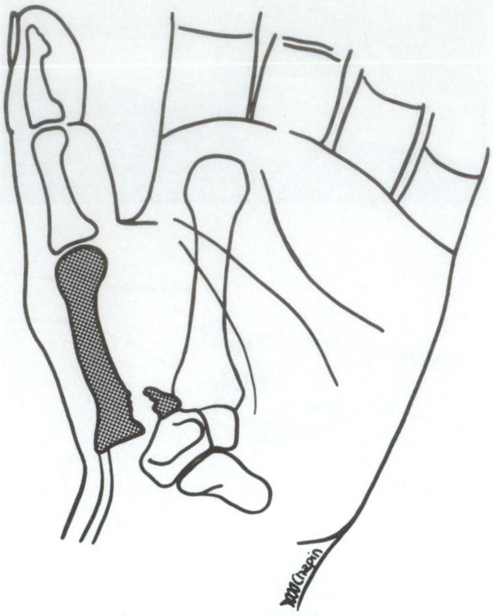

Fig. 72-14. Bennett's fracture.

ulnar fragment of the metacarpal usually remains in its normal position because of the ligamentous attachments in the area. It requires reduction and, often, internal fixation. A similar intraarticular fracture or fracture dislocation can occur at the base of the fifth metacarpal, involving the carpalmetacarpal joint. This fracture also requires reduction and, often, internal fixation.

*Fracture of the scaphoid.* Fracture of the scaphoid usually results from a fall on an outstretched hand. The patient presents with pain and tenderness elicited by palpation in the anatomic snuff-box (Fig. 72-15). Fracture of the scaphoid is the most common fracture of the carpal bones and the most commonly undiagnosed fracture of the upper extremity. When a scaphoid injury is suspected, the wrist should be immobilized despite a negative x-ray and treated for presumed scaphoid fracture. X-ray examination should be repeated in two weeks. A fracture may be visualized at that time. The most common dislocation of the carpals is a volar dislocation of the lunate. It can be associated with acute median nerve compression, requiring immediate reduction.

## Dislocations

Dislocations in the hand occur primarily at the interphalangeal and metacarpophalangeal joint levels. At the interphalangeal level they are a result of hyperextension force or direct trauma on the fingertip and result in a burst wound along the flexor crease at the distal or proximal interphalangeal joint. Closed injuries often can be reduced without difficulty and splinted in slight flexion at the interphalangeal joint level. Metacarpophalangeal joint dislocation usually results from a hyperextension injury. The volar plate is usually disrupted proximally at its metacarpal attachment, and the joint is dislocated so that the proximal phalanx lies dorsal to the metacarpal head. The metacarpal head can become trapped through a buttonhole of tissue. The thumb metacarpophalangeal joint

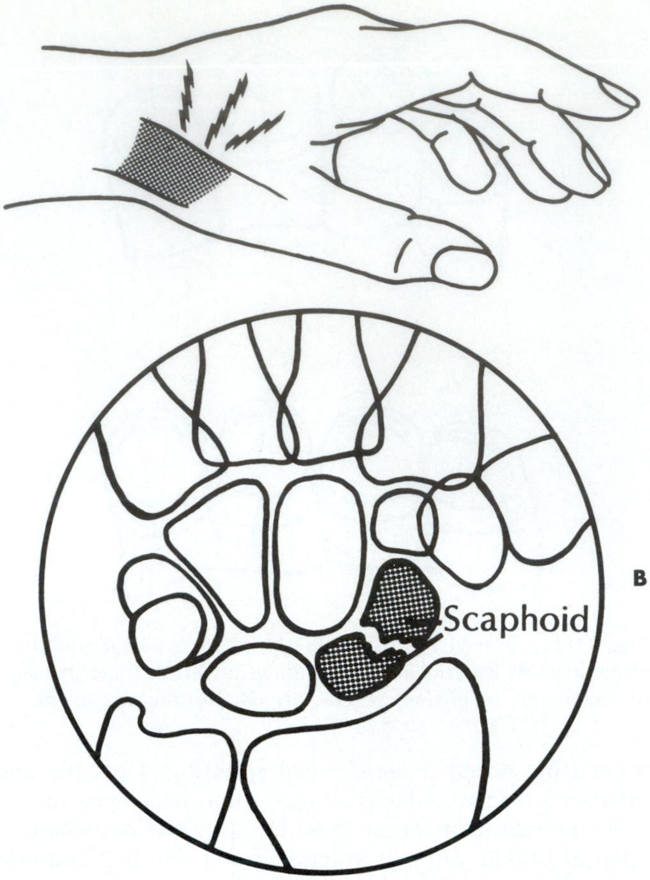


**Fig. 72-15. A,** Pain in the anatomic snuff-box. **B,** Fracture of the scaphoid.

often can be reduced closed, but it occasionally requires open reduction. If the physician is not familiar with techniques of reduction, the patient should be referred.

## Ligamentous injury

Injury to the ulnar collateral ligament at the metacarpophalangeal joint of the thumb usually results from acute radial deviation of the thumb at the metacarpophalangeal joint (Fig. 72-16). This injury usually is caused by a skiing fall and results in a complete or incomplete tear of the ulnar collateral ligament. The patient presents with swelling, pain, and tenderness on the ulnar side of the metacarpophalangeal joint of the thumb. The area should be examined by x-ray, and if no fracture is found, stress testing is recommended. When there is an incomplete lesion and minimal deviation on stress testing, immobilization with a thumb spica cast can be satisfactory treatment. When there is significant laxity associated with a complete disruption of the ulnar collateral ligament, surgical repair of the ligament is indicated.

## Mallet finger

Mallet finger is a flexion deformity of the fingertip at the distal interphalangeal joint secondary to avulsion of the extensor tendon from its insertion on the dorsal surface of the distal phalanx (Fig. 72-17). The patient presents with absent or incomplete active extension at the distal interphalangeal joint. The mechanism of injury is often direct trauma to the fingertip, resulting in an avulsion of

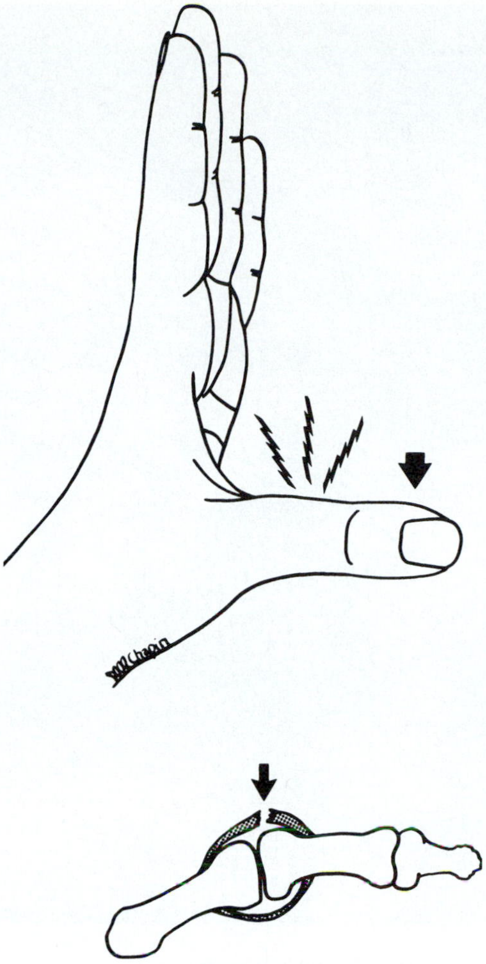

**Fig. 72-16.** Injury to the ulnar collateral ligament at the metacarpophalangeal joint of the thumb.

the extensor tendon. Treatment of a closed injury with a tendon avulsion or a tendon avulsion with a small fragment consists of splinting the distal interphalangeal joint in the neutral position for 6 weeks and night splinting for an additional 2 or more weeks. When a larger fragment representing one third or more of the articular surface is present, or when a fragment is associated with volar subluxation of the terminal phalanx, open reduction and internal fixation are indicated. When assessing these injuries by x-rays it is important to obtain a true lateral view, of the distal interphalangeal joint.

## Boutonnière deformity

Boutonnière deformity is a flexion deformity of the finger at the proximal interphalangeal joint with hyperextension of the distal interphalangeal joint (Fig. 72-18). This injury results from a rupture or laceration of the central slip of the extensor mechanism at or near its insertion into the base of the middle phalanx. The lateral bands of the extensor mechanism progressively dislocate in a volar direction caused by tearing or stretching of the transverse retinacular ligament that normally maintains the position of the lateral bands dorsal to the axis of the proximal interphalangeal joint. As the lateral bands slip volar to the axis of the proximal interphalangeal joint, a flexion deformity of the proximal interphalangeal joint is created;

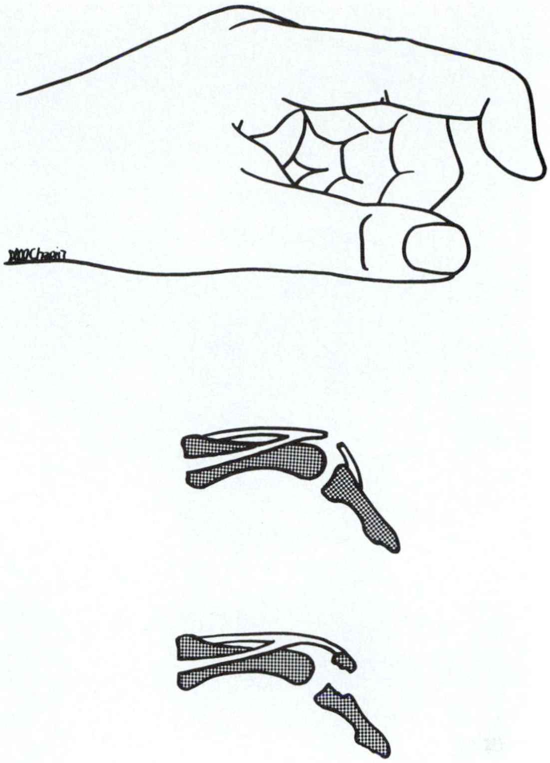

**Fig. 72-17.** Mallet finger.

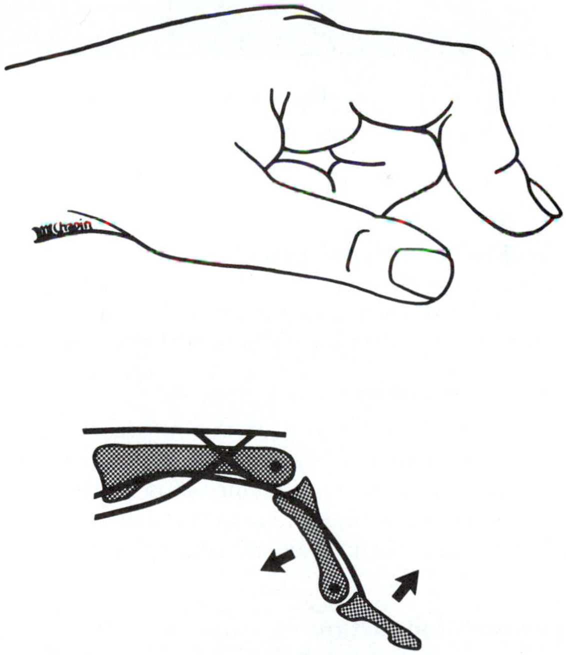

**Fig. 72-18.** Boutonnière deformity.

and because of the shortening of the lateral bands a hyperextension deformity arises at the distal interphalangeal joint. This deformity often is not present at the time of injury but develops slowly over a period of weeks as the lateral bands drift progressively in a volar direction. If the injury is due to an open wound, the central slip should be surgically repaired. The deformity is often seen late, and late closed injuries should be treated by splinting

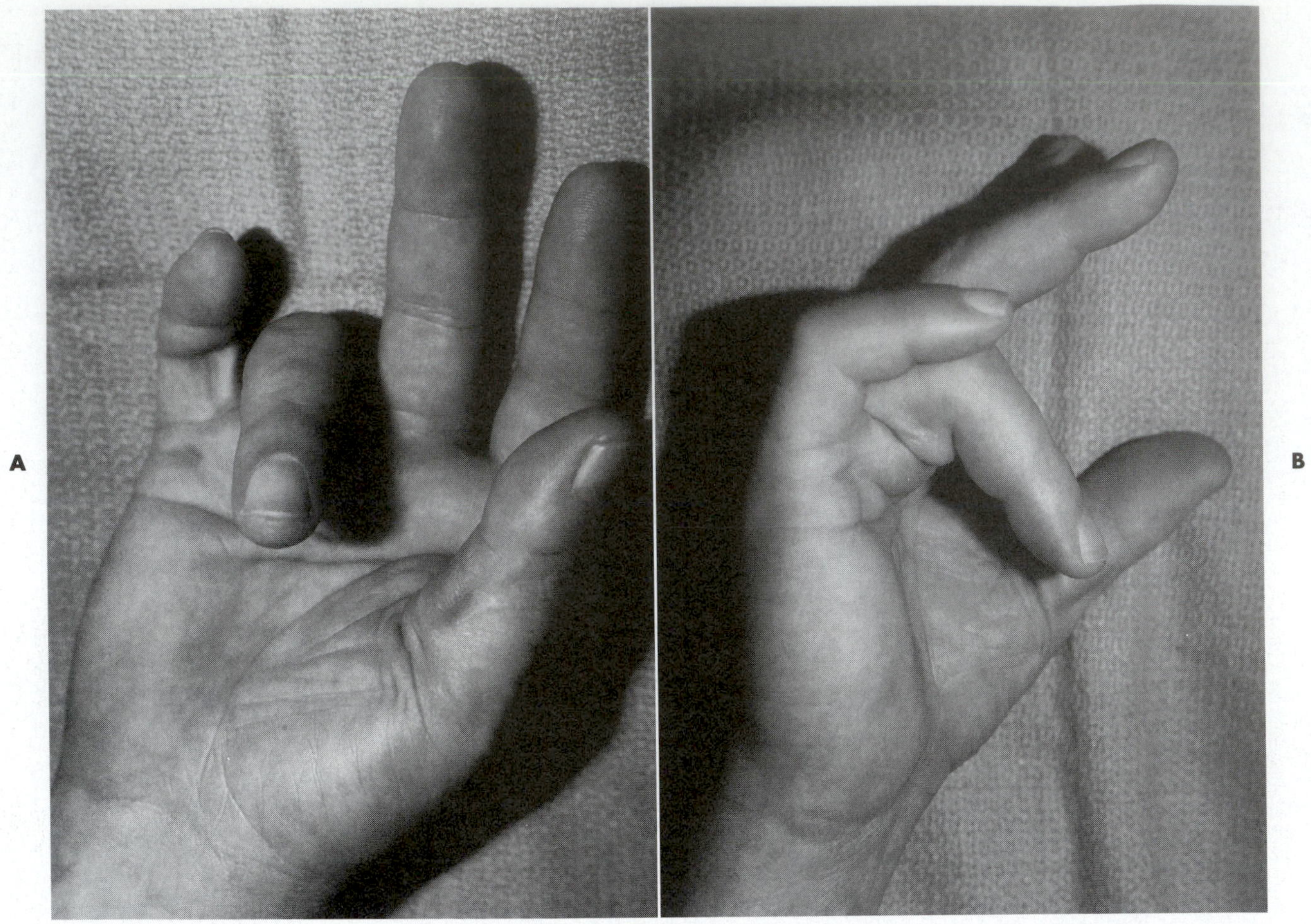

Fig. 72-19. Dupuytren's contracture, anteroposterior (A) and lateral (B) views.

the proximal interphalangeal joint in extension and allowing active flexion at the distal interphalangeal joint to stretch the shortened lateral band. This injury requires a prolonged period of carefully supervised splinting.

## Swan-neck deformity

In a swan-neck deformity of the finger, the proximal interphalangeal joint is in hyperextension and the distal interphalangeal joint is in flexion. This condition can be caused by traumatic injury to the volar plate, an old mallet finger deformity, rheumatoid arthritis, or intrinsic contraction.

## Dupuytren's contracture

Dupuytren's contracture results from a proliferative fibroplasia of the longitudinal band of the palmar aponeurosis that forms in nodules and cords (Fig. 72-19). The area involved is between the skin and the flexor tendon in the distal palm and fingers and can produce contractures at the metacarpal and proximal interphalangeal joints. The flexor tendons are not involved. The cause of this disorder is unknown, although heredity is a factor. The most common areas affected are the ring and little fingers, with occasional involvement of the thumb and long fingers. The condition is sometimes associated with thickened knuckle pads over the proximal interphalangeal joint of the fingers and involvement of the plantar fascia. Surgical intervention is not recommended until definite flexion contracture develops at the metacarpal or proximal interphalangeal joints.

## Trigger finger and thumb

Trigger finger and thumb may be of congenital origin, occurring in infancy, but it usually develops in adulthood as a result of a nonspecific tenosynovitis of the flexor tendon sheath. The inflammation at the level of the proximal pulley of the flexor sheath produces a stenosis of the sheath, causing telescoping of the fibers of the flexor tendon, and results in a discrepancy between the size of the tendon and the opening at the level of the proximal pulley. The patient presents with a locking or snapping of the finger or thumb, with point tenderness and a nodule over the base of the flexor sheath near the metacarpophalangeal joint. The finger may be locked in the flexed or extended position. If the condition is chronic, referral for steroid injection or surgical treatment is often needed.

## Bowler's thumb

Bowler's thumb is an injury to the ulnar proper digital nerve of the thumb at the level of the metacarpophalangeal joint secondary to repetitive trauma while grasping a bowling ball or heavy tools. Repetitive trauma can lead to perineural fibrosis. The patient presents with a tender mass on the ulnar aspect of the thumb just distal to the metacarpal joint, which usually represents a swelling of the nerve. In addition there is decreased sensation on the ulnar tip of the thumb. With early presentation, avoidance of the repetitive trauma usually allows the condition to resolve.

### De Quervain's stenosing tenosynovitis

De Quervain's stenosing tenosynovitis is a nonspecific inflammatory condition involving the abductor and extensor pollicis tendons at the level of the first dorsal compartment. The condition usually affects women 30 to 50 years of age who present with pain and tenderness with palpable thickening in the area of the first dorsal compartment. Finkelstein's test may be positive (Fig. 72-20). This entity must be differentiated from a bony pathologic condition of the distal radius or carpus and from metacarpal joint degenerative arthritis. Recommended early treatment consists of splint immobilization and antiinflammatory medications. Chronic conditions may require referral for steroid injection or surgical intervention.

### Carpal tunnel syndrome

Carpal tunnel syndrome is a median nerve compressive neuropathy that occurs at the level of the wrist where the median nerve passes deep to the transverse carpal ligament. The condition usually affects women 30 to 60 years of age. The patient complains of numbness in the median nerve distribution, which may be exacerbated at night and is associated with some pain on the volar aspect of the forearm. The patient also may note tingling in the thumb, index, and long fingers and may tend to drop small objects. The condition usually involves the dominant hand but can be bilateral. It may be related to trauma, as in Colles' fracture, repetitive activity, or to edema secondary to trauma or infection, or it may be associated with any space-occupying lesion such as lymphoma or ganglion. It is also associated with systemic medical conditions such as diabetes mellitus, thyroid dysfunction, amyloidosis, and pregnancy. Often the cause is nonspecific but accompanies inflammatory conditions and rheumatoid tenosynovitis.

On examination, the patient may have slight atrophic changes of the fingertips in the median distribution and atrophy of the thenar muscles, particularly the abductor pollicis brevis. Sensory testing may indicate abnormal two-point discrimination. Tinel's sign, production of paresthesias in the hand by tapping over the median nerve at the level of the wrist or carpal tunnel, is often present with carpal tunnel syndrome (Fig. 72-21). When a degree of compressive neuropathy exists, Phalen's test, flexing of the wrist for 1 minute, causes increased paresthesias in the median nerve distribution resulting from increased pressure within the carpal tunnel. Patients can be symptomatically improved with a volar carpal splint and antiinflammatory medications. If these measures are not efficacious, the patient should be referred for consideration of steroid injection of the carpal tunnel or surgical release.

### Arthritis

The major forms of arthritis that affect the hand are osteoarthritis and rheumatoid arthritis (see Chapters 78, 79, and 80). Osteoarthritis involves the interphalangeal joints and the carpalmetacarpal joint of the thumb and often presents with swelling, stiffness, pain, and deformity. At the distal interphalangeal joints, osteophytes develop and may be associated with mucous cyst formation dorsally over the distal interphalangeal joint or in the eponychium. Rheumatoid arthritis affects the metacarpal and proximal interphalangeal joints and presents with pain, swelling, and stiffness. The condition may progress to deformity.

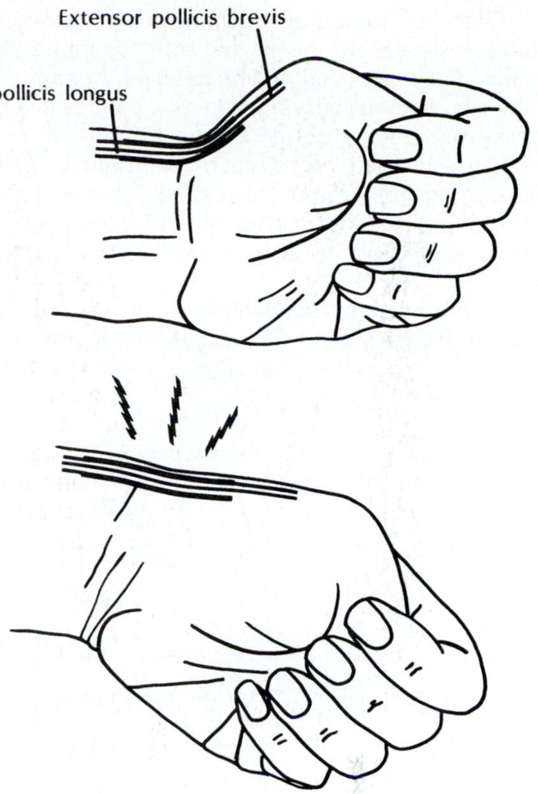


**Fig. 72-20.** Finkelstein's test is positive in de Quervain's stenosing synovitis. Ulnar flexion of the wrist produces pain over the dorsal compartment containing the extensor pollicis brevis and abductor pollicis longus.

### Tumors

***Ganglions.*** Ganglions are the most common soft tissue tumor of the hand. These cystic masses arise from the tendon sheath or joint and may be related to acute trauma or recurrent chronic injury. The most common location is on the dorsum of the wrist over the radiocarpal joint in the area of the scapholunate ligament. Other locations include the volar surface of the wrist near the flexor carpi radialis tendon and the flexor sheaths of the fingers. Ganglions may present as an asymptomatic mass or may be associated with aching, pain, and weakness. They may disappear spontaneously. Persistent symptomatic ganglions may be referred for aspiration or may have to be removed completely through surgical intervention.

***Lipomas.*** Lipomas are unusual soft tissue tumors of the hand that present as a soft, asymptomatic mass. They may be deceptively large, extending deep beneath the fascia of the hand.

***Giant cell tumors of tendon sheath.*** Giant cell tumors of tendon sheath are the second most common tumor in the hand. They can occur at any age and are more common in women. They usually present as a painless, slow-growing mass on the volar or dorsal aspect of the finger. They have been associated with repetitive trauma. These benign lesions may enter joint spaces and create extrinsic pressure defects on the bone. They should be distinguished from giant cell tumors of the bone, which are malignant lesions.

***Inclusion cysts.*** Inclusion cysts of the digits result from penetrating trauma with the implantation of epidermal elements beneath the skin. These painless cystic masses usually occur in the palm or on the volar aspect of the finger in the immediate vicinity of a remote penetrating injury. Glomus tumor is an abnormal growth of an arteriovenous anastomosis, which normally exists in the digits. The tumor usually occurs in the nail beds and fingertips. Patients often complain of severe pain exacerbated by exposure to cold. There may be some alteration in color of the nail bed, associated with point tenderness over the area of the lesion. The lesion is often less than 1 cm in diameter. If it is large enough, it may erode the bone of the terminal phalanx, as can be demonstrated by x-ray examination.

***Bone tumors.*** Bone tumors are usually benign and most often an enchondroma. They may present with posttraumatic pain and a pathologic fracture, or be discovered as an incidental finding on x-ray examination.

## Infections

Infections can result in significant morbidity and functional loss; they are usually caused by a minor injury such as an abrasion. A significant infection can result in edema, tissue necrosis, and fibrosis and contracture. Antibiotics have significantly decreased the rate of mortality from hand infections but have not eliminated the need for incision and drainage. The timing and technique of surgical drainage is important in minimizing the degree of morbidity with infections.

The majority of hand infections are caused by coagulase-positive *Staphyloccocus aureus* and *Streptococcus*. Infections caused by staphylococci require incision and drainage in many instances. Streptococcal infections usually present as cellulitis with lymphangitis and lymphadenopathy. Human bite infections, common in the hand, often present with an injury over the metacarpophalangeal joint and sometimes with septic arthritis. The onset of symptoms resulting from the injury is rapid; classic signs of joint involvement include pain on passive range of motion at the metacarpophalangeal joint and point tenderness over the volar aspect of the metacarpophalangeal joint. The pathogenic organisms include anaerobic

A

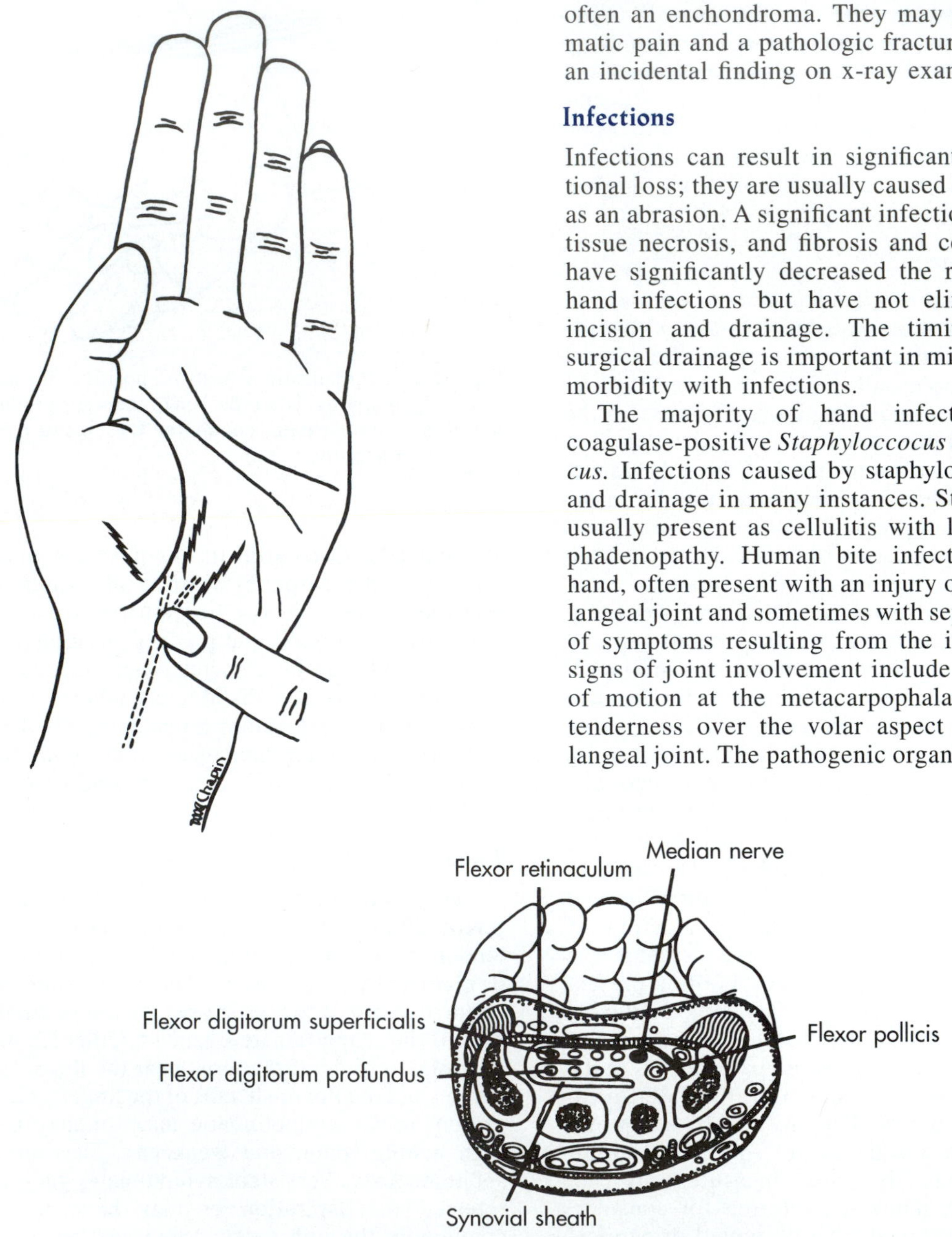


B

**Fig. 72-21. A,** Tinel's sign is often present with carpal tunnel syndrome. **B,** Cross-sectional anatomy of the wrist, showing tendons and the median nerve, which may be compressed by inflammation or infection because they are encompassed by the synovial sheath and flexor retinaculum.

mouth organisms in addition to *S. aureus* and *Streptococcus*. An injury suggestive of a human bite infection with involvement of the metacarpophalangeal joint requires exploration in the operating room. In certain anatomic spaces the organisms may develop a localized abscess requiring surgical incision and drainage.

***Paronychia.*** Paronychia is an infection of the soft tissue around the fingernail. It usually begins as a hangnail (Fig. 72-22). The most common organism is *S. aureus,* with the portal of entry being the eponychium. It may involve one corner of the nail or extend to the opposite side under the eponychium or fingernail. The patient presents with pain, erythema, and tenderness in the area of the eponychium or paronychium. Incision and drainage are indicated when localized collections of pus are present. This may require removing a portion of the nail to obtain adequate drainage. One should be suspicious of a fungal infection with chronic recurrent paronychia.

***Herpetic whitlow.*** Herpes infection can involve the fingertip (herpetic whitlow) and may have the appearance of a bacterial paronychia. Distinction is important because incision does not help and may delay healing. Herpetic whitlow is a viral infection of the finger. Medical and dental personnel are at particular risk. Usual symptoms include pain or pruritus followed by the formation of vesicles, which may coalesce. The pain may become intense and is occasionally accompanied by bacterial infection. Healing usually takes 2 to 3 weeks. Therapy includes analgesia, saline soaks, and local wound care.

***Felon.*** A felon is a digital pulp space abscess. It usually causes significant throbbing pain which develops over a 48- to 72-hour period (Fig. 72-23). The fingertip is extensively involved and may become necrotic, a result of ischemia. Interference with the blood supply to the diaphysis of the terminal phalanx may also result in aseptic necrosis. The bone can become secondarily infected, and osteomyelitis may develop. Treatment consists of incision and drainage after adequate anesthesia. In making the incision, it is important to avoid the digital nerves and not to create painful scars on the contact points of the volar pad of the digit.

***Deep space infections.*** The deep palmar space lies between the fascia covering the metacarpals and the fascia below the flexor tendon sheaths on the volar aspect of the palm (Fig. 72-24). This space is divided into the thenar and midpalmar spaces by a septum that passes from the fascia beneath the index flexor sheath dorsally to the third metacarpal shaft. The adductor muscle of the thumb rises from the entire length of the third metacarpal bone and inserts in the thumb in the area of the metacarpophalangeal joint. This muscle divides the thenar space into anterior and posterior divisions. Both deep space infections cause systemic signs in addition to local pain, tenderness, and decreased active range of motion of the fingers. A thenar space abscess causes tenderness over the thenar half of the palm plus marked swelling of the thumb-index web space (Fig. 72-25). This infection requires drainage through the thumb-index web space. A midpalmar space abscess causes tenderness and swelling over the palm on the ulnar aspect with decreased range of motion of the middle, ring, and little fingers (Fig. 72-26). This space is drained through a transverse incision at the level of the distal palmar crease.

***Tenosynovitis.*** Acute or purulent tenosynovitis is an infection of the flexor sheath that usually results from a penetrating wound over a flexor crease of the finger or palm. The patient usually presents with rapidly developing signs of infection. The cardinal points of tenosynovitis were emphasized by Kanavel (Fig. 72-27). The four signs of flexor sheath infection are uniform swelling of the digit, slight flexion of the involved finger, tenderness over the

A

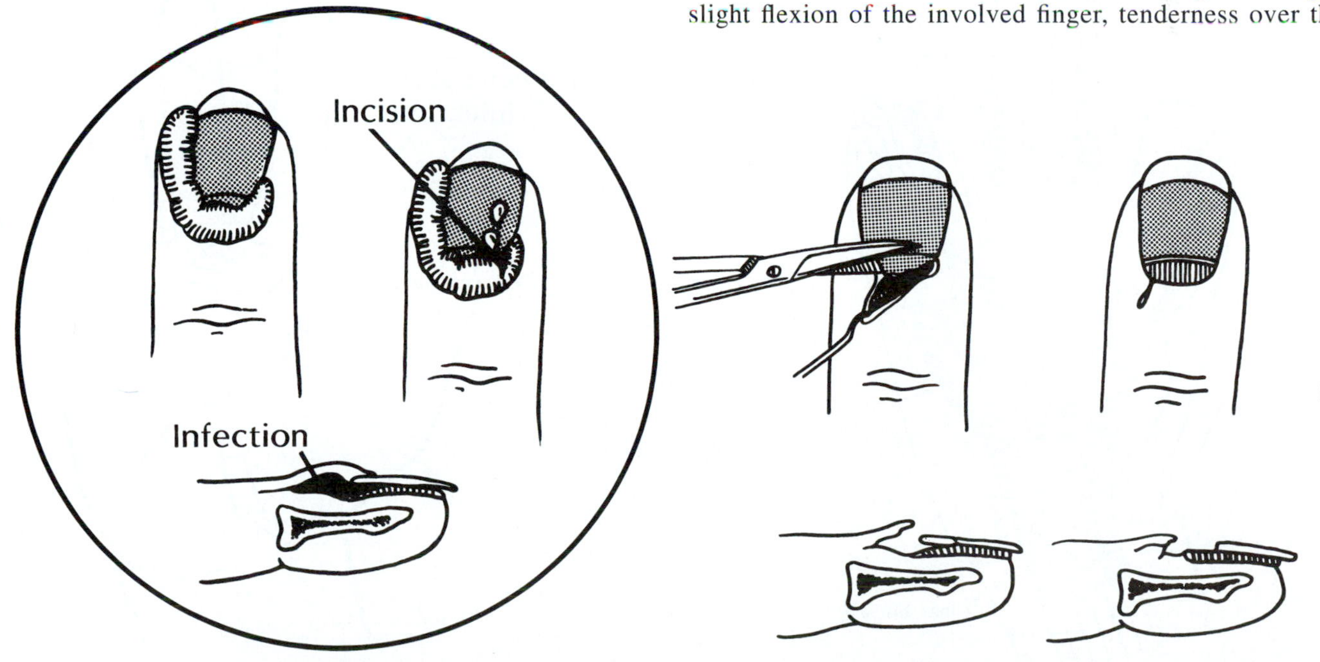


B

**Fig. 72-22.** Paronychia. **A,** Location of infection. **B,** Incision and drainage with removal of a portion of the fingernail.

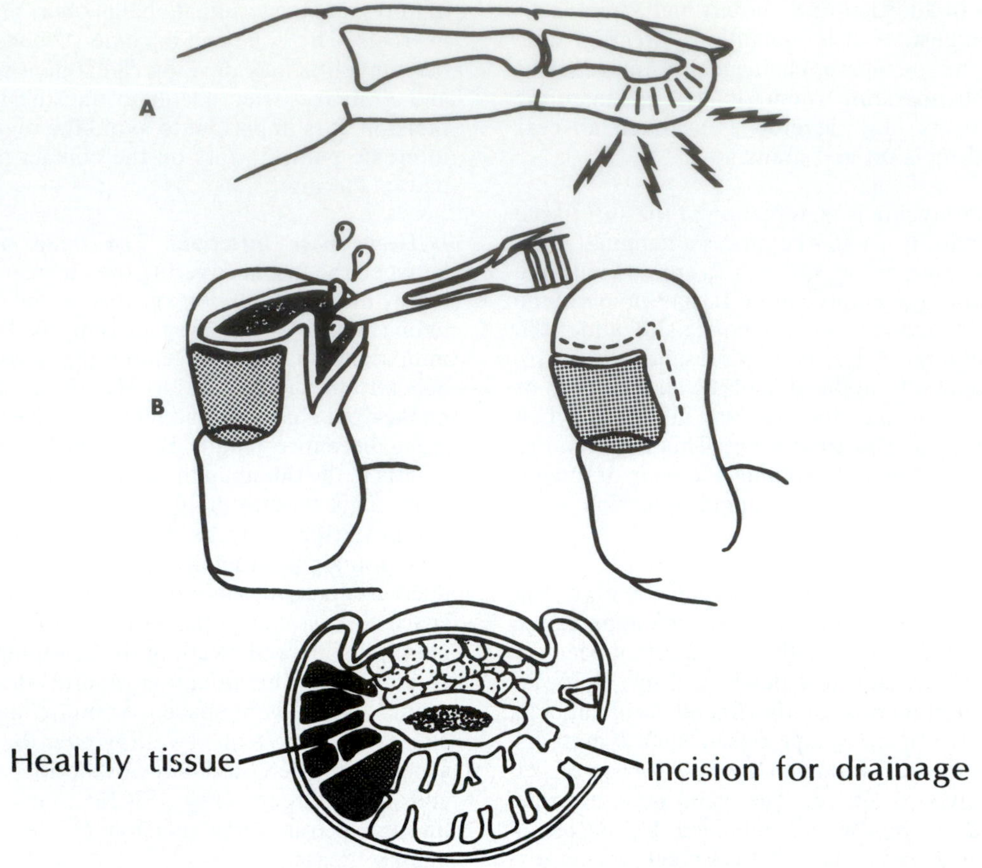


**Fig. 72-23.** **A,** Felon, a digital pulp space abscess. **B,** Treatment requires complete drainage of the infected tissue. **C,** An incision must be made into each of the infected portions of the pulp space.

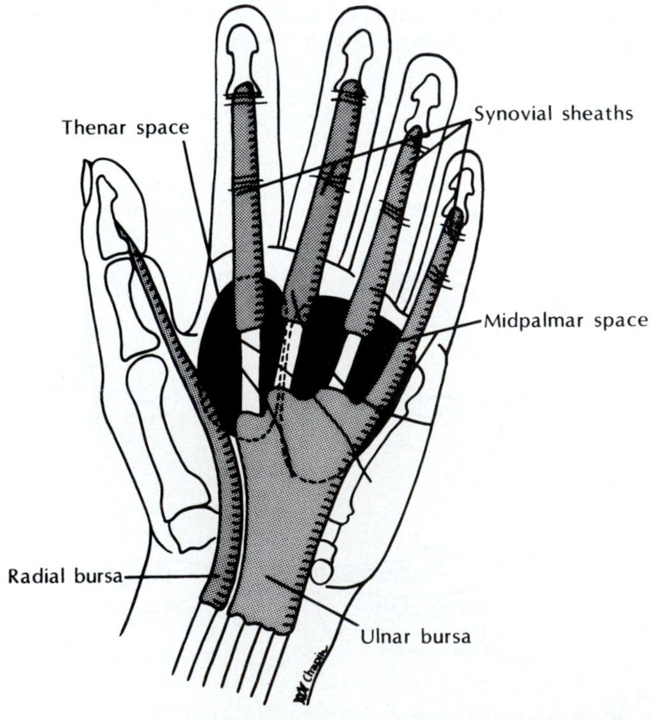


**Fig. 72-24.** Normal bursal anatomy.

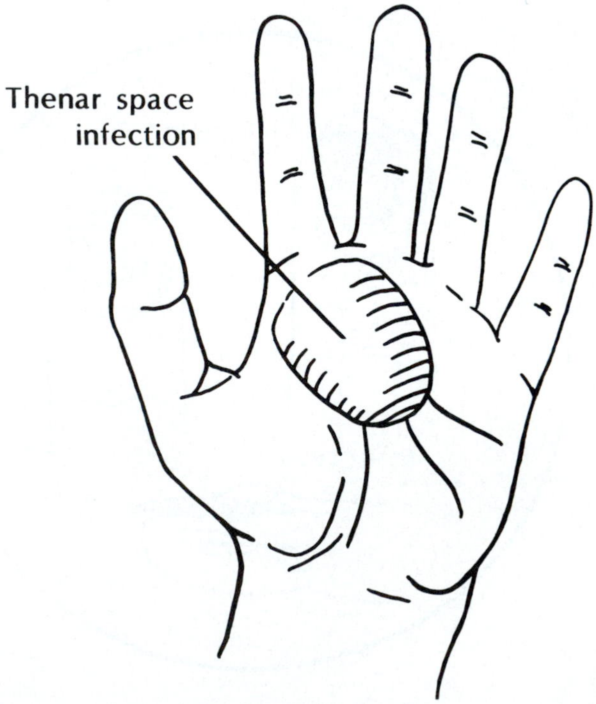


**Fig. 72-25.** Thenar space abscess.

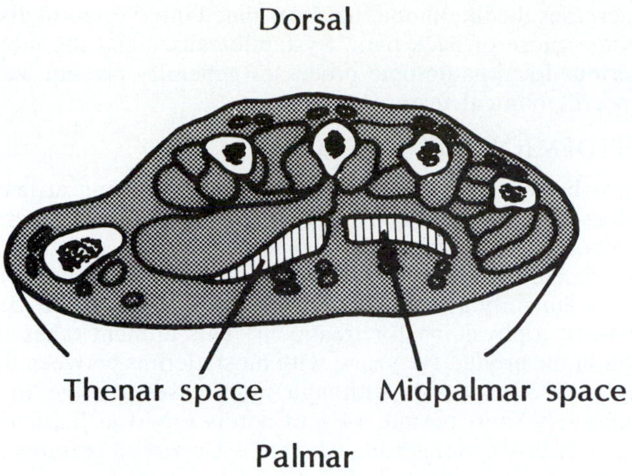


**Fig. 72-26.** Cross-section of the palmar spaces.

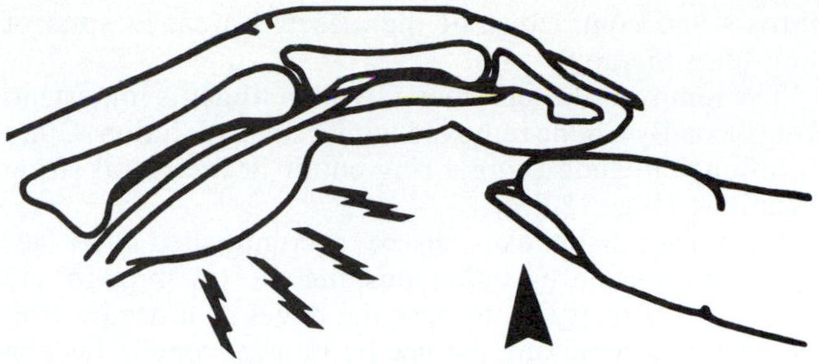

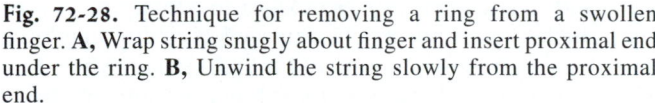

**Fig. 72-27.** The cardinal points of tenosynovitis as emphasized by Kanavel.

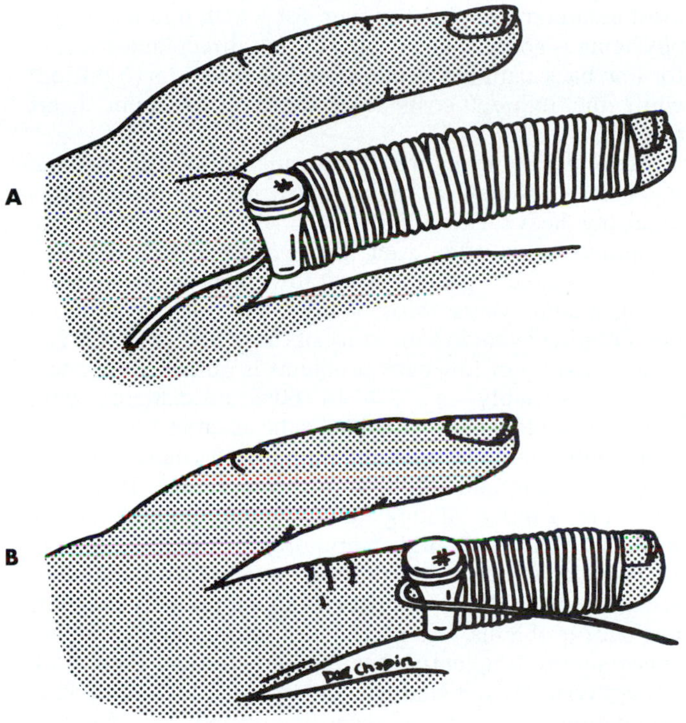


**Fig. 72-28.** Technique for removing a ring from a swollen finger. **A,** Wrap string snugly about finger and insert proximal end under the ring. **B,** Unwind the string slowly from the proximal end.

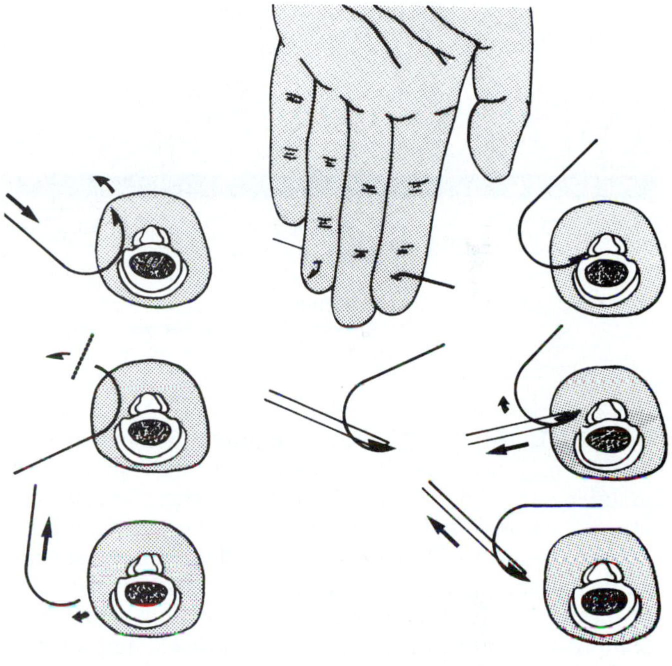

**Fig. 72-29.** Technique for removing fishhooks embedded in tissue by either snapping off the barb or by using the bevel of a needle to minimize further injury (see text).

length of the involved flexor tendon sheath, and increased pain on passive extension of the finger. The patient cannot actively flex the finger and experiences pain on attempting to do so.

Acute purulent tenosynovitis is a closed-space infection and often requires incision and drainage. The flexor sheath of the thumb extends from the tip of the thumb proximally through the carpal canal into the radial bursa on the distal forearm. The flexor sheath of the little finger extends from the tip of the little finger throughout the carpal canal into the ulnar bursa on the distal forearm. The flexor sheaths on the index, long, and ring fingers extend to the level of the proximal palmar crease (see Fig. 72-24). Surgical drainage usually requires an incision in the palm and in the affected digit and, in the case of the thumb and little finger, possibly at the level of the distal forearm.

The general principles for treatment of hand infections are immobilization; incision and drainage when indicated; elevation of the infected part; systemic antibiotics; placing of the wrist, hand, and fingers in the position of function; and treatment of systemic diseases that can be exacerbated by the infection. Surgical intervention for closed space infections of the hand should be carried out in a bloodless field under general or regional block anesthesia. Significant infection with its associated edema may result in fibrosis and contracture of the affected area, in spite of long-term therapy.

The removal of rings from a swollen finger is important. Rings usually can be removed with a soapy solution. Other techniques include using a ring cutter or the spiral string technique (Fig. 72-28).

Removing fishhooks can be accomplished after adequate anesthesia by either pushing the tip through and cutting it off or trying to pass the bevel of a needle over the barb and removing the needle in a retrograde fashion (Fig. 72-29).

## BIBLIOGRAPHY

Green DP: *Operative hand surgery,* ed 3, New York, 1993, Churchill Livingstone.
Lucas GL: *Examination of the hand,* Springfield, Il, 1972, Thomas.
Milford L: *The hand,* St. Louis, 1982, Mosby.

CHAPTER

# 73 Low Back

James J. Heffernan

Low back pain is the most common musculoskeletal complaint among adult patients seen in primary care practice and second only to limb pain (generally related to injury) among patients seen in urgent care settings. Potential causes of low back pain are legion but a specific pathoanatomic diagnosis is established in fewer than 20% of cases. The back is a complex mechanical structure, a composite of vertebrae, intervertebral disks, and apophyseal joints stabilized by ligaments and the paraspinal and abdominal musculature. It supports the trunk and transmits, via the sacroiliac joints, upper body loads to the pelvis and lower extremities. The posterior vertebral elements encase and protect the spinal cord and cauda equina. Connections to the bulk of the body's peripheral nervous system run through the vertebral neural foramina. Moreover, innervation of the spine and its supporting structures is rich: the posterior rami of the lumbosacral spinal nerves supply the apophyseal joints, the interspinous ligament, the paravertebral muscles and associated cutaneous areas; at each vertebral level, the sinuvertebral nerve, joined by a sympathetic branch, innervates the anterior dura mater and dural sleeve, the posterior vertebral periosteum, the posterior longitudinal ligament, epidural blood vessels, and the annulus fibrosus. Most episodes of low back pain arise from regional (i.e., nonsystemic) processes, a result of mechanical derangements to the complex anatomic relationships within and around the spine. About 1% of patients with acute low back pain have sciatica, defined as pain in the distribution of a lumbar or sacral nerve root, with or without associated neurosensory and motor deficits. The presence of sciatica increases the likelihood that a herniated intervertebral disk is the cause of back pain. Systemic causes and the more serious local pathologic processes generally present with specific clinical features.

## EPIDEMIOLOGY/ETIOLOGY

Low back pain is extremely common, producing at least short-term impairment in 70% to 80% of a general population. The point prevalence of low back pain is 5% to 7% among adults. Nearly 2% of adults lose time from work annually as a result of low back pain, and 2% to 5% consult a physician for treatment. This ailment takes its toll in the productive years, with most victims between the ages of 30 and 60. Although most cases resolve in a relatively short period, 14% of adults report at least one episode lasting longer than 2 weeks, 1.6% with features of sciatica.

Among chronic conditions, back and spine impairment is the most common cause of limited activity in individuals under age 45 and ranks third behind heart disease and arthritis in the 45- to 64-year age range. It is the second most common complaint of pain for which treatment by a physician is sought. The annual cost of direct medical care for low back pain has been estimated at $13 to 16 billion, while the indirect costs rival those of ischemic heart disease.

Men and women are comparably affected, but the incidence is somewhat higher for women in occupations requiring heavy exertion. Women also report low back symptoms more often after the age of 60, whereas men more commonly present with low back pain in their younger adult years. Most studies have demonstrated a precipitating event in a minority of cases (6% to 28%). The natural history of low back problems is one of recurrence, reported variably in 33% to 60% of patients with occupational low back pain during the ensuing 1 to 3 years. Symptoms tend to be mild and transient in young workers, more persistent and severe with increased age. Incidence rates are similar among heavy, light, and sedentary workers, although a higher proportion of heavy workers are incapacitated with low back pain. Those bored or dissatisfied with their occupations are more likely to report low back problems. In a given work setting, low back pain appears more frequently in those who consider their work to be physically demanding. Specific risk factors include occupations that require repetitive lifting in a forward bent-and-twisted position, exposure to vibrations caused by vehicles or heavy machinery, and cigarette smoking. Low back pain arises commonly in individuals who either sit or stand for prolonged periods; however, jobs requiring sudden maximal efforts have also been correlated with higher than average incidence rates.

There is no convincing evidence that those with moderate kyphosis, scoliosis, or lordosis are more at risk for low back pain than those with normal spine curvature. Likewise, moderate differences in body habitus do not predict differences in incidence rates, although massive obesity and major skeletal abnormalities are attended by increased rates of low back pain. Isthmic spondylolisthesis, spinal osteochondrosis, and the spinal stenosis associated with achondroplasia appear to predispose affected individuals to low back problems.

Recreational activities have not been associated convincingly with low back pain syndromes, although isthmic spondylolisthesis has reportedly increased fourfold among gymnasts and interior linemen on football teams.

Attempts to characterize the low back pain patient psychologically have produced a variety of profiles. Of note, most such studies have been performed retrospectively on patients already involved in treatment programs, raising questions about cause and effect, and about selection bias. Nonetheless, low back pain patients have demonstrated greater levels of psychopathology than extremity-injured peers or noninjured industrial workers. A tendency toward neurotic depression rather than hysteria has been described, although other data support increased rates of hysteria and hypochondriasis along with anxiety and depression. Increased rates of alcoholism and divorce have also been noted among individuals disabled by low back pain.

## PATHOPHYSIOLOGY

The potential causes of low back pain are myriad (see the box at right). Systemic illness, regional cancer, and local infection account for only a trivial percentage of total cases. Most low back pain arises from uncharacterized regional processes. Although many putative causes have been identified by invasive studies and postmortem examinations, the specific anatomic cause of backache in a given patient most often goes unidentified (Figs. 73-1 and 73-2).

The herniated vertebral disk is probably the best known cause of low back pain (Fig. 73-3). Disk herniations tend to occur in a lateral or central posterior direction. However, posterior prolapse of a herniated vertebral disk accounts for only a small subset of cases and generally declares itself through the classic neural impingement syndrome of sciatica. Herniation of the nucleus pulposus occurs in 95% to 98% of cases at the L4-L5 or L5-S1 disk spaces, with herniation at two levels in 10% of cases. Older individuals have an increased risk of disk herniation at higher lumbar disk levels. Other causes of sciatica include spinal stenosis, synovial cysts, congenital anomalies of lumbar nerve roots, primary neural and osseous tumors, metastatic cancer, and epidural abscesses. Retroperitoneal neoplastic processes and endometriosis may cause sciatica by involvement of the lumbosacral plexus. Sciatica from local pressure to the sciatic nerve may result from toilet seats, especially in thin individuals, or from habitual placement of a wallet in a back pocket.

With aging, the intervertebral disk degenerates, and much low back pain is probably related to small tears in the annulus fibrosus, compression of endplate cartilage, and microfractures of subchondral bone in the end plates, processes that cannot be demonstrated acutely. As these processes continue over time, however, subtle anatomic derangements are integrated, and spondylosis develops, manifested radiographically in thinning of the intervertebral disk with narrowing of neural foramina and bony spurring and lipping, especially apparent at the disk margins. (Spondylolisthesis refers to actual slippage of one vertebra over another, usually at the L5-S1 level.) Studies using fluoroscopically directed injections of (1) hypertonic saline and (2) anesthetic agents with or without corticosteroids have reproduced and relieved low back pain respectively in a variety of patients. Sites injected have included the facet joints, ligamentum flavum, interspinous and supraspinous ligaments, intradiskal space, and epidural space. Derangement of posterior structures may therefore cause or contribute to low back pain in a given patient.

### Causes of low back pain

**Primary mechanical derangements (generally a putative cause)**

Ligamentous strain
Muscle strain/spasm
Facet joint disruption/degeneration
Intervertebral disk degeneration and/or herniation
Vertebral compression fracture
Vertebral endplate microfractures
Spondylolisthesis
Spinal stenosis
Diffuse idiopathic skeletal hyperostosis
Severe scoliosis or kyphoscoliosis
Scheuermann's disease (vertebral epiphyseal aseptic necrosis)

**Infection**

Epidural abscess
Vertebral osteomyelitis
Septic diskitis
Pott's disease (tuberculosis)
Nonspecific manifestation of systemic illness
  Bacterial endocarditis
  Influenza

**Neoplasia**

Epidural and/or vertebral carcinomatous metastases
Multiple myeloma, lymphoma
Primary epidural or intradural tumors

**Metabolic disease**

Osteoporosis
Osteomalacia
Hemochromatosis
Ochronosis

**Inflammatory rheumatologic disorders**

Ankylosing spondylitis
Reactive spondyloarthropathies (including Reiter's syndrome)
Psoriatic arthropathy
Polymyalgia rheumatica

**Referred pain**

Abdominal or retroperitoneal visceral process
Retroperitoneal vascular process
Retroperitoneal malignancy
Herpes zoster

**Paget's disease of bone**

**Primary fibromyalgia**

**Psychogenic pain**

**Malingering**

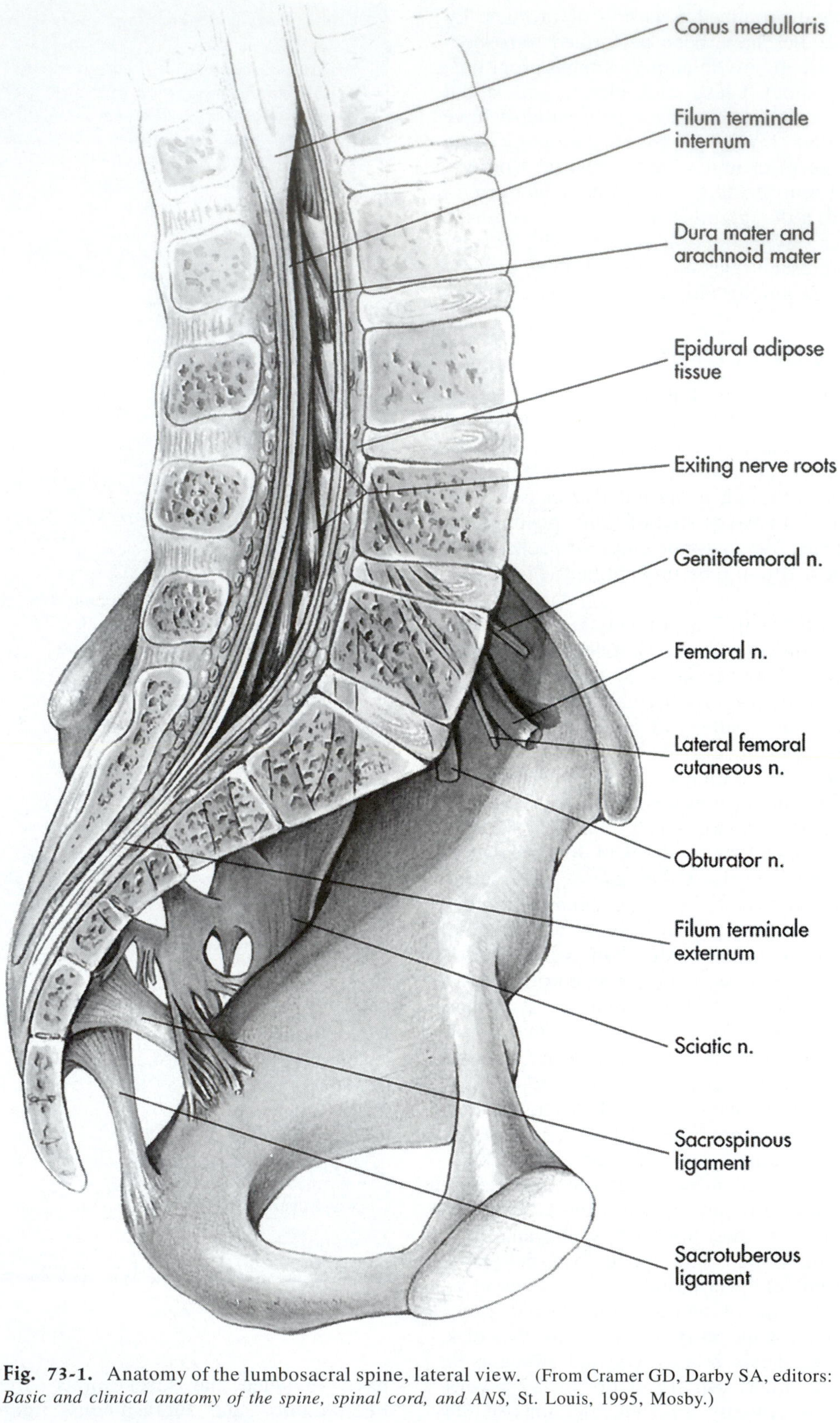


**Fig. 73-1.** Anatomy of the lumbosacral spine, lateral view. (From Cramer GD, Darby SA, editors: *Basic and clinical anatomy of the spine, spinal cord, and ANS,* St. Louis, 1995, Mosby.)

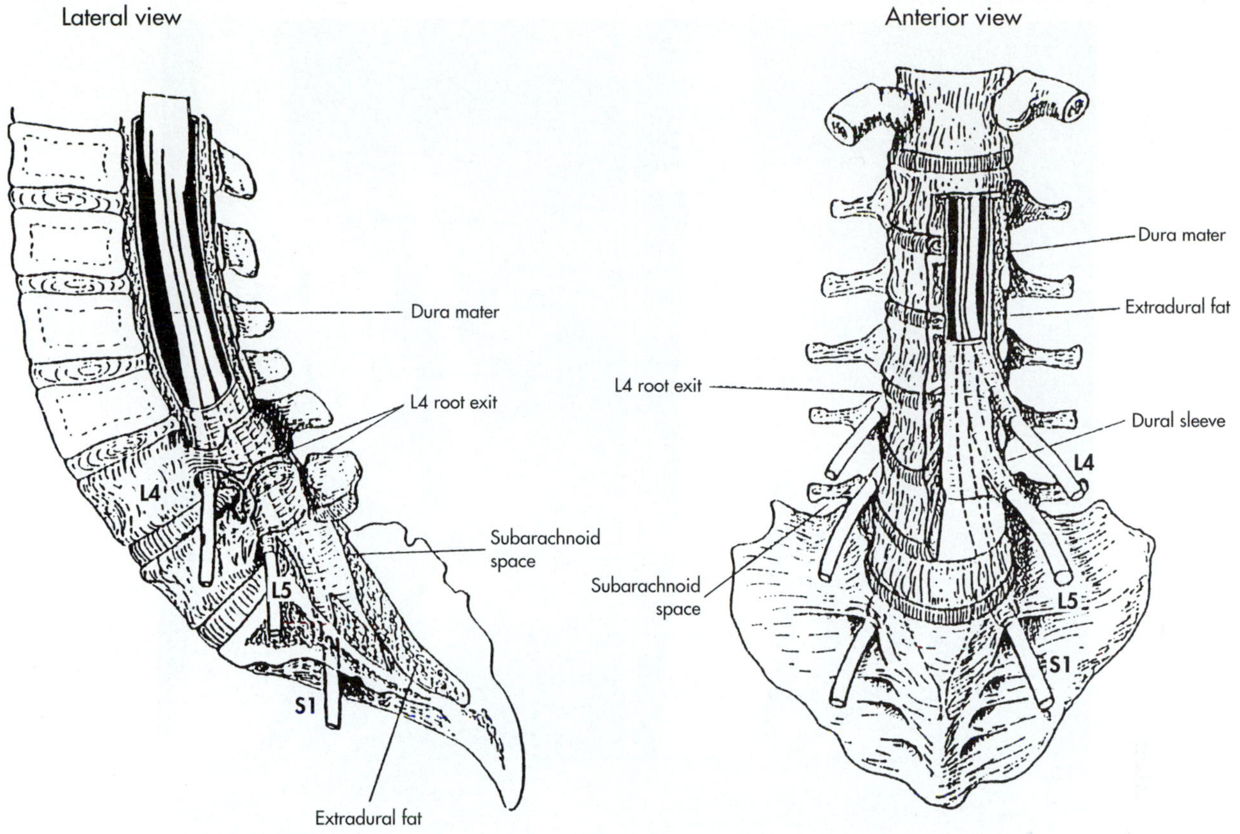


**Fig. 73-2.** The relationships of the lumbar nerve roots to the vertebrae and disk.

Spinal stenosis resulting from bony encroachment by osteoarthritis, generally superimposed on congenital narrowing of the lumbar spinal canal, can result in lumbosacral radiculopathy and neural claudication (or pseudoclaudication) with pain on ambulation or standing, relieved by sitting. The pain of spinal stenosis probably represents reversible cord or root ischemia.

Muscle pain and spasm are common features in low back pain, but a primary role for muscle strain remains uncertain. Axial myalgias associated with polymyalgia rheumatica and the low back pain and tender points associated with idiopathic fibromyalgia (fibrositis) are relatively common syndromes that cause low back pain nonskeletally. An inflammatory spondyloarthropathy may affect as many as 2% of the population, and most often presents as low back pain and stiffness, especially apparent in the morning after sleep. Diffuse idiopathic skeletal hyperostosis, noted predominantly in middle-aged and elderly men, may be dominated by complaints of low back pain and stiffness.

One systemic process that is a major public health problem is osteoporosis (see Chapter 38). This condition can produce back pain by the mechanism of vertebral collapse, albeit more often in the thoracic spine. Chronic, poorly localized back pain associated with osteoporosis in the absence of overt vertebral collapse probably results from multiple microfractures near vertebral end plates and can be a debilitating condition among the elderly population.

The spectrum of causes of back pain differs above and below the lumbosacral area. The thoracic spine is the region most commonly affected by vertebral compression fractures resulting from osteoporosis; the lower thoracic and upper lumbar vertebrae are the most common sites of bony metastatic disease. Middle and upper back pain may result from axial loading of the spine, as in football or jumping injuries, or after strenuous upper extremity trauma, as in the vertebral spinous process avulsion fractures or "clay shoveler's back," a condition noted among manual laborers in whom shear forces are transmitted to the spine from abrupt unloading of upper extremity loads. Sacral fractures, a form of traumatic spondylolisthesis, may result from direct trauma to a flexed hip and extended leg. Coccygeal fracture may likewise result from direct trauma, usually a fall, and rarely from difficult childbirth. Pelvic malignancies may involve coccyx or sacrum by direct extension as well as by lymphatic or hematogenous spread.

The clinical course of low back pain associated with systemic illness is that of the underlying disease. Excluding such patients from consideration, as well as those few with local infections and neoplastic processes whose prognosis depends on the specific cause and available treatment, one is left with the core of typical low back pain

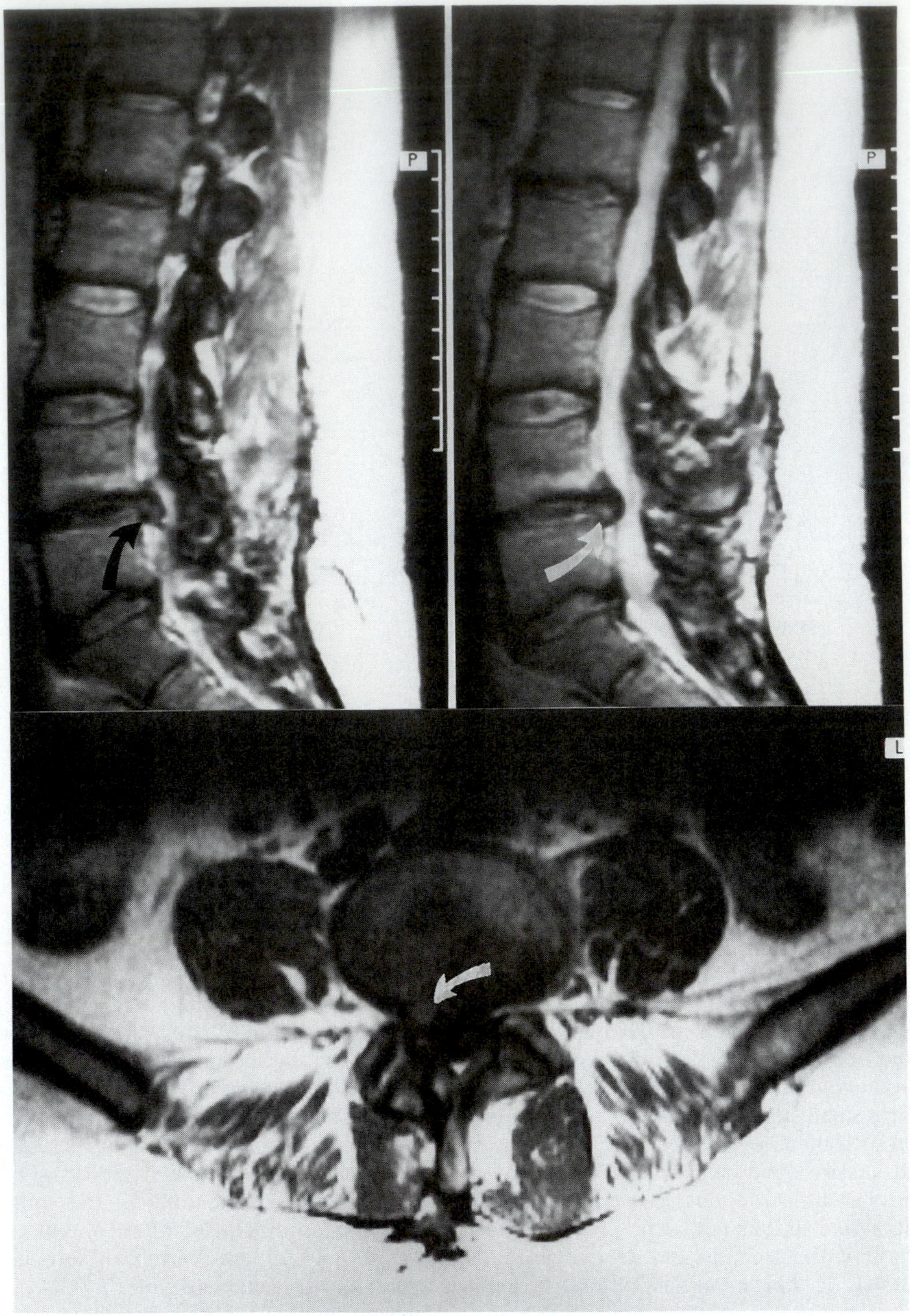


**Fig. 73-3.** Magnetic resonance imaging demonstrating a right posterior herniated L4-5 disk.

patients. Among this group the natural course is one of remittence and recurrence. Acute low back pain is generally a self-limited disease with remittence rates of 40% in one week, 50% to 85% in 3 weeks, and 90% in 2 months. Even when low back pain is considered a work-related, compensable injury, 85% to 90% of patients return to work within 12 weeks. Among patients who have sought medical attention for low back pain, recurrence is noted in 90%; recurrences are generally longer lasting than the initial attack.

## HISTORY

Although a firm anatomic diagnosis is seldom achieved, the history and physical examination are generally discriminating enough to focus attention on the more serious causes of low back pain. Severe backache after serious trauma suggests the possibility of fracture or acute disk herniation. Pain after a pure flexion injury suggests a pathologic condition of the disk or end plate, whereas pain after a torsional injury is more often associated with disruption of posterior structures with facet joint disruption and ligamentous injury. With either such injury, pain may radiate to the buttocks or upper thigh. The pain associated with an acutely herniated intervertebral disk is often sharp or lancinating with radiation down the back of a leg, often to the ankle or foot. Such a patient resists movement and generally finds relief in a fixed, somewhat awkward posture, supine, or in the lateral decubitus position with the leg of the affected side in partial flexion. Bilateral sciatica associated with bowel or bladder dysfunction (either incontinence or retention) and weakness suggests a massive central disk herniation or another epidural (and rarely intradural) mass lesion, especially hemorrhage, abscess, or metastasis. When a patient is writhing in pain, one should suspect a visceral or vascular source such as a rupturing abdominal aortic aneurysm or ureteral colic. Backache, associated with fever, especially when unremitting and/or progressive, may represent vertebral osteomyelitis, septic diskitis, epidural abscess, or Pott's disease. Other febrile processes associated with back pain include early herpes zoster, influenza, or the nonseptic musculoskeletal manifestations of bacterial endocarditis.

Morning back pain and stiffness persisting several months after an insidious onset in a younger man who derives relief from exercise makes a convincing case for ankylosing spondylitis. Similar symptoms coupled with conjunctivitis, urethritis, skin rash, balanitis, and/or diarrheal illness suggest a reactive inflammatory arthropathy (e.g., Reiter's syndrome; see Chapter 83).

Most patients with typical mechanical low back pain present with pain, often severe, and muscle stiffness involving the back, buttocks, and often the thigh. Pain typically arises hours or days after a new or unusual exertion and is generally relieved by assumption of the supine position.

In the patient with chronic sciatica, pain is often confined to the buttocks and leg and is usually described as dull or aching and exacerbated by sitting. Low or midback pain in an elderly patient may result from osteoporosis with or without overt compression fractures, from polymyalgia rheumatica, or from neoplasia. Dull, progressively worsening bone pain in an elderly patient, especially pain that worsens with recumbency, raises the specter of metastatic carcinoma or multiple myeloma. Spinal stenosis may also present as pain in a recumbent or standing position with relief found in a sitting position. Diffuse, poorly localized back pain may be a manifestation of Paget's or Cushing's disease. Associated pelvic or abdominal disease may refer pain to the low or midback.

## PHYSICAL EXAMINATION

A systematic approach to examination of the back complements the history in focusing attention on the identifiable causes of low back pain. Inspection and palpation yield important initial clues. Severe idiopathic kyphoscoliosis is associated with degenerative arthritis; mild scoliosis or loss of lumbar lordosis is a common finding in the acute setting, the result of paravertebral spasm. Prominent dorsal kyphosis in an elderly patient suggests vertebral collapse as a result of osteoporosis or malignancy. Most patients with acute low back pain have restricted vertebral mobility. However, diminished chest expansion (less than 3 centimeters) in association with decreased mobility of the spine, especially when sacroiliac joint tenderness coexists, strongly suggests ankylosing spondylitis (see Chapter 83). Tenderness of the sciatic nerve in the sciatic notch suggests a component of radiculopathy or neuropathy.

A tender spinous process in the setting of fever and backache raises the possibility of vertebral osteomyelitis, septic diskitis, or an epidural abscess; a tender spinous process in the setting of malignancy and backache points towards vertebral or epidural metastatic disease. In both instances, aggressive emergency evaluation is indicated, especially if neurologic deficits are noted.

Simple maneuvers can provide further diagnostic clues. Induction of pain on torsion or hyperextension of the spine suggests ligamentous or facet joint injury, most common at the L4-5 level. Increased discomfort with spinal extension is also suggestive of spinal stenosis. Reduction of lateral flexion is more suggestive of spondyloarthropathy than of a herniated disk or other cause of mechanical low back pain.

The most useful simple maneuver in assessing nerve root impingement is the straight leg raise (SLR) test, which places the lower lumbosacral nerve roots under tension. With the patient supine, the examiner slowly raises the straightened leg of the affected side through the arc of hip flexion. If pain occurs in a radicular distribution with straight leg elevation through an arc of 60 degrees or less, the test is positive. The probability that herniation is the cause of back pain increases as the angle necessary to produce radicular pain decreases, although there is little or no traction on nerve roots with arcs of less than 20 to 30 degrees. This test is quite sensitive (95%) for herniated lumbosacral disks, but not specific. To exclude false positive results, the examiner should attempt repeated trials, some conducted while distracting the patient. The angle associated with pain should be reproducible when one passively flexes the hip of the patient with the knee in flexion, and then slowly extends the foreleg. An important supplement to the direct SLR is the crossed SLR, which entails elevation of the unaffected leg in the patient with sciatica. A positive test results when radicular pain is produced in the unraised leg. The crossed SLR is substantially less sensitive (25%) but strikingly more specific (88%) than the direct SLR. A similar but less well-quantified provocative test for eliciting pain in the setting of L3-4 disk herniation involves forcing full or exaggerated extension of the hip of the affected side while the knee is flexed and the patient is either prone or in the lateral decubitus position.

In most instances deep tendon reflexes are not affected by mechanical low back pain. However, the ankle jerk (Achilles tendon reflex) is subserved by the S1 root and is often diminished or absent in the compression radiculopathy produced by L5-S1 disk herniation. However, the Achilles tendon reflex is frequently absent in normal, elderly individuals. No reflex deficits occur with L4-5 disk herniations. The infrequent occurrence of L3-4 disk herniation with L4 root compression is manifested as a diminished knee jerk (patella tendon reflex).

Motor deficits are often subtle but can usually be demonstrated in the setting of true sciatica. Compression radiculopathy of the S1 root by L5-S1 disk herniation is associated with weakness of plantar flexion, best demonstrated by having the patient walk on his or her toes. Dorsiflexion weakness is associated with L5 radiculopathy from L4-5 disk herniation, and may be made manifest by having the patient walk on his or her heels or dorsiflex the great toe against resistance. Quadriceps weakness results from L4 radiculopathy associated with L3-4 disk herniation.

Sensory deficits with sciatica are also often subtle but demonstrable. Compression of the S1 root by L5-S1 disk herniation may result in sensory deficits of the posterior calf and lateral aspect of the foot. Compression of the L5 root by disk herniation at L4-5 manifests as hypesthesia on the dorsum of the foot and great toe, especially in the first web space. Hypesthesia over the lateral aspect of the thigh is consistent with L4 root compression from L4-5 disk herniation. Saddle anesthesia in the patient with bilateral sciatica and loss of anal sphincter tone raises suspicion of the cauda equina syndrome from massive central disk herniation or of another space-occupying lesion, and warrants further emergent evaluation.

Hallmarks of malingering or of a psychiatric origin for low back pain include overreaction; reproduction of back pain by "tests" that should not elicit such pain on physiologic grounds (such as axial loading by the application of downward pressure on the head of the standing patient); variable results of true provocative tests, such as the SLR, when the patient is distracted; superficial, nonanatomic tenderness; and motor or sensory disturbances that behave nonphysiologically.

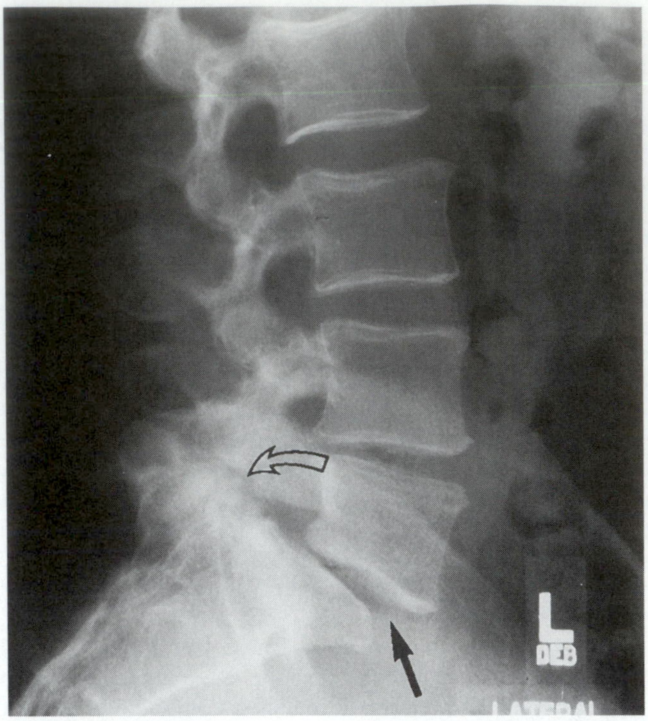


**Fig. 73-4.** Spondylolisthesis.

## LABORATORY STUDIES/DIAGNOSTIC PROCEDURES

Blood tests are of little diagnostic use in most instances of low back pain. Leukocytosis, an elevated sedimentation rate, and anemia are nonspecific markers of possible infection, neoplastic disease, or inflammatory spondyloarthropathy. Serum or urine immunoelectrophoresis may corroborate the suspicion of multiple myeloma. Abnormalities of serum calcium, phosphate, and alkaline phosphatase are crude indices of metabolic bone disease. The diagnosis of spondyloarthropathy usually rests firmly on the history, physical examination, and radiographs of the spine and sacroiliac joints; HLA-B27 determination is corroborative.

Lumbosacral spine radiographs are abnormal in the majority of persons over age 50, and quite frequently in those younger. They are neither sufficiently sensitive nor sufficiently specific to justify routine use in evaluating backache, especially in the acute setting. Findings of degenerative disk disease, osteoarthritis, spina bifida occulta, and transitional or asymmetric vertebrae are common in individuals with and without back pain, and spondylolisthesis (Fig. 73-4) has been noted in 5% to 20% of spinal radiographs.

Radiographs, (anteroposterior and lateral views), however, may be extremely helpful if an inflammatory spondyloarthropathy or a destructive lesion associated with either malignancy or an infectious process is suspected, and they may also provide an overall view of the degree of osteoporosis and associated vertebral collapse. In major trauma, radiographic study may demonstrate the presence of fractures and dislocations. Oblique views are helpful to visualize the facet joint. Selective use of spinal radiographs based on specific criteria may increase the diagnostic yield threefold. Several groups of authors have suggested reasonable indications for spinal radiography in the patient presenting with acute low back pain: (1) age greater than 50; (2) history of serious trauma; (3) known cancer; (4) pain at rest; (5) unexplained weight loss; (6) drug or alcohol abuse; (7) treatment with corticosteroids; (8) temperature above 38° C; (9) suspicion of ankylosing spondylitis; or (10) a demonstrable neuromotor deficit. Spinal radiographs may also be appropriate for a patient with pain that persists beyond 3 to 4 weeks, even in the absence of neurologic findings.

Until the 1980s, contrast myelography was the procedure of choice when epidural compression by tumor or infectious process was suspected, or when neurologic deficits suggested intervertebral disk herniation, especially when a surgical procedure was contemplated. The sensitivity of contrast myelography for herniated lumbar disk is 90%, while the specificity is 70% to 90%. Diskography demonstrates disk herniation reliably at a given level only, is somewhat less sensitive and specific than myelography, and is seldom necessary.

Computed tomographic (CT) scans of the lumbosacral spine achieve sensitivities and specificities comparable to those of myelography for herniated intervertebral disks, and may also reveal bony abnormalities, tumors, and vascular lesions. Unfortunately, CT scans of the lumbosacral spine demonstrate significant abnormalities in over one quarter of asymptomatic individuals, calling into question positive results reported in patients with less than compelling historic features and clinical findings. This technology is now widely available, and sometimes has

**Table 73-1.** Differential diagnosis of common low back pain syndromes

| Clinical entity | History | Physical examination | Supporting studies |
|---|---|---|---|
| Mechanical low back pain | Pain in back, buttocks ± thigh; may be severe<br>Onset following new or unusual exertion<br>No history of major trauma, systemic infection or malignancy<br>Relief of pain in supine position | Paravertebral tenderness/spasm<br>Scoliosis or loss of lumbar lordosis common<br>No neurologic signs (see Table 73-2) | None necessary |
| Herniated intervertebral disk | Acutely, pain in back is severe and lancinating<br>Antecedent flexion strain injury or trauma<br>Sciatica (see Table 73-3)<br>Relief of pain supine with hip flexed<br>Bilateral weakness with bowel and/or bladder dysfunction may be present with massive central disk prolapse<br>With chronic disk herniation, pain, usually dull, may be confined to leg | Striking paravertebral tenderness/spasm with splinting in awkward postures<br>Signs of radicular irritation/injury usually present in acute setting (see Table 73-3) | MRI, CT, or myelogram<br>Electromyography may provide supporting documentation of level of denervation |
| Referred visceral or vascular pain | Patient writhes in discomfort, with no relief in any position<br>Pain may occur in waves | Abdominal findings usually predominate<br>Fever or incipient shock often present | Imaging studies directed at abdomen and retroperitoneum may visualize aortic aneurysm, or abnormality of viscera (e.g., ureteral calculus, pancreatitis, etc.) |
| Metastatic malignancy (or multiple myeloma) | Unremitting or progressive pain at rest<br>Known or suspected malignancy<br>Weight loss, fever, or other systemic symptoms<br>History of weakness, bowel and/or bladder dysfunction may be present | Tender spinous process at level of involvement<br>Variable neurologic findings, up to full paraplegia | Standard radiographs may reveal destructive bony lesions<br>Radionuclide bone scan sensitive for metastatic carcinoma but not for myeloma<br>Epidural impingement of spinal cord or roots best delineated by MRI, myelography, and/or CT<br>Erythrocyte sedimentation rate elevated |
| Epidural abscess, vertebral osteomyelitis, or septic diskitis | Unremitting or progressive pain at rest<br>Fever<br>Drug abuse, diabetes mellitus, immunosuppression<br>Suspected or known systemic infection<br>Previous spinal or genitourinary surgery<br>History of weakness, bowel and/or bladder dysfunction may be present | Tender spinous process at level of involvement<br>Variable neurologic findings, up to full paraplegia<br>Stigmata of systemic infection | Standard radiographs may reveal destructive bony lesions<br>Radionuclide scans may suggest abscess<br>Blood cultures often positive<br>MRI probably best imaging modality to delineate extent of lesion and neural impingement<br>Erythrocyte sedimentation rate elevated |

*Continued.*

**Table 73-1.** Differential diagnosis of common low back pain syndromes—cont'd

| Clinical entity | History | Physical examination | Supporting studies |
|---|---|---|---|
| Ankylosing spondylitis | Insidious onset<br>Progressive morning back pain and stiffness over several months<br>Relief with exercise<br>Age at onset ≤40 y | Painful or ankylosed sacroiliac joints<br>Reduced mobility of spine<br>Reduced chest wall expansion<br>Possible associated uveitis | Sacroiliac joints and lumbosacral spine ankylosed on standard radiographs<br>Erythrocyte sedimentation rate elevated<br>HLA-B27 confirmatory<br>Uveitis may be confirmed on ophthalmologic examination |
| Reactive spondyloarthropathies | As with ankylosing spondylitis<br>Antecedent urethritis, rash, or colitis | As with ankylosing spondylitis<br>Conjunctivitis, balanitis, urethritis, and/or keratoderma blennorrhagicum<br>Psoriasis | As with ankylosing spondylitis<br>Bowel studies may reveal infectious or idiopathic inflammatory bowel disease<br>Infectious urethritis may be confirmed |
| Spinal stenosis | Back pain may vary from severe to absent<br>Pseudoclaudication often prominent, often involving L4 root (anterior thigh)<br>Pain worsens during the day, is aggravated by standing and relieved by rest<br>Weakness, bladder, and/or bowel dysfunction may be present | Neurologic findings vary, but often there is evidence of impairment at multiple spinal levels<br>Findings of osteoarthritis may be prominent | Standard radiographs generally show extensive vertebral osteophytes and degenerative disk disease<br>Imaging with MRI or CT ± myelography supports diagnosis if neurologic and imaging findings are concordant |

*CT*, Computed tomography; *MRI*, magnetic resonance imaging.

**Table 73-2.** Radiculopathies associated with intervertebral disk herniations

| Disk syndrome | Root | Rate* | Pain radiation | Sensory deficit | Motor deficit | Reflex deficit |
|---|---|---|---|---|---|---|
| L5-S1 | S1 | 45-55% | Posterior thigh<br>Posterior and lateral calf<br>Heel | Posterior calf<br>Lateral foot | Plantar flexors | Ankle |
| L4-5 | L5 | 30-40% | Lateral thigh<br>Anterior calf and dorsum of foot<br>± Great toe | Anterior calf<br>Medial foot<br>First web space<br>± Great toe | Dorsiflexors | None |
| L3-4 | L4 | 2-12% | Lateral and anterior thigh<br>Medial calf and foot<br>± Great toe | Medial calf and foot<br>± Great toe | Quadriceps | Knee |
| Cauda equina (massive central anterior prolapse) | Multiple | <1% | Bilateral, including any or all of the above | Saddle anesthesia<br>Any or all of the above, usually bilaterally | Multiple, including any or all of the above<br>Bladder and/or bowel dysfunction | Any or all of the above<br>Anal wink<br>Cremasteric |

*More than one level of involvement in up to 10% of cases.

been employed in place of or in addition to myelography when evaluating patients with low back pain.

Rigorous studies comparing magnetic resonance imaging (MRI) with CT and/or myelography have not been conducted among patients with low back pain; however, uncontrolled data suggest that MRI is equivalent to or more sensitive than CT for the diagnosis of herniated intervertebral disks and spinal stenosis, even when CT is supplemented by myelography or diskography. As with CT, MRI identifies substantial abnormalities (disk herniation and/or spinal stenosis) in up to one third of individuals with no prior low back pain; disk bulging or degeneration at at least one lumbar level is found in nearly all individuals over age 60 (see Fig. 73-3). Where available, MRI has generally become a standard in evaluating patients with suspected epidural abscess or malignancy.

Radionuclide bone scans are more sensitive than standard radiographs in identifying metastatic lesions (other than the plasmacytomas of multiple myeloma) and are also useful in characterizing the spondylolysis associated with isthmic spondylolisthesis. A battery of nuclear medicine studies is sometimes of use in identifying abscesses or osteomyelitis. When there is evidence or suspicion of nerve root compression, electromyography may be confirmatory. "Therapeutic" facet joint injections have been shown to be of no use, and injection studies directed at precisely localizing the source of low back pain are generally not indicated.

## DIFFERENTIAL DIAGNOSIS

See Tables 73-1 and 73-2.

## MANAGEMENT

### Nonpharmacologic interventions

The favorable short-term prognosis of most variants of low back pain supports a standard approach of conservative management for 4 to 6 weeks even with suspected intervertebral disk herniation (see the Managed Care Guide). The generally self-limited course of low back pain has rendered difficult the interpretation of the success of interventions other than in prospective clinical trials. Invasive studies have shown reductions of intradiskal pressure with subjects in the supine position. Bed rest on a firm mattress with or without a bed board has remained a mainstay of therapy for mechanical derangements, including compression fractures and intervertebral disk herniations. A controlled trial among military recruits has demonstrated that strict bed rest is better than none. More recent data have shown that 2 days of bed rest is as effective as 7, and results in 45% less time lost from work. Partial flexion at hips and knees while in the supine or lateral decubitus position further reduces symptoms. Sitting in bed to read or watch television should be prohibited when disk herniation is suspected, because sitting increases intradiskal pressure. Intradiskal pressures are only minimally higher in the standing position than they are lying on the side, and it is reasonable to allow ambulation to the bathroom and brief periods of walking to prevent deconditioning. A recent study among ambulatory patients with milder variants of acute low back pain suggests that continuation of ordinary activities within the limits permitted by the pain may lead to more rapid recovery than either bed rest or back-mobilizing exercises.

In the experimental setting, traction has been shown to reduce intradiskal pressure; however, the weight required to overcome lower segment resistance and produce dimensional changes in the intervertebral disk space approximates 60% of total body weight. Actual clinical trials of "therapeutic" vs. "sham" traction have demonstrated no convincing benefit from the former beyond reinforcement of the need for bed rest. There have been no trials of inversion devices or other gravity traction methods.

Ice massage or local heat may reduce pain from muscle spasm in a given instance, with heat perhaps the more useful modality when there is a major component of muscle stiffness.

Spinal manipulation is of short-term benefit in some patients, particularly those with uncomplicated, acute low back pain. Consensus data, including a large metaanalysis, do not support a role for spinal manipulation in patients with chronic back pain, although several recent prospective trials do suggest benefits from manipulation in the clinical setting of chronic impairment. Several studies have described greater patient satisfaction at the hands of chiropractors than through the prescription pads of physicians.

In experimental situations, corsets and braces can reduce intradiskal pressure, the load on the lumbar spine, and the arc of motion in flexion. There are, however, no clinical data from controlled trials demonstrating their effectiveness, and poorly fitted braces and corsets may result in unpredictable and increased movements of the lumbosacral spine. Their use is also attended by the risk of muscular disuse atrophy. Nonetheless, patients often derive relief from low back pain with binders or braces. Flexion braces are generally most effective for patients with lumbar spinal stenosis or when examination suggests predominantly facet joint injury (with pain on spine extension and torsion). Other patients with less well-defined sources of low back pain may obtain relief with the hydraulic splinting of abdominal binders. The choice of device and restriction of a specific range of motion can perhaps be established most reasonably after a thorough assessment by a physical therapist. Serious injury from the use of back braces has been associated primarily with rigid devices employed in patients with scoliosis. For a list of common back disorders, as well as suggested orthoses and their descriptions and functions, see Table 73-3. Orthopedic consultation is helpful for body positioning when prescribing a custom-fitted, as opposed to "off-the-shelf," back orthosis.

Several exercise regimens have been advocated: (1) spinal mobilization exercises emphasizing flexion, (2) paravertebral strengthening exercises stressing extension, and (3) modified isometric exercises directed at strengthening abdominal muscles and hip extensors. The limited available data suggest the greatest benefit from isometric exercises, although none of these regimens have been compared with simple bed rest. Aerobic exercise programs also have been useful for patients with chronic low back pain. In general, a patient can safely begin a slowly

## Managed Care Guide
## For low back pain

**Typical presentation of acute low back pain ± sciatica**

Diagnostic blood tests or imaging studies not indicated
Anticipate short-term recovery in most patients
- One week: 40%
- Three weeks: 50% to 85%
- Eight weeks: 90%

*Nonpharmacologic interventions*

Enforced bed rest at home for 2 days
- Explicit prohibition against sitting in bed
- Brief periods of standing to use bathroom
- May sit in supportive chair to take brief meals
- Mattress should be firm or supported by bed board

Increasing exercise as tolerated beginning on third day
- Advance to 20-minute walk for each 3 hours supine
- Ability to sit comfortably suggests improvement
- Progress to greater endurance activities: walking, bicycling, swimming
- Explicit time schedule for advancing activity
- Continuation of ordinary activities within limits permitted by pain may be reasonable in selected patients with milder pain syndromes

*Pharmacologic management*

Initial analgesia with acetaminophen (for mild pain) or a nonsteroidal antiinflammatory drug (NSAID) (moderate or severe pain)
- Generic salsalasate, ibuprofen, indomethacin, or enteric-coated aspirin are least expensive options
- Limit initial prescription to two-weeks' supply

Added benefit from adjunctive therapy with muscle relaxant
- Best data support use of carisoprodol or cyclobenzaprine
- Diazepam, orphenadrine, or chlorzoxazone may also be effective
- Limit use to one week
  - These agents are sedating and some are habituating

A short-course (< 7 days) of a narcotic ± acetaminophen is a reasonable alternative for those who fail or are intolerant of NSAIDs

*Follow-up*

By phone, 2 to 3 days after initial presentation
Reexamine in 2 weeks

*Referral*

Consider outpatient physical therapy or chiropractic if significant symptoms persist after 2 weeks
Consider imaging studies and surgical referral if significant neurologic impairments and pain persist beyond 6 weeks, or immediately if symptoms of cauda equina develop

*Other*

No proven benefit from traction, braces, facet joint injection, or transcutaneous nerve stimulation
Treat recurrences as above
Enrollment in "low back school" or an ongoing exercise and educational program may reduce likelihood of recurrence

**Chronic low back pain**

Exclude potential surgically remediable lesions suggested by history and examination
- Repeated imaging not indicated unless clinical situation changes

Treat acute flares as above
Enrollment in aerobic endurance training program may improve functional status substantially
A trial of a tricyclic antidepressant agent may be appropriate

**History of major trauma or suspicion of epidural cancer, epidural abscess, osteomyelitis, or septic diskitis**

Admission to an observation unit or hospital for emergent imaging
- Lumbosacral spine films may reveal gross fractures, dislocations, or destructive lesions to guide further study
- MRI is best single definitive study
- CT and/or contrast myelography are appropriate alternatives
- Radionuclide bone scan occasionally required

Prompt surgical and/or oncologic consultation

**Selective use of lumbosacral spine radiographs in patients with low back pain**

- Age >50
- History of major trauma
- Known cancer
- Pain at rest
- Unexplained weight loss
- Drug or alcohol use
- Treatment with corticosteroids
- Temperature >38° C
- Suspicion of ankylosing spondylitis/reactive arthropathy
- Demonstrable neuromotor deficit

**Table 73-3.** Spinal orthotics

| Disorder | Goals | Suggested orthoses* | Description of orthoses | Function |
|---|---|---|---|---|
| Mechanical low back strain | Rest inflamed tissue; limit bending, lumbosacral motion; reduce abdominal muscles | Dale Binder | A belt in 9 and 12 inch sizes | Reminder to restrict motion and increase intraabdominal pressure |
| | | Neoprene (Richards) | Neoprene corset binder | Anteroposterior compression |
| | | Warm-N-Form or Orthomoid | Elastic binder with posterior-molded plastic insert | Supports while maintaining spinal mobility |
| | | Lumbosacral corset (with rigid posterior paraspinal stays) | Adjustable, flexible cloth/elastic with fitted posterior support, surrounds torso and pelvis | Reminder to restrict motion and increase intraabdominal pressure (greater motion restriction; lumbosacral pad offers additional feeling of support) |
| | | Lumbosacral AP/L control with corset front | Lateral uprights, posterior/thoracic/pelvic bands | Increases abdominal pressure; forces patient into pelvic tilt |
| | | Norton-Brown (AP/L) with trochanteric extensions | Anterior, posterior, lateral support (most like Williams); abdominal pad | Anterior, posterior, lateral stability; abdominal support; regulates twisting and turning |
| | | Williams flexion | (Similar to Norton-Brown) abdominal corset | More stability, more restrictive than Norton-Brown more contact on anterior section |
| | | Williams lumbosacral P/L control | Metal and leather, corset front, open back, pelvic and thoracic, bands, lateral upright, oblique supports (very similar to chair back) | Increases intraabdominal pressure and applies forces to put patient in pelvic tilt; more restrictive than the Norton-Brown; can regulate flexion |
| Osteoarthritis | | | | |
| Facet disease | Stabilize motion at the facet joints | Neoprene (Richards) | As above | As above |
| | | Lumbosacral corset (with rigid posterior paraspinal stays) | As above | As above |
| Spondylolisthesis | Control lordosis; reinforce abdomen; restrict back extension | Lumbosacral AP/L control with corset front | As above | As above |
| | | Norton-Brown (AP/L) with trochanteric extensions | As above | As above |
| | | Williams lumbosacral P/L control | As above | As above |
| | | Clamshell polyethylene back brace | Rigid molded plastic orthosis | Provides maximum immobilization of lower thoracic and lumbar thoracic and lumbar spine; more useful for severe, thoracic lesions |

*Continued.*

**Table 73-3.** Spinal orthotics—cont'd

| Disorder | Goals | Suggested orthoses* | Description of orthoses | Function |
|---|---|---|---|---|
| Lumbar spinal stenosis | Control lordosis; reinforce abdomen; restrict back extension | Lumbosacral corset | As above | As above |
| | | Norton-Brown | As above | As above |
| | | Williams flexion orthosis | As above | As above |
| | | Williams lumbosacral P/L control | As above | As above |
| | | Chair back | Rigid orthosis; apron front, rigid back | Restricts trunk extension, flexion, and lateral motion in addition to increasing intraabdominal pressure; can regulate flexion by adjusting the stays |
| | | Clamshell polyethylene back brace | As above | As above |
| Osteoporotic compression fractures | Control pain; limit motion | Lumbosacral corset | As above | As above |
| | | Cash | Easily adjustable metal and plastic orthosis; sternal, suprapubic, and lumbar pads | Hyperextends thoracic spine |
| Lumbar | | Jewitt | Adjustable metal frame; pads at sternal, suprapubic and lumbar area | Hyperextends thoracic spine |
| Lumbar/thoracic | | Taylor (thoraco-lumbar A/P orthosis) | Metal and leather, apron front, extensive pelvic and interscapular, posterior supports | Restricts motion in flexion and extension and hyperextends thoracic spine |
| | | Clamshell | As above | As above |

*Listed in order of increasing rigidity and stability within each "Disorder."

*A*, Anterior; *P*, posterior; *L*, lateral.

Courtesy Dr. Albert Morin, Dr. Bruce Weinstein, and Dr. David Giansiracusa.

graduated endurance training program when they can sit comfortably.

An effective low-technology intervention for backache is low back school, a multifaceted educational course on body mechanics and back care. Although results have been somewhat variable, low back schools appear to get injured workers back to their jobs quicker than manipulation or detuned diathermy, and may actually reduce the incidence of injuries.

### Pharmacologic interventions

Analgesic agents and muscle-relaxant drugs are commonly prescribed in the treatment for low back pain. Older clinical trials demonstrated no special efficacy over placebo of either first-generation nonsteroidal antiinflammatory drugs (NSAIDs) or muscle relaxants. More recent data have proven a number of NSAIDs effective in reducing pain in general and low back pain in particular. Some patients with mild low back pain respond adequately to therapeutic doses of acetaminophen (1.0 gm PO q4-6h). Since no data support one NSAID as being more effective than any other in treating low back pain, choice of therapy may best be made on the basis of cost and side effects. Generic ibuprofen and salsalasate perhaps best fulfill the balance of efficacy, low cost, and minimal complications. Generic indomethacin is similarly inexpensive, and more potent as an antiinflammatory agent, but produces toxic reactions more frequently than acetaminophen, salsalasate, or ibuprofen. Aspirin is extremely inexpensive but is associated with greater rates of gastritis than is generally seen with other NSAIDs. Patients with moderate or severe low back pain who are either intolerant of or allergic to NSAIDs should take a narcotic such as codeine or oxycodone with acetaminophen, but for no more than 7 days, given the natural history of most low back pain and the potential for abuse of these agents.

The putative muscle relaxant drugs carisoprodol, diazepam, and cyclobenzaprine have also proven beneficial in controlled studies of patients with low back pain, although part of their efficacy is probably related to central nervous system effects. Limited recent data suggest some additive benefit from use of one of these agents in conjunction with an NSAID. Cyclobenzaprine, carisoprodol, and diazepam are all sedating. Carisoprodol and diazepam possess significant addiction potential; cyclobenzaprine, which is similar in structure to the tricyclic antidepressants, has a striking atropine-like effect. As with narcotics, these agents generally should be prescribed to acute low back pain victims for no more than 7 days.

More limited clinical data exist for orphenadrine and chlorzoxazone, two products that demonstrate muscle relaxant capabilities in animals and have reduced discomfort in humans; however, the mechanism appears more likely related to central analgesia and mild sedation than to muscle relaxation.

In the setting of chronic low back pain, tricyclic antidepressant agents have demonstrated efficacy. Response to a tricyclic antidepressant may reflect a combination of mood elevation with improvement in pain threshold, improved sleep pattern with reduction in symptoms of associated fibromyalgia, and a direct effect on neuropathic pain pathways by norepinephrine reuptake blockade. Pain reduction may be noted at doses less than those effective in treating depression.

Injection of long-acting anesthetic agents and/or corticosteroids into facet joints, ligamentous structures, or the epidural space has often been employed as a form of therapy for low back pain. Recent data have shown that corticosteroid injection into facet joints is no better than saline injection. In light of this result, and of the fact that 80% of low back pain sufferers cannot be given definitive anatomic diagnoses, and hence have no specific target for injection, this form of therapy should not be considered part of the standard of care for low back pain.

Chemonucleolysis involves the injection of a chymopapain to dissolve herniated disk material. It was developed as a less invasive and potentially safer intervention than disk surgery in the treatment of sciatica. Although chemonucleolysis proved effective in relieving sciatica in a prospective clinical trial—77% of those treated with chymopapain responded 6 weeks after injection, compared with 47% of controls—both anaphylaxis and severe neurologic complications (e.g., transverse myelitis) have been reported. Morbidity appears to be no better, than that associated with disk surgery, and is perhaps worse, and surgery appears to yield more predictable early relief from sciatica.

### Emotional and behavioral management

Because conservative therapy is usually effective, the initial management of most patients with acute or recurrent low back pain should be at home; this avoids reinforcing illness behavior through hospitalization and reduces health-care costs and inconvenience. A major source of patient dissatisfaction is the failure of health-care providers to give an adequate description of the problem. Because the natural history of low back pain and sciatica is generally favorable, reassurance and education are important, encouraging elements of therapy. Prescriptions for bed rest and graded activity should be explicit, coupled with description of an anticipated time-line for improvement. Medications should be presented as temporary adjuncts to rest and graded exercise. The physician should also discuss the likelihood of recurrence, and encourage lifestyle changes including weight reduction, cessation of tobacco use, and regular exercise in order to minimize long-term risk. Ergonomic changes at work (e.g., work position, lifting posture) and at home (e.g., firm mattress, chairs with firm lumbar support, elevated toilet seat) reduce ongoing discomfort and lower the risk of recurrence.

The individual impaired by chronic low back pain poses a special challenge. Attention must be directed at disruptions in family dynamics caused by this chronic condition, one for which there may be no physical findings. Substance abuse is common among patients with chronic pain, and may include alcohol, prescription medications, and illegal substances. Headache, fibromyalgia, and other somatic complaints may be a proxy for depression, which may benefit greatly from counseling and pharmacologic intervention. Such measures, and explicit programs emphasizing exercise and retraining coupled with psychologic support, may result in a return to work (see the Managed Care Guide).

### Surgery

Emergent surgical referral is clearly indicated when there is suspicion of epidural abscess, malignancy, or hematoma; when neurologic deficits are severe or progressive, as with the cauda equina syndrome; or when the pattern of low back pain suggests referral from an impending infraabdominal or retroperitoneal catastrophe, (e.g., a leaking abdominal aortic aneurysm). Elective surgical referral is also appropriate when neuromotor deficits from sciatica persist despite 4 to 6 weeks of appropriate conservative therapy and are associated with a disk herniation confirmed by anatomic imaging. Persistent pain or neurologic deficits from spondylolisthesis or spinal stenosis are also grounds for surgical consideration.

During the past decade, nearly 200,000 diskectomies were performed annually in the United States, most electively to relieve sciatica. It has been estimated that 5% to 15% of these operations resulted in poor outcomes and reoperation, largely because of inappropriate patient selection. Serious complications are uncommon, occurring in fewer than 1% of cases.

The results of standard diskectomy are excellent for short-term relief from sciatica in appropriately selected patients. Three quarters of such patients are sciatica-free 1 year after surgery, compared with one third of patients treated conservatively. Approximately one half of patients are completely pain-free (i.e., without sciatica or back pain) 1 year after surgery. Standard diskectomy entails a posterior longitudinal incision, removal of laminar bone, incision of the ligamentum flavum, exploration for other abnormalities, and removal of herniated disk material. Complications include dural tears, diskitis, nerve root damage, and spinal instability. Recuperation is often lengthy.

With microdiskectomy, a magnifying scope is employed, allowing smaller incisions with fewer anatomic disruptions. Disk fragments are more likely to be missed than with standard diskectomy, and occasionally the wrong level is entered.

Percutaneous diskectomy involves the use of an automated percutaneous cutting and suction probe to aspirate the nucleus pulposus of the herniated disk with minimal risk to the spinal cord or posterior elements. Only a subset of patients are reasonable candidates for this procedure and recurrent herniation from the same disk is relatively common.

Overall, only a small percentage of those with back pain and sciatica should require surgery. Those who meet criteria for surgery generally do well, with 90% achieving at least partial relief from sciatica and back pain. Preoperative markers of a poor outcome include physical findings suggesting a behavioral disturbance; a distribution and quality of pain that deviates from expected anatomic pain radiation; pending workman's compensation claims; and psychologic tests showing hysteria, hypochondriasis, and somatization. A delay in surgery beyond 12 weeks may compromise the ultimate result, especially in patients with demonstrable weakness.

## BIBLIOGRAPHY


Boden SD et al: Abnormal magnetic-resonance scans of the lumbar spine in asymptomatic subjects, *J Bone Joint Surg* 72-A:403, 1990.

Borenstein D: Low back pain. In Barker LR, Burton JR, Zieve PD, editors: *Ambulatory medicine,* ed 3, Baltimore, 1991, Williams & Wilkins.

Carette S et al: A controlled trial of corticosteroid injections into facet joints for chronic low back pain, *N Engl J Med* 325:1002, 1991.

Deyo RA, Diehl AK: Lumbar spine films in primary care: current use and effects of selective ordering criteria, *J Gen Intern Med* 1:20, 1986.

Deyo RA, Loeser JD, Bigos SJ: Herniated lumbar intervertebral disk, *Ann Intern Med* 112:598, 1990.

Deyo RA, Diehl AK, Rosenthal M: How many days of bed rest for acute low back pain: a randomized clinical trial, *N Engl J Med* 315:1064, 1986.

Deyo RA, Rainville J, Kent DL: What can the history and physical examination tell us about low back pain? *JAMA* 268:760, 1992.

Frymoyer JW: Back pain and sciatica, *N Engl J Med* 318:291, 1988.

Hoffman RM, Wheeler KJ, Deyo RA: Surgery for herniated lumbar discs: a literature synthesis, *J Gen Intern Med* 8:487, 1993.

Jensen MC et al: Magnetic resonance imaging of the lumbar spine in people without back pain, *N Engl J Med* 331:69, 1994.

Liang M, Komaroff AL: Roentgenograms in primary care patients with acute low back pain: a cost effectiveness analysis, *Arch Intern Med* 142:1108, 1982.

Malmivaara A et al: The treatment of acute low back pain–bed rest, exercises, or ordinary activity? *N Engl J Med* 332:351, 1995.

Quinet RJ, Hadler NM: Diagnosis and treatment of backache, *Semin Arthritis Rheum* 8:261, 1979.

Rubin BR: Low back pain, *Prim Care Rheum* 1(3):1, 1991.

Shekelle PG et al: Spinal manipulation for low-back pain, *Ann Intern Med* 117:590, 1992.


CHAPTER

# 74 Hip


**Jerry M. Greene**
**Elinor A. Mody**


Pain in the hip is a frequent complaint of patients seen by primary care physicians. Fig. 74-1 presents some of the regional anatomy of the hip and lower back with notation of the structures from which pain may arise.

## HISTORY

The most important elements of the history include the precise location of the pain, character of the pain, area(s) to which it radiates, severity, activities or other factors that aggravate or alleviate it, and any functional impairment. Causes of pain in the area of a joint are listed in the box on p. 1042.

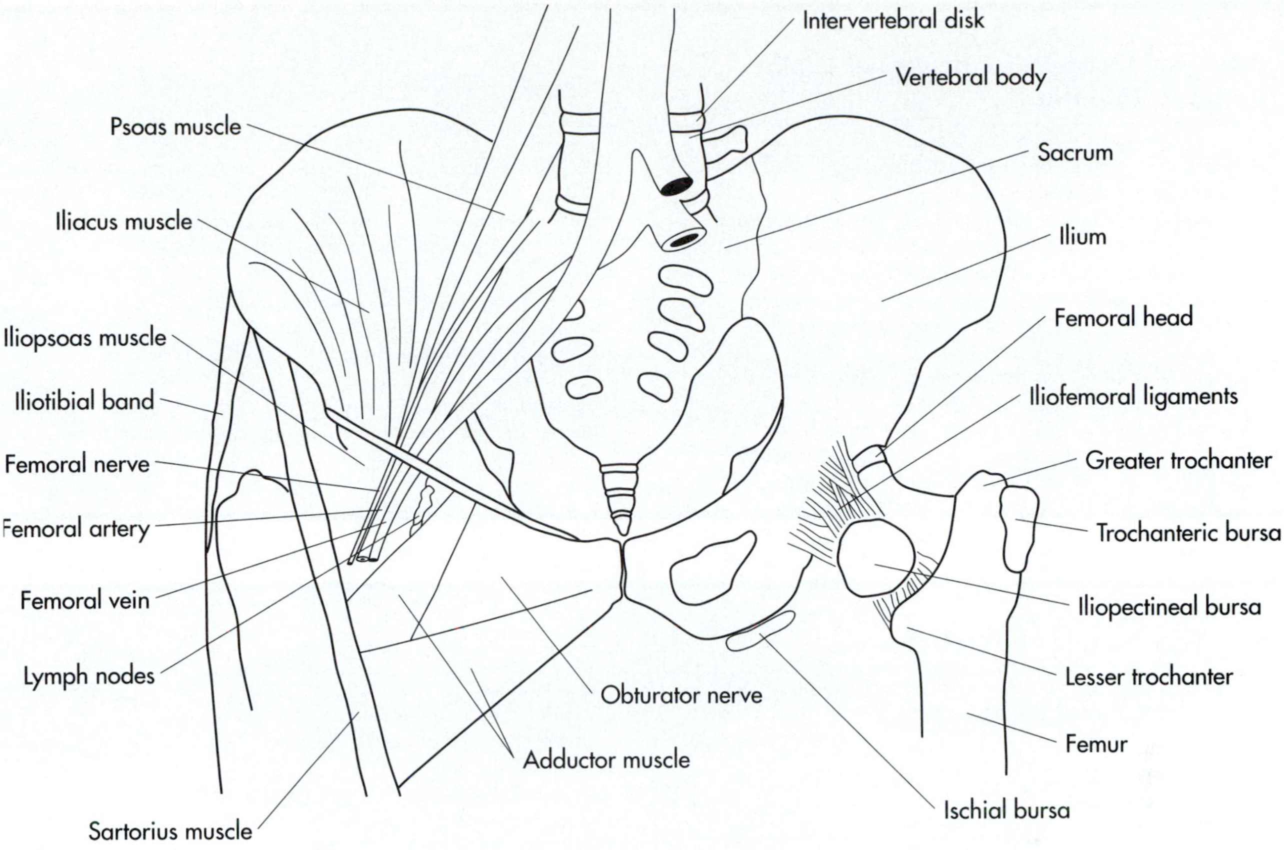


**Fig. 74-1.** Regional anatomy of the hip and lower back.

## Location of pain

Patients use the term *hip* to refer to areas from the lower back to midthigh, and many complaints of hip pain do not arise from the hip joint itself. It is useful to have the patient localize the painful area early in the interview, preferably by pointing. Pain in certain areas suggests particular anatomic structures as the possible sites of the problem (see the box on p. 1042).

Anterior hip, inguinal, proximal thigh, medial thigh, and occasionally knee pain may be due to an intraarticular process. However, pain in these areas may also originate in the iliopectineal bursa, quadriceps, iliopsoas, or adductor muscles, the femoral artery, nerve, or vein, inguinal lymph nodes, the superior and inferior pubic rami, the obturator nerve, or structures within the bony pelvis, especially the adnexa, appendix, and small and large intestines. Inguinal pain may also be referred from the kidney or ureter, be due to upper lumbar radiculopathy, or arise from the facet joints, intervertebral disk, or vertebral bodies in the upper lumbar spine.

Lateral hip pain may arise from the greater trochanter of the femur, the trochanteric bursa, lateral femoral cutaneous nerve, or iliotibial band. Lateral hip pain may be due to a back problem, such as L4 root irritation or L4-5 or L5-S1 facet joint arthritis, intervertebral disk degeneration or infection, vertebral fracture, infection, or neoplasm, or myofascial pain with trigger points.

Posterior hip or buttock pain may also arise from the hip joint. Other structures that may be associated with posterior hip pain include the ischial bursa, sciatic nerve, gluteal muscles, sacroiliac joints, the ischium, and the sacrum. Processes within the pelvis may also cause pain that is experienced in the posterior hip region. Neoplasms or abscesses arising from the rectum, prostate, adnexa, uterus, bladder, and bowel may involve the lumbosacral plexus or cause referred pain. Vascular insufficiency, especially of the external iliac arteries, may cause gluteal claudication. Lumbar spinal stenosis may cause pseudoclaudication (neurogenic) in the buttocks.

## Character of pain

Descriptions of the pain may be helpful in determining the underlying pathophysiology. Dysesthesia, paresthesia, and numbness suggests a neuropathic process. Constant pain, including pain at rest and especially pain that interferes with sleep, is most often seen with neurologic, inflammatory, and neoplastic processes. Pain with use and decreased pain with rest suggests a mechanical process and is classic for osteoarthritis of the hip. Selected causes of hip pain are detailed in Table 74-1.

## Mnemonic for pain in the area of a joint
## Podagra Hot Joint

*P*olyarthritis: rheumatoid arthritis, rheumatic fever, systemic lupus erythematosus
*O*steoarthritis: primary, posttraumatic, postinflammatory
*D*erangements: loose bodies, ligamentous tears, dislocation
*A*vascular necrosis: hemoglobinopathies, decompression
*G*out: pseudogout, apatite crystal–associated arthritis
*R*eactive arthritis: Reiter's syndrome, IBD, psoriatic arthritis
*A*myloid: and other accumulations, e.g., Gaucher's disease

*H*emorrhage: hemophilia, anticoagulation, posttraumatic, tumor
*O*steochondromatosis: also synovial chondromatosis
*T*umors: benign and malignant

*J*uxtaarticular: especially bursitis, tendinitis
*O*steitis deformans: Paget's disease
*I*nfection: including gonococcal and nongonococcal bacterial
*N*europathic: Charcot's disease, referred, radicular
*T*rauma: including fractures, foreign bodies, contusions

*IBD,* Inflammatory bowel disease.

## Causes of pain in the area of a joint

**Anterior hip, medial thigh, knee**
*Acute*
Acute rheumatic fever
Adductor muscle strain
Avascular necrosis
Crystal arthritis
Femoral artery (pseudo) aneurysm
Fracture (femoral neck or intertrochanteric)
Hemarthrosis
Hernia
Herpes zoster
Iliopectineal bursitis
Iliopsoas tendinitis
Inguinal lymphadenitis
Osteomalacia
Painful transient osteoporosis of hip
Septic arthritis

*Subacute and chronic*
Adductory muscle strain
Amyloidosis
Acute rheumatic fever
Femoral artery aneurysm
Hernia (inguinal or femoral)
Iliopectineal bursitis
Iliopsoas tendinitis
Inguinal lymphadenopathy
Osteochondromatosis
Osteomyelitis
Osteitis deformans (Paget's disease)
Osteomalacia (pseudofracture)
Postherpetic neuralgia
Sterile synovitis (e.g., rheumatoid arthritis, psoriatic, systemic lupus erythematosus)

**Lateral hip, lateral thigh**
*Acute*
Herpes zoster
Iliotibial tendinitis
Impacted fracture of femoral neck
Lateral femoral cutaneous neuropathy (meralgia paresthetica)
Radiculopathy: L4-5
Trochanteric avulsion fracture (greater trochanter)
Trochanteric bursitis
Trochanteric fracture

*Subacute and chronic*
Lateral femoral cutaneous neuropathy (meralgia paresthetica)
Osteomyelitis
Postherpetic neuralgia
Radiculopathy: L4-5
Tumors

**Posterior hip, thigh, buttock**
*Acute*
Gluteal muscle strain
Herpes zoster
Ischial bursitis
Ischial or sacral fracture
Osteomalacia (pseudofracture)
Sciatic neuropathy
Radiculopathy: L5-S1

*Subacute and chronic*
Gluteal muscle strain
Ischial bursitis
Lumbar spinal stenosis
Osteoarthritis of hip
Osteitis deformans (Paget's disease)
Osteomyelitis
Osteochondromatosis
Osteomalacia (pseudofracture)
Postherpetic neuralgia
Radiculopathy: L5-S1
Tumors

After characterizing the hip pain, the examiner should determine if any trauma, recent or remote, has occurred to the hip, pelvis, or lower back, and elicit the remaining elements of a general history, especially medication use, habits, occupation, concomitant medical illnesses, prior surgery, any prior episodes of joint pain, sexual history, history of illicit drug use, and episodes of chills, fevers, and rigors. Pertinent historical items for selected disorders that can cause hip pain are listed in Table 74-1.

## PHYSICAL EXAMINATION

The physical examination should be tailored to the acuteness, severity, and complexity of the complaints. The goal is to reproduce the pain through palpation or maneuvers. The essential elements of an examination for hip pain include observing for deformities in those patients who cannot walk. A flexed, externally rotated and shortened leg is seen with hip fracture, whereas an internally rotated, shortened leg suggests posterior dislocation. Patients with either of these deformities should not have any maneuvers of the hip performed until fracture or dislocation has been ruled out by radiographic studies.

The gait of patients who can walk may demonstrate a limp. An antalgic gait is one with a short time spent bearing weight on the affected side. An adductor lurch is noted when the patient shifts upper body weight to the side of the painful hip. Having the patient attempt to stand on one leg at a time, the Trendelenburg test, may demonstrate an inability to bear weight on the affected side or an inability to keep the pelvis level while doing so. It is helpful to observe the patient rising from sitting to standing and to assess whether this movement exacerbates the pain.

Inspect the painful hip for swelling, erythema, and rash. Active range of motion of the hip, knee, and lower back is then assessed.

Palpation is helpful to identify masses and tenderness of the vertebral spines, paravertebral muscles, bursae (especially the greater trochanteric bursa, ischial bursa, and iliopectineal bursa), the inguinal lymph nodes, femoral artery, femoral vein, quadriceps, adductor, and gluteal muscles, superior pubic ramus, symphysis pubis, and sciatic notch.

Limitation of movement can be assessed by passively taking the hip through its range of motion, which normally consists of 90 to 100 degrees of flexion, 30 degrees of extension, and 30 to 45 degrees of rotation, abduction, and adduction. Palpation and passive motion may reproduce the patient's usual hip pain. A regional neurologic examination should be performed if the history or examination suggests a neuropathic process. Provocative testing, including straight leg raising and the Lasègue sign (tensing the sciatic nerve by straight leg raising, then dorsiflexing the foot) for nerve root irritation, are also useful (see Chapter 73). If the history and examination have not led to a definite working diagnosis, a complete physical examination may be necessary, including abdominal, rectal, and pelvic examinations.

## LABORATORY TESTS

Laboratory testing is guided by the findings on the history and physical examination. There is no standard panel of tests that are appropriate for all cases of hip pain. Specific laboratory tests and results for selected disorders are discussed in the sections on diseases that follow and are summarized in Table 74-1.

### Radiography

Depending on the results of the history and physical findings, radiographs may be unnecessary, especially if symptoms are mild, they appear to be due to muscular strain, bursitis, or tendinitis for which conservative therapy is indicated, and the patient can be relied on to return if symptoms persist or worsen. For more severe pain, when conservative therapy has failed, or when local injection of corticosteroids such as a trochanteric bursal injection is anticipated, plain radiographs of the hip and pelvis are indicated to assess for fractures, neoplasm, or infection. Specific findings and special radiographic and imaging studies for selected disorders are listed in Table 74-1.

### Arthrocentesis

Aspiration of fluid from the hip is more difficult than from other more superficial joints. Failure to obtain fluid with blind aspiration is not adequate to rule out an effusion. In cases of suspected septic arthritis or more chronic undiagnosed arthritis of the hip, arthrocentesis should be performed with fluoroscopic guidance and with instillation of contrast medium to confirm the intraarticular location of the needle tip. This procedure is most often performed by interventional or musculoskeletal radiologists or by orthopedic surgeons. Any synovial fluid obtained should be analyzed for glucose, cell count and differential, Gram's stain, and for crystals by compensated polarized microscopy. Joint fluid should be cultured routinely for aerobic and facultative anaerobic bacteria. If there is any suspicion of tuberculosis or opportunistic fungal infection, additional stains and cultures for mycobacteria and fungi should be obtained.

### Other diagnostic tests

If the history, physical examination, routine laboratory tests, plain radiographs, and aspiration (if appropriate) do not provide a diagnosis, other tests may be helpful. Technetium pyrophosphate bone scans may demonstrate increased tracer uptake in neoplastic and infectious foci before they are apparent on plain radiographs. Bone scans can also identify stress fractures that may be difficult or impossible to detect on plain films. Gallium scans may detect infectious foci or tumors around the hip or within the pelvis. Computed tomography (CT) scans are useful for providing more detailed bone and soft tissue images and are particularly useful for evaluating pelvic structures, spinal elements, and the sacroiliac joints. CT scans are also moderately sensitive for avascular necrosis of the femoral head. Magnetic resonance imaging (MRI) is currently the most sensitive tool for early detection of avascular necrosis and is also very useful for evaluating the spinal canal, neural foramina, intervertebral disks, muscles, and bursae. With gadolinium enhancement, MRI is very useful in delineating septic diskitis. Useful tests for individual disorders are listed in Table 74-1.

*Text continued on p. 1055.*

**Table 74-1.** Selected causes of hip pain

| Disorder | Epidemiology | History | Physical examination | Diagnostic tests | Differential diagnosis | Management |
|---|---|---|---|---|---|---|
| Acute rheumatic fever | Children and young adults; poverty and overcrowding, epidemics of arthritogenic strains of streptococci | Preceding pharyngitis (may be asymptomatic) arthralgia, rash, involuntary movements, migratory oligoarthritis | Fever, evanescent salmon-colored rash, synovitis, heart murmur, CHF, chorea, subcutaneous nodules | ASLO titer increased, ESR increased, ECG PR interval prolonged, echocardiogram may demonstrate regurgitation, pericardial effusion | As for rheumatoid arthritis (see p. 1052) | Salicylates in antiinflammatory dosages, steroids for resistant cases at dosages of 1 mg/kg per day, long-term prophylactic use of penicillin |
| Amyloidosis | Hip involvement unusual but may occur with chronic renal dialysis due to $\beta_2$-microglobulin–related amyloid deposition, amyloidosis with chronic infections, chronic inflammatory diseases, and with paraproteinemias | Gradual onset of hip pain, symptoms of carpal tunnel syndrome (numbness, paresthesia, pain in thumb, index, and middle fingers), shoulder pain due to rotator cuff infiltration, easy bruising | Skin: waxy appearance, bruises and echymoses; abdomen: hepatosplenomegaly; musculoskeletal: pseudohypertrophy of deltoid muscles (shoulder pad sign) due to amyloid infiltration, limited shoulder motion; neurologic: peripheral neuropathy and Tinel's sign at wrist common | Plain radiographs demonstrate cysts or erosions in femoral head or neck, hip aspiration; sediment of synovial fluid when stained with Congo red demonstrates apple-green birefringence on polarizing microscopy; needle biopsy of lytic lesions positive for amyloid; serum and urine immunoelectrophoresis; abdominal fat pad aspiration with Congo red staining least invasive biopsy method | In chronic renal failure with patient on dialysis, hyperparathyroidism with brown tumors, other neoplasms (see Tumors on p. 1054) | For amyloid due to familial Mediterranean fever: colchicine prophylaxis may prevent progression; for amyloid secondary to inflammatory or infectious diseases: control of underlying disease may prevent progression; for amyloid related to myeloma or paraproteinemia: chemotherapy may be indicated; for dialysis related amyloid: renal transplantation if possible |

| | | | | | | |
|---|---|---|---|---|---|---|
| Avascular necrosis | Predisposing condition; alcohol, glucocorticosteroids, sickle cell disease, decompression, pancreatitis, trauma, SLE, hyperlipoproteinemias, radiation therapy | Sudden onset of pain, moderate to severe, limits weight bearing, predisposing factors may be present | Despite pain, passive ROM is normal in early disease; motion may be limited once collapse of cartilage and subchondral bone occurs | MRI most sensitive for early disease, demonstrates decreased T1 and increased T2 signal; CT scan also useful; increased density lesional area in femoral head; bone scan decreased uptake early, increased after days to weeks; plain films insensitive until late in course, may show subchondral collapse | Painful transient osteoporosis of hip, bone bruise, pelvic or sacral insufficiency fractures, osteomyelitis, neoplasm | Core decompression with or without vascularized bone or soft tissue grafting for early disease (before collapse of bone and cartilage); rotational osteotomy may be helpful for more advanced disease; total hip replacement for hips with collapse and secondary osteoarthritis |
| Fracture of femoral neck | Increased risk with age; osteoporosis due to postmenopausal status; corticosteroid use; alcoholism; anticonvulsant drugs | Severe hip pain and inability to bear weight following fall | Deformity of hip with external rotation, slight flexion; assess neurovascular integrity; monitor vital signs carefully | Plain radiographs of hip and pelvis with minimal movement of affected leg | Pathologic fracture secondary to tumor or infection of femur; osteomalacia with looser line; impacted fracture; fracture of greater trochanter; avulsion fracture of greater or lesser trochanter; sacral, iliac, or pubic ramus fracture | Motion of affected hip should be minimized while assessment proceeds; if fracture documented: provide analgesia, monitor vital signs, obtain orthopedic consultation |

*ROM*, Range of motion; *ESR*, erythrocyte sedimentation rate; *RF*, rheumatoid factor; *WBC*, white blood cell count; *SLE*, systemic lupus erythematosus; *NSAIDs*, nonsteroidal antiinflammatory drugs; *CHF*, congestive heart failure; *RA*, rheumatoid arthritis; *ARF*, acute rheumatic fever; *ACTH*, adrenocorticotropic hormone; *TSH*, thyroid-stimulating hormone; *DIP*, distal interphalangeal; *SI*, sacroiliac; *ANA*, antinuclear antibodies; *PT*, prothrombin time; *PTT*, partial thromboplastin time; *CPPD*, calcium pyrophosphate deposition disease; *CBC*, complete blood count; *SPEP*, serum protein electrophoresis; *CXR*, chest x-ray; *U/A*, urinalysis; *DTR*, deep tendon reflexes; *LS*, lumbosacral.

*Continued.*

**Table 74-1.** Selected causes of hip pain—cont'd

| Disorder | Epidemiology | History | Physical examination | Diagnostic tests | Differential diagnosis | Management |
|---|---|---|---|---|---|---|
| Gout | Men >> women predominantly after adolescence; drugs may elevate uric acid level, especially hydrochlorothiazide, pyrazinamide, cyclosporin | Prior episodes of self-limited arthritis, severe pain, sudden onset, fever may be noted by patient | Fever may be present, usually <39° C; tophi; markedly limited ROM in all directions | WBC may be elevated; uric acid level elevated in 50% of patients during acute attacks; plain film may suggest effusion; aspiration positive for needle-shaped, brightly birefringent crystals; synovial WBC 10-100,000/$mm^3$; Gram stain negative | Septic arthritis, pseudogout, apatite arthritis, RA, ARF, SLE, Reiter's syndrome, reactive arthritis | For proven gout with low suspicion of sepsis, NSAID, e.g., indocin 50 mg four times daily × 3 days then 25 mg three times a day for a week; colchicine may be used, 0.6 mg every hour for max 10 doses in 24 hr then 0.6 mg twice a day for 7-10 days; ACTH or glucocorticosteroids for some difficult cases |
| Hemorrhage | Children with hemophilia, adolescents with trauma, adults with trauma or anticoagulation | Sudden onset of pain after minor trauma, or no history of trauma; pain at rest and with use, usually severe with antalgic gait or inability to walk, history of prior bleeding diathesis or anticoagulant drug use | Signs of intraarticular process, evidence of bleeding diathesis (bruising, mucosal bleeding) | Plain radiograph to exclude fracture, CBC, PT and PTT, platelet count, aspiration yields frank blood; fat droplets on surface of aspirate (after specimen stands) suggest intraarticular fracture; hematocrit on synovial fluid <5% suggests hemorrhagic effusion rather than hemorrhage | Frank hemorrhage: trauma, excessive anticoagulation or bleeding diathesis; bloody effusion: CPPD and pseudogout, and apatite arthritis, neuropathic joint, pigmented villonodular synovitis, other joint tumors | Replacement of deficient clotting factors for hemophilia or if possible for patients whose anticoagulation can be reversed (e.g., atrial fibrillation); partial correction to therapeutic range for over anticoagulation and clear indication (e.g., mechanical prosthetic valve); aspiration of as much fluid as possible; rest; analgesics; ROM exercises after 48 hours |

| | | | | | | |
|---|---|---|---|---|---|---|
| Hernias | Associated with strenuous lifting, coughing, or Valsalva maneuver | Anterior hip pain; patients sometimes note bulge | Hip motion normal; inguinal or femoral hernia palpated with Valsalva maneuver or cough | If definite hernia, no further tests necessary | Inguinal mass may be tumor, lymphadenopathy, phlebothrombosis, arterial aneurysm, necessitating abscess from pelvis, abdomen, or psoas muscle, or synovial cyst from hip joint | Emergent repair for incarcerated hernia; elective repair for reducible hernia |
| Iliopectineal bursitis | Most frequent in athletic males and dancers | Anterior hip pain; limited hip extension so that running or brisk walking is painful; standing or slow walking does not increase pain | Affected hip may be flexed slightly; extension of hip aggravates pain; tenderness in anterior hip and inguinal region may be present; palpate inguinal area for inguinal or femoral hernia, mass, aneurysm, or lymphadenopathy; examine lower quadrants of abdomen to exclude sigmoid colonic or appendiceal disease; pelvic exam for women to exclude pelvic inflammatory disease, adnexal or other mass | Plain films, negative generally, rarely demonstrate calcific periarthritis or intrabursal calcifications; CBC, ESR, and U/A to exclude infection and ureteral stone | If severe with limited hip ROM: infectious and other hip synovitis; if local anterior pain: iliopsoas tendinitis, psoas abscess, inguinal or femoral hernia, radicular pain, referred pain from kidney, ureter, obturator nerve irritation from pelvic mass or infection, or femoral artery aneurysm | Analgesics, rest, local heat, NSAIDs, therapeutic ultrasound; for refractory cases: local corticosteroid injection (referral may be appropriate if primary physician is not skilled in the technique); refractory pain warrants bone scan, CT scan |
| Iliopsoas tendinitis | Athletes or coexisting osteoarthritis of the hip | Anterior hip pain, active hip flexion may be most painful; stair climbing and putting on shoes and stockings may be difficult | Affected hip may be slightly flexed, anterior hip tenderness may be present; pain reproduced by attempted hip flexion against resistance; hip motion preserved and relatively painless | Plain films negative; CBC, ESR normal | Same for iliopectineal bursitis, above | Same as for iliopectineal bursitis, above; if injection of corticosteroids performed, intratendinous injection should be avoided to prevent tendon rupture (if resistance to injection occurs, reposition needle tip) |

*ROM*, Range of motion; *ESR*, erythrocyte sedimentation rate; *RF*, rheumatoid factor; *WBC*, white blood cell count; *SLE*, systemic lupus erythematosus; *NSAIDs*, nonsteroidal antiinflammatory drugs; *CHF*, congestive heart failure; *RA*, rheumatoid arthritis; *ARF*, acute rheumatic fever; *ACTH*, adrenocorticotropic hormone; *TSH*, thyroid-stimulating hormone; *DIP*, distal interphalangeal; *SI*, sacroiliac; *ANA*, antinuclear antibodies; *PT*, prothrombin time; *PTT*, partial thromboplastin time; *CPPD*, calcium pyrophosphate deposition disease; *CBC*, complete blood count; *SPEP*, serum protein electrophoresis; *CXR*, chest x-ray; *U/A*, urinalysis; *DTR*, deep tendon reflexes; *LS*, lumbosacral.

*Continued.*

**Table 74-1.** Selected causes of hip pain—cont'd

| Disorder | Epidemiology | History | Physical examination | Diagnostic tests | Differential diagnosis | Management |
|---|---|---|---|---|---|---|
| Iliotibial tendinitis | Athletes, overuse with repeated sitting and standing, leg length discrepancy may contribute | Lateral hip pain, aggravated by standing, walking, arising from chair | Tenderness along lateral thigh; pain with forced adduction or resisted abduction of hip; palpable snap of iliotibial band over greater trochanter with hip flexion/extension | History and physical findings; diagnostic injection with local anesthetic of trochanteric bursa to distinguish trochanter bursitis | Same as for trochanteric bursitis (see p. 1054) | Correct leg length discrepancy if present; physical therapy with ultrasound, local heat, stretching of iliotibial band; analgesics and NSAIDs |
| Insufficiency (stress) fractures | Young people after repeated vigorous exercise; anyone after prolonged immobility or limited weight bearing, e.g., following total joint replacement in RA | Onset of pain with activity, aggravated with weight bearing and relieved somewhat with rest; may be severe and prevent weight bearing; pain may radiate widely to thigh or buttock | Passive hip motion usually preserved and does not aggravate pain; active motion may be limited by pain; pelvic compression (anteroposterior or lateral) or rocking may reproduce pain | Plain films of hip and pelvis relatively insensitive for insufficiency fracture of sacrum and ilium; somewhat better for pubic rami; bone scan sensitive and CT scan helps confirm fracture as cause of increased tracer uptake on bone scan | Metastatic and primary bone tumors (see p. 1054); osteomyelitis; lumbar disk disease; referred pain | Analgesics and rehabilitation with partial weight bearing using walker; avoid prolonged bed rest; assess for osteoporosis or osteomalacia of clinical circumstances warrant |
| Ischial bursitis (ischiogluteal bursitis) | Activities that cause repeated trauma to gluteal region predispose to condition, e.g., horseback riding, weaving, skating | Posterior hip pain, increased with forward bending, sitting on hard surface | Tenderness over ischial tuberosity, preserved hip ROM, no sciatic notch tenderness, normal neurologic exam | Plain radiographs usually normal | Pelvic fracture (traumatic or stress related), sciatic nerve compression, pyriformis syndrome, radicular pain, referred pain from within pelvis, bone lesions in ischium | Avoid further repetitive trauma to ischial area; avoid direct pressure when sitting (donut, contoured cushion); analgesics, NSAIDs, local heat, therapeutic ultrasound, local injection with corticosteroids (avoid inadvertent injection of sciatic nerve) |

| | | | | | | |
|---|---|---|---|---|---|---|
| Lateral femoral cutaneous neuropathy | Recent weight loss or weight gain predisposes to pressure on lateral femoral cutaneous nerve as it passes over pelvic brim | Sudden or gradual onset of pain confined to lateral hip and thigh, accompanied by numbness and paresthesia, in absence of back pain or sensory changes below knee | Area of decreased sensation over lateral hip and thigh beginning about at pelvic brim (iliac crest) and ending above or at the knee; preserved DTRs; no tenderness over trochanteric bursa; no exacerbation with hip joint motion | Plain films of pelvis to exclude lytic or blastic lesion of iliac crest | Lumbar radiculopathies should produce neurologic symptoms extending below knee; iliotibial tendinitis or trochanteric bursitis should have local tenderness | Avoid tight-waisted clothing, use suspenders rather than belts; analgesic medications may be necessary; low-dose amitriptyline, imipramine, or desipramine at bedtime; newer serotoninergic antidepressants appear ineffective for pain control |
| Lumbar radiculopathies | May occur in young adults due to herniated disks and in older persons due to lumbar spondylosis (degenerative disk and facet joint disease) with compression of spinal canal (spinal stenosis) or impingement on exiting nerve roots (lateral recess stenosis) | Posterior, lateral, or anterior pain depending on which nerve root compromised; pain extending from back to hip and beyond, usually extending below the knee; loss or change in sensation; pain aggravated by walking for which patient must sit down or lean forward to get relief; suggests lumbar spinal stenosis with neurogenic claudication | Tenderness of lumbar spine, paraspinal muscle spasm, positive straight leg raising, diminished sensation in dermatomal distribution, loss of DTRs, muscle weakness, no exacerbation of pain with hip motion | Lumbosacral spine and pelvic radiographs; if cancer diagnosis and radicular pain without weakness: bone scan and follow-up CT scan of involved area; if weakness, bowel or bladder incontinence: MRI or CT scan of LS spine | See Chapter 73 | See Chapter 73 |

*ROM*, Range of motion; *ESR*, erythrocyte sedimentation rate; *RF*, rheumatoid factor; *WBC*, white blood cell count; *SLE*, systemic lupus erythematosus; *NSAIDs*, nonsteroidal antiinflammatory drugs; *CHF*, congestive heart failure; *RA*, rheumatoid arthritis; *ARF*, acute rheumatic fever; *ACTH*, adrenocorticotropic hormone; *TSH*, thyroid-stimulating hormone; *DIP*, distal interphalangeal; *SI*, sacroiliac; *ANA*, antinuclear antibodies; *PT*, prothrombin time; *PTT*, partial thromboplastin time; *CPPD*, calcium pyrophosphate deposition disease; *CBC*, complete blood count; *SPEP*, serum protein electrophoresis; *CXR*, chest x-ray; *U/A*, urinalysis; *DTR*, deep tendon reflexes; *LS*, lumbosacral.

*Continued.*

**Table 74-1.** Selected causes of hip pain—cont'd

| Disorder | Epidemiology | History | Physical examination | Diagnostic tests | Differential diagnosis | Management |
|---|---|---|---|---|---|---|
| Lyme disease | Children and adults with exposure to ticks in areas with endemic *Borrelia burgdorferi* | Anterior hip pain, decreased ROM, travel or residence in endemic area, history of tick bite or removing ticks, slowly enlarging circular or oval erythematous rash (erythema chronicum migrans), history of painful radiculopathy or cranial nerve palsy, especially Bell's palsy | Fever, usually low grade if present; skin rash may be present, usually polycyclic erythematous eruption; hip motion diminished in all directions; cranial nerve VII weakness or other cranial neuropathy or radiculopathy | If presentation suggests septic arthritis: aspiration of hip reveals inflammatory fluid with lymphocytic predominance; plain films: swelling or normal, CBC normal; ESR: elevated moderately, Lyme titer usually elevated | Other chronic synovitis: as for rheumatoid arthritis (see p. 1052) | For proven Lyme arthritis: ceftriaxone 1 IV every 12 hr for 2 weeks |
| Osteitis deformans (Paget's disease of bone) | Middle-aged to older adults | Pain anywhere in hip; may occur with activity and weight bearing, especially when associated osteoarthritic change of involved hip joint; rest and night pain may be prominent when pain due to bony involvement alone or advanced osteoarthritis | Preserved ROM without exacerbating pain suggests pain from bony involvement; pain with motion suggests concomitant osteoarthritis of hip | Plain films demonstrate coarse trabeculi; may have increase in size of bone, thickening of cortex, areas of lucency; osteoarthritis of hip may be present; alkaline phosphatase elevated; prostate-specific antigen should be checked in men, since metastatic prostate cancer may have similar appearance | Prostate cancer, sclerosing osteomyelitis, other blastic metastatic disease (thyroid, breast, etc.), transformation of Paget's disease to osteogenic sarcoma (suggested by marked change, rise or fall, in alkaline phosphatase unrelated to therapy) | If severe associated osteoarthritis: total hip replacement, treatment with etidronate or calcitonin for 6 weeks to 3 months before surgery to decrease vascularity of bone; if uncertain whether pain is due to Paget's disease or osteoarthritis: trial of etidronate or calcitonin |
| Osteoarthritis | Older > younger; some heritable forms with epiphyseal dysplasias and defined collagen mutations | Pain with use, better with rest, gel phenomenon common, with worsening condition–continuous pain, difficulty sleeping due to pain | Antalgic or adductor lurch, positive Trendelenburg sign, limited ROM, pain reproduced by motion, no tenderness, leg lengths may differ slightly | Plain radiographs show joint space narrowing, osteophyte formation, sclerotic bone, and subchondral cysts | Secondary osteoarthritis (see text), septic arthritis complicating osteoarthritis, crystal disease | Weight loss, moderate low-impact exercise, cane, acetaminophen, NSAIDs, hip replacement for severe symptomatic disease or rotational osteotomy for younger patients |

| | | | | | | |
|---|---|---|---|---|---|---|
| Osteochondromatosis | Rare cause of large joint pain and chronic synovitis | Slowly developing pain, restricted motion in hip | Swelling may be apparent in anterior hip, joint motion restricted | Plain radiographs may demonstrate multiple osteochondral bodies within joint capsule or may suggest joint swelling or effusion when calcification of chondral bodies is not present (synovial chondromatosis); MRI can distinguish multiple cartilaginous bodies from joint fluid | Chronic inflammatory synovitis (see Rheumatoid Arthritis p. 1052), especially with rice bodies, pigmented villonodular synovitis | Synovectomy and removal of all loose bodies is curative, if severe articular cartilage loss due to associated synovitis; hip replacement surgery may be necessary; secondary osteoarthritis may progress following synovectomy |
| Pseudogout | Older persons; men = women; some predisposing conditions, including hyperparathyroidism, hypothyroidism, hemochromatosis, hypomagnesemia | Sudden onset of pain; history suggesting a disorder associated with pseudogout should be sought (see text) | Fever may be present, pain and limited ROM consistent with intraarticular process; features suggesting underlying disease should be sought (see text) | Plain radiographs may be normal, suggest effusion, or demonstrate chondrocalcinosis; WBC normal to mildly elevated; aspiration: weakly birefringent, stubby rhomboidal crystals; elevated synovial WBC 10-100,000/$mm^3$; if suspicion of underlying disease, calcium, magnesium, ferritin; TSH, somatomedin-C, or ceruloplasmin | Same as for gout (see p. 1046) if aspiration proven or if chondrocalcinosis is extensive, consider hyperparathyroidism, hypothyroidism, hemochromatosis, hypomagnesemia, ochronosis, Wilson's disease, and acromegaly | As for gout (see p. 1046; see also Chapter 82) |

*ROM*, Range of motion; *ESR*, erythrocyte sedimentation rate; *RF*, rheumatoid factor; *WBC*, white blood cell count; *SLE*, systemic lupus erythematosus; *NSAIDs*, nonsteroidal antiinflammatory drugs; *CHF*, congestive heart failure; *RA*, rheumatoid arthritis; *ARF*, acute rheumatic fever; *ACTH*, adrenocorticotropic hormone; *TSH*, thyroid-stimulating hormone; *DIP*, distal interphalangeal; *SI*, sacroiliac; *ANA*, antinuclear antibodies; *PT*, prothrombin time; *PTT*, partial thromboplastin time; *CPPD*, calcium pyrophosphate deposition disease; *CBC*, complete blood count; *SPEP*, serum protein electrophoresis; *CXR*, chest x-ray; *U/A*, urinalysis; *DTR*, deep tendon reflexes; *LS*, lumbosacral.

*Continued.*

**Table 74-1.** Selected causes of hip pain—cont'd

| Disorder | Epidemiology | History | Physical examination | Diagnostic tests | Differential diagnosis | Management |
|---|---|---|---|---|---|---|
| Reactive arthritis | Sexually active individuals at risk for postgonococcal arthritis, presence of HLA B27 common, especially with sacroiliac or spinal involvement and in Reiter syndrome; may follow dysentery | Antecedent urethritis, dysentery, inflammatory bowel disease, psoriasis, known HIV infection, previous or current eye pain, photophobia, conjunctivitis, iritis, back pain, back stiffness, skin rash especially on palms or soles or genitalia | Psoriasis or psoriaform lesions on glans penis (circinate balanitis), vesiculopustular hyperkeratotic lesions on palms or soles (keratoderma blennorrhagica), nail pitting or onycholysis, painless oral ulcers, conjunctivitis, irregular pupils (synechiae due to iritis), limited back motion, tenderness over sacroiliac region, tenosynovitis especially Achilles, peripheral arthritis especially asymmetric lower extremity, sausage digits, DIP involvement prominent | If acute gonococcal dermatitis/arthritis suspected appropriate cultures should be obtained (see Infection on p. 1053); if risk factors for HIV infection, counseling and HIV testing; SI joint plain films may demonstrate sacroiliitis, ANA and RF are negative, consider small bowel series for occult Crohn's disease | With evidence of synovitis of the hip, gonococcal arthritis, other septic arthritis; if posterior hip pain and evidence of Reiter's syndrome, sacroiliitis | Indomethacin and naproxen may be more effective than other NSAIDs for Reiter's and spondylitis; phenylbutazone effective but risk of marrow aplasia exists; sulfasalazine or methotrexate for resistant disease; corticosteroids may be needed for severe disease; local injection of involved joint may be helpful |
| Referred pain | | Posterior, lateral, or anterior pain may be referred from many structures, pelvic and retroperitoneal inflammation or tumors, ureteral stones, osteoarthritis of facet joint, and intervertebral disks of spine, pelvic bones | Hip motion usually preserved and does not exacerbate pain; palpable mass may be present in pelvis on abdominal, pelvic, or rectal examination | Plain films of hip and pelvis help to exclude bony pathology; U/A to assess for ureteral stone; consider pregnancy; ultrasound or CT scan of pelvis for pain that remains obscure | Other causes of pain discussed above and below | For pain referred from back; see Chapter 73; pain due to tumors or infections should be treated while underlying problem addressed |
| Rheumatoid arthritis | 1% of population, any age, females > males | Morning stiffness, symmetric pain in hands and feet, fatigue | Limited hip ROM in all directions, nodules, tenderness of small joints of hands and feet | ESR elevated, RF elevated in 80%, joint fluid WBC elevated | Septic arthritis, gout, pseudogout, apatite arthritis, psoriatic and other seronegative arthritis, rheumatic fever, SLE, viral arthritis (parvovirus B19), Lyme disease, sarcoidosis | Rule out septic arthritis with cultures if monoarthritis of hip; NSAIDs, disease modifying drugs, corticosteroids (PO or injected into hip) |

| | | | | | | |
|---|---|---|---|---|---|---|
| Septic arthritis | Children: *Haemophilus influenzae,* staphylococcal streptococcal infection; adolescents and young adults: often gonococcal; older adults: impaired hosts (alcoholic, renal disease, immunosuppressed); staphylococcal, streptococcal, gram-negative bacteria; prior joint damage or chronic inflammation predisposes to infection | Anterior hip pain, usually sudden to subacute onset, generally severe; fever and rigors may occur; skin rash may have been noted; source of sepsis should be sought, e.g., cough, dysuria | Fever in 50%; maculopapular, vesicular, or vesiculopustular rash suggests gonococcal dermatitis arthritis; hip motion reduced in all directions; leathery crepitance may be felt | Blood cultures positive in 50% of nongonococcal bacterial arthritis; synovial WBC usually greater than 50,000/mm$^3$, often greater than 100,000/mm$^3$; peripheral WBC elevated in 50%; synovial Gram stain positive in 50%; presence of crystals does not exclude infection; plain radiographs may demonstrate effusion or adjacent osteomyelitis; if gonococcal arthritis suspected: culture urethra, pharynx, rectum, or cervix as appropriate onto selective media (Thayer Martin); synovial fluid should not be plated on Thayer Martin media | Purulent fluid aspirated: gonococcal and nongonococcal bacterial arthritis, fungal, mycobacterial infectious arthritis, Lyme disease, Whipple's disease, gout, pseudogout, apatite arthritis, rheumatoid psoriatic arthritis, Reiter's syndrome and reactive arthritis, ankylosing spondylitis, septic iliopectenial bursitis, psoas abscess | Drainage: requires arthrotomy or percutaneous placement of drain under CT guidance; antibiotics: ceftriaxone 1 IV every 12 hr for gonococcal arthritis; penicillinase-resistant penicillin (e.g., nafcillin) IV; add aminoglycoside if documented or strongly suspected gram-negative infection, e.g., neutropenic or immunosuppressed patients; analgesics (preferably no antipyretic); physical therapy: passive ROM after about 48 hr |
| Systemic lupus erythematosus | Young women; women > men; African-American and hispanic > white; complement deficiencies especially C2; drugs, especially INH, hydralazine, procainamide | Arthralgia, arthritis, malar skin rash, pleurisy, pericarditis, nephritis, seizures, psychosis, fever, malaise, fatigue | Oral ulcers, fundal hemorrhages or exudates, skin rash, especially malar or photosensitive rash, pleural or pericardial rubs, lymphadenopathy, arthritis of small joints of hands, wrists, feet (symmetric) | Antinuclear antibodies present in 90% of cases, anti-SM more specific as are anti-dsDNA antibodies: anti-ssDNA and antihistone antibodies in drug-induced SLE, Coombs test, VDRL | Pain may be due to avascular necrosis of hip, septic arthritis, synovitis due to SLE, bursitis; most other causes of hip pain may occur in patients with SLE | For arthritis due to SLE, NSAIDs are mainstay, antimalarial drugs, e.g., hydroxychloroquine, may be useful for arthritis; corticosteroids are generally reserved for treatment of life-threatening disease |

*ROM*, Range of motion; *ESR*, erythrocyte sedimentation rate; *RF*, rheumatoid factor; *WBC*, white blood cell count; *SLE*, systemic lupus erythematosus; *NSAIDs*, nonsteroidal antiinflammatory drugs; *CHF*, congestive heart failure; *RA*, rheumatoid arthritis; *ARF*, acute rheumatic fever; *ACTH*, adrenocorticotropic hormone; *TSH*, thyroid-stimulating hormone; *DIP*, distal interphalangeal; *SI*, sacroiliac; *ANA*, antinuclear antibodies; *PT*, prothrombin time; *PTT*, partial thromboplastin time; *CPPD*, calcium pyrophosphate deposition disease; *CBC*, complete blood count; *SPEP*, serum protein electrophoresis; *CXR*, chest x-ray; *U/A*, urinalysis; *DTR*, deep tendon reflexes; *LS*, lumbosacral.

*Continued.*

**Table 74-1.** Selected causes of hip pain—cont'd

| Disorder | Epidemiology | History | Physical examination | Diagnostic tests | Differential diagnosis | Management |
|---|---|---|---|---|---|---|
| Trochanteric bursitis | Bursitis and tendinitis may be due to overuse and may be seen in athletic adolescents; posttraumatic trochanteric bursitis may occur at any age: bursitis and tendinitis may be more common in diabetics and those with chronic inflammatory disorders, especially RA, SLE | Lateral hip pain, often aggravated by weight bearing, rising from a chair, climbing or descending stairs; patients may note increased pain lying on affected side at night; night pain may be prominent; some patients unable to walk due to severe pain | Tenderness over greater trochanter of femur; reproduces pain; hip motion may be decreased by pain but internal and external rotation relatively preserved; forced adduction may aggravate pain | Plain radiographs: calcific deposits superior and lateral to the greater trochanter, irregularity of the trochanter, normal hip joint or early osteoarthritic changes; for severe pain: CBC, ESR may exclude very uncommon septic trochanteric bursitis | Trochanteric fracture or bone bruise due to trauma; impacted fracture of femoral neck; avulsion fracture of greater trochanter (in athletic adolescents); meralgia paresthetica (lateral femoral cutaneous neuropathy); radiculopathy should not produce local tenderness; herpes zoster before appearance of rash | Conservative: local heat, analgesics or NSAIDs, rest, ultrasound with or without 10% hydrocortisone cream (phonopheresis) for 4-6 weeks; local injection: 20 to 40 mg depomethylprednisolone and 2 ml 1% or 2% lidocaine, injected deeply with 1.5-inch 25-gauge or 3.5-inch 22-gauge spinal needle into area of maximal tenderness |
| Tumors | In childhood: leukemia, neuroblastoma most common solid tumor; in adults: metastatic cancer, lymphoma, soft tissue sarcomas | In children: a limp may be noted by parents; in adults: hip pain, may be aggravated by weight bearing but often prominent at night, gradual worsening, may be severe, other constitutional symptoms especially weight loss, review of systems important if no cancer history | If bone lesion: joint motion may be unrestricted and does not reproduce pain; if intrasynovial tumor: restricted joint motion, palpation may detect mass or tenderness of bones or soft tissues; thyroid, chest, breast, rectal, prostate, pelvic examinations for suspected primary | Plain films may demonstrate lytic or blastic lesions within bone or erosion of bone by adjacent intraarticular or juxtaarticular neoplasm; bone scans more sensitive for metastatic deposits (specify total body to assess for other sites); CT helpful to define bone lesions and guide biopsy if necessary; MRI useful for soft tissue tumors; CBC, ESR, SPEP, CXR, U/A, VDRL, liver enzymes (chest CT if documented soft tissue tumor) in preparation for orthopedic/oncologic referral | Benign or malignant neoplasm, infection especially osteomyelitis, gummatous syphillis, histiocytosis, amyloidosis, tophaceous gout, hyperparathyroidism, Paget's disease | Analgesia including narcotics if necessary; tricyclics in low dose may be helpful; local or regional nerve blocks for proven malignant neoplasms; radiation therapy; consider prophylactic pinning if lesion is large and involves the femoral neck or shaft |

*ROM*, Range of motion; *ESR*, erythrocyte sedimentation rate; *RF*, rheumatoid factor; *WBC*, white blood cell count; *SLE*, systemic lupus erythematosus; *NSAIDs*, nonsteroidal antiinflammatory drugs; *CHF*, congestive heart failure; *RA*, rheumatoid arthritis; *ARF*, acute rheumatic fever; *ACTH*, adrenocorticotropic hormone; *TSH*, thyroid-stimulating hormone; *DIP*, distal interphalangeal; *SI*, sacroiliac; *ANA*, antinuclear antibodies; *PT*, prothrombin time; *PTT*, partial thromboplastin time; *CPPD*, calcium pyrophosphate deposition disease; *CBC*, complete blood count; *SPEP*, serum protein electrophoresis; *CXR*, chest x-ray; *U/A*, urinalysis; *DTR*, deep tendon reflexes; *LS*, lumbosacral.

## DIFFERENTIAL DIAGNOSIS

Possible causes of pain in the area of the hip are listed in the boxes on p. 1042 and in Table 74-1.

### BIBLIOGRAPHY

Arlet J: Nontraumatic avascular necrosis of the femoral head: past, present, future, *Clin Orthop* 277:12, 1992.

Dean MT, Cabanela ME: Trans-trochanteric anterior rotational osteotomy for avascular necrosis of the femoral head: long term results, *J Bone Joint Surg* 75B:597, 1993.

Gravallese EM et al: Synovitis of the knee in a 42-year-old man: clinicopathologic conference, *Arthr Rheumat* 36:860, 1993.

Roberts WN, Williams RB: Hip pain, *Primary Care* 15:783, 1988.

Sugioka Y, Hotokebuchi T, Tsutsui H: Trans-trochanteric anterior rotational osteotomy for idiopathic and steroid-induced necrosis of the femoral head: indications and long term results, *Clin Orthop* 277:111, 1992.

CHAPTER

# 75 Knee

Elinor A. Mody
Jerry M. Greene

The knee is one of the most commonly injured joints, and the one most often affected by systemic inflammatory and neoplastic disease. It is necessary to be familiar with the regional anatomy, especially the bony structures, ligaments, tendons, bursae, and cartilage to be able to perform a focused physical examination of the knee, to order the appropriate diagnostic tests, and to be knowledgeable of differential diagnosis of the painful knee. This chapter addresses these issues. The different disorders causing knee pain, and their respective epidemiologies, important historic considerations, physical findings, diagnostic tests, differential diagnoses, and management options are summarized in Table 75-1.

## ANATOMY

The knee, one of the largest joints in the body, is formed from the femur, tibia, fibula, and patella. The femoral condyles and tibial plateaus create a hinge, capped by the patella within its tendon mechanism. The cartilaginous medial and lateral menisci cushion the tibial plateaus and femoral condyles, and distribute the forces across these areas. The medial and lateral collateral ligaments and the anterior and posterior cruciate ligaments provide stability to the knee. External to the synovial membrane and capsule of the knee joint are several bursae described in Chapter 80 and illustrated in Fig. 75-1.

Pathology of any of these structures may contribute to knee pain.

## HISTORY

Important historic features include the temporal course of the knee pain and the nature of onset. Pain tends to be acute in cases of trauma, crystal diseases, sepsis, and hemorrhage. A subacute or insidious onset is more consistent with a systemic inflammatory disease, tumor, or osteonecrosis. The location, character, radiation, aggravating and relieving factors, and severity of the pain, as well as associated local symptoms such as swelling, stiffness, redness, and limitation of motion, are important historic features to elicit. Systemic symptoms such as weight loss, fever, chills, and malaise are also significant.

The hallmarks of inflammatory synovitis are morning stiffness and pain at rest. Pain only during certain activities suggests a mechanical or traumatic disorder. Involvement of other joints should be assessed. In particular, polyarticular involvement of the joints of the wrists, hands, and feet suggests inflammatory disorders such as rheumatoid arthritis. Back pain with morning stiffness suggests spondylitis. A review of systems for rash, myalgias, pleuritic chest pain, mucosal lesions, fever, diarrhea, weight loss, neurologic symptoms, and malaise may suggest other etiologies, such as Lyme disease, inflammatory bowel disease, or systemic lupus erythematosus. Particular conditions may predispose to certain forms of joint disease such as hyperparathyroidism, hypothyroidism, hemochromatosis, and aging for calcium pyrophosphate arthropathies and alcohol abuse for gout. Therefore the interview should include inquiries regarding these predisposing factors. Both sexual and IV drug use histories are important when evaluating for a form of bacterial arthritis such as disseminated gonococcal infection and bacterial arthritis associated with endocarditis. Medication history is especially important, since diuretics may contribute to gouty arthritis and Coumadin poses a risk for intraarticular and intramuscular bleeding. Review of medical problems is important for assessing contraindications to drug therapy, such as peptic ulcer disease or renal disease when considering nonsteroidal antiinflammatory drug therapy. A history of any drug allergies should be elicited. Some rheumatic diseases (e.g., gout, the spondyloarthropathies, osteoarthritis, and the collagen vascular diseases) have a hereditary component, and eliciting a family history is an important part of any evaluation.

## PHYSICAL EXAMINATION

Inspection of the affected knee should include observation for erythema, ecchymosis, swelling, abrasions, puncture wounds, and active range of motion. The physician should palpate the joint line, bursae, muscle, tendons, ligaments, and bones in an attempt to localize tenderness. Joint line tenderness may suggest meniscal or ligamentous injury. An effusion, if present, may be demonstrated by eliciting a "bulge sign" (Fig. 75-2). As the patient lies supine with knees fully extended and the quadriceps muscle relaxed, the medial aspect of the knee is massaged in a cephalad direction. The lateral aspect of the knee is then stroked inferiorly. The presence of a bulge sign or knee effusion as indicated by a medial fluid wave is also called cross

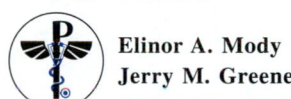

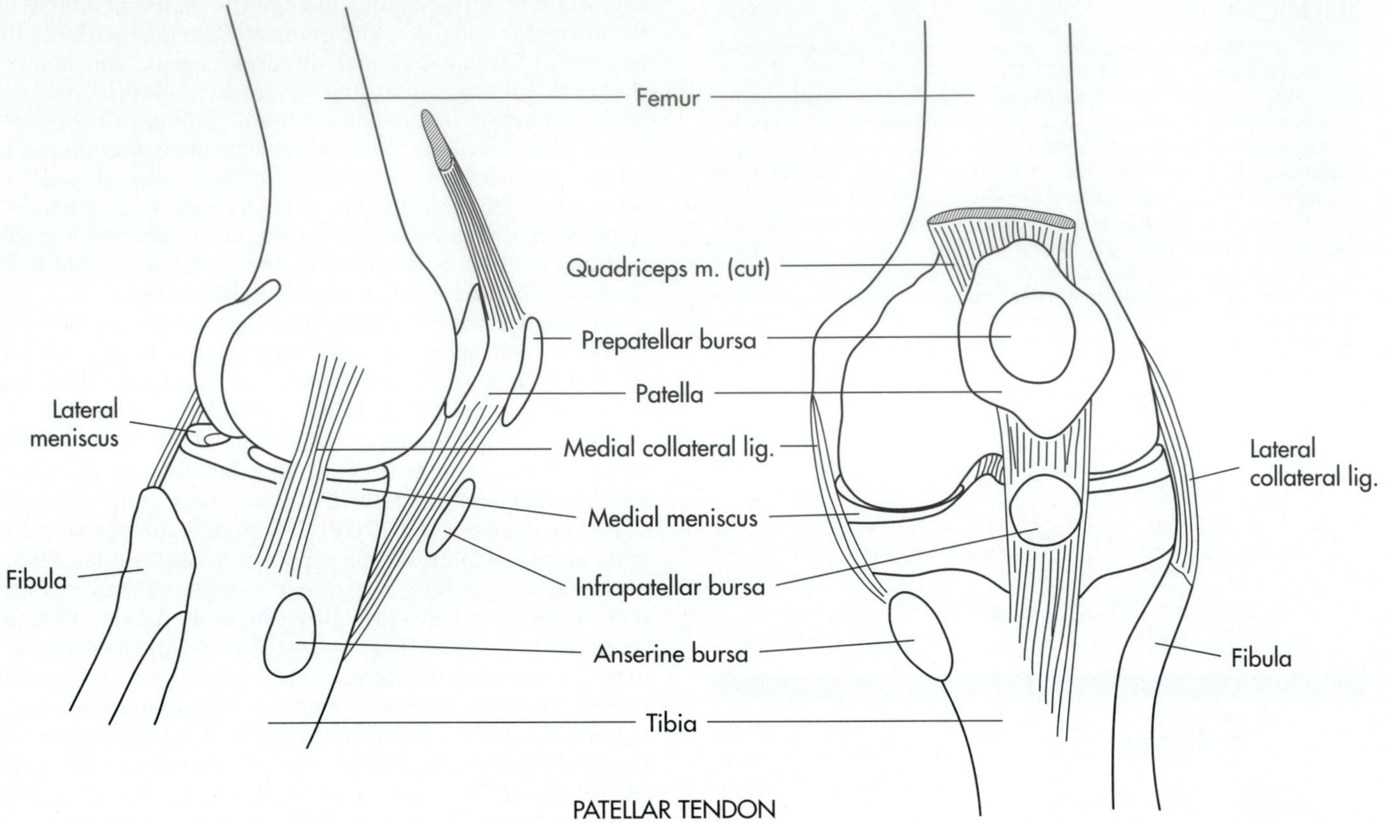


**Fig. 75-1.** Anatomic landmarks of the knee.

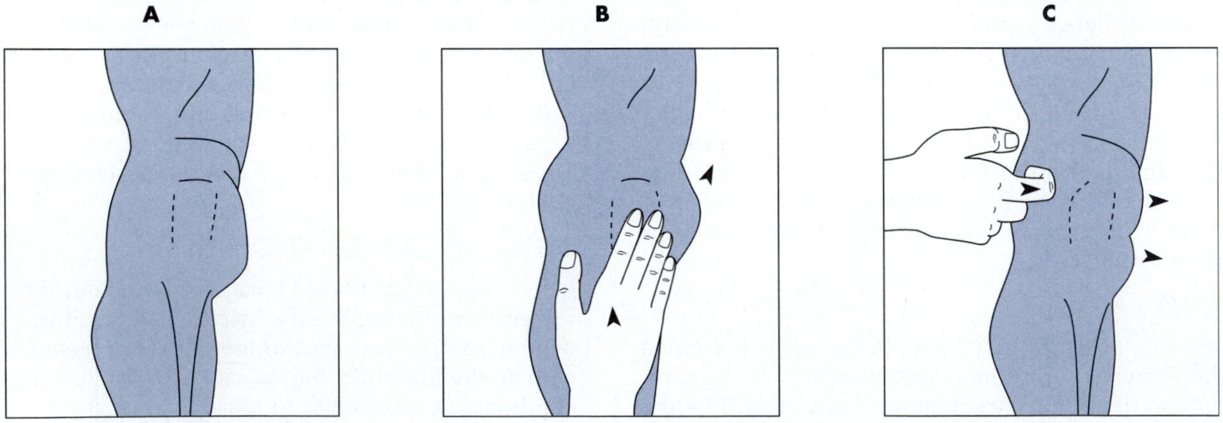


**Fig. 75-2. A,** Bulge sign for knee effusion. **B,** Fluid is balloted into the suprapatellar bursa. **C,** Downward pressure exerted along the lateral aspect of the knee produces a bulge down the medial aspect.

fluctuance. Another maneuver to elicit excessive synovial fluid in the knee is to apply rapid, downward pressure on the patella; if a click is felt as the patella touches the femoral condyle, an effusion is probably present. This is also referred to as patellar ballottement. Occasionally, obesity may result in a false positive ballottement sign. The examiner should also palpate the popliteal space for swelling that may occur with popliteal artery aneurysm, Baker's cysts, and tumors. Passive range of motion of the knee should also be performed.

Several maneuvers may help the clinician elicit mechanical disorders. The McMurray's test is useful for diagnosing meniscal injury. This is performed by passive flexion of the knee with the patient lying supine. The lower leg is externally rotated at full flexion. It is then held in external rotation and the knee is passively extended. A painful click near the top of the extension arc is a positive finding. The maneuver is then repeated with the lower leg in internal rotation. This tests for both medial and lateral meniscal tears or injury. Simply taking the knee through flexion and extension while feeling and listening for crepitation is also helpful in assessing such mechanical problems as a loose body in the knee joint. In the absence of signs of inflammation, crepitation suggests osteoarthritis.

A thorough general physical examination of the patient is also important. It may reveal evidence of a systemic disease associated with knee pathology. The neurologic system, back, and hip merit particular attention because of the possibility of referred pain to the knee. A few examples of cutaneous clues to the cause of arthritis include psoriasis, erythema chronicum migrans, rheumatoid nodules, and tophi.

## DIAGNOSTIC TESTS

Often the first diagnostic test sought after a thorough physical examination is a radiograph, particularly if trauma or a mechanical disorder is suspected. The most useful views are anteroposterior (AP) films, which allow visualization of the medial and lateral femorotibial compartments of the knee and of the patellofemoral joint. If there is no suspicion of fracture, weight bearing anteroposterior radiographs most accurately assess narrowing of the cartilage of the femorotibial joint. The skyline, or sunrise, view allows the clinician to visualize the patella and the patellar surfaces that contact the femoral condyles. Tunnel views may also help, particularly in assessing ligamentous injuries, osteoarthritis, intraarticular loose bodies, and osteonecrosis (osteochondritis dissecans).

Synovial fluid analysis is important in distinguishing noninflammatory conditions from inflammatory joint disease. Arthrocentesis should always be performed under aseptic conditions to prevent infection, and to allow a sterile specimen to be sent for bacterial cultures. In immunocompromised patients, fungal and mycobacterial cultures should be sent as well. Another specimen should be sent for cell count and differential. If the cell count reveals more than 2000 leukocytes per cubic millimeter, the fluid is inflammatory. The cell count may also reveal evidence of intraarticular bleeding. If the synovial fluid is inflammatory, a Gram's stain and culture should be performed to evaluate for joint sepsis. Examination of the fluid with polarizing microscopy should be done to search for birefringent crystals, specifically urate and calcium pyrophosphate. With alizarin red staining of joint fluid smears, hydroxyapatite crystals may be visualized. The presence of fat droplets in synovial fluid suggests fracture of the bone into the marrow space.

Several blood tests may help in evaluation of knee pain. An erythrocyte sedimentation rate (ESR) is a general screen for inflammatory disorders as is the complete blood count, particularly the leukocyte count and differential. A routine chemistry panel is useful to assess for renal disease, particularly since renal insufficiency may affect therapeutic options. Depending on the clinical setting, the serum urate level, rheumatoid factor, or antinuclear antibody may also be helpful. Serum calcium, phosphate, magnesium, alkaline phosphatase, thyroid function and iron studies should be considered in patients with pseudogout or chondrocalcinosis.

A number of imaging techniques are very useful in evaluating knee pain. Magnetic resonance imaging (MRI) allows visualization of joint fluid, synovial swelling, ligaments, menisci, cartilage, and bone (including marrow) structures. If infection is suspected and cannot be completely characterized by the routine methods, gallium scan may be considered as may arthroscopy with synovial biopsy; this is particularly helpful if fungal or mycobacterial arthritis is suspected. Arthroscopy may also be very helpful in the evaluation, and even treatment, of internal derangement of the knee such as meniscal tears. See Chapter 69 for further discussion.

## SELECTED CAUSES OF KNEE PAIN

### Inflammatory arthritis

Any arthritis causing a purulent or exudative effusion is regarded as inflammatory. Although this category includes a number of different diseases, some general patterns occur; frequently more than one joint is affected, and the conditions tend to be chronic or recurrent. Knee arthritis may be a prominent manifestation of the disease. Inflammatory joint diseases that frequently involve the knee include gout, calcium pyrophosphate arthropathy, rheumatoid arthritis, the spondyloarthropathies, septic arthritis, and Lyme disease, as well as mechanical disorders, periarticular disease, osteoathritis, avascular necrosis, and tumors, which are discussed in Table 75-1 and in individual chapters of the musculoskeletal section.

The remainder of this chapter discusses disorders as they specifically affect the knee including mechanical disorders, anserine and prepatellar bursitis, and synovial growths and tumors.

### Mechanical disorders

Mechanical disorders of the knee may involve bone, cartilage, and periarticular structures such as bursae, tendons, and ligaments.

***Fracture.*** Most traumatic fractures within the knee involve the tibial plateaus or patella. The history of trauma followed by acute onset of pain and swelling are typical. Physical examination reveals significant pain on moving or stressing the knee. Swelling and limited range of motion are usually present. It is important to ensure that the neurovascular system of the lower leg is intact. If a fracture is suspected, radiographs (AP, lateral, and sunrise

*Text continued on p. 1062.*

**Table 75-1.** Selected causes of knee pain

| Disorder | Epidemiology | History | Physical examination | Diagnostic tests | Differential diagnosis | Management |
|---|---|---|---|---|---|---|
| Gout | Middle age, elderly, overproducers of urate, transplant patients | Acute onset of pain, often with previous attack in first MTP | Warmth, erythema, effusion, exquisite tenderness | High synovial WBC, urate crystals seen under polarizing microscope, "rat bite" erosions on radiograph | Rheumatoid arthritis, spondylitis, other crystal-induced arthropathy, infection | NSAIDs, colchicine, local corticosteroid injection acutely, allopurinol or uricosuric long-term |
| Pseudogout | Elderly, patients with metabolic disorders such as hypothyroidism, hypomagnesemia, ochronosis, hemochromatosis, Wilson's disease, hyperparathyroidism | Acute onset of pain, if metabolic disease, systemic complaints | Similar to gout | High synovial WBC, calcium pyrophosphate crystals seen under polarizing microscope, chondrocalcinosis on radiograph; if clinically indicated, serum iron studies, magnesium, phosphate, calcium, ceruloplasmin, thyroid studies | Gout, rheumatoid arthritis, spondylitis, infection | NSAIDs, colchicine, local corticosteroid injection acutely, daily colchicine as prophylaxis against further attacks |
| Rheumatoid arthritis | Age varies, usually female | Morning stiffness, involvement of joints of the hand, multiple joint involvement, fatigue, multiple attacks | Warmth, erythema with effusion, if longstanding "boggy" synovium, symmetrical involvement of joints, decreased ROM | High synovial WBC, RF often positive, elevated ESR, anemia, consistent with chronic disease, bone erosions on radiographs | Crystal-induced arthropathy, spondylitis, infection | NSAIDs, local corticosteroid injection, second line agents such as methotrexate and gold |
| Spondyloarthropathy (Reactive arthritis, Reiter's syndrome) | Young adults, male predominance; patients with associated disorders such as IBD, psoriasis, Chlamydia, Yersinia, or Shigella infection, ankylosing spondylitis; acute or subacute onset of pain, often associated with low back pain, and pain in other joints, may have a component of morning stiffness, may have systemic complaints related to underlying condition | Acute or subacute onset of pain, often associated with low back pain, and pain in other joints, may have a component of morning stiffness, may have systemic complaints related to underlying condition | Warmth, erythema, with effusion; may have "boggy" synovium if disease is longstanding; may have evidence of underlying disease, such as oral ulcers, rash, nail changes, decreased ROM of spine | High synovial WBC, erosions on radiograph, sacroiliitis on radiograph, squaring of vertebral bodies, syndesmophytes | Rheumatoid arthritis, crystal-induced arthritis, infection | NSAIDs, local corticosteroid injection, sulfasalazine, methotrexate |

| | | | | | | |
|---|---|---|---|---|---|---|
| Gonococcal infection | Young adults predominantly, but any age if sexually active | Acute onset of symptoms, may complain of GU symptoms, recent menses, general malaise | Warmth, erythema, with very large tense effusion, decreased ROM, maculopapular rash over trunk, fever, urethral or cervical discharge, arthritis of other joints, tenosynovitis | High synovial WBC, positive culture for GC from GU tract, blood, or synovial fluid | Rheumatoid arthritis, spondylitis, crystal-induced arthropathy, nongonococcal infection, Lyme disease | Ceftriaxone, or penicillin G for sensitive strains |
| Nongonococcal infection | IV drug abusers, severely debilitated, patients prone to fulminant sepsis or endocarditis | Acute onset of severe pain, swelling, redness, decreased ROM, may have associated systemic symptoms, may have arthritis in other joints | Warmth, erythema, effusion, decreased ROM, signs of source for bacteremia (e.g., pneumonia, UTI, etc.) | Very high synovial WBC, positive synovial or blood culture or Gram's stain, high ESR, elevated peripheral blood WBC, periosteal elevation on radiograph suggests concomitant osteomyelitis | Rheumatoid arthritis, spondylitis, crystal-induced arthritis, gonococcal infection | IV antibiotic therapy guided by Gram's stain, culture results, and sensitivities; drain with needle aspiration or arthroscopically, ROM exercises, and analgesics |
| Lyme disease | Those who have traveled to or live in endemic areas | Subacute onset of symptoms, swelling, warmth, decreased ROM, pain, history of ECM skin lesion(s), Bell's palsy, other painful joints | Warmth, erythema, effusion, may have "boggy" synovium | Lyme titers, synovial fluid culture rarely positive, radiographs may eventually show erosions | Rheumatoid arthritis, spondylitis, gonococcal and other nongonococcal infection, crystal-induced arthropathy | IV penicillin G or ceftriaxone |
| Fracture | Any age, risk factors include steroid use, osteoporosis or other causes, metastatic malignancy | History of trauma, sudden onset pain, swelling, warmth | Swelling, tenderness over affected area, pain on weight bearing, decreased ROM | Bloody synovial fluid, may show fat droplets under polarizing microscopy, fracture seen on radiograph, bone scan may detect stress fractures inapparent on radiograph | Meniscal tear, ligamentous tear, hemophilia, PVNS, anticoagulant therapy | Splinting to protect against additional neurovascular injury, reduction, and casting |
| Ligamentous injury | Young adults, athletes | Trauma with pivoting or hyperextension, feeling of "giving way" (McCune et al, 1988), acute pain and swelling | Swelling, point tenderness medial or lateral joint line, positive anterior or posterior drawer sign, medial or lateral laxity depending upon ligament disrupted | Bloody or serosanguineous noninflammatory synovial fluid, radiographs to rule out fracture, MRI reveals high $T_2$ signal in area of ligamentous tear | Meniscal tear, fracture, hemophilia, PVNS, anticoagulant therapy | Analgesics, knee immobilizer, orthopedic consultation for possible surgical repair for complete tears in patients who are active |

*MTP*, Metatarsal phalangeal joint; *WBC*, white blood cell; *NSAIDs*, nonsteroidal antiinflammatory drugs; *ROM*, range of motion; *RF*, rheumatoid factor; *ESR*, erythrocyte sedimentation rate; *IBD*, inflammatory bowel disease; *GU*, genitourinary; *GC*, gonococci; *UTI*, urinary tract infection; *ECM*, erythema chronicum migrans; *PVNS*, pigmented villonodular synovitis; *OA*, osteoarthritis; *SLE*, systemic lupus erythematosus; *AVN*, avascular necrosis.

*Continued.*

**Table 75-1.** Selected causes of knee pain—cont'd

| Disorder | Epidemiology | History | Physical examination | Diagnostic tests | Differential diagnosis | Management |
|---|---|---|---|---|---|---|
| Meniscal tear | Two groups: elderly with OA and young adults, athletes | Acute or subacute onset of pain, locking, painful popping | Swelling, tenderness over the lateral or medial joint line, positive McMurray's test | Bloody or serosanguineous synovial fluid, radiograph to rule out fracture, MRI, arthrography, or arthroscopy diagnostic | Fracture, ligamentous tear, hemophilia, PVNS, anticoagulant therapy, worsening osteoarthritis | Initial conservative (rest, NSAIDs), if unsuccessful, orthopedic referral for arthroscopic debridement, or total knee replacement if concomitant severe osteoarthritis |
| Osteonecrosis/ Avascular necrosis | Any age, patients with sickle cell anemia, chronic steroid use, alcoholism, decompression illness, trauma, SLE, dyslipoproteinemia | Acute onset of pain, swelling, rest pain, increased pain with weight bearing | Swelling, tenderness, decreased ROM | Area of subchondral collapse appears after weeks on plain radiograph, MRI most sensitive for AVN prior to subchondral collapse | Tumor, fracture, osteomyelitis, osteoarthritis, meniscal tear (Lotke et al, 1985, Case report, *N Engl J Med,* 1987; Spiera, 1987) | Initial conservative (nonweight bearing, NSAIDs, analgesics); if unsuccessful, tibial osteotomy, hemiarthroplasty, or total knee replacement |
| Osgood-Schlatter syndrome | Young adolescents | Pain at the inferior aspect of the patella, subacute to chronic onset | Tenderness to palpation, occasionally swelling in region of tibial tubercle | None | Fracture, tendinitis of patellar tendon, tumor, osteomyelitis | Reassurance, analgesics |
| Chrondromalacia | Young active persons, either gender | Subacute onset of patellar pain, worse walking stairs, little pain at rest | Reproduction of pain on pressing patella against femoral condyles | Synovial fluid noninflammatory, sunrise radiograph may reveal irregularity of articulating surface of patella | Tendinitis, bursitis, meniscal injury | Quadriceps isometric strengthening exercises, NSAIDs, or pure analgesics |
| Anserine bursitis | Middle age, elderly with OA, young active patients | Subacute onset of pain localized to the posteromedial aspect of the knee | Point tenderness over anserine bursa, rarely palpable swelling | None | Osteoarthritis, medial meniscus injury | NSAIDs, local heat, local corticosteroid injection |
| Pre-patellar bursitis | Those who kneel on hard surfaces, especially carpenters, plumbers, roofers, carpet layers | Subacute onset of pain in prepatellar area, swelling, erythema, desquamation or purulent discharge suggests septic bursitis | Tenderness, erythema, fluctuant swelling of bursa anterior to patella, knee flexion may be limited but full extension possible without increased pain | Bursal aspirate, culture, Gram's stain, crystal search | Cellulitis, gouty bursitis, hemobursa, septic bursitis, patellar fracture, fat necrosis, erythema nodosum | If septic: antibiotics, repeated needle aspiration for drainage; if nonseptic: NSAIDs, local heat, activity modification |

| | | | | | | |
|---|---|---|---|---|---|---|
| Osteoarthritis | Middle aged, elderly, athletes, obese, those with prior knee trauma | Progressive, slowly increasing, pain, stiffness, decreased ROM over years, "cracking" of joint, no rest pain unless very advanced arthritis, short-lived morning stiffness (minutes) | Decreased ROM, swelling, crepitation, bony prominence | Synovial fluid noninflammatory, osteophyte formation, subchondral cysts, sclerosis, joint space narrowing seen on radiograph | Inflammatory arthritis, meniscal tear, anserine bursitis, secondary forms of osteoarthritis: hemochromatosis, Wilson's disease, ochronosis, gout, acromegaly, hypothyroidism, hyperparathyroidism | Analgesics or NSAIDs, quadriceps strengthening exercises, weight loss if appropriate, use of cane<br>Consider surgical intervention (tibial osteotomy or total knee replacement) for unremitting pain |
| Synovial chondromatosis | Wide age range, either gender | Slowly progressing pain, swelling, stiffness | Swelling with effusion, diffuse tenderness | Multiple calcific densities and effusion on plain radiograph, noncalcified chondral bodies may only be apparent on MRI, arthrography, or arthroscopy | Other synovial tumors, inflammatory arthritis, pigmented villonodular synovitis, avascular necrosis with loose osteochondral fragments | Surgical synovectomy, total knee replacement if advanced disease with articular cartilage destruction |
| Pigmented villonodular synovitis | Young adults | Recurrent knee pain and swelling | Erythema, swelling, limited ROM, and tenderness | Synovial fluid reddish-brown, noninflammatory; effusion or soft tissue swelling, joint space narrowing, and erosions may be seen on plain radiograph MRI suggestive, synovial biopsy definitive | Inflammatory arthritis, recurrent hemorrhage, synovial chondromatosis | Surgical synovectomy or radiation synovectomy |
| Malignancy | Metastatic cancer most common, primary bone and soft tissue sarcomas less likely, leukemia, lymphoma, and myeloma | Slowly worsening pain, swelling, stiffness, prominent night pain is suggestive | Decreased ROM, diffuse tenderness, effusion | Synovial fluid with lymphocytic predominance, tumor cells sometimes seen, periosteal disruption or lytic bone lesions on plain radiograph; MRI defines bone and soft tissue involvement; biopsy if no known primary | Inflammatory arthritis, benign tumors, osteomyelitis | Primary tumors: surgical excision or amputation, adjuvant chemotherapy or radiation therapy<br>Metastatic tumors: radiation therapy for pain control, other treatment based upon type of malignancy |

*MTP*, Metatarsal phalangeal joint; *WBC*, white blood cell; *NSAIDs*, nonsteroidal antiinflammatory drugs; *ROM*, range of motion; *RF*, rheumatoid factor; *ESR*, erythrocyte sedimentation rate; *IBD*, inflammatory bowel disease; *GU*, genitourinary; *GC*, gonococci; *UTI*, urinary tract infection; *ECM*, erythema chronicum migrans; *PVNS*, pigmented villonodular synovitis; *OA*, osteoarthritis; *SLE*, systemic lupus erythematosus; *AVN*, avascular necrosis.

views) should be obtained prior to aspiration, since even the small risk of infection associated with needle puncture is best avoided in the presence of a fracture. Occasionally, the diagnosis of fracture is not definite even with radiographs. If the fluid aspirate reveals a bloody effusion or frank blood, a Sudan red stain to detect fat droplets from the marrow should be performed. CT or MRI scanning may help detect fractures not evident on plain films. The differential diagnosis includes other traumatic injuries, such as meniscal tear and ligamentous injury; other causes of hemarthrosis, such as pigmented villonodular synovitis; and bleeding disorders, such as hemophilia and anticoagulant therapy. Management of an intraarticular fracture includes immobilization and orthopedic consultation.

***Ligamentous injury.*** Ligamentous injuries often occur as a result of athletic injuries. The knee is commonly affected. The history is usually one of pivoting on the knee after a jump, excessive extension, or medial or lateral stress. Often the patient describes the feeling of something "giving" within the joint, after which there is the acute onset of pain and swelling (McCune et al, 1988). Joint laxity may be apparent if the ligament tear is complete. Physical examination may reveal swelling and, depending on the ligament involved, point tenderness over the medial joint line (medial collateral ligament) or lateral joint line (lateral collateral ligament). To test for a cruciate ligament tear, instability of the joint may be assessed with the anteroposterior drawer test. This is performed with the knee flexed to 90 degrees. The examiner attempts to pull the tibia forward, away from the femur. If laxity is detected, an anterior cruciate ligament tear is likely. By reversing the force, the posterior cruciate ligament is tested. Medial and lateral collateral ligaments are tested by applying pressure on the lateral aspect of the knee, stressing the medial collateral ligament. These forces are reversed to test the lateral collateral ligament while the patient lies supine with the knee extended. Laxity indicates a collateral ligament injury. Neurovascular examination, as with fractures, is important. Although plain films help rule out fracture, the imaging study of choice to diagnose ligamentous tears is an MRI. Joint aspiration generally reveals either serosanguineous, noninflammatory fluid, or a bloody effusion. Differential diagnosis includes meniscal tear, fracture, or sprain. Management for complete tear in active individuals is usually surgical repair. See Chapter 88 for a more thorough discussion.

***Meniscal tear.*** The two groups of patients who suffer from meniscal tears are young adults with a history of trauma and middle-aged or elderly patients with osteoarthritis. Medial meniscal tears are more common than lateral. A meniscal tear presents with acute or subacute pain. Patients may experience the knee "giving way" and a painful popping or locking. On examination swelling is common, with warmth and point tenderness over either the medial or lateral joint line. Physical examination should include the McMurray's test (see examination section), although a negative test does not exclude meniscal pathology. Diagnostic tests include radiographs to evaluate for fractures, osteoarthritis, and intraarticular loose-bodies. Aspiration generally yields noninflammatory fluid that may be bloody, depending on the extent of the tear. The best imaging study to diagnose a meniscal tear is an MRI scan. This generally should be done only if the diagnosis is in doubt, or if surgical intervention is anticipated. Initial management is conservative and consists of rest, including use of crutches and NSAIDs. If symptoms do not resolve within several weeks, orthopedic referral is appropriate. The differential diagnosis includes fracture, avascular necrosis, intraarticular loose-bodies, and ligamentous injury.

***Osteonecrosis (AVN).*** Any age group is susceptible to osteonecrosis. Several conditions, including sickle cell anemia, corticosteroid therapy, decompression illness, alcoholism, trauma, SLE, and dyslipoproteinemias, predispose to osteonecrosis. When this disease occurs in a young person with a history of trauma and no other predisposing factors, it is often called osteochondritis dissecans. Osteonecrosis presents as acute pain, sometimes accompanied by swelling. Physical examination may reveal an effusion and tenderness over the lateral or medial joint line (Mankin, 1992). Range of motion may vary. If the process has been present for several weeks to months, motion may be limited and painful, and an AP radiograph may reveal an area of sclerosis and collapse of the affected femoral condyle or tibial plateau. Patients who are examined earlier may have normal motion and radiographs. At this stage, the MRI is the diagnostic study of choice. A bone scan may also reveal changes before plain films. The differential diagnosis includes fracture, meniscal tear, neoplasm, osteomyelitis, and osteoarthritis (Lotke et al, 1985; Case report, *N Engl J Med,* 1987; Spiera, 1987). Initial management is conservative (rest, including use of crutches, NSAIDs, and quadriceps strengthening); if this is not effective, orthopedic consultation for possible tibial osteotomy or, in the case of osteoarthritis, hemiarthroplasty or total knee replacement is recommended.

***Osgood-Schlatter syndrome.*** Osgood-Schlatter syndrome is a benign condition seen in adolescents. The patient complains of pain inferior to the patella. On physical examination, pain is elicited by palpation of the attachment of the patellar tendon to the tibial tuberosity. The condition is almost always self-limited and requires no therapy other than avoiding stress to the quadriceps tendon mechanism.

***Chondromalacia.*** Chondromalacia is also a disease of predominantly young, active individuals, particularly women. The condition is also known as the patellofemoral syndrome. It is an overuse syndrome, commonly occurring in the weekend athlete. The onset of knee pain is often subacute and is worse with use, particularly on climbing stairs and standing up after sitting. At rest, pain is generally minimal. Physical examination may reveal an effusion and warmth. Pain may be reproduced by direct downward pressure of the patella against the femoral condyles while the patient lies supine. Routine radiographs may reveal irregularity of the patella's undersurface. Synovial fluid is characteristically noninflammatory. The differential diagnosis includes tendinitis, bursitis, meniscal tear, osteoarthritis, and a plica syndrome (synovial fibrous bond). Management is conservative with quadriceps-strengthening exercises and NSAIDs.

***Anserine bursitis.*** Anserine bursitis generally affects middle-aged and elderly individuals with osteoarthritis of the knee, although it can occur in young, active individuals. Pain is subacute at onset, and is localized to the inferomedial aspect of the knee. Physical examination reveals point tenderness on palpation of the anserine bursa (see Fig. 75-1). Signs of osteoarthritis of the knee may be found. The differential diagnosis includes osteoarthritis and medial meniscal injury. Management includes local corticosteroid injection, NSAIDs, heat, and ultrasound, which may be combined with topical 10% hydrocortisone cream.

***Prepatellar bursitis.*** Prepatellar bursitis, also called housemaid's knee, often results from prolonged kneeling on a hard surface and tends to be an occupational injury. Inflammation occurs in the prepatellar bursa or infrapatellar bursa (see Fig. 75-1). Pain, swelling, and erythema over the patella are often present. Knee extension is generally full, but flexion is limited because of traction on the inflamed soft tissues. Relatively painless motion from full extension to about 90 degrees of flexion helps distinguish prepatellar bursitis from inflammation of the true knee joint. If a bursal effusion is present, aspiration of the bursa should be attempted. If fluid is obtained, the leukocyte count should be performed. If the fluid is inflammatory, septic bursitis must be considered. Since fever, peripheral leukocytosis, and positive bursal fluid Gram's stains are infrequently found, aspirated fluid should be cultured. The differential diagnosis of prepatellar bursitis includes septic bursitis, patella fracture, arthritis of the knee, and cellulitis. Management is conservative and includes NSAIDs, rest, the use of protective knee pads, and avoidance of further trauma. If septic bursitis is likely, empiric antibiotics to cover staphylococcal and streptococcal species should be given after bursal fluid aspiration, Gram's stain, and culture. For a more thorough discussion of prepatellar bursitis, see Chapter 87 on infectious diseases of bones and joints and Chapter 80 on periarthritis.

### Synovial growths and tumors

In general, benign and malignant tumors of synovium and bone are rare causes of knee pain.

***Synovial osteochondromatosis.*** Synovial osteochondromatosis is a benign neoplastic lesion. The history is one of slowly developing pain, swelling, and restricted motion (Varma, 1973). Physical examination is notable for swelling with effusion, decreased range of motion, and tenderness. Routine radiographs may reveal multiple calcific bodies in the region of the knee in longstanding disease. In less advanced disease, plain films may not be helpful; MRI is the definitive imaging study. Differential diagnosis includes other tumors of the synovium and bone, inflammatory arthritis, pigmented villonodular synovitis, and osteonecrosis with loose fragments. Management is surgical synovectomy. Joint replacement may be necessary in cases of severe longstanding disease.

***Pigmented villonodular synovitis.*** A rare, benign neoplastic disorder, pigmented villonodular synovitis primarily affects young individuals. The history is one of recurrent pain and swelling. Physical examination reveals an enlarged, warm joint with an effusion and limited range of motion. Synovial fluid is reddish-brown with noninflammatory characteristics. Routine radiographs reveal soft tissue swelling, effusion, and, if disease is longstanding, joint space narrowing. MRI is the definitive imaging study; it is also necessary to determine the extent of disease. Synovial biopsy is a useful diagnostic procedure. The differential diagnosis includes synovial chondromatosis, hemophilia with recurrent hemarthrosis, and inflammatory arthropathy. Management is a surgical total synovectomy.

***Malignancies.*** The malignancies that involve the knee are diverse, and include chondrosarcoma, synovial sarcoma, lymphoma, osteosarcoma, neuroblastoma, and metastatic carcinomas of many origins. Marrow involvement with leukemia may also produce knee pain, especially in children. Pain from knee involvement is similar, regardless of the underlying neoplasm. It is subacute to chronic, and with progression becomes constant. Swelling of the joint and decreased range of motion are variable. Physical examination may reveal knee warmth, swelling, restricted motion, effusion, and tenderness over the affected area. Routine radiographs may reveal disruption of the periosteum and trabeculae and a soft tissue mass. If plain films do not reveal changes, CT or MRI scans may suggest the disease. Biopsy is necessary for diagnosis, and should be carefully performed to avoid seeding uninvolved tissues. Synovial fluid is usually inflammatory with a lymphocytic predominance. Tumor cells are sometimes seen in synovial fluid. Differential diagnosis includes inflammatory arthropathy and infection with concomitant osteomyelitis, particularly if the leukocyte count is greater than 10,000. Local management includes radiation, surgical debridement and fixation. Systemic management is determined by the nature of the malignancy.

## BIBLIOGRAPHY


Alvarellos A, Spilberg I: Colchicine prophylaxis in pseudogout, *J Rheumatol* 13:804, 1986.

Case report, *N Engl J Med* 316(12):736, 1987.

Lotke P et al: Osteonecrosis of the knee, *Orthop Clin North Am* 16:593, 1985.

Mankin H: Nontraumatic necrosis of bone (osteonecrosis), *N Engl J Med* 326:1473, 1992.

McCune J et al: Evaluation of knee pain, *Prim Care* 15:795, 1988.

Spiera H: Osteoarthritis as a misdiagnosis in elderly patients, *Geriatrics* 42(11):37, 1987.

Varma M: Synovial chrondromatosis of the knee, *Int Surg* 58(6):389, 1973.

CHAPTER

# 76 Foot and Ankle

Robert G. Frykberg

Foot problems, although not frequently serious in nature, can be a significant source of discomfort or morbidity.

In an attempt to quantify the incidence and prevalence of foot disorders in the civilian noninstitutionalized U.S. population, the National Center for Health Statistics designed and conducted the 1990 National Health Interview Survey (NHIS) with a special supplement dealing exclusively with the foot. The results are summarized in Table 76-1 and represent age-adjusted values using the age distribution of the U.S. population as the standard. An estimated 43.1 million people had foot problems during the 12-month period (175 per 1000 people); problems with toenails (e.g., ingrown), foot infections (e.g., athlete's foot and warts), and corns or calluses each afflicted over 11 million individuals. Table 76-2 presents the incidence of specific foot problems stratified by gender and race. Women reported foot problems much more frequently than men, especially bunions, which were 5 times more common in women. Whites generally reported more foot problems than African-Americans, although African-Americans reported 30% more corns and calluses. Incidence of all disorders rose significantly with age (Table 76-3). Collapsing data for all individuals 18 to 44 years old and for all individuals 65 or older, it is apparent that the older adults in the latter category have an overall incidence of foot problems almost 3 times greater than the adults between the ages of 18 and 44.

These data highlight the prevalence and range of foot disorders affecting the population but do not fully enumerate those conditions that might present on a daily basis. Emphasizing the need for early recognition and appropriate treatment or referral, this chapter discusses the etiology, diagnosis, and treatment of most of the common foot disorders presenting to the generalist and primary care podiatrist. Since most surgical procedures of the foot are beyond the scope of practice of the primary care physician, a description of surgical treatments is restricted primarily to nail disorders and verrucae. The section on local anesthetic injection techniques is of interest to practitioners not only for surgical treatments, but also for diagnostic and therapeutic purposes as well. The final portion deals with the most challenging area of foot pathology, the diabetic foot. A full discussion of vascular, neuropathic, and infectious complications attendant with the diabetic lower extremity augments the exposition on foot ulceration and gangrene. The importance of prevention, early intervention, and proper treatment, including correction of underlying structural deformities, is emphasized in concert with the necessity for a multidisciplinary team approach in the overall management of these patients. Since this chapter serves as a general review for the entire scope of foot and ankle disorders, the reader is encouraged to pursue areas of specific interest from the list of references.

## NAIL DISORDERS

### Onychomycosis

Nail pathology is one of the most common of all foot conditions. Fungal infection of the toenails is the most prevalent of such disorders, often involving all 10 toenails in extreme cases. *Onychomycosis* (tinea unguium), albeit a painless and fairly benign disorder, causes considerable concern to the patient and a great deal of frustration to the treating physician because of its recalcitrance to most treatments. The mycotic nail is recognized by its typical yellowish-white opaque appearance on a thickened nail plate. The accumulation of subungual debris is evident, often appearing as a double nail. The infection usually begins at the distal aspect of the nail plate and gradually spreads proximally to involve the nail matrix, nail bed, and entire nail plate. Frequently, there is a history of antecedent injury in the remote past, subungual hematoma, nail loss, and regrowth of the dystrophic nail. A typical chronic plantar and interdigital dermatophytosis are usually found associated with the nail involvement. The most common infecting organisms are *Trichophyton rubrum* and *T. mentagrophytes,* although *Candida albicans* often can be cultured from moist subungual debris. Differential diagnoses include psoriatic nails, lichen planus, or posttraumatic nail dystrophy.

Diagnosis can be confirmed by gathering nail and debris scrapings for dermatophyte culture or potassium hydroxide (KOH) examination. Placing the scrapings in a drop of KOH on a glass slide reveals the fungal hyphae coursing through the epidermal cells.

Definitive treatment for onychomycosis is frequently disappointing; therefore palliation with periodic debridement is most often the treatment of choice. Only early in the course of fungal infection under the nail is topical antifungal treatment effective. Miconazole, clotrimazole, and ketoconazole creams may help in this regard when applied twice daily to a debrided nail for a period of months until improvement is noted. Trials of oral ketoconazole or griseofulvin have met with limited success, recurrence occurring upon their discontinuance. Permanent surgical removal of the nail with a matrixectomy remains the only certain method of eradicating the mycotic nail in severe cases. This is not usually performed, however, unless the nail becomes symptomatic. Although untested by formal clinical trials, carbon dioxide laser vaporization of the nail bed has found some success in eradicating onychomycosis that only partially involves the nail plate. Once the nail is completely infected into the matrix, however, any nail that is permitted to regrow is similarly infected and amenable only to total permanent removal.

### Ingrown toenail

*Onychocryptosis* (ingrown toenail) is, of course, the most symptomatic of nail dystrophies and can range from a simple pinching of a distal skin fold to a severely infected paronychia with granuloma formation. This painful malady is frequently self-inflicted by the patient who has performed "bathroom surgery" on their nail borders. Unfortunately, self-treatment of this disorder commonly leads to an exacerbation of a relatively benign condition. Cryptotic nail borders may therefore be idiopathic, iatrogenic, or secondary to injured matrix tissue,

**Table 76-1.** Incidence and prevalence of foot problems in the United States, 1990

| Problem | People who reported having had this problem in the past 12 months: Number (in millions) | People who reported having had this problem in the past 12 months: Rate per 1000 population | People who reported having this condition now: Number (in millions) | People who reported having this condition now: Rate per 1000 population |
|---|---|---|---|---|
| Ingrown toenails or other toenail problems | 11.3 | 46 | 7.3 | 30 |
| Foot infection, including athlete's foot, other fungal infections, and warts | 11.3 | 46 | 6.2 | 25 |
| Corns and calluses | 11.2 | 45 | 9.2 | 38 |
| Foot injury (sprain, strain, fracture, or dislocation) | 5.6 | 23 | 1.8 | 7 |
| Flat feet or fallen arches | 4.6 | 19 | 4.4 | 18 |
| Bunions | 4.4 | 18 | 3.8 | 16 |
| Arthritis of toes | 3.9 | 16 | 3.5 | 14 |
| Toe and joint deformities (hammer toe, claw toe, missing toes) | 2.5 | 10 | 2.2 | 9 |
| Bone spurs | 0.95 | 4 | 0.67 | 3 |
| Nerve damage to foot | 0.23 | 0.9 | 0.17 | 0.7 |
| Clubfoot | 0.16 | 0.6 | 0.13 | 0.5 |
| Others | 2.7 | 11 | 2.2 | 9 |
| Total number of conditions reported | 58.8 | 239 | 41.6 | 170 |
| Unduplicated number of persons involved | 43.1 | 175 | 31.7 | 129 |

From Greenberg L, Davis H: *J Am Podiatr Med Assoc* 83:475, 1993.

**Table 76-2.** Number of people per 1000 who reported having specific foot problems in the past 12 months, by gender and race, 1990

| Problem | Total US | By gender: Men | By gender: Women | By race: White | By race: African-American |
|---|---|---|---|---|---|
| Toenail problems | 46 | 42 | 49 | 48 | 33 |
| Foot infections | 46 | 61 | 31 | 49 | 28 |
| Corns and calluses | 45 | 30 | 60 | 45 | 56 |
| Foot injuries | 23 | 23 | 22 | 24 | 15 |
| Flat feet | 19 | 19 | 18 | 18 | 25 |
| Bunions | 18 | 6 | 29 | 18 | 17 |
| Arthritis of toes | 16 | 10 | 22 | 17 | 13 |
| Toe and joint deformities | 10 | 6 | 14 | 11 | 5 |
| All foot problems combined | 175 | 163 | 186 | 182 | 144 |

From Greenberg L, Davis H: *J Am Podiatr Med Assoc* 83:475, 1993.

**Table 76-3.** Number of persons per 1000 who reported having specific foot problems in the past 12 months, by age, 1990

| Problem | Age (yr): Under 5 | 5-17 | 18-24 | 25-44 | 45-64 | 65-69 | 70-74 | 75 and over |
|---|---|---|---|---|---|---|---|---|
| Toenail problems | 5 | 20 | 39 | 44 | 59 | 78 | 94 | 123 |
| Foot infections | 5 | 44 | 45 | 52 | 52 | 55 | 46 | 41 |
| Corns and calluses | * | 5 | 23 | 48 | 72 | 90 | 105 | 125 |
| Foot injuries | 3 | 22 | 36 | 28 | 21 | 17 | 14 | 10 |
| Flat feet | 7 | 14 | 20 | 20 | 23 | 25 | 24 | 23 |
| Bunions | * | 2 | 8 | 14 | 29 | 44 | 47 | 66 |
| Arthritis of toes | * | 1 | 3 | 7 | 30 | 47 | 68 | 68 |
| Toe and joint deformities | 2 | 3 | 4 | 6 | 16 | 24 | 39 | 41 |
| All foot problems combined | 26 | 100 | 148 | 179 | 229 | 281 | 316 | 336 |

From Greenberg L, Davis H: *J Am Podiatr Med Assoc* 83:475, 1993.
*Statistically unreliable; fewer than ten observations in the sample.

hypertrophic nail folds, or a subungual exostosis. Tight shoes and injudicious nail care often lead to an inflamed nail fold from an offending nail border or spicule. Patients who dig out the corners of a painful nail often leave a deep portion of the nail intact. This portion acts like a lancet and grows forward into the distal nail groove. A paronychia then develops from the break in the skin, and a granuloma soon appears from the chronic irritation and inflammation (Fig. 76-1). Extremely incurvated or "tented" nails may be the result of the constant deforming pressure from a subungual exostosis on the dorsum of the distal phalanx. In this situation, both the nail disorder and the exostosis need attention.

The primary goal of treatment for any ingrown toenail is removal of the offending nail border from the inflamed skin fold (ungualabia). Antibiotic administration and soaks may be of some value in reducing inflammation and infection when present, but these measures alone do not usually resolve the problem. The severity of the condition usually dictates the treatment. A simple nail debridement of the distal corner of the nail most often is enough to eradicate a minor paronychia. Occasionally, packing the nail groove with cotton after trimming the nail back helps in this regard. In more advanced cases, especially those with granuloma formation, avulsion of the nail or nail border under local anesthesia is required. This allows the process to resolve before the nail's regrowth. For chronic recurrent onychocryptosis, permanent removal of the entire nail or just the offending nail borders with a matrixectomy is needed. A number of matrixectomy techniques can be employed, including phenol or sodium hydroxide chemical cauterization; surgical techniques such as Zadik, Winograd, or Frost procedures; or carbon dioxide laser vaporization. The reader is referred to the appropriate texts for the specific details and indications for these procedures. Since any paronychia can initially be well-treated with a simple total or partial nail avulsion, this useful procedure is described in detail.

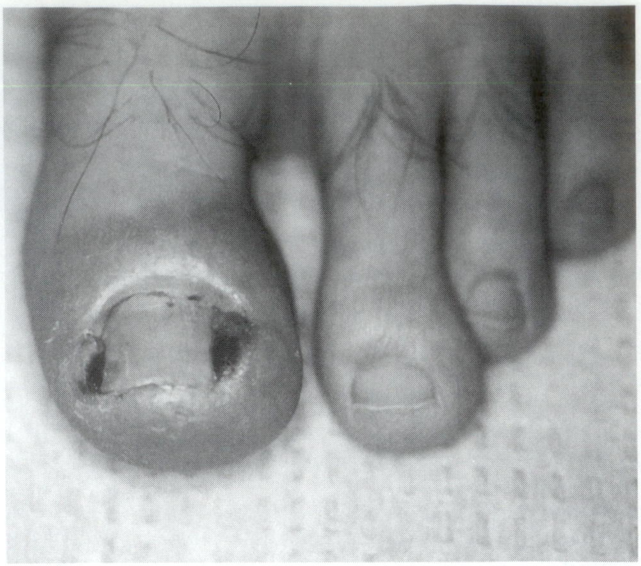

**Fig. 76-1.** Paronychia with granuloma formation.

### Partial and total nail avulsion

***Paronychia.*** For immediate relief and drainage of a paronychia of one or both borders a partial nail avulsion suffices. When the entire nail, both borders, or a deformed nail is involved a total nail avulsion can temporarily remove the entire nail plate, allowing resolution of the drainage. This is also an optimal procedure for traumatically loosened toenails or subungual hematomas that fail to respond to simple drainage procedures and soaks. After performing a digital block with local anesthesia (see anesthesia section) the nail folds should be freed from the nail border(s) and proximal eponychium with a Freer elevator or spatula-like instrument. The nail is then carefully freed from the nail bed using the same instrument or even a hemostat without gouging the nail bed. Starting centrally and distally, the nail is separated from the bed working side to side and back to the matrix area under the proximal eponychium (Fig. 76-2).

Once the nail is adequately loosened a straight hemostat should be used to grasp the entire plate back to its origin. A rolling motion from side to side frees any remaining lateral attachments, while the other hand holds the toe firmly. Finally, the nail is rolled from proximal to distal to remove the nail plate from its attachment to the matrix under the eponychium. If only a partial avulsion of a border is required, the nail should be split with an English anvil nail splitter or other appropriate straight edge nail splitter approximately 1/4″ from the inflamed nail fold. Only this portion of nail needs to be freed and removed using the same basic technique, while the remainder of the nail is left intact. An appropriate antiseptic (e.g., povidone-iodine, bacitracin) is then applied and then a dry, sterile dressing. Bathing is allowed within 24 hours whereupon the dressing should be changed twice daily until the wound heals. Usually these procedures allow a rapid, uneventful recovery with complete healing occurring within one week.

## COMMON SKIN DISORDERS

### Tinea pedis

*Tinea pedis* is a common foot problem not specific to any particular age group, race, sex, or disease status. Often, the patient with chronic dermatophytosis also has chronic onychomycosis, which may be the source of the chronic fungal infection. *T. mentagrophytes, T. rubrum,* and *Epidermophyton floccosum* are the most frequent pathogens; however, *Candida albicans* occasionally appears on fungal culture. The patient has an erythematous, pruritic, desquamating rash usually extending up the medial and lateral borders of the foot (moccasin distribution) and frequently has maceration and peeling between the toes. In the latter circumstance, there is the potential for secondary bacterial infection. Diagnosis is confirmed by KOH examination or culture of skin scrapings from active peripheral vesicular lesions when present. Dermatophytosis must be differentiated from a variety of other skin dermatoses such as contact dermatitis, atopic dermatitis, dyshidrotic eczema, lichen planus, and psoriasis. Interdigital lesions might otherwise be due to simple maceration, white psoriasis, verrucae, or erythrasma.

Treatment consists of drying the moist lesions and eradicating the infection by applying topical antifungal agents. Systemic therapy with griseofulvin or ketoconazole is rarely necessary. Effective topical medications include tolnaftate, miconazole, clotrimazole, econazole, ciclopirox, ketoconazole, and terbinafine when applied

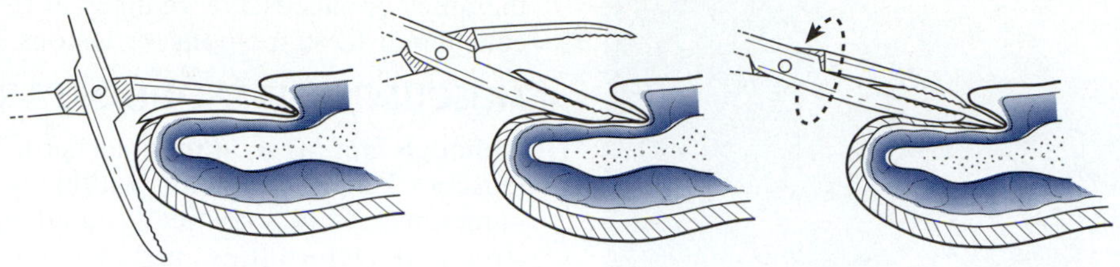

**Fig. 76-2.** Total nail avulsion technique. See text for details. (From McGlamry ED, editor: *Comprehensive textbook of foot surgery,* Baltimore, 1987, Williams & Wilkins, as redrawn from Moschella SL, Pillsbury DM, Hurley HJ: *Dermatology,* Philadelphia, 1975, WB Saunders.)

twice daily. For severely inflamed cases, a combination therapy of clotrimazole with betamethasone is available. Since "athlete's foot" is brought about through a warm, moist environment, efforts must also be directed at proper foot hygiene. The feet should be bathed daily, dried well between the toes, and powder applied routinely or after antifungal application when needed. Antifungal powders are helpful as prophylactic agents, but are not sufficient to treat active cases. When hyperhidrosis is a coexisting and contributing problem, absorbent socks should be worn and changed at least twice daily. Sneakers and other synthetic or rubber-soled shoes are also contributory in this regard and their use must be limited, especially during warmer months.

## Hyperkeratotic lesions

*Hyperkeratotic lesions* (corns or calluses) are the most prevalent of all foot lesions, attributable to their chronicity as well as frequency. Corns and calluses are pressure-induced and, when present, indicate areas of high or sustained pressure. Dorsal, medial, and lateral lesions are almost exclusively the result of shoe pressure. Contracted hammer toes abutting against the top of the shoe are typically the etiology of painful digital corns (clavi). Plantar keratoses can be focal in nature or diffuse callosities. The former are usually termed intractable plantar keratoses (IPK) and are extremely distressing for the patient when walking. As always, pressure is the etiology. A plantarflexed or long metatarsal is the most frequent underlying structural deformity giving rise to the hyperkeratosis. When palpated, the underlying bone is immediately evident, as is pain from the chronic inflammation. Upon debridement no skin lines are visible coursing through the center or core of the lesion. Sometimes this may represent a plugged sweat duct lesion, commonly referred to as a porokeratosis. The opaque core may be the corn so commonly discussed by patients, but is not always present in digital clavi, which are routinely called by the same name. Diffuse plantar calluses (tylomata) are usually biomechanical in nature and are typically not as painful as an IPK, although they may be quite large. This is due to their more superficial nature and lack of a discrete central site of pressure, although one might find an IPK in the center of a diffuse tyloma. Discolored lesions signify capillary hemorrhage with fluid collection under the keratosis and are usually more symptomatic or acute than normal-appearing callosities.

Simple debridement of a hyperkeratotic lesion provides immediate relief in most cases but does not eradicate the problem. This can only be accomplished by correcting the underlying source of the problem, e.g., a bony prominence, structural deformity, tight shoe, or biomechanical imbalance. In patients unwilling or unable to undergo corrective surgery, conservative measures such as shoe and orthotic therapy combined with regular palliative care provides painfree ambulation. Sneakers and cushioned walking shoes with generous toe room usually are advised for daily use. When necessary, cushioned insoles and prefabricated or custom-made orthoses can be beneficial in relieving pressure on the sole of the foot. Although not generally successful in eradicating painful plantar keratoses, such devices provide comfort and extended periods between necessary debridements. If conservative measures fail, consideration should be given to elective reconstructive surgery on the underlying structural deformity in the appropriate patient. Although beyond the scope of this text, such procedures are usually performed on an outpatient basis under local anesthesia. Further discussion of this topic can be found later in the chapter.

## Verrucae

*Verruca plantaris* occurs frequently, especially in children and adolescents who are not particularly prone to callus development. This skin lesion is different from other hyperkeratotic disorders because of its viral etiology (human papovavirus [HPV]). A verruca is distinguished from a callus by its typical pinpoint bleeding on debridement and well-defined borders. The patient often relates a history of a minor puncture wound at the site; this allowed entrance of the virus into the skin. These lesions enlarge in time and frequently develop small satellites near the primary wart. HPV is rather ubiquitous and causes a variety of skin lesions ranging from genital warts to plantar warts to planar warts on the dorsum of the hand. On the foot, HPV causes several types of warts with distinct morphologies probably because of different strains of the virus. The simple plantar verruca as described is the most common. However, this singular verruca can also occur on the dorsum of the foot, on the toes, adjacent to or under the toenails, or in the interdigital areas. The form demonstrating multiple, small disseminated warts across the entire sole of the foot is a difficult type to manage. The most challenging verruca, however, is the mosaic plantar verruca (Fig. 76-3). As its name indicates, this lesion has a mosaic pattern and can consist of hundreds of confluent individual verrucae. Such lesions, usually evolving from longstanding or ineffectively treated single warts, can grow to several centimeters in diameter.

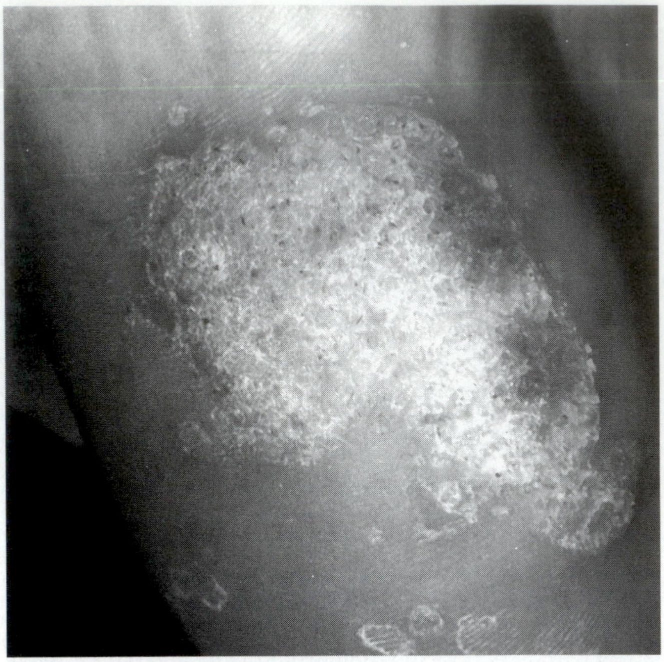

**Fig. 76-3.** Large mosaic verruca of the heel.

Treatments for verrucae are numerous because no one method is successful on all patients for all types of warts. Large clinical trials that contrast multiple therapies currently in use have not been performed. However, case reports and case series of various treatment regimens abound. Salicylic acids (40% or 60%) are perhaps the mainstay of treatment and are applied either once or twice a day in a paste form or as a plaster on an adhesive-backed dressing. Combinations of lactic and salicylic acids are also available as over-the-counter liquids or gels and are similarly applied by the patient each day. Such acid treatments can be effective, but might take many months before noticeable improvement occurs. Other topical therapies include acetic acids, cantharidin, injection of sclerosing agents, formalin, and retinoic acid preparations. Care must be taken with aggressive blistering agents, since they can result in violent skin reactions and attendant pain. Cryotherapy with liquid nitrogen or liquid carbon dioxide is frequently employed by dermatologists especially for singular lesions. Usually applied without the benefit of local anesthesia, this method is uncomfortable and also produces a painful blister. Repeated applications are frequently required as with most modalities. Surgical treatments include electrocautery, blunt dissection, curettage, excision, and carbon dioxide laser vaporization. Although perhaps most effective on smaller, untreated verrucae, such methods are most frequently used on those lesions recalcitrant to other more conservative therapies. I prefer laser vaporization of recurrent or large mosaic verrucae, but success rates only approach 80% for multiple recurrent lesions. Frequently, this treatment also must be repeated to eradicate any lesions that subsequently recur.

These common lesions are notoriously difficult to permanently eradicate; success can take months to years to achieve. Persistence is mandatory in their management as is patience. Early recurrence or recalcitrance to therapy is common; therefore long-term follow-up is required to assess adequacy of treatment. Recurrent lesions should be treated early to prevent entire regrowth. Combinations of therapies or successive changes in therapy should also be considered for unresponsive lesions.

## MUSCULOSKELETAL DISORDERS

Although not as common as skin and nail disorders, musculoskeletal problems within the foot and ankle are numerous and diagnostically challenging. In this regard, structural deformities are usually self-evident either clinically or radiographically. Soft tissue, joint, and functional abnormalities are, however, sometimes difficult to specify and correspondingly difficult to manage. Fortunately, establishing specific diagnoses of related disorders (e.g., tendinitis, bursitis, capsulitis) is not as important as general management, since treatment regimens for the related disorders are the same. When the etiology of a problem is overuse, regardless of the specific source of pain, rest and immobilization generally prove effective. However, diagnostic acumen is still essential in distinguishing between infectious, metabolic, and traumatic etiologies, since the management of each is entirely different. Acquaintance with the more common syndromes and pathologies of the foot enables the generalist to differentiate between them as well as to establish putative differential diagnoses. At the very least, this facilitates initial treatment and directs the course for appropriate referral and future treatment. For organizational purposes, foot disorders are categorized according to the regions of the foot in which they occur. Musculoskeletal disorders, as well as certain neurologic disorders specific to anatomic sites, can be best approached in this fashion. Fig. 76-4 illustrates the major anatomic structures of the foot and ankle pertinent to this discussion.

### Forefoot-digital and metatarsal disorders

Digital disorders become symptomatic primarily because of shoe pressure abutting on dorsal surfaces or squeezing the toes together. By far, the digital deformity causing most distress is the *hammer toe,* which can afflict children and adults alike. Although this term is generally used to denote any toe with a dorsal contracture, it should be distinguished from claw toes and mallet toes. A hammer toe has a dorsal (extensor) contraction at the metatarsal-phalangeal (MTP) joint and a flexion contracture at the proximal interphalangeal (PIP) joint (Fig. 76-5, *A*). The contractures can be the result of a variety of dynamic imbalances of tendinous structures around the joints secondary to hypermobility or neuropathy, as well as to traumatic or arthritic processes. A *claw toe* has a flexion contracture at the distal interphalangeal (DIP) joint (Fig. 76-5, *B*) in addition to the MTP and PIP contractures. A *mallet toe,* however, is characterized by a single flexion contracture at the DIP joint with weight being born on the tip of the toe (Fig. 76-5, *C*). Although the differences are subtle, the effect is such that abnormal pressure is born on dorsal digital surfaces from shoes and the distal toe surface directly. Since these sites are not protected by a fat pad, painful digital keratoses often develop. Contracted toes also can lie under or over adjacent digits causing very painful interdigital corns. Because these deformities progressively worsen over time, patients need to consider corrective surgery when conservative measures fail to provide long-term relief. A simple arthroplasty with resection of the proximal phalangeal head can permanently correct this condition with a generally rapid recovery.

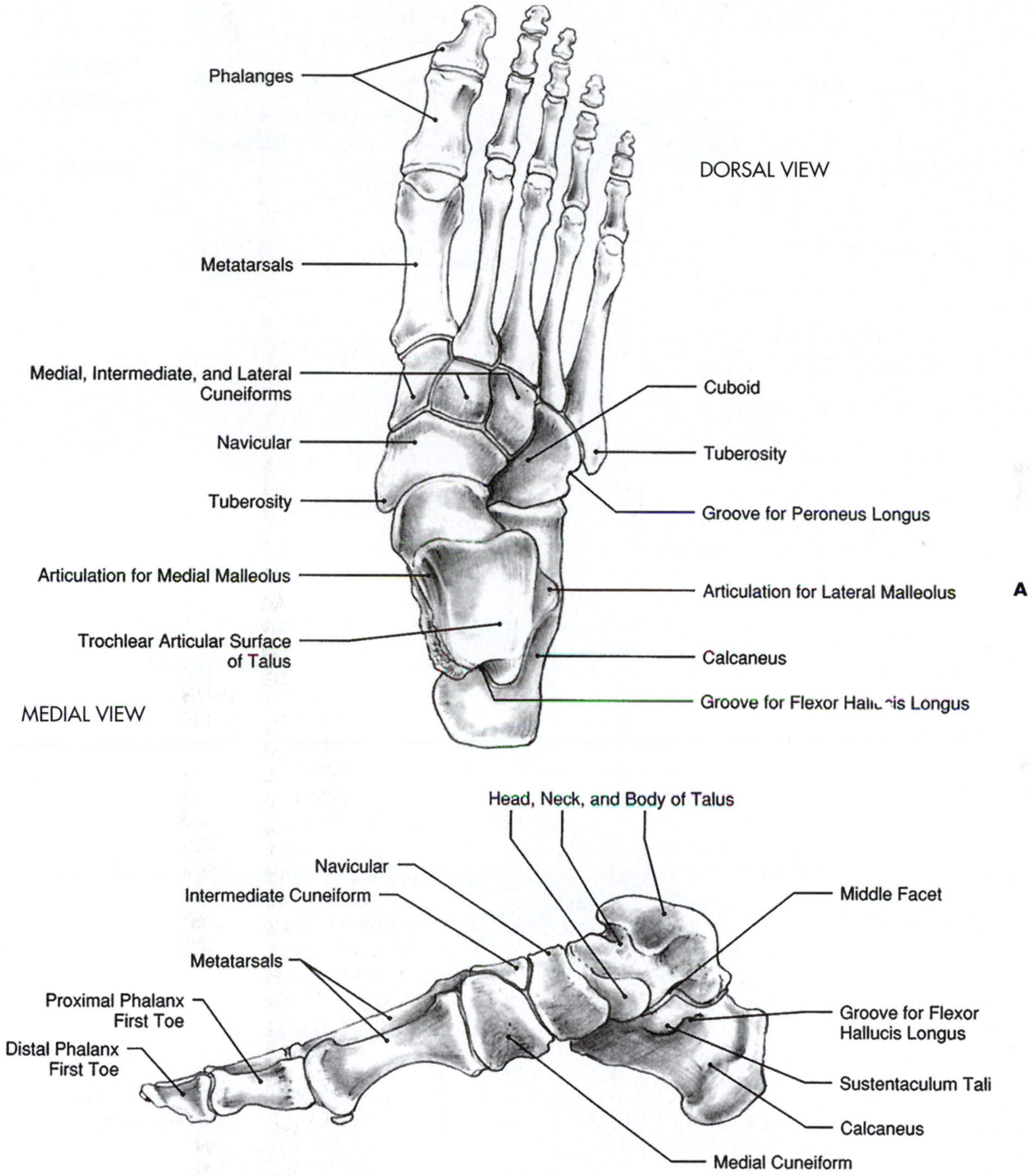


**Fig. 76-4.** Anatomy of the foot. **A,** Osseous structure of the foot.

*Continued.*

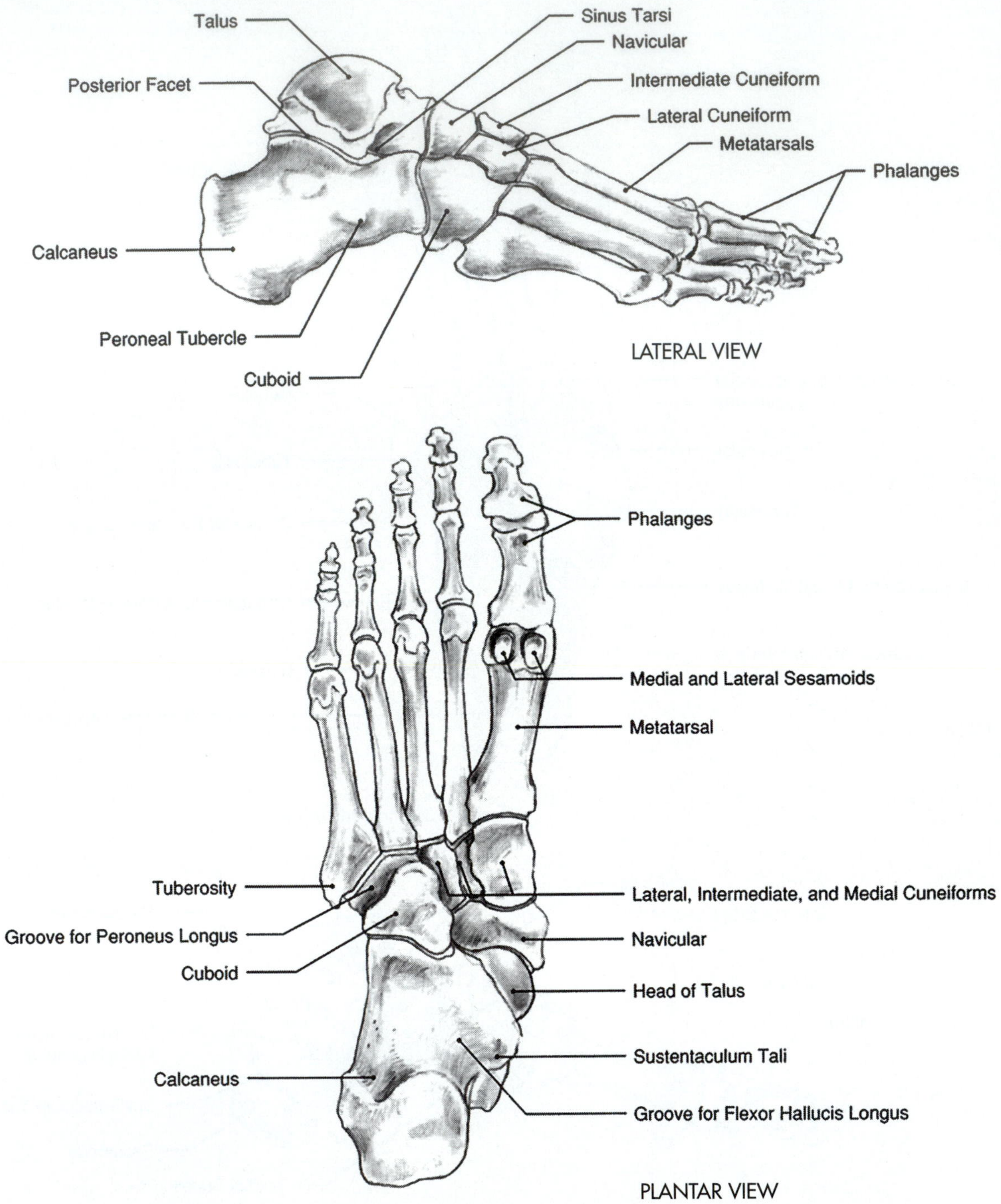
Talus
Posterior Facet
Calcaneus
Peroneal Tubercle
Cuboid
Sinus Tarsi
Navicular
Intermediate Cuneiform
Lateral Cuneiform
Metatarsals
Phalanges
LATERAL VIEW
Phalanges
Medial and Lateral Sesamoids
Metatarsal
Tuberosity
Groove for Peroneus Longus
Cuboid
Calcaneus
Lateral, Intermediate, and Medial Cuneiforms
Navicular
Head of Talus
Sustentaculum Tali
Groove for Flexor Hallucis Longus
PLANTAR VIEW

**Fig. 76-4, cont'd.** For legend see p. 1069.

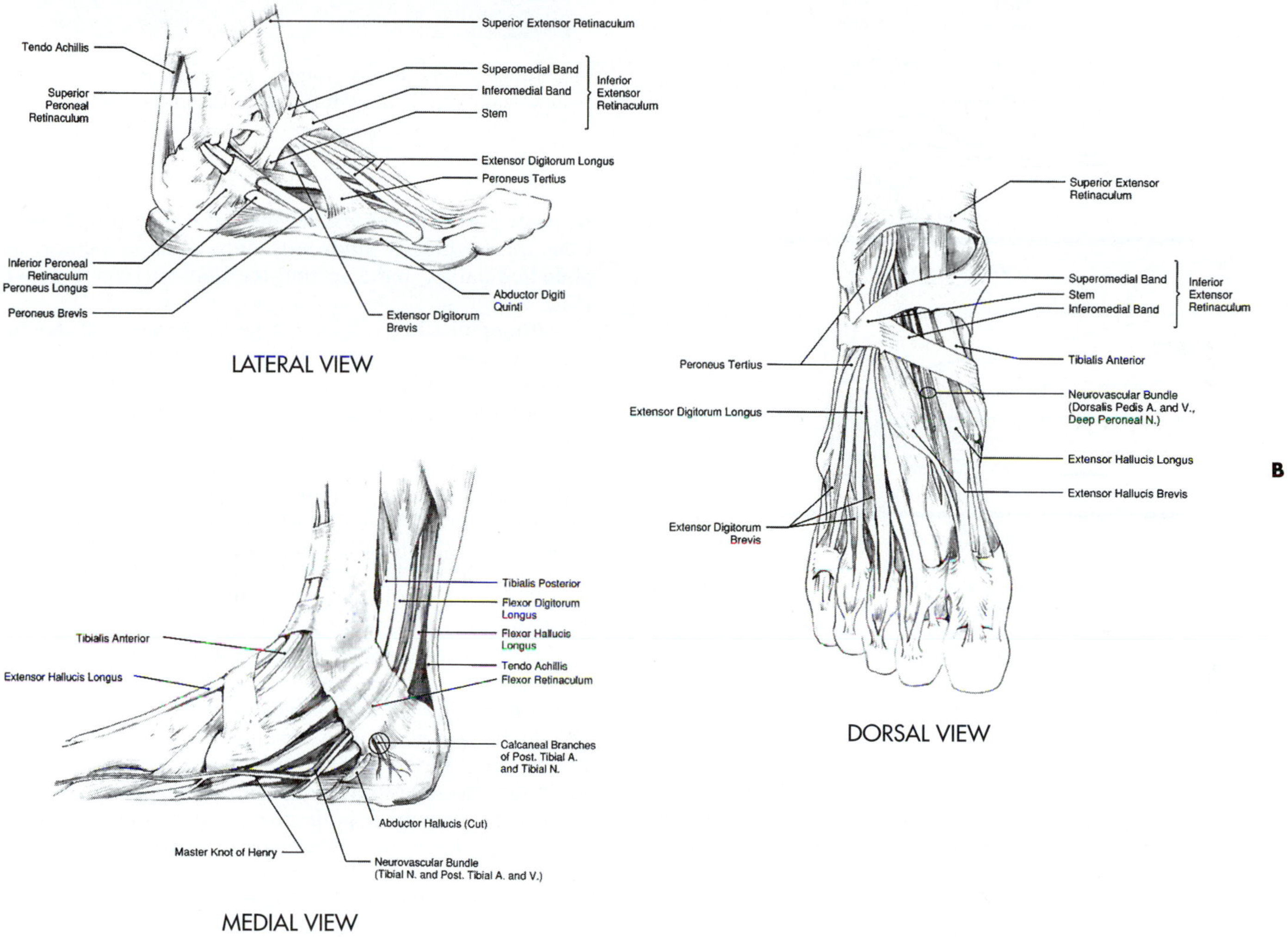


**Fig. 76-4, cont'd. B,** Musculotendinous anatomy. (From Reckling FW, Reckling JB, Mohn MP: *Orthopaedic anatomy and surgical approaches,* St. Louis, 1990, Mosby.)

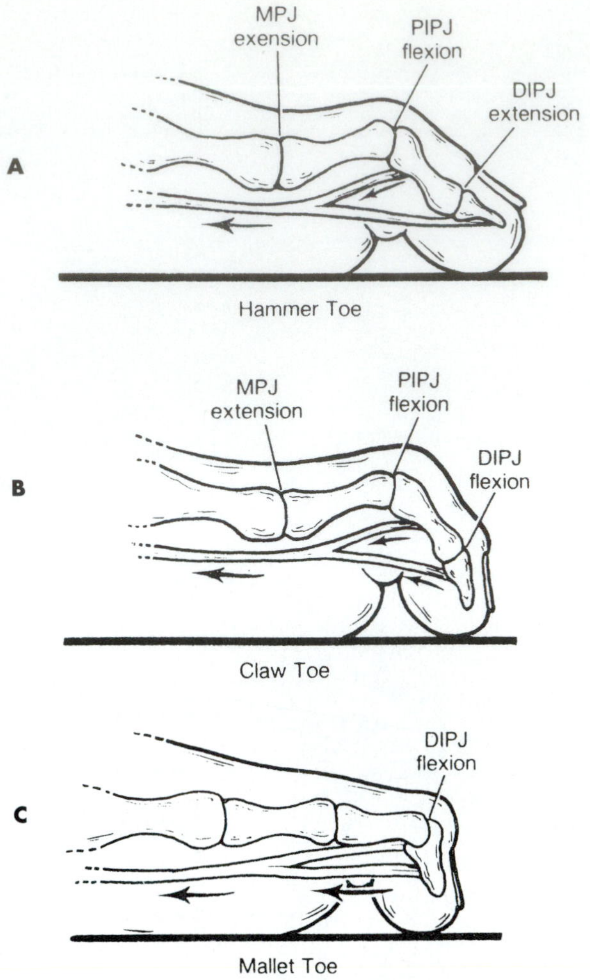


**Fig. 76-5.** Digital deformities. **A,** Hammer toe deformity with extension contracture of the metatarsal-phalangeal joint and flexion contracture of the proximal interphalangeal joint. **B,** Claw toe with additional flexion contraction of the distal interphalangeal joint. **C,** Mallet toe has a single flexion contraction at the distal interphalangeal joint. (From McGlamry ED, editor: *Comprehensive textbook of foot surgery,* Baltimore, 1987, Williams & Wilkins.)

***Hallux valgus and bunions.*** Metatarsal problems are often categorized into first metatarsal and lesser metatarsal disorders because of separate axes of motion as well as distinguishing pathologic entities. First ray deformities comprise the most significant of metatarsal complaints with bunion deformities affecting an estimated 3.8 million individuals annually. *Hallux valgus,* as bunions are more properly called, refers not only to the medial prominence of the first metatarsal head but to the lateral drifting (abduction) and valgus rotation of the great toe as well. The etiology of this condition, aside from its strong familial predisposition, is a hypermobility of the first metatarsal that allows it to progressively drift medially. Hypermobility routinely accompanies, but is not specific to, a pronated foot (flatfoot). Concurrent with the adduction of the metatarsal is a lateral contracture of the hallux caused by a compensatory bowstringing effect of the long and short flexor (with sesamoids) and extensor tendons inserting into the great toe. In severe cases the great toe crowds the second toe, eventually causing a hammer toe of this digit. As the deformity progresses in time, one typically finds not only a large bunion and abducted hallux, but a second toe that overlaps it as well (Fig. 76-6).

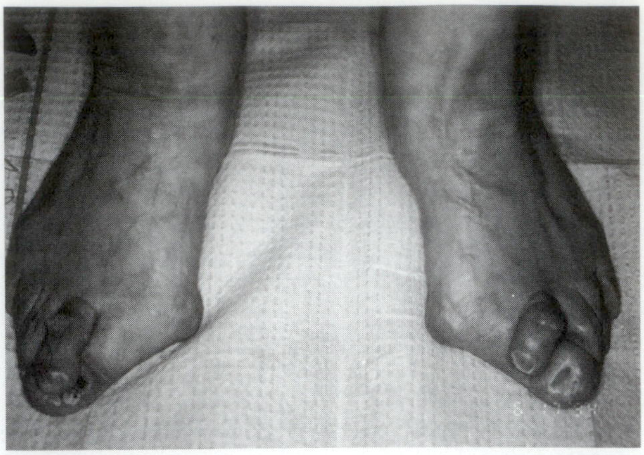

**Fig. 76-6.** Severe hallux valgus deformity with overlapping second hammer toe on both feet result from neglect.

Although hallux valgus can be the sequela of rheumatoid, psoriatic, or gouty arthritis, degenerative joint disease eventually appears after the development of this condition as the joint slowly becomes subluxed. Bunions do not only affect the elderly. Juvenile and adolescent hallux valgus are not rare and, when left unattended, progress to the severe deformities seen so commonly in geriatric patients. Since bunions are not always painful, patients and physicians tend to ignore them if a shoe can be fit over them. They worsen, however, and consideration should be given to correct the deformity before severe degeneration of the joint occurs.

Conservative treatment has not proven effective in arresting the progression of hallux valgus although orthotic therapy has been advocated. Of foremost concern should be footwear with adequate width and depth to prevent compression of the widened forefoot. When the deformity becomes symptomatic or progresses beyond a mild stage, surgery is indicated. A multitude of operative procedures have been described ranging from simple excision of the medial eminence to fusion or prosthetic implantation of the first MTP joint. The specific procedure performed should be based on the degree of deformity, presence of arthritis, age, and activity level of the patient. Surgery should provide pain relief as well as the restoration of normal alignment of the first metatarsal and great toe. Rarely is a simple bunionectomy (Silver, McBride techniques) advisable, since it does not correct the adduction of the first metatarsal. However, when combined with a resection of the proximal phalangeal base (Keller arthroplasty), an excellent correction can be obtained in geriatric patients. Furthermore, most bunionectomies are easily performed under local anesthesia without the need for casts, crutches, or inpatient hospital stays. With much of the morbidity previously associated with these procedures obviated by current techniques, there should be less reluctance to advise reconstruction of moderate or severe deformities.

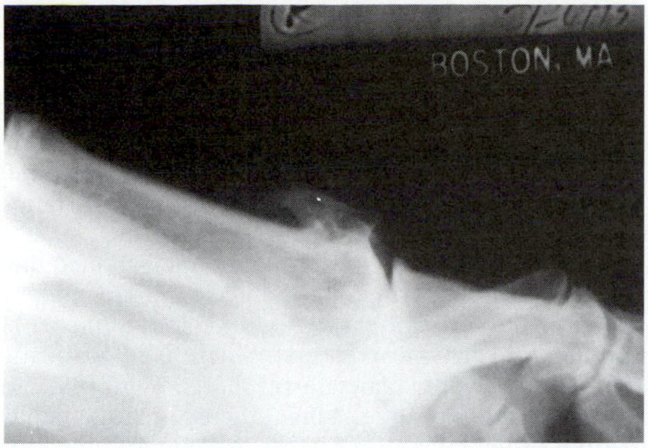


**Fig. 76-7.** Hallux rigidus with dorsal osteophyte and degenerative changes of the first MTP joint.

***Hallux rigidus.*** *Hallux rigidus,* sometimes referred to as hallux limitus, is a similar yet distinct affection of the first MTP joint. The former term implies a rigid great toe at the MTP joint, whereas the latter indicates only a limitation of motion. The bunion in these cases lies dorsal to the metatarsal head and represents dorsal osteophytic proliferation secondary to abnormal function and degenerative changes within the first MTP joint (Fig. 76-7). A previous injury to the great toe is not an uncommon inciting event. This disorder is frequently painful, especially on range of motion, and can significantly restrict normal activity. It can progress from a mild limitation of dorsiflexion to a severe degeneration of the joint with attendant loss of motion. Conservative care in early cases also consists of wearing nonconstricting, rigid-soled footwear with low heels and a trial of orthoses. As the condition progresses, however, surgery is required to provide relief. Relatively mild arthrosis of the joint can be treated with cheilectomy, a debridement of the joint osteophytes. When an elevated first metatarsal is a principal component of the hallux limitus, cheilectomy is often combined with a plantarflexory osteotomy to increase the range of dorsiflexion. If severe arthritic changes are present, Keller arthroplasty, total prosthetic implantation, or arthrodesis procedures should be considered.

***Sesamoiditis.*** *Sesamoiditis* of either the tibial or fibular sesamoid or both can be a painful malady that has an insidious onset and a chronic course if not diagnosed and treated early. The periosteal inflammation usually results from minor repetitive trauma such as aerobic exercises or extended walking in thin-soled dress shoes or high heels. The inflammation may also involve the long flexor tendon whereupon the pain also extends along the central plantar aspect of the great toe. When acute trauma has occurred, sesamoid fracture or stress fracture must be ruled out. The diagnosis of sesamoiditis is made by eliciting maximal tenderness to direct palpation of the sesamoid in question. There is usually no swelling, erythema, or ecchymosis present. Radiographs are negative, but bone scans may show signs of hyperemia and therefore may be falsely read as positive for fracture. Treatment is based on protecting the injured part to avoid exacerbation of the inflammation. Since each step is essentially further trauma to the sesamoids, weight bearing must be limited or modified. Although crutches are rarely necessary, accommodative padding with rest strapping (taping) of the foot frequently provides relief. Nonsteroidal antiinflammatory drugs (NSAIDs) should also be prescribed to expedite resolution of the inflammation. Shoes with cushioned soles and low heels are also required, as is avoiding activities that seem to aggravate the condition. Frequently, soft orthoses are fabricated, which can off-load the sesamoid area during gait. These should be worn on a long-term basis to prevent recurrence once the sesamoiditis has resolved. Recalcitrant sesamoiditis might even require sesamoid excision in the disabled patient.

***Metatarsalgia.*** *Metatarsalgia* is a nonspecific term that commonly refers to pain in the ball of the foot centered around the lesser metatarsal heads. The etiology of this problem can be due to bone, joint, musculotendinous, neurologic, vascular, or dermatologic pathology. The examination of the patient with such a presentation must therefore focus on specific sites, signs, symptoms, and history to differentiate between possible causes of discomfort in the lesser metatarsal region.

***Morton's neuroma.*** *Morton's neuroma* is a classic cause of metatarsalgia, which is usually centered in the third intermetatarsal and web space between the third and fourth toes. It is a benign enlargement of the third common digital branch of the medial plantar nerve as it passes plantar to the deep intermetatarsal ligament and between the metatarsal heads. Compression within this delineated compartment during walking in tight shoes is generally considered to be the etiology of this painful neuralgia. As might be expected, women are affected much more than men. Specific age ranges within the adult population do not appear to be a factor. Symptoms include burning, tingling, sharp, or shooting pains into the third or fourth toe, especially when wearing shoes or upon direct compression of the interspace. Temporary relief is classically provided by removing the shoe and rubbing the foot. Such symptoms are progressive, with an increase in intensity and frequency over the course of months to years. Diagnosis is a matter of excluding osseous or other pathology in the region and is corroborated by negative radiographic findings. At this time, MRI or electrophysiologic examinations are usually not necessary in establishing the diagnosis of Morton's neuroma. Initial treatment consists of a change to comfortable footwear and, occasionally, orthoses. Local corticosteroid injections and a course of NSAID therapy may provide additional relief in acute cases, but these measures are usually only temporizing. In time, most patients require excision of the neuroma when symptoms become too severe to enable normal daily activities. Surgery usually provides immediate relief with a fairly benign postoperative recovery.

***Plantar keratoses.*** Intractable plantar keratoses (IPK) are painful conditions of the forefoot. Underlying these lesions one can usually palpate the plantar surface of a prominent metatarsal head. Because of a plantar displacement, excessive length (or shortened adjacent metatarsal), abnormal plantar prominence, or altered biomechanics the metatarsal head bears more weight than its neighbors during stance and gait. This creates excessive plantar pressure and the IPK develops. As the label suggests, these lesions are intractable unless the underlying bony deformity is addressed. Such problems can be found even in the absence of a keratosis, but are usually more acute in nature. As in the case of sesamoiditis, repetitive moderate stress can result in a capsulitis, tendonitis, or osteitis on the plantar surface of the metatarsal head. On occasion, stress fracture or asceptic necrosis of a lesser metatarsal (Freiberg's infraction) needs to be considered and the diagnoses differentiated through appropriate radiographic techniques. When aberrant functioning of the metatarsal is the cause of this type of metatarsalgia, treatment should begin with custom orthoses to properly redistribute the weight-bearing forces under the foot. This therapy is advisable in concert with footwear modification for almost any type of metatarsal problem. External bars and similar shoe alterations are less frequently employed than orthoses because of patients' resistance to such corrections. In recalcitrant cases, however, a metatarsal osteotomy can often be performed to realign or reconstruct the offending metatarsal so that all the metatarsals lie on the same transverse plane. Care must be taken, however, to prevent excessive shortening or dorsal displacement of the metatarsal head, since such errors can lead to transfer lesions on adjacent metatarsals. Although a variety of techniques are currently practiced, osteotomies are usually performed on the metatarsal neck through a dorsal approach to facilitate postoperative ambulation.

***Stress fractures.*** *Stress fractures* of the lesser metatarsals are fairly common, especially in younger people engaging in activities such as running or aerobics. However, older patients are equally subject to these types of fatigue fractures from rather innocuous occurrences such as missing a step or taking long walks in uncushioned dress footwear. Presenting symptoms include a mild to moderate swelling of the forefoot perhaps with some erythema but a minimum of ecchymosis. Usually there is a localization of the pain to one or two metatarsal shafts. Typically, early radiographs are negative, since there is no complete fracturing of the bone. Bone scans are intensely positive, however, making this the diagnostic modality of choice when early stress fracture is suspected. Plain films become positive approximately 2 weeks after the injury has occurred, whereupon evidence of periosteal proliferation at the site of maximal tenderness appears. Clinically, one can palpate a painful bony prominence usually located on the dorsum of the affected metatarsal at this time. In some cases, the relatively minor stress fracture can propagate to a complete transverse fracture of the metatarsal, especially with delayed or inadequate treatment (Fig. 76-8). Therefore in suspected cases treatment should begin with a discontinuance of recreational activities or extended periods of walking. A standard postoperative shoe should

A B

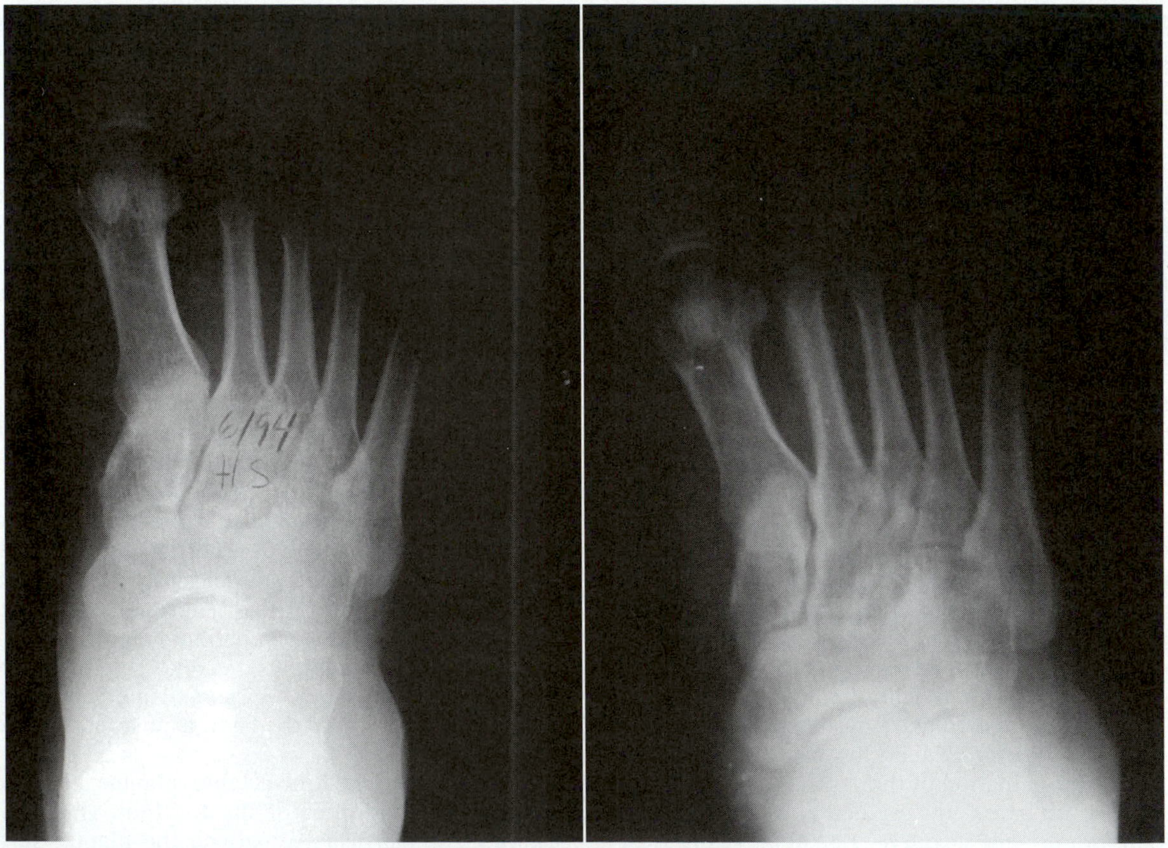

**Fig. 76-8.** Second metatarsal stress fracture. **A,** Initial radiograph does not show evidence of fracture. **B,** At 4 week follow-up x-ray reveals bone callus indicating healing of the fracture, which is now visible.

be prescribed for exclusive use until resolution of symptoms has occurred. Usually, an Unnas boot, rest strapping, or an elastic bandage is applied to provide further support and reduce swelling. Ice, rest, and elevation are also warranted. Crutches are not required in most instances and the patient can return to work if a limitation of walking is possible. Stress fractures respond quickly to these measures, with symptoms resolving within a few weeks. Strenous activities are generally avoided for 4 to 6 weeks and then only after proper conditioning and footwear have been prescribed.

***Bunionette.*** *Bunionette,* or "tailor's bunion," is a lateral prominence or enlargement of the fifth metatarsal head not restricted to any sex or age group. The pathology includes an actual enlargement of the head or a lateral bowing of the fifth metatarsal or both (Fig. 76-9). Painful bunionettes can also rise from chronic shoe irritation over a normal fifth metatarsal head causing only a soft tissue inflammation (adventious bursitis). Similarly, a painful keratosis can develop over the lateral side of the fifth metatarsal head indicating the role of footwear in the symptomatology of this disorder. Therefore treatment must initially be directed at providing relief from lateral shoe pressure; with acute inflammation corticosteroid or NSAID therapy may be of benefit. Orthotic therapy is generally not successful, however. For those patients with significant deformity or whose bunionettes are recalcitrant to conservative measures, a partial metatarsal head resection or adductory fifth metatarsal osteotomy corrects the structural deformity.

## Midfoot disorders

Disorders of the midfoot do not present as frequently as those of the forefoot, but can nonetheless cause considerable discomfort as well as contribute to deformities of the forefoot. In most instances, midfoot structural disorders are related to problems of the rearfoot or leg and represent biomechanical disturbances that can significantly affect normal gait and propulsion. This discussion focuses on the major congenital and acquired affections of the lesser tarsus and arch that comprise the midfoot, with an emphasis on the biomechanical consequences of such alterations of normal anatomy.

***Flatfoot.*** Pes plano valgus, or *flatfoot,* is the most significant of all midfoot disorders with a prevalence of over 4 million people and a rate of 18 per 1000 people in the 1990 NHIS. This chronic structural deformity infrequently has its origin in the midfoot in the absence of trauma, but instead results from more proximal disturbances of function. For example, a tight Achilles tendon (gastrocnemius equinus) causes restriction of ankle joint dorsiflexion. In gait, this is compensated for by an excessive pronation (including dorsiflexion) of the subtalar joint. The pronated subtalar joint allows an unlocking

A

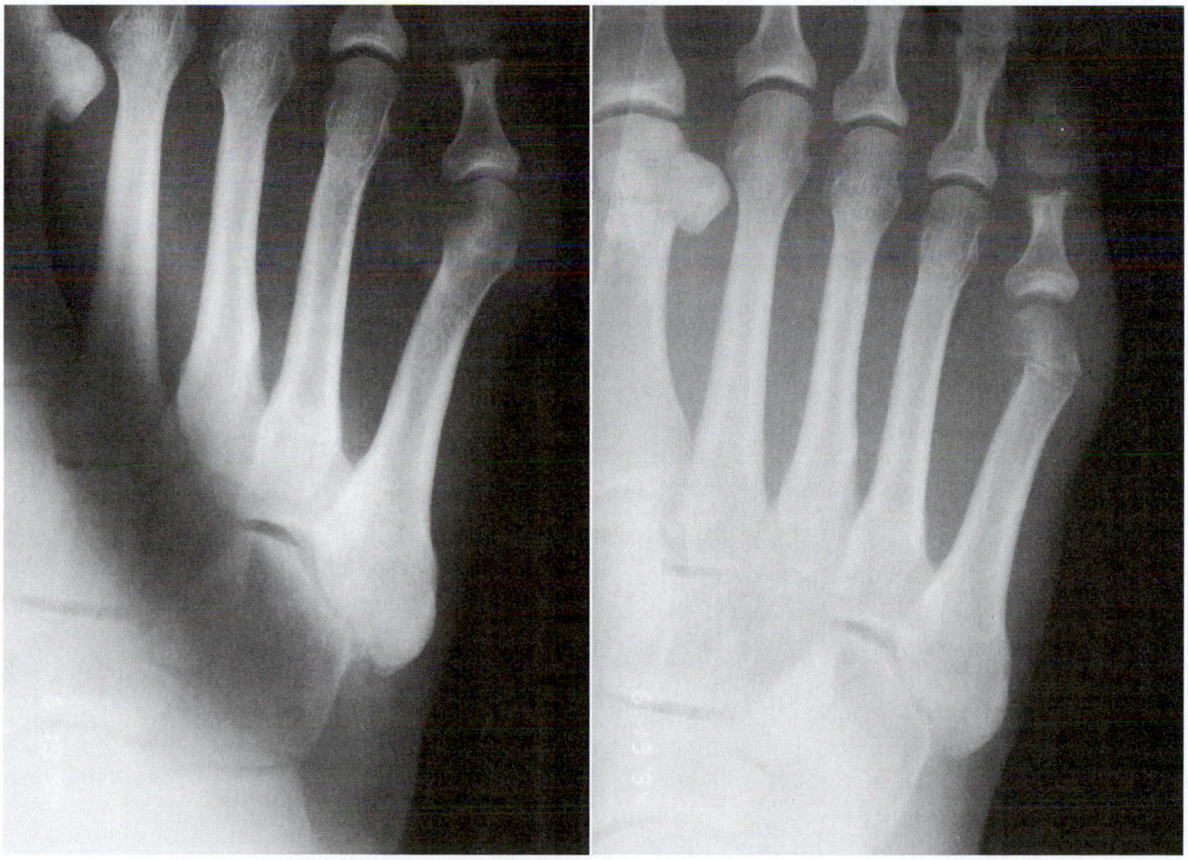

B

**Fig. 76-9.** Tailor's bunion. **A,** Preoperative view demonstrating fifth metatarsal head prominence and lateral bowing of the metatarsal. **B,** Postoperative view after performing a metatarsal head osteotomy.

of the midtarsal joint (talonavicular and calcaneo-cuboid joints), which also results in excessive pronation (flattening of the arch). This general instability is translated into a "hypermobility," which refers to the foot's excessive motion at times when it should be a stable, propulsive organ. The hypermobility contributes to weakness of the foot, fatigue, hallux valgus and hammertoe formation, and inefficient forward propulsion in gait. Aside from symptoms within the foot itself, excessive pronation is a frequent contributor to anterior shin splints or tendonitis, chondromalacia patellae, and chronic low back pain. These problems are particularly relevant to athletes or individuals frequently engaging in exercise programs, since the forces sustained by the weakened feet are exaggerated. Overuse injuries of the lower extremities are therefore more prevalent and more difficult to resolve in those patients with flat feet.

A flatfoot is not a simple deformity, but one that can have multiple etiologies and specific sites of involvement. It can be congenital or acquired, rigid or flexible, and primary or secondary. Pes plano valgus can be the result of a neuromuscular disease, stroke, trauma, arthritis, primary structural deformity, or from a peroneal spasm secondary to a fractured tarsal coalition. Therefore, each patient who has such a finding should be appropriately evaluated with these points in mind. In terms of pathomechanics, neuromuscular disease, peripheral neuropathies, stroke, or other acquired or congenital disorders resulting in weakness, contracture, or paralysis of leg musculature affecting the normal mechanics of the foot can produce a flatfoot deformity. Generally, spasticity of the gastrocnemius-soleus complex results in a flatfoot, whereas flaccidity results in a high-arched foot. Weakness of the posterior tibial muscle also leads to a flatfoot, whereas spasticity of the long flexors can lead to a high arch. Neuromuscular disorders can be complex and must be evaluated on an individual basis to determine muscle groups affected and the qualitative impact of the affection on foot mechanics. Congenital flatfoot also can result from developmental aberrations such as clubfoot (talipes equinovalgus), congenital convex pes valgus, talipes calcaneovalgus, forefoot varus, torsional disturbances of the lower extremities, or ligamentous laxity. These deformities must be properly evaluated for rigidity or flexibility, since nonreducible rigid deformities portend a poor prognosis and require surgical intervention. Minor structural or functional deviations from the norm, such as forefoot varus, accessory navicular with altered insertion of the posterior tibial tendon, flexible calcaneovalgus, or tightened heel cords, are generally considered as nonpathologic or idiopathic causes of flexible pes plano valgus. Acquired flatfoot is usually the result of an acquired neurologic disorder or of trauma to the foot or leg. The most common cause of acquired adult flatfoot is a rupture of the posterior tibial tendon frequently seen in elderly rheumatic patients. This is marked by a unilateral deformity in a patient with a history of injury or prodromal symptoms of chronic posterior tibial tendonitis. (Fig. 76-10).

Treatment of symptomatic hypermobile pes planus should always begin with orthotic therapy, presuming, of course, that potential pathologic causes of flatfoot as previously discussed have been appropriately addressed.

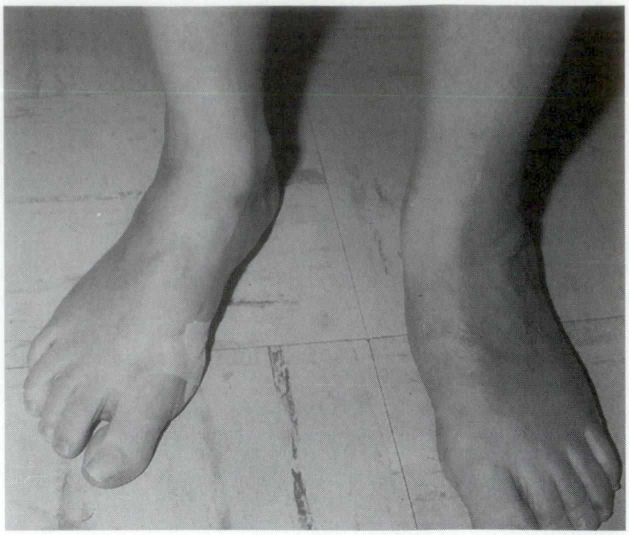

**Fig. 76-10.** Unilateral acquired adult flatfoot caused by posterior tibial tendon rupture of left foot.

In children with nonpathologic deformities, orthotic treatment should be initiated by age 5 even without symptoms. Although not documented by prospective clinical trials, it is rather intuitive that early support of the flat foot in the child can promote better structural development and, at least, fewer symptoms within the feet and legs. It cannot be presumed, however, that orthoses *correct* the structural deformity in either the child or the adult. The purpose of orthoses is generally to relieve symptoms by providing structural support under the weakened foot, by limiting the amount of abnormal pronation, and by allowing more efficient locomotion.

A great variety of foot orthoses exist in the marketplace today. Some are prefabricated devices and others are custom-made by professional laboratories or health professionals. Generally speaking, treatment for pes plano valgus is aimed at functional improvement of the pronated foot, and as such, custom-fabricated "functional" orthoses should be used. Custom orthoses are usually categorized as flexible, semirigid, or rigid designs depending upon the materials used. The specific orthosis used depends in part on the patient's age, weight, and activity level as well as on severity of the deformity and symptoms. Flexible orthoses, often fabricated from softer materials such as plastazote or microcellular rubbers, can provide gentle support and cushioning. They are useful for sports medicine applications and for geriatric or diabetic patients. Semirigid orthoses are traditionally fabricated from leather composites, although newer synthetic materials that are less bulky and more durable can be used. These are a good compromise between flexible and rigid designs and can provide good support with a certain degree of flexibility. Many sports orthoses fabricated in commercial labs come under this category. Rigid orthoses are the "gold standard" of orthotic devices and provide the greatest control over foot function and abnormal pronation (or supination). Although previously made from stainless steel, rigid orthoses are currently fabricated from very durable materials such as polypropylenes and thermoplastics. Often guaranteed

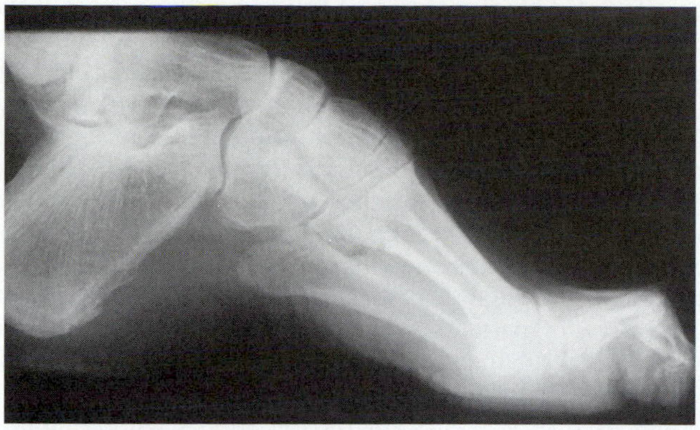

**Fig. 76-11.** Radiograph of pes cavus deformity with anterior metatarsal equinus and clawtoes.

against fatigue and breakage, these low-profile, "high-tech" devices are increasingly computer-generated from digital scanning of plaster cast impressions of the feet. The recent advances in fabrication technology have also resulted in thinner, easier-to-fit designs that are remarkably comfortable as well as more exacting in their correction of abnormal function.

Since orthoses control function and ameliorate symptoms in flatfeet quite well, only the most severe deformities usually require reconstruction. These are the more pathologic entities such as congenital vertical talus, tarsal coalitions, and those resulting from neurologic disorders. Excessive ankle equinus secondary to triceps surae contractures often requires tendo Achillis lengthening in concert with any localized foot procedure. One of the more common flatfoot procedures performed, a Kidner procedure, removes the accessory navicular and tightens the pull of the posterior tibial tendon. Variations of this procedure are also performed in cases of partial or complete rupture of the posterior tibial tendon.

***High-arched foot.*** *Pes cavus,* or a high-arched foot, is not as common as pes planus and more difficult to treat. Classically seen with neurologic disorders such as polio or peroneal muscular atrophy, this foot deformity is generally characterized by a lack of flexibility, an anterior equinus of the forefoot, and clawtoes. Although underlying neurologic disturbances should always be considered in evaluating such patients, idiopathic or nonpathologic pes cavus of a minor degree is certainly the most frequent presentation (Fig. 76-11). Cavus feet are marked by excessive *supination* of the rearfoot and forefoot whereby the plantarflexed first ray (medial column) causes abnormal inversion (supination) of the forefoot to bring the fourth and fifth rays (lateral column) to the ground in stance and gait. Because of the forefoot equinus and attendant exaggeration of metatarsal declination, the toes are usually clawed as a result of a loss of the normal stabilizing mechanism of the intrinsic muscles around the MTP and interphalangeal joints. Hyperactivity of the peroneus longus, posterior tibial, and long flexors, or weakness of the triceps surae, peroneus brevis, anterior crural muscles, and intrinsic foot muscles can all contribute to this foot deformity in varying degrees. Multiple imbalances between agonist and antagonist muscle groups often coexist, especially in patients with documented neuromuscular diseases. Therefore detailed neuromuscular, biomechanical, and gait evaluations are required to properly assess both the etiology of the foot deformity as well as specific pathomechanical attributes.

In the absence of trauma or recent neurologic disease, most patients adapt to their longstanding cavus foot deformities quite well except for repeated ankle sprains, persistent plantar calluses, or painful dorsal digital corns. Periodic debridement and cushioned insoles in shoes with adequate depth for the toes are usually adequate initial measures for relief of hyperkeratotic lesions. However, patients complaining of lateral or postural instability or painful metatarsalgia are best treated with custom functional orthoses to limit supinatory motion during gait. In severe cases that are recalcitrant to these measures, surgery can be performed to realign the forefoot, stabilize lateral ankles, or correct digital deformities.

### Rearfoot disorders

***Heel spur and plantar fascitis.*** *Heel spur* syndrome and its soft tissue analogue, *plantar fascitis,* are certainly the most common disorders of the hindfoot and two of the more frequently presenting complaints to the foot specialist. The painful heel can be attributed to rheumatic diseases such as rheumatoid arthritis, gout, Reiter's disease, ankylosing spondylitis, or other seronegative spondyloarthropathies. These entities are fully discussed elsewhere in this text and are distinguished more by erosive changes to the heel than spur formation. Heel spurs and plantar fascitis, however, are generally considered pathomechanical in nature. With each step the plantar fascia is drawn taut as it resists the collapse of the arch, a function analogous to a windlass mechanism (the stretching of plantar fascia during weight bearing). Concurrently, there is a rather constant traction on the periosteal insertion point on the calcaneus. In the course of time or with overuse, this constant traction results in a spur formation at the anterior inferior aspect of the calcaneus. This enthesopathy is actually an insidious process in many cases, since patients often have rather large asymptomatic calcaneal spurs as incidental findings on radiographs. Conversely, patients with acutely painful heels in the absence of trauma can have negative radiographs. These patients would then be considered to have a heel "bursitis" or localized plantar fascitis at the insertion of the aponeurosis. Typical plantar fascitis as seen in overuse injuries to athletes usually extends more distal along the medial band of the fascia.

Excessive pronation is the underlying etiology of this condition in most instances, except when a cavus foot type is subjected to repetitive heel trauma. Radiographs should routinely be taken to confirm the presence of a spur or to rule out other causes of heel pain when plantar fascitis is suspected. Differential diagnoses that must be considered in patients complaining of heel pain include stress fracture or bone contusion, subtalar joint pathology, tumor, rheumatic disease, nerve entrapment, plantar fascial tear, Achilles tendonitis, calcaneal apophysitis, or Sever's disease (calcaneal avascular necrosis). Treatment for heel spur syndrome (including those with plantar fascitis only) initially requires attenuation of activities, NSAID, and a rest strapping of the foot to limit pronation. Heel cups can be of some use as well as simple heel cushions or cutouts. Corticosteroid injection is reserved only for recalcitrant cases and is limited to three injections from a *medial* approach. Athletic or cushioned walking shoes with a small heel elevation are also beneficial. When improvement is noted from these measures a soft orthosis is usually fabricated that can provide support as well as cushioning for the heel. This should be used on a long-term basis to improve foot function and prevent relapse. Once comfortable, patients can gradually discontinue NSAID therapy while continuing with orthotic therapy. Physical therapy modalities such as ultrasound are prescribed when these prior measures fail to provide relief. Below knee casting or immobilization in ambulatory cast braces with or without crutches must also be considered in severe cases. Inferior calcaneal heel pain usually resolves in a median time of approximately 6 months. Some patients may not improve for a year or longer despite exhaustive efforts. In such patients, heel spur surgery or plantar fasciotomy might be considered. Medial calcaneal nerve entrapment should also be evaluated at this stage and released as necessary. Since the great majority of patients eventually recover from conservative therapy alone, surgery should be the exception to the rule rather than an initial treatment.

***Posterior tibial tendinitis.*** *Posterior tibial tendinitis* is a painful condition of the rearfoot often mimicking a medial ankle sprain or medial arch pain. It most frequently affects individuals past middle age who are moderately active and may have a history of other rheumatic complaints. It is also a common overuse injury in younger individuals or in people with significant degrees of foot pronation. Since the posterior tibial muscle is the major antagonist to the peroneus brevis, it is the major supinator of the foot and primarily functions to resist pronation of the subtalar and midtarsal joints during gait. In the pronated foot, normal anatomic relationships and vectors of force are altered, resulting in inefficiency of this muscle. This inefficiency has the functional consequence of an overuse compensation wherein the muscle functions beyond its usual phasic activity leading to both fatigue and chronic tendinitis. Chronic posterior tibial tendinitis can then lead to partial tearing, internal degeneration, or complete rupture. As previously mentioned, the latter event is a classic cause of adult acquired flatfoot deformity.

Symptoms include pain and mild swelling just below the medial malleolus as the tendon courses below this structure to insert on the navicular and plantar midfoot. Pain is exacerbated by inversion and plantarflexion of the foot, especially when standing on the ball of the foot and toes. With complete rupture, the pain is usually gone but in addition to the unilateral flatfoot, toe stance demonstrates a lack of heel and arch inversion. In stance, the forefoot is markedly abducted and when viewed from behind, the "too many toes" sign is evident. The pain from the chronic tendonitis is usually related to activity, but is persistent from day to day and progressive to the point of becoming almost disabling in its most severe forms. Treatment is based on preventing pronation of the foot, rest, and reducing inflammation of the tendon and tendon sheath. Although rest strapping or resistive ankle taping are often effective, cast or cast bracing with or without the use of crutches might be necessary to provide relief. A prolonged course of NSAID therapy is also necessary and frequently is used in conjunction with physical therapy. Corticosteroid injections are infrequently advisable because of the possibility of subsequent tendon atrophy and rupture. Custom orthotic therapy is always required to support the foot and reduce tension on the posterior tibial tendon. Rigid orthoses are preferable in this regard, but semiflexible or flexible orthoses should be fabricated as an alternative in patients who are unable to tolerate rigid support. Debridement of the degenerated tendon or repair and augumentation of the ruptured posterior tibial tendon should be reserved only for those patients who complain of chronic severe pain or instability. Surgery of this nature on elderly patients requires a prolonged period of immobilization and non–weight bearing, making such procedures inadvisable except for the most severe circumstances.

## Ankle disorders

***Sprains.*** Ankle sprains are common in clinical practice and are the major ankle problem most practitioners treat. *Lateral ankle sprains* of the lateral collateral ligaments are the usual presentation, since medial sprains of the deltoid ligament are frequently accompanied by lateral ankle fractures. The latter two injuries are not discussed, since they usually are attended to in an acute care facility.

There are three separate collateral ligaments of the anterior lateral talocrural joint that are subject to tear or partial tear upon inversion injury (Fig. 76-12). The most anterior and most frequently torn of the three is the anterior talofibular ligament (ATFL). This intracapsular fan-shaped ligament extends from the anterior inferior end of the fibular malleolus and inserts into the lateral surface of the body of the talus. Primarily resisting ankle inversion during plantarflexion, it is usually the first to be ruptured during inversion injuries, since the ankle is least stable when plantarflexed. The calcaneofibular ligament (CFL) is an extracapsular cordlike ligament running from the inferior tip of the fibula to the lateral surface of the calcaneus under the peroneal tendon sheath. It primarily resists inversion during ankle dorsiflexion and usually ruptures only second to the ATFL in severe inversion injuries. The intracapsular posterior talofibular ligament (PTFL), the strongest of the three, runs posteriorly from the fibular malleolus to the posterior lateral surface of the talus. This is infrequently ruptured except in cases of severe trauma with associated osseous injury to the ankle.

Diagnosis of a lateral ankle sprain is rather obvious by history and signs of acute edema, ecchymosis, and pain at the anterior lateral aspect of the ankle. X-rays should always be taken to rule out associated lateral ankle or talar fracture. One must also palpate the base of the fifth metatarsal in such injuries, since ankle sprains can often be accompanied by fracture of the styloid process or proximal fifth metatarsal shaft (Jones fracture). When present, such fractures require a prolonged period of cast immobilization. Crutches should be used in acute cases when symptoms and examination warrant non–weight bearing. Immobilization can be in the form of a simple elastic bandage or tape strapping in minor sprains or, for more severe injuries, below-knee casting, ambulatory-cast

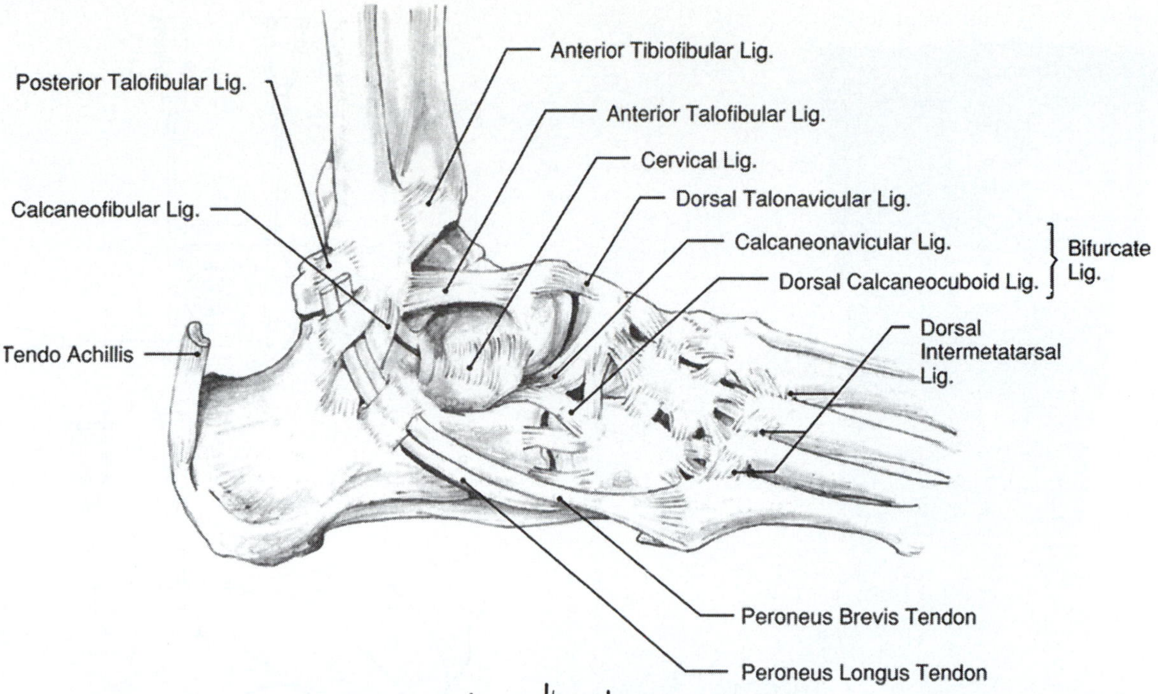


A

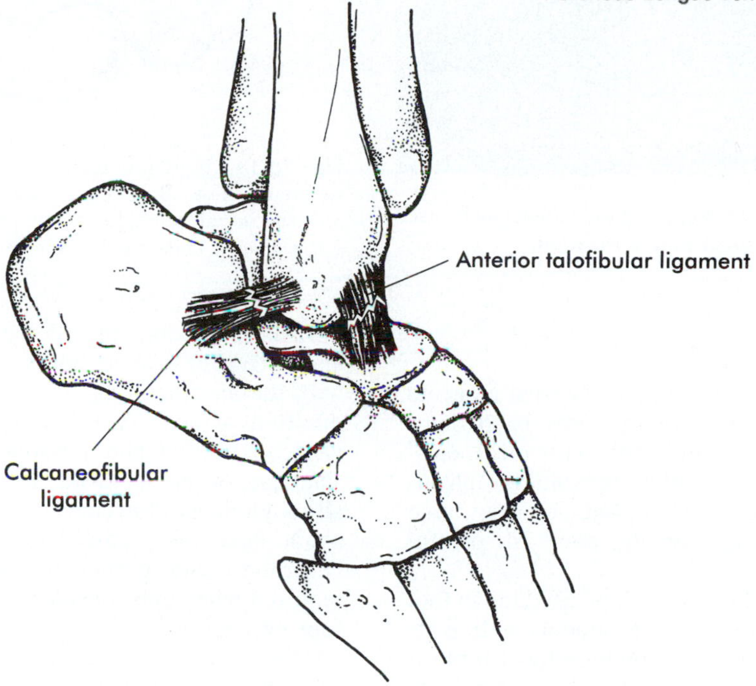


B

**Fig. 76-12.** Lateral ankle sprain. **A,** Ligamentous structures of the lateral foot and ankle. **B,** Inversion sprain demonstrating rupture of the anterior talofibular and calcaneofibular ligaments. (**A** from Reckling FW, Reckling JB, Mohn MP: *Orthopaedic anatomy and surgical approaches,* St. Louis, 1990, Mosby; **B** from Baxter DE: *The foot and ankle in sport,* St. Louis, 1995, Mosby.)

bracing, or ankle stirrup braces (Fig. 76-13). For chronic ankle instability resulting from repeated sprains, an ankle stirrup or taping is advisable when patients engage in athletic activities. Severe instability, especially in competitive athletes, can be corrected with a variety of lateral ankle-stabilization procedures. Such operations attempt to restore ligamentous integrity with direct repair or by augmentation with tendon transfer. In patients with chronic ankle pain and a history of previous sprain in the absence of severe instability, there is the possibility of a talar dome osteochondral lesion (osteochondritis dissecans). This usually can be detected only by CT scan or MRI and rarely heals without intervention. Arthroscopic procedures have been developed to effectively remove or repair these osteochondral fragments as an alternative to open ankle arthrotomy procedures.

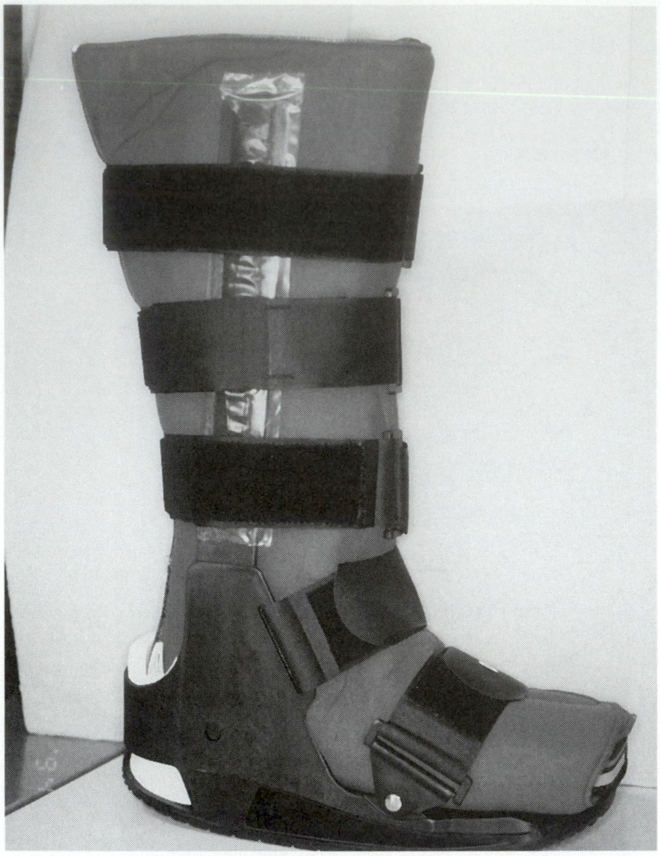

**Fig. 76-13.** Prefabricated removable cast brace that can be used for severe sprains or postsurgical immobilization.

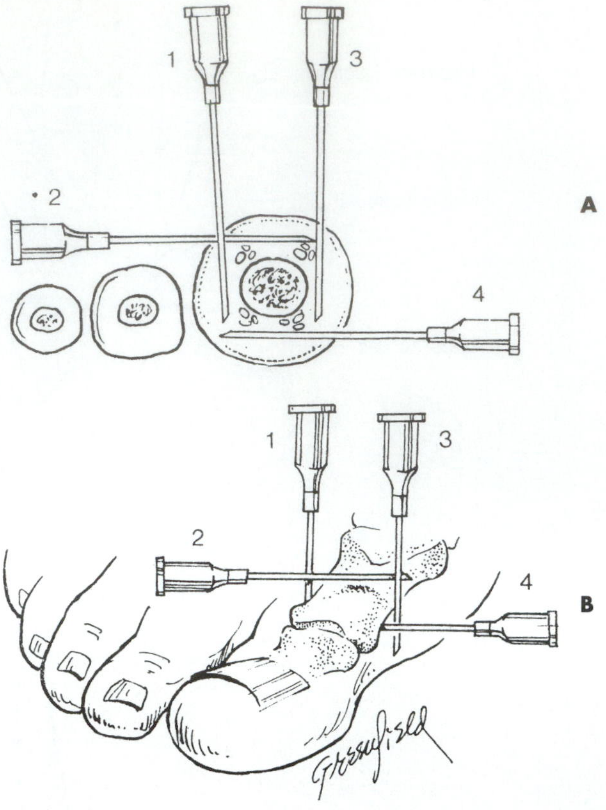


**Fig. 76-14.** Injection technique for the great toe. **A,** Cross-sectional view. **B,** Dorsal view. (From Frykberg RG: Podiatric problems in diabetes. In Kozak GP et al, editors: *Management of diabetic foot problems,* Philadelphia, 1984, WB Saunders.)

## LOCAL ANESTHESIA

The primary care physician may frequently treat an acute paronychia or toenail injury, foreign body, or perhaps fulgurate a plantar verruca. Familiarity with local anesthetic injection techniques not only augments the physician's ability to handle such maladies, but also is a source of comfort to their patients in the face of painful procedures otherwise.

A variety of injection techniques can be used in the foot depending upon the condition being treated as well as its specific location. These techniques include local infiltration, digital block, specific nerve block, or regional anesthesia (ankle block). The basic underlying premise is that the afferent sensory nerves must be blocked *proximal* to the site of the lesion being treated. For example, when dealing with a paronychia it is *always* advisable to perform a digital block at the base of the toe and *never* to inject at the distal pulp of the toe or adjacent to the nail border. Distal toe injections are too painful because of the tautness of the subcutaneous tissues. Conversely, when removing a simple plantar wart it is often easier to infiltrate under and around the lesion than to perform a nerve block. Always keeping the patient's comfort in mind, the excision of multiple plantar lesions is best approached with a posterior tibial nerve block at the medial ankle rather than repeated injections on the sole of the foot.

Lidocaine, 0.5% or 1%, is the most frequently used of the local agents because of its rapid onset. Bupivacaine 0.5% is usually mixed with the lidocaine to provide lasting anesthesia for 8 to 12 hours. Epinephrine in combination with the anesthetic agent can not only provide increased duration of activity through a delay of absorption, but vasoconstriction and intraoperative hemostasis as well. The use of epinephrine in digits is still controversial although many thousands of digital blocks employing this agent have been performed without adverse sequelae. Discretion and proper patient selection are, however, required when one considers the use of epinephrine in any foot procedure.

Digital blocks are easy to perform and can be used in any situation requiring anesthesia of any part of a toe. In fact, most digital operations should be done under local anesthesia unless there is a specific situation requiring general or spinal anesthesia. Usually, all four digital nerves must be infiltrated to produce an adequate block of the entire toe. Either a ring block technique (Fig. 76-14) or an inverted "V" block (Fig. 76-15) can be employed using a 25 gauge 1½-inch needle on a 3-ml syringe. A total of 3 ml for the great toe and 2 ml for the lesser toes usually provides complete digital anesthesia after waiting approximately 5 minutes. When the metatarsal head or MTP joint must be anesthetized, a more proximal "V" block around the metatarsal neck should be used. Bunionectomy procedures usually require a digital block in combination with a circumferential segmental block of the first metatarsal proximal to the metatarsal neck.

Ankle blocks are extremely useful in providing anes-

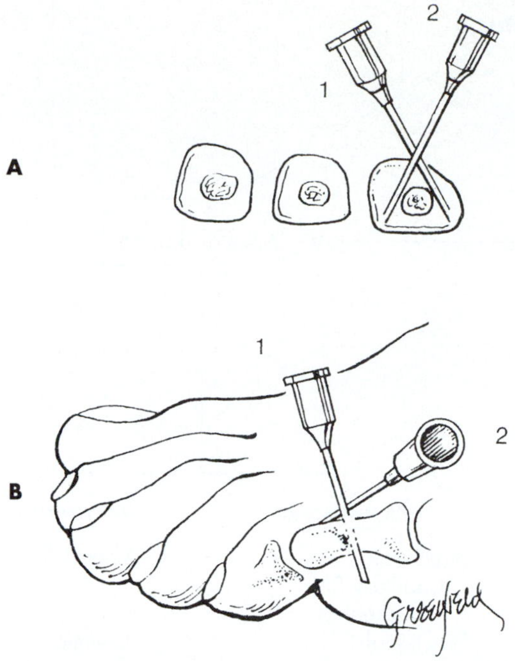


**Fig. 76-15.** Inverted "V" block for lesser toes. **A,** Cross-sectional view. **B,** Dorsal view. (From Frykberg RG: Podiatric problems in diabetes. In Kozak GP et al, editors: *Management of diabetic foot problems,* Philadelphia, 1984, WB Saunders.)

thesia to the entire foot when multiple sites must be approached. The primary care physician rarely needs to perform this technique, but knowledge of the anatomic location and distributions of the nerves crossing the ankle is beneficial when an isolated nerve block is required. The two deep nerves that cross the ankle, the deep peroneal (anterior tibial) and the posterior tibial, run adjacent to the dorsalis pedis and posterior tibial arteries, respectively. The other four nerves are all superficial and, from lateral to anterior to medial, are the sural, intermediate dorsal cutaneous, medial dorsal cutaneous, and saphenous nerves. The sural nerve lies just behind and inferior to the lateral malleolus and innervates the lateral border of the foot and fifth metatarsal. The two branches of the superficial peroneal nerve can often be seen or palpated directly under the skin on the anterior surface of the ankle. They provide sensation to the dorsum of the foot and toes. The saphenous nerve lies anterior to the medial malleolus and runs with the greater saphenous vein, providing sensation to the medial border of the foot. These four superficial nerves are easily blocked with simple subcutaneous infiltration around the nerves. The deep peroneal nerve is blocked by palpating the dorsalis pedis artery and injecting around it deep to the fascia, taking care to aspirate before injection. The large posterior tibial nerve lies deep to the flexor retinaculum and runs adjacent to the posterior tibial artery and veins. The three branches, the medial calcaneal, medial plantar, and lateral plantar nerves, supply the medial and plantar heel, the medial plantar sole and toes, and lateral plantar sole and toes, respectively. Anesthesia of these sites is best obtained concurrently with a block of the posterior tibial nerve behind, deep, and just above the medial malleolus. Once again, the artery should be palpated and the needle inserted so that infiltration occurs around the vessel and nerve without penetrating either structure. Aspiration should always be performed to prevent intraarterial injection. If significant pain and paresthesias occur during the injection, the needle should be very slightly withdrawn to avoid injection directly into the nerve. Approximately 6 to 10 ml are required for this difficult injection and should be delivered with a long 25 gauge needle on a 10-cc syringe.

## THE DIABETIC FOOT

Of the approximately 12 million people with diabetes mellitus in the United States, about 20% develop serious foot lesions during the course of their disease. Nearly two thirds of all nontraumatic amputations in this country are performed on diabetic patients. It is extremely important to prevent foot lesions and, when they are present, to treat them aggressively at an early stage. Since the diabetic foot is often misunderstood in terms of its pathophysiology, many problems are misdiagnosed and inappropriately treated. Many feet and limbs can be salvaged through a better understanding of the pecularities of disorders in diabetic patients, especially those concerning the various etiologies of characteristic foot lesions.

The most characteristic of all diabetic foot lesions is the plantar ulceration, often termed a mal perforans or trophic ulcer. The underlying pathophysiology of this lesion represents a summation of the various systemic alterations occurring in diabetes that have manifestations in the lower extremities. A triad of such intrinsic systemic disorders frequently cited as contributing to diabetic foot disease includes peripheral neuropathy, peripheral vascular disease, and impaired resistance to infection. This "triopathy" does not necessarily need to coexist in order to complete a causal chain to ulceration. Trauma of some sort, when applied to the high-risk diabetic foot, can result in ulceration, even in the presence of a single risk factor when such injuries are neglected or undetected. Usually, however, there are interactions between multiple contributory factors involved in the etiology of diabetic foot ulceration. Fig. 76-16 illustrates these major interrelationships and provides insight into etiopathogenesis of diabetic foot lesions in general.

*Peripheral neuropathy* is an extremely common complication of diabetes mellitus, affecting about 50% of people with longstanding diabetes. Approximately 70% of diabetic foot ulcerations can be attributed primarily to this underlying permissive factor. Neuropathy can be further categorized into motor, sensory, or autonomic components with combinations of these types present in many patients. Motor neuropathy obviously results in muscle weakness, atrophy, dysfunction, and gait disturbance. Clinical manifestations include foot drop from anterior crural muscle atrophy or characteristic hammertoes from intrinsic muscle atrophy ("intrinsic minus foot"). Sensory neuropathy presents in the classic glove-and-stocking distribution, symmetrically affecting the toes first and gradually moving proximally. Loss of deep tendon reflexes, proprioception, vibratory, pain, and light-touch sensation to some degree are the most common findings and can collectively be called negative symptoms. Painful neuropathy, conversely, is a distressing manifestation of peripheral neuropathy consisting primarily of "positive" symptoms such as burning, gnawing, or

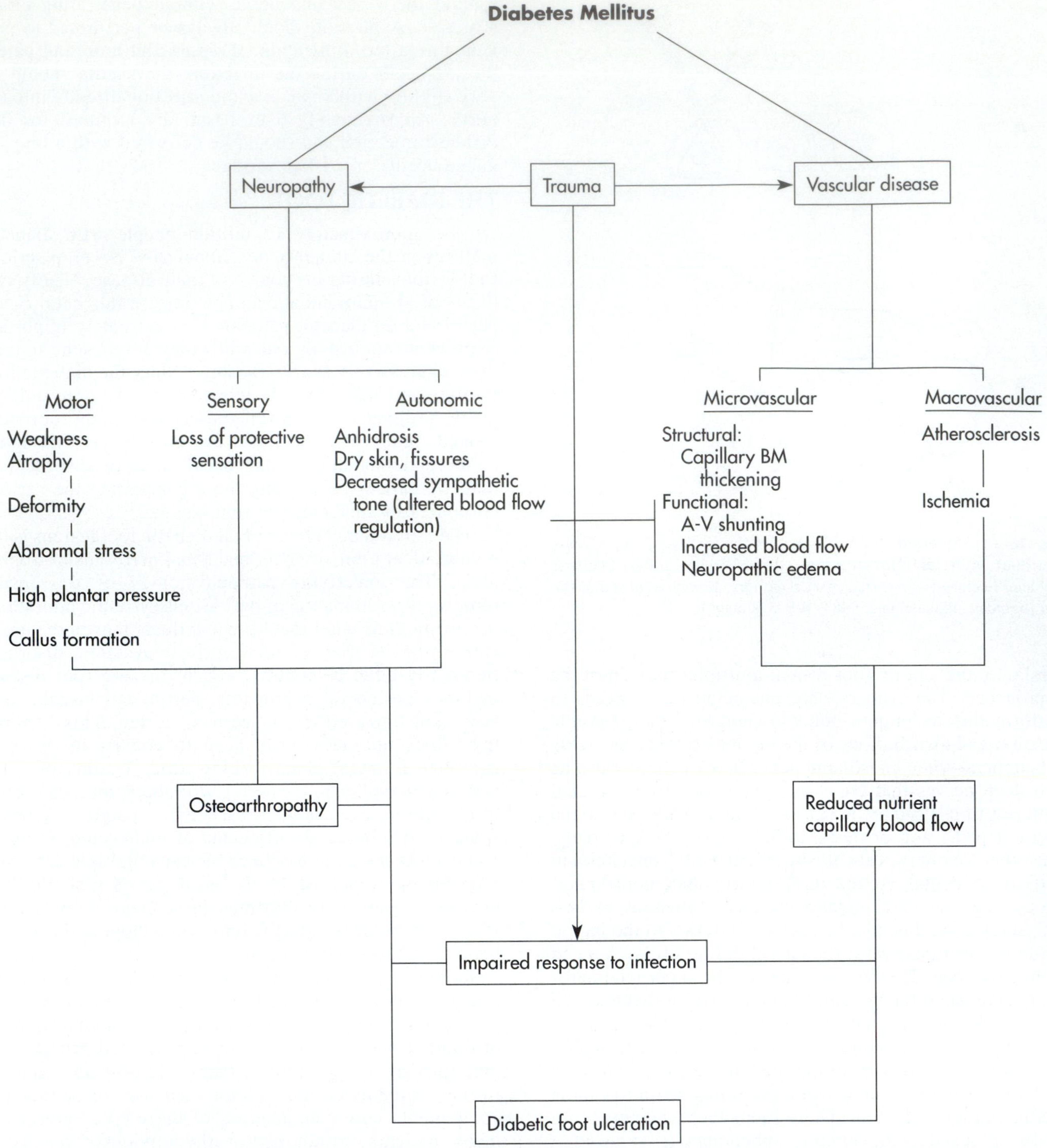


**Fig. 76-16.** Interactions between major contributory factors in the etiology of diabetic foot ulceration. (Modified from Boulton AJM: The diabetic foot, *Med Clin North Am* 72:1513, 1988.)

lancinating pains that seem to become exacerbated at night. The "painful-painless leg" is a descriptive term used to identify patients with positive symptoms of painful neuropathy in concert with negative symptoms characteristic of the insensate foot and limb. Autonomic neuropathy has gained attention in recent years as an early manifestation of neuropathy and significant factor in foot ulceration. Autonomic dysfunction of thermoregulatory mechanisms in the foot results in altered vascular tone and skin blood flow as well as anhidrosis. Arteriovenous shunting is prevalent, diverting blood flow from the nutrient capillary beds and possibly impairing normal responses to injury. Sudomotor dysfunction produces dry skin that is extremely susceptible to cracking and fissuring, common precursors to infection and ulceration.

*Peripheral vascular disease,* long thought to be the

primary etiology of diabetic foot ulcerations, actually plays a dominant role in only one third of such lesions and often coexists with neuropathy. Large vessel atherosclerotic lesions affecting the tibioperoneal trunk of the lower leg are the hallmark of diabetic macrovascular disease, although occlusions of the aortic bifurcation, iliac, and femoral systems are also common. In the typical scenario, a diabetic patient can have a gangrenous foot in the presence of a palpable popliteal artery. A relative absence of atherosclerotic disease in the foot makes distal vascular reconstruction to the dorsalis pedis or posterior tibial arteries the limb-salvaging procedures of choice in most cases. Diabetic microangiopathy refers to disease of the capillaries, the hallmark being a thickening of the capillary basement membrane and a resulting impairment of leukocyte diapedesis and nutrient exchange. There is no intravascular occlusion of these vessels, a longstanding misconception that gave rise to the term "small vessel disease." This term should be abandoned in light of our current understanding of the nature of diabetic vascular disease.

Susceptibility to *infection* and an impairment in one's ability to fight established infections have long been recognized as significant factors in the etiology of diabetic foot infections, ulceration, and gangrene. This "immunopathy" is due to a deficiency in the phagocytic activity of leukocytes, impaired intracellular bacterial killing, and a defect in normal chemotactic mechanisms. In these circumstances even common pathogens can result in overwhelming infections, especially in the presence of neuropathy and ischemia. Bacteria such as Staphylococcus epidermidis or enterococcus, considered rather benign organisms, take on extremely pathogenic roles in the diabetic milieu. Anaerobic infections with *Bacteroides* sp. are characteristic of diabetic foot infections, although they rarely if ever cause infection as isolated organisms. Polymicrobial infection is the rule in most cases of severe diabetic foot infection, with gram-positive cocci, gram-negative rods, and anaerobes being cultured simultaneously from deep specimens. Empirical antibiotic therapy for limb-threatening infections should therefore always attempt to cover a broad spectrum of organisms until final specification and sensitivities are received. Osteomyelitis is an ever-present complication of such infections and must be suspected in deeply probing, longstanding, or recalcitrant ulcerations. Although ulcerations do not completely heal when underlying bone or joint infection exists, local bone debridement with culture-specific antibiotic therapy and vascular reconstruction as necessary are quite successful in eradicating such infections and preserving limb integrity.

*Trauma* is usually the precipitating event in the development of diabetic foot infections or ulcerations. Although such trauma can be acute (sharp, mechanical, thermal, or chemical), most foot lesions in the diabetic patient are due to the minor repetitive trauma of walking and moderate pressures, to the high pressures of a tight shoe, or to any degree of abnormal pressure against a structural deformity. The etiology of any lesion must be investigated with the premise that trauma of some type has played a role in its development. Notwithstanding acute trauma, dorsal, medial, and lateral lesions usually result from tight shoes, whereas plantar lesions are the result of repetitive moderate stress or neglected preexisting hyperkeratoses. Burns are common precursors to ulceration, especially in the insenate foot, and most often result from hot foot soaks or walking barefooted on hot sand or pavement. Acute trauma in the presence of neuropathy and abundant vascular supply can also lead to the onset of another characteristic diabetic foot disorder, the Charcot foot or osteoarthropathy. The ensuing foot deformity creates abnormally high pressures during walking and frequently leads to chronic plantar ulceration (Fig. 76-17).

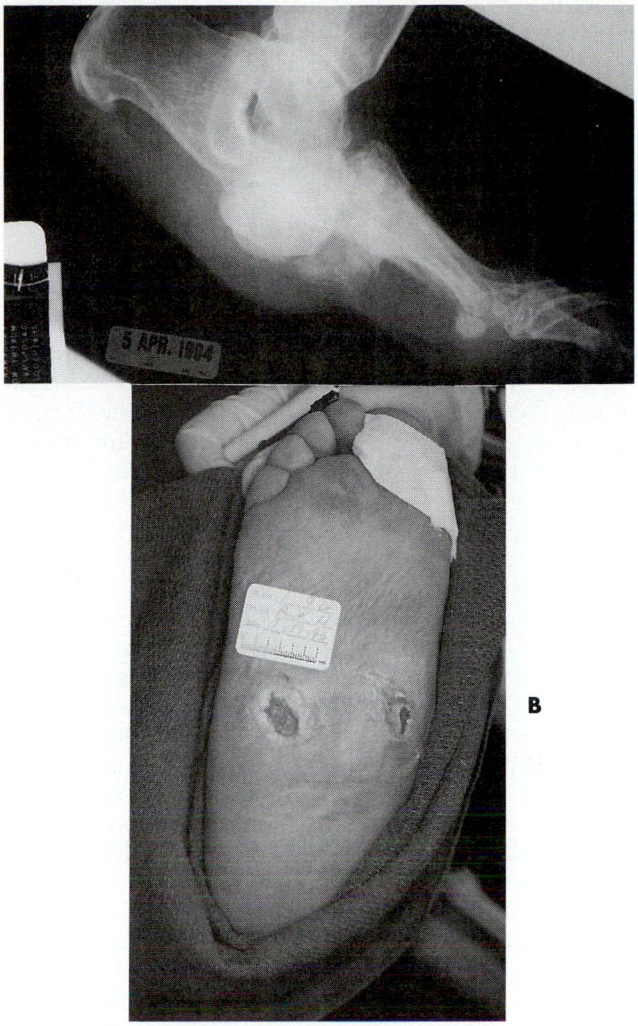


B

**Fig. 76-17.** Charcot foot deformity. **A,** Lateral radiograph demonstrating severe midfoot osteoarthropathy with collapse of the cuboid and medial cuneiform. **B,** Clinical photo of same foot with plantar ulceration underlying the abnormal prominences of the midfoot.

Treatment of foot ulcerations must focus on all of the aforementioned contributory factors and must be appropriately assessed at the onset. Acute infections must be treated by culture-directed antibiotic therapy. Ischemic lesions must be recognized by their atrophic appearance and lack of pedal pulsations and referred for vascular consultation. Such lesions infrequently heal without restoration of pulsatile blood flow. Above all, non–weight bearing or attenuation of weight bearing is essential for the resolution of any type of ulceration. The neuropathic individual, for example, continues to walk on the ulcerated foot because of absent pain sensation or denial of the ulceration. Since walking is a usual causative factor in ulceration, healing does not commence until walking has ceased. Although total non–weight bearing is the ideal situation, pressure-attenuating methods such as foam pressure dispersion dressings, healing sandals, (modified surgical shoes), surgical shoes, total contact casting, and removable cast braces can be used. Local wound care consists of daily or twice daily dressing changes with a topical antiseptic of choice (e.g., ¼ strength povidone-iodine solution, saline, silver sulfadiazine cream). Clinical trials are being conducted to assess the efficacy of topical growth factors in this regard; however, even if proven beneficial, they cannot supplant the need for pressure reduction, treatment of infection, and an abundant blood flow.

Recurrent ulcers usually indicate a persistent bony structural deformity, shoe problem, or functional foot disorder that needs attention in order to resolve the problem. Recalcitrant ulcers can be indicative of the same problem, but also might imply inadequate treatment, noncompliance, or an unrecognized infection and osteomyelitis. Overall treatment of foot ulcers therefore requires not only immediate attention to infection, circulation, and pressure reduction, but to long-term prevention as well. Prevention encompasses proper foot care, patient education, periodic examination, proper footwear, and prophylactic foot surgery as necessary to correct structural deformities. Multiple studies from the United States and abroad indicate that an approximately 50% reduction in ulcer recidivism and subsequent amputation can be realized through appropriate education, regular podiatric care, and appropriate footwear. Education can consist of simple talks or handouts regarding potential diabetic foot problems and how to recognize and avoid them. Regular podiatric care involves bimonthly visits for examination and routine care of toenails and calluses. While serving as forums for constant patient education, such visits also provide a mechanism for early detection of potential problems and appropriate intervention. Shoe therapy involves a variety of footwear, ranging from simple molded insoles in athletic shoes to extra-depth shoes to custom-molded shoes depending upon the severity of foot lesions and the magnitude of foot deformity present. When shoe therapy alone is not effective, corrective surgery is certainly advisable in the appropriate patient and may be the best chance for permanent resolution of a recurrent problem.

As with most complex medical disorders, management of the diabetic foot should ideally be accomplished through a multidisciplinary approach. The primary care physician who regularly attends these patients should serve as the gatekeeper and overseer of the patients' foot health. When problems arise an organized plan for referral to the appropriate service or consultant should commence so that such input is obtained in a timely manner. All consultants should be dedicated to the principles herein outlined and should work as a cohesive service with an emphasis on early aggressive care and concomitant limb preservation. With an organized approach to the high-risk foot in diabetes mellitus the worldwide goal of a 50% reduction in lower extremity amputation can be met or exceeded by the year 2000.

## BIBLIOGRAPHY


Boulton AJM: The diabetic foot, *Med Clin North Am* 72:1513, 1988.

Centers for Disease Control, Public Health Service, US Department of Health and Human Services, Vital and Health Statistics: *Current estimates from the National Health Interview Survey, 1990,* DHHS Publication PHS No. 92-1509, Hyattsville, MD, 1991.

Chan CW, Rudins A: Foot biomechanics during walking and running, *Mayo Clin Proc* 69:448, 1994.

Frykberg RG, editor: *The high risk foot in diabetes mellitus,* New York, 1991, Churchill Livingstone.

Frykberg RG et al: Prophylactic surgery in the diabetic foot. In Kominsky SJ, editor: *Medical and surgical management of the diabetic foot,* St. Louis, 1994, Mosby.

Frykberg RG: Podiatric problems in diabetes. In Kozak GP et al, editors: *Management of diabetic foot problems,* Philadelphia, 1984, WB Saunders.

Greenberg L, Davis H: Foot problems in the US; the 1990 National Health Interview Survey, *J Am Podiatr Med Assoc* 83:475, 1993.

Levy LA: Prevalence of chronic podiatric conditions in the US; National Health Survey 1990, *J Am Podiatr Med Assoc* 82:221, 1992.

McGlamry ED, editor: *Comprehensive textbook of foot surgery,* Baltimore, 1987, Williams & Wilkins.

Regnauld B, editor: *The foot,* Berlin, 1986, Springer-Verlag.

Root ML, Orien WP, Weed JH, editors: *Normal and abnormal function of the foot,* Los Angeles, 1977, Clinical Biomechanics.

Scurran BL, editor: *Foot and ankle trauma,* New York, 1989, Churchill Livingstone.

Wu KK, editor: *Foot orthoses: principles and clinical applications,* Baltimore, 1990, Williams & Wilkins.


CHAPTER

# 77 Idiopathic Inflammatory Myopathies

**Steven R. Ytterberg**

Idiopathic inflammatory myopathies (IIMs) are acquired, inflammatory disorders of skeletal muscle of unknown etiology. They are characterized clinically by muscle weakness that is classically symmetric, involving proximal muscles of the limbs, but that may include the neck and pharyngeal muscles. The chief conditions in this group are polymyositis (PM) and, when accompanied by cutaneous manifestations, dermatomyositis (DM). Several clinically defined subgroups of PM and DM have been described (see the box on p. 1085) that separate adult disease from childhood-onset disease, and, among adults, PM from DM. Additional subgroups identify the association of PM or DM with another connective tissue disease and with malignancy. Recently, inclusion body myositis (IBM) was described as a distinctive member of the IIM group, with more frequent distal weakness and unique inclusions seen on muscle biopsy. Several other less commonly diagnosed disorders have features of inflammatory myositis (see the box on p. 1085). Although the

### Classification of PM and DM

Idiopathic polymyositis
Idiopathic dermatomyositis
Juvenile dermatomyositis or polymyositis
Dermatomyositis or polymyositis with malignancy
Polymyositis or dermatomyositis with another connective tissue disease

### Less common forms of inflammatory myositis

Inclusion body myositis
Eosinophilic myositis
Localized nodular myositis
Proliferative myositis
Infectious myositis

Modified from Strongwater SL, *Mt Sinai J Med* 55:435, 1988.

IIMs have many similarities, they can be distinguished on clinical and histologic grounds. In addition to these IIMs, a number of infectious agents and toxins can cause inflammatory myositis; these are covered later in this chapter in the discussion of differential diagnosis.

## EPIDEMIOLOGY

IIMs are rare disorders, with a combined annual incidence of approximately 5 to 10 per million. In adult patients with IIM, isolated PM and DM are each found in approximately one third of patients. PM or DM is associated with connective tissue disease in approximately 20% of patients, with malignancy occurring in approximately 15%. IBM has probably been underrecognized in the past; it was reported recently in up to 25% of adult patients with inflammatory myositis, although this may be a high estimate because it is from a referral center. PM and DM have a female/male ratio of approximately 2:1. There is a greater female predominance among younger patients and among those patients who have another connective tissue disease, whereas the gender ratio is equal in patients with associated malignancy. In contrast, IBM occurs most often in middle-aged to older men. For PM and DM, there are two peaks of incidence: during childhood and during the fifth to sixth decades. Patients with IIM associated with malignancy have a mean age over 60. PM and DM are three to four times more common in African-Americans than in Caucasians. Seasonal variation in the onset of PM and DM has been reported, suggesting a role for environmental agents in the etiology.

The relationship of IIM with malignancy has prompted much controversy. Early anecdotal observations suggested an increased frequency of malignancy in patients with PM or DM. After a review of several large clinical series, malignancy was found in 20% of adult patients with DM, 13% with PM, and 15% overall. Malignancy is more frequent in patients diagnosed with myositis after age 45. Malignancy has been reported in only a small number of patients with IBM, but experience with this condition is less extensive than with PM and DM. Several recent, well-designed, case-controlled and population-based studies supported the association of DM and PM with malignancy, demonstrating that patients with DM are at greater risk. The data available suggest that the relationship between IIM and malignancy is indirect, not causal. Of patients with IIM associated with malignancy, some develop malignancy first and others develop myositis first. Moreover, no particular type of malignancy has been associated with IIM.

## PATHOPHYSIOLOGY

The etiology of IIMs is unknown. Microorganisms have long been considered to be potential etiologic agents, including *Toxoplasma gondii* and several different groups of viruses, but direct evidence implicating specific microorganisms has been difficult to obtain. Group B coxsackieviruses and encephalomyocarditis virus, members of the picornavirus family, can cause inflammatory myositis with features of human PM in mice. Coxsackievirus A9, adenovirus, echovirus, and influenza virus have been isolated in a few patients with PM and DM. Elevated titers of antibodies to group B coxsackieviruses have been found in children with recent-onset DM. Studies using molecular biologic approaches have demonstrated persistence of coxsackievirus ribonucleic acid (RNA) in some patients with PM and DM, but these findings have not been confirmed by all investigators. The characteristic muscle fiber inclusions in patients with IBM resemble viral inclusions. Early data suggested that mumps virus was present in the inclusions, but this observation was not confirmed in subsequent studies. Recently, PM and DM were found in patients infected with human immunodeficiency virus (HIV). In these cases, HIV is present in the mononuclear cells invading muscle but is not present in muscle fibers.

Although all of the disorders classified as IIMs have clinical weakness and histologic muscle inflammation in common, they have different pathophysiologic mechanisms. Substantial evidence supports a role for cell-mediated immunologic mechanisms in the pathogenesis of PM and IBM. Histologically, T cells, especially $CD8^+$ cytotoxic T cells, predominate in inflammatory infiltrates, typically in the endomysium, in these disorders. Activated $CD8^+$ T cells can be found invading nonnecrotic muscle fibers. Humoral immune mechanisms play a greater role in DM. More $CD4^+$ T cells and a higher proportion of B cells are found, with a perivascular and perifascicular distribution. Mononuclear cells do not invade muscle fibers directly in DM, as they do in PM and IBM. In juvenile DM, vascular damage is apparent. Endothelial cell hyperplasia and vascular infarction are present, with atrophy of muscle fibers at the periphery of the fascicles (perifascicular atrophy). Immunoglobulin and the membrane attack complex of complement are found in areas of muscle necrosis, underscoring the role of humoral mechanisms in disease pathogenesis.

Muscle inflammation results in weakness and muscle tenderness. Muscle fibers demonstrate necrosis, degeneration, regeneration, and phagocytosis. The cause of weak-

**Table 77-1.** Autoantibodies in patients with idiopathic inflammatory myopathies

| Antibody | Approximate frequency in IIM (%) | Clinical associations |
|---|---|---|
| **Antibodies found in other connective tissue diseases** | | |
| Antinuclear (ANA) | 50–90 | SLE, MCTD, scleroderma |
| Anti-Sm | 4 | SLE |
| Anti-nRNP | 10–15 | SLE, MCTD |
| Anti-Ro (SS-A) | 7–12 | SLE, Sjögren's syndrome |
| Anti-La (SS-B) | 2–10 | SLE, Sjögren's syndrome |
| Anti-Scl-70 | 8 | Scleroderma |
| **Myositis-specific antibodies** | | |
| Antisynthetase antibodies | 25 | |
| Anti-Jo-1 (histidyl t-RNA) | 20 | Adult PM; interstitial lung disease, arthritis |
| Anti-PL-7 (threonyl t-RNA) | 2 | Interstitial lung disease |
| Anti-PL-12 (alanyl t-RNA) | 1 | Interstitial lung disease |
| Anti-EJ (glycyl t-RNA) | 2 | Interstitial lung disease |
| Anti-OJ (isoleucyl t-RNA) | 1 | Interstitial lung disease |
| Antisignal recognition particle (SRP) | <5 | Severe PM |
| Anti-Mi-2 | 10–20 | Adult DM |
| Anti-PM-Scl | 8 | PM-scleroderma overlap |
| Anti-Ku | <1 | PM-scleroderma overlap |

*SLE*, Systemic lupus erythematosus; *MCTD*, mixed connective tissue disease.

ness appears to be multifactorial. In addition to loss of muscle fibers and muscle bulk, functional abnormalities of muscle may be involved. Fibrosis and muscle atrophy may be present in later stages, also contributing to muscle weakness.

A variety of autoantibodies can be found in patients with IIM (Table 77-1). They are less common in patients with IBM than in those with PM or DM. Autoantibodies present in other connective tissue diseases may occur, including antinuclear antibodies (ANA), anti-Sm, anti-nRNP, and anti-Ro (-SSA) antibodies. In addition, a number of myositis-specific autoantibodies have been identified in patients with IIM. Most of these antibodies are directed against cytoplasmic ribonucleoproteins involved in protein synthesis. The antigens for one group of these myositis-specific antibodies are the aminoacyl-tRNA synthetases, enzymes that charge the appropriate amino acid onto its corresponding tRNA. Specific antibodies recognized as antisynthetase antibodies in patients with IIM are anti-Jo-1, directed toward histidyl-tRNA synthetase; anti-PL-7 (threonyl-tRNA synthetase); anti-PL-12 (alanyl-tRNA synthetase); anti-OJ (isoleucyl-tRNA synthetase); and anti-EJ (glycyl-tRNA synthetase). Other myositis-specific antibodies are directed against proteins of the signal recognition particle (SRP), translation factors, and other unidentified RNAs and proteins. It is unclear how these autoantibodies come about. Positive-stranded RNA viruses, such as the picornaviruses, use host translation enzymes. In addition, certain viruses, including encephalomyocarditis virus, can substitute for tRNA and be charged by aminoacyl-tRNA synthetases with an amino acid. During such interactions with host proteins, the host proteins might come to be recognized as antigenic and result in autoantibody formation. It is also unclear whether these antibodies can enter cells to disrupt function, although, using in vitro assays, they can inhibit the functions of the target antigens. The myositis-specific antibodies may be markers, rather than causes, of disease. Approximately 50% of patients with PM and DM have myositis-specific antibodies, whereas they are not found in patients with IBM (see Table 77-1).

Genetic factors play a role in disease, presumably through control of immunologic responsiveness. Approximately half of white patients with PM and DM have the HLA-DR3 phenotype, usually linked with HLA-B8. In African-American patients with PM and DM, HLA-DR3 is only slightly increased, but linkage with B8 is increased over the frequency in control populations. These markers are most common in patients with anti-Jo-1 antibodies, regardless of race. In patients with IBM, HLA-DR1 is increased threefold compared with control populations. Familial cases of IBM have been described.

## HISTORY

Muscle weakness is the most frequent presenting complaint of patients with IIM. Weakness is usually insidious in onset and slowly progressive, although at times its onset may be abrupt, with rapid progression. Acute onset may be associated with more severe disease. Weakness is characteristically symmetric and usually affects the legs before the arms. Symptoms are typically progressive and unrelated to exercise. In PM and DM, proximal muscle groups of the limbs are primarily affected. The presence of distal weakness may suggest IBM. Neck, pharyngeal, and, at times, respiratory muscles may be involved. It is helpful to identify specific activities affected by the weakness, such as rising from a low chair or toilet seat, getting out of a car, climbing stairs, or combing the hair. Involvement of pharyngeal or esophageal muscle may result in dysphonia, dysphagia, or aspiration. Muscle tenderness and aching occur in approximately 50% of patients. Muscle atrophy may occur with later disease.

When a patient complains of weakness, it is important to differentiate true loss of muscle strength from fatigue or pain. Fatigue may be present in IIMs, but it is a nonspecific complaint and is seen in a variety of inflammatory diseases, as well as some noninflammatory disorders that may be confused with IIM, such as polymyalgia rheumatica and fibromyalgia. Limitation of activity due to pain from articular or periarticular sources in patients with arthritis may be identified as weakness by some patients. A careful history, followed by careful muscle strength testing with elicitation of maximal effort during the examination are needed to eliminate these possibilities and focus attention on muscle as the source of weakness.

Skin rash may be the presenting complaint of patients with DM. Arthralgia and Raynaud's phenomenon are present in approximately 25% of patients. In patients who have myositis in association with another connective tissue disease, features of the associated condition may be apparent. The most common associated connective tissue or autoimmune disorder is SLE; other relatively frequently associated diseases include Hashimoto's thyroiditis, scleroderma, Sjögren's syndrome, rheumatoid arthritis (RA), insulin-dependent diabetes mellitus, and Graves' disease. Thus arthritis, sclerodactyly, or cutaneous symptoms of SLE may be present. Occasionally, cardiac or pulmonary symptoms lead the patient to seek attention. Pulmonary involvement may lead to diminished chest wall motion or interstitial fibrosis, resulting in complaints of dyspnea or cough. Cardiac involvement may produce conduction disturbances or myocarditis with symptoms from arrhythmia, congestive heart failure, or ischemia. Symptoms of associated malignancy may be found in some patients. Systemic features can include fatigue, morning stiffness, and weight loss.

## PHYSICAL EXAMINATION

Physical examination is aimed at excluding other causes of muscle weakness, especially neuropathic causes, identifying systemic features of myositis, recognizing an associated connective disease, and detecting an associated malignancy. Thus a thorough general physical examination is required, with special attention given to a careful neurologic examination.

Careful examination of muscle strength is important in evaluating a patient suspected of having an IIM. Although strength can be measured using a dynamometer, manual muscle strength testing (see the box below) is used in most clinical situations. Manual muscle strength testing is relatively crude in its sensitivity, but it can be useful to monitor the response to therapy. The timed stands test can also be useful to follow lower extremity strength in patients with IIM. To perform this test, the patient is instructed to stand up and sit down 10 times in a chair of normal height as rapidly as possible. The time it takes to complete this task correlates with muscle testing but offers a more precise measurement than manual muscle strength testing.

Dermatomyositis is present when inflammatory myositis exists with cutaneous manifestations. A variety of skin lesions may be found in patients with DM. Two characteristic lesions are the heliotrope rash and Gottron's papules. A heliotrope rash is a faint, lilac-colored eruption on the upper eyelids. Gottron's papules are raised, red or violaceous, sometimes scaly lesions overlying the metacarpophalangeal (MCP) and proximal interphalangeal (PIP) joints, sparing the phalanges (Fig. 77-1). Gottron's papules may be found over the elbows or knees as well. Other nonspecific lesions, including an erythematous macular rash on the face, neck, upper chest, or shawl distribution, might be present. Vasculitic lesions may be seen at the base of the nails. Some patients have what has been described as machinist's hands. Subcutaneous calcification may be found, most commonly in childhood DM. See Chapters 19-26 for illustrations.

## LABORATORY STUDIES AND DIAGNOSTIC PROCEDURES

### Laboratory studies

Serum creatine kinase (CK) and other muscle-associated enzymes are typically elevated in patients with IIM and can be useful as indicators of response to therapy. CK levels may be modestly or markedly elevated in PM and DM; in IBM they are typically only mildly elevated. Elevation of the MB isoenzyme of CK may occur in patients with IIM in the absence of myocardial involvement. A variety of pathologic and nonpathologic conditions can elevate serum CK values. Men have higher values than do women, reflecting increased muscle mass. CK levels in African-Americans are higher than those in whites; healthy African-American subjects frequently have values that are above normal, as defined by most laboratories. Muscle trauma and jogging are associated

### Manual muscle strength testing

0: No contraction
1: Flicker of muscle contraction but no joint movement
2: Joint movement with gravity eliminated
3: Joint movement against gravity only
4: Joint movement against gravity and resistance
5: Normal power

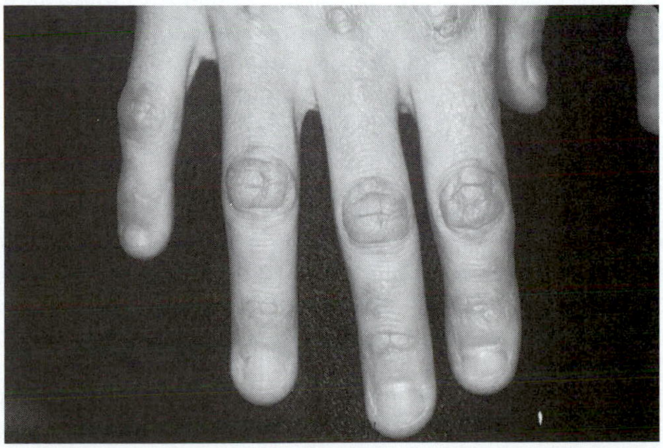

**Fig. 77-1.** Dermatomyositis (Gottron's papules). Note erythematous papules over joints and periungual telangiectasias.

with elevated serum CK values. Drugs can elevate CK levels by damaging muscle or by retarding urinary excretion of CK. In some patients with IIM the CK level may be normal, whereas levels of other muscle-associated enzymes, including aldolase, lactate dehydrogenase (LDH), alanine aminotransferase (ALT), and aspartate aminotransferase (AST), are elevated. Myoglobin and creatine levels may be elevated; myoglobinuria occurs in rare patients. To evaluate patients who have muscle weakness, tests for electrolytes, renal function, thyroid function, calcium, magnesium, and phosphorus are needed to exclude other causes of weakness. These are usually normal in patients with IIM.

The majority of patients with PM and DM have autoantibodies (see Table 77-1). Some are unique to patients with myositis, but many are seen in other connective tissue disorders as well. Serologic testing for autoantibodies can have prognostic significance and can help to categorize patients into subgroups, thereby helping to diagnose a specific connective tissue disorder. Positive ANAs are found in 50% to 90% of patients with IIM. The other non-muscle–specific antibodies may be seen in patients with myositis alone but are most frequent in patients who have an overlap syndrome of another connective tissue disorder. Myositis-specific antibodies are found in approximately 50% of patients with PM or DM and are infrequent in patients with IBM. Sera-containing myositis-specific antibodies may demonstrate cytoplasmic speckling on ANA assays using Hep-2 cell substrates. The most commonly found myositis-specific antibodies are the antisynthetase antibodies, most often anti-Jo-1 (antihistidyl-tRNA synthetase). Anti-Jo-1 antibodies are found in approximately 10% of adult patients with DM and 30% to 40% of those with PM; they are rare in childhood disease. Anti-Jo-1 antibodies are highly specific for IIM. Anti-Jo-1 has a strong association with patients who have interstitial lung disease. Patients with any of the antisynthetases have a higher frequency of interstitial lung involvement and of arthritis. Patients with anti-SRP have the worst prognosis, often having acute onset, severe disease, with myocardial involvement.

A great deal of research on a molecular level is being done to better understand how specific autoantibodies may play a pathophysiologic role in inflammatory muscle disease. From a clinical perspective, the autoantibodies that the primary care physician generally finds most helpful to evaluate patients with weakness and elevated muscle enzymes are the ANAs, the anti-Jo-1 antibody, and the anti-Scl-70 antibody determinations.

*Muscle biopsy* is critical to establish the diagnoses of PM, DM, and IBM and for excluding other neuromuscular disorders. Biopsy can be performed by needle technique, although many pathologists prefer open biopsies. Normal biopsies are found in approximately 7% of patients; the occurrence of normal biopsies is due to the spotty nature of the disease. Despite the possibility of a false-negative result, biopsy is important before committing a patient to a course of therapy that has a significant potential for morbidity. The muscle chosen for biopsy should be carefully selected. Ideally, the muscle should be neither the most nor the least affected muscle. A muscle that has been studied previously by electromyography (EMG) should not be biopsied because of the possibility of finding pathologic changes that were caused by the EMG needle.

The key findings of muscle biopsy in patients with IIM are prominence of inflammatory cells, degeneration, variation in cross-sectional diameter, necrosis, regeneration, and phagocytosis of muscle fibers. Biopsies are usually diffusely abnormal but may show only focal changes in approximately 25% of cases. Capillary damage and increased amounts of connective tissue and fat may be noted. In DM, inflammation tends to be perivascular and around muscle fascicles with fiber atrophy in perifascicular areas. Perifascicular atrophy is not a characteristic finding in PM or IBM. In PM, the inflammation is primarily within muscle fascicles. Necrotic fibers are not grouped as they tend to be in DM and indeed may not be near areas of inflammation. The characteristic histologic finding in IBM is the presence of nuclear and/or cytoplasmic inclusions, with rimmed vacuoles. By electron microscopy, these inclusions show masses of filamentous material.

Although the finding of inflammatory cells on biopsy is a characteristic feature of IIM, their presence alone does not make the diagnosis. Muscle inflammation can be seen in other necrotizing conditions, including Duchenne dystrophy and myasthenia gravis.

EMG can be useful in differentiating myopathic from neuropathic causes of weakness. It can also help to differentiate active from inactive myositis. The myopathic pattern seen in patients with IIM is not diagnostic but can be seen in other forms of active myopathy. Findings include irritability, with increased insertional and spontaneous activity manifested by fibrillations, complex repetitive discharges, and positive sharp waves. With voluntary muscle activity, short-duration, low-amplitude polyphasic motor unit action potentials are observed. Patients with IBM may show neuropathic EMG changes as well. Normal EMGs are present in approximately 5% of patients with active IIM.

Other workup should be directed by specific complaints or physical findings. A chest x-ray study is useful in identifying interstitial fibrosis or associated pulmonary malignancy. If interstitial fibrosis is present, the diffusion capacity is often diminished. The question of how aggressively to look for occult malignancy can be difficult to answer. Because of the cost and potential hazards of performing tests and procedures blindly to try to identify an occult malignancy, it is unreasonable to attempt an exhaustive search for malignancy in all patients who have a new diagnosis of IIM. A patient should undergo a thorough history and physical examination, chemistry panel, blood count, stool guaiac examination, and chest radiograph. A mammogram or prostate-specific antigen test should be performed. Similar screening should probably be performed annually, especially in older patients. Any abnormalities found from these studies should be followed up, but an undirected search for malignancy is not warranted.

## COURSE AND PROGNOSIS

Although older data suggested a gloomier prognosis, survival rates for patients with PM and DM were recently estimated to be approximately 80% 5 years after diagnosis and 73% after 8 years. Several clinical features correlate with a poor prognosis: older age at diagnosis; presence of

## Managed Care Guide
## Treatment of patient with diffuse muscle pain and stiffness

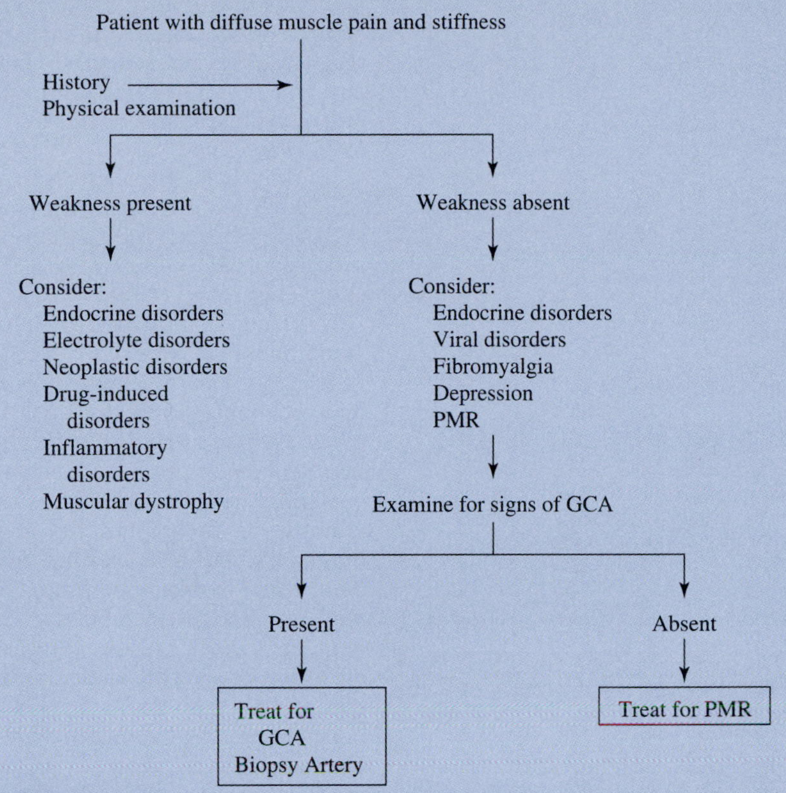


From Maricic MJ: Diffuse muscle pain and stiffness: polymyalgia rheumatica and giant cell arteritis. In Greene HL, Johnson WP, Maricic MJ, editors: *Decision making in medicine,* St. Louis, 1993, Mosby.

cardiac involvement, dysphagia, or malignancy; a long delay between symptom onset and initiation of therapy; and a poor initial response to corticosteroids. Patients with antibodies to SRP or to any of the aminoacyl-tRNA synthetases have been reported to have more severe disease than those without these antibodies. Of patients with PM or DM, approximately half have a complete or near complete recovery. In contrast, patients with IBM often do not respond to therapy and usually follow a gradually deteriorating course.

## DIFFERENTIAL DIAGNOSIS

The diagnosis of PM, DM, or IBM is based on the demonstration of muscle inflammation in a patient with muscle weakness, but it is important to recognize that other diseases can cause weakness and inflammatory myositis, and these must be considered (see the Managed Care Guide). Criteria for diagnosing PM and DM have been proposed and are widely used; preliminary criteria for diagnosing IBM have been suggested as well (see the box at right and on p. 1090). These criteria were established to facilitate classification of patients for study purposes rather than to be specific diagnostic criteria for individuals, but they can be useful when considering the diagnosis of IIM in an individual. Before these criteria are used, other causes of weakness must be excluded. Muscle weakness can result from a variety of different disease processes (see the box on p. 1091). Many of these

### Proposed criteria for the diagnosis of PM and DM

1. Symmetric proximal muscle weakness
2. Elevated serum skeletal muscle enzyme levels
3. Myopathic changes on EMG
4. Muscle biopsy showing inflammatory myositis
5. Skin rash typical of DM

Polymyositis
- Definite: all of criteria 1-4
- Probable: any three of criteria 1-4
- Possible: any two of criteria 1-4

Dermatomyositis
- Definite: criterion 5 plus three other criteria
- Probable: criterion 5 plus two other criteria
- Possible: criterion 5 plus one other criterion

**Proposed criteria for the diagnosis of inclusion body myositis**

**Clinical criteria**

Proximal muscle weakness
Distal muscle weakness
EMG evidence of generalized myopathy
Elevation of muscle enzyme levels
Failure of muscle weakness to improve with high-dose corticosteroids

**Pathologic criteria**

Electron microscopy of muscle showing inclusions containing microtubular filaments
Light microscopy
  Intranuclear and/or intracytoplasmic inclusions
  Lined vacuoles

**Classification of IBM**

Definite: Clinical criterion 1 plus one clinical criterion and pathologic criterion 1
Probable: Clinical criterion 1 plus three clinical criterion and pathologic criterion 2a and 2b
Possible: Any three clinical criteria plus pathologic criteria 2a and 2b

possibilities can be excluded on the basis of the history and physical examination, but laboratory and/or biopsy data may be required.

Neurologic disorders are chief in the differential diagnosis of IIM. The presence of abnormalities other than muscle weakness on the neurologic examination strongly suggests a neuropathic rather than a myopathic etiology. As an exception to this generalization, IBM can have neuropathic features, including diminished deep tendon reflexes. Asymmetric or early distal muscle involvement or muscle hypertrophy may be clues to a diagnosis other than IIM. The presence of facial or ocular complaints and unique EMG findings help identify myasthenia gravis or Eaton-Lambert syndrome. A familial history of weakness and a younger age at onset may suggest a muscular dystrophy, some types of which may increase the serum CK (e.g., Duchenne muscular dystrophy).

Electrolyte abnormalities and metabolic disorders must be excluded. Elevation or lowering of serum sodium, potassium, or calcium levels, as well as hypophosphatemia and hypomagnesemia, should be sought. Hypothyroidism can cause weakness and markedly high CK levels. Hyperthyroidism, hyperparathyroidism, Cushing disease, and Addison disease are other easily excluded endocrine causes of muscle weakness.

A number of drugs can cause weakness, with or without CK elevation. The list of agents that have been implicated is long, but several merit specific mention. Ethanol is probably the most commonly used drug that produces myopathy; it is capable of causing acute muscle swelling and pain after binge drinking or chronic progressive proximal myopathy with longer term use. Corticosteroids can cause proximal muscle weakness, which can be confusing in patients with IIM treated with steroids, but CK levels are typically normal. Clofibrate, colchicine, D-penicillamine, chloroquine, hydroxychloroquine, ϵ-aminocaproic acid, and vincristine can cause weakness with CK elevation. Zidovudine (AZT) has been associated with myalgia and muscle weakness, which may produce diagnostic difficulty because HIV infection itself has been associated with PM. In primary care, one of the most common medications to cause myopathy is lovastatin (HMG-coenzyme reductase inhibitors) *especially* when combined with gemfibrazil, clofibrate, niacin, erythromycin, or cyclosporin. Cocaine may cause an elevated CK and even rhabdomyolysis.

Chronic myositis can result from parasitic infections, including toxoplasmosis, trichinosis, and schistosomiasis, and with certain viral infections, most notably coxsackieviruses and influenza virus. HIV infection has been associated with PM, but muscle is not directly infected by HIV. Bacterial infection of muscle usually causes acute symptoms that are usually not confused with IIM.

Metabolic myopathies may cause muscle weakness and may be confused with IIMs. Several glycogen storage diseases, including McArdle syndrome (myophosphorylase deficiency), can cause elevation of the CK and muscle weakness. Symptoms exacerbated by exercise, muscle cramps, or myoglobinuria may help to suggest these diagnoses. Disorders of fat metabolism (carnitine deficiency and carnitine palmitoyl transferase deficiency), as well as purine metabolism (myoadenylate deaminase deficiency), can present with proximal weakness and CK elevation as well. Ischemic forearm muscle exercise testing can help to identify some of these patients. In normal subjects, venous lactate and ammonia levels rise after ischemic exercise. In patients with glycogen storage disorders, ammonia, but not lactate, rises after such exercise, whereas in myoadenylate deaminase deficiency, lactate levels but not ammonia levels rise. Histochemical studies of muscle biopsy specimens are key to making the diagnosis of a storage disease.

Myositis and muscle weakness may occur with connective tissue disorders that include RA, SLE, and scleroderma. Among the more common disorders considered in the differential diagnosis of IIM are polymyalgia rheumatica (PMR) and fibrositis. Several key features in the workup can eliminate these disorders, however (Table 77-2). Most notable is the presence of pain with normal muscle strength in the latter two conditions. The patient must be urged to maximal effort during the examination to demonstrate normal strength.

## MANAGEMENT

Given the complexity of the differential diagnosis in patients suspected of having an IIM, the need to assess the overlap with other connective tissue diseases, and the potential for complications of therapy, confirmation of diagnosis, and management plans should be made in consultation with a rheumatologist.

Corticosteroids are the mainstay of treatment, although their use has not been tested in controlled studies. Treatment should be started at approximately 1 to 2 mg/kg per day, given in two to three divided doses. Patients with a more acute onset and more severe disease should be treated at the more aggressive end of this range. Clinical and laboratory parameters should be monitored to assess

## Differential diagnosis of idiopathic inflammatory myopathies

**Collagen vascular disease**
Fibrositis
Polyarteritis nodosa
Polymyalgia rheumatica
Rheumatoid arthritis
Scleroderma
Systemic lupus erythematosus
Temporal arteritis

**Neurologic**
Denervation
  Amyotrophic lateral sclerosis
Neuromuscular junction disorders
  Myasthenia gravis
  Eaton-Lambert syndrome
Muscular dystrophies
  Duchenne
  Limb girdle
  Becker syndrome
Neuropathies
  Guillain-Barré syndrome
  Diabetes mellitus
  Porphyria

**Metabolic/Nutritional**
Uremia
Hepatic failure
Malabsorption
Hypercalcemia or hypocalcemia
Hypernatremia or hyponatremia
Hyperkalemia or hypokalemia
Hypophosphatemia
Periodic paralysis
Vitamin E deficiency
Vitamin D deficiency

**Endocrine**
Hyperthyroidism or hypothyroidism
Hyperparathyroidism or hypoparathyroidism
Cushing's disease
Addison's disease
Hyperaldosteronism

**Carcinomatous**
Neuropathy
Neuromyopathy
Myositis
Microembolization

**Drug-induced**
Cimetidine
Clofibrate
Colchicine
Corticosteroids
ϵ-Aminocaproic acid
Emetine
Ethanol
Hydroxychloroquine
Ipecac
Lovastatin
Penicillamine
Vincristine
Zidovudine (AZT)

**Infectious**
Viral
  Influenza
  Epstein-Barr virus
  Coxsackieviruses A and B
  HIV
  Adenovirus
  Echovirus
  Rubella
Parasitic
  Toxoplasmosis
  Trichinosis
  Schistosomiasis
  Toxocariasis
  Cysticercosis
Bacterial
  Staphylococcal
  Streptococcal
  Clostridial
Rickettsia

**Storage diseases**
Glycogen storage diseases
Lipid
  Carnitine deficiency
  Carnitine palmitoyl transferase deficiency
Purine
  Myoadenylate deaminase deficiency

Modified from Wortman RL: In Wyngaarden JB, Smith LHJ, Bennett JC, editors: *Cecil textbook of medicine,* ed 19, Philadelphia, 1992, WB Saunders.

the response to therapy. Muscle enzymes may respond before improvement in muscle strength, but evaluation of functional improvement is most important. Patience on the part of the physician and patient is required; unlike many other inflammatory, autoimmune disorders, IIMs respond slowly. In patients who respond to steroids, strength usually improves in 1 to 2 months but may require 3 months. As the patient responds, the dosing frequency should first be consolidated, ultimately to a single daily dose. High-dose steroids should be continued for 4 to 6 weeks after strength has improved, before tapering is slowly begun. The lowest possible dosage that controls the disease should be used. Attaining a stable condition on the minimal dosage often requires 1 to 2 years. Alternate-day steroids may be effective but should be reserved for patients with mild disease.

A problem in treatment is the patient who responds initially but then has a decrease in strength while on a tapering steroid dosage. Coincident elevation of CK values suggests exacerbation of myositis, but if the serum CK remains normal, steroid myopathy should be considered. The EMG in steroid myopathy may show a myopathic

**Table 77-2.** Findings in IIMs and disorders commonly confused with IIMs

| | Disorder | | | | |
|---|---|---|---|---|---|
| Finding | PM | DM | IBM | PMR | Fibrositis |
| Weakness | Proximal > distal | Proximal > distal | Proximal and/or distal | No | No |
| Pain | No | No | No | Yes | Yes |
| EMG findings | Myopathic | Myopathic | Myopathic or neuropathic | Normal | Normal |
| Muscle enzymes | Elevated, up to 50 × | Elevated, up to 50 × | Elevated, up to 10 × or normal | Normal | Normal |
| Muscle biopsy | Characteristic* | Characteristic* | Characteristic* | Normal or type II fiber atrophy | Normal |
| Skin rash | No | Yes | No | No | No |

*Characteristic features may be seen in these biopsies, as described in the text.

pattern, but the fibrillations seen in IIM are not present. Muscle biopsy can help to show type II fiber atrophy without inflammation in the patient with steroid myopathy, but this is not absolute, given the focal nature of inflammation that may occur in IIM. At times, an educated guess at the direction of the steroid dosage may be necessary, either raising or lowering the dosage and awaiting signs of improvement or worsening. Given the length of time high dosages of steroids are usually required, measures to prevent potential complications of corticosteroid therapy should be instituted. Prophylaxis of steroid-induced osteoporosis with calcium (1 to 2 g per day) and vitamin D (50,000 IU twice weekly) should be undertaken.

For patients who do not respond to corticosteroids, accuracy of the diagnosis should be questioned, giving particular consideration to the possibilities of IBM or an associated malignancy, because both of these groups typically respond less well to treatment. Immunosuppressive agents may be required for patients who do not respond to steroids, flare while the dosage is being lowered, or develop intolerable side effects from steroids. Some authors advocate the early use of immunosuppressives in an attempt to minimize the potential side effects of corticosteroids. The most frequently used immunosuppressive agents are azathioprine and methotrexate, although there are reports of efficacy with 6-mercaptopurine, cyclophosphamide, chlorambucil, and cyclosporin A. A small blinded study suggested that the combined use of azathioprine and steroids for patients with PM from the onset of therapy was beneficial. Methotrexate is reported to be effective in open trials and is used widely. It can be administered intravenously, intramuscularly, or orally; the oral route is preferred to avoid elevation of CK values from the injections. A potential problem of methotrexate therapy that must be considered is that it can cause interstitial pulmonary fibrosis, which is also a potential extramuscular site of pathology in IIM.

For patients who are unresponsive to standard immunosuppressive agents, other immunosuppressive modalities have been attempted, including intravenous gamma globulin, plasmapheresis, and total body irradiation. Of these, intravenous gamma globulin appears to be the most promising. Most patients studied have had PM or DM refractory to conventional treatment with steroids and/or immunosuppressive drugs. The early results reported are encouraging in showing biochemical and clinical response in a population with more severe disease, but they require longer follow-up and confirmation in larger trials. Plasmapheresis was shown to be no more effective than sham pheresis in a controlled, blinded trial. The results of radiation therapy, either total body irradiation or total nodal irradiation, are too preliminary to recommend its use in situations other than study.

Physical therapy and other modalities are important adjuncts to the therapy of patients with IIM. During periods of active muscle inflammation, patients should be kept at bed rest. An exercise program should be initiated to include daily stretching done passively or with therapist assistance to maintain range of motion and prevent contractures. With response to medical therapy, active exercise should be encouraged, but overwork should be avoided because it can damage muscle. Adaptive aids can improve function. A raised toilet seat and grip bars can be helpful. Inspiratory muscle training can help patients with respiratory muscle weakness.

For patients with IIM associated with malignancy, the first step in management is to deal with the malignancy. If the malignancy responds to treatment, the IIM may as well, but this is highly variable. Patients with IBM are considered to be nonresponsive to therapy with steroids, but recent evidence suggests that some patients may respond with improvement or at least stabilization of strength and function. These responses have occurred with steroids, in some cases in addition to azathioprine or methotrexate; thus, an attempt to treat patients with IBM is warranted.

## BIBLIOGRAPHY

Bohan A et al: A computer-assisted analysis of 153 patients with polymyositis and dermatomyositis, *Medicine* 56:255, 1977.

Bunch TW: Polymyositis: a case history approach to the differential diagnosis and treatment, *Mayo Clin Proc* 65:1480, 1990.

Cronin ME, Plotz PH: Idiopathic inflammatory myopathies, *Rheum Dis Clin North Am* 16:655, 1990.

Dalakas MC: Polymyositis, dermatomyositis, and inclusion-body myositis, *N Engl J Med* 325:1487, 1991.

Lotz BP et al: Inclusion body myositis: observations in 40 patients, *Brain* 112:727, 1989.

Love LA et al: A new approach to the classification of idiopathic inflammatory myopathy: myositis-specific autoantibodies define useful homogenous patient groups, *Medicine* 70:360, 1991.

Masi AT, Hochberg MC: Temporal association of polymyositis-dermatomyositis with malignancy: methodologic and clinical considerations, *Mt Sinai J Med* 55:471, 1988.

Plotz PH et al: Current concepts in the idiopathic inflammatory myopathies: polymyositis, dermatomyositis, and related disorders, *Ann Intern Med* 111:143, 1989.

Strongwater SL: Overview and clinical manifestations of inflammatory myositis: polymyositis and dermatomyositis, *Mt Sinai J Med* 55:435, 1988.

Wortman RL: Polymyositis. In Wyngaarden JB et al: editors: *Cecil textbook of medicine,* ed 19, Philadelphia, 1992, WB Saunders.

CHAPTER

# 78 Osteoarthritis

**Eric W. Jacobson**

Osteoarthritis (also known as *osteoarthrosis* or *degenerative joint disease*) is the most common rheumatic disease, affecting more than 50 million people in the United States. The cost to society for treatment and lost earnings is staggering. Recent advances in the understanding of the pathophysiology of osteoarthritis have altered the conception of this disease. Once viewed as a slowly advancing disease with limited possibilities for medical intervention, it is now viewed as a disease that can be modified in regard to immediate treatment and long-term disease outcome. This chapter provides an update on advances in the understanding of osteoarthritis, concentrating on a practical approach to its diagnosis and treatment.

## EPIDEMIOLOGY

Osteoarthritis is a prevalent disease of cartilage that increases steadily with age. Up to 85% of the general population has radiographic evidence of osteoarthritis by the age of 65. There is an equal distribution of this disease among men and women when all age groups are considered. However, in people over the age of 55, women are more commonly affected and tend to have more severe disease. This may be explained by body habitus or genetic predisposition. There may be subtle differences in prevalence patterns of osteoarthritis among different races, but this may relate more to differences in occupations and lifestyles than directly to race. There is some genetic predisposition to osteoarthritis, mainly for osteoarthritis involving the distal interphalangeal (DIP) joint of the hands. Involvement of DIP joints seems to follow an autosomal dominant pattern of inheritance with variable expression. Expression is gender linked and dominant in women.

## ETIOLOGY

The etiology of osteoarthritis is multifactorial (see the box above). Clearly, there is a strong association between osteoarthritis and aging; however, osteoarthritis is not a natural consequence of aging. Biochemical changes in the matrix molecules of cartilage occur with age, but they are different from the biochemical changes that occur in osteoarthritic cartilage. Aging cartilage, however, may be more prone to osteoarthritis if other etiologic factors, such as the genetic predisposition previously noted, are present.

### Important factors in the etiology of osteoarthritis

- Age
- Genetic predisposition (DIP joints)
- Trauma/repetitive stress
- Occupation
- Obesity
- Altered joint anatomy/joint instability
- Changes in cartilage biochemistry
- Secondary inflammation

Trauma plays a significant role in the development of osteoarthritis. Joints that have sustained serious trauma (fractures, ligamentous injuries) are prone to the development of osteoarthritis in later years. Joints exposed to repetitive trauma also are associated with the development of osteoarthritis. This has been related to occupation. Ballet dancers, for instance, have an increased incidence of osteoarthritis in the ankles and feet, supposedly related to repetitive, lifelong trauma across these joints; American football players, on the other hand, are prone to knee osteoarthritis. An exception to this concept is the long-distance runner. Studies have failed to show an increased incidence of osteoarthritis in lower extremity joints in long-distance runners, despite the repetitive stress these joints experience. This may be explained by a self-selected body habitus in runners that, at baseline, may be associated with protection against the development of osteoarthritis.

Obesity may be another etiologic factor associated with the development of osteoarthritis. However, studies evaluating obesity as a risk factor for osteoarthritis show conflicting results. Leach showed a statistically significant increase of knee osteoarthritis in obese women but not in obese men.

Any alteration of normal joint anatomy or of joint stability is associated with an increased risk of the development of osteoarthritis in that joint. This is true for congenital abnormalities (e.g., congenital hip dislocation), as well as for acquired abnormalities (chronic dislocation resulting from trauma). Altered joint anatomy leads to a change in the distribution of force across that joint. In a normal joint, force is distributed uniformly across the cartilaginous surface. If the anatomy is altered, forces across the joint may localize to one area of cartilage, leading to focal damage. This initiates the osteoarthritic process. Therefore any process leading to joint destruction predisposes to secondary osteoarthritis. This includes inflammatory arthropathies (e.g., rheumatoid arthritis [RA], gout, and pseudogout), metabolic conditions affecting joints (hemochromatosis, ochronosis), bleeding diatheses such as hemophilia in which recurrent hemarthrosis occurs, avascular necrosis with subsequent alteration of normal bony contour, and neurologic disorders associated with altered sensation or proprioception around a joint.

### Composition of cartilage

Interstitial fluid
Cellular elements
- Stationary (chondrocytes)
- Circulatory (mononuclear cells)

Proteins
- Type II collagen
- Elastin
- Fibronectin

Complex polysaccharides
- Proteoglycans (glycosaminoglycans plus hyaluronic acid backbone)

Alterations in the molecular composition of cartilage and secondary inflammatory processes, also important etiologic factors in the development of osteoarthritis, are discussed further in the section on pathophysiology.

## PATHOPHYSIOLOGY

To understand the pathophysiology of osteoarthritis, one must first review the composition of normal articular cartilage (see the box above). Cartilage is composed of interstitial fluid, cellular elements, and matrix molecules. Approximately 70% of cartilage is water; this percentage increases with advancing stages of osteoarthritis. Cellular elements may be stationary (such as chondrocytes) or circulatory (such as lymphocytes and other mononuclear cells). The chondrocyte synthesizes matrix molecules, thus possessing reparative capabilities. The major matrix molecules consist of proteins (collagen, mainly type II, elastin, and fibronectin) and complex polysaccharides (proteoglycans). The proteoglycan molecule is made up of a hyaluronic acid backbone with glycosaminoglycan derivatives attached at roughly a 90-degree angle. This composition gives cartilage strength and elasticity. Its function is to absorb impact loading across the joint and to allow smooth gliding of juxtaposed articular surfaces.

The pathogenesis of osteoarthritis involves a dual process of catabolism and repair. In normal cartilage, there is an ongoing remodeling process. Matrix molecules are regularly degraded by autolytic enzymes and then are replaced via production by chondrocytes. In osteoarthritis, this process is altered in a way that causes an overall loss of the matrix molecules despite attempts at repair. The newly synthesized matrix molecules are considered to be mechanically inferior to normal ones; therefore they may be more prone to injury and further damage.

The process may be initiated by a local trauma that leads to chondrocyte injury. Chondrocytes release proteolytic enzymes, such as neutral proteases, acid cathepsins, collagenase, and metalloproteases. These enzymes degrade matrix molecules, including the proteoglycan aggregate, producing smaller, nonaggregating molecules. This leads to thinner, mechanically inferior cartilage. The rate of release of these enzymes and the subsequent rate of matrix molecule destruction are significantly more rapid in osteoarthritic cartilage than in normal cartilage.

With the changes in the cartilage matrix composition there is a loss of tensile strength for load support. This leads to transmission of greater force to chondrocytes and subchondral bone. Chondrocytes sustain greater injury, leading to further release of degrading enzymes. Subchondral bone sustains microfractures, causing stiffening and loss of compressibility. Some of the breakdown products from cartilage and proteoglycans may stimulate a secondary inflammatory response involving polymorphonuclear leukocytes, synovial cells, and macrophages. The whole process is perpetuated in a continuous destructive cycle (Fig. 78-1).

## HISTORY

Osteoarthritis is the prototype of a noninflammatory arthritis. From the history the clinician should begin to differentiate osteoarthritis from inflammatory arthropathies, such as RA. Osteoarthritis typically begins in the later decades of life. It has a slow, insidious onset that is gradually progressive over many years. The joint distribution is quite distinctive, mainly involving the weight-bearing joints, the spine, and the hands. Unless there is a history of trauma or other predisposing factors, osteoarthritis typically spares the wrists, elbows, and shoulders. Involvement of any of these joints without a history of trauma should lead the clinician to look for other causes of the arthritis.

The patient describes classic mechanical joint pain. The pain is typically aching in quality and is brought on by usage of the joint. Early in the disease the pain is relieved by rest. In advanced disease, pain occurs at rest and with exertion. This is in contrast to inflammatory arthritis, in which pain frequently improves with activity. In classic osteoarthritis, patients complain of pain, but there is no obvious swelling, redness, or warmth. With time the patient may describe progressive bony enlargement of joints and restricted joint motion. The patient classically describes short-term stiffness after inactivity and less than 30 minutes of stiffness in the morning. This is in contrast to the classic inflammatory arthritides, in which morning stiffness can be very prolonged and may correlate with disease activity. Patients may also describe a creaking or cracking of joints with motion that may worsen with progressive loss of cartilage. The box below summarizes the classic features of osteoarthritis.

Osteoarthritis may involve the cervical and the lumbosacral spine. This is in contrast to RA, which commonly involves the cervical spine but spares the lumbosacral spine. Nerve root compression may occur with spinal involvement. The patient may then complain of radiating

### Classic features of osteoarthritis

- Aging population
- Insidious onset over many years
- Mechanical pain that worsens with activity
- Bony enlargement, but *no* true swelling, warmth, or erythema
- Progressive loss of joint range of motion
- Short-term morning stiffness (less than 30 minutes)

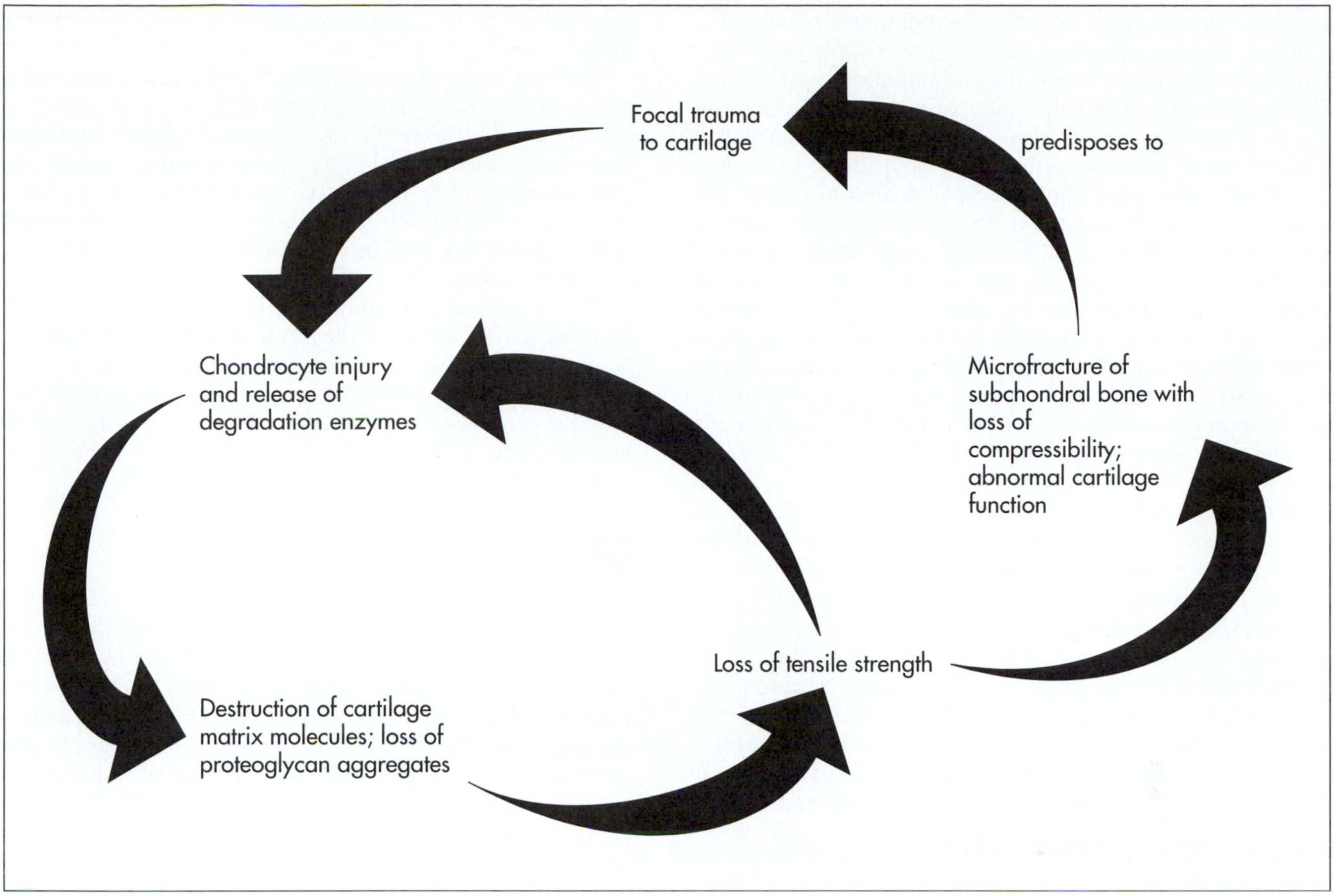


**Fig. 78-1.** Pathogenesis of osteoarthritis.

pain down an extremity, associated with paresthesias and/or focal weakness. These symptoms should present in a dermatomal distribution. Osteoarthritic involvement of the lumbar spine can also lead to spinal stenosis. The classic history of spinal stenosis is that of leg claudication. Pain occurs with ambulation, persists with stopping and standing, but is relieved with sitting or bending forward. Vascular claudication, on the other hand, is relieved with stopping and standing still.

Several subsets of osteoarthritis have been defined. One is inflammatory or erosive osteoarthritis. This form of osteoarthritis also involves hands (proximal interphalangeal [PIP] and DIP joints) but is associated with inflammatory signs and symptoms (i.e., swelling, redness, and warmth). True erosions occur, leading to joint destruction and occasionally bony ankylosis. This arthropathy may be confused with psoriatic arthritis, another erosive arthropathy commonly affecting DIP joints.

### Joint distribution in osteoarthritis

- Weight-bearing joints
  - Hips
  - Knees
- Spine
  - Cervical spine
  - Lumbosacral spine
- Hands
  - CMC joints
  - PIP joints (Bouchard's nodes)
  - DIP joints (Heberden's nodes)
- Feet
  - First MTP joints

## PHYSICAL EXAMINATION

The physical examination of a patient with osteoarthritis requires consideration of the typical joint distribution (see the box at right). Osteoarthritis tends to involve the weight-bearing joints, the spine, and the hands. Hips and knees are commonly affected, usually in a somewhat symmetric fashion. As noted, osteoarthritis involves the cervical and lumbosacral spines. In the hands the classic joint involvement includes the first carpometacarpal (CMC) joint at the base of the thumb, the PIP joints, and the DIP joints. This is in contrast to RA, which involves the metacarpophalangeal (MCP) joints and PIP joints but spares the DIP joints. Osteoarthritis also commonly involves the first metatarsophalangeal (MTP) joints of the feet.

Joint examination in osteoarthritis depends on the area being examined. In general, there is pain with motion and sometimes with palpation, limited range of motion of the joint (related to loss of articular cartilage), and bony enlargement of the joint (related to the proliferative spurs). The capsule may appear thickened. In typical osteoarthritis, there are no signs of active inflammation: warmth, erythema, or true effusions. Lack of these signs helps distinguish osteoarthritis from the inflammatory arthritides.

Examination of the spine may reveal loss of range of motion, depending on the stage of the disease. When spinal involvement is present, a thorough neurologic examination of the extremities should be performed to screen for nerve root impingement syndromes. Hip examination reveals loss of range of motion and pain. Knee examination shows loss of motion, but in addition crepitus (a feeling of crunching when the joint is moved) frequently occurs. Effusions are generally absent. Bony enlargement of PIP and DIP joints leads to a knobby appearance. These changes are referred to as *Bouchard nodes* in the PIP joints and *Heberden nodes* in the DIP joints. CMC involvement is associated with a squaring at the base of the thumb, usually accompanied by marked pain with squeezing. MTP involvement is often associated with bunion formation.

As osteoarthritis progresses, loss of articular cartilage becomes more prominent and the normal anatomy is altered. This changes the distribution of force across the joint, sometimes leading to strain across tendons, bursae, and other periarticular structures. The physician must therefore check for the presence of soft-tissue rheumatism in areas that are in close proximity to osteoarthritic joints. Trochanteric bursitis of the hip and anserine bursitis of the knee are common causes of pain, in addition to the pain caused by the osteoarthritis (see Chapters 74 and 75).

## LABORATORY STUDIES AND DIAGNOSTIC PROCEDURES

Laboratory studies in osteoarthritis are generally unrevealing. Tests checking for systemic inflammation (erythrocyte sedimentation rate [ESR] and C-reactive protein), blood counts, and general chemistries are normal. Ordering rheumatology profiles is not indicated when the history and physical examination are consistent with osteoarthritis.

Routine x-ray films confirm the presence of osteoarthritis (Fig. 78-2). They are helpful in establishing the extent of the disease. X-ray findings include joint-space narrowing, subchondral bony sclerosis, subchondral cysts, and osteophytes (proliferative spurs) (see the box on p. 1097 and Chapter 69). Erosions are not seen in general osteoarthritis but may be seen in the inflammatory subset of osteoarthritis.

Computerized tomography (CT) or magnetic resonance imaging (MRI) scans of the spine may be indicated if the patient has signs or symptoms suggesting a nerve impingement syndrome. These studies rule out neuroforaminal encroachment or disk herniation leading to nerve impingement. They also assess for associated spinal stenosis.

## MANAGEMENT

As with any arthritis, treatment should begin with educating the patient, who should understand the diagnosis, its prognosis, and the treatment options (see the box on p. 1097). In osteoarthritis, it is important to preserve joint cartilage and thus range of motion. This can be accomplished by teaching the patient the concept of joint protection. The patient should avoid activities that lead to repetitive trauma to the joint. For example, jogging is not an ideal exercise for people with osteoarthritis of the knee. Jogging leads to repetitive stress across the knee joints and could predispose cartilage to more rapid deterioration. For similar reasons, weight loss is an appropriate goal for patients with osteoarthritis involving lower extremities and the lumbar spine.

Physical therapy and occupational therapy are useful modalities for patients with osteoarthritis. Basic physical

A

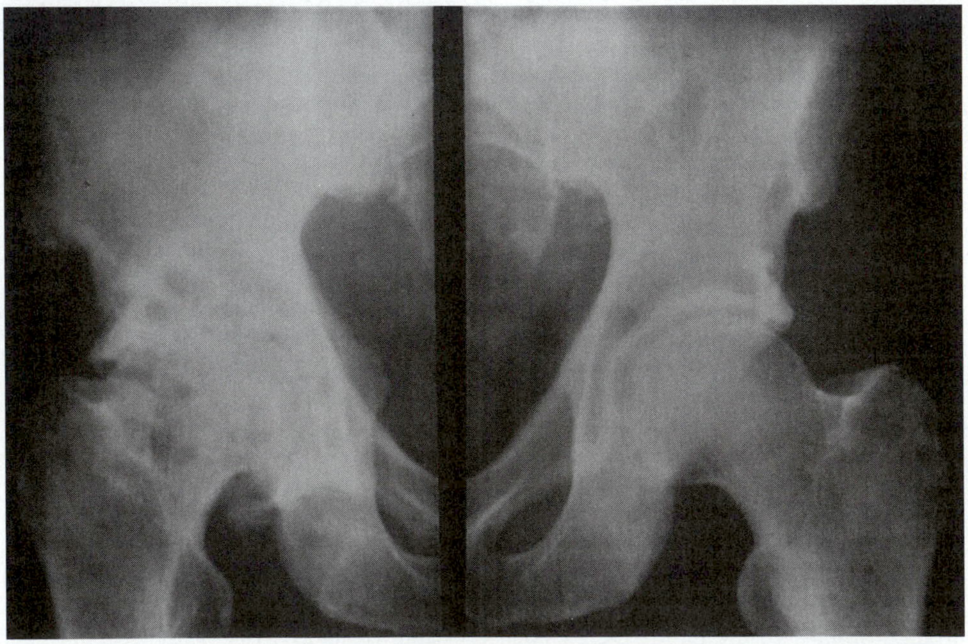

B

**Fig. 78-2.** Comparison of severe osteoarthritis of the hip (**A**) with a normal hip (**B**). (From the American Rheumatism Association.)

### Radiographic changes in osteoarthritis

Joint space narrowing
Subchondral bony sclerosis
Subchondral cysts
Osteophytes (proliferative spurs)

### Treatment options for osteoarthritis

Patient education
Periodic rest
Joint protection
Weight loss
Physical therapy
Occupational therapy
Medications
- Analgesics
- Nonsteroidal antiinflammatory drugs (NSAIDs)
- Topical capsaicin
- Glycosaminoglycan derivatives (experimental)
- Intraarticular corticosteroid injections

Surgery
- Osteotomy
- Joint debridement
- Arthrodesis (fusion)
- Arthroplasty (replacement)

therapy should include education regarding range-of-motion exercises, which may preserve joint mobility. Physical therapists teach patients appropriate strengthening exercises geared at preserving the strength of muscle groups surrounding involved joints. This helps maintain stability of the joints, reduce pain, and prevent injury. Physical therapy can also be used to help with pain control. Heat, ultrasound, and massage techniques may reduce pain. For chronic pain unresponsive to other measures, a transcutaneous electric nerve stimulation (TENS) trial may be appropriate. The patient can be taught how to use a TENS unit and can wear the unit throughout the day. The TENS unit can be adjusted to maximize electrical output when pain increases. This is helpful for some patients with chronic low back, hip, and knee pain related to osteoarthritis. An occupational therapy evaluation is useful in assessing the patient's functional limitations. Occupational therapists can provide patients with assistive devices that allow them to continue to perform home or work tasks that would otherwise be difficult or impossible, as well as teach patients the principles of joint protection and energy conservation.

The main medications used for the treatment of osteoarthritis are analgesics and NSAIDs. Both types of medication reduce pain. NSAIDs have the added advantage of reducing any secondary inflammation that may be present. Bradley and co-workers found little difference between these two types of medications for short-term pain control in symptomatic osteoarthritis of the knee. Further studies are required to assess benefit versus risk of these medications for osteoarthritis in general. In early disease, analgesics may be tried on an as-needed basis. As the disease progresses, regular use of analgesics or NSAIDs may be required to control symptoms. Patients taking NSAIDs chronically must be monitored closely for toxicity, especially gastrointestinal complications (gastritis or peptic ulcer disease) and renal insufficiency.

Topical capsaicin is another medication that may be useful in the treatment of osteoarthritis. Capsaicin has the ability to deplete and prevent reaccumulation of substance P at the sensory nerve terminals, thus reducing pain. It is usually applied four times per day. Local burning may occur initially, but this side effect generally ceases with continued usage.

Glycosaminoglycan derivatives are being studied as potential chondroprotective agents in osteoarthritis. These agents can be injected intramuscularly or intraarticularly. They may slow or prevent progression of cartilage degradation. They are not available for general use.

Another treatment option for osteoarthritis is the judicial use of intraarticular corticosteroid injections. These injections can provide temporary relief of pain in some patients with osteoarthritis. A long-acting corticosteroid preparation (triamcinolone hexacetonide or Depo-medrol) mixed with a local anesthetic (1% lidocaine) is generally used. Patients are instructed to rest the joint for 2 to 3 days after an injection. The main complications include infection (less than 0.001%), bleeding, skin atrophy, and postinjection flare. Frequent injections with corticosteroids may accelerate cartilage deterioration. For this reason the same joint should not be injected more frequently than every 3 months. If a joint is injected at this frequency for more than 1 year, alternate treatment options should be explored.

The final treatment option for osteoarthritis is surgery. Surgical procedures may include osteotomy, joint debridement, arthrodesis (fusion), and arthroplasty (replacement). Joint replacement should be considered for patients who have significant disability related to the osteoarthritis and for whom medical treatment options have failed.

## BIBLIOGRAPHY


Bland JH, Cooper SM: Osteoarthritis: a review of the cell biology involved and evidence for reversibility. Management rationally related to known genesis and pathophysiology, *Semin Arthritis Rheum* 14:106, 1984.

Bradley JD et al: Comparison of an antiinflammatory dose of ibuprofen, an analgesic dose of ibuprofen, and acetaminophen in the treatment of patients with osteoarthritis of the knee, *N Engl J Med* 325:87, 1991.

Kellgren JH: Osteoarthritis in patients and populations, *Br Med J* 2:1, 1961.

Leach RE, Baumgard S, Broom J: Obesity: its relationship to osteoarthritis of the knee, *Clin Orthop* 93:271, 1973.

McCarthy GM, McCarty DJ: Effect of topical capsaicin in the therapy of painful osteoarthritis of the hands, *J Rheumatol* 19:604, 1992.

Moskowitz RW et al: *Osteoarthritis: diagnosis and management,* Philadelphia, 1984, WB Saunders.

Puranen J et al: Running and primary osteoarthritis of the hip, *Br Med J* 2:424, 1975.

Roberts J, Burch TA: *Prevalence of osteoarthritis in adults by age, sex, race and geographic area, United States—1960-1962,* US Public Health Service Pub No 1000, series 11, no. 15, Washington, DC, 1966, US Government Printing Office.

Ryu J, Treadwell BV, Mankin HJ: Biochemical and metabolic abnormalities in normal and osteoarthritic human articular cartilage, *Arthritis Rheum* 27:613, 1984.

CHAPTER

# 79 Rheumatoid Arthritis

Tammi L. Shlotzhauer
James L. McGuire

## EPIDEMIOLOGY AND ETIOLOGY

Rheumatoid arthritis (RA) is an inflammatory arthritis with a prevalence of approximately 1% of the population. It is estimated to affect 3 to 5 million Americans, women are three times as likely as men to develop the condition.

The etiology of RA is unknown. Epidemiologic studies suggest a variety of associations that may be related to a cause or to a disease amplifier. First, the human leukocyte antigen HLA-DR4 has been associated with RA, particularly in patients with more severe or aggressive clinical disease. Second, low formal educational level appears to have a negative influence on the severity of the disease once it is established. Similarly, less education may have a role in the initial development of RA, possibly through behavioral risk factors. Third, a relationship between hormonal and reproductive factors and the development of RA has been reported in several studies. Some studies suggest that a history of previous pregnancy and oral contraceptive use protects women from developing RA, whereas other studies do not show this protective effect. Although the mechanism for this possible protective effect is unknown, the influence of hormones and gender on the development of RA appears to be important. Fourth, numerous infectious agents, particularly Epstein-Barr virus and *Mycobacterium* species, have been associated with RA, perhaps as an environmental trigger without persisting in the host. Therefore it appears that certain environmental, hormonal, and infectious agents may trigger this disease in the genetically susceptible individual. In addition, once the disease is established, some of these same factors can influence the clinical course.

## PATHOPHYSIOLOGY

Previously the pathophysiology within the joint in patients with RA was broadly divided into inflammatory and proliferative phases. It was assumed that the inflammation occurred first, usually in response to a series of external agents (infectious, hormonal, environmental) in the susceptible individual. The inflammatory response became chronic and supported the development of the proliferative phase in the synovium, which resulted in the invasive pannus. A variety of cells, especially lymphocytes (both B and T cells), macrophages, and fibroblasts could be identified in the established lesion. However, this pathophysiologic separation is oversimplified. Both the inflammatory and proliferative components represent a continuum of interrelated events driven by cells and cytokines.

The pathophysiologic processes involved in RA have been correlated with clinical manifestations. The five phases (Table 79-1) incorporate the dominant pathophysiologic events that can be observed during the first few years of established disease. These events could be targeted therapeutically.

**1987 American College of Rheumatology criteria for the classification of rheumatoid arthritis***

1. Morning stiffness lasting at least 1 hour before maximal improvement
2. At least three joint areas simultaneously having had swelling observed by a physician (The 14 possible areas are right and left PIP, MCP, wrist, elbow, knee, ankle, and MTP joints.)
3. Swelling in a wrist, MCP, or PIP joint
4. Symmetric involvement of the same joint areas (as defined in 2); bilateral involvement of the PIPs, MCPs, or MTPs is acceptable without absolute symmetry
5. Subcutaneous nodules observed by a physician
6. Demonstration of positive rheumatoid factor
7. Radiographic changes typical of rheumatoid arthritis, including erosions of unequivocal periarticular bony decalcification, present at least 6 weeks

Modified from Arnett et al, *Arthritis Rheum* 31:315, 1988.
*For the diagnosis of RA, 4 of 7 criteria are required.
*PIP,* Proximal interphalangeal; *MTP,* metatarsophalangeal.

In 1987 criteria for the classification of RA were revised by the American College of Rheumatology (see the box above). To make a diagnosis of RA, criteria 1 through 4 must have been present for at least 6 weeks, and four or more criteria must be met.

RA is a heterogenous disorder that varies in its presentation and clinical course. The onset of RA may be gradual or sudden, involving one or many joints. Most commonly the onset is insidious, presenting as slowly progressive pain and stiffness in the joints over weeks to months. Small joints of the hands and feet are most commonly involved at the onset. Swelling may not be apparent initially despite significant arthralgias. The pain tends to increase slowly, and swelling eventually becomes manifest. This may take months or, rarely, years. In most situations, arthritis presents in a symmetric fashion involving several joints. However, monoarticular or asymmetric arthritis may be the first sign.

In the geriatric population, significant morning stiffness with nonspecific muscle aching, particularly in the shoulders and hips, is a common form of onset, often mimicking polymyalgia rheumatica. It may take weeks to months before joint swelling occurs.

In addition to joint and muscular complaints, fatigue is the most prominent presenting feature of RA, often more debilitating than the arthritis itself.

Fortunately, the acute and intense onset of arthritis presenting with systemic features (e.g., severe fatigue, low-grade fever, anorexia, and weight loss) is rare. RA that presents in this fashion must be differentiated from sepsis, paraneoplastic syndromes, and hypersensitivity reactions. Although impressive in its intensity, this presentation is not predictive of a poor prognosis.

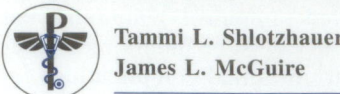

**Table 79-1.** Stages of rheumatoid arthritis

| Pathogenesis | Symptoms | Physical signs | Radiographic changes |
|---|---|---|---|
| **Stage 1** | | | |
| Antigen presentation to T cells | Probably none | — | — |
| **Stage 2** | | | |
| T cell proliferation<br>B cell proliferation<br>Angiogenesis in synovium | Malaise<br>Mild joint stiffness | Possibly, swelling of small joints of hands or wrists | None |
| **Stage 3** | | | |
| PMN leukocyte accumulation in synovial fluid<br>Synovial-cell proliferation without polarization | Joint pain and swelling<br>Morning stiffness<br>Malaise and weakness | Warm, swollen joints<br>Synovial fluid in excess<br>Soft-tissue proliferation within joints<br>Pain and limitation of motion | Soft-tissue swelling |
| **Stage 4** | | | |
| Polarization of synovitis into a centripetally invasive pannus<br>Activation of chondrocytes | Same | Same, but more pronounced swelling | MRI revealing proliferative pannus<br>Periarticular osteopenia indicated by radiographs |
| **Stage 5** | | | |
| Erosion of subchondral bone<br>Invasion of cartilage by pannus<br>Chondrocyte proliferation<br>Stretched ligaments around joints | Same, plus loss of function and early deformity (e.g., ulnar deviation at MCP joints) | Same, plus instability of joints, flexion contractures, and decreased range of motion<br>Extraarticular complications | Early erosions and joint-space narrowing |

From Harris ED Jr, *N Engl J Med* 322(18):1277, 1990.
*PMN*, Polymorphonuclear; *MRI*, magnetic resonance imaging; *MCP*, metacarpophalangeal.

The natural history of RA is also varied and may even change over time in the same person. The presentation in many instances helps predict the subsequent course. RA can take one of four general courses (Table 79-2): spontaneous remission, palindromic or remitting, remitting-progressive, or progressive.

RA can go into a *spontaneous remission* over weeks to months in 10% to 20% of patients. More than 50% of these patients experience a recurrence of RA. Thus the permanent remission rate without treatment is only 5% to 10%.

Physicians often question how long they should wait for potential remission before initiating disease-modifying antirheumatic drugs (DMARDs). Each case should be individualized; however, most rheumatologists begin a DMARD when there is a possibility of impending joint damage. They certainly do so if erosive changes are present on x-ray film. This is particularly important, since DMARDs appear to be most effective early in the course of RA.

Recurrent flare-ups of arthritis with return to normal health between attacks is the hallmark of the *remitting or palindromic course.* These attacks are commonly treated with nonsteroidal antiinflammatory drugs (NSAIDs). DMARDs may not be required if signs of joint damage are absent and the patient returns to normal joint function between flare-ups. If attacks are frequent, protracted, or debilitating, DMARDs should be considered to prevent recurrences.

**Table 79-2.** Clinical course of RA

| Clinical course | Comment |
|---|---|
| Spontaneous remission | Unusual without DMARD exposure |
| Palindromic or remitting | Classic RA developing in 50% of cases |
| Remitting-progressive | No return to normal baseline |
| Progressive | Disability proportional to duration |

*DMARD*, Disease-modifying antirheumatic drug.

In the *remitting-progressive course* complete return to a normal state between attacks does not occur. Ongoing destructive changes develop resulting from persistent active synovitis. DMARD therapy should be strongly considered for patients with this course of disease.

The most common course of RA is characterized by an ongoing synovitis with progressive increase of pain, swelling, and joint damage. The progression of synovitis is generally insidious but may result in a rapid decline of function. Early DMARD therapy is recommended in an attempt to halt the progression of arthritis in this group of patients.

The literature of the past decade has emphasized that patients with chronic RA experience progressive disability and premature mortality. This is in contrast with previous clinical impressions that RA had a relatively benign course. Recent studies suggest that patients who develop more severe disease develop erosive lesions within the first 2 years of diagnosis. Early identification of this subset of patients with more aggressive disease is an area of active investigation. Prognosis is being reevaluated from the perspective of genetics, timing of first exposure to DMARDs, educational level, and articular cartilage damage evidenced on MRI. These factors are being integrated with traditional predictors of disease severity, including positive rheumatoid factor, subcutaneous nodules, insidious onset of joint disease, and erosion of bone on plain radiographs.

### Complications of RA

Musculoskeletal complications of RA can include significant cervical spine involvement with atlantoaxial subluxation and/or impaction and subaxial impaction. Cervical spine involvement should be considered in all rheumatoid patients with painless sensory loss, paresthesias, severe neck or shoulder girdle pain, or weakness in the upper extremities, particularly if deficits increase with neck motion. More serious symptoms of myelopathy, such as loss of sphincter control, dysphagia, vertigo, or syncopal episodes, require immediate intervention. MRI is the radiographic technique of choice to assess for cervical cord compression. Evaluation for cervical spine stability with lateral neck plain radiographs in flexion and extension is recommended for any patient with advanced RA who is being considered for general anesthesia with intubation and concomitant hyperextension of the neck.

The sudden onset or progression of hoarseness should prompt laryngoscopic evaluation for cricoarytenoid joint involvement. Inspiratory stridor may occur and should be considered a medical emergency.

Extraarticular complications of RA may vary in severity. Rheumatoid nodules, generally found on extensor surfaces, are noted in up to one third of patients with RA. Nodules rarely cause more than cosmetic problems but can be painful if traumatized. Other systemic features include sicca syndrome secondary to inflammatory changes in lacrimal and salivary glands and in other exocrine glands. Diffuse lymphadenopathy may also be a feature of RA. Lymph node biopsy should be considered if there is a concern of malignancy.

Hematologic abnormalities that may occur include anemia of chronic disease, eosinophilia, and thrombocytosis. Far less common is the occurrence of Felty's syndrome, a triad of seropositive RA, significant hypersplenism, and granulocytopenia. Such patients may be susceptible to infection. If infections are recurrent, corticosteroid, DMARD, or immunosuppressive therapy may be required after the existing infection is eradicated. Splenectomy has been performed on many patients without clear evidence of utility demonstrated. Drugs used to treat RA may also cause hematologic abnormalities, including anemia from gastrointestinal bleeding and bone marrow suppression.

Systemic vasculitis can occur in patients with severe, deforming RA and high titers of rheumatoid factor. Vascular damage can range from small vessel involvement, causing palpable purpura, to a necrotizing, medium-sized arteritis. Periungual nail infarcts are common and require no specific treatment. In contrast, systemic vasculitis with signs of mononeuritis multiplex, visceral vasculitis, cutaneous ulceration, digital infarction, or other organ involvement requires prompt, aggressive treatment.

Peripheral nerve pathology can occur in addition to the structural cervical neurologic complications previously described. Compressive neuropathies, particularly carpal tunnel syndrome, are common. Peripheral nerve damage can also result from angiopathic, amyloid, and monoclonal antibody-induced inflammatory polyneuropathy.

Pulmonary involvement can take the form of pleural diseases, interstitial fibrosis, nodules, pneumonitis, vasculitis, and airways disease. Pleural involvement is frequent but generally asymptomatic. Large pleural effusions may cause shortness of breath. In rare instances a progressive form of pulmonary fibrosis occurs. The diagnosis can be supported by finding large numbers of polymorphonuclear cells in bronchoalveolar lavage.

Symptomatic cardiac complications are rare. Pericarditis is frequently described but rarely results in cardiac tamponade. Less frequent cardiac involvement includes myocarditis, endocardial changes, arteritis, and conduction defects.

Ocular manifestations range from those that are relatively innocuous to those resulting in blindness. Severity often parallels activity, intensity, and chronicity of RA. Most common is keratoconjunctivitis sicca. Less common and more severe complications include keratitis, episcleritis, scleritis, uveitis, and retinopathy. Visual changes or eye pain should be promptly evaluated by an ophthalmologist who is familiar with RA.

## PHYSICAL EXAMINATION

The physical examination almost always reflects some synovitis. However, early in the disease course, the classic symmetric arthritis involving the hands, wrists, knees, and feet, which is typical of well-established disease, may not be present. The examination may reveal a single swollen joint or an asymmetric pattern of oligoarthritis. Moreover, myalgias are not typically accompanied by obvious weakness early in the course.

Observable changes in the physical examination include warmth, soft tissue swelling, effusion, tenderness, and diminished range of motion of involved joints. Potentially involved joints include the neck, shoulders, elbows, wrists, MCP joints, PIP joints, hips, knees, ankles, MTP joints, and tarsal joints. Less commonly involved joints include the sternoclavicular, acromioclavicular, temporomandibular, and cricoarytenoid joints.

Changes specific to the shoulder include rotator cuff injury with superior migration of the humeral head. Loss of full extension is an early change noted in the elbow. Hand and wrist findings are frequent. Early changes can include diffuse puffiness of the digits with MCP and/or PIP soft tissue swelling (Fig. 79-1). Ulnar deviation at the MCP joint is a result of connective tissue injury and mechanical factors. The swan neck deformity is frequently observed with flexion of the DIP and MCP joints and hyperextension of the PIP joints. Extensor hood damage can result in fixed flexion of the PIP and hyperextension of the DIP, resulting in boutonnière deformity. Evidence of tenosynovitis may also be present, particularly in the wrists and dorsum of the hands. Patients with marked proliferative tenosynovitis may experience tendon rupture.

Lower extremity signs include knee synovitis with

A

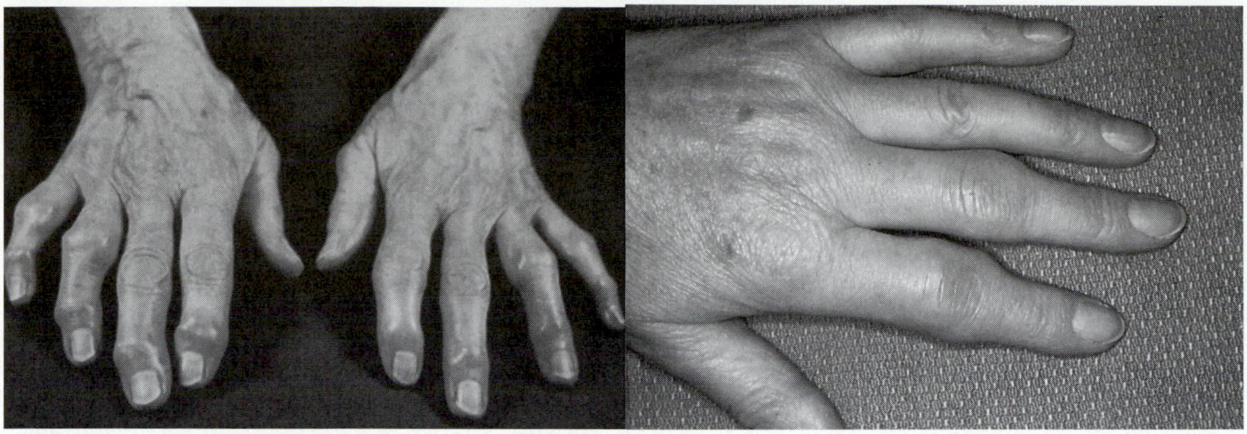

B

**Fig. 79-1.** **A,** Bony proximal interphalangeal (PIP) hypertrophy (osteoarthritis). **B,** Synovial PIP hypertrophy (rheumatoid arthritis). (Courtesy American Rheumatism Association.)

effusion, quadriceps atrophy, and popliteal cysts. Ankle and foot deformities are frequent in RA. Valgus of the ankle, pes planus, and forefoot varus deformity frequently exist simultaneously. MTP joints are often involved with downward subluxation of the metatarsal heads, cock-up deformities, hammer toes, and hallux valgus.

## LABORATORY STUDIES AND DIAGNOSTIC PROCEDURES

Early in the course of RA, clinical history and examination may be more definitive than laboratory analysis. Nonspecific inflammatory indices are commonly present, such as elevations of the erythrocyte sedimentation rate (ESR), C-reactive protein, and gamma globulins, as well as the presence of normocytic anemia, leukocytosis, and thrombocytosis. Rheumatoid factor, frequently absent in the first year of symptoms, eventually converts to a positive status in approximately 80% of patients. Antinuclear antibody (ANA) is frequently present in RA.

Synovial fluid analysis is helpful in the diagnosis of RA and other forms of inflammatory arthritis. Synovial cell counts commonly range from 2000 to 50,000 per $mm^3$ in affected joints, with a predominance of polymorphonuclear cells. Early in the course of RA, counts may be lower with a relative monocytosis. Synovial fluid glucose levels are usually equal to, but can be lower than, serum levels of glucose in chronic, severely inflamed joints. Synovial fluid from these joints, or from those of monoarticular presentation, should also be examined with Gram's stain and culture for bacterial infection. Synovial glucose is routinely extremely low in infected joints.

Synovial tissue biopsy may be useful when the diagnosis of RA is elusive. This is particularly important in chronic monoarticular arthritis of unclear etiology. Tissue is best obtained arthroscopically, but it can also be obtained blindly using needle biopsy.

## DIFFERENTIAL DIAGNOSIS

It is often difficult on initial presentation to differentiate RA from other forms of inflammatory arthritis. Frequently, laboratory analysis is not revealing, and historical clues are particularly important. Four determinants are consistently used in the differential diagnosis of arthritis: the gender of the patient, the age of the patient on presentation, the pattern of joint involvement, and the clinical course of the arthritis. For instance, classic RA occurs in women during their fourth decade, and is a symmetric, progressive arthritis.

The presence of low-back and sacroiliac discomfort should direct the physician toward the HLA-B27–associated diseases, or so-called seronegative spondyloarthropathies. Ankylosing spondylitis in women often is not accompanied by the marked back stiffness and discomfort observed in men. With Reiter's syndrome, questions and examination should be directed toward uncovering evidence of insertional tendinitis, fasciitis, "sausage" digits, conjunctivitis, genital lesions, or urethral symptoms. Reactive polyarthritis can also be associated with psoriasis, inflammatory bowel disease, Whipple's disease, and Behçet's disease, although the association with HLA-B27 is weaker than in ankylosing spondylitis and Reiter's syndrome.

The crystal arthropathies are common and are frequently confused with RA. Chronic gout may mimic RA with symmetric polyarthritis, tophaceous nodules, and recurrent attacks. The abrupt onset and resolution of attacks in early gout, as well as the presence of hyperuricemia, can direct the physician toward the correct diagnosis. Calcium pyrophosphate dihydrate deposition disease (CPPD) or pseudogout may be difficult to differentiate from RA because both conditions can involve similar joints and develop subacutely. Radiographic evidence of chondrocalcinosis is helpful. Definitive diagnosis of gout and pseudogout are usually confirmed by arthrocentesis and examination of synovial fluid for crystals.

Other forms of diffuse connective tissue disease, including systemic lupus erythematosus (SLE), vasculitis, scleroderma, polymyositis, and mixed connective tissue disease, may resemble RA on initial presentation. Primary Sjögren's syndrome is frequently confused with RA clinically and serologically. Significant eye and mouth dryness and the presence of ANA, including SSA and SSB, can provide direction toward the correct diagnosis.

In the systemically ill patient with inflammatory arthritis, the physician should also consider the possibilities of bacterial endocarditis, septic arthritis, Lyme disease, and malignancy if suggestive historical or physical clues are present. Other less acute systemic conditions that can present as polyarthritis include thyroid disease, sarcoidosis, amyloidosis, and paraproteinemias.

Three additional entities are occasionally confused with RA because of patients' similarities in age, gender, morning stiffness, and periodic joint attacks. Fibromyalgia is a clinical syndrome of multiple aches and pains, prominent morning stiffness, and nonrestorative sleep that occurs predominantly in middle-aged women. Synovitis is not present, but classic muscle tender points are present and associated with normal blood counts, ESRs, and blood chemistries. Prominent myalgias and morning stiffness are also characteristic of polymyalgia rheumatica, but this presents almost exclusively after the age of 55. Synovitis can be present in some cases. The ESR is generally significantly elevated, and response to corticosteroids is almost immediate. Palindromic rheumatism may be a presentation of RA, but this can exist as an independent clinical entity. Observation over time, often years, may be necessary to make this differential diagnosis.

## MANAGEMENT

### Pharmacologic

Traditionally, medical treatment for RA was outlined according to a pyramid approach. This entailed therapy that began with nonpharmacologic modalities and NSAIDs at the base of the pyramid. In the distant past, frank destructive changes on radiographs were mandated before physicians moved up the therapeutic pyramid to DMARDs. Most commonly, 2 to 3 years elapsed before DMARDs were even considered. It is now appreciated that cartilage erosions and resultant irreversible damage can occur within 2 years of the diagnosis of RA. Epidemiologic data that suggest progressive disability and premature mortality in RA has resulted in the use of DMARDs earlier in the clinical course. Moreover, combinations of DMARD have been advocated for progressive disease.

Current rheumatology practice supports prompt aggressive intervention with DMARDs in an effort to halt early, irreversible damage in a trend referred to as inverting the pyramid. There have been many suggestions of the best way to reconstruct the pyramid. Usually, a single DMARD is initiated within weeks of a clear diagnosis of RA. If ineffective, serial DMARDs are attempted until control is achieved. Others propose that low doses of multiple DMARDs be initiated simultaneously. Those favoring this strategy suggest that drug synergy may provide rapid improvement with less dose-related toxicity. After control is achieved, therapy is slowly withdrawn, and the patient is maintained on the least toxic DMARD that subdues the inflammatory process. Several randomized trials using combination therapy are under way to determine the risks and outcomes of this treatment regimen.

For the primary care physician, this information could translate into the following therapeutic plan. After 1 to 3 months of arthritis treatment with an NSAID alone, a low-toxicity DMARD such as hydroxychloroquine should be considered if the patient remains symptomatic. If, after an additional 3 to 6 months of an NSAID/hydroxychloroquine combination, evidence of significant synovitis persists, an additional DMARD should be contemplated. If the physician is not comfortable with the second DMARD option, a rheumatology consultation is appropriate, particularly if methotrexate is considered.

This aggressive approach to patients with RA may be difficult to justify because of the potential toxicity of medications and the uncertainty of the disease course. Rheumatoid factor or subcutaneous nodules suggest aggressive disease but are often not present in early disease. HLA-DR4 has been reported to correlate with disease severity, but it is not readily available and has not yet been incorporated into DMARD treatment decisions. Until trial genetic tests are proven to predict severity and become readily available, treatment decisions must rely on physical and radiographic evidence of progressive synovitis and on the presence of acute-phase reactants in early disease when the rheumatoid factor is often negative.

In a managed care system the primary care physician is likely to be expected to make the diagnosis of RA and to initiate the first NSAID and DMARD based on the above clinical features. This is complicated by similarities in the presentations of several different rheumatic disorders. Consultation with a rheumatologist may be helpful for cases that present diagnostic difficulty. Fortunately, some DMARDs have overlapping therapeutic efficacy. For instance, hydroxychloroquine is used to treat the arthritis of SLE, Sjögren's syndrome, and early scleroderma. This makes hydroxychloroquine a reasonable choice for patients with a positive ANA, a negative rheumatoid factor, and frank synovitis. In a similar manner, sulfasalazine has efficacy for the reactive arthritides, such as Reiter's syndrome and inflammatory bowel disease–induced arthritis, as well as for psoriatic arthritis and ankylosing spondylitis. Use of hydroxychloroquine and sulfasalazine should fall easily into the therapeutic arena of the primary care physician for patients with confirmed synovitis.

Agents used for treating RA are divided into three major groups: NSAIDs, DMARDs, and corticosteroids.

***NSAIDs.*** NSAIDs are used as the first-line therapy to decrease pain and inflammation promptly. Because of significant interpatient variability in efficacy, multiple agents may need to be prescribed before the most effective NSAID is discovered for an individual. NSAID efficacy generally requires 1 to 3 weeks to assess. With few exceptions, NSAIDs work by inhibiting the production of inflammatory prostaglandins. Despite their efficacy in reducing the symptoms of arthritis, these drugs probably do not change the natural history of RA. It is important to prescribe antiinflammatory dosages of the NSAID (Table 79-3) and not analgesic dosages, which are generally lower.

Toxicity of aspirin and NSAIDs is well described (see the box on p. 1103). The major toxicity is gastrointestinal with potential gastritis, erosive change, and gastric ulceration. Risk factors for toxicity in RA include advanced age, concomitant corticosteroid use, tobacco use, alcohol use, and a history of ulcers. Patients with prominent risk factors should be strongly considered for

**Table 79-3.** NSAIDs

| Drug | Tablet size available | Antiinflammatory dosages |
|---|---|---|
| **Carboxylic acids** | | |
| Acetylsalicylic acid (aspirin) | 325 mg, 500 mg, 975 mg | Follow serum salicylate levels |
| Choline magnesium trisalicylate | 500 mg, 750 mg, 1000 mg | 750 tid-1000 tid |
| Salsalate | 500 mg, 750 mg | 750 tid-1500 bid |
| Diflunisal | 250 mg, 500 mg | 250 tid-500 tid |
| **Proprionic acids** | | |
| Ibuprofen | 200 mg, 300 mg, 400 mg, 600 mg, 800 mg | 300 qid-800 tid |
| Naproxen | 250 mg, 375 mg, 500 mg | 375 tid-500 bid |
| Naproxen sodium | 275 mg, 550 mg | 275 tid-550 bid |
| Fenoprofen | 300 mg, 600 mg | 300 qid-600 qid |
| Ketoprofen | 25 mg, 50 mg, 75 mg, 200 mg SR | 50 tid-200 qd |
| Flurbiprofen | 50 mg, 100 mg | 100 bid-100 tid |
| Oxaprozin | 600 mg | 1200 qd |
| **Acetic acids** | | |
| Indomethacin | 25 mg, 50 mg, 75 mg SR | 25 qid-50 tid |
| Tolmetin | 200 mg, 400 mg, 600 mg | 400 qid-600 tid |
| Sulindac | 150 mg, 200 mg | 150 bid-200 bid |
| Diclofenac | 25 mg, 50 mg, 75 mg | 50 tid-75 bid |
| Etodolac | 200 mg, 300 mg, 400 mg | 200 tid-300 qid |
| **Fenamic acids** | | |
| Meclofenamate | 50 mg, 100 mg | 50 qid-75 tid |
| **Naphthylkanones** | | |
| Nabumetone | 500 mg, 750 mg | 1000 qd-1000 bid |
| **Enolic acids** | | |
| Piroxicam | 10 mg, 20 mg | 10 qd-20 qd |

prophylactic treatment with the synthetic prostaglandin misoprostol.

***DMARDs.*** DMARDs are aimed at altering the course of rheumatoid synovitis, thus preventing joint damage. These agents often need to be administered for several weeks to months before positive results can be seen. It is postulated that DMARDs are effective in modulating the immune process of RA.

The choice of initial second-line agent depends on the physician's judgment and preference, as well as on the severity of the disease. Patients with severe, aggressive disease should be treated with methotrexate or, less commonly, injectable gold salts by a physician who is familiar with the use and toxicity of these medications. Patients with lesser symptoms may be treated with hydroxychloroquine, auranofin, or sulfasalazine, often by the primary care physician. When the initial DMARD does not result in the expected efficacy, a second agent may be added or may replace the first. As mentioned earlier, initiation of more than one DMARD from the onset of second-line therapy with eventual step-down to a simplified regimen once control is achieved is a treatment strategy under evaluation. Three medications—D-penicillamine, azathioprine, and cyclophosphamide—have efficacy for RA, but these agents should be prescribed only by those most familiar with their toxicities.

### NSAID characteristics

*Time to effectiveness:* Variable, generally at least 2 weeks
*Toxicity*
- Greater than 5%: Ototoxicity, rash, gastric erosions or ulcerations, platelet effect
- Less than 5%: Hypersensitivity, hepatic insufficiency, renal pathology, small bowel ulcerations, central nervous system (CNS), stomatitis, drug fever, pancreatitis, hemolytic anemia, thrombocytopenia, neutropenia, pulmonary infiltrates

*Safety monitoring*
- Initial: CBC, Cr, U/A, AST every 1-3 months
- Stable: CBC, Cr, U/A, AST every 3-12 months

*CBC,* Complete blood count; *Cr,* creatine; *AST,* asparate aminotransferase.

***Injectable gold salts.*** Gold sodium thiomalate (GSTM) (Myochrysine) and gold sodium thioglucose (GSTG) (Solganal) are the two forms of injectable gold used in the United States. GSTM is a water-based solution; GSTG has a sesame oil vehicle (see the box on p. 1104).

Gold was first introduced as a treatment for infections, particularly for tuberculosis, in the early 1900s. Because

## Injectable gold characteristics

Gold sodium thiomalate (Myochrysine)
Gold sodium thioglucose (Solganal)
Generic available: no
*Time to effectiveness:* 6 weeks to 6 months
*Administration:* First week test dose, 10 mg; second week test dose, 25 mg; follow with weekly 50 mg injections to total of 1000 mg; then alternate weekly dosage for 3 months; then every third week for 3 months; then monthly
*Toxicity*
Greater than 5%: Rash, stomatitis, nitritoid reaction*
Less than 5%: Alopecia, thrombocytopenia, granulocytopenia, aplastic anemia, eosinophilia, proteinuria, pulmonary infiltrates, neuropathy, hepatic insufficiency, hematuria, enterocolitis
*Safety monitoring*
Initial: CBC, differential, platelet count, and U/A preinjection for the first 20 weeks
Stable: CBC differential, platelet count, and U/A before every other injection

*Nitritoid reaction may occur with gold sodium thiomalate usage (see text).

tuberculosis was suspected as a cause of RA, rheumatoid patients were treated with high doses of gold, obtaining excellent results but unacceptable toxicity. A period of disfavor ensued until carefully designed studies demonstrated that lower dosages were effective without unacceptable side effects. Although hailed as the DMARD of choice for several years, the efficacy of gold therapy has been questioned in recent studies. Despite this controversy, most rheumatologists still believe that intramuscular gold has a role in the treatment of RA, although its use has largely been replaced by methotrexate.

Initially, intramuscular gold is given in the form of weekly injections. Two test doses are administered; the first is a 10-mg injection, and the second weekly dose is 25 mg. Thereafter the prescribed dosage is 50 mg per week. After improvement is noted or a cumulative dose of 1000 mg is attained, the interval between injections is increased to 2 weeks. If improvement continues, the interval can be further lengthened, generally to a maximum of 1 month. Intramuscular gold therapy frequently requires 6 weeks to 6 months before maximum effectiveness is evident.

Gold therapy is often associated with toxicity, resulting in discontinuation of treatment in approximately 30% of patients. Rash and stomatitis are the most commonly reported problems.

Renal toxicity occurs; the most common problem is proteinuria. In less than 1% of patients treated with parenteral gold, serious renal insufficiency occurs. The major toxicity is nephrotic syndrome. Hematuria may also occur. The vast majority of kidney problems are reversible.

Fortunately, gold-induced hematologic problems are rare. In 1% to 3% of patients, leukopenia or thrombocytopenia may develop. If no other obvious cause is found, gold therapy should be discontinued. Eosinophilia is common in RA, but a marked increase in the eosinophil count may be a warning of impending toxicity, and gold should be at least temporarily withheld until the eosinophilia resolves. In less than 0.5% of patients, aplastic anemia may result; the mortality is in excess of 50%. The most effective therapy for aplastic anemia appears to be antithymocyte globulin.

Nitritoid reaction may occur with GSTM, the water-based gold preparation that is rapidly absorbed. This reaction occurs immediately or within 20 minutes after an injection. It is usually characterized by flushing, fainting, dizziness, and sweating. If this occurs, gold therapy can be changed to the oil-based GSTG.

In view of potential renal and hematologic toxicities, weekly preinjection CBCs and urinalyses (U/As) are suggested for the first 20 weeks. Since toxicity is less likely after the first 6 months, laboratory tests may be obtained before every injection or every other injection.

**Oral gold.** The introduction of auranofin (Ridaura) in the 1980s allowed physicians to prescribe an oral form of gold. Many rheumatologists feel that auranofin is not as effective as injectable gold, but the compound may be more efficacious if used for very early disease. A trial of 6 months may be required before a determination is made that auranofin is definitely not efficacious in a given patient.

The recommended dosage of auranofin is 3 mg twice a day. If no improvement is noted in 6 months, a trial of 3 mg 3 times per day may be considered. Recommended laboratory monitoring for toxicities requires monthly CBCs with manual differential and a U/A.

Unlike injectable gold, auranofin has a low incidence of serious toxicities. The most prominent side effects are abdominal cramps, diarrhea, nausea, and changes in appetite. Most of these problems can be treated by starting with 3 mg a day administered with meals and by prescribing a high-fiber, bulk-inducing agent. Rash and stomatitis are uncommon; renal and hematologic toxicities are rare.

***Antimalarial drugs.*** The medicinal qualities of quinine have been recognized for more than a century. Antimalarial agents include hydroxychloroquine, chloroquine, and quinacrine. Quinacrine was introduced in the 1950s as the first antimalarial used to treat RA. Chloroquine and hydroxychloroquine are used today in the treatment of RA. Hydroxychloroquine has become the antimalarial agent of choice because of its lower toxicity profile (see the box on p. 1105). Hydroxychloroquine is contraindicated in patients allergic to the medication or to quinine.

Hydroxychloroquine is given in initial dosages of 400 mg per day (200 mg orally twice a day). If an excellent response occurs, the dosage can be decreased to 200 mg per day. A trial for a minimum of 6 to 10 weeks is required to determine efficacy.

Hydroxychloroquine is probably the safest DMARDs. Patients should have a baseline ophthalmologic examination before starting hydroxychloroquine. It is estimated that only 5% of patients discontinue the medication because of side effects. The most frequently reported side effects of hydroxychloroquine are gastrointestinal. Thrombocytopenia and other forms of bone marrow suppression are rare. The principal concern regarding antimalarial

### Hydroxychloroquine (Plaquenil) characteristics

Generic available: no
*Dosage:* 200 mg PO bid
*Time to effectiveness:* 6 to 10 weeks
*Toxicity*
Greater than 5%: GI discomfort, rash, headache, irritability, skin hyperpigmentation, corneal deposits
Less than 5%: Tinnitus, retinopathy, neuromyopathy, leukopenia, cardiomyopathy, alopecia, hemolytic anemia with glucose-6-dehydrogenase deficiency
*Safety monitoring*
Initial: Baseline eye examination by ophthalmologist before the start of therapy
Stable: Eye examination every 3 to 6 months; CBC every 6 months

### Penicillamine (Cuprimine, Depen) characteristics

Generic available: no
Cuprimine: capsule 125 mg, 250 mg
Depen: scored tablet, 250 mg
*Administration and dosage:* Initial dose: 125 to 250 mg; incremental dosage increase: 125 to 250 mg; intervals between dosage increase: 3 months; maximum dosage: 750 mg qd in most cases
*Time to effectiveness:* 2 to 9 months
*Toxicity*
Greater than 5%: Hypogeusia, rash, nausea, anorexia, stomatitis, proteinuria
Less than 5%: Thrombocytopenia, leukopenia, autoimmune diseases, gynecomastia, aplastic anemia, liver test abnormalities, pulmonary toxicity, immune complex glomerulonephritis
*Safety monitoring*
Initial: CBC with differential, platelet count, and U/A every 2 weeks for first 6 months
Stable: CBC with differential, platelet count and U/A monthly; CPK every 4 to 6 months

*CPK*, Creatine phosphokinase.

drugs is the risk of retinopathy with long-term use. The risk of retinopathy for patients taking the standard dose of 400 mg per day of hydroxychloroquine is very low. If ophthalmologic evaluation is performed routinely every 3 to 6 months as recommended and hydroxychloroquine discontinued at the earliest sign of retinal change, the risks for permanent eye damage are negligible. When loss of vision is the first sign of damage, continued loss can progress despite drug withdrawal, underling the importance of routine examination. Choloroquine has a higher risk of retinopathy than does hydroxychloroquine. When hydroxychloroquine is initiated, there may be blurring of vision; this is transient and is due to smooth muscle relaxation rather than to retinal pathology. Corneal deposits can also occur but do not present a risk to vision.

***D-Penicillamine.*** D-Penicillamine is an oral preparation with similarities to gold in terms of its delayed onset of action and side effect profile.

Penicillamine therapy (see the box at right) has numerous potential side effects that limit its use to uniquely refractory cases. Toxicity is frequently related to dosage and generally appears in the first year of treatment. Serious side effects are similar to those of injectable gold. The chief concern is the development of hematologic toxicity. Most frequent is the occurrence of thrombocytopenia, which occurs in approximately 4% of patients, and leukopenia, which occurs in approximately 2% of patients. These side effects are largely reversible but can be life threatening in rare situations. Renal toxicity, notably nephritis with proteinuria, can occur but in most circumstances can be halted if detected early. Nephrotic syndrome is more common than with injectable gold. If significant proteinuria (greater than 1 g) is documented by 24-hour urine evaluation, D-penicillamine therapy should be discontinued.

The rare development of other autoimmune conditions, such as myasthenia gravis, pemphigus, Goodpasture syndrome, and SLE, may also result from penicillamine therapy.

D-Penicillamine therapy is initiated very slowly with a starting dosage of 125 to 250 mg per day taken on an empty stomach. Incremental increases of 125 to 250 mg (depending on tolerance) are made every 3 months until the desired beneficial response or a daily maximum of 750 mg is reached. Occasionally higher doses are used, but generally these are discouraged. CBC and U/A should be monitored every 2 weeks for the first 6 months and then on a monthly basis thereafter while the patient is treated with the medication.

***Sulfasalazine.*** Sulfasalazine (see the box on p. 1106) was originally developed in the 1930s specifically for the treatment of RA. Congruent with the notion that RA had an infectious etiology, sulfasalazine was developed to have antibiotic and antiinflammatory properties. It was used throughout the 1940s with proven efficacy until the introduction and promise of corticosteroids and the publication of negative studies that compared sulfasalazine with injectable gold. Since the 1980s, sulfasalazine usage has had a resurgence because several studies demonstrated its effectiveness. Although widely prescribed, it is not approved for use in treating RA by the Food and Drug Administration (FDA).

Sulfasalazine is most frequently prescribed in a dosage of 2 g per day divided into two to four equal doses. The enteric-coated formulation in lower dosages, given initially with an incremental increase over 2 to 4 weeks, limits gastrointestinal intolerance. If no benefit is noted in 3 to 6 months, the dosage can be increased to 3 g per day for an additional 2 to 3 months. Efficacy is generally apparent after 2 to 6 months of therapy. Monitoring for toxicity includes checking CBCs with differentials, platelet counts, and liver function tests within the first 1 to 3 weeks of therapy and then every 8 to 12 weeks thereafter. Sulfasalazine is contraindicated in patients who are

### Sulfasalazine (Azulfidine) characteristics

Generic available: yes
Tablets: 500 mg
Enteric-coated tablets: 500 mg
Liquid form is available
*Dosage:* 2 to 3 tablets bid
*Time to effectiveness:* 2 to 6 months
*Toxicity*
Greater than 5%: Gastrointestinal, rash, headache, macrocytosis
Less than 5%: Leukopenia, thrombocytopenia, megaloblastic anemia, hepatic insufficiency, reduced sperm count, pulmonary toxicity, other hypersensitivities (e.g., arthralgia, angioedema, eosinophilia), hemolytic anemia with glucose-6-phosphate dehydrogenase deficiency
*Safety monitoring:*
Initial: CBC, platelet count
Stable: CBC, platelet count every 3 to 12 months

allergic to sulfa compounds or to salicylates.

The most frequently observed side effect of sulfasalazine is gastrointestinal intolerance, which is reduced with the use of enteric-coated tablets taken with meals. Starting therapy at a low dosage and increasing it slowly also improves tolerance. Rash is another adverse effect. Serious toxicity is rare and generally occurs early in the course of treatment. Most worrisome are severe hypersensitivity reactions, including pneumonitis and hepatitis, and cytopenias, including thrombocytopenia and leukopenia. Spermatogenesis may be affected, causing reversible sterility. The majority of side effects are reversed uneventfully with discontinuation of the medication.

***Methotrexate.*** Methotrexate was introduced in the 1940s as a form of chemotherapy and later became popular in the treatment of psoriasis and psoriatic arthritis. Since the early 1980s, use of methotrexate for treatment of RA has increased dramatically (see the box at right). This increased popularity has many explanations. First, the onset of action of methotrexate is rapid compared with other DMARDs. Clinical improvement may be observed as early as 2 to 3 weeks, with 8 to 12 weeks of therapy required for full evaluation of efficacy. Second, methotrexate is probably the most potent antirheumatic medication since the introduction of corticosteroids. It is as potent as injectable gold and penicillamine, which were previously believed to be the most powerful DMARDs. Third, administration of methotrexate is convenient; it allows a weekly dosage regimen. Routine laboratory monitoring is needed less frequently than that required for gold and penicillamine.

The dosage of methotrexate is 5 to 15 mg per week, with an average weekly dosage of 7.5 mg (three 2.5-mg tablets). Folic acid is often prescribed in a dosage of 1 mg per day to decrease potential toxicity. Safety monitoring requires baseline CBC, platelet count, renal function tests, liver function tests, and chest x-ray studies. A CBC should be performed again within the first 1 to 2 weeks of therapy

### Methotrexate (Rheumatrex), oral or injectable, characteristics

Generic: yes, but not recommended
Tablets: 2.5 mg
Injectable
*Usual dosage:* Two to five tablets 1 day per week or one intramuscular injection per week
*Time to effectiveness:* 6 to 12 weeks
*Toxicity*
Greater than 5%: Gastrointestinal intolerance, stomatitis, headache, liver function test abnormalities, hematologic effects
Less than 5%: Rash, alopecia, hepatitis, cirrhosis, pneumonitis, nodulosis, gastrointestinal ulceration, atypical infection
*Safety monitoring*
Initial: CBC, platelet count every 1 to 2 weeks; liver function tests every 2 to 4 weeks; chest x-ray baseline
Stable: CBC, platelet count every month; liver function tests every 1 to 3 months; creatinine every 3 to 12 months; chest x-ray yearly; need for liver biopsy unclear

and monthly thereafter. Liver function tests, specifically tranaminases and albumin, are checked every 1 to 3 months. Methotrexate is excreted by the kidney and should not be used in the setting of renal function impairment.

As with other immunosuppressants, methotrexate has potential side effects. Those most often reported relate to gastrointestinal intolerance. Nausea, vomiting, and diarrhea can usually be minimized by dividing the weekly dosage throughout the day of administration, taking the medication with food, adjusting the dosage, or using antiemetics. Intramuscular methotrexate is better tolerated.

The most frequent serious side effect of methotrexate is hepatotoxicity. Inflammation and fibrosis of the liver can occur with long-term use. Changes in liver function tests are frequent but do not always correlate with liver damage. Cirrhosis of the liver is rare but has been described, particularly in patients with psoriasis. Fibrosis and cirrhosis appear to be much less common in RA patients who take methotrexate. The risk of liver toxicity can be greatly reduced by eliminating alcohol and staying as close to lean body weight as possible. After 3 to 4 years of use, a liver biopsy may be considered, particularly if abnormalities in liver function tests are persistent.

Like other immunosuppressants, there is a risk of cytopenia with methotrexate. At the dosages used for RA, cytopenia is unusual and almost always reversible with discontinuation of methotrexate. Atypical infections, including pneumocystis pneumonia, due to the immunosuppressive effects of methotrexate have been reported rarely.

Methotrexate may rarely cause pneumonitis, seen most often in smokers. Such patients present with cough, shortness of breath, and interstitial infiltrates on chest x-ray film. This side effect is generally reversible but can be life threatening, requiring treatment with corticosteroids.

### Azathioprine (Imuran) characteristics

Generic: no
*Dosage:* 50 to 150 mg qd (can divide dose)
*Toxicity*
Greater than 5%: Nausea, myelosuppression (thrombocytopenia, granulocytopenia, or lymphopenia), macrocytosis
Less than 5%: Rash, stomatitis, alopecia, atypical infections, hepatotoxicity, pancreatitis
*Safety monitoring*
Initial: CBC, platelet every 1 to 2 weeks
Stable: CBC, platelet every 1 to 3 months

### Cyclophosphamide (Cytoxan) characteristics

*Toxicity*
Greater than 5%: Gastrointestinal intolerance, stomatitis, hemorrhagic cystitis, alopecia, myelosuppression (thrombocytopenia, granulocytopenia, lymphopenia)
Less than 5%*: Atypical infection, hepatotoxicity, infertility, bladder cancer, lymphoproliferative malignancy
*Safety monitoring*
Initial: CBC, platelet count, U/A every 1 to 2 weeks
Stable: CBC, platelet count, U/A every 2 to 4 weeks

*Percentage may be higher with a very high dosage or prolonged use.

***Azathioprine.*** Azathioprine was the first immunosuppressant approved by the FDA for use in RA (see the box above, top). Although effective, toxicity issues may be prohibitive for most primary care physicians. Many rheumatologists reserve this therapy for patients who have failed treatment with other DMARDs. It is, however, a notable component of many of the combination therapies.

Azathioprine requires 6 weeks to 6 months of use to become effective. An initial dosage of 1 mg/kg per day or 100 mg for the first 3 months is generally prescribed. The dosage can be increased every 3 months in increments of 25 mg to a maximum of 150 mg when lower dosages prove ineffective. Safety screening consists of monitoring CBCs monthly and liver function tests every 3 to 4 months.

The toxicities of azathioprine largely depends on the dosage. Of most concern is the development of cytopenias. Most common among these is leukopenia. As with other immunosuppressants, macrocytosis without anemia is frequent. Marked hepatotoxicity is rare, but low-grade liver function abnormalities are not uncommon. Azathioprine therapy increases the risk for atypical infections that may develop without leukopenia. Less common hematologic complications include thrombocytopenia and anemia. These complications are largely reversible. Life-threatening complications are rare when vigilant monitoring is performed.

The potential increased risk of subsequent malignancy, particularly lymphoma, with prolonged use of azathioprine has received much attention. Reports from some recent long-term studies of RA patients taking azathioprine are reassuring. Any additional risk of cancer in patients receiving azathioprine compared with others with RA appears to be small. However, adequate, well-controlled studies are lacking, and patients should be informed of the potential risk when considering this therapy.

### Corticosteroid characteristics

*Toxicity:* Increased appetite, osteoporosis, cataracts, impaired wound healing, diabetes, hypertension, edema, weight gain, increased risk of infection, cushingoid features, acne, easy bruising, suppression of hypothalamic-pituitary-adrenal axis, myopathy, increased intraocular pressure, subcapsular cataracts, avascular necrosis
*Safety monitoring*
Initial: CBC, U/A, blood glucose
Stable: CBC, U/A, blood glucose (at least yearly, but more frequently if symptoms warrant)

***Cyclophosphamide.*** Cyclophosphamide is the most potent and toxic immunosuppressive drug used to treat RA (see the box at left). Although its effectiveness as a disease-modifying agent is undisputed, the potential toxicity of cyclophosphamide prohibits its use in the vast majority of RA patients. Its use is limited to severe complications of RA, such as vasculitis and other severe organ involvement. Cyclophosphamide therapy should be monitored by a rheumatologist because of the seriousness of the rheumatoid and medication complications.

Cytopenias occur and appear to be related to the dosage. Risk of an atypical infection also is increased. Interstitial cystitis may occur, and adequate hydration and taking cyclophosphamide in the morning are crucial to reduce the development of cystitis. Pulmonary toxicity has been observed.

Cyclophosphamide therapy is associated with an increased risk of bladder cancer and hematologic malignancy. Since cyclophosphamide is given almost exclusively for severe, unremitting RA or for life-threatening complications, this increased risk is usually justified.

***Corticosteroids.*** Corticosteroids have been used for patients with RA since the 1940s (see the box above). High-dose corticosteroids were so dramatically effective in the treatment of RA that Hench and Kendall later received a Nobel Prize for their work with these agents. The serious toxicities associated with high-dose therapy soon became apparent.

Corticosteroids have prominent antiinflammatory properties that result in dramatic improvement of symptomatic arthritis and systemic complaints. The ability to modify the rheumatoid disease course with low-dose corticosteroids continues to be debated.

Low-dose corticosteroids, given in a single morning dose, are popular among many rheumatologists as a form of bridge therapy after NSAIDs have been prescribed and before DMARDs become effective. During this period corticosteroids are used to relieve symptoms while

## Joint protection guidelines

Respect pain.
Balance rest with activity to conserve energy.
Maintain muscle strength and tone to increase support to joints.
Avoid prolonged activities that cannot be interrupted.
Avoid positions that promote deformity.
Use the largest joints and the strongest muscles available to complete a task.
Avoid remaining in one position or using muscles in one stationary position for long periods.
Use assistive equipment as needed.

awaiting therapeutic efficacy of DMARD therapy. Corticosteroids should not be used as the sole therapy for RA in most circumstances because of their long-term toxicity. Dosage escalation for the antiinflammatory effects and a shift of dosing to the evening increases the risks of hypercortisolism. Every effort should be made to restrict the dosage to no more than 5 mg of prednisone taken in the morning.

Corticosteroid intraarticular injections are an important adjunct to therapy in RA, particularly in a persistently inflamed joint. "Depo" preparations such as methylprednisolone and triamcinolone hexacinamide may give up to 1 month of relief as sole therapy. Benefits may persist much longer when the steroid injection is combined with systemic therapy. Care must first be taken to rule out a joint infection by aspiration and fluid analysis before injection. Large joints (e.g., knees) can often be easily injected by the primary care physician. Systemic absorption occurs and can temporarily suppress the hypothalamic-pituitary-adrenal axis. This may be clinically relevant in patients who have received multiple recent injections and are undergoing joint replacement or other surgery. Preoperative and postoperative corticosteroid stress dosage should be addressed with the help of the surgeon or anesthesiologist.

### Nonpharmacologic

***Rehabilitation issues: joint protection.*** When joints are inflamed, cartilage is prone to injury and irreversible damage. During this vulnerable period, it is critical that principles of joint protection are understood and practiced. MCP and wrist joints are particularly prone to deformity. Special attention to protecting these joints during daily activities is indicated. An occupational therapist can teach methods of joint protection, giving specific examples of the use of these guidelines as they relate to each joint (see the box above).

Splinting plays an important role in joint protection. Splints can be designed to reduce inflammation through immobilization, to protect a vulnerable joint, or to improve function of a damaged joint. Splints should be worn only if they diminish pain and inflammation or improve function. There is no reliable evidence available documenting that splints prevent deformity, but this is a commonly held notion. Inappropriate or prolonged use of splints may cause increased stiffness, decreased strength, and decreased motion. An occupational therapist with expertise in hand therapy can be particularly helpful in devising appropriate upper extremity splints. There are several types of splints used for the wrist and fingers. Ring splints are often used by persons with swan neck or boutonnière deformities. Hand and wrist splints can be commercially fabricated or custom fit by an occupational therapist or orthotist. The functional wrist splint allows some movement at the fingers while immobilizing the wrist. Resting hand splints can be used at night but are cumbersome and may provide no more benefit than functional wrist splints.

Assistive equipment can facilitate joint protection. Examples of equipment available for upper extremity problems include built-up handles, faucet levers, key adapters, button hooks, elastic shoe laces, the use of Velcro in place of buttons and laces, door-opening levers, and extended handles on utensils. Useful assistive equipment for lower extremity problems includes elevated seats with arm rests, raised toilet seats, shower benches, long-handled reachers, tub grab bars, and walking aids.

Proper footwear is crucial to protect the feet and ankles. RA may cause significant foot deformities and dysfunction. Swelling and secondary ligamentous laxity may result in a broad forefoot with toe deformities. A poorly fit shoe can create foot discomfort and further deformity. With mild arthritis in the feet a good supportive walking shoe or an athletic shoe usually suffices. When choosing shoes, the following features should be considered: light weight, deep enough to clear the top of toes (deeper if an insert is needed), wide enough not to pinch the toes together, 1 inch or less heel, good shock absorption, support along the inside of the shoe with an adequate arch, durable, stiff back for support, and breathable and supple uppers. If deformities of the foot are present, an insert or orthosis may be required. These foot supports can be purchased commercially or can be individually designed by a podiatrist, orthotist, or pedorthist. Orthotic supports are designed to relieve pressure that is secondary to deformities or to correct foot deformity. A metatarsal bar can be applied externally to the sole of the shoe to remove the pressure from the metatarsal heads that is often prominent in RA. If deformity is severe, orthopedic shoes or custom-made shoes can be fabricated from a cast of the feet.

Concepts of energy conservation should accompany principles of joint protection. Activities that cause fatigue in the patient without having an aerobic or strengthening benefit should be eliminated if possible. Discussions on the value of rest during the day are important. An occupational or physical therapist can help to teach methods of task minimization. The Arthritis Foundation has pamphlets available that review energy conservation and joint protection.

***Exercise.*** Appropriate exercise with adequate rest is a mainstay of the treatment of RA. Exercise recommendations have changed significantly over the past 30 years. For many years patients were treated with prolonged bed rest to reduce active arthritis. Since inflammation improves with immobilization, the practice had some merit. However, it has become evident that the negative effects of

### Exercise guidelines for patients

Review exercises in detail with a physician or a therapist who is familiar with RA, particularly if the arthritis is severe.
Perform exercise as part of a daily routine.
Perform a brief series of range-of-motion exercises in the morning, after immobility, and before fitness exercises.
Exercise when the energy level is at its peak.
Balance exercise with adequate rest and sleep.
Always follow principles of joint protection.
Use tactics that make exercise most comfortable:
- Wear loose clothing
- Consider showering before exercise to decrease pain and stiffness and to increase flexibility
- Take medications in advance, timed to be effective during exercise.

Take deep, regular breaths during exercise.
Keep movements smooth and flowing. Avoid jerking or bouncing motions.
Apply ice packs to warm joints for 20 minutes after each exercise session to limit inflammation.
Never perform a painful exercise.
Never exercise to the point of extreme muscle fatigue or weakness.
If joints hurt for more than 2 hours after exercising or if joints hurt or swell the next day, know that the exercise program is too rigorous.
For patients with joint replacements, always review exercises with the orthopedic surgeon before proceeding.
Be adaptable to changes in condition and modify accordingly.
Keep a log of completed exercises.

muscle atrophy, osteoporosis, and generalized deconditioning outweigh the benefits.

Range-of-motion, specific strengthening, and low-impact aerobic fitness exercises can be prescribed with positive effects. Recent studies demonstrated that appropriate exercise can improve stamina, decrease fatigue, reduce time lost from work, and enhance the level of function. Appropriate exercise can also increase joint stability, help prevent joint deformities, decrease pain, improve function, promote self-esteem, improve sleep, and lessen muscle tension and anxiety. Compliance with exercise can be increased and joint damage avoided if guidelines are followed (see the box above).

The recommended amount and type of exercise depend on the degree of inflammation and the pattern of joint involvement. Gentle range-of-motion exercises are prescribed for patients with very active inflammation. Moving affected joints through approximately five repetitions of range of motion helps to maintain motion. Joints should not be stretched to the point of increased pain. Muscle setting can be performed if it does not cause significant discomfort. Muscles surrounding affected joints can be contracted with tension maintained for 6 seconds each day to prevent muscle weakening.

Moderately inflamed or subacute joints should also be taken through range-of-motion exercise. Isometric strengthening exercise with contraction against a fixed resistance can be added. Elastic bands or other forms of fixed resistance can be used. Approximately 75% of maximum strength for 6 seconds should be used with less force when pain occurs. Slow addition of endurance exercises may be appropriate at this stage. Adding a swimming program is often recommended because the buoyancy of water tends to relieve mechanical stress on joints.

In cases of controlled synovitis, exercise recommendations vary depending on the amount of damage in the joints. General guidelines include continuing range-of-motion exercises daily with a maximum of 10 repetitions. Isometric strengthening exercises may be performed as they would with moderately inflamed joints. Once maximum range of motion and strength is achieved, more time can be devoted to aerobic exercise. Endurance exercises are most important at this stage as a means of regaining aerobic conditioning that is lost when the disease is more active. Although swimming is still the best form of exercise, other forms of low-impact aerobics such as walking, bicycling, simulated ski machines, and low-impact dancing, may be considered if lower extremity joints are not severely involved. Thirty minutes of aerobic exercise undertaken three times weekly increases fitness.

***Nutrition.*** There has been considerable interest in determining whether a relationship exists between nutrition and RA. Data suggest that fewer than 5% of patients with predominantly seronegative RA have a food allergy. Improvement in arthritis through elimination diets supports these data. Specific foods to avoid in various reports include milk products, lactose-containing foods, corn, cereals, shrimp, and nitrates.

The foremost nutritional question is whether diet modification can alter the abnormal immune response in RA. There have been studies of hypocaloric diets that show improvement in symptoms of RA. This improvement is usually temporary and is poorly understood. Diets low in saturated fats and high in omega-3 fatty acids have also been shown to have some therapeutic benefit. Supplemental fish oils containing omega-3 fatty acids have been shown to have modest antiinflammatory activity in RA. Clinical studies with $\gamma$-linolenic acid supplementation, an oil derived from borage seeds, have demonstrated antiinflammatory benefit.

A well-balanced diet with total caloric intake calculated to maintain lean body weight and limited stress on weight-bearing joints is recommended. Adequate protein is advised to prevent muscle atrophy. Calcium and vitamin D supplementation, particularly for patients taking corticosteroids, should be considered in view of the increased risk of osteoporosis in patients with RA. Estrogens for postmenopausal women should also be seriously considered. Sodium restriction should be considered to limit fluid retention and secondary hypertension for patients who take NSAIDs or corticosteroids.

## Surgery

RA can result in persistent inflammation and joint deformity, despite timely medical therapy. Surgical techniques provide several alternatives to ensure that patients with RA continue to maintain function. Surgical options are considered to control severe pain resulting from inflammation or damaged joints, to repair ruptured ligaments or tendons, to remove inflamed synovial tissue that has not responded adequately to medical therapy and is threatening joint damage or tendon rupture, and to retain or restore function in an affected joint.

Synovectomy facilitates the removal of proliferating pannus in an effort to preserve cartilage and surrounding soft tissue structures. Synovectomy should not be viewed as a corrective procedure, since complete resection of all synovial tissue is rarely possible and because synovial tissue can regrow. Synovectomy can be performed via arthroscopy or an open procedure. Recovery from arthroscopic synovectomy is generally quite rapid. Although more invasive, open surgical synovectomy has the advantage of improved access, facilitating a more thorough removal of the inflamed synovial tissue.

RA may result in damage to and occasionally rupture of surrounding tendons and ligaments. Rupture of finger extensors secondary to dorsal tenosynovitis is the most common occurrence. If rupture occurs, reconstruction is possible with tendon transfer.

Arthrodesis or joint fusion is performed only on painful and unstable joints, most commonly the wrists, feet, ankles, and thumbs. Although effective in decreasing pain and improving stability, fusion permanently sacrifices motion. For this reason, it is rarely performed on the shoulder or hip.

With long-standing RA, atlantoaxial subluxation and other cervical instability can occur because of ligament and bone loss caused by synovitis. In severe cases with neurologic deficits, fusion may be required to increase stability.

Osteotomy is occasionally performed to improve joint alignment and to compensate for deformity. This procedure is rarely performed because of improved joint replacement procedures.

New techniques for joint replacement have dramatically improved the outlook for even the most severely disabled patients. Traditionally total joint replacement was performed only in older, inactive individuals who had less chance of outliving the replacement. Current trends reveal an increased use of artificial joints in younger, more active patients. Total joint replacement is frequently performed in the knees, hips, and shoulders with excellent results. Replacements for the elbows, wrists, and ankles are available but have more variable outcomes. Newer designs are readily becoming available and will likely provide better and more consistent results.

Cement-adhered replacements can be used. This method is less painful and facilitates easier rehabilitation with faster healing. Potential problems include the cracking of the cement and joint loosening, particularly in very active patients. Recently, surgeons have begun using cementless joint replacements. The replacement stem, designed with small pores, allows the bone to grow into the stem. If successful, the benefits of this replacement are increased strength and durability with theoretically less chance of requiring additional replacement surgery. Disadvantages include prolonged rehabilitation and potential problems with delayed healing, or inadequate bone growth to support and stabilize the new replacement. Bone growth inadequacy may be more common in patients with osteoporosis secondary to chronic RA or corticosteroid use.

Before surgery several precautions must be considered. Ruling out cervical subluxation is imperative if tracheal intubation is anticipated. NSAIDs should be discontinued at least 1 week in advance in most cases; aspirin should be discontinued 2 weeks in advance. Stress doses of corticosteroids should be considered for patients on corticosteroids or for those who recently have had multiple intraarticular injections. Whether to stop methotrexate is controversial, but some evidence indicates a lower postoperative infection rate if methotrexate is stopped for the surgery and held for several weeks after the procedure.

## PSYCHOSOCIAL AND FAMILY ISSUES

RA can have an impact on all aspects of daily living, including interpersonal relationships, family dynamics, and sexuality. The perceived loss of independence and control can create fear, anger, and a loss of self-esteem. This aspect of the patient's care should not be overlooked by the physician. Since depression directly affects outcome negatively, helping the patient cope with these issues is of great use. Sexual issues should be addressed with frankness and sensitivity, since patients are often reluctant to share problems in this area. The Arthritis Foundation provides pamphlets concerning sexual issues, coping strategies, and other practical matters, at no cost to the patient. Other resources include counselors with expertise in chronic disease, self-help groups, social workers, vocational counselors, and nurse educators. Many communities have support groups for RA patients. Meeting times and locations are often published in the newspaper. A list of available community services can be requested from the local chapter of the Arthritis Foundation.

## PREGNANCY AND CHILDBIRTH

Since RA predominantly affects women of childbearing age, counseling of this group is extremely important. Fortunately, there is an ameliorating effect of pregnancy on rheumatoid synovitis in 75% of women with RA. Most remissions occur during the first trimester but can occur at any point during pregnancy. In most situations, medications can be discontinued without adverse sequelae. Methotrexate, with its known teratogenic effects, should be discontinued for a considerable time before pregnancy is attempted. Antimalarials are generally stopped 6 to 12 months before conception because of potential neurotoxicity to the fetus. Postpartum exacerbations unfortunately often occur, most commonly within the first 6 months. This often presents the most significant problem, considering the physical challenges of caring for an infant. If possible, this issue should be addressed with the prospective mother and her partner before pregnancy. Prolonged breastfeeding is not always possible, since antirheumatic medication, most of which is secreted in breast milk, is frequently required in the postpartum period. On a positive note, there is no reported association between RA activity and obstetric complications or adverse fetal health.

## DISABILITY ISSUES

RA can interfere with the ability to work. Stiffness, pain, decreased mobility, and particularly fatigue may present serious obstacles during an 8-hour work day. Practical advice regarding open communication with employers,

**Functional capacity system**

Class I: No restriction of ability to perform normal activities
Class II: Moderate restriction but adequate for normal activities
Class III: Marked restriction, inability to perform most duties of the patient's usual occupation or self-care
Class IV: Incapacitation or confinement to a bed or wheelchair

From *Primer on the rheumatic diseases,* ed 10, Atlanta, 1993, Arthritis Foundation.

increased flexibility of job hours, work-site modifications, energy conservation, and possible job-sharing programs can be a valuable resource to patients trying to remain at work. Continued employment should be encouraged for financial and health insurance benefits, as well as for self-esteem.

The Arthritis Foundation functional capacity evaluation system is listed in the box above. There are situations in which continued employment may prove impossible, especially physically demanding jobs that require repetitive motion of inflamed joints. In such cases, alternative employment, a change of job description, or an application for disability benefits should be considered. This decision is highly individualized and must consider the patient's age, work experience, educational resources, financial responsibilities, and severity of arthritis. Disability benefits vary greatly in eligibility and policy definition of disability. Many private companies offer short- or long-term disability insurance as part of their benefits packages. Some states provide short-term disability benefits.

Patients may be eligible for federal social security benefits. This program is not designed to cover short-term or partial disability and is based on the present and projected inability to perform any kind of work. Social Security standards of disability include the following:

1. Arthritis preventing any gainful employment
2. Condition expected to last for at least 1 year or to result in death

The Social Security reviewers determine whether the arthritis matches disability standards set forth by an objective "listing of impairments." According to social security regulations, to qualify as having disabling RA, the applicant must show proof of persistent joint pain, swelling, or tenderness in multiple joints. Signs of joint inflammation must have existed for at least 3 months despite therapy and must have resulted in decreased function of those joints. It must be expected that arthritis will remain a physical impairment for more than 12 months. ESR, rheumatoid factor, ANA, or biopsy must also be recorded as abnormal. Other factors taken into consideration include pain, fatigue, ability to perform basic work-related activities, age, education, work experience, and transferable skills. The application process may take several months to complete.

Two programs are funded through the Social Security Administration that vary in eligibility requirements: Social Security Disability Insurance Benefits (DIB) and Social Security Income (SSI). DIB is funded through FICA taxes paid by employees and employers. To qualify, the applicant must have accumulated sufficient work credits based on length of employment, time the applicant was employed, and the age at which the disability occurred. The patient cannot be engaged in "substantial gainful activity." Benefits usually begin after 6 full months of disability. The amount of monthly disability benefits is based on lifetime average earnings covered by Social Security. After 24 months of receiving DIB, individuals qualify for Medicare insurance.

SSI is funded through general tax funds. A work history is not required to receive SSI benefits. To qualify, financial need in the form of limited income and resources must be established. Income and assets of a spouse are also taken into consideration. Benefits begin immediately after the application has been approved. The length of time required to qualify varies considerably, depending on the nature of the disability and the availability of medical and financial information to reviewers. The benefit amount varies from state to state. Medicaid benefits may begin immediately upon SSI approval. Medicaid eligibility also varies from state to state.

### Vocational rehabilitation benefits

Vocational rehabilitation (VR) is a jointly funded federal/state program that helps disabled individuals become employable. One eligibility criterion is current unemployment. Recipients of government assistance may automatically be referred to VR. The resources of each state differ markedly, according to state contributions to the program. Potential services include counseling, medical help, job training, educational opportunities, financial assistance, job placement, and on-the-job assistance if problems develop.

## FUTURE DIRECTIONS

Current treatment of RA is multidisciplinary and is likely to remain that way. Future therapies for RA will reflect more than the development of new biologic agents or confirmation that early DMARD therapy is effective. It will depend on the positioning of RA within a managed care and capitated market. Primary care physicians will probably be involved in more of the initial diagnostic and therapeutic decisions, including the timing of DMARDs. There is hope that genetic markers will predict severity of arthritis and help direct aggressiveness of therapy.

Biologic agents are being developed and tested for RA. In general, several cells and cytokines have been targeted for modification. Antibodies to subsets of T lymphocytes, including CD4 cells, have been given parenterally to patients with RA with encouraging but not yet predictable, clinical responses. As more of the critical cellular and cytokine interrelationships involved in the pathogenesis of RA are known, newer biologic agents will be tested. Expense will be a consideration for the use of these parenteral agents for chronic disease. Oral agents, such as collagen fragments, may also be found to induce a clinical response through immunologic tolerance.

In summary, the future therapy of RA will likely emphasize the timing of DMARDs already in widespread clinical practice rather than the use of expensive biologic agents. The primary care physician's familiarity with DMARDs, particularly methotrexate, may become commonplace. The total cost of medications will be scrutinized in the managed care environment and will include the cost of monitoring for adverse effects. Therefore low-cost alternatives, such as low-dose corticosteroids, generic NSAIDs, and less expensive oral biologic agents, may become more popular. As outcome measures become validated and alternatives to office visits, such as repetitive telephone contacts, are shown to be effective in the management of chronic illness, future management may differ considerably from present practices.

## BIBLIOGRAPHY


Arnett FC et al: The American Rheumatism Association 1987 revised criteria for the classification of rheumatoid arthritis, *Arthritis Rheum* 31:315, 1988.

Burmester GR: Hit and run or permanently hit? Is there evidence for a microbiological cause for rheumatoid arthritis? *J Rheumatol* 18:1443, 1991.

Fries J: Reevaluating the therapeutic approach to rheumatoid arthritis: the "sawtooth" strategy, *J Rheumatol* 17:(suppl 22)12, 1990.

Harris ED Jr: Mechanisms of disease: rheumatoid arthritis: pathophysiology and implications for therapy, *N Engl J Med* 322(18):1277, 1990.

Kaufman RL, Baldassare AR, Fiechtner JJ: *Guidelines for reviewers of rheumatic disease care. Council on rheumatic care of the American College of Rheumatology,* ed 3, Atlanta, 1992, American College of Rheumatology.

Kwoh CK: Epidemiology of rheumatic diseases: rheumatoid arthritis, *Curr Opin Rheumatol* 4(2):140, 1991.

Leigh JP, Fries JF: Education level and rheumatoid arthritis: evidence from five data centers, *J Rheumatol* 18:24, 1991.

Pincus T, Callahan LF: Taking mortality in rheumatoid arthritis seriously—predictive markers, socioeconomic status and comorbidity, *J Rheumatol* 13:841, 1986.

Schned E: Future care of rheumatoid arthritis in a managed care environment, *Bull Rheum Dis* 42(7):1, 1993.

Shlotzhauer TL, McGuire JL: *Living with rheumatoid arthritis,* Baltimore and London, 1993, Johns Hopkins University.

Wilske KR, Healy LA: Challenging the therapeutic pyramid: a new look at the treatment strategies for rheumatoid arthritis, *J Rheumatol* 17(suppl 25):4, 1990.


CHAPTER

# 80 Periarticular Rheumatic Disorders


**Nancy Y. N. Liu**
**Juan J. Canoso**


Periarticular rheumatic disorders, also referred to as *soft tissue rheumatism,* include a wide range of musculoskeletal conditions commonly encountered by the primary care physician. In contrast to diseases that primarily affect the joint, these syndromes involve the periarticular region, which includes the tendons, bursae, fascia, nerves, and muscle. Because of the close proximity of these structures to the joint, patients often complain of "arthritis." Similarly, physicians unfamiliar with these conditions may diagnose articular rather than periarticular disease. This confusion may result in delayed or inappropriate therapy.

Accurate diagnosis of periarticular rheumatic conditions remains clinically based. It requires that the physician be knowledgeable about the various periarticular conditions; obtain a history, which may help distinguish between these conditions; and perform an adequate musculoskeletal examination. Once a diagnosis is made, the physician can provide appropriate therapy and advice.

Periarticular rheumatic syndromes typically include the structures depicted in Fig. 80-1. Most of these conditions are localized to one region of the body, although some conditions, particularly fibromyalgia, are diffuse. In addition, systemic diseases, such as rheumatoid arthritis (RA) or the spondyloarthropathies, may have associated periarticular involvement. The following sections discuss regional periarticular conditions with an emphasis on clinical presentation, physical examination findings, differential diagnoses, and treatment. Systemic diseases are mentioned when relevant. Regional myofascial pain is discussed within each anatomic section, and fibromyalgia is in a separate section.

## DEFINITIONS

### Bursitis

Two forms of bursae exist in the body: the superficial bursae and the deep bursae. Superficial bursae (e.g., olecranon and prepatellar bursae) function to enhance the gliding of skin over bone and are not present until after birth. They are not usually filled with fluid unless trauma, infection, or an acute crystal event occurs. Superficial bursae do not communicate with the joint. In contrast, deep bursae (e.g., subacromial, iliopsoas, and gastrocnemius-semimembranosus) often develop communication with joints as they age from constant friction. Deep bursae are formed in utero and facilitate the gliding of one tendon over another tendon or bone. Pathologically, both bursae are composed of synovial lining cells over a loose connective tissue stroma. Thus these bursae can become involved in systemic inflammatory disease.

### Tendinitis

Tendons transmit the tension generated by muscle to move bone. The highly organized type I collagen in tendons provides tremendous tensile strength and elasticity. Some tendons are lined by a sheath that is histologically identical to synovium. Tendinitis occurs with repetitive use, resulting in microscopic fraying of the collagen, fibrosis, and eventual limitation of tendon motion. However, tendinitis may also develop secondary to systemic inflammatory disease such as RA or the spondyloarthropathies. Tendons develop variable pathologic findings of degeneration, fibrosis, or increased vascularity with repetitive local trauma. In systemic inflammatory arthritis the pathology of the tenosynovium is similar to the primary disease.

### Enthesopathy

*Enthesis* is defined as the point of attachment of tendon, fascia, or ligament to bone (see Fig. 80-1). Typical areas include the Achilles tendon attachment to the calcaneus,

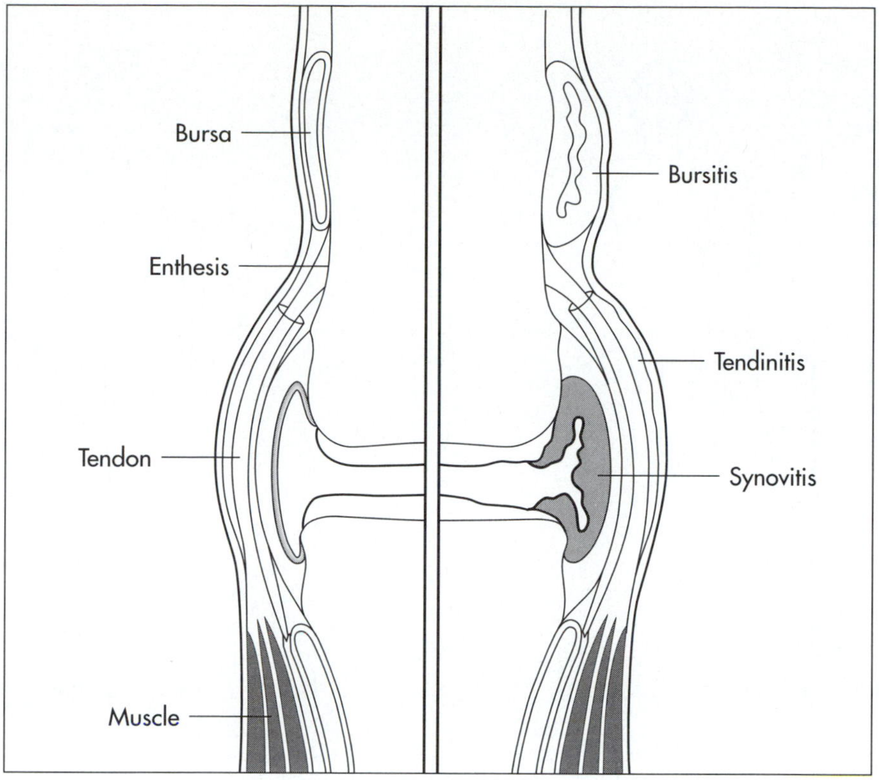


**Fig. 80-1.** Common structures around the joint include the muscle, tendon, enthesis, and bursa.

the plantar fascia to the calcaneus, and the common tendon of the wrist extensor muscles to the lateral epicondyle. These areas are susceptible to spur formation, calcification from hydroxyapatite deposition, and inflammatory changes from the spondyloarthropathies. Clinical findings include asymmetric swelling and pain at or underneath the tendinous insertion.

### Myofascial pain

Regional myofascial syndromes are due to localized areas of pain within muscle that often develop from overt or minor injury. Patients typically describe the pain as a vague, diffuse pain with burning. Clinically, a firm, discrete nodule or taut band, also known as a *trigger point,* can be palpated within the muscle. There is no visible swelling unless muscle spasm is present. When the trigger point is pressed, the pain radiates to a point distant from the trigger point in an atypical dermatome distribution. A twitch response (a sudden contraction of the muscle area that has been palpated) is considered by some authorities to be pathognomonic for a trigger point. In the 1950s, J Travell described and mapped trigger points and their zones of pain referral throughout the body. The most common are in the cervical, shoulder, and lower back regions (Figs. 80-2 and 80-3).

The description of myofascial pain has been mostly anecdotal. Recently, clinical attempts to separate regional myofascial pain from fibromyalgia based on physical findings of trigger points and tender points, respectively, could not be definitively established. However, many experts still feel that the two entities are distinct.

### Nerve entrapment

Nerve entrapment and peripheral neuropathy are discussed in Chapter 103.

## REGIONAL PROCESSES

### Cervical region

Neck pain has many different etiologies, ranging from osteoarthritis to neoplastic disease. Refer to Chapter 70 for a more detailed discussion of various causes of neck pain. Myofascial neck pain, a common primary care problem, is the focus of this section.

Neck pain and stiffness constitute a common complaint even in young adults. By age 45 more than 50% of the working population complains of neck stiffness and pain. History and physical examination are most helpful in differentiating the various diagnostic possibilities from myofascial neck pain.

Typically, myofascial neck pain starts after trauma, often delayed by days to weeks after the event. Sometimes, no specific injury is reported by the patient. The pain is localized to the posterior neck region and is sometimes associated with muscle contraction headaches. Patients may describe the pain beginning after prolonged sitting or sleeping. Activity may improve the pain. No neurologic symptoms are present.

Physical examination reveals well-preserved passive range of motion in the neck, although patients may not be able to actively move the neck well. Palpation of the posterior cervical region reveals trigger points within the trapezius and extensor neck muscles. The ligamentum nuchae may also be very tender (see Fig. 80-2). If multiple

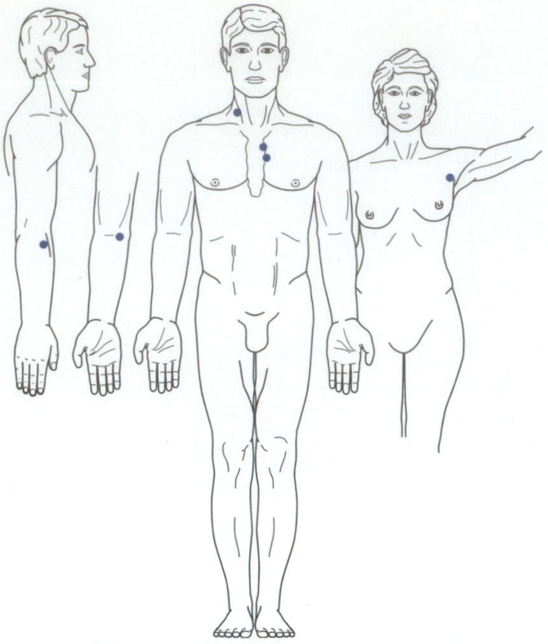

Fig. 80-2. Common myofascial trigger points.

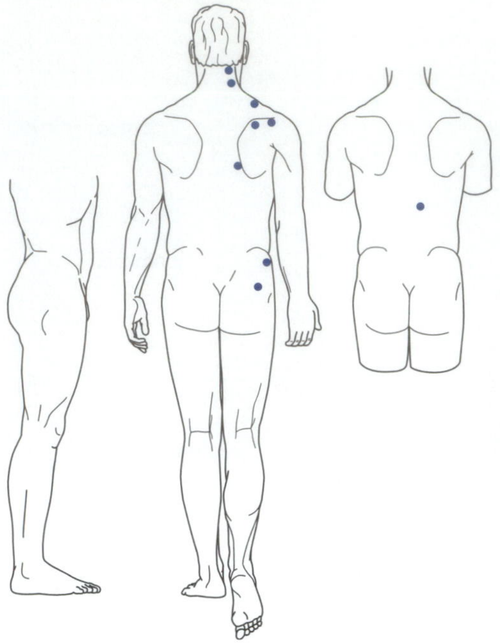

Fig. 80-3. Common myofascial trigger points.

trigger points exist, the referred area of pain can be extensive, although the neurologic examination is completely normal.

Laboratory tests may exclude other diseases but are not specific for myofascial neck pain. Radiographs may be normal or may reveal varying degrees of osteoarthritis. These latter findings, however, may not be responsible for the cervical pain. Further diagnostic tests, such as electromyography (EMG) and nerve conduction studies (NCS), computed tomography (CT) scan of the neck, and magnetic resonance imaging (MRI), are not necessary at the initial stages unless the history or examination suggests other diagnoses.

The differential diagnosis of neck pain is broad and can be divided into inflammatory and noninflammatory processes (see the box at right). Systemic inflammatory diseases include RA, spondyloarthropathies, and systemic juvenile rheumatoid arthritis (JRA). Osteoarthritis, degenerative disk disease, diffuse idiopathic skeletal hyperostosis (DISH), and fibromyalgia are common noninflammatory diseases of the cervical region. Meningitis, osteomyelitis, and infectious diskitis are infectious etiologies. Neoplastic diseases include metastatic lesions, multiple myeloma, and primary spinal cord tumors. In addition, disorders of the temporomandibular joint, heart, and gastrointestinal (GI) tract may cause pain that is referred to the cervical area.

Treatment of myofascial neck pain is similar to that outlined at the end of this chapter. In cervical neck pain, proper working and sleeping positions are crucial to rehabilitation. Appropriate height of desks, computers, and work stations should be established. At night, patients should sleep in a neutral position (lying on back with legs raised) with only a flat or cervical pillow. Appropriate exercises to stretch and strengthen the neck muscles are helpful.

### Differential diagnosis of cervical neck pain

- Inflammatory diseases
  - RA
  - Spondyloarthropathies
  - JRA
- Noninflammatory disease
  - Cervical osteoarthritis
  - Diskogenic neck pain
  - Diffuse idiopathic skeletal hyperostosis
  - Fibromyalgia or myofascial pain
- Infectious causes
  - Meninigitis
  - Osteomyelitis
  - Infectious diskitis
- Neoplasms: primary or metastatic
- Referred pain
  - Temporomandibular joint pain
  - Cardiac pain
  - Diaphragmatic irritation
  - Gastrointestinal sources (gastric ulcer, gallbladder, pancreas)

## Shoulder region

***History and physical examination.*** Shoulder pain may arise from pathology within the true glenohumeral joint, the periarticular structures, or the distant structures that refer pain to the shoulder region. Glenohumeral processes are discussed in detail in Chapter 71. Only adhesive capsulitis is discussed here. The periarticular structures surrounding the shoulder include the rotator cuff complex, subacromial/subdeltoid bursa, and long head of the biceps. Myofascial pain can be misinterpreted by patients as

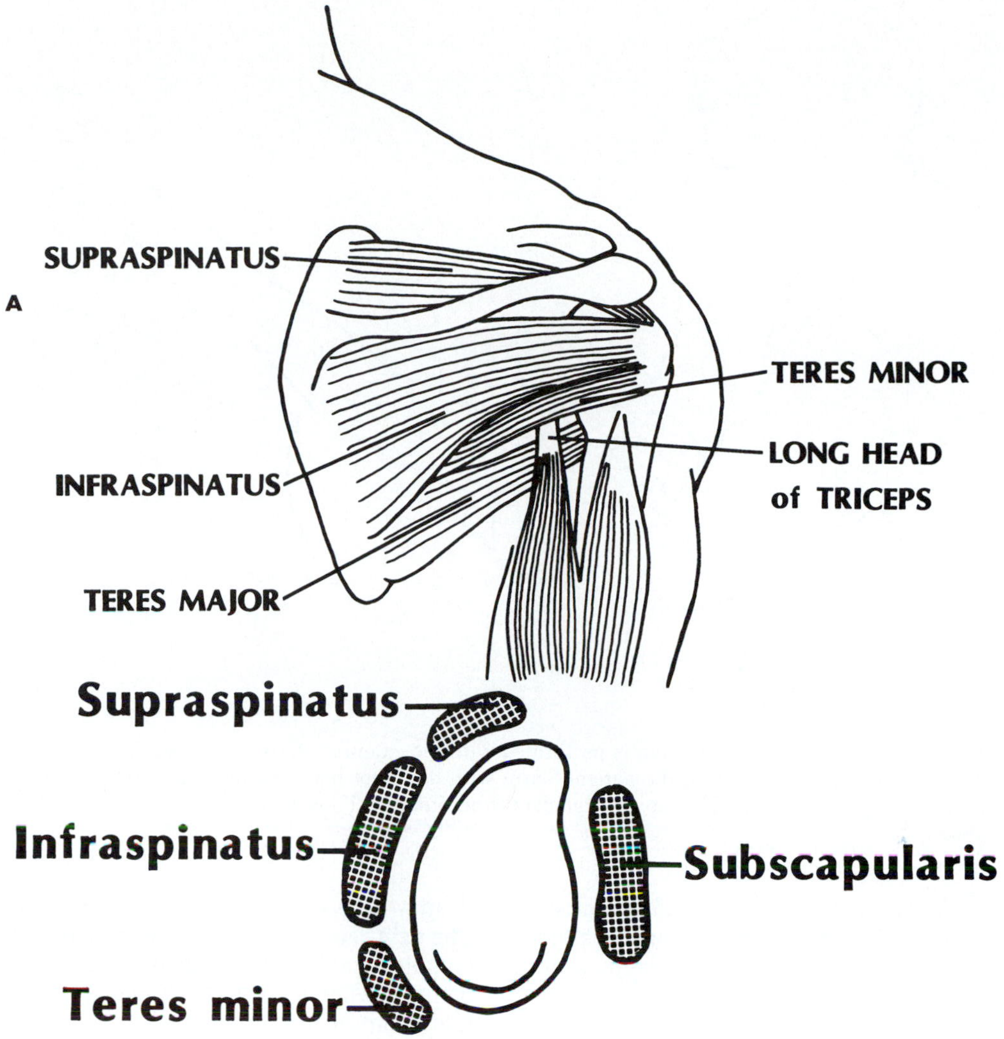


**Fig. 80-4.** Shoulder with the humeral head stabilized in the shallow scapular glenoid by the rotator cuff and capsule. **A,** Posterior view. **B,** Cross-sectional view.

shoulder pain. Thus the history and examination are important to differentiate these entities.

The onset, quality, location, duration, and frequency of pain are important. In addition, factors that exacerbate or improve the pain may help in the diagnosis. Acute pain after trauma suggests a possible tear in the rotator cuff, joint capsule, or intraarticular structures; gradual pain is less specific. Burning or radicular pain may indicate neuropathy or reflex sympathetic dystrophy. Pain localized to the anterior aspect of the shoulder is common in bicipital tendinitis, whereas rotator cuff tendinitis is more subacromial in location. Glenohumeral processes typically have constant pain referred to the lateral aspect of the upper arm. However, constant pain that is not associated with shoulder movement is an ominous symptom for malignancy or referred pain. Systemic features of fever, chills, and weight loss; visible or progressive swelling in the shoulder area; and pain aggravated by neck motion or deep inspiration may indicate nonmusculoskeletal etiologies of pain. Axillary pain is usually not from a shoulder source.

Examination of the shoulder includes inspection for asymmetry between the shoulders and palpation of various anatomic regions of the shoulder, including the common myofascial regions of the rhomboid, trapezius, serratus, and rotator cuff muscles. Joints participating in shoulder movement include the sternoclavicular, acromioclavicular, and glenohumeral joints. Scapulothoracic motion also contributes to shoulder movement. Passive range of motion in abduction and internal and external rotation delineates the integrity of the glenohumeral joint. In contrast, active range of motion provides information not only about the joint, but also about the function of the tendons and muscles surrounding the shoulder. Thus in acute rotator cuff tendinitis the passive range of motion of the shoulder is normal (provided that the patient can relax and avoid guarding), whereas active motion, particularly active motion against resistance, is limited or painful. In adhesive capsulitis, however, both the passive and active ranges of motion are limited.

A general examination also provides clues, particularly if the shoulder examination is relatively normal. Evidence

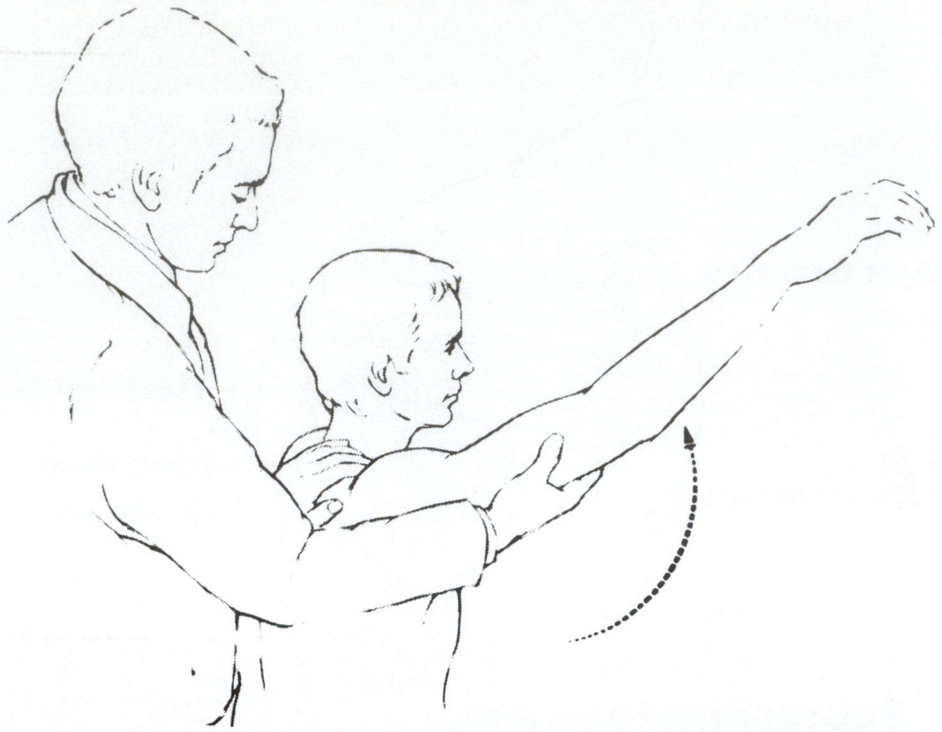

**Fig. 80-5.** The impingement sign is performed with the examiner fixing the scapula with one hand while forward elevating the patient's arm with the other hand. Patient may complain of pain as the greater tuberosity impinge against the acromion. (From Neer CS: *Clin Orthop* 173:73, 1983.)

for other joint involvement may suggest an inflammatory arthropathy. Neurologic deficits point to neuropathic processes. Pain referred to the shoulder may originate in the neck, lungs, heart, or abdomen.

### *Specific disorders*

**Rotator cuff tendinitis/impingement syndrome.** The rotator cuff complex includes the supraspinatus, infraspinatus, and teres minor muscles, which attach to the greater tuberosity of the humerus, and the subscapularis, which attaches to the lesser tuberosity (Fig. 80-4). The rotator cuff is the internal and external rotator of the shoulder and also depresses the humeral head during abduction. Most common shoulder problems are due to rotator cuff pathology that has been categorized into impingement syndrome, acute tendinitis, and rotator cuff tears.

*Impingement syndrome* refers to compression of the rotator cuff (particularly supraspinatus and infraspinatus) and the long head of the biceps against the acromion, coracoacromial ligament, and sometimes the acromioclavicular joint. Neer separated impingement syndrome into three different stages. Stage I usually occurs in patients 15 to 25 years old who perform repetitive overhead activities. Edema and hemorrhage are present in the rotator cuff. Stage II occurs in active individuals between ages 25 and 50 and is typically associated with pathologic changes of fibrosis. Stage III occurs in older individuals when the cuff progressively degenerates or tears, and secondary bony changes develop in the acromion and humerus.

The patient typically complains of pain that is often worse at night and is exacerbated by overhead activity. Pain may be localized to the area of the subacromial region or may diffusely radiate down toward the deltoid region. The pain can be intermittent or constant. In young patients, complete tear, usually resulting from trauma, is acutely painful, whereas in older patients, the condition may be less symptomatic.

Examination reveals normal passive range of motion of the glenohumeral joint. Active motion, however, may be limited because of pain. Patients often use scapulothoracic movement to help in abduction of the shoulder. The impingement sign is useful (Fig. 80-5). The examiner passively forward flexes the arm with one hand while stabilizing the scapula with the other to prevent scapular rotation. Pain occurring near the end of elevation is a positive sign for impingement of the supraspinatus and/or biceps tendon against the greater tuberosity.

In a rotator cuff tear, active abduction, internal rotation, and external rotation against resistance may be weak. The drop sign is positive if the patient's arm suddenly drops or gives way at 90 degrees when the arm is brought down from overhead (180 degrees) along the side.

Radiographs in early impingement are usually normal, whereas advanced stages may reveal sclerosis and cystic changes of the distal acromion or greater tuberosity. If the rotator cuff is torn, the space between the acromion and humeral head (normally measuring greater than 5 mm) is lost, and proximal migration of the humerus occurs. Scalloping or erosions of the acromion are also present. Arthrography alone or in combination with a CT scan is useful to detect a tear. Ultrasound, performed by an experienced radiologist, may be quite sensitive in detecting rotator cuff tears. MRI may be the most sensitive test to identify a tear, whether partial or complete.

Treatment of impingement syndrome depends on the stage. In early disease, conservative therapy with antiinflammatory medications, rest, and physical therapy to strengthen the rotator cuff muscles is usually adequate. In stages I and II, corticosteroid injections into the subacromial space may also be very effective. Job and recreational modifications are necessary to prevent further injury. Patients unresponsive to conservative therapy that has included two or three corticosteroid injections or patients with functional impairment should be referred to an orthopedic surgeon for consultation. Arthroscopic decompression includes the division of the coracoacromial ligament and acromioplasty. The latter is felt to be most successful for patients with an intact rotator cuff. The results of open and arthroscopic decompression are similar.

**Acute tendinitis.** Although supraspinatus and bicipital tendinitis typically result from impingement, they may occasionally occur as separate entities. Supraspinatus tendinitis is more common. This tendon helps abduct the shoulder and maintain the strength of the arm when carrying a heavy load with the shoulder abducted; thus it is susceptible to overuse and eventual degeneration. The biceps muscle functions as a flexor of the elbow, supinator of the forearm, and forward elevator of the upper arm. Again, tendinitis occurs as a result of overuse or repetitive motion.

In supraspinatus tendinitis, pain usually localizes in the region just above the scapular spine and lateral to the acromion, near the greater tuberosity of the humerus. Active abduction against resistance elicits severe pain, but passive motion is entirely normal. In bicipital tendinitis, pain is located anteriorly in the area of the biceps tendon, and discrete swelling is sometimes palpable in the tendon area. Supination of the hand against resistance (Yergason maneuver) is painful at the shoulder. Active and passive motion of the shoulder is normal.

Acute calcific tendinitis occurs secondary to calcium hydroxyapatite deposition in a tendon that has developed degeneration from overuse or impingement. It can involve any tendinous location, but the supraspinatus and bicipital tendons are common areas. Symptoms are usually acute, mimicking gout or pseudogout, and may resolve spontaneously over several days. Calcium deposits within the supraspinatus tendon may eventually rupture into the subacromial bursa, and secondary bursitis develops. Radiographs sometimes reveal amorphous or well-delineated calcific deposits within the subacromial bursa, supraspinatus, or bicipital tendons. Treatment includes nonsteroidal antiinflammatory drugs (NSAIDs), local corticosteroid injection, or intramuscular adrenocorticotropic hormone (ACTH) 40-60 IU. Colchicine, 0.6 mg twice a day, may prevent recurrent flares. Multiple needlings, which manually disrupt the calcific deposits, along with corticosteroid infiltration may help resolve resistant cases. If symptoms recur, surgical intervention may be necessary (see Chapter 71).

**Bursitis.** The terms *subacromial* and *subdeltoid bursitis* have often been misused to describe pain in these regions. Acute bursitis is most likely due to impingement syndrome or calcific tendinitis. Clinical symptoms, physical findings, and treatment are identical to those previously outlined.

**Tears of the rotator cuff or biceps tendon.** In a young patient a tear or rupture of the rotator cuff or biceps tendon occurs only with a traumatic injury. Acute rotator cuff tear often develops after falling with the arm outstretched, whereas acute rupture of the biceps tendon occurs after lifting a heavy object. In older patients minor or no trauma can be associated with rotator cuff tear because of progressive attrition of the tendon from years of overuse or impingement.

It may be difficult to distinguish partial tear of the rotator cuff from acute tendinitis on examination, since weakness of active motion may not be obvious. Chronic tears may be associated with atrophy of the supraspinatus and infraspinatus. The drop sign can be positive. The classic physical finding with rupture of the biceps tendon is the contracted biceps muscle, which fails to move or tighten on active flexion of the elbow.

Diagnosis of tears of the rotator cuff is discussed in the section on stage III impingement. Treatment of acute tears in young patients is surgical. If symptoms of impingement were already present and contributed to the rotator cuff or bicipital tendon rupture, then acromioplasty is indicated. In older patients, if function and pain are not limiting, conservative therapy is adequate.

**Myofascial shoulder pain.** Myofascial pain around the shoulder region is often the result of overuse or poor positioning during work or play. The most common regions include the trapezius, supraspinatus and infraspinatus, and the muscles along the medial border of the scapula (the levator scapulae and rhomboid) (see Fig. 80-3). Pain may be perceived by the patient as diffuse and may include sites distant from the myofascial trigger point. On examination a taut band may be palpable in various regions. Treatment is outlined in the section on therapy.

**Adhesive capsulitis.** Adhesive capsulitis (frozen shoulder) is a slow, insidious loss of shoulder motion accompanied by varying intensities of pain. The condition is usually self-limited and resolves within 1 to 3 years unless there is an underlying disease. Often a patient is left with 20% to 25% residual loss of normal motion. Adhesive capsulitis typically develops after a period of shoulder immobility after acute calcific tendinitis of the shoulder, acute stroke, or myocardial infarction. It is also associated with other diseases such as diabetes, hypothyroidism and hyperthyroidism, tuberculosis, apical lung tumors, and local primary neoplasms (see the box below). Women and middle-aged patients (40 to 60 years old) are at a slightly

### Conditions associated with adhesive capsulitis

Diabetes
Hypothyroidism/hyperthyroidism
Adrenal insufficiency
Pulmonary tuberculosis
Apical lung tumors
Hemiparesis
Complication after brachial cardiac catheterization
Myocardial infarction
Primary local tumors in the humerus, chest wall

greater risk for developing adhesive capsulitis. The pathology of adhesive capsulitis reveals capsular fibrosis and contracture, but it is not clear whether this is a result of inflammation or joint immobility.

Patients complain of slow, gradual onset of shoulder pain that can be severe, even at night. The pain is generalized and referred to the superior lateral aspect of the shoulder and upper arm. On examination, there is no swelling at the glenohumeral joint. Passive and active ranges of motion are markedly limited in all movements.

Diagnosis of adhesive capsulitis is based on the physical findings of limited shoulder motion. The physician should investigate associated diseases such as diabetes and thyroid disease. Laboratory studies and plain radiographs are not helpful except to exclude secondary etiologies. Shoulder arthrography can confirm the reduction of the joint cavity but is not necessary, since the diagnosis is established clinically. Routine arthroscopy is not indicated unless other processes, such as intraarticular pathology, are suspected or patients fail to benefit from conservative therapy.

Numerous treatments for adhesive capsulitis have been described, but most studies are uncontrolled. Prevention is most important. Range-of-motion shoulder exercises should be recommended by the primary care physician for any painful shoulder. The Codman (pendulum) exercise is performed with the patient flexed forward at the waist with most of the body weight supported by the opposite arm on a table or chair back (Fig. 80-6). The affected arm is dangled perpendicular to the ground. The patient then circles the arm clockwise for a set repetition and then counterclockwise. The circles should become bigger, and the patient can progress to holding weights with the affected arm while doing the pendulum exercises.

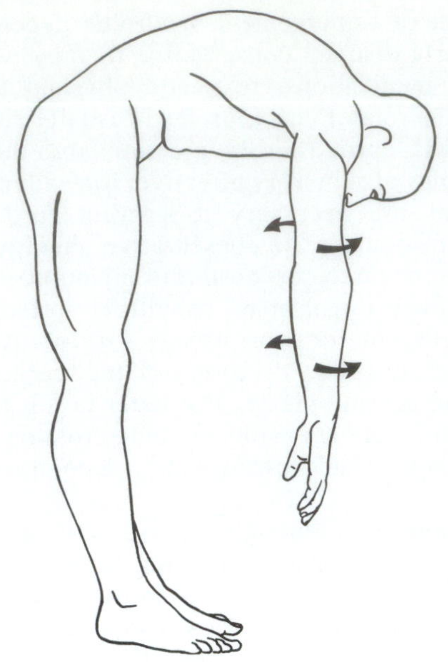

**Fig. 80-6.** Codman (pendulum) range-of-motion exercise for the shoulder.

NSAIDs have inconsistent effects on the pain. Intraarticular steroids and oral prednisone (10 mg at night) appear to be effective in controlling the nocturnal pain on motion in early disease. To regain motion, however, an intensive physical therapy program should be initiated by a physical therapist, followed by a home program. Patients must be informed that improvement is slow. In fact, symptoms may persist for 1 to 2 years.

Some patients have intractable pain unresponsive to conservative therapy; while others have severe shoulder limitation, impairing activities of daily living. Distention arthrography with lidocaine and saline or in combination with manipulation or manipulation under general anesthesia is often performed, but the true efficacy of these interventions has not been proven in well-designed trials. Arthroscopic examination with distention and debridement of capsular adhesions appears comparable to manipulation but offers the advantage of diagnosing and repairing unsuspected rotator cuff tears.

**Reflex sympathetic dystrophy.** Reflex sympathetic dystrophy (RSD) (shoulder-hand syndrome) may present initially as shoulder pain or adhesive capsulitis. Risk factors are similar to those of adhesive capsulitis and range from traumatic soft tissue or bony injury to postmyocardial or cerebrovascular injury. The etiology is unclear, but a disturbance of sympathetic outflow is assumed through the symptoms, physical findings, and response to treatment. RSD may also occur in the lower extremity.

In the earliest stage, patients complain of burning pain, swelling, temperature changes, and excessive perspiration in the extremity. Some 3 to 6 months after the initial stage, the soft tissue swelling progresses to skin induration and muscle atrophy. The late stage is characterized by contractures of the digits; tight, shiny skin; and limitation of motion. Pain may extend proximally from the hand.

Radiographs in early to middle phases may be normal or may reveal patchy osteopenia, whereas late-stage findings have marked osteopenia. Triple-phase technetium bone scan classically demonstrates increased blood flow and pooling, as well as increased uptake in the periarticular structures of the affected extremity. Diagnostically, the improvement of pain and dysesthesia after regional sympathetic block is also characteristic.

The differential diagnosis of RSD includes cervical radiculopathy, carpal tunnel syndrome, the onset of systemic sclerosis, and RA. Treatment in the early phases includes high-dose systemic glucocorticoids (1 mg/kg per day) for 2 weeks. If the patient does not respond, the steroids are rapidly tapered; if improvement occurs, the steroids are tapered gradually over 4 to 6 weeks. Alternative treatments include interruption of sympathetic tone through regional ganglionic block, sympathectomy, and medications. Rigorous physical therapy should follow all interventions to preserve motion. In later stages, physical therapy alone is indicated to help regain function and motion. Full recovery is limited if symptoms have been present for more than 6 months.

***Differential diagnosis.*** The differential diagnosis of shoulder pain is broad and can be separated into four categories (see the box on p. 1119). Intraarticular processes include internal derangement, synovitis, osteoarthritis, infection, osteonecrosis, adhesive capsulitis, and tumor. Periarticular processes primarily involve

### Differential diagnosis of shoulder pain

**Intraarticular processes**

Synovitis secondary to RA or spondyloarthropathies
Infection
Adhesive capsulitis
Osteoarthritis
Internal derangement (labral tears)
Avascular necrosis
Benign or malignant tumors (bone or synovial)

**Periarticular processes**

Impingement syndrome: rotator cuff or bicipital
Calcific tendinitis
Tears of rotator cuff or biceps tendons
Myofascial pain
Acromioclavicular arthritis

**Referred pain**

Sternoclavicular joint processes
Cervical radiculopathy
Pancoast tumors
Subdiaphragmatic processes (abscess or gallbladder disease)
Myocardial infarction
Mediastinal tumors (pain localized to the axilla)

**Others**

Reflex sympathetic dystrophy
Brachial neuritis
Thoracic outlet syndrome
Suprascapular nerve entrapment

Modified from Thornhill TS. In Kelley WN, et al, editors: *Textbook of rheumatology*, ed 5, Philadelphia, 1993, WB Saunders.

### Differential diagnosis of shoulder pain by location

**Top of the shoulder (C4)**

Cervical source
Acromioclavicular
Sternoclavicular
Diaphragmatic

**Superolateral (C5)**

Rotator cuff tendinitis
Impingement
Adhesive capsulitis
Glenohumeral arthritis

**Anterior**

Bicipital tendinitis and rupture
Glenoid labral tear
Adhesive capsulitis
Glenohumeral arthritis
Osteonecrosis

**Axillary**

Neoplasm (Pancoast, mediastinal)
Herpes zoster

rotator cuff pathology, bicipital tendinitis, acromioclavicular arthritis, and localized or generalized myofascial disorders. Referred pain to the shoulder often is associated with cervical radiculopathy, Pancoast tumors, subdiaphragmatic processes, gallbladder disease, and myocardial infarction. Other considerations include RSD, brachial neuritis, suprascapular nerve entrapment, and thoracic outlet syndrome. A differential diagnosis can also be generated by the location of shoulder pain. The box above provides diagnostic possibilities for each region.

## Elbow

True articular causes of elbow pain are extremely rare with the exception of inflammatory processes of the elbow joint. Common soft tissue syndromes include olecranon bursitis, lateral and medial epicondylitis, and nerve entrapment syndromes. Pain often localizes over a particular region.

Passive and active range of motion of the elbow spans 0 degrees (full extension) to 135 degrees (full flexion). With joint inflammation the patient holds the elbow in semiflexion to accommodate inflammatory fluid or cellular infiltrate. Active and passive flexion and extension are limited. However, with periarticular disease, passive range of motion is usually normal.

### *Bursitis*

**Olecranon bursitis.** Systemic diseases such as gout, RA, and, less commonly, pseudogout, oxalosis, and basic calcium phosphate deposition may all involve the olecranon bursa. Traumatic or infectious bursitis, however, is more common in primary care practice. Since the olecranon bursa is a superficial bursa, it is susceptible to repetitive trauma and bacterial infection from direct skin penetration. Patients may not remember a particular event that precipitated the swelling but may have a long-standing habit of bearing pressure on the elbows. In acute crystal or infectious bursitis, pain tends to be severe, and systemic symptoms such as fever, sweats, and chills may be present.

An important physical finding is swelling in a discrete sac at the tip of the olecranon. The region may be warm, erythematous, and painful to palpation. Soft tissue edema distal to the elbow may be present. Occasionally, if septic bursitis is advanced, the olecranon bursa ruptures, resulting in diffuse cellulitis of the elbow and forearm. Pain may be present (sometimes severe) in flexion, but full passive extension of the elbow is possible without pain, suggesting that true elbow joint involvement is unlikely. Rheumatoid nodules or tophaceous deposits may be palpable in the olecranon bursa.

Aspiration and analysis of the olecranon bursa fluid for total and differential white blood cell (WBC) count, crystal search, Gram stain, and culture are important in making the diagnosis. Unlike articular infections, the septic bursal fluid may have deceptively few WBC (less than 10,000 cells/$mm^3$). Infection cannot be excluded until culture results are final. Radiographs typically reveal only soft tissue swelling.

Therapy for traumatic bursitis includes protecting the olecranon region from further trauma by consciously avoiding pressure to the elbow. Corticosteroid injection into the bursa has been successful, but skin atrophy and secondary infections may occur, making it a less-than-optimal treatment. Surgical resection is rarely necessary.

Some 80% of all septic bursitis is due to *Staphylococcus aureus,* followed by *Streptococcus* organisms in 14% of cases. Rarely, gram-negative infection occurs, most often in debilitated or older patients. An oral antibiotic effective against *Staphylococcus* and *Streptococcus* organisms is the initial therapy for septic olecranon bursitis. When final cultures return, the antibiotic can be tailored.

Along with antibiotic therapy, serial needle aspiration of the olecranon bursa fluid is necessary daily until culture results are negative. Antibiotics can be discontinued 5 days after the negative culture. If cultures reveal persistence of the organism despite antibiotic therapy and aspiration, surgical resection of the bursa is necessary. More aggressive initial therapy with intravenous antibiotics may be indicated for patients who are febrile, immunocompromised, or chronically debilitated.

The differential diagnosis for swelling in the olecranon region includes traumatic, septic, gouty, and rheumatoid bursitis. In addition, superficial bursitis sometimes occurs in systemic sclerosis, systemic lupus erythematosus (SLE), and hypertrophic pulmonary osteoarthropathy.

***Lateral and medial epicondylitis.*** Lateral epicondylitis (tennis elbow) results from trauma to the insertion of the common extensor tendon onto the lateral epicondyle. Some investigators report avulsion of the extensor radialis brevis at its insertion onto the lateral epicondyle. Patients typically describe an aching pain in the lateral aspect of the elbow that is aggravated by grasping or turning the wrist. Pain may be present at rest. Onset ranges from acute to subacute or chronic. Despite its name, tennis elbow develops with any occupation or activity that stresses the wrist extensors.

Medial epicondylitis is the counterpart to lateral epicondylitis but results from overuse of the flexor tendons of the wrist. The point of tenderness is located over the medial epicondyle. Although it is given the name *golfer's elbow,* this condition may occur with other sports and occupational activities.

Physical examination reveals focal tenderness in the lateral or medial epicondyle region. In addition, extension of the finger or wrist against resistance produces pain in the lateral epicondyle region, whereas flexion of the wrist against resistance produces pain in the medial epicondyle region.

Bilateral lateral epicondylitis is rare. When present, the physician should consider fibromyalgia. Entrapment neuropathies, particularly the deep branch of the radial nerve, may be confused with lateral epicondylitis, whereas compressive neuropathy of the ulnar nerve may be mistaken for medial epicondylitis. In addition, cervical radiculopathy and carpal tunnel syndrome sometimes manifest as elbow pain. Entrapment neuropathy of the deep branch of the radial nerve should be suspected in chronic refractory tennis elbow. The tenderness is anterior, on the radius, approximately 2 cm distal to the elbow crease.

Treatment of lateral and medial epicondylitis begins with avoiding the aggravating condition and modifying it to prevent recurrent injury. This may require the assistance of a professional in sports medicine or an occupational therapist. Relative rest for 3 to 4 weeks, the use of a forearm compression band, and NSAIDs are the initial steps of therapy. Gentle exercises to stretch the extensor or flexor muscles should progress to strengthening exercises. The success rate of these combined conservative modalities is nearly 75%.

Local corticosteroid infiltration around the lateral and medial epicondyle has been a traditional alternative when conservative therapy fails. However, more recent studies reveal that, although corticosteroid injection is more effective than lidocaine alone for acute pain management, the outcome at 6 months is the same. Thus conservative therapy is recommended for 6 months. If pain persists after that period, surgical consultation is recommended.

## Wrist and hand

The wrist and hand are prone to traumatic injuries as well as to systemic inflammatory disease. Periarticular processes of the wrist include tenosynovitis, median and ulnar nerve entrapment, and ganglions. In the hand, tenosynovitis and Dupuytren contractures are common periarticular conditions.

Wrist flexion normally spans 80 to 90 degrees for flexion and 80 degrees for extension. Ulnar deviation is usually 40 to 45 degrees and radial deviation is 20 degrees. Palpation of the ulnar styloid and radiocarpal joints provides clues for synovitis. Muscle atrophy on examination of the hand may suggest neuropathy. Skin changes, such as tightening and rashes, and nail changes are helpful in diagnosing systemic inflammatory diseases. The range of motion of the fingers can be grossly assessed by the patient's ability to make a complete fist. If the patient cannot, the examination must focus on passive and active range of motion of the fingers to distinguish an articular process from a tendinous one. If the examiner can passively move the metacarpophalangeal (MCP), proximal interphalangeal (PIP), and distal interphalangeal (DIP) joints into full flexion, the pathology resides in the tendon mechanism. However, if passive motion of the joint is limited, articular pathology is present.

***Tenosynovitis.*** Although tenosynovitis is more common in the inflammatory arthritides, such as RA and psoriatic arthritis, stenosing tenosynovitis of the thumb and fingers results more often from overuse or repetitive motion.

**De Quervain tenosynovitis.** Stenosing tenosynovitis of the abductor pollicis longus and extensor pollicis brevis tendons is also known as *de Quervain tenosynovitis.* It is secondary to the thickening of the fibrous sheath over the radial styloid, which impinges on the two tendons. Patients have pain over the radial aspect of the wrist, which is often exacerbated by thumb or wrist motion. Physical findings may include focal soft tissue swelling over the radial styloid region, pain on palpation of the region, or severe pain when the wrist is deviated toward the ulna while the thumb is folded within the fingers (Finkelstein's test) (Fig. 80-7). Differential diagnosis of pain in this region includes carpometacarpal disease from osteoarthritis, tendinitis of the extensors of the wrist, or tendinitis

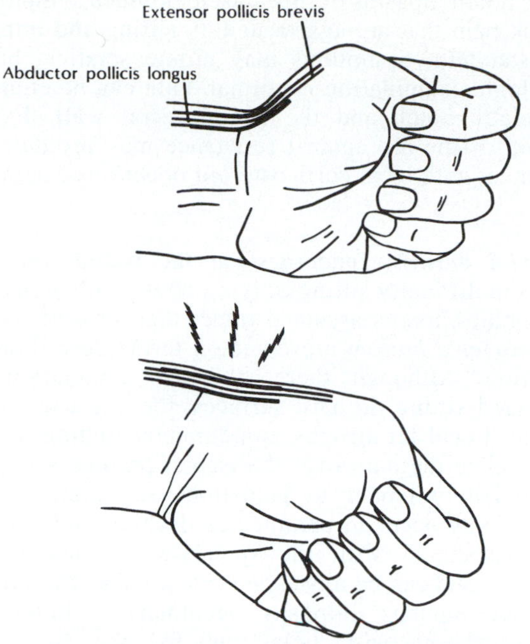


**Fig. 80-7.** Finkelstein's test is positive in de Quervain's stenosing synovitis. Ulnar flexion of the wrist produces pain over the dorsal compartment containing the extensor pollicis brevis and abductor pollicis longus.

associated with systemic disease such as spondyloarthropathies or disseminated gonococcemia. Treatment includes immobilization with a long thumb spica or opponens splint fashioned by an occupational therapist, NSAIDs, and local corticosteroid injection into the tendon sheath. Activities that require repetitive motion of the thumb or wrist should be modified.

**Stenosing tenosynovitis.** Stenosing tenosynovitis of the finger, also known as *trigger finger,* develops secondary to excessive forces at the fibrous rings that affix the flexor tendon in place. As a result of these forces, fibrocartilaginous metaplasia develops and obstructs the normal gliding motion of the flexor tendon. Repetitive motion of the fingers and frequent clutching of the hand are associated with this entity. Patients classically complain of the inability to open a finger from flexion in the morning without active assistance from the other hand. Other patients describe a snapping of the finger from flexion to extension. Examination reveals swelling or nodularity, often tender to palpation, along the tendon sheath in the palmar surface of the hand. If the patient actively flexes and extends the finger, crepitation is palpable in the course of the tendon within the palm.

Differential diagnosis includes suppurative tenosynovitis (an acute syndrome with redness and pronounced tenderness), mycobacterial infections, systemic inflammatory diseases, Dupuytren contracture, and sarcoidosis. If multiple fingers are involved, diabetes mellitus, amyloidosis, and ochronosis should be excluded.

Local corticosteroid injection of the tendon sheath is extremely effective. Most published reports indicate a high percentage of success with local injections. Modification of job or recreational activities is necessary. Referral to a hand surgeon is recommended if symptoms recur.

***Median and ulnar nerve entrapment.*** Entrapment of the median and ulnar nerves at the wrist results in carpal tunnel syndromes, which are described in Chapter 103.

***Dupuytren contracture.*** Dupuytren contracture is a progressive fibrotic condition involving the palmar fascia that leads to fixed flexion deformities at the MCP joint. This entity is painless and does not cause significant disability until the fingers develop contractures that limit function. Pathologically, fibroblasts proliferate in the palmar fascia without an inflammatory component. The flexor tendons, however, are not involved. Taut bands of fibrosis form, typically involving the fourth, fifth, and occasionally the third fingers, but rarely the thumb or index finger. Similar findings may occur in the plantar region. Men are affected more often than women. Previous reports associating Dupuytren contracture with diabetes mellitus and alcoholism have not been consistently documented. Treatment consists of passive extension of the finger in early stages. Surgical intervention at later stages may be necessary, but recurrence is common.

***Ganglions.*** Ganglions are cystic outpouchings of the joint capsule or tendon sheath. They often occur asymptomatically on the dorsum of the wrist and resolve or recur spontaneously. The ganglion is filled with a gelatinous fluid and transilluminates, differentiating it from solid tumors. Lipomas, neuromas, synovial cyst of RA, calcific deposits, giant cell tumor, and sarcomas may have a similar appearance. Management includes observation only, aspiration and injection with corticosteroids, or surgical removal.

### Anterior chest wall pain

Costochondritis or pain in the anterior chest wall along the costosternal junction may mimic acute cardiac or pleuritic pain. Patients describe intermittent pain that lasts for several days, radiates to the chest wall, and is exacerbated by deep breath. Tenderness to palpation of the costosternal junctions at one or more locations and even along the intercostal muscles are common findings. If bilateral tenderness in the costochondral regions is elicited, spondyloarthropathies and fibromyalgia should be considered in the differential diagnosis. In addition, referred pain from cardiac, pulmonary, esophageal, and vascular sources must be excluded.

Tietze's syndrome is a possible diagnosis if swelling is associated with pain in the costochondral regions. The etiology of Tietze's syndrome is unknown, but pathology reveals proliferation of cartilage and increased vascularity in the costochondral region. This syndrome may be acute or chronic. Differential diagnosis includes spondyloarthropathy, infection, and tumor of the bone.

Treatment of both syndromes includes eliminating the factors that may aggravate the pain, administering NSAIDs, instituting physical therapy with ultrasound, or administering local corticosteroid injections. Skin atrophy in the anterior chest wall region can occur secondary to local steroid injections. This complication may be particularly undesirable for some patients.

## Low back and pelvis

Low back pain is one of the most common complaints in a primary care practice. Although it is usually self-limited, loss of productivity in the working population exacts an enormous financial cost to society. Chapter 73 details the causes of low back pain. This section focuses on the soft tissue etiologies, which include myofascial pain, bursitis, and localized muscle syndromes.

***Myofascial low back pain.*** Myofascial low back pain can develop without associated conditions or can be secondary to mechanical back disease, nerve entrapment, and inflammatory diseases of the back. Patients complain of a dull, aching pain that is not well localized. Sometimes muscle spasm is associated with the pain, and nondermatomal radicular symptoms may be present. The pain is exacerbated by activity, prolonged sitting, or cool temperatures. More ominous symptoms that require further evaluation include fever, chills, weight loss, pain unrelated to position, urinary or fecal incontinence, and neurologic deficits.

Inspection of the lower back while the patient is standing may reveal asymmetry that suggests scoliosis or leg length discrepancy. Percussion of the vertebral bodies and palpation of the paravertebral musculature can localize the region of pain. Lower back range of motion includes flexion, extension, lateral bending, and lateral rotation. Numerous myofascial trigger points may be palpable in the lower back. Fig. 80-3 illustrates the most common points, described by Schoen, Moskowitz, and Goldberg. When these points are pressed, the pain is reproduced and can radiate to distant regions.

The diagnosis of myofascial low back pain is based on the exclusion of other etiologies. The major categories include mechanical back pain secondary to degenerative disease, nerve entrapment syndromes, infection, inflammatory back disease, referred pain from abdominal or retroperitoneal sources, neoplasms, and psychogenic causes.

Treatment of myofascial low back pain includes recognition of aggravating factors at home, at work, or in recreational activities. Proper sitting, standing, and sleeping positions should be encouraged. Exercises to strengthen the abdominal musculature and back extensors, improvement of posture, and back protection are the foundation of lifelong back care. Referral to a formal back school or physical therapy program is recommended if patients have chronic pain. NSAIDs may be helpful to patients with myofascial pain secondary to degenerative diseases. Muscle relaxants such as cyclobenzaprine, 10 to 20 mg qhs and 5 to 10 mg in the morning, are helpful if muscle spasms are present. Alternatively, low-dose tricyclic antidepressants (amitriptyline and others) may help patients with chronic back pain. Myofascial trigger-point injections with a long-acting anesthetic followed by muscle stretch provides fairly rapid relief of pain. According to some authors, this can provide lasting benefit without the need for chronic reinjections. Other modalities, including therapeutic massage and the transcutaneous electrical nerve stimulation (TENS) unit, have variable results.

***Piriformis syndrome.*** The piriformis muscle is an external rotator of the hip that occupies the area of the greater sciatic notch. Spasms of this muscle produce symptoms of buttock pain that are aggravated by sitting and improved with standing. Symptoms may mimic sciatica, but the neurologic examination is normal. Pain can be elicited in the sciatic notch and the lateral rectal wall. External rotation of the hip against resistance may produce pain. Treatment with local corticosteroid injections can provide relief.

***Ischial bursitis.*** Tenderness at the ischial tuberosity results in difficulty sitting or lying down. Inflammation of the ischial bursa is assumed rather than proved. *Tailor's* and *weaver's bottom* are common terms describing this condition. Although there is some association with prolonged sitting on hard surfaces, the exact etiology is unclear. Local fat atrophy is a common finding. Patients can localize the pain over the ischial prominence, which is exquisitely tender to palpation. Suppurative ischial bursitis may occur in paraplegics. Ischial tenderness has been associated with the spondyloarthropathies from enthesitis and can be mistaken for low back strain or even herniated nucleus pulposus. Treatment includes using foam cushions with holes cut for the two ischial tuberosities. Local corticosteroid injections should be avoided; they may result in further fat atrophy and pain.

***Osteitis pubis.*** Inflammation of the symphysis pubis has multiple etiologies. Septic seeding of the symphysis occurs most commonly after genitourinary surgery or herniorrhaphy. Spondyloarthropathies, particularly in women, and calcium pyrophosphate dihydrate (CPPD) disease may also affect this region. Trauma from sports, stress fractures, or specific injury to the gracilis or adductor longus muscles may clinically resemble osteitis pubis.

Patients complain of pain in the lower anterior pelvis that may radiate into the medial thighs. Walking may be painful, and palpation over the symphysis pubis produces exquisite pain. Initial radiographs may be normal, but with advanced stages, erosions, widening of the joint space, and sclerosis are present. In CPPD disease, linear calcification in the symphysis is present.

Treatment includes the use of NSAIDs during evaluation for other underlying diseases. The pain may resolve spontaneously. If infection is suspected, percutaneous aspiration must be performed. Local corticosteroid injection may be beneficial. Surgical intervention is reserved for intractable cases.

## Hips

Periarticular structures and referred pain cause hip pain more commonly than true articular processes. In the latter, pathology in the joint results in pain localized to the groin or referred anatomically to the knee. Patients often use the term *hip pain* to refer to any area in the lower back, buttock, and lateral hip regions.

Inspection of the hips during weight bearing detects scoliosis or leg length discrepancy. The gait should be observed. An antalgic gait is characterized by the patient leaning over the painful hip during weight bearing to avoid contraction of the hip abductors. Alternatively, the pelvis may drop down on the opposite side when bearing weight on the affected hip (Trendelenburg gait).

Measurement of leg lengths is performed in the supine position from the anterior superior iliac crest to the medial malleolus. Up to 1 cm of difference in length between the legs is considered normal. Passive range of motion of the hip includes flexion (120 to 135 degrees), extension (20 degrees; it is performed with the patient prone or supine with the leg off the side of the table), internal rotation (35 to 45 degrees), and external rotation (45 degrees). The hips can also abduct to 60 to 70 degrees and adduct to 25 to 30 degrees. The Patrick or Fabere test involves placing the foot (ipsilateral to the hip being examined) onto the knee of the other leg; then the thigh is further abducted toward the table. If pain exists, intrinsic hip disease or sacroiliac disease is present. The Thomas test can detect hip contractures. With the patient supine, both hips are flexed initially and the hip of concern is then extended toward the table; the other hip remains flexed to fix the pelvis and flatten the lumbar lordosis. Limitation of full extension indicates a hip contracture on that side. Examination of the periarticular structures is detailed later.

#### *Bursitis*

**Trochanteric bursa.** The trochanteric bursa is located between the tendon of the gluteus maximus muscle and the posterior aspect of the greater trochanter. Bursitis classically develops from overuse or stress of the hip abductors due to hip disease, degenerative disease of the lumbar spine, leg length discrepancy, and other lower extremity conditions. The trochanteric region is a common tender point for fibromyalgia. Thus any patient with bilateral trochanteric bursitis should be examined for other tender points associated with fibromyalgia (see the section on fibromyalgia).

Patients typically complain of localized lateral hip discomfort exacerbated by rising from a chair or car seat and walking and difficulty sleeping on the affected side. Sometimes the pain is diffuse, involving the lateral hip and thigh, buttock, and even the groin and/or knee.

Localized point tenderness on or posterior to the greater trochanter is the classic finding. Occasionally, the fascia lata is also tender. Active hip abduction against resistance and passive external rotation of the hip produce pain. Passive internal rotation is normal.

Differential diagnosis of lateral hip pain includes referred pain from the spine, particularly the upper lumbar region (L2 to L4) secondary to spinal stenosis, disk herniation, and facet syndromes. Entrapment of the cutaneous branches of the iliohypogastric or subcostal nerve can produce burning pain in the lateral hip. Occult stress fractures of the femoral neck in older patients may present as lateral hip pain. Fascia lata fasciitis may mimic trochanteric bursitis, but the pain usually extends below the trochanteric region along the tensor fascia lata.

Treatment of trochanteric bursitis includes moist heat and correction of associated pathology, such as leg-length discrepancy or gait abnormalities. Physical therapy referral for ultrasound is sometimes beneficial. Local corticosteroid injection mixed with lidocaine (Xylocaine) is most effective. Patients requiring frequent injections (more than three) warrant reevaluation and surgical consultation if no underlying cause is identified.

**Iliopsoas bursitis.** The iliopsoas bursa is a deep bursa located between the iliopsoas and the hip joint capsule. This bursa is in direct communication with the hip joint in approximately 15% of the patients. It is not a common site for inflammation unless underlying hip pathology exists. Patients typically complain of groin pain or anterior hip pain. Examination may reveal a palpable mass in the middle third of the inguinal ligament. Extension of the hip produces pain. Occasionally a patient may have a pelvic mass, venous compression, secondary varices, or compression neuropathy of the femoral nerve resulting from the mass effect of the expanding bursa.

Differential diagnosis of inguinal pain and/or mass includes intrinsic hip pathology, iliopsoas tendinitis, psoas abscess, hernias, adenopathy, femoral artery aneurysm, and tumor. Treatment is directed at the underlying hip pathology when inflammation is present. Local corticosteroid injections are effective but may require radiologic guidance. Surgical resection is sometimes necessary.

***Meralgia paresthetica.*** See Chapter 103.

### Knee

Periarticular structures of the knee contribute substantially to knee complaints in the primary care setting. Intraarticular knee pathology can be divided into inflammatory processes, degenerative processes, and internal derangement. Chapter 75 discusses sports injuries that commonly produce internal derangement; Chapters 78 and 79 cover RA and osteoarthritis. The periarticular structures of the knee include the prepatellar and infrapatellar bursae, the anserine bursa, the gastrocnemius and semimembranosus bursae, which may become a popliteal cyst, and the iliotibial band.

Examination of the knee begins with the patient standing while the physician looks for evidence of genu recurvatum (hyperextension of knee, suggestive of hyperlaxity), valgus or varus deformities, posterior or anterior knee swelling, and patellar malalignment. The knee joint is palpated medial and lateral to the patella for evidence of synovitis, anterior for prepatellar bursitis, and posterior for popliteal cysts. Range of motion includes flexion to 140 degrees and extension to 0 degrees. Instability of the knee can be detected by several maneuvers, described in Chapter 75.

Pain in the knee may be diffuse or localized. Referred pain from the hip typically is perceived medially. The differential diagnosis of knee pain according to location is shown in the box on p. 1124.

#### *Bursitis*

**Prepatellar bursitis.** The prepatellar bursa is a superficial bursa that is easily infected from direct penetration of skin surface bacteria. It can be chronically thickened by constant trauma from kneeling, particularly in occupations such as carpentry and housecleaning. Although gout or RA may occur in this bursa, inflammation in this region is usually infectious. Patients complain of sudden onset of redness, warmth, and swelling, accompanied by variable symptoms of fever or chills. Examination reveals erythema and swelling over the patella with surrounding soft tissue edema. Palpation of the joint reveals no synovitis or fluid. Passive extension of the knee is painless and full, which is in marked contrast to a septic knee joint. End flexion may produce discomfort resulting from

### Differential diagnosis of knee pain based on location

**Diffuse**
Articular

**Anterior**
Prepatellar bursitis
Patellar tendon enthesopathy
Chondromalacia patella
Patellofemoral osteoarthritis
Cruciate ligament injury
Medial plica syndrome

**Medial**
Anserine bursitis
Spontaneous osteonecrosis
Osteoarthritis
Medial meniscal tear
Medial collateral ligament bursitis
Referred pain from hip and L3
Fibromyalgia

**Lateral**
Iliotibial band syndrome
Meniscal cyst
Lateral meniscal tear
Collateral ligament
Peroneal tenosynovitis

**Posterior**
Popliteal cyst (Baker cyst)
Tendinitis
Aneurysms, ganglia, sarcoma

tautness of the skin over the prepatellar bursa.

Diagnosis is based on bursal fluid aspiration for cell count, crystal search, and culture. The WBC count in septic prepatellar bursal fluid may be deceptively low (similar to septic olecranon bursitis). Fluid cultures are therefore important to exclude infection. Blood may be present in traumatic prepatellar bursitis. Occasionally the prepatellar bursa ruptures before the patient visits the office. Aspiration of the cellulitic region near the prepatellar bursa is still indicated, since even a drop of fluid may provide the microbiologic diagnosis.

Treatment of septic prepatellar bursitis requires appropriate antibiotics to cover staphylococcal and streptococcal species (similar to treatment of olecranon bursitis) and serial drainage until fluid cultures become sterile. Although oral antibiotics and close monitoring are initially appropriate, this area is more difficult to treat successfully on an outpatient basis. Thus if patients do not improve within several days (diminution of swelling, erythema, and sterile cultures), hospitalization and intravenous antibiotics may be necessary. In addition, the knee must be immobilized to prevent constant irritation of the bursa, but the patient should be instructed on isometric exercises to maintain quadriceps muscle tone.

Early orthopedic consultation is advised so that debridement or more extensive drainage can proceed if medical therapy fails. Pigtail catheter drainage of the bursa, inserted under ultrasound or CT guidance, is an effective alternative approach to surgery.

Chronic prepatellar bursitis that is noninfectious should be treated by protection of the knee with pads and avoidance of kneeling. Most cases require surgical excision.

**Infrapatellar bursitis.** The infrapatellar bursa is located between the patellar tendon and the tibia. It is commonly associated with the spondyloarthropathies but can also be septic or associated with gout. Diagnosis and management are similar to those for prepatellar bursitis.

**Anserine bursitis.** The pes anserine bursa is located in the medial aspect of the knee, approximately 5 cm below the medial joint line and under the tendons of the sartorius, gracilis, and semitendinosus muscles as they attach to the tibia medially. Irritation of this region is often secondary to overexertion from running, valgus knee deformities, osteoarthritis, and fibromyalgia. Patients complain of medial knee pain with weight bearing and at night if the knees touch each other. Examination reveals exquisite tenderness over the anserine region. In obese patients, there may be overlying fat that is also painful. The knee joint is normal unless osteoarthritis is present. Differential diagnosis includes the various causes of medial knee pain listed in the box at left. Treatment includes NSAIDs or local corticosteroid injections with an anesthetic.

***Baker cyst (popliteal cyst).*** Baker cysts occur with any intrinsic pathology of the knee, including mechanical derangement, osteoarthritis, and all inflammatory arthritides, such as RA. Fluid from the knee enters the connecting gastrocnemius-semimembranosus bursa but is unable to return easily to the joint space, thus mimicking a one-way valve mechanism. Patients complain of fullness or swelling in the posterior aspect of the knee with pain in the calf. The pain is aggravated by walking and relieved by rest. If the cyst has ruptured or, if by mass effect, blocks venous or lymphatic drainage, peripheral edema of the lower extremity may be mistaken for deep venous thrombosis.

Swelling may be evident on inspection of the popliteal fossa. The Foucher sign (hardening of the mass in extension and softening of the mass in semiflexion of the knee) separates Baker cyst from popliteal aneurysm or tumor, in which consistency is unchanged. Edema of the lower extremity with calf tenderness and a positive Homans' sign may be present if the cyst has leaked or ruptured (pseudothrombophlebitis). Other findings associated with a Baker cyst may include secondary varices, ischemia, compressive neuropathies, and posterior compartment syndrome.

The differential diagnosis of a mass in the popliteal fossa includes popliteal artery aneurysm or cystic degeneration of the vessel wall, ganglia, lipoma, and sarcoma. Diagnosis is based on the physical examination. Ultrasonography visualizes the cyst, even if rupture has occurred, since residual fluid usually remains in the cyst. This technology has replaced the arthrogram, which was previously used to document extravasation of dye from the joint into the cyst and calf.

Treatment of a Baker cyst is based on treatment of the

underlying knee condition. Intraarticular steroids are effective if fluid is present in the knee and septic arthritis is excluded. Bed rest, heat, and elevation of the leg are necessary if the cyst has ruptured. True thrombophlebitis can develop secondary to prolonged compression, preventing venous return, and patients then need anticoagulation.

*Iliotibial band syndrome.* The iliotibial band is the extension of the fascia lata as it attaches to Gerdy tubercle, located on the lateral aspect of the tibia. Runners often develop pain over the lateral aspect of the knee because of tightness of this band as it rubs against the lateral femoral condyle during flexion and extension of the knee. Pain is reproduced over the lateral femoral condyle. Treatment includes the use of NSAIDs, ice, and ultrasound. Exercises to stretch the hip abductors and fascia lata, as well as correction of any mechanical factors, are also important.

## Ankle and foot

Foot and ankle problems are common in the ambulatory population. The principal motions of the ankle and foot complex include dorsiflexion, plantarflexion, inversion, and eversion. The small bones of the foot also accommodate various terrains. The true ankle joint functions in dorsiflexion (10 degrees) and plantar flexion (30 degrees). The subtalar joint allows for inversion (30 degrees) and eversion (10 degrees). The metatarsal phalangeal (MTP) joints provide the greatest motion in the foot, since their major role is in the push-off action of the foot. Thus dorsiflexion of the MTP joint is at least 70 degrees. In addition, the Achilles, posterior tibialis, and peroneal tendons function to plantarflex, invert, and evert the ankle and foot, respectively.

Examination of the ankle and foot begins with inspection of the area anteriorly and posteriorly while the patient is standing. The loss of the medial longitudinal arch is a common problem for valgus deformities. If swelling or pain is present, isolation of specific joints of the ankle is important. In true ankle arthritis, the dorsum of the ankle along the joint line is diffusely swollen. In contrast, asymmetric swelling over the medial or lateral malleolus suggests tenosynovitis of the posterior tibialis or peroneal tendon, respectively. Limitation of passive motion suggests true joint involvement. Active motion, particularly against resistance, tests the function of the tendons. The insertion of the Achilles tendon and plantar fascia should be palpated. Vascular and neurologic status completes the examination.

### *Tendinitis*

**Achilles tendinitis.** The Achilles tendon is susceptible to acute injury, rupture, calcification, and inflammation associated with the spondyloarthropathies and RA. Recently, Achilles tendon inflammation and rupture were described with fluoroquinolone treatment. Common symptoms are pain localized to the posterior aspect of the heel and pain exacerbated by dorsiflexion of the ankle. Acute injury usually occurs in running sports, and tendon rupture is possible. When rupture occurs, the patient describes a snapping sensation followed by the inability to stand on the toes. Acute swelling and erythema may be present in calcific tendinitis. In systemic inflammatory processes, the tendon may be diffusely tender and swollen and the retrocalcaneal bursa may also be involved. Treatment consists of rest, NSAIDs, heel inserts, and an ankle splint used at night in neutral position to prevent tendon contractures. In acute ruptures, immobilization and surgical intervention are necessary. Corticosteroid injections into the Achilles tendon are not recommended since this predisposes the patient to subsequent tendon rupture.

**Posterior tibialis tendon.** The posterior tibialis tendon inverts the foot and maintains the medial longitudinal arch. RA and the spondyloarthropathies often involve this tendon. Younger patients commonly injure the tendon while participating in high-stress activities, such as running and dancing. Older patients may note progressively flat arches and pain in the medial ankle secondary to gradual attrition of the tendon from microtrauma or degeneration. In cases of RA or other processes, acute rupture may suddenly result in a flat arch.

Diagnosis is based on physical findings of swelling and pain near the medial malleolus, pain or weakness on active inversion of the foot against resistance, and in late stages as a result of tendon rupture, flattening of the longitudinal arch on weight bearing with associated hindfoot valgus deformity (Fig. 80-8). MRI scans delineate the various stages of tendon degeneration. Treatment for initial stages includes rest, NSAIDs, and medial heel lift. If these approaches are ineffective, casting for a short time or local corticosteroid injection into the tendon sheath is necessary. Persistent inflammation, pain, and swelling may require surgical intervention.

**Peroneal tendon.** The peroneal tendon is susceptible to various inflammatory conditions as well as mechanical injury. This tendon everts the ankle. Examination reveals localized swelling and pain just posterior to the lateral malleolus. Active eversion against resistance is weak or painful. Therapy is similar to that for posterior tibialis tendinitis.

### *Bursitis*

**Retrocalcaneal bursa.** The retrocalcaneal bursa is located posterior to the calcaneus and anterior to the Achilles tendon at its insertion site onto the calcaneus. This bursa is usually associated with systemic inflammatory diseases such as the spondyloarthropathies, RA, and gout. Pain arises in the heel at the Achilles tendon's insertion. Focal swelling may be visible in this area. Therapy is similar to that for Achilles tendinitis. Intrabursal injection or surgery may be required if symptoms persist.

*Plantar fasciitis.* Inflammation of or strain on the plantar fascia is a common cause of foot pain. The plantar fascia is a thick, bandlike structure that attaches at the calcaneus and to each toe. Causes of plantar fasciitis include pes planus, prolonged standing, obesity, aerobic exercises that require jumping or bearing weight on the toes, fluoride or retinoid therapy, and the spondyloarthropathies. Patients complain of pain localized to the plantar surface of the foot that is exacerbated by pushing off with the toes. Examination with the dorsiflexed foot reveals tenderness along the plantar fascia or at the insertion of the fascia into the calcaneus. Heel spurs may be palpable or evident on

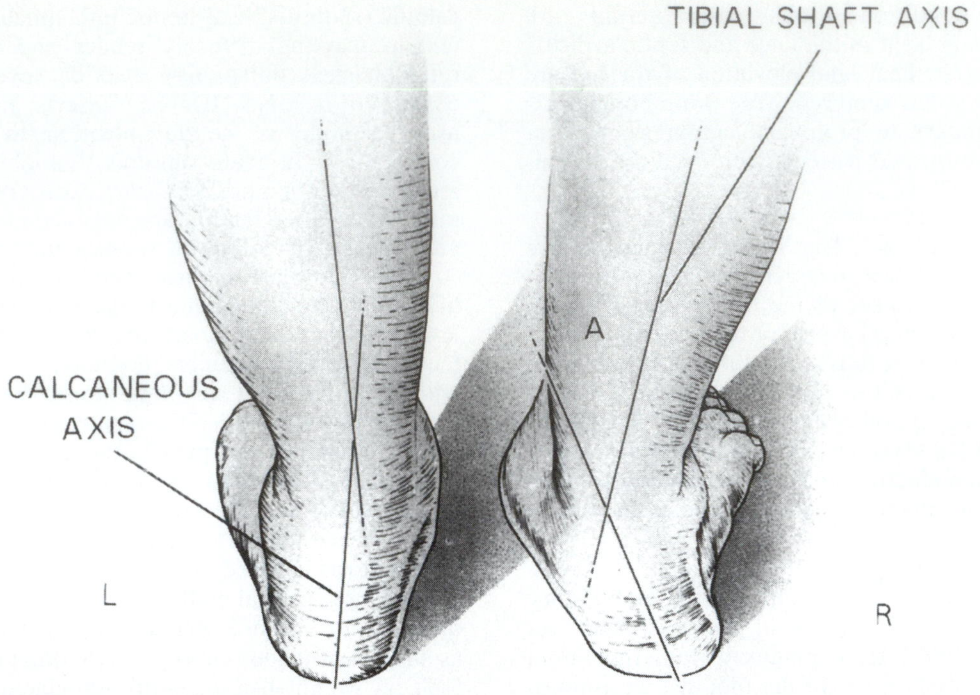


**Fig. 80-8.** Posterior view of the feet with normal on the left and hindfoot valgus on the right. The right foot also has forefoot abduction with "too many toes" seen lateral to the ankle. (From Supple KM et al: *Semin Arthritis Rheum* 22:107, 1992.)

radiographs. If fasciitis is associated with systemic inflammatory disease, plain films may demonstrate periostitis at the calcaneal insertion or even erosions. If clinically suspected, stress fractures of the metatarsals can be evaluated with serial radiographs or bone scan and Morton neuroma by clinical examination.

Treatment includes correction of underlying processes and the use of a plastic heel cup that maintains the soft tissue of the heel pad under the weight-bearing portion of the heel. Longitudinal arch support may also help. Local corticosteroid injection of the plantar fascia is also effective but must be cautiously given to avoid extensive fat pad atrophy at the heel.

*Nerve entrapment or compression*

**Tarsal tunnel syndrome.** See Chapter 103.

**Morton neuroma.** See Chapter 76.

## Fibromyalgia

Fibromyalgia is a generalized musculoskeletal pain syndrome characterized by diffuse soft tissue pain associated with physical findings of multiple tender points. Although the American College of Rheumatology has established criteria for the classification of fibromyalgia (see the box on p. 1127), some physicians still do not accept fibromyalgia as a distinct syndrome that is separate from generalized musculoskeletal pain syndromes or somatic pain disorders. Adding to the controversy, symptoms of fatigue and musculoskeletal pain overlap with fibromyalgia and chronic fatigue syndrome. These similarities led some investigators to propose that the conditions are the same. Until the true etiopathogenesis of either disease is known, these conflicting opinions will continue.

Fibromyalgia affects primarily women between the ages of 20 and 50 years. The female/male ratio is approximately 8 to 20:1. Approximately 2% to 5% of patients in general medical practice and 10% to 25% of patients in rheumatology practices have fibromyalgia by the American College of Rheumatology criteria. Fibromyalgia has also been described in the pediatric and geriatric populations.

The pathogenesis of fibromyalgia is unknown. Various physiologic factors have been described in fibromyalgia patients, but these factors are not unique to the syndrome. Nonrestorative sleep, the most typical feature, is defined as an interrupted sleep pattern or feeling unrefreshed on awakening. Moldofsky characterized this sleep abnormality as alpha wave intrusion on stage IV (NREM) sleep. Normal volunteers in whom alpha wave intrusion on stage IV sleep was experimentally induced developed tender points and musculoskeletal pain. Decreased serotonin in the brain may be responsible for this form of sleep disturbance. Alpha wave intrusion on NREM sleep, however, is not specific for fibromylagia and is found in patients with various medical conditions, as well as in some normal subjects. Sleep apnea, stress, noise, alcohol, myoclonus, and chronic pain are other factors that may contribute to these sleep abnormalities.

The prominent complaints of myalgia and subjective muscle weakness have led researchers to investigate muscle electrophysiology, histopathology, and metabolism in fibromyalgia patients. EMG demonstrates no consistent abnormalities and creatine phosphokinase (CPK) levels are normal. Muscle biopsies have no distinctive changes on histopathology. Muscle metabolism, when studied in detail, is also normal. Bennet proposes that muscle

### The American College of Rheumatology 1990 criteria for the classification of fibromyalgia*

History of widespread pain
*Definition.* Pain is considered widespread when all of the following are present: pain in the left side of the body, pain in the right side of the body, pain above the waist, and pain below the waist. In addition, axial skeletal pain (cervical spine or anterior chest or thoracic spine or low back) must be present. In this definition, shoulder and buttock pain is considered as pain for each involved side. "Low back" pain is considered lower segment pain.
Pain in 11 of 18 tender point sites on digital palpation.
*Definition.* Pain, on digital palpation, must be present in at least 11 of the following 18 tender point sites:
*Occiput:* bilateral, at the suboccipital muscle insertions
*Low cervical:* bilateral, at the anterior aspects of the intertransverse spaces at C5-C7
*Trapezius:* bilateral, at the midpoint of the upper border
*Supraspinatus:* bilateral, at origins, above the scapula spine near the medial border
*Second rib:* bilateral, at the second costochondral junctions, just lateral to the junctions on upper surfaces
*Lateral epicondyle:* bilateral, 2 cm distal to the epicondyles
*Gluteal:* bilateral, in upper outer quadrants of buttocks in anterior fold of muscle
*Greater trochanter:* bilateral, posterior to the trochanteric prominence
*Knee:* bilateral, at the medial fat pad proximal to the joint line
Digital palpation should be performed with an approximate force of 4 kg.
For a tender point to be considered positive the subject must state that the palpation was painful. "Tender" is not to be considered "painful."

From FW Wolfe et al, *Arthritis Rheum* 33:160, 1990.
*For classification purposes patients are said to have fibromyalgia if both criteria are satisfied. Widespread pain must have been present for at least 3 months. The presence of a second clinical disorder does not exclude the diagnosis of fibromyalgia.

### Differential diagnosis of fibromyalgia

**Fibromyalgia symptoms secondary to other diseases**
Hypothyroidism or hyperthyroidism
Hypoparathyroidism or hyperparathyroidism
RA
SLE
Sjögren's syndrome
Lyme disease
Parvovirus B19 infection
HIV infection
Metastatic carcinoma

**Fibromyalgia versus other diseases**
Polymyositis or other inflammatory myopathies
Polymyalgia rheumatica
RA
Spondyloarthropathies
Multiple sclerosis
Major psychiatric disorders
Alcoholic myopathy

microtrauma from various factors (deconditioning, genetic predisposition, disturbed hypothalamic pituitary axis secondary to sleep abnormalities, and exertion at low levels) result in muscle pain.

The role of psychologic and psychiatric factors in the pathogenesis of fibromyalgia remains controversial. Although many fibromyalgia patients report stress or anxiety precipitating or exacerbating their illness, only 20% to 30% of patients in a tertiary setting formally fulfill DSM-IV diagnosis for major depression, anxiety states, panic attacks, or somatization disorders. The severity of these patients' pain, however, may depend on psychologic factors. Some studies suggest that somatization is more frequent in patients with fibromyalgia than in normal controls or in patients with RA.

The major symptoms are diffuse musculoskeletal pain in articular and muscular regions. Some patients describe joint swelling and complain of nonrestorative sleep, fatigue, or morning stiffness. Exercise, cold or humid weather, inactivity, poor sleep, anxiety, and stress exacerbate symptoms, whereas hot showers, baths, warm or dry temperatures, and restful sleep help. In addition, the patient's medical history may include chronic headaches, atypical chest pain, irritable bowel syndrome, paresthesias, Raynaud's phenomenon, or female urethral syndrome.

Physical examination is usually unremarkable and reveals no evidence of synovitis or abnormalities in muscle strength. Multiple symmetric tender points are palpable and are sometimes exquisitely tender (Fig. 80-9). A complete blood count (CBC), erythrocyte sedimentation rate (ESR), CPK, antinuclear antibodies (ANA), rheumatoid factor, and radiographs are normal or absent. EMG and NCS, muscle biopsy, and radionucleotide bone scans are equally unremarkable. For general evaluation, CBC, ESR, CPK, and thyroid-stimulating hormone (TSH) are reasonable. Further laboratory investigations may depend on clinical suspicion of other diseases.

The box above lists the differential diagnosis for fibromyalgia. Hypothyroidism, SLE, Sjögren's syndrome, RA, HIV infection, and Lyme disease are possible causes of secondary fibromyalgia. Muscle weakness on examination, elevated CPK levels, myopathic EMG findings, and abnormal muscle biopsies differentiate polymyositis from fibromyalgia. Polymyalgia rheumatica, which occurs in patients over age 55, is associated with systemic symptoms of fever, weight loss, and an elevated ESR. Multiple tender points may mimic enthesitis of spondyloarthropathies. Finally, psychiatric illnesses, particularly major affective and somatoform disorders, should be excluded.

Multidisciplinary treatment of fibromyalgia begins with educating patients about factors that contribute to symptoms and reassuring patients that progressive joint destruction and muscle weakness do not occur. There is also a need to correct the factors mentioned that may contribute to sleep abnormalities.

Very few controlled studies exist on the treatment of fibromyalgia. Tricyclic antidepressants (e.g., amitrip-

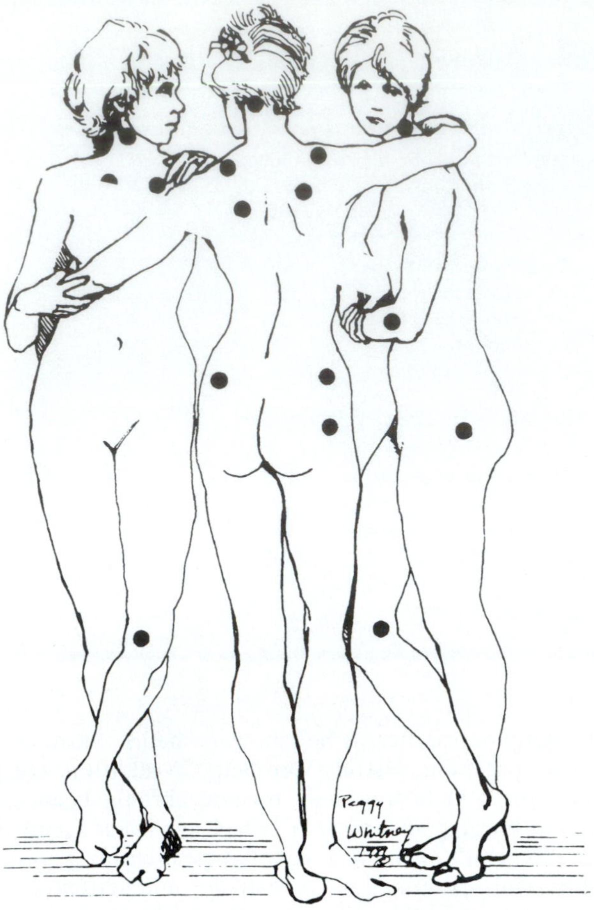

**Fig. 80-9.** Tender point locations for the 1990 classification criteria for fibromylagia. (From Wolfe FW et al: *Arthritis Rheum* 33:160, 1990.)

tyline, 10 to 150 mg qhs) and cyclobenzaprine at 5 to 40 mg qhs have been somewhat effective in well-controlled studies. Both medications are slowly titrated from the lowest dosage upward until the patient sleeps well or through the night. Possible mechanisms of action include direct beneficial effects on stage IV sleep and increased brain serotonin and other neuropeptides. Fluoxetine, however, which raises CNS serotonin exclusively, has no benefit for fibromyalgia or chronic neuropathic pain. Anticholinergic and antihistamine effects produce dry mouth, constipation, palpitations, and sedation. NSAIDs alone generally have very little effect, and systemic corticosteroids are generally ineffective for patients with fibromyalgia.

Slow reconditioning through low-impact aerobic exercises, which also improve cardiovascular fitness, is beneficial. Walking, swimming, and bicycling are alternative forms of exercise. However, patients need to advance slowly, since excessive exercise may exacerbate symptoms. EMG biofeedback training may also be effective.

Treatment of underlying psychiatric disorders is crucial, along with stress reduction. Some rheumatologists advocate heat, massage, and local tender point injection followed by stretching.

Fibromyalgia's course varies from periods of improvement to flares but tends to be chronic. Even with symptomatic improvement, the tender points persist on examination. Regularly scheduled office visits rather than urgent unscheduled ones may optimize the control of patients' symptoms and minimize emergency visits. The majority of patients with fibromyalgia continue with their work and function at home. Patients who develop fibromyalgia after trauma or surgery have a higher incidence of disability, loss of employment, and compensation for disability than do other fibromyalgia patients. Although 17% of fibromyalgia patients viewed themselves as disabled, only 5.75% actually received disability benefits.

## PRINCIPLES OF TREATMENT

### Rehabilitation

Although treatment of the various periarticular rheumatic disorders seems quite diverse, some underlying principles are applicable to tendinitis, bursitis, and myofascial pain. Throughout this chapter, a recurrent theme of overuse and injury predominates in the etiology of these processes. Thus a major focus of treatment is identifying the cause of overuse or injury and adjusting work or recreation to prevent further injury.

An occupational therapy consultation is often extremely helpful and cost effective. An occupational therapist assesses a patient's needs and then establishes a program that maximizes joint protection, prevents disability, and optimizes joint function. Industrial rehabilitation may be required if a patient has significant limitations at work. Work hardening programs have been established to help employees with various regional soft tissue problems to return to work.

Physical therapy includes modalities that initially control pain, followed by passive and active exercises to stretch or move a joint or periarticular structure. The final step is muscle strengthening around the region to prevent reinjury or further damage.

Heat and cold are common modalities to treat various soft tissue pain. Heat from moist heating packs and ultrasound provide relief, although it is usually short lived, for some patients. Since range of motion improves after heat application, use of heat may be a useful adjunct and may allow patients to exercise. Cold, usually reserved for acute injuries, reduces swelling.

TENS has been used for chronic pain of the back, neck, and other regions. The mechanism of action is postulated to be interference of pain impulses to the brain by its own impulses (or the gate control theory of pain). The cost of a TENS unit may not be reimbursed by third-party insurance.

Exercises, both passive and active, are important to maintain range of motion, strength, and function. In passive exercises the therapist or machine moves the muscle while the patient makes no muscle contraction. Active motion requires the patient to contract the muscle in an isometric (no joint motion) or isotonic (joint motion against resistance) fashion. The optimal program for each individual's soft tissue problem is best gauged by a physical therapist. However, if the primary care physician wishes to prescribe or supervise an exercise program, Schoen, Moskowitz, and Goldberg provide extensive exercises for each regional problem (see Bibliography).

Splints or orthotics immobilize an affected area to reduce pain, hold a particular region in an optimal position for function, or redistribute stress from a painful region to surrounding structures. Examples of each of these functions include a neutral wrist splint for carpal tunnel syndrome, a hindfoot orthosis to reduce valgus deformities secondary to posterior tibialis tendon dysfunction, or a forearm band for lateral epicondylitis. Properly fitting shoes are crucial in many of the periarticular disorders, and a consultation with an orthopedic surgeon or a podiatrist may be necessary.

*Medications*

**NSAIDs.** The use of NSAIDs in rheumatic diseases is discussed in detail in Chapter 79. For the periarticular entities, NSAIDs provide analgesic and antiinflammatory effects. Numerous NSAIDs are available and differ in metabolism, dosing, and toxicity profile (see Table 79-3). The efficacy and toxicity of NSAIDs vary among individuals. The principles in choosing NSAIDs are outlined in Chapter 79. A particular NSAID should be prescribed for at least 10 to 14 days before the medication is discontinued for lack of efficacy. Common toxicities include GI intolerance, gastritis, and superficial ulceration. Other toxicities include renal insufficiency, elevated liver enzyme levels, hyperkalemia, headaches, mood changes, and other CNS alterations. NSAIDs are not as effective for fibromyalgia and myofascial pain as they are for inflammatory musculoskeletal disorders.

**Tricyclic antidepressant medications.** Tricyclic antidepressant medications are important in the treatment of fibromyalgia and chronic neck or low back pain. Possible mechanisms of action include their effect on brain neuropeptides, the direct role on stage IV sleep, endogenous opioids, and reduction of brainstem-mediated muscle spasm. In addition, these medications are helpful if there is component of depression.

**Parenteral corticosteroids.** Parenteral corticosteroids may be useful in the early stages of reflex sympathetic dystrophy or adhesive capsulitis. ACTH can be an alternative to NSAIDs in acute calcific tendinitis. The protocol is similar to the treatment of acute gouty arthritis. Patients receive 40 to 60 IU of ACTH intramuscularly; this is repeated each day for a total of 3 days if necessary.

***Corticosteroid injections.*** Corticosteroid injections are a major form of treatment for the various soft-tissue disorders. The principles of corticosteroid injections and their complications are discussed in Chapter 69. Common areas that the primary care physician should be able to inject include the subacromial, trochanteric, and anserine regions, along with the true knee joint. Utmost care is needed when injecting the tendon sheaths, carpal and tarsal tunnels, plantar fascia, and retrocalcaneal bursa. Injection of these regions should be referred to a rheumatologist or orthopedist if the primary care physician has not learned to perform them. The true glenohumeral or hip joint is difficult to enter and injection should be performed by a specialist or even a radiologist under fluroscopic guidance.

After an injection, the area is rested or splinted for the subsequent 48 to 72 hours. Patients should be informed about possible postinjection flare and its treatment with ice and analgesics. If a tendon sheath is injected, strenuous activity of that tendon should be avoided for up to 2 weeks.

Injection of trigger points in myofascial pain is based on the theory of mechanical disruption of the trigger point by saline or an anesthetic, followed by passive stretch of the muscle. Some studies have reported a longer duration of improvement if corticosteroids are combined with the local anesthetic. Most studies have been uncontrolled; thus corticosteroids are not recommended for injection of trigger points.

## SUMMARY

Periarticular rheumatic disorders are a group of diverse but common problems in primary care practice. Physicians should be familiar with the diagnosis and management of these problems. Subspecialty referrals are indicated only if patients do not respond to initial management that includes avoidance of aggravating factors, pain control, and further strengthening exercises.

## BIBLIOGRAPHY


Bennet R: Fibromyalgia and the facts: sense or nonsense, *Rheum Dis Clin North Am* 19:45, 1993.

Bennet R: The fibromyalgia syndrome: myofascial pain and the chronic fatigue syndrome. In Kelly W et al, editors: *Textbook of rheumatology* ed 4, Philadelphia, 1993, WB Saunders.

Block S: Fibromyalgia and the rheumatism, *Rheum Dis Clin North Am* 19:61, 1993.

Fu F, Harner C, Klein A: Shoulder impingement syndrome: a critical review, *Clin Orthop* 269:162, 1991.

Goldenberg D: Treatment of fibromyalgia syndrome, *Rheum Dis Clin North Am* 15:61, 1989.

Goldenberg D: Do infections trigger fibromyalgia? *Arthritis Rheum* 36:1489, 1993.

Goldman L, Rosenberg N: Myofascial pain syndrome and fibromyalgia, *Semin Neurol* 11:274, 1991.

Janisse D: The art and science of fitting shoes, *Foot Ankle* 13:257, 1992.

Moldofsky H et al: Musculoskeletal symptoms and non-REM sleep disturbance in patients with "fibrositis syndrome" and healthy subjects, *Psychosom Med* 37:341, 1975.

Nakano K: Neck pain. In Kelly W et al, editors: *Textbook of rheumatology,* Philadelphia, 1993, WB Saunders.

Neer C: Impingement lesions, *Clin Orthop* 173:70, 1983.

Raddatz D, Hoffman G, Franck W: Septic bursitis: presentation, treatment, and prognosis, *J Rheumatol* 14:1160, 1987.

Schoen R, Moskowitz R, Goldberg V: The low back. In Schoen R, Moskowitz R, Goldberg V, editors: *Soft tissue rheumatic pain: recognition, management, prevention,* ed 2, Philadelphia, 1987, Lea & Febiger.

Supple K et al: Posterior tibial tendon dysfunction, *Semin Arthritis Rheum* 22:106, 1992.

Szabo R, Madison M: Carpal tunnel syndrome, *Orthop Clin North Am* 23:103, 1992.

Travell J, Rinzler S: The myofascial genesis of pain, *Postgrad Med* 11:425, 1952.

Underwood P, McLeod R, Ginsburg W: The varied manifestations of iliopsoas bursitis, *J Rheumatol* 15:1683, 1988.

CHAPTER

# 81 Systemic Lupus Erythematosus

Leslie E. Kahl

Systemic lupus erythematosus (SLE) is a chronic systemic inflammatory disorder of unknown etiology. With an unpredictable clinical course and manifestations ranging from troublesome rashes and alopecia to life-threatening cerebritis and nephritis, lupus is among the most challenging disorders to treat. Moreover, the clinician must not only treat acute flares of disease to minimize end-organ damage, but also must distinguish manifestations of lupus from those related to adverse drug effects.

The hallmark laboratory feature of idiopathic lupus is the presence of both tissue-specific and nonspecific autoantibodies. Immunoglobulin and complement deposits have been identified in involved tissues, including the skin, kidney, and brain, and are thought to be pathogenic. For this reason, many investigators consider lupus the prototypic autoimmune disease.

## EPIDEMIOLOGY

Idiopathic SLE is predominantly found in women of childbearing age. There are approximately 25 to 150 cases per 100,000 people, with higher rates seen in urban areas, and among African-Americans and Asians. The ratio of female to male lupus victims is between 8:1 and 13:1 during the childbearing years, but only approximately 2:1 to 5:1 in children and older adults. This gender discrepancy is thought to be due to hormonal effects, as evidenced by the relative rarity of the disease before menarche and after menopause, the apparent association of disease flares with pregnancy and oral contraceptive use, and the presence of altered estrogen kinetics among women with SLE.

## ETIOLOGY

SLE is a heterogeneous disorder that appears to have a complex etiology rather than a single cause. Current theory suggests that in the genetically predisposed host some stimulus (or stimuli) triggers aberrant function of T and B cells and, ultimately, increased immunoglobulin and autoantibody production. Genetic markers of the major histocompatibility complex (MHC), including HLA-DR2 and HLA-DR3 as well as genes producing deficiencies of complement components, are associated with an increased risk of lupus in certain ethnic groups and populations. Moreover, the specific type of antibodies produced also seems to be influenced by MHC genes.

The stimulus that triggers SLE probably differs from patient to patient. The potential role of sex hormones, either endogenous or exogenous, is outlined above. Environmental triggers such as ultraviolet radiation, infections, certain drugs, chemicals, and foods may play a role. Some patients associate stress, either physical or emotional, with disease onset or with flares of established disease.

SLE is characterized by the presence of a variety of autoantibodies. Although many of the protein antigens against which these antibodies are directed play a critical role in cellular functions such as ribonucleic acid (RNA) processing and cell division, there is little evidence that the autoantibodies impede these functions. Complexes of antibodies and their antigens (immune complexes) may have a pathogenic role in SLE. These complexes are normally cleared from the circulation by the complement system. In lupus, however, they may be found deposited along with complement at sites of tissue injury, contributing to the inflammatory response. Complement components are consumed during either immune complex clearance or tissue deposition, producing a characteristic fall in serum complement levels during disease flares.

Although most of the clinical manifestations of lupus are inflammatory in origin, some patients develop problems related to apparent hypercoagulability. Vascular occlusions in both the arterial and venous systems have been associated with the presence of antiphospholipid antibodies. Whether these antibodies are pathogenic or simply laboratory markers for this complication is unclear.

## CLINICAL COURSE

Both the presentation and clinical course of SLE are highly variable. The initial symptoms may be nonspecific and resolve spontaneously, leading to a considerable delay in diagnosis. In many patients, only the gradual unfolding of a pattern of disease over several months leads to the correct diagnosis. In others, however, the disease is fulminant and easily recognizable at the onset.

Lupus generally has remissions interspersed with acute or chronic relapses. In a given patient disease flares may involve the same organ systems each time, producing a characteristic and predictable pattern of disease. This is useful when trying to distinguish symptoms of active SLE from other conditions such as acute infection or adverse drug reactions. However, many patients do not have such a reproducible profile of their disease flare, and present a continuing diagnostic challenge.

Most SLE patients have fairly mild disease characterized by constitutional symptoms, arthralgias or arthritis, and rash. These individuals often lead a relatively normal life and have a normal or near-normal life span. Patients with more aggressive disease may suffer considerable morbidity. The 10-year survival rate for SLE victims is 75% to 90%. Deaths early in the course of disease usually result from active SLE or acute infections, whereas those occurring later tend to be related to cardiovascular disease.

### History

The clinical presentations of lupus are remarkably diverse. A series of classification criteria for SLE (Table 81-1) has been produced by the American College of Rheumatology as a guideline for researchers. These criteria are also commonly employed by clinicians to assign the diagnosis of SLE. The individual criteria were specifically selected for their ability to distinguish patients with lupus from those with other connective tissue diseases and do not include many common but nonspecific features of lupus, such as arthralgias and alopecia.

**Table 81-1.** 1982 Revised criteria for the classification of systemic lupus erythematosus

| Criterion | Definition |
|---|---|
| Malar rash | Fixed erythema, flat or raised, over the malar eminences, tending to spare the nasolabial folds |
| Discoid rash | Erythematous raised patches with adherent keratotic scaling and follicular plugging; atrophic scarring may occur in older lesions |
| Photosensitivity | Skin rash as a result of unusual reaction to sunlight, noted by patient history or physician observation |
| Oral ulcers | Oral or nasopharyngeal ulceration, usually painless, observed by a physician |
| Arthritis | Nonerosive arthritis involving two or more peripheral joints, characterized by tenderness, swelling, or effusion |
| Serositis | Pleuritis—convincing history of pleuritic pain or rub heard by a physician or evidence of pleural effusion<br>**OR**<br>Pericarditis—documented by ECG or rub or evidence of pericardial effusion |
| Renal disorder | Persistent proteinuria >0.5 g/day or greater than 3+ if quantitation is not performed<br>**OR**<br>Cellular casts may be red cell, hemoglobin, granular, tubular, or mixed |
| Neurologic disorder | Seizures in the absence of offending drugs or known metabolic derangements (e.g., uremia, ketoacidosis, or electrolyte imbalance)<br>**OR**<br>Psychosis in the absence of offending drugs or known metabolic derangements (e.g., uremia, ketoacidosis, or electrolyte imbalance) |
| Hematologic disorder | Hemolytic anemia with reticulocytosis<br>**OR**<br>Leukopenia $<4000/mm^3$ total on two or more occasions<br>**OR**<br>Lymphopenia $<1500/mm^3$ on two or more occasions<br>**OR**<br>Thrombocytopenia $<100{,}000/mm^3$ in the absence of offending drugs |
| Immunologic disorder | Positive LE cell preparation<br>**OR**<br>Anti-DNA: antibody to native DNA in abnormal titer<br>**OR**<br>Anti-Sm: presence of antibody to Sm nuclear antigen<br>**OR**<br>False positive serologic test for syphilis known to be positive for at least 6 months and confirmed by *Treponema pallidum* immobilization or fluorescent treponemal antibody absorption test |
| Antinuclear antibody | An abnormal titer of antinuclear antibody by immunofluorescence or an equivalent assay at any point and in the absence of drugs known to be associated with drug-induced lupus syndrome |

Although nonspecific constitutional symptoms including fatigue, fever, and weight loss provide few clues to the diagnosis of SLE, they may dominate the clinical picture. The fatigue that occurs in SLE can be particularly overwhelming; patients may barely be able to get up, eat, or dress themselves. Fatigue is the chief complaint of many lupus patients whose disease is otherwise in remission.

Musculoskeletal symptoms, including myalgias, arthralgias, and frank arthritis, occur at some point in nearly all SLE patients. The arthritis is inflammatory, with prominent morning stiffness, although the symptoms are frequently out of proportion to the findings on physical examination. Joint involvement is usually symmetric and may include the small joints of the hands and feet, wrists, elbows, knees, and ankles. The patient may describe swelling of the joints that waxes and wanes over the space of a few hours, a feature rarely found in other forms of arthritis.

Mucocutaneous features of SLE are nearly as common as those involving the joints. The characteristic butterfly rash on the cheeks and nose is present at some point in up to 50% of patients. Approximately one third note photosensitivity, with exacerbation of the rash after sun exposure. Patients may also give a history of nonscarring alopecia or unusual breakage of hair, particularly along the hairline. This history must be interpreted with caution in women using harsh coloring or curling treatments on their hair or having a tightly-braided hairstyle. Although oral or nasal ulcers occur in up to 40% of patients, they are frequently asymptomatic. Raynaud's phenomenon is present in approximately 30% of patients, but also commonly occurs in other connective tissue diseases including scleroderma and polymyositis. Patients usually describe aching and white or bluish discoloration of the digits on exposure to cold, and may also note erythema during rewarming.

Pleurisy or pericarditis (serositis) occurs in about one half of SLE patients. Although occasionally manifest only as an asymptomatic pleural effusion or globular cardiac contour on chest x-ray, serositis generally produces a characteristic sharp or stabbing pain on one or both sides of the chest. Pain referred to the left shoulder or relieved by leaning forward is more suggestive of pericarditis, whereas exacerbation of the chest pain on deep inspiration is more common with pleurisy. Pulmonary parenchymal involvement is much rarer than pleurisy in SLE. Patients with pneumonitis usually develop dyspnea suddenly, and are acutely ill. They may also give a history of hemoptysis. Cough with sputum production is not typical of lung disease in lupus, and should raise the possibility of a superimposed infection.

Central nervous system manifestations of SLE may be either functional or organic. Among the most common symptoms are mild depression and subtle cognitive deficits. Headaches are also a frequent complaint. These range from simple tension-type headaches to classic migraines, and in some patients may present with short-lived focal neurologic deficits in a "migraine equivalent" form. Migraine headaches appear to be more common among patients experiencing Raynaud's phenomenon. More serious neurologic problems are less common, and include major affective disorders, seizures, and strokes. Patients with antiphospholipid antibodies are at particular risk for stroke.

Some of the most serious complications of lupus may be silent or present with nonspecific symptoms. Nephritis, which occurs in up to 40% of patients, may be manifest as fatigue, peripheral edema, or weight gain. Hypertension associated with nephritis is also frequently silent. Patients with hemolytic anemia may also have fatigue or may develop jaundice or dark urine. Thrombocytopenia is usually asymptomatic, but may produce petechiae, bruising, or more serious bleeding complications.

### Physical examination

The classic physical finding in SLE is the malar or butterfly rash (Fig. 81-1). Along with the cheeks, the forehead, chin, and bridge of the nose may also be involved, but the nasolabial folds are generally spared. Involved skin is erythematous and may be slightly indurated. A maculopapular eruption with fine scaling may also be present. Unlike the classic butterfly rash that resolves without sequelae, discoid lupus erythematosus (DLE) involves deeper layers of the dermis and produces residual scarring. Discoid lesions are most common on the face, scalp, and ears, but can also occur on the palms and soles (Figs. 81-2 and 81-3). Acute discoid lesions are annular, erythematous, indurated plaques that may be covered by an adherent scale with follicular plugging. Chronic lesions generally show central atrophy and depigmentation, with an erythematous or hyperpigmented circular border (Fig. 81-4). Discoid lesions occurring in the scalp may produce well-defined areas of scarring alopecia. In contrast, the nonscarring alopecia that occurs in the absence of discoid lesions is diffuse and may be associated with breakage of hairs at the hairline or fine lanugo-like hair growth. Patients with antibodies to the Ro or SS-A antigen may have annular or psoriasiform (nonscarring) rashes, termed *subacute cutaneous lupus erythematosus* (SCLE). Some patients, particularly those with antiphospholipid antibodies, have livedo reticularis, a violaceous netlike pattern of vessels in the skin of the extremities.

The musculoskeletal examination may be normal in lupus, even when the patient relates a history of joint pain conducive with inflammation. Joint swelling, tenderness, and erythema may be present, but synovial effusions are usually not large. Chronic arthritis may produce deformi-

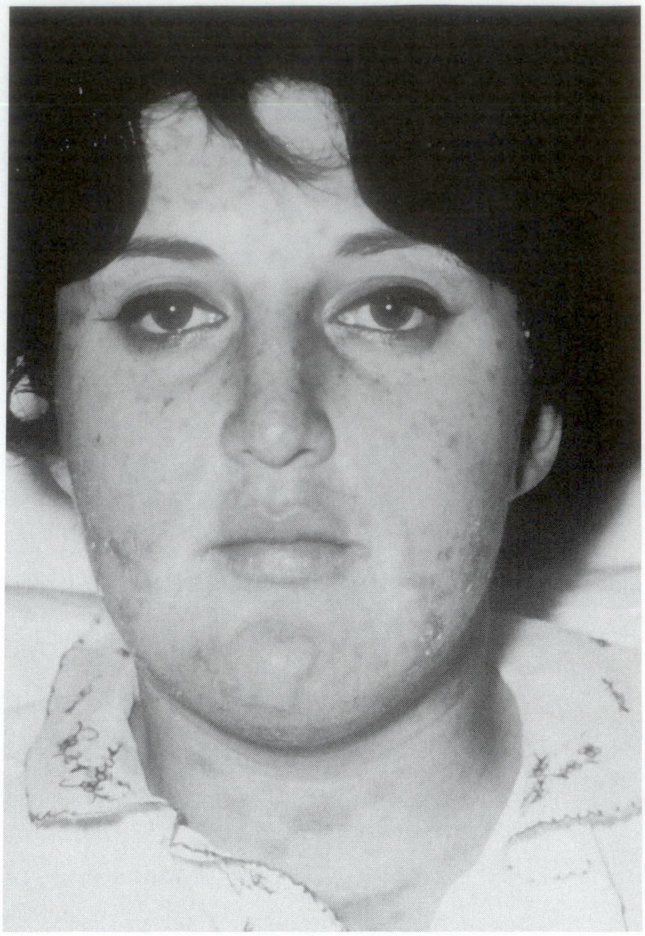

**Fig. 81-1.** The characteristic erythematosus facial rash in SLE may involve the forehead and chin along with the cheeks. The nasolabial fold is usually spared. (From American College of Rheumatology: *Clinical slide collection on the rheumatic diseases,* 1991, The College.)

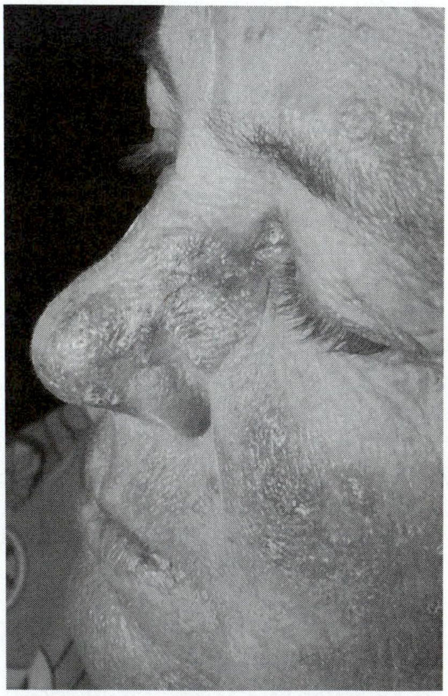

**Fig. 81-2.** Discoid lupus erythematosus. Note photodistribution of erythematous plaques. (Courtesy Frank W. Crowe, M.D.)

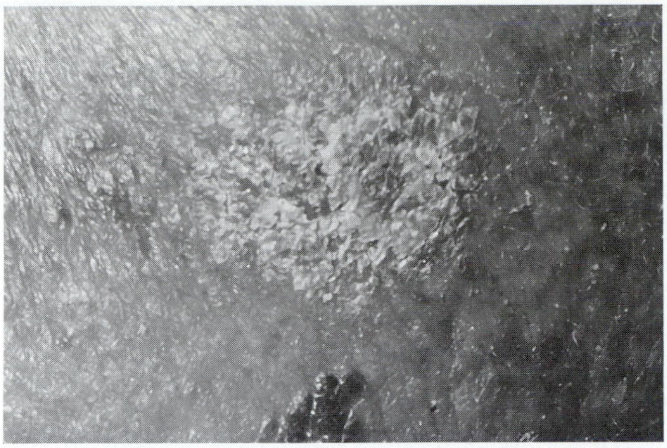

**Fig. 81-3.** Discoid lupus erythematosus. Note erythema and adherent scale.

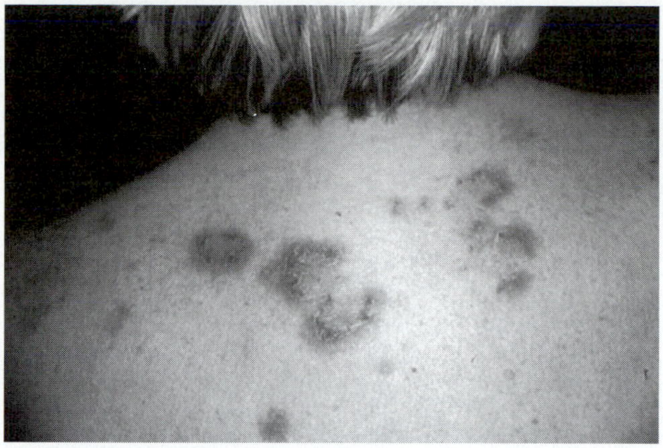

**Fig. 81-4.** Subacute cutaneous lupus erythematosus. Note the arcuate configuration of raised erythema and scaling.

ties, particularly in the hands. Ulnar deviation of the metacarpophalangeal (MCP) joints and flexion or swan-neck deformities of the fingers are most common. However, in contrast to the joint abnormalities seen in rheumatoid arthritis, those in SLE are usually reducible.

Patients with serositis may have no abnormal physical findings; a friction rub is sometimes heard. Atelectasis may occur, producing localized findings of consolidation at the lung bases. Dullness at the lung bases may be detected if pleural effusions are large. Pericardial effusions are rarely of hemodynamic significance and signs of congestive heart failure are not generally seen.

The neurologic examination is normal in most patients with lupus, despite the high frequency of neuropsychiatric symptoms. However, the disease may affect virtually any portion of the central or peripheral nervous system. Stroke occurs in up to 15% of patients, producing focal deficits in the distribution of any of the cerebral vessels. Similarly, transverse myelitis may occur at any level of the spinal cord, although it is much less common than stroke. Patients with a history of headaches generally have a normal neurologic examination, but papilledema may occasionally be seen with pseudotumor cerebri. Neuropathies occur in up to 15% of patients. Cranial nerve involvement is usually in the optic or trigeminal distribution. Peripheral nerve involvement may present as either a distal sensory neuropathy or a mononeuritis multiplex. Patients with a history of seizure generally have normal examinations between seizure events. Among patients with mood disturbances, findings consistent with an affective disorder, usually anxiety or depression, may be present. Formal testing may be necessary to detect some of the more subtle cognitive defects that may occur.

In addition to the above findings, which would most likely be detected by using a symptom-based approach to the patient, several potential asymptomatic abnormalities should also be sought. Adenopathy occurs in up to 25% of patients, usually in the setting of active disease elsewhere, and may be a clue that the other symptoms are a manifestation of lupus rather than of some unrelated problem. The blood pressure must be measured each visit. Hypertension may be the first indication of occult renal disease. The prognosis of nephritis is worse for patients with persistent hypertension; this manifestation should be treated aggressively. Similarly, the patient should be checked regularly for peripheral edema, which may be the presenting sign of proteinuria.

## Laboratory studies

The laboratory is useful in establishing a diagnosis of SLE when the clinical picture is suggestive. The classic serologic finding for SLE is the presence of antinuclear antibody (ANA). Since ANA is present in virtually all lupus patients, it serves as a reasonable screening test for the disease. A negative ANA test makes SLE extremely unlikely. However, ANA is by no means specific for lupus, and can be seen in healthy elderly individuals as well as in patients with rheumatoid arthritis, other connective tissue diseases, and inflammatory conditions such as interstitial lung disease and chronic active hepatitis.

A positive ANA should be interpreted on the basis of the clinical setting and the titer. Titers of less than 1:160 are more likely to be false positives or manifestations of nonspecific immune reactivity than are higher titers. In contrast, ANA titers of 1:1280 or greater usually indicate a connective tissue disease, though not always SLE. The screening ANA detects antibody to a variety of antigenic substrates that, in turn, may give a good clue to the exact type of connective tissue disease. For this reason a positive screening ANA in a reasonable titer should be followed by more specific testing, including assays for Sm, RNP, SS-A/Ro, and SS-B/La. Patients with SLE frequently demonstrate several different types of autoantibodies in their sera, whereas a single autoantibody is usually seen in other connective tissue diseases (Table 81-2).

Additional laboratory studies that may be useful in making the diagnosis of SLE are listed in Table 81-3. The presence of antibody to double-stranded (native) DNA is pathognomonic for lupus and in some patients may also be a marker of active disease, particularly nephritis. Anti-Sm is also virtually specific for SLE. Reduced serum complement levels may be seen in any disorder mediated by immune complexes, but are highly suggestive of SLE when found in the presence of a positive ANA. A positive direct Coombs' test is found in up to 60% of SLE patients, but clinically evident hemolytic anemia is usually absent.

**Table 81-2.** Percentages of frequency of autoantibodies in connective tissue diseases

| | SLE | Drug-induced SLE | Rheumatoid arthritis | Sjögren's syndrome | MCTD | Systemic sclerosis | CREST syndrome | Polymyositis or dermatomyositis |
|---|---|---|---|---|---|---|---|---|
| Antibody: | | | | | | | | |
| Native DNA | **60** | R | R | R | R | R | R | R |
| Histone | 70 | **95** | 30 | 20 | R | R | R | R |
| Sm | **30** | R | R | R | R | R | R | R |
| RNP | 40 | R | R | R | **95** | 15 | 10 | 15 |
| SS-A/Ro; SS-B/La | 30 | R | 20 | **70** | R | R | R | R |
| Scl-70 | R | R | R | R | R | **35** | 10 | R |
| Centromere | R | R | R | R | R | R | **70** | R |
| Jo-1 | R | R | R | R | R | R | R | **25** |

Frequencies of autoantibodies with high diagnostic utility are shown in **bold** type. *R* indicates that the antibody occurs rarely.

**Table 81-3.** Laboratory studies useful in diagnosing SLE

| Finding | Cumulative frequency (%) |
|---|---|
| ANA | 99 |
| anti-DNA | 40-60 |
| anti-Sm | 15-30 |
| ↓ C3 or C4 | 50-70 |
| Lymphopenia, leukopenia | 60-80 |
| Direct Coombs' test | 40-60 |
| Antiphospholipid antibodies | 20-40 |
| Thrombocytopenia | 20-40 |
| Proteinuria | 30-50 |
| Cellular urinary casts | 20-30 |

Although the normochromic normocytic anemia commonly seen in lupus is a nonspecific manifestation of chronic diseases, the lymphopenia is usually mediated by antilymphocyte antibodies, and serves as another indicator of the diffuse immunologic hyperreactivity that characterizes SLE. Similarly, thrombocytopenia in this setting is immune mediated. The greater the number of antibodies present, the more likely the patient has SLE.

Antiphospholipid antibodies, which may be associated with thrombosis, are detected by any of three tests (see box on right). The classic false positive syphilis serology has long been recognized as a marker for SLE. The lupus anticoagulant test, in which a prolonged partial thromboplastin time (PTT) does not correct by the addition of normal plasma, is also thought to reflect antiphospholipid antibody activity. The more recently developed anticardiolipin antibody test is the third assay for antiphospholipid activity. These antibodies may be accompanied by venous or arterial thrombosis, presenting with phlebitis, stroke, or miscarriage. Antiphospholipid antibodies are not specific for SLE, but can also be seen in the primary antiphospholipid syndrome, with similar vascular events. A few patients with this syndrome have low titers of ANA and thrombocytopenia, and may be misdiagnosed with SLE.

A urinalysis and determination of the serum creatinine level should be performed on all new patients suspected of having SLE, to screen for occult renal disease. A renal biopsy may be indicated by a rising serum creatinine, new onset proteinuria of over 500 mg/dl, or a urinary sediment containing cellular casts or red blood cells. In this setting, new onset hypertension, reduced serum complement levels, or a positive anti-DNA antibody test should strongly increase the clinical suspicion for nephritis, and lead to consultation with a nephrologist or rheumatologist. Percutaneous renal biopsy may reveal a variety of histologic patterns that cannot be accurately predicted by routine laboratory studies. The renal biopsy also reveals information regarding both the chronicity and activity of renal disease, which may have both prognostic and therapeutic implications.

### Antiphospholipid antibodies and their clinical associations

**Assay**

False positive syphilis serology
Lupus anticoagulant
Anticardiolipin antibody

**Clinical manifestations**

Arterial or venous thrombosis (i.e., thrombophlebitis, stroke)
Miscarriage
Livedo reticularis
Thrombocytopenia

**Disease associations**

SLE
Drug-induced lupus
Primary antiphospholipid syndrome

## Differential diagnosis

The clinical manifestations of SLE are so diverse that some clinicians have dubbed it one of the "great imposters." When the initial presentation includes the malar rash along with any of the more serious organ system manifestations, serologic testing is performed and

**Table 81-4.** Differential diagnosis of SLE

| Disease | Cutaneous | Extracutaneous | Laboratory |
|---|---|---|---|
| SLE | Widespread photoaccentuated | Multisystem renal, neurologic arthritis, serositis | ANA 98%<br>Anti-dsDNA 60%-80%<br>Low C3 90%<br>High ESR 90% |
| SCLE | Widespread photoaccentuated | Less systemic involvement than SLE | ANA 60%<br>Anti-dsDNA 30%, low titer<br>Anti-Ro 30% |
| DLE (discoid LE) | Localized or rarely widespread photoaccentuated | None | ANA 5% |
| Drug-induced LE | Widespread | Can be multisystem | ANA 100%<br>Antihistone Ab 80%-100% |
| Dermatomyositis | Can be widespread photoaccentuated | Multisystem or rarely cutaneous only; associated malignancy | ANA 50%-75%<br>Elevated muscle enzymes (CPK, Ald, SGOT)<br>Muscle biopsy |

the diagnosis is relatively straightforward. More commonly, however, the patient may complain of nonspecific symptoms such as low-grade fever, fatigue, or arthralgias, and the clinical suspicion for lupus is not as high. SLE should always be in the differential diagnosis of a multisystem disease presenting in a young woman, particularly a young black woman, and in the setting of an apparent infection in a young woman where cultures are negative and there has been no response to antibiotics.

A lupus diagnosis is most likely to be missed when the disease presents in a single organ system. Pleurisy or pericarditis is usually attributed to a viral infection unless the ANA test is performed. The pleural fluid in SLE is typically an exudate with lymphocytic predominance in the cell count, which may be helpful in the differential diagnosis. Isolated thrombocytopenia or hemolytic anemia is generally considered idiopathic unless an ANA test is done. Involvement of the central nervous system is particularly challenging to diagnose, since it often occurs without other signs or symptoms of SLE. In this setting, seizure or stroke may be thought to be idiopathic, and optic neuritis or transverse myelitis may be attributed to multiple sclerosis. Isolated synovitis may be misdiagnosed as rheumatoid arthritis. The articular findings in the two disorders have a similar character and distribution, and up to 30% of patients with rheumatoid arthritis may have positive ANA tests. The true nature of the diagnosis in any of these clinical scenarios may not be revealed until, with time, the multisystemic nature of the disease is revealed.

Although the most common diagnostic error involving SLE is its being overlooked as a clinical possibility, cutaneous lesions are probably overdiagnosed as lupus. The erythematous rash of acne rosacea may assume a malar distribution, but can be differentiated from SLE by the presence of pustules. Seborrheic dermatitis also commonly occurs in a malar distribution but, unlike SLE, involves the nasolabial folds. Superficial fungal infections may resemble cutaneous lupus but give positive results on examination of skin scrapings with potassium hydroxide. Photoallergic contact dermatitis and polymorphous light eruption may be difficult to distinguish from lupus clinically, but they have distinctive histopathologic pictures. Similarly, the rash of dermatomyositis may closely resemble lupus; however, dermatomyositis' color is more purple than red and its scaling lesions (Gottron's papules) occur over the knuckles, whereas those of lupus occur on the dorsum of the hand between the joints (Table 81-4).

Lupus must also be differentiated from other systemic inflammatory disorders such as necrotizing vasculitis. Although cutaneous vasculitis may be a manifestation of SLE, widespread vascular involvement is unusual. Serologic studies are generally negative in vasculitis. The arthralgias or arthritis, fever, malaise, and cutaneous lesions of bacterial endocarditis may also be confused with SLE. Again, serologic studies, along with blood culture results, should clarify the issue. Among the connective tissue diseases, lupus shares cutaneous features with dermatomyositis, synovitis with rheumatoid arthritis, serositis with rheumatoid arthritis and Sjögren's syndrome, and Raynaud's phenomenon with all of these disorders. In general, the clinical picture and active serologic profile of lupus are sufficient to make the distinction between these disorders. Occasionally, a patient has features characteristic of several of these diseases but diagnostic of none. Antibodies to RNP are generally present, and this constellation of findings is termed mixed connective tissue disease or overlap syndrome.

After making the lupus diagnosis, the clinician is often faced with deciding whether a new symptom represents SLE, an adverse drug effect, or some other unrelated problem. For example, a patient with longstanding lupus who develops fever and pleuritic chest pain may have lupus-related serositis, but might also have pneumonia or a pulmonary embolus. The presence of signs or symptoms of active SLE in other organs may help clarify the diagnosis, along with judicious use of the laboratory and radiographs. Similarly, a rise in the serum creatinine or new onset hypertension is probably related to the development of nephritis, but nephrotoxicity from nonsteroidal antiinflammatory drugs (NSAIDs) must also be considered.

### Agents implicated in drug-induced lupus

**Definite**

Hydralazine
Procainamide
Isoniazid
Methyldopa
Chlorpromazine

**Possible**

***Anticonvulsants***

- Diphenylhydantoin
- Mephenytoin
- Ethosuximide
- Trimethadione

***Beta blockers***

- Practolol
- Acebutolol
- Atenolol
- Metoprolol

***Miscellaneous***

- Penicillamine
- Captopril
- Quinidine
- Sulfonamide
- Tartrazine
- Lithium carbonate
- Propylthiouracil

In a patient who appears to have SLE the distinction must also be made between spontaneous and drug-induced lupus. Medications implicated in drug-induced lupus are listed in the box above. These drugs do not cause exacerbations of spontaneous lupus. Patients with drug-induced lupus are older, and more likely to be men. They usually present with fever, malaise, serositis, and arthralgias or arthritis. Weight loss may be a prominent feature, raising the diagnostic suspicion for malignancy. More serious organ system involvement such as cerebritis, nephritis, thrombocytopenia, or hemolytic anemia is rare. Serologic abnormalities are usually limited to a positive ANA test in a homogenous pattern and an elevated erythrocyte sedimentation rate; hypocomplementemia and the plethora of autoantibodies typically seen in spontaneous SLE are absent. When the offending medication is discontinued, the signs and symptoms of lupus generally resolve over several weeks, although the ANA may persist for much longer. Patients who develop a positive ANA test during treatment with a lupus-inducing drug but who remain asymptomatic may continue taking the medication.

## MANAGEMENT

Because lupus is not well understood by the public, treatment must begin with education. Common misconceptions about lupus include that it is always fatal, either contagious or strongly familial, and a form of AIDS. Reassuring lupus patients and their families about these issues may relieve many unspoken anxieties. SLE patients often look quite well despite overwhelming fatigue and arthralgias. Frequently, this disparity leads to a lack of understanding and unrealistic expectations on the part of family, friends, and coworkers. Educating them may be helpful. Both the Arthritis Foundation and the Lupus Foundation of America, Inc., are excellent sources for educational materials regarding SLE. Many chapters also sponsor patient support groups, allowing individuals with this disease and their families to come together and share their fears, frustrations and successful strategies.

### Nonpharmacologic approaches

Although medications are frequently indicated in the management of lupus, several nonpharmacologic approaches also have merit. Many patients link flares of their disease with periods of excessive fatigue. Rest is important in the daily management of this disease. Patients must learn to prioritize their daily schedules, plan ahead, and pace themselves. Because the disease tends to vary from day to day, many patients save up their chores or activities until they feel well, overdo it on that day, and are exhausted for the next several days. Other patients observe that emotional rather than physical stress is a disease precipitant. For these individuals, counseling for stress management may be particularly useful.

Environmental manipulations may also help some lupus patients. Only 30% to 40% of patients are photosensitive but, for them, avoidance of the sun by staying indoors during the midday or by wearing long sleeves and a hat can be a good preventive strategy. Topical sunscreens also provide considerable protection. Patients with Raynaud's phenomenon need to avoid the cold. Most patients do not realize, however, that they must keep the whole body warm, and not just the digits. Using pot-holder mitts for handling cold items from the refrigerator and insulated holders for cold drinks can be helpful. Obviously, they must also refrain from smoking.

### Pharmacologic approaches

There is no single medication appropriate for all SLE patients. Rather, the disease is managed in a problem-oriented fashion. Medications commonly used in SLE are listed in Table 81-5, along with their indications and common toxicities. NSAIDs are the medications most widely prescribed for this disease. The efficacy and toxicity of a particular drug in an individual patient is unpredictable. NSAIDs should generally be prescribed at the upper end of the recommended dose range. If one preparation does not provide relief after a 2- to 3-week trial, another may be tried. Lupus patients are subject to all of the toxicities of the NSAIDs seen in other patients, but also have a few peculiarities. Because of the presence of subclinical or undiagnosed nephritis, they are at increased risk for NSAID-induced nephrotoxicity. This usually presents with a rise in serum creatinine, and may be accompanied by hyperkalemia and hypertension. These abnormalities are reversible once the drug is stopped, but do occur with sufficient frequency to merit monitoring of the serum creatinine in any patient after an NSAID is begun. Lupus patients are also probably at increased risk of mild hepatitis from NSAIDs, particularly salicylates, and serum transaminases should be monitored along with the creatinine. Aseptic meningitis, a rare complication of

**Table 81-5.** Drug treatment for SLE: medications, indications, and toxicities

| Drug | Indication | Adverse effects |
|---|---|---|
| NSAIDs | Arthritis<br>Pleurisy<br>Pericarditis | Gastritis, ulceration<br>Nephrotoxicity<br>Fluid retention |
| Hydroxychloroquine | Photosensitivity<br>Rash<br>Alopecia<br>Arthritis<br>Oral ulcers | Gastrointestinal upset<br>Retinal toxicity |
| Corticosteroids | Nephritis<br>Cerebritis<br>Thrombocytopenia<br>Hemolysis<br>Skin lesions | Hypertension<br>Glucose intolerance<br>Weight gain<br>Osteoporosis<br>Infection<br>Accelerated atherosclerosis<br>Avascular necrosis |
| Cyclophosphamide, azathioprine | Nephritis<br>Vasculitis<br>Steroid-resistant severe disease | Bone marrow suppression<br>Infection<br>Malignancy<br>Infertility |
| Heparin, warfarin | Thrombosis (usually with antiphospholipid antibodies) | Hemorrhage |

NSAID use, appears to be much more common in SLE, and may also be caused by use of sulfa-containing antibiotics in these patients.

The antimalarial drug hydroxychloroquine is useful in the management of photosensitivity, rash, articular symptoms, alopecia, and oral ulcers in lupus. Some patients also experience less fatigue. The usual starting dose is 400 mg daily. Clinical response may not occur for 3 months. Once symptoms are under control, the drug may be continued at a lower dose. The most common toxicity, gastrointestinal upset, may be better tolerated if the drug is taken before bedtime. The most worrisome toxicity is retinal damage, occurring in approximately 1% of patients. Patients should be monitored every 6 months by an ophthalmologist, who can discover early retinal changes before they are symptomatic. Although these lesions are generally not reversible, they usually do not progress once the drug is discontinued.

The treatment of cutaneous lupus centers on the use of topical corticosteroids. Mild to potent topical steroids may be used depending on the severity and thickness of the lesions and their location. Intralesional injections of betamethasone 6 mg/ml or triamcinolone 5 mg/ml may be required in well-established lesions of DLE. Antimalarial drugs are the second line of treatment of cutaneous lupus.

Systemic corticosteroids should be reserved for the more serious manifestations of lupus; however, they are also effective for milder symptoms if other therapies prove unbeneficial or intolerable. Fig. 81-5 provides a general guideline to the appropriate dose of prednisone according to disease manifestation. The lowest dose that provides control of the problem at hand should be used. Once the manifestation comes under control, the dose of prednisone should be gradually tapered and, if possible, discontinued. A schedule reducing the dose by 25% every 3 to 4 weeks is generally appropriate. If the disease flares during this process, the next higher dose that controlled symptoms should be resumed, and a taper reattempted once the disease has stabilized. The addition of topical steroids, hydroxychloroquine, or an NSAID may be steroid-sparing in certain circumstances. Some manifestations of lupus, including thrombosis, end-stage or pure membranous nephritis, and occasionally thrombocytopenia or hemolytic anemia, do not respond to steroid therapy.

Rarely, when the illness is particularly fulminant or life-threatening, high-dose "pulse" intravenous steroid therapy is used. This approach has met with some success in nephritis, cerebritis, pneumonitis, vasculitis, and thrombocytopenia. Methylprednisolone is generally given in a single intravenous dose of 500 to 1000 mg daily for 3 to 6 days, followed by 60 mg oral prednisone daily. Patients requiring this aggressive approach should generally be managed with the consultation of an appropriate specialist.

Although corticosteroids may be lifesaving treatment in SLE, their use, particularly at high doses, is fraught with complications. Hypertension, weight gain, glucose intolerance, and acne are among the most common adverse effects. Osteoporosis is also a major problem, especially during prolonged use. Many lupus patients also avoid the sun, and some experience premature menopause resulting from cytotoxic use, placing them at particular risk for osteoporosis. Calcium supplementation of 1000 mg daily should be used, along with a vitamin D–containing multivitamin.

Lupus patients are at particular risk of three potentially serious adverse effects of steroid use. Infections of all types occur more frequently in patients taking prednisone, particularly at higher doses. Infection is a primary or contributing factor in 30% to 50% of all deaths in SLE patients. Bacterial infections are most common, but fungal and opportunistic infections also occur and must be aggressively sought. The second unusual toxicity of steroid use in SLE is atherosclerosis. Both peripheral vascular and ischemic cardiac diseases occur at substan-

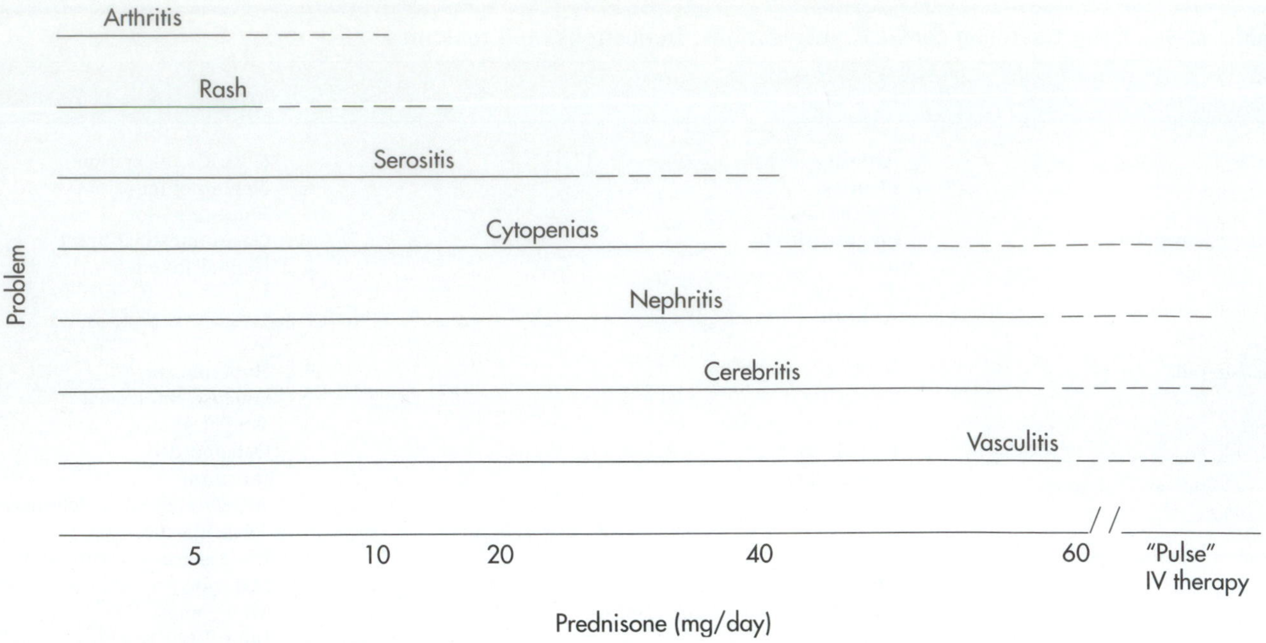


**Fig. 81-5.** Problem-oriented guide to corticosteroid dosage. Suggested minimal steroid doses are shown in solid lines, with ranges indicated by broken lines. Arthritis, rash, and serositis can often be managed without steroids.

tially increased frequency in SLE, even in young female patients, and appear to be related to long-term steroid use. Ischemic necrosis of bone, also referred to as avascular or aseptic necrosis, is the third type of steroid toxicity that is a particular problem in SLE. The femoral head is most commonly involved. However, many patients have multiple sites, including the humeral heads, femoral condyles and tali. The pain of avascular necrosis, unlike that of lupus-related synovitis, is exacerbated by use and relieved by rest. Joint stiffness is minimal.

Cytotoxic drugs are generally reserved for serious or potentially life-threatening manifestations of disease. They should be prescribed in consultation with an appropriate specialist experienced in their use. Cyclophosphamide is probably more effective than azathioprine in this setting, but also more toxic. Monthly boluses of intravenous cyclophosphamide are used primarily for diffuse proliferative glomerulonephritis. The initial dosage of 500 to 750 mg/m$^2$ is adjusted to achieve a nadir white blood cell count of 3500 to 4500, 10 to 14 days postinfusion. Although this route of therapy is associated with less bladder toxicity and a lower risk of malignancy than daily oral therapy, the risk of serious infection is similar. Either cyclophosphamide or azathioprine can be used in a daily oral dose of 1 to 3 mg/kg when the clinical situation is serious enough to warrant the toxicity. Patients must be monitored for marrow suppression, and are at risk of infection, malignancy, infertility, and menopause.

Anticoagulants are used in the subset of patients whose disease manifestations can be attributed to thrombosis. These patients usually have one or more forms of antiphospholipid antibody. Initial therapy of the thrombosis is with intravenous heparin, followed by oral warfarin. Patients with antiphospholipid antibodies who have had clear-cut thrombotic episodes are at increased risk of recurrent thrombosis. Lifelong anticoagulation must be considered, particularly if the initial event was a stroke or large vessel occlusion. Management in this setting is the same whether the patient has SLE or the primary antiphospholipid syndrome.

### Monitoring

Several laboratory tests useful in making the diagnosis of lupus are also helpful in monitoring patients with established disease. Some patients have their own distinctive pattern of laboratory abnormalities that track with clinical disease activity. For example, levels of anti-DNA antibodies may rise with flares of disease and return to negative when disease is under control. ANA titers, in contrast, are rarely useful in monitoring disease activity. Some patients reproducibly demonstrate a fall in serum complement levels just before a disease flare. In others, the erythrocyte sedimentation rate may rise, or quantitative immunoglobulin levels may become elevated. These markers should be surveyed when the lupus is quiescent to establish each patient's baseline normal profile. When a disease flare is suspected the studies may be repeated and compared with original values. As long as the lupus is inactive it is unnecessary to repeat these measurements. A urinalysis, serum creatinine, and complete blood count should, however, be performed at least twice yearly, even if the lupus appears to be in remission, in order to screen for occult disease.

### Reproductive issues

One of the most problematic management areas in lupus involves issues of reproduction. Patients with active SLE should avoid becoming pregnant; there are clearcut risks to both the mother and fetus. Use of estrogen-containing oral contraceptive preparations for birth control may induce a disease flare. Patients taking them without difficulty are generally permitted to continue, but most rheumatologists are reluctant to allow their lupus patients to begin oral contraceptives. Barrier methods of contraception, including the diaphragm and condom with contraceptive spermicide, may be preferable, and the newer progesterone-based implantable contraceptive devices also appear safe from the standpoint of the lupus.

If pregnancy occurs when the disease is under control, there is controversy regarding the risk of lupus flare. Hypertension, proteinuria, or thrombocytopenia developing in a pregnant woman with lupus may be difficult to distinguish from preeclampsia. Serial monitoring of renal function and serum complement levels may be useful in tracking the course of the lupus. Lupus patients should be observed through their pregnancy in consultation with a high-risk obstetrician or perinatologist.

The fetus is also subject to potential dangers related to the mother's lupus. When the mother has antiphospholipid antibodies there is an increased frequency of second-trimester miscarriage and stillbirth. Early miscarriages may also be increased. Some women suffer multiple recurrent miscarriages and are unable to carry a pregnancy to term. Trials with aspirin, steroids, and heparin anticoagulation in this setting have given conflicting results, and should be undertaken only with the guidance of an experienced perinatologist.

The other major risk to the fetus is neonatal lupus. This occurs when maternal anti-SS-A/Ro, an IgG immunoglobulin, crosses the placenta to the fetus. In roughly one half of affected fetuses congenital heart block occurs, generally becoming evident between weeks 20 and 22 of the pregnancy. Structural cardiac defects may also occur and carry a poorer prognosis. Infants of mothers with lupus may also experience a temporary neonatal lupus syndrome manifest as a positive ANA and photosensitive dermatitis, with malar erythema and discoid or annular skin lesions. The rash and serologic abnormalities gradually disappear over the first few months of life as the infant metabolizes the maternal immunoglobulins.

## SUMMARY

SLE is an exceptionally challenging clinical disorder. The physician caring for a patient with suspected lupus may need to call on a variety of consultants both to confirm the diagnosis and to assist in treatment decisions. In a patient with probable lupus including a rash, a dermatologist may be able to provide clinical or histologic information to clarify the diagnosis. For patients with more generalized problems, or in whom the serologic picture is confusing, a rheumatologist may be more appropriate. Consultation should also be sought when serious or potentially life-threatening complications such as cerebritis, nephritis, thrombocytopenia, or hemolysis develop. Any patient in whom high-dose steroid therapy or cytotoxic use is being contemplated should also be referred for subspecialty input into management.

## BIBLIOGRAPHY

Callen JP: Treatment of cutaneous lesions in patients with lupus, *Dermatol Clin* 8:355, 1990.

Carette S: Cardiopulmonary manifestations of systemic lupus erythematosus, *Rheum Dis Clin North Am* 14:135, 1988.

Ginzler EM, Schorn K: Outcome and prognosis in systemic lupus erythematosus, *Rheum Dis Clin North Am* 14:67, 1988.

Klippel JH: Systemic lupus erythematosus. Treatment-related complications superimposed on chronic disease, *JAMA* 263:1812, 1990.

Love PE, Santoro SA: Anti-phospholipid antibodies: anticardiolipin and the lupus anticoagulant in systemic lupus erythematosus (SLE) and in non-SLE disorders. Prevalence and clinical significance, *Ann Intern Med* 112:682, 1990.

Steinberg AD: Concepts of pathogenesis of systemic lupus erythematosus, *Clin Immunol Immunopathol* 63(1):19, 1992.

Steinberg AD, Steinberg SC: Long-term preservation of renal function in patients with lupus nephritis receiving treatment that includes cyclophosphamide versus those treated with prednisone alone, *Arthritis Rheum* 34:945, 1991.

Tan EM: Antinuclear antibodies: diagnostic markers for autoimmune diseases and probes for cell biology, *Adv Immunol* 44:93, 1989.

Tan EM et al: The 1982 revised criteria for the classification of systemic lupus erythematosus, *Arthritis Rheum* 25:1271, 1982.

CHAPTER

# 82 Crystal-Induced Rheumatic Disorders

**David F. Giansiracusa**

## CRYSTAL DEPOSITION DISEASE: GOUT

### Epidemiology and etiology

Gout occurs as a result of elevated serum levels of monosodium urate that cause the deposition of urate crystals in joints and soft tissues and/or excessive urinary excretion of uric acid. Clinical manifestations of gout include (1) recurrent attacks of acute arthritis; (2) chronic, deforming, erosive arthritis related to deposition of large deposits of monosodium urate (tophi) in and around joints; (3) deposition of monosodium urate crystals in the kidneys, causing urate nephropathy; (4) uric acid kidney stones; and (5) uric acid crystallization in renal tubules, termed *acute hyperuricemic* (or *uric acid*) *nephropathy.*

Hyperuricemia is a requisite for the development of gout. Statistically, hyperuricemia can be defined as a serum urate level greater than 2 S.D. above the mean. However, since gout represents a group of diseases that result from excessive amounts of monosodium urate, hyperuricemia is better defined in physicochemical terms as the level above which urate concentration exceeds the saturation point. Since the solubility of urate in plasma at 37° C is approximately 7 mg/dl, which by most chemical and automatic analyzer techniques corresponds to a serum urate level of approximately 7.5 to 8 mg/dl, *hyperuricemia* can be defined as a serum urate level that exceeds this concentration. Hyperuricemia may result from overproduction of urate and/or diminished urinary excretion of uric acid. The term *primary gout* refers to the clinical disease that is due to hyperuricemia caused by a genetically determined metabolic error of excessive de novo biosynthesis and/or impaired excretion of uric acid.

The overproduction of uric acid is determined when a patient is put on a purine-restricted diet for 5 days and excretes more than 600 mg of uric acid in 24 hours. This group of patients constitutes fewer than 15% of individuals with gout. In a very small fraction of patients who produce too much uric acid, a primary enzymatic abnormality such as hypoxanthine guanine phosphoribosyltransferase (HG-PRTase) deficiency or increased phosphoribosylpyrophosphate (PRPP) synthetase activity is responsible for excessive biosynthesis of uric acid.

In approximately 75% to 90% of individuals with primary gout, hyperuricemia is the result of diminished renal clearance of uric acid. These individuals require serum urate levels 2 to 3 mg/dl higher than normal to achieve comparable uric acid excretion rates.

*Secondary gout* results from an acquired disease state or a drug that causes an overproduction or impaired excretion of uric acid. Secondary causes of hyperuricemia include myeloproliferative and lymphoproliferative diseases, multiple myeloma, hemolytic anemia, polycythemia vera, and psoriasis. Acquired renal disease, acidosis, and drugs (particularly low-dose salicylates, nicotinic acid, ethambutol, cyclosporine, and any diuretic that causes volume contraction, but especially thiazides, which also compete with urate secretion by the renal tubule) are the most common causes of secondary hyperuricemia resulting from diminished renal excretion of uric acid. Lead-induced renal tubular injury also impairs uric acid excretion. Alcohol consumption elevates serum urate levels because of the generation of organic acids, which compete with tubular secretion of uric acid and enhance uric acid production secondary to accelerated conversion of adenosine triphosphate to adenosine monophosphate, which is metabolized in uric acid.

## Pathophysiology

Urate crystals are virtually always present in synovial fluid in cases of acute gouty arthritis. Laboratory studies of crystal growth indicate that the saturation concentration varies with temperature, so that in temperatures below 37° C, as occurs in the extremity joints, the saturation point for uric acid is significantly below 7 mg/dl. This biochemical phenomenon correlates well with the clinical observations that gouty arthritis characteristically affects the joints of the feet, ankles, knees, hands, and elbows and that tophi deposit in cool sites, such as the cartilaginous helix of the external ear, the olecranon bursae, and the peripheral joints.

Acute gouty arthritis occurs when monosodium urate crystals appear in the synovial fluid as a result of either shedding from articular cartilage or synovium or from precipitation of new crystals. Mechanical stresses, such as twisting an ankle or stubbing the great toe, may dislodge urate crystals. Crystal shedding may also occur as a result of rapid changes in urate concentration, as in the institution of uric acid–lowering therapy such as allopurinol and uricosuric agents or the ingestion of alcohol or salicylates. Once in the joint fluid, a series of processes, including coating of the crystals with immunoglobulins, occurs. Polymorphonuclear leukocytes ingest the crystals, releasing lysosomal enzymes and other inflammatory mediators, including toxic superoxide radicals, prostaglandins, leukotrienes, kinins, and components of the complement pathways, causing inflammation and, with repeated attacks, joint damage.

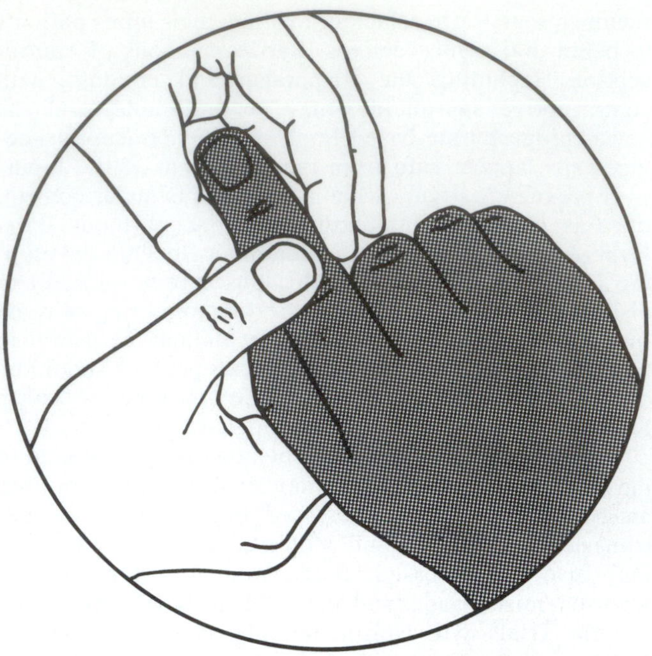

**Fig. 82-1.** Palpation of interphalangeal joints.

## Clinical features

***History and physical examination.*** After a period of prolonged asymptomatic hyperuricemia (often 20 to 30 years), some individuals (approximately 5% to 10%) may develop acute gouty arthritis characterized by the abrupt onset of exquisite pain, tenderness, swelling, and erythema that most commonly affects a single joint (Fig. 82-1). Approximately 50% of individuals experience their first attack in the metatarsophalangeal (MTP) joint of the great toe. Other peripheral joints, including the joints of the midfoot, ankles, knees, fingers, wrists, and elbows, may be involved in a monoarticular fashion. Approximately 10% to 15% of individuals afflicted with acute gouty arthritis present initially with polyarticular gout. Gouty arthritis most frequently affects men in the fourth through sixth decades of life and, less commonly, postmenopausal women. Attacks often occur at night and may be associated with inflammation of the surrounding tendons, bursae, and skin, raising the differential diagnosis of joint infection and cellulitis. Even if untreated the acute attack is self-limited, generally lasting 3 to 7 days, after which the patient is completely asymptomatic. The attacks may become more frequent and more prolonged, to the point that the individual may eventually develop chronic, persistent gout, with increasing accumulation of urate deposits clinically evident as palpable tophi on examination, or erosions and soft tissue swelling on radiographs.

***Laboratory studies and diagnostic procedures.*** Characteristic bone radiographic features of chronic tophaceous gout include cortical indentations or erosions with sharply defined sclerotic margins resulting from tophi in adjacent soft tissues, cortical erosions with an overhanging or hooklike margin as a result of tophaceous deposits in the periosteum or cortical bones, and round or oval cysts generally with sclerotic margins in medullary bone near

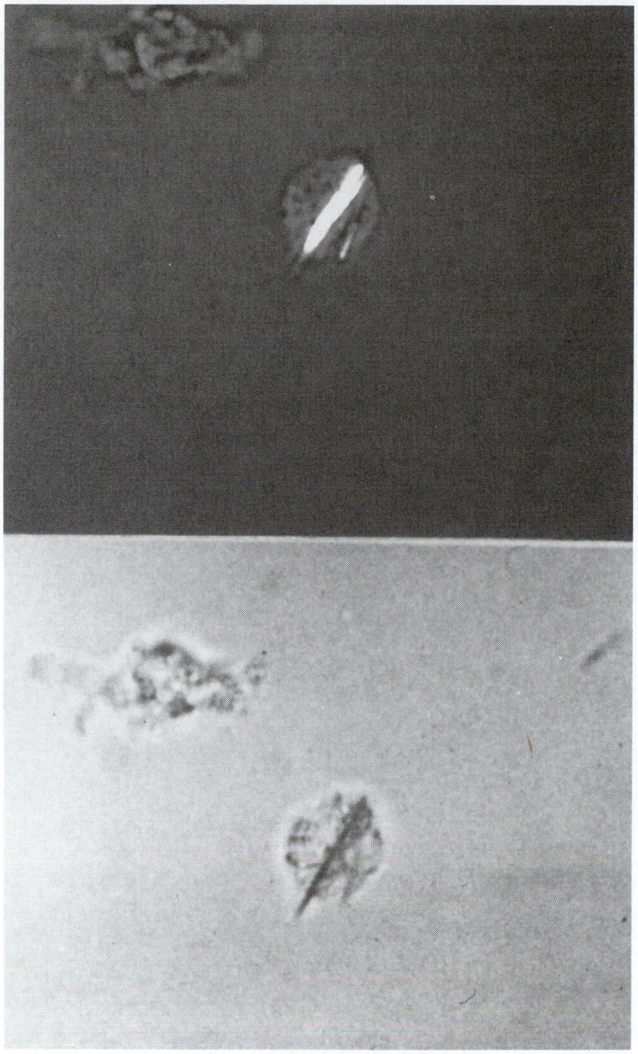

**Fig. 82-2.** Monodosium urate crystals phagocytosed by a synovial fluid polymorphonuclear leukocyte. In the top section, compensated polarized light clearly demonstrates two longer crystals and one shorter one. The bottom section shows the same field under ordinary light. Comparison of the two views demonstrates the superiority of compensated polarized light over ordinary light microscopy when evaluating joint fluid for crystals. (From American College of Rheumatology: *Clinical slide collection on the rheumatic diseases,* slide 11-9 [1981 numbering system], 1991, The College.)

joints. Relative preservation of joint space, absence of profound periarticular demineralization, and eccentric location of soft tissue swelling are features that help differentiate tophaceous gouty arthritis from rheumatoid arthritis.

A definitive diagnosis of gouty arthritis is established by the demonstration of needle-shaped monosodium urate crystals within synovial fluid polymorphonuclear leukocytes aspirated from clinically affected joints (Fig. 82-2). Because of birefringent characteristics, urate crystals (and, in the case of pseudogout, the calcium pyrophosphate crystals) are more readily visualized by polarizing microscopy than by plain light microscopy. The monosodium urate crystal appears as a bright needle-shaped object on a dark background. With the use of a red compensator, the negatively birefringent urate crystals are yellow when they lie parallel to the axis of the light coming through the microscope, whereas the positively birefringent, rhomboid, or square calcium pyrophosphate crystals are blue when parallel to the microscope's plane of light. The more acute the attack of gout, the more likely it is that monosodium urate crystals are visualized within synovial polymorphonuclear leukocytes.

### Differential diagnosis of acute monoarticular and oligoarticular arthritis

- Septic arthritis
- Crystalline-induced arthritis
  - Gout
  - Pseudogout (calcium pyrophosphate arthropathy)
  - Hydroxyapatite and other basic calcium/phosphate crystals
  - Calcium oxalate
- Traumatic joint injury
- Hemarthrosis
- Monoarticular or oligoarticular flare of an inflammatory polyarticular rheumatic disease (rheumatoid arthritis, psoriatic arthritis, Reiter's syndrome, systemic lupus erythematosus)

***Differential diagnosis of gout.*** The differential diagnosis of gout is that of an acute monoarticular or oligoarticular (four or fewer joints) arthritis (see the box above).

## Renal complications of hyperuricemia and hyperuricaciduria

Excesses of serum urate and urinary uric acid may affect the kidneys and cause a variety of medical problems, specifically urate nephropathy, acute hyperuricemic (uric acid) nephropathy, and uric acid urolithiasis.

Urate nephropathy manifests in the development of proteinuria, loss of maximal tubular concentrating ability, hypertension, and azotemia related to the deposition of monosodium urate crystals within the medullary and pyramidal interstitium of the kidney as a result of long-standing hyperuricemia. This condition rarely occurs in the absence of gouty arthritis and generally correlates with the severity of the joint disease. Urate nephropathy is diagnosed clinically. Pathologically the condition is characterized by urate crystal deposition in the medullary interstitium and pyramids with surrounding giant cell reaction. In the majority of gouty patients, hypertension, heart disease, peripheral atherosclerosis, aging, diabetes mellitus, nonsteroidal antiinflammatory drug (NSAID) use, analgesic abuse, lead exposure, other intrinsic renal disease (such as glomerulonephritis, pyelonephritis, and interstitial nephritis), and urinary obstruction are generally more important contributors to renal function impairment than urate nephropathy.

Acute hyperuricemic nephropathy (acute uric acid nephropathy) is characterized by oliguria and renal failure related to the precipitation of massive amounts of uric acid within renal tubules and collecting ducts, causing tubular

### Evaluation of patient with asymptomatic hyperuricemia

Obesity
Alcohol consumption
Use of salicylate, thiazide, or other diuretics
Use of nicotinic acid, ethambutol, and cyclosporine
Volume depletion
Renal disease
High cell turnover state such as leukemia, hemolytic animia, and severe psoriasis
Evidence of hypertension or cardiovascular disease
History of renal stones
Previous acute attacks of arthritis
Presence of tophi
Family history of gouty arthritis, renal stones, and renal disease

obstruction. This condition most commonly develops during cytotoxic therapy for myeloproliferative disorders as a result of massive cell death and an increased release of uric acid. Therapy to prevent uric acid nephropathy includes vigorous hydration and the use of the xanthine oxidase inhibitor, allopurinol, generally in a dosage of 600 mg per day begun 2 to 3 days before the institution of cytotoxic radiation or chemotherapy.

Approximately 10% to 25% of individuals with gouty arthritis develop urolithiasis, usually with stones composed of a mixture of uric acid and calcium oxalate. The incidence of nephrolithiasis increases with the degree of hyperuricemia but more closely correlates with the amount of uric acid excreted in the urine (i.e., the degree of uric aciduria). One large epidemiologic study indicated that approximately 50% of individuals who excrete more than 1100 mg of uric acid in 24 hours develop stones. Other factors that predispose to uric acid urolithiasis include high urine concentration, low pH, and possibly urinary solubility factors. Therapeutic measures to prevent uric acid calculi include adequate hydration, alkalinization to maintain a urine pH more than 6, moderation of dietary intake of alcohol and protein, control of infection, and reduction of uric acid production with allopurinol and hence reduction in the amount of uric acid excreted.

### Purine content of foods

**Foods to avoid**

These foods contain between 150 and 800 mg purines per 100-g (3-oz) portion.
Sweetbreads
Anchovies
Sardines
Liver
Gravies
Kidney
Brain
Meat extracts

**Foods to use in moderation**

These foods contain 50 to 150 mg of purine per 100-g (3-oz) portion. One serving of each may be used each day.
Meat
Poultry
Lentils, dried
Meat soup and broth
Oatmeal
Peas, dried
Spinach
Wheat germ and bran
Beans, dried
Shellfish
Fish, fresh and saltwater

**Foods allowed in unlimited quantities**

These foods contain between 0 and 15 mg of purine per 100-g (3-oz) portion.
All fruits
Vegetables (except those listed above)
Most breads, cereals, and cereal products (except whole wheat)
Milk
Cheese
Eggs
Fish roe
All nuts
Sugar, syrup, sweets
Gelatin
Milk and fruit desserts
Vegetable and cream soup
Textured vegetable protein
Coffee, tea, chocolate, cocoa
Fats (allowed in limited amounts)

## Management of hyperuricemia and gouty arthritis

Asymptomatic hyperuricemia is an elevated serum urate level without gouty arthritis, tophi, urate nephropathy, or uric acid renal calculi. Evaluation of a patient with asymptomatic hyperuricemia includes items in the box above.

Treatment of asymptomatic hyperuricemia with pharmacologic agents is rarely indicated. Arguments against treating asymptomatic hyperuricemia include the following: (1) Although as many as 5% of the population in the United States may have hyperuricemia, the majority (approximately 80% to 90%) never develop recognizable consequences; (2) gouty arthritis is a treatable condition; (3) urate nephropathy and tophaceous gout rarely develop in the absence of a history of acute gouty arthritis; (4) renal function is not adversely affected by hyperuricemia, and its normalization has little effect on renal function; and (5) treatment with an agent that lowers uric acid requires lifelong therapy, which is expensive and may be associated with potentially serious side effects. The risk of uric acid stone formation is more closely related to uric acid excretion rates than to the degree of serum urate elevation. Detailed studies on cardiovascular disease indicate that hyperuricemia does not appear to be an independent risk factor for coronary artery disease but rather is associated with other risk factors such as obesity, hypertension, and hyperlipidemia. Conversely, there is no evidence to support the contention that lowering serum urate to normal levels independently reduces the risk of coronary artery disease. Appropriate management of asymptomatic hyper-

### Suggested meal plan for gout patients

**Morning**
Fruit or juice
Bread
Meat or substitute
Fat
Beverage

**Noon and evening**
Meat or substitute
Potato or substitute
Vegetable(s) (except those listed above)
Fruit
Bread
Fat
Dessert
Beverage

### Restricted purine sample menu

**Morning**
Orange juice
Rice Krispies
Hard-cooked egg
Toast
Margarine/jelly
Skim milk
Tea or coffee

**Noon**
Turkey breast
Mashed potatoes
Green beans
Cranberry sauce
Tossed salad/Mayonnaise
Roll
Margarine
Sugar cookies
Pineapple
Iced Tea
Sugar

**Evening**
Swiss steak with tomatoes and onions
Noodles
Broccoli
Roll
Peaches
Skim milk
Tea or coffee

uricemia consists of weight reduction for the obese patient, moderation in the consumption of alcohol, protein, and foods high in purine content, cessation of smoking, and treatment of hypertension and hypercholesterolemia. A diet low in purine content allows patients to reduce their serum urate levels by 1 mg/dl and the 24-hour urinary uric acid excretion by 200 to 400 mg per day. See the boxes on pp. 1142 and 1143 for the purine contents of foods, a suggested meal plan, and a restricted purine sample menu. Diuretics and other drugs that contribute to hyperuricemia should be avoided if possible. Any primary condition that contributes to hyperuricemia, such as renal disease and high cell turnover states, should be treated.

### Treatment options for acute gouty arthritis

Nonsteroidal antiinflammatory drugs (NSAIDs)
  (See Table 79-3 for a list of agents, doses, and side effects)
Colchicine
  Oral
  Intravenous
Glucocorticosteroids
  Oral
  Intravenous
  Intramuscular
  Intraarticular
Adrenocorticotropic hormone (ACTH)
  Intramuscular
  Intravenous

## Treatment of gout

The goals of the treatment of gouty arthritis are termination of the acute attack, prevention of recurrent attacks, and prevention or resorption of tophi in joints and soft tissues. Pharmacologic agents used to treat gouty arthritis can be divided into antiinflammatory drugs, drugs used for prophylaxis against episodes of acute gouty arthritis, and drugs to lower urate (and uric acid) levels (see the box above).

The earlier an acute attack of gouty arthritis is treated, the more rapidly the inflamed joints respond. Medications used to treat acute gouty arthritis include colchicine (taken orally or given intravenously); NSAID; and corticosteroids given orally, infused intravenously, or injected into the involved joints. NSAIDs are generally given in high dosages for the first 2 to 3 days (pulse therapy) and then tapered to a lower dosage (e.g., indomethacin, 50 mg three to four times a day for 1 to 2 days with meals, followed by a taper to 25 mg three to four times a day with meals for 5 to 7 days). Other NSAIDs, including tolmetin sodium, naproxen, ibuprofen, piroxicam, sulindac, ketoprofen, fenoprofen, and meclofenamate, may also be effective. Because of the potential adverse effects of phenylbutazone and the availability of other NSAIDs, it is recommended that primary care physicians do *not* treat patients using phenylbutazone. All NSAIDs may cause gastrointestinal and central nervous system side effects as well as gastrointestinal bleeding, inhibition of platelet function, fluid retention, aggravation of congestive heart failure, hypertension, and renal function impairment.

If the treatment of acute gouty arthritis is begun within several hours of the onset of the attack, oral colchicine, 0.6 mg every hour for a maximum of 8 to 10 tablets or until gastrointestinal side effects develop, followed by a maintenance therapy of 0.6 mg twice daily, may be effective. The efficacy of oral colchicine is markedly reduced the longer that treatment is delayed after onset of the arthritis; therefore, oral colchicine is not the ideal drug for the treatment of acute attacks.

Colchicine may also be delivered intravenously, a particularly useful mode of therapy for the patient who cannot take oral medications or who has a diarrheal illness such as viral gastroenteritis, inflammatory bowel disease, or medication- or dietary-induced diarrhea. Intravenous colchicine may also be a useful option in the patient who should avoid NSAIDs because of other medical problems, such as peptic ulcer disease, anticoagulation, or congestive heart failure. A total of 2 to 3 mg may be infused initially, followed by an infusion of 0.5 to 0.1 mg 8 to 12 hours later for a total dose of intravenous colchicine not to exceed 4 mg in 24 to 48 hours. No more colchicine should be administered for at least 7 days. Colchicine is extremely irritating to soft tissues and may cause tissue necrosis and cutaneous slough if extravasation occurs. Colchicine should be diluted in 20 ml of normal saline and infused over 10 to 20 minutes in a well-running intravenous line. Although intravenously administered colchicine does not tend to cause the gastrointestinal side effects associated with oral administration, it may result in myelosuppression. Excessive dosing of intravenous colchicine may also cause disseminated intravascular coagulation, shock, renal shutdown, hepatocellular necrosis, and central nervous system dysfunction.

Colchicine excretion is reduced in patients with chronic liver disease and impaired renal function, including older individuals who appear to have normal serum creatinine levels. Myopathy and neuropathy associated with long-term colchicine therapy have been reported in patients with renal insufficiency; therefore colchicine either should *not* be used or should be used very carefully (including a reduction in the dosage) in patients with significant liver or renal disease. Colchicine should *not* be used in the presence of combined renal and liver dysfunction, biliary obstruction, or severe renal disease (creatinine clearance less than 10 ml per minute).

Corticosteroids may be required in patients with particularly severe or prolonged attacks or in patients who have contraindications to treatment with other agents. After joint sepsis has been excluded, corticosteroids may be administered directly into the inflamed joint or given systematically, such as 30 to 40 mg of prednisone or its equivalent on day 1, tapered by 5 mg per day or 40 to 80 USP units of adrenocorticotropic hormone (ACTH) intramuscularly (or slow intravenous infusion of 20 USP units of ACTH) repeated every 6 to 12 hours for 1 to 3 days as needed.

See the boxes on pp. 1143 and 1144 for treatment options of acute gout and options to consider when treating acute gout in patients with other medical problems.

After an acute attack of gout has subsided, chronic maintenance therapy with colchicine, 0.6 mg twice daily in patients with normal renal and hepatic function or NSAIDs with meals may act as a prophylaxis against subsequent gouty attacks.

The issue of chronic uric acid–lowering therapy after one attack of gouty arthritis remains controversial. Definite indications for uric acid–lowering therapy are (1) repeated attacks of disabling gouty arthritis, (2) the presence of tophaceous deposits on physical examination or by radiographic studies, (3) clinical or radiographic signs of chronic gouty joint disease, (4) evidence of renal damage (glomerular filtration rate less than 60 ml per minute), (5) recurrent urolithiasis caused by pure uric acid stones or mixed stones in the setting of hyperuricosuria, (6) gross overproduction of uric acid (urinary uric acid excretion greater than 1000 mg per day), and (7) prevention of hyperuricemia and uricosuria in patients with lymphoproliferative and myeloproliferative disease before cytotoxic therapy.

Allopurinol should be used for indications 4 through 7 and for indications 1 through 3 if urinary uric acid excretion on a low-purine diet (see box on p. 1143) exceeds 600 mg in 24 hours. Allopurinol should be instituted only after the resolution of an acute attack of gout and with the concurrent administration of NSAIDs or maintenance colchicine, 0.6 mg once to twice daily to prevent an attack of acute gout. Colchicine or NSAIDs should be continued for approximately 6 months after allopurinol has resulted in the resolution of all palpable tophi or, for the patient without tophi, for approximately 6 months after serum urate levels are suppressed below 6 mg/dl. Allopurinol is generally begun with a dosage of 100 mg a day and increased every 2 to 4 weeks by 100 mg to the dosage necessary to depress the serum urate level below 6 to 7 mg/dl. The dosage of allopurinol must be kept low in the setting of renal failure. This may mean as

### Agents to consider when treating gouty arthritis in patients with other medical problems

Patients with renal disease with normal liver function
- Consider: Corticosteroids (including ACTH)
- Avoid: NSAIDs
- Avoid: Colchicine

Patients with liver disease with normal renal function
- Consider: Ibuprofen
- Consider: Dexamethasone (avoid steroids with mineralocorticoid effects)
- Avoid: Colchicine

Patients with renal disease and liver disease
- Consider: Corticosteroids (including ACTH)
- Avoid: NSAIDs
- Avoid: Colchicine

Patients with peptic ulcer disease
- Consider: Intravenous colchicine or intraarticular corticosteroids
- Try to avoid: Systemic steroids, including ACTH
- Avoid: NSAIDs
- Avoid: Oral colchicine

Patients with congestive heart failure but good renal and hepatic function
- Consider: Corticosteroids without mineralocorticoid effect (e.g., dexamethasone)
- Consider: Intravenous colchicine
- Avoid: NSAIDs

Patients on anticoagulation:
- Consider: Colchicine
- Consider: Oral corticosteroids
- Consider: Intravenous corticosteroids or ACTH
- Avoid: NSAIDs
- Avoid: Intramuscular corticosteroids or ACTH

little as 100 mg every other day or every third day. Since allopurinol reduces the metabolism of warfarin, 6-mercaptopurine, and azathioprine, the dosage of these medications must be appropriately reduced. In the case of azathioprine the dosage is generally reduced to approximately 25% of the usual dosage when given in the setting of allopurinol therapy. Potential toxicities of allopurinol include nausea, diarrhea, drug fever, leukopenia, hepatotoxity, interstitial nephritis, vasculitis, and a rash that may evolve into toxic epidermal necrolysis. Serious side effects most commonly occur when allopurinol is prescribed to patients with renal insufficiency, particularly with concomitant thiazide therapy.

Uricosuric agents may be prescribed in hyperuricemic patients with gout who excrete less than 700 mg of uric acid per day. Patients must have normal renal function for the agents to be effective (the glomerular filtration rate should be greater than 60 ml per minute) and should maintain good urine volumes to minimize the risk of urolithiasis. The commonly used uricosuric agents are probenecid given initially in a dosage of 250 to 500 mg twice a day and increased to 1.5 g twice a day as needed and sulfinpyrazone 100 mg twice a day and increased to 400 mg twice a day. Similar to allopurinol therapy, prophylaxis against acute gouty arthritis should be administered when a uricosuric agent is prescribed, and the prophylactic medication should be continued for at least 6 months after the serum urate level is controlled below 6 mg/dl or for 6 months after resolution of all clinically apparent tophi. Side effects of probenecid include headache, nausea, anorexia, skin rash, and, rarely, nephrotic syndrome, hepatic necrosis, and aplastic anemia. Sulfinpyrazone may cause bone marrow suppression.

If a patient experiences an attack of gouty arthritis while taking allopurinol or a uricosuric agent, the dosage of the agent to lower uric acid level should *not* be changed until after resolution of the attack.

## CALCIUM PYROPHOSPHATE DEPOSITION DISEASE

Calcium pyrophosphate dihydrate (CPPD) crystal deposition disease, also referred to as *pyrophosphate arthropathy,* is a calcium crystal-induced form of joint disease that is characterized by diverse clinical manifestations associated with the deposition of calcium pyrophosphate dihydrate crystals in and around joints. The crystals most commonly deposit in fibrocartilage, such as menisci of the knee, intervertebral disks, and symphysis pubis and in hyaline articular cartilage of the knees, wrists, and other joints. These deposits may also occur in tendons, ligaments, synovial membranes, and joint capsules. The deposition of CPPD increases with aging and in osteoarthritic joints; thus calcium pyrophosphate arthropathy is fairly common in older individuals, particularly in the acute form, called *pseudogout.* Even more common is the asymptomatic radiographic presence of articular cartilage calcifications that may occur in as many as 15% of individuals 65 to 75 years of age and more than 40% of those 85 years of age and older.

### Clinical features

CPPD is best known for causing acute arthritis (pseudogout) because of its similarities to acute gouty arthritis. Pseudogout most commonly affects the knees of older women, in contrast to gout, which most commonly affects the joint at the base of the great toe (first MTP joint) and the joints of the instep and ankle in middle-aged men. Pseudogout may also involve the wrists and, less frequently, metacarpophalangeal (MCP) joints, ankles, shoulders, and elbows.

In addition to the acute arthritis or pseudogout presentation, deposition of calcium pyrophosphate crystals may cause a more subacute, polyarticular presentation similar to rheumatoid arthritis (the so-called pseudorheumatoid form), a pseudoosteoarthritis form, and a destructive form as is seen with severe neuropathies, the so-called pseudoneuropathic form. CPPD crystals may be detected radiographically in an asymptomatic individual as articular chondrocalcinosis.

### Associated diseases

The most common association with CPPD deposition is aging, but a number of other conditions are associated with deposition of calcium pyrophosphate crystals in articular and periarticular structures. These include disorders associated with elevated calcium levels, specifically hyperparathyroidism, and metabolic disorders characterized by diminished activity of pyrophosphatases, such as familial hypophosphatasia and hypomagnesemia. In addition, familial hypocalciuric hypercalcemia, hemochromatosis, hypothyroidism, and Bartter syndrome are associated with CPPD. Osteoarthritic degeneration of cartilage also facilitates calcium pyrophosphate crystal deposition.

### Diagnosis and management

Although the diagnosis of pseudogout is suggested by an acute arthritis that occurs in the setting of radiographic evidence of articular chondrocalcinosis, definitive diagnosis requires joint aspiration with synovial fluid examination and visualization by compensated polarized microscopy of the rhomboid or square, positively birefringent calcium pyrophosphate crystals within synovial fluid leukocytes (Fig. 82-3). Joint fluid aspirated from inflamed joints should also be examined and cultured for infectious agents. See Chapter 69 for joint aspiration technique.

### Treatment

A fundamental component of the management of acute CPPD crystal-induced arthritis (pseudogout) is joint aspiration and synovial fluid examination to identify the crystal and exclude joint sepsis. Management of pseudogout and other forms of calcium pyrophosphate arthropathy include the evaluation and treatment of underlying medical disorders and the administration of antiinflammatory medications. NSAIDs, intravenous colchicine, and intraarticular and systemic steroids, including ACTH, may be used. Screening laboratory studies may include those for calcium, phosphorus, albumin, magnesium, thyroid function, alkaline phosphatase, iron and total iron-binding capacity, and ferritin levels. The most cost-effective approach to the metabolic evaluation is to examine for hyperparathyroidism and hemochromatosis, since CPPD arthropathy may be the first clinically apparent manifestation of these conditions. Other associated metabolic diseases generally manifest with other signs and symptoms, such as liver disease in the case of Wilson's disease.

Chronic forms of calcium pyrophosphate arthropathy

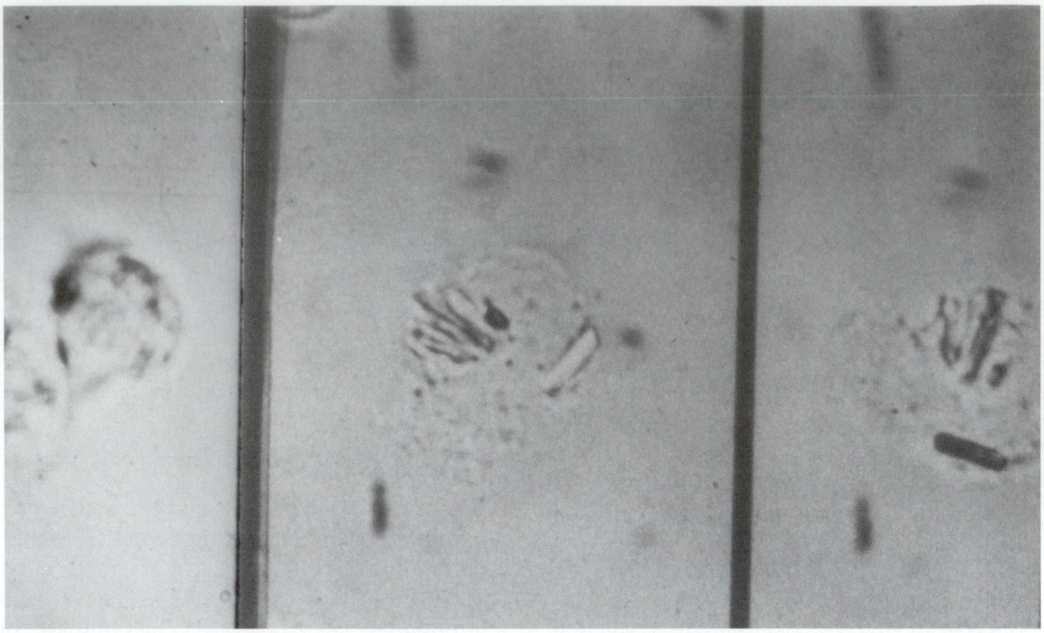

**Fig. 82-3.** Calcium pyrophosphate crystals phagocytosed by polymorphonuclear leukocytes in synovial fluid. Their rectangular or rhomboid shapes are demonstrated. (From American College of Rheumatology: *Clinical slide collection on the rheumatic diseases,* slide 91 [by 1972 numbering system], 1991, The College.)

are generally treated similarly to osteoarthritis, with NSAIDs, nonnarcotic analgesics, joint splinting as appropriate, and range-of-motion and strengthening exercises. Joint lavage and arthroscopic irrigation may occasionally be beneficial. In severe, destructive cases of CPPD arthropathy, particularly those involving the hips and knees, joint replacement for alleviation of pain and deformity may be necessary.

## HYDROXYAPATITE ARTHROPATHY

Hydroxyapatite, another calcium phosphate–containing crystal, is now well recognized to deposit in and around joints, causing acute and chronic arthropathy and periarticular inflammation.

### Periarthritis

The most familiar clinical form of hydroxyapatite-induced disease is supraspinatus tendinitis and/or calcific subacromial bursitis, presenting as shoulder pain aggravated by abduction and the presence of amorphous calcium deposits in the region of the greater tuberosity of the humerus on radiographic studies. The deposition of hydroxyapatite in periarticular structures (tendons, bursae, and joint capsules) may cause acute calcific periarthritis at multiple sites. The most commonly affected areas are the subacromial and trochanteric bursae, the supraspinatus tendon, the Achilles tendon, tendons of the wrists, capsules of the knees, and MCP joints. The clinical features of periarticular hydroxyapatite disease are quite variable, ranging from no symptoms to severe pain, tenderness, localized edema, and restricted motion. On plain radiographs, hydroxyapatite appears as amorphous, soft tissue, calcium-dense deposits or clumps, often in the anatomic sites of bursae, tendon sheaths, or joint capsules. The absence of trabeculae and the presence of the amorphous, homogenously dense deposits help to radiographically distinguish these hydroxyapatite deposits from avulsion fractures. Conditions that may predispose to calcific periarthritis include repetitive motion, diabetes mellitus, hyperthyroidism, and chronic renal failure, particularly in the setting of chronic hemodialysis.

Treatment of calcific periarthritis may include analgesics, NSAIDs, intravenous colchicine, aspiration and local injection of a depot steroid preparation once the possibility of an infectious process has been excluded, ACTH, and physical measures including the application of heat, cold, diathermy, and ultrasound. During the initial acute stage, joint rest, including splinting, may help in conjunction with gentle range-of-motion exercises progressing to a full, active range-of-motion program to prevent the development of joint contractures and adhesive capsulitis. In recurrent and refractory cases, surgical removal of the calcium deposits may be necessary.

### Hydroxyapatite crystal–induced arthritis

The presence of hydroxyapatite crystals may cause acute flares of osteoarthritis in joints, such as those of the knees and fingers. Hydroxyapatite crystals also cause a destructive arthritis, which was initially described in the shoulders, called *Milwaukee shoulder syndrome.* This form of hydroxyapatite arthropathy tends to occur most commonly in older women and results in the destruction of the rotator cuff and a degenerative arthritis of the glenohumeral joint. The synovial fluid is characterized by a paucity of white cells but high concentrations of prostaglandins and destructive enzymes in the setting of hydroxyapatite crystals. Since hydroxyapatite crystals are not birefringent, they cannot be detected easily by polarized microscopic examination but can be screened for using calcium phosphate stains (alizarin red or von Kossa) or by examining synovial fluid with techniques of x-ray diffraction and electron microscopy. The destructive process initially described as Milwaukee syndrome may also involve other joints, such as the knees and hips.

Treatment of hydroxyapatite crystal–induced arthritis consists primarily of controlling inflammation with NSAIDs and colchicine, and the use of analgesics. Intraarticular "depo" corticosteroid preparations may provide transient benefit (see Chapter 103).

## OTHER INTRAARTICULAR CRYSTALS

In addition to monosodium urate, calcium pyrophosphate, and hydroxyapatite crystals, cholesterol and calcium oxalate crystals and iatrogenically injected steroid crystals may play a role in rheumatic diseases. Patients with renal failure, particularly those on hemodialysis, may develop acute arthritis or periarthritis from the presence of calcium oxalate crystals. These crystals may appear on radiographs as amorphous calcifications similar to those of hydroxyapatite. The calcium oxalate crystals may be visualized under polarized light microscopy as positively birefringent crystals, thereby creating confusion with calcium pyrophosphate dihydrate.

Injection of the intraarticular "depo" corticosteroid preparation may also result in an inflammatory arthritis termed *postinjection flare.* This occurs in approximately 5% of the patients who receive such injections and generally begins within 3 to 6 hours after the injection, lasting up to 3 days. Aspiration of synovial fluid from these patients may reveal positively or negatively birefringent crystals, thus causing confusion with calcium pyrophosphate or monosodium urate crystals, respectively.

In some cases the identification of crystals in synovial fluid is simply the result of synovial fluid having been placed in tubes containing calcium oxalate or lithium heparin as the anticoagulant. Since these materials are birefringent crystals, their presence may be incorrectly interpreted as diagnostic of a crystal-induced process that is the cause of joint inflammation.

Cholesterol crystals have a platelike appearance with a notch in one corner and tend to be seen in fluid aspirated from chronic joint and bursal effusions, most commonly in patients with longstanding rheumatoid arthritis.

## BIBLIOGRAPHY


Alexander GM et al: Pyrophosphate arthropathy: a study of metabolic associations and laboratory data, *Ann Rheum Dis* 41:377, 1982.

Axelrod D, Preston S: Comparison of parenteral adrenocorticotropic hormone with oral indomethacin in the treatment of acute gout, *Arthritis Rheum* 31:803, 1988.

Diamond HS: Control of crystal-induced arthropathies, *Rheum Dis Clin North Am* 15:557, 1989.

Faller J, Fox IH: Ethanol-induced hyperuricemia: evidence for increased urate production by activation of adenine nucleotide turnover, *N Engl J Med* 307:1598, 1982.

Fudman FJ, Fox IH: When clinical clues point to gout, *J Musculoskel Med* 10(2); 64, 1993.

Halverson PB et al: "Milwaukee shoulder." II. Synovial fluid studies, *Arthritis Rheum* 24:747, 1981.

Kuncl RW et al. Colchicine myopathy and neuropathy, *N Eng J Med* 316:1562, 1987.

Liang MH, Fries JF: Asymptomatic hyperuricemia: the case for conservative management, *Ann Intern Med* 88:666, 1978.

Lin HY et al. Cyclosporine-induced hyperuricemia and gout, *N Engl J Med* 321:287, 1989.

McCarty DJ et al: "Milwaukee shoulder" association of microspheroids containing hydroxyapatite crystals, active collagenase, and neutral protease with rotator cuff tears. I. Clinical aspects, *Arthritis Rheum* 24:464, 1981.

Paul H, Reginato AJ, Schumacher HR: Alizarin red S staining as a screening test to detect calcium compounds in synovial fluid, *Arthritis Rheum* 26:191, 1983.

Reginato AJ, Kurnik B: Calcium oxalate and other crystals associated with kidney diseases and arthritis, *Semin Arthritis Rheum* 18:198, 1989.

Resnik LS, Resnick D: Crystal deposition disease, *Semin Arthritis Rheum* 12:390, 1983.

Rubenstein J, Pritzker KPH: Crystal-associated arthropathies, *AJR* 152:685, 1989.

Schumacher HR et al: Erosive arthritis associated with apatite crystal deposition, *Arthritis Rheum* 24:31, 1981.

Schumacher HR et al: Osteoarthritis, crystal deposition and inflammation, *Semin Arthritis Rheum* 11:116, 1981.

Schumacher R: The role of inflammation and crystals in the pain of osteoarthritis, *Arthritis Rheum* 18:81, 1989.

Tam S, Carroll W: Allopurinol hepatotoxicity, *Am J Med* 86:357, 1989.


CHAPTER

# 83 Seronegative Spondyloarthropathies


**Nancy Y. N. Liu**
**Bruce R. Weinstein**


The term *seronegative spondyloarthropathies* refers to a group of rheumatic diseases that share a number of clinical, radiologic, and pathogenetic features. These disorders are characterized by (1) inflammatory arthritis with a predilection for involvement of the axial skeleton and sacroiliac joints; (2) enthesopathy, defined as inflammation at sites of insertion of tendon, ligament, or fascia to bone; (3) asymmetric, peripheral oligoarthritis; (4) extraarticular features, most notably ophthalmologic, mucocutaneous, and urogenital involvement; (5) familial predisposition; (6) a strong association with the class I HLA-B27 antigen; and (7) seronegativity for rheumatoid factor.

This group of disorders includes ankylosing spondylitis, reactive arthritis/Reiter's syndrome, psoriatic arthritis, and the arthropathy of inflammatory bowel disease (IBD), as well as less common entities such as Whipple's disease, Behçet's syndrome, undifferentiated spondyloarthropathies, and uveitis associated with the HLA-B27 haplotype.

The pathogenesis of this group of diseases is unclear. A very strong association exists between the class I antigen HLA-B27 and the spondyloarthropathies. The prevalence of B27 in the white population is 8%, but nearly 90% of white patients with ankylosing spondylitis, Reiter's syndrome, reactive arthritis, or juvenile ankylosing spondylitis are HLA-B27 positive. The significance of this association, however, remains to be elucidated. Researchers have developed several hypotheses based on the HLA-B27 association and other clinical observations. The first theory is that the B27 antigen may be merely a marker, closely linked to the true causative gene. The second is that the HLA-B27 antigen has a structural homology with certain bacteria that results in cross-reacting antibodies. The third hypothesis, and probably the most likely, is that HLA-B27 binds arthritogenic bacterial peptides and elicits a cytotoxic T cell response; subsequently the cytotoxic T cell cross-reacts with structurally similar self-peptides in articular tissue, which are also presented by HLA-B27. Recently researchers reported the spontaneous development of colitis, arthritis, psoriasiform skin lesions, and genitourinary inflammation in B27 transgenic rats. These experiments support the direct role of HLA-B27 in the manifestation of disease.

The onset of arthritis after a urogenital or enteric infection by particular organisms *(Chlamydia, Salmonella, Shigella, Yersinia,* and *Campylobacter)* suggests that bacterial agents can initiate arthritis in a genetically susceptible host. Viable organisms, however, have not been cultured from the joint fluid or synovium. Instead, bacterial antigens have been detected in the synovial white blood cells or tissue. These findings lead some researchers to postulate that the persistence of such antigens may induce specific synovial immune responses, particularly a cell-mediated one.

The close association of the gastrointestinal tract with the spondyloarthropathies has been supported by the presence of asymptomatic, microscopic intestinal inflammation in patients with ankylosing spondylitis, reactive arthritis, and undifferentiated spondyloarthropathies. Ileocolonoscopies and random biopsies performed on patients with these diseases revealed that 65% of the patients had subclinical IBD. Researchers therefore postulate that chronic inflammation in the intestinal tract may increase mucosal permeability and facilitate entrance of exogenous antigens into the circulation. Subsequently, these antigens initiate joint inflammation through various immunologic mechanisms.

It is likely that genetics (particularly HLA-B27), bacterial infections, and increased intestinal mucosa permeability make variable contributions to the pathogenesis of the spondyloarthropathies. Other possible pathogenetic mechanisms are mentioned in the sections on specific spondyloarthropathies.

## ANKYLOSING SPONDYLITIS

Ankylosing spondylitis (AS) is often considered the prototype of the seronegative spondyloarthropathies. It is characterized by symmetric sacroiliitis and a progressive inflammatory arthritis of the axial skeleton.

It is a common, although often unrecognized, disease with an overall prevalence of approximately 0.2%. The disease usually begins in adolescence or young adulthood, with a threefold incidence in men compared with women. Men often experience more severe axial manifestations. It is a race-related disease, affecting whites and some Native Americans more frequently than African-Americans. Some 90% of patients with AS have the HLA-B27 antigen, although only approximately 2% of B27-positive individuals have a clinically detectable disease. Familial aggregation is quite pronounced. Roughly 10% to 20% of HLA-B27–positive first-degree relatives of HLA-B27–positive patients with AS have or will develop AS.

### Pathology

Ankylosing spondylitis is a chronic arthritis involving the sacroiliac (SI) joints and the axial skeleton and an enthesitis, which is inflammation at ligamentous insertions into bone. In 90% of cases the spine tends to be involved in an ascending manner, from the lumbar to the cervical region. Inflammation is followed by the formation of granulation tissue, calcification, and eventual ossification around the intervertebral disk margins, the apophyseal joint capsule insertion on bone, and the ligamentous insertions on the spine, such as the ligamentum flavum, interspinal and supraspinal ligaments, and the costovertebral joints.

Peripheral arthritis frequently affects the larger, weight-bearing joints, particularly the hips. Synovitis is pathologically similar to the abnormalities seen in rheumatoid arthritis, although it is usually less destructive. The enthesopathy includes Achilles and supraspinatus tendinitis, plantar fasciitis, and digital tenosynovitis.

Extraarticular manifestations often occur and are sometimes the only clue to disease onset. Acute anterior uveitis, the most frequent extraarticular lesion, is present in 25% of cases. It is usually unilateral, recurrent, and associated more frequently in HLA-B27–positive AS patients. Cardiac, pulmonary, renal, and neurologic involvement is decidedly less common. Aortic regurgitation and conduction abnormalities, such as complete heart block, are seen in fewer than 5% of cases. Restrictive lung disease, secondary to ossification of rib and sternal articulations limiting maximal chest expansion, is often detected on pulmonary function tests but often is not clinically important. Upper lobe pulmonary fibrosis and cavitation occur in less than 1% of patients. Cauda equina syndrome, atlantoaxial subluxation, spinal stenosis, and spinal fractures total fewer than 5% of all individuals with AS.

### Clinical manifestations

Patient symptoms provide the most important clues for suspecting diagnosis. The most common early complaint relates to SI and lower axial skeleton pathology and consists of chronic, insidious lower back pain and stiffness. The pain is dull and often localized in the gluteal or lower lumbar region as well as the proximal posterior thigh. The pain can also be difficult to localize. Mechanical stresses aggravate the pain.

Morning stiffness is an important feature. In contrast to lower back syndromes from mechanical causes, this stiffness tends to be exacerbated by inactivity and immobility and improved with exercise. Typically, it takes 30 to 60 minutes for the morning stiffness to subside, and patients often complain that the stiffness worsens after prolonged sitting. Sleep may be interrupted by discomfort and stiffness so that the patient needs to get out of bed to stretch and walk around.

Sometimes, nonaxial symptoms provide the first clue to diagnosis. A young man presenting with synovitis in a large lower extremity joint or tenosynovitis unrelated to overuse or another mechanical cause should prompt the physician to consider AS in the differential diagnosis. Other joints, including the temporomandibular joint, can be affected. The patient may describe a pleuritic-like chest pain that represents the enthesopathy at the costosternal and costovertebral joints.

Uveitis is the most important extraarticular manifestation that should raise the physician's index of suspicion. Approximately 25% of all patients with uveitis eventually develop a spondyloarthropathy. Uveitis has a distinct presentation. The onset is usually acute, starting with a 1- to 2-day prodrome of mild eye discomfort or headache, followed by rather severe eye pain and redness. The patient may also complain of photophobia, blurry or cloudy vision, and increased lacrimation. Episodes are usually unilateral, lasting several weeks to several months. Recurrences can occur in either eye.

Though usually not prominent, constitutional symptoms may develop, consisting of fatigue, weight loss, and a low-grade fever. A family history of a spondyloarthropathy or HLA-B27 positivity should be sought.

Physical findings reflect the predilection of this disease for the axial skeleton, including the SI joints, large peripheral joints, and the entheses. The apophyseal joints, which have the principal role in spinal flexion, are involved early in this disease. The Shober test (Fig. 83-1) can detect limitation in flexion of the lumbar spine. The ability to touch the floor with the fingers while the knees are extended is not a reliable examination technique because the hip joints can compensate for spinal immobility. Lateral flexion, extension, and rotation of the back also diminish. Their measurement is part of the initial evaluation and subsequent follow-up. Limitation of neck movement tends to occur somewhat later in the disease. The occiput-to-wall test helps detect the decrease in cervical extension (Fig. 83-2). Chest expansion, measured by the difference in chest circumference between full inspiration and end expiration, is often diminished in AS. Normal measurement is greater than 5 cm, but this measurement can be difficult to interpret because it is age and gender dependent.

Inflammation of the SI joints can be assessed in several ways (Fig. 83-3). Direct pressure over the joints with the thumbs may elicit tenderness, and various maneuvers that stress the SI joints may cause pain in that region.

Palpation of inflamed enthesis may elicit pain. Typical tender areas include the spinous processes, ischial tuberosities, greater trochanters, iliac crest, costovertebral and costochondral junctions, Achilles tendons, and plantar fascia attachments. Since the hips or shoulders are involved in one third of cases, range-of-motion measurements of these joints should be part of the physical examination.

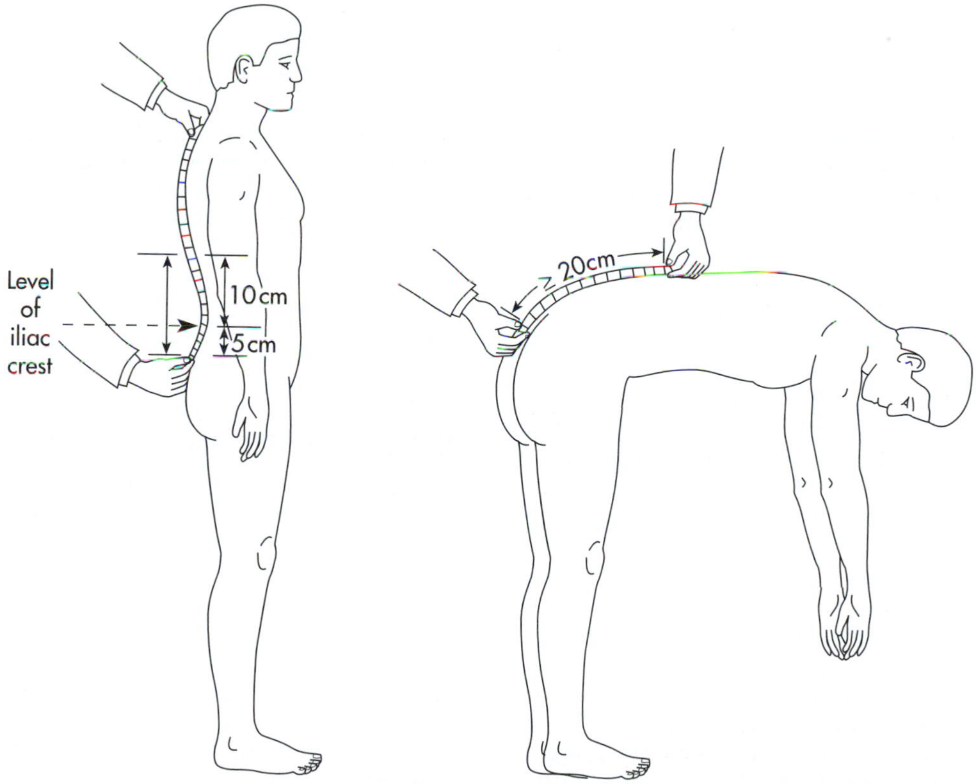


**Fig. 83-1.** The Shober test measures forward flexion of the lumbar spine and the degree of separation of the spinous processes. The midpoint between the posterior iliac crests is marked, and measurement is made 10 cm above and 5 cm below this mark with the patient in an upright position. Marks are then made at the upper and lower portions. In normal individuals performing forward flexion, this 15-cm distance should lengthen by at least 5 cm. In patients with AS, distraction of this distance is often reduced. (From Wise CM: In Turner RA, Wise CM, editors: *Textbook of rheumatology,* New York, 1986, Elsevier Science Publishing. Adapted from Moll JMH, Wright V: *Ann Rheum Dis* 30:381, 1971.)

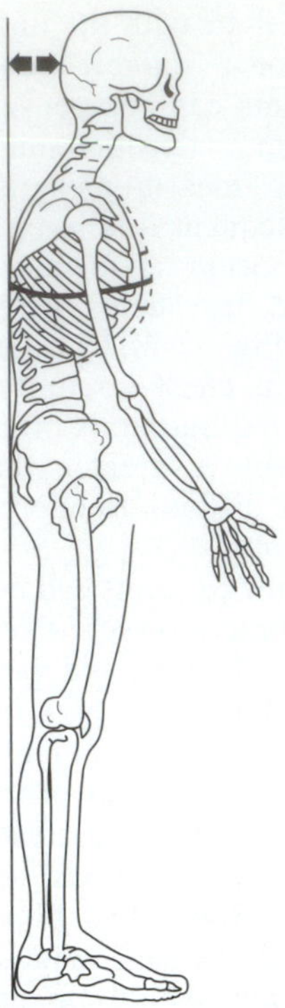

**Fig. 83-2.** The occiput-to-wall test helps detect a decrease in cervical extension.

Symptoms of uveitis are usually more helpful than the physical examination in differentiating it from conjunctivitis. During an acute attack, a circumcorneal flush is present. The pupil tends to be small, and there is no discharge. A slit-lamp examination is required to make the definitive diagnosis.

The other extraarticular manifestations are relatively uncommon and are usually seen after the disease is well established. The history and physical examination need to be directed toward these potential complications during routine follow-up. Auscultating for aortic insufficiency and remaining alert to symptoms that suggest conduction disturbances are part of this follow-up. Perhaps the most catastrophic complication of AS involves neurologic sequelae, which are, fortunately, rare. Minor trauma can fracture the spine; the cervical region is the most vulnerable. Spontaneous anterior atlantoaxial subluxation can present as occipital pain. Spinal cord compression and cauda equina syndrome, often unrecognized, may start with urinary and fecal incontinence. Similar to rheumatoid arthritis, general anesthesia can pose a degree of risk for neurologic injury when cervical spine disease is present. The primary care physician may need to assess cervical spine stability before surgery. Lateral x-ray studies of the neck in flexion and extension are useful to evaluate the range of motion of the neck as well as the infrequent occurrence of cervical subluxations. If cervical instability or marked limitation of range of motion is noted, the anesthesiologist should be informed. Nasotracheal intubation may be preferred over oral intubation in these circumstances because the former requires less neck movement.

### Radiographic findings

A routine anteroposterior x-ray study of the pelvis usually suffices in demonstrating symmetric sacroiliitis. Early in the illness, radiologic abnormalities may be only unilateral or sometimes are not apparent. SI joint views can sometimes better demonstrate these findings in mild cases. Computed tomography (CT) and magnetic resonance imaging (MRI) scans have the greatest sensitivities but are considerably more costly. Both plain SI joint views and CT scan views are associated with greater radiation exposure to the gonads than are routine pelvis x-ray studies.

X-ray studies of the spine and inflamed entheses can reveal bony erosions, osteitis, ossification, or syndesmophytes. Bony ankylosis is a characteristic, albeit late, finding. Osteoporosis of the spine, kyphosis, and symmetric joint space narrowing of the hips and shoulders may be present.

### Laboratory findings

There are no diagnostic laboratory tests. Nonspecific evidence of systemic inflammatory disease frequently includes an elevated erythrocyte sedimentation rate (ESR) and a normochromic normocytic anemia. The HLA-B27 is most useful as a diagnostic adjunct when the probability of disease is 50%. It is generally not indicated as a screening or routine diagnostic test because of the prevalence of this antigen in the general population as well as the prevalence of AS.

### Natural history

Expression of AS is highly variable. The course tends to progress slowly and intermittently. Severe, unrelenting AS resulting in complete ankylosis of the spine and hips is uncommon. It is more characteristic to see a milder, progressive disease punctuated with acute flares. Life expectancy is not reduced. Most patients maintain good functional capacity and continue to work. Frequently, the first 10 years of AS can serve as a rough barometer of disease severity over a patient's lifetime. If the hips and other peripheral joints are not involved within the first decade of disease, they are unlikely to become affected later.

## REITER'S SYNDROME/REACTIVE ARTHRITIS

Reiter's syndrome is probably the most common cause of asymmetric inflammatory arthritis of the lower extremities in young men. The term *Reiter's syndrome* is gradually being supplanted by *reactive arthritis.* This latter term encompasses a broader group of patients, in whom inflammatory arthritis develops after an infection, usually in the genitourinary or gastrointestinal tract. It is also common to distinguish reactive arthritides on the basis of antecedent infection sites by referring to them as *postvenereal* and *postenteric,* respectively. Khan has used the term *B27-associated reactive arthritis* to emphasize the heterogeneity of these diseases and to differentiate them from other postinfectious diseases, such as rheumatic fever. Reiter's syndrome is still used to describe postvenereal reactive arthritis.

### Epidemiology

Approximately 1% of patients develop reactive arthritis after nongonococcal urethritis. *Chlamydia trachomatis* is

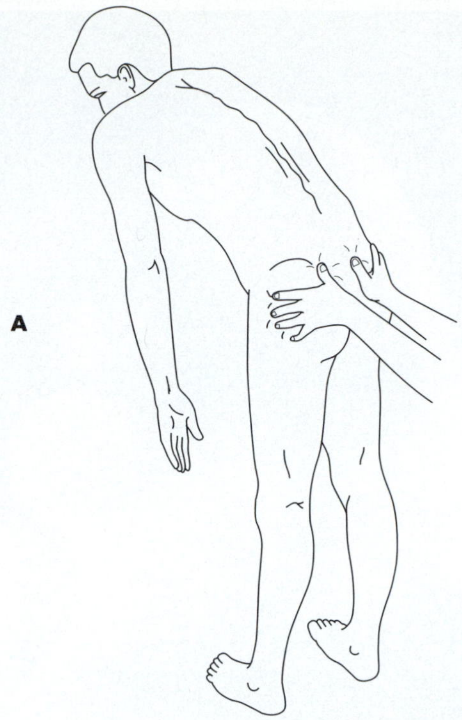


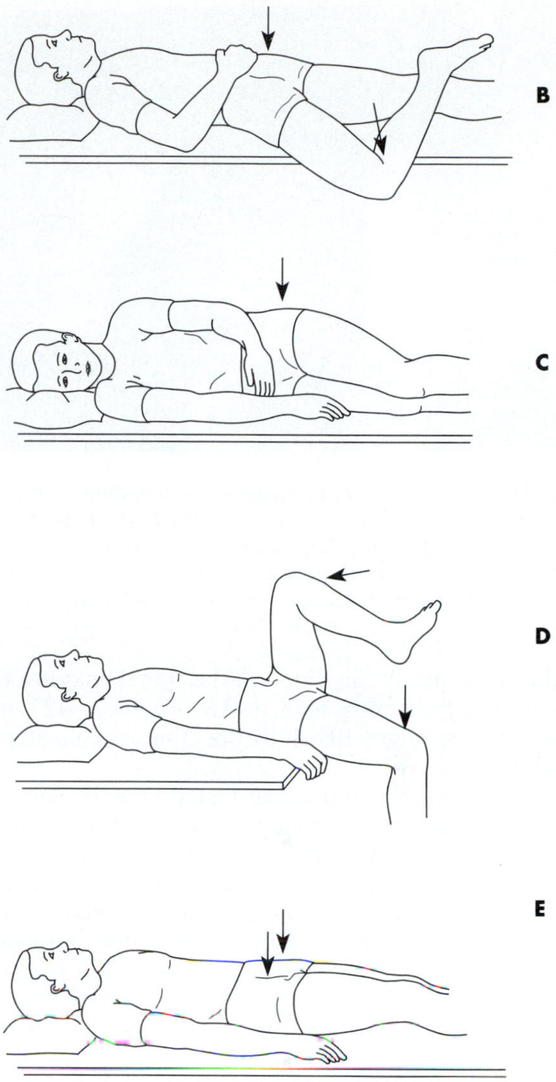


**Fig. 83-3.** Clinical tests for sacroiliitis: **A,** Application of direct pressure by thumbs over the sacroiliac joints to elicit tenderness. **B,** With knee flexed and hip flexed, abducted, and externally rotated, downward pressure applied on the flexed knee and the contralateral anterosuperior iliac spine. **C,** Compression of the pelvis with patient lying on the side. **D,** Patient lying supine, with flexed knee pushed maximally toward the opposite shoulder. **E,** Anterosuperior iliac spines forced laterally apart. (Adapted from Khan MA. In Calin A, editor: *Spondyloarthropathies,* Orlando, 1984, Grune & Stratton.)

the primary urogenital pathogen associated with Reiter's syndrome. After an enteric infection with one of the *Salmonella* species, *Shigella flexneri,* or *Campylobacter jejuni,* 2% to 3% of patients develop reactive arthritis. Another bowel pathogen, *Yersinia,* has been associated with a much higher occurrence of reactive arthritis in other countries, but it is rare in the United States.

As in AS, there is a strong association with the HLA-B27 antigen in reactive arthritis. Approximately 60% to 80% of patients with reactive arthritis have HLA-B27 antigen, and approximately 20% of these patients develop reactive arthritis after exposure to the appropriate stimulus. The postenteric form displays equal gender distribution, whereas the postvenereal type has a male predominance.

## Clinical manifestations

Reiter's syndrome/reactive arthritis is a multisystem disorder, often unrecognized, and difficult to diagnose. The classic Reiter's syndrome triad of arthritis, urethritis, and conjunctivitis is frequently not present or is not identified.

The arthritis typically develops 1 to 3 weeks after the urogenital or gastrointestinal infection. Urethritis symptoms may be quite subtle and, in women are often absent. Constitutional symptoms of fever and weight loss may be present, particularly during the early acute phase, but are usually mild.

The hallmark of reactive arthritis is the development of a sterile synovitis and enthesitis similar to that seen in AS. There is a predilection for the joints of the lower extremities, especially the knees, ankles, and feet. The upper extremities may also be affected. Early in the illness, the patient complains of joint stiffness, myalgias, and low back pain. Initial physical findings may be quite scant. The enthesitis commonly involves the Achilles, peroneal, and posterior tibial tendons, and the plantar fascia, causing ankle, foot, and heel pain. The combination of tenosynovitis, periostitis, and arthritis affecting the fingers or toes may give rise to a characteristic diffuse swelling known as *sausage digits* (Fig. 83-4). The physician should strongly consider a spondyloarthropathy in the differential diagnosis if a patient presents with sausage digits, especially reactive arthritis if the toes are involved and psoriatic arthritis when the fingers are affected.

Sacroiliitis and axial involvement occur less often in reactive arthritis than in AS. Back and buttock discomfort are common manifestations. Sacroiliitis is frequently unilateral and often is not identified by conventional

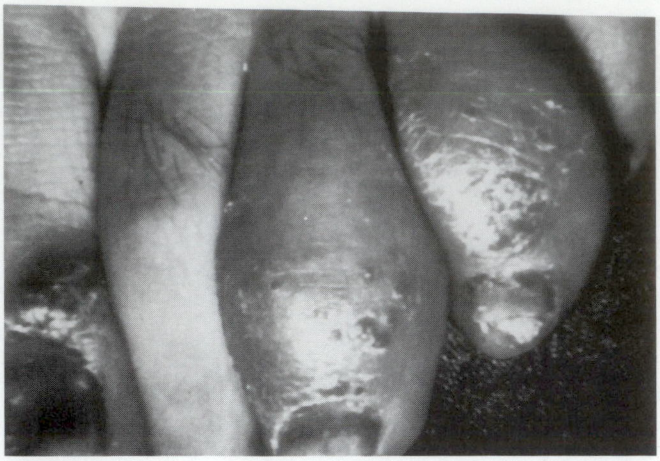

**Fig. 83-4.** Sausage toes or dactylitis in a patient with psoriasis. The sausage swelling is a combination of tenosynovitis, periostitis, and arthritis. It can also occur in patients with reactive arthritis. (From American College of Rheumatology: *Clinical slide collection on the rheumatic diseases,* slide 4-46, 1991, The College.)

radiology early in the illness. True spinal ankylosis occurs much less frequently than in AS. An HLA-B27–positive individual is more likely to develop inflammatory back symptoms.

Urethritis is the initial manifestation in the postvenereal form and can be a secondary feature in the postenteric form. Dysuria and urinary frequency are the usual complaints of men. The urethral meatus can be erythematous and edematous. Prostatitis is commonly seen. In women urethritis and cervicitis are often unrecognized.

Approximately 20% of patients with the postvenereal form of reactive arthritis develop the classic skin lesion, keratoderma blennorrhagicum (Fig. 83-5). It has an appearance strikingly similar to pustular psoriasis and typically affects the soles of the feet but can also involve the genitalia, scalp, and trunk. Nails may show onycholysis and thickening. Circinate balanitis produces small, usually painless superficial erosions on the glans penis (Fig. 83-6). The oral mucosa is also frequently affected by painless, superficial ulcerations.

Conjunctivitis, which can be mild and asymptomatic, occurs commonly. Acute anterior uveitis, another ocular manifestation, is strongly associated with the presence of the HLA-B27 antigen. Cardiac, pulmonary, renal, and neurologic complications may occur, and they are similar in type and frequency to those encountered in AS.

## Laboratory evaluation

Like in AS, no definitive tests establish a diagnosis of reactive arthritis. There is evidence, however, that the natural history of postchlamydial reactive arthritis can be improved with aggressive treatment to eradicate the organism. This suggests that diligent efforts should be undertaken to identify *Chlamydia* organisms and treat them accordingly. This intracellular microbe is difficult to culture. Proper collection and transport are imperative. It is necessary to obtain cellular material from an affected mucous membrane. This is best done through the use of a swab or cytobrush. Culture of discharge material is not

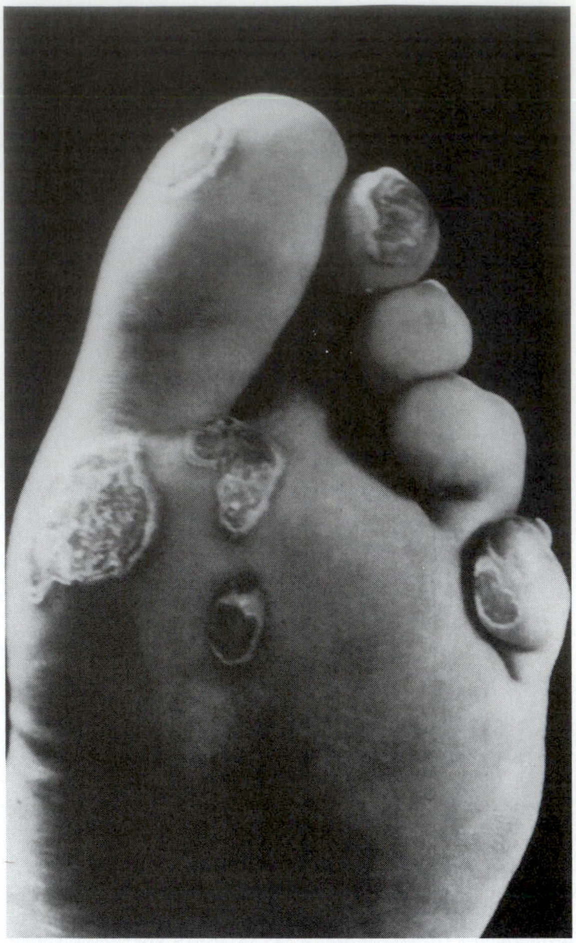

**Fig. 83-5.** Keratoderma blennorrhagica on the sole of a patient with Reiter syndrome. The lesions are discrete, papular, or plaquelike. They may resemble psoriatic plaques. (From American College of Rheumatology: *Clinical slide collection on the rheumatic diseases,* slide 4-68, 1991, The College.)

satisfactory. Serologic methods can also be used but often there is a considerable delay in obtaining results. It is still not clear whether aggressive treatment of the responsible bowel pathogens have the same beneficial effect on the natural history of the postenteric form.

The synovial fluid from an inflamed joint is usually inflammatory but is otherwise nondiagnostic. Analysis of the fluid is important to exclude infection and crystal disease. The ESR is often elevated. Leukocytosis and normochromic normocytic anemia may occur.

HLA-B27 determination may help diagnostically in difficult cases, particularly in the evaluation of an uncharacterized chronic monoarticular or pauciarticular arthritis without other distinguishing features. This antigen can also provide prognostic information about the development of acute anterior uveitis and axial disease. The role of HIV testing is discussed later.

## Radiographic findings

The enthesopathic features of this disease may cause periostitis, erosions, and reactive new bone formation. Periosteal spurs occur most frequently in the feet and heels. Axial disease, including sacroiliitis, may be seen,

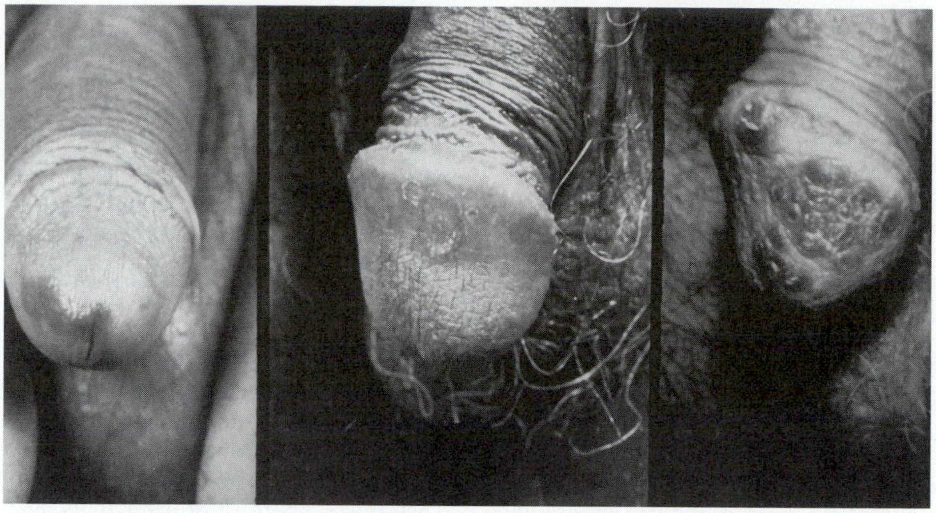

**Fig. 83-6.** Circinate balanitis in Reiter's syndrome. The lesion is painless, regardless of the stage. On the left, the earliest lesion is erythematous and moist. Other lesions may be pustular or vesicular initially and then progress to discrete circumscribed lesions. The late changes are dry, scaly, hyperkeratotic as demonstrated on the right. (From American College of Rheumatology: *Clinical slide collection on the rheumatic diseases,* slide 4-615, 1991, The College.)

although it is often not radiographically evident early in the disease.

### Course and prognosis

Reactive arthritis is marked by bouts of exacerbations and remissions. Severity varies considerably among individuals. The postvenereal form has a greater propensity for chronicity of arthritic manifestations than the postenteric form. This difference may be related to degrees of arthritogenicity of the various organisms, to the difficulties involved with completely eradicating *Chlamydia* organisms from the genitourinary tract, or to the greater likelihood of repeated episodes and recurrent antigen exposure in the postvenereal type.

The prognosis of postvenereal reactive arthritis is difficult to predict. This disease was once considered typically self-limiting. However, it has become increasingly apparent that many patients do not follow this path. Many patients experience recurrent arthropathy. These acute flares may be associated with significant functional impairment. A significant minority develop persistent joint symptoms as well as chronic axial involvement similar to AS.

## REITER'S SYNDROME/REACTIVE ARTHRITIS AND HUMAN IMMUNODEFICIENCY VIRUS DISEASE

Human immunodeficiency virus (HIV) infection has been associated with a broad spectrum of cutaneous and musculoskeletal disorders (see Chapter 68), including arthritis and enthesopathies. Controversy still exists about the significance of these rheumatic associations, however. Reiter's syndrome was the first rheumatic disease to be linked with HIV infection. It can develop before, simultaneously, or after signs of immunodeficiency. That Reiter's syndrome may antedate signs of HIV infection by up to one to two years has important implications for the treatment of Reiter's syndrome with immunosuppressive agents; these agents may inadvertently accelerate the development of frank acquired immune deficiency syndrome (AIDS).

Reiter's syndrome associated with HIV disease is likely to be more severe, with pronounced constitutional symptoms and more aggressive arthritis and enthesitis. Involvement of the foot and ankle is common and often debilitating, altering the gait and interfering with ambulation, leading to the sobriquet AIDS foot. Enthesopathy also affects the upper extremities. Hip and axial skeleton involvement is uncommon. Severe muscle atrophy may be prominent. Standard therapy with nonsteroidal antiinflammatory drugs (NSAIDs) is often inadequate.

The importance of HIV's association with reactive arthritis is twofold. First, it is necessary for the physician to consider early HIV infection in a patient presenting with Reiter's syndrome, psoriatic arthritis, or other unexplained monoarticular or pauciarticular arthritis. The physician must inquire about HIV risk factors. Second, it is essential that HIV infection be excluded before administering immunosuppressive therapy for refractory disease. Because of the frequent severity of musculoskeletal and cutaneous manifestations in these patients, as well as the difficult treatment issues, it is often desirable to seek consultation with a rheumatologist, dermatologist, and infectious disease expert to help with management.

## PSORIATIC ARTHRITIS

Psoriasis affects 1% to 2% of the North American white population but is less prevalent in the African-American and Native American populations. Since psoriasis is a common disease, it is possible that coexisting inflammatory or noninflammatory arthritis develops in psoriatic patients and may not be directly related to psoriasis. Thus the true incidence of psoriatic arthritis (PsA) in patients with psoriasis is unknown, and various estimates have ranged widely, from 6% to 42%. In addition, a small percentage of patients (approximately 15%) develop arthritis that may precede the onset of skin disease. Several studies have weighed these variables. The most recent estimate of PsA frequency in patients with psoriasis is 20% to 34%. Men and women are equally affected, but in the subsets of PsA, male predominance occurs in the spondylitic form, whereas female predominance occurs in the rheumatoid arthritis–like form. Onset occurs usually in the second or third decade of life, but can be as late as the sixth decade. Earlier onset, however, is associated with a poorer prognosis.

### Etiology and pathogenesis

The etiology of psoriasis and PsA is unknown. As in the case of many rheumatic diseases, the causes are likely to be multifactorial. Genetic predisposition is suggested by studies that document familial aggregates, concordance in monozygotic twins compared with dizygotic twins, and variable disease expression in different races. HLA-B13, HLA-B17, HLA-B38, HLA-B39, and HLA-Cw6 antigens are more common in patients with psoriasis alone and in those with PsA. In the subset of psoriatic patients who develop spondylitis or sacroiliitis HLA-B27 is present in 50%.

Humoral and cellular abnormalities contribute to immune mechanisms. The presence of immunoglobulins in the skin and synovial tissue, detection of autoantibodies in the sera, and evidence of complement activation support a humoral pathogenesis. Cellular mechanisms include abnormal suppressor or helper T cell function. This latter mechanism is indirectly implicated by the improvement in skin and joints when psoriatic patients receive cyclosporin or by the onset of severe psoriasis as the initial manifestation of HIV infections. Cytokines such as IL-1, IL-6, IL-8, leukotriene B4, or various growth factors may also contribute to the pathogenesis of PsA.

Trauma and other environmental factors may exacerbate joint disease with the development of acroosteolysis. Infections, whether related to streptococci found in the skin or to HIV, may also have some role in the pathogenesis of PsA.

### Clinical manifestations

Skin disease precedes the onset of articular manifestation in 75% of patients with PsA. Concomitant presentation of skin and joint disease occurs in 10% to 15%. The remaining patients develop skin disease after the onset of inflammatory arthritis.

Five major forms of PsA have been described (see the box above). The most common form is an asymmetric, oligoarticular arthritis, which affects 60% to 70% of PsA patients. Oligoarticular arthritis is arthritis affecting fewer than five joints. Large and small joints may be affected. A single joint (metacarpal phalangeal [MCP], proximal interphalangeal [PIP], and distal interphalangeal [DIP]) may be involved. Dactylitis, or sausage digits, is another common feature (see Fig. 83-4). Although the majority of patients are initially categorized into this group, many progress to develop asymmetric polyarthritis.

Symmetric polyarthritis, which is clinically indistinguishable from rheumatoid arthritis, is the second most common form. It affects 15% to 25% of PsA patients. Patients are rheumatoid factor negative and have no rheumatoid nodules. DIP joint involvement, not typically described in rheumatoid arthritis, occurs in this form of PsA. In addition, radiographic evidence of PIP or DIP ankylosis helps to differentiate between the two diseases.

#### Patterns of psoriatic arthritis

- Asymmetric, oligoarticular arthritis (60% to 70%)
- Symmetric polyarticular arthritis (15% to 25%)
- Pure DIP disease (5%)
- Arthritis mutilans (5%)
- Isolated sacroilitiis and spondylitis (5%)

Isolated DIP involvement occurs in only 5% of PsA patients. This form of arthritis is associated with nail bed changes, including multiple nail pits and onycholysis (Fig. 83-7).

Arthritis mutilans, a progressively destructive form of arthritis, also occurs in a small minority of patients (5%). Starting as DIP joint disease, the arthritis progresses with osteolysis of the phalanges, resulting in telescoping of digits or pencil-in-cup deformities on radiographs. Many of these patients also have sacroiliitis and severe skin involvement.

The fifth form of PsA is isolated spondylitis or sacroiliitis. Again, this is rare, affecting only 5% of PsA patients. Inflammatory back symptoms include prolonged morning stiffness that improves with activity and pain that persists for more than 3 months. Psoriatic spondylitis may be difficult to distinguish from AS except for the presence of psoriasis. Sacroiliitis is more often radiographically asymmetric than is AS. In addition, the syndesmophytes are usually nonmarginal and asymmetric, in contrast to the marginal, symmetric pattern of AS.

As with all classification schemes, some patients cannot be categorized easily into one of the five subsets. Others may evolve from one pattern to another or may overlap between subsets. Often, axial involvement is silent. Some 20% to 40% of PA patients have sacroiliitis on plain x-ray film, but nearly two thirds of these patients are asymptomatic. Enthesitis also occurs in PsA, contributing to the sausage deformities, plantar fasciitis, heel spurs, and syndesmophyte formation in the axial spine.

### Extraarticular features

Skin involvement is the predominant extraarticular feature of PsA. Since the majority of patients have skin diseases that antedate or parallel the onset of their arthritis, the diagnosis is not difficult. However, patients who present with only asymmetric arthritis, tenosynovitis, or inflammatory back pain require a careful search for occult skin lesions that should include examining the scalp, umbilicus, intergluteal fold, groin, external acoustic meatus, and perineum. Extensive nail pitting (greater than 20 pits per nail) and subungual hyperkeratosis are present in 80% of PsA patients, similar nail changes are found in only 20% to 30% of patients with isolated skin disease.

Aortic insufficiency and apical pulmonary fibrosis are rare complications and are associated only with patients who have spondylitis. Inflammatory eye disease occurs in

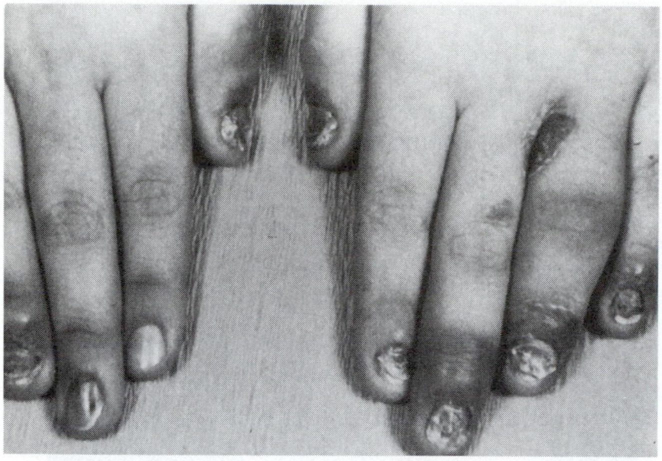

**Fig. 83-7.** PsA with nail, skin, and joint involvement. DIP joint involvement in both hands are characterized by swelling and erythema. There is prominent soft tissue swelling or sausage-like changes at the fourth PIP joint. Nail changes include fragmentation and lifting of the nail away from the base resulting from hyperkeratosis. (From American College of Rheumatology: *Clinical slide collection on the rheumatic diseases,* slide 4-65, 1991, The Colleges.)

### Radiographic features common to psoriatic arthritis and reactive arthritis

- Erosions without periarticular osteopenia
- Distal phalangeal tuft resorption
- Soft tissue swelling
- Pencil-in-cup deformities
- Periostitis

approximately 30% but usually consists of conjunctivitis rather than nongranulomatous uveitis.

### Laboratory and radiographic features

No specific laboratory studies can confirm the diagnosis of PsA. Nonspecific indicators of inflammation include an elevated ESR and C-reactive protein, anemia, and leukocytosis. Rheumatoid factor or positive antinuclear antibodies (ANA) are present in a small percentage of patients, but these findings are likely to reflect the baseline positive rate in the general population.

Radiographic features help distinguish PsA from some of the other inflammatory arthritides (see the box above). In the peripheral joints the asymmetric pattern of joint involvement, along with DIP disease, are important clues. Periarticular osteopenia, a classic finding in RA, is absent in PsA despite erosive changes. Tuft resorption, bony ankylosis, and periostitis are other common features of PsA that are uncommon in RA.

Axial involvement in PsA is similar to that of reactive arthritis and can usually be distinguished from AS (Table 83-1). Asymmetric, nonmarginal syndesmophytes in the thoracolumbar region, paravertebral ossification, vertebral fusion, and disk space calcification are features of psoriatic spondylitis.

**Table 83-1.** Radiographic features of the spondyloarthropathies

| | Ankylosing spondylitis/IBD | Reactive arthritis/PsA |
|---|---|---|
| Sacroiliitis | Bilateral | Unilateral |
| Syndesmophytes | Marginal | Nonmarginal |
| | Symmetric | Asymmetric |
| | Continuous | Skip levels |
| Vertebral bodies | Squaring | Less squaring |
| Apophyseal fusion | Common | Less common |

## IBD

The first associations between bowel disease and arthritis were described in the early 1900s. Despite these descriptions, however, the distinct entity of inflammatory arthritis occurring in patients with IBD was not accepted in the medical community until after 1960. Today, musculoskeletal involvement is the most common extraarticular manifestation of IBD.

Two distinct patterns of arthropathy are associated with IBD. A peripheral, oligoarticular arthritis may occur in patients with Crohn's disease or ulcerative colitis. Other patients may develop axial skeletal involvement. This latter pattern can be further divided into two subsets: asymptomatic sacroiliitis and symptomatic axial disease clinically indistinguishable from idiopathic AS.

The incidence of peripheral arthropathy in IBD patients is between 15% and 20%, with a more frequent occurrence in Crohn's disease than in ulcerative colitis patients. In addition, peripheral arthritis is more frequently associated with colonic than with ileal involvement in Crohn's disease. The incidence of asymptomatic sacroiliitis may be as high as 29%, but frank AS occurs in only 2% to 8% of IBD patients.

The genetics of the various clinical subsets also differ. No HLA-B27 association has been established in patients with peripheral arthritis or asymptomatic sacroiliitis. In contrast, 50% to 75% of IBD patients with symptomatic spondylitis are HLA-B27 positive.

### Etiology and pathogenesis

The etiology of IBD arthropathy is unknown. Given the genetic and clinical differences among the various subsets, researchers believe that a different pathogenesis may exist for each group. Since there is an association with HLA-B27 in patients with spondylitis, the pathogenesis in this group may be similar to theories previously outlined for idiopathic AS. As for the peripheral arthritis subset, since clinical disease is parallel to the activity of bowel disease, mechanisms directly related to gut inflammation may be more applicable.

### Clinical manifestations

***Peripheral arthritis.*** Peripheral joint involvement classically begins with or after the onset of bowel disease. Subsequent flares also parallel disease activity in the bowel. Men and women are equally affected. Joint involvement is typically oligoarticular, is often migratory, and lasts for weeks to months but rarely becomes chronic.

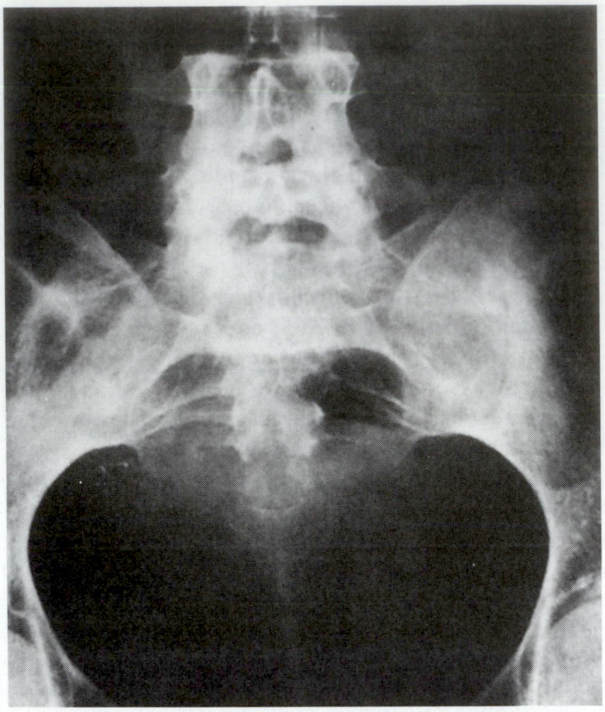

**Fig. 83-8.** Ankylosing spondylitis. Note the total ankylosis of right sacroiliac joint and moderate change in left joint. Juxtaarticular sclerosis, joint space narrowing, and irregularity are seen, with partial fusion. (From Stein JH: *Internal medicine,* St. Louis, 1994, Mosby.)

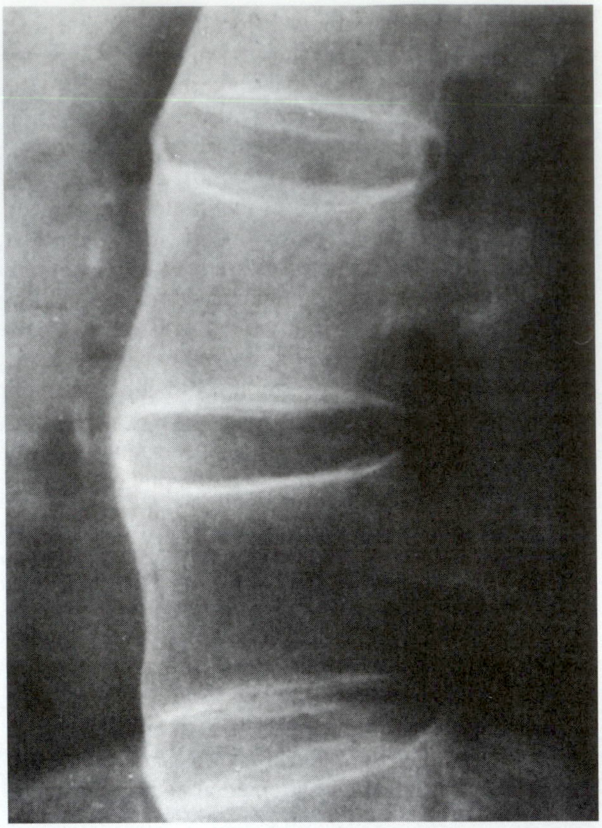

**Fig. 83-9.** Same patient as shown in Fig. 83-8. Note ossification in the anterior fibers of anulus fibrosus between the lumbar vertebrae. (From Stein JH: *Internal medicine,* St. Louis, 1994, Mosby.)

The most commonly affected joint is the knee, followed by the ankle, elbow, and wrist. Smaller joints are less commonly affected. Enthesopathy, such as tendinitis, may develop. Often, other extraarticular features of IBD, including the skin, mucous membranes, and eyes, are concurrently active. Progressive deformities rarely develop. In the few cases of erosive arthropathy, granulomatous synovitis may be responsible.

***Axial arthropathy.*** In contrast to peripheral arthropathy, axial skeletal disease does not correlate with the activity of IBD. Spondylitis often precedes the development of active bowel disease by many years, thus making the diagnosis difficult. Unfortunately, even when IBD is under control or in remission, axial disease may persist or progress. Men are slightly more affected than are women, but not to the degree that occurs in idiopathic AS. Classically, the symptoms of inflammatory back pain develop insidiously. Hip and shoulder involvement also occurs. Extraarticular features include iritis.

### Laboratory and radiographic features

Laboratory tests are, again, nonspecific. Rheumatoid factor is usually negative and the ESR and other indicators of inflammation are elevated. Chronic anemia may exist. Synovial fluid is mildly inflammatory, with white blood cell counts (WBCs) of 5000 to 15,000/mm$^3$.

Radiographs of peripheral joints usually reveal only soft tissue swelling without erosive changes. The axial findings may include shoulder and hip joint space narrowing, vertebral body squaring, symmetric sacroiliitis, osteitis pubis, marginal syndesmophytes, and progressive bony bridging cephalad, beginning in the lumbar region. All of these features are indistinguishable from idiopathic AS (Figs. 83-8 and 83-9 and Table 83-1).

### Treatment

The management of peripheral arthropathy is aimed at treating the underlying bowel disease. Thus although the use of sulfasalazine and oral corticosteroids seems to control the joint disease, this is probably related more to the control of the bowel disease. If a total colectomy is necessary for ulcerative colitis, the peripheral arthritis completely disappears. However, joint disease may not resolve after total colectomy in Crohn's disease, perhaps because of residual or occult disease in the small intestine. NSAIDs and intraarticular corticosteroids are also useful adjuncts. Since the axial arthropathy does not correlate with bowel disease activity, management is very similar to that of idiopathic AS (see the following section).

## UNDIFFERENTIATED SPONDYLOARTHROPATHY

The current categories of spondyloarthropathies are often inadequate to encompass a spectrum of patients who may have oligoarthritis, enthesopathy, or inflammatory back symptoms without antecedent infection or dermatologic abnormalities. Thus the term *undifferentiated spondyloarthropathies* encompasses those patients with one or more of the features of spondyloarthropathy but who do not fulfill the criteria for established disease categories. Long-term follow-up of these patients reveals that 50% develop a defined spondyloarthropathy, 40% obtain remission, and only 10% continue with recurrent oligoarticular arthritis.

## DIFFERENTIAL DIAGNOSIS

When a patient presents with classic inflammatory back symptoms and extraarticular features, the primary care physician can easily establish the diagnosis. However, if the disease presents insidiously and the various symptoms and signs span many years, the diagnosis is less obvious and may elude the physician.

The differential diagnosis of spondyloarthropathies can be separated into three categories: back pain, peripheral arthritis, and peripheral arthritis with back pain (see the box at right). Low back pain is extremely common and has a broad differential that is discussed in Chapter 73. Some of the unique features of inflammatory low back pain have been previously described.

SI joints can be affected by osteoarthritis, infection (particularly in intravenous drug users), hyperparathyroidism, paraplegia and quadriplegia, and osteitis condensans ilii (seen mostly in multiparous women). These can usually be distinguished clinically and radiologically. Diffuse idiopathic skeletal hyperostosis (DISH) may be initially confused with AS, but the former is a condition of older individuals and both disorders have characteristic radiographic features that differentiate them.

Peripheral arthritis may be the initial or only manifestation of a spondyloarthropathy. The arthritis is classically monoarticular or oligoarticular but is sometimes polyarticular. Early rheumatoid arthritis, acute crystal disease such as gout and pseudogout, acute or chronic infections (particularly Lyme disease arthritis), osteoarthritis, sarcoidosis and synovial neoplasia are within the differential diagnosis. Synovial fluid analysis, including crystal search and cultures, is crucial. Serologies may be helpful in the evaluation. Occasionally synovial biopsy is necessary to exclude tuberculous arthritis.

Disseminated gonorrheal infection (DGI) can closely resemble reactive arthritis in its articular and nonarticular features. The epidemiology of the two diseases is similar, occurring in the sexually active population. However, the rash of DGI is usually vesiculopustular and can be easily distinguished from keratoderma blennorrhagicum. Appropriate sites (i.e., blood, joint, skin, vagina, urethra, throat, and rectum) should be cultured if DGI is suspected. It is also possible for the diseases to coexist in the same individual.

The symmetric pattern of PsA may be confused with rheumatoid arthritis. However, the lack of rheumatoid factor, rheumatoid nodules, swan neck and boutonnière deformities differentiates the two diseases. The involvement of DIP joints, absence of periarticular osteopenia, presence of bony ankylosis, periostitis, acroosteolysis, and bony resorption are typical for PsA or reactive arthritis but are unusual for rheumatoid arthritis. Osteoarthritis of the DIP or PIP joints, especially erosive osteoarthritis, may be confused with PsA or reactive arthritis. The presence of Bouchard nodes (osteoarthritic involvement of the PIP joints) and carpametacarpal joint disease are more consistent with osteoarthritis. Radiographically, osteophyte formation or the central erosions of erosive osteoarthritis help distinguish osteoarthritis from PsA and reactive arthritis.

The physician may not initially suspect enthesitis when a patient complains of pain or swelling in a tendon or ligamentous area. Tender areas are common in fibromyalgia. Mechanical overuse or calcific tendinitis resembles enthesopathy, particularly in the shoulder, Achilles tendon, and plantar fascia. Drugs, including retinoids or fluoride, may produce plantar fasciitis or ossification, respectively. Achilles tendinitis has been associated with fluoroquinolone therapy. However, recurrent or persistent tenosynovitis with inflammatory features or in atypical

### Differential diagnosis for spondyloarthropathies

- Axial arthritis
  - Discogenic back pain
  - Osteoarthritis
    - Facet disease
    - Diffuse idiopathic hypertrophic osteoarthropathy
    - Osteoarthritis of SI joints
  - Osteitis condensans ilii
  - Infection (sacroiliitis)
    - Tuberculosis, brucellosis*
    - Bacteremia from intravenous drug abuse
  - Others
    - Whipple's disease*
    - Behçet's syndrome*
    - Relapsing polychondritis
    - Secondary hyperparathyroidism
- Peripheral arthritis
  - Other inflammatory arthritides
    - Rheumatoid arthritis
    - Crystals
  - Infections
    - *Borrella burgdorferi* (Lyme disease)
    - Gonococcal
    - Poststreptococcal, acute rheumatic fever*
    - HIV
    - Chronic fungal or tuberculous
  - Noninflammatory arthritides
    - Osteoarthritis, particularly inflammatory osteoarthritis
    - Mechanical derangement
  - Synovial neoplasia
    - Pigmented villonodular synovitis*
    - Osteogenic sarcoma*
    - Synovial osteochondromatosis*
  - Others
    - Sarcoidosis
- Axial and peripheral arthritis
  - Osteoarthritis
  - Rheumatoid arthritis
  - Whipple's disease*
  - Behçet's syndrome*
  - Relapsing polychondritis*
  - Familial Mediterranean fever*

*Rare occurrences.

locations, such as the toes, fingers, or heels, should alert the physician to include spondyloarthropathies in the differential diagnosis.

Osteoarthritis and rheumatoid arthritis are common diagnoses for low back pain and peripheral joint disease. More unusual diseases that can involve both areas include Whipple's disease, Behçet's syndrome, relapsing polychondritis, and familial Mediterranean fever.

AIDS must be considered in the differential diagnosis of patients with reactive arthritis or PsA who also have risk factors for HIV infection. Fulminant psoriasis with or without arthritis and reactive arthritis have been reported as an initial presentation of HIV infections.

Finally, given the similarities among the spondyloarthropathies, each disease must be included in the differential diagnosis of the other. The separation of Reiter's syndrome from PsA can be extremely difficult. The skin lesions of keratoderma blennorrhagicum may be indistinguishable clinically and pathologically from psoriatic skin lesions. The patterns of joint involvement and radiographic findings are also similar. However, oral lesions, circinate balanitis, and urethritis are not features of PsA. Reports of an evolution of one spondyloarthropathy into another with time (e.g., the patient with urethritis and arthritis who later develops the skin disease of psoriasis) make the distinction between diseases less clear.

## TREATMENT

Treatment for spondyloarthropathies begins with educating patients, since many of these diseases are chronic, often affecting young people during their most active and productive years. Although the pathogenesis of the disease is unknown, patients' understanding of the disease course, the potential factors that may aggravate and improve their arthritis, and the prevention measures are of utmost importance. National associations, patient newsletters, and support groups can provide educational, social, and emotional support. The Spondylitis Association of America is a national organization that provides mutual support and promotes research and education. Their quarterly newsletters provide information extremely useful to patients and their physicians.

Control of the associated medical conditions may have a direct benefit for the various spondyloarthropathies. The peripheral arthritis of IBD parallels the activity of bowel disease. Some studies of psoriasis suggested a correlation between improvement of joint disease when the skin disease is aggressively treated (treatment of skin disease is discussed in Chapter 21). In patients with acute urethritis or infectious diarrhea, appropriate antibiotic therapy should be instituted, but it does not prevent the development of reactive arthritis. Recently patients with reactive arthritis caused by *Chlamydia* organisms received long-term therapy with lymecycline, an antibiotic similar to tetracycline but unavailable in the United States. Improvement in the patients' arthropathy occurred. However, it is not clear if this response is due to lymecycline's antibacterial actions or to some other mechanism.

### NSAIDs

NSAIDs are the mainstay of pharmacologic intervention in the spondyloarthropathies. More than 20 NSAIDs are available (Table 83-2) and differ in their half-lives, routes of excretion, and interaction with other drugs. The mechanism of action for all NSAIDs is based on the inhibition of prostaglandin synthesis as well as the inhibition of neutrophil function.

### Factors influencing NSAID choice

- Age
- Preexisting medical conditions
- Active or history of peptic ulcer disease
- Renal or hepatic insufficiency
- Congestive heart failure
- Asthma
- Bleeding diathesis or chronic anticoagulation
- Concurrent medications
- Ease of drug dosing
- Cost (limits of managed care formulary)

Various factors influence the choice of an NSAID in a particular patient (see the box above). NSAIDs are contraindicated for patients with active peptic ulcer disease or chronic anticoagulation (sometimes nonacetylated salicylates can be used if needed). Concurrent medical problems, such as history of peptic ulcer disease, congestive heart failure, renal insufficiency, hepatic insufficiency, or bleeding diathesis, make NSAIDs relatively contraindicated. The decision about the necessity of the NSAID must be weighed against the patient's other medical problems. Drug interactions occur between some NSAIDs and sulfonylureas, antihypertensives, and anticoagulants. Patients taking these medications require careful monitoring of their glucose level, blood pressure, and prothrombin time (PT). High-dose nonacetylated salicylates may increase the PT in patients on warfarin when starting an NSAID. Asthmatic patients or patients with a known allergy to aspirin can develop allergic reactions to NSAIDs. Patients' lifestyles may also be a consideration. A young, busy individual may not remember to take a drug that requires a dose three times a day, whereas another patient may find two or three times a day more effective. Drug cost is another major factor for many patients who must pay for their own prescriptions. The NSAIDs available generically (ibuprofen, sulindac, salicylate, piroxicam, tolmetin, meclofenamate, indomethacin, and naproxen) tend to be less expensive than the newer NSAIDs.

Although rheumatologists traditionally prefer indomethacin to aspirin for reactive arthritis, many other NSAIDs are equally effective. High dosages are typically necessary to control the inflammatory process (e.g., indomethacin at 150 to 200 mg per day or naproxen at 1500 mg per day). Specific toxicities of indomethacin include gastrointestinal distress and central nervous system effects. Indomethacin is also available as a rectal suppository.

Treatment with one NSAID should continue for at least 2 to 4 weeks before the drug is discontinued for a lack of efficacy. When one NSAID fails, another should be chosen from a different chemical class. Frequently, several different NSAIDs are prescribed before the most effective

**Table 83-2.** Nonsteroidal antiinflammatory drugs: physiologic properties, dosing, and toxicities

| Drug | Metabolism/ excretion | Half-life (hours) | Total daily dosage (mg) | Dosing frequency | GI* | Adverse effects: CNS | Adverse effects: Others |
|---|---|---|---|---|---|---|---|
| **Propionic acid** | | | | | | | |
| Fenoprofen | Liver | 2-3 | 1200-3200 | 3-4 | ++ | | Interstitial nephritis<br>Papillary necrosis |
| Flurbiprofen | Liver, kidney | 6 | 200-300 | 2-3 | | | |
| Ibuprofen | Liver, kidney (1% to 14%) | 2 | 1600-3200 | 3-4 | ++ | Confusion<br>Aseptic meningitis | Drug-induced lupus |
| Ketoprofen | Liver | 2-4 | 150-300 | 3-4 | ++ | | |
| Naproxen | Kidney | 13 | 500-1000 | 2-3 | ++ | Confusion | |
| Oxaprozin | Liver | 21 | 600-1800 | 1-2 | ++ | | |
| Ketorolac† | Kidney | 4-9 | 120 (IM) | 4-6 | ++ | Sedation, headaches, somnolence (IM and PO) | |
| | | | 40-60 (PO) | 4-6 | ++ | | |
| **Indoleacetic acid** | | | | | | | |
| Indomethacin | Liver | 2 | 75-200 | 3-4 | +++ | Headaches<br>Confusion | Thrombocytopenia |
| Sulindac | Enterohepatic circulation | 8 | 300-400 | 2 | +++ | Aseptic meningitis | |
| Tolmetin | Liver | 1-2 | 600-1600 | 3-4 | ++ | Aseptic meningitis | |
| Etodolac | Kidney, bile | 6-8 | 400-600 | 2 | ++ | | |
| **Phenylacetic acid** | | | | | | | |
| Diclofenac | Bile 35%, kidney 65% | 2 | 150-200 | 2-4 | | | |
| **Enolic acid** | | | | | | | |
| Piroxicam | Liver | 30-86 | 10-20 | 1 | +++ | | |
| **Pyrazole** | | | | | | | |
| Phenylbutazone | Liver, kidney | 40-80 | 300-400 | 3-4 | ++ | | Drug-induced lupus<br>Aplastic anemia<br>Thrombocytopenia<br>Hepatotoxicity |
| **Mefenamic acid** | | | | | | | |
| Meclofenamate | Liver | 2-3 | 300-400 | 3-4 | | | Diarrhea<br>Coombs-positive hemolytic anemia |
| **Salicylates** | | | | | | | |
| Aspirin | Liver | 4-15 | 1000-6000 | 2-4 | +++ | | Tinnitus, hepatitis, thrombocytopenia |
| Choline magnesium trisalicylate | Liver | 4-15 | 1500-4000 | 2-4 | + | | Tinnitus, hepatitis, thrombocytopenia |
| Salicylsalicylate | Liver | 4-15 | 1500-5000 | 2-4 | + | | Tinnitus, hepatitis, thrombocytopenia |
| Diflunisal | Liver | 7-15 | 500-1500 | 2 | +++ | | Tinnitus, hepatitis, thrombocytopenia |
| **Others** | | | | | | | |
| Nabumetone | Liver | 21 | 1000-2000 | 1 | ++ | | |

*+, Mild; ++, moderate; +++, severe and may require discontinuation of drug.
†Ketorolac is approved *only* for *short-term management* of *acute* pain. It has all the potential gastrointestinal, renal, and hematologic toxicities as other NSAIDs.
From Liu NY, Giansiracusa DF, Strongwater SL: Collagen vascular disease in the intensive care unit. In Rippe JM et al, editors: *Intensive care medicine,* Boston, 1995, Little, Brown.

one is established for an individual. Patients should be informed of this rationale, since they often perceive this method as haphazard.

Phenylbutazone is quite effective for intractable cases of spondyloarthropathies; however, because of its potentially fatal toxicities, it is rarely used by primary care physicians.

NSAIDs' toxicities are secondary to their antiprostaglandin effects; gastrointestinal intolerance is the most common. *NSAID gastropathy,* a term that includes superficial gastric erosions, diffuse gastritis, and frank ulcer craters, has greater morbidity. Some 2% to 5% of patients taking NSAIDs for more than a year may develop ulcers, bleeding, or perforation.

Advanced age, additional medical problems, and a history of peptic ulcer disease are risk factors for NSAID gastropathy. Misoprostol, a prostaglandin $E_1$ analogue, can reduce the incidence of gastric and duodenal mucosal damage from NSAIDs. Recently, NSAID-induced colitis has been reported.

Renal toxicities include renal insufficiency from decreased renal blood flow, interstitial nephritis, and hyperkalemia. Reversible impairment of platelet aggregation may result in prolonged bleeding. Central nervous system toxicities include headaches, dizziness, mental-status changes, and depression. Aseptic meningitis has been reported with ibuprofen, sulindac, naproxen, and tolmetin. Cutaneous reactions are varied. Certain NSAIDs have been reported to exacerbate psoriasis, particularly ibuprofen, indomethacin, and meclofenamate.

### Corticosteroids

Intraarticular corticosteroids may be judiciously used in the peripheral joints of patients with spondyloarthropathies (see Chapter 69). Occasionally, injection of the plantar fascia, tendon sheath, or deep bursae is helpful if rest, NSAIDs, and orthotics have been ineffective. Systemic steroids have been used for short-term control of severe AS; however, this therapy is not recommended for routine treatment.

### Second-line agent

When NSAIDs and physical measures are ineffective in controlling symptoms or if progressive erosive disease develops in the peripheral joints, a rheumatologic referral to assist with decisions for second-line agents and monitoring for potential toxicities should be considered. Unfortunately, effective therapy to prevent ankylosis in the axial arthropathy has not been established.

Sulfasalazine, a drug initially developed for rheumatoid arthritis and subsequently used for IBD, has been studied for treatment of patients with AS, reactive arthritis, and undifferentiated spondyloarthropathies. Results reveal some benefit to patients' spondylitis symptoms in the short term, but whether the drug modifies the long-term outcome of AS is unknown. However, sulfasalazine appears to be more effective in peripheral arthritis of AS or reactive arthritis. Its mechanism of actions may include reduction of intestinal mucosal inflammation and permeability or direct reduction of mediators of inflammation. Sulfasalazine has also been used in psoriasis and PsA on a limited basis. Sulfasalazine dosages range from 2 to 3 g daily. Enteric-coated tablets given with food may reduce gastrointestinal upset. Other toxicities include leukopenia, thrombocytopenia, and, rarely, hepatic dysfunction. Laboratory monitoring of CBC and liver function tests should be performed every 2 to 4 weeks initially, then every 2 to 3 months after a stable dosage has been established.

Methotrexate, a folate antagonist, has been used as an effective agent for PsA since the 1960s. Initially dermatologists used methotrexate for skin diseases, but beneficial effects on joints were coincidentally noted. Methotrexate is administered orally or intramuscularly on a weekly basis, beginning with dosages of 7.5 to 15 mg per week and titrated upward to 20 to 30 mg per week based on response. Mucositis, gastrointestinal intolerance, dizziness, and headaches are common toxicities. More severe toxicities include bone marrow suppression, acute pneumonitis, and hepatotoxicities that can result in fibrosis. Patients who abuse alcohol and those who have diabetes mellitus, obesity, or renal or hepatitic insufficiency are at greatest risk for developing hepatotoxicity. Laboratory monitoring initially includes baseline liver function tests (asparate aminotransferase [AST], alanine aminotransferase [ALT], alkaline phosphatase, bilirubin, and albumin), CBC with platelets, creatinine, and chest radiography. Monitoring of ALT, AST, albumin, and CBC with platelets should be performed every 4 to 6 weeks. Baseline liver biopsies are recommended for patients with a history of alcohol consumption, abnormal liver functions, and chronic hepatitis B or C infection. Dermatologists routinely request yearly liver biopsies on psoriatic patients who have received more than 1.5 g of methotrexate. No consensus has been reached about the necessity or frequency of liver biopsies in patients on methotrexate for various forms of arthritis. However, if persistent liver function abnormalities exist (e.g., if 6 of 12 AST are out of the normal range or if serum albumin falls below the normal range), then liver biopsies should be obtained. Methotrexate has also been used for intractable Reiter's syndrome. Before instituting methotrexate, HIV infection must be excluded. Reports exist documenting the onset of AIDS in patients after methotrexate was started for severe psoriasis or reactive arthritis. Trimethoprim is contraindicated for patients who take methotrexate because of its additive antifolate effects.

Parenteral gold is also effective in the treatment of PsA. Although most studies have not been prospectively controlled, 60% to 75% of the patients improved on parenteral gold therapy. When compared to a rheumatoid population, drug intolerance was less in PsA. Patients with peripheral arthritis responded best. Gold had no effect on the spondylitic patients. It also had no beneficial effects on the skin, although it did not exacerbate underlying skin disease. Toxicities of gold include allergic dermatitis, mucositis, diarrhea, bone marrow suppression, proteinuria, and pneumonitis. Weekly CBC, platelet count, and urinalysis are required while patients receive weekly injections and can be extended to every month when injections are monthly.

Hydroxychloroquine, a drug often used to treat rheumatoid arthritis and systemic lupus erythematosus (SLE), has been prescribed for PsA and Reiter's syndrome. Exacerbation of psoriasis was reported anecdotally, in the old literature with hydroxychloroquine use. In recent studies, skin reaction has not been a significant problem,

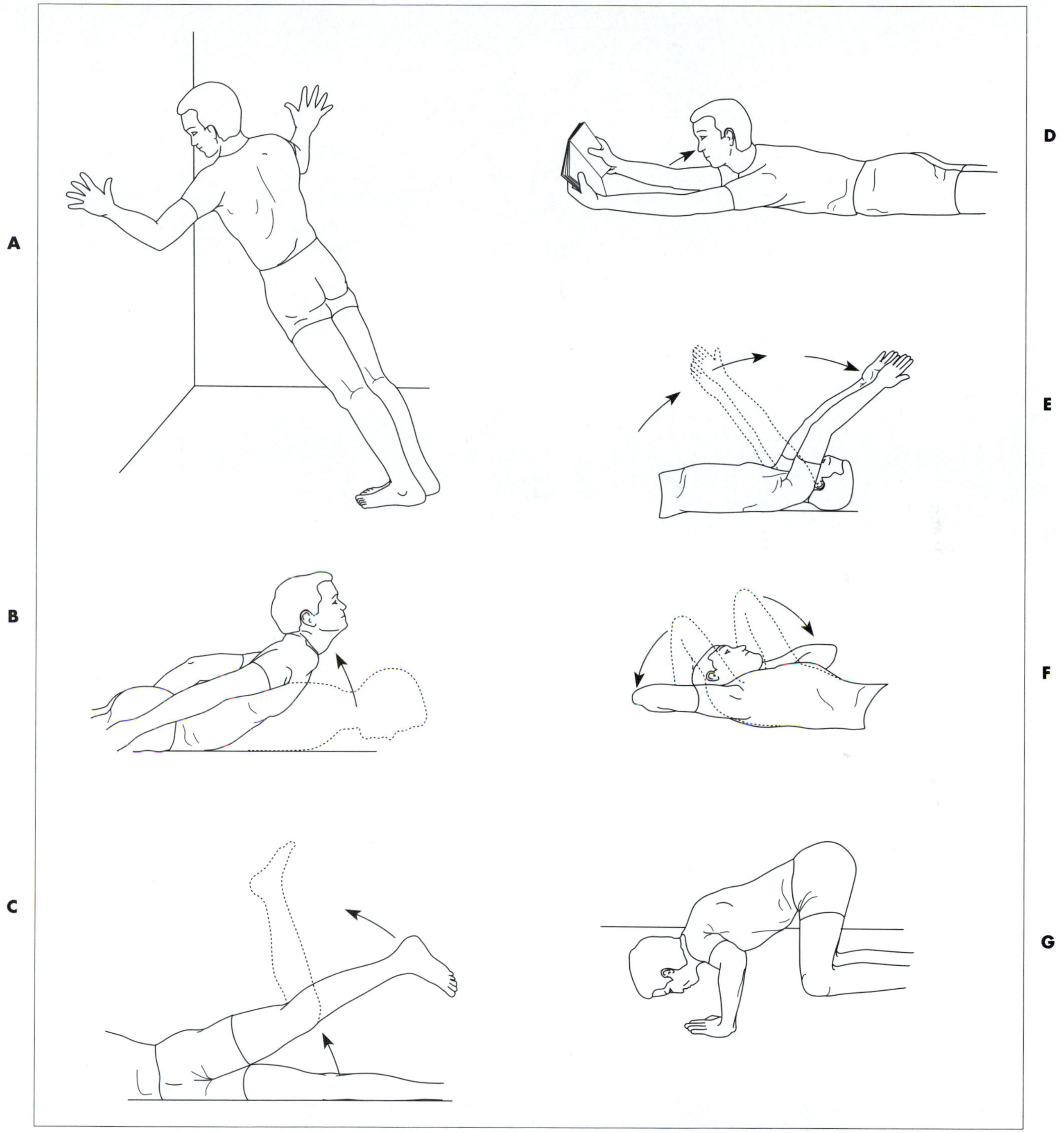


**Fig. 83-10.** Regular exercises for patients with AS. Most of these exercises do not require further explanation, except the "corner push-up" exercise **(A).** It is performed with the patient standing 2 feet or more from the corner; both hands are placed on the wall about 2 feet from the corner, and the patient then gently leans forward toward the corner, keeping the heels on the ground. The patient is asked to inhale (expand the chest) and try to straighten the spine when leaning toward the corner and exhale when returning to the starting position. (Adapted from Khan MA. In Calin A, editor: *Spondyloarthropathies,* Orlando, 1984, Grune & Stratton.) *Continued.*

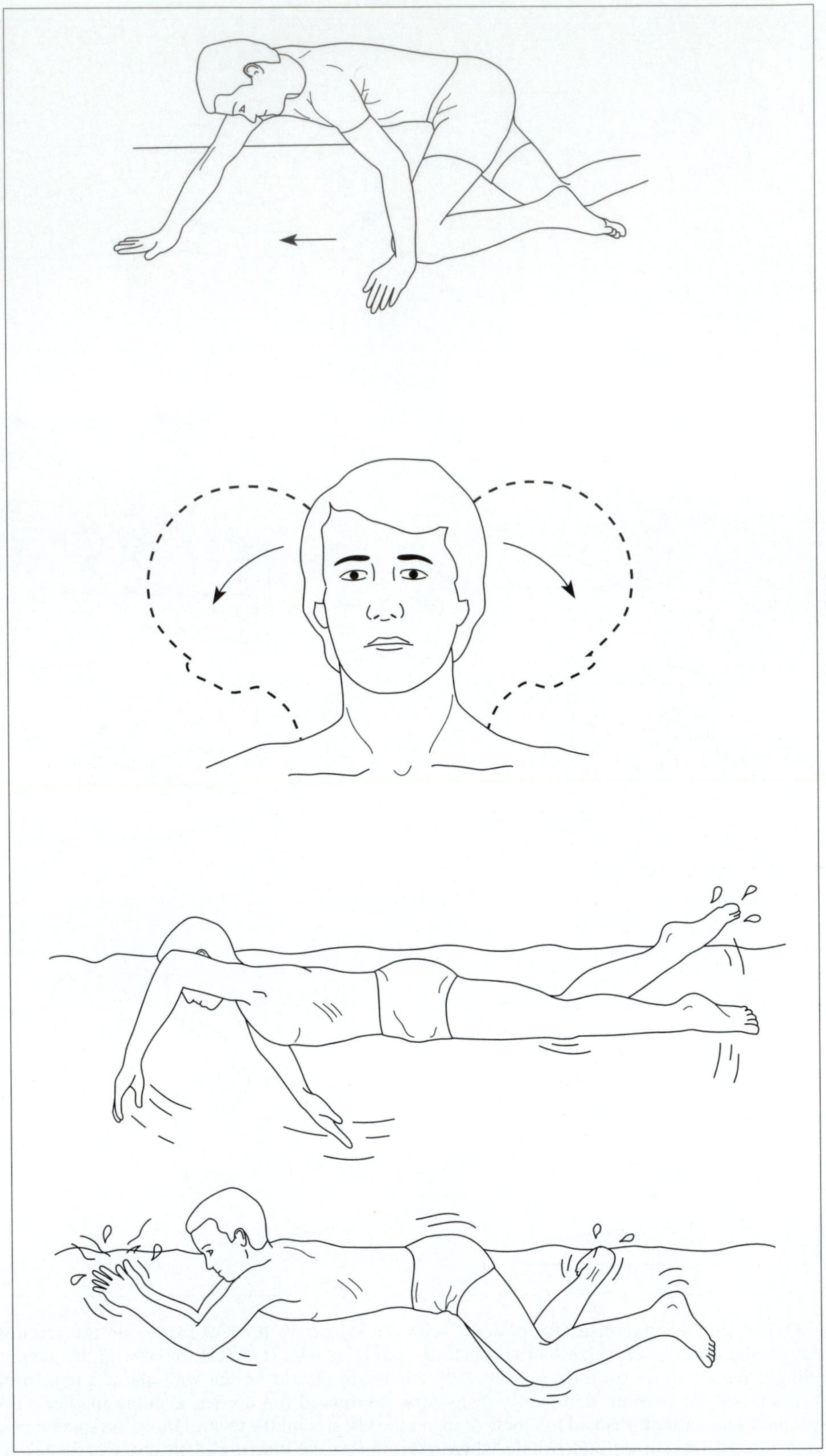

H

I

J

**Fig. 83-10, cont'd.** For legend see p. 1161.

but any antimalarial agent should be used cautiously in psoriatic patients. Toxicities include nausea, allergic dermatitis, headache, dizziness, and retinal toxicities. After a baseline opthalmologic examination, monitoring every 6 months is recommended.

Retinoid (vitamin A) derivatives, particularly etretinate, has been studied extensively for the treatment of psoriasis; smaller studies have demonstrated etretinate to be extremely effective in treating PsA. Cyclosporin A, a potent immunosuppressive agent, can successfully treat severe psoriasis unresponsive to other drugs. Concurrent improvement in joint disease was reported for patients with arthritis. However, cyclosporin's current toxicities are too significant for Food and Drug Administration (FDA) approval of its use in the treatment of psoriasis or PsA. Etretinate and cyclosporin A are considered experimental therapies at this time.

## Rehabilitative management

Exercise to maintain muscle tone and function is of utmost importance for patients with inflammatory arthritis. A programed routine set by a physical therapist should be the initial step. Often, because of lower extremity disease, even low-impact weight-bearing exercises are not possible. Exercises performed in a heated pool or walking in a pool may be ideal alternatives.

Judicious use of splints during acute inflammatory periods may preserve function and alignment of involved joints. Referral to an occupational therapist for upper extremity splints and assessment of activities of daily living are important for patients with upper extremity involvement.

Patients with reactive arthritis or PsA often have foot and ankle involvement. Dactylitis, metatarsophalangeal (MTP), and interphalangeal involvement cannot be accommodated by regular shoes. Prescription shoes with extra depth or a toe box can help. Soft shoe inserts with metatarsal bars redistribute weight away from the MTP joints. Plantar fasciitis may also respond to soft inserts or to local corticosteroid injections. Heel cups provide extra cushioning for symptomatic heel spurs. If multiple midfoot or hindfoot joints are involved, limited periods of casting (less than 7 days) for immobilization can be ordered. However, since these patients tend to ankylose joints rapidly, prolonged immobilization without diligent range-of-motion exercises is not advisable. Management of Achilles tendinitis is difficult. NSAIDs are the mainstay, with cautious corticosteroid injections. Ice and immobilization may also help.

Axial involvement in any of the spondyloarthropathies should begin with referral to a physical therapist to maintain functional capacity. However, daily back and chest expansion exercises must become ingrained in patients' routines (Fig. 83-10). To minimize spinal flexion deformities, patients should sleep on a firm mattress and thin pillows. Patients should also be instructed to lie for least 30 minutes each day or night in a prone position (belly down). In addition, protection from injury should be emphasized, since spinal fractures with minimal trauma occur in the osteoporotic spondylitic spine. Thus patients need to avoid prolonged periods of non–weight bearing, maintain adequate dietary intake of calcium and vitamin D, and refrain from sports that can result in spinal injury.

### Surgery

Orthopedic intervention may be necessary for patients who have persistent peripheral arthritis despite the various interventions described. Arthroscopic or surgical synovectomy is an option in persistent synovitis of the knee. Total joint replacement for severe hip or knee arthritis can be successful, although heterotopic bone formation may influence surgical outcome.

Psoriatic patients with aggressive, small joint arthritis should be referred to hand surgeons early for possible procedures to prevent the mutilans state. Surgical fusion of the wrist may reduce pain and preserve function. Persistent tendinitis of the fingers or synovitis at the wrist despite medical therapy may require synovectomy.

In AS, cervical fractures at C6-7 and other levels may require stabilization. Rarely, severe flexion deformities of the spine can be corrected by osteotomies, but the procedure carries great risk.

### Referral

The seronegative spondyloarthropathies are multisystem disorders. The need for consultations for individual patients depends on numerous factors. These include questions regarding the diagnosis, the severity of the clinical manifestations, the response to treatment, the particular organ system involvement, and the primary care physician's familiarity and proficiency in treating these disorders (see the Managed Care Guide).

Rheumatology consultation remains the cornerstone referral. It should usually be sought if the diagnosis is established or suspected. It may be possible, however, for the primary care physician to provide most of the day-to-day management, as well as the long-term follow-up. If the disease is refractory to standard treatment with physical therapy and NSAIDs, or if second-line agents are being considered, a rheumatologist's input becomes even more important.

Patient education, exercise, and physical therapy are mainstays of therapy. A physical therapy consultation is highly recommended when the diagnosis is made. Most programs can be performed at home. A single consultation may be all that is needed.

Acute anterior uveitis, especially if unrecognized and untreated, can lead to severe ocular sequelae, including

#### Managed Care Guide
#### Pointers on management of seronegative spondyloarthropathies

1. Consultation with a rheumatologist for complex or suspicious cases, and for the consideration of second-line agents for treatment and consultation of other specialists
2. Patient education, physical and occupational therapy may significantly improve and preserve function
3. Ophthalmologic evaluation for the development of acute anterior uveitis.

blindness. It is imperative that a referral be made urgently to an ophthalmologist if the history or examination suggests the occurrence of this extraarticular manifestation. The primary care physician must also provide information about uveitis so that the patient recognizes the symptoms and seeks help immediately if they occur.

Consultations with an orthopedist, podiatrist, dermatologist, cardiologist, or pulmonologist may be necessary, depending on each patient's disease manifestations.

## BIBLIOGRAPHY


Benjamin R, Parham P: HLA-B27 and disease: a consequence of inadvertent antigen presentation, *Rheum Dis Clin North Am* 18:11, 1992.

Calin A: Reiter's syndrome. In Calin A, editor: *Spondyloarthropathies,* Orlando, 1984, Grune & Stratton.

Carette S et al: The natural disease course of ankylosing spondylitis, *Arthritis Rheum* 26:186, 1983.

Espinoza LR et al: Rheumatic manifestations associated with human immunodeficiency virus infection, *Arthritis Rheum* 32:1615, 1989.

Eulderink F: Pathology of ankylosing spondylitis. In Khan MA, editor: *Spine: state of the art reviews,* Philadelphia, 1990, Hanley & Belfus.

Fan PT, Yu DT: Reiter's syndrome. In Kelly WN et al, editors: *Textbook of rheumatology,* ed 4, Philadelphia, 1993, WB Saunders.

Fox R et al: The chronicity of symptoms and disability in Reiter's syndrome, *Ann Intern Med* 91:190, 1979.

Gerber LH: Psoriatic arthritis: pharmacologic, surgical and rehabilitative management. In Gerber LH, Espinoza LR, editors: *Psoriatic arthritis,* Orlando, 1985, Grune & Stratton.

Gladman DD: Psoriatic arthritis: recent advances in pathogenesis and treatment, *Rheum Dis Clin North Am* 18:247, 1992.

Gravallese EM, Kantrowitz FG: Arthritic manifestations of inflammatory bowel disease, *Am J Gastroenterol* 83:703, 1988.

Inman RD: Reiter's syndrome and reactive arthritis. In Khan MA, editor: *Spine: state of the art reviews,* Philadelphia, 1990, Hanley & Belfus.

Kaye BR: Rheumatologic manifestations of infection with human immunodeficiency virus *(HIV), Ann Intern Med* 111:158, 1989.

Keat A: Reiter's syndrome and reactive arthritis in perspective, *N Engl J Med* 309:1606, 1983.

Keat A, Rowe I: Reiter's syndrome and associated arthritides. In Winchester R, editor: *Rheumatic disease clinics of North America,* Philadelphia, 1991, WB Saunders.

Khan MA: Ankylosing spondylitis. In Calin A, editor: *Spondyloarthropathies,* Orlando, 1984, Grune & Stratton.

Khan MA: Spondyloarthropathies. In Khan MA, editor: *Rheumatic disease clinics of North America,* Philadelphia, 1992, WB Saunders.

Khan MA, van der Linden SM: Ankylosing spondylitis and other spondyloarthropathies, *Rheum Dis Clin North Am* 16:551, 1990.

Lauhio A, et al: Double-blind, placebo-controlled study of three-month treatment with lymecycline in reactive arthritis, with special reference to chlamydia arthritis, *Arthritis Rheum* 34:6, 1991.

Leirisalo-Repo M, Repo H: Gut and spondyloarthropathies, *Rheum Dis Clin North Am* 18:23, 1992.

Rahman MU, Hudson AP, Schumacher HR: Chlamydia and Reiter's syndrome (reactive arthritis). In Khan MA, editor: *Rheumatic disease clinics of North America,* Philadelphia, 1992, WB Saunders.

Rosenbaum JT: Acute anterior uveitis and spondyloarthropathies. In Khan MA, editor: *Rheumatic disease clinics of North America,* Philadelphia, 1992, WB Saunders.

Silveira LH, et al: Psoriatic arthritis, *Arthritis Rheum Prim Care Rev* 2:1, 1990.

Solomon G, Brancato L, Winchester R: An approach to the human immunodeficiency virus–positive patient with a spondyloarthropathic disease. In Winchester R, editor: *Rheumatic disease clinics of North America,* Philadelphia, 1991, WB Saunders.

Sparling M et al: Association of uveitis with systemic or rheumatic diseases in a community-based population (abstract), *Arthritis Rheum* 32:38, 1989.

Veys EM, Mielants H: Enteropathic arthritis, uveitis, Whipple's disease, and miscellaneous spondyloarthropathies, *Curr Opin Rheumatol* 5:420, 1993.

Weiner SR et al: Rheumatic manifestations of inflammatory bowel disease, *Semin Arthritis Rheum* 20:353, 1991.

White RH: Preoperative evaluation of patients with rheumatoid arthritis, *Semin Arthritis Rheum* 14:287, 1985.

Winchester R et al: The co-occurrence of Reiter's syndrome and acquired immunodeficiency, *Ann Intern Med* 106:19, 1987.

Wollheim FA: Ankylosing spondylitis. In Kelley WN et al, editors: *Textbook of rheumatology,* ed 4, Philadelphia, 1993, WB Saunders.

Zeidler H, Mau W, Khan M: Undifferentiated spondyloarthropathy, *Rheum Dis Clin North Am* 18:187, 1992.


CHAPTER

# 84 Vasculitis

**David W. Puett**
**John S. Sergent**

Vasculitis refers to a disease group that is characterized by inflammation of blood vessels. The inflammation can affect vessels of any size and distribution and is thus responsible for a wide spectrum of disease states. Complications most commonly result from vessel obstruction and the consequent organ ischemia, but aneurysm formation with rupture can occur. Although the first case of vasculitis was reported in 1866, it was not until 1952 that Zeek proposed a classification scheme, based primarily on pathologic appearance. Since then many schemes have been proposed. However, because the pathophysiology of most vasculitis syndromes is either incompletely understood or unknown, the current classification schemes remain descriptive. Distinguishing features include clinical presentation, the size of involved vessels, histopathology, associated serologic abnormalities, and the presence of an underlying disease (see the box on p. 1165). If an underlying disease can be found, the vasculitis is referred to as secondary. Otherwise, it is termed primary. A clinically useful classification scheme of the primary vasculitis syndromes is shown in Table 84-1.

## EPIDEMIOLOGY

Incidence figures are unavailable for most types of vasculitis and, when available, demonstrate marked variability based on patient demographics, such as age and ethnic origin. For example, Behçet's disease is rare in Americans, but its prevalence has been estimated at 1 per 10,000 people in some areas of Japan. In the United States leukocytoclastic vasculitis (LCV) is probably the most common type. Henoch-Schönlein purpura is estimated to affect 14 per 100,000 children, and hypersensitivity responses to drugs or infections are probably more common. At the other end of the age spectrum the prevalence of temporal arteritis in people 50 years or older

**Table 84-1.** Classification of primary vasculitis by histopathology and vessel size

| Histopathology | Vessel size | Syndrome/disease |
|---|---|---|
| Granulomatous angiitis | Large arteries | Temporal arteritis<br>Takayasu's arteritis |
| Necrotizing vasculitis | Medium arteries | Polyarteritis nodosa |
| Granulomatous angiitis | Small arteries | Wegener's granulomatosis<br>Churg-Strauss vasculitis |
| Leukocytoclastic vasculitis | Arterioles, venules | Hypersensitivity vasculitis<br>Henoch-Schönlein purpura<br>Essential cryoglobulinemia |
| Cellular infiltrate with limited necrosis | Diffuse sizes<br>Prominent venulitis | Behçet's disease<br>Buerger's disease |

was 12 per 100,000 in Olmstead County, Minnesota.

Secondary vasculitis is more common. Rheumatoid arthritis affects approximately 1% of the population, and, of the rheumatoid factor–positive patients, 5% to 10% develop vasculitis. Similarly, systemic lupus erythematosus (SLE) is a common inflammatory disease, and some form of vasculitis occurs in approximately 30% of patients with this illness.

## PATHOPHYSIOLOGY

Research into the mechanisms of serum sickness and hepatitis B–associated vasculitis has demonstrated that immune complex formation and deposition in blood vessel walls is involved. Complement is activated, resulting in direct cellular injury, the recruitment of inflammatory cells, and depression of the circulating levels of the complement components. Hypocomplementemia is seen in 20% of patients with primary polyarteritis nodosa and in many cases of LCV. However, although low levels of circulating immune complexes can be detected in other vasculitic syndromes, hypocomplementemia is rarely seen, and immunofluorescence detects little immunoglobulin or complement in areas of vessel inflammation. Clearly the pathogenesis of such "pauciimmune" vasculitis is different.

The discovery of the antineutrophil cytoplasmic antibody (ANCA) family has provided not only a valuable serologic marker but may also shed light on the pathogenesis of some types of pauciimmune vasculitis. Two staining patterns are recognized by immunofluorescence of alcohol-fixed neutrophils. These include a diffuse cytoplasmic pattern (C-ANCA), in which proteinase 3 is the primary antigen, and a perinuclear pattern (P-ANCA), in which the antibody recognizes myeloperoxidase (MPO-ANCA) or other diffusable granule proteins. It has been hypothesized that these antibodies may react with neutrophils, resulting in vessel wall injury.

## HISTORY

Vasculitis should be suspected in any patient who presents with an unexplained systemic illness or signs and symptoms of organ ischemia. The coincident involvement of several organs or the presence of organ ischemia in a young person suggests vasculitis. Although any organ system may be involved, the presence of mononeuritis multiplex and palpable purpura is highly suggestive of an underlying vasculitis.

The primary vasculitis syndromes differ in their tendency to affect people of a particular sex, age, and ethnic background (Table 84-2). Although much overlap

### Distinguishing features of vasculitis syndromes

**Clinical presentation**

Distribution of organ involvement

**Vessel size**

Large vessels, including the aorta and its major branches
Medium vessels that lie outside of, but supply, organs
Small vessels found within organs and in subcutaneous tissue
Precapillary arterioles and postcapillary venules

**Histopathology**

Granulomatous arteritis: predominant mononuclear cell infiltrate with giant cell and granuloma formation
Necrotizing vasculitis: predominant polymorphonuclear infiltrate with fibrinoid necrosis
Leukocytoclastic vasculitis

**Underlying illnesses**

- Systemic inflammatory disease
  - Rheumatic disease
    - Rheumatoid arthritis
    - Systemic lupus erythematosus
    - Sjögren's syndrome
  - Inflammatory bowel disease
- Malignancy
- Infection (e.g., hepatitis B and C)

**Serologic abnormalities**

Hypocomplementemia
Cryoglobulinemia
Antineutrophil cytoplasmic antibodies
Antinuclear antibodies
Rheumatoid factor

**Table 84-2.** Demographics of primary vasculitis

| Age group | Vasculitis | Background or ethnic origin | Sex |
|---|---|---|---|
| Child | Kawasaki disease | Asian >> European | M = F |
| | Behçet's disease | Asian >> European | M > F |
| | Henoch-Schönlein purpura | | F > M |
| Young adult | Takayasu's arteritis | Asian >> European | F > M |
| | Polyarteritis nodosa | | M > F |
| Middle age | Wegener's granulomatosis | | M > F |
| | Churg-Strauss vasculitis | History of allergy | M = F |
| | Buerger's disease | Smoker | M > F |
| Elderly | Temporal arteritis | White >> African-American | M = F |

exists, such demographic clues can be helpful. Clearly, the demographics of secondary vasculitis reflect that of the underlying disease.

## PHYSICAL EXAMINATION

When approaching treatment of a patient with systemic vasculitis, it is important to determine the distribution of organ involvement through history, physical examination, laboratory tests, and imaging studies. This assessment suggests the size of the involved vessels and thus helps to categorize the vasculitis. Table 84-3 lists the more common manifestations of vasculitis and their frequency of occurrence in the different syndromes. Constitutional symptoms, such as fever, fatigue, and weight loss, as well as muscle and joint aches, are present in most patients with vasculitis. However, frank inflammatory arthritis is unusual unless the vasculitis accompanies a systemic rheumatic disease.

### Laboratory evaluation

Laboratory studies typically demonstrate nonspecific evidence of inflammation, including leukocytosis, anemia of chronic disease, and an elevated erythrocyte sedimentation rate (ESR). In contrast, serologic tests help to establish the diagnosis and categorize the type of vasculitis. Rheumatoid factors, antinuclear antibodies (ANA), complement levels, cryoglobulins, and ANCA are often helpful in evaluating patients with suspected vasculitis.

C-ANCA is associated with small vessel granulomatous vasculitis; it is present in 90% of patients with Wegener granulomatosis at the time of diagnosis, and is also found in other diseases that behave similarly, such as microscopic polyarteritis nodosa. The MPO-ANCA is associated with necrotizing vasculitis of medium-sized vessels, such as polyarteritis nodosa, and is also found in 70% of patients with idiopathic, crescentic glomerulonephritis. ANCAs, which recognize undetermined antigens, are commonly found in inflammatory bowel disease (IBD) and immune liver disease.

Cryoglobulins are immunoglobulins that precipitate in the cold. Three classes are recognized. Type I consists of a single monoclonal immunoglobulin. Type II is defined by the presence of a mixed cryoglobulin population, including a monoclonal IgM rheumatoid factor and polyclonal IgG immunoglobulins. In type III, a mixed population of one or more classes of polyclonal immunoglobulins that possess rheumatoid factor activity are present without a monoclonal component. The different cryoglobulin types are associated with various underlying illnesses (see below).

### Biopsy and arteriography

The diagnosis of vasculitis usually requires confirmation with biopsy or arteriography. Biopsy of a fresh skin lesion, an inflamed temporal artery, or the kidney in a patient with an active urinary sediment has the highest yield. A sural nerve biopsy is indicated if symptoms of weakness or numbness suggest a peripheral neuropathy and if nerve conduction studies confirm nerve injury. The yield of a muscle biopsy in a patient without clinical evidence of muscle involvement (blind biopsy) may be as high as 80% for patients with polyarteritis nodosa and hepatitis B vasculitis but lower in other forms of vasculitis.

Arteriography is useful in several clinical situations. An abdominal angiogram with selected visualization of the renal, celiac, and mesenteric arteries shows vascular aneurysms or vessel occlusions in approximately 75% of patients with polyarteritis nodosa. In patients with suspected Takayasu's arteritis, arteriography of the aortic arch and its branches is the diagnostic procedure of choice. However, with the exception of Buerger's disease, arteriography is otherwise of limited benefit.

### Diseases associated with secondary vasculitis

- Involvement of large muscular arteries (the aorta and its branches)
  - Syphilis
  - Seronegative spondyloarthropathies
- Involvement of small to medium muscular arteries
  - Hepatitis B and C
  - Systemic rheumatic diseases
    - Rheumatoid arthritis
    - Systemic lupus erythematosus
    - Sjögren's syndrome
- Involvement of arterioles and venules (leukocytoclastic vasculitis)
  - Drug reactions
  - Infections
  - Malignancy
  - Systemic inflammatory diseases

**Table 84-3.** Common manifestations of vasculitis

| Manifestation | Vasculitic syndrome | | | | | | | |
|---|---|---|---|---|---|---|---|---|
| | Temporal arteritis* | Takayasu's arteritis* | Polyarteritis nodosa† | Churg-Strauss vasculitis‡ | Wegener's granulomatosis‡ | Hypersensitivity vasculitis§ | Henoch-Shönlein purpura§ | Essential cryoglobulinemia§ |
| Rash | | | ++ | ++ | + | +++ | +++ | +++ |
| Peripheral neuropathy | | | +++ | +++ | + | | | ++ |
| Glomerulonephritis | | | +++ | +++ | +++ | | +++ | ++ |
| Respiratory symptoms | | | | +++ | +++ | | | |
| Gastrointestinal pain | | | ++ | ++ | + | | +++ | + |
| Claudication | ++ | +++ | + | + | | | | |
| Headache | +++ | ++ | + | + | + | | | |

*Large vessel granulomatous disease.
†Medium vessel granulomatous disease.
‡Small vessel granulomatous disease.
§Leukocytoclastic vasculitis.
+, Occasionally seen; ++, commonly seen; +++, frequently seen.

## DIFFERENTIAL DIAGNOSIS

It is important to distinguish vasculitis look-alikes from true vasculitis and to establish the presence of an underlying disease when a diagnosis of vasculitis is confirmed. As noted in the box on p. 1166, vasculitis involving any vessel size may be associated with another illness. The systemic rheumatic diseases account for many cases of secondary vasculitis, and, since it is unusual for vasculitis to be the sole presenting manifestation in rheumatic disease, the presence of the underlying illness is usually known or easily detected (see the box below). However, vasculitis may be associated with a clinically silent hepatitis.

LCV may represent a hypersensitivity response to a drug or infection (see the box on p. 1168). An attempt to identify the triggering agent should be made, although a cause is found only in the minority of cases. LCV is also seen with systemic inflammatory conditions and rarely malignancy (see the box on p. 1168).

Monoclonal cryoglobulinemia (type I) is associated with multiple myeloma and Waldenström macroglobulinemia. The mixed cryoglobulinemias can occur in the setting of lymphoproliferative disease, systemic rheumatic disease, or chronic infections (see the box on p. 1168). Recent studies suggest that previously unrecognized hepatitis C viral infection may be responsible for many cases of essential cryoglobulinemia.

Vascular injury from any source may be clinically indistinguishable from vasculitis. Examples include embolic disease, noninflammatory vessel wall disruption, and coagulopathies (see the box below). A detailed history may suggest a vasculitis simulator and should include a careful drug list, with attention to over-the-counter medications (many cold remedies contain phenylpropanolamine) and

### Vasculitis simulators

- Embolic disease
  - Infectious or marantic endocarditis
  - Cardiac mural thrombus
  - Atrial myxoma
  - Cholesterol embolization syndrome
- Noninflammatory vessel wall disruption
  - Atherosclerosis
  - Arterial fibromuscular dysplasia
  - Drug effect: ergotamines, phenylpropanolamine, cocaine, warfarin
  - Radiation
  - Genetic disease: neurofibromatosis, Ehlers-Danlos syndrome
  - Amyloidosis
  - Intravascular malignant lymphoma
- Diffuse coagulation
  - Disseminated intravascular coagulation
  - Thrombotic thrombocytopenic purpura or hemolytic uremic syndrome
  - Deficiencies of anticoagulants: proteins S and C
  - Antiphospholipid antibodies

### Exposures associated with hypersensitivity vasculitis

Drugs
- Anticonvulsants: phenobarbital and phenytoin
- Antibiotics: penicillins and sulfonamides
- Antiarrhythmics: quinidine and procainamide
- Nonsteroidal antiinflammatory drugs
- Allopurinol
- Vaccines
- Many others

Infections
- Acute bacterial infections
  - Group A streptococci
  - *Neisseria*
- Chronic bacterial infections
  - Subacute bacterial endocarditis
  - Chronic sinusitis
- Mycobacterial infections
  - Tuberculosis
  - Leprosy
- Viral infections
  - Hepatitis B and C
  - Cytomegalovirus (CMV)
  - Human immunodeficiency virus (HIV)
- Fungal infections

### Diseases associated with leukocytoclastic vasculitis

Systemic inflammatory disease
- Rheumatic disease
  - Rheumatoid arthritis
  - Systemic lupus erythematosus
  - Sjögren's syndrome
- Gastrointestinal disease
  - Inflammatory bowel disease
  - Primary biliary cirrhosis

Malignancy
- Multiple myeloma and Waldenström macroglobulinemia
- Lymphoma
- Leukemia
- Carcinomas

illicit drugs (cocaine). Laboratory studies may show a coagulation disorder, and, because several illnesses located within the heart may simulate vasculitis, consideration should be given to performing an echocardiogram.

Cholesterol embolization syndrome deserves special attention because it is probably the most common vasculitis simulator. It should be suspected in all elderly patients, especially if there is a known history of atherosclerotic vascular disease. Although cholesterol emboli produce many different clinical pictures, livedo reticularis (a nonpalpable, lacy, red to purple rash, most commonly on the legs) is an almost universal finding. Finally, antiphospholipid antibodies are now recognized more commonly in patients with ischemic syndromes, and, as mentioned above, livedo reticularis is almost always present.

### Diseases associated with cryoglobulinemia

Malignancy
- Multiple myeloma or Waldenström macroglobulinemia (type I)
- Lymphoma or leukemia (types II and III)

Systemic rheumatic diseases (type III > type II)
- Rheumatoid arthritis
- Systemic lupus erythematosus
- Sjögren's syndrome

Chronic infections (type III > type II)
- Bacterial
  - Subacute bacterial endocarditis
  - Abscesses
- Viral: hepatitis B and C

## MANAGEMENT

The aggressiveness of therapy depends upon the type of vasculitis and its severity at presentation.

### Vasculitis of the aorta and its major branches

Temporal arteritis is corticosteroid responsive. Therapy is initiated at a prednisone dosage of 1 mg/kg per day, roughly 60 mg per day in the typical patient. The dosage is divided and administered at least twice daily until the inflammation has been suppressed, as determined by the disappearance of constitutional symptoms, the resolution of specific symptoms such as headache or extremity claudication, and normalization of the ESR. This is often achieved in 4 to 6 weeks. The prednisone can then be consolidated into a single morning dose and slowly tapered by roughly 5 mg per day every 1 to 2 weeks as permitted by the patient's disease. Most patients can be tapered to a low dosage (5 to 15 mg per day) by 3 to 4 months. This dosage should be continued for 6 to 12 months. Steroid-resistant or chronically active disease is unusual but occurs, and methotrexate has shown promise in such patients. A variety of immunosuppressive agents have been used in Takayasu's arteritis with mixed results.

### Vasculitis of small to medium muscular arteries

Patients with small to medium artery vasculitis (polyarteritis nodosa, Wegener's granulomatosis, and Churg-Strauss vasculitis) require more aggressive immunosuppression. Although many drugs have been tried, alkylating agents appear to be the most effective. Cyclophosphamide has been used extensively and is the treatment of choice. One to 2 mg/kg per day is given orally as a single morning dose. Since alkylating agents may take 3 to 4 weeks for maximum immunosuppression, a divided dosage of prednisone at 1 mg/kg per day is also started. After 3 to 4 weeks the prednisone can be consolidated into a single morning dose and tapered by 5 mg per day every 1 to 2 weeks as tolerated. The cyclophosphamide dosage is adjusted as necessary to achieve disease suppression while maintaining a total white blood cell count (WBC) above 3000. The alkylating agent is usually continued for 1 to 2 years after disease remission. Azathioprine and methotrexate are alternatives if patients are unable to tolerate alkylating therapy, but these agents are less effective.

### Leukocytoclastic vasculitis

The therapy of LCV depends on its type and presentation. Hypersensitivity vasculitis and Henoch-Schönlein purpura typically require symptomatic and supportive care only. However, LCV can involve organ- and life-threatening visceral disease that may require aggressive immunosuppressive therapy with corticosteroids and other drugs. Plasmapheresis has been lifesaving in instances of cryoglobulinemic crises.

## PROGNOSIS

### Vasculitis of the aorta and its major branches

The prognosis of the different vasculitis syndromes is quite variable. Patients with temporal arteritis have a good prognosis. The disease resolves within 6 to 12 months in approximately 50% of cases, and the remainder are usually disease free by 3 to 4 years. Sequelae are unusual if adequate therapy is administered, although 25% of untreated patients go blind from ciliary or ophthalmic artery occlusion. The natural history of Takayasu's arteritis in the United States is poorly understood. Most patients have an inflammatory state for the first several years that may be corticosteroid responsive. However, it is the secondary phase of slow, fibrosis-producing vessel stenosis that accounts for most of the morbidity and mortality. Strokes, cardiac dysfunction from coronary artery involvement or aortic valve incompetence, accelerated hypertension from aortic coarctation or renal artery stenosis, aneurysm rupture, and extremity claudication may occur.

### Vasculitis of small to medium arteries

Polyarteritis nodosa, Wegener's granulomatosis, and Churg-Strauss vasculitis involve small to medium muscular arteries and carry a poor prognosis. Most untreated patients with Wegener's granulomatosis die within several months of diagnosis, typically from pulmonary hemorrhage or renal disease. Corticosteroids and cyclophosphamide result in clinical improvement in many patients, producing a remission in up to 75%. However, disease recurrence is seen in 50%, and 80% of patients suffer severe morbidity from their disease or its therapy. The mortality remains in the range of 10% to 25%. Polyarteritis nodosa and its pulmonary variant, Churg-Strauss vasculitis, are also life-threatening illnesses. Without treatment, most patients die within the first year of diagnosis. Corticosteroids improve the 5-year survival to approximately 50%, and cyclophosphamide may provide additional benefit. However, as in the case of Wegener's granulomatosis, morbidity is common.

### Leukocytoclastic vasculitis

The prognosis of primary LCV depends on its severity at presentation. Hypersensitivity vasculitis to a drug and Henoch-Schönlein purpura in children are usually self-limited. In contrast, cryoglobulinemia is more often associated with chronic visceral disease and has a wide variability of prognosis.

## BIBLIOGRAPHY


Brovet JC et al: Biologic and clinical significance of cryoglobulins: a report of 86 cases, *Am J Med* 57:775, 1974.

Calabrese LH, Clough JD: Hypersensitivity vasculitis group (HVG), *Cleve Clin J Med* 49:17, 1982.

Fan PT et al: A clinical approach to systemic vasculitis, *Semin Arthritis Rheum* 9:248, 1980.

Hoffman GS et al: Wegener's granulomatosis: an analysis of 158 patients, *Ann Intern Med* 116:488, 1992.

Huston KA et al: Temporal arteritis: a 25-year epidemiologic, clinical and pathologic study, *Ann Intern Med* 88:162, 1978.

Ilan Y, Naparstek Y: Schönlein-Henoch syndrome in adults and children, *Semin Arthritis Rheum* 21:103, 1991.

Jennette JC, Charles LA, Falk RJ: Antineutrophil cytoplasmic autoantibodies: disease associations, molecular biology, and pathophysiology, *Int Rev Exp Pathol* 32:193, 1991.

Lanham JC et al: Systemic vasculitis with asthma and eosinophilia: a clinical approach to the Churg-Strauss syndrome, *Medicine* 63:65, 1984.

Lie JT: Vasculitis, 1815 to 1991: classification and diagnostic specificity, *J Rheumatol* 19:83, 1992.

Schneider HA et al: Rheumatoid vasculitis: experience with 13 patients and review of the literature, *Semin Arthritis Rheum* 14:280, 1985.

Sergent JS et al: Vasculitis with hepatitis B antigenemia: long-term observations in nine patients, *Medicine* 55:1, 1976.

Shelhamer JH et al: Takayasu's arteritis and its therapy, *Ann Intern Med* 103:125, 1985.

Travers RL et al: Polyarteritis nodosa: a clinical and angiographic analysis of 17 cases, *Semin Arthritis Rheum* 8:184, 1979.


CHAPTER

# 85 Systemic Sclerosis

**Virginia D. Steen**
**James C. Shaw**

Systemic sclerosis (SSc) is a chronic, multisystem disorder of connective tissue characterized by degenerative and inflammatory changes that subsequently lead to intense fibrosis. The skin, blood vessels, synovium, skeletal muscle, and certain internal organs are affected, including the gastrointestinal tract, lungs, heart, and kidneys.

## EPIDEMIOLOGY

SSc has a worldwide distribution. There are approximately 20 new cases of SSc per million population yearly and a prevalence of 300,000 patients in the United States. Women are affected 3 to 4 times more than men. The onset of disease usually occurs between ages 30 and 50, but it is not uncommon in young adults and older people. Childhood SSc is rare, although localized forms of scleroderma, i.e., linear scleroderma and morphea, are more common in children. Familial cases have rarely been

**Characteristics of limited cutaneous and diffuse cutaneous scleroderma early in their course that are helpful in classifying patients in these categories**

| Limited | Diffuse |
|---|---|
| Long history of Raynaud's phenomenon | Recent or absent Raynaud's phenomenon |
| Minimal constitutional symptoms except fatigue | Acute onset with fatigue, weight loss, polyarthritis, feeling ill |
| Puffy fingers | Puffy fingers, hands, and lower legs |
| Calcinosis and telangiectasias common | Carpal tunnel syndrome |
| Old "CREST" syndrome | Tendon rubs |
| Skin thickening restricted to distal extremities | Skin thickening progresses up arms, legs to trunk |
| Pulmonary hypertension | Renal crisis |
| Anticentromere antibody | Antitopoisomerase and RNA polymerase III |

reported and no strong genetic relationships have been found. It is not infrequent for different connective tissue diseases to be encountered, however, among first-degree relatives of individuals with SSc.

The American College of Rheumatology's criteria for the classification of SSc require skin thickening proximal to the metacarpal phalangeal joints or two of the following: sclerodactyly, digital pitting scars, or interstitial pulmonary fibrosis. It is important to understand that these criteria have no relationship to the major clinical subsets of systemic sclerosis, limited cutaneous and diffuse cutaneous scleroderma.

These two subsets are different in their disease onset and overall courses (see the box above). The classic form of diffuse scleroderma has a rapid onset of symptoms including Raynaud's phenomenon, polyarthritis, carpal tunnel syndrome, swollen hands and legs, and fatigue. Skin thickening progresses up the patient's arms and over the trunk, resulting in contractures and disability. Visceral involvement, including gastrointestinal, lung, heart, and kidney, is common, particularly in the first 4 years of disease.

Limited scleroderma, or the old CREST syndrome, is at the other end of the spectrum (Fig. 85-1). Limited scleroderma patients have a much less progressive disease. They usually have Raynaud's phenomenon for a prolonged period before developing other symptoms. Thus a careful search for associated findings in patients with Raynaud's phenomenon can be important. Puffy fingers, heartburn, and telangiectasias may be the only other symptoms. Severe intestinal hypomotility and pulmonary hypertension are the most deadly complications of limited scleroderma. Severe digital ischemia and calcinosis can cause troublesome disability. Anticentromere antibody is found in the majority of these patients.

The natural history of SSc varies considerably between the different subsets (Fig. 85-2). Even within the subsets, survival varies significantly, depending on the extent of internal organ involvement. Overall, the 10-year cumulative survival rate after first diagnosis is approximately 65%. Both death and disability are much more frequent early in the course of diffuse scleroderma, especially in those patients with lung, heart, or kidney involvement. Pulmonary hypertension and intestinal malabsorption are frequent causes of mortality in patients with the limited cutaneous scleroderma.

## PATHOPHYSIOLOGY

The pathophysiology of SSc is not completely understood; however, many interactions occur between vascular and immunologic factors with connective tissue, causing an excessive amount of normal collagen production by fibroblasts (Fig. 85-3). A skin biopsy shows a striking increase of compact collagen fibers in the reticular dermis (Fig. 85-4). Small arterioles show subintimal hyperplasia and hyalinization. In patients with early diffuse disease focal collections of lymphocytes, most of which are T-cells, can be identified in the deep dermis. Activated T-cells produce cytokines, particularly interleukin-2 (IL-2) and transforming growth factor-β (TGF-β), that stimulate fibroblast proliferation and collagen production. γ Interferon has the potential of turning off the fibroblast production of collagen. Inadequate amounts of γ interferon have been noted in scleroderma.

The endothelial cell plays an important role in SSc. There is probably a cytotoxicity factor that can incite injury in endothelial cells. This results in increased permeability and the release and activation of cell growth factors. Platelet activation, platelet derived growth factors (PDGF), and mast cells also have major effects of stimulating the fibroblast.

The humoral immune system with B-cell activation is involved in SSc, although its relationship to endothelial cells and increased collagen production remains obscure. Autoantibodies specific to SSc, i.e., antitopoisomerase or anticentromere antibodies, are commonly found. These antibodies are not believed to play a role in the development of fibrotic tissues or abnormal vessels. Because of the many toxin-induced scleroderma-like illnesses, it is intriguing to hypothesize that a toxin or environmental factor is responsible for triggering scleroderma. Thus far, none have been identified.

## HISTORY

The first symptoms of scleroderma are usually Raynaud's phenomenon, puffy fingers, and/or polyarthritis involving the small joints of the hands. Within several months, progressive skin thickening occurs. Rarely, polymyositis or symptoms referrable to the esophagus, small bowel, or lungs are the earliest manifestations. SSc is a multisystem disease and patients can have many symptoms and findings. Reviewing the symptoms and findings for each organ system results in a better understanding of the

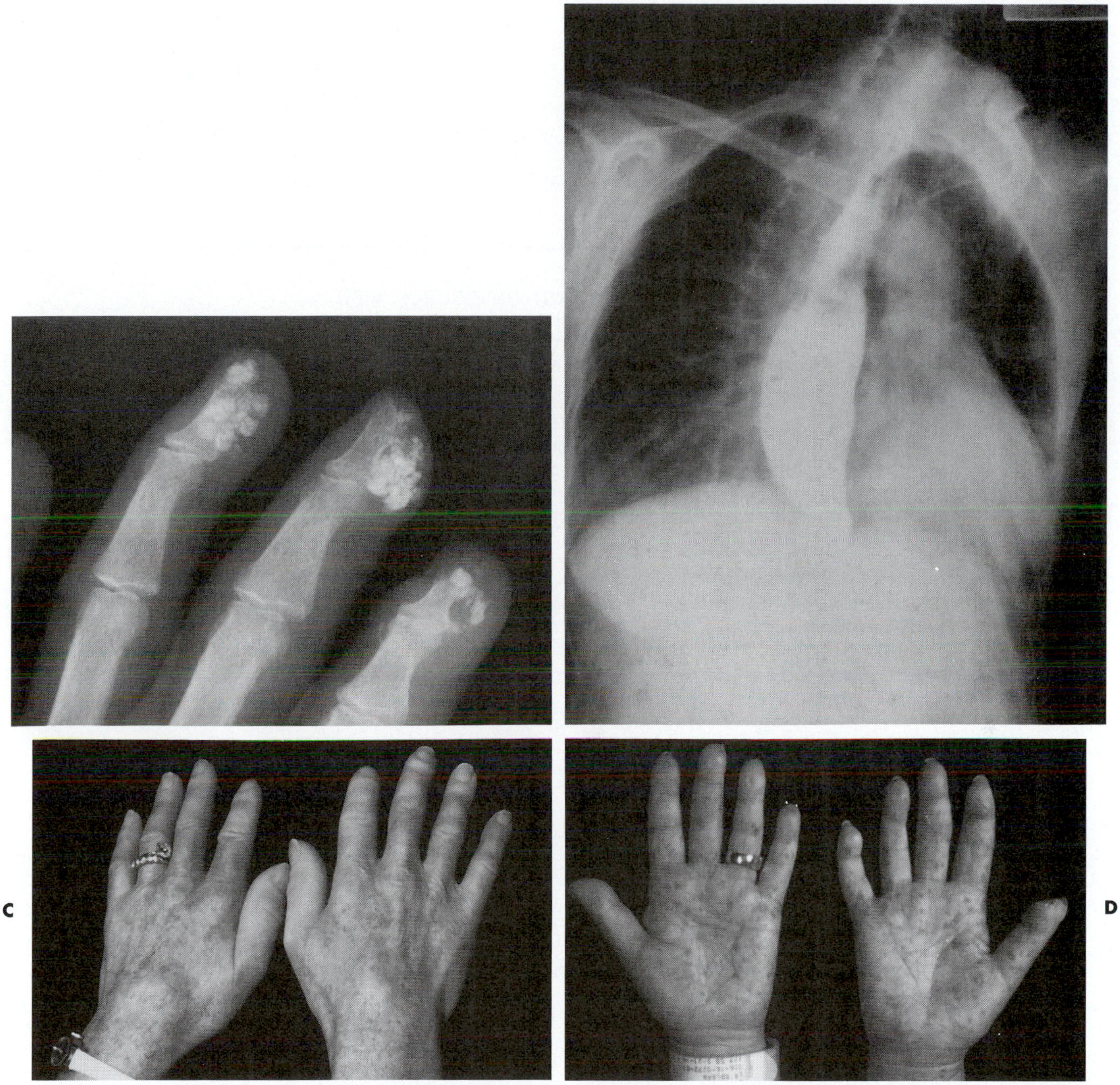

**Fig. 85-1. A,** Calcinosis primarily occurs in fingers after many years of Raynaud's phenomenon. **B,** Distal esophageal hypomotility is commonly seen in all scleroderma patients. **C** and **D,** Sclerodactyly and telangiectasias in a patient with limited scleroderma.

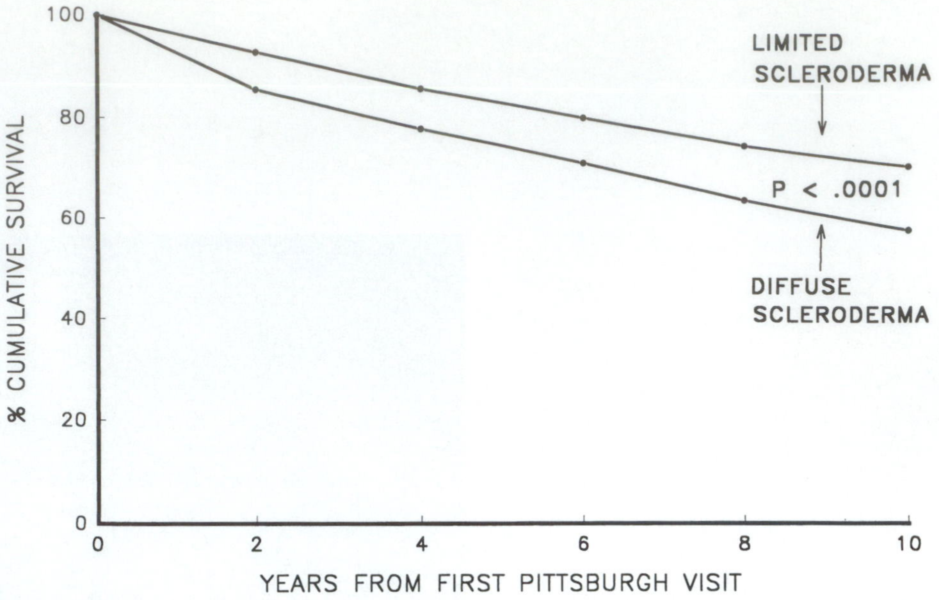


**Fig. 85-2.** The percent cumulative survival from first Pittsburgh evaluation in patients with limited and diffuse scleroderma. Five-year survival is 85% vs. 75%, $p < 0.0001$.

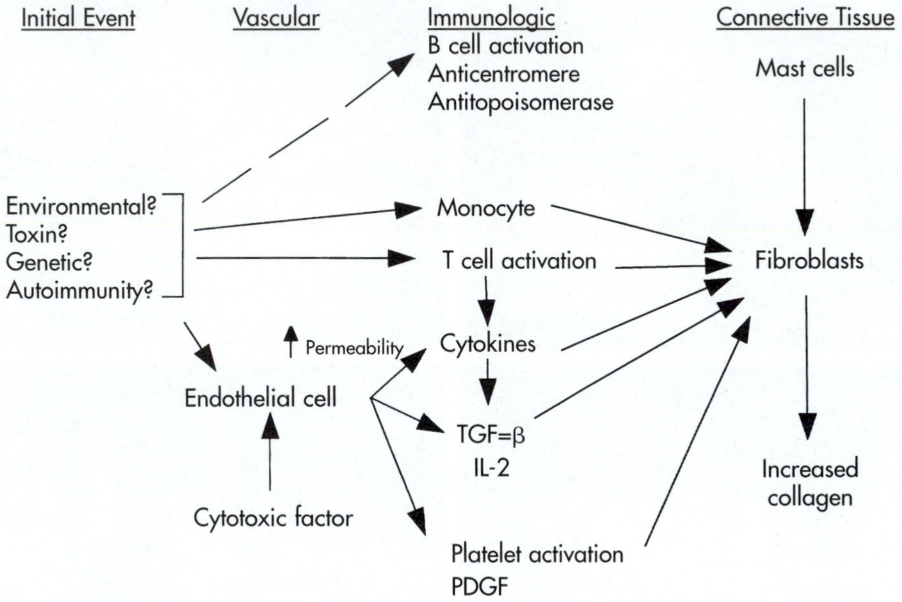


**Fig. 85-3.** Possible interactions in vascular and immunologic factors that result in increased collagen.

patient's disease. It is unlikely that the same presentation occurs in more than a few patients. Management needs to be directed at the individual's specific problems.

## Clinical manifestations

***Raynaud's phenomenon.*** Cold exposure and emotional stress may induce vasospasm, causing characteristic episodes of bilateral blanching or cyanosis of the digits (see Chapter 18). Infarction of tissue at the fingertips may lead to painful ulcerations or frank gangrene. In limited cutaneous disease, Raynaud's phenomenon is almost universally present, often antedating other evidence of SSc by years or even decades. In contrast, Raynaud's phenomenon is initially present in only 75% of patients with diffuse scleroderma.

The finding of dilated nailfold capillaries with capillary dropout is typical for scleroderma and is a helpful differential finding in patients with Raynaud's phenomenon. Digital pitting scars in the fingertips from chronic ischemia is specific for systemic sclerosis.

***Skin.*** In diffuse scleroderma, an early manifestation is often bilateral symmetric swelling of the fingers and hands and the legs and feet (Fig. 85-5). Patients frequently get evaluated for cardiac, endocrine, or protein-losing illnesses because of striking peripheral edema. After a few weeks to several months, edema is replaced by induration, resulting in thick, hard skin. A pinching of the skin to elicit a wrinkle is a reliable method for determining the presence of skin thickening. Skin thickness spreads rapidly up the arms and onto the trunk, particularly the upper anterior chest and abdomen. The skin becomes increasingly thick for several years and then stabilizes. In many patients the skin eventually spontaneously softens to some degree. Improvement typically begins centrally in the last areas to become clinically involved (anterior chest, abdomen) and progresses distally down the arms and legs. Fingers rarely show any significant improvement. This skin thickening is pathognomonic of systemic sclerosis and occurs only rarely in other conditions (Fig. 85-6).

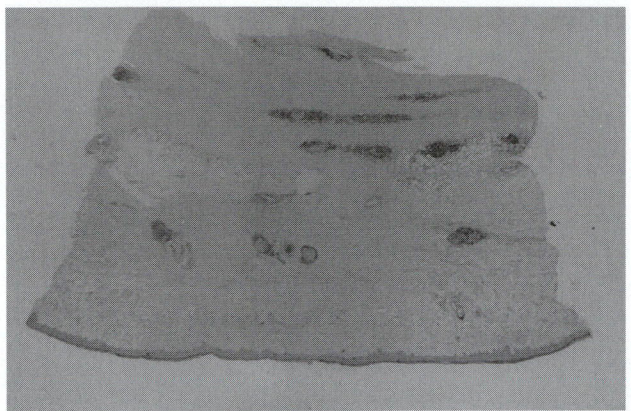

**Fig. 85-4.** A skin biopsy of a patient with diffuse scleroderma showing an excessive amount of collagen, "thick skin," and islands of lymphocytes.

In contrast, limited scleroderma patients tend to have puffiness of only the fingers which may be present for years before skin thickening occurs. As the term limited scleroderma implies, skin thickening is limited to the distal extremities and face, and rarely changes significantly throughout the illness. Accompanying changes include loss of normal skin folds, a shiny appearance, and hyperpigmentation and hypopigmentation, often in areas where the skin is of normal thickness.

After many years of the illness, numerous small macular punctate telangiectasias appear on the fingers, face, lips, and tongue (see Fig. 85-1). They are most frequently encountered in patients with limited scleroderma, but can also be found in those patients with late stage diffuse scleroderma who have survived the first 5 to 10 years of their disease. Their skin thickness may have regressed so that they only have limited skin changes and numerous telangiectasias. This may result in their being

A B C D

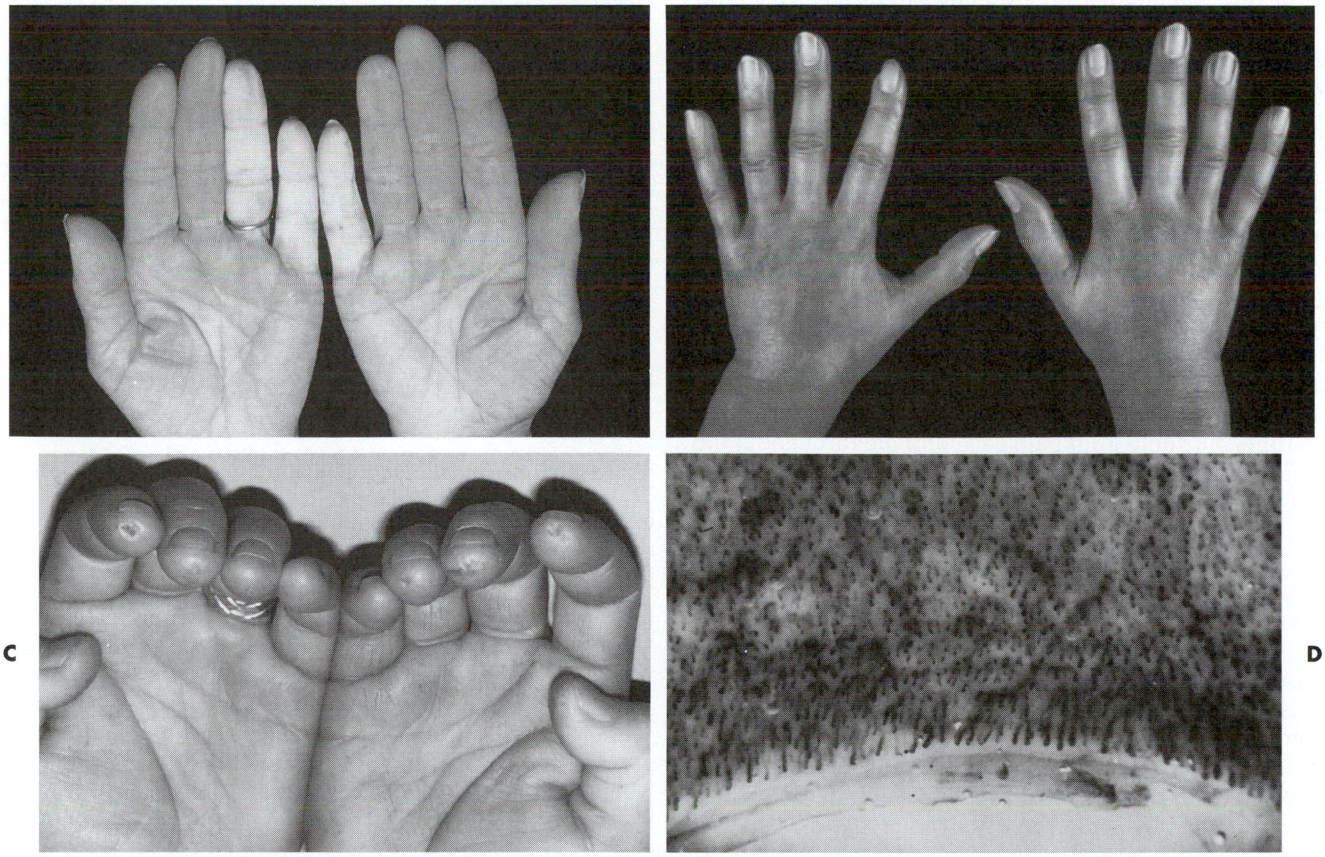

**Fig. 85-5.** **A,** Pallor from vasoconstriction in primary Raynaud's phenomenon. **B** and **C,** Puffy, swollen fingers and digital pitting scars in patients with early systemic sclerosis. **D,** Normal nailfold capillaries using nailfold capillaroscopy (4x). Note even distribution of uniform capillaries without a dilatation or capillary dropout.

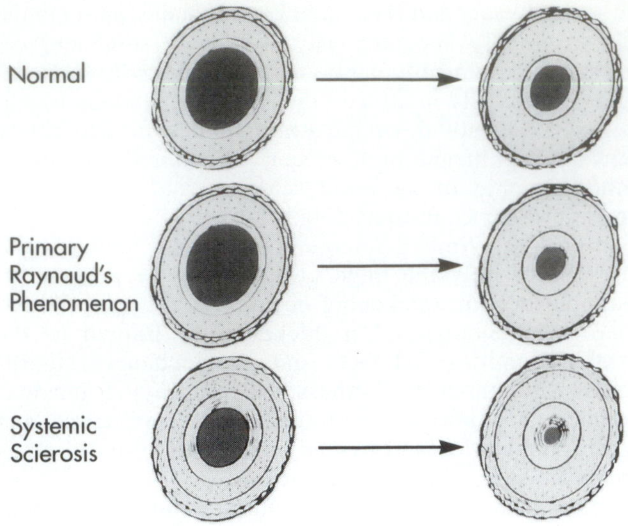


**Fig. 85-6.** Digital vessel vasoconstriction in response to cold exposure. The vessels of patients with primary Raynaud's phenomenon are normal but have exaggerated vasoconstriction in response to the cold. Systemic sclerosis patients have thickened vessels with a decreased lumen even before vasoconstriction occurs.

misdiagnosed as having a limited variant. An early history of an acute onset of symptoms and the presence of significant hand contractures are clues to the classification of late stage diffuse scleroderma even if diffuse skin thickening is no longer apparent (see the box at right).

Subcutaneous calcinosis is a late-developing complication that is more frequent in limited than diffuse scleroderma (Fig. 85-1). Sites of minor trauma are often affected, such as the fingers, forearms, elbows, and knees. Calcifications may vary from tiny punctate deposits to large masses ulcerating the overlying skin.

*Joints and tendons.* Polyarthralgias affect both small and large joints and are especially frequent early in diffuse scleroderma. Joint pain, swollen fingers, and polyarthritis often lead to the premature diagnosis of rheumatoid arthritis. The inflammatory polyarthritis usually improves with time, but some joint pain can continue throughout the disease. In diffuse scleroderma, rapid development of hand swelling and skin tightening often leads to severe flexion contractures with clawlike hands and serious disability. Limited scleroderma patients get only mild, if any, contractures because the disease process is slower. Acroosteolysis, thought to be due to hypovascularity, causes bone resorption primarily of the distal phalanges, but sometimes affects other sites including the distal radius and ulna, mandibular ramus, and superior portion of the posterior ribs ("notching").

Carpal tunnel syndrome is commonly seen early in diffuse scleroderma and often is the symptom that brings the patient to a physician. Coarse, leathery tendon friction rubs palpated during active and even passive motion of the extensor and flexor tendons of the fingers, distal forearms, knees, and ankles are found almost exclusively in patients with diffuse cutaneous disease. Their presence can foreshadow the subsequent development of widespread scleroderma.

## Sclerodermoid skin changes: diseases other than scleroderma

**Undifferentiated connective tissue disease (UCTD)**

Also called mixed connective tissue disease (MCTD)
Features of scleroderma, polymyositis, and SLE
Antibodies to RNP
Responds to corticosteroids
Prognosis better than systemic sclerosis

**Eosinophilic fasciitis**

Resembles scleroderma, but without Raynaud's phenomenon and usually spares hands
Follows physical exertion in 50% of cases
Skin and fascia of extremities involved
Rarely has systemic features
Responds to corticosteroids

**Chronic graft versus host disease**

History of bone marrow transplant

**Scleredema**

Induration and edema of skin on the upper back, neck
Follows upper respiratory infection
Idiopathic form seen in diabetics

**Porphyria cutanea tarda (PCT)**

Sclerodermoid changes rarely
May improve with PCT treatment

*Skeletal muscle.* Patients with diffuse scleroderma may have some mild muscle atrophy but two other forms of myopathy exist. The most frequent is a bland, nonprogressive process characterized by mild proximal weakness, minimal elevation of serum creatine kinase, and a noninflammatory fibrotic replacement of myofibrils on muscle biopsy. A second type is seen in patients with overlap connective tissue syndromes who have impressive weakness, markedly increased creatine kinase, and a classic inflammatory myopathy indistinguishable from polymyositis.

*Intestinal tract.* Gastrointestinal involvement occurs in most patients and differs little between the diffuse and limited subgroups. Distal esophageal motor dysfunction results from weakness and incoordination of esophageal smooth muscle and leads to a distal dysphagia. The lower esophageal sphincter musculature is similarly affected, resulting in reflux of gastric contents into the distal esophagus and peptic esophagitis. This may be complicated by ulcerations and stricture, which are particularly common in longstanding limited cutaneous disease. Symptomatic gastric emptying malfunction is much less common, although the duodenum is frequently affected, leading to postprandial abdominal pain and bloating.

Hypomotility of the jejunum and ileum is similar to hypomotility of the esophagus (loss of smooth muscle function). Fortunately, clinically meaningful syndromes such as malabsorption or pseudoobstruction are infrequent. Intestinal malabsorption occurs in some patients because the small bowel hypomotility results in bacterial overgrowth that interferes with normal fat absorption. Symptoms of malabsorption and bacterial overgrowth include persistent diarrhea and impressive weight loss. Intermittent episodes of abdominal distention may occur and lead to vomiting after meals. More severe, prolonged painful episodes of pseudoobstruction mimic mechanical obstruction and can lead to unnecessary surgery.

Patchy smooth muscle atrophy of the large intestine leads to the development of characteristic wide-mouthed diverticula, which are unique to systemic sclerosis. Colonic hypomotility may result in obstipation. Some patients experience incontinence or rectal prolapse resulting from rectal sphincter incompetence.

A cine-esophagram in the supine position demonstrates decreased peristaltic activity of the lower two thirds of the esophagus, often with wide open reflux. Later the organ may be grossly dilated and completely nonfunctioning. Roentgenograms may also demonstrate evidence of duodenal atony and dilatation *(loop sign)* or dilatation and hypomotility of the small bowel.

***Lungs.*** Clinical evidence of pleural involvement, including pleuritic pain or a pleural friction rub, is infrequent. Clinical or radiographic evidence of pulmonary interstitial fibrosis develops in most SSc patients. Abnormalities on pulmonary function tests also are common. The most frequent of these abnormalities are a decline in forced vital capacity (restrictive lung disease) and a reduced diffusing capacity for carbon monoxide (DLCO). There is a wide variability in the severity and course of the interstitial fibrosis. Many patients do not complain of dyspnea, even with mild to moderate decreases in the forced vital capacity. Progression is variable; the majority of patients maintain mild dysfunction without progressing to a severe, terminal illness. The few patients who become incapacitated usually have a rapid reduction in forced vital capacity during the first several years of disease. Death may occur after 5 to 10 years of scleroderma symptoms. Bronchoalveolar lavage and high resolution CT scan can help to determine if alveolitis is present early in the course of the disease.

In addition to a restrictive pattern on pulmonary function tests, patients may demonstrate an isolated decrease in the DLCO with the forced vital capacity remaining normal or near normal. Unless the DLCO is less than 50%, this is not a worrisome finding. Most people do not have progressive lung disease. Patients with a low DLCO are at high risk of developing isolated pulmonary arterial hypertension, which develops in a small proportion of patients, nearly all of whom have limited cutaneous involvement. This condition is heralded by rapidly progressive dyspnea and marked reduction of diffusing capacity (usually less than 50% of predicted normal). Other pulmonary function test results are normal or only mildly abnormal. Interstitial fibrosis on chest radiograph is absent or mild and is not nearly severe enough to result in such dramatic pulmonary hypertension. Histologically, the small pulmonary arteries show intense subintimal hyperplasia without inflammation. The prognosis is grave with the mean survival only 2 years.

***Heart.*** Clinical evidence of myocardial involvement is uncommon (less than 15%) and is more frequent in patients with diffuse scleroderma. In contrast, cardiac tests including electrocardiogram, echocardiogram, Holter monitor, and nuclear cardiac studies show evidence of asymptomatic left ventricular dysfunction, conduction abnormalities, arrhythmias, or pericardial effusions in a high proportion of patients. The symptomatic manifestations of myocardial disease include recalcitrant congestive heart failure and a variety of atrial and ventricular arrhythmias. The mortality rate is high. Patchy replacement of the myocardium and conducting system by fibrous tissue is the rule in such cases. Interestingly, the vascular changes that occur in most other organs are not found in similar-sized blood vessels in the heart.

Acute pericarditis or pericardial tamponade is also unusual, but echocardiographic and pathologic evidence of asymptomatic pericardial involvement with effusion is considerably more frequent. The right ventricle is secondarily affected in the end-stage pulmonary diseases of either interstitial fibrosis or pulmonary arterial hypertension.

***Kidneys.*** Renal involvement is manifested by scleroderma renal crisis, a potentially deadly process. This dramatic complication once was the major cause of death in patients with the diffuse cutaneous involvement. It affects approximately 20% of individuals with diffuse disease and typically occurs early (less than 4 years after disease onset) and during the phase of rapidly progressive skin thickening. In contrast, renal crisis is rare in patients with limited cutaneous involvement, and a more slowly progressive chronic renal process rarely, if ever, occurs.

Without warning, the patient develops malignant arterial hypertension with hyperreninemia and oliguric acute renal failure. Fatigue, headache, and shortness of breath may be present. This is occasionally accompanied by hypertensive encephalopathy or acute congestive heart failure. At presentation, the urinalysis usually shows small amounts of protein and microscopic hematuria. The serum creatinine may be normal or elevated. If not treated promptly, these patients rapidly develop progressive renal insufficiency. Occasionally, the blood pressure remains normal; in these instances microangiopathic hemolytic anemia with thrombocytopenia is generally prominent. This type of hemolysis may also occur with the malignant hypertension, and is an intravascular rather than an immune-mediated problem.

The primary targets in renal crisis are interlobular and arcuate arteries and arterioles. Severe mucoid subintimal hyperplasia is evident histologically, and blood vessel walls may undergo fibrinoid necrosis. An inflammatory component and immune complex deposition are lacking.

***Other organs.*** Sjögren's syndrome has been confirmed in 20% or more of SSc patients, but symptoms of Sjögren's syndrome, including dry eyes and dry mouth, may also be due to glandular fibrosis. Both lymphocytic inflammation *(Hashimoto's thyroiditis)* and fibrous replacement of the thyroid have been observed and are commonly associated with clinical evidence of hypothyroidism. Biliary cirrhosis is found in a few women with limited scleroderma, but hepatic involvement is otherwise rare. Trigeminal sensory neuropathy has been described.

### Laboratory findings

The routine laboratory tests from a typical SSc patient are generally unremarkable. The erythrocyte sedimentation

**Table 85-1.** Autoantibody subsets in scleroderma

| Antibody | Staining pattern | Clinical subset | Specificity |
|---|---|---|---|
| Antinuclear | Varied | 80% of all patients | Some other connective tissue diseases |
| Anticentromere | Centromere | Limited scleroderma | Sometimes in Raynaud's phenomenon |
| Antitopoisomerase (Scl-70) | Speckled | ¾ diffuse, ¼ limited<br>Peripheral vascular pulmonary fibrosis | Highly specific for SSc |
| Anti-Th | Nucleolar | Limited scleroderma | Rarely Raynaud's phenomenon |
| Anti-RNA polymerase III | Speckled/nucleolar | Diffuse scleroderma<br>Severe skin disease<br>Renal crisis | Highly specific |
| Anti-U1 RNP | High-titered<br>Speckled | Overlap with lupus and myositis (mixed connective tissue disease) | Not for SSc alone |
| Anti-U3 RNP | Nucleolar | Diffuse > limited<br>Black race | Highly specific |
| Anti-PM/Scl | Nucleolar | Overlap with myositis | Polymyositis |

rate is generally normal or slightly elevated. Anemia may result from peptic esophagitis, malabsorption, or microangiopathic hemolytic anemia associated with renal crisis, but otherwise the hemoglobulin is normal.

Nearly all patients with SSc have serum antinuclear antibodies. These antibodies are frequently associated with a distinct clinical subset of patients (Table 85-1). Anticentromere antibody (centromeric staining on routine immunofluorescence) is highly specific for limited cutaneous scleroderma. Antitopoisomerase I (or Scl-70) tends to identify individuals with diffuse cutaneous disease with more frequent pulmonary fibrosis and peripheral vascular difficulties, although about one quarter remain with limited skin thickening. Anti-Th (nucleolar staining) accounts for a small number of limited disease patients and some primary Raynaud's phenomenon patients. Anti-RNA polymerase III (speckled and nucleolar staining) identifies a large group of diffuse disease patients at the greatest risk of developing severe skin thickening and renal crisis. Finally, several autoantibodies appear to correlate with SSc in overlap syndromes, especially with polymyositis. They include anti-U1 RNP (speckled pattern), associated with the classic mixed connective tissue disease, anti-U3 RNP (nucleolar), and anti-PM Scl (nucleolar).

## DIFFERENTIAL DIAGNOSIS

The diagnosis of SSc is usually not difficult because of the characteristic findings in scleroderma. Early diffuse scleroderma can be confused with other forms of arthritis or some endocrine, cardiac, or renal diseases that result in similar types of edema. There are many scleroderma-like diseases (see the box at right) that, although infrequent, can mimic scleroderma; localized forms of scleroderma, including morphea and eosinophilic fasciitis, are the most common. The absence of Raynaud's phenomenon and atypical distribution of skin thickening are helpful clues. The chemically-induced scleroderma-like illnesses, including toxic oil syndrome, bleomycin, and tryptophan-induced eosinophilic myalgia syndrome are particularly interesting from a pathogenetic standpoint.

### Disorders that resemble scleroderma (pseudoscleroderma)

**Primary cutaneous disease**

Scleredema
Porphyria cutanea tarda
Scleromyxedema
Lichen sclerosus et atrophicus

**Systemic diseases**

Amyloidosis
Juvenile onset diabetes mellitus
Acromegaly
Carcinoid syndrome
Phenylketonuria
Werner syndrome
Graft vs. host disease

**Chemically induced**

Polyvinyl chloride
Organic solvents, epoxy resins
Bleomycin
Contaminated L-tryptophan (eosinophilic myalgia syndrome)
Rapeseed oil (toxic oil syndrome)

## TREATMENT

Treatment of SSc has been a major challenge. The relative rarity of the disease makes performing double-blind, controlled trials difficult. There also is a wide spectrum of manifestations, severity, and disease courses. In addition, spontaneous improvement may occur, rendering interpretation of the results of therapeutic intervention impossible without untreated comparison groups.

### Disease modifying agents

Many drugs are being studied for SSc treatment, since no single agent has proven convincingly effective. Fig. 85-7 summarizes the pathogenesis of SSc and the potential sites of drug actions. Vascular abnormalities, immune mechanisms, and collagen production are all possible areas for therapeutic intervention, but thus far no effective agent has been found.

D-penicillamine, an immunomodulating agent that also interferes with crosslinking of collagen, is the most

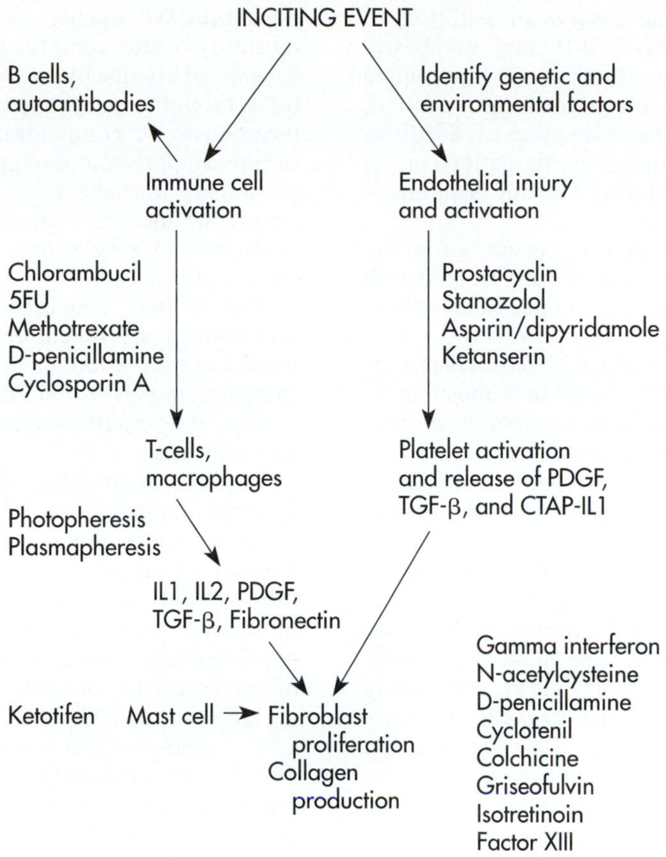


**Fig. 85-7.** Hypothetical pathogenesis of systemic sclerosis and the location of the possible sites where drugs might be useful for therapeutic intervention. Identification of inciting events, the alteration of T-cell function, and endothelial cell activity may interfere with the stimulation of the fibroblasts' production of collagen. There are a variety of ways in which drugs can interfere with collagen production directly. Further investigation will greatly influence the future of the treatment of systemic sclerosis.

widely used drug in the treatment of scleroderma. A large retrospective study showed that patients receiving D-penicillamine had a significant improvement in skin thickening after two years of therapy and an improved 5-year survival compared with similar untreated patients. Methotrexate, cyclosporin A, extracorporeal photopheresis, and γ interferon are currently being evaluated.

## Management of affected organ systems

Although no cure or remittive drug for this disease exists, there are many ways patients can be treated to improve or stabilize different aspects of their disease. Raynaud's phenomenon is the most common symptom in SSc patients. Abstinence from smoking, avoidance of cold temperatures, and commonsense measures are usually effective for mild to moderate symptoms. Raynaud's phenomenon associated with scleroderma is more frequently accompanied by digital tip ulcers, requiring the use of vasodilators. Calcium channel blockers (especially nifedipine, which relaxes vascular smooth muscle) have been effective in decreasing the frequency and severity of Raynaud's phenomenon in double-blind studies. The slow release preparation has improved tolerance, with fewer patients experiencing headaches or hypotensive symptoms. Other agents, including prazosin and topical nitroglycerin, have also helped some patients.

Local management of digital tip ulcers includes soaking the affected fingers in antiseptic fluid such as half-strength hydrogen peroxide, air drying, and then covering only the ulcer with antibiotic ointment and a bandage. This occlusive type of dressing promotes wound healing and protects from trauma and infection. When an ulcer becomes infected, a trial of oral antistaphylococcal antibiotics should be given. For deeper infections, surgical debridement of devitalized tissue and intravenous antibiotics may be necessary. Avoidance of amputation preserves the greatest amount of tissue.

Local skin care for dryness includes avoiding excessive bathing, which dries skin, and using moisturizing creams containing lanolin. Pruritus, often a serious problem early in the course of diffuse disease, has no effective treatment. Fortunately, it usually disappears with time. Likewise, calcinosis cannot be prevented or dissolved. The inflammatory process associated with hydroxyapatite crystal deposition may be controlled with a brief course of colchicine or another antiinflammatory agent.

Joint and tendon sheath involvement is common. Treatment with nonsteroidal antiinflammatory drugs (NSAIDs) is helpful, but relief is often more difficult to achieve than in other connective tissue diseases. In early diffuse disease, tenosynovitis can be painful, limiting joint movement. When NSAIDs fail to control pain, low dose corticosteroids (prednisone less than 10 mg/day) and/or narcotic analgesics may be necessary. In addition to medication, early aggressive physical therapy emphasizing stretching is important to prevent or to minimize contractures. Active and passive stretching exercises themselves can be quite painful. The use of adequate analgesia is required to optimize participation in an exercise program. Dynamic splinting has not been effective.

Carpal tunnel symptoms, which often occur before the diagnosis of scleroderma, can be successfully treated with resting wrist splints and/or local steroid injections without requiring surgery.

Inflammatory myositis is treated with corticosteroids and sometimes requires the addition of immunosuppressive drugs, but the bland, fibrotic myopathy is best managed with strengthening exercises alone.

Esophageal dysmotility most commonly causes heartburn and lower dysphagia. In some patients, symptomatic relief may be achieved by having the patient elevate the head of the bed on 4 to 8 inch blocks, eat frequent small meals in an upright position, abstain from nocturnal eating, and use antacids frequently. However, the mainstay of therapy is histamine blockade. The newest and most potent of those agents is omeprazole, which completely eliminates heartburn in most patients; however, it is only recommended for intermittent use. Calcium channel blockers, which decrease lower esophageal sphincter pressure, and NSAIDs often aggravate reflux symptoms. Prokinetic drugs such as metaclopramide are used to stimulate esophageal muscle contraction but have limited effectiveness. Distal esophageal stricture is managed with periodic dilatations. Surgical procedures for reflux have not achieved general acceptance because of their high failure rate.

Primary small bowel involvement with delayed transit and bacterial overgrowth may result in abdominal distention (or bloating), diarrhea, weight loss, and malabsorption. Broad spectrum antibiotics, such as ampicillin, tetracycline, trimethoprim-sulfamethoxazole, metronidazole, or ciprofloxacin, given in tandem in 2-week courses or continuously in low doses may produce a dramatic effect on these symptoms. Metaclopramide or cisapride also may be useful. Poor nutrition may require hyperalimentation. The first approach to patients with pseudoobstruction should be conservative (nonsurgical decompression) with nasogastric suction, bowel rest, and observation.

Pulmonary interstitial disease has become a major therapeutic problem in SSc. Fortunately, most patients have mild, nonprogressive involvement that does not require treatment. Attempts to reverse advanced, fixed fibrosis have been unsuccessful. In contrast, treatment of inflammatory alveolitis identified by bronchoalveolar lavage may prevent further fibrosis. Corticosteroids, and more recently cyclophosphamide, have had variable success in altering the progression of lung disease in such patients. The best hope for patients with advance end-stage pulmonary interstitial fibrosis is a single- or double-lung transplant; however, few have been performed.

Isolated pulmonary arterial hypertension without significant interstitial fibrosis has the worst prognosis of all scleroderma visceral problems. No therapy, including potent vasodilators, antiinflammatory agents, and immunosuppressive agents, has altered the progression or mortality of this complication; it is uniformly fatal within 5 years of its discovery. Most patients die from arrhythmias brought on by hypoxia, pulmonary arterial *in situ* thrombosis, or cor pulmonale resulting from respiratory failure. Supplemental oxygen, anticoagulation (to prevent pulmonary thromboembolism), and control of right heart failure are the best supportive measures available. Again, heart-lung or single-lung transplant is the only effective therapeutic option.

Pericarditis, congestive heart failure, and serious arrhythmias are potential complications of SSc. All are treated as they would be independent of scleroderma. Mild to moderate pericardial effusions and other asymptomatic cardiac abnormalities usually do not progress and require no treatment.

In previous decades, renal crisis was the most feared visceral complication of SSc. Renal failure typically occurred since there was no effective pharmacologic method of managing malignant hypertension. With the introduction of angiotensin-converting enzyme (ACE) inhibitors, which are capable of reversing underlying hyperreninemia and controlling hypertension, the outcome of renal crisis has dramatically changed. Patients now have an 80% 1-year and 60% 5-year survival in contrast to a 15% 1-year survival without the use of ACE inhibitors. The key to successful treatment is early detection and rapid normalization of the blood pressure. ACE inhibitors are the most reliably effective agents, but other new and potent antihypertensives may be added if necessary. In some cases, renal failure ensues despite early and vigorous intervention. However, approximately 50% of those patients progressing to dialysis who remain on ACE inhibitor therapy have enough improvement in renal function to discontinue dialysis 6 to 18 months later. Although there still is no effective cure for scleroderma, important advances in the management of visceral involvement have led to improved survival.

## LICHEN SCLEROSUS ET ATROPHICUS

***Epidemiology/etiology.*** Lichen sclerosus et atrophicus (LSA) is a chronic skin disease of unknown etiology although recent evidence has suggested a possible etiologic role for the spirochete *Borrelia burgdorferi.* LSA has a predilection for genital areas. Women are thought to be affected more than men, although one study of 76 patients with LSA showed no sex difference. A subset of patients with LSA is that of prepubertal girls with involvement of the vulva and perineum. Most commonly, LSA develops in postmenopausal women and in men 40 to 60 years old.

***History/physical examination.*** Pruritus and burning sensation are the most common symptoms associated with LSA, especially with genital involvement. The characteristic feature of LSA is the development of ivory white papules that gradually evolve into plaques and patches of slightly sclerotic (indurated) skin with atrophy and wrinkling of the epidermis. Small hyperkeratotic follicular plugs are also characteristic. The atrophic patches can become bullous and hemorrhagic, or can erode repeatedly, resulting in scarring. In men, the distribution of lesions is most often on the glans penis (balanitis xerotica obliterans) although other cutaneous involvement can be seen. In women, genital involvement can include labia majora and minora, clitoris, perineum, and perianal skin. The term kraurosis vulvae applies to vulvar involvement with LSA. Other cutaneous involvement is commonly truncal or on distal extremities.

***Differential diagnosis/laboratory evaluation.*** The differential diagnosis of LSA includes localized scleroderma (morphea), atrophic lichen planus, and cutaneous discoid lupus erythematosus. Skin biopsy for routine staining usually shows characteristic findings of sclerosis in the upper dermis that confirm the diagnosis.

***Management.*** Mild cases are best treated with medium or low potency topical corticosteroids (Group IV, V for extragenital, Group VI or VII for genital, see Table 20-1). The use of topical testosterone propionate 2% has also been successful. Twice daily application is best, and some patients benefit from alternating the use of corticosteroids and testosterone. The goal of treatment is palliation, since the disease tends to be chronic. The majority of prepubertal girls with LSA improve spontaneously at menarche. In older patients with LSA, squamous cell carcinoma can develop within the lesions in up to 10% of cases. Periodic examination and biopsy of suspicious areas is indicated.

## BIBLIOGRAPHY

Clements PJ et al: Muscle disease in progressive systemic sclerosis: diagnostic and therapeutic considerations, *Arthritis Rheum* 21:62, 1978.

Follansbee WP: The cardiovascular manifestations of systemic sclerosis (scleroderma), *Curr Probl Cardiol* 11:245, 1986.

Kahaleh MB: The role of vascular endothelium in the pathogenesis of connective tissue disease: endothelial injury, activation, participation and response, *Clin Exp Rheumatol* 8:595, 1990.

Kovalchik MT et al: The kidney in progressive systemic sclerosis: a prospective study, *Ann Intern Med* 89:881, 1978.

LeRoy EC: A brief overview of the pathogenesis of scleroderma (systemic sclerosis), *Ann Rheum Dis* 51:286, 1992.

LeRoy EC et al: Scleroderma (systemic sclerosis): classification, subsets and pathogenesis, *J Rheumatol* 15:202, 1988.

Maricq H: Diagnostic potential of in vivo capillary microscopy in scleroderma and related disorders, *Arthritis Rheum* 23:183, 1980.

Masi AT et al: Preliminary criteria for the classification of systemic sclerosis (scleroderma), *Arthritis Rheum* 23:581, 1980.

Okano Y, Steen VD, Medsger TA Jr: Novel human serum autoantibodies reactive with RNA polymerase III: a major autoantigen in systemic sclerosis with diffuse cutaneous involvement, *Ann Intern Med* 119:1005, 1993.

Reimer G: Autoantibodies against nuclear, nucleolar and mitochondrial antigens in systemic sclerosis (scleroderma), *Rheum Dis Clin North Am* 16:169, 1990.

Roumm AD et al: Lymphocytes in the skin of patients with progressive systemic sclerosis: quantification, subtyping and clinical correlations, *Arthritis Rheum* 27:645, 1984.

Silver R et al: Cyclophosphamide and low dose prednisone therapy in systemic sclerosis (scleroderma) patients with interstitial lung disease, *J Rheumatol* 20:838, 1993.

Smith C: Controlled trial of nifedipine, *Lancet* 1:76, 1982.

Steen VD: Epidemiology of rheumatic disease: systemic sclerosis, *Rheum Dis Clin North Am* 16:641, 1990.

Steen VD et al: Clinical associations of anticentromere antibody (ACA) in patients with progressive systemic sclerosis, *Arthritis Rheum* 27:125, 1984.

Steen VD et al: Outcome of renal crisis in systemic sclerosis: relation to availability converting enzyme (ACE) inhibitors, *Ann Intern Med* 113:352, 1990.

Steen VD et al: Isolated diffusing capacity reduction in systemic sclerosis, *Arthritis Rheum* 35:765, 1992.

Steen VD, Medsger TA Jr, Rodnan GP: D-penicillamine therapy in progressive systemic sclerosis (scleroderma), *Ann Intern Med* 97:652, 1982.

Stupi AM et al: Pulmonary hypertension (PHT) in the CREST syndrome variant of progressive systemic sclerosis (PSS), *Arthritis Rheum* 29:515, 1986.

CHAPTER

# 86 Sjögren's Syndrome

**Ann L. Parke**

## EPIDEMIOLOGY AND ETIOLOGY

Sjögren's syndrome (SS) is defined as the presence of xerostomia (dry mouth) and xerophthalmia (dry eyes). Unfortunately, there are many reasons for patients to complain of dry eyes and dry mouth (see the box on p. 1180), and this has led to confusion in defining a specific, separate disease entity. Therefore the diagnosis of SS should be limited to patients who have a specific pathologic disease process, namely, an autoimmune exocrinopathy demonstrated by the infiltration of T helper cells into exocrine glands. In this chapter this pathologic disease process is called Sjögren's disease (SD).

SD may be found in patients who have a well-defined rheumatologic disease, such as rheumatoid arthritis or systemic lupus erythematosus (SLE), and these patients are defined as having secondary SS/SD. Patients with sicca complaints who do not have an additional rheumatologic disease are defined as having primary SS/SD.

The difficulties that arose from the original definition of SS led to the development of several sets of criteria, the most recent being the European criteria for SS. Each of these sets of criteria has its limitations because they are all based primarily on investigations designed to evaluate glandular function. The California and the Greek criteria require pathologic changes that demonstrate an autoimmune exocrinopathy (i.e., a positive lip biopsy). However, as many as 30% of lip biopsies may be falsely negative, which means that, although these criteria may be very specific, they are not sensitive.

Manthorpe and colleagues commented on four sets of criteria and stated that the prerequisite for a positive lip biopsy overemphasizes the oral component of the disease. There is some disagreement with this opinion considering that a positive pathologic specimen (either salivary or lacrimal) is necessary to understand this disease process

### Causes of xerostomia and xerophthalmia

**Xerostomia**

Medications:
- Tricyclic antidepressants: amitriptyline (Elavil), doxepin (Sinequan)
- Antihistamines: diphenhydramine (Benadryl), chlorpheniramine (Chlor-Trimeton), promethazine (Phenergan), and many cold and decongestant preparations
- Anticholinergic agents: antiemetic agents such as scopolamine, antispasmodic agents such as oxybutynin chloride (Ditropan)

Dehydration due to
- Debility
- Fever

Polyuria due to
- Alcohol intake
- Arrhythmias
- Diabetes

Previous head and neck irradiation

Systemic diseases
- Sjögren's syndrome
- Sarcoidosis
- Amyloidosis
- HIV infection
- Graft-versus-host disease

**Xerophthalmia**

See medications and systemic diseases listed above

Abnormalities of eyelid function
- Neuromuscular disorders
- Aging
- Thyrotoxicosis

Abnormalities of tear production
- Hypovitaminosis A
- Stevens-Johnson syndrome
- Familial diseases affecting sebaceous secretions

Abnormalities of corneal surface
- Previous scarring: old injuries, herpes simplex infection

and to identify the clinical and laboratory features associated with it.

The lack of a precise definition makes it difficult to assess the prevalence of true SS/SD. Previous estimates based on the assumption that at least 50% of patients with rheumatoid arthritis have SS/SD and 50% of patients with SS/SD have primary disease as opposed to secondary, have led to the conclusion that SS/SD is the most common connective tissue disease, with more than 4 million afflicted Americans. True SS/SD is probably more common in postmenopausal women, for unknown reasons.

### Genetic factors

Although etiology of SS/SD is unknown, there is now considerable evidence demonstrating the abnormal expression of autoantigen, activation of infiltrating lymphocytes, and local synthesis of autoantibodies at the primary site of pathology (i.e., the exocrine glands). These findings are all evidence of a local immune response.

HLA antigens play a vital role in individualizing the immune response by virtue of their function of presenting antigen to T cells, and the presence of specific HLA markers dictate the host's ability to respond to specific environmental triggers. There are now many diseases associated with the presence of specific HLA antigens. Some autoimmune diseases in particular are associated with the presence of HLA-A1, B8, and DR3. SD has also been reported to be associated with B8 DR3 antigens, but is most closely associated with the DRw52 antigen. It has also been demonstrated that the production of antibodies to the Ro and La nuclear antigens is associated with Dr3 and DR2. DR3 is in linkage disequilibrium with DQ2, and DR2 with DQ1. Subsequent studies have demonstrated that Sjögren patients who are heterozygous for both DQ1 and DQ2 alleles are more likely to produce these autoantibodies. Antibodies to Ro and La have been shown to be associated with more severe systemic SD and may be useful to test for prognosis. See the section on laboratory studies for recommendations.

### Environmental factors

Viruses have been implicated in the pathogenesis of a variety of autoimmune diseases, but the evidence for this association remains inconclusive. Interest in this area has been renewed recently, however, because of the autoimmune complaints associated with HIV infection. Some patients infected with HIV develop xerostomia and xerophthalmia. Biopsies of the salivary glands of these patients demonstrate lymphocytic infiltrates, but these are predominantly T suppressor cells, as opposed to the T helper cells that are found in patients with SD.

Some retroviruses are trophic for the ductal epithelium of salivary and lacrimal glands. Epstein-Barr virus, a DNA virus that belongs to the herpes virus family, is excreted in saliva and is known to be associated with the development of nasopharyngeal carcinoma. This virus infects B cells and promotes B cell proliferation.

A variety of studies have suggested an association between EB virus and SS. Peripheral blood mononuclear cells taken from Sjögren's patients are more likely to contain EB virus DNA than are cells from normal controls, and it is easier to establish B cell lines expressing EB nuclear antigen when the B cells are taken from Sjögren's patients than when taken from control subjects. However, not all studies agree with these findings.

Most recently attention has been directed to an association between SS/SD and hepatitis C infection. Hepatitis C is excreted in saliva, and some patients with hepatitis C infection have been noted to develop sicca complaints. A recent study has also demonstrated that more than 50% of patients with chronic hepatitis C liver disease have focal lymphocytic infiltrates in salivary gland biopsies. If this is confirmed, it would mean that hepatitis C is one of the few diseases capable of producing a falsely positive lip biopsy.

## PATHOPHYSIOLOGY

### Infiltrates of T cells into glandular tissues

Histopathologic changes found in the salivary glands of SD patients include a benign lymphoepithelial lesion and focal lymphocytic sialoadenitis. Benign lymphoepithelial lesions (BLEL) are found in approximately 40% of *major* salivary glands from patients with SS, and this term defines a pathology where the salivary epithelium is replaced and infiltrated with lymphocytes. Epimyoepithe-

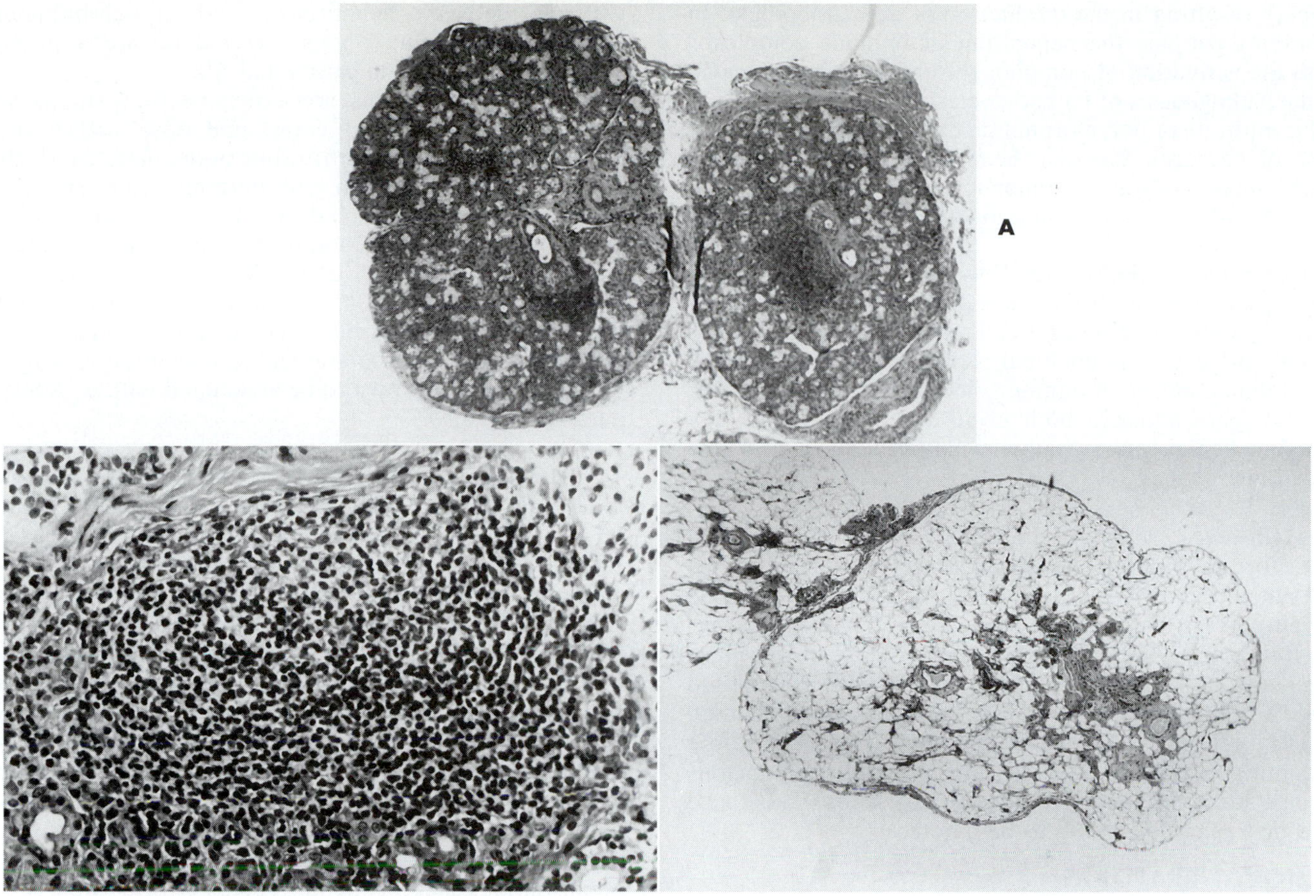

A

B

C

**Fig. 86-1.** **A,** Salivary gland biopsy magnified ×40 showing foci of lymphocytes. **B,** High power view of lymphocytic focus (×250). **C,** Salivary gland biopsy magnified ×40 showing loss of glandular tissue and atrophy with no lymphocytic foci.

lial islands, remnants of ductal epithelium, are found, which help to distinguish this lesion from overt lymphoma. A pathologic feature found in the *minor* salivary glands of these patients is a focal lymphocytic infiltrate that consists primarily of an infiltrate (Fig. 86-1) of T helper cells. This pathology, however, is not specific for SD. Other disease entities, such as sarcoidosis and more recently the diffuse infiltrative lymphocytosis syndrome (DILS) found in patients infected with HIV-1, may show similar pathologic changes.

Xerophthalmia and xerostomia may be consequences of senescence. Studies suggest that glandular fibrosis and atrophy are a feature of aging. Fatty change with some slight nonspecific inflammatory cell infiltrate may occur in normal, healthy salivary glands.

### B cell hyperactivity

***Autoantibody production.*** Autoantibody production is a feature of SS/SD. Most commonly organ-nonspecific antibodies are produced, including antinuclear antibodies (ANAs) and rheumatoid factor. There are numerous nuclear antigens, and therefore a variety of autoantibodies can give positive immunofluorescence when reacting with nuclei. The pattern of the produced reaction can vary and to some extent depends on the antigenic specificity of the antibody. Sjögren's patients most frequently produce a speckled ANA with the major antibody reactivity directed toward the extractable nuclear antigens Ro and La (SSA and SSB). Approximately 60% of primary SS/SD patients have the antibody to Ro, but this is not specific for SS/SD, and patients with SLE (30%) and subacute cutaneous SLE (60%) may also produce this antibody. Recent work has suggested that Sjögren's patients and SLE patients produce antibodies to different fractions of the Ro antigen. Antibodies to the 52 kiloDalton (kD) band occur more commonly in Sjögren's patients, whereas antibodies to the 60-kD band occur more commonly in patients with SLE.

Ro antibodies are reported to be associated with the more severe complaints of SD (e.g., vasculitis). Antibodies to La rarely occur alone and are nearly always associated with antibodies to Ro. The finding of La antibodies in saliva suggests that there is local glandular production that it is antigen driven.

Rheumatoid factor is an autoantibody that is much less specific for SS/SD. It has been suggested that IgA rheumatoid factor may occur more commonly in both the blood and saliva of patients with SS/SD than in patients with other autoimmune diseases. Mixed cryoglobulinemia may also be found in patients with SS/SD and is more commonly found in patients who produce autoantibodies, in particular, Ro antibodies. Cryoglobulinemia may be associated with the development of vasculitis (as can any disease resulting in the production of autoantibodies). In Sjögren's patients the deposition of immune complexes with the activation of complement has been incriminated in the pathogenesis of leukocytoclastic vasculitis (perivascular infiltrate of polymorphonuclear leukocytes). Another type of vasculitis has also been described in which the predominant infiltrate is mononuclear. The pathogenesis of this type of vasculitis is unknown.

*Hypergammaglobulinemia.* Polyclonal hypergammaglobulinemia is another marker denoting B cell hyperactivity. In some individuals B cell reactivity becomes oligoclonal or even monoclonal with the production of monoclonal spikes on immune electrophoresis and monoclonal light chains in both urine and serum. This may remain a benign gammopathy or may be associated with a B cell malignancy.

*Malignancy.* Patients with SS/SD are at an increased risk for developing non-Hodgkin's lymphoma. It is estimated that fewer than 10% of Sjögren's patients develop overt malignancy. The majority of these lesions are low-grade lymphomas, and some of these lesions have been noted to regress spontaneously. It has been suggested that B cell hyperactivity may progress from benign reactivity through a phase called pseudolymphoma before becoming overtly malignant. This pseudolymphomatous change must be managed aggressively if progression to true malignant change is to be averted.

## CLINICAL FEATURES

### Glandular disease

The predominant site of pathology in SD is the exocrine gland. The previously described lymphocytic infiltrate results in acinar destruction, and it is only when this process has progressed sufficiently that the patient becomes clinically dry. The most frequent complaints are those of xerostomia and xerophthalmia, but exocrine glands throughout the body are frequently affected, leading to the complications of dry skin, dry airways, and a dry vagina. These patients also have an increased predisposition to develop autoimmune thyroiditis and pancreatitis.

### Extraglandular disease

It must be remembered that SD is a systemic disease; therefore it is not surprising that lymphocytic infiltrates have been identified in tissues other than exocrine glands (kidneys, lungs, liver, skin, and muscles). It is unclear whether the abnormal physiology of these affected organs is due to the lymphocytic infiltrate, the deposition of immune complexes, or the local synthesis of $\gamma$-globulin.

*Gastrointestinal and hepatic disease.* More than 70% of patients with primary biliary cirrhosis and 40% of patients with chronic active hepatitis complain of dry eyes or dry mouth. The relationship of SD to these autoimmune hepatic diseases, which have fairly specific autoantibody production, is unclear, but the liver is an exocrine gland and it has been suggested that all features can be explained as consequences of damage to the ductal epithelium.

With recent interest directed once again toward a viral etiology for connective tissue diseases, and the known association between hepatitis B and the vasculitides as well as between hepatitis C and cryoglobulinemia, attention has recently been directed toward a possible association between hepatitis and SS.

Nutritional problems are extensive for patients with SS/SD. Rampant dental caries and oral candidiasis (a consequence of dry mouth) result in the inability to chew and a sore painful mouth with burning mouth syndrome. The lack of saliva makes it difficult to form a bolus of food. Dysphagia is further complicated by a dry esophagus, esophageal dysmotility, or esophageal candidiasis. Atrophic gastritis, pancreatitis, and small bowel malabsorption have all been described. There are several reports documenting the association of celiac disease with SS. Celiac disease is known to be associated with a variety of autoimmune diseases.

*Renal disease.* Renal tubular acidosis (RTA) may occur in as many as 30% of SS/SD patients. Type I RTA (distal RTA) occurs most commonly, but both distal and proximal RTA have been described in association with SS/SD. These abnormalities are frequently subclinical and detected only when the patient cannot produce an acidic urine, even when challenged. In some patients, however, hypokalemia, polyuria, metabolic acidosis, nephrocalcinosis, and renal stones are overt manifestations of the disease.

Glomerulonephritis may occur in any disease that results in the production of increased levels of circulating immune complexes. Patients with SS/SD are no exception, and proliferative, membranoproliferative, and membranous glomerulonephritis have been described. Glomerulonephritis may also occur in patients with cryoglobulinemia. Any glomerulonephritides must be treated aggressively to preserve renal function.

*Pulmonary disease.* Pleurisy may occur in patients with SLE and rheumatoid arthritis, but it is comparatively rare in patients with SS/SD. Recurrent pulmonary infection is an expected feature of patients with SS/SD, but some studies suggest that this is not the case. Lymphocytic infiltrate may occur in the pulmonary interstium, however, making SS/SD one of the causes of lymphocytic interstitial pneumonitis (LIP).

*Neonatal lupus syndrome.* An immune-mediated disease of neonates has been described that is considered to be due to the transplacental passage of the maternal antibody. The clinical features of this syndrome are a transient photosensitive rash and/or primary congenital complete heart block that is permanent. Children with primary congenital complete heart block have an overall mortality rate of 30%, and 50% require pacemakers. Maternal antibody to the 52-kD fraction of Ro antigen and to the 48-kD La antigen carries an odds ratio of 35 for developing the permanent features of this syndrome. However, not all mothers with these antibodies produce abnormal infants, and a fetal factor determining infants at risk must play a role. The same mother can produce both normal and abnormal children with no variation in maternal antibody status. Some of these mothers are clinically normal even though the antibodies are present.

*Other extraglandular involvement.* Recent interest has been directed toward the neurologic manifestations of

SS/SD. It has been suggested that 25% of patients have central nervous system (CNS) manifestations, some presenting with features suggestive of multiple sclerosis. Other investigators have been unable to substantiate these reports, leading to the impression that, although patients with autoimmune disorders may develop a variety of neurologic complaints, CNS disease is rare in Sjögren's patients.

Other features commonly associated with autoimmune connective tissue diseases may occur. Thirty percent of patients with primary SS/SD may complain of Raynaud's phenomenon. Arthritis and arthralgias are a common complaint, but boggy synovitis is rare. Patients with primary SS/SD rarely complain of photosensitivity, even though they may have the antibody to Ro antigen, which appears to predispose lupus patients to photosensitive rashes. This may be due to the fact that Sjögren's patients appear to have the antibody to a separate fraction of Ro antigen. The most common skin complaint in primary SS/SD is a petechial rash (hypergammaglobulinemia purpura), most commonly found on the legs. Biopsy of these lesions reveals vasculitis. In time the legs become pigmented because of constant hemosiderin deposition in the skin. Other skin complaints include dryness, urticarial-like lesions, erythema multiforme, and necrotizing panniculitis.

## EVALUATION

### Clinical history

A full history must be taken looking for complaints that are compatible with xerostomia and xerophthalmia. Fatigue often is a dominant symptom. Features suggestive of an underlying connective tissue disease must be sought, and direct questioning must therefore include questions about photosensitivity, alopecia, mucosal ulceration, and Raynaud phenomenon as well as a family history of connective tissue diseases. It is also important to take a full obstetric history because it is now evident that abnormal pregnancies may be one of the earliest presentations suggesting a potential for developing a connective tissue disease (e.g., the neonatal lupus syndrome).

### Physical examination

***Oral component of Sjögren's syndrome.*** The examination for the presence of oral dryness includes an examination of the tongue for redness, dryness, and loss of papillae. An evaluation should be performed of sublingual pooling and overall moistness of the oral cavity. Evaluating saliva production can be done using the Saxon test, which requires chewing on a 4 × 4 gauze swab for 2 minutes. The difference in weight of the swab before and after chewing is a measure of the saliva produced in those 2 minutes (normal in our institution is over 1 g or 1 ml per minute).

Patients with dry mouths are at risk for the development of oral candidiasis. These patients frequently do not show the usual white plaques that are commonly associated with oral candidiasis. It is therefore very important to culture for *Candida* even if an oral inspection is not typically performed for this problem.

Patients who complain of xerostomia should have a lip biopsy performed. This can be done in an outpatient setting using local anesthesia with epinephrine to minimize blood loss. Patients who take nonsteroidal drugs are usually not troubled by excessive bleeding but patients who take anticoagulants may have additional blood loss that requires suturing. Routinely, however, the mouth heals well and the wound does not require sutures. All patients requiring antibiotic coverage for prophylaxis to prevent bacterial endocarditis must be covered with antibiotics when having a minor salivary gland biopsy. The biopsy involves the removal of 5 to 10 small salivary glands from the inside of the lower lip, according to the technique of Daniels. Lip biopsies should be evaluated according to the method described by Greenspan and colleagues. A focal score greater than 1; i.e., more than 50 cells/4 mm$^2$ area of gland is considered a positive biopsy, suggesting an autoimmune exocrinopathy.

***Ocular component of Sjögren's syndrome/Sjögren's disease.*** Evaluating the ocular component of SS/SD can be done in the clinic with a Schirmer test. This involves placing filter papers inside the lower lid at the junction of the nasal and middle thirds of the lid for 5 minutes and measuring the length of the filter paper that is made wet by tears (normal is considered greater than 5 mm of wetting per 5 minutes).

All other testing should be done by an ophthalmologist and include the Rose bengal test (any residual staining is abnormal), examination of the tear film and height, examination for the presence of cells and/or cellular debris as well as mucus and mucous debris, fluorescein staining and a tear breakup time.

Rose bengal staining can be done in the clinic but some patients react adversely to the preservative used in this stain. We generally choose not to do this test in our clinic. Other tests, including tear osmolality and tear lactoferrin levels, are available only in specialized centers.

***Glandular function and glandular inflammation.*** Scintigraphy is used to evaluate these parameters. Technetium scanning measures glandular function. The glandular uptake is evaluated by scanning the patient for 20 to 25 minutes. The patient is then given a lemon stimulus to promote glandular emptying and is then scanned for an additional 20 to 25 minutes. Glandular uptake and glandular secretion can therefore be measured.

Gallium scanning is a useful test for inflammation and has been found to be positive in approximately 70% of patients with sarcoidosis, a disease that can cause false positive biopsies when evaluating patients for SS/SD. Some centers prefer to use sialography, claiming that scintigraphy with either gallium or technetium is too insensitive. However, we are concerned about the long-term consequences of instilling contrast into chronically inflamed tissues and prefer to use scintigraphy methods.

### Laboratory studies

Autoantibody tests include those for rheumatoid factor and ANA, FARR (antibody to native double-stranded DNA), and extractable nuclear antigens (ENA) that includes Ro, La, Sm, and RNP. In patients with Ro antibodies additional studies can be done to determine if the Ro antibodies are directed against the 60-kD or the 52-kD component of the Ro antigen, since this has been shown to be useful in differentiating between patients with SLE and patients with SS/SD.

These patients may also have antibodies to thyroid tissue as well as antimitochondrial antibodies and anti-liver–kidney microsomal antibodies, both of which are associated with autoimmune liver disease. However, these tests should not be included in the initial evaluation.

Routine laboratory tests include complete blood count (CBC) differential, erythrocyte sedimentation rate (ESR), platelet count, urinalysis, electrolytes, alanine aminotransferase (ALT) and aspartate aminotransferase (AST), amylase, lipase immunoglobulin levels, complement levels, and cryoglobulins. If cryoglobulins are found, patients should be screened for hepatitis C infection. Immunoglobulin levels plus immunoglobulin electrophoresis must be done to look for a monoclonal spike. Low complement levels may signify complement consumption and indicate the potential for vasculitis. We order blood work and a chest x-ray annually. This is done primarily as a screening for occult lymphoma along with a full examination for lymphadenopathy and hepatosplenomegaly. It has been suggested that a fall in the titre of autoantibodies (ANA and rheumatoid factor) may herald the onset of premalignant or malignant changes.

## DIFFERENTIAL DIAGNOSIS

The differential diagnosis of xerostomia and xerophthalmia includes all of the diseases listed in the box on p. 1180.

Patients with obvious extraglandular disease and other features suggestive of an autoimmune disease are sometimes difficult to differentiate between primary and secondary SS/SD, especially patients with SLE. The diagnosis of SLE generally requires the presence of four of 11 ARA criteria, although some patients may have SLE even though at a particular time, they do not meet criteria.

Sicca complaints are the end stage of this disease. These patients probably have had their autoimmune exocrinopathy for many years before they developed symptoms of dryness. Patients therefore may not complain of dryness but may present with other complaints. Hence it is important to remember SS/SD in patients presenting with any of the extraglandular complaints listed previously, especially patients who have major organ damage, such as immune-mediated liver disease and renal tubular acidosis.

Diseases that can give a false positive lip biopsy include sarcoidosis and DILS, a syndrome that is associated with HIV infection. These HIV-positive patients are more likely to be young males than elderly, postmenopausal women. Patients with DILS frequently have massive glandular swelling with numerous extraglandular manifestations. The autoantibody production that commonly occurs in classic SD is infrequent in these patients and HLA associations are different with DR5 and DR6 occurring in African-American DILS patients and DR6 in white patients.

The usual pathology of sarcoidosis is noncaseating granulomas. Sarcoid patients may also produce rheumatoid factors and have elevated immunoglobulin levels (IgG). However, the chest x-ray is usually abnormal in these patients, revealing either bilateral hilar adenopathy or diffuse parenchymal disease. Gallium scanning is positive in approximately 65% to 70% of these patients, with a positive panda sign detected as the gallium is taken up by the parotid, lacrimal, and submandibular glands. An identical pattern may be seen in patients with SS/SD (Fig. 86-2), but Sjögren's patients do not develop the lambda sign outlining the trachea and its bifurcations that is frequently found in sarcoid patients.

### Artificial tears and ointments

**With preservative**

***Tears***

Hypotears
Tears naturale
Adsorbotear
Murocel
Tears plus
Liquifilm

***Ointments***

Duratears
Lacrilube

**Without preservative***

***Tears***

Hypotears PF
Tears naturale free
Cellufresh
Refresh

***Ointments***

Duolube
Lacriserts
Refresh PM

* Some patients develop reactions to the preservatives in artificial tears, but those preparations without preservatives are generally more expensive. Different patients find different preparations useful.

## MANAGEMENT

### Nonpharmacologic

Artificial tears and artificial saliva are mainstays of treatment for SS. Such therapy often reduces, but does not eliminate, the symptoms of dryness. Artificial eyedrops appear to be more effective than artificial saliva. Various preparations are now available (see the box above), including a long-acting substitute eyedrop that can last up to 12 hours. One problem is that some patients are sensitive to the preservatives used to make artificial tears. Patients frequently have to experiment to find out which product they can tolerate and which suits them best. Eyedrops produced without preservatives are more expensive.

Other measures that are used to protect the dry eye include the use of moisture chamber glasses. These glasses look like protective goggles, with a protective screen extending down the arms of the glasses. This minimizes the effects of wind and automobile heating and cooling systems blowing onto the dry eye surface. Those patients who have continuing sicca problems with the cornea and who are at risk for ulceration may benefit from the use of soft contact lenses. Such patients should consider punctal occlusion in an attempt to preserve more of a tear film on

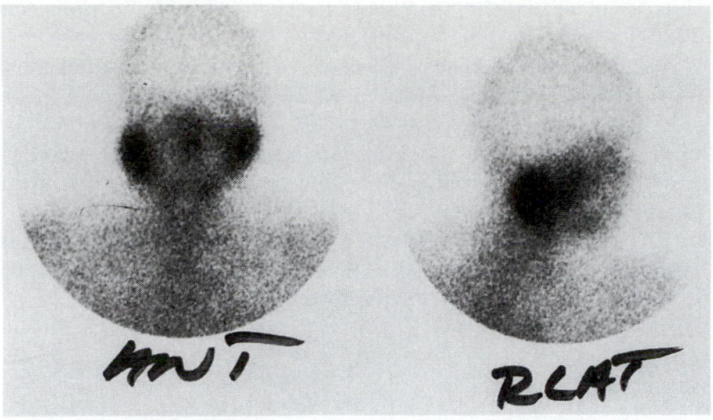


**Fig. 86-2.** "PANDA SIGN" in a patient with Sjögren's disease demonstrated by the uptake of gallium-67 citrate in the parotid and submandibular glands. In this particular patient, uptake by the lacrimal glands is not marked.

the eye surface. Stents can be inserted as a temporary measure to determine if there is a benefit to the patient before surgical ablation of the punctum is performed.

Saliva substitutes are less effective at maintaining moisture in the mouth than artificial tears are for maintaining moisture in the eyes. This is because they do not last long enough. Patients frequently carry water bottles with them, and some find that mixing water with a little glycerin and lemon and using a spray bottle to apply the solution is more palatable and feels better than simply sipping water. Constant chewing or sucking helps to stimulate saliva secretion, but a major problem with this approach is rampant dental caries if sugarless products are not used. Fluoride-containing gel used twice a day is essential.

Oral candidiasis is another problem, resulting in a sore, painful mouth that further hinders eating. The usual oral preparations for treating candidiasis frequently contain sugar, and for this reason we prefer to prescribe vaginal suppositories to treat this problem in patients who are not edentulous. Patients should be treated for at least 1 month. We also recommend that patients eat live culture yogurt daily. Studies have demonstrated that yogurt containing lactobacilli can prevent recurrent vaginal candidiasis, and this may also help to prevent yeast colonizing the mouth and esophagus.

Skin dryness may respond to moisturizers, whereas vaginal dryness may be improved with KY jelly or replens.

### Dietary

Other approaches that are currently being developed are the use of polyunsaturated fatty acids, such as γ-linoleic acid (the major constituent of oil of evening primrose). Ingesting these fats results in the synthesis of fewer inflammatory prostanoids, and studies have demonstrated that these agents may be useful in the management of rheumatoid arthritis.

### Pharmacologic

The pharmacologic approach to managing these patients can be divided into two groups: the agents used for promoting secretions (sialogogues and mucolytic agents) and antiinflammatory agents.

Agents that promote the production of natural secretions have been tried, and most recently pilocarpine (a cholinomimetic alkaloid) has been reported to be useful. However, the only currently approved use for pilocarpine is as eyedrops for the treatment of glaucoma. Side effects from pilocarpine include bronchospasm, abdominal cramping, diarrhea, bradycardia, and hypotension.

Mucolytic agents, such as bromhexine and acetylcysteine, have been reported to be useful but some controlled studies have not found a benefit. Many patients report finding relief with bromhexine. This agent is not available in the United States, and patients go to extreme lengths to obtain it.

Hydroxychloroquine (Plaquenil) is a very good agent for treating arthritis and skin disease in patients with rheumatoid arthritis and SLE. Recent work suggests that it may also be beneficial to patients with SS/SD, although this has not been confirmed by all studies. Some patients feel that hydroxychloroquine not only improves their arthralgias and arthritis but also reduces the overwhelming fatigue that is often a major component of this disorder.

Corticosteroids and immunosuppressive agents should be reserved for patients with severe extraglandular disease where end-organ failure is a potential problem. Such patients may need high-dose corticosteroids as well as additional immunosuppression. Methotrexate is not a well-recognized agent for managing SS/SD. However, some patients with SS/SD secondary to rheumatoid arthritis also experienced an improvement in their sicca complaints as well as in their underlying arthritis when treated with methotrexate. The use of azathioprine (Imuran) should be discouraged, since these patients are already at an increased risk of developing lymphoma. Cyclophosphamide should be used only as intermittent boluses due to the risk of bladder toxicity, including hemorrhagic cystitis or malignancy with daily oral therapy.

### Psychosocial/family approach

The constant fatigue and difficulty of eating and talking are severely debilitating for SS/SD patients. This sicca complex can lead to major psychosocial and family problems. It is therefore vital that these patients have access to support groups through the Arthritis Foundation, the Sjögren's Syndrome Foundation, or the National Sjögren's Syndrome Association, (see box on p. 1186) where patients can benefit from the experience of others and take comfort in the knowledge that they are not alone in coping with this disease. The Sjögren's Syndrome Foundation also publishes *The Moisture Seekers Newsletter,* which discusses the condition and treatments while the National Sjögren's Syndrome Association publishes the *Sjögren's Digest.*

### Continuing follow-up and care

Patients with SS/SD must have regular follow-up with an ophthalmologist who specializes in the dry eye, a dentist who has expertise in the dry mouth, and either a rheumatologist or an internist. Preventing the major medical problems associated with SS/SD is an essential aspect of care. An awareness of other exocrine glandular involvement is essential because some patients require pancreatic supplementation and others become thyrotoxic or diabetic.

## Resources

Arthritis Foundation
P.O. Box 19000
Atlanta, GA 30326
1-800-283-7800

Sjögren's Syndrome Foundation, Inc.
382 Main Street
Port Washington, NY 11050
516-767-2866
FAX: 416-767-7156

*The Moisture Seeker's Newsletter*
Published by the Sjögren's Syndrome Foundation, Inc.
382 Main Street
Port Washington, NY 11050

National Sjögren's Syndrome Association
3201 West Evans Drive
Phoenix, AZ 85023
602-516-0787
FAX: 602-516-0111

*Sjögren's Digest*
Published by the National Sjögren's Syndrome Association
3201 West Evans Drive
Phoenix, AZ 85023

### Indications for consultation and hospitalization

Patients with extraglandular diseases pose additional problems. These patients generally have a more severe disease and require aggressive therapy with corticosteroids or immunosuppressive agents. The development of major-organ damage and/or associated vasculitis are of particular concern and require consultation with a rheumatologist.

## BIBLIOGRAPHY

Alexander EL et al: Sjögren's syndrome: association of anti-Ro-SS-A antibodies with vasculitis, hematologic abnormalities, and serologic hyperreactivity, *Ann Intern Med* 98:155, 1983.

Alexander EL: Neuromuscular complications of primary Sjögren's syndrome. In Talal N, Kassan SS, editors: *Sjögren's syndrome. Clinical and immunological aspects,* Berlin, 1987, Springer-Verlag.

Buyon JP et al: Acquired congenital heart block. Pattern of maternal antibody response to biochemically defined antigens of the SSA/Ro-SSB/La system in neonatal lupus, *J Clin Invest* 84:627, 1989.

Flescher E, Talal N: Do viruses contribute to the development of Sjögren's syndrome? *Am J Med* 90:283, 1991.

Fox PC et al: Pilocarpine treatment of salivary gland hypofunction and dry mouth (xerostomia), *Arch Intern Med* 151:1149, 1991.

Fox RI et al: Treatment of primary Sjögren's syndrome with hydroxychloroquine, *Am J Med* 85(suppl 4A): 62, 1988.

Greenspan JS et al: The histopathology of Sjögren's syndrome in labial salivary gland biopsies, *Oral Surgery* 37:217, 1974.

Kohler PF, Winter ME: A quantitative test for xerostomia: the Saxon test, an oral equivalent of the Schirmer test, *Arthritis Rheum* 28:1128, 1985.

Leventhal LJ, Boyce EG, Zurier RB: Treatment of rheumatoid arthritis with gammalinoleic acid, *Ann Intern Med* 119:867, 1994.

Manthorpe R et al: Sjögren's syndrome: comments on the proposed criteria for classification, *Arthritis Rheum* 30:954, 1987.

Pavlidis NA et al: Lymphoma in Sjögren's syndrome, *Med Pediatr Oncol* 20:279, 1992.

Silverman ED: Congenital heart block and neonatal lupus erythematosus: prevention is the goal, *J Rheumatol* 20(7):1101, 1993.

Sjogren H: Keratoconjunctivitis sicca, *Hygie* 82:829, 1930.

Talan N et al: Detection of serum antibodies to retroviral proteins in patients with primary Sjögren's syndrome (autoimmunity exocrinopathy), *Arthritis Rheum* 33:774, 1990.

Vitali C et al: Preliminary criteria for the classification of Sjögren's syndrome. Results of a prospective concerted action supported by the European Community, *Arthritis Rheum* 36(3):340, 1993.

CHAPTER

# 87 Infectious Agents and the Musculoskeletal System

**Bernard Zimmermann III**
**Edward V. Lally**
**Nancy Y.N. Liu**

Musculoskeletal infections constitute an important group of illnesses for which patients commonly seek primary care. Acute inflammation of a joint, bursa, or tendon must be identified as either infectious or noninfectious to institute proper treatment. The history and physical examination are of paramount importance to the initial diagnosis of these syndromes, whereas confirmation is provided by the appropriate use of laboratory data. This chapter reviews the diagnosis and treatment of the most common bacterial infections that affect the musculoskeletal system: septic arthritis, septic bursitis, and osteomyelitis. In addition, viral arthritis, HIV-associated musculoskeletal syndromes, and Lyme disease are discussed.

## SEPTIC ARTHRITIS

### Epidemiology and etiology

Acute bacterial septic arthritis is an urgent medical emergency because of the potential for joint destruction and mortality if the diagnosis and treatment are delayed or overlooked. The most common presentation of septic arthritis is that of an acutely painful and swollen joint in the setting of preexisting arthritis. In most cases septic arthritis is caused by the hematogenous spread of bacteria to a joint that was previously damaged by arthritis or injury. More than half of the patients with septic arthritis have preexisting arthritis, usually osteoarthritis or rheumatoid arthritis. Skin flora are the most common sources of infection, but upper respiratory, gastrointestinal, and genitourinary portals of entry are also found. Rarely septic arthritis may follow a penetrating injury or may be related to contiguous osteomyelitis, especially in children. The knee is the joint most commonly affected by septic arthritis followed, in decreasing order of frequency, by the shoulder, hip, elbow, wrist, ankle, and small joints of the hands and feet.

Seventy-five percent to 80% of cases of nongonococcal bacterial septic arthritis in adults are caused by gram-positive bacteria, (usually *Staphylococcus* or *Streptococ-*

**Table 87-1.** Microbiology of bacterial septic arthritis related to age of patient*

| | Children (6 mo-5 yr) | Young adult | Adult | Elderly |
|---|---|---|---|---|
| *Staphylococcus aureus* | 10% - 20% | 15% - 20% | 60% - 70% | 45% - 65% |
| *Streptococci* | 5% - 10% | 1% - 5% | 15% - 20% | 10% - 15% |
| Gram negative | 1% - 5% | Rare | 10% - 15% | 15% - 35% |
| *Haemophilus influenzae* | 30% - 50% | 1% - 5% | 1% - 5% | Rare |
| *Neisseria gonorrhoeae* | 1% - 5% | 60% - 80% | 1% - 5% | Rare |

*Percentages compiled from several studies.

*cus*), but 15% to 20% of these infections are caused by gram-negative organisms (Table 87-1). The incidence of gram-negative septic arthritis, particularly *Escherichia coli,* has risen somewhat in the past 20 years. These infections occur notably in elderly, debilitated patients; intravenous drug users; and young children. Anaerobic joint infections, although still rare, have also increased in frequency and are most commonly found in association with postoperative wound infections, especially following total joint replacement. A variety of unusual organisms, including fungi and mycobacteria, have been reported to cause septic arthritis. These usually present as chronic insidious infections.

## History

Risk factors for septic arthritis in addition to a preexisting joint disorder include intravenous drug use, chronic systemic illnesses such as cancer, diabetes mellitus, systemic connective tissue diseases, and sickle-cell disease, and the presence of a remote focus of infection. The patient usually complains of several days of progressive pain and swelling in one or more joints. There may be fever, sweats, or shaking chills indicative of systemic infection and cough or dysuria suggestive of an extraarticular source of bacteremia. Acute migratory polyarthritis with tenosynovitis in a young, sexually active adult suggests septic arthritis from disseminated gonococcal infection.

## Physical examination

The physical examination may yield findings of a source of infection such as pneumonia, otitis, pharyngitis, or cutaneous abscess. A synovial effusion is invariably present but may be difficult to discern in the obese patient. There is swelling, erythema, warmth, and limited range of motion of the affected joint. A complete musculoskeletal examination should be performed to investigate the possibility of polyarticular septic arthritis, which may be found in 20% of cases.

## Diagnosis

The definitive diagnosis of septic arthritis depends on the analysis of synovial fluid obtained by arthrocentesis. Septic synovial fluid appears cloudy or purulent. Essential laboratory studies are shown in the box below. The Gram stain demonstrates bacteria in 50% to 75% of cases of nongonococcal bacterial septic arthritis and should be used to guide the initial choice of antibiotic therapy. Synovial fluid white blood cell (WBC) counts greater than 50,000 signify a high probability of infection, although gout and acute flares of rheumatoid arthritis may produce this degree of inflammation. Bacterial septic arthritis, particularly with disseminated gonococcal infection, may occasionally present with a lower synovial fluid WBC count. Radiographs of the affected joints should be obtained to assess underlying arthritis, investigate for contiguous osteomyelitis, and establish a baseline for future compari-

### Essential laboratory studies in septic arthritis

**Synovial fluid**

| | |
|---|---|
| Gram stain | Positive in 50% to 75% of cases (less in gonococcal arthritis) |
| Culture | Essential for diagnosis and treatment (may be negative in patients taking antibiotics) |
| White blood cell count | >50,000 is indicative of infection (lower in gonococcal arthritis) |
| White blood cell differential | >95% polymorphonuclear leukocytes is indicative of infection |
| Crystal analysis | Presence of crystals does not exclude infection |

**Blood**

| | |
|---|---|
| Peripheral | |
| White blood cell count | Elevated in most cases |
| Blood cultures | Positive in 50% of cases |

**Radiology**

X-ray of affected joint evaluates for preexisting arthritis and possible osteomyelitis son. Blood cultures are also necessary to determine the presence of bacteremia. Clues to the presence of extraarticular sources of infection should be pursued with appropriate diagnostic studies.

The differential diagnosis includes crystalline arthritis, acute viral arthritis, and nonseptic inflammatory arthritis. The patient with preexisting rheumatoid arthritis or another chronic inflammatory arthritis presents a particular diagnostic challenge, since septic arthritis may initially be mistaken for a flare of the underlying disease. A history of pain and swelling of one joint that is out of proportion to the others, or the presence of fever or systemic signs, should raise the suspicion of joint infection. The demonstration of monosodium urate or calcium pyrophosphate crystals by polarized microscopy establishes the diagnosis of acute crystalline arthritis in the appropriate clinical setting. However, care must be taken not to overlook the possibility of coexistent bacterial arthritis.

### Gonococcal arthritis

Disseminated gonococcal infection may present with manifestations of acute septic arthritis. Dermatitis-arthritis syndrome is usually seen in sexually active adults, often in females within 1 week of menstruation or in the postpartum period. Two thirds of patients have tenosynovitis that affects the tendon sheaths of the wrists, fingers, ankles, and toes. Approximately 50% of patients have frank arthritis that is commonly monoarticular but may progress to migratory or additive polyarthritis. Skin involvement occurs in as many as two thirds of patients with disseminated gonococcal infection. Cutaneous papules or pustules with an erythematous base are usually noted on the extremities and may have a necrotic center. The diagnosis must often be made on clinical grounds, since the synovial fluid WBC counts are lower than those seen with nongonococcal bacterial infections (range 30,000 to 60,000), the Gram stain is often nondiagnostic, and even careful cultures plated on chocolate agar are positive in only 25% of cases. To increase the yield of positive cultures, urethral, cervical, blood, and, when appropriate, rectal and pharyngeal cultures should be performed if disseminated gonococcal infection is suspected. Many skin and joint manifestations of the syndrome are mediated by circulating immune complexes rather than direct microbial infection. The emergence of penicillin-resistant strains of gonococci requires third-generation cephalosporins in geographic areas where resistance is common.

## Management and outcome

The treatment of nongonococcal bacterial septic arthritis requires hospitalization for initiation of intravenous antibiotic therapy and joint drainage. Adult patients with synovial fluid revealing gram-positive cocci should be treated initially with nafcillin, 2 g intravenously every 4 hours. Alternatives include cefazolin, 1 g intravenously every 8 hours, vancomycin, 1 g intravenously every 12 hours, or clindamycin, 600 mg intravenously every 6 hours. If gram-negative bacilli are the only organisms found in the aspirate, two antibiotics with gram-negative activity should be initiated, such as ceftriaxone, 1 to 2 g intravenously every 24 hours, and gentamicin, 1.5 mg/kg intravenously every 8 hours. Alternative agents for ceftriaxone include ciprofloxacin, imipenem-cilastatin, or aztreonam. If the Gram stain is unrevealing or equivocal, initial antibiotics should broadly cover gram-positive and gram-negative organisms. Empiric therapy with an antistaphylococcal agent, such as nafcillin, combined with an aminoglycoside or other antibiotic active against gram-negative organisms is appropriate.

**Table 87-2.** Antibiotic therapy of presumed bacterial arthritis in adults (pathogen unknown)

| Gram stain | Presumed organism(s) | Antibiotic(s) |
|---|---|---|
| **Positive** | | |
| Gram-positive cocci | *Staphylococcus aureus* | Oxacillin or nafcillin (alternatives: cefazolin or vancomycin) |
| Gram-positive cocci (prosthetic joint) | *Staphylococcus epidermidis, Staphylococcus aureus* | Vancomycin |
| Gram-negative cocci | *Neisseria gonorrhoeae* | Ceftriaxone |
| Gram-negative bacilli | *Escherichia coli, Serratia marcescens, other Enterobacteriaceae* | Third-generation cephalosporin, imipenem, aztreonam, or ciprofloxacin* (in cases of bacteremia or severe infection the addition of an aminoglycoside) |
| Gram-negative bacilli (thin) | *Pseudomonas aeruginosa* | Ceftazidime, piperacillin, imipenem, or aztreonam, plus tobramycin |
| **Negative** | | |
| Noncompromised host | *Staphylococcus aureus, Enterobacteriaceae*† | Nafcillin plus gentamicin or a third-generation cephalosporin (ceftriaxone or cefotaxime) plus vancomycin |
| Compromised host | *Staphylococcus aureus, Enterobacteriaceae, and Pseudomonas aeruginosa*† | Nafcillin plus gentamicin or a third-generation cephalosporin (ceftriaxone or cefotaxime) plus vancomycin and imipenem, ceftazidime, piperacillin, or aztreonam plus tobramycin |

Modified from Upchurch KS, Giansiracusa DF. In Rippe JM et al, editors: *Intensive care medicine,* ed 3, Boston, 1995, Little, Brown.
*Ciprofloxacin is available for parenternal use (400 mg IV q12h).
†Treatment for both gram-positive and gram-negative pathogens must be continued until cultures return.

Table 87-2 presents recommendations for the initial choice of antibiotics for adults based on the Gram stain and clinical setting. Results of culture and sensitivity analysis determine the final antibiotic selection (Table 87-3). Thorough drainage of the joint to remove inflammatory cells producing proteolytic enzymes must be accomplished by one of several techniques. In many cases, such as uncomplicated knee infections, satisfactory drainage may be achieved by daily closed-needle arthrocentesis. A poor clinical response is indicated by a rising WBC count and/or persistent culture positivity despite several days of antibiotic treatment. Under these circumstances more invasive methods of drainage, such as arthroscopy or open arthrotomy, should be employed.

When the inflammation subsides, physical therapy with passive mobilization followed by active strengthening of periarticular structures prevents joint contracture. Parenteral antibiotic therapy should continue for at least 3 to 4 weeks to ensure complete eradication of bacteria and prevent recurrence. Home intravenous therapy may be an effective alternative to prolonged hospitalization, particularly in the patient with an infection in a non–weight-bearing joint who has had a good initial response to antibiotics and drainage.

The outcome of treatment for septic arthritis depends on many variables, including the duration of the infection, the virulence of the organism, and the age and comorbidities of the patient. Virtually all patients with gonococcal arthritis recover completely, and infections with group A streptococci have a good outcome in 70% to 85% of cases. However, up to 50% of patients who have septic arthritis from *Staphylococcus aureus* or gram-negative infections have residual joint damage. Patients with rheumatoid arthritis who develop polyarticular infection have less than a 50% chance of survival.

## SEPTIC BURSITIS

Septic bursitis is a common soft-tissue infection encountered in the outpatient arena. Features of the history and examination readily distinguish septic bursitis from other causes of periarticular inflammation, such as septic arthritis, traumatic bursitis, and tendinitis. The diagnosis is confirmed by bursal fluid analysis and culture. Treatment with oral antibiotics and appropriate drainage usually results in a good functional outcome.

### Activities predisposing to the development of septic bursitis

**Prepatellar bursitis**

Carpet-laying
Plumbing
Wrestling
Crawling

**Olecranon bursitis**

Hemodialysis (dialysis elbows)

### Pathophysiology

The pathophysiology of septic bursitis differs from septic arthritis in that bacterial seeding is almost always via the transcutaneous route, and it is rarely associated with bacteremia. The subcutaneous olecranon and prepatellar bursae, located in the superficial tissue overlying the olecranon process and the patella, respectively, are the most frequently infected bursae. Local trauma may lead to superficial lacerations and abrasions, resulting in local cellulitis and bursal infection (see the box above). Infections of deep bursae, such as the subacromial and iliopectineal bursae, have occasionally been reported, but they are most often found in conjunction with infection of the contiguous joint.

The vast majority (80% to 100%) of cases of septic bursitis are caused by gram-positive organisms, with *Staphylococcus* being the most common. Streptococcal organisms, especially β-hemolytic streptococcus, account for 5% to 30% of infections. Case reports have described

**Table 87-3.** Antibiotic therapy of acute bacterial arthritis in the critically ill adult (known pathogen)

| Organism | Antibiotic choice | Alternatives |
|---|---|---|
| *Staphylococcus aureus* | Nafcillin, 9-12 g/day (q4h) or oxacillin, 9-12 g/day (q4h) | Cefazolin, 4.5-6 g/day (q8h), or vancomycin, 2 g/day (q12h) |
| *Staphylococcus aureus, methicillin resistant* | Vancomycin, 2 mg/day | None |
| *Streptococcus pyogenes, Streptococcus pneumoniae* | Penicillin G, 12-18 million U/day (q4h) | Cefazolin or vancomycin |
| *Neisseria gonorrhoeae* | Ceftriaxone, 1-2 g/day (q12h) | Tetracycline, aztreonam, or ciprofloxacin, or penicillin-G if sensitive |
| *Pseudomonas aeruginosa* | Piperacillin, 12 g/day (q4h), plus tobramycin, 4-5 mg/kg/day (q4h) | Ceftazidime, 3-6 g/day (q8h), or imipenem-cilastin Aztreonam, 3 g/day (q8h), or ciprofloxacin* plus gentamicin or amikacin |
| Enterobacteriaceae | Third-generation cephalosporin plus gentamicin, 4-5 mg/kg/day (q8h) | Aztreonam, 3 g/day (q8h) or ciprofloxacin* plus gentamicin or amikacin |

*Ciprofloxacin is available for parenteral use, 400 mg IV q12h.

Modified from Upchurch KS, Giansiracusa DF. In Rippe JM et al, editors: *Intensive care medicine,* ed 3, Boston, 1995, Little, Brown.

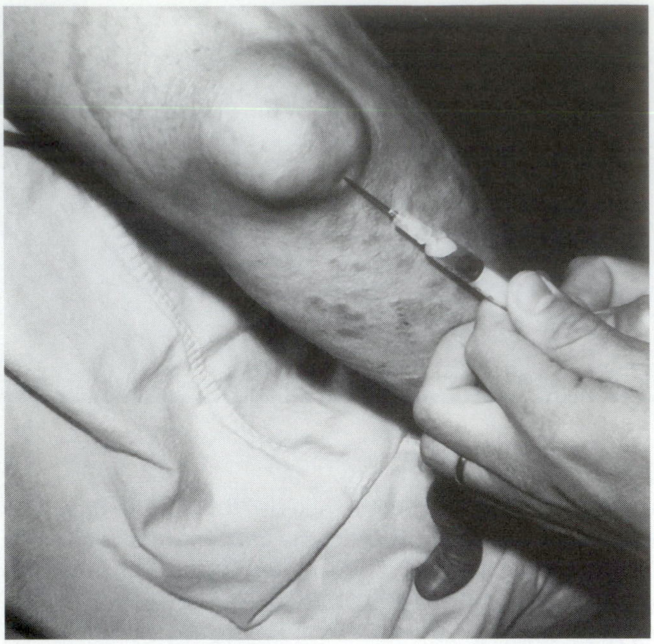

**Fig. 87-1.** Demonstration of technique for aspirating olecranon bursa. (From Ho G Jr, Mikolich D: *Clin Rheum Dis* 12:445, 1989.)

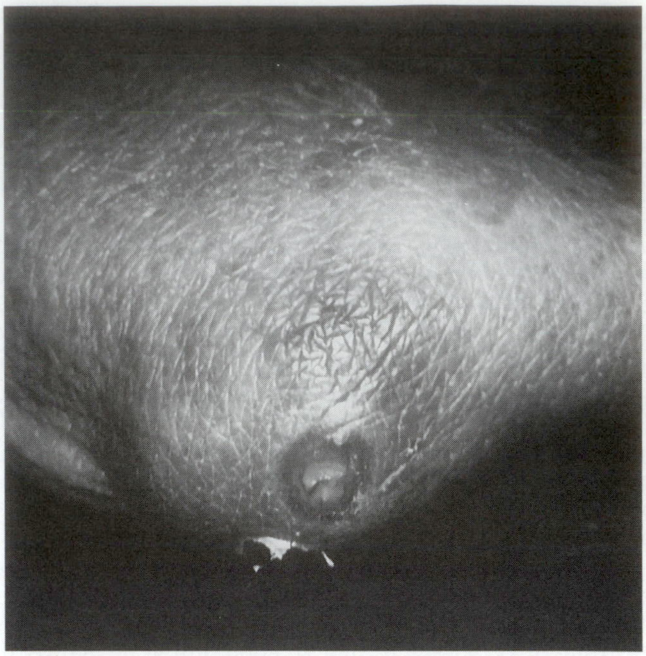

**Fig. 87-2.** Septic olecranon bursitis with large central abrasion and surrounding cellulitis. (From Ho G Jr, Mikolich D: *Clin Rheum Dis* 12:454, 1986.)

a variety of gram-negative, anaerobic, and fungal infections, but these are rare.

### History and physical examination

The presenting symptoms of septic bursitis are usually those of gradually progressive pain, warmth, and swelling around the elbow or knee. A history of acute or chronic antecedent trauma should be sought. Fever, chills, or systemic symptoms should raise the suspicion of a more serious infection. The physical examination often reveals discrete tenderness and swelling of the bursal sac, but there may be extensive surrounding erythema and cellulitis, which obscures the source of the infection. The absence of joint involvement can be inferred if there is a full passive range of joint motion. Articular fluid, if present, should be investigated for the possibility of septic arthritis, but in some cases arthrocentesis demonstrates a sterile sympathetic effusion.

### Laboratory studies and differential diagnosis

Needle aspiration of the inflamed bursal fluid provides both diagnostic information and relief of symptoms. The technique employs a large-bore (18- or 20-gauge) needle inserted into the bursal sac parallel to the long axis of the extremity with the joint extended. The insertion point should be away from the apex of the bursa in an area of more normal skin, if possible, to avoid poor wound healing and a chronic draining sinus tract (Fig. 87-1). Aspirated fluid should be sent for a WBC count with differential, Gram stain, and crystal analysis. Superficial septic bursitis is often less inflammatory than septic arthritis. The bursal fluid WBC count is less than 20,000 cells/mm$^3$ in 50% of cases, but the range may be as high as 100,000 cells/mm$^3$. The Gram stain reveals organisms in approximately 75% of cases, which serves to direct initial antibiotic treatment while culture results are pending. As in the diagnosis of the inflamed joint, the presence of intrabursal crystals does not rule out the possibility of a coexistent infection.

### Management

The proper treatment of septic bursitis includes appropriate antibiotic therapy, bursal drainage, and local care. An oral penicillinase-resistant antibiotic such as dicloxacillin, or a first-generation cephalosporin (cephalexin, 500 mg orally every 6 hours, or clindamycin, 300 mg every 6 hours) treats the most common pathogens and penetrates well into the inflamed bursa. Daily needle aspiration should be performed until the fluid is sterile and no longer reaccumulating. Clinical situations that require hospitalization for intravenous antibiotics include the presence of extensive cellulitis (Fig. 87-2), a debilitated or immunocompromised host, and evidence of systemic infection. Some authors recommend inpatient therapy for all cases of septic prepatellar bursitis because of the difficulty of eradicating organisms in the thick skin overlying the knee. In cases of recurrent or resistant infection surgical consultation is advised to obtain open drainage and to consider bursectomy for definitive therapy.

The outcome of therapy for septic bursitis is generally favorable, but some individuals have recurrent infections, especially if the behavior leading to the local trauma in the predisposed area is not modified.

## OSTEOMYELITIS

The clinical spectrum of osteomyelitis varies considerably depending on the age of the patient, the duration of infection, the anatomic location of bone involvement, a variety of host factors, the rapidity of diagnosis, and the

**Table 87-4.** Osteomyelitis in adult and pediatric age groups

| Parameter | Pediatric | Adult |
|---|---|---|
| Transmission | Hematogenous | Traumatic, contiguous focus (hematogenous) |
| Site | Growth plate—long bones | Diaphysis, vertebrae |
| Microbiology | *Staphylococcus aureus* | *Staphylococcus aureus* |
| | β-Hemolytic streptococci | *Staphylococcus epidermidis* |
| | | Gram-negative rods |
| | | Mixed (contiguous) |
| | | Fungi (IV drugs) |
| Risk factors | Indwelling catheters | Penetrating trauma |
| | Remote infection | Soft-tissue infection |
| | Bacteremia | Diabetes mellitus |
| | | Peripheral vascular disease |
| | | IV drug abuse |
| | | Immunosuppression |
| | | Sickle-cell disease |

adequacy of initial treatment. The ability to diagnose and adequately treat bone infections is a difficult exercise at best, but a clearer understanding of this disease has emerged in recent years.

## Pathophysiology

Osteomyelitis is generally divided into adult and pediatric categories and is considered in acute, subacute, and chronic forms (Table 87-4). Furthermore, vertebral osteomyelitis is a distinctly different entity from infections of the nonaxial skeleton.

In neonates and children hematogenous osteomyelitis most often results from a bacteremia or septicemia. Adult osteomyelitis is less likely to be hematogenous in origin and is usually associated with trauma or a contiguous focus of infection. The duration of infection (acute, subacute, or chronic), whether in the neonate, child, or adult, depends on the severity of the initial infection and the host's response to it.

In adults hematogenous osteomyelitis is much less common, but when it occurs it tends to affect the diaphysis and, if not adequately treated, the medullary canal. Osteomyelitis in the adult develops secondary to trauma; surgical procedures, including interosseous prosthetic devices; and contiguous soft-tissue infections.

Osteomyelitis in the adult may develop by hematogenous spread (although uncommon) and occurs most often in the vertebrae, particularly in the lumbar region. An apparent focus of infection at another site or a history of intravenous drug use is usually present. In the adult the arterial blood supply to the vertebrae ends at the vertebral endplate, and thus vertebral osteomyelitis is confined to the vertebral body and involves the disk only secondarily.

In adults, osteomyelitis most commonly develops secondary to trauma, contiguous infection, or surgical instrumentation. Bacteria are directly seeded into the bone at the level of the periosteum or medullary canal and produce an acute inflammatory reaction that often becomes subacute or chronic. In patients with vascular insufficiency the small bones of the feet are commonly involved with contiguous infection osteomyelitis.

The microbiology of osteomyelitis varies with the mode of transmission. Aerobic bacteria or fungi are most often associated with hematogenous osteomyelitis. In this setting a single pathogen is almost always responsible in both pediatric and adult cases. *S. aureus* is the most common organism in all age groups. In adult hematogenous osteomyelitis aerobic gram-negative rods and fungal species are frequently causative, particularly in elderly patients with an extraosseus focus of infection or in intravenous drug users.

In contrast to the single pathogens that are responsible for hematogenous osteomyelitis, patients with trauma-related or contiguous infection osteomyelitis are typically infected with mixed microbial species, although *S. aureus* and *S. epidermidis* are frequent participants. Aerobic gram-negative bacilli and anaerobic organisms are frequently isolated from these mixed microbial infections. Unique pathogens are found under certain clinical circumstances. *Pseudomonas* species are found commonly in drug addicts. Osteomyelitis in patients with SC (sickle cell–hemoglobin C disease) and SS (sickle cell anemia) hemoglobinopathies is often caused by *Salmonella.* In immunocompromised patients fungal species, particularly *Candida,* may be the causal agents.

## History

The symptoms of osteomyelitis may reflect an acute localized infection of abrupt onset or a smoldering infectious process that is poorly localized and is associated with a paucity of systemic symptoms. Osteomyelitis is categorized as acute, subacute, or chronic based on the historical duration of relevant symptoms. Overall, acute osteomyelitis is the most common form of the disease. The presentation is that of an acute febrile illness of a few days' duration. Localized pain in the axial or appendicular skeleton, accompanied by symptoms of acute infection, is the most common history obtained in adult osteomyelitis. Subacute or chronic osteomyelitis is usually a result of traumatic inoculation or transmission from a contiguous focus of infection. Pain is usually of longer duration, is less well localized, and frequently is not associated with systemic signs of infection.

In hematogenous osteomyelitis, risk factors are those

associated with bacteremia and include recent surgical or dental procedures, indwelling intravenous catheters, distant foci of infection (particularly of the skin and respiratory and urinary tracts), intravenous drug use, and an immunocompromised host. A history of localized or generalized trauma, including penetrating soft-tissue injuries, should be elicited. Patients with comorbid cardiovascular disease or diabetes mellitus are at increased risk for chronic osteomyelitis. A major risk factor for chronic osteomyelitis is inadequate treatment of acute osteomyelitis.

### Physical examination

The physical examination of acute osteomyelitis reveals signs of infection, including fever and warmth, erythema, swelling, and tenderness over the affected site. The clinical picture may be confused with cellulitis, but the localized nature of bony tenderness should raise the suspicion of underlying osteomyelitis. With vertebral involvement, the spine is often rigid and there is localized tenderness over involved vertebrae. Signs are frequently lacking in subacute or chronic osteomyelitis. Tenderness in the axial or appendicular skeleton is often poorly localized. In cases associated with trauma or contiguous soft-tissue infection, signs of osteomyelitis may be obscured by overlying inflammation. In patients with osteomyelitis contiguous with a joint, there may be evidence of acute septic arthritis. Careful neurologic examination should be performed, since patients with sensory peripheral neuropathies may have impaired pain perception.

### Laboratory and imaging studies

The ability to diagnose osteomyelitis depends on the host's ability to mount an appropriate localizing response to the osseous infection, as well as a high index of suspicion on the part of the physician. An accurate diagnosis requires the documentation of a microbial species from a culture of blood or infected bone. In acute, untreated hematogenous osteomyelitis, blood cultures are positive in approximately 50% of cases, but the offending organism can be cultured from involved tissue in a much higher percentage. In chronic osteomyelitis it is usually necessary to obtain bone tissue for culture, since blood cultures are usually negative.

Radiographic abnormalities may support a diagnosis of osteomyelitis but are usually not conclusive. Plain x-rays in acute osteomyelitis usually demonstrate no bony pathology. Subacute osteomyelitis may require 2 to 3 weeks for x-ray changes to appear. These include periosteal elevation, cortical erosions, or large lytic areas. X-rays of suspected osteomyelitis adjacent to joints may be confused in patients with preexisting erosive arthritis, such as rheumatoid arthritis or gout.

Radionuclide imaging has been advocated as an adjunctive method to assist in the diagnosis. $^{99m}$Tc, $^{67}$Ga citrate, or $^{111}$In chloride scans may become positive within 48 to 72 hours of infection, but false positive and false negative results are common. It is particularly difficult to interpret such scans in the presence of overlying soft-tissue infection or adjacent inflammatory arthritis. Most recently, the $^{111}$In-labeled leukocyte scan has been noted to have significant discriminatory capacity for osteomyelitis, particularly in diabetics and in patients with overlying soft-tissue infection. Computed tomography (CT) and magnetic resonance imaging (MRI) hold promise as diagnostic tests to define areas of osteomyelitis more accurately.

The standard method of diagnosing osteomyelitis demands a positive culture result from a tissue specimen involved with infection; arriving at a diagnosis using any other method is presumptive. Practically speaking, it is often difficult to make a culture-proven diagnosis, and management strategies are developed based on a high diagnostic probability for osteomyelitis. Culture of a single pathogen from blood or an overlying soft-tissue infection combined with high-probability radionuclide or plain x-ray imaging studies may warrant presumptive antibiotic therapy. Less specific therapy results when diagnostic data are inconclusive. It is recommended that, wherever possible, a surgical or a radiographically directed needle biopsy specimen of involved bone be obtained for culture and sensitivity before initiating antibiotic therapy.

## Management

Optimal treatment for osteomyelitis results from the early detection of bone infection and the isolation of a specific pathogen with known antibiotic sensitivities. Under these circumstances specific antibiotics can be administered. In early acute osteomyelitis intravenous antibiotics can be administered for a few days and then switched to oral antibiotics for up to 6 weeks. As initial therapy, antibiotics directed at *S. aureus* and β-hemolytic streptococci should be administered pending the results of culture sensitivities. Oxacillin (100 to 200 mg/kg per day), nafcillin, or benzylpenicillin (1 to 4 million Units per day) are reasonable choices. In penicillin-allergic patients a third- or fourth-generation cephalosporin is indicated. If the diagnosis of acute osteomyelitis is delayed for up to 2 weeks following symptoms, or if the patient has chronic osteomyelitis, drainage of pus and debridement of infected bone are essential adjuncts to antibiotic therapy. Treatment of overlying soft-tissue infection or the removal of prosthetic devices is also necessary in most cases to eradicate infection.

Chronic osteomyelitis requires antibiotic therapy directed at identified organisms with appropriate sensitivities. In blood culture–positive adult osteomyelitis antibiotics should be administered intravenously for at least 2 weeks and usually for 4 to 6 weeks. In osteomyelitis that is secondary to contiguous infection the microbial flora is usually mixed, and a single pathogen is unlikely to be isolated. Under these circumstances broad-spectrum antibiotics that target gram-positive cocci, aerobic gram-negative organisms, and, where appropriate, anaerobic or fungal species should be administered.

An issue of recent interest is the ability to treat chronic osteomyelitis with oral antibiotics after an initial treatment phase of parenteral medication. This approach has been advocated largely due to the availability of newer antibiotics, in particular the fluoroquinolones (ciprofloxacin, ofloxacin), that achieve excellent bone penetration and inhibit most strains of bacteria that cause osteomyelitis. It has been demonstrated that many patients with osteomyelitis may be treated entirely with prolonged oral courses of such agents. Exceptions to this include patients with diabetes mellitus and severe peripheral vascular disease. Such oral therapy is directly dependent on the ability to isolate the microbial pathogen (with appropriate antibiotic sensitivities) and to achieve a complete surgical debridement or excision of necrotic tissue. Nonetheless, in most cases of chronic osteomyelitis it is probably prudent to treat the patient with intravenous antibiotics for at least 2 weeks before considering a course of oral antibiotic medication. For patients in whom the bacteriology is unknown or uncertain, a full course of broad-spectrum intravenous antibiotics is still recommended.

The outcome in osteomyelitis depends directly on the ability to isolate a causative organism, initiate appropriate antibiotic therapy, and, where necessary, accomplish adequate surgical drainage. In adults with chronic soft-tissue infection, underlying diabetes, or peripheral vascular disease a cure frequently is not achieved. Progressive bone loss may occur and antibiotic therapy may only accomplish disease suppression.

## VIRAL ARTHRITIS

### Pathophysiology

Viruses have been implicated in a variety of musculoskeletal syndromes and rheumatic disorders. Chronic rheumatic disease, such as rheumatoid arthritis, may be triggered by viruses or viral antigens, although the exact etiologic role of these agents remains uncertain.

During an acute infection viremia is commonly associated with severe myalgias and arthralgias, irrespective of the causative viral species. Much less commonly frank arthritis or tenosynovitis is associated with an acute viral infection. Acute viral arthritis may be caused by direct viral replication in the joint or synovial tissue or, more commonly, by promoting an immune complex formation that serves to initiate an inflammatory cascade within the joint. The vast majority of acute articular syndromes (arthralgias and arthritis) are of short duration and do not lead to chronic arthritis or joint damage. However, certain viruses (human parvovirus, for example) often produce polyarthritis that is subacute or chronic.

An array of viruses has the potential to cause acute articular syndromes (see the box above), although frank arthritis has most often been associated with human parvovirus, hepatitis B virus, and rubella. The other viruses listed in the box are associated most often with transient polyarthralgias and no long-term joint damage.

### History

Patients who develop viral arthritis initially have features of a typical viral syndrome: fever, headache, malaise, myalgias, arthralgias, nausea, pharyngitis, or coryza. Such viral symptoms may occur sporadically or in association with a defined outbreak. Frequently clusters of similar viral prodromes are apparent in a defined social or geographic area. Historically, generalized arthralgias are commonly associated with viremia from diverse viral species. However, joint swelling, severe stiffness, and redness should raise the suspicion of frank arthritis. In many viral syndromes polyarthralgias may be the only prodromal symptom. In viruses associated with characteristic rashes articular symptoms frequently appear at or near the time of the viral exanthem. Concomitant findings associated with arthralgias include rash, oral ulcers, swollen glands, and cough. It is also necessary to determine a history of underlying medical problems, particularly those associated with immune suppression.

#### Arthritogenic viruses

Human parvovirus
Hepatitis B
Rubella (natural and vaccine)
Mumps
Coxsackievirus
Echovirus
Smallpox
Vaccinia
Adenovirus
Varicella zoster
Herpes simplex
Cytomegalovirus
Epstein-Barr
Hepatitis A
Retroviruses (HTLV-I)
Alphaviruses

### Physical examination

Physical examination of patients with viral arthritis frequently reveals signs of an acute viral infection, including rash, pharyngitis, lymphadenopathy, hepatosplenomegaly, and oral ulcers. Viral arthritis may be monoarticular or oligoarticular, but it is most often symmetric and polyarticular. Most viruses lead to an arthropathy that involves large and small joints, which develops in an additive or migratory fashion. With all of the viruses involvement of the small finger joints and knees is most common. Other joints frequently involved include wrists, ankles, feet, elbows, and shoulders. Some viruses (notably hepatitis B and rubella) may involve the tendon sheath and produce a tenosynovitis with swelling, erythema, and tenderness across the joint (typically the wrist or ankle), corresponding to the distribution of extensor tendons.

### Specific viruses that cause musculoskeletal disease

The three viruses that most commonly cause articular syndromes are human parvovirus, hepatitis B virus, and rubella virus. It is worth considering each of these separately.

*Human parvovirus B19,* a DNA virus, is the causal agent of erythema infectiosum (fifth disease of childhood). Parvovirus is a ubiquitous virus, with 30% to 40% of adults having serologic evidence of prior exposure. In children parvovirus infection is characterized by an evanescent rash (often a slapped face appearance) with low-grade fever and occasional mild arthralgias (Fig. 87-3). In adults the rash is not a prominent feature of the

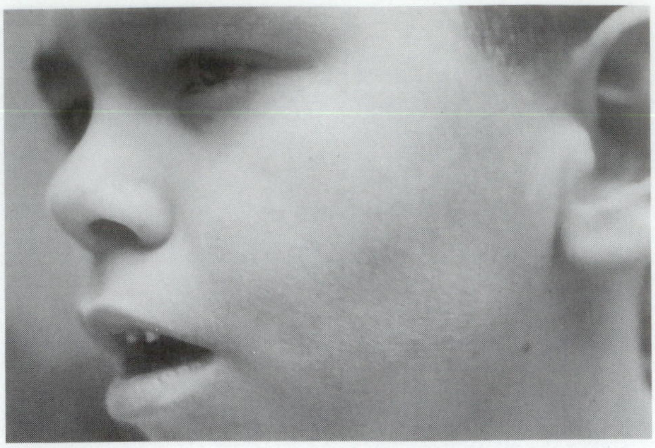

**Fig. 87-3.** The slapped cheeks appearance of fifth disease.

illness. However, it has been recognized recently that adults exposed to parvovirus B19 may develop severe arthralgias with or without an acute polyarthritis.

Arthralgias occur in up to 77% of patients with this infection. Joints most often affected include the small finger joints, wrists, and knees, although the ankles, feet, and elbows may also be affected. The arthritis may resemble acute rheumatoid arthritis, although rheumatoid factor is usually not detected. Unlike most other forms of viral arthritis, parvovirus-associated arthritis may persist for months or even years. To date no evidence of chronic erosive arthritis or permanent joint damage has been documented. Parvovirus arthritis is usually documented by the identification of IgM anti-B19 antibodies for up to several weeks following the initial exposure.

*Hepatitis B virus* is a well-known cause of articular syndromes, particularly during the prodromal phase of the illness. The incubation period for the hepatitis B virus is 40 to 180 days. Several features of the illness are mediated by hepatitis B surface antigen (HBsAg) and the humoral response to this agent. Prodromal symptoms include fever, headaches, malaise, anorexia, nausea, vomiting, and abdominal pain. These symptoms precede the icteric phase by 2 to 14 days.

Articular symptoms are a common feature of the clinical prodrome of hepatitis B infection, occurring in 10% to 25% of cases. Immune complexes with hepatitis B surface antigen and antibody are felt to mediate this process. Arthralgias or arthritis usually precede clinical jaundice by days to weeks and resolve before the icteric phase of the infection. Joint symptoms are often associated with urticarial, petechial, or maculopapular skin rashes, usually on the lower extremities. Tenosynovitis of the wrist or ankle may be noted on physical examination. Articular involvement is usually symmetric and additive and involves the large and small joints. Arthritis usually resolves completely by the onset of jaundice but persists in 5% of cases. Chronic hepatitis B antigenemia is associated with additional rheumatic syndromes, including polyarteritis nodosa.

*Rubella virus* infection produces a characteristic maculopapular eruption and lymphadenopathy. In children, there is no typical prodrome. However, in adults sore throat, headache, fever, swollen glands, and myalgias may precede the rash by 1 to 5 days. Adult patients with rubella infection who develop joint symptoms tend to be women between the ages of 20 to 40. One study found that 30% of women and 6% of men with rubella infection manifested joint symptoms. Articular symptoms may develop before or after the appearance of the rash. Most commonly polyarthralgias develop, but frank arthritis is not infrequent. The joint involvement is usually bilaterally symmetric with small and large joints affected in an additive or migratory fashion. Arthritis and arthralgias usually evolve over 7 to 10 days and most often are short lived with complete resolution. A similar articular syndrome has been associated with rubella vaccine virus. Women are also predominantly affected in this setting. Severe arthralgias with stiffness, particularly of the hands and knees, usually develop approximately 2 weeks after the vaccination. Unlike the articular symptoms associated with natural rubella infection, those seen with the vaccine virus may recur. However, permanent joint damage does not develop.

### Diagnosis and management

The diagnosis of viral arthritis is usually presumptive when it develops in the setting of a clear viral syndrome. Confirmatory tests include the demonstration of acute and convalescent viral antibody titers of the IgM and IgG classes. It is usually not necessary to accurately identify the offending virus, since the course of the joint disease is usually self-limited and specific antiviral treatment is not indicated. Synovial fluid from joints involved with viral arthritis usually has a mild leukocytosis, although there is a wide range of synovial fluid WBCs. There is typically a mononuclear cell predominance.

The treatment of viral arthritis includes standard supportive treatment for the acute viral syndrome. Inflamed joints and tendons should be splinted in the acute setting. If arthritis persists after the resolution of the viral infection, nonsteroidal antiinflammatory drugs (NSAIDs), administered for a short course, are indicated. More substantial treatment in the form of second-line antirheumatic drugs is rarely necessary.

The prognosis of viral arthritis is usually excellent. In genetically predisposed individuals a viral infection may trigger an immune response that leads to chronic arthritis. The details of such a mechanism have not been elucidated. In such cases treatment is directed at the suppression of chronic joint inflammation.

## HIV-ASSOCIATED MUSCULOSKELETAL SYNDROMES

Since 1987 a variety of rheumatic syndromes has been reported in association with HIV infection (Table 87-5). It is still not established that HIV itself is directly responsible for the association of these syndromes or even that there is a statistically significant association with these conditions (see Chapter 68 for further discussion).

### Epidemiology and pathogenesis

The incidence and prevalence of musculoskeletal syndromes in the HIV-infected population are unknown. A number of studies have tried to establish these figures but suffer from ascertainment bias. Estimates vary depending on the gender, ethnicity, and risk profile of the population

**Table 87-5.** HIV-associated rheumatic syndrome

| Syndrome | Incidence | Patterns of involvement | Severity | Associated features |
|---|---|---|---|---|
| Arthralgias | 33% | Intermittent; occurs at any stage; usually resolves in weeks to months | May be severe | Bone pain |
| Reiter's syndrome (RS) | 1% to 10%; unknown if HIV predisposes patient for RS | Usually develops around transformation to symptomatic AIDS; prominent peripheral arthritis, usually asymmetric, oligoarticular; predilection for lower extremity joint and entheses | Often peripheral oligoarthritis and cutaneous manifestations are more severe than RS not associated with HIV | Severe axial involvement (sacroiliitis and spondylitis), conjunctivitis, and uveitis are uncommon. Hyperkeratotic skin lesions, particularly keratoderma blennorrhagicum, may be indistinguishable from pustular psoriasis |
| Psoriatic arthritis | Less common than RS | More often polyarticular than is RS; involvement of distal interphalangeal (DIP) joints | | Pitting of nails, particularly those adjacent to affected DIP joints; severe psoriasis of skin |
| HIV-associated arthritis | Unknown | Oligoarthritis involving knees and ankles; short lived, lasts 1 to 6 weeks | Severe, incapacitating symptoms; often more severe than objective findings | Synovial fluid and synovial histology mildly inflammatory |
| Septic arthritis/ osteomyelitis | Not as common as might be expected | Includes opportunistic organisms | | |
| Sicca complex | Unknown | Dry eyes and mouth may occur at any stage of HIV infection; when associated wtih parotid gland enlargement and lymphocyte infiltration of salivary glands, may resemble Sjögren's syndrome; referred to as diffuse infiltrative lymphocytosis syndrome (DILS) | | Many genetic, pathologic, and serologic differences between DILS and primary Sjögren's syndrome (see Chapter 86) |
| Polymyositis | Unknown | Myopathy may develop at any time during course of HIV infection; indistinguishable from idiopathic polymyositis | | Must be distinguished from the myopathy associated with zidovudine |
| Vasculitis | Unknown | Inflammatory vascular disease may resemble polyarteritis (necrotizing, medium-sized arteritis), leukocytoclastic vasculitis, and granulomatous vasculitis | | |

studied as well as the clinical stage of the HIV infection. Probably the most common rheumatic manifestations of HIV infection are polyarthralgias and bone pain, which occur in up to one third of patients. Frank arthritis is noted at some time during the course of infection in approximately 5% to 10% of cases. True Reiter's syndrome or psoriatic arthritis probably occurs in fewer than 5% of patients. Sporadic cases of septic arthritis, osteomyelitis, vasculitis, Sjögren's-like syndrome, and inflammatory myopathy have been described, but incidence figures are currently indeterminate.

Several possible mechanisms may explain the relationship between HIV infection and rheumatic disease. The HIV itself, during a phase of viremia, could produce polyarthralgias and bone pain, as is seen in other viral infections. HIV could produce a direct viral synovitis, and this may be an explanation for AIDS-associated arthritis syndrome. AIDS virus has been isolated from synovial fluid, but this does not confirm an etiologic role for it in arthritis. Immune complexes can be found in HIV-infected individuals, but whether or not these mediate arthritis (as is the case in hepatitis B virus) is unknown. Infection with HIV may lead to an enhanced role for CD8-positive cytotoxic T cells, which may have a pathogenetic role in the seronegative spondyloarthropathies (especially Reiter's syndrome) (see Chapter 83).

### History

When obtaining a history from an individual with known or suspected HIV infection and musculoskeletal symptoms, it is important to consider the spectrum of multisystemic rheumatic disease. In addition to questions about the symptoms of joint pain and swelling, patients with HIV should be questioned about low back and heel pain, rashes, genital ulcers, ocular inflammation, dry eyes, dry mouth, and muscle weakness.

### Physical examination

Physical examination should include inspection for signs of ocular inflammation, lymphadenopathy, oral ulcers, skin rashes, mucocutaneous and genital ulcers, and nail changes. In addition to signs of arthritis, patients with seronegative spondyloarthropathies may have dactylitis (swelling and tenderness along an entire digit) or sausage digits. Evidence of inflammation at the entheses (points of ligamentous attachment to bones) may be particularly apparent in the heels, the plantar surface of the foot, and the pelvic brim. Signs of sacroiliac inflammation should also be sought on physical examination.

### Diagnosis

The diagnosis of rheumatic syndromes in AIDS patients requires the documentation of HIV infection by the usual serologic parameters and T cell subset analysis. Most rheumatic syndromes are diagnosed on the basis of clinical findings. Analysis of synovial fluid obtained from involved joints demonstrates a mild to moderate inflammatory reaction with a monocytic predominance. Rheumatic serology is generally not helpful. Rheumatoid factor and antinuclear antibodies (ANAs) are typically not found in these patients and do not help to establish a specific diagnosis.

### Management

The treatment of the rheumatic manifestations of AIDS requires treatment of the underlying infections. Antiviral therapy with zidovudine (AZT) should be instituted when indicated. AZT itself does not appear to treat the arthritis syndromes that are associated with AIDS but may improve skin manifestations. Some of the rheumatic syndromes (arthralgias, AIDS-associated arthritis) may be transient and require only analgesic medications. Syndromes associated with frank arthritis (Reiter's syndrome, psoriatic arthritis, AIDS-associated arthritis) usually require NSAIDs. Physical therapy measures may also be helpful. When these modalities are ineffective, sulfasalazine may be used for chronic arthritis. Caution should be exercised in the use of methotrexate or other immunosuppressive agents for Reiter's syndrome or psoriatic arthritis associated with AIDS, since this form of treatment may convert AIDS-related complex or mild AIDS to a fulminant syndrome, including malignant transformation. Septic arthritis/osteomyelitis is treated similarly to that occurring in non-AIDS patients.

The prognosis of AIDS-related rheumatic syndrome is directly related to the underlying disease. Reiter's syndrome may lead to chronic arthritis with deformity and disability. There are not enough cases with long-term data to evaluate the natural history of these conditions (see Chapter 68 on the primary care of the HIV patient).

## LYME DISEASE

Lyme disease is a multisystem spirochetal infection secondary to *Borrelia burgdorferi.* The organism is transmitted to humans from infected deer and white-footed mice by the tick vector *Ixodes dammini* (in the Northeast and North Central regions of the United States) or *Ixodes pacificus* (in the Pacific Northwest). Although nearly every state has reported cases of Lyme disease, the most endemic areas include the northeast, north central, and Pacific northwest states.

The clinical manifestations of Lyme disease have been divided into three stages: early localized, early disseminated, and late or persistent infection (see the box on p. 1197). Initial infection usually occurs in the late spring or early summer when the nymphal tick is 1 to 2 mm in size. Thus the tick or tick bite may not be detected until the symptoms of early localized infection occur, usually within 3 to 32 days. Fevers, malaise, myalgias, arthralgias, headache, and localized lymphadenopathy may mimic viral infections. Erythema migrans (EM), the classic skin lesion that develops at the site of tick bite, occurs in 60% to 80% of patients. Characteristically it is an erythematous macule or papule with expanding borders, reaching a mean size of 15 cm and often accompanied by central clearing (Fig. 87-4). The lesions resolve spontaneously without antibiotic therapy.

The early disseminated stage, representing the hematogenous spread of the spirochete, develops days to weeks after infection. Secondary skin lesions may develop and are typically smaller than the initial EM lesion. Neurologic manifestations are common (15% to 20%) and include aseptic meningitis, encephalitis, Bell palsy (often bilateral), and radiculoneuritis that can be sensory, motor,

## Clinical stages of Lyme disease*

**Early localized infection (stage 1)**

Skin: Erythema migrans (EM)
Systemic: Fever, malaise, lymphadenopathy (localized)

**Early disseminated infection (stage 2)**

Skin: Secondary EM lesions
Musculoskeletal: Migratory arthritis or periarthritis
Neurologic: Meningitis, facial palsy or other cranial neuritis, and radiculoneuritis
Cardiac: Atrioventricular block, myopericarditis
Systemic: Severe malaise, fatigue
Others (rare): Hepatitis, myositis, inflammatory eye diseases

**Late or persistent infection (stage 3)**

Skin: Acrodermatitis chronica atrophicans (rare in the United States)
Musculoskeletal: Oligoarticular arthritis—intermittent or chronic
Neurologic: Polyradiculoneuropathy, subacute encephalopathy, meningoencephalomyelitis
Others: Keratitis, dilated cardiomyopathy

Modified from Steere AC, *N Engl J Med* 321:586, 1989.

*Some patients may be totally asymptomatic after infection, present at stage II, or even stage III without other manifestations of earlier stages.

or mixed. Cardiac involvement occurs in 4% to 8% and manifests as fluctuating degrees of atrioventricular block or myopericarditis. Migratory arthralgias in large and small joints may accompany these symptoms.

Late or persistent infection may present months to years after the initial infection. The spirochete appears to persist in selected organs, particularly the central nervous system, joints, and rarely the skin, heart, and eyes. Neurologic disease includes chronic sensorimotor polyradiculopathy, subacute encephalopathy, and rarely a meningoencephalomyelitis. The encephalopathy is characterized by cognitive abnormalities, headache, and fatigue. Cerebrospinal fluid (CSF) may reveal mild pleocytosis, elevated protein, and intrathecal production of antibodies to *B. burgdorferi.*

Joint disease occurs in 62% of untreated patients and manifests as inflammatory, monoarticular or oligoarticular arthritis of the knees, ankles, and elbows. The small joints and bursae are rarely affected. Temporomandibular joint, hip, shoulder, back, and neck pain are common. Initially the pattern of joint inflammation is intermittent, lasting days to several weeks. Chronic arthritis, defined as persistent inflammation for 1 or more years, develops in 10% of untreated patients. Joint effusions may be massive; synovial fluid WBCs range from 10,000 to 20,000/mm$^3$ with predominantly polymorphonuclear cells. Cultures are usually negative.

Acrodermatitis chronica atrophicans, a late skin manifestation, is rare in the United States.

Since culture of the spirochete from EM lesions, blood, synovial fluid, or CSF is rare, the diagnosis of Lyme disease is based on the clinical manifestations and

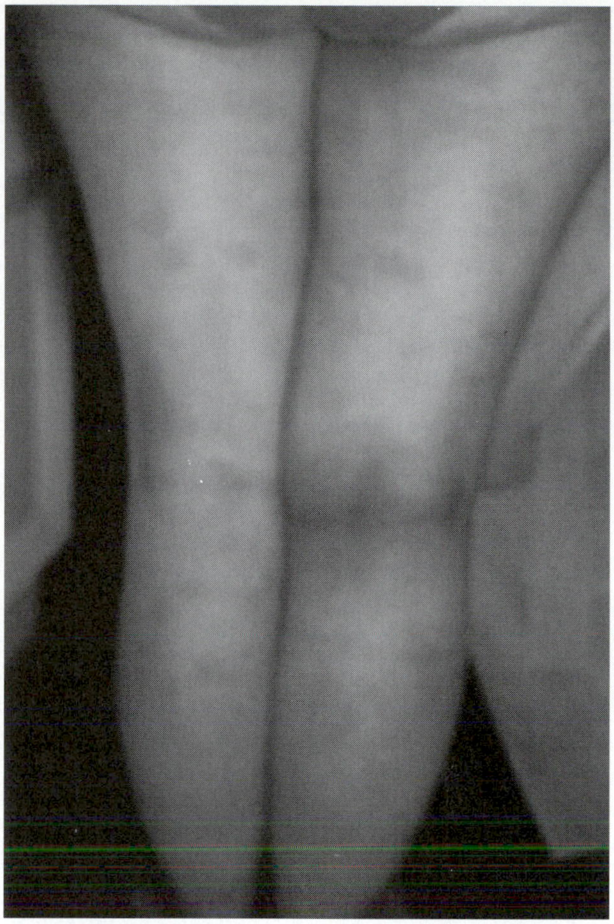

**Fig. 87-4.** Primary erythema migrans (EM) lesion of Lyme disease behind the knee, with multiple secondary lesions. (Courtesy Dr. Howard Keller, Infectious Disease Division, Massachusetts General Hospital.)

serologic studies that detect antibodies to *B. burgdorferi.* The IgM response occurs 2 to 4 weeks following the infection, whereas IgG is rarely detected before 4 to 8 weeks. The enzyme-linked immunosorbent assay (ELISA) is the most commonly used assay; however, its sensitivity and specificity vary widely due to the lack of standardization among commercial laboratories, as well as the patient population tested. False negative results occur due to (1) serum obtained too early in the disease course to detect even IgM or (2) prior antibiotic therapy for early Lyme disease, which can abort the immune response. False positive results may be seen in healthy individuals, autoimmune diseases, and other spirochetal and viral infections. Immunoblotting (Western blot) may be used in borderline cases or to distinguish the true from the false positive results. Recently polymerase chain reaction (PCR) was used to detect the presence of *B. burgdorferi* DNA in the synovial fluid, CSF, urine, and serum of Lyme disease patients. Although currently not available through commercial laboratories, the PCR technique may eventually help to identify patients who are infected and to determine whether antibiotics have eradicated the infection.

Other tests that may support the diagnosis of Lyme

**Table 87-6.** Recommendations for treatment of Lyme disease

| | Drug dosage | Duration |
|---|---|---|
| **Localized infection** | Doxycycline, 100 mg PO bid<br>Amoxicillin, 500 mg PO tid<br>Cefuroxime axetil, 500 mg PO bid<br>Erythromycin, 250 mg PO tid (may be less effective than other oral regimens) | 10-30 days depending on clinical response |
| **Early disseminated** | | |
| Isolated facial palsy (without other neurologic symptoms)<br>First-degree AV block (PR interval <0.3 sec) | Oral regimen as above may be adequate | 10-30 days depending on clinical response |
| Meningitis, encephalitis, radiculoneuritis, or other cranial neuritis<br>High-degree AV block | Ceftriaxone, 2 g IV daily<br>or<br>Penicillin G, 20 million U IV daily in divided doses | 14-21 days |
| **Late (persistent) infection** | | |
| Arthritis (intermittent or chronic) | Amoxicillin, 500 mg PO qid, and probenecid, 500 mg PO qid<br>or<br>Doxycycline, 100 mg PO bid<br>Ceftriaxone, 2 g IV daily<br>or<br>Penicillin G, 20 million U IV daily in divided doses | Oral regimen for 30 days<br>IV dosage for 14 days |
| Late neurologic symptoms | Ceftriaxone, 2 g IV daily<br>or<br>Penicillin G, 20 million U IV daily in divided doses | 30 days |
| **Pregnancy** | | |
| Tick bite or early disease | Amoxicillin, 500 mg PO tid<br>or<br>Erythromycin, 250 mg-500 mg PO tid-qid (may be less effective than amoxicillin) | 21 days |
| Disseminated early or late | Ceftriaxone, 2 g IV daily<br>or<br>Penicillin G, 20 million U IV daily in divided doses | 14 days |

Modified from Steere AC, *N Engl J Med* 321:586, 1989.

disease include synovial fluid analysis, lumbar puncture with CSF analysis and antibody studies, and electromyography and nerve conduction (EMG/NCS) tests. MRIs may have nonspecific abnormalities in 25% of patients. Neuropsychiatric testing is useful to differentiate subtle encephalopathy from depression.

Antibiotics are the major treatment for Lyme disease. Currently prophylactic therapy for tick bites is not indicated unless the patient is pregnant. Table 87-6 outlines the current recommendations for treating various stages of Lyme disease. Oral antibiotic therapy is adequate for early disease and arthritis. Doxycycline is contraindicated in children and in pregnant or lactating women. Parenteral antibiotics are recommended for meningitis, carditis, arthritis that is unresponsive to oral antibiotics, and other neurologic manifestations. Patients with early neurologic symptoms improve quickly, whereas late neurologic symptoms improve slowly over months. Empiric courses of intravenous antibiotics are recommended for patients with classic manifestations but not for those who have symptoms of chronic fatigue or fibromyalgia and only positive Lyme titers. Similarly, patients with treated Lyme disease may have persistent fatigue or fibromyalgia symptoms that remain unresponsive to repeated courses of antibiotics.

In addition to antibiotics, management of high-degree atrioventricular block may require a temporary pacemaker. Joint aspiration and corticosteroid injections for chronic arthritis are effective but should be performed only after antibiotic therapy.

A minority of patients may not respond to antibiotic therapy. Repeated courses of antibiotics are not indicated. Surgical synovectomy is often successful in chronic arthritis. In patients with fatigue, headaches, or cognitive deficits other modalities such as tricyclic antidepressants, antiinflammatory medications, cognitive retraining, and behavioral modifications are useful.

In pregnant women with early disease or tick bites amoxicillin, 500 mg three times a day, or erythromycin, 250 to 500 mg three or four times a day for 3 weeks, is recommended by the American College of Obstetrics and Gynecology. Parenteral therapy with ceftriaxone or penicillin can be used safely for disseminated or late manifestations. Maternal exposure to Lyme disease before conception or during pregnancy has not been associated with fetal death, congenital malformations, or premature birth.

Prevention of Lyme disease should be stressed to patients traveling to endemic areas. Since most experts feel that the spirochete is not transmitted until 36 to 48 hours after tick attachment, a careful, daily body check for ticks is crucial. If a tick is found, gentle pulling with tweezers in a steady fashion is best. In addition, wearing long sleeves, tucking pants into socks, and using insect repellent containing diethyltoluamide (deet) are effective measures against tick attachment. A human vaccine for Lyme disease is currently under development.

## BIBLIOGRAPHY


Cooper C, Cawley MID: Bacterial arthritis in the elderly, *Gerontology* 32:222, 1986.

Coyle PK: Neurologic complications of Lyme disease, *Rheum Clin North Am* 19:993, 1993.

Espinoza LR et al: Rheumatic manifestations associated with human immunodeficiency virus infection, *Arthritis Rheum* 32:1615, 1989.

Gentry LO: Oral antimicrobial therapy for osteomyelitis, *Ann Intern Med* 114:980, 1991.

Goldenberg DL, Cohen AS: Acute infectious arthritis, *Am J Med* 60:369, 1976.

Ho G Jr: Bacterial arthritis. In McCarty BJ, Koopman WJ, editors: *Arthritis and allied conditions,* ed 12, Philadelphia, 1993, Lea & Febiger.

Malane MS et al: Diagnosis of Lyme disease based on dermatologic manifestations, *Ann Intern Med* 114:490, 1991.

Naides SJ et al: Rheumatologic manifestations of human parvovirus B19 infection in adults: initial two-year clinical experience, *Arthritis Rheum* 33:1297, 1990.

Newman LG et al: Unsuspected osteomyelitis in diabetic foot ulcers: diagnosis and monitoring by leukocyte scanning with indium In 111 oxyquinoline, *JAMA* 266:1246, 1991.

O'Brien JP, Goldenberg DL, Rice PA: Disseminated gonococcal infection: a prospective analysis of 49 patients and a review of pathophysiology and immune mechanisms, *Medicine* 62:395, 1983.

Schauwecker DS: The scintigraphic diagnosis of osteomyelitis, *Am J Roentgenol* 158:9, 1992.

Sharp JT et al: Infectious arthritis, *Arch Intern Med* 139:1125, 1979.

Soderquist B, Hedstrom SA: Predisposing factors, bacteriology and antibiotic therapy in 35 cases of septic bursitis, *Scand J Infect Dis* 18:305, 1986.

Steere AC: Lyme disease, *N Engl J Med* 321:586, 1989.


CHAPTER

# 88 Common Sports Injuries


**Lisa Rowland Callahan**
**Michael F. Dillingham**
**Kathryn M. Peuvrelle**
**James L. McGuire**


## ACKNOWLEDGMENTS


The authors would like to thank Gerald P. Keane, MD, and George Thabit III, MD, of Sports, Orthopedic and Rehabilitation in Menlo Park, California, for their contributions to this chapter.


An increasing awareness of the health benefits of fitness and the pleasure of competing in sports has also increased demand for state-of-the-art sports medicine. An injured athlete desires a timely return to normal function. The primary care physician is in a position to provide not only treatment and rehabilitation, but also fitness evaluation, exercise programs, and injury prevention counseling. At the office-based level of care the clinician needs to provide proper evaluation of injuries, understand the sequelae of chronic injuries, and delineate the risks of overtraining. This chapter helps the primary care physician blend the best of current aggressive and conservative approaches to treatment of the athlete with appropriate timing of subspecialty referral.

Physicians should be prepared to guide patients in three areas. First, a regular exercise program should be encouraged for its psychologic benefits, such as better work performance and decreased stress levels. Second, nutritional advice is important, especially for weight maintenance or reduction through exercise. This is particularly true for young women who have not yet attained maximal bone mass. Third, cardiac and arthritic risk monitoring is also an important element of total care.

## GUIDELINES FOR FITNESS TRAINING

### Exercise

Exercise, like a medication, should be prescribed properly to attain maximum benefit. During the history and physical examination, consideration should be given to the individual's current level of fitness, history of medical illnesses, medications, family history, and review of any past injuries. Laboratory testing may be necessary, including lipid screening for cholesterol levels and electrocardiogram (ECG). Formal exercise testing is generally recommended for those with known or suspected cardiovascular or pulmonary disease and should at least be considered in any sedentary patient over 35 before initiating an exercise program.

Upon completion of the appropriate tests, recommendations concerning exercise should be made. The basic recommendations, summarized in the box on p. 1200, include consideration of the frequency, intensity, and duration of exercise, as well as the type of activity. In addition, the updated recommendations acknowledge the need for some resistance training to achieve minimum fitness levels.

**Guidelines for exercise prescription**

| | |
|---|---|
| Frequency: | 3 to 5 days/week |
| Intensity: | 60% to 90% of HRmax or 50% to 80% of $\dot{V}O_2$ max |
| Duration: | 20 to 60 minutes |
| Mode: | Any continuous aerobic activity using large muscle groups (e.g., running, cycling, swimming) |
| Resistance training: | One set, 8 to 12 repetitions of 8 to 10 exercises (minimum recommendation) |

*HRmax,* Maximum heart rate. This may be estimated by the formula 220 − Age = HRmax. Variation ± 10% is common.
*$\dot{V}O_2$ max,* Maximum oxygen uptake.

Each exercise session should consist of three phases: warm-up, aerobic activity, and a cool-down period. The warm-up and cool-down may simply be the same aerobic activity performed with less intensity. The warm-up usually includes stretching and activation of the aerobic mechanism, and the cool-down attempts to minimize both postexercise myalgia and the risk of cardiac events.

The goals and methods for attaining fitness in children differ significantly from those outlined for adults. Children have a relatively inefficient metabolism, less anaerobic capacity, and less heat tolerance. Moreover, children are generally motivated by the idea of having fun rather than by increasing fitness. These factors should guide the physician's recommendations for achieving fitness in children. The type of exercise recommended should be determined by the child's individual interests and strengths. It is clear that the more active the child, the better the gain in bone density as young adulthood is reached.

Weight training in children is controversial. Recent studies suggest that children probably can achieve increases in strength through resistance training. Much work still needs to be done in this area before the primary care physician will have clear guidelines for prescribing weight training for children. Adolescents may generally use the same fitness training guidelines as adults. If an adolescent's goal is to achieve excellence in a particular sport, exercise prescription should focus particularly on developing skills relative to the chosen sport (such as drills to develop hand-eye coordination) in addition to achieving aerobic fitness and muscular strength and endurance. This idea of sport-specific conditioning is also applicable to adults.

The opportunity to prescribe appropriate exercise for the school-age athlete may come as a preparticipation physical examination. Growing numbers of children participate in organized athletics; physicians are often asked to screen these students for conditions that might limit participation or predispose to injury. This type of examination should consist of a directed history as well as medical and orthopedic evaluations.

## Nutrition and fluid intake

Good nutrition is essential for good health, as well as for athletic success. Athletes, like their sedentary counterparts, frequently do not practice proper eating habits. The primary care physician's role is to review and explain sound nutrition principles.

Generally, a healthy diet should consist of 60% to 70% carbohydrate, 20% to 30% fat, and approximately 15% protein. Furthermore, the physician should be aware that some athletes are too restrictive with their diets, consuming minimal amounts of fats and calories. Once identified, these athletes should be screened carefully for possible eating disorders, counseled in proper nutrition, and if necessary referred for appropriate psychologic care. In contrast, one should be aware that young athletes, especially those engaged in vigorous activity, require high caloric intakes to build and maintain appropriate muscle mass. For example, high school football players training twice daily have caloric needs of 5000 to 6000 kcal per day.

Adequate fluid intake is an essential and frequently neglected aspect of sports nutrition. Exercise greatly increases heat production. The body's thermoregulatory system dissipates this excess heat primarily by evaporation of sweat. If the fluids and electrolytes lost through sweat are not replaced, the athlete will become dehydrated. This can lead to both cardiovascular and thermoregulatory compromise, which directly affects the athlete's health and performance. To prevent this state from occurring, athletes should be encouraged to drink adequate fluids before, during, and after competition. Adequate intake can be estimated by having the athlete monitor weight and urine color. A pound of weight lost is roughly equivalent to 2 cups of sweat and should be replaced accordingly. If the urine volume is low and the color becomes dark yellow, dehydration probably exists and increased fluid intake is immediately warranted.

Questions concerning fluid replacement with water versus sports drink often arise. In general, water is sufficient for the recreational athlete and exercise sessions lasting 90 minutes or less. For longer exercise sessions and endurance events, a sports drink or diluted fruit juice is recommended, since it provides both glucose (carbohydrate source) and electrolytes. Cold concentrations of 2% to 6% carbohydrate are absorbed most quickly. The physician should encourage the athlete not to rely on thirst as an indicator of fluid loss because enough body water can be lost as to adversely affect performance before the athlete becomes thirsty.

## Androgenic steroids and other ergogenic aids

Maximal athletic performance depends on a complex combination of physical and psychologic factors. Competitors have always tried a variety of methods to enhance performance, including psychologic techniques, vitamins, food supplements, and androgens and other illicit drugs. Currently athletes are experimenting with anabolic steroids. Because these substances are banned by all official sporting organizations, the true prevalence of their use is difficult to quantify. Despite some highly publicized suspensions and loss of Olympic medals, the use of anabolic steroids in certain sports continues to increase. Furthermore, androgen use has unfortunately found its way beyond the well-publicized professional and world class amateur athlete to the high school and community health clubs. Physicians need to be aware of the extensive risks of androgen use so that they can convey these risks, especially because of the belief among athletes that androgens provide a competitive advantage in some sports.

It is generally accepted that anabolic steroids improve muscle strength through increased lean muscle mass and exercise tolerance. However, many hormone-related side effects result from their use. Anabolic steroids, related to the naturally produced testosterone, are available to athletes in both injectable and oral forms. Androgenic effects in males have been reported to include testicular atrophy, abnormal sperm counts, cystic acne, gynecomastia, decreased sex drive, liver adenomas, and aggressive behavior. In females, masculine secondary sexual characteristics develop and are thought to be largely irreversible. These include growth of facial hair, deepening of the voice, male pattern baldness, and enlargement of the clitoris. In prepubertal athletes anabolic steroids have been reported to cause premature epiphyseal closure, which arrests growth. Chronic androgen use typically results in lower high-density lipoprotein (HDL) cholesterol levels, whereas exercise usually increases this beneficial cholesterol. These serious side effects, coupled with psychologic and cardiac risks, underline the danger of steroid use in athletes.

It should be noted that the terms *steroids, androgens,* and *anabolic steroids* are used interchangeably by athletes, coaches, and some sports physicians, whereas for primary care physicians the word *steroids* usually refers to glucocorticoids.

Other substances used by athletes to enhance performance include human growth hormone (HGH) and erythropoietin (EPO), two naturally occurring hormones. Some users of HGH report an increase in muscular size and strength, but others do not. EPO is used by endurance athletes to increase the hemoglobin concentration, thereby increasing the amount of oxygen that may be delivered to working muscles. As the concentration of red blood cells rises (enhanced also by dehydration), so does the risk of clot formation and stroke. Death following blood doping, as use of EPO is also known, has been reported. Androgens can be readily detected in urine, but illicit HGH and EPO injections may be difficult to detect in serum.

### Specificity of training

Proper conditioning demands specificity in training. This means that the exercise done for the sporting contest somehow mimics the event itself in aspects of required endurance, motion, velocity, movement, and load. Weight training and other types of resistance training encourage development of metabolic systems that are specific to the overload and muscle size. Specificity of motion encourages neural coordination, not only among muscle groups but also within the actual muscles themselves. Untrained persons cannot fully activate muscles, particularly their high threshold muscle motor units. Specificity of training allows complete and coordinated activation of muscle with a specific task in mind. Given two muscles of equal size, the better coordinated muscle will be stronger. Thus muscular strength gains in any particular activity are achieved not only through hypertrophy of muscle but through better coordination of muscle activity. Practice must be proper so that the athlete develops appropriate neural patterning and habits.

### Overtraining

Overtraining is a very real syndrome that affects athletes of all ages and abilities. It occurs when an athlete's training program exceeds the body's ability for recovery. Muscle growth occurs primarily as a response to muscle breakdown during bouts of exercise. In addition, adequate rest and recovery are necessary or muscular gains are not made. Exercise programs that emphasize endurance with high-frequency, low-resistance activity can be done relatively frequently, perhaps every other day. Exercise programs that are primarily oriented toward strength and building of muscle mass with low-repetition, high-load resistance training are generally done only every fourth day. This is true even for highly conditioned Olympic athletes. However, overtraining, both in weight training and in aerobic conditioning, is a common error made primarily by recreational athletes.

Overtraining manifests itself both psychologically and physiologically. Probably the most universal complaint is fatigue, often referred to by the athlete as staleness or burnout. Apathy, sleep disturbances, loss of appetite, irritability, heavy legs, sore muscles, and decreased ability to concentrate are other common complaints. Physiologic changes include a rise in resting heart rate and blood pressure for the particular athlete. The primary care physician should attempt to distinguish this syndrome from other causes of medical conditions that accompany fatigue, such as depression, anemia, asthma, mononucleosis, or other viral illness. A complete history and physical examination should be performed. Screening complete blood counts and serum chemistries should be obtained. The physician should pay careful attention to details of the training regimen, and sometimes a discussion with the coach or athletic trainer is helpful. If the cause of the athlete's symptoms are determined to be secondary to overtraining, rest is the best treatment. The bottom line of overtraining is that the desired gains will not be made, and in fact in some cases less adequate conditioning, injury, and psychologic imbalance are the end result.

## ATHLETIC INJURIES

### Head injuries

Most athletic injuries involve the musculoskeletal system. However, virtually all contact sports and many so-called noncontact sports such as basketball, baseball, and soccer, may also produce head and thoracoabdominal injuries. The attending physician should examine the severely injured athlete for airway and hemodynamic stability and perform any necessary stabilization and resuscitation. In addition, whenever a head injury has occurred, associated neck injury must also be considered. Moreover, the physician should evaluate for a concussion, a temporary disturbance of brain function with or without loss of consciousness. No permanent structural injury is implied.

The physician may refer to several different methods for assessing and grading concussions. Probably the single most important indicator of severity is the athlete's level of consciousness. When a head injury has occurred, five historical points are pivotal to the evaluation:

1. Was there loss of consciousness?
2. Is there retrograde amnesia?
3. Is headache persistent?

4. Is nausea present?
5. Is there blurring of vision?

In general, the athlete can return to the competition if the duration of the loss of consciousness was under several minutes and the athlete can remember all events or plays up to injury. Although a headache may be present shortly after the head injury, it should not persist. The physical examination, with careful emphasis on the neuromuscular evaluation, should be completely normal. If the answer to any of the above questions is yes and there is not total resolution, a magnetic resonance image (MRI), or computed tomography (CT) with contrast is probably indicated before resumption of play. Postconcussion headaches, especially when exercising, may occur for several weeks after the injury.

During an athletic contest the primary care physician should generally feel comfortable allowing a patient to reenter the game if there is no retrograde amnesia and no headache in the presence of a normal neurologic examination. When there is clinical doubt, many sports physicians are extremely cautious about letting the athlete resume play following a concussion.

Fig. 88-1 delineates steps to be taken in evaluating head injuries on the playing field or soon thereafter. Decisions regarding the athlete's return to play can be made based on this brief summary.

## Musculoskeletal injuries

Evaluation of musculoskeletal injuries should include examination of joint stability, deformity, and function. The most accurate examination is obtained if conducted as soon as possible after the injury occurs. With time, muscle spasm, joint effusion, and discomfort increase, making ligamentous laxity more difficult to detect and dislocations more difficult to reduce. Therefore a primary care physician with knowledge of sports medicine working on the sidelines can facilitate the athlete's return to play, as safely and as soon as possible, by providing an expedient and accurate assessment.

Ligamentous injury is commonly called a sprain. Sprains are generally classified as mild, moderate, or severe, depending on the degree of disruption of the ligament's fibers. The greater the degree of disruption of the fibers, the more severe and potentially unstable the injury. A simple grading system from I to III is used to signify the degree of instability (Table 88-1 and Fig. 88-2).

An injury to a musculotendinous unit is termed a strain. These are generally classified as acute or chronic, again with a grading system from I to III to describe the severity of the injury (see Table 88-1).

Athletic injuries may be acute (traumatic, such as an anterior cruciate ligament tear in a football player), chronic, or related to overuse (such as a stress fracture in a runner). A careful history delineates which type of injury has occurred. In addition, the primary care physician must remember that medical illnesses, such as rheumatologic disease, may masquerade as an athletic injury. At the first manifestation of an acute or subacute rheumatic disease, patients often attribute their joint symptoms to a recent injury. At times there may be a cause and effect relationship. For example, the first manifestation of rheumatoid arthritis may follow a knee or ankle injury. Premature osteoarthritis is a well-established sequela of internal derangement of the knee. On the other hand, some patients attribute the early phases of a pseudogout or gout attack to a strained knee or ankle, respectively. At other times an adolescent may attribute a swollen knee to an athletic injury. A radiograph may demonstrate a more severe bony abnormality, such as osteomyelitis or osteosarcoma. Thus the primary care physician must consider all medical possibilities when diagnosing an athletic injury.

Before examining the athlete with an acute musculoskeletal injury, the examiner should elicit a directed history. The athlete should be questioned about the mechanism of injury. Was a pop or snap heard or felt? Was there immediate or delayed onset of pain or swelling? Was the athlete able to continue activity? Is there a history of injury? If the injury is to the lower extremity, the relationship to weight bearing should be determined. If the injury is to the upper extremity, it is helpful to know if the injured limb is the dominant one. The responses to these questions help the examiner form a working differential diagnosis and direct the physical examination.

Table 88-2 outlines many common sports injuries, both acute and overuse in nature. In addition to the history, symptoms, and physical examination findings associated

**Table 88-1.** Classification of musculoskeletal injury

| Grade | Classification | Description | Treatment |
|---|---|---|---|
| **Sprains (injury to ligament)** | | | |
| I | Mild | Minimal disruption of fibers, minimal or no instability | Symptomatic |
| II | Moderate | Mild to moderate instability | Symptomatic; consider protection with brace |
| III | Severe | Complete disruption of fibers, gross instability | Symptomatic; consider surgery |
| **Strains (injury to musculotendinous unit)** | | | |
| I | Mild | No gross disruption of fibers | Symptomatic |
| II | Moderate | Partial disruption of fibers | Symptomatic; consider protection with brace/splint or surgery for tendon tear |
| III | Severe | Complete disruption of fibers | Symptomatic; consider surgery for tendon tear |

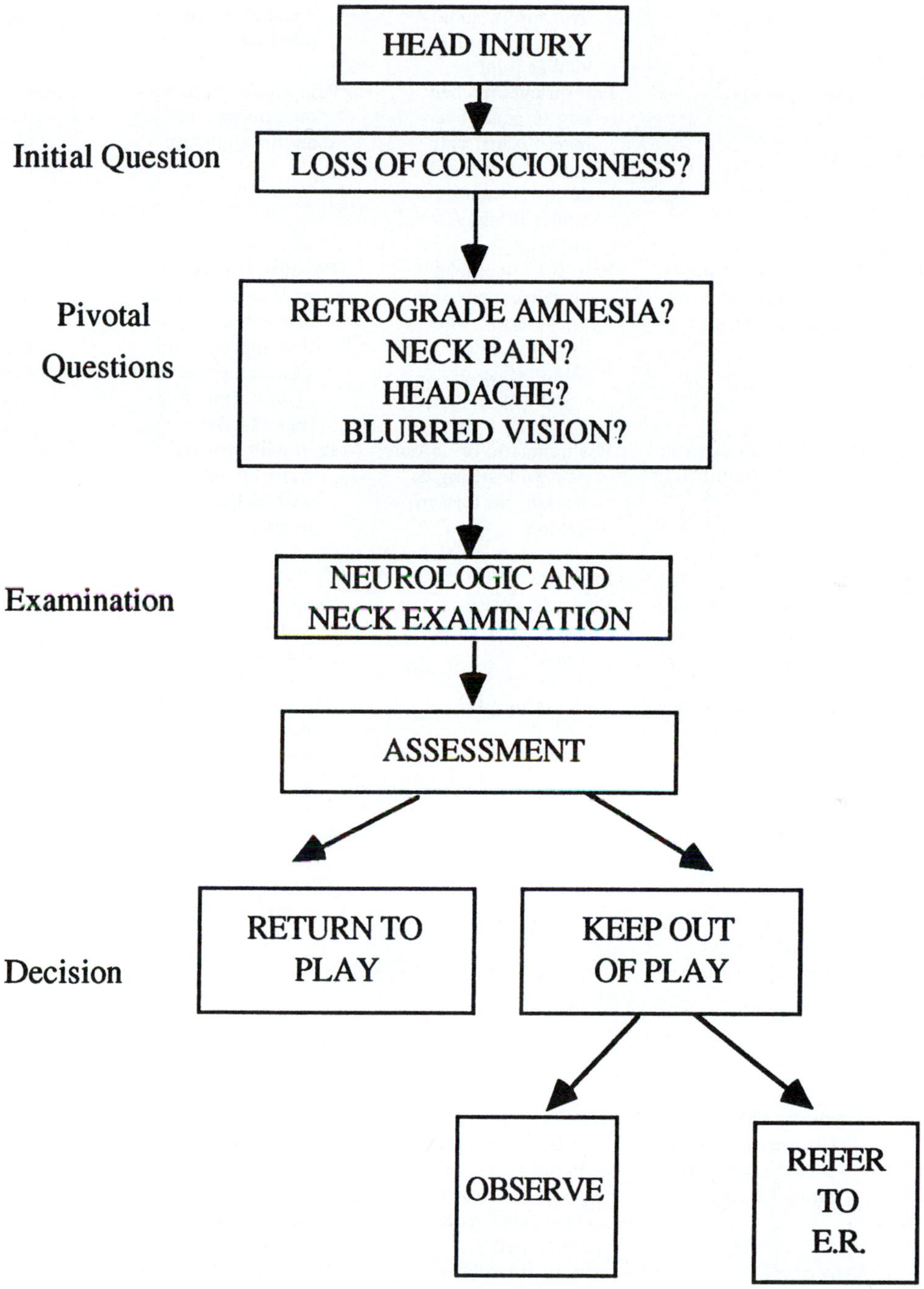


**Fig. 88-1.** Flowchart to assess head injury without neck complaints.

**Table 88-2.** Common sports injuries

| Region and injury | Sport | History/symptoms | Physical examination | Initial tests/treatment |
|---|---|---|---|---|
| **Shoulder** | | | | |
| Acromioclavicular separation | Cycling, falls | Acute injury; pain and possible deformity over top of shoulder at acromioclavicular joint | Localized tenderness, possible deformity, distal clavicle displacement | X-ray; grade II: symptomatic treatment; grade III or greater: orthopedic consult |
| Rotator cuff tear | Contact sports | Fall on outstretched arm or acute overload of cuff; pain over lateral shoulder, occasional difficulty in abducting arm | Pain and/or weakness on external rotation and/or abduction | X-ray to rule out fracture, MRI; if complete tear, surgical repair required |
| Instability, anterior or posterior/subluxation | Overhead and throwing sports, serving and swimming | Pain with overhead maneuver, possible "dead arm" when throwing, occasional sense of instability | Possibly consistent with cuff irritation or weakness; positive apprehension sign, either anterior or posterior; findings of joint laxity | Orthopedic consult to determine further treatment, including possible rehabilitation and/or surgical treatment |
| Biceps tendinitis | Contact and overhead sports, weightlifting | Posttraumatic or chronic; pain with lifting or working in forward flexion | Pain with resisted forward flexion and/or with palpation of tendon | Diagnostic block; rest, injection, rehabilitation; rarely requires surgery |
| **Elbow** | | | | |
| Epicondylitis (medial or lateral) | Throwing and racquet sports, golf | Pain with use of the forearm, wrist, or hand | Tenderness to palpation and with resistance of the involved musculotendinous unit | Rest, rehabilitation, NSAIDs, possible injection |
| Medial ligament sprain | Throwing and racquet sports, javelin | Pain during play | Tenderness over the ligament and with valgus stress; possible clinical instability | Stress x-rays, MRI; grade I and II: rehabilitation and rest; grade III (complete or near complete tear): orthopedic consult and surgery |
| Navicular fracture | Contact sports | Fall on outstretched hand | Tenderness in anatomic snuffbox | X-ray; consider immobilization; if fracture present, orthopedic referral; if no fracture, but symptoms present, orthopedic referral |
| **Lumbar spine** | | | | |
| Spondylolysis | Gymnastics, football (linemen), weight training, dancing, figure skating | Low back pain and stiffness; occasional buttock, leg, or thigh pain; occasionally associated with radiculopathy | Tenderness to palpation, occasional muscle spasm; pain with rotation and extension, increased lordosis | X-ray; if results equivocal, bone scan and/or MRI; if positive, orthopedic consult |
| Diskogenic pain (annular tear, disk protrusion) | Any sport | Any of the following: low back pain, buttock pain, thigh and/or leg pain, possible radicular pattern | Midline tenderness to palpation; possible increased pain with forward flexion; possible positive straight leg raise | X-rays, rest, ice, NSAIDs; if symptoms are severe or persistent, orthopedic or physiatry referral |

**Table 88-2.** Common sports injuries—cont'd

| Region and injury | Sport | History/symptoms | Physical examination | Initial tests/treatment |
|---|---|---|---|---|
| **Knee** | | | | |
| ***Injury to ligament*** | | | | |
| Anterior cruciate ligament | All sports involving change of direction, jumping, or contact | A sense of giving way, often with associated pop, subsequent swelling and pain | Effusion, positive Lachman test; positive anterior drawer test; frequent joint line pain | Non–weight bearing and immobilization briefly for symptoms, possible MRI, and/or acute arthroscopy |
| Posterior cruciate ligament | All sports involving change of direction, jumping, or contact | Generally a fall onto the proximal tibia, acute or subacute onset, posterior (popliteal space) knee pain | Positive posterior drawer test, (may evolve over hours or days); possible effusion, possible popliteal area pain | Initial treatment is symptomatic; orthopedic consult, generally nonsurgical |
| Medial and lateral collateral ligaments | All sports involving change of direction, jumping, or contact | Occasional sense of tearing with a sense of acute tibial displacement and subsequent pain | Local tenderness, instability on stress testing, frequent hamstring guarding | Immobilization and/or crutches for comfort, possible MRI; grade I: symptomatic treatment; grade II or III: orthopedic consult |
| ***Injury to cartilage*** | | | | |
| Meniscal tear (medial or lateral) | All sports | Usually joint line pain, occasionally clicking, popping, or locking | Joint line pain, possible effusion, possible positive McMurray test | MRI, symptomatic treatment and possible orthopedic consult for arthroscopy |
| **Leg** | | | | |
| Shin splints | Running, jumping, diving | Pain with activity | Localized tenderness if bone stress reaction or periostitis; possible muscle tenderness if compartment syndrome | X-ray; if necessary, bone scan or MRI; rest, ice, orthotics; if persistent, orthopedic referral |
| **Foot/ankle** | | | | |
| Achilles tendinitis | Running, jumping, dancing, and diving | Pain with activity, subacute onset | Tenderness and possible swelling and edema over involved segment of tendon | If symptoms persist, MRI (to rule out tear); rest, rehabilitation, occasional immobilization, occasional surgery |
| Plantar fasciitis | Running, jumping, dancing | Usually insidious onset, occasionally acute, atraumatic onset, pain at proximal arch | Tenderness along plantar fascial insertion on calcaneus; occasionally tight Achilles and/or hindfoot | Taping, orthotics, stretching, antiinflammatory modalities and NSAIDs; rarely surgery |
| Ankle sprain (medial-syndesmodic) | Any sport involving running or jumping | Ankle inverted, everted, and/or forcibly plantar flexed or dorsiflexed | Swelling and pain to palpation over involved ligaments | X-ray to rule out fracture, ice, crutches, compression, possible acute immobilization; if severe, orthopedic consult |

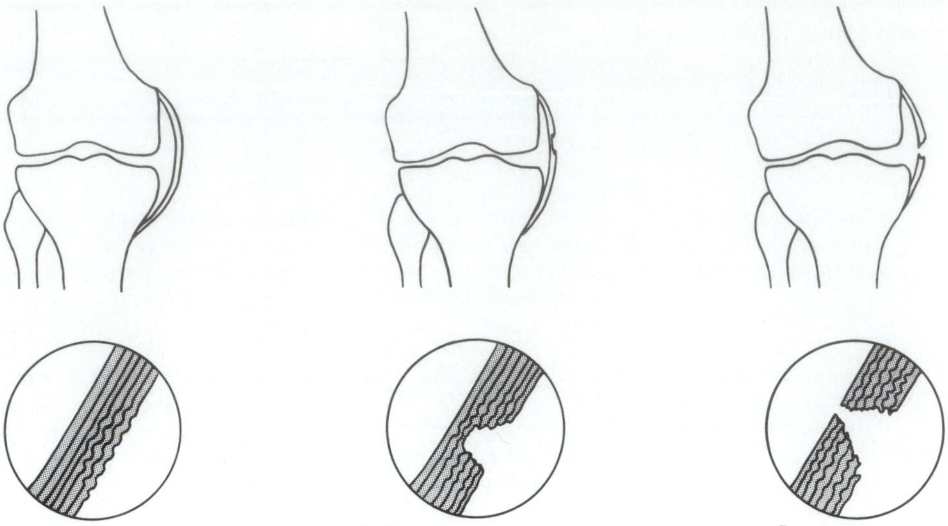


**Fig. 88-2.** Ligamentous sprains vary in severity. **A,** First degree. **B,** Second degree. **C,** Third-degree sprain, which indicates complete rupture.

with each injury or condition, potentially appropriate initial tests and treatment are discussed.

Radiographs can be useful when evaluating musculoskeletal injury. A few general principles can guide the primary care physician's decisions when ordering radiographs. At least two views—anteroposterior (AP) and lateral—should always be obtained, since injuries are not always apparent on a single view. In some instances it is helpful to obtain comparison views of the contralateral extremity. This is true for children who have epiphyseal areas of radiolucency. Moreover, anatomic variations of normal or subtle dislocations of carpal bones can be identified by comparison images.

In general, AP and lateral views are done when standard x-rays are indicated. However, additional radiographs of a specific area sometimes require special views that will help the sports medicine specialist at the time of referral (see the box at right). Other radiographic techniques, including MRI, CT, and bone scan, are also valuable in certain settings. Because they are expensive, their use is best limited to specialists.

***Overuse injuries.*** Overuse syndromes result from repetitive microtrauma to bones, ligaments, and musculotendinous units. Intrinsic factors include either structural (e.g., leg length discrepancy) or biomechanical (e.g., poor flexibility, muscular weakness, and especially eccentric weakness) abnormalities. Extrinsic factors relate to equipment (worn-out running shoes) and training errors (increasing mileage too rapidly). The history taken from an athlete with a suspected overuse injury should incorporate questions about each of these factors. A detailed account of training schedules and techniques often illustrates the reason for injury. Specifically, the type, intensity, and duration of training workouts should be evaluated for the all too common "too much too soon" phenomenon. This is especially apparent in high school and college athletes who enter a specific sport season without being conditioned. It is also a pattern seen in many recreational runners. If the treating physician remembers to consider these different factors, the etiology of the overuse injury is usually apparent. This gives the physician the opportunity both to treat the injury and to counsel the athlete to prevent recurrence.

### Additional radiographic views

- Acromioclavicular joint
  - Axillary
  - Oblique
  - Flexion
- Shoulder/elbow
  - Oblique
  - Flexion
- Wrist/hand
  - Oblique
  - Navicular view
- Cervical spine
  - Obliques
  - Odontoid views for C1-C2
- Lumbar spine
  - Lumbosacral spot
  - Bilateral obliques
- Hip
  - None
- Knee
  - Tunnel
  - Oblique
  - Merchant or sunrise (patella)
- Ankle
  - Bilateral stress views
  - Mortise
- Foot
  - Standing comparison AP
  - Obliques

Bone has the ability to constantly remodel and repair. However, if the degree of repetitive microtrauma exceeds the bone's capability for repair, an overuse injury in the form of a stress fracture occurs. Stress fractures occur most commonly in the weight-bearing bones of the lower extremity, such as the tibia and metatarsals, but have also been seen in the upper extremity of the throwing athlete. The athlete presents with pain in the area of the fracture and often gives a history compatible with overuse. The physician should ask specifically about training errors, such as changes in the length, intensity, or duration of exercise. There may be swelling and point tenderness in the area of the fracture. Radiographs are frequently negative initially. However, the fracture may be apparent on repeat radiographs in 2 weeks when healing has begun. Although not usually advised in the initial evaluation, a bone scan and special MRI (fat suppression) may be positive before the radiograph. Treatment of the uncomplicated stress fracture consists of relative rest, generally of at least 3 weeks' duration, and antiinflammatory therapy with nonsteroidal antiinflammatory drugs (NSAIDs) and periodic ice. It should be noted that athletes frequently have difficulty complying with rest; the reason for rest needs to be explained carefully and reemphasized. As healing occurs, substituting another activity may be a method to increase rest compliance (e.g., swimming instead of running for an athlete with a metatarsal stress fracture). Following the resolution of the stress fracture, a careful program should be started to prevent overtraining and repetition of the injury.

In young athletes the physician should be aware of the overuse syndrome known as traction apophysitis. This condition results from repeated stress at the insertion of a tendon into a growth plate center. It is most commonly seen at the insertion of the infrapatellar tendon on the tibial tubercle, a condition known as Osgood-Schlatter disease. The young athlete presents with pain and swelling over the tubercle, which is usually enlarged and tender. It frequently appears during a period of rapid growth in association with tight hamstrings and quadriceps muscles. As in stress fractures, the cornerstone of treatment is rest. NSAIDs may be helpful as well. To prevent occurrence, the athlete should be screened for contributing factors, such as tight muscles, and instructed in a stretching program, especially for the warm-up session.

Repetitive trauma at the site of tendon attachment to bone causes a common overuse syndrome of tendinitis. This is probably due in part to the relatively poor blood supply of the tendon combined with tension overload. Commonly affected are the patellar tendon, wrist flexors, elbow extensors, the supraspinatus tendon, and the biceps tendon of the shoulder. Ligaments may be the tissue affected by overuse, such as in breaststroker's knee, an overuse strain of the medial collateral ligament. Similarly, pitchers, golfers, and javelin throwers experience overuse strains of the medial collateral ligament of the elbow. A complete history should discover the contributing factors that resulted in the athlete's development of tendinitis and ligament strains. Treatment is similar to that for other types of overuse syndromes, with a similar emphasis on prevention.

Overuse injuries essentially occur in all sports. See the box above for a brief listing of common overuse syndromes and the sports in which they are most commonly encountered.

### Common overuse syndromes and the sports in which they commonly occur

- Stress fracture or epiphyseal slip/proximal humerus: throwing sports, particularly in children and adolescents
- Rotator cuff tendinitis: throwing and lifting sports
- Lateral epicondylitis (tennis elbow): tennis, golf, and throwing sports
- Medial epicondylitis: tennis, golf, and throwing sports
- Strained medial collateral ligament (elbow): throwing sports
- Little leaguer's elbow: baseball
- Radiocapitellar degenerative change: throwing sports, particularly in children and adolescents
- Spondylolysis/spondylolysthesis: gymnastics and football
- Trochanteric bursitis: running and weightlifting
- Stress fracture (femoral neck): running and jumping sports
- Distal iliotibial band tendinitis: running sports, cycling, hiking, and climbing
- Patellar tendinitis (jumper's knee): running and jumping sports, diving
- Breaststroker's knee: swimming
- Tibial stress fracture: running and jumping sports, diving
- Tibial tubercle apophysitis (Osgood-Schlatter disease): running and jumping sports
- Achilles tendinitis: running and jumping sports
- Plantar fasciitis: running sports
- Calcaneal apophysitis (Sever's disease): running sports

***Running injuries.*** Special mention should be made of a group of common overuse injuries often found in runners. Most injuries incurred by runners are overuse rather than acute and can primarily be attributed to training errors. Generally, injuries are seen in those who run more than 30 miles per week or increase their mileage by more than 10% per week. The type and grade of the running surface in addition to fatigue and lack of strength are factors that may contribute to injuries. Other predisposing factors include muscle tightness and accelerated training schedules.

Not surprisingly, most running injuries occur in the lower extremity. Tendinitis of the quadriceps, patellar, and Achilles tendons are common. A strain of the hamstring muscle group also can occur. The runner complains of localized pain, which usually increases during the run. On examination pain is reproduced with palpation or contraction of the involved musculotendinous unit. The physician should be reminded that posterior leg or thigh pain may be radicular. Treatment depends on accurate diagnosis, a search for exacerbating factors, and symptomatic treatment, emphasizing rest. Compliance with rest should improve if the patient understands that acute tendinitis and strains respond most favorably to this therapy. If allowed to become chronic, these injuries often take months to resolve.

If the runner complains of anterior or medial knee pain, one should evaluate for patellofemoral syndrome with medial facet arthritis and a synovial plica (medial shelf). A plica is a remnant of an embryologic wall that divides the knee into compartments and remains present in an estimated 15% to 20% of the adult population. It may become symptomatic with repetitive flexion and extension of the knee, such as in running. Often bilateral, it is frequently the source of pain in runner's knee and growing pains. It causes medial parapatellar pain, often on palpation. In a minority of cases it is palpable in flexion and extension of the knee. Symptomatic treatment of a plica is often unsuccessful, therefore arthroscopic release may be indicated.

Lateral patellofemoral pain develops in the setting of joint overload. It is a common cause of bilateral knee pain, especially in females. Risk factors include a relatively greater angle from hip to knee, called the Q angle (Fig. 88-3). The Q angle increases the lateral forces on the patella. Consequently the patella moves out of the normal femoral groove, and the undersurface compresses against the femoral condyles in a reduced area, increasing stress. Biomechanical abnormalities, including pes planus (flatfoot) and genu valgum (knock-knee) also contribute to the development of patellofemoral pain syndrome by increased lateralization. In a young athlete it may be due to inflexibility. Physical examination findings may be quite variable; there is frequently apprehension on the part of the athlete when the examiner's hands are placed on the knee, and even greater apprehension when gentle pressure is applied during lateral parapatellar palpation. Once the diagnosis is suspected and underlying causes identified, a treatment plan addressing the predisposing factors can usually be made. This generally involves NSAIDs and quadriceps stretching and strengthening. The rehabilitation program should stress eccentric strengthening and closed chain exercises. Biomechanical factors may be addressed by using devices such as braces and orthotics. Occasionally surgery is indicated, with arthroscopic lateral release or other procedures.

Included in the differential of a runner with lateral knee pain is the iliotibial band syndrome. Common in cyclists and runners, this syndrome is an inflammatory condition caused by chronic friction of the iliotibial band with the bony prominence of the lateral femoral condyle. Runners with varus deformities (bowlegs) or those who run on sloped surfaces are likely to complain of lateral knee pain in association with a popping sensation. Again, treatment is symptomatic and emphasizes stretching, strengthening, and adequate warm-up exercises.

The runner complaining of foot pain should be evaluated for plantar fasciitis, an inflammation and strain at the origin of the plantar fascia on the calcaneus. Patients describe pain on the bottom of the heel, especially upon first awakening in the morning, which is relieved with activity. Frequently associated with tight heelcords of the foot and hyperpronation, plantar fasciitis can usually be controlled by heelcord stretching and orthotics. In recalcitrant cases injection or, rarely, surgical release may be considered.

Anterior lower leg pain is common in runners and is frequently diagnosed as shin splints. Shin splints commonly refers to one of three syndromes: chronic compartment syndrome, chronic periostitis, or tibial stress fracture. Pain is generally at the medial distal tibia. Bone scan or special MRI can differentiate between stress fracture and periostitis. Factors that predispose runners to shin splints include training errors, anatomic variations, and poor running techniques or equipment. Patients develop localized tenderness, which increases during running and subsides after activity. Treatment consists of rest, ice, stretching, and careful warm-up, antiinflammatories, and correction of predisposing factors, such as the use of orthotics. Shin splints must be differentiated from stress fractures of the anterior tibia.

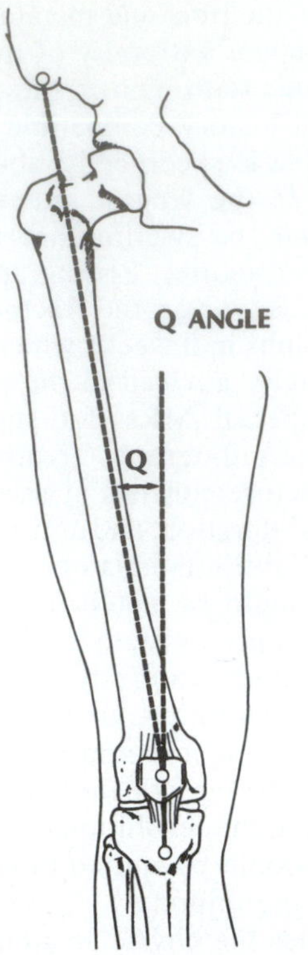


**Fig. 88-3.** Q angle. (From Insall J, Falvo KA, Wise DW: *J Bone Joint Surg* 58(A):1, 1976.)

In addition to tibial stress fractures, other stress fractures occur in virtually all sports but are particularly common in runners. This overuse injury is suggested when the runner complains of a persistent, dull pain while weight bearing. Although the metatarsals and tibia are probably the most common sites, the fibula, femoral neck, and pelvic bones may also sustain this type of fracture.

***Shoulder injuries.*** Injuries to the shoulder are common in sports. Examination should include evaluation of the bony structures, musculotendinous units, and neurovascular system. The purpose of the examination is to evaluate deformity, limitation of function, and instability. Referred pain should be considered when movement of the affected joint does not change the symptom or elicits no pain. For instance, consider the case of an amateur hockey player involved in a collision who complains of severe left shoulder pain with full range of motion. A referred pain syndrome could result from a range of problems from cervical disk herniation to a ruptured spleen with diaphragmatic irritation.

One of the most common injuries to the shoulder is a sprain of the acromioclavicular (AC) joint. This type of injury is common in contact sports such as football. It frequently follows a blow to or fall onto the shoulder, forcibly separating the acromion from the clavicle, or arises from a fall on an outstretched arm. The athlete usually complains of well-localized pain over the AC joint and difficulty with abduction or cross-body motion of the shoulder. The findings on examination and treatment differ with the degree of sprain. In general, grade I (nondisplaced) and grade II (minimally displaced) reveal little or no deformity and are managed easily with NSAIDs and a compression sling. Grade III or IV (complete AC displacement) should be referred to an orthopedist for possible surgical management.

A fracture of the clavicle results from a direct blow to the bone. Suspect this injury when the athlete complains of pain directly over the clavicle; radiographs easily confirm the diagnosis. Unless complicated, this fracture can usually be managed with a figure-of-eight bandage and pain medication. If the injury involves the AC joint, referral is advised. Similarly, occasional nonunion occurs and also requires orthopedic referral.

Another injury that may result from a fall onto an outstretched arm is a tear of the rotator cuff. The athlete complains of pain and weakness of the shoulder; examination confirms the weakness of the rotator cuff muscles on abduction and external rotation. This injury is generally best managed by surgical intervention and requires referral to an orthopedist.

Dislocation of the glenohumeral joint is another commonly encountered athletic injury. These are usually anterior but can be inferior or posterior. Anterior dislocation generally results from forcible external rotation of the abducted shoulder, such as a quarterback who, with his arm abducted horizontally, ready to throw a pass, is hit in the arm by an opponent. The dislocation is usually quite apparent, since the athlete complains of severe pain in association with deformity. Examination should include evaluation of the axillary nerve, which innervates the deltoid, before attempting reduction. A popular method for reduction is a traction-countertraction maneuver with steady pulling on the arm while pressuring the glenohumeral head into the joint. In this case an assistant anchors the patient's trunk with a sheet around the chest.

Impingement is an overuse condition, resulting in cuff tendinitis with associated bursitis and compression against the overlying acromion. It is especially common in swimmers and throwers (see Chapter 71).

***Elbow, wrist, and hand injuries.*** Most of the injuries to the elbow are from overuse, whereas wrist and hand injuries result from small microtraumas to the affected area. One of the more acute injuries that deserves mention is a fracture of the navicular bone of the wrist. It is frequently seen after a fall on the outstretched hand in sports such as in-line skating. The examiner should suspect this type of fracture in a patient with tenderness in the anatomic snuffbox of the radial wrist. There may be no other physical findings, and radiographs may be negative initially. It is wise for the primary care physician to splint the patient's wrist and refer the case to an orthopedist.

Gamekeeper's or skier's thumb is an acute sprain of the ulnar collateral ligament (UCL) of the thumb (see Chapter 72). This injury occurs when the skier or other athlete falls, and the thumb is forced into abduction. The metacarpophalangeal joint may appear swollen, and there is tenderness over the UCL. If radiographs reveal no fracture, the examiner may assess stability by stressing the UCL and evaluating for laxity. If the sprain is partial, treatment can be with a special thumb cast and NSAIDs. If a complete tear is suspected, referral to an orthopedist is advised. For an athlete with persistent wrist pain that was thought initially to indicate a simple sprain, consider the possibility of ligamentous injury with associated instability and refer for orthopedic evaluation.

***Knee injuries.*** The knee is perhaps the most frequently injured joint with which the primary care physician may be confronted. Working knowledge of the basic anatomy, function, and topography of the knee is essential to making an accurate diagnosis and treatment plan. As with the shoulder, the knee should be evaluated for deformity, loss or limitation of function, stability, and localization of tenderness. Assessment should also be made for effusion, although aspiration is rarely recommended in the acute knee injury (see Chapter 75 for further information on the knee).

One of the most commonly injured structures of the knee is the anterior cruciate ligament (ACL). The ACL may be injured by a valgus stress with external rotation or by hyperextension and internal rotation. Injury to this ligament frequently occurs in sports requiring jumping and quick directional change (cutting), although skiing is also a common cause. The athlete usually complains of a pop and may feel as if the knee is going to give way. Swelling usually occurs within 2 hours. If the examiner evaluates the knee before swelling has occurred, the examination is usually more diagnostic. One anticipates findings of positive Lachman test, anterior drawer test, and pivot shift test (see Glossary). Once swelling has occurred, and it usually occurs rapidly, the examination is less reliable. It is important to have the athlete as comfortable as possible while examining the injury; a pillow placed under the knee to encourage muscular relaxation is often helpful. Radiographs are necessary to rule out associated fractures. If an ACL injury is suspected, NSAIDs, ice, immobilization, compression, and acute referral to an orthopedist for diagnostic testing (MRI) and possible ligament reconstruction are recommended. Ligament reconstruction usually uses a portion of the patellar ligament, although some surgeons prefer to use one of the hamstring tendons. Allografts are occasionally used.

An injury to the meniscus may accompany a tear of the ACL or may occur as an isolated injury. This frequently results from a twisting injury. The simple finding of joint line tenderness in the athlete complaining of knee pain, especially if associated with a pop or click, supports this diagnosis. The McMurray test alone is often inconclusive; the key to this diagnosis is joint line tenderness. Radiographs are not generally helpful. Arthroscopic surgery and possible repair are indicated for athletes with a meniscal tear. It is important to note that a repair may reduce the future possibility of clinical osteoarthritis.

Injuries to the medial (MCL) and/or lateral (LCL) collateral ligaments are also frequent athletic injuries. The MCL is injured by a lateral (valgus) force to the knee, especially common in sports such as football and soccer. The athlete complains of pain and swelling medially, and the ligament is tender to palpation at the site of injury. Applying valgus stress to the knee in 30 degrees of flexion confirms laxity and may exacerbate the pain. Radiographs may demonstrate an associated avulsion fracture if the sprain represents a complete tear. If the tear is grade I or

II, immobilization in flexion or protected mobilization with bracing, ice, and NSAIDs is indicated. Crutches may be used as needed. Grade III may or may not require surgical repair, so referral to an orthopedist is advisable. Virtually all clinically significant knee ligament injuries require physical therapy as part of the treatment.

***Foot and ankle injuries.*** One of the most common athletic injuries is ankle sprain; however, the prudent examiner should remember that several other injuries may mimic this condition (see Chapter 76 for other conditions affecting the foot and ankle).

A true sprain is a stretching or tearing of the ligaments. The most common type of ankle sprain is an inversion sprain, where the plantar surface of the foot rolls in, resulting in damage to the lateral ligaments, especially the anterior talofibular. This occurs frequently in running and jumping sports, such as basketball, where one player might jump for a rebound and land unevenly on another player's foot. The athlete complains of pain over the lateral ankle, and swelling usually develops quickly in the area anterior to the lateral malleolus. If there is prominent swelling or difficulty with weight bearing, radiographs should be obtained to evaluate for a fracture. On examination the most important finding is point tenderness over the injured ligament. Tests for stability, including the anterior drawer and talar tilt maneuvers, can be gently performed but are not critical to acute diagnosis. Initial treatment should consist of elevation, ice, and compression. If the sprain is determined to be mild, this treatment, followed by appropriate rehabilitation, should be sufficient. More severe sprains, especially if unstable, require referral.

Braces are available for use while a sprain is acute and also during rehabilitation. Any type of immobilization used should effectively brace the injury while accommodating the patient's lifestyle. Three phases characterize subsequent rehabilitation to return to sport: immobilization and rest to control swelling and pain, training to increase strength and range of motion, and finally the athlete's return to the desired activity.

Less commonly, sprains to the deltoid ligament (medial) and tibiofibular ligament (syndesmosis) occur. The mechanism is an eversion injury, as opposed to the more common inversion injury. Both are significant and often require immobilization and prolonged treatment. Some severe syndesmosis sprains (tender at tibiofibular) require surgery to prevent arthritis from instability. If this type of injury is suspected, consultation with an orthopedic surgeon is warranted.

As mentioned previously, some ankle injuries initially thought to be sprains are not. Two injuries the physician needs to be aware of are those affecting the Achilles tendon and the peroneal tendons. An injury to the Achilles may be suspected in a basketball or tennis player who forcefully pushes off the foot. Frequently the athlete hears a pop. Pain may be variable, and continued walking is possible. However, attempts to stand on the toes are unsuccessful with a complete tear. Thompson test confirms the diagnosis. To perform this maneuver, the athlete either sits with the leg dangling or lies prone while the examiner gently grasps and squeezes the calf muscle. If the tendon is intact, the foot passively plantar flexes. Lack of this passive flexion signals rupture of the Achilles, in which case referral for casting or surgical repair is recommended.

A second injury that masquerades as an ankle sprain is subluxation of the peroneal tendon, which runs posteriorly to the lateral malleolus. This injury is seen in instances where the foot is fixed and the leg is forcibly rotated, as in cross-country skiing. The peroneal tendon tears free of its anchoring retinaculum and subluxates over the malleolus. The athlete complains of signs and symptoms similar to an ankle sprain. If the examiner holds the foot in neutral position and asks the athlete to resist eversion, the tendon may subluxate and the athlete complain of pain along the tendon. If the diagnosis is made promptly, before further damage occurs, treatment may consist of several weeks of casting without surgery. If diagnosis is delayed or the disorder recurs, surgery may be required.

The acute onset of pain in the middle to lower calf can represent a tear, not of the Achilles tendon, but of the musculotendinous junction of the gastrocnemius. The very sharp onset of pain behind the knee often represents a rupture of the plantaris tendon. Both injuries are treated symptomatically.

In general, acute athletic injuries of the foot are much less common than overuse injuries. However, an injury that deserves mention is a hyperextension injury of the metatarsophalangeal joint of the great toe, commonly known as turf toe. This is commonly seen in football players, especially those playing on artificial turf. The athlete complains of pain; tenderness and swelling of the joint confirm the diagnosis. Radiographs are usually normal. Treatment is symptomatic with NSAIDs and rest; shoe inserts are useful in recurrent or severe cases. Also important is the midfoot sprain, often a partial subluxation of the tarsometatarsal joints. This may require prolonged metatarsal immobilization, rest, and possibly surgery. Comparison standing AP radiographs may be diagnostic. If necessary, the MRI is definitive.

Foot and ankle fractures are relatively uncommon and are not addressed here.

***Spine injuries.*** Athletic injuries of the spine fall into two major groups: the neck and lower back. Neck, or cervical spine, injuries are potentially the most serious and life-threatening of athletic injuries. The most severe injuries occur with the neck in flexion, as in the now-banned tackling technique known as spearing. This can lead to quadriplegia and death. Any question of a possible severe neck injury should be treated as a medical emergency, even if this involves suspension of the athletic event until the neck can be protected and the patient safely transported.

More commonly, injury to the cervical spine results in transient neurapraxia, most often seen in football. The athlete may complain of altered sensation and motor function in the upper extremity, although the lower extremity may also be involved. Radiographs are negative. The paresthesias resolve spontaneously, usually within minutes.

The burner or stinger syndrome is commonly seen in contact sports. This is a stretching injury of the brachial plexus or a compression of nerve roots at the foramen. The athlete complains of burning pain radiating into the shoulder, upper arm, and hand, associated with weakness of muscles such as the deltoid and biceps. Symptoms generally resolve spontaneously, over minutes or hours.

The athlete may not be allowed to return to play until normal strength and sensation are returned (see Chapter 70 for other conditions of the cervical spine).

Myofascial sprains occur but are overdiagnosed. Many neck and trapezial pain syndromes are facet or neurogenic with associated disk or root pathology. Frequently the mechanism of such injuries is hyperextension in contact athletes. They are treated symptomatically, usually with NSAIDs, rest, and physical therapy. Occasionally the electromyograph (EMG) and MRI are useful in refractory cases.

The lumbar spine is frequently a site of pain and injury for athletes and nonathletes alike. Participants in virtually every sport, including gymnastics, football, weightlifting, wrestling, and figure skating, are at risk for low back injury. Lumbar injury is frequently diagnosed as muscle strain; although muscle strain does occur, it is important to look for other common causes of pain. Disk herniation or annular tears have been reported in athletes of all ages. They are frequently associated with radiculopathy. There may be pain on flexion or with midline palpation of the spine at the involved level. Patients with spondylolysis, thought to occur as a stress fracture of the pars interarticularis, may have acute low back pain. This is most common in teenage athletes involved in gymnastics, football, or weightlifting. The onset of pain is associated with a specific activity and is often nonradicular. Physical findings may include pain on spinal extension, while standing on the single leg on the side of the defect (positive one-legged hyperextension test), on rotation, and during palpation over the irritated area. Radiographs confirm a defect of the pars interarticularis in spondylolysis seen on oblique view (fracture of the neck of the "Scotty dog"). Rest is the treatment of choice, and occasionally immobilization is required. If the defect has progressed to become a spondylolisthesis, consultation with a spine specialist is advised (see Chapter 73 for further information on the diagnosis and management of low back pain).

***Hip and thigh injuries.*** Acute injuries to the hip and thigh are most often contusions or muscle strains. For example, a groin pull usually involves the adductors of the thigh; a commonly encountered contusion is the hip pointer, resulting from a direct blow to the ilium, causing pain and swelling. Examination may be difficult due to painful range of motion. The affected area is markedly tender. Immediate application of pressure then ice and rest are the cornerstones of treatment. A syndrome known as osteitis pubis may occur, involving a combination of groin or abductor rectus strain, pubic ramus stress, and/or pubic symphysis osteolysis. Treatment consists of rest, NSAIDs, and orthopedic referral. Fractures of the pelvis and femur are rare in athletics and are not addressed here (see Chapter 74 for conditions affecting the hip).

## REHABILITATION

Once an injury has occurred and the initial treatment plan has been instituted, the physician should think ahead to the need for rehabilitation. No matter how insignificant an injury may appear, if it results in time lost from activity, rehabilitation needs to be considered. The primary goal of rehabilitation should be to return the athlete to activity as soon and as safely as possible.

In the initial 24 to 48 hours following an athletic injury, acute treatment may be carried out according to the mnemonic PRICE:

**P**rotection from further injury is accomplished by keeping the athlete from playing while injured and using a splint for immobilization.

**R**est prevents further injury and allows the injury to begin healing.

**I**ce is a potent antiinflammatory by decreasing swelling, pain, and muscle spasm. Ice should be applied for periods of 10 to 30 minutes, with an equal period without ice.

**C**ompression, usually in the form of an elastic bandage, limits swelling and may provide some support to the injured tissue.

**E**levation helps to decrease swelling.

After definitive diagnosis and acute therapy, the actual rehabilitation process begins. Rehabilitation should be sport and athlete specific. In other words, a program should be individually designed for each athlete depending on the sport in which he or she participates. The physician must remember that, when an athlete is injured, it is not a "knee injury" or "shoulder injury," but rather an athlete with a specific knee injury or shoulder injury. Therefore attention needs to be paid to general conditioning as well as local rehabilitation of the injured limb. Flexibility, strength, proprioception, and endurance must be addressed. Modalities that may be employed include ice and heat, ultrasound, electrical stimulation, and iontophoresis. An athlete's return to play depends on progress during rehabilitation and should be delayed until the athlete is symptom free and has regained confidence in the injured limb.

## SPECIAL NEEDS

### Female athletes

Women are participating in athletics in increasing numbers. The primary care physician should keep in mind a few special considerations when evaluating and treating female athletes.

There are considerable differences in the male and female anatomy and physiology that affect exercise. Females have less dense bone, less muscle mass, a lower center of gravity, shorter limbs, and a gynecoid pelvis. These and other factors affect body mechanics and influence the ability to perform exercise. The female pelvis, because of its relative width, results in different running biomechanics than in males and has been associated with knee injury and overuse syndromes. Female bone is possibly at greater risk for stress fracture because it is less dense than male bone.

Nutritional considerations also differ for women. Because of menstruation, women have a greater need for iron than men. Because of estrogen effects, they also have a greater need for vitamin C. Competitive female athletes often have a diet that is restrictive in calories, leading in its extreme to a host of complications, including the recently described syndrome *female athlete triad,* characterized by disordered eating, amenorrhea, and osteoporosis. Inadequate calorie intake reduces peripheral fat, which can result in decreased conversion of androgens to estrogen. This hypoestrogenic state contributes to amenorrhea and is associated with osteoporosis. Inadequate calcium intake exacerbates the effects of this syndrome.

The primary care physician should also be aware of the prevalence and appropriate treatment of eating disorders in athletes. Although most common in females, it is estimated that 5% of those suffering from eating disorders are male. Between the ages of 10 and 20, young women must maintain sufficient caloric intake to ensure adequate bone density. Surveys do indicate that about one third of female athletes suffer from eating disorders and/or obsessions about food. An uninformed coach, especially in sports such as gymnastics, figure skating, and diving, which are scored in part on appearance, may actually contribute to the dietary problem and increase the athlete's risk of further psychologic and physiologic damage.

For the pregnant woman, exercise is generally agreed to be safe, although there is significant controversy regarding the degree of recommended endurance and intensity. Certain anatomic and physiologic changes may affect the pregnant athlete's ability to perform exercise, and it is therefore prudent for the physician to individualize each patient's exercise prescription and consult the obstetrician as appropriate. In general, exercise should be carefully monitored for exacerbation of back pain, some degree of which is common to virtually all pregnant women.

## Young athletes

The notion that children are not small adults applies also in the field of sports medicine. Children and adolescents have rapidly changing anatomic and physiologic characteristics that affect their ability to participate in various sports as well as their predisposition to certain injuries. Discussion here is limited to orthopedic concerns.

The young athlete's skeletal immaturity predisposes to injuries not encountered in the older athlete. The epiphyseal plate, the cartilaginous growth center, is the weakest portion of growing bone and is commonly injured. It is important for the primary care physician to understand that such injuries are common and can affect growth, so careful evaluation is required. Physical examination should always include palpation of the epiphysis. Epiphyseal injuries are generally described by the Salter-Harris classification system. Depending on the type of and extent of epiphyseal injury, therapy ranges from closed reduction with excellent prognosis to open reduction and potential growth impairment.

In response to injury or trauma, young children and adults generally sustain ligament injuries, whereas fractures most often appear in adolescent patients. These injuries are a reflection of the maturity of the musculoskeletal system and the relative strength of ligament or epiphysis, not the patient's chronologic age. The box above lists the most common injuries or conditions, in no exact order of prevalence, that require referral to a pediatric orthopedist.

### Common pediatric orthopedic injuries

- Ankle sprains and fractures
- Osgood-Schlatter disease (tibial tubercle)
- Shoulder instability (more likely in teenagers)
- Elbow tendinitis and osteochondritis (little leaguer's elbow)
- Clavicle fractures (typical playground injury)
- AC joint separation
- ACL tears
- Distal radius fractures
- Patellofemoral and plica syndromes (anterior knee pain syndromes)
- Spondylolysis

As in the adult athlete population, tennis elbow, AC separations, and ACL tears are seen in athletic children. However, certain fractures, such as those of the distal radius and clavicle, are seen more commonly. Additionally, developmental abnormalities, including patellofemoral dysplasia, Osgood-Schlatter disease, spondylolysis, and shoulder instability can result in injuries or symptoms during participation in sports. Injury may precipitate these conditions, but there appears to be some predisposition based on preexisting abnormalities of growth and connective tissue, such as joint laxity in shoulders and patellar dislocations.

## Older athletes

The athlete over 65 years has the same injury profile as younger athletes, except in three areas. First, active weight-bearing exercise such as jogging is associated with better bone density in the general skeleton. This in turn offers some protection against compression fractures of the vertebral spine and hip, especially when compared to the risks of fracture encountered by a sedentary age-matched group. However, fractures of the wrist and sprained ankles are more common in the geriatric running population due to falls. To avoid falls, every effort should be made to run on completely level surfaces, such as tracks, rather than on the side of the road.

Second, a warm-up period is mandatory for the older population to minimize tendon injuries. The combination of degenerative processes may predispose to higher rates of muscle tendon type injuries when compared to those of younger athletes. This is particularly applicable to sports where sudden acceleration and deceleration occur, such as tennis. The same sort of degenerative predisposition probably accounts for some of the back injuries seen in golf. A complete warm-up is essential to facilitate injury prevention.

Third, exercise can aggravate existing osteoarthritis of the knee, hip, and lower spine. However, this is usually offset by exercise-induced weight control and increased muscle strength, which ultimately serve to protect the joints. As discussed earlier, the cardiovascular system needs to be carefully evaluated before beginning any incremental exercise regimen.

## Sports-specific injuries

Primary care physicians may treat patients participating in a variety of sports. Table 88-3 outlines the risk of injury to specific joint regions that occur in sports most common in high school. Primary care physicians need to pay particular attention to the incidence of previous neck injuries in wrestlers, gymnasts, and football players. This information is most relevant during a preparticipation examination, where athletes can be screened for these

**Table 88-3.** Approximate frequency distribution of selected injuries within individual sports

| Sport | Wrist/hand | Shoulder | Elbow | Lumbar spine | Knee | Foot/ankle | Neck |
|---|---|---|---|---|---|---|---|
| Football/rugby | +++ | +++ | + | ++ | +++ | +++ | +++ |
| Baseball/softball | ++ | +++ | + | + | + | ++ | + |
| Soccer/field sports | + | + | + | | +++ | +++ | |
| Volleyball | + | +++ | | + | + | ++ | + |
| Basketball | + | + | | + | ++ | +++ | + |
| Swimming | | +++ | | + | + | | + |
| Gymnastics | +++ | ++ | + | +++ | +++ | ++ | +++ |
| Tennis/racquet sports | + | ++ | +++ | | ++ | + | ++ |
| Weight training | + | +++ | + | ++ | ++ | | + |
| Running | | | | + | ++ | +++ | |
| Wrestling | + | ++ | | + | ++ | | +++ |
| Skiing/snowboarding | ++ | + | | | +++ | + | |
| Ice hockey | + | + | + | ++ | +++ | + | + |
| Cycling | + | ++ | | ++ | ++ | | + |

+, Mild concern; ++, moderate concern; +++, high concern.

types of injuries. Continued participation in sport might expose them to further neck injury.

## MEDICAL CONSIDERATIONS

The primary care physician is in the unique position of integrating the total care of the athlete. Although athletes are susceptible to the same illnesses as the general population, treatment of an athlete may require special considerations. Communicability of an infectious disease, control of asthma and diabetes, and risks imposed by certain conditions such as cardiovascular arrhythmias may have special implications for an athlete's health and subsequent return to safe participation.

### Infectious disease

One of the most common infectious diseases is an acute febrile illness, such as an upper respiratory tract infection, which affects athlete and nonathlete alike. Although treatment of an athlete's acute infection does not differ, the athlete will have questions about ability to practice and return to play. It is generally advisable to avoid strenuous activity while acutely ill, febrile, and experiencing myalgias, although the athlete does not need to be symptom free before returning to play. Adequate fluid intake is especially important for an athlete recovering from illness. For an athlete with infectious mononucleosis, contact sports should not be resumed until the spleen has returned to normal size. Resolution of splenomegaly can be confirmed with palpation.

In wrestlers, transmission of herpes simplex virus type I (HSV-I), known as herpes gladitorium, occurs primarily through skin-to-skin contact. Coaches and parents should be advised to exclude any wrestlers with active skin lesions from competition or practice. Similarly, skin lesions of impetigo caused by streptococci should also preclude athletic participation.

The physician involved with the treatment of athletes may be questioned about communicability of certain diseases, such as the human immunodeficiency virus (HIV). It is essential to understand and communicate to patients that the risk of contracting HIV through intact skin by infected blood or saliva is extremely low. Moreover, in the asymptomatic HIV-positive patient there is little or no evidence that exercise activates HIV into clinical acquired immune deficiency syndrome (AIDS). In addition, the primary care physician should stress safe sexual techniques through condom use in all sexually active patients. All health personnel, including trainers, should use universal precautions (e.g., gloves) when treating injured athletes despite the extremely low risk of contracting HIV through intact skin. In fact, regulatory agencies, including the National Collegiate Athletic Association (NCAA), are recommending the immediate changing of blood-stained uniforms in basketball. These highly publicized communications in the media urge physicians to transmit realistic information and precautionary guidelines to their patients.

### Diabetes

Study of the many diabetics active in athletic events has provided much knowledge about the positive effects of fitness on diabetes. Training seems to improve glucose tolerance, aid in weight control, and decrease insulin requirements in diabetics. Monitoring of glucose levels in insulin-dependent diabetics is crucial, since insulin requirements vary with exercise. One must be aware of the possibility of hypoglycemia and have glucose readily available should the insulin-dependent athlete require it. Although exercise is generally beneficial, the poorly controlled diabetic may become more hyperglycemic and ketotic with activity. It is therefore generally advisable that diabetes be fairly well controlled with diet and insulin before initiating an exercise program. On rare occasions the type II diabetic patient (adult onset) taking oral hypoglycemic agents can lower his or her blood sugar during sustained exercise over hours, such as golf. It is wise to carry a glucose source while playing this sport.

### Asthma

Asthma is common among athletes, especially in the form of exercise-induced asthma (EIA). EIA does not interfere with ability to perform, provided that a few precautions are followed.

Those with EIA complain of cough, dyspnea, or wheezing after several minutes of moderately intense exercise. Symptoms are worse in cold, dry air but improved by warm, humid air. Swimming, therefore, may be a better activity to recommend to a patient with EIA than running. In cold weather sports such as downhill and cross-country skiing, cold-induced bronchospasm can be observed. Its relationship to EIA has been debated.

Prophylaxis includes a warm-up period before vigorous exercise as well as a number of medications. The two most important medications are the β-agonists and cromolyn, which should be administered 10 to 15 minutes before exertion. One must be careful to comply with prescribing and disclosure guidelines of the applicable athletic organization. The list of medicines that are allowed by the NCAA and the United States Olympic Committee (USOC) include NSAIDs, antihistamines, antibiotics, insulin, topical steroids, and antiulcer medicines.

### Cardiovascular conditions

There has been a great deal of interest in cardiac disease in the athlete in the past few years, largely stemming from a few incidences of sudden death among high-profile athletes. Sudden death can be defined as that which is unexpected, nontraumatic, and instantaneous. Over the age of 30 the most common etiology is coronary artery disease. Before the age of 30 the most common etiology is a congenital condition such as abnormal coronary arteries, valve disease, or hypertrophic cardiomyopathy. Hypertrophic cardiomyopathy is suggested by a midsystolic crescendo-decrescendo murmur heard best at the left sternal border without an accompanied ejection sound that increases in duration and intensity with maneuvers that reduce ventricular filling, such as a standing Valsalva's maneuver.

It is also important to consider Marfan syndrome, which is associated with thoracic aortic aneurysm/dissection. Family history or typical physical features, including long limbs and fingers, may suggest this diagnosis. Although these entities are relatively uncommon, they are emphasized because of their potential for fatal outcomes. Thus the primary care physician should be aware of their characteristics. More common cardiac problems such as mitral valve prolapse can be associated with exercise-induced arrhythmias. A history of troublesome palpitations, syncope, or pre-syncope should raise concern of a preexcitation syndrome, which should warrant a formal cardiac evaluation.

The most important clues to a cardiac abnormality include history of syncope, chest pain, and family history of sudden death. The physical examination may reveal a murmur. Although cardiac disease in a young athlete is an uncommon finding, one must consider the possibility when the situation arises and ensure that the athlete is referred for appropriate evaluation.

The physician should be aware of a condition known as the athletic heart syndrome. This is a constellation of physiologic adaptations of the heart to exercise. It provides improved cardiac function and is a benign condition characterized by bradycardia, an irregular pulse, and a flow murmur. This is an asymptomatic syndrome not associated with syncope or other ominous findings and does not place the athlete at risk for cardiac events.

## SUMMARY

Primary care sports medicine is a rapidly expanding field, incorporating many facets of medical care. As their role in managing the total health care of the competitive athlete develops, primary care physicians need to feel comfortable with the variety of issues presented in this chapter. These issues include exercise prescription, medical conditions affecting athletes, anticipation and prevention of athletic injuries, and effective treatment when injury does occur. In addition, provision of high-quality, cost-efficient care to address these injuries depends on timely and appropriate specialty referral. The trend toward a more complete approach to care of the injured athlete should be encouraged as an opportunity for primary care physicians to positively influence patients in making healthy lifestyle choices.

## GLOSSARY

**Anabolic Steroids ("Steroids"):** Testosterone and its derivatives, having pronounced anabolic properties. They are commonly used by athletes to improve muscle strength and increase muscle mass and exercise tolerance.

**Closed Chain Exercises:** When applied to the limbs, the term describes exercises done with the limb in contact with a surface. Leg presses and pushups are examples of this type of strengthening, which requires contraction of all muscles in the limb in a coordinated manner (cocontraction).

**Concentric Strengthening:** The musculotendinous unit shortens during contraction. Biceps curls and leg extensions (quadriceps) are examples of this type of strengthening.

**Concussion (of the brain):** A temporary disturbance of brain function without permanent macrostructural injury as the result of a blow to the head. The degree of loss of consciousness and amnesia varies from mild to severe.

**Eccentric Strengthening:** The musculotendinous unit lengthens during contraction. Squats (quadriceps) and elbow extensions (biceps) are examples of this type of strengthening exercise.

**Hamstring Muscle:** Thigh muscles that flex the knee. The biceps femoris, semitendinosus, and semimembranosus are collectively termed the hamstring muscle group.

**Lachman Test:** Test to determine ACL competence. It is performed with the patient supine on the examining table and the knee at 15 degrees of flexion. The examiner stands on the side of the affected extremity; the thigh is held immobile in one hand while the opposite hand grasps the proximal tibia and attempts to move it anteriorly, avoiding rotation. The examiner looks and feels for anterior tibial translation compared with the opposite normal knee. Quality of end point should also be evaluated; it should be firm, not soft or mushy.

**McMurray's Test:** Examination to determine meniscal injury. Positive test produces increased joint line pain with forced flexion and rotation of the knee; there may be an audible or palpable click or pop along the joint line in conjunction with the motion. Its presence is not necessary to diagnose meniscal derangement. Joint line pain to palpation is a more sensitive means of diagnosing meniscal injury.

**Meniscus:** C-shaped fibrocartilaginous structure of the knee, which helps distribute load and stabilize the joint. Cartilage tear refers to an injury of this structure.

**Osgood-Schlatter Disease:** Tension overload of the bone and soft tissue at the insertion of infrapatellar tendon on the tibial tubercle. This disease is seen in adolescents. Pain found only over the midtendon or at the distal pole of the patella is not indicative of Osgood-Schlatter disease.

**Overtraining:** A syndrome that occurs when an athlete's training program exceeds the body's ability for recovery, physically or mentally.

**Plica Band or Medial Shelf:** A remnant of an embryologic elastic tissue wall remaining on the medial capsule of the knee near the medial rim of the patella.

**Pivot Shift Test:** Test used to assess integrity of the ACL. Beginning with the knee fully extended and the foot internally rotated, the examiner applies a valgus stress while progressively flexing the knee. Watch and feel for translation of the tibia on the femur, which is, in fact, the actual type of luxation that occurs when a knee gives way in an episode of anterior cruciate incompetence or anterior cruciate tearing.

**Shin Splints:** A term implying pain in the leg after exercise. It applies most commonly to three distinct syndromes: compartment syndrome, periostitis, and stress reaction or stress fracture of the tibia.

**Spondylolisthesis:** Forward luxation of one vertebra over the one below it as a result of a stress fracture of the pars interarticularis.

**Spondylolysis:** Stress fracture of the pars interarticularis without displacement. Radiographs confirm a defect of the pars interarticularis (fracture of the neck of the Scotty dog).

**Sprain:** A ligament injury in which some or all of the fibers of a ligament are torn.

**"Stacking":** Taking combinations of anabolic steroids in a certain series to maximize strength gains.

**Stinger/Burner:** A stretching injury of the brachial plexus or a compression injury to the nerve roots giving similar clinical pictures. The patient complains of burning pain radiating into the arm and hand. It may be associated with weakness of muscles in innervated areas.

**Strain:** A tension injury to the muscle fiber that can result in tearing of the muscle.

## BIBLIOGRAPHY

American Academy of Family Practice (AAFP), American Academy of Pediatrics (AAP), American Medical Society for Sports Medicine (AMSSM), American Orthopedic Society for Sports Medicine (AOSSM), American Osteopathic Academy of Sports Medicine (AOASM): *Preparticipation physical evaluation,* Swander H, editor, 1992.

American College of Sports Medicine: Position stand on the recommended quantity and quality of exercise for developing and maintaining cardiorespiratory and muscular fitness in healthy adults, *Med Sci Sports Exerc* 22(2):265, 1990.

American College of Sports Medicine: Position stand on the use of anabolic-androgenic steroids in sports, *Med Sci Sports Exerc* 19(5):534, 1987.

Belongia EA et al: An outbreak of herpes gladitorium at a high school wrestling camp, *N Engl J Med* 325(13):906, 1991.

Clark N: How to approach eating disorders among athletes, *Top Clin Nutr* 5(3):41, 1990.

Fuentes RJ, Rosenberg JM, Davis A: *Allen and Hanbury's athletic drug reference '94,* Durham, NC, 1994, Glaxo.

Grana WA, Kalenak A, editors: *Clinical sports medicine,* Philadelphia, 1991, WB Saunders.

Greenspan A: *Orthopedic radiology: a practical approach,* ed 2, New York, 1992, Raven Press.

Hoppenfeld S: *Physical examination of the spine and extremities,* East Norwalk, CT, 1976, Appleton-Century-Crofts.

Johnston CC Jr et al: Calcium supplementation and increases in bone mineral density in children, *N Engl J Med* 327(2):82, 1992.

Lane NE et al: The risk of osteoarthritis with running and aging: a 5-year longitudinal study, *J Rheumatol* 20(3):461, 1993.

Lane NE et al: Running, osteoarthritis and bone density: initial 2-year longitudinal study, *Am J Med* 88(5):452, 1990.

Strauss RH, editor: *Sports medicine,* ed 2, Philadelphia, 1991, WB Saunders.

Thabit G III, Micheli L: Orthopedic disorders of the extremities. In Burg FD, Ingelfinger JR, Wald ER, editors: *Current pediatric therapy,* Philadelphia, 1993, WB Saunders.

# IX Nephrology

CHAPTER

# 89 Diagnostic Testing and Assessment of Renal Function

James A. Delmez

## GLOMERULAR FILTRATION RATE

### Concepts

The concept of plasma clearance by the kidneys, developed in the 1920s, refers to the volume of plasma freed of a substance by renal activity per unit time (usually 1 minute). Depending on the substance studied, the renal clearance may be achieved by glomerular filtration, net tubular secretion, or a combination of the two. For clinical purposes the focus of interest is the volume of plasma cleared per minute of a substance solely by the process of glomerular filtration. If a substance is freely filtered by glomeruli and not subsequently altered by tubular reabsorption or tubular secretion, its plasma clearance represents the glomerular filtration rate (GFR). Accurate measurement of GFR is probably the most critical index of renal function; it is also one of the most difficult.

### Measurements

A number of substances fulfill the criteria as accurate markers of GFR. These include inulin, $I^{125}$-iothalamate, and $Tc^{99m}$–diethylenetriaminepentaacetic acid (DPTA) (I, iodine; Tc, technetium). The disadvantages of these are that they must be administered exogenously as an intravenous (IV) bolus, usually followed by a constant infusion to maintain steady-state plasma levels. During the infusion, four urine collections are obtained over 30-minute intervals to calculate the GFR. These are costly and labor-intensive tests whose use is usually restricted to research protocols at major medical centers.

### Estimations

The endogenous substance used most often in the clinical assessment of GFR is *creatinine*. It is a waste product that is derived from the spontaneous degradation of creatinine and creatine phosphate. The body content of these substances is proportional to muscle mass, and therefore the amount of creatinine requiring excretion per day is also proportional to muscle mass. Accordingly, muscular athletes and males produce more creatinine than inactive females, children, and elderly persons. Widespread acute necrosis of skeletal muscle from any cause will also increase the production rate of creatinine. Generally, however, the daily production rate of creatinine in an individual subject is constant.

Creatinine is freely filtered by the kidneys. However, there is also proximal tubular secretion that results in an overestimation of the true GFR. In those with normal GFR, the overestimation is only 5% to 10%. As renal function deteriorates, the contribution of creatinine secretion to creatinine clearance assumes a major role. In some subjects with renal insufficiency, creatinine clearance may exceed GFR by 70%. Unfortunately, the magnitude of tubular secretion of creatinine varies from patient to patient and even within a given patient at different times. Another potential problem in assessing creatinine clearances is the use of drugs that interfere with the tubular secretion of creatinine. Such drugs, including cimetidine and trimethoprim, may decrease creatinine clearances without affecting GFR. Some investigators have advocated administering cimetidine to patients to improve the accuracy of creatinine clearances. The drug is usually given for 3 to 6 days, with the 24-hour urine collection saved during the last day. Because cimetidine is removed via renal excretion, the dose must be altered according to renal function. The usual dose is 400 mg four times a day.

Despite its limitations, creatinine clearances continue to be widely measured in the evaluation of renal function, largely because of the test's simplicity. Nonetheless, it is critical that the test be performed by collecting the urine sample in a complete and precisely timed fashion. The patient should be instructed to void on awakening and discard the urine sample. All voided specimens should then be collected for the next 24 hours, with care to ensure that the bladder is emptied at exactly 24 hours and that the final urine specimen is included in the collection. The normal daily creatinine excretion is 18 to 21 mg/kg body weight for males and 15 to 18 mg/kg for females. Values less than these may represent an inadequate urine collection, except in individuals with either decreased muscle mass or advanced renal insufficiency. The urine container should be refrigerated during this period to avoid overgrowth of bacteria, which may promote the conversion of creatinine to creatine and therefore spuriously lower the creatinine clearance. The patient's serum may be analyzed for the concentration of creatinine either at the start or end of the urine collection (see the box below). The results should be expressed per 1.73 $m^2$ (body surface area). The normal ranges depend on the chemical assay used for creatinine. In general, they are:

Females: 75 to 115 ml/min/1.73 $m^2$

Males: 85 to 125 ml/min/1.73 $m^2$

Measurement of the serum creatinine is probably the first and easiest test in estimating renal function. The wide range of normal values (usually 0.6 to 1.4 mg/dl) reflects differences in muscle mass from subject to subject. The "rule of thumb" is that for every doubling of serum

#### Formula for creatinine clearance

Urine creatinine (mg/dl) × Urine flow rate (dl/min)/Serum creatinine

Or for a 24-hour collection period:

Urine creatinine (mg/dl) × Urine volume (dl)/Serum creatinine (mg/dl) × 14.4

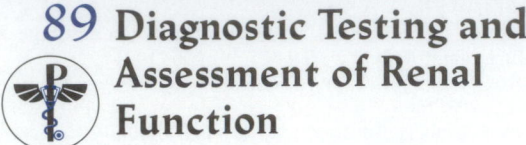

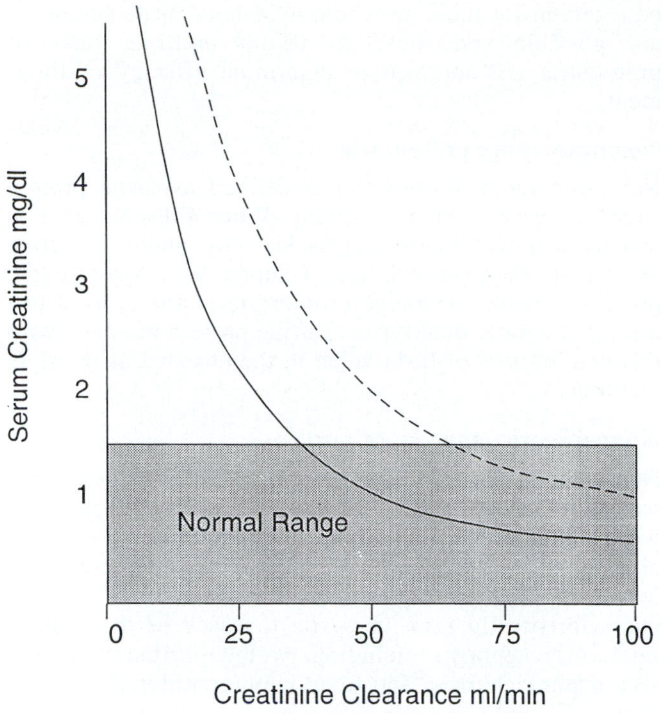


**Fig. 89-1.** Relationship between serum creatinine and creatinine clearance in two patients with different baseline values for serum creatinine.

creatinine, the GFR will decrease by 50%. Thus, a healthy but frail subject may have a baseline serum creatinine of 0.6 mg/dl. If half the renal function is subsequently lost, the corresponding serum creatinine would be only 1.2 mg/dl, still within the normal range. This relationship is illustrated by the solid line in Fig. 89-1. In this example, a further rise to 2.4 mg/dl would represent a loss of 75% of renal function. In contrast, the dashed line shows this relationship in a subject with a baseline serum creatinine of 1.0 mg/dl. Loss of half the renal function results in a serum creatinine of 2.0 mg/dl, a value that is outside the normal range. Because of enhanced tubular secretion of creatinine and increased extrarenal metabolism of creatinine with renal failure, the rule of thumb may greatly underestimate the decline in GFR. If any question exists that renal function may be impaired despite a normal serum creatinine, a creatinine clearance should be done. Although creatinine levels are not as affected by protein intake as much as urea values, a protein meal will increase serum creatinine levels by as much as 0.4 mg/dl for up to 10 to 12 hours. To avoid misinterpretation of changes in serum creatinine levels, it is preferable to measure values after an overnight fast. Another potential source of error in interpreting creatinine values is the presence of substances in the serum that falsely elevate the values. These include acetoacetate, which is elevated in ketoacidosis, and certain cephalosporins, such as cephalothin, cefazolin, cefoxitin, and cefamandole.

Approximately 1 ml/minute GFR is lost per year after age 30. However, the serum creatinine does not increase with age because of the decreased muscle mass accompanying aging. Thus, perceived minor abnormalities in the serum creatinine in the elderly person may represent severe impairment of renal function.

### Formula for estimating creatinine clearance

Creatinine clearance = (140 − age) × Weight/(Creatinine × 72) × (Men)
Creatinine clearance = (140 − age) × Weight/(Creatinine × 85) (Women)

Various nomograms have been published that attempt to estimate creatinine clearance from the levels of serum creatinine. The most accepted formulas are those of Cockcroft and Gault, which incorporate the variables of age, gender, and weight (see the box above).

In these equations, age is in years, weight in kilograms, and creatinine in mg/dl. Limitations to these equations include (1) they will overestimate creatinine clearance if the subject is obese or edematous; (2) the patient must have relatively stable renal function; (3) they are of no value in those with acute renal failure; and (4) they are estimates of creatinine clearance, which, as discussed, is itself an estimate of GFR.

Measurement of serum *urea* as an index of renal function has largely been supplanted by creatinine, since urea levels are more affected by dietary protein intake. In addition, urea levels may rise with gastrointestinal (GI) bleeding and states of accelerated protein catabolism. Nonetheless, many nephrologists believe that urea levels correlate better than creatinine with uremic symptoms and monitor both values.

It is of interest to know, as well as possible, the GFR in those with severe renal failure. This allows for the orderly planning of transplantation or dialysis. As discussed, creatinine clearances may greatly overestimate GFR in this situation. Alternatively, one may measure simultaneously creatinine and urea clearances and average the values. This ploy uses the properties of both substances in that they are freely filtered. Creatinine, however, is secreted, whereas urea is reabsorbed by the tubules. The two errors tend to offset each other, and the maneuver is fairly accurate when the GFR is less than 30 ml/minute.

Occasionally, it is important to determine if the function of one kidney is significantly different from the other. This issue is usually raised when the consequences of a surgical nephrectomy are being weighed. A renal scan is the test of choice, but no agreement exists concerning the best radiopharmaceutical agent. $Tc^{99m}$–DTPA, $Tc^{99m}$–glucoheptonate (GHA), and $Tc^{99m}$–dimercaptosuccinic acid (DMSA) are widely used. The general procedure is to inject the agent by vein and compare the radioactivity of the two kidneys, usually within the first 3 minutes of the scan.

## MEASUREMENTS OF URINE PROTEINS

Plasma proteins are prevented from entering the urine because of the permselectivity and negative charge of the glomerulus. In addition, much of the protein traversing the glomerulus into the urine space is reabsorbed by the renal tubules. Thus, the kidneys normally excrete less than 150 mg/day of proteins. Approximately 60% are derived from plasma, with the remainder produced by the kidneys and lower tract. The measurement of urine proteins is often helpful in determining the presence, severity, and prognosis of renal diseases. In addition, a decline in proteinuria may indicate response to therapy.

The *urine dipstick* is the simplest and most common measurement of urine proteins. It is fairly sensitive to the presence of negatively charged proteins such as albumin. However, it is insensitive to positively charge proteins such as some immunoglobulin light chains. The limit of detection of standard dipsticks is 10 to 20 mg/dl. Assuming a 24-hour urine output of 2 L/day, the dipsticks may not detect proteinuria of up to 200 to 400 mg/day. In patients with nephrotic range proteinuria (greater than 3.5 g/day) and no paraproteinuria, the dipstick should always be positive. Because the dipstick measures only the concentration of proteins in the urine, it is not a useful quantitative test of proteinuria.

The "gold standard" for quantitating proteinuria is the measurement of a *24-hour urine collection* performed in the same manner as a creatinine clearance. The interpretation of proteinuria should always be in the context of renal function. As renal function deteriorates, there is decreased delivery of protein available for filtration, and proteinuria often declines with moderate to severe renal failure. A very low serum albumin may also cause a decline in proteinuria by similar mechanisms.

An alternative to collecting a 24-hour urine for protein determination is a *spot urine* measuring the protein/creatinine ratio. In the presence of stable renal function, a protein/creatinine ratio more than 3.5 (mg/mg) indicates nephrotic range proteinuria, whereas a ratio less than 0.2 is within normal limits. The best correlation is found when samples are collected after the first morning void and at bedtime. Estimation of proteinuria by this method should be reserved for those in whom a 24-hour urine sample is not possible and those in whom multiple tests of proteinuria are obtained to determine efficacy of treatment.

### Nephrotic range proteinuria

Nephrotic range proteinuria is defined as urine protein excretion greater than 3.5 g/day. When present, there is usually a defect in the permselectivity and/or negative charge of the glomeruli (see Chapter 93). Most of the protein in nephrotic range proteinuria is albumin. Determining the individual types of urine protein in adults with this condition is of little value in the absence of multiple myeloma.

### Nonnephrotic range proteinuria

Nonnephrotic range proteinuria is defined as urine protein excretion between 150 mg and 3.5 g/day. Proteinuria within this range renders little information about the etiology of the defect. However, urine protein excretion of less than 2 g/day suggests a tubulointerstitial disease, characteristically seen in cystic diseases of the kidney, interstitial nephritis including pyelonephritis, hypertensive nephrosclerosis, and toxic nephropathies.

### Microalbuminuria

Microalbuminuria is defined as an elevated rate of urinary albumin excretion with a total protein excretion less than 150 mg/day. The excretion rates may be determined by timed specimens or a 24-hour urine collection, with the albumin measured with an assay that is very sensitive to small amounts of albumin. The upper range of albumin excretion usually ranges from 15 to 30 μg/minute, but it varies between laboratories. A dipstick test also is

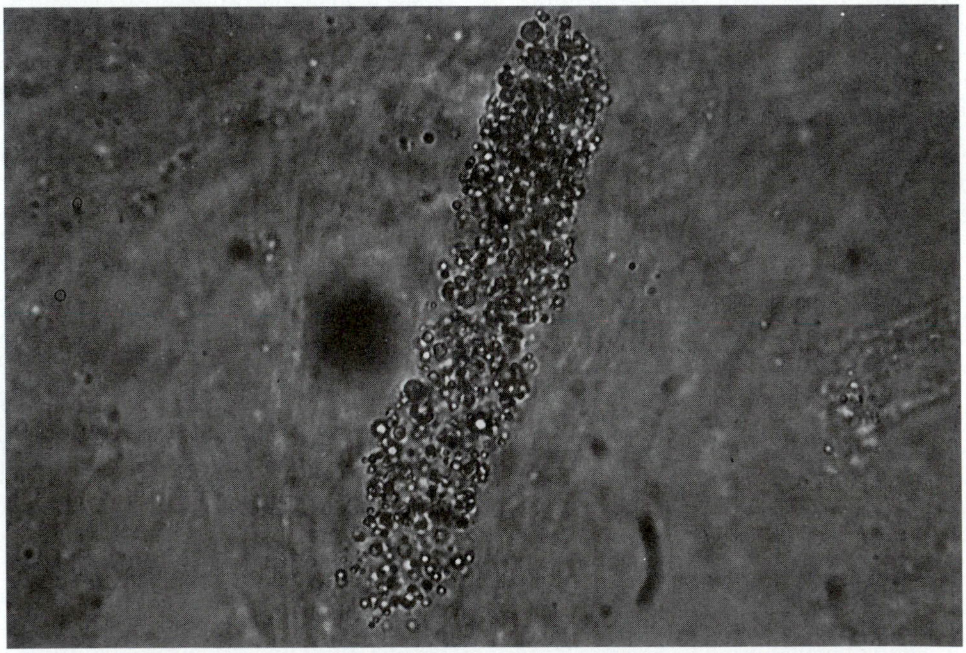

**Fig. 89-2.** Hyaline cast with fatty inclusions. The microscopic finding of this suggest presence of the nephrotic syndrome. (×400.) (From Piccoli G, Varese D, Rotunno M: *Atlas of urinary sediments: diagnosis and clinical correlations in nephrology,* New York, 1984, Raven.)

available for testing microalbuminuria that can detect concentrations as low as 2 mg/dl. These tests are primarily used to determine which patients with a relatively recent onset of diabetes are at risk to develop overt diabetic nephropathy (see Chapter 33).

### Paraproteinuria

The normal excretion of immunoglobulin light chains is 1 to 7 mg/day. The presence of an increased amount of light chains in the urine always results from their overproduction and warrants a search for a lymphoproliferative disorder. Immunofixation electrophoresis is the most sensitive test to detect urinary paraproteins.

## URINALYSIS

A careful examination of the urine often provides useful information about diseases of the urinary tract as well as metabolic or systemic diseases not directly related to the kidney. As with all laboratory procedures, the tests should be carefully performed in a standardized fashion. For chemical (dipstick) and microscopic examination, a *clean-catch, midstream urine collection* is optimal. The urine should be visually assessed for color and clarity. The unspun urine should then be subjected to a dipstick analysis done according to the manufacturer's specifications. A sample of the urine (10 to 15 ml) should then be centrifuged in a capped urine tube for 5 minutes at 450 × *g*. The supernatant is poured out, and the bottom pellet resuspended by gentle-suction pipetting. Cellular elements begin to break down within 2 hours at room temperature. The microscopic examination using a high-power lens should therefore be done promptly. It is important to identify the type and number of cells and casts per high-power field (HPF) as well as the presence of microorganisms and crystals. Cells may originate from any tissue in the urinary system. Casts are formed only in the renal tubules because of gelation of Tamm-Horsfall glycoprotein and are most easily seen at the edge of the coverslip. The type of cast refers to the material (cells, fat, filtered proteins) trapped within the cast at the time of formation. The presence of casts of any type strongly suggests significant renal disease. For example, if fatty inclusions are found within a hyaline cast (Fig. 89-2), it is likely that the patient has nephrotic syndrome. Epithelial cell casts (Fig. 89-3) are comprised of desquamated renal tubular cells embedded in a protein matrix. Their presence suggests an active renal process, such as glomerulonephritis, interstitial nephritis, or acute tubular necrosis. Cellular casts may degenerate into granular casts (Fig. 89-4), wherein the outlines of the cells are lost. It should be emphasized that urine should be considered a hazardous material, and gloves should be worn when handling any specimens.

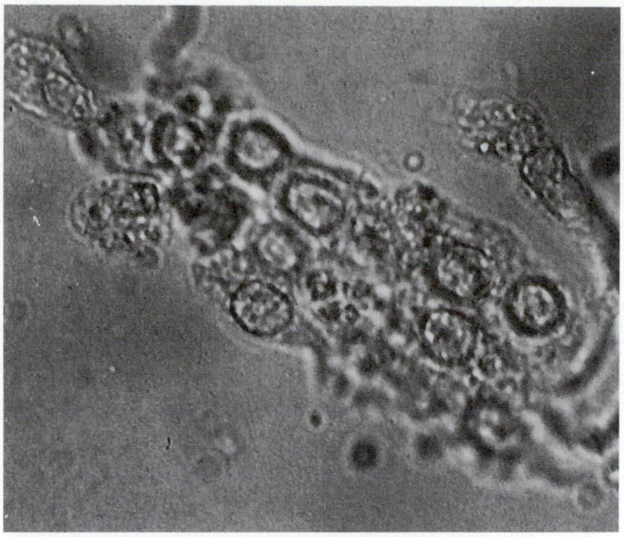

**Fig. 89-3.** Epithelial cell cast. (×400.) (From Piccoli G, Varese D, Rotunno M: *Atlas of urinary sediments: diagnosis and clinical correlations in nephrology,* New York, 1984, Raven.)

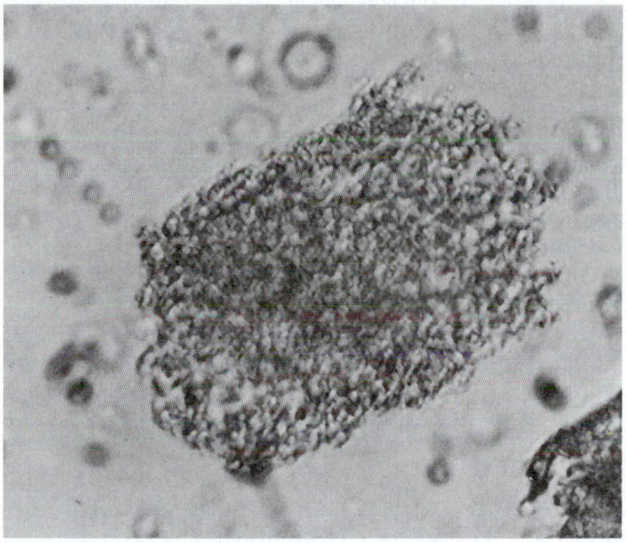

**Fig. 89-4.** Granular cast. (×400.) From Piccoli G, Varese D, Rotunno M: *Atlas of urinary sediments: diagnosis and clinical correlations in nephrology,* New York, 1984, Raven.)

### Hematuria

Gross hematuria is the most frequent cause of an alteration in the urine color. The color may range from pink to black. The lower the pH and the longer the hemoglobin is in contact with the urine, the darker is the color. Hemoglobinuria and myoglobinuria also may cause a red-tinged urine. The presence of hemoglobin turns the urine dipstick blue or green in two different patterns. Spotted activity indicates intact erythrocytes, whereas a uniform pattern signifies free hemoglobin. Free hemoglobin in the urine is usually the result of lysis of erythrocytes in the urine because of a high pH or low specific gravity. The dipstick also detects urine myoglobin. The normal spun urine contains less than one erythrocyte per HPF. The presence of more than three per HPF suggests bleeding anywhere along the urinary system. It has been suggested that erythrocytes of glomerular origin have a more distorted (dysmorphic) appearance than those arising elsewhere, but this is controversial. The finding of an erythrocyte cast (Fig. 89-5), however, almost always suggests that the hematuria is caused by a glomerulonephritis or vasculitis (see Chapter 93). The urine is often contaminated with blood during menses.

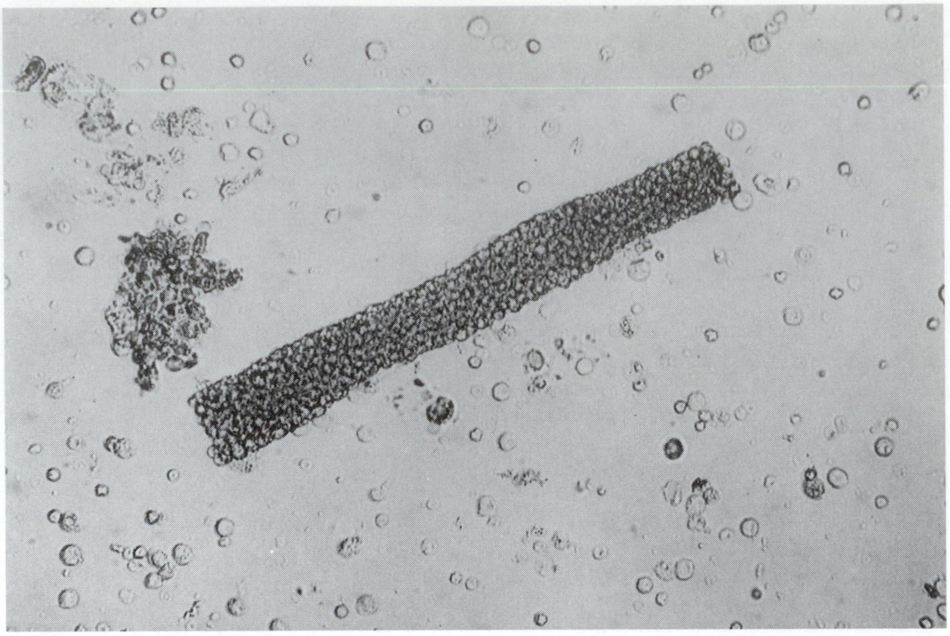

**Fig. 89-5.** Red cell cast. This strongly suggests a glomerulonephriti or vasculitis. (×160.) (From Piccoli G, Varese D, Rotunno M: *Atlas of urinary sediments: diagnosis and clinical correlations in nephrology,* New York, 1984, Raven.)

## Pyuria and bacteriuria

The dipstick measures the esterase enzyme of neutrophils and correlates well with the number of these cells in the urine. The presence of cephalexin or cephalothin or high concentrations of oxalic acid may decrease the test result. The most common contamination is vaginal discharge. Overall, however, false-positive and false-negative results are quite low. A positive nitrite test by dipstick indicates bacteria that reduce urinary nitrate to nitrite are present in significant numbers. Most (90%) Enterobacteriaceae bacteria are able to form nitrite from nitrate, but some bacteria, especially enterococcus, cannot. In addition, because it takes up to 4 hours for the conversion to nitrite in the bladder, a first morning specimen is preferable. Thus, a positive nitrite test by dipstick, especially when accompanied by pyuria, is very suggestive of a urinary tract infection (UTI). A negative test, however, does not rule out the diagnosis.

The normal number of leukocytes is probably less than one per HPF. When present in greater numbers, inflammation is probably occurring somewhere in the urinary system. If leukocytes are found in casts (Fig. 89-6), the inflammation originates in the renal parenchyma. Leukocyte casts can be differentiated from epithelial cell casts by the lobulation of the nuclei. Most leukocytes in the urine are neutrophils; however, in certain conditions such as allergic interstitial nephritis, pyelonephritis, vasculitis, and atheroemboli to the kidneys, the cells may be eosinophils. A Hansel stain (see Chapter 93) of the sediment should be done if pyuria is present and one of these diagnoses is suspected. Bacteria are often seen with unstained urine specimens in the presence of infection. The presence of squamous epithelial cells that are large and flat and have a small central nucleus (Fig. 89-7) in women suggests vaginal contamination. Transitional epithelial cells (Fig. 89-8) lining the bladder and ureter are smaller with a relatively larger nucleus. These may be normally present or may represent some form of irritation of the urinary tract.

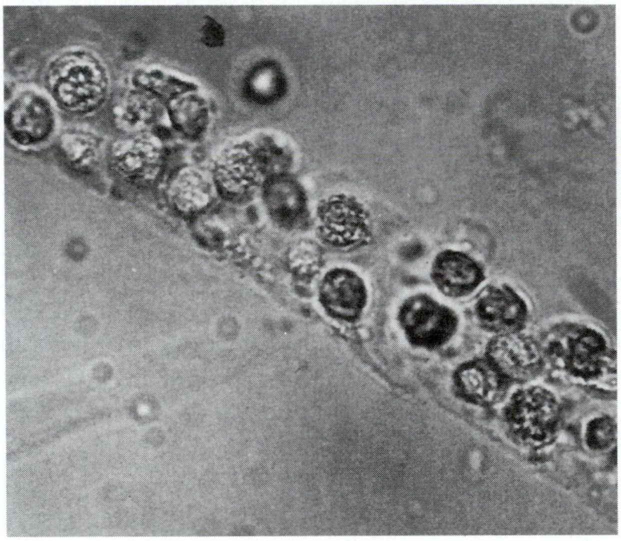

**Fig. 89-6.** Granulocyte cast. This indicates inflammation within the renal parenchyma. (×400.) (From Piccoli G, Varese D, Rotunno M: *Atlas of urinary sediments: diagnosis and clinical correlations in nephrology,* New York, 1984, Raven).

## Glycosuria

Glucose does not usually appear in the urine until the serum glucose levels exceed 180 to 200 mg/dl. Thus, diabetes is by far the most common cause of glycosuria. In pregnancy, however, glycosuria with normal glucose

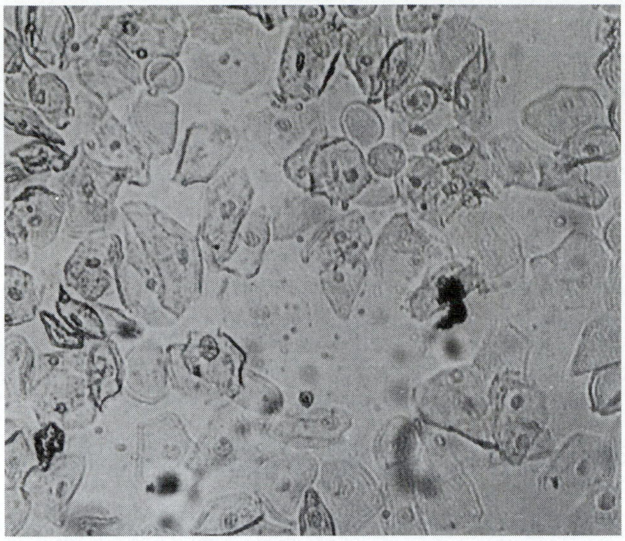

**Fig. 89-7.** Vaginal squamous cells. This indicates that the urine sample was not collected properly and that the diagnosis of a urinary tract infection cannot be made with certainty. (×100.) (From Piccoli G, Varese D, Rotunno M: *Atlas of urinary sediments: diagnosis and clinical correlations in nephrology,* New York, 1984, Raven).

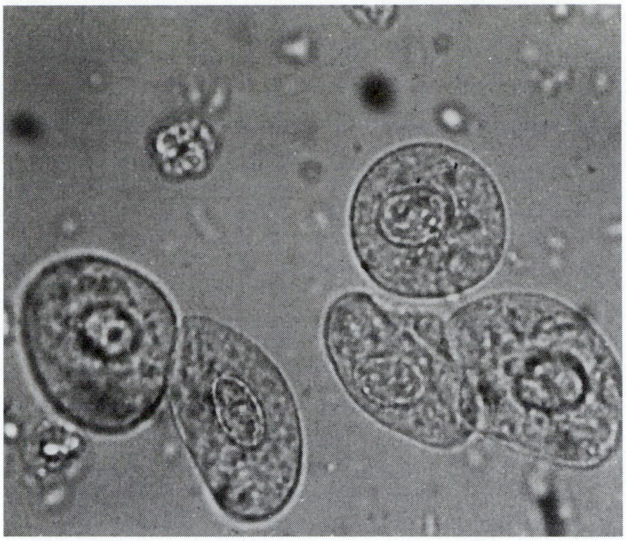

**Fig. 89-8.** Transitional epithelial cells. (×400.) (From Piccoli G, Varese D, Rotunno M: *Atlas of urinary sediments: diagnosis and clinical correlations in nephrology,* New York, 1984, Raven).

levels may occur. In addition, disorders that disrupt the proximal tubular reabsorption of glucose may lead to glycosuria; these include lead poisoning, myeloma, galactosemia, and cystinosis. Finally, glycosuria may occur as part of a more generalized disorder of tubular transport. With Fanconi syndrome, there is also impaired reabsorption of sodium, amino acid, bicarbonate, phosphate, and water. The assay for glucose varies according to the manufacturer, but most can detect a urine glucose concentration of 100 mg/dl.

## Crystaluria

A wide variety of crystals may be seen in the urine. However, only the crystals of cystine (Fig. 89-9), leucine, tyrosine, and cholesterol have pathologic significance. In recurrent stone formers, urinary crystals may assist in predicting the type of stone being produced (see Chapter 92). This is particularly true with magnesium ammonium phosphate crystals (Fig. 89-10) when their presence suggests struvite stones made by urease-producing bacteria such as Proteus.

## Measurement of urine acidity

The dipstick measures the urine pH usually within the range of 5.0 to 8.5. A urine pH greater than 6.5 indicates bicarbonaturia, whereas a urine pH less than 5.5 indicates an absence of bicarbonate in the urine. At times, urine pH determination assists in the evaluation of acid-base disorders (see Chapter 90) and renal stone diseases (see Chapter 92).

## Urinary concentrating ability

The volume and concentration of the urine reflects the renal adaptation to maintain normal water and solute balance. A urine specific gravity of 1.010 corresponds to an osmolality of about 285 mOsm/L, that is, the same osmolality as that normally measured in plasma. For this reason, urine samples whose osmolalities are about 1.010 are referred to as *isosthenuric.* Those less than 1.007 are termed *hyposthenuric.* Adults ingesting a normal diet generally produce a urine specific gravity of 1.016 to 1.022. The urine specific gravity after a 12-hour overnight fast should be 1.022. If the diagnosis of central or nephrogenic diabetes insipidus is suspected, more sophisticated tests of urine and plasma osmolality may be necessary (see Chapter 36).

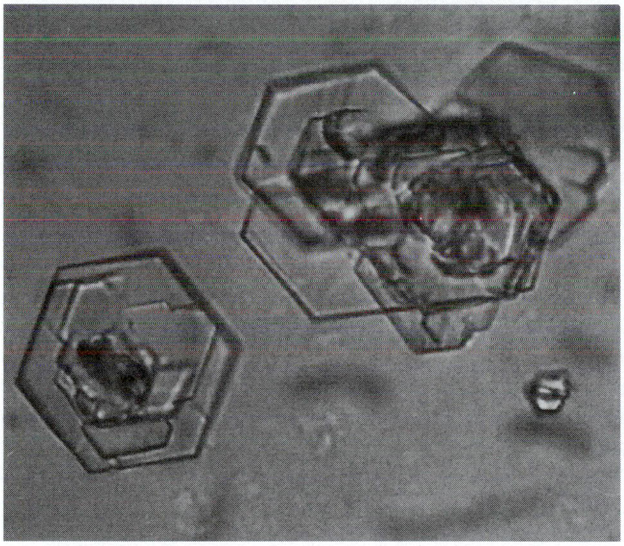

**Fig. 89-9.** Hexagonal cystine crystals. This is indicative of cystinuria. (×400.) (From Piccoli G, Varese D, Rotunno M: *Atlas of urinary sediments: diagnosis and clinical correlations in nephrology,* New York, 1984, Raven).

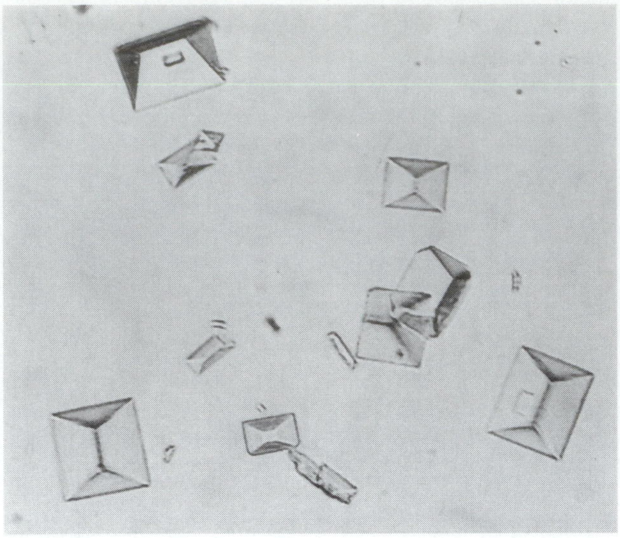

**Fig. 89-10.** Magnesium ammonium phosphate crystals with typical "coffin-lid" appearance. (×400.) (From Piccoli G, Varese D, Rotunno M: *Atlas of urinary sediments: diagnosis and clinical correlations in nephrology,* New York, 1984, Raven).

### Ultrasound and urinary tract obstruction: causes of false-positive and false-negative tests

**False positive**

1. Cystic diseases of kidneys
2. Full bladder
3. States of increased urine output
4. Extrarenal pelvis
5. Vesicoureteral reflux
6. Renal sinus lipomatosis
7. Papillary necrosis

**False negative**

1. Acute obstruction without dilatation
2. Hypovolemia
3. Staghorn calculi
4. Renal cysts and obstruction, interpreted only as renal cysts
5. Intermittent obstruction

## IMAGING STUDIES

### Renal ultrasonography with Doppler echography

In some institutions, ultrasound (US) has supplanted intravenous pyelography (IVP) as the most common imaging test in evaluating urologic structures. The advantages of US over IVP are that it requires no IV injection of contrast and does not expose the patient to radiation. The longitudinal and transverse lengths of the kidneys are easily determined by US. The normal renal length varies according to body size and age, with the right kidney ranging from 8 to 14 cm and the left 7.5 to 12.5 cm. Large kidneys are associated with poorly controlled diabetes, acromegaly, acute glomerulonephritis, human immunodeficiency virus (HIV) infection, and infiltrative processes such as amyloidosis, leukemia, and lymphoma. The presence of small kidneys suggest that irreversible renal damage has occurred, and further evaluation may not be warranted. The finding of increased echogenicity of the renal cortex relative to the that of the liver is an abnormal but nonspecific finding. The degree of hypoechogenicity correlates with the extent of glomerular sclerosis and interstitial fibrosis. Doppler flow studies can often detect patency and direction of flow of the main renal arteries and veins. Although Doppler studies may detect thrombosis of the main renal arteries and veins, they are not reliable tests of renal artery stenosis.

Unlike some other imaging tests (e.g., IVP), US relies exclusively on structural changes such as dilated calyces to detect obstructive uropathy. Hydronephrosis is diagnosed with a sensitivity rate of 98% to 100% and specificity rate of 90% to 93%. The box above lists causes for false-positive and false-negative test results.

Renal US is also the first-line test in evaluating inherited and acquired cycts of the kidneys. With well-established autosomal dominant polycystic kidney disease, the renal size is large because of the multiple cysts destroying the normal renal parenchyma. The early diagnosis of autosomal dominant polycystic kidney disease may be missed before age 30 years because the cysts may be too small to be detectable. Benign cortical cysts are the most frequently encountered renal masses. Cysts must meet four criteria to be considered benign (see the box above). If these criteria are fulfilled, the accuracy of diagnosis of a benign cyst is greater then 95% and no further workup is warranted. Cysts that do not meet the criteria have a 37% chance of being a neoplasm and must be further evaluated, often by computed tomography (CT). Suggested criteria for the CT diagnosis of a simple cyst include homogenous attentuation value of water density, no enhancement with IV contrast, no measurable thickness of the cyst wall, and smooth interface with renal parenchyma. The probability of a correct diagnosis with a CT is quite high. Therefore, if these criteria are not met, many centers do not do further testing (e.g., percutaneous cyst puncture, angiogram) but proceed with a surgical exploration. Structures that are poorly evaluated by US include solid renal masses and nondilated ureters.

### Ultrasound criteria for classification of benign renal cysts

1. No internal echoes
2. Round or oval in shape
3. Clearly demarcated far wall
4. Acoustic enhancement of tissue next to far wall

### Intravenous pyelography

An IVP may be helpful in evaluating the location of the obstruction in a patient passing a renal stone. For routine imaging of a renal stone, a plain x-ray of the abdomen is often satisfactory, since 85% of stones are radiopaque. It is controversial whether US or IVP should be chosen for the initial renal imaging evaluation of persistent, isolated hematuria.

An IVP requires the administration of IV contrast. This may lead to idiosyncratic reactions ranging from mild urticaria (up to 10%) to severe anaphylaxis (1:3000 to 1:4500). Up to 10% of patients also report nausea and a transient sensation of warmth. In patients with impaired renal function, acute renal failure may result from contrast, particularly in the setting of volume depletion or multiple contrast studies. Cardiac arrhythmias may also occur. The newer, lower-osmolar contrast agents may decrease the incidence of adverse events.

### Computed tomography and magnetic resonance imaging

If a solid renal mass has been suggested by prior US or IVP, a CT scan should be considered. In CT-proven solid lesions less than 1 cm in diameter, US detects only 26%. In lesions 3 cm or larger, 85% are detected. The overall accuracy of CT is 95% to 99% for solid renal mass. This is higher than that of magnetic resonance imaging (MRI). However, with the addition of Gd-DTPA for contrast-enhanced MRI, the accuracy is similar to CT (Gd, gadelinium). MRI is of little value in evaluating renal stones.

### Renal scans

Renal scans may be of some value in evaluating renovascular disease, in determining if mild obstruction is physiologically significant, or in assessing leakage of urine from the urinary system. They, however, provide little structural information about the kidneys that cannot be obtained by US. They also provide little valuable information about renal function except when marked differences exist between the two kidneys.

## RENAL BIOPSY

Percutaneous renal biopsies have been routinely performed on patients with renal diseases for more than 25 years. They have greatly increased our knowledge of the classification, prognosis, epidemiology, and treatment of a variety of renal disorders (see the box above).

The usual procedure is to have the patient lie prone and localize the lower pole of either kidney with the guidance of US. After the establishment of a sterile field and the administration of local anesthesia, two cores of renal cortex may be obtained by the use of different types of biopsy needles. The specimens are then analyzed by light, immunofluorescence, and electron microscopy. It should be emphasized that a renal biopsy is an invasive procedure that should only be performed by an experienced nephrologist or invasive radiologist.

Several indications exist for a renal biopsy. Probably the most common is the nephrotic syndrome in adults in whom the etiology is not obvious after a thorough clinical and laboratory investigation (see Chapter 93). The renal biopsy provides information concerning the type of primary glomerular disease, as well as its severity and degree of irreversible scarring. The extent of interstitial damage correlates better with the level of GFR than does the severity of the glomerular lesion. Among the various glomerular diseases, in some (e.g., minimal change nephrotic syndrome) patients respond well to daily oral steroids. In others (e.g., membranous) patients are thought to be best treated with steroids and cytotoxic agents. For still others (e.g., focal segmental glomerulonephritis) patients generally respond poorly to all treatments.

### Information gained from renal imaging studies and biopsies

A. Ultrasound (US)/Doppler flow studies
   1. Size
   2. Structural changes
      a. Stones
      b. Obstruction
      c. Masses
      d. Cysts
      e. Abnormal vascularity
   3. Thrombosis of main renal artery or vein
B. Intravenous pyelography (IVP)
   1. Size and structure
   2. Site of obstruction
C. Computed tomography (CT) and magnetic resonance imaging (MRI)
   Evaluation of suspicious renal masses and adjacent structures noted on previous US or IVP
D. Renal scan
   1. Renovascular disease
   2. Leakage of urine (renal trauma)
   3. Differential renal function
E. Renal biopsy
   1. Diagnosis of primary glomerular disease
      a. Severity
      b. Degree of irreversibility
   2. Diagnosis of systemic disease
   3. Evaluation of unexplained decline in renal function

The kidneys are affected by a variety of systemic illnesses. Occasionally, a renal biopsy is warranted to make the diagnosis of the systemic disease, such as in amyloidosis. In other situations, a renal biopsy assists in determining the aggressiveness with which one wishes to treat a systemic disease, such as systemic lupus erythematosus. Patients with signs and symptoms of a vasculitis may undergo a renal biopsy. The findings of focal necrotizing glomerulonephritis is very suggestive of a vasculitis but does not indicate which type. Finally, some patients' renal function deteriorates acutely or chronically for no obvious reason. A renal biopsy should be considered after carefully evaluating the risk/benefit ratio.

The kidneys are highly vascular organs, and it is not surprising that the major complication of a renal biopsy is hemorrhage. Although almost 90% of patients have evidence of perirenal hemorrhage shown by CT scanning, less than 5% require a transfusion. Severe renal hemorrhage is usually successfully treated by selective embolization of the involved vessels. Less than 1% of patients require an emergency nephrectomy. Some patients complain of pain at the site of the biopsy, but this usually resolves within 1 week. Gross hematuria may be observed in about 5% of patients, but this, too, usually resolves without specific treatment.

The major contraindication for a renal biopsy is a coagulopathy. Criteria for exclusion vary but generally include a platelet count less than 100,000, an elevated prothrombin time or partial thromboplastic time, or a history of ingesting aspirin-containing compounds within the previous week. Other contraindications include a solitary kidney, an active UTI, uncontrolled hypertension, and uncooperativeness of the patient.

An open (surgical) renal biopsy is considerably more invasive than a closed (percutaneous) renal biopsy. It should never be considered when a percutaneous biopsy is possible.

## BIBLIOGRAPHY


Ginsberg JM et al: Use of single voided urine samples to estimate quantitative proteinuria, *N Engl J Med* 309:1543, 1983.

Hilbrands LB et al: Cimetidine improves the reliability of creatinine as a marker of glomerular filtration, *Kidney Int* 40:1171, 1991.

King AJ, Levey AS, Dietary protein and renal function, *J Am Soc Nephrol* 3:1723, 1993.

Kohler H, Wandel E, Brunck B: Acanthocyturia—a characteristic marker for glomerular bleeding, *Kidney Int* 40:115, 1991.

Levey AS: Measurement of renal function in chronic renal disease, *Kidney Int* 38:167, 1990.

MacKenzie W, Drew HH, LaFrance ND: Creatinine measurements often yield false estimates of progression in chronic renal failure, *Kidney Int* 34:412, 1988.

Nolan CR III, Anger MS, Keheller SP: Eosinophiluria—a new method of detection and definition of the clinical spectrum, *N Engl J Med* 315: 1516, 1986.

O'Reilly PH, George NJR, Weiss RM, editors: *Diagnostic techniques in urology,* Philadelphia, 1990, Saunders.

Piccoli G, Varese D, Rotunno M: *Atlas of urinary sediments: diagnosis and clinical correlations in nephrology,* New York, 1984, Raven.

Roubenoff R et al: Oral cimetidine improves the accuracy and precision of creatinine clearance in lupus nephritis, *Ann Intern Med* 113:501, 1990.

Shemesh O et al: Limitations of creatinine as a filtration marker in glomerulopathic patients, *Kidney Int* 28:830, 1985.


CHAPTER

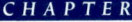

# 90 Acid-base and Fluid and Electrolyte Disorders

**Saulo Klahr**

## ACID-BASE DISORDERS

### Acid-base balance in health

The pH of the blood is normally maintained within the narrow range of 7.37 to 7.42. The range of plasma pH compatible with life is approximately 6.8 to 7.8. The pH of body fluids in humans is maintained despite the normal production of large amounts of acid from two major sources: (1) volatile carbonic acid ($H_2CO_3$), derived from carbon dioxide ($CO_2$), the end product of oxidative metabolism; and (2) a variety of nonvolatile acids produced from dietary substances, mainly protein. The pH of plasma represents the ratio of bicarbonate to carbonic acid (dissolved $CO_2$), as formulated in the Henderson-Hasselbalch equation:

$$\text{pH} = \text{pK} + \log \text{ of } \frac{HCO_3^-}{H_2CO_3 \text{ } or \text{ } \alpha \cdot P\text{CO}_2}$$

where α, the solubility constant for $CO_2$, has a value of 0.03 at 37°C (98.6°F). In a normal individual the above expression has the following numeric values:

$$7.4 = 6.1 + \log \text{ of } \frac{26 \text{ mmol/L}}{1.3 \text{ mmol/L}}$$

The denominator of the Henderson-Hasselbalch equation, the plasma carbon dioxide tension ($P\text{CO}_2$), is maintained within narrow limits by the excretion of $CO_2$ by the lungs. Although pH changes are minimized through changes in extracellular fluid (ECF) $P\text{CO}_2$, the integrity of plasma pH depends on the availability of bicarbonate ions ($HCO_3^-$) in the extracellular fluid. The kidneys participate in stabilizing the concentration of $HCO_3^-$ in plasma (the numerator of the Henderson-Hasselbalch equation). A normal individual ingesting 1 to 2 g of protein per kilogram of body weight generates daily approximately 60 mmol of nonvolatile acid. The same amount of $HCO_3^-$ is consumed in the ECF to buffer this surplus acid. Restoration of serum $HCO_3^-$ consumed in buffering either metabolically produced or exogenous acid loads occurs both by virtually complete reabsorption of filtered $HCO_3^-$ (reclamation) and by the regeneration of $HCO_3^-$ formed in conjunction with the excretion of titratable acid and ammonium (de novo synthesis of $HCO_3^-$). Both the reabsorption and the regeneration of $HCO_3^-$ result from the secretion of hydrogen ions ($H^+$) into the nephron's tubular lumen. When ECF $HCO_3^-$ rises, this is corrected by the renal excretion of a larger-than-normal fraction of the filtered $HCO_3^-$.

### Laboratory considerations

In evaluating a patient's acid-base status, it is necessary to measure two of the three values (pH, $P\text{CO}_2$, $HCO_3^-$) in the Henderson-Hasselbalch equation. The third value can then be calculated or read directly from a nomogram (Fig. 90-1). The initial screening test traditionally used to evaluate a patient's acid-base status is the measurement of the total $CO_2$ content of plasma or serum. This measurement reflects the total number of moles of $CO_2$ liberated from both $HCO_3^-$ and $H_2CO_3$. Because of the relatively small amounts of $H_2CO_3$ (1.3 mmol at a $P\text{CO}_2$ of approximately 40 mm Hg), the value for the $CO_2$ content approximates the $HCO_3^-$ concentration of plasma. Normal values for $CO_2$ content are 26 to 28 mmol/L and can be measured in venous blood. Because the $H_2CO_3/HCO_3^-$ pair is the ECF's principal buffer system, measurement of the two components provides a meaningful and convenient expression of the organism's acid-base status. The pathophysiologic events that tend to alter pH are of two general types, metabolic and respiratory. *Metabolic* acid-base disturbances result from processes that alter fluid pH primarily by changing the concentration of plasma $HCO_3^-$ (numerator of the Henderson-Hasselbach equation). *Respiratory* acid-base disorders result from primary changes in the respiratory component (denominator of the equation), which is measured as $P\text{CO}_2$. A series of overlapping defense mechanisms tends to maintain the pH of the ECF within narrow limits. The defense mechanisms consist of

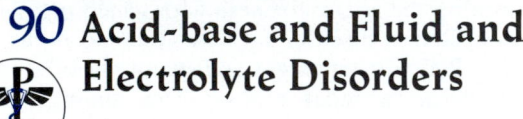

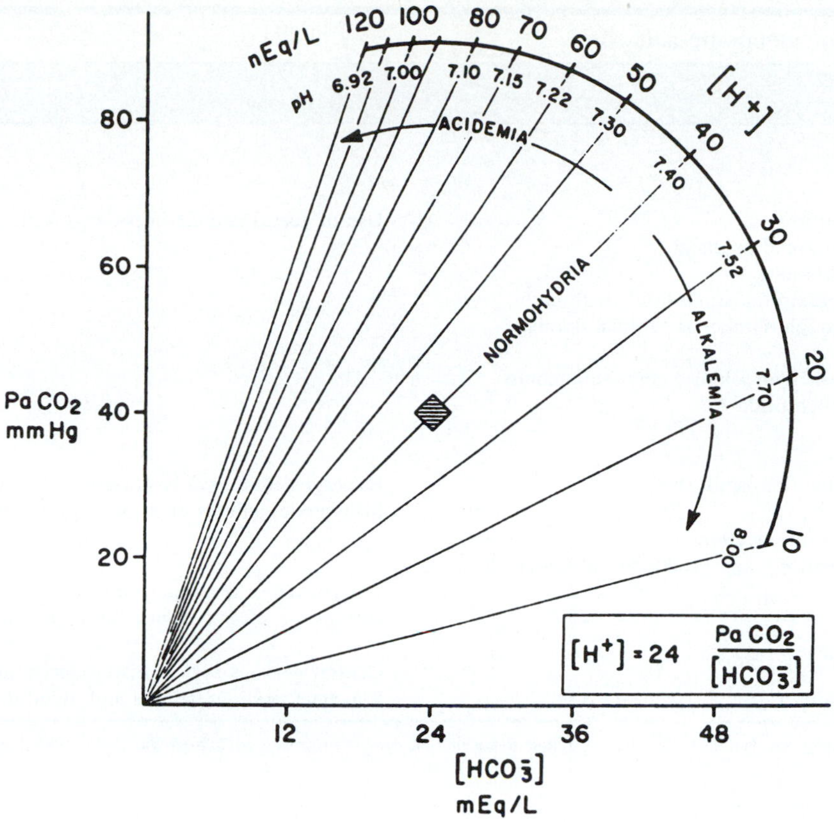


Fig. 90-1. Acid-base nomogram.

at least three well-defined systems:

1. Extracellular and intracellular buffers provide an almost instantaneous, first line of defense against changes in pH.
2. Respiratory compensation of fairly rapid onset constitutes a secondary defense in metabolic disorders.
3. The kidneys not only maintain plasma $HCO_3^-$ constant under normal circumstances, but also modify $HCO_3^-$ excretion in respiratory acid-base disorders. The renal compensatory mechanism is slower to respond (several hours).

## Metabolic acidosis

***Clinical features and systemic effects.*** The clinical manifestations of metabolic acidosis in part may reflect the primary disorder responsible for the acidosis. The manifestations directly attributable to severe metabolic acidosis include depressed left ventricular function and decreased peripheral vascular resistance. This may lead to hypotension, pulmonary edema, arrhythmias (particularly ventricular fibrillation), and tissue hypoxia. The depth and rate of respiration increase, sometimes referred to as Kussmaul's respiration, which is especially prominent when plasma $HCO_3^-$ levels are less than 15 mEq/L. Central nervous system manifestations may include changes in mentation, confusion, and sometimes convulsions. Prolonged chronic metabolic acidosis may cause osteopenia and osteoporosis as a result of the buffering of $H^+$ by calcium carbonate ($CaCO_3$) in bone. This may contribute to bone disease, particularly in conditions such as chronic renal failure and renal tubular acidosis.

***Laboratory findings.*** Metabolic acidosis occurs when the addition rate of $H^+$ to the extracellular space exceeds the rate of excretion of $H^+$ or when base is lost from the body in excess of its rate of replenishment. The hallmark of metabolic acidosis is a high $H^+$ concentration (low pH and low $HCO_3^-$ in plasma). Metabolic acidosis may also be suspected by the finding of a wide plasma anion gap (greater than 15 mEq/L) even in the absence of a pH or $HCO_3^-$ change. The anion gap is calculated by subtracting the sum of chloride plus $HCO_3^-$ concentrations from the sodium concentration in plasma or serum:

$$\text{Anion gap} = Na^+ - (Cl^- + HCO_3^-)$$

Normally a difference of 8 to 12 mEq/L exists, made up predominantly by plasma proteins, phosphate, and sulfate.

***Causes.*** Metabolic acidosis caused by a gain of $H^+$ is usually manifested by an increased anion gap (Table 90-1). Quantitatively the increase in the plasma anion gap equals the decrease in the plasma $HCO_3^-$ concentration. Metabolic acidosis resulting from loss of $HCO_3^-$ is characterized by a normal anion gap. In metabolic acidosis, the expected physiologic response is a lowering of plasma $P_{CO_2}$ to minimize the decrease in pH. This is accomplished by an increase in the depth and rate of respiration. Quantitatively, the decrease in $P_{CO_2}$ from 40 mm Hg should equal the decrease in plasma $HCO_3^-$ from 26

**Table 90-1.** Causes of metabolic acidosis

| Cause | Clinical comments |
|---|---|
| **Normal anion gap** | |
| Renal loss of bicarbonate | |
| Carbonic anhydrase inhibitors | Use of acetazolamide in patients with glaucoma |
| Renal tubular acidosis, proximal or distal | |
| Gastrointestinal loss of bicarbonate | |
| Diarrhea or loss of other gastrointestinal fluids with high bicarbonate content through fistulas or surgical drainage | |
| Ileal loop conduit | |
| Administration or ingestion of hydrochloric acid, ammonium chloride, or arginine hydrochloride | |
| **Increased anion gap** | |
| Uncontrolled diabetes mellitus (ketoacidosis) | Hyperglycemia usually present |
| Lactic acidosis | In hypoxic patients or those with decreased hepatic blood flow |
| Administration, ingestion, or intoxication | |
| Ethyl alcohol, with "starvation" and production of ketoacids | |
| Salicylate | Initial event a respiratory alkalosis |
| Methyl alcohol | Increase in plasma osmolality (osmolal gap) |
| Paraldehyde | |
| Ethylene glycol | Central nervous system disturbances, acute renal failure |
| Renal failure (acute and chronic) | Elevated serum creatinine and blood urea nitrogen |

Modified with permission from Klahr SK, Hamm L. In Klahr S, editor: *Renal and electrolyte disorders*, ed 2, Norwalk, Conn, 1984, Appleton-Century-Crofts.

mmol/L. Compensation at the level of the kidneys involves the excretion of increased amounts of ammonium to increase the de novo synthesis of $HCO_3^-$. Normally the kidneys excrete 40 mmol of ammonium daily. During metabolic acidosis, ammonium excretion is at least as copious as dietary acid production, 1 mmol/kg/day, and can reach 200 mmol daily.

### *Metabolic acidosis associated with normal anion gap*

#### Renal loss of bicarbonate

***Use of carbonic anhydrase inhibitors.*** Carbonic anhydrase inhibitors increase $HCO_3^-$ excretion in the urine by inhibiting the enzyme responsible for the hydration of $CO_2$. This process is key in the secretion of $H^+$ and consequently in $HCO_3^-$ reabsorption from the renal tubule. The most frequently used drug in this group is acetazolamide (Diamox), a diuretic often prescribed to decrease intraocular pressure in patients with glaucoma.

***Renal tubular acidosis.*** Renal tubular acidosis (RTA) is a metabolic hyperchloremic acidosis that occurs in patients with a nonazotemic renal acidification defect. RTA is characterized by decreased $H^+$ excretion in the urine. The two major types of RTA are proximal and distal with several admixtures and hybrids.

*Distal,* or *classic,* RTA is characterized by an inability of the distal nephron to excrete $H^+$ normally. The normal kidney can lower urine pH to 4.7, which represents a urine-to-plasma concentration ratio for $H^+$ of approximately 800:1. By contrast, kidneys of patients with classic RTA cannot lower urine pH below 6 regardless of the severity of the systemic acidosis. A urine pH of 6 limits the amount of $H^+$ that can be excreted as ammonium or titratable acid ($H^+$ bound mainly to phosphate). The inability to excrete $H^+$ at a rate comparable to the rate of formation and consequently the failure to regenerate the $HCO_3^+$ consumed daily in the buffering process causes metabolic acidosis. Distal RTA is characterized by increased urine excretion of cations (sodium, potassium, calcium) and anions (sulfate, phosphate). This results in depletion of these cations with reduction of the ECF volume, hypokalemia, and rickets or osteomalacia. The increased calcium and phosphate excreted into the alkaline urine often causes renal stones or nephrocalcinosis. Distal or classic RTA is seen in (1) a sporadic congenital primary form; (2) certain hypergammaglobulinemic states; (3) nephrocalcinosis, which may result from various genetic and metabolic disorders; (4) distal tubule nephrotoxicity caused by drugs such as amphotericin B, vitamin D, and toluene; (5) medullary sponge kidney; and (6) interstitial renal disease (pyelonephritis, collagen disorders, etc.). Distal RTA may also develop after renal transplantation.

*Proximal* RTA is characterized by a large excretion of $HCO_3^-$ in the urine. Alkaline urine is excreted, and hyperchloremic metabolic acidosis develops. Proximal RTA may be suspected by the presence of concomitant defects in proximal reabsorption, such as aminoaciduria, glycosuria, and phosphaturia. The hallmark of proximal RTA is normal acidification of the urine in the presence of normal renal function when plasma $HCO_3^-$ concentrations are low, and excretion of an alkaline urine as plasma $HCO_3^-$ is raised by the administration of exogenous $NaHCO_3^-$.

**Gastrointestinal loss of bicarbonate.** $HCO_3^-$ loss through the gastrointestinal tract may lead to normal-anion-gap metabolic acidosis. *Diarrhea* may result in loss of fluid containing $HCO_3^-$ in excess (30 to 50 mmol/L) of the concentrations present in plasma. Large amounts of potassium may also be lost, and metabolic acidosis with hypokalemia may occur. Secretions from *fistulas, the small bowel, the pancreas,* or *biliary tract* may be rich in $HCO_3^-$.

Losses of such fluids to the exterior may cause hyperchloremic acidosis. Patients with complete cystectomies, especially caused by bladder malignancies, require the construction of artificial bladders in the form of an *ileal loop conduit.* Although hyperchloremic acidosis is uncommon in patients with ileal bladders, it may occur when the ileal segment is extremely long, when an antiperistaltic loop has been constructed, or when the stoma of the ileal loop is obstructed. Prolonged exposure of the urine to the ileal mucosa probably results in exchange of chloride for $HCO_3^-$, leading to loss of $HCO_3^-$ from body fluids.

Other causes of normal-anion-gap metabolic acidosis include expansion of the extracellular space with solutions not containing $HCO_3^-$ (dilutional acidosis) and the administration of hydrochloric acid, ammonium chloride, arginine, or lysine hydrochloride. Sometimes during hyperalimentation, amino acid infusions containing inorganic cations in a significant excess of organic anions may cause a metabolic acidosis with hyperchloremia.

***Metabolic acidosis associated with increased anion gap.*** An excess of acid is characterized by an increase in the anion gap. The major acids that may accumulate under these conditions are (1) keto acids, as in insulin-deficiency diabetes; (2) lactic acid, in conditions characterized by tissue hypoxia; (3) acetylsalicylic acid (aspirin); or (4) intoxicant acids or substances that can be metabolized to them, such as methanol; which leads to the formation of formic acid; ethylene glycol, which results in the formation of glioxalic acid; paraldehyde, which is converted to acetic acid; or toluene, which is converted to hippuric acid. Patients with renal failure have increased-anion-gap metabolic acidosis (mainly caused by phosphate and sulfate), not because acid production is increased, but because the kidney fails to regenerate enough $HCO_3^-$.

When an increase in the anion gap occurs with metabolic acidosis, the diagnosis of ketoacidosis can be made if there is hyperglycemia, large serum ketones, and a wide anion gap. Patients who fulfill these criteria usually have ECF volume contraction, hyperventilation, and the smell of acetone on their breath. The treatment includes insulin to decrease the production of $H^+$ and sodium chloride to restore ECF volume.

Lactic acid, the end product of glycolysis, may accumulate in several conditions, some of which have hypoxia as a common denominator (circulatory insufficiency, hypotension, etc.). Lactic acidosis can also occur during extreme exercise and with the administration of phenformin or other uncouplers of oxidative phosphorylation. Destruction or replacement of liver tissue may increase lactic acid because of the decreased conversion of lactic acid to glucose. The same is true when gluconeogenesis is impaired as a result of drugs or inborn errors of metabolism.

The finding of an increased osmolar gap in the plasma of patients with metabolic acidosis should raise the suspicion of methanol, isopropyl alcohol, or ethylene glycol intoxication. These substances and ethanol increase the osmolar gap. The osmolar gap is the difference between the measured serum osmolality and the calculated osmolality.

$$\text{Calculated osmolality} = 1.87\ ([\text{Na}] + [\text{K}]) + \text{BUN}/2.8 + \text{glucose}/18$$

## Treatment

The ideal treatment of metabolic acidosis corrects or ameliorates the cause. Only when the acidosis is responsible for severe physiologic disturbances is treatment of the acidosis itself required. Historically, the therapy has involved the administration of sodium bicarbonate ($NaHCO_3$). At present, this modality of treatment is somewhat controversial, although judicious use of $NaHCO_3$ has been advocated. It is appropriate to administer $HCO_3^-$ if the blood pH is less than 7.1.

Chronic metabolic acidosis, as in RTA or chronic renal failure, requires treatment in children to allow normal growth and in adults to ameliorate or prevent gastrointestinal or neurologic symptoms of acidosis and bone disease. $NaHCO_3$ can be given to maintain plasma $HCO_3^-$ at about 20 mmol/L. Sodium overload should be avoided. In chronic metabolic acidosis, $NaHCO_3$ may be given orally as tolerated. One-gram tablets contain 12 mmol of $NaHCO_3$.

## Metabolic alkalosis

The hallmark of metabolic alkalosis is an elevated blood pH caused by a primary increase in the concentration of plasma $HCO_3^-$. The increased plasma $HCO_3^-$ concentration may result from (1) net loss of $H^+$ from the extracellular space or (2) net addition of $HCO_3^-$ or its precursors to the extracellular space or loss of ECF-containing chloride in a concentration greater than $HCO_3^-$. Therefore metabolic alkalosis results from abnormal loss of acid or excessive retention of base or both. Normally, uncomplicated metabolic alkalosis is short-lived because the kidneys promptly excrete the excess $HCO_3^-$. In established metabolic alkalosis, two mechanisms should be considered: the events responsible for the development of metabolic alkalosis (i.e., the *generation* of such an acid-base disorder) and the factors that allow this disorder to persist (i.e., the *maintenance* of metabolic alkalosis). The maintenance of metabolic alkalosis relates to inability of the kidney to excrete $HCO_3^-$. The factors that promote the renal tubular reabsorption of $HCO_3^-$ include contraction of the ECF volume, chloride deficit, decreased levels of plasma and intracellular potassium, and increased mineralocorticoid levels in plasma.

***Clinical features and systemic effects.*** No specific symptoms or signs indicate the diagnosis of metabolic alkalosis. The disorder should be suspected in patients with a history of vomiting, surgery and gastric drainage, diuretic therapy, muscle cramps, and weakness and hypertension (primary hyperaldosteronism). Physical examination may reveal the presence of neuromuscular irritability such as tetany or hyperactive reflexes. These signs are more prominent if hypocalcemia is present, since ionized calcium decreases further as the pH rises.

***Laboratory findings.*** Blood pH is elevated, and plasma $HCO_3^-$ is increased with increased arterial $P_{CO_2}$ as a compensatory mechanism. The $P_{CO_2}$ values, however, seldom exceed 50 mm Hg. This is not surprising because the hypoventilation required to elevate the $P_{CO_2}$ also would reduce arterial $P_{O_2}$. The increased $P_{CO_2}$ and reduced $P_{O_2}$ in arterial blood stimulate the respiratory center, thereby tending to restore ventilation and blood gases toward normal. Occasional patients with metabolic alkalosis have marked hypercapnia ($CO_2$ retention) that cannot be ascribed to accompanying pulmonary disease or neuromuscular weaknesses. The elevated $P_{CO_2}$, which is sometimes in excess of 75 mm Hg, may be caused by alveolar hypoventilation from depression of the respiratory center.

Patients with metabolic alkalosis are characterized by an elevated total $CO_2$ content, hypochloremia, and almost invariably, hypokalemia, which is multifactorial. Renal loss of potassium, however, is the predominant event and partly results from accelerated distal potassium secretion. Volume depletion may lead to increased blood urea nitrogen (BUN) and creatinine concentrations in metabolic alkalosis. The hematocrit may be increased from hemoconcentration. The anion gap may be increased by as much as 5 to 6 mmol/L, partly because of elevations of lactic acid concentrations and increased concentrations of undefined anions. However, this change has no diagnostic significance, unlike in metabolic acidosis.

The concentration of chloride in the urine is an important test in the differential diagnosis of the causes of metabolic alkalosis. It may help distinguish metabolic alkalosis with volume expansion, mainly related to pathologic conditions of the adrenal gland, from metabolic alkalosis with volume depletion, mainly related to loss of fluid, such as through vomiting and use of diuretics. A spot urine chloride concentration less than 10 mmol/L suggests avid reabsorption of NaCl by the renal tubule. A urine chloride concentration greater than 20 mmol/L in a patient with metabolic alkalosis indicates that neither ECF volume depletion nor chloride availability is a critical factor in perpetuating the metabolic alkalosis and points to excess mineralocorticoid activity as the cause of the disorder. A word of caution: in analyzing chloride concentrations in patients who received diuretics 24 to 48 hours preceding such a spot urinalysis, the validity of the previous assumptions is questionable.

## Causes of metabolic alkalosis

**ECF volume contraction (urinary Cl <10 mmol/L)**

Gastrointestinal loss of $H^+$: vomiting, gastric drainage, villous adenoma of the colon, diarrhea with high chloride content

Renal loss of $H^+$: diuretic therapy—current or remote; other—Bartter's syndrome

**ECF volume expansion with mineralocorticoid excess (urinary Cl >20 mmol/L)**

Primary or secondary aldosteronism, Cushing's syndrome, licorice abuse, Liddle's syndrome

**Excessive $HCO_3^-$ loads (particularly with advanced renal insufficiency)**

Excessive intake of $HCO_3^-$ or alkalinizing salts

Conversion of accumulated or administered organic acids (lactate, acetate) to $HCO_3^-$

Glucose-induced alkalosis during fasting

Posthypercapnic state

Modified with permission from Klahr SK, Hamm L. In Klahr S, editor: *Renal and electrolyte disorders,* ed 2, Norwalk, CT, 1984, Appleton-Century-Crofts.

***Causes.*** The box above presents the causes of metabolic alkalosis. Clinically, it is helpful to divide metabolic alkalosis into two major categories, one characterized by ECF volume contraction and the other by ECF volume expansion, usually the result of excessive mineralocorticoid secretion. The latter form is often accompanied by hypertension. This hypertension may be accompanied by high plasma levels of renin and aldosterone, low renin and high aldosterone levels, or even low renin and low aldosterone levels (in this case, other mineralocorticoids play a primary role in expansion of the ECF and increased excretion of potassium and hydrogen in the urine). Patients with ECF volume contraction, except possibly for those with Bartter's syndrome, are characterized by low chloride concentrations in their urine. Excessive $HCO_3^-$ loads may cause metabolic alkalosis, but this occurs mainly in the setting of advanced renal insufficiency.

Several important questions must be answered in evaluating a patient with metabolic alkalosis: Is the ECF volume contracted? Why is the ECF volume contracted? If ECF volume contraction exists, is the renal response appropriate? If ECF volume is normal or expanded, what should be done?

***Treatment.*** The underlying disease process causing the metabolic alkalosis should be treated. Treatment should also be directed at increasing renal $HCO_3^-$ excretion. Restoration of ECF volume in the form of NaCl plus potassium will increase the excretion of $HCO_3^-$ and retain NaCl and potassium in most varieties of metabolic alkalosis. Treatment of the excess mineralocorticoid varieties of metabolic alkalosis requires removal or ablation of secretory tumors or blockade of renal tubular effects of the mineralocorticoids with spironolactone. Patients with severe potassium depletion and NaCl-resistant alkalosis require administration of large amounts of KCl before NaCl can be effective in correcting the alkalosis.

### Respiratory acidosis

Respiratory acidosis is a disorder characterized by an increase in $P_{CO_2}$ and a decrease in blood pH. This disorder represents an imbalance between $CO_2$ production and $CO_2$ excretion by the lungs. The rise in $P_{CO_2}$ increases the concentration of $H_2CO_3$ in body fluids. Since $CO_2$ production from metabolism (13,000 to 15,000 mmol/day) tends to be constant, the increase in $P_{CO_2}$ is usually related to decreased excretion of $CO_2$ via the lung. The first line of defense in respiratory acidosis is a chemical reaction in which the increased $H_2CO_3$ resulting from increased $P_{CO_2}$ is buffered mainly by intracellular proteins and phosphate to mitigate a marked fall in pH. The second line of defense relates to increased $H^+$ excretion by the kidney and thus an increase in the production of $HCO_3^-$. In the initial phases of respiratory acidosis, the increased $P_{CO_2}$ stimulates the generation and secretion of $H^+$. Increased excretion of titratable acid and particularly ammonium results in de novo generation of $HCO_3^-$.

***Clinical features and systemic effects.*** Respiratory acidosis can be acute or chronic. In acute respiratory acidosis, there is a marked and sudden decrease in the excretion of $CO_2$. The acute onset of hypercapnia (increased $PCO_2$) is usually accompanied by hypoxemia. The patient may have signs or symptoms of acute respiratory distress with marked restlessness, tachypnea, and dyspnea. As the process progresses, further manifestations include fatigue, weakness, confusion, hyperactivity and even manic periods, and headache. Coma occurs at levels of $PCO_2$ from 70 to 100 mm Hg, depending on arterial pH and on the rapidity of elevation of $PCO_2$. Physical signs include tremor, asterixis (similar to hepatic encephalopathy), weakness, incoordination, occasional cranial nerve signs, abnormal pyramidal tract signs, papilledema, and retinal hemorrhages.

Patients with chronic respiratory acidosis have few if any signs or symptoms related directly to hypercapnia. The signs and symptoms of chronic pulmonary disease with or without cor pulmonale usually predominate.

***Laboratory findings.*** The arterial blood profile reveals a marked increase in $PCO_2$ and sometimes a moderately elevated plasma $HCO_3^-$. In acute respiratory acidosis, plasma $HCO_3^-$ rarely exceeds 30 mmol/L. However, in chronic compensated respiratory acidosis, levels of $HCO_3^-$ may be as high as 40 mmol/L. In both chronic and acute varieties, the $PO_2$ is generally decreased. Total plasma $CO_2$ content is increased, usually with normal concentrations of sodium and potassium. Urine pH is usually acidic. In chronic respiratory acidosis, plasma chloride is greatly decreased.

### Causes of respiratory acidosis

**Acute respiratory acidosis**

Airway obstruction
- Aspiration (vomiting, food), foreign body
- Severe bronchospasm, laryngeal edema

Suppression of respiratory center: hypnotics, sedatives, other drugs

Hypoventilation from muscular or neuromuscular disorders: myasthenia gravis, brainstem or high cord injury, Guillain-Barré syndrome, botulism, hypokalemia

Disease of lung or thoracic wall
- Flail chest, pneumothorax, pneumonia, smoke inhalation
- Severe cardiogenic pulmonary edema, massive pulmonary embolization

**Chronic respiratory acidosis**

Lung disease: chronic obstructive lung disease and chronic bronchitis, end-stage interstitial lung disease

Neuromuscular abnormalities: poliomyelitis, diaphragmatic paralysis, myasthenia gravis

Chronic suppression of respiratory center
- Chronic use of narcotics
- Obesity with decrease in alveolar ventilation (pickwickian syndrome)
- Primary or idiopathic alveolar hypoventilation

Modified with permission from Klahr SK, Hamm L. In Klahr S, editor: *Renal and electrolyte disorders*, ed 2, Norwalk, CT, 1984, Appleton-Century-Crofts.

***Causes.*** The box at right summarizes the causes of respiratory acidosis. The differential diagnosis of acute versus chronic respiratory acidosis relies on both the clinical and the laboratory criteria discussed earlier.

***Treatment.*** The main goal in the treatment of acute respiratory acidosis is the restoration of effective ventilation. If some delay prevents achieving this goal, oxygen should be given at once. Modest amounts of $NaHCO_3$ may be given intravenously to mitigate severe acidosis (blood pH less than 7.2).

Chronic respiratory acidosis can be treated effectively only by restoring or improving the lung's ability to excrete $CO_2$. This is often impossible because of irreversible lung changes. However, airway drainage (clearing secretions, etc.), relief of bronchospasm, and treatment of pulmonary infections and congestive heart failure may result in significant improvement.

## Respiratory alkalosis

Increased alveolar ventilation causes increased $CO_2$ excretion, resulting in decreases in $PCO_2$, $HCO_3^-$ concentration, and in $H^+$ concentration (reflected in a rise in blood pH). Since the production of $CO_2$ from metabolism is usually constant, a negative $CO_2$ balance can only be achieved through increased alveolar ventilation. Hyperventilation can result from two main processes: (1) increased neurochemical stimulation of the respiratory center and (2) iatrogenically assisted or controlled mechanical ventilation. To maintain blood pH within normal limits as arterial $PCO_2$ and thus $H_2CO_3$ decreases, plasma $HCO_3^-$ must decrease. Release of $H^+$ from body buffers reduces plasma $HCO_3^-$. Changes in cellular metabolism also contribute by increasing the production of lactic acid and probably other organic acids. In general, plasma $HCO_3^-$ levels decrease by approximately 2.5 mmol/L for each decrement of 10 mm Hg in arterial $PCO_2$ below normal. In respiratory alkalosis, $HCO_3^-$ values may occasionally decrease to as low as 15 mmol/L or arterial $PCO_2$ to as low as 15 mm Hg, but one should always suspect metabolic acidosis when plasma $HCO_3^-$ is less than 18 mmol/L. The other line of defense in respiratory alkalosis relates to diminished rate of $H^+$ secretion into the tubular fluid, leading to an $HCO_3^-$ diuresis that tends to restore pH toward normal. Ammonium excretion decreases, with resulting decreased de novo synthesis of $HCO_3^-$. This renal adaptation to respiratory alkalosis occurs rapidly and is probably complete within 24 hours.

***Clinical features and systemic effects.*** Respiratory alkalosis may be manifested by symptoms and signs of neuromuscular irritability. Vasoconstriction of the cerebral circulation occurs, with reduced blood flow to the brain. Blood pressure and pulmonary vascular resistance are decreased, and pulmonary flow and cardiac output are increased. Patients may complain of paresthesias in the perioral region and extremities, muscle cramps, and tinnitus. In some patients, tetany and seizures occur, and an increase in deep tendon reflexes is present. Marked alkalosis may result in cardiac arrhythmias.

***Laboratory findings.*** The hallmark of respiratory alkalosis is a decrease in the $P_{CO_2}$ of body fluids. As a consequence, the arterial pH is elevated and plasma $HCO_3^-$ decreases as a compensatory mechanism. The serum electrolyte levels remain within normal limits unless another disorder is also present. The electrocardiogram (ECG) may show flattening or inversion of ST segments or T waves. Impaired release of oxygen from hemoglobin, caused by the shift in the oxyhemoglobin dissociation curve, may account for the ECG abnormalities in hypocapnia. A rise in blood concentrations of lactic acid and pyruvic acids in response to the reduction in $P_{CO_2}$ has been observed frequently. One should consider the development of an $HCO_3^-$ deficit in the presence of a simultaneous rise in lactic and pyruvic acids in patients with respiratory alkalosis, since it may be confused with the findings seen in metabolic acidosis with an increased anion gap.

***Causes.*** The box below lists the causes of respiratory alkalosis. It is important to note that the acid-base disorder produced by pulmonary disease depends on the severity of that disease.

***Treatment.*** Effective therapy corrects or ameliorates the basic disorder responsible for the hyperventilation. Correction of hypoxemia is critical to the patient's well-being. If the respiratory alkalosis is related to mechanical ventilation, decreasing the minute ventilation or increasing the dead space may be effective. If this cannot be done without compromising oxygenation, the use of an inhaled mixture containing 3% $CO_2$ may be helpful.

### Causes of respiratory alkalosis

**Central nervous system**

Voluntary hyperventilation, anxiety-hyperventilation syndrome
Cerebrovascular accident, infection, trauma, tumor

**Hypoxia**

High altitude, hypotension
Inequality of ventilation-perfusion ratio

**Drugs or hormones**

Salicylates, nicotine, xanthines
Pressor hormones
Progesterone

**Pulmonary diseases**

Interstitial fibrosis, pneumonia, pulmonary edema, pulmonary embolism

**Miscellaneous**

Anemia
Pregnancy
Hepatic failure
Gram-negative septicemia
Exposure to heat
Mechanical overventilation

Modified with permission from Valtin H, Gennari EJ. In *Acid-base disorders: basic concepts and clinical management,* Boston, 1987, Little, Brown.

### Mixed acid-base disorders

The entities described, metabolic acidosis, metabolic alkalosis, respiratory acidosis, and respiratory alkalosis, represent simple acid-base disturbances. They denote the presence of one primary process and its appropriate physiologic response. A mixed acid-base disturbance refers to the coexistence of two or more primary processes. Since these processes may have either additive or nullifying effects on plasma pH, mixed acid-base disturbances may produce dramatically extreme deviations of hydrogen concentration or disarmingly minor or undetectable deviations.

The coexistence of two or more simple acid-base disturbances is quite common in hospitalized patients. A mixed acid-base disturbance is frequently suspected from a careful analysis of the acid-base values. When the magnitude of the secondary change in $P_{CO_2}$ or $HCO_3^-$ concentrations (in metabolic and respiratory disorders, respectively) is inappropriate with respect to the magnitude of the initiating process, the presence of a mixed disturbance should be considered (Table 90-2). Even when a seemingly appropriate relationship exists between an initiating disturbance and an anticipated secondary response, such a relationship may merely be the consequence of a dual or even a triple acid-base abnormality. To avoid this diagnostic pitfall, clues to the presence of complicating acid-base disturbances should be sought from a close examination of other laboratory data and particularly from the patient's history.

Chronic respiratory acidosis may coexist with metabolic alkalosis, particularly in patients with pulmonary insufficiency and cor pulmonale treated with diuretics and a low-salt diet. This disturbance can also emerge when longstanding hypercapnia is partially corrected by mechanical ventilation or other means.

A combination of chronic and acute respiratory acidosis may be seen in patients with moderately severe $CO_2$ retention caused by chronic obstructive lung disease who also experience a sudden worsening of pulmonary function from the use of sedatives capable of depressing the respiratory center, correction of their hypoxia by oxygen therapy, or concomitant acute pulmonary infections.

Metabolic acidosis plus acute respiratory acidosis is common in patients with acute cardiopulmonary arrest and results from lactic acidosis (triggered by poor tissue perfusion) and $CO_2$ retention. A similar picture may be seen in patients with severe, acute pulmonary edema. Extreme decreases in plasma pH may be seen under these conditions.

## FLUID AND ELECTROLYTE DISORDERS

### Disorders of potassium homeostasis: general discussion

Potassium is an essential cation located predominantly in the intracellular space. Total body potassium approximates 3600 mmol, with the extracellular space containing only 65 to 70 mmol. Approximately 100 mmol of potassium is ingested daily in the average American diet. Under normal circumstances, 90% of this amount is excreted in the urine (80 to 90 mmol daily) and 10% in the stools (8 to 15 mmol daily). Because potassium is located primarily in the intracellular space (98%), it is difficult to monitor accurately any changes in body stores of this cation. Distribution of potassium between the intracellular and extracellular fluids affects potassium concentration in plasma. Potassium homeostasis is regulated mainly by the kidney. Potassium excretion by the kidney is influenced by acid-base status, anion excretion, urine flow rate, potassium intake, and levels of mineralocorticoids.

## Hypokalemia

Hypokalemia is usually defined as a condition marked by a plasma potassium concentration of less than 3.5 mEq/L. Hypokalemia may be relative or absolute. Changes in acid-base balance may shift potassium into cells, causing relative hypokalemia (depressed plasma concentration), when in fact total body potassium may be normal. Absolute hypokalemia, on the other hand, reflects a fall in both intracellular and extracellular potassium concentrations. For a 1 mmol/L decline in plasma potassium, the total potassium deficit may be 100 to 400 mmol.

***Clinical features and systemic effects.*** The organ systems most significantly affected by hypokalemia include skeletal muscle, heart, kidneys, and gastrointestinal tract. Clinical manifestations of mild hypokalemia may be subtle. A high degree of suspicion about the clinical setting (history of vomiting, diuretics, laxative use, diarrhea) helps to identify patients at risk. Most patients with plasma potassium levels less than 2.5 mmol/L complain of moderate muscle weakness. As the plasma levels fall below 1.5 mmol/L, areflexic paralysis may occur, and respiratory depression may be an immediate threat to survival. Potassium also significantly affects cardiac function. Acute potassium losses may cause hyperpolarization, since intracellular potassium may remain normal as extracellular potassium falls. This situation may cause premature ventricular contractions, frequent ectopic tachycardias, and widening of the QRS complex. With small changes in intracellular potassium concentration, which is related to myocardial contractility, cardiac output begins to fall. Significant changes in the ECG may be present, including early depression of the ST segment, with a decreased amplitude of the T wave. U waves may also be present, as well as first-degree atrioventricular block. As intracellular potassium decreases further, contractility progressively decreases, leading to marked ventricular irregularity and profound heart failure. Potassium depletion also decreases gastric and small intestinal motility and may cause paralytic ileus. Severe prolonged potassium depletion causes histologic changes of the kidney and an inability to concentrate the urine, resulting in polyuria, polydipsia, and nocturia.

***Causes.*** The box on p. 1232 lists the causes of hypokalemia. In hypokalemic patients, it is important to assess blood pressure and the ECF volume status. Also, when hypokalemia is severe (plasma potassium less than 3 mmol/L), one must consider causes other than or in addition to diuretic therapy. The determination of potassium excretion in the urine is extremely important. Usually, individuals with hypokalemia related to losses of potassium via the gastrointestinal tract will have a urine potassium concentration less than 15 mmol daily. Magnesium depletion also may cause hypokalemia. Fig. 90-2 outlines the evaluation of hypokalemia.

***Treatment.*** In most patients, judicious correction of the potassium deficit is most appropriate. Since potassium is located mainly intracellularly, it is difficult to judge the total deficit of potassium. The rapidity of potassium replacement depends on the chronicity of the disorder, the presence of other fluid and electrolyte abnormalities, and the presence and severity of end-organ sequelae of the hypokalemia. Specific salt use to replace a potassium deficit is important. With alkalosis, potassium must be replaced as potassium chloride. When hypokalemia is associated with metabolic acidosis, as in RTA or diabetic ketoacidosis, potassium replacement by potassium bicarbonate ($KHCO_3$) or a $KHCO_3$ equivalent (potassium citrate or gluconate) can be effective. Since many derangements that occur with hypokalemia are not life-threatening, oral replacement of potassium is usually indicated. When intravenous potassium replacement is required, one should remember that a rate of 10 mmol hourly without monitoring is safe. However, doses of 40 mmol hourly or higher should be given only with close monitoring of the ECG. Hypokalemia related to diuretic use, when diuretic therapy is necessary, may require the administration of potassium-sparing drugs, such as triamterene or amiloride. These are usually more effective in correcting hypokalemia than potassium supplementation alone.

**Table 90-2.** Usual magnitude of compensatory mechanism in acid-base disorders

| Disorder | Compensatory mechanism |
|---|---|
| Metabolic acidosis | $P_{CO_2}$ should decrease by 1.0-1.5 mm Hg for every 1 mEq/L fall in $HCO_3^-$. |
| Metabolic alkalosis | $P_{CO_2}$ should increase by 0.5-1.0 mm Hg for every 1 mEq/L rise in $HCO_3^-$. |
| Acute respiratory acidosis | $HCO_3^-$ concentration increases but seldom above 30 mEq/L. |
| Chronic respiratory acidosis | $HCO_3^-$ concentration should increase by 4 mEq/L for every 10 mm Hg rise in $P_{CO_2}$. |
| Respiratory alkalosis | $HCO_3^-$ concentration should decrease by 2.5 mEq/L for every 10 mm Hg fall in $P_{CO_2}$; $HCO_3^-$ seldom falls below 16-18 mEq/L. |

From Klahr S, Hamm L. In Klahr S, editor: *Renal and electrolyte disorders,* ed 2, Norwalk, Conn, 1984, Appleton-Century-Crofts.

## Causes of hypokalemia

### Gastrointestinal causes

Decreased potassium intake: starvation, anorexia nervosa
Loss of hydrochloric acid: vomiting from pyloric stenosis or gastroenteritis, gastric aspiration without adequate replacement
Defective potassium absorption
- Fistulas: biliary, pancreatic, gastrocolic
- Zollinger-Ellison syndrome, malabsorption
- Postgastrectomy dumping syndrome
- Inflammatory bowel disease: regional enteritis, ulcerative colitis

Increased intestinal secretion of potassium: diarrhea (usually infectious), villous adenomas
Iatrogenic lesions: laxative use, repeated enemas, use of exchange resins

### Renal causes

Diuretic therapy: furosemide/ethacrynic acid, thiazides, carbonic anhydrase inhibitors
Antibiotic therapy: carbenicillin, gentamicin, amphotericin B
Renal tubular or parenchymal diseases: renal tubular acidosis: proximal and distal types; Fanconi's syndrome; chronic pyelonephritis

### Renal causes

Magnesium depletion
Adrenal steroids
- Primary hyperaldosteronism (aldosteronism): adrenal adenomas, adrenal hyperplasis, 17-α-hydroxylase or 11-β-hydroxylase deficiencies, dexamethasone- or glucorticosteroid-suppressible hyperaldosteronism
- Secondary hyperaldosteronism: associated with decreased "effective plasma volume" cirrhosis, congestive heart failure, or hypoalbuminemia; Bartter's syndrome; associated with malignant hypertension
- Cushing's syndrome: excessive adrenocorticotropic hormone (ACTH) production from anterior pituitary gland, exogenous ACTH production (malignancy), exogenous cortisol production (malignancy)
- Adrenal steroid therapy
- Licorice ingestion

### Miscellaneous causes related to intracellular shifts of potassium

Systemic alkalosis, either respiratory or metabolic
Infusion of large amounts of glucose or insulin therapy
Familial hypokalemic paralysis
Ingestion of barium salts
Vitamin $B_{12}$ therapy in patients with pernicious anemia

Modified with permission from Harter H. In Klahr S, editor: *Renal and electrolyte disorders,* ed 2, Norwalk, CT, 1984, Appleton-Century-Crofts.

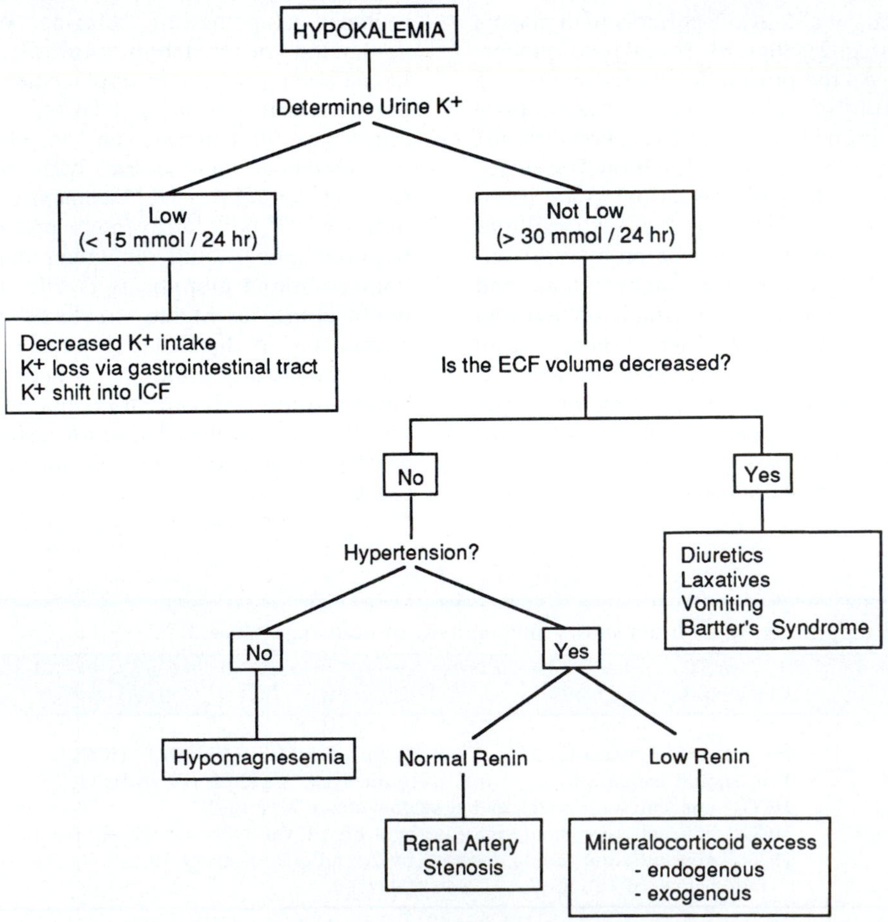


**Fig. 90-2.** Evaluation of hypokalemia.

## Hyperkalemia

Hyperkalemia is defined as a condition marked by a plasma potassium level greater than 5 mmol/L. It is a relatively uncommon clinical entity but has potentially lethal consequences. Hyperkalemia can be classified as relative or absolute. *Relative* hyperkalemia occurs with shifts of intracellular potassium to the extracellular fluid space without an increase in total body potassium. *Absolute* hyperkalemia is present when both intracellular and extracellular potassium concentrations are increased.

***Clinical manifestations and systemic effects.*** Patients with hyperkalemia have abnormalities of the cardiovascular and neuromuscular systems. Cardiac contractility is not affected by hyperkalemia, but significant arrhythmias may occur because of changes in conduction. ECG changes usually occur when plasma potassium levels exceed 7 mmol/L. Initially, usually with modest increases in plasma potassium, tall peaked T waves are seen with a normal QT interval, and decreased amplitude of the P waves occurs with a prolonged PR interval. As hyperkalemia progresses, atrial asystole is seen, with widening of the QRS complex leading to a sine wave. Finally, plasma potassium concentrations greater than 10 mmol/L lead to ventricular standstill. The effects of hyperkalemia on cardiac function can occur with smaller increases in plasma potassium when hyponatremia, hypocalcemia, or acidosis are present. Changes in muscle strength or nerve conduction velocity also occur, particularly with potassium levels exceeding 8 mmol/L. Muscular weakness develops, usually beginning in the lower extremities and ascending to the upper extremities. Respiratory depression also may occur.

### Causes of hyperkalemia

**Acute or severe chronic renal failure**

Continued potassium intake, acidosis, increased catabolism, administration of potassium-containing solutions, gastrointestinal bleeding, hemolysis, volume depletion

**Translocation of potassium from intracellular to extracellular fluid space**

Acidosis, severe catabolism, rhabdomyolysis, familial hyperkalemic periodic paralysis, depolarizing muscle paralysis (succinylcholine therapy)

**Mineralocorticoid deficiency states**

Addison's disease, hyporeninemic hypoaldosteronism

**Aldosterone antagonists or potassium-sparing diuretics**

Spironolactone, triamterene

**Other medications**

Nonsteroidal antiinflammatory drugs (NSAIDs), β-blockers, angiotensin converting enzyme (ACE) inhibitors, trimethoprim

**Miscellaneous**

"Pseudohyperkalemia" of myeloproliferative disorders (hyperkalemia associated with thrombocytosis or granulocytosis), hemolysis at blood sampling, intravenous potassium

Modified with permission from Harter H. In Klahr S, editor: *Renal and electrolyte disorders*, ed 2, Norwalk, Conn, 1984, Appleton-Century-Crofts.

***Causes.*** The box at right lists the most common causes of hyperkalemia. Acute and chronic renal failure account for most cases of hyperkalemia. Since the kidney is the major organ responsible for potassium excretion, a marked and sudden loss of renal function would lead to hyperkalemia if dietary intake of potassium is not curtailed. Increased catabolism also plays a role in the development of hyperkalemia in patients with acute renal failure. Hyperkalemia is usually not seen with chronic renal failure unless excessive potassium is administered. Hyperkalemia may occur as a consequence of translocation of potassium from the intracellular to the extracellular space. This may be related to acidosis, severe tissue catabolism, muscle breakdown (rhabdomyolysis), and certain entities such as familial hyperkalemic periodic paralysis. Since aldosterone is a major regulatory hormone of potassium homeostasis, its absence may lead to hyperkalemia. While isolated aldosterone deficiency is exceedingly rare, primary adrenal insufficiency (Addison's disease) may be associated with severe depression of plasma aldosterone levels.

Addison's disease caused by hypopituitarism is not associated with hyperkalemia, since aldosterone secretion rates remain normal. Addison's disease from adrenal gland pathology may lead to hyperkalemia. In addition, patients with this condition may have hyperpigmentation, decreased appetite, hypoglycemia, and hypotension. Hyponatremia and renal sodium wasting may also be observed. In hyporeninemic hypoaldosteronism, hyperkalemia may occur because of a deficiency of aldosterone secretion and a decrease in the secretion of potassium in the distal tubule. Approximately 50% of patients with hyporeninemic hypoaldosteronism have associated diabetes. About 50% of these patients will achieve lowered potassium levels by improved diabetic control. Drugs such as spironolactones, which are aldosterone antagonists, or potassium-sparing diuretics may also cause hyperkalemia.

***Treatment.*** The treatment of hyperkalemia differs based on the level of plasma potassium, the chronicity of the hyperkalemic state, and clinical manifestations. In acute hyperkalemia, if the potassium concentration is less than 6.5 mmol and there are no ECG changes, potassium intake should be decreased and drugs that compromise potassium excretion discontinued. With greater levels of potassium or pertinent ECG changes, other measures are necessary. Calcium administration may reverse several of the effects of hyperkalemia. Calcium therapy has an onset of action within minutes, but the action is short-lived, about half an hour. Redistribution of potassium from the extracellular space to the intracellular space is also an effective treatment for hyperkalemia. This can be accomplished with $NaHCO_3$, one or two ampules (44 to 88 mmol) given intravenously, or by the infusion of glucose and insulin. A solution of 500 ml of 10% glucose with 10 units of regular insulin is an adequate dose for the latter treatment. Glucose and insulin therapy has an onset of action within 30 minutes, and the action lasts for several hours. A

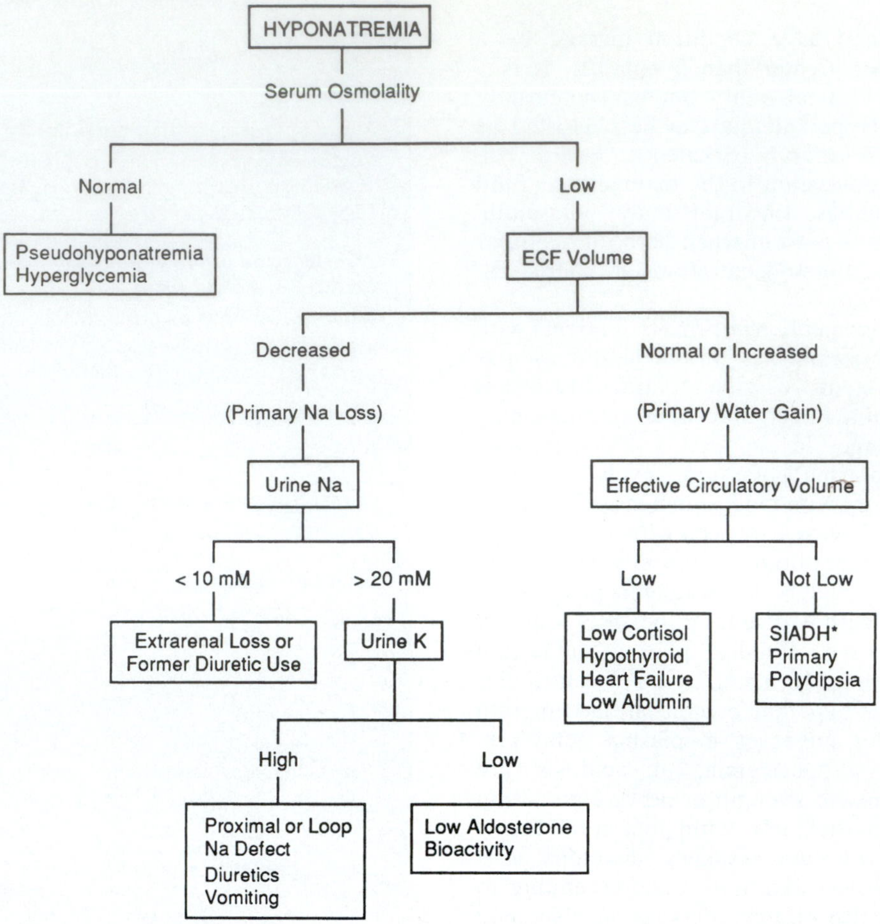


**Fig. 90-3.** Evaluation of hyponatremia. *SIADH,* Syndrome of inappropriate antidiuretic hormone (ADH) release.

β-agonist such as albuterol used as a nebulizer at doses of 10 to 20 mg lowers serum potassium concentration by approximately 0.6 mmol/L. The effect of albuterol is apparent within 30 minutes and persists for at least 2 hours. Potassium can be removed from the body using exchange resins such as Kayexalate, which can be administered orally or rectally. Hemodialysis or peritoneal dialysis can also be employed to remove potassium. The effect of dialysis on plasma potassium is seen within hours, and its duration depends on the rate of endogenous release of potassium.

### Hyponatremia

Hyponatremia is defined as a condition marked by a serum sodium concentration less than 135 mmol/L. Hyponatremia does not necessarily indicate a decrease in total body sodium. Since the concentration of sodium depends on the relative amounts of sodium and water in the ECF, a low serum sodium concentration only indicates that there is relatively more water than sodium in this space. This may occur when ECF sodium content is decreased, such as with diarrhea, in which losses of both sodium and water occur, but the sodium losses are greater than those of water. When the ECF sodium content is normal (e.g., with excess administration of water) or when ECF sodium content is increased (e.g., with edema), increases in both sodium and water content occur. Fig. 90-3 summarizes an approach to the patient with hyponatremia.

Hyponatremia can occur in the setting of an expanded, normal, or contracted ECF volume. Excess water in the ECF may result from excessive intake of water or reduced excretion of water. Increased ingestion of water may be related to compulsive polydipsia, acute psychosis, excessive parenteral administration of fluids, use of tap water enemas, or postoperative irrigation of the prostatic bed with hyponatremic solutions. Reduced excretion of water may result from intrinsic renal disease or extrinsic factors that modify the kidneys' ability to excrete water, such as the syndrome of inappropriate antidiuretic hormone (SIADH) (see Chapter 39), congestive heart failure, and cirrhosis. The first step in the evaluation of hyponatremia is to rule out hyperglycemia, hyperproteinemia, and hyperlipidemia as potential causes of pseudohyponatremia. With true hyponatremia, the osmolality of plasma is low. If sodium loss is the reason for the hyponatremia, urine sodium and chloride concentrations will be less than 20 mmol/L. If the major reason for the hyponatremia is water excess, excretion of a volume of 1 L hourly of the most dilute urine, 50 to 75 mOsm/kg water, is to be expected.

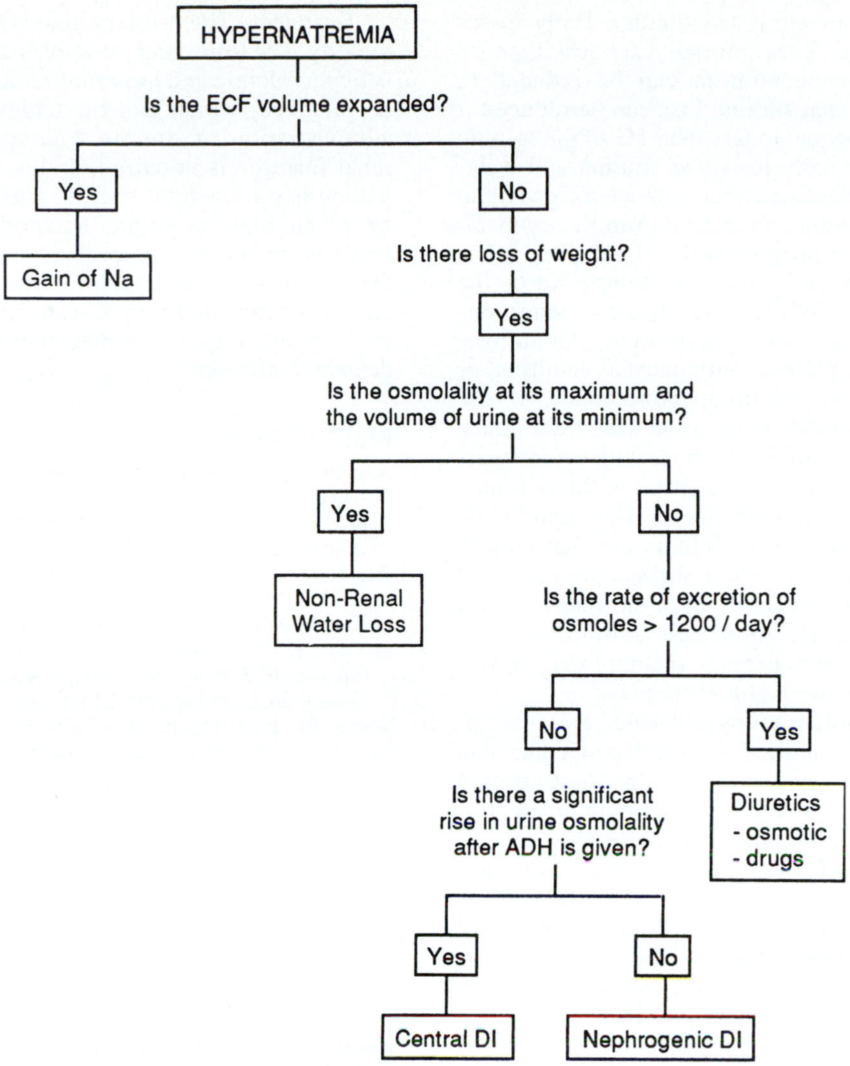


**Fig. 90-4.** Evaluation of hypernatremia.

***Clinical manifestations and systemic effects.*** Patients with hyponatremia rarely have symptoms unless the plasma sodium is less than 125 mmol/L and especially with rapid development of hyponatremia. There is some evidence that symptomatic hyponatremia is more common in women. The typical symptoms relate to osmotic swelling of brain cells, and vary from mild lethargy to convulsions and coma. There may additionally be gastrointestinal symptoms such as anorexia and nausea.

***Treatment.*** Treatment depends on whether the condition is acute or chronic. In acute hyponatremia, neurologic symptoms are more often seen in young females in the postoperative state, in elderly persons receiving thiazide diuretics, and in patients with psychogenic polydipsia. These patients should be treated promptly to prevent cerebral edema and seizures. Rapid correction through intravenous administration of sodium, 1.5 to 2.0 mM/L/hour in this setting, may be associated with a lower mortality than slower correction (0.6 mM/L/hour). The correction can be accomplished with hypertonic saline, preferably given with furosemide to prevent sodium overload and to enhance water excretion. The symptomatic patient with chronic hyponatremia is best managed conservatively by water restriction even when the serum sodium is very low. Long-time water restriction may be difficult to enforce, and therefore agents that antagonize the renal action of ADH have been employed. Demeclocycline is safer and more effective than lithium in the treatment of SIADH.

## Hypernatremia

Hypernatremia is marked by plasma sodium concentrations in excess of 145 mmol/L. Disturbances of either sodium or water metabolism are responsible for hypernatremia. This usually results from sodium gain or water loss. Physiologically, hypernatremia results in a decrease in cell volume. Hypernatremia is not a specific clinical entity. The clinician should look for the underlying cause of the increase in serum sodium concentration. Most often, hypernatremia is caused by water loss from renal or extrarenal sources. Daily obligatory fluid loss is related to evaporative losses through the lungs and skin plus the amount of water necessary to excrete the solutes in the urine. These obligatory fluid losses amount to about 1300 ml daily or approximately 10% of the ECF volume.

Obligatory sodium losses are much smaller. Daily losses of sodium in sweat and feces normally are less than 20 mmol. Urine sodium concentration can be reduced to below 5 mmol daily so that sodium loss can be reduced if necessary to an amount equal to less than 1% of the sodium pool in the ECF. If the daily losses of sodium and water are not replaced, the negative water balance exceeds that for sodium, and the sodium concentration in the extracellular space will increase progressively. If the patient has fever or is in a high environmental temperature, the situation will be aggravated because all these conditions increase evaporative water losses more than sodium loss. Water is not replaced in patients with nausea, vomiting, or dysphagia, who experience thirst consequent to the hypernatremia and are unable to increase their fluid intake appropriately. Comatose patients or those with cerebrovascular accidents (strokes) may not be aware of thirst or may not be able to communicate their needs. They depend on others for adequate fluid intake. Infants are particularly susceptible to hypernatremia. Their surface area per unit of body mass is much greater than that of the adult, so their evaporative water losses are greater. In addition, infants' ability to concentrate their urine is incompletely developed, increasing obligatory water losses.

When the major problem is loss of water in excess of sodium loss, volume contraction usually occurs, and laboratory studies show evidence of hemoconcentration with increasing hematocrit and serum protein concentrations. BUN and serum creatinine concentrations may be elevated. Unless the patient has coexistent renal disease, urine output will be low, less than 500 ml daily, and the urine will be hyperosmolar, in excess of 1000 mOsm/kg water, with a very low urine sodium concentration. Failure to find a very low urine volume and a maximally concentrated urine suggests a renal problem.

The major renal causes of hypernatremia are diabetes insipidus (see Chapter 36) or an osmotic diuresis. These two disorders can be distinguished by appropriate measurement of urine osmolality. When thirst is absent in patients with hypernatremia, a central nervous system lesion should be considered. Hypernatremia caused by sodium gain is rare. Usually, it is characterized by ECF volume expansion, thirst, and the excretion of small volumes of very concentrated urine. If the hypernatremia results from water loss of extrarenal origin and the patient does not have access to water, he or she will be thirsty and excrete a minimal volume of maximally concentrated urine. If the cause of the hypernatremia is loss of water via the kidney, the urine will not be concentrated and the urine volume will not be decreased. In this setting, two major diseases may be present: diabetes insipidus (central or nephrogenic) or diuretic-induced water loss (usually osmotic diuresis from glucose or urea). Fig. 90-4 summarizes an approach to the patient with hypernatremia.

***Clinical manifestations and systemic effects.*** As with hyponatremia, the principal clinical manifestations relate to osmotic effects on the brain. In hypernatremia there is dehydration of brain cells, which leads to symptoms ranging from confusion to convulsions and coma. The intensity of the symptoms correlates with both the severity and rapidity of development of the hypernatremia.

***Treatment.*** The primary goal is the restoration of serum tonicity. The following principles are helpful. If the patient is hypervolemic and hypernatremic, excess sodium should be removed, which can be achieved by the intravenous administration of diuretics along with 5% dextrose. If renal function is impaired, dialysis may be needed. If the patient has a low total body sodium, isotonic NaCl should be given until systemic hemodynamics are stabilized. Hypernatremia is then treated with half-normal saline or 5% dextrose. The patient who is hypernatremic but euvolemic, and therefore has sustained water losses almost exclusively, requires replacement of water with a 5% dextrose infusion.

## BIBLIOGRAPHY


Anderson RJ: Hospital associated hyponatremia, *Kidney Int* 29:1237, 1986.

Berl T: Treating hyponatremia: damned if we do and damned if we don't, *Kidney Int* 37:1006, 1990.

Gabow PA: Disorders associated with an altered anion gap, *Kidney Int* 27:472, 1985.

Harrington JT: Metabolic alkalosis, *Kidney Int* 26:88, 1984.

Madias NE, Perrone RD: Acid-base disorders in association with renal disease. In Schrier RW, Gottschalk CW, editors: *Diseases of the kidney,* ed 5, Boston, 1993, Little, Brown.

Tannen RL: Potassium metabolism, *Semin Nephrol* 7:173, 1987.

Teitelbaum I, Kelleher SP, Berl T: Diabetes insipidus and the syndrome of inappropriate antidiuretic hormone secretion. In Schrier RW, Gottschalk CW, editors: *Diseases of the kidney,* ed 5, Boston, 1993, Little, Brown.

Valtin H, Gennari FJ: *Acid-base disorders: basic concepts and clinical management,* Boston, 1987, Little, Brown.


CHAPTER

# 91 Urinary Tract Infections

**Bahar Bastani**

Urinary tract infection (UTI) is the most common bacterial infection affecting humans in their life span. Up to one third of all females experience at least one episode of UTI in their life. UTIs occur in all ages, neonatal to geriatric, with a particular impact on females, males at the two extremes of life, and anyone with functional or structural abnormalities of the urinary tract. The infection may be limited to one part or extend throughout the urinary tract and may involve the perinephric tissues. Although the bacteriology and pathogenesis of UTI may be the same, the clinical features, the risk of acute or chronic complications, and the treatment vary depending on the location of infection and whether or not functional or structural abnormalities are present.

## EPIDEMIOLOGY AND ETIOLOGY

### Definitions and terminologies

Despite the pitfalls and difficulties in determining bacte-

## Classification of urinary tract infections (UTIs)

Lower UTI: cystitis, urethritis, prostatitis
Upper UTI: acute or chronic pyelonephritis, renal or perirenal abscess
Uncomplicated lower or upper UTI
Complicated lower or upper UTI (risk of renal damage, urosepsis, abscess formation): presence of functional or anatomic abnormalities, obstruction, calculi/catheter/stent, pregnancy, hospitalization, immunosuppression, diabetes mellitus, sickle cell disease, analgesic/NSAID abuse
Acute urethral syndrome: dysuria/frequency with less than $10^5$ bacteria/ml of urine
Asymptomatic bacteriuria: asymptomatic with greater than $10^5$ colonies of the same bacteria/ml of clean-catch midstream urine

*NSAID*, Nonsteroidal antiinflammatory drug.

riologic localization, the UTIs have conventionally been classified into those involving the upper versus the lower urinary tract. Each category is further divided into uncomplicated versus complicated UTI, depending on the absence or presence of host conditions known to promote infection, account for persistence of infection, or promote recurrence of infection. Although the vast majority of the *uncomplicated* UTIs occur in young women and are community acquired, *complicated* UTIs occur in patients with anatomic or urologic abnormalities or with recent urinary catheterization or instrumentation, involve both sexes, and are often hospital acquired. The complicated UTIs are associated with a higher incidence of antimicrobial resistance, a poorer response to therapy, and a higher risk of renal damage, urosepsis, and abscess formation.

The *lower* UTIs include cystitis, prostatitis, and urethritis (see the box above). Atrophic vaginitis; sexually transmitted diseases caused by *Chlamydia trachomatis, Neisseria gonorrhoeae,* or herpes simplex; and vaginal infections caused by *Candida albicans* or *Trichomonas* species can also present with dysuria and urinary frequency but are not considered UTIs (see Chapter 65).

The *upper* UTIs, which are much less common, include acute or chronic pyelonephritis, focal or multifocal acute bacterial interstitial nephritis, and renal or perirenal abscess. Acute pyelonephritis is a clinical diagnosis based on the presence of fever, flank tenderness, and bacteriuria. However, diagnosis of chronic pyelonephritis is based on radiologic demonstration of calyceal clubbing and deformity associated with renal scarring, typically a sequela of bacterial infection superimposed on an anatomic abnormality of the urinary tract (e.g., obstruction, more often vesicoureteral reflux).

The term *acute urethral syndrome* (also called the dysuria-pyuria syndrome) describes women with signs and symptoms suggestive of lower UTI but less than $10^5$ bacteria/ml of urine. Between 30% and 50% of all patients with dysuria have this condition. *Asymptomatic bacteriuria* refers to presence of greater than $10^5$ of the same bacterial species/ml of urine in two consecutive midstream urine cultures, in the absence of any signs or symptoms of UTI.

### Incidence and prevalence

Except during the newborn period, when the incidence of UTI in both symptomatic and asymptomatic infants is much greater in males than in females, in all other age groups, UTIs occur much more frequently in females. The incidence of UTI, which only occasionally occurs in prepubertal girls, greatly increases in late adolescence and during the second and third decades of life. Approximately one third of women 20 to 40 years of age develop signs and symptoms suggestive of UTI. During the reproductive years, women are 20 to 50 times more likely to acquire UTI than men. It is more common in sexually active women, and its incidence increases with age. The difference in the incidence of UTI between men and women diminishes in later life. Use of a diaphragm and spermicides for contraception may also increase the risk. The spermicides may promote colonization of *Escherichia coli* in the vagina by altering the vaginal pH.

In the older age group, hospitalization for other illness is frequently associated with urinary catheterization and acquisition of nosocomial UTI. Up to 10% of all hospitalized patients have a urinary catheter, 20% of whom subsequently develop bacteriuria. Catheter-associated UTI accounts for 40% of all nosocomial infections. Predisposing factors for UTI in women include sexual intercourse, use of a diaphragm and spermicides, and presence of receptors to *E. coli* and in men include lack of circumcision (infants and sexually active young adults), rectal intercourse, and benign prostatic hyperplasia. Hospitalization and catheterization increase the risk of infection in both sexes.

### Uropathogenic bacteria

Most UTIs are caused by bacteria that originate from flora in the lower gut. *E. coli,* normally present in large quantities in the feces, accounts for 80% to 90% of uncomplicated community-based UTIs. The same strain of *E. coli* recovered from infected urine is usually also recovered from the patient's periurethra, vagina, and rectum. However, not all *E. coli* strains are uropathogenic, and a relatively small number of strains that possess certain virulence factors cause most UTIs.

Other enteric gram-negative bacteria, such as *Klebsiella pneumoniae, Enterobacter aerogenes,* and *Proteus* species, as well as gram-positive bacteria such as *Enterococcus faecalis, Staphylococcus epidermidis,* and *S. saprophyticus,* are also common uropathogens. However, anaerobic bacteria, which are present in much greater abundance in the gut flora, only rarely produce UTI.

Although the urethra, periurethra, introitus, and vagina do not normally contain significant quantities of the uropathogenic bacteria, it has been shown that in women with recurrent UTI, a heavy colonization with the uropathogenic bacteria precedes or is associated with the episodes of UTI. Table 91-1 shows the frequency of different uropathogenic bacteria in uncomplicated community-acquired and complicated hospital-associated UTIs.

*S. saprophyticus* is the second most common pathogen

**Table 91-1.** Prevalence of different microorganisms in uncomplicated outpatient vs. complicated hospital-associated UTIs

| Microorganism | Uncomplicated (%) | Complicated (%) |
|---|---|---|
| *Escherichia coli* | 80.0 | 32.0 |
| *Klebsiella* species | 2.0-5.0 | 7.5 |
| *Enterobacter* species | 2.0 | 4.5 |
| *Proteus* species | 2.0 | 7.5 |
| *Pseudomonas aeruginosa* | 0 | 12.5 |
| *Citrobacter* species | 0 | 1.5 |
| *Serratia* species | 0 | 1.0 |
| Enterococci | 1.0 | 15.0 |
| *Staphylococcus epidermidis* | 0 | 3.5 |
| *Staphylococcus saprophyticus* | 10.0-15.0 | 0 |
| *Staphylococcus aureus* | 0 | 1.5 |
| Group B streptococci | 0 | 1.0 |
| *Bacteroides* and other anaerobes | 0 | Very rare |
| *Candida* species | 0 | 5.0 |

isolated from young women. It accounts for 10% to 15% of uncomplicated lower UTIs, especially during summer and fall. The bacterial counts with this organism are often less than $10^5$/ml of urine. Its pathogenic role at this low titer has been supported by the finding of $10^2$ to $10^4$ colonies of this organism/ml in bladder urine, obtained via suprapubic aspiration, of symptomatic young women.

Among gram-negative microorganisms, *Proteus mirabilis* is particularly important because it produces the enzyme urease, which splits urea into carbon dioxide and ammonia. This process results in alkalinization of urine and leads to the formation of struvite stones that entrap the bacteria, protecting them from antimicrobial agents (see Chapter 92). The continued growth of bacteria leads to further urinary alkalinization and precipitation of struvite crystals, resulting in formation of massive staghorn stones.

Since contamination of urine samples by bacteria normally present in the anterior urethra or periurethra occurs often, especially in women, a bacterial count of greater than $10^5$ colonies/ml of clean-catch midstream urine has been used to distinguish genuine bladder bacteriuria from contamination. Therefore, *significant bacteriuria* is traditionally defined as the presence of more than $10^5$ colonies of the same organism/ml in clean-catch midstream urine. In men, since contamination of carefully collected urine is less common, a count greater than $10^4$/ml of urine with the same organism has been considered adequate for diagnosing bladder bacteriuria. However, prospective studies of women with recurrent UTI have shown that bacterial counts less than $10^5$/ml may be responsible for symptoms on some occasions. Moreover, some recent studies have demonstrated that about one third of women with acute lower UTI caused by *E. coli, S. saprophyticus,* and *Proteus* have colony counts, in midstream urine, of $10^2$ to $10^4$/ml. Similarly, acute pyelonephritis has been reported in association with low bacterial counts in voided urine. Many cases of the acute urethral syndrome are in fact bacterial UTIs with low colony counts and respond to the usual antibiotics. In addition, viruses, chlamydia, mycoplasma, and other sexually transmitted diseases have been implicated.

Genuine mixed infections with a significant number of different microorganisms occurs infrequently except in catheterized patients and those with ileal conduit, stones, neurogenic bladder, or vesicocolonic fistula. Presence of mixed infection is best confirmed by culture of urine samples obtained via sterile catheterization or suprapubic aspiration.

### Host susceptibility and bacterial virulence factors

Several systemic and local factors increase host susceptibility to develop UTI. Malnutrition, diabetes mellitus, an altered immune system, local receptor characteristics of uroepithelial cells, presence of foreign bodies (stone, stent, catheter), urine stasis (obstruction or neuromuscular dysfunction such as neurogenic bladder), and congenital or acquired abnormalities (ureterovesical reflux, bladder diverticula) all predispose patients to develop UTI. Other risk factors include insertive anal intercourse and lack of circumcision in infants and young sexually active men, resulting in colonization of the glans and prepuce with uropathogenic *E. coli.*

Bacterial virulence factors are bacterial characteristics that facilitate infection of the urinary tract. These include bacterial adherence, capsular K antigens, endotoxins, resistance to serum bactericidal effects, hemolysin production and iron-binding proteins, and finally the ability to produce urease enzyme.

Bacterial selective adherence to genitourinary mucosal surfaces can influence the degree of colonization by rendering the organisms resistant to being washed away by the urinary flow. Different fimbriate surface proteins (pili) present on the surface of gram-negative bacteria and the presence of specific receptors for them in some humans' uroepithelial cells may play an important role in bacterial adherence and colonization leading to infection.

*E. coli* elaborates a capsular antigen also called K antigen. Certain K antigens, when expressed in high quantities, can determine the degree of virulence of the strain. For example, strains of *E. coli* that produce pyelonephritis in humans have been shown to have three to five times more K-2a and K-2c capsular antigens than strains that cause only cystitis.

The toxic properties of gram-negative bacteria relate to the endotoxins present in the bacterial wall called lipopolysaccharide-containing lipid A. Lipid A is immunogenic and induces antibodies that cross-react among different gram-negative bacteria. Presence of antibody in the host against lipid A decreases the frequency of shock and death in patients with gram-negative sepsis.

Many strains of gram-negative bacteria are killed in the presence of fresh human serum via a process that involves activation of the complement pathways. *E. coli* strains isolated from patients with acute pyelonephritis or acute cystitis have been found to be significantly more serum resistant than strains normally found in the feces.

Since bacteria require iron, their ability to release hemolysin, resulting in hemolysis of the host erythrocytes and release of hemoglobin, and their iron-binding proteins' content are the other two important virulence factors.

### Normal defense mechanisms of urinary tract

A variety of mechanisms, some of which are nonspecific, protect against microbial invasion in general. Others are specific immunologically based mechanisms directed against the antigenic structures of particular microorganisms. One of the nonspecific resistant mechanisms is the lactobacilli of the normal vaginal/introital flora, which interfere with the adhesion of *E. coli,* resulting in the elimination of colonization with the uropathogenic *E. coli.* Another mechanism is a hydrophilic glycocalyx protein on the surface of the bladder epithelium, rendering it resistant to bacterial adherence. Tamm-Horsfall glycoprotein, which is produced in the kidney and excreted in the urine, binds to *E. coli* receptors and facilitates the removal of *E. coli* in the urine. Normal slow shedding of bladder epithelial cells is greatly increased during episodes of UTI, resulting in removal of a greater number of organisms from the urinary tract.

The specific immune responses in the urinary tract consist of urinary secretory immunoglobulin A (IgA), half of which originates in the urethra and may provide a barrier to the ascent of microbacteria, and IgG excretion, which is increased during acute pyelonephritis.

## PATHOPHYSIOLOGY

### Routes of infection

Bacteria generally do not enter the urinary system by filtration. The three well-recognized routes of infection are (1) ascending infection, as with fecal microorganisms colonizing the periurethral area and subsequently entering the bladder via the urethra; (2) hematogenous spread, as in *Staphylococcus* bacteremia and bacterial seeding of the renal cortex resulting in abscess formation; and (3) direct extension, as with enterovesical fistula.

*Ascending transurethral infection* is the most common route. The short female urethra offers little obstacle to the passage of uropathogenic bacteria, which have colonized the periurethral area, to the bladder. Massage of the urethra and sexual intercourse force bacteria into the bladder, accounting for the increased incidence of UTIs in sexually active women. In males, the length of the urethra, the distance between the external urethral orifice and the perianal area, and the presence of antibacterial factors in prostatic secretions are all responsible for the reduced risk of infection. The presence of a foreskin, fecal incontinence, and poor toilet habits promote colonization by the fecal bacteria and contribute to the higher prevalence of infection seen in uncircumcised infants, young sexually active men, and the elderly with poor anal sphincter control. Catheterization or other instrumentation in either sex increases the risk of UTI, which has been reported to occur with a frequency of 1% after an acute bladder catheterization. In patients with indwelling bladder catheters and an open drainage system, infection invariably occurs within a few days.

*Hematogenous spread* of bacteria, fungi, and mycobacteria from a distant focus of infection may invade the kidneys, bladder, or prostate. Renal cortical and perirenal abscesses caused by staphylococci or group A streptococci are frequently the result of bacteremia with a primary focus of infection in another organ.

*Direct extension* of bacteria from the gut into the bladder may occur via a colovesical fistula, secondary to diverticulitis or colon cancer, or an enterovesical fistula, as in Crohn's disease. These infections are usually recurrent, polymicrobial (high titers of several different species of enteric bacteria present), and accompanied by pneumaturia (air in the urine) or fecaluria (fecal material in the urine).

## HISTORY AND PHYSICAL FINDINGS

### Symptoms and signs of lower vs. upper UTI

Acute bacterial cystitis produces inflammation of the bladder and urethra. The typical symptoms of uncomplicated lower UTI include dysuria, frequency, urgency, nocturia, voiding of small urine volumes, incontinence, and suprapubic or pelvic pain. Hematuria may occur and is usually at the termination of voiding; however, women may have total gross hematuria and may even pass clots. Patients may also complain of a foul smelling or cloudy urine. Fever and flank tenderness occur infrequently in these patients.

With acute pyelonephritis, patients are generally sicker with flank or low back pain, chills, fever, sweats, nausea, vomiting, headache, and malaise. Patients may or may not have symptoms of cystitis. Gross or microscopic hematuria is present in 10% to 15% of patients. Acute pyelonephritis may cause either a mild or a very severe illness that may include gram-negative septicemia, papillary necrosis, oliguric or anuric acute renal failure, and intrarenal or perirenal abscess formation. In 20% of these patients, bacteremia can be documented.

With complicated UTI, such as in hospitalized patients or those with indwelling catheters, the clinical manifestations can range from asymptomatic bacteriuria to a severe gram-negative sepsis with shock. Most of the catheter-associated UTIs are asymptomatic. Similarly, a high percentage of elderly patients who are institutionalized or community based without an indwelling bladder catheter may have asymptomatic bacteriuria. Complicated UTI can also present with signs and symptoms of acute cystitis or acute pyelonephritis. The hallmark of complicated UTI is the broader spectrum of microorganisms involved, which are generally more virulent and antibiotic resistant, have a lower clinical response rate to antimicrobial therapy, and tend to recur. It should be emphasized that in hospitalized patients who suddenly develop signs and symptoms of septic shock with fever and hypotension, urosepsis should be considered, even in the absence of urinary symptoms, particularly if the patient has a history of a recent instrumentation or catheterization. Patients with complicated UTI are particularly prone to develop urosepsis, papillary necrosis, and renal or perirenal abscess.

Although clinicians usually use patients' signs and symptoms to differentiate upper from lower UTI, diagnosing the site of infection based on clinical signs can be quite inaccurate. Approximately one half of women with asymptomatic bacteriuria may have infection originating in the upper tract. Also, as many as one third of women with characteristic symptoms of uncomplicated acute cystitis may have subclinical infection of the upper urinary tract. On the other hand, in some studies, flank pain and tenderness with fever were present in up to one third of patients documented to have lower UTI.

In some patients with recurrent infection, particularly

the elderly, symptoms may be much less obvious, and the patient may only notice a slight change in frequency or "smelly urine" or may develop urinary incontinence or some vague abdominal pain.

Both acute and chronic bacterial prostatitis are associated with UTI. The diagnosis is often made on the basis of symptoms of dysuria; frequency; perineal, groin, or low back pain; and difficulty in urination and the finding of an enlarged, tender prostate gland. Relapsing UTI in men is highly suggestive of chronic bacterial prostatitis.

### Physical examination

In patients with acute cystitis, the abdomen is usually found to be normal. Although about 10% of patients may have some suprapubic tenderness, there is generally no flank tenderness.

With acute pyelonephritis, the patient's temperature may rise to 104° F (40° C), the abdomen may be distended with hypotonic bowel sounds, and there is severe tenderness in the lumbar region. In bacteremic patients, signs of septic shock may be evident.

Except for women with clear-cut signs and symptoms of upper or lower UTI associated with significant pyuria and bacteriuria and a prompt response to the appropriate antimicrobial treatment, all other women need a careful pelvic examination to rule out other conditions presenting with acute dysuria and frequency or as acute pyelonephritis (see Differential Diagnosis).

In men with UTI symptoms, physical examination should include inspection and palpation of the genitals (including retraction of the foreskin in an uncircumcised man) for evidence of urethral discharge, meatal erythema, inflammation of the glans penis, penile lesions, enlarged or tender epididymis or testicle, and inguinal lymphadenopathy. It is emphasized that a rectal examination with palpation of the prostate gland should be a standard part of the physical examination in all men with UTI symptoms. Evidence for prostate infection has been found in one half of men with relapsing UTI. In patients with acute bacterial prostatitis, the prostate gland is swollen, warm, and tender, whereas in those with chronic bacterial prostatitis, the gland is usually but not always tender and may feel slightly irregular. Massage of the prostate gland in patients with acute bacterial prostatitis may result in bacteremia and should be avoided.

### Natural course

In most women, acute cystitis is an isolated event which may never or rarely be repeated. The onset of sexual activity or change in sexual partner may coincide with the attack(s). In a small proportion of women, UTI may be recurrent and the episodes may or may not chronologically coincide with coitus. In many women, symptoms may disappear spontaneously as a result of high fluid intake. The response to antimicrobial agents is usually prompt. Acute symptoms disappear within 2 to 3 days. If untreated, in some patients, especially pregnant women or patients with obstruction, the infection may extend to the upper tract. Although lower UTI does not predispose the patient to kidney damage, the quality of life of the affected women can be seriously impaired.

With upper UTI, the presence or absence of complicating factors is critical in defining the natural course and renal sequelae. Uncomplicated upper UTI generally leaves no residual damage and can easily be treated with antimicrobial agents. Although severe renal infection can result in cortical scars, its long-term functional significance is not clear. Presence of complicating factors such as obstruction, particularly with diabetes, sickle cell disease or trait, or analgesic/NSAID abuse, can result in severe bacterial nephritis, papillary necrosis, life-threatening septicemia, and renal or perirenal abscess.

## LABORATORY STUDIES AND DIAGNOSTIC PROCEDURES

A number of biochemical screening tests have been developed to detect significant bacteriuria. The most frequently used, the Griess test, depends on the bacterial reduction of nitrate normally present in the urine into nitrites, the latter being detected by a chemical reaction. Preferably, first-morning urine specimens should be used. This test is reasonably accurate in identifying Enterobacteriaceae but does not detect gram-positive organisms and *Pseudomonas*. False-negative results may be caused by lack of dietary nitrate, low urine pH, ascorbic acid, or urobilinogen or may occur during diuresis, since bacteria require some time to reduce nitrate into nitrites in the bladder urine. False-positive results usually result from contamination of urine with the vaginal flora. This test and the leukocyte esterase test (detects pyuria), combined on a single inexpensive dipstick test, have greatly increased the usefulness of this approach. Bacterial counts greater than $10^5$ Enterobacteriaceae/ml of urine with concomitant pyuria can be detected by this method. Overall, the combined test has a sensitivity and specificity of approximately 85% and 75%, respectively.

Microscopic examination of centrifuged urine can detect the presence of significant pyuria ( greater than four white blood cells per high-power field) and/or hematuria (greater than four red blood cells per high-power field). This provides further support for the diagnosis of UTI. While presence of pyuria does not differentiate upper from lower UTIs, leukocyte casts strongly support the diagnosis of pyelonephritis. Documentation of pyuria is especially valuable in supporting the diagnosis of UTI in symptomatic patients who have low bacterial counts ($10^2$ to $10^4$/ml of urine). Vaginitis may result in significant pyuria because of contamination of vaginal secretions with the voided urine and should be ruled out in abacteriuric symptomatic patients who demonstrate pyuria.

Pyuria alone is not specific for bacterial infection. It can occur with nephrolithiasis, allergic interstitial nephritis, papillary necrosis, and renal tuberculosis. Persistence of pyuria after a UTI or genital infection has been eradicated requires further investigation. Presence of a significant number of squamous epithelial cells in the urine of women highly suggests that the white blood cells may be of vaginal origin. Although pyuria is present in all patients with UTI, microscopic hematuria is present in only one half of them. Pyuria in the absence of bacteriuria (sterile pyuria) should raise the possibility of renal tuberculosis or allergic interstitial nephritis. Demonstration of significant eosinophiluria would support the latter diagnosis.

Urine culture remains the "gold standard" in documenting significant bacteriuria and the presence of UTI, as well as identifying the pathogenic microorganism. To reduce the chance of contamination, clean-catch midstream urine samples should be used for culture purposes.

Casual collection of urine samples often leads to heavy contamination, which makes the interpretation of microbiologic findings very difficult, if not impossible. In a few, often obese, women it may be almost impossible to obtain uncontaminated urine samples. To minimize the chance of contamination in males, the urine sample should be collected after retraction of the foreskin. To obtain a clean-catch midstream urine, the female patient with a full bladder should stand legs apart over the toilet, separate the labia with the left hand, and clean the vulva front to back with a sterile swab. The patient should then void downward into the toilet until half through without interrupting the stream, catch urine in a sterile cup, and complete voiding. In symptomatic patients with low bacterial counts in midstream urine samples, the first-morning urine sample after awakening may increase the yield, since overnight stasis of urine in the bladder allows bacteria to proliferate and be present in higher concentrations. The presence of more than one bacteria per high-power field on a Gram-stained film of uncentrifuged urine correlates with greater than $10^5$ bacteria / ml in 90% of patients. Aproximately 50% of patients with dysuria have fewer than $10^5$ bacteria/ml, and in 30% the urine is sterile, leading to the diagnosis of acute urethral syndrome.

Suprapubic aspiration and bladder catheterization should only be used in patients in whom it is impossible to obtain uncontaminated urine samples or in symptomatic patients with low ($10^2$ to $10^4$/ml) bacterial counts. For suprapubic aspiration of urine, the bladder should be full and percussible. This can be facilitated by oral administration of 300 ml of fluids and 20 mg of furosemide given 1 hour before the procedure. In very obese patients, localization of bladder by ultrasound may be helpful. With the patient in supine position and after appropriate sterilization of the area, at the midline one inch above the symphysis pubis, the skin is penetrated with a 21-gauge, 4½-inch-long needle.

Catheterization of the bladder should be avoided if possible, since it can introduce bacteria into the bladder resulting in false-positive cultures, as well as a 1% chance of developing UTI.

Radiologic imaging techniques have undergone major technologic improvement in the last decade especially in regards to the study of the genitourinary tract. Whereas the intravenous pyelogram was formerly the gold standard, computed tomography (CT) and ultrasound (US) are now the preferred modalities for assessing GU infections. US is sensitive in detecting obstruction, perinephric and intrarenal abscesses, tumors, and cysts. Patients with pyelonephritis should have CT with contrast or US to assess the presence of foci of pyelonephritis in the renal cortex or cortical or perinephric abscesses. Although US is extremely sensitive, it is operator dependent. Thus CT with contrast may be the preferred modality in centers that do not have special competence in US. Immediately following a CT with contrast, it is possible to obtain the equivalent of an IVP by taking a KUB film in the prone position and observing the anatomy of the collecting system and ureters as the contrast is cleared into the bladder.

Intravenous pyelography (IVP) is essential for visualizing ureters, the details of calyceal anatomy, and the presence of stricture, calyceal dilatation, stones, or obstruction. Demonstration of calyceal details is required for an accurate diagnosis of reflux nephropathy as well as papillary necrosis. Pyelonephritis complicated by intrarenal or perinephric abscess formation is best studied by US, followed by US-guided aspiration and drainage. Coupled with appropriate antibiotic therapy, this is often a lifesaving procedure for many patients.

An US is generally indicated in patients who are hospitalized because of severe bacteremic pyelonephritis, especially if they have a slow response to intravenous antibiotic therapy. In this setting, it is imperative to rule out obstruction. In patients with septic shock caused by presumed urosepsis, an US should be performed on an emergency basis because these patients often do not respond to therapy unless obstruction, if it is the underlying pathology, is relieved by a drainage procedure. In centers that do not have special competence in US, a CT with contrast may be the preferred imaging study, which similarly allows CT-guided abscess drainage. IVP is rarely indicated during an acute episode of pyelonephritis because of the poor quality of the results. Patients with clinical pyelonephritis not requiring hospitalization should have an US examination or IVP (the IVP should be deferred at least 4 weeks to optimize its quality).

Most men with bacterial UTI have some anatomic abnormality in their urinary tract. Obstruction at the prostate level may be caused by benign hypertrophy, prostate cancer, cysts or stones in the ejaculatory ducts or vas deferens, or other prostatic problems (see Chapters 138 and 140). Transrectal US is the procedure of choice for imaging these pathologies in the prostate and for abnormalities in the bladder. New US technology permits a quantitative assessment of prostatic enlargement, detailed imaging of anatomic abnormalities, and the option to perform biopsy at the same time. An IVP may demonstrate prostatic enlargement and postvoiding residuals. It is also useful in diagnosing abnormalities in the bladder.

In women, it is generally accepted that the first episode of UTI does not require any urologic evaluation. However, the management of recurrent infection remains controversial. Multiple studies indicate lack of cost-effectiveness of urologic studies in the evaluation of women, even with recurrent UTIs (Table 91-2). Therefore, the routine anatomic evaluation of women with recurrent UTI cannot be strongly recommended. However, the patient's response to antimicrobial therapy may be used as a guide. Patients with relapsing infection who are cured by a 6-week course of an antibiotic and patients with recurrent reinfection who are successfully managed with a low-dose prophylactic regimen do not require anatomic evaluation. By contrast, those who fail to respond to these regimens require radiologic imaging, typically an ultrasound. An-

**Table 91-2.** Comparison of the cost of radiologic investigations in a university hospital

| Test | Cost ($) |
|---|---|
| Intravenous pyelogram (IVP) | 313 |
| Ultrasound | 352 |
| Computed tomography (CT) scan (without contrast) | 415 |
| CT scan (with contrast) | 719 |

other indication for radiologic imaging is persistence of pyuria and flank pain. IVP should not be carried out during pregnancy because of the risk of irradiation to the fetus, or within 6 weeks after delivery because of the pregnancy-related changes of the urinary excretory system.

When gross hematuria occurs there is a significant risk of genitourinary cancer. US is particularly sensitive for identifying small renal cell carcinomas, especially when performed in conjunction with Doppler flow analysis, which may identify tumor vascularity in the lesion.

In children with the first or second episode of UTI, particularly in those younger than 5 years old, IVP or ultrasonography as well as a voiding cystourethrogram should be obtained to detect obstruction or other abnormalities such as vesicoureteral reflux, renal scarring, or posterior urethral valve. Since active infection itself can produce some degree of transient vesicoureteral reflux, the test has traditionally been delayed by 4 to 6 weeks after eradication of the infection. However, it has recently become a more common practice to perform a voiding cystourethrogram as soon as the infection is resolved and the infant is documented to have a negative urine culture.

Cystoscopy is only rarely indicated. It should be reserved for the workup of older patients with gross hematuria in whom bladder cancer may be suspected. Cystoscopy may also be used in patients with recurrent or persistent unexplained urinary frequency and dysuria who have no bacteriuria on repeated testing.

## DIFFERENTIAL DIAGNOSIS

Although several techniques such as ureteral catheterization, bladder washout, serum antibody response, and the antibody-coated bacteria test have been used to differentiate upper versus lower UTI, lack of sensitivity of most of these procedures and the associated morbidity and cost have precluded their routine use in clinical practice. As mentioned earlier, the clinical signs and symptoms are not accurate to distinguish between the two entities. Thus, it is generally accepted that distinction between upper and lower UTI is better assessed by the response to treatment. Since uncomplicated UTIs do not produce kidney damage, emphasis has recently swayed from localization studies toward distinguishing between complicated and uncomplicated infections.

Between 10% and 30% of women with sexually transmitted diseases or other forms of vaginitis have frequency and dysuria. Therefore, acute bacterial cystitis should be differentiated from vulvovaginitis caused by yeast, *Trichomonas,* or bacterial infections, as well as sexually transmitted infections that involve the urethra and the cervix, such as *Chlamydia trachomatis, Neisseria gonorrhoeae,* or herpes simplex virus.

In patients with vulvovaginitis, the discomfort on urination is generally felt externally (external dysuria) when urine flows over the inflamed labia. These patients may also complain of soreness of the vulva, malodorous vaginal discharge, pruritus, and dyspareunia. In these patients, pyuria and hematuria are very rare, and the urine culture typically reveals less than $10^2$ colonies of bacteria/ml.

Urethritis caused by sexually transmitted pathogens usually causes milder symptoms with a more gradual onset of dysuria without other urinary symptoms. These patients may also complain of vaginal discharge or bleeding (from concomitant cervicitis) or lower abdominal pain. They usually have pyuria but only rarely hematuria, and their urine culture shows less than $10^2$ bacterial colonies/ml. Presence of gross hematuria suggests bacterial cystitis.

In postmenopausal women, atrophic changes in the mucosa of the vulvovagina and urethra caused by hormone deficiency may result in persistent or recurrent frequency and dysuria. These patients generally respond to hormone replacement creams.

Renal and other genitourinary neoplasms must also be seriously considered in differential diagnosis of the older individual who presents for the first time with symptoms of a UTI and hematuria.

In young sexually active men, the uropathogenic strains of *E. coli* can result in an acute uncomplicated cystitis. However, some patients may develop urethral discharge and urethral leukocytosis, which mimic *N. gonorrhoeae* urethritis and *C. trachomatis* infections.

Acute pyelonephritis in a young female should be differentiated from other intraabdominal conditions such as pelvic inflammatory disease, appendicitis, atopic pregnancy, and ruptured ovarian cyst.

## MANAGEMENT

The treatment of UTI depends on the patient's symptomatology, whether the infection is located in the upper or lower urinary tract as judged by clinical signs and symptoms, and whether it is an isolated episode or a recurrent problem.

A young woman with the first episode of seemingly an acute uncomplicated cystitis does not require urinalysis or urine culture and may be treated with a short course of antibiotics on an empiric basis. No follow-up visit or culture after therapy is recommended unless symptoms persist or recur. In recent years, there has been considerable interest in the use of single-dose therapy on the basis of convenience, cost, compliance, and reduction in side effects. Trimethoprim-sulfamethoxazole (TMP-SMZ, 320 mg/1600 mg, two double-strength tablets), amoxicillin (3 g), cephaloridine (2 g), gentamicin (5 mg/kg), and doxycycline (300 mg) have all been used as a single-dose regimen. In general, cure rates of 85% to 90% or even higher have been reported. Among these agents, TMP-SMZ is the preferred drug. With single-dose therapy, urinary symptoms may persist for 1 to 2 days, and a higher incidence of early recurrent infection occurs compared with a short-course treatment using the same antibiotics (see the Managed Care Guide).

A more common practice is a short-course (3 to 5 days) treatment with either trimethoprim (100 to 200 mg every 12 hours), TMP-SMZ (160 mg/800 mg every 12 hours), nitrofurantoin, (100 mg every 8 or 6 hours), amoxicillin (250 mg every 8 hours), ciprofloxacin (250 to 500 mg every 12 hours), or norfloxacin (400 mg every 12 hours) (Table 91-3). Among these regimens, TMP-SMZ is considered the drug of choice because it effectively reduces the fecal, vaginal, and periurethral colonization. There has been an increasing trend in using less ampicillin, amoxicillin, and first-generation cephalosporins because of frequent in vitro resistance, as well as their not being

### Managed Care Guide
### For single-dose therapy of UTI

1. The patient is female
2. The infection is likely to be uncomplicated and is clinically confined to the lower urinary tract
3. Less than 48 hours have elapsed between the onset of symptoms and treatment
4. There has not been a UTI in the past several weeks

very effective in elimination of vaginal and periurethral colonization. Nitrofurantoin should not be used in patients with renal impairment because effective urinary concentrations may not be achieved and because of the increased risk of peripheral neuropathy in these patients. Symptomatic improvement is usually obtained within 1 to 2 days of therapy. Recurrence of symptoms after short-course therapy indicates the need for a urine culture and retreatment of the patient for a longer period (10 to 14 days), with the choice of antibiotic based on the urine culture results. Empiric treatment with TMP-SMZ may be instituted until the culture result is available (see the box above).

Pregnant women with acute uncomplicated cystitis may be treated for 7 to 10 days with oral amoxicillin (250 mg every 8 hours), ampicillin (250 mg every 6 hours), macrocrystalline nitrofurantoin (100 mg every 6 hours), or an oral cephalosporin.

Young healthy men with acute cystitis and no discernible complicating factor can be treated with a 7- to 10-day regimen of TMP-SMZ (160 mg/800 mg every 12 hours), trimethoprim (100 to 200 mg every 12 hours), or a fluoroquinolone (norfloxacin, 400 mg every 12 hours, or ciprofloxacin, 250 to 500 mg every 12 hours). A pretreatment urine culture is recommended in these patients. A urologic evaluation is usually unrewarding in those who respond to treatment.

About 20% of young women with an initial episode of acute cystitis will develop recurrent infections. In patients with recurrent lower UTI, it is critical to distinguish between relapse and reinfection.

## RECURRENT URINARY TRACT INFECTIONS

*Relapses* with the same microorganism highly suggest that the source of bacteriuria is the upper tract and are usually

### Supportive measures

High fluid intake of more than 2 L daily and complete voiding at 2- to 3-hour intervals during the daytime

Alkalinization of urine with sodium bicarbonate or potassium citrate

Voiding at bedtime and after sexual intercourse, and avoiding bubble baths or chemical additives in bath water (to decrease chance of future infections)

Patients with diabetes mellitus, those with UTI symptoms longer than 7 days, patients over 65 years old, and those who use a diaphragm are recommended to take a longer course (7 to 10 days) of antibiotic therapy

associated with renal stones, scars, or polycystic kidneys. A relapse would be suggested if the same microorganism is recultured and has the same antibiotic sensitivities. In men, a high chance exists that a concomitant chronic bacterial prostatitis may be responsible for these relapses. In patients who relapse despite a 2-week course of appropriate antimicrobial therapy, the treatment should be extended to 4 to 6 weeks with the hope of eradication of the microorganisms from the kidney, while at the same time determining potential complicating factors, such as stones, papillary necrosis, or partial obstruction, with an IVP or ultrasound.

*Reinfection* causes more than 90% of recurrent lower UTI in women. When one or two episodes occur per year, each acute attack should be treated with either a single dose or a short course of antibiotic therapy, as with a single infection. However, if attacks of infection are more frequent, the patient may be treated with short-course antibiotic therapy followed by a long-term (12-month), low-dose, prophylactic antibacterial regimen.

Antibiotics frequently used for low-dose prophylaxis are trimethoprim (100 mg), TMP-SMZ (40 to 80 mg/200 to 400 mg), nitrofurantoin (50 to 100 mg), norfloxacin (200 mg), and cephalexin (250 mg) taken at bedtime (Table 91-4). Trimethoprim with or without sulfamethoxazole has been a preferred regimen because it reduces the development of periurethral colonization. Side effects and emergence of resistant strains are unusual. Patients with recurrence of infection after sexual intercourse should be encouraged to void and to use a single prophylactic dose of an antibiotic (TMP-SMZ, 40 mg/200 mg; cephalexin,

**Table 91-3.** Cost comparison of 3-day or 10-day treatment course for uncomplicated cystitis

| Antibiotic | Regimen | 3 day ($)* | 10 day ($)* |
|---|---|---|---|
| Trimethoprim | 100-200 mg q12h | 0.95-1.90 | 3.20-6.40 |
| Trimethoprim-sulfamethoxazole | 160 mg/800 mg q12h | 1.20 | 3.90 |
| Nitrofurantoin | 100 mg q8h/q6h | 0.23/0.31 | 0.78/1.00 |
| Amoxicillin | 250 mg q8h | 1.39 | 4.63 |
| Ciprofloxacin | 250-500 mg q12h | 8.90-17.80 | 29.70-59.40 |
| Norfloxacin | 400 mg q12h | 14.00 | 46.80 |

*Average wholesale price per *Red Book,* Montvale, NJ, 1993, Medical Economics Data Production.

**Table 91-4.** Cost comparison of 12 months of low-dose prophylactic antibiotic regimen

| Antibiotic | Regimen (bedtime) | Cost ($)* |
|---|---|---|
| Trimethoprim | 100 mg | 73 |
| Trimethoprim-sulfa-methoxazole | 40-80 mg/200-400 mg | 23.50-47.00 |
| Nitrofurantoin | 50-100 mg | 20-48 |
| Norfloxacin | 200 mg | 880 |
| Cephalexin | 250 mg | 164 |

*Average wholesale price per *Red Book,* Montvale, NJ, 1993, Medical Economics Data Production.

250 mg; or nitrofurantoin, 50 to 100 mg) after each sexual intercourse. They should also be informed that use of a diaphragm and spermicides may predispose them to recurrent UTI and that other forms of birth control would be available to them if they so desire. In general, all the patients with recurrent UTI should also be encouraged to maintain a high fluid intake and to void completely at 2 to 3 hour intervals during the daytime.

Postmenopausal women may develop recurrent lower UTIs (reinfections), which may result from residual urine after voiding (often associated with bladder or uterine prolapse) or from lack of estrogen resulting in changes in the vaginal flora (loss of lactobacilli and increased colonization by *E. coli*). Prophylactic antibiotic treatment or topical estradiol cream/hormone replacement therapy is beneficial in these patients.

## ACUTE URETHRAL SYNDROME

Patients with the acute urethral syndrome may have fewer than $10^5$ colonies on routine bacterial cultures. They may have positive isolates when viral, gonococcal, chlamydia, or other special cultures are obtained. Vaginitis and sexually transmitted diseases, including trichomoniasis, must be considered (see Table 91-5 and Chapter 65) for treatment recommendations.

No obvious cause is found for the acute urethral syndrome in 10% to 30% of women with dysuria. Suggestions for management include the following:

1. Wear cotton underwear to decrease moisture in perineal area.
2. Sitz baths followed by careful drying off of perineum.
3. Weight loss and exercise.
4. Urinary tract analgesia—with phenazopyridine (Pyridium), 200 mg Tid for 5 to 10 days. Advise patient that the urine will have an orange color.
5. Arrange for a urologic consult if symptoms persist.

## ASYMPTOMATIC BACTERIURIA

Patients with *asymptomatic bacteriuria,* with or without an indwelling catheter, do not require antimicrobial treatment. The indication for treatment in these patients is development of clinical symptoms and signs of UTI, presence of leukopenia, renal transplantation, urea-splitting bacteria (particularly *Proteus mirabilis,* which can cause infectious stones), presence of some degree of upper urinary tract obstruction, or conditions predisposing to papillary necrosis (e.g., diabetes mellitus, sickle cell disease or trait, analgesic/NSAID abuse). As many as 40% of elderly men and women have asymptomatic bacteriuria, especially in nursing homes. However, since it only rarely leads to symptomatic infection, including pyelonephritis or sepsis, routine screening and antibiotic treatment are not advocated for these patients. Asymptomatic bacteriuria in pregnant women is an exception and should always be treated. There is an approximately 30% risk of developing acute pyelonephritis in the second or third trimester, with attendant complications for both mother and fetus (prematurity and low birth weight). Moreover, asymptomatic bacteriuria by itself has been suggested to increase the incidence of premature labor. All pregnant women should be screened for bacteriuria in the first trimester, and if present, they should be treated with a short course (3 to 5 days) of amoxicillin (250 mg every 8 hours), ampicillin (250 mg every 6 hours), macrocrystalline nitrofurantoin (100 mg every 6 hours), or an oral cephalosporin. After successful treatment, monthly urine cultures should be performed to detect recurrent bacteriuria. Pregnant women with recurrent asymptomatic bacteriuria can be managed safely with low-dose nitrofurantoin prophylaxis.

## ACUTE PYELONEPHRITIS

Acute uncomplicated pyelonephritis can generally be treated on an outpatient basis if the patient does not have nausea or vomiting, is not severely volume depleted, has no evidence of septicemia, and is reliable. All other patients with acute uncomplicated upper UTI, including pregnant women, should be hospitalized for an initial 2 to 3 days of parenteral therapy. A urine culture should be obtained in all patients with suspected pyelonephritis. In 20% of patients, the culture will show less than $10^5$ bacterial colonies/ml of urine. A blood culture should be obtained in patients who are hospitalized. A positive blood culture is obtained in 15% to 20% of these patients. For outpatient management, a 2-week course of TMP-SMZ (160 mg/800 mg every 12 hours), trimethoprim (200 mg every 12 hours), amoxicillin (500 mg every 8 hours), norfloxacin (400 mg every 12 hours), or ciprofloxacin (500 mg every 12 hours) is recommended. For inpatients, empiric parenteral therapy with TMP-SMZ (160 mg/800 mg every 12 hours), ciprofloxacin (200-400 mg every 12 hours), gentamicin (1 mg/kg every 8 hours) with or without ampicillin (1 g every 6 hours), or a third-generation cephalosporin (e.g., intravenous [IV] or intramuscular [IM] ceftriaxone, 1 to 2 g daily) should be initiated until the patient becomes afebrile and there is evidence of clinical improvement, usually within 48 to 72 hours. Subsequently, the patient may be switched to oral therapy based on sensitivity of the microorganism. Patients with uncomplicated upper UTI, with or without documented bacteremia, are best treated with a 2-week course of antibiotics, and in those who show evidence of relapse, a longer course (6 weeks) should be adopted. If fever and flank pain persist after 72 hours of therapy, blood and urine cultures should be repeated and ultrasonography or computed tomography of the kidneys obtained to rule out obstruction, urologic abnormalities, and renal or perirenal abscesses. A follow-up urine culture 2 weeks after completion of antibiotic therapy is indicated. In patients with UTI complicated by stones, renal scars, diabetes, or papillary necrosis, a 6-week course of antibiotic treatment is usually necessary. However, these

**Table 91-5.** Recommended empiric therapy for bacterial urinary tract infections (UTIs)*

| Condition | Circumstances | Empiric treatment† | Duration |
|---|---|---|---|
| Acute uncomplicated cystitis | Young woman, first episode | TMP-SMZ preferred over amoxicillin, cephaloridine, doxycycline | Single dose |
| | | TMP ± SMZ, amoxicillin, nitrofurantoin, ciprofloxacin, norfloxacin | 3-5 days |
| | Diabetes mellitus, symptoms >7 days, age >65 yr, diaphragm | TMP ± SMZ, amoxicillin, nitrofurantoin, ciprofloxacin, norfloxacin | 7-10 days |
| | Pregnancy | Amoxicillin/ampicillin, nitrofurantoin, oral cephalosporin | 7-10 days |
| | Young healthy man | TMP ± SMZ, ciprofloxacin, norfloxacin | 7-10 days |
| Recurrent cystitis | Relapses | Based on sensitivity results; rule out renal stone/scar/cyst or chronic bacterial prostatitis | 14 days; if relapse, 4-6 wk |
| | Reinfection: | | |
| | ≤2 episodes/yr | Treat each episode as first episode in young woman | Single dose or 3-5 days |
| | ≥3 episodes/yr | TMP ± SMZ, amoxicillin, nitrofurantoin, ciprofloxacin, or norfloxacin, followed by low-dose antibiotic prophylaxis | 3-5 days, then 1 yr of prophylaxis |
| | Temporally related to coitus | TMP ± SMZ, nitrofurantoin, cephalexin; void after intercourse | Postcoital prophylaxis |
| | Postmenopause | Topical estradiol cream ± low-dose antibiotic prophylaxis | |
| Asymptomatic bacteriuria | With/without catheter | Do not treat unless symptomatic, neutropenic, renal transplant, urea-splitting bacteria, obstruction, diabetes mellitus, sickle cell disease/trait, NSAID/analgesic abuse | 10-14 days |
| | Pregnancy | Amoxicillin/ampicillin, nitrofurantoin, oral cephalosporin | 3-5 days |
| Acute uncomplicated pyelonephritis | Very sick or septic | Parenteral: TMP-SMZ, ciprofloxacin, ceftriaxone, or gentamicin ± ampicillin until afebrile, then oral regimen | 14 days; if relapse, 6 wk |
| | Not very sick | Oral: TMP ± SMZ, amoxicillin, ciprofloxacin, norfloxacin | 14 days; if relapse, 6 wk |
| | Pregnancy | Parenteral: ceftriaxone, gentamicin ± ampicillin, aztreonam, or TMP-SMZ until afebrile, then oral regimen | 14 days |
| Symptomatic complicated upper UTI | Very sick or septic | Parenteral: gentamicin + ampicillin, ceftriaxone, aztreonam, imipenem-cilastatin, ciprofloxacin, ticarcillin-clavulanate | 2-3 wk; if relapse, 6 wk |
| | Not very sick | Oral: ciprofloxacin, norfloxacin, or TMP-SMZ (if sensitive) | 2-3 wk; if relapse, 6 wk |

TMP, Trimethoprim; SMZ, sulfamethoxazole.
*Therapy should be targeted to infecting organism as soon as it is identified.
†For more details on antibiotics and their doses, see text.

patients may initially be treated for only 2 weeks, and only those who show evidence of relapse may be retreated for an extended 6-week course.

All pregnant women with acute pyelonephritis should be hospitalized and initially treated with parenteral antibiotics. The choice of antibiotic may be ceftriaxone (1 to 2 g IV or IM daily), gentamicin (1 mg/kg every 8 hours) with or without ampicillin (1 g every 6 hours, aztreonam (1 g every 8 to 12 hours), or TMP-SMZ (160 mg/800 mg every 12 hours), until fever resolves. The patient should subsequently be treated with oral amoxicillin (500 mg every 8 hours), TMP-SMZ (160 mg/800 mg every 12 hours), or a cephalosporin for 14 days. The antimicrobial therapy should be specifically targeted to the infecting microorganism as soon as the results of urine culture and antimicrobial sensitivity tests become available. Fluoroquinolones should not be used in pregnancy. TMP-SMZ is not approved for use in pregnancy, especially in the third trimester because sulfonamides reduce the binding of bilirubin to albumin and may precipitate kernicterus, but it is widely used. Gentamicin should be used with caution because of its possible toxicity to eighth-nerve development in the fetus.

In patients with symptomatic complicated upper UTI, the relatively broad array of bacterial species responsible for the infection and the severity of the patient's illness should be considered while choosing the appropriate empiric antimicrobial agent(s). For septicemia in hospitalized patients, IV broad-spectrum antibiotics covering *Pseudomonas* and enterococci should be initially instituted. Ampicillin (1 g every 6 hours) and gentamicin (1 mg/kg every 8 hours), a third-generation cephalosporin with anti-*Pseudomonas* activity (e.g., ceftriaxone, 1 to 2 g IV or IM daily), aztreonam (1 g every 8 to 12 hours), ticarcillin-clavulanate (3.2 g every 8 hours), ciprofloxacin (400 mg every 12 hours), or imipenem-cilastatin (250 to 500 mg every 6 to 8 hours) are reasonable initial choices. After the cause of infection has been identified, antimicrobial therapy should be specifically targeted to the infecting agent. In patients who are less ill, outpatient oral therapy with ciprofloxacin or norfloxacin is appropriate. If the infecting pathogen is known to be susceptible, TMP-SMZ is a reasonable and less costly choice.

The duration of initial therapy for complicated upper UTI is 2 to 3 weeks depending on the clinical circumstances. A follow-up urine culture should be obtained 1 to 2 weeks after completion of therapy. With symptomatic relapse of the infection, a longer course (6 weeks) of appropriate antimicrobial therapy should be instituted. It should be emphasized that (1) complicated UTIs tend to recur unless the underlying anatomic or functional defect is corrected, (2) infections with *Pseudomonas* and enterococci are more prone to recur, and (3) chronic or recurrent complicated upper UTIs result in renal damage with loss of renal function. Patients with a chronic indwelling bladder catheter typically develop many recurrences of bacteriuria and UTI despite treatment of individual infections. Use of aseptic techniques, a closed catheter system, and continuous downhill gravity drainage can reduce the incidence of catheter-associated UTI. Antimicrobial prophylaxis has no value for the chronically catheterized patients. It has been suggested that intermittent catheterization results in lower rates of bacteriuria than a long-term indwelling catheter. Oral nitrofurantoin or TMP-SMZ prophylaxis may reduce the incidence of bacteriuria in patients undergoing intermittent catheterization but not in those with a long-term indwelling catheter.

Table 91-5 summarizes empiric therapy of different UTI syndromes.

## BIBLIOGRAPHY


Boscia JA, Abrutyn E, Kaye D: Asymptomatic bacteriuria in elderly persons: treat or do not treat? *Ann Intern Med* 106:764, 1987.

Carlson KJ, Mulley AJ: Management of acute dysuria: a decision-analysis model of alternative strategies, *Ann Intern Med* 102:244, 1985.

Johnson JR, Stamm WE: Urinary tract infections in women: diagnosis and treatment, *Ann Intern Med* 111:906, 1989.

Lipsky BA: Urinary tract infection in men: epidemiology, pathophysiology, diagnosis and treatment, *Ann Intern Med* 110:138, 1989.

Roberts JA: Pyelonephritis, cortical abscess and perinephric abscess, *Urol Clin North Am* 13:637, 1986.

Rubin RH, Tolkoff-Rubin NE, Cotran RS: Urinary tract infection, pyelonephritis, and reflux nephropathy. In Brenner BM, Rector FC, editors: *The kidney,* ed 4, Philadelphia, 1991, WB Saunders.

Sant GR: Urinary tract infections in the elderly, *Semin Urol* 5:126, 1987.

Schaeffer AJ et al: Urinary tract infection. In Jacobson HR, Striker GE, Klahr S, editors: *The principles and practice of nephrology,* ed 1, Philadelphia, 1991, Decker.

Stamm WE, Hooton TM: Management of urinary tract infection in adults, *N Engl J Med* 329:1328, 1993.

Sussman M, Cattell WR, Jones KV: Urinary tract infection. In Cameron S et al, editors: *Oxford textbook of clinical nephrology,* ed 1, New York, 1992, Oxford University Press.


CHAPTER

# 92A Nephrolithiasis


**Jay R. Seltzer**
**Saulo Klahr**


## EPIDEMIOLOGY

Nephrolithiasis is defined as the formation of stones or calculi inside the kidney or urinary tract. Stones may occur at any location from the renal pelvis to the urethra, but most stones form in the kidney and then travel down the urinary tract. The four regions where stones typically lodge are the renal calyx, ureteropelvic junction, pelvic brim, and ureterovesical junction. Stones that form in the ureter are usually associated with an anatomic abnormality (ureterocele, proximal to a stricture). Bladder calculi, although prevalent in some parts of the world, are uncommon in the United States.

Kidney stones form in about 500,000 people in the United States each year, and these stones account for 1 of every 1000 hospital admissions. Although kidney stones are two to three times more common in men than women and are distinctly uncommon in African-Americans, Asians, and American Indians, up to 10% of Americans will have a kidney stone in their lifetime. The age and sex distribution of 571 patients referred for evaluation of nephrolithiasis at The Jewish Hospital of St. Louis Kidney Stone Center shows a 1.6:1.0 ratio of male to female patients and a maximal incidence in the 30- to 50-year-old group (excluding patients with cystinuria and infection stones).

Risk factors for development of nephrolithiasis include geographic location, occupation, family history, and diet. The incidence of nephrolithiasis is highest in the southeast, northwest, and southwest United States, with peak incidence in the late summer months. A relatively low incidence of kidney stones is seen in Africa and Central and South America. White-collar workers, who are sedentary, are more likely to form kidney stones than active blue-collar workers. Some forms of nephrolithiasis are familial; distal renal tubular acidosis and cystinuria are two important hereditary diseases that usually cause nephrolithiasis. Diet remains the most important risk factor in the formation of kidney stones, and a careful dietary history is essential in the evaluation of patients with nephrolithiasis. Prevention is the most important aspect of the management of nephrolithiasis and involves determination of the factors that lead to stone formation and specific treatment of those abnormalities.

## MECHANISM OF STONE FORMATION

Kidney stone formation results from an imbalance in the physicochemical composition of the urine. A delicate balance exists in urine among the concentrations of solutes, crystal inhibitors, and solvent. When the concentrations of certain solutes (calcium, oxalate, uric acid, cystine, phosphate) in the urine exceed their limits of solubility (and/or the solubility changes with pH), crystallization may occur. Crystal formation is most likely to occur in areas of relatively decreased urine flow or stagnation. Thus stones tend to form with increased urinary excretion of calcium, oxalate, uric acid, or cystine; decreased citrate; decreased urinary water volume; or impaired urine flow. Although this is a simplistic view, and other substances that act as crystallization promoters or inhibitors are involved in this process, it serves to illustrate the general mechanism of initial crystal formation. The process of stone formation involves supersaturation and crystal formation (precipitation of crystals from solution), nucleation (the early crystal lattice formation), and crystal growth and agglomeration (the formation of larger groups of crystals and nuclei) and may involve epitaxy (the growth of one crystal type on the surface of another, e.g., the growth of calcium oxalate crystals on a nucleus of uric acid). Table 92A-1 summarizes the frequency and composition of various types of kidney stones.

Although it remains to be shown exactly why stones form, overexcretion of stone constituents or underexcretion of stone inhibitors are important factors in stone formation. Less is known about crystal growth and agglomeration, and their role in stone formation is not well quantified.

The following sections describe the various disorders associated with stone formation.

**Table 92A-1.** Kidney stone composition

| Crystal composition | Percent of stones analyzed |
|---|---|
| Calcium oxalate | 60 |
| Calcium phosphate | 20 |
| Uric acid | 10 |
| Cystine | 3 |
| Struvite | 7 |

### Hypercalciuria

Defined as increased urinary calcium excretion (exceeding 225 mg/24 hours in women, 250 mg/24 hours in men, or 4 mg/kg/24 hours), hypercalciuria is present in 50% to 70% of patients evaluated for nephrolithiasis. It may occur as the sole abnormality in 15% to 20% of patients but is usually found in combination with other metabolic abnormalities in the urine (Table 92A-2). Because the etiology of many of the causes of hypercalciuria remains unknown, it is appropriate to categorize hypercalciuria as either idiopathic or secondary.

***Idiopathic hypercalciuria.*** Idiopathic hypercalciuria is usually a familial disorder and accounts for most cases of hypercalciuria. The disorders that make up this category include absorptive hypercalciuria, fasting hypercalciuria, renal hypercalciuria, and renal phosphaturia. Absorptive hypercalciuria is familial in most patients and is characterized by intestinal hyperabsorption of dietary calcium. There is an increased filtered load of calcium and suppression of parathyroid hormone (PTH) leading to hypercalciuria. The etiology of intestinal hyperabsorption is unknown, and most patients have normal 1,25-dihydroxycholecalciferol (1,25-$[OH]_2$–vitamin $D_3$) levels; however, some have elevated levels, suggesting a possible role for this vitamin in absorptive hypercalciuria. Fasting hypercalciuria is characterized by increased urinary calcium excretion unrelated to dietary calcium intake; calcium is mobilized from skeletal sites. Renal hypercalciuria is characterized by increased urinary calcium excretion resulting from impaired renal tubular reabsorption of calcium. There are reflex increases of PTH and 1,25-$(OH)_2$–vitamin $D_3$ levels but no hypercalcemia. Renal phosphaturia is presumably caused by impaired tubular phosphate reabsorption leading to elevated 1,25-

**Table 92A-2.** Urinary chemistries in patients evaluated for nephrolithiasis

| Diagnosis | Percent of total: Sole occurrence | Percent of total: Combined occurrence |
|---|---|---|
| Hypercalciuria | 14 | 51 |
| Male: >250 mg/24 hr | 8 | 34 |
| Female: >225 mg/24 hr | 6 | 17 |
| Hyperuricosuria | 8 | 42 |
| Male: >0.75 g/24 hr | 6 | 30 |
| Female: >0.70 g/24 hr | 2 | 12 |
| Hypocitraturia | 9 | 34 |
| Male: <250 mg/24 hr | 5 | 18 |
| Female: <300 mg/24 hr | 4 | 16 |
| Hyperoxaluria (>40 mg/24 hr) | 8 | 34 |
| Hypomagnesuria (<5 mEq/24 hr) | 5 | 26 |
| Low urinary volumes (<1500 ml/24 hr) | 26 | 61 |
| No diagnosis | — | 2 |

Data from The Jewish Hospital of St. Louis Kidney Stone Center. Diagnostic categories of 587 patients evaluated for nephrolithiasis from 1987 to 1993 (excludes patients with cystinuria and infection stones).

### Causes of secondary hypercalciuria

**With hypercalcemia**
Primary hyperparathyroidism
Sarcoidosis
Granulomatous diseases
Lymphoma
Multiple myeloma
Paget's disease of bone
Metastatic bone disease
Prolonged immobilization

**Endocrine disorders**
Hyperthyroidism
Cushing's syndrome

**Medications**
Furosemide
Acetazolamide
Excessive calcium ingestion
Vitamin D intoxication
Milk-alkali syndrome

**Renal tubular acidosis**

**Medullary sponge kidney**

$(OH)_2$–vitamin $D_3$ levels. The number of patients fulfilling the criteria for renal hypercalciuria and renal phosphaturia is extremely small, and it is doubtful that these entities are significant in explaining the many patients with recurrent calcium stone formation. These generalized definitions are useful for classification but may also be important in certain cases for therapeutic decisions; but, as already stated, the exact etiology of these disorders is not known.

***Secondary hypercalciuria.*** Hypercalciuria is caused by an identifiable secondary disorder in less than 10% of patients evaluated for nephrolithiasis (see the box above). Primary hyperparathyroidism, at one time a common cause of kidney stones, now accounts for less than 1% of calcium stone disease because of early diagnosis of hyperparathyroidism. These stones may be composed of calcium oxalate alone or in combination with calcium phosphate. Primary hyperparathyroidism causes increased absorption of calcium in the gut, increased resorption of calcium from bone, and increased tubular reabsorption of calcium in the kidneys. The net result is an increase in the serum calcium, which tends to inhibit tubular calcium reabsorption, and an increased filtered load of calcium. Thus hypercalciuria occurs despite effects of increased PTH levels on the renal tubular reabsorption of calcium.

Distal renal tubular acidosis (RTA) causes stones composed mainly of calcium phosphate through three mechanisms: (1) metabolic acidosis leads to skeletal calcium loss and hypercalciuria; (2) persistently alkaline urine pH favors calcium phosphate precipitation; and (3) metabolic acidosis and hypokalemia lead to reduced urinary citrate excretion. Nephrolithiasis is generally not seen in patients with proximal RTA or hyporeninemic hypoaldosteronism.

Granulomatous diseases (including sarcoidosis, tuberculosis, histoplasmosis, histiocytosis, coccidioidomycosis, and berylliosis) and lymphomas can cause hypercalciuria and nephrolithiasis. The mechanism involves increased calcium absorption from the gut caused by elevated levels of 1,25-$(OH)_2$–vitamin $D_3$.

Medullary sponge kidney is a benign disorder characterized by anatomic defects in the collecting ducts that cause various degrees of dilatation in the pericalyceal region of the renal medulla. Patients with this disorder often form kidney stones composed of calcium phosphate with or without calcium oxalate. Stone formation probably occurs from stasis of urine in the dilated collecting ducts and from hypercalciuria (through impaired renal tubular calcium reabsorption). An increased incidence of urinary tract infection (UTI) in these patients may also lead to formation of infection stones composed of struvite. The box at left lists other causes of secondary hypercalciuria.

### Hyperoxaluria

The 24-hour urinary excretion of greater than 40 mg oxalate leads to stone formation by increasing the urinary saturation of calcium oxalate. An increase in urinary oxalate concentration is at least as important as a rise in urinary calcium concentration in causing calcium oxalate stone formation. Hyperoxaluria is detected in as many as one third of patients evaluated for nephrolithiasis but is the sole abnormality in only 8% (see Table 92A-2). Hyperoxaluria occurs with increased intestinal oxalate absorption, increased oxalate substrate, or decreased oxalate metabolism; the major cause is hyperabsorption.

Gastrointestinal (GI) absorption of oxalate depends on the amount ingested, the amount bound by dietary calcium and magnesium, and the permeability of the colon to oxalate. Foods with a relatively high concentration of oxalate include teas, chocolate products, spinach and other greens, rhubarb, beans, and nuts. GI diseases with absent or dysfunctional small bowel and intact function of the large bowel (Crohn's disease, pancreatitis, nontropical sprue, ileal bypass or resection) can cause hyperoxaluria through several mechanisms. Malabsorption of bile acids causes increased colonic permeability to oxalate. Fat malabsorption causes saponification (soap formation) of fats with calcium and magnesium. This decreases the amount of calcium and magnesium able to bind with oxalate and allows free oxalate to be readily absorbed in the colon. Whether subclinical abnormalities in the intestinal tract lead to increased absorption of oxalate has not been determined but remains a possibility, since most hyperoxaluria associated with stones is through intestinal absorption.

Sources of excess oxalate synthesis include vitamin C and ethylene glycol. Vitamin C is metabolized to oxalate, and even modest doses of vitamin C supplements (500 mg daily) may cause significant hyperoxaluria in some patients. Ethylene glycol ingestion may cause severe oxalosis.

Causes of disordered oxalate metabolism include pyridoxine deficiency and the rare inborn errors of metabolism called *primary* hyperoxaluria. Pyridoxine is a cofactor necessary for the conversion of glyoxalate to glycine. Pyridoxine deficiency leads to an accumulation of glyoxalate and increased oxalate production. In type I primary hyperoxaluria (glycolic aciduria), there is a deficiency of alanine glyoxylate aminotransferase, which leads to accumulation of oxalate. Type II primary hyperoxaluria (L-glyceric aciduria) is caused by a deficiency of the enzyme D-glyceric dehydrogenase.

### Hyperuricosuria

Hyperuricosuria, the 24-hour urinary excretion of greater than 700 mg uric acid in women or 750 mg uric acid in men, is found in about 40% of patients evaluated for stones. It may occur as the sole abnormality in 8% of patients but is usually found in combination with other abnormalities (see Table 92A-2). Increased urinary excretion of uric acid under conditions of acidic urine pH and low urine volumes may lead to formation of uric acid stones. However, hyperuricosuria is also important in the formation of calcium oxalate stones, since it is thought that monosodium urate may act as a nidus for nucleation of calcium oxalate through epitaxy (see earlier). The box below lists clinical conditions that may be associated with hyperuricosuria. One clinical setting worth special mention is chronic diarrhea. These patients may form uric acid stones, even in the absence of hyperuricosuria, if they have a persistently low urine pH and low urine volumes (as usually occurs with chronic diarrhea).

### Hypocitraturia

Hypocitraturia is present in 30% to 50% of patients evaluated for nephrolithiasis and is an important contributor to stone formation. Citrate is a crystallization inhibitor and acts by complexing with calcium, thus reducing the concentration of calcium salts in the urine. Citrate inhibits precipitation, crystallization, and aggregation of calcium oxalate and is a potent inhibitor of calcium phosphate crystallization and growth. Urinary citrate concentration is affected mainly by acid-base status. Intracellular acidosis, such as occurs in metabolic acidosis and hypokalemia, causes decreased citrate excretion. The box at right summarizes potential causes of hypocitraturia.

### Hypomagnesuria

Magnesium decreases the saturation of calcium oxalate by complexing with oxalate. Hypomagnesuria is present in up to 25% of patients evaluated for kidney stones and may be an important risk factor for stone formation. The causes of hypomagnesuria usually reflect decreased magnesium intake and/or impaired GI magnesium absorption. The box below lists the causes of hypomagnesuria. (For more information on magnesium metabolism see Chapter 37.)

### Low urine volumes

By far the most common abnormality detected during evaluation for nephrolithiasis is inadequate urine volume. As many as 60% of patients tested have 24-hour urine volumes less than 1500 ml. Urine volume is important because it is a key determinant of solute concentration and saturation; the greater the urine water volume, the less the concentration of a given solute. Factors that may affect urine volume include inadequate fluid intake, increased insensible fluid losses, increased GI fluid losses, and volume depletion.

### Idiopathic stone formation

No biochemical abnormality is detected in less than 3% of patients evaluated for kidney stones. This small group of patients may have an unidentifiable inhibitor deficiency or the presence of an unknown promoter substance.

### Cystinuria

Cystinuria is an autosomal recessive inherited disorder characterized by an amino acid transport defect. The result is increased urinary excretion of *c*ystine, *o*rnithine, *a*rginine, and *l*ysine (COAL). The solubility of ornithine, arginine, and lysine is sufficiently high not to cause clinical crystal precipitation, but cystine is much less soluble and does cause nephrolithiasis. Homozygous

#### Clinical conditions associated with hyperuricosuria

Gout
Increased purine intake: excess dietary purine
Increased turnover of nucleic acids
  Hematologic malignancies: leukemia, lymphoma, myeloma
  Hemolytic anemias
  Polycythemia
  Psoriasis
Increased uric acid synthesis: alcohol consumption
Inborn errors of metabolism
Uricosuric agents

#### Causes of hypocitraturia

Metabolic acidosis (distal renal tubular acidosis)
Thiazide use (hypokalemia)
Chronic diarrhea
Idiopathic
Animal protein intake
Acute urinary tract infection

#### Causes of hypomagnesuria

**Decreased dietary intake**

Low-oxalate diet (also low in magnesium)
Alcohol abuse
Starvation

**Gastrointestinal malabsorption**

Inflammatory bowel disease
Nontropical sprue
Pancreatitis
Chronic diarrhea

expression occurs in about 1:20,000 Americans; heterozygotes occur in 1:200 people. Clinically, nephrolithiasis is only seen in those who are homozygous for the defect.

Cystine solubility and the risk for stone formation depends on three factors: cystine excretion, urine volume, and urine pH. Cystine excretion is affected both by dietary methionine and sodium intake. Methionine is essential for cystine production, and sodium intake appears to correlate well with cystine excretion, although the exact mechanism responsible for this is not known. High urine volumes are important in decreasing the urinary saturation of cystine. Cystine solubility is pH dependent; however, the pH must increase to more than 7.0 to 7.5 to have a clinically significant effect on cystine solubility.

### Infection stones

Struvite stones are composed of magnesium ammonium phosphate and carbonate apatite and form only in the presence of persistently alkaline urine pH (greater than 7.0) and ammonia. These conditions arise when the urinary tract is infected with organisms that produce urease, especially if the infection is chronic and untreated. Urease-producing bacteria include *Proteus, Klebsiella, Citrobacter,* and *Staphylococcus aureus. Escherichia coli* does not produce urease. Struvite stones account for less than 10% of all stones and occur most often in women and paraplegic or quadraplegic patients because of their increased frequency of UTIs. Struvite grows rapidly and typically extends to involve more than one renal calyx, forming "staghorn calculi."

## PATIENT EVALUATION

### History and physical examination

The first step in the evaluation of patients with nephrolithiasis is a complete history and physical examination. The history should include the present and past medical history, family history, social history, and most importantly an accurate dietary history. Physical examination focuses on detecting conditions associated with nephrolithiasis.

Stones cause symptoms of pain and hematuria only when they become lodged at some point in the urinary tract. When a stone is impacted in a renal calyx, it can cause calyceal distention with pain and hematuria. A stone impacted in the ureter causes ureteral spasm and may cause obstruction with ureteral dilatation proximal to the stone. Renal colic occurs suddenly as excruciating pain in the flank or back, which tends to radiate anteriorly and down into the groin. Stones lodged in the ureterovesical junction may also cause symptoms of urinary frequency and urgency. The role of the autonomic nervous system in the pain process may also cause nausea, vomiting, and ileus.

Obtain a detailed history of each stone episode, including the date, size and location of each stone, chemical composition, symptoms, treatment/outcome, and any complications. Note any previous workup or treatment, and obtain a genitourinary review of systems. Review all medications, including any over-the-counter preparations. Antacid consumption may represent a significant calcium intake, vitamin C supplements can cause hyperoxaluria, and excess vitamin A or D supplements may cause hypercalciuria. Triamterene has been reported to cause triamterene stones, and furosemide increases urinary calcium excretion. Acetazolamide increases urine pH, increases urinary calcium excretion, and decreases urinary citrate excretion. Uricosuric agents such as probenecid can cause uric acid stones. The remainder of the medical history should focus on determining if any history suggests diseases known to cause nephrolithiasis: symptoms of GI disease (especially diarrhea or malabsorption), granulomatous disease, or diseases known to cause hypercalcemia. Note any family history of kidney stones or diseases known to cause stones, and determine any environmental risk factors for nephrolithiasis (e.g., high ambient temperature or humidity causing dehydration, occupation, lifestyle).

In the diet history, note any excess intake of dairy products or seafoods high in calcium content, and assess the intake of oxalate-containing foods such as spinach and other green leafy vegetables, rhubarb, beets, nuts, tea, and chocolate products. Determine any intake of purine-rich proteins (Table 92A-3), and assess average daily fluid intake, including what types of fluids are consumed because some bottled or well waters may be especially rich in calcium and sodium.

The physical examination should be directed toward detecting any underlying conditions that may be associated with nephrolithiasis. Specific attention should be given to the presence of pulmonary, cardiac, or renal insufficiency. Any alterations in the function of a major organ system will have a great impact if a surgical approach for stone removal is necessary. Therefore patients with a history of coronary artery disease, pulmonary insufficiency secondary to asthma or smoking, and renal insufficiency should be adequately evaluated and properly treated before the stone removal procedure. The detection and appropriate management of hypertension is especially important in those patients undergoing extracorporeal shock wave lithotripsy (ESWL). Recent studies have found the incidence of perirenal hematomas may increase by as much as 60% if the patient has uncontrolled hypertension.

### Radiologic evaluation

Specific radiologic and imaging studies are presented in Chapter 92B.

### Laboratory evaluation

The laboratory evaluation of patients with nephrolithiasis includes measurement of serum electrolytes, urea nitrogen, calcium, phosphorus, magnesium, uric acid, and creatinine, as well as urine chemistries. Laboratory testing should not be performed within 3 to 4 weeks of an acute stone episode or in the presence of UTI, since the results may not accurately reflect the patient's baseline urine chemistry (the acute stone episode or UTI may alter the urinary excretion of various substances). Urine chemistries ("stone battery") should include volume, pH, calcium, phosphorus, uric acid, creatinine, urea nitrogen, sodium, potassium, magnesium, citrate, and oxalate. As noted in the following discussions, the evaluation should be tailored to the individual patient after taking into consideration the clinical setting. Certain medications must be held at least 1 week before urinary testing because

**Table 92A-3.** Low-purine diet

| Foods allowed | Foods to avoid |
|---|---|
| Meats: A total of 4 oz daily | All meats, including red meat, chicken, liver, organ meats; fish; gravies and broth soups |
| Vegetables: all vegetables except as noted | Spinach, mushrooms, asparagus, cauliflower, most beans, peas |
| Dairy products: eggs and cheese, milk, ice cream | None |
| Fats: butter or margarine | None |
| Breads: most cereals, breads and bread products, all pastas | Oatmeal and whole-grain products (may have two servings per week) |
| Fruits: all | None |
| Desserts: cake, pie, jello, puddings | None |
| Beverages: milk, water, decaffeinated coffee | Coffee, tea, cocoa, or chocolate-containing beverages; all alcoholic beverages |

they may interfere with the results. These include thiazides, loop diuretics, nonsteroidal antiinflammatory drugs, acetazolamide, theophylline, uricosuric agents, antacids, and any health food or vitamin supplements.

### Evaluation of patients with first stone

Approximately 50% of patients who form their first kidney stone will have another stone over the next 5 years. On the other hand, half these patients will not have another stone in 5 years. For this reason it is important to determine which patients are at higher risk for recurrence. Patients at high risk for recurrent stone formation are those with a positive family history of stone disease and those with chronic diarrhea or other illness known to cause stones. In these patients it is appropriate to perform a complete metabolic evaluation. In those patients at low risk for recurrent stone disease, it is reasonable to perform a more limited evaluation. (See following discussions.) An alternative approach is to perform a history and physical examination and provide conservative therapy (increased fluid intake; low-sodium, low-oxalate, and low-purine diet), not performing any further evaluation unless the patient forms another stone. In either approach, a KUB film should be obtained to look for evidence of any radiopaque stones. This x-ray also serves as a baseline to compare future films.

### Limited evaluation of patients at low risk for recurrent stones

In patients at low risk for stone recurrence (those with no obvious predisposing factors or family history), a thorough history and physical examination (with review of the urine sediment) are performed. Also, a general laboratory screening evaluation is aimed at detecting any abnormalities that may predispose the patient to form another stone in the near future. Serum chemistries and a 24-hour urine chemistry evaluation allow detection of hypercalcemia, hyperuricemia, hypercalciuria, hyperuricosuria, hypocitraturia, and hyperoxaluria. Any significant abnormalities can then be treated (Table 92A-4) and investigated further if indicated. Patients who do not demonstrate any significant abnormalities with limited testing and who form recurrent stones should undergo complete metabolic testing.

### Complete metabolic evaluation

The complete metabolic evaluation involves examination of urine chemistries with the patient's usual diet, after a controlled diet, and after an oral calcium load. Serum chemistries and any necessary x-rays are performed as well. The evaluation starts with the history and physical examination, including urinary sediment, and the patient is instructed in detail on the collection of 24-hour urine samples. The patient collects two consecutive 24-hour specimens with the usual diet and returns for the second visit. Then the patient is instructed on a low-sodium, low-calcium, low-purine (see Table 92A-3), low-oxalate diet (see Hyperoxaluria). After following the diet for 1 week, the patient collects another 24-hour urine specimen and returns for the third visit, when the serum chemistries are drawn, (including electrolytes, creatinine, uric acid, calcium, phosphorus, magnesium, albumin, and PTH). After collecting a 2-hour fasting urine sample after overnight fasting, the patient drinks an oral calcium load (NeoCalglucon). Urine is again collected at 2 hours and 4 hours. The urine is analyzed for calcium and creatinine, and the calcium/creatinine ratio is calculated. (See Interpretation of Laboratory Data.)

### Limited evaluation through outside laboratories

Some laboratories in the United States offer testing of 24-hour urine samples similar to that already described. These "stone batteries" usually measure volume, pH, calcium, phosphorus, uric acid, creatinine, potassium, magnesium, sodium, oxalate, and citrate. Some laboratories can also measure the relative supersaturation of calcium oxalate, brushite, and uric acid. These services are valuable to physicians located in areas where these complex tests are not available.

### Interpretation of laboratory data

Interpretation of data collected during evaluation should take into consideration two important factors. *Compliance* with the protocol (review medications and verify dietary compliance during testing) and *accurate collection* of 24-hour urine specimens (rule out incomplete or excessive urine collection) are crucial to accurate diagnosis. Poor dietary compliance with the testing protocol may cause erroneous values, especially during the oral calcium load test. Evidence suggesting compliance with the diet is a 24-hour sodium excretion test (after following the prescribed diet) significantly lower than that obtained on the two consecutive 24-hour specimens with the patient's usual diet. Inaccurate urine collection for 24-hour testing

**Table 92A-4.** Treatment of specific metabolic abnormalities in patients with nephrolithiasis

| Disorder | Treatment | Comments |
|---|---|---|
| Idiopathic hypercalciuria | Thiazide (HCTZ/amiloride)<br>Potassium citrate | Consider sodium cellulose phosphate in patients with intestinal hyperabsorption or neutral phosphate in patients with renal phosphaturia |
| Hypocitraturia | Potassium citrate<br>Treat underlying disorders | |
| Hyperoxaluria | Avoid calcium-restricted diet<br>Treat underlying disorders<br>Strict low-oxalate diet | Consider calcium supplement with meals<br>Consider pyridoxine in patients with moderate to marked hyperoxaluria |
| Hyperuricosuria | Dietary purine restriction<br>Potassium citrate | Allopurinol if diet alone not effective<br>Especially in patients with uric acid stones |
| Hypomagnesuria | Magnesium preparation with meals<br>Treat underlying disorders | |
| Cystinuria | Strict low-sodium diet<br>Potassium citrate<br>Marked increase in fluid intake<br>MPG | Decreases urinary cystine excretion<br>To achieve urine pH 6.5-7.0<br>To achieve urine volumes of 3000-4000 ml/day<br>Pyridoxine supplement; monitor serum iron and zinc<br>Consider captopril |
| Infection stones | Treat underlying infection<br>Remove infected stone material<br>Consider AHA | <br><br>If other modalities contraindicated or unsuccessful |

*HCTZ,* Hydrochlorothiazide; *MPG, N*-(2-mercaptoproprionyl)glycine; *AHA,* acetohydroxamic acid.

**Table 92A-5.** Categories of idiopathic hypercalciuria

| Category | Distinguishing features |
|---|---|
| Absorptive hypercalciuria (AHC) | Calcium/creatinine ratio 2 or 4 hours after oral calcium load >0.20 |
| Fasting hypercalciuria (FHC) | Fasting calcium/creatinine ratio >0.13 |
| Renal hypercalciuria | FHC, normal serum calcium, and elevated parathyroid hormone |
| Renal phosphaturia | FHC and/or AHC, hypophosphatemia, elevated 1,25-$(OH)_2$–vitamin $D_3$ |

may significantly alter the test results, possibly causing erroneous diagnoses. Therefore it is important to assess the accuracy of urine collection by calculating the expected creatinine excretion rate for the patient and comparing it with the actual amount. Males should excrete 18 to 21 mg/kg lean body weight (LBW) of creatinine daily (10 to 18 mg/kg LBW/day in patients over 50 years old). Females should excrete 15 to 18 mg/kg LBW/day (7 to 15 mg/kg LBW/day in patients over 50). If the 24-hour urinary creatinine excretion is less than the expected range, one should consider incomplete urine collection; if it is greater than the expected range, one should consider excessive urine collection. Table 92A-5 summarizes the categories composing idiopathic hypercalciuria; Table 92A-6 lists the diagnostic findings associated with various stone-forming conditions.

## MANAGEMENT

The management of patients with nephrolithiasis involves treatment of the acute stone episode and prevention of further stone formation.

### When to consult a nephrologist or urologist

Patients with an acute stone episode, those unable to pass the stone with conservative treatment, and all patients with nephrolithiasis complicated by UTI (fever, dysuria, signs of systemic infection) should be seen by a urologist. Patients with impaired renal function should have a nephrologist consulted as well. Although the outpatient evaluation of many patients can be performed without consultation, some patients, particularly those with recurrent nephrolithiasis, may benefit from testing under the guidance of a nephrologist and/or urologist experienced in metabolic evaluation of stone disease.

### Acute stone episode

The most cost-effective approach to diagnosis and management of the acute stone episode in patients with "classic" signs and symptoms (flank pain with radiation to groin, colicky nature, hematuria, and absence of pyuria) is to perform a KUB. The KUB shows the size and location of any radiodense stones. IVP is not necessary in these patients unless intervention is required. IVP should be performed when patients lack the classic signs and symptoms and when intervention may be required. This approach obviates the need for an initial KUB and provides an efficient and cost-effective evaluation in the acute setting. Sonography will accurately assess the presence of intrarenal calculi and hydronephrosis without

**Table 92A-6.** Diagnostic findings associated with stone-forming conditions

| | Fasting HC | Absorptive HC | Primary HPT | Renal HC | RP | UAN | HUCN | Hypocitraturia | Hyperoxaluria | RTA |
|---|---|---|---|---|---|---|---|---|---|---|
| **Serum chemistry** | | | | | | | | | | |
| Calcium | N | N | ↑ | N | N | N | N | N | N | N |
| Phosphorus | N | N | N or ↓ | N | ↓ | N | N | N | N | N |
| Parathyroid hormone | N | N | ↑ | ↑ | N | N | N | N | N | N or ↑ |
| $1,25(OH)_2$–vitamin $D_3$ | N | N or ↑ | N or ↑ | N | ↑ | N | N | N | N | N or ↑ |
| **Urine chemistry** | | | | | | | | | | |
| Fasting calcium | ↑ | N | ↑ | ↑ | N | N | N | N | N* | ↑ |
| Post-OCL calcium | N or ↑ | ↑ | N or ↑ | N or ↑ | ↑ | N | N | N | N* | N or ↑ |
| Uric acid | N | N | N | N | N | N or ↑ | ↑ | N | N or ↓ | N |
| Citrate | N | N | N | N | N | N | N | ↓ | ↓ | ↓ |
| Oxalate | N | N | N | N | N | N | N | N | ↑ | N |
| pH | N | N | N | N | N | ↓ | N | N | N or ↓ | ↑ |

*OCL,* Oral calcium load; *HC,* hypercalciuria; *HPT,* hyperparathyroidism; *RP,* renal phosphaturia; *UAN,* uric acid nephrolithiasis; *HUCN,* hyperuricosuric calcium nephrolithiasis; *RTA,* renal tubular acidosis; *N,* normal; ↑, increased; ↓, decreased.

*Urinary calcium excretion may be low in patients with enteric hyperoxaluria.

## Managed Care Guide
## Approach to the acute stone episode

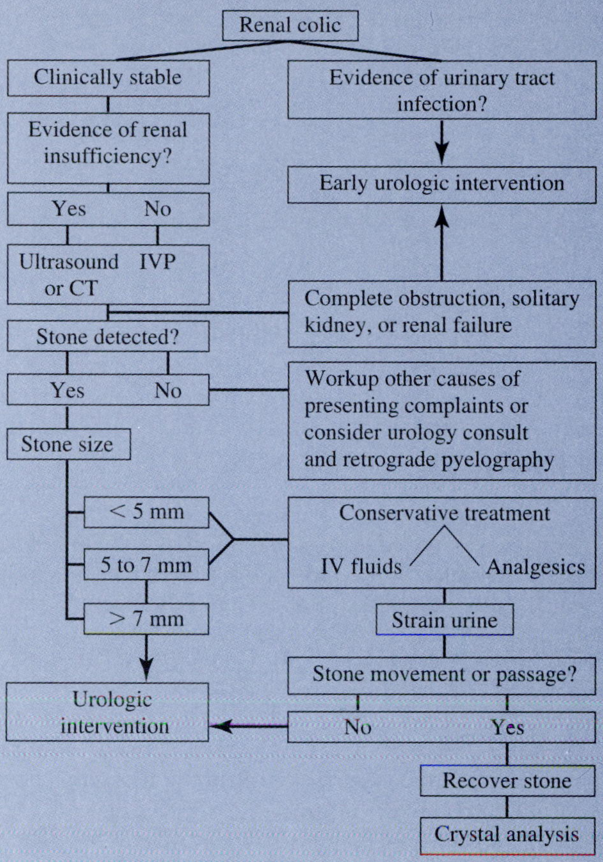


exposing the patient to diagnostic radiation.

Evaluation proceeds as described previously, and any signs of systemic infection (fever, hypotension, leukocytosis with a left shift) should be taken seriously (see Managed Care Guide). An infection proximal to an obstruction in the urinary tract is a true emergency and must be treated aggressively with drainage and antibiotics. If there are no signs of systemic illness and the patient is hemodynamically stable, treatment of the acute stone episode is aimed at pain relief and stone passage. The pain of renal colic can usually be relieved, at least partially, by narcotic analgesics. The nonsteroidal antiinflammatory drugs (NSAIDs) may also provide relief, since prostaglandins probably mediate some of the pain response in renal and ureteral colic. However, NSAIDs should not be used in patients with renal insufficiency or in those with a history of chronic liver disease with cirrhosis, volume depletion, congestive heart failure, or other prerenal states. Stone passage may be facilitated by the administration of intravenous fluids at rates sufficient to increase urine flow, but it is important to achieve adequate analgesia first, since the transient increase in pressure in the urinary tract proximal to an obstruction may cause marked worsening of pain symptoms. All urine specimens must be strained and any recovered calculi sent for crystal analysis.

Stones less than 5 mm in diameter tend to pass spontaneously; those greater than 7 mm usually will not pass. Indications for early aggressive intervention include UTI or urosepsis, complete ureteral obstruction, solitary kidney, or significant renal insufficiency. In patients with small stones without indications for more aggressive therapy, it is appropriate to provide conservative treatment with intravenous fluids and analgesics and close observation for stone passage. If there is no evidence of stone movement or passage with conservative treatment, urologic intervention is warranted.

Surgical management of urinary calculi is presented in Chapter 92B.

### Prevention of further stone formation

Prevention of recurrent stone formation usually requires dietary modification and/or pharmacologic treatment. Dietary modifications may include any combination of the following: low-oxalate diet, low-sodium diet, low-calcium diet, low-protein/low-purine diet, and increased fluid intake.

***Dietary modification.*** Low-oxalate intake decreases the amount of oxalate potentially absorbed by the intestinal tract and excreted by the kidneys. It is important not to restrict calcium intake, since decreased binding of oxalate by calcium in the gut may allow what little oxalate is ingested to be readily absorbed and excreted, thus defeating the purpose of low-oxalate intake. Foods that should be avoided or restricted include beets, rhubarb, spinach, chard, greens, endive, okra, all teas, all chocolates and cocoa, and all nuts.

A low-sodium diet decreases the urinary excretion of cystine and calcium and probably also decreases urate excretion.

Although low-calcium intake has been historically advocated in the treatment of various types of nephrolithiasis, the benefits of decreased calcium intake are not clear at this time. In fact, evidence suggests that a low-calcium diet not only may cause significant long-term bone loss, but may also increase the incidence of recurrent stone formation. The role of calcium-restricted diets in the treatment of kidney stones remains to be determined.

Low-protein/low-purine diets (see Table 92A-3) restrict the intake of meat products (which, if consumed in large amounts, could lead to hyperuricosuria) and animal proteins (a potential source of high acid content, which can cause hypocitraturia and hypercalciuria).

The goal of increased fluid intake is to achieve daily urine volumes greater than 2000 ml. Since the average insensible losses amount to 800 to 1000 ml daily, about 3000 ml of fluids must be consumed a day to achieve adequate urine volumes. Increased insensible losses from perspiration can amount to an additional 1000 ml. Many patients find it difficult to change their fluid consumption habits, and the easiest method for many patients is to keep a 2 L plastic bottle (e.g., empty soft drink bottle) filled with water in the refrigerator and make sure to drink it all every day. This at least guarantees a minimum fluid intake of 2 L a day. Patients should be advised to increase their fluid intake when active and during the summer months if exposed to high ambient temperatures. Also, since stones may often form overnight, patients should be advised to drink a glass or two of water at bedtime and again during the night if they awake to urinate. A good hint for patients follows: if they urinate and their urine is not as clear as tap water, they are not drinking enough fluid.

***Pharmacologic treatment.*** Pharmacologic treatment should selectively treat metabolic abnormalities that may predispose to recurrent stone formation.

**Citrate.** Potassium citrate is used to correct hypocitraturia (idiopathic or secondary to RTA or chronic diarrhea) and as an alkalinizing agent to treat cystine and uric acid stones. As mentioned earlier, citrate is a crystallization inhibitor and acts by complexing with calcium to reduce the concentration of calcium salts in the urine. Citrate inhibits precipitation, crystallization, and aggregation of calcium oxalate and is a potent inhibitor of calcium phosphate crystallization and growth. The potassium salt of citrate is the preferred form for treatment for several reasons. It is consistent and more effective in providing an increase in urinary citrate levels than potassium bicarbonate. Compared with sodium citrate, potassium citrate causes a decrease in urinary calcium in addition to a more pronounced effect on increasing urinary citrate in patients with hypokalemia. The goal of treatment with potassium citrate is to increase the urinary citrate concentration and, in some patients, to raise the urine pH to 6.5 to 7.0. The usual starting dose for adults is a 40 to 60 mEq a day in two or three divided doses. Potassium citrate is available as a wax matrix tablet for oral use in 5 and 10 mEq strengths and also as a crystalline powder and liquid. The potential side effects of potassium citrate include nausea and diarrhea (more common with liquid forms than tablets) and hyperkalemia (in patients with renal insufficiency).

**Thiazide diuretics.** These are used in the treatment of idiopathic hypercalciuria to decrease urinary calcium excretion and the saturation of calcium oxalate and brushite. The mechanism of action of thiazides initially involves increased distal tubular reabsorption of calcium; then, with the development of mild volume depletion, there is enhanced proximal tubular calcium resorption as well. This mechanism requires dietary sodium restriction, and an increase in urinary sodium excretion will negate the thiazide effect on urinary calcium excretion. The clinical effectiveness of thiazides may be limited to a few years (in treatment of absorptive hypercalciuria but probably not renal hypercalciuria), since evidence suggests that long-term thiazide use can lead to a low bone turnover state and recurrent hypercalciuria. Thiazide treatment is frequently complicated by hypokalemia and hypocitraturia. Hypokalemia causes an intracellular acidosis in the renal tubules that leads to increased tubular reabsorption of citrate and decreased urinary citrate excretion. For this reason, most patients treated with thiazides should also receive potassium citrate supplementation.

Complications of thiazide use include hypokalemia, hypomagnesemia, hyperuricemia, impotence, and adverse effects on lipids. Alternative agents include indapamide and the combination of hydrochlorothiazide and amiloride, which decreases the risk of hypokalemia and hypocitraturia.

**Sodium cellulose phosphate.** A nonabsorbable ion exchange resin, sodium cellulose phosphate binds calcium in the GI tract, preventing it from being absorbed. The potential benefits are decreased GI calcium absorption and decreased urinary calcium excretion. Adverse long-term effects of sodium cellulose phosphate are more likely when used in patients with idiopathic hypercalciuria not caused by intestinal hyperabsorption (renal hypercalciuria, primary hyperparathyroidism). The common side effects are important and include negative calcium balance (with potential long-term bone loss), hypomagnesemia (from magnesium binding in the gut), and hyperoxaluria. The increase in urinary oxalate excretion occurs as a result of the increased binding of calcium and magnesium in the gut, which decreases the amount of free calcium and magnesium able to bind with oxalate, thus allowing free oxalate to be readily absorbed in the colon. These adverse effects are best avoided by prescribing sodium cellulose phosphate only for patients with hypercalciuria caused by intestinal hyperabsorption (when other measures are not effective), prescribing an oxalate-restricted diet, and giving a magnesium supplement (not at the same time as the exchange resin).

**Potassium phosphate (neutral phosphate).** This is used by some clinicians to treat idiopathic hypercalciuria caused by renal phosphate leak (renal phosphaturia). Potassium phosphate may act by suppressing synthesis of 1,25-$(OH)_2$–vitamin $D_3$ but can also increase urinary pyrophosphate and citrate (crystallization inhibitors). The usual dose is 500 mg three times daily. Neutral phosphate is contraindicated in patients with renal insufficiency.

**Allopurinol.** Allopurinol decreases the production of uric acid by inhibiting the enzyme xanthine oxidase. A clinically significant lowering of urinary uric acid excretion occurs after 3 to 4 days of therapy. The usual dose is 300 mg once a day, but a lower dose should be used in patients with renal insufficiency. The potential adverse effects include allergic reaction, interstitial nephritis, and rarely, hepatitis. Allopurinol should be used with great caution in patients taking 6-mercaptopurine.

**Magnesium.** Oral magnesium supplements are useful in patients with hypomagnesuria, especially those with chronic diarrhea or other disorders associated with chronic magnesium deficiency. It acts by complexing with oxalate in the gut to decrease the urinary saturation of calcium oxalate. Magnesium supplements (magnesium oxide, magnesium gluconate, magnesium citrate) should be taken with meals three or four times a day; the only side effect encountered with any frequency is diarrhea or GI upset.

**Calcium.** Calcium supplements in the form of calcium carbonate or calcium citrate may occasionally be useful in the treatment of patients with hyperoxaluria related to bowel disease. When taken with meals, the calcium binds any free oxalate, preventing its absorption.

**Pyridoxine (vitamin $B_6$).** Pyridoxine is useful in the treatment of primary hyperoxaluria (see Hyperoxaluria). The usual dose is 25 mg once or twice daily.

***N*-(2-mercaptoproprionyl)glycine (MPG).** MPG is a complexing thiol compound that forms a soluble disulfide complex with cystine. MPG replaces D-penicillamine in the treatment of cystinuria because it is equally effective and has far fewer side effects. Because MPG is more effective in alkaline urine, and because cystine solubility increases with a urine pH greater than 7.0, MPG is usually used in conjunction with potassium citrate. Dosage is titrated to achieve a reduction in urinary cystine excretion to levels less than 250 mg/L. MPG binds pyridoxine, zinc, and iron, and it is important to prescribe pyridoxine supplements and periodically monitor serum levels of zinc and iron.

**Captopril.** Captopril may form a soluble disulfide complex with cystine, but its use in the treatment of cystinuria has not been fully evaluated.

**Acetohydroxamic acid (AHA).** AHA is a urease inhibitor used in the treatment of infection stones. AHA in large doses has been shown to be carcinogenic and has frequent side effects. It should be used only in conjunction with treatment of any underlying infections and when other therapies are contraindicated. The usual dose is 250 mg three times a day.

## Specific treatment recommendations

All patients with nephrolithiasis should be advised to increase their fluid intake and follow a diet low in oxalate, sodium, and purine-containing proteins. Table 92-4 summarizes the treatment of specific metabolic abnormalities in patients with nephrolithiasis.

## Patient follow-up

After completion of all laboratory investigations, arrange to meet with the patient to discuss the results of the evaluation and to formulate a treatment plan. The most important aspect of this encounter is patient education. Patients are more likely to comply with the prescribed treatment if they have insight into the disease process and the reasoning behind any treatments. The most effective and consistent method of patient education is the use of patient handouts or brochures that summarize diagnoses and treatments. Clinical dietitians can also help educate patients about any prescribed dietary changes.

Three to four weeks after initiation of therapy, repeat the 24-hour urine "stone battery" to assess for compliance and to verify a favorable response to treatment. A lack of response to thiazides usually results from poor compliance with sodium restriction. Persistent hypocitraturia may be caused by ongoing metabolic acidosis or hypokalemia, and persistent hyperoxaluria may be related to dietary noncompliance, inadequate dietary calcium intake, or increased activity of bowel disease (if present). If urinary uric acid is not decreased acceptably with purine restriction alone, the addition of allopurinol may be necessary.

Patients who remain asymptomatic should be seen again at 3 months. If they remain stone free and have a favorable response to therapy, they can be followed at 6-month to 1-year intervals. It may be appropriate, especially in recurrent stone formers, to check a 24-hour urine stone battery before each follow-up visit to assess the urine chemistry. Examine the urine sediment for any crystalluria or evidence of UTI, and obtain a brief diet history to verify compliance with any prescribed diet.

## BIBLIOGRAPHY

See end of Chapter 92B for bibliography.

CHAPTER

# 92B Surgical Management of Urinary Calculi

Glenn M. Preminger

Considerable progress has been made in the management of nephrolithiasis over the past 10 years. This progress has been particularly noteworthy in the surgical area. Recently, the innovative surgical techniques of percutaneous nephrostolithotomy, ureterorenoscopy, and extracorporeal shock wave lithotripsy (ESWL) were introduced, allowing efficacious stone removal with a significant reduction in pain and postoperative convalescence compared with open surgical procedures. In fact, probably 95% of all renal and ureteral calculi can be successfully removed using these therapeutic modalities.

## PREOPERATIVE EVALUATION

The goal of all surgical procedures for urinary calculi, including open surgery, endourology, and all forms of lithotripsy, should be complete stone removal, repair of anatomic defects, and preservation of renal function. However, even the most skillfully performed open surgical or endourologic procedure may fail if the patient has not been properly evaluated or medically prepared for surgery. Therefore careful evaluation and planning are the key to successful stone management. This chapter describes a comprehensive approach toward the patient with symptomatic urinary calculi.

### Medical history and physical examination

A thorough medical history, as presented in Chapter 92A, should be obtained.

### Preoperative laboratory evaluation

***Blood.*** A multichannel blood screen followed by specific blood tests (see Chapter 92A and Table 92A-6) can be helpful in identifying certain systemic problems that may account for recurrent stone disease.

***Urine.*** Voided urinary specimens should be obtained for comprehensive analysis and culture and sensitivity (see Chapter 92A and Table 92A-6).

***Renal function.*** Assessment of renal function is important during the evaluation of a patient with nephrolithiasis especially if a patient has had a history of multiple stones and/or stone removal procedures. Differential renal function studies can suggest whether a stone-laden kidney is worth salvaging and can allow educated decisions on the appropriate time of stone surgery in patients with bilateral nephrolithiasis. The most convenient test for accurately determining the total renal function with the least expense is the 24-hour creatinine clearance.

***Stone composition.*** Any available stone should be analyzed to determine its crystalline composition (see Chapter 92A).

## PREOPERATIVE RADIOLOGIC EVALUATION

A thorough radiologic evaluation is one of the most important parts of the overall investigation of urinary stone disease. Multiple roentgenographic examinations can be used to assess the three major questions that must be answered before selecting an appropriate stone removal procedure: stone burden, urinary tract anatomy, and renal function.

### Kidney, ureter, and bladder (KUB) x-rays

Over 90% of stones within the urinary tract are radiopaque. Calcium phosphate and calcium oxalate are the most radiodense stones, and struvite, especially when it complexes with calcium phosphate, is also visible with a characteristic multilobulated shape and laminated appearance. Cystine stones are often poorly visualized on plain films and have what has been termed a *ground glass* appearance with radiodensity only slightly greater than surrounding soft tissue. Pure uric acid stones are radiolucent and usually only visualized by CT scanning or intravenous pyelography (IVP). Therefore a plain film of the abdomen (KUB) should be the initial radiographic examination obtained in all patients with nephrolithiasis. A KUB should be performed before any subsequent films that employ contrast media, since the contrast may obscure the presence of even large calculi.

Abdominal films are obtained to document the number, size, and location of all stones within the urinary tract. The radiopacity of any existing stones may suggest the type of stones present. The plain abdominal film is also useful in identifying nephrocalcinosis (suggestive of renal tubular acidosis, sarcoidosis, hyperparathyroidism, or primary hyperoxaluria) and staghorn calculi (likely due to infection lithiasis).

It is important not to overlook stones that may be obscured when they overlie bony structures, such as the sacrum or transverse processes of the lumbar vertebrae. These stones can be more easily identified using oblique or AP views. In addition, nephrotomograms can also be employed to assist in the identification of small, less radiopaque calculi within the kidneys.

### Intravenous pyelogram

The IVP is instrumental in defining the relationship of the calculus to the pyelocaliceal system and the ureter. The exact location of the stones, the presence or absence of obstruction, hydronephrosis, caliectasis, and renal/ureteral anomalies are all important bits of information that must be gleaned from the IVP. In addition, the IVP can approximate the renal function of an affected or "normal" contralateral kidney as suggested by the promptness of contrast excretion, thickness of renal parenchyma, and amount of pyelocaliectasis.

The IVP should be performed as an *individualized* test for each patient with a renal/ureteral calculus. This means that after obtaining a KUB, plain tomographic cuts should be performed if necessary. After injection of the contrast media, a 1-minute and a 5-minute film should be able to discern the promptness of contrast excretion, as well as the possibility of obstruction somewhere along the urinary tract. Oblique views may be necessary during the course of the IVP to help define the presence of renal/ureteral stones, which may overlie bony structures, or to help identify the presence of ureteral obstruction. It is imperative that delayed films be obtained as long as necessary to specifically identify the cause of delayed contrast excretion in patients with small obstructing calculi.

Finally, the IVP may confirm the presence of radiolucent stones and also identify anatomic abnormalities that may be responsible for stone formation such as a ureteropelvic junction obstruction or calyceal diverticulum.

### Ultrasound

Ultrasonography can be utilized as a screening tool for hydronephrosis or stones within the collecting system. Sonograms are useful for uncovering perirenal extravasation or perirenal abscesses in patients with infection lithiasis. If a perirenal process is identified, definitive stone therapy probably should be delayed until this problem has been adequately treated.

Additional information provided by sonographic examination of the kidneys is the amount of parenchyma present in an obstructed kidney, as well as identifying radiolucent calculi. The classic "sonographic shadow" will clearly identify stones that may not be visualized on radiographic examinations.

Although not part of the preoperative evaluation, sonography has proved useful in identifying retained or residual stone fragments during open stone surgery. This technique has been proven quite useful in identifying residual stone fragments as small as 1 to 2 mm.

In the future, sonographic examination will become part of the urologist's diagnostic armamentarium to help identify the presence of renal pathology. Therefore more and more renal calculi will be first identified by sonography as ultrasound technology becomes more available to the urologist.

### Computerized tomography

Although not considered as useful a screening examination as the IVP and ultrasound, computerized tomography (CT) scan can provide extremely useful information in the diagnostic assessment of the stone patient. CT scanning is particularly useful in helping to identify the etiology of radiolucent filling defects within the renal pelvis or ureter. In addition, anatomic abnormalities and obstruction can be easily identified.

CT scanning is especially useful to delineate the presence of perirenal, renal, or periureteral fluid collections. Extravasation of urine or contrast material, as well as the presence of an abscess cavity, is extremely important information that will ultimately dictate the appropriate management of these complicated stone patients. In addition, CT–directed needle aspiration of various masses or fluid collections have both diagnostic and therapeutic implications.

### Magnetic resonance urography

Magnetic resonance urography provides excellent visualization of the obstructed genitourinary tract. It is useful for examining patients who are allergic to contrast media or are too obese for other imaging modalities.

### Retrograde pyelogram

Retrograde pyelography may be utilized in patients who are "allergic" to contrast media to identify stones within the urinary tract, as well as uncover evidence of obstruction or other anatomic abnormalities. In patients with borderline renal function, a retrograde pyelogram obviates the need for an intravascular bolus of contrast medium, which may further insult the renal function. In patients with high-grade obstructions as a result of impacted ureteral calculi, a retrograde pyelogram will help to define the exact anatomy and may also prove useful in defining the necessity for preoperative drainage with a ureteral catheter or percutaneous nephrostomy tube.

In some cases where the exact anatomy is difficult to define or a radiolucent filling defect can be identified but its etiology remains obscure, placement of a catheter into the renal pelvis or to the level of obstruction may be helpful before the patient is transferred to the radiology suite. On the more sophisticated fluoroscopy table, the radiologist may then inject contrast through the ureteral catheter and obtain multiple exposures in varying projections to help further define the etiology of a filling defect.

One other instance where retrograde pyelography proves useful is immediately before open surgery when one or more stones have already been identified, but the distal ureter has not been well visualized. This preoperative study performed in the operating room allows the exclusion of unsuspected additional ureteral calculi and allows the assessment of coexistent ureteral disease, such as stricture or retroperitoneal fibrosis, which may complicate the operative or postoperative course of the patient.

### Antegrade pyelogram

In the case of profound obstruction or impaired renal function, intravenous pyelography may be inadequate to delineate renal/ureteral anatomy. In some cases, retrograde pyelography may be either unsuccessful or contraindicated and those patients may benefit from antegrade pyelography.

Placement of percutaneous nephrostomy tube can be accomplished under fluoroscopic or sonographic guidance. In fact, in patients with large renal calculi occupying the renal collecting system, one may actually pass the needle directly onto the stone to gain percutaneous access to the collecting system.

The percutaneous nephrostomy tube not only allows adequate visualization of the urinary tract through an antegrade fashion, but it also provides adequate and safe drainage to the obstructed collecting system. The nephrostomy tube may serve as a useful adjunct for either endoscopic or lithotripsy procedures for stone removal.

### Radionuclide evaluation

Renal radionuclide tests provide rapid and safe information about total and differential renal function. These tests are specifically advantageous since the radionuclide evaluation is not invasive, requires no bowel prep or specific preoperative preparation, subjects the patient to only minimal radiation exposure, and is apparently free of allergic complications.

Glucoheptonate and dimercaptosuccinic acid (DMSA) are useful radiopharmaceuticals for the evaluation of renal morphology. However, for the diagnostic evaluation of the renal stone patient, radionuclide scans that evaluate renal blood flow, tubular function, and assess the presence of renal obstruction are probably more useful.

Alterations in renal function can be easily measured utilizing $^{131}$I-orthoiodohippurate (OIH). This radionuclide can be used to determine the effective renal plasma flow that has been shown to be more accurate than serum creatinine as an indicator of total renal function. In addition, quantitative measurements can be made between different segments of an affected kidney or between a stone-bearing and apparently normal contralateral kidney to gain access to the appropriate approach for stone removal. Knowledge of poor function may significantly alter the approach for stone removal and in some cases may suggest that partial or total nephrectomy may be a more appropriate procedure.

A radionuclide evaluation can also help to determine the presence of obstruction in the face of hydronephrosis. Both $^{131}$I-OIH or $^{99}$Tc-DTPA (diethylenetriaminepentaacetic acid) can be used to perform a "Lasix (furosemide) wash-out scan." This diuretic renal scan can help differentiate between hydronephrosis and functional obstruction either at the level of the ureteropelvic junction or further along down the ureter. This finding, of course, would alter the approach for stone removal since surgical or endourologic repair of the obstruction may be necessary.

### Renal arteriogram

Although not routinely used as a screening test during the initial evaluation of patients with renal calculi, renal arteriography is usually reserved in those patients with large branched calculi or to patients with renal anomalies such as a horseshoe kidney. When planning a procedure that will require temporary occlusion of an arterial segment, partial nephrectomy, or surgical approach of an anomalous kidney, arteriography should be considered an essential diagnostic tool.

In some instances, digital subtraction angiography may provide vascular anatomic information with less risk and morbidity than standard angiography procedures.

## EVALUATION OF THE SURGICAL PLAN

Before embarking on the removal of symptomatic renal/ureteral calculi utilizing either open, endourologic, or lithotripsy procedures, many of the aforementioned diagnostic techniques should be employed to assist the surgeon in identifying the most appropriate plan of action. Determination of the stone burden, composition, and location are all important factors in planning the appropriate approach for stone removal. The fact that ESWL may have been overused in the past is evidenced by the 10% to 20% incidence of adjunctive endourologic procedures necessary to render some patients free of stones. ESWL appears ideally indicated for stones less than 2 cm in size, with success rates ranging from 90% to 94%. These figures are comparable to the 90% to 98% success rates for most percutaneous procedures for small renal calculi. Lithotripsy procedures appear preferable since they offer the patient less pain and hospitalization time with a comparable cost.

However, for larger renal calculi, shock wave lithotripsy monotherapy has been plagued by a high incidence of residual fragments (upwards of 60%), as well as the necessity for multiple lithotripsy and ancillary procedures. Therefore consideration should be given to a combined percutaneous debulking of large calculi followed by lithotripsy therapy of residual fragments or an open surgical procedure, most commonly an anatrophic nephrolithotomy.

As with renal calculi, the location and size of stones within the ureter will be the most important factors in planning the approach for ureteral stone removal. Upper ureteral calculi can be approached by direct shock wave lithotripsy therapy, antegrade percutaneous stone extraction, or ureteroscopy. Current experience reveals that lower ureteral calculi may be best approached by ureteroscopy.

## SURGICAL MANAGEMENT

Surgical therapy for urinary tract calculi has changed significantly over the previous ten years. In the past, symptomatic stone removal required an open surgical procedure. However, advances in fiberoptics with the subsequent development of flexible instruments as well as small caliber rigid endoscopes have allowed the development of the subspecialty of endourology ("the closed, controlled manipulation of the entire urinary tract").

### Percutaneous nephrostolithotomy

The indications for percutaneous stone removal are the same as those for open procedures, i.e., symptomatic stones, obstruction or danger of obstruction, hematuria, and recurrence of infection. In addition, establishment of a percutaneous nephrostomy tract allows access to the renal pelvis for chemolysis of residual or recurrent uric acid or struvite (infection) stones.

The technique of percutaneous nephrostolithotomy relies on access to the intrarenal collecting system through a percutaneous nephrostomy tract (Fig. 92B-1). In this procedure, a hollow needle is passed into the renal pelvis under x-ray guidance. A flexible guide wire is then passed through the hollow needle and manipulated down the ureter. The nephrostomy tract is then formed by dilating the skin, muscles and renal tissues over the guide wire. Nephrostomy tract dilation can be performed using graduated plastic dilators or a balloon catheter. After the nephrostomy tract has been dilated up to a 30 French (10 mm diameter) size, a hollow plastic sheath is placed into the renal pelvis. Fiberoptic telescopes can now be directly passed into the renal pelvis where stones are then located, and if small enough, extracted directly through the plastic sheath. If the stones are too large to be extracted intact, ultrasonic lithotripsy is employed which allows fragmentation of the stone into small pieces which can then be extracted manually or evacuated by suction (Fig. 92B-2).

For stones that are located in calyces that cannot be reached using rigid fiberoptic telescopes, a flexible fiberoptic endoscope can be employed. Certain instruments, such as stone baskets, grasping forceps and electrohydraulic lithotripsy probes can be passed through

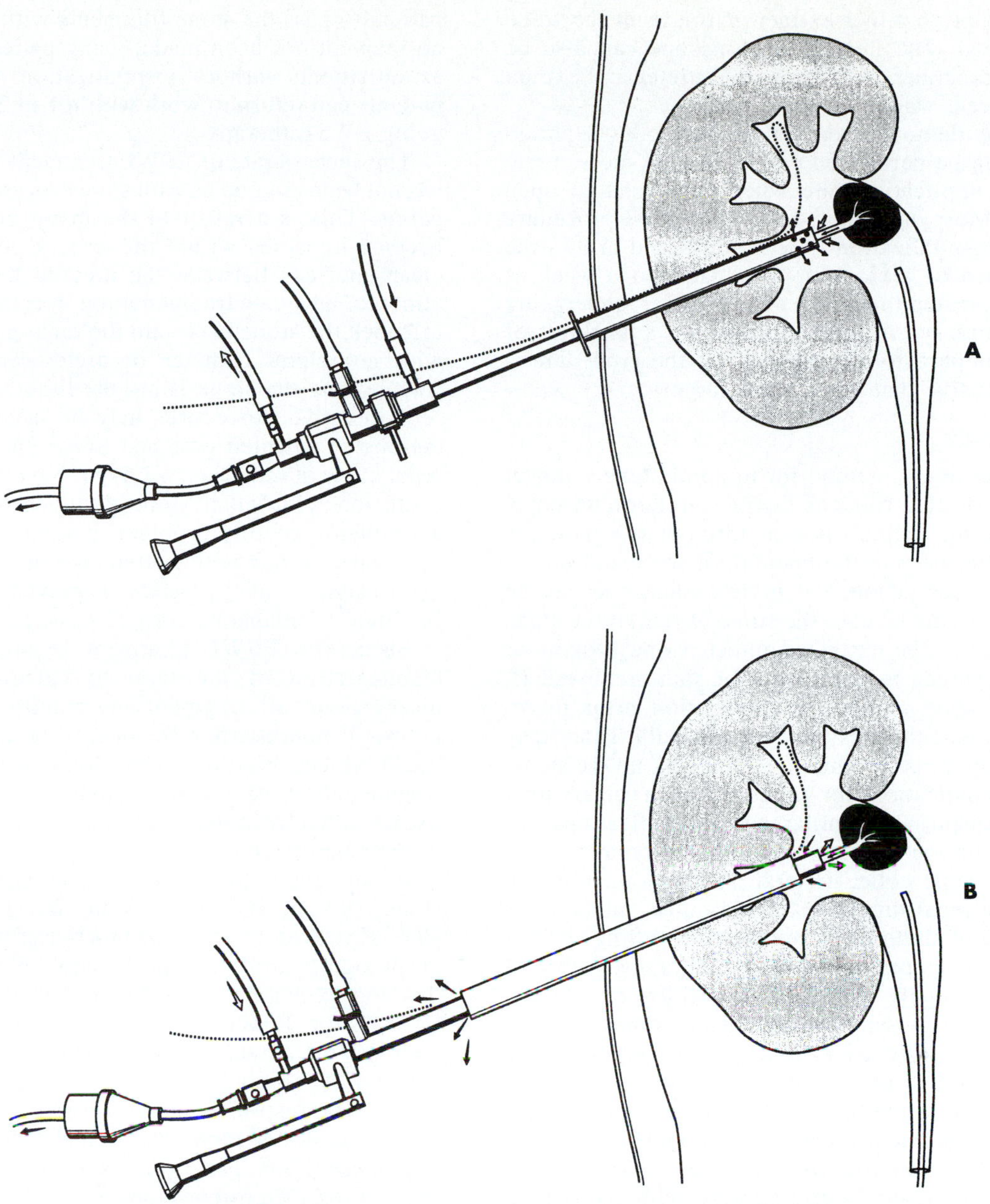


**Fig. 92B-1.** Percutaneous ultrasonic stone disintegration. **A,** Nephroscope sheath with a closed continuous flow irrigation system: using the working channel as an outflow port *(open arrows)* keeps the fragments around the tips of the sonotrode, even if the latter is clogged. **B,** Open system with a nephrostomy sheath; debris is flushed out continuously alongside the nephroscope. (From Krane R, Siroky M, Fitzpatrick J, editors: *Clinical urology,* Philadelphia, 1994, JB Lippincott.)

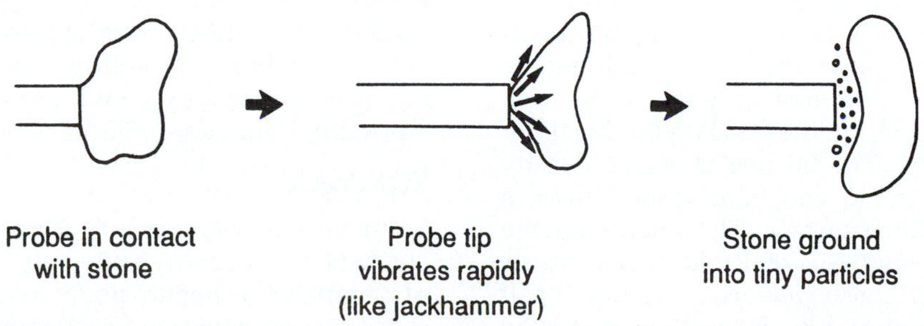


**Fig. 92B-2.** Schema of stone fragmentation by ultrasonic lithotripsy. The probe vibrates at 23-27 kHz and acts as a jackhammer at the surface of the stone. Direct contact is necessary between the probe and the stone. (From Krane R, Siroky M, Fitzpatrick J, editors: *Clinical urology,* Philadelphia, 1994, JB Lippincott.)

the flexible scope to either extract or fragment the stone prior to removal. The flexible nephroscope can also be used to localize stones in the proximal ureter and extract them under direct vision.

Studies have demonstrated that percutaneous nephrostolithotomy can be performed with a similar success rate and similar complication rate when compared to open renal surgery. More important, this less invasive procedure shortens the hospitalization time by 60% and allows the patient to return to work in approximately one week as compared to greater than three weeks after undergoing open renal surgery. Another significant advantage of percutaneous nephrostolithotomy is that the procedure is 40% less expensive than open renal surgery.

### Ureterorenoscopy

Another endourologic method for ureteral stone removal employs the use of a rigid or flexible ureterorenoscope. These instruments can be passed through the patient's urethra, bladder and into the opening of the distal ureter. Then, under direct vision, the ureterorenoscope can be passed directly to the level of the stone. Again, if the stone is small enough to be extracted intact, stone baskets or grasping forceps can be employed for stone removal. If, however, the stone requires fragmentation prior to removal, ultrasonic lithotripsy, electrohydraulic lithotripsy or laser lithotripsy can be employed to break up the stone.

The current indications for ureteroscopy in urinary tract stone management are similar to the indications for surgical intervention in both ureteral and renal calculi. These include renal colic, ureteral obstruction, infection and decreasing renal function. An additional indication is the evaluation of ureteral or renal pelvic filling defects seen on intravenous or retrograde pyelography. Apparent lesions can be visually inspected, sometimes revealing a soft tissue mass or possibly a radiolucent stone.

While ureterorenoscopy is somewhat time consuming and requires specific expertise, the major advantage is the decreased morbidity and trauma to the patient undergoing the stone extraction. In most cases of uncomplicated direct vision stone extraction utilizing the ureterorenoscope, the procedure is performed in day surgery with the patient returning to work within 1 to 2 days. Again, this is a significant improvement when compared to open surgery for ureteral stone removal which requires 5 to 6 days of hospitalization and 3 to 4 weeks of recuperation at home.

### Extracorporeal shock wave lithotripsy

Perhaps the most significant advance in the removal of renal and ureteral stones has been the development of ESWL. This procedure employs the use of high energy shock waves that are transmitted through water and directly focused onto renal/ureteral stones with the aid of fluoroscopy or ultrasound. The change in tissue density between the soft renal tissue and hard stone causes a release of energy at the stone surface. This energy release will cause stone fragmentation. Multiple shock waves applied to the stone will cause pulverization into small pieces (between 2 and 3 mm), which can then be passed down the ureter and out of the body with the urine.

***Efficacy of ESWL.*** The major advantage of ESWL is the noninvasive nature of stone fragmentation allowing the patient to pass the stone fragments without surgery. Since no incision has been made, many patients can be treated as outpatients without hospitalization. In addition, many patients can return to work within 1 to 2 days after undergoing EWSL therapy.

The success rate of ESWL treatment for ureteral stones has not been as good as with stones located within the renal pelvis. This is a result of the many ureteral stones that become impacted within the ureteral wall; there is not a clear interface between the ureteral tissue and stone to allow for adequate fragmentation. It is therefore preferable to knock the stone back into the renal pelvis by pushing it with a ureteral catheter or ureterorenoscope and then fragmenting the stone using the lithotripsy machine.

Adjunctive procedures may be needed before ESWL therapy in selected patients. Some patients with a large renal stone burden (i.e., >2.5 cm) have developed ureteral occlusion with small stone particles after treatment. In anticipation of this problem, patients with large stones may have an indwelling ureteral stent or a percutaneous nephrostomy tube placed to prevent obstruction and facilitate spontaneous particle passage.

Successful ESWL treatment requires both complete disintegration of the targeted calculus and complete discharge of all fragments as monitored by roentgenograms 3 months after treatment. As one would expect, larger stones require more shock waves for complete fragmentation. In addition, stones composed of calcium oxalate monohydrate and cystine are difficult to break due to their hardness.

Experience in the United States reveals that for smaller stones (≤2 cm) the overall stone-free rate at 3 months is 87%. However, as stone size increases, the stone-free rate drops significantly to approximately 65%. It now appears that approximately 70% of nonselected stone patients are eligible for ESWL monotherapy. This group includes patients with single or multiple stones in the kidney (stone mass <2.5 cm) and in selected patients with ureteral stones. The rest of the patient population presenting with more complex symptomatic stone disease will probably require auxiliary procedures such as percutaneous stone removal or ureterorenoscopy.

While controversy still exists concerning the most appropriate treatment for large, branched calculi, the consensus view is that these stones should be treated with a combined approach of percutaneous stone removal and ESWL. The advantage of a combination percutaneous ESWL approach over ESWL monotherapy is that the combined technique offers a significant reduction in residual stone rates from approximately 60% to almost 10% of patients. In addition, initial percutaneous stone removal followed by ESWL has been shown to have less morbidity than anatrophic nephrolithotomy.

## SUMMARY

Surgical management of urinary calculus disease has changed dramatically in the past decade. The development of percutaneous nephrostomy techniques has allowed new access to upper tract stones. Percutaneous removal of large calculi was made possible by the development of ultrasonic and electrohydraulic lithotripsy. All upper tract calculi can now successfully be removed in 70% to 100% of cases with minimal complications. Percutaneous techniques have reduced transfusion rates and hospital costs and markedly shortened convalescence periods when compared with open surgery.

Ureteroscopy followed percutaneous stone procedures as advanced fiberoptic technology allowed the development of small caliber instruments required for this procedure. With experience, successful stone retrieval has occurred in upwards of 90% of cases, again with minimal complications. As percutaneous nephrostolithotomy and ureteroscopy have become available, the subspecialty of endourology has emerged and significantly changed the management of urinary tract calculi.

Perhaps the most significant advance in stone therapy has been the design and implementation of ESWL. With this noninvasive technique, most renal and proximal ureteral calculi can be effectively treated with minimal morbidity and convalescence. Research in lithotripter design is ongoing with more advanced and effective machines on the horizon. The applicability of ESWL for urinary and biliary tract calculi is currently under investigation.

## BIBLIOGRAPHY


Bleyer A, Agus ZS: Approach to nephrolithiasis, *Kidney* 25(2), 1992.

Coe FL, Parks JH: *Nephrolithiasis: pathogenesis and treatment,* ed 2, Chicago, 1988, Mosby.

Coe FL, Parks JH, Asplin JR: The pathogenesis and treatment of kidney stones, *N Engl J Med* 327(16):1141, 1992.

Drach GW: Urinary lithiasis: etiology, diagnosis, and medical management. In Walsh PC et al, editors: *Campbell's urology,* ed 6, Philadelphia, 1992, WB Saunders.

Dyer RB, Zagoria RJ: Radiological patterns of mineralization as predictor of urinary stone etiology, associated pathology, and therapeutic outcome, *J Stone Dis* 4(4):272, 1992.

Goldfarb S: Dietary factors in the pathogenesis and prophylaxis of calcium nephrolithiasis, *Kidney Int* 34:544, 1988.

Johnson CM et al: Renal stone epidemiology: a 25 year study in Rochester, Minnesota, *Kidney Int* 16:624, 1979.

Lingeman JE et al: Extracorporeal shock wave lithotripsy: the Methodist Hospital of Indiana experience, *J Urol* 135:1134, 1986.

Liong ML et al: Treatment options for proximal ureteral urolithiasis: review and recommendations, *J Urol* 141:504, 1989.

Preminger GM: Sonographic, piezoelectric lithotripsy: More bang for your buck, *J Endourology* 3:321, 1989.

Preminger GM: The metabolic evaluation of patients with recurrent nephrolithiasis: A review of comprehensive and simplified approaches, *J Urol* 141:760, 1989.

Preminger GM et al: Percutaneous nephrostolithotomy versus open renal surgery: A comparative study. *JAMA* 254:1054, 1985.

Preminger GM, Kennedy TJ: Ureteral stone extraction utilizing nondeflectable, flexible fiberoptic ureteroscopes. *J Endourology* Vol 1, 1:31, 1987.

Preminger GM: Renal calculi: pathogenesis, diagnosis, and medical therapy, *Semin Nephrol* 12(2):200, 1992.

Resnick MI, Pak CYC: *Urolithiasis: a medical and surgical reference,* Philadelphia, 1990, WB Saunders.

Sakhaee K et al: Contrasting effects of potassium citrate and sodium citrate therapies on urinary chemistries and crystallization of stone-forming salts, *Kidney Int* 24:348, 1983.

Segura JW et al: Percutaneous removal of kidney stones: review of 1,000 cases. *J Urol* 134:1077, 1985.

Uribarri J, Oh MS, Carroll HJ: The first kidney stone, *Ann Intern Med* 111:1006, 1989.

Williams HE: Oxalic acid and the hyperoxaluric syndromes, *Kidney Int* 13:410, 1978.


CHAPTER

# 93 Glomerular and Tubulointerstitial Disease

**Paul G. Schmitz**

## ETIOLOGIC CLASSIFICATION

Glomerular and tubulointerstitial diseases are the most common causes of chronic renal insufficiency. A combination of clinical and pathologic attributes has been used to classify these diverse disease processes. A precise understanding of the relationship between clinical features and histopathology is necessary to classify glomerular and tubulointerstitial renal disease correctly.

### Glomerular disease

The clinical hallmark of glomerular disease is proteinuria and/or hematuria. Proteinuria in the nephrotic range or the presence of red blood cell (RBC) casts in the urine sediment is virtually pathognomonic for significant glomerular inflammation. Importantly, most glomerular diseases can be conveniently classified into those presenting with a "nephrotic" urine sediment versus those with a "nephritic" urine pattern (Tables 93-1 and 93-2). In some instances, combined proteinuria, hematuria, and RBC casts are the presenting features (e.g., membranoproliferative glomerulonephritis). Thus, examination of the urine is a crucial initial step in the clinical evaluation of glomerular disease. Glomerular disease can be further classified into primary (idiopathic) and secondary (e.g., systemic lupus erythematosus [SLE], amyloidosis) causes. Since the clinical presentation may not accurately predict the underlying histology, a renal biopsy is often indicated in the evaluation of suspected glomerular involvement.

### Tubulointerstitial disease

Although scarring of the tubules and interstitium often occurs with glomerular disease, primary tubulointerstitial injury can occur as the principal manifestation of a variety of toxic, metabolic, and genetic diseases (see the box on p. 1262). Acute tubular necrosis secondary to ischemic or toxic injury is the most common cause of hospital-acquired acute renal insufficiency. Other common causes of tubulointerstitial disease include allergic interstitial nephritis, polycystic kidney disease, analgesic nephropathy, and chronic pyelonephritis. In contrast to glomerular involvement, tubulointerstitial disease is characterized by mild proteinuria (usually greater than 1 g/24 hours) and impaired distal or proximal tubular function (renal tubular acidosis, glucosuria, aminoaciduria, impaired urinary concentration). Although, *acute* tubulointerstitial injury is often characterized by an active urinary sediment (white blood cells [WBCs], WBC casts, and RBCs), a "bland" urinalysis is the rule in *chronic* tubulointerstitial disease.

**Table 93-1.** Clinical classification of the nephrotic syndrome

| Principal causes | Associated histology |
|---|---|
| Idiopathic (75%) | Membranous glomerulonephritis<br>Focal segmental glomerulosclerosis<br>Membranoproliferative glomerulonephritis<br>Minimal change disease<br>Rapidly progressive glomerulonephritis |
| Diabetes | Nodular glomerulosclerosis |
| Systemic lupus erythematosus | Membranous glomerulonephritis |
| Amyloidosis (myeloma) | Amyloid deposition |
| Malignant disease (lymphoma, solid tumors) | Membranous glomerulonephritis or minimal change lesion |
| Intravenous drug abuse and HIV infection | Focal segmental glomerulosclerosis |
| Drugs and toxins (captopril, NSAIDS, gold, penicillamine) | Varying, usually minimal change lesion or focal segmental glomerulosclerosis |
| Infectious disease (hepatitis B, occasionally postinfectious such as endocarditis, infected arteriovenous shunt) | Membranous glomerulonephritis or proliferative glomerulonephritis (diffuse or focal) |

*HIV,* Human immunodeficiency virus; *NSAIDs,* nonsteroidal antiinflammatory drugs.

## Classification of tubulointerstitial nephritis

**Toxic**
Acute tubular necrosis (aminoglycosides)
Chronic pyelonephritis (analgesics, lithium, lead)
Cyclosporine nephrotoxicity

**Ischemic**
Acute tubular necrosis

**Allergic interstitial nephritis** (see the box on p. 1272)

**Cystic renal disease**
Simple renal cysts
Acquired cystic disease
Medullary sponge kidney
Polycystic kidney disease

**Infectious**
Acute and chronic pyelonephritis (reflux nephropathy)

**Miscellaneous**
Acute urate nephropathy
Multiple myeloma
Hypercalcemia
Sarcoidosis
Hematologic malignancy (lymphoma)
Transplant rejection

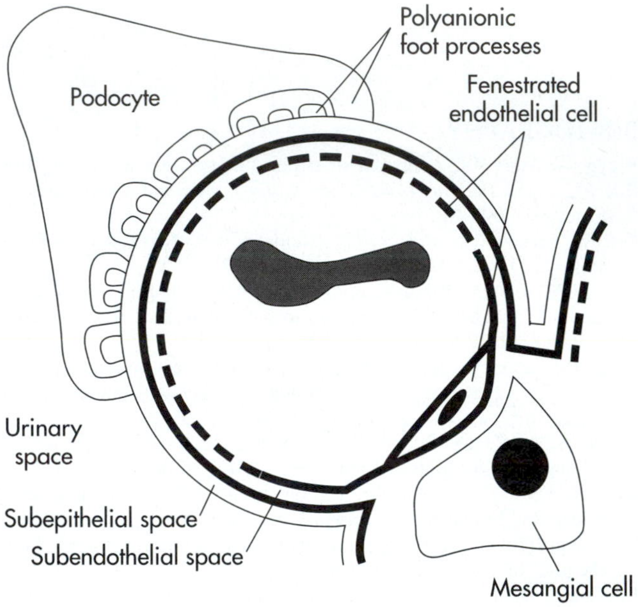


**Fig. 93-1.** Schematic depiction of normal glomerular anatomy.

# PATHOPHYSIOLOGY

## Normal anatomy and function

The glomerulus is a specialized vascular structure that functions as the basic filtering unit of the kidney (Fig. 93-1). Glomerular cells are comprised of endothelial cells, epithelial cells (podocytes), mesangial cells, and resident macrophages. These cells serve differential functions, including regulation of renal blood flow and intraglomerular pressure, synthesis and degradation of extracellular matrix, modulation of glomerular permeability for various macromolecules, and phagocytosis. An important function of the normal glomerulus is to restrict passage of certain plasma constituents while allowing filtration of endogenous waste products. The glomerular filtration barrier is composed of three layers: an inner fenestrated endothelium, a middle basement membrane, and an outer visceral epithelial cell. These elements form a physical barrier limiting the passage of molecules with molecular weights exceeding 50,000 daltons. Moreover, the visceral epithelial cell lining contains negatively charged sialoglycoproteins and thus impedes filtration of negatively charged substances (e.g., albumin).

The renal interstitium is composed of interstitial cells embedded within extracellular matrix. Interstitial cells provide physical support for the renal tubules embedded within the interstitium. Certain toxins (analgesics), drugs

**Table 93-2.** Clinical classification of the nephritic syndrome

| Principal causes | Associated histology |
|---|---|
| Rapidly progressive glomerulonephritis | Crescentic (>60% of glomeruli) glomerulonephritis |
| Type 1 (Goodpasture's syndrome) | |
| Type 2 (immune complex: SLE, postinfectious) | |
| Type 3 or pauci-immune (Wegener's granulomatosis, systemic vasculitis) | |
| Systemic lupus erythematosus (SLE) | Diffuse or focal proliferative glomerulonephritis |
| Immunoglobulin A (IgA) nephropathy | Mesangioproliferative glomerulonephritis with deposits of IgA |
| Vasculitic syndromes (microscopic polyarteritis, polyarteritis nodosa, SLE, Wegener's, essential mixed cryoglobulinemia) | Focal segmental necrotizing glomerulonephritis with or without crescents |
| Membranoproliferative glomerulonephritis (idiopathic, immune disorders: SLE, endocarditis, cryoglobulinemia) | Type 1: "tram tracking"<br>Type 2: dense linear deposits in basement membrane |
| Postinfectious (endocarditis, infected arteriovenous shunt) | Diffuse proliferative glomerulonephritis with immune deposits |
| Thrombotic microangiopathies | Endotheliosis and platelet microthrombi |

(antibiotics), and genetic diseases (polycystic kidney disease) predominantly affect the renal interstitium and/or tubules. However, since glomeruli and tubules fundamentally depend on one another, diseases affecting one structure will inevitably lead to destruction of its associated structure.

## Pathogenesis of glomerular and tubulointerstitial injury

A variety of factors have been implicated in the pathogenesis and progression of glomerular and tubulointerstitial disease. Glomerular injury is frequently accompanied by deposition of immunoglobulins within the glomerulus. Experimental models of autoimmune glomerulonephritis have greatly advanced our understanding of the pathogenesis of immune glomerular injury. For example, induction of antibody in rats with the tubular specific antigen, $FXA_1$, results in a lesion that is indistinguishable from human membranous glomerulonephritis. Glomerular subepithelial immune deposits are present on electron microscopic examination of renal tissue. Antibody deposition presumably leads to recruitment of inflammatory cells, activation of serum complement components, and release of a variety of mediators of cell injury (interleukins, tumor necrosis factor, reactive oxygen metabolites) (Fig. 93-2). T lymphocyte activation may also contribute to glomerular injury in classic autoimmune glomerulonephritis. Two mechanisms may explain antibody deposition within the glomerulus: (1) circulating antibody bound to a fixed glomerular antigen or (2) passive glomerular entrapment of circulating immune complexes. Similar mechanisms of immune renal injury have been described in tubulointerstitial disease. An appreciation of the importance of immune injury in the pathogenesis of glomerular disease provides the basis for its treatment with immunomodulatory therapy.

A variety of nonimmune mechanisms may contribute to the initiation and progression of chronic renal insufficiency. The significance of nonimmune-mediated renal injury is underscored by the absence of immune deposits in such common renal diseases as diabetic nephropathy and hypertensive nephrosclerosis. Animal models of experimental renal disease have demonstrated that a significant reduction in nephron mass leads to adaptive changes in the remaining (remnant) glomeruli, which may

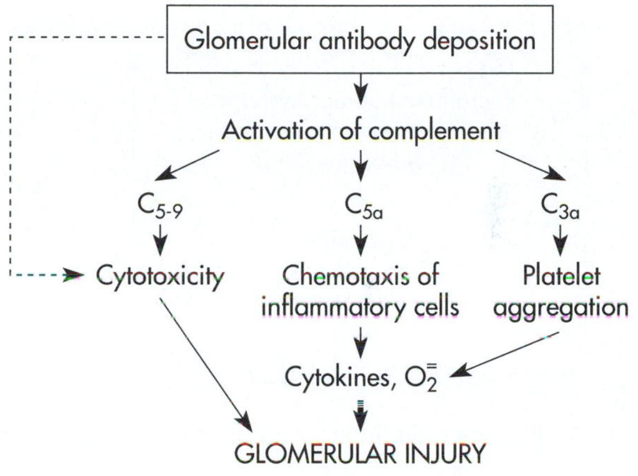


**Fig. 93-2.** Immunopathogenesis of glomerular injury. (See text for discussion.)

serve to potentiate the progression of renal disease. For example, removal of five sixths of the renal mass in the rat results in glomerular capillary hypertension and progressive renal injury. Recent studies in nonprimates have demonstrated that dietary reduction in protein and converting-enzyme inhibition (captopril) attenuate the glomerular hemodynamic and ultrastructural changes occurring in remnant nephrons. Whether such therapeutic strategies can be extrapolated to human renal disease is currently being investigated.

Although hemodynamic mechanisms of renal injury have received the greatest attention, a variety of other factors have also been postulated to be important in the progression of renal injury (Fig. 93-3). These include: (1) abnormalities in circulating lipids and hormones, (2) perturbations in tissue lipid composition, (3) enhanced renal synthesis of eicosanoids, (4) mesangial cell proliferation, (5) enhanced matrix deposition, (6) platelet aggregation, and (7) secretion of growth factors and other biologically active substances (interleukins, tumor necrosis factor, growth factors). Treatment strategies aimed at correcting these factors may provide a novel approach to treating medical renal disease.

### Pathophysiology of the nephrotic syndrome

The nephrotic syndrome is defined as a urine protein excretion rate in excess of 3.5 g/24 hours. Frequently, hypoalbuminemia, edema, and hyperlipidemia accompany nephrotic range proteinuria (Fig. 93-4). The mechanism(s) underlying the nephrotic syndrome remain poorly understood; however, an abnormality of glomerular permselectivity is the hallmark of patients with this syndrome. The altered glomerular permselectivity may be due to injured epithelial cells and loss of sialoglycoproteins (minimal change disease) or physical disruption of the glomerular filtration barrier (necrotizing glomerulonephritis). The magnitude of proteinuria is influenced by changes in glomerular filtration rate (GFR), plasma albumin concentration, and dietary intake of protein.

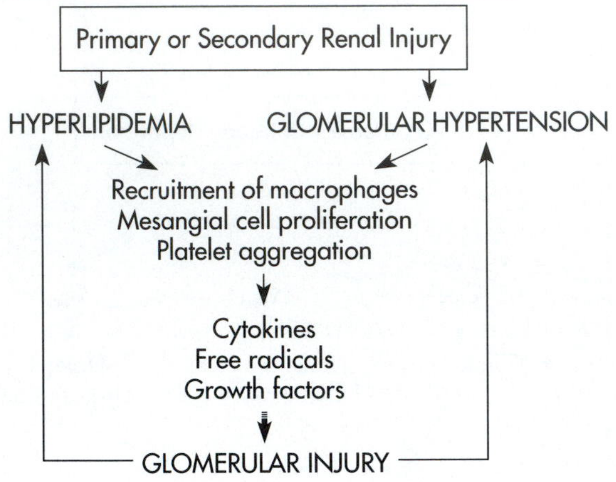


**Fig. 93-3.** Possible nonimmune basis of progressive renal injury.

Renal sodium and water retention leading to edema formation occurs often in patients with the nephrotic syndrome. The mechanism of enhanced tubular sodium and water reabsorption has been attributed to a reduced effective circulating volume caused by vascular redistribution of fluid. However, recent evidence suggests that plasma volume is not contracted in the nephrotic syndrome. Furthermore, the gradient of plasma to interstitial oncotic pressure is unchanged. Other studies suggest that disturbances in intrarenal physical factors, atrial natriuretic peptides, or sympathetic nervous system activity may account for the changes in tubular sodium and water reabsorption in the nephrotic syndrome.

Since hepatic synthesis of albumin can normally increase several fold (up to 30 g/day), the mechanism of hypoalbuminemia in the setting of nephrotic range proteinuria has generated much debate. Possible factors contributing to hypoalbuminemia include (1) enhanced degradation of albumin by the kidney, (2) impaired hepatic synthesis of albumin, and (3) extrarenal changes in albumin catabolism. Hyperlipidemia also accompanies urinary loss of protein and is thought to be secondary to increased hepatic synthesis of very-low-density lipoproteins (VLDLs). An increase in low-density lipoproteins (LDLs) is also common in patients with the nephrotic syndrome and is probably the result of VLDL catabolism. Not surprisingly, an increase in serum cholesterol and triglycerides is frequently noted in patients with the nephrotic syndrome. Whether the increased incidence of cardiovascular disease noted in patients with the nephrotic syndrome is independently modified by changes in serum lipids is unclear. Although insufficient data exist to permit precise recommendations, the results of preliminary studies suggest that patients at high risk for cardiovascular disease may benefit from treatment of hyperlipidemia.

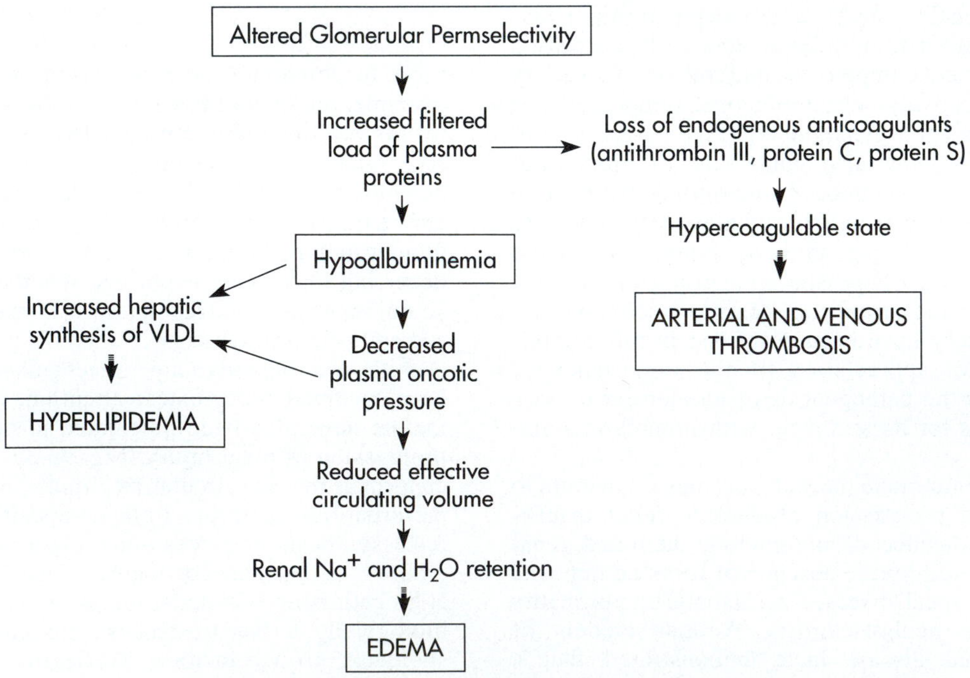


**Fig. 93-4.** Pathophysiology of the nephrotic syndrome. (See text for discussion.)

There is an increased incidence of arterial and venous thrombosis in the nephrotic syndrome. Urinary loss of endogenous anticoagulants, particularly antithrombin III, protein C, and protein S, may account for the hypercoagulable state. Indeed, plasma levels of these substances are often decreased in patients with the nephrotic syndrome. Nonetheless, considerable overlap exists in normal patients and patients with the nephrotic syndrome. Whether systemic anticoagulation should be initiated prophylactically in all patients with severe proteinuria remains controversial.

## HISTORY AND PHYSICAL EXAMINATION

A careful history is important in the differential diagnosis of glomerular or tubulointerstitial injury. For example, childhood nephrotic syndrome is most likely secondary to minimal change disease, whereas idiopathic adult nephrotic syndrome is frequently a consequence of membranous glomerulonephritis. A careful drug history may provide a clue to the presence of nephrotoxic renal injury. Intravenous (IV) drug abuse (heroin) has been described in association with focal glomerulosclerosis and the nephrotic syndrome. Eliciting the duration of the illness is helpful in establishing the chronicity of the process. The presence of comorbid conditions such as diabetes, cancer, SLE, or chronic active hepatitis may also provide an important clue to the underlying renal histology (e.g., membranous glomerulonephritis and malignant disease). Finally, obtaining a detailed family history to evaluate for the presence of hereditary nephritis or polycystic kidney disease is invaluable.

The physical examination may also provide important information in the evaluation of patients with renal disease. Hypertension and edema are frequently noted and are often the presenting signs in patients with significant renal disease. All patients should be carefully examined for the presence of edema, skin rashes, arthritic changes, adenopathy, and neuropathy. The presence of a malar rash in a patient with renal insufficiency, proteinuria, and hematuria strongly suggests renal involvement secondary to SLE. In contrast, peripheral neuropathy in an elderly patient with proteinuria and an elevated serum globulin should prompt an investigation for systemic amyloidosis. The presence of livedo reticularis in a patient recently undergoing cardiac catheterization should raise the possibility of cholesterol embolization. Abdominal pain and a purpuric rash in an adolescent with renal failure would strongly support the diagnosis of Henoch-Schönlein purpura. In addition, palpation of the abdomen may reveal the presence of irregular or enlarged kidneys consistent with polycystic kidney disease or renal cell carcinoma.

## LABORATORY STUDIES AND DIAGNOSTIC PROCEDURES

### Examination of urine

Patients with clinically significant renal disease most often have an abnormal urinalysis (hematuria, proteinuria, casts) and/or a decrease in GFR. Therefore, examination of the urine specimen and determination of the serum creatinine provide the basis for the initial evaluation of renal disease. Isolated or transient abnormalities in the urinalysis must be distinguished from abnormalities secondary to glomerular or tubulointerstitial disease. Moreover, false-positive elevations in the serum creatinine must be differentiated from a true reduction in GFR.

*Transient proteinuria* may occur in up to 10% of otherwise healthy individuals. The magnitude of proteinuria is typically mild but can rarely be severe (more than 3 g/24 hours). Transient proteinuria is particularly common in patients with congestive heart failure and infection. Other stresses, such as fever and exercise, may induce proteinuria. The mechanism responsible for the induction of transient proteinuria is poorly understood but may involve changes in the circulating levels of stress hormones (angiotensin II, epinephrine). These hormones have been shown to alter glomerular permeability for protein and to modulate intrarenal blood flow and glomerular pressure. Importantly, transient episodes of proteinuria are not associated with the presence of significant glomerular diseases and thus are considered benign.

*Postural,* or *orthostatic, proteinuria* is noted only during upright posture and not during recumbency. The magnitude of proteinuria is generally mild (less than 1 g/day) but can occasionally exceed 3 g/day. It is much more common in adolescents and is rare in patients over 30 years old. The diagnosis rests on establishing the relationship of posture to the presence of protein in the urine. However, it is important to keep in mind that postural changes in urine protein excretion can sometimes occur in serious renal diseases. Therefore, benign orthostatic proteinuria should only be diagnosed when the recumbent protein excretion rate is less than 50 mg/day.

In contrast to proteinuria, *hematuria* can arise anywhere within the urinary tract. The most common cause of hematuria in an adult is urinary tract disease (e.g., prostatitis, renal calculi, cystitis). In the absence of RBC casts, a thorough urologic evaluation (intravenous pyelography [IVP], cystoscopy) should be performed before consideration of a renal biopsy. Recently, RBC morphology has been used to distinguish a renal parenchymal from a nonparenchymal source of hematuria. Typically, extrarenal hematuria is characterized by uniform red blood cell morphology, whereas glomerular hematuria is usually accompanied by dysmorphic cells as a result of their passage through the glomerular basement membrane and the hypertonic medullary interstitium.

### Measurement of glomerular filtration rate

The hallmark of significant renal disease is a reduction in GFR. The assessment of GFR generally begins with a serum creatinine determination. At steady state the serum creatinine measurement inversely correlates with GFR. Thus, a doubling of the serum creatinine (e.g., 1 mg/dl to 2 mg/dl) indicates a 50% reduction in the GFR. Since the rate of creatinine production largely depends on muscle mass, changes in serum creatinine may occur with changes in lean body mass. Therefore, a random serum creatinine determination only provides an estimate of the absolute GFR (see Chapter 89).

The clearance of endogenous creatinine is the most widely used method of determining GFR. The endogenous creatinine clearance tends to overestimate GFR, however, since approximately 10% of urine creatinine is derived from tubular secretion. The endogenous creatinine clearance may grossly overestimate the GFR when renal function is reduced by more than 75%. Under these conditions the percentage of creatinine undergoing tubular secretion may exceed 50%. To circumvent this problem, some investigators have pretreated patients with cimetidine, a competitive inhibitor of tubular creatinine secretion, for 3 days, followed by a 24-urine collection for creatinine clearance. Alternate methods of measuring GFR using radionuclide plasma disappearance curves are becoming increasingly available in hospital laboratories. Whether these methods will replace traditional methods of measuring GFR remains to be determined.

### Serologic studies

Determination of serum complement components (C3, C4, CH50) constitutes an important step in the evaluation of patients with suspected glomerular disease. Quantitating serum complement components may also provide a useful biologic index of disease activity and response to therapy. Other serologic markers useful in the evaluation of glomerular disease include serum cryoglobulins (essential mixed cryoglobulinemia), hepatitis serologies (membranous glomerulonephritis), human immunodeficiency virus (HIV) screening (focal glomerulosclerosis), serum and urine immunoelectrophoresis (myeloma, amyloidosis), and quantitative determination of antinuclear antibodies (SLE).

Recently, the presence of circulating antibodies to specific cytoplasmic antigens (antineutrophil cytoplasmic antibodies, or ANCAs) has been described in association with renal vasculitis. These antibodies appear to have several different antigenic specificities, but two major classes have been reported using indirect immunofluorescence staining. Antibodies with a cytoplasmic pattern of staining on indirect immunofluorescence (C-ANCA) are directed toward a serine protease. In contrast, antibodies with specificity to myeloperoxidase demonstrate a perinuclear staining pattern. Interestingly, the C-ANCA is more frequently associated with Wegener's granulomatosis, whereas the P-ANCA is more often noted in patients with systemic vasculitis (e.g., polyarteritis nodosa) (Fig. 93-5). Determination of the presence or absence of ANCA is particularly helpful in establishing the renal diagnosis in the setting of a rapidly progressive glomerulonephritis (see later discussion).

### Radiologic studies

The usefulness of radiologic procedures in establishing the etiology of glomerular or tubulointerstitial disease is limited. However, ultrasonic determination of kidney size can be useful in the evaluation of unexplained renal insufficiency. Kidneys measuring less than 10 cm in length are highly suggestive of a chronic process and would tend to mitigate against further evaluation. Asymmetric kidney size suggests the possibility of renal vascular disease. Renal angiography, however, should be undertaken with great caution in patients with serum creatinine levels greater than 2.0 mg/dl. Abnormal renal scintigraphy is seen in virtually all patients with significant glomerular or tubulointerstitial disease and thus adds little in establishing the correct diagnosis. Magnetic resonance imaging (MRI) may be used to evaluate the presence of renal vein thromboses.

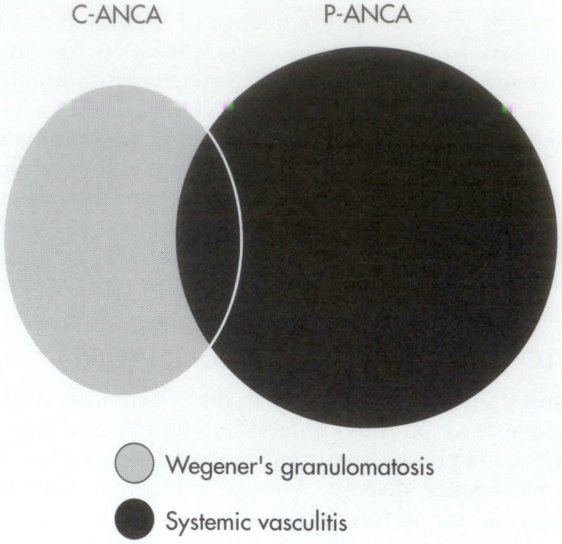


**Fig. 93-5.** Relationship of C-ANCA and P-ANCA in renal vasculitis and Wegener's granulomatosis. *ANCA,* Antineutrophil cytoplasmic antibody.

### Renal biopsy

The renal biopsy remains the "gold standard" for establishing the diagnosis of significant glomerular and tubulointerstitial renal disease. Often the clinical description and laboratory features of renal disease may be insufficient to arrive at a definitive diagnosis. In these circumstances, a renal biopsy is necessary to delineate the underlying disease (see Chapter 89).

## DIFFERENTIAL DIAGNOSIS

### Glomerular disease associated with a nephrotic pattern

Classifying glomerular disease according to the urinary findings (nephrotic versus nephritic) is a useful way of formulating a differential diagnosis (Fig. 93-6). Five entities account for most cases of the nephrotic syndrome in an adult: (1) diabetic nephropathy, (2) membranous glomerulonephritis (MGN), (3) focal segmental glomerulosclerosis (FSGS), (4) amyloidosis, and (5) minimal change disease (MCD).

***Diabetic nephropathy.*** Diabetic nephropathy accounts for the majority (up to 40%) of patients receiving dialysis for end-stage renal disease (ESRD). The incidence of diabetic renal disease is greater in Mexican and African-Americans and in some Native American populations. The presence of microalbuminuria (greater than 30 mg/day) is the hallmark of incipient diabetic renal disease and is predictive of inexorable progression to ESRD. "Hyperfiltration" (GFR greater than 140 ml/minute) is usually present in insulin-dependent diabetes mellitus (IDDM) in the early stages of the disease and precedes the development of microalbuminuria, which occurs in less than 40% of the patients, especially in those with poor glycemic control and hyperlipidemia. With the advent of microalbuminuria, renal function slowly deteriorates over 15 to 20 years, ultimately progressing to ESRD (Fig. 93-7). Whether patients with non-IDDM evolve through similar

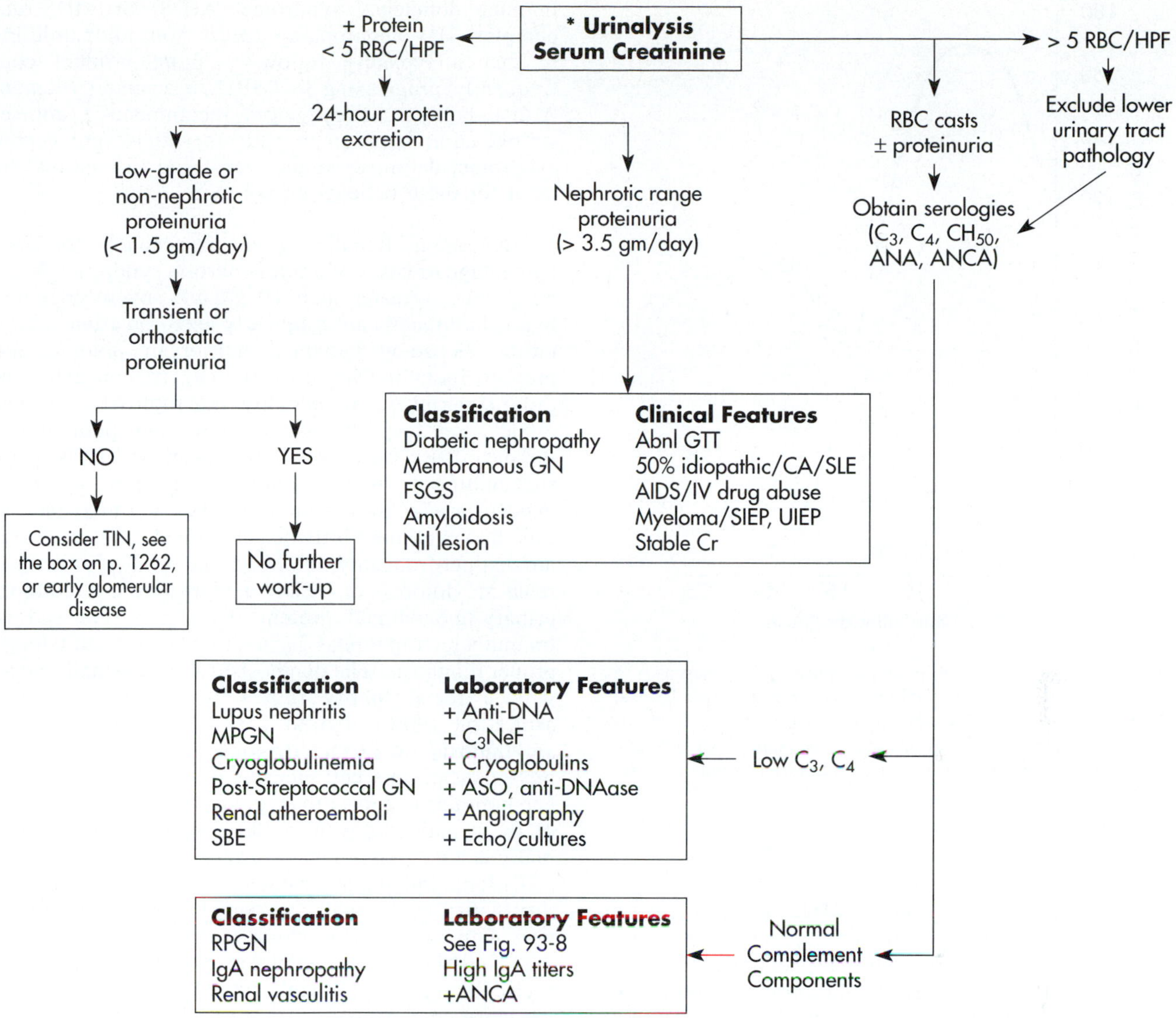


**Fig. 93-6.** Approach to the differential diagnosis of suspected glomerular disease. *RBC,* Red blood cells; *ANA,* antinuclear antibodies; *ANCA,* antineutrophil cytoplasmic antibodies; *GTT,* glucose tolerance test; *CA,* cancer; *SLE,* systemic lupus erythematosus; *SIEP* and *UIEP,* serum and urine immunoelectrophoresis; *C3NeF,* C3 nephritic factor; *ASO,* antistreptolysin O antibody. A renal biopsy is frequently required to establish the clinical diagnosis.

stages of hyperfiltration and microalbuminuria is unclear. Nephropathy appears to be strongly associated with other complications of diabetes (e.g., retinopathy, neuropathy). Indeed, in the absence of retinopathy, one should question the diagnosis of diabetic nephropathy.

Systemic hypertension plays an important role in the progression of diabetic nephropathy, since antihypertensive therapy can significantly attenuate the progression of renal disease. Angiotensin converting-enzyme inhibitors appear selectively to alter intrarenal hemodynamics and ameliorate renal injury and proteinuria in humans independent of alterations in systemic blood pressure. A general strategy for managing hypertension in diabetic patients with renal disease is to initiate therapy with converting-enzyme inhibitors in patients with mildly to moderately compromised renal function (creatinine greater than 2.0 mg/dl). The initiation of converting-enzyme inhibitors demands careful monitoring for renal functional deterioration and hyperkalemia. In patients intolerant of converting-enzyme inhibitors, the use of diltiazem or verapamil may be reasonable alternatives based on preliminary studies. A protein-restricted diet (0.6 g/kg/day) has also been shown to slow the rate of progressive renal disease in diabetic renal disease. However, many patients find these diets unpalatable, and frequent assessment of nutritional status is necessary with extremely low protein intakes (less than 40 g/day). See Chapter 33 for more details.

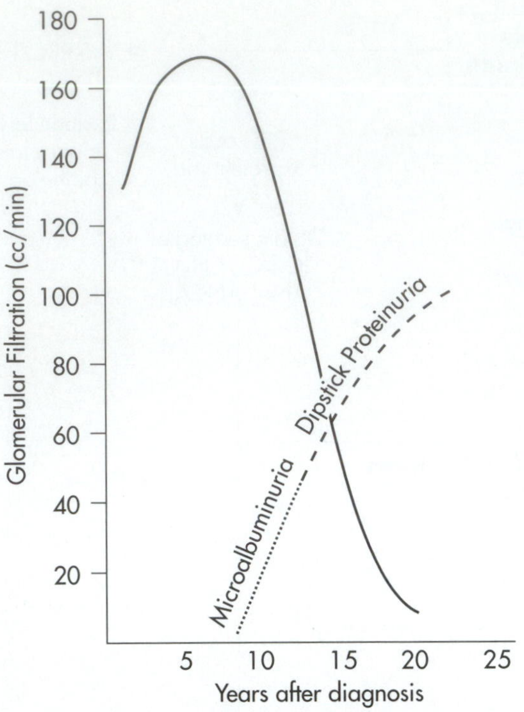


**Fig. 93-7.** Stages of diabetic nephropathy. An increase in glomerular filtration rate (hyperfiltration) is noted within several years of the diagnosis. Hyperfiltration is followed by microalbuminuria, which precedes frank proteinuria by 3 to 5 years. Microalbuminuria is the precursor of end-stage renal disease.

***Membranous glomerulonephritis.*** MGN accounts for up to 40% of adult patients with the idiopathic nephrotic syndrome. The pathologic hallmark of MGN is the presence of glomerular subepithelial immune deposits on electron microscopic examination of renal tissue. A variety of underlying conditions have also been described in association with this clinicopathologic syndrome. These include chronic hepatitis B, SLE (lupus nephritis type V), malignancies, and some drugs (gold, penicillamine). For unknown reasons, the incidence of thrombotic events is more common in MGN than other causes of the nephrotic syndrome. The natural history of MGN varies depending on the underlying cause, but in idiopathic MGN, up to 50% of patients remain in partial or complete remission 10 to 15 years after the original diagnosis. Less than 25% will succumb to ESRD. Because of the variable clinical course, considerable controversy exists regarding the optimal treatment for these patients. Some series report striking benefits with a combination of chlorambucil and prednisone, whereas other investigators have been unable to confirm these findings.

***Focal segmental glomerulosclerosis.*** FSGS accounts for up to 10% to 15% of cases of adult nephrotic syndrome. Unfortunately, many of these patients progress to ESRD within 5 years of the diagnosis. Although most cases appear to be idiopathic, many have been reported in patients after IV drug abuse (heroin) and with acquired immune deficiency syndrome (AIDS) or AIDS-related complex. HIV nephropathy differs from idiopathic FSGS in that it typically follows a more virulent course, frequently progressing to ESRD in a matter of months. Although some investigators recommend a course of steroid administration in patients with severe nephrotic syndrome, definitive studies regarding the optimal treatment for these patients do not exist.

***Amyloidosis.*** Renal amyloidosis accounts for a small percentage of cases of adult nephrotic syndrome. Massive proteinuria (greater than 10 g/day), severe edema, and hypoalbuminemia are frequently noted on clinical presentation. In some patients, multiorgan involvement is present, including hepatosplenomegaly, congestive heart failure, peripheral neuropathy, macroglossia, and carpal tunnel syndrome. The overall prognosis is poor, and often the mean survival is less than 1 year, with most patients succumbing to renal failure or infection. *Light chain deposition disease* (LCDD) involves a similar pathogenesis; however, the fibrils detected on electron microscopy are distinct from amyloid. More than 80% of patients with renal amyloidosis or LCDD demonstrate a circulating or urinary monoclonal protein. Thus, a serum and urine immunoelectrophoresis is invaluable in establishing the proper diagnosis. The diagnosis can occasionally be made with a rectal biopsy (60%) or a transcutaneous fat aspiration (90%). Up to 25% of patients with renal amyloidosis or LCDD demonstrate the presence of a malignant plasma cell clone (e.g., myeloma). Melphalan and prednisone appear to offer promise in the management of these patients, even in the absence of a plasma cell malignancy.

Chronic inflammatory disorders such as rheumatoid arthritis may occasionally be complicated by renal deposition of amyloid. The amyloidogenic protein in these disorders is distinct from light chains and may be derived from a circulating protein synthesized in the liver. Treatment for these conditions is directed at the underlying disease process.

***Minimal change disease.*** The most common histology detected in the childhood nephrotic syndrome is MCD, also known as *lipoid nephrosis* or *nil disease.* Up to 25% of adults with the nephrotic syndrome may also present with MCD. Generally, only "fusion" of the glomerular epithelial cell foot processes are observed with electron microscopy. Light microscopy and immunofluorescent studies are unremarkable. The pathogenesis appears to be secondary to diffuse injury of the epithelial cell foot processes and loss of polyanionic sialoglycoproteins. Patients with this syndrome typically have edema, hypoalbuminemia, hyperlipidemia, and a *normal GFR.* Rarely, patients may develop acute renal failure, presumably secondary to profound volume depletion. Although most cases are idiopathic, MCD has occasionally been noted in association with hematologic malignancy (Hodgkin's disease) or drug administration (NSAIDs, gold, lithium). Most patients with idiopathic MCD respond to corticosteroid therapy, although remissions are less frequent in adults. Although an excellent response is usually detected within 2 weeks of initiating therapy, some individuals may require up to 12 weeks to respond. Frequent relapses and resistance may occur in some individuals, and long-term administration of low-dose steroids (up to 1 year) may be required to induce a permanent remission. An occasional patient with refractory disease may respond to immunotherapy with either cytotoxic agents (cyclophosphamide and chlorambucil) or cyclosporine.

### Glomerular disease associated with a nephritic urinary sediment

***Hereditary nephritis.*** Hereditary nephritis, or Alport syndrome, is characterized by lenticular opacities, renal insufficiency, and sensorineural hearing loss. Three modes of inheritance have been described: X-linked dominant, autosomal dominant, and rarely autosomal recessive. The differing modes of inheritance are associated with the expression of different phenotypes. For example, X-linked dominant families present with renal insufficiency and deafness, which is usually less severe in females. In contrast, autosomal dominant or recessive inheritance results in renal insufficiency but usually no auditory or eye involvement. The pathologic hallmark in the kidney consists of thinning and splitting (lamination) of the glomerular basement membrane. Urinary findings frequently include hematuria and proteinuria; the latter can be severe. Most males with this disorder progress to ESRD by age 40. Females typically follow a less virulent course, although some may progress to ESRD by age 30. The pathogenesis of this disorder is poorly understood, although recent evidence suggests that patients have a deficient basement membrane antigen. Unfortunately, no specific therapy exists for hereditary nephritis.

***Postinfectious glomerulonephritis.*** Poststreptococcal glomerulonephritis (PSGN) is the most common form of postinfectious glomerular injury. Certain strains of "nephritogenic" streptococci are more frequently associated with glomerular inflammation (type 12 β-hemolytic streptococci and type 49 β-hemolytic streptococci). Electron microscopy reveals granular deposits of immune complexes (IgG and complement) in the subepithelial space. Affected glomeruli usually show diffuse proliferation of inflammatory cells and crescent formation. Epidemiologic studies suggest that glomerulonephritis may occur in up to 25% of patients infected with nephritogenic strains of group A β-hemolytic streptococci. Serum complement components, particularly C3, are low, and circulating antibodies to antistreptolysin O (ASO) and DNAase B are usually elevated. The clinical manifestations of PSGN range from florid nephrotic syndrome to asymptomatic hematuria and proteinuria. Although most patients spontaneously recover, some may exhibit mild urinary abnormalities for several years. Sporadic reports of patients with chronic renal insufficiency and severe intrarenal scarring occurring 30 to 40 years after an acute episode have been described. The mechanism of progression to ESRD is uncertain in these patients. Other infectious causes of diffuse proliferative glomerulonephritis and immune complex deposition include infected ventriculoatrial shunts and subacute bacterial endocarditis. These disorders typically resolve after appropriate antimicrobial therapy and/or removal of the infected shunt.

***Membranoproliferative glomerulonephritis (MPGN).*** MPGN is classically associated with a combination of hematuria and nephrotic range proteinuria. The clinical course of renal disease ranges from a fulminant, rapidly progressive glomerulonephritis to a slowly progressive course characterized by the nephrotic syndrome. Two histologic subtypes have been characterized: type 1 MPGN is associated with mesangial and subendothelial immune deposits resulting in the characteristic "tram track" appearance on light microscopy; and type 2 MPGN (dense deposit disease) is characterized by heavy deposits of immune complexes along the entire length of the glomerular basement membrane. Both types of MPGN are associated with hypocomplementemia, although type 1 is characterized by activation of the classic pathway (low C3 and C4) while type 2 is characterized by activation of the alternate pathway (low C3). The latter is thought to occur as a consequence of persistent activation of C3 via an antibody (C3 nephritic factor, C3NeF), which stabilizes and prolongs the half-life of C3 convertase. Although most cases of MPGN are idiopathic, an association with SLE, chronic hepatitis B, chronic lymphocytic leukemia, cryoglobulinemia, IV drug abuse, and transplant rejection has also been reported.

The treatment of idiopathic MPGN is controversial. An investigation in childhood MPGN demonstrated a beneficial effect of long-term low-dose administration of corticosteroids. However, there is no evidence in adults that steroid use is of benefit. A controlled trial of aspirin and dipyridamole for 1 year in adult MPGN appeared to slow the progression of renal injury when compared to placebo. However, other studies did not confirm the benefits of antiplatelet drugs.

***Systemic lupus erythematosus.*** Renal disease in the setting of SLE is extremely common. Approximately 90% of patients have abnormalities on a renal biopsy. In many instances, pathologic abnormalities are present in the absence of clinical or urinary findings. Five histologic subtypes of renal disease have been described in patients with SLE:

Class I: normal
Class II: mesangioproliferative
Class III: focal glomerulonephritis
Class IV: diffuse proliferative glomerulonephritis
Class V: membranous glomerulonephritis

Hypocomplementemia frequently accompanies active SLE nephritis. Serum complement levels are used to follow disease progression and response to treatment. Rarely, lupus nephritis may present without systemic involvement (e.g., renal-limited SLE). The natural history of lupus nephritis is poorly understood. Spontaneous conversion from one histologic subtype to another is often the rule rather than the exception. The uncertain natural history has complicated treatment strategies and the interpretation of interventional studies. Treatment has been best defined for the diffuse proliferative class of SLE nephritis, where response rates to a combination of prednisone and cyclophosphamide are clearly superior to placebo or steroids alone. However, it is uncertain whether treatment for other histologic subtypes of SLE nephritis offers similar benefits.

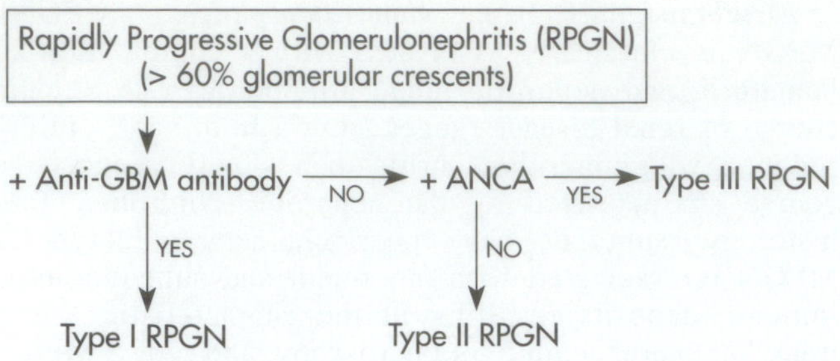


**Fig. 93-8.** Serologic evaluation of a rapidly progressive glomerulonephritis (RPGN). (See text for discussion.)

***Rapidly progressive glomerulonephritis (RPGN).*** The pathologic hallmark of RPGN is the presence of cellular crescents in greater than 60% of the glomeruli examined in a renal biopsy specimen. Three major subtypes of RPGN have been described based on the pathologic distribution of immune deposits.

Type 1 RPGN has linear deposits of immunoglobulin G (IgG) along the glomerular capillary basement membrane. Anti–glomerular basement membrane antibodies (anti-GBM Ab) are also detected in serum. Pulmonary hemorrhage may also occur (classic Goodpasture syndrome), or the immune deposits may be limited to the kidneys.

Type 2 RPGN is characterized by immune complex deposition along the glomerular capillary basement membrane. In most cases the inciting antigen is unknown; however, some individuals may have an underlying malignancy, SLE, or an infectious process.

Type 3 RPGN (pauci-immune) is characterized by the absence of immune deposits within the kidney. Many patients have an underlying systemic vasculitis. Interestingly, type 3 RPGN is frequently characterized by the presence of circulating ANCAs. Serologic evaluation in patients with RPGN can provide an important clue to the pathogenesis of the underlying disease process (Fig. 93-8).

The prognosis and treatment for all three subtypes of RPGN is similar. Early initiation of cytotoxic therapy (500 mg/m$^2$ IV) and prednisone (1000 mg methylprednisolone each day for 3 days followed by 1mg/kg prednisone daily) has led to significant improvement in renal function in most patients. However, response rates are substantially less when patients have severe renal dysfunction (creatinine greater than 5.0 mg/dl). Plasma exchange therapy may be beneficial in patients with high titers of circulating anti-GBM Ab.

***IgA nephropathy.*** Immunoglobulin A (IgA) nephropathy is the most common cause of glomerulonephritis worldwide. Its pathogenesis remains poorly understood, but the presence of increased circulating levels of IgA suggests an abnormal regulation of IgA synthesis or degradation. Although elevations in circulating levels of IgA are found in up to 50% of affected patients, the relative nonspecific nature of this finding precludes its usefulness as a diagnostic test. The presence of mesangial deposits of IgA is pathognomonic. Gross or microscopic hematuria is the most common presenting feature and is often preceded by a viral syndrome. In some individuals a secondary cause of IgA mesangial deposits appears likely (e.g., hepatic disease). Most patients have normal renal function and follow a benign course. However, progression to ESRD with nephrotic range proteinuria may occur in up to 20% of affected individuals. Treatment remains controversial, although some studies suggest that corticosteroid administration may be helpful. A large multicenter trial assessing the efficacy of marine oils in IgA nephropathy is currently underway. Preliminary data suggest that these agents may ameliorate the progression of renal disease in IgA nephropathy.

***Systemic vasculitis.*** The classification of vasculitis is frequently perplexing, partly because of the varying causes of this syndrome and a lack of understanding of the underlying pathophysiology. A reasonable classification system is based on the typical site of involvement and the size of the artery involved. Although systemic vasculitis can frequently present with multiorgan involvement, renal-limited forms are increasingly recognized. Renal vasculitis can be conveniently classified into three major categories: (1) Wegener's granulomatosis, (2) polyarteritis nodosa syndromes, and (3) hypersensitivity vasculitis.

*Wegener's granulomatosis* affects the small and medium-sized arteries and is associated with granuloma formation in the respiratory tract. A sinus biopsy in a patient with sinusitis and renal disease can often yield a diagnosis. Renal biopsy specimens are characterized by segmental necrotizing glomerulonephritis with or without granuloma formation. Immune deposits are conspicuously absent. Affected patients may either have renal-limited disease or pulmonary hemorrhage and/or sinusitis. Response rates as high as 90% are obtained with a combination of cyclophosphamide and prednisone.

*Polyarteritis nodosa* (PAN) is a systemic vasculitis that typically involves the small and medium-sized arteries. There are at least four major subclassifications of PAN, including classic PAN, microscopic PAN, Churg-Strauss syndrome, and the overlap syndrome. Classic PAN affects the medium-sized arteries and often leads to aneurysm formation, which can be demonstrated by angiography. Microscopic PAN is similar in its clinical presentation with the exception of less involvement of other organs and less severe systemic findings. However, renal disease is typically more severe in patients with the microscopic variant of PAN. Churg-Strauss syndrome is characterized by granuloma formation and eosinophilic infiltration of the arteries and veins. Affected patients characteristically have bronchospasm secondary to lung involvement.

*Hypersensitivity vasculitis* affects the small arterioles and venules. Several subtypes have been described, including Henoch-Schönlein purpura, essential mixed cryoglobulinemia, and serum sickness. Henoch-Schönlein purpura is characterized by purpuric lesions of the lower extremities, arthralgias, abdominal pain, and renal failure. Classically, this syndrome is seen in children and resolves spontaneously with supportive care. Adults appear to have less favorable outcomes. Deposits of IgA in the mesangium and mesangial cell proliferation are the hallmarks of this disorder.

Circulating cryoglobulins consist of an antigen, an antibody of the IgG type to the antigen, and a rheumatoid factor IgM antibody to the IgG. The inciting event that stimulates the synthesis of these antibodies is uncertain. In many cases there is an underlying hepatitis B or C infection. Up to 60% of patients with circulating cryoglobulins will present with renal involvement. Characteristic findings include arthralgias, fatigue, purpuric rash, lymphadenopathy, Raynaud's phenomenon, and hepatosplenomegaly. Hypocomplementemia frequently accompanies disease activity. Pathologically, essential mixed cryoglobulinemia is characterized by the presence of intraluminal thrombi consisting of precipitated cryoglobulins. Treatment is similar to other vasculitic syndromes (cytotoxic agents and corticosteroids) but may also include plasmapheresis to remove circulating cryoglobulins. Administration of interferon-α may result in disease remissions.

***Serum sickness.*** Serum sickness is rarely observed in clinical practice. Classically reported after administration of heterologous antisera, most cases occur after the administration of an antibiotic (commonly a penicillin) or an acute viral syndrome. For example, acute viral hepatitis has been associated with a serum sickness-like syndrome. Circulating antibody-antigen complexes are the hallmark of these disorders. Clinical manifestations include fever, urticaria, rash, and lymphadenopathy. In renal involvement, the urinalysis is dominated by red blood cells and cellular casts. Infrequently a rapidly progressive glomerulonephritis may ensue. Virtually all patients respond to removal or treatment of the inciting event (e.g., discontinuance of drugs, resolution of viremia, or effective treatment of underlying viral hepatitis).

***Renal atheroemboli.*** Renal atheroembolic disease may occur in association with invasive angiographic procedures. Virtually all patients with atheroemboli will have an ulcerated atherosclerotic aorta. Clinical findings that distinguish renal atheroemboli from contrast nephropathy include embolic findings in the lower extremities, livedo reticularis, hypocomplementemia, and peripheral eosinophilia. Many individuals also experience labile hypertension. The mechanism of hypertension appears to be renin mediated, perhaps due to occlusion of small renal vessels. A biopsy of the affected tissue may disclose the presence of a microthrombus, with needle-shaped crystals representing dissolved cholesterol. Occasionally, examination of the retina will reveal refractile bodies consistent with cholesterol embolization. Systemic anticoagulation may exacerbate atheroemboli and thus should be avoided.

***The thrombotic microangiopathies.*** These syndromes are characterized by thrombocytopenia, microangiopathic hemolytic anemia, and renal insufficiency. In adults, neurologic complications secondary to thrombotic occlusion of the cerebral vessels may also occur (thrombotic thrombocytopenic purpura). In contrast, renal insufficiency is typically severe in the childhood form of the disease (hemolytic uremic syndrome). Indices of disseminated intravascular coagulation (thrombin time, fibrin split products, fibrin monomers, prothrombin time, partial thromboplastic time) are not increased in these syndromes.

Thrombotic microangiopathy may occur in the setting of cyclosporine administration, combination chemotherapy (especially mitomycin C), malignant hypertension, vasculitis, postpartum acute renal failure, and HIV infection. Recent outbreaks of hemolytic uremic syndrome have been associated with the verotoxin-producing *Escherichia coli* (serotype 0157:H7). The pathologic hallmark of these syndromes includes endothelial cell injury and swelling (endotheliosis) with platelet and fibrin thrombi of the microvasculature. The pathogenesis remains poorly understood, but recent studies suggest that endothelial injury results in abnormalities in circulating von Willebrand factor that predispose patients to platelet aggregation. Children with the disorder frequently recover spontaneously with supportive care alone. In adults or children who do not recover within 1 to 2 weeks, treatment should be initiated without delay because the mortality rate can exceed 90%. Infusions of fresh-frozen plasma alone can induce a remission in up to 50% of patients. If no response is noted within 24 hours, plasma exchange therapy should be instituted. Occasional patients with refractory disease respond to IV infusions of IgG and administration of aspirin and dipyridamole.

## Tubulointerstitial disease

Tubulointerstitial disease represents a broad group of renal diseases that predominantly affect the tubules and interstitium (see the box on p. 1262). In contrast to glomerular disease, heavy proteinuria (more than 2 g/day), RBC casts, lipiduria, and oval fat bodies are usually not found. More often the urine sediment is either normal or demonstrates pyuria and WBC casts (allergic or infectious interstitial nephritis). In some instances, discrete tubular defects such as renal tubular acidosis may be the presenting feature (e.g., multiple myeloma).

***Allergic interstitial nephritis (AIN).*** The most common cause of tubulointerstitial disease is drug-induced AIN. A variety of drugs have been implicated in the pathogenesis of AIN (see the box on p. 1272), although the exact mechanism responsible for renal injury is uncertain. An immune basis for injury seems likely because antibody deposition, complement activation, and infiltration of inflammatory cells (especially eosinophils) are frequently noted in the renal interstitium. The clinical features of AIN include peripheral eosinophilia, rash, fever, renal insufficiency, and pyuria. The urine sediment may also demonstrate WBC casts and hematuria. The presence of eosinophils in the urine can be helpful in establishing the correct diagnosis. In this regard, Hansel stain of the urine sediment appears to offer greater sensitivity for detecting the presence of eosinophils (about 90%) compared with the traditional Wright stain (about 25%). Although a renal biopsy may be required for a definite diagnosis, in many patients with AIN the classic symptoms of a rash, fever, eosinophilia, and renal insufficiency after exposure to a known offending agent would favor a short trial of discontinuing the likely offending agent. Unfortunately, the classic clinical syndrome above is noted in fewer than 60% of patients with AIN. Gallium scintigraphy has been used to determine noninvasively the presence of interstitial inflammation. Unfortunately, radiologic evaluation of AIN with gallium is highly subjective, and considerable overlap exists among various renal diseases. Nonetheless, it is imperative to establish the proper diagnosis of AIN, since the clinical and laboratory findings are largely reversible on removal of the offending agent. Several uncontrolled reports suggest more rapid resolution of symptoms and improved recovery of renal function with corticosteroid therapy. However, randomized controlled clinical trials have yet to establish definitively the role of corticosteroids in the treatment of AIN.

*Analgesic nephropathy.* Analgesic-induced chronic renal insufficiency probably accounts for less than 1% of all cases of ESRD. There are geographic variations in the incidence of this disorder. In some European countries, such as West Germany, the incidence may be as high as 18%. In the southeastern regions of the United States the incidence may be as high as 10%. The specific analgesic or combination of analgesics necessary to initiate this process remains controversial. Epidemiologic data suggest that a combination of phenacetin with an NSAID such as ibuprofen or aspirin may be the most nephrotoxic combination. Classic descriptions of this disorder include a middle-aged female with chronic somatic pain (headaches or arthritic complaints) who has been ingesting large doses of nonnarcotic analgesic agents for many years. Most patients have ingested at least 1 g of analgesic per day for a minimum of several years before the advent of significant renal disease. Renal biopsy specimens reveal severe interstitial fibrosis associated with mild infiltration of inflammatory cells. Papillary necrosis is the hallmark of analgesic nephropathy. Its pathogenesis is uncertain, but, inhibition of vasodilator prostaglandins may lead to

## Drugs associated with allergic interstitial nephritis

**β-Lactam antibiotics**

*Methicillin
Penicillin G
Ampicillin
Flucloxacillin
Oxacillin
Nafcillin
Carbenicillin
Amoxicillin
Mezlocillin
Cephalothin
Cephalexin
Cephradine
Cephaloridine
Cefotaxime
Cefoxitin
Cefaclor

**Other antibiotics**

*Sulfonamides
*Trimethoprim-sulfamethoxazole
*Rifampin
Polymyxin sulfate
Ethambutol
Vancomycin
Chloramphenicol
?Gentamicin
?Isoniazid
Minocycline
Aminosalicylic acid
Ciprofloxacin
Norfloxacin
Piromidic acid
Erythromycin
Spiramycin

**Diuretics**

*Thiazides
Furosemide
Chlorthalidone
Ticrynafen
Triameterene

**Nonsteroidal antiinflammatory drugs**

*Fenoprofen
Indomethacin
Naproxen
Ibuprofen
Benoxaprofen
Phenazone
Mefenamic acid
Tolmetin
Diflunisal
Zomepirac
Piroxicam
Diclofenac
Ketoprofen
Suprofen

**Other drugs**

*Phenindione
*Glafenine
*Phenytoin
*Cimetidine
*Sulfinpyrazone
Allopurinol
Aspirin
Carbamazepine
Clofibrate
Azathioprine
Phenylpropanolamine
Methyldopa
Phenobarbital
Leukocyte A interferon
Floctafenine
Haloperidol
Warfarin sodium
Imipramine
Diazepam
Valproate sodium
Chlorprothixene
Captopril
Propranolol
Amphetamines
Doxepin
Quinine

*Most common offending agents.
From *Scientific American Medicine* Table 2, Section 10, Subsection VIII.

ischemia of interstitial cells and surrounding tubules. Papillary necrosis also occurs in association with diabetes, sickle cell disease, and some infections.

***Reflux nephropathy and chronic pyelonephritis.*** Reflux nephropathy results from the abnormal backflow of urine from the urinary bladder to the renal parenchyma. It is unclear whether the mechanism of tubulointerstitial scarring is a direct consequence of high-pressure reflux or is secondary to chronic repeated urinary tract infections (UTIs). Children with chronic reflux usually have symptoms and signs of UTI, such as dysuria, pyuria, flank pain, and fever. In later stages, glomerular involvement may occur, manifested by focal scarring and heavy proteinuria (more than 3.5 g/day). The diagnosis of urinary tract reflux can be readily made with a voiding cystourethrogram. Management of reflux nephropathy depends on the severity of the reflux. Mild abnormalities generally respond to conservative measures such as long-term administration of low-dose antimicrobial agents. Many patients have spontaneous remission with time. More severe grades of reflux may require surgical intervention. The hallmark of advanced reflux nephropathy is interstitial scarring, tubular atrophy, and mild inflammatory cell infiltration (e.g., chronic pyelonephritis). Although chronic pyelonephritis is most frequently described in association with chronic UTI with or without reflux, it has also been reported with chronic lithium exposure, cisplatin administration, cyclosporin use, hyperoxaluria, cadmium exposure, hypercalcemia and hypercalciuria, chronic hypokalemia, and hyperuricemia.

***Polycystic kidney disease (PKD).*** PKD is a clinical disorder with two distinct inheritance patterns. The infantile variety is transmitted via an autosomal recessive gene, whereas adult PKD is transmitted in an autosomal dominant fashion. Infantile PKD usually follows a fulminant course, resulting in ESRD early in childhood. More than 90% of patients with adult PKD have an abnormal gene on the short arm of chromosome 16 ($PKD_1$). Most of these patients have a family history of PKD. A sporadic form of adult PKD (non-$PKD_1$) infrequently may occur. Interestingly, non-$PKD_1$ patients appear to have a more favorable prognosis than patients with the $PKD_1$ locus. Significant renal cyst formation may occur in up to 50% of affected patients. The mechanism of cyst formation in this disorder remains poorly understood. However, cyst enlargement results in compression of adjacent normal tissue, resulting in scarring and progressive renal insufficiency. Demonstration of multiple renal cysts with ultrasonography confirms the diagnosis. Most of these patients develop ESRD by age 55 to 60. Cysts may also occur in the liver, pancreas, and spleen.

Significant cystic involvement of the kidney may not be apparent until early adulthood. Thus, screening high-risk patients with ultrasonography may be negative early in the course of PKD. However, by age 30 virtually all patients have multiple cysts on ultrasonography. The natural history of this disease is variable and seems to depend on a combination of genetic and environmental factors. Approximately 35% of patients present with hematuria.

Complications of PKD include infection and bleeding into cysts, usually accompanied by severe pain. Infections can be treated symptomatically with antimicrobial therapy, but cyst drainage may be necessary for resolution of symptoms. The most ominous complication of PKD is a ruptured intracerebral berry aneurysm. This complication has been reported in up to 4% of affected patients. Guidelines for screening patients for intracranial aneurysms have not been clearly established, although patients with a family history of intracranial aneurysm should undergo routine testing with either CT or MRI angiography. Patients at high risk for development of a ruptured aneurysm (previous rupture, large aneurysms, bleeding diathesis) should be considered for invasive repair. Other complications of PKD include renal calculi (20%), colonic diverticuli (70%), cardiac valvular abnormalities (25%), and hepatic cysts (75%). No specific therapy exists for this disorder.

## MANAGEMENT

### General measures

Several nonspecific measures can be used in the management of patients with progressive renal injury. These include some degree of dietary protein restriction, treatment of hypertension, and management of associated metabolic disorders (hyperphosphatemia, hypocalcemia, metabolic acidosis, hyperlipidemia). Recent evidence also suggests that angiotensin-converting enzyme inhibition (ACE-In) may be renoprotective independent of its antihypertensive effect.

Several studies have examined the role of protein-restricted diets in chronic renal insufficiency. Dietary restriction of protein (0.6 to 0.8 g/kg/day) has been shown to retard the rate of progressive renal disease and lessen proteinuria. However, severely restricting the protein intake must be balanced against its effect on nutritional status and patient acceptance. A prudent approach is to initiate protein restriction (about 0.8 g/kg/day) when the serum creatinine exceeds 2.0 mg/dl.

The role of hypertension in accelerating the progression of renal disease is well established. Moreover, antihypertensive therapy appears to delay the onset of ESRD. In diabetic nephropathy, ACE-In offers a selective advantage over other antihypertensive agents. It seems prudent to initiate antihypertensive therapy with ACE-In when renal function is not severely compromised (creatinine less than 3.0 mg/dl). However, rapid deterioration of renal function or significant hyperkalemia would mitigate against the use of these agents.

Other metabolic complications contributing to renal injury include hyperlipidemia, hyperphosphatemia, and secondary hyperparathyroidism. Treatment of these complications may attenuate progressive renal scarring in addition to reducing the risk of various comorbid events such as atherosclerotic vascular disease and renal osteodystrophy. Clinical trials to establish the efficacy of lipid-lowering agents in the management of progressive renal injury are currently lacking; however, animal studies provide evidence linking lipid reduction to preservation of renal function and structure. Since the cardiovascular risk of hyperlipidemia is well established, it seems prudent to initiate antihyperlipidemic therapy in patients with renal disease who are at high risk for cardiovascular events (e.g., those with high-risk profiles).

**Table 93-3.** Probable benefit of specific treatment in medical renal disease*

| Disease | Effectiveness |
|---|---|
| Allergic interstitial nephritis | + |
| Amyloidosis | ± |
| Diabetic nephropathy ‖ | 0 |
| Focal segmental glomerulosclerosis | + |
| Hereditary nephritis | 0 |
| IgA nephropathy | ± |
| Membranoproliferative glomerulonephritis† | + |
| Membranous glomerulonephritis | + |
| Minimal change disease | +++ |
| Polycystic kidney disease | 0 |
| Poststreptococcal glomerulonephritis | 0 |
| Rapidly progressive glomerulonephritis | ++ |
| Renal atheroemboli | 0 |
| Systemic lupus erythematosus‡ | ++ |
| Systemic vasculitis§ | ++ |
| Thrombotic microangiopathy | ++ |

0, Ineffective; +++, very effective.
*Removal of offending agents or treating associated disorders (malignant disease) may ameliorate renal injury.
†Perhaps better in children.
‡Especially diffuse proliferative.
§Especially Wegener granulomatosis.
‖ ACE inhibitors ± protein restriction may slow progression.

### Approach to management of specific renal disease

Specific approaches to the management of individual glomerular or tubulointerstitial disorders have been delineated earlier and are not reiterated here. Perhaps the most important aspect of establishing the proper diagnosis in clinical renal disease is the development of effective treatment strategies. The risks of using immunotherapy (cytotoxic agents, corticosteroids) must be weighed against the benefits. This requires an understanding of the natural history of the specific renal disorder and the effects of treatment on the course of the disease. Unfortunately, only a few renal diseases have established treatment guidelines (Table 93-3). Until clinical trials clearly establish treatment recommendations for other renal disorders, the clinician/nephrologist must carefully balance the benefits of treatment with the risks.

## BIBLIOGRAPHY

Balow JE, Fauci AS: Vasculitic diseases of the kidney: polyarteritis, Wegener's granulomatosis, necrotizing and crescentic glomerulonephritis and other disorders. In Schier, R, Gottschalk C, editors: *Diseases of the kidney,* ed 5, Boston, 1992, Little, Brown.

Couser WG: Mediation of immune glomerular injury, *J Am Soc Nephrol* 1:13, 1990.

Falk RJ, Jennette JC: The Third International Workshop on Antineutrophil Cytoplasmic Autoantibodies, *Am J Kidney Dis* 18:145, 1991.

Gabow PA: Polycystic kidney disease: clues to pathogenesis, *Kidney Int* 40:986, 1991.

Garella S: Drug-induced renal disease, *Hosp Pract,* April 1993, p 129.

Harris RC, Ismail N: Extrarenal complications of the nephrotic syndrome, *Am J Kidney Dis* 23:477, 1994.

Klahr S et al: The effects of dietary protein restriction and blood-pressure control on the progression of chronic renal disease, *N Engl J Med* 330:877, 1994.

Lewis EJ et al: The effect of angiotensin-converting–enzyme inhibition on diabetic nephropathy, *N Engl J Med* 329:1456, 1993.

Piccoli A et al: Therapy for idiopathic membranous nephropathy: tailoring the choice by decision analysis, *Kidney Int* 45:1193, 1994.

CHAPTER

# 94 Renal Failure

Kevin J. Martin

## EPIDEMIOLOGY AND ETIOLOGY

*Acute renal failure* occurs often and is characterized by a sudden reduction in kidney function that limits the kidney's ability to maintain the body's internal environment. The possible causes of acute renal failure are multiple and can occur in a variety of clinical conditions discussed later. Severe cases of ischemic or nephrotoxic acute renal failure are often associated with acute tubular necrosis.

*Chronic renal failure* is a syndrome characterized by a slow, progressive decline in glomerular filtration rate (GFR) and other kidney functions. Various adaptations of the diseased kidney serve to limit the clinical manifestations until the loss of kidney function is severe. In practice it is convenient to divide chronic renal failure into stages such as *mild,* representing GFRs between 70 ml/min and the normal 120 ml/min; *moderate* renal insufficiency, representing GFRs from 30 to 70 ml/min; *severe* renal failure, with GFRs less than 30 ml/min; and *end-stage renal disease* (ESRD), representing GFRs less than 10 ml/min.

*Uremia* is the clinical syndrome associated with the retention of the end products of nitrogen metabolism that occurs with severe reductions in renal function. Symptoms of uremia are unusual before the blood urea nitrogen (BUN) reaches 60 mg/dl or with a serum creatinine level of 8 mg/dl. Uremic symptoms are more frequently associated with a BUN level greater than 100 mg/dl and a serum creatinine greater than 12 mg/dl; the BUN level typically correlates most strongly with uremic symptoms. Many organ systems are abnormal with severe renal failure and may be encountered whether the renal failure is acute or chronic.

The overall incidence of new cases of ESRD in the United States is approximately 150 patients per million population annually. Approximately 300 to 350 patients per million population are receiving chronic dialysis treatment. Fig. 94-1 depicts the most common causes of ESRD in the United States. Diabetes mellitus has become the most common cause of ESRD in the United States, accounting for 34% of new cases, and is followed closely by hypertension, which accounts for 29% of new cases. Polycystic kidney disease, urologic disorders, and other known diseases account for approximately the same incidence as glomerular diseases. In approximately 10% of patients, the cause of the ESRD remains obscure.

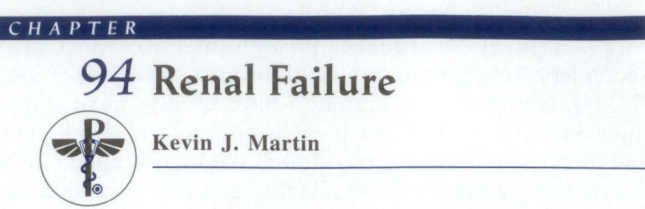

## Causes of acute renal failure

**Prerenal causes**

Decreased intravascular volume: hemorrhage, vomiting, diarrhea, burns
Increased intravascular capacity: sepsis, vasodilators, anaphylaxis
Myocardial failure: myocardial infarction, pulmonary embolism, congestive heart failure
Hepatorenal syndrome

**Intrinsic renal causes**

Ischemic: conditions above, postoperative shock
Nephrotoxic: aminoglycosides, contrast agents, heavy metals
Pigment release: rhabdomyolysis, hemolysis
Inflammatory: interstitial nephritis, acute glomerulonephritis, vasculitis
Pregnancy related: septic abortion, abruptio placentae, eclampsia, postpartum hemorrhage
Renovascular disease: renal artery thrombosis and embolism, dissecting aneurysm
Miscellaneous: uric acid nephropathy, hypercalcemia, myeloma

**Postrenal causes**

Obstruction to ureters: stones, papillary necrosis, tumors, lymph nodes, retroperitoneal fibrosis
Obstruction to bladder outlet: prostatic hypertrophy, carcinoma

# PATHOPHYSIOLOGY

## Acute renal failure

Classically in acute renal failure, the GFR is reduced to 1 to 5 ml/min and is associated with a marked fall in urine output to less than 500 ml in 24 hours. Many patients, however, do not have such severe reductions in renal function. Urine output of less than 500 ml daily is termed *oliguria.* It is important to emphasize that severe acute renal failure may occur without such marked reductions in urine output, giving rise to the term *nonoliguric acute renal failure.* The term *anuria,* which literally means no urine output, is usually applied to urine volumes less than 100 ml daily.

The principal causes of acute renal failure (see the box at left) are considered under the categories of prerenal causes, intrinsic renal causes, and postrenal causes. Differentiation into these three broad groups is of extreme importance, since the prognosis and treatment are radically different for the specific causes. Thus severe acute renal failure from obstruction of the urinary tract requires relief of the obstruction. Acute renal failure from a marked reduction in intravascular volume requires treatment with replenishment of the extracellular fluid volume. Analysis of the specific intrinsic renal causes of acute renal failure is also important, since various conditions may be associated with this type of renal failure and require specific evaluation and treatment.

Most cases of acute renal failure occur in the hospital setting and are related to losses of extracellular fluid volume, the use of nephrotoxic drugs or radiographic contrast diagnostic agents, or the effects of surgery or anesthesia. Cases of acute renal failure that occur outside the hospital setting often produce a great diagnostic

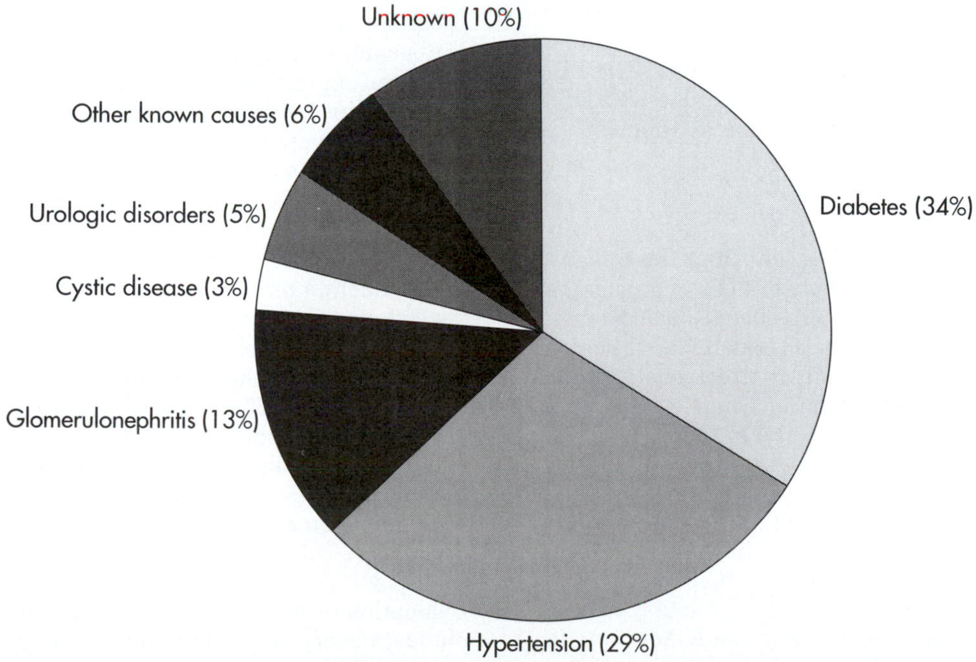


**Fig. 94-1.** Causes of end-stage renal disease (ESRD).

**Table 94-1.** Urine chemistries in acute renal failure*

| Test | Prerenal | Renal |
|---|---|---|
| Urine sodium concentration | <20 | >20 |
| Urine creatinine/plasma creatinine ratio | >20 | <20 |
| Fractional sodium excretion | <1 | >1 |

*Although these laboratory tests are extremely useful, urine chemistries are not diagnostic in these conditions: urinary tract obstruction, acute glomerulonephritis, prior administration of diuretics, preexisting chronic renal disease, and metabolic alkalosis.

challenge; these cases are often serious and if a definite cause is not readily identifiable (see following discussion) or if the clinical course cannot be easily monitored, prompt referral to a nephrologist for detailed evaluation is required.

Laboratory assessment of acute renal failure is important to distinguish between prerenal and intrinsic renal causes. In the presence of oliguria, the measurement of the concentrations of sodium and creatinine in serum and urine can lead to valuable information regarding the cause of the renal insufficiency. In prerenal acute renal failure, the kidney's normal response is to conserve salt and water. Conservation of salt is manifested by a low concentration of salt in the urine. Water conservation is manifested by an elevated concentration of the nonreabsorbable solute creatinine in the urine compared with the concentration of this solute in plasma; that is, the ratio of urine creatinine to plasma creatinine (U/P creatinine) is high. In the presence of intrinsic renal disease, these adaptations may not occur. Thus the finding of a relatively high sodium concentration and a low U/P creatinine ratio usually are indicative of intrinsic renal disease but are not invariable findings. These two parameters can be combined to yield the fractional sodium excretion ($FE_{Na}$), which has improved diagnostic value and is extremely useful in supporting the diagnosis of prerenal azotemia. The $FE_{Na}$ is calculated from measurements of serum and urine concentrations of sodium and creatinine as follows:

$$FE_{Na} = \frac{\text{Urine sodium} \times \text{Serum creatinine} \times 100}{\text{Serum sodium} \times \text{Urine creatinine}}$$

As illustrated in Table 94-1, an $FE_{Na}$ less than 1 suggests prerenal conditions, whereas an $FE_{Na}$ greater than 1, in the presence of oliguria, indicates intrinsic renal insufficiency. These values are occasionally misleading in the circumstances noted. In urinary tract obstruction a wide range of sodium concentrations may be found, so obstruction must be excluded directly. In acute glomerular disease, urinary excretion of sodium may be low, reflecting the marked decrease in GFR with preservation of tubular reabsorption of sodium. Prior administration of diuretics increases urine sodium and renders the value of such determinations useless. If there is preexisting renal disease, the diseased kidney may not be able to reduce the concentration of sodium maximally, and therefore the results may be misleading. Finally, in metabolic alkalosis with an alkaline urine, sodium bicarbonate excretion may cause urine sodium to be high, and measurement of urine chloride may yield more useful physiologic information in this circumstance. Some cases of acute renal failure from allergic interstitial nephritis or secondary to radiographic contrast toxicity may have low values for $FE_{Na}$.

Imaging of the urinary tract, usually with sonography, is important to evaluate the possibility of obstruction. Further examination with radionuclide techniques, computed tomography (CT), or angiography may be indicated in special circumstances. Since acute renal failure is a serious condition that carries an appreciable mortality, prompt referral for specialized care may be indicated.

### Chronic renal failure

Although chronic renal failure may occur as a result of many disorders, the same signs and symptoms occur irrespective of the primary cause of nephron loss, and many of the pathophysiologic adaptations are similar. As the nephrons become damaged, the remaining nephrons undergo compensatory hypertrophy. Thus each tubule undergoes several adaptations in an effort to maintain the composition of the extracellular fluid. Although these adaptations serve to maintain the constancy of the internal environment, the capacity of the residual nephrons to cope with the extremes of salt, water, or potassium excess or deficiency is limited. Thus until renal insufficiency is severe, adaptations of tubular function can allow the excretion of relatively normal amounts of salt and water.

Serum potassium can be maintained within the normal range until renal insufficiency is severe (GFR less than 10 ml/min), and phosphorus excretion can be maintained by increasing the levels of parathyroid hormone (PTH). Although the increases in PTH serve to maintain the levels of phosphorus within the normal range, there are additional consequences of the high levels of PTH on the skeleton, such as the development of hyperparathyroid bone disease (renal osteodystrophy), which may occur as a result of this adaptation.

As renal function decreases, the kidney's endocrine functions also become limited. Erythropoietin, which is essential for normal red blood cell (RBC) production, is produced in the kidney. The development of anemia is associated with progressive renal disease as erythropoietin production diminishes. Anemia may occur with reductions of renal function of 30% to 50% of normal values and tends to be progressive unless treated with recombinant erythropoietin.

An additional major endocrine function of the kidney is the production of calcitriol, the active form of vitamin D. As calcitriol levels decrease during progressive renal insufficiency, further stress is placed on efforts to maintain calcium and phosphorus homeostasis, which exaggerates the development of secondary hyperparathyroidism. Calcitriol may be supplemented in the course of chronic renal insufficiency, but this is not without risk, and careful dose monitoring is essential to avoid complications of therapy such as hypercalcemia.

## HISTORY

Evaluation of the patient should include a comprehensive clinical history of not only the present complaint, but also a previous history of systemic diseases, including those of childhood; a history or family history of hypertension or

**Table 94-2.** Occupational nephrotoxins

| Site of action | Nephrotoxin | Industrial setting |
|---|---|---|
| Glomerulus | Silica | Stone cutting, sandblasting |
| | Solvents | Paints, degreasers, fuels |
| Proximal tubule | Lead (inorganic) | Battery manufacture, smelter, lead abaters |
| | Cadmium | Manufacture of alloys, glass, paints, electrical equipment, smelting |
| | Mercury (inorganic) | Manufacture of mirrors, batteries, alloys, scientific instruments; mines; dental offices |
| | Halogenated aliphatic hydrocarbons (e.g., carbon tetrachloride) | Solvent usage, dry cleaning, fumigants |
| Interstium | Uranium | Mining, refining |
| Acute tubular necrosis | Cadmium | Welding of cadmium-plated metal (may also be seen with heavy materials such as chromium, mercury, ranadium) |
| | Arsine gas | Coal or metal processing, semiconductor manufacture (secondary to hemoglobinuria) |
| Bladder (cancer) | Aromatic amines | Manufacture and use of synthetic dyes |

From Dr. John Burris and Dr. David Christiani.

diabetes; and a careful history of drug ingestion, including over-the-counter medications such as analgesics, nonsteroidal antiinflammatory drugs (NSAIDs), and other potential nephrotoxins. In women a full gynecologic and obstetric history is also required, including hypertension, proteinuria, or preeclampsia during pregnancy. Occupational history for exposure to potential nephrotoxins may be relevant in certain instances (Table 94-2).

Both acute and chronic renal insufficiency may present in a variety of ways, and the initial manifestations are often mistaken for primary problems in the affected organ system (see the box at right). Thus patients may have nausea and vomiting that may be evaluated as primary peptic ulcer disease, which sometimes might represent manifestations of uremia. Presentations with such vague symptoms such as weakness and tiredness can easily be attributed to anemia, the basis of which could be renal insufficiency. Difficulties with salt and water homeostasis, such as edema or dyspnea on exertion, may be mistaken for a primary cardiac problem. At the other end of the spectrum, significant renal disease may be present without significant clinical manifestations and may only be detected by routine urinalysis, which may reveal the presence of hematuria or proteinuria and should prompt further evaluation. It is important to emphasize that moderate to severe renal insufficiency may occur in the absence of symptoms. The patient should be asked questions to determine the etiology of acute renal failure (see the box on p. 1275), as well as its systemic effects.

### Symptoms of renal insufficiency

**Symptoms referable to the urinary tract**

Nocturia
Polyuria
Hematuria
Anuria/oliguria

**General symptoms**

Nausea/vomiting
Dyspepsia
Malaise
Lassitude
Confusion
Weakness
Pruritus
Bruising/bleeding
Halitosis
Muscle twitching

**Presence or history of systemic disease associated with renal insufficiency**

Hypertension
Diabetes
Connective tissue disorders
Multiple myeloma
Amyloidosis
Hereditary renal diseases

## PHYSICAL EXAMINATION

A complete physical examination should be performed to evaluate the patient with regard to the etiology of the renal disease and the assessment of complications (see the box on p. 1278). Clues to the etiology of renal disease may be elicited by searching for manifestations of systemic problems such as dehydration, diabetes, vasculitis, or leukemia/lymphoma. Hearing impairment may be associated with the hereditary Alport syndrome. Large bilateral abdominal masses may indicate polycystic kidney disease. Peripheral vascular disease or the presence of abdominal bruits may raise the possibility of atheroembolic renal disease. An enlarged bladder or abnormal prostate or pelvic examination may suggest obstructive uropathy.

Physical examination should strive to assess complications of the chronic renal disease. Assessment of the extracellular fluid volume is important; the patient should be examined for elevation of neck veins, the presence or absence of edema, and ascites. Determination of blood pressure should be performed, lying and standing, and cardiac and lung examinations performed. The optic fundi

### Clinical consequences of advanced renal failure

**Signs of renal failure**
***Cardiovascular***
Expansion of extracellular fluid
Pulmonary edema
Hypertension
Cardiac arrhythmias
Peripheral edema
Pericarditis

***Hematologic***
Anemia
Platelet dysfunction

***Gastrointestinal***
Bleeding

***Neurologic***
Asterixis
Seizures
Coma

***Infectious***
Pneumonia
Urinary tract infection
Septicemia

***Miscellaneous***
Corneal calcifications
Skin abnormalities
Uremic frost
Carpal tunnel

**Laboratory abnormalities**
Abnormal urinalysis: proteinuria, hematuria, casts
Hyponatremia
Hypocalcemia
Hyperphosphatemia
Hyperuricemia
Hyperkalemia (BUN, creatinine)
Azotemia
Anion gap metabolic acidosis

should be examined for evidence of hypertension or diabetes, the skin for bruising or signs of vasculitis, the bones for tenderness or fracture, and joints for swelling or arthritis. Pericarditis, asterixis, Kussmaul's respirations, ecchymoses, and encephalopathy are manifestations of severe uremia.

Some of the presentations of renal disease are serious and require emergency management. Examples of such emergencies would include malignant hypertension, marked decreases in urine output, severe abnormalities in serum chemistries, the presence of systemic vasculitis, cardiovascular or respiratory emergencies, severe flank pain, or development of fever in the presence of urinary tract obstruction.

## LABORATORY STUDIES AND DIAGNOSTIC PROCEDURES

If renal insufficiency is suspected, laboratory evaluation is indicated to assess the degree of renal insufficiency and to monitor complications. Microscopic examination of the urine may reveal the presence of moderate numbers of hyaline and finely granular casts in prerenal azotemia. The presence of RBC casts is indicative of glomerular diseases such as glomerulonephritis or vasculitis. The presence of large amounts of cellular debris or brown muddy casts is suggestive of ischemic or nephrotoxic acute renal failure. The principal means by which renal function is assessed is by measurement of GFR. Although the "gold standard" procedure is the measurement of inulin clearance, for practical purposes it is more convenient to use endogenous creatinine clearance. The normal range is 90 to 150 ml/min/1.73 $m^2$ surface area. At low levels of GFR, creatinine clearance may overestimate GFR because of secretion of creatinine by the kidney tubules. (See Chapter 89 for details of measuring GFR.)

Further laboratory evaluation should include a chemistry profile to evaluate serum electrolytes, calcium, phosphorus, uric acid, serum proteins, cholesterol, and creatine kinase (CK, CPK). Anemia should be assessed with a complete blood count and evaluated further as appropriate. As noted earlier, in acute renal failure the $FE_{Na}$ provides insight into the likely type of renal failure.

Imaging of the kidneys and urinary tract, initially by ultrasound, is often helpful to evaluate the size of the kidneys and to exclude the possibility of urinary tract obstruction, which can be reversed with appropriate intervention. Small kidneys are indicative of chronic renal insufficiency with little possibility of reversal of renal dysfunction, whereas normal-size kidneys in the presence of severe renal insufficiency should prompt urgent further evaluation for the possibility of reversal of renal dysfunction. Specific diagnoses such as polycystic kidney disease may be revealed by these techniques. In certain patients, renal biopsy is indicated for the specific diagnosis, particularly if consideration for a specific treatment has a significant possibility of improving or stabilizing renal function.

## DIFFERENTIAL DIAGNOSIS AND DIAGNOSTIC EVALUATION

When a patient is found to have renal insufficiency, the initial consideration should be to decide if it is acute or chronic renal failure. This may be difficult in certain patients, and previous history/laboratory determinations may be useful. Factors that suggest chronicity include long duration of symptoms, nocturia, absence of symptoms with a very high BUN or creatinine, severe anemia, bone disease (renal osteodystrophy), sexual dysfunction, skin pigmentation or calcification, neurologic complications, and small kidneys on imaging.

In any patient with acute or chronic renal failure, one needs to search for factors that may aggravate the degree of renal insufficiency and especially those that may be potentially reversible (see the box on p. 1279). Such reversible factors may represent the activity of the primary renal disease, which may require specific treatment. A common problem is related to contraction of the extracellular fluid volume because of overdiuresis or fluid loss from vomiting or diarrhea. The development of congestive heart failure as a result of primary cardiac disease or as a manifestation of expansion of the extracellular fluid volume may result in decreases in cardiac output, leading

### Factors that may aggravate renal insufficiency

Active primary renal disease
Extracellular fluid volume contraction
Congestive heart failure/volume overload
Drugs
Radiographic contrast
Infections
Obstruction
Acute interstitial nephritis
Hyperuricemia
Hypercalcemia
Renal vein thrombosis
Atheroembolic disease/cholesterol embolism

### Risk factors for contrast nephrotoxicity

Underlying renal insufficiency (serum creatinine >2 mg/dl)
Diabetes mellitus, especially with renal insufficiency
Congestive heart failure
Volume contraction
High doses of contrast
Multiple myeloma
Advanced age

to decreases in renal perfusion and worsening of renal insufficiency.

A careful drug history is always essential so that possible nephrotoxicity may be discovered. NSAIDs may decrease renal blood flow, especially in the diseased kidney, by blunting the production of vasodilatory prostaglandins, which play a role in the maintenance of renal blood flow. The use of aminoglycoside antibiotics should also be avoided because of their well-known nephrotoxicity. It is also important to be aware of the nephrotoxicity of radiographic contrast procedures, which may be performed for a variety of reasons, such as cardiac catheterization or CT examinations of head or abdomen with the use of intravenous contrast. Although the incidence of nephrotoxicity of the radiographic contrast agents is small with normal renal function, toxicity may be enhanced and the consequences more severe in certain circumstances. The box above lists factors that appear to increase the risk of nephrotoxicity.

Urinary tract infections may lead to pyelonephritis and decreased renal function. Obstruction to the urinary tract may result from stones or sloughed renal papillae, in addition to the development of obstruction from prostatic disease. Allergic interstitial nephritis as a result of drug therapy may also cause decrements in renal function in the presence of preexisting renal disease (see Chapter 93). The development of blood chemistry abnormalities, such as hyperuricemia or hypercalcemia, may also result in a worsening of renal function. The final group to be considered is vascular complications, such as the persistence of atheroembolic disease or cholesterol emboli to the kidneys, often associated with generalized vascular disease and also the possible development of renal vein thrombosis in those patients with heavy proteinuria. These factors must be evaluated in any patient with a sudden or unexpected decrement in renal function, since prompt correction of the abnormality may be successful in returning renal function to baseline.

## MANAGEMENT

### Acute renal failure

Acute renal failure is a serious condition that carries considerable mortality, ranging from 30% to 50%. If acute renal failure is suspected, prompt referrals should be made to specialized centers for specific diagnosis and management if resolution does not occur promptly or if the etiology is in doubt. Since the course of acute renal failure ranges from 7 to 21 days, dialysis may be required until renal recovery can occur. Absolute indications for prompt referral include volume overload with congestive heart failure, hyperkalemia, severe acidosis, bleeding, and uremic symptoms. If hyperkalemia is present with electrocardiographic (ECG) changes of peaked T waves, flattened P waves, prolongation of the PR interval, or widening of the QRS complex, urgent treatment is required. Immediate therapy should include the administration of calcium gluconate intravenously, followed by correction of acidosis with intravenous bicarbonate. Additional therapy should include 50 ml of 50% dextrose with 10 units of regular insulin to shift potassium intracellularly. Potassium removal from the body can be accomplished by the use of Kayexalate given orally or as a retention enema. If renal failure is severe, arrangements should be made for the institution of dialysis.

In patients with oliguric renal failure, it is advisable to attempt to convert this situation to nonoliguric failure through the use of loop diuretics. In this way, fluid balance can be improved and there may be some therapeutic benefit by continuously flushing the kidneys.

### Chronic renal failure

The general principles for the management of chronic renal failure involve efforts to monitor the progression of the primary disease and to evaluate the response to specific treatment. In addition, one should monitor the progression of renal failure with regard to the response to various treatments that may also be useful to slow the progression of renal impairment. The patient should also be followed for the management of any intercurrent illnesses and for the detection of any complications of renal failure so that they may be appropriately assessed and treated. The final goal of management should deal with anticipation of the need of dialysis or transplantation (see below). Appropriate referral should be made early in the course of chronic renal insufficiency so that the management of ESRD may be planned, including patient education and consideration for dialysis modality and renal transplantation.

As already discussed, the mainstay of monitoring for the progression of renal failure is the measurement of serum creatinine and the calculation of GFR, supplemented with occasional determination of creatinine clearance of GFR. Some have advocated the use of plots of the reciprocal of the serum creatinine over time to monitor progression of renal failure, since a linear relationship often is found, making it possible to predict the time at which dialysis might be required and to evaluate deviations from the predicted course.

Serial serum chemistry determinations are important in the assessment of complications to evaluate compliance with the diet and to monitor the levels of potassium, bicarbonate, serum albumin, cholesterol, and uric acid and parameters of renal function. This is also important in evaluating the efficacy of efforts to control serum phosphorus and to maintain the levels of serum calcium. In diabetic patients, serial assessment of glycosylated hemoglobin determination is useful to obtain an index of the efficacy of blood sugar control between office visits. It is important to realize that renal insulin clearance decreases with increasing renal insufficiency. Therefore diabetic patients typically have decreasing insulin requirements.

General guidelines for the management of progressive renal insufficiency, after GFR reaches 75% of normal, include detailed attention to diet with modest restriction of dietary protein to 0.8 g/kg/day, phosphorus to 700 to 800 mg/day, and potassium to 70 mmol/day according to specific clinical indications. Sodium retention with signs of volume overload and sodium depletion with signs of dehydration and volume contraction are common in patients with chronic renal failure; therefore, attention to salt and water intake is extremely important in their management. In general, only moderate salt restriction should be prescribed except with clear evidence of volume overload. Patients with chronic renal failure are usually able to maintain normal serum potassium levels until the GFR falls below 10 ml/min.

The importance of control of blood pressure in patients with renal disease is not only to prevent further deterioration in renal function, but also to prevent the development of vascular complications of hypertension. Measurements of blood pressure, both lying and standing, are useful in diabetic patients and for the evaluation of potential postural hypotension in patients receiving drug therapy. This may also be valuable in patients with suspected water depletion. Measurements of blood pressure at office visits should be supplemented by careful examination of the retina to detect hemorrhages, exudates, and papilledema, which may indicate how well blood pressure is being controlled between visits. Although lowering systemic blood pressure has beneficial effects on the progression of renal disease, evidence also suggests that angiotensin-converting enzyme (ACE) inhibitors may have additional beneficial effects. It is important to note that blood pressure should be followed closely after the institution of antihypertensive therapy so that excessive reductions in renal blood flow do not further compromise renal function, especially in the presence of renal vascular disease. This may be seen with any agent that effectively lowers the blood pressure, but the use of ACE inhibitors has been particularly implicated in such effects. An additional caution with the use of ACE inhibitors is the development of hyperkalemia. Serum potassium should be checked several days after the start of therapy with ACE inhibitors to exclude hyperkalemia. This is particularly important in diabetic patients and those using β-blockers and NSAIDs, who may be particularly prone to the development of hyperkalemia.

In general, thiazide diuretics are ineffective as antihypertensive agents at GFRs less than 25 ml/min. Loop diuretics may be useful for the control of volume overload. The use of potassium-sparing diuretics is contraindicated in the presence of chronic renal failure. Potassium supplementation should be used only with extreme caution in such patients. Similar to ACE inhibitors, some evidence indicates that certain calcium channel blockers (specifically, diltiazem and verapamil) decrease intraglomerular pressures. Although data showing that these agents preserve renal function are lacking, many clinicians use these agents as second-line antihypertensives for patients intolerant of ACE inhibitors.

Hyperlipidemia is often associated with chronic renal failure and is often more severe in patients who have nephrotic syndrome and in diabetic patients. Since cardiovascular complications are common in chronic renal disease and since experimental evidence shows that hyperlipidemia may have a deleterious effect on the progression of renal disease, one should attempt to limit hypercholesterolemia. This can be done by attention to the diet, but many patients require drug intervention.

Attention should also be given to the prevention of progressive hyperparathyroidism. The mainstays of therapy include dietary phosphorus restriction, supplementation of the diet with phosphorus binders such as calcium carbonate or calcium acetate, and judicious use of calcitriol. These therapeutic modalities are best guided by those familiar with their use. The use of aluminum-containing antacids as phosphorus binders is no longer recommended.

Acidosis should be treated, if possible, with the awareness that bicarbonate supplementation may also lead to excessive sodium intake. Citrate-containing alkali salts should be avoided in advanced renal failure because of the possibility of enhancing the absorption of aluminum from the intestine.

The patient should also be followed for the development of anemia. Appropriate intervention includes the institution of therapy with recombinant erythropoietin when necessary, usually when the hematocrit falls below 30%. Such therapy requires careful supervision because aggravation of hypertension and development of polycythemia may occur.

Since many drugs required for general medical management are handled by the kidneys for excretion, it is imperative that the dosing of any prescribed drug be verified for the degree of renal insufficiency.

***End-stage renal disease.*** It is usual to initiate dialysis when the creatinine clearance is less than 5 to 8 ml/min, which would usually correlate with a serum creatinine concentration of 8 to 12 mg/dl. Often, however, the initiation of dialysis depends upon the development of symptoms of uremia. Excessive delay in starting dialysis can potentially result in malnutrition and delay the ultimate recovery and rehabilitation. Most facilities provide hemodialysis and peritoneal dialysis and either perform transplantation or can refer to a transplantation center. The involvement of the nephrologist is important in the choice of dialysis modality and in the consideration for renal transplantation. Although it is desirable to consult a nephrologist early in the course of renal disease to formulate a plan for therapy as renal disease progresses, it is appropriate to again refer patients to a nephrologist when the creatinine clearance has fallen to 20 to 30 ml/min. Thus the patient may become both educated about the various forms of therapy and acquainted with the personnel involved in the management of the ESRD program.

For hemodialysis it is necessary to obtain vascular access. The preferred access is through a primary arteriovenous fistula, which can usually be inserted under local anesthesia. The fistula requires 1 to 3 months maturation before use. If the patient's vessels are inadequate, synthetic grafts can be inserted in the arm. These grafts can generally be used within 3 weeks of placement. The major complications of such vascular access procedures are clotting and infection. It is usual to perform hemodialysis 3 times per week with each session lasting approximately 4 hours. As a group, there is an approximately 20% to 25% annual mortality for hemodialysis patients that varies according to co-morbid conditions (e.g., diabetes or cardiovascular disease).

Continuous ambulatory peritoneal dialysis (CAPD) is an alternate treatment in which dialysis fluid is inserted through a catheter into the abdominal cavity where exchange of solute occurs between blood and fluid. The fluid is then removed through the catheter. The techniques of peritoneal dialysis have improved in recent years and have increased its popularity among patients. A modified form of such therapy is to use an automated cycling machine during the night. This continuous cycling peritoneal dialysis (CCPD) can be helpful to patients with limited mobility. CAPD requires a minimum of four dialysis exchanges per day. The advantages of this form of dialysis is that it provides greater flexibility to the patient, enabling them to work or travel and set their own schedule. The major problem with peritoneal dialysis is the development of peritonitis. Strict attention to sterile technique is necessary. Since repeated connections of tubing are required, it is desirable that the patient's vision be satisfactory; however, there are devices that can facilitate these connections in the absence of good vision. Although strict comparative survival statistics between hemodialysis and peritoneal dialysis are somewhat difficult to interpret in view of the unmatched patients, it would appear that under most conditions survival rates are comparable.

Of the therapies for ESRD, a successful renal transplant provides the most complete correction of the uremic syndrome. Kidney transplantation from living related donors now has one-year success rates in excess of 85% to 90%, and transplantation with cadaveric kidneys now routinely exceeds 80%. Long-term success rates are somewhat lower and some kidneys fail from the process of chronic rejection; 30% to 50% of successfully transplanted kidneys may show severe deterioration in renal function after 5 years. Nonetheless, in selected patients, excellent outcomes are achievable with renal transplantation.

## BIBLIOGRAPHY

Bakris GL, Stein JH: Diabetic nephropathy, *Dis Mon* 39:573, 1993.

Brazy PC, Fitzwilliam JF: Progressive renal disease: role of race and antihypertensive medications, *Kidney Int* 37:1113, 1990.

Brazy PC, Stead WW, Fitzwilliam JF: Progression of renal insufficiency: role of blood pressure, *Kidney Int* 35:670, 1989.

Cameron S et al, editors: *Oxford textbook of clinical nephrology,* 3 vols, New York, 1992, Oxford University Press.

Kasiske BL et al: Effect of antihypertensive therapy on the kidney in patients with diabetes: a meta-regression analysis, *Ann Intern Med* 118(2):129, 1993.

Keane WF et al: Hypertension, hyperlipidemia and renal damage, *Am J Kidney Dis Suppl* 21(5):43, 1993.

Klahr S: Low-protein diets and angiotensin-converting enzyme inhibition in progressive renal failure, *Am J Kidney Dis* 22(1):114, 1993.

Klahr S, Schreiner G, Ichikawa I: The progression of renal disease, *N Engl J Med* 318:1657, 1988.

Klahr S et al: The effects of dietary protein restriction and blood pressure control on the progression of chronic renal disease, *N Engl J Med* 330:877, 1994.

Lewis EJ et al: The effect of angiotensin-converting-enzyme inhibition on diabetic nephropathy, *N Engl J Med* 329:1456, 1993.

Neuringer JR, Brenner BM: Glomerular hypertension: cause and consequence of renal injury, *J Hypertension* 10:391, 1992.

Neuringer JR, Brenner BM: Hemodynamic theory of progressive renal disease: a 10-year update in brief review, *Am J Kidney Dis* 22(1):98, 1993.

O'Donnell MP, Schmitz PG: Dietary and pharmacologic manipulations of lipids: impact on progression of experimental renal disease. In Keane WF, editor: *Lipids & renal disease: contemporary issues in nephrology,* 1991, Churchill Livingstone.

Parfrey PS et al: Contrast material induced renal failure in patients with diabetes mellitus, renal insufficiency or both, *N Engl J Med* 320:143, 1989.

# X NEUROLOGY

CHAPTER

# 95 Headaches

John R. Graham

EDITORS' NOTE: Dr. Graham passed away before he was able to redo this chapter for the present edition of this text. Dr. Graham was an internist who devoted most of his career to the study and care or patients with headache. The editors found the original chapter so rich with his personal wisdom and knowledge on this common problem that they were loathe to present an entirely new chapter on this topic. This chapter therefore has been somewhat shortened in keeping with the crisper style of the present edition but with effort to retain the personal style and voice of experience so useful for the primary caregiver. The discussion relating to the use and complications of methysergide has been truncated, since the drug is now only rarely used by primary care physicians because of the availability of other prophylactic agents for migraine, paticularly the calcium channel blockers and sumatriptin. Dr. Graham's original but somewhat shortened version of his work on headache follows and includes some of his own charming drawings.

What does the headache patient want? This question is particularly important for the physician to ask when dealing with the patient who presents with headache as the chief complaint. Experience shows that headache patients, even before relief of symptoms, want attention to and respect for their symptoms. They want the physician to take time to grasp its nature and explain its meaning, to make a thorough investigation, and to treat the headache with the same seriousness with which he or she treats other important medical symptoms.

People live by their wits, and they know it. When they hurt, this is important for them, whether the cause is organic, emotional, or just "overload," as in other forms of "angina." Headache or "cranial angina" deserves care, time, and understanding by the physician *and* the patient. Very few headache problems brought to the physician are solved by one treatment in one visit. A minor headache can indicate serious problems. A major headache may arise from functional disturbances. Hundreds of diseases present as headaches somewhere during their course. The persons with this confusing and complicated problem, which may kill them or just make them miserable while alive (Fig. 95-1), deserves intelligent study, explanation, and dedicated treatment by the physician. Many effective treatments are now available. Most need to be tailored to the nature of the headache and the individual's lifestyle. Patient and physician need to cooperate in solving such problems, and it usually takes considerable time and often repeated visits to work out a satisfactory solution. This requirement must be made clear at the first visit.

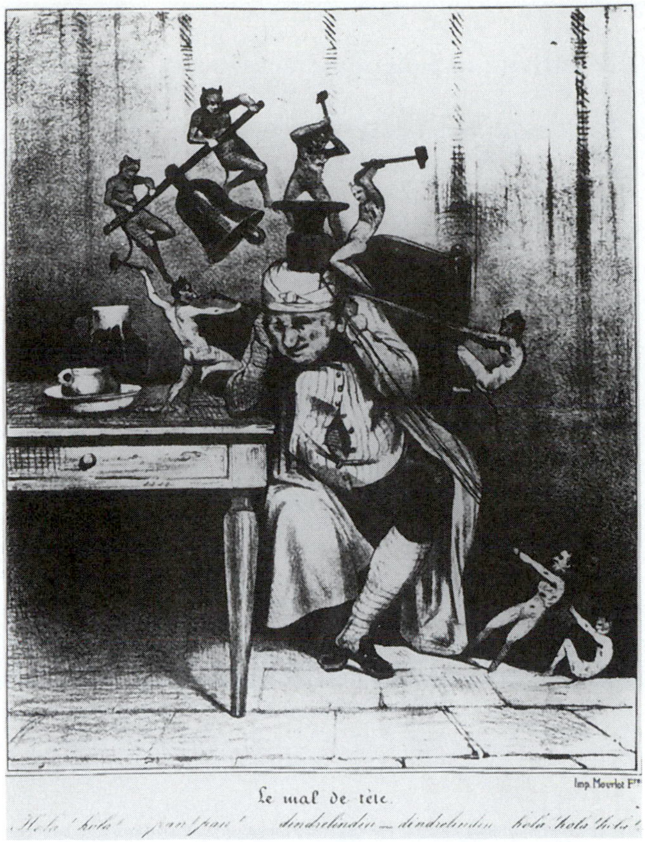


**Fig. 95-1.** *Le mal de tête.* Honoré Daumier, 1841.

## SOURCES, PATHWAYS, AND MECHANISMS OF CRANIAL PAIN

Faced with a headache patient in the office, the physician needs to ask the following questions:

Which structures in the head are sensitive to pain?

Where is the pain from these structures felt?

Which sensory tracts carry the painful messages to the brain?

What are the mechanisms responsible for the pain?

Which and how many structures may be involved when pain is reported from a given location?

Extracranial structures that are and are not sensitive to pain are summarized in the box on p. 1284. The intracranial structures sensitive and not sensitive to pain are shown in the box on p. 1284. Cranial structures project their pain to the cranial surface, as near the source of pain as possible in most cases. Because many such sources register their pain in the same general surface area, it is important to bear in mind that a pain in a given location may represent disordered function of several structures, some intracranial and some extracranial.

Although some pains in the head are referred from intracranial structures to somewhat distant extracranial areas, pain arising from malfunction or damage of most superficial structures, (e.g., teeth, turbinates, eyes) is usually felt in the immediate region of those structures as well as at some distant point of referral. When the source of pain is deeper (e.g., sphenoid sinus, internal carotid artery, tentorium), the pain is usually referred to a superficial area as close as possible to the source. When such referral is suspected to be the case, every effort is

## Sensitivity to pain of extracranial structures

**Extracranial structures sensitive to pain**

1. Skin, scalp, periosteum, fascia
2. Sensory nerves
3. Arteries and veins
4. Muscles of the head, face, and jaws and their ligamentous attachments
5. Eyes, ears, teeth
6. Nasal cavity contents, especially turbinates, septum, ostia and canals to sinuses, and to a lesser degree sinus linings when inflamed
7. Membranes of mouth, pharynx, and nasopharynx; tongue; eustachian tube
8. Temporomandibular joint

**Extracranial structures not sensitive to pain**

1. Bones of the skull
2. Diploic veins
3. Linings of noninflamed sinuses and extraocular muscles, except when stretched, show limited reaction to most painful stimuli

## Sensitivity to pain of intracranial structures

**Intracranial structures sensitive to pain**

1. Meningeal blood vessels
2. Major venous sinuses and tributary veins leading into them, including those crossing the subarachnoid space from the brain just as they lead into the sagittal sinus; sylvian vein and inferior cerebral veins leading to the lateral sinus and superior petrosal sinus
3. Dura immediately adjacent to blood vessels and in most areas in the floor of the anterior and posterior fossae
4. Large arteries leading into the brain (common carotid, vertebrals, basilar, and its cerebellar branches)
5. Circle of Willis
6. Anterior, middle, and posterior cerebral arteries for an inch or two along their course into the brain, after which, as pial vessels, they lose sensitivity to pain
7. Most of the upper surface of the tentorium and the edges of the lower surface of the tentorium directly adjacent to its venous sinuses
8. Falx, for only a few centimeters above its attachment to the crista galli
9. Sensory nerves and ganglia

**Intracranial structures not sensitive to pain**

1. Much of the dura covering the convexities of the cerebrum and cerebellum except, as noted, immediately adjacent to major blood vessels
2. Substance of the brain itself
3. Much of the falx
4. Pia arachnoid except possibly near great vessels
5. Pial vessels
6. Walls of the lateral, third, and fourth ventricles
7. Choroid plexuses

made to discover damage or malfunction at the suspected source before specific medical or, especially, surgical treatment is initiated. Some common sites at which cranial pain is felt and the anatomic structures that may be the source of referral to these areas are shown in Fig. 95-2.

In general, pain arising from disordered function, damage, or inflammation of structures located anterior to and above the tentorium is felt in the front half of the head. This pain sensation is conveyed to the brain over the fifth nerve and is ipsilateral to the lesion. Similarly, pain arising from structures below the tenorium is usually felt in the back half of the head and is carried over the three upper cervical nerves. Pain from structures in the throat, ear, and middle fossa is carried over the ninth and tenth nerves and, occasionally, over some sensory fibers in the seventh nerve. It is felt in the posterior pharynx or the region immediately around, in, and just behind the ear. Exceptions to this general principle are found with occasional lesions below the tentorium that register their pain in the anterior half of the head, carried there by the recurrent nerve of Arnold, a branch of the fifth nerve, which passes directly backward into the posterior fossa. Pain in the eye and temple also may result from ipsilateral lesions causing irritation of the posterior roots of the cervical nerves C1, C2, and C3, or even cervical disturbances as low as C4-5, C6, and C7. The sensory pathways responsible for pain from various areas of the cranium are shown in Fig. 95-3.

There are eight well-recognized mechanisms for pain in the head that create conscious pain only after the message of their disordered function has reached centers in the brain at least as high as the thalamus. Some sources of pain in the head may lie in the brain itself rather than in more peripheral structures. Rapidly developing knowledge about the nociceptive system, its receptor sites for pain in the central gray matter of the spinal cord and brain, and the pain-relieving capacity of endorphins, enkephalins, and other neuropeptides is bringing new concepts about the central control of pain impulses originating either within the brain or in the periphery. Such modulation of pain thresholds by changes in the central nociceptive areas may provide explanations for pain syndromes in the head for which no demonstrable pathology exists at this time.

There are several mechanisms of cranial pain (Fig. 95-4).

1. *Conversion or hysterical pain.* This is head pain for which no pathology or biochemical abnormality is as yet known but that is very "real" to the patient.

2. *True neuralgia pain,* as in tic douloureux. An abnormal process takes place in the ganglion of a given cranial nerve or its central connections that produces pain in the distribution of that nerve.

3. *Direct pressure on a pain-sensitive structure.* Pressure is exerted on a pain-sensitive structure by an anatomic mass or inflammation such as a tumor, cyst, or aneurysm, such as an acoustic neuroma growing to distort the pain-sensitive tentorium.

4. *Traction on pain-sensitive structures* (Fig. 95-4, *B*). Space-occupying lesions such as cysts or tumors may distort or drag on pain-sensitive structures, tributary veins, or venous sinuses.

5. *Excessive generalized vasodilatation or pulsation of pain-sensitive intracranial vessels.* Examples of this are excessive vasodilatation of areas of vascular structures

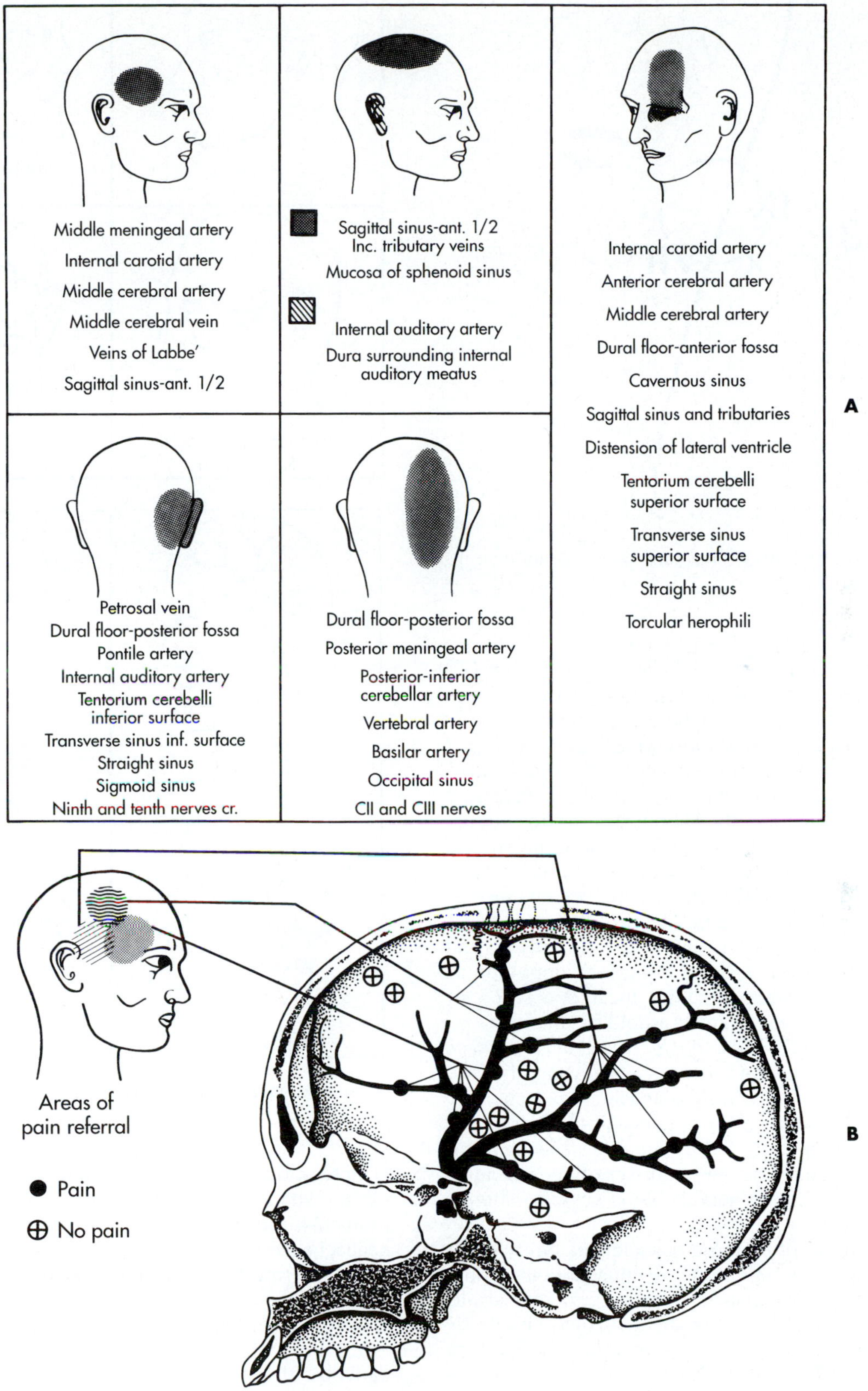


**Fig. 95-2.** Some areas of the head to which pain is referred **(A)** by stimulation of certain cranial structures **(B).** (From Wolff HG: *Headache and other head pain,* New York, 1948, Oxford Press.)

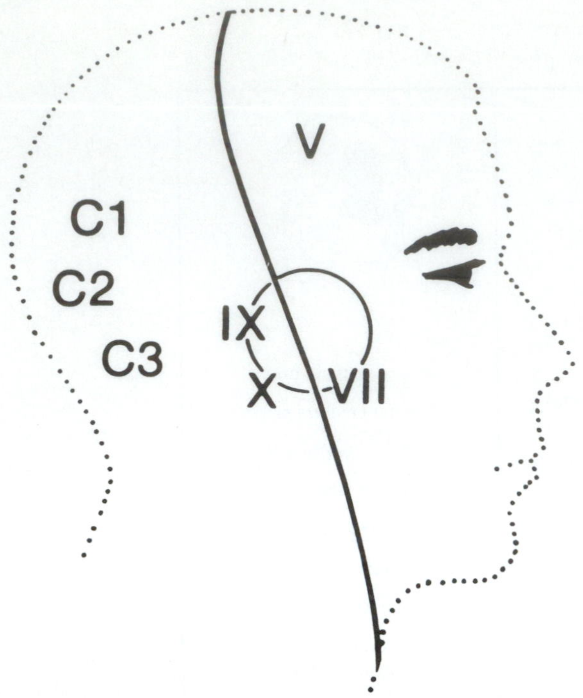


**Fig. 95-3.** Sensory pathways for cranial pain. (Courtesy of the American College of Physicians.)

that are caused to dilate and pulsate unduly by anoxia, hypercapnea, fever, histamine injection, nitroglycerine ingestion, and sudden rises in blood pressure.

6. *Excessive localized vasodilatation and increased amplitude of pulsation of certain intracranial and extracranial vessels.* Such pain may be caused by excessive amplitude of pulsation chiefly in branches of the external carotid arteries, which include the middle meningeal arteries. It may also include reaction of the main stem branches of some of the major intracranial vessels, such as basilar, circle of Willis, internal carotids, and lower reaches of the branches of the anterior, middle, and posterior cerebral arteries. Such excessive amplitude of pulsation may be accompanied by local deposition of substances that lower the pain threshold in that area.

7. *Prolonged contraction of face, head, and neck muscles.* This is at least one of the mechanisms involved in so-called muscle contraction or tension headache.

8. *Inflammation of any pain-sensitive cranial structure.* Inflammation of any sort—viral, bacterial, biochemical, autoimmune, or otherwise—of pain-sensitive structures such as meninges, sensory nerves, blood vessels, sinuses, eyes, and teeth.

Headaches produced by these mechanisms rarely occur in "pure culture." Combinations of muscle contraction, vasodilation, or inflammation may occur in various headache syndromes. These are distinguished chiefly by what is considered the most important or primary mechanism at work at the time.

## WORKUP OF THE HEADACHE PATIENT

Taking the headache history is the most important step in the management of a headache patient. This step serves not only to garner details of the characteristics of the headache symptom, but also to learn as much as possible about the person who has the headache, his or her life situation and problems, and concerns and expectations regarding the headache problem.

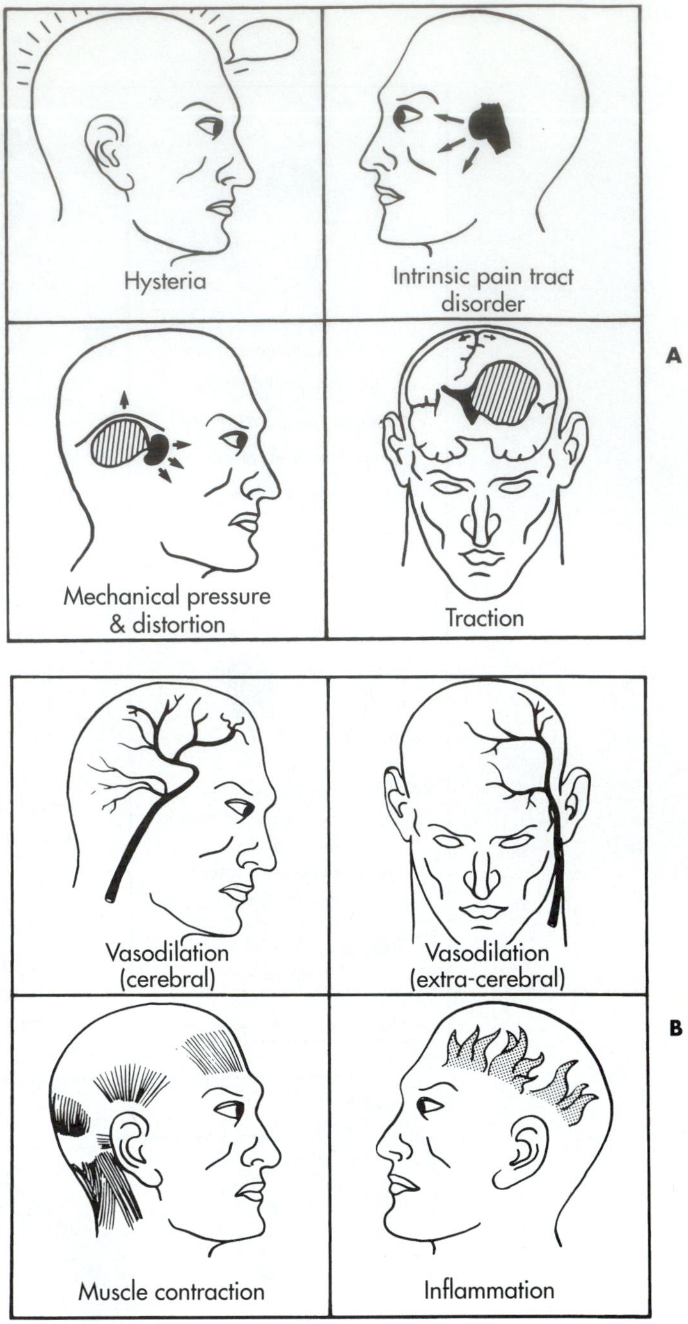


**Fig. 95-4.** **A** and **B,** Mechanisms of cranial pain.

It is during this interview that patients find out if the physician is really interested in *them* as well as their *symptom* and what sort of a "therapeutic alliance" can be made. If the physician appears to be in a hurry and makes patients stick to only the exact medical details of the illness, they quickly sense that discussion of the emotional aspects of the problem that may provide the basic background of the illness is not welcomed. Therefore, patients do not proffer such material even if they wish they could.

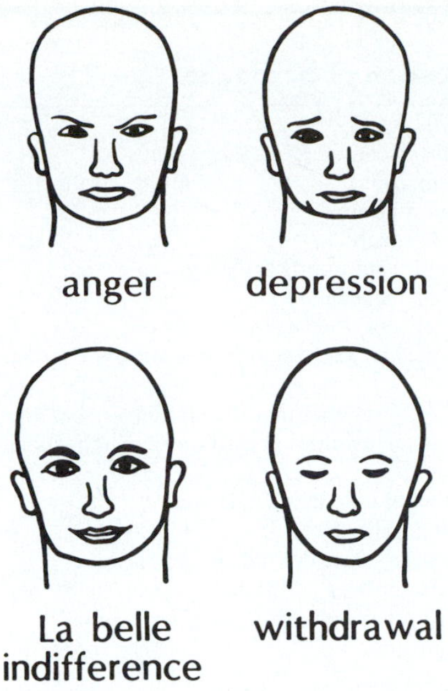


**Fig. 95-5.** Patient affect. The patient's mood may reveal the diagnosis.

At the same time, the physician needs to obtain many details that are especially important in discriminating between the different diagnostic categories of headache, since successful therapy depends greatly on such differential diagnosis. Headache history taking taxes the best in the art of medicine in dealing with both the disease and the patient as a whole.

Headache histories are divided into two major parts: a profile of an individual attack and a profile of the behavior of this form of headache over years. If the patient has more than one type of headache, separate profiles for each must be formulated. Such profiles may be formed in the mind of the physician or may also be outlined on paper in the record, along with a quickly and roughly composed diagram of the head, demonstrating areas in which the pain is located. The patient may assist in filling in some of the details. Such a "portrait" is of considerable use for future reference (Fig. 95-5).

The *attack profile* includes the time of onset; prodromal symptoms, if any, and their nature; the time the headache takes to reach its peak of severity; its duration in seconds, minutes, hours, or days; factors that precipitate and relieve the headache; other symptoms that accompany the pain, (e.g., nausea, vomiting, fever or weakness, neurologic dysfunction); and the patient's behavior during the headache episode.

A *life profile* of the patient's headache may also be constructed in written or diagrammatic form. It starts with headaches in the patient's family, childhood forerunners of headache (e.g., carsickness), cyclic vomiting attacks, and the subsequent frequency and severity of headaches in relation to milestones of development and state of responsibility of the patient. Important correlations to be observed include the relation of the headache to school, puberty, job, family problems, marriage, pregnancy, travel, vacations, sickness and surgery, major losses, and occurrence of other diseases of special interest in headache sufferers. Some of the latter are exemplified by vascular disease, collagen disorders, hypertension, cerebrovascular accident (CVA, stroke), psychiatric disease, head injuries, infections, toxemia of pregnancy, mitral valve prolapse, and seizure disorders. Examples of such attack and life profiles of headache are given in relation to the discussion of several of the subsequent categories of headache in this chapter.

The patient's physician must be acquainted not only with the details of the patient's headache history, but also with the details of the regular medical history and physical examination, since many diseases may cause or contribute to headache problems.

A few points of special interest in headache patients are (1) observation of the patient's affect and behavior; especially during attacks; (2) palpation and auscultation of the head and its major vessels; (3) overall appearance of the patient, which may suggest an underlying disease presenting as headache, such as Cushing's disease, hypothyroidism, Paget's disease, acromegaly, Raynaud's phenomenon of lupus or scleroderma, leonine facies suggesting cluster headache, and vascular malformations on the surface suggesting possible intracranial arteriovenous (AV) malformations. Other underlying disorders include tender, pulseless, painful temporal or other cranial arteries; cervical disease or previous head or neck injury; anemia; and swollen lymph nodes.

If the patient is observed during an attack, special attention is paid to the presence and location of certain physical findings, such as flushing, pallor and sweating, unilaterality or bilaterality of symptoms and findings, Horner's syndrome, tearing, salivation, and nasal congestion.

The compression of superficial arteries such as the temporal, occipital, and carotid arteries is tested relative to its effect on the headache. Manual head traction may be attempted to study any cervical involvement with the pain. The effect of properly used ergotamine tartrate on the headache may be of diagnostic significance, pointing toward a diagnosis of migraine.

In the process of reviewing the headache problem in the manner suggested, the physician is usually mentally stacking up facts from the history and findings that either point to organic causes for the symptoms, demanding further neurologic or medical investigation, or suggest that the disorder is a functional one not requiring such further investigation, at least at this time.

Worth noting are a few points that indicate organicity (see the box on p. 1288). When such signs and symptoms are noted in the history or physical examination, the physician may wish to employ certain investigative techniques that are of special value in identifying or ruling out sources of headache in doubtful situations that suggest the possibility of specific organic disease. Their selection may be enhanced by the guidance of a neurologist and include skull x-ray films, neck and sinus x-ray films, electroencephalograms (EEGs), neuroimaging, and lumbar puncture.

Features of the history and physical examination may indicate important psychogenic factors behind the patient's headache problem. At times, serious disturbances of mood, (e.g., depression or suicidal thoughts) may demand consultation with a psychiatrist. Uncontrolled anxiety or anger, disturbances of memory, and confusion about facts or their interpretation may suggest a need for mental

### Warnings of organic disease

**Headaches associated with:**

1. Unconsciousness or seizure
2. Sudden onset—no previous history
3. Neurologic signs during and following headache
4. Stiff neck, fever
5. Monocular blindness
6. History of recent head or neck trauma
7. First appearance after age 50
8. Change in response to usual treatment
9. Change in personality and personal habits
10. Presence of hypertension
11. Bruits in the head or neck
12. Endocrine abnormalities

**Headaches that:**

13. Are precipitated by the Valsalva maneuver: lifting, coughing, straining, coitus
14. Goes its own way; does not follow the usual course of migraine or tension headaches
15. Appears for no good reason

### Classification of headache

Vascular headache of migraine type
- Classic migraine
- Common migraine
- Cluster headache
- Hemiplegic and ophthalmoplegic migraine
- Lower-half headache

Muscle contraction headache
Combined headache: vascular and muscle contraction headaches
Headache of nasal vasomotor reaction
Headache of delusional, conversion, or hypochondriacal states
Nonmigrainous vascular headaches
Traction headache
Headache from overt cranial inflammation
Headache from disease of ocular, aural, nasal, and sinusal, dental, or other cranial or neck structures
Cranial neuritides
Cranial neuralgias
Chronic posttraumatic headache

testing, cognitive testing, and advice from a psychologist or psychiatrist. The MMPI (Minnesota Multiphasic Personality Inventory), although somewhat out of date in some of its questions, has a wealth of sound experience behind it and is still useful as a screen for depression, hysteria, and neurasthenia that may not be overtly present in the patient. Sometimes discussion of the patient's problem with a spouse or other family member may be indicated, especially when the patient seems hesitant or unable to describe the nature of the illness.

Patients with chronic headache problems often have used many drugs and sometimes are continuing to do so. It is important to obtain information on this subject and to evaluate it in relation to the conduct of treatment.

## CLASSIFICATION OF HEADACHE

Although many classifications of headache have been devised, the box above right lists the one used here.

In general, this chapter focuses on identification and management of headaches of a functional type—those occurring spontaneously and not those based on specific overt pathology (e.g., acute sinusitis, brain tumor, brain abscess, meningitis) for which the treatment of the headache is the treatment of the recognizable disease process.

## MIGRAINE

Migraine appears to be a disorder that consists of an abnormal pattern of response to a variety of stimuli in the external, physiologic, and psychological environments. Heredity plays a powerful role in setting the physiologic and psychologic stages for these outbursts of head pain. Environmental influences and experiences undoubtedly condition the use of this reaction pattern by the patient in certain circumstances.

### Classic migraine

Classic migraine (Fig. 95-6, *A*) is so called because it is the same entity that was described in the "classic age" of Galen and Hippocrates. Its hallmark is the succinct, relatively short neurologic prodrome that takes place before the headache phase begins or, sometimes, all by itself without any succeeding headache. The prodrome may take many forms but usually has a sharp beginning and ending, lasts for 10 to 60 minutes (most often 20 to 25 minutes) and usually is followed, as it is disappearing, by the beginning of a headache. By far the most common prodrome is visual in the form of a scintillating scotoma. This starts as a small, twinkling, corrugated circle of tiny white, golden, or colored lights that form a castellated or fortification spectrum (Fig. 95-6, *B*). The lights appear in an elliptic form in one homonymous field of vision, spreading further and further toward the periphery, followed by a blackout of vision in the area of the visual field where the scintillating lights have passed. Gradually the whole strange apparition disappears, vision returns, and headache, usually but not always, begins.

The next most common and equally diagnostically characteristic prodrome is the development of a prickling in the fingers of one hand which creeps up the arm to the face, especially around the mouth, followed by hypoanesthesia and/or complete anesthesia of the same area that has been "prickled," until the whole process clears and headache begins.

Less frequent forms of the classic migraine prodrome include many bizarre events, including spots of flashing lights, "seeing through heat waves," aphasia, confusion, fuguelike states, distortion of the size of objects seen (micropsia), and even sensations of another person being present at one side or the other of the patient.

These classic prodromes are usually homonymous hemisensory effects but occasionally affect both sides of

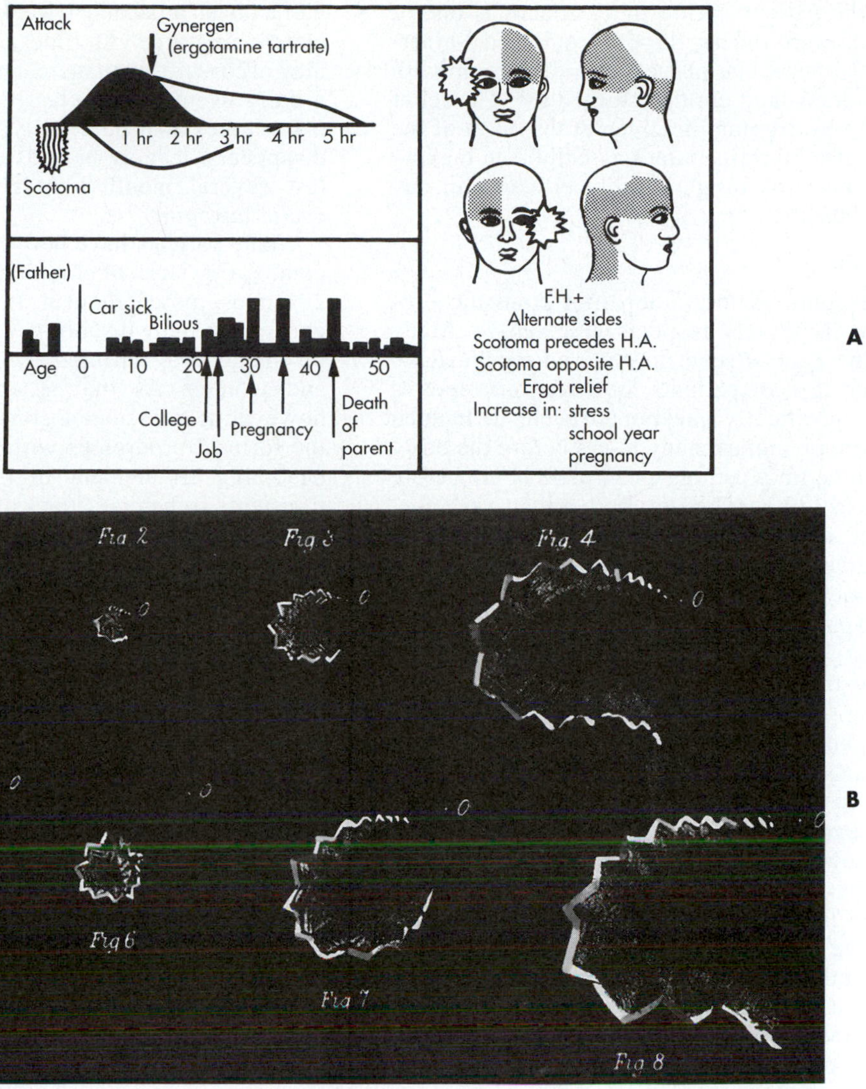


**Fig. 95-6. A,** Classic migraine. Profile of attack, profile of life history of headache, and "portrait." On this and similar diagrams the physician may register (above the line) the attack profile—duration, speed of onset and offset, severity, effect of therapy on the attack—and (below the line) the accompaniments of the attack—prodromes, nausea and vomiting, polyuria, etc. In the life profile the frequency and severity of attacks are recorded in relation to milestones in the patient's life (including family history). The portrait shows the location of the symptoms on a diagram of the patient's head and (*bottom right*) a list of key points in diagnosis. It is suggested that each physician create a similar diagram for patients. **B,** Scintillating scotomas tend to enlarge and occupy a central portion of the field of vision. This progression was drawn by P.W. Latham for his description of the "Nervous or Sick Headache" in 1873.

the body at once. The headache following the prodrome is usually on the opposite side of the head, but it may be bilateral, especially in children, and at times is on the same side as the prodrome. On rare occasions, prodromes recur during the headache phase, and occasionally rare neurologic disturbances continue after the patient's headache has ceased. When this happens, it is important that thorough neurologic testing be carried out to rule out organic disease.

The painful phase, or headache, during attacks of classic migraine tends to last for "a few hours" (e.g., 2 to 6) and is often accompanied by photophobia, hyperacousis, and hyperosmia. Nausea and vomiting frequently occur as prominent symptoms. The quality of the pain is usually steady; it frequently has a throbbing character and is worse on bending over or performing the Valsalva maneuver in any form. Attacks may recur consistently on one side of the head but more often swap sides from one attack to another. Persistence always on one side may raise the index of suspicion for organic causes and stimulate more neurologic testing to rule out angioma, vascular malformation, or other organic disease.

Behavior of the patient during these attacks is one of annoyance and concern during the prodrome and "hibernation" during the headache phase—in a dark room with light, noise, problems, and children turned off. The relief of such head pain by ergotamine given at the onset of the headache phase of a migraine attack is helpful in making the diagnosis, since this drug is rarely effective in any other type of headache.

## Common migraine

The profiles for common migraine differ from those of classic migraine in several respects (Fig. 95-7). Many common migraine attacks seem to have no recognizable prodrome. About 25% of patients, however, do report a prodrome when specifically questioned about it. In such patients the prodrome comes many hours before the onset of a headache, sometimes as long as 24 to 48 hours before but more often 6 to 12 hours before. Rather than a succinct neurologic event, it is more apt to be a vague change in mood or vegetative behavior, such as depression, euphoria, unusual hunger, irritability, or physical weight gain.

The headache phase is similar to that of classic migraine but tends to last longer and be more prostrating. It is accompanied by more nonheadache symptoms, such as nausea, vomiting, diuresis, diarrhea, "faint" spells, and generalized weakness and debility. The attack of pain frequently arises during sleep or on awakening, lasts until the patient goes to sleep, and may be present each day on awakening for several days.

In its "life profile" it shows a tendency to begin or to be accentuated by milestones of increased responsibility and stress in the patient's life. Unlike classic migraine, which tends to be recurrent or reactivated during pregnancy, common migraine disappears significantly during pregnancy in about 80% of patients.

Common migraine tends to recur as single episodes during the course of a year rather than in short flurries of half a dozen attacks in a week or two, as is the custom with classic migraine. At times, however, common migraine may occur with ever-increasing frequency until it becomes a daily event and is classified as "migraine status." At other times it occurs daily for several weeks and then disappears, leaving periods of freedom from attacks that last several months, thereby gaining the terminology *cyclic migraine*.

Many patients have both types of migraine, classic and common. Attacks of common migraine are probably about 20 times more frequent than classic migraine and in general are more disabling. Classic migraine tends to clear up and go away during the years before age 40 in both men and women. As the patient enters the 60s and 70s, however, it may stage a comeback, reappearing largely in the form of prodromes without subsequent headache and becoming an element in the differential diagnosis of transient ischemic attacks (TIAs) and minor CVAs. Recurrence of the phenomenon repeatedly at the same site and with the characteristic homonymous zigzag scintillating scotomas usually serves to identify it as the "return of the native," rather than as a new embolic or ischemic process. Occasionally, however, the transient migrainous scotomas which return in older years cause a fixed, permanent lesion in the area of their activity.

Common migraine during middle life may be associated with the development of essential hypertension. It tends then to become a daily "wake-up" headache and acquires the new name "hypertensive" headache. Even under these designations, it responds to antimigraine medication.

### *Mechanisms*

**Prodromal phase.** Theories regarding the mechanisms at work in the prodromal phase of migraine range between origins in the brain parenchyma and primary disturbances in the cranial circulation. Local and generalized changes in blood supply, usually related in their greatest severity

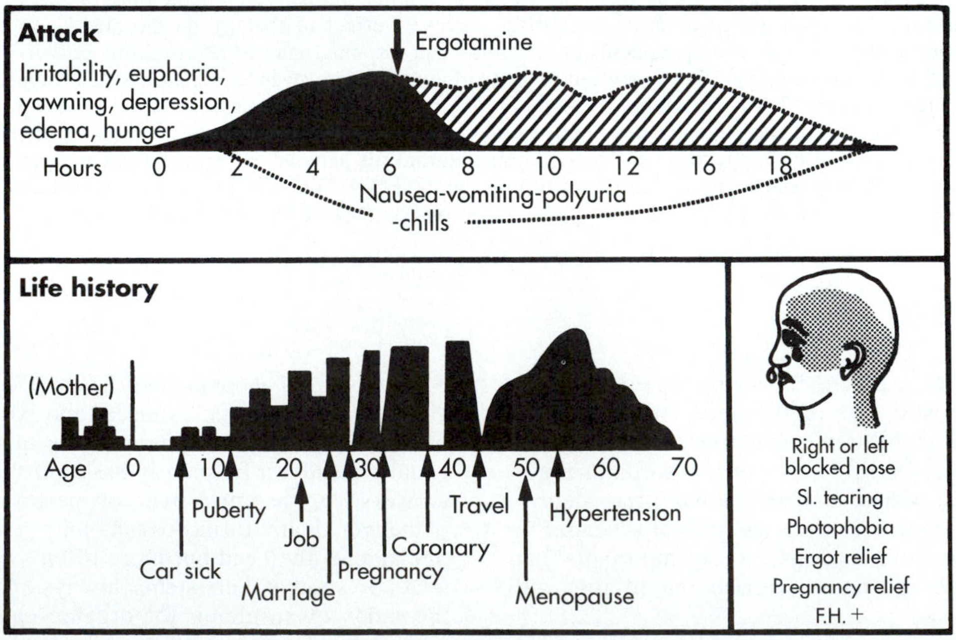


**Fig. 95-7.** Profile of common migraine.

to the area from which the symptoms arise, are well documented. It is not known, however, whether these changes are caused by local and/or generalized spasm of cerebral vessels, by sludging in these vessels as a result of platelet aggregation or other causes of increased blood viscosity, or by primary metabolic or membrane alterations in the brain cell circuitry that result in the circulatory changes. Cellular metabolic disturbances may precipitate a wave of excitation in the brain parenchyma accompanied by a sudden, short peak in local cerebral blood flow. The excitatory stage is followed by a prolonged period of brain cell electric inhibition and decreased blood flow, followed by increased intracranial and extracranial blood vessel pulsation and blood flow associated with the painful phase of the attack.

The latter sequence of events is consistent with what happens in experimental animals (and can be created in vitro in human brain slices) in the "spreading depression" of Leão. *Editorial update:* The spreading depression of Leão is a transient reduction in electrical activity in gray matter of animals that advances contiguously over the cortical surface. In a remarkable study of blood flow with positron-emission tomography in a human subject who happened to develop a migraine headache (see Plate 50), the rate of the advance of electrical depression and vascular hypoperfusion were consistent with the spread of symptoms during the migraine and aura. This spreading cerebral hypoperfusion is demonstrated in Plate 50 by cerebral blood-flow measurement using an intracarotid xenon-133 technique. Plate 49 artistically depicts the visual distortions and scintillating scotoma during the aura of a migraine headache that may relate temporally with the spreading cerebral hypoperfusion.

**Painful phase.** Much evidence still supports the early observations of Wolff and his group during the late 1930s that a great deal of the pain in migraine arises from excessive amplitude of pulsation of the branches of the external carotid artery plus the local presence of a pain-threshold-lowering substance in the tissues surrounding the excessively pulsating vessels. "Neurokinin," probably related to bradykinin, and substance P created at the site of headache, in the presence of vasodilation, may have a role in relaying pain to the central nervous system (CNS) via sensory nerves and ganglia.

During many but not all observations on migraine attacks, a decrease in plasma serotonin has been noted relative to the painful phase of the migraine attack. Many other observations of altered behavior of vasoactive amines have been documented in migraine attacks. However, it is still not clear whether these are the cause or effect of the migraine event and if they are really different from what happens in control subjects who have been subjected to similar headache-provoking events.

Another theory involves the concept that temporary abnormalities in the central pain regulation centers produce failure or inadequate behavior of the endorphin-enkephalin systems that results in lowering the pain threshold to stimuli from peripheral structures (e.g., "misbehaving" cranial blood vessels).

In general, for both classic and common migraine, the patient, by inheritance, seems to be endowed with a very sensitive, physiologically irritable nervous system that reacts to stress—whether from environmental, physiologic, or psychologic stimuli—in an excessive or abnormal manner. This leads to transient functional impairment of nerve cells, cranial blood flow disturbances, vascular "misbehavior," and abnormalities in the central nociceptive control of head pain: the migraine attack.

## Management

Management of migraine is divided into three areas: (1) elimination or avoidance of stimuli, (2) prophylactic treatment of the patient to increase resistance to the migraine stimuli, and (3) treatment of the attack. The physician needs to learn the details of the environment and the psychologic climate in which the migraine occurs (Fig. 95-8). Information regarding the details in a typical day in the patient's life during the week and, separately, on weekends and on vacations is important. The school situation, the in-laws, the domineering relatives, the annoying telephone calls, the deadlines, the mealtimes, and the diet need to be understood to have a good picture of the stimuli to migraine. Failure to explore the stresses and strains in a patient's life situation is the most common reason for failure to achieve successful headache therapy.

***Elimination or avoidance of stimuli.*** The stimuli that trigger an attack in a genetically susceptible migraine individual arise in three environments: the *external,* the *physiologic,* and the *psychologic.* It is essential for the physician to recognize them and to teach the patient what they are. This usually involves several visits and periods of trial and error rather than a simple prescription or a "magic pill." The patient needs to be warned about this from the beginning.

The vulnerability of the patient to these stimuli varies from time to time in relation to the cyclic behavior of migraine itself and the life stress situation of the patient. Thus, at one time a single stimulus from any one of the three major areas mentioned may set off the explosion of an attack, whereas at other times several stimuli from more than one category may need to appear together to precipitate an attack.

**Common stimuli from external environment**

1. Weather: hot, humid days
2. Major shifts in weather fronts
3. Special well-known "weathers," such as the Foehn (Switzerland), the Sirrocco (Mediterranean), the Shavan (Israel); hot, muggy August (New England)
4. Sudden major shifts in altitude (e.g., traveling by plane from Florida to Mexico City)

**Local environmental factors**

1. Loud noise, bright light (especially flickering), penetrating smells including pleasant smells (e.g., perfume)
2. Toxic fumes (as in some buses, garages; carbon monoxide in cars and cabins), smoke-filled rooms

**Ingested substances**

1. Alcohol (in any form), even in small amounts
2. Chocolate
3. Foods containing tyramine and nitrates (cheeses, fermented foods, pickles, some citrus fruits, cured meats)
4. Monosodium glutamate (Chinese food, Accent)

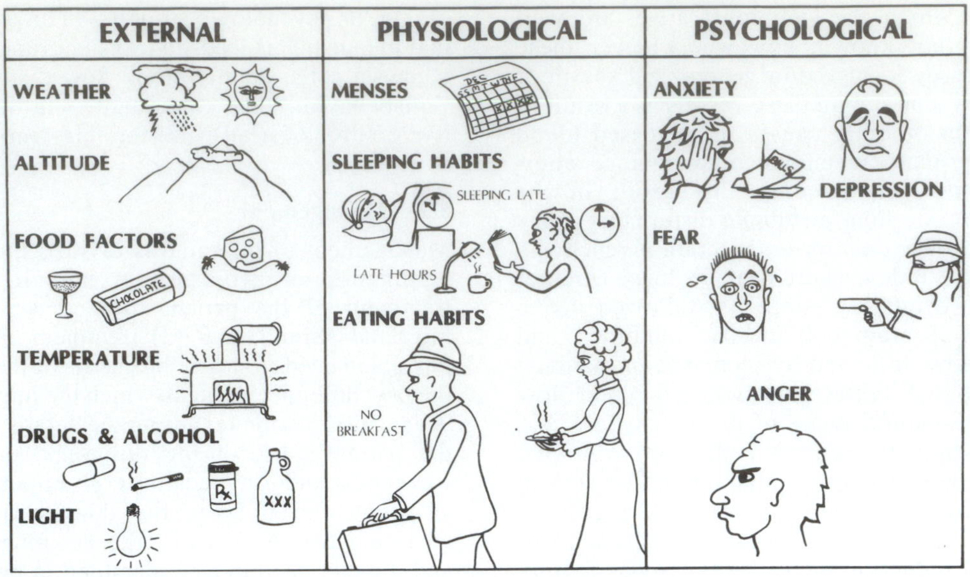


**Fig. 95-8.** Factors influencing the onset of migraine headaches from the external, physiologic, and psychologic environments.

5. Medicines causing vasodilation, such as nitroglycerine (pills and ointment); isosorbide dinitrate (Isordil); occasionally calcium channel blockers; large doses of reserpine, nicotinic acid, theophylline

Almost all migraine patients are sensitive to alcohol products. Many are sensitive to chocolate, especially during youth, and to monosodium glutamate. Only 5% to 10% of migraine patients are sensitive to the other foods. A food should be eliminated from the diet only by trial and error rather than as a blanket dietary restriction.

**Physiologic stimuli to migraine**

1. Menstrual cycle. Many women with migraine are more susceptible to headache before or at the time of their period and/or at ovulation.
2. Major changes of pace (from very busy to very relaxed, and vice versa: busy week followed by a relaxed weekend)
3. Failing to eat on time: no breakfast, delayed lunch
4. Sleeping too late (Saturdays, Sundays, holidays)
5. Prolonged mental strain
6. Severe exercise
7. Sleep abnormalities (sleep apnea, insomnia)

**Psychologic stimuli**

1. Depression
2. Repressed anger (at the boss, spouse, relative, world)
3. Poststress anxiety, especially about personal accomplishments
4. Deadlines; fear of personal failure

Not all these stimuli can be eliminated, but they can often be diminished, avoided, or not allowed to accumulate to unbearable peaks. For instance, a dinner party need not be planned at the time of a menstrual period; the desire to succeed in two adult education courses can be reduced by taking one at a time; and the number of committee appointments and chairpersonships may be checked.

***Improving the patient's resistance to headache.*** When headaches, by their frequency or severity, are causing disruption of family, social, or work life, the physician and patient may want to take steps not only to relieve attacks by manipulation of migraine stimuli, but also to toughen the patient's resistance to attacks. Such prophylactic activities may take the form of pharmaceutical therapy, behavioral techniques, and psychotherapy. More and more in this day and age, emphasis on prophylaxis of this sort is shifting from drug and hormone therapies to behavioral and relaxation techniques, as well as various forms of psychotherapy.

Some patients are not interested in or susceptible to behavioral and psychotherapeutic approaches and may prefer the pharmaceutical route and the support of an understanding physician. Other patients may want and need formal psychiatric help. A third group of patients, becoming more widespread in recent years, is anxious to learn techniques that help their minds and bodies to function better together. Biofeedback and behavioral counseling techniques, although psychiatrically more superficial, are also more acceptable and practical for this group of patients who cannot afford or face formal psychotherapy. As physician and patient become better acquainted with each other over several visits, decisions can be made regarding the best route to success. Physicians often fail to recognize how effective they may be in this regard by spending as much time at each visit discussing the patient's life situation and style as in prescribing more and more medicines. Provision by the physician for a "telephone hour" in which patients may call in reports or seek advice is a powerful support to the "therapeutic alliance" between patient and physician.

***Pharmaceutical prophylaxis.*** The usual precautions and contraindications for medications must be recognized and observed. Only some special precautions regarding their use in the treatment of headache are mentioned in this text.

**β-Adrenergic blockers.** Propranolol in long- or short-acting form is probably the most effective β-adrenergic agent against migraine and in some patients with "mixed-type" or "combined" headache. Patients whose anxiety has overt physical manifestations (e.g., rapid pulse, arrhythmias, sweating, flushing, tremor) seem to benefit particularly well from this agent, which "cools" the activity of the β-adrenergic system. Dosages may range from 20 to 320 mg/day. If even mild hypertension is present, the addition of small doses of hydrochlorothiazide (25 to 50 mg/day) is a useful adjunct. The concomitant daily usage of β-adrenergic blockers and vasoconstrictors (e.g., ergotamine, methysergide) may lead to compromise of the peripheral circulation. (Intermittent use of ergotamine during β-blockade is usually well tolerated, but chronic daily use of the two is inadvisable.)

The use of β-blockers with tricyclic compounds is permissible and sometimes helpful. Concomitant use of β-blockers with calcium channel blockers must be monitored very closely because of possible hypotension. Also, the use of β-blockers may be unwise in the presence of Raynaud-like peripheral vasoconstriction, which at times is present in migraine patients. β-Blockers may be especially useful in a double role in migraine patients who also have mitral valve prolapse or coronary disease.

β-Blockers have been associated in very rare instances with fibrous peritonitis and Peyronie disease, examples of localized systemic scleroses related to those caused by methysergide in headache patients. A migraine patient who has experienced any of these scleroses probably should not be given β-blockers (see Methysergide).

β-Blockers designed especially for their effect on blood pressure or the heart are also useful for migraine, although they may not be as specific as propranolol, which is also effective in these other situations.

**Antidepressant drugs.** The antidepressant agents are sometimes effective in migraine but are more often useful in patients with "mixed" or "combined" headache. They may be clearly indicated by overt signs and a history of depression, although they also may prove useful when depression is not clinically evident. Amitriptyline, imipramine, desipramine (Norpramin), and trazodone in small, medium, and full dosage schedules, usually at bedtime, may be very helpful.

The monoamine oxidase (MAO) inhibitors phenylethylhydrazine (Nardil) and isocarboxazid (Marplan) are similarly useful but carry more risk of side effects, such as postural hypotension and liver toxicity. During their use, one must be careful to give supplemental pyridoxine (50 mg orally [PO] daily) and avoid foods and drugs containing tyramine, ephedrine and meperidine, and barbiturates. It is important to check cross-reactions between these and many other drugs used for headache when starting and stopping the use of these drugs.

**Tranquilizers.** Agents such as diazepam (Valium), chlordiazepoxide (Librium), alprazolam (Xanax), hydroxyzine (Atarax), and other antianxiety agents may be somewhat helpful for short, tense periods but in general are not of much use specifically in migraine prevention. Their long-term use, to cover up the effects of anxiety rather than to get at its source, is to be avoided except in unusual situations.

**Anticonvulsants.** Agents such as phenytoin (Dilantin), primidone (Mysoline), mephobarbital (Mebaral), phenobarbital, and carbamazepine are beneficial in a small number of patients, especially those who demonstrate spike and wave activity in the EEG, focal lesions of sharp activity, or localized temporal and olfactory lobe symptoms and EEG abnormalities.

In a rare form of migraine the features of both epilepsy and migraine are present simultaneously. Patients with this syndrome have such prodromes as classic migraine plus headache, seizures, and unconsciousness. Anticonvulsant drugs are very useful in managing them.

**Antihistamines, antiserotonin, antiacetylcholine drugs.** One of the earliest antihistamine drugs, diphenhydramine (Benadryl), taken at bedtime in 50 to 100 mg doses, has a beneficial effect on migraine in a few patients. Cyproheptadine also is helpful for some patients and is especially useful in children who have migraine frequently enough to be missing school. For children of school age, a dose of one tablet (4 mg) at bedtime and 2 mg (½ tablet) at breakfast may be well worth trying.

Pizotyline (Sandomigran) is used in Canada, Scandinavia, and other European countries but is not available in the United States. It holds a good record of reducing migraine attacks with few serious side effects (sedation, weight gain).

Many over-the-counter preparations contain antihistamines as decongestants along with analgesic medication. Such combinations are helpful in mild migraine attacks if nasal congestion is a feature but usually do not suffice for major attacks and are not very effective as prophylactic medication.

**Antiinflammatory agents**

***Aspirin.*** Aspirin in small doses (300 mg three to seven times/week) is as useful as any other agent, chiefly for its action in diminishing the aggregation of platelets, which seems to be a feature of migraine pathophysiology. This approach may be particularly effective in patients with classic migraine and especially in older patients whose migraine scotomas return during middle or old age. Small amounts of aspirin designed to inhibit prostaglandin activity are better than large amounts, which may also affect prostacyclin activity, which helps to keep blood vessels open. Aspirin prophylaxis combined with persantine, 50 mg PO one to three times daily, may be useful in "basilar artery migraine," during which major impairment of blood flow in the basilar system appears to create major impairment of function. Patients with basilar artery migraine, usually young women, must also avoid taking oral contraceptives, and they must stop smoking.

***Indomethacin.*** Indomethacin (Indocin) may be useful in prophylaxis of certain types of migraine, such as exercise-induced migraine and cyclic migraine (common migraine appearing in cycles of daily occurrence for several weeks followed by no headache for several weeks or months). It also seems to be specifically helpful for migrainelike syndromes of pain arising from or aggravated by injuries or lesions in the neck. Doses of 25 mg four times daily or slow-release indomethacin (75 mg twice daily) are worth a trial in these situations. Effectiveness may not be achieved until doses of 150 or 200 mg/day have been reached. At these doses, however, relief is obtained in 2 to 3 days if the drug is going to be worthwhile. Because of gastrointestinal (GI) side effects, antacids or gastric acid–suppressing drugs (ranitidine, 150 mg twice daily) or cimetidine (Tagamet), 300 mg four times daily, may be needed. When indomethacin proves useful, it works quickly and specifically. If a few days' trial does not produce marked benefits, the drug should be changed. (See also Chronic Paroxysmal Hemicrania, for which indomethacin is specifically and dramatically effective.)

*Other Agents.* Ibuprofen (Motrin), fenoprofen (Nalfon), and naproxen (Naprosyn), given in their usual antiarthritic doses, may prove worthwhile in some patients with migraine, used prophylactically either constantly or just at the time of the menstrual period. All nonsteroidal antiinflammatory drugs (NSAIDs) can cause renal function impairment. Therefore, when these agents are used chronically, this possibility, as well as GI and hematopoietic complications, must be carefully monitored.

**Antihypertensive medications.** When even mild hypertension complicates migraine, the attacks become more frequent and severe. The presence of the headaches may incline the physician to treat even these lesser degrees of hypertension because such therapy often benefits both conditions. Hydrochlorothiazide in doses of 25 to 50 mg/day in addition to a long- or short-acting β-Blocker, (e.g., propranolol [Inderal]) in doses ranging from 40 to 160 to 240 mg/day are suggested.

**Reserpine.** Reserpine in very small amounts (e.g., 0.1 mg daily or every other day) in combination with hydrochlorothiazide (25 mg/day) may slowly create significant improvement in headache. Larger amounts may lead to depression and should be avoided. Attention is also drawn to the persisting concern that reserpine may have a carcinogenic effect, especially on the breast, through prolactin stimulation. Clonidine (Catapres) may prove useful to some migraine patients with or without hypertension. Antihypertensive agents that depend for their effect on suppression of angiotensin-releasing enzymes may also be helpful in migraine but have not been specifically tested. Guanabenz (Wytensin), a centrally acting antihypertensive agent, has been found to be effective prophylactically. The antihypertensive hydralazine is to be avoided in headache patients because it tends to increase headache.

**Calcium channel blockers.** Calcium channel blockers are used prophylactically in the treatment of migraine. In Europe, flunarizine has been tested and used to advantage. Verapamil, diltiazem, and nimodipine may be effective in preventing both migraine and cluster headache. Doses may need to be carried to the high levels used in other cardiovascular conditions, and continued use for at least 3 to 4 weeks may be necessary to determine their usefulness for a given patient's migraine or cluster headache. If they are used simultaneously with antihypertensive or β-blocking drugs, the patient's blood pressure must be monitored carefully for fear of hypotension.

**Ergotamine-containing drugs.** Although usually not recommended for prolonged prophylactic therapy, ergotamine in small amounts over circumscribed periods may be very useful. In children who are sick enough with migraine to miss school frequently, the use of half a Bellergal-Spacetab at bedtime may be justified. In such circumstances, interruption of constant use should occur for several days at monthly intervals. Such use should be very rare. Cyproheptadine or preferably behavioral therapy and biofeedback, if available, are preferred.

Ergotamine tartrate may be used daily by adults as short-term prophylaxis at times when headaches are most apt to appear and are particularly undesired, such as at times of weddings, funerals, graduations, anniversaries, or the menstrual cycle, when a particular patient's headaches tend to occur with recognized regularity. It may be very useful if taken on the nights before such events, at breakfast on the day of the event, and again that evening.

Some migraine patients have a "vague" prodrome hours before a headache. Such prodromes are usually changes in mood, (e.g., euphoria, depression, hunger, irritability) and are well recognized by the patient. Use of an ergotamine product at this time is sometimes effective in preventing further development of an attack.

The same principle may be applied to other migraine medicine, such as ergonovine maleate, dihydroergotamine mesylate (D.H.E. 45), and corticosteroids, usually considered to be useful only at the time of an attack.

*The "Ergot Cycle."* Some patients begin to take ergotamine with increasing frequency so they can continue to perform at a level that is perhaps beyond their capability. Gradually, ergotamine becomes a daily need. If it is not taken for even 1 day, a vascular "rebound" phenomenon takes place that brings about another headache. Thus, headaches continue to occur daily over long periods because of this ergot rebound cycle, even when other causes of headache may have cleared up. "St. Anthony's fire," the ergot poisoning of previous centuries, arose from the prolonged use of moldy rye in times of famine. *Claviceps purpurea,* the mold that provides ergot on the contaminated rye, causes marked vasoconstriction, gangrene, CNS symptoms, and hallucinations. Some think the girls who testified against the "witches" in Salem during the 1700s were suffering from delusion caused by famine and ergot poisoning.

Some patients may have to be hospitalized for a week while all ergot is stopped and the resulting severe headaches are managed by pain and antinausea medicine as well as intravenous (IV) fluids because of the nausea and vomiting until the headaches stop. The patient may then be discharged with strict orders not to let the level of stress become so heavy again and, preferably, to use medicines other than ergot for treatment of the condition. A return to the same prehospital level of life performance usually leads to a return to the same level of ergot abuse. Changes in behavior may render the patient headache free.

**Methysergide.** Methysergide (Sansert) is highly effective against migraine. Because of serious side effects in certain subjects, it seems wise to reserve its use for patients whose lives are seriously altered by frequency or severity of migraine and who are reliable in following the rules of therapy and reporting to their physician. They must be willing to stop the use of the drug every 3 months for a 2- to 4-week period. During this interval, other migraine prophylactic agents may be employed. The drug is best administered as a 2 mg tablet at bedtime. Subsequent increases in dosage up to a total of four 2 mg tablets daily may be made at intervals as seems clinically necessary.

Side effects of this drug include nausea; abdominal pain; edema; weight gain; vasoconstriction of abdominal, carotid, peripheral, and coronary arteries; and localized areas of sclerosis in the retroperitoneal, pleuropulmonary, and endocardial spaces. The fibrotic lesions related to the use of this drug usually regress in whole or in part when it is discontinued but at other times can require major surgery for correction of impaired function of important body structures, such as the aorta, iliac arteries and celiac axis, coronary orifices and heart valves, and kidneys.

Intermittent use of the drug has prevented these complications but leaves the patient subject to rebound headache when the drug is temporarily stopped. The patient taking methysergide needs to be examined regularly by the physician about three times a year so he or she can check all peripheral pulses, listen for cardiac murmurs and arterial bruits and pleural rubs, and check for any symptoms suggesting fibrotic compromise of any organ or system in the body. Patients with such complications should never again be given methysergide or its "first cousin" ergotamine.

**Hormones.** Deficiency of thyroid, pituitary, gonadal, and adrenal hormones may singly or in tandem cause the beginning or the increasing of migraine. Hypothyroidism that occurs "idiopathically" or secondarily as a result of previous thyroid surgery, disease, or radioactive iodine therapy accentuates migraine. Substitution therapy brings significant relief.

Migraine headaches may appear for the first time or be accentuated by hypoadrenocortical states that occur either "spontaneously" or, more often, as an aftermath of corticosteroid therapy for some other condition. For example, a patient who has previously had migraine but has not had any attacks for several years may have a series of migraine attacks after the conclusion of several weeks' or months' treatment with corticosteroids for asthma or regional enteritis. Such a return of migraine may be controlled by reinstitution of steroid therapy and a more gradual reduction of the doses.

Major changes in the level of ovarian hormones may also affect the occurrence of migraine. A sharp drop in estrogen at the time of the menstrual period is related in some women to the occurrence of migraine but is usually not helped by prescribing estrogen at the time, since such a maneuver may merely "postpone the evil day." Some patients with migraine just before the monthly period have been found to lack progesterone. Replacement by oral or parenteral progesterone during the week before the period is occasionally helpful (medroxyprogesterone [Provera], 10 mg PO daily for a week, or hydroxyprogesterone [Delalutin], 250 mg intramuscularly [IM] in one dose a week before the period is due).

When menopause occurs and hot flashes appear, migraine may increase for a while in both frequency and severity. Modifying the change by giving low doses of estrogen may make this transition easier. When periods stop and hot flashes do not appear and yet headaches increase, a search for correction of the endocrine imbalance is directed to the pituitary and hypothalamus. Usually the help of an endocrinologist is indicated in this search. Too much estrogen apparently is as frequent a cause for migraine exacerbation as too little. Thus, accentuation of migraine may be a result of estrogen dosage that is more than the body requires, and reduction of the dosage may relieve the headache problem.

The use of oral contraceptives may be dangerous for women who have migraine. Transient and even permanent cerebral and retinal vascular accidents have been reported to be unusually frequent in patients with migraine. Increase in headache and the development of hypertension are also noted. In general, a good rule seems to be that women with classic migraine and other forms accompanied by neurologic symptoms should not take oral contraceptives; women with common migraine should preferably avoid oral contraceptives but may be allowed a trial period of close observation for 3 to 4 months, during which blood pressure and headache incidence are observed. If there is an increase in either, birth control pills are stopped. Low-level estrogen content of the oral contraceptive is advisable in the migraine patients who are allowed to take it.

Hysterectomy is not good therapy for migraine, even in patients whose headaches occur chiefly at the time of menstrual periods. Experience has shown that as many headache patients are made worse by this procedure as are made better or remain the same. Hysterectomy, with rare exceptions, is reserved for complaints directly related to gynecologic lesions.

Migraine headaches, in rare instances, may also be accentuated by adrenocortical, parathyroid, pituitary, and thyroid tumors that cause hyperactivity of the glands involved.

***Psychosomatic therapy.*** Many patients and their physicians now are striving to find forms of therapy other than pharmaceutical programs for the relief of chronically recurring headache such as migraine and tension headaches. Such a search is useful for those who want to avoid the hazards of the chronic use of drugs and to maintain a sense of personal control of their problems. It is to be hoped that the physician can supply the various elements of headache therapy for many such patients, but there may be a problem of finding the time, or the physician may not be inclined to handle situations involving the patient's psychosomatic relation to life stresses that contribute heavily to headache incidence and severity.

In any event, the physician must make sure that recommendations for referral of the patient to those who can supply these forms of therapy are made after the "therapeutic alliance" with the patient has been established and the patient's capacity to use the various levels of therapy available are assessed. Such referrals are apt to be useful to patients if they understand the reasons for this approach, know what the method chosen will entail, and want to participate in an elected program. The patients should make the appointment as an indication of their positive approach to this form of therapy.

The options open to the patient and the physician in seeking this kind of help are affected greatly by the availability of time, money, the patient's desire to participate, and the patient's capacity to examine, express, and relate emotional feelings to life situations and symptoms.

Thus, some patients with little ability to comprehend and use deep psychic concepts may profit from practical programs that demonstrate some of the body's physical reactions during tension states and teach methods of improving them. Others with more psychogenic "savvy" and ability to identify and relate their feelings to clinical situations may find more help in forms of psychotherapy that examine these areas directly. There are several categories of this type of therapy.

*1. Behavioral modification* (useful for patients with limited insight into feelings but logical thinking about behavior). Patients learn to recognize behavior that produces headaches and ways to modify it to reduce pain. This modification is often provided by psychologists.

*2. Somatic relaxation therapy.* This form is suitable for patients who become tense in reaction to emotional and physical stress but have difficulty recognizing the feelings that create this reaction. These techniques teach the patient how to recognize and change the physiologic components involved in experiencing stress and to practice techniques that keep such responses at a low level. They do not attempt to discover *why* a patient becomes tense or to find the underlying cause of the headaches. These techniques are provided most often by psychologists, physical therapists, psychiatrists, and physicians. They include the use of biofeedback from machines that indicate to patients when they are being successful in altering key physiologic functions in a favorable direction.

*3. Meditation, relaxation tapes, hypnosis.* These methods are useful in helping the patient to achieve favorable physical and physiologic responses to stress.

A combination of these techniques in a manner that not only provides the patient with training of body responses to stress but also achieves a relationship between the patient and the therapist seems to be more productive than simple "lonesome" use of a biofeedback machine or relaxation tapes. In general, young people tend to respond slightly better than older ones to these therapy forms. Children are particularly interested, adept, and flexible.

***Psychodynamic therapy.*** Psychodynamic therapy techniques depend on patients' ability to relate their feelings to their life experiences. The therapist and patient attempt to uncover and treat emotional conflicts and trauma that are producing somatic symptoms such as headache. These services are provided by clinical social workers, psychologists, physicians, and psychiatrists. They may be provided (1) as emotional support through stressful periods, (2) in an effort to unravel a particular problem over long- or short-term therapy, or (3) in rarer instances as psychoanalytic techniques devoted to in-depth excursions into the emotional roots of behavior patterns and attitudes.

A joint interview among the physician, patient, and psychiatrist to evaluate which of these routes to follow is often helpful to the patient and physician. The psychiatrist in this situation comes to the physician's office and sees the patient with the physician present. (The patient pays only the psychiatrist, since the interview is for the benefit of both the patient and the physician.)

### Treatment of attacks

***Prodromal stage.*** Reliable, effective treatment of the prodrome is not at hand. Some patients have found "tricks" that seem to work for them. These include:

1. Vigorous exercises at the onset of the prodrome for 5 minutes
2. Taking 1/200 gr of nitroglycerine under the tongue
3. One or two whiffs of an amyl nitrite ampule at the very onset of the scotoma
4. Taking papaverine in the form of a Pavabid capsule at the onset of the scotoma
5. Putting a plastic bag over the head and down to the shoulders, and breathing within the plastic bag to increase carbon dioxide accumulation in the bloodstream, thereby causing cerebral vasodilatation with relief of the symptom
6. Breathing 100% oxygen at 7 L/minute for 15 minutes at onset of prodrome

***Headache phase.*** A good spot for "hibernation" helps stop the headache. A quiet, semidark area free from interruptions and problems helps eliminate the pain and avoids the overuse of medication.

If migraine pain can be controlled by simple analgesics such as aspirin or acetaminophen, there is no need to turn to more powerful drugs (see Managed Care Guide to acute migraine therapies). For more severe attacks, isometheptene mucate (Midrin), pentazocine (Talwin), or propoxyphene (Darvon) compounds may be used; at times it is justifiable to add codeine. Rarely, the more powerful narcotics are indicated but only in limited, well-monitored amounts and preferably in noninjectable form. Only under very unusual circumstances should narcotic medications be placed in the hands of the patient's spouse to administer on an as-needed basis (especially in the family of a physician). Occasional patients respond to the use of indomethacin in 50 to 100 mg doses at the onset of a headache and at 4- to 6-hour periods thereafter.

In general, rather than resort to narcotic medication, the physician may wish to give the ergot drugs a thorough trial. Their administration is tailored to the individual patient's situation, bearing in mind that ergotamine products work better the earlier they are taken and are more efficacious by the rectal or parenteral routes than by the oral, sublingual, or inhalational routes.

The main ergotamine products currently available are shown in Table 95-1. It is wise to start any patient with half the recommended dose, since some patients, especially women, are very sensitive to the action of these drugs. It is helpful to suggest that the patient ultimately take two thirds of the dose that works effectively at the onset and take the other third an hour or two later, but only if the headache is not clearing. After three doses, further ergotamine usually is not useful and may only make the

#### Managed Care Guide
#### Acute migraine therapies

| Drug | Daily dose range | Cost for 30 days at minimum dose |
|---|---|---|
| Ibuprofen | 400-3200 mg | 1.13 |
| Acetaminophen | 500-4000 mg | 1.53 |
| Aspirin | 1000-3000 mg | 3.10 |
| Midrin (isomemethep./ dichloraphen/ acetamin.) | 2-5 capsules | <11.30 |
| Ergostat (ergotamine) | 2-4 mg max 5 tabs/week | 14.13* |
| Cafergot (ergotamine/ caffeine) | 2-6 tabs, max 10 tabs/week | <40.48* |
| Anaprox (naproxen sodium) | 500-1000 mg | <42.78 |
| DHE 45 (dihydroergotamine) | 2-4 mg. max 6 mg IV/week | 212.90* |
| Imitrex (sumatriptan) | 6 mg SQ. 6 syringes max/ month | 204.48* |

From PSC—Prescribing guidelines, 1994-95.
*Maximum/month.

**Table 95-1.** Common commercial products containing ergotamine for migraine

| Name | Route | Ergotamine (mg) | Caffeine (mg) | Other (mg) | Dosage (tablets): Initial dose | Dosage (tablets): After 1 hour PRN | Dosage (tablets): After 2 hours | Dosage (tablets): Top dose in 24 hours | Comment |
|---|---|---|---|---|---|---|---|---|---|
| Cafergot pill | PO | 1 | 100 | | 1-2 | 1-2 | 1 | 5 | Note total caffeine* |
| Cafergot P-B pill | PO | 1 | 100 | Pentobarbital 30<br>Bellafoline 0.125 | 1-2 | 1-2 | 1 | 4 | Note total caffeine and pentobarbital* |
| Wigraine pill | PO | 1 | 100 | | 1-2 | 1-2 | 1 | 5 | Note total caffeine* |
| Bellergal tablets | PO | 0.3 | | Pentobarbital 20<br>Bellafoline 0.1 | 1-2 | 1 | 0 | 3 | For attacks and prophylaxis† |
| Bellergal-S | PO | 0.6 | | Pentobarbital 40<br>Bellafoline 0.2 | | | ½-1 tid | | For prophylaxis only‡ |
| Ergomar | SL | 2 | | | 1 | 1 | 1 | 3 | * |
| Ergostat | SL | 2 | | | 1 | 1 | 1 | 3 | * |
| Wigrettes | SL | 2 | | | 1 | 1 | 1 | 3 | * |
| Medihaler ergotamine | Inhalation | 0.36/whiff | | | 1-2 whiffs | 1 | 1 | 4 | * |
| Cafergot suppository | Rectal | 2 | 100 | | ½-1 | ½-1 | ½ | 2 | * |
| Cafergot P-B suppository | Rectal | 2 | 100 | Pentobarbital 60<br>Bellafoline 0.25 | ½-1 | ½-1 | ½ | 2 | * |
| Wigraine suppository | Rectal | 2 | 100 | | ½-1 | ½-1 | ½ | 2 | * |
| Dihydroergotamine | Intramuscular or deep subcutaneous | 1 (1 ml) | | | 1 ml | ½-1 ml | ½ ml | 2 ml | For attacks* |

PO, oral; SL, sublingual.
*To be used for attacks not more than 3-4 days weekly.
†Used for children during attacks and prophylactically for adults and children.
‡For prophylaxis only.

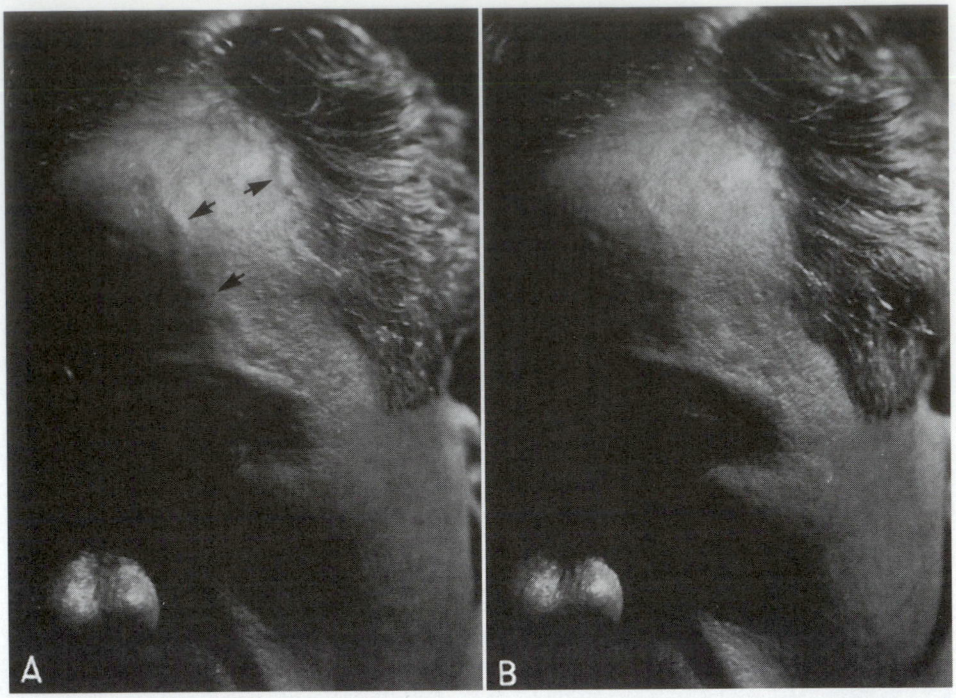


**Fig. 95-9.** Patient experiencing a left temporal migraine headache. **A,** During headache. **B,** Note constriction of temporal vessels (*arrows* in **A**) after head pain has been stopped by an injection of ergotamine tartrate. (From Wolff HG. In Dalessio DJ, editor: *Headache and other head pain,* ed 4, New York, 1980, Oxford University.)

patient sicker. Because both migraine and ergotamine can create significant nausea, it is wise to have the patient start treatment of the attack by using at the onset metoclopramide (Reglan, 10 to 20 mg PO), prochlorperazine (Compazine), or trimethobenzamide (Tigan) by rectum about 30 minutes before taking the first dose of ergotamine to avoid nausea and vomiting. It is traditional to say that, after 3 to 4 hours of the attack have passed, the use of ergotamine is never effective. This is not true. This drug may still be very helpful even if taken late, but the sooner it is taken, the better it works (Fig. 95-9).

Although the effectiveness of ergotamine on migraine may be related to some of its actions on the CNS, it seems more likely and demonstrable that this relates to its specific capacity to contract the branches of the external carotid artery, which certainly participate in the etiology of the pain by their excessive dilatation and amplitude of pulsation. Ergotamine constricts vessels throughout the body as well as those in the head and therefore is avoided in patients who have a known vascular problem or who are of an age to be candidates for potential trouble in this regard. It is not used in the presence of hepatic or renal disease or during pregnancy. It is unwise to use ergotamine on more than 3 days a week for fear of developing "the ergot cycle," as described earlier.

Among the other advances that should be mentioned is the recent approval of sumatriptan for the treatment of acute migraine attacks. This is a serotonin blocking agent that has proved quite effective in terminating migraine with or without aura even after the headache has become established. The drug is inconvenient because the present preparation requires subcutaneous self-injection. The patient may experience injection site reactions, dizziness, and vertigo. The agent is contraindicated in patients with ischemic heart disease, particularly Prinzmetal angina, because of its potential ability to cause coronary vasospasm. It also has to be used with great care in hypertensive patients, since it can increase blood pressure. Some patients experience sensations of pressure in the chest and neck or have mild confusion, tingling, or heat. For these reasons, it may be prudent to have patients first inject themselves in the clinician's office to see how well they tolerate this agent. Sumatriptan can be given to those patients who are taking the usual migraine prophylactic drugs such as the calcium channel blockers, β-blockers or tricyclics, but it should not be administered to patients using any form of ergot because of the potential for additive side effects.

Prednisone is useful in stopping unusually prolonged or severe attacks of migraine or for those who may not take ergotamine. Doses over 2 to 3 days may be effective in amounts of 30 mg PO on day 1, 20 mg on day 2, and 10 mg on day 3. It is advisable that not more than twenty 5 mg tablets of prednisone be used during any 1 month for fear of long-term prednisone side effects.

In general, it is important to convey to the patient that successful use of such medications as ergotamine or steroids to stop an attack of migraine does not represent a license to disregard the basic rules for migraineurs: they must not exceed their own limits of energy and should recognize that a migraine headache has a biologic meaning, that is, they have been exceeding their own limits.

**Case report.** A 33-year history of migraine headache is outlined in Fig. 95-10. This chart reveals the gradual relentless increase in headache frequency and severity,

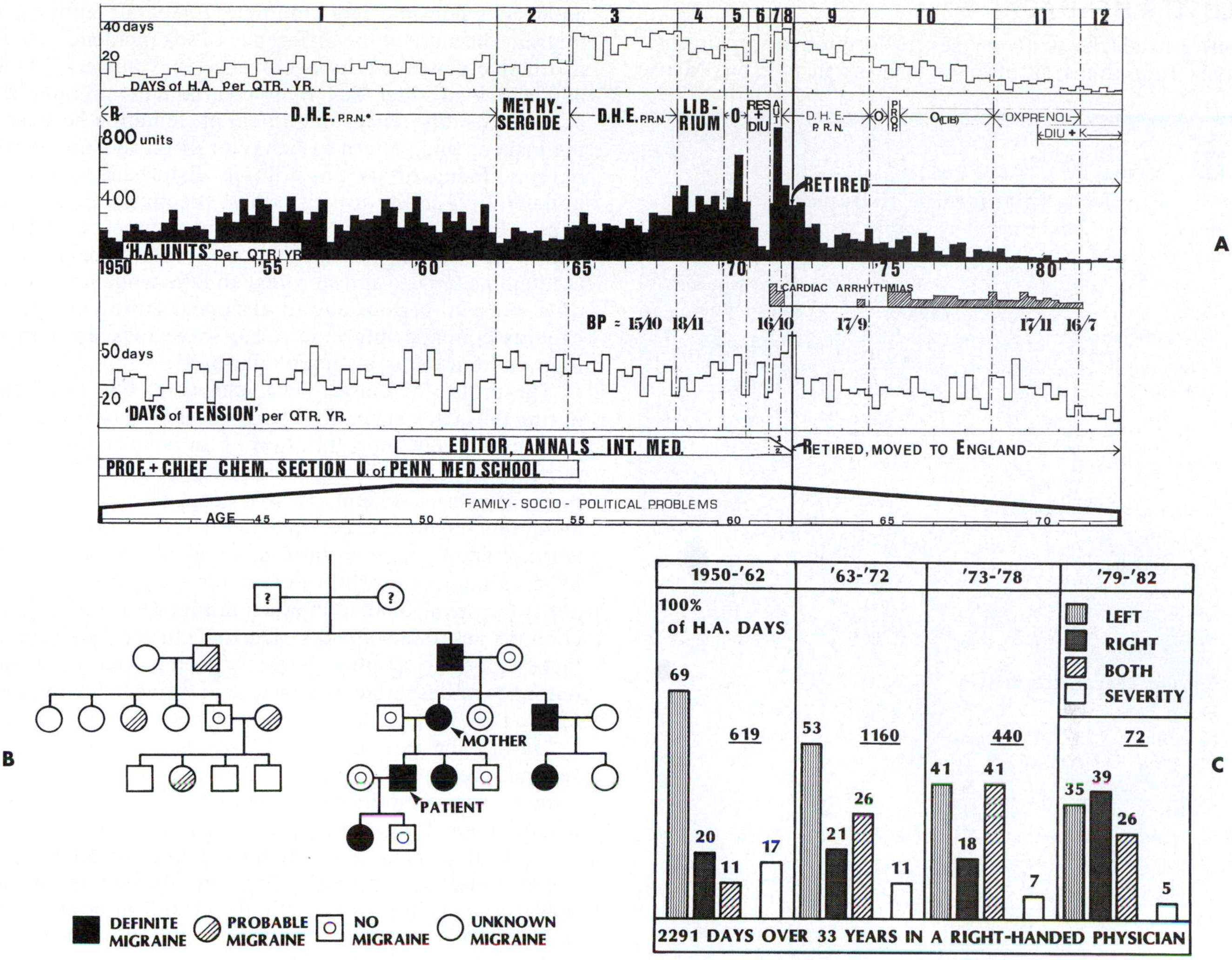


**Fig. 95-10.** **A,** A 33-year record of migraine headache related to family history, therapy, days of tension, occupation, life situation, medical condition, and retirement. D.H.E. p.r.n. = dihydroergotamine, as necessary; Res + Diu = reserpine 0.1 mg daily, hydrochlorothiazide 25 mg daily; 0 = no drug treatment; Aut = autogenic exercises; Prop = propranolol; Lib = Librium; Oxprenol = oxprenolol; DIU + K = diuretic and potassium. **B,** Migraine in the family of the patient's mother. One daughter of the patient's daughter—a very lively young lady—is beginning to have headaches in her teens. **C,** Laterality of this right-handed patient's migraine switched slowly over the years from predominance on the left side to predominance of headache on the right and/or both sides. Speculation is current regarding the possible relation of the side of the brain involved in certain types of activity to the laterality of the headache: the patient suggested that his right-sided headaches (on weekends) were related to the pressure of physical weekend tasks around the house for which he was responsible. (From Elkinton JR and Graham JR. Presented at first meeting of International Headache Society, Munich, 1983.)

despite occasional mitigation by specific therapies, as life stresses stacked higher and higher. Relief of headache by methysergide permitted an increased number of "days of tension." The most effective medical therapy was a combination of small doses of reserpine and hydrochlorothiazide, which was stopped because of cardiac arrhythmias. Moderate hypertension appeared at around age 55. The marked decline in headache severity and frequency, however, seems to have been related not to correction of hypertension, but to retirement and decrease in total life stress.

Note that during period two, 2½ years of methysergide therapy made a marked difference in headache frequency and severity (note the change in total units of headache). Days of tension during this period increased, however, suggesting that headache relief may provide a license for overwork. Headache units quickly rose after 1965, when methysergide was stopped because of possible fibrotic complications, since this possibility became apparent during the mid-1960s.

## Prophylaxis of migraine headache

There are a number of different medications that may be taken prophylactically to decrease the frequency of migraine headaches. These are summarized in the Managed Care Guide for prophylactic migraine therapies.

## CLUSTER HEADACHE

Cluster headache is a very severe form of head pain that occurs four times as often in men as in women. Many authorities consider it a completely separate entity from migraine because of the difference in sex incidence and the distinctive pattern of its occurrence in "clusters." Other authorities consider that it is a variant of migraine that achieves its differences in clinical presentation because of the makeup and pattern of behavior of those patients who have it. Many of its physiologic disturbances, such as unilaterality; ability to shift sides; precipitation by sleep, naps, alcohol, nitroglycerin, and histamine; association with distended extracranial blood vessels; response to ergotamine tartrate and steroids; and the tendency to occur *after* stressful periods and to disappear during pregnancy, even as common migraine does, serve to keep it in the migraine family as a "poor relation."

The profile of cluster headache (Fig. 95-11) reveals, during the attack stage, the sharp onset of very severe pain with a relatively short duration of an hour or two, one or more times per day or night usually at points of relaxation or rapid eye movement (REM) sleep, as well as marked autonomic features of ipsilateral sweating, flushing, tearing, enophthalmos, miosis, nasal blocking, and ultimately rhinorrhea. All these features are prominent in this entity but are also noted in much diminished degree during common migraine attacks. During cluster headache attacks, patients display restless pacing and occasional outbursts of desperate or angry, aggressive behavior, quite unlike the "hibernation" of the common migraine patient.

During the periods of a "cluster," which may last several weeks or months, the patient is extremely vulnerable to vasodilating stimuli (e.g., alcohol, nitrites, histamine) and great changes in pace (e.g., weather, time and activity), such as occur during naps or REM sleep, travel, seasons, and work. Once the cluster has passed, however, and the patient is "in the clear," these stimuli no longer serve to precipitate attacks. A few unfortunate individuals may remain in a constant or chronic cluster

### Managed Care Guide
### Prophylactic migraine therapies

| Drug | Daily dose range | Cost for 30 days at minimum dose |
|---|---|---|
| ***Beta-antagonists*** | | |
| Propranolol | 80-32 mg | *0.70 |
| Timolol | 20-60 mg | *13.03 |
| Atenolol | 50-100 mg | *17.53 |
| Lopressor (metoprolol) | 100-300 mg | <21.80 |
| Corgard (nadolol) | 80-160 mg | 39.44 |
| ***Tricyclic antidepressants*** | | |
| Amitriptyline | 50-200 mg | *0.54 |
| Imipramine | 75-300 mg | *2.10 |
| Doxepin | 75-300 mg | *3.26 |
| Desipramine | 75-300 mg | *5.51 |
| Nortriptyline | 75-200 mg | *42.26 |
| ***Calcium channel blockers*** | | |
| Verapamil | 80-240 mg | *2.01 |
| Nifedipine | 30-120 mg | *30.04 |
| Cardizem (diltiazem) | 180-240 mg | <53.21 |
| ***Other*** | | |
| Depakene (valproic acid) | 750-2000 mg | <93.35 |
| Sansert (methysergide) | 2-6 mg | 44.71 |

From PSC—Prescribing guidelines, 1994-95.
*Maximum allowable cost of generic medications.
<Cost is decreased further due to volume discount contracts.

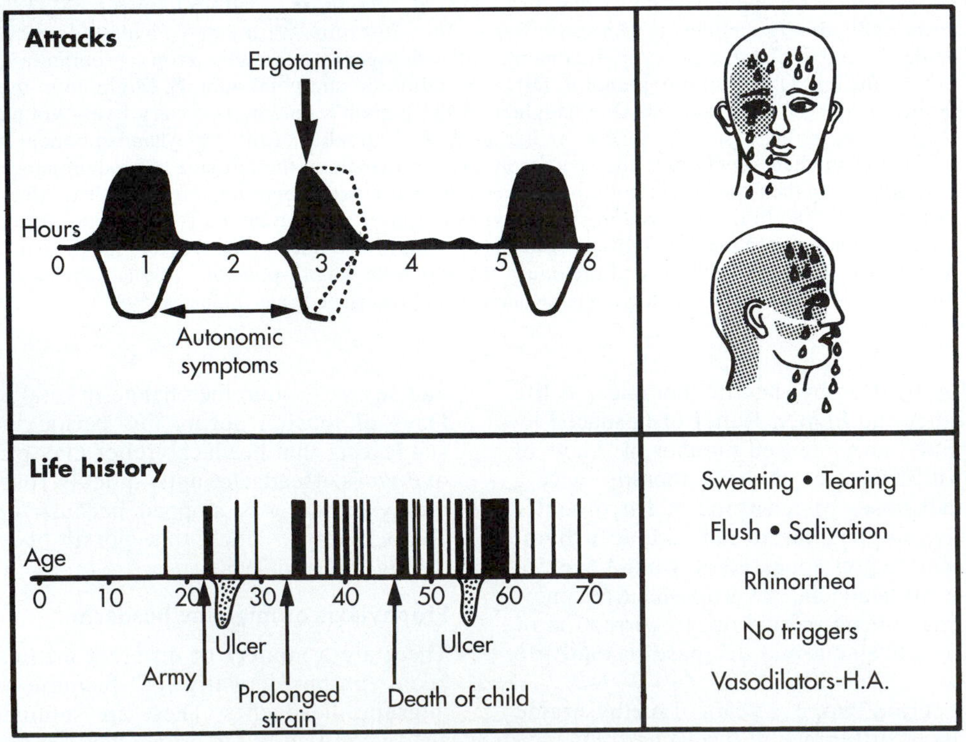


**Fig. 95-11.** Profile of a cluster headache.

state almost daily for more than a year or even for several years. Usually, chronic clusters result from the gradual compression of periodic clusters closer together until a continuous or chronic state results. Rarely, clusters are chronic or classified as primary chronic cluster from the beginning.

Cluster headache patients, mostly men, tend to have an athletic build, including increased height, a leonine facies characterized by thick "orange peel" skin, deep furrows in forehead, cheeks, and chin, and telangiectasia, especially on the cheeks and bridge of the nose (Fig. 95-12).

Despite this "macho" leonine appearance, these individuals seem to have emotional dependency needs that are not consistent with their bold appearance. They are often brought to the physician by a petite wife who makes the appointments and takes the prescriptions while "Leo" sits by obediently. The patients are usually hard-working men who strive to improve their status in life, take too few vacations, often have two jobs, or are in a one-man business or family business in which there is a frustrating relationship with a father or older brother. They tend to work hard and long until they drop exhausted into a letdown or vacation and are rewarded by a cluster of headaches. About 25% of them at some period have a peptic ulcer, and they may be more susceptible than normal people to cardiovascular disease, especially coronary disorders. They tend to drink and smoke cigarettes more than other headache patients, especially during clusters, and they also dream very actively.

Attacks frequently originate during or immediately after REM sleep. During the attacks the patients may behave in a bizarre manner. They almost always are up and about, pacing, stamping, locking themselves into bathrooms or cellars, violently resisting help, at times screaming, begging God or Heaven for relief, occasionally going into a "trance" for short or, rarely, long periods. Their behavior may be mistaken for drunkenness, "hysteria," "seizure," or a drug reaction. Sometimes patients threaten suicide during an attack, but they rarely if ever perform it. Many patients explain that the pain is worse than that experienced with a fracture, surgery, or delivery or that associated with passing a kidney stone. These symptoms are so unbearable that patients develop great anxiety about attacks that have not yet occurred.

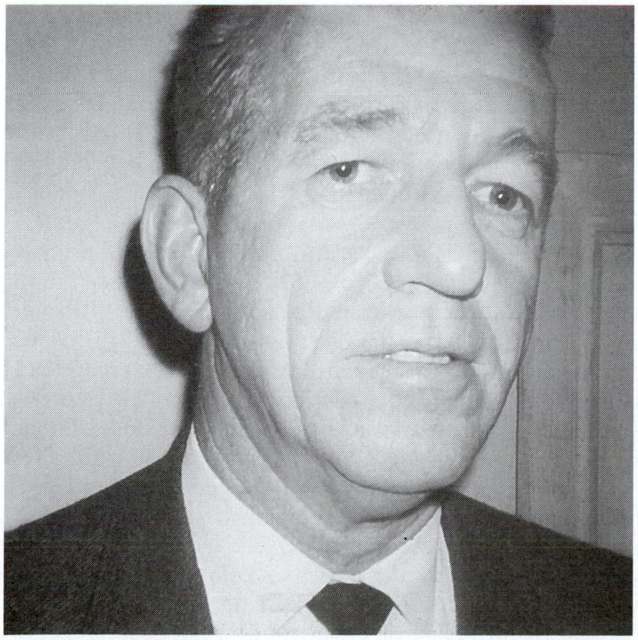

**Fig. 95-12.** Leonine facies of a cluster headache patient. Note the thick vertical and horizontal furrows, extra crease in the cheek, thick "orange peel" skin, and telangiectasis on the nostril.

Individual attacks and whole clusters are precipitated by (1) great changes in pace between working hard and "letting down," (2) extreme changes in weather from cold to warm or sunny to rainy, (3) emotional letdowns after solving a major problem or making a major decision, (4) sudden changes in barometric pressure such as occur during plane trips, (5) great shifts in time rhythms as in jet lag on or after long air trips, or (6) the end of a school year or special season (as in the ministry after Easter). Individual attacks may also be precipitated by a drink of any alcoholic beverage, certain foods such as monosodium glutamate or chocolate, or the use of nitroglycerin by mouth, inhalation, or transdermally.

At times, infection in the upper respiratory tract seems to precipitate a cluster, whether by action of the infectious agent or by virtue of the letdown called for by the infection. In a number of patients, herpes simplex infections have been associated with the onset of clusters, a fact of considerable investigative interest, since this virus has been found in the fifth, sympathetic, and parasympathetic ganglia of the head, suggesting the possibility that its presence, possibly altered by changes in the individual's immune state, may affect the pain thresholds in the nerve supply of the affected areas.

At times the individual attacks occur with clocklike regularity at certain times of day or night, only to shift these fixed times to a different period at some point as the cluster progresses. Although the attacks of pain usually remain limited to a given side of the head and face during a given cluster, in some patients the attacks may switch to the other side before the cluster is over and, in a few rare instances, may involve both sides at once during one or several individual attacks.

Clusters may begin during childhood or more often in young adulthood, or they may not occur until middle and late middle age. They may persist over a lifetime into the 70s and 80s but more often tend to decrease during the 60s. Intervals between clusters may range from a few weeks to a few months or a few years. The headaches recur occasionally after 10, 15, or even 35 years of freedom.

One receives the impression that attacks and clusters of headache in these individuals tend, as with common migraine, to come on the descending limb of stressful periods when either inner or external pressures shift from high to low levels, and the setting of the body's "physiologic thermostat" is significantly changed. The pattern and timing of such changes may be related to the individual's patterns of behavior and may result from the manner in which the person uses his or her energies.

## Differential diagnosis

Cluster headache is most often confused with tic douloureux or trigeminal neuralgia. Important differences are as follows:

1. *Age of onset.* Tic, unless secondary to multiple sclerosis or tumor, usually first appears in patients over 60

years of age, whereas cluster headache begins even during childhood and most frequently during the second, third, and fourth decades of life.

2. *Nature of pain.* Tic pain is a succession of lightning jabs of pain that occur in quick succession in bursts lasting minutes to hours. Cluster pain is steady, severe pain, burning, pulling, and twisting, like the constant grinding of a screwdriver deep in the temple or behind the eye. Rarely, cluster pain is accompanied by short shocks or jolts of pain similar to that of tic superimposed on the constant steady pain, thereby creating the so-called cluster-tic syndrome.

3. *Location of pain.* Tic douloureux confines its pain to the territory supplied by the three branches of the fifth nerve, whereas cluster headache pain frequently involves not only the area of the fifth nerve distribution, but also the occipital, upper neck, and carotid areas on the side of the headache.

4. *Trigger mechanisms.* Precipitating factors for tic douloureux are sensory stimuli, such as touching the face, brushing the teeth, and applying hot or cold to the face or mouth. Triggers for cluster headache are vasodilating events, such as the effect of alcohol, nitroglycerin, histamine, and changes in the state of arousal of the CNS.

5. *Response to treatment.* Tic responds to phenytoin (Dilantin), carbamazepine (Tegretol), and nerve-blocking procedures, but not to ergotamine, lithium, or prednisone. Cluster headache responds to ergotamine, lithium, and prednisone, but only in special cases to nerve-blocking procedures.

Other disorders that must be differentiated include vernal keratitis and recurrent scratched cornea, in both of which extreme pain and redness of the eye may simulate cluster headache. Corneal examination and the constancy of the pain indicate the ocular source.

Raeder syndrome and the Tolosa-Hunt syndrome sometimes present with recurring steady pain in the eye and face lasting days, weeks, or occasionally months. These and other syndromes involving the orbit, orbital fissure, and cavernous sinus vascular connections also create similar pain syndromes. They are all characterized by varied involvement of cranial nerves II, III, IV, V, and VI, causing definite organic sensory and/or motor dysfunction. Several of these syndromes are related to stress and may involve inflammation that responds favorably to steroid therapy. When neurologic complications of this sort are present, consultation with a neurologist is advisable regarding the exact nature, location, and treatment of the lesion.

Malignant growths of the nose and throat may also mimic the pain of cluster headache, even presenting at first with intermittent bouts of pain associated with Horner's syndrome, pain in the cheek and eye, and nasal blocking. X-ray films and computed tomography (CT) scans of the nasofacial bones and sinuses may reveal organic lesions in the nasopharynx and sinus areas, with destructive lesions in the hard palate and floor of the skull. The pain of such lesions does not usually respond to the medicines effective in other functional sources of pain, such as those of cluster headache and the neuralgias (Fig. 95-13).

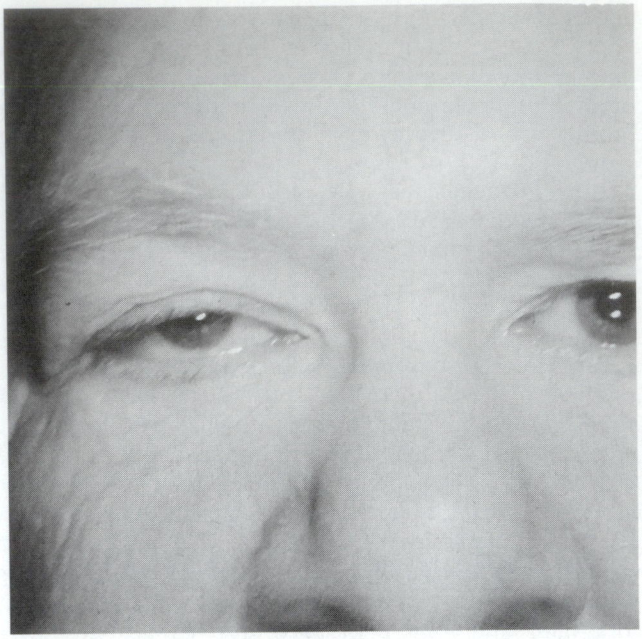

**Fig. 95-13.** Horner's syndrome, causing drooping eyelid and small pupil in the right eye of a 60-year-old woman with a history of cluster headaches increasing in intensity over 3 months. Sinus x-rays revealed destruction of the floor of the maxillary sinus by a nasopharyngeal carcinoma.

## Mechanism

The basic mechanism of cluster headache is unknown, although several current theories exist. Cluster headache could be explained by dilatation or swelling of the walls of the internal carotid artery in its bony canal, resulting in changes in distribution of blood flow in the anterior areas of the cranium and compression of the autonomic fibers in the wall of the carotid artery that lead to a partial Horner's syndrome. Whether the attacks occur in relation to changes in vascular "tone" or to local edema in the carotid canal is unknown. Angiography has shown narrowing of the carotid with return in its canal during one attack of cluster headache, with return to normal at the end of the attack. Changes in the setting of vascular tone may correlate well with periods of greater and lesser patient activity. Under such circumstances, exposure to substances such as alcohol that cause further vasodilatation and possible swelling in numerous cranial narrow spaces containing arteries and nerves might precipitate attacks. Changes in immune states, as influenced by long periods of stress and their relief, may also be hypothesized as a cause of changed cranial blood vessel–foramen–nerve relations, or local nerve–virus symbiosis. Because the herpes simplex virus has been demonstrated in ganglia of the fifth nerve and sympathetic and parasympathetic chains in the neck and head, changes in the activity of the virus could lead to periods of increased reaction of regional nerves to vasodilatory substances and so result in clusters of attacks of pain. Reversed direction of blood flow and altered reaction to carbon dioxide and oxygen ($CO_2$ and $O_2$) in cranial blood flow studies during cluster attacks suggest an altered state of vascular reactivity in general that may affect mechanically the nerve vascular supply in patients with certain anatomic features of the head.

Patterns of behavior governed by very basic vegetative activity in the limbic system affecting the body's response to stress, time, seasons, environment, hormonology, and mental and emotional activity seem to offer some basic concepts of how the hard-working, dependent, or counterdependent patient with cluster headache manages the cranial circulation, which at times slips into a low-energy, hyperrelaxed state leading to physiologic "misbehavior." Underneath the handsome, bold face of the cluster "lion," who often maintains a prolonged superhigh level of activity, may lie fatigue, anger, and volcanic outbursts of physiologic and half-contained emotional responses that end up in a series of eruptions until the pressure chamber is empty and normal activity may be resumed. If a person of this type (type A) who works and pushes for as long or longer than he or she can stand also tends to have migraine, which is the pressure release, the clinical behavior of the headache problem may manifest in a series of terrible outbursts, followed by long headache-free intervals before the pressure chamber of the migraine is refilled.

### Treatment of attacks

Any treatment for the pain of the individual acute attack of cluster headache must be *immediately available* and quick in its action. Patients should always have their treatment with them or within easy reach because the pain develops rapidly; although it does not last long, it is devastating. Several suggestions are made, each of which is to be tested by trial and error:

1. Breathing 100% oxygen by nasal mask at 7 to 10 L/minute for 10 to 15 minutes at onset of attacks
2. Strenuous exercise for 5 to 10 minutes at onset
3. Ice-cold applications or very hot applications to the affected area
4. Immediate use of the most effective ergotamine-containing drug
   a. Wigrettes, Ergomar, Ergostat: sublingual
   b. Medihaler ergotamine, two or three whiffs
   c. Rectal suppository (Wigraine or Cafergot)
   d. Injection of D.H.E. 45, 1 ml IM immediately
   e. Analgesic medication by itself or in addition to the above

### Prophylactic treatment of cluster headaches

Several prophylactic regimens have been found useful for prevention of the *attacks* during a cluster period. Some of them may also be useful in the prophylaxis of *clusters* as well as in warding off individual attacks. Their selection may depend on the patient's age and contraindications for some therapies, such as ergot for patients with vascular disease or steroids for patients with peptic ulcer.

1. Ergotamine tablets, 1 mg three or four times daily
2. Ergotamine and caffeine tablets three or four times daily
3. Ergotamine rectal suppositories one or two times daily
4. D.H.E. 45 by injection once daily
5. Methysergide, 2 mg tablets one to four times daily. This therapy must be stopped at 3-month intervals for at least 2 weeks.
6. Steroid therapy. With prednisone (or equivalents); 40 to 60 mg prednisone/day, reduced by 5 mg/day every 2 or 3 days; total period of therapy to be no longer than 6 to 8 weeks, preferably 4 weeks. Reduction may be held for more than 3 days, depending on progress, but patient must agree to stop at end of 6 to 8 weeks because of possible chronic steroid side effects. Ergot therapy, if necessary, may be combined with this. When this episode of therapy is stopped, the mildly hypoadrenal state following its cessation may allow a few headaches to return. It is advisable to tolerate these for a week or more before starting a new type of prophylactic therapy.
7. Lithium therapy. This may be used for episodic or chronic cluster headache. The usual dose is 900 mg lithium carbonate/day in three divided doses, striving to achieve a blood lithium level of 0.5 to 1.0 mEq/L. Thyroid function, blood counts, and renal function are followed as in other patients taking lithium. As the patient improves, the dose may be gradually reduced. In chronic cluster headache, it may be wise to continue one dose of lithium per day for many months—or permanently. When headache cycles break through, the dosage may be raised appropriately. Ergot or steroids may be added to the lithium regimen, with care, if severe recurrence takes place. Dosage levels of lithium may have to be decreased in patients who have had gastrectomy, a procedure that may be used in cluster headache patients. Blood lithium levels must be appropriately monitored.

The calcium channel blocking drugs (e.g., verapamil, diltiazem, nimodipine) have been the subject of favorable reports in the prophylactic treatment of cluster headache. They must be taken in full dosage over at least a month to gain their full effect. Cluster headache patients are extremely sensitive to vasodilators and may actually develop headaches if given nifedipine because of its greater vasodilatory effects.

Other pharmaceutical regimens have occasionally proved useful for cluster headache:

Cyproheptadine (Periactin), 4 mg doses PO one to four times daily
Reserpine, 0.1 mg PO daily
Delalutin (for male and female patients), 250 mg IM every 5 days
Estrogens, especially in menopausal female patients
MAO inhibitors: isocarboxazid (Marplan), phenylethylhydrazine (Nardil)
Tricyclic antidepressants: amitriptyline (Elavil), doxepin (Sinequan), trazodone (Desyrel)

During cluster periods, patients are advised to avoid alcohol, monosodium glutamate, large amounts of cheese and chocolate, and pickled and spicy foods. Regular exercise is helpful, and maintaining activity in general, if possible, is helpful after a break has provided some rest.

Patients with cluster headache are usually not good candidates for psychotherapy. They profit more from the continued interest, guidance, and reassurance of a conscientious general physician. In the same way that coronary patients have to be taught new lifestyles, so cluster headache patients who have this cranial counterpart of cardiac angina have to learn to modify behavior, a difficult task that takes time.

### Surgical procedures

Consideration may be given to surgical relief for cluster headache under a few unusual circumstances. For the most part, surgery remains at the bottom of the list of potential therapies largely because of the uncertainty of results and, in some instances, the addition of seriously unpleasant sensations as side effects. Situations in which surgery may be advisable include the following:

1. Intractable cluster headache that has failed to respond to any medical treatment and that is seriously affecting the patient's life
2. Patients who have allergies or medical conditions that make the use of the usual medical therapies impossible (prednisone may be interdicted in patients with active peptic ulcer, ergotamine in patients with vascular disease, lithium in patients with serious electrolyte and metabolic problems, etc.)
3. Cluster headache that is always on the same side

Whenever surgery is undertaken for cluster headache, two consultations are requested. The first is with a psychiatrist acquainted with pain problems who considers the usefulness and likelihood of success of the procedure and also makes some evaluation of how the particular patient will manage its undesired side effects should they occur. The other consultation is with a neurosurgeon well acquainted not only with head and neck surgery for pain, but also with the disease, cluster headache, itself.

The types of surgery employed with variable degrees of success have been excision of a portion of the temporal artery or other branches of the external carotid; sphenopalatine ganglion block or excision; greater superficial petrosal neurectomy; nervus intermedius neurectomy; manipulation of the ganglion of the fifth nerve, whether by radiofrequency or surgical transection; steroid, novocaine, and/or glycerol deposition in the Meckel cavity; separation of posterior fossa–trapped arteries from adhesions involving branches of the cerebellar arteries by the Janetta procedure; medullary tractotomy of pain tracts in the medulla; or placing of electronic implants in the central gray areas of the brain.

All these procedures are limited by one's inability to predict with reasonable certainty what the positive and negative results may be and how long they will last. On the other hand, in desperate attempts to alleviate cluster headache by medical means, one may forget the ravages of long-term suffering, the addiction possibilities of pain-relieving drugs, and the serious side effects of some of the potent medicines used for this disease, such as serious impairment of thyroid, renal, liver, hematopoietic, vascular, and bone function, as well as the long-term stress and suffering of the disease itself.

Cluster headache patients are willing to do almost anything to relieve even 5 minutes of the dreadful cluster pain that makes them cry in fear and break down before their family into a shaking, pacing, crying, screaming "jelly."

Three physicians tried applying a transcutaneous pain-suppressing instrument that theoretically helps stop clinical pain by producing superficial pain signals of a lesser degree than the clinical headache pain. A stoic cluster headache patient had previously been asked to wear this machine and turn it up (on a maximum scale of 10) to create the degree of pain he experienced during one of his cluster headaches. He reported that when the instrument was at about 9, the pain equaled his clinical headache. Of the three physicians who tried wearing the instrument themselves and turning it up to 9, one could not go higher than 6 or 7; the other two made it to 9 but after 30 seconds had to remove it because of the severity of the pain. The thought of suffering such a pain for 5 minutes, not to mention 90 minutes, seemed inconceivable.

## CHRONIC PAROXYSMAL HEMICRANIA

In 1974, Sjaastad and Dale described a variant form of cluster headache characterized by its occurrence most often in women (in contrast to the male predominance in the usual cluster headache incidence). This syndrome also differed in the short duration of the attacks and their frequent occurrence—up to 15 or more attacks in 24 hours. The pain followed the same distribution as cluster headache pain in its unilaterality; its involvement of the eye, cheek, temple, and occipital region; and in the associated autonomic symptoms of ipsilateral sweating, Horner syndrome, and nasal block. A remarkable feature of this condition was its specific rapid response to indomethacin. Within a few hours of the first dose, the attacks ceased completely. Doses of up to 150 to 200 mg of indomethacin daily were required. Some patients with this syndrome had these multiple daily attacks for several years without relief from any of the ordinary cluster headache remedies. Indomethacin has not proved useful in ordinary cluster headache.

Some 50 or more patients of this type have now been described, of whom 80% to 90% are women. Both chronic and periodic varieties of this disorder have occurred. In some patients the dosage of indomethacin may be gradually decreased and stopped, and the patient may remain free of attacks for many months only to have them recur and then respond well, again, to indomethacin. A 2-day trial of indomethacin in a dose of 150 to 200 mg may be worth prescribing as a starter when treating any patient who is a woman and/or has more than five attacks per day. In some of these patients, thumb pressure in the suboccipital space precipitated an attack.

## HEMIPLEGIC MIGRAINE

A severe and fortunately uncommon form of migraine is called hemiplegic migraine because motor paralysis of central origin takes place during headache attacks in addition to striking sensory, mood, orientation, and speech phenomena. This disorder often, but not always, has a familial incidence of similar attacks or of classic and/or common migraine.

Recurrent, usually widely spaced attacks tend to begin with headache, followed by dramatic neurologic symptoms, an order of events that is the reverse of the usual classic migraine attack and that, by this token, requires thorough neurologic investigation to make sure it is not caused by an organic lesion. In addition to the usual array of sensory neurologic phenomena experienced in classic migraine, motor paralysis of all or parts of one side of the body may take place. Dysarthria, aphasia (motor and sensory), ataxia, tinnitus, vertigo, transient global amnesia, confusion, and fever may occur. Unlike the other types of migraine, these dramatic neurologic phenomena usually outlast the headache, at times for days and weeks. EEG abnormalities may persist several weeks in the area of the brain related to the symptoms. Many patients who have marked sensory disturbances during classic migraine report that they are "paralyzed" during the attacks, but careful questioning and observation, when possible, provide evidence that actual motor paralysis is not present. In hemiplegic migraine, motor weakness may be demonstrated.

Hemiplegic migraine is distinguishable from so-called basilar artery migraine only by the neurologic components that are disturbed. In basilar artery migraine, symptoms are related to malfunction of posterior portions of the brain (occipital lobe, cerebellum, brainstem) areas supplied primarily by the basilar artery and its branches, the cerebellar arteries, and the posterior cerebral arteries. Symptoms resulting from disturbances in these areas include vertigo, ataxia, total blindness, total sensory and motor paralysis ("locked-in syndrome"), and unconsciousness. Hemiplegic migraine tends to involve higher centers, including motor areas, either primarily or secondarily.

As in other forms of migraine, the question arises as to whether the initial disturbance that sets off the attack arises in the brain itself and is similar to the spreading depression of Leão or arises in its blood supply. Perhaps this should be called "brainstem" migraine rather than "basilar artery" migraine.

Hemiplegic migraine and/or brainstem or basilar artery migraine tend to occur in young people, often young women, usually those who smoke. They happen in rather widely spaced attacks, often several weeks or even months apart. Menstrual periods, tense life situations, prolonged mental strain, and use of oral contraceptives seem to bear some relation to their frequency and severity. The attacks usually tend to disappear or decrease over the years; however, in a few patients, after months or even years of freedom, they reappear during middle and old age. Occasionally in such instances, severe episodes may end in a fixed organic lesion, such as a cerebral infarction in the involved area. These attacks, at any age, are very frightening and in some instances dangerous. Global amnesia and the locked-in syndrome, in which the patient is conscious but can move only the eyes (the rest of the body being paralyzed), is related usually to organic lesions in the pons and may be fatal. One episode with spontaneous recovery has been reported in a migraine patient.

Suggestions for treatment are based chiefly on anecdote rather than on extensively studied and controlled trials. They may be categorized as follows:

1. Treatment of attacks
   a. Attendance by a friend or relative during attack
   b. Propranolol, 20 mg PO
   c. Inhalation of one or two whiffs of amyl nitrite ampules
   d. Repeated record of blood pressure and pulse
   e. Use of papaverine (Pavabid) capsule at 4-hour intervals
   f. Breathing of $O_2$-$CO_2$ mixture (90% $O_2$, 10% $CO_2$) for 5- to 10-minute intervals
   g. Ingestion of 15 mg prednisone PO immediately and repeated twice at 4-hour intervals (or, if patient is unable to take PO medication, parenteral steroid therapy)
   h. Use of a calcium channel blocker is theoretically useful.
2. Prophylaxis of attacks
   a. Aspirin, 300 mg PO once daily *and/or*
   b. Dipyridamiole (Persantine), 50 mg PO three times daily
   c. ? Calcium channel blockers
   d. Avoidance of smoking
   e. Avoidance of oral contraceptives
   f. Avoidance of ergotamine during attacks
   g. Revised, less stressful lifestyle

## OPHTHALMOPLEGIC MIGRAINE

Ophthalmoplegic migraine is an unusual form of headache that occurs in families often reporting common migraine and occasionally ophthalmoplegic migraine in other family members. It is apt to occur in infants and very young children and to recur over many years at intervals. It is characterized by attacks of headache associated simultaneously and during the postheadache period for days or weeks with third nerve paralysis or paresis. Occasionally, over the years this third nerve paralysis becomes permanent. In all cases an early, thorough neurologic workup is necessary to make sure an aneurysm or other organic lesion is not present. Arteriography may be required to rule out a small vascular lesion in the circle of Willis or anterior or posterior communicating artery that may cause repeated painful attacks of third nerve paralysis.

Some believe that ophthalmoplegic migraine is caused by migrainous vascular swelling pressing on the third nerve. These headaches are associated with third nerve paralysis *and* dilatation of the pupil. They may be distinguished from diabetic ophthalmic neuropathy or intrinsic pathology *in* the third nerve that does not involve paralysis of the pupillary fibers.

CT scans immediately after an episode of headache with third nerve paralysis may demonstrate local bleeding or an actual vascular anomaly. However, scans may miss a small aneurysm that may be detected only by traditional angiography, magnetic resonance angiography (MRA), and spinal fluid examination.

Once organic causes have been ruled out, attacks of ophthalmoplegic migraine may be treated symptomatically and prophylactically similar to common migraine. Occasionally, if paralysis persists after the headache is over, steroids (prednisone tapered from 40 mg daily over several days) may relieve this part of the experience and may be indicated for subsequent attacks at the very onset of the symptoms.

## LOWER-HALF HEADACHE (ATYPICAL FACIAL NEURALGIA)

A lower-half headache is included by some, but not by others, under the category of vascular headaches of the migraine type. It is characterized by unilateral, constant, ever-present, steady, and at times throbbing pain in the lower half of the face, the carotid sheath, and suboccipital areas.

Its first appearance may be in the form of intermittent attacks resembling common migraine. These attacks gradually become increasingly frequent and prolonged until they reach a continuous state in which the patient reports dull or moderate pain at all times while awake.

In the beginning it may respond to ergotamine, but this effect tends to wear off. Its pulsatile quality and response to pressure on branches of the carotid artery and to ergotamine, *and* its unilaterality and occasional association with nausea and a partial Horner syndrome, maintain its resemblance to common migraine. As the disease progresses and the pain becomes a continuum, however, associated symptoms of anxiety and depression become more and more prevalent. Addiction to pain-relieving drugs is a common result. The patient's personality changes. All the problems of the patient's life seem to be rolled up together into this one painful experience, which begins to dominate the patient's whole life and whole spectrum of activities.

In some instances this type of pain begins after an injury to the cheek, face, neck, or teeth, especially if at the time of injury the patient is under psychogenic strain or has a background of hysteria. An example of this situation is a young woman who developed lower-half headache of this type after a tooth extraction and a "dry socket." The pain of this phenomenon made it impossible for her to continue to play the clarinet in a group whose professionalism was superior to hers and one of whom was a desired boyfriend. Another patient whose life as a child and adolescent had been lived in a series of unhappy foster homes developed a pain in the face that never went away after a board from a sawmill flipped out and struck him a painful blow in the cheek. Some physical damage and an entrapment syndrome were found at a high cervical level at surgery, but relief of this failed to relieve his face and neck pain, which had led to the use of 20 to 30 analgesic medications per day. Three patients with basic psychic disturbances related to this type of facial pain and upper neck pain (of some 15 or so) had a major schizoid breakdown when their pain was relieved by surgical and pharmaceutical means.

It is clear from these remarks that great care must be taken with patients of this sort to control drug use before addiction sets in and to approach surgical relief with great caution and only after expert psychiatric opinion and the advice of a conservative neurosurgeon experienced in this field have been obtained. Procedures on maxillary and other sinuses, extraction of healthy teeth, turbinectomies, and nasal septum surgery are usually not helpful and often aggravate the syndrome of lower-half headache.

A positive approach consists in that most difficult of physician-patient relationships, the art of keeping the patient out of trouble and supporting him or her in every personal way possible, with a limited goal, over years of care. Antidepressant drugs of the tricyclic or quadricyclic type or MAO inhibitors can be very helpful for such patients, especially when combined with visits to the physician at appropriately planned intervals. This sort of therapy may keep the patient out of the way of addiction, cults, and other harm.

At times, physical therapy, neck collars, traction, and techniques such as transcutaneous nerve stimulation or NSAIDs are useful. When it is impossible for the physician to carry out such long-term, time-consuming measures, referral of the patient to the increasingly prevalent "pain centers" may be a suitable alternative. It is important to search diligently at the beginning for remediable physical causes of pain. The most recent generation of CT scans and the magnetic resonance imaging (MRI) techniques can be of great value in locating organic soft tissue lesions that, until now, have been difficult to observe by other radiation techniques. A search for hysteria early in the patient's life is also worthwhile and revealing when found.

Keeping patients with lower-half headache or atypical facial neuralgia away from drug addiction and overenthusiastic, damaging surgery that may produce new symptoms is a major achievement of which the physician may be proud, although the patient's pain may continue.

## MUSCLE CONTRACTION (TENSION) HEADACHE

The most frequently used term for muscle contraction headache (Fig. 95-14) is *tension headache.* This name was changed in 1962 because at that time it had been shown that exaggerated contraction of the muscles of the face, head, and neck occurred during the symptoms and were thought to be their cause. Since then it has been shown that muscle contraction is not always a physiologic feature of this headache and may be only one of many factors involved in its etiology. Factors such as pressure on sensory nerves, interference with blood supply of muscles and other tissues, alterations in the threshold to pain from changes in the central nociceptive system, or others still unrecognized may play roles in muscle contraction headache.

The symptoms of this disorder frequently do not include actual pain or ache if the patient is questioned closely about their nature in detail. More often the headache is actually described as a "tight band" on the head, a pressure, a feeling that the head is in a vise, a fullness, a tightness, or a feeling that the head will explode. The patient states that these symptoms change to a "real pain or ache" if they become very severe or persist for a long time. Such symptoms usually involve the whole head and often the neck and upper shoulders. At times, however, they may be just bitemporal or involve the face and jaws bilaterally or both sides of the neck and upper trapezius areas only. Occasionally the disturbance appears unilaterally in any or all of these regions and may be the causative mechanism in the production of the temporomandibular joint syndrome.

Attacks of muscle contraction or tension headache most often develop while the situation causing the disturbance exists (in contrast to migraine headache, which tends to follow the etiologic event). The responsible situation may be one in which physical strain alone, emotional strain alone, or more often both are operative. The anxious driver of a car bends his head and neck forward to see better through a snow-spattered windshield against the blinding lights of approaching traffic in an effort to get himself and his family safely home after a long trip. His head and neck and shoulders soon are painfully "tight, exploding, clamped in a vise." The secretary whose chair is not at the right height for her typewriter and who is stationed in a noisy, brightly lit, crowded office begins to feel a pressure and tightness in her eyes and head and neck as the day unfolds. It is not helped by the increasing pressure exerted on her by the boss who is under pressure from above to get the critical report out and copied for distribution before closing. The "discomfort" ultimately turns into a growing interfering pain until in a moment of overt frustration she bursts into tears and gives up.

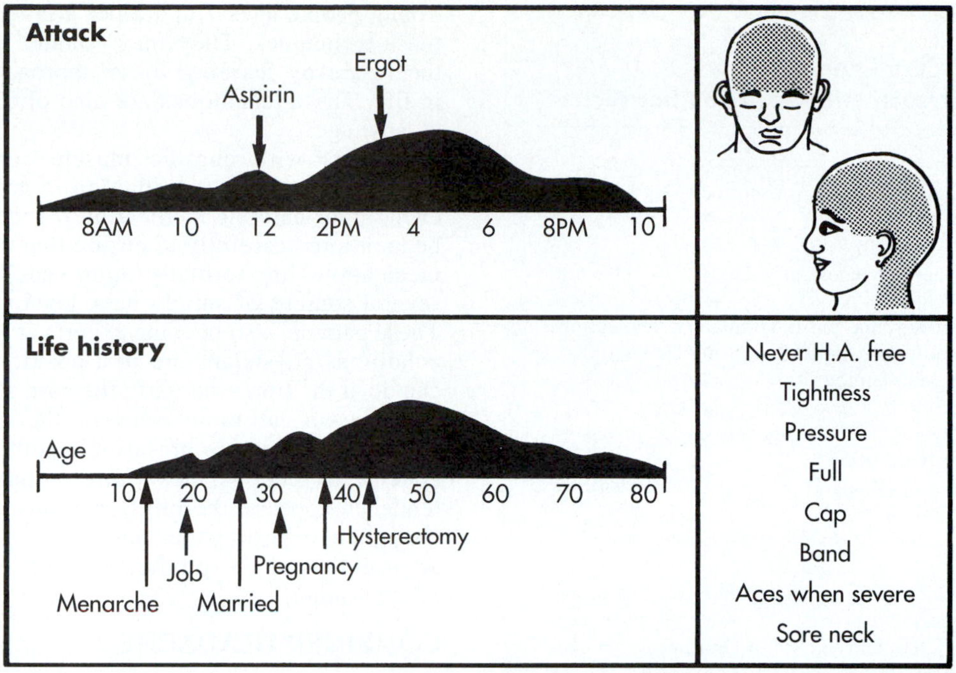


**Fig. 95-14.** Profile of muscle contraction headache.

In such situations, one can readily detect how physical and emotional pressures lead to "pressure" on that most important part of the patient, the head, where most of such burdens have to be negotiated. Most frequently, such situations are episodic and appear as individual "attacks" of muscle contraction (tension) headache. Some patients, however, live in prolonged states of anxiety that lead to episodes of this type of headache, which may go on day after day for weeks or months or, in extreme cases, become a chronic state that continues for years. These more protracted forms of tension headache usually are rooted in personal life situations that are very difficult to unravel and that may be hidden from the patient in his or her own subconscious mind.

Such episodes of headache are often successfully treated by one or more types of therapy, including physical measures, electric or ultrasonic counterstimulation, relaxation techniques, and drugs. Physical measures that may prove useful are hot applications to the neck, head, and shoulders; hot baths; massage; and gentle muscle and joint manipulation. Ultrasonic or electric stimulation or, in some patients, acupuncture may prove helpful. Relaxation techniques provided by courses of instruction and aided by tapes and biofeedback are often useful.

The use of pharmaceutical products is often a convenient and effective way to gain control over this form of headache (see Managed Care Guide to the stepwise treatment of tension headache). This route depends mostly on muscle relaxants, sedatives, analgesics, and all too frequently caffeine-containing mixtures of these substances. The intermittent use of these drugs is appropriate, but more and more frequently headache and pain centers are becoming involved in detoxifying patients from the results of increasing daily dosing with these medicines in ever-increasing amounts. The medicines then create the vicious cycle of drug-dependency headache and caffeine withdrawal headaches, which often require hospitalization or treatment in a detoxifying unit.

Phenacetin has been considered to be the most important component of these antiheadache agents in creating "analgesic nephritis," a nonreversible and serious source of renal failure. The constant use of phenacetin-containing drugs amounting to a total of about 3 kg over 3 years may cause this condition. Tumors of transitional cell type in the genitourinary tract have also been related to such use, as well as to the chronic use of acetaminophen. In some patients the latter is known also to be capable of causing liver damage, as shown by changes in the prothrombin time and in alkaline phosphatase, aspartate aminotransferase (AST, SGOT) and alanine aminotransferase (ALT, SGPT) levels. The NSAIDs useful in correcting some of the pain of chronic muscle contraction headache may also have an adverse effect on renal function when used over weeks and months. These drugs thus require monitoring.

The caffeine often found in tablets for headache relief may have a "boomerang" effect: it picks patients up at the time but drops them down a few hours later into what is called a *caffeine withdrawal headache.* Sedatives and tranquilizers, which are often included in antiheadache medications, also lead to dependency states and sometimes depression.

Patients with muscle contraction (tension) headache obtain easy relief from these over-the-counter and other prescription antiheadache medications. They have a great tendency to depend on them in increasing amounts to solve problems that require much deeper and basic attention related to the patient's life situation, habits, job, feelings, and mood.

Interestingly, many such patients who do not manifest depression outwardly benefit greatly from the use of tricyclic or quadricyclic antidepressant drugs such as

## Managed Care Guide
### Stepwise treatment of tension headaches*

I. Over-the-counter antiinflammatory medications
   A. Ibuprofen (Advil and others), 400-800 mg initially up to 2400 mg daily
   B. Aspirin, 650 mg q4h as needed
   C. Acetaminophen (Tylenol and others), 650-1000 mg q4h as needed
II. Prescription nonsteroidal antiinflammatory medications
   A. Naproxen sodium (Anaprox), 550 mg bid
   B. Ketorolac tromethamine (Toradol), 10 mg qid as needed
   C. Diflunisal (Dolobid), 1000 mg initially followed by 500 mg bid as needed
   D. Mefenamic acid (Ponstel), 500 mg initially followed by 250 mg q6h as needed
III. Combination analgesic-sedative medications (1 or 2 tablets or capsules q4h as needed up to 8 daily)
   A. Acetaminophen, caffeine, and butalbital (Esgic, Floricet, Medigesic)
   B. Aspirin, caffeine, and butalbital (Fiorinal)
   C. Aspirin and butalbital (Axotal)
   D. Acetaminophen and butalbital (Bancap, Phrenilin)
   E. Isometheptene mucate, dichloralphenazone, and acetaminophen (Midchlor, Midrin)
IV. Prophylactic medications
   A. Tricyclic antidepressants†
      1. Amitriptyline HCl (Elavil, Endep), 10-50 mg tid
      2. Nortriptyline HCl (Aventyl, Pamelor), 25 mg tid
      3. Desipramine HCl (Norpramin, Pertofrane), 25 mg tid
      4. Doxepin HCl (Adapin, Sinequan), 10-50 mg tid (often, daily dose given at bedtime to avoid sedation)
      5. Imipramine HCl (Janimine, Tofranil), 10-50 mg tid
   B. Beta-adrenergic blockers
      1. Propranolol HCl (Inderal), 160-240 mg daily in divided doses or single time-released dose
      2. Nadolol (Corgard), 20-240 mg daily

Adapted from Trachtenbarg DE: Headache: home study self assessment, No. 138. Kansas City, Mo: American Academy of Family Physicians, 1990.
*Agents listed in order of the author's preference.
†Daily dose may also be given once at bedtime.

amitriptyline or doxepin in full doses. Because all these measures have their own set of side effects, other approaches to the basic problems are recommended in the form of psychotherapy or behavioral modification, aided by biofeedback or social counseling or the interested discussion about life problems with the patient's own physician. For the busy physician who may find it impossible to provide the attention necessary to explain and manage the problems arising in the life of chronic headache patients, the services of a psychiatric social worker may be helpful to both patient and physician.

Behavioral modification therapy associated with relaxation instruction and tapes, the therapist's counsel, and monitoring of progress by biofeedback techniques is especially useful in the tension form of headache. Young people ages 7 and older are very good at learning these techniques. They may counter many headaches in the future by learning these approaches to stress early in life. These techniques are also often useful for people at any age.

Patients with chronic muscle contraction (tension) headache are prone to addiction in any form. The use of even minor narcotic medication for them therefore has to be monitored carefully to ensure that the numbers of such medications are formally approved. One may find that several sources of supply have been used by the patient. These patients also become experts at learning under what conditions physicians are in a position in which all they can do at the time (the party they are at, the weekend they are to be off-call to an assistant, the day they are leaving for vacation) is to prescribe another consignment of codeine, oxycodone, meperidine, or barbiturate. When this tendency appears, the physician must talk seriously with the patient regarding the "rules of the game" and often the advisability of hospitalization for detoxification at a proper center.

## COMBINED HEADACHE

Combined headache refers to a form of headache that is also known as *mixed headache* or, in Europe, as *vasomotor headache*. Its mechanism is thought to be related to both vascular and muscle contraction abnormalities working together, prominently, at the same time in the same person. This headache is present constantly, during every waking hour, and has the symptoms of tightness, pressure, and discomfort of the muscle contraction (tension) headache plus the pulsatile, painful quality of the migraine headache, which at times leads to nausea and vomiting. Patients with this type of headache may have a family history of migraine. Severe attacks may be relieved by ergotamine, and prophylaxis may be provided by other antimigraine drugs (e.g., propranolol, methysergide, NSAIDs). The ordinary analgesics described earlier for muscle contraction (tension) headache also bring significant relief. Full doses of tricyclic and quadricyclic agents help sometimes in a striking fashion, even in combination with β-blocking drugs.

Patients with combined headache tend to go from one physician to the next, clinic to clinic, to seek help. As with severe muscle contraction (tension) headache patients, they tend to accumulate drugs and develop dependency-addiction syndromes that may demand pain center or hospital withdrawal treatment before real progress can be made. An antitherapy process may take place in these patients that creates a vicious circle spinning down hill: pain leads to tests. Negative tests equal "Nothing is wrong." This means "It's all in your head," which equals "You must be neurotic." This indicates "It's all your fault." This means "You don't need all this medicine," and that statement equals "You're a fake or a weakling." This sequence leads the patient to think "No one believes me . . . . They don't know what a real headache is. . . . I wish they just had one of my headaches. . . ." "This is all making me angry—in fact, it is giving me a worse headache. I need some more medicine."

Another vicious headache circle is slightly different: "No matter how hard I try, Joe doesn't pay any real attention to me—you know, it makes me mad. When I have been mad a long time, I get a headache. When I have a headache, he's *nice* to me. One is starting now."

Both these situations and almost all chronic headache problems that have similar or other vicious circles involved require a knowledge of the total situation for solution. Some of these situations have been described as "diseases caused by being caught in a trap." The physician, the psychiatric social worker, or a psychiatric consultant may be able to help the person in a "human trap." It is not often that the caregiver can release the patient from the trap, even when the trapped person wants to get out (which is not always the case). The counselor may need to help make living in the trap more comfortable. Learning the elements of such traps and being able to discuss them with the patient take time and interest but can be very useful even though not curative. Understanding the trap may also save the patient some troubles from addiction, unnecessary surgery, and inadvisable decisions and behavior.

In these trapped patients the use of multiple drugs for relief leads to a continual state of headache. The agents that bring relief lead to rebound headache when their effect has worn off. It is not just the heavy narcotic pain relievers that have this effect, but also those common concoctions containing combinations of several substances—aspirin, caffeine, sedatives, tranquilizers, decongestants—and more powerful agents such as barbiturates, propoxyphene (Darvon), pentazocine (Talwin), bromides, codeine, and oxycodone. When the physician finds that the patient is using more and more of these substances, supplied by the physician or sometimes by several physicians, the physician should have a frank confrontation with the patient in an effort to find better solutions before the situation becomes fixed and severe. The first step in such situations may be to eliminate these substances either by a definite outpatient office program or by detoxification in a pain center or hospital. Inpatients may be surprised to find how much less headache they have and how much better they feel when they have been relieved of the "headache-relieving" substances.

The editors also must emphasize the increasing problem to which Dr. Graham alludes: dependency on analgesics or ergotamine. Such patients may have daily "rebound" headaches and enter a vicious cycle of dependency, even with simple analgesics such as acetaminophen or ASA with caffeine. These patients experience daily withdrawal from these agents and ergotamine, craving escalating doses. Since headache is a major feature of these withdrawal symptoms, such patients are classified as having chronic headache, but it is vital that they be withdrawn from these agents. This may require inpatient hospitalization or the help of a multidisciplinary team of a headache clinic or pain center to confront this difficult problem.

The follow-up period after detoxification is important. It must be continued for months and at times years, during which attention is paid to the life situations and habits of behavior that have led to this serious habituation. Meditation, behavioral modification with biofeedback, hypnosis, social service counseling, and formal therapy with a psychologist or psychiatrist can be very useful in helping to remodel lifestyles that are detrimental to the continued benefits of eliminating excessive medication.

## HEADACHE OF NASAL VASOMOTOR REACTION

The nose and its various complicated passages, ostia, turbinates, sinuses, septum, and delicate highly reactive membranes can become the source of major acute pain and headache when affected by acute trauma, infection, inflammation, structural pressures, atmospheric pressure changes, and tumor growth. Allergic disturbances such as hay fever may cause marked swelling of the nasal mucous membrane, which causes much discomfort from "pressure and obstruction" but rarely *pain.* So-called chronic sinusitis and even mucous cyst formation infrequently cause pain, which behooves physicians to seek very conservative otolaryngologic advice before embarking on surgery for relief of face and head pain alleged to be related to these diagnoses (see Chapter 28). The painful phase of migraine is often associated with nasal congestion and blocking on the affected side. This is part of the vasodilatory phase of migraine and is not a "sinus condition" causing the attack of pain. On closely examining the migraine patient's statement that "my father had 'sinus headaches' all his life," one usually finds that father had migraines like his daughter.

However, a form of headache is associated with marked painful swelling of the nasal mucous membrane that is not related to infection or allergy but rather seems to have its roots in deeply based emotional reactions. This consists of obnoxious obstruction of the nasal passages and chronic, continuous pain in the nose, forehead, and central area of the face. Although usually bilateral, it may be unilateral and related to an injury or surgery on one side of the nose. Symptoms such as these are often kept alive by the constant use of decongestant nose drops or pills, which results in a "rebounding" chronic state. Surgical procedures to alter nasal structures and passages usually tend to aggravate the problem in the long term. Sphenopalatine blocks, cauterizations, and procedures to separate the nasal mucous membranes from their autonomic nerve supply may make matters worse as well as improve them. They should be undertaken only after psychiatric evaluation and carried out, if at all, by very conservative ear, nose, and throat (ENT) surgeons.

Lying behind persistent psychosomatic symptoms and signs, hidden emotional conflicts of considerable severity may or may not respond to psychotherapy. Relief of these symptoms by medical means may lead to new symptoms elsewhere or to psychotic breaks, suggesting that these painful changes in physiology preserve the patient from a more dangerous life state.

In one case a middle-aged mother of a closely treasured son was about to lose him in marriage to a very beautiful girl. Before the wedding the mother, who was also very attractive, decided to have surgery on her nasal septum to remove the crook in her nose despite her son's protests. Postoperatively, her nose became blocked and her whole face was painful. The discomfort was not relieved by further surgery or by multiple drug therapies. After 2 years of psychotherapy, her symptoms were much relieved as she adjusted to her son's marriage.

Antidepressant medication, psychotherapy, and avoidance of narcotics and further surgery may be helpful in managing patients with symptoms such as those previously listed and keeping them away from damaging treatments that reinforce the symptom.

## HEADACHE OF HYPOCHONDRIACAL OR CONVERSION STATES

Hypochondriacal or conversion state headaches are psychogenic headaches in which a peripheral pain mechanism is nonexistent or minimal. Headache may be a symptom if a patient reacts to life problems in a hypochondriacal manner. Headaches arising in this way may have some basis in organic pathology, such as cervical arthritis or myositis of a degree not sufficient in most people to produce symptoms that so insistently demand medical attention. Not infrequently the nature of the headache may be revealed by its association with multiple system involvement causing discomfort of one sort or another. A long list of ineffective medications and another long list of "ineffective doctors" should arouse suspicion that the headache is mostly a request for attention, sympathy, and a justification for disability.

It tends to be a mistake in therapy for physicians to approach the problem of "the chronic complainer" with the concept in mind that they will "cure or completely relieve" this symptom. Rather, this is the time and place for physicians to do what they can to help bring relief of sorts and permit a sequence of visits that may never "fix" the complaint but that serve the more basic need for the patient to establish a relationship with the physician. This offers a chance for ventilation of troubles and support in special times of need, a limited but very useful goal. One may be dismayed to observe that such a patient's symptoms are little changed in severity or frequency over some years. Because many physicians consider their "mission" to be to cure people, they may wonder if they are really doing anything good by this prolonged association. The question may be answered by asking oneself, "Why does the patient come back?"

*Conversion* or *hysterical headache* may take several forms. One may be a sudden, severe, acute onset of headache and at times being localized in one half or one area of the head. Such an onset of headache simulates the onset of a subarachnoid hemorrhage or another vascular accident or a "cough Valsalva" headache if related to strain, coitus, or coughing. When organic causes have been eliminated, the physician may find that such an acute headache occurred in response to a thought or sudden emotion usually coming out of the unconscious or a headache precipitated by a sudden event that created an association with very disturbing psychogenic material.

Single events of this type may occur or at times headaches of an intermittent sort may recur in relation to a chronically recurring emotional disturbance. Such headaches are helped significantly by psychiatric consultation and treatment.

A more chronic form of conversion headache may take the form of a "cap, hood, or vise" enclosing the whole head and compressing it with baffling discomfort during every waking moment of the day for weeks, months, and years. The extreme persistence, vague description, and absolutely continuous tenacity of this symptom is unlike even the persistence of muscle contraction headache and combined headache. The patient always has "his head on his mind" to the exclusion of being able to concentrate and at times to perform daily activities of living. The symptoms may be complicated by visual disturbances that are revealed by visual fields to be characteristic of the tunnel vision of the hysteric patient.

In young or relatively young patients, psychotherapy may be successful in determining the root of such symptoms. In older patients, supportive therapy from a social worker or physician may be more practical and successful. Avoidance of overmedication and invasive procedures and surgery is important. The nature of the symptoms may be revealed by finding a history of definite hysteric symptoms in other areas of the body at an earlier age.

A third form of semiconversion headache is found occasionally, especially in cluster headache patients. Patients present themselves as going through one of their typical attacks, with all the behavior that goes with it, even after they had long since stopped having "real" attacks. Such episodes are related in some cases to an attempt to obtain medication and seem to be well within the patient's conscious control. The eye may be reddened by rubbing it for such occasions and held half shut. Genuine tearing of the eye is usually not present.

In other patients the "recurrence" of the attack seems to be as genuine to the patient as to the physician and seems to come from a psychiatric "no man's land" somewhere between the subconscious and the real world. In one patient a series of such somewhat "unreal" cluster headaches (which had been a cause for hospitalization and parenteral medication) suddenly stopped when the patient was asked to see a psychiatrist. Another patient had been going through a very severe cluster series in the hospital with meperidine (Demerol) relief for several attacks. He confessed after he was out of the cluster that at times he could not distinguish between the real pain of a cluster attack and the pain that developed when he yearned for another shot of meperidine, during which his dramatic behavior was similar to that in "real" cluster headaches.

## VASCULAR HEADACHE ASSOCIATED WITH VARIOUS MEDICAL DISORDERS

A variety of medical conditions cause headaches by distorting cranial vascular function. A list of some of these is worth considering as a reminder of some of the physiologic disturbances that may lead to significant headache. Special attention is called to a few medical situations associated with headache that tend to have special features.

### General list

1. Systemic infections, usually with fever
2. Miscellaneous disorders: hypoxic states; carbon monoxide poisoning; effects of nitrites and nitrates; caffeine withdrawal reaction; cranial circulatory insufficiency; postconcussive and postconvulsive states; foreign protein reactions; hypoglycemia; hypercapnia; acute pressor reactions (during MAO inhibitor treatment and with pheochromocytoma); headache associated with arterial hypertension, renal failure, and dialysis

### Special situations

***Withdrawal from steroids.*** Withdrawal from prolonged steroid therapy being taken for a variety of medical conditions may be accompanied by the first appearance of migrainous or cluster headaches in a patient who has never had them before. Return to a slower reduction of the steroid dose is the best solution to this problem.

***Syphilis.*** Syphilis in its secondary stage tends to be a forgotten cause of headache. Low-grade fever and constant headache may be the only indicators of this specific fever and headache.

***Headache related to hypertension.*** Hypertension is well known to be related to the occurrence of headache. Certain specific hypertensive states (e.g., hypertensive encephalopathy) and sudden increases in blood pressure related to pheochromocytoma crises and toxemia of pregnancy are special cases in which either a sudden rise in blood pressure or cerebral edema associated with hypertensive crises lead to headache. Hypertension associated with Cushing syndrome or with aldosterone-producing tumors may present with headache of a vascular type resembling migraine in a few patients.

Ordinary essential hypertension is also associated with headache of a vascular sort related to increased amplitude of pulsation in the branches of the external carotid artery strongly resembling migraine and relieved by migraine medicines. Such hypertension and its accompanying headache have been found to occur more frequently in migraine patients. As with migraine, the headache comes not while vessels are constricted and the pressure is high, but rather afterward in a state of rebound vasodilatation. This situation often arises after periods of tension and vasoconstriction as blood vessels (and the patient) relax during sleep, only to awaken in the morning with lowered blood pressure *and* headache.

Headache of this type responds to ergotamine and methysergide, both of which should be used with caution in patients with hypertension, as well as to β-blockers, reserpine, and chlorothiazide drugs. The degree of headache is related to a drop from high to low pressure in the blood pressure cycle; the headache tends to appear as pressure is falling, being greater depending on the amount of change in blood pressure from high to low. The daily wake-up headache of these patients is usually greatly helped by measures that improve the blood pressure, even though in itself it is not threatening or necessarily requiring treatment.

β-Blockers plus chlorothiazides in moderate doses are indicated. Reserpine in 0.1 mg daily or every-other-day doses, along with 25 mg hydrochlorothiazide (Hydrodiuril), followed for at least 2 to 3 months is another therapeutic approach. Guanabenz (Wytensin) and clonidine (Catapres) are other centrally acting antihypertensive drugs useful in preventing headache. Hydralazine effectively lowers blood pressure but produces headache in the process and so should be avoided as a treatment for hypertensive headache.

An unusual type of headache resembling migraine (but without the family history or earlier life occurrence) has been noted to occur in patients whose renal disease is beginning to become significantly decompensated. This may represent the beginning of the need for dialysis.

***Dialysis headache.*** Almost all patients who have had problems with headache of the migraine variety or "headaches associated with renal decompensation" tend to have headaches as a prominent symptom of each dialysis when they come to that form of therapy. Headache is reduced during their dialyses by increasing the $Na^+$ in the dialysate and by avoiding "negative pressure" during dialysis if possible and otherwise advisable. Dialysis headache is related chiefly to significant changes in osmolality caused by large $Na^+$ decreases; it is also greater as blood pressure drops, and its severity is proportional to the degree of decrease during the procedure (Fig. 95-15). These dialysis headaches occur with both machine and peritoneal dialysis. Removal of "sick" kidneys and successful transplant usually stops dialysis and renal disease headache. Headache, however, is one of the first symptoms of transplant rejection disease.

***Headache from dissection of the carotid artery.*** Sudden, severe, unilateral headache may be caused by acute dissection of a carotid artery. When unilateral neck and head pain in the region of the carotid sheath and radiating to the region of the ear, temple, and eye suddenly takes place "out of the blue" in a patient unaccustomed to having such attacks, this diagnosis must be suspected. Most patients with this condition hear a bruit inside their own head, have ipsilateral disturbance of vision, and develop a Horner syndrome on the side of the lesion. After an initial episode, recurrent episodes may occur in a "stuttering" fashion over some weeks or months as further dissection takes place. Embolic episodes above the lesion may also cause CNS deficits. During the acute phase the

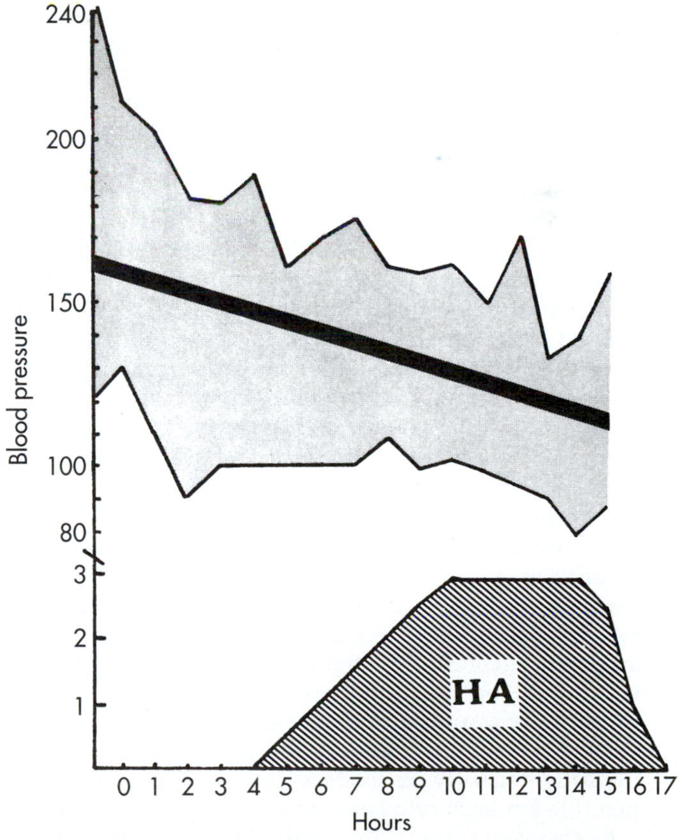


**Fig. 95-15.** Dialysis headache. Headache (*HA*) appears as blood pressure (*BP*) *falls* during renal hemodialysis. (From Graham JR, Bara DS, Yap AU: *Res Clin Stud Headache* 6:147,1978.)

carotid sheath is tender, the pulse is poorly felt, and a bruit may be heard by the physician as well as the patient. The situation should be investigated as soon as suspected and the help of noninvasive and angiographic techniques applied to make the diagnosis and govern treatment by surgery or medical means.

*Migraine and mitral valve prolapse (Barlow syndrome).* A strong suggestion exists, as yet unproved statistically, that patients with migraine have an increased incidence of mitral valve prolapse. Such a coincidence may be responsible for the frequency of paroxysmal cardiac arrhythmias in migraine patients, since they are common to both conditions. In some migraine patients, episodes of cardiac arrhythmias may become "migraine equivalents" and take the place of "migraine in the head" over weeks or months. When this possible combination is suspected by auscultatory findings of a late systolic murmur and click, or even in their absence, echocardiography is used to make the diagnosis. When mitral valve prolapse is present in a migraine patient, propranolol may serve a double therapeutic purpose. These patients also need to be instructed in penicillin prophylaxis before and after dentistry and certain surgical procedures. Small cerebral embolizations in patients with mitral valve prolapse may simulate classic migraine attacks. Aspirin and dipyridamole (Persantine) may be useful prophylactically for both conditions. Some of these patients may have anticardiolipin antibodies and require specialized assessment and treatment.

*Headache from spinal fluid drainage.* Whenever about one fourth of the total volume of cerebrospinal fluid (CSF) has leaked or drained out of the meningeal sac around the brain and spinal cord, headache may manifest when the patient remains in a vertical position for minutes or hours. This simple form of headache from CSF loss, most frequently of iatrogenic origin and occurring in the course of the performance of a lumbar puncture, disappears when the patient lies flat, only to recur when the patient stands up for a while again, until at last the needle hole in the dural sac has healed and no longer leaks. This type of headache may be avoided by using a small needle with a conified rather than a beveled tip and by requiring that the patient lie flat 6 to 8 hours after the procedure. Raising the foot of the bed on 4-inch blocks for the first 2 of these hours may also be helpful, the main object being to give the needle hole time to heal before fluid is forced through it by the increased CSF pressure that occurs in the patient's vertical position.

Headache that occurs after spinal anesthesia may be of the drainage type. It is present only when patients assume a vertical position and disappears when they lie flat, or it may result from an allergic inflammatory reaction to the anesthetic agent. In the latter case, the headache is present whether the patient is horizontal or vertical. Fever and occasionally a stiff neck are present. It is to be hoped that a repeat lumbar puncture will reveal a sterile pleocytosis. The patient usually responds well to the use of steroids (if infection has been ruled out) and/or to the passage of time.

Occasionally, true "drainage" headaches persist over many days. The most important therapeutic maneuver is to require patients to stay flat until headache no longer occurs when they lift the head. In very exceptional cases, this type of headache persists for weeks. In such instances, one therapeutic maneuver that has met with some success is the injection of a few milliliters of the patient's own blood into the lumbar spinal canal to put a "patch" on the unhealed leaking hole. The artificial inflammation thus caused may support the observation that "drainage" headache rarely occurs after neurosurgical entrance to the spinal canal (with some resulting inflammation from trauma and blood) or when the CSF protein level is elevated because of an underlying lesion or bleeding or infection within the meningeal envelopes.

CSF leaks resulting in chronic, posturally related headache occur also as a result of trauma, a congenital defect, or neoplastic invasion of the meninges. The patient who has a persistent headache related to being upright, cured by lying flat, and resistant to most ordinary types of therapy may be found at lumbar puncture to have very low, undetectable pressure and very little fluid to draw out through the lumbar puncture needle even though the examiner is sure it is in the proper place. Such a patient must be closely questioned regarding the possibility of a dural tear during vigorous athletics, produced by a leak at the base of the skull and opening a passage between cranial and nasal sinus chambers. If the patient gives a history of sudden dripping of clear fluid from the nose at unexpected moments for no obvious reason, some of this fluid needs to be collected for examination. If the fluid does not give a positive test for glucose, it is not CSF. If it tests positively for glucose, it is highly suspect but is not necessarily CSF, and further examination is required for its chloride and protein contents. When a CSF leak is strongly suspected, injection of radioactive material intraspinally (radioimmunosorbent assay [RISA] scan) is performed with pledgets in place in the nose and sinus areas to detect where radioactive fluid collects outside the cranial cavity.

Patients with congenital defects in the cribriform plate and other areas of the skull where CSF can escape into the nasopharynx may have repeated bouts of meningitis, often of a mild but nevertheless dangerous type. Prophylactic antibiotic therapy may be indicated for these patients if the defect cannot be closed.

*Iatrogenic headache from vasodilating agents.* Some older patients who have long since recovered from their attacks of migraine may have a recurrence of common migraine attacks shortly after a heart attack when nitroglycerine, isosorbide dinitrate (Isordil), or nitroglycerine ointment therapy is started. Nitrites are a specific precipitant of typical unilateral migraine in susceptible patients and cause "ordinary" headache in many other nonmigrainous patients. Reduced doses or substitution of calcium channel blockers may be useful in eliminating this effect. Occasionally, calcium channel blockers *cause* headache instead of relieving it, especially if their action includes peripheral vasodilatation. Because patients with coronary disease and older patients in general are not good subjects for treatment with ergot products, calcium channel blockers are worth a careful selective trial. One female patient had a return of her former migraines when exposed to the nitroglycerin ointment on her husband's chest during his recovery from heart attack. Some patients become desensitized to the effect of nitroglycerin ointment as smaller doses are used and time passes.

Other drugs may cause localized or general headache by directly causing undue cranial vasodilatation or by creating it as an aftereffect or rebound of their vasoconstricting action. These include indomethacin, hydralazine (Apresoline), alcohol, histamine, and nicotinic acid; the rebound headache may also follow excessive use of caffeine, ergotamine, or methysergide. Propranolol may be useful in reducing the effect of such "rebound" headache producers.

***Headache associated with attacks of flushing.*** Headaches of a vascular sort and pulsating in character are produced rarely by mastocytosis, the carcinoid syndrome, pheochromocytoma, and GI conditions in which vasoactive peptides are involved. All these are characterized by attacks of flushing associated with headache. Mastocytosis may masquerade as common freckles, and biopsy of newly acquired freckles may provide the diagnosis. Carcinoid tumor needs to be considered when flushing, wheezing, diarrhea, and headache join in a clinical picture. Alcohol, epinephrine, and histamine in small amounts may quickly bring headache into action in the carcinoid or mastocytosis syndromes. Bronchogenic carcinoids may cause these attacks before metastasis to the liver, whereas liver metastasis usually must be present for GI carcinoid to produce these symptoms. Carcinoid syndrome of the bowel may be a part of a multiple-lesion syndrome in which gastrin-producing tumors, responsible for the Zollinger-Ellison syndrome, are also present. Syndromes presenting with headache, attacks of flushing, asthma, and diarrhea demand thorough investigation, often with the help of a gastroenterologist.

Headaches associated with flushing or pallor attacks with sweating and sudden rises in blood pressure require investigation for pheochromocytoma by blood and urinary catechol tests and appropriate scanning studies in search of the tumor. It is important to examine the patient during such episodes at the time they occur so that blood pressure measurements may be recorded and the physician can make sure that the urine in the patient's bladder at the time of the hypertensive episode is included in the collection to be tested for vanillylmandelic acid (VMA), catechols, and metanephrine.

***Endocrine conditions that may present as headache.*** Hypothyroidism for any reason—primary, secondary, or tertiary—may produce migrainelike headaches that are corrected by appropriate treatment. Cushing syndrome is another condition that may present as a "headache problem."

Pituitary tumors also may masquerade as unilateral headaches of a vascular type and pass for migraine for long periods until acromegaly is noted, menstruation ceases, or hypoglycemia and fatigue become apparent. Patients with Addison disease may also go first to the physician's office for treatment of headache.

In each of these endocrine syndromes, the physician should remember that one look "is worth a thousand words" of description. The appearance of the whole patient may reveal the diagnosis of the disease that is the cause of the specific headache syndrome.

***Headache from traction on intracranial structures, mainly vascular, by masses.*** Masses, whether a primary or metastatic tumor, hematoma, abscess, or general cerebral swelling (e.g., pseudotumor cerebri), cause head pain by distorting, stretching, or dragging on pain-sensitive structures in the head, mostly vascular structures (Fig. 95-16). Their recognition, investigation, and management are discussed in detail in other chapters of this book, but a diagram of their profile, compared with that of other, more frequent "functional" headaches, is worth presenting because, as usual, the history points to the diagnosis.

An important feature of the headache history of a tumor or other intracranial mass may be that it *fails to follow the pattern* of migraine, tension headache, and other headache syndromes that have rather characteristic profiles over both a day and months or years. This fact should point toward its potential organicity and call for thorough investigation. Traction lesions tend to be accentuated or

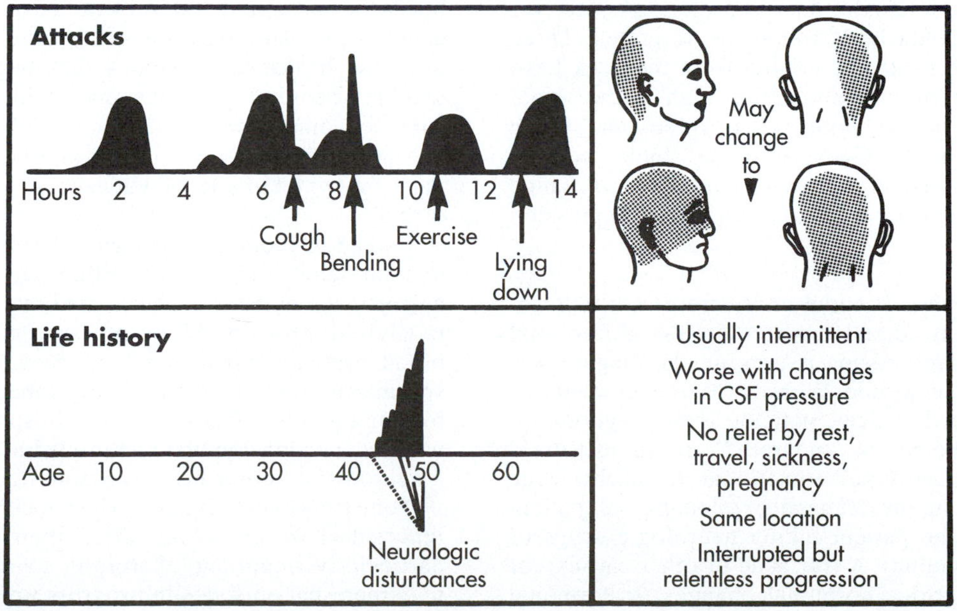


**Fig. 95-16.** Profile of a brain tumor.

relieved by physical changes rather than by response to emotional or physiologic vicissitudes or patterns. Such features include change in position; change in CSF dynamics; change in coughing, straining, or coitus; onset during exertion; short bursts or jabs with changes in physical activity; and association with recurrent increasing nausea and vomiting or, especially, blackouts or seizures recurring in an intermittent but gradually more frequent and serious fashion. All these may point to an organic lesion gradually impinging on pain-sensitive structures in the head or causing obstructive local abnormalities in CSF pressure and venous damage. Local disturbances of brain function in thinking, concentration, balance, gait, vision, hearing, continence, and patterns of living point toward organic lesions of this kind. A history of head and/or neck injury during recent months, especially in elderly patients, should raise suspicion of subdural hemorrhage. It is easy to think of a space-occupying lesion as a cause for headache in a patient who develops a history such as this who had had no significant headache history in the past. However, when a patient has had a long history of recurrent headaches of the migrianous or tension type, as change in this form, in which the headache seems to go its own way, unmindful of the person who has it, may go unnoticed unless the history indicates, in great detail, the nature, location, and behavior of the headache. Moreover, its responses to previous therapy should draw attention to this organic possibility.

During a migraine headache the performance of the Valsalva maneuver (as in coughing or straining) often accentuates the already existing headache. If, however, a headache is precipitated "out of the blue" every time the Valsalva maneuver is performed, and especially if it becomes more and more easily produced and longer in duration when it occurs, a thorough investigation is indicated for an organic, space-occupying or space-crowding lesion within the cranium or in the neck, where the free flow of CSF from one area to another may be compromised by a narrowing lesion. The new CT head and neck scans and especially the newest MRI scans can be very helpful in finding such lesions. Lesions are typically sought in the posterior fossa, but the neck as a source for such "Valsalva" headache is frequently forgotten. Three examples of cough headache arising from the neck have been seen: (1) a syringomyelia lesion high in the spinal cord, (2) a disk in the midcervical spine, and (3) a metastatic lesion in the C4-5 vertebrae. Such "cough" headache may be transient, however, and related to change in vasomotor tone during transitory periods of depression or anxiety.

***Pseudotumor cerebri.*** Pseudotumor cerebri is the headache-causing lesion often forgotten in the differential diagnosis. When papilledema is present, the diagnosis is readily and quickly explored. Without external evidence of increased pressure, however, patients with pseudotumor can easily be labeled as "neurotic" or subject to a "combined or mixed-type" functional headache. One should suspect it in the teenage or menopausal patient (usually female), the patient taking neurologic drugs or large amounts of vitamin A (for acne or other causes), or one undergoing various hormonal changes or hormonal therapy. Before undertaking lumbar puncture to determine if CSF pressure is increased, the patient is hospitalized and consultation with a neurologist obtained to ensure no local cause of obstruction and increased pressure might lead to "coning" of the brainstem after lumbar puncture.

***Headache from overt cranial inflammation.*** Inflammation of any sort involving pain-sensitive cranial structures produces headache as a prominent symptom. The inflammation may be caused by infectious agents (bacterial, viral, parasitic) or chemical or autoimmune processes. Without recalling all the common causes of inflammation that may create such headaches and that can be treated successfully by specific antibiotics or antiinflammatory agents, selected entities that present clinically as *headache* problems are discussed next.

**Inflammation caused by bleeding from vascular malformations.** The profile of an attack of headache resulting from intracranial hemorrhage from vascular malformations such as aneurysms or AV malformations is shown in Fig. 95-17. Such lesions rarely cause headache except when they bleed. Early in their history, they may present with seizures. In some exceptional cases, constant headache may result from gradual enlargement of an aneurysm that leads to pressure on another pain-sensitive structure. A change in response to usual therapy for recurring headaches always on the same side of the head may indicate hemorrhage or thrombosis in a vascular lesion that has been involved in determining the location of previous headaches.

The characteristic clinical picture of these events reveals a sudden hammer-blow onset in most patients, with headache coming "out of the blue" without apparent cause, although occasionally related to physical strain, the Valsalva maneuver, or severe emotional stress. Such episodes rarely if ever occur during sleep, whereas migraine and cluster headache frequently do. Headache may be localized in small episodes of bleeding and recur in several stepwise progressions leading to major, often fatal events. Depending on the location of the malformation, the bleeding may occur into the subarachnoid space, leading to stiff neck, fever, backache, and severe, sudden headache, or it may extend into intracerebral tissue and cause local neurologic deficits that develop during and after the headache. Episodes that begin with headache and local cerebral symptoms may suddenly extend into the subarachnoid or ventricular spaces with resulting spread of the headache. Stiff neck, fever, and development of back pain are symptomatic of widespread subarachnoid hemorrhage.

Spread of blood into ventricles is often the forerunner of fatal demise. Early recognition and treatment of these episodes are essential. The immediate use of propranolol is advised, provided blood pressure is adequate, to keep blood pressure down and help prevent cerebrovascular spasm caused by the presence of blood in the CSF or later by angiography. Transport to a hospital for a CT scan *without* and *with* contrast and immediate consultation with a neurologist and/or neurosurgeon are indicated.

Sometimes such events, when localized or minor, are reported days or weeks after their occurrence. It is particularly important, therefore, to recognize that they may represent episodes in progress toward a major bleed. Full, prompt investigation is indicated.

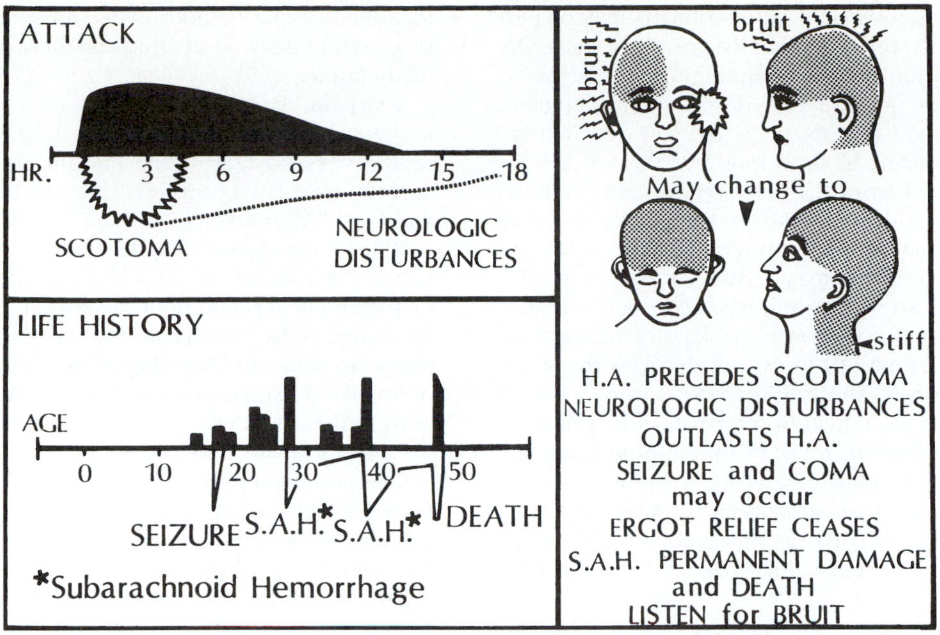


**Fig. 95-17.** Profile of subarachnoid hemorrhage from a vascular anomaly.

There are other sources of sudden headache "out of the blue," but a history of the type just described demands full investigation to rule out aneurysmal or vascular malformation bleeding. Other sources of sudden headache may be onset of meningitis, pheochromocytoma episodes, embolism, cerebral thrombosis, cysts in the lateral ventricles, and sudden onset of migraine or psychogenic headache of a conversion type. A CT scan *without* contrast taken within a few days of the event may show the presence of extravasated blood; *with* contrast the scan may show the lesion. Alternatively, angiography may be required.

The rapid development of imaging as it applies to headaches should also be mentioned because of the new and constantly improving software for magnetic resonance angiography. Thus the possibility of visualizing aneurysms and vascular malformations noninvasively has been greatly enhanced in the past year.

**Inflammation from foreign chemical agents in cerebrospinal space.** The most common foreign chemical agents are spinal anesthetics that cause an allergic or chemical inflammation in the CNS in a few patients. Headaches of this type are accompanied by sterile pleocytosis in the CSF, some stiff neck, and low-grade fever. Examination of CSF may be necessary to rule out bacterial infection. The headache in this patient is present in *both* horizontal and vertical positions, as differentiated from the simple lumbar puncture headache, which is defined by its *absence* in the horizontal position and *presence* when the patient sits or stands upright. Analgesics and antihistamines such as diphenhydramine (Benadryl) may be useful in treating this type of headache. At times, corticosteroids are needed, when it is ensured that bacterial infection is not present. Other substances (e.g., air, contrast media of various types, antibiotics), when injected into the subarachnoid space, may lead to this sort of inflammatory headache.

**Vasculitis.** Vasculitis of autoimmune origin, such as that associated with periarteritis nodosa, lupus, scleroderma, Wegener granulomatosis, and Takayasu disease, is a rare source of headache.

**Cranial arteritis.** Cranial arteritis is an important entity to consider in patients complaining of headache for the first time after age 55. Depression, menopause, hypertension, cervical spondylitis, and recurrent migraine may also be causes of headache in this age group. It is particularly important to recognize cranial arteritis, since steroid therapy may prevent the development of monocular or binocular blindness caused by retinal artery thrombosis or other cerebral artery thromboses that may occur with this disease.

Patients may have a mild to moderate headache that is constant and that may move slowly from one area of the head to another. In addition to head pain, there is frequently soreness and tenderness of the scalp where the inflammatory process is active. Forerunners or accompaniments of the actual headache may be painful "angina" on chewing or swallowing or dental pain that may have led to misguided extractions. "Angina" of the tongue while talking may be described, arising from narrowing of the lingual arteries. Confusion, impaired concentration, and aphasia may arise from cerebral artery involvement. Repeated small episodes of blurry or blotted-out areas of vision may be a prelude to complete loss of vision in one or both eyes. The patient often feels poorly, usually has a low-grade fever, and has loss of appetite, malaise, and weight loss. A significantly elevated erythrocyte sedimentation rate (ESR) and positive antinuclear antibody (ANA) titers are almost always found to be present. Prominent tender temporal or other superficial cranial vessels may be easily demonstrated. Usually, despite the enlarged size of the affected vessels, the patient's pulse is diminished or absent because of the obliterating process involving the lumina of both arteries and veins. This is often a differentiating point between arteritis and the tender, swollen cranial vessels associated with headache in migraine and hypertension headache, in which the amplitude of pulsation is *increased*. Cranial arteritis may be part of a larger, more generalized vasculitis (e.g., periarteritis nodosa) or, more often, with polymyalgia rheumatica.

When the clinical picture just described is detected, treatment with corticosteroids is, with very few exceptions, started at once. It is important that a biopsy specimen be obtained from the most tender and inflamed area of artery available to confirm the diagnosis. The biopsy may be done after treatment has been started because delay in therapy may allow serious vascular events (e.g., retinal artery thrombosis) to occur, whereas the biopsy will remain positive in the face of therapy for several days. Prednisone, 40 to 60 mg daily, is the usual starting dose and brings rapid relief of symptoms. Gradual tapering of this dose is indicated over weeks and months (and occasionally years) in relation to symptoms and the decreasing ESR. The value of having a biopsy may be greatly appreciated after several months, when potential complications of steroid therapy threaten and questions arise as to the veracity of the diagnosis and the need for treatment.

When the biopsy is done, the surgeon should select the most tender or inflamed spot(s) that needs to be excised and to take several samples, which should be examined longitudinally. Doppler flow studies, when available, may help identify areas in the superficial cranial circulation where occlusion is taking place and the process is active. If for some reason steroidal therapy is contraindicated (active infection, active GI ulceration or perforation, serious CNS reaction to steroids), other NSAIDs may be tolerated and prove useful.

In some patients the arteritis may continue to be active over 3 to 4 years, with symptoms recurring whenever the steroid dose falls below a certain level. In long-term patients, alternate-day steroid therapy may prove practical and necessary.

***Headache from disease of eyes, ears, nose, sinuses, and dental and neck structures.*** Most of these headaches are discussed in chapters devoted to these special areas. Only a few points of special relevance to headache problems are mentioned here.

**Refractive errors.** When headache is caused directly by refractive errors, it usually occurs *while* the patient is engaged in using the eyes for reading or other fine work, not hours later. Strain and fatigue from prolonged use of the eyes, especially if their refraction is imperfect, may become a source of tension or migraine headache, as with any other stress, in susceptible individuals. Correction of refractive errors is important in patients with headache as part of a total program of stress management. Many children with migraine are first taken to an ophthalmologist for relief. Correction of refractive errors often brings improvement but misses or masks the underlying migrainous condition, which ultimately is revealed under conditions other than use of the eyes.

**Glaucoma.** In mild form, glaucoma may be missed by internists and general practitioners because ocular tension is not often measured by them. More and more often the simple test of intraocular pressure is being included as part of the practicing physician's annual checkup of patients. Mild glaucoma, before the stage of halos around lights and impairment of vision, can be a cause of recurring headache localized in one or both eyes and forehead and is related to general stress or at times to the use of anticholinergic medications.

**Eye pain.** Pain in the eye may be related to a migrainous process involving the temporal artery or other more deeply seated vessels such as the middle meningeal or common carotid artery. Digital pressure on the carotid tree may make this obvious.

**Cluster headache.** Cluster headache may occur in the site of an enucleated eye, accompanied by tearing.

**Recurrent scratching of the cornea.** Certain individuals are subject to recurrent corneal scratching. This may mimic attacks of cluster headache in the mutual symptoms of recurrent severe attacks of unilateral eye pain associated with redness and tearing of the eye, which often occur as the patient awakens from sleep.

**Temporomandibular joint pain.** Headache resulting from disorders of temporomandibular joint (TMJ) requires evaluation by very conservative oral surgeons and dentists. Abnormalities of the bite and of the joint itself and its meniscus can be a source of local pain around the TMJ in the cheek, mouth, ear, and temple in some patients who, under stress and tension, clamp their jaw muscles together unduly or have bruxism as a habit or a reaction to anxiety. The question often arises as to whether disease in the joint causes the pain or is caused by the muscle contraction habits of the anxious patient, or if both are required to produce symptoms.

Before implementing prolonged, expensive forms of jaw and dental manipulation, patients may be advised to have thorough medical and at times psychiatric evaluation of their headache problem. The enthusiasm, interest, money, and effort applied to some TMJ problems have such a powerful placebo effect on pain that it is sometimes difficult to judge which therapeutic factors are responsible for improvement. At times it seems as though some neurotic patients use this approach to avoid being labeled neurotic and to escape into health. When the success is durable, one cannot complain about the results, no matter how they are obtained. When this is not the case and symptoms recur or shift to other areas, serious questions arise about the value of prolonged and expensive courses of therapy and implementation of this type, unless the indications for this course are very clear. When definite abnormalities of the TMJ and its mechanics can be demonstrated to be clearly related to head pain, conservative help from experienced, capable dental practitioners may be indicated.

**Nasopharyngeal tumors.** Tumors of the nasopharynx arising in the fossa of Rosenmüller and involving the eustachian tube or the hard palate may simulate atypical facial neuralgia and even cluster headache for weeks or months until finally detected by CT scans or x-ray techniques. Pain in the ear, obstruction of hearing, Horner syndrome, and changing levels of facial and temple pain may simulate functional facial pain for months before their true nature is revealed. Prolonged episodes of this sort require consultation with ENT specialists.

**Trapezius canal syndrome resembling migraine.** A syndrome has been described in a number of patients in whom trauma, fibrosis, or lymphadenopathy have created an entrapment syndrome in the canal containing the occipital artery and posterior branch of the first cervical nerve (when present) as they pass through the trapezius muscle from the spine to the surface of the cranium. In patients with this syndrome, repeated attacks of pulsating head pain radiating from the occipital region forward to the ipsilateral temple and eye region may occur, simulating attacks of common migraine.

Blocking this canal area with procaine hydrochloride may bring relief during an attack. Surgical exploration of the area may reveal either a lymph node pressing on the area of emergence of this nerve-artery combination or fibrosis from previous infection or injury at the opening of the canal, both of which can be removed. Presumably, the intermittence of such attacks may be related to the periodic migrainously produced dilatation of the artery compromising the associated nerve in a narrow space.

**Head pain of neck origin.** When considering pain in the head, one must always bear in mind its possible origin in the neck. Because the upper three cervical nerves are responsible for carrying pain sensations felt in the posterior half of the head and in some instances the ipsilateral temporal and eye areas, the neck must be carefully considered in any head pain problem. Also, it is not only the irritation of the three upper cervical nerves that may convey or cause the pain. Disturbances in one neck area often cause spasm and physical alterations of positioning of other neck areas. The descending tract of the fifth nerve may be affected by irritating lesions low in the neck in its descending course. Even cervical ribs, scalenus lesions, and disease involving the disks and foramina and joints of the entire neck may combine to cause head pain syndromes.

Attention may be especially called to the neck when motion of the neck causes head pain, downward pressure on the head precipitates head pain, upward traction of the head brings relief, and head pain extends into the neck and down the arm, as well as when it is associated with ipsilateral Horner's syndrome.

In the past, x-ray studies have been used to search for lesions in the neck. CT and MRI scans, which can demonstrate soft tissue lesions, are now available to demonstrate soft tissue lesions that may not have been detectable in the past.

Physical therapy, traction-orthopedic, and neurosurgical approaches to these problems need to be considered. NSAIDs, especially indomethacin, are often useful. Properly fitted plastic cervical collars may be useful for patients with cervical arthritis, those with a neck injury, and in some who wake up with headache in the morning. The prolonged use of cervical collars may create weakness of cervical muscles and in neurotic individuals promote "invalidism." Neck lesions also may be responsible for "Valsalva" headache, which responds to treatment for the neck lesion. One must remember that almost any injury of consequence to the head frequently also causes damage not only to bone, disks, and joints in the neck, but also to muscles, ligaments, blood vessels, and sensory nerves, which may participate actively in the painful experience.

**Cranial neuralgias.** The three true neuralgias related to head pain are trifacial, glossopharyngeal, and occipital neuralgia. Each is related to injury or malfunction of the individual sensory nerve that gives its name. The pain in each condition is limited to the terrain subserved by its particular nerve and is characterized by repeated short bursts of sharp jabs or jolts of lancinating pain lasting a second or two that are repeated at a few seconds' interval over minutes or hours. They are frequently initiated by peripheral sensory stimuli to the involved nerves supplying the area (e.g., touching the face, swallowing, rubbing the face). The most important and common of these is the trifacial (trigeminal) neuralgia or tic douloureux. Usually this disease affects patients over 55 years of age. When it occurs in younger patients, a careful search is needed for multiple sclerosis, tumors or other lesions near the foramen ovale, or dental lesions such as abscesses or cracked teeth.

The nature of the pain is profiled in Fig. 95-18. It is distinguished from the profile of cluster headache, which it is confused with at times, by its triggers and its limitation to the areas of distribution of the branches of the fifth nerve (especially II and III). The cluster headache patient demonstrates the location of the pain by pressing firmly or deeply into the temple or cheek. The tic patient may not wish to touch the face at all. Tic is usually helped by anticonvulsants such as phenytoin (Dilantin), carbamazepine (Tegretol), or chlorphenesin carbamate (Maolate) and is not helped by ergotamine or steroids. Cluster headache occurs at earlier ages, is set off by alcohol, and is helped by ergotamine and steroids but not by anticonvulsants. It is a steady pain that often involves several nerve areas; it persists for an hour or two and is associated with tearing, red eye, blocked nose, and Horner's syndrome—quite different from the tic pain which comes in lightning jabs in older patients. Tic is not affected by alcohol but is affected by sensory stimuli. The distinction between the two disorders is important because their therapies differ greatly.

Drug treatment for tic douloureux consists in the prophylactic use of phenytoin, carbamazepine, or chlorphenesin carbamate or combinations of these agents during periods of recurrent pain. In cases not well controlled by these measures, surgical approaches are considered. Treatment for cluster headache is different and is described in the cluster headache section of this chapter.

For tic douloureux, phenytoin in doses ranging from 100 to 400 mg/day is often very effective in treating tic of the fifth nerve (and glossopharyngeal neuralgia). Skin reactions, fever, and adenopathy are side effects that may prevent its continued use. Anemia of a "pernicious" type may also result from phenytoin therapy.

Carbamazepine may be used instead of phenytoin in doses of 200 mg one to four times a day. Blood counts and blood levels need to be followed.

Chlorphenesin carbamate (400 mg PO two or three times daily) may be added to either of these two agents when either one is not fully effective. Alternately, one may decide to use surgical therapy, which is frequently very successful for tic (in contrast to surgery for cluster headache, which is unpredictable, often unsuccessful, and at times damaging).

Whenever surgical therapy is considered for treatment of head pain, experienced neurosurgical consultation should be obtained. Trifacial, glossopharyngeal, and occipital neuralgias deserve a trial of medical therapy, as described. If medical therapy fails, neurosurgery is apt to be successful.

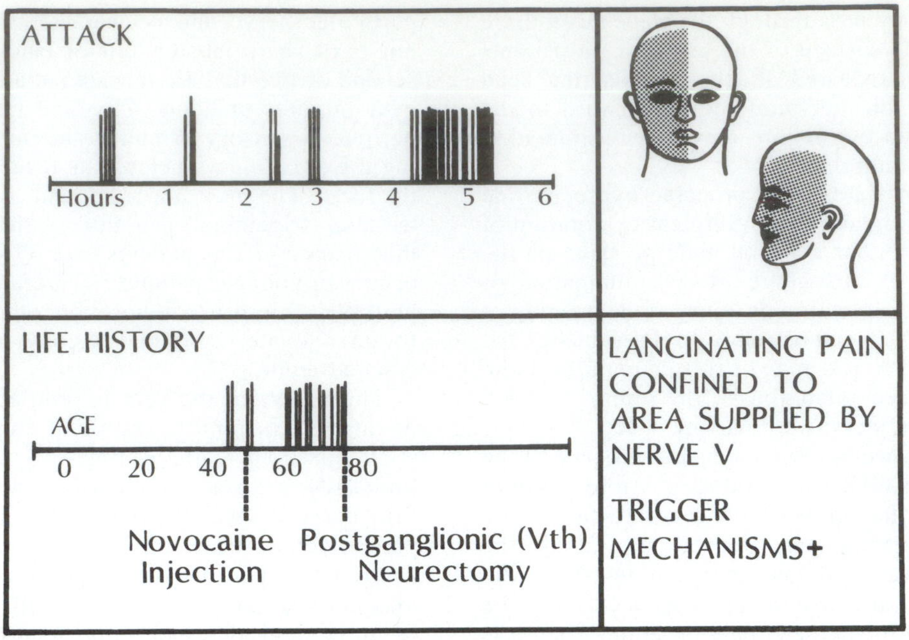


**Fig. 95-18.** Profile of trigeminal neuralgia.

With other forms of head pain in which medical measures have failed, psychiatric evaluation is advisable in addition to or before neurosurgical consultation. This is because results depend greatly on the patient's personality, especially if the surgery is unsuccessful and the patient's condition is worse rather than better.

**Postherpetic neuralgia.** Postherpetic neuralgia involving the cranial nerves can be a formidable problem in terms of treatment. The painful neuralgia and eruption that occurs in herpes zoster syndrome over the distribution of a sensory nerve anywhere in the body is a source of serious suffering. It is particularly intense and dangerous when it involves the branches of the trigeminal nerve, especially the fifth nerve and the nerve endings involving the eye. Advances in the treatment of herpetic lesions with antiviral agents such as acyclovir systemically or locally bring hope to the therapy of this condition. Ointment containing acyclovir may be applied to the affected areas of skin and even the cornea with the expectation of considerable benefit.

With severe infections, especially if vesicles begin to appear unilaterally on the tip of the nose as a warning of approaching corneal and uveal tract involvement, one may consider systemic use of acyclovir. Evidence is accumulating that such use may be beneficial in minimizing eye damage and the duration of postherpetic pain. Current consultation about the state of this therapy at the time of the infection may be indicated regarding this development. Many other approaches to the problem exist, but there is strong indication that none is consistently successful. Many analgesic medications, as well as antidepressant and tranquilizing drugs, have been tried with varying degrees of success. Surgical approaches to this disease should be the last, desperate move.

## POSTTRAUMATIC HEADACHE

This discussion does not cover the details of major forms of "neurologic" posttraumatic headache, such as cerebral contusion, laceration, epidural and subdural hematomas, and major intracerebral hemorrhages. Rather, this section discusses the headache syndromes that appear after head and neck injuries and that may form new headache problems for the accident victim or aggravation of headache syndromes existing before the injury. The simplest of these results from local injury to a specific nerve or nerve-artery complex in which local damage leads to causalgic pain or neuroma formation in a given area, often denoted by tenderness or paresthesia. These headaches are subject to reversal by procaine hydrochloride infiltration and relief by surgical extirpation of the offending damaged localized area. Unfortunately, such simple lesions are not common. Others are more complicated because the ingredients of their painful experience are many and often hidden and difficult to manage.

Posttraumatic headache is influenced greatly in its course by the circumstances of the accident, the life situation and personality of the patient, and the antitherapy factors that surround such events. It is important to realize that posttraumatic headache involves not only a blow to the head, but also a blow to the person and to the state of his or her life. Accidents that happen at home or because of one's own carelessness or foolishness are much less likely to produce significant prolonged headache syndromes than those related to circumstances in which someone else is at fault or in some way responsible. The time required for recovery and return to work is much shorter with home accidents than with industrial or motor vehicle accidents. This shorter interval results from not only litigious aspects of the incident, but also from what has been called the "antitherapy factors" that surround industrial accidents and those caused by someone else's neglect.

Head injuries, especially when the precipitating cause is seen, although briefly, before the blow, are very threatening by themselves and often are followed by weeks or months of anxious dreams of catastrophe, fear of driving or working again in similar circumstances, and a significant lack of confidence in oneself. These features are sufficient to cause tension or "combined" headache in anyone, especially a person already lacking in confidence or living in a difficult life situation.

To this important component of headache arising directly from the accident and causing a degree of disability are frequently added the antitherapy factors of anger at the assailant or factory owner, anxiety over the litigation urged by friends and relatives, the "law's delay" and complications, the wish to have it all done and over with, the fear about losing the job and income, and the depression that results from all these anger-producing losses that seem so unfair. These feelings are in addition to the pain, the effects of drugs taken to relieve the headache, and some of the impaired cerebral controls that techniques (e.g., BEAM [brain electric activity mapping] evoked potential tests) show to be somewhat damaged by certain types of injury.

This type of generalized "combined" headache arising from injury, anxiety, depression, and vascular disturbance responds to analgesics and tranquilizing drugs such as chlordiazepoxide (Librium) to some extent but may respond better to antidepressant medicines such as amitriplyline (Elavil), doxepin (Sinequan), trazodone (Desyrel), desipramine in full doses, or MAO inhibitors such as isocarboxazid (Marplan) and phenylethylhydrazine (Nardil). Encouragement to return to daily exercise and to work helps to make this syndrome shorter and more bearable.

Sources of anxiety are discussed with patients to help them ventilate their feelings. Settlement should be sought as early as possible. The more prolonged the period of disability, the more loss of ego occurs and the more difficult it is for the patient to pull out of the "slough of despond."

When an industrial accident was caused by work in certain circumstances or with certain machinery, the patient should return to the same situation should have a lead-in time and perhaps experience in another department or situation to allow regaining of confidence. Settlement of the "case," although highly desired, may not end the problem because much has happened to this injured individual. The person has been knocked off his or her perch in life, not just "hit on the head." Such factors are difficult for some physicians, juries, and judges to understand, partly because some individuals with personal gain as an objective take advantage of these situations and provide fuel that leads to distrust of others who have really had a major blow to themselves as well as their head.

Whiplash injuries resulting in sprain and injury to multiple tissues in the neck (regardless of x-ray findings that show no significant abnormalities) sometimes precipitate bouts of cluster headache or accentuate previous vascular headaches of the migraine type. Short-term use of physical therapy, a Thomas collar, and repeated visits at 2-week intervals to encourage gradually but definitely increasing activity and return to work, preferably with as little litigation as possible, seem advisable. Indomethacin may be useful prophylactic medication in these patients, along with antidepressant therapy if the symptoms do not respond within a few weeks.

At times, patients who have had serious damage in accidents may require prolonged rehabilitation in a center for such purposes, where staff may encourage and provide activity, discourage extensive use of analgesics, and provide alternative relief of pain by ice, heat, traction, ultrasound, transcutaneous nerve stimulation, exercise, and group therapy. If no progress is made following head and neck injuries after 2 to 3 months of physician-guided therapy on a personal basis, it may be wise to recommend entry to a rehabilitation center before chronic depression, loss of ambition and desire to return to work, and major discouragement have set in. Families may need to be informed of this positive approach and taught, if possible, not to promote invalidism by special care and privilege in the home or elsewhere.

## BIBLIOGRAPHY


Ad Hoc Committee on Classification of Headache, *Cephalalgia* 8(suppl 7):1, 1988.

Cady RK et al: Treatment of acute migraine with subcutaneous sumatriptan, *JAMA* 265:2831, 1991.

Gardner-Medwin AR, Skelton JL: Leão's spreading depression: evidence supporting a role in the migraine aura. In Rose FC, Amery WK, editors: *Cerebral hypoxia in the pathogenesis of migraine,* London, 1982, Pitman.

Graham JR: Pathophysiology of headache for behavioral therapists. In Surwit RS et al, editors: *Behavioral treatment of disease,* New York, 1982, Plenum.

Graham JR, Bana DS, Yap AU: Headache, hypertension and renal disease, *Res Clin Stud Headache* 6:147, 1978.

Heyck H: Pathogenesis of migraine, *Res Clin Stud Headache* 2:1, 1969.

Leão AAP: Spreading depression of activity in the cerebral cortex, *J Neurophysiol* 7:359, 1944.

Sakai F, Meyer JS: Abnormal cerebrovascular reactivity in patients with migraine and cluster headache, *Headache* 19:257, 1979.

Sjaastad O, Dale I: Evidence for a new treatable headache entity, *Headache* 14:105, 1974.

Sulkava R, Kovanen J: Locked-in syndrome with rapid recovery: a manifestation of basilar artery migraine? *Headache* 23:238, 1983.

Wolff HG: Migraine. In Dalessio DJ, editor: *Headache and other head pain,* ed 4, New York, 1980, Oxford University.


CHAPTER

# 96 Alterations in Mental State: Coma and Acute Confusional States


**Harold B. Schiff**
**Thomas D. Sabin**


## COMA

### Definition

Coma is defined as a disturbance of consciousness in which the patient cannot be aroused by any stimulus, no matter how vigorous. With the return of any form of responsiveness, coma ends. The recovering patient then progresses through various levels of disordered consciousness until finally attaining a clear sensorium. An understanding of the pathogenesis is essential to the clinical management of the comatose patient. A brief discussion of the criteria for brain death appears in Chapter 128.

## Pathogenesis

The ascending reticular activating system (RAS) is a highly complex polysynaptic region in the core of the upper pons and midbrain. These isodendritic fibers extend from the midbrain into the thalamic regions bilaterally and ultimately become widespread within the hemispheres. Specific afferent systems contribute some portion of their neuronal activity to the RAS as they pass through these brainstem structures. Specific neurotransmitter function in the RAS is not fully understood. GABAergic fibers and cholinergic systems play a role in controlling consciousness (GABA, $\gamma$-aminobutyric acid). A pathologic decrease in consciousness results from either a local anatomic or a general biochemical disturbance of the RAS.

If the brainstem is sectioned below the level of the upper pons, a disturbance in alertness does not occur. Once the ascending RAS has reached the level of the thalamus and becomes bilaterally distributed, a unilateral destructive lesion does not cause obtundation. Although extramedullary distortion of the ascending RAS in the midbrain is the major anatomic basis for disordered arousal, critically located small focal lesions from the upper pons to the mesencephalic-diencephalic junction may also produce this clinical picture. Thus, small infarcts that destroy the reticular core of the brainstem may cause states of prolonged coma. In unilateral supratentorial space-occupying lesions, the medial or uncal portion of the temporal lobe is forced through the tentorial notch beside the midbrain. This distorts the reticular-activating substance in the core of the midbrain and thereby causes a decrease in alertness. The herniated uncus also causes compression of the oculomotor nerve. Parasympathetic pupillomotor fibers are superficially placed, and the compression may result in an ipsilateral dilated pupil that is unresponsive to light.

When the herniated uncus forces the midbrain against the rigid, contralateral tentorial margin, motor fibers within the midbrain may be affected, and signs of upper motor neuron deficits appear on the same side as the supratentorial mass lesion. Pupillary dilatation, however, is a more accurate predictor of the side of supratentorial mass lesion than the side of the hemiparesis. When there is bilateral herniation of supratentorial structures, the midbrain is forced caudally and elongated in the anteroposterior direction.

The pharmacologic and biochemical vulnerability of the RAS is also well recognized. This vulnerability is reflected in the appearance of obtundation in almost every variety of severe metabolic disturbance. The most common causes of obtundation are endogenous or exogenous toxins. The numerous synapses in the ascending RAS may be the basis for the striking vulnerability of the RAS to so many classes of drugs and toxins.

Making the distinction between an intracranial structural lesion and an extracranial toxic-metabolic encephalopathy is the primary diagnostic step in evaluating the comatose patient.

## Early management of the comatose patient

If patients with transient loss of consciousness are excluded and coma persists for 6 hours or more, the chance of either a sedative/toxic or a hypoxic/ischemic etiology is 40%; of a cerebrovascular etiology (stroke, hemorrhage, or subarachnoid bleed), 35%; and of a metabolic etiology (diabetes, infection, renal/hepatic, etc.), 25%. The overriding concern in the early management of the comatose patient is the immediate treatment of any remedial cause of brain damage. Several steps should be taken even before a full diagnostic assessment is made.

The patient must be guaranteed an adequate airway, respiratory exchange, circulation, and metabolic substrate, glucose, and thiamine (which acts as a cofactor in the metabolism of glucose). After blood is obtained for various diagnostic studies (including glucose levels), the patient should be given 100 mg thiamine intravenously followed by a 50 ml 50% glucose solution. Thiamine must be administered before the glucose, since a glucose load in a thiamine-deficient patient may precipitate acute Wernicke encephalopathy and cause sudden death from circulatory collapse. If narcotic ingestion is suspected, naloxone (Narcan) should be administered. The patient should be positioned so as to prevent aspiration but nevertheless should be handled as though a cervical spinal fracture is present until further history and diagnostic studies can be performed. As soon as these initial urgent needs are satisfied, a rapid general medical and neurologic examination should be performed.

## Evaluation of the comatose patient

The neurologic examination of the comatose patient is quite different from the routine neurologic evaluation. In most common conditions associated with coma, a rostral-caudal deterioration in nervous system function tends to occur as the process worsens. This is generally the case for both structural intracranial processes and toxic metabolic encephalopathies. A rostral-caudal deterioration refers to the sequential loss of certain functions, beginning with the cerebral cortex and followed by the diencephalon, midbrain, pons, and finally the medulla. A rapid assessment of the anatomic level of a given patient can be made by examination of the state of consciousness, pupils, eye movements, respirations, and remaining motor functions. Before this evaluation, one should make a quick assessment for evidence of head trauma. An ecchymosis that surrounds the eye ("raccoon sign"), a hemotympanum, and "bogginess" with or without ecchymosis on the mastoid process just behind the ear (Battle sign) are evidence of a basal skull fracture. The importance of looking for subtle signs of head injury must be emphasized. Slight bogginess with an area of petechiae on the scalp, which can only be identified if the patient's hair and scalp are carefully searched, may be the sole evidence for head trauma. Certain injuries, such as a blow to the head from a stocking filled with sand, can create devastating brain lesions with minimal external signs.

The level of consciousness is evaluated by repeated efforts to wake the patient and gain his or her attention. Terms such as *light coma, semicoma,* and *stupor* as defined in the literature are of little value in clinical practice and are best avoided. A clear description of the patient's behavior and clinical status is preferred.

Examination of the pupils should include size, symmetry, and response to light. In the diencephalic stage of the rostral-caudal deterioration, both pupils tend to be small. This may be noted in an expanding supratentorial mass or with widespread edema that causes midline herniation. A magnifying glass may be necessary to see if the pupillary response to light has been preserved. A unilateral supratentorial mass that causes the uncus to herniate through the tentorial notch is signaled by compression of the parasympathetic motor fibers surrounding the third cranial nerve, producing a loss of constriction and thus progressive pupillary dilatation and finally a widely dilated, unreactive pupil. The pupillary signs of third nerve dysfunction appear before the paralysis of extraocular muscles. The diencephalic stage is thus characterized by either unilateral pupillary dilatation (with unilateral herniation syndromes) or symmetric, small pupils that respond to light (in midline herniation or most toxic metabolic encephalopathies).

Once the deterioration involves the midbrain, the pupils are no longer reactive to light; they tend to be in the midposition and may not change with progression of the syndrome to the pontine and medullary phases of deterioration. The agonal dilatation of unresponsive pupils has been attributed to a widespread release of norepinephrine throughout anoxic body tissues.

Examination of the state of extraocular movements is another valuable way of establishing the level of remaining nervous system function. Drowsiness may cause phorias to become manifest tropias. Divergence squints are most common and are exaggerated with upward deviation of the eyes. These signs reflect a decreased level of consciousness but do not have specific anatomic localization value. In the diencephalic stage of coma, the so-called doll's-head eye maneuvers become overly facile (Fig. 96-1). When a normal conscious individual has the head passively turned to the right, the eyes move to the right. In an obtunded individual, they move to the left. This release of vestibular reflexes is believed to be the basis for the doll's-head maneuver, and a stronger stimulus may be necessary. Conjugate deviation of the eyes to the stimulated side can be induced by instilling ice water to the external ear canal. The maximal stimulus consists of 40 ml ice instilled over a 30 seconds. One should be careful that no perforation of the drum or other process in the external ear is present that might be adversely affected by this irrigation. In the mesencephalic stage of dysfunction, the eyes can still be conjugately drawn to the side of the stimulation, although if third nerve connections are sufficiently damaged, there may be a deficit in adduction.

Once the pons and medulla have been destroyed, the lateral eye movements do not respond to the doll's-head maneuver or ice water caloric stimulation. When the patient's head is at 35 degrees to the horizontal and both ears are simultaneously stimulated with warm water at 44° C (111° F), conjugate upward deviation of the eyes occurs if the midbrain centers for vertical gaze are intact.

The comatose patient may have tonic conjugate deviation of the eyes. In an acute hemispheric lesion, destruction of the fibers from the frontal gaze center occurs; for contralateral conjugate gaze, this results in a relative overactivity of the contralateral intact center, causing

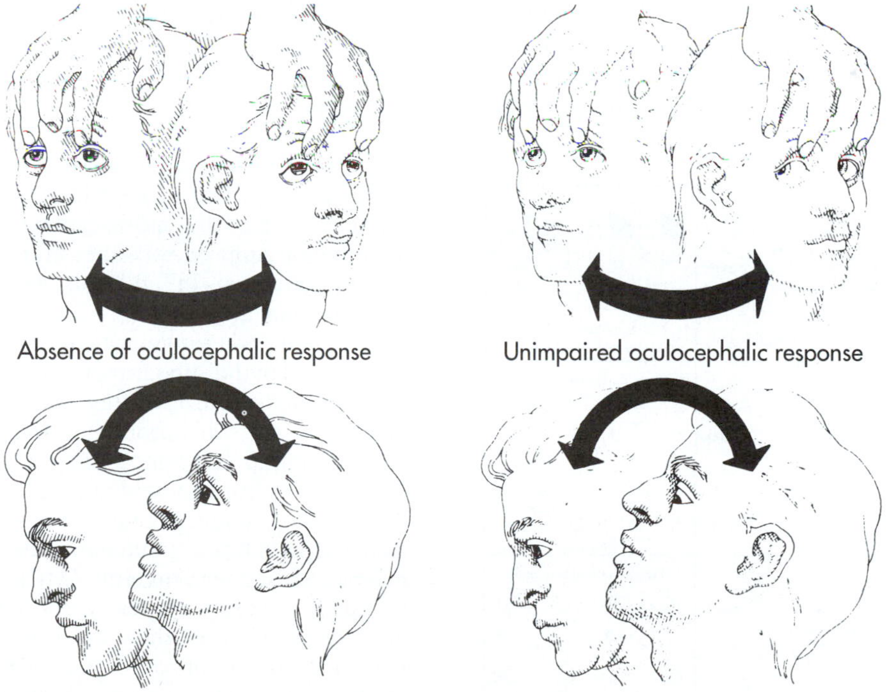


**Fig. 96-1.** Doll's-head maneuver. This maneuver consists of rapidly turning the head from side to side or by flexion-extension of the neck. Conjugate movement of the eyes to the side opposite the direction of head movement demonstrates that brainstem centers for eye movement are intact. In the bottom drawing, as in the top drawing, the eyelids are held open because the patient is comatose. (From Geller AE, Sabin TD, *Med Times* 106:47, 1978.)

deviation of the eyes toward the injured hemisphere. If an associated hemiplegia exists, the eyes deviate away from the side of the hemiplegia and toward the side of the lesion (Fig. 96-2). With lesions in the brainstem, these fibers have already crossed in the midbrain, and the eyes may conjugately deviate away from the side of the lesion and toward the hemiplegia.

The respiratory pattern is another useful marker for determining the level of remaining nervous system function. Respirations at the diencephalic stage of rostral-caudal deterioration may be normal or show periodic respiration, including Cheyne-Stokes respirations. Central neurogenic hyperventilation with continued respiratory rates of about 40 breaths/minute (with appropriate changes in blood gases) may occur with midbrain dysfunction. When pontine damage is superimposed on the midbrain syndrome, central neurogenic hyperventilation disappears and may be replaced by breathing that is apparently more normal. A pause at inspiration (apneustic breathing) is characteristic of pontine-level lesions. As the pons is destroyed, breathing becomes ataxic, irregular, and unpredictable. At this point, respiratory arrest is imminent.

Testing of motor system function in obtunded patients is different from the usual neurologic examination. Simple observation of spontaneous movements or the movements in relation to painful stimuli is done. In the diencephalic stage an associated hemiplegia is easily recognized, and bilateral decorticate posture may rarely be seen. A stage occurs before decorticate posturing in which fairly facile movement is away from painful stimuli, but the range of passive movement in these limbs is often limited by counterholding (gegenhalten or paratonia). Decorticate posturing consists of adduction at the shoulder and flexion at the elbows, wrists, and fingers, with extensor posturing of the lower extremities.

In the midbrain state of deterioration, decerebrate postures appear. Decerebration rarely appears in a florid, full-blown form but is seen more often as only fragments of the posture in response to noxious stimulation. The examiner should place the semiflexed upper extremities across the patient's abdomen and then provide a painful stimulus to the sternum. If the patient consistently reacts to the painful stimulus with only one limb, one can determine that the opposite side is hemiplegic. If the patient's forearms extend away from the painful stimulus or pronate even slightly, one should suspect decerebration and thus dysfunction at the mesencephalic level. When the patient moves the limb toward the painful stimulus at the sternum, a second stimulus at the iliac crest confirms that the patient is not simply demonstrating decorticate posturing but is actually reaching for the noxious stimuli.

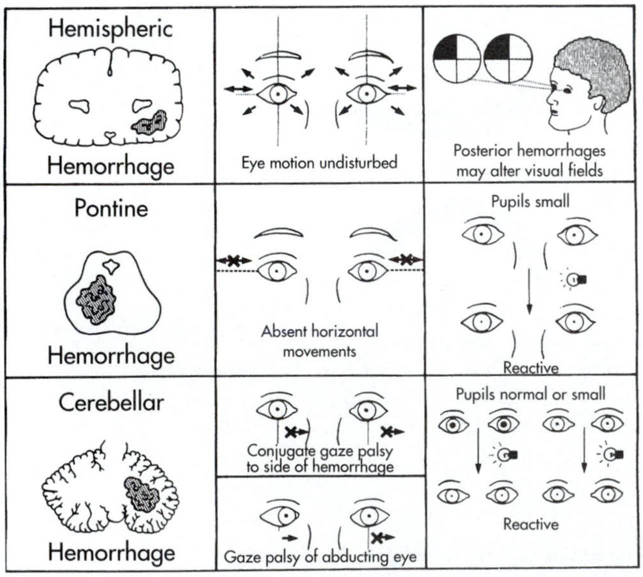


**Fig. 96-2.** Schematic illustration of hemispheric, pontine, and cerebellar hemorrhage demonstrating the accompanying eye movement and pupillary responses.

As the midbrain is destroyed and pontine dysfunction appears, decerebration disappears and the limbs become flaccid. No movement appears with noxious stimulation. Disappearance of decerebration is often mistaken for improvement. The limbs remain flaccid in the medullary phase of deterioration.

With these parameters of examination in mind, one can quickly localize the level of nervous system dysfunction and begin consideration of the major diagnostic categories.

## Differential diagnosis

The initial diagnostic consideration is to determine whether the alteration in consciousness is caused by a primarily intracranial structural lesion or a systemic toxic or metabolic disorder.

***Structural central nervous system lesions.*** The intracranial processes are subdivided into those in which focal signs are likely versus those in which no focal signs may be anticipated. The major categories of intracranial processes with focal brain dysfunction include trauma, intraparenchymal hemorrhages, tumors, certain forms of infection, and brain infarction.

**With focal signs**

***Trauma.*** *Concussion* refers to a transient loss of consciousness. If there is associated brain contusion, unconsciousness may be more lasting. Focal signs such as hemiplegia, aphasia, or other signs of cortical injury are usually obvious. In addition, blood may be found in cerebrospinal fluid (CSF).

Frequent consequences of closed-head trauma are hematomas in the subdural or epidural space or in the brain parenchyma. Neuroimaging has greatly simplified the diagnosis of this problem. However, an apparently negative computed tomography (CT) scan in an appropriate clinical setting should not dissuade the physician from diagnosis of subdural hematoma, since this lesion may be isodense with brain tissue but is seen on the more sensitive magnetic resonance imaging (MRI). Since the mass lesion produces a widely dispersed force over the convexity of one side of the brain, there are often no focal cortical signs. However, the distortion of the ascending RAS, secondary to the mass effect, causes abnormal drowsiness, which may be the only feature present.

***Hemorrhage.*** Spontaneous hemorrhages into brain parenchyma are occurring less frequently as the assiduous treatment of hypertension becomes more widely practiced. Brain hemorrhages may occur in a variety of disorders, such as anticoagulation, end-stage leukemias, hepatic disease, amyloid angiopathy, and intracranial aneurysms; however, the major association is still with hypertension. Symptoms and signs usually appear suddenly, but occasionally the onset of these hemorrhagic syndromes may progress in severity, taking several days to develop.

Hypertensive hemorrhages tend to occur in five sites (see Fig. 96-2). The lateral ganglionic or putaminal areas of the hemisphere are most often affected. Hemorrhage at these sites results in severe headache, hemiplegia, conjugate deviation of the eyes away from the hemiplegia, and signs of progressive uncal herniation with rostral-caudal deterioration.

The thalamus is a second common site of hypertensive hemorrhage and also produces headache and hemiplegia. The hemorrhage frequently dissects into upper midbrain structures, which may explain why the eyes are often conjugately deviated toward the hemiplegia. A rarer but highly characteristic tonic downward convergence of the eye has also been reported with thalamic hemorrhage (see Fig. 96-2).

Pontine hemorrhage is usually fatal within 48 hours. Since the initial lesion is in the pons, the clinical picture is different from that seen with rostral-caudal deterioration. There is bilateral flaccid paralysis of the limbs, and the doll's-head maneuver or the ice water caloric test fail to cause lateral conjugate eye deviation, although some vertical gaze may remain because of intact midbrain centers. Peculiar vertical conjugate eye movements known as "ocular bobbing" may be witnessed. The eyes drift downward and then more rapidly elevate upward, slightly above the resting level, before descending once again to the resting level. The movements often occur in brief bursts. Pontine hemorrhage is usually also associated with pinpoint pupils, resulting from destruction of the descending sympathetic fibers at a time when midbrain parasympathetic fibers are still functioning. The pinpoint pupils respond to light but so minimally that a magnifying glass may be necessary to see the constriction (see Fig. 96-2).

The prompt diagnosis of hypertensive cerebellar hemorrhage is most important because of the urgency of surgical intervention as a lifesaving procedure. Cerebellar hemorrhage presents with acute ataxia, nausea, vomiting, and severe headache. On examination, both truncal ataxia and hemiataxia may be present. Nystagmus usually occurs, and there may be forced deviation of gaze opposite the side of the hematoma (see Fig. 96-2). An acute cerebellar mass can compress medullary respiratory centers and cause sudden death. Surgical evacuation of cerebellar hemorrhages can be lifesaving.

***Tumors.*** Most intracranial tumors are now diagnosed early enough so that patients do not present with coma. However, one should keep in mind certain situations.

Tumors in the midline of the neuraxis either within or outside the ventricular system may cause minimal neurologic symptoms or signs until CSF flow is obstructed, and then obtundation occurs with acute hydrocephalus and a rapid deterioration in clinical status. Patients with posterior cranial fossa lesions may have respiratory arrest as the first manifestation of foramen magnum herniation. The evaluation of patients suspected of having posterior fossa mass lesions should reflect this possibility. Papilledema is usually present in these patients. Since papilledema takes about 24 hours to develop fully, it is not seen in massive acute hemorrhages, but if the patient has a slowly growing tumor, he or she is more apt to have papilledema when seen with an acute deterioration in level of consciousness. Midline posterior fossa or intraventricular tumor-associated hydrocephalus should be treated with emergency ventricular drainage or ventriculostomy.

Patients with pituitary adenomas can lapse into acute coma when spontaneous hemorrhagic necrosis of the tumor occurs. Patients with pituitary apoplexy have headaches, visual loss, stiff neck, obtundation, extraocular palsies, and acute hypotension. The recognition and treatment of the acute hypoadrenal state caused by the failure of adrenocorticotrophic hormone (ACTH) production are essential lifesaving maneuvers. An enlarged sella seen on plain skull films serves as an important clue to the diagnosis of pituitary apoplexy. MRI or CT scans have proved to be extremely useful in diagnosing most intracranial tumors.

Cerebellar abscess usually presents as a mass lesion. The appearance is often characteristic on MRI or CT scan. A small bubble of air in the low-density center of a lesion with a ringlike enhancement is diagnostic of abscess. Brain abscesses alone do not necessarily result in fever, and the CSF may be normal.

***Infarction.*** Hemispheric infarcts may produce lethargy or confusion acutely, but unilateral lesions seldom cause complete coma. An exception occurs when a massive, acute hemispheric infarction results in severe brain edema; herniation and fatal rostral-caudal deterioration of brain function can occur in 1 to 2 hours. Small infarcts of the brainstem can interrupt the RAS and produce lasting coma. In the "locked-in" syndrome, extensive paralysis occurs because of bilateral destruction of the motor pathways in the basis pontis. The patient is conscious, but the medical staff may not realize it. These patients are able to develop a code, using eye blinks to communicate.

**Without focal signs.** In certain other intracranial processes that cause coma, such as meningitis, encephalitis, and subarachnoid hemorrhage, no focal signs may be present. The physician depends greatly on careful examination of the spinal fluid for the correct diagnosis. Focal signs may be present but are a bonus for the diagnostician. Aneurysms of the posterior communicating artery often cause an acute third nerve palsy. Bacterial meningitis may cause cerebral thrombophlebitis with hemiplegias and focal seizures. Similarly, the predilection of the herpes simplex virus for the temporal lobe often assists in the diagnosis of that variety of viral encephalitis.

This category of intracranial processes without obvious focal signs should serve as a forceful reminder that every comatose patient must have a CSF examination performed unless lumbar puncture is contraindicated. If the patient is deemed too ill for a lumbar puncture, some other diagnostic procedure must be substituted on an emergency basis. An MRI or CT scan before lumbar puncture is advisable in many circumstances. Standard CSF studies may be complemented by brain creatine kinase (CK, CPK) and neuron-specific enolase tests, which may be useful in prognostication.

***Toxic-metabolic causes.*** The differential diagnosis of endogenous metabolic derangement is extensive and includes disturbances in all organ systems. The box below presents a logical schema for the approach to the differential diagnosis of endogenous metabolic encephalopathies.

The toxic encephalopathies are most often caused by drug overdose, and some patients, especially elderly ones, may be unusually sensitive to the side effects of many drugs, even at standard dosages.

Some sedative drugs have special effects on the eyes that may help with the diagnosis. Glutethimide (Doriden) may cause large pupils that are unresponsive to light. Morphine produces pupilloconstriction. Atropine-like effects cause dilated fixed pupils. Severely obtunded patients with drug overdose may be capable of brushing away painful stimuli and even muttering a few sounds but may have no eye movements even with ice water caloric stimulation. This disparity of rostral-caudal localization is highly suggestive of sedative drug overdose. A toxic screen and an electroencephalogram (EEG) that shows characteristic effects of sedative medication are useful in confirming the diagnosis.

Patients with endogenous metabolic encephalopathies usually have no focal signs, but exceptions occur when clinically inapparent, earlier neurologic lesions once again become manifest as metabolic derangement occurs. A patient who has had a previous cerebral infarct with complete recovery may have hemiplegia reappear when he or she begins to develop, for example, carbon dioxide narcosis of chronic pulmonary disease. Focal seizures apparently arising from the supplementary motor area, with fencing postures and groping movements of the extended arm, have proved to be highly suggestive of nonketotic hyperglycemic coma.

One of the most important practical distinctions between the toxic-metabolic encephalopathies and the structural intracranial processes relates to the pupillary light response. In all the toxic-metabolic encephalopathies except anoxic encephalopathy and those caused by drugs that have specific effects on the pupil, pupillary response to light is spared regardless of the rostral-caudal involvement. The clinical differentiation of structural from metabolic causes of coma pivots around a clearly progressive anatomic localization of the rostral-caudal syndrome. Intracranial mass lesions usually follow this syndrome exactly, whereas the signs of the toxic-metabolic encephalopathy may be much more patchy, such as pontine involvement without prior mesencephalic involvement and no clear-cut rostral-caudal progression.

Decerebration does occur in the toxic-metabolic encephalopathies and should not be considered diagnostic of structural brain disease. Metabolic encephalopathy is often accompanied by widespread, involuntary, small-amplitude myoclonic jerks. The patient should be examined with an oblique light for several minutes, since the muscle twitches are often not otherwise apparent.

Clearly, a full discussion of all the causes of coma is beyond the scope of this chapter, which serves only as a model for an approach to the comatose patient.

### Outcome and prognostication

A body of literature exists on the outcome of coma, but the most reliable data stem from studies of posttraumatic coma. The Glasgow Coma Scale and the Glasgow Outcome Scales are most helpful in the monitoring and prognostication of traumatic coma but are less reliable in other forms of coma. Only 10% of patients with nontraumatic coma, who do not demonstrate spontaneous eye movements at 6 hours, will make a moderate to good recovery. Eye opening to painful stimuli at 6 hours raises the chances

### Toxic-metabolic causes of coma

**Exogenous intoxications**

Alcohol, barbiturates
Tranquilizers
Belladonna derivatives
Psychotomimetics
Others: ergot, salicylates, caffeine, heavy metals
Withdrawal syndromes

**General medical diseases**

Disturbances of hydration, electrolytes, osmolarity
Cardiovascular disturbances (hypotension, congestive heart failure, hypertensive encephalopathy)
Pulmonary failure (carbon dioxide narcosis, anoxia)
Hepatic encephalopathy
Uremia and the postdialysis syndrome
Endocrine disorders: hypoglycemia; thyroid, adrenal, and pituitary syndromes
Porphyria
Vasculitides
Acute infections outside the central nervous system
Toxemia of pregnancy

### Managed Care Guide
### Brain death in adults*

I. Cessation of all function of the entire brain
  A. Unresponsive coma
  B. Absent brainstem reflexes
    1. Pupillary light reflex
    2. Corneal reflex
    3. Cephalic (caloric) reflexes
    4. Oropharyngeal (gag) reflex
    5. Respiration (apnea testing)
II. Irreversibility
  A. Coma of known cause without potential for reversibility
  B. Exclusion of contributory, reversible conditions
    1. Drug intoxication
    2. Neuromuscular blockade
    3. Hypothermia (<32.2° C, 90° F)
    4. Shock
    5. Major metabolic disturbance
  C. Persistence for an appropriate period of observation (6-24 hours, depending on cause of coma and local practice)
III. Confirmatory investigations (may be optional or required)
  A. Electrocerebral silence (isoelectric EEG)
  B. Absence of circulation to the brain

Adapted from *JAMA* 246:2184, 1981.
*Local and institutional rules are superseding.

of moderate to good recovery. Eighty-five percent will die, remain in a vegetative state, or recover to a state of significant dependency.

## BRAIN DEATH

Guidelines for the determination of brain death recommended by the President's Commission in 1981 are now used widely; however, state and local laws or practices may modify their applications. (See the Managed Care Guide).

Patients are not brain dead if they have reactive pupils, corneal or gag reflexes, decerebrate or decorticate posturing (see the box below). The pupils are generally midposition and dilated in brain death. Small pupils are uncommon, and should be checked for reactivity because of possible drug overdose. Spinal reflexes (deep tendon and Babinski's) may persist in the presence of brain death. And, in the 15 to 30 minute interval after ventilatory assistance is withdrawn, unusual movements of the extremities may occur, most likely resulting from terminal ischemia of the spinal cord.

Hypothermia, drug intoxication and viral encephalitis may all produce an isoelectric EEG. Thus, the presence of an isoelectric EEG alone is not sufficient to serve as a criterion for brain death.

## ACUTE CONFUSIONAL STATES

Acute confusion, also known as *acute encephalopathy, acute toxic psychosis,* or *delirium,* can be thought of as an acquired incapacity to think with customary speed and clarity. The major feature of this syndrome is the failure to maintain normal, sequential thought, reflecting an inability to rank the priority of stimuli. Patients thus are unable to maintain a coherent stream of thought. The consequent failure in the designation of behavioral priorities causes an immediate and drastic disintegration of the adaptational interaction with the environment. Patients' general behavior and speech reflect an inappropriate sequencing of ideas, and patients present a wide range of abnormal behaviors, including assaultiveness, motor hyperactivity, hallucinations, somnolence, and extreme states of panic or fear.

The diagnosis of an acute confusional syndrome is often not entirely objective, and most physicians rely to some degree on intuition. A clear definition has not been established, but the fourth edition of the *Diagnostic and Statistical Manual of Mental Disorders* (DSM-IV) does provide specific diagnostic criteria that may serve as a point of departure in defining the clinical features of this syndrome (see the box below).

### Clinical features

The diagnosis of confusion depends on the recognition of specific disturbances in the processes of attention, thought, and perception.

***Attentional deficits.*** Disordered attention is a major feature of confusion. Disturbances include difficulty in attaining and maintaining attention. This disturbance is apparent in the evaluation of patients with confusion; it is often very difficult to attract the attention of these individuals, who may appear relatively unresponsive to external stimuli. Furthermore, maintaining their attention may also prove difficult. Patients respond equally to all auditory, visual, and kinesthetic stimuli and are unable to filter out irrelevant stimuli. They may be extremely distractible and thus unable to sustain any goal-directed behavior.

***Thought disorder.*** Disordered thought is most frequently recognized as an incoherent stream of thought. The patient may be aware of this and complain of being "confused," "unable to think straight," or "unable to get it together." Some patients, however, may be unaware of their deficit.

The term *thought disorder* is used here to encompass the various cognitive deficits that result in an incoherent stream of thought. Although memory disturbance and disorientation are invariably present, the patient may respond appropriately on formal memory and orientation testing. The patient does have significant difficulty in organizing recent and remote memories into an orderly

### Clinical features of brain death

Hemisphere death
- Deep coma
- Absence of purposeful movement, well-defined posturing, or convulsions
- Can be corroborated by EEG, brain scan, or angiography*

Brainstem death
- Unreactive midposition or enlarged pupils
- Absent eye movements with oculocephalic ("doll's eyes") and oculovestibular (caloric) stimulation
- Absent corneal responses
- Absence of spontaneous breathing with apnea testing

Exclusions
- Sedative drugs
- Severe hypothermia
- Immediately preceding circulatory arrest

*Brain death is a clinical diagnosis; laboratory confirmation may be used in special circumstances.

### Diagnostic criteria for acute confusional syndrome

1. Clouding of consciousness, that is, a reduced capacity to shift, focus, and sustain attention to environmental stimuli
2. At least two of the following: (a) perceptual disturbances (i.e., misinterpretations, illusions, hallucinations), (b) incoherent speech, (c) disturbances of the sleep-wake cycle, or (d) increased or decreased psychomotor activity
3. Disorientation and memory disturbance
4. Clinical features that develop over a short period and tend to fluctuate over the course of the day
5. Elements from the history and physical examination and laboratory tests that suggest a specific organic factor, judged to be etiologically related to the disturbance

sequence. Thus, features of spatial disorientation may be expressed as symptoms of reduplicative paramnesia. This usually involves the reduplication of place; for example, the patient insists that the hospital room is duplicated and shifted in place so "a branch of the main hospital is in my home." Temporal disorientation is obvious when events from the past are directly related to the present. This association of unrelated events may lead to a diagnosis of confabulation. Indeed, the patient may exhibit frank confabulation; this may be concrete and obviously related to surrounding visual and auditory cues; alternatively, it may be quite bizarre, apparently generated from inner thought processes.

Thought content may have a dreamlike quality. The patient may find it difficult to separate fact from fantasy or dreams from reality. Delusions may occur, are usually fleeting, and may be modified by environmental stimuli. Vague feelings of apprehension are often crystallized into persecutory delusional beliefs. Delusions are often concrete; the classic schneiderian delusions of thought insertion, withdrawal, control, and broadcasting are only rarely seen.

***Perceptual disturbances.*** Perceptual disturbances are perhaps the most dramatic manifestations of acute confusion. Illusions range from simple to more complex misinterpretations of environmental stimuli. For example, markings on the wall are interpreted as crawling insects, folds in the bedclothes as snakes or wild animals, and sounds as fire alarms or gunshots. In more complex illusions the hospital room might be mistaken for a prison or the door for a window. The patient may act on these misinterpretations, resulting in inadvertent accident or death.

Hallucinations may occur in all sensory modalities. Visual and auditory hallucinations are more frequent than tactile, kinesthetic, olfactory, and gustatory hallucinations. However, no characteristic type of hallucination exemplifies the acute confusional state. The content of these hallucinations varies greatly and is usually interpreted by the patient as real.

***Language disturbances.*** Language is often vague, circumlocutory, and perseverative. Word-finding difficulty may take the form of approximations. A pitcher may be called a glass or a bedrail a gate. Reading is often preserved, whereas writing is very abnormal. The patient demonstrates poor penmanship, starting off well but ending with micrographia. The patient characteristically shows no regard for paper space or lines and neglects to dot the i's and cross the t's (Fig. 96-3). Misspellings and perserverations or overdrawings on letters and words are common.

***Disturbance in the sleep-wake cycle.*** Disturbance in the sleep-walk cycle is an invariable feature of confusional states. Some patients are hypersomnolent, whereas others remain awake for days at a time. The patient may not offer this information, but it is the most common complaint of family or friends.

***Fluctuations in symptomatology.*** The patient shows fluctuations in cognitive function over a 24-hour cycle and also from day to day. The patient usually functions worse in the early morning, after a nap, or at sundown. However, the patient has periods of surprising lucidity. Such fluctuation is rarely seen in any other disorder of the mental status.

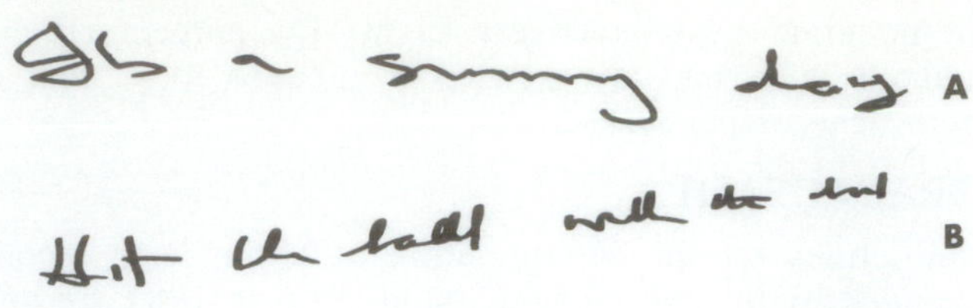

**Fig. 96-3.** **A,** "It's a sunny day." The down-slant of the sentence, the "t" uncrossed, and the preservation on the "n" of "sunny" illustrate the dysgraphic features of the confusional state. **B,** "Hit the ball with the bat." The up-slant of the sentence, the "t" uncrossed, and the generally sloppy orthography further illustrate the dysgraphic features of the confusional state.

***Arousal; psychomotor and autonomic activity.*** The degree of psychomotor activity in acute confusion varies. Two distinct syndromes have been described. In the *hypoactive syndrome,* patients have diminished psychomotor activity and are generally quiet and withdrawn. Verbal output is restricted, varying from complete mutism to empty, vague speech. In the *hyperactive syndrome,* on the other hand, patients appear to be hyperaroused, and there is psychomotor and autonomic overactivity. These patients tend to require minimal sleep and constantly thrash about in bed or pace the halls. Speech output is increased and emotional tone heightened. Most often, however, one encounters a clinical syndrome that contains elements of both the hyperactive and the hypoactive variants, with unpredictable changes over the course of the day. No evidence indicates that the hypoactive syndrome is a milder form of, and will progress to, the hyperactive variant, and no obvious relationship exists between the specific cause of acute confusion and a particular variant of this syndrome.

## Pathophysiology

The pathophysiologic mechanisms underlying the confusional states remain to be established. Some researchers have suggested that acute confusional states may result from a decrease in cerebral metabolism. However, in studies of patients with delirium tremens and delirium associated with hyperthermia, the cerebral metabolic rate has been shown to be normal. Likewise, regional cerebral blood flow studies have thus far been inconclusive.

Studies of endocrine function and delirium tremens have shown abnormalities of thyroxine ($T_4$), ACTH, and growth hormone; however, these disturbances are not considered to be of clinical significance. Similarly, EEG and polygraphic sleep studies have not been helpful in understanding the pathophysiology of acute confusional states. The most common EEG abnormality is general slowing with activity in the theta and delta ranges. Bifrontal delta activity and triphasic waves have also occasionally been noted. However, the EEG is not invariably abnormal in confusion and is not directly correlated to mental status or behavior abnormalities.

In studies of the CSF metabolites of confused patients, abnormalities of 5-hydroxyindoleacetic acid (5-HIAA), homovanillic acid (HVA), serotonin, and dopamine breakdown products have been documented. Also, an acute confusional state associated with infarction in the area of the right middle cerebral artery, involving the parietal and frontal lobes, has been reported. Similarly, other case reports have demonstrated lesions associated with confusion in the right fusiform and calcarine regions, the hippocampal formation, and the fusiform and lingual gyri.

No unified hypothesis for the pathophysiology of confusional states has yet emerged from these diverse observations. However, a discussion on consciousness and selective attention postulated a central nervous system (CNS) network, involving a disturbance in the integration of stimuli at one or more of several specific sites, the reticular activating system (RAS), the limbic system, and the polymodal association areas of the cortex. Such an elaborate network might be vulnerable to the wide range of etiologic agents reported to result in acute confusional states. The biochemical disturbances that are by far the most common causes of confusional states would probably act at the RAS level. This hypothesis would also encompass the less common focal cortical lesions associated with this disorder. This theory is an attractive one and could explain various issues concerning the etiology, clinical signs, treatment, and outcome of confusional states.

## Etiology

Acute confusional states can be divided into those of CNS origin and those caused by toxic-metabolic disorders. The common CNS disorders are trauma, seizures, infections, dementing diseases, nutritional problems, and mass lesions.

In head trauma a period of loss of consciousness may be followed by an agitated confusional state, even in the absence of obvious focal deficit.

A variable period of confusion may follow a seizure. In most instances, however, the duration of this confusional state is short. Occasionally, continuous psychomotor seizures manifest as an acute behavioral syndrome with profound confusion. Close observation of the patient may reveal clonic twitches, mouthing, or lip-smacking movements; an EEG may be needed to elucidate the diagnosis.

Encephalitis, especially when caused by herpes simplex and purulent meningitis, is an important infectious cause of the acute confusional syndrome and is one reason for performing a lumbar puncture in all patients with acute confusion in whom no clear contraindication exists.

Elderly patients or patients with dementia seem particularly prone to episodes of acute confusion. Acute confusion occurs in elderly patients most often when they develop congestive heart failure, a slight electrolyte imbalance, mild carbon dioxide retention, or constipation with fecal impaction. A relatively asymptomatic pyelonephritis or pneumonia may also manifest with acute confusion as the presenting problem.

Nutritional disorders such as Wernicke-Korsakoff syndrome (encephalopathy) are not rare. Patients with this syndrome have acute confusion, ataxia, bilateral sixth nerve palsies, and nystagmus. The disorder is most common in alcoholics, but food faddists and recluses may also develop thiamine deficiency. The policy of discharging increasing numbers of patients from state mental institutions has resulted in an increased incidence of Wernicke-Korsakoff encephalopathy in nonalcoholic patients. Some of these patients become recluses and severely neglect their nutrition. Pellagra caused by niacin deficiency is much rarer in our society; confusion, irritability, insomnia, and photosensitive rash with diarrhea suggest this diagnosis.

Intracranial space-occupying lesions may cause confusional states as a nonfocal manifestation of distortion of the intracranial contents. The mass may be a neoplasm, hematoma, cyst, or granuloma. In all these instances, gadolinium-enhanced MRI or contrast CT is the major diagnostic test to sort out these possibilities.

As previously discussed, an occasional patient with an acute, agitated confusional state may have only a small area of infarction, presumably in one of the multimodal cortical areas.

Drug intoxication is the most common cause of the acute confusional state in older adolescents and young adults. Amphetamines, lysergic acid, cocaine, and phencyclidine (angel dust) often produce an excited, hyperalert confusion with hallucinations (see Chapter 131). The belladonna alkaloids can cause a dramatic acute confusion in the elderly patient being treated for parkinsonism. Many prescription drugs in common use can cause acute confusional states, and this should be a prime consideration in any individual recently beginning medical treatment. Cimetidine has been found to be a fairly common cause of confusion in recent years, but many other frequently used drugs also seem capable of producing acute confusion.

The paradigm of the hyperalert, acute confusional state is that associated with alcohol withdrawal. In this condition, confusion, tremulousness, illusions, and hallucinations with restlessness appear within 10 to 72 hours after cessation of drinking (see Chapter 130). Withdrawal seizures consistently occur before the onset of the mental symptoms.

The range of alcohol withdrawal syndromes is wide. The most severe form is delirium tremens, in which simultaneous mental, motor, and autonomic abnormalities occur. It is a life-threatening disorder with a significant mortality rate. Major withdrawal syndromes and seizures with confusion may also develop from 2 to 8 days after withdrawal from chronic use of many sedatives and tranquilizers, including the barbiturates, glutethimide, and paraldehyde.

The metabolic encephalopathies are partially listed (see the box on p. 1328). The clinical appearances of the mental syndrome in almost all disorders may be indistinguishable from one another. The distinction must be based on a careful, general medical evaluation and appropriate laboratory investigations for these disorders. The encephalopathy caused by endogenous derangements in metabolism usually causes a hypoalert or sleepy confusion with progression to coma. Some interesting exceptions to this rule include the hyperalert, agitated mental syndromes that may be seen in acute porphyria and hyperthyroidism. The finding of asterixis (metabolic flaps) or widespread, small-amplitude myoclonic jerks is characteristic of the metabolic encephalopathies.

## Etiologic agents in acute confusional states

A. Injury by physical agents
 1. Head trauma
 2. Heatstroke
 3. Radiation
 4. Electrocution
B. Infections
 1. Systemic pneumonia, typhoid, typhus, acute rheumatic fever, malaria, influenza, diphtheria, brucellosis, infectious mononucleosis, infectious hepatitis, subacute bacterial endocarditis, bacteremia, septicemia, Rocky Mountain spotted fever, legionnaires' disease
 2. Intracranial: acute, subacute, and chronic
  a. Viral encephalitis, aseptic meningitis, rabies
  b. Bacterial meningitis: meningococcal, pneumococcal, *Haemophilus influenzae,* etc.
  c. Postinfectious and postvaccinial encephalomyelitis
  d. Tuberculous meningitis
  e. Neurosyphilis
  f. Fungal infections: cryptococcosis, coccidioidomycosis, histoplasmosis, candidiasis (moniliasis), mucormycosis
  g. Protazoal infections: *Toxoplasma* encephalitis, cerebral malaria
  h. Trichinosis
C. Intoxication by drugs and poisons and withdrawal syndrome
 1. Drugs: anticholinergics, sedative-hypnotics, digitalis derivatives, opiates, corticosteroids, salicylates, antibiotics, anticonvulsants, antiarrhythmics and antihypertensives, antineoplastic agents, cimetidine, lithium, antiparkinsonian agents, disulfiram, indomethacin, bismuth salts, phencyclidine
 2. Alcohol: ethyl and methyl
 3. Addictive inhalants: gasoline, glue, ether, nitrous oxide, nitrates
 4. Industrial poisons: carbon disulfide, organic solvents, methyl chloride and bromide, heavy metals, organophosphorus insecticides, carbon monoxide
 5. Snakebite
 6. Poisonous plants and mushrooms
D. Metabolic disorders: nutritional and hormonal
 1. Hypoxia
 2. Hypoglycemia
 3. Hepatic, renal, pancreatic, and pulmonary insufficiency (encephalopathy)

D. Metabolic disorders: nutritional and hormonal—cont'd
 4. Avitaminosis: nicotinic acid, thiamine, cyanocobalamin (vitamin $B_{12}$), folate, pyridoxine
 5. Hypervitaminosis: intoxication by vitamins A and D
 6. Hormonal disorders: hyperinsulinism, hyperthyroidism, hypothyroidism, hypopituitarism, hyperparathyroidism
 7. Disorders of fluid and electrolyte metabolism
  a. Dehydration, water intoxication
  b. Alkalosis, acidosis
  c. Hypernatremia, hyponatremia, hyperkalemia, hypercalcemia, hypocalcemia, hypermagnesemia, hypomagnesemia
 8. Errors of metabolism
  a. Porphyria
  b. Carcinoid syndrome
  c. Hepatolenticular degeneration (Wilson disease)
E. Vascular disorders
 1. Migraine
 2. Cerebrovascular disorders
  a. Transient ischemic attacks
  b. Hypertensive encephalopathy
  c. Thrombosis, embolism
  d. Subarachnoid hemorrhage
 3. Cardiovascular disorders
  a. Myocardial infarction
  b. Congestive heart failure
  c. Cardiac arrhythmias
 4. Vasculitis
  a. Polyarteritis nodosa
  b. Systemic lupus erythematosus
  c. Rheumatoid vasculitis
  d. Temporal arteritis
 5. Hematologic disorders
  a. Pernicious anemia
  b. Erythema
  c. Thrombotic thrombocytopenic pupura
F. Cerebral degenerative disorders: multiple sclerosis
G. Extracranial neoplasms and intracranial space-occupying lesions
H. Hypersensitivity and autoimmune disorders
 1. Serum sickness
 2. Food allergy

Modified from Lipowski ZJ: *Delirium,* Springfield, Ill, 1980, Charles C Thomas.

A full discussion of the psychiatric disorders that may be associated with acute confusional states is beyond the scope of this chapter. Acute schizophrenia and manic-depressive illness in the manic phase are the two most common problems. Physicians should be very wary of making the diagnosis of a psychiatric disorder in a somnolent or obtunded, confused patient.

The cause of confusional states appears to be nonspecific. Almost any disturbance of body function may result in this syndrome. The box above presents an etiologic classification as an example of the long list of agents associated with confusional states.

## Differential diagnosis

The differential diagnosis of acute confusional states includes both "organic" and "functional" disorders. Although acute confusion is a distinctive syndrome, the varied symptomatology may cause difficulty in differentiating it from closely related disturbances.

***Dementia.*** Dementia is an important consideration in the differential diagnosis of confusional states (see Chapter 97). The two conditions are similar in that they both involve a diffuse impairment of intellectual functioning. The confused patient, however, has what appears to be a specific disturbance of consciousness, whereas dementia occurs in the context of a "clear sensorium." The nature of onset and course of the illness are most valuable in separating these two conditions. Dementia is usually insidious in onset with a progressive deterioration, whereas confusion usually begins abruptly and shows little progression. Confusional states are relatively short-lived. If treated appropriately, and in some patients even if left untreated appropriately, spontaneous clearing may occur. Most cases of dementia, on the other hand, will not improve unless a specific treatable cause exists. Other features that help to differentiate the two conditions are (1) fluctuation in symptoms, (2) disruption of the sleep-wake cycle, and (3) autonomic overactivity. These features, if present, usually favor a diagnosis of acute confusion. Periods of acute confusion, however, may be noted in the course of dementia. Demented patients sometimes deteriorate greatly, and a stable patient may exhibit a sudden deterioration. Frequently, this deterioration in the mental status is the result of a superimposed confusional state for which a reversible cause may be identified and corrected.

***Korsakoff psychosis.*** Korsakoff psychosis is an amnesic syndrome associated with features of disorientation and confabulation and dominated by memory disturbance. Confusional states should be easily differentiated, since Korsakoff psychosis occurs in the setting of a clear sensorium.

***Psychiatric disorders.*** If the criteria in the DSM-IV are followed, the physician should have no difficulty in differentiating delirium from illnesses such as schizophrenia, mania, or depression.

### Laboratory investigations

The workup of the acutely confused patient is similar to that of the patient in coma: routine chest x-ray; complete blood count; sedimentation rate, along with determination of serum glucose, electrolytes, calcium, and blood urea nitrogen; and a toxic screen serve as the core laboratory evaluation. Arterial blood gases, serum ammonia, liver function studies, serum cortisol and $T_4$ levels, antinuclear antibodies, serum protein electrophoresis, and a urine test for porphyrins and heavy metals may be required in certain patients. An EEG may offer important evidence of a continuous complex partial seizure disorder or demonstrate the widespread symmetric slowing with triphasic activity that characterizes metabolic encephalopathies (e.g., hepatic encephalopathies). Rapid, frontally distributed EEG activity may signify the presence of sedative drugs.

A lumbar puncture should be performed on every patient who is acutely confused unless a distinct contraindication exists. Contraindications consist of two possibilities: (1) the patient may be seen in a phase marked by extremely rapid, ongoing improvement, as in the treatment of a bout of hypoglycemia, or (2) a lumbar puncture may be deferred, a circumstance that arises in a patient with signs of increased intracranial pressure from a mass lesion. In this second situation, it is not satisfactory simply to defer a lumbar puncture; urgent alternative diagnostic measures, usually neuroimaging, should be performed.

Neurologic and neurosurgical consultation should be obtained for advice and guidance regarding the selection of procedures or further diagnostic tests. The role of other noninvasive examinations, such as isotope brain scanning, flow scans, and the EEG, remain a matter of judgment that must take into account both the rate of progression of the patient's clinical status and the likelihood of diagnostic yield. Both EEG and neuroimaging may be difficult if the patient is restless or combative.

## Management

Treatment largely depends on correcting the specific underlying abnormality. Since medication is frequently a cause of confusional states, the most effective approach is to discontinue the medication whenever possible while correcting any underlying metabolic disturbance. In most instances the etiology is clear, but in the more difficult cases a full workup is essential because attempts at simply controlling the behavior may result, for example, in not recognizing a case of fatal meningitis.

The management of the behavior disturbance could be accomplished by pharmacotherapy; however, most confused patients benefit much more from specialized nursing care. For the more belligerent patients, geriatric chairs, padded bedrails, and gloved and partially restrained limbs are often necessary. Generally, however, patients do best unrestrained but contained in an environment where strict limits are set. Large calendars, constant reassurance, and positive reinforcement from the staff are invaluable orienting stimuli and often improve behavior. The bedside lamp and radio are helpful aids when the patient awakens at night. Only when these measures have failed should pharmacotherapy be used.

Antipsychotics are the most popular drugs in the treatment of confusional states. No evidence has shown that one is superior to any other. Haloperidol is frequently used. Loxapine is more sedating and, in some patients, might be preferable. Most of the sedative-hypnotics, such as barbiturates, chloral hydrate, and flurazepam, are less helpful and may even exacerbate the confusional state. The anxiolytics are sometimes effective. Chlorazepam and oxazepam have relatively short half-lives with little buildup of active metabolites. β-Adrenergic blockers such as propranolol have been reported to be effective in agitated and belligerent patients and may be particularly effective in elderly patients. Antihistamines are sedating and sometimes useful. Initial dosages of all drugs should be low with gradual increments, since all these medications may precipitate a paradoxical reaction with greatly increased behavioral disturbances. Disturbances in the sleep-wake cycle are often difficult to correct. Prevention of "catnaps" during the day may help promote a full night of sleep. Sedation, however, is rarely effective; the sleep-wake cycle usually normalizes only as the confusional state clears.

## BIBLIOGRAPHY

Adams RD, Victor M: Delirium and other acute confusional states. In Adams RD, Victor M, editors: *Principles of neurology,* New York, 1981, McGraw-Hill.

Adams RD, Victor M: *Principles of neurology,* ed 4, New York, 1989, McGraw-Hill.
ANA Committee on Ethical Affairs: Persistent vegetative state: report of the American Neurological Committee on Ethical Affairs, *Ann Neurol* 33:386, 1993.
Defeudis FV: Cholinergic roles in consciousness. In Defeudis FV, editor: *Central cholinergic systems and behavior,* London, 1974, Academic.
Horenstein S, Chamberlain W, Conomy J: Infarction of the fusiform and calcarine regions: agitated delirium and hemianopia, *Trans Am Neurol Assoc* 92:85, 1967.
Jouvet M: The role of monoamines and acetyl choline containing neurons in the regulation of the sleep/wake cycle, *Rev Physiol* 64:166, 1972.
Levy DE et al: Prognosis in non-traumatic coma. *Ann Intern Med* 94:293, 1981.
Lloyd GG: Acute behavior disturbances, *J Neurol Neurosurg Psychiatry* 56:1149, 1993.
Mesulam M: A cortical network for directed attention and unilateral neglect, *Ann Neurol* 10:309, 1981.
Plum F, Posner JB: *The diagnosis of stupor and coma,* ed 3, Philadelphia, 1980, FA Davis.
Sabin TD: Coma and the confusional state in the emergency room, *Med Clin North Am* 65:15, 1981.
Teasdale G: Prognosis of coma after head injury. In Turnbridge WMG, editor: *Advanced medicine,* London, 1981, Pittman Medical.
Tinuper P: Idiopathic recurring stupor: a case with possible involvement of the gamma aminobutyric acid (GABA)ergic system, *Ann Neurol* 31:503, 1992.

CHAPTER

# 97 Dementing Illnesses

**Claire A. Levesque**
**Thomas D. Sabin**

*Dementia*
*Mind fields*
*Once untilled and fertile soil,*
*Lie quiet.*
*Memories stand,*
*Leafless as winter trees*
*Bare monuments of accumulation.*
*Intellect decays*
*Thorny brambles of overgrowth,*
*Remnant of complexity.*
*Emotions spoil*
*Fallen like overripe fruit,*
*Discarded nourishment.*
*Spinal fluid circulates*
*Crystalline and unspeaking,*
*In purposeless motion.*

**Jane A. Hawes**
*N Engl J Med* 305:290, 1981

Dementing illnesses occur often, particularly in elderly persons, and are major causes of devastating losses of function, leading to institutionalization. Dementia, a syndrome resulting from many etiologies, is defined as a slow loss of previously acquired intellectual or behavioral function without alteration in level of awareness. At least two areas of cognitive function, such as memory, language, personality, visuospatial abilities, or judgment, are impaired in dementia, and the disabilities affect independent daily living.

Dementia differs from delirium. *Delirium,* or an acute confusional state, is an acute or subacute onset of disorientation with alterations in levels of awareness, including hyperalert and drowsy states. It often disrupts day/night cycles and can be accompanied by delusions (see Chapter 96). Delirium may coexist with dementia. Dementia also differs from normal aging. In elderly persons, short-term memory may be impaired in tasks requiring manipulation of material, such as digit spans backward, or in memory tasks requiring divided attention. Response time can increase, and memory for proper names may be affected. This "benign senescent forgetfulness" is a gradual process that does not impair daily living or disrupt social skills.

Dementia is a common disorder in elderly persons, occurring in all ethnic groups. The underlying etiology seems to differ based on heritage. Whites are prone to Alzheimer disease (AD), and Asians and African-Americans tend to develop vascular dementia. However, patients in all ethnic groups show an increasing prevalence of dementia with increasing age, with one study showing an estimated prevalence of probable AD of 47.2% in those over 84 years old. These statistics are sobering in the context of a predicted population of 4.6 million over age 85 in the United States in the year 2000.

Dementia is truly a devastating disease that robs patients of the very qualities that make them human. It is also a killer disease and is the fourth or fifth most common cause of death, although it rarely appears on death certificates. The economic impact of this problem is staggering. The annual cost of the formal and informal care for one patient with AD is estimated at $47,000 in 1990 dollars, with the annual cost for all forms of dementia at $58 billion. In a brief survey of Massachusetts Nursing Homes, more than 95% of the occupants were found to reside there primarily because of dementia. The cost of a full diagnostic evaluation (usually less than $2000) is clearly cost-effective even if only an occasional patient is found to have a treatable form of dementia. Also, the difference in the quality of life is vast. Unfortunately, many are found to have progressive irreversible forms of dementia. Families, especially in the minority community, keep their loved ones in the home in the face of staggering caregiver burden. Behaviors most likely to lead to institutionalization include wandering, aggressive outbursts, sleep disturbances, and especially incontinence. Home care is practical and cost-effective in the early stages of dementia. In later stages, nursing home care provides relief to the overburdened caregiver and can also be less costly than formal and informal home care costs.

Multiple studies have been done on the risk factors for development of dementia. Many have focused on the most common progressive neurodegenerative cause called AD. Some studies have implicated factors such as history of head trauma or lower educational level, but no definitive risk factors have been identified. Hypertension and diabetes are major risk factors for vascular forms of dementia, such as multiinfarct dementia and Binswanger disease, and are particularly prevalent in minority populations. Since the differential diagnosis of dementia is so broad, other risk factors can be found specific to particular etiologies, such as alcohol abuse and subdural hematomas or exposure to the transmissible agent and development of Creutzfeldt-Jakob's disease. Genetic factors also play a role in some dementing illnesses, such as Huntington's disease and the familial form of AD.

Most causes of dementia lead to death or metabolic dysfunction of neurons producing losses in cognitive function. The location of the cell loss is a critical factor. In AD the cell loss is most prominent in the cortex, hippocampus, and amygdala, disrupting connections critical for memory and other cognitive function. In multiinfarct dementia, small cerebrovascular accidents (CVAs, strokes) placed in strategic locations can lead to loss of memory, visual spatial abilities, language, and personality. Disturbances of primary and secondary sensory modalities can also distort interpretations of the environment and produce a clinical syndrome that may be confused with dementia. Dementia can also occur because of a change in the overall chemical milieu of the brain; common examples include endocrine disturbances such as hypothyroidism and toxic encephalopathies resulting from medications. These and other "reversible" dementias are less common but are critically important to diagnose. Patients with a definitive neurodegenerative cause of dementia often have a coexisting treatable factor at initial presentation or later in the course of the disease. For instance, a patient with AD may have severe functional deterioration caused by minor nonneurologic diseases such as urinary tract infections (UTIs) and electrolyte abnormalities.

### HISTORY

In a dementing illness, it is critically important to obtain a major portion of the history from the caregiver. In addition to open-ended questions about the changes in the patient's behavior, specific questions should be asked about difficulties with activities of daily living such as eating, dressing, and toileting. Some standardized questions have been developed to assist in this history taking, such as the Blessed Dementia Scale (see the box on p. 1332). Another less detailed but widely utilized assessment is the Folstein mini-mental status role described in Chapter 6. All medications should be carefully reviewed, including inquiry about use of over-the-counter (OTC) medications, folk remedies, alcohol, and "street" drugs. A change in drinking pattern may go unnoticed by family members, especially if the patient lives alone, and may represent "self-treatment" of involutional depression. Currently, a history of street drug use occurs infrequently in elderly persons but may be expected to increase in prevalence in the ensuing years and is a risk factor for dementia related to acquired immune deficiency syndrome (AIDS). A medical review of systems should focus on a history of hypertension, diabetes, thyroid disease, vitamin $B_{12}$ deficiency (including history of gastric surgery), syphilis, and an evaluation of the risk factors for disease related to the human immunodeficiency virus (HIV). The family history of dementia is vital for certain diagnoses such as Huntington disease and familial AD. Prior psychiatric illnesses in the patient or other family members should be recorded. The patient's educational and occupational history allows estimation of premorbid cognitive functioning.

### PHYSICAL AND NEUROLOGIC EXAMINATION

In addition to a general medical examination, orthostatic blood pressures are indicated in any patient with vascular risk factors. The mental status examination should include a range of questions to assess multiple cognitive spheres. The Blessed Dementia Scale (see the box on p. 1332) includes a scale of information, memory, and concentration. Further tests of language and visuospatial abilities should be added. This can include writing a sentence, copying a complex geometric figure, following one-step and two-step commands (verbal and written), and naming objects and parts of objects. Testing for apraxia can include imitation of gestures and demonstrations of complex movements, such as saluting or brushing hair. Vision should be tested with a hand-held card with patients wearing their eyeglasses, if applicable. Hearing can be tested by whispering numbers in each ear. The remainder of the neurologic examination should focus on finding focal abnormalities. Hemiparesis, reflex asymmetries, and sensory changes may be signs of previous CVAs. Patterns of sensory loss may represent peripheral neuropathy suggestive of vitamin $B_{12}$ deficiency, alcohol-related causes of dementia, neurosyphilis, and multiple other reversible causes. These focal signs suggest the need for further neurologic consultation.

## DIFFERENTIAL DIAGNOSIS

The evaluation of the patient with dementing illness, particularly in the mild to moderate stages, must emphasize a search for potentially reversible causes. Patients may also have causes for dementia, and even when the clinical impression strongly suggests a neurodegenerative process, coexisting reversible causes should be investigated. The primary care physician should consider neurologic consultation when the dementing process is accompanied by elementary neurologic findings or when atypical features emerge. The differential diagnoses listed here emphasize the most common and the most treatable causes.

#### Alzheimer's disease and familial Alzheimer's disease

AD is the most common cause of devastating progressive dementia in elderly white patients and occurs in all other ethnic groups. The characteristic neuropathologic change consists of senile plaques (Fig. 97-1), neurofibrillary tangles (Fig. 97-2), and atrophy. Although some of these changes can be seen with normal aging, both the distribution and the extent of the senile plaques and tangles are different.

Many neurotransmitters are decreased in brains of AD patients, but these changes are unlikely to be the initiating factor. The cholinergic system shows consistent involvement and has been a target of various therapeutic approaches, including the recently released drug tacrine, which have been minimally effective at best. Multiple lines of research implicate β-amyloid or its processing as a key event in causation. The β-amyloid protein is a major constituent of the plaque seen in brains of AD patients (see Fig. 97-1), and mutations have been found in pedigrees of familial AD on chromosome 21 near the gene encoding amyloid precursor protein. However, other pedigrees have mutations in other loci on chromosomes 14 and 19. These genetic data, plus the variability in age at presentation and

## Blessed dementia scale

Name ________________________________
Total incompetence = 1
Variable incapacity = ½

**Changes in performance of everyday activities**

| | | | |
|---|---|---|---|
| 1. Inability to perform household tasks, handle money | 1 | ½ | 0 |
| 2. Inability to cope with small sums of money | 1 | ½ | 0 |
| 3. Inability to remember short list of items, (e.g., in shopping) | 1 | ½ | 0 |
| 4. Inability to find way about indoors | 1 | ½ | 0 |
| 5. Inability to find way about familiar street | 1 | ½ | 0 |
| 6. Inability to interpret surroundings (e.g., to recognize whether in hospital or at home, to discriminate among patients, physicians, nurses, relatives, hospital staff) | 1 | ½ | 0 |
| 7. Inability to recall recent events (e.g., recent outings, visits of relatives or friends to hospital) | 1 | ½ | 0 |
| 8. Tendency to dwell in the past | 1 | ½ | 0 |

**Changes in habits**

| | |
|---|---|
| 9. Eating | |
| a. Cleanly with proper utensils | 0 |
| b. Messily with spoon only | 1 |
| c. Simple solids, (e.g., biscuits) | 2 |
| d. Has to be fed | 3 |
| 10. Dressing | |
| a. Unaided | 0 |
| b. Occasionally misplaced buttons , etc. | 1 |
| c. Wrong sequence, often forgetting items | 2 |
| d. Unable to dress | 3 |
| 11. Complete sphincter control | 0 |
| a. Occasional wet beds | 1 |
| b. Frequent wet beds | 2 |
| c. Doubly incontinent | 3 |

**Changes in personality, interests, drive**

| | |
|---|---|
| No change | 0 |
| 12. Increased rigidity | 1 |
| 13. Increased egocentricity | 1 |
| 14. Impairment of regard for feelings of others | 1 |
| 15. Coarsening of affect | 1 |
| 16. Impairment of emotional control (e.g., increased petulance and irritability) | 1 |
| 17. Hilarity in inappropriate situations | 1 |
| 18. Diminished emotional responsiveness | 1 |
| 19. Sexual misdemeanor (appearing de novo in old age) | 1 |
| 20. Hobbies relinquished | 1 |
| 21. Diminished initiative or growing apathy | 1 |
| 22. Purposeless hyperactivity | 1 |

Subtotal ______________

**Information-Memory-Concentration test**

*Positive score for each correct item; 37 points maximum (intact)*

| | |
|---|---|
| Name ______________ | 1 |
| Age ______________ | 1 |
| Time (hour) ______________ | 1 |
| Time of day ______________ | 1 |
| Day of week ______________ | 1 |
| Date ______________ | 1 |
| Month ______________ | 1 |
| Season ______________ | 1 |
| Year ______________ | 1 |
| Place: Name ______________ | 1 |
| Street ______________ | 1 |
| Town ______________ | 1 |
| Type of place (home, hospital, etc.) ______________ | 1 |
| Recognition of persons (cleaner, physician, nurse, patient, relative; any two available) ______________ | 1 |

***Memory***

| | |
|---|---|
| 1. Personal | |
| a. Date of birth | 1 |
| b. Place of birth | 1 |
| c. School attended | 1 |
| d. Occupation | 1 |
| e. Name of siblings/spouse | 1 |
| f. Name of any town where patient had worked | 1 |
| g. Name of employer | 1 |
| 2. Nonpersonal | |
| a. Date of WWI | 1 |
| b. Date of WWII | 1 |
| c. President | 1 |
| d. Vice-President | 1 |
| 3. Name and address (5-minute recall) Mr. John Brown 42 West Street Cambridge, MA | 5 |

***Concentration***

| | | | |
|---|---|---|---|
| Months of year backward | 2 | 1 | 0 |
| Counting 1 to 20 | 2 | 1 | 0 |
| Counting 20 to 1 | 2 | 1 | 0 |

Subtotal ______________

Total dementia score ______________

Modified from Blessed G et al, *Br J Psychiatry* 114:797, 1968.

extrapyramidal features, point to heterogeneity in familial cases. A potential genetic link for sporadic cases has been identified with an association with the E4 allele for apolipoprotein E, which is involved in lipoprotein metabolism and binds to the β-amyloid protein. Environmental toxins have also been considered in AD, and studies have demonstrated aluminum in the neurofibrillary tangles.

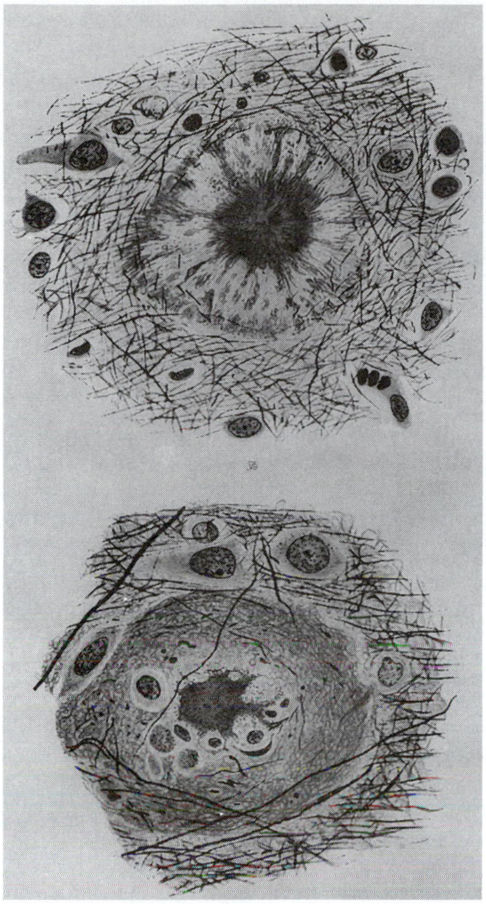

**Fig. 97-1.** Senile plaque appears to be made up of degenerating neural processes with central accumulation of amyloid. (From Spielmeyer W: *Histopathologie des Nervensystems,* Berlin, 1922, Springer.)

In patients with both sporadic and familial AD, mental changes are gradual and progressive. Sometimes, they are first noted by family members or health care providers after a major event in the patient's life, such as death of a family member, surgery, or other medical illness. The mental change usually begins with impaired recall of recent events, word-finding difficulty, and inability to perceive spatial relationships. A series of words may be correctly done with immediate repetition if the patient is attentive, but the patient is unable to perform accurately if an interval of 3 to 4 minutes is interposed. Complaints by family members that the patient is "living in the past" reflect the relative preservation of remote memory. Stories of early adult life may be recounted with painfully accurate detail, but the events of a recent shopping trip are totally forgotten. The attentive examiner often is able to detect difficulty in word finding as the patient makes word substitutions in circumlocutory phrases that characterize the early anomia. Asking the patient to name a series of common objects and their parts confirms this finding. Difficulty in drawing a simple map of a familiar intersection, an outline map of the United States, or a geometric shape reveals the associated difficulty with spatial relationships. A patient with this problem often becomes lost when driving alone or walking even in a familiar area.

These three features—retentive memory, spatial difficulties, and anomic aphasia—are usually well established before frontal lobe dysfunction supervenes. With progression, inappropriate behavior with neglected personal hygiene develops, sometimes with coarsening of the sense of humor. Other patients appear to be euphoric with crude, punning humor. Both the humor and the irritability are shallow emotional states and do not evoke empathy in the family or examiner. The episodic outburst, sometimes called a *catastrophic reaction,* can involve aggressive behavior toward family members. These outbursts by a demented patient are very frightening to caregivers and sometimes lead to institutionalization. Wandering is another behavior that is very difficult for family members.

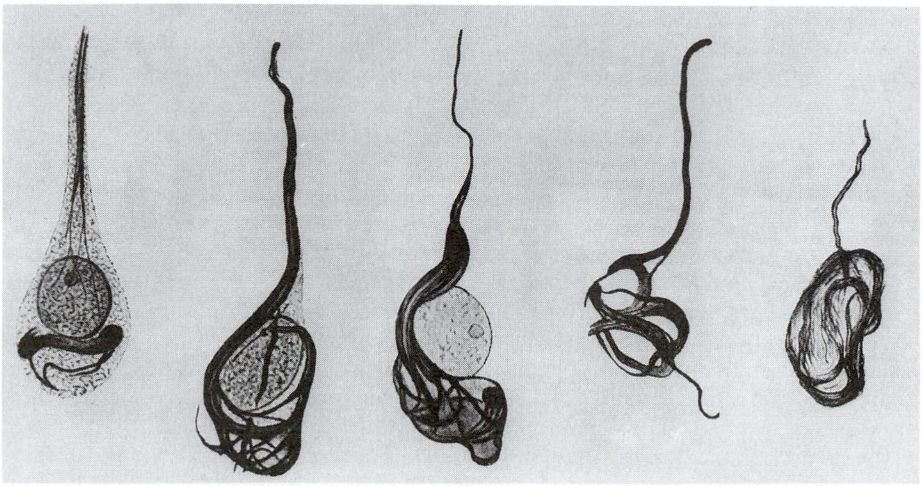

**Fig. 97-2.** Neurofibrillary tangles consist of intraneuronal bundles of filomentous material that progressively amass in swirls within the perikaryon and neurites. (From Spielmeyer W: *Histopathologie des Nervensystems,* Berlin, 1922, Springer.)

Patients may leave the home inappropriately attired and lose their way. Wandering demented patients unfortunately are often found dead because of exposure to the environment or traumatic injury. Sleep disturbances also occur, and patients wake in the middle of the night and wander in the home. This can be particularly dangerous, since the patient can drop burning cigarettes, turn on the gas stove, or engage in other potentially dangerous activities while the caregiver sleeps.

Even the most severe abnormalities in these higher functions are not ordinarily accompanied by elementary neurologic findings. Upper motor neuron signs, cortical blindness, cortical deafness, and cortical sensory loss are not found in AD. The motor abnormalities occur only in advanced cases and include hyperreflexia, spasticity, or upgoing toes. Most patients have paratonic rigidity with a tendency toward flexed immobility in the upper and lower extremities. A state of paraplegic inflexion of cerebral origin develops with suck, snout, and grasp reflexes (frontal lobe reflexes). This state is preceded by a deterioration in gait, which has been attributed to grasp reflexes in the feet. Initiating gait becomes difficult, and the patient takes many small steps before moving forward, the so-called slipping-clutch syndrome. Seizures may occur very late in the course of AD. A patient with focal neurologic signs or early onset of seizures should be evaluated by a neurologist because other causes of dementia may be present.

Patients with AD usually die 2 to 10 years after diagnosis, although some live longer. Pneumonia is a common cause of demise. No specific test is available to prove this diagnosis. The only definitive test is neuropathologic evaluation of the brain at brain biopsy or postmortem examination. Since no effective treatment currently exists for AD, brain biopsy is not recommended. Computed tomography (CT) or magnetic resonance imaging (MRI) of the head shows widespread atrophy with a predilection for the temporal lobes and assists in exclusion of other causes. Biparietal hypoperfusion is seen on single-positron emission computed tomography (SPECT) scanning, although this finding is not specific and has not been well documented pathologically. Potential peripheral markers in blood, including platelets and skin, are being investigated as potential diagnostic tests, but currently none of them can be recommended for routine clinical use. CSF studies of breakdown products of neurotransmitters and of amyloid precursor protein do not yet have proven clinical utility. Genotypes for the E4 allele of apolipoprotein E are commercially available but the association of this genotype with AD needs further investigation in larger studies before this test can be used as a predictor of risk of development of the disease.

Although no "gold standard" test exists for AD, clinicopathologic correlations have shown that clinicians are correct in most cases. This accuracy is improved by an initial evaluation by a clinician specializing in dementia and a clinical reevaluation about 6 to 12 months after the diagnostic evaluation. Although previously underdiagnosed, AD may now be overdiagnosed, and reversible causes may be missed. In addition, AD sometimes does not occur in isolation. Overlap of AD and vascular dementia is relatively common, and treatable causes such as depression, drug effects, vitamin $B_{12}$ deficiency, or coexisting chronic infections can occur. AD is slowly progressive, and rapid deteriorations in function or additional focal neurologic signs should always prompt evaluation for other causes, such as intercurrent pneumonias, UTIs, or chronic subdural hematomas.

### Other neurodegenerative diseases

Frontal lobe dementias are syndromes characterized by frontal atrophy with prominent behavioral features. The most common is **Pick's disease**, a neurodegenerative disorder that is sometimes difficult to differentiate from AD. The temporal and frontal lobes are selectively involved in this disease. Features that support a diagnosis of Pick's disease include early onset of personality change, disinhibition, increased oral behaviors (e.g., eating, smoking, drinking), and onset before age 65. A very severe and unusual form of aphasia may be an early manifestation and is often combined with behavioral disturbances. This disorder may occur more often than previously thought. The course of Pick's disease appears to be more rapid than AD. Imaging studies may show preferential enlargement of the temporal horns with focal frontal and temporal atrophy. SPECT scanning also shows a preferential hypoperfusion of the frontal lobes with relative sparing of parietal lobes. Definite diagnosis requires examination of the brain, which reveals "knife edge" atrophy of the superior temporal gyrus, absence of the characteristic plaques and tangles of AD, and the presence of Pick cells and Pick bodies. No known treatment exists for Pick's disease, and patients with this condition often require earlier nursing home placement because of the behavioral disturbances.

Other primary neurologic causes of dementia have associated elementary neurologic findings accompanying the changes in mental status. **Huntington's disease** is an autosomal dominant disorder with dementia, chorea, and psychiatric changes. The average age of onset is the fourth decade, although dementia may appear more than a year before any movement disorder is present. During this time, diagnosis may be difficult if a positive family history is not available. CT or MRI shows marked atrophy of the caudate nucleus. **Wilson's disease** is an autosomal recessive disorder of copper metabolism characterized by behavioral disturbances, tremors, other abnormal movements, Kayser-Fleischer rings, and liver disease. Onset is usually in adolescence or young adulthood but may be as late as the fifth decade of life.

**Multiple sclerosis** may present as a dementing disease because of the development of bilateral periventricular demyelination. The evaluation of demented patients should include a detailed search of the medical history for evidence of a previous demyelinating episode in an atypical cause of dementia, especially with early, severe, frontal lobe features. Examination of the spinal fluid for oligoclonal banding and for immunoelectrophoresis and MRI of the brain showing the characteristic white matter changes are diagnostic in the appropriate clinical setting.

The tremor, rigidity, and bradykinesias present in **Parkinson's disease** eliminate diagnostic difficulties in this cause of dementia. Treatment of Parkinson's disease and any associated depression often temporarily improves these patients' intellectual function. The CT appearance of atrophy correlates with the mental state in dementia of Parkinson's disease. Olivopontocerebellar degeneration is a progressive disorder and is often associated with very slowly progressive dementia. Characteristic shrinkage of the pons and cerebellum can be best seen on MRI and is always present at the time mental changes supervene. No effective treatment is available for this disorder. A mild dementia, compounded by extreme slowness in expression, language, and movement, accompanies progressive supranuclear palsy. Loss of vertical eye movements and development of truncal rigidity are characteristic features of this rare disease. These patients do not respond to dopaminergic drugs, but some appear to have amelioration of some symptoms with low-dose amitriptyline.

## Cerebrovascular disease

In the past, dementia was commonly thought to result from "hardening of the arteries." This misconception resulted in the widespread use of cerebrovasodilators for dementia, a treatment of dubious value. Cerebrovascular disease, however, does produce dementia if lesions are strategically placed. A recent series demonstrated a 38.7% prevalence of vascular dementia in a white Northern European cohort of 85-year-old persons, which is even higher than previously reported. As noted earlier, vascular causes of dementia can also coexist with AD. A patient who has several CVAs in areas important for cognitive function (e.g., deep temporal lobe, frontal lobes) can be easy to diagnose. However, in other patients, multiple small lacunar infarcts can occur, often in "silent" areas of the brain. Hypertension or diabetes significantly increases the risk for lacunar infarctions. A careful history often elicits several episodes of clear-cut deterioration in function. Since multiinfarct dementia can be difficult to distinguish from AD, a scoring system has been developed called the Hachinski ischemic score (Table 97-1). MRI can also be helpful in this diagnosis because very small infarctions can be found with the high resolution now available. This diagnosis is important to make, since careful control of hypertension while maintaining adequate perfusion and avoiding episodic hypotension may be the key to preventing further deterioration in these patients.

**Table 97-1.** Hachinski ischemic score to distinguish cerebrovascular dementia from Alzheimer's disease

| Feature | Score |
|---|---|
| Abrupt onset | 2 |
| Stepwise deterioration | 1 |
| Fluctuating course | 2 |
| Nocturnal confusion | 1 |
| Relative preservation of personality | 1 |
| Depression | 1 |
| Somatic complaints | 1 |
| Emotional incontinence | 1 |
| History of hypertension | 1 |
| History of CVAs (strokes) | 2 |
| Evidence of associated atherosclerosis | 1 |
| Focal neurologic symptoms | 2 |
| Focal neurologic signs | 2 |

A total score less than 4 means vascular dementia is unlikely, while scores greater than 7 indicate vascular dementia is probable.

Modified from Hachinski VC et al: Cerebral blood flow in dementia, *Arch Neurol* 32:632, 1975.

Another dementing cerebrovascular disorder is Binswanger encephalopathy. The dementia in this case is accompanied by bilateral pyramidal signs (weakness, increased reflexes) and intense frontal lobe signs. The patient may appear abulic and have diffusely increased muscle tone. Prominent palmar and plantar grasp reflexes are often present, and urinary incontinence with a slow, unsteady gait is common. Variability in blood pressure appears to be a risk factor for this syndrome. MRI shows multiple white matter infarcts in a periventricular distribution becoming confluent. Unfortunately, MRI also shows this pattern in patients who do not exhibit a clinical syndrome. This diagnosis is in the process of evolution, and more definitive criteria need to be developed.

## Depression

Depression can cause a syndrome termed *pseudodementia,* which can be difficult to distinguish from other causes of dementia. Depression can also coexist in AD, usually in the early stages in patients with enough retained insight. A depressed affect may be present in some of these patients but is not universal. As with other forms of depression in elderly patients, agitation or psychotic features can occur. During cognitive testing, these patients have a high frequency of "I don't know" responses and often give up easily. The examination reveals inconsistencies in performance. One missed question often leads to complete failure on subsequent tasks, even though the questions may be less complex than previous satisfactorily completed testing. The failures tend to occur in all areas of testing, unlike the more selective deficit seen in AD. For instance, in depression, remote, recent, retentive, and playback memory may all be equally defective. A previous history of depression in the patient or a positive family history can be helpful. Patients with mild or moderate dementia can still answer questions about their mood, and statements can be corroborated by caregivers. Formal testing by a qualified neuropsychologist may be helpful, but even then, the patient's condition may be indistinguishable from that of true dementia. Extensive and repeated interdisciplinary assessments may be necessary.

If depression is a serious consideration, a trial of antidepressant treatment should be given. However, this treatment should have clear end points with reevaluations because long-term use of antidepressants, particularly those with anticholinergic side effects, can cause confusion. The pharmacologic options for treatment of depression include tricyclic antidepressants and related compounds and serotonin reuptake inhibitors (fluoxetine, sertraline). The medication chosen should have the least potential for serious side effect and the most potential for improvement. Methylphenidate, a stimulant drug, may be helpful in depressed elderly patients with psychomotor retardation, but again, it should be started at low doses, gradually increased, and continued only if improvement is noted. In some patients, electroconvulsive therapy (ECT) is beneficial and safe even in the fragile elderly patient, especially when medication side effects prohibit drug use (see Chapter 133).

### Normal-pressure hydrocephalus

In normal-pressure hydrocephalus (NPH) the clinical triad of dementia, incontinence, and gait disorder is associated with enlarged cerebral ventricles out of proportion to any atrophy present. This is a disorder of cerebrospinal fluid (CSF) circulation or absorption, with normal or high-normal opening pressure on lumbar puncture. The syndrome may develop after inflammatory states within the subarachnoid space, such as meningitis, encephalitis, or subarachnoid bleeding, but most are idiopathic. The dementia associated with NPH does not appear to have any characteristic features. CT or MRI of the head shows enlargement of ventricles out of proportion to the amount of atrophy, transependymal fluid, and rounding of the ventricular horns. On MRI, a signal void caused by moving CSF has been described in the third ventricle. Radioisotope cisternography demonstrates absence of isotope flow in the subarachnoid space over the hemispheric convexities. Another test that may be helpful is removing a high volume (20 to 30 ml) of CSF, followed by a careful observation for transient improvements in cognitive status and gait. Cognitive and timed-gait testing is then repeated after the lumbar puncture at intervals over several days. An improvement in clinical status after a high-volume lumbar puncture may be predictive of the response to shunting. Patients with the appropriate clinical syndrome and evidence of NPH on confirmatory tests are referred to neurosurgery for possible shunting of spinal fluid. Lumboperitoneal shunting can be performed even on fragile elderly patients with minimal risk. Unfortunately, none of the diagnostic tests has been effective in demonstrating a high probability of favorable response to shunting.

### Nonconvulsive status

Most seizures are dramatic events with sudden alteration in consciousness, stereotyped behaviors, and jerking movements. However, in some instances, subclinical seizures can occur and may be almost continuous, resulting in a state called nonconvulsive status or complex partial status. This state of continuous nonclinical seizures can continue for prolonged periods. It is readily diagnosed by electroencephalography (EEG), with a characteristic ictal pattern. This syndrome occurs infrequently but is treatable with anticonvulsants. It may occur with metabolic or toxic disruptions or with no apparent precipitant. A prior seizure history is not necessary.

### Infections

At the turn of the 20th century, neurosyphilis would have been one of the most common reasons for chronic progressive dementia. Although the widespread use of penicillin has made central nervous system (CNS) syphilis a rare disorder, a case is discovered at the Boston City Hospital every 2 to 3 years. The CSF in active cases always contains increased white cells. The patients tend to have a progressive frontal-type dementia associated with bilateral pyramidal signs and distal and perioral tremors, along with delusions of grandeur and Argyll Robertson pupils.

Several diseases traditionally classified as degenerative are now known to be caused by slow viral infections; the prime example is Creutzfeldt-Jakob disease. This disorder affects middle-aged individuals, who develop severe dementia, widespread myoclonic jerking, and rigidity, with a fatal outcome usually in weeks to months. Some patients have survived for several years and have had a more chronic course. This disease has been transmitted to nonhuman primates, and human-to-human transmission has been documented via corneal transplants, injection with growth hormone extracted from human pituitary glands, and indwelling brain electrodes. Usual methods of sterilization are not adequate to destroy the agents responsible for this disease; common household bleach is most effective. Tissue may remain infectious for years. The infectious agent appears to be a prion. Brain biopsy is required to prove the diagnosis. The clinical syndrome and an EEG showing characteristic periodic complexes support the diagnosis of Creutzfeldt-Jakob disease. Antiviral agents have been tried in a small number of patients and do not seem to be effective. Rare familial forms of prion diseases (e.g., Gerstmann-Straussler disease) appear to represent a situation in which the genome can manufacture an infectious polypeptide.

Other infectious causes of dementia include frontal or temporal lobe brain abscesses and chronic meningitides, such as cryptococcal meningitis, which is spread by ubiquitous spores. Although most common in immunosuppressed patients, cryptococcal meningitis is one of the only fungal meningitides that occurs in an otherwise healthy adult.

The AIDS-related dementia complex must also be considered in the initial evaluation of dementia. Inquiries about risk factors for HIV disease are often neglected in elderly persons. Consent for HIV testing can be difficult to obtain in patients with dementia. Low T cell counts are surrogate markers of HIV disease but can raise ethical questions if performed without consent. Neuroimaging such as MRI or CT with contrast delineates many of the mass lesions associated with deterioration in cognitive function in this population, but HIV-related dementia is a clinical diagnosis without clear-cut radiologic or pathologic correlation.

### Metabolic disorders

Metabolic disorders may cause gradual changes in mental status, and the aged brain is extremely vulnerable to a host of changes in the metabolic state. Mild degrees of pulmonary, renal, hepatic, or cardiac failure that would not cause mental changes in younger individuals seem capable of causing mental disease in older persons. Small imbalances in endocrine function, particularly hypothyroidism and the apathetic form of hyperthyroidism, are frequently associated with change in mental status as the dominant clinical feature. Disturbances in electrolyte balance, acid-base balance, and mild anemia or anoxia may also present with mental changes. Laboratory examinations are available to confirm or deny clinical suspicion of most of these metabolic, endocrine, or deficiency states. Even chronic constipation causes decreased mental acuity and confusion in elderly persons. Hepatic encephalopathy, common in alcoholic patients but found in patients with other forms of liver disease, produces a drowsy confusional state that sometimes may be misinterpreted as dementia.

Nutritional deficiencies are a prominent problem in elderly persons, who may lead isolated lives on inadequate incomes. This, combined with depression, may result in severe neglect of dietary intake of vitamins. The most common vitamin disorder that can produce dementia is vitamin $B_{12}$ deficiency. Most traditional American diets are rich in vitamin $B_{12}$, but occasionally, strict vegetarians can become deficient. More often, gastric surgery or pernicious anemia are the cause. Signs of a peripheral neuropathy and myelopathy are often present. Neuropsychiatric manifestations of $B_{12}$ deficiency can occur in the absence of anemia or macrocytosis. A vitamin $B_{12}$ level should be performed routinely in evaluation of dementia. In patients with other signs of $B_{12}$ deficiency, it is important to remember that tissue stores can be depleted before the serum level falls. If $B_{12}$ deficiency is strongly suspected, a normal $B_{12}$ level should prompt a request for methylmalonic acid assay, a metabolite of vitamin $B_{12}$ that is increased in $B_{12}$ deficiency.

Thiamine deficiency can produce an acute Wernicke encephalopathy, sometimes followed by Korsakoff psychosis, also known as alcoholic amnestic syndrome. Although most often seen in alcoholic patients, patients with thiamine malabsorption caused by surgery (e.g., gastric plication) or severe malnutrition have occasionally been reported to develop thiamine deficiency with neurologic effects. The classic patient is apathetic and has marked impairment of immediate and short-term memory and relative preservation of more distant memory. These patients repeat three objects, then cannot recall them after a 10-second distraction. Confabulation may occur but is not necessary for the diagnosis, and it can be induced in some patients who want to please the examiner. Recovery of memory function is variable and slow. Peripheral neuropathy, cerebellar degeneration, and other signs of neurologic damage from alcoholism are often present.

Dialysis encephalopathy refers to a syndrome characterized by dementia, language disturbance, myoclonus, asterixis, and an abnormal EEG. Evidence links it to aluminum in dialysate, and the disease has been largely eliminated by changes in dialysis procedures. Rare cases have still been reported in renal failure patients who use aluminum-containing phosphate binders. Pathologic studies show spongiform changes in superficial layers of cerebral cortex. Patients with renal failure are prone to other dementing illnesses, such as coexisting metabolic disorders or cerebrovascular disease.

### Tumors

Dementia can be a presenting feature of certain tumors that develop in the frontal or temporal lobes, especially when they are situated medially and impinge on the limbic system without causing elementary neurologic signs. Some are benign and easily resected, even in elderly persons. A subfrontal meningioma that distorts and compresses the frontal lobes in the olfactory tracts causes anosmia and lends itself to surgical treatment. Certain tumors in the midline fail to cause lateralizing signs but often result in deterioration of behavior, which may be caused by direct effects on the limbic, hypothalamic, or endocrine system or by hydrocephalus. Mental status of patients in the latter situation improves dramatically with CSF shunting, even if the tumor cannot be removed. Neoplasms can also cause dementia through more distant effects. Meningeal carcinomatosis with spread of neoplastic cells to CSF can present as dementia. Neoplasms also produce multiple metabolic disturbances that can affect mental status. Limbic encephalitis can occur as a result of antibody to neuronal cells produced as part of a paraneoplastic syndrome. In tumors involving the brain, imaging studies may provide a diagnosis. In some cases, stereotactic biopsy of the mass may be necessary for a definitive answer. Indirect effects of tumors can be more challenging. CSF studies with cytology, serum samples for neuronal antibodies, and metabolic studies should be considered in the evaluation and may need to be repeated to establish a diagnosis.

### Trauma

Trauma to the nervous system occurs frequently, particularly in patients with a history of alcoholism. Traumatic injuries to the brain are easy to diagnose near the time of the event if the patient remembers it. However, minor head injuries can produce chronic subdural hematomas, particularly in elderly and alcoholic patients. The normal loss of brain volume in aging causes a slight stretching of the veins that bridge the subdural space, allowing relatively trivial trauma to tear a vein with accumulation of blood in the subdural space. When the accumulation is unilateral, early herniation distorts the ascending reticular activating system and causes somnolence, sometimes without other focal neurologic deficits. Bilateral subdural hematomas (about 20% of cases) may not present with focal signs, and mental changes often occur without drowsiness. These patients may show an extreme degree of apathy and immobility, sometimes mistaken for advanced depression. These chronic subdural hematomas can be missed because they are isodense with brain tissue on a CT scan of the head. This is a particular problem when the hematomas are bilateral and do not produce a shift of the brain. MRI of the head can be extremely helpful in these cases (Fig. 97-3).

### Toxic causes

The most important toxic cause of dementia is prescription or over-the-counter (OTC) medications. A good dementia workup must include complete cataloging of the patient's medications and careful consideration of their possible adverse effects on the brain. There is widespread use of phenothiazines, benzodiazepines, and other mind-altering agents among elderly persons. The aged brain is particularly sensitive to such drugs. Some patients end up in chronic nursing home settings because the acute confusional state that accompanied a general medical illness was treated with a phenothiazine and/or benzodiazepine to prevent disruption of the hospital ward. The patient still receives this medication on transfer to a long-term care setting, where efforts at reducing the medications result in withdrawal states and the assumption by health care providers that the patient needs the drug. In these situations, very slow reduction of the agents allows successful withdrawal with potential clearing of sensorium.

In addition to these drugs that were developed to alter mental function, various drugs often used for general medical illnesses are capable of causing mental changes. Some examples are antihypertensives, analgesics, and $H_2$ blockers. In addition, drugs that may be well tolerated as monotherapy have prolonged half-lives, and their side effects are potentiated when used in combination with

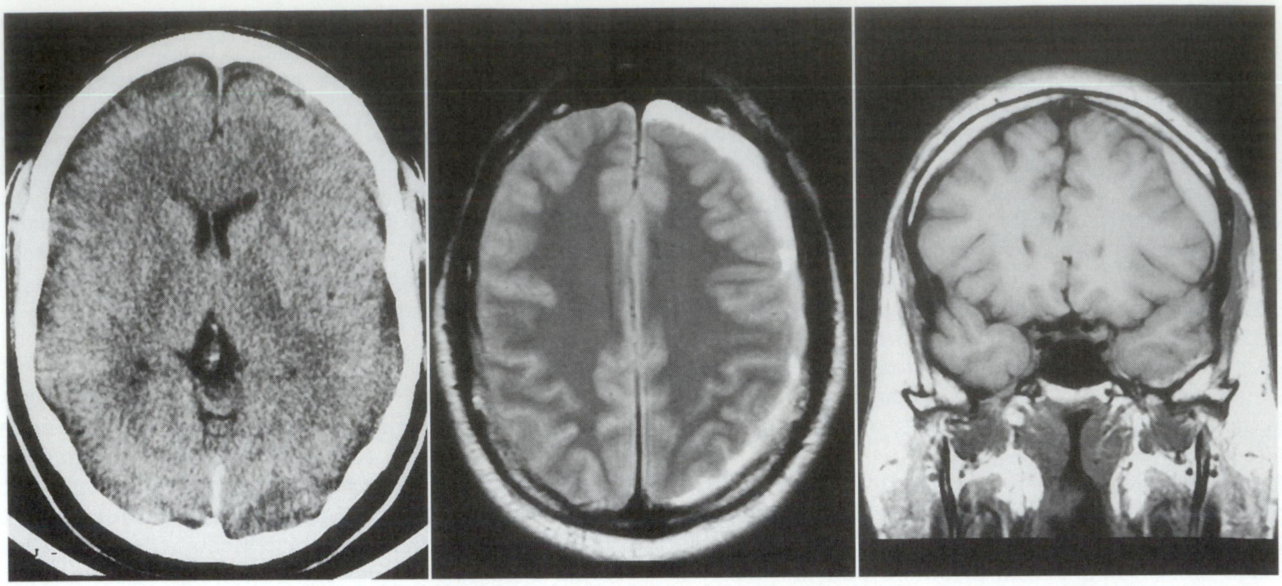

A B C

**Fig. 97-3.** Subacute subdural hematoma. **A,** Head computed tomography (CT) shows a nearly isodense subdural hematoma. **B** and **C,** With magnetic resonance imaging (MRI) the hematoma is much more apparent. **C,** Sagittal image demonstrates the mass effect of the lesion.

other medications. The average elderly patient takes multiple medications and has a higher likelihood of experiencing significant side effects. After careful review of medications, all potentially unnecessary drugs should be discontinued. In those medications deemed necessary, the lowest possible dose should be given. It is important to remember that low doses in elderly patients may produce the intended result and dramatically reduce side effects.

OTC medicines, home remedies, and folk remedies must also be considered during evaluation of patients. Patients and their families often neglect to mention the use of OTC antihistamines, sleeping preparations, and analgesics that may alter sensorium. A home visit by health care providers can be helpful if the patient allows a review of the medicine cabinet. This may also reveal a stash of expired medications that the patient may use intermittently. Patients with dementia may also use overdoses or underdoses of their medications. Calendar-type drug boxes may be helpful, but often the caretaker must dispense medications.

### Alcohol-related dementia

In addition to Wernicke-Korsakoff syndrome, which is specific to thiamine deficiency, another less clearly delineated disorder is called alcohol-related dementia. This disorder is likely a result of the combined effect of alcohol on the brain, poor nutrition, and multiple traumatic insults. The cognitive disabilities are more varied than in Wernicke-Korsakoff syndrome, including loss of memory function, visuospatial abilities, and naming. Head CT or MRI shows diffuse cerebral atrophy. Abstinence from alcohol and good nutrition may result in essentially complete recovery of cognitive function in some of these patients. The cognitive losses in the active alcoholic patient can pose considerable challenges for the clinician. The patient may be essentially incompetent while drinking and highly functional when abstinent. Alcohol rehabilitation services are critical to treatment of these patients. In the acute phases, retention of material related to alcohol avoidance is minimal because of cognitive impairment, and patient education sessions need to be repeated later in the hospital stay and in the community.

### Vasculitis

Systemic vasculitides, such as systemic lupus erythematosus, can involve the brain and cause a confusional state. These patients can be diagnosed by the systemic signs and symptoms. Vasculitis involving the brain occurs infrequently in other systemic illnesses, such as sarcoidosis and AIDS. Less often, isolated CNS vasculitis occurs without involvement of other organs and without increases in sedimentation rate or antibody titers. Cerebral angiography may show beading of blood vessels and other changes in vessel caliber but often is normal. Biopsy of meningeal vessels can show vasculitic changes in some cases. Although CNS vasculitis is a challenging diagnosis, patients do respond, at least transiently, to immunosuppressive agents.

### Sensory deprivation

Losses in hearing ability and visual acuity are common in elderly persons and, when undetected or minimized by the patient, can present as confusion. Treatment can be gratifying, with improvements noted even in those with neurodegenerative disease.

## LABORATORY INVESTIGATIONS

The evaluation of any patient with dementia should be tailored to the patient's clinical history, risk factors, and examination. The evaluation must stress the search for the most probable disorder but must also contain an evaluation for less common but highly treatable etiologies (Table 97-2). It is also important to remember that dementia can be multifactorial.

### Laboratory studies

In mild to moderate dementia, all patients should have a complete blood count (CBC) with differential, thyroid-stimulating hormone (TSH) level, vitamin $B_{12}$ level, syphilis testing (VDRL), and liver function tests. Erythrocyte sedimentation rate (ESR) and urinalysis should also be performed. These laboratory tests should be supplemented by analysis of other endocrine functions, if necessary, or arterial blood gas (ABG), ceruloplasmin, or antinuclear antibody (ANA) testing. The physician should consider HIV testing, remembering that this disease occurs in elderly as well as young persons.

### Lumbar puncture

A lumbar puncture is an appropriate examination for all patients with dementia except for those severely affected. Although positive studies occur infrequently, they often reveal the presence of a treatable etiology. The spinal tap should be deferred until imaging is performed to avoid possible brain herniation and to guide any special CSF studies. CSF should be collected with careful note of the opening pressure and the fluid's appearance. Cell count, protein, glucose, VDRL, cryptococcal antigen, and cultures should be performed. If multiple sclerosis is suspected, oligoclonal bands should also be sent. High-volume lumbar puncture is indicated in NPH.

### Imaging studies

All patients should have an imaging study at the time of the initial diagnosis of dementia. A repeat of the imaging study should be considered in patients with acute deterioration in function, particularly with development of new focal neurologic signs or any history of head trauma. CT scan of the head or MRI should be performed (see Fig. 97-3). The determination of the most appropriate test depends on the likely diagnosis, the level of patient cooperation, and consideration of any contraindications. CT scan of the head, particularly with contrast, demonstrates most mass lesions, CVAs, subdural hematomas, and atrophy. However, isodense subdural hematomas may be missed or underestimated (see Fig. 97-3), and small lesions of all types may also be inapparent. Head CT with contrast carries the risk associated with the contrast agent and cannot be performed in patients who have renal insufficiency.

For the evaluation of dementia, MRI can usually be performed without contrast. However, the MRI procedure is very difficult for claustrophobic patients and requires a higher level of cooperation than CT scanning. MRI cannot be performed in patients who have any metal in their body, including many surgical clips and metal fragments from occupational injuries (e.g., welding-related eye injuries). Pacemakers are also an absolute contraindication for MRI. The anxiety associated with MRI can be ameliorated by reassurance by the technologists, but this may sometimes need to be supplemented by a low dose of a sedating agent (e.g., a benzodiazepine) with a short half-life.

SPECT scanning may also have a role in the evaluation of patients with dementia. Characteristic patterns have been described in AD and Pick disease but have not been fully substantiated with clinicopathologic correlations. The test involves the infusion of a radionucleotide followed by a relatively brief period of imaging. It again requires some patient cooperation, but most patients can tolerate the procedure. At this stage, results should be considered supportive but not diagnostic. SPECT scanning should not be part of a routine evaluation at this stage.

### Electroencephalography

An EEG should be considered in some patients with dementia. This test is diagnostic in nonconvulsive status, showing a pattern of continuous ictal discharges. Also, a characteristic pattern is usually present in Creutzfeldt-Jakob disease. In other cases the EEG may suggest a mass lesion by showing high-voltage slow-wave activity in the area involved. However, imaging studies make this indication rarely useful. The low-voltage fast activity present with the use of sedatives may indicate a toxic encephalopathy. The EEG in certain metabolic derangements shows slowing and highly suggestive triphasic waves. However, in both these instances, other hints from the history or laboratory studies are more definitive in making the diagnosis. EEG should be considered with an abrupt deterioration in a patient with dementia if other evaluations are unrevealing.

### Neuropsychologic testing

Formal neuropsychologic testing consists of a battery of standardized tests of cognitive functions such as memory, visuospatial abilities, and language function. Intelligence quotient (IQ) testing is a well-known example. Neuropsychologists can be particularly helpful in establishing a diagnosis of dementia in early cases and in patients with high premorbid IQs. They can sometimes be helpful in supporting a diagnosis of depression by demonstrating variability in performance and patterns of losses inconsistent with a neurodegenerative process. Neuropsychologic evaluations are sometimes also performed before and after a course of treatment to help determine its usefulness.

• • •

Dementia is the result of many common and uncommon disorders. The clinician's skills and judgment are important in delineating the most likely cause and in evaluating for all potentially present, treatable causes.

## MANAGEMENT

A full account of treatments for disorders that may cause dementia would be inappropriate. These treatments may range from penicillin for neurosyphilis to shunting for NPH to discontinuation of medications. Some of these therapies are described in the section on differential diagnosis. This section presents common treatable features and an approach to the neurodegenerative disorders.

Therapy for all treatable causes must be maximized. One must remember, however, that treatable causes often do not totally reverse but can be arrested. In all patients, medications known to cause confusion should be discontinued if at all possible. The essential medications should

**Table 97-2.** Causes of dementia

| Disease | Laboratory aids to diagnosis |
|---|---|
| **Primary neurologic disease** | |
| Alzheimer's disease and senile dementia | — |
| Pick's disease | CT or MRI, SPECT |
| Huntington's disease | CT or MRI |
| Progressive supranuclear palsy | — |
| Olivopontocerebellar degeneration | MRI |
| Parkinsonism | — |
| Brain tumors | CT with contrast or MRI |
| Multiple sclerosis | CSF γ-globulin, oligoclonal banding, basic myelin protein, evoked potentials |
| Wilson's disease | Serum ceruloplasmin, urinary copper, slit-lamp examination for Kayser-Fleischer rings |
| Ceroid lipofuscinosis | Brain biopsy |
| **Vascular disease** | |
| Multiinfarct dementia | MRI |
| Lacunar state | CT or MRI |
| | CT or MRI |
| Binswanger encephalopathy | Erythrocyte sedimentation rate, specific antibodies (e.g., antinuclear antibody) |
| Cerebral vasculitis (as in systemic lupus) | |
| **Traumatic central nervous system lesions** | |
| Multiple contusions | MRI |
| Dementia pugilistica ("punch-drunk" syndrome) | — |
| Chronic subdural hematoma | CT or MRI |
| **Normal-pressure hydrocephalus** | |
| Idiopathic or following meningitis or subarachnoid hemorrhage | CT or MRI, isotope cisternography, high-volume lumbar puncture |
| **Seizures** | |
| Nonconvulsive status | EEG |
| **Metabolic disturbances** | |
| Anoxia-hypoxia | Arterial blood gases |
| Chronic hypercapnea | Arterial blood gases |
| Hyperammonemic encephalopathy | Liver function studies, serum ammonia, CSF glutamine |
| Chronic electrolyte-calcium or acid-base imbalance | Serum Na, K, Cl, $CO_2$, Ca, pH, alkaline phosphatase |
| Endocrine dysfunction, hypothyroidism, apathetic form of hyperthyroidism, Cushing disease, Addison disease | Thyroid-stimulating hormone, timed serum cortisol levels |
| Vitamin $B_{12}$ deficiency | Serum $B_{12}$ level, methylmalonic acid |
| Thiamine or niacin deficiency | — |
| Azotemia | Serum creatinine, blood urea nitrogen |
| **Toxic encephalopathies** | |
| Alcohol-related dementia | Alcohol level, aspartate aminotransferase, mean corpuscular volume (MCV) |
| Heavy metals (lead, arsenic, mercury) | 24-hour urine collection |
| Dialysis dementia | — |
| Psychiatric drugs | Blood levels where available |
| Barbiturates, bromides, benzodiazepines, phenothiazines, haloperidol, lithium, especially certain combinations (e.g., thioridazine/lithium, haloperidol/methyldopa) | Urine toxicology screening |
| Drugs used in general medicine | |
| Analgesics, antihypertensives, antidiabetic agents, digitalis preparations, cimetidine, methyldopa, propranolol, reserpine, OTC medications | |
| **Infectious-inflammatory** | |
| General paralysis | Blood and CSF tests for syphilis |
| Chronic basilar meningitis (with/without hydrocephalus) | — |
| Fungal (especially cryptococcal) | CSF cryptococcal antigen and fungal cultures |
| Syphilitic | Blood and CSF tests for syphilis |
| Sarcoid | Angiotensin-converting enzyme level, lymph node biopsy |
| Carcinomatous-leukemic | CSF cytology |
| Whipple disease of brain | Brain biopsy, periodic acid–Schiff staining of CSF cells, small bowel biopsy |
| Creutzfeldt-Jakob disease | EEG, brain biopsy |
| Brain abscess | CT with contrast or MRI |
| Progressive multifocal leukoencephalopathy | MRI |
| Limbic encephalitis | Search for occult carcinoma (usually small cell carcinoma of lung) |
| Acquired immunodeficiency syndrome encephalopathy | Human immunodeficiency virus antibodies |
| **Psychiatric** | |
| Pseudodementia of depression | Neuropsychologic testing |
| | Dexamethasone suppression test |
| Sensory deprivation | Hearing/vision testing |

*CT*, Computed tomography; *MRI*, magnetic resonance imaging; *CSF*, cerebrospinal fluid; *EEG*, electroencephalography.

be used in the lowest possible dose. Alcohol use should be discouraged in patients who have a long history of daily alcohol use; even small amounts may require detoxification in an inpatient or outpatient setting. Hearing and vision correction should be prescribed when necessary, even for patients with neurodegenerative causes such as AD, which may be worsened by visual or auditory misperceptions.

Multiple nonpharmacologic interventions are helpful for patients and their caregivers. One of the first measures is to ensure safety at home by making sure outside doors cannot be opened by the patient and stoves can be disconnected intermittently when necessary. Home visits by nurses who have trained as dementia specialists can provide valuable assistance to the family by providing safety hints and activity suggestions. Patients with wandering habits should be enrolled in the National Alzheimer Wanderers Alert Registry* sponsored by the Alzheimer's Association, which enters patients into a national data bank, provides labels for them and their clothing, and ensures access to recent, high-quality photographs of patients. Driving by the patient can be a concern. Families may hide the keys or disable vehicles if the patient has moderate dementia. In early dementia the patient and caregiver can avoid adversarial roles by finding an objective third party to arbitrate. Some state motor vehicle departments or rehabilitation hospitals will retest patients at the request of a physician or family member. In other cases the patient can be referred to a driving school for a safety evaluation.

Some general measures are also helpful in improving the level of functioning of patients with AD. Patients with dementia do better if their environment and daily routines are stable. In nursing homes, color coding of the room, stripes leading along the hallway to various shared areas, and large-print calendars with a single day on each page are all simple measures that help the patient retain orientation. "Sundowning" is a term often used to describe the agitated, confused state that may be brought on in demented patients when the level of light is reduced in their room. This problem is sometimes resolved by leaving the light on. Even during the day, many patients do better if present in a room where some activities are occurring. Frequent recreational activities keep the patient occupied, decrease catastrophic reactions, and increase positive interactions between the patient and caregiver. Activities may include reminiscence sessions, singing old favorites, art activities, and continued involvement in household duties. For instance, many patients with neurodegenerative dementia can perform tasks such as folding clothes. In these activities, it is important to tailor the task to the level of the patient's cognitive abilities. When frustration occurs over inability to perform the task, a simpler activity should be substituted.

Activities of daily living eventually deteriorate, and the patient gradually requires more and more assistance. Eating with silverware deteriorates, and substitution of finger foods is helpful. Bath time may be stressful, with the patient becoming fearful of the running water. Preparing the bath in advance may help, and sponge baths can be substituted. Dressing can be facilitated by providing each item in a stepwise fashion and eliminating choices. Incontinence is a significant stress for caregivers and often prompts nursing home referrals. Frequent trips to the bathroom can minimize accidents in early stages, and adult diapers can be used later in the course. A workup for UTIs and benign prostatic hypertrophy in males is indicated for new onset of incontinence.

Support groups are important for the patient in the early stages and for the caregiver throughout the disease. Responsible family members must be told about the features and progression of the disease. Arrangements for protection of the patient's financial affairs should be made. Early in the course of the disease, a health care proxy form should be filled out so that the decision maker in future health issues is clearly delineated. If the family understands the symptoms to be expected, the patient can often be maintained in the home setting for much longer. This is particularly true when an interdisciplinary approach is available, including access to nurses, social workers, and physicians. Literature available from the Alzheimer's Association and books written specifically for families of patients (e.g., *The 36-Hour Day* by Mace and Rabins) can be of enormous value. A recent book called *Living in the Labyrinth,* written by a person with dementia, also provides insight. Adult day-care programs can allow family members to continue working or provide them with free time for other errands and respite. Overnight respite programs are unfortunately rare, and the financial burden for these usually falls on the family. As the disease progresses, the focus becomes the caregiver, who now needs additional assistance with care and emotional support, especially when the often heart-rending decision about nursing home placement approaches.

### Pharmacologic interventions

In many patients a trial of antidepressants may be worthwhile and is outlined in the previous section on depression. Only one medication has been released for the treatment for AD—tacrine, a long-acting anticholinesterase inhibitor developed to increase availability of acetylcholine. In studies a subset of patients appear to benefit marginally according to subjective scales of quality of life and sometimes standardized cognitive testing. The starting dose of tacrine is 10 mg four times a day, increasing every 6 weeks to 20 mg, then 30 mg, and finally 40 mg four times a day. The major side effect is liver toxicity. A trial of the medication is reasonable in any patient with early to moderate AD. As with all medications, repeat cognitive testing should be performed after tacrine is started, along with questions about quality of life. If no improvement is seen, the medication should be stopped.

Medications are also used to control behaviors in patients with various forms of dementia. One of the most common medications is haloperidol, which can be used to decrease aggressive behaviors. Although haloperidol should be used with caution, a low dose can sometimes maintain a patient in the home for longer periods. Aggressive outbursts resulting in injury to family members are common reasons for placement in a nursing home.

*National Alzheimer Wanderers Alert Registry and educational materials, Alzheimer's Association National Headquarters, 919 North Michigan Ave., Suite 1000, Chicago 60611-1676, (800) 272-3900.

Benzodiazepines are also used in some patients to ameliorate aggressive behaviors. With both haloperidol and benzodiazepines, the potential for buildup of the drug must be considered, and frequent reevaluation of the dose is essential. Sleep disruptions may also require drug treatment (e.g., benzodiazepines) but can sometimes be treated by establishing a bedtime routine.

## INDICATIONS FOR NEUROLOGIC CONSULTATION

Any patient with an unclear diagnosis should be referred to a neurologist for further evaluation. If the dementing process is accompanied by elementary neurologic findings such as hemiparesis, asymmetric reflexes, and visual field disturbances, the patient should be seen in consultation. An atypical course of the dementia, particularly unexpectedly rapid decline, should also prompt referral. Referrals to interdisciplinary settings that specialize in the evaluation and treatment of dementia can also be helpful in the initial diagnostic workup and in behavioral management. These centers can provide the patient and family members with additional support.

• • •

The evaluation of a patient with dementia can be disheartening to a physician. Although it may be difficult to deliver the bad news to the patient and family, it often comes as a relief to them. Knowing the reason for the deterioration lets them know that they are not "going crazy." Nonpharmacologic treatments, particularly the support of a knowledgeable and caring physician, can make tremendous improvements in quality of life for both the patient and the caregiver.

## BIBLIOGRAPHY


Clark RF, Goate AM: Molecular genetics of Alzheimer's disease, *Arch Neurol* 50:1164, 1993.

Consensus Conference: Differential diagnosis of dementing diseases, *JAMA* 258:3411, 1987.

Evans DA et al: Prevalence of Alzheimer's disease in a community population higher than previously reported, *JAMA* 262:2251, 1989.

Friel McGowin D: *Living in the labyrinth,* San Francisco, 1993, Elder Books.

Kemper TL: Neuroanatomical and neuropathological changes in normal aging and dementia. In Albert M, editor: *Clinical neurology of aging,* Oxford, 1984, Oxford University.

Larson EB et al: Diagnostic evaluation of 200 elderly outpatients with suspected dementia, *J Gerontol* 40:536, 1985.

LeMay M: CT changes in dementing disease: a review, *Am J Neuro Rad* 7:841, 1986.

Mace NL, Rabins PV: *The 36-hour day,* Baltimore, 1981, Johns Hopkins University.

Max W: The economic impact of Alzheimer's disease, *Neurology* 43(suppl 4):S6, 1993.

McKhann G et al: Clinical diagnosis of Alzheimer's disease: report of the NINCDS-ADRDA Work Groups under the auspices of Department of Health and Human Services Task Force on Alzheimer's Disease, *Neurology* 34:939, 1984.

Sabin TD, Vitug AJ, Mark VH: Are nursing home diagnosis and treatment inadequate? *JAMA* 248:321, 1982.

Simon RP: Neurosyphilis, *Arch Neurol* 42:606, 1985.

Skoog I et al: Population based study of dementia in 85-year-olds, *N Engl J Med* 328:153, 1993.

Wells CE: Pseudodementia, *Am J Psychiat* 136:895, 1979.


CHAPTER

# 98 Cerebrovascular Disease


**Kinan K. Hreib**
**Nagagopal Venna**


## EPIDEMIOLOGY

Stroke (CVA) is the third leading cause of death in the United States, accounting for about 150,000 deaths a year. Approximately 500,000 new strokes occur each year, accounting for substantial disability and enormous health care cost. It is estimated that in 1993, the cost of medical care of acute stroke, rehabilitation, and loss of productivity was about $18 billion. As many as 70% of survivors of CVA have impaired work capacity 7 years after the ictus; approximately 28% of these patients are under age 65. These persons, who form a productive part of the work force, suddenly become disabled and are often unemployable after their recovery.

Cerebrovascular disease affects men and women and people of all ages. Data from several stroke registries and from long-term follow-up of patients participating in the Framingham Study reveal that in the population under age 30, the incidence of CVA is similar in men and women, estimated at 0.10:1000 per year. In those under age 44 the incidence increases to approximately 0.15:1000 per year in both men and women. With increasing age the incidence in men surpasses that in women. From ages 45 to 55 the incidence of CVA in men, 2.2:1000 per year, is approximately double that in women. Between ages 55 and 65 the annual incidence is 4.5:1000 for men and 2.8:1000 for women. The incidence in women approaches that in men between ages 65 and 74, with an approximate annual incidence of 9.0:1000. In elderly persons ages 75 to 84 the annual incidence of CVA in men increases again to approximately 19:1000 versus 15:1000 in women. The type of strokes that affect women is similar to that affecting men, but certain types are more prevelant in certain age groups. For example, arterial dissection and subarachnoid hemorrhages are more common in the younger population, whereas atherothrombotic and embolic CVAs are more common in older people. Incidence of CVA is approximately 60% higher in African-Americans than in the white population. Death from CVA also appears to be higher in men and African-Americans. The box at right lists types of CVAs and their incidence.

Advances on several fronts of medical science, including new diagnostic techniques, better long-term follow-up, and reliable epidemiologic data, have provided opportunities to expand our knowledge of stroke mechanisms and treatments. Each type of CVA demands a different diagnostic and treatment approach. The aim of this chapter is to enable the physician to identify the different types of CVAs, to design an approach to treatment based on the known pathophysiology, and to review the known benefits of medical and surgical interventions of the different CVAs.

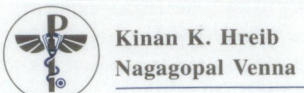

**Types of cerebrovascular accidents (CVAs, strokes) and their incidence**

| | |
|---|---|
| **Infarction** | |
| Atherothrombotic and lacunar | 45% |
| Embolic | 25% |
| Transient ischemic attacks (TIAs) or minor strokes | 20% |
| **Hemorrhage** | |
| Aneurysmal | 4%-44% |
| Intraparenchymal | 10% |

These data were compiled from the literature (see Bibliography). The incidence varies significantly depending on the population studied and their ages.

## PATHOPHYSIOLOGY OF CEREBRAL ISCHEMIA: HEMODYNAMICS

The degree of hemodynamic instability resulting in a neurologic deficit depends on multiple factors, including the degree of stenosis, the presence of collaterals, and autoregulation. Cerebral blood flow (CBF) depends on cerebral perfusion pressure and cerebrovascular resistance. Under normal circumstances, the cerebral perfusion pressure is equal to arterial pressure. Therefore, when the cerebral perfusion pressure is normal, changes in CBF depend on changes in the cerebrovascular resistance. This resistance, in turn, depends on several factors, including the blood's viscosity and the blood vessel's length and radius. Although the length of a given blood vessel is constant, other factors are influenced by a variety of physiologic changes, such as a change in hydrogen ions. The effect of viscosity on CBF is uncertain. Most studies of hyperproteinemia suggest that, at least in the large vessels, hyperviscosity has little effect on CBF.

The role of arterial endothelium in cerebral autoregulation has become better appreciated in recent years. The endothelium produces endothelium-derived relaxing and constricting factors. Damage to the endothelium may occur during periods of hypoxia, chronic hypertension, atherosclerotic disease, or hyperglycemia, resulting in inappropriate response to changes in cerebral perfusion. Compounded by arterial stenosis, the loss of autoregulatory mechanisms may become deleterious. However, the degree of carotid artery stenosis that may result in significant CBF abnormalities distally is not known. Using positron emission tomography (PET) scans, researchers have investigated the relationship of carotid artery stenosis to cerebral hemodynamics and the association with CVAs. During a 1-year follow-up of 30 symptomatic patients with carotid artery disease, the investigators were unable to demonstrate a relationship among the degree of stenosis, hemodynamic changes, or the rate of CVAs. However, these studies revealed that a decrease in blood flow to the brain may be compensated for by the extraordinary ability of the neurons to increase oxygen and glucose extraction from the remaining blood. Therefore, it seems that the failure of these compensatory mechanisms, especially the loss of local dilatation of blood vessels and reduced oxygen extraction, ultimately leads to the development of neurologic symptoms.

The brain has the unique capacity for collateral circulation through the circle of Willis, connecting the carotid arteries with vertebral basilar arteries and the contralateral counterparts. Similarly, a complex anastomotic network among the pial vessels of the anterior, middle, and posterior cerebral arteries provides another mechanism of compensation for inadequate CBF. Extensive collaterals also can develop between the extracranial and intracranial vessels. These collaterals can be so efficient that if occlusion develops gradually, total occlusion of both internal carotid arteries may be asymptomatic. The occurrence of symptoms or signs of cerebral ischemia therefore depends not only on fixed arterial lesions, but also on an intricate interplay among several of these dynamic factors.

## TRANSIENT ISCHEMIC ATTACKS

### Pathophysiology

In 1955, Millikan and colleagues outlined the symptoms associated with transient ischemic attacks (TIAs) of the internal carotid and vertebral arteries. Their observations indicated that carotid artery TIAs are often stereotyped; episodes consist of abrupt, temporary, focal neurologic deficits that typically last 2 to 15 minutes but occasionally as long as 24 hours. More prolonged symptoms, often lasting up to 6 weeks, have been referred to as *reversible ischemic neurologic deficit* (RIND). Recent studies have shown that in 50% of TIAs, the symptoms resolve within 1 hour. In patients with neurologic symptoms lasting more than 60 minutes, the likelihood that the symptoms will completely resolve is less than 2%. These observations are supported by a significant number of patients with TIAs having a demonstratable CVA in areas appropriate to the symptoms on computed tomography (CT) or magnetic resonance imaging (MRI).

The time limit initially imposed on the definition of TIAs may have confounded our understanding of the mechanisms of transient ischemia and complicated the interpretation of outcome after interventional therapy. The importance of TIAs and RINDS is that they reflect the presence of occlusive vascular pathology sufficiently severe to alter brain function, which needs to be recognized so that treatment to prevent permanent ischemia can be instituted.

Emboli and hemodynamic crises are suspected to be major causes of TIAs. Other plausible explanations include platelet, cholesterol, and fibrin emboli or focal sensitivity to changes in hemodynamics; the latter is especially important when both carotid arteries have severe stenosis. Temporal arteritis and hypercoagulable states are often overlooked causes of amaurosis fugax.

### Clinical features

The most common symptoms reported during carotid artery TIAs (see box on left on p. 1344) include painless loss of vision in one eye (amaurosis fugax); a motor deficit such as weakness, clumsiness, or paralysis; sensory abnormalities such as tingling or numbness affecting half the body or restricted to the face or arm or leg; and dysarthria or aphasia. Usually the symptoms of weakness

### Symptoms associated with carotid artery disease

Monocular blindness: sudden and painless
Aphasia
Dysarthria
Motor symptoms: clumsy hand, transient hemiparesis or monoparesis
Sensory symptoms: hemibody numbness or tingling, or arm and face paresthesias

and sensory changes accompany dysarthria or aphasia, depending on the hemispheric dominance, but amaurosis fugax usually occurs in isolation. The visual symptoms accompanying amaurosis vary. The best known is the "shade" dropping in front of the eye; however, this description is clinically the least common. "Looking through ground glass" is perhaps a more common description by patients when part or all of their visual field is affected. Rarely, scintillating visual images may be described and may easily be confused with symptoms accompanying migraine. Sunlight-induced dimming of vision occurs even more rarely.

TIAs in the vertebrobasilar artery area are more complex (refer to the box at right) and often poorly described by the patient. Some of these symptoms include transient episodes of vertigo, nausea, vomiting, unsteadiness, headaches, loss of vision in one half of the visual field or bilateral blindness with or without scintillations, sensory changes, and dysarthria. The repertoire of clinical presentations reflects the structures supplied by the basilar artery, which include the cerebellum, ascending and descending sensory and motor pathways of the brainstem, cranial nerve nuclei, medial temporal lobes, occipital lobes, and thalami. Vertebrobasilar ischemia has several distinctive features. Bilateral or crossed limb weakness with or without paresthesias and paresthesias affecting the face, especially the gums, cheeks, and tongue, are especially suggestive of vertebrobasilar TIAs. Diplopia and disequilibrium from involvement of the cerebellum or the vestibuloocular centers are also common features of posterior circulation ischemia.

Vertigo or "dizziness" is a common complaint in any medical practice and usually not related to TIAs unless other neurologic features are present (see Chapter 10 for discussion of syncope). A typical TIA often has sudden onset of diplopia, vertigo, and unsteady gait, usually accompanied by an occipital headache, and lasts for few minutes or few hours. The symptoms are usually nonpositional and not replicated by any maneuvers. However, occasional TIAs may be induced by neck extension, which reduces the flow in the posterior circulation. During the rare symptom of "drop attacks," patients suddenly loose body tone and drop to the floor abruptly, without loss of consciousness.

## Natural history

The highest risk for CVA is immediately after an episode of TIA. A prospective study of 469 patients diagnosed with TIAs followed for an average of 4 years revealed that the risk of CVA was 6.6% in the first year and 3.4% per year on average over the first 5 years. The strokes occurred in the same vascular territory as the initial TIAs in about two thirds of patients. The type of strokes was variable, including lacunar strokes, hemorrages, and infarcts. In addition, the risk of coronary events during the first 5 years after a TIA was similar to the risk of CVA, and the mortality rate from either was 6.5% per year. Therefore, it appears that the risk of vascular disease and death is higher in patients who first present with TIAs and that TIAs represent a warning of more serious cerebral events as well as silent coronary artery disease. The recognition of TIA as ischemia to the brain is critical in preventing future disabling strokes. The primary care physician should recognize TIAs as "angina" of the brain and act quickly to prevent further complications. Unfortunately, only a third of patients who have CVAs experience warning TIAs.

### Symptoms associated with vertebral artery disease

Vertigo: usually associated with diplopia, dysarthria, or disequilibrium
Motor difficulties: clumsiness or paresis, usually bilateral or crossed limb weakness
Sensory abnormalities: such as perioral paresthesias, bilaterally on face and/or limbs
Visual symptoms: visual scintillations, "floating clouds," or loss of vision, usually bilateral in the corresponding visual fields
"Drop attacks": very rare, with no loss of consciousness

## Diagnosis

It is important to realize that TIAs describe symptoms and that the diagnosis is based on clinical grounds because laboratory tests only provide supportive evidence. One cannot diagnose TIAs by angiography, and similarly, not all patients with anatomic vascular lesions experience TIAs. The location of the event should be related to the vascular distribution of the anterior and posterior circulation. The tempo of the onset, the duration, and any associated symptoms should be recorded so that TIAs can be differentiated from other causes of transient neurologic difficulties (see the box at right). For example, focal sensory seizures may be difficult to differentiate from TIAs. However, seizures are often shorter in duration than TIAs, lasting only a few seconds. Hypoglycemia can cause similar symptoms but is usually accompanied by other systemic signs. The neurologic symptoms of complicated migraine often have a characteristic deliberate evolution over 20 to 30 minutes and regression over a similar period. Subdural hematomas may be difficult to differentiate from TIAs and should be considered routinely in this context. A detailed history of the symptoms and a search for cardiovascular risk factors provide supportive evidence. Examination of the patient should focus on vascular abnormalities that may contribute to symptoms, such as the presence of carotid bruits, atrial fibrillation, cardiac

### Other disorders mimicking TIAs

Focal seizures: paroxysmal, brief, usually only few seconds to 1 minute, mainly seen with structural brain lesions such as tumors
Subdural hematomas: usually in elderly persons; symptoms indistinguishable from TIAs reported with this condition
Migraines: especially complicated migraines
Multiple sclerosis: usually in young persons
Hypoglycemia: usually in patients with insulin-dependent diabetes mellitus (IDDM), accompanied by other systemic symptoms such as diaphoresis, hunger, and tremulousness

murmurs, evidence of cardiomegaly or congestive heart failure, baseline blood pressure, and asymmetry in limb pulses. Once a diagnosis of TIAs has been established, the appropriate supportive test should be obtained to document the nature and extent of the arterial lesions to help in planning treatment and determining prognosis.

## Laboratory investigations

The tests of choice are rapidly changing. At present, for suspected carotid artery ischemic attacks, a carotid Doppler study is a reasonable first test. In many centers, magnetic resonance angiography (MRA) of the neck vessels is emerging as the test of choice. MRA noninvasively and rapidly provides information regarding both carotid and vertebral vessels. Furthermore, it is capable of evaluating distal flow in the intracranial vessels, especially at the circle of Willis. One of the major limitations of MRA at present is its sensitivity to motion. In an uncooperative patient, the information obtained from an MRA may be severely compromised by artifact. Other disadvantages are that MRA does not reveal the extent of collateral circulation, the precise morphology of the abnormality, and does not differentiate between severe stenosis and complete occlusion.

The rapid pace of improvement in MRA technology, however, will soon make this test the first step in evaluating patients with TIAs. An increasing number of vascular surgeons are making decisions about surgical intervention based on the MRA. Once carotid artery disease, on the appropriate side, has been established, either by Doppler studies or by MRA, digital substraction angiography (DSA) may still be required. This procedure has some risk, but it remains the "gold standard" for defining intracranial disease. The complications associated with the procedure include permanent neurologic deficits, which may occur in 4% of patients, a reaction to the contrast material, and the development of a local hematoma. The need for DSA depends on the quality of the noninvasive studies and the preference of the vascular surgeon, as well as the individual circumstances in any given patient.

## Treatment

The principal modes of therapy are carotid endarterectomy, antiplatelet treatment, and anticoagulation.

*Carotid endarterectomy.* The effect of surgery in high-grade carotid artery stenosis (greater than 70%) was evaluated for the first time in a multicenter randomized trial, the North American Symptomatic Carotid Endarterectomy Trial (NASCET). Surgery was shown to reduce the risk of ipsilateral CVAs at 2 years by 17%. However, this study had several strict inclusion criteria that selected the surgeons with the lowest overall complications, patients who had an ischemic event less than 120 days before surgery, and those who did not have tandem lesions. Based on the NASCET study, carotid endarterectomy combined with best medical treatment has become the treatment of choice for patients with recently symptomatic carotid atherostenosis greater than 70%, but short of total occlusion, and provided it is done by an experienced team with low morbidity in their patients. The importance of selecting a surgical team with a good track record in carotid endarterectomy cannot be overemphasized. Even with these appropriate indications, systematic evaluation of other common variables in each patient is needed so that the presence of tandem intracranial lesions, occlusion of the contralateral carotid artery, and severe systemic disease are taken into account. In asymptomatic patients and in those with less than 70% stenosis, the benefits of surgical intervention have not yet been determined but are being actively investigated. Therefore, at this point, patients with carotid artery stenosis less than 70% are treated medically.

*Medical treatment.* The most frequently used medical treatments are intravenous (IV) heparin, coumadin, aspirin, or ticlopidine.

**Heparin and Coumadin.** The anticoagulant effect of heparin depends on its ability to bind to antithrombin III, which then inactivates several clotting factors, primarily thrombin and activated factor X. In addition, heparin binds to the endothelium and prevents the binding of platelets to the blood vessel wall. Even though heparin is widely used in the treatment of TIAs, its efficacy has never been evaluated properly. In a small trial, 27 patients were assigned to IV heparin and 28 to aspirin. During a mean treatment period of 6 days, TIAs occurred in 30% in the two groups, but CVAs occurred in 4% of the heparin group and 14% of the aspirin group. Although this trial demonstrated some benefit to heparin, the small sample size prevents meaningful conclusions. Furthermore, there is an inherent limitation to the use of heparin because of such local factors as fibrin binding to thrombin, which causes heparin to lose its ability to inactivate thrombin. Similarly, thrombin bound to the subendothelial surface is also protected from inactivation by heparin. The efficacy of heparin in the treatment of TIAs has not been proved, but heparin continues to be widely used in the immediate and short-term treatment of transient ischemia in the hope of preventing major CVAs. At our institution, heparin is used during the acute management and evaluation of TIAs.

The precise role of coumadin in TIAs has not been delineated. Coumadin is effective in diminishing or sometimes abolishing atherosclerosis-related TIAs, but it has not been conclusively shown to prevent subsequent cerebral infarctions. Neurologists with experience in this area empirically suggest coumadin as having a particular role in patients with TIAs as a result of vertebrobasilar stenotic disease and in those who continue to experience TIAs despite antiplatelet agents. In addition, coumadin is indicated in patients in whom TIAs are caused by a cardiogenic or aortic source of embolism. Because of potential serious bleeding complications during long-term treatment with coumadin, several factors, such as concurrent bleeding diathesis, reliability of the patient in monitoring bleeding parameters, and propensity for falls, have to be systematically considered before embarking on this path.

**Antiplatelet Agents.** Aspirin interferes with the synthesis of prostaglandins by inhibiting the enzyme cyclooxygenase. This leads to reduced production of thromboxane $A_2$ and thus the impairment of platelet aggregation. This platelet inhibition, however, is not absolute because exposed collagen and increased levels of circulating thrombin may still induce platelets to aggregate via alternate pathways.

Several clinical trials have evaluated the benefits of aspirin in patients with TIAs or minor CVAs. The first large-scale randomized landmark clinical trial used 1300 mg of ASA a day. Other studies since then have tested the efficacy of different doses of aspirin, attempting to define the optimal smallest dose to decrease overall vascular mortality. In 1991 the Dutch TIA Trial randomized patients to receive 30 mg or 283 mg of ASA a day. In all these studies, there was an overall reduction of CVA and death by 18%. However, the only study that directly measured the efficacy of aspirin against strokes was the UK-TIA Study Group, in which 300 mg was compared with 1200 mg of aspirin daily or a placebo. In that study, there was a 15% reduction in all vascular events and deaths, but only a 7% reduction in disabling CVAs and death. Similarly, the Swedish Aspirin Low-dose Trial investigated the efficacy of 75 mg of ASA compared with a placebo. The researchers' conclusion was similar to that in the UK-TIA Study Group. The aggregate evidence from these large trials demonstrated that large-dose aspirin is as effective as low-dose aspirin in reducing fatalities from vascular deaths or disabling CVAs. Interestingly, the use of ASA in asymptomatic patients demonstrated no benefits in the reduction of strokes but did demonstrate a substantial reduction in myocardial infarctions (U.S. Physicians' Health Study, 1989). At present, aspirin is the most widely used agent for carotid and vertebrobasilar atherosclerotic TIAs, with or without carotid endarterectomy. Although minidoses (80 mg/day) and conventional doses (1300 mg/day) of aspirin are effective, it is not clear whether they are equally effective, and the optimal dose for the individual patient remains controversial.

Ticlopidine is a newly introduced antiplatelet agent that inhibits the adenosine diphosphate pathway of the platelets, a mechanism that is distinct from that of aspirin. Its efficacy in stroke prevention was studied in two large clinical trials. In the first trial, patients with TIAs or minor CVAs were randomized to receive ticlopidine or aspirin. The overall event rates at 3 years for a nonfatal stroke or death was 10% for ticlopidine and 13% for aspirin. In the second trial, patients with a recent CVA were randomized to receive either ticlopidine or placebo. The treatment with ticlopidine resulted in 30% reduction in vascular events. These trials demonstrated some benefit to ticlopidine over aspirin and a significant benefit over placebo. However, the rare side effect of leukopenia and its cost have prevented its widespread use. In our institution, enterically coated aspirin, supplied only in 325 mg tablet, is used first. If the patient develops unacceptable side effects to the aspirin and or recurrent TIAs, ticlopidine at a dose of 250 mg twice a day is used, assuming no change in the underlying pathology. Some evidence also suggests that ticlopidine may be more efficacious than aspirin in preventing TIAs in women. We also recommend coumadin in those with TIAs or minor CVAs who demonstrate a recurrence of symptoms despite antiplatelet drugs or who have had embolic CVAs from a fixed lesion in the appropriate internal carotid artery or an aortic or a cardiac source of embolism. See Managed Care Guide for TIAs with CVAs.

**Managed Care Guide**
**TIA/minor CVAs (in carotid artery distribution)***

Single or multiple episodes
↓
Stabilize blood pressure and anticoagulate
↓
Carotid Doppler studies and/or magnetic resonance angiography
↓
Four-vessel digital substraction angiography
↓
- More than 70% stenosis (in symptomatic artery) → Surgery
- Less than 70% stenosis
  - Ulcerating plaque → Surgery (controversial)
  - Stable stenosis → Medical drug therapy

*These are general guidelines. Therapy should be dictated by each patient's condition and other systemic problems.

*Modification of risk factors.* Since TIAs are usually caused by atherosclerosis, which is a multiorgan disease, modification and treatment of the factors that aid and accelerate the progression of atherosclerosis is important. These include optimal long-term control of elevated blood pressure, cessation of tobacco smoking, and control of diabetes. The beneficial effects of controlling hyperlipidemias are expected but not yet proved in relation to symptomatic cerebral atherosclerotic disease. One more fundamental advance would be finding ways to cause regression of the underlying atheroma itself.

## CEREBRAL INFARCTIONS

### Embolic infarction

Embolic CVAs (strokes) account for at least one fourth of all strokes. Patients may present with sudden onset of symptoms, some may complain of a prodrome, and others may have transient symptoms climaxing with a CVA. Seizures are a more common presentation in embolic strokes than other strokes because of involvement of the cortex, especially in patients with diabetes. The symptoms

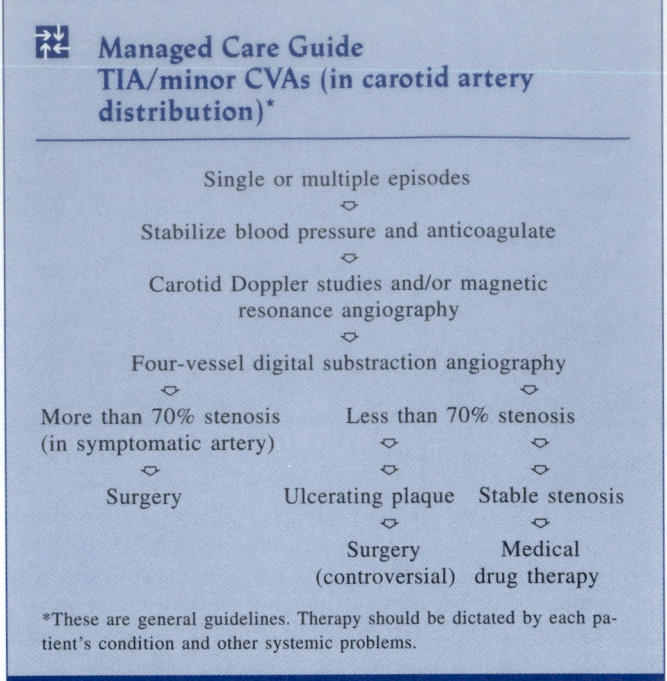

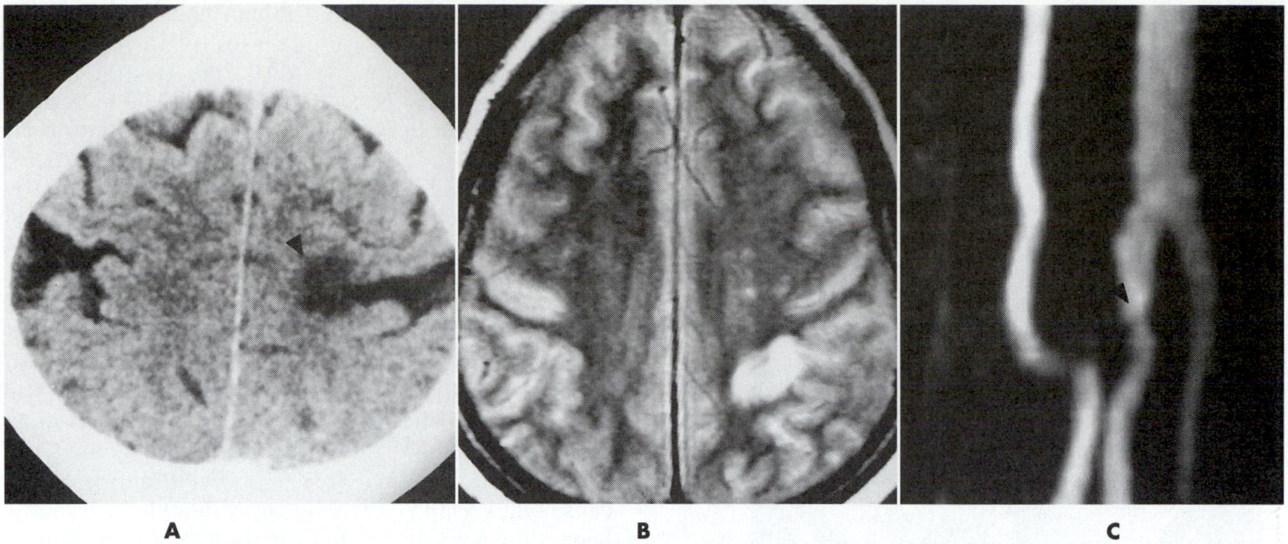


**Fig. 98-1.** Embolic stroke (cerebrovascular accident, CVA). **A,** Computed tomography (CT) image demonstrating a small area of hypodensity in the depth of the sulcus *(arrowhead)*. **B,** Magnetic resonance imaging (MRI) of the same patient demonstrates an obvious area of increased signal in the left parietal area. The source of the embolus was from the left internal carotid artery. **C,** Magnetic resonance angiography (MRA) shows good flow in the common carotid artery and a moderate amount of disease in the left internal carotid (*arrowhead*). The vertebral artery is also visualized in this image.

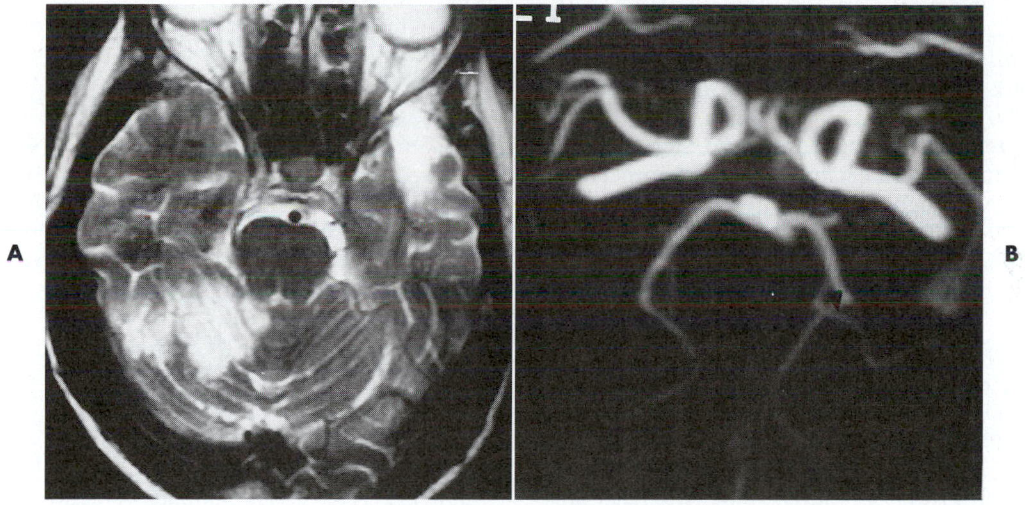


**Fig. 98-2.** Embolic stroke. **A,** MRI demonstrates an area of increased signal in the cerebellar hemisphere. **B,** MRA in the same patient demonstrates an occlusion of the right superior cerebellar artery. The arrowhead points to the intact left superior cerebellar artery.

depend on the size of the embolus and the vascular territory involved. The infarctions tend to be hemorrhagic. These hemorrhages reflect reperfusion of infarcted brain matter. Reperfusion may also be documented on angiography, since initially the blood vessel(s) involved will be occluded, but within 72 hours, repeat angiography usually will demonstrate patency of the same vessel, reflecting fragmentation or dissolution of the embolus. Although most emboli go to the middle cerebral artery territory, any vascular territory may be involved, and some emboli are large enough to occlude the internal carotid artery. Furthermore, contrary to previous assumptions, most posterior circulation strokes are embolic, either from the heart or from a proximal arterial source.

Figs. 98-1 to 98-3 show CT and MRI images of embolic CVAs (infarctions).

***Clinical presentation and diagnosis of cerebral embolism.*** The differentiation of embolic from thrombotic CVAs is based on clinical findings in embolic stroke. The symptoms are usually abrupt, with maximal deficit at onset followed by improvement. The embolus may involve

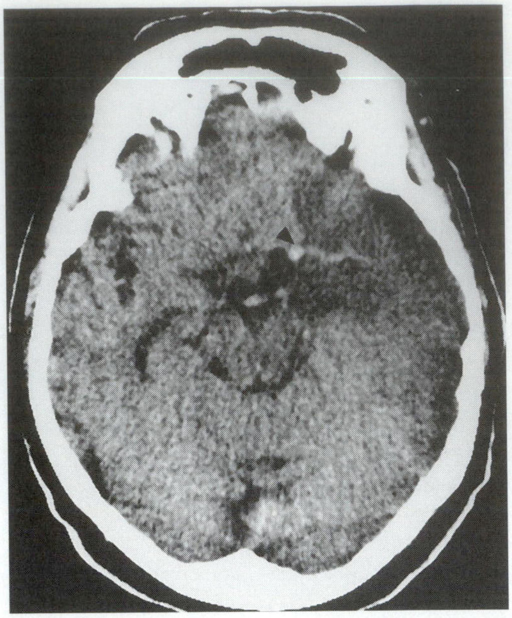

**Fig. 98-3.** Early CT image of a left middle cerebral artery infarct showing a clot/thrombus in the artery (*arrowhead*).

branches of major vessels, and multiple vascular territories may be involved. Clinicoradiologic evidence of superficial infarctions within the cortical arterial branch territories are particularly characteristic of embolism. Evidence of limb or visceral embolism and source of the embolism (e.g., atrial fibrillation) strengthen the diagnosis of cerebral embolism.

As most physicians can appreciate, the source of an embolus can be elusive. Fisher and Adams examined 179 brains of patients with cerebrovascular disease at Boston City Hospital in 1949. The diagnosis of embolus was made in 57 but only clearly demonstrated pathologically in 26. The source of the embolus was from the left atrium in four patients, a mural thrombus in the left ventricle in three, atheromatous ulcer in the ascending aorta in one, and atrial fibrillation in the remaining patients. Therefore, in more than 50% of autopsy cases, an embolus was never found or the source identified. More recent studies have suggested that the most common source of emboli is from the extracranial arteries, a source that was perhaps underestimated in previous studies (see the box on the left on p. 1349).

The search for the source of the embolus can be extensive. Often the history, neurologic examination, and basic admission laboratories help in explaining the etiology of the CVA and guide further investigations. Electrocardiography may demonstrate anterior wall myocardial infarction (MI), atrial enlargement, or atrial fibrillation. Hematuria or unexplained renal impairment may represent systemic emboli. Transesophageal echocardiography (TEE) has increased the detection of cardiac and thoracic aortic sources of embolism.

***Cardiac emboli.*** Atrial fibrillation has been recognized as a major cause of emboli in the elderly population. The estimated risk for CVAs in patients with atrial fibrillation who do not have valvular disease is one in three. The incidence of strokes in those who have atrial fibrillation with mitral valve disease increases by 18-fold. Similarly, in the presence of endocarditis, the risk of neurologic complications may be as high as 30%. The increased risk of embolization in patients with atrial fibrillation and or mitral stenosis results from left atrial blood stasis, which may be detected on TEE as spontaneous echo contrast or "smoke." Smoke reflects microaggregates of erythrocytes or platelets. In one study, 9 of 42 patients with spontaneous contrast had CVAs or peripheral embolisms, compared with 1 of 40 control subjects. More importantly, that study demonstrated that 6 of 12 patients in atrial fibrillation and with demonstrable spontaneous echo contrast had strokes versus 1 of 28 patients with atrial fibrillation but without echo contrast. The presence of echo contrast is clearly a high risk for embolization. Other cardiac sources include mitral valve prolapse. This is probably an overestimated cause of CVAs in young women. Although the prolapse has been shown to result in formation of fibrin deposits or annular thrombus, it has rarely been associated with strokes. Ventricular wall dyskinesia has been known to be associated with embolic CVAs, but the true incidence of mural thrombi was not known until the introduction of echocardiograms. Left ventricular mural thrombi occur in at least 38% of patients with MI, especially with anterior wall infarction. Risk of embolization from left ventricular thrombi has been estimated at 20%. Studies of patients with ventricular aneurysm reveal a very low risk for embolization.

Studies and case reports have emphasized the importance of atrial septal defect (ASD) as a source of paradoxical emboli responsible for strokes in patients under age 55. A 1986 CVA study demonstrated that at least 40% of patients with a CVA of presumed embolic etiology had a right-to-left shunt, compared with 10% of patients without a CVA. Pulmonary hypertension and the Valsalva maneuver may promote embolization via a right-to-left shunt. However, more recent studies have demonstrated no relationship between right-to-left shunt and CVAs. Therefore, at this time, ASD as a source of emboli remains controversial, and further clinical studies are warranted.

***Artery-to-artery emobilization.*** Arterial dissection had been considered a rare cause of CVAs, but a recent review of the literature suggests that it may be responsible for one in every four CVAs in patients under age 45. Arterial dissection usually presents with either transient neurologic symptoms or minor strokes and may evolve to cause a complete occlusion of an artery. Dissection is most often associated with pain in the involved area and, depending on the proximity of the dissection to the carotid bifurcation, Horner syndrome. The process is usually associated with some trauma, which may be very minor. Significant aortic arch disease is usually present in the elderly population. Necropsy studies have revealed significant aortic arch disease in 60% of patients with CVAs (see Fig. 98-2).

### Thrombotic infarction

A thrombus usually results in occlusion of the stem of the artery or, much less frequently, one of its major branches. The occlusion may be slow, resulting in progressive neurologic deficits, or may be preceded by TIAs. The

### Source of emboli

**Cardiac disease**

Myocardial infarction: usually with anterior wall myocardial infarction; (MI), echocardiogram used, (ECG), with echocardiography for hypokinesis
Atrial fibrillation: very high risk, especially in the presence of spontaneous echo contrast on transesophageal echocardiography; ECG used, with Holter monitoring.
Atrial septal defect/patient foramen ovale: controversial; paradoxical emboli in patients with pulmonary hypertension or peripheral venous thrombosis
Atrial septal aneurysm
Valvular disease: bacterial endocarditis, valvular heart disease, nonbacterial thrombotic endocarditis

**Arterial**

Atherosclerosis: of carotid or vertebral arteries with or without an ulcerating plaque; stenosis of intracranial arteries may also promote formation of emboli
Aortic disease: Arch and/or ascending aorta
Dissection: TIA-like prodrome, pain in the area of dissection; Horner syndrome present if dissection is at carotid bifurcation

pathophysiology of the thrombotic process is poorly understood. By far the most common cause of cerebral arterial thrombosis is atherosclerosis. The extracranial carotid and vertebral arteries are now recognized as the major sites of atherothrombosis. Intracranially, the basilar artery and stem of the middle cerebral artery are other common locations for atherosclerosis. It appears that intracranial atherothrombosis is more prevalent among blacks. Less common causes of arterial thrombosis are dissection, hypercoagulable states, and arteritis. A complete occlusion of a major artery may lead to a large infarction, extensive cerebral edema, and even cerebral herniation syndromes.

***Clinical presentation and diagnosis of cerebral thrombosis.*** Clinically, preceding TIAs strongly indicate a thrombotic process. A "stuttering" course or a stepwise accumulation of focal neurologic deficits characteristically occurs over 24 to 48 hours with carotid artery disease. However, the thrombosis may evolve over 4 to 6 days, as seen in basilar artery thrombosis. Risk factors such as arterial bruits, hypertension, and other systemic signs of vascular disease provide supportive evidence. MRA may demonstrate atherostenosis of the carotid, vertebral, basilar, or other intracranial arteries. Fig. 98-3 shows a CT image of a cerebral artery infarct.

## Treatment of cerebral infarction

***Anticoagulation.*** The efficacy of anticoagulation in the prevention of CVAs has only been studied in association with a few selected cardiac diseases (see the box above). The benefit of anticoagulation in patients with left ventricular thrombus is still not known. However, warfarin therapy should be considered, especially during the first four months after an anterior wall MI, when the risk of embolic CVA from the thrombus is highest. Clear

### Anticoagulation in acute CVAs (strokes): indications and contraindications

Indications: small to moderate-size embolic stroke, by clinical examination; atrial fibrillation, anterior wall MI, arterial dissection, cervical or intracranial arterial atherosclerosis, aortic arch disease, arterial thrombosis and progressing stroke, well-documented paradoxical emboli
Contraindications: large stroke, by clinical examination; uncontrollable hypertension, bleeding tendency from underlying systemic disease (e.g., thrombocytopenia)

beneficial effect for anticoagulation in atrial fibrillation has been shown in three large-scale studies. The Boston Area Anticoagulation Trial for Atrial Fibrillation, completed in 1990, randomized patients to warfarin or placebo. This study demonstrated an 86% reduction in relative risk of major embolic events. In another study, from the Veterans Administration, the risk reduction in the warfarin group was 79%. The role of aspirin in atrial fibrillation was evaluated by the Stroke Prevention in Atrial Fibrillation Trial, completed in 1991. Patients were randomized to receive 325 mg of aspirin daily, warfarin, or placebo. This study demonstrated an incidence of major strokes in the placebo group of 6% per year; those receiving aspirin, 3.6% per year; and those taking warfarin, 2.3% per year. Finally, the Copenhagen AFASAK Study demonstrated no benefit to 75 mg of aspirin daily compared with coumadin or placebo. Therefore, although aspirin seems to have some effect of reducing the risk of embolic CVAs in patients with atrial fibrillation, coumadin therapy is superior. The treatment of dissection is anticoagulation with heparin followed by coumadin. The appropriate regimen of anticoagulation in an actively dissecting artery is not known, but we have tended to maximize the effect by adding aspirin and by maintaining the partial thromboplastin time (PTT) above 1.5 times normal.

Most medical centers tend to anticoagulate patients with carotid atherothrombosis, although the benefit in that setting is not known. In fact, a recent report of prolonged transcranial Doppler ultrasonography monitoring of patients with minor CVAs demonstrated that despite anticoagulation, cerebral embolization occurred in all patients at a frequency of 4.1 per hour. Similarly, anticoagulation is frequently used in "progressing" strokes. A substantial number of patients demonstrate some progression of their symptoms within the first 4 days of CVA onset, which may be as high as 30% in vertebrobasilar CVAs. Again, the use of heparin in progressing strokes, at least for now, has not been shown to be of clear benefit. It is possible that a subset of patients do benefit from heparin, as suggested by the empiric experience of many stroke specialists. However, this subgroup of patients has not yet been defined. Therefore, using anticoagulation in the acute management of stroke should be guided by the underlying pathology and the predicted risks and benefits.

Clearly, one of the major potential complications of anticoagulation is uncontrollable bleeding. As discussed earlier, embolic CVAs or border-zone infarcts often develop hemorrhagic transformation. The incidence of

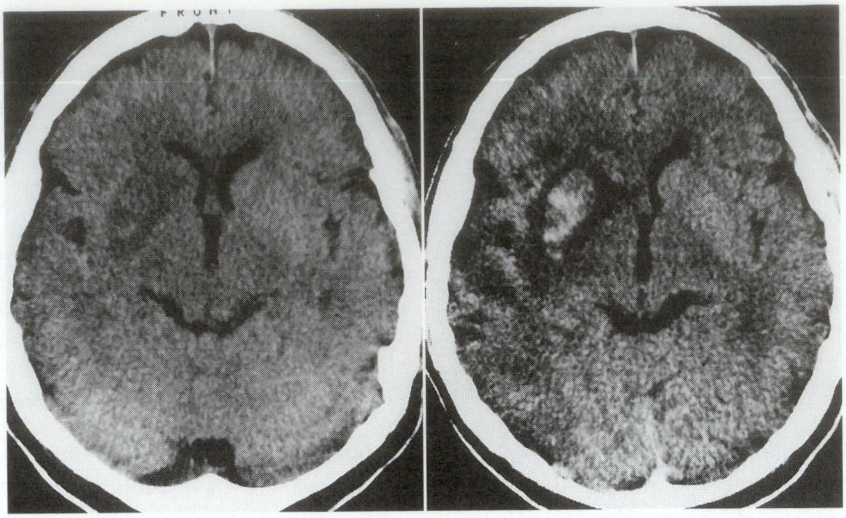

A B

**Fig. 98-4.** Two CT images demonstrating the hemorrhagic transformation of an infarct. **A,** Effect of a deep middle cerebral artery infarct with a hypodense area in the right basal ganglia. **B,** Blood with some mass effect in the same area 2 days later.

such change was not known until the introduction of CT scanning, which has revealed that many embolic strokes exhibited changes in signal on CT consistent with delayed bleeding. With the introduction of MRI, it was soon discovered that approximately 70% of patients with presumed embolic CVAs demonstrate some evidence of delayed hemorrhage. It was feared that in this setting, in which a "white" infarct becomes a "red" infarct, anticoagulation may be deleterious. This notion received some support from a study of 28 patients who were anticoagulated with heparin for presumed cardioembolic strokes. Three of those patients developed cerebral hemorrhage. This and other scattered case reports, as well as anectodal experience of some clinicians, suggested that anticoagulation of patients with embolic CVAs may promote bleeding and therefore should be contraindicated. Several investigators have retrospectively analyzed data from patients who received anticoagulation at the onset of their stroke. These reports have suggested that the poor outcome was the result of the development of hematomas in association with large infarcts, a PTT time greater than twice the control, and excessively elevated blood pressure. In patients with a high risk for recurrent embolization, anticoagulation should be weighed against the risk of cerebral hemorrhage. Uncontrollable severe hypertension, which in isolation increases the risks of cerebral hemorrhage, is a relative contraindication for anticoagulation. The size of the ischemic area is more controversial, but clinical experience suggests that the larger the infarction, the more likely that immediate anticoagulation will induce cerebral hemorrhage. The exact intensity of anticoagulation is being reexamined. With atrial fibrillation but without valvular disease, low-intensity anticoagulation (1.2 times the control) seems adequate. On the other hand, more intense anticoagulation (2.0 to 2.5 times the control) is indicated in patients with valvular heart disease or an artificial valve. The duration of anticoagulation is indefinite if the underlying cardiac abnormality is persistent but may be much more limited (6 to 12 months) in patients with MIs (Fig. 98-4).

Antithrombolytic therapy was introduced to treat patients with embolic or thrombotic CVAs in the hope of reestablishing blood flow and restoring function to previously ischemic areas. Streptokinase and urokinase were the first agents to be used for this purpose. They act systemically by converting plasminogen into plasmin. Early trials using this approach were associated with serious hemorrhagic complications. Therefore, more selective antithrombolytic agents with a shorter half-life were developed. Tissue-type plasminogen activator (t-PA) is now undergoing multicenter clinical trial for the treatment of strokes within 4 hours of onset of the ictus but remains as an experimental treatment at this time.

Our practice, at the Boston City Hospital, has been to anticoagulate patients who are in atrial fibrillation, who have evidence of arterial dissection or ventricular thrombus; have demonstrated evidence of repeated embolic events, even if the source cannot be found; and in the presence of a right-to-left shunt. With a large infarct, we to repeat the CT scan 48 to 72 hours after the ictus to determine whether hemorrhaging has occurred. The risks and benefits of anticoagulation are then reevaluated.

***Surgery.*** Surgery plays a small role in acute brain infarctions, whether embolic or thrombotic. In very rare cases of large right cerebral hemispheric infarction with cerebral herniation, life may be saved by hemicraniectomy with decompression of the swollen hemisphere. However, surgery has a very important role in cerebellar infarctions, which, if large, can cause sudden death by tonsillar herniation, obstructive hydrocephalus, and brainstem compression. Early recognition and neurologic consultation can lead to shunting, to relieve the hydrocephalus, and posterior fossa decompression. The outcome from prompt surgical intervention in cerebellar CVAs is often excellent, with minimal deficits 6 months after the infarction, as long as the cerebellar roof nuclei are not excised.

***Antiedema agents.*** Despite their widespread use, no evidence indicates that dexamethasone and mannitol have any lasting benefit or make a clinically significant difference in the treatment of ischemic brain edema. This is in contrast to the well-documented benefits of these agents in edema caused by metastatic disease or brain abscess.

## Lacunar infarction

Small vessel infarcts, or "lacunar strokes," are the most common complication of untreated hypertension. These CVAs are in the territory of the small penetrating arterioles supplying subcortical structures. Two basic abnormalities in the small vessels of patients with lacunar strokes were first described by Fisher, lipohyalinosis and microatheromatous disease. Lipohyalinosis, which is more often found in hypertensive patients, is characterized by the presence of atheromas in the arteries as well as hyaline and connective tissue in the arterioles. For many years, lacunar strokes have been synonymous with hypertensive strokes. This unfortunate relationship was never intended when this entity was first described. Since then, other investigators have found that the relationship between hypertension and lacunar infarcts is not exclusive and that less than 50% of patients with lacunar CVAs have hypertension. Other mechanisms for lacunar strokes include emboli, atherosclerosis, thrombosis, hypercoagulable states, and vasospasms.

***Clinical presentation and diagnosis.*** The usual presentation of lacunar CVAs is the sudden onset of unilateral paresis associated with dysarthria and facial weakness. However, since most of the white matter, thalamus, and pons could potentially be affected by this pathology, the clinical syndromes are heterogenous. The clinical course varies, but approximately 20% of patients worsen within the first 24 hours. The reason for this exacerbation is not fully understood but may reflect excessive iatrogenic lowering of blood pressure or local dysfunction of hemodynamics. Progression may also reflect that the pathology underlying lacunar strokes is heterogenous.

MRI is the most sensitive imaging technique that readily detects acute lacunar infarct on T2 imaging. Typically in a patient with a lacunar CVA, several other silent lacunes (lacunae) are also revealed by MRI, indicating preexisting vascular disease secondary to hypertension. It is probably prudent to evaluate the larger arteries in the neck noninvasively as well because of frequent coexistence of large and small vessel disease. With brainstem lacunes, syphilis should also be ruled out, especially in young patients and patients positive for the human immunodeficiency virus (HIV). Deep infarcts, especially in the basal ganglia territory, may also result from tuberculous meningitis and should be considered in the appropriate setting.

## Complications of hypertension

Hypertension is the major risk factor in approximately 50% of all patients with CVAs. Untreated hypertension increases the risks for intraparenchymal and possibly subarachnoid hemorrages and causes deep, small vessel strokes. Longstanding hypertension has been shown to result in accelerated atherosclerosis in the carotid and vertebral arteries as well as in the penetrating intracerebral vessels. Disease of the penetrators is most frequently seen in the white matter, putamen, thalamus, and pons. Therefore, it is not surprising to find that most CVAs in hypertensive patients are located in these areas.

Hypertension results in loss of autoregulation and thus the ability of the cerebral vasculature to adjust to hemodynamic changes. Autoregulation is most effective when the mean blood pressure is 60 to 150 mm Hg. Initially, uncontrollable hypertension leads to upward adjustment of autoregulatory mechanisms. Eventually these mechanisms begin to fail as the endothelium becomes less responsive to circulating factors. The combination of local pathology of the small penetrating vessels as well as loss of the autoregulatory mechanism can cause diffuse white matter ischemia or focal infarcts. Untreated hypertension results in several distinct syndromes, including hypertensive encephalopathy, multiinfarct dementia, small vessel infarcts, and lacunar strokes.

Hypertensive encephalopathy may result from untreated idiopathic hypertension or from abuse of sympathomimetics. It is associated with a sudden increase in blood pressure that exceeds the upper limit of cerebral autoregulation. This syndrome is characterized by headache, confusion, lethargy, seizures, and papilledema. MRI may reveal superficial cortical infarcts, focal subcortical infarcts, and diffuse edema. The treatment is aimed at gradually reducing the blood pressure and maintaining the mean at 120 mm Hg.

Ischemic dementia (Binswanger disease) results from chronic and poorly controlled hypertension. MRI shows abnormal confluent white matter signals most prominent in the periventricular areas and centrum semiovale. These changes may be the result of small infarcts, deficient blood supply to the distal penetrators, or chronic extravasation of circulating factors through damaged endothelium. Some evidence suggests that wide fluctuations in blood pressure, often induced by hypotensive drugs, may play an important role in the genesis of this condition. The boxes below and on p. 1352 list consequences of hypertension and outline common lacunar syndromes (Fig. 98-5).

***Treatment.*** Several studies have now clearly demonstrated the beneficial effects of treating hypertension. Studies of the population of Rochester, Minn, and Minneapolis–St. Paul revealed approximately a 50% decline in the incidence of CVAs that coincided with the introduction of effective antihypertensive medications. Treatment of isolated systolic hypertension in patients over age 60 is also associated with significant reduction of

### Consequences of hypertension

Basal ganglia hemorrhage
Lobar hemorrhage
Thalamic hemorrhage
Cerebellar hemorrhage
Pontine hemorrhage
Lacunar infarcts
Hypertensive encephalopathy
Vascular dementia/Binswanger disease
Accelerated atherosclerotic disease

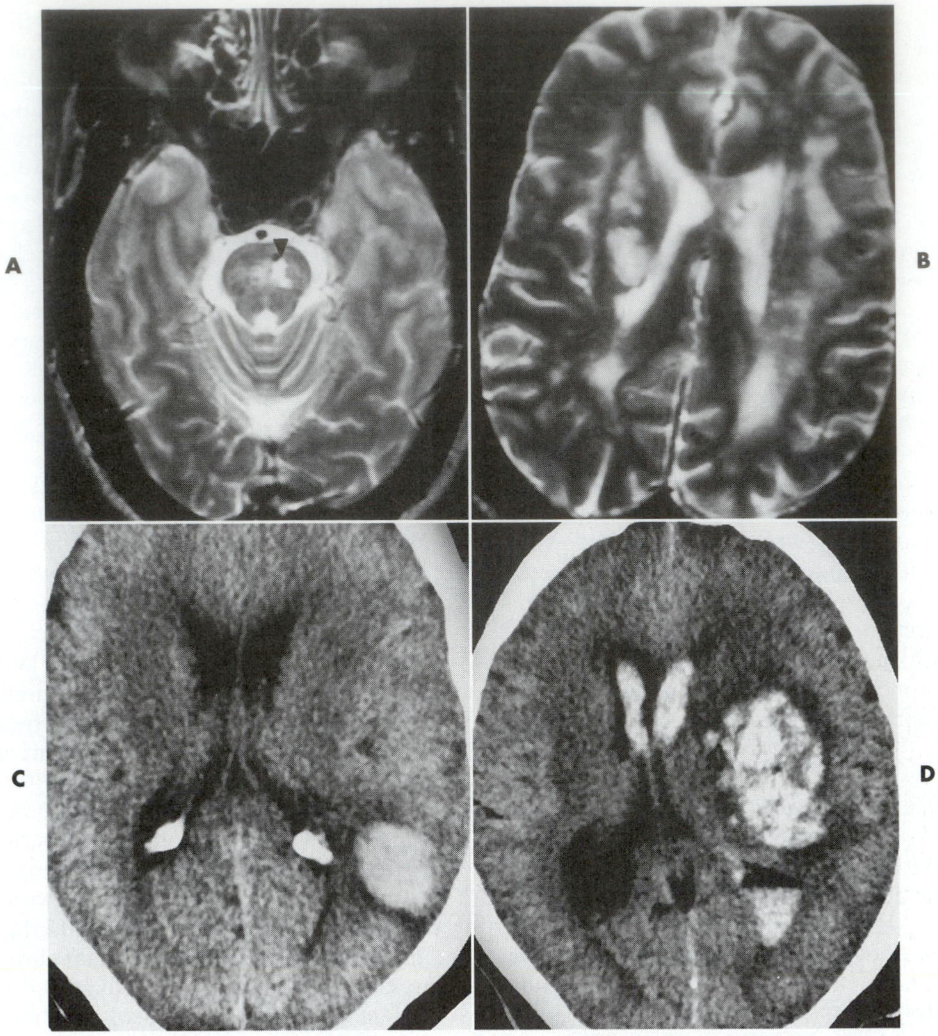


**Fig. 98-5.** Complications of hypertension. **A,** T2-weighted MRI scan demonstrating a lacunar infarct in the left pons (*arrowhead*). **B,** T2-weighted MRI scan showing extensive paraventricular white matter disease. **C,** CT image showing a small cortical aneurysmal bleed. **D,** CT image of large basal ganglia bleed with extension into the ventricles.

### Clinical presentation of common lacunar syndromes

Internal capsule: symptomatic if in the posterior limb; usually results in contralateral hemiparesis or hemiplegia

Thalamus: symptomatic if in the posterior thalamic nuclei; usually results in contralateral hemisensory loss to all modalities

Pons: base of pons—monoparesis or dysarthria with clumsy hand; small penetrators in the pons—internuclear opthalmoplegia, leg weakness, and ataxia

strokes and cardiovascular events (SHEP Cooperative Research Group, 1991). A lacunar infarction is a sign of longstanding hypertension with target organ injury and offers the opportunity for long-term, systematic treatment of hypertension to prevent further CVAs. The role of anticoagulation and particularly antiplatelet agents, in addition to the treatment of hypertension, for lacunar infarction has not been studied. Poorly controlled severe hypertension has been considered a relative contraindication for anticoagulation.

### Border-zone infarcts

These types of infarcts, also known as *watershed infarcts,* result from severe ischemia to areas bordering on major vascular territories where the terminal branches of blood vessels meet. A landmark study by Romanul and Abramowicz (1964) investigated the underlying pathology of border-zone infarcts. One group of patients had severe

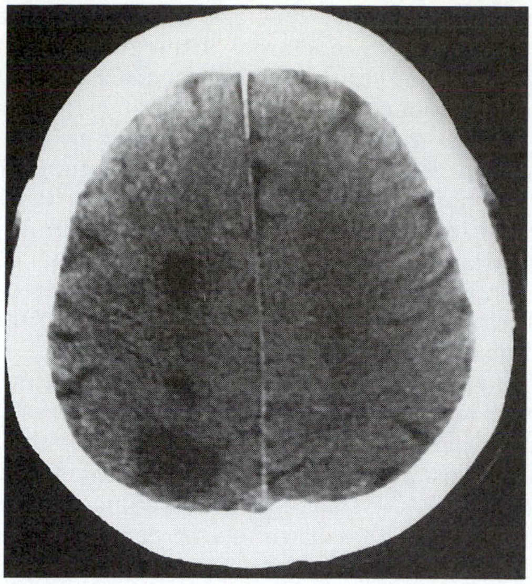

**Fig. 98-6.** CT image of deep border-zone infarct after cardiac surgery. The small hypodense areas in the white matter of the right hemisphere are in small penetrating vessels vulnerable to sudden changes in perfusion pressure.

bilateral carotid artery disease and previous episodes of TIAs or minor CVAs. The border-zone infarct in these patients was preceded by a significant drop in blood pressure during hospitalization or after surgery. The infarcts involved the cortex and the underlying white matter, usually triangular in shape and most often located between the terminal branches of the anterior and middle cerebral arteries. The second group of patients had severe intracranial atherosclerotic disease and the onset of ischemia resulted in slow neurologic deterioration. The infarcts in these patients were in the depth of the sulci involving deep layers of the cortex and the white matter. Several symptoms have been reported preceding watershed infarcts including TIAs, and in some patients, TIAs were clearly induced by a drop in blood pressure. Other symptoms at presentation include syncope in 37%, focal myoclonic jerks in 12%, and headaches in 8%. Severe unilateral stenosis or obstruction may be found in 90% of the patients and severe bilateral carotid disease in 55% of the patients. In the group of patients with severe carotid artery disease, the blood flow to the cerebrum may be supplied by collaterals via anastomoses of the ophthalmic artery with the external carotid artery or from collateral flow via the circle of Willis. The capacity of these collaterals to continue to provide sufficient blood flow becomes severely compromised during sudden drops in perfusion pressure, directly affecting pial vessels and their anastomoses. Similarly, in those patients with patent carotid arteries, the distal branches of the middle cerebral artery and its anastomoses with the anterior cerebral artery are most vulnerable to sudden changes in cerebral perfusion pressure.

Management of these patients depends largely on the time of presentation. TIAs clearly warrant evaluation of the neck vessels, as discussed earlier. Syncope without neurologic deficits is usually not related to carotid artery

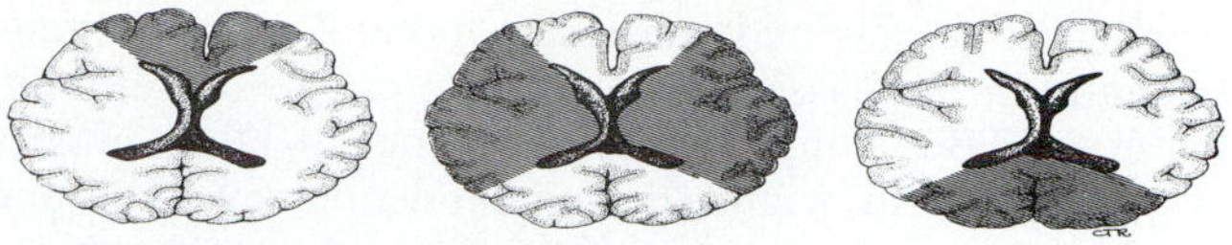

**Fig. 98-7.** Border-zone territories as seen on horizontal cuts of the brain.

disease, and a cardiogenic source should be investigated (see Chapter 10). Preventing significant drops in blood pressure is probably the most important part of management, and anticoagulation with heparin may prevent the complete occlusion in severely stenotic vessels.

Figs. 98-6 and 98-7 show a CT image of a border-zone infarct and border-zone territories.

### Nonatherosclerotic cerebral infarctions

***Vasculitis.*** Vasculitis is a rare cause of CVAs. A large variety of diseases may cause vascular inflammation; some may cause systemic disease such as hypersensitivity vasculitis, polyarteritis nodosa, and Wegener granulomatosis; and others cause isolated central nervous system (CNS) disease. The vascular pathology may be diffuse, causing multiple cerebral infarcts in the gray and white matter, but usually the vasculitis causes focal cerebral infarcts or subarachnoid or cerebral hemorrhages. The clinical manifestations vary from radiculopathy and polyneuropathy, as may be seen with Wegener granulomatosis, to intracerebral hemorrhages, as may be seen in Behçet disease. The onset may be acute to subacute, and manifestations may include altered mental function, headaches, hemiparesis, stupor, and seizures.

The most common inflammatory disorder resulting in isolated CNS disease is referred to as *granulomatous angiitis.* Characteristically, the vasculature of the leptomeninges and the cortical mantle is segmentally affected and infiltrated by lymphocytes, plasma cells, and macrophages. Patients typically have subacute behavioral and cognitive changes, with seizures and stroke syndromes steadily progressing over a few weeks to months without signs of systemic illness. Cerebrospinal fluid (CSF) mononuclear pleocytosis and elevated protein are present in most patients. Cerebral angiography is abnormal in approximately 50% of patients demonstrating "beading," which indicates focal narrowing and poststenotic dilatation. Brain and meningeal biopsy may be positive in 70% of patients.

Treatment includes a course of cyclophosphamide and prednisone. Small-scale studies have shown that this approach produces clinical remission.

***Infections and strokes.*** Several infectious diseases may lead to cerebral infarction by causing inflammation of the blood vessels. Syphilis, before the age of antibiotics, was the most important cause of CVAs in the young. A characteristic endarteritis obliterans affects penetrating vessels, causing small infarctions in the tertiary stage of syphilis. Meningovascular syphilis is reemerging as an important cause of strokes in HIV-infected patients. Clinically, CVAs are quite similar to lacunar infarctions in the brainstem or cerebral hemispheres. Tuberculous (TB) meningitis can cause an obliterative arteritis of the basal meningeal vessels and can result in cerebral infarctions, typically in the basal ganglia. Stroke can be a presenting feature of TB meningitis. The resurgence of TB meningitis in patients with acquired immunodeficiency syndrome (AIDS) and in those with resistant TB strains make this an important but an unusual cause of CVA in modern practice. AIDS patients develop cerebral infarctions without a definite secondary cause; these have been attributed to HIV vasculopathy, an entity that as of yet is not well defined. Aspergillosis and mucormycosis are also important infectious agents that may cause CVAs in the immunocompromised patient.

***Drug-induced strokes.*** The use of alkaloidal cocaine, or "crack," has been associated with a variety of strokes, including intraparenchymal and subarachnoid hemorrhages as well as infarcts. Vasculitis, although less common in cocaine users, has now been reported in several cases of infarcts and hemorrhages. This is in contrast to an inflammatory vasculopathy that is well described with amphetamine use. In cocaine users, another mechanism of CVA is cardiogenic embolism secondary to MIs with subsequent development of mural thrombi or cardiomyopathy with severe hypokinesis.

The use of oral contraceptives has been linked for many years to CVAs in young women. The underlying mechanism causing strokes is not known. However, it is believed that the use of oral contraceptives prevents or limits the deformability of red blood cells, therefore promoting thrombogenesis. However, it is likely that the tendency to promote clot formation is augmented by a substrate of procoagulant tendency, such as a protein C deficiency. The combination of tobacco smoking with oral contraceptives seems to increase substantially the risk for cerebral thrombosis.

***Antiphospholipid antibody syndrome.*** Antiphospholipid antibodies refer to antibodies directed against several phospholipids containing proteins that form an essential part of hemostasis. The estimated prevalence of antiphospholipid antibodies in healthy people is 2% to 5%. The neurologic disorders associated with these antibodies are variable but include TIAs, retinal vascular disease, cerebroarterial thrombosis, seizures, headaches, and encephalopathy. The anticardiolipin antibody assay includes testing for IgG, IgA, and IgM. All are associated with venous or arterial thrombosis or the generation of emboli. Although venous thrombosis is prominent peripherally, arterial thrombosis usually affects the cerebral vasculature. Screening for the anticardiolipin antibody is indicated in patients who have early onset of cardiovascular disease or systemic venous thrombosis and in those under age 55 who have a CVA, early dementia, or retinal hemorrhages.

Treatments of antiphospholipid antibody syndrome are controversial and include a combination of coumadin and aspirin and, in more severe cases with recurrent cerebral infarctions, prednisone and even plasma exchange.

### Venous infarcts

Venous infarcts are rare and are caused by thrombosis of the venous sinuses and/or the cortical veins, most often in the superior sagittal sinus. The factors that predispose to thrombosis include head trauma, brain tumors, meningitis, hypercoagulable states, oral contraceptives, postpartum period, paroxysmal nocturnal hemoglobinuria, Crohn disease, ulcerative colitis, and Behçet disease. Headache is the most common presenting symptom. However, the symptoms are quite heterogenous, including acute-onset of focal and generalized seizures, obtundation, motor or sensory abnormalities, and gait difficulties. Particularly characteristic complaints are visual scintillation accompanied by cortical blindness, reflecting the predilection of venous infarction to the occipital lobes. Infarcts in the frontal parasagittal area cause focal seizures of the lower extremities and weakness of one or both legs.

CT may show the empty delta sign, present in 20% of patients. The delta sign is seen after injection of contrast material, which fills patent veins surrounding the nonfilling, thrombosed sinus. MRI clearly provides a major advantage over CT. The T1 and the T2 images reveal lack of flow void as well as surrounding parenchymal hemorrhages.

The long-term prognosis varies, depending primarily on the underlying etiology, the level of consciousness at presentation, and the mass effect, but in most patients the prognosis is excellent because the arterial supply is spared. The acute management is aimed at limiting the increased intracranial pressure, controlling seizures, and correcting the underlying cause. Heparin has been shown to be beneficial in the acute treatment of sinus thrombosis, and coumadin is usually necessary for long-term management of the condition.

## INTRACRANIAL HEMORRHAGE

### Cerebral hemorrhage

Recent studies indicate that cerebral hemorrhage (CH) accounts for 10% to 30% of all CVAs (strokes). Hypertension is the single most important cause, responsible for approximately 45% of all CHs. The most common areas of the brain that develop CHs in hypertensive patients are the putamen, the thalamus, the cerebellum, the pons, and the subcortical white matter of the cerebral hemispheres (lobar hemorrhages).

Lobar hemorrhages deserve special attention because the underlying pathology of these bleeds is heterogenous. The most common causes of lobar hemorrhages are hypertension, amyloid angiopathy, venous malformation, tumors, and vasculitis (see the box on left on p. 1355). Amyloid infiltration of cerebral vessels is common in elderly persons and has been estimated to be responsible for as many as 40% of lobar hemorrhages. The most common site for these bleeds is in the occipital area. However, multifocal lobar hemorrhages have also been reported. It is well recognized that arteriovenous malformations (AVMs) have a high rate of recurrent bleeding. Hypertension may also lead to lobar hemorrhages. Bleeding from tumors accounts for approximately 10% of all intracerebral hemorrhages. The most common metastatic tumors that can hemorrhage include lung cancer, melanoma, choriocarcinoma, and hypernephroma. Glioblastoma is associated with CH in 6.4% of patients. Vasculitis is a rare cause of lobar hemorrhages. Bleeding diathesis may cause brain hemorrhages, which tend to be multifocal, small, and widespread, especially those related to thrombocytopenia and disseminated intravascular coagulation (DIC). Anticoagulant-related hemorrhages can be unifocal and large.

### Common causes of cerebral hemorrhage (CH)

Hypertension: most often seen in the basal ganglia and thalamus, but also in the pons, cerebellum, and subcortical white matter
Amyloid angiopathy: in the elderly, usually in the occipital area, may be multifocal
Arteriovenous malformation: in young patients, may be in any part of the brain
Tumors: most common tumors to bleed are metastatic melanoma, bronchogenic carcinoma, choriocarcinoma, and renal cell carcinoma. Primary tumors of the brain such as glioblastoma and pituitary adenoma may also present as a CH.
Bleeding diathesis: thrombocytopenia, DIC, anticoagulation
Drug induced: cocaine, amphetamine, phenylpropanolamine (diet pills)

### Symptoms of CHs at different locations

Lobar: headaches, seizures, hemiplegia, aphasia, conjugate eye deviation to the side of the lesion and away from the hemiparesis
Thalamic: headaches, hemisensory loss, hemiparesis, small pupils, obtundation, "wrong-way eyes"—conjugate deviation of eyes toward the hemiparetic side, "down and in" deviation of eye on the side of the thalamic hemorrhage
Basal ganglia: headaches, obtundation, hemiplegia
Cerebellar: headaches, dizziness, inability to walk, hemiataxia, nystagmus, obtundation; midline cerebellar hemorrhage may only develop headaches and a gait ataxia without limb ataxia and therefore may be missed if gait is not tested
Pontine: headaches, coma, quadriparesis, pinpoint pupils, neurogenic hyperventilation

***Clinical presentation and diagnosis.*** The presentation of these CVAs varies with the size and location of hemorrhage. Patients with small hemorrhages may only have a mild headache, especially patients with lobar bleeds. At the other extreme the patient may suddenly lapse into coma. Putamenal hemorrhage encroaches on the internal capsule, which results in contralateral hemiparesis and gaze paresis with eyes deviated away from the hemiplegia. Hemorrhage in the thalamus tends to result in both hemisensory and motor deficits, since thalamic hemorrhages encroach on the adjacent internal capsule; conjugate deviation of the eyes to the paretic side and down and inward deviation of the ipsilateral eye with small pupils are characteristic findings. Similarly, pontine hemorrhages produce pinpoint pupils, hyperventilation, and coma with bilateral motor deficits as well as gaze abnormalities. Expanding hematomas within the brainstem damage the reticular activating system and may lead to obstruction of the fourth ventricle and death. Similarly, cerebellar hemorrhages also may result in early ventricular obstruction and death unless promptly diagnosed and treated. In most patients the onset of neurologic symptoms is catastrophic, with steady worsening over a few hours to 48 hours rather than stepwise. The box at right lists symptoms of CHs at different locations.

CT is extremely sensitive to acute CH and readily differentiates ischemic CVA from hemorrhage. MRI of the brain is often difficult to obtain acutely, but in the diagnosis of acute CH, MRI is not as sensitive in demonstrating acute blood. However, MRI is helpful in determining the etiology of the bleed. For example, MRI may reveal the classic appearance of a glioblastoma or the venous and arterial network of an AVM.

***Prognosis.*** The prognosis of the different bleeds depends most importantly on the volume of blood and the level of consciousness at presentation. Small lobar hemorrhages, especially high convexity, are associated with a good prognosis. Blood in the deeper structures such as the thalamus or the basal ganglia, depending on the size, may result in coma. Under pressure, deeper hematomas may dissect through the surrounding tissue and leak into the ventricles. The overall mortality from large intracerebral hemorrhage with extension into the ventricles has been estimated at over 80% within 30 days. Interestingly, if patients survive the hemorrhage, the eventual neurologic recovery is much better than in patients with infarctions in the same regions of the brain. Hemorrhages under pressure tend to dissect through the fiber system, and unless the local oxygen supply is compromised, the neurons and their fiber system near the focus of the bleed may be affected minimally (Fig. 98-8).

***Treatment.*** Medical treatment is designed to prevent brain herniation and to reduce the mass effect on adjacent brain structures while the edema and the blood are being resorbed by the brain. This subject has been extensively reviewed by Ropper and Rockoff. Based on the level of consciousness at presentation, free-water restriction may be sufficient to prevent further edema. However, water restriction does not imply fluid restriction, and IV fluid in the form of normal saline is usually given. Normal saline has been chosen because it will remain in the vascular space and has higher osmolarity than serum, which minimizes fluid shifts into the CNS. If there is evidence of increasing intracranial pressure and decreasing consciousness, it becomes necessary to intubate the patient and begin hyperventilation. The optimal arterial partial pressure of carbon dioxide is 28 to 35 mm Hg. Osmotic diuretics may be used intravenously to lower intracranial pressure. Mannitol is the diuretic of choice for controlling increasing intracranial pressure. The initial dose is usually 1g/kg, then 0.25 g/kg every 4 to 6 hours.

The role of urgent control of blood pressure in the context of acute CH is controversial because a moderate increase in blood pressure often normalizes with watchful rest alone. No good evidence suggests that the high blood pressure in this setting is the driving force for continued expansion of the hematoma. On the other hand, aggressive control of blood pressure to normal levels can be detrimental, especially if the patient has premorbid chronic hypertension. Rapid reduction of blood pressure may cause "brain shock" when the vascular bed is unable

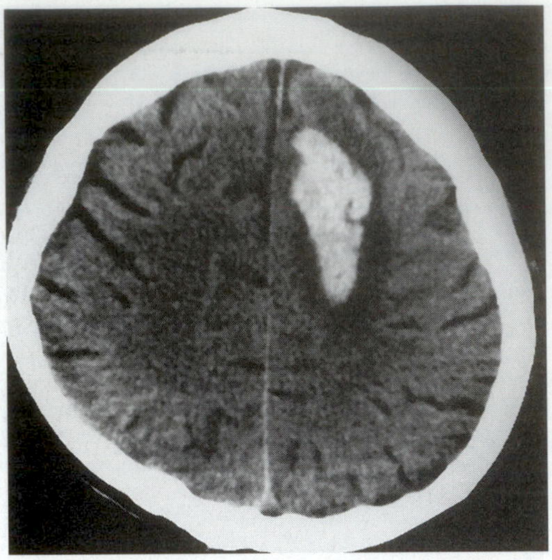

**Fig. 98-8.** CT image in a patient with thrombocytopenia demonstrating a lobar, high-convexity hemorrhage with minimal mass effect. This type of bleed is also seen in patients with amyloid angiopathy.

to autoregulate, consequently causing diffuse ischemic brain injury. Thus a moderate approach seems best in these circumstances, and slow reduction of blood pressure is advisable. Seizures are another potential complication of CHs. Although earlier reports have suggested no evidence of seizures in patients with lobar hemorrhages, several recent reports have provided evidence to the contrary. The estimated risk of seizures in these patients has ranged from 15% to 25%. Most seizures occur immediately after the onset of the hemorrhage and are usually associated with small hematomas, 2.5 to 3.8 cm. Phenytoin is the most widely used medication for controlling seizures caused by a focal hemorrhage.

***Role of surgery.*** The presence of intraventricular blood results in the development of clots that obstruct normal flow or drainage of the CSF. Depending on the patient's neurologic status, the appearance of early hydrocephalus in the presence of intraventricular blood may necessitate shunting of the CSF. Surgical evacuation of CH has been controversial. Most neurologists and neurosurgeons agree that medical treatment should be the mainstay of therapy in lobar hemorrhages. However, bleeding from AVMs or tumors present a different kind of a problem that necessitates individualized diagnostic and treatment approaches. Lobar hemorrhages may benefit from decompression and drainage if initial medical treatment fails and if the affected hemisphere is nondominant for language. This aggressive approach may only be beneficial when an AVM is suspected, since AVMs have a high rate of rebleeding. Hemorrhages in deeper structures such as the putamen and the thalamus are surgically difficult to drain without causing additional damage to the adjacent structures. Nevertheless, evacuation has been advocated in patients with putamenal hemorrhage who show evidence of rapid progression. However, no good documented studies have shown that surgical evacuation of hypertensive deep CHs has been beneficial.

A special situation, from the therapeutic viewpoint, is cerebellar hemorrhage. In patients with acute onset of cerebellar signs, it is imperative that a diagnosis of hemorrhage in the posterior fossa be excluded. Because of the potential for the development of obstructive hydrocephalus and compression of the brainstem, cerebellar hemorrhages are often fatal unless diagnosed early. The mainstay of therapy is surgical evacuation. Temporary external ventricular shunting while awaiting surgery is often lifesaving. Surprisingly, after extensive debridement of infarcted or hemorrhagic cerebellar tissue, patients do extremely well with minimal residual, if roof nuclei are spared. Therefore, it cannot be overemphasized that diagnosis of cerebellar CVAs should be taken seriously and surgical intervention considered early. Advances in microsurgical and stereotactic techniques have encouraged some neurosurgeons to reintroduce evacuation of deep hematomas as a possible mode of treatment. The benefits of this surgical approach remain to be properly evaluated. At our institution, we advocate surgical decompression in patients with cerebellar hematomas and in those with large lobar hemorrhages in the nondominant hemisphere with progressive clinical deterioration.

### Subarachnoid hemorrhage caused by cerebral aneurysm

The exact prevalence of congenital cerebral aneurysm is not known, but autopsy studies suggest a 2% incidence. Subarachnoid hemorrhage (SAH) accounts for approximately 45% of all strokes in patients under age 44 and 4% of strokes in those over age 65. The most significant risk factors for the development of SAH are smoking and high blood pressure, although the exact relationship of the latter is still unsettled. However, a strong relationship exists between congenital aneurysms and the rare conditions of polycystic kidney disease and pseudoxanthoma elasticum. Most clinicians recognize that the sudden onset of severe headache, or "thunderclap headache," sometimes accompanied by vomiting, raises the specter of aneurysmal SAH. However, the clinical presentation is variable and may not be always as dramatic. Loss of consciousness only occurs in 50% of patients, and at least 2% of patients with SAH have no headaches. Some patients may report having milder headaches that may precede rupture of the aneurysm; this is considered to represent a "warning leak." Localizing signs, when present, are helpful; however, in two thirds of patients, neck stiffness may never develop, and motor deficits may only be present in 15%. Some of the more common localizing signs include third nerve palsy in posterior communicating artery aneurysm and aphasia in middle cerebral artery aneurysm.

Fig. 98-9 illustrates the major arteries and common locations of congenital aneurysms.

***Diagnosis.*** It is surprising that even with the heightened awareness of SAH, many cases are still missed. Diagnostic confusion occurs with migraine, hypertensive crisis, gastroenteritis (because of prominent vomiting), and alcohol intoxication. The diagnosis of SAH is based on the history and laboratory evaluations, especially brain CT scan. Acute blood on CT is seen as hyperdense areas in the subarachnoid space at the base of the brain. The value of CT in the diagnosis of SAH depends greatly on the

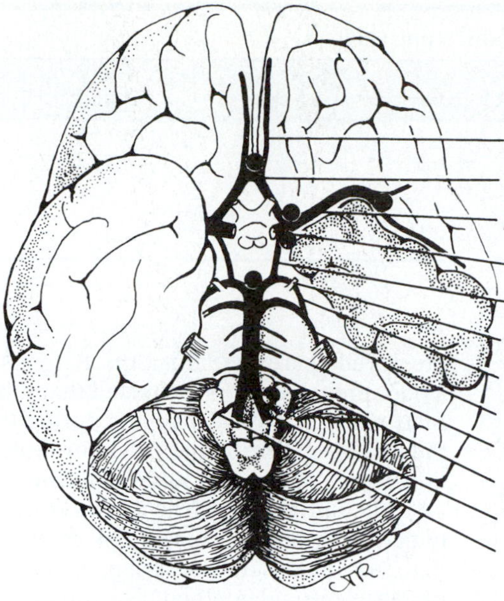

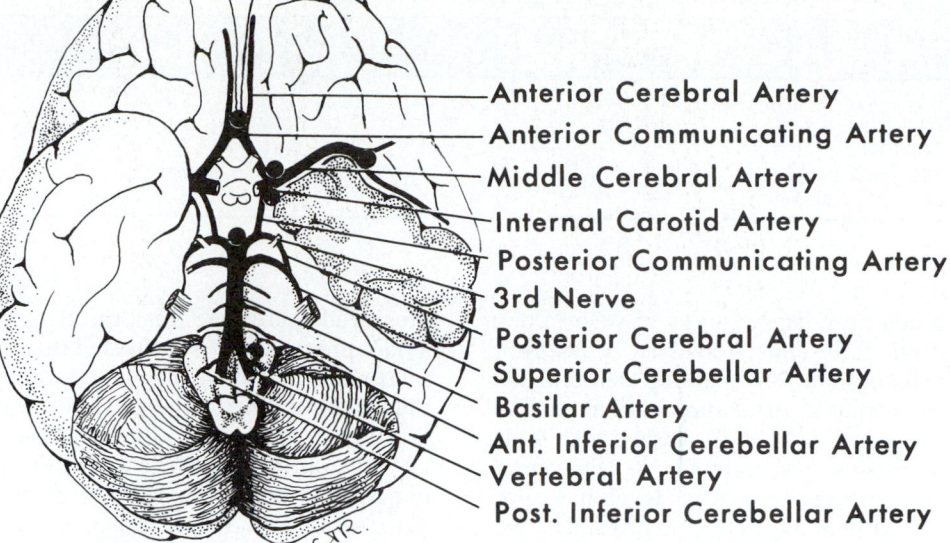

**Fig. 98-9.** Location of the major arteries as seen from the base of the brain. The illustration also demonstrates the most common location of congenital aneurysms.

observer and the timing and quality of the CT. The reported proportion of "positive" CTs in patients with SAH varies from 50% to 100%. This significant variability results from inability to detect blood on the brain CT after a few days of the ictus. Blood changes signal characteristics over time and becomes "isodense" after 3 days of the onset of the event. The trained eye should still be able to detect changes in the anatomic appearance of the cistern. Depending on the location of the aneurysm, an intraparenchymal hematoma may also be present, which is slower to resolve. When a CT scan is obtained for evaluation of SAH, it should be scrutinized with an experienced neuroradiologist or neurologist or neurosurgeon before accepting it as normal. Small amounts of blood in the basal cisterns or the sylvian fissure recognized by experienced physicians are often missed by others, with catastrophic results. Conventional angiography is indicated in all patients with positive head CT/MRI or CSF who are likely to benefit from surgery. In patients who present late, 2 weeks after the onset, conventional angiography should be done, since the CT scan and the CSF are often negative and MRI/MRA may be unrevealing.

Exhaustive diagnostic efforts of most "thunderclap headaches" usually reveal no evidence of SAH. "Crash migraine," benign coital headache, or vascular headaches may have similar presentation. Nevertheless, ruling out SAH when it is suspected is always prudent. Lumbar puncture is always indicated when the presentation is suggestive and the brain CT is read as negative for SAH. MRI has now become widely available and can be very useful in the diagnosis of SAH, especially in cases of delayed presentation. Blood breakdown products, oxyhemoglobin and methemoglobin, are quite evident on the T1-weighted images and may last up to 2 weeks. In addition, MRI can reveal the presence of aneurysm as a signal void. Most centers with MRI facilities are now also able to perform MRA, which may be able to reveal aneurysms. Therefore, MRI and MRA are the best methods for evaluating SAH in patients with delayed presentation.

Mass lesions and intracerebral hematoma from SAH must be ruled out before lumbar puncture is performed. Lumbar puncture performed by inexperienced clinicians is often traumatic, which unfortunately leads to diagnostic uncertainty. The only reliable method of differentiating a traumatic tap from SAH is to examine the supernatant fluid in a specimen that is spun immediately after the tap. Examination of the CSF for xanthochromia with the naked eye is unreliable, and spectrophotometry of CSF in patients with SAH is the most reliable method for the detection of blood breakdown products. Unfortunately, spectrophotometry is not readily available in all institutions for routine use in CSF analysis. Fibrin degradation products can be detected in patients with SAH but not in those with traumatic lumbar punctures.

Table 98-1 outlines the diagnosis of SAH at different stages.

***Complications.*** SAH results in cerebral ischemia usually 7 days after the event. The ischemia is typically widespread in more than one vascular territory and in large and small vessels. Vasospasm has been suggested as the cause of the diffuse ischemia. However, a definite association among vasospasm, ischemia, and neurologic deficits has not been established, since vasospasm can be detected in at least half the patients with a recent SAH, but only half of those may have neurologic deficits. The best method for diagnosing vasospasm is conventional angiography. Transcranial Doppler fails to detect almost half the patients with documented vasospasms on angiography. Detecting early signs of ischemia may be difficult, and therefore valuable "abortive" treatment may be delayed until the onset of more serious neurologic deficits. This has lead some investigators to advocate the use of single-photon emission computed tomography (SPECT) scans to

**Table 98-1.** Diagnosis of subarachnoid hemorrhage at different stages

| Diagnostic test | <12 hours | >12 hours | 3-5 days | >7 days | >10-14 days |
|---|---|---|---|---|---|
| Computed tomography | + | + | +/– | – | – |
| Magnetic resonance imaging | +/– | + | + | + | + |
| Red blood cells (cerebrospinal fluid) | + | + | – | – | – |
| Xanthochromia (cerebrospinal fluid) | –/+ | + | + | + | +/– |

+, Positive; –, negative.

detect changes in blood flow. The etiology of vasospasms is complicated and not fully understood, but it has been proposed that oxyhemoglobin surrounding cerebral arteries within the subarachnoid space may initiate a chain reaction that leads to free-radical formation and infiltration of the blood vessel wall with leukocytes damaging the endothelium. The patients typically develop a subacute evolution of focal deficits such as hemiparesis and aphasia over a few hours to days, usually with recurrent headache. CT or MRI may show evolving focal ischemia.

***Management.*** The acute medical management of SAH demands that the patient be in an intensive care setting to allow frequent monitoring of fluid changes, electrolytes, and blood pressure and frequent neurologic examinations. The management of SAH is best accomplished by a team of intensive care specialists, neurosurgeons, and neurologists who understand the complexity of this illness. The aim of medical management preoperatively and postoperatively is to minimize and preferably prevent contradicting goals of both rebleeding and cerebral ischemia in the presence of failed cerebral autoregulatory mechanisms. This can be accomplished by maintaining the patient in a relative hypervolemic state. A common complication of SAH is polyuria resulting in hypovolemia. This is due to sodium wasting, probably from hypothalamic damage, and must not be mistaken for inappropriate antidiuretic hormone secretion, since their management is quite different.

Nimodipine, a calcium channel blocker, has become a standard part of the management of SAH. In large trials, nimodipine has been shown to improve the outcome after SAH. The effects of nimodipine on the cerebral circulation are poorly understood, but it has been suggested that it promotes collateral flow into ischemic areas, compensating for decreased oxygen delivery. Other medical complications in patients with SAH include neurogenic pulmonary edema and electrocardiographic (ECG) abnormalities suggestive of subendocardial ischemia. These topics are beyond the scope of this chapter.

Hydrocephalus, as seen by CT scan, is common in SAH, often of moderate degree without clinical deterioration. However, the patient may become progressively obtunded. CT may show rapid development of hydrocephalus secondary to blood in the aqueduct of the fourth ventricle. In selected cases, acute shunting of the ventricle may be beneficial.

***Rebleeding from aneurysms.*** This phenomenon is probably the most ominous event in a patient who has preserved neurologic function. Patients who rebleed have a poor prognosis. It is estimated that rebleeding may occur in as many as 30% of patients during the first month after the first bleed. The highest risk for rebleeding is during the first week, and many rebleed during the first few hours after the initial bleed. The causes of rebleeding are poorly understood, but two major risk factors have been identified, loss of consciousness at presentation and the presence of intraventricular blood. No direct relationship to fluctuation of blood pressure has been identified. Furthermore, it is now well recognized that the blood in the subarachnoid space interacts with the pia, which has fibrinolytic activity to dissolve the blood. This fibrinolysis ultimately spreads through the CSF and may lyse the clot. To prevent rebleeding, clipping of the aneurysm as soon as possible is the most desired intervention. However, the timing of surgery is also critical and somewhat controversial. Recent studies have suggested that the morbidity and mortality of early versus late surgery are similar, but many neurosurgeons still prefer the later approach. Two antifibrinolytic agents have been introduced to combat rebleeding. ϵ-Aminocaproic acid and tranexamic acid were introduced in the late 1960s and early 1980s, respectively. Several clinical trials have demonstrated the overall reduction in rebleeding when these antifibrinolytic agents were given early. However, the overall outcome was not modified because it seems that tranexamic acid increased the incidence of ischemia. Therefore, additional clinical studies combining the aggressive medical treatment used to prevent ischemia with the antifibrinolytic therapy should be performed to exploit fully the potential benefits and reduce the known complications.

Surgical treatment of aneurysms has advanced technically to a remarkable degree with developments in microscopic surgery and neuroanesthesia. The single most important factor for good outcome is the neurologic status at the time of surgery. Thus, it is extremely important to recognize patients with mild sentinel hemorrhages, for which modern management should lead to excellent outcome. On the other hand, surgery in comatose patients, although technically successful, actually does not improve neurologic function. An exciting development is the use of endovascular obliteration of aneurysm by using coils released in the aneurysm that induce thombosis and occlusion of the aneurysm. This technique currently is being pursued and refined.

## Medical complications of strokes

One of the most important reasons for admitting a patient to the hospital after a CVA is to prevent or minimize the medical and psychosocial complications associated with such an event. The acute complications may be simply related to an element of denial or neglect when the patient may attempt to ambulate while suffering from a hemiplegia. Therefore, it is our policy to order strict bed rest or to supervise the patient out of bed to a chair for at least the first 3 days after the ictus.

One of the major medical complications of a stroke is aspiration pneumonia, which potentially may be fatal if not promptly diagnosed and treated. Although the risk of aspiration is clearly highest in patients with CVAs affecting the swallowing reflex (e.g., brainstem), supratentorial CVAs also cause similar problems either by indirectly influencing the swallowing mechanisms or by depressing the level of alertness. Therefore, it is prudent that patients be restricted from any oral intake for at least the first 48 hours and possibly longer depending on the degree of deficits. During this period of restricted oral intake, dehydration must be prevented by providing IV fluid in the form of normal saline without glucose. The amount of normal saline given should be appropriate for body weight and as tolerated by the patient's other underlying medical problems (e.g., congestive heart failure). It is preferable that the head of the bed be elevated to 30 degrees with two goals in mind: (1) to prevent brain edema from high venous pressures and (2) to prevent aspiration from the patient's own secretions. Often, a formal swallowing evaluation is necessary. The value of such a test is to determine the capacity of the swallowing reflexes and the type of foods that may be tolerated. Another major complication in patients with restricted movements is the development of deep venous thrombosis. This can be prevented using compression boots or small doses of subcutaneous heparin.

## Prevention of strokes

In addition to primary prevention by modifying risk factors, secondary prevention has a very important role. The recognition of TIAs provides an opportunity to intervene to reduce the risk of CVAs. The primary care physician should be as educated in recognizing TIAs as in recognizing angina, since both reflect ischemia and warn of potential permanent tissue damage. The risk factors involved in increasing the risks for strokes have been studied in large populations of different countries and communities. From these extensive epidemiologic studies, the risk factors for atherosclerotic disease have been identified. The most important determinants of carotid artery disease are hypertension, smoking, male sex, low high-density lipoproteins, high triglycerides, low folate levels, and to a lesser extent diabetes. These are the same risk factors that are responsible for other vascular diseases, although diabetes seems to contribute significantly more to coronary artery and peripheral vascular disease. Despite the overall concern regarding our dietary habits and the aggressive public drive against smoking, the prevalence of CVAs has remained unchanged since 1980. This, however, does not necessarily reflect failure of prevention as much as the reduction of one risk factor in isolation possibly not being sufficient. Nevertheless, medical intervention in controlling hypertension has been shown to reduce the risk of strokes in elderly persons, a benefit that should not be underestimated when almost half the CVAs may be directly related to hypertension.

## Rehabilitation after strokes

Disability from stroke varies and depends on a variety of cultural and psychosocial considerations. The enormous cost associated with loss of productivity and the impact on families justify aggressive approaches to rehabilitation. The goals of rehabilitation are (1) to lessen the dependence on others for activities of daily living (ADLs) and (2) to return to work. The most difficult part of rehabilitation is to motivate the patient to participate in an aggressive program. Initially the patient's ability to participate may be hindered by other nonsomatic deficits. For example, patients with CVAs involving the right parietal lobe exhibit severe spatial and sensory neglect as well as constructional apraxia, whereas those with global aphasia tend to have difficulties following instructions.

Patients with left hemispheric strokes are more likely to exhibit depression. Depression is probably the most treatable effect of CVAs that is frequently underrecognized. In a 3-year longitudinal study in Sweden, depression after a stroke was identified in 25% of patients. Patients who lived alone before their CVA, dependence in ADLs, and the presence of dysphasia after a CVA were related to a higher risk for developing depression. Therefore, to identify those patients at the highest risk for depression and to determine the degree, the benefits, and the goals of rehabilitation, the premorbid lifestyle of patients involved in rehabilitation must be evaluated.

Early mobilization of paretic limbs with physical therapy by active and passive exercises is very important to prevent frozen shoulder and the painful shoulder-hand syndrome, which is similar to reflex sympathetic dystrophy. Shoulder subluxation is common in hemiplegia but often unrecognized. Protection of the limb by a sling should prevent periarticular tissue injury. Physical and occupational therapies have a valuable role in maximizing functional response and should be used from early on. For many years the effects of long-term rehabilitation were thought to be limited to 6 months. However, recent studies have demonstrated benefits up to 3 years. Whether this recovery reflects the continuous ability of the damaged brain to "heal" or whether rehabilitation contributes to learning of adaptive mechanisms is not known. Regardless of the mechanism, however, continuous improvement should be expected and encouraged.

In patients with aphasia, speech therapists have a useful role, although specific benefits in reversing the language disturbance are not established. However, speech therapy is especially helpful in patients with nonfluent aphasias with good comprehension to enable them to maximize their limited speech repertoire. The psychologic support provided by dedicated speech therapists may be the most beneficial part of the treatment.

A neglected area in stroke medicine is poststroke pain syndromes. These occur characteristically a few weeks to a few months after thalamic infarction and less often with infarctions in the parietal cortex. Pain is most excruciating, poorly localized, deep, and intense, with spontaneous flare-ups often accompanied by electric jolt–like sensations. Pain occurs spontaneously in the hemibody affected but can be initiated by sensory stimuli to the limb. The pain is poorly responsive to analgesics and opioids but responds well to anticonvulsants such as carbamazepine and phenytoin.

### New and future treatments for strokes

This section introduces new treatments that focus on protecting neurons and salvaging them from ischemia. Most of these treatments are based on basic concepts of cellular injury, which are reviewed briefly. During periods of reduced cerebral blood flow (CBF) to approximately 20 ml/100 g/minute, reversible deficits may be demonstrated. At levels of 15 ml/100 g/minute, electric silence on EEG develops. If CBF continues to decrease to 8 ml/100 g/minute, permanent deficits will develop. At the cellular level, CBF at approximately 18 ml/100 g/minute results in adenosine triphosphate depletion and induction of anaerobic glycolysis, which then results in the buildup of lactate. As the energy-requiring pumps fail, the electrochemical balance is offset. This electrochemical disequelibrium results in an increase in the concentration of sodium and calcium intracellularly and an increase in potassium concentration extracellularly. An increase in the release of glutamate and aspartate accompanies the electrochemical changes. These neuroactive substances are considered excitatory, acting as local neurotoxins by causing further influx of calcium. The degree of neuronal damage is gradated, with decreasing cellular dysfunction away from the core of ischemia. The outer boundaries of the ischemic area are known as the penumbra. The preserved flow is presumed to result from collateral flow or preservation of local autoregulatory mechanisms. Based on these basic observations, investigators have attempted to intervene during an acute ischemic episode to restore blood flow, to limit the size of infarcts, and to prevent cell death.

A logical interventional approach is to prevent the influx of calcium, which leads to cell death, or to limit the release of excitatory neurotransmitters by blocking their ability to bind to membrane receptors. Among the calcium channel blockers available, nimodipine is considered the most specific to the CNS. Earlier clinical trials demonstrated some beneficial effect by reducing the mortality and improving the outcome in patients with ischemic CVAs. However, larger-scale trials in the United Kingdom were disappointing. Nevertheless, nimodipine is still used in some institutions empirically in all types of strokes.

Another approach to blocking calcium influx is to block the receptors of the excitatory neurotransmitters. Several receptor subtypes have been described for the glutamate neurotransmitter. The most important of these receptors are the NMDA and AMPA receptors. Animal studies using a noncompetitive antagonist to the NMDA ionophore, such as MK-801, revealed that in severe ischemia, these blockers were not beneficial. However, NBQX, an AMPA antagonist, has been shown in several animal models to be extremely effective in reducing cellular injury even when given 90 minutes after the onset of ischemia. Whether these promising results from animal experiments will be replicated in humans is unknown at this point.

In summary, stroke remains one of the most frustrating medical problems to treat. However, advances in pharmacology, neurochemistry, and neurophysiology have made it possible to begin serious consideration for interventional and salvaging treatments. The complexity of the pathophysiology of strokes and the importance of acute intervention require that patient management be highly coordinated by a stroke team that has the interest and the resources to evaluate and treat patients acutely. In addition, it is essential that the public becomes aware of the signs and symptoms of early CVAs so that their treatment not be delayed.

## BIBLIOGRAPHY


Astrom M, Adolfson R, Asplund K: Major depression in stroke patients: a 3-year longitudinal study, *Stroke* 24:976, 1993.

Biller J et al: A randomized trial of aspirin or heparin in hospitalized patients with recent transient ischemic attacks, *Stroke* 20:441, 1989.

Boston Area Anticoagulation Trial for Atrial Fibrillation Investigators: The effect of low-dose warfarin on the risk of stroke in patients with nonrheumatic atrial fibrillation, *N Engl J Med* 323:1505, 1990.

Canadian Cooperative Study Group: A randomized trial of aspirin and sulfinpyrazone in threatened stroke, *N Engl J Med* 299:53, 1978.

Caplan LR: Brain embolism, revisited, *Neurology* 43:1281, 1993.

Chimowitz MI et al: Left atrial spontaneous echo contrast is highly associated with previous stroke in patients with atrial fibrillation or mitral stenosis, *Stroke* 24:1015, 1993.

Fisher CM: Unusual vascular events in the territory of the posterior cerebral artery, *Can J Neurol Sci* 13:1, 1986.

Hankey GJ, Slattery JM, Warlow CP: The prognosis of hospital-referred transient ischaemic attacks, *J Neurol Neurosurg Psychiatry* 54:793, 1991.

North American Symptomatic Carotid Endarterectomy Trial Collaborators: Beneficial effect of carotid endarterectomy in symptomatic patients with high-grade carotid stenosis, *N Engl J Med* 325:445, 1991.

Powers WJ, Tempel LW, Grubb RL Jr: Influence of cerebral hemodynamics on stroke risk: one year follow-up of 30 medically treated patients, *Ann Neurol* 25:325, 1989.

Ropper AH, Kennedy SK: Neurological and neurosurgical intensive care. In Ropper AH, Rockoff MA, editors: *Treatment of intracranial hypertension,* ed 2, Rockville, Md, 1988, Aspen.


CHAPTER

# 99 Infections of the Nervous System


**Elcinda L. McCrone**
**Nagagopal Venna**
**Peter R. Bergethon**


The infectious syndromes of the central nervous system (CNS) can be some of the most life-threatening in clinical practice. Most CNS infections can be categorized in one of the following groups: acute meningitis, chronic and subacute meningitis, acute encephalitis, and space-occupying lesions. The cardinal signs of CNS infection are headache, fever, alterations in mental state, and focal neurologic signs. Seizures can be seen with infections of the cortical tissues. This chapter focuses on the infections that affect adults and the patterns most likely to be seen in general practice. HIV infection of the nervous system is presented in Chapter 68.

## MENINGITIS

The cerebrospinal fluid (CSF) and the leptomeningeal membranes enveloping the brain, spinal cord, and nerve roots are often the focus of a variety of infections that cause serious neurologic sequelae and death. The clinicopathologic syndromes of meningitis form a spectrum from the acute benign self-limited viral meningitis to the chronic meningitis of tuberculosis and fungi that are fatal without treatment. The ultimate morbidity and mortality of these CNS infections often depend on the temporal course of their diagnosis and the initiation of treatment. Therefore, because many of these diseases can be effectively treated, timely diagnosis and treatment are of major practical importance.

Based on the clinical presentation and the CSF profiles, the meningitides can be divided into the acute pyogenic, the acute "aseptic," and the chronic meningitides. This classification system is useful in formulating a differential diagnosis and in determining the urgency of treatment. Acute bacterial pyogenic meningitis is a medical emergency that threatens brain function and life, whereas the acute aseptic forms are usually benign self-limiting diseases. The more chronic infections lack the urgency of immediate therapy, but clinical response to treatment is much slower, and therefore errors in diagnosis and treatment regimen may not be as apparent.

## Acute bacterial pyogenic meningitis

***Epidemiology and etiology.*** *Streptococcus pneumoniae* and *Neisseria meningitidis* are the major causes of bacterial meningitis in adults (Table 99-1). The remaining important pathogens are gram-negative bacilli, *Staphylococcus aureus* and *S. epidermidis, Listeria monocytogenes,* and *Haemophilus influenzae.* The incidence of each of these bacterial pathogens varies with age, even in the adult population (Fig. 99-1). The frequency of nosocomial meningitis, especially gram-negative meningitis, has been increasing; predisposing factors include a previous neurosurgical procedure and CSF leak. With the exception of CNS shunt infections, which are predominantly caused by staphylococci, 70% of postsurgical infections result from gram-negative bacilli: *Klebsiella pneumoniae, Acinetobacter calcoaceticus,* and *Escherichia coli.*

An increased risk of meningitis exists with underlying conditions such as diabetes, alcoholism, dialysis, sickle cell disease, splenectomy, malignancy, transplantation, and steroid therapy. Individuals with defects in humoral immunity are more susceptible to infection with the encapsulated organisms. *S. pneumoniae, H. influenzae* type B, and *N. meningitidis. L. monocytogenes* is more common in individuals with defects in cell-mediated immunity. Neutropenic patients are more likely to acquire *Pseudomonas* meningitis.

***Pathophysiology.*** In most patients, bacterial meningitis begins with nasopharyngeal colonization by the pathogen. Following mucosal colonization, a primary bacteremia occurs, thus leading to CNS infection. Bacterial encapsulation may be important for colonization and mucosal invasion. The mechanisms of CNS invasion across the intact blood brain-barrier are not known, but entry through the dural venous sinuses or choroid plexus into the subarachnoid space has been postulated. Pathologically, an acute outpouring of purulent exudate into the CSF spills over the cerebral convexities. This process may cause a secondary bacteremia, or in protracted cases, a basilar inflammatory exudate may cause hydrocephalus. The cranial nerves, especially the eighth, may be injured by the inflammation. Subarachnoid space inflammation leads to many of the consequences of meningitis, such as cerebral edema and increased intracranial pressure. Cerebral edema may be cytotoxic, vasogenic, or interstitial and result in

**Table 99-1.** Bacterial etiology of meningitis in adults

| Organism | Percent |
|---|---|
| *Streptococcus pneumoniae* | 30-50 |
| *Neisseria meningitidis* | 10-35 |
| Staphylococci | 5-15 |
| Gram-negative bacilli | 1-10 |
| Streptococci | 5 |
| *Listeria monocytogenes* | 5 |
| *Haemophilus influenzae* | 1-3 |

Data from Schlech WF III et al: *JAMA* 253:1749, 1985.

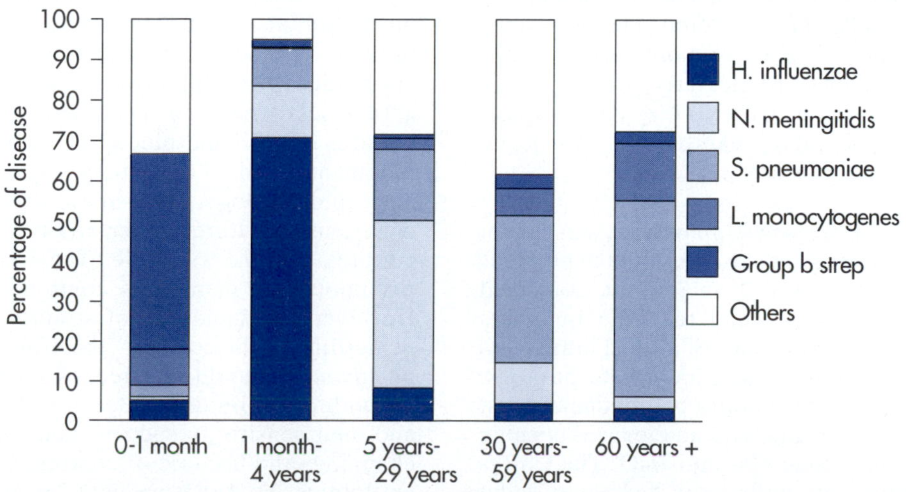


**Fig. 99-1.** Bacterial etiology of meningitis by age group. (From Wenger JD et al: *J Infect Dis* 162:1316, 1990.)

life-threatening herniation. The blood vessels traversing through the subarachnoid space may be severely affected, resulting in narrowing and thrombosis and leading to ischemia or infarction of the underlying brain. Infarction of large arteries at the base of the brain may lead to hemiparesis or quadriparesis. Cortical thrombophlebitis may produce focal deficits and result in seizure activity. Formation of a brain abscess secondary to purulent meningitis is extremely rare, although an abscess rupturing into the cerebral ventricles may present as an acute pyogenic meningitis. Ventriculitis leading to loculated ventricular empyema is an occasional complication.

***History and physical examination.*** The illness evolves rapidly over just several to 48 hours, with fever, chills, myalgias, severe headache, photophobia, and pain and stiffness of the neck. A rapid deterioration of mental status progresses from drowsiness with confusion to stupor and coma. Seizures are frequently seen. In elderly, alcoholic, and malnourished patients, the presentation may be less dramatic, with only a febrile, confusional state. In patients with a ventricular shunt, bacterial meningitis may only appear with a subtle decrease in alertness and a low-grade fever. Occasionally with meningococcal meningitis, acute aggressive, irrational behavior may herald the infection. The patient may be found in febrile coma.

Physical examination shows an ill-looking person with fever, neck stiffness, Kernig sign, photophobia, and various degrees of alertness ranging from an agitated confusional state to stupor and coma. Neck stiffness is often absent in comatose patients. There are remarkably few focal neurologic deficits. Papilledema is so exceptional in its acute form that its presence should alert the physician to a preexisting mass lesion, such as a brain abscess or a more subacute meningitis. Petechial skin rash is highly suggestive of meningococcal disease and may appear during the physical examination. Rarely, such a rash may occur in *Haemophilus* and pneumococcal meningitis. *H. influenzae* meningitis often presents with sepsis and pneumonia. Furuncles, skin abscesses, or needle marks should alert the physician to staphylococcal infection. Signs of sinusitis, mastoiditis, otitis, pneumonia, and endocarditis should be sought and may be found, especially in patients with pneumococcal meningitis. Elderly patients typically have altered mental status, progressing rapidly to coma, and are more likely to have focal deficits and seizures, particularly with *Listeria* meningitis. Immunosuppressed patients may have atypical presentation because of their inability to mount an adequate inflammatory response.

***Laboratory studies and diagnostic procedures.*** An urgent lumbar puncture is mandatory in patients with the previous signs and should not be delayed awaiting a computed tomography (CT) scan of the head to "rule out mass lesion" unless there is clear evidence of a focal brain mass such as hemiplegia, decorticate or decerebrate postures, unilateral unreactive pupil, or definite papilledema. Most cases show a typical CSF profile with an elevated opening pressure, sometimes more than 400 mm $H_2O$. The CSF is cloudy or frankly purulent, with total leukocyte count greater than 1000 cells/mm$^3$ with more than 90% polymorphonuclear leukocytes. The protein is greater than 150 mg/dl, and the sugar is less than 40 mg/dl, often less than 20 mg/dl. Gram stain of the centrifuged sediment identifies the causative organism in 70% to 80% of patients. Atypical profiles may be seen; in fulminant pneumococcal infection, the cell count in CSF may be less than 100/mm,$^3$ but a smear of the sediment may be packed with gram-positive diplococci—a profile of grave prognosis. Early cases may show only mild polymorphonuclear leukocytosis of CSF. The Gram stain may not be diagnostic, especially in patients partially treated with antibiotics. Regardless of the Gram stain findings, the CSF should be cultured and sensitivities determined. Particle agglutination tests, such as latex agglutination and staphylococcal coagglutination, are available to detect pneumococcal, meningococcal, and *H. influenzae* type B antigens. The particle agglutination tests have replaced counterimmunoelectrophoresis (CIE) as the rapid diagnostic test of choice because of their simplicity and their greater or equal sensitivity.

Peripheral blood leukocytosis with a shift to the left is regularly seen. Blood cultures should be routinely obtained and are frequently positive in meningococcal, pneumococcal, and *Haemophilus* meningitis. X-rays of the chest, skull, sinuses, and mastoids may reveal other foci of infection. Brain imaging is not routinely indicated unless complications arise during the course of the disease.

***Differential diagnosis.*** Patients with many other infectious processes have headache, fever, and some alteration in mental status. The differential diagnosis is broad and includes CNS infections (e.g., parameningeal foci, aseptic meningitis, encephalitis) and noninfectious disorders (e.g., intracranial tumors, subarachnoid hemorrhage, neuroleptic malignant syndrome). These disorders can be distinguished from bacterial meningitis by a careful history and physical examination, particularly with detailed attention to the neurologic examination for signs of increased intracranial pressure and focal deficits. Neuroimaging can evaluate for mass lesions.

***Management.*** Appropriate antibiotics are the keystone of treatment and should be started as soon as blood and CSF samples are obtained. Any delay increases the morbidity and mortality. Tables 99-2, 99-3, and 99-4 provide a guide for empiric as well as organism-specific antibiotics to be administered intravenously. The choice of antibiotics when no organism is identified, pending cultures of CSF and blood, is a matter of careful clinical judgment based on the patient's age, predisposing factors, and epidemiology. The initial treatment is subject to change after culture and sensitivity results of CSF or blood cultures become available. The treatment of choice for pneumococcal meningitis continues to be penicillin G. However, the incidence of strains relatively resistant to penicillin is increasing; therefore, all isolates of *S. pneumoniae* should be screened for penicillin susceptibility with oxacillin disks. Because the causative organisms and their sensitivity and resistance to antibiotics are ever changing, and because of continuous introduction of new antibiotics, consultation with an infectious disease specialist is highly recommended. However, initial treatment should not be delayed.

**Table 99-2.** Empiric therapy for acute bacterial meningitis

| Age (years) | Probable organisms | First-choice antibiotic | Alternative antibiotic |
|---|---|---|---|
| 18-50 | *Streptococcus pneumoniae*<br>*Neisseria meningitidis* | Penicillin G or ampicillin | Third-generation cephalosporin* |
| >50 | *S. pneumoniae*<br>*N. meningitidis*<br>Gram-negative bacilli<br>*Listeria monocytogenes* | Ampicillin plus third-generation cephalosporin* | Ampicillin plus an aminoglycoside |

*Cefotaxime or ceftriaxone.

**Table 99-3.** Recommend therapy for bacterial meningitis in adults

| Organism | Antibiotic of choice |
|---|---|
| *Streptococcus pneumoniae* | Penicillin G or ampicillin |
| *S. pneumoniae* (penicillin-resistant) | Third-generation cephalosporin* |
| *Neisseria meningitidis* | Penicillin G or ampicillin |
| *Staphylococcus aureus* (methicillin sensitive) | Nafcillin or oxacillin |
| *S. aureus* (methicillin resistant) | Vancomycin |
| *S. epidermidis* | Vancomycin† |
| Enterobacteriaceae | Third-generation cephalosporin* |
| *Pseudomonas aeruginosa* | Ceftazidime‡ |
| *S. agalactiae* (group B) | Penicillin G or ampicillin‡ |
| *Listeria monocytogenes* | Ampicillin or penicillin G‡ |
| *Haemophilus influenzae* (β-lactamase negative) | Ampicillin |
| *H. influenzae* (β-lactamase positive) | Third-generation cephalosporin* |

*Cefotaxime or ceftriaxone.
†Rifampin may be considered if no improvement in 48 hours.
‡Addition of aminoglycoside may be considered.

**Table 99-4.** Recommended doses of antibiotics for bacterial meningitis in adults (normal renal function)

| Antibiotic | Total daily dose (dosing interval) |
|---|---|
| Penicillin G | 20-24 million units (divided q4h) |
| Ampicillin | 12 g (divided q4h) |
| Cefotaxime | 8-12 g (divided q4h) |
| Ceftriaxone | 4-6 g (divided q12h) |
| Ceftazidime | 6-12 g (divided q8h) |
| Nafcillin, oxacillin | 9-12 g (divided q4h) |
| Vancomycin | 2 g (divided q12h) |
| Chloramphenicol | 4-6 g (divided q6h) |
| Metronidazole | 30 mg/kg (divided q6h) |
| Gentamicin, tobramycin | 3-5 mg/kg (divided q8h) |
| Amikacin | 15 mg/kg (divided q8h) |
| Trimethoprim/sulfamethoxazole | 10 mg/kg (divided q8h) (based on trimethoprim component) |

The duration of antibiotic therapy is based on clinical experience, which suggests 7 to 10 days for *H. influenzae,* 7 days for *N. meningitidis,* 10 to 14 days for *S. pneumoniae,* and 3 to 4 weeks for gram-negative meningitis. Studies on the use of dexamethasone in adults are limited, but given the demonstrated benefit in children, it could be considered initially in cases of meningitis associated with severe CNS dysfunction. Supportive therapy for septic shock and other severe medical illness is essential. Clinical follow-up is also critical for ensuring satisfactory outcome. As long as clinical improvement progresses, repeated lumbar puncture for CSF analysis is not necessary. Lack of satisfactory improvement, occurrence of seizures, or focal neurologic deficits should be investigated by brain imaging, ideally MRI, which may reveal suppurative sinusitis or subdural or ventricular empyema requiring surgical intervention.

Chronic neurologic sequelae include cranial nerve dysfunction, especially nerve deafness and facial palsy, as well as dementia, seizures, hemiparesis, cortical blindness, ataxia, and hydrocephalus. With early recognition and prompt therapy, the incidence and severity of these complications can be expected to be minimized. Despite appropriate antibiotic therapy, the mortality from meningitis remains high, with a 30% rate for pneumococcal meningitis.

***Prophylaxis.*** Person-to-person transmission does not occur in pneumococcal meningitis, and chemoprophylaxis is not indicated. For *N. meningitidis* meningitis, prophylaxis is indicated for all household members of the patient and for hospital personnel with intimate, but not casual, contact with the patient (as in mouth-to-mouth respiration). A 2-day course of rifampin at 600 mg twice daily for adults and 10 mg/kg twice daily for children is recommended. For *H. influenzae,* prophylaxis is indicated for household members only if at least one household member is less than 4 years of age. A 4-day course of rifampin at 600 mg daily for adults and 20 mg/kg daily for children is recommended.

### Acute aseptic meningitis

***Epidemiology and etiology.*** The etiologies of acute aseptic meningitis include enteroviruses, mumps, herpes simplex virus type 2 (HSV-2), and lymphocytic choriomeningitis (LCM). Greater than 80% of cases of acute viral meningitis in the United States are caused by enteroviruses, especially coxsackievirus and echovirus. Enteroviruses are transmitted by the fecal-oral route and are more common in summer and early fall. LCM virus is acquired through contact with rodents or their excreta. HSV-2 meningitis may be seen in association with primary genital infections. Since the widespread use of mumps vaccine, mumps occurs less frequently; it is spread by the respiratory route, generally in late winter or spring. Aseptic meningitis may be associated with the acute human immunodeficiency virus (HIV) syndrome (see Chapter 68).

### Pathophysiology

Primary infection with the enteroviruses occurs in the gastrointestinal (GI) tract. Viral replication occurs in the Peyer patches, followed by a minor primary viremia with seeding of the CNS, liver, lungs, and heart. Additional replication is followed by a major secondary viremia with the signs and symptoms of a viral syndrome; spread to the CNS may also occur during the secondary viremia. The mechanism of spread from the blood into the CNS is not known, although spread to the CNS by neural transport has been postulated.

*History and physical examination.* The clinical syndrome is characterized by an acute febrile illness with malaise, headache, photophobia, and neck stiffness. Mental status is not affected beyond a confusional state, and elementary neurologic functions are normal. The illness is mild; the patient looks relatively well and does not show the worsening of mental state characteristic of acute pyogenic meningitis. There may be a morbilliform skin rash, genital herpes, or parotitis, although these occur infrequently.

*Laboratory studies and diagnostic procedures.* CSF examination reveals a leukocyte count of usually less than 1000 cells/mm$^3$ with a predominance of mononuclear cells and a protein level less than 100 mg/dl, whereas the sugar level is normal and the Gram stain negative. However, many cases show an early preponderance of polymorphonuclear leukocytes, especially with enteroviruses; a shift to mononuclear cells occurs if the lumbar puncture is repeated in 12 hours. In meningitis from mumps, HSV-2, or LCM, the CSF sugar level is mildly diminished. Peripheral leukocyte count is usually normal.

*Differential diagnosis.* The importance of this otherwise benign self-limited syndrome lies in the problems of differential diagnosis it poses (see the box at right).

**Partially treated bacterial meningitis.** A predominance of polymorphonuclear leukocytes and depression of glucose in the CSF raise the possibility of early purulent bacterial meningitis. If the clinical diagnosis is of viral meningitis and the patient is not particularly ill appearing or deteriorating by the hour, antibiotics can be withheld and lumbar puncture repeated in 8 to 12 hours. A shift to mononuclear cells, which is suggestive of a viral etiology, is reassuring. Patients with similar CSF profiles need to be distinguished from patients who have been partially treated with antibiotics for acute bacterial pyogenic meningitis. About 60% of such patients show organisms in a Gram-stained smear of CSF sediment. They tend to have CSF leukocyte counts of more than 1000 cells/mm,$^3$ a protein level of greater than 150 mg/dl, and a more severe reduction of the CSF sugar level (less than 30 mg/dl) than in viral meningitis. Such patients should be treated for acute bacterial meningitis.

**Causes of acute aseptic meningitis syndrome**

- Acute viral meningitis
- Partially treated acute bacterial pyogenic meningitis
- Tuberculous meningitis
- Acute spirochetal meningitis
  - Secondary syphilis
  - Lyme disease
  - Leptospirosis
- Parameningeal suppurative foci
- Acute noninfectious meningitis
  - Vasculitis (systemic lupus erythematosus)
  - Drug induced
- Acute viral encephalitis

**Tuberculous meningitis.** An important consideration in the acute aseptic meningitic syndrome, tuberculous meningitis often presents with elevated polymorphonuclear leukocyte counts in the CSF. The initial CSF sugar level may be normal, and acid-fast staining of CSF is often negative. This diagnosis should be considered if the patient is more ill looking than the usual patient with viral meningitis and fails to improve as expected, or if neurologic deterioration occurs in the form of increasing lethargy or third cranial nerve palsies. Serial CSF examinations are essential and show a characteristic fall in sugar level and an increase in protein levels, often to more than 200 mg/dl.

**Spirochetal meningitis.** Acute aseptic meningitis is sometimes a manifestation of secondary syphilis. A characteristic desquamative rash involving the soles and palms and alopecia are strongly suggestive of syphilis. Strongly positive Venereal Disease Research Laboratories (VDRL), fluorescent treponemal antibody absorption (FTA-ABS), or treponemal hemagglutination tests of blood and VDRL test of CSF establish the diagnosis. Lyme disease is recognized to have a similar CSF profile and clinical picture in the second stage of the illness. A history of antecedent skin rash (erythema chronicum migrans) and the accompanying cranial and peripheral nerve palsies are highly suggestive of Lyme disease in an individual from an endemic area. Bell palsy is particularly common, and some patients have a widespread radiculoneuritis. The diagnosis is confirmed by serologic tests for specific antibodies. Leptospiral infections can have a similar appearance. A history of contact with water or soil contaminated with infected animal urine is suggestive, and diagnosis is confirmed by culturing the organisms from blood, urine, or CSF and by serologic agglutination tests. Neurosyphilis and Lyme disease are discussed in more detail in the section on subacute and chronic meningitis.

**Parameningeal focus of suppuration.** Patients with a parameningeal focus of pus, such as a spinal epidural abscess, brain abscess, or subdural empyema, often have a CSF profile of aseptic meningitis. Clinical suspicion and appropriate investigations such as brain and spinal imaging with contrast magnetic resonance imaging (MRI) are essential to identify these important disorders, since they can be successfully treated and, if unrecognized, can lead to death or severe neurologic disability.

**Aseptic meningitis in vasculitis.** This is a fairly common occurrence in systemic lupus erythematosus (SLE) and may be accompanied by neuropsychiatric or other peripheral manifestations of SLE. Serum antinuclear antibody (ANA) helps establish the diagnosis.

**Aseptic meningitis syndrome from drugs.** An acute meningitis syndrome has been reported with nonsteroidal antiinflammatory drugs (NSAIDs) such as ibuprofen, sulindac, and tolmetin, as well as with azathioprine, isoniazid, and trimethoprim. Most patients have had collagen vascular disease. Otherwise healthy people have also been affected. The illness occurs within hours to days after starting the drug. The CSF shows a predominance of polymorphonuclear leukocytes, but the sugar level is usually normal. The associated symptoms of pruritus, facial edema, and conjunctivitis, and rapid resolution after stopping the drug, help in the diagnosis.

***Management.*** No specific treatment exists for viral meningitis. Intravenous acyclovir for herpes simplex may be considered for primary genital herpes or significant bladder symptoms. The course of aseptic meningitis is steady improvement in fever and signs of meningeal irritation over 1 or 2 weeks, although malaise may linger. Most patients have no neurologic sequelae. Some degree of pleocytosis may persist for several weeks and, in some cases of LCM, for several months; however, the CSF profile is one of decreasing cell counts and protein level, as well as increasing sugar level if it was initially low.

### Subacute and chronic infectious meningitis

Various pathogens infect the subarachnoid spaces with much slower progressive course than seen in the acute meningitides. The insidious progress of these diseases may mask the significiant morbity and mortality that they cause. These chronic syndromes include tuberculous, treponemal, and fungal meningitis (see the box at right). Many similarities exist in the pathophysiology of the TB and fungal meningitides, and these are discussed together. The spirochetal meningitides are discussed separately under Differential Diagnosis and Management.

***Pathophysiology.*** Tuberculosis and a variety of fungi cause a subacute or chronic progressive inflammation of the subarachnoid spaces. The pathologic processes and the core clinical and CSF abnormalities of all these diseases are quite similar. An adhesive exudate develops at the base of the brain, entrapping the cranial nerves early, especially the sixth, seventh, and eighth nerves. CSF flow is often obstructed, resulting in hydrocephalus. A CSF block can occur in the basal cisterns, at the outlet of the fourth ventricle, or at the aqueduct of the midbrain. The arteries branching from the circle of Willis may become entrapped in the adhesive exudate and become inflamed and occluded, leading to brain infarction. The brain itself may be directly infected with formation of focal granulomas, including tuberculomas, cryptococcomas, and aspergillomas. The resulting clinicopathologic picture is a complex meningoencephalitis with serious neurologic sequelae.

#### Etiologies of subacute and chronic meningitides

**Infections**

Tuberculosis
Fungal infections (generally associated with immunocompromise)
- *Cryptococcosus*
- *Coccidioides*
- *Candidia*
- *Aspergillus*
- *Blastomyces*
- *Histoplasma*
- Zygomycetes
- *Pseudoallescheria*
- *Sporothrix*

**Noninfectious causes**

Meningeal carcinomatosis or lymphomatosis
Sarcoidosis
Systemic lupus erythematosus
Behçet's disease
Vogt-Koyanagi-Harada syndrome

***History and physical examination.*** Clinically, a subacute illness is found with low-grade fever, malaise, headache, and neck pain that progresses over several weeks. The syndrome progresses with increasing alterations in mental status, including lethargy, apathy, and psychosis. In some patients the clinical presentation may be similar to that of aseptic meningitis; occasionally, meningeal symptomatology may be obscured by subacute evolution of dementia. Cranial nerve palsies appear, especially bilateral sixth nerve palsies, and the seventh and eighth nerves may be affected as well. Progressive visual impairment may occur because of chiasmatic invasion and entrapment. The mental state deteriorates, and focal neurologic deficits are superimposed as a result of hydrocephalus, cerebrovascular accident (CVA, stroke), and intracerebral granulomas. The course is generally relentlessly downhill but may be relapsing and remitting. Death usually occurs in untreated patients; thus, early diagnosis is essential.

***Laboratory studies and diagnostic procedures.*** The CSF shows moderate lymphocytic pleocytosis of 100 to 500 cells. The protein is greatly elevated, sometimes up to 1 g/dl. The glucose is moderately to severely decreased. Progressive increase in protein level and decrease in sugar level on serial CSF examinations are characteristic. The Gram stain is negative, acid-fast stain rarely reveals mycobacteria, but India ink preparations may show cryptococci. The demonstration of organisms in the CSF can be enhanced by acquiring large volumes of CSF and using serial

**Table 99-5.** Classification of neurosyphilis

| Clinical stage | Clinical syndrome |
|---|---|
| **Early** | |
| Asymptomatic | Unknown |
| Meningitis | Acute aseptic meningitis |
| **Late** | |
| Asymptomatic | Chronic meningitis |
| Meningovascular | |
| Cerebral | Chronic meningitis, endarteritis with or without cerebral infarction |
| Spinal | Chronic meningitis, infarction of spinal cord |
| Parenchymal | |
| General paresis | Chronic meningoencephalitis and brain atrophy with dementia |
| Tabes dorsalis | Chronic meningomyelitis, spinal cord atrophy |
| **Gummatous** | Syphilitic granuloma |

Modified from Tramont EC: Syphilis of the central nervous system. In Lambert HP, editor: *Infections of the central nervous system,* Philadelphia, 1991, Decker.

specimens. Atypical clinical presentations and laboratory profiles are often found. Both tuberculosis and cryptococcal meningitis may first present as an acute aseptic meningitis, with the CSF initially showing a predominance of polymorphonuclear leukocytes. This usually progresses in time to the more typical lymphocytic pleocytosis; a change to mononuclear cells may occur later. Usually, cryptococci and *Candida* can be seen on smears or cultured from the CSF. Other fungi are difficult to obtain from the CSF, and occasionally the organisms may be cultured only from the CSF obtained from cisternal or ventricular tap. Cryptococcal antigen and complement-fixing antibodies to certain fungi can be identified in the CSF.

Unlike in acute meningitides, brain imaging is important in understanding the extent and complications of subacute and chronic infectious meningitis. MRI is optimal, but CT can also be useful. The basal meninges show diffuse enhancement with contrast. Hydrocephalus is well seen, and intracerebral granulomas can be identified.

### *Differential diagnosis and management*

**Neurosyphilis.** The incidence of syphilis in the United States is rising after a nadir in the mid-1960s. Spirochetemia occurs soon after primary inoculation, during which the CNS can be infected. Success in controlling the infection is directly related to the vigor of the host's cellular immune response; more widespread disease is seen in individuals with malnutrition, HIV infection, and late pregnancy. CNS involvement occurs at all stages of the illness (Table 99-5). Individuals with asymptomatic disease are at risk of developing clinically apparent disease at any time if untreated. Syphilitic meningitis generally occurs within 1 to 2 years of acquiring the infection and presents as an acute aseptic meningitis, often with cranial nerve palsies, especially seventh and eighth.

**Table 99-6.** Antibiotic therapy for neurosyphilis

| Therapy | Dose/Route | Duration |
|---|---|---|
| Aqueous penicillin G | 2-4 million units IV q6h | 10-14 days |
| Procaine penicillin plus | 2.4 million units IM qd | 10-14 days |
| Probenecid | 500 mg PO qid | |
| Amoxicillin plus | 3 g PO bid | 14 days |
| Probenicid | 1 g PO bid | |
| Ceftriaxone | 1 g IM qd | 14 days |
| Benzathine penicillin plus | 2.4 million units IM weekly | 3 weeks |
| Any of the above regimens | | |

Data from Center for Disease Control and Prevention: *MMWR* 42(RR-14):30,1993; and Lambert HP, editor: *Infections of the central nervous system,* Philadelphia, 1991, Decker.

The peak incidence of meningovascular syphilis occurs 5 to 7 years after the primary infection and is characterized by focal neurologic deficits resulting from vasculitis. General paresis and tabes dorsalis are very late sequelae of disease and result from irreversible neuronal damage. Individuals who have HIV infection often have accelerated disease and are more likely to progress to symptomatic neurosyphilis. Ocular involvement in the HIV patient is common. The CSF VDRL or FTA-IgM is positive in 80% of neurosyphilic patients but is less sensitive with HIV infection. Table 99-6 lists the treatment regimens for neurosyphilis.

**Lyme disease.** Although Lyme disease has been found throughout the United States, it is most frequently seen in southern New England and New York, New Jersey, Minnesota, and Wisconsin; it is widespread throughout Europe. Neurologic involvement with *Borrelia burgdorferi* infection has an incidence of nearly 40%. It frequently occurs early in Lyme disease but can be seen in all stages of the disease. Four neurologic syndromes have been described: meningitis, cranial neuritis, radiculoneuropathy, and meningoencephalitis (Table 99-7). Bell palsy is one of the most common and earliest neurologic manifestations of Lyme disease, and Lyme disease is the most frequent cause of bilateral Bell palsy. Meningitis can develop up to 6 months after initial infection; it can remit spontaneously or become chronic or relapsing. The diagnosis of Lyme disease should be considered in individuals with concurrent cranial or peripheral neuropathy, a history of travel to an endemic area, or a history of the characteristic rash of erythema chronicum migrans. Carditis or migratory arthritis may also be seen. The late neurologic complications of Lyme disease can occur months or years after exposure.

Serologic testing remains the most reliable method of diagnosis but may be negative early in disease. The specific IgM response peaks during the third to sixth week of the disease; the IgG response rises over months to years and may remain elevated despite clinical remission. Acute and convalescent serum demonstrates an IgM response in 90% of patients with early disease; however, only IgG antibody is seen in late disease. CSF IgA, IgM, and IgG

**Table 99-7.** Neurologic manifestations of Lyme borreliosis

| | Stage I | Stage II | Stage III |
|---|---|---|---|
| Central nervous system | Meningismus | Meningitis, encephalitis, myelitis, hemiparesis, chorea, cerebellar ataxia | Subacute encephalopathy, encephalomyelitis, stroke (CVA) |
| Peripheral nervous system | — | Cranial neuritis, radiculitis, plexitis, mononeuritis, Guillain-Barré syndrome | Polyneuropathy |

Data from Lambert HP, editor: *Infections of the central nervous system,* Philadelphia, 1991, Decker; and Scheld WM, Whitley RJ, Durack DT, editors: *Infections of the central nervous system,* New York, 1991, Raven.

**Table 99-8.** Recommendations for treatment for neurologic manifestations of Lyme disease

| Stage | Treatment | Duration |
|---|---|---|
| Facial nerve palsy alone | Doxycycline 100 mg PO bid | 2-4 weeks |
| | Amoxicillin 500 mg PO qid plus Probenecid 500 mg PO qid | 2-4 weeks |
| Stage II or III | Ceftriaxone 2 g IV qd | 2-4 weeks |
| | Penicillin G 20-24 million units IV qd in divided doses | 10-21 days |
| | Doxycycline 100 mg PO bid or Doxycycline 200 mg IV, then 100 mg IV | 10-30 days<br>2 days, then 8 days |

Modified from Reik L Jr: Lyme disease. In Scheld WM, Whitley RJ, Durack DT, editors: *Infections of the central nervous system,* New York, 1991, Raven.

titers are found in individuals with meningitis. There are several pitfalls to serologic testing. False-positive IgM can be seen, especially in other spirochetal infections. In highly endemic areas, seropositivity may reflect past resolved infection.

CSF studies may be normal in peripheral neuropathy syndromes, and nerve biopsy can assist a clinical diagnosis. Biopsy of the characteristic skin rash may be diagnostic. If a high index of suspicion exists for the diagnosis of Lyme disease on a clinical basis, treatment should be initiated (Table 99-8).

**Tuberculous meningitis.** Tuberculous (TB) meningitis affects both the native and the immigrant populations of the United States. Early diagnosis and empiric institution of anti-TB therapy based on clinical suspicion is important to minimize the serious sequelae of this disease. Although a positive purified protein derivative (PPD), recent conversion of PPD reaction, and pulmonary or extrapulmonary disease should be carefully sought, lack of these should not be interpreted as evidence against the diagnosis. Many patients have normal chest x-rays. If miliary spread is suspected, biopsy and culture of bone marrow or liver are indicated.

An atypical presentation with an acute aseptic meningitis picture followed by progressive worsening should arouse suspicion of TB meningitis, even when the initial

**Table 99-9.** Antimicrobial therapy for treatment of tuberculosis meningitis

| Agent | Usual daily dose | Length of therapy |
|---|---|---|
| Isoniazid | 300 mg | 6 months |
| Rifampin | 600 mg | 6 months |
| Pyrazinamide | 15-30 mg/kg | 2 months |

CSF glucose level is normal. Serial CSF analyses are crucial to the successful diagnosis; a progressive decline in sugar level and rise in protein level are strong evidence of TB meningitis. The yield of growing organisms from the CSF is increased by culturing the sediment of large volumes of CSF (greater than 10 ml). With the increase in incidence of multidrug-resistant TB in the United States, it is important to obtain CSF cultures for both diagnosis and susceptibility testing.

Prompt initiation of therapy is essential without waiting for CSF culture results, which take 4 to 6 weeks. The American Thoracic Society recommends initial therapy with the tuberculocidal agents isoniazid, rifampin, and pyrazinamide for 2 months, followed by isoniazid and rifampin for an additional 6 months (Table 99-9). If pyrazinamide cannot be used, ethambutol (25 mg/kg/day) or streptomycin (1 g/day) can be substituted. If drug resistance is suspected, an initial four-drug regimen may be chosen or the length of therapy extended to 9 to 12 months.

In the presence of hydrocephalus, adhesive meningitis causing visual failure, or cerebral infarction, a course of prednisone (40 to 60 mg/day) is sometimes recommended for 4 to 6 weeks, although no clear benefit has been proved. The relief of severe hydrocephalus may require ventricular shunt placement. Microsurgical lysis of adhesions around the optic chiasm may restore vision.

**Fungal meningitis.** The clinical and CSF profiles of cryptococcal, coccidioidal, *Blastomyces,* and *Histoplasma* meningitis are quite similar to the pattern subacute and chronic meningitis outlined earlier. Normal host defense mechanisms are usually extremely effective in preventing fungi from invading the CNS; therefore, most patients with fungal meningitis have an immunologic deficit, even if subtle. Table 99-10 lists immunologic defects that predispose to specific fungal infections.

**Table 99-10.** Some factors predisposing to fungal infections of the central nervous system

| Predisposing factor | Examples | Typical organisms |
|---|---|---|
| Inherited immune defects | CGD* | *Candida, Cryptococcus, Aspergillus* |
| Acquired immune defects | Corticosteroids | *Cryptococcus, Candida* |
| | Cytotoxic agents | *Aspergillus, Candida* |
| | HIV infection | *Cryptococcus, Histoplasma* |
| | Alcoholism | *Sporothrix* |
| Iron chelator therapy | Desferoxamine | Zygomycetes |
| Intravenous drug abuse | | Zygomycetes, *Candida* |
| Diabetic ketoacidosis | | Zygomycetes |
| Trauma, surgery, foreign body, near-drowning | | *Candida, Pseudoallescheria,* dematiaceous fungi |

Modified from Perfect JR, Durack DT: Pathogenesis and pathophysiology of fungal infections of the central nervous system. In Scheld WM, Whitley RJ, Durack DT, editors: *Infections of the central nervous system,* New York, 1991, Raven.
*Chronic granulomatous disease.

*Cryptococcus neoformans* is ubiquitous. Cryptococcal meningitis is a common opportunistic infection associated with HIV infection; it also occurs in patients with reticuloendothelial malignancy, sarcoidosis, organ transplantation, and collagen vascular disease and those receiving corticosteroid therapy. Initial infection is acquired via a respiratory route that seeds the lymph nodes, with subsequent dissemination through the blood. Cryptococci have a predilection to infect the subarachnoid space. Cryptococcal meningitis can be remarkably indolent, relapsing and remitting over years, or may be fulminant. The estimation of cryptococcal antigen in the CSF has greatly aided in the rapid diagnosis of this most common of the fungal meningitides. CSF cultures are positive in 75% of patients, whereas the antigen is detected in more than 90%.

*Coccidioides immitis* is endemic to the semiarid portions of the southwestern United States. Dissemination to the meninges generally occurs within 6 months of its initial acquisition by inhalation. Immunocompromise is less clearly associated with coccidioidal meningitis than with other mycoses; dissemination has been associated with extremes of age, male sex, nonwhite race, late pregnancy, and immunosuppression, especially HIV infection. The diagnosis is confirmed by complement-fixing antibodies in the CSF and blood. Direct cultures of CSF are positive in about 50% of cases.

*Histoplasma capsulatum* is endemic to the Ohio, Mississippi, and St. Lawrence river valleys and along the Appalachian mountains. The disease is acquired by inhalation and can disseminate latently in individuals with reticuloendothelial malignancies or HIV infection. The meningitis is usually accompanied by hepatosplenomegaly and lymphadenopathy. Culture of CSF is only positive in 25% to 50% of patients; cultures of bone marrow, blood, urine, and sputum are more likely to be positive. Serologic testing of complement-fixing antibodies of blood and CSF may be helpful in establishing the diagnosis. A urinary antigen test under development looks promising.

*Blastomyces dermatitidis* is endemic to the Ohio, Mississippi, and St. Lawrence river valleys and southeastern United States. Disseminated disease involves the skin, bone, prostate, and only rarely the CNS. CSF cultures are positive only in 25% of patients and may take 30 days to grow. Biopsy of prostate, cutaneous or subcutaneous lesions, and cultures of blood, urine, and sputum may have greater yield. There is no serologic test.

Less often, other mycoses cause meningitis in immunocompromised patients, including patients with acquired immunodeficiency syndrome (AIDS). Candidal meningitis may be acute or subacute and may be accompanied by microabscesses or macroabscesses in the brain parenchyma. *Candida* may be grown from culture of CSF. *Aspergillus* and the Zygomycetes produce a subacute progressing meningitis with a prominent polymorphonuclear leukocyte reaction and propensity for vascular invasion causing cerebral infarction or hemorrhage. The diagnosis is difficult to establish except by biopsy of the granulomatous tissues.

With few exceptions, amphotericin B is the mainstay of treatment for all the fungal meningitides and is given intravenously over 6 weeks. Intrathecal therapy is needed in coccidioidomycosis. Flucytosine may be used in combination with amphotericin in the treatment of some of the fungal meningitides. Fluconazole may be useful as primary therapy for mild cryptococcal meningitis in AIDS patients, but it is predominantly used for suppressive therapy. Itraconazole, a new azole, may prove promising for aspergillosis and histoplasmosis. Lifelong suppressive therapy may be indicated for immunosuppressed patients with fungal meningitides.

## ACUTE VIRAL ENCEPHALITIS

### Epidemiology and etiology

The parenchyma of the brain as well as the leptomeninges may be invaded by certain viruses, causing an acute febrile meningoencephalitis of substantial mortality and serious neurologic morbidity. In the United States, diffuse encephalitides are caused most often by the mosquito-borne arboviruses. The epidemiology of the different viruses is characteristic. Most occur in the summer and early fall. California encephalitis occurs in the rural midwest, St. Louis encephalitis affects the rural and urban midwestern and eastern states, eastern equine encephalitis affects the urban and rural areas of the eastern seaboard, and western equine encephalitis occurs across the country. A diffuse encephalitis also occurs as an immune reaction of the brain to viral infections or viral vaccination (postinfectious/postvaccinal diffuse encephalomyelitis) such as measles, mumps, and chickenpox. Herpes simplex virus type-1 (HSV-1) causes the most common endemic viral encephalitis of adults in the United States.

### Pathophysiology

In the arthropod-borne encephalitides, a primary viremia follows viral replication at the local skin site and involves the reticulendothelial system (RES). A secondary viremia occurs after viral replication in the RES, infecting the CNS. The brain shows various degrees of neuronal necrosis and perivascular mononuclear cell infiltration, chiefly in the gray matter. In the postinfectious encephalomyelitides, demyelination of the cerebral white matter with perivenous lymphocytic cuffing is the characteristic pathology. In contrast, HSV-1 causes a focal encephalitis of the inferior frontal and temporal lobes with severe necrosis and intraneuronal inclusion bodies. HSV-1 enters the brain by peripheral intraneuronal routes. Pathologically, Cowdry type A inclusion bodies may be seen.

### History, physical examination, and diagnosis

The clinical syndrome of acute viral encephalitis consists of a febrile illness with headache, vomiting, photophobia, and rapid evolution over a day or two of progressive stupor, convulsions, and a combination of upper motor neuron, cerebellar, and brainstem derangements. The CSF profile is similar to that described for acute viral meningitis. Virologic diagnosis is based on epidemiology and the retrospective identification of a specific virus by a fourfold increase in serum viral antibodies.

Because of focal brain destruction, HSV-1 encephalitis presents with focal neurologic abnormalities in addition to a febrile illness. The demonstration of focal brain injury is the key to diagnosis. Clinical signs of behavioral change, aphasia, hemiparesis or convulsions, focal slowing on the electroencephalogram (EEG), and low-density brain swelling of the temporal and frontal lobes that evolves over a few days on serial brain imaging scans are characteristic. The diagnosis is established by brain biopsy examined by electron microscopy for intraneuronal intranuclear inclusions, identification of viral antigen by immunofluorescence, and finally by culture of the organisms from the biopsy. Results of the immunofluorescence study are available in 2 to 3 hours, electron microscopy in 24 hours, and isolation of virus in 1 to 3 days. There is a recent trend to make a probable diagnosis of this encephalitis without brain biopsy because of the availability of acyclovir, a relatively nontoxic therapy. However, each case should be reviewed carefully with neurologic and infectious disease specialists so that alternative but treatable brain lesions are not overlooked.

The postinfectious encephalomyelitis has a similar clinical and CSF picture except that it evolves monophasically, usually 1 to 2 weeks after vaccination, or as the viral exanthem is subsiding. Widespread low-density lesions of white matter and brainstem swelling on CT scan provide supportive evidence.

### Management

The treatment of acute diffuse viral encephalitis is symptomatic. The mortality rates and disabilities depend on the specific virus. With California encephalitis, the mortality rate is 2%, but a third of survivors experience sequelae, including behavioral and emotional difficulties, or seizures. Western equine encephalitis has a mortality rate of 3% and minor long-term neurologic disability in 5% of patients. The mortality rate from St. Louis encephalitis is 10%, with 5% showing late sequelae. In contrast, eastern equine encephalitis is a much more aggressive infection, with a 50% mortality and severe neurologic sequelae. Acyclovir is the antiviral agent of choice for treatment of HSV-1 encephalitis at a dose of 10 mg/kg every 8 hours for 10 to 14 days. In postinfectious encephalitis, corticosteroids have been used with apparent benefit; prognosis for good recovery is better than in viral encephalitis except in postmeasles encephalitis, which has a 25% mortality.

## INFECTIONS CAUSING MASS LESIONS

### Brain abscess

***Epidemiology and etiology.*** Sophisticated neurologic imaging has enhanced the recognition of brain abscesses, although the true incidence is decreasing as a result of the decrease in the prevalence of diseases often complicated by brain abscesses, such as chronic mastoiditis, bronchiectasis, and thoracic empyema. Brain abscess as a complication of otitis media demonstrates a bimodal distribution with peaks in the pediatric age group and in those over age 40 years. Abscesses secondary to paranasal sinusitis occur in patients who are between the ages of 10 to 30 years. An increased incidence of brain abscess occurs in immunocompromised patients, who are at risk for opportunistic infections such as fungi and parasites. Table 99-11 lists the microbiology of the most common brain abscesses.

***Pathophysiology.*** Brain abscesses are the result of contiguous spread from a nearby focus of infection, hematogenous spread from a distant focus, or direct inoculation by penetrating cranial trauma or surgery. The most common site for a solitary abscess is in the temporal lobe, followed by the frontoparietal, parietal, cerebellar, and occipital lobes. Hematogenously acquired infections are more likely to be multiple and occur in the distribution of the middle cerebral artery at the junction of the gray and white matter. A brain abscess begins as a cerebritis accompanied by significant edema, which develops a necrotic center. Capsule formation usually begins by the second week.

***History and physical examination.*** The clinical presentation of a brain abscess is insidious and may occur after the original focus has resolved. With advancing size, symptoms of brain compression develop. Headache and altered levels of consciousness may become apparent with seizures or focal neurologic deficits. In nearly half the patients the clinical syndrome is indistinguishable from brain tumor, without evidence of systemic illness such as fevers, foci of infection, elevated erythrocyte sedimentation rate (ESR), or leukocytosis. Abscesses near the meningeal or ventricular surfaces may produce meningismus, fever, and a leukocytic CSF pleocytosis. Abscesses that rupture into the ventricular or subarachnoid space may lead to coma and death.

**Table 99-11.** Microbiology and most common conditions associated with brain abscesses

| Predisposing condition | Site of abscess | Microbiology |
|---|---|---|
| Otitis media and mastoiditis | Temporal lobe or cerebellum | Streptococci, *Bacteroides fragilis,* Enterobacteriaceae |
| Frontoethmoidal sinusitis | Frontal lobe | Streptococci, *Bacteroides,* Enterobacteriaceae, *Staphylococcus aureus, Haemophilus* |
| Sphenoidal sinusitis | Frontal or temporal lobe | Same as for frontoethmoidal sinusitis |
| Dental procedures | Frontal lobe | Mixed *Fusobacterium, Bacteroides,* and streptococci |
| Postsurgery or trauma | Related to wound | *S. aureus,* streptococci, Enterobacteriaceae, *Clostridium* species |
| Congenital heart disease | Multiple abscesses, middle cerebral artery distribution | Streptococci, *Haemophilus* |
| Lung abscess, empyema, bronchiectasis | Same as for congenital heart disease | *Fusobacterium, Actinomyces, Bacteroides,* streptococci, *Nocardia* |
| Bacterial endocarditis | Same as for congenital heart disease | *S. aureus,* streptococci |
| Compromised host | Same as for congenital heart disease | *Toxoplasma,* fungi, Enterobacteriaceae, *Nocardia* |

Modified from Wispelwey B, Dacey RG Jr, Scheld WM: Brain abscess. In Scheld WM, Whitley RJ, Durack DT, editors: *Infections of the central nervous system,* New York, 1991, Raven.

***Laboratory studies and diagnostic procedures.*** A CT or MRI scan with contrast enhancement is the procedure of choice for diagnosis of an intracranial abscess. MRI is the procedure of choice for posterior fossa lesions. The specificity of the diagnosis is increased with MRI, which can differentiate brain abscess from the similar CT-appearing lesions of neoplasm, hematoma, granuloma, and infarction. MRI is also more useful in following the response to therapy. Chest x-ray and CT scan of paranasal and mastoid sinuses searching for a primary focus should also be obtained. Blood and urine cultures may provide a microbiologic diagnosis. Cardiac echocardiography may be performed if the diagnosis of endocarditis is suspected. A peripheral leukocytosis and elevated ESR may be seen. A lumbar puncture is contraindicated.

***Differential diagnosis.*** The diagnosis of brain abscess may be difficult because of the nonspecific presentation and lack of fever. Meningitis, viral encephalitis, epidural abscess, subdural empyema, mycotic aneurysms in association with endocarditis, and noninfectious etiologies such as intracerebral hemorrhage, cerebral venous sinus thrombosis or infarctions, and CNS malignancies may all have similar presentations. A high clinical suspicion is an important key to diagnosis.

***Management.*** Optimal management requires prompt consultation with neurosurgical and infectious disease specialists. Biopsy and/or drainage of encapsulated accessible lesions is required for microbiologic diagnosis and may be therapeutic. Empiric therapy should be initiated promptly despite a small risk that it may interfere with the recovery of microorganisms from a subsequent surgical procedure. Antibiotics should be chosen based on the likely pathogens (see Table 99-11). Penicillin, chloramphenicol, metronidazole, nafcillin, vancomycin, trimethoprim/sulfamethoxazole, and perhaps some third-generation cephalosporins have demonstrated clinical efficacy against susceptible organisms (see Table 99-4 for antibiotic dosing in CNS infections). Antibiotic therapy alone is recommended for cerebritis, with a good outcome. Medical management alone may also be necessary for inaccessible or multiple lesions and in individuals at high risk for surgery. Length of therapy is based on clinical response, and a prolonged course of therapy is likely to be required. The use of corticosteroids is controversial but may be beneficial in patients with impaired mental status from increased intracranial pressure. Poor outcomes are associated with advanced age, large abscesses, delay in appropriate therapy, and ventricular rupture. Neurologic sequelae, especially seizures, occur often. Cortical thrombophlebitis is a common complication of subdural abscesses.

## Epidural abscess

***Epidemiology and etiology.*** Paraspinal infections are relatively uncommon. Most epidural abscesses occur in individuals with an underlying condition and a source for hematogenous spread. Predisposing conditions include prior spinal surgery, degenerative joint disease, trauma, or underlying conditions such as diabetes, alcoholism, or cirrhosis. Sources of bacteremia include skin, urinary tract, sepsis, and catheter infections. *Staphylococcus aureus* is the etiologic agent in 60% to 90% of patients. Other etiologies include streptococci, gram-negative bacilli, tuberculosis, fungi, and a few parasites.

***Pathophysiology.*** Epidural abscesses are most often acquired via hematogenous spread from the bloodstream, from Batson's plexus, or through the lymphatics. They can also be a consequence of contiguous spread from vertebral osteomyelitis or from extension of infection from a retroperitoneal or intraabdominal site. An expanding abscess can cause cord compression or thrombosis of the surrounding vessels with infarction of the spinal cord. The abscess generally spans the length of several vertebrae.

The infection may spread to the subarachnoid space, producing a meningitis.

***History and physical examination.*** The clinical onset is either acute (less than 7 days) or chronic (progressing over weeks to months), although paralysis from cord compression occurs rapidly. Individuals have fever and intense, persistent, localized back pain; a radiculopathy may be present. Headache and meningismus may occur if the subarachnoid space becomes involved. The neurologic examination may be abnormal. Individuals with a chronic presentation are less likely to have fever. Weight loss is likely in patients with a tuberculous abscess.

***Laboratory studies and diagnostic procedures.*** A leukocytosis and elevated ESR are often present. Blood cultures are positive in up to 70% of nontuberculous epidural abscesses. The diagnostic procedures of choice are MRI or myelography with CT scan; CT scanning alone lacks sensitivity. Until the advent of MRI, a myelogram performed at the level of the first and second cervical vertebrae was important to define better the extent of the abscess. A plain x-ray is useful only with tuberculous abscesses and may demonstrate soft tissue calcifications not detectable by MRI. An isolated lumbar puncture should be avoided, but if CSF is obtained during myelography, it usually demonstrates a protein level greater than 100 mg/dl, normal glucose, and moderate pleocytosis.

***Differential diagnosis.*** Delay in diagnosis of this otherwise curable condition often leads to permanent paraplegia or quadriplegia. A high index of suspicion for epidural abscess must be maintained in any individual with back pain, since either the subtleness of the presentation or overwhelming sepsis may divert attention away from making an accurate diagnosis. The broad differential diagnosis includes other infectious etiologies (e.g., vertebral osteomyelitis, spinal subdural abscess) and noninfectious etiologies (e.g., back strain, disk herniation, transverse myelitis, neoplasm, sarcoidosis, hematoma, epidural lipomatosis).

***Management.*** The mainstay of treatment for epidural abscess has been specific antibiotic therapy combined with surgery to prevent mechanical compression. Some evidence suggests that some infections may respond to antibiotic therapy alone. The decision not to perform surgery must be made cautiously and with very close follow-up; any progression in the neurologic examination, which can occur within hours, should prompt immediate surgery. Empiric therapy should contain an antistaphylococcal agent plus additional agent(s), depending on the presumed site of the original infection, which can be modified when a specific etiologic diagnosis is made. Antibiotic therapy should be continued for 3 to 4 weeks or 6 to 8 weeks if vertebral osteomyelitis is also present. Complete recovery is expected if neurologic dysfunction is present for less than 24 hours. Patients who have cervical or posterior lesions may have a more limited recovery. At the present time, no role exists for corticosteroid therapy.

## BIBLIOGRAPHY


Centers for Disease Control and Prevention: Sexually transmitted diseases treatment guidelines, *MMWR* 42(RR-14):30, 1993.

Darouiche RO et al: Bacterial spinal epidural abscess: review of 43 cases and literature survey, *Medicine* 71:369, 1992.

Lambert HP, editor: *Infections of the central nervous system,* Philadelphia, 1991, Decker.

Scheld WM, Wispelwey B, editors: Meningitis, *Infect Dis Clin North Am* 4:4, 1990.

Scheld WM, Whitley RJ, Durack DT, editors: *Infections of the central nervous system,* New York, 1991, Raven.

Schlech WF III et al: Bacterial meningitis in the United States 1978 through 1981: the National Bacterial Meningitis Surveillance Study, *JAMA* 253:1749, 1985.

Tunkel AR, Scheld WM: Pathogenesis and pathophysiology of bacterial meningitis, *Clin Microbiol Rev* 6:118, 1993.

Wenger JD et al: Bacterial meningitis in the United States, 1986: report of a multistate surveillance study, *J Infect Dis* 162:1316, 1990.

Wheeler D et al: Medical management of spinal epidural abscess: case report and review, *Clin Infect Dis* 15:22, 1992.

Whitley RJ: Viral encephalitis, *N Engl J Med* 323:242, 1990.


CHAPTER

# 100 Multiple Sclerosis and Related Disorders

**Nagagopal Venna**

Multiple sclerosis and related disorders share the common pathologic condition of demyelination affecting the white matter fiber systems of the brain and spinal cord. However, their etiologies and natural course are diverse, as shown in the box below.

## MULTIPLE SCLEROSIS

Multiple sclerosis (MS) is the most common chronic neurologic disease among young adults and causes substantial chronic and recurring neurologic disability. It has a prevelance of 30 to 80 cases per 100,000 population in the northern United States and Canada, in contrast to a rate of about 5 per 100,000 in Japan, Asia, and Africa.

### Demyelinating diseases of the central nervous system

**Idiopathic**

Multiple sclerosis

**Related to infections**

Parainfectious acute disseminated encephalomyelitis
Progressive multifocal leukoencephalopathy
HTLV-1 myelopathy (tropical spastic paraparesis)

**Related to metabolic derangements**

Central pontine myelinolysis

Women and whites have an incidence twice that of white men and blacks in the United States. A 15-fold increase occurs among first-degree relatives of patients. Persons with the HLA-DR2 antigen have a sevenfold increased risk of MS. Its long course involves widespread disturbances of neurologic function, including motor, sensory, and gait abnormalities and impaired bladder, bowel, and sexual control. Various pain syndromes, fatigue, and affective and cognitive mental disturbances also occur. These diverse conditions demand the understanding and expertise of the primary physician as well as of many specialists to provide comprehensive care and support to patients.

### Pathology

The hallmark of MS is the multifocal inflammatory demyelination of the white matter fiber systems in the brain and spinal cord, which occurs in bouts over years. The axons are spared, as is the myelin of peripheral nerves. The optic nerves and tracts, cerebellar peduncles, medial longitudinal fasciculus of the brainstem, areas around the ventricles, and motor and sensory tracts of the cervical and thoracic spinal cord are preferentially affected. The acute lesions consist of focal demyelination with dense perivenular infiltration by activated T lymphocytes, B lymphocytes, macrophages, plasma cells, and inflammatory edema. In the chronic phase, these are replaced by dense gliosis (sclerosis).

### Etiology and pathogenesis

The etiology of this common disease remains obscure, but autoimmune mechanisms clearly are critically involved in the pathogenesis of MS. Activated circulating T lymphocytes enter the central nervous system (CNS) through the blood-brain barrier, secrete interleukins that stimulate a few clones of B lymphocytes, which in turn produce antibodies in the CNS. Interleukins also activate macrophages. The antibodies, cytokines, and activated macrophages thus produced are involved in a cascade that results in the inflammatory demyelination. The triggers to this autoimmune attack are not understood. Extensive epidemiologic studies have demonstrated that the increased risk of MS is acquired by living in the high-prevalence areas for the first 15 years of life, indicating the role of an environmental factor although it remains elusive.

The demyelinated axons within the brain, spinal cord, and optic nerves interfere with neurologic function by delay, dispersion, and blockage of electric impulses greatly decreasing the efficiency of central neural transmission. Certain features (e.g., pain, paresthesia, neuralgia) are probably related to abnormal generation of impulses by the injured fibers.

### Clinical features

The symptoms of MS are protean, depending on the locations of the demyelinating lesions, although surprising numbers of lesions are asymptomatic (see box at right). Typically, focal neurologic symptoms occur episodically, lasting several days to a few weeks, and abate. An abrupt decrease of vision in one eye, with a particular decline in color perception accompanied by a dull ache behind the eye, signals optic neuritis, which heralds the disease in nearly 25% of patients. Two thirds of such patients experience an excellent recovery of vision from the first episode. Only a third of all patients with monosymptomatic optic neuritis go on to develop clinical MS.

#### Clinical features of multiple sclerosis

**Episodic, but lasting days to weeks**

Cranial nerves: monocular decrease of vision, double vision

Limbs/trunk: Paresthesias/dysesthesias, Lhermitte sign, limb weakness and spasticity, limb/gait ataxia

Bladder: urinary urgency/frequency, incontinence (rarely retention)

Mental functions: depression, mania, euphoria; lability of emotional expression; cognitive decline

**Episodic, lasting minutes**

Trigeminal neuralgia

Tonic seizures

Episodes resembling transient ischemic attacks (TIAs)

**Chronic progressive syndrome**

Progressive spastic paraparesis with onset in middle age

**Hyperacute form**

Rare; encephalopathy with predilection for brainstem; tends to occur in adolescents and young adults

Manifestations of spinal cord demyelination are common initial complaints; lesions in the dorsal sensory columns cause episodes of tingling and numbness and a feeling of tightness as if the body part is wrapped in a cast or a tight garment. Paresthesias encircling the trunk (girdle sensations), brief numbing paresthesias in the genital and perineal region, and electric jolt–like sensations spreading down the body with neck flexion (Lhermitte sign) are characteristic. Fluctuating weakness of the limbs, often exacerbated by exercise, occurs frequently. Urgency of urination is an early symptom because of the development of spastic bladder. Occasionally the patients may have lumbar pain and sciatica closely mimicking disk herniation syndromes, probably related to demyelinating plaques affecting the root entry zones in the lumbar cord. Intermittent pain in the whole limb or trunk may also occur because of involvement of the spinothalamic tracts. A presentation similar to peripheral neuropathy, with tingling and numbness beginning in toes and spreading up the legs and trunk to affect the fingers, occurs because of an enlarging lesion in the posterior columns of the cervical cord (see Chapter 104 for additional information).

Prolonged episodes of double vision, dysarthria, body disequilibrium, clumsiness, and unsteadiness of limbs occur often and indicate foci of brainstem-cerebellar system demyelination. Lancinating unilateral facial pain identical to idiopathic trigeminal neuralgia may occur. Less frequently, acute bouts of vertigo or even deafness may occur from involvement of vestibular and auditory connections in the brainstem.

Increasingly, disorders of mental function are being recognized in MS even in the early stages of the disease. These may appear as depression, mania, and psychoses, as well as cognitive decline because of the lesions affecting the limbic and frontal areas of the cerebral hemispheres. However, seizures and aphasia are rare.

Neurologic symptoms that occur in brief paroxysms are less familiar. These are identical to transient ischemic episodes and episodes of painful spasms of one side of the body lasting minutes ("tonic seizures"), in which the arm, leg, and sometime head and neck undergo a tonic, painful flexion spasm. Sometimes patients experience numerous daily episodes of these symptoms.

A particularly suggestive aspect of the neurologic disturbances of MS is the transient exacerbation of visual, motor, or sensory symptoms caused by an increase in body temperature from exposure to a hot bath, hot weather, or high fever. A common and insidiously disabling symptom is fatigue.

## Physical signs

Neurologic examination is usually abnormal and typically reveals more findings than symptoms suggest. For example, a young woman seeking advice regarding numbness in one leg may be found to have bilateral upper motor neuron signs and nystagmus and an afferent pupillary defect. On the other hand, some patients have recurrent fleeting paresthesias and pains in the limbs for months or years with no abnormal physical signs on examination until an unequivocal episode of optic neuritis or acute transverse myelopathy declares the disease. Optic neuritis is manifest by decreased visual acuity. Color vision may be diminished even when visual acuity is normal. When light is shone in each eye alternately, the pupil on the side of optic neuritis fails to constrict and appears to dilate paradoxically. This afferent pupillary defect is caused by impaired optic nerve conduction into the pupillary light reflex arc. Another tell-tale sign is internuclear ophthalmoplegia; with attempted lateral gaze, there is paresis of adduction of one eye, and the abducting eye shows horizontal nystagmus because of involvement of the medical longitudinal fasciculus in the brainstem. Bilateral internuclear ophthalmoplegia in a young person is almost pathognomonic of MS.

Scanning dysarthria, ataxia of limbs, ataxia of trunk and gait, and head titubation reflect the disease's predilection for cerebellar tracts. Various combinations of upper motor neuron signs of spasticity, a pyramidal pattern of weakness, Babinski reflexes, and abnormalities of different modalities of sensation in the limbs and trunk reflect injury to the corticospinal, dorsal column, and lateral spinothalamic tracts. Superficial abdominal reflexes are lost early. Passive neck flexion may evoke the Lhermitte sign of electric jolt down the body. Mental alterations are common; most patients are appropriately concerned about their disability, whereas a few show prominent euphoria. More often, patients may experience major depression, but mania is rare. In some more advanced cases, cognitive decline of dementia proportions may occur. Lability of emotional expression of the "pseudobulbar palsy" type may accompany bilateral subcortical cerebral lesions, with crying or laughing inappropriate to the situation or out of synchrony with the person's mood.

## Natural course

The remitting and relapsing form is the most common clinical subgroup of the MS, in which multifocal CNS dysfunctions appear, regress, and relapse over several years. Most of these patients eventually enter into a progressive phase because of the cumulative effects of widespread lesions, with moderate to severe disability.

In about 20% to 30% of patients, the disease runs a benign course, with mild remitting symptoms and no significant impairment of function.

Rarely, MS with onset in middle age follows a slowly progressive form of spastic paraparesis.

A hyperacute form of MS is rare but is especially likely to occur in adolescents and may cause a "locked-in" syndrome because of transmural pontine demyelination.

## Diagnosis

The diagnosis of MS is based on a characteristic clinical picture assisted by certain laboratory tests and exclusion of other causes of a similar clinical picture. No pathognomonic laboratory test exists, and the tests should be evaluated in the clinical context.

Magnetic resonance imaging (MRI) scans provide good supportive evidence. The T2-weighted images are sensitive to areas of demyelination and appear as high-intensity signals in the brain and spinal cord (Figs. 100-1 and 100-2). They have characteristic topography in the periventricular white matter, cerebellar peduncles, and brainstem. Scanning after injection of the paramagnetic contrast agent gadolinium reveals even more lesions in the

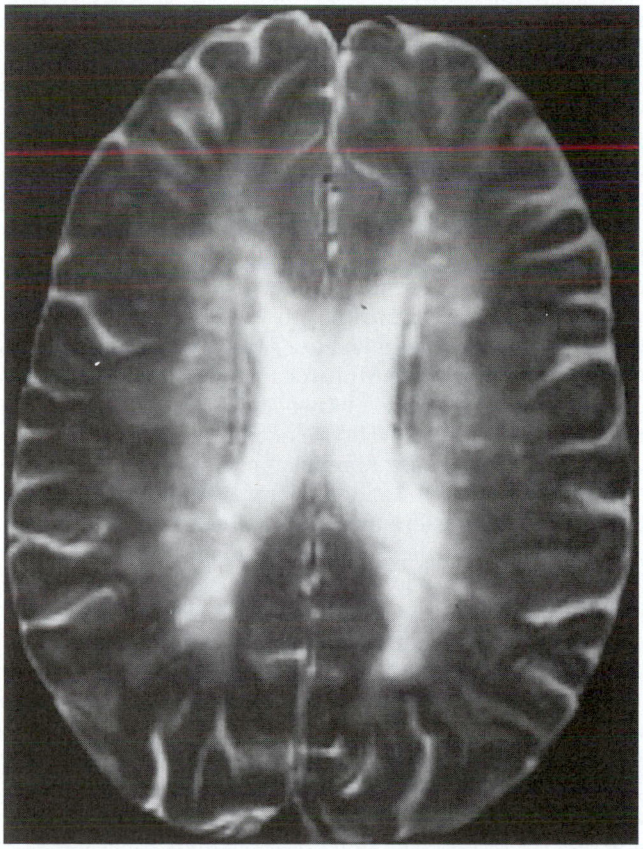

**Fig. 100-1.** Multiple sclerosis. Axial T2-weighted MRI brain scan shows extensive punctate and confluent periventricular bright signals in the white matter at the level of the lateral ventricles' bodies.

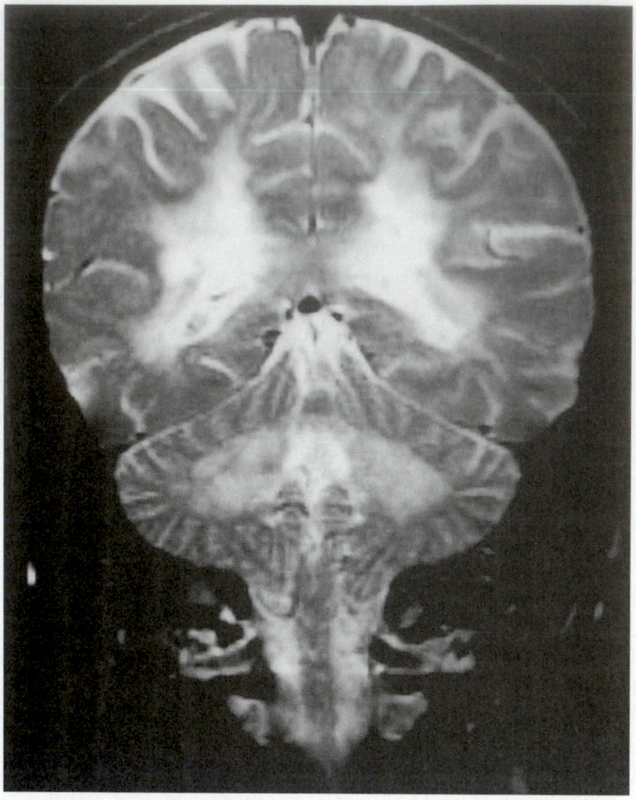

**Fig. 100-2.** Multiple sclerosis. Coronal T2-weighted MRI brain scan shows periventricular bright signal surrounding the occipital horns of the lateral ventricles and in the deep white matter of the cerebellar hemispheres (same patient as in Fig. 100-1).

white matter and may show enhancement of the lesions, possibly correlating with the plaque's inflammatory activity. The MRI scans are especially helpful in demonstrating the widespread, multifocal nature of the neurologic illness. For example, a patient with a clinical picture of cervical spinal cord lesion may have numerous cerebral white matter hyperintensities on the scan that are asymptomatic and even "asignamatic." However, the images are not specific for MS. Multifocal ischemia, sarcoidosis, progressive multifocal leukoencephalopathy, human immunodeficiency virus (HIV) encephalopathy, and leukodystrophies may cause similar appearances.

Visual- auditory-, and somatosensory-evoked potentials help detect asymptomatic involvement of the appropriate systems. Of these, the visual responses are the most useful clinically because of the frequent subclinical involvement of the optic nerves in MS. These tests are not specific for MS and are most useful to detect abnormalities not clinically evident.

The cerebrospinal fluid (CSF) may be acellular or show up to about 50 mononuclear cells/$mm.^3$ Higher counts should arouse suspicion of other diseases. Pleocytosis may correlate with activity of MS. CSF protein may be normal or mildly elevated, usually to less than 80 mg/dl, whereas glucose is normal. The detection of oligoclonal bands of immunoglobulin G (IgG) on electrophoresis of the CSF is a useful adjunct supporting the diagnosis because of their occurrence in about 80% of MS patients. Again, oligoclonal immunoglobulins are not specific for MS and may occur in systemic lupus erythematosus (SLE), sarcoidosis, neurosyphilis, and viral meningoencephalititis—all conditions that may mimic MS at some stage. CSF analysis is especially indicated and helpful in differentiating MS from other conditions that mimic it rather than in confirming the diagnosis.

## Differential diagnosis

A small group of unifocal lesions can resemble MS by producing a complex combination of neurologic disturbances because of their location and, moreover, may show the apparent fluctuations in symptoms. Arteriovenous malformations of the brainstem and Chiari malformation at the skull base are particularly relevant examples.

Certain remitting-relapsing systemic diseases can similarly affect the CNS; the notable ones include sarcoidosis and SLE. It is worth remembering that not every neurologic syndrome that remits and relapses and that is multifocal is MS. Patients with myasthenia gravis have been misdiagnosed as having MS because of fluctuating symptoms and asymmetric oculomotor weakness that mimics internuclear ophthalmoplegia, a similarity enhanced by the patient's response to corticosteroids.

## Treatment

In the absence of knowledge about the etiology of MS, treatment so far has been aimed at suppressing or modulating the immunopathogenic mechanisms with slight to modest benefit. A variety of symptomatic and supportive treatments are available to help patients cope with the illness better.

### *Specific treatment*

**Corticosteroids.** Adrenal steroids are useful in the treatment of disabling exacerbations of paraplegia, bulbar paresis, or *recurrent* optic neuritis by shortening the period of disability. However, they do not prevent recurrences or alter eventual neurologic disability. A currently popular, widely used, and quite safe method is an intravenous dose of 1g of methylprednisolone daily for 5 days. Others have used adrenocorticotropic hormone (ACTH, corticotropin), 80 units intravenously for a week followed by another week intramuscularly. When parenteral drugs are not acceptable, a 10-day course of prednisone at 60 mg daily may be given. However, in patients with idiopathic acute optic neuritis without other evidence of MS, steroids should be avoided, since a recent study indicated that steroid therapy may increase the risk of subsequent MS.

**β-Interferon.** A recent multicenter, double-blind, clinically controlled MRI brain study showed, for the first time, that the immunomodulator β-interferon is beneficial in the 2-year course of MS. This was measured by number of exacerbations, time to first relapse, severity of relapse, and decrease in the brain plaque load, as measured by serial MRI scans. Although the benefit seemed to taper off in the third year, the study is the first to show a clinically significant effect on the long-term disease activity and is a promising beginning. Genetically engineered β-interferon is given at 8 million units subcutaneously 3 days a week for an indefinite period in patients with remitting and relapsing MS. It is now approved by the U.S. Food and Drug Administration for general use, but its final place and

**Table 100-1.** Symptomatic therapies in multiple sclerosis

| Condition | Therapy |
|---|---|
| Urinary disturbances | Urologic evaluation for precise definition of bladder pathophysiology and to rule out nonneurologic structural causes of symptoms |
| | Anticholinergic drugs |
| | Oxybutinin: 2.5-5.0 mg tid |
| Urgency/incontinence | Propantheline: 7.5-15 mg qid |
| | Imipramine: 10-75 mg/day |
| | Mechanical assistance |
| | Intermittent self catheterization |
| Urinary retention | Bethanecol: 10-50 mg tid or qid |
| | Intermittent self catheterization |
| Spasticity | Needs treatment if associated with flexor spasms or is dysfunctional |
| | Baclofen: start at 10 mg bid; increase up to 80 mg/day |
| | Diazepam: 5 mg bid; increase up to 10 mg tid |
| Fatigue | Drugs moderately useful |
| | Amantadine: 100 mg once or twice a day |
| | Pemoline: 18.75 mg once or twice a day |
| Tonic seizures | Drugs very effective |
| | Carbamazepine: 100-200 mg tid |
| | Clonazepam: 0.5-1.0 mg tid |
| Trigeminal neuralgia | Drugs very effective |
| | Carbamazepine: 100-200 mg tid |
| | Baclofen: 10-40 mg bid |
| Emotional disturbances | |
| Pathologic crying or laughing | Amitriptyline: 10-50 mg qhs |
| Oscillopsia | Clonazepam: 0.5-1.0 mg tid |
| Vertigo | Scopolamine: transdermal patches |
| | Meclizine: 25 mg tid prn |

indications and limitations will become apparent only with more widespread experience. The drug probably interferes with the immunopathologic cascade in an as yet poorly understood manner. It is noteworthy that *gamma* interferon consistently increased exacerbations.

**Other immune therapies.** The benefits of immunosuppressive therapy with periodic intravenous infusions of cyclophosphamide and methylprednisolone in slowing MS in its chronic progressive forms remain controversial and ambiguous. However, this therapy appears to stabilize neurologic decline in some patients. Wide-ranging and increasingly targeted immune therapies are being tried and tested in many centers based on expanding and sophisticated knowledge about the immunopathogenesis of MS. It is hoped clinically relevant results will be forthcoming.

***Symptomatic treatment.*** Symptomatic treatments are available to enhance the quality of life of MS patients and can be remarkably effective (Table 100-1).

***Supportive measures.*** The lack of a cure or a specific treatment that halts progression, the long and unpredictable course, and accumulating neurologic and neuropsychologic disabilities, with the attendant dislocations of work, recreation, and family life in young adults, make the care of MS patients complex and at times daunting. Pharmacologic therapies form only a small, but significant, part of the treatment. The physician needs to anticipate and coordinate extremely helpful support from physical and occupational therapists to enable the patient to adapt to the disabilities at home and work. Psychologic support is often of paramount importance and is available through support groups and other organizations such as the MS Society. Consultations are often needed with psychiatrists, physiatrists, urologists, and nutritionists for specific complications and needs. Patients need expert information on a variety of issues that arise in the long course of the disease.

Since many patients are young women, the question of pregnancy and its impact on MS arises regularly. The findings of systematic studies will help patients in their personal decisions. Pregnancy actually diminishes flare-ups, but exacerbations are more frequent in the 6-month postpartum period. However, the long-term course and disability are not affected by pregnancies and childbirths. Because of the potential for worsening in the postpartum period, proper planning for additional help in caring for the newborn is needed.

Finally, the informed physician has an important role in guiding the patient away from unproven fads that are often costly and potentially harmful besides being useless. Physical and occupational therapy evaluation and treatment are frequently invaluable in maximizing the patient's neurologic function.

## DEMYELINATING DISORDERS RELATED TO INFECTIONS

### Acute parainfectious disseminated encephalomyelitis

Acute disseminated encephalomyelitis is an uncommon but serious sequela to exanthems such as measles, chickenpox, rubella, mumps, and influenza. It may follow vaccinations, especially against rabies, and complicate administration of serum. At present, however, the most frequent antecedent is a nonspecific upper respiratory infection. Pathologically, there are small, widespread, multifocal, periventricular lymphocytic infiltrations surrounded by foci of demyelination of white matter tracts throughout the brain and spinal cord. The disorder appears to be a cell-mediated immune hypersensitivity reaction to viruses similar to experimental acute allergic encephalomyelitis, which can be readily induced in animals by inoculating them with extracts of brain with adjuvants.

Clinically, this serious illness evolves rapidly in a monophasic course 1 to 3 weeks after the inciting event with abrupt onset of fever, headache, neck stiffness, drowsiness, seizures, and various focal cerebral symptoms, including confusion, hemiparesis, hemianopsia, choreoathetosis, or myoclonus. Myelopathy may be manifest by paraparesis or quadriparesis. Computed tomography (CT) or MRI of the brain shows multifocal, small, abnormal white matter signals widespread in cerebral, cerebellar, and brainstem areas, sometimes with brain swelling. CSF may be normal but often shows predominantly lymphocytic pleocytosis with normal glucose. Oligoclonal immunoglobulins are often present in CSF. Electroencephalography (EEG) shows prominent, widespread, but nonspecific slowing. The diagnosis is clinical through the combination of an acute, monophasic encephalomyelitis syndrome occurring in the appropriate context of a latent period after the inciting event and supported by brain imaging and CSF abnormalities.

Acute parainfectious disseminated encephalomyelitis causes substantial mortality and morbidity, with a rate of about 20% for each. Survivors may have epilepsy, focal residual neurologic deficits, and chronic behavioral disorders, although complete recovery also occurs. High-dose steroid therapy is widely used, with dexamethasone or methylprednisone for 1 week to 10 days, and seems to ameliorate the condition. However, no controlled trials have been done.

### Progressive multifocal leukoencephalopathy

This once rare disorder has entered into everyday clinical practice with the acquired immunodeficiency syndrome (AIDS) epidemic. In the pre-AIDS era, progressive multifocal leukoencephalopathy (PML) was a rare neurologic complication arising in the course of lymphomas, during antineoplastic treatment of cancers, in myeloproliferative disorders, during immunosuppressive treatment of autoimmune disorders and organ transplants, and in association with sarcoidosis, Whipple disease, and nontropical sprue. All these conditions are accompanied by deficient cellular immunity. AIDS now is the leading cause of this disease, occurring in up to 5% of patients. PML is caused by an extraordinarily specific infection of the brain oligodendrocytes (which normally produce the CNS myelin) by the papova JC virus, with resulting extensive patches of demyelination scattered throughout the brain with remarkably little inflammatory response. The white matter of the cerebral hemispheres, cerebellum, and brainstem is affected in various combinations, with lesions accumulating over a few months.

The clinical picture of PML is characterized by subacute evolution of various focal neurologic deficits depending on the location of the lesions. Progressive hemiparesis, hemianopsia, hemisensory impairments, cerebellar and brainstem abnormalities, and cognitive and behavioral abnormalities appear and accumulate in a stepwise manner over months without headaches, impaired alertness, or seizures. MRI of the brain shows highly characteristic lesions (Figs. 100-3 and 100-4). Multifocal abnormal signals are seen in the subcortical white matter of the cerebral and cerebellar hemispheres and brainstem tracts. Lesions appear "punched out," without mass effect and with little if any enhancement with contrast agent. CSF is unremarkable, without inflammatory response. Presumptive diagnosis may be made by the characteristic clinical and MR images along with a negative CSF analysis. Confirmation is by stereotactic brain biopsy, which reveals focal demyelination, bizarre astrocytosis, and intranuclear inclusions in the oligodendrocytes on electron microscopy. Recently, the papova JC virus deoxyribonucleic acid (DNA) has been identified by polymerase chain reaction (PCR) techniques from the blood and CSF and may provide supportive evidence.

PML is an aggressive disease that usually results in severe disability over a few months and death in about 6 months to a year. In the AIDS era, however, cases have been reported with unexpected stabilization or even spontaneous regression of the disease. No specific effective treatment is documented in controlled trials, although a few case reports indicate an apparent response to

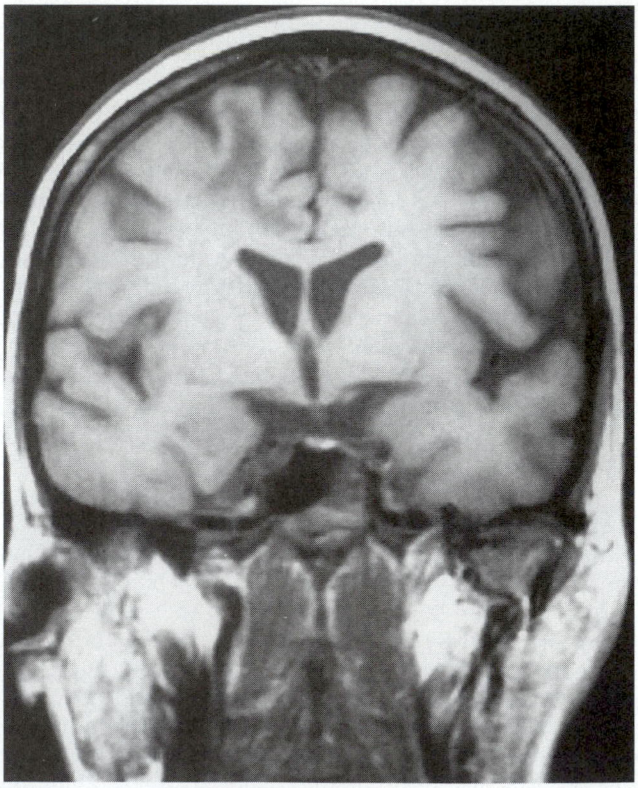

**Fig. 100-3.** Progressive multifocal leukoencephalopathy (PML). Coronal T1-weighted MRI brain scan shows a "punched-out" area of low signal undercutting the medial frontal lobe cortical gyri above the right frontal horn. There is no mass effect.

α-interferon and/or cytarabine. With the increased incidence of PML, a great need exists for systematic therapeutic trials of antiviral and immunomodulatory treatments for this devastating condition.

### HTLV-1 myelopathy

With the advances in our understanding of retroviruses over the last decade, a chronic myelopathy of unknown cause that was known to be endemic to many parts of the world and called *tropical spastic paraparesis* has been shown to be caused by the virus HTLV-1 (human T cell lymphotrophic virus type 1). The endemic areas are southwestern Japan, the Caribbean region, and western Africa. Increasing numbers of patients are recognized in the United States among immigrants as well as in the native population. The predominant pathologic change is diffuse demyelination of the lateral and posterior columns of the spinal cord accompanied by perivascular lymphocytic infiltrations, astrocytosis, and chronic meningitis. Evidence suggests that immunopathogenic mechanisms mediate the spinal cord damage and that less than 1% of the patients with HTLV-I antibodies in the serum develop the neurologic complication. The virus is spread by transfusion, intravenous drug use, breastfeeding, and less often by sexual intercourse.

Clinically, patients have an insidious, chronic, slowly worsening spastic paraparesis beginning about age 40 years, with women affected much more often than men. Symptoms of bladder spasticity, constipation, impotence, and back pain are common. The neurologic functions tend to stabilize after a few years of gradual decline and only rarely progress to paraplegia. Patients regularly survive 10 to 40 years after onset of myelopathy. The relationship of this myelopathy to other viral myelopathies including HIV and CMV is described in Chapter 104.

The CSF shows mild lymphocytic pleocytocis and oligoclonal immunoglobulins with normal glucose. About 1% of the CSF and blood lymphocytes have a characteristic multilobulated appearance of their nuclei similar to the appearance of T cell leukemia. Spinal cord MRI may be normal or may show mild diffuse enlargement of the cord and increased signals on T2 images similar to those seen in MS. Confirmation is provided by serum and CSF, which show high titers of HTLV-1 antibodies.

Empiric therapies have been tried with oral and intravenous steroids, plasmapheresis, and AZT (azidothymidine) and interferon, with minimal results and short-lived improvements. No systematic clinical trials have yet been reported.

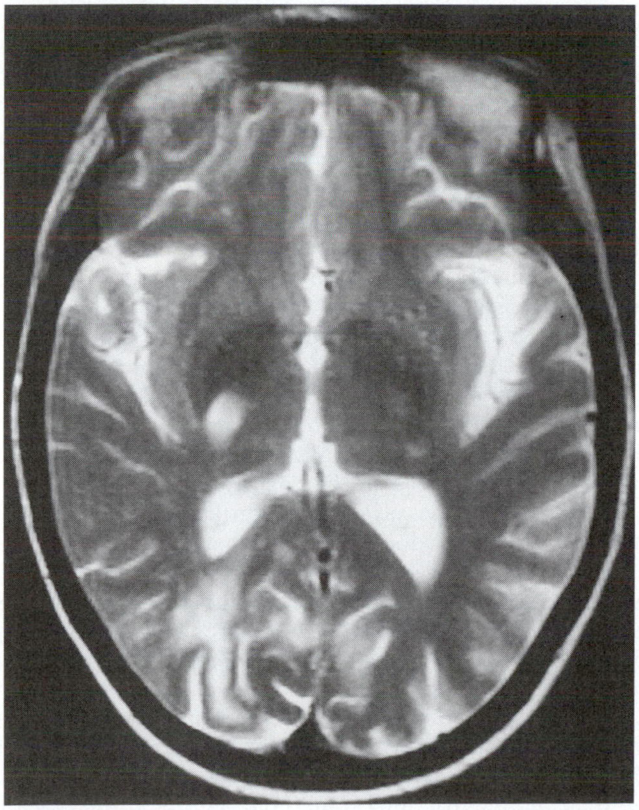

**Fig. 100-4.** PML. Axial T2-weighted MRI brain scan shows patches of bright signal in the subcortical white matter of the parietooccipital area and in the internal capsule on the right (same patient as in Fig. 100-3).

## DEMYELINATING DISORDER RELATED TO METABOLIC DERANGEMENTS: CENTRAL PONTINE MYELINOLYSIS

This uncommon and unique disorder is characterized by a monophasic, subacute, discrete demyelination of the pontine white matter tracts composed of corticospinal, corticobulbar, and pontocerebellar fibers. Central pontine myelinolysis is a hospital-acquired demyelinating disorder occurring typically in malnourished patients with alcoholism admitted for an intercurrent illness such as liver failure or gastrointestinal bleeding and treated intensively. The critical pathogenic factor is hyponatremia and its rapid correction to eunatremia. However, the disorder has been described without hyponatremia and in patients with hyponatremia without alcoholism.

Clinically, patients develop paradoxical worsening while recovering from their intercurrent illness. Spastic

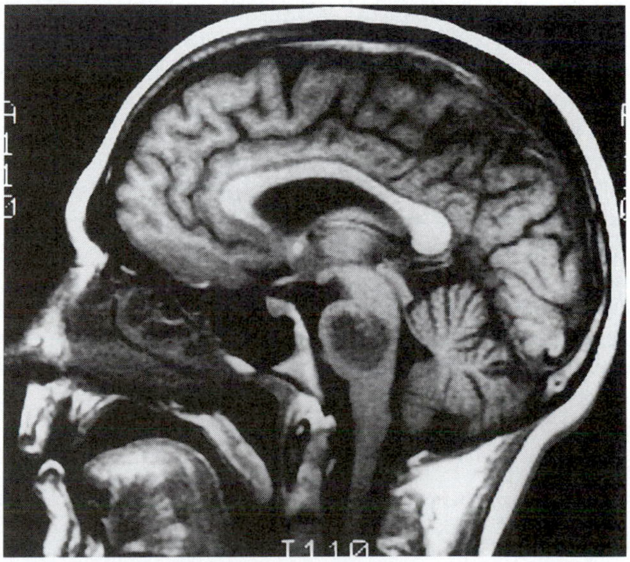

**Fig. 100-5.** Central pontine myelinolysis. Midsagittal T1-weighted MRI brain scan shows a clearly demarcated large area of low signal occupying the pons without causing mass effect.

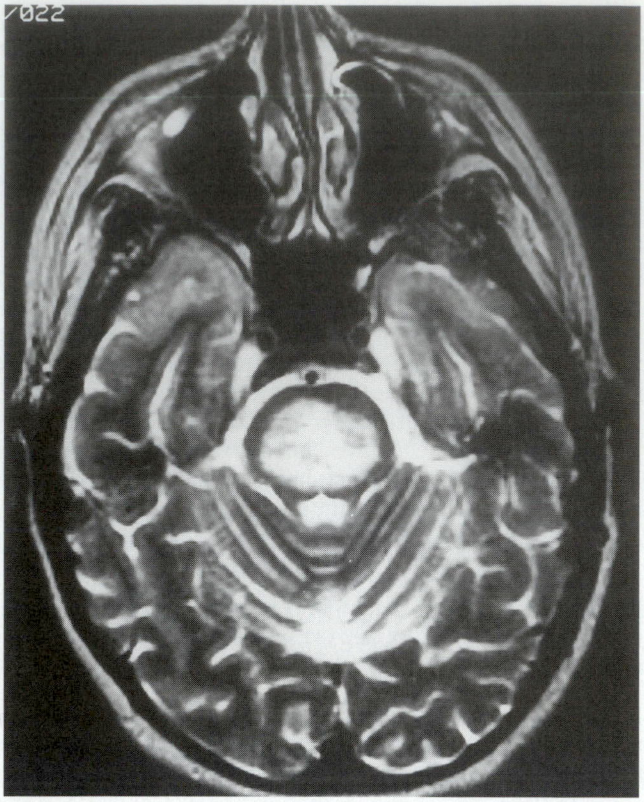


**Fig. 100-6.** Central pontine myelinolysis. Axial T2-weighted MRI brain scan shows bright signal occupying almost the entire cross section of the pons without mass effect on the adjacent fourth ventricle (same patient as in Fig. 100-5).

quadriparesis, dysarthria and difficulty swallowing, and lability of emotional expression with facile crying and laughing occur and in severe cases may worsen to "locked-in" syndrome with stupor. Occasionally, cerebellar dysfunction of speech and of limbs and trunk predominates. The best laboratory aid for diagnosis is MRI of the brain, which shows a large "punched-out" area of abnormal signal in the basis pontis without mass effect, sometimes associated smaller foci of abnormal signal in the cerebral white matter as well (Figs. 100-5 and 100-6). CSF is normal. Presence of hyponatremia and its correction usually provide the tell-tale diagnostic clue.

Despite the catastrophic appearance of the brainstem syndrome, central pontine myelinolysis is reversible in most patients with supportive therapy of protecting the airway and maintaining nutrition. Most patients make an astonishingly complete recovery over a few months. Prevention of this condition is even more important by being aware of this disorder in the correct context and deliberately slowing correction of hyponatremia.

## BIBLIOGRAPHY

Berger JR et al: Progressive multifocal leukoencephalopathy associated with human immunodeficiency virus infection, *Ann Intern Med* 107:78, 1987.

Birk K, Smeltzer SC, Rudick R: Pregnancy and multiple sclerosis, *Semin Neurol* 8:205, 1988.

Blaivas JG, Kavcan SA: Urologic dysfunction in patients with multiple sclerosis, *Semin Neurol* 8:159, 1988.

Canadian MS Research Group: A randomized controlled trial of amantadine in fatigue associated with multiple sclerosis, *Can J Neurol Sci* 14:273, 1987.

Gout O et al: Chronic myelopathy associated with HTLV-1, *Arch Neurol* 46:255, 1989.

IFNB Multiple Sclerosis Study Group: Interferon beta-lb is effective in relapsing-remitting multiple sclerosis. I. Clinical results of a multicenter, randomized, double-blind, placebo-controlled trial, *Neurology* 43:655, 1993.

Johnson RT, Griffin DE, Gendelman HE: Postinfectious encephalomyelitis, *Semin Neurol* 5:180, 1985.

McFarlin DE, McFarland HF: Medical progress: multiple sclerosis, *N Engl J Med* 307:1183, 1246, 1982.

Messert B et al: Central pontine myelinolysis—consideration on etiology, diagnosis and treatment, *Neurology* 29:147, 1979.

Milligan NM, Newcombe R, Compston DAS: A double-blind controlled trial of high dose methylprednisolone in patients with multiple sclerosis. I. Clinical effects, *Neurology* 50:511, 1987.

Olsson T: Immunology of multiple sclerosis, *Curr Opin Neurol Neurosurg* 5:195-202, 1992.

CHAPTER

# 101 Seizure Disorders

**Marianne E. Giuffra**
**Fereydoun Shahrokhi**

A seizure can be one of life's most frightening experiences, both for the individual and the observer. The sudden, violent motion of a motor seizure or the noxious odor that heralds the helpless, twilight state of a complex partial episode each cause trepidation in the person that does not diminish even after years of stereotyped repetition. The panic that a "fit" provokes in the onlookers has resulted in bizarre interpretations, such as possession by evil spirits. Even among physicians, the liberal prophylactic treatment of seizures is testimony to our desire to avoid this phenomenon that epitomizes loss of control. However, seizures are one of the most common neurologic symptoms, occurring in millions of people each year.

The original assertion of Hughlings Jackson in the mid-19th century, that seizures are an abnormal electric discharge of the gray matter of the brain, still characterizes much of our concept of the nature of seizures today. "Seizure" encompasses a great variety of clinical phenomena, many of which are not generally recognized as such. *Partial* seizures begin in a discrete area of the brain and have symptoms that reflect the functions of that area and related areas. *Generalized* seizures can immediately produce unconsciousness and convulsions. Thus a seizure can be symptomatic of focal brain damage, such as a contusion, or a transient metabolic disturbance, such as hypoglycemia. If the first seizure of a patient's life occurs during medical illness, the seizure probably is a symptom of that illness. An important goal of the primary care physician is to recognize, investigate, and ameliorate the causes of symptomatic seizures.

However, if despite identifying and eliminating known causes of seizures, they occur repeatedly over years, the designation *epilepsy* is sometimes used. "Epileptic" has many negative connotations and tends to identify the illness with the person, isolating that person from his or her peers. The seizures that constitute epilepsy may be *secondary* to a structural or metabolic derangement (e.g., congenital malformation, aminoaciduria) and may have associated mental retardation and neurologic deficits. Primary or idiopathic epilepsies of genetic origin have no identifiable gross structural pathology but may have altered synaptic architecture or neurotransmitter chemistry that predisposes members of a kindred to have seizures.

Classification of seizure types by phenomenology is valuable because it can suggest the location of the brain disturbance, the likelihood of a correctable cause, and the most promising forms of pharmacotherapy. The largest division in the classification is between seizures that are generalized at the onset and seizures that begin focally. Sometimes, seizures that appear clinically to be generalized will be found on an electroencephalogram (EEG) to begin locally and spread promptly to both hemispheres of the brain, resulting in a generalized convulsion. This can occur with partial seizures of many types and is referred to as *secondary generalization.* Partial seizures of temporal lobe or frontal lobe origin, in which consciousness is incompletely affected, can be particularly difficult to recognize as such. The patient appears to be in a dreamlike state, although the EEG shows a focal seizure discharge. These patients frequently also have secondarily generalized seizures. A vague malaise or emotional dysphoria may be present for several days preceding a seizure, referred to as the *prodrome.* Immediately before the seizure, sensations such as fear, sensory hallucinations such as an unpleasant odor, visual obscurations, or other lightning-fast warnings of seizure are referred to as the *aura.* A few patients may perceive that they can abort the seizure by sensory stimulation or intense mental concentration at this stage. In the vast majority, however, the aura is simply a signal to sit or lie down to avoid injury.

Table 101-1 provides one classification system for seizures and associated EEG abnormalities.

## TYPES OF SEIZURES

### Generalized seizures

The most familiar seizure has loss of consciousness at onset and is often referred to as a *grand mal seizure.* The procession of motor phenomena follows a somewhat predictable pattern. Beginning with a sudden muscular stiffening, the tonic phase causes the patient to fall to the ground like a board rather than a rag doll. With the muscles locked in contraction, respiration stops, the jaw clenches (causing involuntary tongue biting), and the bladder is emptied as the eyes roll upward and the neck and back extend. In short succession, clonic movements (i.e., repetitive flexion of the arms, neck, and hips) begin to occur simultaneously throughout the body. After a few minutes the clonic movements slow their rate and finally cease, but the patient remains unconscious for several minutes. As consciousness is regained, the person is confused, has no memory for the seizure or its onset, and feels tired, with headache and muscle soreness *(postictal state).* The individual may defensively push people away who are in physical proximity in the first moments of awakening. Variants of generalized seizures include pure clonic or tonic seizures or initial clonic activity followed by a tonic phase that becomes clonic again. Generalized seizures of the tonic-clonic type can be occur in many settings: as symptoms of systemic disease, metabolic disturbances, and drug reactions, as well as the manifestation of idiopathic epilepsy.

Uninterrupted, generalized seizure activity or frequent, repeated activity that does not permit the recovery of consciousness between seizures is called *status epilepticus.* Status is an emergency from both a general medical and a neurologic standpoint. Besides the effects of prolonged autonomic dysfunction and the possibility of aspiration, there are severe, unmet metabolic demands in brain tissue during continuous seizures that can lead to permanent dysfunction. The treatment of status epilepticus is discussed later in this chapter.

### Simple partial seizures

Simple partial seizures refer to those that occur in a discrete part of the brain, also referred to as the *seizure focus.* Therefore, their symptomatology relates to the normal neuronal function of that region. By definition, simple partial seizures are not associated with impairment of consciousness; however, the initial discharge may spread and give rise to other symptoms, even a generalized tonic-clonic seizure. The earliest symptoms generally give the best localizing information regarding any possible structural abnormality in the brain.

The partial *somatosensory* seizures that originate from the parietal sensory area give rise to paresthesias such as a "pins and needles" sensation or a feeling of numbness. In a simple partial *motor* seizure, twitching or jerking can be seen in an extremity or in one side of the face. A hand or foot may begin shaking, and the seizure may progressively include the more proximal portion of the extremity and then that side of the body, in what is referred to as a *Jacksonian march.* Partial seizures of the *special senses* may occur. Occipital seizures may manifest with lights, colors, flashes, or other unformed visual phenomena, including partial visual obscuration. More well-formed visual hallucinations may follow from progressive involvement of the adjacent temporal lobe. Auditory seizures are rare but may manifest in an analogous manner, with phenomena ranging from crude sounds to music. Distinct auditory hallucinations, however, especially voices, are much more frequently a manifestation of psychiatric disease. Olfactory, gustatory (taste), and vertiginous seizures may occur, although infrequently. Seizures also may have *autonomic* features, such as nausea, pallor, pupillary dilatation, sudden diarrhea, abdominal cramps, sweating, piloerection, and skin redness or blanching. These symptoms rarely occur alone, however, and are usually a part of the complex partial seizures of temporal or orbitofrontal origins, as discussed next.

### Complex partial seizures

Complex partial seizures are also commonly referred to as "psychomotor" or "temporal lobe" seizures, although they can also arise from the frontal lobes. The term "petit mal" is sometimes erroneously used to refer to complex partial seizures; however, neurologists reserve this term for the peculiar seizure of childhood called *absence.*

Complex partial seizures are associated with partial impairment of awareness and various psychic symptoms such as memory flashbacks, dreamlike states, or intense feelings, such as the feeling that a given new experience has occurred before (déjà vu) or of strangeness in a familiar environment (jamais vu). The mind may become fixed on a single thought, memory, tune, or "vision," or the patient may even have the feeling that he or she has moved out of the body and is observing his or her own life from outside the body (depersonalization). Distortion of perception in visual (micropsia, macropsia) or auditory (hypoacusis, hyperacusis) sensations may occur. Unprovoked affective sensations, such as laughter, rage, terror, intense sadness, elation, or a feeling of omniscience, have been reported as part of complex partial seizures. These same patients may develop automatisms, in which they repeatedly carry out an elaborate learned motor task such as lip smacking, chewing, picking at clothing, swallowing, dressing, undressing, eating, running, or more complex motor behavior. Directed violent behavior is not attributable to seizure activity. Although patients may repel the attempts of helpful passersby by pushing or struggling, particularly in the postictal stage, purposeful aggression involving pursuit or a weapon is not an unconscious act.

The most prevalent pathologic and radiologic correlate of the tendency toward complex partial seizures in adults and children is *hippocampal sclerosis.* This refers to alterations in certain cellular components of a phylogenetically older portion of the medial temporal lobe, believed to result from a prenatal or perinatal insult.

### Myoclonic seizures

*Myoclonus* is a quick jerk of one or more extremities, the trunk, or the face and can occur in many clinical contexts. The most familiar form of myoclonus is the sudden jolt that can occur in the first stages of drowsiness or sleep, frequently awakening us. Another form of myoclonus, especially with intentional movement, is sometimes present in individuals who have anoxic brain damage. Multiple small and large jerking movements can be prominent in acute renal failure. Myoclonus can also be either the predominant clinical manifestation of a seizure or a prelude to a generalized seizure. Idiopathic familial myoclonic epilepsies usually begin in early childhood and may be benign and easily controlled. Juvenile myoclonic epilepsy presents with a series of myoclonic jerks, occurring in the morning and sometimes, but not always, progressing to a generalized tonic-clonic seizure. More malignant syndromes, the progressive myoclonic epilepsies, are usually accompanied by other seizure types, are associated with intellectual and motor deterioration, and result from genetic or metabolic abnormalities. Myoclonic jerks occur frequently in patients with Creutzfeldt-Jakob disease and in 15% of those with end-stage Alzheimer disease.

### Atonic seizures

Atonic seizures consist of a sudden loss of tone in the muscles of the jaw, neck, extremities, or the entire body, which may cause the patient to drop suddenly to the ground. Most seizures of this type have some associated myoclonic jerks or generalized seizures. Atonic seizures are differentiated from the cataplexy of the narcoleptic patient by the epileptiform discharges on the EEG and from the "drop attacks" of posterior circulation ischemia by the associated symptoms of brainstem ischemia. Atonic seizures usually occur in children and rarely occur in adults.

### Febrile convulsions

When an infant or child age 6 months to 5 years has a brief, generalized seizure during a fever of 38°C (100.4°F) or more, without any evidence of intracranial infection or other predisposing cause, it is said to be a *simple febrile* convulsion. In children under age 6 months, who may not manifest typical signs of meningitis, a lumbar puncture is strongly indicated. If any possibility of trauma or electrolyte disturbance exists, the appropriate diagnostic tests (imaging or blood chemistries) should be performed. *Complex febrile* seizures last more than 15 minutes, begin focally, are accompanied by neurologic abnormalities, recur within 24 hours, or progress to status epilepticus. These also should be more thoroughly investigated.

### Absence seizures

Absence (pronounced with a French accent), also referred to as *petit mal,* is a generalized seizure disorder of childhood. It is distinct from general tonic-clonic seizures clinically and has a unique EEG pattern and most likely a different pathophysiology. Attacks usually consist of a brief interruption of motor and mental activity, often without a change in posture or tone. The child has a blank stare and does not respond when spoken to for several seconds. At other times, the lapse of consciousness may be associated with minimal myoclonic movements around the eyelids or mouth or a mild increase or decrease in muscular tone. Children may realize that they had an episode because there is no postictal confusion. The ictal EEG in absence shows a characteristic three-per-second generalized spike-and-wave discharge (Fig. 101-1), and spells can frequently be elicited by hyperventilation. The attacks are sometimes accompanied by automatisms, including lip smacking or fumbling movements with the fingers, but these are less common and elaborate than those of complex partial seizures. Other differentiating factors include the shorter duration of the absence attack, which lasts less than 30 seconds, in contrast to 1 or more minutes for complex partial seizures. Furthermore, absence seizures rarely persist into adulthood.

### Reflex epilepsy

In certain susceptible patients, seizures can be regularly evoked by simple sensory experiences, the most common and familiar being flashing lights or shifting patterns. The phenomenon occurs in a small percentage of all epileptic patients, but particularly in those with the benign, primary, generalized epilepsies of childhood. Routine stimulation during an EEG with flashing light at various frequencies attempts to take advantage of this to demonstrate epileptiform activity. However, very rare cases have been described in which seizures can be elicited by more complex sensory or mental phenomena, such as mental arithmetic, listening to music, reading, and even simply moving, which serves as a proprioceptive stimulus. Seizures thus evoked are usually partial, and the seizure focus corresponds to the cortical area responsible for the evoking

**Table 101-1.** Classification of seizures

| Clinical types | EEG abnormalities |
|---|---|
| I. Partial (focal) seizures | |
| A. Simple partial seizures (consciousness or awareness not impaired) | Focal contralateral paroxysmal discharge (spikes, sharp waves, other abnormal bursts) in ictal or interictal states |
| 1. Motor seizures | |
| a. Focal without march | |
| b. Jacksonian march | |
| c. Versive (usually contraversive seizures with head and eyes deviated to opposite side from seizure focus) | |
| 2. Sensory seizures | |
| a. Somatosensory (i.e., paresthesia over opposite side of body) | |
| b. Visual (e.g., light flashes or formed hallucinations) | |
| c. Auditory, olfactory (usually as part of complex partial seizures) | |
| 3. Autonomic seizures (usually as part of complex partial seizures) | |
| B. Complex partial seizures (mainly psychomotor or temporal lobe epilepsy) | Unilateral or bilateral paroxysmal discharges, usually in temporal regions in ictal or interictal states |
| Level of awareness always impaired; ictal symptoms include some of following: | |
| 1. Cognitive or perceptive impairment (e.g., dreamy state, déjà vu, depersonalization, illusions, or hallucinations) | |
| 2. Affective symptoms (e.g., fear, rage, sadness, elation) | |
| 3. Automatic and repetitive behavior (e.g., chewing, smacking) | |
| C. Partial seizures evolving to secondary generalized convulsions | |
| II. Generalized seizures (convulsive or nonconvulsive) | |
| A. Petit mal (absence) seizures | Rhythmic, symmetric three cycles/second and slow waves in ictal or interictal states |
| 1. Impairment in level of awareness always present | |
| 2. Small clonic movements in some patients | |
| 3. Tonic or atonic components in some patients | |
| 4. Automatic behavior in some patients | |
| B. Tonic-clonic (grand mal) seizures | Rhythmic 10 or more cycles/second polyspike activity during tonic phase, interrupted by slow waves during clonic phase; low voltage or slow activity in postictal state; fragments of paroxysmal discharges in interictal state |
| C. Clonic seizures | |
| D. Tonic seizures | |
| E. Myoclonic seizures (or jerks): single or multiple myoclonic jerks | Polyspike and wave or at times spike wave or sharp wave in ictal or interictal states |
| F. Atonic seizures: "drop attacks," head drop, slackening of the jaw, with brief or no loss of consciousness | Polyspikes and slow wave or repetitive fast activity or flattening of EEG background in ictal state; fragments of these, but usually polyspike and slow waves, in interictal state |
| III. Addendum | |
| A. Status epilepticus (no complete recovery between attacks) | |
| 1. Grand mal status | |
| 2. Petit mal (absence) status | |
| 3. Focal status (e.g., Jacksonian, sustained ictal confusion, periodic lateralized epileptiform discharges, epilepsia partialis continua) | |
| B. Precipitated seizures | |
| 1. Reflex epilepsy | |
| a. Evoked by simple sensory stimuli (e.g., tactile, proprioceptive, flashing lights, noise) | |
| b. Evoked by complex sensory stimuli (e.g., visual patterns, voice, music) | |
| c. Evoked by complex cognitive or affective functions (e.g., decision making, reading) | |

Modified from Dreifuss FE et al: *Epilepsia* 22:489, 1981.

stimulus. If the technologist is aware of phenomena that are suspected of eliciting the seizure, the conditions can often be duplicated during recording of the EEG.

### Pseudoseizures

The differential diagnosis of seizurelike spells, as for many phenomena in medicine, includes either purposeful or psychogenic spells resembling seizures. Disturbances of consciousness, however, can be caused by a variety of potentially life-threatening events, including ingestions and cardiopulmonary disease. The seriousness of these conditions, as well as seizures themselves, compels physicians to hesitate in making the diagnosis of hysteria or malingering. Pseudoseizures can be difficult for even an experienced neurologist to diagnose safely, requiring simultaneous recording of the EEG and clinical manifestations during prolonged monitoring. A surface EEG in as many as 20% of persons may not reveal the electric discharges responsible for complex partial seizures.

Malingering is usually aimed at some tangible result, such as favorable settlement of a lawsuit or respite from lawful detention. Nevertheless, the prison population also includes verifiable epileptic patients. Some individuals have both true seizures and pseudoseizures. Simple somatosensory or motor seizures may be embellished by other behaviors that serve to prolong or enhance the attention that the patient receives. Psychologic conflicts, as well as past and current mistreatment or abuse, are

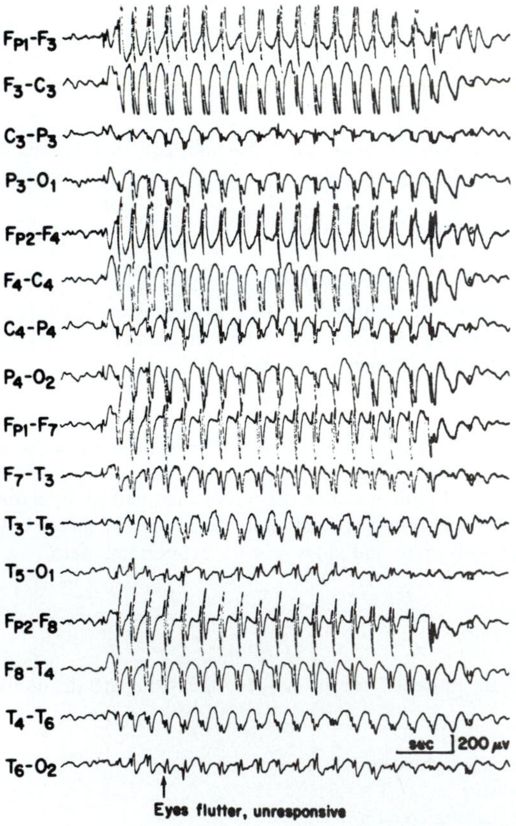


**Fig. 101-1.** Typical three-cycles-per-second spike-wave paroxysm in a 7-year-old girl with absence (petit mal) seizure. (From Klass DW, Daly DD: *Current practice of clinical EEG,* New York, 1979, Raven. Reproduced by permission.)

usually significant contributors. After determining that an individual is having pseudoseizures, one needs to approach the patient carefully, without reproach, using all the counseling and support resources available. Suddenly removing the psychologic defense that pseudoseizures may provide can cause extreme vulnerability and depression. Psychiatric counseling should be readily available.

## DIAGNOSIS AND EVALUATION

The box below outlines a comprehensive evaluation of patients to determine if they have a seizure disorder.

### History

Many types of paroxysmal spells need to be differentiated from seizures to guide diagnostic testing appropriately. The proportion of seizures caused by metabolic, toxic, cerebrovascular, and cardiopulmonary disorders is higher in the adult population, since most primary idiopathic epilepsies present in childhood. The history of the primary care provider should be directed toward predispositions to these secondary seizures.

In determining the type of seizure, the description of the event by the patient and witnesses is critical. Details of experiences that occurred hours or days earlier may seem unrelated until perspective is provided by a seizure. Emotional or sensory phenomena that might indicate a focal origin may have been dismissed but now should be reviewed. Memory for the initial events of the seizure is usually poor, and only a witness may recall focal motor activity or the clouding of consciousness and automatisms that indicate a partial seizure preceded a generalized seizure. The most able witness is one who describes events meticulously without any premature conclusion as to their nature. Description should include the best discernible level of consciousness that was exhibited before and during the seizure, movements and changes in muscle tone, injuries, tongue or cheek biting, and behavior at each stage. One should ask whether, after the seizure apparently subsided, the patient behaved in a confused manner, had residual paralysis, fell asleep, or became combative. If

#### Outline for comprehensive seizure evaluation

Complete history
General medical and neurologic examinations
Electroencephalography (EEG)
Magnetic resonance imaging (MRI) or computed tomography (CT) of the head, with measurement of hippocampal volume on MRI
Lumbar puncture when no signs of increased intracranial pressure present
Blood tests, including glucose, electrolytes, $Ca^{2+}$, $Mg^{2+}$, complete blood count, erythrocyte sedimentation rate, blood urea nitrogen, and creatinine; when pertinent, liver function tests, toxic screens, and laboratory tests for porphyria
Chest x-ray and other studies for the evaluation of a primary tumor or other pertinent medical problem

there have been repeated spells, then duration and frequency of seizures, family history, anticonvulsant response, and compliance should be reviewed in detail and tabulated.

## Physical and neurologic examination

The general physical examination is obviously of paramount importance in detecting the causes of secondary seizures. Signs of infection, organ failure, poisoning, neoplasia, or rheumatologic disease should be carefully sought. Seizures may also be the first recognized symptom of an underlying neurologic disorder, and the neurologic examination is the critical step leading to the discovery of important additional signs, such as confusion, hemiparesis, sensory change, or reflex asymmetry. If the neurologic examination suggests the presence of structural abnormalities of the nervous system, the diagnostic evaluation is appropriately focused there.

## Electroencephalography

EEG performed during a seizure is exquisitely useful as a diagnostic test in epilepsy, establishing the diagnosis and indicating the type of seizure in many cases. Even in the interictal period, electric discharges can often be seen that suggest the epileptic nature of the episode. A positive EEG is a specific, although not sensitive, test for seizures. The usefulness of EEG, however, extends beyond epilepsy to the localization and characterization of other abnormalities of the brain predisposing to seizures, as well as the differentiation of focal or structural lesions from generalized disturbances.

*Epileptiform discharges,* the interictal electric discharges that indicate a seizure tendency, include spikes and sharp waves, often followed by slow waves, and paroxysms (bursts) of other abnormal rhythmic or nonrhythmic discharges (Fig. 101-2). Seizures are repetitive discharges with a temporal correlation to clinical seizure activity.

The chances of recording interictal epileptiform activity are increased by performing a portion of the recording during drowsiness and sleep, by stimulating the patient with strobe flashes, and by having the patient hyperventilate (contraindicated in myocardial infarction, cerebrovascular accident, subarachnoid hemorrhage, or severe cardiac or respiratory compromise). Sleep deprivation before the EEG can help provoke epileptiform activity when a routine EEG has been negative or equivocal. Split-screen video monitoring of the patient and the EEG is useful when the nature of the clinical episode is unclear. Ambulatory EEG and other forms of prolonged monitoring may record spells that occur infrequently or are provoked by settings difficult to duplicate in the laboratory.

## Laboratory tests

Abnormalities of glucose and blood chemistry tests; the detection of infectious, hematologic, renal, or hepatic disease; and the discovery of drug use or toxins are all important. Seizures can be part of the syndrome of certain systemic disorders, such as porphyria, which can be tested for with blood and urine chemistries, and systemic lupus erythematosus, which can be identified with tests for autoantibodies. The measurement of levels of anticonvulsants is important in patients taking these chronically.

No clinical laboratory test exists for epilepsy, per se. In specialized settings with meticulous technique, measurements of prolactin have been shown to be somewhat useful in differentiating true complex partial seizures from pseudoseizures.

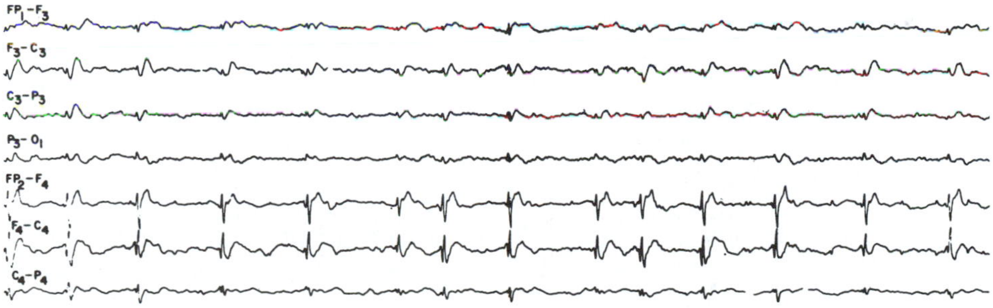

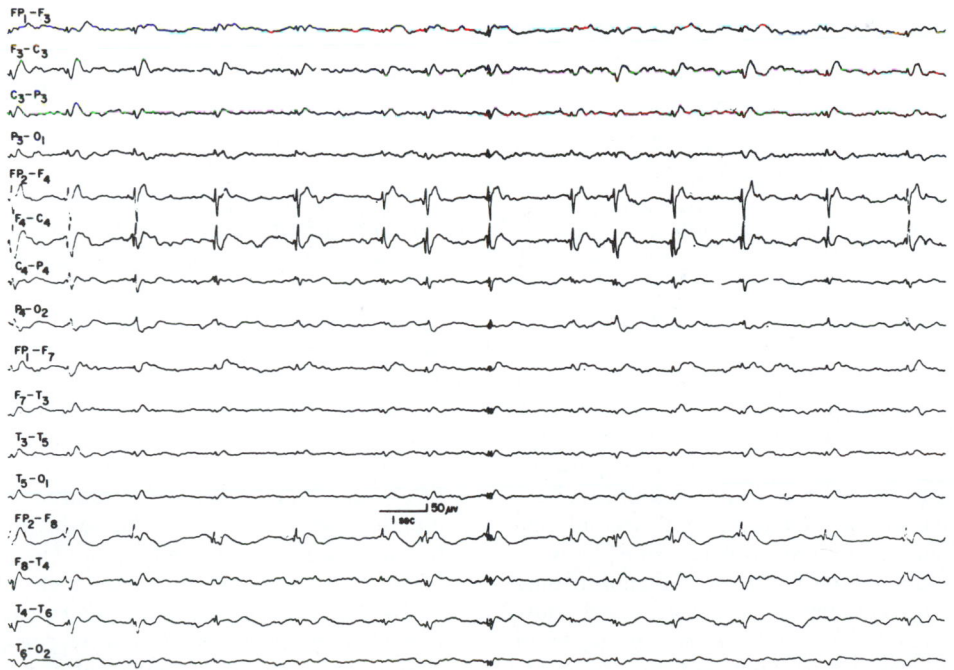

**Fig. 101-2.** Right-sided periodic lateralized epileptiform discharges (PLEDs) in an obtunded 65-year-old man with left face and arm focal motor seizures every 15 to 60 minutes and left hemiparesis caused by an acute right cerebral infarct. (From Klass DW, Daly DD: *Current practice of clinical EEG,* New York, 1979, Raven. Reproduced by permission.)

### Brain imaging studies

The need for brain imaging after a seizure is determined by the seizure phenomenology, the patient's age and the circumstances surrounding the seizure, and the presence of abnormalities in the neurologic examination. The seizure phenomenology, especially in the childhood epilepsies such as absence, can indicate the essential nature of the syndrome and the unlikely possibility of finding an evident structural cause. With increasing age in adults, the incidence of supratentorial brain tumors and cerebrovascular disease rises, increasing the need for imaging. The known abuse of alcohol can either obviate or indicate the need for imaging, depending on the time since abstinence, the seizure type and duration, and again, most importantly, the presence of abnormalities on neurologic examination. After the first seizure, *any* indication of focal neurologic abnormality, whether the focal onset of the seizure, a Todd paralysis (resolving hemiparesis after seizure), or focal neurologic abnormality on examination, warrants scanning with magnetic resonance imaging (MRI) or computed tomography (CT).

MRI is of value in detecting a change in the medial temporal lobe and hippocampus that suggests *mesial temporal sclerosis* in patients with complex partial epilepsy. Single-photon emission computed tomography (SPECT) contributes information about the location and activity of a seizure focus when comparisons are made of scans performed during, immediately after, and between seizures. The information can aid in the detection of occult complex partial epilepsy in combination with EEG and MRI. Both MRI and SPECT are used to select patients likely to benefit from surgical resection of a seizure focus in intractable epilepsy.

## DIFFERENTIAL DIAGNOSIS

Paroxysmal events that can be confused with seizures are generally caused by transient cardiopulmonary or cerebrovascular compromise, metabolic or toxic disorders, or psychiatric or confusional states. The most common differential diagnoses include syncope, hyperventilation syndrome, transient ischemic attacks, migraine, and cataplexy.

*Syncope* is one of the most common events to be misdiagnosed as a seizure. Vasodepressor and other types of syncope can be accompanied by myoclonic jerking and even tonic-clonic seizure activity with incontinence if the duration of cerebral anoxia is prolonged. This is especially likely when the patient is forced to maintain an upright posture during the vasovagal decrease in the cerebral blood flow, as may occur if the patient is in a telephone booth or dentist's chair. Stokes-Adams attacks, paroxysmal atrial tachycardia, other transient arrhythmias, heart disease, and orthostatic hypotension, if profound, can result in syncope. The distinction can sometimes be made between seizures and syncope because of the prodromal symptoms related to decreased cerebral blood flow: lightheadedness, weakness, blurred vision, and hypotension. Seizure patients tend to become stiff and fall to the ground like a board, whereas in syncope the patient slumps to the ground. Syncope usually resolves rapidly (as long as the patient is able to assume the horizontal position), and the patient has minimal postictal confusion. Generalized seizures characteristically cause more postictal confusion, and patients tend to sleep afterward.

*Hyperventilation syndrome* is most often seen in young adults and presents with numbness and tingling in the hands and feet and around the mouth. The episode may proceed from a perception of shortness of breath and progress to lightheadedness, blurred vision, tachycardia, and syncope. Carpal-pedal spasm or tetanic muscular cramping may be mistaken for focal seizure activity.

*Transient ischemic attacks* (TIAs) can cause repeated episodes of focal neurologic symptoms. Usually these are negative symptoms (paralysis, numbness, visual field defects, aphasia) in a fully conscious patient, suggesting the focal absence of blood flow to a specific region of the brain. The symptoms of seizure are more often positive symptoms (twitching or jerking, spontaneous sensations, visual phenomena) with subsequent loss of consciousness corresponding to generalization of the seizure. TIAs of the posterior cerebral circulation, also known as vertebrobasilar attacks or "drop attacks," are characterized by loss of muscular tone in the legs and a fall to the ground without a change in the level of consciousness. If the posterior circulation is further deprived, a confusional state can develop, with later amnesia for events. Some confusion results from the occasional seizure at the onset of an embolic cerebrovascular accident (CVA, stroke). Careful serial examination is required to detect the presence of the more protracted neurologic deficits resulting from the ischemic disease.

*Migraine* frequently begins with neurologic symptoms (aura), both positive and negative, such as homonymous hemianopsia, visual phenomena (flashes, lightning bolts, fortification-like hallucinations), or spreading sensory changes in the opposite side of the body (see Chapter 95). The development of the aura in migraine can take up to 30 minutes to develop, which is considerably longer than the duration of a focal seizure, usually a few seconds or minutes. However, in certain individuals there is pathophysiologic and clinical overlap among seizure, migraine, and cerebral ischemic disease, and the assignment of a single diagnosis may lead to inattention for the important symptoms of the other, such as when migraine patients have a CVA. A tentative diagnosis may be the most prudent one in some of these patients.

*Cataplexy* occurs in narcoleptic patients and consists of a sudden change in muscle tone precipitated by the extremes of emotion. The knees may buckle or the head or jaw drop, or the whole body may jerk so suddenly that it seems to throw the patient to the ground, without loss of consciousness. Narcolepsy has other features and symptoms that distinguish it from seizure disorders, including daytime sleep attacks, sleep paralysis (brief paralysis on awakening), and hypnagogic hallucinations (vivid hallucinations just before falling asleep). Blood testing of highly associated human lymphocyte antigen (HLA) types is available, which can confirm the clinical impression.

*Metabolic and toxic disorders* may infrequently be mistaken for seizures. Alcoholic persons can experience prolonged periods of apparently normal behavior for which they have no memory, called *alcoholic blackouts*. Psychosis with confusion and hallucinations can be the presentation of acute intermittent porphyria. Adding to the diagnostic confusion, approximately 15% of patients with porphyria can have seizures, as well as worsening of porphyria from antiepileptic medications. Ingestion of hallucinogens, anticholinergics, and stimulants can cause seizures as well as mimic them.

*Psychiatric disorders* are usually distinct from seizures in that alertness and consciousness are maintained despite a profound disturbance of thought content and behavior. Nonetheless, complex partial status epilepticus often enters into the differential diagnosis of psychosis, especially the first presentation of schizophrenia. Similarly, acute confusional states may be caused by absence status epilepticus in children or complex partial status in adults. The EEG is an appropriate diagnostic test for any unexplained confusion or change in mentation, since it can indicate the presence of occult seizures or suggest encephalopathy, degenerative disease, ischemia, or intoxication.

## SECONDARY CAUSES OF SEIZURES

The common causes of seizures include metabolic and toxic disorders, drugs, posttraumatic epilepsy, intracranial and central nervous system (CNS) neoplasms, cerebrovascular disease, and intracranial infections (Table 101-2). Table 101-3 lists causes of seizures according to age groups, from neonates to elderly persons. Primary generalized epilepsies are discussed in the next section.

### Metabolic and toxic disorders

Seizures resulting from metabolic abnormalities need to be recognized because they are best treated by correction of the cause rather than by administration of anticonvulsants. Indeed, in specific instances, these secondary seizures will be refractory to anticonvulsants or even exacerbated by them. Hypoglycemia may be associated with seizures, usually from use of insulin or oral hypoglycemic agents in diabetic patients. Nonketotic hyperglycemia is associated with a peculiar type of focal seizure that may be produced by certain postures of the extremity. These seizures are resistant to anticonvulsants, and the use of phenytoin may antagonize insulin, increase hyperglycemia, and exacerbate seizures. Ketotic hyperglycemia is generally not associated with seizures. Hyponatremia can result from sodium depletion, water intoxication, or both and is often seen in malnourished alcoholic patients, with the syndrome of inappropriate antidiuretic hormone (SIADH), in hypoadrenalism, and rarely with carbamazepine use. Levels of hyponatremia sufficient to cause seizures usually cause diminished levels of consciousness as well. Hypocalcemia, hypomagnesemia, and hypophosphatemia are occasionally the cause of seizures at profound levels of depletion. Seizures occur frequently, however, in identified individuals with hypoparathyroidism, who respond only to correction of the metabolic abnormality.

Uremia is often associated with generalized seizures, muscular irritability, and myoclonus. In renal failure, seizures occur in patients already manifesting confusion, asterixis, tremulousness, and paratonia. The contributing pathophysiologic factors in these patients include the uremia itself, hypocalcemia, electrolyte imbalance, and hypertension. Amelioration of any of these factors will aid in the control of the seizures. The acute dialysis disequilibrium syndrome, believed to result from rapid shifts in solutes and electrolytes across the neuronal membrane during and after dialysis, is characterized by headache and nausea; progresses to encephalopathy, seizures, and coma; and may be fatal.

**Table 101-2.** Common causes of seizures

| General cause | Specific disorders |
|---|---|
| Idiopathic epilepsy | |
| Primary generalized epilepsies with hereditary tendency | Grand mal epilepsy, complex partial epilepsy, or bilateral massive myoclonic epilepsy |
| No cause found or recorded | Focal or generalized recurrent seizures |
| Head trauma | Brain contusions, intracerebral hematomas, open-head injuries, birth injuries |
| Cerebral vasoanoxia | Pulmonary or cardiac arrest, perinatal hypoxia |
| Intracranial infections | Meningitis, brain abscess, subdural empyema, viral encephalitis, granulomas, Creutzfeldt-Jakob disease, cytomegalic inclusion body disease, toxoplasmosis |
| Brain tumors | Primary, metastatic |
| Cerebrovascular diseases | Intracerebral hemorrhage; acute cerebral embolism; arteriovenous malformation, occasionally in previous ischemic cerebrovascular accidents; lupus cerebritis; cortical vein thrombosis |
| Congenital, hereditary, and developmental disease of central nervous system (CNS) | Porencephaly, cerebral palsy, tuberous sclerosis, neurofibromatosis, encephalotrigeminal angiomatosis |
| Degenerative CNS disease | Rarely in Alzheimer disease |
| Metabolic and toxic | Hypoglycemia, hyponatremia, hypocalcemia, uremic myoclonic twitch syndrome, dialysis, toxemia of pregnancy, hepatic encephalopathy, porphyria, acute lead poisoning in children, Reye syndrome, aminoacidopathies, neurolipidosis, pyridoxine deficiency, hyperbilirubinemia |
| | Withdrawl from alcohol, barbiturates, or benzodiazepines; administration of phenothiazines, haloperidol, theophylline, or aminophylline |

**Table 101-3.** Common age-related causes of seizures

| Age group (years) | Causes |
|---|---|
| Neonatal | Perinatal hypoxia and birth injury, intracranial hemorrhage, congenital malformations, metabolic abnormalities (hypoglycemia, low sodium, low calcium, low magnesium, vitamin $B_6$ deficiency or dependency, amino acidopathies, hyperbilirubinemia), intracranial infections (meningitis, subdural empyema) |
| Neonatal-3 | Perinatal hypoxia and birth injury, acute intracranial infections (meningitis, subdural empyema, encephalitis, abscess), battered child syndrome, congenital malformations, metabolic abnormalities including electrolyte imbalance, Reye syndrome, congenital and hereditary disturbances, febrile convulsions |
| 3-10 | Perinatal hypoxia and birth injury, idiopathic epilepsy, intracranial infections (meningitis, encephalitis, abscess), primary generalized epilepsy, cerebrovascular pathologies, congenital hereditary and developmental disease (porencephaly, cerebral palsy, tuberous sclerosis, arteriovenous [A-V] malformations) |
| 10-16 | Primary generalized epilepsy, acute intracranial infections, congenital hereditary and developmental defects including A-V malformation, head trauma |
| 16-25 | Primary generalized epilepsy, head trauma, drug and alcohol withdrawl, intracranial infections, neoplasms, congenital hereditary and developmental malformations including A-V malformation |
| 25-40 | Trauma, alcohol and drug withdrawl, brain tumors |
| 40-65 | Trauma, alcohol withdrawl, brain tumors, cerebrovascular accidents (CVAs) |
| >65 | Cerebrovascular disease (intracerebral hemorrhage, cerebral embolism, and occasionally previous ischemic CVAs); brain tumors, degenerative disease |

Hepatic porphyria is associated with seizures, psychosis, and abdominal pain and can be caused or exacerbated by medications, especially anticonvulsants. If porphyria is the cause of seizures, benzodiazepines are preferable to phenytoin, phenobarbital, or carbamazepine to control seizures.

Systemic lupus erythematosus has CNS manifestations in nearly one fifth of patients, most often seizure, but also cranial nerve signs, altered mentation, and CVA.

### Drug-induced seizures

Drug-induced seizures are usually generalized, rarely focal motor, and status epilepticus can occur. The toxicity of tricyclic antidepressants, one of the most common drugs used in suicide attempts, includes a hyperadrenergic state with seizures and anticholinergic delirium, but seizures can occur at reasonable doses in the therapeutic range. Studies have shown that antipsychotic drugs, which also lower seizure threshold, are also frequently used in overdose. Cocaine is associated with a variety of severe neurologic complications, including ischemic CVA, subarachnoid and intraparenchymal hemorrhage, and in approximately 10% of patients, seizures. Seizures usually occur within hours after use of intravenous or "crack" cocaine and are brief and generalized. Status epilepticus, focal seizures, or multiple seizures are more often associated with neurologic complications (CVA, hemorrhage) and an abnormal neurologic examination. The use of injectable drugs and abused substances of other types, such as heroin, amphetamines, and phencyclidine, can also be complicated by seizures. In hospital populations, theophylline and aminophylline typically have convulsant effects, and seizures appear to be dose related. Isoniazid, penicillin, sympathomimetics, antihistamines, and anticholinergics are examples of frequently used medications having seizures among their potential side effects. Treatment with high-dose pyridoxine (milligram dose equal to the dose of isoniazid) has been found to antagonize some convulsant properties of isoniazid. Lidocaine used as an antiarrhythmic is convulsant, in a dose-related fashion, and thus has a particular tendency to cause seizures after 24 hours of infusion when accumulation occurs. Insulin is a frequent cause of seizures in diabetic patients.

### Posttraumatic epilepsy

Trauma is an infrequent cause of first seizure, accounting for less than 10%. Seizure as a sequela of head trauma can occur early or be delayed. Approximately 5% to 15% of individuals with closed-head trauma have been observed to have a seizure in the first week, usually on the first day. The likelihood is increased if there is evidence of structural brain damage (e.g., depressed skull fracture, intracranial hematoma) on CT or MRI or focal neurologic deficit on examination. Delayed or recurrent seizures are unusual in closed-head trauma without evident structural brain damage. However, penetrating injuries, especially those that go beyond the dura mater and invade the substance of the brain, are associated with delayed-onset epilepsy in 30% to 50% of patients. The onset is usually within 2 years; thus, some neurosurgeons routinely give anticonvulsants. Evidence indicates that prophylactic treatment does not prevent the development of a posttraumatic seizure disorder, and in fact, inconsistent compliance with anticonvulsants may be responsible for more seizures than would occur with no treatment at all. In a large study, phenytoin was only effective in reducing the number of seizures during the first week after severe structural or penetrating head injury. Whether the seizures of late posttraumatic epilepsy can be successfully treated by strict compliance with any of the other major anticonvulsants is still being studied.

### Intracranial and central nervous system neoplasms

Seizure can be a symptom of intracranial neoplasms, both primary and metastatic. However, contrary to the common fears of patients, brain tumors only account for a small percentage of patients with a first unprovoked seizure. Personality change or altered mentation is more likely to signal a brain tumor. The occurrence of either a focal seizure or an abnormal neurologic examination, especially in a patient with a past history of cancer of the skin, breast, lung, or thyroid gland, is the most significant indicator. Incidence rises with age. Several types of primary CNS tumors, both malignant and benign, can cause seizures.

### Cerebrovascular disease

Seizures can complicate cerebral infarction as well as cerebral or subarachnoid hemorrhage in 5% to 15% of patients. Seizures are sometimes a presenting or early feature of CVA, usually a brief focal seizure without recurrence and thus not requiring chronic anticonvulsant therapy. When seizures occur for the first time or continue months or years after a CVA, and when they may be related by symptomatology to the specific area of infarcted cerebral cortex, long-term anticonvulsant therapy is likely to be required. The probability of a seizure does not appear to be related to the size of the infarct or other features of the acute morbidity but is significantly related to the location of the infarct in the cortex as opposed to subcortical structures. Similarly, seizure is seen with frontal, temporal, or parietal parenchymal brain hemorrhage caused by an aneurysm, tumor, or vascular malformations and infrequently with deep subcortical hemorrhages, usually from hypertension. Childhood CVA, associated with persistent hemiparesis, is complicated by recurrent seizures in as many as 18% of patients.

### Intracranial infections

Seizures can result from space-occupying infectious lesions (e.g., abcess, cyst, empyema) that irritate the cortex. One of the most common causes of seizures in tropical areas of the Western Hemisphere such as Mexico is the endemic infection *cysticercosis,* which can result in many small calcified brain cysts. Acute purulent meningitis and encephalitis are occasionally complicated by seizures during the acute phase of the illness. Systemic infection can also be complicated by seizure as a result of metabolic or electrolyte abnormalities.

### Secondary seizure syndromes in children

*West syndrome* is a severe disorder occurring in infancy with a characteristic type of seizure, infantile spasms, and characteristic EEG pattern (hypsarrhythmia). Frequently associated with mental retardation, it is notoriously difficult to treat in most patients. *Lennox-Gastaut syndrome* is another epileptic disorder that presents in early childhood with a variety of generalized seizures types and a characteristically slow spike-and-wave discharge on the EEG. Mental retardation almost invariably occurs, especially with onset before age 3 years.

The *progressive myoclonus epilepsies* are a heterogenous group of rare, inherited disorders that manifest with myoclonic seizures and variable degrees of intellectual and neurologic decline, depending on etiology. Baltic myoclonus, or Unverricht disease, an autosomal recessive disorder recognized in Finland, presents with progressive ataxia, photosensitive action-induced myoclonus, and generalized myoclonic seizures. Mitochondrial genomic transmission is thought to be responsible for the varied symptoms of mitochondrial encephalomyopathy with ragged red fibers (MERRF), in which neurologic and intellectual decline, myopathy, and ataxia accompany myoclonus. Myoclonic and generalized tonic-clonic seizures and intellectual deterioration are the presenting symptoms of Lafora disease, a degenerative disorder diagnosed by the widespread presence of characteristic amyloid bodies in tissues. Various metabolic diseases of infancy and childhood, including ceroid lipofuscinosis and sialidosis, can present as progressive myoclonus epilepsies.

## PRIMARY (IDIOPATHIC) GENERALIZED EPILEPTIC SYNDROMES

Most seizure disorders result from acquired changes in the nervous system. Several familial syndromes of primary generalized epilepsy occurring in childhood or adolescence appear to be autosomally inherited, single-locus genetic disorders. These are juvenile myoclonic epilepsy (JME), benign familial neonatal convulsions, and some forms of progressive myoclonus epilepsy. Benign Rolandic epilepsy and absence are also likely inherited as autosomal disorders, since there are high rates of concordance in monozygotic as opposed to dizygotic twins and a higher incidence of epilepsy in the relatives of those with these primary idiopathic epilepsies. In each syndrome, one type of generalized seizure (tonic-clonic, absence, or myoclonic) predominates, but more than one type of generalized seizure can develop during the course, and members of an affected family can have more than one type of seizure. Signs of focal neurologic abnormality and intellectual impairment are absent in the primary generalized epilepsies, and the EEG is often characteristic.

### Absence

Absence, formerly petit mal, develops in childhood, although a few patients have onset in their teens. Typical attacks are very brief staring spells, sometimes with eye fluttering or elementary automatisms such as chewing, that can occur up to hundreds of times a day. Generally, no postictal confusion occurs, and the possibility of *absence status epilepticus* should be considered in a child with this disorder who displays prolonged periods of apparent unawareness. The EEG pattern of the classic syndrome is a three-per-second spike and wave, often predictably occurring during hyperventilation. Ethosuximide is the medication specifically effective for this disorder and is used in children, but most childhood absence attacks eventually disappear and are quite rare in adults. (Absencelike attacks in adults are usually secondary complex partial seizures rather than absence.) However, about a third of those with childhood-onset absence and half of those with juvenile-onset absence will develop generalized tonic-clonic seizures as they age. When generalized seizures are superimposed, both seizure types are treated with valproic acid. Absence can occur in the syndrome of JME as well, but the faster frequency of spike-wave discharge and polyspike discharges on the EEG, as well as the associated early-morning myoclonus, should distinguish this entity.

### Juvenile myoclonic epilepsy (of Janz)

One of the most common benign epileptic syndromes, JME is characterized by myoclonic jerking of the arms and shoulders early in the morning on awakening, with generalized tonic-clonic seizures ultimately occurring in most patients. One third of patients can have absence seizures as well. Age of onset of early-morning myoclonus is usually around age 14 or 15 and can be precipitated by fatigue or alcohol. The EEG shows bursts of bilateral high-amplitude polyspike discharges that may be precipitated by photic stimulation. Patients with a first generalized tonic-clonic seizure in early adulthood should be specifically questioned about jerking movements interfering with early-morning activities, since many may have become accustomed to this and do not see an association. Benign JME should be distinguished from the various progressive myoclonus epilepsies associated with intellectual and neurologic deterioration.

### Benign Rolandic epilepsy

Benign Rolandic epilepsy manifests as a hemifacial focal motor or somatosensory seizure while awake, with three fourths of the children experiencing secondarily generalized seizures during sleep. Centrotemporal sharp waves can be seen on the interictal (between seizures) EEG. Hypersalivation, speech arrest, and gurgling noises are other associated seizure phenomena, and hemibody jerking is sometimes seen. A proportion of these adolescents have one or a few seizures only, and only a small percentage of patients require lengthy treatment. A similar prognosis is associated with the epilepsy that occurs in childhood with high-voltage occipital spikes and waves that appear on the EEG when the eyes are closed. Seizure symptomatology is characteristically visual. Field defects or hallucinations are followed by clonic movements or generalized seizure and culminate in a migrainelike headache, further evidence of the overlapping pathophysiology of epilepsy and migraine.

The symptomatology in each of these benign focal epilepsies could be mimicked by a specific structural lesion in the sylvian fissure or the occipital cortex, and any static or progressive neurologic or intellectual impairment requires further evaluation by a neurologist.

### Benign neonatal convulsions

Some convulsions in the first few days of life in neonates with a family history are genetic, associated with more than one genotype. However, the likelihood of treatable causes such as meningitis, hypoglycemia, and hyperammonemia, as well as pyridoxine (vitamin $B_6$) or biotin dependency, requires further evaluation in all patients with neonatal seizures.

## MANAGEMENT

### General considerations in drug treatment

Antiepileptic treatment is most likely to be successful in reducing seizure frequency in the many patients who respond to a single drug. A significant research effort has gone into the determination of which medications are most likely to be successful in which seizure types and patient circumstances (see the box at right). Anticonvulsants have evolved from a family of compounds related chemically to barbiturates and bromides to a group of dissimilar drugs with unique mechanisms of action, pharmacokinetics, and side effect profiles. Attempts at treatment may require weeks or months, during which frequent seizure activity and the attendant loss of income or school time can damage the rhythm of the patient's life as well as the therapeutic relationship. Since it is difficult to know which patients will respond, it is advisable to involve a neurologist early to assist in making informed choices among the many drugs available. Those who have persistent seizures in sequential trials of monotherapy, assuming that adequate doses were used for adequate periods of time with documented compliance, are considered refractory to treatment and become candidates for combination therapy or surgery.

The principles of therapy with anticonvulsants differ from other common therapeutic regimens, such as with antibiotics, and more closely resemble cardiovascular drugs or anesthetics, in that the range of blood levels associated with the desired therapeutic effect is closely flanked by the two highly undesired states of no effect at the lower end and exponentially increasing side effects at the higher end. Measurable plasma levels have aided considerably in the ability to ensure that the drug is behaving in the individual patient in the same manner as it does in the population at large. When a patient takes the standard 300 mg maintenance dose of phenytoin, for example, a blood level of 10 to 20 mg/dl indicates intact absorption, conventional metabolism, and predictable elimination in this individual. The loading and maintenance doses determined for the population are therefore extrapolatable to this individual. Occasionally, a patient is identified who requires different dosing, and measuring

### Choice of antiepileptic drugs for various seizures

Grand mal seizures
- Phenytoin, phenobarbital, carbamazepine, primidone, valproic acid, IV diazepam for status epilepticus (not used for maintenance therapy)

Simple partial (focal) seizures
- Phenytoin, phenobarbital, carbamazepine
- Valproic acid rarely effective
- Adjunctive therapy: felbamate, gabapentin, lamotrigine

Complex partial seizures (psychomotor seizures, temporal lobe epilepsy)
- Carbamazepine, primidone, phenytoin
- Phenobarbital not as effective in complex partial seizures*
- Phenytoin does not prevent development of secondary seizure foci, i.e., mirror focus*

Myoclonic seizures
- Valproic acid, clonazepam, diazepam, phenytoin, felbamate (adjunctive therapy)

Myoclonus as part of infantile spasms
- Valproic acid, adrenocorticotropic hormone (ACTH), diazepam, clonazepam, felbamate

Myoclonus associated with absence (petit mal)
- Ethosuximide, valproic acid

Absence (petit mal)
- Ethosuximide, valproic acid

*According to some reports.

the steady-state levels assists in choosing the proper dose. The most useful function of plasma drug levels in practice, subsequent to these intitial determinations, turns out to be the assessment of *compliance* and effects of *drug interactions.*

In accordance with principles of pharmacokinetics, it is important to wait until a new steady state is reached before checking the plasma level after the maintenance dose of the drug is changed. The appropriate period to wait is four to six half-lives ($4$ to $6 \times t½$), which for phenytoin is at least 7 days. Toxicity can result when the maintenance dose is increased because of an apparently low plasma level that has simply not reached a steady state. Adjustments in dose and frequency of administration are needed for renal, hepatic, and pulmonary failure as well as for the unique characteristics of metabolism in neonates, children, and elderly persons.

Considerable differences exist among anticonvulsants in whether they should be loaded or should be initiated at their maintenance dose. Many drugs are given as intravenous (IV) loading doses for treatment of status epilepticus; however, oral administration in less serious situations is indicated in terms of safety and patient tolerance. The pharmacokinetics of phenytoin is such that oral loading is necessary to achieve therapeutic blood levels even in nonemergency situations. However, carbamazepine and valproate cannot be effectively loaded either orally or intravenously.

The dose and associated plasma level that are optimal for the patient receiving chronic therapy is the dose and level that *controls the seizures.* For some individuals, this dose is slightly above or below the published laboratory normative therapeutic range. However, if the treatment is efficacious and the side effects are minimal and acceptable to the patient, it should not be a concern. Those who require higher levels or appear to be controlled with lower levels are best treated in consultation with a neurologist.

Side effects of anticonvulsants are both dose related and idiosyncratic. Sedation is a property of virtually all CNS active agents. Similarly, ataxia and confusion potentially complicate higher-dose therapy. Gastrointestinal distress is often reported. There are differences of degree among drugs. Phenobarbital, for example, is considered more acutely sedating than carbamazepine. Valproate is more often associated with stomach upset than phenytoin. Some side effects can be avoided by introducing the medications at lower doses and increasing gradually toward the maintenance dose. Tolerance develops to the sedative and ataxic side effects over several weeks of therapy.

Life-threatening idiosyncratic adverse effects are possible with most major anticonvulsants and must be avoided by careful surveillance during their introduction. The incidence of Stevens-Johnson syndrome with phenytoin, agranulocytosis with carbamazepine, and fulminant hepatic failure with valproate is low, but it is impossible to predict which patients will be affected. Recommendations exist for frequent hematologic and hepatic laboratory tests with these drugs. Valproic acid should not be used in children under age 3 years and should be avoided in children under age 7 because of the high incidence of hepatic failure.

Newer anticonvulsant medications, such as felbamate and gabapentin, appear to have fewer adverse effects than the major anticonvulsants but correspondingly lower activity. Their indications are for adjunctive treatment of certain seizure types and for epilepsy refractory to phenytoin, carbamazepine, and valproate.

The addition of a second drug can provoke immediate and evolving complex interactions, risking diminished effectiveness and increased side effects from either drug. This is true of both a second anticonvulsant and unrelated medications. Phenytoin, carbamazepine, and valproate are inducers of hepatic microsomal metabolism and decrease the effectiveness of drugs such as coumadin and oral contraceptives. Beginning an anticonvulsant may therefore result in pregnancy, and stopping it could lead to hemorrhage.

The decision to discontinue seizure medications is complex, requiring explicit knowledge of the nature of the seizure disorder and the EEG, a certain seizure-free interval of 2 to 5 years, and a thorough understanding of the risks of recurrent seizures. Once discontinuation is decided, the medications should be slowly tapered off, one by one, each over 2 to 4 months.

### Specific therapy for specific seizure types

In absence seizures of childhood and adolescence, ethosuximide and valproate are the drugs of choice. If absence is complicated by generalized seizures, or if ethosuximide is ineffective, valproate is used. Clonazepam may also be useful, but carbamazepine and phenobarbital can exacerbate absence. Valproate is indicated for JME and is often used in the childhood-onset, presumably inherited primary epilepsies, although phenytoin and carbamazepine have been shown to be equally effective. The two syndromic epilepsies of childhood that are notoriously refractory to treatment are Lennox and West syndromes. Valproate and felbamate are indicated in the Lennox syndrome, and some success has resulted from the use of adrenocorticotropic hormone (ACTH) in West syndrome.

Adults with primary generalized or secondary generalized seizures or with complex partial seizures are likely to be treated effectively by either phenytoin, carbamazepine, valproate, or primidone. Most often the decision is based on consideration of the side effect profile for a particular agent, the frequency of dosing required, and other medications the patient is taking. Phenytoin is the only single-dose-per-day medication, if compliance is an issue. A significant proportion of patients with complex partial seizures are refractory to treatment and require combination therapy. Monotherapy should be painstakingly explored in these individuals, but if unsuccessful, a promising combination would be either phenytoin or carbamazepine with valproate.

### Single, apparently unprovoked, seizures

Controversy surrounds the necessity of chronic anticonvulsant therapy for a single seizure or an isolated cluster of seizures. The overall chance of recurrence is approximately one in three within 3 to 5 years. The risk is highest in the first year and diminishes with time. Patients with an identifiable provocation such as hypoglycemia or water toxicity have a lower risk of recurrence and can be spared long-term anticonvulsant therapy. The possibility of recurrence is highest in those with a previous insult to the CNS such as a CVA, infection, or significant previous head injury; the cumulative risk for these patients is 50% at 5 years. Risk of recurrence is also significantly increased in those with a family history of seizures or generalized epileptiform activity on an EEG.

### Alcoholic patients with seizures

Alcohol withdrawal seizures ("rum fits") occur 2 or 3 days into abstinence, are usually brief and generalized, and can be single or multiple. Status epilepticus can occur, particularly in patients with polysubstance abuse. However, other serious causes of secondary seizures, such as head trauma, hypoglycemia, meningitis, SIADH (with hyponatremia), or idiopathic epilepsy can also be present in alcoholic persons. Clusters of withdrawal seizures can be acutely treated with anticonvulsants, but these seizures are often more responsive to benzodiazepines, phenobarbital, and paraldehyde than to phenytoin. Long-term treatment of alcoholic patients with the major anticonvulsants for the prevention of withdrawal seizures is ineffective and not advised. Alcoholic persons tend to take anticonvulsants erratically, and this predisposes them to withdrawal seizures from the anticonvulsants themselves, the leading cause of status epilepticus in this patient population.

The seizures that are provoked by withdrawal from barbiturates or benzodiazepines are best treated with the same category of medication. The usual daily dose is determined and reinstituted in divided doses for a few days, followed by a slow tapering of the medication in concert with psychologic support and counseling.

### Pregnancy

The pregnant woman with epilepsy who takes anticonvulsant medications is subject to risks that must be discussed with her as early in the process as possible. The incidence of seizures is slightly increased in about half of pregnant epileptic patients. The incidence of complications of pregnancy, such as stillbirth, eclampsia, hemorrhage, and premature labor, are reported to be twofold higher in epileptic patients. The antiepileptic drugs are suspected of being teratogenic, causing cleft palate, cleft lip, and heart defects. These defects are about two or three times higher (4% to 6%) in babies born to mothers taking these drugs than in the general population. The other contributing factors to congenital malformation may include folic acid deficiency aggravated by the use of anticonvulsants. On the other hand, generalized seizures themselves can cause trauma to the fetus and produce metabolic or vasoanoxic injuries. Since a correlation exists between the incidence of birth defects and the serum concentration of anticonvulsants, a single drug should be used at the lowest effective dose, when possible.

It is not known which anticonvulsants are more teratogenic, making their choice dependent on the clinical appropriateness. When the mother is receiving phenobarbital, obstetricians should be made aware of the possibility of withdrawal symptoms in the newborn. These include overactivity, tremors, hypercapnia, vomiting, and rarely convulsions, which, because of phenobarbital's long half-life, occur around the sixth postnatal day. In pregnant women taking anticonvulsants, especially valproate, supplemental folic acid is an especially important prenatal vitamin in the prevention of neural tube defects.

During pregnancy, dynamic changes in the absorption, metabolism, clearance, and catabolism of anticonvulsant drugs cause lower but at times unpredictable plasma levels. Hormonal changes, weight gain, retention of water, and sodium can change the distribution of the protein-bound fraction and free fraction (the active drug). In addition to the total plasma drug level, the free fraction can be followed monthly for several months postpartum.

Anticonvulsant drugs are transferred to the fetus through the placenta, producing fetal blood levels equal to that of the mother, but lower levels in the milk and colostrum. Since metabolism of these drugs is slower in the newborn, large doses of sedative drugs given to the mother before labor may cause a poor sucking reflex, floppiness, shallow respiration, and subnormal body temperature in the newborn. A pause in breastfeeding can improve the newborn's symptoms when the mother is still receiving higher doses of sedative anticonvulsants. Breastfeeding by epileptic mothers taking anticonvulsants remains controversial and should be individualized.

### Febrile convulsions

The treatment of a simple febrile seizure is the control of fever. Prophylactic treatment of simple febrile seizures is rarely indicated because they do not affect intellectual or physical development. Recurrent simple febrile seizures are common, however, occurring in one third of infants and two thirds of children. Factors such as the duration of seizures (more than 15 minutes), focal seizures, presence of any abnormal neurologic signs, abnormal EEG, and a family history of nonfebrile seizures suggest a slight predisposition to later epilepsy. However, even in children with one or two complicated features, there is no indication that prophylactic administration of anticonvulsants for the prevention of further febrile seizures has any effect on the later development of epilepsy.

When status epilepticus occurs in infants and children, the measurement and administration of glucose is an important immediate intervention. In neonates, pyridoxine (100 mg) rapidly reverses the seizures in autosomal recessive pyridoxine dependency. Pharmacologic management of status is accomplished by slow IV loading with phenobarbital, diazepam, or phenytoin. Phenobarbital and phenytoin are used in neonates in adult doses (up to 20 mg/kg) but somewhat lower doses in children (5 to 15 mg/kg). Diazepam (0.1 to 0.5 mg/kg) can be given by slow IV injection or rectally. Neuromuscular blockade, continuous EEG monitoring, and even pentobarbital coma may be required in refractory status epilepticus, as for adults. Further investigation of metabolic, infectious, or other conditions requiring intervention is essential to the prevention of recurrence. Treatment of status epilepticus is discussed in the next section.

## STATUS EPILEPTICUS

Status epilepticus consists of prolonged (20 to 30 minutes) or frequent seizures without recovery between attacks. The seizures are most often generalized. Prolonged or closely spaced simple partial or complex partial seizures can also be considered status and constitute as much as 25% of the incidence. Partial status may have specific antecedents and treatments that need to be addressed. The occurrence of generalized tonic-clonic convulsive status is a serious emergency that occurs in up to 16% of all patients with epilepsy, with a mortality rate of about 10% to 12%. Seizures that last for only a few hours can cause permanent neuronal damage despite meticulous maintenance of oxygenation and other vital functions, especially in children. Factors contributing to the neuronal damage include excessive metabolic demands, noxiously high calcium influx, brain edema, lactic acidosis, hyperthermia, late hypoglycemia, and hypotension. The main causes of death include cardiovascular and respiratory failure, renal failure from myoglobulinuria and/or hypotension, and the IV administration of anticonvulsants. Death may occur during seizures or after they are controlled. In addition, serious complications such as the persistent vegetative state may occur among the survivors. Other sequelae include cognitive impairment, permanent focal neurologic deficits, and future recurrent seizures.

The reasons for status epilepticus in a general hospital population include all the causes of seizures: idiopathic seizure disorder, withdrawal from anticonvulsant medications, alcohol and drug toxicity, intracranial infection, trauma, CVA, tumor, and febrile convulsions. Withdrawal from anticonvulsants, including benzodiazepines, is overrepresented as a cause of status.

## Management

Management of generalized status epilepticus should swiftly be undertaken by a team of physicians, when possible in a medical intensive care unit. In the management of status, three broad goals should be achieved simultaneously: (1) maintain the patient's vital functions, (2) diagnose and treat the precipitating factors, and (3) stop the seizures with antiepileptic medications. The practical steps for treatment are listed next.

***Immediate steps and maintenance of vital functions.*** Insert a plastic oral airway, open the patient's collar, remove dentures, position the patient to optimize respiration, quickly evaluate the overall cardiac and respiratory condition, and monitor the blood pressure and electrocardiogram (ECG).

Draw blood for glucose, electrolytes, blood urea nitrogen, creatinine, calcium, magnesium, blood gases, antiepileptic drug levels, and toxic screens when pertinent.

Give 50 or 100 ml of a 50% glucose solution, and administer IV thiamine if the patient is alcoholic or malnourished.

Continuous maintenance of oxygenation, blood pressure, hydration, electrolytes, and management of the acidosis by IV sodium bicarbonate should be done vigorously throughout the course of the seizure and during the following comatose state.

Intubation during generalized status epilepticus is difficult and may cause injuries to the patient but may be needed when large amounts of medications are used or there are signs of respiratory depression. A neuromuscular blocker may be necessary to accomplish the intubation. These agents have the disadvantage of masking clinical seizure activity despite the continuation of the cerebral electric discharges that are, per se, harmful to the brain. However, these drugs can be used when there is a danger of cardiorespiratory failure caused by continued seizures or of renal failure by myoglobulinuria. In such patients, continuous EEG monitoring can be used as a guide throughout the course of anticonvulsant therapy.

***Anticonvulsant therapy.*** The anticonvulsant drugs may be given intravenously, with a couple of rare exceptions mentioned below. Several drug combinations can be used. Diazepam is a very-fast-acting medication whose anticonvulsant effects rapidly diminish over about 20 minutes. Phenytoin is a slow-acting drug but is effective for many hours. Phenobarbital is somewhat slower, but its anticonvulsant effects remain for more than 24 hours. Lorazepam is a benzodiazepine with a longer anticonvulsant effect than diazepam, but again causes significant sedation. The main problems with the IV use of the anticonvulsants are respiratory depression and persistent hypotension. IV phenytoin may additionally cause bradycardia or cardiac arrest. The latter side effects are especially troublesome in elderly patients and with signs of heart block.

Generally recommended anticonvulsant therapy regimens in status epilepticus include (1) combined use of diazepam and phenytoin, (2) phenobarbital with or without phenytoin, and (3) lorazepam with or without phenytoin. Diazepam, because of its rapid onset but short duration of action, is used in the earliest stages of status to allow time to load IV phenytoin, which can take up to 20 minutes depending on the patient's weight. Lorazepam is a less-rapid-onset benzodiazepine that has a longer duration of action than diazepam. However, lorazepam is only useful in the initial management of status because tolerance develops to its anticonvulsant effects with repeated use. An alternative procedure is to administer a loading dose of phenobarbital. The combined use of diazepam and phenobarbital should be avoided unless the patient is intubated, since their side effects are additive and can cause respiratory arrest or severe hypotension. The secondary drugs used in status epilepticus include paraldehyde, lidocaine, and pentobarbital to induce coma in refractory status.

**Starting with diazepam combined with phenytoin**

1. Give IV infusion of diazepam at 2 mg/minute or slower up to 10 to 20 mg or until the seizures stop (0.15 to 0.5 mg/kg or up to 10 mg total in children). Watch closely for respiratory depression or hypotension. Diazepam is fully effective in a few minutes. However, because of its wide and rapid distribution, its half-life is only about 20 to 40 minutes. In infants and small children with inaccessible veins, the rectal administration of 0.25 to 1.0 mg/kg diazepam solution provides very fast absorption, with EEG effect and the control of seizures appearing within 5 minutes.
2. In another vein, infuse 14 to 18 mg/kg phenytoin at 50 mg/minute or slower in normal saline using an infusion pump. Dilution by dextrose solution may cause precipitation. The ECG and blood pressure should be closely monitored. Stop the infusion if significant bradycardia occurs. Phenytoin may be used in smaller doses at a slower infusion rate in one-half normal saline when one is unsure of the patient's cardiac condition or in older patients. Contraindications for the use of phenytoin include significant bradycardia, second- or third-degree atrioventricular block, sinoatrial block, and severe myocardial insufficiency. The use of IV

phenytoin in older patients is associated with a significant incidence of cardiac side effects. Phenytoin becomes fully effective after about 20 to 30 minutes from the start of infusion, but its initial effect begins in a few minutes. Plasma levels remain therapeutic for 12 to 24 hours.

3. If the seizures are not controlled after 20 to 30 minutes from the start of infusion of phenytoin, IV loading of phenobarbital can be undertaken. Intubation is required when phenobarbital is used or these drugs are used together.
4. Other secondary choices of drugs include lorazepam, lidocaine, and paraldehyde. Lorazepam is a benzodiazepine that has been used in a single IV dose of 2.5 to 10 mg with good results. Respiratory depression has been reported, but its therapeutic effects last for many hours. Seizures have been suppressed for 2 to 72 hours at these doses. Lidocaine, 50 to 100 mg, can be given by slow IV push initially, followed by a 1 to 2 mg/minute brief IV infusion. Paraldehyde is often useful in alcohol withdrawal status but can also be used in status from other causes when the primary anticonvulsants have failed. The dosage is 0.1 to 0.15 ml/kg, which can be repeated every 2 to 4 hours. However, paraldehyde is an intensely corrosive drug and decomposes the plastic syringes and tubing in less than 2 minutes. It can also produce acidosis, pulmonary edema, and azotemia. Paraldehyde can be used intramuscularly (IM), about 5 ml in each buttock, away from the sciatic nerves. The IM route gives peak plasma levels in 15 to 20 minutes. The safety of IV paraldehyde is questionable. Paraldehyde can be used rectally diluted 2:1 in oil or in 200 ml normal saline. The absorption via this method is somewhat slower than the IM route.

**Persistent status epilepticus.** When seizures persist for more than 1 hour, and in patients with recent myocardial infarction, orthopedic surgery, or massive myoglobulinuria, general anesthesia with pentobarbital or halothane and neuromuscular blockers is required.

**The phenobarbital alternative.** Phenobarbital is an effective antiepileptic drug for status epilepticus that can be used alone or with phenytoin. Phenobarbital's great advantage is its long duration of effectiveness. It can be used instead of diazepam from the beginning of management. Some authors recommend an IV dose of 8 to 15 mg/kg given slowly at 100 mg or less/minute. Others recommend an initial IV dose of 250 to 300 mg given in 2 or 3 minutes, to be repeated once or twice at 20- to 30-minute intervals if the seizures have not stopped. Respiratory depression may occur with high doses of phenobarbital but is usually of a slower onset than that associated with diazepam. Phenobarbital can be used only with extreme caution in conjunction with diazepam, and always after intubation has been accomplished, since their respiratory depression and hypotensive effects are additive.

***Neuroimaging and maintenance dose of anticonvulsants.*** A head CT scan or MRI scan should be obtained at some point if the cause of status epilepticus is unclear. The timing of this procedure should be individualized. Often it can be done after status epilepticus has been reasonably controlled and when the patient's vital signs are stable. The patient should *never* be left unattended in the corridors of the radiology department. Lumbar puncture should also be delayed until a reasonable control of convulsive seizures is achieved. If it is needed sooner to establish the diagnosis of meningitis or encephalitis, lumbar puncture can be performed after administration of a neuromuscular blocker. Once status epilepticus is controlled, high maintenance doses of phenytoin and/or phenobarbital can be given starting in a few hours. Repeat blood level measurements of anticonvulsants (e.g., about twice a day) can be done for the purpose of dose adjustment. Plasma levels should be maintained in the high therapeutic range. If the levels of phenytoin fall below the therapeutic range, reloading will likely be required.

## COMMON ANTIEPILEPTIC DRUGS

### Phenytoin

Phenytoin is one of the primary antiepileptic drugs for generalized, simple partial, and complex partial seizures but is ineffective in absence. Phenytoin blocks the spread of seizure activity but does not raise the seizure threshold.

Phenytoin's gastrointestinal (GI) absorption is slow. A single oral dose produces peak plasma levels in 8 to 12 hours. The suspension is better absorbed in some patients, but IM injection is slowly and incompletely absorbed and may cause muscle necrosis. The IV infusion of 14 to 18 mg/kg phenytoin in normal saline is used for the emergency treatment of status (see Status Epilepticus).

The usual adult oral dosage of phenytoin is about 300 to 500 mg daily (three to five capsules) and can be given in single or divided doses. Phenytoin is a long-acting drug with a plasma half-life of about 24 hours. The plasma steady-state level is achieved in about 7 to 10 days with the usual maintenance dose. An oral loading dose of 1000 to 1500 mg can be given within the first 24 hours in divided doses. The therapeutic blood levels are 10 to 20 μg/ml.

Renal failure reduces phenytoin's protein binding, which in turn leads to lower plasma levels and consequently a higher dose requirement. Hepatic failure may lower hepatic cytochrome activity, leading to a decreased metabolism and a lower dose requirement. In the liver, phenytoin is metabolized to its inactive by-products, which are conjugated and excreted in the urine.

The plasma levels of phenytoin are increased by oral anticoagulants, tricyclic antidepressants, isoniazid (INH), and disulfiram. Its plasma levels are decreased by valproic acid (transient), folic acid, and sporadic heavy consumption of alcohol. Phenytoin decreases the efficacy of oral anticoagulants (its withdrawal may cause hemorrhage), digitoxin, thyroxine, vitamin D, guanidine, and dexamethasone.

Phenytoin's side effects include (1) nystagmus with blood levels more than 20 μg/ml, cerebellar ataxia with more than 30 μg/ml, and confusion with more than 35 or 40 μg/ml; (2) allergic rash, gingival hyperplasia (common), hirsutism, coarse facial features, probable teratogenicity, peripheral polyneuropathy, and folate deficiency megalobastic anemia; and (3) rarely, a lupuslike syndrome, pseudolymphoma, pancytopenia, Stevens-Johnson syndrome, and myasthenic syndrome.

### Phenobarbital

Phenobarbital is a primary anticonvulsant in generalized, simple partial, and complex partial seizures but is ineffective in absence. Phenobarbital both increases the seizure threshold and suppresses its spread.

The GI absorption of phenobarbital is complete and fairly rapid. A single oral dose produces peak plasma levels in 4 to 7 hours. It can be used orally or by IM or IV injection. Although some phenobarbital is excreted unchanged in the urine, most is parahydroxylated in the liver. Renal failure may reduce its dose requirement, in contrast to that of phenytoin.

Phenobarbital's usual adult daily dosage of 60 to 150 mg can be given in single or divided doses. The plasma half-life is 3 to 4 days, and plasma steady-state level is achieved in about 2 to 3 weeks.

Valproic acid and other drugs that lower the urinary pH can significantly increase the plasma levels of phenobarbital by reducing its elimination. Conversely, phenobarbital decreases the level of valproic acid and the efficacy of oral anticoagulants and digitoxin. Drugs such as sodium bicarbonate that alkalinize the urine significantly increase the renal elimination of phenobarbital and can be used in the treatment of its overdose.

Phenobarbital's most common side effects include drowsiness in the first few weeks of treatment and occasionally hyperactivity in children.

### Carbamazepine

Carbamazepine is one of the major anticonvulsant drugs in generalized, simple partial, and complex partial seizures. Many recommended it as the drug of choice in complex partial seizures, but it is ineffective in absence. Carbamazepine suppresses the transmission of discharges from the amygdala, hippocampus, thalamus, and reticular formation.

The GI absorption of carbamazepine is slow because of its poor solubility. Most carbamazepine becomes protein bound, but unlike phenytoin, the binding is not altered by renal failure. Carbamazepine's metabolites have anticonvulsant effects.

The usual daily dosage of carbamazepine is about 600 to 1200 mg, which must be given in divided doses because of the rather short half-life of about 8 to 20 hours. Its therapeutic plasma level is about 4 to 12 μg/ml.

Carbamazepine and phenytoin slightly reduce each other's efficacy. Carbamazepine reduces the effect of anticoagulants, and its sudden withdrawal may cause hemorrhage.

Carbamazepine's side effects include a transient drowsiness, GI irritation, dizziness, diplopia, and ataxia initially or with toxic blood levels. Because of these effects, the drug should be started at a small dosage of about 100 mg two or three times per day and gradually increased by 100 mg to 200 mg increments every few days. Carbamazepine has been implicated in several cases of aplastic anemia and therefore is contraindicated in patients with a previous history of bone marrow depression. A complete blood count should be done before initiation of treatment, weekly or biweekly at the beginning of treatment, and monthly later. An allergic rash similar to that seen with phenytoin can occasionally occur.

### Valproic acid

Valproic acid is a major antiepileptic drug for generalized, complex, partial, and myoclonic seizures. Another major use is treatment of absence. It is less effective against simple partial seizures. Valproic acid prevents seizure spread without suppressing the seizure focus. It suppresses thalamocortical excitability.

The GI absorption of valproic acid is rapid, producing peak plasma levels in about 1 to 4 hours. Because of the transient side effects of GI irritation and a subjective feeling of fatigue, the drug should be started slowly at about 250 mg (one tablet) three times a day. The dosage is then gradually increased by one to two tablets per week to the full dosage of about 1000 to 3000 mg daily in divided doses. Its therapeutic plasma level is about 50 to 100 μg/ml. A long-acting, slowly absorbed, and more frequently used formulation of the drug is valproate sodium.

Valproic acid's combined use with clonazepam may rarely cause absence status epilepticus. Valproic acid increases the plasma levels of phenobarbital significantly. Its own plasma levels, however, are somewhat decreased by phenobarbital, as well as by phenytoin and primidone.

Valproic acid's side effects include some initial GI irritation, sedation, and rarely alopecia, all of which are transient. There may also be a transient elevation of the hepatic enzymes (alanine aminotransferase, aspartate aminotransferase, lactic acid dehydrogenase, and occasionally bilirubin), which return to normal by reduction of the dose. However, severe hepatotoxicity in the first 6 months of treatment has also been reported, and therefore the liver function tests should be performed before the initiation of treatment and monitored. Children under age 3 years and those with significant hepatic dysfunction should not receive valproic acid. In patients receiving this drug, the liver function tests should be periodically measured starting about 1 week after the initiation of treatment and later at gradually increasing intervals.

### Primidone

Primidone is a primary antiepileptic drug in generalized, simple partial, and complex partial seizures but is not effective in absence. Primidone decreases the seizure spread and raises the seizure threshold.

The GI absorption of primidone is rapid, giving peak plasma levels in 2 to 4 hours. It is metabolized in the liver to phenobarbital and phenylethyl malonamide (PEMA), both of which are powerful anticonvulsants.

Primidone's half-life is rather short (6 to 18 hours), as with carbamazepine and valproic acid, and requires that it be given in divided doses. Sedative effects can be minimized by starting at a low dosage of about 125 mg (half a tablet) three times a day, then gradually increasing at 3- to 7-day intervals to the full dosage of 500 to 1000 mg.

Primidone's main side effects are those of phenobarbital: drowsiness and occasionally hyperactivity in children.

### Clonazepam

Clonazepam is effective in myoclonic seizures. It improves absence and photosensitive epilepsy. It is an adjunctive drug for generalized, complex partial, and

**Table 101-4.** Common antiepileptic medications

| Drug | Seizure type | Usual adult daily dosage | Children's daily dosage | Therapeutic plasma level | Half-life | Days to achieve steady state plasma levels |
|---|---|---|---|---|---|---|
| Phenytoin (Dilantin) | Grand mal, simple focal, complex partial, grand mal status epilepticus | 300-500 mg in single or divided doses | 5-10 mg/kg | 10-20 μg/ml | 1 day | 7-10 |
| Phenobarbital | Same | 60-150 mg in single or divided doses | 4-6 mg/kg | 15-50 μg/ml | 3-4 days | 14-21 |
| Carbamazepine (Tegretol) | Same (not used for status epilepticus) | 600-1200 mg in divided doses; start from low dosage | 10-15 mg/kg | 4-12 μg/ml | 8-20 hours | 3-4 |
| Primidone (Mysoline) | Same (not used for status epilepticus) | 500-1000 mg in divided doses; start from low dosage | 10-25 mg/kg | 5-15 μg/ml | 6-18 hours | 4-7 |
| Valproic acid (Depakene) | Absence (petit mal); atonic and myoclonic seizures, epilepsia partialis continua | 1000-3000 mg in divided doses; start from low dosage | Start 15 mg/kg, increase by 5-10 mg/kg/week to 15-60 mg/kg/day | 50-100 μg/ml | 6-18 hours | 4 |
| Clonazepam (Klonopin) | Primary drug for myoclonus and epilepsia partialis continua; secondary drug for other seizures | 1.5 to 5-10 mg in divided doses; start from low dosage | Start 0.05 mg/kg, gradually increase to 0.05-0.2 mg/kg | 20-80 ng/ml | 1-2 days | 5-7 |
| Ethosuximide (Zarontin) | Absence (petit mal) | 750-1500 mg in divided doses; start from low dosage | 15-35 mg/kg | 40-100 μg/ml | 1-3 days | 7-10 |
| Diazepam (Valium) | Grand mal status epilepticus, absence status epilepticus, myoclonus | IV 5-20 mg status epilepticus | 0.15-0.5 mg/kg or up to 10 mg total for status epilepticus | | See text | |
| **Adjunctive therapies** | | | | | | |
| Felbamate (Felbatol) | Refractory partial seizures, Lennox-Gestaut syndrome, infantile spasms | 2400-3600 mg in divided doses | 30-45 mg/kg | 20-80 μg/ml | 14-20 hours | 3-5 |
| Gabapentin | Refractory partial seizures in adults | 900-1800 mg in divided doses | None | 2-3 μg/ml | 5-7 hours | 1-2 |
| Lamotrigine | Refractory partial seizures in adults | Start with low doses 300-500 mg (in two doses) when not in combination with valproate 100-500 mg (in two doses) in combination with valproate | None | 2-4 μg/ml | 12-48 hours | 3-12 |

simple partial seizures. It is effective in some cases of epilepsia partialis continua.

Clonazepam's daily dosage is about 1.5 to 5-10 mg. However, because of its sedative effect, it should be started at a low dosage of 1.0 to 1.5 mg daily in divided doses. The dosage is then gradually increased by weekly increments of 0.25 mg in children and 0.5 mg in adults. Its therapeutic blood levels are 20 to 80 ng/ml.

### Diazepam

Diazepam is a powerful drug for status epilepticus of either convulsive, partial complex, or absence type. It is effective in single seizures of all types, including that of eclampsia. However, because of its very rapid drop in blood levels, diazepam cannot be used as a maintenance anticonvulsant medication. Diazepam increases seizure threshold and blocks seizures from thalamic stimulation. It also enhances GABAergic synaptic inhibition (GABA, $\gamma$-aminobutyric acid).

The drug's absorption is rapid from the IV, oral, and rectal routes. Diazepam has a biophasic plasma level decay curve with a phase I half-life of 15 to 90 minutes, corresponding to its fast distribution, and phase II half-life of 27 to 57 hours or longer, related to slow elimination. Diazepam's half-life is increased in liver failure and in elderly patients, leading to prominent and prolonged sedative effects. The plasma steady state is reached in about 4 to 10 days with common oral therapeutic dosages.

Diazepam's metabolites have anticonvulsant effects. Its major side effects are drowsiness and physical dependence. Diazepam's withdrawal after prolonged use may cause seizures and therefore should be done slowly.

### Ethosuximide

Ethosuximide is one of the two frequently used major antiepileptic drugs for absence (the other is valproic acid). It is ineffective in other seizures.

The drug is rapidly and completely absorbed from the oral route and metabolized in the liver to inactive metabolites. The half-life of 1 to 3 days does not significantly vary between ages 5 and 15 years. Its usual daily dosage is 750 to 1500 mg.

Ethosuximide may transiently cause nausea, fatigue, drowsiness, dizziness, euphoria, or photophobia, which usually disappear with the continuation of the treatment.

### Felbamate

Felbamate is a recently approved drug for the treatment of the severe and refractory multiple seizures associated with the Lennox syndrome, a childhood encephalopathy. It may also be effective as an adjunctive treatment for refractory partial seizures in adults and children.

The drug is well absorbed orally and is available only by this route. Peak serum concentrations occur in 1 to 3 hours, and felbamate is only 25% protein bound, with a half-life of 20 hours.

Felbamate decreases plasma concentrations of carbamazepine by almost 30%; however, it increases carbamazepine's active metabolite. Felbamate increases phenytoin and valproate levels.

Adverse effects are few and mild, with headache, insomnia, anorexia, fatigue, and GI distress reported most often. Rash is reported in a few patients, and fever and transaminase elevations have been seen. Safety in pregnancy has not been determined.

Rare but fatal aplastic anemia and severe hepatic dysfunction have been reported since marketing of felbamate, which likely will be similar in incidence to that of carbamazepine and valproate. As with all anticonvulsant medications, risks should be compared with benefits and clinical monitoring should be more frequent after the initiation of new pharmacotherapy.

Recommended starting dose is 15 mg/kg/day in divided doses, increased weekly by another 15 mg/kg/day to a maximum of 45 mg/kg/day. In adults, 1200 mg in divided doses is increased to a maximum of 3600 mg daily. A concurrent lowering of the dose of phenytoin, carbamazepine, or valproate may preclude the side effects resulting from drug metabolism interactions.

### Gabapentin

Gabapentin is another recently approved adjunctive antiepileptic medication. It is marketed for partial seizures in adults with or without secondary generalization. Its small GABA-like molecule is water soluble and is totally and directly excreted through the urine without being metabolized in the liver.

Gabapentin's elimination half-life is 5 to 7 hours, and it should be taken in three divided doses. It comes in 100, 300, and 400 mg capsules. The usual dosage is one 300 mg capsule on the first day, two capsules the second day, and one capsule three times a day after that. The efficacy increases with a higher dose of 600 mg three times a day.

Gabapentin has no known drug interaction with other anticonvulsants. Its blood levels are difficult to measure and are not currently practical to report.

The adverse effects have been some initial somnolence, dizziness, ataxia, nystagmus, and fatigue.

### Lamotrigine

Lamotrigine is another anticonvulsant medication with a favorable side effect profile recently marketed in the United States for the treatment of refractory partial seizures in adults. Lamotrigine is approximately 55% protein bound, 90% metabolized, and has significant interactions with other anticonvulsants. Phenytoin, phenobarbital, and carbamazepine reduce lamotrigine's half life to 12 hours, whereas valproate increases it to 48 hours, necessitating a decrease in dose when used together.

Side effects include ataxia, dizziness, sedation, diplopia, and rash. Widespread use in other countries attests to the safety of this drug, which has broad-spectrum anticonvulsant activity.

• • •

Table 101-4 lists the common antiepileptic drugs, their dosages, therapeutic levels and days to achieve, half-lives, and the seizures they treat.

## BIBLIOGRAPHY

Brodie MJ: Lamotrigine, *Lancet* 339:1397, 1992.

Commission on Classification and Terminology of the International League Against Epilepsy: Proposal for classification of epilepsies and epileptic syndromes, *Epilepsia* 30:389, 1989.

Delgado-Escueta AV, Fe Enrile-Bacsal: Juvenile myoclonic epilepsy of Janz, *Neurology* 34:285, 1984.

Efficacy of felbamate in childhood epileptic encephalopathy (Lennox Gastaut syndrome), *N Engl J Med* 328:29, 1993.

Ettinger AB, Shinnar S: New-onset seizures in an elderly hospitalized population, *Neurology* 43:489, 1993.
Hauser WA et al: Seizure recurrence after a first unprovoked seizure, *Neurology* 40:1163, 1990.
Lowenstein DH, Alldredge BK: Status epilepticus at an urban public hospital in the 1980's, *Neurology* 43:483, 1993.
Messing RO, Closson RG, Simon RP: Drug-induced seizures: 10 year experience, *Neurology* 34:1582, 1984.
Salazar AM et al: Epilepsy after penetrating head injury, *Neurology* 35:1406, 1985.
Shorvon SD: *Status epilepticus: its clinical features and treatment in children and adults,* New York, 1993, Cambridge University Press.
Temkin NR et al: Randomized double-blind study of phenytoin for the prevention of post-traumatic seizures, *N Engl J Med* 323:497, 1990.

CHAPTER

# 102 Movement Disorders

**Nagagopal Venna**
**Marianne E. Giuffra**

The readily identifiable cortical motor strip, the large efferent corticospinal pathway descending into or near the lower motor neurons of the anterior horn cells, has lent itself so well to medical school anatomic and physiologic teaching that most medical students are left with the idea that all movement consists of on-off switching within this system. If one were to analyze all an individual's movements in a day, however, it must be a miniscule portion that depends entirely on the pyramidal system. Various postures basic to complex movements are maintained through an elaborate series of reflexes and reactions that do not come to consciousness. These reflexes and reactions require continuously acting feedback circuits operating at multiple levels within the nervous system. Antigravity postures are maintained unconsciously despite changing circumstances of comfort and other types of input. Within the lower portion of the brainstem, powerful vestibular influences have special effects in the orientation of the head and eye movements with other body postures. The cerebellum and associated pontine structures appear to provide the flowing synergy to normal movements, whereas rostral midbrain centers have important roles in the influence of sound, vision, posture, and movement. Basal ganglia situated between cortex and brainstem structures appear to be involved in the involuntary integration of movement, sampling a widespread area of cortex and projecting indirectly to motor neurons by polysynaptic systems.

The characterization and classification of abnormal movements are extensive, but our knowledge of the precise mechanisms producing them is sparse. Movement disorders formerly associated with specific damage in one anatomic region are increasingly attributed to dysfunction in any of several areas. Current approximations of the functional architecture of the basal ganglia suggest that the cortex sends afferent information to the corpus striatum (caudate and putamen), which, via the globus pallidus and subthalamus, projects to the thalamus and back to the cortex. Multiple overlapping, reciprocal connections of these centers with others in the brainstem and spinal cord modulate in this concert of brain activity. With increasing knowledge of the specific neurotransmitters and neuromodulators for these pathways, they are being probed with drugs and lesioned with toxins to elucidate their interrelationships. The potential exists in the near future for both specific new drug therapies and precise surgical intervention.

The neuronal "poundage" and phylogenetic priority speak powerfully for the importance of the extrapyramidal system. The clinician must recognize a series of disorders of this system in which the essential feature is a problem in nonvolitional motor function. This disorder may be expressed as a deficit in movement, a postural bias, or an involuntary movement.

## HYPOKINETIC MOVEMENT DISORDERS

### Parkinson's disease

***Epidemiology.*** Parkinson's disease (PD) is one of the most common neurologic diseases of advancing age. The disease is sporadic, has its greatest incidence in the 50s and 60s decades of life, but can be seen in all ages. Many speculated in the past that PD was caused by a toxic or infectious environmental agent. Parkinsonism haunted survivors of the encephalitis lethargica epidemic of the 1920s. California designer-drug users in the 1980s accidentally synthesized a compound, methylphenyltetrahydropyridine (MPTP), which causes both human and primate parkinsonism and has subsequently been developed into an animal model of the disease. Neither of these forms of parkinsonism matches PD pathologically or clinically. Although PD has occurred in geographic clusters, no clear relationships have emerged among pesticide exposure, diet, or smoking. A rare familial form of parkinsonism exists; however, the sporadic form is the more common type. The classic symptoms described by James Parkinson in 1817 remain the bulwark of the diagnosis of *idiopathic Parkinson's disease,* a neuronal degenerative disease with distinctive pathologic features. Table 102-1 lists clinical manifestations, differential diagnosis, tests, and treatment for parkinsonian syndromes.

***Symptoms.*** The most common symptom of PD, a complaint of most patients, is *tremor.* Frequently present when the hands are in the patient's lap, as well as during posture holding, tremor tends to abate during arm movement. The tremor usually occurs with a frequency of 3 to 7 Hz. A pronating and supinating motion of the arm can occur, as well as flexion-extension of the fingers, with the thumb tending to rub the forefinger in a motion referred to as "pill rolling." Tremor is an important symptom in the diagnosis of PD but can occur in several other pathologic conditions and, by itself, does not constitute the diagnosis.

*Rigidity* is another cardinal manifestation of parkinsonism, with resistance to both flexion and extension occurring evenly throughout the range of motion at both distal and proximal joints. The performance of reinforcing maneuvers in the opposite limb, such as opening and closing of the fist, enhances rigidity. While rotating the wrists to check for rigidity, the examiner may feel a

**Table 102-1.** Parkinsonian syndromes

| Disorder | Clinical manifestations | Differential diagnosis | Tests | Treatment |
|---|---|---|---|---|
| Parkinson's disease (PD) | Tremor: prerequisite for PD; present at rest; chiefly in fingers and hands at 3-7 Hz<br>Bradykinesia: paucity of spontaneous movements of face, giving "masklike" appearance; scarcity of natural limb and trunk movements is less obvious.<br>Disturbed body posture and gait: stooped posture; slowed, shuffling gait, sometimes festination and "freezing." Postural instability, causes falls<br>Rigidity: shoulder girdle rigidity presents as "frozen shoulder." Neck and trunk rigidity contributes to stooped posture. Lower trunk rigidity manifests as low back pain syndrome.<br>Micrographia<br>Speech: low volume | Essential tremor: tremor is only on activity such as holding arms outstretched; voice and head tremor frequent accompaniments. Neurologic examination shows no other abnormalities. Family history of tremor; tremor is dampened by propranolol or small doses of alcohol.<br>Symptomatic parkinsonism: structural brain lesions such as frontal lobe meningioma, sub dural hematoma, normal-pressure hydrocephalus, Binswanger disease, multiple basal ganglionic infarcts; rarely, infiltrating lesions of midbrain, traumatic (boxer's) encephalopathy<br>"Metabolic parkinsonism": toxins such as meperidine-related MPTP, carbon monoxide, manganese<br>Drug induced: phenothiazines, haloperidol, metoclopramide, reserpine<br>Hypocalcemia of hypoparathyroidism<br>Degenerative brain disorders (parkinsonism plus syndrome): Steele-Richardson-Olszewski syndrome, Shy-Drager syndrome, corticobasal ganglionic degeneration | Diagnosis is primarily clinical.<br>Brain computed tomography/magnetic resonance imaging: to exclude structural brain lesions but show no abnormalities pathognomonic of PD<br>Serum calcium: for rare cause of hypoparathyroidism<br>Positron emission tomography scan using radioactive fluorodopa shows hypometabolism in basal ganglia but is research tool at present.<br>Therapeutic test with L-dopa: dramatic improvement of bradykinesia, rigidity, and sometimes tremor with L-dopa strongly suggests PD. Response may take a few weeks. Lack of response casts doubt on diagnosis of idiopathic PD. | See Table 102-2. |
| Steele-Richardson-Olszewski syndrome (progressive supranuclear palsy) | Resembles PD because of rigidity, bradykinesia, gait disorder, and falls. Cardinal distinguishing feature is supranuclear gaze palsy with early paresis of downward gaze, which can deteriorate to total gaze paralysis. Tremor is minimal or absent; dysarthria/dysphagia early; neck held in extension dystonia. | | Diagnosis is clinical. | No specific therapy at present. L-dopa is temporarily beneficial in early stages; tricyclic antidepressants ameliorate pseudobulbar emotional lability. |

*Continued.*

**Table 102-1.** Parkinsonian syndromes—cont'd.

| Disorder | Clinical manifestations | Differential diagnosis | Tests | Treatment |
|---|---|---|---|---|
| Shy-Drager syndrome (multiple-systems atrophy) | Bradykinesia and rigidity mimic PD. Distinctive features: progressive autonomic failure with orthostatic hypotension, impotence, anhidrosis, neurogenic bladder, obstipation, dry mouth, impaired pupillary reflexes. Vocal cord paralysis and sleep apnea are rare. | | Diagnosis is clinical. Autonomic function tests clarify the clinical dysautonomia. | No specific treatment; pharmacologic and physical treatments available for various aspects dysautonomia. |
| Corticobasal ganglionic degeneration | Increasingly recognized disorder; progressive limb and trunk rigidity, bradykinesia; distinctive features: apraxia, cortical-type sensory loss | | Diagnosis is clinical and confirmed by brain biopsy. | In early stages, slight benefit from L-dopa; no specific treatment |

ratcheting superimposed on the motion of the joint, known as "cogwheeling."

One of the more distressing symptoms of parkinsonism involves the inability to move briskly or to perform sequential or simultaneous movements easily. Delays in initiating movements *(bradykinesia),* difficulty reaching a target with a single continuous movement *(hypokinesia),* and delayed reaction times, especially for planned movements, are major sources of disability. The patient experiences slowing in gait as well, periodically being "glued to the floor" when attempting to walk or "freezing" in midaction.

In addition, postural control is affected; patients lose their balance easily and fail to make the proper adjustments to remain standing. The gait is described as "festinating," with small, shuffling steps steadily increasing in velocity until the patient appears to be running. Small handwriting, reduced facial expressivity, infrequent eyeblinks, inaudible and inarticulate speech, and diminished habitual and associated movements such as arm swinging while walking are frequently seen. To demonstrate the postural instability, the patient can be pulled backward lightly at the shoulders from behind after being instructed to be ready to maintain the upright posture (i.e., "I'm going to pull you backward, but don't let yourself fall").

Neuropsychologic abnormalities, ranging from slowed cognitive processing to frank dementia, can occur, especially in older individuals. Depression also occurs more frequently in PD. Every patient does not manifest all the symptoms, especially at onset, but a gradual and relentless progression of symptoms occurs over years. The eventual tendency toward a permanent flexion posture of the neck, trunk, and limbs and the resulting immobility invites infectious complications.

The box at right lists symptoms of Parkinson's disease.

### Symptoms of Parkinson's disease

Pill-rolling tremor
Lead-pipe rigidity
Slowness of movement
Postural imbalance
Small handwriting
Arising slowly from chair
Absent arm swing
Festinating gait
Cogwheeling
Reduced facial expressivity
Diminished blinking
Inaudible speech

Diagnosis rests on history, physical examination, and clinical judgment, since no electrophysiologic or radiologic tests can confirm the diagnosis of idiopathic PD (Fig. 102-1).

***Pathophysiology.*** Degeneration of the pigmented nucleus of the midbrain called the substantia nigra is the hallmark of idiopathic PD. The characteristic pathologic marker seen at autopsy is the Lewy body, a microscopic eosinophilic neuronal inclusion.

***Genetics.*** Studies of identical and fraternal twins have concluded that no autosomal pattern of inheritance exists in PD. Recently, researchers have speculated on possible abnormalities in the mitochondrial genome, in part because the pattern of maternal inheritance in mitochondrial disorders could resemble that of a sporadic disorder. Furthermore, there is evidence of dysfunction of mitochondrial respiratory chain enzymes in the autopsied

CLINICAL TESTS IN MONITORING PATIENTS WITH PARKINSON'S DISEASE

Writing sample ________________________________

Draw a spiral

right hand    examiner    left hand

A

Timed motor performances

turn over in bed
sit up in bed
get up out of chair
drink from a cup with both hands
take off and put on a shoe
walk the length of the room

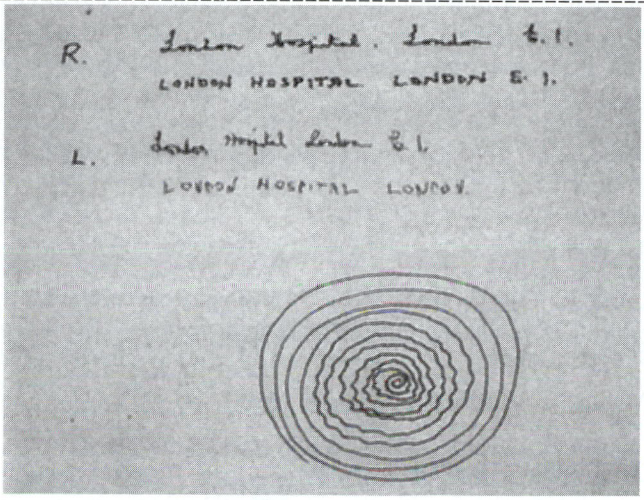


B

**Fig. 102-1. A,** Clinical tests in monitoring Parkinson's disease. **B,** The handwriting of a patient with Parkinson's disease shows micrographia and the tremulous spiral. (From Trend P et al: *Neurology: colour guide,* Edinburgh, 1992, Churchill Livingstone.)

substantia nigra of PD patients. The significance of these findings is being debated.

***Differential diagnosis.*** A distinction should be made between idiopathic PD, which is exquisitely sensitive to dopaminergic replacement therapy, and *parkinsonism* secondary to drug or toxic exposure, brain damage, or atherosclerosis, since these suggest different interventions.

**Iatrogenic causes.** Of particular concern among the causes of parkinsonism should be the reversible disorder caused by dopamine-blocking or dopamine-depleting medications. Frequently used agents of this type are the neuroleptic antipsychotics, metoclopramide, reserpine, and α-methyltyrosine. In addition to flexion posture, akinesia, and other signs of parkinsonism, these agents may cause tardive dyskinesia or akathisia. Although the clinical situation may require use of these agents, reducing the dose, switching to an agent causing fewer side effects, or adding an anticholinergic agent can frequently improve symptoms. The use of replacement dopaminergic agents when parkinsonism is caused by therapy with dopamine blocking drugs is illogical.

**Atherosclerotic causes.** Some individuals with hypertension have many small brain infarctions slowly over years, a few of which may be recognized as individual cerebrovascular accidents (CVAs, strokes). Damage to the connections of the extrapyramidal and pyramidal motor systems results in slowness and rigidity, flexion posture, and abnormal speech. Clues to the diagnosis of so-called atherosclerotic parkinsonism are the infrequent occurrence of tremor, the presence of moderate to severe dementia, and an abnormal neurologic examination, including brisk deep tendon reflexes and Babinski signs (see the box below). A history of hypertension and strokelike episodes, the absence of a response to dopaminergic medications, and radiologic evidence of multiple, bilateral basal ganglia and white matter infarctions are additional evidence.

**Dementia.** Individuals with a degenerative dementia such as Alzheimer disease can manifest changes in muscle tone, posture, and gait and have concurrent senile tremor. Information regarding use of neuroleptic medications to control behavior should be sought. Since dementia occurs in a proportion of idiopathic PD patients, the distinction rests on the severity, neuropsychologic features, and course of the dementia, which is usually more prominent in Alzheimer disease. Those with primary dementia have a greater variety of behavioral abnormalities than idiopathic PD patients and are not responsive to dopaminergic medications.

**Miscellaneous causes.** Repeated trauma (e.g., boxing), subacute hypoxia (e.g., carbon monoxide), chronic exposure to manganese (e.g., mining or chemical manufacturing), hypoparathyroidism, or a frontal lobe tumor can include symptoms of parkinsonism. A careful history and neurologic examination are required in these situations.

**Other differential diagnoses.** The differential diagnosis of PD includes other rigid, akinetic degenerative diseases such as progressive supranuclear palsy (Steele-Richardson-Olszewski syndrome), Shy-Drager syndrome (multiple systems Atrophy), olivopontocerebellar atrophy, Wilson disease, and the juvenile form of Huntington chorea (disease), all of which occur much less frequently and have a different course and prognosis.

*Progressive supranuclear palsy* (PSP) presents with rigidity and dementia at approximately the same age as idiopathic PD. However, PSP patients have a striking tendancy to extend the neck and have difficulty with voluntary vertical gaze, especially downward gaze, with some preservation of reflexive vertical gaze. Emotional disturbances and severe dysphagia are more common in PSP, but tremor is infrequently seen. Patients do not respond to either levodopa (L-dopa) or anticholinergics. PSP is generally more rapidly progressive than PD, with an average of 4 years from symptoms to diagnosis and 6 years from diagnosis to complete disability or death.

**Suggested timed motor performances in patients with Parkinson's disease**

- Turn over in bed
- Sit up in bed
- Get up from chair
- Drink from cup with both hands
- Take off and put on shoe
- Walk length of room

*Shy-Drager syndrome* is the eponym for parkinsonism occurring in association with significant autonomic dysfunction, such as orthostatic hypotension, bradyarrhythmias, impotence, anhidrosis, urinary problems, dry mouth, and blurred vision. L-Dopa and other dopaminergic drugs are also a common cause of orthostasis, and anticholinergic medications can cause dry mouth and other symptoms, so their effects should be considered before this diagnosis is made.

*Olivopontocerebellar atrophy* (OPCA) is a rare and sometimes familial progressive neurologic disease that can begin at any age, with prominent cerebellar ataxia and dysarthric, scanning speech. Atrophy of the pons, cerebellum, and olivary nuclei of the medulla may be seen on anatomic brain scanning in OPCA patients. No treatment is effective.

*Wilson disease* usually presents with a high-amplitude, "flapping" tremor prominent in proximal rather than distal extremities. However, patients may exhibit a variety of presentations, including parkinsonism.

*Adult-onset Huntington chorea* is rarely confused with PD, although the juvenile form presents with rigidity, immobility, and dementia (not tremor). Family history and age of onset distinguish this autosomal dominant disease entity.

Although PD typically causes tremor in association with other symptoms, the clinician should consider systemic disease such as hyperthyroidism, essential tremor, or a cerebellar syndrome in a patient who has tremor as an isolated symptom.

The prevalence of postencephalitic parkinsonism, seen in the survivors of the flu epidemic of the 1920s, has declined significantly.

***Management.*** Treatment of idiopathic PD is aimed at symptomatic improvement of the tremor, rigidity, and bradykinesia. The assessment of benefit is important for diagnosis as well as therapy; therefore, careful, reproducible quantitation of the effect of treatment is necessary. The dopaminergic agents have euphoric and mood-elevating effects in some patients, so their subjective impression of benefit may not be entirely reliable. Tasks such as walking, arising from a chair, or picking up a certain number of coins can be timed with a stopwatch and repeated at each visit. Writing samples and the drawing of a spiral highlight tremor and illustrate the patient's small handwriting (see Fig. 102-1). Even with adequate doses of medication, the effect of L-dopa in previously untreated patients may be delayed for several weeks. Therefore, a lengthy therapeutic trial is advised. Table 102-2 outlines pharmacologic, surgical, and symptom management of PD.

**L-Dopa therapy.** The mainstay of treatment is to replace dopamine, using either L-dopa, the amine precursor, or dopamine agonist drugs. The development of L-dopa therapy has been of significant benefit in the treatment of PD. In the early stages, patients have a relatively rapid and prolonged improvement in motor function with small doses of L-dopa three or four times daily. Side effects are usually few, tolerable, and dose related but can include nausea, vomiting, postural hypotension, and rarely, car-

**Table 102-2.** Management of Parkinson's disease

**Pharmacologic treatment**

| Medication | Dosage | Side effects |
|---|---|---|
| ***Dopaminergic drugs*** | | |
| Carbidopa/levodopa (L-dopa) | 25/100 mg qid; maintenance usually up to 500 mg L-dopa daily | Orthostatic hypotension; nausea, confusion, especially in elderly; visual hallucinations, nightmares, myoclonus, dyskinesias |
| Bromocriptine | 2.5 mg tablets; start with half tablet, increase gradually; bid or tid dosage; maintenance: 7.5-30 mg | Hypotension, visual hallucinations, confusion, livedo reticularis, cryomelalgia of feet |
| Pergolide | 0.05 mg/day; increase up to 1 mg tid or qid | Same as for bromocriptine |
| Amantadine | 100 mg bid | Nausea, confusion, livedo reticularis |
| ***Anticholinergic drugs*** | | |
| Trihexyphenidyl (Artane) | 2 mg/day; increase to 2 mg up to tid | Dry mouth, blurred vision; can precipitate narrow-angle glaucoma |
| Benztropine (Cogentin) | 0.5-1.0 mg/day; increase up to 4-6 mg/day | Urinary hesitancy (can precipitate urinary retention), confusion |
| ***Monoamine oxidase inhibitor*** | | |
| Deprenyl | 5 mg bid | Nausea, nervousness, insomnia |

**Surgical treatment**

| Procedure | Indication | Comment |
|---|---|---|
| Stereotactic thalamotomy | Intractable, unilateral | A few patients with disabling tremor but without severe bradykinesia or rigidity experience marked relief. |
| Fetal adrenal medulla and substantia nigra transplants into caudate nuclei | | These treatments remain experimental at present. |
| Stereotactic pallidotomy | | |

**Symptom management**

| Symptom | Intervention |
|---|---|
| Activities of daily living, frozen shoulder prevention, prevention of falls | Physical therapy |
| Low-volume speech | Speech therapy |
| Dysarthria | Clonazepam: 0.5-1 mg tid |
| Spastic bladder | Oxybutynin: 5-10 mg tid |
| Constipation | High-fiber diet: Metamucil, Colace |
| Action tremor (frequently coexists with PD) | Propranolol: 40-80 mg tid |
| Painful dystonia of limbs | Baclofen: 5-10 mg tid |
| Paroxysmal drenching sweats | β-Blockers |
| Depression | Tricyclic antidepressants, electroconvulsive treatment |

diac arrhythmias. Many patients experience vivid dreams and even occasional hallucinations without disturbing emotional import; however, others have agitation and frank psychosis. If reduction in dose does not reverse the mental changes, discontinuing L-dopa and/or dopamine agonists may be necessary. The newer generation of antipsychotic agents, the prototype of which is clozapine (Clozaril), do not have the same propensity to antagonize the motor benefits of L-dopa and have been used in treatment-related psychosis in PD. L-Dopa can theoretically accelerate the growth of melanotic tumors, and the initial evaluation should include a precautionary skin examination.

Initially used alone, L-dopa was effective only in large, side effect–producing doses. The subsequent addition of an inhibitor of peripheral metabolism, carbidopa, permitted larger proportions of the L-dopa to be taken up by the central nervous system (CNS). The commercially available form of L-dopa contains a 4:1 ratio of L-dopa to carbidopa. A minimum of approximately 100 mg carbidopa is required to saturate the peripheral enzymatic systems. A longer-acting preparation of the same ingredients is also available to use once the effectiveness of the treatment has been established with some certainty using the standard preparation.

***Timing and side effects.*** Controversy exists over the optimal time to begin L-dopa therapy, since the effectiveness of replacement L-dopa therapy has been seen to diminish over 3 to 7 years in a somewhat predictable pattern. Initially, substantial therapeutic effect and prolonged duration of action occur. The first change is the appearance of "wearing off," in which a single dose of medication has an increasingly short duration of action and the patient begins to increase the frequency of dosing. L-Dopa is taken up by the brain by a membrane transport system for large neutral amino acids, and evidence suggests that a diet rich in protein may result in diminished transfer of L-dopa into the CNS. A "protein redistribution diet" with the bulk of daily protein in the evening meal minimizes the effect of competition for transport.

As patients begin taking increased amounts of L-dopa, they may experience unwanted, involuntary movements known as dyskinesias and dystonias. *Dyskinesia* resembles a writhing movement of the extremities, neck, or face; *dystonia* is a painful twisting or cramping in an extremity. They are common at the peak of medication effect, although they can occur at any time. Dystonias may also be a presenting complaint in younger PD patients. Eventually, the time and frequency of dosing seems to become completely dissociated from the clinical effect. Most patients progress to this stage after 5 to 7 years of treatment. There are periods of sudden and severe akinesia ("freezing"), unresponsive to further oral doses of L-dopa, alternating in an unpredictable pattern with either reasonable motor function or dyskinetic movements.

**Dopamine agonists.** Acting at the postsynaptic dopamine receptor, bromocriptine and pergolide are two agents that increase dopaminergic activity, although not providing quite as complete an effect as L-dopa. Each agent can be used alone or as adjunctive treatment, alternating with doses of L-dopa/carbidopa. Postural hypotension, psychosis, and nausea neccessitate beginning these drugs at low doses, then titrating slowly over weeks or months to the desired clinical effect.

**Anticholinergics.** Anticholinergics (benztropine, trihexyphenidyl, biperiden, ethopropazine), once the only available treatment for PD, have become secondary because of the availability of L-dopa and dopamine agonists. Anticholinergics tend to cause confusion and worsening of dementia in elderly patients but can be particularly useful as first-line therapy when tremor is the most prominent symptom. Their use is limited in many patients by side effects such as urinary retention, constipation, dry mouth, lightheadedness, and blurred vision. Anticholinergics should not be given to patients with untreated increased intraocular pressure because they may precipitate acute glaucoma.

**Other drugs.** *Amantadine* is an antiviral agent incidentally discovered to have antiparkinsonian effects and presumed to enhance L-dopa release, although it is also mildly anticholinergic. Usually regarded as benign, amantadine has an effect that may not persist over time, although rapid withdrawal causes apparent short-term worsening of symptoms. Side effects are those of the anticholinergics, including delirium, as well as congestive heart failure, livedo reticularis, and edema.

*Deprenyl,* a monoamine oxidase (MAO) inhibitor, as well as antioxidants and free radical scavengers, have been under investigation to determine their potential to delay progression of the degeneration that constitutes PD. Clinical trials are ongoing; however it appears that deprenyl has a symptomatic effect (diminishes breakdown of dopamine) but not a clear neuroprotective effect. In addition, the antioxidant vitamin E has been ineffective in delaying progression of the disease at doses of 400 IU daily.

**Surgery.** Fetal adrenal medulla and substantia nigra implants remain experimental procedures with advocates and detractors but there is no clear consensus regarding their effectiveness. Thalamic surgery was a more common intervention for PD and tremor in general before the advent of dopaminergic drugs. Recently, because of increasing information on the anatomy of basal ganglia pathways as well as the refinement of surgical techniques, surgical treatment such as stereotactic pallidotomy is being discussed and investigated anew.

***Lifestyle and emotional problems.*** The diagnosis of a progressive degenerative disease, coming at a time of life when the patient is still physically capable and anticipating continued activity, is significant. In addition to offering continuing medical care, the physician should suggest the beneficial effects of lifestyle changes and emotional support. Regular physical exercise, especially stretching or yoga, and avoidance of concomitant morbidity from alcohol, tobacco, and obesity can increase the quality of life considerably. Patients should not relinquish control of their bodies because of the diagnosis of PD. Support groups, information, and other services are provided by the Parkinson's Disease Society. Depression can be a reaction to the situation as well as a feature of the neurotransmitter disorder itself. If persistent or disabling, treatment of depression is indicated.

## HYPERKINETIC MOVEMENT DISORDERS

Disorders characterized by excess movement can be seen in association with systemic illness, as a result of medications, or as part of an inherited, degenerative, or other neurologic syndrome (Table 102-3).

***Types of abnormal movements.*** *Fasciculation* is the contraction of all the muscle fibers innervated by a single anterior horn cell. Individuals with the syndrome of benign fasciculations may become convinced that they have a serious, progressive neurologic disorder. Benign fasciculations tend to occur in bursts of 5 to 50, with each twitch precisely like the preceding one. They are most common in the muscles of the thigh and around the eye and may be brought on by anxiety, excessive caffeine, sudden change from a sedentary to an active lifestyle, and anticholinergic and anticholinesterase medications. Fasciculations that represent denervation or anterior horn cell disease (amyotrophic lateral sclerosis) are more scattered and less stereotyped, tend not to occur in bursts, and are almost always associated with weakness and atrophy of the affected muscles.

**Table 102-3.** Hyperkinetic movement disorders

| Disorder | Clinical manifestations | Differential diagnosis | Tests | Treatment |
|---|---|---|---|---|
| Chorea, choreoathetosis, tardive dyskinesia | Continuum of abnormal involuntary movements; jerky, nonrhythmic, semipurposive, predominantly in limbs; may affect head, neck, trunk; lips and tongue may participate (buccolingual dyskinesia); often mixed with writhing (choreoathetosis) | Drug induced<br>Phenothiazines<br>L-dopa<br>Phenytoin<br>Cocaine<br>Amiphetamines<br>Tricyclics<br>Oral contraceptives | Urine toxic screen | Withdrawal of toxic drug<br>Symptomatic treatment: clonazepam: 0.5 mg bid up to 4-16 mg/day<br>Haloperidol: 0.5-1.0 mg tid up to 5-15 mg/day |
| | | Liver failure | Liver function tests | Treatment of hepatic encephalopathy |
| | | Wilson's disease: dyskinesia accompanied by dystonia, cerebellar ataxia, dysarthia, proximal limb tremor, emotional lability | Slit-lamp examination for Kayser-Fleischer rings; serum ceruloplasmin, serum copper | Penicillamine |
| | | Thyrotoxicosis | Serum thyroxine, TSH | Antithyroid drugs |
| | | Polycythemia | Hematocrit | Phelbotomy |
| | | Systemic lupus erythematosus | Antinuclear antibody | Steroids |
| | | Sydenham's chorea | — | Symptomatic |
| | | Huntington's chorea | Brain CT/MRI, DNA analysis | Symptomatic |
| Hemiballismus | Large, flinging, ballistic limb movements; predominates in arm or leg | Lacunar CVA in vicinity of subthalamic nuclei in basal ganglia; other focal lesions: metastases and toxoplasmosis (in AIDS) | Brain CT/MRI | Therapy of underlying lesion<br>Symptomatic treatment same as for chorea |
| Focal dystonia | Spasmodic torticollis | Idiopathic | Clinical | Anticholinergics (high dose): trihexyphenidyl (Artane), 2 mg bid up to 10-40 mg/day<br>Benzodiazepines: clonazepam as above; diazepam, 5 mg bid up to 20-60 mg/day<br>Botulin A toxin: focal injections<br>Surgery: peripheral muscle denervation |
| | Spasmodic dysphonia (laryngeal) | Idiopathic | — | Botulin A toxin: injection into vocal muscles |
| | Essential blepharospasm: dystonia of obicularis oculi muscle is principal feature; if accompanied by dystonia of facial, tongue, and neck muscles, called Meige syndrome | Idiopathic | — | Clonazepam as above<br>Botulin A toxin: injection into appropriate muscles |

*Continued.*

**Table 102-3.** Hyperkinetic movement disorders—cont'd.

| Disorder | Clinical manifestations | Differential diagnosis | Tests | Treatment |
|---|---|---|---|---|
| Segmental and generalized dystonia | May affect different segments of body or be generalized or multifocal | Idiopathic<br>Hereditary<br>Drug induced:<br>Phenothiazines<br>L-dopa<br>Calcium channel blockers | — | Symptomatic treatment: anticholinergics, clonazepam<br>Baclofen: 10 mg bid up to 50-100 mg/day<br>Carbamazepine: 100 mg bid up to 600-1200 mg/day |
| | | Wilson's disease | Same as for chorea | Penicillamine plus symptomatic treatment |
| | | Diurnal dystonia: childhood-onset (Segawa disease type) may have parkinsonian features | Familial | Dramatic response to L-dopa<br>Carbidopa/L-dopa: 25/100 mg bid or tid |
| Acute dystonic reaction | May be segmental or generalized with oculogyric crisis, torticollis, tongue protrusion, opisthotonus; children more susceptible | Drug induced<br>Prochlorperazine<br>Metoclopramide | — | Benztropine (Cogentin): 1-2 mg IM<br>Diphenhydramine: 50 mg IM |
| Paroxysmal dystonia | Kinesigenic: brief attacks of dystonia triggered by sudden movements | Idiopathic or familial | — | Carbamazepine: 100-200 mg tid<br>Phenytoin: 100 mg tid |
| | Nonkinesigenic dystonia: prolonged paroxysm of dystonia unrelated to activity | Idiopathic or familial | — | Carbamazepine, clonazepam<br>Acetazolamide (Diamox): 250 mg tid |

*TSH,* Thyroid-stimulating hormone; *CT,* computed tomography; *MRI,* magnetic resonance imaging; *DNA,* deoxyribonucleic acid; *CVA,* cerebrovascular accident; *AIDS,* acquired immune deficiency syndrome.

*Athetosis* consists of writhing-type movements. The arm alternates between a posture of extreme adduction and flexion to one of abduction and extension. The face and voice are often affected by similar slow involuntary movements.

In mild cases of *chorea,* the observer often simply notes that the patient appears restless or nervous. The patient may conceal movements by combining them with a purposeful movement. Thus a movement that begins as involuntary flexion of the arm might be continued into one in which the patient brushes back the hair. Chorea is often most prominent in the fingers and wrists.

*Myoclonus* consists of sudden, lightninglike movement or a series of such movements. It is one of the most nonspecific terms in neurology. Myoclonus may arise from cortical, basal ganglia, cerebellar, brainstem, or spinal lesions. Movements may involve small muscle bundles or large postural muscles, giving massive myoclonic jerks, in which the whole body suddenly contracts and the patient may be thrown to the floor. *Tremor* implies a small-amplitude, rhythmic, alternating movement that may be regular or irregular, that may be associated with the maintenance of a posture, or that may be brought on by movements.

*Dystonia* is a torsion and cramping of a muscle group or the trunk itself. The patient assumes fixed, unnatural postures that cannot be voluntarily averted.

## Disorders associated with systemic diseases

Hyperkinetic movement disorders related to systemic conditions represent a significant diagnostic category for the primary care physician. Some patients with *polycythemia vera* show a choreoathetosis once their hematocrit reaches a critical level, which promptly disappears with the reduction of the hematocrit. Some patients with *hypoparathyroidism* may become rigid with flexed posture or have choreoathetosis. These patients often have calcifications of the basal ganglia, as seen on computed tomography (CT) scan.

*Hyperthyroidism* may present with chorea, especially in children and in elderly persons. Chorea can also be a manifestation of cerebral *systemic lupus erythematosus* (SLE). The exact cause of *chorea gravidarum,* or chorea in pregnancy, is uncertain. Many of these patients are found to have SLE, although some cases of chorea have been associated recently with oral contraceptives. Phenytoin (Dilantin) has also produced chorea. *Sydenham's chorea* is rare but is one of the major diagnostic signs of rheumatic fever. A personality change with irritability and difficulty in concentration is associated with Sydenham's chorea and sometimes overshadows it as a presenting problem. Chorea responds to rest and mild sedation. In severe cases, haloperidol has been used to suppress movements, which can be violent enough to fling a child off the bed.

In *nonwilsonian hepatocerebral degeneration,* there is chronic portocaval shunting, most often caused by surgery or hepatic cirrhosis. Symptoms include choreoathetosis of the face, lips, and tongue; dementia; and ataxia with axial tremors. The movements can be suppressed with haloperidol, and treatment is aimed at reducing ammonia production with lactulose, a low-protein diet, and a nonabsorbable antibiotic such as neomycin.

Myoclonus is often a dominant feature in certain *metabolic encephalopathies,* especially those associated with severe hyponatremia. Patients who have had a *severe cerebral anoxic episode* may chronically have myoclonus whenever reaching out to grasp an object. Abnormalities in serotonin neurotransmitter precursors have been described, and tryptophan has been used in postanoxic myoclonus with some success.

## Drug-induced disorders

Various drugs, including phenothiazines, butyrophenones, antihistamines, α-methyl-L-dopa, phenytoin, oral contraceptives, reserpine, metoclopramide, lithium, and L-dopa have been associated with movement disorders. The most frequent offenders are the neuroleptics. Five syndromes that may be seen with these drugs are (1) acute dystonic reactions, (2) parkinsonism, (3) akathisia, (4) tardive dyskinesia, and (5) neuroleptic malignant syndrome.

*Acute dystonic reactions* may occur with the first dose of a phenothiazine. They consist of paroxysmal, violent movements of torticollis or retrocollis, sometimes with sustained dystonic posture after a single dose, and can appear to be tetanus. We have seen cases in which the patient has a midline dystonia and is unable to speak or swallow. He or she comes to the emergency room with a towel under the chin to catch saliva and is panicked. These reactions respond to a small dose of anticholinergic medication (benztropine, 1 to 2 mg intramuscularly) or intravenous diphenhydramine (Benadryl), 1 mg/kg in divided doses over 24 hours.

*Neuroleptic parkinsonism* consists of rigidity and akinesia without typical tremor. *Akathisia* involves compulsive movement of the limbs, especially feet. The patient paces so much that the increased activity is mistaken for anxiety, and the offending medication is increased. To meet the full definition of akathisia, the movement must be accompanied by a conscious, irrepressible desire to continue to move. Treatment consists of discontinuing the medication.

The most troubling category of drug-induced movement disorders is *tardive dyskinesia.* Symptoms include involuntary repetitive movements, especially of the orofacial muscles, with tongue protrusion, lip smacking, chewing, grimacing, and grunting movements in the face, as well as writhing or choreiform movements in the limbs and axial musculature. These involuntary movements usually appear after prolonged therapy, particularly with phenothiazines, but can even appear when the medication is reduced or stopped. Once established, these tardive dyskinesias are extremely difficult to treat, and various drugs have been tried with limited and sporadic success. If the offending drug is removed, the movements may eventually quiet, but it may take years. Prevention is the best intervention and is accomplished by the judicious, conservative use of phenothiazines and other powerful dopamine-receptor blockers. Anticholinergic medication should not be given automatically as part of an antipsychotic regimen. Certain antipsychotics, such as thioridazine (Mellaril), may have less tendency to produce tardive dyskinesia. Tardive dyskinesia sometimes responds to drugs that reduce the amount of dopamine present. Reserpine, 2 to 5 mg daily, is effective in depleting dopamine by preventing intraneuronal storage. However, the side effect of depression may not be well tolerated in psychiatric patients. Dopamine antagonists such as pimozide, 2 mg daily and gradually increasing to 20 mg daily, or haloperidol have been used. Clonazepam, a benzodiazepine, is sometimes effective in suppressing the movements when doses of 1 to 3 mg daily are used.

*Neuroleptic malignant syndrome* (NMS) is an idiosyncratic response to neuroleptics that has been reported to occur not only in patients receiving dopamine blockers, but also in those acutely withdrawn from dopamine agonists, such as during a L-dopa "drug holiday" in PD. The syndrome is unusual but can be fatal and deserves prompt recognition. High fever, muscular rigidity, tremors, confusion, delirium, and dysautonomia in a patient who has recently received dopamine-blocking or dopamine-depleting agents should arouse suspicion. The presence of rhabdomyolosis with elevated creatine kinase (CK, CPK) and myoglobinuria are confirmatory. Infectious, toxic, and metabolic disorders, as well as other neurologic syndromes caused by neuroleptics, have overlapping symptoms, and strict criteria for the diagnosis of NMS have not been established. Septicemia and meningitis need to be ruled out. Treatment of NMS is largely symptomatic. The goal is preventing the complications of severe hyperthermia, myoglobinuria, and the septic complications of immobility. Neuroleptics need to be discontinued, but not dopamine agonists. Diazepam and dantrolene have been used in high doses to diminish muscular tension. Intensive medical support is required, since fatalities have been reported in as many as 11% of the cases.

### Huntington's chorea

The prototype neuronal degenerative disorder associated with excess movement is dominantly inherited Huntington's chorea (disease).

***Epidemiology.*** The prevalence of Huntington's disease is 5 per 100,000 population in the United States. Since this is a familial disorder, clustering of cases may occur in one geographic region, and there are communities in South America with extremely high prevalence.

***Presentation.*** Average age at onset is in the late 30s. Individuals that present younger usually have a phenotypically different or more severe symptomatology, whereas those that present older are sometimes less severely affected. Depression and cognitive difficulties may precede the movement disorder, which can be difficult to recognize initially. Personality disorders, typically irritable apathy, may lead the patient to substance abuse or criminal activity. Psychosis and paranoia can occur at any stage. Movements may be minor at first and appear as a restlessness or jitteriness. Fleeting movements of the fingers or shoulders are merged into common mannerisms such as adjusting one's glasses. Choreatic movements in the face can appear as an expression of interest, but the eyebrow raising, grimacing, and puckering are soon observed to occur too quickly and too often and are not coupled to the content of the conversation. The patient may sweep the chin across the clavicle. Eventually, the gait has a grotesque, waltzing character.

Individuals who come from intact families and have witnessed the slow decline of a parent often deny that they notice chorea and reject the diagnosis. Persons with Huntington's disease have an increased risk of suicide. The time between diagnosis and death varies, but institutionalization usually occurs 12 years after diagnosis. When the patient approaches the final stages of the disorder, the movements subside and are replaced by flexion postures, with only fragments of choreoathetosis remaining.

***Diagnosis.*** Observation of the characteristic signs and symptoms in an individual with a family history of the disorder makes the diagnosis. An imaging study, preferably a magnetic resonance imaging (MRI) scan, showing atrophy of the caudate nucleus and putamen and genetic testing are confirmatory.

***Genetics.*** The abnormality is caused by a gene on the long arm of chromosome 4. Previously, all affected individuals were members of a kindred, but some evidence now indicates that a vanishingly small number of cases may result from new mutations. The occurrence of mutations is so rare that family history should be considered a requirement for diagnosis. The gene for Huntington's chorea contains an unstable "triplet repeat sequence," similar to the genes for other neurologic diseases such as fragile X and myotonic dystrophy. The length of this repeating sequence of base pairs coding for the same amino acid (glutamine) varies from one individual to another has been correlated with disease severity. This variation may be responsible for the phenomenon of *amplification,* in which the disease appears to worsen or occur at an earlier age in successive generations. The detection of triplet repeats in the genome has permitted the development of a test that does not rely on comparison with a known Huntington's patient's deoxyribonucleic acid (DNA) and is available to those without a large or surviving family.

***Pathophysiology.*** The primary sites of neurodegeneration are the medium-sized neurons of the striatum, whose transmitter is $\gamma$-aminobutyric acid (GABA) in association with the opiate peptide enkephalin. *Excitotoxicity,* the hypothesis that cell death may occur in neuronal degenerative diseases through excess stimulation of neurotransmitter receptors, has made Huntington's chorea especially interesting to researchers. The neurons affected in Huntington's disease have a high proportion of receptors for the NMDA (*n*-methyl-D-aspartate) glutamate receptor.

***Management.*** Currently, no effective specific treatment is available for the degeneration. Chorea is somewhat alleviated by haloperidol, although evidence suggests that the optimal dose for chorea is usually 5 mg daily or less. Other indications, such as psychotic depression, may warrant higher doses, but dementia is not alleviated by dopamine blockade.

### Other hyperkinetic movement disorders

***Wilson's disease.*** Wilson's disease is a very rare autosomal recessive disease that has many nonneurologic manifestations. The disease is associated with a specific decrease in ceruloplasmin (ferroxidase), a globulin that binds 98% of serum copper. This results in an increase in free or loosely bound serum copper, and copper is deposited in the tissues, which are ultimately damaged. Neuronal loss, necrosis, and astrocytosis occur in the brain, and actual cavitation may occur in the putamen, globus pallidus, cerebellum, and cerebral cortex. Cirrhosis, aminoaciduria, and a ring of copper deposition in the limbus of the cornea result in the diagnostic Kayser-Fleischer ring, seen on slit-lamp examination. The childhood form of Wilson's disease presents mostly with dystonia, whereas in adults, tremor predominates. The characteristic proximal tremor can be enhanced by having the patient abduct and flex the arms. The limbs move with a wing-beating, irregular tremor. Patients have dysarthria, a peculiar fixed smile, and difficulty in walking and writing. Personality change is characterized by poor judgment and bizarreness. The untreated disease shows a progressive downhill course to fixed postures and complete dementia.

Diagnosis is based on the Kayser-Fleischer ring and on an abnormally low serum ceruloplasm. Liver function tests are often abnormal. Family members should be screened and abnormalities found before the disease is evident. Current treatment is penicillamine, 1 to 2 g daily, an active chelating agent that binds copper and results in increased urinary copper excretion. Oral potassium sulfide binds dietary copper in the gastrointestinal tract and prevents some absorption into the bloodstream. Early detection and treatment are most helpful in this disorder.

***Hemiballismus.*** Hemiballismus is an unusual but dramatic and unique movement disorder that usually appears in a patient over age 50 with diabetes or hypertension. Most cases are caused by a small infarction or hemorrhage in the region of the subthalamic nucleus. Relentless, high-amplitude, proximal, flinging movements occur that are so violent that the patient can be injured or thrown to the ground. Speech and swallowing can be impaired. The movements are exacerbated by anxiety, can only be volitionally suppressed for a short time, and disappear during sleep. There is a high spontaneous remission rate for hemiballismus, and the prognosis is usually determined by the underlying disease.

***Dystonia.*** Dystonia has been defined as the simultaneous contraction of antagonist (flexor and extensor) muscles. It is the mechanism of a variety of clinical phenomena, from "writer's cramp" to "wryneck." Dystonia can result from drug ingestion (oculogyric crisis), metabolic or toxic disorders, neurodegenerative disease, or rarely, structural brain lesions. Primary, or idiopathic, dystonia is mainly an inherited disorder with incomplete penetrance. The twisting and cramping of dystonia can be slow or rapid and can result in fixed postures that are extremely difficult to correct by the examiner applying force. Sometimes, however, the patient may use a so-called sensory trick and return the contorted limb or head to the natural position through the precise placement of a single finger. Dystonia may involve the vocal cords and laryngeal musculature, resulting in stridorous and unintelligible speech *(spasmodic dysphonia).* The syndrome of craniocervical dystonia (Meige syndrome) consists of facial, oromandibular, lingual, laryngeal, and pharyngeal dystonias, often with twisting of the neck *(torticollis).* Generalized dystonia occurs in *dystonia musculorum deformans,* an autosomal dominant disorder with onset in childhood or adolescence that does not respond to pharmacotherapy and causes extreme contortionist postures that fix the joints in permanent contractures. *Hemidystonia* can be caused by a structural lesion in the putamen.

*Focal dystonias,* such as blepharospasm, hemifacial spasm, torticollis, and spasmodic dyphonia, are now successfully treated in one half to two thirds of patients using local injections of botulin toxin. Side effects are transient, occurring when large doses are required. Thus, this therapy is confined to localized dystonias affecting one or a few muscles only. Anticholinergic drugs are occasionally effective in primary dystonias of the trunk or axial musculature or in multisegmental dystonia. The dose should be slowly but systematically increased as tolerance develops to the side effects, since the best results are obtained at high doses (20 to 50 mg or more of trihexyphenidyl).

***Essential tremor.*** Essential tremor is a common movement disorder for which patients infrequently seek medical attention. Occurring as an isolated symptom, sporadically, or in families, with onset at any age but increasing prevalence in all ages over 40, it can remain static or progress. The beating movement of the hands, head, and voice varies in frequency (typically 6 to 12 per second) and is often mistaken for PD, although the rigidity, bradykinesia, and postural imbalance of PD are not present. The tremor is observed on maintenance of a posture, such as outstretched arms, and can persist during intentional movement, with deterioration of writing and dexterity. Patients report that the tremor is lessened by alcohol. Treatment of essential tremor is palliative and frequently incomplete. β-Blockers can reduce tremor amplitude in one half to two thirds of patients; however, doses up to 240 mg daily of propranolol may be required for optimal effect. Long-acting preparations are equivalent to divided doses. Other β-blockers have shown inconsistent effects. Another incidentally discovered medication for essential tremor is the anticonvulsant primidone, 50 to 250 mg daily. If tolerated, primidone has equal or superior palliative effects to β-blockers.

Tremor should not be considered an inevitable feature of aging. It can be a symptom of other neurologic diseases (e.g., cerebellar degeneration, Wilson's disease), a side effect of medications (e.g., lithium, valproate), or a feature of thyrotoxicosis or renal failure.

***Tourette's syndrome and tic disorders.*** The genetically inherited disorder Tourette's (Gilles de la Tourette) syndrome is one of a spectrum of interesting and varied conditions with abnormal movements and psychiatric features. In Tourette's syndrome, quasivoluntary movements and vocalizations, as simple as a grunt or as complex as genuflecting, occur with stereotyped precision many times each minute or hour. Patients report a sensation of emotional or sensory dysphoria that is satisfied by the performance of tics. Suppression is possible for minutes or hours but provokes a rebounding series of tics in compensation. Some patients display compulsive and obsessive tendencies that are congruent with their tics. Checking, arranging, disinfecting, and other rituals merge with the tics and serve as their apparent justification. Rarely, individuals can also have sleep disturbances, sexual aggressiveness, or self-destructiveness. Obssessive-compulsive disorder occurs more often in female relatives and attention deficit disorder more often in male relatives of Tourette syndrome patients.

Dopamine receptor blockers (neuroleptics) have been used as symptomatic treatment, although they often provide limited relief and unwanted side effects. Amphetamine, an indirect dopamine agonist, can aggravate tics and is suspected of precipitating Tourette's syndrome in susceptible individuals when given for attention deficit disorder and hyperactivity. Tics usually resolve spontaneously but can persist into adulthood.

Treatment should be directed at the symptoms that are most distressing to the patient. Tics and vocalizations are frequently misinterpreted as intentional mimicry of the observer and can lead to embarrassment. These often intelligent and sensitive individuals deserve respect and compassion, which can be enhanced by the education of family, friends, and teachers.

Therapeutic interventions for tics include haloperidol, 0.25 to 2.5 mg daily, or pimozide, 0.5 to 10 mg. The cardiovascular side effects require electrocardiographic monitoring, and the possibility of neuroleptic side effects necessitates careful clinical monitoring. Dopamine-depleting agents (reserpine, tetrabenazine), benzodiazepines, and clonidine have not been successful. The newer dopamine receptor blockers have not been investigated. Obsessive-compulsive symptoms may respond to fluoxetine (Prozac) and possibly other serotonergic antidepressants. Attention deficit disorder with hyperactivity has been treated with neuroleptics and clonidine when coexistent with Tourette's syndrome rather than with stimulants (methamphetamine, methylphenidate, pemoline), which may unmask tics. Investigation of other neurotransmitter or endogenous opioid abnormalities may result in more specific treatments in the future.

## BIBLIOGRAPHY


Benabid AL et al: Long-term suppression of tremor by chronic stimulation of the ventral intermediate thalamic nucleus, *Lancet* 337:403, 1991.

Boshes B: Sinemet and the treatment of parkinsonism, *Ann Intern Med* 94:364, 1981.

Calne DB: Treatment of Parkinson's disease, *N Engl J Med* 329:1021, 1993.

Clinicopathological Conference: Huntington's disease, *N Engl J Med* 326:117, 1992.

Gusella JF et al: Molecular genetics of Huntington's disease, *Arch Neurol* 50:1157, 1993.

Hallett M: Classification and treatment of tremor, *JAMA* 266(8):1115, 1991.

Jankovic J, Brin MF: Therapeutic uses of botulinum toxin, *N Engl J Med* 324(17):1186, 1993.

Shoulson IB et al: Effects of tocopherol and deprenyl on the progression of disability in early Parkinson's disease, *N Engl J Med* 328:176, 1993.

Singer HS, Walkup JT: Tourette's syndrome and other tic disorders: diagnosis, pathophysiology and treatment, *Medicine* 70:15, 1991.


CHAPTER

# 103 Peripheral Neuropathies

**Nagagopal Venna**

A knowledge of diseases of peripheral nerves is essential to identify and treat the diverse neuropathies that the primary care physician is likely to encounter in day-to-day practice. *Mononeuropathies* such as the carpal tunnel syndrome are the most common, cause substantial pain and disability, and are eminently treatable. Familiarity with these conditions helps to avoid misdiagnosis of benign conditions, such as acute radial nerve palsy as stroke and the entrapment neuropathy of ulnar nerve as early amyotrophic lateral sclerosis. The awareness that diabetes can cause localized pain over the trunk as a result of intercostal neuropathy is important in the differential diagnosis of painful conditions of the abdomen and chest. Moreover, the mononeuropathies are occasionally the presenting symptoms of systemic disease, as exemplified by carpal tunnel syndrome in hypothyroidism or amyloidosis. In addition, the mononeuropathies may evolve as treatable complications of known diseases, as illustrated by the occurrence of carpal tunnel syndrome in rheumatoid arthritis or systemic lupus erythematosus. *Mononeuropathy multiplex* is a syndrome of exceptional diagnostic value because it points to a disseminated vasculitic process and is often the first clue to an otherwise puzzling clinical picture.

*Generalized polyneuropathy* is another common clinical entity and forms a major facet of certain chronic systemic diseases such as diabetes mellitus and acquired immune deficiency syndrome (AIDS). The somatic and autonomic neuropathy of this disease has important impact on the complications of diabetes such as foot infection and gangrene and sudden cardiorespiratory arrest, as well as on the control of hyperglycemia. The physician should be aware of the many drugs in daily use that can produce peripheral neuropathy and of the ways to avoid or minimize such damage. The occurrence of a generalized neuropathy without apparent cause should alert the physician to toxic exposure, occult malignancy, or plasma cell dyscrasia. Over the past decade, AIDS has become a leading cause of the whole spectrum of peripheral neuropathies, from mononeuropathies to generalized polyneuropathies. This chapter also highlights some of the advances in the management of chronic painful states caused by nerve lesions.

No completely satisfactory classification of neuropathies exists. This chapter uses an essentially clinical classification that can be readily used in practice. Only selected areas are discussed, mostly in emphasizing common conditions. A few rare disorders are also considered because they illustrate important principles.

## MONONEUROPATHIES

Palsies of individual peripheral nerves are seen regularly in clinical practice (see the box on p. 1409). They occur

## Clinical classification of mononeuropathies

**Acute mononeuropathies**
Radial nerve palsy
Ulnar neuropathy
Peroneal neuropathy
Femoral neuropathy
Bell's palsy

**Chronic mononeuropathies**
Carpal tunnel syndrome (median nerve)
Cubital tunnel syndrome (ulnar nerve)
Tarsal tunnel syndrome (posterior tibial nerve)
Meralgia paresthetica (lateral cutaneous nerve of thigh)

**Acute asymmetric proximal neuropathies**
Diabetic amyotrophy
Neuralgic amyotrophy
Diabetic truncal radiculopathy

**Mononeuropathy multiplex**
Vasculitides
- Polyarteritis nodosa
- Systemic lupus erythematosus
- Vasculitis limited to the peripheral nerves

Sarcoidosis
Macroglobulinemia/cryoglobulinemia
Leprosy

most frequently in the extremities but are being increasingly recognized over the trunk. Their clinical features are well defined, and results of treatment are rewarding in most patients. Moreover, in certain situations the palsies are preventable.

### Acute compression mononeuropathies

The sudden appearance of a wristdrop from radial nerve palsy or a footdrop from peroneal nerve palsy are familiar examples of acute mononeuropathies.

***Pathogenesis.*** The nerve is injured by external pressure where it lies against bone in a subcutaneous position. The radial nerve as it transverses the spiral groove of humerus, the ulnar nerve as it passes behind the elbow, and the common peroneal nerve winding around the neck of the fibula are especially vulnerable. In most cases the pressure is the weight of the patient's body on the limb for a prolonged period because of a state of stupor from alcoholic or drug intoxication or coma of any cause. An iatrogenic form results from pressure on these nerves because of improper positioning of the limbs under general anesthesia for major surgery. Cachexia with the loss of the cushion of subcutaneous fat and generalized polyneuropathy from any cause increase the susceptibility to pressure palsies, and rarely the tendency is inherited.

***Pathology.*** The change is limited to the short segment of the nerve at the site of compression and preferentially affects the large fibers with thick myelin sheaths. The myelin is initially deformed and telescoped away from the nodes of Ranvier and may progress to segmental loss of myelin. In most patients, recovery occurs by remyelination as the axons are preserved.

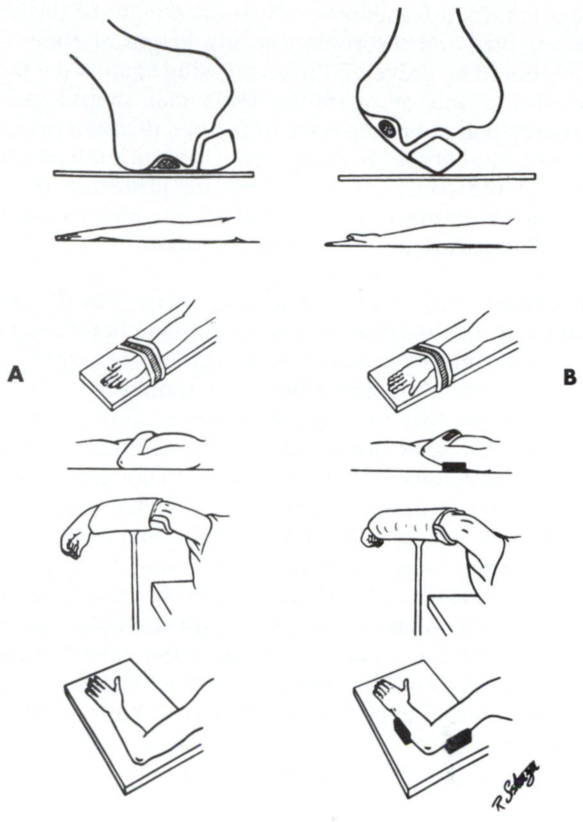


**Fig. 103-1.** Ulnar nerve compression. **A** illustrates positions that put the ulnar nerve behind the elbow at risk for external compression. **B** illustrates positioning of the upper extremity that minimizes this risk. (From Wadsworth TG: *Anesth Analg* 53:303, 1974.)

***Diagnosis.*** Diagnosis is made by clinical examination. Nerve conduction velocity (NCV) measurements are not routinely needed but demonstrate a block or marked slowing of conduction across the injured segment, whereas conduction in the nerve distal to injury is normal. One should look for evidence of a generalized polyneuropathy and inquire carefully into the circumstances in which the palsy occurred to understand its mechanism.

***Prevention.*** Awareness of the possibility of nerve injury and careful technique should obviate this complication resulting from the application of tourniquet or plaster casts to limbs. Every effort should be made to prevent (Fig. 103-1) or minimize pressure palsies in patients undergoing prolonged general anesthesia and patients in coma. The regions of the limbs where nerves are vulnerable to pressure are protected. If the upper extremity is to be immobilized on an arm board for intravenous (IV) infusion, it should be held in a supine position. If it is not immobilized, it should be kept half-flexed at the elbow and across the chest so that elbows are clear off the bed. If the arm is to be kept by the side, soft pads under the arm and forearm take the pressure off the nerve. The unconscious patient is turned frequently so that the weight of the body does not press on the limbs for any length of time. The elbow should be prevented from pressing against the metal edge of the bed or operating table and should not be allowed to hang over the edge of the bed to avoid pressure over the radial nerve. In the lower extremities the peroneal nerves at the backs of the knees are protected by soft cushions, avoiding crossing of the legs, and by care in using stirrups for the lithotomy position.

*Treatment.* No specific treatment exists, but disability resulting from the palsy can be minimized before natural recovery occurs in 4 to 8 weeks. The use of appropriate splints for wristdrop and a brace for footdrop are helpful for patient comfort and for prevention of contractures. In some patients with ulnar neuropathy, a minor causalgia syndrome develops, with burning pain in the hand that can last for weeks or months and can be quite distressing. This condition is treated by nonnarcotic analgesic drugs, transcutaneous electrical nerve stimulation (TENS), and in recalcitrant cases with carbamazepine or tricylic antidepressant drugs. There is little indication for surgery because in the vast majority of cases the palsies recover spontaneously. An occasional patient with postoperative ulnar neuropathy may continue to have severe palsy 1 to 2 years after onset. Surgical transposition of the nerve to an anterior position should be carried out.

*Acute radial nerve palsy.* In this well-known syndrome the radial nerve is compressed in the posterior aspect of the upper arm as it lies in the spiral groove (Fig. 103-2). It occurs typically as the patient lies on the arm in a state of alcoholic intoxication ("Saturday night palsy"). It may occur from pressure of a partner's head on the abducted arm in sleep ("bridegroom's palsy") as well as from improper positioning under anesthesia with the arm hanging over the edge of the operating table. Rarely, it may appear after heavy exertion in a very muscular individual.

The patient complains of weakness of the hand without pain, noted on awakening and often misconstrued as a stroke. The chief abnormality is weakness of dorsiflexion of the wrist and fingers while sensation and triceps reflex are usually normal.

A common pitfall is the apparent weakness of the ulnar and median innervated muscles of the hand in addition to those supplied by the radial nerve so that the entire hand appears weak. This pseudoparesis is caused by the lack of normal fixation of the wrist and fingers by the extensor muscles necessary for the optimal use of other hand muscles. The confusion can be readily resolved by demonstrating that these movements are in fact normal when the wrist and fingers are supported by laying them on a firm, flat surface.

When the radial nerve palsy is bilateral or appears subacutely, the possibility of lead poisoning should be considered. In patients with rheumatoid arthritis, symptoms should be differentiated from those of rupture of the extensor tendons.

*Acute ulnar neuropathy.* The ulnar nerve is vulnerable in its subcutaneous position in the ulnar groove behind the elbow. The most common setting for development of neuropathy is during general anesthesia for surgery, at which time the forearm is immobilized on a board in a prone position for IV infusion, putting the nerve directly in the line of pressure. It may also be compressed against the steel edge of the operating table. A similar mechanism of injury applies in the course of nursing the patient in a coma.

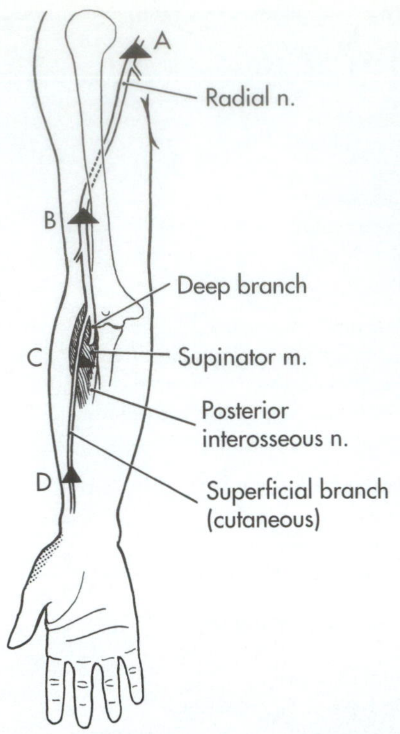


**Fig. 103-2.** Radial nerve compression. The radial nerve can be compressed in the axilla *(A)* or, more often, as it winds around the humerus *(B)* in the spiral groove. Its deep motor branch may become entrapped at the supinator muscle *(C)*, whereas the superficial cutaneous branch *(D)* may be injured along the forearm or wrist, causing sensory symptoms over the dorsum of the hand *(stippled area)*. (From Dyck PJ, Thomas PK, Lambert EH: *Peripheral neuropathy*, Philadelphia, 1975, WB Saunders.)

Symptoms appear within days of anesthesia or as the patient recovers from coma and are predominantly sensory at the outset. Tingling paresthesias and numbness and decreased sensation affect the little and ring fingers, sometimes accompanied by pain in the forearm. In more severe cases, weakness and later wasting of the interossei and hypothenar muscles occur.

*Acute common peroneal nerve palsy.* Peroneal neuropathy results from pressure on the nerve as it winds around the neck of the fibula in a subcutaneous plane (Fig. 103-3). It usually occurs in the course of stupor or general anesthesia. Occasionally, it results from prolonged squatting or "duck walking," as in farm workers ("strawberry picker's palsy"). The chief symptom is the acute onset of painless footdrop. Examination reveals weakness of dorsiflexion of the ankle and toes and of eversion of the foot with little sensory impairment. The patient with severe weakness has steppage gait, and bilateral footdrop can greatly impair walking.

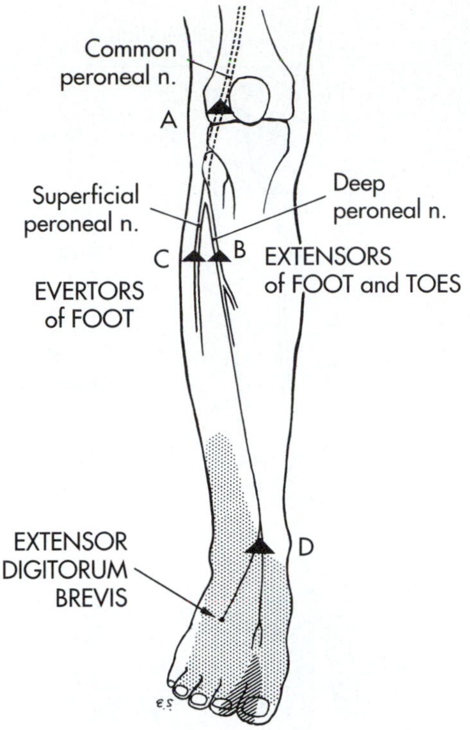


**Fig. 103-3.** Common peroneal nerve palsy. The common peroneal nerve may be compressed at the level of the knee *(A)*. When only the deep peroneal branch *(B)* is injured, dorsiflexion of the foot and toes is weak and sensory loss occurs between the first and second toes *(hatched area)*. Damage of the superficial branch *(C)* causes weakness of the evertors and more extensive sensory impairment over the foot *(stippled area)*. In compression of the deep peroneal branch at the ankle *(D)*, only the extensor digitorum brevis is weak and little sensory impairment occurs *(hatched area)*. (From Dyck PJ, Thomas PK, Lambert EH: *Peripheral neuropathy,* Philadelphia, 1975, WB Saunders.)

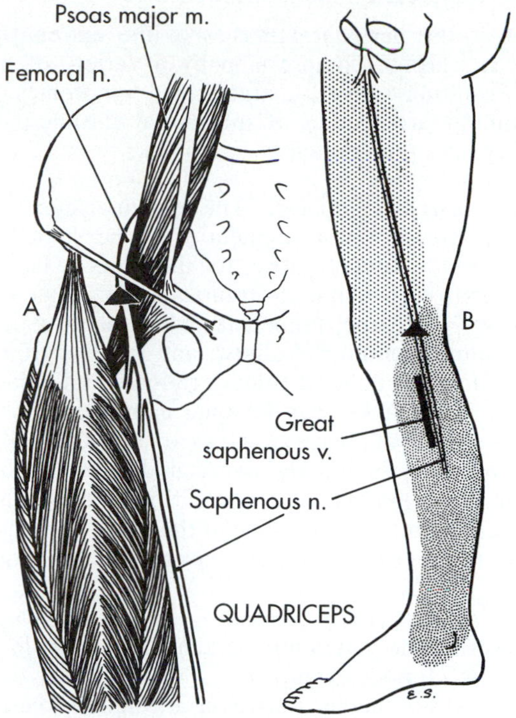


**Fig. 103-4.** Femoral nerve compression. This nerve has a close anatomic relation with the psoas muscle and inguinal ligament *(A)*. Compression at the groin may cause quadriceps weakness and sensory impairment in the nerve's distribution at the thigh *(lightly stippled area)* and in the saphenous branch *(heavily stippled area)*. Pressure at the knee *(B)* or surgery to the saphenous veins may affect the saphenous nerve. (From Dyck PJ, Thomas PK, Lambert EH: *Peripheral neuropathy,* Philadelphia, 1975, WB Saunders.)

The diagnosis can usually be made readily by clinical examination. If footdrop is pronounced, there may be apparent weakness of inversion and plantar flexion of the foot caused by lack of fixation of the ankle, a situation analogous to that in severe radial palsy. On occasion the ankle reflex may be diminished, which does not necessarily mean that a first sacral vertebra (S1) root lesion is present. An acute fifth lumbar vertebra (L-5) root lesion causes back pain, and straight-leg raising is painfully restricted. Pin sense is impaired in the L5 dermatome over the outer aspect of the leg and dorsum of the foot, but weakness is usually not profound. In doubtful cases, NCV and electromyography are helpful; peroneal nerve conduction can be measured readily, and marked slowing can be demonstrated across the knee. When an L5 root lesion is suspected, evidence of denervation is sought in muscles supplied by L5 but not by the peroneal nerve, such as the posterior tibial, hamstring, and gluteus medius muscles.

***Acute compression femoral neuropathy.*** In femoral neuropathy the femoral nerve is compressed by a hematoma in the iliopsoas muscle (Fig. 103-4), although rarely the bleeding occurs directly into the nerve. Most often it affects patients receiving anticoagulant treatment or those who have hemophilia.

Pain in the thigh and weakness of flexion of the hip and extension of the knee rapidly evolve over hours or days. The knee reflex is diminished or lost. Sensation is diminished over the anterior aspect of the thigh, and bluish discoloration may be seen in the inguinal region.

The diagnosis of acute femoral neuropathy is made by clinical evidence. In patients with coagulation disorders, there should be a high degree of suspicion for this complication, and computed tomographic (CT) scan of the retroperitoneal region is a ready means of visualizing iliopsoas hematoma.

With conservative therapy of rest, discontinuation of anticoagulation, or correction of bleeding disorder in hemophiliac patients, the neuropathy improves and recovers fully in a few weeks, although mild residual disability may remain in some patients.

The role of early surgical evacuation of hematoma is controversial. Some have advocated its use, claiming that ensuing recovery of nerve function is more rapid and more complete. This has to be weighed against the risk of performing surgery on patients with bleeding disturbances. When no clot is seen on CT scan and bleeding has occurred into the nerve itself, surgery is not indicated.

### Chronic compression mononeuropathies

Several of the peripheral nerves of the extremities are subject to chronic compression by a variety of mechanisms, resulting in well-characterized syndromes. Many are common, are sources of substantial chronic pain and disability, and are eminently treatable.

*Pathogenesis and pathology.* The basic mechanism is one of chronic pressure on a segment of the nerve that lies in a fibroosseous tunnel close to the joint where it is vulnerable to recurrent microtrauma. The median nerve as it traverses the carpal tunnel, the ulnar nerve within the cubital tunnel behind the elbow, and the posterior tibial nerve as it passes under the flexor retinaculum or laciniate ligament at the ankle can become entrapped. The compressed segment of the nerve shows areas of demyelination chiefly affecting the thickly myelinated fibers, although in time the fibers may show degeneration of axons as well. Moreover, the interstitial tissue of the nerve also shows an increase in proteinaceous fluid and eventual disorganization.

*Diagnosis.* The *anatomic* diagnosis is made fairly reliably by clinical examination. Measurement of NCV, however, is a valuable, sensitive, and readily performed laboratory test and shows slowing across the entrapped nerve segment. In general, sensory conduction is impaired earlier than motor conduction, although the latter is more easily tested. Electromyographic examination of the muscles supplied by the affected nerve is a useful supplement because presence of denervation of the muscle indicates a substantial degree of compression. However, on occasion, these tests may be normal despite a typical clinical picture.

The *etiologic* diagnosis is usually evident by comprehensive clinical evaluation, including local examination of the nerve and regional and systemic examination for clues such as hypothyroidism or generalized polyneuropathy, which are then confirmed by selected laboratory tests. However, as mentioned earlier, in the largest group of idiopathic entrapment, a careful analysis of occupation and habitual or hobby-related trauma to the nerve should be made.

*Treatment.* It is gratifying to treat these neuropathies. In a few patients, specific medical therapy is available and may be sufficient. For instance, treatment of hypothyroidism, acromegaly, or gout often relieves the associated carpal tunnel syndrome but in most patients, therapy is nonspecific. Conservative therapy is attempted in most instances; it is the rule in certain self-limited neuropathies such as the carpal tunnel syndrome of pregnancy. Occupational and habitual modification is important. Rest from heavy work with hands and wrists in a patient with carpal tunnel syndrome is helpful. In some patients, this may call for a change of jobs. Industry has become more aware of this in recent years, and it is possible that switching to power tools will lessen this problem. The avoidance of habitual trauma is essential. For instance, the patient with ulnar entrapment should be asked not to lean on the elbows. Physical medicine has a useful role. A splint to the wrist may abolish severe nocturnal pain in carpal tunnel syndrome. A soft pad behind the elbow may ease the pain and paresthesias of mild ulnar neuropathy.

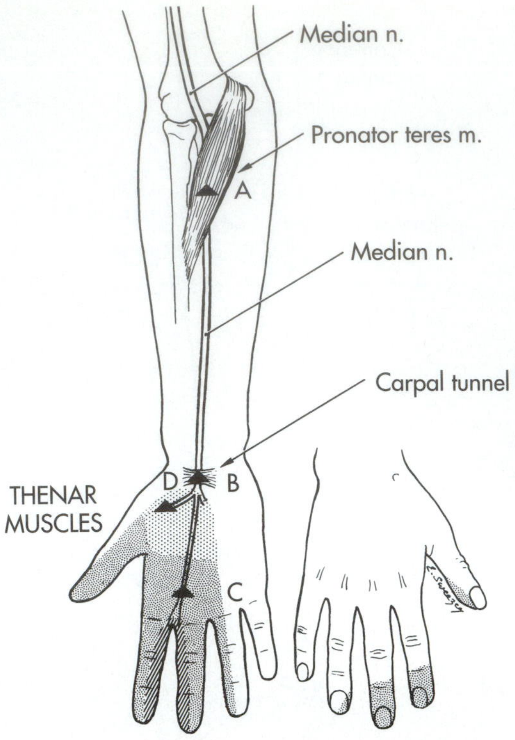


**Fig. 103-5.** Carpal tunnel syndrome. *B* points to the level where the median nerve is compressed in the carpal tunnel. The pronator teres muscle *(A)* and the transverse intermetacarpal ligaments *(C)* are less common sites of median nerve compression. The motor branch innervates the thenar muscle *(D)*. The lightly stippled area shows the sensory supply of the palmar cutaneous branch, which arises proximal to the carpal tunnel and thus is spared in the carpal tunnel syndrome. The densely stippled zone represents the cutaneous sensory area of the median nerve distal to the carpal tunnel. The hatched area shows the sensory supply of the interdigital branch of the nerve. (From Dyck, PJ, Thomas PK, Lambert EH: *Peripheral neuropathy,* Philadelphia, 1975, WB Saunders.)

Local injection of steroids is a time-honored and frequently effective treatment that presumably acts by decreasing the interstitial edema of the nerve and of the tendons in their synovial membranes surrounding the nerve. The steroid is injected in the vicinity of the entrapped nerve segment, *not into* the nerve itself. The techniques of injecting the carpal tunnel, for which it is most frequently used, can be learned quickly and performed in the clinic. When successful the injection can be repeated, but if it is required more than every 2 or 3 months, surgery should be considered.

Surgery is indicated for failure of conservative measures and the presence of enduring sensory loss or weakness. The procedures are simple and direct and in principle involve decompressing the affected nerve segment by sectioning the flexor retinaculum for the carpal and tarsal tunnel syndromes. Surgery for ulnar nerve entrapment is more extensive because transposition of the nerve to a protected position in the anterior compartment of the forearm is required. Care is taken to avoid surgical trauma to the nerve and its branches. Surgery effectively relieves pain and paresthesias and in most cases leads to gradual recovery of sensation. Muscle weakness, if already established before surgery, is the last to recover.

**Some causes of carpal tunnel syndrome**

Idiopathic (often in middle-aged women)
Endocrine
  Hypothyroidism
  Acromegaly
  Pregnancy
Repetitive occupational wrist trauma
Connective tissue diseases
  Rheumatoid arthritis
  Gouty arthritis
  Systemic lupus erythematosus
  Polymyalgia rheumatica
  Amyloidosis
Regional disorders
  Arteriovenous shunt in the arm for renal dialysis
Local diseases of the wrist
  Ganglion

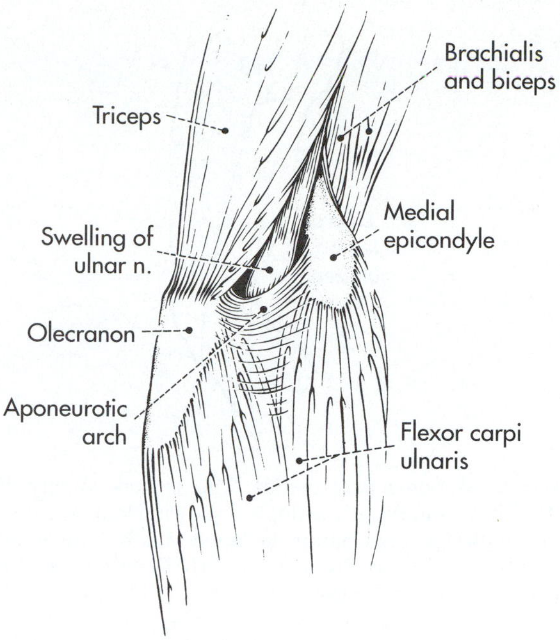


**Fig. 103-6.** Cubital tunnel syndrome. The anatomy of the cubital tunnel from the posterior aspect of the elbow. Note the arch of aponeurosis of flexor carpi ulnaris overlying the ulnar nerve. Its sharp edge may be important in compression of the nerve. (From Feindel W, Stratford J: *Can J Surg* 1:287, 1958.)

***Carpal tunnel syndrome.*** Carpal tunnel syndrome is the most common and best known chronic compression mononeuropathy and the most important because of the disability of the hand it causes. The median nerve is entrapped in the carpal tunnel at the wrist under the flexor retinaculum, where it is surrounded by the tendons and synovial sheaths of long flexors of the fingers (Fig. 103-5).

Recurrent painful numbness in the hand and fingers that usually intensifies at night is the outstanding symptom. It often affects all fingers rather than being restricted to the thumb, index, and middle fingers. The pain frequently spreads to the forearm and even the shoulder, and patients may complain of dropping objects from the hand. A patient may rarely have painless wasting of the thenar muscles. The syndrome is frequently bilateral, in which case it is worse in the dominant hand. In the early stages, examination may be normal despite prominent symptoms. There may be decreased two-point discrimination over the tips of the thumb, index, and middle fingers (greater than 6 mm in noncalloused hands) or decreased sensation to pinprick. In more severe cases there is wasting and weakness of the thenar muscles, especially of the muscles of opposition and abduction of the thumb. The causes of the syndrome are numerous and some of them are listed in the box above. The principles of diagnosis and management are outlined in the introductory section on chronic compression neuropathies.

***Cubital tunnel syndrome (ulnar nerve entrapment at the elbow).*** Cubital tunnel syndrome is another common entrapment neuropathy, although less spectacular than the carpal tunnel syndrome. It arises from chronic compression of the ulnar nerve in the cubital tunnel formed by the medial epicondyle and the origin of the flexor carpi ulnaris (Fig. 103-6). The subcutaneous position of the nerve at the posterior surface of the elbow makes it vulnerable to recurrent occupational and habitual pressure.

Patients may present with tingling and numbness on the inner aspect of the palm and on the little and ring fingers. However, a common presentation is gradual onset of wasting of the muscles of the hand, with clawlike deformity of the fingers and little pain or paresthesias. Wasting and weakness of dorsal and palmar interossei and hypothenar muscles and decreased sensation over the little finger and ulnar half of the ring finger are found. The nerve may be tender at the elbow and may be enlarged above the ulnar groove.

*Tardy ulnar palsy* appears years after an injury to the elbow such as supracondylar fracture of the humerus. The elbow is deformed and its movements restricted.

*Idiopathic ulnar palsy* is the most common variety and occurs with a normal elbow. Recurrent trauma to the nerve during movement of the elbow (as may happen with frequent and vigorous "arm curls" with weights for fitness training) may cause the neuropathy.

*Recurrent subluxation of ulnar nerve,* in which the nerve snaps out of the ulnar groove frequently with elbow flexion, is usually asymptomatic but may cause pain and paresthesias.

The principles of diagnosis and treatment are outlined in the introductory section on chronic compression neuropathies.

***Meralgia paresthetica.*** Meralgia paresthetica is a common but innocuous syndrome caused by entrapment of the lateral femoral cutaneous nerve of the thigh as it dips under the lateral part of the inguinal ligament, beyond which it supplies sensation to the skin of the anterolateral part of the thigh to just above the knee. The chief symptom is a persistent burning, prickly sensation and numbness over the anterolateral aspect of the thigh that may be bilateral (Fig. 103-7). It often occurs in relation to recent weight gain or weight loss, as may happen with pregnancy, accumulation of ascites, as well as wearing tight garters or abdominal binders, although frequently none of these

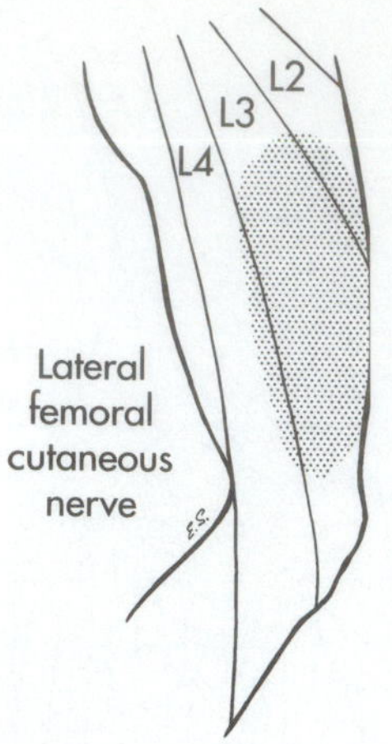


**Fig. 103-7.** Meralgia paresthetica. The sensory supply of the lateral cutaneous nerve of the thigh is shown. Note how this area overlaps with the distribution of upper lumbar innervations. (From Dyck PJ, Thomas PK, Lambert EH: *Peripheral neuropathy,* Philadelphia, 1975, WB Saunders.)

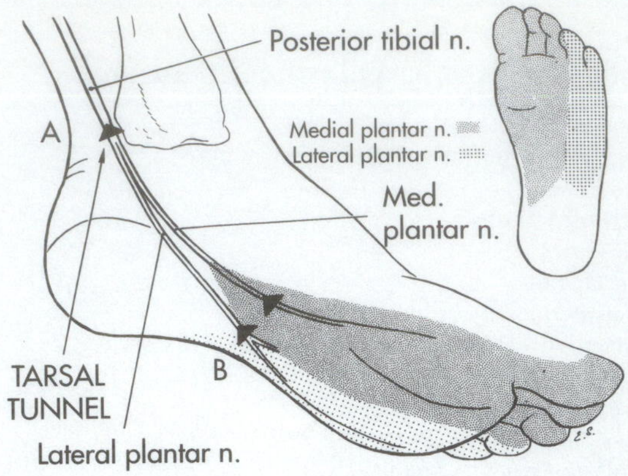


**Fig. 103-8.** Tarsal tunnel syndrome. Compression of the posterior tibial nerve in the tarsal tunnel behind the medial epicondyle *(A)* or of the plantar nerves *(B)* causes sensory impairment in the sole of the foot and weakness of the intrinsic pedal musculature. (From Dyck PJ, Thomas PK, Lambert EH: *Peripheral neuropathy,* Philadelphia, 1975, WB Saunders.)

factors is apparent. The diagnosis is entirely clinical, based on the characteristic distribution of paresthesias accompanied by a patch of decreased sensation over the anterolateral aspect of the thigh.

An explanation and reassurance as to the benign nature of the otherwise baffling symptoms constitute the most important step. Tight garments should be avoided, and in most patients the symptoms subside in weeks or months spontaneously. Occasionally, injections of lidocaine and corticosteroids at the site of the entrapment may be helpful.

***Tarsal tunnel syndrome.*** Tarsal tunnel syndrome is the rather uncommon condition that is the lower-extremity counterpart of the carpal tunnel syndrome and results from chronic entrapment of the posterior tibial nerve in the tarsal tunnel formed by the medial malleolus and laciniate ligament at the ankle (Fig. 103-8). Pain, tingling, and numbness in the sole of the foot are the main manifestations, often with nocturnal exacerbations. It may be bilateral and present as the "burning feet" syndrome. The posterior tibial nerve is usually tender behind the medial malleolus, and the Tinel's sign may be elicited on tapping it, diminishing sensation over the sole of the foot. In established cases there is wasting of the abductor hallucis brevis, causing a hollowing out of the normal bulge on the medial margin of the foot. Symptoms may often be prominent, with little in the way of objective findings.

The diagnosis rests primarily on an awareness of this syndrome and its clinical features, but motor NCV across the ankle of the posterior tibial nerve is a valuable confirmatory test.

Many cases occur without apparent cause. In others there is a previous fracture with deformity of the ankle or a generalized polyneuropathy. Rarely, it may be accompanied by carpal tunnel syndrome. A ganglion or neurofibroma is an occasional cause.

Treatment is outlined in the preceding section. In many patients, definitive relief is obtained by decompression of the tunnel by surgical sectioning of the laciniate ligament.

***Bell's palsy.*** Bell's palsy is the most common cranial mononeuropathy seen in general practice, but the etiopathogenesis of this self-limited disorder remains unclear. Weakness of one side of the face appears abruptly manifested by inability to close the eye and deviation of the mouth to the unaffected side on talking or smiling. The weakness is often preceded by pain behind the ear or in the upper neck. Many patients complain of a feeling of numbness in the affected side of the face. Excessive sensitivity to noise and decreased sensation of taste to sweet and salt may accompany the weakness and result from involvement of the nerve to the stapedius muscle and the chorda tympani branches, respectively. Examination shows equal involvement of both the upper and the lower halves of the face as well as of the platysma. A few patients report a decrease in touch and pinprick sense over the affected face and external ear, but corneal sensation is intact. Taste on the anterior two thirds of the tongue may be decreased. Diagnosis is based on characteristic clinical picture. Well-lighted examination of the throat and external ear canal may reveal vesicles of herpes zoster (Ramsay Hunt syndrome). A history of tick bite, outdoor activities in an endemic area, fleeting skin rash, and polyarthritis should arouse suspicion of Lyme disease, which often presents with facial palsy. Typically, however, it progresses to bilateral facial nerve involvement and to more widespread mononeuropathy multiplex. Bell's palsy may be the presenting feature of human immunodeficiency virus type 1 (HIV-1) seroconversion. It may also be a manifestation of sarcoidosis, especially if bilateral or recurrent. In the appropriate clinical setting tests for Lyme disease, HIV-1 antibodies, and chest x-ray for mediastinal adenopathy of sarcoidosis are appropriate, although in most patients these tests are not needed.

Prognosis for spontaneous full recovery is excellent in idiopathic Bell's palsy as well as those of HIV-1 infection and sarcoidosis. Reassurance that the palsy is caused by a self-limited affection of the nerve and not a cerebrovascular accident (CVA, stroke) often brings relief to the patient. In palsies of moderate to severe degree, a brief course of prednisone at 60 mg a day orally for 5 days seems to minimize the low risk of long-term sequelae such as abnormal reinnervation of facial muscles leading to synkinetic movements. When the jaw moves, the eyelid may close ("jaw winking"); eating spicy food may cause tears ("crocodile tears"). Recovery of strength is the rule even without any treatment. About 50% of patients make brisk and full recovery beginning within 10 days and completely by 6 weeks. Patients who begin to recover after 2 months tend to show incomplete resolution, stabilizing within about 9 months. About 10% of patients have clinically relevant residual abnormalities. The benefit of surgical decompression of the nerve in the stylomastoid foramen has not been established. In palsy caused by zoster, treatment with acyclovir and prednisone seems beneficial, although controlled studies are not available.

Prompt treatment with oral doxycycline at the stage of Bell's palsy is appropriate for Lyme disease.

### Acute asymmetric proximal neuropathies

These form a group of disorders with distinctive clinical syndromes of rapidly evolving painful weakness in the arm and shoulder or thigh and hip caused by involvement of the brachial or lumbrosacral plexus. The pathology and pathogenesis, however, are not well understood. The conditions are frequently misdiagnosed because of lack of awareness of these entities.

***Diabetic amyotrophy.*** Diabetic amyotrophy is the most common of the syndromes in which microinfarcts have been demonstrated in the lumbrosacral plexus, but the pathogenesis is not fully understood. Patients are usually middle aged or elderly with undiagnosed or mild diabetes who present with severe, persistent deep pain in the thigh accompanied by marked weakness and wasting of the hip and thigh muscles. It is usually unilateral and when bilateral, it is asymmetric. There is severe weakness of the iliopsoas and quadriceps femoris; careful examination, however, usually reveals milder weakness out of femoral nerve distribution often in gluteal and obturator innervated muscles. The knee reflex is lost, but sensation is normal. There is often much weight loss, which raises the suspicion of malignancy.

The diagnosis is based on the characteristic clinical picture. The condition, however, is regularly misdiagnosed as an L4 root lesion caused by disk prolapse. *L4 root lesion* does not produce such profound weakness of the iliopsoas and quadriceps, and sensory impairment over the inner aspect of the leg is notable, whereas in diabetic amyotrophy, weakness spills over to muscles supplied by obturator and sciatic nerves, outside the territory of the L4 root. The condition needs also to be distinguished from acute femoral neuropathy from retroperitoneal hematoma in patients with bleeding disorders.

Treatment is symptomatic, with reassurance that the dysfunction will resolve over 3 to 18 months. The main problem is to provide relief from the pain. Diphenylhydantoin and carbamazepine are helpful for some patients. Others respond to amitriptyline; in intractable cases this is combined with fluphenazine. These agents are given along with nonnarcotic analgesics such as aspirin or ibuprofen. Aspirin is probably preferable whenever tolerated because it has the theoretic advantage of inhibiting platelet aggregation, which might be involved in the pathogenesis. When paralysis is severe, the patient may benefit from bracing the knee.

***Neuralgic amyotrophy or idiopathic brachial plexus neuropathy (Parsonage-Turner syndrome).*** This syndrome has been well characterized clinically, although the cause and pathogenesis are not known. It may follow immunizations and rarely is familial.

The process seems to cause an acute dysfunction of multiple nerves of the brachial plexus or more distal nerve branches, usually unilaterally but occasionally bilaterally. Otherwise healthy patients between 20 and 40 years of age are usually affected. The onset is abrupt, with intense pain over the shoulder and upper arm that persists for days or a few weeks. As pain abates, weakness and atrophy appear rapidly, most often affecting the serratus anterior, deltoid, supraspinati and infraspinati, rhomboids, sternomastoids, biceps, triceps, brachioradialis, and extensors of the wrist in various combinations. Sometimes only one or two of these muscles are affected. If any sensory impairment occurs, it is confined to an area over the deltoid in the distribution of axillary nerve.

The diagnosis is clinical. Cerebrospinal fluid (CSF) is usually normal. In the acute phase of pain, the diagnosis is difficult with referred pain from gallbladder disease, local disease such as bursitis of the shoulder, or cervical disk prolapse entering into the differential diagnosis. Unlike acute disk protrusions, there is no neck spasm or limitation of neck movement.

No specific treatment is available. It is a clinical impression that a short course of steroids decreases the duration of pain but does not seem to alter the course of the disease otherwise. Recovery occurs in most instances but may take up to 2 or 3 years.

***Diabetic truncal radiculopathy.*** Diabetic truncal radiculopathy is a recently recognized syndrome of diabetic neuropathy that can cause diagnostic confusion with many medical and surgical disorders and in which the thoracic nerve roots are affected in an asymmetric fashion. A deep burning pain is the chief symptom. It is felt predominantly unilaterally over the upper abdomen or side of the chest and may be present for some weeks. Curiously, it is often associated with anorexia and weight loss, which raise the specter of cancer, and most patients are indeed extensively investigated for occult malignancy.

Diagnosis is made primarily by an awareness of this syndrome in diabetic patients. Electromyography of thoracic and lumbar paraspinal muscles is the most important test and shows extensive signs of denervation, usually bilaterally. A myelogram may occasionally be required to rule out compressive or inflammatory lesions of the roots. This neuropathy is different from the painless truncal neuropathy, which is bilateral, symmetric, and causes sensory impairment over the anterior abdominal wall. In these patients there is invariably a severe sensory loss in the extremities up to the thigh and arms. There is accompanying evidence of visceral autonomic neuropathy, and these cases represent a very advanced stage of the common diabetic distal symmetric polyneuropathy.

The painful condition resolves spontaneously over months, but pain may be alleviated as outlined under the treatment of diabetic amyotrophy.

### Lumbosacral polyradiculopathy in AIDS (Cauda Equina syndrome)

A rapidly evolving cauda equina syndrome is now recognized as a distinct clinical entity in patients with AIDS. The condition is caused by necrotizing vasculitis of the lumbar and sacral nerve roots of the cauda equina from cytomegalovirus (CMV) infection. Clinically, the patients in the advanced stages of HIV-1 infection have numbness in feet or sacral areas, beginning asymmetrically and progressing rapidly to areflexic, hypotonic paraparesis and urinary retention. CSF shows brisk, predominantly granulocytic pleocytosis of up to 1000 cells/cm with elevation of protein and decreased glucose. CMV can usually be cultured from the CSF. The clinical picture is strongly suggestive, supported by evidence of other foci of CMV infection such as retinitis, pneumonitis, or encephalitis. Diagnosis and prompt therapy with gancyclovir based on the clinical and CSF picture while awaiting confirmations by CSF cultures are critical to prevent worsening to paraplegia.

A similar syndrome may evolve in a slower, subacute fashion in patients with AIDS and can be caused by leptomeningitis localized to the cauda equina from cryptococcosis, syphilis, and tuberculosis.

A rare cause of a similar syndrome but with CSF abnormalities has been recognized in otherwise normal persons resulting from industrial exposure to dimethylaminoproprionitrite (DMAPN), which is used as a catalyzer in polyurethane foam manufacture.

### Mononeuropathy multiplex

In this rather striking clinical syndrome, palsies of individual peripheral nerves appear scattered over the body in an irregular pattern. Each nerve lesion may rapidly evolve in a matter of hours or days to be followed by others at varying intervals. In some cases they develop more gradually. For instance, a wristdrop appears from radial nerve palsy followed in a few days by a footdrop from peroneal nerve injury and later an ulnar neuropathy or cranial nerve palsy such as facial paralysis. It is this scattered multiple nerve involvement that gives the title of mononeuropathy multiplex.

This syndrome is highly characteristic of certain vasculitides, especially polyarteritis nodosa and Wegener's granulomatosis, and is a rare manifestation of rheumatoid arthritis and systemic lupus erythematosus. In polyarteritis nodosa or Wegener's granulomatosis, it is often a presenting manifestation or the feature that finally suggests the diagnosis in a patient with other poorly defined symptoms. In rheumatoid arthritis or systemic lupus erythematosus, the neuropathy occurs against the background of established disease. It has been described in patients with amphetamine-induced arteritis. In recent years, increasing numbers of cases of this syndrome are being described where the vasculitis remains limited to the peripheral nervous system without evidence of systemic vasculitis. The essential lesion is angiitis of the vasa nervorum causing nerve infarctions. Mononeuropathy multiplex also occurs in Waldenström's macroglobulinemia and cryoglobulinemia, but nerve ischemia in these disorders is caused by hyperviscosity of the blood. It is now recognized as a manifestation of HIV-1 infection and Lyme disease.

Mononeuropathy multiplex may evolve more gradually over months or years. In the Western world, it is most often caused by diabetes mellitus vasculitis or sarcoidosis. However, worldwide, it probably most frequently results from leprosy.

The diagnosis is aided substantially by the relatively limited number of causes and by nerve biopsy, which shows vasculitis of the vasa nervora, granuloma of sarcoidosis, or the bacilli of leprosy. In the appropriate clinical and epidemiologic circumstances, serologic tests for HIV-1 infection and Lyme disease should be obtained. A mononuclear CSF lymphycytosis is common to both disorders.

The treatment and prognosis are of the underlying diseases. In the acute vasculitides of polyarteritis nodosa, the neuropathy may respond to corticosteroids although the overall prognosis is poor. In Wegener's granulomatosis, modern treatment with steroids and immunosuppressive drugs is very helpful in improving neurologic function. Neuropathy resulting from vasculitis limited to peripheral nerves responds well to immunosuppressive treatment with prednisone and cyclophosphamide. In macroglobulinemia and cryoglobulinemia, patients with mononeuropathies may recover fully. Antibiotic therapy is critical for Lyme disease, whereas plasmaphoresis and IV immunoglobulin may alleviate HIV-related neuropathies.

### Long thoracic nerve injury

Long thoracic nerve injury may produce pain in the shoulder that is referred to the scapula and parascapular muscles. Injuries include shoulder trauma, carrying heavy weights, and neuritis following viral respiratory illness such as coxsackievirus and pleurodynia infections. The patient may complain of pain when moving the neck to extreme rotation or extension. The long thoracic nerve innervates the serratus anterior muscle, which fixes the scapula to the chest wall when forward pressure is exerted on the upper limb. It also brings the scapula forward when the arm is thrust forward, as in a fencer's lunge. Paralysis of the serratus anterior does not cause a deformity at rest. When the patient is asked to push the arm forward against resistance, the inner border of the scapula assumes a winged position. The patient is also unable to raise the arm over the head in the forward position.

Conservative treatment with rest leads to a resolution of symptoms in most cases. Restorative surgery is possible in patients with persisting deficits.

## ACUTE SYMMETRIC POLYNEUROPATHIES

Numerous etiologic factors can affect the peripheral nervous network from roots to terminal branches resulting in widespread, more or less symmetric loss of motor, sensory, and reflex functions, sometimes accompanied by autonomic derangement (see the box on p. 1417). The neuropathy may evolve with alarming rapidity over a matter of hours or days and may be life-threatening because of respiratory paralysis.

### Acute symmetric polyneuropathies

Guillain-Barré syndrome
Acute toxic polyneuropathies
  Biologic toxins
    Diphtheria
    Shellfish, ciguatera fish
  Chemical toxins
    Triorthocresyl phosphate poisoning
    Thallium intoxication
Acute infectious polyneuropathies: Lyme disease
Acute metabolic neuropathies: porphyric neuropathy

The pathogenic mechanisms are varied. While Guillain-Barré syndrome is mediated by an autoimmune attack on peripheral nerve myelin, others are caused by biologic or chemical neurotoxins acting on the axonal membrane or axoplasmic transport, blocking certain aspects of neuronal metabolism, or combinations of these.

## Guillain-Barré syndrome

Guillain-Barré syndrome is by far the most common form of acute polyneuropathy encountered in clinical practice. The outstanding process is widespread, symmetric segmental demyelination of the nerve roots, brachial plexus, and lumbosacral plexus, and distal nerves and of cranial nerves accompanied by mononuclear inflammatory cell infiltration. Acute infections by a variety of viruses and mycoplasmal agents and, rarely, connective tissue diseases such as systemic lupus erythematosus and polyarteritis nodosa and malignancies such as Hodgkin's disease are known to trigger this autoimmune destruction. The syndrome has heralded HIV-1 seroconversion. However, a specific cause is not identifiable in most patients.

Persons of any age group may be affected. The chief presenting feature is acute onset of weakness of the lower extremities, progressing over hours or a day or two to the upper extremities and facial, bulbar, and sometimes respiratory muscles. The weakness is often accompanied by paresthesias in the limbs. The neurologic syndrome is usually preceded by a febrile "viral" illness by 1 to 3 weeks. An uncommon but misleading presentation is the acute onset of ataxia of gait and limbs without weakness or sensory loss, presumably from denervation of muscle spindles. Examination reveals symmetric weakness of upper and lower extremities, often with proximal predilection and universal loss of tendon reflexes. Sensory abnormalities are relatively minor but may follow a stocking-and-glove pattern, with position and vibratory sense especially affected. Bilateral facial paralysis is the most common cranial neuropathy, but bulbar and extraocular muscles are affected in severe cases. Respiratory paralysis is the dreaded feature in severe cases. A variety of autonomic disturbances have also been documented, mostly in the acute phase of the illness. Sinus tachycardia, postural hypotension, and excessive sweating are the most common, but paroxysmal atrial or ventricular tachycardia and various bradyrhythmias and wide swings of blood pressure have been documented. Sphincter control and mental clarity are usually retained.

The diagnosis is based on the characteristic clinical picture and evolution. The acute ataxic forms without weakness are often misdiagnosed as hysterical. Universal areflexia should alert the physician to this syndrome. The CSF is normal at the outset but shows increasing amounts of protein on subsequent taps to over 1 g/ml without elevation of white cells. In the cases associated with HIV-1 seroconversion, moderate lymphocytosis also occurs. Nerve conduction studies show marked slowing of velocity in multiple nerves both distally and proximally, although in some documented cases, they remain unimpaired despite extensive paralysis. In these cases the demyelination is limited to the roots.

A distinctive aspect of Guillain-Barré syndrome is the temporal profile of its evolution. In general the neurologic deficits progress for 2 weeks, stabilize for 2 to 4 weeks, and thereafter improve gradually. Most patients recover fully, but about 30% have significant residual disability at the end of 2 years.

The mainstay of treatment is support of vital functions, especially of respiration. Support is achieved by treating the patient in an intensive care unit, monitoring pulmonary function with vital capacity, inspiratory force, and blood gases. Endotracheal intubation should be performed promptly when the pulmonary function shows deterioration or bulbar paralysis occurs. Even with modern endotracheal tubes, tracheostomy may be necessary if the ventilatory weakness persists beyond 10 days. Other measures include maintenance of fluid, electrolyte, nutritional, and hemodynamic balance. Subcutaneous heparin is used to prevent venous thrombosis. Pressure areas including those over nerves must be protected by proper positioning of the limbs and soft pads. Constant psychologic support is required for these understandably anxious patients. Some device by which the paralyzed patient can signal the nursing staff is vital.

Plasmapheresis has been established as an effective and safe treatment wherever the technology and expertise are available (Table 103-1). It has become the standard in all except the mildest cases. Benefit is seen in the form of briefer periods of ventilatory assistance and better functional recovery in the long term. However, about 30% of patients do not respond to the therapy. A recent study from the Netherlands indicated similar benefit with IV immunoglobulin infusion. If replicated, this would be a good alternative and easily administered. As the immunopathogenesis is more precisely defined, more targeted therapies are likely to emerge. Patients with an HIV-1–related syndrome also seem to respond to this treatment.

## Acute toxic polyneuropathies

***Biologic toxins: shellfish and ciguatera fish.*** The ingestion of certain shellfish and ciguatera fish in endemic coastal areas can cause severe acute peripheral neuropathy. The fish accumulate potent flagellate-elaborated neurotoxins but are themselves unaffected by them. The usual offenders among ciguatera are barracuda and red snapper along the reefs off Florida, Hawaii, and the West Indies. Among the shellfish, oysters, mussels, clams, and scallops along the coasts of New England, Alaska, and the West Coast have been implicated. The toxins directly affect the axonal nerve membrane (see Chapter 4G).

Ingestion is followed by nausea and vomiting, and

**Table 103-1.** Treatments for neuropathies

| Treatments | Neuropathies |
|---|---|
| **Immunotherapies** | |
| Plasmapheresis | Guillain-Barré syndrome<br>Chronic inflammatory demyelinating polyneuropathy (CIDP) |
| Intravenous immunoglobulin | Guillain-Barré syndrome<br>Demyelinating neuropathies associated with HIV-1 infection |
| Cytotoxic immunosuppressive drugs | |
| Prednisone | Bell's palsy<br>CIDP<br>Vasculitic neuropathies |
| Cyclophosphamide (often in combination with prednisone) | Vasculitic neuropathy of polyarteritis nodosa<br>Wegener's granulomatosis<br>Motor neuropathy associated wtih multifocal conduction block and anti-GM1 ganglioside antibodies |
| Antiinfectious agents | |
| Penicillin, ceftriaxone, doxycycline | Lyme-associated neuropathies |
| Gancyclovir | Cytomegalovirus lumbosacral radiculitis in AIDS |
| Dapsone, rifampin, clofazimine | Leprosy |
| **Replacement therapies** | |
| Thyroxine | Hypothyroid carpal tunnel syndrome<br>Hypothyroid meralgia paresthetica |
| Vitamin $B_1$ | Nutritional neuropathies |
| Vitamin $B_6$ | Nutritional neuropathies<br>INH-induced neuropathy (preventive) |
| Vitamin $B_{12}$ | Pernicious anemia myeloneuropathy |
| Vitamin E | Malabsorption syndrome with myeloneuropathy |
| **Toxic-metabolic modulations** | |
| Identification, chelation, and prevention of reexposure | Alcohol<br>Heavy metal neuropathies of arsenic, mercury, and lead<br>Drug-induced neuropathies |
| Hematin | Neuropathy of acute intermittent porphyria |
| Low phytanic acid diet and plasmapheresis | Refsum disease |
| Hemodialysis/renal transplantation | Uremic polyneuropathy |
| Local corticosteroid injection | Carpal tunnel syndrome |
| **Surgical treatment** | Entrapment neuropathies: carpal tunnel syndrome, cubital tunnel (ulnar nerve) syndrome, tarsal tunnel syndrome |
| **Radiation therapy** | Polyneuropathy associated with plasmacytoma |

within a few hours neuropathy explosively evolves. Paresthesias occur around the face and spread to the limbs and are accompanied in severe cases by quadriparesis and bulbar and respiratory weakness. Bizarre sensations such as the "feeling that teeth are coming loose" or "the body is floating away" have been noted.

The diagnosis is based on clinical evidence of rapid evolution of a neuropathy shortly after ingestion of marine food in endemic areas. One should be aware that respiratory paralysis can occur swiftly. No specific treatment exists, but supportive therapy is lifesaving and neuropathy recovers over many months.

***Acute neuropathy of triorthocresyl phosphate poisoning.*** Triorthocresyl phosphate (TOCP) is a synthetic organophosphate compound used worldwide in the manufacture of hydraulic fluids, lubricants, and plastics. It is a potent neurotoxin, and thousands of cases of neuropathy have occurred from its consumption. Most outbreaks have resulted from contamination or adulteration of foods, cooking oils, or alcohol with TOCP. One of the best-known examples is the Jamaica ginger paralysis, which affected thousands in the United States in Prohibition years, when TOCP adulterated illicit liquor. Similar neuropathies occur with organophosphates used as pesticides in agriculture such as chlorophos and Mipafox (see Chapter 4H).

A predominantly motor neuropathy evolves in a few days, leading in severe cases to flaccid quadriplegia. A distinctive feature is the latency of 1 to 2 weeks from the time of ingestion of organophosphate to the onset of neuropathy. In the case of pesticides, the neuropathy is preceded by cholinergic crisis immediately after ingestion with diarrhea, sweating, fasciculations, and convulsions. Although the acute neurologic picture is one of severe generalized polyneuropathy, as patients recover over months, signs of upper motor neuron dysfunction emerge.

No specific therapy is available. Patients with mild or moderately severe disease make a gradual and often complete recovery. Severely involved patients are left with spastic weakness.

***Acute polyneuropathy of thallium poisoning.*** Poisoning with thallium, a heavy metal, is distinctly unusual today but does occur. The most common sources are the thallium-containing rodenticides such as Gizmo mouse killer, Zelio paste, or Senco corn mix, ingested accidentally by children or for suicidal purposes.

The neuropathy that evolves closely resembles the Guillain-Barré syndrome and includes autonomic disturbances. Nausea and vomiting may precede the neuropathy. Some patients are encephalopathic with clouded consciousness and seizures. Alopecia, the telltale sign of thallium intoxication, appears 2 to 4 weeks after ingestion. The diagnosis is established by detecting thallium in a 24-hour collection of urine, but it can also be found in the blood or even in the saliva.

Vigorous supportive therapy is the mainstay of treatment, as outlined in the section on the Guillain-Barré syndrome. Chelating agents that are helpful in poisoning with other heavy metals are not effective for thallium. However, Prussian blue (potassium ferric ferrocyanote II), an ion exchange resin, is said to help prevent or minimize evolution of the neuropathy, although it is not useful once the neuropathy is established. The Prussian blue forms a complex with thallium in exchange for potassium, and the complex is excreted in the gut, thus decreasing the absorption of thallium. This treatment should be combined with a good laxative. Early treatment with Prussian blue has decreased severe residual neurologic disability. Alopecia recovers fully and spontaneously.

### Acute infectious polyneuropathies: Lyme disease

A variety of peripheral nerve abnormalities occur often in the course of Lyme disease, typically following the phase of erythema marginatum and polyarthropathies but sometimes without such recognized antecedents (see Chapter 87). Neuropathy may sometimes be associated with encephalitis. In a subgroup of patients, facial palsy similar to Bell's palsy appears and may become bilateral and spread to involve the sixth, fifth, and eighth cranial nerves (cranial polyneuritis). Widespread peripheral neuropathy often appears about 6 weeks after a tick bite or erythema marginatum with prominent pain, paresthesias, and dysesthesia in the limbs and trunk, followed in days to weeks by asymmetric, spreading, multifocal areflexic paralysis in the limbs in a pattern of mononeuropathy multiplex or monoradiculopathy multiplex. Sometimes the picture evolves into a Guillain-Barré syndrome. The CSF shows prominent mononuclear pleocytosis, unlike in idiopathic Guillain-Barré syndrome. Electrophysiologic tests show a combination of axonal and demyelinating multifocal neuropathy. The diagnosis is strongly supported or confirmed by antibodies to *Borrelia burgdorferi* in the serum and CSF in the course of disease or a fourfold increase in the acute and convalescent titers in the appropriate clinical context.

Neurologic abnormalities can be halted and improved in most patients by early diagnosis and prompt antibiotic therapy. In the stage of Bell's palsy alone, oral therapy with doxycycline, 100 mg four times a day for 4 weeks, is recommended. With more generalized neuropathy, IV therapy with penicillin, ceftriaxone, or doxycycline is needed. Improvement occurs gradually and may take up to 6 months.

### Acute metabolic polyneuropathies: porphyric neuropathy

Although rare, porphyric neuropathy is discussed because of the principles of prevention and treatment involved. Recurrent bouts of acute polyneuropathy are a major and serious facet of the autosomal recessively inherited, inducible hepatic porphyrias—the acute, intermittent, variegate coproporphyric types. The principal pathologic abnormality is axonal degeneration, affecting the nerve roots and proximal parts of nerves as well as the autonomic fibers. The pathogenesis of nerve injury is not known, although it has been suggested that the large amounts of δ-aminolevulinic acid (ALA) and porphobilinogen (PBG) produced in the acute attack may be neurotoxic.

An attack of neuropathy is heralded by prominent and persistent abdominal and limb pain and constipation followed by weakness of the limbs that eventually becomes quite symmetric and mainly proximal. In severe cases, bulbar and respiratory paralysis occurs. General areflexia is present, although curiously, ankle reflexes may remain intact. The most distinctive feature of the neuropathy is sensory impairment, which often takes the form of broad bands around the thighs or arms or the shape of an old-fashioned bathing suit affecting the trunk. Autonomic disturbance is a constant feature, manifested by persistent tachycardia, ileus, hypertension, postural hypotension, and cardiac arrhythmias. The neuropathy is often accompanied or preceded by neuropsychiatric disturbances in the form of emotional lability, intense anxiety, depression, or frank psychosis with seizures.

A matter of great importance is the precipitation of acute attacks of porphyria by drugs, the most notorious of which are barbiturates. Other precipitants include starvation, acute infection, and possibly menstrual periods.

Because of emotional changes associated with acute attacks, patients in the early phases of neuropathy with bilateral limb pain are often misdiagnosed as hysterical. Another common and potentially tragic setting is of a patient with acute abdominal pain in whom an exploratory laparotomy is performed under anesthesia using barbiturates, and as the patient recovers from the anesthesia, a catastrophic barbiturate-induced neuropathy develops. Diagnosis is established by examining urine for PBG and ALA, both of which are present in great abundance in the acute phase. The urine typically turns port-wine color on standing in light. Relatives must be screened.

Symptomatic therapy is needed for maintenance of respiratory autonomic and metabolic functions. Propranolol has been found to be a well-tolerated, effective therapy for tachycardia and hypertension and may also suppress the overproduction of porphyrins. Specific therapy consists primarily of avoidance of drugs that are known to exacerbate porphyria (Table 103-2). Second, an adequate amount of carbohydrates is given because they seem to suppress porphyria precursor production and to have a protective effect on neuropathy. Dextrose or levulose is given by nasogastric tube or IV route. Recently, hematin has been advocated early in the course of acute attack and has been shown to consistently suppress the overproduction of ALA by feedback inhibition of ALA synthetase. Individual case reports indicate that it is of major benefit in minimizing neurologic damage.

The recovery from severe attacks of porphyric neuropathy is slow and often leaves substantial chronic neurologic disability. Thus prevention and early treatment assume great importance. This is especially true because the patient with porphyria is at continual risk of attacks of neuropathy throughout life. It is vital to identify relatives and caution them against factors that could induce attacks of porphyria, especially anesthesia and drugs.

**Table 103-2.** Drugs in porphyria

| Drugs to be avoided | Drugs that are safe |
|---|---|
| **Analgesics** | |
| Pentazocine (Talwin) | Codeine |
| | Meperidine |
| | Methadone |
| | Morphine |
| | Propoxyphene |
| **Sedatives** | |
| Barbiturates | Chloral hydrate |
| Chlorodiazepoxide | Diazepam |
| Glutethimide | Diphenhydramine (Benadryl) |
| Meprobamate | |
| **Psychotropics** | |
| Imipramine (Tofranil) | Chloropromazine (Thorazine) |
| Amphetamines | Meclizine |
| | Promazine (Sparine) |
| | Promethazine (Phenergan) |
| | Trifluoperazine (Stelazine) |
| | Prochlorperazine (Compazine) |
| | Valproic acid |
| **Anticonvulsants** | |
| Barbiturates, including primidone | |
| Phenytoin (Dilantin) | |
| Mephenytoin | |
| Methsuximide | |
| **Antibiotics** | |
| Sulfonamides | Ampicillin |
| Griseofulvin | Cloxacillin |
| | Nitrofurantoin |
| | Penicillin |
| | Tetracycline |
| | Streptomycin |
| **Cardiovascular** | |
| Ergot | Digoxin |
| Methyldopa (Aldomet) | Propranolol |
| | Reserpine |
| | Warfarin sodium (Coumadin) |
| **Endocrine** | |
| Estrogen | |
| Progesterone | |
| Tolbutamide (Orinase) | |
| Chlorpropamide (Diabinase) | |

## CHRONIC SYMMETRIC POLYNEUROPATHIES

The entity of subacute or chronic symmetric polyneuropathy is one of the most common neurologic syndromes in general medical practice. A bewildering variety of diseases result in a rather stereotyped clinical picture, although in many instances the cause cannot be identified (see the box on p. 1421). The manifestations range from mild asymptomatic abnormalities such as loss of tendon reflexes to quadriplegia, severe disabling pain, profound sensory loss, chronic autonomic disturbance, and secondary trophic change in the limbs.

Sensory symptoms consist of paresthesias and numbness, beginning in the feet and spreading to the legs and hands. There may be dysesthetic sensations in the same distribution in the form of burning, prickling, coldness, and heaviness. Considerable pain may develop in the limbs. The pain is poorly localized, often lancinating, and especially severe at night. At times, however, severe sensory loss may develop silently.

Sensory loss develops according to axonal length, and therefore examination reveals sensory impairment, chiefly over the extremities in a symmetric fashion in a stocking-and-glove distribution. Cutaneous sensory loss extends to about the knee before it appears in fingers and hands. In more advanced stages it extends to the trunk so that there is hypesthesia to pinprick on either side of the midline of the abdominal wall and lower part of the anterior chest in the configuration of a teardrop (Fig. 103-9).

Motor abnormalities generally follow the same distribution, with weakness or clumsiness appearing in the feet and extending to the legs and hands and, in the most severe cases, involving the proximal muscles; however, as a rule, muscles innervated by cranial nerves are spared. There is wasting and weakness of affected muscles, disabling bilateral footdrop, and bilateral wristdrop.

In the longstanding cases of polyneuropathy with sensory loss, as illustrated by those of diabetes mellitus of many years' duration, trophic changes appear in the feet and less often in the hands. The best known are Charcot's joints or neuroarthropathy, in which the joints undergo insidious, painless disorganization, leading to a swollen, grossly deformed but essentially painless foot. The joints of foot and ankle are most frequently affected, but neuroarthropathy can also occur in the knee, wrist, elbow, and shoulder. Much more common than neuroarthropathy are consequences of recurrent injury to insensitive parts of the body; corns and calluses break down to punched-out chronic ulcers over the feet that may penetrate down to the bone, setting the stage for serious infection of foot spaces and gangrene. Cigarette burns are a telltale sign in the hands.

Tendon reflexes are, as a rule, lost early and symmetrically. In some instances the trunks of peripheral nerves

## A classification of chronic symmetric polyneuropathies

- Acquired neuropathies
  - Toxic
    - Drugs
    - Industrial toxins
    - Heavy metals
    - Abused substances
  - Metabolic/endocrine
    - Diabetes
    - Chronic renal failure
    - Hypothyroidism
    - Polyneuropathy of critical illness
  - Nutritional deficiency
    - Vitamin $B_{12}$ deficiency
    - Alcoholism
    - Vitamin E deficiency
  - Paraneoplastic
    - Carcinoma
    - Lymphoma
  - Plasma cell dyscrasia
    - Myeloma, typical, atypical, and solitary forms
    - Primary systemic amyloidosis
  - Idiopathic chronic inflammatory demyelinating polyneuropathies
  - Polyneuropathies associated with peripheral nerve autoantibodies
  - AIDS
- Inherited neuropathies
  - Neuropathies with biochemical markers
    - Refsum disease
    - Bassen-Kornzweig disease
    - Tangier disease
    - Metachromatic leukodystrophy
    - Krabbe's disease
    - Adrenomyeloneuropathy
    - Fabry's disease
  - Neuropathies without biochemical markers or systemic involvement
    - Hereditary motor neuropathy
    - Hereditary sensory neuropathy
    - Hereditary sensorimotor neuropathy

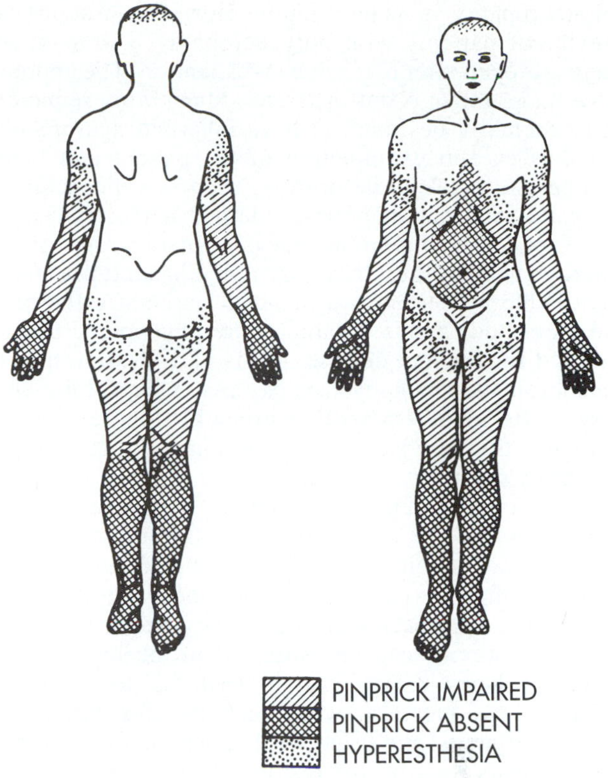


**Fig. 103-9.** Sensory map from 67-year-old man with 18-year history of diabetes mellitus. There is sensory loss in distal (stocking-and-glove) distribution in limbs and in band over anterior trunk. Autonomic dysfunction is also present. (From Sabin TD, Geschwind N, Waxman SG: Patterns of clinical deficits in peripheral nerve disease. In Waxman SG, editor: *Physiology and pathology of axons,* New York, 1978, Raven Press.)

may be enlarged. This is best appreciated by palpating the greater auricular nerve across the lateral side of the neck, the superficial cutaneous branch of radial nerve in the distal forearm, or the ulnar and peroneal nerves.

Autonomic disturbances are being more widely recognized as integral facets of many chronic polyneuropathies with major impact on complications and prognosis. They are well known to occur with chronic diabetic neuropathy and with many forms of hereditary as well as primary systemic amyloidosis. The dysautonomia is often asymptomatic and needs to be sought by careful examination. Postural hypotension, urinary retention or incontinence, impotence, generalized or regional anhidrosis, cardiac irregularities, gastroparesis, diarrhea, and impaired pupillary motility are some of the myriad manifestations. The recent development of a battery of tests that can be performed at the bedside by the clinician makes it relatively easy to document autonomic impairment in any comprehensive evaluation of a neuropathy.

The diagnosis of chronic polyneuropathy is readily made on clinical grounds, although it is clear that in many patients it is subclinical. The preservation of ankle reflexes in what appears otherwise to be symmetric polyneuropathy should arouse suspicion that one is dealing with a myelopathy. Exceptionally, ankle reflexes are preserved in some familial polyneuropathies and others that preferentially affect the small-diameter fibers subserving pain and temperature sensation, as in neuropathy of amyloidosis, rare cases of diabetes, and porphyric neuropathy. NCV and electromyography are useful adjuncts to the diagnosis, not so much to prove the presence or absence of neuropathy, but to give an indication as to whether the neuropathy is predominantly axonal or demyelinating. In demyelinating neuropathy, NCV is greatly slowed, whereas it is only minimally decreased in predominantly axonal neuropathies, in which the electromyography shows denervation. Most patients show a combination of such changes.

The etiologic diagnosis of chronic symmetric polyneuropathy may be obvious on clinical examination and a limited routine biochemical screening. The common causes are diabetes, chronic renal failure, alcoholism, and nutritional deficiencies. In the last decade, AIDS has become the most common cause of chronic symmetric polyneuropathy in young adults. However, a significant number of patients with polyneuropathy lack a specific diagnosis even after extensive investigation. The approach to such a problem is outlined later. Many of these patients will eventually be found to have inherited neuropathies, and thus careful examination of the patient and family members for skeletal deformities such as kyphoscoliosis, pes cavus and hammer toes, enlarged nerve trunks, and NCVs provides important clues. A small group of rare inherited neuropathies may appear first in adult life and are identifiable by certain biochemical markers in the blood and other body fluids. Examples are phytanic acid levels in blood for Refsum disease, levels of arylsulfatase A for metachromatic leukodystrophy, and serum long-chain fatty acids in adrenomyeloneuropathy. These tests are available through laboratories specializing in inherited metabolic disorders.

A major group of polyneuropathies whose cause may be obscure is the *toxic neuropathies*. Careful analysis of occupational, habitual, or hobby-related exposure to environmental toxins is essential and, although time-consuming, may be rewarding. Only a small number of these neurotoxins can be estimated in the body tissues, examples being heavy metals such as lead, arsenic, thallium, and mercury, which can be measured in the blood, hair, nails, and urine. With most other neurotoxins, the diagnosis rests on the history of exposure.

*Paraneoplastic syndromes* are another well-known group of polyneuropathies in which the cause may not be obvious because the malignancy is occult. The neuropathies associated with solitary plasmacytoma are especially difficult to identify. Careful survey of the entire skeleton, a radionuclide bone scan, and immunoelectrophoresis of blood and urine will uncover these conditions. Primary systemic amyloidosis is being increasingly recognized as a cause of severe chronic polyneuropathy in middle-aged and elderly patients. The diagnosis is established by biopsy of skin, fat pad, or rectal mucosa. In the last decade an interesting group of neuropathies associated with circulating peripheral nerve autoantibodies have been delineated.

An important group of rare disorders are the *chronic/relapsing inflammatory demyelinating polyneuropathies,* which may be thought of as chronic forms of Guillain-Barré syndrome. The neurologic picture is quite similar to that of Guillain-Barré syndrome except it evolves gradually and tends to remit and relapse over years. This has been described with early phases of HIV infection. The NCV is greatly slowed and areas of conduction block are identified, indicating a demyelinating process, and CSF protein is regularly elevated. These polyneuropathies tend to respond to corticosteroids, immunosuppressants, and plasmapheresis.

Nerve biopsy is a useful, if rather overrated, procedure in identifying the cause of some polyneuropathies. Amyloidosis, leprosy, sarcoidosis, certain toxic neuropathies that cause giant swellings of axons, and vasculitic neuropathies may be identified by biopsy, even when other investigations are negative.

### Principles of treatment

***Specific therapy*** *(see Table 103-1).* The most impressive results perhaps occur in toxic polyneuropathies, where the identification and removal from toxic exposure leads to gradual recovery. Glue sniffing by a teenager, surreptitious inhalation of nitrous oxide by a dentist, or medical use of nitrofurantoin are examples of remediable situations. Chelating agents such as calcium–ethylenediaminetetra-acetic acid (Ca-EDTA) or penicillamine can accelerate the elimination of lead, arsenic, and mercury, whereas Prussian blue functions as an ion exchanger to decrease absorption of ingested thallium.

Gratifying improvement occurs by good nutrition with multiple and specific vitamin supplements in vitamin deficiency and nutritional neuropathies. Endocrine polyneuropathies are rare but respond to appropriate treatment of the endocrinopathy. Replacement of thyroxin in hypothyroidism or correction of thyrotoxicosis leads to rapid amelioration of the associated polyneuropathy. Polyneuropathy associated with plasma cell dyscrasia is rare but important because the syndrome of severe neuropathy in association with solitary plasmacytoma usually regresses with excision or radiation therapy to the plasmacytoma. Immunosuppressive drugs improve the rare neuropathy associated with benign monoclonal gammopathy. In metabolic polyneuropathies, the early use of hemodialysis has made severe uremic neuropathy a rarity. Even when severe neuropathy has developed, remarkable recovery is the rule after renal transplantation. The most common chronic polyneuropathy in medical practice is caused by diabetes mellitus. It is resistant to current modalities of treatment. Recently, several studies have indicated that rigorous control of hyperglycemia improves nerve function as measured by conduction velocities.

Interestingly enough, some inherited polyneuropathies can be substantially alleviated by specific therapy. Refsum disease is the outstanding example where long-term modification of diet with low content of phytols, combined with intermittent plasmapheresis to remove large quantities of plasma phytanic acid, definitely ameliorates the neuropathy. Recent evidence suggests that the neuropathy and myelopathy of the rare Bassen-Kornzweig syndrome (abetalipoproteinemia) respond to large doses of vitamin E. Lastly, the substantial group of chronic inflammatory demyelinating polyneuropathies with recurrent and relapsing course over many years often responds to treatment with corticosteroids or azathioprine combined with intermittent plasmapheresis and IV immunoglobulin therapy.

***Symptomatic therapy.*** Symptomatic therapy is the mainstay of the long-term management of many chronic polyneuropathies for which no specific therapy exists and helps the patient to cope with the disorder, adds comfort, and most importantly, serves to prevent certain serious complications of the neuropathy.

Management of loss of sensation in the limbs is vital because the consequences are insidious and grave. Insensitivity of the feet and to a lesser extent of the hands leads to recurrent minor trauma that goes unnoticed but eventually results in corns and calluses that break down to form penetrating ulcers. Moreover, they provide a portal of entry to infection of deep fascial planes of the foot or hand and serious cellulitis. This complication is most sinister in diabetes mellitus because the associated obliterative vascular disease and hyperglycemia appear to impede wound healing. Similar complications occur in

## Pharmacotherapy of neuropathic pain

Antidepressant drugs
- Amitriptyline
- Desipramine
- Trazodone
- Fluoxetine

Anticonvulsant drugs
- Carbamazepine
- Phenytoin
- Clonazepam

Antiarrhythmic drugs
- Tocainide
- Mexiletine
- Nifedipine
- Baclofen (trigeminal neuralgia)

Antiserotonin agent
- Cyproheptadine

Anti–substance P agent
- Topical capsaicin (Zostrix, Axsain)

Opioids
- Morphine, codeine, and analogues
- Transdermal opioids

other neuropathies with anesthetic limbs, especially in leprosy, amyloidosis, and hereditary sensory neuropathies. In addition to recalcitrant ulcers, there is often autoamputation and resorption of toes and fingers.

Prevention is the key to the management of trophic changes and their complications. Patients should be educated that their hands and feet are vulnerable to mechanical and thermal injury that is likely to go unrecognized because of lack of pain sensitivity. The need for long-term deliberate steps to avoid this problem should be emphasized so that they become a routine to the patient. The feet should be kept clean and inspected daily for abrasions and other injuries. When feet are dry because of loss of sweating, they should be soaked for 15 minutes in tepid water daily, lightly dabbed, and petroleum jelly applied so that moisture is kept in and cracking of skin is prevented. The use of properly fitting shoes with leather tops is essential because poorly fitting shoes are the most common cause of ischemic ulcers of the feet. Corns and calluses should not be pared by the patient, keratolytic agents should be avoided, and the patient should be referred to a podiatrist. Precautions are necessary to avoid thermal injury by, for instance, wearing gloves in the kitchen, using pots with long wooden handles, and avoiding cigarette smoking.

Once a foot ulcer develops, it should be vigorously treated from the outset. If there is evidence of acute ulceration or infection, bed rest with elevation of the foot and appropriate antibiotics are necessary. Once the acute phase subsides, walking can be allowed, but it is crucial to avoid weight bearing on the foot. Although this is a self-evident principle and patients with normal sensation will not bear weight on an ulcerated foot, much exhortation is needed for the patient with anesthetic limbs to follow this direction. A total-contact cast to the foot and leg is the best method, but in conscientious patients who decline the cast, crutches may be used. It is remarkable that with such care even patients with severe, inherited sensory neuropathies can protect their limbs for years.

***Management of motor disabilities.*** Physical medicine and rehabilitation departments can help the patient make the best use of remaining strength. Braces for dropped feet, special shoes, and attachments to utensils, tools, and cutlery can aid disabled patients in activities of daily living.

***Management of chronic neuropathic pain.*** Persistent pain is a relatively uncommon problem but is difficult to treat and requires special strategies. Chronic pain may be a distressing feature of some cases of diabetic, alcoholic, and uremic polyneuropathy. It is a common manifestation of amyloid neuropathy and an outstanding aspect of the rare sex-linked Fabry's disease.

The first step is to make sure that the pain is indeed neuropathic and not ischemic. Musculoskeletal and joint pain secondary to weakness and uneven distribution of body weight should be excluded. Depression may frequently masquerade as chronic pain.

Narcotic analgesics should be avoided because of the danger of addiction in these chronic situations. Treatment should be initiated with simple analgesics such as aspirin or with nonsteroidal antiinflammatory drugs (NSAIDs) such as ibuprofen (see the box above). The next choice is a trial of diphenylhydantoin or carbamazepine. In resistant cases, amitriptyline or other tricyclic antidepressant drugs are generally effective. Occasionally they may need to be combined with a neuroleptic drug such as fluphenazine (Prolixin). The use of neuroleptics should be a last resort because of the risk of tardive dyskinesia. Occasional case reports have indicated success with an assortment of drugs such as propranolol, cyproheptadine, small doses of levodopa (L-dopa), and clonazepam-mexiletine. Topical application of 10% xylocaine ointment or ointment of capsaicin (Axsain, Zostrix) may bring modest relief in some cases. TENS is helpful in some instances. No single drug is consistently effective in every patient, and one must work to find a suitable agent for a given patient. The painful states usually remit, although it takes several months.

***Management of chronic autonomic neuropathy.*** This challenging therapeutic problem is typically encountered in diabetic and amyloid polyneuropathy. Elastic thigh-length stockings and elevation of the head end of the bed while the patient is recumbent may suffice in mild cases of symptomatic postural hypotension. In more severe postural hypotension, the most consistently effective treatment is fluorocortisone, although it is far from ideal. Many patients may still be disabled by orthostatic symptoms. A variety of pharmacologic agents have been tried singly or in combination and include indomethacin, ephedrine, propranolol, monoamine oxidase (MAO) inhibitors, and in desperate cases even atrial tachypacing. Holter monitoring of the heart rhythm may identify intermittent heart block that requires a pacemaker. Gastrointestinal autonomic dysfunction is occasionally symptomatic. Gastroparesis of diabetes may be eased by metoclopramide. Small-bowel dysautonomia may cause intermittent diarrhea, which responds to antidiarrheal agents or courses of tetracyclines. Neurogenic bladder is of major importance because it predisposes to bladder and upper urinary tract distention and infection and eventual renal impairment. Pharmacotherapy tailored to physiologic abnormalities found on cystometrography is helpful. The detrusor stimulant bethanechol (urecholine) is the mainstay. In selected cases, resection of the bladder neck is effective. The vexing problem of impotence can now be proved to be neuropathic and not primarily psychogenic, ischemic, or endocrinologic by flow studies and measures of nocturnal penile tumescence. Neuropathic impotence is permanent, and the recently developed penile prostheses are a significant advance for this condition in selected patients.

### Diabetic polyneuropathy

Diabetic polyneuropathy is the prototype of chronic, symmetric polyneuropathy and affects both type I and type II diabetics. The peripheral nerves show a combination of nonspecific segmental demyelination, axonal degeneration, and sometimes a vasa nervorum plugged with platelets. The pathogenesis of this common neuropathy is not known but seems primarily related to metabolic derangement. However, there are gross disparities between hyperglycemia and the presence or absence and severity of the neuropathy, pointing to many factors that are not yet understood.

The neuropathy is predominantly sensory and varies in severity from asymptomatic loss of ankle reflexes to severe sensory loss and weakness of all limbs. A rare variant is the painful "small-fiber neuropathy" in which there is dissociated loss of pain and temperature sensation with relative preservation of touch and proprioception and intact tendon reflexes. Other patients may have proprioception impairment that is so severe that combined with diminished pupillary light reflexes, it has been called *diabetic pseudotabes*. Persistent pain in the limbs with nocturnal exacerbation can be troublesome in a few patients.

Autonomic neuropathy occurs frequently and in some forms is the major disabling feature of the disease. Recently, several cases of sudden cardiorespiratory arrests have been reported in diabetic patients with autonomic neuropathy in association with pulmonary infections, respiratory depressant drugs, and anesthesia. Because patients with diabetic neuropathy frequently live for many years, trophic changes in the feet and hands are typically seen. Autonomic neuropathy can abolish the awareness of hypoglycemia by blunting the anxiety, tremor, sweating, and hunger mediated by the autonomic systems. These patients rapidly pass into hypoglycemic coma. The combination of gastroparesis, which makes the absorption of food and serum glucose erratic, and neurogenic bladder, which causes urinary stasis, may make urine sugars an unreliable test, and the patient may be considered "brittle."

The CSF may show a moderate elevation of protein to about 100 to 200 mg/dl but is otherwise normal.

Treatment of established polyneuropathy is unsatisfactory. Present evidence, meager as it is, suggests that control of hyperglycemia should be as tight as practical in each individual circumstance for as long as possible. Preliminary evidence indicates that aldose-reductase inhibitors may improve nerve function to a small extent. Otherwise, treatment is symptomatic for pain, insensitivity, and autonomic dysfunction, as outlined in the introductory section on chronic symmetric polyneuropathies.

### Uremic polyneuropathy

With the advent of hemodialysis, patients lived with chronic renal failure longer and many developed a symmetric polyneuropathy, often severe enough to cause quadriplegia. However, with improved methods of dialysis, a serious degree of neuropathy is now rare. The nerves show predominant axonal degeneration. Pathogenesis of nerve damage is not known though it is clear that some bloodborne dialyzable toxin(s) are responsible.

The neuropathy is symmetric, distal, and sensorimotor. Mild autonomic dysfunction is manifest by postural hypotension. Whereas some patients have troublesome limb pains, others experience the "restless legs" syndrome, which compels them to move the legs or walk about because of a peculiar distress in the legs. The CSF is usually normal.

Early and adequate modern hemodialysis is effective in mild or moderate cases. However, severe established neuropathy responds only to renal transplantation and then often remarkably well. Curiously, the neuropathy may also be improved by bilateral nephrectomy performed to control malignant hypertension of renal failure. Nitrofurantoin, which can cause severe neuropathy especially in the presence of renal failures, should be avoided.

### Polyneuropathy associated with malignancy and Sjögren's syndrome

A symmetric polyneuropathy is frequently seen in patients with known malignancy. In the overall context of the cancer, the neuropathy is significant chiefly as a side effect of cancer chemotherapy. Vincristine, procarbazine, cisplatin, and mesonidazole regularly produce distal symmetric polyneuropathy. The drug-induced nerve dysfunction is a dose-related limiting factor in the treatment. The second major cause of polyneuropathy is neoplastic infiltration of multiple nerve roots, both of spinal and cranial nerves, by meningeal carcinomatosis or lymphomatosis; this infiltration produces an asymmetric patchy monoradiculopathy multiplex syndrome. The true *paraneoplastic polyneuropathies* are rare but do occur and have special significance as heralding a previously undiagnosed cancer.

The most distinctive of these syndromes is the rare *subacute sensory neuropathy,* in which a unique selective neuronal loss affects the dorsal root ganglia in a generalized symmetric fashion. The condition is most often associated with bronchogenic carcinoma, which may be occult or not be evident until 1 or 2 years later. The patient presents with subacute onset of pain, paresthesias, and dysesthetic sensations in the limbs and face along with severe ataxia of gait and limbs. There is a striking loss of all modalities of sensation over the limbs, sometimes extending to face and buccal mucosa. Sensory ataxia of gait is present with a prominent Romberg's sign. Weakness is absent or minimal, whereas areflexia is universal. A similar syndrome has been highlighted over the last 10 years in association with Sjögren's syndrome, often as its presenting features.

Unfortunately, the prognosis is poor. In the rare cases associated with lymphoma, treatment of the lymphoma produced remarkable remission of neuropathy.

*Subacute motor neuropathy* is an equally rare disorder that is a mirror image of the sensory neuropathy and is associated with lymphoma rather than lung cancer. It has also been described with Waldenström's macroglobulinemia. A subacute weakness appears affecting distal and proximal muscles of limbs and sometimes of the neck with areflexia but without sensory impairment. In contrast to the bleak prognosis of the sensory form, this neuropathy often spontaneously recovers over 1 to 3 years, independent of the activity of the underlying neoplasm.

### Polyneuropathies associated with peripheral nerve antibodies

Much interest has surrounded the recent ongoing delineation of several chronic neuropathic syndromes associated with high levels of antibodies to peripheral nerves in the serum. Several cases of a chronic sensorimoter polyneuropathy affecting middle-aged men have been described, with predominant demyelination and marked sensory and motor nerve conduction slowing. High serum titers of antibodies against peripheral nerve myelin-associated glycoprotein (anti-MAG) appear to be involved in its pathogenesis. Improvement occurs with combinations of plasmapheresis, IV immunoglobulin, and immunosuppressive drugs.

A syndrome resembling motor neuron disease has also been defined in young adults caused by multifocal nerve conduction block, affecting exclusively the motor nerves and associated with high serum levels of antibodies against GM1 ganglioside (anti-GM1 antibodies). Unlike the usual motor neuron disease, there are no upper motor neuron or bulbar signs and the course is indolent. IV cyclophosphamide therapy has produced significant improvement.

These antibody titer measurements are currently available through commercial laboratories.

### Polyneuropathy associated with plasma cell dyscrasias

Polyneuropathy is well known to occur in multiple myeloma but is overshadowed by the many systemic derangements of this disease of rather poor prognosis. However, in recent years, there has been much interest in the group of disorders in which a chronic, unremitting, severe sensorimotor polyneuropathy evolves as an outstanding manifestation with little systemic impairment. The CSF protein is often strikingly elevated to 1 to 2 g/ml, sometimes in association with papilledema. The general examination is remarkably normal. Careful investigation by radiologic survey of the entire skeleton will reveal a solitary plasmacytoma in the vertebral body, pelvis, or clavicle. It may be osteoblastic, osteolytic, or mixed. This entity is important to diagnose because moderate and sometimes marked regression of the neuropathy follows on surgical or radiation therapy of the solitary plasmacytoma.

Another relatively recently described rare and extraordinary syndrome is called the *POEMS syndrome* (polyneuropathy, organomegaly, endocrinopathy, monoclonal gammopathy, and skin changes), originally described in Japan but later found in the United States. A severe subacute or chronic polyneuropathy is associated with pigmentation of skin, hypertrichosis, hypogonadism, hypothyroidism, and hepatosplenomegaly. Immunoelectrophoresis shows monoclonal gammopathy, and a skeletal survey reveals solitary or multiple areas of myeloma. Radiotherapy of the tumors ameliorates the neuropathy as well as the skin and endocrine changes.

*Atypical myeloma* is much more common than either of the syndromes just described and may also be associated with a severe polyneuropathy, high CSF protein, and monoclonal gamma globulin in serum. Compared with classic multiple myeloma, however, the condition is less aggressive, patients are not systemically ill, and the degree of plasmacytosis in bone marrow is mild. Unfortunately, the neuropathy does not respond to therapy.

A chronic sensorimotor polyneuropathy is a significant clinical problem in *Waldenström's macroglobulinemia.* Chemotherapy with chlorambucil may improve the neuropathy.

*Primary systemic (nonhereditary) amyloidosis* is now considered a plasma cell dyscrasia. Most patients have a monoclonal gammopathy or immunoelectrophoresis of serum and/or urine. An infiltration of the peripheral nervous system with amyloid is the microscopic hallmark of the disease, which also affects the gastrointestinal, cardiovascular, and renal organs. There is a relatively selective loss of thinly myelinated fibers (small-fiber neuropathy). A disabling, and in some cases distinctive, chronic polyneuropathy is a major early or late aspect of this progressive disease. Pain and paresthesias in the lower extremities are prominent. Carpal tunnel syndrome is a common presenting feature. In many instances there is a dissociated loss of sensation in stocking-and-glove distribution with loss of pinprick and temperature sensation, whereas touch and proprioception are intact although eventually all modalities are lost. As the disease progresses, motor impairment occurs and is severe. Neuropathic ulcers and Charcot's joints may occur. A prominent feature is autonomic neuropathy, which causes impotence, bowel and bladder incontinence, intractable postural hypotension, and cardiac denervation. Unfortunately, no specific treatment exists, and death results usually from renal failure. The effects of liver transplantation in the course of amyloidosis and neuropathy are just emerging and appear promising.

### Polyneuropathy of endocrine disease: hypothyroidism

In hypothyroidism, a common disease, paresthesias and cramps in the feet and legs suggesting peripheral neuropathy frequently occur but without objective evidence of neuropathy. However, a rare, predominantly sensory, clinically significant polyneuropathy has been documented. It may be accompanied by evidence of mild myelopathy (myeloneuropathy). Pathologically, segmental demyelination occurs. A common accompaniment is unilateral or bilateral carpal tunnel syndrome. Although rare, the diagnostic search is rewarded by dramatic response to thyroid replacement.

*Polyneuropathy of vitamin $B_{12}$ deficiency.* Peripheral neuropathy is one aspect of the neurologic syndrome resulting from vitamin $B_{12}$ deficiency. The initial symptoms are sensations of pins and needles and numbness in the feet and later in the hands that tend to be prominent. Occasionally, paresthesias may appear first in the hands. Because of these presenting symptoms, the initial diagnostic impression is usually one of a peripheral neuropathic syndrome. One finds evidence of this in the form of depressed or absent ankle reflexes and even a stocking-distribution impairment of touch and pinprick. However, examination also reveals signs of myelopathy with loss of proprioception in the lower extremities and upper motor neuron dysfunction in the form of brisk knee reflexes and Babinski responses. Romberg's sign is positive. It is probable that most of the symptoms in fact are related to the posterior column and corticospinal tract involvement. The myeloneuropathic syndrome may occur in an otherwise well-looking person without clinical evidence of anemia.

The diagnosis is established by low plasma $B_{12}$ levels, and macrocytic megaloblastic anemia is usual. However, neuropathy can undoubtedly occur with normal blood and bone marrow examination.

The response to injections of vitamin $B_{12}$ is truly dramatic except in long-established cases. These paresthesias may improve within days of injection, and the neuropathy recovers completely if therapy is started within a few weeks of onset of symptoms. Vitamin $B_{12}$ injections must be lifelong.

### Drugs that cause polyneuropathy

- Drugs in oncology
  - Vincristine
  - Procarbazine
  - Cisplatin
  - Mesonidazole
  - Metronidazole (Flagyl)
  - Taxol
- Drugs in infectious diseases
  - Isoniazid
  - Nitrofurantoin
  - Dapsone
  - ddC (Dideoxycytidine)
  - ddI (Dideoxyinosine)
- Drugs in cardiology
  - Hydralazine
  - Perhexiline maleate
  - Procainamide
  - Disopyramide
- Drugs in rheumatology
  - Gold salts
  - Chloroquine
- Drugs in neurology and psychiatry
  - Diphenylhydantoin
  - Glutethimide
  - Methaqualone
- Miscellaneous
  - Disulfiram (Antabuse)
  - Vitamin: pyridoxine (megadoses)

*Polyneuropathy in steatorrhea (vitamin E deficiency neuropathy).* A chronic myeloneuropathic syndrome similar to that caused by vitamin $B_{12}$ deficiency may develop insidiously in patients with longstanding fat malabsorption caused by biliary atresia, chronic liver diseases, familial intrahepatic cholestasis, and following ileal resection in Crohn's disease or for small bowel obstruction. The recent discovery of therapeutic significance is that these patients have very low or undetectable blood levels of vitamin E. Supplementation with large doses of vitamin E to obtain normal blood levels of the vitamin has been associated with encouraging improvement in neurologic function.

## Toxic polyneuropathies

*Drug-induced neuropathies.* Many drugs in common use cause subacute or chronic polyneuropathy of varying severity (see Table 103-1). In AIDS patients, neuropathy caused by retroviral nucleosides, ddI, and ddC has become common. Axonal degeneration is the rule, except only with the neuropathy of procainamide and perhexiline maleate (a European antianginal drug), in which demyelination predominates. The drugs are chemically disparate. Although the mechanisms of injury are known in some cases, they are obscure in most. For instance, isonicotinic acid hydrazide (INH) neuropathy is mediated by the pyridoxine deficiency that it induces, especially in those persons who are genetically slow acetylators. *Vinca* alkaloids seem to interfere with axonal microtubules and nerve cell body metabolism. Some drugs cause neuropathy in a predictable dose-related fashion, as exemplified by vincristine. In others, such as INH, the risk of neuropathy is substantial in high-dose therapy and in slow acetylators. With certain drugs, the neuropathy is rare and unpredictable. The newly introduced antineoplastic agent taxol has been associated with dose-related dysesthetic polyneuropathy.

The clinical picture is one of symmetric sensorimotor polyneuropathy evolving in a subacute or chronic manner and can be severe and disabling or mild and asymptomatic. Autonomic neuropathy is an added feature with certain drugs such as vincristine. Moreover, vincristine may cause facial palsies, ophthalmoplegia, and recurrent laryngeal nerve palsy, whereas cisplatin regularly causes sensorineural hearing loss.

The diagnosis rests on clinical awareness of drug-induced neuropathies. The physician should also be alert to this complication in relation to the variety of newly introduced drugs. Improvement of neuropathy with discontinuation of the suspect drug and relapse when the drug is reintroduced provide the only confirmation under these circumstances. Large doses of pyridoxine dispensed by health food stores can cause disabling sensory polyneuropathies.

The crucial step in treatment is recognition and withdrawal of the culprit drug. In most patients, neuropathy will gradually recover. When the neurotoxicity is dose related (e.g., vincristine), the drug may be continued or resumed at a lower level.

Certain drug-induced polyneuropathies are preventable. For instance, supplementation of INH with daily pyridoxine obviates the danger of neuropathy, whereas

**Table 103-3.** Sources and modes of exposure to industrial chemicals

| Occupational | Abuse/accidental |
|---|---|
| ***N*-Hexane** | |
| Hexacarbon solvent widely used in adhesives, glues, laminated products, shoes, cabinet finishing | Glues containing *n*-hexane inhaled in enormous quantities, principally by teenagers ("glue sniffing") |
| **Methylbutylketone (MBK)** | |
| Hexacarbon used as an industrial solvent in color printing, furniture finishing, plastic-coated fabrics | Cleaning and washing with lacquer thinner containing MBK |
| **Solvent mixtures** | |
| Lacquer thinners containing several solvents such as acetone, methylisobutylketone, methylethylketone | Abused for euphoriant effect ("Huffer neuropathy") |
| **Nitrous oxide** | |
| Used in dental offices as anesthetic; food propellant | Abused by dentists and related health workers for euphoriant effects and as an unconventional remedy for hangover |
| **Acrylamide** | |
| Widely used chemical grouting agent for waterproofing in tunnels, water conduits, sewers | Outbreaks possible from contamination of water supplied from sewers recently grouted with acrylamide |
| **Dimethylaminoproprionitrile (DMAPN)** | |
| Catalyzer in polyurethane foam manufacture | |

nitrofurantoin should be avoided in patients with renal failure.

The boxes on pp. 1423 and 1426 list drugs for neuropathic pain and drugs that cause neuropathy.

***Polyneuropathy caused by industrial chemicals.*** Over the past 2 decades, a few of the large numbers of chemicals introduced into industry have been found to produce severe peripheral neuropathy. It is a matter of great importance that exposure to these chemicals is *not* limited to the industrial environment. For example, the widely utilized industrial solvent *n*-hexane is abused by teenagers in glue sniffing, which results in severe neuropathy. The grouting agent acrylamide may contaminate water sources, causing outbreaks of neuropathy. Even within industry the nature and source of responsible toxic chemicals may take a painstaking search to identify. The pathologic changes are often distinctive. For instance, in cases of neuropathy caused by *n*-hexane, methylbutylketone, acrylamide, and solvent mixtures, the nerves show characteristic giant swellings of the axons (Table 103-3).

Clinically, the general pattern is one of a subacutely developing, symmetric, distal sensorimotor polyneuropathy. However, some toxins display characteristic variations on this theme. The most remarkable is the cauda equina syndrome with urinary retention, impotence, and paresthesias in the limbs progressing to paraparesis, which is seen with dimethylaminoproprionitrile poisoning. A neuropathy with prominent sensory ataxia associated with blisters on the hands suggests acrylamide poisoning.

The diagnosis rests on a high degree of suspicion and careful occupational, hobby, and abuse history. Unfortunately, none of these chemicals can be measured in the body as proof of exposure. In the case of volatile hydrocarbons and acrylamide poisoning, nerve biopsy may provide strong supportive evidence for the diagnosis.

Treatment is by removal from further exposure. The neuropathy may continue to worsen for a few months after the last exposure but gradually improves to a large extent in most cases.

***Polyneuropathy caused by heavy metal intoxication.*** In modern times, intoxication with heavy metals occupationally or by accident has become distinctly uncommon in western countries but is by no means extinct (Table 103-4). Lead, arsenic, and thallium continue to cause occasional cases of florid neuropathy. The metals cannot be rapidly excreted and thus accumulate in tissues, including those of the peripheral and the central nervous system as well as in skin, hair, nails, and other organs. They cause a multisystem illness by interfering with cellular enzymes. Axonal degeneration is the principal pathologic change.

Clinically, a sensorimotor polyneuropathy appears subacutely or chronically. Arsenic and thallium polyneuropathy may also develop acutely and resemble the Guillain-Barré syndrome. Intermittent exposure to the toxin causes a puzzling neuropathy that may remit and relapse. Each of these toxins tends to produce a different pattern of neuropathy. For instance, neuropathy of lead poisoning in adults is predominantly motor and often asymmetric, frequently presenting with bilateral radial nerve or peroneal palsies. Arsenical neuropathy tends to be predominantly sensory and painful. Thallium neuropathy is associated with autonomic disturbances. Diagnostic clues are also provided by changes in skin, hair, and nails. Transverse white lines (Mees' lines) occur in arsenic and thallium poisoning. Hyperkeratosis of the palms and soles and hyperpigmentation of the skin suggest arsenical intoxication, whereas alopecia, often generalized and striking, is the hallmark of thallium toxicosis. Another characteristic and often confounding feature of metal poisoning is the occurrence of encephalopathy as well as of multiple system dysfunction simulating many other endogenous diseases.

Fortunately, the intoxications can be reliably and readily diagnosed by estimation of the metals from hair, urine, and blood. The identification of the source of the poison may require difficult sleuthing in many cases.

Identification and removal from exposure usually lead to a gradual recovery. The accumulated toxin can be eliminated more rapidly by chelating agents such as Ca-EDTA, dimercaprol, or penicillamine, and in the case of thallium by Prussian blue, an ion exchanger that complexes with thallium and prevents absorption of the metal from the gut.

## POLYNEUROPATHY OF CRITICAL ILLNESS

In the last decade a severe generalized axonal polyneuropathy has been identified among patients critically ill with prolonged period of sepsis, multiple organ failure, and hypoalbuminemia. Failure to wean the patient off the ventilator often brings the weakness to attention. Examination reveals generalized areflexic quadriparesis with muscle atrophy, and nerve conduction studies show an axonal neuropathy while CSF remains normal. With supportive therapy, surprisingly good recovery of the neuropathy is the rule, although improvement may take several months. The pathogenesis is uncertain but appears related to complex toxic-metabolic systemic derangements.

### Nutritional and vitamin deficiency neuropathies

***Polyneuropathy of alcoholism.*** Alcoholism is an important worldwide cause of chronic polyneuropathy. The principal pathologic change in the peripheral nerves is axonal degeneration. Deficiencies of multiple B complex vitamins and especially vitamin $B_1$ seem critical, although other nutritional deficiencies and direct toxic effects of alcohol may contribute to the neuropathy. Other toxic neuropathies to which the alcoholic patient is likely to be exposed must also be considered. These include lead, triorthocresyl phosphate from drinking illicit liquor, and disulfiram (Antabuse), which is used in rehabilitation of alcoholics.

The neuropathy is symmetric, distal, and predominantly sensory. Painful hypersensitivity of the feet to contact is common. In severe cases there is weakness of the distal parts of the limbs. Pressure palsies are often superimposed, causing footdrop or wristdrop unilaterally or bilaterally. Proximal neuropathy manifest by hoarseness, dysphagia, and postural hypotension has been rarely described. Cerebellar ataxia and Wernicke-Korsakoff's syndrome often accompany the neuropathy.

Abstinence from alcohol, supplementation with B-complex vitamins, and a well-balanced diet are essential and lead to gradual improvement of the neuropathy. Superimposed pressure palsies in the care of bedridden or restrained patients should be assiduously avoided.

**Table 103-4.** Sources and modes of exposure to heavy metals

| Occupational | Abuse/accidental |
|---|---|
| **Lead** | |
| Use of lead-based paint in automobile industry; manufacture of storage batteries and printing | Drinking of bootleg whiskey distilled in lead-containing pipes; burning of batteries as cheap fuel; hand mixing of lead-based paints by artists |
| **Arsenic** | |
| Exposure in farming to arsenic-containing sprays, pesticides, weed killers | Accidental ingestion of arsenic-containing rodenticides such as Antrol, Paris Green, Rat-Doom; rare source is old medicinal solutions such as Fowler's; still occasionally abused for suicidal and homicidal purposes |
| **Thallium** | |
| Manufacture of optic glass, prisms, industrial diamonds, fuel additive in internal combustion engines | Accidental ingestion still occurs from thallium-containing rodenticides such as Gizmo mouse killer, Zelio paste, etc. |

### Polyneuropathy of AIDS

With the AIDS epidemic, HIV-1 infection has rapidly become the leading cause of chronic polyneuropathy in young adults. The pathogenesis of this predominantly axonal neuropathy is not established but appears to be parainfectious rather than directly related to HIV-1 infection. It appears in the advanced phase of immunodeficiency with prominent pain and intolerable dysesthetic sensations aggravated by standing, walking, and pressure. The course is indolently progressive but may stabilize after months. Treatment remains symptomatic, and many patients require long-term narcotic analgesics to alleviate the neuropathic pain. Various other neuropathic syndromes have been described in association with HIV-1 infection (see the box on p. 1429).

### Inherited polyneuropathies

The inherited polyneuropathies are a large group of a bewildering variety of disorders that have not yet been satisfactorily classified. Recent studies of polyneuropathies of obscure cause have shown that nearly half of them are eventually found to be inherited forms.

The following is a partial categorization that provides a clinical approach to these neuropathies.

***Group A.*** Polyneuropathy is the cardinal feature. Systemic examination is normal except for pes cavus, hammertoes, or kyphoscoliosis, and no biochemical lesion can be identified. The nomenclature and identification of

### Peripheral neuropathies of AIDS

- Mononeuropathies
  - Bell's palsy
  - Peroneal nerve palsy
- Lumbosacral radiculopathy: cauda equina syndrome
  - Cytomegalovirus radiculitis
  - Cryptococcosis, tuberculosis, syphilis
- Mononeuritis multiplex
- Generalized symmetric polyneuropathies
  - Acute Guillain-Barré syndrome
  - Chronic inflammatory demyelinating polyneuropathy (CIDP)
  - Chronic polyneuropathies
    - AIDS-related painful neuropathies
    - Drug-induced neuropathy (e.g., ddI, ddC, vincristine)
- Autonomic neuropathy

the different entities under this group have been a source of much confusion because the clinical expression of the disease can vary greatly within a family, there is no specific clinical or biochemical marker, and authors have not used universal criteria. The Mayo Clinic classification attempts to bring some order but is still imperfect.

**Hereditary motor neuropathy (peroneal muscular atrophy, progressive muscular atrophy, Charcot-Marie-Tooth disease).** This autosomal recessively inherited neuropathy causes wasting and weakness chiefly in the feet and legs and later in the hands without sensory changes, causes little disability, and is associated with a normal life expectancy.

**Hereditary sensory neuropathy (HSN)**

***HSN type I (hereditary sensory neuropathy of Denny-Brown, dominantly inherited sensory neuropathy).*** HSN type I is autosomal dominantly inherited and presents in the second and third decade of life with painless foot ulcers and distal dissociated sensory loss. With good preventive care, life expectancy can be normal.

***HSN type II (congenital sensory neuropathy, recessive hereditary sensory neuropathy).*** HSN type II is a rare autosomal recessively inherited neuropathy that presents with mutilation of feet and hands from loss of all modalities of sensation and is established by the first decade.

***HSN type III (Riley-Day syndrome, familial dysautonomia).*** HSN type III is a rare autosomal recessively inherited neuropathy that affects Ashkanazi Jews and appears in infancy with autonomic dysfunction in the form of labile blood pressure, labile sweating, and dissociated sensory loss.

***HSN type IV (congenital insensitivity to pain).*** HSN type IV is an exceedingly rare autosomal recessive disorder that causes dissociated sensory loss and mental retardation.

**Hereditary motor and sensory neuropathies (HMSN)**

***HMSN type I (dominant hypertrophic Charcot-Marie-Tooth disease, Roussy-Lévy syndrome and peroneal muscular atrophy).*** Probably the most common of this group of inherited neuropathies, HMSN type I appears in the second or third decade with peroneal muscular atrophy, distal sensory impairment and enlarged peripheral nerves, and greatly slowed NCV. Most patients can lead active lives with a normal span.

***HMSN type II (peroneal muscular atrophy, neuronal Charcot-Marie-Tooth disease).*** HMSN type II is a rare disorder that is clinically similar to type I but does not have enlargement of peripheral nerves and the NCVs are only mildly prolonged.

***HMSN type III (Déjerine-Sottas disease, hypertrophic neuropathy of infancy).*** The characteristics of HMSN type III are similar to those of HMSN type I except it begins in infancy and patients are severely disabled by midlife.

Diagnosis of HSN and HMSN disorders may be easy when distinctive clinical features are present as in Riley-Day or Déjerine-Sottas disease. In others, nerve biopsies show hypertrophic neuropathy with onion-bulb formation (this is characteristic but *not* pathognomonic of inherited neuropathy). Careful clinical and electrophysiologic testing of family members for evidence of neuropathy, pes cavus, hammertoes, or kyphoscoliosis is essential. No specific treatment is available other than genetic counseling. However, in many of the common forms, symptomatic and supportive therapy for motor disabilities and insensitivity can enable patients to live active lives often with a normal life span.

*Group B.* Group B includes inherited neuropathies with which a specific biochemical lesion has been identified. The neuropathy, moreover, is part of a multisystem disorder. Most of these diseases are inherited by autosomal recessive mode through sex-linked recessive inheritance, as occurs in Fabry's disease and adrenomyeloneuropathy. This group of diseases, although rare, is of exceptional significance because biochemical manipulations of therapeutic benefit are already known for some and others are likely to develop in the near future.

**Refsum disease.** A nonspecific sensorimotor polyneuropathy, Refsum disease appears in the second to fourth decades, is sometimes associated with enlarged nerves, and follows a chronic or relapsing course over years. Bilateral nerve deafness, retinitis pigmentosa, ichthyosis, corneal and lens opacities, cardiomyopathy, and epiphyseal dysplasia complete the picture, although only retinitis pigmentosa invariably occurs. Diagnosis is established by the finding of elevated levels of serum phytanic acid. Lowering of the phytanic acid content of blood and tissues by long-term low–phytanic acid diet perhaps combined with plasmapheresis is of major benefit for the disease, including neuropathy.

**Bassen-Kornzweig disease.** A chronic sensorimotor polyneuropathy associated with ataxia, Bassen-Kornzweig disease begins in childhood or adolescence and is preceded by steatorrhea in infancy. Retinitis pigmentosa is universal. Plasma lipoprotein analysis shows the diagnostic abnormality of very low cholesterol and low triglycerides; betalipoprotein is absent. Another characteristic abnormality is the presence of spiculated red blood cells in peripheral blood (acanthrocytosis). A promising development has been the identification of severe deficiency of vitamins A and E in this condition. Treatment with large doses of these vitamins improves the neuropathy.

**Tangier disease.** The neuropathy of this rare disease is

clinically distinctive and resembles syringomyelia, with dissociated sensory loss for pain and temperature and segmental atrophy and areflexia that affect the face, upper extremities, and/or lower limbs. Eventually the whole body may be involved in the anesthesia. The telltale sign of this disease is the presence of unique orange discoloration and enlargement of the tonsils. Plasma lipoprotein analysis establishes the diagnosis by showing very low cholesterol levels combined with normal or high triglycerides and absence of alphalipoproteins.

**Fabry's disease.** Neuropathy of this extraordinary syndrome of boys is evident by curious and disabling episodes of pain in the extremities and abdomen with few signs on examination. The paroxysms of excruciating burning or lightninglike pains are often precipitated or aggravated by fever or hot weather. Progressive anhidrosis may occur. Clusters of dark-red punctate telangiectases around the umbilicus, buttocks, groin, knees, and elbows are diagnostic. Decreased activity of $\alpha$-galactosidase in serum or leukocytes or skin fibroblasts establishes the diagnosis. The enzyme deficiency leads to the tissue accumulation of the lipid ceramide. No specific treatment is yet available, but the disabling pain can be relieved or suppressed by diphenylhydantoin.

**Adrenomyeloneuropathy.** The spectrum of the sex-linked recessive adrenoleukodystrophy has been expanded to include patients with a chronic neuromyelopathic syndrome but without the cerebral manifestations. The neuropathy is chronic, symmetric, sensorimotor, and associated with spastic paraparesis (neuromyelopathy). Primary hypoadrenalism may be subclinical, and hypogonadism often accompanies this syndrome. The diagnosis is usually established by testicular or adrenal biopsy and less consistently by sural nerve or conjunctival biopsies, which show specific cytoplasmic inclusions on electron microscopy. The recent finding of marked increase in serum long-chain fatty acids seems to be a specific biochemical marker. It is not yet clear whether treatment of hypoadrenalism by steroids ameliorates the neuropathy. The role of bone marrow transplantation and efforts to decrease blood levels of long-chain fatty acids are currently being investigated.

**Metachromatic leukodystrophy.** Polyneuropathy is a universal feature of this disease but is overshadowed by cerebral dysfunction in most of the infantile and juvenile forms. The identification of metachromatic material in nerve biopsies and demonstration of deficiency of arylsulfatase A enzymes in serum, white blood cells, and skin fibroblasts establish the diagnosis. Unfortunately, no effective treatment is available.

## NEUROPATHIC PAIN SYNDROMES

Neuropathic pain syndromes are a group of syndromes in which chronic intense pain is the outstanding manifestation. The pain arises from injury to one or more nerves such as the trigeminal, glossopharyngeal, intercostal, or any limb nerve. In some patients the cause of the nerve injury is clear, such as infection by herpes zoster virus, herpetic neuralgia, or a partial injury to a major nerve trunk in causalgia. In others, such as tic douloureux, the etiology is obscure. Diagnosis rests chiefly on the characteristic features of the pain itself, and therefore these conditions are often misdiagnosed. The treatment of these disorders is challenging and difficult, but considerable advances have recently been made.

### Causalgia

Causalgia is one of the most dramatic chronic pain syndromes in medical practice. It occurs most often from partial injury to major nerve trunks, especially of the sciatic and median nerves and the lower and medial cords of the brachial plexus. Most cases are the result of high-velocity missile injuries of wartime, but knife and gunshot wounds of civilian life can produce the same syndrome. The pathogenesis is not well understood, although it is clear that regional sympathetic neural dysfunction plays a major role.

The clinical picture is unique and dominated by pain of burning quality felt diffusely in the limb with the injured nerve. This pain is spontaneous, continuous, excruciating, and characteristically intensified by emotional upset, light touch, exposure to cold, manipulation of the limb, or even by noise. Patients often go to extraordinary lengths to protect the limb and resent physical examination. The deterioration of behavior secondary to chronic intense pain often leads to a psychiatric diagnosis. The skin of the affected part is shiny, moist, either warm or cool, and often edematous. Enforced immobility often leads to contracture. Light touch and pinprick may induce excruciating diffuse pain, but proper neurologic examination other than the observation of any obvious weakness and atrophy may be impossible.

The diagnosis is clinical. In most cases the syndrome resolves spontaneously in 6 months to a year but occasionally persists for several years.

The treatment of this disorder is truly difficult. Simple analgesics are ineffective. Narcotic drugs may relieve the pain temporarily but should not be used for more than a few weeks. A variety of other measures are available and need to be tried step by step. The principal aim is to suppress the pain and begin exercising the limb so that no permanent changes occur from disuse. TENS of the nerve trunk proximal to injury is a simple, safe, and sometimes remarkably effective method. Sympathectomy is undoubtedly the most consistently effective measure and should be done as early as possible to avoid the sequelae of causalgia. A sympathetic block is first performed, with local anesthetic aimed at the stellate ganglia for upper extremity and lumbar ganglia for lower limb causalgia. Repeated injections occasionally may be sufficient. In many cases, surgical sympathectomy is needed. Physical therapy is of the utmost importance; it should be instituted from the earliest stage and pursued with perseverance by an increasingly vigorous program of massage, range of movement, and active exercises. Squeezing a ball of putty is a helpful way of encouraging active exercises for the hand.

#### Minor causalgia and reflex sympathetic dystrophy

These are much more common in civilian practice than full-blown causalgia. Minor causalgia refers specifically to the syndrome associated with a nerve injury and, while a reflex sympathetic dystrophy is a similar syndrome that results from soft tissue injury to the limb such as a sprain or fracture, there is no particular affliction of the nerve.

The predominant symptom is burning pain in the

distribution of the injured nerve. The nerve injury itself is often trivial, such as mild ulnar compression caused by improper positioning of the arm under general anesthesia. Compared with causalgia, the pain is less profound and less intensified by various emotional, tactile, and temperature stimuli. The affected limb shows signs of partial nerve injury. In addition, there is sympathetic dysfunction seen as reddened, smooth, shiny skin with excessive sweating and marked increase of pain by manipulation of the limb. Reflex sympathetic dystrophy shows similar features but without neurologic deficit.

The diagnosis is again clinical. The pain is distressing, lasts a few weeks to a few months, and impedes rehabilitation of the limb. Narcotic drugs are avoided. TENS has proved effective in many instances and may be sufficient. In some, carbamazepine significantly ameliorates the pain. When these conservative measures fail, sympathectomy is consistently effective. Recently regional postganglionic sympathetic blockade has been used effectively by an IV technique identical to that commonly used for anesthesia. Both IV guanethidine and reserpine have been used with success. On occasion, patients have responded to oral propranolol. Vigorous physical therapy is important.

***Trigeminal neuralgia.*** Trigeminal neuralgia is described in Chapter 95.

***Glossopharyngeal neuralgia.*** Glossopharyngeal neuralgia is described in Chapter 95.

***Postherpetic neuralgia.*** The pain of acute herpes zoster usually subsides in a few weeks. In about half the patients over age 60 years, a prolonged, persistent painful state appears in the wake of zoster. The pain is felt in the dermatomal distribution of the affected nerve root. Herpes zoster ophthalmicus and zoster of the upper thoracic roots are the most common sites for the development of neuralgia. The pain is spontaneous, continuous, and burning with paroxysms of stabbing pain superimposed. The affected skin may be hyperesthetic to touch or the friction of clothes. Many patients become insomniac and depressed and may contemplate suicide.

Because elderly persons are at such a high risk for this distressing complication, attempts are being made to *prevent* its emergence. A 3-week course of oral steroid therapy may decrease this risk and is indicated in selected patients without malignancies, immune deficiency, severe diabetes, or active peptic ulcer disease. There is evidence that treating acute zoster with the antiviral drugs acyclovir or famciclovir decreases postherpetic neuralgia.

There is no single consistently effective therapy for established postherpetic neuralgia. Use of different methods and combinations tailored to individual patient requirements with realistic expectation of alleviation but not abolition of pain is necessary. TENS is simple and effective in some patients. Local injection of corticosteroids subcutaneously in the area of zoster is helpful. When local measures fail, the most consistently useful medical therapy is the use of tricyclic antidepressant drugs such as amitriptyline beginning in small doses. If not sufficient by itself, it may be combined in disabling cases with fluphenazine, carbamazepine, and phenytoin. These drugs are very useful in trigeminal neuropathy but are of little benefit for postherpetic neuralgia by themselves, although they may be useful in combination with tricyclic drugs.

Throughout the illness, one should provide psychologic support, be aware of suicidal potential, and reassure the patient that eventually the pain will resolve.

## BIBLIOGRAPHY


Barohn RJ et al: Chronic inflammatory demyelinating polyradiculoneuropathy: clinical features, course and prognosis, *Arch Neurol* 46:878, 1989.

Dyck PJ et al: *Peripheral neuropathy,* ed 3, Philadelphia, 1993, WB Saunders.

Leger JM et al: The spectrum of polyneuropathies in patients infected with HIV, *J Neurol Neurosurg Psychiatry* 52:1369, 1989.

Limpton RB et al: Taxol produces a predominantly sensory neuropathy, *Neurology* 39:368, 1989.

Maciewicz R, Bouctoma A, Martin JB: Drug therapy of neuropathic pain, *Clin J Pain* 1:39, 1985.

McKhann GM: Guillain-Barré syndrome: clinical and therapeutic observations, *Ann Neurol* 27(suppl):513, 1990.

Miller RG, Storey JR, Greco CM: Gancyclovir in the treatment of progressive AIDS-related polyradiculopathy, *Neurology* 40:569, 1990.

Pachner AR, Steeve AC: The triad of neurological manifestations of Lyme disease, meningitis, cranial neuritis and radiculoneuritis, *Neurology* 35:47, 1985.

Pestronk A et al: A treatable multifocal motor neuropathy with antibodies to GM1 ganglioside, *Ann Neurol* 24:73, 1988.

Sabin TD, Geschwind N, Waxman SG: Patterns of clinical deficits in peripheral nerve disease. In Waxman SG, editor: *Physiology and pathology of axons,* New York, 1978, Raven Press.

Schwartzman RJ, McLellan TL: Reflex sympathetic dystrophy: a review, *Arch Neurol* 44:555, 1987.

Sun SF, Sterib EW: Diabetic thoracoabdominal neuropathy: clinical and electrodiagnostic features, *Ann Neurol* 9:75, 1981.

Zochodone DW et al: Critical illness polyneuropathy: a complication of sepsis and multiple organ failure, *Brain* 110:819, 1987.


CHAPTER

# 104 Diseases of the Spinal Cord

**Jeremy D. Schmahmann**

## CLINICAL ANATOMY OF THE SPINAL CORD

The central nervous system (CNS) continues within the spinal canal as the spinal cord, which reaches from the caudal end of the medulla oblongata in the foramen magnum to a level corresponding to the first or second lumbar vertebra in adults. In children the cord may extend to as low as the fourth lumbar vertebra. The spinal cord is divided into segments according to the paired nerve roots that exit from each level and comprises eight cervical (C1 to C8), 12 thoracic (T1 to T12), five lumbar (L1 to L5), and five sacral roots (S1 to S5), as well as some vestigial coccygeal roots. The tapered terminal end, the conus medullaris, has an anatomic organization sufficiently different from the remainder of the cord that it is associated with distinct clinical syndromes. The exiting nerve roots traverse the appropriate intervertebral foramina to reach their destination, and because the spinal cord is shorter than the spinal canal, the roots exit their segment of the cord at levels different from the corresponding vertebral level (Fig. 104-1). The roots that leave the lower spinal cord have a longer intraspinal course than those at more rostral levels. The lumbar and sacral nerve roots make up the cauda equina, which is formed below the conus medullaris, and travel some distance before exiting through the vertebral neural foramina.

The spinal cord is maintained in a relatively stable position by the filum terminale, which attaches the conus medullaris to the lowest reaches of the spinal canal, and by the dentate ligaments, which attach the lateral aspects of each spinal cord segment to the dura. As with the cerebral hemispheres, the cord is invested by pia mater and is separated from the arachnoid by the circulating cerebrospinal fluid (CSF). A potential space exists between the arachnoid and dura mater. A layer of fatty areolar tissue and the internal vertebral venous plexus occupy the epidural space between the spinal dura and the vertebral periosteum.

The blood supply of the spinal cord (Fig. 104-2) is derived from multiple sources: cervical levels from the vertebrobasilar system and branches of the subclavian arteries, thoracic and lumbar segments from radicular branches of the aorta, and sacral divisions from the internal iliac arteries. Certain regions of the spinal cord are particularly vulnerable to ischemia because vascular border zones exist in the cord, just as they do in the cerebral hemispheres.

The spinal cord contains neurons and fiber tracts (Fig. 104-3). Neurons occupy the gray matter in the middle of the cord, grouped into anatomically and functionally organized nuclei lying within 10 cell layers, or laminae. Anterior horn cells, the motor neurons of the peripheral nervous system (lower motor neurons), lie within the ventral half (ventral horn) of the gray matter zone, mostly in lamina IX. Internuncial neurons, which receive most of the descending motor impulses from the cerebral hemispheres before passing the information to the anterior horn cells, lie within the central region of the gray matter in laminae V to VII. Sensory neurons, including the pain-recipient zone (substantia gelatinosa, lamina II), lie within the posterior horn of the gray matter (laminae I to V).

Numerous tracts ascend and descend in the spinal cord. Those tracts important for understanding most clinical situations are readily identifiable and their properties reasonably well appreciated. Ascending systems immediately relevant for clinical purposes are the spinothalamic tracts, posterior columns, and spinocerebellar tracts. The spinothalamic tracts convey information concerning pain, temperature, and pin sense. Laterally situated afferents within the dorsal root ramify within one to three segments of the cord in Lissauer's tract and terminate mostly on neurons in the substantia gelatinosa of the dorsal gray zone. Axons from these neurons then cross to the other side of the cord, passing anterior and adjacent to the central canal, and form the spinothalamic tracts, which are laminated; the sacral segments are found externally and more rostral segments internally. The spinothalamic tracts terminate within the thalamus. Medially situated dorsal nerve root axons enter the ipsilateral dorsal columns

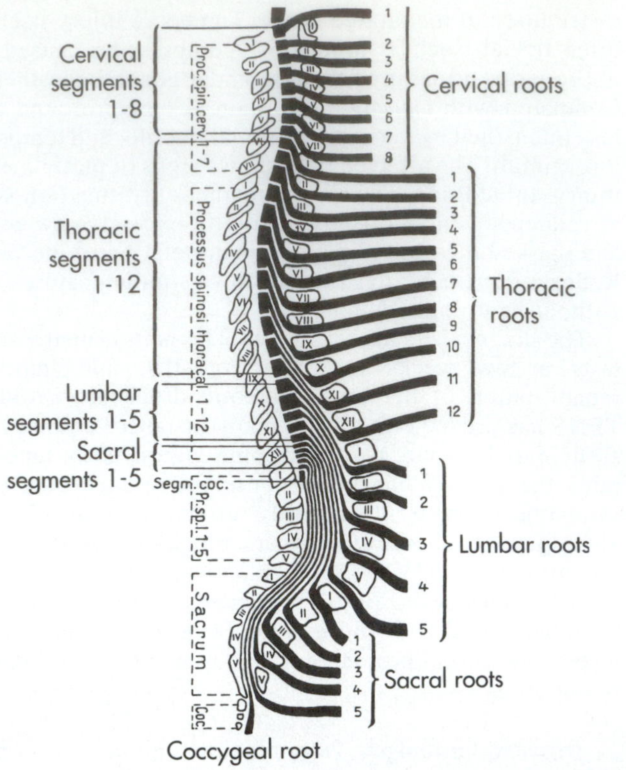


**Fig. 104-1.** Relative positions of the spinal cord and cauda equina with respect to the vertebral column are represented, as well as the relationships between the nerve roots and the foramina through which they exit the spinal canal. The original drawing showing this relationship was by Gowers in 1880. (From Haymaker W, editor: *Bing's local diagnosis in neurologic diseases,* ed 15, St Louis, 1969, Mosby.)

directly or indirectly after synapsing on neurons in the dorsal horn. The dorsal columns convey touch, position, and vibratory information to the ipsilateral cuneate and gracile nuclei in the medulla. Axons from these nuclei cross in the medial lemniscus to end on neurons in the contralateral thalamus. The sensory afferents in the gray matter of the cord are intricately arranged and are important for the appreciation and modulation of pain at the spinal cord level. Spinocerebellar tracts, some crossed and others not, lie most laterally within the cord and convey proprioceptive and kinesthetic information from the trunk and extremities to the cerebellum.

The descending spinal tract of most immediate clinical significance is the corticospinal tract, which decussates at the cervicomedullary junction and carries motor impulses from the opposite cerebral hemisphere to the spinal cord. Disruption of this tract results in the upper motor neuron syndrome described in the next section. Other descending motor pathways are relevant to spinal cord physiology and perhaps for recovery of function after brain and spinal cord injury, including the rubrospinal, vestibulospinal, reticulospinal, and interstitiospinal tracts. The clinical results of disruption of these pathways in the spinal cord are not well established.

Descending autonomic pathways control bladder, bowel, and sexual function as well as blood vessel and sweat

A
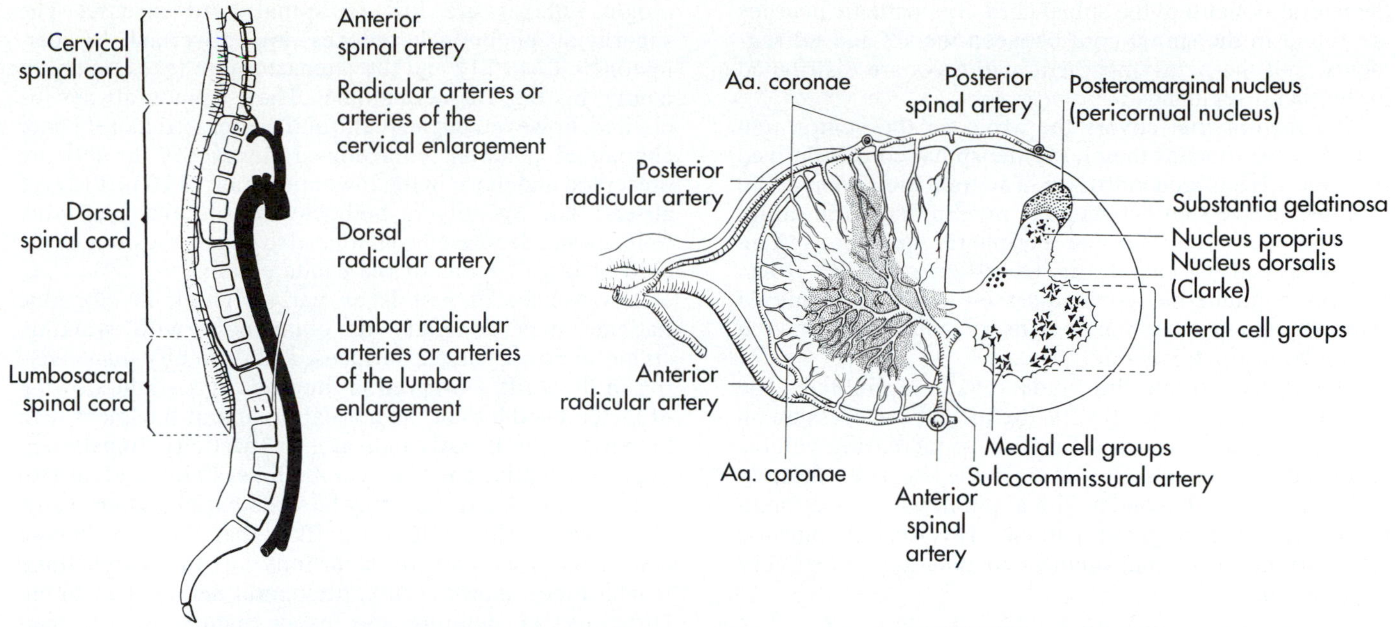

B

**Fig. 104-2.** **A,** Principal sources of the blood supply to different levels of the spinal cord. Arteries from the iliac vessels to the sacral cord are not shown here. The border zones lie at the junctions of the different territories. **B,** Arterial supply of the cord as seen in cross section reveals the single anterior spinal artery, dual posterior spinal arteries, and the plexus of vessels encircling the cord (perimedullary or coronal vessels). The major nuclear groups within the gray matter are seen on the right. (**A** from Lazorethes G et al: *Neuro-Chirurgie* 4:3, 1958; **B** from Haymaker W, editor: *Bing's local diagnosis in neurologic diseases,* ed 14, St Louis, 1956, Mosby.)

A
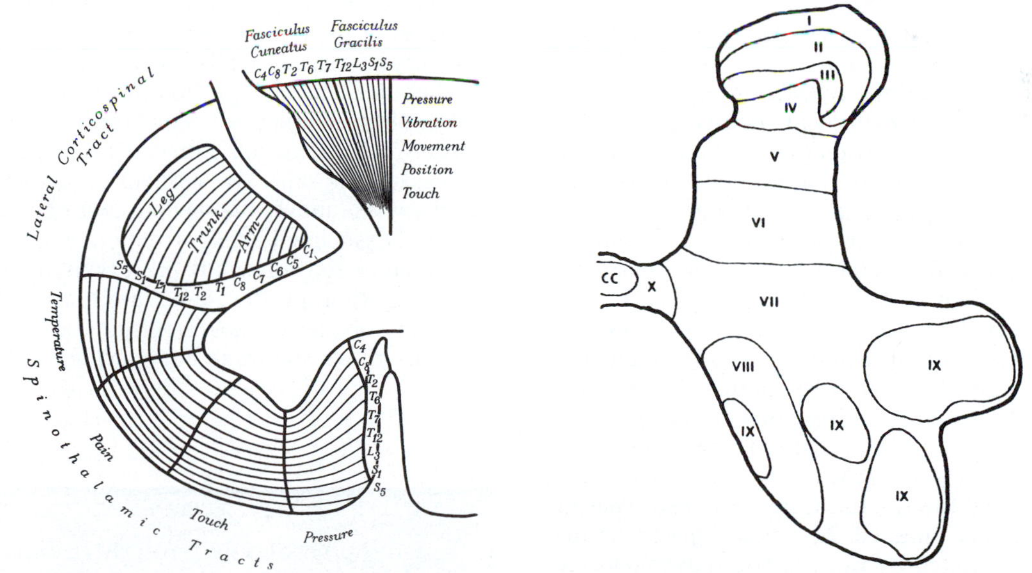

B

**Fig. 104-3.** **A,** Cervical-to-sacral lamination of the major tracts relevant for clinical purposes. Note that the sacral and lower extremity regions are represented laterally in the spinothalamic and corticospinal tracts but are found medially in the posterior columns. **B,** Gray matter of the cord was subdivided on anatomic grounds into 10 layers, or lamellae, by Rexed in 1952, as shown here. Each lamella has identified physiologic, functional, and connectional properties (see text). (**A** from Williams PL, Warwick R, editors: *Gray's anatomy,* ed 36, New York, 1980, Churchill Livingstone; **B** from Woolsey RM, Young RR: *Neurol Clin* 9:535, 1991.)

gland reactivity. These tracts are loosely distributed within the lateral funiculi of the spinal cord. Sympathetic neurons are found in the spinal cord between the C8 and L2 segments, and the parasympathetic pathways are distributed in the sacral segments.

The myelin that covers the axons in the ventral and dorsal nerve roots as they leave the spinal cord is derived from the CNS oligodendrocyte. The transition point at the proximal nerve root between the myelin of central origin and that derived from the peripheral nervous system Schwann cell is called the Obersteiner-Redlich zone. Certain immune-mediated diseases such as multiple sclerosis and paraneoplastic sensory neuropathy have a predilection for this site.

The space within the spinal canal is limited. The pressure-volume curve, that is, the increase in pressure on a spinal cord segment as a function of increasing volume produced by a compressive lesion at the site, rises abruptly and dramatically beyond a critical point, which is difficult to predict in any given patient. This has therapeutic implications in the management of potential spinal cord compression.

## IMPORTANT CLINICAL MANIFESTATIONS

Diseases of the spinal cord affect motor, sensory, and autonomic functions; reflex changes are detected on examination; and patients may be afflicted with pain. If one is aware of where the major spinal pathways decussate, how to differentiate upper from lower motor neuron lesions, and what is the pattern of abnormalities in a given patient, it is a relatively straightforward matter to make an accurate anatomic diagnosis at the bedside and to delineate a narrow differential diagnosis that can be tested with a limited set of special investigations.

### Lower motor neuron syndrome

Lesions affecting the anterior horn cells produce the lower motor neuron syndrome, characterized by weakness, diminished tone, fasciculations at rest, atrophy, and loss of deep tendon reflexes. The pattern of involvement of the affected muscles is a major component of the anatomic localization of the lesion in focal myelopathies or radiculopathies. Lesions affecting the descending motor pathways but not the anterior horn cells, in contrast, produce weakness with increased tone or spasticity, minimal atrophy (if at all), and exaggeration of deep tendon reflexes with extensor plantar responses. In addition, various release phenomena occur, including spread of reflexes from one joint to another, Hoffmann's sign, and crossed adductor reflexes. Flexor spasms are a peculiar feature of involvement of the descending spinal pathways, characterized by prominent, tonic, and often painful flexion of the lower extremities. Extensor spasms are less frequently encountered. Myoclonic spasms of the limbs can be precipitated by even subtle movement, are often distressing, and interfere with attempted ambulation when the spinal lesion is subtotal.

### High cervical myelopathy

A critical feature differentiating high cervical myelopathy from lesions of the brain or brainstem above the level of the fifth nerve nucleus is the preservation of the normal jaw jerk reflex in myelopathy, as well as heightening of this reflex in lesions above the midpons. Several physiologic reflexes are lost in spinal cord disease. The superficial abdominal reflexes are governed by dermatomes T7 to T12 and the cremasteric reflexes predominantly by the L1 dermatome. They cannot always be elicited, however, but are helpful if asymmetric, or if upper abdominal quadrant cutaneous reflexes (T7 to T9) are preserved and those in the lower quadrant (T10 to T12) are absent. The loss of the bulbocavernosus and anal wink reflexes and decreased anal tone also suggest lesions of the cord or large lesions of the cauda equina.

Disturbance of gait is an early sign in myelopathy. Patients may complain of clumsiness with walking, stumbling over uneven surfaces, and difficulty maneuvering in the dark. Observation may reveal a slight slowing of the gait and loss of the normal flexion of the knees with locomotion as an early indicator of spasticity. Impairment of proprioceptive and spinocerebellar systems leads also to a clumsiness of gait that may be wide based and unsteady. The myelopathy gait is unlike that of the classic disturbances arising from lesions of the cerebellum, frontal lobes, motor cortex, peripheral nerves, and so on. Difficulty in defining the exact nature of the gait disturbance should alert the clinician to the possibility of a spinal cord disorder.

### Pattern of sensory loss

Certain patterns of sensory loss strongly implicate the spinal cord (see the box below). A distinct sensory level on the trunk is essentially diagnostic of a myelopathy. It is often too late to save the acutely compressed spinal cord by the time the sensory loss has become complete, and thus it is worth looking for the subtle changes that are the harbinger of such a development. Mild discrepancies in appreciation of sensation on the trunk, loss of vibration sense (but normal pin sense) at the vertebral spines below the level of the lesion, and a gradient on the trunk to any modality of sensation, all may be indicative of an incipient myelopathy. The change from normal to abnormal sensation on the trunk may not occur abruptly, and there is often a transition zone of either diminished sensation or increased pin sense (hyperpathia) between the normal dermatomes above the lesion and the affected region below. Dissociated sensory deficit with loss of pin and temperature sensation but preservation of vibration and proprioception in the same area usually indicates an intrinsic cord lesion. Loss of spinothalamic sensation in the extremities and trunk but sparing of the saddle region

#### Sensory phenomena strongly indicating spinal cord disease

Sensory level on the trunk
Dissociated sensory loss
Sacral sparing
Brown-Séquard pattern
Suspended band of bilateral spinothalamic sensory loss

compose the clinical scenario of sacral sparing, implying also an intrinsic cord lesion sparing the laterally placed sacral fibers in the spinothalamic tracts. The classic Brown-Séquard syndrome caused by hemisection or asymmetric extrinsic compression of the spinal cord produces ipsilateral upper motor neuron signs and loss of vibration and position sense, with contralateral loss of pin and temperature appreciation. Early lesions of the cord and some metabolic derangements such as pernicious anemia may present only with subjective complaints of burning, sometimes intense paresthesias, and difficulty with urination and gait. Even advanced chronic compressive myelopathies, such as cervical spondylotic myelopathy, may not have convincing sensory abnormalities on examination until well into the late stages despite the patient's complaints of paresthesias. The central cord syndrome, resulting most often from hemorrhage within the cervical cord, is a peculiar entity because it seems at first to be counterintuitive, the arms being weaker than the legs; however, the clinical-anatomic basis is sound. Trauma to the anterior horn cells and disruption of the crossing spinothalamic fibers produce lower motor weakness and a suspended band of spinothalamic sensory loss to the modalities of pin and temperature sense at the level of the lesion (usually the arms). Relative sparing of the white matter tracts, however, means that leg strength and sensation are spared.

### Cord transection

Complete acute transections cause spinal shock with flaccid paralysis, areflexia, sensory loss, and autonomic dysfunction at and below the level of the lesion. Sphincters are contracted because of loss of descending inhibitory control, and constipation and urinary retention with overflow incontinence result. Gastric dilatation, ileus, and systemic hypotension can be life-threatening. Disturbance of cutaneous integrity results from immobility and loss of autonomic regulation, and pressure necrosis and infection can set in rapidly. Transection above the C3 level paralyzes all muscles of respiration and without ventilatory support is not compatible with life. Spinal shock can persist for 1 to 6 weeks before maturing into a chronic myelopathy. Some patients with a nonpenetrating injury and a clinical picture consistent with spinal shock recover fully within days. This reversible entity of spinal concussion is not well understood.

### Pattern of motor loss

Chronic lesions below the T1 segment cause leg weakness of upper motor neuron type and variable involvement of the trunk muscles, depending on the level of the lesion. Spinal injury at the C5 to T1 region causes lower motor neuron weakness at the level of the lesion and upper motor neuron weakness below. Signs may ascend proximally over time with a single thoracic or cervical lesion by virtue of lamination of the fiber tracts within the cord, and this clinical progression does not necessarily signify the presence of new or separate lesions. Sexual dysfunction varies according to the site and severity of the lesion but is often impaired to some extent. Autonomic dysreflexia refers to the constellation of hypertension, bradycardia or tachycardia, sweating and flushing above the level of the lesion, pounding headache, and often painful muscle spasms precipitated in patients with spinal injury by mildly noxious stimuli, including infections. The mass action reflex affects regions below the level of the lesion, is essentially an exaggerated withdrawal reflex, and consists of flexor spasms, sweating, piloerection, and emptying of bowel and bladder. It can be precipitated by mildly noxious stimuli or intercurrent infections.

### Horner's syndrome

A Horner's syndrome may result from damage to the sympathetic neurons of the intermediolateral cell column in the C8 to T1 levels of the spinal cord (see the box below). Ipsilateral meiosis, anhidrosis, and ptosis can occur as a result of lesions of many different sites along the course of the sympathetic chain (including the cervical plexus, carotid plexus, lateral medulla, hypothalamus), so the associated signs and symptoms are important in establishing the correct anatomic diagnosis.

### Pain in spinal cord disease

The presence and nature of pain in spinal cord disease can be helpful in suspecting and arriving at the correct diagnosis (Table 104-1). Localized back pain is an essential clue in the diagnosis of metastatic or infectious disease of the spinal column. Local pain in the spine with radiation of the pain anteriorly to the abdomen is a common complaint in patients with transverse myelitis.

#### Horner's syndrome

Meiosis: Small pupil
Ptosis: Drooping upper lid
Anhydrosis: Diminished sweating on same side of face
Enophthalmos: Eye appears slightly sunken into orbit

**Table 104-1.** Patterns of pain in spinal cord disorders

| Disorder | Cause |
|---|---|
| Localized back pain | Epidural tumor or abscess, diskitis |
| Back pain radiating anteriorly to abdomen | Transverse myelitis |
| Back pain radiating around abdomen | Dorsal root lesions (syphilis, multiple sclerosis, varicella, diabetes) |
| Leg pain with walking, relieved by rest and forward flexion, but normal pedal pulses | Spinal stenosis |
| Lhermitte's sign | Cervical spondylotic or other compressive myelopathy, multiple sclerosis |
| Intense foot paresthesias | Vitamin $B_{12}$ deficiency myelopathy and/or neuropathy |

Pain that radiates around the abdomen or chest in a bandlike distribution is encountered in diseases that affect the dorsal nerve root, including syphilis, multiple sclerosis, diabetes, and herpes zoster. Epidural masses also produce nerve root symptoms with pain, burning paresthesias, and shooting pain that radiates down an arm or leg or around the abdomen and is worsened by coughing or sneezing. Localized back pain that is worsened by lying and relieved by sitting or standing is encountered in patients with tumors arising within the spinal cord. Pain and weakness in the legs with exertion may represent neurogenic claudication accompanying spinal stenosis. The Lhermitte's sign, typically associated with multiple sclerosis but first described in the setting of cervical spondylotic myelopathy, is the "electric shock" paresthesia that shoots down the spine precipitated by flexion of the neck.

### Disorders mimicking myelopathy

Bilateral medial cerebral hemisphere convexity lesions (bilateral anterior cerebral artery infarction, giant anterior communicating artery aneurysm, falx cerebri meningioma)
Hydrocephalus
Foramen magnum tumors
Guillain-Barré syndrome
Proximal neuropathy (bilateral lumbosacral plexus lesions, as in diabetic amyotrophy)
Proximal myopathy (paraneoplastic, polymyositis, hypothyroidism, alcohol)
Conversion reaction/hysteria/malingering

## Conditions that can mimic spinal cord disease

Certain diseases and other anatomic sites in the nervous system can superficially mimic spinal cord patterns of involvement, although sometimes with surprising clinical overlap (see the box above). Bilateral lower extremity weakness, gait disturbance, and incontinence suggest spinal cord disease, but this may also be seen following bilateral medial convexity lesions of the cerebral hemispheres after anterior cerebral artery infarction, with compression by falx meningioma or giant anterior communicating artery aneurysm, and in hydrocephalus. The cerebral syndromes may have similar motor deficits, but the behavioral changes and the lack of appropriate sensory findings are ready distinguishing features. Primary muscle diseases and acute ascending polyneuropathy (Guillain-Barré syndrome) often present with leg weakness, but the clinical evolution and the peripheral nervous system features set them apart. Lumbosacral plexopathies such as diabetic amyotrophy cause leg weakness and sensory loss, but they are painful and asymmetric and characterized by lower motor neuron findings. Lesions of the foramen magnum produce myelopathy, but they are frequently accompanied by other signs, including lower cranial neuropathies, ataxia, nystagmus, and dysarthria. The exaggerated jaw jerk is a helpful sign in these patients, as already discussed. At the other end of the spinal canal, it is important to distinguish between lesions affecting the conus medullaris (truly a spinal cord syndrome) and those of the cauda equina (peripheral nervous system, outside the spinal cord but within the spinal canal). Conus medullaris lesions produce a mixed picture of upper and lower motor neuron signs within the limited theater of the lumbosacral nerve roots (Table 104-2). The pattern of involvement is usually bilateral. Strength is lost in both legs without a clearly discernible myotomal pattern. The deep tendon reflexes may be exaggerated or absent despite bilateral extensor plantar responses. Sensation is often impaired, not clearly corresponding to a dermatomal pattern. Integrity of bowel and bladder is compromised, and there may be urge incontinence suggesting an upper motor neuron bladder or overflow incontinence from a large, atonic, lower motor neuron bladder. Lesions of the cauda equina mimic the conus syndrome because there is weakness, sensory loss, areflexia, and sphincter disturbance. However, the cauda equina lesion is more often asymmetric and is not associated with extensor plantar responses, and the patterns of weakness and sensory loss more closely fit radicular patterns. When the sacral nerve roots are affected bilaterally, decreased anal tone and a lower motor neuron bladder develop (hypotonic, enlarged, with overflow incontinence).

**Table 104-2.** Differentiation of conus medullaris lesions from large cauda equina lesions, both of which produce leg weakness and sensory loss in legs and perineum

| | Conus medullaris | Cauda equina |
|---|---|---|
| Symmetry | + | − |
| Extensor plantar responses | + | − |
| Hyperreflexia | Variable | − |
| Incontinence | + | Variable |
| Dermatomal sensory loss | − | + |
| Myotomal pattern of weakness | − | + |

More than a few patients later proved to have myelopathy have been discharged home from emergency rooms with a diagnosis of conversion reaction, hysteria, malingering, and other psychiatric terminologies marshaled by stumped clinicians when the presentation does not seem to add up completely. The reason for this is apparent from the foregoing discussion. Myelopathy does not always present as expected. Odd peripheral paresthesias, an atypical gait that does not fit a clear pattern immediately recognized and vague complaints of trouble with bladder function are all that may be present in the early stages of cord compression, infection, or noninfectious myelitis. As long as one is aware of the subtleties involved in the presentation of early myelopathy, and if the level of suspicion for the diagnosis is raised on learning of such an array of complaints, the likelihood of missing the opportunity to save a patient's spinal cord is lessened.

**Table 104-3.** Classification of spinal cord disorders

| Category | Cause |
|---|---|
| Congenital | Friedreich's ataxia and spinocerebellar degenerations |
| | Diastematomyelia |
| | Tethered cord |
| | Spina bifida |
| | Craniocervical junction anomalies (Klippel-Feil syndrome, Morquio syndrome) |
| | Inherited metabolic diseases (adrenoleukomyeloneuropathy) |
| | Klippel-Trenaunay-Weber syndrome |
| Traumatic | Gunshot wounds |
| | Penetrating stab wounds |
| | Blunt trauma (including falls) with or without spinal fractures |
| | Hematomyelia |
| | Post–spinal tap epidural hematoma |
| Infectious | Bacterial: epidural abscess, endocarditis |
| | Viral*: HIV, HAM-TSP, CMV, HSV, VZ, LCM, polio |
| | Spirochetal: syphilis, Lyme disease |
| | Mycobacterial: tuberculosis (Pott disease) |
| | Fungal: cryptococcosis, histoplasmosis, coccidioidomycosis, blastomycosis, aspergillosis |
| | Parasitic: schistosomiasis, hydatid disease, paragonimiasis |
| | Protozoal: toxoplasmosis |
| Neoplastic: | Benign: schwannoma, meningioma, neurofibroma, neurilemoma, chordoma, lipoma |
| | Malignant |
| | Intramedullary: primary—astrocytoma, ependymoma, oligodendroglioma, melanoma |
| | Intradural extramedullary: secondary—astrocytoma, meningeal carcinomatosis (e.g., lymphoma, breast) |
| | Extradural: invasive (sarcoma of bone/muscle, eosinophilic granuloma, myeloma), metastatic (colon, breast, lung, prostate) |
| | Paraneoplastic: myelopathy, motor neuron disease |
| Acquired metabolic toxic | Vitamin $B_{12}$ deficiency |
| | Clioquinol: subacute myeloopticoneuropathy (SMON) |
| | Organic solvents (*n*-hexane, benzene derivatives) |
| | Carbon disulfide |
| | Lathyrism |
| | Intrathecal drugs (e.g., methotrexate) |
| | Radiographic contrast agents |
| | Chymopapain |

*See text for viral abbreviations.

*Continued.*

## DIFFERENTIAL DIAGNOSIS

The history of the patient's symptoms leads to consideration of the appropriate category of illness to be considered. A systematic review is helpful in organizing the approach to diagnosis, and Table 104-3 lists many of the major causes of spinal cord disease.

### Congenital and inherited diseases

Various congenital myelopathies have their first clinical presentation in childhood or early adulthood, often with orthopedic difficulties (see the box on p. 1438). Friedreich's ataxia, for example, is inherited in an autosomal recessive or autosomal dominant pattern and manifests in the teenage years with symptoms and signs attributable to the cerebellar system (ataxia, clumsiness). Examination further reveals extensor plantar responses, variable or absent deep tendon reflexes, and loss of posterior column sensation initially in the legs. Weakness and atrophy of the extremities accompany the progressive, debilitating disorder, and patients do not often survive beyond the third decade. Musculoskeletal deformities include kyphoscoliosis and pes cavus. Cardiac arrhythmias are common and account for death in many instances. The slow onset and gradually progressive course, positive family history, and associated findings are all central to the diagnosis. The spinal cord is involved in other predominantly ataxic inherited disorders, and weakness, exaggerated deep tendon reflexes, and extensor plantar responses are seen in adults as part of the late-onset spinocerebellar degenerations.

The presence of a persistent bony spur in the spinal canal during development impinges on and disrupts the caudal aspect of the elongating spinal cord (diastematomyelia). In childhood and teenage years, patients present with what are often misinterpreted as orthopedic problems of the feet, including pes cavus and high arches, and there may be evidence of upper motor neuron signs in the legs and a hyperactive bladder. A related condition is tethered spinal cord, which may occur concomitantly with other conditions such as diastematomyelia or spina bifida or as an isolated phenomenon. The filum terminale is shortened, and the spinal cord extends as low as the L5 vertebral level in the adult. One of my patients had several corrective

**Table 104-3.** Classification of spinal cord disorders—cont'd

| Category | Cause |
|---|---|
| Vascular | Infarction |
| | Border zone infarct in global hypoperfusion |
| | Compression or obstruction of aorta |
| | Atherosclerosis at ostium of radicular arteries |
| | Embolism: from aorta, endocarditis, disk embolism |
| | Extrinsic compression (in pachymeningitis) |
| | Vasculitis: systemic lupus erythematosus, Wegener's granulomatosis |
| | Arteriovenous malformation: "steal" phenomenon, hemorrhage, thrombus |
| | Hemorrhage |
| | Coagulopathy (disseminated intravascular coagulation, thrombotic thrombocytopenic purpura, coumadin, liver disease) |
| | Focal (tumor, vascular malformation, trauma) |
| | Decompression sickness myelopathy |
| Immune mediated | Postinfectious myelopathy/transverse myelitis |
| | Hemorrhagic (encephalo) myelopathy |
| | Multiple sclerosis |
| | Paraneoplastic myelopathy and motor neuron disease |
| Degenerative | Osteoarthritic spondylosis |
| | Intervertebral disk herniation |
| | Disseminated idiopathic sclerotic hyperostosis |
| | Rheumatoid arthritis |
| | Paget's disease |
| | Motor neuron disease (amyotrophic lateral sclerosis; progressive spinal muscular atrophy, primary lateral sclerosis) |
| | Syringomyelia |
| Idiopathic | Sarcoidosis |
| | Electrical injury |
| | Chronic adhesive arachnoiditis |
| Iatrogenic | Spinal tap–induced epidural hematoma |
| | Radiation myelopathy |
| | Fluorosis |
| | See acquired metabolic/toxic category |

orthopedic interventions of the feet before she was evaluated and found to have extensor plantar responses, absent ankle reflexes, exaggerated knee jerks, myoclonic spasms of the legs, and a tethered cord on magnetic resonance imaging (MRI) (Fig. 104-4). The development of foot deformities in a previously healthy child or young adult should alert the physician to the possibility of a progressive disorder secondary to a congenital anomaly of the spinal cord.

The varying degrees of severity of spina bifida with or without cranial involvement, hydrocephalus, and syringomyelia present little diagnostic challenge when obvious at birth. Early intervention has dramatically changed the prognosis of the disease. Less severe forms of the spinal dysraphism may affect only the conus medullaris or may be associated with other spinal deformities such as tethered cord. Spina bifida occulta is a radiologic diagnosis not associated with neurologic disability. The characteristic patch of hair or nevus over the lumbar spine is a helpful clue to congenital spinal anomalies.

Klippel-Feil syndrome of absent or fused cervical vertebrae presents a typical appearance of a neck that is short and often webbed. Neurologic complications of this bony entity include cervical myelopathy from deformity and compression of the cord and hydrocephalus by virtue of obstruction of the fourth ventricle outflow foramina. The patients with this condition I have encountered have been mentally deficient, in agreement with the general experience. Other bony developmental anomalies of the craniocervical junction that are associated with high cervical cord compression include fusion of the atlas and the foramen magnum, platybasia (flattening of the base of

### Developmental myelopathies that may present with primarily orthopedic complaints

Diastematomyelia
Tethered cord
Friedreich's ataxia
Klippel-Feil syndrome
Klippel-Trenaunay-Weber syndrome

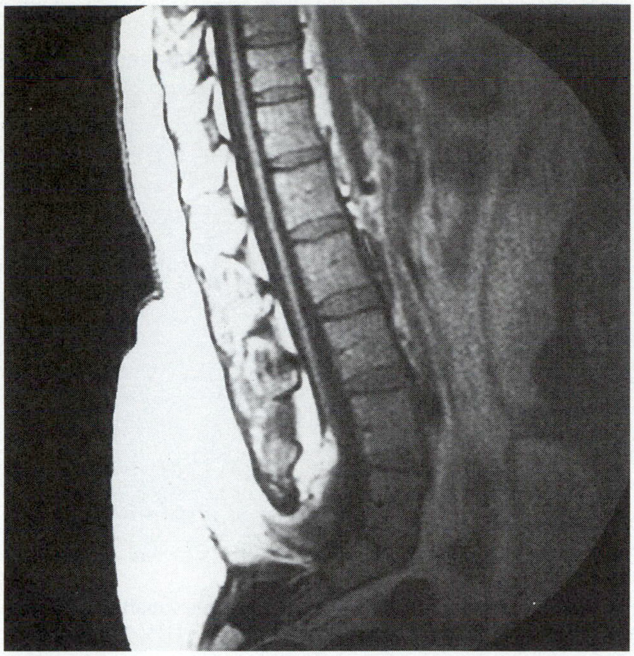

**Fig. 104-4.** T1 weighted magnetic resonance (MR) image demonstrating a tethered spinal cord. The cord terminates at the level of the L5 vertebral body, more than three vertebral segments below its normal position. The patient presented in young adulthood with pes cavus and scoliosis, which were orthopedically corrected. Severe tonic spasms of the legs were controlled more recently with benzodiazepine derivatives.

the skull), and hypoplasia of the odontoid process with atlantoaxial subluxation, which occurs in mucopolysaccharidosis type IV (Morquio syndrome). Achondroplastic dwarfism may be associated with vertebral bony thickening, narrowing of the spinal canal particularly at thoracolumbar regions, and slowly progressive myelopathy as a consequence. Rare inherited metabolic disorders affecting the spinal cord include X-linked adrenoleukodystrophy, which produces adrenal insufficiency and degeneration of myelin in brain, spinal cord, and peripheral nerves, and manifests as myelopathy and peripheral neuropathy. Patients with the Klippel-Trenaunay-Weber syndrome of vascular malformations, hemihypertrophy of limbs, and high-output cardiac failure have spinal cord vascular malformations that are complicated by cord compression, hemorrhage, or infarction. The two patients I have seen with this condition were similar to those in the literature, with prominent hemihypertrophy of an extremity and associated cutaneous nevi.

## Traumatic diseases

Spinal cord trauma is a leading cause of disability, particularly in the younger population, with an annual incidence in the United States of 5 per 100,000 population. Spinal cord injury occurs following direct penetrating trauma from gunshots and stab wounds. Fractures of the spine in a variety of circumstances result in compressive or shearing injury to the cord, as encountered in automobile, diving, and skiing accidents, and in falls from heights. Significant spinal cord injury may occur in the absence of a detectable vertebral fracture. Extreme flexion or extension of the spine, with or without bony dislocation, can produce compression and contusion of the cord. This is most liable to occur in the cervical spine region, where mobility is greatest. Cervical spine injuries are a frequent accompaniment of blunt head injury and should always be looked for specifically. The level of the cord at which the trauma is maximal dictates the clinical presentation, and the findings on examination correspond to the principles outlined in the introductory section of the chapter. The central cord syndrome discussed earlier is most often seen in hyperextension injuries of the neck in the setting of underlying cervical spondylosis. Detection at the bedside or in the emergency ward can substantially alter management.

Hematomyelia refers to hemorrhage within the spinal cord. It is frequently associated with cord contusion after trauma, in which patients have a myelopathy with features suggestive of both syringomyelia and central cord syndrome. Weakness and sensory deficit are noted in the upper extremities, long tract signs may develop in the legs, and there is variable loss or heightening of reflexes in the arms, depending on the extent and level of the lesion. A static posttraumatic myelopathy may become worse late in the course because of development of a syrinx, or the expansion of an existing syrinx, as discussed later.

## Infectious diseases

Concurrent fever and back pain should alert the physician to the possibility of an epidural abscess or disk space infection, which has the potential for cord compression or direct cord infection. This occurs in the setting of endocarditis or intravenous drug abuse, and I have seen it both as the heralding manifestation of the disease and as a late complication in an otherwise uncomplicated course and seemingly adequate response to therapy. Sources of systemic infection other than the heart should also be considered. Epidural abscess can also occur after direct trauma to the back, as a complication of surgical intervention, and rarely, after spinal tap. For this reason, lumbar puncture is avoided if there are potentially infected skin lesions over the lumbar spine. In such circumstances, if CSF is critically needed, cisternal puncture by a neurosurgeon is the preferred approach.

Myelopathy in the setting of infection with the acquired immune deficiency syndrome (AIDS) virus is now common. The offending agent is frequently the human immunodeficiency virus (HIV) itself, presumed responsible for vacuolar changes and loss of myelin and nerve cells, particularly in the posterior columns and the corticospinal tracts (Fig. 104-5). The corresponding impairment of vibration and position sense and weakness, spasticity, gait disturbance, and hyperreflexia with extensor plantar responses are seen usually in the later stages of the illness. The clinical constellation is often not "pure," however, since these patients often have other neurologic impairments, including peripheral neuropathy, primary muscle disease, or any of a number of cerebral hemisphere diseases that complicate the presentation. Infection with cytomegalovirus (CMV), also seen in the patient with AIDS, produces a less selective transverse myelitis, affecting multiple levels and not confined to the posterior and lateral columns. Elevated titers of CMV antibody in the CSF help in the differentiation of the two entities, although this distinction is not always possible, and therapeutic intervention must of necessity be broad based. A more slowly evolving myelopathy caused by the first of the human T cell lymphotrophic retroviruses to be described (HTLV-I) has received the rather cumbersome eponym HAM-TSP (HTLV-I-associated myelopathy—tropical spastic paraparesis [see Chapter 100]). Described initially in equatorial regions but seen with increasing regularity in the continental United States, this is a gradually progressive myelopathy with motor features predominant, characterized by signs of upper motor neuron disability. Pathologically there is axon loss with demyelination, vacuolization of the cord parenchyma, and gliosis. There have been rare reports of infection with the lymphocytic choriomeningitis virus (LCM), an arenavirus acquired by inhalation from exposure to rodents in the winter, resulting in a chronic pachymeningitis causing obliteration of spinal vessels and spinal cord infarction. This unusual entity may be suspected in the correct clinical setting and if there are many lymphocytes and a very high globulin concentration in the CSF.

Myelitis with extensive inflammation and necrosis has been described following infection with herpes simplex virus (HSV) types I and II, varicella zoster (VZ), CMV, Epstein-Barr virus (EBV), echovirus, coxsackieviruses A and B, and arenaviruses such as Lassa fever virus and dengue virus. White matter tracts may be disproportionately involved with infection by rabies virus and the B virus transmitted from monkeys. In all these instances the severity of the myelopathy ranges from mild to devastating, and the entire clinical picture and viral serology are important in establishing the diagnosis. Before the development of the highly effective oral vaccines, poliovirus was widespread and produced a severe, sometimes fatal, polio-(gray matter)-myelitis. This condition is still encountered in countries where vaccination is underutilized, and it has reappeared in the United States in populations who have not been immunized and who have come in contact with carriers from elsewhere. A similar syndrome can also result from infection with coxsackieviruses A and B and echovirus. During the febrile stage of poliomyelitis, patients develop lower motor neuron weakness in one or more extremities accompanied by local pain and cramping. Fasciculations are prominent, and atrophy occurs rapidly. There is a predilection for muscles that are overused or subjected to local trauma. For these reasons, rest and avoidance of intramuscular injections have long been emphasized in the care of these patients. When polio is widespread, it paralyzes muscles of respiration, and consequently in the worldwide pandemic of the 1950s, iron lung wards were established in most major hospitals. A late complication, postpolio syndrome, is now occurring decades after the original infection. Limbs that had recovered substantial function become weak again, most likely a consequence of failure, or age-related attrition, of the compensatory giant motor units that were responsible for the initial recovery. The key to the treatment of poliomyelitis is clearly prevention. Currently, no adequate way exists to reverse the postpolio syndrome, and some have recommended limiting patients' activities to prevent its development. This issue is yet to be resolved.

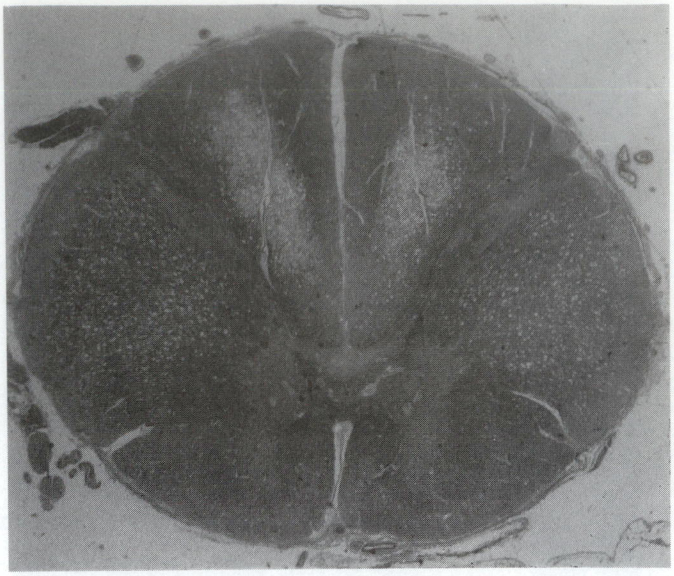

**Fig. 104-5.** Histologic features of the myelopathy caused by human immunodeficiency virus type 1 (HIV-1) consist of vacuolar degeneration of the posterior columns and the lateral corticospinal tracts, as shown in this photomicrograph of a transverse section of the cervical spinal cord stained with luxol fast blue, hematoxylin, and eosin. (Magnification ×10.) (Courtesy Dr. E.T. Hedley-Whyte.)

**Differential diagnosis of combined systems disease of the cord (corticospinal tract and posterior column involvement)**

Vitamin $B_{12}$ deficiency
Syphilis
HIV vacuolar myelopathy

The Romberg test was initially offered as a clinical method for detecting the posterior column involvement of the spinal cord in patients with tabes dorsalis, a form of neurosyphilis. The association of corticospinal tract signs with posterior column sensory loss is a discrete combination with a limited differential diagnosis among syphilis, vitamin $B_{12}$ deficiency, and HIV vacuolar myelopathy (see the box above). Sensory ataxia from loss of position and vibration sense, weakness, spasticity, and extensor plantar responses with exaggerated tendon reflexes are detected, whereas pin and temperature sensation are relatively preserved. When severe, the loss of position sense leads to development of a Charcot's joint, which is now something of a rarity. Syphilitic meningeal infiltration leads to a chronic inflammatory and fibrosing hypertrophy of the dura, called pachymeningitis, described more fully later, with secondary manifestations that are themselves debilitating. Syphilitic vasculitis also causes obliterative endarteritis with resultant thrombosis of medium and small blood vessels. Infarction of the spinal cord (and other brain regions) therefore occurs as a direct complication of neurosyphilis. The resurgence of syphilis, in the AIDS population particularly, has led to both an increasing number of affected patients as well as earlier and more severe manifestations of the infection.

Lyme disease, as with syphilis, is another great imitator and has been described as a cause of chronic myelitis. History of exposure to the organism (*Borrelia burgdorferi*) through tick bites is not always elicited, and the typical spreading erythematous rash of Lyme disease may be missed. The clinical setting, epidemiologic factors, spinal fluid formula, and culture of the organism are required to establish the diagnosis.

Tuberculosis is a cause of major morbidity and mortality throughout the underdeveloped world and is increasingly common in the United States partly as a consequence of AIDS. Tuberculoma of the spinal cord itself is rare. Pott's disease is a more common cause of spinal cord manifestations and is characterized by tuberculous infection of the spine with subsequent collapse of vertebrae and compression of the spinal cord. Orthopedic management as well as antimycobacterial regimens are critical in these patients to prevent the complications. The clinical adage that the earliest symptom of tuberculous spine disease is back pain, the earliest physical finding is tenderness to palpation, and the earliest radiographic feature is narrowing of the joint space still holds true in this era of sophisticated neuroimaging. Fever is usually absent because the disease is subacute or chronic, and there may not necessarily be clinical stigmata of tuberculous disease elsewhere because of the natural history of the illness. A high level of suspicion is required to perform the requisite tests (most notably a purified protein derivative [PPD] and radiographic studies) that lead to the diagnosis. Thoracolumbar regions are most often affected, but cervical spine infection also occurs.

Schistosomiasis (bilharziosis) is another disease uncommon in developed countries but rampant still throughout much of the world. Spinal cord infestation with this blood fluke is more common with *Schistosoma mansoni* and *S. haematobium* and brain involvement with *S. japonicum.* The presentation of spinal cord infestation is usually abrupt because of massive necrosis. Schistosomal ova obstruct arteries and veins and produce ischemic necrosis, sometimes corresponding to an anterior spinal artery syndrome. A more insidious course corresponds to the development of granulomas that produce focal cord compression. The disease should be suspected in patients recently immersed in slow running water in endemic areas. Katayama fever (with diarrhea, urticaria, lymphadenopathy, splenomegaly) occurs in patients infected with *S. mansoni,* characteristically after the initial febrile illness but before the myelopathy. An acute febrile illness with eosinophilia followed by myelopathy should raise the suspicion for this diagnosis. The CSF shows an eosinophilic pleocytosis, schistosomal ova may be detected in the stool, and complement fixation tests and biopsy of liver or rectal mucosa are confirmatory. Treatment with praziquantel effectively controls the infestation.

Bacterial infection of the cord is rare and usually devastating. It may occur after hematogenous dissemination or direct invasion from an adjacent epidural abscess. Even less common is necrotizing myelitis caused by *Listeria monocytogenes* or *Mycoplasma pneumoniae.*

Fungal myelitis is usually confined to patients who are immunocompromised. The diagnosis can be made in patients found to have a focal inflammatory process in the spinal cord and in whom the CSF evaluation is diagnostic. A more common scenario is chronic fungal meningitis with resultant adhesive arachnoiditis, described later.

Parenchymatous toxoplasmosis produces a heavy toll on the nervous system in patients with AIDS, and some cases of *Toxoplasma* myelitis have been recorded.

Parenchymatous or racemose neurocysticercosis, caused by the cysts of the pork tapeworm, *Taenia solium,* can seed throughout the spinal cord as it can the rest of the brain. If cysts are slow growing, they may not have an overtly destructive effect, but their mass and the overall burden of disease can produce localized or multifocal spinal cord symptoms. The racemose form, in which cysts protrude into or float within the CSF, can cause symptoms by obstruction of flow. A history of exposure to possibly infested meat is not necessary to make the diagnosis, since most patients seem to acquire the organism through unclean water supplies. Neuroimaging studies reveal the multiple cysts, the scolex of the organism is often visible, and immunoassays can confidently establish the diagnosis in most instances. Rare cases have been reported of infestations of the cord by cysts of the dog tapeworm, *Echinococcus granulosus* (hydatid disease), and by the lung fluke *Paragonimus westermani.*

### Neoplastic diseases

Tumors can arise within the spinal cord itself, in the meninges, or from the surrounding soft tissue and bones. They can infiltrate from adjacent sites, disseminate by CSF from within the nervous system, or metastasize from elsewhere. As with other organ systems, tumors are primary or secondary, benign or malignant. The spinal cord accounts for 15% of all CNS tumors. Tumors arising outside the dura account for about half of the total (usually metastatic or locally invasive); those within the dura but outside the spinal cord account for 40% (usually neurofibromas or meningiomas, as well as meningeal cancers); and intramedullary tumors (primarily gliomas, rarely metastases) make up the remaining 5% to 10% of the total. A central feature of management is to prevent the spinal cord compression that can occur rapidly and without notice in seemingly indolent situations.

The most common benign tumors arise from the investing sheaths of the cord or the nerve roots, namely, neurofibroma, meningioma, and schwannoma. These intraspinal, extramedullary tumors produce a slowly progressive myelopathy with signs attributable to the particular level of the tumor. Neurofibromas tend to be located in the region of the thoracic cord, whereas menigiomas are more evenly distributed throughout the spinal cord. The clinical presentation may be asymmetric between the extremities, depending on the site of the lesion. Motor features may be more striking than objective sensory deficit, or the opposite may be true if the compressive lesion is predominantly posterior. Local back pain may be associated with radiation along the course of a nerve root, exacerbated by the Valsalva maneuver, worsened with

**Table 104-4.** Differentiating features among intramedullary lesions, extramedullary intradural lesions, and extradural lesions with added focal radiculopathy

| | Intramedullary (intrinsic myelopathy, e.g., spinal cord glioma, syringomyelia) | Extramedullary intradural (e.g., meningeal lymphoma) | Extradural (e.g., disk herniation, epidural abscess, bony metastases) |
|---|---|---|---|
| Lower motor neuron weakness | Present at the level, not in nerve root distribution | Variable; depends if nerve root invasion is present | Present at the level, confined to nerve root distribution |
| Dissociated sensory loss | + | – | – |
| Sacral sparing | + | – | – |
| Suspended band of bilateral pin sense loss | + | – | – |
| Horner's syndrome with cervicothoracic myelopathy | + | – | – |
| Ascending clinical presentation | Common | Usually not | Usually not |
| Flexor/extensor spasms | Common | Uncommon | Uncommon |

All patients may have upper motor neuron weakness with variable symmetry, a sensory level or Brown-Séquard syndrome, and incontinence.

recumbency, and relieved by sitting or standing. "Dumbbell" tumors invaginate themselves through the neural foramina, lying partly within the spinal canal and partly outside, thus giving rise to their name. They may produce focal radiculopathy as well as myelopathy by virtue of their location within the neural foramen, where they compress nerve roots. Patients with neurofibromatosis type II (those with bilateral acoustic neuromas) are at risk for developing spinal neurofibromas or meningiomas, and a tendency exists in this population for the initially benign tumors to undergo malignant transformation. Benign tumors at the lowest end of the spinal cord include chordomas, which also occur also at the base of the skull; lipomas; hamartomas; and epidermoids. These tumors produce conus medullaris or cauda equina syndrome or combinations of the two.

Malignant tumors can metastasize to the spinal cord directly, but this occurs infrequently. In general, metastatic tumors achieve their destructive effect on the cord by invasion or pressure from surrounding structures, usually bone. Those arising locally but outside the dura are notably sarcomas of bone or muscle and vascular tumors such as hemangioblastoma. Rarely, a retroperitoneal or mediastinal tumor (pancreas, esophagus) or a localized eosinophilic granuloma of bone invades the spinal cord and produces neurologic compromise. More often, metastatic disease of bone, arising from carcinoma of the colon, breast, lung, and prostate, as well as myeloma and extraosseus lymphoma, impinge on the epidural space and threaten the spinal cord, sometimes decompensating acutely. Radicular symptoms may also occur in this setting because of distortion of the nerve roots by the tumor. The development of localized back pain in a patient with known carcinoma, either active or remote, should be investigated on an urgent basis because of the potentially devastating effect on management of superimposed paraplegia or tetraplegia, lifestyle, and life expectancy. It is not sufficient to wait for the signs of spinal cord compromise to develop before embarking on an evaluation. The time to intervene to best advantage is when the disease is confined to the epidural space and not yet compressing the cord.

Certain primary nervous system tumors can spread to distant sites within the nervous system, including to the spinal cord. Medulloblastomas and ependymomas seed the CSF and manifest at far removed sites such as the spinal cord. Astrocytomas may seed the CSF but can also spread along nerve pathways. These features have implications for treatment options such as radiation.

Tumors arising within the spinal cord itself (intraspinal, intramedullary) tend most often to be astrocytomas or ependymomas, the latter being more common at the filum terminale. Oligodendrogliomas seldom arise within the cord. Primary melanoma of the cord is a rarity. Intramedullary tumors are often associated with pain, particularly when located at the filum terminale. Their manifestations differ from the extrinsic compressive lesions (Table 104-4). The clinical picture of a single lesion may suggest an ascending process because of the lamination of the fiber tracts within the cord. Sacral spinothalamic sensation may be spared early. There is likely to be evidence of a lower motor neuron lesion at the site of the tumor because of local destruction of the anterior horn cells. This is more appreciable when the level is at the cervical or lumbar enlargements than at the thoracic level, where asymmetries of the abdominal musculature are not always noted.

There is also likely to be a band of bilateral pin sense loss at the level of the lesion because of the destruction of the crossing spinothalamic fibers. The location of the root pain, sensory loss, and atrophic paralysis may be of greater help in defining the location of the tumor than the upper level of the sensory loss on the trunk. Intramedullary tumors may themselves produce a syringomyelic syndrome, but in addition, and for reasons that are not clear, they may be associated with acquired syringomyelia elsewhere in the cord. The expansion of the cord by the intrinsic mass can produce blockage of the flow of CSF with a Froin's syndrome (elevated protein, decreased glucose, xanthochromia, clotting of CSF) and an absent Queckenstedt phenomenon (digital pressure on the jugular venous pulse does not produce a rise in the measured CSF pressure). The absence of tumor burden elsewhere, normal imaging of the vertebral column, and often characteristic features in the spinal cord on contemporary neuroimaging

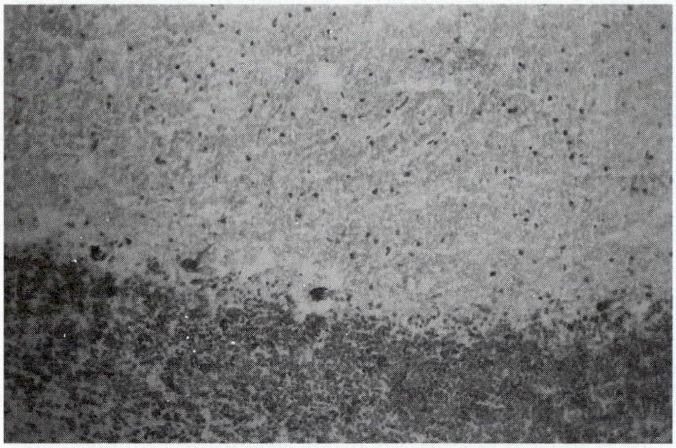

**Fig. 104-6.** Photomicrograph of the cerebellar Purkinje's cell reactivity (and some granule cell reactivity as well) against a 70 kd antibody found in the serum of a woman with paraneoplastic myelopathy (see text). (Magnification ×75.) (Courtesy Dr. Jerome Posner.)

procedures are important in arriving at a diagnosis.

Certain tumors have a predilection for invading the CSF and spreading along the surface of the cord. Tumors of the breast and lung and lymphoma are prime culprits. The tumors infiltrate and destroy nerve roots and less often produce cord compression. Multiple radiculopathies cause widespread clinical deficit, including loss of strength, sensation, and reflexes in arms and legs, and abolition of sphincter control.

Paraneoplastic myelopathy, a remote effect of cancers, mostly of the ovary and breast, and oat cell carcinoma of the lung, is characterized by a subacute course of motor and autonomic findings, with variable sensory loss. The clinical constellation suggests compressive myelopathy, but pain is seldom present, and evaluation fails to disclose the expected anatomic features of a compressive lesion. The thoracic spinal cord is most frequently involved. The serologic evaluation for antineuronal antibodies may be positive, and CSF evaluation is essentially benign except for mild elevation of protein content and a small number of reactive lymphocytes. In one such patient whom I examined, the serum contained a 70 kd antibody that reacted against both cerebellar Purkinje's cells (Fig. 104-6) and cortical neurons, providing confirmation of the diagnosis. Treatment has not been available to date. New experience with addition of the protein A column to plasmapheresis in certain types of paraneoplastic syndromes, notably the opsoclonus-myoclonus syndrome, leads to some cause for optimism.

A rare form of paraneoplastic motor neuron disease has been described. In the one patient I saw with this condition, the clinical features and electromyographic findings were similar to the more familiar sporadic or inherited forms of amyotrophic lateral sclerosis. In this patient, however, the onset was unusually rapid and occurred in association with oat cell carcinoma of the lung. Fortunately, the neurologic syndrome regressed with surgical removal of the lung tumor.

## Acquired metabolic/toxic disorders

Pernicious anemia, or vitamin $B_{12}$ deficiency, produces a variety of neurologic syndromes, including dementia, peripheral neuropathy, and subacute combined degeneration of the spinal cord. The posterior columns and corticospinal tracts undergo axonal degeneration and demyelination. Patients often complain initially of intense burning paresthesias in the feet, then unsteadiness of gait, falling, and inability to keep their balance in the dark. The story of the patient falling into the washbasin as he holds a cloth up to his face in the morning is a typical one for posterior column position sense loss. The findings on examination reveal the loss of vibration and position sense and upper motor neuron dysfunction, which is first noted in the lower extremities. Hematologic abnormalities are not a prerequisite for making this diagnosis. The complete blood count and peripheral smear typically may be unaffected at the same time that neurologic manifestations and deficient vitamin $B_{12}$ levels are evident. The differential diagnosis is limited but important (see the box on p. 1440). Treatment with intramuscular vitamin $B_{12}$ injections needs to be instituted immediately on suspicion of the diagnosis because these patients can decompensate rapidly. This does not interfere with later diagnosis of the cause of the vitamin deficiency, since replenishment of vitamin $B_{12}$ stores is a requirement for the performance of the Schilling test.

Chronic exposure to the drug clioquinol is toxic to the spinal cord and optic nerves, producing a subacute myeloopticoneuropathy. Volatile gases such as benzene derivatives and *n*-hexane are associated with demyelination of the peripheral and central nervous systems, and the spinal cord is not immune to such attack. I have seen one woman who sustained acute, disseminated demyelination of the brain and spinal cord after inhalation of toxic levels of a number of gases, including carbon disulfide. Her recovery was slow but almost complete over 2 years. Lathyrism is a progressive spastic myelopathy with paresthesias, sensory loss, impotence, and incontinence that is caused by ingestion of the grass pea, *Lathyrus sativus*. A toxic neuroexcitatory amino acid appears to be responsible for this syndrome, which occurs in selected regions of Africa and India. Intrathecal injection of methotrexate, particularly in combination with radiation therapy, can produce an acute and permanent myelopathy or a progressive necrotizing myelopathy, often with cerebral involvement as well. Injection of chymopapain for the treatment of intervertebral disk herniation has produced some cases of transverse myelitis. Myelopathy has been associated with the intrathecal injection of contaminants of anesthetics and steroids; it has been documented as a consequence of vascular spasm precipitated by the injection of previously available toxic contrast agents used for myelography and aortic angiography; and it has been reported after excessive exposure to fluorine.

## Vascular diseases

Spinal cord infarction occurs relatively infrequently. The rich anastomotic vascular supply and the lower metabolic requirements of the cord compared with the cerebral hemispheres serve to protect it from ischemic insult. The cord contains longitudinally oriented vascular border zones at rostrocaudal levels, as well as transverse border zones within segments (see Fig. 104-2). These border zones are at particular risk during periods of hypoperfusion. The border zone at the cervicothoracic junction lies between the vascular supply of the anterior spinal artery and the radicular arteries of the thoracic aorta. Consequently, low flow states may produce low cervical or high thoracic lesions. This should be suspected if a patient is unable to move the legs but does not have the findings expected after infarction in cerebral border zones, such as impaired mental state and weakness of the proximal upper extremities. The vessel of Adamkiewicz, the major radicular branch of the aorta that supplies the cord around the T10 level, and lumbar branches of the abdominal aorta are at risk during surgical clamping of the aorta for such procedures as repair of aortic aneurysms or surgery on renal vessels. The cord can withstand about 30 minutes of ischemia, but longer durations produce infarction. Patients with this complication come out of anesthesia with flaccid paraplegia but normal upper extremity function. The single anterior spinal artery is at greater risk of producing clinical disease when it is occluded than are the dual posterior spinal arteries. Relative preservation of vibration and position sense but paralysis and loss of pin and temperature sense represent a striking disparity in selective infarction in the anterior spinal artery territory (Fig. 104-7). Embolism rarely arises from systemic sources (e.g., endocarditis, meningococcemia, thrombotic thrombocytopenic purpura). More usual scenarios include atheromatous occlusion of the ostium of a radicular vessel at the aorta, dissecting aortic aneurysm, selective catheterization of aortic vessels, and use of intraaortic balloon pumps. Artery-to-artery embolism arising within the aorta is thought to be rare. A growing number of case reports describe acute infarction of the spinal cord caused by fibrocartilaginous embolism arising from extruded intervertebral disk material. The pathophysiology of this condition is speculative. Patients often present after a minor injury with pain and a fulminant myelopathy that may lead to death. Systemic vasculitides, such as systemic lupus erythematosus and periarteritis nodosa, involve spinal arteries and produce disseminated and multifocal cord ischemia. Chronic pachymeningitis obliterates spinal vessels from without, meningeal tumors produce compression or infiltration, and syphilis provokes an obliterative endarteritis with obstruction of the lumina of arteries or veins.

Spinal arteriovenous malformations (AVMs), angiomas, and arteriovenous fistulas account for 20% to 40% of vascular malformations of the CNS. The thoracolumbar cord is most often involved, but no site is immune. The malformations are generally dural based and are formed between the radicular arteries derived from the aorta and the draining veins of the cord. They generally lie outside the cord's substance, although an intramedullary location is noted occasionally. These malformations produce problems in several different ways. The sheer mass of the vessel tangle can produce a compressive myelopathy. The AVM produces a "vascular steal" phenomenon with a resultant ischemic myelopathy that may progress in a stepwise fashion. Thrombosis of low-flow components of the AVM and development of embolism from within the AVM are potential sources of cord infarction. The disease may manifest with acute and recurrent subarachnoid and intramedullary hemorrhage. Intradural AVMs in later life tend to cause a more chronic, progressive radiculomyelopathy. This entity has received several names, including Foix-Alajouanine syndrome or subacute necrotizing my-

A

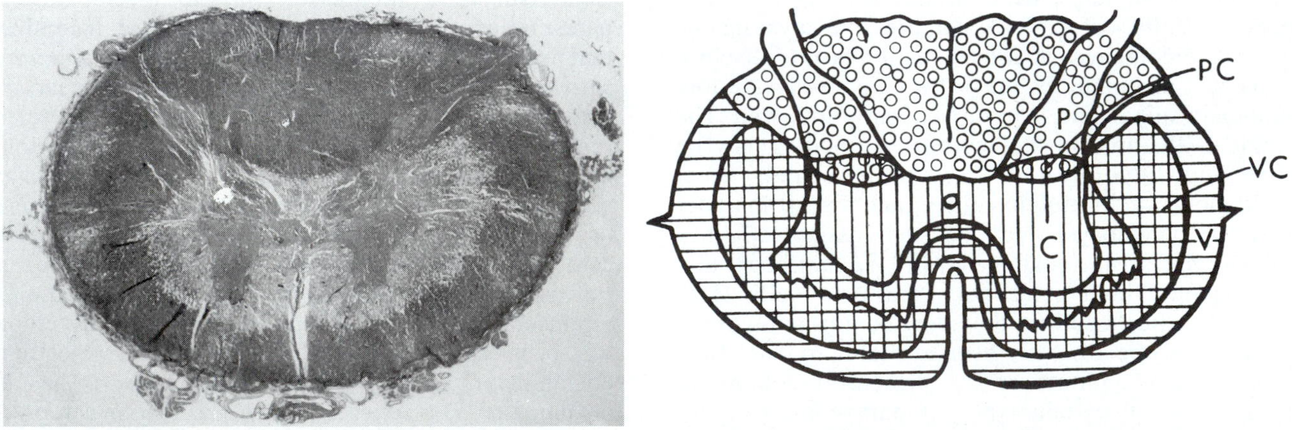


B

**Fig. 104-7. A,** Low-power photomicrograph showing a transverse section of the rostral thoracic spinal cord from a patient with infarction confined to the territory of the anterior spinal artery. Note that the posterior columns are entirely spared. Also, the rim of the spinal cord is spared, illustrating the importance of the collateral supply received from the coronal vessels. (Hematoxylin-eosin stain; magnification ×10.) **B,** Source of blood supply to a segment of the spinal cord. *C,* Region supplied by the central artery (branch of the anterior spinal artery); *P,* region supplied by penetrating arteries from the plexus formed by the paired posterior spinal arteries; *PC,* region supplied by either central or posterior penetrating arteries; *V,* region supplied by penetrating arteries of the lateral and ventral pial plexuses; *VC,* region supplied by either central or ventral and lateral penetrating arteries. (**A** courtesy of Dr. E.T. Hedley-Whyte; **B** from Austin GM, editor: *The spinal cord,* ed 3, New York, 1983, Igaku-Shoin.)

elopathy. Diagnosis in most of these patients can be difficult, and a combination of imaging modalities (MRI, selective spinal angiography) may be required before certainty is achieved. Currently recommended therapeutic approaches include endovascular embolization or excision.

Hemorrhage within the spinal cord (hematomyelia) often occurs after trauma but also in conditions of disseminated coagulopathy, including that caused by anticoagulant use (see the box below). It also occurs in spinal cord lesions, such as AVMs, venous angiomas, and vascular tumors (hemangioblastoma), and in conditions in which the spinal cord is involved along with multiple other sites, such as hereditary hemorrhagic telangiectasia (Osler-Weber-Rendu disease). Massive cord hemorrhage, as with complete infarction of the cord, is abrupt and catastrophic. More restricted hemorrhagic lesions after trauma can resolve with good clinical recovery, although long-term complications may result, as discussed later.

The rapid phase change of nitrogen from liquid to gas in the bloodstream that is the pathologic underpinning of the clinical syndrome of decompression sickness, or caisson disease, has a dramatic effect on the CNS. Nitrogen bubbles trapped in spinal arteries produce ischemic changes ranging from minor neurologic manifestations, such as paresthesias and headache, to major syndromes, including acute encephalopathy (progressing to coma) and myelopathy. The white matter of the upper thoracic cord appears to be most affected. In the correct clinical setting (too rapid emergence from a deep underwater dive), confusion, dysarthria, joint and abdominal pains, and painful tingling paresthesias of the extremities are signs of imminent disaster. Urgent reinstitution of elevated atmospheric pressures is required, either by resubmersion or by use of decompression chambers managed by a nation's coast guard.

### Transverse (noninfectious) myelitis

Any inflammation of the spinal cord may be considered a myelitis, including the many viral, bacterial, and other diseases already covered, but this overly inclusive approach is not especially helpful in categorizing and thinking about spinal cord disease. The term *transverse myelitis* used here includes acute inflammatory diseases in which an infectious agent cannot be detected within the spinal cord. The great majority of these cases are immune mediated in some manner. Besides trauma, immune-mediated diseases account for most of the previously well individuals who develop myelopathy.

#### Causes of hematomyelia

- Trauma
- Anticoagulant use and other systemic coagulopathies
- Arteriovenous or other vascular malformations of the cord
- Vascular tumors (e.g., hemangioblastoma)
- Hereditary hemorrhagic telangiectasia (Osler-Weber-Rendu disease)

Inflammation of the cord often occurs after an antecedent viral infection or vaccination, although such a precipitant cannot always be elicited in the history. The onset may be abrupt, occurring within hours or more often over a few days. Back pain radiating through to the abdomen is a frequent accompaniment, and urinary retention is noted early. Sensory loss to all modalities and weakness are manifest to varying degrees, depending on the attack's severity. The clinical setting and loss of posterior column sensation mitigate against anterior spinal artery infarction, and a sensory level and the nature of the progression argue against ascending polyneuropathies or diseases principally affecting muscle. The association of myelopathy with optic neuritis is known as Devic's disease. This is frequently but not exclusively seen in multiple sclerosis and does not automatically imply this diagnosis at first presentation. The CSF formula in transverse myelitis reveals elevated protein and lymphocytes and decreased glucose in as many as half the patients. Blood or xanthochromia in the CSF is unusual, and all cultures are necessarily negative to make the diagnosis. Elevation of the CSF globulin, oligoclonal bands in the CSF but not the serum, and presence of myelin basic protein may all be observed, but with the acute inflammation these features do not confirm a diagnosis of multiple sclerosis. Parasagittal and transverse MRI views reveal contrast-enhancing lesions in a considerably swollen cord. The prognosis for recovery from a single attack of transverse myelitis depends on the severity of the illness at presentation. The long-term outlook has been considerably improved by limiting the damage at the time of the attack by immunosuppressive agents. About 5% to 10% of patients with transverse myelitis go on to develop multiple sclerosis.

When transverse myelitis is suspected but the investigations, including MRI and CSF evaluation, suggest a major hemorrhagic component in addition to inflammation, the entity of acute hemorrhagic myelopathy with or without a cerebral and encephalopathic component should be considered. Also most likely a postinfectious complication, the hemorrhagic encephalomyelopathy is life-threatening and should be treated aggressively with immunosuppressives early in the course, as long as direct infection of the cord has been excluded. Such infections are referred to earlier and include herpes zoster, herpes simplex, and cytomegalovirus. Hemorrhagic infections of the CNS by arenaviruses (e.g., Lassa fever virus) also enter this category, but these are rare.

Spinal cord involvement in multiple sclerosis is common, although the exact incidence is not known. It can vary from the predominant or only clinical manifestation (Fig. 104-8) to a subclinical entity detected incidentally on MRI (see Chapter 100 on multiple sclerosis for further information). Myelin produced by the oligodendrocyte is the principal target of attack in this immune-mediated disease. Plaques of demyelination occur at multiple sites, most frequently the cervical and high thoracic regions. The patchy nature of the plaque distribution leads to the ubiquitous manifestations, including unusual subjective sensory phenomena with minimal objective findings, stiffness and unsteadiness of gait, hemicord syndromes, and incapacitating spastic paraparesis or tetraparesis with flexor spasms. A presentation difficult to diagnose is

A

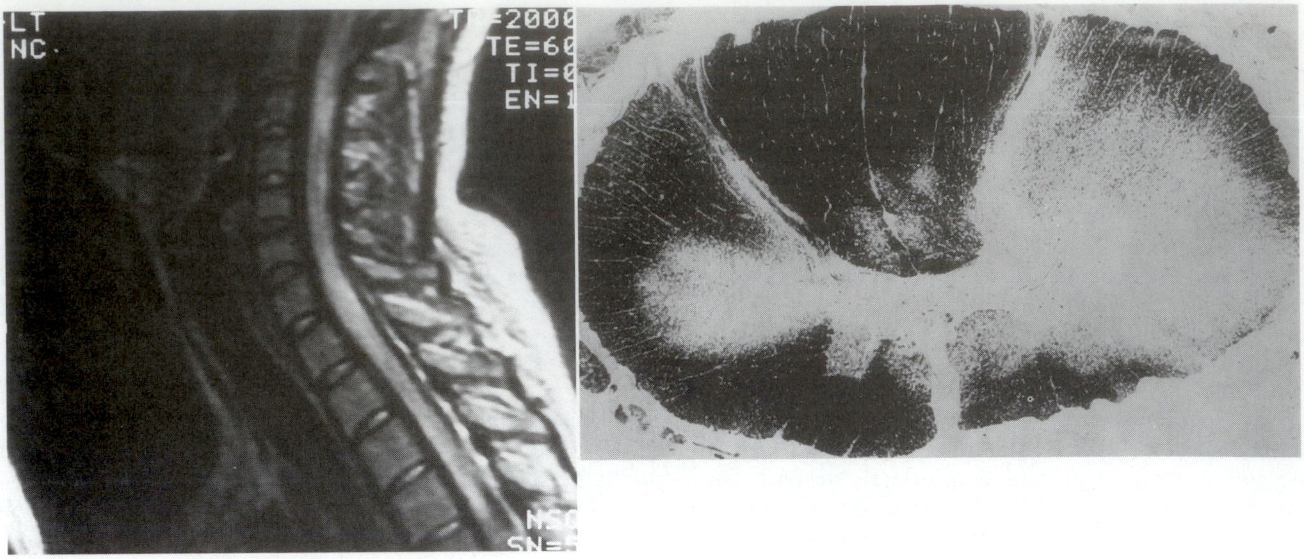


B

**Fig. 104-8. A,** Parasagittal view of the cervicothoracic spine with a T1-weighted MR image after gadolinium injection in a patient with multiple sclerosis. The diameter of the spinal cord is seen to be enlarged in two areas, both of which show diffusely increased signal. This patient had a pure spinal cord syndrome that responded well to a 10-day course of intravenous methylprednisolone. Her cranial MR image showed multiple, subclinical, white matter, T2-weighted hyperintensities, and the cerebrospinal fluid demonstrated elevated immunoglobulins and oligoclonal bands that were not present in the serum. She has had a relapsing and remitting course but remains fully ambulatory. **B,** Photomicrograph of a transverse section of thoracic spinal cord in a 6-year-old girl with acute spinal cord multiple sclerosis. (Loyez myelin stain; magnification ×10.) (Courtesy Dr. E.P. Richardson; see also *N Engl J Med* 273:760, 1965.)

demyelination of the proximal part of the dorsal root entry zone, which is invested with myelin derived from the oligodendrocyte. Subjective symptoms and sensory loss may be restricted to a single or adjacent dermatomal levels, resembling herpes zoster without the rash, or the dermatomal pain and sensory loss of conditions such as syphilis, diabetes, and Lyme disease. The detection by MRI of multiple patches of demyelination in the cord and elsewhere in the CNS is central to making the diagnosis. The Lhermitte's sign of shocklike paresthesias shooting down the spine precipitated by neck flexion is helpful in reaching a diagnosis of myelopathy, but it is not specific for multiple sclerosis or for other demyelinating diseases. The course of spinal multiple sclerosis waxes and wanes, but when the plaque burden reaches a critical level, recovery of function becomes less likely and ambulation is lost. Promising new developments in the treatment of demyelinating diseases include the role of interferons and the potential for oral vaccination.

Paraneoplastic myelopathy is discussed earlier. The mechanism of disease is presumed to be attack by antibodies produced by the tumor against neuronal elements within the cord; thus it may rightly be considered an immune-mediated disease.

### Degenerative diseases

Compression of the spinal cord or thecal sac by overgrowth of bone in osteoarthritic spondylosis and by rupture and herniation of a degenerated intervertebral disk occurs frequently and causes considerable morbidity. Compression of lumbosacral nerve roots in the cauda equina or at the intervertebral foramina is more appropriately considered in the discussion of the peripheral nervous system. Suffice it to mention here that large intervertebral disk herniations at the lumbosacral level produce compression of multiple nerve roots in the cauda equina, and as discussed earlier, this can simulate conus medullaris lesions.

Cervical radiculomyelopathy is the constellation of compression of a nerve root as well as of the spinal cord in the neck (Fig. 104-9). The resulting clinical manifestations include pain in the neck with radiation into the arms, limitation of neck motion, focal radiculopathy in the upper extremity, myotomal weakness and diminished deep tendon reflex, and dermatomal sensory loss that often includes a triangle of paraspinal numbness with its base at the vertebral spines. Myelopathy usually commences insidiously with gait instability, irritable bladder, and paresthesias. Spasticity and hyperreflexia in the legs are more prominent than weakness and out of proportion to the findings in the arms. If the myelopathy is high cervical and the reflexes are diffusely exaggerated, preservation of the jaw jerk is helpful in eliminating cerebral disease. The distribution of pain in the upper extremity helps localize the site of the cervical lesion. Irritation of the C5 nerve root produces pain radiating from the neck to the region of the deltoid muscle; C6 lesions produce pain accompanied by paresthesias in the thumb and index finger; C7 lesions produce pain in the middle three fingers as well as around the pectoral region and the scapulae; and C8 lesions affect the fifth finger, resembling an ulnar neuropathy but less well localized on examination. Despite considerable motor

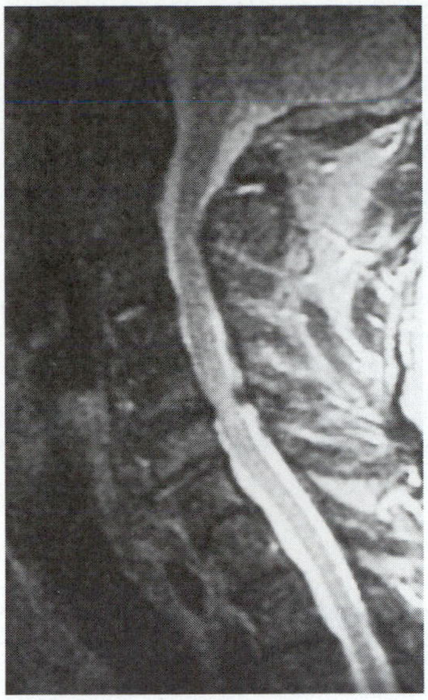

**Fig. 104-9.** Parasagittal T2-weighted MR image of the cervical spine in a 68-year-old man with slowly evolving spastic paraparesis, weakness in the proximal upper extremities, and urinary frequency. The study demonstrates focal bony encroachments anteriorly and posteriorly impinging on the spinal cord at the C5 level. After resection of the bony spurs by an anterior approach, the patient made a full recovery.

findings, prominent paresthesias and dysesthesias, loss of vibration sense in the feet, and sometimes striking cord compression on neuroimaging procedures, pin sense loss in the legs is often not present on examination. Cord compression should therefore not be excluded because of this disparate finding, because by the time the sensory loss or a sensory level to pin have appeared in patients with extrinsic cord compression, complete recovery of function is unlikely even after surgical decompression.

Cervical osteoarthritis and spondylosis are the background for some stereotypic clinical scenarios. Elderly individuals who fall down stairs or somehow experience hyperextension injuries of the neck are prone to develop the central cord syndrome. The combination of lower motor neuron pattern weakness and loss of pin and temperature sensation in the arms with relative sparing of leg strength should alert suspicion for this diagnosis. A patient with a history of such a fall and transient difficulty using the arms may develop the late complication of posttraumatic syringomyelia, heralded by progressive atrophic paralysis (lower motor neuron type) and dissociated sensory loss in the region of and usually above the prior injury. Intervertebral disk herniation, bony spur and bar protrusion into the extramedullary space, progressive spinal stenosis, and compression fractures of the cervical or thoracic spines are potential accompaniments of osteoarthritic spondylosis with or without osteoporosis affecting the vertebral column. These can all produce an extrinsic compressive myelopathy. Disk herniations tend to produce radiculopathies when they encroach on the neural foramina. Myelopathy results when a large disk component is extruded or a disk fragment breaks loose from the nucleus pulposus and occupies the central aspect

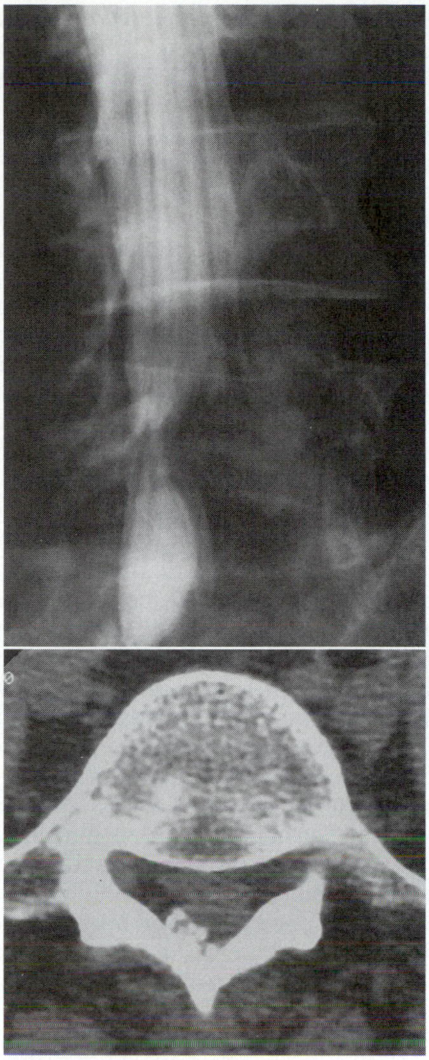

**A**

**B**

**Fig. 104-10.** A 36-year-old woman with a nonspecific past history of low back pain slipped on the floor at home and experienced sudden onset of excruciating lower back pain, weakness in the legs, perineal sensory loss, and urinary retention over a few hours. Myelography revealed the massive L5-S1 disk herniation compressing the cauda equina **(A),** a finding even more dramatically illustrated by the postmyelogram CT scan taken at the L5-S1 level **(B).** Emergency surgery produced a resolution of most of her symptoms and signs, but recovery to normal was gradual over a year.

of the epidural space (Fig. 104-10). This is an uncommon complication despite the frequency of disk herniation with neurologic compromise, but it needs to be recognized early because of the need for urgent surgical intervention to prevent irreversible damage.

Rheumatoid arthritis produces degeneration of the odontoid ligament with subluxation of the atlantoaxial joint and places the patient at risk for sudden death from compression at the cervicomedullary junction. Dynamic radiographs and possibly cervical spine MRI are prudent investigations in a patient with rheumatoid arthritis who complains of neck pain and has signs that could be consistent with a myelopathy.

Paget's disease of bone can be particularly troublesome

because of fragile and enlarged vertebrae that crowd the spinal column and intervertebral foramina, producing symptoms of spinal stenosis, compressive myelopathy, and radiculopathies. Plain x-rays and elevated alkaline phosphatase levels help establish the diagnosis, and effective therapy includes analgesics, calcitonin, etidronate, and in some patients cytotoxic agents.

Syringomyelia refers both to a cystic cavity within the spinal cord and a characteristic clinical syndrome (see the box at right). The cervical spinal cord is almost universally involved, with or without extension up to the brainstem or down to lower cord levels. Postulated to result from altered fluid dynamics around the outflow of the fourth ventricle and the central canal, syringomyelia occurs as an isolated phenomenon or together with brainstem involvement (syringobulbia). Associated conditions include Chiari malformations at the base of the brain, obstructive lesions of the foramen magnum, spinal dysraphism (spina bifida, meningomyelocele), pachymeningitis, and intramedullary tumors (see the box at right). Radiation necrosis, ischemia or hemorrhage within the cord, and rarely, extramedullary compressive lesions can also produce the clinical picture of syringomyelia. The pattern of syrinx enlargement around the central core of the spinal cord leads to the clinical picture of dissociated anesthesia with loss of pin and temperature sense in a capelike distribution affecting the C4-5 dermatomes down to about the C8 or T1 level, lower motor neuron dysfunction at this level, and preservation of posterior column sensation until rather late in the disease course. Similarly, long tract signs in the legs do not usually develop until late in the course. Patients complain of being unable to feel hot items with their hands, and so coffee, cigarette, and stove top burns of the digits may be presenting problems. Patients may report that they have to use their feet rather than hands to test the temperature of bath or shower water. This entity must be distinguished from intramedullary tumors of the cord. The time course of the two diseases is different, with syringomyelia tending to be slower in onset. The distinction has been made easier by MRI, which demonstrates the diameter and rostrocaudal extent of the intramedullary cystic cavity (Fig. 104-11). Rarely a patient may present with abrupt onset of syrinx cavity expansion, as occurred in a nurse whom I saw in the recovery stages after a rapid onset of syringomyelia-syringobulbia while lifting a patient off a bed. Acute neurosurgical intervention was required in her case. However, treatment is usually elective and includes decompression of the foramen magnum and rostral cervical cord and placing a shunt between the cyst cavity and the spinal subarachnoid space, with generally good outcomes.

### Diseases presenting with a syringomyelia syndrome

Syringomyelia
Hematomyelia
Intramedullary tumor
Chronic diffuse pachymeningitis
Subtotal spinal cord ischemia
Delayed effects of radiation therapy
(Extramedullary compressive lesions)

### Syringomyelia subtypes

With obstruction at foramen magnum and dilatation of central canal
With no obstruction at foramen magnum
With other spinal cord diseases (e.g., tumor, trauma)
With hydrocephalus and no other discernible pathology

## Amyotrophic lateral sclerosis

Motor neuron diseases are degenerative, genetically mediated, sometimes inherited diseases affecting the spinal cord and/or cerebral motor cortex. Sensation and mental functions are typically spared. These diseases in adults include amyotrophic lateral sclerosis (ALS), primary lateral sclerosis, and progressive spinal muscular atrophy. ALS has its onset usually after age 40, is characterized by a combination of both upper and lower motor neuron signs, and affects all skeletal muscles except extraocular muscles. Weakness, atrophy, and often prominent fasciculations with complaints of muscle cramps early in the course indicate loss of anterior horn cells in the cord's gray matter. However, concomitant hyperreflexia and extensor plantar responses result from the death of motor neurons in the cerebral cortex, with wallerian degeneration of myelinated fibers in the corticospinal tracts. ALS may commence asymmetrically, for example, in one hand or one leg, and the diagnosis may not be readily apparent. Careful inspection for fasciculations and brisk or pathologic reflexes in subclinically affected extremities is important, and the presence of extensor plantar responses should also raise suspicion for this diagnosis. A characteristic dysarthria occurs in ALS, which is dominated by an atrophic, fasciculating, and flabby tongue. When a patient with a nasal dysarthric voice and dysphagia complains of weakness in one or more extremities, the suspicion for ALS should immediately be raised.

It is important to exclude treatable diseases that can mimic ALS. I had the fortunate experience of examining a woman in her 50s who had slowly progressive atrophy and weakness in a leg, an extensor plantar response, and a brisk quadriceps reflex, but absent ankle reflex. The finding of hyperreflexia is such an integral component of ALS that even though this person had both upper and lower motor neuron findings in one extremity, a workup was pursued that revealed two separate lesions: a chronic S1 radiculopathy accounting for the lower motor neuron signs and a superior convexity motor cortex cavernous hemangioma accounting for the upper motor neuron signs. Other diseases may resemble ALS (see the box on p. 1449), including, most notably, cervical radiculomyelopathy and lumbar polyradiculopathies in patients with

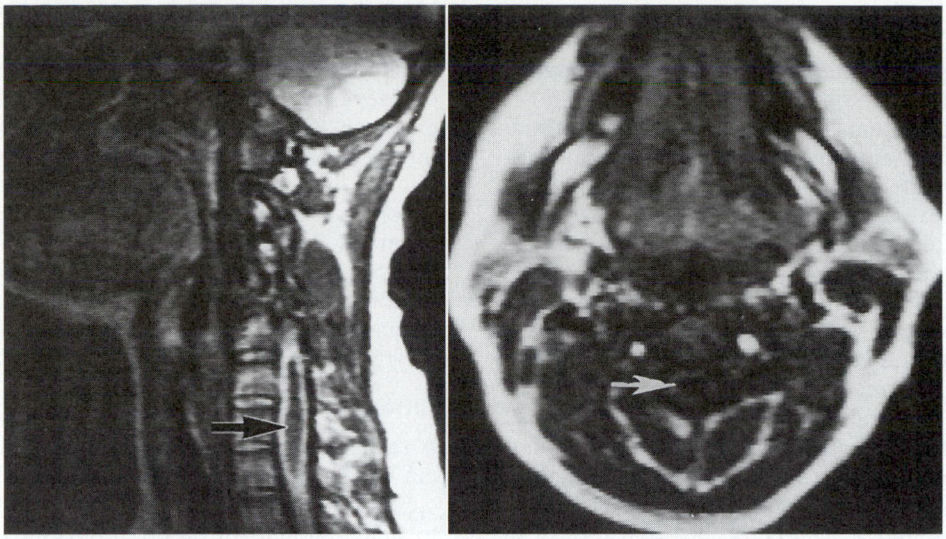

**Fig. 104-11.** This 32-year-old nurse was lifting a patient when she developed symptomatically acute-onset syringomyelia-syringobulbia that clinically resembled a major brainstem cerebrovascular accident (stroke), including a mental state that was near coma. The parasagittal MR image in 1988 demonstrated the large cystic expansion in the cord, which is seen on both parasagittal **(A)** and axial **(B)** views. The Chiari I malformation (low-lying cerebellar tonsils in the foramen magnum) can also be seen on the parasagittal view. After emergency decompression of the foramen magnum, rostral cervical spine laminectomy, and placement of a shunt between the syrinx and the subarachnoid space, the patient greatly improved, although she is left with the signs and symptoms of syringomyelia.

### Diseases with clinical presentations that mimic amyotrophic lateral sclerosis (ALS)

- Multifocal motor neuropathy with conduction block
- Lead axonal neuropathy
- Multifocal polyradiculopathy with spondylotic myelopathy
- Unrelated lesions causing combination of both upper and lower motor neuron findings
- Paraneoplastic ALS that regresses with treatment of tumor
- Spinal cord glioma without sensory features
- Syphilitic myelitis with amyotrophy
- Chronic fibrosing pachymeningitis
- Delayed effects of electrical injury to spinal cord

predisposing factors such as disseminated idiopathic sclerotic hyperostosis and other conditions discussed previously. An insidious glioma of the ventral aspect of the spinal cord may produce destruction of anterior horn cells and impairment of corticospinal tract function without sensory loss in the early stages and thus may simulate ALS. Such a patient would benefit from radiation therapy and would most likely have a better prognosis. Syphilitic infection of the cord and meninges is said to produce a pure motor syndrome in some patients. The resulting combination of spastic lower extremity weakness and segmental upper extremity amyotrophy (lower motor neuron weakness with atrophy) would clearly need to be differentiated from ALS here as well. It is thus critical in establishing a possible diagnosis of ALS to obtain serum and CSF for analysis, as well as neuroimaging and electrodiagnostic evaluations to ensure that the nerve conductions and electromyographic findings conform to established guidelines for the diagnosis of this unremitting entity.

Apparently new categories of motor neuron disease include a condition I have seen affecting two young men in their 20s, of progressive upper and lower motor neuron devastation including muscles of respiration but sparing extraocular muscles, sensation, and mentation, and a paraneoplastic motor neuron disease, discussed earlier. Motor neuron diseases are not confined to adults. Infants are afflicted by the rapidly progressive Werdnig-Hoffmann disease and children and young adults by the more indolent and less invariably fatal Kugelberg-Welander disease.

Motor neuron disease manifests less often as primary lateral sclerosis, a disease of the corticospinal tracts but not of the anterior horn cells or motor neurons in the cerebral cortex, and thus the presentation is upper motor neuron in type. Progressive spinal muscular atrophy is essentially the inverse disease, in that the anterior horn cells in the spinal cord degenerate but the corticospinal tracts and motor cortex are not involved. The presentation is a lower motor neuron disorder resembling and to be differentiated from an axonal motor neuropathy (e.g., that seen in lead poisoning) or the multifocal motor neuropathy with conduction block associated with the presence in the blood of antibodies to the $GM_1$ component of the neuronal membrane. Nerve conduction studies and electromyography are central in the diagnostic workup of these patients. The presentation is more complex in some families who have a combination of both progressive muscular atrophy and a peripheral axonal polyneuropathy.

### Idiopathic disorders

Some diseases affecting the spinal cord are not easily categorized in terms of their etiology or the mechanism by which they inflict damage on the cord. When sarcoidosis affects the nervous system, its most common manifestations include cranial nerve palsies, peripheral polyneuropathy, primary muscle disease, and recurrent meningitis. Additionally, however, sarcoidosis involves the CNS parenchyma, including the spinal cord. The clinical manifestations are difficult to separate from other intrinsic mass lesions affecting the cord (most notably tumors), and associated features are necessary to suspect and then establish the diagnosis. Lesions scattered in different parts of the neuraxis (brain and spinal cord involvement in the same patient) or a combination of both central and peripheral manifestations (myelopathy, Bell's palsy, meningeal inflammatory reaction) should alert the clinician. Hilar adenopathy, elevated levels of angiotensin-converting enzyme, and if necessary, positive biopsy of affected sites are all useful diagnostically. The response to steroid therapy can be most gratifying.

Chronic fibrosing pachymeningitis is known by a number of vague and suboptimal names. It is a serious spinal condition with an unclear pathophysiology and only occasionally definite initiating pathology, and it is often refractory to treatment (see the box below). A prominent fibrosis of the meninges, particularly the dura mater, produces multiple nerve root compressions, strangulation of the cord because of the crowding within the limited confines of the spinal canal, and cord infarction from external compromise and obliteration of radicular arteries. Diagnosis is suggested by finding the thickened and usually contrast-enhancing dura on MRI and is confirmed by biopsy, which may provide clues to the etiology. This entity occurs following bacterial infections such as pneumococcal meningitis, after the infection has been eradicated. Tuberculosis, fungal disease, cryptococcosis, and syphilis are typically associated, and sarcoidosis, vasculitis, and other chronic infections may also produce this result. Intrathecal injection of contaminants of procaine (no longer used for anesthesia) and steroids have been implicated. Lymphocytic choriomeningitis virus has been described in this connection in the literature. I have encountered such an entity in the setting of a clinicopathologic conference, although the definitive viral studies on serum and CSF were not available to confirm the clinical picture in that patient. Two recent patients with chronic diffuse pachymeningitis were treated with steroids and cyclophosphamide at our institution with limited success. One patient's disease occurred after a chronic bacterial paranasal sinus infection, and the other against a background of Crohn's disease, systemic hypercoagulability, and cerebral vasculitis diagnosed by arteriography. A third patient, whose pachymeningitis occurred in the setting of AIDS and cryptococcal meningitis, responded slowly to chronic intraventricular antifungal therapy (ketoconazole).

Electrical injury to the spinal cord, whether by lightning or electrical appliances or outlets, can cause an acute myelopathy, a delayed and chronic myelopathy, and a gradually progressive, late-onset, segmental amyotrophy. The pathology is characterized predominantly by demyelination, but axonal disruption and neuronal loss are also observed. The cord segment that lies in the current's path is most affected, with the cervical spinal cord being most often involved. The clinical syndrome varies according to the severity, extent, and location of the insult. Some evidence suggests that treatment of acute electrical spinal injury with high-dose steroids affects the long-term clinical outcome. Patients who sustain considerable electrical injury but seem well initially should be closely observed for at least a few days because of delayed demyelination, which may be aggressive and widespread. Steroids appear to be indicated here as well. No evidence indicates that electricity-induced demyelination leads to the remitting and relapsing course of multiple sclerosis.

### Iatrogenic disorders

A recognized but fortunately rare complication of spinal tap is the possibility of producing a clinically important epidural hematoma. Penetration of dural vessels may lead to small amounts of blood in the epidural space, but when bleeding is extensive, a rapid compressive myelopathy may develop. This development is unlikely to be missed given the clinical setting, and the emergency use of available neuroimaging modalities, osmotic agents, steroids, and possibly acute surgical decompression should all be expedited. Spinal epidural or subdural abscess or iatrogenic meningitis after spinal tap can generally be prevented by avoiding infected skin regions when attempting to obtain CSF.

Radiation of the head and neck, mediastinum, retroperitoneum, or spinal cord itself may lead to the delayed complication of arteriolar fibrosis and obliteration, which produces a progressive, ischemic myelopathy. The process usually begins 6 to 18 months after the radiation therapy and is gradually progressive over months. Usually no pain occurs at the site, but patients complain of distal paresthesias and sensory loss, and a Lhermitte's sign may be seen. The precise clinical presentation varies according to the site of involvement. Motor findings and sphincter incontinence are early problems. The history and absence of other etiologic factors lead to the diagnosis. Treatment options are limited, although immunosuppressive agents have been reported to be effective in some patients. This entity is less common now that the total dose and frequency of irradiation have been limited to no more than 6000 rad over approximately 2 months. The very late

#### Major known causes of chronic diffuse pachymeningitis

Syphilis
Tuberculosis
Cryptococcosis
Pneumococcal meningitis
Vasculitis
Lymphocytic choriomeningitis virus
Foreign substances
Contaminants of procaine/steroids/penicillin
Repeated lumbosacral surgery (produces a focal process, not diffuse)

development (after 15 to 20 years) of progressive neurologic syndromes has been described after radiation therapy and is unrelated to recurrent cancer after a careful search. The pathophysiology of this syndrome is not known, but it may relate to progressive fibrosis of neural tissue and/or surrounding structures. I have seen this in patients in whom radiation affected the spinal cord, brachial plexus, and sciatic nerve. Toxic myelopathies resulting from medical interventions and cord infarction during clamping of or surgery on the aorta are discussed earlier.

## MANAGEMENT

A few central themes govern the management of spinal cord disease and are reiterated and emphasized here. The spinal cord recovers poorly if at all from acute destructive or compressive lesions. It is therefore imperative to differentiate compressive from noncompressive lesions as rapidly as possible. Situations that may lead to such an emergency need to be recognized, including the patient with cancer and back pain (metastases), fever and back pain (epidural abscess), or bone disease (rheumatoid, osteoarthritis with spondylosis, osteoporosis, Paget's disease) and new symptoms referable to the spinal cord. The liberal use in these settings of whatever neuroimaging technique is most readily available can substantially alter the patient's course. MRI is optimal, but if not immediately available in a given patient setting, computed tomographic (CT) scanning, with or without myelography, should be performed. Indeed, a postmyelography CT scan may be more informative than MRI in determining patency of the subarachnoid space surrounding a focal obstructive lesion. Even a plain x-ray of the spine can be helpful in documenting metastatic disease. The key to this issue, however, is not to wait for the "better" study but to obtain the best neuroimaging study available as urgently as possible. Decompressive surgery or palliative radiation therapy needs to be done even in the early morning hours in patients with acute spinal cord compression, because once function is lost, it is difficult to regain.

Certain neurologic manifestations of spinal cord disease must be managed directly. Common examples include the following: flexor spasms respond to antispasticity agents (baclofen, clonazepam); autonomic dysreflexia is treated successfully with α-adrenergic blocking agents (tolazoline, phentolamine); urinary urgency is lessened with anticholinergic agents (propantheline, oxybutynin, dicyclomine), and a flaccid bladder is strengthened with cholinergic agents (urecholine). Some features, such as flexor spasms and autonomic dysreflexia, can be exacerbated by otherwise silent medical conditions, including urinary tract infections, pressure sores, and bowel obstructions. The exaggerated spinal reactions improve once the superimposed medical condition has resolved, and it is therefore worth excluding these possibilities before directly treating the neurologic manifestations. Another central issue with respect to management is that patients with abrupt loss of spinal cord function, such as after trauma, develop complications astonishingly fast. Urinary obstruction facilitates infection, impaired cough encourages pneumonia, and immobility leads to pressure necrosis of the skin and deep venous thrombosis sometimes within hours. Skilled nursing management of these patients is a critical feature of their care and prognosis, and prophylactic heparinization is usually instituted unless a clear contraindication exists. If there is no concomitant cerebral insult, patients are aware of their predicament and need to be counseled through the acute stages of their illness and involved as much as possible in the decision-making processes.

## ACKNOWLEDGMENT

The author is grateful to Dr. E. Tessa Hedley-Whyte for her critical review of the manuscript.

## BIBLIOGRAPHY

Adams RD, Victor M: *Principles of neurology,* ed 5, New York, 1992, McGraw-Hill.

Atlas SW: *Magnetic resonance imaging of the brain and spine,* New York, 1991, Raven Press.

Austin GM: *The spinal cord,* ed 3, New York, 1983, Igaku-Shoin.

Guttman L: *Spinal cord injuries: comprehensive management and research,* ed 2, London, 1976, Blackwell.

Pia HW, Djindjian R: *Spinal angiomas: advances in diagnosis and therapy,* New York, 1978, Springer-Verlag.

Spillane JD, Spillane JA: *An atlas of clinical neurology,* ed 3, Oxford, 1982, Oxford University Press.

William PL, Warwick R, editors: *Gray's anatomy* British ed 37, New York, 1989, Churchill Livingstone.

Woolsey RM, Young RR, editors: Disorders of the spinal cord, *Neurol Clin* 9:535, 1991.

Zejdlik CP: *Management of spinal cord injury,* ed 2, Boston, 1992, Jones and Bartlett.

# XI Ophthalmology

CHAPTER

## 105 The Eye in Systemic Disease

David D. Bogorad

### ANATOMIC AND EMBRYOLOGIC CONSIDERATIONS

The eye and the visual system are the most complex and highly developed sensory mechanisms of the body. Of all the organs, the eye is uniquely accessible to study. The transparent cornea functions as a window through which the effects of systemic disease on ocular tissue can be seen directly. For example, the direct inspection of the retina and its associated vascular tree can provide insights into the condition of the central nervous system (CNS) and vascular system that cannot be obtained by physical examination elsewhere in the body.

In the development of the eye, the neural ectoderm, surface ectoderm, and neural crest are all major contributors. Given this broad embryologic base, it is not surprising that the eye is involved in a wide range of systemic disorders.

### HOW TO USE THIS DATA

This chapter provides the generalist clinician with a listing of specific systemic disease entities associated with ocular findings. The disease entities are organized within larger, general classifications. The list does not claim to be exhaustive, but it is quite comprehensive. The depth of the discussion is intended to be adequate for a general introduction to the subject matter and to assist in differential diagnosis. Only minimal attention is directed to the treatment of the ocular conditions outlined here; medical and surgical management of ophthalmic disease is beyond the scope of this book. Standards of care dictate that patients with ocular manifestations of most of the disorders included here be evaluated and treated by an ophthalmologist. More general presentations of many of these disease entities appear elsewhere in this volume.

If a patient's systemic disease is known, the generalist may choose to obtain an ophthalmologic consultation for diagnostic confirmation and any necessary treatment of the associated ocular pathology. On the other hand, eye findings in some systemic disorders can offer diagnostic insight that will aid in identifying the systemic disease. In these cases, an ophthalmic examination can aid the generalist in arriving at the correct diagnosis. Finally, the generalist should refer a patient who presents with primary eye symptoms without known systemic disease to an ophthalmologist for a specific ocular diagnosis. This might in turn lead to consideration of an underlying, unsuspected systemic disease.

### CATEGORIES OF SYSTEMIC DISEASES AND THEIR OCULAR MANIFESTATIONS

#### Allergic diseases (Table 105-1)

*Asthma.* Asthma can be associated with allergic conjunctivitis (see Hay Fever). Conjunctival allergic reactions may result from local exposure to allergens or as part of a generalized hypersensitivity. The prolonged systemic corticosteroid treatment often required in severe asthma can lead to posterior subcapsular cataract and secondary glaucoma. Thus a patient who requires the prolonged administration of systemic steroids for any reason should have periodic examinations by an ophthalmologist.

*Atopic dermatitis.* Allergic dermatoconjunctivitis, or contact allergy of the eyelids and conjunctiva, is the most common form of ophthalmic allergic reaction. Cosmetics, animal or vegetable material, or ophthalmic drugs are usually etiologic. The primary symptom is severe itching. Diagnostic findings include papillary conjunctivitis, eczema of the skin of the eyelids (see Atopic Eczema), and conjunctival eosinophilia. Treatment consists of eliminating the sensitizing agent and possible short-term use of topical corticosteroids.

*Atopic eczema.* Eczema is a general term used for allergic inflammation of the skin of the eyelid. The epidermis is primarily involved. In addition to the symptoms of itching and erythema, signs may include papules, oozing, vesicles, crusting, induration, and scaling. Associated conjunctivitis or keratoconjunctivitis can result in opacification of the superficial cornea in extreme cases. When these problems occur, patients require ophthalmic referral. There is an association between keratoconus, anterior cortical cataract, and atopic disease.

*Hay fever.* The acute atopic conjunctivitis associated with hay fever is mediated by IgE. Airborne dust, spores, and pollen are the usual offending agents. Hyperemia, edema, and a watery discharge are the hallmarks. These findings may be limited to the eye, or they may be part of a broader hay fever reaction with respiratory and nasal symptoms.

*Urticaria.* Periorbital edema can occur as part of a generalized allergic reaction of the atopic or type I variety. Urticaria or angioneurotic edema are etiologic, although local contact sensitivity can cause allergic swelling. The natural laxity and thinness of the eyelid skin allow alarming edema to occur in the eyelids that would be minor elsewhere.

#### Cardiovascular disorders (Table 105-2)

*Aortic arch syndrome (Takayasu).* Ocular findings in aortic arch disease vary according to the site of occlusion and the pattern of blood flow. Ocular manifestations include characteristics of the specific diseases in addition to the nonspecific changes of poor ocular circulation.

Nonspecific changes in ocular hypoperfusion include retinal venous dilation, beading, cotton-wool spots, and microaneurysms in the early stages. Subsequently, periph-

**Table 105-1.** Allergic diseases

| Disease entity | Lids and adnexa | Conj. & sclera | Cornea | Cataract | Glaucoma | Retina & opt. nerve | Extra-oc muscles | Orbit | Uveitis | Visual CNS |
|---|---|---|---|---|---|---|---|---|---|---|
| Asthma | | XX | | | | | | | | |
| Atopic dermatitis | XX | XX | | | | | | | | |
| Atopic eczema | XX | XX | XX | XX | | | | | | |
| Hay fever | | XX | | | | | | | | |
| Urticaria | XX | | | | | | | | | |

**Table 105-2.** Cardiovascular disorders

| Disease entity | Lids and adnexa | Conj. & sclera | Cornea | Cataract | Glaucoma | Retina & opt. nerve | Extra-oc muscles | Orbit | Uveitis | Visual CNS |
|---|---|---|---|---|---|---|---|---|---|---|
| Aortic arch syndrome | | XX | | XX | XX | XX | | | XX | |
| Arteriosclerosis | | | XX | | | XX | | | | |
| Endocarditis | | | | | | XX | | | | XX |
| Hereditary hemorrhagic telangiectasia | | XX | | | | | | | | |
| Hypertension | | | | | | XX | | | | |
| Occlusive vascular disease | | | | | | | | | | |
| Cranial arteritis | | | | | | XX | | | | |
| Thrombi and emboli | | | | | | XX | | | | |
| Carotid artery disease | | | | | | XX | | | | |
| Sickle cell disease | | | | | XX | XX | | | | |

eral retinal hemorrhages and nonperfusion of the peripheral retina can occur. The dreaded complications of retinal neovascularization and iris neovascularization (rubeosis) can follow. In turn, uncontrolled iris neovascularization leads to the development of neovascular glaucoma, which is extremely difficult to treat. Therefore any patient who reveals retinal vascular changes, hemorrhages, and exudates on examination should be referred to an ophthalmologist for evaluation. Additional nonspecific signs of ocular vascular insufficiency include cataract and chronic low-grade ocular inflammation.

Aortic arch abnormalities are associated with vasculitis, granulomatous diseases, collagen vascular diseases, and atherosclerosis. If the aortic arch widens, the associated aortic valvular insufficiency may produce embolic retinal vascular manifestations.

Takayasu's disease (pulseless disease) typically occurs in young women. In addition to the preceding general eye findings, Takayasu's disease may be associated with scleritis.

***Arteriosclerosis.*** A general term referring to hardening and thickening of the arteries, arteriosclerosis is subclassified into atherosclerosis and arteriolosclerosis according to the location of the changes within the arterial wall. The retinal vasculature is most commonly affected by intimal atherosclerosis (changes in the intima) and arteriolosclerosis (pathology in the intima and/or the media). The corneal arcus senilis is often associated with systemic atherosclerosis. Retinal arteriolosclerosis is specifically associated with systemic hypertension. The nomenclature is confusing, and atherosclerosis and arteriolosclerosis have often been used interchangeably in the literature. Arteriosclerosis is clearly the most important systemic condition related to central retinal vein occlusion (CRVO). Also etiologic in CRVO is arterial hypertension, which accelerates arteriosclerosis.

***Endocarditis.*** The classic ocular manifestation of infective endocarditis is Roth's spots, a focal intraretinal hemorrhage with a white center. The white center is thought to be either a platelet and fibrin clot or an area of focal retinitis caused by an infected embolus. Other ocular complications include petechial hemorrhages on the conjunctiva, cotton-wool spots in the retina, capillary nonperfusion, and central or branch artery obstruction. Papillitis and metastatic endophthalmitis also can occur. Visual symptoms can vary from transient visual obscuration to complete loss of vision. If the CNS is invaded by the bacterial embolic process, eye signs such as ocular muscle palsies, nystagmus, and anisocoria may occur.

Nonbacterial thrombotic endocarditis usually is seen in the terminal stages of chronic debilitating disease, such as malignancy, tuberculosis, and uremia.

***Hereditary hemorrhagic telangiectasia (Rendu-Osler-Weber disease).*** An autosomal dominant disorder, hereditary hemorrhagic telangiectasia involves the skin as well as the mucous membranes of the GI tract, lungs, mouth, nose, and eyes. In the eye, dilated conjunctival vascular lesions, which may bleed, are seen. These patients require ophthalmologic evaluation.

*Hypertension.* Three specific changes occur in the retinal arterial tree during the evolution of chronic hypertension. First, generalized attenuation of the arterioles occurs in the presence of long-term significant elevation of the diastolic pressure. Second, arterioles respond to the constant elevation of intraluminal pressure by developing arteriolosclerosis. Arteriolosclerosis is manifested by progressive changes in the appearance of the retinal arteriolar walls, from so-called copper wiring, to silver wiring, to the end stage where the arterioles are seen as fibrous cords, with no visible blood column. The ophthalmoscopic picture is thought to parallel the general state of the arterioles elsewhere in the body. Third, focal constriction, localized waistlike narrowing of the arterioles, can occur. The severity of this process appears related to the acuteness of the rise in pressure and the height of the diastolic pressure.

Arteriolovenous crossing changes (AV nicking) appear to be secondary to a compression and deflection of the vein at the crossing point. Such changes are characteristic of chronic hypertension and evolve over many years.

Flame-shaped hemorrhages, located in the nerve fiber layer, are commonly seen in chronic hypertension. Due to a loss in the integrity of the capillary endothelium, scattered intraretinal hemorrhages of this type usually have no significant effect on vision.

Cotton-wool spots are areas of focal nerve-fiber layer ischemia due to local arteriolar occlusion. They occur suddenly and usually disappear ophthalmoscopically within a few weeks.

Microaneurysms probably arise at points of localized weakness in the capillary walls. Most frequently seen in diabetics, they occur next most commonly in patients with hypertensive retinopathy.

Hard exudates, yellowish white deposits usually located in the posterior pole, result from focal leakage of terminal arterioles. They are composed of residual lipid material that remains trapped in the extravascular retina.

Malignant hypertension is not a separate entity but rather a more severe, rapidly progressive form of systemic hypertension. An encephalopathic picture with headache, vomiting, convulsions, or coma can occur. All of the retinal changes described previously can be seen in severe form. In addition, papilledema is common. Although papilledema may be a result of increased intracranial pressure, the more common underlying cause in malignant hypertension is the ischemia of arteriolar occlusion and leakage from the damaged peripapillary vasculature.

Retinal vascular changes in toxemia of pregnancy are correlated with the severity of the rise in the blood pressure. Diffuse retinopathy and the development of exudative retinal detachment, while rare, are grave signs and are indications for the termination of pregnancy.

### *Occlusive vascular disease*

**Cranial arteritis.** Cranial arteritis, also known as giant cell arteritis or temporal arteritis, is almost never seen in patients younger than 50 years of age. All vessels may be affected, although the temporal arteries are most frequently involved. Headache is the most common symptom, often presenting as tenderness over the temporal artery or scalp. Polymyalgia rheumatica, jaw claudication, anorexia, and malaise are other common presenting clinical features. More than 90% of patients with cranial arteritis have an elevated erythrocyte sedimentation rate. Temporal artery biopsy has long been the method for making the diagnosis; however, false-negative biopsies may occur about 5% of the time.

The most frequent ocular manifestation of cranial arteritis is ischemic optic neuropathy due to involvement of the posterior ciliary arteries supplying the optic nerve. Clinically, it presents as a painless, sudden loss of vision with an altitudinal visual field defect. Prompt institution of systemic corticosteroids is essential to minimize the risk of ischemic optic neuropathy.

**Thrombi and emboli.** Acute arterial obstructive disease of the eye is commonly encountered in clinical practice. Patients with central retinal artery occlusion present with sudden, severe, but painless loss of vision. The acute ophthalmoscopic picture of the cherry-red spot on the fovea of the macula is pathognomonic. An afferent pupillary defect is almost always present. Acutely, the arterial tree is narrow and irregular. Note that retinal hemorrhages are not characteristic of CRA occlusion. Branch arterial occlusions also can occur.

Arteriosclerosis is the most commonly associated systemic condition. Other conditions in order of frequency are hypertension, carotid artery disease, diabetes, and valvular heart disease. Other causes include emboli from a mural thrombus following myocardial infarction, cardiac myxoma, subacute bacterial endocarditis, coagulopathies, and collagen vascular diseases.

Acute CRVO presents with a distinctly different fundus picture than CRAO. Some degree of intraretinal hemorrhage is always present; according to the degree of ischemia present, the hemorrhage can vary from moderate and scattered to severe, diffuse hemorrhaging. Engorgement of the venous tree is always prominent, with tortuosity. Disc edema may be present.

Nonischemic CRVO generally presents with less severe visual loss than the ischemic variety. Eyes that have sustained a CRVO are at risk for the subsequent development of retinal and/or iris neovascularization. Referral to an ophthalmologist is essential.

As with CRAO, the most commonly associated systemic condition with CRVO is arteriosclerosis. Also closely related is arterial hypertension, which is associated in about 60% of cases of CRVO. Diabetes is a significant risk factor as well.

Any patient who presents with acute loss of vision should be evaluated by an ophthalmologist on an emergent basis.

**Carotid artery disease.** The major cause of chronic ocular arterial obstruction is carotid artery disease. Atherosclerosis, in turn, is by far the most common cause of carotid artery disease. The eye is commonly involved in atheromatous disease of the carotid artery bifurcation because the ophthalmic artery is one of the first branches of the internal carotid artery in the neck. Ocular symptoms are often the first indication of carotid artery disease. Symptoms can occur acutely or in an insidious, slowly progressive manner. These symptoms include partial or complete visual loss due to arterial obstruction, transiently decreased vision (amaurosis fugax), or pain resulting from the ocular ischemic syndrome.

It is essential to recognize that amaurosis fugax is a type of transient ischemic attack because about 30% of all patients with an untreated transient ischemic attack can be expected to have a cerebral vascular accident. On the other hand, not all amaurosis fugax is due to carotid disease; other causes include cranial arteritis, pseudotumor cerebri, and migraine.

Various symptomatic ocular manifestations of chronic arterial obstruction can result from carotid artery disease; these result from hypoperfusion of the eye secondary to stenosis or complete obstruction of the carotid artery. The pathology can be confined to the retina, producing the picture of hypotensive retinopathy, or more generalized, as in the ocular ischemic syndrome. On the other hand, another group of patients with carotid artery disease is asymptomatic; signs of the disease may be found during a routine fundus examination as part of a general physical examination. Specifically, two types of microemboli may be observed in the retinal arterial tree. The first type is cholesterol emboli, which are a bright yellow color, often called Hollenhorst plaques. The second type, grayish white, platelet-fibrin emboli, are seen less frequently, as they do not persist in the arteriole as long as the cholesterol plaques.

**Sickle cell disease.** Sickle cell disease in its various forms can produce a retinopathy of variable severity and chronic course. Ocular complications are most severe in the SC and SThal types. Most of the retinal abnormalities can be attributed to vascular occlusion. In some cases, neovascularization occurs secondary to ischemia caused by vascular occlusion. The neovascular or vasoproliferative process, in turn, can lead to vitreous hemorrhage, retinal detachment, and neovascular glaucoma. The nonproliferative retinal findings are highly characteristic, but usually asymptomatic; they include venous tortuosity, black sunbursts, salmon-patch hemorrhages, and refractile deposits. Finally, the occlusive process associated with sickling can predispose to CRAO. Patients with the ocular manifestations of sickle cell disease should be followed by an ophthalmologist.

## Collagen diseases (Table 105-3)

***Ankylosing spondylitis.*** The main ocular manifestation of ankylosing spondylitis is a recurrent, acute iridocyclitis. Between 25% and 33% of patients with ankylosing spondylitis will experience at least one attack of uveitis; 90% or more of patients will be HLA-B27 positive.

***Cranial arteritis.*** See Occlusive Vascular Disease.

***Dermatomyositis.*** The most common ocular manifestation of patients with dermatomyositis is a heliotrope rash affecting the eyelids. Occasionally, ophthalmoplegia due to involvement of the extraocular muscles by myositis may be seen. Nerve fiber layer infarcts (cotton-wool spots) also have been reported.

***Polyarteritis nodosa.*** Ocular findings are seen in 10% to 20% of patients with polyarteritis nodosa. Manifestations usually are due to the vascular disease and include hypertensive retinopathy in patients with renal disease, retinal vasculitis, and retinal arterial occlusive disease. Anterior or posterior scleritis has been described, as has marginal corneal ulceration. Central CNS lesions can lead to visual field defects, and choroidal ischemia with secondary serous detachment of the retina has occurred.

***Reiter's syndrome.*** Conjunctivitis was one of the original triad of findings described by Reiter and is most commonly seen during the initial attack. More serious, however, is recurrent, acute iridocyclitis, which occurs in up to 50% of patients with long-term follow-up.

***Rheumatoid arthritis.*** The most common ocular manifestations of rheumatoid arthritis (RA) are keratoconjunctivitis sicca (secondary Sjögren's syndrome), scleritis, and rheumatoid corneal melting.

Sjögren's syndrome is characterized by lymphocytic infiltration of the lacrimal and salivary glands resulting in progressive destruction of the glands and secondary lacrimal insufficiency. About 12% of patients with RA have secondary Sjögren's syndrome. Occasional severe cases require aggressive ophthalmic management to preserve corneal integrity.

Scleral inflammation is the second most common ocular finding in RA, occurring in about 1% of patients. Episcleritis is more superficial and less severe and is usually self-limiting. Scleritis, on the other hand, is more likely to

**Table 105-3.** Collagen diseases

| Disease entity | Lids and adnexa | Conj. & sclera | Cornea | Cataract | Glaucoma | Retina & opt. nerve | Extra-oc muscles | Orbit | Uveitis | Visual CNS |
|---|---|---|---|---|---|---|---|---|---|---|
| Ankylosing spondylitis | | | | | | | | | XX | |
| Cranial arteritis | | | | | | XX | | | | |
| Dermatomyositis | XX | | | | | XX | XX | | | |
| Polyarteritis nodosa | | XX | XX | | | XX | | | | XX |
| Reiter's syndrome | | XX | | | | | | | XX | |
| Rheumatoid arthritis (adult) | | XX | XX | | | | | | | |
| (juvenile) | | | XX | XX | | | | | XX | |
| Sarcoidosis | XX | | | | | XX | | | XX | |
| Scleroderma | XX | XX | XX | | | | | | | |
| Systemic lupus erythematosus | XX | | XX | | | XX | | | | XX |
| Wegener's granulomatosis | XX | XX | XX | | | XX | | XX | | |

present with pain and can be anterior or posterior in location.

Rheumatoid corneal melts are usually peripheral. If necrotizing, they can become an ophthalmic emergency. Even aggressive systemic therapy with corticosteroids and immunosuppressives is not always effective in preventing progressive corneal melting, leading to sight-threatening perforation. In these situations, the case should be comanaged with an anterior segment ophthalmic surgeon.

Patients with RA who are being treated with hydroxychloroquine should be referred for ophthalmic evaluation and follow-up. The drug is accumulated in the retinal pigment epithelium and may produce a "bull's eye" pigmentary retinopathy, which is reversible if discovered early.

The ocular manifestations of juvenile rheumatoid arthritis are two different types of iridocyclitis. The more severe, chronic variety is seen in the antinuclear antibody-(ANA) positive pauciarticular subgroup. Although it is usually only minimally symptomatic, severe visual disability may develop, with band keratopathy and cataract occurring in one third of these patients.

***Sarcoidosis.*** Sarcoidosis, a systemic granulomatous disease of unclear etiology, is placed in this section somewhat arbitrarily. Sarcoidosis presents with ocular symptoms in 7% of patients. Once the diagnosis is made and a systemic search performed, the globes are found to be involved in 20%, the lacrimal gland in 7%, and the CNS in 4% of patients.

Uveitis is both the most common and most serious form of intraocular involvement in sarcoidosis. It may be granulomatous or nongranulomatous, acute or chronic, diffuse or localized. Chronic iridocyclitis in sarcoidosis can be associated with chronic cystoid macular edema. Midperipheral retinal periphlebitis is a common retinal finding in sarcoidosis, as are "candle wax drippings," small exudates near retinal veins.

The skin of the lids and mucosa of the conjunctiva may have easily biopsied sarcoid nodules. A biopsy of an enlarged lacrimal gland demonstrating noncaseating granulomas can differentiate sarcoidosis from other causes of lacrimal gland enlargement, such as systemic lupus erythematosus (SLE), lymphoma, tuberculosis, pseudotumor, and Sjögren's syndrome.

***Scleroderma.*** The most common ocular involvement in patients with scleroderma is progressive tightness of the skin of the eyelids, resulting in blepharophimosis. This problem occurs in 30% to 60% of patients. Lacrimal insufficiency with a Sjögren's-like picture has been described. Conjunctival telangiectasias are frequently reported. Severe corneal decompensation is rare.

***Systemic lupus erythematosus.*** The ocular effects of SLE can be divided into four areas: eyelid skin changes associated with cutaneous disease, lacrimal insufficiency with associated ocular surface abnormalities secondary to Sjögren's syndrome; retinal vascular changes, and neuro-ophthalmic pathology.

Retinal vascular manifestations are the most common form of ophthalmic damage in SLE. The underlying microangiopathy of SLE appears to be etiologic in the development of cotton-wool spots and intraretinal hemorrhages. Severe retinal vasoocclusive disease is less common, but can present as central or branch artery or vein occlusion, or as a diffuse vasculitis. Secondary retinal neovascularization can develop.

The CNS involvement in SLE includes cranial nerve palsies, lupus optic neuropathy (1% to 2% of patients), and central visual pathway disorders.

***Wegener's granulomatosis.*** Ocular disease occurs in about 50% of patients with Wegener's granulomatosis. Orbital involvement is probably the most common form of ophthalmic pathology, presenting as an extension of

**Table 105-4.** Dermatologic and mucous membrane disorders

| Disease entity | Lids and adnexa | Conj. & sclera | Cornea | Cataract | Glaucoma | Retina & opt. nerve | Extra-oc muscles | Orbit | Uveitis | Visual CNS |
|---|---|---|---|---|---|---|---|---|---|---|
| Acne rosacea | XX | XX | XX | | | | | | | |
| Albinism | | | | | | XX | XX | | | XX |
| Atopic dermatitis | XX | XX | | | | | | | | |
| Behçet's disease | | | | | | XX | | | XX | XX |
| Cicatricial pemphigoid | XX | XX | XX | | | | | | | |
| Ehlers-Danlos syndrome | XX | XX | XX | XX | | XX | | | | |
| Epidermolysis bullosa | | XX | XX | | | | | | | |
| Erythema multiforme | XX | XX | XX | | | | | | | |
| Ichthyosis | XX | XX | XX | | | | | | | |
| Incontinentia pigmenti | | XX | | XX | | XX | XX | | | XX |
| Nevus of Ota | XX | XX | XX | XX | XX | XX | | | | |
| Pemphigus | XX | XX | XX | XX | | | | | | |
| Psuedoxanthoma elasticum | | | | | | XX | | | | |
| Psoriasis | XX | XX | XX | | | | | | | |
| Vogt-Koyanagi-Harada syndrome | XX | | | | | XX | | | XX | |
| Xeroderma pigmentosum | XX | | XX | | | | | | | |

granulomatous inflammation from the paranasal sinuses into the orbit. Sinus superinfection may extend into the orbit, causing orbital cellulitis. Dacryocystitis can develop if the nasolacrimal drainage system is obstructed due to changes in the nasal mucosa. Separate from the sinus inflammation, orbital pseudotumor can be seen.

Scleritis of any type is almost as common as orbital involvement in Wegener's granulomatosis. Marginal necrotizing corneal ulcers are associated with the scleritis, but can occur without it. Finally, retinal vascular and optic nerve lesions occur in perhaps 15% of patients.

## Dermatologic and mucous membrane disorders (Table 105-4)

***Acne rosacea.*** Ocular manifestations of acne rosacea include blepharitis, recurrent chalazion, and hyperemic conjunctivitis that can have associated small, marginal corneal ulcerations. About 5% of patients develop the most severe ocular complication, rosacea keratitis, an initially asymptomatic inferior vascularization of the cornea that can progress to erosion and scarring of the central cornea. Systemic tetracycline, along with local measures, often controls the condition.

***Albinism.*** The term *albinism* can be applied to any congenital hypopigmentation; here, it refers to those forms of albinism that involve the eye.

Oculocutaneous albinism is divided into four subtypes, all inherited as autosomal recessive traits. The ocular findings are identical in all four subtypes. Hypoplasia of the macula is a constant feature. The resulting absence of the development of foveal fixation in infancy causes the emergence of a coarse, pendular nystagmus. Best corrected visual acuity is in the 20/80 to 20/400 range. Diffuse transillumination of the iris and globe, and a blond, hypopigmented fundus also are present. Other findings are photophobia and a high incidence of strabismus and astigmatism.

In ocular albinism, cutaneous pigmentary dilution is much less notable, but the ocular features are similar to those of oculocutaneous albinism. The pigmentary dilution seen in the eye also may be more subtle. In general, the more nearly normal the degree of ocular pigmentation, the better the visual acuity; however, some degree of foveal hypoplasia is always present. Ocular albinism is inherited as either an X-linked or autosomal recessive trait.

Albinoidism is a group of autosomal dominant disorders that are differentiated from ocular albinism by the lack of nystagmus and the presence of normal visual acuity. Patients with albinoidism are mildly hypopigmented, and may manifest iris transillumination defects.

***Atopic dermatitis.*** See Allergic Diseases.

***Behçet's disease.*** Originally described as a triad of painful oral and genital ulcers and hypopyon uveitis, Behçet's disease also has significant skin involvement and arthritis. CNS disease occurs less often. The disease is most common in the Middle and Far East; there is a strong association with the HLA-Bw51 antigen. The most frequent ocular manifestation is anterior uveitis, with or without a hypopyon. Retinal vasculitis in Behçet's disease can involve both the arterial and venous sides, leading to arterial occlusion and retinal necrosis with detachment and neovascularization. The majority of patients with Behçet's disease have severe visual loss within 5 years of diagnosis, despite aggressive treatment with corticosteroids and immunosuppressives.

***Cicatricial pemphigoid.*** Ocular involvement in cicatricial pemphigoid is characterized by progressive conjunctival shrinkage, symblepharon, entropion, lacrimal insufficiency, and progressive corneal decompensation leading to opacity. Fibrosis beneath the conjunctiva is a constant pathologic feature. The process is invariably bilateral, with a mean age at presentation of about 70 years.

***Ehlers-Danlos syndrome.*** Of autosomal dominant inheritance, Ehlers-Danlos syndrome is associated with the following ocular manifestations: lens subluxation, keratoconus, angioid streaks, thin blue sclera, and high myopia due to posterior staphyloma formation. Marked epicanthal folds are commonly present. This connective tissue disorder also has a high incidence of retinal detachment.

***Epidermolysis bullosa.*** Having both hereditary and acquired forms, epidermolysis bullosa is associated with conjunctival scarring, symblepharon formation, and recurrent corneal erosions.

***Erythema multiforme (Stevens-Johnson syndrome).*** Erythema multiforme major, also known as Stevens-Johnson syndrome, presents with skin lesions, necrotizing inflammation of mucous membranes, and systemic toxicity. The most frequent precipitating factors are drugs and infections. The process may last up to 6 weeks.

The acute ocular disease can last 2 to 3 weeks. The eyelids become swollen, ulcerated, and crusted. Conjunctival involvement varies from a mild process that resolves without sequelae to a severe membranous conjunctivitis that results in scarring, symblepharon, entropion, and lacrimal insufficiency, with secondary corneal decompensation. Severe cases require early, aggressive intervention by the anterior segment ophthalmic specialist.

***Ichthyosis.*** Ichthyosis is a group of inherited disorders that produce thickening and scaling of the skin. Eyelid involvement in ichthyosis can cause secondary changes in the conjunctiva and cornea due to exposure.

***Incontinentia pigmenti.*** A disorder of skin pigmentation, incontinentia pigmenti is transmitted as an autosomal-dominant or sex-linked trait. About 35% of patients with the Bloch-Sulzberger type have ocular involvement, which includes cataracts, optic atrophy, strabismus, and nystagmus. Retinal dysplasia and exudative retinal detachment have been reported, as have conjunctival pigmentary changes.

***Nevus of Ota.*** Also called oculodermal melanocytosis, nevus of Ota is a blue-gray pigmentation of the skin of the cheek, temple, eyelids, and nose associated with a similar pigmentation of the sclera in the ipsilateral eye. Associated ocular findings include unilateral glaucoma, a retinitis pigmentosa picture, and congenital cataract. It may be congenital or appear in childhood or adolescence.

In addition to the scleral changes, pigmentation has been seen in the conjunctiva, cornea, iris, choroid, optic disc, and optic nerve sheath. Malignant change does occur in the nevus of Ota, but has been reported only in white patients.

*Pemphigus.* Pemphigus is a group of vesiculobullous eruptions of the skin and mucous membranes seen primarily in mid-life. Ocular involvement in pemphigus is not as severe as in cicatricial pemphigoid, but the disease may affect the lids, conjunctiva, cornea, lens, and iris. Progressive scarring and blindness, however, do not occur.

*Pseudoxanthoma elasticum.* An autosomal recessive condition, pseudoxanthoma elasticum is associated with the development of angioid streaks in the fundi of about 85% of patients. Angioid streaks are cracks in an abnormal Bruch's membrane. In 70% of the patients with angioid streaks, fibrovascular proliferation occurs through the cracks into the subretinal space, leading to disciform macular degeneration and subsequent loss of central vision.

*Psoriasis.* Ocular findings occur in about 10% of cases of psoriasis and are twice as prevalent in men. Most often, the skin of the eyelids is involved, and lesions can occur in the palpebral and bulbar conjunctiva. Photophobia is a common symptom. Plaquelike lesions can occur in the corneal epithelium, which can affect vision.

*Vogt-Koyanagi-Harada syndrome.* Vogt-Koyanagi-Harada syndrome (VKH) occurs more frequently in Asians and is a condition that combines poliosis, vitiligo, and alopecia with ocular and CNS signs. The ocular process may begin with deep orbital pain, which evolves into a panuveitis with optic disc swelling and exudative retinal detachment. Appropriate management with systemic steroids improves the otherwise poor visual prognosis in untreated cases.

*Xeroderma pigmentosum.* Xeroderma pigmentosum is a rare premalignant condition of the skin where there is a high incidence of the development of basal and/or squamous cell carcinoma; 70% or more of these patients develop ocular complications. The most common ocular problem is a progressive atrophy of the lower eyelid. Severe corneal disease, with opacification, ulceration or perforation, can occur. The corneal limbus is a site of malignant transformation, usually squamous cell carcinoma. Close follow-up and prompt surgical excision of any malignancies are required.

### Endocrine diseases (Table 105-5)

*Hyperadrenalism (Cushing's disease).* Hypertensive retinopathy can appear as an ocular complication of hyperadrenalism. Exophthalmos has been reported in 6% to 8% of patients, and elevated intraocular pressure may occur in as many as 25% of patients.

*Hypoadrenalism (Addison's disease).* Ocular involvement is not usually a feature of Addison's disease, but the skin hyperpigmentation may involve the lids and conjunctiva. Papilledema and optic atrophy have been reported.

*Hyperparathyroidism.* The ocular sign of hyperparathyroidism, band keratopathy, can occur in prolonged hypercalcemia of any etiology. Band keratopathy is a metastatic calcification of the surface of the cornea that creates a diffuse, granular, white, superficial opacity in the area of the palpebral fissure. The ophthalmologist can remove the band by mechanically denuding the corneal epithelium and then irrigating the exposed calcium with the chelating agent ethylenediaminetetraacetic acid (EDTA).

*Hypoparathyroidism.* The main ocular manifestation of hypoparathyroidism is cataract, which is seen in about 50% of patients. With therapy the progression of these cataracts can be halted. Papilledema and increased intracranial pressure also may occur.

*Hyperthyroidism.* Ocular signs can be seen in thyrotoxicosis of any etiology. These include upper lid retraction and lid lag. Graves' disease is the most common cause of hyperthyroidism. Its ocular effects are highly variable and can range from mild lid retraction to severe proptosis, with major visual loss due to corneal decompensation and/or optic nerve involvement. Diplopia and gaze limitation are among the most debilitating symptoms of Graves' disease. The mechanism of the relationship between thyroid dysfunction and Graves' ophthalmopathy is unclear, and the typical orbitopathy may be present in patients who are clinically euthyhroid, or even hypothyroid. In any event, the physical result is an increase in the mass of orbital tissue. The process is generally self-limited, and the thyroid ophthalmopathy burns out after months to years.

The treatment of the ocular manifestations of Graves' disease is complicated by the fact that control of the primary disease frequently does not improve and may exacerbate the ocular findings. Thus management must be coordinated between the endocrinologist and ophthalmologist.

*Hypothyroidism.* In hypothyroidism, myxedema can be especially prominent in the eyelids. Loss of the outer third of the eyebrows is another well-recognized sign. Ocular changes per se, however, are not a major feature.

*Diabetes mellitus.* See Chapter 33.

### Gastroenterologic diseases (Table 105-6)

*Pancreatitis.* Acute pancreatitis may give rise to the release of fat emboli into the circulation. Such emboli may produce retinal arterial obstruction. If damage to the pancreas is sufficient to cause maldigestion and malabsorption, ocular complications secondary to deficiency of fat-soluble vitamins can result. Inadequate vitamin A levels lead to impaired dark adaptation and in extreme cases to xerophthalmia.

*Regional enteritis and ulcerative colitis.* The most common ocular complication of these diseases is uveitis, especially iritis, which occurs in 0.5% to 12% of patients with ulcerative colitis (UC) and in about 2% of patients with regional enteritis (RE). Among patients with UC and RE who also manifest sacroiliac arthritis, the incidence of uveitis approaches 50%. The uveitis is usually bilateral and responds to topical corticosteroids. It does not flare up in synchrony with exacerbations of the colitis. The posterior uveitis is occasionally associated with exudative retinal detachments.

***Whipple's disease.*** A rare disorder occurring primarily in white men, Whipple's disease produces widespread CNS lesions that can lead to ophthalmoplegia. Other ocular findings include keratitis, uveitis, retinal hemorrhage with cotton-wool spots, and optic disc edema.

### Hematologic diseases (Table 105-7)

***Anemias.*** Patients with anemia have a greater tendency to manifest retinal hemorrhages when both the platelet and red cell counts are depressed. When anemia is significant, the fundus appears pale and the retinal vessels appear less deeply red than normal. Subconjunctival hemorrhages also can occur.

***Leukemias.*** The frequency of ocular involvement in leukemia varies depending on the study cited. Autopsy frequencies vary from 31% to 80%. The eye appears to be somewhat more frequently involved in acute than in chronic leukemia. In one series, 42% of patients with recently diagnosed acute leukemia had some form of ocular involvement. The initial changes in the retina include pallor from the associated anemia and increased venous tortuosity. Later, exudates, hemorrhages, and cotton-wool spots can be seen. Occasionally, orbital leukemic infiltration can cause proptosis.

***Lymphomas.*** Lymphomatous hyperplasia can occur in the conjunctiva, the lacrimal gland, and lids. The clinical appearance of benign lymphoid hyperplasia and malignant lymphoma can be similar; therefore a biopsy is essential to establish a diagnosis. A patient who presents with a

**Table 105-5.** Endocrine diseases

| Disease entity | Lids and adnexa | Conj. & sclera | Cornea | Cataract | Glaucoma | Retina & opt. nerve | Extra-oc muscles | Orbit | Uveitis | Visual CNS |
|---|---|---|---|---|---|---|---|---|---|---|
| Diabetes mellitus | | | | XX | | XX | | | | XX |
| Hyperadrenalism | | | | | XX | XX | | XX | | |
| Hypoadrenalism | XX | | | | | XX | | | | |
| Hyperparathyroidism | | | XX | | | | | | | |
| Hypoparathyroidism | | | | XX | | XX | | | | |
| Hyperthyroidism | XX | | | | | | XX | XX | | |
| Hypothyroidism | XX | | | | | | | | | |

**Table 105-6.** Gastroenterologic diseases

| Disease entity | Lids and adnexa | Conj. & sclera | Cornea | Cataract | Glaucoma | Retina & opt. nerve | Extra-oc muscles | Orbit | Uveitis | Visual CNS |
|---|---|---|---|---|---|---|---|---|---|---|
| Pancreatitis | | | | | | XX | | | | |
| Colitis | | | | | | | | | XX | |
| Whipple's disease | | | XX | | | XX | | | XX | XX |

**Table 105-7.** Hematologic diseases

| Disease entity | Lids and adnexa | Conj. & sclera | Cornea | Cataract | Glaucoma | Retina & opt. nerve | Extra-oc muscles | Orbit | Uveitis | Visual CNS |
|---|---|---|---|---|---|---|---|---|---|---|
| Anemias | | XX | | | | XX | | | | |
| Leukemias | | | | | | XX | | XX | | |
| Lymphomas | XX | XX | | | | | | XX | | |
| Multiple myeloma | | | | | | XX | | | | |
| Polycythemia vera | | | | | | XX | | | | |
| Sickle cell disease | | | | | XX | XX | | | | |
| Thrombocytopenia | | | | | | XX | | XX | | |
| Waldenström's macroglobulinemia | | XX | | | | XX | | | | |

conjunctival lymphoma is unlikely to have a systemic lymphoma, but should still be evaluated for systemic involvement, as it occasionally does occur. Orbital lymphomas are the third most common cause of proptosis after orbital inflammation and hemangiomas. The presentation of orbital lymphoid tumors is usually subtle; overt inflammatory clinical signs are usually absent. The superior orbit is affected most frequently.

*Multiple myeloma.* Up to 66% of patients with multiple myeloma have some form of retinopathy, and peripheral microaneurysms are the most common form, although hemorrhages and exudates are also seen. Cysts can develop in the iris, ciliary body, and pars plana.

*Polycythemia vera.* At hematocrits greater than 50%, blood viscosity increases rapidly. The resulting retinal manifestations include venous dilation and tortuosity and intraretinal hemorrhages. The fundus can take on an overly red hue. Disc hyperemia and papilledema can occur, and patients may complain of amaurosis fugax.

*Sickle cell disease.* See Occlusive Vascular Disease.

*Thrombocytopenia.* As expected, patients with thrombocytopenia can present with retinal or orbital hemorrhages. Retinal edema and exudates also have been reported.

*Waldenström's macroglobulinemia.* In Waldenström's macroglobulinemia, the retinopathy is secondary to the serum hyperviscosity that occurs as a result of the large size of the IgM molecule. The result is venous dilation and tortuosity, with flame-shaped hemorrhages. Sludging of the conjunctival blood flow and retinal vascular occlusion may occur. These findings may resolve with treatment of the hyperviscosity.

## Infections (Table 105-8)

### *Bacterial*

**Brucellosis.** *Brucella* species are gram-negative bacilli that cause undulant fever. Ocular findings include keratitis, recurrent iridocyclitis, and cataract. Papilledema and multifocal choroiditis can be seen. In the United States, the disease is seen mostly in slaughter-house workers.

**Chlamydia.** An obligate intracellular parasite, *Chlamydia trachomatis* is the most frequent cause of neonatal conjunctivitis. If either erythromycin or tetracycline ointment is used within 1 hour of delivery, the risk of chlamydial neonatal inclusion conjunctivitis becomes minimal. On the other hand, silver nitrate prophylaxis is ineffective against *Chlamydia.* In adults, inclusion conjunctivitis presents as an acute follicular conjunctivitis with a mucopurulent discharge. Usually transmitted by oral-genital sexual activity, keratitis may develop the second week after onset, with infiltrates and superficial vascularization. Chronicity is the rule, and *Chlamydia* is the most common cause of chronic follicular conjunctivitis.

The syndrome called trachoma begins as a chronic follicular conjunctivitis, but as the disease progresses scarring of the conjunctiva occurs with secondary tear deficiency, lid deformation with trichiasis, and entropion. The result is corneal ulceration and scarring. Blinding trachoma is still a major public health problem in many parts of the world.

**Diphtheria.** Ocular infection with diphtheria presents with a membranous or pseudomembranous conjunctivitis with discharge, lid edema, and regional lymphadenopathy. The organism is unusual in that it can penetrate intact corneal epithelium and invade the stroma. Toxic demyelinating neuritis can affect peripheral motor and cranial nerves. A classic ocular finding is accommodative paralysis.

**Gonorrhea.** One of the sites of primary infection of *Neisseria gonorrhea* is the conjunctiva of the eye. The infection produces a striking, hyperacute conjunctivitis with lid edema, chemosis, and copious mucopurulent discharge. Like diphtheria, the organism can invade the intact corneal epithelium, allowing rapid stromal ulceration with perforation and endophthalmitis. In adults, the eye disease often occurs after self-inoculation from genital infection.

**Leprosy (Hansen's disease).** Caused by the acid-fast bacillus *Mycobacterium leprae,* leprosy affects the skin of the ocular adnexa, the cornea and conjunctiva, the sclera, and the uvea. Brow and eyelash loss are common manifestations, as is seventh nerve paralysis. Involvement of the fifth nerve causes corneal anesthesia, which increases the risk of corneal ulceration. The lid deformities that often develop also predispose to corneal decompensation. The organism can directly invade the cornea, causing white, punctate subepithelial opacities. In about 16% of leprosy patients, episcleritis, scleritis, and uveitis are the presenting findings.

**Septicemia.** Hematogenous spread of bacterial organisms from extraocular sites can cause endogenous endopthalmitis. Any cause of immunodeficiency is a predisposing cause of this uncommon condition. Meningitis, endocarditis, and urinary and abdominal infections are the most common causes of septic embolization to the eye. Anterior and posterior segments of the eye may be involved in a focal or diffuse fashion. About 25% of cases are bilateral.

**Syphilis.** The eyes may be involved in the secondary or tertiary stages of acquired and congenital syphilis. Acute bilateral interstitial keratitis is common in congenital disease, most often associated with eighth nerve deafness and Hutchinson's teeth. A salt-and-pepper fundus is associated with congenital disease. An active chorioretinitis can occur in acquired disease. Motility problems, ptosis, and optic atrophy are seen with neurosyphilis.

**Tularemia.** A gram-negative coccobacillus causes tularemia. The oculoglandular form is the least common, accounting for 1% to 4% of cases. Also known as Parinaud's syndrome, it presents with a granulomatous conjunctivitis and enlarged preauricular, parotid, submaxillary, and cervical lymph nodes. Less often, dacryocystitis, corneal ulceration, and preseptal or orbital cellulitis can be seen.

**Tuberculosis.** Ocular tuberculosis is seen in less than 2% of patients. Among the many ocular findings are conjunctivitis, phlyctenular keratoconjunctivitis, interstitial keratitis, scleritis, anterior and/or posterior uveitis, direct orbital infection, retinal periphlebitis, and choroidal tuberculoma.

**Table 105-8.** Infectious diseases

| Disease entity | Lids and adnexa | Conj. & sclera | Cornea | Cataract | Glaucoma | Retina & opt. nerve | Extra-oc muscles | Orbit | Uveitis | Visual CNS |
|---|---|---|---|---|---|---|---|---|---|---|
| Bacterial | | | | | | | | | | |
| Brucellosis | | | XX | XX | | XX | | | XX | |
| *Chlamydia* | XX | XX | XX | | | | | | | |
| Diphtheria | XX | XX | XX | | | | | | | XX |
| Gonorrhea | | XX | XX | | | | | | | |
| Leprosy | XX | XX | XX | | | | | | XX | |
| Septicemia | | | | | | XX | | | XX | |
| Syphilis | | | XX | | | XX | | | | XX |
| Tularemia | XX | XX | XX | | | | | XX | | |
| Tuberculosis | | XX | XX | | | XX | | XX | XX | |
| Fungal | | | | | | | | | | |
| *Candida albicans* | XX | XX | XX | | | XX | | | | |
| Coccidiodomycosis | | XX | XX | | | XX | | | XX | |
| Cryptococcus | | | | | | XX | | | | XX |
| Histoplasmosis | | | | | | XX | | | | |
| Parasitic | | | | | | | | | | |
| Cysticercosis | XX | XX | | | | XX | | | | |
| Echinococcosis | | | | | | XX | | XX | | |
| Loiasis | XX | | | | | | | | | |
| Onchocerciasis | | XX | XX | | | XX | | | XX | |
| Toxocariasis | | | | | | XX | | | XX | |
| Trichinosis | XX | XX | | | | | XX | | | |
| Protozoal | | | | | | | | | | |
| Malaria | | XX | | | | XX | | | | |
| Toxoplasmosis | | | | | | XX | | | XX | |
| Viral | | | | | | | | | | |
| Adenoviris 3 | | XX | | | | | | | | |
| Adenoviris 8 | | XX | XX | | | | | | | |
| Cytomegalovirus (adult) | | | | | | XX | | | | |
| (congenital) | | | | XX | | XX | | | XX | |
| Herpes simples (primary) | XX | XX | | | | | | | | |
| (recurrent) | | XX | | | | XX | | | XX | |
| Herpes zoster | XX | XX | XX | | | XX | | | XX | |
| Infectious mononucleosis | XX | XX | XX | | | XX | | | | XX |
| Influenza | | | XX | | | | XX | | | |
| Mumps | XX | XX | XX | | | XX | XX | | | |
| Rubella | | | XX | XX | XX | XX | | | | |
| Rubeola | | XX | XX | | | XX | | | | XX |
| Vaccinia | | XX | XX | | | | | | | |
| Varicella | XX | XX | | XX | | XX | | | | |

### *Fungal*

**Candida albicans.** *C. albicans* is the most common cause of infectious endogenous endophthalmitis and is seen most often in immunocompromised individuals. Other predisposing conditions include prolonged systemic antibiotic and/or corticosteroid therapy, intravenous drug abuse, hemodialysis, and malignancy. The most common presenting symptoms of *Candida* endophthalmitis are blurred vision with floaters, cobwebs or veils, pain, photophobia, and a red eye. The most characteristic ophthalmologic finding is a well-circumscribed, creamy-white lesion in the posterior pole, which can be single or multiple. Yellow-white vitreous opacities can have a "fluff ball" appearance.

*Candida* also can cause marginal granulomatous ulcers of the eyelids. Conjunctivitis and corneal ulcers have been described.

**Coccidioidomycosis.** Endemic to the southwestern United States, this soil saprophyte primarily causes pulmonary disease. Ocular lesions include conjunctivitis, episcleritis, keratitis, anterior and posterior uveitis, and chorioretinitis. Papilledema and endophthalmitis also can occur.

**Cryptococcus.** A saprophytic yeastlike fungus, *Cryptococcus* is found in high concentrations in soil that contains pigeon droppings. About 40% of patients with cryptococcal meningitis have ocular complications, which include papilledema, optic atrophy, and extraocular muscle paresis. Endogenous endophthalmitis can occur.

**Histoplasmosis.** The Ohio and Mississippi river valleys are endemic regions for *Histoplasma capsulatum,* where inhalation of spores causes infection. The presumed ocular histoplasmosis syndrome includes midperipheral chorioretinal "punched-out" scars, peripapillary scarring, and subretinal neovascularization, the latter causing disciform maculopathy. About 50% of patients have bilateral disease. The risk of visual loss from macular subretinal neovascularization may be reduced by laser photocoagulation.

### *Parasitic*

**Cysticercosis (tapeworm).** After they penetrate the intestinal wall, the embryos of *Taenia solium* are distributed throughout the body via the circulatory system. After metamorphosis into the larval form, the cysticercus can be found in the lids, conjunctiva, anterior chamber, retina, choroid, and vitreous. The parasite can be seen moving inside a grayish-white, semitransparent cyst.

**Echinococcosis (hydatid cyst).** Caused by the larval state of the canine tapeworm, most infections occur in children who ingest the eggs while playing with infected dogs. The incidence of ocular involvement is low. The main predilection is the vitreous cavity or between the choroid and retina. Proptosis may be produced by intraorbital cysts, and papilledema can occur secondary to enlarging intracranial cysts.

**Loiasis.** *Loa loa,* the African eyeworm, can cause swollen eyelids as the microfilaria migrate through that area.

**Onchocerciasis.** "River blindness" is endemic across equatorial Africa and in areas of Central and South America. The microfilariae enter the cornea from the skin via the conjunctiva. Vascular spread can lead to organisms in the aqueous and uvea. The death of microfilariae causes local inflammation and scarring. Corneal opacity, uveitis, optic neuritis, and chorioretinitis lead to the blindness that afflicts 2 million persons. The drug ivermectin has revolutionized the treatment of onchocerciasis.

**Toxocariasis.** In ocular toxocariasis, the nematodal infection usually is limited to the posterior segments of the eye. Usually seen in children and contracted by playing with infected dogs, the ocular infection may present with decreased vision, leukocoria, strabismus, or uveitis. The most common intraocular presentation is an elevated subretinal granuloma in an otherwise quiet eye. The granuloma may evolve into a well-defined chorioretinal scar with a central granuloma. At this stage the process is self-limited. Remains of larvae are found within the granulomas, which contain dense collections of histiocytes and eosinophils. On the other hand, an exudative endophthalmitis with retinal detachment can be the presenting picture, which must be distinguished from retinoblastoma.

**Trichinosis.** Trichinosis is myositis caused by larvae of the *Trichinella spiralis* nematode; periorbital edema occurs in about 90% of patients. Associated with the ingestion of undercooked pork, trichinosis commonly involves the extraocular muscles causing pain on eye movements. Conjunctivitis and subconjunctival hemorrhage are frequent features.

### *Protozoal*

**Malaria.** *Plasmodium vivax* and *P. falciparum* account for 95% of the infections of this parasitic infection which is endemic throughout the tropics and subtropics. The most common ocular manifestations are conjunctival hyperemia and subconjunctival hemorrhage. Retinal hemorrhages and edema can be seen as a result of vasoocclusion and diffuse retinitis. Papilledema and optic neuritis also occur. Chloroquine, the drug of choice for acute attacks and prophylaxis, can cause a toxic maculopathy with a classic "bull's-eye" fundus picture.

**Toxoplasmosis.** Cats are the definitive host for the obligate intracellular protozoan *Toxoplasma gondii.* The developing human fetus can acquire toxoplasmosis if the mother becomes acutely infected during pregnancy. In cases of congenital toxoplasmosis, the ocular finding is a bilateral macular chorioretinitis, leaving behind large, atrophic chorioretinal scars that often reveal bare sclera centrally, with hyperpigmented borders.

It is thought that reactivations of congenital infections are almost always the cause of acute *Toxoplasma* chorioretinitis in adults. These repeat attacks occur at the edge of old atrophic lesions and are believed to be caused by the opening of toxoplasma cysts in the retina that developed at the time of the original congenital infection.

### *Viral*

**Adenoviris 3 (pharyngoconjunctival fever).** The most common manifestation of ocular adenovirus infection, pharyngoconjunctival fever (PCF) is characterized by pharyngitis, fever, and nonpurulent follicular conjunctivitis. The infection is transmitted by airborne respiratory droplets and by contact with the lids and conjunctiva. Hospitals and physicians' offices are known sites for the spread of infection. There is an incubation period of 5 to 12 days. The watery discharge is usually unilateral at first. In general the cornea is only minimally affected, and infiltrates do not occur. The virus is shed from the conjunctiva and throat for about 14 days after onset, although fecal excretion may persist for up to 1 month. Although most cases of PCF are caused by adenovirus 3, various other serotypes, including 2, 6, and 7, are also etiologic.

**Adenoviris 8 (epidemic keratoconjunctivitis).** Unlike PCF, epidemic keratoconjunctivitis (EKC) usually does not have associated respiratory symptoms, but is distinguished by the corneal involvement. About 5 days after onset of the conjunctivitis, patients with EKC develop slightly elevated focal epithelial lesions associated with a foreign body sensation. Virus has been shown to be replicating in these epithelial lesions. Subsequently, nummular subepithelial opacities develop, which slowly disappear over several months in most patients, but can persist for as long as 2 years in some individuals. These opacities consist of collections of lymphocytes in the superficial corneal stroma.

During the acute phase, some patients develop conjunctival membranes and marked swelling of the lids. Like PCF, EKC is highly contagious, and virus can be recovered from the eyes and throat for up to 14 days after onset. Other adenovirus serotypes, including 19, 29, and 37, also can cause EKC. During the acute phase, the only treatment is supportive. The late subepithelial opacities can cause reduced visual acuity and persistent irritation. Topical steroids can suppress the opacities and these symptoms, but they will tend to recur if the steroids are withdrawn. Steroids appear to provide only symptomatic relief; the natural course of the disease does not appear to be altered. Therefore because topical steroids can have adverse effects, they should be used only in those patients who are persistently symptomatic.

**Cytomegalovirus.** A herpes virus, cytomegalovirus (CMV) causes a mononucleosis syndrome in young adults, congenital malformations, and multiple lesions in immunosuppressed persons, especially those with acquired immune deficiency syndrome (AIDS). In the adult eye CMV causes a necrotizing, hemorrhagic retinitis with perivasculitis and exudate. Often, there is little reaction in the anterior segment or vitreous. Congenital CMV also can cause retinitis, anterior uveitis, cataract, and optic atrophy. CMV retinitis in AIDS patients is a poor prognostic sign.

**Herpes simplex.** Herpes simplex virus (HSV) type 1 accounts for the majority of ocular herpetic infections. Primary exposure to HSV type 1 usually occurs in childhood, and by puberty 60% to 80% of the population is seropositive. Primary infection with HSV type 1 is often asymptomatic, but may produce oral, eye, or skin lesions. In primary ocular HSV infections, a severe follicular conjunctivitis can occur with regional adenopathy and often vesicles on the eyelid or lid margin. After the primary infection, HSV survives in latent form inside sensory nerve ganglia and may reactivate at any time, producing recurrent disease.

Recurrent ocular herpes may take the form of dendritic or geographic ulcers, recurrent erosions, interstitial or disciform stromal keratitis, and anterior uveitis. Attacks tend to be more frequent in autumn and winter. Stromal keratitis can cause permanent structural damage to the cornea, which is of particular concern because the disorder is chronic and difficult to treat. HSV may also cause an acute retinitis with retinal necrosis.

**Herpes zoster.** Herpes zoster (HZ) is a reactivation of varicella-zoster virus, usually in adults, causing an eruption of vesicles, with pain in a dermatome distribution (shingles). The incidence of HZ increases with age and is greater in immunocompromised persons. Therefore the presentation of HZ in a young adult should raise the possibility of an underlying systemic illness. The thoracic nerves are most frequently involved, followed by the trigeminal and cervical nerves. In uncomplicated HZ, the skin lesions and pain resolve within 4 weeks. Postherpetic neuralgia, with persistent pain, is more common in people over the age of 60.

Development of HZ in the first division of the trigeminal nerve is often referred to as herpes zoster ophthalmicus, regardless of whether the eye is inflamed. Of patients with vesicular eruptions on the side of the tip or midportion of the nose, 85% will have ocular involvement. A wide range of ocular manifestations can be seen, including keratitis, episcleritis, scleritis, conjunctivitis, uveitis, retinal vasculitis, choroiditis, and optic neuritis. Corneal complications are most frequent, the earliest and most common of which are superficial punctate keratitis and pseudodendrite formation. In more severe cases, stromal infiltrates and disciform keratitis can occur. With loss of corneal sensation, neurotrophic ulceration, corneal melting, and even perforation may follow.

**Infectious mononucleosis.** Facial paralysis presenting unilaterally or bilaterally is an uncommon manifestation of infectious mononucleosis caused by the Epstein-Barr virus. Nummular interstitial keratitis, unilateral tarsal conjunctival granuloma, dacryocystitis, and retinal periphlebitis also have been reported.

**Influenza.** Extraocular muscle myalgia and superficial punctate keratitis can occur with influenza.

**Mumps.** Ocular involvement in mumps may present as conjunctivitis, keratitis dacryoadenitis, optic neuritis, scleritis, and extraocular muscle palsies.

**Rubella (German measles).** Congenital heart disease, cataracts, and deafness are the classic triad of the congenital rubella syndrome. The incidence of cataracts in patients with congenital rubella is about 20%. Other ocular complications include microphthalmia, corneal clouding, congenital glaucoma, and a classic "salt and pepper" retinopathy.

**Rubeola (measles).** Measles usually produces a nonspecific conjunctivitis with follicles or an occasional Koplik's spot. Subepithelial infiltrates of the cornea may appear. Measles encephalitis is associated with optic neuritis, neuroretinitis, and extraocular muscle palsies.

**Vaccinia.** Vaccinia is associated with central deep disciform keratitis and vascularization. Blepharitis and conjunctivitis also have been described.

**Varicella (chickenpox).** Varicella is the primary infection of the varicella-zoster virus. Ophthalmic involvement is usually mild. A nonspecific papillary conjunctivitis and pocks on the eyelids are the common findings. Occasionally, a dendritic, geographic, or disciform keratitis can occur. Rarely, necrosis of the eyelids, corneal melting, cataract, and optic neuritis are seen.

### Injuries (Table 105-9)

*Chemical.* The prognosis for a chemically burned eye depends not only on the severity of the burn, but also on how rapidly the therapy is initiated. Therefore chemical burns are among the most urgent of ocular emergencies. Immediate flushing with water should be the initial treatment for every chemical eye burn. Delay of even a few minutes allows longer contact time and increases the risk of more serious injury. Irrigation should be continued for

**Table 105-9.** Ocular injuries

| Disease entity | Lids and adnexa | Conj. & sclera | Cornea | Cataract | Glaucoma | Retina & opt. nerve | Extra-oc muscles | Orbit | Uveitis | Visual CNS |
|---|---|---|---|---|---|---|---|---|---|---|
| Chemical | XX | XX | XX | XX | | | | | | |
| Infared radiation | | | | XX | | | | | | |
| Ultraviolet radiation | XX | XX | XX | XX | | | | | | |

**Table 105-10.** Metabolic diseases

| Disease entity | Lids and adnexa | Conj. & sclera | Cornea | Cataract | Glaucoma | Retina & opt. nerve | Extra-oc muscles | Orbit | Uveitis | Visual CNS |
|---|---|---|---|---|---|---|---|---|---|---|
| Albinism | | | | | | XX | XX | | | XX |
| Alkaptonuria | | XX | XX | | | | | | | |
| Amyloidosis | XX | XX | XX | | | | | XX | | XX |
| Chédiak-Higashi syndrome | | | | | | XX | XX | | | XX |
| Cystinosis | | XX | XX | | | | | | | |
| Fabry's disease | | | XX | XX | | XX | | | | XX |
| Galactosemia | | | | XX | | | | | | |
| The gangliosidoses | | | | | | XX | | | | |
| Gaucher's disease | | XX | | | | XX | XX | | | |
| Gout | | XX | XX | | | | | | | |
| Hemochromatosis | XX | XX | | | | XX | | | | |
| Histiocytosis | XX | XX | XX | | | | | XX | | |
| Homocystinuria | | | | XX | | XX | XX | | | |
| Lipid metabolism disorders | XX | | XX | XX | | XX | | | | XX |
| Mucopolysaccharidoses | | | XX | | | XX | | | | |
| Niemann-Pick disease | | | | | | XX | | | | |
| Refsum's disease | | | XX | XX | | XX | | | | XX |
| Wilson's disease | | | XX | XX | | | | | | |

at least 30 minutes, or until litmus paper indicates neutrality of the fornices. During the irrigation process, 0.5% proparacaine should be instilled and the fornices swabbed to remove any trapped particles of caustic material. After irrigation and debridement are concluded, topical antibiotics and cycloplegics should be initiated. The patient is then referred to the ophthalmologist for additional management. Severe cases may require close medical and surgical ophthalmic follow-up for many months. The extent of vascular injury to the perilimbal area is the most important factor in determining the prognosis for recovery.

**Acid.** In general injuries from weak acids are less extensive than alkali burns, although strong acids can produce severe damage. The intact corneal epithelium provides moderate protection against dilute or weak acids, but damage increases when the pH is 2.5 or less. Acids form complexes with proteins in the corneal stroma, which tend to retard additional penetration. Automotive battery acid burns are the most common type of acid burn, secondary to battery explosions.

**Alkali.** With rising pH, emulsification of lipids in cell membranes occurs, allowing easy penetration of alkali cations. These in turn cause rapid break-up of corneal mucoproteins. Ammonium hydroxide is fat soluble and penetrates most rapidly, producing the most severe burns, with deep stromal injury and cataract formation. Sodium hydroxide, potassium, and calcium hydroxide penetrate more slowly.

***Infrared radiation.*** Solar infrared radiation is not considered harmful to the eye. Long-term, relatively high level exposure, as occurs in industrial environments, has been associated with a higher incidence of the development of wedge-shaped cortical spoke cataracts.

***Ultraviolet radiation.*** The cornea absorbs all radiation of wavelengths less than about 300 nm. Such absorbed radiation causes the clinical condition "snow blindness," also known as photokeratitis. It is usually correlated with facial sunburn. "Welder's flash" is the same entity, caused by momentary direct corneal exposure during arc welding. While permanent damage is rare, sunbathers and skiers should be instructed to wear UV absorbing eye protection. Corneal pterygium has clearly been associated with UV exposure. The lens of the eye absorbs most UV radiation below about 400 nm. UV radiation has been implicated in the development of cataracts.

### Metabolic diseases (Table 105-10)

***Albinism (cutaneous and ocular).*** See Dermatologic and Mucous Membrane Disorders.

***Alkaptonuria (ochronosis).*** Alkaptonuria is a rare, autosomal recessive metabolic disease in which the enzyme homogentisic acid oxidase is missing. Ocular involvement is seen in 79% of these patients. The ochronotic pigment build-up is seen in the sclera, conjunctiva, and corneal limbus. Vision usually is not impaired.

***Amyloidosis.*** Amyloidosis is classified according to the absence or presence of underlying disease (primary or secondary amyloidosis), genetic association (familial or nonfamilial) and whether the process is systemic or localized. Ophthalmic manifestations are not a feature of secondary systemic or localized amyloidosis. Primary amyloidosis, on the other hand, can have various ocular findings. The stromal lesions of lattice corneal dystrophy contain amyloid. Nonfamilial amyloidosis confined to the conjunctiva is another example of primary nonsystemic amyloidosis. Primary systemic amyloidosis commonly has lesions in the skin of the eyelids and deposits in the orbits, causing proptosis. Opacities in the vitreous also have been described. Various neuroophthalmic manifestations, associated with amyloid deposition in nerves, have been reported.

***Chédiak-Higashi syndrome.*** A rare autosomal recessive disorder, Chédiak-Higashi syndrome is characterized by partial oculocutaneous albinism, increased susceptibility to viral and bacterial infections, anemia, leukopenia, thrombocytopenia, and peripheral and central neurologic changes.

***Cystinosis.*** A rare metabolic disorder characterized biochemically by an abnormally high intracellular content of free cystine, cystinosis results in cystine crystal deposition in various organs, including the eye. The striking ocular clinical feature is iridescent corneal and conjunctival cystine crystal deposition, causing secondary photophobia. The material also builds up in the iris, choroid, and sclera. The unique ocular findings of cystinosis are sufficiently characteristic that they form one of the criteria for the diagnosis of the disease.

***Fabry's disease.*** Transmitted as an X-linked recessive trait, Fabry's disease is a metabolic defect, resulting in the accumulation of the glycosphingolipid trihexosyl ceramide. The ocular deposition of this material is highly distinctive; whorl-like corneal opacities develop in the superficial corneal stroma. Referred to as corneal verticillata, these opacities do not degrade visual acuity. A cataract with narrow feathery spokes radiating from the posterior pole of the lens is pathognomonic. Dilatation and corkscrew tortuosity of the retinal vessels are seen. Neurologic complications include cerebral thrombosis, hemorrhage, and hemiplegia.

***Galactosemia.*** Galactosemia is a recessively inherited disorder that manifests itself in infancy within a few days after the onset of milk ingestion. Caused by deficiency of galactose-1-phosphate uridyl transferase, it presents with vomiting, diarrhea, hepatomegaly, cataracts and mental retardation. Galactitol, the reduced sugar conjugate of galactose, accumulates in the lens of the eye, which in turn results in an influx of water, swelling of the lens fibers, and eventual opacity. Galactokinase deficiency also is characterized by elevated blood galactose, but is clinically much less severe, with slower development of cataract being the only major adverse effect.

Galactosemia is one of the few treatable inborn errors of metabolism if the diagnosis is made early and lactose and galactose are removed from the diet. If the cataract changes and other manifestations are still mild, they may regress. However, more advanced cataracts and mental retardation do not regress if treatment is begun too late.

***The gangliosidoses.*** The gangliosidoses are a group of autosomal recessive disorders of which Tay-Sachs disease is the most common. In each condition an enzymatic defect results in the deposition of excessive amounts of sphingolipid in the CNS neurons. The classic ophthalmic finding in these disorders is the cherry-red spot of the macula, due to the accumulation of ganglioside in the retinal ganglion cells, which are absent in the fovea. The parafoveal area, therefore, takes on an opaque, whitish haze, whereas the foveal zone maintains its normal reddish color.

***Gaucher's disease.*** An autosomal recessive sphingolipidosis, the disease leads to an accumulation of glucosylceramide in reticuloendothelial cells. Three subtypes have been distinguished. The major ocular finding in Gaucher's disease, pigmented pingueculae, are present in about 25% of cases. They are bilateral, yellow-brown, wedge-shaped patches on the bulbar conjunctiva in the palpebral fissure. Type III juvenile neuropathic Gaucher's disease is associated with an eye movement disorder affecting mainly horizontal and occasionally vertical gaze. Enzyme studies are necessary to distinguish the disorder from congenital ocular motor apraxia.

***Gout.*** A clinical disorder of hyperuricemia, primary gout is thought to be the result of an inborn error of metabolism. Secondary gout is associated with conditions where there is a high rate of breakdown of cell nuclei, as in lymphomas, leukemias, and hemolytic anemia. The ocular manifestations include chronic hyperemic conjunctivitis, scleritis, episcleritis, and tenonitis. Monosodium urate crystals may be deposited in the corneal epithelium. Allopurinol, the most common agent used to treat gout, is cataractogenic in some patients.

***Hemochromatosis.*** A rare disorder of iron metabolism, hemochromatosis results in widespread deposition of hemosiderin in many tissues. Primarily seen in men over the age of 40, the major ocular findings are hyperpigmentation of the eyelid margins and perilimbal bulbar conjunctiva. A diffuse, slate-blue hyperpigmentation of the fundus, most prominent in the peripapillary region, also has been described.

***Histiocytosis.*** The histiocytic disorders, a group of related disorders that present with a variable clinical picture, involve the proliferation and activation of mononuclear phagocytes. From an ophthalmic perspective, eosinophilic granuloma, also called histiocytosis X, is an uncommon cause of orbital tumors and secondary proptosis. Hand-Schüller-Christian disease, a subset of eosinophilic granuloma, presents as a triad of lytic skull lesions, proptosis, and diabetes insipidus.

Juvenile xanthogranuloma is a benign histiocytic inflammatory condition occurring in infants and children. The skin, including the eyelid, and the eye make up the most common sites of involvement. The clinical hallmark is the development of a spontaneous hyphema in infants, secondary to lesions of the iris and ciliary body.

Recurrent bleeding in the anterior chamber will lead to secondary glaucoma and loss of sight. The iris lesions can be nodular or diffuse. Epibulbar lesions involving the sclera, conjunctiva, and cornea, are less frequent.

***Homocystinuria.*** An autosomal recessive inheritance pattern characterizes homocystinuria, which follows phenylketonuria as the second most common inborn error of amino acid metabolism. Due to enzymatic deficiency, homocystine precursors accumulate. The most common ocular manifestation is ectopia lentis, with the lens usually displaced inferonasally, in contrast to what is seen in Marfan's syndrome, where the lens tends to shift superiorly and temporally. Lens subluxation is found in about one third of homocystinuric patients by the age of five and in almost all by age 25. If the subluxed lens causes pupillary block glaucoma, then emergency treatment is required. Other common ocular findings in homocystinuria include myopia, strabismus, and retinal detachment.

***Lipid metabolism disorders.*** The ocular manifestations of the hyperlipoproteinemias include xanthelasma of the lids, corneal arcus, and lipemia retinalis. In the rare disorder abetalipoproteinemia (Bassen-Kornzweig syndrome), atypical retinitis pigmentosa is the main ocular finding; but cataract, choroiditis, and ophthalmoplegia are also associated. Another rare disorder, Tangier disease (familial high-density lipoprotein [HDL] deficiency) often includes diffuse corneal clouding as one of its manifestations. Vision is not usually affected.

***Mucopolysaccharidoses.*** A group of conditions with specific enzymatic defects, all of these disorders are characterized by excretion of mucopolysaccharides in the urine. The major ocular findings are corneal clouding and pigmentary retinopathy.

***Niemann-Pick disease.*** Although several variants of this autosomal recessive condition are recognized, all of them are characterized by storage of lipids in the viscera, nervous, and reticuloendothelial systems of the body. The macular cherry-red spot (see Gangliosidoses) is seen in about 50% of patients with Niemann-Pick disease.

***Refsum's disease.*** An autosomal recessive disorder, Refsum's disease is due to a defect in fatty acid oxidation. The major ophthalmic feature is pigmentary retinopathy, which first presents as night blindness. Posterior subcapsular cataracts, corneal clouding, and ophthalmoplegia also are seen.

***Wilson's disease.*** Transmitted as an autosomal recessive trait with variable expressivity, Wilson's disease is a defect in copper metabolism. The striking and pathognomonic feature of Wilson's disease is the Kayser-Fleischer ring, a green-brown pigment deposit located just inside the corneal limbus. Although it is often visible grossly, biomicroscopy with gonioscopy, performed by the ophthalmologist, is required to verify its presence. Also seen in Wilson's disease is the "sunflower" cataract, which is a central pigmented lens opacity with tapering peripheral petals.

### Musculoskeletal diseases (Table 105-11)

***Apert's disease.*** Apert's disease is a usually sporadic congenital anomaly affecting bones throughout the body. The cranial malformation is a premature synostosis of the coronal suture and hypoplasia of the midbase of the skull and the sphenoethmomaxillary complex. The ocular findings include an antimongoloid palpebral slant. Proptosis secondary to the anatomically shallow orbit can lead to severe exposure keratitis. Optic atrophy with visual loss is common, as is exotropia.

***Conradi's syndrome.*** A rare autosomal recessive disorder, Conradi's syndrome commonly has craniofacial anomalies. Hypertelorism, bilateral dense cataracts, and bilateral optic atrophy are characteristic.

***Craniofacial syndromes.*** Craniofacial syndromes are a group of disorders that share premature closure of one or more suture lines in the developing calvarium. Optic atrophy is common, as is exophthalmos and exotropia.

***Facial deformity syndromes.*** This group of syndromes includes the Treacher Collins syndrome, Pierre Robin syndrome, Goldenhar's syndrome, and Hallermann-Streiff syndrome. All include multiple congenital anomalies of the head and face, including coloboma of the lower lids, antimongoloid slant, and microphthalmos.

***Marfan's syndrome.*** Marfan's syndrome, an autosomal dominant disorder, has a classic triad: subluxated lenses, skeletal anomalies, and cardiovascular disease. Great variability of expression is possible. Subluxation of the lenses is usually bilateral and most often superior or superonasal. Myopia, ptosis, strabismus, and blue sclera are all common in Marfan's syndrome. Retinal degeneration and detachment also occur.

***Muscular dystrophy.*** Two forms of muscular dystrophy have specific eye findings. The first type, ocular muscular dystrophy, usually begins with ptosis and progresses to

**Table 105-11.** Musculoskeletal diseases

| Disease entity | Lids and adnexa | Conj. & sclera | Cornea | Cataract | Glaucoma | Retina & opt. nerve | Extra-oc muscles | Orbit | Uveitis | Visual CNS |
|---|---|---|---|---|---|---|---|---|---|---|
| Apert's disease | XX | | | | | XX | XX | XX | | |
| Conradi's disease | | | | XX | | | XX | XX | | |
| Craniofacial syndromes | | | | | | XX | XX | XX | | |
| Facial deformity syndromes | XX | | | | | | | XX | | |
| Marfan's syndrome | XX | XX | | XX | | | XX | | | |
| Muscular dystrophy | XX | | | | | | XX | | | |
| Myasthenia gravis | XX | | | | | | XX | | | |
| Myotonic dystrophy | XX | | | XX | | XX | XX | | | |
| Osteogenesis imperfecta | | XX | XX | XX | | | | | | |
| Paget's disease | XX | | | | | XX | XX | | | |

bilateral external ophthalmoplegia. Although the facial, neck, trunk, and limb muscles also are affected, the orbicularis oculi muscles are most profoundly involved. This disorder usually presents itself in the second or third decade of life. The second type, oculopharyngeal dystrophy, is seen in individuals of French-Canadian descent. Its clinical features resemble myotonic dystrophy.

*Myasthenia gravis.* The clinical manifestations of myasthenia gravis are often initially ocular in nature and may be the only signs of the disease. Myasthenia gravis has a relationship with thymic tumors or hyperplasia, thyroid abnormalities, and autoimmune disorders. About 40% of patients present with diplopia, and 30% to 40% present with unilateral or bilateral ptosis. Therefore myasthenia gravis must be ruled out in any patient who presents with new onset of ptosis or diplopia. As with other symptoms of myasthenia gravis, the ocular findings are often more severe later in the day and after exertion. Ocular manifestations of myasthenia are among the most difficult to treat. The intravenous Tensilon test is most commonly used in the diagnosis of myasthenia gravis. It should be performed by the ophthalmologist or neurologist.

*Myotonic dystrophy.* An autosomal dominant disorder, myotonic dystrophy is characterized by progressive muscular atrophy with excessive contractility and difficulty of relaxation. Nearly pathognomonic is the handshake with the inability to release the grasp. Multiple ocular abnormalities are noted. Cataracts are seen in almost all patients. Upper lid ptosis, reduced ocular range of motion, and exotropia or exophoria are commonly seen. Lacrimal insufficiency and retinal degenerative changes have been reported.

*Osteogenesis imperfecta.* Usually autosomal dominant, osteogenesis imperfecta presents with a triad of brittle bones, deafness, and blue sclera. The blue coloration of the sclera is due to increased translucency, which allows the uveal pigment to be seen. Often both cornea and sclera are reduced in thickness by 50% or more. Megalocornea, keratoconus, hyperopia, and cataracts also have been reported.

*Paget's disease.* Paget's disease of bone, also known as osteitis deformans, has multiple inheritance forms. Some of the ocular manifestations of Paget's disease are caused specifically by the bone disease, whereas others occur in association with Paget's disease.

The symptoms caused by bony interference with nerves and blood vessels can produce significant ocular and periocular morbidity. Compression of the seventh nerve can cause painful blepharospasm. In the same way, painful trigeminal neuralgia can occur. Extraocular muscle palsies are seen, and gradual optic nerve compression can lead to progressive visual field loss and optic atrophy.

The major internal ocular findings associated with Paget's disease are choroidal sclerosis and angioid streaks. Angioid streaks are, in turn, associated with an increased risk of disciform macular degeneration due to the development of subretinal neovascularization. The end result can be a severe loss of central vision.

### Neoplastic diseases metastatic to the eye and orbit (Table 105-12)

About 25% of patients who present with symptoms secondary to intraocular or orbital metastasis have no prior history of carcinoma. The uveal tract is the most common site of metastasis; such tumors occur six to nine times more frequently than tumors metastatic to the orbit. About 50,000 new cases of cancer metastatic to the uvea are diagnosed each year in the United States as compared to only about 1900 new cases of primary intraocular malignancy. Thus metastatic disease represents the vast bulk of intraocular cancer, almost always arriving via hematogenous spread. Therefore a comprehensive systemic survey should be given to all patients presenting with malignancy of the eye and orbit to identify a primary source.

The choroid is the most common portion of the uveal tract to be invaded by metastatic carcinoma. The usual complaint is painless loss of vision. The ophthalmoscopic appearance is usually a posteriorly located gray or creamy yellow, dome-shaped lesion with a surrounding area of retinal detachment. Much less commonly involved are the iris and ciliary body; a metastatic lesion to the iris most often appears as a gelatinous, pink or yellow mass with anterior uveitis. Up to 11% of patients with metastatic cancer to the uvea have scleral involvement, usually by direct extension.

Cancer metastatic to the orbit represents less than 10% of all orbital tumors. The presenting signs and symptoms include proptosis with or without orbital pain, lid swelling, ptosis, and ophthalmoplegia with diplopia.

Breast cancer is the most common malignancy metastatic to the uvea and orbit in women, representing more than 66% of cases in a large series. Lung cancer is the second most common source in women, representing about an additional 9% of cases.

In men, lung cancer is the most common source, producing about 55% of cases; GI tumors are second, accounting for about 16% of cases. Other, less common causes include metastatic cutaneous melanoma, accounting for about 4% of cases in men and women combined,

**Table 105-12.** Metastatic neoplasms

| Disease entity | Lids and adnexa | Conj. & sclera | Cornea | Cataract | Glaucoma | Retina & opt. nerve | Extra-oc muscles | Orbit | Uveitis | Visual CNS |
|---|---|---|---|---|---|---|---|---|---|---|
| Metastatic neoplasms | | XX | | | | XX | | XX | | |

plus renal, thyroid, and reproductive primary tumors.

The eye and orbit also may be involved by systemic hematologic and lymphoproliferative disorders such as the leukemias, lymphomas, and plasma cell dyscrasias. Orbital infiltration is common. Vitreous cells and retinal vascular lesions also are associated.

### Nutritional diseases (Table 105-13)

***Generalized malnutrition.*** Lack of adequate protein intake results in the kwashiorkor syndrome, the ocular manifestations of which are nonspecific and include lid edema, chemosis, decreased resistance to external infection, and keratopathy.

***Hypervitaminosis A, B, and D.*** Excessive dietary intake of vitamin A is associated with increased intracranial pressure, which in turn causes papilledema and diplopia. Exophthalmos also has been described. Vitamin B, nicotinic acid, is sometimes used in large doses to lower serum cholesterol and triglyceride levels. Diminished visual acuity, apparently secondary to cystoid macular edema, has been reported. Large doses of vitamin D can cause calcium to deposit in the perilimbal conjunctiva and in a horizontal band across the cornea known as band keratopathy.

***Nutritional hepatic insufficiency.*** The visual system can be affected secondarily by the malabsorption and malnutrition associated with liver disease. Jaundice may first be noted by examination of the eyes, the elevated bilirubin pigment highlighted against the white sclera. Night blindness can be a feature of acute hepatitis and also cirrhosis due to marked drop in plasma vitamin A levels. Impairment of color vision has been associated with cirrhosis. Malabsorption of the fat-soluble vitamins, which occurs in chronic diffuse liver disease, and biliary obstruction can lead to the vitamin A and D deficiency syndromes discussed later.

***Vitamin A deficiency.*** Vitamin A deficiency results in night blindness and xerophthalmia. Vitamin A is a key element in the formation of the visual pigments of the retinal rods and cones. It is thus fundamental to the visual process. It is also necessary for the synthesis of mucous gland secretions, and its lack causes xerosis of the conjunctiva and cornea. The presence of Bitot's spots, triangular patches of foamy conjunctival epithelial debris in the interpalpebral space, is a classic sign of vitamin A deficiency. Severe cases lead to progressive degeneration of the cornea, which can lead to perforation, as well as keratinization of the conjunctiva.

***Vitamin B deficiency.*** The term *vitamin B* refers to a group of dietary factors with certain common features. Thiamine, riboflavin, and nicotinic acid play a key role in intracellular oxidative phosphorylation. The ocular manifestations of thiamine deficiency (beriberi) include central visual field defects and external ophthalmoplegias, especially of cranial nerves III and VI. Thiamine deficiency is also a factor in the toxic amblyopias of alcohol and tobacco and Wernicke's encephalopathy. Corneal neovascularization is one of the earliest signs of lack of riboflavin. The corneal stroma is invaded by vessels from the limbus. Pellagra is the lack of nicotinic acid (niacin).

**Table 105-13.** Nutritional diseases

| Disease entity | Lids and adnexa | Conj. & sclera | Cornea | Cataract | Glaucoma | Retina & opt. nerve | Extra-oc muscles | Orbit | Uveitis | Visual CNS |
|---|---|---|---|---|---|---|---|---|---|---|
| Generalized malnutrition | XX | XX | XX | | | | | | | |
| Hypervitaminosis A, B, and D | | | XX | | | XX | | XX | | XX |
| Nutritional hepatic insufficiency | | XX | | | | XX | | | | |
| Vitamin A deficiency | | XX | XX | | | XX | | | | |
| Vitamin B deficiency | XX | | XX | | | XX | XX | | | XX |
| Vitamin C deficiency | | XX | | | | XX | | XX | | |
| Vitamin D deficiency | | | | XX | | | | | | |

**Table 105-14.** Phacomatoses

| Disease entity | Lids and adnexa | Conj. & sclera | Cornea | Cataract | Glaucoma | Retina & opt. nerve | Extra-oc muscles | Orbit | Uveitis | Visual CNS |
|---|---|---|---|---|---|---|---|---|---|---|
| Angiomatosis retinae | | | | | | XX | | | | XX |
| Ataxia-telangiectasia | | XX | | | | | XX | | | |
| Encephalotrigeminal angiomatosis | XX | | | | XX | XX | | | | |
| Neurofibromatosis | XX | | XX | | XX | | | XX | | |
| Tuberous sclerosis | XX | | | | | XX | | | | XX |
| Wyburn-Mason syndrome | | | | | | XX | | XX | | XX |

It is associated with a distinctive dermatitis that can involve the skin of the eyelids. External ophthalmoplegia, optic neuritis, and pigmentary maculopathy also have been described.

***Vitamin C deficiency.*** The ocular manifestations of scurvy consist of subconjunctival hemorrhages, with hyphemas and retinal and orbital hemorrhages seen in severe cases.

***Vitamin D deficiency.*** Vitamin D is involved in the control of plasma calcium levels. The ocular manifestation of vitamin D deficiency is a distinctive zonular cataract, with white and colored crystals in layers in the lens cortex. The same type of cataract is seen in hypoparathyroidism.

### Phacomatoses (Table 105-14)

***Angiomatosis retinae (von Hippel-Lindau disease).*** A rare syndrome with no sexual or racial predilection, angiomatosis retinae usually presents sporadically, with no familial grouping. Presenting symptoms usually relate to the eyes or CNS. A cerebellar hemangioblastoma, the classic CNS lesion, can present with the usual signs of increased intracranial pressure. Spinal cord tumors also occur. Cysts and tumors of the kidney, epididymis, and other viscera are often seen. The ocular manifestations include retinal angiomas, which are often multiple and are bilateral in over 50% of cases. On ophthalmoscopic examination a smooth, dome-shaped tumor with an engorged vascular supply is seen. An exudative retinal detachment can develop around these lesions, which may become total and, if untreated, lead to absolute glaucoma and a blind, painful eye.

***Ataxia-telangiectasia (Louis-Bar syndrome).*** An autosomal recessive disorder, Louis-Bar syndrome can involve the skin and CNS, and ocular, hematologic, and lymphatic systems. Neurologic dysfunction includes a progressive and ultimately severe cerebellar ataxia with mental retardation. The immune system of these patients is incompetent, and thus they are subject to an increased rate of infections, lymphomas, and leukemias. The classic ocular finding is marked telangiectasia of the conjunctiva. Various oculomotor abnormalities also are seen.

***Encephalotrigeminal angiomatosis (Sturge-Weber syndrome).*** The hallmarks of the Sturge-Weber syndrome are a facial port-wine stain (nevus flammeus) and leptomeningeal angiomas. The syndrome also includes characteristic intracerebral calcifications, seizures, mental retardation, and ocular dysfunction. The three major eye findings are glaucoma ipsilateral to the port-wine stain, choroidal hemangiomas, and an ipsilateral darker iris (heterochromia).

Glaucoma is seen in 30% of patients and is often thought to be secondary to increased episcleral venous pressure due to the vascular malformations. The choroidal hemangiomas, seen in about 40% of patients, can be confused with metastatic lesions. Secondary retinal detachments with severe ocular complications can develop.

***Neurofibromatosis (von Recklinghausen's disease).*** Probably the most common of the phacomatoses, neurofibromatosis occurs in about 1 in 3,000 births. It is autosomal dominant, with a highly variable penetrance. The skin, CNS, and eye are the primary sites of abnormality. The presence of more than five cutaneous café au lait spots is pathognomonic; the neurologic hallmark of the disorder is the neurofibroma, which can occur anywhere in the peripheral or central nervous system.

Numerous possible ocular and orbital findings are possible. A marked distortion of the upper lid can occur if a neurofibroma develops inside it. This distortion in turn produces ptosis and a typical S-shaped contour to the upper lid. Proptosis and pulsatile exophthalmos can occur secondary to congenital bony malformations of the skull, particularly the absence of the orbital roof or the greater wing of the sphenoid bone. The herniation of brain tissue into the orbit causes proptosis, which can also occur secondary to neurofibromas or meningiomas arising from any of the orbital nerves, optic nerve, or meninges. Therefore any child presenting with proptosis should be evaluated for neurofibromatosis.

Up to 50% of patients with lid and facial involvement in neurofibromatosis develop glaucoma on the ipsilateral side due to various mechanisms. Also characteristic are thickened corneal nerves and neurofibromas on the surface of the iris.

***Tuberous sclerosis (Bourneville's syndrome).*** Both autosomal dominant and sporadic forms of tuberous sclerosis exist. About 60% of patients are mentally retarded. Epilepsy and skin lesions are also key findings. Fifty percent of patients have intracranial astrocytic hamartomas containing calcium. Hamartomas in the kidneys, heart, lungs, and liver have been reported. The classic cutaneous finding is the adenoma sebaceum, which are angiofibromas that appear as small nodules on the sides of the nose and across the face.

About 50% of patients have ocular findings, the most common being a large astrocytic hamartoma of the optic disc, with a multinodular appearance resembling fish eggs, tapioca, or mulberries. Bilateral in about 15% of cases, visual field defects can be seen.

***Wyburn-Mason syndrome.*** A syndrome of unknown etiology, Wyburn-Mason can present with either ocular or neurologic symptoms. The major pathology is arteriovenous malformations (AVM) in the retina and the brain. AVMs can occur in the orbit, leading to pulsatile exophthalmos. The retinal AVMs can vary from small vessels in a localized area to extensive, racemose lesions covering the retina and creating a "bag of worms" fundus appearance. Cranial nerve palsies also have been reported.

### Pulmonary diseases (Table 105-15)

***Asthma.*** See Allergic Diseases.

***Bacterial pneumonia/sepsis.*** See Septicemia.

***Bronchogenic carcinoma.*** See Neoplastic Diseases Metastatic to the Eye.

***Cystic fibrosis.*** A generalized abnormality of the exocrine, eccrine, and some endocrine glands, cystic fibrosis has an autosomal recessive inheritance and occurs in about

**Table 105-15.** Pulmonary diseases

| Disease entity | Lids and adnexa | Conj. & sclera | Cornea | Cataract | Glaucoma | Retina & opt. nerve | Extra-oc muscles | Orbit | Uveitis | Visual CNS |
|---|---|---|---|---|---|---|---|---|---|---|
| Asthma | | XX | | | | | | | | |
| Bacterial pneumonia/sepsis | | | | | | XX | | | XX | |
| Bronchogenic carcinoma | | XX | | | | XX | | XX | | |
| Cystic fibrosis | | | | | | XX | | | | |
| Tuberculosis | | XX | XX | | | XX | | XX | XX | |

**Table 105-16.** Renal diseases

| Disease entity | Lids and adnexa | Conj. & sclera | Cornea | Cataract | Glaucoma | Retina & opt. nerve | Extra-oc muscles | Orbit | Uveitis | Visual CNS |
|---|---|---|---|---|---|---|---|---|---|---|
| Alport's syndrome | | | | XX | | XX | | | | |
| Lowe's syndrome | | | | XX | XX | | | | | |
| Medullary cystic disease | | | | | | XX | | | | |
| Nephroblastoma | | | Aniridia | | | | | | | |
| Nephrotic syndrome | | | | | | XX | | | | |
| Pyelonephritis | | | | | | XX | | | | |
| Renal transplantation | | | | XX | | | | | | |

1 in 2000 births. Mucus secretion becomes abnormal, and mucin-producing cells become obstructed. The pancreas, lungs, and biliary tree are directly affected; and gastric malabsorption with secondary vitamin deficiency occurs.

The most common ocular findings are retinal venous dilation, tortuosity, and hemorrhages. These appear to be attributable to the hypercapnia associated with the pulmonary insufficiency. Xerophthalmia and night blindness may occur secondary to vitamin A deficiency. Fortunately, the lacrimal glands have minimal or no involvement in the secretory defect of cystic fibrosis.

***Tuberculosis.*** See Infections.

## Renal diseases (Table 105-16)

***Alport's syndrome.*** An autosomal dominant disorder with variable penetrance, Alport's syndrome has progressive renal interstitial inflammation and fibrosis, with eventual renal failure. Nerve deafness is often seen as part of the syndrome. The major ophthalmic findings are anterior lenticonus and anterior polar cataracts. Retinal pigmentary changes and drusen of the optic nerve head also are associated.

***Lowe's syndrome.*** Lowe's oculocerebrorenal syndrome is a recessive X-linked characteristic. The renal abnormalities emerge during the first year of life. The most common ocular finding in Lowe's syndrome is the presence of congenital cataracts; posterior lenticonus is often present. Congenital glaucoma is present in the majority of cases of Lowe's syndrome.

***Medullary cystic disease.*** Also called familial juvenile nephrolithiasis, medullary cystic disease causes an inability to concentrate urine. Ocular findings include decreased visual acuity and a retinitis pigmentosa fundus picture.

***Nephroblastoma (Wilms' tumor).*** Wilms' tumor, or nephroblastoma, a malignant embryonic connective tissue tumor, is associated with aniridia. Genital abnormalities and mental retardation are also seen. A partial deletion of chromosome 11p appears to be the cause.

***Nephrotic syndrome.*** Patients with nephrotic syndrome have only mild retinal edema and normal retinal arterioles. The absence of azotemia apparently causes the retinal manifestations of renal failure to be less severe than in pyelonephritis.

***Pyelonephritis.*** Azotemic renal failure includes the components of hypertensive retinopathy. In addition diffuse retinal and disc edema can be seen. Extensive cotton-wool exudates, papilledema, and retinal detachment are seen.

***Renal transplantation.*** The most common ocular complication in patients who have had renal transplantations is posterior subcapsular cataract, secondary to systemic prednisone therapy. Steroid-induced elevation of intraocular pressure is also seen. The immunosuppression makes these patients more prone to CMV retinitis and other opportunistic infections such as Candida.

## BIBLIOGRAPHY

Albert DM, Jakobiec FA, editors: *Principles and practice of ophthalmology,* 5 vols, Philadelphia, 1994, WB Saunders.

Gold DH, Weingeist TA, editors: *The eye in systemic disease,* Philadelphia, 1990, JB Lippincott.

Ryan SJ, editor: *Retina,* vol 1, *Basic science and inherited retinal disease,* vol 2, *Medical retina,* St Louis, 1989, Mosby.

Spalton DJ, Hitchings RA, Hunter PA, editors: *Atlas of clinical ophthalmology,* Philadelphia, 1984, JB Lippincott.

Yanoff M, Fine BS: *Ocular pathology, a text and atlas,* ed 3, Philadelphia, 1989, JB Lippincott.

CHAPTER

# 106 Glaucoma

G. Robert Lesser
Deborah A. Darnley-Fisch
Talya H. Kupin
Rhett M. Schiffman

Glaucoma is a name used for a group of diseases characterized by damage to the optic nerve and visual field loss, usually associated with an elevated intraocular pressure (IOP). The optic nerve may become pale and cupped, and other abnormalities may be noted as well (Fig. 106-1). Once the optic nerve has been damaged, the visual loss is irreversible. For this reason early detection and prompt treatment are essential.

There are two distinct patterns of visual field loss in glaucoma: (1) an overall depression of the visual field, presumably from diffuse axonal damage, and (2) focal areas of field loss, usually associated with corresponding focal areas of damage to the optic nerve. The defects usually begin in the periphery and gradually move closer to the center of vision. Common patterns of field loss are shown in Fig. 106-2.

## INTRAOCULAR PRESSURE ELEVATION

The key risk factor for losing vision is elevated IOP. The mean IOP (± S.D.) in the general population is 15.5 ± 2.57 mm Hg. The normal range is arbitrarily defined as 11 to 21 mm Hg, which represents 2 S.D. from the mean. The normal pressure curve in the general population is not a normal gaussian distribution, but is skewed toward the higher pressures (Fig. 106-3).

Almost 80% of patients with glaucoma have documented elevation of IOP. Although a direct prospective study of treated versus untreated glaucoma patients has not been formally conducted, there does appear to be a direct correlation between the magnitude and duration of IOP elevation and subsequent visual loss.

Up to 20% of patients with typical optic nerve and field changes have IOP measurements completely in the normal range. It is believed that there must be other unknown factors that contribute to the optic nerve damage. These factors might include vascular or structural abnormalities of the optic nerve.

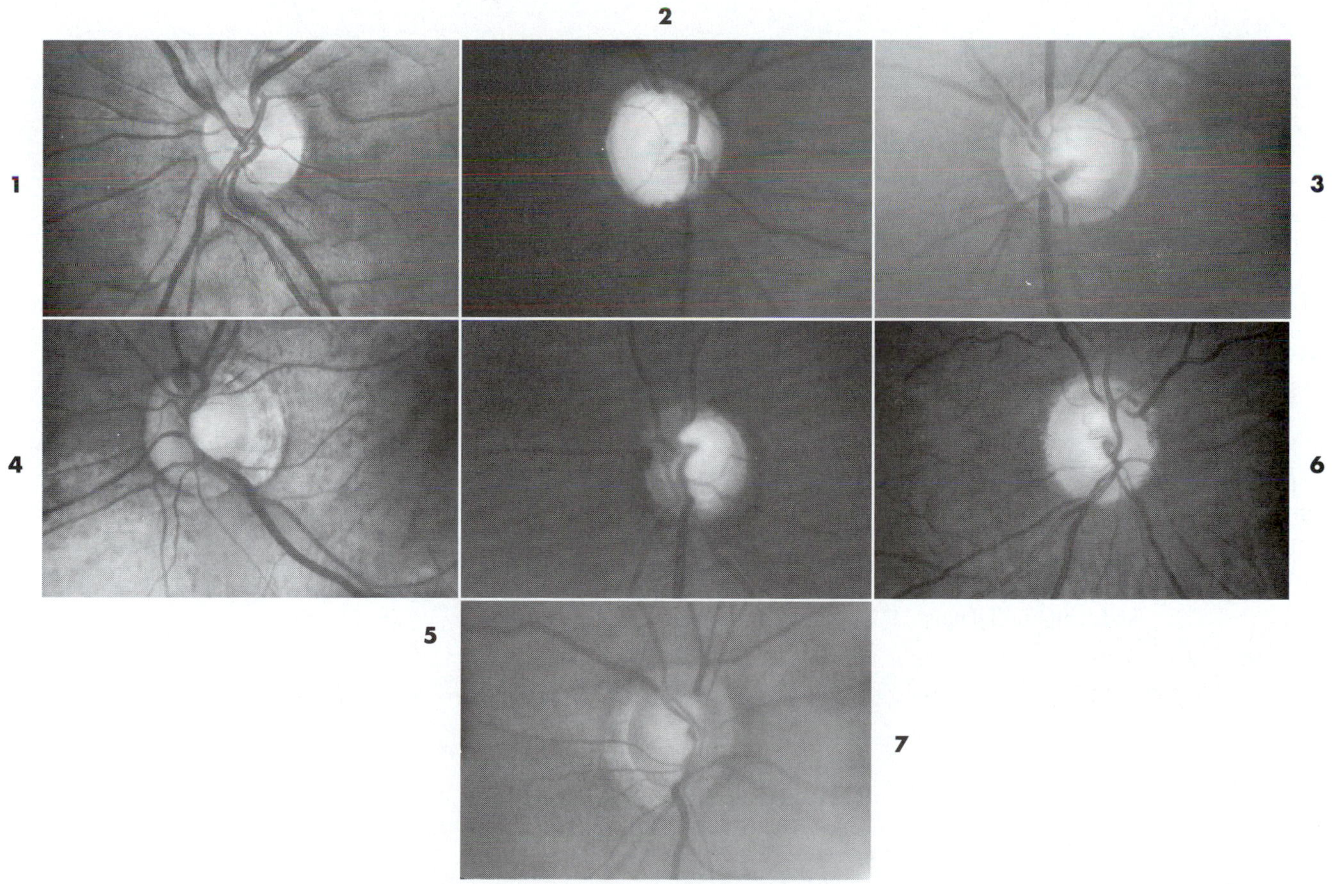


**Fig. 106-1.** Optic nerve damage from glaucoma. *1,* Normal optic nerve; *2,* enlarged cup and pallor; *3,* eccentric cupping; *4,* superficial nerve fiber layer hemorrhage; *5,* focal notching; *6,* verticalization cup; *7,* peripapillary atrophy.

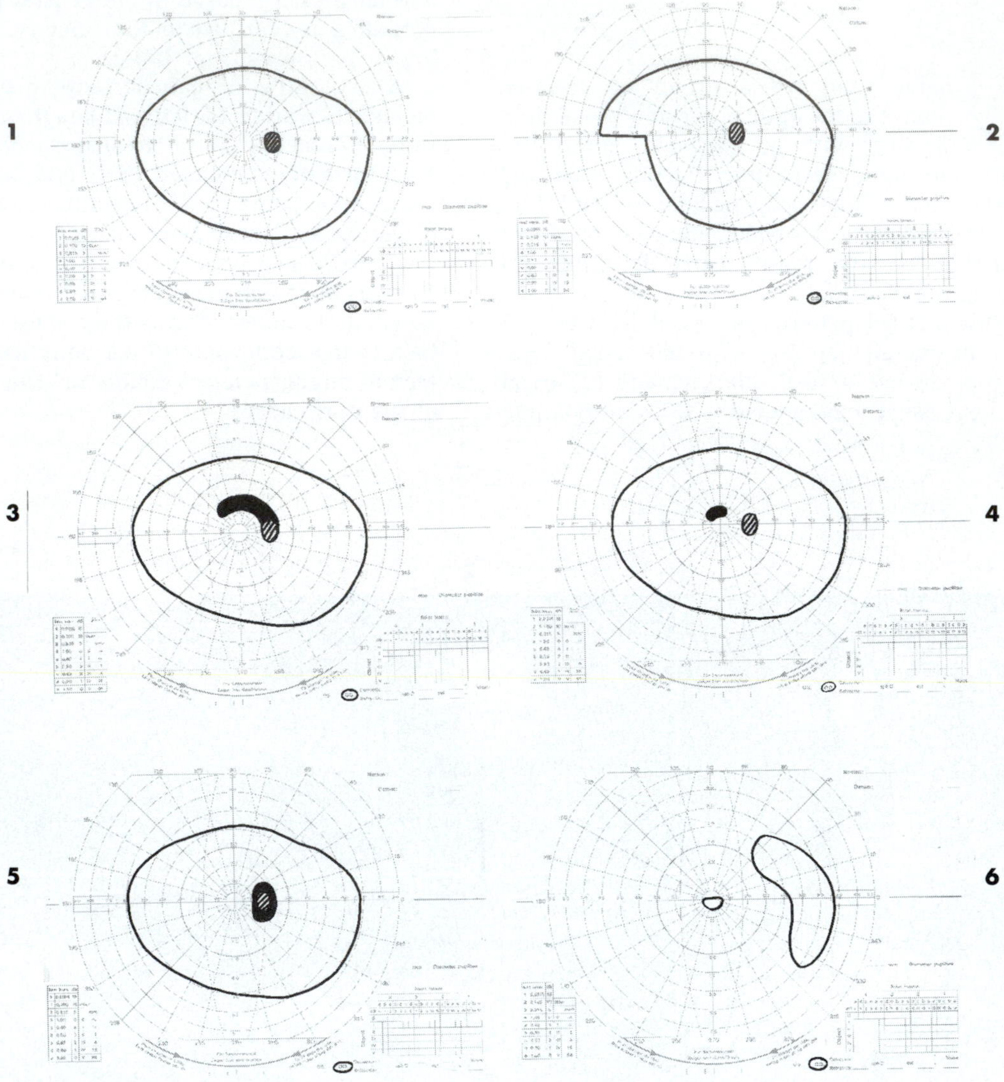


**Fig. 106-2.** Patterns of visual field loss (right eye only shown). *1,* Normal visual field; *2,* nasal step; *3,* arcuate scotoma; *4,* paracentral scotoma; *5,* enlargement blind spot; *6,* remaining central and temporal islands.

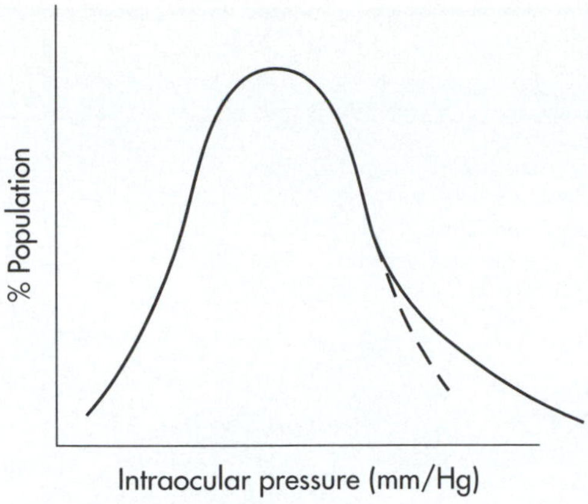


**Fig. 106-3.** Normal IOP.

### Risk factors for glaucoma

Family history
African-American
Increasing age
Diabetes
Myopia
Vascular disease
Elevated IOP

Around 5 to 10 million Americans have elevated IOP without optic nerve or visual field damage, a condition called ocular hypertension. It is not known how many of these people with ocular hypertension progress to actual glaucoma, but current estimates are approximately 1% per year. The rate of conversion of ocular hypertension to glaucoma, as well as the benefit of prophylactic treatment to lower IOP, is being studied in a 5-year prospective trial by the National Institutes of Health (NIH).

Many factors influence the IOP. It varies throughout the day and is often higher early in the morning. This pressure fluctuation is subject to the individual's diurnal rhythm and may vary greatly between patients. The IOP increases slightly when the patient is supine but may be lowered during sleep. Mean IOP increases with age and is higher in African-Americans.

Although IOP rises only slightly with increased systemic hypertension, it may be lowered by medications administered systemically to lower blood pressure, such as β-blockers and calcium channel blockers. There are conflicting reports with respect to the effect of caffeine, smoking, and exercise on IOP. There is also a small group of people who are steroid responders. In these individuals there can be a large elevation of IOP in response to systemic steroids, topical ocular steroids, and in rare instances the use of topical dermatologic steroid preparations close to the eyes.

This marked variability in IOP makes an isolated measurement a poor indicator in predicting the presence or absence of glaucoma, and seriously limits any screening process that relies on IOP alone.

## RISK FACTORS

Investigators now think there is a strong genetic component to many of the glaucomas, and glaucoma should be suspected in patients over age 40 with a positive family history. The disease is also more common in patients with diabetes, high myopia, and vascular disease (see the box at left). The risk of optic nerve damage increases with age, and there may be additional risk factors that make elderly patients more susceptible to optic nerve damage. African-Americans are at particularly high risk because they tend to develop visual loss at an earlier age (30s), and their disease is very aggressive. It has been estimated that one in 10 elderly African-Americans has glaucoma, a rate five times higher than elderly white patients.

## PATIENT HISTORY

Patients with early and moderate primary open-angle glaucoma are asymptomatic. Only when there is advanced optic nerve damage may they notice dimmed or blurred vision. Rarely can they detect peripheral vision loss, and usually monocular patching is necessary for patients to be aware of their visual defect. Conjunctival injection, ocular pain, or halo vision may be noted by patients with intermittent angle-closure glaucoma. In addition to the latter symptoms, nausea and vomiting can be dramatic during acute angle-closure attacks.

Because symptoms may be lacking, subtle, or generalized, it is important to obtain a careful ocular and general medical history. Ocular history may reveal recent or remote ocular trauma or intraocular surgery. Previous ocular inflammatory diseases such as herpes zoster ophthalmicus or uveitis also indicate patients at higher risk for glaucoma.

The general medical history may reveal associated systemic diseases such as diabetes, hypertension, herpes zoster, sarcoidosis, and ankylosing spondylitis.

A review of patient medications is necessary, since steroids may cause a marked elevation of IOP in susceptible individuals. Anticholinergics, such as atropine, tropicamide, and scopolamine, may precipitate acute angle-closure glaucoma. Other relatively common medications have some anticholinergic effects as well, including antihistamines, antipsychotics, and antiparkinsonism medications (see the box on p. 1474).

Finally, a family history of glaucoma needs to be sought in every patient in whom the disease is suspected. The risk for glaucoma is at least 10 times higher in individuals with a first-degree relative with the disease.

## IOP DETERMINATION

IOP is measured by determining the force needed to indent the eye. The most common device available to the general practitioner for measurement of IOP has been the Schiøtz tonometer (Fig. 106-4). With the patient in the supine position, a metal footplate plunger is gently placed on the anesthetized cornea and the IOP is determined by the displacement of a weighted plunger that protrudes through the footplate. The displacement of the plunger is read on a scale at the top of the device. The actual IOP is calculated by converting the scale reading to millimeters of mercury

### Drugs that may precipitate angle-closure glaucoma

Phenothiazines
Antihistamines—$H_1$ antagonists
Stimulants
- Amphetamines
- Caffeine
- Methylphenidate

Vasodilators
Sympathomimetic agents
- Epinephrine
- Ephedrine
- Norepinephrine
- Dopamine
- Naphazoline
- Tetrahydrozoline
- Methoxamine
- Hydroxyamphetamine

Parasympathomimetic agents
Parasympatholytic agents
- Cyclopentolate
- Tropicamide
- Atropine
- Homatropine
- Scopolamine

Cocaine
Clonidine
Antiparkinsonism agents

Modified from Mandelkorn RM, Zimmerman TJ. In Ritch R, Shields MB, editors: *The secondary glaucomas,* St Louis, 1982, Mosby.

using a nomogram chart, which comes with the device. The advantage of this technique is the durability and portability of the device. It is, however, sometimes difficult to apply and may be uncomfortable for the patient. Moreover, it underestimates IOP in highly myopic patients due to the decreased scleral rigidity.

Optometrists often use a noncontact air puff tonometer in which the eye is indented with a rapid impulse of air. This technique has the advantage of not requiring topical anesthetic drops and has a minimal chance of cross-contamination between patients, since only the stream of air actually touches the cornea. It is somewhat uncomfortable for patients, requires moderately expensive equipment, and tends to give measurements higher than actual. Many public health screenings are conducted with this device, and the results should not be used to establish a diagnosis or follow a patient.

Ophthalmologists usually use Goldman applanation tonometry, in which a small plastic device mounted on a slit lamp indents the cornea, and the pressure is determined by displacement of the tear film. This requires a topical anesthetic and is very accurate and reproducible. The technique requires special equipment and training.

A newer device for measuring IOP is the Tonopen (Fig. 106-5), a hand-held device in which a 1.02-mm central plunger is connected to a microprocessor to measure the applied force. This device and its successors offer the general practitioner a convenient way of screening for elevated IOP. The device is portable and battery operated, and pressures may be taken with the patient in any position. After instillation of a topical anesthetic, proparacaine HCl (Alcaine), the tip of the Tonopen is gently applied to the central cornea until an audible tone is heard, and the pressure measurement is immediately available on a small display within the handle. A disposable sterile cap is used on the tip of the Tonopen. Although significantly more expensive than a Schiøtz tonometer, the Tonopen is easy to use with limited training and much more comfortable for both the patient and physician. The Tonopen tends to overread pressures below 5 mm Hg and underread pressures over 30 mm Hg, but for screening purposes these limitations are not significant.

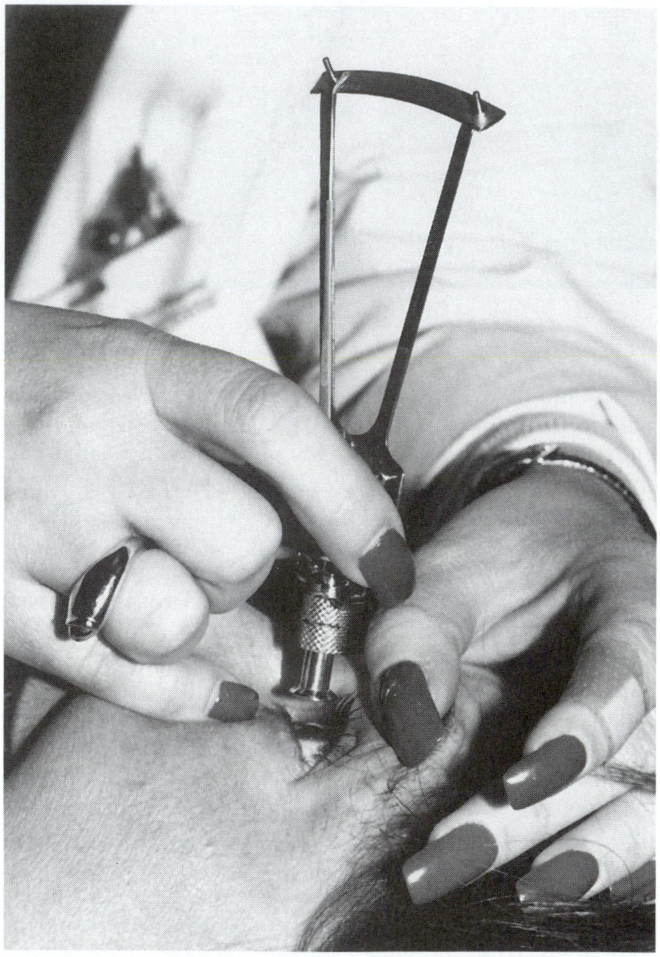

**Fig. 106-4.** Use of Schiøtz tonometer.

A home device for IOP measurement is currently undergoing Food and Drug Administration (FDA) evaluation and may play a role in future glaucoma diagnosis and management.

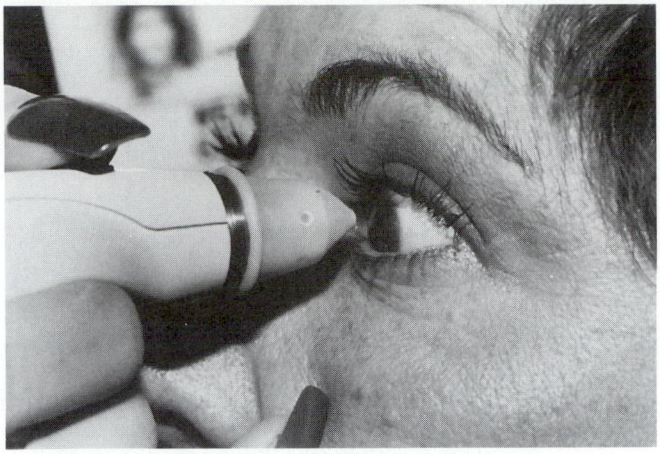

**Fig. 106-5.** Tonopen device.

## GLAUCOMA SCREENING

Glaucoma is one of the leading causes of blindness in the United States, affecting at least 2 million people, and is the leading cause of blindness among African-Americans. Studies indicate a prevalence of almost 0.7%, with over 2 million people affected and another 5 to 10 million at risk of developing the disease. The medical and financial implications of the disease and its treatment are staggering, and delayed diagnosis is a major component of glaucoma-induced blindness. The general practitioner needs to screen for this disease during routine physical examinations. If the IOP is elevated (see Fig. 106-3) or the optic nerve appears abnormal (see Fig. 106-1), a patient should be referred for formal ophthalmologic testing. If either factor cannot be assessed adequately or if the patient has additional risk factors (see Fig. 106-4), the patient should also be referred.

## DIFFERENTIAL DIAGNOSIS

The general practitioner may encounter patients with glaucoma in two clinical settings. The first is a patient with a white, quiet eye, in whom the disease is suspected because of high risk factors, elevated IOP found during screening examination, optic disc cupping and pallor found during routine funduscopic examination, or painless visual loss. Commonly encountered glaucomas in this setting are shown in the box above. In the second setting the patient presents with an inflamed red eye, and an elevated IOP is found during the evaluation (see the box above). The treatment varies according to which setting is encountered.

### Elevated IOP and the white eye

Chronic open-angle glaucoma
Steroid-induced glaucoma
Chronic angle-closure glaucoma
Old trauma or previous inflammation

### Elevated IOP and the red eye

Angle-closure glaucoma
Neovascular glaucoma
Herpes zoster and other uveitic glaucomas
Acute ocular or orbital trauma

### Therapy for primary open-angle glaucoma

Topical β-blockers (e.g., timolol maleate [Timoptic])
Topical epinephrine (e.g., Propine)
Topical miotics (e.g., pilocarpine [Isopto Carpine])
Argon laser trabeculoplasty
Carbonic anhydrase inhibitors (e.g., acetazolamide [Diamox])
Glaucoma surgery

## PRIMARY OPEN-ANGLE GLAUCOMA

### Pathophysiology

Primary (chronic) open-angle glaucoma is the most common form of glaucoma. Patients initially have no symptoms until the disease is far advanced, at which time they have sustained significant field loss close to fixation. Anatomically the angle and trabecular meshwork appear normal, but there is a blockage of aqueous outflow in the trabecular meshwork. The pressure is usually elevated above 21 mm Hg and is often over 30 mm Hg. There can be much individual variation in the amount of damage to the optic nerve for a given pressure. This is also true for normal tension glaucoma, in which the IOP is consistently in the normal range but the patients sustain optic nerve and field change identical to that seen with primary open-angle glaucoma.

### Therapy

Treatment consists of a stepwise progression of drops, pills, laser surgery, and filtration surgery, modified to take into account the overall health of an individual and side effects from the medications (see the box above). β-Blockers are usually the first line of therapy in the United States, and the order of additional therapy varies among physicians.

## ACUTE ANGLE-CLOSURE GLAUCOMA

### Pathophysiology

Acute angle-closure glaucoma occurs when the pupillary margin of the iris is pushed against the surface of the lens, a configuration called pupillary block. Aqueous fluid can no longer flow forward through the pupil, resulting in an increase in the pressure behind the iris. The iris is then pushed forward, blocking the trabecular meshwork. This results in a raised IOP. As the IOP increases, the iris is then pushed further forward, increasing the pupillary block, resulting in an upward spiral of increasing IOP over several hours.

Pupillary block is often precipitated in predisposed individuals by pupillary dilatation. This can occur several hours after they have been pharmacologically dilated for examination, when their pupils dilate in the dark, or as a result of dilatation from medications with anticholinergic effects such as antihistamines and some cold remedies (see the box on p. 1474). This sudden rise in intraocular pressure often results in severe ocular pain and can be accompanied by referred gastrointestinal pain with nausea and vomiting. The vision is often very blurred, and patients may complain of halos around lights.

When examined with a handlight, the cornea appears cloudy or steamy from corneal edema and the anterior chamber is often very shallow. The pupil is commonly middilated, fixed, and can be slightly eccentric. The sclera is injected and there can be profuse reflex tearing. The eye may feel firm to touch, and the IOP is very elevated; pressures of greater than 50 mm Hg are often seen. The fundus is difficult to see through the cloudy cornea. Examination of the opposite eye should demonstrate shallowing of the anterior chamber as well (Fig. 106-6).

Untreated, acute angle closure glaucoma can lead to permanent blindness. The optic nerve may be severely damaged and a secondary retinal vascular occlusion can occur. Damage to the corneal endothelium may result in thickening and clouding of the cornea (bullous keratopathy), and cataract formation is accelerated.

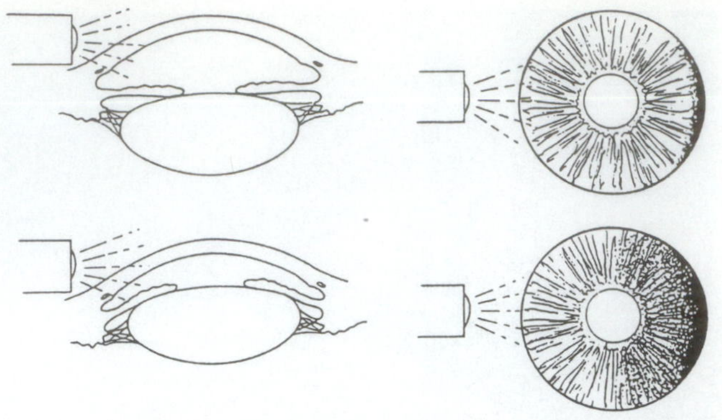

**Fig. 106-6.** Angle-closure glaucoma. Anterior chamber depth can be estimated using oblique illumination with a handlight.

### Medical therapy for angle-closure glaucoma

- Miotics (pilocarpine [Isopto Carpine 2%])
- β-Adrenergic blockers (timolol maleate [Timoptic 0.5%])
- α-Adrenergic agonists (apraclonidine [Iopdine 0.5%])
- Carbonic anhydrase inhibitor (acetazolamide [Diamox] 500 mg PO or IV)
- Hyperosmotic agents (Osmoglyn, mannitol)

### Therapy

When the patient is first seen, the immediate goal is to reduce the IOP. Corneal indentation with an anesthetic (proparacaine)-soaked cotton applicator may help break the pupillary block. Medications to acutely lower IOP are shown in the box above. Definitive treatment for angle-closure glaucoma is an iridectomy to bypass the mechanical blockage of the iris. This usually can be achieved with a YAG or argon laser, although occasionally a surgical iridectomy is necessary. Following an acute attack a patient may have persistently elevated pressures despite adequate iridectomies as a result of damage to the trabecular meshwork and may require medications on a chronic basis.

## NEOVASCULAR GLAUCOMA

### Pathophysiology

Patients with extensive ischemia to the retina from diabetic retinopathy or following a central retinal vein occlusion are at risk for developing neovascular glaucoma, a particularly devastating disease that often results in blindness and is difficult to treat. The ischemic retina releases an unidentified angiogenic factor(s), which causes proliferation of new vessels in the retina and on the surface of the iris (rubeosis iridis). These vessels eventually grow across the trabecular meshwork, resulting in mechanical closure of the angle and elevation of the IOP.

The eye may initially be white and quiet, but eventually it becomes inflamed with bulbar injection, corneal edema, and elevated IOP. Fine vessels are invariably present on the surface of the iris but may be difficult to see with a handlight. Occasionally the fibrovascular membrane on the surface of the iris contracts, pulling the darker posterior layer of the iris through the pupil, which is easily visible as ectropion uvea.

### Therapy

Treatment is directed toward reducing IOP and inflammation and removing the underlying stimulus to neovascularization with retinal laser photocoagulation (see the box on p. 1477). In addition to the poor visual prognosis, patients with this diagnosis have a higher incidence of death than age-matched controls, often from cerebral vascular and cardiac causes within 6 to 12 months from the time of diagnosis.

## HERPES ZOSTER OPHTHALMICUS

Herpes zoster affecting the first division of the trigeminal nerve has a high incidence of ocular involvement and is frequently found when there are lesions on the tip of the nose (Hutchinson's sign). Secondary glaucoma often occurs with ocular involvement. The pressure elevation may be asymptomatic. Therefore IOP should be checked in every patient during the acute phase of the disease and probably rechecked 1 to 2 weeks later. The mechanism of the glaucoma is probably direct inflammation of the trabecular meshwork, and the treatment includes systemic acyclovir, topical steroids, and antiglaucomatous medications (see the box on p. 1477).

### Treatment for neovascular glaucoma*

β-Adrenergic blockers (e.g., Timoptic and/or apraclonidine [Iopidine])
Carbonic anhydrase inhibitors (e.g., acetazolamide [Diamox])
Topical atropine 1%
Topical prednisolone acetate 1%
Filtration surgery with adjunct antimetabolites and/or glaucoma valves
Panretinal photocoagulation ASAP

*Do not use miotics.

### Treatment for glaucoma in association with herpes zoster

β-Adrenergic blockers and/or apraclonidine (e.g., Timoptic and/or apraclonidine [Iopidine])
Carbonic anhydrase inhibitors if necessary
Topical atropine 1%
Topical prednisolone acetate 1%
Acyclovir (Zovirax)

## ACUTE TRAUMA

Blunt and penetrating trauma to the eye may cause elevated IOP and glaucoma acutely by several different mechanisms. Bleeding directly into the orbit can cause acute proptosis and a very high IOP. The fundus should be visualized immediately to rule out spontaneous arterial pulsations (best seen on the optic nerve), which indicates impending vascular occlusion from the high IOP. The orbit needs to be decompressed immediately, usually with a lateral canthotomy or a controlled fracture of the orbital floor into the maxillary sinus.

Intraocular bleeding may also cause an acute elevation of IOP. Blood and inflammatory debris can plug the trabecular meshwork, and a large clot in the anterior chamber (hyphema) can result in pupillary block glaucoma. The pressure is usually controlled with aqueous suppression (β-blockers and/or carbonic anhydrase inhibitors) and if necessary osmotic agents (Osmoglyn, mannitol). If the pressure is persistently elevated, the anterior chamber can be washed out in the operating room. Patients with sickle cell trait or disease are at increased risk from these anterior segment bleeds, and early surgical intervention is often recommended.

After the acute episode patients with ocular trauma are at long-term risk for secondary glaucoma. The trabecular meshwork may be permanently damaged, and a laceration into the ciliary body (angle recession) is associated with an elevated IOP. These patients are often completely asymptomatic with white, quiet eyes and as in chronic open-angle glaucoma, may not be aware of their visual loss until it is far advanced.

## MANAGEMENT

Although there are many different types of glaucoma, there are only a limited number of modalities currently available to lower IOP. They are used in a stepwise progression, analogous to the treatment of systemic hypertension.

### Pharmacologic agents

In the United States, the initial treatment for glaucoma is usually the use of drops to lower the IOP. These drops work by decreasing aqueous production and/or increasing aqueous outflow, and they may be used in combination. When these drops are applied to the eye, a significant portion flow through the nasal lacrimal duct, where they may be absorbed through the mucous membranes into the systemic circulation. The clinician therefore needs to be aware of the potential side effects of these medications (Table 106-1). The most commonly prescribed antiglaucomatous medications used are β-blockers, which may have adverse cardiovascular and bronchopulmonary effects, such as worsening chronic obstructive pulmonary disease (COPD) and congestive heart failure, precipitation of asthmatic attacks, and increasing sinus bradycardia or heart block. These medications may also raise serum triglycerides and lower high-density lipoprotein (HDL) cholesterol, which may have serious cardiovascular implications, since these medications could be taken for decades. Less obvious effects include impotence in men and confusion in elderly patients.

A second class of drops are the parasympathomimetics (e.g., pilocarpine), which increase aqueous outflow and cause pupillary constriction. Patients taking these medications often complain of dimming of vision from the miosis and can have severe frontal headaches from the medication.

When drops fail to adequately lower IOP, carbonic anhydrase inhibitors may be added, such as acetazolamide (Diamox) and methazolamide (Neptazane). They decrease aqueous production in the ciliary body and commonly cause side effects such as generalized fatigue, loss of appetite, and paresthesias in the hands and feet. They may also be associated with renal stones and aplastic anemia and should not be used for patients with a sensitivity or allergy to sulfonamides. Of particular interest to the general practitioner is a transient hypokalemia, which can be severe and may require adjustment of a concurrent diuretic or other antihypertensive medications, as well as potassium replacement.

### Lasers

When the pressures are not controlled with medications, argon laser trabeculoplasty may be used to lower pressure. The procedure is done in an outpatient setting and consists of using a mirrored contact lens to place 80 to 100 small burns on the trabecular meshwork. The exact mechanism by which argon laser trabeculoplasty works is not known, but the procedure is initially effective in almost 80% of patients. Unfortunately, at 5 years almost 50% of those patients who responded to the laser are no longer controlled. Some ophthalmologists have advocated using the procedure before drops, but a clinical trial to study this is still under way.

**Table 106-1.** Medication actions and side effects

| Medication | Strength | Frequency | Action | Side effects |
|---|---|---|---|---|
| **β-Blockers** | | | Reduces aqueous secretion | Local allergy and irritation, bradycardia, heart block, bronchospasm, decreased libido, depression |
| Timolol (Timoptic) | 0.25%-0.5% | qd-bid | | |
| Levobunolol (Betagan) | 0.25%-0.5% | | | |
| Carteolol (Ocupress) | 1% | | | |
| Metipranolol (Optipranolol) | 0.3% | | | |
| Betaxolol (Betoptic) | 0.25%-0.5% | | | |
| **Sympathomimetics** | | | Improves aqueous outflow | Ocular irritation and allergy, adrenochrome deposits, rebound hyperemia, mydriasis, cystoid macular edema in aphakia, hypertension, extrasystoles, headache |
| Epinephrine (Glaucon) | 1%-2% | bid | | |
| Dipivefrin (Propine) | 0.1% | bid | | |
| **α-Adrenergic agonist** | | | Reduces aqueous secretion | Ocular irritation and allergy, upper lid elevation, mydriasis, bradycardia, dry mouth |
| Apraclonidine (Iopidine) | 0.5% | tid | | |
| **Direct- and indirect-acting parasympathomimetics** | | | | |
| Pilocarpine (Isopto Carpine) | 0.5%-6% | qid | Improves aqueous outflow | Miosis, decreased night vision, variable induced myopia, brow ache, exacerbation of cataract, induced-angle closure, retinal tear or detachment |
| Carbachol (Isoptocarbachol) | 0.75%-3% | tid | Improves aqueous outflow | Intense miosis, iris pigment epithelial cysts, induced myopia, cataract, retinal detachment, paradoxic angle closure, punctal stenosis, intense bleeding and inflammation with ocular surgery, abdominal cramps, diarrhea, enuresis, prolonged recovery from succinylcholine |
| Echothiophate iodide (Phospholine Iodide) | 0.03%-0.25% | bid | | |
| **Carbonic anhydrase inhibitors** | | | Reduce aqueous secretion | Paresthesias, malaise, lethargy, abdominal cramps, diarrhea, nausea, renal stones, loss of libido, anorexia, depression, hypokalemia, acidosis, aplastic anemia, thrombocytopenia |
| Acetazolamide (Diamox) | 125-250 mg | qid | | |
| Acetazolamide (Diamox Sequels) | 500 mg | bid | | |
| Methazolamide (Neptazane) | 25-50 mg | bid-tid | | |
| **Hyperosmotic agents** | | | Reduces vitreous volume | Congestive heart failure, headache, subdural and subarachnoid hemorrhages, diabetic ketoacidosis (glycerol) |
| Mannitol | 1-2 g/kg | IV or PO q8-12h | | |
| Isosorbide (Ismotic) | 1.5 g/kg | | | |
| Glycerin (Oxmoglyn) | 2-3 ml/kg | | | |

## Surgery

The IOP can be effectively controlled with glaucoma filtration surgery, in which a fistula is created between the anterior chamber and the subconjunctival space. The procedure is 85% to 90% effective but does carry significant potential complications, including increased cataract formation. When successful, the procedure may reduce or eliminate the need for glaucoma medications and does not depend on the compliance of patients with their medications. In the United States surgery is done when medications and lasers are not effective. The English have questioned this premise and are conducting clinical studies on the efficacy of surgery versus medical therapy as the initial treatment for glaucoma.

### Preoperative and postoperative surgical management

The glaucoma patient may be sent to a general practitioner before glaucoma filtering surgery for medical evaluation. Unlike cataract surgery, these procedures are often not elective, and prolonged delays may be vision threatening.

The surgery may be done under local anesthesia, particularly in elderly patients with significant cardiovascular and/or pulmonary disease. Lidocaine (Xylocaine) and bupivacaine (Marcaine) are often used for the regional blocks, and epinephrine may be added for hemostasis and prolongation of the block. Allergies to these medications need to be noted, and contraindications to epinephrine use need to be explicitly conveyed to the operating surgeon.

Since vascular disease is one of the risk factors in glaucoma, it is not surprising that some of these patients may be taking anticoagulation medication. Anticoagulation can create several problems during glaucoma surgery, including a retrobulbar hemorrhage during the local block and an increased risk of an intraoperative sudden massive hemorrhage of a suprachoroidal blood vessel, which usually results in blindness. Therefore, if possible, anticoagulation medications such as aspirin and coumadin should be discontinued, if medically safe, before surgery. The IOP may be very low for several days following the surgery, and the anticoagulation medications can be safely restarted once the IOP returns to the normal range.

Close attention needs to be taken to control systemic hypertension and to suppress severe coughing during the procedure. Identifiable sources of infection such as an active upper respiratory tract infection need to be cleared if possible before surgery.

Occasionally general anesthetics are used. A particular problem arises if the patient has been using long-acting parasympathomimetics such as echiothiophate iodide (Phospholine Iodide) to control glaucoma. If succinylcholine is used as a paralyzing agent during intubation, there may be prolonged apnea because of the pseudocholinesterase inhibition by the echiothiophate. In addition, succinylcholine may also cause a transient rise in IOP due to sustained extraocular muscle contraction.

Postoperatively, patients often have very blurred vision until the IOP stabilizes. The eye is often patched or covered with a protective metal shield, and care needs to be taken to avoid falls. Strenuous activity such as heavy lifting should be avoided. Other activities such as a physical rehabilitation program might need to be modified for a limited time.

## BIBLIOGRAPHY

Hoskins HD Jr, Kass M: *Becker-Shaffer's diagnosis and therapy of the glaucomas,* ed 6, St Louis, 1989, Mosby.

Ritch R, Shields MB, Krupin T: *The glaucomas,* St Louis, 1989, Mosby.

CHAPTER

# 107 Diseases of the Orbit and Ocular Adnexa

Murray D. Christianson

## OCULAR ADNEXA

### Infections, infestations, and inflammations

***Viral infections.*** Common viral infections include those with pox viruses (molluscum contagiosum), wart viruses (verruca vulgaris, plana, digitata, and filiformis), and the herpes viruses (herpes simplex, varicella-zoster).

Molluscum contagiosum is mildly contagious, presenting with one or, more often, multiple dome-shaped, skin-colored, umbilicated nodules, 1 to 3 mm in diameter, from which a cheesy, sebum-like material can be expressed. If found on the lid margin, a follicular conjunctivitis can result. Treat by incision, gentle curettage, and swabbing with alcohol.

Verruca (from human papillomaviruses) are circumscribed growths appearing on the lids after autoinoculation, occasionally causing a conjunctivitis and keratitis. The excrescences can be round and hyperkeratotic (verruca vulgaris), flat and sessile (verruca plana), digitate with several projections with horny caps grouped on a narrow base (verruca digitata), or filiform, slender, and threadlike, covered with apparently normal skin (verruca filiformis). They should be excised.

Herpes simplex is usually spread by kissing and has two peaks of infection: between ages 6 months and 4 years, and between 16 and 25 years. The primary infection may be subclinical or associated with a unilateral crop of pinhead-sized vesicles on a swollen, slightly red base, usually on the lower lid. Sometimes associated with fever, they resolve in about 7 days, leaving no scars. The infection may cause a conjunctivitis or keratitis and occasionally, usually in atopic patients, gives a severe systemic infection—Kaposi's varicelliform eruption (eczema herpeticum). Recurrent herpes infection (cold sores) may affect the eyelids but is usually benign unless the eye itself is infected. Treat lid lesions with acyclovir, 300 mg by mouth five times daily, and topical vidarabine 0.1% eye drops five times daily.

Varicella-zoster virus causes chickenpox and herpes zoster. The former is a highly contagious but usually mild childhood epidemic infection with a papular or vesicular rash that is widespread, but often attacks the lid margins and the conjunctiva. It usually regresses without sequelae. Herpes zoster typically affects the eyelids and eyes of adults and the aged, but can attack the young. Immunosuppressed patients are at special risk. Virus latent in the ganglion replicates and migrates down, usually affecting the first and more rarely the second trigeminal nerve division. It gives sudden onset of fever, malaise, and preherpetic neuralgic pain in the nerve distribution. Usually 3 or 4 days later the skin blushes, then swells, and then develops vesicles filled with initially clear, then turbid fluid. These quickly burst, giving an eschar in the nerve distribution, inviting secondary infection, and healing over a week or two. Ocular inflammation may be marked. Pain is often severe and may persist (postherpetic), particularly in the elderly, for years afterward. The skin is often left mildly anesthetic, yet giving pain on the slightest provocation (anesthesia dolorosa). If diagnosed within the first few days, treat immunocompetent patients with oral acyclovir, 600 mg five times daily for 10 days, topical corticosteroid/antibiotic ointment, and oral prednisone, 60 mg daily for 7 days. Postherpetic neuralgia may be helped with antidepressants.

***Bacterial infections.*** Bacterial infections can be uncommon but serious, such as anthrax, or more common, such as hordeolum. External hordeola, often secondary to staphylococcal blepharitis, are purulent inflammations of lash follicles and adjacent glands. Internal hordeola involve meibomian glands. Both present with pain and lid margin redness and swelling that rapidly localize to form a small abscess that may point and drain. Treat with hot compresses, systemic penicillinase-resistant antibiotics, and surgical drainage when necessary.

***Fungal infections.*** Although they are rare, fungal infections of the eyelid include blastomycosis, coccidioidomycosis (valley fever, San Joaquin fever), cryptococcosis, and sporotrichosis. North American blastomycosis often affects lid skin, producing gradually enlarging, hyperkeratotic, verrucous plaques that may become confluent, ulcerate, and crusted. After confirmation by biopsy, treat with oral itraconazole, 100 to 200 mg twice daily, or intravenous amphotericin, 0.3-0.6 mg daily. Coccidioidomycosis, acquired only in southwestern North America, cryptococcosis, and sporotrichosis may produce chronic lid margin and periocular ulceration.

***Infestations.*** Lid infestations include phthiriasis palpebrarum (crab lice), demodicosis (*Demodex* blepharitis), myiasis, subcutaneous dirofilariasis, leishmaniasis, and cysticercosis. The examination of chronic, itchy crab lice blepharitis may reveal multiple nits (eggs) glued to the lash bases and several lice gripping the lash bases or crawling about the shafts, or only one or two nits. Treat by washing all clothes and bed linen in hot, soapy water, by using an antilice shampoo on all affected individuals, and picking off the nits and lice.

*Demodex folliculorum,* the hair follicle mite, and *Demodex brevis,* the sebaceous gland mite, may infest the lid margin pilosebaceous units and contribute to chronic blepharitis and meibomianitis. Diagnosis is difficult. Treat as for marginal blepharitis.

Myiasis, infestation with fly larvae, is rare but in endemic areas (Central and South America) may result from bites by insects carrying *Dermatobia hominis* (human botfly, warble fly). Excise the furuncle-like mass.

*Dirofilaria tenuis,* a racoon parasite, common in the southeastern United States, may be transferred to the eyelid by a mosquito bite and produce a solitary, subcutaneous nodule. It should be excised.

"Oriental" sores from leishmaniasis commonly affect the face and uncommonly the eyelids. Slowly growing, painless, subcutaneous eyelid nodules from cysticercosis are rare and should be excised.

***Inflammations.*** Lid inflammations include marginal blepharitis and associated disorders, dermatitis, and foreign body granulomas.

Marginal blepharitis is a common, chronic, poorly understood condition associated with staphylococcal infection, seborrhea, acne rosacea, and dry eyes. It eventually produces secondary lid margin scarring with misdirection of lashes, causing corneal damage. Patients complain of chronic burning, itching, and redness of their lids, often worse in the morning. Symptoms are often out of proportion to signs. Though often a mixed staphylococcal/seborrheic condition, each type has its hallmarks.

Staphylococcal marginal blepharitis usually begins in childhood and may last a lifetime, affecting mostly females. It produces dilated skin vessels (rosettes) and at the lash roots brittle yellow crusts that, when removed, leave a bleeding ulcer. Recurrent hordeolum may occur. Chronic inflammation deforms the lid margin, producing cicatricial entropion or ectropion, thickening (tylosis), or notching. Lashes are lost (madarosis) or misdirected (trichiasis) or lose their color (poliosis). Hypersensitivity to staphylococcal exotoxins may cause secondary chronic papillary conjunctivitis, inferior corneal epithelial punctate erosions, marginal corneal ulcers, and phlyctenules (rare).

Seborrheic marginal blepharitis is usually associated with seborrheic dermatitis of the scalp, nasolabial folds, brow, retroauricular area, and sternum. It produces reddened lid margins with soft, greasy scales, not clustered at the lash roots, and not giving bleeding microulcers when removed. Meibomian glands hypersecrete, giving a foamy tear meniscus, meibomian orifices swollen or plugged by oil globules, and chalazia. Conjunctival and corneal irritation with excess lipids and free fatty acids produce secondary chronic papillary conjunctivitis and interpalpebral corneal epithelial punctuate erosions.

Treatment, usually lifelong, is aimed at relieving irritation and minimizing scarring and secondary changes. It includes baseline facial and lid hygiene with more aggressive treatment of exacerbations. If the condition is seborrheic, begin with a dandruff shampoo. In both types use twice daily face washes with a facecloth and warm, soapy water, augmented with eyelid scrubs with warm water, using either a facecloth or cotton-tipped applicators to remove all crusts. For flare-ups or resistant cases, after scrubbing massage into the lid margin sulfacetamide, bacitracin, erythromycin, or gentamicin ointment. A combination antibiotic/corticosteroid ointment may speed resolution of severely inflamed lids. In severe cases and if acne rosacea is suspected, add oral tetracycline. Artificial tears help relieve the commonly associated dry eye symptoms.

A hordeolum (stye) is a furuncle at the lid margin. An external hordeolum involves a lash follicle and gland of Zeis or Moll; an internal hordeolum involves a meibomian gland. It presents with painful lid swelling that becomes localized, often pointing through the skin at the lash line (external) or through the tarsal conjunctiva (internal). Treat with hot compresses, oral dicloxacillin, and incision and drainage when necessary.

A chalazion is a localized, lipogranulomatous inflammation of eyelid sebaceous glands, secondary to duct obstruction, sometimes caused by inflammatory, infectious, and neoplastic lid margin disease, but usually arising spontaneously, often associated with seborrheic dermatitis or acne rosacea. A meibomian gland chalazion is usually a painless, rounded, slowly enlarging, subcutaneous lid mass that may wax and wane in size. It may rupture posteriorly, giving a polypoid mass of granulation tissue on the conjunctiva or rarely anteriorly, producing a subcutaneous mass. Treat acne rosacea or seborrheic dermatitis if present, and recommend hot moist compresses for 15 minutes four times daily. For resistant or chronic chalazia advise incision and curettage. In recurrent cases add intralesional triamcinolone. Marginal chalazia are resistant to conservative treatment.

Eyelid dermatitis is common, since eyelid skin is thin and often rubbed and exposed to irritants. Acute dermatitis produces burning and itching, redness, swelling, scaling, and in severe cases blistering. Chronic dermatitis produces itching, thickening, and scaling. Contact dermatitis results from cosmetics, nail polish, chemicals in soaps, aerosols such as hair sprays, and topical ophthalmic antibiotics (especially neomycin). To treat, stop topical use of all products and any aerosols, nail polishes, or new laundry soaps, fluff agents, or water softeners, and recommend cool compresses four times daily. Once improvement begins, add hydrocortisone 0.5% in Unibase massaged into the skin three or four times daily until resolution. Then judiciously reintroduce the products the patient must have, monitoring carefully for recurrence. Atopic eyelid dermatitis occurs in those with a personal or family history of asthma, hay fever, or atopic dermatitis (often in the lateral neck folds and antecubital and popliteal fossae). Treat with hydrocortisone 0.5% in Unibase four times daily and dermatologic referral if more widespread.

### Other eyelid lesions

Foreign body granulomas after injury produce slowly growing eyelid lumps that require excision.

Xanthelasma (eyelid xanthoma), the most common cutaneous xanthoma and the only common lid xanthoma), occurs in the middle aged and elderly, two thirds of whom are normolipemic. Usually bilateral and at the inner canthi, they are flat or slightly raised, yellowish tan, soft plaques. Excise for cosmetic improvement.

Hidrocystomas, retention cysts either of the apocrine (Moll) gland or eccrine sweat glands, are common, appearing occasionally as multiple, but usually as a solitary, translucent lid margin cystic nodule, often with a bluish hue that transilluminates. They should be excised.

Pilosebaceous cysts include milia and sebaceous cysts. Milia are asymptomatic, rounded, white, sharply circumscribed, pinhead-sized, pearly nodules. Treat with excision, diathermy, or electrolysis.

Sebaceous (pilar) cysts are globular, subcutaneous masses, closely attached to the skin, often of the brow, often with preservation of the plugged pore at the summit. They may be stable or grow slowly. Treat by excision.

Epidermal inclusion cysts, often resulting from trauma or surgery, are slowly progressive, firm, globular, painless, mobile dermal or subcutaneous masses covered by intact epidermis.

### Malpositions

See Table 107-1 for diagnosis and management of eyelid malpositions.

### Injuries

See the box below for management of eyelid lacerations.

## LACRIMAL SYSTEM

### Dry eyes

Treat any treatable systemic diseases. Change any contributing systemic medication. Recommend avoiding wind, fans, low humidity, smoking, and all air pollutants.

#### Eyelid lacerations

**Repair**

Nonmarginal lacerations that do not involve:
- Canthal tendons
- Levator
- Lacrimal drainage system
- Extensive tissue loss

Close:
- Clean carefully
- Debride conservatively
- Repair meticulously
- 6-0 or 7-0 nonabsorbable sutures
- Do not fix the lid to the orbital rim by including orbital septum in the repair

**Refer to an ophthalmologist***

Nonmarginal eyelid lacerations involving canthal tendons
Nonmarginal eyelid lacerations involving levator or aponeurosis
Eyelid lacerations involving eyelid margin
Lacerations with significant tissue loss
Canalicular lacerations
Any eyelid laceration about which there is any doubt

*Cover with a light, moist dressing and refer.

**Table 107-1.** Eyelid malpositions

| Malposition | Symptoms | Signs | Management |
|---|---|---|---|
| Trichiasis: normal lid position, but lashes directed posteriorly | Irritation, tearing red eye | Eyelid: no entropion, scarring, inflammation<br>Eyelash: against the eye<br>Eye: red, corneal ulcer | Lid scrubs, hot compresses, antibiotics<br>For lash: temporary epilation, permanent epilation<br>Electroepilation: excision of root(s), cryodestruction |
| Entropion: can be congenital, acquired, cicatricial, mechanical, senile | Intermittent (?), irritation, tearing, red eye | Eyelid: lid flipped in lashes and skin against the eye<br>Eye: red, corneal ulcer | For lid: temporary or permanent tape, restore anatomy<br>For eye: lubricate |
| Ectropion: can be congenital, acquired, cicatricial, paralytic, senile | Irritation, tearing, red eye, red lid | Eyelid: eyelid flipped out, irritated, exposed conjunctiva<br>Eye: dry, irritated | For lid: surgically restore anatomy |
| Blepharoptosis<br>Neurogenic<br>Neuromuscular junction: myogenic, aponeurotic, mechanical | Upper lid droop | Frontalis contraction, brow elevation, excess skin, high lid crease, droopy lid | Surgically restore, suspend lid |
| Retraction: Graves' disease ? | Stare, eye too big, irritation, tearing | Lid: upper > up, lower > down<br>Eye: red, exposed | Surgically lower upper and/or raise lower |
| Blepharospasm | Eyes close involuntarily | Lid spasms, facial twitches | Botulinum toxin, surgery |

Suggest artificial tears during the day and lubricant ointment at night. Consider temporary lacrimal punctal occlusion with punctal plugs or permanent occlusion with cautery.

### Epiphora or tearing

Identify and treat the cause by surgically correcting lid laxity, punctal atresia, punctal ectropion, canalicular disease or obstruction, or lacrimal sac and nasolacrimal duct disease (dacryocystorhinostomy [DCR]). A DCR has a 97% success rate in primary cases, can be done as an outpatient case under local anesthetic, and usually leaves little scarring.

### Infections

Dacryoadenitis may be acute (viral or bacterial) or chronic (bacterial). Acute viral dacryoadenitis produces a fullness or pain in the upper outer orbit with an inflammatory, abscesslike, firm, tender, lateral lid swelling, an S-shaped upper lid margin, a mechanical ptosis, sometimes inferonasal proptosis, and preauricular lymphadenopathy. Lid eversion shows gland swelling with localized chemosis. Resolution takes a week or two. Causes include mumps, infectious mononucleosis, herpes zoster, measles, influenza, and dengue fever. Acute bacterial dacryoadenitis is very rare, more severe, and may suppurate, draining through the conjunctiva (palpebral lobe) or skin (orbital lobe). Causes include staphylococci, streptococci, pneumococci, and gonococci. Chronic bacterial dacryoadenitis produces a superotemporal orbital mass with diplopia on looking toward it, inferonasal proptosis, and often dry eye. Causes include trachoma, tuberculosis, leprosy, syphilis, and actinomycosis. Canaliculitis, usually due to *Actinomyces israelii* or similar organism, presents with chronic unilateral tearing and irritation, with redness and swelling of the area over the canaliculus. It is resistant to all topical medicines. Treat with canaliculotomy, stone removal, and painting with iodine solution. Dacryocystitis, a common condition due to nasolacrimal duct obstruction, presents usually in middle-aged adults (female/male ratio is 3:1) with acute or chronic lacrimal sac swelling (below the medial canthal tendon), irritation, and tearing. Often recurrent, the usual infecting organisms are *Staphylococcus aureus, Streptococcus pneumoniae,* and *Streptococcus pyogenes.* Titrate the treatment to the clinical picture, with appropriate systemic antibiotics (oral or intravenous), hot compresses, abscess drainage, and dacryocystorhinostomy.

## ORBIT

### Idiopathic sclerosing inflammation

This entraps orbital structures in scar. Sometimes part of multifocal fibrosclerosis, usually unilateral, it produces diplopia, proptosis, progressive visual loss, lid retraction, mild inflammation, and pain. Computed tomography (CT) shows homogenous dense lesions, often contrast enhancing, with regular margins, infiltrating orbital fat, and muscles. Histopathology shows scarring with scattered inflammatory cells. Differential diagnosis includes chronic inflammations (Wegener's and other granulomatous inflammations), secondary and metastatic cancers (especially sclerosing types), and lymphomas. Initial response to steroids may be good, but later relentless progression is the rule. After assessment by biopsy, treat with prednisone (80 mg daily) plus radiotherapy (2500 to 3000 Gy).

### Idiopathic noninfectious granulomatous inflammation

This is defined by its histopathology (nonnecrotizing granuloma or lipogranuloma), affecting orbital soft tissues without specific localization or systemic associations. It presents with mild inflammation, a palpable mass, and a slow onset. Treat with excision or prednisone, 80 mg daily.

### Thyroid-associated ophthalmopathy

This is the most common cause of both unilateral and bilateral proptosis. The ophthalmopathy associated with Graves' hyperthyroidism and, less often, with Hashimoto's thyroiditis, it is an organ-specific, autoimmune-mediated inflammation of the extraocular muscles and perhaps the periorbital connective tissue. Behind the globe the orbit becomes a three-sided pyramid narrowing to its apex at the optic foramen. This crowded posterior third contains the optic nerve and bellies of the extraocular muscles. Here, in Graves' disease, the muscles swell, pushing the globe forward, tethering the levator and rectus muscles, and squeezing the optic nerve.

Of those who develop thyroid disease, 30% have a positive family history. Thyroid-associated ophthalmopathy (TAO) involves both divisions of the immune system: the humoral, mediated by antibodies secreted by B lymphocytes, and the cellular, mediated by T lymphocytes. TAO is probably initiated by a primary abnormality of immune surveillance or by an intrinsic cellular disorder with secondary autoimmune phenomena. Signs of autoimmune derangement include the presence of autoantigens, autoantibodies, sensitized T lymphocytes, and other autoimmune diseases such as myasthenia gravis in the patient and family (see Chapter 34 for further discussion).

### Sarcoidosis

Sarcoidosis is a multisystem, immunologic disorder, with noncaseating granulomas involving many tissues (in particular, the hilar lymph nodes and pulmonary parenchyma), with symptoms dependent on the site and degree of involvement. Ophthalmic findings include eyelid nodules or papules, uveitis, chorioretinitis, keratoconjunctivitis sicca, lacrimal gland enlargement, conjunctival nodules, neuropathies, and very rarely deep orbital disease. Diagnosis should be based on the clinical presentation with bilateral hilar lymphadenopathy and characteristic biopsy. With significant disease treat with prednisone, 80 mg daily, and tapering depending on response. Relapses are frequent; prognosis is usually good.

### Sjögren's syndrome

Sjögren's syndrome is a chronic, systemic inflammatory disorder of unknown cause, with dry mouth, eyes, and other mucous membranes associated with rheumatoid arthritis (most common), systemic lupus erythematosus, polymyositis, vasculitis, scleroderma, mixed connective tissue disease, autoimmune liver disease, and hemolytic anemia. It produces dry eyes, filamentary keratopathy, enlarged tender lacrimal and parotid glands, dry mouth, epistaxis, reduced sense of smell, hoarseness, recurrent bronchitis, and increased risk of pseudolymphoma and malignant lymphoma. There is often evidence of other autoimmune diseases and, in the primary disease, highly specific antinuclear antibodies. Biopsy of lacrimal or salivary glands may be diagnostic. Differential diagnosis includes Mikulicz syndrome—involvement of the lacrimal and salivary glands with sarcoidosis, lymphoma, leukemia, tuberculosis, syphilis, and other specific and nonspecific inflammations. Manage local symptoms with lubricants and the systemic disease with systemic steroids and immunosuppressives. The risk of malignant lymphoma precludes radiotherapy.

### Vasculitides

These include periarteritis nodosa (classic polyarteritis nodosa, allergic angiitis, and granulomatosis [Churg-Strauss syndrome], and systemic necrotizing vasculitis overlap syndrome); hypersensitivity (leukocytoclastic) angiitides (orbital vasculitis, vasculitides with connective tissue disorders, Cogan's syndrome); Wegener's granulomatosis; other respiratory vasculitides; and giant cell arteritis. Early cases mimic nonspecific inflammations. Diagnosis can be difficult; treatment must be specialized.

### Other granulomatous and histiocytic diseases

These include eosinophilic granuloma (histiocytosis-X), juvenile xanthogranuloma, Erdheim-Chester disease, necrobiotic xanthogranuloma, pseudorheumatoid nodules, and fibrous histiocytoma.

### Orbital inflammations secondary to ocular disease

These include endophthalmitis, severe uveitis, and scleritis. The diagnosis is usually clear, but posterior scleritis can mimic other acute and subacute orbital inflammations. Suspect it in older patients, usually those with collagen vascular diseases, presenting with orbital inflammation, severe aching pain, and typical ultrasound and CT findings.

### Viral infections

Acute viral dacryoadenitis produces a fullness or pain in the upper outer orbit with an inflammatory, abscesslike, firm, tender, lateral lid swelling, an S-shaped upper lid margin, a mechanical ptosis, sometimes inferonasal proptosis, and preauricular lymphadenopathy. Lid eversion shows gland swelling with localized chemosis. Resolution takes a week or two. Causes include mumps, infectious mononucleosis, herpes zoster, measles, influenza, and dengue fever.

### Bacterial infections

Acute bacterial dacryoadenitis is very rare and severe; the orbit may suppurate, draining through the conjunctiva (palpebral lobe) or skin (orbital lobe). Causes include staphylococci, streptococci, pneumococci, and gonococci.

Chronic bacterial dacryoadenitis produces a superotemporal orbital mass with diplopia on looking toward it, inferonasal proptosis, and often dry eye. Causes include trachoma, tuberculosis, leprosy, syphilis, and actinomycosis.

Acute orbital cellulitis is usually due to a bacterial sinus infection; it threatens vision and life. Nonsinus sources include the face, teeth, meninges, ear, conjunctiva, eye, lacrimal sac or gland, bacteremia, or a foreign body. Infected abrasions, impetigo, erysipelas, and facial cellulitis may spread to the orbit, as may dental abscesses, especially in infants with rudimentary antra. Maxillary tooth bud infection may give maxillary osteoperiostitis with orbital floor destruction. Abscesses (extradural, cerebral, from otitis media) may infect the orbit. *Haemophilus influenzae* conjunctivitis, sinusitis, and orbital cellulitis occur in children under 3 years, producing upper respiratory tract infection, fever, and malaise. Bacteremia is common and the progression rapid. Obtain local and blood cultures and treat with chloramphenicol eye drops and systemic ampicillin or chloramphenicol. Panophthalmitis, dacryocystitis, and dacryoadenitis can produce orbital cellulitis. Bacteremia may seed the orbit or eye, especially in an immunocompromised patient. Suspect, localize, and remove foreign bodies to avoid persistent cellulitis, fistula formation, and scarring.

Cellulitis may be preseptal or postseptal (orbital), cavitate to form a subperiosteal or orbital abscess, or spread and cause cavernous sinus thrombosis, intracranial abscess or thrombophlebitis, or temporalis fossa abscess. Diagnosis requires clinical suspicion and CT or MRI, serially, if indicated.

Younger children have viral coryza, spread from the ethmoid and maxillary sinuses (the frontal developing after the fifth year), and infection with aerobes *(H. influenzae).* Adults often have a history of sinusitis, polyps, allergy, trauma, or recent dental extraction, spread from the frontoethmoidal sinuses, and multiple microbial infection, often anaerobic. Preseptal cellulitis (usually *Staphylococcus aureus* or *Streptococcus pyogenes*), produces pain, lid swelling, chemosis, and systemic toxicity with fever and leukocytosis. To the preseptal presentation orbital (postseptal) cellulitis adds proptosis, limited eye movement, and decreased vision. Radiologic subclasses include subperiosteal, extraconal, and intraconal. Subperiosteal infections—medial, from the ethmoid sinus, or superior, from the frontal—displace the eye laterally and inferiorly. Spread into the extraconal and intraconal spaces produces increased fat density and obscures normal tissue planes. Abscesses, usually superior or retrobulbar, are poorly defined masses showing homogenous, heterogenous, or ring enhancement on CT with contrast. Subperiosteal abscesses, infrequent in children, when treated, usually resolve without drainage or sequelae. More common in adults, their treatment often requires sinus drainage, and sequelae are more severe. Osteomyelitis may result.

For adult preseptal cellulitis consider an outpatient trial of hot compresses and oral antibiotics. Treat more severe adult cases, all children, and all postseptal cellulitis with careful, in-hospital, systemic, visual and neurologic monitoring, bacterial isolation, high-dosage intravenous antibiotics (infectious diseases consultation), and with progressive deterioration drainage of sinuses or abscesses. Increases in proptosis, chemosis, venous engorgement, cranial nerve palsies, and headache with onset of bilateral signs and varying consciousness suggest progression to cavernous sinus thrombosis, a life-threatening disease.

Orbital tuberculosis presents as periostitis or orbital tuberculoma. Periostitis usually occurs before age 20 years, involves the zygomatic bone, and produces a painless, indolent, red swelling that points and drains. After confirmation with biopsy, treat with drugs and generous debridement. Tuberculoma, most common in women in the fifth and sixth decade who have had tuberculosis elsewhere, produces a painless, slowly enlarging mass. After biopsy, debulk and treat with antituberculosis drugs, expecting steady improvement.

Orbital syphilis, in tertiary disease, presents as a diffuse hyperplastic periostitis involving the margin, walls, or apex. Marginal periostitis most commonly involves the superior rim with an indolent inflammatory swelling, tenderness, intractable headache, and radiating neuralgia most marked at night. Bony thickening may be marked, or the gumma may break down, leaving a persistent fistula with a depressed scar leading down to softened bone. Bony absorption may be marked, especially in congenital cases. Periostitis of the orbital walls is similar, with the addition of proptosis, eye movement restriction, anesthetic cornea, and neuropathy. Gummatous apical periostitis adds the orbital apex syndrome. Treat with antisyphilitic antibiotics and expect rapid improvement.

Orbital glanders, anthrax, and metastatic lesions from typhoid have been reported.

### Mycotic infections

These include phycomycoses (rhinoorbital mucormycosis), aspergillosis, actinomycosis, and much less commonly sporotrichosis, maduromycosis, cryptococcosis, blastomycosis, coccidioidomycosis, rhinosporidiosis, African histoplasmosis, and candidiasis.

Rhinoorbital mucormycosis or phycomycosis occurs almost exclusively in immunocompromised patients with diabetic ketoacidosis or AIDS, or those receiving corticosteroids systemically or as nasal sprays. In such patients who develop sinusitis, pharyngitis, and nasal discharge, it presents with a boring orbital pain, dramatic cellulitis, proptosis, cranial nerve pareses, visual loss, and general deterioration. The mold causes thrombosing arteritis with gangrene of the nasal mucosa, turbinates, and palate, septal perforation, and intraluminal spread into the brain. CT shows the sinus and orbital disease with or without bony destruction. If suspected, treat the predisposing disease, perform a biopsy immediately, ask for rapid histologic processing, and start intravenous amphotericin B. When the large, nonseptate, branching hyphae are demonstrated on hematoxylin-eosin–stained sections, generously debride the involved tissues, ensure postoperative drainage, and consider local irrigation with amphotericin B or hyperbaric oxygen treatment. The prognosis is grave.

Orbital aspergillosis usually occurs in immunocompromised patients living in hot, humid climates and presents as a slowly enlarging mass that spreads to the orbit from a paranasal sinus or the lacrimal sac. It takes two forms: allergic and invasive. If suspected, perform a biopsy, confirm the diagnosis by identifying the long septate filaments with dichotomous branches that stain with hematoxylin-eosin as well as Gomori methenamine silver, excise the lesion, and treat with amphotericin B.

Actinomycosis spreads into the orbit from the mouth, nose, paranasal sinuses, conjunctiva, lids, or canaliculus, produces a slowly growing mass with proptosis, and gradually spreads to involve more orbital structures. Treat with debridement and penicillin.

## BIBLIOGRAPHY

Albert DM, Jakobiec FA, editors: *Principles and practice of ophthalmology,* Philadelphia, 1994, WB Saunders.
Collin JRO: *A manual of systematic eyelid surgery,* Edinburgh, 1983, Churchill-Livingstone.
Duke-Elder S, MacFaul PA: *The ocular adnexa.* In Duke-Elder S, editor: *System of ophthalmology,* London, 1974, Kimpton.
Duke-Elder S, MacFaul PA: *Injuries.* In Duke-Elder S, editor: *System of ophthalmology,* London, 1972, Kimpton.
Hart WM, editor: *Adler's physiology of the eye,* ed 9, St Louis, 1992, Mosby.
McCord CD, editor: *Oculoplastic surgery,* New York, 1981, Raven Press.
Spencer WH, editor: *Ophthalmic pathology: an atlas and textbook,* ed 3, Philadelphia, 1986, WB Saunders.
Stewart WB, editor: *Ophthalmic plastic and reconstructive surgery,* San Francisco, 1984, American Academy of Ophthalmology.
Whitnall SE: *Anatomy of the human orbit and accessory organs of vision,* facsimile of 1921 edition, Huntington, NY, 1979, Robert E Krieger.

CHAPTER

# 108 Cornea

**Thomas J. Byrd**

Although only 12 mm across and less than 1 mm thick, the cornea is full of mysteries that even a lifetime of study cannot solve. The structure is optically transparent and has no blood supply, but it is far more complex than a simple "watch crystal" crowning the globe.

## CORNEAL ANATOMY

The cornea is composed of five layers: epithelium, Bowman's layer, stroma, Descemet's membrane, and endothelium. The epithelium is 5 or 6 cell layers thick and richly supplied with free nerve endings only, as specialized receptors would compromise corneal clarity. Bowman's layer is an 8 to 10 μm thick collagenous layer to which the basal epithelial cells adhere via hemidesmosomes.

The stroma constitutes about 90% of the total corneal thickness. It consists almost entirely of an extracellular matrix of collagen (and other glycoproteins) interspersed with occasional fibroblasts and keratocytes. The regularity and organization of the collagen fibril orientation is responsible for corneal clarity. The cornea becomes cloudy when edema or new collagen synthesis alter the spacing of these fibrils.

The endothelium is a monolayer of hexagonal cells rich in cytoplasmic organelles, especially mitochondria. These cells actively pump fluid across an osmotic gradient from the corneal stroma to the aqueous cavity and are thus primarily responsible for maintenance of corneal clarity. These cells do not replicate and therefore steadily decrease in number with advancing age or disease.

Cellular mediators of infection must migrate in from adjacent limbal vessels unless the cornea has been vascularized by an earlier process. Corneal physiology may be best summarized briefly by quoting the renowned corneal specialist Dr. Herbert E. Kaufman: "The cornea breathes air and eats aqueous."

## DIAGNOSTIC APPROACH

As with all ocular disease, a thorough history and eye examination as outlined in Chapter 105 are the keys to accurate diagnosis. Particular attention should be paid to document the presence of protective eyewear, contact lens type and wearing schedule, photophobia, decreased vision, or type of foreign body. Unilaterality, bilaterality, and time course can be important. Lids matted shut in the morning argues for conjunctivitis. Autoimmune disease can cause lacrimal insufficiency. Severe pain on opening the eyes in the morning is diagnostic of recurrent erosion.

Visual acuity with optical correction must be measured, as well as noting any improvement from looking through a pinhole. A pinhole compensates for uncorrected refractive errors and can limit visual degradation due to diffraction from corneal (or lens) opacities or irregularities. Improved acuity through a pinhole therefore suggests the cornea or lens as the etiology for visual disturbance. Intraocular, inflammatory, hemorrhagic, retinal, optic nerve, or cortical causes of decreased acuity are not correctable with a pinhole.

Conjunctival injection is noted because it helps to define the process as either inflammatory or noninflammatory. The lids should be evaluated for signs of inflammation and the lash bases examined for dried scales that indicate staph infection. Fingertip pressure at the lid margin should elicit clear oily meibomian gland secretions, not white strands that resemble toothpaste.

Although gross corneal foreign bodies or opacities can be visible with a penlight, a slit lamp is essential for any detailed examination of the cornea. The optical cross-section combined with high magnification allows comprehensive assessment of the multiple layers of the cornea. Contour irregularities, stromal thinning, and epithelial hypertrophy are readily detected. Fluorescein dye highlights areas where the epithelium is disrupted or missing. Useful information can be difficult to obtain if one makes the common mistake of applying too much dye. Decreased corneal sensation can be measured using a wisp of cotton if herpes simplex virus is suspected.

For clinical simplicity, the text subdivides corneal disorders based on whether they generally cause a red eye (Fig. 108-1).

## THE RED EYE

### Anterior blepharitis

Bacteria (overwhelmingly *Staphylococcus*) colonize the lash bases, form a crusty scale where lash meets skin, secrete toxins into the tear film, and can cause a red eye and possible corneal infiltrates. It is usually bilateral, with the chief complaint of itching of lid margins that may be injected. Lash whitening (poliosis) or loss (madarosis) can occur. Foam often forms on the lid margins as the toxins saponify the tear lipids, and conjunctival injection is common. When a sebaceous gland at the base of a lash becomes acutely infected and forms a painful localized purulent abscess, it is known as a hordeolum or stye.

Initial treatment is simple hygiene twice daily. A 5-minute hot washcloth soak softens the scales. Next, scrubbing the lash bases with a cotton ball soaked in a 50:50 mixture of baby shampoo and water, followed by a rinse and patting dry, cleanses the area. For initial treatment, local or systemic antibiotics usually are not warranted (although severe styes may require incision and drainage). If significant debris persists for 2 months, erythromycin ointment to the lash bases is added to the end of the regimen. This chronic problem usually requires chronic treatment.

### Allergic blepharitis

The predominant symptom of ocular allergy is itching, often accompanied by lid edema, mucoid discharge, conjunctival hyperemia, burning, lacrimation, and conjunctival edema (chemosis). Eosinophils are seen on Giemsa staining of conjunctival scrapings except in mild cases.

Short-lived episodes of these symptoms accompanied by nasal involvement are often seen in hay fever conjunctivitis after exposure to airborne allergens. Acute treatment consists of cool compresses, topical vasoconstrictor-antihistamine combinations, or topical nonsteroidal antiinflammatory drugs (NSAIDs). Prophylactic treatment may include topical mast-cell stabilizing agents such as cromolyn sodium or lodoxamide tromethamine. Topical steroids may be indicated in severe cases.

Vernal conjunctivitis causes severe itching, photophobia, and a heavy, ropy mucus discharge. Symptoms begin in the first 2 decades of life, are bilateral, and typically recur in the spring months in nontropical climates. About 90% of patients have a history of atopy. Giant cobblestone papillae are characteristically found on the superior tarsal conjunctiva and can cause corneal complications in severe cases. Environmental control of allergens is the best initial treatment, followed by the therapy for hay fever conjunctivitis as discussed above. Treatment seldom eradicates symptoms altogether, and the practitioner must be cautious to avoid steroid-induced ocular complications in this generally self-limited disease.

The incidence of ocular involvement in atopic dermatitis is approximately 25%. Atopic keratoconjunctivitis causes a moist, erythematous skin eruption that becomes vesicular and then crusts. The lid skin ultimately becomes scaly and excessively wrinkled. Although sometimes difficult to differentiate from vernal conjunctivitis, atopic symptoms are perennial, the tarsal conjunctival papillae are smaller, and corneal involvement tends to be more severe. Treatment is similar to that of vernal conjunctivitis, with the same caution to avoid chronic steroid use.

The delicate and distensible lid tissues are particularly susceptible to irritants, including environmental allergens, cosmetics, topical medications, and some chemicals. Eczematoid inflammation of the lids is characteristic of contact dermatitis. Topical steroid ointment is used to treat the acute inflammation, while elimination of the offending agent is the definitive treatment.

### Posterior blepharitis

Meibomian glands are responsible for secreting the oil layer of the tear film. When they become inspissated and plugged, an acute chalazion may develop if the lipid is extruded into the surrounding tissues. In most cases, the secretions are merely thick and of poor quality, causing tear film instability and ocular irritation symptoms.

Initial treatment is simple hygiene twice daily. A 10-minute hot soak is needed to heat the meibomian glands sufficiently to thin the secretions. Vigorous fingertip

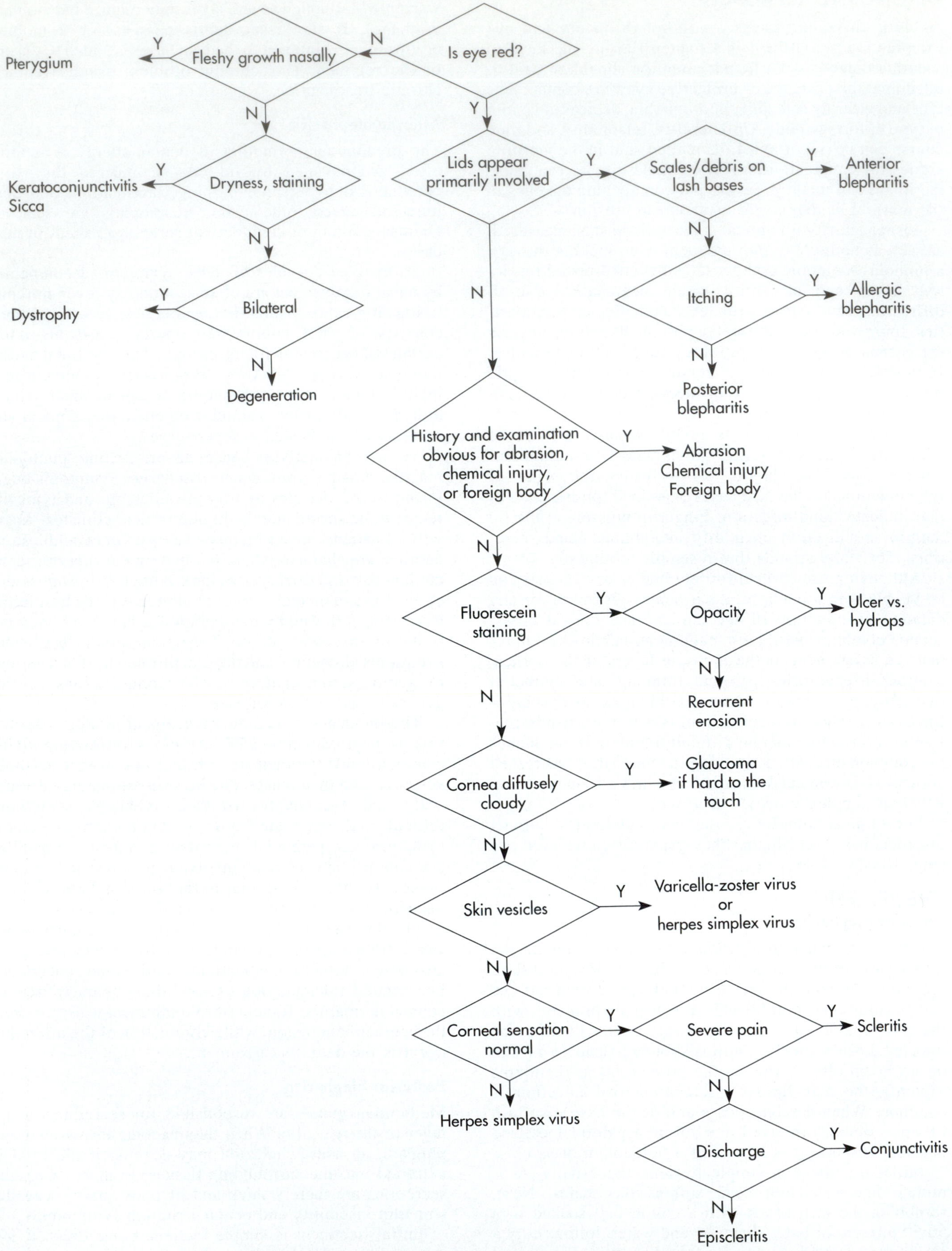


**Fig. 108-1.** Approach to the patient with corneal disorders.

compression of the eyelid against the globe then forces the fluids to flow and avoid stagnation. If symptoms are not relieved after 2 months of this hygiene regimen, oral tetracycline is added to the plan. It is used not for its antibiotic effect, but rather for its poorly understood effect on lipid metabolism; 250 mg are given four times daily for a month, then once daily. The thinner secretions then cause fewer symptoms.

## Conjunctivitis

Conjunctival injection is a nonspecific indicator of inflammation. Follicles are small white bumps in the conjunctiva that represent collections of lymphocytes that have displaced adjacent blood vessels. They suggest a viral or chlamydial cause of conjunctivitis. Papillae are velvety red conjunctival bumps with a central vessel that are nonspecific indicators of conjunctival inflammation. Papillary conjunctivitis is more likely bacterial in origin. Examination also should note the presence of preauricular adenopathy. Because the lower conjunctiva drains there, the presence of tender preauricular nodes suggests adenoviral conjunctivitis.

Conjunctivitis is approximately 50% bacterial and 50% adenoviral in children. The bacterial cases tend to have a more mucopurulent discharge, less adenopathy, and no other viral symptoms. The three most common agents are *Staphylococcus aureus, Streptococcus pneumoniae,* and *Haemophilus influenzae,* with the latter most commonly affecting young children.

Because adenoviral conjunctivitis is self-limiting and topical antibiotics are safe, virtually all cases of pediatric conjunctivitis are treated as bacterial. Either sulfacetamide 10% or trimethoprim sulfate and polymyxin B sulfate (better *H. influenzae* coverage) is given four times a day for a week to 10 days.

Patients should be advised that they may get worse for 1 or 2 days before they get better. The infection may spread to the other eye. Family members should use separate washcloths to avoid transmission, and frequent hand washing is advised. Infected children should not attend school and adults who deal with the public should not attend work. Hot or cool compresses may provide symptomatic relief.

Conjunctivitis in adults is approximately 85% adenoviral and 15% bacterial, so routine antibiotic treatment of all patients is unnecessary. A better approach is to use antibiotics for patients with a more purulent discharge, no nodes, and no follicles, since the presence of the latter two suggests a viral etiology. The prognosis, hygiene, and infection control advice listed earlier applies to these patients as well. Any conjunctivitis that is not improving by 7 to 10 days merits ophthalmologic evaluation.

## Episcleritis

Ocular redness without irritation is characteristic of episcleritis. Transient and self-limited, it is a disease affecting adults and lasting approximately 1 to 3 weeks with spontaneous resolution. It is generally not related to systemic immunologic disease. The redness is often in the interpalpebral zone with inflammation of the straight episcleral vessels that run perpendicular to the limbus. Unlike the vascular injection of scleritis, these vessels are salmon pink in natural sunlight, can be moved over the underlying sclera with a cotton tip applicator, and blanch with topical phenylephrine 10% solution.

Simple episcleritis usually requires no treatment, although the nodular form is more severe, lasts longer, and requires topical steroids. The redness of simple episcleritis may be treated with topical vasoconstrictors. When present, pain may be relieved with topical NSAIDs or mild topical steroids.

## Scleritis

Scleritis is a far more serious disease than episcleritis and is usually associated with a systemic immunologic disease (see Chapter 105). Affected patients complain of a severe, deep pain, and the eye is often tender to palpation. Examination in natural sunlight reveals a blue or violet hue to the affected sclera. The vessels are not straight and radial, cannot be moved with a cotton tip applicator, and do not blanch with topical phenylephrine 10% solution. There can be significant visual morbidity.

Scleritis is divided anatomically into anterior and posterior forms. Anterior scleritis is further divided into three clinical subtypes that carry prognostic and therapeutic significance: diffuse, nodular, and necrotizing.

Diffuse anterior scleritis is the most benign form of the disease. The vascular injection is nonfocal without nodularity or avascularity. It is associated with connective tissue disease in approximately 30% of cases. Heavy topical steroids are often enough to control the inflammation. As in all scleritis, subconjunctival steroid injunction is contraindicated because of the propensity for the sclera to melt at the injection site.

Nodular anterior scleritis consists of single or multiple deep red or purple nodules of immobile scleral tissue with overlaying edematous episclera. One half of patients have an autoimmune disorder.

Vision and life-threatening complications can occur in the setting of necrotizing anterior scleritis. The lesion is usually inflammatory with a rather pale center, but scleral necrosis without inflammation (scleromalacia perforans) can also occur, usually in patients with longstanding rheumatoid arthritis. In most cases, symptoms of severe, boring pain are out of proportion to inflammatory signs. The sclera thins and the dark underlying uveal tissue becomes visible as the disease progresses. About 60% of necrotizing scleritis patients develop bilateral disease, and approximately 30% die within 5 years of diagnosis, usually from complications of vasculitis.

Only 10% of patients with posterior scleritis have had an associated systemic disease. The diagnosis can be easily missed in the absence of anterior inflammation, especially if the pain is referred elsewhere in the head. Pain, proptosis, and visual loss are common complaints. Visual consequences may ensue from exudative retinal detachment and optic disc edema.

Topical steroids are seldom sufficient to control more severe scleritis. Systemic NSAIDs are often enough to control the inflammation in diffuse or nodular scleritis. Control of the pain is a useful guide to therapy. Oral corticosteroids should be employed in severe or necrotizing cases with the addition of systemic cytotoxic immunosuppressive therapy (often cyclophosphamide, azathioprine, or methotrexate) as needed. In patients with systemic autoimmune disease, prednisone is often used for quick effect when waiting a week or more for an immunosuppressive to work.

## Chemical injury

Chemical injury is one of only two true ophthalmic emergencies, the other being central retinal artery occlusion. Minutes or even seconds delay in treatment can result in irreparable tissue damage and loss of vision. Chemical injury is the *only* condition when treatment may be initiated before obtaining a visual acuity.

The first priority is immediate and copious irrigation with any noncaustic liquid. Although sterile irrigating solution or saline is preferable once the patient arrives at the office, tap water is usually most practical at the time of injury. Fifteen minutes of continuous irrigation at home or 1 liter of fluid irrigation in a medical setting is recommended, with the emphasis on rapid dilution of the offending agent. Topical anesthetic drops and a lid speculum make irrigation far more comfortable and effective. Tears should be tested with pH paper a few minutes later. If not within the 7.2 to 7.8 range, another liter of irrigation should be administered after inspection of the everted lids to detect retained particulate matter.

A good history with an exact description of the agent should be obtained after irrigation. The container that identifies the chemical is helpful. Documentation of protective eyewear is important, particularly for work-related accidents.

Alkali burns are generally worse than acid, although either can be blinding. Acid is precipitated and inactivated by the tissue proteins it destroys, whereas alkali saponifies collagen and damages underlying tissue. Hydrocarbons can be quite irritating but usually cause far less tissue damage.

The epithelium should be assessed with fluorescein stain, but it is important to realize that "all off" is easily confused with "all on" when no clear demarcation line is present. Prophylactic topical antibiotics are used three or four times a day, and some practitioners omit a patch for the first 24 hours to permit additional clearing of any retained chemical.

Steroid-antibiotic combinations are often used to help decrease inflammation. "Clean" chemical injuries and bilateral ocular allergies are two of very few indications for topical ocular steroid use by the nonophthalmologist. Note that aminoglycoside antibiotics retard epithelial healing and should be avoided. Oral analgesia and sedatives enhance patient comfort, whereas topical nonsteroidals such as ketorolac provide effective pain control in an unpatched eye when used four times a day for up to 4 days.

Healing of epithelial defects (when present) is of paramount importance, and daily examinations to rule out infection and monitor progress are mandatory. Healing will be slower than a comparable abrasion for the first day or two because the remaining epithelium also has been chemically damaged. The practitioner should apply ointment and patch an epithelial defect daily. Having the patient remove and reapply the patch at home is not effective, so patients should not apply topical medications when patching. Steroid-antibiotic drops to reduce inflammation are continued for approximately a week after epithelialization is complete.

Severe chemical burns, large epithelial defects, any suspicion of infection or tissue thinning, slow healing, and the development of conjunctival adhesions are all indications for immediate referral to an ophthalmologist. Ultimate prognosis is related to the degree of limbal ischemia as well as symblepharon (conjunctival adhesion) formation.

## Foreign body

A thorough history, including the wearing of protective eyewear, should be obtained. As always, visual acuity is then obtained before other examination or placement of any eyedrops. Proparacaine drops will then be used to facilitate further examination.

Both upper lids should always be everted to look for additional foreign bodies, and their absence should be documented, as patching over a retained foreign body is inexcusable. Multiple vertical, linear, superficial abrasions are a clue to a foreign body trapped under the upper lid. Eversion is quite simple and painless when performed properly and with consideration of the tarsal plate. This structure makes the inferior 10 mm of the upper lid quite rigid, so it is fruitless to attempt to fold this region. The patient is asked to look down and the upper lashes are grasped with your fingers. A cotton-tipped applicator (or any small blunt instrument) is then placed 10 to 12 mm superior to the lash margin, and the lid is everted using the applicator as a fulcrum. When the examination is completed, the lid will right itself if the patient is asked to look up and blink.

Although using a slit lamp is preferable, a hand light may be used to look for a corneal foreign body. If not readily visible, a small particle can sometimes be detected by observing its shadow cast on the iris. Vigorous irrigation or a moistened cotton-tipped applicator are the only methods that should be used to remove a superficial foreign body without the assistance of a slit lamp.

Many ophthalmologists routinely dilate such patients with a mid-acting mydriatic such as homatropine 5% or scopolamine ¼% to prevent pain from iritis. The presence of "consensual photophobia" (pain in the injured eye when a light is shone only in the opposite eye) is a good indication for dilation.

Daily follow-up and patching are the norm, and healing should be steady and rapid over 1 or 2 days. No steroids are used. Inability to remove the particle, the presence of a rust ring or infiltrate, worsening vision, or failure to heal are all indications for immediate ophthalmologic evaluation.

## Corneal abrasion

The examination begins with a thorough history, including the presence of protective eyewear. Visual acuity measurement is followed by proparacaine drops to ease the examination. The lid is everted to detect a foreign body. A small quantity of fluorescein outlines the defect, and charting a diagram with a size estimate simplifies follow-up.

The general principles of monitoring and facilitating epithelial healing are identical to those used in treating chemical injuries as outlined earlier. Daily patching and follow-up with or without cycloplegia are routine. Antibiotic ointment without steroid use is appropriate for these presumably contaminated wounds. The presence of an infiltrate, worsening vision, or failure to heal are all indications for immediate ophthalmologic referral.

Nonhealing epithelial defects are one of the most frustrating ophthalmologic maladies. Treatment options restricted to ophthalmologists and corneal subspecialists include bandage soft contact lenses, placement of collagen shields, mechanical or excimer laser debridement, anterior stromal micropuncture, tarsorrhaphy, and placement of a conjunctival flap.

### Recurrent corneal erosion

A good history is the key to diagnosis and treatment of recurrent corneal erosions. Patients present with symptoms (and often signs) of a corneal abrasion but without acute trauma. Patients almost always report being asymptomatic when going to bed and awakening with severe pain as the eye is first opened. Symptoms subside gradually over several hours, but recur another morning several days or weeks later.

The pathophysiology is based on a defect of epithelial adhesion. Patients often have a history of prior traumatic abrasion, classically a paper cut or fingernail injury. The injury causes defects in Bowman's layer. During the 6 to 8 weeks required for reformation of hemidesmosomal complexes, the epithelium is often separated from the underlying Bowman's layer by a thin fluid layer. This separation happens at night when evaporative loss is diminished by closed lids. The epithelium then sticks to the inside of the upper lid and is torn off when the eyes open in the morning. Treatment therefore must focus on eliminating the fluid layer, so that hemidesmosomes may form, and preventing adhesion between the epithelium and lid.

Clinically, this corneal erosion often appears identical to a corneal abrasion on hand light examination. The edges often are more loose and ratty. Initial treatment is that of an abrasion with patching, pain control, and optional cycloplegia. Once epithelialized, hyperosmotics become the mainstay of treatment. Five percent sodium chloride ointment is used at bedtime for a full 8 weeks after the most recent erosive episode. This agent both dehydrates the subepithelial space and lubricates the epithelial surface. Simple lubricating ointment often works but is less effective because it does not have a dehydrating effect. Concomitant use of 5% NaCl drops four times a day for 2 weeks after an acute episode is also helpful. Patients must know why they must use ointment for 8 weeks so they will not stop treatment and precipitate another erosion.

Recurrent erosion sufferers without a prior history of trauma usually have map-dot-fingerprint corneal dystrophy, an abnormality of Bowman's layer that includes reduplication of the layer and the presence of epithelial inclusion cysts. Fortunately, their initial treatment is identical to that of traumatic erosion sufferers because the dystrophy cannot be detected without a slit lamp.

Referral indications are recurrence during hyperosmotic treatment or any of those listed under corneal abrasion. Ophthalmologic treatment options include all those used for corneal abrasions.

### Corneal ulcer

Corneal ulcer is a keratitis accompanied by an overlying epithelial defect. Most are bacterial with *Staphylococcus, Streptococcus,* and *Pseudomonas* the most common agents. This medical urgency requires ophthalmologic evaluation and initiation of treatment within hours of diagnosis, as permanent visual loss may easily ensue. Because the cornea has no blood supply and is less than 1 mm thick, certain virulent collagenolytic organisms can penetrate the full thickness and perforate in less than 24 hours. The nonophthalmologist's role is early diagnosis, differentiation from nonurgencies, and immediate referral once the diagnosis is suspected.

A good history includes questions about trauma and contact lens wear. Patients who sleep in lenses have approximately an eightfold increased risk of ulceration compared to those who do not sleep with them; the latter are at increased risk over nonlens wearers. They complain of pain, tearing, and photophobia similar to abrasion patients.

A bacterial ulcer causes a red eye and a localized corneal opacity containing bacteria, inflammatory cells, and edema. Although there are other noninfectious causes of a corneal opacity in a red eye, they cannot be differentiated without a slit lamp, considerable experience, and often diagnostic testing. Any such lesion is a bacterial ulcer until proven otherwise.

Patients should be instructed to bring their contact lenses and the case (for culture) on referral. Antibiotic treatment *should not* be started without prior approval of the consultant. The antibiotics commonly used by nonophthalmologists are seldom adequate for treatment and usually only prevent obtaining good cultures. If consultation must be delayed, treatment should consist of ciprofloxacin 0.3% every half hour around the clock until the patient can be evaluated.

Ophthalmologic treatment of corneal ulceration consists of thorough culturing (directly onto culture plates) followed classically by frequent doses of specially formulated topical cephalosporin and aminoglycoside antibiotics. Recent reports of effective monotherapy with commercially available fluoroquinolones are the rationale for the ciprofloxacin recommendation, and many ophthalmologists still treat small ulcers with such monotherapy. Emerging concern about the effectiveness of these agents against *Streptococcus* species (common causes of ulceration) have prompted most ophthalmologists to stay with the cephalosporin/aminoglycoside combination in severe cases.

### Herpes simplex virus

The possibility of herpetic keratitis is the reason why no practitioner should ever treat a red eye with steroids without first performing a slit lamp examination. Such unwitting treatment can hasten the demise of an eye with an already severe and recurrent problem. The medicolegal consequences can be severe as well.

More than 95% of cases of clinical herpetic disease are recurrences that develop long after the primary infection. Although primary infection usually occurs by 5 years of age, most adults do not have a history of clinical herpetic disease. The cervical and trigeminal ganglia become host to the latent virus, which is reactivated intermittently and travels via the neuronal network to the end organ. Corneal nerves are thought to shed reactivated virus into the tears, which may cause corneal disease.

Herpetic blepharitis is most likely to occur with a primary infection, exhibiting classic vesicles on the eyelids and surrounding skin. Although most patients will not develop ocular disease, many ophthalmologists recommend prophylactic treatment with an ocular antiviral agent.

Recurrent follicular conjunctivitis can be caused by herpes simplex virus, even in the absence of corneal disease. One should consider this possibility before initiating steroid treatment of a chronic conjunctivitis of undetermined etiology.

Herpetic epithelial and stromal keratitis (HSV) are potentially blinding disorders that require care by an ophthalmologist. Dendritic staining patterns with fluorescein or rose bengal as well as decreased corneal sensation are classic signs of HSV keratitis, but they are not always present. Like syphilis, HSV is "the great mimic" in the eye and must be included in a great many differential diagnoses. Epithelial, endothelial, and various stromal forms of herpetic keratitis all have been described. Treatment with assorted combinations of topical and systemic antivirals and corticosteroids is complicated and often chronic.

### Varicella-zoster virus

Ocular involvement during primary varicella infection is uncommon but may occur. Lid lesions begin as papules, become vesicular and pustular, and then crust. Conjunctivitis is the most common ocular involvement.

Recurrent varicella-zoster infection in the trigeminal distribution is more likely to cause corneal disease. The ophthalmic division is most commonly involved (herpes zoster ophthalmicus). Because the nasociliary branch of the trigeminal nerve innervates both the tip of the nose and the cornea, the presence of herpetic vesicles on the tip of the nose (Hutchinson's sign) often suggests corneal disease.

Lid edema that impairs proper closure (lagophthalmos) leads to the most common cause of permanent ocular damage from zoster. Liberal use of lubricating ointments can prevent this unfortunate complication.

Epithelial dendrites are the next most common type of ocular involvement. These eyes lose sensation far more often than those with herpes simplex, and they frequently have chronic surface problems that are challenging to manage. Antivirals are of little use in treating active varicella-zoster corneal infections, although oral acyclovir decreases the incidence and severity of dendritiform keratopathy, stromal keratitis, and uveitis when taken within 72 hours of onset of the skin lesions. Acyclovir therefore should be given to any patient with herpes zoster ophthalmicus as early as possible.

### Acute glaucoma

Acute glaucoma can overwhelm the endothelial ability to maintain corneal stromal deturgescence in the presence of an elevated intraocular pressure. A hot red eye and cloudy cornea (with or without epithelial defects) may ensue. In these cases, palpation of the globe through the closed lid will reveal a unilateral increase in intraocular pressure, which establishes the underlying diagnosis of acute glaucoma.

Treatment is focused on the glaucoma, as discussed in Chapter 106. The corneal problems usually resolve spontaneously, with restoration of normal intraocular pressure.

### Acute hydrops

Keratoconus is a degenerative corneal ectasia characterized by noninflammatory corneal stromal thinning that is most pronounced at the apex of the cone. Patients suffer from progressive myopia and increasing astigmatism that becomes irregular and uncorrectable with glasses. Hard or gas permeable lenses are required to correct vision adequately, and corneal transplantation is required when lenses can no longer be worn or when central scarring prevents useful vision.

Acute corneal hydrops can cause a red painful eye, with corneal clouding in a patient with keratoconus. Tears in Descemet's membrane can violate the endothelial barrier and lead to acute stromal edema (hydrops) in the region of the cone. The clinical scenario is that of a contact-lens-wearing patient who presents with a unilateral red, painful, photophobic eye with decreased acuity and a corneal opacity.

This presentation is similar to that of an infectious corneal ulcer. Because keratoconus patients are at increased risk of ulceration from epithelial instability at the cone apex, such patients must be assumed to have an infectious ulcer and should be referred immediately to an ophthalmologist. Once ulceration has been ruled out, watchful waiting will allow the edema to clear in about 4 months.

## THE WHITE EYE

### Keratitis sicca

Keratoconjunctivitis sicca (dry eye) is seen frequently in the setting of connective tissue disease. Keratoconjunctivitis sicca plus xerostomia has been classified as a primary Sjögren's syndrome; the addition of a connective tissue disease is secondary Sjögren's syndrome. A wide variety of drugs (including antihistamines, nasal decongestants, analgesics, sedatives, and tricyclic antidepressants) decrease lacrimation. Patients complain mainly of chronic "dryness" and foreign body sensation. A dry cornea can cause blurring of vision. Many patients report increased mucus in the cul-de-sacs.

Examination reveals decreased tear strips along the lower lid margins, as well as punctate staining of the ocular surface with fluorescein. Tear film deficiency can cause severe problems (including ulceration and perforation) for an ocular surface designed to function as a wet system.

Artificial tear substitutes (drops by day and ointments at night) are the mainstay of treatment for these patients. Referral to an ophthalmologist is indicated if symptoms persist with artificial tears used four times daily. Plugging of the lower lacrimal punctae (tear drains) with silicone plugs or hot cautery can provide dramatic relief. Heavier ointments or partial lid closure (tarsorrhaphy) can be used in severe cases.

### Corneal dystrophies

As the anatomy suggests, there are a variety of dystrophies of the corneal epithelium, basement membrane, Bowman's layer, stroma, Descemet's membrane, and endothelium. They are inherited, bilateral abnormalities of the cornea unassociated with systemic disease or prior inflammation. Most dystrophies present in the first few decades of life and demonstrate autosomal dominant inheritance.

Basement membrane and Bowman's layer dystrophies manifest themselves clinically via the faulty epithelial adhesion of recurrent erosion. Stromal dystrophies generally cause blurriness and glare trouble, although some anterior stromal dystrophies cause epithelial adhesion problems. Endothelial dystrophies lead to corneal decompensation via failure of the pump function.

The history may reveal a family member with similar complaints. Penlight examination may reveal (at most) a vague loss of corneal luster or clarity. An experienced observer using a slit lamp is necessary to make the diagnosis, so any patient suspected of having a dystrophy should be referred for complete ophthalmologic evaluation.

### Corneal degenerations

Several corneal stromal degenerations lead to corneal thinning (e.g., keratoconus, keratoglobus, and pellucid marginal degeneration). The resulting ectasia causes visual disturbance due to irregular astigmatism. They tend to have a later onset, more rapid progression, and unilateral occurrence to distinguish them from the dystrophies.

Because physical findings are unremarkable on penlight examination, all patients must be referred to an ophthalmologist for slit lamp evaluation. In some early cases, changes are not visible on slit lamp examination. New computerized topographic mapping systems can diagnose many more subtle disorders of corneal contour in these patients.

### Pterygium

Pterygium is a triangular wedge of fibrovascular tissue that begins on the epibulbar conjunctiva and grows slowly onto the cornea. Its unsightly appearance and propensity to become inflamed on occasion often bring it to a physician's attention.

The incidence of pterygium is directly related to the proximity to the equator; the incidence is negligible beyond the 40th parallel. Ultraviolet exposure seems to be the primary factor; with such exposure only surgery can arrest growth. The variety of available surgical techniques and reported recurrence rates, ranging from 3% to 40% is testament to the stubborn propensity for pterygium to recur. Because growth often stops spontaneously and surgery may stimulate a fast-paced regrowth, surgeons are wise to delay excision until necessary.

Clear indications for excision are a lesion that is encroaching upon the visual axis, one that is inducing significant irregular astigmatism causing loss of acuity, and a lesion that tethers eye movement enough to cause double vision. A "soft" but valid indication is cosmesis. Any lesion causing concern to the patient should be referred to an ophthalmologist for a detailed discussion of prognosis and treatment options.

## BIBLIOGRAPHY


Brightbill FS: *Corneal surgery: theory, technique and tissue*, ed 2, St. Louis, 1993, Mosby.

Casey TA, Sharif KW: *A colour atlas of corneal dystrophies & degenerations*, Aylesbury, England, 1991, Wolfe Publishing.

Grayson M: *Diseases of the cornea*, St. Louis, 1979, Mosby.

Kaufman HE, Barron BA, McDonald MB, Waltman SR: *The cornea*, New York, 1988, Churchill Livingstone.

Roy FH: *Ocular differential diagnosis*, ed 5, Philadelphia, 1993, Lea & Febiger.

Tasman W, Jaeger EA: *Clinical ophthalmology*, vol 4, rev ed, Philadelphia, 1993, JB Lippincott.

CHAPTER

# 109 Retinal and Choroidal Diseases

Uday R. Desai
Julian J. Nussbaum

Because this book is geared toward primary care specialists, this chapter must meet their demands. These physicians see problems from all organ systems. They must be able to diagnose conditions and refer certain patients to the appropriate specialty clinics. Frequency of referrals to the ophthalmologist is relatively high because of the need for specialized examination modalities including slit lamp biomicroscopy, tonometry, and ophthalmoscopic examinations. In patients with vitreoretinal or choroidal disease, adequate examination requires the indirect ophthalmoscope and may also include ophthalmic ultrasonography; therefore suspected vitreoretinal or choroidal disease always mandates a referral to a vitreoretinal specialist. Awareness of the more common vitreoretinal abnormalities allows the primary care physician to better understand diagnoses and prognoses and thus be better equipped to judge the urgency of different referrals. Moreover, by identifying the patient's condition as vitreoretinal in nature, the physician may be able to refer the patient directly to the retinal specialist.

This chapter is organized into two sections: general topics such as anatomy, physiology, and signs and symptoms and specific entities that occur in the vitreous, retina, and choroid.

## ANATOMY

The adult human eye averages 24 mm in diameter and consists of the anterior segment and posterior segment (Fig. 109-1). The posterior segment contains the retina, choroid, sclera and vitreous. The three layers of the posterior segment are the retina, choroid, and sclera (Fig. 109-2). The retina consists of the neurosensory retina, which is the sensory component of the ocular system, and the retinal pigment epithelium, which provides metabolic support. The retina has a vascular supply that provides for the inner three fourths of the neurosensory retina. The choroid is composed of Bruch's membrane, choriocapillaris, middle and outer choroidal vascular layers, and the suprachoroidal space. Bruch's membrane is located adjacent to the retinal pigment epithelium and is composed of basement membrane, collagen, and elastic layers. The vascular layers proceed outward from the choriocapillaris to the outer choroidal layer. This vascular supply is responsible for the outer one fourth of the neurosensory retina and the retinal pigment epithelium. The choroid contains connective tissue and melanocytes. It also contains the short posterior ciliary nerves, which are responsible for pain sensation in this portion of the globe. Outside the choroid lies the sclera.

These three layers encompass the vitreous body, which averages a volume of 4 ml. The vitreous is a gel-like substance, the composition of which is 99% water. Its other components include hyaluronic acid, which provides for the vitreous' elasticity, and collagen, which provides for its strength. The vitreous is attached to the overlying retina early in life. The strongest attachments are at the vitreous base, which attaches to the peripheral retina, optic nerve, macula, and retinal vessels.

The vitreous can be visualized with slit lamp biomicroscopy. The retina and choroid are seen with direct and indirect ophthalmoscopy (Fig. 109-3). The most prominent structure is the optic nerve, which is 1.5 mm wide and 1.75 mm high. It is seen as the yellow-red oval structure located nasal to the visual axis. From this nerve emerge the retinal arterioles and venules. Four pairs of vessels extend to each one of the following quadrants: superonasal, inferonasal, inferotemporal, and superotemporal. The superotemporal and inferotemporal arcades outline the retinal structure known as the macula. Within the macula is a 1500 μm wide depression called the fovea centralis. Within the fovea is a 350 μm wide area called the foveola, which contains only cone photoreceptors. Because cone photoreceptors have potential for good vision, the foveola is the only area of the retina with 20/20 visual potential.

The choroid lies deep to the retinal structures. The most visible of the choroidal structures are the four to seven vortex veins, which are the efferent arm of the choroidal circulation (Fig. 109-4). These orange-colored vessels are located 2 to 3 disc diameters (1 disc diameter = approximately 1.5 mm) posterior to the equator of the eye. The other vascular structures of the choroid can be seen in patients who are lightly pigmented or in patients who have atrophy of the retinal pigment epithelium.

## PHYSIOLOGY

The sensory function of the eye is performed by the neurosensory retina. The eye is capable of photopic and scotopic vision. Photopic vision is used in bright illumination and includes the recognition of colors. This vision is a function of the cone photoreceptors. Scotopic vision

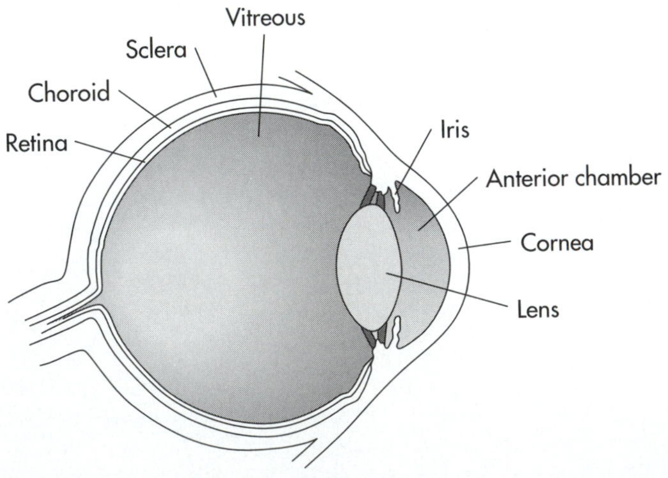


**Fig. 109-1.** Sagittal section showing the major structures of the eye.

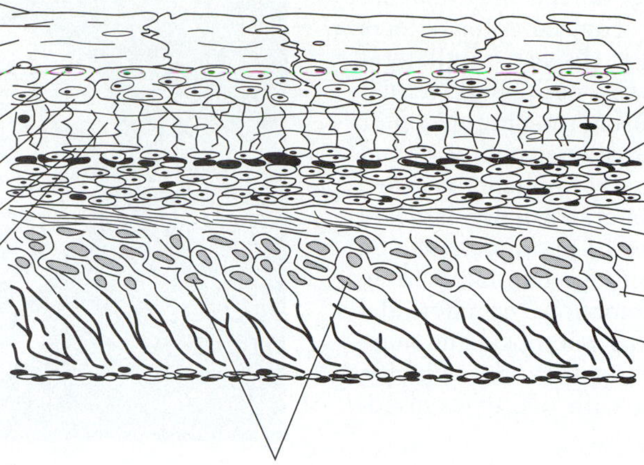

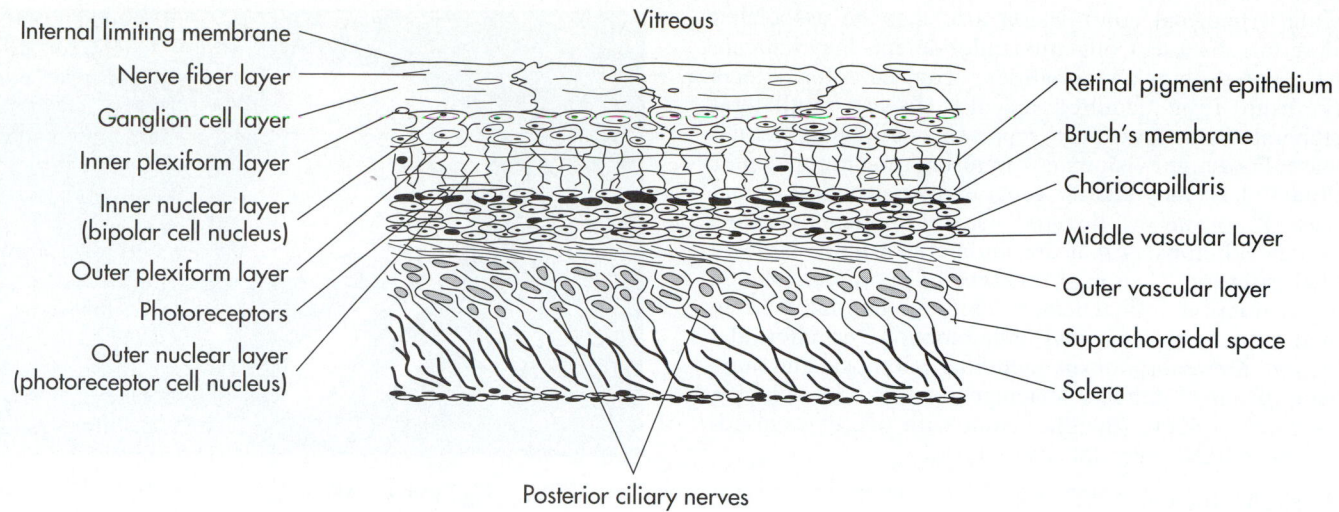

**Fig. 109-2.** High magnification view of posterior segment layers.

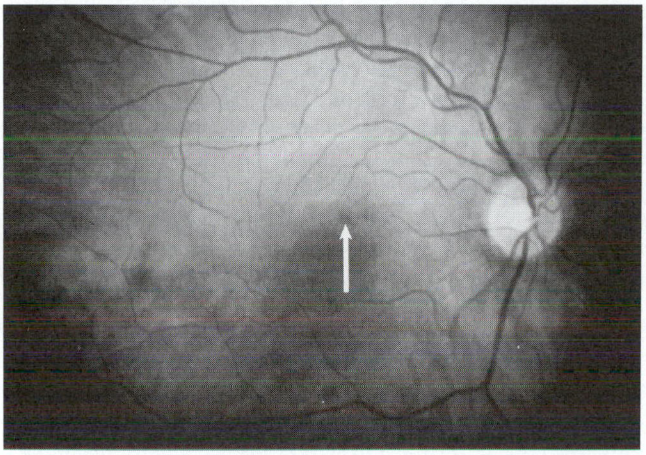

**Fig. 109-3.** Macular region of retina. The arrow identifies the area of the fovea and the foveola.

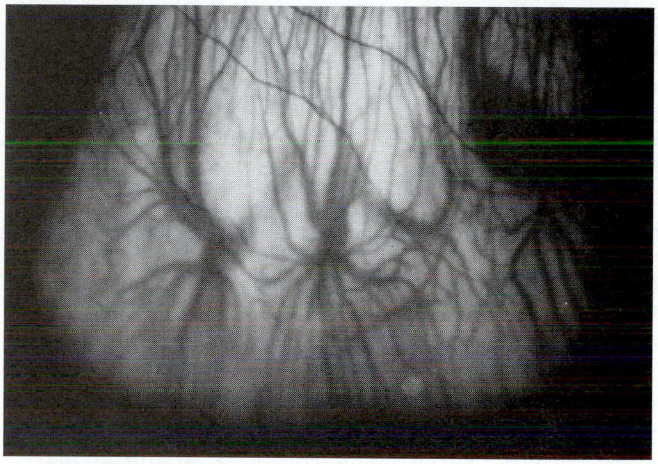

**Fig. 109-4.** Vortex veins.

is used in dim illumination and does not include color recognition. This vision is a function of the rod photoreceptors.

Cone photoreceptors are located primarily within the macula; rod photoreceptors are located in the peripheral retina. The macula therefore provides color vision as well as central visual acuity; the peripheral retina is responsible for peripheral vision and night vision.

The photoreceptors are located in the deepest portion of the retina. They contain light-sensitive pigment molecules in the 11-*cis*-retinal configuration. Once stimulated, they convert to the *trans* configuration, which initiates an electrical potential that spreads from the photoreceptor cell to the bipolar cell. The bipolar cells stimulate the ganglion cells, the axons of which form the nerve fiber layer. This nerve fiber layer exits the eye as the optic nerve. The optic nerve transmits the visual information back to the brain. The information that began at the photoreceptors ultimately ends in the visual cortex of the occipital lobe (Fig. 109-2).

## HISTORY

Symptoms that include painless visual disturbance point to retinal pathology. Disorders of the peripheral retina would impair peripheral vision and night vision. Disorders of the central retina would affect central visual acuity and color vision.

Decreased visual acuity may represent an abnormality within the macula. It also may represent a media opacity (e.g., hemorrhage, inflammation) that is obscuring the macula. Abnormal color vision also may be associated with retinal disease. Congenital color defects may indicate cone photoreceptor abnormalities; acquired color defects may result from acquired macular disease. Unilateral peripheral field loss may represent peripheral retinal disease. Poor night vision may represent rod photoreceptor dysfunction or may signify generalized peripheral retinal disease. Entopsias or "floaters" usually implicate vitreous opacities. Photopsias that are unilateral usually indicate retinal irritation. Causes of this type of photopsia include vitreous traction, retinal detachment, retinal inflammation, retinal infection, choroidal inflammation, or choroidal infection. Metamorphopsia, including micropsia and macropsia, usually indicate macular dysfunction. Finally, monocular diplopia (double vision with one eye closed) also can indicate macular dysfunction.

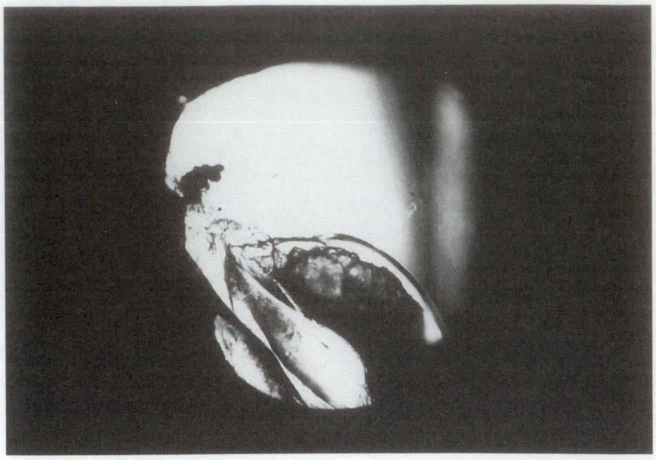

**Fig. 109-5.** Abnormal red reflex.

## PHYSICAL EXAMINATION

Media opacities in the vitreous cavity can be visualized by the direct ophthalmoscope. Retroillumination of the fundus will disclose dark opacities within the red reflex. A partially absent or completely absent red reflex may indicate a retinal detachment, vitreous opacity, or intraocular tumor (Fig. 109-5).

Abnormalities in the retina or choroid may be differentiated by the color of the lesions. Most abnormalities are red, yellow, white, gray-white, brown, or black.

Red lesions in the retina typically represent hemorrhage. The location of the hemorrhage, both topographically on the retina and depth within the retina, helps narrow the differential diagnosis. For example a sector of retina that exhibits hemorrhages may contain a branch vein occlusion, whereas mid peripheral and macular hemorrhages point more to a systemic vasculopathy such as hypertensive retinopathy or diabetic retinopathy. In addition, the depth of the hemorrhages suggests different entities. An intraretinal hemorrhage would be characteristic of diabetic retinopathy, whereas a subretinal hemorrhage is classic for a choroidal neovascular membrane. Vascular tumors such as hemangiomas and vascular abnormalities such as telangiectasias also appear red.

Yellow-colored lesions also may be seen in the retinal examination. The most common lesions are probably the deep subretinal lesions known as drusen. Seen in elderly patients, drusen are a risk factor in the development of age-related macular degeneration. Hard exudates also are a common yellow lesion seen in the retina. They have numerous causes, but the common pathophysiology is the presence of incompetent vasculature, which allows the exudation of extracellular material into the outer plexiform layer of the retina. Because the outer plexiform layer forms a radiating pattern from the central foveola, lipid exudates may form a so-called "macular star" if the incompetent vessels are located close to the macula. Atrophic chorioretinal scars also may appear yellow. Finally, heredo-degenerative conditions may present with retinal or subretinal yellow lesions within either the macula, periphery, or both.

White lesions include "soft" exudates or cotton-wool spots. These areas represent focal areas of retinal ischemia, which block the retrograde axoplasmic flow resulting in the accumulation of axoplasmic material. Cotton-wool spots suggest different diagnoses but are not a diagnosis themselves. They usually occur in retinal diseases characterized by retinal ischemia. Another white lesion consists of myelinated nerve fibers, myelin sheathing of the nerves in the nerve fiber layer. They are usually adjacent to the optic nerve and have feathering borders. Although they may be confused with cotton-wool spots, they are whiter than cotton-wool spots and the lesions are persistent, whereas cotton-wool spots are transitory. Colobomas, which are a congenital absence of retinal and choroidal structures, also appear as white lesions. Fibrosis, which occurs with disciform scars, causes a white-appearing retinal lesion. Gliosis also can appear white and is impossible to differentiate from fibrosis without histology. Tumors such as astrocytic hamartomas and retinoblastomas can appear white. Finally, infectious retinitis or chorioretinitis can lead to the accumulation of inflammatory cells, which can give the retina a whitish appearance.

Gray-white lesions of the retina occur with edema or elevation of the retina. These lesions are usually associated with loss of the choroidal details. A retinal arterial occlusion can cause edema of the retina with a resultant gray-white discoloration. In addition, vascular leakage (e.g., diabetic maculopathy, retinal telangiectasia) can cause edema of the retina before the development of lipid exudation. Elevation of the retina can occur with retinal detachment from a tractional, rhegmatogenous, or exudative cause. Any of these etiologies of retinal detachment can cause the retina to appear gray-white in color.

Brown and black lesions indicate alterations in the pigment of the retina and choroid. Normally, pigment is seen only in the retinal pigment epithelium and the choroidal stroma. Migration of pigment into the retina can occur with hereditary conditions such as retinitis pigmentosa. Migration also can be caused by retinal trauma or intraocular inflammation. Chorioretinal scarring can result in retinal pigment epithelial hyperplasia, which appears as irregular brown-black lesions in areas that usually have adjacent pigment epithelial atrophy. Well-demarcated areas of dark black pigmentation usually signify congenital pigment epithelial hypertrophy. When pigmented lesions occur within the choroid, the lesions may have a

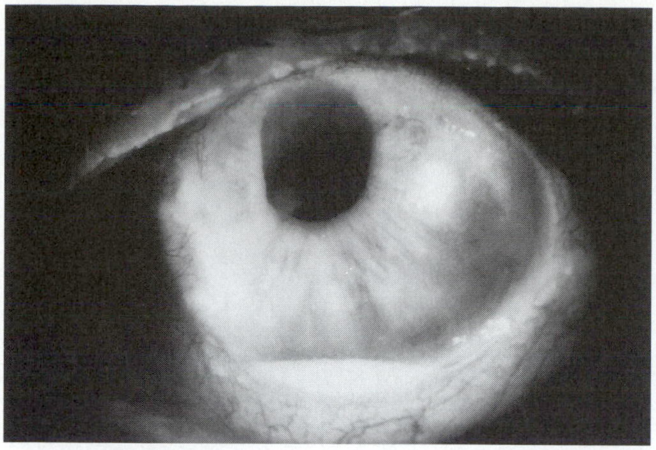

**Fig. 109-6.** Bacterial endophthalmitis.

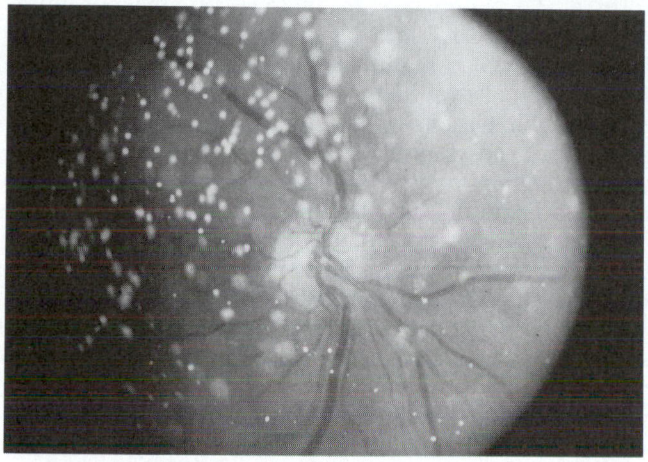

**Fig. 109-7.** Asteroid hyalosis.

subtle greenish hue. The most common lesion is a choroidal nevus. Another serious lesion is a choroidal melanoma, which is also quite elevated.

The retina and choroid respond in only a few ways to different pathologic insults. These signs, however, may vary considerably in their location, duration, fluctuation, and associated history.

## VITREOUS ABNORMALITIES

The vitreous body is normally attached to the retinal surface early in life. The consistency of the vitreous changes from gel-like to liquid with age. As this change occurs, condensations of collagen can present to the patient as floaters. These structures may be described as hairlike or cobweb shaped. They also may appear to the patient as insectlike. Floaters, although annoying, are not a threat to vision.

With increasing liquefaction, liquid vitreous may work its way between the posterior vitreous surface and the inner retinal surface, a condition known as a posterior vitreous detachment. An acute presentation would be associated with photopsias. As the vitreous surface separates from the retina, the stimulated retinal surface produces the sensation of flashing lights. As the separating vitreous moves anteriorly, the collagen fibers condense even further, producing a more noticeable vitreous floater. A vitreous detachment by itself is not a visual risk, but because vitreous detachments can be associated with retinal tears and vitreous hemorrhage, a referral within the week is warranted.

Vitreous detachments can be associated with vitreous hemorrhage when the retina or superficial retinal vessel is torn. More common causes of vitreous hemorrhage include diabetic proliferative disease and sickle cell disease. The bleeding comes from active neovascular tufts on the retinal surface. The patient presents with painless loss of vision. Initially, the patient sees numerous floaters. The patient may even see a "waterfall," which would represent a stream of blood. The blood would then clot and the patient may complain of seeing a "cobweb" or a dense floater if the bleeding is not excessive. If there is a large amount of blood, the complaint may be acute loss of vision. The patient should be told to avoid aspirin and aspirin-like medicines and to remain in a strict head-up position. The patient should sleep with the head elevated at least 45 degrees to allow the blood to settle in the inferior vitreous cavity. A retinal specialist should be consulted within 24 hours.

Floaters and loss of vision also may be associated with vitritis, an inflammation of the vitreous. In actuality, the inflammation spills into the vitreous from either the retina or posterior uvea (choroid or ciliary body). Any infectious or noninfectious inflammation of the choroid or retina produces similar symptoms. Generally, this posteriorly located inflammation does not produce pain. The eye also does not look inflamed externally. The red reflex is dulled and ophthalmoscopy reveals obscured or absent details. Vitritis seen in association with recent ocular surgery may be indicative of bacterial endophthalmitis (Fig. 109-6) and warrants immediate referral to an ophthalmologist. Vitritis not associated with previous ocular surgery may be referred to the ophthalmologist within 24 hours.

Other uncommon vitreous conditions include asteroid hyalosis (Fig. 109-7) and synchisis scintillans. These two conditions are characterized by the presence of crystals within the vitreous cavity. Asteroid hyalosis is a primary condition that presents with calcium crystals in the vitreous cavity. Synchisis scintillans is a secondary condition in which old vitreous hemorrhage results in the deposition of cholesterol crystals in the vitreous cavity.

## VITREORETINAL INTERFACE ABNORMALITIES

The vitreoretinal interface may be the location or the cause of ocular pathology. Vitreous separation is the primary cause for these abnormalities. In the process of posterior vitreous separation, certain areas of tight vitreoretinal adhesion may be sites of retinal tear formation (Fig. 109-8). The symptoms of tears are not different from symptoms of posterior vitreous separation. Floaters and photopsias are commonly noted. Decreased vision related to vitreous hemorrhage also may be present. As retinal tears may be a cause of retinal detachment, patients with

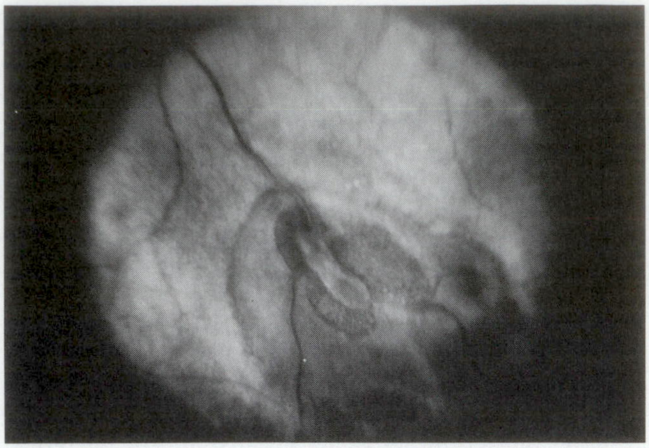

Fig. 109-8. Retinal tear.

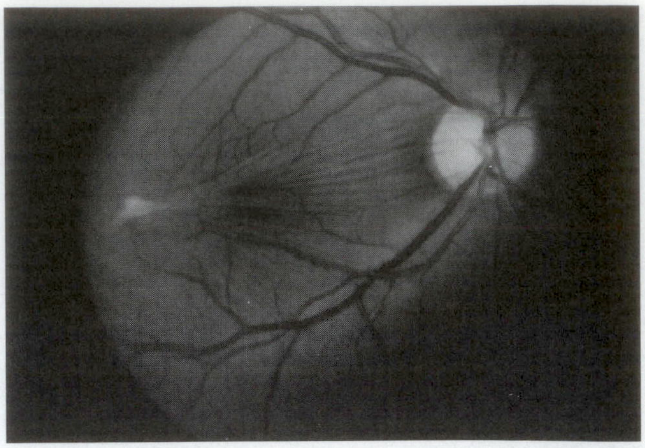

Fig. 109-9. Epiretinal membrane.

such symptoms should be seen within 24 hours.

Vitreous separation also may be a cause of epiretinal membranes. The separation of the posterior hyaloid may cause a microscopic dehiscence of the retinal internal limiting membrane. This dehiscence may allow glial cells, metaplastic pigment epithelial cells, and fibrocytes to have access to the inner surface of the internal limiting membrane. The growth and ultimate contraction of this tissue result in distortion of the retinal surface (Fig. 109-9). Patients may complain of decreased vision as well as metamorphopsia. These complaints are chronic, as the epiretinal membranes are slow growing. Visual impairment may be mild. If the visual acuity is better than 20/60 Snellen visual acuity, intervention is not warranted. For vision worse then 20/60, pars plana vitrectomy with removal of the epiretinal membrane is recommended. Because the progression of epiretinal membranes is slow and because many cases do not have significant visual impairment, the referral does not have to be on an urgent basis. An appointment within 3 weeks is reasonable.

When vitreous liquefaction causes retention of posterior cortical vitreous, this layer may exert horizontal traction on the retina. This horizontal or tangential traction may cause a full-thickness foveal dehiscence called a macular hole (Fig. 109-10). The formation of a macular hole may be associated with a rapid drop in visual acuity, which may not be appreciated by the patient because vision in the other eye remains good. On discovering the affected eye, the patient will notice a central scotoma with poor acuity.

Certain macular holes may be treated surgically to remove the posterior cortical vitreous. As this procedure can be attempted even years after the formation of a macular hole, an ophthalmic referral is not urgent. Consultation within 3 weeks is appropriate.

## RETINAL ABNORMALITIES

### Vascular abnormalities

Systemic hypertension can cause ocular changes that primarily affect the neurosensory retina. Fundus examination may reveal focal or generalized attenuation of the retinal arterioles. Breakdown of the endothelial tight junctions may result in intraretinal hemorrhages and exudation. Hard exudates may be seen within the neurosensory retina. In severe cases, these hard exudates may form a star within the macula. Focal areas of retinal ischemia may be seen as cotton-wool spots. Severe hypertension also may cause edema of the optic nerve. Recognition of hypertensive retinopathy may allow better control of hypertension and thereby lessen ocular complications such as retinal vascular occlusions, as well as systemic complications such as coronary artery disease and neurologic disease. The primary goal after diagnosis of hypertensive retinopathy is control of blood pressure. Once this is established, an ophthalmic referral may be made to rule out ocular complications.

Diabetic retinopathy has many of the retinal findings seen in hypertensive retinopathy because both cause similar breakdown in the retinal vascular endothelial tight junctions. Intraretinal hemorrhages, hard exudates, cotton-wool spots, and retinal vascular microaneurysms may be seen on fundus examination. These findings indicate background diabetic retinopathy (Fig. 109-11). With worsening retinal ischemia, growth of neovascular tissue can be seen on the optic nerve or elsewhere on the retina; this clinical picture is known as proliferative diabetic retinopathy (Fig. 109-12). Because bleeding may occur from these neovascular fronds, recognition of such vessels by the primary physician should be followed by prompt referral within 24 hours; otherwise, referral within 3 weeks is appropriate.

Sickle cell disease can be associated with retinal neovascular fronds, which primarily occur in the retinal periphery. These areas are generally asymptomatic unless vitreous hemorrhage occurs. Because of the potential for hemorrhage, patients should be seen urgently by the retinal physician, even if the patient is asymptomatic. When vascular occlusions occur in the retina, the patient should be referred to an ophthalmologist within 24 hours.

Retinal venous occlusion can occur in either the central retinal vein or one of its branches (Figs. 109-13 and 109-14). If the fovea is involved, the patient presents with acute visual loss. Funduscopic examination reveals venous dilation, tortuous retinal veins, intraretinal hemorrhages, hard exudates, and cotton-wool spots in the affected quadrants. If the fovea is not involved, the patient may be

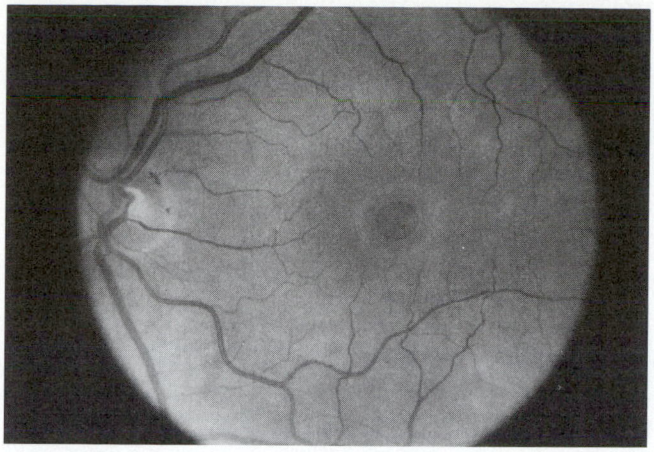

**Fig. 109-10.** Macular hole.

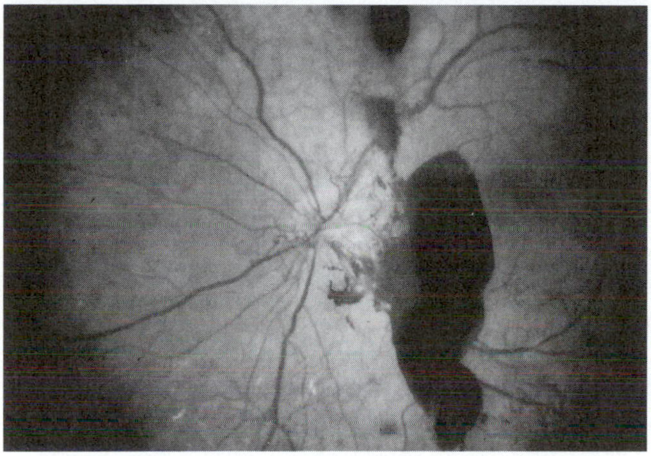

**Fig. 109-12.** Proliferative diabetic retinopathy.

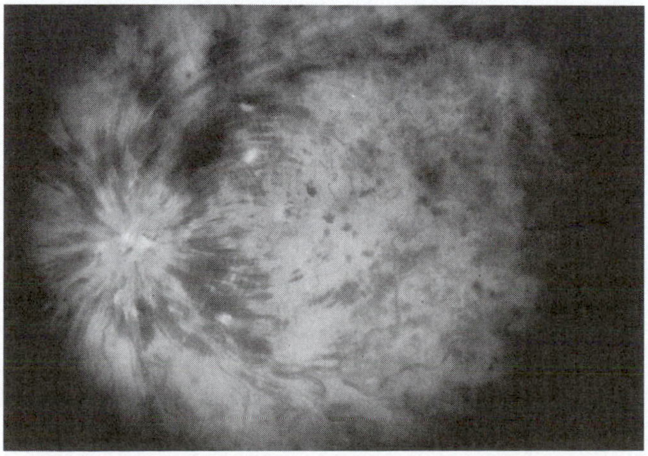

**Fig. 109-14.** Central retinal vein occlusion.

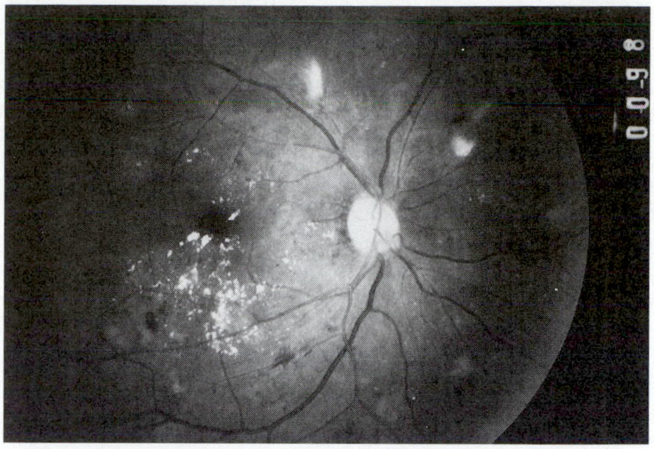

**Fig. 109-11.** Background diabetic retinopathy.

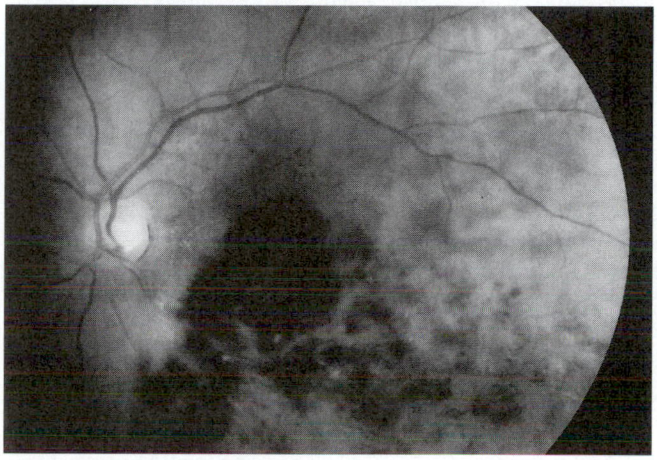

**Fig. 109-13.** Branch retinal vein occlusion.

asymptomatic or may present with only peripheral visual field loss. This diagnosis does not require acute intervention, but to confirm the diagnosis, referral should be made within 24 hours.

Retinal arterial occlusions also may occur within the central retinal artery or any of its branches. The manifestation of arterial occlusion is the presence of ischemic, opaque retina in the affected quadrants, which may be associated with visible emboli within the retinal arterial circulation as well as a cherry-red spot (prominent red color in the fovea) (Fig. 109-15). If the fovea is involved, vision drops acutely, creating one of the few extreme emergencies in ophthalmic practice. Once this diagnosis is suspected, the patient should be referred immediately to the ophthalmic specialist. A delay of even a few minutes may adversely affect visual outcome.

### Retinal pigment epithelial abnormalities

Two conditions of the retinal pigment epithelium are central serous retinopathy and age-related macular degeneration. Central serous retinopathy generally occurs in patients less than 50 years of age, whereas macular degeneration occurs in patients who are older. The

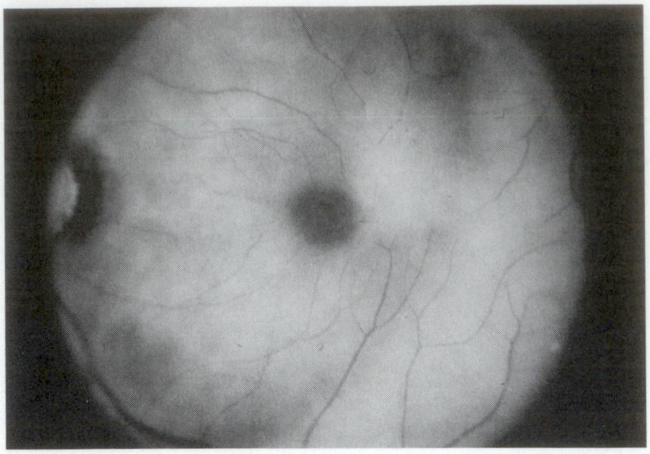

Fig. 109-15. Central retinal artery occlusion.

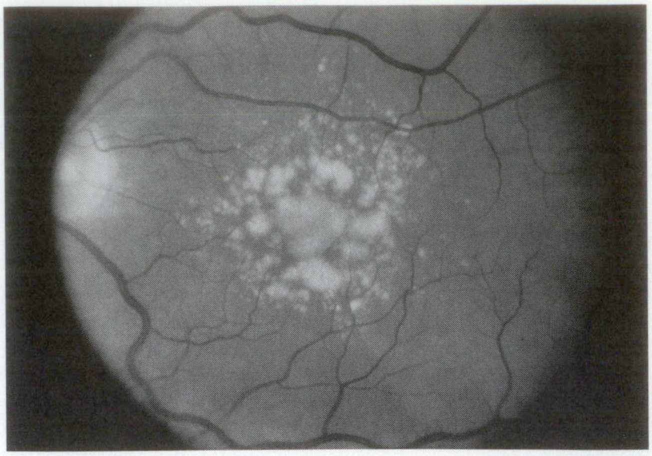

Fig. 109-16. Dry macular degeneration.

pathogenesis of central serous is not completely understood, but it probably involves misdirected fluid transport by the pigment epithelium. The epithelium transports fluid underneath the neurosensory retina causing a neurosensory retinal elevation. The patient complains of acute loss of vision with metamorphopsia, usually in the form of micropsia. Examination of the fundus reveals a dulled foveal reflex and also neurosensory retinal elevation. This condition is generally self-limited. Within 4 months the neurosensory elevation resolves. If resolution does not occur, laser photocoagulation may be necessary. Referral can be made within 3 weeks.

Macular degeneration also is probably a disease of the pigment epithelium. Dry macular degeneration (Fig. 109-16) results from loss of pigment epithelial cells, giving the macula a mottled appearance. The retinal pigment epithelium has atrophic as well as hypertrophic regions. There are also subretinal accumulations of waste products called drusen, which appear yellow-white in color and primarily occur in the macula. Dry macular degeneration causes gradual central visual loss.

In 10% of cases of macular degeneration, there is a growth of new vessels underneath the retina called choroidal neovascular membranes, abnormal extensions of choroidal vasculature. These new vessels change the diagnosis from dry macular degeneration to wet macular degeneration. The vessels have a propensity to grow close to the fovea and predispose the eye to subretinal exudation and subretinal hemorrhage (Fig. 109-17), both of which can cause rapid decrease in central visual acuity with accompanying metamorphopsia. If the choroidal neovascularization is not immediately under the fovea, laser photocoagulation may allow closure of the vessels with retention of good visual acuity. Because the vessels show continued growth without treatment, urgent referral within 24 hours is mandated.

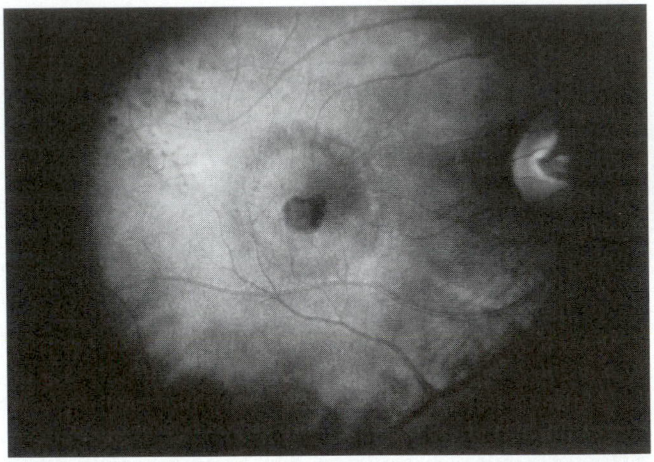

Fig. 109-17. Wet macular degeneration.

## Retinal inflammatory conditions

Retinal inflammatory conditions cause inflammation of the retinal pigment epithelium or inner retina. They include retinal pigment epitheliitis, acute posterior multifocal placoid pigment epitheliopathy (Fig. 109-18), multiple evanescent white dot syndrome, acute macular neuroreti-

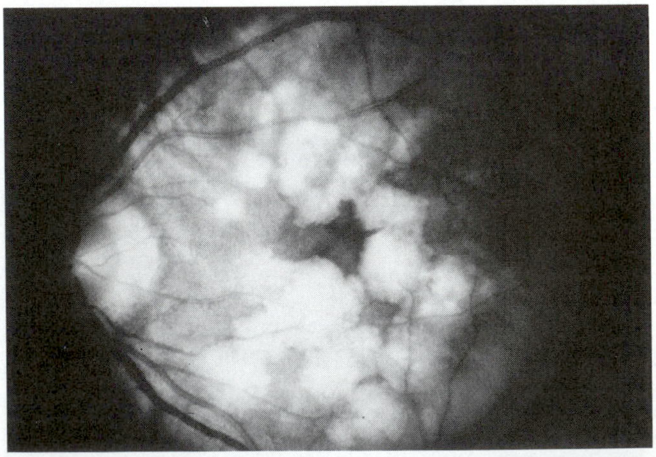

Fig. 109-18. Acute posterior multifocal placoid pigment epitheliopathy.

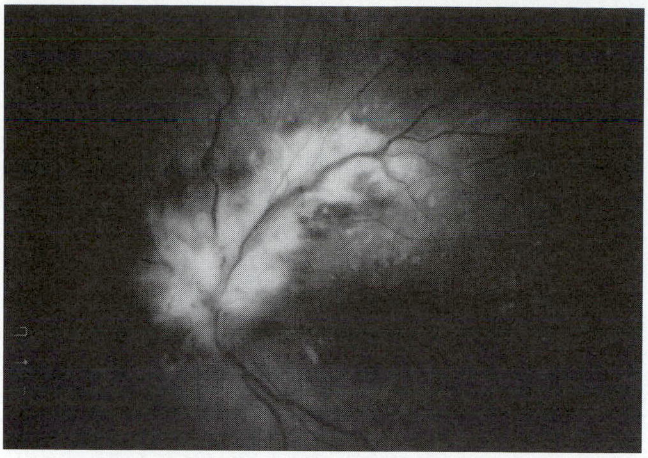

**Fig. 109-19.** CMV retinitis.

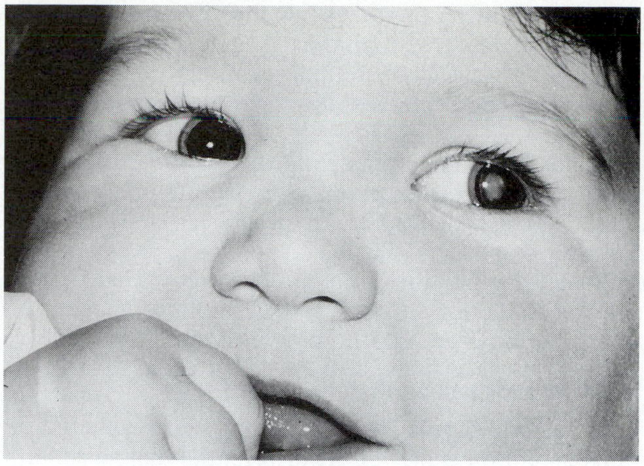

**Fig. 109-20.** White pupil.

nopathy, and birdshot chorioretinopathy. These conditions primarily are acute in onset and occur in younger patients. The etiologies are unknown but are presumed to be viral. They are usually self-limiting and treatment is not warranted. Referral would be semiurgent as no immediate therapy would be necessary. Patients have an acute loss of vision, with the affected eyes displaying yellow-colored retinal inflammatory lesions.

### Retinal infectious conditions

The more common infectious agents that infect the retina include the parasites *Toxoplasmosis gondii* and *Toxocara canis,* as well as the human immunodeficiency virus (HIV) and the cytomegalovirus (CMV). Toxoplasmosis is acquired congenitally and results in large pigmented and depigmented chorioretinal scars that occur bilaterally. These scars contain the dormant organism that may reactivate later in adolescence or young adulthood. Reactivation results in marked inflammation that involves the retina and vitreous and causes floaters and decreased vision.

Toxocariasis also occurs in younger children and results in granuloma formation, primarily affecting the optic nerve, macula, or peripheral retina. The granulomas that affect the optic nerve and the macula usually are associated with decreased vision and a white pupillary reflex. They may result in the formation of a retinal detachment, as well as cause significant vitreal inflammation.

Viruses also may result in infectious retinitis. HIV may result in the formation of cotton-wool spots in the retina, which are white in color with soft margins. Cotton-wool spots are transitory and are not associated with a decrease in vision.

When patients who are HIV positive present with a white retinal lesion, the most devastating etiology is CMV retinitis, which initially may be indistinguishable from a cotton-wool spot. With time, the retinitis, which begins around retinal arterioles, acquires a cheeselike consistency and becomes associated with intraretinal hemorrhages (Fig. 109-19). The retinitis spreads rapidly and, if it involves the optic nerve or macula, is associated with sudden visual loss. HIV retinopathy necessitates every 2- to 3-month examinations for the detection of CMV retinitis. Once CMV retinitis is diagnosed, the patient needs lifelong treatment with ganciclovir, foscarnet, or a combination of the two. When CMV retinitis is suspected, immediate referral for confirmation is necessary.

### Retinal neoplastic conditions

Retinal neoplasms may be pedunculated or sessile. The shape, color, and associated findings may help differentiate them. Because of its potentially fatal outcome, retinoblastoma should be ruled out immediately. Retinoblastomas are pedunculated white vascular tumors that may grow into the vitreous cavity or outward toward the choroid. It is the most common intraocular malignancy of childhood, being diagnosed mainly between the ages of 12 and 18 months. This condition is diagnosed when a young child presents with a white pupil (Fig. 109-20) or new onset of ocular misalignment (strabismus). Because of the risk of metastatic spread, the child should be referred immediately for the possibility of enucleation.

Retinal astrocytomas may be mistaken for retinoblastomas. Astrocytomas are pedunculated white lesions that extend into the vitreous cavity. They are benign growths of glial astrocytes and are primarily avascular. They have a "mulberry" shape, may be unilateral or bilateral, and may be multifocal. Patients with tuberous sclerosis and neurofibromatosis may manifest retinal astrocytomas, but this tumor most commonly is unassociated with any systemic syndrome.

Retinal capillary hemangiomas are pedunculated vascular lesions that begin as small red-colored intraretinal lesions. With time they grow and can be recognized by the presence of a feeding retinal vessel. These hemangiomas may result in bleeding, exudation, and tractional retinal detachment. They may occur as a part of the autosomal dominant transmitted von Hippel-Lindau syndrome or on a nonfamilial basis. Because the larger tumors are harder to treat, attempts should be made to diagnose all hemangiomas when they are small and can be treated with laser photocoagulation or retinocryopexy.

Retinal cavernous hemangiomas are sessile lesions that

appear as a "cluster of grapes" on the retinal surface. They may be associated with similar skin and central nervous system lesions. Unlike retinal capillary hemangiomas, these lesions do not exhibit marked hemorrhage or exudation.

Congenital retinal pigment epithelial hypertrophy (Fig. 109-21) is a jet-black lesion with well-defined margins. Retinal pigment epithelial hyperplasia is an acquired condition that has a mottled appearance; it occurs as a result of inflammation, trauma, or vitreoretinal traction. With the exception of suspected retinoblastomas, retinal tumors can be seen on a nonurgent basis.

## Hereditary retinal conditions

Three factors should be considered when a hereditary retinal condition is part of the differential diagnosis. First, the condition tends to occur in younger patients, with most entities manifesting changes in adolescence or young adulthood. Second, the condition is usually bilateral and the extent of involvement is symmetrical. Finally, the patient may have other affected family members, and a specific genetic transmission pattern may be discovered. These entities may affect primarily the periphery and result in decreased peripheral vision and night vision or may affect the macula and result in early central visual loss. The most common peripheral entity would be retinitis pigmentosa, whereas the most common central entity would be cone dystrophy.

## Retinal detachments

Three pathogenic mechanisms can result in the retina being elevated off the retinal pigment epithelium. Detachments that occur as a result of a break in the retina are called rhegmatogenous. Those that occur because of tractional fibrosis within the vitreous cavity are called tractional. Finally, conditions that result in the exudation of fluid under the retina result in exudative detachments.

Rhegmatogenous retinal detachments, the most common type (Figs. 109-22 and 109-23), result from a posterior vitreous separation that causes a retinal break. This break allows liquid vitreous to enter the subretinal space and cause a retinal detachment. The patient generally presents with photopsias and "floaters." With detachment of the fovea, the central vision markedly

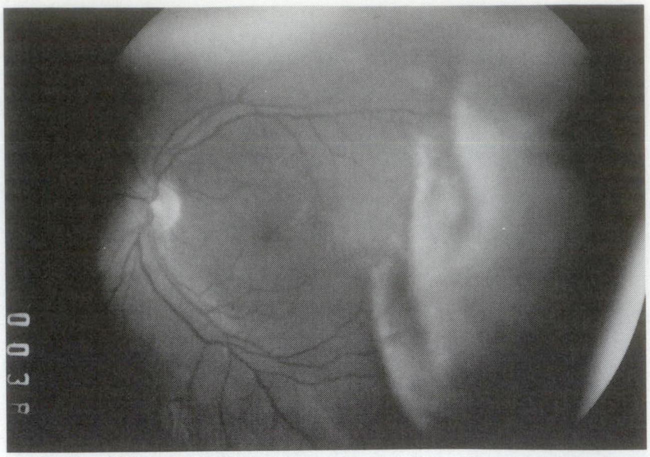

**Fig. 109-22.** Retinal detachment.

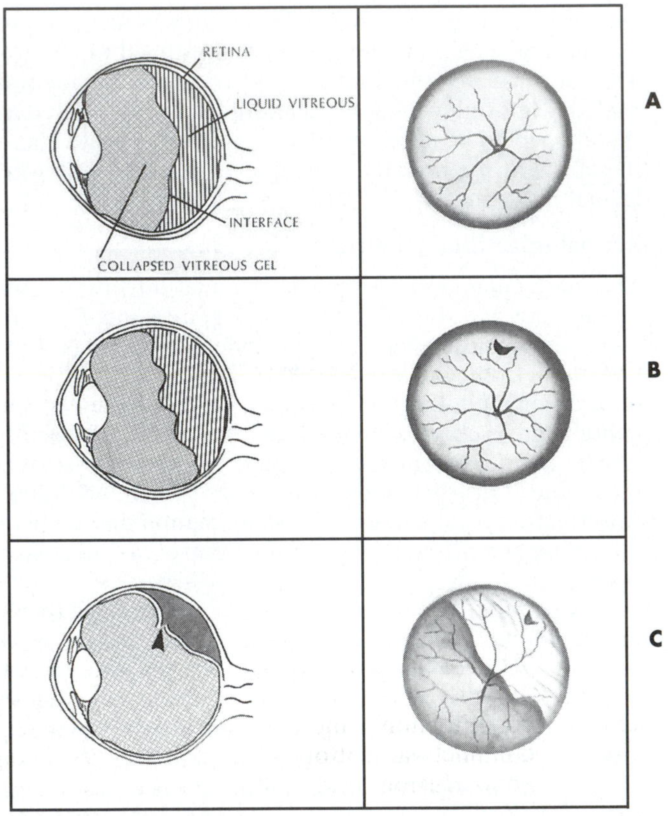


**Fig. 109-23.** Vitreous detachment, retinal hole, and retinal detachment. **A,** The vitreous body has collapsed and has pulled away from the retina in the posterior half of the eye. The retina remains intact. **B,** The vitreous body has collapsed and pulled away from the retina in the posterior portion of the eye. Superiorly, a strong adhesion between the vitreous and retina remains and has led to tearing of the retina due to the vitreous detachment. The retinal tear usually takes a "horseshoe" appearance when viewed through the ophthalmoscope. **C,** The vitreous has detached as in **A** and **B** and has caused a retinal tear as in **B.** Fluid from the area of liquid vitreous posteriorly has worked its way through the retinal hole, and the retina itself has now become detached from the wall of the eye. It takes a balloon shape when seen with the ophthalmoscope.

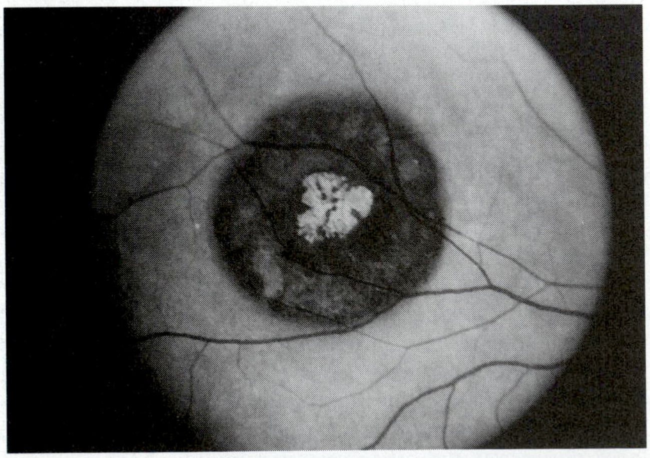

**Fig. 109-21.** Congenital retinal pigment epithelial hypertrophy.

decreases. When the fovea is not detached, the central vision can be quite good even though the peripheral vision is limited. When a patient presents with symptoms of a detachment and good vision, the referral should be made urgently. If vision is decreased, the patient can be seen semiurgently. The primary goal should be to prevent foveal detachment. Once the fovea detaches, surgery to reattach the retina may be performed within the following week for equivalent results.

The most common cause of tractional retinal detachment is a diabetic retinal detachment. The proliferative stage of diabetic retinopathy results in the growth of vascular and fibrous components into the vitreous cavity. The fibrous component may cause tractional forces to develop between the retina and vitreous. These forces may cause the retina to be pulled off the underlying retinal pigment epithelium. Unlike rhegmatogenous detachments, tractional detachments do not produce acute symptoms, and the earliest detectible symptom may be visual loss once the fovea detaches. Tractional detachments are slow to form and thus referral should be semiurgent. Treatment involves vitrectomy surgery to remove the tractional components; this procedure is performed only if the fovea is detached or if a foveal detachment appears imminent.

Exudative retinal detachments result from subretinal inflammatory and neoplastic conditions that cause the accumulation of fluid under the retina. The fluid has the ability to "shift" under the retina, with different portions of the retina detaching with alterations in position. Once the fluid reaches the fovea, vision decreases. These detachments tend to be inferior in primary position because of gravity. Consultation should be on an urgent basis.

## CHOROIDAL ABNORMALITIES

### Choroidal neovascular membranes

Choroidal neovascular membranes occur when normal choroidal vasculature extends into the subretinal space through breaks in Bruch's membrane. Several conditions may result in such a break. Angioid streaks result in Bruch's membrane cracks that radiate from the optic nerve. These orange-red streaks may occur in patients with pseudoxanthoma elasticum, sickle cell disease, and Paget's disease. High myopia may result in attenuations of Bruch's membrane, *lacquer cracks,* which occur primarily in the macula. Trauma can result in ruptures of the choroid including Bruch's membrane. These ruptures usually occur concentrically around the optic nerve. Presumed ocular histoplasmosis syndrome results in circular, yellow-white chorioretinal scars. These scars have breaks in the overlying Bruch's membrane. All these conditions can result in green-gray extensions of the choriocapillaris under the retina that may result in subretinal exudation and hemorrhage. Depending on the location of these membranes, central visual acuity may be markedly affected. If none of the predisposing factors are present, the neovascular membrane would be considered idiopathic. Once the diagnosis is suspected, referral is made urgently for the possibility of laser photocoagulation to obliterate the neovascular membrane.

### Choroidal inflammatory conditions

Like retinal inflammatory conditions, choroidal inflammatory conditions have unknown etiologies. The entities are diagnosed because of the constellation of signs that accompany each particular disorder. All of the choroidal inflammatory disorders may present with photopsias and decreased vision that is sudden in onset. Serpiginous choroidopathy occurs in a peripapillary location. The choroid is actively inflamed, and the leading edge has a snakelike shape, from which the condition gets its name. Multifocal choroiditis and punctate inner choroidopathy both have characteristic inflammatory inner choroidal lesions. The eye usually has lesions that are in differing stages of evolution. The acute lesions have a yellowish, thickened appearance, whereas the chronic lesions look like typical chorioretinal scars that are circular with a pigmented and a depigmented component. The difference between the two conditions is that multifocal choroiditis has intravitreal inflammation, whereas punctate inner choroidopathy does not.

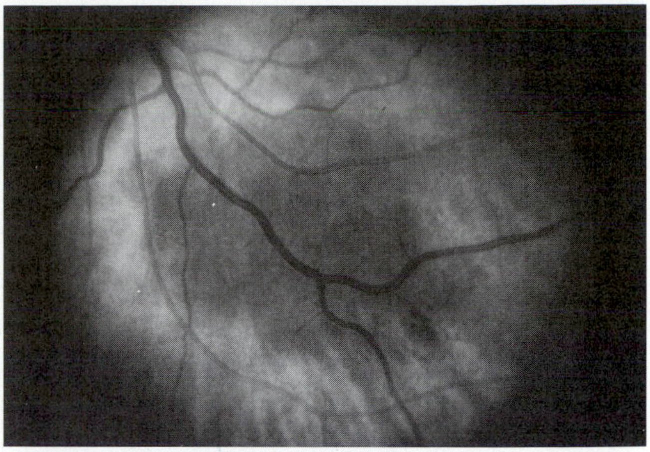

**Fig. 109-24.** Nevus.

### Choroidal neoplastic conditions

Choroidal neoplastic conditions present to the clinician as either melanotic or amelanotic subretinal lesions that may be unifocal or multifocal. The most common entity is the choroidal nevus (Fig. 109-24). This benign accumulation of melanocytic cells presents as a flat, greenish-brown lesion. It is a congenitally present lesion which may become more pigmented with time. The lesion may be unifocal or multifocal, and the size varies from less than 1 mm to many millimeters. There is no overlying retinal involvement and the patient is totally asymptomatic. These patients should be referred semiurgently; follow-up consists of yearly observation because of the small risk of malignant transformation into a malignant melanoma.

A choroidal malignant melanoma (Fig. 109-25) may arise from a choroidal nevus or may arise de novo. Although amelanotic melanomas are present, the more common presentation is a melanotic subretinal lesion. The color may range from green to brown; a jet-black lesion is most uncommon. It is differentiated from a choroidal nevus by its height, which is more than 2 mm and can be as large as 10 to 15 mm. It can be associated with neurosensory retinal elevation, subretinal exudation, and subretinal hemorrhage. Large melanomas can show extension through the sclera. Metastatic spread of a choroidal

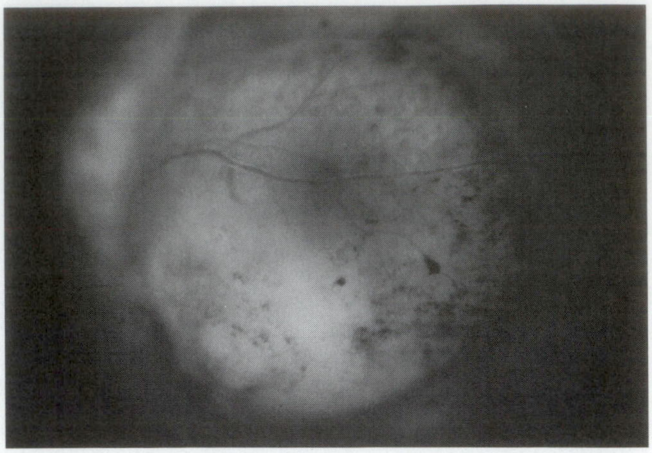

**Fig. 109-25.** Choroidal melanoma.

melanoma occurs primarily to the liver and lungs. Once metastasis occurs, life expectancy is less than 1 year. The best treatment modality for choroidal melanoma is unknown. Treatments include observation, laser photocoagulation, cryopexy, radiation, surgical resection, or enucleation. Urgent referral while the tumor is still small may afford the patient and retina specialist more treatment options, which may save some sight as well as the patient's life.

Another malignant condition of the choroid is metastatic disease. Choroidal metastases are primarily amelanotic, multifocal lesions that occur in the posterior pole and result in visual decline. Bilateral involvement is common. The condition affects men and women equally. The most common primary tumors are the breast and lungs. Other less common sites include the kidney, testicle, prostate, and gastrointestinal tract. Ocular involvement may be the first sign of lung cancer, whereas patients with choroidal metastases from breast cancer usually have already been diagnosed. Although systemic treatment is of prime importance in metastatic disease, ocular radiation may be beneficial in patients whose vision has decreased from choroidal metastases.

## SUMMARY

This chapter has introduced the primary care physician to diseases that affect the vitreous, retina, and choroid. The most important aspect of this introduction is the anatomy of this area and how its alteration leads to symptoms. Once symptoms implicate a possible abnormality in one of these structures, examination can be directed appropriately. If a confident diagnosis can be made, referral should be made urgently or semiurgently. If the diagnosis cannot be made confidently, referral should be made emergently, within minutes, to the ophthalmologist if the symptoms are acute or urgently, within 24 hours, if the symptoms are chronic.

## BIBLIOGRAPHY


Basic and Clinical Science Course: Section 4, Retina and Vitreous. American Academy of Ophthalmology, 1987.

Hilton GF, McLean EB, Chuang EL: Retinal detachment. American Academy of Ophthalmology, 1989.

Kini MM: Retina and vitreous. In Pavan-Langston D, editor: *Manual of ocular diagnosis and therapy,* Boston, 1985, Little, Brown.

Newell FW, editor: *Ophthalmology: principles and concepts,* St Louis, 1986, Mosby.

Schlaegel TF Jr, Pavan-Langston D: Uveal tract: iris, ciliary body and choroid. In Pavan-Langston D, editor: *Manual of ocular diagnosis and therapy,* Boston, 1985, Little, Brown.

Vaughn D, Asbury T, editors: *General ophthalmology,* Los Altos, CA, 1983, Lange Medical Publications.


CHAPTER

# 110 Neuro-Ophthalmology

**Barry Skarf**

Vision, and hence the discipline of ophthalmology, involves more than just the eyes and their supporting structures. The eyes form extensive connections with the brain, and normal visual function depends on the development and maintenance of connections to visual, sensory, and motor centers. The field of neuro-ophthalmology deals with those disorders of neurologic function that can affect vision: diseases of the central nervous system (CNS) and of the cranial nerves as well as systemic conditions that affect the nervous system. Representative conditions that affect vision by their action on the nervous system are multiple sclerosis, cerebral vascular disease, intracranial and intraorbital tumors, and generalized systemic diseases such as syphilis and sarcoidosis.

Neuro-ophthalmology is divided into two broad divisions: sensory and motor. The sensory visual system directly subserves sight; disorders affecting it can cause profound visual disturbances. This system is made up of the retinas, the optic nerves and chiasm, the optic tracts, both lateral geniculate nuclei of the thalamus, the optic radiations (which connect the lateral geniculate nucleus to the visual cortex), and those regions of cerebral cortex, primarily in the occipital lobe, that subserve vision. Neuro-ophthalmology deals with diseases that affect all portions of this pathway, excluding disorders that involve only the eye and retina. The second division of neuro-ophthalmology involves the ocular motor system and its disorders. Essential to the normal function of vision is the ability to execute appropriate, coordinated eye movements. Disturbances of eye movements and of ocular alignment can seriously degrade vision and visual function. The ocular motor system includes the eye muscles and the nerves that control them, as well as the brainstem and cortical centers, which direct eye movements. The principal symptoms that result from ocular motor system disorders are blurring of vision, diplopia, and difficulty achieving or maintaining appropriate fixation.

The neuro-ophthalmologist is concerned with conditions causing visual disturbances for which there is no obvious intraocular pathology. Included in this category are a variety of transient visual disturbances, functional complaints, and factitious visual loss, as well as conditions that cause optic nerve swelling (edema) and systemic conditions that affect vision and nervous system structures.

This chapter describes neuro-ophthalmic disturbances of the visual sensory system and conditions that affect the ocular motor system. Each section outlines the major presenting symptoms likely to confront the primary care physician. Associated clinical findings and their evaluation are discussed. A topographic description of the common neuro-ophthalogic disorders that cause these visual disturbances is presented.

## THE SENSORY VISUAL SYSTEM

### Evaluating visual loss from retrobulbar (nonocular) disease

***History.*** Visual loss is the principal manifestation of disease involving the sensory visual system. Patients who note an unexplained change in vision will present to their primary care physician, optometrist, or ophthalmologist. When the change in vision is sudden and/or dramatic, or when it is accompanied by a headache or other systemic disturbance, the primary care physician is consulted preferentially. Usually the visual loss is spontaneous, but a history of trauma and antecedent ocular, neurologic, or systemic disease should be elicited.

A patient's visual loss may be transient or persistent and may affect one or both eyes. Loss of central vision and/or a decrease of peripheral vision may occur. Most important, visual loss may be acute, having occurred instantaneously or over a few days, or it may have developed much more gradually.

Patients with true sensory pathway dysfunction often complain of blurred vision, dim vision, or a decrease in the brightness of colors. Although a detailed history is essential, care must be taken in its interpretation, as patients are often unclear or even incorrect about the nature of their visual loss. For example, a patient with a right homonymous hemianopsia may describe visual loss in the right eye. In fact, the patient has lost vision in the right hemifield of both eyes, but this can be determined only through appropriate examinations. Or a patient claiming acute visual loss in one eye may have been unaware of a gradual loss of vision in the eye until this loss is "discovered" when the good eye is inadvertently covered. The nature of the visual loss, whether transient or permanent, can be invaluable in making a diagnosis and determining suitable management.

Frequently, patients present with transient photopsias or complaints of seeing flashing lights or various other positive visual phenomena not associated with visual loss. These complaints must be taken seriously, as they could relate to incipient retinal detachment or retinal tear, migrainous visual auras, or more serious CNS diseases such as arteriovenous malformations and brain tumors.

***Examination.*** Objective clinical findings may be difficult to obtain in neuro-ophthalmic disease. The most reliable sign of monocular visual loss due to neuro-ophthalmic disease is the relative afferent pupillary defect (Marcus Gunn pupil) as determined by the swinging flashlight test. When this clinical sign is absent in a patient complaining of persistent uniocular visual loss, the examiner should look for an abnormality of the eye itself (e.g., a refractive error, media opacity, or mild retinal edema). If tests for these conditions are negative, one must consider the possibility of factitious visual loss. The presence of a relative afferent pupillary defect, however, confirms the patient's visual deficit and is usually indicative of a serious problem.

The primary care physician should determine visual acuity in any patient who presents with a visual complaint. If a patient does *not* have normal acuity, looking through a pinhole (pinhole test) will diminish the effect of uncorrected refractive error. Evaluation of the patient's color perception is useful in diagnosing diseases of the retrobulbar visual pathway. The patient is asked to compare the brightness of colors seen with either eye in the temporal and nasal hemifields of each eye. This test offers invaluable information as long as the colored object is held at positions equidistant from fixation under uniform lighting conditions. Finally, a funduscopic examination, preferably through dilated pupils, is essential to determine intraocular pathology and, more specifically, to establish the presence of optic nerve swelling in one or both eyes.

***Visual fields.*** The primary care physician can quickly evaluate the patient's visual fields by using simple confrontation testing. The physician asks the patient to count fingers held in each quadrant while the patient alternately covers one eye and fixates on the examiner with the other eye. This simple test can be diagnostic when evaluating patients with hemifield defects due to a silent stroke or a slowly progressive tumor even when the remainder of the examination is normal.

The visual field examination is useful in topographically localizing the cause of visual disturbances. Retinal diseases often produce discrete geographic defects located in the central portion of the visual field. When the primary pathology is at the optic disc, visual field defects tend to be sectoral, arcuate, or altitudinal, radiating from the blind spot. Retrobulbar optic nerve disease usually produces central visual loss, but also can produce any of the visual field defects described previously. The hallmark of chiasmal involvement is bilateral visual field defects. Although these defects classically involve temporal hemifields of both eyes, several variations can occur. Retrochiasmal lesions involving the optic tract, geniculate, optic radiations, and occipital cortex produce complete or partial homonymous hemianopsias. In these situations there is always bilateral involvement, but the defects in each eye may be congruous or incongruous. Generally, the more posterior the lesion (farther back from the chiasm) the more congruous it will be. Complete homonymous hemianopsias, however, are nonlocalizing.

### Optic nerve diseases

Funduscopic examination of the optic nerve heads is an established part of any complete medical examination. It is especially critical to perform this examination in patients who complain of headaches, other neurologic problems, or visual disturbances. Abnormal optic nerves can reflect a variety of local, neurologic, and systemic diseases. It is important to emphasize, however, that the optic nerve head may be *abnormal* in only one of three ways:

1. It may be swollen (edematous)
2. It may be pale in color, which is usually a sign of optic atrophy
3. It may be morphologically or structurally abnormal or anomalous, for example, optic disc cupping in glaucoma and optic disc drusen (calcific bodies embedded within the optic nerve substance)

The primary care physician must determine whether the appearance of each optic nerve is normal or abnormal and categorize them appropriately. When visual loss is due to retrobulbar optic neuropathy (neuritis), the optic nerve head may appear normal. Because optic nerve pathology can be difficult to recognize, consultation with an ophthalmologist or neuro-ophthalmologist should be obtained whenever there is doubt concerning the appearance of the optic nerve heads.

*Optic nerve disorders associated with optic disc swelling.* Disorders associated with optic disc swelling can be divided into two groups:

1. Optic disc swelling without significant visual loss
2. Optic disc swelling with visual loss

**Optic disc swelling without significant visual loss.** Patients complaining of headache associated with transient visual disturbances may have bilateral disc swelling or edema. Bilateral disc edema usually implies *papilledema,* a term reserved exclusively for disc edema secondary to elevated intracranial pressure. Visual function is usually preserved, except for enlarged blind spots. Patients may describe shadows or photopsias in the temporal portion of the visual field. There may be a slight disturbance of central vision, but patients can usually achieve normal or near-normal acuity.

Although true papilledema is usually bilateral, it may be asymmetric. *Papilledema should be considered a medical emergency requiring computed tomography (CT) or magnetic resonance imaging (MRI) to rule out an intracranial mass lesion.* The patient's medical history must include detailed information on trauma, illness, infection, and other neurologic symptoms. Because papilledema can be the result of severe hypertension, it is necessary to check blood pressure. Another common cause of papilledema is pseudotumor cerebri or benign intracranial hypertension (BIH). BIH commonly affects middle-aged, overweight women who have had children.

Patients with BIH often complain about frequent headaches; however, the condition may occur without headache and may be discovered only when a routine examination reveals papilledema. Because BIH is a diagnosis of exclusion, patients must have MRI or CT to rule out an intracranial mass. If a space-occupying lesion is not found, the patient should have a lumbar puncture to obtain cerebral spinal fluid (CSF) for laboratory studies as well as to determine CSF pressure.

Unfortunately, many normal optic nerves appear elevated with blurred margins, giving them a "swollen" appearance. When exaggerated, prominent disc elevation and blurred disc margins represent *pseudopapilledema,* a congenital variation that mimics true papilledema. This anomaly is often associated with intrapapillary calcium deposits known as *optic disc drusen.* The examining physician must distinguish between pseudopapilledema, a benign condition, and papilledema, as well as other causes of disc edema.

True disc edema, including papilledema, can be recognized because the swollen edge of the optic disc obscures some of the small- and medium-sized vessels that transverse the disc margin. This clinical picture can occur relatively early in the development of disc edema before elevation of the disc is obvious. If there is marked elevation of the optic discs with blurred margins, but all vessels traversing the optic disc margin (including small capillaries) are well defined and are not obscured by edema, the patient probably has pseudopapilledema. Fluorescein angiography of the fundus, which results in leakage of dye into and around the optic disc, can help distinguish true edema.

Occasionally, unilateral disc swelling, indistinguishable from papilledema, is noted; in rare cases, this can be true papilledema due to elevated intracranial pressure. More frequently, however, it is caused by localized optic nerve disease. Unilateral causes of optic disc edema in the absence of significant visual loss include (1) compressive optic neuropathies (i.e., tumor compression of the optic nerve obstructing venous drainage and causing disc swelling) and (2) papillophlebitis, an idiopathic condition that usually causes only slight visual loss and mild to moderate disc swelling, mainly in young, otherwise healthy patients.

Finally, unilateral optic disc swelling may be the result of ocular hypotony, which can occur after a perforating injury of the globe, including ocular surgery. This condition is seen most frequently after cataract extraction.

**Optic disc swelling associated with visual loss.** Patients presenting with visual loss (usually in one eye) and mild to moderate swelling of the optic disc may have a number of different disorders. *Papillitis* is the most common cause of visual loss associated with disc swelling in patients younger than 40. In this form of optic neuritis, the anterior portion of the optic nerve becomes inflamed and the optic nerve head is swollen. Occasionally, the disc swelling may be accompanied by retinal swelling and exudates, a condition known as neuroretinitis. Retrobulbar optic neuritis presents acutely without any change in the appearance of the nerve head. It must be emphasized, however, that neuroretinitis, papillitis, and retrobulbar optic neuritis are essentially the same type of inflammatory condition involving different segments of the optic nerve. All forms of optic neuritis are discussed below.

*Anterior ischemic optic neuropathy (AION)* is the most common cause of visual loss associated with optic disc swelling in patients older than 50. This condition represents an acute infarction of the optic nerve head. Typically, patients present with sudden, painless loss of vision in one eye, but mild orbital pain may precede or be associated with the event. Both eyes are rarely involved simultaneously. Usually the visual loss is central or altitudinal, but patients may complain of seeing a shadow to one side, above, or below their fixation. The typical fundus appearance shows a swollen optic disc; a portion of the disc is hyperemic, with the remaining portion somewhat paler in appearance. Frequently, one or a few streaky nerve fiber layer hemorrhages surround the disc.

The two major pathologic types of AION are the idiopathic, nonarteritic form and the arteritic form,

### Conditions causing anterior ischemic optic neuropathy

Giant cell arteritis
Hypertension
Diabetes mellitus
Atherosclerosis
Migraine
Systemic lupus erythematosus
Polyarteritis nodosum
Syphilis
Carotid occlusive disease
Buerger's disease
Allergic vasculitis
Postviral vasculitis
Postimmunization
Radiation necrosis
Takayasu's disease
Polycythemia vera
Sickle cell disease (trait)
Acute hypotension (shock)
G-6-P-D deficiency

associated with temporal arteritis. In addition, a variety of vasculitides, coagulopathies, and systemic diseases can contribute to the development of this condition (see the box above). Occasionally, ischemic optic neuropathy develops within a few days of cataract surgery. All patients with ischemic infarction of the optic disc should undergo the following laboratory tests: complete blood count (CBC), platelets, erythrocyte sedimentation rates (ESR), glucose, antinuclear antibodies (ANA), venereal disease research laboratory (VDRL), prothrombin time (PT), partial thromboplastin time (PTT), cardiolipin antibodies. Neuroimaging studies are not indicated.

Idiopathic AION is more common than the arteritic form and generally occurs in patients older than 45. Hypertension is an accepted risk factor, but there is also a relationship to diabetes, and it tends to occur more frequently in persons with small, crowded optic discs. AION affects men more than women and results in a permanent visual deficit. Approximately one third of patients experience progressive visual loss and another one third improve. When recovery occurs, it is usually modest, although if central vision is involved, substantial improvement in visual acuity can occur.

Although no treatment for AION has proved successful, patients should be advised to take one tablet of aspirin daily. Risk factors such as hypertension should be treated appropriately.

With time, optic disc swelling subsides but the patient has residual sectoral optic atrophy. Once visual loss stabilizes, there is little chance of recurrent infarction of the same optic nerve head. Bilateral involvement occurs in approximately 25% of affected individuals, although the second eye may not succumb for months or years.

AION associated with temporal (giant cell) arteritis is a treatable medical emergency; without appropriate medi-

### Symptoms and signs of temporal arteritis

Visual loss
Amaurosis fugax
Diplopia
Headache
Scalp tenderness
Jaw claudication
Tongue claudication
Difficulty talking
Numbness, burning dysesthesias of tongue
Intermittent arm claudication
Myalgias
Anorexia
Weight loss
Fever
Malaise
Vertebrobasilar insufficiency causing:
- Vertigo
- Deafness
- Tinnitus
- Ataxia

Dementia
Angina pectoris
Ischemic optic neuropathy
Central retinal artery occlusion
Ocular motor paresis
Cyanosis, blanching necrosis of tongue
Swollen, tender temporal artery
Absent temporal artery pulse
Decreased upper extremity blood pressure or pulse

cal management, visual loss can progress rapidly in both eyes, resulting in blindness. This arteritic form of AION occurs in elderly patients who often appear cachectic. Although known to occur in younger individuals, temporal arteritis is unusual in patients younger than 65. Visual loss in the arteritic form of AION frequently develops in stages and becomes catastrophic with severe reduction in field and acuity. The entire optic disc is swollen and pale. In untreated cases, the risk of rapid progression with involvement of the second eye is great.

In order not to miss this treatable condition and to help establish the diagnosis, the primary care physician should obtain an immediate ESR on every patient over 50 who presents with sudden visual loss and a swollen optic disc. In addition the patient should be questioned carefully about constitutional symptoms suggesting temporal arteritis (see the box above). Persons in their seventies or eighties are particularly vulnerable, and it is always best to obtain an ESR, even when the diagnosis of AION is uncertain. If temporal arteritis is suspected based on the ESR or clinical history, immediate therapy with oral prednisone (1 mg/kg per day) must be initiated. If the diagnosis is uncertain, it is best to begin treatment (unless steroids are contraindicated) and arrange for a temporal artery biopsy. Histopathologic examination of a segment of the superficial temporal artery usually confirms the diagnosis; in rare situations, however, a normal biopsy may be obtained in a patient with temporal arteritis. Once again, clinical judgment is crucial.

The principal goal of therapy is to prevent further visual loss and to preserve vision in the second eye. Unfortunately, high-dose corticosteroids do not promote recovery once vision is lost.

Several features of *retinal vein occlusion,* which occurs mainly in patients over 40, resemble those seen in anterior ischemic optic neuropathy. Acute visual loss is common, although patients often complain of a "sputtering" of their vision before they develop a persistent visual deficit. Fundus examination reveals a swollen disc with peripapillary hemorrhages. The veins are markedly dilated, but unlike ischemic optic neuropathy, the hemorrhages extend along the affected vascular tree outward toward the periphery. If the central vein is involved, multiple hemorrhages are scattered along both upper and lower arcades of the fundus. If a branch vein is occluded, hemorrhage is found only in the territory of the involved branch.

*Papillophlebitis* is a milder form of vein occlusion that occurs in younger individuals. It is characterized by moderate swelling of the optic discs, moderate engorgement of the veins, and a few hemorrhages. Visual deficits are usually minimal.

All patients with retinal venous occlusive disease should be examined for causes of increased serum viscosity, including dysproteinemia, polycythemia, hemoglobinopathy, diabetes, and leukemia. These patients are at risk for developing a secondary form of glaucoma and must be followed closely by an ophthalmologist.

*Neoplasms* can cause optic nerve swelling and loss of vision through a variety of mechanisms. Externally, they compress the optic nerve causing venous congestion, which, in turn, leads to disc swelling. Primary optic nerve tumors (meningiomas or gliomas) can produce the same effect (see later). Leukemia, lymphoma, and meningeal carcinomatosis may infiltrate the optic nerve causing optic disc swelling either by direct tumor extension into the optic nerve head or by producing venous congestion. Visual loss occurs rapidly with optic nerve infiltration, but may be gradual and insidious when there is optic nerve compression. Optic nerve swelling and visual loss also can occur in advanced dysthyroid ophthalmopathy when markedly enlarged extraocular muscles compress the optic nerve at the apex of the orbit. Any patient with optic nerve swelling and visual loss who does not fit a typical description of optic neuritis or ischemic optic neuropathy should undergo neuroimaging studies, as should any patient who gives a history of slowly progressive visual loss over weeks to months.

*Leber's hereditary optic neuropathy* superficially resembles papillitis. It tends to occur in young healthy individuals who present with subacute visual loss and optic nerve swelling. Several features, however, differentiate this condition from optic neuritis. Visual loss is always painless and optic nerve hyperemia is marked, with engorgement of the peripapillary capillaries and small retinal vessels. The contralateral optic nerve may appear swollen as well, even when visual function is normal. At the very least, there is prominence of the small vessels in the contralateral peripapillary region.

This condition is transmitted by mitochondrial DNA from mothers to their children (never through the paternal line). Men are twice as likely to be affected as women. Recently, several markers on mitochondrial DNA linked to Leber's hereditary optic neuropathy have been identified. Patients who suffer bilateral visual loss from optic neuropathy have tested positive for these markers, even in the absence of the characteristic fundus appearance.

In Leber's hereditary optic neuropathy, the second eye is almost always affected within weeks to months; however, the visual loss may be asymmetric. Patients tend to have permanent central visual loss, although some improve several years after the acute episode. Patients may have a cardiac myopathy, and an electrocardiogram (ECG) should be obtained to rule out a preexcitation syndrome. No effective treatment exists for this condition.

***Optic nerve disorders resulting in optic atrophy.*** *Retrobulbar optic neuritis* is one of the most common causes of subacute visual loss in young adults, although it also can occur in older individuals. It is especially common in young women between the ages of 18 and 45. Pain and/or discomfort in or around the affected eye, often exacerbated by eye movements, are common symptoms. Within a few days of the onset of ocular discomfort, the patient generally notes progressively decreasing visual acuity. This disturbance can vary from mild blurring or dimming of vision, with colors taking on a somewhat "washed out" appearance, to complete blindness. Visual field deficits and an afferent pupillary defect are present in the affected eye.

In acute retrobulbar optic neuritis, examination of the fundus is completely normal, with no evidence of swelling or pallor of the optic disc. Papillitis and neuroretinitis are also forms of optic neuritis, but in adults those forms occur much less frequently than the retrobulbar form. Clinically, however, all forms of optic neuritis have similar natural histories. After a few weeks most affected individuals begin to notice improving vision followed by a slow protracted recovery, which can continue for up to 1 year. Optic atrophy usually develops after a few weeks.

A high rate of association with multiple sclerosis is present with retrobulbar optic neuritis. Frequently, directed questioning reveals a relationship to systemic demyelinating disease. On other occasions, there will be no previous history, but MRI shows multiple small lesions scattered in the brain's white matter. A positive MRI can forewarn the development of multiple sclerosis in otherwise idiopathic cases of optic neuritis.

Treatment of this condition is still controversial. The results of the Optic Neuritis Treatment Trial sponsored by the National Institutes of Health (NIH) have shown that oral steroids are of no value, but that intravenous methylprednisolone can promote a more rapid recovery and may delay the development of multiple sclerosis. The established dose is 250 mg of intravenous methylprednisolone every 6 hours for 3 days followed by 11 days of oral prednisone, 1 mg/kg per day. The prednisone is then tapered. Vision usually begins to improve within 1 month with or without treatment. Patients who do not improve within 6 weeks or who continue to worsen after the first 2 weeks should be investigated fully for other causes of optic neuropathy.

*Gliomas* of the visual pathway, including optic nerve and chiasm, are primarily childhood phenomena frequently associated with neurofibromatosis. Proptosis, visual loss, disc swelling, or optic atrophy may occur; however, not all optic nerve and chiasmal gliomas produce visual deficits. Some cause asymptomatic optic nerve enlargement that can remain stable for many years.

*Optic nerve sheath meningiomas* are the second major primary tumor of the optic nerve. They are most prevalent in young to middle-aged women, but can occur in older individuals. Although they tend to occur in an older population than gliomas and usually have a distinct radiologic appearance, occasionally it may be difficult to differentiate between the two types of tumors. Patients with optic nerve sheath meningiomas usually present with proptosis and slowly progressive visual loss. Optic disc swelling, optic atrophy, and optociliary shunt vessels on the optic disc are common.

Treatment of primary optic nerve tumors remains controversial and depends on the extent of visual loss and location of the tumor. Management of these tumors is best left to a neuroophthalmologist or neurosurgeon familiar with current treatment.

*Intracranial meningiomas* growing along the sphenoid ridge or the planum sphenoidal frequently involve the chiasm and optic nerves. They may infiltrate the orbit along the optic nerve sheath and can compress optic nerve causing swelling and visual loss similar to that seen with primary optic nerve sheath meningiomas. En plaque meningiomas are particularly common in women between 40 and 60 years of age. They may be associated with hyperostosis, which can lead to proptosis, often the presenting sign. Neuroimaging is mandatory, and the patient should be referred to a neurosurgeon once the diagnosis is made.

*Dominantly-inherited optic atrophy* is thought to be present from birth. Mild to moderate reduction in visual acuity and decreased color vision are common. Both eyes usually are affected symmetrically, but there may be some degree of variation. Family members are affected in a dominantly inherited pattern. Expression of the abnormality is quite variable, with some individuals manifesting only a mild color vision deficit and better than 20/100 vision. More severely affected individuals may develop nystagmus.

*Nutritional optic neuropathy* is typically associated with an inadequate supply of B-complex vitamins and folate in the diet. These nutritional factors are frequently exacerbated by excessive consumption of alcohol and use of tobacco products, producing classical tobacco alcohol amblyopia. Most significant, however, is the nutritional inadequacy that usually accompanies a diet in which most calories are obtained from alcohol. Resultant visual loss, usually central, can be rapid or insidious.

*Toxic optic neuropathy* can result from exposure to a variety of drugs and toxic substances. The list of medications and environmental substances that can produce toxic optic neuropathy is long and includes many chemotherapeutic agents such as vincristine, mevatricate, and BCNU. Other drugs frequently implicated are ethambutal, fluoroquinolones, isoniazid, quinine, streptomycin, and sulfacetamides. Among the environmental toxins are ethylene glycol mercury and methylalcohol. To diagnose toxic optic neuropathy, patients must be questioned carefully about their working environment, medications, and about drug and alcohol use.

Toxic and nutritional optic neuropathies are typically bilateral and symmetrical. If unilateral involvement occurs, another diagnosis should be suspected. In addition to central visual loss, there may be generalized constriction of the visual field. Optic atrophy can develop, color vision is lost, and visual acuity may decrease to recognition of hand movements only. In nutritional amblyopia, visual acuity can improve if proper diet is restored.

*Traumatic optic neuropathies* occur after closed head injuries or skull fractures. Although the ocular examination may be normal, sudden or subacute visual loss occurs. Visual loss in closed head injury is attributed to shearing forces at the optic canal or microfractures in the skull base that produce optic nerve ischemia and swelling in the canal. When visual loss is sudden, recovery usually does not occur. There is a greater potential for visual recovery with subacute visual loss, which can develop within hours to days after injury. Aggressive treatment with intravenous corticosteroids or surgical decompression of the optic canal can be beneficial in cases where progression of visual loss over time is documented.

*Radiation optic neuropathy* occurs months to years after radiotherapy treatment for primary or secondary intracranial tumors. Because a delay in development of visual loss is common, a relationship to radiation therapy is not always apparent. Usually, the only finding is decreased vision, with a field defect and mild optic disc pallor indicating atrophy. In acute cases, disc pallor may be absent initially. Practitioners should be aware of the possibility of radiation optic neuropathy in any patients with a history of radiotherapy to the head. When the eyes have been included in the irradiated field, the diagnosis becomes easier because characteristic radiation retinopathy with neovascularization, microaneurysms, soft exudate, and arteriolar narrowing likely occurs along with optic disc pallor. Usually, the dose of radiation must exceed 5000 cGy. There is no effective treatment to reduce radiation injury to the optic nerves.

**Optic nerve anomalies.** Congenital anomalies that alter the typical appearance of the optic nerve head can create diagnostic confusion. Some of these anomalies are associated with reduced vision or visual field defects, complicating the diagnosis even more. The most common and important anomaly is pseudopapilledema in which the optic nerve head appears elevated and enlarged with blurred margins. Moderate blind spot enlargement and subtle field defects also may be present. Unlike papilledema, however, pseudopapilledema is not associated with elevated intracranial pressure, the retinal venules are not distended, and spontaneous venous pulsations are frequently present. In pseudopapilledema, hemorrhages around the optic nerve are very unusual.

Pseudopapilledema is usually, but not always, bilateral. Generally, it is completely benign, reflecting a local process at the optic nerve head and not intracranial pathology. Often, refractile crystalline bodies (optic disc drusen) can be seen on or beneath the surface of the optic disc. When drusen are noted, the diagnosis is straightforward; when they are not apparent, however, distinguishing pseudopapilledema from papilledema can be difficult. An expert opinion should be obtained before proceeding with an extensive neuroradiologic investigation.

Other congenital anomalies that affect the shape and size of the optic disc develop at the time the eye and optic nerve are formed. These include tilted optic discs, optic nerve colobomas and pits, and hypoplasia (congenitally underdeveloped optic nerves). Each anomaly has a characteristic morphology and a spectrum of severity. Eyes with the worst anomalies also may be associated with developmental abnormalities of the CNS and usually have poor vision. Mildly anomalous optic nerves are compatible with normal acuity and mild to moderate peripheral visual field defects.

An optic disc anomaly should be suspected when the optic discs appear abnormal in an otherwise healthy individual with no complaints, especially when the rest of the examination is unremarkable and the condition is bilateral and fairly symmetrical. Except for the unusual optic disc appearance, the fundus is quiet, with no evidence of swelling, hemorrhage, infarct, or edema.

### Optic chiasm and the chiasmal syndrome

***Chiasmal compression.*** Most lesions at the chiasm are compressive, producing visual loss in both eyes. The most common cause of chiasmal compression is a pituitary tumor arising from within the sella turcica and extending upward to stretch and compress the chiasm.

Most pituitary tumors are adenomas. In premenopausal women they cause amenorrhea and are discovered early, usually before producing any visual loss. In contrast, nonsecreting pituitary tumors and those in men and in postmenopausal women are usually not detected until they produce visual loss. Other tumors such as craniopharyngiomas, meningiomas, gliomas, and aneurysms also can cause a similar pattern of visual loss by compressing the chiasm.

Pituitary tumors cause slowly progressive, painless visual loss, usually occurring asymmetrically, and characteristic bilateral visual field defects, which are typically bitemporal and asymmetric, but which assume several forms. Occasionally, if hemorrhage or infarction occurs within a pituitary tumor, visual loss can be rapid and associated with severe headache and even loss of consciousness (pituitary apoplexy).

Patients with pituitary tumor often present with endocrinologic disturbances such as amenorrhea and galactorrhea (women) and impotence or decreased libido (men). A hormonal workup, particularly for prolactin levels, is critical in evaluating patients with suspected pituitary tumor. Patients must be asked about endocrine functions such as menstrual cycles, symptoms of acromegaly, and thyroid dysfunction.

When the condition has evolved slowly, the optic nerves appear atrophic, and occasionally a characteristic horizontal band of atrophy may be noted across the optic disc. Not infrequently, changes in the optic nerve may be subtle, even in the presence of a large visual field defect. A relatively normal appearing optic nerve suggests a fairly good potential for visual recovery, which often occurs after surgical decompression in patients with a chiasmal syndrome. Occasionally, tumors of this region may extend into the patient's cavernous sinus causing palsies of the third, fourth, and sixth cranial nerves, which results in diplopia.

All patients suspected of having chiasmal syndrome must undergo formal perimetry. If perimetry confirms a characteristic pattern of visual field loss—normally bitemporal field loss—with some portion of the field deficit in at least one eye respecting the vertical meridian, the next step is to proceed with neuroimaging. MRI is generally more effective than CT in evaluating lesions of the chiasmal region. If a pituitary tumor is demonstrated, management depends on tumor size and whether it secretes prolactin. Prolactin-secreting adenomas can be treated with bromocriptine, which should shrink the tumor and improve symptoms. When this treatment is inappropriate or inadequate, however, a neurosurgeon should be consulted. Most pituitary tumors, even those with marked suprasellar extension, can be decompressed via a transphenoidal approach. Depending on the degree of optic atrophy and type of tumor involved, visual improvement often occurs after treatment. Some patients, however, require lifetime hormonal replacement.

Although chiasmal compression by extrinsic tumor is the most common cause of the chiasmal syndrome, visual loss at the chiasm can be due to compression by an aneurysm, mucocele, abscess, or glioma (chiasmal or hypothalamic). Demyelinating lesions of the optic chiasm, ischemic and traumatic lesions, traction due to chiasmal arachnoiditis, postradiation neuropathy, and prolapse of the chiasm into an empty sella may also be associated with visual loss.

### Visual loss due to postchiasmatic disease

Retrochiasmal lesions involving the optic tract, optic radiations, and cerebral cortex produce homonymous hemianopsia. These lesions can be caused by stroke, tumor, vascular malformations, demyelinating lesions, and abscesses.

Patients who develop a partial or complete homonymous hemianopsia may be unaware of the extent of their visual loss. They may have a vague sense of visual disturbance on the affected side, which they may attribute to a problem with the ipsilateral eye. They may complain of difficulty reading or of bumping into objects on that side. Visual acuity is unaffected in unilateral hemispheric lesions. Occasionally, patients with a tumor or an arteriovenous malformation will experience visual hallucinations contralateral to the affected hemisphere. These may resemble migrainous aura, but are always present on the same side.

Visual field examination is mandatory in the diagnosis of retrochiasmal disease. Thus patients with normal visual acuity should be referred for visual field testing if they complain of difficulty reading and/or difficulty with vision to one side. A visual field obtained on confrontation often can establish the diagnosis with minimal effort.

Although a complete homonymous hemianopsia is nonlocalizing, partial hemianopsias can localize the lesion to the temporal, parietal, or occipital lobes. Visual field defects produced by occipital lesions are exquisitely congruent in both eyes. Patients with occipital lobe lesions also may demonstrate macular sparing; that is, they may have a complete hemianopsia except for a small region of the hemifield extending from central fixation into the hemianopic field. This condition occurs when an infarction of the occipital cortex spares the most posterior portion of the occipital lobe, which is quite common in strokes of this region. Macular sparing is virtually pathognomonic for an infarction of the occipital cortex. Cortical blindness can result from bilateral occipital lobe lesions. When the patient denies blindness, the condition is termed Anton's syndrome. Temporal lobe lesions tend to produce visual field defects that are more dense superiorly in the visual field; parietal lobe lesions tend to produce defects that are denser inferiorly. Temporal and parietal defects are less congruent than those produced by occipital lobe lesions and are usually associated with other neurologic deficits. The least congruent homonymous hemianopsias result from lesions of the optic tract. These lesions occur relatively infrequently.

CT, or preferably MRI, is required in any patient who has a complete or partial homonymous hemianopsia. These examinations usually demonstrate an infarct, tumor, or other CNS lesion. Appropriate management of these neurologic conditions can then be arranged.

### Transient and subjective visual disturbances

Patients frequently complain of transient, temporary, and/or vague visual disturbances that frighten or concern them. It is important to distinguish potentially serious disturbances from the multitude of symptoms that are usually benign. Because objective signs are rare and the symptoms have frequently passed, physicians must rely on the patient's history of the event or events.

The duration of the visual disturbance is critical. Momentary spots or flashes of light indicate vitreous traction or a retinal tear, but are not characteristic of pathology along the retrobulbar visual pathway. Transient visual obscurations lasting less than a minute can occur in papilledema. Transient monocular visual loss that develops as a result of vascular occlusion of the retinal or optic nerve circulation (amaurosis fugax) usually lasts several minutes, but can be prolonged up to one-half hour. The positive and negative visual disturbances that accompany migraine typically last 15 to 20 minutes. They rarely last less than 5 minutes or more than 45 minutes.

Although it is crucial to determine whether the visual loss is monocular or binocular, patients often are unable to make this determination. Patients may also attribute visual loss in one hemifield to a visual disturbance in the ipsilateral eye. For these reasons, care must be taken in interpreting patient descriptions.

The mode of onset and evolution of the visual disturbance, as well as the recovery, further define the pathophysiology. Common symptoms in patients with visual disturbances include dimming or darkening of vision in all or part of the visual field, photopsias, shimmering lights, rings, and arcs of light that can obscure vision. The patient's activity at the time of onset, the nature of onset, changes that occurred during the period of visual loss, and the nature and duration of the recovery help define the visual disturbance. Also, neurologic symptoms such as light-headedness, weakness, numbness, paresthesias, dizziness, and unsteadiness can help localize the disturbance to the anterior or posterior visual pathway.

Amaurosis fugax usually is due to carotid artery stenosis, which produces decreased vascular perfusion of the retina and optic nerve. The carotid artery also can be a source of platelet-fibrin emboli, which may obstruct the central retinal artery or any of its branches. Patients complain of "darkening" or dimming of vision. They often describe a curtain or shade that may rise or fall to obscure part or all of the vision in the affected eye. The onset is usually rapid, and the episode may last seconds or minutes. On examination, whitish Hollenhorst plaques may be seen in the retinal circulation.

When amaurosis fugax is suspected, patients should be asked if they have experienced symptoms suggestive of other transient ischemic attacks, with or without visual loss. Frequently, vascular risk factors, including stroke, are present. Transient neurologic symptoms (paresthesia or weakness) or a carotid bruit may indicate a high-grade stenosis of the carotid artery. These patients are at significant risk of stroke and permanent visual loss. Management requires a complete cardiovascular and cerebrovascular workup and possible treatment with antiplatelet agents, anticoagulants, or endarterectomy.

When similar episodes of transient monocular visual loss occur in a young person in the absence of any risk factors, they can be attributed to retinal migraine. Transient visual loss in retinal migraine is thought to be produced by vasospasm of the retinal artery and is rarely associated with risk of permanent deficit. It is important, however, to determine that the history does not suggest carotid artery dissection, which can cause similar transient visual loss.

Patients presenting with transient photopsias describe flashing lights or spots of light in one eye that last moments but occur sporadically. They should be asked whether their symptoms are more noticeable in the dark and whether they are aggravated by head or eye movement. Movements of the eyes or head that induce flashes or photopsias suggest the possibility of vitreous traction on the retina or, more seriously, retinal tear or detachment. These patients should be referred immediately for dilated ophthalmologic examination, even when they have normal vision and no other complaints.

Photopsias that last from 5 to 45 minutes more typically represent migrainous phenomena. They usually are binocular, but can be monocular if due to retinal migraine. Patients typically refer binocular photopsias occurring in one hemifield to the ipsilateral eye.

A history of a scintillating scotoma or fortification scotoma that expands or contracts, lasts from 15 to 40 minutes, and is followed by a headache is typical of migraine. It is important to ask patients who do not currently experience headache whether they have ever had migraine-like headaches. In older patients, migraine-like symptoms can be caused by vertebrobasilar insufficiency, although this problem is usually associated with other neurologic symptoms such as dizziness, ataxia, or diplopia. If the episodes are always unilateral, an arteriovenous malformation or other intracranial pathology must be suspected, and neuroimaging studies should be ordered.

Patients who complain of blurred vision that changes from day to day may have diabetes with a fluctuating blood sugar level that is not under good control. Other causes of bilateral blurred vision are vasculopathies, hyperviscosity syndromes, hypercoagulation syndromes, and seizures.

Patients may report a variety of visual experiences in which they see distorted or illusory objects as well as hallucinations. Visual illusions and distortions are the altered visual perception of real objects. These phenomena can arise from optical as well as central mechanisms. Hallucinations, on the other hand, are visual perceptions that have no basis in reality. They are generated centrally, although they may be triggered by an external sensory stimulus. They may be related to seizure disorders, intake of a variety of medications and toxic substances, various disease processes, or altered states of consciousness.

Occasionally, a patient presents with factitious visual loss, which may be psychogenic or may represent outright malingering. Differentiation of factitious visual loss from genuine deficits caused by organic disturbances can be difficult. It rests primarily on demonstrating that the pattern of visual loss is inconsistent with normal physiologic constraints by uncovering various inconsistencies in the pattern and degree of visual dysfunction. It is essential to rule out the possibility of an underlying organic defect and to demonstrate that visual function exceeds that claimed by the patient.

## THE OCULAR MOTOR SYSTEM

### Functions of the ocular motor system

An intact ocular motor system is essential for normal vision. Eye movements are responsible for capturing and locking onto a visual object of interest and for maintaining fixation on that object even during head and body movements. To accomplish this an elaborate supranuclear control system has developed involving extensive connections among the visual, vestibular, and ocular motor centers. Disturbances of this system profoundly affect vision and bring patients to their physicians with complaints of double vision, blurred vision, jumpy vision, and more general complaints of unsteadiness, dizziness, and vertigo.

The functions of the ocular motor system can be categorized into five subgroups.

1. Saccades are rapid eye movements that are used to refixate from one object of regard to another. They rapidly execute a foveation reflex, which captures items of interest onto the fovea.
2. The fixation mechanism enables the maintenance of foveation or fixation on an object once it has been "captured."
3. Smooth pursuit movements are slow movements that allow an object to be followed as it moves from place to place.
4. The vestibuloocular mechanism produces reflex eye movements driven by the semicircular canals, which detect head movement. A combination of the smooth pursuit, fixation, and vestibuloocular mechanisms allows continued steady fixation of moving targets during head or whole body movement. All of these mechanisms generate conjugate eye movements; that is, they move both eyes equally and symmetrically in the same direction.
5. In contrast, the vergence mechanism produces disconjugate movement, principally horizontal, which adjusts the position of the two eyes with respect to each other so that fixation is maintained by both eyes on the object of interest.

During normal activity, all of these mechanisms operate simultaneously to produce a seamless pattern of eye movements. To evaluate ocular motor function clinically, it is best to test each of these mechanisms separately.

***Clinical evaluation of ocular motor function.*** Fixation maintenance and smooth pursuit mechanisms are tested by asking the patient to fixate on a target, while slowly moving the target to extreme positions of gaze. During this process, it is important to observe the steadiness of eye position and fixation. If the target motion is slow and steady, any instability in eye movement is abnormal, except in the most extreme positions where physiologic nystagmus can occur. Saccades can be tested by having patients refixate back and forth from a central to a peripheral target held successively up, down, and to each side. The vestibuloocular reflex can be tested by having the patient make rapid head movements (side to side and up and down) while fixating on a distant target. This test does not rely only on the vestibuloocular reflex because visual feedback exists; however, if head movements are rapid, the principal mechanism driving the eye movements is vestibular. Vergence mechanisms can be tested by having a patient refixate between distant and near targets.

When evaluating the ocular motor system, ocular alignment must also be tested by covering first one eye and then the other while looking for movement of the uncovered eye. This test should be performed with the eyes in the primary position and to the left, right, up, and down.

### Symptoms relating to ocular motor disease

Double vision or diplopia is one of the most frequent complaints related to the ocular motor system. Diplopia can be monocular or binocular; therefore when examining a patient with diplopia, it should be determined whether double vision disappears when one eye is covered. If double vision persists with monocular viewing, the patient has monocular diplopia, which is never due to an ocular motor disturbance. Various optical and ocular diseases can combine to cause monocular diplopia; infrequently it can result from CNS pathology. True binocular diplopia always disappears when either eye is covered. Occasionally, patients do not recognize diplopia and simply complain of blurred vision or of letters, print, or sentences running together. Once it is determined that a patient has true binocular diplopia, the patient should be asked the following:

- Whether two perceived images are displaced horizontally, vertically, or obliquely
- Whether one image is tilted with respect to the other
- Which direction of gaze results in the greatest separation of the images and which produces the least
- Whether the diplopia is worse at distance or at near

Typically, lateral rectus muscle weakness produces an esodeviation (inturning eye), which is worse at distance; weakness of the medial rectus muscle produces an exodeviation (outturning eye), which is worse at near. Note, however, that patients may be troubled more by double images that are close to each other than by those that are widely separated.

Diplopia is most frequently due to a benign process and often resolves spontaneously; however, it also can be a medical emergency. Therefore any patient who presents with acute diplopia must be evaluated immediately by a neuro-ophthalmologist or neurologist.

Nystagmus (an involuntary rhythmic oscillation of the eyes) is a cardinal sign of ocular motor dysfunction. Often, patients do not recognize that they have nystagmus; instead, it is discovered by friends or family. Commonly, these patients complain of blurred vision or actual jumpiness of objects, a phenomenon termed oscillopsia.

Ocular motor dysfunction and diplopia also can lead to unsteadiness or a sense of dizziness, or it may be associated with true vertigo. In certain oculomotor disorders patients may have difficulty looking to either side or up or down, and they may complain of difficulty looking at their feet or at a plate of food. Not infrequently, a history of this type of disorder will be revealed only on appropriate questioning.

The patient with an ocular motor disorder may complain of difficulty reading, but when tested visual acuity at distance and near will be perfect. Reading is adversely affected by the patient's inability to make precise movements from one word to another. This problem can occur with ocular motor disturbances that affect saccadic eye movements.

## Disorders of ocular motility

Disturbances of eye movement can be divided topographically into two categories: infranuclear disorders and central or supranuclear disorders. Infranuclear disorders result from lesions in the cranial nerves, extraocular muscles, or the tissue supporting the eyes and their muscles. They frequently affect only one eye and generally present with diplopia. Central disorders upset the control of eye movements and create problems with conjugate gaze. That is, they affect the saccadic, pursuit, or convergence movements of both eyes and may upset the balance or alignment between them.

### *Infranuclear disorders of ocular motility*

**Orbital and systemic diseases.** Diseases that involve the orbital contents can cause disturbances in ocular motility. They can restrict the range of normal eye movements both mechanically and physiologically, producing diplopia.

Thyroid ophthalmopathy is the most common disease affecting orbital tissues, and results in ocular motor symptoms. This condition occurs in a high percentage of patients with Graves' disease. It should be noted, however, that approximately 10% of patients with thyroid ophthalmopathy are clinically euthyroid. Typical signs of thyroid ophthalmopathy include exophthalmos, lid retraction, lid lag, and limitation of eye movement, particularly on attempted upgaze. Patients may or may not have a previous history of thyroid disease. Thyroid ophthalmopathy may simulate other causes of ophthalmoplegia. Typically, however, the abnormal eye movement cannot be explained on the basis of a single or even multiple oculomotor nerve palsies. The diagnosis is established by endocrine investigation, by the presence of other signs of hyperthyroidism, and by demonstrating restriction of eye movements and enlargement of the eye muscles on CT of the orbits. Thyroid ophthalmopathy can pose difficult management problems. Sensory visual function and diplopia must be monitored carefully by an ophthalmologist with experience in managing and treating this condition.

Besides thyroid disease, there are many other causes of mechanically restricted eye movements. Orbital trauma most frequently results in an orbital floor fracture and entrapment of the inferior rectus muscle. The medial rectus muscle also can be caught in a medial wall fracture. Infiltrative diseases (inflammatory or neoplastic) can enlarge one or more orbital muscles causing limitation of eye movement. Orbital myositis can involve one muscle or several muscles and is associated with pain and discomfort. Orbital pseudotumor is a more extensive inflammatory condition affecting the eye muscles, as well as other orbital soft tissue, causing severe pain and limitation of movement. Less frequently, the muscles and soft tissues of the orbit may become infiltrated with lymphoma or an inflammatory process such as sarcoidosis, polymyositis, or Wegener's granulomatosis. Neoplasm can infiltrate the orbit by direct extension from adjacent sinuses and periorbital tissues or by metastatic spread from distant sites.

**Chronic progressive external ophthalmoplegia (CPEO).** CPEO is a group of syndromes that result in a slow gradual loss of eye movements. Progressive bilateral ptosis is an early sign, with affected individuals gradually developing a generalized ophthalmoplegia over many years. Diplopia may not occur because the eyes can remain aligned in the primary position, although their movements become extremely limited. A variety of associated conditions coexist with CPEO including heart block, pigmentary retinopathy, ataxia, myopathy, and weakness elsewhere. Patients may complain only of bilateral ptosis and may have a vague sense of difficulty looking to the side. Most forms of chronic, progressive external ophthalmoplegia are related to mitochondrial disease, and muscle biopsy reveals ragged red fibers characteristic of mitochondrial myopathy. Because the risk of heart block and sudden death is not insignificant, CPEO can be potentially life-threatening.

**Myasthenia gravis.** Myasthenia gravis, a condition that can affect all skeletal muscles, is prone to affect the extraocular muscles, particularly those that elevate the eyelids. Isolated ocular myasthenia occurs in 20% of patients and can pose a diagnostic challenge to clinicians. Myasthenia gravis can mimic almost any ocular motor disorder—from single nerve palsies to complete ophthalmoplegias. Its distinguishing characteristics, however, are fatigability and variability. The ptosis that occurs in myasthenia varies with the time of the day and usually worsens toward evening. Patients often relate that their lids open normally in the mornings, but become increasingly ptotic as the day progresses. Diplopia, when present, may also worsen later in the day. Fatigue is demonstrated when the clinician has the patient look steadily upward for several minutes, without blinking. The eyelids will gradually descend over the globe in affected individuals. Diplopia, when present, may also worsen later in the day.

Myasthenia gravis results from defective synaptic transmission at the motor end plates due to the presence of antibodies to the acetylcholine receptors. The diagnosis can be confirmed by demonstrating an elevation of circulating acetylcholine receptor antibodies; by testing with Tensilon, which produces a transient improvement in lid position; or by having the patient rest his or her eyes for a half hour and noting improvement in lid position and ocular alignment. Further confirmation can be obtained by demonstrating characteristic electromyographic disturbances in skeletal or ocular muscles.

Definitive diagnosis and treatment are best handled by a neurologist. Treatment is usually oral pyridostigmine bromide (Mestinon), but in resistant cases corticosteroids or azathioprine can be added. A CT of the chest determines whether the thymus gland is enlarged. If it is, surgical resection is recommended.

**Ocular motor palsies.** Three paired cranial nerves are responsible for innervating the extraocular muscles and producing eye movements. A dysfunction in any of these nerves can cause diplopia in one or more positions of gaze. There are numerous causes of such dysfunction; some affect more than one of the nerves, whereas others are specific for a particular nerve. Patients may present with single or multiple nerve palsies that affect movements in one or both eyes.

***Sixth nerve palsy.*** The most easily recognized isolated ocular nerve palsy involves the sixth cranial nerve producing weakness in the ipsilateral lateral rectus muscle. Patients complain of horizontal double vision that worsens when they look toward the side of the affected nerve. On examination a limitation of abduction is seen when the patient looks in the direction of the weak lateral rectus muscle. Lateral rectus weakness can be caused by any of the orbital diseases already described; however, if there is no evidence to suggest orbital involvement, a diagnosis of sixth nerve palsy can be made.

The sixth nerve passes through the cavernous sinus and can be compromised by diseases of this region. Conditions such as an intracavernous carotid artery aneurysm or fistula, meningioma, or metastatic disease, as well as infection and inflammation such as the Tolosa-Hunt syndrome, can cause sixth nerve dysfunction. Nasopharyngeal carcinoma and pituitary tumors also can invade the cavernous sinus from adjacent regions. Tracing the course of the sixth nerve proximally, it turns caudally to descend down the clivus toward the pons. This segment of the nerve can be compromised by tumor, head trauma, or by elevated intracranial pressure. Carcinomatosis meningitis can also involve the sixth nerve in the prepontine portion of its course. Gradenigo's syndrome, which develops when an otitis media spreads to involve the sixth nerve, occurs principally in children. Finally, CNS disease such as tumor, stroke, and multiple sclerosis can affect the sixth nerve fasciculus within the pons; usually other brainstem structures are involved so that additional oculomotor and neurologic abnormalities coexist.

The most common etiology of an acute isolated sixth nerve palsy is idiopathic. Presumably, these cases result from small vessel infarction along the course of the sixth nerve, most probably in its intracavernous portion. This infarction occurs more frequently in patients with vasculopathic histories, including diabetes and hypertension. Usually, idiopathic sixth nerve palsies resolve spontaneously within 2 to 3 months.

Congenital abnormalities and those acquired early in childhood can sometimes be confused with sixth nerve palsies. Patients with Möbius' syndrome may appear to have bilateral sixth nerve palsies, but they also have facial diplegia, clubbed foot, branchial malformations, and abnormalities of their pectoral muscles. Patients with Duane's syndrome have unilateral or occasionally bilateral absence of the sixth nerve, with limitation of abduction and sometimes adduction. The globe retracts on attempted adduction.

***Fourth nerve palsy.*** The fourth nerve is the only cranial nerve to exit from the dorsal surface of the brain. It leaves the posterior midbrain, crosses to the opposite side, and travels beneath the tentorium and then through the cavernous sinus to innervate the contralateral superior oblique muscle.

Patients with fourth nerve palsy complain of vertical or oblique double vision, which becomes worse when they look downward. They may assume a characteristic head posture in which their head is turned and titled away from the affected side. Because of its relationship to the tentorium, the fourth nerve is subject to physical injury during head trauma. For this reason, fourth nerve palsies are most frequently associated with trauma.

Idiopathic fourth nerve palsies, attributed to microvascular infarction along the nerve, also are common. They usually resolve spontaneously with time. Tumors rarely cause fourth nerve palsies, although myasthenia and orbital disease can occasionally mimic this disorder. Patients with congenital fourth nerve palsies have a long history of abnormal head posture, which can be revealed by examining old photographs. The fourth nerve also can be compromised by the same cavernous sinus and brainstem diseases that produce sixth nerve palsies.

***Third nerve palsies.*** The third nerve is the largest and most important cranial nerve involved with eye movements. It innervates the superior, inferior, and medial rectus muscles, as well as the inferior oblique and levator palpebrae. It also innervates the pupil and ciliary body, producing pupillary constriction and accommodation. Thus a complete third nerve palsy immobilizes most eye movements. Nevertheless, patients often develop a partial third nerve palsy that does not affect all of its components. Thus third nerve palsies present with a variety of symptoms and findings. Patients usually complain of horizontal or oblique diplopia, but they may not complain of diplopia if the ptotic eyelid covers the eye. In partial third nerve palsies consideration must be given to the possibility of myasthenia gravis or orbital disease, especially if the pupil is spared.

Orbital or cavernous sinus diseases can cause third nerve palsies, but typically one or more of the fourth, fifth, or sixth cranial nerves are also involved. Of greatest concern, third nerve palsies may arise as a result of compression by an aneurysm of the posterior communicating artery or as a result of uncal herniation. Strokes and demyelinating disease, as well as brainstem tumors, can cause lesions of the third nerve nucleus or fasciculus in the midbrain. These lesions usually produce other neurologic abnormalities. Nuclear lesions produce bilateral ptosis and weakness of the contralateral superior rectus muscle.

One of the most common causes of third nerve palsy is microvascular infarction, which typically spares the pupil; however, some of these patients can have partial pupillary involvement. Small vessel infarction tends to affect the interpeduncular or intercavernous portions of the nerve and generally resolves within 2 to 3 months. It is much more common in patients with diabetes, hypertension, and other vasculopathies.

***Multiple ocular motor nerve palsies.*** As previously stated, diseases affecting the cavernous sinus and orbital apex frequently cause multiple ocular motor nerve palsies. The optic nerve and trigeminal nerve also may be involved. These diseases may mimic myasthenia gravis and other orbital diseases that cause multiple extraocular muscle dysfunction. However, in the absence of clinical signs of these diseases, careful investigation of the cranial nerves traversing the cavernous sinus and neuroimaging of that region are mandatory when a combination of ocular motor palsies occur. If there is associated pain, inflammatory disease of the cavernous sinus (Tolosa-Hunt syndrome) should be suspected.

Another condition that may produce multiple ocular motor nerve palsies is the Fisher variant of the Guillain-Barré syndrome. Patients develop acute onset of diplopia and ptosis often after an upper respiratory tract infection, resulting from involvement of multiple extraocular muscles bilaterally. Pupillary involvement is variable and when present distinguishes this condition from myasthenia gravis. Associated neurologic abnormalities include ataxia and loss of the deep tendon reflexes. The condition resolves spontaneously, but may last several months.

***Investigation of ocular motor palsies.*** Isolated fourth and sixth nerve palsies are rarely emergencies. Microvascular infarction is the most frequent cause in the absence of a history suggesting trauma. A blood glucose test to rule out diabetes and an ESR to check for temporal arteritis in patients older than 50 should be obtained. If myasthenia gravis is considered in the differential diagnosis, a Tensilon test should be arranged and acetylcholine antibodies measured. Neuroimaging studies should be performed only on those patients who have other cranial nerve involvement or other neurologic abnormalities, or in whom orbital disease is suspected. Acute third nerve palsies, on the other hand, can be much more serious, particularly when they are caused by aneurysm. If the pupil is involved, neuroimaging studies and cerebral angiography should be obtained immediately in acute cases. If the pupil is spared, and particularly if the patient has a history of diabetes or hypertension, the patient may be observed and a broader differential diagnosis can be considered. As already indicated, multiple ocular motor nerve palsies are virtually synonymous with cavernous sinus disease. Multiplanar MRI with gadolinium will uncover cavernous sinus involvement that is otherwise difficult to demonstrate. Consideration also must be given to myasthenia gravis and thyroid disease, which mimic multiple ocular motor nerve palsies.

*Central (supranuclear) disorders of ocular motility.* CNS disorders such as stroke and brain tumor affect the conjugate movements of both eyes and also may disturb the balance or alignment between the eyes and the coordination of eye movements. In contrast, peripheral ocular motor nerve disorders generally affect one eye or, if they involve both eyes, tend to affect them asymmetrically. Eye movement abnormalities produced by lesions in the CNS include disorders of both horizontal and vertical conjugate gaze, skew deviations, ocular dysmetria, and many forms of nystagmus.

**Disorders of conjugate gaze.** Conjugate gaze depends on a flow of impulses from centers in the brain including the cerebral hemispheres, midbrain, pons, and cerebellum, as well as the pathways that connect them. Thus lesions of the CNS frequently produce disorders of eye movement.

The inability to move both eyes to one side is called a horizontal gaze palsy; it results from a lesion in the pons that damages either the ipsilateral paramedian pontine reticular formation (PPRF) or the ipsilateral sixth nerve nucleus. Bilateral lesions in the pons can cause a complete bilateral horizontal gaze palsy, while leaving vertical movements preserved. Less complete lesions in this region may result in partial horizontal gaze palsies or in gaze evoked nystagmus, i.e., nystagmus on attempted gaze with rapid beats in the direction of gaze. Usually, other neurologic deficits are present.

Hemispheric disorders and those involving the upper brainstem can produce similar horizontal gaze palsies, but these are typically transient and usually can be overcome by reflex horizontal eye movements generated by the vestibular nuclei with head movement (doll's head maneuver) or by caloric stimulation.

Vertical gaze depends on intact centers in the midbrain. Diseases that affect the dorsal midbrain produce upgaze paresis and may also produce light/near dissociation of the pupils and characteristic convergence-retraction nystagmus. In the young patient this condition is commonly due to a pinealoma or hydrocephalus, whereas in older patients infarction is more usual. Down-gaze paresis occurs less frequently than upgaze and results from a bilateral midbrain lesion in the region of the red nuclei. While infarction may precipitate a sudden down-gaze palsy, difficulty with down-gaze frequently develops slowly in association with Parkinson's disease, progressive supranuclear palsy, and a variety of diffuse neurodegenerative diseases.

Midbrain lesions also can cause a vertical misalignment between the two eyes (skew deviation). *Skew deviation* is a term reserved for vertical ocular motor imbalances that result from supranuclear (i.e., central) disorders. A skew deviation may resemble a fourth nerve palsy superficially, but usually does not include all the characteristic features of a fourth nerve palsy. In addition, skew deviations rarely occur in isolation and are usually accompanied by other central disorders of ocular motility and other neurologic signs.

Internuclear ophthalmoplegia (INO) is a common central disorder of ocular motility that results from a lesion of the medial longitudinal fasciculus between the pons and midbrain. It causes weakness of the medial rectus muscle on the ipsilateral side and produces a partial or complete adduction palsy accompanied by abducting nystagmus of the contralateral eye. INO can be unilateral or bilateral and may occur in relative isolation. In young adults and especially women, acute bilateral INO is highly suggestive of multiple sclerosis. Unilateral INO in elderly patients is more typical of a small lacunar infarct and is frequently associated with diabetes, vasculitides such as systemic lupus erythematosus, aneurysm, and a variety of other conditions.

Central disorders can selectively disrupt rapid or slow eye movements. Disturbances of rapid refixation eye movement (saccades) produce ocular dysmetria, which can cause the affected person to undershoot or overshoot the intended visual target. More severe disorders of saccadic movement can generate ocular flutter (brief bursts consisting of reversing saccades) and, in the worst cases, opsoclonus (back-to-back, continuous unrestrainable saccades, "saccadomania"). Saccadic dysmetria, flutter, and opsoclonus occur in cerebellar and brainstem disease. Specifically, opsoclonus can be a component of a paraneoplastic syndrome such as neuroblastoma in children or oat-cell carcinoma in adults. Loss of rapid eye movements occurs in a variety of degenerative disorders such as Wilson's disease, spinocerebellar degenerations, and progressive supranuclear palsy.

Children can manifest a congenital absence of rapid eye movements called congenital ocular motor apraxia. During the first 2 years of life, these children develop head thrusts that compensate for their inability to make normal refixation movements. As indicated earlier, saccadic palsies that occur with lesions in the cerebral hemispheres and brainstem, whether partial or incomplete, also may result in an inability to initiate refixation movements or in slowed or hypometric saccades.

Disorders impairing slow eye movements used in smooth pursuit result in jerky movements termed saccadic pursuit. This finding is not always indicative of disease, but may be caused by fatigue, drugs, or lack of attention. When asymmetric, saccadic pursuit is likely due to an organic disease of the brainstem, cerebellum, or parietooccipital junction of the cerebrum.

Vergence system dysfunction is frequently psychogenic, and it may be difficult to separate organic disease from a factitious abnormality. A paresis of convergence can occur after infarction, demyelination, or head trauma. Patients complain of diplopia occurring at near range only and have no obvious limitation or abnormality in their eye movements, except for the inability to converge. When this symptom has been present for a long time and is associated with longstanding reading difficulties, it may be a true convergence insufficiency, which is congenital and not due to neurologic disease.

Patients who continue to converge, even when attempting to fixate at a distance, may have spasm of the near reflex, which includes convergence spasm, excessive accommodation, and pupillary constriction. Excessive accommodation causes these patients to complain of blurred vision. While convergence spasm is associated with organic diseases, such as neurosyphilis, trauma, and encephalitis, it is related to stress and psychogenic causes.

Divergence palsy occurs rarely and results in the acute onset of esotropia and diplopia, with full preservation of eye movements. It may follow systemic illness and is usually benign and self-limited; however, it also can be caused by demyelinating disease, neurosyphilis, encephalitis, and trauma.

**Evaluation of patients with central disorders of ocular motility.** Patients may present with vague symptoms that may not easily characterize their ocular motor disturbance. While diplopia may be a prominent symptom, other patients may complain of blurred vision, difficulty looking to one side, difficulty reading, running together of words, blurred vision when looking to one side, difficulty focusing at near gaze, or jumpiness of targets (oscillopsia).

Any time a patient's symptoms suggest a central disorder affecting eye movements, the attending physician should try to uncover other neurologic symptoms. A complete ocular motor examination is essential. Fixation must be observed in all positions and a cover test performed to evaluate ocular alignment. The range of eye movements in all directions, steadiness of fixation, saccadic refixations, smooth pursuit movements, and convergence should be tested. Finally, reflex eye movements should be evaluated by observing the doll's head response to head rotation and Bell's phenomenon: Elevation of the globe during forced eye closure.

### Nystagmus

The term *nystagmus* describes a group of involuntary ocular movements that are rhythmic and oscillatory. The two major categories of nystagmus are jerk nystagmus, which consists of a slow phase in one direction followed by a fast phase in the opposite direction, and pendular nystagmus in which movements in both directions are equal in velocity. Ocular oscillations that are involuntary and recurrent but not rhythmic also occur; these are called nystagmoid movements.

***Physiologic nystagmus.*** These following situations will evoke nystagmus in normal individuals:

- Extreme gaze in any direction can result in *end-point nystagmus,* a jerk nystagmus with fast phase in the direction of gaze.
- *Optokinetic nystagmus* is a jerk nystagmus that develops when a subject views a repetitive visual stimulus. The slow phase of the nystagmus occurs when the subject follows the moving target; this phase is interrupted by fast phases as the eyes return to refixate on to another target entering the visual field.
- *Vestibularly induced nystagmus* can result from the effect on the semicircular canals of whole body rotation or caloric stimulation.

***Congenital motor nystagmus.*** Congenital motor nystagmus results from a primary ocular motor system abnormality. The nystagmus may be pendular or jerk. Typically, complex cycles of repetitive eye movements are generated. The amplitude of the nystagmus decreases with convergence. Acuity is mildly reduced, and patients do not complain of oscillopsia.

An early infantile form of nystagmus can result from sensory (visual) deprivation. This sensory form of "congenital" nystagmus usually develops between 2 and 3 months of age in a child with abnormally decreased central vision. Sensory deprivation nystagmus is typically pendular and also may decrease with convergence.

***Latent nystagmus.*** Latent nystagmus is demonstrated only when one eye is occluded; it is a jerk nystagmus that beats away from the occluded eye. It is seen frequently in children with strabismus and amblyopia and may be bilateral or unilateral.

It is important to note that the physiologic, congenital, and latent forms of nystagmus are benign and that they differ from the pathologic forms. Patients with congenital or physiologic nystagmus may be unaware of their condition and do not have symptoms of oscillopsia. They may have decreased central vision, but this is longstanding.

***Acquired types of nystagmus.*** Most forms of acquired nystagmus produce ocular oscillations that involve both eyes fairly equally; however, some forms of nystagmus may produce asymmetric nystagmus or exclusive involvement of only one eye. Acquired nystagmus is usually of the jerk form and can be divided into two major subcategories: nystagmus due to disorders of the peripheral vestibular apparatus and nystagmus due to disorders of the CNS.

Peripheral nystagmus develops when there is a loss of vestibular function. It is usually purely horizontal, or horizontal and rotatory. Purely vertical or tortional nystagmus is unusual with peripheral vestibular disease. Peripheral nystagmus is frequently acute in onset and associated with severe vertigo. Symptoms can be recurrent, transient, and last days to weeks; but they usually resolve with time. Postural effects and hearing deficits are not uncommon. The common causes are infectious disease involving the labyrinth (labyrinthitis) or the vestibular nerve (neuronitis), Meniere's disease, or trauma.

Central nystagmus is much more variable and usually is not associated with severe vertigo. Symptoms may be transient or permanent. The nystagmus may beat in both directions depending on eye position, and in some forms the direction may change over time. Central nystagmus often is a result of a brainstem or cerebellar lesion caused by demyelinating disease, vascular infarction, or tumor.

The pattern of nystagmus has many variations, some of which have particular pathognomonic or localizing significance. Acquired nystagmus should always be investigated by a neurologist, ophthalmologist, or otolaryngologist familiar with its variations. A multiplicity of rhythmic ocular oscillations, many of them vertical, can affect the eyes and are usually pathognomonic for lesions in specific regions of the brainstem. These special forms of nystagmus include up-beating and down-beating vertical nystagmus, ocular myoclonus, ocular bobbing, convergence-retraction nystagmus, rebound nystagmus, and periodic alternating nystagmus. Some forms of nystagmus respond to medications, but most are resistant to any therapy.

## The pupil

***Evaluating the pupillary response.*** Observation of the pupillary responses is one of the most important components of the routine physical and ophthalmic examinations. Pupil size should be evaluated in both bright and dim illumination while the patient fixates on a distant object. Any difference in pupil size (anisocoria) should be noted, with particular attention to whether the difference increases in bright or dim light.

The light response of each pupil should then be evaluated independently. Next, the pupils are examined for a relative afferent pupillary defect (Marcus Gunn pupil) by swinging a flashlight back and forth from one eye to the other while noting pupillary responses. Both eyes must be stimulated equally and symmetrically. If the pupils are unequal to begin with, it may be helpful to observe the reaction of one pupil to stimulation of the ipsilateral and contralateral eyes during the swinging flashlight test.

Finally, the pupillary reaction when the eyes converge and accommodate onto a near target should be observed. It is important to ask the patient about the use of eye drops and oral medications, as they may affect pupillary response and size.

***The dilated or nonreacting pupil.*** If a patient's larger pupil does not constrict well to a light stimulus and the anisocoria increases with greater light levels, the patient has a form of pupillary sphincter palsy. Once local disease in the eye (e.g., history of trauma, ocular inflammation) is ruled out, only three causes for dilated pupil remain: (1) compression or other lesion of the third cranial nerve, (2) parasympathetic denervation of the pupil due to injury or lesion in the ciliary ganglion that produces an Adie's pupil, and, (3) pharmacologic block of the pupillary sphincter. Therefore when confronted with a dilated pupil, the physician must search for other signs of a third nerve palsy such as ptosis, diplopia, or ocular motor paresis. Even when these conditions are not present, a dilated, sluggish, or nonreactive pupil can be a sign of third nerve compression, which can result from uncal herniation or posterior communicating artery aneurysm. Therefore if recent in onset or acute, a dilated pupil is considered a medical emergency, particularly when accompanied by headache or other neurologic signs. However, if the pupil has been dilated for at least a few weeks and the reaction to a near stimulus produces slow constriction, followed by an even slower redilation after the near stimulus is removed, the diagnosis is likely to be *Adie's pupil.* This benign condition is usually unilateral, but may be bilateral. Adie's pupil is supersensitive to dilute solutions of pilocarpine and can be positively identified if 0.1% pilocarpine constricts the pupil. Patients with Adie's pupil may complain of difficulty reading because of accommodative paresis, but usually the dilated pupil is an incidental finding. The condition is believed to be a result of damage to the ciliary ganglion due to infectious (viral) or vascular disease.

Sometimes patients introduce substances into the eye that dilate the pupil pharmacologically. These pupils react poorly to both light and near stimulation and do not react to 1% pilocarpine. Thus they can be distinguished from Adie's pupil and the dilated pupil seen with lesions of the third nerve, both of which constrict with pilocarpine. A dilated pupil may also result from direct or indirect trauma. The pupillary sphincter may be damaged during surgery or as a result of penetrating injury to the globe or indirectly by blunt trauma to the globe. Trauma to the iris usually can be detected by slit lamp examination. Depending on the extent of damage, the pupil may constrict to pilocarpine. Occasionally, the pupil remains dilated as a result of previous intraocular disease such as inflammation, rubeosis, trauma, or surgery. Other less common causes of an unreactive pupil are congenital anomalies, central iris atrophy, and tumors involving the anterior chamber of the eye.

***The constricted or small pupil.*** If the two pupils are unequal in size and the pupillary light reaction appears normal, the anisocoria is either physiologic or the patient may have Horner's syndrome. Physiologic anisocoria occurs in 20% of the normal population. Additionally, many elderly individuals have involutional ptosis, which also may be asymmetric. Horner's syndrome is characterized by a slight ptosis of the ipsilateral upper lid and a minor elevation of the lower lid causing narrowing of the palpebral fissure. Patients may complain that their eye appears smaller. In addition to the ptosis and miosis, patients with Horner's syndrome may have anhydrosis (decreased sweating on the ipsilateral forehead region). Horner's syndrome is suspected by observing an increase in anisocoria in dim light and a decrease in bright light. Pharmacologic testing for Horner's syndrome is performed by instilling 4%, 5%, or 10% cocaine drops in both eyes. Normal pupils dilate over 40 minutes, but in Horner's syndrome the pupil dilates much less, if at all. Thus the anisocoria increases. Care must be taken, however, in patients with dark irides, as the response to cocaine may be minimal in both eyes. If the anisocoria does not increase with the cocaine test, the patient does not have Horner's syndrome. If the anisocoria increases after instillation of cocaine, the diagnosis of Horner's syndrome is confirmed, implying a lesion of the sympathetic pathway. Hydroxyamphetamine, 1%, drops can be used on a subsequent visit to determine whether the lesion in the sympathetic pathway is preganglionic or postganglionic. Postganglionic lesions are distal to the superior cervical ganglion, whereas preganglionic lesions are more proximal or central. Hydroxyamphetamine does not dilate a miotic pupil resulting from a postganglionic lesion, but does dilate the pupil if there is a preganglionic lesion.

Horner's syndrome is frequently observed in asymptomatic patients and may be longstanding. It is helpful to review old photographs of the patient to determine the duration of the ptosis and the anisocoria. Congenital Horner's syndrome can arise as a result of birth trauma, but it is also associated with a lightly pigmented iris on the affected side. In the absence of a history of birth trauma, a child with Horner's syndrome should undergo radiologic studies to exclude the presence of a tumor in the mediastinum or cervical region. In adults a postganglionic Horner's syndrome is almost always benign and is frequently associated with a history of migraine headaches. Preganglionic lesions are more ominous and are often a result of neoplasm affecting the cervical region or brainstem. Because preganglionic lesions can be a sign of internal carotid dissection, a high order of suspicion is appropriate when a patient presents with severe radiating neck pain, headache, and new onset Horner's syndrome.

When caused by a central lesion, Horner's syndrome usually is associated with other neurologic abnormalities. Patients with preganglionic lesions therefore require a complete neurologic examination including a careful examination of the neck and thyroid gland. Imagining studies of the mediastinum, neck, and brain are recommended to rule out neoplasm. If carotid dissection is suspected magnetic resonance angiography and/or selective cerebral arteriography will be required. If old photographs establish that the Horner's syndrome has been present for years, however, investigation is not indicated, even in preganglionic cases.

***Other abnormalities of the pupil.*** Episodic dilation of the pupil lasting minutes to hours can occur in otherwise healthy patients. It may be associated with headache, blurred vision, or photophobia. Patients are rarely seen during episodes, and when examined they usually are normal. In such cases, the condition is considered benign and further investigation is not indicated.

Patients with severe neurologic lesions or on certain drugs may have small, but reactive pupils. Light/near dissociation (i.e., a good response to an accommodative target, but a poor response to light stimulation) occurs in any patient with severe visual impairment; but in the presence of normal vision, it occurs in patients who have midbrain lesions, a long history of diabetes, alcoholism, or late syphilis (Argyll-Robertson pupils).

## BIBLIOGRAPHY


Burde RM, Savino PJ, Trobe D: *Clinical decisions in neuro-ophthalmology,* ed 2, St Louis, 1992, Mosby.

Hedges TR III: *Consultation in ophthalmology,* Philadelphia, 1987, BC Decker.

Heuven WAJ, van Zwaan JT: *Decision making in ophthalmology.* Philadelphia, 1992, BC Decker.

Newman NM: *Neuro-ophthalmology: a practical text,* New York, 1992, Appleton & Lange.

# XII Pulmonary Disease

## Chapter 111 Common Cold

Barry M. Bernstein

The common cold is believed to result in more physician visits, more lost days of work, and more school absences than any other infectious disease. Over 200 agents have been identified as causative, including rhinoviruses, coronaviruses, parainfluenza and influenza viruses, adenoviruses, and respiratory syncytial virus. *Mycoplasma pneumoniae, Chlamydia pneumoniae,* and group A β-hemolytic streptococci have also been implicated as causing similar clinical syndromes. Despite improved understanding of the etiology of this clinical syndrome, much of the epidemiology, pathophysiology, and treatment is unknown. This chapter discusses the clinical manifestations of the common cold, including those features which are suggestive of specific etiology and those which imply possible complications.

### ETIOLOGY

As mentioned above, the etiologies of the common cold have only recently been identified. Most studies have suggested that the most common identifiable cause of the common cold is the rhinovirus, accounting for 30% to 40% of cases. Other identified etiologies include coronavirus, parainfluenza, influenza, respiratory syncitial virus, adenovirus, and enterovirus. Nonviral etiologies of the common cold syndrome include group A β-hemolytic streptococci, *Mycoplasma pneumoniae,* and *Chlamydia pneumoniae* (Table 111-1). Syndromes often overlap significantly, making differentiation on clinical grounds alone very difficult. Nonviral etiologies for similar symptoms should be carefully considered in the differential diagnosis, since some are treatable, and some, such as group A β-hemolytic streptococcal infection, may result in serious sequelae. The specific clinical syndromes associated with these etiologies are discussed in the clinical manifestations section.

**Table 111-1.** Etiology of common cold symptoms

| Etiology | Percent (%) |
|---|---|
| **Viruses** | |
| Rhinovirus | 30-40 |
| Coronavirus | 5-10 |
| **Other** | |
| Respiratory syncitial virus, adenovirus, enterovirus, influenza, parainfluenza | 10-20 |
| **Bacteria** | |
| Group A β-hemolytic streptococci | 10 |
| **Unknown** | 20-45 |

### EPIDEMIOLOGY

The common cold occurs with greater frequency than any other infectious disease. The National Health Interview Surveys conducted in the early 1980s have shed light on the overall impact of the common cold in the United States. In these surveys 30,000 to 50,000 households were selected to complete extensive health history questionnaires. The 1980 survey estimated 75 million visits to office physicians were prompted by symptoms of the common cold. The 1981 survey estimated 112 million influenza-like infections in the United States during the preceding 12 months. The common cold was second, with 93 million episodes in the prior year, an attack rate of 41.1 per 100 persons per year. The enormous morbidity of these infections was noted as well. Over 250 million days of restricted activity were attributed to the common cold alone, with almost 150 million days of lost work in 1981 attributed to upper respiratory tract infections.

The annual incidence of infections by age and sex was reported by Monto in a study of 14,600 respiratory tract illnesses in the 4905 residents of Tecumseh, Michigan. The highest incidence of infection occurred in those less than 1 year of age (6.1 per year). With increasing age the incidence gradually fell to 1.3 per year in those patients over 60 years old. Of note, a slight increase in cases was seen in young adults (ages 20 to 29), probably due to greater exposure to young children. This increase is most marked in women. Seasonal variation in the incidence of the common cold has also been noted, with adults averaging six to eight colds per 1000 persons per day in the peak respiratory disease season. This level falls to only two to three colds per 1000 persons per day in the summer months. A number of possible explanations for this seasonal variation have been proposed. Crowding of children in schools and increased indoor activity of adults probably accounts for some of this variation. However, other variables may play a significant role. Relative humidity has been postulated to affect survival of viruses, particularly enveloped viruses. These viruses have greater survival in low humidity, as found in colder months of the year. Seasonal variation may also be virus specific. Influenza and coranovirus infections are more common in the winter, adenovirus in the spring and early summer, rhinovirus in the early fall and late spring, and coxsackievirus in the late summer and early fall.

The major determinant of the incidence of the common cold is risk of exposure. Although patients with underlying respiratory tract disease, including smokers, may have more severe colds, they occur no more frequently than in the general population. Tonsillectomy has not been shown to decrease the incidence of the common cold. Exposure to cold, damp conditions had, for years, been felt to be a risk factor for more frequent and severe colds. Douglas, in a carefully controlled study, evaluated the effect of cold temperature exposure at the time of experimental inoculation, incubation, illness, and recovery from rhinovirus infection. The results were compared to those from volunteers exposed to the same virus, but without cold temperature exposure. Infection rates, incubation period, clinical illness, and recovery were similar in the two groups.

## TRANSMISSION

The exact mode of transmission of the common cold is the subject of much misunderstanding and in many ways is not well understood. In part this reflects the multiple etiologies of cold symptoms, and in part the paucity of well-controlled trials to document spread in the natural environment. Most information on spread relates to rhinovirus, the most frequent identifiable cause of the common cold.

Rhinovirus transmission occurs most commonly in the home, where up to 50% of contacts develop infection. Frequent transmission also occurs in the school. The principal reservoir is the nose of the schoolchild. Clinical studies of rhinovirus transfer have suggested prolonged, close contact is essential for transmission. Transmission occurs most often on the third day after inoculation of the donor, usually within the first 24 hours of symptomatic disease. Gwaltney studied the efficiency of several methods of transmission, including hand contact, exposure by air across a double wire partition, and exposure by air around a small table. The most efficient mode of transmission was hand to hand, a system where the donor deliberately contaminated the hands immediately before hand-to-hand contact with the recipient. In this model 11 of 15 volunteers were infected. The wire barrier exposure group of patients were together in the same air space for 72 hours. No infections occurred among 10 recipient patients. In the small table model donors attempted to shower recipients with secretions by coughing and singing. Again, little transmission occurred (1 of 10 infected).

The reason aerosol spread of rhinovirus appears uncommon is unknown. Studies have demonstrated that sneezing and nose blowing produce large particle aerosols, whereas coughing produces more small particle aerosols. Although rhinovirus is present in the nasal secretions of patients, attempts to isolate the virus by coughing or sneezing onto Petri dishes were largely unsuccessful. Both failure of incorporation of rhinovirus into an aerosol and dilution of the virus in the aerosol have been proposed as explanations for the relative lack of infectivity via this route.

The duration of infectivity of the common cold depends, in part, on the specific etiology of the symptom complex. Cold viruses are generally not present in asymptomatic individuals. Rhinovirus shedding may persist for up to several weeks, with maximum concentration of virus in the first 2 to 4 days of symptoms. The coronavirus may be detectable in secretions for only 1 to 4 days, and influenza for 5 to 10 days after viral shedding begins.

## PATHOGENESIS

Although infection of the upper respiratory tract with the agents responsible for the common cold underlies the pathophysiology of these infections, the mechanisms of infection, host response, and subsequent symptom formation are poorly understood. As with studies on transmission of common colds, most information available on pathogenesis also relates to rhinoviruses. Receptor sites for human rhinovirus type 16 have been identified on an intercellular adhesion molecule known as ICAM-1. Subsequent infection results in shedding of ciliated epithelial cells. It is interesting that no correlation is seen between numbers of shed cells and severity of symptoms. The infection appears to begin in the posterior nasopharynx and spreads anteriorly. Shedding of virus may occur after symptoms have resolved, suggesting that viral replication may not correlate with symptom development. Inflammatory mediators may also play a role in symptom severity. Although histamines seem to play only a minor role in severity of symptoms, the presence of kinins may significantly exacerbate symptoms. Proud measured kinin levels in nasal lavages from 16 patients with naturally acquired rhinovirus infections. In 11 of 16 subjects increases in kinin levels were noted during infection. These levels were significantly greater than levels in subjects with asymptomatic infections. Studies in volunteers have also shown that intranasal challenge with bradykinins results in upper respiratory tract symptoms.

Control of infection may be related to local production of interferons. The cellular immune response to rhinovirus infections has also been examined. A mild increase in peripheral white blood cell count associated with a slight decrease in circulating lymphocyte counts has been noted. Edema and hyperemia of the submucosa are the predominant histopathologic findings and may be focal. Local cellular response to infection includes increases in both lymphocytes and polymorphonuclear neutrophil leukocytes (PMNs) in nasal secretions. Mucosal biopsies show infiltration with PMNs but not lymphocytes. The relative role of each in host defense and symptom production is unknown. However, the PMN infiltrative changes do correlate with symptomatic disease. Overall, little histopathologic damage to nasal epithelium can be demonstrated. Both the influx of PMNs and local kinin production contribute to development of symptoms in patients with the common cold.

## CLINICAL MANIFESTATIONS

### General

The classic clinical manifestations of the common cold are well known. An initial incubation period of 1 to 4 days is followed by prodromal symptoms of chills, low-grade fevers, myalgias, and arthralgias. These are followed by scratchy throat, dry cough, and rhinorrhea. Sneezing, nasal stuffiness, headache, and hoarseness are also seen. Fever is almost always low grade. Varying severity of each of these symptoms may be seen, depending in part on the underlying cause of the syndrome. Reports on large series of infections led to some generalizations regarding the relationship between specific symptom complexes and specific etiology. Excessive nasal discharge is more frequent with rhinovirus and enterovirus and relatively uncommon with group A β-hemolytic streptococcal infections. Constitutional symptoms are more common with influenza, enteroviral, and adenoviral infections than in rhinoviral-associated disease. Cough is seen in the majority of patients with respiratory syncytial virus (RSV) and influenza infections but is less common in enteroviral, rhinoviral, and streptococcal infections. Despite these differences in clinical presentation, diagnosing a specific etiology may be difficult. Exposure history, season, age of patient, and local epidemiology all provide important clues to the differential diagnosis.

### Rhinovirus

Rhinoviruses are single-stranded RNA viruses of the picornavirus family. These viruses infect only humans and produce clinical symptoms characteristic of the common cold. In reviewing the clinical manifestations of rhinovirus infections, Gwaltney reported 139 consecutive cases of infection confirmed by culture technique. Rhinorrhea and sneezing were the most common symptoms occurring in almost two thirds of patients by the second day. Sore throat was noted in 50% of patients by day 2. Fevers and rigors were distinctly uncommon. Cough and hoarseness were less common although more persistent. Overall, the median length of illness was 7.4 days. However, almost one fourth noted persistent symptoms for as long as 2 weeks. In particular, coughing was noted as a persistent symptom in smokers, an effect that was even more pronounced in female smokers. Other studies that compare the relative frequency of symptoms related to the common cold have found similar results. The localization of rhinovirus illness to the upper respiratory tract may be due to the preferential growth of this virus at the lower temperatures of the nasal passages.

### Coronavirus

Coronaviruses are also single-stranded RNA viruses. Little is known about the clinical presentation of infections due to the coronavirus. Bradburne studied infection of volunteers with coronavirus and compared their clinical syndromes to other volunteers infected with rhinoviruses. The incubation period was slightly longer than for rhinovirus (3.3 days versus 2.1 days), but the duration of illness was shorter (6 to 7 versus 9 to 10 days). Low-grade fever, malaise, nasal discharge, and sore throat were seen with similar frequency in the two groups. Rarely, coronaviruses may cause pneumonia, with outbreaks noted in infants and military recruits, or excerbations of chronic bronchitis.

### Influenza

Influenza virus may produce a clinical syndrome which overlaps that of the common cold. The typical influenza syndrome includes sudden onset of fever, dry cough, and retrosternal discomfort. Major complaints also include headache, myalgias, and malaise. Slight nasal obstruction and scratchy throat may be present and, if they precede other constitutional symptoms, may mimic rhinovirus or coronavirus infection. Symptoms typically resolve in 3 to 7 days. Cough and weakness may persist, but actual pneumonia is rare, occurring with increasing frequency in older patients (Fig. 111-1). Cases tend to occur in epidemics, usually in the winter, with small particle aerosols responsible for transmission (talking, coughing, sneezing). Severe headache, fevers, and myalgias help to differentiate influenza infections from more typical causes of the common cold. Patients at risk for pneumonia, including those with chronic pulmonary or cardiac disease, residents of chronic care facilities, those over 65 years old, patients with diabetes or renal disease, and the immunosuppressed should be carefully followed.

### Group A β-hemolytic streptococci

Approximately 10% of common cold syndromes are due to group A β-hemolytic streptococci. With an incubation period of 2 to 4 days, onset is typically abrupt. Fever (over 101° F), sore throat, tender cervical adenopathy, malaise, and myalgias may be similar to symptoms seen with the common cold. However, relative lack of coryza, cough, hoarseness, and conjunctivitis helps to distinguish streptococcal infections from viral upper respiratory tract infections. In infants, symptoms are less localizing and may include rhinorrhea and abdominal pain. Diagnosis on clinical grounds is difficult. Although the presence of exudative pharyngitis, fever, and tender cervical adenopathy suggests streptococcal disease, other pathogens, including Epstein-Barr virus and *Corynebacterium haemolyticum* may produce similar symptoms. Throat culture and rapid group A carbohydrate antigen detection remain the diagnostic tests of choice. Further discussion of streptococcal infections, differential diagnosis, and approach is reviewed in Chapter 30.

### *Mycoplasma pneumoniae*

Mycoplasma infections are caused by the smallest free-living organisms (Fig. 111-2). Although often thought of as a common cause of community-acquired pneumonia, only 3% of infections result in pneumonia, and 77% result in tracheobronchitis or pharyngitis. Infection is most common in the first two decades of life but may occur at any age. The incubation period is 3 weeks, with a high likelihood of transmission in close living quarters such as dormitories. Onset occurs over several days. Constitutional symptoms are frequent, including fevers, myalgias, sore throat, and malaise. Clinical features include nasal symptoms in 29% to 69% of patients. Sinus pain or fullness is seen in 50% of patients, with ear pain seen less frequently. Physical findings include fever (96% to 100%), pharyngeal erythema without exudate (12% to 73%) and cervical adenopathy (18% to 27%). Rales or wheezes are common (80% to 84%) and help to differentiate mycoplasma infections from other causes of the common cold syndrome.

### *Chlamydia pneumoniae*

Chlamydial infections have only recently been recognized as a cause of both upper and lower respiratory tract infections. The majority of adults have serologic evidence of prior infection. Sore throat is present in the majority of patients and may precede development of lower respiratory tract symptoms by several weeks. Symptoms of sinusitis may also be present. Differentiation from mycoplasma may be difficult. However, the prolonged cough, especially when preceded by sore throat, helps to exclude viral etiology as a diagnostic consideration.

## DIAGNOSIS

The diagnosis of the common cold in clinical practice is based on identification of symptoms of rhinorrhea, sore throat, hacking cough, and low-grade fevers. Knowledge of local epidemiology and the seasonal patterns of various viral infections may help to identify a likely specific viral etiology. Further investigation focuses on diagnosis of those diseases with similar presentation that require specific therapy. Most commonly this focus is on the

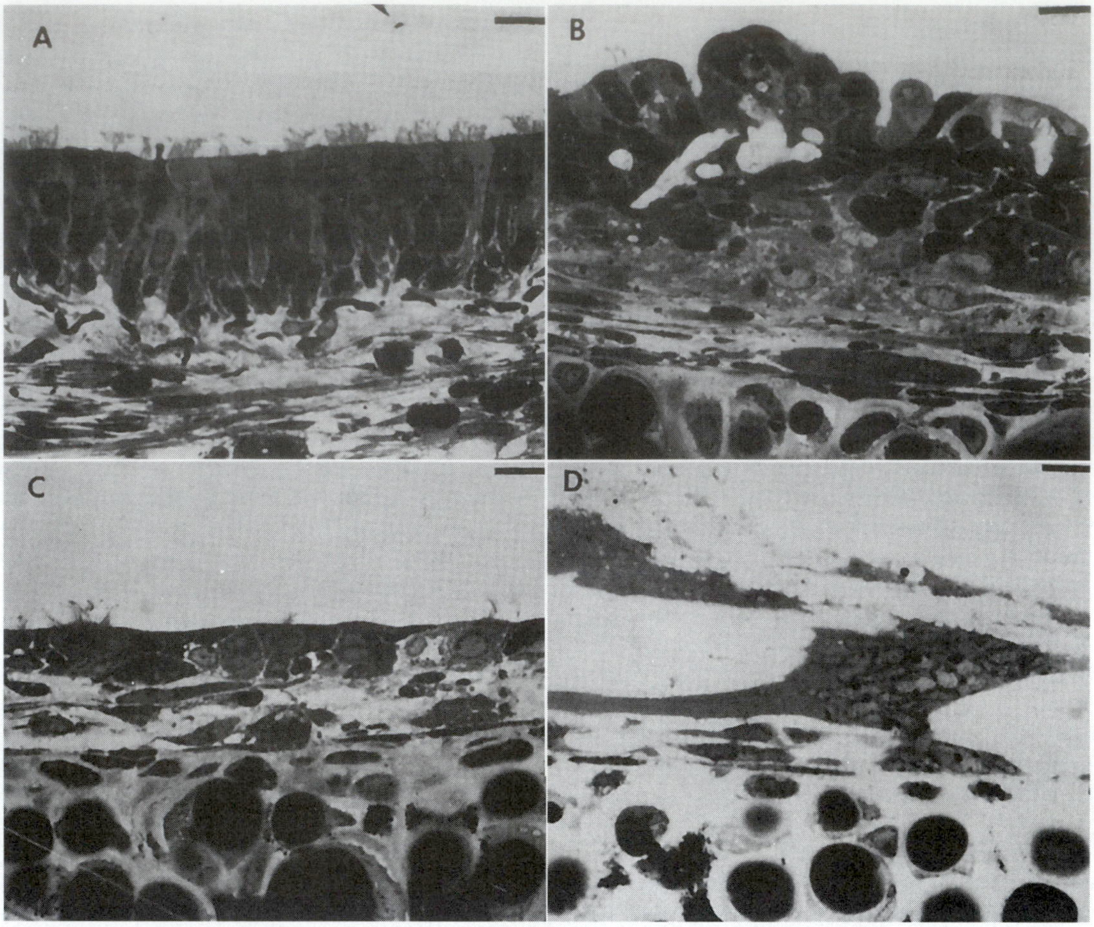

**Fig. 111-1.** Human parainfluenza type 3 infection. Results of infection of hamster tracheal cells in organ culture with human parainfluenza virus. **A,** Control trachea maintained in organ culture for 14 days, demonstrating normal cells with intact cilia. **B,** Disorganized respiratory epithelium with multinucleated cells in the lamina propria at day 7 postinfection. **C,** Fusion of respiratory epithelial cells and loss of cilia, also at 7 days postinfection. **D,** Replacement of respiratory epithelium with multinucleated synctium at 14 days postinfection. (× 2150 with bar in each photograph = 5 μm.) (Courtesy of Dr. A. M. Collier. From Klein JD, Collier AM: Pathogenesis of human parainfluenza type 3 virus infection in hamster tracheal organ culture. *Infect Immun* 10(4):883, 1974.)

A

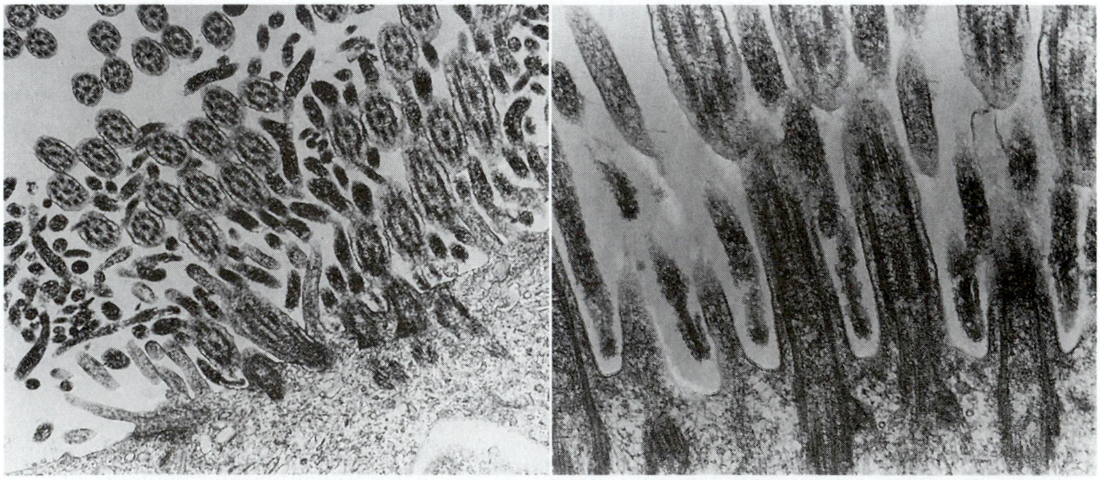

B

**Fig. 111-2.** Orientation of *Mycoplasma pneumoniae* organisms with respect to ciliated epithelial cells of human fetal tracheas in organ culture for 24 h. **A,** The *Mycoplasma* organisms are the darker filamentous structures seen parallel to the cilia, which are the "striped"-appearing structures that insert down into the membrane × 25,500. **B,** In a higher-power photograph of the same preparation, one can see the mycoplasmas aligned in between the cilia, with a specialized terminal structure oriented toward the cell membrane × 50,000. (From Collier AM: Pathogenesis of *Mycoplasma pneumoniae* Infection as Studied in the Human Foetal Trachea in Organ Culture. In Elliott K, Birch J, editors: *Pathogenic Mycoplasmas,* A Ciba Foundation Symposium, Jan. 25-27, 1972. Amsterdam: Elsevier, 1972, Pp. 307-320.)

exclusion of streptococcal pharyngitis. When severe sore throat, pharyngeal exudate, fever, cervical adenopathy, and leukocytosis are present, a diagnosis of streptococcal pharyngitis is likely. However, when pharyngitis is milder or associated with rhinorrhea, clinical diagnosis is unreliable. In these situations either culture or rapid antigen detection should be employed. Other diagnostic studies are usually reserved for identification of complications of the common cold, such as sinusitis (see further).

## TREATMENT

Treatment of the uncomplicated common cold is symptomatic. An enormous number of over-the-counter (OTC) preparations are available, but only a few have been carefully studied. Smith presented a critical review of clinical trials of OTC medications and found no good evidence of the effectiveness of these medications in preschool children. In this age group serious toxicity from OTC medications may be seen, especially with combination therapies. If OTC medications are used, single-ingredient preparations should be prescribed. Antihistamines, whose effectiveness may be more related to their drying action on mucous membranes than their inhibition of histamine, did reduce symptoms, especially sneezing, and nasal mucus amount. This result was seen most consistently with chlorpheniramine. Studies of other antihistamines showed less conclusive benefits. In a large study of terfenadine involving almost 100 patients with rhinitis symptoms related to the common cold, no difference was noted in symptoms when placebo was compared to drug. Similar results were noted when diphenhydramine was reviewed. Decongestants, whose effects are primarily sympathomimetic, result in vasoconstriction of the nasal mucosa with subsequent lessening of discharge and blockage. Several were reviewed by Smith, with findings suggesting more reliable activity than antihistamines. Oral pseudoephedrine resulted in a "dramatic" reduction in nasal symptoms. Oxymetazoline and phenylpropanolamine were also found to be effective. Few data supported the effectiveness of expectorants or antitussives.

The effects of aspirin and acetaminophen on the common cold have also been extensively evaluated. Early work by Stanley suggested that aspirin may impair host response to rhinovirus infection, resulting in more prolonged viral shedding. In a carefully controlled trial of 60 patients inoculated with rhinovirus type 2, Graham reported the effects of aspirin, acetaminophen, and ibuprofen on a variety of microbiologic, immunologic, and clinical markers. Both aspirin and acetaminophen were found to impair antibody response and increase symptoms of nasal congestion and discharge. No significant effect on viral shedding was noted.

Relatively few studies have addressed the effects of specific antiviral therapy for the common cold. Of the agents tested, interferon α-2 has been shown to provide prophylaxis against rhinovirus infections and may reduce nasal symptoms. Side effects of nasally administered interferon included stuffiness, dryness, and ulcerations. Combination approaches, especially when using short-course interferons, may minimize side effects and maximize therapeutic benefits. Such an approach was reported by Gwaltney. In this study a combination of interferon α-2, ipratropium, and naproxen was begun 24 hours after experimental rhinovirus infection. Viral shedding, rhinorrhea, cough, and malaise were all reduced in treated patients. Only six of 16 treated patients developed colds, compared to seven of eight control patients. These combination studies suggest that, with carefully selected and dosed agents, reduction of incidence and severity of the common cold is achievable. Cost and toxicity of therapy, however, may continue to limit widespread application.

## COMPLICATIONS

The most common complications of the common cold include maxillary sinusitis in 0.5% and otitis media in 2% of patients. Although sinus radiology and computed tomography (CT) are highly sensitive for diagnosis of sinusitis, expense limits usefulness in clinical practice. A number of clinical signs have been correlated with bacterial sinusitis and may be of value in distinguishing complicated from uncomplicated colds. Duijn compared ultrasonography with clinical findings to determine predictive value of various symptoms and signs for diagnosis of fluid in the maxillary sinus. In this review five symptoms were found to be predictive of fluid, including onset with the common cold, purulent rhinorrhea, pain at bending, unilateral maxillary pain, and pain in teeth. The presence of these symptoms, prolonged symptoms, leukocytosis, or high fever should alert the clinician to the possibility of sinusitis associated with the common cold. Williams compared radiographs to clinical findings in 247 consecutive patients presenting with rhinorrhea or facial pain. As in prior reviews, the presence of maxillary toothache, purulent secretions, poor response to decongestants, abnormal transillumination, and colored nasal discharge correlated with abnormal x-rays of the sinus. The presence of multiple symptoms was even more suggestive of sinusitis. If all five symptoms are present, the likelihood ratio rises to 6.4. In summary, the history and physical examination can be strongly suggestive of complications of the common cold and may limit the need for more expensive diagnostic tests such as radiographs. See Chapter 28 for evaluation and treatment.

## BIBLIOGRAPHY


Breese BB, Disney FA: The accuracy of diagnosis of beta streptococcal infections on clinical grounds, *J Pediatr,* 44:670, 1954.

Cate TR: Clinical manifestations and consequences of influenza, *Am J Med* 82 (suppl 6A):15, 1987.

Clyde WA: Clinical overview of typical *Mycoplasma pneumoniae* infections, *Clin Infect Dis* 17 (suppl 1):S32, 1993.

Gadomski A, Horton L: The need for rational therapeutics in the use of cough and cold medicine in infants, *Pediatrics* 89(4):774, 1992.

Garibaldi RA: Epidemiology of community-acquired respiratory tract infections in adults—incidence, etiology, and impact, *Am J Med* 78 (suppl 6B):32, 1985.

Graham NM et al: Adverse effects of aspirin, acetaminophen, and ibuprofen on immune function, viral shedding, and clinical status in rhinovirus-infected volunteers, *J Infect Dis* 162:1277, 1990.

Gwaltney JM Jr: Airborne contagion—epidemiology of the common cold, *Ann N Y Acad Sci* 353:54, 1980.

Gwaltney JM Jr: Combined antiviral and antimediator treatment of rhinovirus colds, *J Infect Dis* 166:776, 1992.

Gwaltney JM Jr et al: Rhinovirus infections in an industrial population—characteristics of illness and antibody response, *JAMA,* 202(6):158, 1967.

Panusarn C et al: Prevention of illness from rhinovirus infection by a topical interferon inducer, *N Engl J Med* 291(2):57, 1974.

Perlman PE, Ginn DR: Respiratory infections in ambulatory adults—choosing the best treatment, *Resp Tract Infect* 87(1):175, 1990.

Smith MBH, Feldman W: Over-the-counter cold medications—a critical review of clinical trials between 1950 and 1991, *JAMA* 269(17):2258, 1993.

Turner RB: The role of neutrophils in the pathogenesis of rhinovirus infections, *Pediatr Infect Dis J* 9(11):832, 1990.

VanDuijn NP, Brouwer HJ, Lamberts H: Use of symptoms and signs to diagnose maxillary sinusitis in general practice: comparison with ultrasonography, *Br Med J* 305:684, 1992.

Williams JW, Simel DL: Does this patient have sinusitis? *JAMA* 270:1242, 1993.

CHAPTER

# 112 Asthma and Other Allergic Disorders

**Richard M. Effros**
**Jack Kaufman**

## BRONCHIAL ASTHMA

Bronchial asthma is a clinical disorder in which the airways are hyperreactive to a variety of stimuli. Following exposure to these stimuli, airway resistance increases because of smooth muscle contraction, increased secretions, and inflammation of the bronchial walls. In contrast to the relatively fixed airway obstruction encountered in emphysema, increased airway resistance in asthma is episodic and improves between attacks. During remissions the patients may be essentially asymptomatic, but in more severe forms of the disease some bronchospasm may persist even between attacks. There is no evidence that asthma progresses to irreversible airway disease, though pulmonary mechanics may decline in asthmatics at a somewhat more rapid rate with aging than in the nonasthmatic population.

### Pathogenesis

Although it had formerly been assumed that asthma was due to an abnormal immune response of the lungs, it is now recognized that multiple inflammatory factors play an important role in the etiology of this disease (Fig. 112-1). The primary immune mechanism of asthma involves the association of antigen with IgE bound to the cell surfaces, which triggers the release of histamine and a variety of other factors that promote both bronchospasm and local inflammation. Histamine increases leakage of protein and fluid from venules, increases airway secretions, and can stimulate irritant receptors in the airway walls. This in turn leads to reflex vagal release of acetylcholine near smooth muscles, promoting further bronchoconstriction. Although antihistamines are useful in the treatment of other allergic disorders such as allergic rhinitis, they have not proven helpful in asthma.

Many factors in addition to histamine undoubtedly play an important role in the pathogenesis of bronchial asthma. Among these are the lipoxygenase products of arachidonate, the leukotrienes (formerly known as slow reacting substance of anaphylaxis). Other mediators that may play a role in bronchospasm include platelet activating factor, bradykinin, substance P, oxidants, complement fragments, and a variety of other substances. Agents that inhibit these mediators may eventually prove useful in the treatment of asthma.

It has also become clear that virtually all types of inflammatory cells may play a role in the complex inflammatory events that occur during an asthmatic attack (see Fig. 112-1). The intensity of the eosinophilia observed in patients with asthma appears to be correlated with the severity of airflow obstruction, and eosinophil counts are increased in bronchoalveolar lavage fluid obtained from asthmatics. Response to steroids is marked by a decrease in both airway resistance and eosinophil counts. Mast cells within the lung tissues of asthmatics appear to be activated and probably play an important role in the early events preceding an asthmatic attack.

Bronchospasm can be induced by cholinergic nerves that travel in the vagus nerve and may release acetylcholine in a reflex manner when irritant receptors in the airways are stimulated. Stimulation of these same receptors is also responsible for cough. Although not as effective as β-adrenergic agents (see further), anticholinergic drugs can relieve airway obstruction in some asthmatics.

### Epidemiology

Bronchial asthma is a common clinical problem in the United States, affecting perhaps 10 million people, or about 4% of the population. Males predominate over females by a factor of 1.5 to 2.0 below the age of 10, but the incidence of disease becomes approximately equal at age 12 to 14, and the incidence in women becomes greater thereafter. Airway hyperresponsiveness is almost always present in asthmatic persons, but this observation is also seen among many asymptomatic subjects. Perhaps 20% of these individuals eventually develop clinical asthma. Atopy is associated with more severe asthma and appears to be in part an inherited disorder that may contribute to the common occurrence of asthma in a number of family members. Viral upper respiratory tract infections (e.g., respiratory syncytial virus disease in infancy) are commonly associated with increased airway hyperreactivity, but the relation of this event to either acquiring or worsening asthma remains uncertain. Air pollutants such as sulfur dioxide can initiate attacks in asthmatic persons, but it is not known if they contribute to the incidence of the disease. Both active and passive smoking may also predispose subjects to the development of asthma. Perhaps 50% of children with asthma improve or become symptom free upon reaching early adulthood, but a very early onset of disease is associated with a less favorable prognosis. Mortality is uncommon in the United States, averaging 3.2 per 100,000 in 1986, but higher mortality frequencies have been observed elsewhere (e.g., England and New Zealand). There has been some concern that mortality in the United States and elsewhere has increased over the last 20 years.

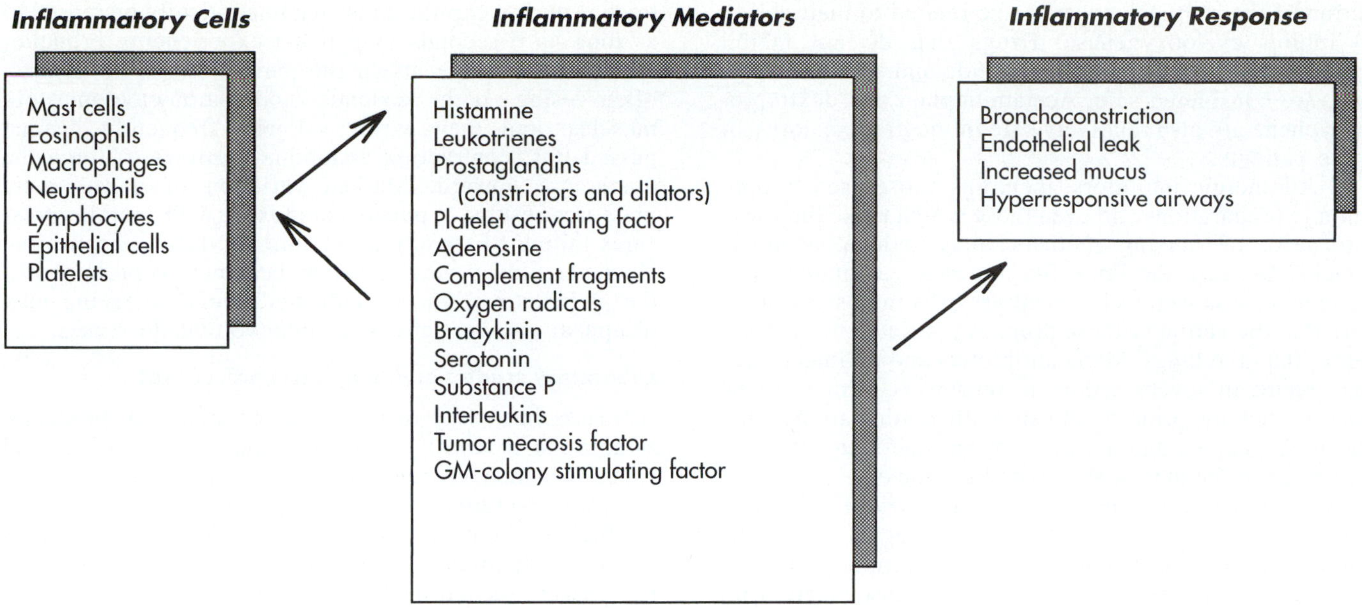


**Fig. 112-1.** The complex interplay of inflammatory cells and mediators and their actions to promote bronchial asthma is illustrated in a simplified schematic diagram.

## Agents and circumstances that induce asthma

The airways of asthmatics can become exquisitely sensitive to a wide variety of chemical and physical stimuli. Atopic patients tend to develop immediate sensitivity of the anaphylactic type I immune reaction to one or more antigens. This form of asthma is sometimes referred to as extrinsic asthma, whereas asthma unrelated to an atopic predisposition or to specific environmental antigens is designated as intrinsic. These patients are generally younger and may have a personal or family history of associated disorders such as allergic rhinitis, infantile eczema, and atopic dermatitis. Pollens, molds, house dust, and animal dander are common antigens. Because the pollens are too large to reach the bronchi, it is assumed that fragments of the pollens are responsible for asthmatic attacks. Antigens associated with the skin mites *Dermatophagoides pteronyssinus,* especially the feces of these arthropods, are the principal factors in housedust that are allergenic. Cockroaches are a common cause of asthma, particularly in high-density inner city apartments. An important antigen associated with cats is derived from the saliva with which they groom themselves. True asthmatic attacks related to foods are much less common than those induced by inhaled antigens, but exposure to specific foods and additives such as metabisulfites (sometimes used as a preservative for salads) can induce serious attacks.

A careful occupational history is essential in the evaluation of adults with bronchial asthma. Substances that can cause asthma in the workplace can be divided into low–molecular weight substances and proteins. Toluene diisocyanate is an important ingredient of polyurethane foams that can cause the development of asthma in workers who may have had no previous reaction to the substance over a period of many months. Platinum salts and a variety of anhydrides may cause development of both IgE antibodies and asthma. Among the proteins that can cause asthma are enzymes used in detergents, which can result in hypersensitivity in approximately one fourth of workers exposed to these substances. A variety of wood dusts, particularly cedar, can also cause occupational asthma. Exposure to cotton and other organic fibers can provoke bronchospasm by stimulating release of histamine, a condition referred to as byssinosis (see Chapter 116). Although formaldehyde appears to have been responsible for asthma in a few workers exposed to heavy concentrations, evidence on the small amounts released from fiberboard or foam in homes is not considered persuasive.

The hyperreactivity of the airways of asthmatics extends to a wide variety of nonspecific stimuli, including cold air, perfume, smoke, and sulfur dioxide. Vigorous exercise is not infrequently followed by bronchospasm in asthmatics, and hyperventilation, either voluntary hyperventilation or that associated with laughing and crying, can initiate an asthmatic attack. Exercise-induced asthma can be avoided by prior inhalation of cromolyn or a β-adrenergic agent (see further). Other nonspecific factors that can contribute to asthma are esophageal reflux and chronic sinus disease.

It has been estimated that drugs are responsible for approximately 10% of acute asthmatic attacks. Nonsteroidal antiinflammatory drugs (NSAIDs), and in particular the innumerable preparations that contain aspirin, have been implicated in more than half of these cases. Hypersensitivity to aspirin and other NSAIDs typically appears in the third and fourth decades of life and does not appear to be inherited. Intense vasomotor rhinitis frequently precedes asthmatic symptoms, and nasal polyps and sinusitis are commonly present. Within an hour of ingesting aspirin, the patients experience rhinitis and wheezing and may develop nausea, vomiting, facial edema, angioedema, and life-threatening anaphylaxis. The action of these drugs appears to be related to their ability to inhibit cyclooxygenase. Drugs that do not inhibit cyclooxygenase, such as salicylamide and sodium salicylate, are considered safe. Acetaminophen and dextropropoxyphene are also relatively safe in the great majority of these patients.

β-Adrenergic inhibitors, including those used in ophthalmic preparations and even those which make their way into milk of nursing mothers, may induce asthmatic attacks. Because the lung, like the heart, contains some $\beta_1$-receptors as well as $\beta_2$-receptors, it is impossible to be sure that the action of these drugs is restricted to the heart rather than the lungs. Many antibiotics and iodinated dyes may result in severe asthmatic responses, which can be ameliorated by prior treatment with antihistamines and steroids. Cocaine and a variety of anesthetic agents have also been associated with asthmatic attacks.

Any of the angiotensin converting enzyme inhibitors may result in a persistent cough that begins soon after administration or as late as 1 year after initiating therapy; however, these reactions are rarely associated with bronchospasm or changes in bronchial hyperreactivity and are relieved within weeks after the drug is discontinued.

### History

In no other respiratory disease does the history play such an important diagnostic role as it does in bronchial asthma. The patient usually gives a history of dyspnea with recurrences and remissions. Often the dyspnea worsens at night and may be initiated by viral infections or exposure to irritants or antigens, such as those already listed. Although intrathoracic obstruction leads to greater resistance during expiration, patients commonly complain more of inspiratory distress. Fatigue of the inspiratory muscles is probably related to the fact that they remain tonically contracted throughout the respiratory cycle and are disadvantaged by the high volumes at which the lungs are maintained. Wheezing is apparent to both the patient and physician but may disappear when tidal volumes become sufficiently compromised in severe asthma. Not only is cough a common manifestation of asthma, it may be the only complaint given by the patient, and response to bronchodilators may reveal the cause of the cough. Frequently a cough productive of intrabronchial plugs may herald relief during an attack. Symptoms of asthma usually occur within 10 to 30 minutes of exposure to an irritant or antigen. However, late responses are also very common, occurring several hours after exposure. Usually an early response precedes the late response, but there may be no early phase in some patients with occupational asthma. Whereas the early response appears to be due to bronchospasm, edema, and vascular congestion, the late response is associated with the appearance of inflammatory cells in the tissues.

### Physical examination

Wheezing is the most common physical finding in asthma and, more often than not, is audible during both inspiration and expiration rather than just expiration. If these sounds are audible only during inspiration, extrathoracic obstruction with stridor is probably present rather than intrathoracic obstruction due to bronchial asthma. The time required for airway sounds to disappear over the trachea during expiration is characteristically increased to as long as 6 seconds in patients experiencing bronchospasm. In a severe attack the patient strains to inspire, often using both scalenus and sternocleidomastoid muscles, and then expires slowly, frequently against pursed lips, contracting abdominal muscles to force the diaphragm upward. Marked variation of intrathoracic pressures results in pulsus paradoxus, with systolic pressures falling by more than 15 mm Hg during inspiration. However, pulsus paradoxus may become less prominent if the patient tires, and as indicated above wheezing may disappear in severe attacks as tidal volume decreases.

### Laboratory studies and diagnostic procedures

Increases in airway resistance associated with bronchial asthma can be readily detected by spirometry. Forced vital capacity maneuvers reveal decreased flow rates: the forced expiratory volume ($FEV_1$) and peak expiratory flow rate (PEFR) are the most commonly used to assess alterations in airway obstruction. It is common practice to determine responsiveness to bronchodilators during the evaluation of pulmonary function, but failure to document a response is not particularly helpful, since patients who showed no improvement in the laboratory may respond outside of the laboratory; a clinical trial of bronchodilator therapy should generally be given regardless of the laboratory response. Decreases in flow to between 60% to 80% of predicted rates can be interpreted as mild, those between 40% and 60% as moderate, and airflows below 40% as severe obstruction. It is important to assess the $FEV_1$/FVC (forced vital capacity) ratio, since a reduction of this ratio from expected values is specific for obstructive rather than restrictive disease. Differentiation between intrathoracic and extrathoracic obstruction is facilitated by obtaining a flow-volume loop. The total lung capacity and, during remission, the carbon monoxide diffusion test are frequently increased in asthmatic patients. Between bronchospastic episodes pulmonary function may be completely normal, and it is helpful under these circumstances to obtain bronchoprovocative studies. These are generally conducted by having the patient inhale an aerosol containing methacholine. Patients who have hyperreactive airways experience a decrease in airflow with very low concentrations of this agent in comparison to normal subjects. Documentation of a normal challenge test argues against bronchial asthma, but many normal subjects who have airway hyperreactivity as judged by a bronchoprovocation test may have no history of asthma, and bronchoprovocation tests may become abnormal for several months following a viral infection in nonasthmatic individuals.

Arterial blood gases must be carefully followed in patients with severe asthma. Mild hypoxia and hypocapnia are commonly observed in mild and moderate asthma. With more severe episodes, hypoxia worsens and the $PCO_2$ may rise to normal or greater than normal levels, resulting in a respiratory acidosis. If oxygen delivery to the tissues becomes inadequate, lactic acidosis ensues. If a rise in $PCO_2$ to normal or elevated levels occurs in a patient in distress, the possibility of respiratory failure is present and mechanical ventilation may become mandatory.

Eosinophilia is common in all forms of allergic diseases, including asthma, drug reactions, allergic rhinitis, angioedema, and eczema. As noted above, the number of eosinophils tends to reflect the severity of asthma and may indicate whether steroid therapy is adequate.

The lungs are characteristically hyperinflated on x-rays. Chest x-rays should be obtained in patients with severe asthma, since they may reveal unexpected findings such as pneumothorax, atelectasis, and pneumonia, which require immediate attention. The detection of central bronchiectasis with mucous plugs strongly suggests bronchopulmonary aspergillosis, which is usually accompanied by asthmatic symptoms.

### Complications

Status asthmaticus, generally defined as life-threatening asthma that does not respond to standard medication, is one of the most serious complications in asthmatic patients. A patient who shows signs of respiratory failure with severe hypoxia and rising $P_{CO_2}$ must be admitted to an intensive care unit where mechanical ventilation can be properly managed (see Chapter 117). Other complications of acute asthma include pneumothorax, pneumomediastinum, and atelectasis due to bronchial plugging.

## Differential diagnosis

Many clinical disorders can mimic bronchial asthma (see the box below). Not uncommonly, manifestations of extrathoracic obstruction due to lesions of the upper airways are confused with those of intrathoracic obstruction due to asthma. Because of injuries sustained to the larynx and trachea during intubation and tracheostomies, extrathoracic obstruction is becoming increasingly common in general practice. Careful examination should make it possible to detect inspiratory stridor, which is loudest over the larynx and trachea. In some cases laryngeal dysfunction may be a manifestation of psychiatric disorders. Wheezing is also commonly associated with early congestive heart failure with edema of the airways, and congestive heart failure may cause a cough that worsens when the patient is recumbent. An increased incidence in bronchial hyperreactivity has been described in patients with congestive heart failure. Bronchial asthma must also be distinguished from hypersensitivity pneumonitis, which is related to inhalation of fungi or proteins. Unlike bronchial asthma, this condition is more often manifested by rales than wheezing, is frequently associated with pulmonary infiltrates and fever, and recurrent exposure may lead to chronic pulmonary fibrosis.

Bronchiolitis is a common disease in infants, in whom it is frequently associated with respiratory syncytial virus infections. It is also seen in adults following viral infections and may present with chronic cough and wheezing, which subside over a period of weeks or months. Bronchiolitis obliterans is a more serious form of small airway obstruction in which granulation tissue fills the smaller bronchioles. This disease may be idiopathic or it may be caused by a variety of factors such as toxic fume exposure, connective tissue disorders such as rheumatoid arthritis, and bone or organ transplantation (graft-versus-host disease). Early inspiratory crackles are common, and chest x-rays may be normal or show patchy overinflation. Bronchiolitis obliterans with organizing pneumonia (BOOP) is characterized by small airway obstruction with plugs of granulation tissue and accumulation of fibrinous exudates and foamy macrophages in inflamed alveoli. Patchy infiltrates are visible in chest x-rays, and the illness frequently responds favorably to steroid therapy.

### Diseases that can mimic or be associated with bronchial asthma

Chronic obstructive lung disease
Upper airway obstruction
Congestive heart failure
Bronchopulmonary aspergillosis
Pulmonary infiltration with eosinophilia
Churg-Strauss syndrome
Endobronchial sarcoid or tuberculosis
Angioedema
Carcinoid syndrome
Gastroesophageal reflux
Bronchiolitis
Cystic fibrosis
Factitious asthma
Pulmonary embolism

## Management

Although considerable effort has been devoted to development of more effective treatment of asthma, progress has been slow and many of the drugs now in use represent variants of agents that have been used for many centuries. The complexity of the inflammatory events responsible for hyperreactive airways suggests that it is necessary to block multiple mediators and effectors to prevent and treat asthma more effectively than is now possible. It is therefore not surprising that many of the more effective drugs tend to have multiple biologic actions. Treatment should be graded in accordance with the severity and chronicity of the disorder. Therapeutic strategies (based upon recent NIH recommendations) that can be used by the patient and physician are provided in Tables 112-1 to 112-4. Asthma is frequently a very unpredictable disease, and the clinician must use considerable judgment and ingenuity in designing a regimen for individual patients. There is good evidence that the frequency of hospitalization of these patients can be reduced if they are closely followed by their physicians, are instructed carefully in the use of their medications, and in more labile patients are taught to keep a record of their own pulmonary function with a peak flowmeter.

***Sympathomimetic agents.*** Recognition that there are a number of different adrenergic receptors in different tissues has led to the development of $\beta_2$-adrenergic drugs that are more specific in their action to promote bronchodilation and less likely to be associated with side effects. $\alpha$-Agonists cause vasoconstriction, whereas $\beta_1$-adrenergic agents increase cardiac contractility and heart rate, effects that are undesirable in patients undergoing therapy for asthma. In addition to promoting bronchodilation, $\beta_2$-adrenergic agents also increase secretion of electrolytes by the airways and enhance mucociliary

**Table 112-1.** Therapeutic staging: instructions for adult patient with exacerbation

| Severity | Symptoms | Peak flow* | Treatment |
|---|---|---|---|
| Mild | Mild wheeze, cough, dyspnea on exercise | 70%-90% | Inhaled bronchodilator |
| Moderate | Wheeze, cough, tightness, dyspnea at rest | 50%-70% | Inhaled bronchodilator every 20 min for 1 hour, then every 3-4 hr × 24-48 hr. If no improvement in 2-6 hr start or increase prednisone, and call physician |
| Severe | Severe dyspnea, wheeze may disappear if very severe, cough, chest tightness, difficulty walking and talking, muscle retraction | <50% | 4-6 puffs of MDI every 10 minutes up to 2 or 3 times or 1 nebulized dose; begin or increase prednisone; call physician; if no improvement in 20 min, seek emergency care |

Adapted from Guidelines for the Diagnosis and Management of Asthma, Publication No. 91-3042. National Institutes of Health. U.S. Department of Health and Human Services.

*MDI*, Metered dose inhaler.

*PEFR or $FEV_1$: % baseline or predicted.

**Table 112-2.** Therapeutic staging: chronic maintenance therapy

| Severity | Duration | Peak flow* | Treatment |
|---|---|---|---|
| Mild | Symptoms for <1 hr up to 2 × per week | >80% or >20% variation | Inhaled bronchodilator prn if asymptomatic or 2 puffs every 3-4 hr during episode |
| Moderate | >2 × per week | 60%-80% or 20%-30% variation | Inhaled bronchodilator 2 puffs qid; inhaled steroids 2-4 puffs bid or cromolyn 2 puffs qid and/or sustained release theophylline or oral $\beta_2$-agonist; if worsens, begin short course of oral prednisone |
| Severe | Continuous symptoms, limited activity, many exacerbations, nocturnal problems, hospitalizations | <60% or >50% variation | Same as moderate; up to 6 puffs of steroids qid and/or inhaled cromolyn and oral theophylline and/or oral β-agonist; burst of oral prednisone, 40 mg/day tapered for week or longer; may require chronic prednisone therapy (?alternate day) |

Adapted from Guidelines for the Diagnosis and Management of Asthma. Publication No. 91-3042. National Institutes of Health. U.S. Department of Health and Human Services.

*PEFR or $FEV_1$: % baseline or predicted. Both the absolute value of peak flow and variability are monitored chronically.

**Table 112-3.** Emergency management of asthmatic attack after initial therapy*

| Classification | Response | Peak flow† | Management |
|---|---|---|---|
| Good response | Symptoms returned to baseline | >70% | Discharge, consider prednisone course |
| Incomplete response | Moderate shortness of breath persists with wheezing | 40%-70% | Hourly $\beta_2$-agonists, begin intravenous corticosteroids, ?SC epinephrine, ?IV theophylline |
| Poor response | Severe symptoms and signs | <40% | Continue $\beta_2$-agonist every hr; if respiratory failure ($Pco_2$ rising to 40 mm Hg or above and flow <25%), consider intubation and ventilation |

Adapted from Guidelines for the Diagnosis and Management of Asthma. Publication No. 91-3042. National Institutes of Health. U.S. Department of Health and Human Services.

*Initial treatment: inhaled $\beta_2$-agonist × 3 in 60-90 minutes (less frequently, subcutaneous agonist; see text), supplemental $O_2$, consider systemic steroids.

†PEFR or $FEV_1$: % baseline or predicted.

**Table 112-4.** Oral and parenteral agents frequently used in treatment of asthma

| Agent | Form/clinical circumstance | Dosage |
|---|---|---|
| **Beta adrenergics** | | |
| ***Subcutaneous*** | | |
| Epinephrine HCl | 1:1000 aqueous solution | 0.2-0.5 mg every 20 min × 3 |
| Sus-Phrine | 1:200 aqueous suspension | 0.1-0.3 mg every 6 hr or more often |
| Terbutaline | 1 mg/ml aqueous solution | 0.25 mg × 2 within 4 hr |
| ***Oral administration*** | | |
| Metaproterenol | 10-, 20-mg tablets | 10-20 mg every 6 hr |
| Terbutaline | 2.5-, 5-mg tablets | 2.5-5.0 mg every 6 or 8 hr |
| Albuterol | 2-, 4-mg tablets | 2-4 mg every 6-8 hr |
| **Glucocorticoids** | | |
| ***Parenteral*** | | |
| Hydrocortisone | 100-, 1000-mg vials | 4 mg/kg IV every 4-6 hr |
| Methylprednisolone | 100-, 1000-mg vials | 1-2 mg/kg IV every 4-6 hr |
| Prednisone | Tablets, syrup, suspension | 10-50 mg/day |
| Prednisolone | Tablets, syrup, suspension | 10-50 mg/day |
| **Theophylline** | | |
| ***Parenteral*** | | |
| Loading dose | Not on therapy | 5 mg/kg in 20 min |
| | On therapy | 2.5 mg/kg in 20 min |
| Maintenance dose | Young smoker | 700 μg/kg/hr |
| | Nonsmoking adult | 430 μg/kg/hr |
| | Older adult, cor pulmonale | 260 μg/kg/hr |
| | Adult, CHF or liver failure | 200 μg/kg/hr |
| ***Oral maintenance dose*** | | |
| Immediate release | Smokers | 6-8 mg/kg |
| | Nonsmokers | 3 mg/kg |
| | Older, CHF and liver disease | 2 mg/kg |
| Sustained release | All patients | 200-400 mg bid adjusted to condition and blood level |

*CHF*, Congestive heart failure.

activity. Protein kinase A levels increase within the smooth muscle cells, resulting in inhibition of myosin phosphorylation and smooth muscle cell relaxation.

$\beta_2$-Agonists are not free from side effects, such as skeletal muscle tremor, hyperglycemia, and hypokalemia as well as dilatation of the vasculature of skeletal muscles. A transient decrease in oxygen saturation is sometimes observed following administration of adrenergic agents. This paradoxic effect is related to the effect of increased cardiac output, which can result in perfusion of underventilated regions of the lungs and is not a contraindication to continued use of these drugs.

Epinephrine was introduced in 1910 and continues to be administered subcutaneously, and less frequently by intravenous injections, in the treatment of severe asthmatic or anaphylactic attacks (see section on anaphylaxis). Cardiac necrosis has been described following administration of parenteral epinephrine, and if at all possible such injections should be avoided in older patients and those with histories of coronary artery disease. Because it is the only aerosolized agent available without prescription, many patients continue to use it. However, epinephrine is associated with potent $\alpha$-adrenergic and nonspecific $\beta$-adrenergic activity and has a very limited half-life, and its use in aerosols has been largely replaced by newer, more specific agents. Ephedrine, an oral drug with weak properties similar to those of epinephrine, is of largely historical interest, since it was used for millennia in herbal form and was popular in various proprietary combinations for many years. Isoproterenol became popular after its introduction in the 1940s because it lacked $\alpha$-adrenergic activity. Unfortunately, it is relatively nonspecific for $\beta_1$-adrenergic and $\beta_2$-adrenergic effects, and the former may have been responsible for an increase in the incidence of sudden death when it was widely used as a metered aerosol. It is still occasionally used intravenously in children with status asthmaticus to avoid the need for intubation and ventilation, but terbutaline is safer for this purpose.

At this time the three most popular drugs for bronchial asthma in the United States are metaproterenol, which retains some $\beta_1$-adrenergic activity; terbutaline, which can currently be purchased in oral and subcutaneous forms; and albuterol, which can be purchased for aerosol and oral administration but not parenteral therapy. These drugs remain active for relatively longer periods of time than the earlier preparations and are less likely to cause unwanted cardiovascular effects. Other selective $\beta_2$-adrenergic drugs used in metered dose inhalers (MDIs) include biloterol and pirbuterol. Salbuterol has a particularly long duration of action and is useful for preventing nocturnal bronchospasm. However, the onset of bronchodilation is also delayed and it should not be used to treat acute bronchospasm.

There is consensus that $\beta_2$-adrenergic agents are best prescribed in aerosol form because much higher concentrations can be reached locally within the lungs than can be achieved with oral and parenteral administration, and systemic effects can be minimized. However, it can be argued that the latter routes may permit the drug to reach areas of the lung which are inaccessible to aerosols because of severe bronchoconstriction and mucous plugging, and oral and occasionally parenteral administration is helpful. A number of studies have been published which suggest that MDIs are just as effective as aerosol generators, particularly if the patients are properly trained in inhaling during administration of a nebulized dose. For those who have difficulty with the MDI inspiratory maneuver, spacers can be used to permit administration of medication during tidal breathing. However, considerably more medication is delivered with the aerosol generators, and they continue to be popular for patients with episodes of very severe asthma that has not responded to the MDIs.

There has been concern over the years that patients tend to develop tachyphylaxis to β-adrenergic therapy. Although laboratory evidence for such an effect can be shown in experimental models, the clinical significance of this phenomenon is not clear. Nevertheless, the physician must be alerted if the patient finds it necessary to use the medication more frequently, since this may signal worsening of the disease and mandate additional therapy. It has been common practice to recommend that β-adrenergic aerosols be given on a regular basis (for example, two breaths four times a day), but concern that this may be associated with increased cardiac events or tachyphylaxis has led to the recommendation that, in patients with relatively mild asthma, MDIs can be used on a less frequent, as needed basis. The frequency of administration of aerosols is commonly increased to as often as every 15 minutes in patients receiving therapy in the Emergency Room, but chronic administration of high doses should probably be avoided, since it is possible that an increase in overall asthma mortality may be related to overuse of these agents.

***Corticosteroids.*** The widespread effects, both beneficial and deleterious, of the glucocorticoids in the treatment of asthma are related in part to the specific cytoplasmic receptors for these agents that are present in both inflammatory cells and many parenchymal cells, including those of the lungs. Subsequent activity requires interaction with regulatory elements of DNA, so the antiinflammatory actions of corticosteroids are not seen for 6 to 12 hours. Chronic administration can reduce nonspecific airway hyperresponsiveness, and single doses inhibit the late, inflammatory response to antigen exposure.

Intravenous administration is particularly valuable in patients with severe episodes of asthma (see Tables 112-1 to 112-3). Because the effects of these agents may not be clinically evident for as long as 12 hours and the course of the illness is so unpredictable, it has become accepted practice to administer these drugs as early as possible to patients who require hospitalization. Recommended dosages are indicated in Table 112-4. High dosages of steroids may be continued in oral form until flow returns toward baseline levels, and then tapering may proceed over a period of 1 or 2 weeks, with adjustment if peak flows begin to deteriorate. Concomitant use of steroid aerosols is recommended both during and after tapering (see further). Oral glucorticoids can be used for recurrences in the home environment with appropriate tapering schedules. In a minority of patients oral steroids must be used on a chronic basis with attempts at as slow a taper as possible. Of course longer exposure entails increased risks of the innumerable side effects of steroids. Administration of more than the physiologic levels of glucocorticoids (7.5 to 10 mg per day) leads to suppression of the hypothalamic-pituitary-adrenal axis. This effect can be reduced by administering all of the medication in the morning when adrenocorticotropic hormone (ACTH) levels are maximal rather than in multiple doses throughout the day. Alternate day dosing is even more effective in preventing hypothalamic-pituitary-adrenal axis suppression and, by allowing recovery of some of the inflammatory function, may reduce the incidence of infection, but it is difficult to control asthmatic symptoms in many patients with this regimen. Following prolonged glucocorticoid administration, weaning should be done slowly (e.g., by decreasing dosage by 1 mg per day for a month). Hypothalamic-pituitary function may remained suppressed for as long as a year, and the patient should keep steroids at hand for stressful circumstances and carry a card indicating possible need for steroid administration if stress or surgery occurs during the year following discontinuation of steroids.

Like the $\beta_2$-adrenergic drugs, aerosolized steroids have gained considerable popularity in the treatment of asthma. These have been designed to exert maximal local activity while minimizing absorption and systemic effects. They have proven helpful in permitting withdrawal of oral steroids in patients chronically receiving them and may reduce dependence on frequent administration of $\beta_2$-adrenergic agents and the incidence of exercise dyspnea. Oropharyngeal candidiasis can be ameliorated or avoided by thoroughly rinsing the mouth after administration of aerosolized steroids. Dysphonia, manifested as hoarseness, is usually related to the effect of the drugs on the skeletal muscles of the larynx. It may respond to less frequent administration or use of spacers to improve more distal delivery of medication.

High dosages of inhaled steroids may have systemic effects such as suppression of the hypothalamic-pituitary-adrenal axis, and bone formation can be decreased; use of a spacer can decrease absorption through the membranes of the mouth and upper airways; patients should rinse their mouths after administration. It should be emphasized to the patients that these aerosolized steroids do not provide immediate relief and must be taken on a regular basis for some weeks before improvement may occur and some months before maximal effect is observed.

***Methylxanthines.*** The popularity of methylxanthines for the treatment of asthma has waxed and waned dramatically over the past few decades. On the one hand, they cannot be considered primary drugs for the treatment of asthma because of a less favorable ratio of benefits to complications than aerosolized $\beta_2$-adrenergic agents, but they can be very helpful as ancillary therapy in many patients with asthma. Of the three most common derivatives of methylxanthine, namely theophylline, caffeine, and theobromine, only the first is used for treatment of asthma. Theophylline is frequently formulated with ethylenediamine (aminophylline) to improve solubility by making the diluent solution more alkaline. The mode of action of this group of compounds remains something of a mystery. Although it had long been thought that the actions of methylxanthines are mediated by inhibition of phosphodiesterases, this requires concentrations well above those encountered clinically. In addition to bronchodilatation, theophylline appears to increase diaphragmatic contractility, decrease pulmonary artery resistance, and act as a respiratory stimulant.

During acute attacks aminophylline is commonly administered intravenously at a rate designed to keep blood levels between 10 and 20 μg/ml. Lower blood levels are less effective but may be of help in patients who cannot tolerate higher concentrations. Chronic therapy is generally given in the form of one or another sustained release oral medication. As blood concentrations increase, patients develop anorexia, nausea, and vomiting because of the central action of theophylline. The patient may also develop more serious symptoms such as cardiovascular toxicity with tachycardia, tachyarrhythmias, and hypotension. Nervousness, insomnia, headache, and refractory seizures are central nervous system manifestations of toxicity. Drugs, illnesses, and smoking can have a profound effect on blood levels, complicating therapy (see the box below). Dosage should be reduced by one third when a patient is given ciprofloxacin or erythromycin and by one half when fever develops or the patient is given cimetidine or oral contraceptives. Blood levels should be determined after the onset of therapy or a change in dosage and when bronchospasm worsens or symptoms are consistent with toxicity, and patients should be advised to refrain from taking their next dose and to contact their physicians when these symptoms appear. Theophylline is often recommended in patients with nocturnal asthma resistant to bedtime β-adrenergic agonists.

**Some agents and illnesses that interact with theophylline metabolism**

**Increased metabolism**

- Carbamazepine
- Children
- Cimetidine
- Cystic fibrosis
- Hyperthyroidism
- Phenobarbital
- Phenytoin
- Rifampin
- Sulfinpyrazone
- Terbutaline
- Tobacco, marijuana

**Decreased metabolism**

- Allopurinol
- Chronic obstructive pulmonary disease
- Cimetidine
- Ciprofloxacin
- Troleandomycin
- Old age
- Erythromycin
- Oral contraceptives
- Propranolol
- Congestive heart failure
- Liver disease

***Other medications.*** Cromolyn (disodium cromoglycate) is useful in inhibiting both the immediate and delayed bronchoconstriction that follows exposure to antigens. Although its exact mode of action is unclear, it does inhibit release of mediators such as histamine and leukotrienes from mast cells and has a number of other antiinflammatory properties. Recently the drug has been reformulated in liquid aerosol, which is less irritating than the powder formerly used. It has proven particularly helpful in children and adults in whom asthma appears to be related to specific allergic responses but may also be helpful in others. It is effective in both the immediate and delayed bronchospasm that follows airway challenges and exposure to animals and substances encountered at work, and it is somewhat less effective than $\beta_2$-adrenergic agonists in preventing bronchospasm induced by exercise or exposure to cold. Response may take up to 2 months, and the medication provides no relief in an acute asthmatic attack. Side effects are quite rare, though some local irritation and hoarseness and a variety of other minor complications have been described. Nedocromil sodium is a recently released agent for inhalation that appears to have antiinflammatory effects in the airways. It may also inhibit reflex reactions to exercise and cold.

Although aerosolized anticholinergic drugs such as ipratropium bromide are used primarily for chronic obstructive disease, some asthmatics appear to respond to this medication. Antibiotics are indicated only if there is evidence for bacterial infection associated with asthma.

Desensitization may have a role in the treatment of asthma related to specific pollens and to mites if patients do not respond adequately to routine pharmacotherapy, but it is more effective in the treatment of allergic rhinitis.

A variety of other drugs have been tried in the treatment of asthma, such as magnesium, gold, methotrexate, and cyclosporin, but these drugs are potentially toxic and must be considered experimental at this time. Bronchoalveolar lavage has been tried in status asthmaticus but can worsen bronchospasm and should probably be avoided. Newer inhibitors of leukotrienes are currently under investigation.

## ANAPHYLAXIS

### Pathophysiology

Anaphylaxis is the most dreaded complication of immediate hypersensitivity. Like other disorders of immediate hypersensitivity, anaphylaxis is initiated by binding of antigen to IgE attached to the surfaces of mast cells, with the subsequent release of agents that mediate vascular leak of protein, smooth muscle contraction, and mobilization of inflammatory cells. The relationship of anaphylaxis to prior atopy remains unclear: the incidence of anaphylactic reactions to both penicillin and bee stings is no more common in subjects with atopy than those without. Antigenic substances include proteins and smaller solutes that combine with proteins. Some drugs, such as nonsteroidal antiinflammatory drugs, cause anaphylactic-like reactions that may be due to direct effects on mast cells rather than IgE-mediated events.

### Etiology

Stings of bees, yellow jackets, wasps, and hornets (all of which are members of the order Hymenoptera) can induce reactions varying from local cutaneous symptoms to the characteristic manifestations of anaphylactic shock. Penicillin is the most common cause of drug-related anaphylaxis, and cross-reaction with cephalosporins is common. Other antibiotics, local anesthetics, and specific foods, such as eggs, seafood, nuts, beans, and chocolate, can also be associated with anaphylaxis. Blood products can cause anaphylactic reactions as well as more common complications such as hemolysis. Patients with an inherited absence of IgA may develop severe anaphylaxis following administration of blood or plasma containing this protein.

### History and physical examination

Within seconds to minutes after exposure to the offending agent, the patient who has been stung may experience symptoms related to both upper and lower airway obstruction, with hoarseness, stridor, chest tightness, wheezing, and shortness of breath. Pruritic, raised, and erythematous urticaria typically appear in either a local or diffuse distribution over the skin. Angioneurotic edema is also common, with localized swelling that does not pit and may or may not be accompanied by local burning or stinging. Angioedema of the larynx and/or epiglottis may result in asphyxiation. Intense bronchospasm with mucosal swelling, intense bronchospasm, and bronchial edema are found at autopsy with secondary emphysematous overdistention of the lungs. The patient may experience severe hypotension and syncope.

### Laboratory studies and diagnostic procedures

Skin tests and radioallergoabsorbent tests are available for both bee stings and penicillin allergies.

### Management

Subcutaneous injection of epinephrine (0.2 to 0.5 ml of 1:1000, repeated twice at 20 to 30-minute intervals if needed) remains the cornerstone for immediate treatment of anaphylaxis and should be given as early as possible. Antihistamines and steroids seem to have relatively little effect in the acute episode. Aerosolized bronchodilatation and theophylline may be needed as well as oxygen if the patient is hypoxic. If the patient is in profound shock, 5 ml of 1:10,000 epinephrine should be administered intravenously every 5 minutes as needed; if no response is observed, 2 to 50 μg/kg dopamine is indicated. Patients should wear bracelets indicating agents to which they are allergic, and if use of a drug is essential, desensitization with increasing doses of medication administered intradermally, subcutaneously, and then intramuscularly can be tried with the assistance of an allergist. Immunotherapy is particularly effective in preventing anaphylactic reactions to insect stings but may have to be continued indefinitely if the skin test remains positive. Allergic patients should carry kits for self-administration of epinephrine if they are not receiving immunotherapy.

## ALLERGIC RHINITIS

### Etiology and epidemiology

Interaction of IgE on mast cells and basophils in the nasal mucosa with antigens is responsible for the manifestations of allergic rhinitis, which affects at least 15 million Americans. Pollens are the most common antigens involved, and the disease is frequently seasonal. Many of the same antigens that cause asthma (see previously) can also cause allergic rhinitis. However, many patients have perennial symptoms or vasomotor rhinitis unrelated to specific antigens but aggravated by changes in temperature, humidity, spicy foods, and inhaled irritants.

### History and physical examination

The cardinal manifestations of allergic rhinitis are nasal obstruction and secretions, sneezing, and itching of the mucous membranes of the nose, eyes, posterior pharynx, and conjunctivae. When symptoms are severe, patients complain of fatigue, loss of appetite, and irritability. The nasal mucous membranes tend to appear blue with swollen turbinates, and the conjunctivae are injected. Nasal polyps are uncommon unless the patient has aspirin-type allergy (see further), but serious otitis media is quite common and may lead to hearing defects, especially in young children. Chronic sinusitis may occur and result in throbbing pain over the sinus areas.

### Diagnostic procedures

A variety of scratch, prick, and intradermal skin tests are available, and if negative they argue against allergic rhinitis. Radioallergoabsorbent and other in vitro tests are available.

### Management

Avoidance of antigens (e.g., those associated with animals) is frequently possible, and levels of pollens can be decreased by remaining indoors and using electrostatic precipitators. The $H_1$–histamine receptors can be blocked with a variety of antagonists. Many of the older agents crossed the blood-brain barrier and caused sleepiness, but agents introduced more recently do not have this effect (terfenadine and astemizole). Overdoses of either of these new drugs may cause potentially fatal arrhythmias. Liver disease, hypokalemia, and concomitant usage of ketoconazole, macrolide antibiotics, ciprofloxacin, cimetidine, and disulfiram are all considered contraindications to the use of terfenadine, since they interfere with the metabolism of this drug. Antihistamines should be given on a regular basis, since they are more effective if administered before exposure to the antigen than afterward. α-Adrenergic agents are very effective when applied to the nasal mucosa and are available in both short- and long-acting forms. However, continued use for more than a few days results in rebound nasal congestion and reliance on the medication (rhinitis medicamentosa). Oral preparations are also effective but have systemic effects. Nasal steroid aerosols have proven very effective in the treatment of allergic rhinitis, though they may not relieve ocular symptoms. In addition, nasal cromolyn can be effective both for prevention and treatment, though a beneficial response may require some weeks to occur. Immunotherapy, utilizing increasing doses of the offending antigen, can also help but requires prolonged therapy. Administration of antigen is believed to result in the development of IgG antibody, which binds to the antigen and limits access to IgE, but other mechanisms have also been proposed.

## URTICARIA AND ANGIOEDEMA

Hives (urticaria) are commonly encountered in clinical practice and may or may not be a manifestation of an allergic reaction. These pruritic, raised lesions are due to local vasodilatation and accumulation of fluid in the superficial layers of the skin. When fluid enters the deeper tissues, it causes a nonpitting edema with erythema over a more diffuse area and is referred to as angioedema. Angioedema and urticaria may appear together or independently and are more frequent in young adults. Interaction of IgE on cutaneous mast cells with antigens is responsible for the allergic forms of these disorders. Histamine is released from the mast cells and interacts with receptors in the venules, which dilate and leak fluid and inflammatory cells. If the symptoms persist for more than 6 weeks, then the disorder is considered to be chronic. In the great majority of cases no cause is ever found for chronic urticaria-angioedema. In addition to recurrent reactions to defined antigens, urticaria may be initiated by physical stimuli such as cold exposure (which can be acquired or inherited and can actually result in life-threatening anaphylaxis), heat, stroking (dermatographism), vibration, and pressure. Inherited and acquired deficiencies of the inhibitor (C1NH) of the activated form of the first component of complement (C1) can result in angioedema unassociated with urticaria. Antihistamine therapy may be of some help in treating patients with these disorders, and attenuated androgens (e.g., oxymetholone) have also proven effective in some cases (see Urticaria on p. 358).

## BIBLIOGRAPHY

Clark TJH. *Asthma,* ed 3, London, 1992, Chapman and Hall Medical.

Guidelines for the Diagnosis and Management of Asthma. Publication No. 91-3042. National Institutes of Health. U.S. Department of Health and Human Services.

McFadden ER: Evolving concepts in the pathogenesis and management of asthma, *Adv Intern Med* 39:357, 1994.

Weiss EB: Bronchial asthma: mechanisms and therapeutics, ed 3, Boston, 1993, Little Brown.

CHAPTER

# 113 Pneumonia

Randolph J. Lipchik

More than two million cases of community-acquired pneumonia occur each year in the United States, with more than 800,000 hospitalizations and approximately 50,000 deaths. As the number of microorganisms identified as pathogens has increased and the number of patients with altered immune status due to underlying disease and/or medications has grown, the diagnosis and treatment of pneumonia have become more complicated. It is essential that a careful history and physical examination are obtained so that the range of diagnostic possibilities can be narrowed and optimal therapy initiated. It is the aim of this chapter to provide a rational approach for the evaluation and treatment of pneumonia. Common pathogens are discussed separately at the end of the chapter.

## EPIDEMIOLOGY AND ETIOLOGY

The actual incidence of pneumonia in ambulatory patients is difficult to estimate because the etiologic agent is rarely identified except in clinical trials, and it is not currently considered a reportable disease. Traditionally, *Streptococcus pneumoniae* was thought to be responsible for 60% to 70% of pneumonias; however, its prevalence has decreased with the identification of other agents (Table 113-1). The likelihood of each of these agents causing disease in a given patient is not certain, although certain host factors (Table 113-2) and geographic location may favor one infection rather than another. Travel to the Southwestern United States (Arizona, California, Texas) and contiguous areas of Mexico raises the possibility of infection by *Coccidioides immitis. Histoplasma capsulatum* is endemic in states bordering the Mississippi and Ohio rivers. *Blastomyces dermatitidis* is endemic in the southeast United States but also in Wisconsin, Minnesota, and neighboring Canadian provinces. Exposure to birds necessitates the addition of psittacosis to the differential diagnosis, and exposure to parturient cats, cattle, or sheep makes Q fever *(Coxiella burnetii)* a possibility.

Annual vaccination against influenza should reduce its incidence and that of secondary bacterial pneumonias. Vaccination against pneumococcal infection is recommended for patients 65 years and older and for younger persons at increased risk (i.e., anatomic or functional asplenia including sickle cell disease, cardiovascular disease, pulmonary disease, diabetes mellitus, alcoholism, cirrhosis, and cerebrospinal leaks). The current vaccine is a 23-valent preparation that provides coverage against approximately 90% of the most frequently reported capsular types. Although the duration of effect is unknown, routine revaccination of adults is not currently

**Table 113-1.** Causes of community-acquired bacterial pneumonia

| Pathogen | Prevalence (%) |
|---|---|
| *Streptococcus pneumoniae* | 30-75 |
| *Mycoplasma pneumoniae* | 5-35 |
| *Haemophilus influenzae* | 6-12 |
| *Staphylococcus aureus* | 3-10 |
| *Legionella pneumophila* | 3-30* |
| Gram-negative organisms | 3-10 |
| *Chlamydia pneumoniae* | 5-12† |
| *Moraxella catarrhalis* | 0.5-1 |
| Viruses | 2-10 |

*High prevalence in specific geographic locations.
†High prevalence in University of Washington student population.

**Table 113-2.** Association of host factors with particular pathogens

| Condition | Pathogen(s) |
|---|---|
| Chronic obstructive pulmonary disease | *Streptococcus pneumoniae, Haemophilus influenzae, Moraxella catarrhalis* |
| Alcoholism | *S. pneumoniae, Klebsiella pneumoniae, Staphylococcus aureus* |
| Diabetes | *S. aureus, S. pneumoniae* |
| Sickle cell anemia, asplenism | *S. pneumoniae, H. influenzae, S. aureus* |
| After influenza | *S. aureus, S. pneumoniae* |
| Neutropenia | *S. aureus, S. pneumoniae,* enteric gram-negative bacteria |
| Intravenous drug use | *S. aureus, S. pneumoniae* |
| HIV infection | *Pneumocystis carinii, S. pneumoniae* |

recommended unless the patient is at high risk for pneumococcal infection (asplenic) and originally received the 14-valent vaccine. Revaccination should also be considered for high-risk patients who received the 23-valent preparation more than 6 years previously and for those who have shown a rapid fall in pneumococcal antibody levels. It is less certain if this vaccine is efficacious in cases of immunocompromise, such as lymphoma, organ transplant, and infection with HIV.

## PATHOPHYSIOLOGY

The respiratory tract is a unique system in that it is open to the external environment and therefore continuously exposed to microorganisms, particulate matter, and fumes. In addition to all the organisms that are coughed or sneezed into the environment by other humans, we regularly aspirate nasopharyngeal flora during sleep. That pneumonia is rare in the face of constant microbial exposure is remarkable. There are multiple defense mechanisms to counteract these continuous exposures, including mechanical, anatomic, and immunologic barriers. The cough reflex, the mucociliary transport mechanism, and secretory immunoglobulins remove and neutralize microbes in the upper and central airways. In the alveoli the alveolar macrophages, immunoglobulins, and complement combine to clear organisms from the distal areas of the lung. Alterations in mental status may reduce the cough reflex, mucus production and ciliary function can be overcome by viral illness or tobacco smoke, and the immune response can be blunted by many illnesses or medications. Loss of these defenses in the setting of a large inoculum or particularly virulent organism can produce a significant infection.

Whether or not colonization of the upper airway is necessary before the development of pneumonia is unclear. In the outpatient population the carrier rate for *S. pneumoniae* is quite high, yet the incidence of pneumonia is quite low. In hospitalized patients, however, there is good evidence that colonization by gram-negative organisms occurs before the development of pneumonia. In a minority of cases pneumonia may result from hematogenously spread infection.

## HISTORY

Because of the multiple potential pathogens that cause pneumonia, the history becomes especially important in the evaluation of a patient with pneumonia. The presence or absence of fever, a dry or productive cough, an acute or gradual onset, the presence of chest pain and dyspnea may help distinguish upper from lower respiratory tract infection and a typical from an atypical pneumonia. In contrast to typical (pneumococcal) pneumonia, atypical pneumonia is characterized by lack of sputum production, lack of chest pain, and radiographic infiltrates that are not evident on physical examination. Agents causing atypical pneumonia are *Mycoplasma pneumoniae, Chlamydia pneumoniae,* viruses, and C. *burnetii.* As already discussed, information regarding concomitant medical conditions, recent travel, and animal exposure helps to direct the evaluation and therapy of the patient.

## PHYSICAL EXAMINATION

Attention to all aspects of the physical examination is crucial to determining severity of illness, whether the patient should be hospitalized, and possibly what treatment should be instituted. Fever is nonspecific, but a pulse-temperature disparity (normal pulse in the setting of high fever) favors pneumonia due to *Mycoplasma, Legionella,* or *Chlamydia* species or virus. Tachypnea and/or cyanosis suggests significant respiratory compromise and thus careful consideration before considering outpatient, rather than inpatient, therapy. Examination of the thorax may be unremarkable, show evidence of consolidation (dullness to percussion, increased tactile fremitus, and egophony), suggest interstitial infiltrates (crackles), or show evidence of a pleural effusion (dullness to percussion, decreased tactile fremitus, and decreased breath sounds). Extrapulmonary findings should not be overlooked and can offer clues to the underlying pathogen (Table 113-3). Neurologic disease, altered level of consciousness, and recent seizures suggest aspiration pneumonia. Periodontal disease makes an anaerobic infection more likely. Bullous myringitis is associated with *Mycoplasma* infection, and findings of encephalitis suggest *Mycoplasma, Legionella,* or *Coxiella.* Erythema multiforme is associated with *Mycoplasma, Histoplasma,* and *Coccidioides* species and some viruses. Erythema nodosum has also been associated with tuberculosis, chlamydial infection, histoplasmosis, and coccidioidomycosis.

## LABORATORY STUDIES AND DIAGNOSTIC PROCEDURES

The chest x-ray is the gold standard for determining the presence or absence of pneumonia. For many years the radiographic pattern was felt to be useful in determining the etiology of the pneumonia, but with more pathogens

**Table 113-3.** Extrapulmonary findings and causes of pneumonia

| Finding | Organism(s) |
|---|---|
| Bullous myringitis | *Mycoplasma pneumoniae* |
| Erythema multiforme | *M. pneumoniae, Histoplasma capsulatum, Coccidioides immitis,* some viruses |
| Erythema nodosum | Tuberculosis, *Chlamydia* species, *H. capsulatum, C. immitis* |
| Absent gag, due to seizure activity, CNS disease | *Bacteroides* species, aerobic and anaerobic streptococci; include *Staphylococcus aureus,* gram-negative organisms for institutionalized patients |
| Periodontal disease | Anaerobes |
| Encephalitis | *Legionella pneumophila, M. pneumoniae, Coxiella burnetii* |

and more elderly and immunocompromised patients this has become less reliable. The presence of an abscess, a central mass, or a pleural effusion is, however, very helpful in management decision making. Because of the lack of specificity of the chest x-ray, supplemental studies are necessary to determine an etiology. Examination of a sputum sample provides data that are available at the time of presentation and may help guide therapy. Unfortunately, most patients cannot produce a sample, and if they do it is often contaminated by oral flora. Nonetheless, a sputum smear with fewer than 10 squamous cells and greater than 25 neutrophils per high-power field should be representative of the secretions in the lung. Sputum culture requires 24 to 48 hours and may not provide diagnostic information. For example, the sensitivity for pneumococcus is only about 50%.

There are several invasive methods that can be employed when sputum is unobtainable, but the risks must be considered and compared to the use of empiric antibiotics, a safe and usually successful treatment. Transtracheal aspiration consists of passing a catheter via a large-bore needle through the cricothyroid membrane to allow aspiration of material distal to the oropharynx, thus avoiding contamination by oral flora. Its sensitivity has been questioned, and the potential for complications is real. Bronchoscopy can be employed to obtain distal samples, but passing through the upper airway makes contamination difficult to avoid. Quantitative cultures obtained during bronchoscopy with a protected brush or by bronchoalveolar lavage may distinguish infection from colonization or contamination; however, if the patient has already received antibiotics, the results have poor predictive value. This approach does have a useful role in evaluating the immunocompromised patient and cases of nonresolving pneumonias. Routine use, however, is not justified because standard antibiotics are quite effective and of low risk.

In addition to sputum cultures, blood cultures should be obtained, although on average only 10% to 15% of patients hospitalized for pneumonia have bacteremia. A thoracentesis should be performed if a pleural effusion is present to obtain material for Gram staining as well as culture. Infections with *Mycoplasma, Legionella, Chlamydia,* and *Coxiella* organisms and some viruses can be proven with serologic assays, but because convalescent titer samples must be drawn at least 3 weeks after onset of illness, empiric therapy is still necessary. Cold agglutinins may rise after 7 to 14 days of infection in *Mycoplasma* infections but are nonspecific, and similar increases can also be seen with influenza. *Legionella* species can be detected in sputum, pleural fluid, or tissue by direct immunofluorescent staining with a specificity of 90% to 100% but a sensitivity of only 25% to 50%. Detection of *Legionella* antigen in the urine has recently been demonstrated to be more useful, with sensitivity as high as 86%. Blood chemistries and leukocyte count with differential are nonspecific. An elevated leukocyte count with a left shift is common in any infection, and a low leukocyte count does not rule out a bacterial infection. Although hyponatremia, hypophosphatemia, and liver function abnormalities are associated with *Legionella* infection, these abnormalities can be seen with other severe infections.

## DIFFERENTIAL DIAGNOSIS

Pulmonary infiltrates on chest x-ray, cough, dyspnea, and fever are the presenting features of not only pneumonia, but also a substantial list of noninfectious conditions including pulmonary embolism, congestive heart failure, malignancy, vasculitis, collagen vascular disease, hypersensitivity, and idiopathic processes (Table 113-4). Often the presentation and clinical clues help distinguish these from a community-acquired infection, but the failure to respond to standard empiric therapy or progression of the process in an unexpected manner should alert the clinician to reconsider the initial diagnosis. Pulmonary embolism is usually characterized by the sudden onset of dyspnea, often in the setting of immobilization, the perioperative period, congestive heart failure, or malignancy. Chest pain and hemoptysis, which signify pulmonary infarction, occur in a minority of cases. The chest x-ray is usually normal in cases without infarction but may show evidence of atelectasis or a small pleural effusion. Congestive heart failure is usually not difficult to distinguish from pneumonia because of elevation of jugular venous pressure, lack of fever, and lack of a productive cough. In patients with chronic obstructive lung disease pulmonary edema may produce infiltrates that are asymmetric or focal. Resolution within hours to a day with diuresis confirms the presence of pulmonary edema.

Malignancy may present as a segmental consolidation, atelectasis, or diffuse interstitial pattern but presents clinically with a subacute development of cough or dyspnea. Fever, if present, is usually low grade and the cough is frequently dry. Often radiographic abnormalities are present without significant symptoms. The abrupt onset of dyspnea, hypoxemia, radiographic infiltrates, variable degrees of hemoptysis, and a falling

**Table 113-4.** Differential diagnosis of pneumonia and noninfectious pulmonary diseases

| Disease | Clinical features | Radiographic appearance |
|---|---|---|
| Pulmonary embolism | Sudden dyspnea, low-grade fever; cough not characteristic | Usually normal, but can see atelectasis or small pleural effusion; peripheral consolidation with infarct |
| Congestive heart failure | Increased jugular venous pressure, $S_3$ gallop, no fever or purulent sputum | Large cardiac shadow, bilateral infiltrates; can be asymmetric in COPD |
| Lymphangitic carcinomatosis | Insidious but progressive dyspnea | Resembles pulmonary edema |
| Alveolar hemorrhage | | |
| Rapidly progressive glomerulonephritis; systemic vasculitis: Wegener's granulomatosis, microscopic polyarteritis, systemic lupus erythematosus | Abrupt dyspnea, falling hematocrit, hemoptysis (50%), abnormal urinalysis | Bilateral infiltrates |
| Hypersensitivity pneumonitis | Flulike illness, relevant exposure history | Diffuse bilateral reticulonodular infiltrates |
| Bronchiolitis obliterans organizing pneumonia (BOOP) | Indistinguishable from pneumonia | Bilateral consolidation |

*COPD*, Chronic obstructive pulmonary disease.

hematocrit are seen in alveolar hemorrhage. This can occur in the setting of rapidly progressive glomerulonephritis or systemic necrotizing vasculitis (e.g., Wegener's granulomatosis, microscopic polyarteritis, or systemic lupus erythematosus). The rapid progression of renal abnormalities and extrapulmonary evidence of vasculitis should suggest a noninfectious process. Symptoms of hypersensitivity pneumonitis (e.g., farmer's lung and humidifier lung) include fever, dry cough, and pulmonary infiltrates within 4 to 6 hours of exposure to inhaled organic antigens, in these instances thermophilic actinomyces. Eliciting the history of inhalational exposure is the only way to distinguish this illness from community-acquired pneumonia.

Several medications have been associated with an acute onset of a pneumonia-like illness. Nitrofurantoin use can result in fever, dry cough, dyspnea, and infiltrates. A detailed history and peripheral blood eosinophilia provide clues to the diagnosis. Amiodarone can also produce pulmonary infiltrates. The diagnosis is often one of exclusion, since there are no distinguishing diagnostic features specific for this process. Last, an idiopathic process such as bronchiolitis obliterans organizing pneumonia (BOOP) may be initially confused with infectious pneumonia because of cough, dyspnea, alveolar infiltrates, and constitutional symptoms. Failure to respond to antibiotics may lead to open lung biopsy, the definitive way to confirm the diagnosis.

## SPECIFIC PATHOGENS

### *Streptococcus pneumoniae*

The classic presentation of pneumonia caused by *S. pneumoniae* is an abrupt onset of shaking chills, high fever, and dyspnea in the winter or early spring. About 75% of patients develop pleuritic chest pain and a cough productive of blood-streaked, or rusty, sputum. Physical examination demonstrates an ill-appearing patient with fever, tachypnea, tachycardia, and evidence of pulmonary consolidation. The white blood cell count usually demonstrates a polymorphonuclear leukocytosis between 12,000 and 25,000 cells/$mm^3$, but a normal or low white count can sometimes be seen in patients with overwhelming infection and bacteremia. Characteristically, a homogenous consolidation in the affected part of the lung with air bronchograms is visible on the x-ray, but findings can be diverse, from a patchy bronchopneumonia to diffuse bilateral infiltrates. In an emphysematous lung the consolidation can appear to be interstitial (Fig. 113-1). The organism is a gram-positive, encapsulated, lancet-shaped diplococcus that in sputum is seen singly or in pairs. Sputum cultures are helpful when positive; however, in one study of patients with pneumonia and blood cultures positive for *S. pneumoniae* the sputum culture was positive in only 45% of cases. Blood cultures are positive in 20% to 30% of cases.

Penicillin is the drug of choice for this pneumonia, but erythromycin should be substituted for penicillin-allergic patients. Penicillin resistance is a problem in some parts of the world, so culture with sensitivities should not be omitted. With the institution of antibiotics rapid clinical improvement is the rule, with 71% of patients afebrile within 5 days. Treatment should continue for at least 2 to 3 days after defervescence. Potential complications include pleural effusion with a 15% chance of empyema, endocarditis, meningitis, and septic arthritis. The latter three are seen rarely today, but the mortality remains significant at 5% for pneumonia and 20% with bacteremia.

The 23-valent pneumococcal vaccine is recommended for some patients (see previously and Chapter 3).

### *Mycoplasma pneumoniae*

*Mycoplasma* species differ from other bacteria because of the lack of a rigid cell wall structure. This results in absolute insensitivity to penicillins and lack of staining by Gram stain. Infection can occur at any time of the year and affects predominantly children and young adults. Attack rates are high with close indoor contact such as in households, dormitories, and barracks. Most often it produces a flulike respiratory illness with gradual onset of headache, malaise, fever, and dry cough. Physical examination is often remarkable only for fever. The white blood

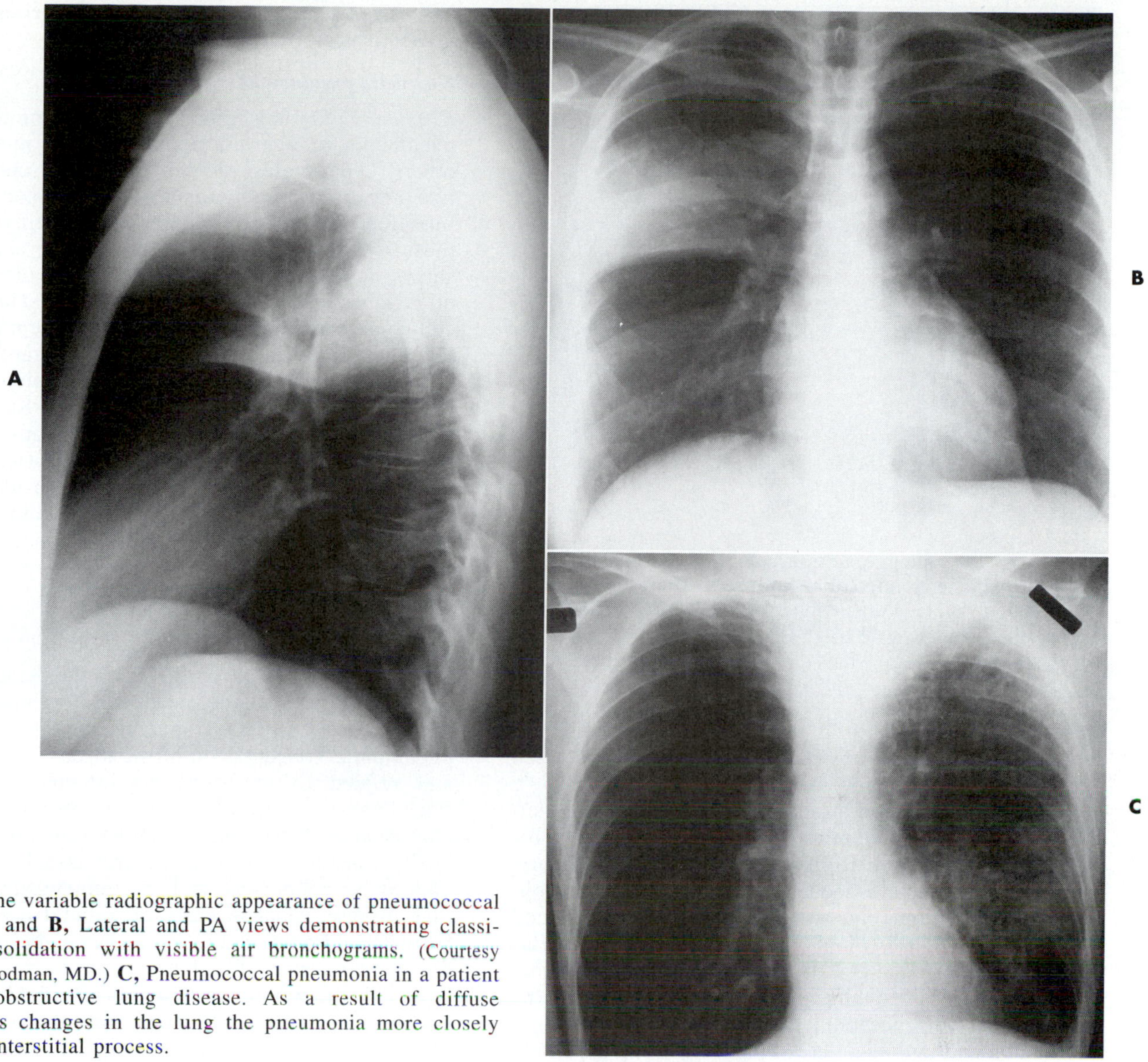


**Fig. 113-1.** The variable radiographic appearance of pneumococcal pneumonia. **A** and **B,** Lateral and PA views demonstrating classical lobar consolidation with visible air bronchograms. (Courtesy Lawrence R. Goodman, MD.) **C,** Pneumococcal pneumonia in a patient with severe obstructive lung disease. As a result of diffuse emphysematous changes in the lung the pneumonia more closely resembles an interstitial process.

cell count and differential are usually normal. Cold agglutinins may be present but nonspecific. Cultures of sputum or serologic studies are possible but do not provide information in time to assist in clinical decision making. The chest x-ray may show an interstitial infiltrate or small areas of atelectasis or small nodular densities (Fig. 113-2).

Treatment with erythromycin, clarithromycin, or doxycycline shortens the duration of illness. Antibiotics should be given for 14 days. Relapses after therapy are not unusual but respond to reinstitution of antibiotics. Complications such as bullous myringitis, erythema multiforme, meningoencephalitis, myocarditis, pericarditis, disseminating intravascular coagulation (DIC), and hemolytic anemia are rare, as is mortality.

### *Haemophilus influenzae*

*H. influenzae* are small pleomorphic gram-negative bacteria that appear as coccobacilli in culture. The upper respiratory tract of children is colonized by nonencapsulated strains at an early age; however, it is the type b encapsulated strain that is associated with virulent childhood infections such as epiglottitis, meningitis, and pneumonia. Because of the high prevalence of β-lactamase–producing type b strains in the United States, empiric therapy must take this into account. For household contacts of these patients rifampin (20 mg/kg per day for children, 600 mg daily for adults) is given in a single daily dose for 4 days to eliminate nasopharyngeal carriage and thus secondary infections. Vaccination against the type b strain is now recommended for all children as part of the standard immunization schedule. Nonencapsulated strains of *H. influenzae* have been associated with otitis, sinusitis, bronchitis, and pneumonia in the adult population, and alcohol abuse, asplenism, and immunoglobulin deficiency predispose to infection. The clinical features of pneumonia are indistinguishable from other bacterial pneumonias, although the chest x-ray frequently shows multilobar involvement. Successful aerobic culture requires both X and V factors to ensure growth. Isolation of the organism from infected tissues and body fluids confirms the diagnosis, but the

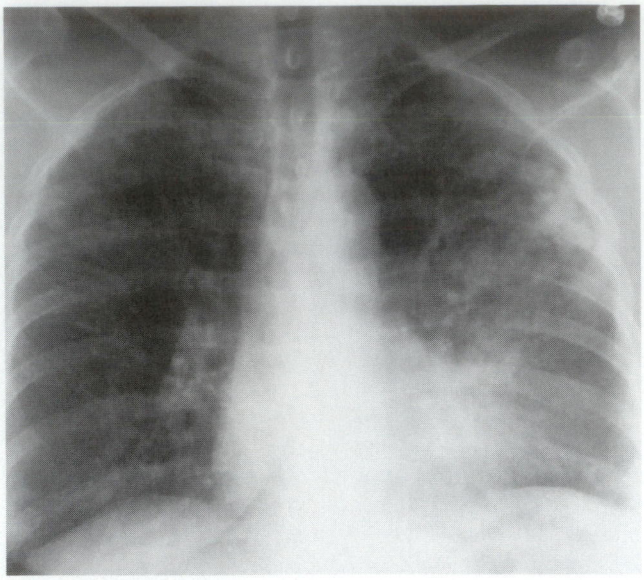

**Fig. 113-2.** The radiographic appearance of mycoplasma pneumonia with bilateral interstitial infiltrates. There are areas of consolidation visible in the periphery of the left upper lung zone. (Courtesy Lawrence R. Goodman, MD.)

presence of the organism in nasopharyngeal secretions of patients with chronic obstructive lung disease is often related to the high carrier rate in this population.

The nonencapsulated strains of *H. influenzae* are usually susceptible to conventional antibiotics, but assays for β-lactamase and sensitivity studies are mandatory. Ampicillin-clavulanate, second- or third-generation cephalosporins, azithromycin, and ciprofloxacin are all good choices for empiric therapy. Trimethoprim/sulfamethoxazole (TMP/SMX) is often effective for less severe infections such as bronchitis and otitis but should not be used for treating pneumonia. Complications such as pleural effusion and empyema are sometimes seen, and rarely other suppurative complications such as pericarditis and osteomyelitis have occurred.

### *Staphylococcus aureus*

An occasional cause of community-acquired pneumonia, this gram-positive coccus is most often seen following influenza infection. After or during a typical influenza syndrome the onset of prostration, high fever, chest pain, cough productive of purulent sputum, and hemoptysis suggests staphylococcal pneumonia. The chest x-ray often shows bilateral patchy infiltrates that may cavitate. Pleural effusion is common. The white blood cell count is usually elevated but can be depressed in severe cases. Blood cultures are positive in 20% to 30% of cases. Sputum cultures are only suggestive of the diagnosis because the organism frequently colonizes the upper airway. Therapy requires an intravenous semisynthetic penicillin such as dicloxacillin or nafcillin. First-generation cephalosporins are useful for patients with mild allergic manifestations to penicillin. When methicillin-resistant organisms are present, vancomycin is the drug of choice. Duration of therapy is 14 days, but for endocarditis 4 to 6 weeks of therapy may be necessary. Complications such as lung abscess, empyema, and bacteremia are common, and the subsequent mortality rate is significant.

### *Klebsiella pneumoniae*

*K. pneumoniae* is a minor cause of community-acquired pneumonia, and certain populations are more prone than others. Older males, alcohol abuse, and chronic obstructive lung disease are factors frequently associated with this infection. The clinical features are indistinguishable from those of pneumococcal pneumonia. The chest x-ray film shows a segmental consolidation that often spreads to other lobes if it is not properly treated. The white blood cell count can be elevated but is often depressed. Sputum Gram stain reveals short, plump, encapsulated gram-negative rods. Blood cultures and pleural fluid are potential sources for positive cultures. Susceptibility to antibiotics is variable, so empiric therapy with a third-generation cephalosporin is indicated. Ticarcillin-clavulanate is another option. An aminoglycoside is added for severely ill patients. Lung abscess and empyema are more common complications than with pneumococcal pneumonia. Therapy should last 10 to 14 days but longer if complications develop.

### *Legionella pneumophila*

Since its recognition in 1976 at the American Legion convention in Philadelphia, this organism has been identified as a cause of epidemic and sporadic cases of pneumonia. Transmission of the disease is environmental and related to proximity to infected water sources. Pneumonia is most often seen in the middle-aged and elderly population, and although occurring in previously healthy persons, most cases are associated with other underlying conditions such as immunosuppression, cardiac disease, renal disease, or general debilitation. The typical prodrome includes headache and myalgias followed by the onset of high fever and shaking chills. Cough is usually minimally productive. Confusion or delirium may be seen in up to half of patients and diarrhea in 25%. Physical examination reveals an ill patient often with a relative bradycardia in the face of high fever. There is usually no evidence of consolidation on lung examination. Laboratory studies are remarkable for leukocytosis and frequent transaminase elevation, hypophosphatemia, and hyponatremia. The chest x-ray often shows patchy infiltrates that can progress. Although suggestive, most of these findings are nonspecific so confirmation of the diagnosis must be pursued. Gram stain of sputum is unrevealing, but culture on selective media is possible. Direct immunofluorescent staining (DFA) of sputum or tissue is a rapid diagnostic tool, but it has only 25% to 50% sensitivity. A recently described assay of *Legionella* antigen in the urine appears to be rapid and much more sensitive. A fourfold rise in titer between acute and convalescent sera confirms the diagnosis but is not helpful in initial management decisions. Erythromycin is the drug of choice and is continued for 21 days to prevent relapse. In severe cases rifampin can be added to improve efficacy. In vitro studies have shown that clarithromycin, azithromycin, and ciprofloxacin may be effective alternatives for erythromycin-intolerant patients. Complications include respiratory failure, shock, rhabdomyolysis, DIC, and renal failure. Mortality can be as high as 25%.

### *Moraxella catarrhalis*

For many years *Moraxella catarrhalis* was felt to be a harmless colonizer of the upper airway. In recent years it has been recognized as a cause of acute bronchitis and pneumonia in ill and elderly patients with chronic obstructive lung disease. Chest pain, hemoptysis, and high fever are unusual, and the physical examination is dominated by signs of the underlying obstructive lung disease. The white cell count can be mildly elevated but is usually normal. The chest x-ray usually reveals scattered patchy infiltrates. Diagnosis is suggested by gram-negative kidney-shaped diplococci that resemble *Neisseria* organisms and is confirmed by culture. Most species produce β-lactamase and are resistant to penicillins. Ampicillin-clavulanate, TMP/SMX, clarithromycin, and ciprofloxacin are all effective drugs. If β-lactamase is not present, treatment with penicillin or ampicillin is adequate.

### Chlamydial infections

*Chlamydia psittaci* is the classic etiologic agent for the atypical pneumonia that develops after exposure to birds (e.g., parrots, parakeets, pigeons, ducks, turkeys). It is characterized by a severe dry cough, high fever, and severe back and neck muscle pain. Delirium, hepatitis, and splenomegaly are common extrapulmonary findings. The chest x-ray usually reveals patchy infiltrates, but any pattern can occur. The diagnosis is usually confirmed by serologic studies because culture is hazardous and requires special expertise. Doxycycline is effective therapy and should be continued for 7 days after defervescence. Mortality is approximately 1%, but before the development of adequate antibiotics it was 20% to 40%.

More recently, *Chlamydia pneumoniae* has been identified as a distinct species. From serologic studies it appears that infections by this organism are ubiquitous and range from pharyngitis and sinusitis to bronchitis and pneumonia. The pneumonitis resembles that caused by *M. pneumoniae.* Diagnosis is difficult because culture methods are too insensitive and serologic studies are not universally available. Treatment with erythromycin or doxycycline for 10 to 14 days is recommended.

### *Histoplasma capsulatum*

*H. capsulatum* is a dimorphic fungus that is found worldwide. In the soil it is in the mycelial phase, but within a mammalian host it replicates in the yeast phase. States with the highest infection rates border the Mississippi and Ohio rivers, particularly Ohio, Kentucky, Indiana, Illinois, Tennessee, Missouri, and Arkansas. The concentration of fungus is variable within these states, with heavy concentration in bird excrement. Any disturbance of soil results in airborne organisms that, if inhaled, may result in infection. Most cases have minimal or no symptoms. Approximately 2 weeks after a large exposure a flulike illness with fever, chills, myalgias, and dry cough may develop. With or without symptoms there is systemic hematogenous spread of organism until the development of cell-mediated immunity in 7 to 14 days, which rapidly limits the infection in the lung and elsewhere. Physical examination is usually unrevealing, although the presence of erythema nodosum is suggestive of the diagnosis. The chest x-ray may show a patchy bilateral bronchopneumonia with hilar adenopathy that usually resolves spontaneously. It is not unusual for residual nodules and hilar lymph nodes to calcify after several years. In older smokers with emphysema, histoplasmosis can result in chronic upper lobe cavitary disease, which resembles tuberculosis.

Symptoms include chronic cough and eventual weight loss with variable fever as the infection progresses. Disseminated histoplasmosis is rare but can be a fulminant illness in infants and immunosuppressed adults. This is manifest by fever, lymphadenopathy, hepatosplenomegaly, pancytopenia, and interstitial pulmonary infiltrates. In most adult cases the disseminated form of infection can be more indolent, with chronic fever, weight loss, skin lesions, and possible adrenal insufficiency. Less than half of these cases will have pulmonary symptoms or an abnormal chest x-ray. A definitive diagnosis is made by isolation of the fungus from sputum, blood, or tissue but may take several weeks. If possible, direct visualization of the organism provides rapid information that helps determine therapy. With complement fixation a fourfold rise in titer is diagnostic of recent infection, and a single titer of 1:32 or greater is suggestive in the proper clinical setting.

Treatment is indicated for disseminated and progressive chronic cavitary histoplasmosis. Ketoconazole or itraconazole is indicated for immunocompetent patients with nonmeningeal disease who are not critically ill. All other cases require intravenous amphotericin B.

### *Blastomyces dermatitidis*

*B. dermatitidis* is a dimorphic fungus that grows in the yeast phase when in tissue, with characteristic broad-based budding. This fungus is endemic in the southeastern United States and along the western shore of Lake Michigan, as well as in Minnesota, North Dakota, and bordering Canadian provinces. Infection follows inhalation of spores and may be symptomatic. Symptomatic infection appears as an acute pneumonia with fever, productive cough, pleuritic chest pain, and myalgias.

Symptoms range from mild to severe and last a few days to several weeks. The chest x-ray often shows patchy consolidation, which can be bilateral. Hilar adenopathy is not unusual, but pleural effusion is rare. Infection is usually self-limited. A chronic form of infection is also recognized with weeks of cough, low-grade fever, sweats, and weight loss. The chest x-ray may show fibrocavitary disease, as in tuberculosis, or a large mass that appears like a bronchogenic carcinoma. Disseminated disease involving skin, bone, and the genitourinary tract is not unusual in the chronic form of disease. Meningeal involvement is rare. Diagnosis is made by visualization of characteristic budding yeast in sputum, tissue, and sometimes prostatic secretions. Culture confirms the diagnosis but may take up to 3 weeks.

Acute blastomycosis often requires no specific therapy. For severe pulmonary involvement, progressive chronic disease, or disseminated disease, treatment with oral ketoconazole or itraconazole is usually effective. Amphotericin B is the drug of choice for severe life-threatening infections, meningeal disease, or failures of oral therapy.

### *Coccidioides immitis*

*C. immitis* is a dimorphic fungus endemic to southern California, Arizona, Nevada, New Mexico, Texas, and northern Mexico. Airborne spores are very infectious, and inhalation results in high rates of primary infection. Although usually asymptomatic, 40% of cases develop fever, malaise, dry cough, dyspnea, chest pain, pharyngitis, and rash. The chest x-ray may show variable infiltrates that are transient, migratory, or cavitary. Pleural effusion is seen in fewer than 10% of cases. Symptoms and radiographic abnormalities lasting more than 6 to 8 weeks are categorized as persistent coccidioidal pneumonia. Disseminated infection is rare in the immunocompetent host; however, for unclear reasons African-Americans are 10 to 15 times more likely to develop extrapulmonary manifestations than are whites. There have also been suggestions that Filipinos and Asians are also at higher risk, but the evidence for this is circumstantial. Patients with lymphoma or AIDS or taking immunosuppressive medications are also at risk.

Disseminated disease most commonly involves skin, bones, soft tissue, and the meninges, but it can involve any organ. Diagnosis is reliably made by the demonstration of the characteristic spherules, containing multiple endospores, in secretions or infected tissues. Growth in culture is relatively rapid, requiring only 5 to 7 days. In addition, complement fixation titers tend to be higher for more severe disease, but a low titer does not rule out disseminated disease. Amphotericin B is the drug of choice for severe, life-threatening disseminated disease. Oral ketoconazole as well as itraconazole have been used for less severe chronic pulmonary, skin, and soft tissue infections with reasonable results, but failures of therapy and relapses occur in up to 45% of cases. Primary coccidioidal infection ordinarily requires no therapy, but in high-risk patients therapy to prevent dissemination is reasonable.

## MANAGEMENT

Management of pneumonia must include both antibiotic therapy directed against the causative organism and supportive measures. The latter include rest, adequate hydration to correct for fever-induced fluid loss and poor intake, supplemental oxygen for saturation less than 90%, and analgesia for chest pain. Chest percussion and postural drainage may be useful in selected patients with bronchiectasis or those too weak to generate an adequate cough. Routine use of this time- and labor-intensive modality has not been beneficial in uncomplicated pneumonias.

Antibiotic therapy should be administered as quickly as possible once the diagnosis has been confirmed radiographically. In the ideal situation the choice of antibiotic should be guided by a Gram stain of sputum. Many polymorphonuclear neutrophil leukocytes, no epithelial cells, and a predominant organism allow more specific therapy. More often the choice is empiric, and all the clinical data must be considered before deciding on a regimen. Unless the presentation or history suggests a particular pathogen, erythromycin is the drug of first choice because it is effective for the agents causing the vast majority of community-acquired pneumonias (i.e., *S. pneumoniae* and *M. pneumoniae*). Therapy can be altered or narrowed, when there are positive cultures of sputum or blood, with sensitivity studies. Extended spectrum macrolides such as clarithromycin can be substituted for patients with *Mycoplasma* infection and erythromycin-

**Table 113-5.** Recommended antibiotics for initial empiric therapy

| Pneumonic process | Pathogens | Outpatient* | Inpatient |
|---|---|---|---|
| Acute community-acquired pneumonia | *Pneumococcus, Mycoplasma, H. influenzae, S. aureus, Legionella, Chlamydia* | Erythromycin or clarithromycin<br>Amoxicillin-clavulanate<br>Cephalexin or cefaclor | Erythromycin, 0.5 g IV q6h *and/or*<br>Cefuroxime, 0.75-1.5 g IV q8h<br>Ceftriaxone, 1-2 g IV q24h |
| Atypical community-acquired pneumonia | *Mycoplasma, Legionella, Chlamydia* | Erythromycin or clarithromycin<br>Doxycycline | Erythromycin, 0.5-1 g IV q6h<br>Doxycycline, 200 mg IV day 1, then 100 mg IV daily |
| Community-acquired aspiration | *Bacteroides* species, aerobic/anaerobic streptococci | Clindamycin<br>Amoxicillin-clavulanate | Clindamycin, 600-900 mg IV q8h<br>Ampicillin-sulbactam, 1.5-3 g IV q6h<br>Cefoxitin, 0.5-2 g IV q4-8h |
| Nosocomial aspiration (nursing home) | As above, plus enteric gram-negatives and *S. aureus* | Clindamycin and ciprofloxacin | Ticarcillin-clavulanate, 3.1 mg IV q4-6h<br>Imipenem, 0.5-1 g IV q6-8h<br>Ceftazidime/clindamycin, 1-2 g IV q8h/600-900 mg IV q8h (add aminoglycoside if *Pseudomonas* present) |
| Neutropenia | Gram-positives from community including *S. aureus,* and enteric gram-negatives | | Ticarcillin/piperacillin, 3-4 g IV q4-6h or ceftazidime plus aminoglycoside |
| Chronic steroids +/− cytotoxic drugs | Gram-positives, gram-negatives, *Pneumocystis carinii* | | As above, plus high-dose TMP/SMX, 15-20 mg/kg/d in 3-4 divided doses (based on TMP content) |
| AIDS | *S. pneumoniae, P. carinii* | | High-dose TMP/SMX plus erythromycin or clarithromycin |

*See Table 113-6 for dosages.
*TMP/SMX,* Trimethoprim/sulfamethoxazole.

induced nausea or in patients with streptococcal or *H. influenzae* infections who are allergic to penicillins or cephalosporins. Although most community-acquired pneumonia is due to *S. pneumoniae,* the empiric use of penicillin may no longer be appropriate given the increasing reports of penicillin resistance. The prevalence of this problem varies from 1.3% in Canada to near 50% in South Africa and has been reported sporadically in the United States. Clinicians should be aware of the local prevalence. Penicillin is still the drug of choice for sensitive *S. pneumoniae.* Suggestions for empiric and specific antibiotic therapy are listed in Tables 113-5 and 113-6. The narrowing or simplification of therapy to treat a particular organism should be guided by the results of diagnostic laboratory studies, especially cultures and sensitivities.

The diagnosis of pneumonia and therapy for the geriatric population deserve special attention, particularly if the patient is a resident of a nursing home. Classic symptoms of cough, sputum production, chest pain, and fever are much less frequent in weak, debilitated patients. Coughing requires adequate muscle strength, and pleuritic pain and fever result from a vigorous inflammatory response. These may be lacking in elderly patients who have poor nutrition or poor general health. Confusion and mental status changes may be the predominant clinical findings. Although *S. pneumoniae* is the most common pathogen, other agents such as *H. influenzae* (which produces β-lactamase in greater than 15% of cases) and *M. catarrhalis* must be considered, particularly in the setting of chronic obstructive lung disease. Gram-negative bacilli are also more common, particularly in the chronically institutionalized patient. *M. pneumoniae* is an uncommon pathogen in the older patient. *Legionella* incidence is variable, being more prevalent in certain regions of the country and during epidemic outbreaks.

A second group of patients that requires special consideration consists of those with altered immunity. This can result from infection with HIV, the presence of leukemia or lymphoma, chemotherapy-induced granulocytopenia, or treatment for a variety of illnesses with long-term steroids and/or cytotoxic agents. A detailed discussion of each of these conditions is beyond the scope of this chapter, but some important issues must be considered. First, the evaluation and treatment of a pneumonia in these patients should be in hospital. Because the morbidity and mortality of infections are much higher than in the general population, prompt empiric therapy along with diagnostic procedures is essential. Second, initial empiric antibiotic therapy must cover multiple potential pathogens; and last, because of the possibility of unusual and/or multiple pathogens (Table 113-7), invasive diagnostic procedures such as bronchoscopy with bronchoalveolar lavage are considered in the first 24 to 48 hours in addition to cultures of sputum, blood, and other fluids. Although pulmonary infiltrates may also represent drug or radiation toxicity or an underlying leukemia/lymphoma, these can be considered only after an infectious etiology has been ruled out.

Once therapy has been initiated, patients should be monitored for fever, respiratory and cardiovascular status, and general features such as energy and appetite. Most patients taking appropriate antibiotics improve within 48 to 72 hours. Fever that continues 24 hours into therapy does not necessarily indicate a failure of antibiotics. A gradual decrease in the maximum daily temperature is the usual response to therapy. Persistent fever, with worsening clinical status, may herald the development of a suppurative complication such as an empyema, an inappropriate choice of antibiotics, the wrong diagnosis, or drug fever. Therapy should be continued for 7 to 14 days. *M. pneumoniae* infections should be treated for 14 days, whereas confirmed cases of *Legionella* infection require 21 days of therapy. For hospitalized patients intravenous

**Table 113-6.** Antibiotic choices for specific pathogens

| Pathogen | Antibiotic of choice | Alternative |
|---|---|---|
| *S. pneumoniae* | Penicillin, 250-500 mg PO qid, 1-4 million U IV q 4-6h | Erythromycin, 250-500 mg PO/IV qid<br>Clindamycin, 300-600 mg PO tid, 600-900 mg IV q8h |
| *Mycoplasma* | Erythromycin<br>Clarithromycin, 250 mg PO bid<br>Azithromycin, 500 mg PO day 1, then 250 mg/day × 4 days | Doxycycline, 200 mg PO/IV day 1, then 100 mg/day |
| *H. influenzae* | Ampicillin-clavulanate, 250-500 mg PO tid<br>Cephalosporins (second/third generation) | TMP/SMX, 80/400 mg PO bid<br>Clarithromycin<br>Ciprofloxacin, 500 mg PO bid |
| *S. aureus*<br>Methicillin sensitive | Dicloxacillin, 125-250 mg PO qid<br>Nafcillin, 0.5-1 g IV q4h | Cefazolin, 0.5-2 g IV q8h<br>Erythromycin<br>Clindamycin |
| Methicillin resistant | Vancomycin, 1-2 g IV daily | |
| *M. catarrhalis* | Ampicillin-clavulanate<br>TMP/SMX | Clarithromycin<br>Ciprofloxacin |
| *K. pneumoniae* | Cephalosporin (third generation)<br>Ciprofloxacin, 500-750 mg PO bid, 400 mg IV q12h | Ticarcillin-clavulanate, 3.1 g IV q4-6h |
| *Legionella* | Erythromycin, 1g IV/PO q6h | Clarithromycin, 500 mg PO bid |

*TMP/SMX,* Trimethoprim/sulfamethoxazole.

**Table 113-7.** Pneumonia in the immunocompromised host

| Condition | Pathogen(s) |
|---|---|
| Leukemia/lymphoma, high-dose prolonged steroids, organ transplants | CMV, PCP, *Cryptococcus, Nocardia, Legionella* |
| Neutropenia (<500/mm³) | Gram-negative bacteria, *Aspergillus, Mucor, Candida* |
| Immunosuppressive drugs; steroids and/or cyclophosphamide, methotrexate | Gram-positive and gram-negative bacteria, PCP, CMV |

*CMV*, Cytomegalovirus; *PCP*, *Pneumocystis carinii* pneumonia.

antibiotics are continued until the patient has been afebrile for a minimum of 48 hours; then oral medication can begin. In the outpatient setting additional chest x-rays may be repeated at the end of therapy. It is important to note that radiographic infiltrates may completely clear only after many weeks, particularly with pneumococcal pneumonia. Slow radiographic resolution does not mean a failure of therapy in the face of clinical response, and frequent chest x-rays are not necessary. Consultation by a pulmonary or infectious diseases specialist should be considered for immunocompromised patients, those who fail to respond in a typical manner, those in whom suppurative complications develop, or when there is respiratory compromise.

### Indications for hospitalization

Indications for hospitalization must be carefully considered, since inadequate therapy can lead to increased morbidity and mortality (see Managed Care Guide).

The majority of patients with pneumonia do not meet the criteria in the Managed Care Guide and can be managed as outpatients without complication; however, more than a third of these patients may suffer a more complicated course. Independent predictors of a complicated course include age greater than 65 years, comorbid illness, fever greater than 38.3°C (101°F), and immunosuppression. If any of these are present, careful evaluation is mandatory before deciding upon outpatient therapy. If the pneumonia requires inpatient therapy, a good outcome is not assured. Current mortality ranges between 6% and 24%. Several features have been found to be predictive of subsequent mortality. In one study a discriminant rule based on a respiratory rate of 30 per minute or more, a diastolic blood pressure of 60 or less, and a blood urea nitrogen of 20 mg/dl or more predicted mortality with an accuracy of 82%.

**Managed Care Guide**
**Indications for hospitalization in the treatment of pneumonia**

1. Inability to take oral medications
2. Multilobar involvement on chest x-ray
3. A severe vital sign abnormality (pulse more than 140 beats/min, systolic blood pressure less than 90 mm Hg or a respiratory rate more than 30 per minute)
4. Acute mental status changes
5. Arterial hypoxemia (room air oxygen tension less than 60 torr)
6. A secondary suppurative infection such as empyema, meningitis, or endocarditis
7. A severe acute electrolyte, hematologic, or metabolic abnormality (serum sodium less than 130 mEq/L, hematocrit less than 30%, absolute neutrophil count less than 1000/mm³, blood urea nitrogen more than 50 mg/dl, or creatinine greater than 2.5 mg/dl)
8. Acute coexistent medical conditions such as a suspected acute myocardial infarction, renal insufficiency, liver disease, or malignancy

## BIBLIOGRAPHY

Caputo GM, Appelbaum PC, Liu HH: Infections due to penicillin-resistant pneumococci-clinical, epidemiologic, and microbiologic features, *Arch Intern Med* 153:1301, 1993.

Farr BM, Sloman AJ, Fisch MJ: Predicting death in patients hospitalized for community-acquired pneumonia, *Ann Intern Med* 115:428, 1991.

Fein AM, Feinsilver SH, Niederman MS: Atypical manifestations of pneumonia in the elderly, *Clin Chest Med* 12(2):319, 1991.

Fine MJ, Smith DN, Singer DE: Hospitalization decision in patients with community-acquired pneumonia: a prospective cohort study, *Am J Med* 89:713, 1990.

Gross TJ, Chavis AD, Lynch JP: Noninfectious pulmonary diseases masquerading as community-acquired pneumonia, *Clin Chest Med* 12(2):363, 1991.

Marrie TJ, Durant H, Yates L: Community-acquired pneumonia requiring hospitalization: 5-year prospective study, *Rev Infect Dis* 11:586, 1989.

Pennington, JE, editor: *Respiratory infections: diagnosis and management,* ed 2, New York, 1989, Raven Press.

Rosenow EC, Wilson WR, Cockerill FR: Pulmonary disease in the immunocompromised host. Part I, *Mayo Clin Proc* 60:473, 1985.

Wilson WR, Cockerill FR, Rosenow EC: Pulmonary disease in the immunocompromised host. Part II, *Mayo Clin Proc* 60:610, 1985.

CHAPTER

# 114 Tuberculosis and Nontuberculous Mycobacterial Diseases

David Rosenzweig

## TUBERCULOSIS

### Epidemiology

In the past century and until the past decade the incidence of tuberculosis in the United States had continuously declined, and efforts against this formidable scourge appeared to be one of medicine's substantial success stories. Between 1900 and 1985 tuberculosis mortality declined from 200 per 100,000 to fewer than 2 per

100,000, a decrease of over a hundredfold. The worldwide picture was never quite so promising. Declines have occurred, but tuberculosis remains the most important fatal infection worldwide, accounting for 3 million deaths annually; those who have been infected by *Mycobacterium tuberculosis,* (i.e., tuberculin reactors) number over 2 billion, nearly half of humankind (Table 114-1). About 2.5 million tuberculosis deaths occur in developing nations annually, where tuberculosis accounts for 6.7% of all deaths, 18.5% of deaths among persons 15 to 59 years of age, and 26% of all preventable deaths.

Over the past decade tuberculosis has been resurgent both in the United States and throughout the world, especially in Africa and Asia. Fueled by the AIDS epidemic as well as other factors, including immigration, poverty, homelessness, and deterioration of public health programs, substantial increases in tuberculosis have occurred. In the United States, these increases or outbreaks have been focused in larger cities and particularly in closed institutions: shelters, penal institutions, nursing homes, and hospitals. Another worrisome trend has been the shift of the age incidence of tuberculosis cases from the elderly to peaks in younger adults, especially in the minority populations, implying greater recent infection in these groups (Fig. 114-1). The problem has been compounded by an increase in drug-resistant cases, so a more intense, individualized approach to treatment is needed.

Robert Koch in 1882 first demonstrated that tuberculosis is an infectious disease caused by *M. tuberculosis.* The bacillus is a rod 1 to 4 μm in length with a waxy cell wall that accounts for its resistance to acid stain decoloring, referred to as acid fastness. The organism is hardy, requiring minimal nutrients for culture and able to survive adverse conditions for long periods. A closely related organism, *M. bovis,* can cause bovine tuberculosis, a similar illness, but this infection has virtually disappeared from the United States due to elimination of its source in infected dairy herds and pasteurization of milk products.

Tuberculosis disease is characteristically chronic or recurrent, but its manifestations range from an inapparent or subclinical infection in the majority of those affected to an acute and rapidly progressive illness, especially in immunocompromised hosts or small children.

## Natural history

Airborne spread from an infected person, the usual mode of infection, is especially likely to occur during aerosolization of droplets in speaking, singing, coughing, or sneezing. Such droplets quickly evaporate to droplet nuclei, which are capable of penetrating deeply into the respiratory tract. Large droplets, if inhaled, are likely to settle in or be trapped by mucous linings of the upper respiratory tract or larger airways and are harmlessly excreted by the mucus escalator. However, infected droplet nuclei of 1 to 5 μm will penetrate and be deposited at the alveolar level, where infection is more likely to occur. Since this mechanism is uncertain, repeated exposure and close household contact constitute the most usual pattern of spread.

Initially the host mounts no defense and the mycobacteria multiply, but within days cellular and humoral defense mechanisms develop. At first organisms are lysed within macrophages, and mycobacterial antigens become accessible to T lymphocytes and B lymphocytes. Sensitized T lymphocytes secrete lymphokines, which attract and enhance macrophage activity, making phagocytosis and bacterial killing far more effective. This process takes 4 to 6 weeks to become effective and parallels the development of tuberculin reactivity. This reaction, which depends on activated T lymphocytes, appears at a mean of 6 weeks after inoculation with a range of 3 to 12 weeks.

The stage of primary tuberculosis also appears at about this time. It may be subclinical and is usually nonspecific with symptoms of fever and cough, which subside over 2 to 3 weeks. If tuberculosis is suspected and the patient is evaluated, there are few, if any, signs on physical examination, but the chest x-ray may show a middle or lower zone segmental infiltrate and enlarged hilar lymph nodes. In children atelectasis from lymph node compression may be present. Mycobacterial stains and cultures of respiratory specimens, sputa, or bronchial lavage may be negative in over half of the cases because the organisms

**Table 114-1.** World Health Organization and Centers for Disease Control recent epidemiologic estimates for tuberculosis

| | United States | World |
|---|---|---|
| Infected (tuberculin reactors) | 10 million (4%) | >2 billion (30%-50%) |
| New disease cases (annual) | 26,000 | 8 million |
| Deaths (annual) | 2000 | 3 million |

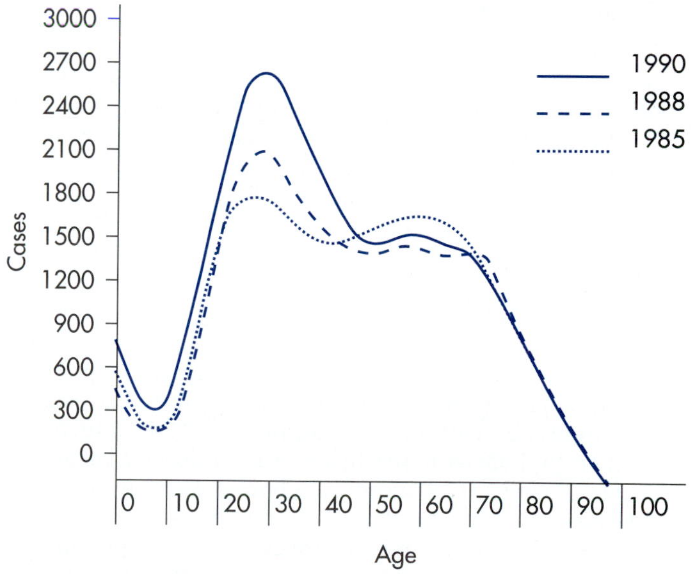


**Fig. 114-1.** Age distribution of reported tuberculosis cases by year of report, United States, 1985-1990. (From Jereb JA, Kelley GD et al: Tuberculosis morbidity in the United States. *MMWR* 40:55-3, 23-27, 1991.)

are still relatively few at this stage. However, transient mycobacteremia occurs during primary tuberculosis, seeding distant sites and setting the stage for potential later reactivation of disease at such sites, most commonly the pulmonary apex, renal cortex, epiphyses of long bones, and meninges.

Primary tuberculosis can then spontaneously subside or lead to several outcomes: (1) no further disease and no residual lesions, or only a calcified primary complex on x-ray, a calcified parenchymal nodule, and ipsilateral hilar lymph node calcification; this is the most common scenario; (2) manifestations of progressive primary infection with development of pleural effusion or mediastinal and cervical lymphadenitis (see section on extrapulmonary tuberculosis); (3) more serious life-threatening dissemination with the development of miliary or meningeal tuberculosis; or (4) a dormant phase with the development of reactivation disease years or decades later in distant sites, most frequently the lung apex, less commonly in the extrapulmonary sites of hematogenous spread noted above. The immunocompromised host, especially the HIV infected, is far more likely to develop progressive primary and disseminated stages of disease than is the otherwise healthy host.

Conventional wisdom and historical data indicate that, once an individual is infected, he or she is relatively immune from subsequent new infection, and that later recurrences or relapses are due to endogenous reactivation of the original strain. However, recent data show that this relative immunity can be overcome. In certain situations of closed institutions, such as nursing homes and prisons where exposure may be heavy, exogenous new infection with different strains may be identified. An immunocompromised host is more prone to new infection than others. Indeed, in AIDS patients *during treatment* for drug-susceptible tuberculous disease, new drug-resistant strains with different DNA fingerprints have emerged with reversal of a previously favorable course.

## Clinical features

***Pulmonary tuberculosis.*** Systemic manifestations are usually present. Fever occurs in 50% to 80% of cases, and other symptoms of malaise and weight loss are also frequent. Night sweats are often noted as a manifestation of fever; the sweating occurs during defervescence following daily afternoon fever spikes.

Other notable laboratory abnormalities include leukocytosis in 10% to 20% of cases, anemia in at least 10%, and hyponatremia in 10% to 15%. Anemia is more likely in more advanced disease and may be a sign of dissemination. Occasionally, anemia or pancytopenia may result from direct bone marrow involvement. Hyponatremia is usually of the normovolemic type and is a result of inappropriate antidiuretic hormone (ADH) secretion marked by hyperosmolar urine in the presence of hyposmolar plasma. It is more commonly seen in advanced disease.

Over 85% of all forms of tuberculosis are pulmonary, so respiratory symptoms, especially cough, are common. The cough may be nonproductive in early stages, but later patients may produce sputum and, less commonly, they may experience hemoptysis. Pleuritic pain is occasionally seen even if overt pleural effusion is absent. Dyspnea, if present, is an ominous feature seen with widespread advanced disease. Spontaneous pneumothorax is quite rare. The physical examination is usually not helpful and disappointing. Crackles and bronchial breath sounds may be present, but more often there are no abnormal findings even in well-developed pulmonary disease.

Because these manifestations are nonspecific and often insensitive, a high index of suspicion may be needed for diagnosis. The box below lists groups at high risk for tuberculosis in whom screening and a careful diagnostic approach are justified.

***Extrapulmonary tuberculosis.*** Tuberculosis can involve almost any organ, but only the more common types are mentioned here. Extrapulmonary involvement is present in about 15% of all cases but is far more likely in the immunocompromised host.

**Pleuritis.** Tuberculous pleural effusion is thought to result from a breakdown of a subpleural focus of tuberculosis into the pleural space or as the result of a delayed hypersensitivity reaction to tuberculous antigens. The chest radiograph demonstrates an underlying parenchymal infiltrate representing active pulmonary tuberculosis in only a minority of cases of tuberculous pleuritis. A purified protein derivative (PPD) skin test may be positive in only a minority of patients with tuberculous pleuritis if the test is performed before the patient has developed an immune response to the mycobacteria. Therefore, in cases where tuberculous pleuritis is suspected despite a negative PPD, the PPD should be repeated in 6 to 8 weeks. Evaluation of patients with suspected tuberculous pleural effusions includes sputum smear and culture, smear and culture of pleural fluid, and percutaneous pleural biopsy analyzed by smear, culture, and histopathology. The analysis of the pleural fluid and pleural biopsy specimens diagnoses more than 90% of the cases of tuberculous pleural effusions, although the yield of pleural fluid culture alone is less than 25% (see Chapter 118). Untreated, most tuberculous pleural effusions spontaneously resolve in several weeks, although 65% of patients develop active pulmonary tuberculosis within 5 years—hence the importance of diagnosis and treatment.

**Lymphadenitis.** Hilar lymph node involvement with enlargement is a frequent sequela of primary tuberculosis. In children it can cause bronchial compression with atelectasis. Hilar and mediastinal lymphadenitis is also

### High-risk groups for tuberculosis

Racial/ethnic minorities: 70% of all U.S. cases
Foreign born: 24% of all U.S. cases
Substance abusers (drugs and alcohol): Relative risk 5 to 20 times normal
HIV infection: Relative risk 40 to 100 times normal
Predisposing medical condition (diabetes, immunosuppressive drugs, silicosis, cancer): Relative risk 3 to 5 times normal
Residents of prisons, nursing homes, shelters: Relative risk 2 to 10 times normal
Contacts of an active case: Risk 3% within first year

frequent in the immunocompromised adult, especially in the HIV-infected host.

Cervical lymphadenitis, or scrofula, presents as a firm group of supraclavicular or anterior nodes that are usually nontender and matted. Ulceration with sinus tracts is a later development. Diagnosis is usually made by aspiration or excision of the involved area. Granulomatous cervical lymphadenitis in younger children is rarely due to tuberculosis in the United States. Most such cases now are caused by *M. avium* complex (see further).

**Genitourinary tuberculosis.** This may take several forms. Renal involvement may present as proteinuria, hematuria, or pyuria and should be suspected in the presence of persistent sterile pyuria. Discrete involvement of renal papillae and distortion of the collecting system are seen. Genital involvement in women is usually in the uterus or salpinx and may be a cause of menstrual disorders or infertility. In men the prostate and seminal vesicles are more typical sites of infection, and thickening of the vas deferens may be noted on physical examination.

**Tuberculosis of bone.** This may involve the spine (Pott disease) or the epiphyses of larger long bones, especially at the knees or hips, and occasionally the wrists or elbows. The lumbar spine is more frequently involved than the dorsal spine, and involvement of the cervical spine is rare. Manifestations include pain, compression fracture and deformity, and radiculopathy from compression. The gibbous deformity with sharp spinal angulation is characteristic. Diagnosis is usually suspected from the clinical and radiographic features. Early x-ray changes include soft tissue swelling, subchondral osteoporosis, cystic sclerosis, and later involvement of the synovial space. Diagnosis is best made by needle aspiration and occasionally by open biopsy.

**Meningitis.** Meningitis is the most common type of central nervous system tuberculosis. This dreaded disease was uniformly fatal before chemotherapy was available, and even with prompt and adequate treatment today permanent sensory, motor, and cognitive impairment may be unavoidable; mortality may reach 40%. Usual features are basilar meningitis and cranial nerve involvement with headache, stiff neck, and obtundation. Lumbar puncture shows 100 to 1000 leukocytes with lymphocytes predominant in two thirds of cases. Protein concentrations are high, and glucose concentrations are usually low. Acid-fast stains are positive in only 10% to 20% of cases with later culture confirmation in 50% to 75% of cases. Evidence indicating pulmonary or other forms of tuberculosis may often be present and should be sought as an aid for diagnosis. If the diagnosis is suspected, early empiric therapy is prudent and may be lifesaving.

**Disseminated or miliary tuberculosis.** This also carries a grave prognosis if unrecognized or untreated. Systemic manifestations are prominent with fever, weakness, and malaise. Anemia or pancytopenia is frequent because of marrow involvement. The name *miliary* is derived from the characteristic innumerable fine nodules of uniform size (millet seeds) that appear on chest x-ray or on cut section of the lung at autopsy. However, in its earlier stages the x-ray shadows may be inapparent. High-resolution computed tomography (CT) scanning can demonstrate such shadows more sensitively than plain films. Diagnosis can be made in half of cases by sputum examination, but invasive procedures, especially transbronchial lung biopsy and bone marrow biopsy, give a much more reliable yield and should be sought early.

In addition to increased frequency of disseminated or extrapulmonary disease, the immunocompromised host, especially the HIV infected, exhibits many features of tuberculosis that differ from those in the immunocompetent host (Table 114-2).

## Diagnostic testing

***Microbiology.*** The microbiology laboratory is essential for confirming the diagnosis by identification of *M. tuberculosis* as well as for following the course of disease and documenting the disappearance of organisms with successful therapy.

In pulmonary disease expectorated first morning sputum is the preferred specimen, usually on 3 successive days. If such sputum is unobtainable, sputum induction using hypertonic 3% saline aerosol is an alternative. The next step, should these be unrewarding, is fiberoptic bronchoscopy with sampling by bronchoalveolar lavage, brushing, or biopsy of affected segments.

The initial examination is the standard Ziehl-Neelsen acid-fast stain. Specimens generally give best results if they are predigested and centrifuged, and then the sediment is examined. Fluorescent stains using auramine-rhodamine improve the sensitivity and rapidity with which the slide can be examined, but false positives do occur, so

**Table 114-2.** Host response differences in tuberculosis

| | Normal host | Immunocompromised host (especially HIV) |
|---|---|---|
| Pathologic response | Granuloma with caseation | Nonspecific inflammation or poorly organized granulomas |
| Tuberculin sensitivity | Usually reliable except in the aged or in advanced disease | Unreliable |
| Chest x-ray | Nodular infiltrates, cavitations | Lymphadenopathy, diffuse infiltrates, sometimes no infiltrates |
| Chronicity | May appear after many years of dormancy | Frequently progressive within 3 to 12 months of infection |
| Extrapulmonary spread | 15% | 30%-50% |

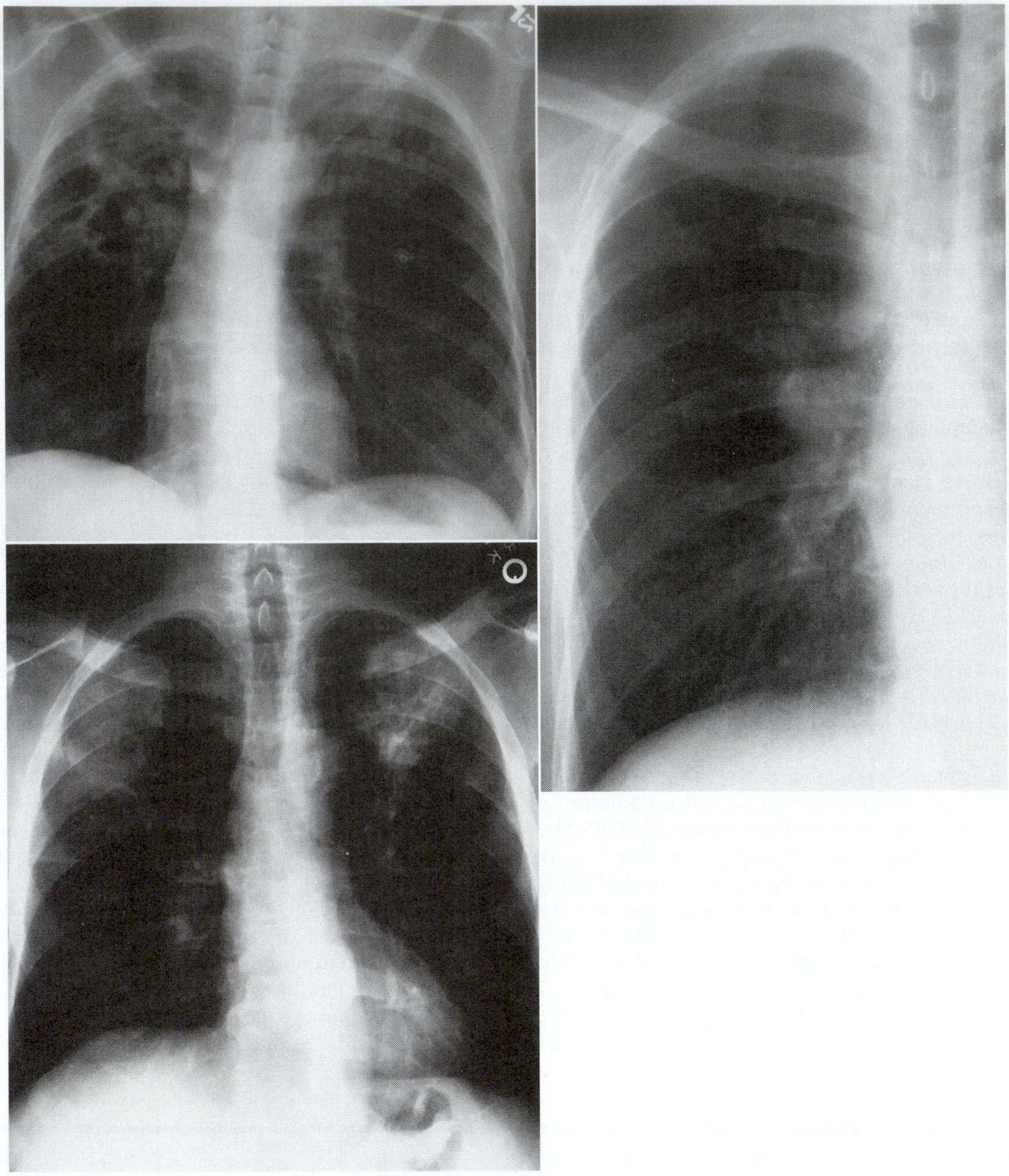

A

B

C

**Fig. 114-2.** **A,** Common features of pulmonary tuberculosis with bilateral upper zone nodular infiltrates and cavitation. The small air-flow level in the right mid-zone cavity is unusual. Target shadows are ECG lead artifacts. **B,** Tuberculosis in AIDS. Hilar and paratracheal lymph node enlargement is prominent and there is a faint infiltrate in the lung apex. **C,** Tuberculosis in AIDS. Bilateral infiltrates resembling segmental pneumonitis with moderate hilar node enlargement.

a positive fluorescent specimen must be confirmed by the standard Ziehl-Neelsen stain. A positive acid-fast stain does not identify *M. tuberculosis,* since all other mycobacteria as well as *Nocardia* species are acid fast. Acid-fast stains require a fairly heavy population of organisms for detection so consequently may be falsely negative. Culture methods increase sensitivity so that 40% to 60% of eventual isolates may be negative on initial stains.

Classic culture methods require 3 to 8 weeks for identifiable growth. Because of this inordinate delay posed by these classic culture methods, a number of techniques, especially the Bactec method, are now being developed to accelerate growth and identification. However, these new techniques are currently only available in larger reference laboratories. Other genetic techniques that show great promise are polymerase chain reactions, which can greatly amplify antigenic detection allowing rapid results in hours or days, and restriction fragment length polymorphism analysis for DNA typing of *M. tuberculosis* and particular strains of subspecies.

Drug susceptibility studies go hand in hand with culture techniques. Standard methods are proportion plates in which growth inhibition is measured against concentrations of drugs. With recent increases in drug-resistant strains it is strongly recommended by the Advisory Council for the Evaluation of Tuberculosis, Centers for Disease Control, American Thoracic Society (CDC-ATS) that susceptibility studies be conducted on all initial isolates and that these studies be repeated if organisms are still recovered after 2 to 3 months of treatment.

### Important differential diagnoses for radiography of tuberculosis

**Multinodular infiltrates**

Other mycobacterial or fungal granulomatous infections
Hematogenous or lymphogenous metastases
Collagen vascular or vasculitic diseases
Sarcoidosis

**Cavitations**

Lung abscess
Neoplasm
Septic infarction
Necrotizing pneumonia, especially staphylococcal or gram-negative organisms
Vasculitis

**Lymphadenopathy**

Neoplasm, especially lymphoma
Sarcoidosis

**Pleural effusion**

Transudate
Malignant effusion
Parapneumonia effusion
Thromboembolism
Collagen vascular disease

***Radiography.*** Routine chest radiography is highly sensitive for recognition of pulmonary tuberculosis. Supplementary x-ray techniques, especially CT scans, can give additional information in areas that are difficult to visualize with conventional x-rays such as the mediastinum, retrocardiac, or apical zones, which can be obscured by overlying structures. The characteristic features are nodular infiltrates and cavitation. Air-fluid levels are uncommon in cavities and if seen would suggest another problem such as lung abscess. In later stages, when healing occurs, signs of fibrosis with loss of volume, linear shadows, and traction deformities of the hilum and mediastinum may appear. The most common areas of involvement are the apical and posterior segments of upper lobes and superior segments of lower lobes. Adjacent pleural thickening is frequent (Fig. 114-2, *A*). A normal chest x-ray can occur rarely in pulmonary tuberculosis, as in an isolated endobronchial lesion or a very early miliary stage.

In primary tuberculosis the x-ray picture is different and less specific. Infiltrates without nodularity, usually in the middle or lower zones, are seen. Hilar lymph node enlargement is also a frequent feature. Lymphadenopathy is also a prominent feature in patients who are immunosuppressed, especially those with AIDS, and parenchymal infiltrates may be poorly defined without nodularity or cavity formation (Fig. 114-2, *B* and *C*). Tuberculosis in AIDS can also have an interstitial pattern and be confused with pneumocystis pneumonia (see the box at right).

***Histology.*** The characteristic lesion of tuberculosis is the formation of granulomas, which represent aggregations of inflammatory cells, principally macrophages, many of which assume epithelioid forms and join to create giant cells. Necrosis is a prominent feature with a relatively solid caseation rather than liquefaction. These features are not specific for tuberculosis and may be seen in infectious granulomas due to fungi or other mycobacteria. Granulomas without caseation may be found in sarcoidosis, foreign bodies, or as an adjacent reaction to a variety of neoplastic and inflammatory diseases. Specific recognition of the tuberculous granuloma rests on demonstration of the organism by stain or culture of this tissue, as well as on clinical circumstances.

In the immunocompromised host, granulomas may not be seen or may be poorly formed, and the inflammatory response may be modest. In such cases the organisms may be abundant on tissue stains.

***The tuberculin test.*** The tuberculin reaction is the classic example of delayed hypersensitivity immune response. Tuberculin, an extract of killed tubercle bacilli, is now well standardized as purified protein derivative (PPD), and its activity is measured in units by bioassay. The standard test is the intradermal administration in the volar forearm of 5 units (5 TU) diluted to 0.1 ml, the Mantoux technique.

The reaction is read at 48 to 72 hours as diameter of induration, not erythema. A positive reaction can be interpreted as infection with *M. tuberculosis.* The infection may be recent or remote, since persistence of reactivity is the rule. However, up to 10% of reactors may become negative on retest a decade or more later.

The tuberculin test is plagued by uncertainties related to both sensitivity and specificity. In diagnostic testing

### Conditions predisposing to false negative tuberculin reactions

Age: Newborns and the aged, over 60 years
Acute infection: Measles, mumps, chickenpox, typhoid fever, brucellosis, typhus, pertussis
Live virus vaccines: Measles, polio, mumps
Immunosuppressive states: HIV, chronic renal failure, drugs (corticosteroids, anticancer agents)
Overwhelming tuberculosis itself
Sarcoidosis
Neoplasm: Especially lymphomas and lymphoid leukemias
Errors in test administration or interpretation

### Thresholds for positive tuberculin test interpretation recommended by American Thoracic Society-CDC Advisory Committee

*5 mm:* Recent close TBC contacts, those with fibrotic or healed x-ray lesion, the HIV infected
*10 mm:* Special medical conditions (diabetes, silicosis, corticosteroid therapy); foreign born from Asia, Africa, or Latin America; underserved or low-income groups, or minorities, including African-American, Hispanic, and Native American; IV drug users; residents of long-term care facilities
*15 mm:* All others

sensitivity is as low as 70%, and false negatives are likely when the diagnosis is most important—in overwhelming disease, in immunocompromised hosts, in the aged, and in sarcoidosis (see the box above). Cutaneous anergy may be present in such cases. Anergy is assessed by simultaneous intradermal testing with common antigens such as mumps, tetanus toxoid, *Candida,* and *Trichophyton.* Anergy, the failure to react to any of these, makes a nonreactive tuberculin result indeterminate. In those infected with HIV, anergy is inversely related to CD4 counts and is present in two thirds of those with CD4 under 200/mm$^3$.

In epidemiologic testing of healthy populations tuberculin sensitivity is more reliable. In case contact surveys or employment screening programs the test is uniquely valuable.

Specificity problems occur due to cross-reactivity to other mycobacterial infection, a common regional problem especially in the southeast United States, or to prior bacille Calmette-Guérin (BCG) vaccination. Such cross-reactivity usually gives weak reactions of 5 to 10 mm.

Another difficulty is the booster phenomenon. A host who is weakly reactive may get an enhanced reaction on retesting a month or a year later. Since the implication is newly acquired versus remote infection, interpretation can be confusing. This phenomenon is often seen in the aged and is encountered in annual surveys in nursing homes. One technique for clarifying the booster phenomenon is double testing, or repeating a negative test after 1 week. A positive reaction on second test represents a boost rather than a true conversion. This method is useful in screening persons over 60 years old.

Because of these difficulties, the American Thoracic Society has proposed a scaled interpretation of tuberculin tests based on clinical circumstances (see the box at right). Although this interpretation formula does offer improvement over the previous standard of 10 mm induration as the uniform positive threshold, there are still intrinsic defects in the test (e.g., 10% to 25% of AIDS patients have false negative tests even at the 5 mm induration threshold).

## Management

Comprehensive management of any contagious disease includes effective treatment of the source case as well as evaluation, prevention, and treatment of contacts. The cornerstone of effective treatment is multiple drug chemotherapy, but the public health measures of contact surveys, isolation methods, and ensuring that the patient completes treatment are no less important and need to be addressed at the outset.

Tuberculosis is a reportable disease. Every case must be reported to the local health department when the diagnosis is made, but it is good policy to report cases even when tuberculosis is suspected but not proved. The public health officer should serve as a consultant to primary care and is helpful in initiating the contact surveys of the patient's household and, if necessary, the patient's place of employment. Contact surveys begin as tuberculin testing followed by chest x-ray studies for reactors to evaluate them for active disease. A second round of tuberculin testing after 6 to 8 weeks is prudent for nonreactors to detect those who may have been very recently infected but who were not yet reactive on initial survey. Preventive treatment is appropriately offered for contact reactors without evidence of clinical or radiographic disease. The health department also helps promote the successful completion of a prolonged course of patient treatment.

The decision for hospitalization is based on clinical circumstances. If the patient has pronounced symptoms and is seriously ill, if he or she requires extensive expedited diagnostic testing, or if drug resistance is suspected, hospitalization is indicated. On the other hand, many mildly ill patients can be managed at home. The hazard to household contacts is greatest before the diagnosis is made. Once effective treatment is begun, contagiousness rapidly decreases.

***Chemotherapy.*** Successful chemotherapy is based on the prolonged use of multiple effective drugs. The earliest lesson in treatment of tuberculosis with streptomycin in 1946 was that early success but late relapse occurred because of the spontaneous emergence of resistance of the organisms to a single drug. With the use of multiple drugs, and especially since the use of isoniazid-rifampin (INH-RIF) combinations, this risk of acquired drug resistance has been minimized. Prolonged uninterrupted treatment is needed because persistent slowly growing or dormant bacilli can only be eliminated slowly, even though the main population of rapidly dividing organisms quickly responds to therapy.

Several large drug trials sponsored by the U.S. Public Health Service and the British Medical Research Council showed that the ideal course of therapy can be as short as 6 months, if it has an intensive early three-drug phase followed by 4 months of INH-RIF. In the intensive phase daily treatment is needed, but later the schedule may be daily or twice weekly. Demonstrated success in these drug trials included 95% or higher initial clearance of the disease, as well as freedom from relapse over 1 to several years after treatment. For the past decade the standard of treatment has been an initial 2 months of daily INH-RIF and pyrazinamide (PZA) followed by 4 months of INH and RIF either daily or 2 to 3 times weekly. If PZA cannot be tolerated, an alternative is INH-RIF for a 9-month course. Intolerance or drug resistance to either of the major drugs would then require addition of two other drugs, usually ethambutol and streptomycin, and a more prolonged course of 12 to 18 months. These treatment programs need not be altered for extrapulmonary tuberculosis. In HIV-infected hosts a minimum of 9 months is customary, though standard courses are likely to be effective. Table 114-3 lists the features of the major drugs.

Unfortunately the increasing problem of drug-resistant strains has undermined the effectiveness of the above approaches. In New York state resistance to a single major drug is now 33%, and combined INH-RIF resistance is 19%. High levels of drug resistance have also been reported from New Jersey and Florida, and a trend of increasing resistance has been found in all reporting regions of the United States. National figures from 1991 indicate 3% resistance to both INH and RIF in new cases and 6.9% resistance in recurrent cases. Recognizing the trend, the CDC-ATS now advises the addition of an initial fourth drug, ethambutol or streptomycin, in any region where INH resistance rates of greater than 4% have been found. (This would include at least cities on the east, west, and Gulf coasts of the United States, as well as the southern border states at present.) Treatment would then be later modified based on susceptibility results, with reversion to standard regimens if resistance is not found, and prolonged 18-month regimens given if INH or RIF resistance is confirmed.

Retreatment of failed cases or treatment of multi-drug–resistant cases is not the province of primary care, and cases should be referred. Treatment of diseases resistant to both INH and RIF is difficult and largely unknown. These forms of tuberculosis occur most frequently in patients with HIV infections in whom they have a rapid devastating course with a median survival of 4 to 16 weeks and mortality of 70% to 90%.

Treatment monitoring is necessary to ensure the safety and effectiveness of treatment. The patient should be seen at least monthly to discuss symptoms of the disease as well as side effects of therapy. For pulmonary tuberculosis sputum studies should be done at monthly intervals for 3 months or until negative, at conclusion of treatment, and 3 to 6 months after treatment. Chest x-rays during the course of therapy are desirable but not imperative because symptomatic and bacteriologic status indicators are more valuable. X-rays should, of course, improve during treatment, but signs such as closure of cavities are not essential for success. Initial baseline complete blood count, blood urea nitrogen (BUN), liver enzymes, visual testing (for ethambutol), and uric acid (for PZA) are recommended. Since the three standard drugs are all potentially hepatotoxic, periodic monthly liver enzymes should be measured. Modest elevations (alanine aminotransferase [ALT] 100 U) are quite frequent but are often nonsignificant and subside with continued therapy. Such enzyme elevations need careful follow-up but do not mandate discontinuance of treatment.

The most important and common reason for therapeutic failure is patient noncompliance. Patient education can be quite helpful. The patient should understand the nature of the disease and the need for adhering to prolonged treatment, long after he or she is feeling well. Another measure of proven effectiveness is supervised or directly observed therapy. This means having a caregiver or dedicated family member dispense each dose and observe the patient ingesting it. The method is most conveniently adapted for intermittent, thrice weekly dosing. It is appropriate to use directly observed therapy for anyone who is reasonably likely to be noncompliant. Although it might seem that alcoholics and drug users would be noncompliant, there is actually no known basis for predicting compliance from any social, economic, or educational group. Given the gravity of the reemergence of tuberculosis, the recommendation that all therapy be routinely given as directly observed therapy is now the policy of CDC-ATS. This advice is for anywhere that compliance is less than 90% or is unknown, which really includes everywhere. Other coercive measures such as involuntary confinement and reopening of sanatoria for long-term care are undergoing serious discussion but are not policy at this time.

Any measure that simplifies treatment can improve compliance. Twice or thrice weekly dosing is such a simplification. Another is fixed combination tablets containing INH-RIF or INH-RIF-PZA to discourage taking only part of the regimen. Pyridoxine is often routinely given to prevent the rare INH-induced peripheral neuropathy. However, the patient may then opt only for the vitamins rather than also taking the tuberculosis medication, so routine use of pyridoxine can be counterproductive. The best tactic is keep it simple.

Drug toxicity or intolerance accounts for a far smaller number of treatment failures than does patient compliance. Hepatotoxicity, even with three potentially toxic drugs (INH-RIF-PZA), occurs in less than 4% of cases but is seen more frequently in patients with preexisting liver disease. PZA usually produces hyperuricemia but rarely symptomatic gout. Optic neuritis due to ethambutol is quite rare if the initial dosage of 25 mg/kg per day is reduced to 15 mg/kg per day after the first 6 weeks of use.

Adjunctive surgery has a very small role in tuberculosis treatment today. Resection of healed cavities or other residuals is not needed. Occasional cases may require drainage of tuberculous empyema, decompression of constrictive pericarditis, or relief of neurocompression in spinal tuberculosis, but these are performed for specific reasons to improve organ function. Surgery could have a renewed role in multi-drug–resistant disease, but this has yet to be demonstrated because successful surgery is not an alternative to effective chemotherapy, but an adjunct to it.

**Table 114-3.** Recommended drugs for the treatment of tuberculosis

| Drug | Dosage forms | Daily dosage | | Maximum daily dose in children and adults | Twice weekly dosage | | Adverse reactions |
|---|---|---|---|---|---|---|---|
| | | Children | Adults | | Children | Adults | |
| Isoniazid | Tablets: 100 mg*,† 300 mg<br>Syrup: 50 mg/5 ml<br>Vials: 1 g | 10-20 mg/kg, PO or IM | 5 mg/kg, PO or IM | 300 mg | 20-40 mg/kg, max 900 mg | 15 mg/kg, max 900 mg | Hepatic enzyme elevation, peripheral neuropathy, hepatitis hypersensitivity |
| Rifampin | Capsules: 150 mg*,† 300 mg<br>Syrup formulated from capsules: 10 mg/ml<br>Vials: 600 mg | 10-20 mg/kg, PO | 10 mg/kg, PO | 600 mg | 10-20 mg/kg, max 600 mg | 10 mg/kg, max 600 mg | Orange discoloration of secretions and urine; nausea, vomiting, hepatitis, febrile reaction, purpura (rare) |
| Pyrazinamide | Tablets: 500 mg† | 15-30 mg/kg, PO | 15-30 mg/kg, PO | 2 g | 50-70 mg/kg | 50-70 mg/kg | Hepatotoxicity, hyperuricemia |
| Streptomycin | Vials: 1 g, 4 g | 20-40 mg/kg IM | 15 mg/kg,‡ IM | 1 g‡ | 25-30 mg/kg, IM | 25-30 mg/kg | Ototoxicity, nephrotoxicity |
| Ethambutol | Tablets: 100 mg, 400 mg | 15-25 mg/kg, PO | 15-25 mg/kg, PO | 2.5 g | 50 mg/kg | 50 mg/kg | Optic neuritis (decreased red-green color discrimination, decreased visual acuity), skin rash |

Data from *Core curriculum on tuberculosis*, CDC-ATS, 1990.

*Isoniazid and rifampin are available as a combination capsule containing 150 mg isoniazid and 300 mg rifampin.

†A combination of isoniazid, rifampin, and pyrazinamide in a single tablet is being introduced.

‡In persons above age 60 the daily dosage of streptomycin should be limited to 10 mg/kg with a maximum dose of 750 mg.

### Indications for preventive treatment of tuberculosis

**Skin test–positive persons in the following high-risk groups, *regardless of age:***

Persons with HIV infection
Close contacts of infectious tuberculosis cases
Recent tuberculin skin test converters
Previously untreated or inadequately treated persons with abnormal chest radiographs
Intravenous drug users
Persons with medical conditions that increase the risk of tuberculosis

**Skin test–positive persons in the following high-risk groups who are less than *35 years of age*:**

Foreign-born persons from high-prevalence countries
Low-income populations, including high-risk minorities
Residents of long-term care facilities (including prisons)

From *Core curriculum on tuberculosis,* CDC-ATS, 1990.

***Treatment of children and pregnant women.*** Treatment of children is similar to that for adults in combinations and duration of treatment. Dosage adjustments are shown in Table 114-3. Treatment of tuberculosis in pregnant women is essential and should not be deferred. The preferred initial treatment is INH-RIF and ethambutol. The teratogenicity of PZA is undetermined, so it is unwise to use this drug unless resistance to other drugs is demonstrated or likely. Streptomycin is ototoxic to the fetus and should not be administered unless lack of other options forces its use.

***Preventive treatment.*** Approximately 10% of persons who have been infected by the tubercle bacillus but have no disease (i.e., tuberculin reactors who have no active disease seen on x-ray) develop tuberculous disease at some time during their lifetime. This risk is considerably greater within the year after infection occurs and in persons with immunosuppression, such as those taking corticosteroids or chemotherapy, and patients with diabetes or cancer. The risk is extremely high in the HIV infected, perhaps 100 times that of the normal population.

Several large field trials conducted in the 1960s have shown that INH given daily for 6 to 12 months gives effective protection of 80% to 90% against this risk and that the protection endures in follow-up over at least a decade. Subsequently the hepatotoxic hazard of INH has been recognized to temper our enthusiasm for its use in this setting. INH hepatotoxicity risk increases with patient age. The incidence is 2% to 3% in those over age 60 and 1% in younger adults and is virtually never seen in children. However, INH is still clearly recommended for most tuberculin reactors without disease, except those at lowest risk. The box above lists indications for INH preventive treatment.

INH preventive treatment in the HIV-infected tuberculin reactor is strongly recommended. Other indications for such treatment in the HIV infected include anergy and no apparent disease but high risk shown by a previous positive reaction, exposure to a patient with tuberculosis, a chest x-ray compatible with healed tuberculosis, or high likelihood of exposure (e.g., Haitian or Mexican immigrants or IV drug users).

Alternatives to INH have never been studied in a controlled way. If INH is indicated but cannot be given because of intolerance or suspected INH resistance, RIF would be the next drug of choice. Other inferior options include ofloxacin and ethambutol.

BCG vaccine has a checkered history and is of uncertain and variable effectiveness. It is not used for tuberculin reactors and indeed has no clear role for tuberculosis prevention in the United States. In addition, it is a live vaccine capable of causing progressive disease in immunocompromised patients, so it is clearly contraindicated in HIV disease.

### Managed Care Guide Prevention of tuberculosis

1. *Identification and effective treatment of active tuberculosis cases.* An undiagnosed, untreated active case will infect 10 to 14 other people in 1 year. Once a patient has been started on effective treatment, the risk of spread of disease diminishes rapidly, usually within the first 1 to 2 weeks.
2. *Reduction of infected aerosols.* Patients should be taught to cover their coughs. Effective masks capable of filtering particles as small as 0.1 μm are now available for patients and personnel.
3. *Ventilation.* Ventilation is clearly valuable. It should be of negative pressure with exhaust to the outside and not recirculated. Air change capacity of six times per hour is recommended.
4. *Ultraviolet air sterilizers.* These are inexpensive and relatively effective. They are mounted high in a room and directed upward to avoid possible visual damage.
5. *Tuberculin testing of personnel at risk of exposure.* This should be done at the start of employment and periodically at 6 to 12-month intervals. Additional testing should follow known exposure to untreated active cases. Preventive treatment is recommended for all tuberculin convertors.

### Preventive measures in the control of tuberculosis

With the reemergence of heightened risk of tuberculous infection, it is important that health care facilities and other close environments be aware of and implement the effective surveillance and preventive measures in the Managed Care Guide.

## DISEASES DUE TO NONTUBERCULOUS MYCOBACTERIA

Several dozen species of mycobacteria have been identified in the century since the tubercle bacillus itself was discovered. Most are found in the environment. Many are saprophytes, and some are pathogenic for fish, amphibia, or birds. Only a handful are important to humans, however. All are less virulent than *M. tuberculosis* and are most often seen as opportunistic infections. Of these, the commonest and most important group is the *M. avium-intracellulare* complex (MAC). Noteworthy others are *M. kansasii, M. marinum,* and the rapid growers, the *M. fortuitum-chelonei* complex. Laboratory differentiation is based on colonial morphology, a biochemical test battery, and growth rates.

### Diseases due to MAC

***Chronic pulmonary disease.*** This form usually occurs in middle aged men more often than women and may mimic pulmonary tuberculosis but with the following distinctive features. Respiratory symptoms are frequent, but systemic symptoms are uncommon. Disease and progression are indolent, and radiographic features are usually limited to lung parenchyma with thin-walled cavities and thickening of overlying pleura but rarely pleural effusion. Primary stages are rarely seen, and it is most usual that involvement occurs in a portion of the lung previously damaged by chronic bronchitis or bronchiectasis, emphysema, healed tuberculosis, or silicosis. Another form seen in older women without preexisting lung disease and showing interstitial involvement in the middle and lower zones has more recently been described. Extrapulmonary involvement is rare, but occasional cases of bone and joint disease occur.

Because the MAC organisms may be casual isolates rather than disease producers, a firm diagnosis requires several criteria, including repeated isolates of the same organism over days or weeks in more than scanty numbers, as well as a compatible radiographic and clinical picture.

Because of drug resistance, treatment is often of uncertain benefit. In mild disease observation alone may be the best choice. In symptomatic cavitary disease effective treatment often requires four or more drugs and a prolonged course of up to 2 years. If possible, the choice of drugs should be guided by susceptibility studies. Drugs exhibiting substantial susceptibility include rifampin, ethambutol, streptomycin, amikacin, ciprofloxacin, clofazimine, rifabutin, clarithromycin, and azithromycin. Adjunctive surgical resection can be valuable if disease is well localized and the patient is an acceptable surgical risk.

***Cervical lymphadenitis.*** This disease presents in children ages 1 to 5 as chronic nontender enlarged lymph nodes in the anterior or posterior chain. It is probably acquired by oral ingestion of contaminated materials from floors. It is a far more common cause of granulomatous lymphadenitis in children than is tuberculosis. Diagnosis is made by identification of the organisms from aspirated or resected material. The preferred treatment is complete surgical excision. Drugs are weakly effective, and untreated disease often progresses to draining fistulae or disfiguring scars.

***Disseminated MAC disease.*** This devastating disease occasionally occurs in immunosuppressed transplant or cancer patients, but its chief importance is in the late stages of AIDS. It is a disease marked by high fever, weakness, diarrhea, and pancytopenia that carries a grave prognosis. It is seen when marker CD4 T lymphocyte counts are below $50/mm^3$ and often below 10. It is quite common if searched for and may occur in 20% to 40% of such late-stage AIDS cases. Diagnosis is most reliably made by blood or marrow culture. Stool cultures are usually positive as well, but a positive stool culture is inconclusive only for diagnosis. If untreated, the median life expectancy is 4 months. Life expectancy can be doubled with multiple drug treatment, usually involving rifampin, clarithyromycin, ethambutol, and ciprofloxacin. Rifabutin has shown some efficacy as single drug prophylaxis for MAC in AIDS.

### Infections due to *M. kansasii*

Although MAC can be widely found in the environment in soils and bodies of water, *M. kansasii* is rarely found in nature but can be found sporadically in tap water. The organism is larger than other mycobacteria on stained preparations, so an experienced microscopist can identify it from acid-fast bacillus stains alone. It shows the peculiar culture characteristic of pigmentation only if grown in light (photochromogen).

*M. kansasii* shows limited virulence for humans. Like MAC, it can cause chronic pulmonary disease and disseminated disease in AIDS as well as the rare bone or joint disease. It differs from MAC most importantly in its favorable response to therapy. Rifampin is highly effective in treatment, and the recommended current regimen is RIF, INH, and ethambutol for a minimum of 9 months.

### Cutaneous infections due to *M. marinum*

These infections present as nodular ulcerations that occur in swimmers (swimmers itch), in fish processors, or can be derived from cleaning fish tanks (fish tank granuloma). Diagnosis is made by skin biopsy and identification of the organism. The disease may heal spontaneously, but deep infection should be treated for at least 3 months. The organism is usually susceptible to sulfonamides, tetracycline, rifampin, and ethambutol, and monotherapy or a RIF-EMB combination is appropriate.

### Infection due to rapid growing mycobacteria, especially the *M. fortuitum-chelonei* complex

These organisms have their greatest importance in wound infections and in contamination of implanted prosthetic materials. Notable problems have been found with breast implants, long-term catheters, porcine heart valves, and bone wax. Occasional occular or cutaneous infections are also seen. Diagnosis is usually evident if suspected, since the organisms are easy to grow and cultures mature quickly in 3 to 7 days. Successful treatment usually involves removal of prosthetics and wide excision of infected tissue. Chemotherapy is of variable effectiveness, but drugs, including amikacin, tobramycin, cefoxitin, sulfamethoxazole, imipenem, and ciprofloxacin, are likely to show some effectiveness.

## BIBLIOGRAPHY

Advisory Council for the Elimination of Tuberculosis: Initial therapy for tuberculosis in the era of multi-drug resistance, *MMWR* 42:1, 1993.

American Thoracic Society / CDC: Treatment of TB and TB infection in adults and children, *Am J Respir Crit Care Med* 149:1359, 1994.

American Thoracic Society / CDC: Diagnostic standards and classification of tuberculosis, *Am Rev Respir Dis* 142:725, 1990.

Division of Tuberculosis Control, Centers for Disease Control and American Thoracic Society (CDC-ATS): *Core curriculum on tuberculosis,* June 1990.

Farer LS, Snider DE Jr: Tuberculosis: current recommendations for cure and control, *Postgrad Med* 84:58, 1988.

Styblo K: The global prospects of tuberculosis and HIV infection, *Bull Int Union Tuberc Lung Dis* 65:28, 1990.

Sunderam G et al: Tuberculosis as a manifestation of the acquired immunodeficiency syndrome, *JAMA* 256:362, 1986.

Wallace RJ et al: Diagnosis and treatment of disease caused by non-tuberculosis mycobacteria (ATS statement), *Am Rev Respir Dis* 142:940, 1990.

CHAPTER

# 115 Chronic Obstructive Pulmonary Disease

**Ralph M. Schapira**
**Lynn F. Reinke**

The term *chronic obstructive pulmonary disease* (COPD) refers to a spectrum of pulmonary disorders that have in common an impairment to expiratory airflow, termed airways obstruction. It is diagnosed spirometrically by a permanent reduction in the ratio of the forced expiratory volume at one second (FEV$_1$) to forced vital capacity (FVC). The major disorders recognized to be a part of the clinical spectrum of COPD are emphysema and chronic bronchitis. There are many definitions of chronic bronchitis and emphysema, leading to confusion among clinicians. *Chronic bronchitis* is defined clinically as a disease characterized by cough and mucus hypersecretion (phlegm production) for at least 3 months of the year for 2 consecutive years with airways obstruction defined by spirometry. Some authors use the term *simple chronic bronchitis* to differentiate those patients with mucus hypersecretion who do not have airways obstruction; therefore simple chronic bronchitis is not a part of the spectrum of COPD. In contrast to the clinical definition of chronic bronchitis, *emphysema* is an anatomic abnormality of the lung defined by abnormal permanent enlargement of the airspaces distal to the terminal bronchiole, accompanied by destruction of their walls, and without obvious fibrosis. Although emphysema is an anatomic diagnosis, there are characteristic clinical features associated with it. Chronic bronchitis and emphysema should not be considered isolated disorders, since most patients with COPD have clinical features of coexistent chronic bronchitis and emphysema. Clinical features of patients with predominant chronic bronchitis (blue bloater) and predominant emphysema (pink puffer) allow general qualitative differentiation between the two forms of COPD. Pure forms of chronic bronchitis and emphysema are exceptions.

Cigarette smoking is the most important factor in the development of COPD. Some patients with classic smoking-related COPD have clinically pronounced bronchial responsiveness manifested by episodes of wheezing and worsening of expiratory airflow superimposed on the permanent airways obstruction. This form of COPD must be differentiated from *asthma,* which is characterized by intermittent airways obstruction that completely normalizes between episodes. Thus asthma is not part of the spectrum of COPD. However, some individuals who initially have asthma develop irreversible obstruction to airflow even in the absence of smoking, a form of COPD termed *chronic asthmatic bronchitis.* Chronic asthmatic bronchitis can mimic the classic smoking-induced COPD with bronchial responsiveness, although clinical features can help differentiate these two entities.

## EPIDEMIOLOGY AND ETIOLOGY

Approximately 15 million people in the United States are believed to have COPD. In 1989, COPD ranked fifth as a cause of death in the United States, accounting for nearly 4% of all deaths. COPD is a common disorder seen in outpatient settings, accounting for 17 million annual office visits in a recent survey. The prevalence of COPD, as well as hospitalization for it, is directly related to increasing age. Males are affected much more often than females, reflecting the fact that the percentage of males who smoke is higher than that of females. However, recent data have shown that the percentage of current male cigarette smokers has dropped dramatically from about 50% in the mid-1960s to about 35% in the late 1980s. In contrast, the percentage of current female smokers among has remained at about 30% during the same period.

The risk of developing COPD is related to the number of cigarettes smoked and the duration of smoking. Cigar or pipe smoking also increases the risk of developing COPD, but to a much lesser extent than does cigarette smoking. Individual host susceptibility to the effect of smoking is believed to be a key factor in the development of COPD, since only about 15% of smokers develop COPD. Smokers who develop COPD have a much greater annual decline in the FEV$_1$ than do nonsusceptible smokers or nonsmokers. This rate of decline normalizes to that of nonsmokers with smoking cessation. The role of passive smoking as a cause of COPD is unknown, although passive smoking has been associated with lung cancer.

People with homozygous $\alpha_1$-protease inhibitor ($\alpha_1$-PI) deficiency (usually PiZZ phenotype) are at risk for the development of emphysema, although this condition represents fewer than 2% of patients with emphysema. Certain chronic occupational exposures, particularly to inorganic dusts (coal, cement), grain dusts, or acid fumes (sulfuric acid), may result in chronic bronchitis. The role of indoor air pollution, ambient outdoor air pollution and recurrent childhood respiratory tract infections in causing COPD in the absence of smoking has not been clearly established.

## PATHOPHYSIOLOGY

Emphysema is an anatomic abnormality of the acinus, the portion of the lung parenchyma supplied by and distal to a terminal bronchiole (the respiratory bronchiole, alveolar ducts, and alveolar sacs). Emphysema is characterized by destructive changes of the acinus. In contrast, chronic bronchitis is a functional abnormality defined by clinical criteria but is associated with pathologic changes in the airways.

The pathogenesis of emphysema is a subject of debate, although there is considerable evidence that emphysema is caused by an imbalance between proteinases and antiproteinases in the lung. Neutrophils are believed to be a major source of proteinases, such as elastase. It is believed that cigarette smoking causes a chronic inflammatory response in the lung characterized by a migration of neutrophils. The neutrophils in the lung release elastase, which overwhelms the local natural antiproteinase activity, resulting in the destruction of lung elastin. Cigarette smoke may inactivate $\alpha_1$-PI, a major antiproteinase found in the epithelial lining fluid of the lung. In addition, some people with $\alpha_1$-PI deficiency develop emphysema on the basis of inadequate antiproteinase protection. The resulting proteinase-antiproteinase imbalance in the lung leads to the destruction of elastin, an integral component of the structural framework of the lung parenchyma. Loss of elastin is associated with airspace enlargement and reduction in the elastic recoil of the lung. Several forms of emphysema have been described. Centriacinar emphysema is the type of emphysema strongly associated with cigarette smoking. It predominantly involves the respiratory bronchiole, is very irregular in severity, and most commonly involves the upper lobes. In contrast, panacinar emphysema is characteristic of $\alpha_1$-PI deficiency but may be seen in patients who do not have this disorder. The entire acinus is uniformly enlarged and destroyed. The factors that determine why some smokers develop emphysema and others do not are not known.

In contrast to emphysema that involves the pulmonary parenchyma (acinus), the pathologic lesions of chronic bronchitis involve the airways. Morphologic changes in chronic bronchitis include hypertrophy of the submucosal glands and goblet cells of the large airways, clinically manifested as mucus hypersecretion and cough. In addition, infiltration of the submucosa by chronic inflammatory cells is common. Involvement of the small airways (bronchioles) is manifested by the abnormal presence of mucus-secreting cells, frequently accompanied by chronic inflammation. Smooth muscle hyperplasia and edema may also be present in the airways. The mucus hypersecretion seen in chronic bronchitis may be complicated by bacterial colonization and infection, potentially aggravating the underlying chronic inflammation.

Chronic bronchitis is believed to represent the airway epithelial response to chronic irritation by tobacco smoke or other agents. The pathogenesis of chronic bronchitis is less well understood than that of emphysema. In animal models the induction of airway injury by irritant gases, proteinases, and acids results in the pathologic changes in the airways seen in chronic bronchitis.

The final common pathway of the pathologic changes in COPD is chronic airflow obstruction. In emphysema the loss of radial support produced by a decrease in elastic recoil results in airflow obstruction. In chronic bronchitis the obstruction to airflow is believed to result from chronic inflammatory changes and muscle hyperplasia of the airways. In addition to airway obstruction, major abnormalities of gas exchange occur in COPD. Ventilation-perfusion ($\dot{V}/\dot{Q}$) relationships are deranged due to destruction of pulmonary parenchyma (emphysema) and airway abnormalities (chronic bronchitis). The changes in $\dot{V}/\dot{Q}$ relationships are highly complex but can result in hypoxemia and hypercapnia. Patients with COPD who develop hyperinflation (predominant emphysema) develop a mechanical disadvantage of the muscles of respiration and respiratory muscle dysfunction. These changes increase the work of breathing, leading to respiratory muscle fatigue and potential respiratory failure. Hypoxemia results in pulmonary arterial hypertension and right ventricular failure.

## HISTORY

COPD is usually a disease of smokers or exsmokers (one pack per day for greater than 20 years), usually above the age of 50. The diagnosis of COPD is suggested by the history and confirmed by the criterion standard, spirometry. The cardinal symptom of COPD is progressive dyspnea, frequently accompanied by cough and phlegm production and episodes of wheezing. The cough usually precedes or accompanies the onset of dyspnea. Phlegm is whitish gray and expectorated in the morning but may continue intermittently during the day. A history of productive cough with relatively less prominent dyspnea suggests predominant chronic bronchitis.

In contrast, patients with predominant emphysema usually give a history of minimal productive cough but with marked dyspnea. Asthmatic bronchitis is suggested by a history of typical paroxysmal asthma, especially occurring at rest or during sleep, with no or minimal smoking history. Changes in the quality of expectorated sputum, from whitish gray and mucoid to purulent, suggest acute bacterial bronchitis. A history of wheezing may suggest a beneficial response to inhaled bronchodilators. A family history of COPD suggests $\alpha_1$-PI deficiency, particularly if the onset is during the fourth or fifth decade of life. Hemoptysis in patients with COPD usually results from acute bacterial bronchitis or pneumonia, but an underlying lung cancer must always be considered. A patient who presents with progressive dyspnea and a history of asthma, particularly a nonsmoker, may have asthmatic bronchitis, a form of COPD. A detailed occupational history, including exposure to dusts and fumes, should be obtained.

## PHYSICAL EXAMINATION

Patients with predominant chronic bronchitis are usually of normal body weight or obese. The physical examination may reveal cyanosis and peripheral edema due to right ventricular failure (blue bloater). The respiratory rate is usually normal with no use of the accessory muscles of respiration. Chest percussion note is usually resonant, and auscultation may demonstrate wheezes and coarse rhonchi that change in location and intensity following a cough. Physical findings compatible with allergic rhinitis or nasal polyps may be noted in patients with asthmatic bronchitis.

In contrast, patients with predominant emphysema are frequently asthenic with weight loss. Tachypnea, the use of accessory muscles of respiration, retraction of the lower intercostal spaces with inspiration, and the use of pursed lips during expiration are common. Cyanosis is uncommon until the disease becomes very advanced because the increased minute volume maintains a sufficient hemoglobin oxygen saturation to prevent cyanosis and hypercapnia (pink puffer). The chest percussion note is usually resonant. Auscultation reveals diminished breath sounds.

A useful bedside diagnostic test for COPD is the forced expiratory time (FET) measured by timing a full exhalation of the vital capacity during chest auscultation. In a large clinical study evaluating the performance of the FET, the sensitivity and specificity of the FET at a value of 6 seconds or more for the diagnosis of airways obstruction were 74% and 75%, respectively. The FET measurement is most useful in subjects older than 60 years.

## LABORATORY STUDIES AND DIAGNOSTIC PROCEDURES

Pulmonary function testing is the criterion standard that demonstrates an obstructive ventilatory defect, the hallmark of COPD. An obstructive defect is defined spirometrically by a reduction in the ratio of the forced expiratory volume at one second ($FEV_1$) to the forced vital capacity (FVC) below the predicted value. Alternatively, some pulmonary function laboratories do not utilize a predicted $FEV_1$/FVC ratio but rather a $FEV_1$/FVC as <70 to indicate obstruction, although this practice is not recommended. The severity of the obstructive abnormality is graded by the patient's percentage of predicted $FEV_1$ (70% or greater, mild; between 60% and 70%, moderate; between 50% and 60%, moderately severe; between 34% and 50%, severe; and less than 34%, very severe). Patients with COPD have an irreversible obstructive impairment as demonstrated by a persistently abnormal $FEV_1$/FVC ratio, although there may be variation in the $FEV_1$ and FVC between bouts of wheezing or pulmonary infection and clinical stability during optimal therapy. Any changes in spirometry, either improvement or worsening, should be viewed cautiously unless serial tests show a consistent trend. In contrast, asthmatics have a reversible obstructive impairment with normalization of the $FEV_1$/FVC ratio between clinical episodes of asthma. The 5-year survival of patients with COPD begins to decrease at an $FEV_1$ between 1.15 and 1.5 L. At $FEV_1$ ranges of 0.75 to 1.15 L, 5-year survival decreases to 66% and is even lower in this group if chronic hypercapnia is present. The functional ability of a patient with COPD is better assessed by a formal pulmonary exercise evaluation than by the $FEV_1$ alone, since the functional impairment of patients with COPD varies for any given $FEV_1$, although in general functional ability decreases as the $FEV_1$ decreases. Exercise testing can differentiate between limitations due to gas exchange, ventilation, or cardiovascular abnormalities. Many patients with COPD are limited due to cardiovascular deconditioning and not by a gas exchange or ventilation impairment.

Spirometry typically includes measurement of the $FEV_1$ and FVC immediately following the administration of an inhaled bronchodilator—the bronchodilator response. The criteria for and clinical relevance of a significant bronchodilator response are controversial, but a recommended guideline is the presence of both a 12% *and* an absolute increase of 200 cc in the $FEV_1$ or FVC. Patients with a significant bronchodilator response are believed to derive the greatest benefit from inhaled bronchodilators and corticosteroids, although there is no clinical proof of this observation. The lack of a significant bronchodilator response does not preclude clinical benefit, since the one-time administration of a bronchodilator during spirometry does not necessarily predict response with regular use. Inhaled bronchodilators should not be withheld from a patient with COPD who does not exhibit a significant bronchodilator response during spirometry.

Patients with predominant chronic bronchitis or asthmatic bronchitis tend to have a mild reduction in diffusing capacity for carbon monoxide, since the principal abnormality is in the airways. In contrast, patients with predominant emphysema, a parenchymal abnormality, have a greater reduction in diffusing capacity for carbon monoxide. The lung volumes in predominant chronic bronchitis tend to show a normal or slightly increased total lung capacity (TLC). However, in predominant emphysema the lung volumes often show hyperinflation as manifested by a marked increase in TLC and residual volume (RV). The increase in RV may compromise the vital capacity. Arterial blood gas (ABG) results in patients with predominant bronchitis demonstrate marked hypoxemia and, in advanced cases or during exacerbations, hypercapnia. However, ABG abnormalities may be relatively modest in patients with predominant emphysema, demonstrating only mild hypoxemia without hypercapnia except in advanced cases. Significant ABG abnormalities in patients with COPD tend to be unusual until the $FEV_1$ drops below 1.5 L. Exercise may worsen hypoxemia in patients with preexisting abnormalities, and secondary polycythemia may ensue in severely hypoxemic patients.

Standard chest radiographs can suggest the diagnosis of emphysema. Marked overdistention of the lungs, as manifested by flattened diaphragms and an enlarged retrosternal airspace, is highly suggestive of emphysema. A small and vertically oriented heart contour and hyperlucent lung fields due to oligemia are also suggestive of emphysema. Localized radiolucencies and upper lobe bullae may be visible on the radiograph of the chest. Lower lobe bullae are highly suggestive of emphysema associated with $\alpha_1$-PI deficiency. It should be stressed that, although the chest radiograph can provide only a rough approximation of the severity of emphysema, it is most useful in suggesting the presence of severe emphysema.

## DIFFERENTIAL DIAGNOSIS

Chronic bronchitis and emphysema must be distinguished from other lung diseases that cause an obstructive ventilatory impairment on spirometry. Patients with an exacerbation of *asthma* may present with an obstructive ventilatory impairment and radiographic abnormalities suggestive of emphysema. However, by definition the airways obstruction in asthma is reversible between acute exacerbations. Patients with *cystic fibrosis* (CF) may have an obstructive ventilatory impairment due to airway inflammation and obstruction by secretions. CF is differentiated from chronic bronchitis and emphysema by its numerous systemic nonpulmonary manifestations and early age of onset. *Bronchiectasis,* the persistent dilatation and destruction of bronchi, represents the sequelae of other lung processes such as granulomatous infections and an array of genetic defects. The spirometric results in patients with bronchiectasis vary, but in diffuse bronchiectasis there may be an obstructive ventilatory defect. The history, underlying disease process, and the CT scan can help differentiate bronchiectasis from chronic bronchitis and emphysema.

## MANAGEMENT

### Pharmacologic therapy

The aim of pharmacologic treatment of emphysema and chronic bronchitis is to achieve both an improvement of symptoms and a measurable improvement of lung function. This section describes the major categories of pharmacologic agents currently prescribed for the management of COPD and provides the primary care physician with practical information to facilitate clinical decision making (see Managed Care Guide).

The use of inhaled medications (parasympatholytics, β-adrenergic agonists, and inhaled steroids) delivered by a metered dose inhaler (MDI) are preferred in the pharmacotherapy of COPD, since this route of administration allows direct deposition of medication in the airways and helps to minimize systemic side effects (Table 115-1). The optimal method of delivery of all inhaled medications from an MDI involves the use of a spacer device. Spacer devices function as a holding chamber reservoir that eliminates the need for coordination of simultaneous inhalation and depression of the MDI canister to deliver the dose. Several reports have demonstrated that the use of a spacer device with an MDI provides greater drug deposition to the smaller airways, less impaction in the oropharynx, and a greater overall bronchodilator effect. Spacer devices are of particular benefit to patients with poor eye-hand coordination. To maximize drug deposition in the airways from the MDI, it is imperative that the patient be educated as to the proper use of the MDI. The patient should take a slow and complete inhalation from the end of a normal tidal breath (full exhalation to residual volume is not necessary) and hold the breath for up to 10 seconds to allow for adequate drug deposition (see the box at right). The use of a nebulizer to deliver inhaled medications should be reserved for patients with severe disease who are unable to hold their breath when using MDI or who are unable, even with a spacer device, to coordinate the use of a MDI, since the combination of a properly used spacer device and MDI has been shown to be equally effective.

*Anticholinergics (parasympatholytics).* Anticholinergic drugs antagonize the effect of the parasympathetic system on the airways, which mediates bronchoconstriction and is believed to be heightened in COPD. Recent evidence suggests that ipratropium, a quaternary anticholinergic bronchodilator available by MDI, is more efficacious than inhaled β-agonist therapy and should supplant β-agonists as first-line therapy in COPD. Several recent reports recommend that the traditional dosage of ipratropium (2 puffs, four times a day) is suboptimal and should be increased to 3 to 6 puffs four times a day. Ipratropium is appropriate for use as a maintenance treatment of COPD and is not indicated in the initial treatment of acute exacerbations due to its slow onset of action (about 20 minutes) compared to β-agonists. Ipratropium is poorly absorbed from the airways and thus has few systemic adverse effects, unlike β-agonists. Potential side effects include dry mouth and cough. Ipratropium is the only anticholinergic bronchodilator available by MDI in the United States.

*β-Adrenergic agonists.* β-Agonists have been the traditional cornerstone in the management of COPD. However, the role of β-agonists in the pharmacotherapy of COPD continues to evolve, particularly since the efficacy and safety of the anticholinergic agent ipratropium have become more clearly established. Most authorities recommend that β-agonists be used as second-line therapy, either to supplement or replace ipratropium in patients who do

#### Proper use of a metered dose inhaler (MDI)

- Shake the inhaler.
- Tilt the head back slightly and exhale normally. Forced exhalation to residual volume is not necessary.
- Hold the mouthpiece 1 to 1½ inches away from open mouth. However, if using a spacer, seal lips around the mouthpiece of the spacer.
- Activate the MDI while simultaneously taking a slow, deep inhalation.
- Hold breath at the end of inspiration for 5 to 10 seconds. Slowly exhale through mouth.
- Wait 1 minute between puffs.
- If using a steroid inhaler, rinse mouth after use to avoid thrush or dysphonia.

**Table 115-1.** Commonly prescribed metered dose inhalers (MDIs) for COPD

| Commercial name | Chemical name | Action | Dose per inhalation |
|---|---|---|---|
| Proventil, Ventolin | Albuterol | $\beta_2$-Agonist | 90 μg |
| Alupent | Metaproterenol | $\beta_2$-Agonist | 650 μg |
| Maxair | Pirbuterol | $\beta_2$-Agonist | 200 μg |
| Brethine, Brethaire | Terbutaline sulfate | $\beta_2$-Agonist | 200 μg |
| Atrovent | Ipratroprium bromide | Anticholinergic (parasympatholytic) | 18 μg |
| Azmacort | Triamcinolone acetonide | Antiinflammatory corticosteroid | 100 μg |
| Aerobid | Flunisolide | Antiinflammatory corticosteroid | 250 μg |
| Vanceril or Beclovent | Beclomethasone dipropionate | Antiinflammatory corticosteroid | 42 μg |

## Managed Care Guide
## Algorithm for management of COPD

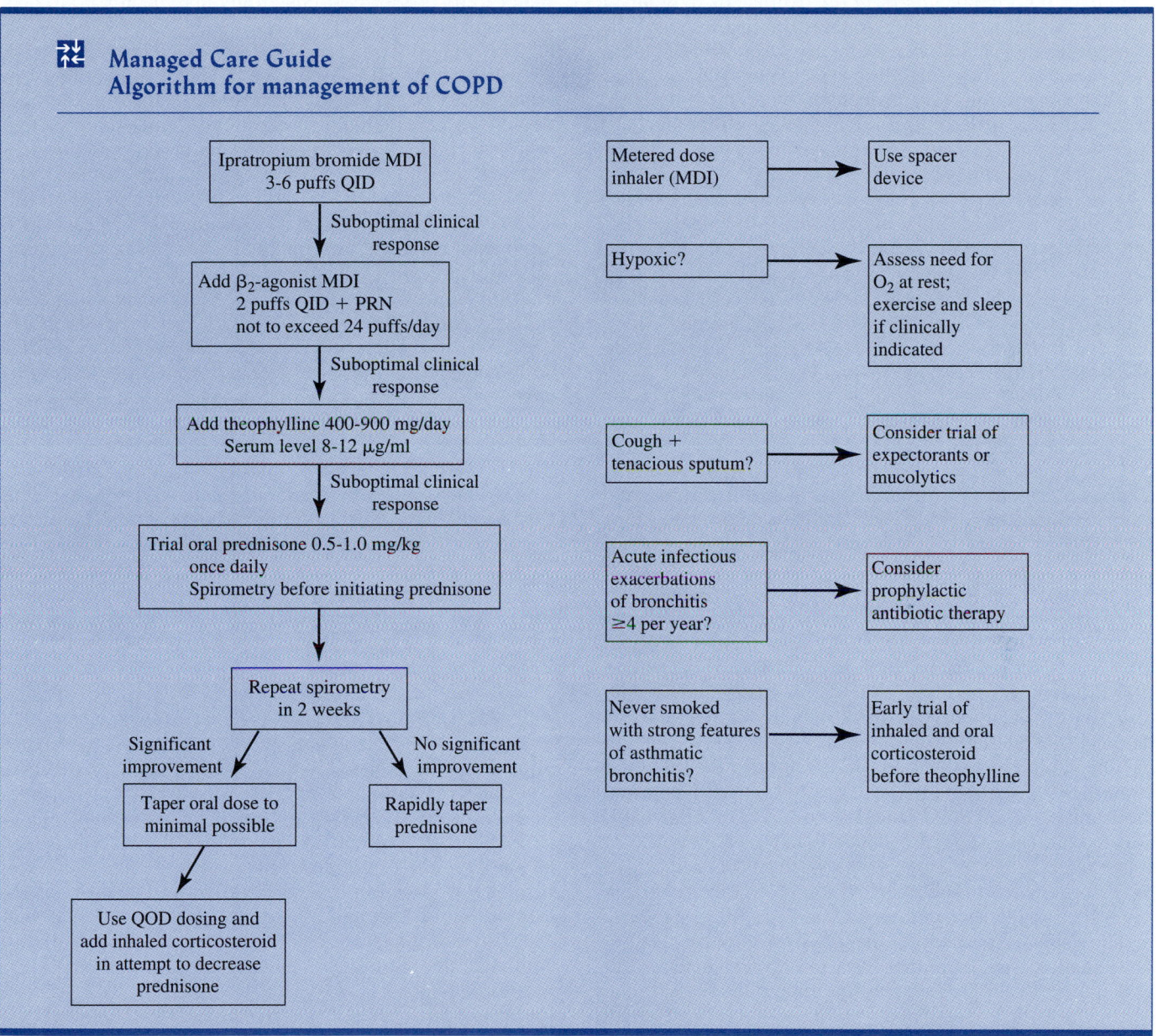

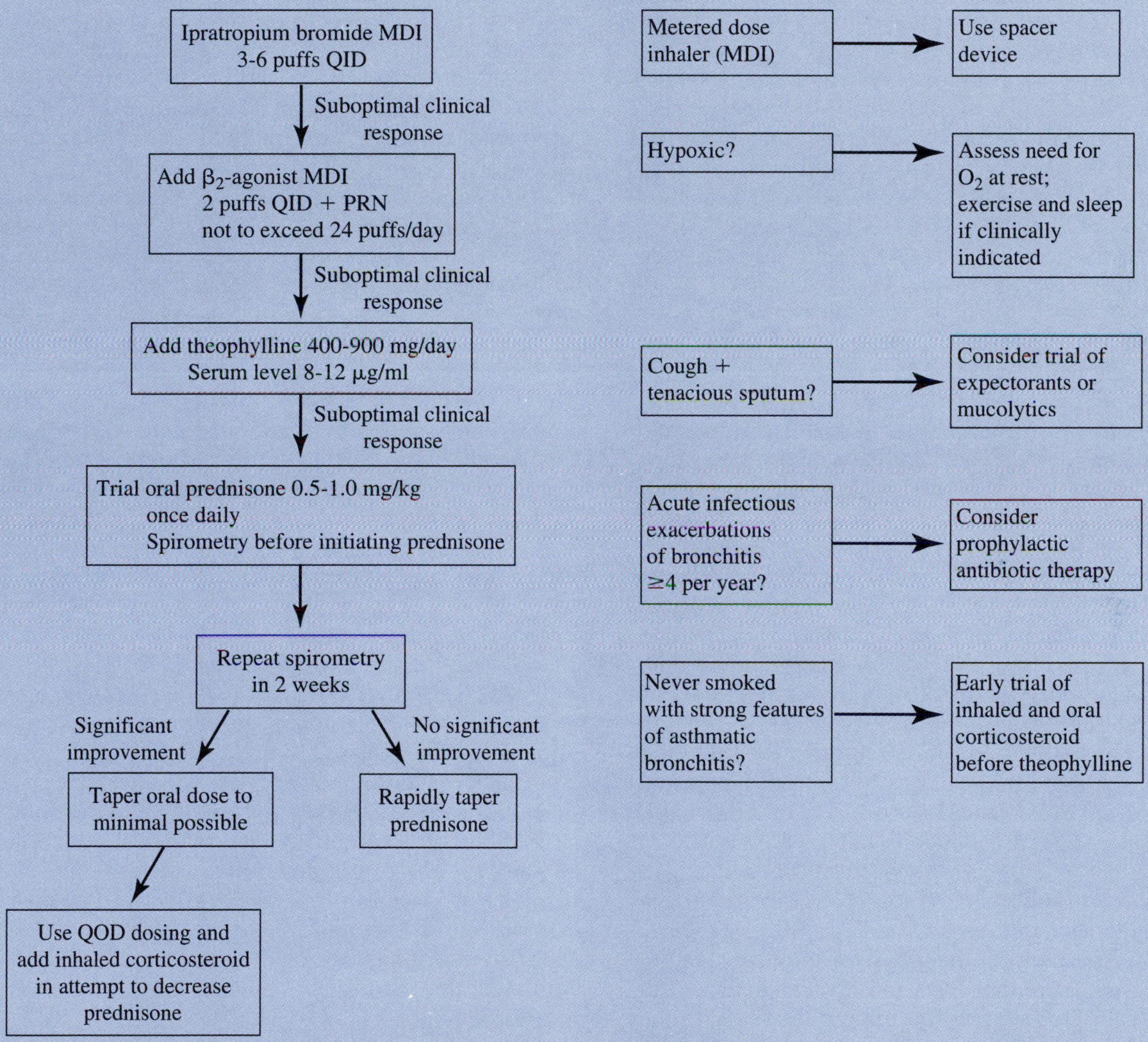

not obtain satisfactory clinical benefit from ipratropium alone.

The use of β-agonist bronchodilators has been demonstrated to increase airflow, improve mucociliary clearance, and reduce dyspnea in patients with COPD. Recent reports in the literature suggest that administering higher dosages of β-agonists (2 to 6 puffs four to six times a day) may result in greater achievement of airway bronchodilation without additional side effects than the traditional dosage of 2 puffs four times a day. However, recent concern has risen over reported deaths from the overuse of β-agonists in patients with asthma, though there are insufficient data to suggest that β-agonists are directly responsible for this increase in mortality. In addition, tachyphylaxis, rebound bronchoconstriction, and bronchial hyperreactivity may occur with use of β-agonists. Patients should be encouraged to limit the dosage of β-agonists to no more than 24 puffs per day depending on symptoms. Although the inhaled route helps to minimize systemic side effects, β-agonists can result in tachycardia, palpitations, tremor, and metabolic derangements such as hypokalemia. β-Agonists can be prophylactically administered before engaging in physical activity known to provoke bronchospasm. The use of oral β-agonists is discouraged, since they are no more effective than MDIs, and the incidence of systemic adverse effects is higher than with MDIs.

***Theophylline.*** Theophylline, a methylxanthine derivative, has been shown to act as a bronchodilator, improve gas exchange, decrease dyspnea, improve mucociliary clearance, enhance respiratory muscle performance, have a positive inotropic effect, and increase neuroinspiratory drive. The precise role of theophylline in the management of COPD has been controversial.

The toxicity of theophylline and its interactions with other drugs make it a relatively complex drug to dose. Common side effects of theophylline include nausea, diarrhea, tremor, anxiety, and insomnia and even include life-threatening side effects such as seizures and cardiac arrhythmias. A number of drugs reduce the clearance of theophylline including antibiotics such as erythromycin and the quinolones. The therapeutic range for theophylline levels has been debated in the clinical literature. The usual therapeutic serum level ranges from 10 to 20 μg/ml. However, most potential bronchodilatation is believed to occur once levels of 10 to 15 μg/ml have been reached. Therefore a serum level of 8 to 12 μg/ml has been suggested as the therapeutic goal.

The decision to institute theophylline therapy must be individualized and should not be universally made in all patients with COPD. Theophylline should be added to the treatment plan in patients who have not achieved an optimal clinical response to β-agonist and ipratropium MDIs. Theophylline should be continued only if there is a clinical benefit to the patient, such as an objective improvement in spirometry or a decrease in dyspnea. The usual dosage of theophylline is 400 to 900 mg/day of a long-acting preparation, but the precise dosage is determined by concurrent drug administration, the patient's medical problems, and the metabolism of the drug. Upon initial prescription of theophylline, serum levels must be checked in 1 to 2 weeks and dosages adjusted to achieve and maintain an adequate clinical response without side effects. Subsequent serum levels should be monitored twice annually and dosages adjusted.

***Systemic corticosteroids.*** Unlike ipratropium, β-agonists, and oral theophylline, which are bronchodilators, corticosteroids are antiinflammatory agents that appear to benefit about 10% of clinically stable outpatients with COPD. Corticosteroids are thought to increase the clinical response to β-agonists, possibly by increasing β-adrenergic responsiveness of the airways. In addition, the antiinflammatory property of corticosteroids may decrease airways inflammation in COPD.

The role of oral corticosteroids therapy in stable outpatients with COPD is not well defined, due in part to the serious adverse effects of steroids. Oral corticosteroids should be considered in outpatients with stable COPD whose symptoms are not optimally controlled by a regimen of β-agonists, ipratropium, and theophylline. Although it can be difficult to predict which patients with COPD will respond to corticosteroids, factors such as a significant response to bronchodilators during spirometry and clinical features of asthmatic bronchitis suggest that a trial of steroids is warranted. A therapeutic trial of corticosteroids must be preceded by spirometry to verify objective improvement in pulmonary function ($FEV_1$) following the initiation of therapy. Prednisone (approximately 0.5 to 1 mg/kg daily) is started and spirometry repeated 2 weeks after the start of therapy. Although there are no formal criteria, most authorities recommend that prednisone be continued only if there is significant improvement in $FEV_1$ (generally defined as greater than 20%), otherwise corticosteroids should be discontinued. Subjective improvement in dyspnea without objective improvement in spirometry generally does not support the continuation of corticosteroids. Since oral corticosteroids are associated with significant toxicity, if a patient demonstrates a significant objective response to oral corticosteroids, the dosage should be tapered to identify the lowest possible dosage that continues to provide objective spirometric benefit. Subjective worsening such as an increase in dyspnea during a corticosteroid taper should not be equated with a worsening of the $FEV_1$. Spirometry should be repeated to determine whether a correlation exists between subjective worsening and a decrement in pulmonary function. Alternate-day oral therapy and the use of an inhaled corticosteroid alone can also help to minimize side effects. Patients taking corticosteroids should continue to receive maximal therapy with inhaled bronchodilators and theophylline to minimize the requirement of oral corticosteroids.

***Inhaled corticosteroids and cromolyn sodium.*** Inhaled corticosteroids and cromolyn sodium are antiinflammatory drugs that can be delivered by MDI. The role of inhaled corticosteroids in the pharmacotherapy of COPD is still evolving, although these agents have become an established part of asthma therapy. Two recent studies suggest that adding inhaled corticosteroids to bronchodilators can have a beneficial response on airways obstruction in patients with COPD, although the long-term benefits are unknown. Inhaled corticosteroids used in conjunction with oral corticosteroids may allow a decrease in the dosage of oral corticosteroids. Additional studies are needed to clarify the role of inhaled corticosteroids in COPD and identify the subset of COPD patients who would be most likely to benefit. The role of cromolyn sodium in COPD has not been studied, and it is not recommended as an antiinflammatory agent at this time.

***Mucolytics and expectorants.*** The benefits of mucolytics and expectorants in the management of secretions are not well documented. Mucolytics, such as iodinated glycerol and acetylcysteine, are postulated to work by helping to liquefy tenacious mucus in the bronchial tree. The results from the National Mucolytic Study indicate that, although patients with chronic bronchitis treated with iodinated glycerol reported subjective improvement in chest symptoms, pulmonary function was not affected. In contrast to mucolytics, oral expectorants such as guaifenesin may help to loosen bronchial secretions possibly by stimulating the flow of respiratory tract fluid and facilitating the movement of secretions by ciliary motion and coughing. Patients with chronic bronchitis often subjectively report that these expectorants help them to raise their secretions more readily; however, the efficacy of such products has not been demonstrated. There is no standard role for expectorants or mucolytics in the symptomatic treatment of COPD.

***Antibiotics.*** Antibiotics are frequently prescribed to patients with COPD as therapy for or to prevent an acute infectious exacerbation of COPD. Three organisms—*Haemophilus influenzae, Streptococcus pneumoniae,* and *Branhamella catarrhalis*—have emerged as the major bacterial pathogens in the setting of infectious exacerbations in patients with COPD. Acute infectious exacerbations, which are characterized by worsening dyspnea, increased cough, sputum production, and sputum purulence, may worsen pulmonary function during the infection, although there is controversy as to whether pulmonary function is permanently altered. Antibiotic prophylaxis with alternating agents administered 1 week a month may reduce the frequency of exacerbations in the subset of patients with COPD who have four or more exacerbations a year.

Although there is controversy regarding the role of antibiotics in managing exacerbations of COPD, it has become standard practice to prescribe a course of antimicrobial therapy when a patient presents with an acute exacerbation of COPD, particularly if the exacerbation appears infectious (characterized by an increase in sputum volume and purulence). The most common antimicrobial agents used in the treatment of patients with acute infectious exacerbations of COPD include amoxicillin, amoxicillin/clavulanate, tetracycline, erythromycin, and trimethoprim-sulfamethoxazole.

***$\alpha_1$-PI replacement.*** Patients with COPD and a documented homozygous $\alpha_1$-PI deficiency with serum levels under 11 μM may potentially benefit from intravenous $\alpha_1$-PI replacement. However, although replacement therapy can increase serum and bronchoalveolar lavage fluid levels of $\alpha_1$-PI, it remains to be proven that therapy slows the progression of airways obstruction. Replacement therapy is expensive and requires frequent intravenous infusions (once weekly to once monthly).

***Prevention of influenza and pneumococcal pneumonia.*** Since pulmonary infection is a common complication in COPD that can lead to worsening pulmonary function and respiratory failure, an annual prophylactic vaccine against influenza is recommended in those individuals who are not sensitive to egg protein. This vaccine is associated with a 60% to 80% protection rate. Amantadine can be considered in patients with COPD who have not received the vaccination and who are at risk for influenza A or in patients with early influenza A. The polyvalent pneumococcal vaccination, administered one time, is also recommended for people over 50 who have COPD.

***Supplemental oxygen therapy.*** Oxygen ($O_2$) is a component of the pharmacotherapy of COPD because it is a potent pulmonary arterial vasodilator. Since hypoxemia leads to pulmonary arterial hypertension and right ventricular failure (cor pulmonale), supplemental oxygen would be expected to blunt pulmonary arterial hypertension and prevent cor pulmonale. The importance of supplemental oxygen (termed long-term oxygen therapy, or LTOT) in a subset of patients with COPD has been derived from two clinical trials conducted in the early 1980s. The trials demonstrated that the use of supplemental $O_2$ therapy significantly decreased morbidity and mortality in COPD patients with chronic hypoxemia. Additional benefits included an improvement in neuropsychiatric functioning, possibly related to an increase in oxygen delivery to the brain, an increase in exercise tolerance, and a fall in hematocrit in patients with secondary polycythemia from hypoxemia.

The three criteria for the initiation of LTOT are listed in the box below. It is recommended that an arterial blood gas on room air sample be obtained from an approved laboratory for the initial evaluation of the need for LTOT. Pulse oximetry is easily obtained, noninvasive, and less expensive but is less accurate and gives no information regarding arterial $P_{CO_2}$. The identification of patients with hypercapnia is extremely important, since hypercapnia may worsen with the institution of LTOT.

A subset of patients with COPD may be at risk for desaturation during exercise or sleep even if the patient does not meet the criteria for LTOT based on resting

### Indications for long-term supplemental oxygen therapy*

1. A resting room air $Pa_{O_2} \leq 55$ mm Hg or $Sa_{O_2} \leq 88\%$
2. A resting room air $Pa_{O_2}$ 56 to 59 mm Hgor $Sa_{O_2} \leq 89\%$ if there is polycythemia (hematocrit ≥ 52%) or clinical or electrocardiographic evidence of cor pulmonale
3. $Pa_{O_2} \leq 55$ mm Hg or $Sa_{O_2} \leq 88\%$ during exercise (documented by a 6- or 12-minute walk test) or sleep (documented by a sleep study) regardless of the resting room air $Pa_{O_2}$

*All assessments for the need of long-term oxygen therapy must be done during a stable clinical state and not during an acute illness. When long-term oxygen therapy is initiated, arterial blood gases on room air, in a resting state, should be repeated within 3 months to confirm a continued need for oxygen.

arterial blood gas levels (criterion 1 or 2 in the box on p. 1557). Room air resting arterial $Po_2$ levels between 60 and 65 mm Hg or complaints of dyspnea on exertion warrant consideration of a 6- or 12-minute standardized walk test with pulse oximetry to evaluate the need for supplemental $O_2$ during exercise (criterion 3 in the box). However, there is no clinical proof that supplemental oxygen during exercise alone has any long-term clinical benefit. Some investigators also recommend a sleep study in the same group of patients to evaluate for nocturnal desaturation that would warrant supplemental $O_2$ therapy during sleep (criterion 3 in the box), particularly in patients who are obese, hypercapnic, or polycythemic (hematocrit of 52% or higher), or who have cor pulmonale.

The majority of patients who meet the indications for LTOT warrant the use of $O_2$ therapy on a continuous basis unless $O_2$ was prescribed solely for exercise- or sleep-induced desaturation. In these two instances $O_2$ should be prescribed only during the times of desaturation. Dyspnea without evidence of significant hypoxemia at rest or exercise is not an indication for LTOT.

**Flow.** The majority of patients with COPD can attain a $PaO_2$ of 60 torr or greater (corresponding to an oxyhemoglobin saturation of about 90%) on 1 to 2 L per minute of supplemental $O_2$. A small subset of patients with hypoxemic COPD develop hypercapnia with oxygen supplementation, and careful titration in these patients is essential.

**Routine delivery devices.** The most commonly used $O_2$ delivery device for LTOT is the nasal cannula. It is easy for patients to use and has few side effects (dryness of the nasal membranes, facial irritation). A disadvantage of the nasal cannula is that the amount of $O_2$ inspired is variable due to variations in the breathing pattern, including breathing through the mouth. In addition, since $O_2$ flow is continuous, even during expiration, $O_2$ is wasted. LTOT can also be delivered through a tracheostomy mask in patients with a tracheostomy. Unlike delivery through a nasal cannula, humidification should be provided with a tracheostomy mask.

**Oxygen-conserving delivery devices.** LTOT oxygen is expensive. Therefore oxygen-conserving devices have been developed that decrease the waste of oxygen so as to cut costs and maximize the duration of use of portable systems. A conserving device should be considered for patients who require flow rates of over 2 L per minute, use liquid oxygen, or are active and spend over 6 hours per day away from the stationary $O_2$ delivery system. Examples of conserving devices include reservoir nasal cannulas, demand $O_2$ delivery systems, and transtracheal oxygen therapy. The reservoir nasal cannula allows for $O_2$ conservation by storing $O_2$ delivered from the equipment system in a reservoir during exhalation. These techniques have been demonstrated to result in an $O_2$ savings of 50% or more during rest. The demand $O_2$ delivery system, which allows for $O_2$ flow only during inhalation, can be built into an ambulatory $O_2$ unit or function as an accessory on stationary units. The transtracheal (TT) catheter delivers $O_2$ directly into the trachea via an 18-gauge catheter. This delivery method is very efficient and decreases the amount of $O_2$ usage by 33% to 50%. Oxygen delivered by TT catheter may increase exercise tolerance more than other methods of $O_2$ delivery. The TT catheter can be easily concealed under a scarf or necktie. However, insertion of a TT catheter is an invasive procedure: catheters may become obstructed and infection may occur.

**Equipment systems.** There are three major types of $O_2$ systems for use in the home: the $O_2$ concentrator, compressed $O_2$, and liquid $O_2$. The $O_2$ concentrator separates atmospheric $O_2$ from nitrogen ($N_2$) and delivers $O_2$. This system operates by electrical power and is not portable. Therefore it is the most acceptable system for the homebound or less active patient. The concentrator is economical, requires low maintenance, and does not need refills. Compressed $O_2$ is usually prescribed in conjunction with the $O_2$ concentrator as a portable source of $O_2$ therapy for when the patient is away from home (Fig. 115-1). Compressed $O_2$ tanks of various sizes are provided on a stroller. These compressed sources need to be exchanged for full tanks when they are empty. Delivery schedules are usually arranged between the $O_2$ vendor and the patient. Liquid $O_2$ is 100% pure and provided to the patient in cylinders filled with frozen cryogenic $O_2$ (Fig. 115-2). When the system is turned on, the $O_2$ is warmed to room temperature before delivery to the patient. For portability the patient can fill a shoulder bag portable-type tank by attaching the portable tank to the main liquid $O_2$ reservoir. This portable liquid system weighs approximately 8 to 10 pounds and allows about 6 hours of $O_2$ at 2 L per minute. The liquid $O_2$ system requires frequent refills by the $O_2$ vendor, depending on the prescribed liter flow. This makes the liquid $O_2$ system the most expensive $O_2$ delivery

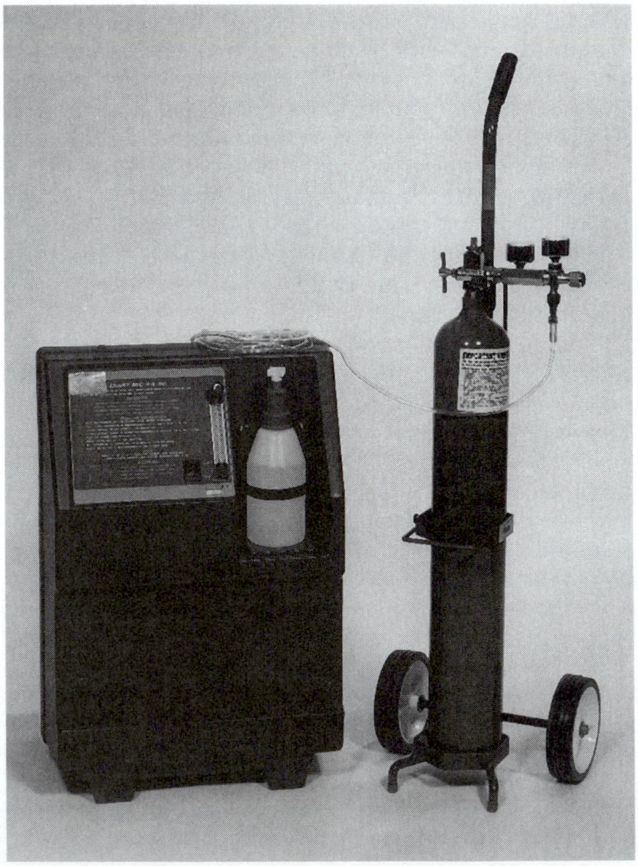

**Fig. 115-1.** Oxygen Concentrator (left) with a portable "E" tank cylinder (right).

system and should be reserved for active, mobile patients.

**Follow-up evaluations.** LTOT is frequently initiated before discharge from an acute care facility before the patient's clinical pulmonary status has returned to baseline. Patients may no longer meet the criteria for LTOT after discharge. Therefore it is recommended that arterial blood gases be repeated on room air, in a resting state, within 1 to 3 months after initiation of LTOT to reevaluate the need for LTOT. If LTOT is continued, then annual documentation of arterial blood gases or oxyhemoglobin saturation by pulse oximetry is recommended to assess the patient's clinical and physiologic status. In contrast, if LTOT is discontinued, we recommend repeat arterial blood gases on room air 1 to 2 weeks after cessation to verify continued adequate oxygenation.

**Air travel.** At altitude the pressure of inspired oxygen falls considerably due to a decrease in total barometric pressure, since cabins are not pressurized to sea level. All travelers develop some degree of arterial oxygen desaturation during flight due to the decrease in inspired oxygen, but patients with lung disease, including COPD, are particularly prone to develop significant hypoxemia during flight. Patients with ground-level room air $PaO_2$ levels of less than 70 mm Hg should be referred to a pulmonary function laboratory for an evaluation to determine the need for and amount of $O_2$ supplementation during flight.

### Nonpharmacologic therapy

***Lung transplantation and bullectomy.*** Lung transplantation has been utilized with success for patients with severe COPD, although clinical follow-up has been limited to a few years. In 1990 over 100 lung and heart-lung transplants were performed in the United States for COPD, including 50 for $\alpha_1$-PI deficiency-related COPD. Patients being considered for lung transplantation should be referred to specialized centers. The resection of large bullae may improve gas exchange and improve symptoms in selected patients with bullae of sufficient size to compress normal lung parenchyma.

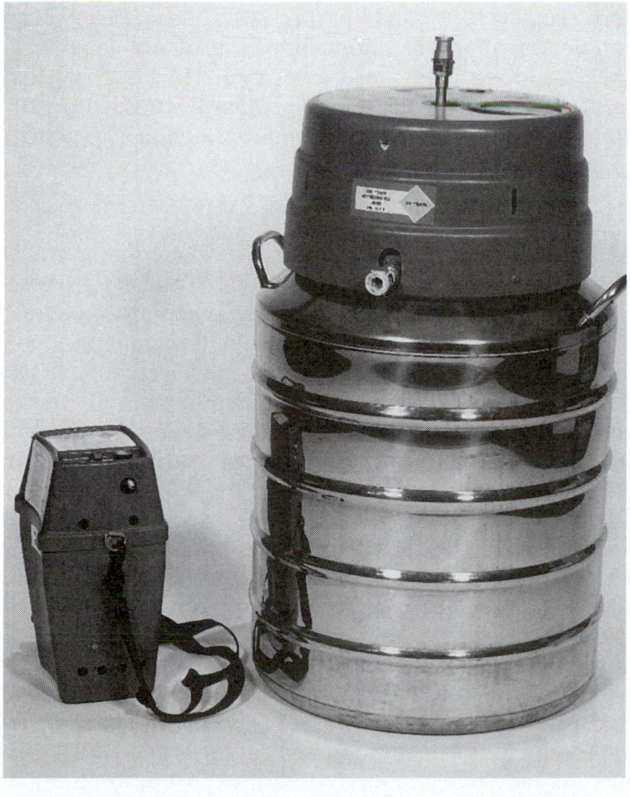

**Fig. 115-2.** Liquid Oxygen Stationary Reservoir (right) with a portable liquid system (left).

***Smoking cessation.*** Most patients diagnosed with COPD are or were cigarette smokers. Several investigations have clearly shown that smoking cessation slows the annual decrement of $FEV_1$ to the level of a nonsmoker. In addition, the nonpulmonary benefits include improved cardiovascular status and a reduced risk of developing lung cancer. The optimal method for nicotine replacement is the transdermal patch, which has supplanted the nicotine chewing gum (see Chapter 124). The patch is available in three doses, which are tapered over 2 to 3 months during the smoking cessation program. Some clinicians initiate therapy with a low-dose patch in patients with coronary artery disease. Both the short-term and long-term effects of the nicotine patch have been studied in controlled trials. The results from the short-term trials indicate that the patch is associated with a rate of smoking cessation that ranges from 18% at 3 weeks to 77% at 6 weeks. A study evaluating patients 6 months after completion of smoking cessation programs demonstrates that nicotine patch users have a higher rate of smoking cessation than do users of a placebo patch, although the cessation rate at 6 months is considerably lower than that at 6 weeks. In addition to temporary nicotine replacement, it is imperative that smoking cessation programs address the psychologic aspects of smoking to achieve long-term success at smoking cessation.

### Pulmonary rehabilitation

Patients with COPD have many objective and subjective barriers to living an active and productive life. Comprehensive, multidisciplinary pulmonary rehabilitation programs offer patients education, exercise training and reconditioning, proper nutrition, and psychosocial interventions to decrease anxiety and other emotional disturbances related to the effects of COPD. Although pulmonary rehabilitation does not improve spirometry, it has been demonstrated to reduce respiratory symptoms, anxiety, depression, and the need for medical care as well as to improve exercise tolerance and quality of life. The functional improvement a patient derives from pulmonary rehabilitation can be followed by serial pulmonary exercise testing.

## BIBLIOGRAPHY

American Thoracic Society: Lung function testing: selection of reference values and interpretative strategies, *Am Rev Respir Dis* 144:1202, 1991.

Cherniak NS: *Chronic obstructive pulmonary disease,* Philadelphia, 1991, WB Saunders.

Dompeling E et al: Slowing the deterioration of asthma and chronic obstructive pulmonary disease observed during bronchodilator therapy by adding inhaled corticosteroids, *Ann Intern Med* 118:770, 1993.

Ferguson GT, Cherniak RM: Management of chronic obstructive pulmonary disease, *N Engl J Med* 328:1017, 1993.

Gross NJ: The influence of anticholinergic agents on treatment for bronchitis and emphysema, *Am J Med* 91(4A):11S, 1991.

Huib AM et al: A comparison of bronchodilator therapy with or without inhaled corticosteroid therapy for obstructive airways disease, *N Engl J Med* 327:1413, 1992.

Murphy TF, Sethi S: Bacterial infection in chronic obstructive pulmonary disease, *Am Rev Respir Dis* 146:1067, 1992.

Schapira RM et al: The value of the forced expiratory time in the physical diagnosis of obstructive airways disease, *JAMA* 270:731, 1993.

Skorodin MS: Pharmacotherapy for asthma and chronic obstructive pulmonary disease, *Arch Intern Med* 153:814, 1993.

Vaz Fragoso CA, Miller MA: Review of the clinical efficacy of theophylline in the treatment of chronic obstructive pulmonary disease, *Am Rev Respir Dis* 147:S40, 1993.

CHAPTER

# 116 Interstitial Lung Diseases

**Donald P. Schlueter**

More than 130 acute and chronic diseases can involve the interstitium of the lung either as a primary disorder or as a secondary manifestation of a systemic disease. Some of the more common interstitial lung diseases are listed in the box below. They constitute a heterogenous group of disorders in which often no cause can be identified. The interstitium of the lung or connective tissue structure includes the connective tissue of the pleura, blood vessels and bronchi, and the alveolar walls. Interstitial lung disease has been defined as an inflammatory process involving all of the components of the alveolar wall that may go on to heal completely or that may result in the development of an excess of connective tissue with gross distortion of the lung architecture. The initial event involves a focal or diffuse alveolitis due to the accumulation in the alveolar walls of pulmonary macrophages, circulating lymphocytes, monocytes, and neutrophils that mediate acute and chronic inflammation. This inflammatory process results in the release of mediators that stimulate collagen production by fibroblasts and may eventually progress to interstitial pulmonary fibrosis, also known as fibrosing alveolitis. The clinical course depends on the pathologic diagnosis, and prognosis is quite variable. In some cases where a specific etiologic agent has been identified, simply removing the individual from exposure results in gradual recovery; others respond to steroid therapy, but the condition progresses in many despite treatment.

### Interstitial lung diseases

**Acute**

- Infection (e.g., viral, mycoplasmal, fungal)
- Acute interstitial pneumonitis (Hamman-Rich syndrome)
- Drug induced
- Organic dust– or chemical-induced hypersensitivity pneumonitis
- Adult respiratory distress syndrome (ARDS)
- Toxic gas exposure (chlorine, nitrogen dioxide)
- Radiation therapy
- Eosinophilic pneumonia
- Bronchiolitis obliterans organizing pneumonia (BOOP)
- Pulmonary vasculitis syndrome

**Chronic**

- Usual interstitial pneumonitis (UIP)
- Idiopathic pulmonary fibrosis (IPF)
- Sarcoidosis
- Pneumoconiosis due to inorganic dust
- Connective tissue disorder
- Chronic hypersensitivity pneumonitis due to organic dust
- Carcinomatosis and alveolar cell carcinoma
- Drug induced
- Goodpasture syndrome
- Lymphangioleiomyomatosis
- Eosinophilic granuloma histiocytosis X

## CLINICAL PRESENTATION

The most common presenting complaint of patients with interstitial lung disease is dyspnea. Initially it may be present only with exertion, but as the disease process progresses it may occur at rest. Since the loss of lung function may be gradual (since there is a substantial functional reserve in the lung), the disease may progress significantly before the patient seeks medical attention. A nonproductive, irritating cough frequently aggravated by exertion and deep breathing and a feeling of chest tightness or heaviness may be present, especially as the fibrosis develops and progresses. Wheezing, sputum production, anorexia, and weight loss are not usually seen until the disease is more advanced. However, systemic symptoms may be present in patients whose interstitial lung disease is secondary to another condition such as a connective tissue disorder.

## HISTORY AND PHYSICAL EXAMINATION

A thorough and accurate history is extremely important in the evaluation of a patient with interstitial lung disease. This should involve potential environmental exposures at work. The occupational history should include a detailed listing of all jobs held by the patient, the specific tasks performed, and materials used. Where potentially hazardous materials are utilized, the employer must provide the worker with the pertinent material safety data sheets (MSDS). This information should be helpful in considering the possible contribution of this source to the patient's problem. Since there is a long latent period, usually 10 to 20 years, for some exposures such as asbestos to produce clinically apparent disease, it may require considerable perseverance to obtain the appropriate information. The home environment should not be neglected, since contaminated humidifiers and air conditioning systems can be a cause of interstitial lung disease in the form of hypersensitivity pneumonitis. Prolonged low-level exposure, as may be encountered with exposure to an organic dust in the home environment, may not produce sufficient acute symptoms to cause the patient to seek medical attention and therefore results in a delay in diagnosis. With the acute form of hypersensitivity pneumonitis symptoms of malaise, fever, dyspnea, and cough develop 4 to 8 hours after exposure to the offending agent. Because of this delay, the patient often does not recognize the causal relationship. Early recognition is essential, since avoidance of further exposure can result in resolution or at least stabilization of the interstitial process. A number of drugs, particularly cancer chemotherapeutic agents and illicit street drugs, have been implicated as causative agents in this disease, and their use should be carefully evaluated. A geographic history may be helpful in suggesting or excluding a chronic infectious process. Symptoms consistent with a connective tissue or vascular disorder should be sought.

In the early stages of interstitial lung disease the physical examination, including auscultation of the chest, may be entirely normal. As the disease process progresses and dyspnea develops, basilar crackles (Velcro rales) signal the presence of interstitial pulmonary fibrosis. However, the absence of crackles does not exclude the diagnosis. Later cyanosis and, in about 10% to 15% of patients, finger clubbing develop. The latter is more common in patients with idiopathic pulmonary fibrosis (IPF) and asbestosis. With advanced disease cardiac involvement is common with pulmonary hypertension and right-sided heart failure. With the exception of sarcoidosis and the collagen vascular diseases, the physical findings are generally limited to the chest.

## LABORATORY STUDIES

The chest radiograph is the most important piece of information in the initial evaluation of a patient with suspected interstitial lung disease and may be abnormal in the absence of significant respiratory symptoms. However, some patients with dyspnea and interstitial lung disease may have a normal chest x-ray. Eplar and colleagues reported a series where 13% of patients with IPF, 37% with hypersensitivity pneumonitis, and 10% with sarcoidosis had normal chest x-rays. The introduction of high-resolution computed tomography (HRCT) scanning of the lung has increased the sensitivity for detecting minimal interstitial disease not evident on the conventional chest radiographs. Early in the disease process radiographic changes may be limited to an increase in interstitial markings, more prominent in the lower lung fields. Every effort should be made to obtain any existing chest radiographs, since subtle changes may become more obvious when previous chest films are available for comparison. They may also provide information on the onset and progression of the disease. Hilar and mediastinal lymphadenopathy are usually associated with sarcoidosis, silicosis, and some lymphomas. Pleural disease is uncommon in interstitial lung disease. Pleural effusion and pleural thickening may occur with collagen vascular disease, lymphoma, asbestos-related disease, and a small percentage of patients with sarcoidosis. As the disease progresses, a more clearly defined reticulonodular pattern becomes evident along with a decrease in lung volume, as indicated by elevation of the diaphragms (Fig. 116-1).

Pulmonary function studies reflect the structural changes that cause a stiff noncompliant lung. There is a reduction in all lung volumes consistent with a restrictive

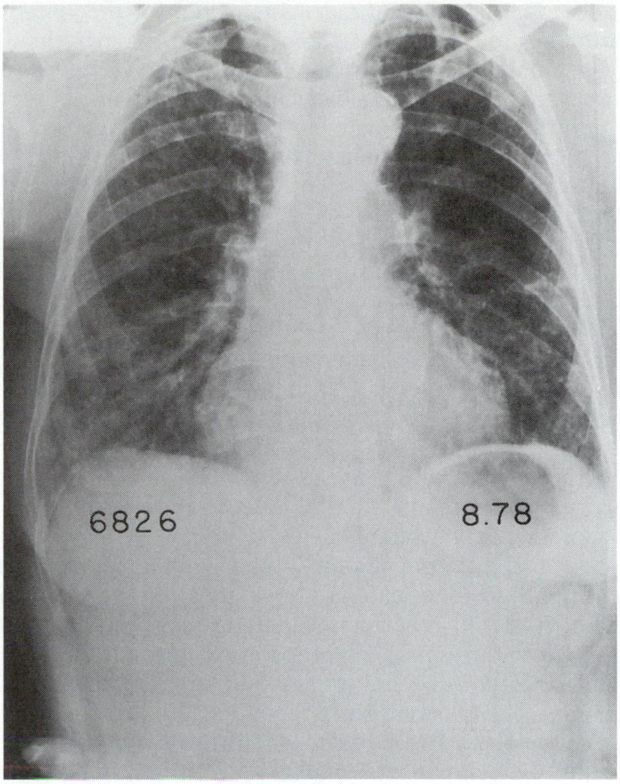


**Fig. 116-1.** Radiograph of a 73-year-old woman shows diffuse linear opacities with honeycombing and early cor pulmonale. She had progressive dyspnea for 3 years, bilateral end-inspiratory crackles and physiologic studies showing a decreased vital capacity, very low single-breath diffusing capacity, and oxygen desaturation at rest that became more severe with exercise. The lung biopsy shows usual interstitial pneumonia.

ventilatory impairment. Spirometry shows a decrease in forced vital capacity (FVC) and forced expiratory volume in 1 second ($FEV_1$) but a normal $FEV_1$/FVC ratio. Usually flow rates are not significantly decreased unless the restriction is severe, although evidence for small airways obstruction has been reported in interstitial lung disease. Lung volume measurements show a decreased total lung capacity (TLC), functional residual capacity (FRC), and residual volume (RV), with a normal to low RV/TLC ratio. Most patients have a disturbance in gas exchange manifested by a significantly diminished single breath carbon monoxide diffusing capacity. Although arterial oxygenation may be normal at rest, arterial hypoxemia is usually present with exercise. Carbon dioxide retention does not occur, and despite hypoxemia erythrocytosis and elevated hematocrits are uncommon.

Routine blood tests and serology may be helpful but relatively nonspecific, such as an increased erythrocyte sedimentation rate (ESR) or serum angiotensin converting enzyme (ACE) level, which is elevated in about 29% to 93% of patients with active sarcoidosis. Serologic tests for collagen vascular disease are necessary to exclude these diagnoses, although low titers of antinuclear antibodies (ANA) and rheumatoid factor (RF) have been reported in patients with IPF. Antineutrophil cytoplasmic antibody (ANCA) determinations appear helpful in diagnosing and assessing the activity of some of the necrotizing vasculitides. The demonstration of high titers of precipitating antibodies to organic dusts known to cause hypersensitivity pneumonitis, such as the thermophilic *Actinomyces*, may support this diagnosis when accompanied by an appropriate history. This is not a definitive diagnostic test for hypersensitivity pneumonitis, since 40% to 50% of exposed individuals may have antibodies in their serum without developing disease.

Bronchoalveolar lavage (BAL) provides a relatively simple and safe means of obtaining fluid samples for culture and cytologic evaluation in patients with interstitial lung disease. BAL has been particularly helpful in characterizing the inflammatory process in the lungs by providing viable cells for analysis of functional and secretory activity. Analysis of the cellular constituents has been suggested not only as a means for diagnosing the specific interstitial disease process, but also as guide for instituting and monitoring the effectiveness of therapy. A predominance of lymphocytes is found in sarcoidosis, hypersensitivity pneumonitis, and lymphoma, whereas neutrophils predominate in idiopathic pulmonary fibrosis, histiocytosis X, asbestosis, cigarette smokers, and obviously in the presence of infection. At present the use of BAL for diagnosing and staging of interstitial lung disease remains controversial, since the procedure is invasive, the technique is not standardized, and results show significant variability. Lymphocytes tend to predominate in BAL fluid obtained from patients with sarcoid and hypersensitivity pneumonitis, whereas polymorphonuclear cells (PMNs) are more frequent in those with idiopathic pulmonary fibrosis and asbestosis.

Radioactive gallium scanning has been used to evaluate patients with interstitial lung disease. Its role remains somewhat controversial because of its nonspecificity; varied types of pulmonary inflammation as well as neoplasms can produce a positive result. Gallium is most likely taken up by activated alveolar macrophages or PMNs in the areas of inflammation, and the uptake may be a marker of alveolitis. This is supported by the finding of a better correlation of gallium uptake with the extent of inflammation on open lung biopsy compared with conventional chest radiographs. Gallium scanning has been used to follow the course of disease during treatment, but it has proven to be disappointing in predicting responsiveness to corticosteroid or immunosuppressive therapy. One study found that only 10% to 30% of patients with increased uptake respond to therapy. In fact, favorable responses to therapy have been noted even when the gallium scans are normal. However, gallium scanning may be helpful in planning a biopsy procedure by identifying areas of active inflammation and increase the probability of a positive result.

Despite the large number of causes, it is frequently possible to make a definitive diagnosis of interstitial disease on the basis of the history, clinical findings, and laboratory data. Some examples include pneumoconiosis, hypersensitivity pneumonitis, and drug-induced lung diseases. Sarcoidosis could be included, particularly if organs other than the lung are involved. However, in most cases of interstitial lung disease histologic examination of lung tissue is the most effective method of obtaining a definitive characterization of the extent and pattern of diseases, and the presence or absence of organisms might be responsible. Fiberoptic bronchoscopy with transbronchial biopsy is the initial procedure of choice when the suspected diagnosis includes sarcoidosis, hypersensitivity pneumonitis, pulmonary alveolar proteinosis, eosinophilic granuloma/histiocytosis X, and malignancy.

Open lung biopsy remains the gold standard for a histologic diagnosis when the transbronchial biopsy is nondiagnostic or with a suspected disease process that is not likely to yield a definitive result by this procedure. In addition, it excludes other etiologies and directly assesses the inflammatory and fibrotic lesions. It also provides enough tissue to perform a variety of special tests, including electron microscopy, energy-dispersive x-ray analysis, and immunofluorescence. Tissue can be obtained from several lobes and areas with different degrees of involvement. Recently video-assisted thoracoscopic lung biopsy has been introduced in the diagnosis and staging of interstitial lung disease. This procedure involves the introduction of two or three endoscopic trocars and instruments, requiring single-lung ventilation with the lung to be biopsied collapsed. Hospital stay and postoperative pain are reduced, and adequate tissue can be obtained in most patients.

## ACUTE INTERSTITIAL PNEUMONIAS

Acute interstitial pneumonia, or diffuse alveolar damage, can result from a variety of insults to the lung. This response can be seen in viral pneumonias, adult respiratory distress syndrome (ARDS), toxic chemical exposures, antineoplastic drugs, active connective tissue diseases, radiation injury, and fat embolism syndrome. In most cases the pathologic changes of diffuse alveolar damage gradually resolve with minimal residual effect. In ARDS the chest x-ray shows a diffuse infiltrate consistent with pulmonary edema, whereas in the other conditions the infiltrates may be more patchy. The diagnosis usually can be suspected from the clinical setting, and usually biopsy is resorted to only when an infectious process is suspected. For the majority of these conditions treatment is supportive, but corticosteroids may accelerate recovery with acute interstitial pneumonia associated with connective tissue disorders or due to chemical exposure, radiation therapy, or antineoplastic drugs.

## CHRONIC INTERSTITIAL PNEUMONIAS

Idiopathic pulmonary fibrosis (IPF), or cryptogenic fibrosing alveolitis (a term preferred by the British), is one of the more commonly occurring interstitial lung diseases of unknown etiology. It is a chronic progressive lung disorder associated with both inflammation and fibrosis of the lung parenchyma. Confusion has arisen concerning IPF and its relation to the morphologic classification of interstitial pneumonias, including desquamative interstitial pneumonitis (DIP) and usual interstitial pneumonitis (UIP) as defined by Liebow and colleagues. Crystal has recommended that this terminology not be applied to IPF, even though lung tissue from patients with IPF may show morphologic changes typical of DIP or UIP, since they are nonspecific and found in other interstitial lung diseases. However, this suggestion has not been generally accepted. The distinction between DIP and UIP has some prognostic significance, since patients with DIP are more likely to respond to corticosteroids. This has led to the conclusion that DIP is probably an early stage of UIP. In addition, Liebow described certain subgroups of interstitial pneumonias based on the types of predominating inflammatory cells in the lung biopsy. These include lymphocytic interstitial pneumonia LIP, giant cell interstitial pneumonia (GIP), and plasma cell interstitial pneumonia (PIP).

IPF typically occurs in people 50 to 80 years old but may affect all age groups and is more common in men and in smokers. It occurs with a prevalence rate of three to five cases per 100,000 population. In 1935 Hamman and Rich first described five patients with rapidly progressive dyspnea, diffuse infiltrates in chest radiographs, and death occurring in 6 months of presentation. Recent studies suggest that this more fulminant type of pulmonary fibrosis occurs more often in connective tissue diseases, particularly rheumatoid arthritis. Although the course of IPF is quite variable, progressive deterioration in pulmonary function and exercise capacity, increasing hypoxemia, and radiographic evidence of extensive fibrosis and honeycombing over a period of 2 to 8 years are typical. Periods of stabilization may occur, but spontaneous improvement is rarely seen. Mean survival ranges from 3 to 5 years with mortality exceeding 40% within 5 years of onset of symptoms.

Patients with IPF typically present with a history of an insidious onset of progressive dyspnea on exertion and nonproductive cough. The cough often occurs with prolonged paroxysms and responds poorly to antitussives. Examination of the chest in the majority of the patients reveals bilateral late inspiratory crackles (Velcro rales) predominantly over the lower lung fields. Wheezing is not a feature of IPF. Finger clubbing is relatively common, occurring in 40% to 75% of patients. Cardiac examination usually yields normal results, except in the later stages of the disease when signs of pulmonary hypertension and cor pulmonale may become evident. Cyanosis is also a late manifestation indicative of severe disease.

The chest radiograph is abnormal in the majority of patients with IPF, and often it is these changes that alert the physician to the presence of interstitial lung disease. The most common abnormalities are a reticular or reticulonodular pattern diffusely involving the lower lung fields along with volume loss. With advanced disease multiple cystic or honeycombed areas may be seen. Although the correlation between the radiographic pattern and the stage of disease (clinical or histopathologic) is generally poor, chest radiographs and HRCT of the lungs are important in gauging progression or regression of disease in response to therapy. The HRCT may show the presence of interstitial fibrosis in a small percentage of patients with IPF who have a normal chest radiograph. A variety of abnormal laboratory tests have been noted in IPF, including an elevated ESR, circulating immune complexes, RF, and ANA. However, serologic parameters fail to correlate with activity of disease or predict responsiveness to therapy. Recently Nakos and colleagues reported that serum anticollagen antibodies could be a marker of IPF activity. The typical pulmonary function changes are consistent with a restrictive impairment, with reduction in all lung volumes including FVC, $FEV_1$, TLC, FRC, and RV. Airways obstruction is not usually present unless there is complicating chronic obstructive lung disease. A major physiologic abnormality is a disturbance in gas exchange due to ventilation-perfusion ($\dot{V}/\dot{Q}$) inequality and contraction of the pulmonary capillary volume. As a result the diffusing capacity ($D_LCO$) is reduced, a change that may precede the reduction in lung volume. Although arterial oxygenation at rest may be normal, desaturation almost always can be demonstrated with exercise. Exercise testing is more sensitive in the detection of abnormalities in oxygen transfer and provides a more sensitive parameter for following the clinical course.

The clinical, physiologic, and radiographic manifestations of IPF are similar to a variety of other interstitial lung diseases; therefore in most cases open lung biopsy is required to substantiate the diagnosis and exclude other etiologies. The lung biopsy in IPF shows a wide spectrum of histologic changes depending on the stage of the disease. The early stages involve an alveolitis characterized by an accumulation of mononuclear cells (lymphocytes, alveolar macrophages, and type II alveolar cells) in the alveolar spaces, with relative preservation of the alveolar walls, referred to as desquamative interstitial pneumonitis. As the disease progresses, there is distortion of the alveolar walls with edema, mononuclear cell infiltration, and fibroblast proliferation or usual interstitial pneumonitis. In the advanced stages alveolar walls are markedly thickened, and much of the alveolar architecture is destroyed and replaced by connective tissue and fibrosis. Large cystic spaces, forming the honeycomb lung and minimal inflammatory cells, represent the end stage of this disease. Because of the small amount of tissue obtained by transbronchial biopsy (TBB), it is difficult to assess the degree of inflammation and fibrosis and therefore it provides little prognostic information. Thoracoscopic lung biopsy may provide a compromise between TBB and open lung biopsy by minimizing operative risks and yet providing adequate tissue for diagnosis.

BAL is not specific enough to provide a definitive diagnosis of IPF but may predict therapeutic responsiveness, since the presence of BAL lymphocytosis has been associated with a greater responsiveness to corticosteroid therapy.

The most effective treatment for IPF is corticosteroids, but response to therapy is inconsistent. In general, patients with the shortest duration of symptoms, BAL fluid showing greater than 5% lymphocytes and less than 10% neutrophils, and a lung biopsy demonstrating more inflammation with less fibrosis have the greatest potential for a response to corticosteroids and a more favorable prognosis. Usually an initial dose of oral prednisone at 40 to 60 mg daily is given for several months, and, if a favorable response is obtained, prednisone is tapered slowly to 15 to 20 mg daily or an equivalent alternate-day dosage. Corticosteroids should be continued for at least 1 year. If no response is observed in the initial therapeutic trial of corticosteroids, they should be rapidly tapered and discontinued. Cytotoxic agents, such as azathioprine and cyclophosphamide, are used as second-line drugs usually in combination with oral corticosteroids. However, the number of subjects in the few controlled prospective studies is small; thus the efficacy of these treatments has not been definitively demonstrated, and they carry a considerably greater risk of adverse effects than corticosteroids alone. Colchicine has been suggested as a potentially useful agent in the treatment of IPF because of its antifibrotic properties. No controlled prospective clinical studies are available to evaluate the efficacy of this therapy. Finally, single-lung transplantation is now a consideration for patients with end-stage pulmonary fibrosis refractory to medical therapy. Through 1990 there were over 170 single-lung transplants with a 2-year survival approaching 55% and a number of recipients exceeding 5 years. Survival time has increased significantly in the past several years to around 75% in some centers. Unfortunately, due to the shortage of donor organs, many patients with IPF die while awaiting transplantation.

## HYPERSENSITIVITY PNEUMONITIS

Hypersensitivity pneumonitis, or extrinsic allergic alveolitis, is an immunologic-induced interstitial pneumonitis characterized by predominantly mononuclear cell inflammation of the pulmonary parenchyma, terminal bronchioles, and alveoli. The antigenic agents include organic dusts derived from fungal, bacterial, or serum protein sources, as well as some reactive organic chemicals (Table 116-1).

Because of the very small particle size, usually less than 5 μm, a large quantity of antigenic material can be delivered to the alveolar level. The clinical response to antigen exposure depends on the individual's immunologic reactivity, the nature of the dust or chemical, the size of the particles, and the intensity of the exposure, particularly whether it is regular or intermittent. The immunologic reactivity appears to be an important predisposing factor in the development of hypersensitivity pneumonitis, since large surveys of farmers and workers exposed to bagasse, the spent sugar cane after the sugar has been removed, and a number of organic chemicals reveal a high percentage with serum precipitating antibody against specific antigen, but a low incidence of lung disease. The immunologic hallmark of hypersensitivity pneumonitis is the presence of serum IgG and/or IgA precipitating antibody to the inhaled antigen, precipitins usually being present in over 90% of patients. This finding of precipitating antibody in studies of farmer's lung disease suggested the possibility of a hypersensitivity reaction. Subsequent investigations have provided evidence that multiple immunologic reactions are involved predominantly with cell-mediated delayed hypersensitivity, with or without amplification by immune complexes, lymphokines, and other biologic modifiers. Recently the predominance of CD8+ T lymphocytes in BAL fluid in farmer's lung disease has been shown to shift toward the CD4+ predominance after removal from exposure.

Although exposure in the workplace has most often been the focus of reports of hypersensitivity lung disease, more recently the home environment and even the family automobile have been implicated as a source of respiratory problems. Air conditioning systems, furnace and room humidifiers, cold steamers, saunas, and hot tubs can cultivate a variety of organisms that have been identified as etiologic agents in hypersensitivity pneumonitis. Alleviation of symptoms when away from home with recurrence on return, or changes in symptoms during the heating or cooling season, may also offer clues. Thus it is evident that a patient's total environmental exposure must be considered when a hypersensitivity lung disease is suspected.

The clinical manifestations of hypersensitivity pneumonitis are similar, regardless of the organic dust or chemical inhaled, and these diseases should be considered as a syndrome with a spectrum of clinical features. The patient with hypersensitivity pneumonitis may present with three different clinical pictures—acute, subacute, or chronic.

### Acute form

The classic and most readily recognized form of hypersensitivity pneumonitis results from intermittent exposure to antigen and resembles an acute viral or bacterial infection. Symptoms include chills, fever, malaise, headache, nonproductive cough, chest tightness, and dyspnea without wheezing. Symptoms develop 4 to 6 hours after exposure and resolve spontaneously in 12 to 24 hours but recur on reexposure. Fatigue and weight loss may follow frequent or severe episodes. Physical findings include fever, tachypnea, tachycardia, cyanosis, and late bibasilar inspiratory crackles; wheezing is rarely heard. Laboratory studies reveal a leukocytosis without eosinophilia and elevated immunoglobulin levels. High titers of precipitating antibody against the offending antigen is characteristic. However, since precipitins are also common in exposed individuals without disease, this finding is not sufficient to make a diagnosis of hypersensitivity pneumonitis.

The chest radiograph may be normal after a brief exposure, but with an intense or more prolonged exposure a diffuse pattern of small, somewhat discrete, nodules or a diffuse, soft, stringy or patchy interstitial infiltrate may be seen.

The typical physiologic change is restrictive in type with a decrease in vital capacity and lung volumes without airways obstruction. In some patients, particularly with severe reactions, small airways obstruction can be demonstrated. Bronchial hyperreactivity is found in a significant number of individuals, particularly following an acute attack. This enhanced responsiveness may be due to mediators released in the inflammatory response. Hypoxia is usually present, and the carbon monoxide–diffusing capacity is invariably reduced, particularly at the height of the reaction. This abnormality may persist for some time after other parameters have returned to normal. Long-term follow-up studies in patients who continue to have only brief and infrequent exposure to the antigens usually do not show a significant decrement in pulmonary function.

### Subacute form

This form of hypersensitivity pneumonitis is considerably less common and tends to develop with more chronic exposure. Symptoms develop insidiously with features of progressive chronic bronchitis, including productive cough, dyspnea, easy fatigue, anorexia, and weight loss. Typical acute attacks, although infrequent, can be precipitated by heavy exposure. The chest radiograph may show diffuse nodulation or change consistent with interstitial fibrosis, but normal radiologic findings are not unusual.

**Table 116-1.** Occupational hypersensitivity pneumonitides

| Disease | Exposure | Specific inhalant |
|---|---|---|
| Farmer's drug | Moldy hay | *Thermoactinomyces vulgaris* |
| | | *T. candidus* |
| | | *T. viridis* |
| | | *Micromonospora faeni* |
| Bagassosis | Moldy sugar cane | *T. vulgaris* |
| | | *T. sacchare* |
| Maple bark–stripper's lung | Contaminated maple logs | *Cryptostroma corticale* |
| Bird-breeder's lung | Avian droppings | Serum protein |
| Air-conditioner, humidifier lung | Contaminated water | *T. vulgaris* |
| | | *T. candidus* |
| | | *Amoeba* sp. |
| | | Endotoxin |
| Mushroom-worker's lung | Mushroom compost | *T. vulgaris* |
| | | *M. faeni* |
| Malt-worker's lung | Moldy barley | *Aspergillus clavatus* |
| | | *A. fumigatus* |
| | Flour | |
| Detergent-worker's lung | Detergent powder | *Bacillus subtilis* |
| Grain-weevil (miller's) | Grain dust | *Sitophilus granarius* |
| | Flour | |
| Suberosis | Oak bark | *Penicillium frequentans* |
| | Cork dust | |
| Furrier's lung | Fox | Hair protein |
| Coffee-worker's lung | Coffee-bean dust | Coffee bean protein |
| Vineyard-sprayer's lung | Spray solution | Copper sulphate |
| | | *T. viridis* |
| Sequoiosis | Redwood sawdust | *Graphium* sp. |
| | | *Aureobasidium* |
| | | *Pullulans* spores |
| Cheese-washer's lung | Cheese mold | *Penicillium caseii* |
| | | *P. roqueforti* spores |
| Fish meal–handler's lung | Fish meal (pet food) | Fish proteins |
| Wood-dust disease | Mahogany and oak dust | Unknown |
| Wood pulp–worker's lung | Moldy logs | *Alternaria tenuis* |
| Paprika-slicer's lung | Moldy paprika pods | *Mucor stolonifer* |
| Fog fever | Cattle | *T. candidus* |
| Feather-plucker's lung | Chicken products | Chicken proteins |
| Tobacco-grower's lung | Tobacco plants | Unknown |
| Tea-grower's lung | Tea plants | Unknown |
| Bible-printer's disease | Moldy typestting water | Unknown |
| Plastics and resin makers | Plastics industry | Toluene diisocyanate |
| | Polyurethane | Methylene diphenyl-diisocyanate |
| | Paints | Hexamethylene-diisocyanate |
| Painters and paint makers | Sand binders | Trimellitic anhydride |

Both restrictive and obstructive defects in pulmonary function are seen, with the former predominating. The diffusing capacity is reduced, along with hypoxemia, at least with exercise if not at rest. Long-term avoidance of exposure and administration of corticosteroids usually result in a reduction of symptoms and physiologic abnormalities. This is the most difficult form of the disease to diagnosis because of the insidious nature and nonspecific clinical findings.

## Chronic form

Recurrent intense exposure to antigen, or prolonged low-level exposure, can lead to the chronic form of hypersensitivity pneumonitis, with the gradual development of disabling respiratory symptoms and irreversible physiologic changes. Progressive dyspnea is the most common symptom along with nonproductive cough and easy fatigue.

Physical findings include tachypnea, bibasilar crackles (Velcro rales), and wheezing, which are heard in some patients with a predominantly obstructive profile. With advanced disease, signs of pulmonary hypertension and cor pulmonale may be present.

The chest radiograph in this predominantly fibrotic phase shows contraction of the lungs particularly in the upper lobes, more peripheral involvement, and the development of a honeycomb appearance. Some nodulation may persist but probably does not represent active granulomatous disease. Avoidance of exposure for prolonged periods and the administration of corticosteroids and bronchodilators afford only slight improvement.

### Pathology

The histologic pattern found in the lung in hypersensitivity pneumonitis depends at what stage of disease the biopsy is obtained. In the acute stage the primary process is an interstitial granulomatous pneumonitis with foreign body giant cells, large numbers of lymphocytes, and macrophages with abundant foamy cytoplasm. Eosinophilia may be seen in the perivascular areas; vasculitis is rare. In the subacute stage there is moderate interstitial thickening, with only slight fibrosis, along with changes consistent with chronic bronchitis. In the chronic stage interstitial fibrosis is the predominant feature and may be focal or diffuse. Intraalveolar septa are infiltrated with lymphocytes, and collections of dust-laden macrophages may be seen in the alveolar spaces. Bronchiolitis obliterans, cystic changes, or honeycombing is found in association with densely fibrotic areas. Confluent fibrosis tends to occur predominantly in the upper lobes. It should be emphasized that, regardless of the stage of the disease, these changes are not specific for hypersensitivity pneumonitis, but have to be interpreted in the context of all of the associated clinical information.

### Diagnosis

The diagnosis of hypersensitivity pneumonitis requires a high index of suspicion on the part of the physician, a thorough and accurate history focusing on potential exposures in both the work and home environment, and the temporal relationship between the development of symptoms and the exposure. Some familiarity with the variety of organic dusts and chemicals that are capable of causing this disorder is particularly helpful (see Table 116-1). However, frequently a specific antigen is not readily identified, and environmental sampling and culturing are necessary to isolate the offending agent. This isolate can then be used to prepare an antigen to test the patient's serum for precipitating antibodies. The demonstration of precipitating antibody against a particular organic antigen reflects exposure and is not sufficient evidence of itself to make a diagnosis of hypersensitivity pneumonitis. About 40% to 50% of exposed individuals may have antibodies present in their serum without developing disease. In addition, serum precipitins may disappear after exposure ceases. BAL studies show a predominance of lymphocytes reflecting an active alveolitis, but this finding is not limited to hypersensitivity pneumonitis. The most specific diagnostic test at the present time, if the suspected antigen can be identified, is controlled inhalation challenge in the laboratory followed by serial pulmonary function tests and monitoring the clinical response. In the sensitized individual the signs, symptoms, and physiologic changes are accurately reproduced.

### Treatment

The major therapeutic approach to treatment is removal from exposure to the offending antigen. In the case of an affected farmer, for example, this could cause significant economic hardship. Efforts to reduce the intensity of antigen exposure by changes in work practices and the use of personal protection with a respirator have been of some benefit. Cromolyn is capable of blocking the immediate and late reaction in some individuals, whereas corticosteroids block only the late reaction. However, it is not certain that continued exposure to antigen and control of the symptoms with medication will prevent subsequent lung damage. Recent studies have reported that in some cases continued antigen exposure may not lead to clinical deterioration.

## INORGANIC DUST DISEASE—PNEUMOCONIOSIS

The word pneumoconiosis literally means dust in the lungs; however, not all dusts deposited in the lungs cause disease, and a more widely accepted definition is that of the International Labor Organization (ILO), which states that "pneumoconiosis is the accumulation of dust in the lungs and the tissue reaction to its presence." Inorganic dusts that do not disrupt the alveolar architecture or produce fibrosis when retained in the lung are classified as inert dusts or nuisance particulates, provided that they are free from toxic impurities and contain less than 1% quartz. These dusts ordinarily do not cause respiratory symptoms or functional abnormalities and may be cleared from the lung over time with avoidance of exposure; the term *benign pneumoconiosis* has been applied to this condition. The box below lists agents causing benign pneumoconiosis. The most common benign pneumoconiosis is siderosis, occurring primarily in welders and in workers mining and crushing iron ores.

The inhalation of inorganic dusts, which elicit a response in the lungs that eventually leads to irreversible fibrosis and structural and functional alterations, causes the fibrosing or collagenous pneumoconioses. The box below lists the more commonly encountered etiologic agents, with silica and asbestos being the most important.

### Inorganic dusts causing pneumoconiosis

**Dusts causing benign pneumoconiosis**

Iron oxide (siderosis)
Tin ore (stannosis)
Barium compounds (baritosis)
Antimony ore
Zirconium compounds
Chromite ore
Cerium dioxide
Titanium dioxide

**Dusts causing a fibrosing pneumoconiosis**

Silica
- Quartz
- Cristobalite
- Tridymite

Diatomaceous earth
Beryllium
Asbestos
Coal dust
Graphite
Carbon black
Aluminum
Talc

### Silicosis

Silicosis is a chronic fibrotic disease of the lungs resulting from prolonged and intense exposure to free crystalline silica. Industrial sources of free silica include mining, quarrying and tunneling, foundry work, sandblasting, stone cutting and polishing, glass manufacturing, ceramics, and vitreous enameling. Several different clinical forms of silicosis are seen. The most common is chronic classic silicosis, which occurs with moderate exposure over a period of 20 to 45 years, usually involving respirable dust with less than 30% quartz. The lesions are usually nodular with a predominance in the upper lobes, probably due to better clearance of dust from the lower lobes. This simple stage of silicosis is associated with nodules generally 5 mm or less and usually normal pulmonary function. However, silicosis may be complicated by coalescence of the nodular lesions into conglomerate or confluent lesions, called massive fibrosis, usually in the upper lobes (progressive massive fibrosis) (Fig. 116-2) . It would appear that high quartz content is the primary factor in the pathogenesis of massive fibrosis in silicosis.

Accelerated silicosis occurs most frequently in sandblasters and silica flour workers. It results from moderately high exposure to dust containing 40% to 80% quartz and appears 5 to 15 years after the initial exposure. The nodular lesions tend to be smaller than in chronic silicosis, and the massive fibrosis favors the midzones of the lungs.

Acute silicosis (silicoproteinosis) is a rare form of silicosis occurring in workers with intense exposure to dust with very high concentrations of silica. It has been reported primarily in sandblasters. The disease develops over a period of 1 to 3 years and progresses rapidly to death from respiratory failure. The characteristic histopathologic finding is a lipid-proteinaceous material filling the alveoli, which gives a strongly positive reaction to periodic Schiff reagent similar to that in idiopathic pulmonary alveolar proteinosis. Since acute silicosis is frequently associated with occupations in which freshly fractured crystalline silica of respirable size is generated, it has been suggested that fracture-generated silicon-based radicals may play a significant role in the pathogenesis of this disease.

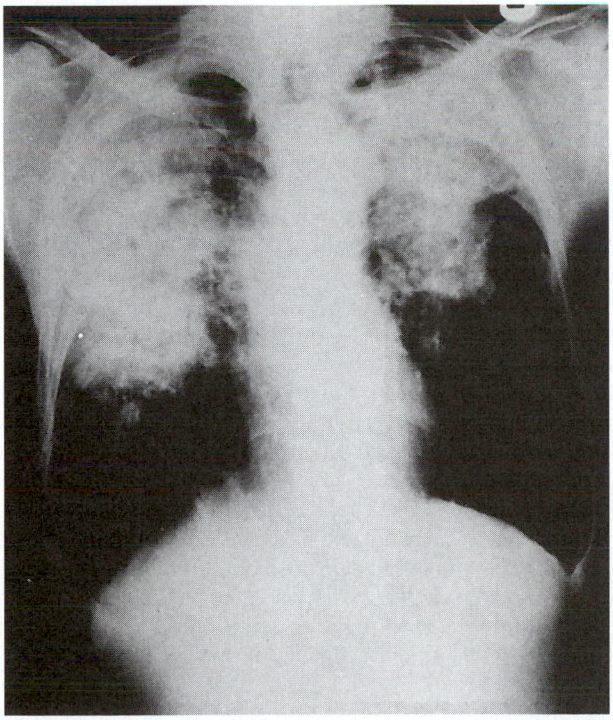

**Fig. 116-2.** Chest x-ray of coal worker 2 weeks before his death. The appearance is classic for progressive massive fibrosis (PMF), with larger conglomerate masses in both lung fields. (Courtesy JC Wagner.)

***Pathogenesis.*** Inhalation of silica particles small enough to reach the alveolar level induces a series of events resulting in the activation and persistence of inflammatory cells, with the alveolar macrophage playing a central role in the development of pulmonary inflammation. Earlier studies in the pathogenesis of silicosis suggested that ingestion of silica particles by the macrophages resulted in an interaction of silica-containing phagosomes with lysozymes releasing enzymes, which caused rupture of the phagosome and freed the silica particles in the cell cytoplasm. This process eventually leads to death of the cell due to the release of lysosome enzymes. The cycle of cell destruction is perpetuated by ingestion of the silica particles by other macrophages. However, more recent studies have shown that silica-laden macrophages can maintain normal viability but may be activated to produce proinflammatory mediators such as cytokines, interleukin 1 (IL-1), and tumor necrosis factor alpha ($TNF_{\alpha}$) that can participate in numerous inflammatory processes. Repeated inhalation of silica and slow clearance of silica-laden macrophages would keep the inflammatory mediators chronically activated and would perpetuate the inflammatory process, resulting in the development of granulomatous inflammation and fibrosis in the lung. Alveolar macrophages have also been shown to produce fibronectin and macrophage-derived growth factor, which would also contribute to the subsequent progressive fibrosis.

The typical lesion of silicosis is the silicotic nodule. These well-circumscribed nodules consist of whorled zones of acellular hyalin surrounded by a moderately cellular collagenous capsule. The majority of the silica particles are found in the outer layers of the nodules. The silica can be demonstrated as birefringent particles when the tissue sections are viewed under polarized light. The nodules are usually associated with adjoining parenchymal fibrosis.

***Clinical features.*** Silicosis is a disease with a long latent period and usually requires 15 to 20 years of exposure before the chest film shows significant abnormality, except where very intense exposure has occurred. With simple silicosis, although a nodular infiltration may be seen on the chest radiograph, the worker is usually asymptomatic, and no functional impairment is evident. With progression of disease to a more advanced stage, shortness of breath with exertion is the major symptom. It is important to point out that there is often poor correlation between the radiographic findings and the degree of functional impairment. Cough and sputum may develop, especially in smokers, as the disease progresses, but wheezing is not usually present. With the development of progressive massive fibrosis there is distortion of the normal lung structure due to contraction of the upper lobes, and emphysematous changes develop in the lower lobes, resulting in airways obstruction. Silicosis is the only pneumoconiosis that predisposes to the development of tuberculosis and is most likely to occur after the age of 50 in association with moderate to severe silicosis. There is also an increased incidence of atypical mycobacteriosis primarily due to *Mycobacterium avium intracellulare* (MAC), which can be difficult to treat due to resistance to most of the antituberculosis drugs.

Physical findings in simple silicosis are nonspecific unless complicated by heart or other lung disease, such as congestive heart failure, chronic obstructive pulmonary disease, and tuberculosis. With complicated silicosis there are signs of fibrotic or obstructive lung disease. Finger clubbing is not a feature of this disease, even though significant hypoxemia may be present.

***Lung function.*** In simple nodular silicosis lung function is usually normal. With progression of disease there is a gradual increase in a restrictive impairment with a reduced FVC, $FEV_1$, and TLC. There is gradual decrease in diffusing capacity, and although hypoxemia may be absent at rest, it usually can be demonstrated during exercise. In the absence of progressive massive fibrosis, hypoxemia at rest is rare. Associated airways obstruction may also be present, particularly in smokers with advanced disease. The latter suggests a synergistic effect between silica dust exposure and cigarette smoke.

***Diagnosis.*** With an occupational history of significant silica exposure and a chest radiograph showing a discrete nodular infiltrate, a diagnosis of simple silicosis can be made with reasonable certainty. Obtaining old chest x-rays is helpful in establishing the stability and progression of the disease. Although a restrictive impairment and abnormal diffusing capacity may be demonstrated in some cases at this stage, pulmonary function studies are usually normal. A lung biopsy is rarely indicated to make a diagnosis. Where the diagnosis is in question, a biopsy may be utilized to rule out a potentially treatable disease. If tissue is available, it can be examined under light and electron microscopy. Examination under polarized light can identify birefringent foreign material. Spectroscopy and x-ray diffraction have been used for the qualitative and quantitative analysis of lung tissue. However, these techniques require a rather large amount of lung tissue. More recently the use of energy-dispersive x-ray analysis (EDXA) permits simultaneous multielemental analysis while examining the tissue in the scanning electron microscope (SEM) without destruction of the tissue sample.

***Treatment.*** There is no specific treatment for silicosis. When a diagnosis has been made, the worker should be removed from further silica exposure. Although even simple silicosis may progress in the absence of further exposure, it is more likely to do so if exposure continues. In certain selected situations it may be possible for the worker to continue working with the use of an external air–supplied airstream helmet, which does offer excellent dust protection. With advanced disease treatment is supportive with oxygen, bronchodilators, cardiac medications, and antibiotics for infections.

### Asbestos-related disease

The term *asbestos* is given to a group of naturally occurring fibrous silicates with the unique property of great resistance to heat and chemical destruction. There was little commercial use of asbestos until the industrial revolution, when the need arose to insulate the steam engine. Between 1877 and 1967 the world production of asbestos increased from 50 tons to 4 million tons per year. Of the various types of asbestos fibers only chrysotile, crocidolite, and amosite are of economic importance. More than 90% of all asbestos used in the United States is chrysotile. With the wide use of asbestos in this country, it is estimated that about 2.5 million workers had potential exposure to asbestos by 1976.

Asbestosis is a pneumoconiosis resulting from the inhalation of asbestos fibers and is characterized by diffuse interstitial fibrosis of the lung. These parenchymal changes may be associated with pleural fibrosis and parietal pleural plaques. The first detailed epidemiologic study of asbestos workers in the United States was undertaken by the U.S. Public Health Service in 1937. This study demonstrated a relationship between the extent of exposure and clinical symptoms, prompting the recommendation of an exposure limit of 5 million particles per cubic foot of air. In 1965 Selikoff and colleagues published a landmark survey of 1500 asbestos insulation workers. They found that nearly half of those examined had asbestosis and concluded that asbestosis and its complications were significant hazards among insulation workers. This was subsequently corroborated by a number of other investigators.

***Pathogenesis.*** Deposition of inhaled particles, in this case asbestos fibers, depends on the aerodynamic behavior of the fibers, the dimensions of the respiratory tract entered, and the pattern of breathing. Since the fibers tend to align with the airstream, large fibers (even greater than 50 μm) can reach peripheral locations. Longer fibers are retained and eventually gain access into the interstitium of the lung. Smaller fibers are cleared by the alveolar macrophages. Exposure to asbestos results in the accumulation of macrophages in the area of deposition, which may serve a protective role. However, since alveolar macrophages are able to release a variety of mediators capable of injuring the alveolar walls and stimulating fibroblast proliferation, the alveolar macrophage may play the central role in the production of fibrosis and asbestosis. Studies in animals and in humans exposed to asbestos, using bronchoalveolar lavage, have demonstrated an inflammatory process (alveolitis) preceding the development of pulmonary fibrosis. Alveolar macrophages contribute to the alveolitis and fibrosis by the direct release of tissue-destructive metabolites, release of growth factors that stimulate fibroblast to replicate and synthesize collagen, such as alveolar macrophage-derived growth factor and fibronectin, and the release of neutral proteases. The presence of active alveolitis appears to be predictive of disease progression and can be evaluated by bronchoalveolar lavage or gallium scan. Despite a clear understanding of the mechanisms involved in the development of lung fibrosis resulting from asbestos exposure, it is not clear why individuals with similar exposure may have very different responses in terms of the fibrotic process.

***Pathology.*** In the early stages of asbestosis only microscopic changes, manifested by fibrosis at the level of the respiratory bronchiole, are observed. As the disease evolves, the fibrosis extends peripherally, resulting in diffuse interstitial fibrosis most prominent in the lower lobes. Fibrous wall cysts may form, giving the lung a honeycomb appearance. Pleural fibrosis and circumscribed pleural plaques, involving the parietal pleura with or without calcification, may be present. Asbestos bodies are an indicator of asbestos exposure that differentiates it from other forms of lung fibrosis. They are considered an essential feature for the histologic diagnosis of asbestosis. Asbestos bodies tend to form a yellow-brown structure on the larger fibers that measures 20 to 150 µm in length. These bodies result from the deposition of an iron protein complex on the core fiber by alveolar macrophages. Asbestos body content has been quantitated by counting asbestos bodies in tissue sections, by digesting lung tissue and extracting the bodies, and more recently by examination of bronchoalveolar lavage fluid. By employing a combination of ultrastructural morphology, electron microscopy, and EDXA it is possible to identify almost every asbestos fiber found in the lung. From a medicolegal standpoint the number of fibers present would provide some estimate of the asbestos exposure, and data on the fiber type might allow identification of a source of exposure if the worker was thought to have been exposed to a specific type of asbestos.

***Clinical features.*** Asbestosis develops insidiously many years after the initial exposure, so the association may not be recognized. Symptoms and signs are not specific for asbestosis, since they do not differ from those found in diffuse interstitial fibrosis from a variety of other causes. The most common symptom is shortness of breath, particularly with exertion, which slowly progresses to breathlessness at rest. The dyspnea may be out of proportion to the radiographic abnormality, and cough is often present and may be productive, especially among smokers, due to coexisting chronic bronchitis. The most characteristic physical sign is the presence of bibasilar inspiratory crackles and is believed by many to be an early finding in asbestosis. Finger clubbing has been noted in a frequency varying from 20% to 84%. With advancing disease cyanosis may become apparent along with signs of pulmonary hypertension and cor pulmonale.

***Lung function.*** A characteristic functional change in asbestosis is that of restrictive lung disease. All lung volumes are reduced, particularly the vital capacity, inspiratory capacity, and TLC. Lung compliance is reduced due to the pulmonary fibrosis. Airways obstruction is uncommon, except in cigarette smokers. However, varying degrees of small airways obstruction have been demonstrated in nonsmoking asbestos workers, which was attributable to distortion of the small airways with bronchiolar fibrosis. The diffusing capacity is frequently reduced, and although hypoxemia may be absent at rest, it may first become evident only under the stress of exercise. In general, the effects of asbestos on lung function are dose related, but functional abnormalities can be demonstrated in some asbestos-exposed individuals in the absence of definite radiologic change.

The radiographic appearance is characterized by linear and irregular opacities predominant in the lower half of the lung fields, as opposed to the nodular changes seen in silicosis and coal worker's pneumoconiosis. The early changes of asbestosis consist of linear shadows of varying thickness, between 1 and 3 mm, most marked in the lower lung fields. As these lesions increase in profusion, there is gradual obscuring of the cardiac and diaphragmatic borders. Irregular opacities may be seen, but discrete rounded opacities are not a feature of asbestosis. As the fibrotic process progresses, the linear and irregular opacities become thicker and spread into the middle zones but rarely reach the upper zones. There is a gradual decrease in the lung volume. The basilar fibrotic changes are bilateral, and although they tend to be more prominent in one side, they are never unilateral.

***Diagnosis.*** A clinical diagnosis of asbestosis can be reached on the basis of a history of asbestos exposure and the presence of one or more of the following: radiographic changes of parenchymal and/or pleural fibrosis, basilar crackles, dyspnea on exertion, and abnormal pulmonary function that demonstrates restrictive impairment, low diffusing capacity, and hypoxemia at rest or with exercise. With all criteria present the diagnosis would be certain, but for most purposes a history of exposure and a chest x-ray consistent with asbestosis are sufficient. A lung biopsy is rarely indicated, but it is important to emphasize that the pathologist cannot make a definite diagnosis of asbestosis in cases that show characteristic fibrosis in the absence of asbestos bodies or other evidence of asbestos fibers.

***Treatment.*** There is no specific treatment for asbestosis, although corticosteroids have been used with some symptomatic improvement but without evidence that they affect the course of the disease. Removal from further exposure to asbestos is an accepted approach, since it seems reasonable that eliminating further asbestos burden on the lungs, at an early stage, would favor arresting the disease. However, despite removal from further exposure, it has been well demonstrated that the disease can continue to progress, albeit very slowly.

### Asbestos-related pleural disease

See Chapter 118.

***Lung cancer.*** The association between lung cancer and asbestos exposure was reported as early as 1935, and in 1964 Selikoff and colleagues firmly established the relationship in a study of insulation workers. Their data indicated that the effects of smoking and asbestos are multiplicative and result in a cancer risk over 50 times greater for a smoking asbestos worker compared with a nonsmoker with no asbestos exposure. The risk for nonsmokers exposed to asbestos is also slightly increased. Epidemiologic surveys indicate that the risk of lung cancer is dose related. Lung cancers tend to arise in relation to areas of fibrosis and therefore occur chiefly in the lower lobes and in the periphery. All major tumor cell types are seen, but adenocarcinoma is predominant. In the absence of asbestosis it is difficult to establish an asbestos etiology for the lung cancer, particularly in a smoker.

*Clinical features.* Clinical findings are those of the underlying asbestosis. A rapid increase in respiratory symptoms, appearance of hemoptysis, loss of appetite, and weight loss should alert the physician to the possibility of lung cancer. Chest x-rays should be taken and compared to previous radiographs. Since the changes of asbestosis progress slowly, any abrupt change should prompt further studies to include sputum cytology and a diagnostic bronchoscopy and biopsy. Once the cell type has been determined, appropriate therapy can be instituted. It cannot be emphasized too strongly that the most effective measure is to convince the worker to discontinue cigarette smoking.

*Mesothelioma.* The incidence of mesothelioma in the United States is estimated to be about 12 per million persons per year. The association of pleural mesothelioma and asbestos exposure was first demonstrated by Wagener and colleagues in 1960. The latency period from first exposure to diagnosis is long, ranging from 20 to 40 years with a mean around 35 years. Although a dose effect response has been shown in some groups, there is no threshold below which asbestos exposure is safe with regard to mesothelioma. In addition, mesothelioma may occur without radiologic evidence of asbestosis. In contrast to bronchogenic carcinoma, cigarette smoking does not play a synergistic role in the development of mesothelioma. Fiber type appears to be important, since a much higher mesothelioma death rate is seen in those individuals exposed to crocidolite.

*Pathology.* A diagnosis of mesothelioma can be difficult for the pathologist, not only to recognize that the tumor is a mesothelioma, but also to distinguish it from metastatic adenocarcinoma or sarcoma. A thoracotomy and open biopsy are invariably required to obtain an adequate specimen for histologic evaluation.

*Clinical features.* The major presenting symptoms in patients with mesothelioma is chest pain of insidious onset. The pain is nonpleuritic, aching, persistent and may be referred to the upper abdomen or shoulder. Progressive shortness of breath and cough may accompany the pain. The chest pain gradually becomes an incapacitating symptom along with dyspnea, anorexia, and weight loss. Physical findings vary with the stage of disease, but patients usually present with signs of fluid in the involved hemithorax. The fluid often is hemorrhagic. A chest x-ray may show a pleural effusion and/or thickened pleura on the affected side. A CT scan may be helpful in determining the extent of the disease and separating fluid from tissue densities. Most patients with mesothelioma die within 12 to 15 months from the onset of symptoms. Radical surgery, chemotherapy, and megavolt therapy have had only minimal beneficial affects on survival and have not been curative.

## BIBLIOGRAPHY


Crystal RG et al: Interstitial lung disease of unknown cause. Disorders characterized by chronic inflammation of the lower respiratory tract, *N Engl J Med* 310:154, 1984.

Daniels RP et al: Bronchoalveolar lavage: role in the pathogenesis, diagnosis and management of interstitial lung disease, *Ann Intern Med* 102:93, 1985.

Dement JM, Merchant JA, Green FHY. In Merchant JH, editor: *Occupational respiratory diseases,* Washington, DC, 1986, US Department of Health and Human Services (NIOSH).

Epler GR, McLoud TC, Gaenslar EA: Normal chest roentgenogram in chronic diffuse infiltrating lung disease, *N Engl J Med* 298:934, 1978.

Fink JN, Banaszak EF, Barboriak JJ: Interstitial lung disease due to contamination of forced air systems, *Ann Intern Med* 84:406, 1976.

Fink JN, Deshazo R: Immunologic aspects of granulomatous and interstitial lung disease, *JAMA* 258:2938, 1987.

Fulmer JD, Roberts WC: Small airways and interstitial pulmonary disease, *Chest* 77:470, 1980.

Funahashi A et al: Value of in situ elemental microanalysis in the histologic diagnosis of silicosis, *Chest* 85:506, 1984.

Gelb AF et al: Immune complexes, gallium lung scan and bronchoalveolar lavage in idiopathic interstitial pneumonitis-fibrosis: a structure-function clinical study, *Chest* 84:148, 1983.

Grossman RF et al: Results of single-lung transplantation for bilateral pulmonary fibrosis, *N Engl J Med* 322:727, 1990.

Hodges GR, Fink JN, Schlueter DP: Hypersensitivity pneumonitis caused by contaminated cool mist vaporizer, *Ann Intern Med* 80:501, 1984.

Kilburn KH et al: Airway disease in non-smoking asbestos workers, *Arch Environ Health* 40:293, 1985.

Liebow AA, Carrington CB: The interstitial pneumonias. In Simon M, Potchen EJ, LeMay M, editors: *Frontiers of pulmonary radiology,* New York, 1969, Grune & Stratton.

Muller NL, Miller RR: State of the art: computed tomography of chronic diffuse infiltrative lung disease. Part 2, *Am Rev Respir Dis* 142:1440, 1990.

Nakos G, Adams A, Andriopoulos N: Antibodies to collagen in patients with idiopathic pulmonary fibrosis, *Chest* 103:1051, 1993.

Parkes WR: *Occupational lung disorders,* Boston, 1988, Butterworths.

Pratt DS et al: Rapidly fatal pulmonary fibrosis: the accelerated variant of interstitial pneumonitis, *Thorax* 34:587, 1979.

Rennard SI et al: Colchicine suppresses the release of fibroblast growth factors from alveolar macrophages in vitro: the basis of a possible therapeutic approach to the fibrotic disorders, *Am Rev Respir Dis* 137:181, 1988.

Rom WN, Travis WD, Brody AR: State of the art cellular and molecular basis of the asbestosis-related diseases, *Am Rev Respir Dis* 143:408, 1991.

Rose C, King TE Jr: Controversies in hypersensitivity pneumonitis, *Am J Rev Respir Dis* 145:1, 1992 (editorial).

Schlueter DP: Infiltrative lung disease hypersensitivity pneumonitis, *J Allergy Clin Immunol* 70:50, 1982.

Schlueter DP: Response of the lung to inhaled antigens, *Am J Med* 57:476, 1974.

Selikoff IJ, Churg J, Hammond EC: Asbestos exposure and neoplasia, *JAMA* 188:22, 1964.

Selikoff IJ, Churg J, Hammond EC: The occurrence of asbestosis among insulation workers in the US, *Ann NY Acad Sci* 132:139, 1965.

Sheppard MN, Harrison NK: Lung injury, inflammatory mediators, and fibroblast activation in fibrosing alveolitis, *Thorax* 47:1064, 1992.

Snider GL: Interstitial lung disease: pathogenesis, pathophysiology, and clinical presentation. In Schevary MJ, King TE Jr, editors: *Interstitial lung disease,* Philadelphia, 1994, BC Decker.

Specks U et al: Anticytoplasmic autoantibodies in the diagnosis and follow-up of Wegener's granulomatosis, *Mayo Clin Proc* 64:28, 1989.

Trentin L et al: Longitudinal study of alveolitis in hypersensitivity pneumonitis patients: an immunologic evaluation, *J Allergy Clin Immunol* 82:577, 1988.

Wagner JC, Sleggs GA, Marchand P: Diffuse pleural mesothelioma and asbestos exposure in the Northwestern Cape Province, *Br J Ind Med* 17:260, 1960.

Wall GP et al: Comparison of transbronchial and open biopsies in chronic infiltrative lung diseases, *Am Rev Respir Dis* 123:280, 1981.

Walters LC et al: Idiopathic pulmonary fibrosis: pretreatment bronchoalveolar lavage cellular constituents and their relationships to lung histopathology and clinical response to therapy, *Am Rev Respir Dis* 135:696, 1987.

Winterbauer RH: The treatment of idiopathic pulmonary fibrosis, *Chest* 100:233, 1991.

Ziskind M, Jones RN, Weill H: State of the art silicosis, *Am Rev Respir Dis* 113:643, 1976.

CHAPTER

# 117A Respiratory Failure

Kenneth W. Presberg

Respiratory failure is defined as the failure of the respiratory system to provide for adequate gas exchange, that is, adequate oxygenation of the circulating blood for sufficient oxygen ($O_2$) delivery to tissues and adequate elimination of carbon dioxide ($CO_2$) produced by cellular metabolism. Arterial oxygen tensions ($PaO_2$) less than 50 mm Hg and arterial carbon dioxide tensions ($PaCO_2$) greater than 50 mm Hg are generally accepted criteria for the presence of respiratory failure. However, severe abnormalities of the respiratory system's capacity may occur that can imminently lead to respiratory failure, but these are not always reflected in an initial measurement of an arterial blood gas (ABG).

Patients may present with the signs and symptoms attributable to the primary process causing the gas exchange abnormality or may have manifestations secondary to the adverse end-organ effects of hypoxemia and hypercapnia. When confronted with a patient with evidence of respiratory failure, one needs to first ascertain whether the process is *acute* or *chronic* and then further delineate the cause and initiate treatment. The acute causes will require expeditious evaluation and treatment that is best handled in the inpatient setting. An acute process is often apparent early in the evaluation because of an obvious insult or symptoms that indicate a recent deterioration. *Chronic respiratory failure* is often suggested by an insidious progression of limitation along with evidence of a chronic thoracic or neuromuscular disorder. At times the patient may not mention any specific complaints, and respiratory failure is apparent after an ABG determination is performed for other reasons. Hypoxemia can be judged to be chronic if no history suggests a recent event, evaluation discloses signs and symptoms of a chronic cardiopulmonary disorder, and other findings of chronic hypoxemia are present (see later discussion). Chronic hypercapnia is easier to judge because it is accompanied by respiratory acidosis that is mild due to renal compensation. When chronic respiratory failure is discovered, evaluation and therapy can often proceed in the outpatient setting. However, daytime hypoxemia should be corrected early. *Acute on chronic* respiratory failure refers to the acute deterioration in the patient who previously had well-compensated chronic impairment. Severe, life-threatening hypoxemia and worsening hypercapnia with severe respiratory acidosis often occur in this setting.

Many of the chronic pulmonary and neuromuscular disorders are discussed in other chapters. Therefore more attention is given here to the causes of the acute decompensation in chronically impaired patients and the acute, fulminant processes leading to respiratory failure.

## CHRONIC RESPIRATORY FAILURE

### Pathophysiology: overview of gas exchange abnormalities leading to respiratory failure

The lung can be considered conceptually as an alveolar-capillary gas exchange unit and the respiratory pump. The pump is driven by an integrated control center, the central nervous system (CNS). The pump (muscles of respiration) directs the bulk flow of gas through the airways to the gas exchange unit. Gas exchange failure caused by the respiratory system results from the malfunction of one or more of these many components. Disorders causing respiratory failure are often further categorized by the predominant gas exchange abnormality that is present. Mechanisms for these gas exchange abnormalities are discussed next.

***Tissue oxygenation failure.*** Inadequate tissue oxygenation can result from other well-known mechanisms quite distinct from the respiratory system. These causes of tissue hypoxia need to be well understood for an expeditious and directed approach to the patient with oxygenation failure (Table 117A-1). Failure to correct severe hypoxemia *within minutes* can result in irreversible organ damage. The CNS and cardiovascular system are particularly affected by hypoxemia. Treatment may require the rapid implementation of mechanical ventilatory and cardiac resuscitative support. Measurement of oxygenation is essential.

Mechanisms of hypoxemia caused by ambient hypoxia, hypoventilation, and lung diseases are covered in Chapter 112. Chronic lung disorders usually cause hypoxemia by ventilation/perfusion (V/Q) inequality. In contrast, acute lung injuries are associated with severe hypoxemia that is most often secondary to physiologic shunting or increased venous admixture and that responds poorly to supplemental $O_2$. Table 117A-2 summarizes and contrasts these various mechanisms of hypoxemia in terms of frequently measured and calculated variables. The degree of hypoxemia is often described by the ratio of $PaO_2$ to fractional inspired $O_2$ concentration ($FiO_2$). Values less than 150 are usually due to significant degrees of physiologic shunting.

Patients with chronic hypoxemia may be relatively asymptomatic until pulmonary vascular, cardiac, and other end-organ sequelae ensue. These include cognitive impairment, weight loss, left-sided heart dysfunction, pulmonary hypertension with cor pulmonale, edema, cyanosis, and polycythemia. Hypoxemia should always be expeditiously corrected when found. If the pulmonary parenchyma appears normal and evaluation is also negative for the common cardiac abnormalities, one should consider the possibility of an intracardiac right-to-left shunt, pulmonary arteriovenous malformations, or the hepatopulmonary syndrome.

***Mechanisms of hypoventilatory respiratory failure.*** The failure of ventilation to eliminate the $CO_2$ produced by cellular metabolism ($VCO_2$) can lead to hypercapnia and respiratory acidosis. Virtually all $CO_2$ is eliminated from

**Table 117A-1.** Causes of tissue hypoxia

| Condition | Measured abnormality |
|---|---|
| Hypoxemia caused by pulmonary disorders (see Table 117-2) | Decreased $Pao_2$ |
| Decreased oxygen delivery | Low $Do_2 = Cao_2 \times$ cardiac output |
| Low cardiac output | Increased a-v $O_2$ content difference = $Cao_2 - Cvo_2$ |
| Decreased Hgb-bound oxygen (e.g., anemia, carbon monoxide poisoning) | Low $Cao_2 = Sao_2 \times$ g% Hgb $\times$ 1.34 |
| Increased oxygen consumption | High $Vo_2$ and high a-v $O_2$ content difference |
| Defects of oxygen extraction and utilization (e.g., cyanide poisoning, sepsis) | Low $Vo_2$ and low a-v $O_2$ content difference |

*$Do_2$*, Oxygen delivery; *$Vo_2$*, oxygen consumption; *$Pao_2$*, arterial oxygen tension; *$Cao_2$*, arterial oxygen content; *$Cvo_2$*, mixed venous oxygen content; *$Sao_2$*, hemoglobin oxygen saturation of arterial blood; *a-v $O_2$ content difference*, arterial-to-mixed-venous oxygen content difference; *Hgb*, hemoglobin.

**Table 117A-2.** Mechanisms of hypoxemia caused by pulmonary disorders

| Condition | $Fio_2$ | $PAo_2$ | $Pao_2$ | $Sao_2$ | $Paco_2$ | A-a gradient |
|---|---|---|---|---|---|---|
| Normal | 0.21 (room air) | 100 | 90 | 95% | 40 | Normal |
| Hypoventilation | 0.21 | 70 | 60 | 90% | 70 | Normal |
| Ambient hypoxia (low ambient $Po_2$) | 0.21 | 75 | 60 | 90% | 40 | Normal |
| Shunt | 0.21 | 100 | 45 | 75% | 40 | Increased |
| | 1.00 | 650 | 50 | 80% | 40 | Increased |
| Ventilation/perfusion (V/Q) inequality | 0.21 | 100 | 50 | 85% | 40 | Increased |
| | 0.50 | 300 | 75 | 93% | 40 | Increased |

*$Fio_2$*, Fractional inspired oxygen concentration; *$PAo_2$*, alveolar $Po_2$; *$Pao_2$*, arterial $Po_2$; *$Sao_2$*, hemoglobin oxygen saturation of arterial blood; *$Paco_2$*, arterial $Pco_2$; A-a gradient = ($PAo_2 - Pao_2$). All pressures in mm Hg. Note the different responses to supplemental oxygen between conditions with shunt and those with V/Q inequality.

the body via the lungs. $Paco_2$ is tightly controlled by the regulation of alveolar ventilation under the control of the central chemoreceptors. The failure of the combination of respiratory drive and the respiratory pump to meet the ventilatory requirement for adequate elimination of $CO_2$ results in hypoventilatory failure. Acute hypercapnia can lead to severe dyspnea, flushing of the skin, and vasodilatation of the cerebral vessels with an increase in intracranial pressure that may result in headache, papilledema, depressed consciousness, and frank coma. For every *acute* increase in $Paco_2$ of 10 mm Hg, there is a corresponding pH decrease of 0.08 pH units. Respiratory acidosis leading to a pH less than 7.20 or failure of ventilation to compensate for a metabolic acidosis to a pH greater than 7.20 can adversely affect myocardial function, predisposing the patient to hypotension and arrhythmias. The respiratory acidosis from *chronic* hypoventilatory respiratory failure associated with ongoing $CO_2$ retention is mild because of renal compensation. However, the renal compensation with the retention of bicarbonate does not totally correct the acidosis under these circumstances. No specific symptoms are related to chronic hypercapnia, and these patients can tolerate marked elevations in $Paco_2$ without experiencing adverse consequences. Many of the patients with chronic hypoventilation due to central or extrapulmonary disorders, such as hypothyroidism or sleep apnea, have a blunted respiratory drive response to elevations in $Paco_2$. Nevertheless, these patients also experience chronic hypoxia because of the alveolar gas relation described previously and V/Q inequalities. Therefore, patients with chronic hypoventilation often have the symptoms and signs related to coexistent hypoxemia described earlier.

$Paco_2$ is determined by three key factors: $CO_2$ production ($Vco_2$), total minute ventilation ($V_E$), and the physiologic dead space (Vd/Vt). Their relationship is described by the following equation, where *k* is a constant:

$$Paco_2 = k\ Vco_2\ [1/V_E\ (1 - Vd/Vt)]$$

$Vco_2$ can be increased in hypermetabolic states, such as acute illness, which also increase $Vo_2$. Therefore the acute increase in $Paco_2$ and decrease in $Pao_2$ in a patient with respiratory failure who develops a high fever is not necessarily caused by any change in pulmonary gas exchange efficiency or a new mechanical problem. Rather, the increase in $Paco_2$ and the decrease in $Pao_2$ may be secondary to changes in the patient's metabolic state. Dead space is increased in patients with underlying lung disease and particularly in patients with chronic obstructive pulmonary disease (COPD). The increase in Vd/Vt increases the basal ventilatory requirement ($V_E$) needed to maintain a normal $Paco_2$. Vd/Vt is also increased when positive-pressure ventilation is used and tends to increase as mean airway pressure increases. This increase in Vd/Vt can be mitigated if careful attention is paid to limiting mean airway pressure. Therefore the effect of ventilatory settings on Vd/Vt needs to be considered if the $Pco_2$ is not responding in the usual way to adjustments of $V_E$. At times it is not possible to normalize the $Paco_2$ with mechanical ventilation without incurring prohibitive risks of complications.

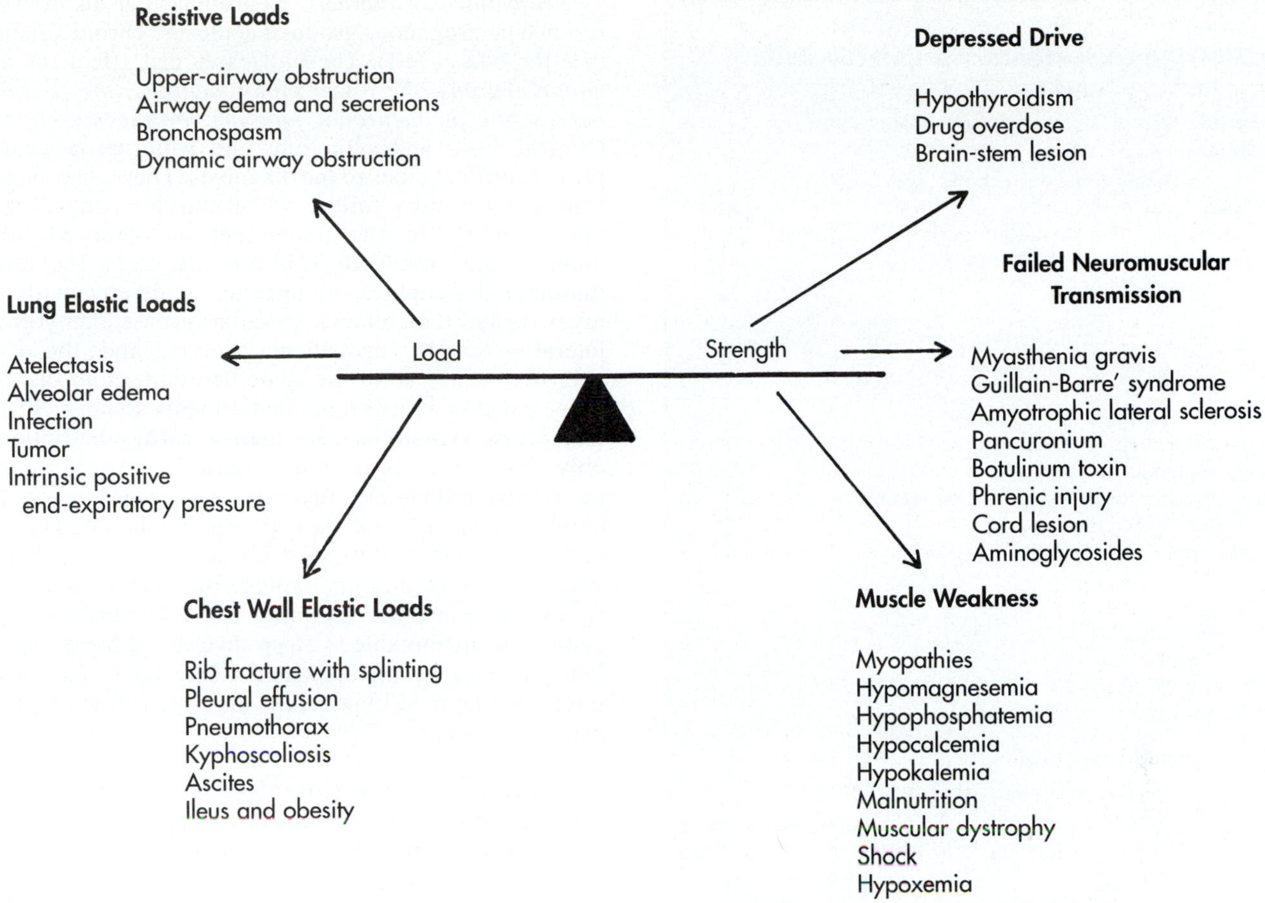


**Fig. 117A-1.** Abnormalities that can increase the normal respiratory resistive and elastic workloads are listed on the left. Defects of the normal respiratory capacity are noted on the right. Unless respiratory capacity remains sufficient to counterbalance these workloads, respiratory failure will ensue. (From Schmidt GA, Hall JB: *JAMA* 261:3444, 1989. Reproduced by permission.)

Certain strategies for mechanical ventilation of patients with severe adult respiratory distress syndrome (ARDS) and asthma have incorporated *permissive hypercapnia* to avoid barotrauma-related complications (see discussion under Acute Respiratory Failure). However, the safe threshold below which a graded elevation of $Pa{CO_2}$ does not lead to adverse CNS or other organ effects has not been determined.

Hypoventilatory respiratory failure occurs when the normal or increased ventilatory requirement of the patient cannot be met. It results from an imbalance between the work of breathing imposed by *respiratory loads* and the *respiratory capacity,* which is determined by the respiratory drive and the respiratory pump (Fig. 117A-1). Normally, the respiratory capacity reserve is sufficient to accommodate modest increases in respiratory loads, such as bronchospasm, without leading to hypoventilatory failure. Acute hypoventilatory failure with an underlying lung or muscular disease is usually caused by *respiratory muscle fatigue,* which reflects a *reversible* defect of strength. Treatment strategies for patients with respiratory failure critically depend on reversing respiratory muscle fatigue while reducing respiratory workloads.

## Pathophysiology and differential diagnosis of chronic disorders causing respiratory failure

The box on p. 1574 lists the common causes of hypoventilatory respiratory failure. A further classification within this group distinguishes between disorders with normal and abnormal respiratory workloads. Those with *normal respiratory workloads* involve *impaired respiratory capacity.* These diseases include disorders of CNS control and intrinsic neuromuscular disorders. On the other hand, patients with *abnormal respiratory workloads* have pulmonary disorders or extrapulmonary thoracic disorders. Fig. 117A-1 shows a classification of the abnormalities of respiratory loads and capacity. Table 117A-3 further describes these abnormalities of respiratory mechanics, strength, and gas exchange for specific chronic disorders.

***Chronic central hypoventilation syndromes.*** Chronic central hypoventilation syndromes include acquired processes that result in an abnormal central respiratory drive to common stimuli, including hypoxemia and hypercapnia. This abnormal central regulation can result from specific vascular or anatomic insults, such as midbrain cerebrovascular accidents (CVAs, strokes) and *multisystem atrophy syndrome (Shy-Drager syndrome).* Metabolic abnormali-

## Causes of hypoventilatory respiratory failure

**Abnormal respiratory capacity (normal respiratory workloads)**

Acute depression of central nervous system
- Various causes, see text

Chronic central hypoventilation syndromes
- Obesity-hypoventilation syndrome
- Sleep apnea syndrome
- Hypothyroidism
- Shy-Drager syndrome (multisystem atrophy syndrome)

Acute toxic paralysis syndromes
- Botulism
- Tetanus
- Toxic ingestion or bites
- Organophosphate poisoning

Neuromuscular disorders (acute and chronic)
- Myasthenia gravis
- Guillain-Barré syndrome
- Drugs
- Amyotrophic lateral sclerosis
- Muscular dystrophies
- Polymyositis
- Spinal cord injury
- Traumatic phrenic nerve paralysis

**Abnormal pulmonary workloads**

Chronic obstructive pulmonary disease (COPD)
- Chronic bronchitis
- Asthmatic bronchitis
- Emphysema

Asthma and acute bronchial hyperreactivity syndromes

Upper airway obstruction

Interstitial lung diseases

**Abnormal extrapulmonary workloads**

Chronic thoracic cage disorders
- Severe kyphoscoliosis
- After thoracoplasty
- After thoracic cage injury

Acute thoracic cage trauma and burns

Pneumothorax

Pleural fibrosis and effusions

Abdominal processes

ties (hypothyroidism being the most common) can also lead to hypoventilation. Some patients with morbid obesity can also experience chronic daytime hypoventilation, for which the exact cause is unknown. Some of these individuals have associated severe *obstructive sleep apnea syndrome.* In these patients, daytime hypoventilation may improve with treatment of the sleep abnormalities alone. In other individuals with *obesity-hypoventilation syndrome,* the $PCO_2$ can be voluntarily decreased with forced tachypnea. Some clinical investigators suggest that these are the individuals who may benefit from respiratory stimulants. In all these disorders, respiratory abnormalities and gas exchange may worsen during sleep. These aggravating sleep abnormalities may require specific evaluation and treatment (see the Managed Care Guide).

***Neuromuscular disorders.*** Neuromuscular disorders represent a heterogenous group of acute and chronic disorders (see the box at left). These diseases can affect *the upper motor neurons, the lower motor neurons, the peripheral nerves, the myoneuronal junction, or the muscle itself.* Clinical signs and symptoms and patterns of weakness provide critical clues to the diagnosis. These disorders will lead to respiratory failure when muscles controlling the upper airway or the diaphragm or other respiratory muscles are involved. *Chronic disorders* include the muscular dystrophies, myopathies associated with polymyositis and the collagen vascular diseases, amyotrophic lateral sclerosis, myasthenia gravis, and those with persistent sequelae of the acute neuromuscular disorders. Some patients with chronic impairments do not experience respiratory symptoms with their everyday activities and only show evidence of mild respiratory muscle weakness on formal pulmonary function testing. However, these chronic, compensated patients are predisposed to early respiratory muscle fatigue with acute illnesses that may lead to acute respiratory failure. In contrast, others have significant exertional dyspnea, exercise intolerance, and symptoms attributable to sleep-disordered breathing. This latter group of patients would likely have chronic $CO_2$ retention, daytime hypoxemia, and little to no respiratory capacity reserve.

***Obstructive and restrictive thoracic disorders.*** These diseases are discussed in preceding chapters. Certain common diseases are readdressed here with regard to the specific mechanisms leading to their presentation with respiratory failure.

**Chronic obstructive pulmonary disease.** It is estimated that more than 10 million Americans have COPD and that the majority of these patients will die of progressive respiratory failure. Patients with COPD can experience, on average, one to four exacerbations per year. An *exacerbation* is generally defined as an increase in dyspnea that is persistent for a few days and is not readily reversed with acute bronchodilatory treatment. An exacerbation is usually accompanied by increased sputum production, sputum purulence, cough, and wheezing. In those with the most severe forms of disease, these episodes may lead to acute on chronic respiratory failure. Patients with COPD have a number of abnormalities that predispose them to respiratory pump failure (see Chapter 115 and Table 117A-3). As a result, the patient with COPD has a limited and often precarious reserve of respiratory capacity.

The box on p. 1576 lists common causes of a COPD exacerbation and other aggravating conditions that can lead to acute respiratory failure. Overall, more than 50% of COPD patients over age 50 have a coexistent cardiovascular disease. Therefore early recognition of cardiac disease and cor pulmonale is important for directing other specific therapy. Signs of pulmonary hypertension are often difficult to discern in the patient with COPD. Edema is more readily apparent and suggests decompensated cor pulmonale in this patient population.

The severity of the patient's condition can be assessed by evaluating pulmonary function tests, exercise capacity, and arterial blood gases (ABGs); examining for the presence of cor pulmonale; and documenting the frequency of exacerbations and hospital admissions. Recent

**Table 117A-3.** Basic physiologic abnormalities encountered in patients with disorders associated with hypoventilatory respiratory failure

| Clinical disorder | Mechanical abnormality | Gas exchange |
|---|---|---|
| Central nervous system (CNS) insult | Depressed CNS drive | Secondary hypoventilation and hypoxemia |
| Neuromuscular disease | Respiratory muscle weakness | Same as above |
| Chronic obstructive pulmonary disease (COPD) | Increased inspiratory resistance<br>Increased expiratory resistance<br>Increased compliance<br>Dynamic hyperinflation and intrinsic positive end-expiratory pressure (PEEPi)<br>Abnormal respiratory muscle length-tension relationship | Increased dead space (Vd/Vt)<br>Hypoxemia from ventilation/perfusion (V/Q) inequality |
| Asthma | Increased large airways resistance<br>Dynamic hyperinflation<br>Acute change in respiratory muscle configuration | Hypoxemia from V/Q inequality<br>Increased Vd/Vt |
| Interstitial lung disease | Increased elastic loads from parenchymal fibrosis | Increased Vd/Vt<br>Hypoxemia from V/Q inequality |
| Thoracic cage deformity | Increased elastic loads from atelectasis and chest wall malformations | Secondary hypoventilation<br>Hypoxemia from V/Q inequality and hypoventilation |

## Managed Care Guide
## Sleep apnea

**History and physical**

History of snoring and excessive daytime somnolence
Obesity with body mass greater than 20% of normal, ENT examination, measure $T_4$ and TSH levels

**Documentation**

Syndrome confirmed by greater than 15 apneic episodes per hour with desaturation of at least 4% by oximetry
Syndrome ruled out by normal overnight oximetry test or if $S_aO_2$ level is less than 90%, less than 1% of total sleep time

**Treatment**

Weight loss
Nighttime treatment with continuous positive airway pressure (CPAP) as necessary to overcome desaturation

From Burk JR et al: *Sleep Res* 21:182, 1992; Matheson JK: Sleep and its disorders. In Stein JH: *Internal medicine*, St. Louis, 1994, Mosby.

reports indicate that the mortality rate for COPD patients requiring an intensive care unit (ICU) is only approximately 10%. Furthermore, mortality among patients with COPD who require ICU care for acute respiratory failure is no greater than that observed in patients matched for comparable degrees of respiratory impairment. Nevertheless, previous studies reported a 40% 2-year survival after patients with COPD experienced their first episode requiring mechanical ventilation. Consequently, decisions about when to forego or limit mechanical ventilation remain difficult. Nevertheless, a rational decision can often be made with patients using the previous information in conjunction with their beliefs and attitude toward their illness.

**Interstitial lung disease.** Patients with interstitial lung disease, especially idiopathic pulmonary fibrosis (IPF), often experience life-threatening respiratory complications, and many will unfortunately die of primary respiratory failure. Right ventricular failure due to pulmonary hypertension and cor pulmonale also contribute to the morbidity and mortality of these patients. Nevertheless, some patients with certain forms of interstitial lung disease may exhibit mild to severe restrictive functional impairment and have a very stable respiratory status over a period of years. This latter course has been frequently described in patients with collagen vascular diseases. (See Chapter 116 for further discussion of the interstitial lung diseases and their courses and specific therapy.)

The physiologic abnormalities encountered in these patients include predominantly *increased elastic loads* that encroach on their respiratory capacity, and these patients adopt breathing patterns that seek to decrease the work of breathing (see Table 117A-3). Consequently, they function with little respiratory capacity reserve, and events that increase the work of breathing or compromise respiratory muscle strength can quickly lead to respiratory failure.

Common causes of deterioration in patients with interstitial lung disease are similar to those nonspecific conditions listed in the box for patients with COPD and include pulmonary infection, worsening pulmonary hypertension, decompensated cor pulmonale, and pneumothorax. This latter complication can be recurrent and troublesome in these patients. Cardiovascular complications, bronchogenic carcinoma, and pulmonary embolism also need to be considered. Other specific causes of deterioration in these patients include adverse reactions to treatment with corticosteroids or cytotoxic agents and

### Causes of acute on chronic respiratory failure in patients with chronic obstructive pulmonary disease (COPD)

Exacerbation of COPD (see text for definition)
- Nonspecific bronchial irritants (dusts, air pollution, cigarette smoke, etc.)
- Viral and bacterial respiratory infections
- Gastroesophageal reflux disease

Acute bronchospasm
- Occupational exposures
- Environmental exposures
- Inhaled allergens (in "asthmatic bronchitis" patients)
- Pharmacologic agents

Pneumothorax: spontaneous or iatrogenic

Pulmonary embolism

Worsening coexistent cardiovascular disease
- Decompensated cor pulmonale
- Ischemic heart disease
- Worsening left ventricular failure
- Cardiac arrhythmias

Bronchogenic carcinoma

Fungal or mycobacterial infections

opportunistic infections. Fortunately, opportunistic infections still occur infrequently in this patient population despite the frequent use of corticosteroids and immunosuppressive agents. Many of these complications are associated with a more insidious disease process. Others, such as pulmonary embolism, pneumothorax, arrhythmias, and infection, can be associated with abrupt clinical deterioration. Diagnostic evaluation and treatment need to be approached accordingly.

***Thoracic cage abnormalities.*** Patients with severe kyphoscoliosis or thoracic cage deformities from trauma or surgery have decreased thoracic compliances primarily because of chest wall abnormalities and associated atelectasis. Given the abnormal configuration of the chest wall, cough and secretion clearance are also compromised. The high-energy cost of breathing from the *increased elastic loads* results in a pattern of rapid, shallow respirations. Chronic hypoventilation and secondary hypoxemia are common in these patients. Secondary cor pulmonale from hypoxemia and pulmonary vascular remodeling are frequently present. These disorders are also associated with many different *respiratory abnormalities during sleep.* These patients may have severe central apneas and hypopneas or obstructive events. These abnormalities are worse during rapid eye movement (REM) sleep and can be prolonged and associated with severe $O_2$ desaturation. These patients can be quite stable for years and then present with respiratory failure after minor insults such as a viral upper respiratory infection or illnesses that lead to mild decreases in muscle strength.

## Diagnostic evaluation

***Arterial blood gases and pulse oximetry.*** Early evaluation of gas exchange by ABG analysis is important. The initial measurement of $O_2$ saturation by pulse oximetry is not sufficient in patients with a chronic respiratory disorder. Accuracy of these devices can vary by up to 5%, and falsely elevated arterial hemoglobin $O_2$ saturation ($SaO_2$) values obtained by pulse oximeters can be seen in smokers with elevated carboxyhemoglobin levels. Furthermore, $SaO_2$ tells the clinician nothing about ventilation and the level of $PaCO_2$. Attention to the pH associated with changes in $PaCO_2$ is essential to make correct assessments of the acute gas exchange abnormalities. A pH that cannot be expeditiously corrected to above 7.20 with treatment often signals the need for mechanical ventilatory support. Hypoxemia in these chronic disorders is usually caused by V/Q inequality and can be corrected with supplemental $FiO_2$ gas delivered at a sufficient flow. More severe hypoxemia heralds a complicating pneumonia or cardiac failure.

***Radiologic studies.*** A chest x-ray should be obtained early in all patients to rule out a pneumothorax, confirm the presence of a pneumonia, or detect signs of cardiogenic pulmonary edema. Additionally, the chest x-ray can provide evidence of pulmonary hypertension if there is increased dilatation of the pulmonary arterial tree. The value of chest x-ray, computed tomography (CT) scan, and high-resolution CT scan of the thorax in patients with interstitial lung disease is discussed in Chapter 116. In the patient with severe kyphoscoliosis, the chest x-ray can be difficult to interpret, and a chest CT scan may be occasionally necessary to evaluate adequately the lung parenchyma. There should be a low threshold to initiate imaging studies for the evaluation of deep vein thrombosis and pulmonary embolism if no other apparent cause of respiratory failure is readily discernible (see Chapter 119). If necessary, lower extremity duplex Doppler ultrasound and lung perfusion scan can be done at the patient's bedside in most institutions.

***Other studies.*** An electrocardiogram (ECG) is necessary to rule out an arrhythmia or cardiac ischemia early. Multifocal atrial tachycardia (MAT) is one of the arrhythmias encountered in this patient group. Correct early recognition of MAT may lead to a reversal of its metabolic causes and may avoid potentially harmful and ineffective therapy typically used for other supraventricular arrhythmias. Unfortunately, the ECG is not sensitive (approximately 33%) in detecting cor pulmonale in the COPD patient population. An echocardiogram is more accurate in this regard and is also sensitive for the detection of pulmonary hypertension and cor pulmonale in other chronic cardiopulmonary disorders.

Measurements of respiratory muscle strength, spirometry, and lung volumes can be useful if the patient is able to cooperate and reproducible values can be obtained. However, emergency clinical decisions are made without these measurements, and one must rely more on an assessment of the patient's clinical status and gas exchange.

Evaluation for bronchitis and pneumonia should follow the guidelines in Chapter 113. Sputum Gram stain and culture and blood cultures before antibiotic therapy are essential initial studies. Bronchoalveolar lavage (BAL) and perhaps transbronchial biopsy or open lung biopsy should be undertaken when opportunistic infection needs to be ruled out. This question most often arises in the patient with interstitial lung disease who is receiving immunosuppressive therapy. Other indications for BAL, transbronchial biopsy, and open lung biopsy in the patient with interstitial lung disease are discussed in Chapter 116.

***Nocturnal oximetry and sleep studies.*** Nocturnal oximetry alone is most often used to detect significant nocturnal desaturation during sleep in patients with chronic pulmonary disorders. Patients with severe limitation or evidence of pulmonary hypertension or cor pulmonale are the best candidates for screening. Desaturation in these conditions usually occurs from worsening V/Q inequality or hypoventilation during REM sleep and is readily treated with supplemental $O_2$. However, in patients with suspected primary or secondary severe respiratory abnormalities during sleep, a four-channel or full polysomnogram is indicated. These studies also include pulse oximetry.

## Treatment

***Oxygen therapy.*** *Acute* $O_2$ therapy is often mismanaged in patients with chronic pulmonary disorders because of the concern about the known association between supplemental $O_2$ and further hypercapnia and respiratory acidosis. However, ongoing hypoxemia can result in severe end-organ damage and lead to rapidly progressive deterioration in respiratory muscle and cardiac function. Therefore $O_2$ should be provided in sufficient amounts to achieve an $SaO_2$ of at least 85% and preferably 90% saturation. Care must be taken not to decrease abruptly or to discontinue supplemental $O_2$ if $PCO_2$ is high, since this may result in a precipitous fall in $PO_2$. In most instances the $PCO_2$ will not rise more than 20 mm Hg, and therefore the pH will likely remain above the 7.20 to 7.25 range. If adequate $O_2$ saturation cannot be met without resulting in severe hypercapnia and acidosis, the patient should be assessed for the need for assisted ventilation.

*Long-term* $O_2$ therapy has been well studied in the COPD patient population and increases quality of life and survival. The specific guidelines for prescribing chronic $O_2$ therapy to the patient with COPD are included in Chapter 115. These guidelines are also generally used for patients with other conditions causing chronic hypoxemia. However, no similar multicenter trials have documented increased survival in these other groups. Intermittent $O_2$ therapy for desaturations that occur only at night or during exertion is more controversial, and its benefits are not well studied. However, most clinicians agree that nocturnal and exertional desaturation should be treated in patients with chronic pulmonary disorders, especially if there are any signs of pulmonary hypertension, cor pulmonale, or other coexistent cardiovascular disorder.

***Selected pharmacologic treatments.*** The standard accepted treatment approach for the patient with an exacerbation of COPD includes (1) maximal inhaled bronchodilator therapy with $\beta_2$-agonists and ipratropium bromide alone or in combination; (2) intravenous (IV) corticosteroids in initial doses equivalent to methylprednisolone, 0.5 mg/kg every 6 hours; (3) empiric antibiotics to cover common bacterial pathogens; (4) titrated $O_2$ therapy; and (5) electrolyte and nutritional supplementation. Theophylline is generally avoided acutely because of its other associated toxicities. Some discussion has surrounded the true efficacy of corticosteroids in this situation, but little harm has been attributable to therapy with the previous doses.

Specific pharmacologic treatment for progressive interstitial lung disease in the patient with acute on chronic respiratory failure has not been shown to be of benefit. Those patients who are likely to respond to therapy are usually at a less precarious stage of their disease, and improvement is usually noticed after only weeks of treatment. Corticosteroids and cyclophosphamide are typically prescribed for these patients. High-dose corticosteroids are indicated in the patient who experiences rapid deterioration soon after discontinuing or tapering corticosteroids. Other causes of respiratory failure that may mimic progressive interstitial lung disease need to be pursued and treated accordingly. These conditions most often include bacterial, viral, and opportunistic infections or left ventricular failure. Specific treatments for decompensated cor pulmonale can be offered and may allow stabilization and significant improvement of the patient's condition. Treatments for cardiovascular complications often need to be given in the ICU with the aid of a pulmonary artery catheter and arterial blood pressure monitoring to ensure safety and allow interpretation of response to therapy.

***Noninvasive ventilation and long-term respiratory aids.*** "Noninvasive" positive-pressure ventilatory assistance delivered by a facial or nasal mask has been used in a limited number of patients with acute exacerbations of COPD. Experience is too limited to make general recommendations for use of these devices on these patients. However, these strategies offer promise as useful adjuncts to ventilatory care. Negative-pressure ventilation systems using a poncho wrap device have also been studied in patients with acute exacerbations of COPD. Tolerance was highly variable, but benefits in $PaCO_2$ and muscle strength were observed. Clear outpatient indications for these assist devices are not available at present.

On the other hand, respiratory assist devices and "noninvasive" ventilator strategies have been extensively used in patients with chronic neuromuscular impairments and are of proven benefit. These treatments can improve daytime $PaCO_2$, decrease dyspnea, and resolve symptoms attributed to sleep-disordered breathing. Chronic support is frequently provided by positive-pressure assist devices. These include intermittent positive-pressure ventilation, conventional positive-pressure ventilation by a tracheotomy or nasal mask, and more recently by a bilevel positive-airway-pressure (BiPAP) device also delivered by a nasal mask. These machines are used intermittently throughout the day or just nocturnally. Other assist devices include rocker beds and externally applied negative-pressure respiratory devices. Guidelines for use of these "noninvasive" devices in the acute care setting have not been formalized. Their use should be highly individualized and directed with the assistance of a pulmonary or other experienced consultant.

Patients with thoracic cage disorders also can benefit from "noninvasive" respiratory assistance with positive-pressure ventilation typically delivered via a nasal mask.

Occasionally, the patient must undergo a tracheotomy and the intermittent ventilatory support must be delivered via the tracheotomy tube. Prolonged improvement in compliance and gas exchange has been reported after brief intermittent pressure-assisted inflations, which appear to reverse underlying atelectasis. Improvement in daytime gas exchange and symptoms and mitigation of nocturnal desaturation have been reported with long-term use of nocturnal or intermittent ventilatory assistance.

*Pulmonary rehabilitation.* A comprehensive discussion of the proven benefits and costs of pulmonary rehabilitation is beyond the scope of this chapter. Despite being considered essential and routine at some centers, this therapy has not been uniformly accepted by the medical community. However, these programs are integral to any lung transplantation program. Briefly, pulmonary rehabilitation programs may "self-select" for the most motivated patients, who in turn derive benefit in terms of increased exercise tolerance and physical conditioning, along with an improved quality of life and increased sense of well-being. However, there are often no other systematic improvements in pulmonary function, and no survival benefit has been shown. Variabilities in application and reimbursement and the failure of many patients to quit smoking are important obstacles that impede uniform utilization of pulmonary rehabilitation programs for the patient with a chronic pulmonary disorder.

*Lung transplantation.* Heart-lung, double-lung, and single-lung transplantation are now options for patients with end-stage respiratory failure. Patients who are candidates are generally less than 60 years of age, are free of any significant systemic disorder, and have a poor prognosis related primarily to their underlying lung disease. Patients with COPD, end-stage emphysema from $\alpha_1$-antitrypsin deficiency, cystic fibrosis, IPF, primary pulmonary hypertension, and pulmonary hypertension secondary to congenital heart defects have accounted for the vast majority of recipients to date. Detailed guidelines for recipient selection have been proposed. Patients with IPF, primary pulmonary hypertension, and cystic fibrosis have the highest mortality rates while awaiting transplantation; early referral of these patients is recommended. The average time on the waiting list is now approaching 1 year. Therefore prolonged mechanical ventilatory support is not recommended for potential recipients. However, some patients are now receiving transplants after being maintained on mechanical ventilation immediately before transplant.

The 1- and 2-year posttransplant survival of these patients is about 70% and 60%, respectively. Early mortality is related to immediate postoperative complications and infections. Later mortality is seriously complicated by rejection and bronchiolitis obliterans. Recurrence of the underlying disease has been reported. The number of lung transplants being performed is increasing worldwide, but experience is more limited with lung transplantation relative to other common organ transplants. This limited experience is due to (1) more limited donor acceptability because of pulmonary infection and other environmental exposures, (2) complications related to the bronchovascular blood supply and anastomotic healing, and (3) the limited time that has elapsed since programs have been able to proceed successfully after achieving some solutions to previous problems. Despite these limitations and the involved posttransplant medical regimen, lung transplantation has allowed for a meaningful improvement in quality of life with a prolonged survival for many recipients. It is hoped that experience, research, and technical advancements will make this a more successful and less costly option for patients in the future.

## ACUTE RESPIRATORY FAILURE

### Pathophysiology and differential diagnosis

Acute respiratory failure is often discussed in terms of the predominant gas exchange abnormality that occurs in the affected patient, that is, acute hypoventilatory respiratory failure and acute hypoxemic respiratory failure. The chronic lung disorders most often lead to *hypoventilatory* failure because of acute on chronic respiratory failure, as discussed earlier. In addition, diseases that acutely impair respiratory capacity (CNS drive, neuromuscular strength) also lead to hypoventilation and respiratory acidosis. In contrast, acute *hypoxemic* respiratory failure most often results from an acute parenchymal lung insult that may lead to life-threatening hypoxemia even in the normal host. A discussion of the most common clinical disorders leading to these types of acute respiratory failure follows.

*Acute hypoventilatory respiratory failure.* A failure of ventilation with acute respiratory acidosis represents the predominant abnormality in a number of disorders. In patients with chronic restrictive or obstructive disorders, respiratory muscle fatigue ensues because of further increases in respiratory workloads or from causes that impair the respiratory muscles themselves. Acute asthma will also lead to respiratory muscle fatigue and hypoventilatory failure if the acute, severe bronchospasm cannot be expeditiously reversed. Neuromuscular disorders are not associated with any increased workloads but rather with a decreased capacity. Furthermore, diseased muscles are more prone to early failure leading to hypoventilation. In all these disorders, hypoxemia is often present as well. However, hypoxemia in these instances is caused by V/Q inequalities and is often easily corrected with supplemental $O_2$ at low $FiO_2$ concentrations.

**Acute on chronic respiratory failure.** The common causes of acute deteriorations in patients with chronic obstructive and restrictive thoracic disorders are discussed in the section on chronic failure. Most often, these patients present with hypoventilatory failure and hypoxemia. However, the hypoventilatory failure is usually the predominant abnormality and is the reason most require mechanical ventilatory support. If the hypoxemia is not readily reversible, causes of hypoxemic respiratory failure, such as pneumonia and cardiac failure, should be suspected.

**Asthma.** Fortunately, only a minority of patients with asthma will develop respiratory failure requiring mechanical ventilatory support. However, an estimated 4% of asthmatic patients admitted to the hospital will require observation in the ICU. Additionally, recent reports have indicated an increased incidence of near-fatal and fatal asthma in the United States and other countries. Patients with chronic severe disease, steroid dependency, undertreatment, and prior intubation are at particular risk for a severe exacerbation of their asthma. Underuse of corticosteroids and frequent daily treatment with inhaled $\beta_2$-agonists have also been associated with near-fatal and fatal presentations. Nevertheless, any asthmatic patient can develop a severe, life-threatening episode of acute bronchospasm. At times these severe attacks can be linked to acute exposures to specific agents (see Chapter 112). These patients are known to experience significant morbidity and mortality from positive-pressure ventilation. However, more recent reports indicate that ventilator strategies designed to minimize barotrauma and adverse cardiopulmonary interactions have resulted in a very low mortality rate but significant remaining morbidity. Therefore it is important to optimize immediately the treatment during a severe exacerbation, carefully monitor the patient for signs of compromise, and judiciously use mechanical ventilation only when required.

Physiologic abnormalities encountered in asthmatic patients are listed in Table 117A-3. Common findings in the patient with an asthma exacerbation are covered in Chapter 112. Diaphoresis, tachycardia greater than 120 beats/min, a pulsus paradoxus greater than 15 mm Hg, persistent dyspnea at rest, agitation and frequent repositioning, fragmented speech, and delirium are alarming signs of a severe exacerbation of asthma. Barotrauma is a feared complication and is indicated on physical examination by subcutaneous emphysema, tracheal deviation on palpation, and a mediastinal crunch or focal absence of breath sounds on auscultation. When signs and symptoms of a severe attack persist after early aggressive treatment, the condition is often referred to as *status asthmaticus*.

**Upper airway obstruction.** It can be difficult for the primary practitioner to distinguish asthma from mechanical obstruction of the large airways. However, the consequences of this missed diagnosis can be severe for the patient. *Stridor,* or a high-pitched inspiratory wheeze during inspiration, is a critical finding for the patient with a variable, *extrathoracic* lesion or a fixed trachea or major airways abnormality. If the large airways obstruction is *intrathoracic* and is variable, or if it only occurs with expiration, it is often difficult to distinguish from common expiratory wheezing. Often these intrathoracic lesions are caused by bronchogenic carcinoma and occur in patients with underlying obstructive disease. Clues to a major airways obstruction in these instances include focal wheezes and wheezes that are heard best in the upper lung fields relative to the more peripheral areas. Gas exchange abnormalities usually only occur when these lesions are advanced and the narrowing is quite severe. Therefore early diagnosis based on clinical findings is required to avoid acute complications and the need for an emergency surgical airway.

Acute infectious processes leading to stridor from extrathoracic airway obstruction include epiglottitis, supraglottitis, and parapharyngeal abscesses. Symptoms and signs accompanying these acute processes help distinguish them from other causes of upper airway obstruction, which predominantly include tumors of the thyroid, trachea, and major bronchi. Vocal cord paresis, vocal cord dysfunction, and tracheal stenosis from prior intubation are other notable causes.

**Depressed central nervous system drive and acute neuromuscular disorders.** Acute insults to the CNS can impair the respiratory control and integrating center, resulting in ineffective transmission of efferent neurologic impulses to the muscles of respiration. Additionally, cranial nerve function and reflexes may be impaired, leading to aspiration of oropharyngeal secretions. The result is acute hypoventilation, atelectasis, and aspiration pneumonia. Drug overdoses, metabolic encephalopathies, CVAs, and trauma are common causes of hypoventilatory failure. Seizures can also lead to respiratory insufficiency by central depression of the respiratory drive and by respiratory muscle dysfunction. Generalized or partial status epilepticus may also present with generalized, flaccid paralysis or a confusional state, respectively. Furthermore, the pharmacologic agents used to treat convulsions often suppress respiratory drive.

Disorders leading to acute neuromuscular failure are listed in the box on p. 1574. These patients may have a history that points to a definite process, such as a bite or ingestion, or they may show a characteristic pattern of weakness that can aid the clinician to identify a specific disorder. Symptoms and signs of cholinergic excess can be seen with organophosphate poisoning and cholinergic crisis in patients with myasthenia gravis who are taking cholinesterase inhibitors. Signs include miosis, nausea and vomiting, excess salivation and diaphoresis, bronchorrhea, and bronchoconstriction. *Clostridium tetani* toxin causes local or generalized muscle rigidity and painful spasms. Sensory deficits should alert the clinician to a spinal cord injury or compression or a generalized myelitis. An urgent workup should be undertaken to rule out these latter possibilities and circumvent further neurologic damage. Acute CVAs causing hemiparesis, including the muscles of respiration, do not usually lead to respiratory failure unless there is coexistent cardiopulmonary disease.

***Acute hypoxemic respiratory failure.*** The box below lists disorders associated with acute hypoxemic respiratory failure. In contrast to the causes of hypoventilatory respiratory failure, these disorders are often the result of an acute, severe, pulmonary insult. These insults are sufficient to cause respiratory failure even in patients

## Causes of acute hypoxemic respiratory failure

**Diffuse pulmonary abnormalities**

Cardiogenic pulmonary edema
Adult respiratory distress syndrome (ARDS)
Diffuse infectious pneumonitis
Alveolar hemorrhage
Pulmonary alveolar proteinosis

**Focal pulmonary lesions**

Lobar pneumonia
Atelectasis
Pulmonary contusion
Alveolar and pulmonary hemorrhage
Reperfusion pulmonary edema
Reexpansion pulmonary edema

A

B

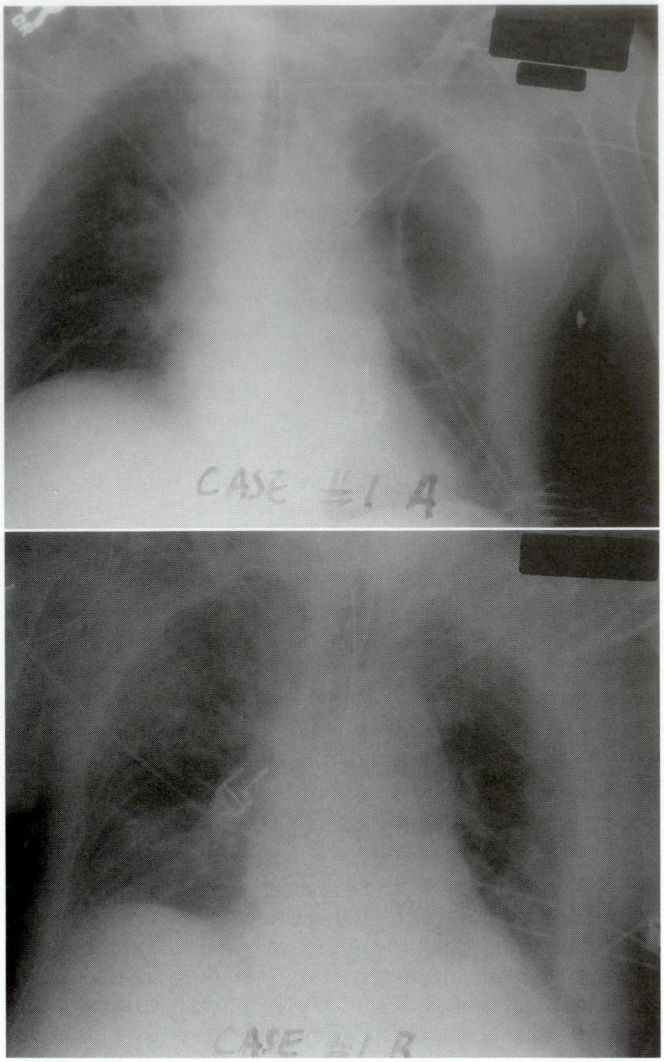


**Fig. 117A-2.** **A,** Admission anteroposterior chest x-ray of a man being monitored for an exacerbation of COPD. He required intubation and later developed acute hypoxemia. **B,** Repeat chest x-ray revealed a silhouette sign of the left hemidiaphragm consistent with left lower lobe atelectasis. Oxygenation improved quickly with reversal of the atelectasis.

with previously normal pulmonary function, and life-threatening hypoxemia is often present. Hypoxemia may not be readily corrected with supplemental $O_2$ by face mask because it is often the result of "shunting." Therefore these patients may require prompt mechanical ventilation with settings that reduce the "shunt" and increase $PaO_2$ to mitigate the adverse effects of tissue hypoxia. Because of the occasional prolonged need for high-$FiO_2$ supplementation, the potential for oxygen toxicity arises. However, it is not a serious consideration when $FiO_2$ is less than 0.60 or if levels as high as 1.00 are given for less than 48 hours.

These disorders can be further divided into diffuse and focal processes. This distinction quickly directs the clinician's attention to different sets of causes, diagnostic strategies, and treatment. The *diffuse* lung lesions are usually associated with more pronounced hypoxemia and mechanical abnormalities. Once cardiogenic pulmonary edema is ruled out, ARDS or diffuse lung infection must be considered. Diffuse alveolar hemorrhage is much less common but must not be overlooked. *Focal* lesions often result from obvious causes. Although hypoxemia is usually less severe than in the diffuse lesions, it may be disproportionate to the degree of lung involvement. Atelectasis is a common focal lesion that can complicate any of these respiratory disorders and should always be considered in any patient with a sudden decline in oxygenation (Fig. 117A-2).

**Diffuse processes**

***Adult respiratory distress syndrome.*** ARDS has many different causes. It is estimated that 150,000 cases occur annually in the United States. Table 117A-4 shows the variation in incidence and mortality among predisposing disorders. Twenty percent of patients with ARDS will experience a primary respiratory death. Recent reports indicate that the mortality rate associated with ARDS may be decreasing and that younger patients (less than 60 years old) do much better. Many patients who die from ARDS will succumb to infectious complications and multiorgan system dysfunction. The need for prolonged mechanical ventilation is a likely contributor to the increased incidence of infectious complications and death in these individuals.

ARDS is clinically defined by a limited number of diagnostic criteria that have been slightly modified since the early description of the syndrome. Current criteria for ARDS include:

- Compatible clinical history and presentation of a severe lung injury
- Signs of respiratory distress (tachypnea, dyspnea)
- Severe hypoxemia ($PaO_2$ less than 50 mm Hg with an $FiO_2$ greater than 0.6 or $PaO_2/FiO_2$ less than 150
- Chest x-ray findings with bilateral, widespread infiltrates with consolidation (Fig. 117A-3)
- Exclusion of other causes (cardiogenic edema, progressive chronic respiratory failure)
- Normal pulmonary capillary wedge pressure (PCWP)

Given the variability in presentation, severity, and course of ARDS, an expanded definition has been proposed that includes (1) a predisposing condition, (2) a lung injury score using physiologic parameters (chest x-ray, $PaO_2/FiO_2$, PEEP, compliance), and (3) the phase of the lung injury (acute or chronic).

The criteria reflect a common injury response of the lung to a variety of insults. The box on p. 1582 lists these common pathophysiologic processes and the phases of ARDS. The key pathophysiologic abnormality is an *increase in alveolar-capillary permeability.* The Starling equation (see below) describes the forces governing capillary fluid filtration. Under normal circumstances, the hydrostatic forces favor fluid flux out of the capillary and into the perivascular tissues. This movement is usually counterbalanced by the oncotic forces that keep colloid in the vessels and favor fluid movement into the vascular space. The lung injury of ARDS results in an increase in the filtration coefficient, *Kf.*

$$\text{Capillary fluid flux (edema formation)} = Kf[(P_{vascular} - P_{tissue}) - (\pi_{vascular} - \pi_{tissue})\sigma]$$

where *Kf* is the filtration coefficient; σ is the reflection

**Table 117A-4.** Selected causes of ARDS

| Cause | Incidence* | Mortality† |
|---|---|---|
| Infections | | |
| Bacterial sepsis syndrome | High | High |
| Bacteremia | Low | High |
| Pneumonia treated in ICU | Moderate | High |
| *Pneumocystis carinii* pneumonia | High | High |
| Miliary tuberculosis and fungal disease | Low | High |
| Aspiration syndromes | | |
| Acidic gastric aspiration | High | High |
| Near-drowning | High | Low |
| Coagulation and hematologic disorders | | |
| Disseminated intravascular coagulation (various causes) | Moderate | High |
| Transfusion reactions | Low | Low |
| Thrombotic thrombocytopenic purpura | Low | N/A |
| Drugs | | |
| Narcotics | Low | Low |
| Acetylsalicylic acid | Low | Low |
| Chemotherapy agents | Low | Low |
| Noninfectious embolic disorders | | |
| Fat embolism | Low | Low |
| Amniotic fluid and venous air | Low | Low |
| Inflammatory and metabolic disorders | | |
| Pancreatitis | Low | N/A |
| Acute fulminant liver failure | High | High |
| Vasculitis, collagen vascular disease‡ | Low | N/A |
| Neurogenic pulmonary edema | | |
| After grand mal seizure | Low | Low |
| After intracranial injury | Low | High |
| Toxic inhalational injuries | Low | N/A |

*Rate among predisposed groups.
†N/A, Not available.
‡Only alveolar hemorrhage reported; see the box on p. 1579 and text below.

coefficient; $P$ is the hydrostatic pressure; and $\pi$ is the oncotic pressure.

Increases in $Kf$ encourage the flow of fluid into the interstitium and alveolar spaces. ARDS is also associated with a decrease in the reflection coefficient, $\sigma$, from almost 1 to near 0. This parameter measures the efficiency with which proteins in the plasma return fluid to the vasculature; $\sigma$ decreases as the capillary membrane becomes more permeable to protein. These effects of ARDS result in the formation of *exudative* pulmonary edema at *normal* hydrostatic pressures.

In contrast, *cardiogenic edema* is caused by an increase in capillary hydrostatic pressure that results in the transudation of fluid into the tissues and air spaces of the lungs. $Kf$ and $\sigma$ remain normal under these conditions. Furthermore, with cardiogenic edema the excess filtered fluid is initially located in the peribronchial tissue space and causes alveolar flooding only if this compartment is overwhelmed. This provides an additional safety factor with cardiogenic edema, in contrast to increased permeability states, since gas exchange and mechanical abnormalities are only appreciable when edema causes alveolar flooding. When cardiogenic edema results in respiratory failure, the gas exchange and mechanical abnormalities are similar to those seen in *early* ARDS.

A number of mediators have been implicated in the cellular injury, the interstitial inflammation and fibrosis, and the pulmonary and systemic hemodynamic changes seen in ARDS. The box on p. 1582 lists some of these mediators. A discussion of the possible pathophysiologic importance of these various mediators is beyond the scope of this chapter.

Survivors of ARDS often recover remarkably. Some patients with the most severe lung injury can recover pulmonary function to within their normal predicted limits. Others may sustain a decrease in diffusing capacity, and some may be predisposed to secondary bronchial hyperreactivity. Fortunately, the vast majority of survivors are not troubled by symptomatic respiratory insufficiency.

***Alveolar hemorrhage syndromes.*** Alveolar hemorrhage can lead to hypoxemia and can be associated with *diffuse* or *focal* hemorrhage (Fig. 117A-4). Diffuse, fulminant alveolar hemorrhage can quickly lead to respiratory failure and death. The triad of hemoptysis, pulmonary infiltrates, and anemia is well described. However, since the hemorrhage is distal to the ciliated central airways, hemoptysis may be scant or even absent. Patients also often have constitutional or other symptoms suggestive of a systemic disorder. Early recognition is important to allow early treatment to obviate the potential severe morbidity from fulminant alveolar hemorrhage, progressive renal failure, and severe anemia. Increasing infiltrates in the face of a rapidly declining hematocrit with no other source of bleeding affords good presumptive evidence of pulmonary

A

B

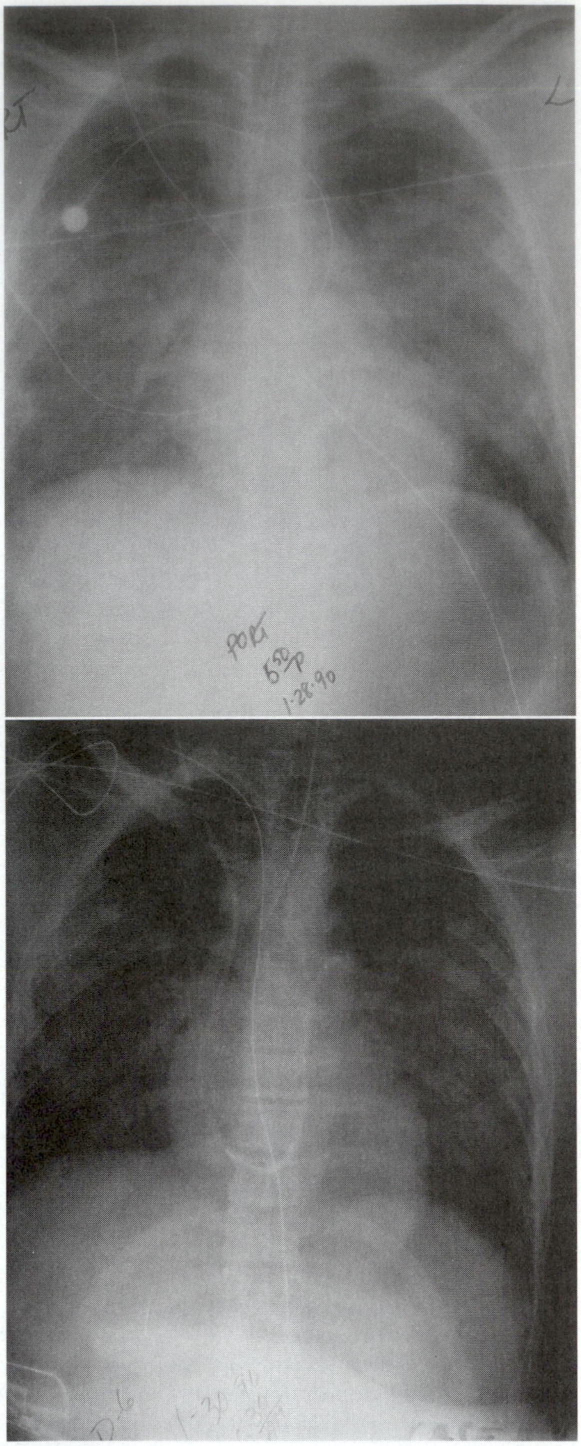

**Fig. 117A-3. A,** Chest x-ray of a 26-year-old male who developed confusion and ARDS 48 hours after an intramedullary rodding procedure for a femur fracture. **B,** Pulmonary artery catheter was placed to aid hemodynamic management. With diuresis the calculated shunt decreased from 35% to 20% over 48 hours, and the patient was extubated shortly thereafter.

hemorrhage. Patients are often misdiagnosed as having an unresolving pneumonia with associated mild hemoptysis and are often treated with repeated antibiotic courses if their disease is mild at onset. Hypoxemia from shunt or increased venous admixture is quite common. If the process is diffuse, patients have the constellation of gas

### Key pathophysiologic features and the phases of ARDS

**Pathophysiologic hallmarks**

Increased alveolar-capillary permeability leading to edema formation at normal capillary hydrostatic pressures
Severe hypoxemia from shunt due to alveolar flooding
Decreased pulmonary compliance due to alveolar exudative edema and surfactant dysfunction
Increased pulmonary vascular resistance

**Phases**

Exudative and edemagenesis
Proliferative and reparative
Fibrotic and organizational

### Some postulated mediators of acute lung injury

Products of complement activation
- C5a and related peptides

Oxygen-reactive species
Products of arachidonate-containing phospholipid metabolism
- Cyclooxygenase products
- Lipooxygenase products
- Platelet-activating factor

Proteolytic enzymes from neutrophils and macrophages
Cytokines, including growth factors
- Interleukins 1, 2, and 6
- Tumor necrosis factor
- Fibroblast growth factors

Intravascular, extravascular, and intraalveolar coagulation abnormalities
Endotoxin

exchange and mechanical abnormalities that also affects patients with ARDS. The causes of alveolar hemorrhage include anti–basement membrane antibody disease (Goodpasture's syndrome), idiopathic pulmonary hemosiderosis, immune complex–mediated vasculitides, Wegener's vasculitis, other ANCA-associated (antineutrophil cytoplasmic antibody) and pauci-immune–associated vasculitides, hematologic disorders (coagulopathies, thrombocytopenia, bone marrow transplantation), and ingestion or exposure to certain exogenous agents.

**Focal processes**

***Lobar pneumonia.*** Patients with lobar or multilobar pneumonia can have life-threatening hypoxemia without developing ARDS. Hypoxemia can be particularly pronounced when the pneumonia is most extensive in the well-perfused, gravity-dependent lung units. In addition, the venous admixture or shunt can be disproportionately elevated relative to the percentage of lung involved if hypoxic pulmonary vasoconstriction is reversed by other vasoactive mediators of inflammation. Bacterial infection is, by far, the most likely cause of these consolidative processes (see Chapter 113).

A
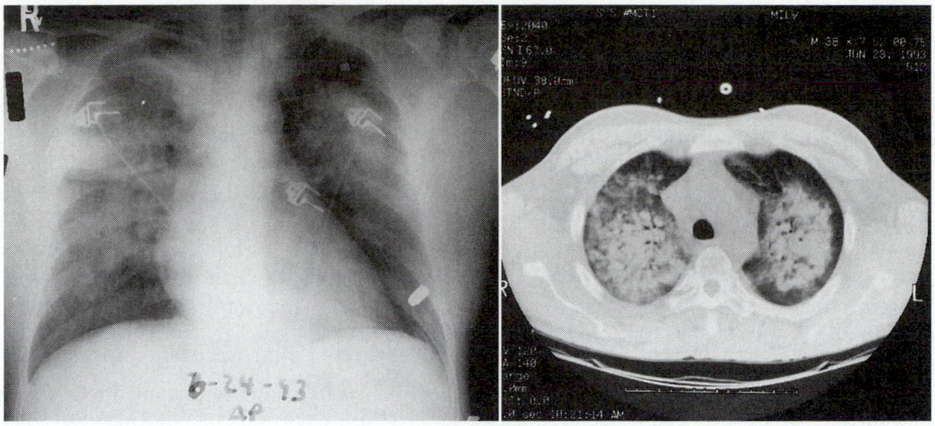
B

**Fig. 117A-4.** Anteroposterior chest x-ray **(A)** and a select view of the computed tomography (CT) scan of the lung **(B)** of a 37-year-old male with acute, severe alveolar hemorrhage from limited Wegener's vasculitis. Note the widespread dense consolidations, with an upper zone predominance in this instance. These infiltrates were greatly increased from the previous 36 hours, and the patient's hematocrit also decreased by 10% in the interim. The patient had severe hypoxemia that was able to be corrected by using 60% $FiO_2$ gas by face mask.

*Atelectasis.* This occurs frequently in patients receiving mechanical ventilation with higher $FiO_2$ gas. Problems with secretion clearance and prolonged supine positioning often lead to left and right lower lobe atelectasis. These changes can often be appreciated on routine daily chest x-rays (see Fig. 117A-2). *Resorption* atelectasis is promoted by high $PAO_2$ values in alveolar gas and low V/Q ratios in the lung units at risk. At high levels of $FiO_2$, atelectasis of large lung unit areas can be radiographically apparent within minutes and cause hypoxemia from shunting. This needs to be considered in any patient with an abrupt change in $PaO_2$ without any other apparent clinical cause. By accurate recognition and treatment, one can quickly reverse the deterioration in $PaO_2$, avoid using prolonged higher levels of $FiO_2$ that further predispose to atelectasis, and obviate the need for investigations into other potential causes of sudden $O_2$ desaturation, such as pulmonary embolus.

## Diagnostic evaluation

Arterial blood gases are necessary to determine the severity of hypoxemia and adequacy of ventilation. Once the patient is stable and has achieved an acceptable $SaO_2$, pulse oximetry can be used to assess the adequacy of oxygenation. The pulse oximeter needs to be intermittently correlated to ABGs. The $PaCO_2$ needs to be measured independently according to the patient's clinical course. Serial ABGs are often necessary for the early evaluation of the patient with a severe asthma exacerbation or acute on chronic respiratory failure. Most patients initially have a respiratory alkalosis. A normal $PaCO_2$ in a patient with persistent signs of respiratory distress indicates the potential for impending respiratory muscle fatigue and exhaustion. However, as the patient's clinical status improves, the $PaCO_2$ will also naturally normalize. Therefore, interpretation of laboratory data always requires close correlation with the patient's clinical condition. A progressively rising $PaCO_2$ in the face of increasing respiratory efforts or signs of fatigue and exhaustion are common indications for intubation and mechanical ventilation. However, no specific $PCO_2$ value is sufficient to make a decision regarding mechanical ventilation without clinical correlation. The ABG may also show evidence of a metabolic acidosis, and the patient's ventilatory requirement is increased accordingly.

An initial chest x-ray is warranted to delineate the pattern of abnormal pulmonary parenchymal processes, evaluate for pleural abnormalities, and provide information regarding any coexistent cardiac abnormality. Further thoracic imaging is usually not needed in the vast majority of cases. In addition to direct visualization, fluoroscopy and CT imaging of the thorax and neck are helpful in patients with upper airway lesions. Magnetic resonance imaging (MRI) or CT scans of the head are required for patients who have persistent, unexplained focal neurologic abnormalities and depressed CNS drive as the cause of their respiratory failure. Abdominal imaging may be necessary in the patient with ARDS and a likely undiagnosed infection. The lungs and abdomen are the most common sites of infection associated with ARDS.

For the acute neuromuscular disorders, the history and clinical pattern of presentation are critical. In some instances, such as tetanus, they may provide the sole means for diagnosis. *Early assessment of respiratory function is essential,* and respiratory failure represents the most life-threatening abnormality in these patients. Respiratory muscle weakness does *not* directly correlate with peripheral muscle strength and needs to be directly assessed (see following discussion). Some patients with Guillain-Barré syndrome may develop apnea at any time during their acute presentation. Therefore these patients require 24-hour monitoring until they start to improve. Early ICU care is justified in other conditions if there are signs of significant respiratory muscle involvement. ICU care has been clearly shown to decrease mortality in these patients, and a pulmonary or critical care consultant should be contacted early for assisting with respiratory care. Acute ABG abnormalities are a *late* sign of respiratory insufficiency in these patients. Therefore measurements of strength and mechanics should also be used to determine the need for ICU care. Acute hypercapnia and hypoxemia signal the need for ventilatory assistance.

Bedside measurements of respiratory muscle strength can be performed reproducibly by trained respiratory therapy personnel (see Chapter 112). Abnormalities of maximal inspiratory and expiratory pressures (MIP, MEP) are the most sensitive tests for respiratory muscle weakness. A MIP less than 15 to 20 cm $H_2O$ is often incompatible with adequate ventilation. The MEP is generated by those muscles that can be recruited for active expiration and cough. A MEP less than 40 cm $H_2O$ is associated with abnormal cough and clearance of respiratory secretions. Inability to clear respiratory secretions and an inadequate cough are common reasons for continued ventilation and reintubation in these patients. The forced vital capacity (FVC) determination is also useful. Values less than 30 ml/kg predispose to atelectasis; values less than 10 ml/kg, or approximately 1 L, are associated with inadequate ventilation. Bedside measurements of strength and volume should be done frequently throughout the day in the patient with an acute illness. Once the patient is at a stable, predictable level of function, treatments can be continued with less monitoring. The edrophonium test is recommended for the diagnosis of myasthenia gravis, but it can be positive in botulism as well.

Peak expiratory flow rates can be useful in the patient with acute asthma, but these data only complement careful clinical assessment (see Chapter 112). Values less than 100 L per minute or decreased peak flow rates that increase by less than 10% after initial inhaled bronchodilator therapy indicate a severe attack. Patients who do not show significant improvement within the first 1 to 2 hours of treatment require close observation until consistent clinical improvement is noted on a stable treatment regimen. This observation may need to occur in the ICU setting. The flow-volume loop and airways resistance measurements can be helpful in identifying upper airway obstruction. Spirometry and ABGs alone will not identify lesions that cause variable obstruction only during inspiration.

In patients with pneumonia and risk factors or exposures that suggest an opportunistic infection or atypical pneumonia, more definitive diagnostic studies can be pursued. Bronchoalveolar lavage (BAL) can help to diagnose *Pneumocystis carinii* pneumonia and mycobacterial and fungal infections. Careful examination of the sputum and BAL results in a high yield for the diagnosis of blastomycosis when it leads to ARDS. The yield of sputum and BAL for other fungal infections and for miliary tuberculosis (TB) is less certain, and histologic tissue analysis may need to be pursued. Transbronchial biopsy carries a substantial risk of a complicated pneumothorax in a patient supported with mechanical ventilation and high cycling pressures. Open lung biopsy may need to be pursued to confirm or exclude these opportunistic and atypical pulmonary infections.

Fingerstick and serum glucose, basic chemistry and electrolyte panel, urine and blood toxicology screens, and specific serum drug levels are particularly valuable soon after the patient with depressed CNS drive arrives at the hospital. The ABG and electrolyte panel may provide early evidence of a severe underlying metabolic problem with life-threatening acid-base abnormalities. In patients with pulmonary or alveolar hemorrhage syndromes, serial blood counts, urinalysis, and biopsy of a suspicious skin lesion are studies that can be done promptly. Serologic tests should include the antinuclear antibody (ANA), anti–basement membrane antibody, and ANCA. The ANCA can be very helpful in confirming a diagnosis of Wegener's vasculitis or an ANCA-associated vasculitis. Transbronchial biopsy is usually *not* helpful in making a specific histologic diagnosis with the immune alveolar hemorrhage disorders, but an open procedure can be considered for diagnosis.

### Treatment: pharmacologic and supportive care

*Acute hypoventilatory respiratory failure*

**Acute CNS and neuromuscular disorders.** Treatment of ingestions may promptly restore consciousness and correct respiratory insufficiency. Rapid recovery may follow the administration of glucose, naloxone, and flumazenil for hypoglycemia, narcotic overdose, and benzodiazepine overdose, respectively. Flumazenil is useful for documenting benzodiazepine overdose. However, it is not recommended in this general patient population because of its propensity to cause seizures. Other toxicology and critical care sources should be consulted for additional guidelines for treatment of these disorders.

The most immediate life-threatening abnormality in these conditions is respiratory insufficiency and hypoventilation. If patients have not responded promptly to a specific antidote or treatment, they should be expeditiously evaluated for airway protection and respiratory support (see section on mechanical ventilation) (see the box below). Neurologic consultation is needed for all patients in whom a specific diagnosis is not readily apparent. Pulmonary or critical care consultation should be obtained for patients who require prolonged mechanical ventilation, have pulmonary complications, or have persistent problems requiring more expert management in the ICU.

Plasmapheresis for Guillain-Barré syndrome and other specific treatments for these disorders are covered elsewhere in this textbook. Adjunctive preventive therapies are very important for support of these patients. Deep venous thrombosis prophylaxis is essential. Combination

#### Indications for intubation and mechanical ventilation in patients with CNS abnormalities and neuromuscular insufficiency

- Severely depressed or absent respiratory efforts
- Aspiration or high risk for aspiration of oropharyngeal secretions or gastric contents
- Persistent atelectasis with uncorrected gas exchange abnormalities
- Acute decrease in maximal inspiratory pressure (MIP) to less than 20 cm $H_2O$
- Acute decrease in forced vital capacity (FVC) to less than 10 ml/kg
- Acute hypercapnia with or without hypoxemia (often a late finding)

therapy with sequential compression devices and subcutaneous heparin should be strongly considered in patients who cannot raise their legs against gravity. Additional treatments include stress ulcer prophylaxis, prevention of infectious complications, and management of autonomic dysfunction.

**Asthma.** The patient's response to aggressive pharmacologic treatment must be carefully monitored. Specific treatments include aggressive treatment with inhaled bronchodilators and high doses of corticosteroids (see Chapter 112). IV aminophylline is generally avoided in the initial treatment of these patients, although ongoing debate surrounds this topic. IV magnesium sulfate, even with normal magnesium levels, may be helpful in improving the status of the patient with an acute exacerbation. However, this reported benefit has not been routinely reproduced. In refractory cases, inhaled general anesthetics and other agents have been employed.

### *Acute hypoxemic respiratory failure*

**ARDS.** The vast majority of patients with ARDS require mechanical ventilation because of the associated abnormalities (see the box on p. 1582). The intense supportive treatment needed by these patients requires expertise in mechanical ventilation, management of complications from barotrauma, hemodynamic management, and comprehensive care to avoid infection, gastrointestinal bleeding, and thromboembolic disorders. If these needs cannot be *readily* met at a certain medical center, it is strongly recommended that the patient be transferred to a center that is so equipped.

Appropriate hemodynamic and fluid management is crucial for the care of ARDS patients. Mechanical ventilation with the associated high levels of positive end-expiratory pressure (PEEP) and mean airway pressure can lead to impaired cardiac filling and a depressed cardiac output (CO). $O_2$ delivery may fall and tissue hypoxia may ensue even if $SaO_2$ has been normalized. Volume expansion could lessen the potential for this adverse consequence. However, increases in fluid administration and PCWP are associated with increases in edema formation and ventilatory requirements. Diuresis should be initiated and a negative fluid balance targeted if feasible. Strong consideration should be given to placement of a pulmonary artery catheter to guide fluid and hemodynamic management. The goals for using the pulmonary artery catheter can be simply stated as achieving the lowest PCWP associated with an adequate CO and $O_2$ delivery. CO can be augmented by vasoactive agents to maintain an adequate $O_2$ delivery. Inotropic agents, such as dobutamine, should be the first-line agents. Increasing CO may increase mixed-venous $O_2$ saturation and $SaO_2$ if shunt and $O_2$ consumption remain constant. However, this needs to be attempted on a trial-and-error basis because increases in CO may also increase shunt.

Pharmacologic treatments are being actively sought for ARDS and sepsis syndrome in general. Early administration of short-course, high-dose corticosteroids has been tested in various disorders leading to ARDS. The current consensus is *not* to give corticosteroids to patients early in their course. Nevertheless, case reports indicate that there may be some benefit to prolonged administration of lower doses of corticosteroids during the fibroproliferative phase of established ARDS in selected patients. Administration of $PGE_1$ to patients with ARDS initially appeared to decrease mortality in preliminary studies. Unfortunately, appreciable toxicities but no benefits were observed in a subsequent multicenter trial. Other approaches being investigated in sepsis (antioxidants, cyclooxygenase inhibitors, anticytokine agents, antiendotoxin agents) have not yet proved to be effective. Preliminary data from surfactant replacement trials in adult patients with ARDS indicated that this agent can be safely administered and may confer a survival benefit. However, results from a multicenter study of aerosolized sufactant in ARDS patients failed to show any survival benefit. Inhaled nitric oxide has been given to patients with severe ARDS, in whom it decreased shunting, improved oxygenation, and decreased pulmonary artery pressure without systemic hemodynamic effects. This therapy may improve $PaO_2$ and save some patients with severe lung injury who cannot otherwise be oxygenated or who develop severe pulmonary hypertension.

**Alveolar hemorrhage syndromes.** High-dose IV methylprednisolone can ameliorate the ongoing alveolar hemorrhage within 24 hours in most patients with these disorders. Correction of any coagulopathy and thrombocytopenia is an obvious priority. Cyclophosphamide and plasmapheresis can be added for other specific conditions. Prolonged supplemental $O_2$ may be required for the hypoxemia. If these patients require intubation and mechanical ventilation, they often have widespread hemorrhage, and their ventilator management can follow the guidelines given for the patient with ARDS. If the patient requires mechanical ventilation, a pulmonary artery catheter is also recommended to guide fluid management and hemodynamic assessment and treatment. Careful attention needs to be given to aiding the patient in the clearance of secretions. In particular, large blood clots may obstruct major airways and endotracheal tubes and may require emergency attention and therapy.

**Atelectasis.** Mechanical and pharmacologic strategies that promote lung inflation and secretion clearance should be vigorously pursued. Previous investigations showed no clear benefit to bronchoscopic treatment versus these approaches. However, bronchoscopic clearance of tenacious mucus and other materials can be used early in those patients with severe hypoxemia and in those with unresolving large areas of atelectasis.

**Focal lesions.** Prolonged administration of supplemental tal $O_2$ may be required in these patients. If the shunt is greater than 25%, mechanical ventilation may be necessary to provide adequate oxygenation. The patient can also be positioned more often with the most normal lung units in a gravity-dependent fashion in an attempt to improve V/Q matching, but this may lead to atelectasis of these areas. Aggressive chest physiotherapy should be instituted to augment clearance of secretions and inflammatory debris.

## Treatment: mechanical ventilation

***Modes.*** Once the basic physiologic abnormalities of various disorders causing respiratory failure and the general features of the various modes of mechanical ventilation are understood, it becomes apparent that different modes of therapy may be suitable for the same patient. Common methods of mechanical ventilation are listed in Table 117A-5, and appropriate machine settings for

**Table 117A-5.** Common modes of mechanical ventilation

| Ventilator mode | Breath initiated by | Set parameters | Monitored parameters |
|---|---|---|---|
| **Volume controlled modes ("conventional modes")** | | | |
| Controlled mandatory ventilation (CMV) | Ventilator | Vt, $V_E$, peak flow and waveform | Airway pressures (peak, plateau, mean) |
| Assist-control ventilation (ACV) | Ventilator or patient | Vt, *minimum* $V_E$, peak flow and waveform (spontaneous effort *assisted* by ventilator to *set* Vt) | Airway pressures, RR, total $V_E$; flow limitation of patient effort with *assisted* breath |
| Synchronized intermittent mandatory ventilation (SMV) | Ventilator or patient | Machine Vt, *minimum* $V_E$, peak flow and waveform, *synchronized* spontaneous breath assisted to *set* Vt, (other spontaneous breaths not assisted) | Airway pressures, RR, total $V_E$, spontaneous Vt (unassisted); flow limitation on *assisted* breaths |
| **Pressure controlled modes** | | | |
| Pressure-support ventilation (PSV) | Patient only | Inspiratory pressure (above set PEEP) during inspiratory flow only | Vt, $V_E$, RR, mean airway pressure (no mandatory ventilation) |
| Continuous positive airway pressure (CPAP) | Patient only | Set positive pressure maintained during respiratory cycle | Vt, $V_E$, RR (no mandatory ventilation) |
| Pressure-control ventilation (PCV) | | Peak inspiratory pressure set; flow (pressure cycled) or inspiratory time (time cycled) set | Vt, $V_E$, RR, mean airway pressure, inspiratory/expiratory ratio, intrinsic PEEP (at longer inspiratory times) |
| With CMV (PC-CMV) | Ventilator | | As above |
| With ACV (PC-ACV) | Ventilator or patient | Spontaneous effort also *assisted* to *set* inspiratory pressure | As above |
| With SIMV (PC-SIMV) | Ventilator or patient | *Synchronized* spontaneous breath assisted | As above; also *unassisted* spontaneous Vt |
| **Inverse-ratio ventilation** | | | |
| Volume control (VC-IRV) or pressure control (PC-IRV) | Ventilator | See ARDS discussion | Also mean airway pressure and intrinsic PEEP |

*Vt,* Tidal volume; *$V_E$,* minute ventilation; *RR,* respiratory rate; *PEEP,* positive end-expiratory pressure.

different conditions are indicated in Table 117A-6. The first principle of using any mode of ventilation is that it should be one that all the operators are familiar with and can apply and monitor safely.

***Complications.*** Some of the complications of mechanical ventilation are discussed throughout this chapter. The box on p. 1588 gives a succinct list of the common complications of mechanical ventilation. Appreciation of pressure-related and volume-related lung injury and occult intrinsic PEEP with its associated cardiac and respiratory complications have significantly impacted the approach to ventilation and monitoring in these patients. The risk of pneumothorax is not clearly defined, and certain conditions clearly predispose the patient to these complications. Peak airway pressures in excess of 45 cm $H_2O$ have been associated with an increased incidence of pneumothorax in some retrospective reviews. In certain conditions the plateau pressure and mean airway pressure are more indicative of the alveolar pressure. In general, it is desired to keep the transpulmonary pressure below 30 cm $H_2O$ and the plateau pressure below 35 cm $H_2O$. PEEP can have a number of effects on cardiovascular function. These include decreasing venous return (as occurs with other forms of positive intrathoracic pressure), decreases in right and left ventricular preload, increases in pulmonary vascular resistance, and alterations of venous admixture.

#### *Indications and guidelines for specific disorders*

**CNS disorders and neuromuscular insufficiency.** The box on p. 1584 lists common indications for intubation and mechanical ventilation for this patient group. Mechanical ventilation in these patients is straightforward, since they have only a deficiency in capacity and otherwise normal respiratory mechanics and gas exchange. A mandatory volume-controlled mode is necessary initially. Other recommended machine settings can be found in Table 117A-6. These settings are intended to *prevent atelectasis and barotrauma while providing for adequate gas exchange.* An abnormal thoracic compliance and the need for an $FiO_2$ greater than 40% may signal an acquired pulmonary abnormality. Expeditious extubation of the patient once the condition has resolved will avoid complications of self-extubation and the paradoxical use of other sedative drugs. For patients with neuromuscular disorders who require more prolonged ventilatory support, daily measurements of respiratory muscle strength (MIP, MEP) and FVC are helpful. The patient can be evaluated for liberation from the ventilator once these parameters have sufficiently improved and the patient is able to clear secretions

**Table 117A-6.** Common ventilator machine settings for various disorders

| Condition | Mode | Vt, $V_E$ | PEEP (cm $H_2O$) | Pressure targets | $Fio_2$ |
|---|---|---|---|---|---|
| Depressed CNS drive | Mandatory ACV, SIMV | Vt = 10 ml/kg<br>$V_E$ = 6-8 L/min | 0-5 | Peak usually <35 cm $H_2O$ | Minimum for $Sao_2$ >90% |
| Neuromuscular insufficiency | Acute: mandatory ACV, SIMV<br>Mild, recovering: SIMV and PSV, PSV alone | Vt = 8-10 ml/kg<br>$V_E$ = 6-8 L/min<br>Guarantee Vt >350 ml with PSV breaths | 0-5<br>0-5 | Peak usually <35 cm $H_2O$ | As above |
| COPD | Early: ACV, SIMV<br>Late: see text | Vt = 8 ml/kg<br>$V_E$: minimize, usually 8-10 L/min<br>Peak flow ≥60 L/min | 0* | Plateau <30 cm $H_2O$; monitor for intrinsic PEEP (auto PEEP) | As above |
| Asthma | Early: ACV, SIMV | Vt = 8-10 ml/kg<br>$V_E$ = approximately 8 L/min<br>Peak flows variable for sufficient expiratory time | 0 | Plateau <35 cm $H_2O$; peak dependent on peak flow; monitor for intrinsic PEEP; neuromuscular blockade often needed early | As above |
| Interstitial lung disease | ACV, SIMV, PSV or PCV | Vt = 6-8 ml/kg<br>$V_E$ = 8-10 L/min, peak flow ≥60 L/min | 5 | Plateau <35 cm $H_2O$ | As above |
| ARDS | ACV or PCV<br>Severe, early: IRV (see text)<br>Mild: consider PSV | Vt = 6-8 ml/kg<br>$V_E$ > 10 L/min | Minimum: 7.5; maximum: 15 | Peak <45 cm $H_2O$; (plateau-PEEP) <35 cm $H_2O$<br>Adjust to minimum mean airway pressure for adequate $Sao_2$ | $Fio_2$ of 1.00 for 48 hours acceptable; attempt to decrease to ≤0.60 |

See Table 117A-5 for abbreviations. *$Fio_2$*, Fractional inspired oxygen concentration; *CNS*, central nervous system; *COPD*, chronic obstructive pulmonary disease; *ARDS*, adult respiratory distress syndrome.
*PEEP added to obstructive disease only in special circumstances.

adequately and avoid significant problems with atelectasis.

**COPD.** The box on p. 1588 lists indications for intubation and initiating mechanical ventilation in the patient with severe obstructive lung disease. Patients who are confused and agitated or those unable to clear secretions from the central airways due to weakness are the individuals most at risk for an imminent crisis. Intubation and mechanical ventilation should be promptly initiated under these circumstances. These indications are not objective in all cases, and the decision to proceed with intubation and mechanical ventilation needs to be individualized. The Managed Care Guide lists important principles of mechanical ventilation for the patient with COPD. Serious adverse consequences may occur with the initiation and subsequent titration of mechanical ventilation in this patient group. Therefore, any clinician who will be responsible for choosing any ventilator machine settings for these patients should be familiar with these considerations. Table 117A-6 lists recommended initial ventilatory settings.

Nasal and face mask ventilation has been used in COPD patients with respiratory failure. It has been used more extensively in Europe and is now being delivered outside the ICU in some cases because of limited ICU resources at some centers. The studies reporting the use of this ventilatory strategy are difficult to interpret because of variable control groups and varying treatment in the control groups, among other design problems. Furthermore, less experienced centers reported that nursing and monitoring requirements may be substantial. Therefore no clear recommendations can be made for use of these alternative ventilatory treatments at this time. Nevertheless, they offer promise as a potentially useful treatment modality for patients with COPD in the future.

**Asthma.** Indications for intubation and mechanical ventilation are again highly individualized; however, the indications in the box on p. 1588 are commonly accepted criteria. When the clinician decides that intubation is necessary, it is imperative that it proceed in a controlled, expert, and expeditious manner. The most experienced clinician with airway management should be the individual in charge of securing the airway. Losing the airway after initial placement can be disastrous. Therefore, heavy sedation and neuromuscular relaxants are often required initially. Patients should continue receiving heavy sedation until signs of significant airways resistance abates. Once asthmatic patients are intubated and mechanically ventilated, they require frequent assessments and adjust-

### Complications from mechanical ventilation

Alveolar injury from increased alveolar pressure and distention
Oxygen toxicity
Atelectasis
Barotrauma
- Pulmonary interstitial emphysema
- Pneumomediastinum and pneumopericardium
- Pneumothorax (often with tension)
- Systemic air embolism
- Gastric distention and pneumoperitoneum

Mechanical ventilator malfunctions
Endotracheal tube complications
- Mucus plugging
- Improper tube placement
- Tracheal injury and stenosis
- Laryngeal edema
- Bronchospasm and cough paroxysms

Adverse cardiopulmonary interactions
- Decreased venous return
- Impaired cardiac filling
- Increased pulmonary vascular resistance

Infections
- Nosocomial pneumonia
- Tracheotomy site infections
- Paranasal sinus infection

Prolonged diffuse muscular weakness
- Associated with neuromuscular blocking agents, especially with corticosteroids

### Managed Care Guide
### Principles of mechanical ventilation in patient with COPD

1. Provide *initial* total respiratory muscle rest.
2. Do not overventilate. Correct *acute* elevations in $PaCO_2$ gradually (target patient's chronic compensated $PaCO_2$ level).
3. Minimize ventilator requirement. Select ventilator settings with careful attention to intrinsic PEEP.
4. Provide minimal level of $FiO_2$ to achieve $SaO_2 \geq 90\%$.
5. Avoid deep sedation after 48 hours. Use paralysis only if essential.
6. Increase patient's work of breathing (weaning) as soon as tolerable.
7. Add PEEP *only* in specific circumstances to decrease patient work.
8. Provide periods for patient respiratory muscle rest until ready for focused trials of liberation from ventilator.
9. Attempt to treat true "panic" attacks while avoiding alteration of mechanical ventilation treatment plan.
10. Maintain nutrition and electrolyte balance.
11. Move to liberation from ventilation when:
    a. Reversible physiologic abnormalities are optimally treated.
    b. Patient has tolerated spontaneous or minimally assisted ventilation with signs of stable strength and gas exchange.

(See Table 117A-6 for common ventilator machine settings.)

### Indications for intubation and mechanical ventilation in patient with COPD

Hypoxemia that is unable to be corrected to an $SaO_2 \geq 85\%$
Increasing $PaCO_2$ despite therapy and with increased respiratory efforts
Persistent increase in respiratory rate to >40/min
Confusion, agitation, and altered sensorium
Increasing dyspnea with sense of exhaustion and fragmented speech
Inability to clear pooled secretions in central airways
Evidence of ongoing cardiac ischemia or failure
Need to pursue diagnostic or therapeutic procedures that place patient at risk for a respiratory crisis

ments to machine settings to avoid complications from barotrauma. Further adjustments are best directed by a pulmonary or critical care specialist. The use of nondepolarizing neuromuscular relaxants in asthmatic patients has been associated with myopathy and prolonged muscular weakness on recovery. This may result from an adverse interaction between neuromuscular relaxants and high doses of corticosteroids. Therefore, these drugs should be continued only when key therapeutic goals are not being met.

Table 117A-6 lists initial recommended ventilatory settings for patients with asthma. It is recommended that the clinician adhere to the recommended plateau pressure limits and be less scrupulous about the peak airway pressure for these patients. Asthmatic patients also develop intrinsic PEEP, and settings should provide for prolonged expiration and a limited $V_E$. This latter guideline often necessitates higher inspiratory flows and peak pressures, but plateau pressure can still be maintained. More conservative limits on peak pressure have been associated with hypotension and other adverse consequences consistent with increased intrinsic PEEP. If the patient does develop hypotension, the ventilator should be disconnected for a time (30 to 60 seconds) to release the trapped gas and relieve the intrinsic PEEP. A chest x-ray should be obtained to rule out a pneumothorax as well. Monitoring these airway pressures and the degree of intrinsic PEEP is essential for assessment of the patient's response to treatment while being supported on the ventilator. When ventilation to a normal $PaCO_2$ is not compatible with pressure targets, permissive hypercapnia has been used in an attempt to mitigate the risk of barotrauma and adverse cardiopulmonary interactions. This approach is controversial, and the reader is referred to other sources for further information. When the patient's clinical status improves, airway pressures fall toward normal, gas exchange normalizes, and the patient requires less sedation to coordinate with the ventilator. Since the patient may have labile airways resistance, the

Vt may vary greatly on a pressure-controlled mode of ventilation (pressure support, pressure control), so Vt and $V_E$ must be monitored. Mechanical ventilation can be discontinued when the bronchospasm is well controlled and gas exchange, respiratory muscle strength, electrolyte balance, and nutritional status have returned to normal.

**Restrictive diseases (interstitial lung diseases, thoracic cage deformities).** The causes of acute respiratory failure in these patients are generally not readily reversible. Therefore a decision to intubate does not have to be prolonged pending serial evaluations during acute therapy. However, patients with thoracic cage deformities may show a prompt, dramatic response to acute maneuvers that reverse atelectasis. Table 117A-6 lists recommended ventilator settings. Once reversible physiologic abnormalities are optimally treated and the patient has regained muscle strength, the patient's work of breathing can be increased while on the ventilator. This strategy can be continued until the patient's respiratory status is optimized and the patient is ready for focused attempts to be liberated from the ventilator. These patients normally breathe with a relatively *rapid, shallow pattern,* and a low Vt and FVC should be expected when "weaning parameters" are measured. A near-normal MIP (50 to 60 cm $H_2O$) suggests that the patient may be able to sustain ventilation in the face of the increased elastic loads when spontaneous breathing is resumed. Pressure support is a well-tolerated mode of ventilation for increasing these patients' work of breathing. Patients can be liberated from the ventilator once they have sustained prolonged assisted ventilation with a pressure-support level that is just sufficient to overcome the resistance of the ET tube.

**ARDs and other diffuse lung lesions.** The general goals of mechanical ventilation are to reverse life-threatening hypoxemia quickly, limit the potential for oxygen toxicity, provide adequate ventilation to specific goals of $Paco_2$ and pH, limit barotrauma and alveolar damage by carefully monitoring airway pressure limits, and avoid adverse cardiopulmonary interactions. Table 117A-6 lists guidelines for machine settings. Important settings in these patients include *lower physiologic tidal volumes with higher respiratory rates.* A high $V_E$ (greater than 10 L/minute) almost always is required, and PEEP needs to be employed at a minimal level of 7 cm $H_2O$ and adjusted judiciously according to important pressure targets. To avoid oxygen toxicity, it is important to attempt to reduce the $Fio_2$ to less than 0.60 within 48 hours. However, an $Sao_2$ greater than 90% and pressure targets must be met before this $Fio_2$ goal is sought. Permissive hypercapnia may be allowed if an adequate ventilation cannot be achieved while meeting the key pressure targets with the desired lower physiologic Vt. The recommended limits of this approach are a $Paco_2$ less than 65 mm Hg and a pH of greater than 7.20. It has been reported that this alternative approach may improve survival compared with *historic* controls.

The initial choice of the mode of mechanical ventilation should be one that the clinician and personnel coordinating mechanical ventilation know well and can monitor closely. The rationale for choosing a particular mode for the patient with ARDS is briefly discussed in the general section on mechanical ventilation. *The minimum mean airway pressure that is needed to achieve an adequate oxygenation is an important precept of ventilator management in these patients.* These maneuvers may include inverse-ratio ventilation. This mode is usually most successful early in the course of ARDS and should be abandoned if no benefit is seen within a few hours of implementation. Since pressure targets are prominent goals in the current ventilatory management of these patients, pressure-controlled modes are typically used at many centers. However, these pressure targets may also be achieved with the conventional volume-controlled modes as well. When pressure targets are easier to achieve, the volume-controlled modes may be desirable to prevent hyperinflation and "volutrauma." Sedation and neuromuscular blockade should be used initially in almost all patients. Prolonged neuromuscular blockade should only be used when the patient is not meeting other prominent therapeutic goals, including pressure targets. The patient's assistance with ventilation can be increased as physiologic abnormalities resolve. Once the $Fio_2$ is less than 0.4 with a PEEP of 5 cm $H_2O$ or lower and a compliance greater than 25 ml/cm $H_2O$, patients can be evaluated for more specific trials to liberate them from the ventilator. *Extracorporeal $CO_2$ removal* ($ECCO_2R$) allows for very low Vt and $V_E$ in these patients. However, recent studies failed to demonstrate a survival benefit from this very invasive treatment compared with patients who were treated with more contemporary ventilatory strategies and other supportive care.

**Focal lesions causing hypoxemic respiratory failure.** Mechanical ventilation maneuvers used in the patient with ARDS and a more widespread pulmonary process may not be beneficial in patients with focal lesions. Therefore PEEP should be applied carefully and reversed if no benefit occurs. The clinician may need to use high and potentially toxic $Fio_2$ levels of inspired gas until the process subsides. Cyclooxygenase inhibitors have been shown to improve shunt fraction and improve $Pao_2$ in animal models and during short administration periods in adults with pneumonia. The benefits and hazards of prolonged administration of these compounds are not known. Other causes of focal lesions, such as reperfusion edema and lung contusion, can be handled similarly.

***"Weaning" and "liberation" from mechanical ventilation.*** Given the previously listed complications, certain clinicians have taken exception to using the term *weaning* to refer to removing a therapy that poses such hazards to the patient. To emphasize that patients should be removed from mechanical ventilation as soon as feasible, they have proposed to refer to the process as *liberation.* Perhaps the judicious use of both terms can better describe the process by which patients increase their work of breathing while still being assisted on the ventilator and later are successfully removed from mechanical ventilation. The initial part of the process, when the patient can assist with ventilation but is not self-sufficient, is conceptually congruous with the notion of weaning. When the patient's capacity is adequate and the loads on the system have been reasonably reversed to suggest that the patient can independently resume spontaneous respiration, focused trials for true discontinuation or liberation from the ventilator can proceed.

In the patient who has a clear, acute process that is reversed, and when respiratory loads and capacity are normal, a very expeditious approach to liberation from

### Factors that impede liberation from mechanical ventilation

**Abnormalities that increase ventilatory demand**

Underlying acute and chronic pulmonary disease (increased resistive and elastic loads)
Atelectasis
Endotracheal tube resistance and the ventilatory circuit
Fever, infection
Metabolic acidosis
Overfeeding

**Abnormalities that decrease ventilatory capacity**

Respiratory muscle weakness
Reversible respiratory muscle fatigue
Nutritional deficiency
Electrolyte imbalance
Infection
Central nervous system dysfunction
Excessive sedation
Cardiac dysfunction
Psychologic dependence

mechanical ventilation is warranted. For the patient who requires a more gradual approach, the weaning process should begin as soon as the patient has regained a sufficient amount of neuromuscular capacity and can coordinate with mechanical ventilation to achieve adequate gas exchange. Patients with mechanically disadvantaged respiratory muscles that are prone to atrophy should commence with some work of breathing as soon as fatigue has been initially reversed. Additionally, it is generally accepted that these periods of work should be intermixed with periods of near-total respiratory muscle rest, including rest overnight, until the patient is ready for a focused trial of liberation from the ventilator.

No particular method of weaning has been proved to be superior in terms of shortening the time to liberation from the ventilator. Nevertheless, certain modes of ventilation are more easily tolerated by patients and allow for a more uniform amount of work to be performed by the patient for a prolonged period. T-piece "sprints," progressive lowering of the respiratory rate on SIMV, and trials on CPAP are strategies that have been used for a longer time. Patients can be liberated when they have resumed near-spontaneous respiration for a period that is appropriate for the cause of respiratory failure and the likelihood of failure. The clear disadvantage of these methods is that not every patient can tolerate these approaches even for a very short time. Therefore many clinicians have opted for using PSV in concert with the spontaneous breaths during SIMV or alone as a mode where patients can *gradually* increase their work of breathing. Also, PSV provides more coordination with the patient and an option whereby the patient can at least be provided with a minimal level of support to overcome the flow-related resistive load of the ET. It is necessary to observe carefully the patient's tolerance, Vt, and respiratory rate on any mode chosen for weaning. If the initial observation at the bedside clearly indicates that the patient is distressed or exhibits rapid, shallow breathing (generally a respiratory rate greater than 30 per minute with a Vt less than 300 ml), the patient will probably fail quickly. Adjustments can be made immediately or another method chosen, and the patient can then proceed with the intended increase in work of breathing. Failures that are primarily caused by problems with psychologic dependence on the ventilator can potentially be overcome with reassurance or other adjustments to a better-tolerated mode. Monitoring systems are now available that continuously measure and trend patient work of breathing. No data are available, as yet, to show that this system can lead to a shorter time to liberation from the ventilator. The box at left lists common processes that impede weaning from mechanical ventilation.

After successfully progressing with weaning, the patient can be evaluated for the final process, liberation from the ventilator. Predicting the success of liberation from mechanical ventilation has been extensively studied. However, the methods used mainly rely on "static" indices with respect to time in order to predict long-term patient endurance. Furthermore, these methods have been certainly less helpful for patients who have been on mechanical ventilation for a prolonged period (longer than 7 to 10 days). No substitute exists for comprehensive, ongoing assessment of the patient's respiratory loads and capacity and vigorous correction of reversible abnormalities before trials of liberation from ventilation. Of the indices studied, the simple parameters of respiratory rate, average Vt, and the [frequency (respiratory rate)/average Vt (liters)] index have been the most helpful. The *frequency/Vt index* during spontaneous or minimally assisted ventilation quantitates the well-known bedside observation for rapid, shallow breathing. Recent investigations have found that a frequency/Vt index less than 105 was effective in predicting a successful outcome from liberation from ventilation in patients who were mechanically ventilated for less than 8 days. MIP, MEP, FVC, $V_E$, and other indices are important for ongoing evaluation of the patient. Certain parameters will be more important for specific patient problems. However, they have been less useful as an index to predict endurance once the patient is liberated from the ventilator.

## BIBLIOGRAPHY


Hall JB, Wood LDH: Acute hypoxemic respiratory failure. In Hall JB, Schmidt GA, Wood LDH, editors: *Principles of critical care,* New York, 1992, McGraw-Hill.

Hill NS: Noninvasive ventilation: does it work, for whom and how? *Am Rev Respir Dis* 147:1050, 1993.

Leatherman JW: Immune alveolar hemorrhage, *Chest* 91:891, 1987.

Lipchik RJ, Presberg KW, Jacobs ER: Pulmonary normobaric oxygen toxicity, *Prob Crit Care* 6:375, 1992.

Marcy TW, Marini JJ: Modes of mechanical ventilation, *Curr Pulmonol* 13:43, 1992.

Marini JJ: Ventilatory management of COPD. In Cherniak NS, editor: *Chronic obstructive pulmonary disease,* New York, 1991, WB Saunders.

Panos RJ et al: Clinical deterioration in patients with idiopathic pulmonary fibrosis: causes and assessment, *Am J Med* 88: 396, 1990.

Pingleton SK: Complications of acute respiratory failure, *Am Rev Respir Dis* 137:1463, 1988.

Said SI, Foda HD: Pharmacologic modulation of lung injury, *Am Rev Respir Dis* 139:1553, 1989.

Yang KL, Tobin MJ: A prospective study of indexes predicting the outcome of trials of weaning from mechanical ventilation, *N Engl J Med* 324:1445, 1991.

CHAPTER

# 117B Sarcoidosis

Richard A. DeRemee

Sarcoidosis is a relatively common problem in a pulmonary disease practice. At the Mayo Clinic, approximately 100 new cases are evaluated each year. Among the diffuse interstitial pulmonary diseases, the two major entities are sarcoidosis and idiopathic pulmonary fibrosis. Worldwide, the incidence of sarcoidosis ranges from 11 to 640 cases per 100,000 population. The mean age of affected patients is approximately 40 years, although the age range is broad and includes some patients in their 70s. Although many published series report a larger proportion of women than of men, data from the Mayo Clinic (unpublished) suggest that this seeming preponderance may be inaccurate because of a higher incidence of symptoms in women that probably leads to more frequent medical attention. Furthermore, sarcoidosis is often more symptomatic and aggressive in African-Americans than in Caucasians. Thus drawing firm conclusions from studies that combine data from African-American and Caucasian cohorts is unwise.

## PATHOPHYSIOLOGY

Because the cause of sarcoidosis is unknown, a somewhat lengthy and descriptive definition is necessary. In a sense, sarcoidosis is a syndrome—a collection of signs, symptoms, and laboratory, radiologic, and pathologic data that presumably identify a group of patients for whom the prognosis and management are predictable. Authorities may offer various definitions, all of which should include four major points. First, a noncaseous or nonnecrotizing (the more modern parlance) granuloma is the characteristic pathologic finding. This finding is not specific for sarcoidosis but can be caused by specific agents or conditions, such as mycobacteria, fungi, beryllium, or syphilis. It may also be associated with Crohn's disease (regional enteritis). Thus the finding of noncaseous granuloma alone is nondiagnostic but must be assessed in the context of the total clinical framework, and reasonable efforts should be exerted to exclude these alternative causes. The second point is that, thus far, the cause of sarcoidosis is unknown. Continued investigations may ultimately elucidate specific etiologic mechanisms. Third, sarcoidosis should be considered a systemic disease. For example, noncaseous granuloma isolated to skin in a foreign body reaction or in regional lymph nodes that drain areas of a malignant lesion represents a local "sarcoid reaction" and is not sarcoidosis. Fourth, sarcoidosis should have clinical consistency. This concept is the most difficult to convey but should be clarified by the subsequent discussion.

This chapter is modified from *Mayo Clin Proc* 70:177, 1995.


## CLINICAL MANIFESTATIONS

In general, the initial manifestations and clinical picture are a function of the predominant organ involvement (see the box below). In more than 90% of patients the lungs or intrathoracic lymph nodes are affected. Paradoxically, few (if any) symptoms are attributable to lung involvement, at least in the early phase of the disease. In Caucasian cohorts, pulmonary symptoms such as dyspnea and cough may be absent, even with extensive lung disease manifested on a chest x-ray. Symptoms, particularly dyspnea, usually occur when the disease is in a late fibrotic phase associated with obstruction of the airways. This characteristic contrasts with idiopathic pulmonary fibrosis, which has dyspnea as a cardinal, early symptom.

Sarcoidosis may be diagnosed because of involvement of the eyes with uveitis, iritis, conjunctivitis, or perhaps dry eyes from involvement of the lacrimal glands. Twenty-five percent of Mayo patients have such involvement. In approximately 20% of patients, characteristic skin involvement, such as erythema nodosum, lupus pernio, or salmon-colored to brown plaques, may be the first manifestation that leads to further investigations for sarcoidosis. In patients with a seventh cranial nerve palsy (Bell's palsy), an obscure peripheral neuropathy, or perhaps even a mass lesion in the central nervous system that proves to be noncaseous granuloma, sarcoidosis should be included in the differential diagnosis. Approximately 10% of patients with sarcoidosis have neurologic involvement. A physician may suspect sarcoidosis in patients with pituitary gland dysfunction or an increased serum calcium concentration. Other sundry manifestations include hepatosplenomegaly, cystic or erosive lesions of bones (particularly in the hands), or a symmetric ascending polyarthritis. Clinically significant heart involvement occurs infrequently, but sarcoidosis is a possible cause of conduction disturbances, arrhythmias, and cardiomyopathies. Fever may be present in up to 10% of affected patients, particularly those with extensive involvement of retroperitoneal lymph nodes (as may be assessed by a computed tomographic scan of the abdomen).

In summary, intrathoracic involvement is often asymptomatic but may be accompanied by cough or dyspnea, particularly in late phases of the disease. Other symptoms are dictated by specific organ involvement, such as the eyes, skin, nervous system, bones, or joints, and by the presence of hypercalcemia.

### Sites of manifestation of sarcoidosis

Lymph nodes (especially intrathoracic)
Lungs
Liver
Spleen
Eyes
Bones (especially small bones of hands and feet)
Salivary and lacrimal glands
Central nervous system
Skin
Heart (infrequently)

## RADIOLOGIC STAGING SYSTEM

For more than 30 years a radiologic staging system has been used in the classification of sarcoidosis. This system is based solely on the appearance of the plain chest x-ray and has no foundation in data from computed tomography, gallium scanning, or other findings.

Stage I consists of bilateral hilar adenopathy, often in conjunction with a right paratracheal node (Fig. 117B-1). In stage II sarcoidosis, patients have bilateral hilar adenopathy and diffuse parenchymal infiltration, which usually is interstitial but occasionally is finely nodular or miliary (Fig. 117B-2). Parenchymal infiltration without hilar adenopathy constitutes stage III (Fig. 117B-3). Some authorities use a stage IV classification to indicate irreversible fibrosis, but this category must be based on information other than that available from the plain chest x-ray and probably is not helpful.

More than simply transmitting radiologic visual information, the staging system also provides information on prognosis, frequency of symptoms, and degree of derangement of pulmonary function. Relative to prognosis, the probability of spontaneous remission is approximately 80% in patients with stage I sarcoidosis, 50% in those with stage II, and 30% in those with stage III. In a study of 256 Mayo patients, only 1 of 125 with stage I sarcoidosis, 6 of 48 with stage II, and 30 of 83 with stage III complained of dyspnea. The complaint of dyspnea was correlated with the finding of airways obstruction. In another study of pulmonary function, only 1 of 32 patients with stage I sarcoidosis had an abnormal finding, a mild obstructive change. Of 21 patients with stage II disease, seven had abnormalities (one obstructive and six restrictive patterns). Of 21 patients with stage III disease, 15 had abnormalities of pulmonary function, including 12 restrictive and three obstructive patterns (three had a combination of obstruction and impairment of diffusing capacity).

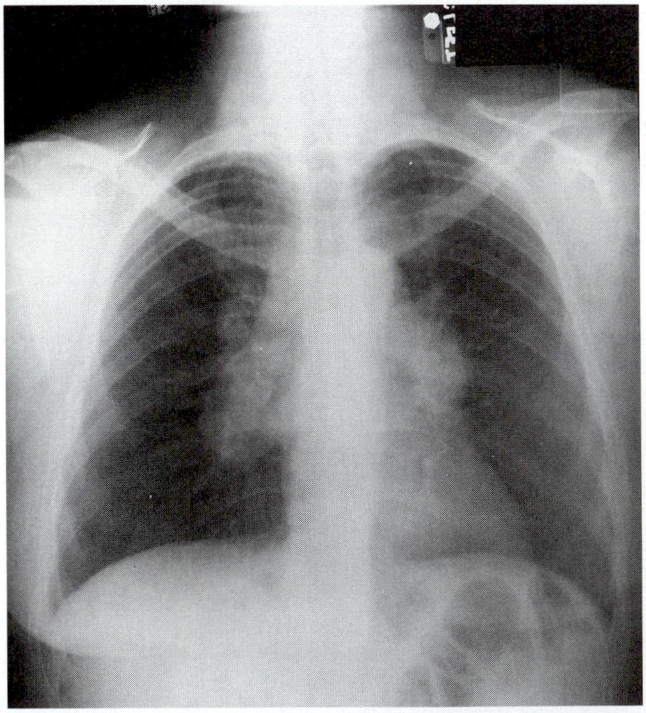

**Fig. 117B-1.** Chest x-ray appearance of stage I sarcoidosis: bilateral hilar adenopathy without parenchymal infiltration.

Thus the radiologic staging system effectively reflects not only the prognosis but also the frequency of symptoms and pulmonary function abnormalities. Many patients with stage II or stage III sarcoidosis may have no symptoms and may have pulmonary function variables within normal limits at the initial assessment.

## LABORATORY STUDIES AND DIAGNOSTIC PROCEDURES

Because more than 90% of patients have intrathoracic disease often as the sole manifestation of sarcoidosis,

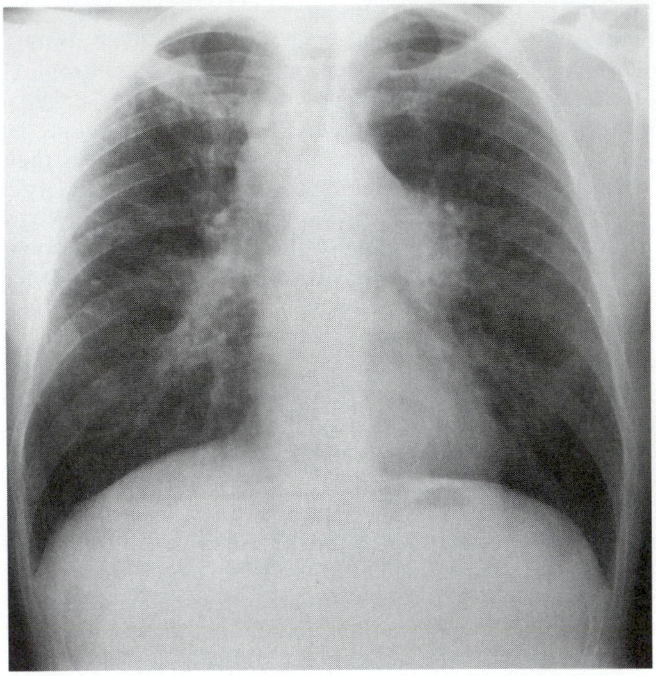

**Fig. 117B-2.** Chest x-ray appearance of stage II sarcoidosis: bilateral hilar adenopathy with parenchymal infiltration.

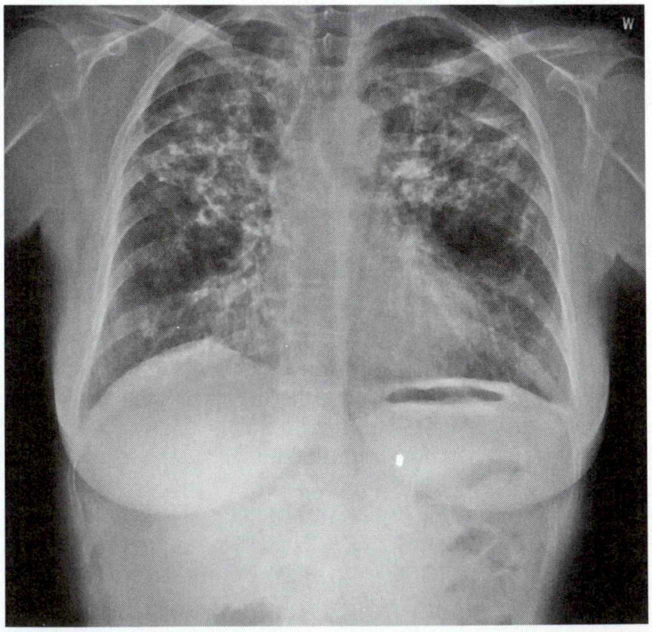

**Fig. 117B-3.** Chest x-ray appearance of stage III sarcoidosis: parenchymal infiltration without hilar adenopathy. Note preponderant upper zone involvement.

many will likely be asymptomatic and are brought to medical attention only because of abnormal findings on a chest x-ray. Chest x-rays may have been performed during a mass screening program (infrequent today), a routine physical examination, or an investigation of other problems or seemingly unrelated symptoms. As previously mentioned, other organ system involvement may have prompted clinical attention. Once the diagnosis of sarcoidosis is considered, tissue confirmation should be sought. In patients with stage I sarcoidosis, mediastinoscopy is recommended. Some clinicians might argue that an asymptomatic patient without physical findings but with stage I x-ray abnormalities needs no tissue confirmation. This may be a reasonable approach, but because the diagnosis necessitates tissue confirmation, the patient cannot be given a firm diagnosis or prognosis. If the patient is comfortable with this degree of uncertainty, tissue confirmation may be postponed, but careful follow-up is imperative, that is, chest x-rays every 3 to 6 months until the course is clarified. For patients with stage II or stage III sarcoidosis, bronchoscopy in conjunction with bronchial and transbronchial lung biopsy is recommended. With experienced investigators, tissue confirmation should be achieved in more than 80% of cases. Should these measures fail, open-lung biopsy can be considered; however, before such a biopsy is done, a diligent search should be made for possible sarcoidal lesions in the skin or conjunctiva. A conjunctival biopsy is unlikely to reveal sarcoidosis if no gross abnormalities of the conjunctiva are evident on visual inspection. Open-lung biopsy should be resorted to infrequently. In a series of 99 consecutive Mayo patients, only five required open-lung biopsy for final diagnosis. All biopsy material should be cultured for mycobacteria and fungi, and the diagnosis of sarcoidosis cannot be confirmed until a specific cause for the noncaseous granuloma has been excluded. The Kveim test is primarily of historic interest. Although it may still be used, the antigen is not commercially available, and few centers are actively engaged in its production and validation.

## MANAGEMENT

After sarcoidosis has been diagnosed, the next challenge is management and treatment. The treatment of lung manifestations remains controversial more than 40 years after the introduction of glucocorticoids. On the basis of a large experience, use of glucocorticoids is advocated in all patients with stage II or stage III sarcoidosis if, after a period of observation of 6 to 12 months, the disease either shows no evidence of spontaneous clearing or has worsened, as determined by serial x-rays and pulmonary function studies. Alternate-day regimens of prednisone, usually beginning at 40 mg, are uniformally effective. The recommended management approach is outlined in the algorithm depicted in the Managed Care Guide. Stage I disease rarely is an indication for treatment unless symptoms of erythema nodosum and arthritis must be alleviated. If nonsteroidal agents such as indomethacin, 25 mg three times a day, are ineffective, a short course of alternate-day prednisone therapy beginning at 20 mg can be used. Although some authorities view pulmonary

### Managed Care Guide
### A method of treatment of pulmonary sarcoidosis

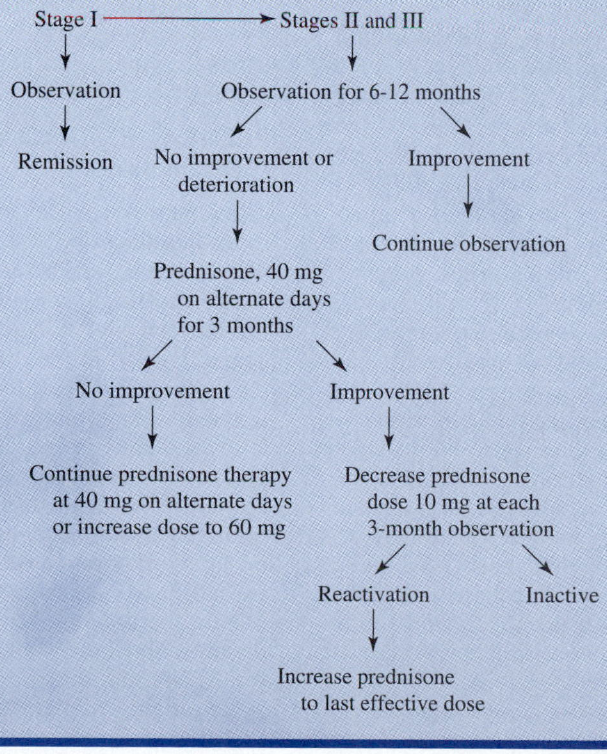

symptoms as an indication for treatment, research has found that dyspnea is a strong indicator of irreversible disease. Therefore, glucocorticoid treatment is best administered in the presymptomatic phase of sarcoidosis to stave off irreversible changes.

Most authorities agree on the following indications for glucocorticoid treatment: (1) uveitis (local treatment may be attempted first), (2) hypercalcemia, (3) myocardial involvement (particularly cardiomyopathy), and (4) neurologic disease. If glucocorticoids cannot be used, other agents are available, but they are second-line drugs, seldom as effective as glucocorticoids, or have equally consequential side effects. These second-line agents include methotrexate, chloroquine, azathioprine, and oxyphenbutazone.

## MONITORING COURSE AND EFFECT OF TREATMENT

Serial chest x-rays and pulmonary function studies are essential in the management of sarcoidosis. Their intervals are dictated by either the individual patient's course or the personal preferences of the managing physician. In addition, serum angiotensin converting enzyme (SACE) determinations are of considerable value in monitoring the course. The level of SACE is thought to reflect the mass or "load" of granuloma in the individual patient. Mayo studies have shown that the level of SACE is increased more than two standard deviations from the mean in 67% of patients with stage I sarcoidosis, in 87% with stage II, and in 95% with stage III. A substantial number of patients deemed to have active sarcoidosis had SACE levels in the "normal" range. Therefore, one should not use an individual SACE determination in assessing a patient's clinical activity; the serial profile is indicative of activity. Patients with SACE levels in the normal range manifest appreciable decreases either in the course of spontaneous remission or under the influence of glucocorticoid treatment. Thus, SACE levels can be used to detect the degree of granulomatous activity and, consequently, the adequacy of the glucocorticoid suppression. Increasing levels should raise concern about an impending relapse or an inadequate glucocorticoid dose. The levels of SACE should never be used as the sole indication for treatment.

Involvement of additional sites necessitates assessment of changes pertinent to the organs affected. Relapse is common after effective treatment, occurring in as many as 25% of patients with stage II or stage III sarcoidosis. Thus, physicians must be vigilant in maintaining periodic surveillance for years after treatment. If stability of the condition and signs of inactivity have been maintained for longer than 1 year after cessation of treatment, the possibility of relapse is considerably diminished.

Only a few laboratory studies other than those previously mentioned are helpful in the diagnosis and management of sarcoidosis. Some basic studies are reasonable, such as a complete blood cell count, serum creatinine and calcium concentrations, and urinalysis. A few patients with hypersplenism may have leukopenia and even mild anemia. Every patient should be tested for hypercalcemia, a prime indication for treatment. A urinalysis and serum creatinine determination can reveal the presence of hypercalcemic nephropathy and renal stones.

In the early 1980s, bronchoalveolar lavage and gallium citrate lung scanning were touted as important in determining the clinical course and need for treatment. Although bronchoalveolar lavage has led to important discoveries about the humeral and cellular mechanisms involved in the pathogenesis of sarcoidosis, neither of these procedures yields practical information for the day-to-day management of sarcoidosis.

## BIBLIOGRAPHY


DeRemee RA: The roentgenographic staging of sarcoidosis: historic and contemporary perspectives, *Chest* 83:128, 1983.

DeRemee RA: Sarcoidosis: current perspectives on diagnosis and treatment, *Postgrad Med* 76:167, 1984.

DeRemee RA: The treatment of sarcoidosis. In Lieberman J, editor: *Sarcoidosis,* Orlando, Fla, 1985, Grune & Stratton.

DeRemee RA: *Clinical profiles of diffuse interstitial pulmonary disease,* Mount Kisco, NY, 1990, Futura.

DeRemee RA, Offord KP: The treatment of pulmonary sarcoidosis: the house revisited, *Sarcoidosis* 9(suppl 1):17, 1992.

DeRemee RA, Rohrbach MS: Normal serum angiotensin converting enzyme activity in patients with newly diagnosed sarcoidosis, *Chest* 85:45, 1984.

Wurm K, Reindell H, Heilmeyer L: *Der Lungenboeck im Röntgenbild,* Stuttgart, Germany, 1958, Thieme.


CHAPTER

# 118 Disorders of the Pleural Space


**Basil Varkey**

**Ralph M. Schapira**


An estimated 1 million cases of pleural effusions are diagnosed annually in the United States. Pleural effusion is an abnormal accumulation of fluid in the pleural space due either to an intrinsic abnormality of the pleura (exudative pleural effusion) or to an imbalance in oncotic or hydrostatic pressures (transudative pleural effusion) (see the box on p. 1595). Other pleural disorders discussed in this chapter are fibrothorax, asbestos-related pleural disease, and pneumothorax.

## PLEURAL EFFUSION

### Pathophysiology

The pleura is a serous membrane made of a single layer of mesothelial cells. The visceral pleura covers the lung parenchyma, and the parietal pleura covers the remaining structures of the thoracic cavity. The airless space between the parietal and visceral pleurae is known as the pleural space. Due to a net gradient favoring movement of fluid through the parietal pleura into the pleural space, a nearly indetectable amount of clear, colorless pleural fluid with a low protein concentration (less than 1.5 g/dl) is normally present, estimated to be on the order of about 10 ml in humans. The fluid in the pleural space is believed to be removed by the lymphatics of the parietal pleura, which normally maintain an equilibrium between the physiologic formation of pleural fluid and the removal of pleural fluid. (The visceral pleural lymphatics are poorly developed and do not contribute significantly to the removal of pleural fluid.) The parietal pleura receives its blood supply from systemic arteries of the adjacent chest wall, and the visceral pleura is supplied by the bronchial circulation.

### Causes of pleural effusions

**Transudates**

- Common
  - Congestive heart failure
  - Cirrhosis
- Less common
  - Nephrotic syndrome
  - Peritoneal dialysis
  - Urinothorax
  - Pulmonary embolism
  - Atelectasis
  - Superior venal caval obstruction

**Exudates**

- Common
  - Parapneumonic
  - Malignancy
  - Pulmonary embolism
- Less common
  - Tuberculosis
  - Nonbacterial infections: viral, fungal, parasitic
  - Pancreatitis, pseudocyst
  - Esophageal rupture
  - Endoscopic sclerotherapy
  - Subphrenic/liver abscess
  - Collagen vascular diseases
  - Dressler's syndrome
  - Drugs, including those causing drug-induced lupus
  - Benign asbestos effusion
  - Chylothorax
  - Uremia
  - Sarcoidosis
  - Meigs' syndrome
  - Yellow nail syndrome
  - Trauma

### Clues to the cause of pleural effusion

**History**

- Smoking
- Asbestos exposure
- Trauma
- Drugs
- Tuberculosis exposure
- Cough with purulent sputum
- Hemoptysis
- Chills, fever
- Joint pains, swelling, stiffness
- Urinary obstruction
- Present or recent subclavian venous line insertion
- Recent abdominal surgery, orthopedic surgery, parturition, vomiting, abdominal pain, upper gastrointestinal endoscopy, sclerotherapy
- History of congestive heart failure, nephrotic syndrome, cirrhosis, deep venous thrombosis, any malignant disease, cardiac surgery

**Physical examination**

- Clubbing of fingers
- Yellow nails
- Superior vena cava syndrome
- Horner's syndrome
- Cervical/supraclavicular/other lymphadenopathy
- Rheumatoid subcutaneous nodules, joint swelling, deformity
- Sclerodactyly, malar rash, Raynaud's phenomenon
- Putrid breath, purulent sputum
- Herpes labialis, fever
- Jugular vein distention, $S_3$, rales, leg edema
- Ascites
- Abdominal tenderness, mass

Much of the venous drainage of the visceral pleura is into the pulmonary veins; that of the parietal pleura is the bronchial veins and inferior vena cava.

Pleural effusions are caused by increased pleural fluid formation, decreased pleural fluid lymphatic drainage, or a combination of the two mechanisms. Transudative pleural effusions are noninflammatory and are caused by oncotic or hydrostatic factors that favor increased formation of pleural fluid, the most common cause being congestive heart failure. Exudative pleural effusions are caused by factors that increase the permeability of the pleural surfaces. Examples of exudates include malignant pleural effusions (usually caused by direct tumor invasion of the pleura) and pleural effusions associated with bacterial pneumonia (parapneumonic effusion).

The presence of a pleural effusion limits full expansion of the lung and may cause diaphragmatic dysfunction. Consequently, a restrictive ventilatory impairment is noted on pulmonary function testing. The dyspnea associated with some pleural effusions, particularly those of large size, is believed to result mainly from the mechanical disadvantage of the diaphragm. Hypoxemia in patients with a pleural effusion frequently results more from the underlying lung disease than from the mechanical effects of the effusion on the lungs.

## History

The three cardinal symptoms of a pleural effusion are dyspnea, chest pain (either pleuritic or nonpleuritic), and a nonproductive cough. However, even large pleural effusions can be asymptomatic. The underlying disease producing the pleural effusion may play an important role in the production of symptoms. For example, a patient with bilateral pleural effusions from left ventricular failure may have symptoms from pulmonary edema rather than from the pleural effusions. Aspects of history and physical examination provide diagnostic clues (see the box above).

## Physical examination

The findings on physical examination usually correlate with the volume of pleural fluid that is present. Inspection of the thorax in a patient with a large pleural effusion may reveal bulging intercostal spaces on the side of the effusion and a shift of the trachea away from the side of the effusion. Palpation reveals a decrease in tactile fremitus over the effusion. The percussion note is dull. Auscultation over the pleural effusion reveals a decrease or absence of breath sounds. Palpation, percussion, and auscultation are useful in delineating the superior border of the effusion, since the physical signs are normal above this level.

## Laboratory studies and diagnostic procedures

The presence of an effusion is confirmed by chest radiographs. A small effusion (about 100 ml) obliterates the normally sharp posterior costophrenic angle on a lateral view. A moderate effusion (500 to 1000 ml) typically obliterates the lateral costophrenic angle and shows a meniscus-shaped border laterally on a posteroanterior (PA) view. Subpulmonic effusions, loculated effusions, and underlying lung disease may alter the typical radiographic pattern. When a pleural effusion is suggested on a PA or lateral chest radiograph, the clinician must decide whether there is a need to obtain pleural fluid for analysis. If the cause of a pleural effusion is clearly evident, such as bilateral effusions in a patient with heart failure or asymptomatic effusions within 48 hours of parturition or abdominal surgery, the effusions may be observed and resolution documented on serial radiographs during treatment. However, if a patient presents with a pleural effusion of unknown cause, an evaluation is mandatory. The first goals are to obtain a sample of the pleural fluid by thoracentesis and define the effusion as a transudate or an exudate.

To safely perform a thoracentesis, a lateral decubitus chest x-ray with the effusion dependent should be taken to determine whether the suspected pleural fluid is free flowing. If the fluid layers along the inner chest wall, and if the distance between the inner chest wall and the superior surface of the effusion is at least 10 mm, a diagnostic thoracentesis can be performed on the location of the effusion as determined by physical examination. However, if the pleural effusion does not layer on the lateral decubitus film, or if the distance is less than 10 mm, it suggests three possibilities: (1) that the effusion is small in volume; (2) that it is loculated; or (3) that the abnormalities on the chest x-ray represent pleural thickening and not a pleural effusion. An ultrasound of the pleural space can help to differentiate between these possibilities and, if pleural fluid is indeed present, can guide a simultaneous diagnostic thoracentesis. A common error is for a patient's chest wall to be marked in ink by the ultrasonographer for subsequent thoracentesis. Unless the patient is in precisely the same position as at the time of marking, the effusion may have shifted, making thoracentesis unsuccessful and prone to complications. Computed tomography (CT) of the chest is usually not necessary in attempting to define the presence of a pleural effusion. However, CT does give additional information regarding the underlying lung parenchyma and mediastinum that is not derived from ultrasound, such as the presence of a mass or lymphadenopathy. Magnetic resonance imaging (MRI) of the chest is considered to have less utility than CT or ultrasound.

In contrast to a therapeutic thoracentesis (the removal of as much pleural fluid as possible to improve patient symptoms or induce chemical pleurodesis), a diagnostic thoracentesis is performed to differentiate a transudative pleural effusion from an exudative effusion and to find the cause of the effusion. Therefore only a small volume (50 ml) of pleural fluid needs to be obtained. The major complications are pneumothorax in about 10%, pleural space infection, hemothorax, and reexpansion pulmonary edema. An end-expiratory PA chest radiograph should be performed after thoracentesis to check for the presence of a pneumothorax. Pleural fluid in patients with suspected or confirmed infections such as human immunodeficiency virus (HIV) or hepatitis B should be handled with special precautions to avoid transmission of these agents to health care workers.

Invasive procedures are selectively employed to determine the cause of a pleural effusion should thorocentesis fail to provide a definitive answer. These invasive procedures include percutaneous parietal pleural biopsy (PPB), thoracoscopy (pleuroscopy), fiberoptic bronchoscopy (FOB), and thoracotomy with open pleural biopsy.

## Differential diagnosis

To define an effusion as a transudate or an exudate, the protein and lactate dehydrogenase (LDH) concentrations of the pleural fluid must be compared with those of simultaneously obtained serum. An exudative effusion has at least one of the following characteristics: (1) a pleural fluid/serum protein ratio of more than 0.5, (2) a pleural fluid/serum LDH ratio of more than 0.6, or (3) an absolute LDH greater than two thirds the upper limits of normal for the serum LDH. Transudative pleural effusions meet none of these three criteria. Additional tests depend on the clinical suspicion of the clinician.

***Transudative pleural effusions.*** Congestive heart failure is the most common cause of pleural effusions. Typically the effusion is bilateral, the pleural fluid is serous in appearance, and chemical analysis reveals a transudate. Recent evidence suggest that biventricular failure is a requirement for the development of a pleural effusion and that right ventricular failure alone does not cause a pleural effusion. Diuresis usually does not convert a transduative pleural effusion from cardiac failure into an exudate. A patient who presents with typical clinical features of left-sided cardiac failure, a radiograph demonstrating cardiomegaly, and bilateral effusions usually does not need to have the pleural effusion analyzed. However, the clinician must keep in mind that some patients with cardiac failure are at risk for pulmonary embolism; if a patient with cardiac failure presents with a unilateral pleural effusion or atypical features such as a fever or pleuritic chest pain, other causes of the pleural effusion such as pulmonary embolism or pneumonia should be considered.

Another common cause of a transudative pleural effusion is cirrhosis of the liver. The pleural effusion of cirrhosis arises in large part because of movement of ascitic fluid from the peritoneal cavity through the diaphragm. The chemical characteristics of the pleural and ascitic fluid are usually similar. The chest radiograph typically shows a right-sided pleural effusion (70%) and a normal sized heart. The patient usually has evidence of chronic liver disease and ascites, although if enough of the fluid in the peritoneum has traversed the diaphragm, clinical evidence of ascites may be lacking, and an abdominal ultrasound should be considered.

Although frequently associated with an exudative bloody pleural effusion, pulmonary thromboembolism can cause a typically unilateral transudative pleural effusion in up to 20% of patients. Therefore in a patient with a pleural effusion the finding of a transudative pleural effusion does not rule out the possibility of a pulmonary embolism, and further diagnostic evaluation should be pursued if clinically indicated.

Other less common causes of transudative effusions include the nephrotic syndrome (due to decreased oncotic pressure), urinothorax (due to retroperitoneal urinary leakage associated with urinary obstruction), and peritoneal dialysis in patients with renal failure (due to movement of dialysate from the peritoneal to pleural space). Collapse of an entire lobe or lung by an endobronchial tumor or foreign body can cause a transudative pleural effusion due to a further decrease in the negative pleural pressure, which favors an increase in the formation of pleural fluid. The cause of these transudative effusions is usually readily apparent by clinical history.

***Exudative pleural effusions.*** A pleural effusion associated with bacterial pneumonia, termed a parapneumonic effusion, is the most common cause of an exudative pleural effusion. Parapneumonic effusions occur in about 40% of cases of bacterial pneumonia, are ipsilateral to the pneumonia, and have leukocyte counts over 10,000/μl with a predominance of polymorphonuclear leukocytes. Parapneumonic effusions are termed uncomplicated if they resolve with appropriate antibiotic therapy alone without sequelae and complicated if they require chest tube drainage to avoid complications such as persistent pleural space infection, bronchopleural fistula, or pleural adhesions. Typically the differentiation between a complicated and an uncomplicated parapneumonic effusion is based on the gross characteristics of the pleural fluid, a Gram stain and culture of the pleural fluid, and biochemical characteristics of the pleural fluid. Complicated parapneumonic effusions consist of empyemas (gross pus, a Gram stain demonstrating bacteria or a positive culture) or effusions characterized by a pH under 7.0 or a glucose level under 40 mg/dl. The pleural fluid LDH concentration alone is not used to define a parapneumonic effusion as complicated, although effusions with a pH value under 7.0 or glucose levels under 40 mg/dl are frequently accompanied by an LDH greater than 1000. Bacterial organisms vary vastly in their potential to cause complicated parapneumonic effusions. *Streptococcus pneumoniae,* although a common cause of pneumonia, seldom causes complicated parapneumonic effusion. In contrast, anaerobic bacteria, gram-negative bacteria, *Staphylococcus aureus,* and *Streptococcus pyogenes* are often associated with complicated parapneumonic effusions.

Malignant pleural effusions, usually due to pleural invasion by malignant cells, are the second major cause of exudative pleural effusions. Carcinomas of the lung and breast are the leading causes of malignant pleural effusions and along with lymphomas account for about 75% of the cases of malignant pleural effusions. A malignant pleural effusion may be the presenting clinical evidence of cancer and implies an advanced stage and poor prognosis.

Cytopathologic examination of pleural fluid is positive in 60% to 80% of cases of malignant effusions, which has led to some confusion over terminology regarding malignant pleural effusions. The pleural effusions associated with malignancy that do not contain malignant cells may be caused by tumor invasion of mediastinal lymph nodes, atelectasis, or pneumonia and not by direct pleural invasion by tumor. Some authors do not consider these cytologically negative effusions true malignant effusions but instead utilize the term *paramalignant effusion.* The differentiation of a true malignant effusion (an effusion that contains malignant cells) from a paramalignant effusion can be very important clinically. For example, in the case of lung cancer a malignant effusion (cytologically positive) implies surgical unresectability. However, a patient with a lung malignancy and a paramalignant effusion (cytologically negative) should be considered for surgery if the cancer is otherwise resectable.

The third most common type of pleural effusion is that due to pulmonary thromboembolism (PE), which is an exudate about 80% of the time. Pleural effusions occur in up to 50% of patients with PE. The effusion usually is unilateral and may be bloody. An underlying pulmonary infiltrate may be present. However, it must be stressed that the history, physical examination, pleural fluid, and chest radiographic characteristics are nonspecific and variable in the case of PE. Therefore the clinician should always consider PE in the differential diagnosis of a patient presenting with a pleural effusion with symptoms or signs suggestive of a PE or risk factors for PE.

Disease caused by *Myocobacterium tuberculosis* can cause pleuritis with an associated unilateral exudative pleural effusion and should always be considered in the case of a lymphocyte-predominant exudative pleural effusion (see Chapter 114).

Upper abdominal disease can also cause a pleural effusion. A subphrenic abscess due to perforation of an abdominal structure, a hepatic or splenic abscess, or viral hepatitis may cause upper abdominal or lower thoracic pain, fever, and a pleural effusion. Amebic abscess of the liver may cause right-sided pleural effusions as an inflammatory response to the abscess or, more commonly, as a result of rupture of the abscess, through the diaphragm, into the pleural cavity. These causes may mislead the clinician into looking for pleuropulmonary disease, delaying early recognition of an intraabdominal problem. Acute and chronic pancreatitis may result in a high amylase exudative pleural effusion, which is usually left sided. A pleural effusion with or without an associated pneumomediastinum or pneumothorax in a patient presenting with a history of vomiting, chest pain, and dyspnea should lead the clinician to consider spontaneous esophageal rupture. The exudative effusion in esophageal rupture typically has a high salivary amylase and a low pH in the range of 6.0. In addition, the pleural space may be infected with oropharyngeal anaerobes. Early diagnosis and management are essential.

Collagen vascular diseases, particularly systemic lupus erythematosus (SLE) and rheumatoid arthritis (RA), may be complicated by effusions. Although pleural effusions usually complicate previously defined SLE and RA, an effusion may be the presenting clinical manifestation. Glucose levels in the pleural fluid are very often markedly reduced in rheumatoid effusions, and physical examination almost invariably shows joint abnormalities. Another immunologically based cause of pleural effusions is Dressler's syndrome, also known as postcardiac injury syndrome (PCIS). PCIS can occur following myocardial injury such as myocardial infarction, cardiac trauma, or surgery. The syndrome includes pericarditis, pleural effusions, and pulmonary infiltrates associated with fever or chest pain, usually a few weeks to several months after myocardial injury. PCIS should be considered in any patient presenting with a pleural effusion, unilateral or bilateral, following a myocardial infarction or cardiac surgery.

### Drugs that can cause a pleural effusion

Drugs that induce SLE (diphenylhydantion, hydralazine, isoniazid, procainamide)
Sclerosing agents for esophageal varices
Chemotherapeutic agents (e.g., procarbazine, methotrexate)
Tocolytics used for premature labor
Bromocriptine
Dantrolene
Methysergide
L-Tryptophan
Nitrofurantoin
Amiodarone

Exudative pleural effusions may be due to medications, either directly or as a part of the drug-induced lupus syndrome (see the box above). The clinician should always consider drugs as a potential cause of an exudative pleural effusion. Other rare causes of exudative effusions include sarcoidosis, yellow nail syndrome, Meigs' syndrome (benign ovarian tumors with ascites and pleural effusion), uremia, chylous effusion, and hemothorax.

***Utility of tests in diagnosing the cause of a pleural effusion.*** The clinician should avoid ordering unnecessary tests and should not fail to order the appropriate tests, since both actions add to the cost of care. The key to striking the right balance is to integrate all clinical information to form a pretest clinical diagnosis.

Pleural fluid tests can be divided into four groups based on their relative usefulness (Table 118-1). Observation of gross characteristics (group A) costs nothing yet may provide a specific diagnosis or lead to individual tests that are diagnostic. Foul-smelling, yellow-green thick fluid is pus (empyema). Chocolate-colored (anchovy sauce) fluid strongly suggests a ruptured amebic liver abscess. White milky pleural fluid indicates a chylous or chyliform effusion and the need for triglyceride level and cytologic evaluation. A grossly bloody fluid suggests hemothorax, and the pleural fluid hematocrit must be checked. Protein and LDH along with serum protein and LDH separate transudates and exudates with a 99% accuracy. A two-step approach in one study reduces costs without missing important diagnoses. This entails keeping some pleural fluid in reserve pending protein and LDH determination. If the fluid is a transudate, no further tests are done; if it is an exudate, further tests are ordered. In cases where a transudate is suspected, this would be an appropriate approach.

Group B tests are those which have the potential to provide a definite diagnosis of empyema or malignant effusion. Although about 40% of bacterial pneumonias may be associated with a parapneumonic effusion, only a small percentage develop into an empyema. In contrast, cytologic examination proves malignancy in the majority of cases of malignant effusions. In either case negative studies do not exclude the diagnosis of a parapneumonic effusion or a malignancy.

Group C tests are those which have a high specificity for diagnosing uncommon causes of pleural effusion. These tests should be selectively ordered based on one's clinical suspicion and the gross appearance of the pleural fluid. Pleural fluid cultures for mycobacteria and fungi have a low sensitivity but should be obtained if the clinician believes that these organisms may be the cause of the exudative effusion. Pleural effusions are present in 16% to 37% of patients with SLE. These patients are symptomatic with pleuritic chest pain, and the majority of them have arthralgias or arthritis before the pleuritis. Measurement of the antinuclear antibody (ANA) level in pleural fluid and serum helps in diagnosing lupus pleuritis. Pleural fluid ANA titer is usually 1:160 or greater, and the pleural fluid/serum ANA ratio is 1 or greater. The finding of LE cells in pleural fluid is considered to be diagnostic of lupus pleuritis.

Pleural fluid amylase determination is indicated when pancreatitis or esophageal rupture is suspected. Pleural fluid amylase is above the upper limits of normal for serum and above the amylase level of a simultaneously sampled serum in pancreatitis. In chronic effusions due to pancreatic pseudocyst abdominal symptoms may be minimal, and chest symptoms may predominate. In large left-sided effusions of unknown cause the possibility of an effusion of pancreatic origin must be considered. Pleural fluid amylase is also elevated in esophageal rupture, but unlike pancreatitis the amylase is of salivary origin. Pleural fluid amylase may also be elevated in some malignant effusions, but the levels of amylase usually do not reach the levels seen in pancreatic disease and esophageal rupture, and the amylase is of salivary origin.

A triglyceride level of over 110 mg/ml in the pleural fluid indicates chylothorax. If the level is indeterminate—between 50 and 110—lipoprotein analysis needs to be done; the detection of chylomicrons confirms the diagnosis of chylothorax. A chylothorax indicates disruption of the thorax duct, which allows chyle to enter the pleural space. The commonest causes to consider are malignancy, particularly lymphoma, and trauma.

The hematocrit of a bloody pleural effusion should be measured. A pleural fluid hematocrit approaching that of blood indicates the presence of a hemothorax and suggests trauma is the cause; chest tube drainage should be strongly considered. A hematocrit over 1% suggests malignancy, trauma, or pulmonary embolism. A hematocrit of less than 1% is a relatively nonspecific finding.

Group D tests do not by themselves provide specific diagnoses, but integrated with clinical information they often help the clinician narrow the range of possible disorders. Red blood cell (RBC) count of pleural fluid should be interpreted with great caution, and RBC counts generated by an automated counter may not be reliable. RBC counts of over 5000 cells/mm$^3$ may impart a bloodlike color (serosanguineous) to the fluid but are not very helpful, since 40% of exudative effusions and some transudates may be blood tinged. Effusions with RBC counts of over 100,000 cells/mm$^3$ suggest the same diagnostic possibilities as those with a hematocrit of less than 1%.

A white blood cell (WBC) count of above 10,000/mm$^3$ is most commonly seen in parapneumonic effusions but may also be seen in other conditions such as pulmonary embolism, malignancy, tuberculosis, pancreatitis,

**Table 118-1.** Diagnostic utility of pleural fluid tests

| Group | Tests | Utility |
|---|---|---|
| A (useful in all) | Observation of gross characteristics | May be diagnostic, e.g., empyema |
| | LDH | Allows separation of transudates and exudates |
| | Protein | Allows separation of transudates and exudates |
| B (useful in exudates) | Stains, cultures for bacteria | Diagnostic if positive |
| | Cytology for malignant cells | Diagnostic if positive |
| C (selectively useful) | Stains, cultures for mycobacteria, fungi | Diagnostic if positive |
| | Antinuclear antibody and LE cells | ANA titer ≥1:160 and pleural fluid/serum ANA ratio ≥1 are strongly suggestive of lupus pleuritis; LE cells in the pleural fluid are diagnostic of lupus pleuritis |
| | Amylase | Increased and above serum level in pancreatic effusion; amylase of salivary origins is elevated in esophageal rupture and may be increased in malignancies |
| | Triglycerides, chylomicrons | More than 110 mg/ml indicates chylothorax<br>Presence of chylomicrons is diagnostic of chylothorax |
| | Hematocrit | High hematocrit, approaching that of blood, indicates hemothorax<br>Hematocrit over 1% suggests malignancy, trauma, or pulmonary embolism |
| D (useful when combined with a strong prethoracentesis clinical diagnosis) | Red cell count | $>100,000/mm^3$ suggests same diagnosis as hematocrit >1% |
| | White cell count, differential count | $>10,000/mm^3$ in parapneumonic effusions, pulmonary embolism, malignancy, tuberculosis, Dressler's syndrome, lupus pleural effusion<br>Neutrophilic predominance indicates acute inflammation<br>Lymphocyte predominance suggests malignancy or tuberculosis |
| | Glucose | <60 mg/ml suggests rheumatoid arthritis and parapneumonic and malignant effusions |
| | pH | <7.2 due to a variety of causes<br><7.0 in a parapneumonic effusion is a strong indication for chest tube drainage<br><6.0 accompanied by elevated amylase strongly suggests esophageal rupture |

*LE*, Lupus erythematosus; *ANA*, antinuclear antibody.

Dressler's syndrome, and SLE. Neutrophilic predominance indicates acute pleural inflammation. A predominance of small lymphocytes in an exudative effusion is very suggestive of tuberculosis or malignancy. Eosinophilic effusions (over 10% eosinophils) have a variety of causes. The presence of air or blood in the pleural space often causes pleural fluid eosinophilia. In one report half of benign asbestos pleural effusions showed eosinophilia. The generally held opinion that eosinophilia is unlikely in malignancy has been challenged. Drug-induced pleural effusions are frequently eosinophilic, as are effusions due to parasitic and some fungal diseases. Mesothelial cells are sparse (under 5%) in tuberculous pleural effusions. However, this finding is not specific, since any extensive inflammatory process may diminish the number of mesothelial cells in the pleural fluid.

A low pleural fluid glucose level (less than 60 mg/ml) suggests a short list of possible causes of the effusion. Chief among these are RA and parapneumonic and malignant effusions. Often the pleural fluid glucose in rheumatoid pleural effusions is strikingly low. In one study 78% of the patients had pleural fluid glucose levels under 30 mg/ml. In comparison, lupus pleuritis is less commonly (in one study, only 14%) associated with low glucose pleural effusions, and the levels are not as low as in effusions associated with RA.

Pleural fluid acidosis (pH less than 7.2) can have a variety of causes, including infection, esophageal rupture, rheumatoid effusion, tuberculosis, malignancy, hemothorax, lupus pleuritis, and urinothorax. In combination with high pleural fluid amylase, a low pH (under 6.0) suggests esophageal rupture as a cause. At present the best use of pH testing is for parapneumonic effusions to decide if chest tube drainage is necessary, since effusions with pH under 7.0 generally need tube drainage to avoid serious pleural space complications such as the formation of loculations and adhesions. Although helpful in this regard, pleural fluid pH is by no means foolproof in its predictive value.

***Indications and utility of other invasive procedures.*** Consideration should be given to other invasive procedures when the cause of a pleural effusion remains unknown despite thoracentesis and pleural fluid tests.

Percutaneous pleural biopsy (PPB) is particularly useful in the diagnosis of tuberculous pleuritis or pleural malignancy (see Chapter 114). The predominance of lymphocytes in pleural effusion is predictive of a high diagnostic yield by PPB. The diagnostic yield of PPB in tuberculous pleuritis is 75% when the tissue is sent for both histologic analysis and culture and approaches 90% when pleural fluid is also cultured. The yield of PPB alone in pleural malignancy is lower—46% in a major study. Lower yields in malignancy are thought to be due to several factors, including a nonuniform distribution of pleural metastasis, which makes blind sampling less successful. The yield of pleural fluid cytopathologic analysis is 60% to 80% in malignant pleural effusions, and the gain from adding PPB to a negative cytologic study is 7.1%. Thus it has been recommended that PPB be performed only after a series of negative cytologic studies of pleural fluid in a suspected malignant effusion. Both pleural fluid analysis and pleural biopsy are insensitive tests in the diagnosis of malignant pleural mesothelioma. The most common complication of PPB is pneumothorax usually due to the entry of atmospheric air into the pleural space (3% to 15%). An end-expiratory PA chest radiograph should be performed after the procedure. PPB is most safely performed in a cooperative patient when a sufficient amount of pleural fluid is present in the area of the biopsy so as to minimize the chance of penetrating the underlying lung during the biopsy.

A PPB that yields a histologic diagnosis of nonspecific pleuritis is not helpful and forces the clinician to decide whether to take the conservative approach of observing the effusion without further diagnostic tests or proceeding with thoracoscopy, fiberoptic bronchoscopy, or open pleural biopsy.

Thoracoscopy has replaced thoracotomy and open pleural biopsy as the preferred procedure in pleural diseases that are difficult to diagnose. In a study of thoracoscopy in 102 patients with undiagnosed pleural disease a diagnosis of malignancy was established in 38 patients, yielding a sensitivity of 91% and a specificity of 100%. The four cases of malignancy that were missed by thoracoscopy were all malignant mesothelioma. Thoracoscopy is also useful in the diagnosis of tuberculous pleuritis. However, some controversy remains on the role of thoracoscopy, since it may not add much to the diagnosis of metastatic pleural malignancy or tuberculous pleuritis compared to thoracentesis and PPB. In addition, biopsy from other causes of exudative pleural effusions such as rheumatologic disease and pulmonary embolism demonstrate a nonspecific pleuritis. Thus thoracoscopy should be considered when the clinician feels that a diagnosis of tuberculous pleuritis has been missed despite a negative pleural fluid and pleural tissue mycobacterial culture and a nondiagnostic pleural histopathology, or if the diagnosis of a malignant pleural effusion has not been established following cytopathologic analysis of at least three pleural fluid samples obtained by thoracentesis. Thoracoscopy is also useful in the case of a suspected malignant mesothelioma because of the relatively low yields of PPB and thoracentesis.

Fiberoptic bronchoscopy (FOB) following a nondiagnostic thoracentesis and PPB is indicated only when the chest radiograph or CT scan demonstrates an underlying lung parenchymal abnormality, such as a mass or collapse, or if the patient has a history of hemoptysis. In the absence of these features FOB has a very low diagnostic yield.

Even after an extensive workup including invasive procedures the cause remains unknown in about 15% of pleural effusions. However, the course and outcome are often favorable. In a study of 51 patients 31 (60.8%) had spontaneous resolution of the effusion, two died of unrelated cause, and 18 (35.3%) had the cause of the effusion become apparent during the follow-up period. The major causes included malignancy in 13 (25%) patients and collagen vascular diseases in three.

### Management

The long list of causes of pleural effusions (see the box on p. 1595) makes it obvious that treatment should be directed at the cause of the pleural effusion. However, in some cases the pleural fluid needs to be drained for therapeutic or palliative reasons.

An empyema should be promptly drained by closed chest tube drainage. A similar approach is needed in other types of "complicated" parapneumonic effusions that have a pH under 7.0 or a glucose level under 40 mg/ml. Parapneumonic effusions with a pH over 7.2 usually respond to an appropriate antibiotic alone; a repeat thoracentesis in 5 to 7 days should be done only if fever or leukocytosis persists or the effusion is unchanged or enlarging. In parapneumonic effusions with pH of 7.0 to 7.2 a thoracentesis should be repeated within 12 to 24 hours and chest tube drainage instituted if the pleural fluid pH has dropped further.

Pleural fluid drainage using a chest tube followed by chemical pleurodesis with talc, tetracycline, or bleomycin is frequently effective in providing symptomatic relief for patients with dyspnea from a recurrent malignant effusion. An 80% success rate has been reported with tetracycline instillation. The decision to perform these interventions depends on the overall condition and life expectancy of the patient.

There are a few caveats to note in the management of other conditions causing pleural effusions. In pulmonary embolism neither the bloody character of the pleural fluid nor hemoptysis is a contraindication to anticoagulation treatment. A patient with an undiagnosed lymphocyte-predominant exudative effusion who has a positive intermediate strength tuberculin skin test (PPD) should be considered for antituberculosis drug therapy. Pleural effusion and pleuritis due to PCIS respond to nonsteroidal antiinflammatory agents. In severe cases of PCIS glucocorticoids are also effective. In effusions due to esophageal rupture or a pancreatic pseudocyst, thoracic surgical consultation should be promptly obtained.

## FIBROTHORAX

Deposition of fibrous tissue results in a thick fibrotic visceral pleura that impairs the mobility of the pleura and the expansion of the underlying lung. This condition, fibrothorax, is commonly caused by pleural empyema, hemothorax, or tuberculous pleural disease. Other conditions that induce pleural inflammation, including uremia, collagen vascular disease and pancreatitis, can also cause fibrothorax.

Dyspnea on exertion is a common symptom, and examination may reveal diminished expansion and narrowed intercostal spaces in the involved side. A tracheal shift toward the involved side may be noted by palpation of the suprasternal notch. Radiographic findings are ipsilateral mediastinal shift and a dense pleural peel surrounding the lung. Calcification may be noted in the inner peel. Pulmonary function tests show restrictive ventilatory impairment. The only effective treatment is decortication with removal of the fibrous peel from the visceral pleura. The degree of impairment caused by the fibrothorax and the status of the underlying lung are the main factors to consider in deciding whether decortication will be beneficial. In patients without significant lung disease, especially fibrosis, improvement after decortication can be expected.

## ASBESTOS-RELATED PLEURAL DISEASE

Asbestos is a naturally occurring, fibrous silicate that is recognized as a cause of a variety of pleural and pulmonary parenchymal diseases. Asbestos enters the respiratory tract through inhalation. Because of its size and shape it is only minimally cleared by the normal host defense system of the lungs. The retained fibers are found both in the lung parenchyma and the pleura, where they are believed to generate a chronic inflammatory response that causes tissue injury. There are five pleural disorders associated with asbestos exposure: benign pleural effusions, pleural plaques, pleural fibrosis, rounded atelectasis, and malignant mesothelioma.

Benign pleural effusion (BPE) is the most common asbestos-related disorder occurring within 10 years of asbestos exposure. In some cases the latency period may be longer. BPE may be incidentally discovered on a chest radiograph or may simulate a pneumonia with pleuritic pain and fever. The effusions more often are unilateral, and the natural history is one of spontaneous resolution with a tendency to recur. The pleural fluid may be blood tinged and often eosinophilic. The diagnosis of BPE is made by excluding other causes in a patient with a history of asbestos exposure.

Pleural plaques, the most common manifestation of asbestos exposure, are discrete areas of the parietal pleura that consist of an abnormal accumulation of mesenchymal cells and connective tissue matrix. They often become calcified. Asbestos can be found in plaques using electron microscopy. Pleural plaques are located on the parietal pleura, usually on the lateral and inferior aspects, frequently involve the diaphragmatic pleura, and may be bilateral. Plaques are a manifestation that usually occurs at least 20 years after asbestos exposure, and the presence of pleural plaques usually does not lead to pulmonary function abnormalities. CT scanning is much more sensitive in demonstrating pleural plaques than is the conventional chest radiograph. No therapy is needed for pleural plaques, and they do not evolve into malignant mesothelioma. In contrast to pleural plaques, diffuse pleural fibrosis (which involves both the visceral and parietal pleura) is a rare manifestation of asbestos exposure than can cause a severe restrictive ventilatory impairment.

Rounded atelectasis is actually a pleuropulmonary process that usually occurs in patients with asbestos exposure. It is believed that an inflammatory process in the visceral pleura causes underlying lung parenchyma to collapse. On chest radiograph rounded atelectasis can simulate a lung carcinoma from which it must be differentiated. The CT scan is helpful in this situation, since the appearance can be diagnostic; however, a biopsy is necessary if doubt remains.

Patients with malignant pleural mesothelioma frequently complain of chest pain or dyspnea. About 80% of cases of malignant pleural mesothelioma occur in patients who have had asbestos exposure. The latency period from exposure to the development of disease is usually 35 to 40 years. Chest radiographs demonstrate a unilateral pleural effusion and thickening. The diagnosis of malignant pleural mesothelioma usually requires thoracoscopy or thoracotomy, since needle biopsy and cytologic specimens do not yield enough material for analysis, so confusion with other malignant or inflammatory processes is possible. The use of electron microscopy and advanced staining techniques has helped to make the diagnosis of malignant pleural mesothelioma more accurate. The prognosis of patients with malignant pleural mesothelioma is poor, although pleuropneumonectomy combined with chemotherapy shows some promise. In contrast to malignant pleural mesothelioma, fibrous mesothelioma is a benign disease unrelated to asbestos exposure.

## PNEUMOTHORAX

A pneumothorax is an accumulation of air in the normally airless pleural space between the lung and chest wall. Pneumothorax can be divided into spontaneous or traumatic causes. Spontaneous pneumothoraces can be further subdivided into primary spontaneous or secondary spontaneous pneumothoraces. Primary spontaneous pneumothorax occurs in healthy persons without preexisting lung disease, whereas a secondary spontaneous pneumothorax occurs as a complication of underlying pulmonary disease. A primary spontaneous pneumothorax occurs more commonly in young, tall, asthenic men. A reasonable theory for this predisposition is that, because of the configuration of the thoracic cage, traction on the alveolar walls is increased, causing rupture of subpleural apical blebs. The most common underlying disease responsible for secondary pneumothorax is obstructive airways disease. Infections that cause necrosis—pulmonary tuberculosis, necrotizing pneumonias, lung abscess—can cause a pneumothorax. Other diseases that predispose to secondary pneumothorax include histiocytosis X, sarcoidosis, tuberous sclerosis, cystic fibrosis, pulmonary infarction, and primary lung carcinoma. Catamenial pneumothorax is an uncommon entity that recurs at the time of menstrual periods. Although the exact pathogenesis of this disorder is unknown, it may be related to pleural and diaphragmatic endometriosis. Traumatic (noniatrogenic) pneumothorax is caused by penetrating or nonpenetrating chest trauma. Iatrogenic pneumothorax, the most common type of pneumothorax diagnosed in the hospitalized patient, is a complication of procedures such as transthoracic needle aspiration, subclavian vein puncture, thoracentesis, pleural biopsy, and transbronchial lung biopsy. Another iatrogenic cause is positive pressure mechanical ventilation, and pneumothorax is particularly liable to occur when airway pressures are high or when airway obstruction is present.

Normally the pressure in the pleural space is negative with reference to the atmospheric pressure and the alveolar pressure. Therefore, if there is a communication between the pleura and the atmosphere (e.g., following penetrating

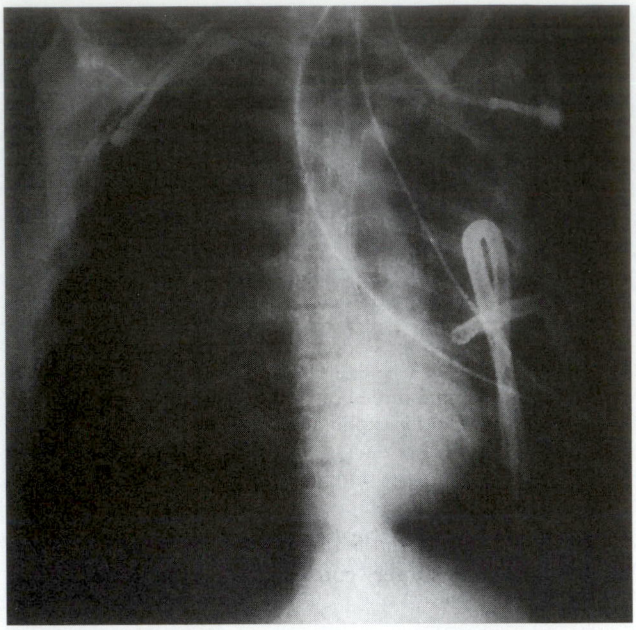

**Fig. 118-1.** Tension pneumothorax. Chest radiograph of a 34-year-old woman with noncardiac pulmonary edema following a tricyclic antidepressant overdose. The two chest tubes present on the right side were placed to treat a pneumothorax. This chest x-ray was taken to evaluate the sudden onset of hypotension due to the tension pneumothorax on the left. Notice the depressed left hemidiaphragm; the heart shadow and mediastinum are shifted toward the right.

trauma) or if there is communication between the pleura and the lung (e.g., following rupture of an emphysematous bulla), air continues to enter the pleural space until pleural pressure becomes atmospheric. This increased pleural pressure collapses the lung. In some instances a ball-valve communication is formed in which air can enter but cannot leave the pleural space. Intrapleural pressure may then exceed atmospheric pressure throughout expiration and often during inspiration as well. This *tension pneumothorax* is life threatening because it compromises ventilation by shifting mediastinal structures, impairing venous return, and diminishing cardiac output (Fig. 118-1). Tension pneumothorax more commonly develops as a complication of mechanical ventilation or other secondary pneumothoraces rather than as a complication of primary spontaneous pneumothorax.

The main symptoms of pneumothorax are chest pain and dyspnea, and in most patients the symptoms start abruptly. The severity of the symptoms depends on the volume of air in the pleural space and the degree of underlying disease. The physical signs are hyperresonance on percussion and diminished or absent tactile fremitus and breath sounds on the affected side. Patients with tension pneumothorax are in distress with dyspnea, tachypnea, and tachycardia often accompanied by distended neck veins, thready pulse, and hypotension. Bulging of the ipsilateral intercostal spaces is sometimes observed, and mediastinal shift may be signaled by tracheal deviation to the contralateral side. The chest radiograph is diagnostic because the margin of the collapsed lung is separated from the parietal pleura by air.

The management options are observation only, small-catheter pleural aspiration or chest tube drainage to evacuate the air, and chemical pleurodesis or open thoracotomy or thoracoscopy with pleural abrasion to prevent a recurrence of pneumothorax. The choice of a particular option clearly depends on the severity of the pneumothorax, predisposing state, and underlying disease.

Asymptomatic, unilateral, small (10% to 20% of the lung volume) primary spontaneous pneumothoraces can be observed, since most resolve within 10 days. A repeat chest radiograph in 6 to 12 hours should be done to check for progression of the pneumothorax. Supplemental oxygen is believed to hasten the resorption of air in the pleural space, since supplemental oxygen increases the gradient between nitrogen in the pleural space and nitrogen in the pleural capillary blood, favoring movement of nitrogen out of the pleural space. Progressively increasing spontaneous pneumothorax and large symptomatic pneumothoraces should be treated by evacuation of the pleural air. The preferred method is insertion of a small catheter (7 to 9 French) in the second anterior intercostal space in the midclavicular line using either a trochar or the Seldinger technique. Air is aspirated using a stopcock and a 60-ml syringe until a mild resistance is felt, and a Heimlich valve is attached to permit continued air evacuation. In large symptomatic pneumothoraces suction can be added through the exhaust port of the Heimlich valve. After the pneumothorax is evacuated and there is no evidence of reaccumulation of air by chest radiograph, the catheter can be removed. Chest tube insertion and drainage are indicated in a few cases of primary spontaneous pneumothorax when the initial volume of air evacuated is large (about 4 L) or when there is a persistent pneumothorax after catheter evacuation. Small-catheter pleural aspiration can also be used in iatrogenic pneumothoraces or very selectively in some minor trauma cases.

Chest tube drainage is the preferred method in tension pneumothorax, hydropneumothorax, hemopneumothorax, and in pneumothorax with underlying pulmonary disease. Tension pneumothorax is a medical emergency; if the diagnosis is suspected, a large-bore needle should be immediately inserted into the second anterior intercostal space to evacuate the air in the pleural space. A large amount of air coming through the needle confirms the diagnosis. The needle should be left in place until a chest tube is inserted and the air drained under water seal.

The recurrence rate of primary spontaneous pneumothorax is about 50% in 2 years. An ipsilateral recurrence should be treated with chest tube drainage and chemical pleurodesis. If there is a subsequent recurrence, open thoracotomy or thoracoscopy with pleural abrasion is indicated.

## BIBLIOGRAPHY

Collins TR, Sahn SA: Thorentesis: clinical value complications, technical problems and patient experience, *Chest* 91:817, 1987.

Light RW: *Pleural diseases,* ed 2, Philadelphia, 1990, Lea & Febiger.

Peterman TA, Speicher CE: Evaluating pleural effusions in a two-stage laboratory approach, *JAMA* 252:1051, 1984.

Prakash UB, Reiman HM: Comparison of needle biopsy with cytologic analysis for the evaluation of pleural effusion: analysis of 414 cases, *Mayo Clin Proc* 60:158, 1985.

Ryan CJ et al: The outcome of patients with pleural effusion of indeterminate cause at thoracotomy, *Mayo Clin Proc* 56:145, 1981.

Sahn SA: The pleura, *Am Rev Respir Dis* 138:184, 1988.
Schwartz DA: New developments in asbestos-induced pleural disease, *Chest* 99:191, 1991.
Smyernios NA, Jederline PJ, Irwin RS: Pleural effusion in an asymptomatic patient: spectrum and frequency of causes and management considerations, *Chest* 97:192, 1990.
Varkey B: Pleural effusions caused by infection, *Postgrad Med* 80:213, 1986.
Wiener-Kronish JC et al: Relationship of pleural effusion to pulmonary hemodynamics in patients with congestive heart failure, *Am Rev Respir Dis* 132:1253, 1985.

CHAPTER

# 119 Venous Thromboembolism and Other Pulmonary Vascular Diseases

**Randolph J. Lipchik**
**Kenneth W. Presberg**

## VENOUS THROMBOEMBOLISM

### Epidemiology and etiology

Venous thromboembolism (VTE) is a common and serious problem that can lead to premature mortality and long-term morbidity. Physicians in almost all areas of patient care encounter patients at risk for this disease. VTE often occurs in patients with significant underlying medical problems. In recent studies the overall, all-cause, 1-year mortality for patients who developed VTE was 20% to 40%. Cardiac disease, chronic lung disease, and malignancy accounted for the majority of deaths. Therefore the diagnosis of pulmonary embolism can be difficult if the signs and symptoms are masked by the presentation of the patient's underlying condition. Over 5 million cases of deep venous thrombosis (DVT) are estimated to occur per year in the United States. Of these patients approximately 500,000 have a clinically apparent pulmonary embolism (PE), and approximately 10% of these individuals die of this complication. The Prospective Investigation of Pulmonary Embolism Diagnosis (PIOPED) study indicated that 2.5% of patients who survive to hospitalization will die of PE and 8% will experience a recurrence in the ensuing months. A small percentage of those who survive will fail to resolve the pulmonary vascular clots and will develop chronic pulmonary hypertension (Fig. 119-1). The major conceptual advance concerning this problem stipulates that *pulmonary embolism is a complication of venous thrombosis*. Furthermore, venous thrombosis is preventable and amenable to early diagnosis and treatment.

Despite the advances in understanding, diagnosis, and treatment, it is not apparent that the overall incidence of VTE has been substantially decreased. This may be due, in part, to the increase in age of the population. Indeed, the majority of the patients enrolled in the PIOPED study were older than 60 years. An additional study in the elderly noted that the VTE incidence of 1 per 1000 at 65 years rose to approximately 3 per 1000 at 85 years of age. However, it is also evident that a number of practitioners are not providing proven, preventive therapy for their patients. Certain groups, such as orthopedic surgery patients, now uniformly receive prophylaxis and develop VTE much less frequently.

Approximately 90% of clinically significant pulmonary emboli arise from the deep veins of the lower extremities. Recent investigations reported a 40% incidence of high-probability ventilation/perfusion (V/Q) scans in patients with DVT but without any symptoms of PE. These data are in agreement with prior clinical and pathologic studies and confirm that DVT and PE are manifestations of the same disease. However, not all venous thrombi of the lower extremities or other venous systems pose such a significant risk. Thrombi that *remain* confined to the calf veins do not cause significant pulmonary emboli, but if calf thrombi are left untreated there may be a risk of local recurrence at a later date. Diagnostic methods and management approaches appropriately concentrate on the larger veins of the lower extremities; however, 30% of patients with acute PE have a negative noninvasive evaluation of the lower extremities. Therefore confirmation of the diagnosis of VTE may require testing for both PE and DVT.

Thrombi may also originate in the pelvic veins, but these veins are smaller and the emboli are less of a hazard to the patient. Axillary and subclavian vein thrombosis are more commonly recognized, and central venous catheterization is a major risk factor for the development of this abnormality. This problem may also arise spontaneously or related to effort in a young adult. In this instance there is usually a thoracic outlet venous compression, and the condition is called the Paget-Schroetter syndrome. Clinically significant pulmonary embolism occurs less often from thromboses involving these sites. However, all the complications of DVT of the lower extremities have been described for thrombosis in these locations.

Data from studies looking at the natural history of VTE indicate that the vast majority of patients who die of complications of a PE do so within the first few hours of the event. Furthermore, recent data from the PIOPED study strongly support the previous tenet that death due to PE after the first few hours of the event is likely due to a recurrent embolism. Inadequate early anticoagulation was reported as one of the risks for recurrence. Other risks for recurrence, including proximal extent of thrombus, have yet to be clarified. The vast majority of fatal recurrences

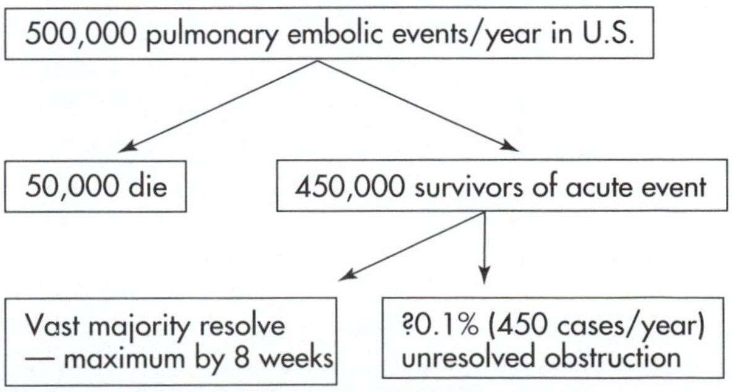


**Fig. 119-1.** Estimated incidence of venous thromboembolism and associated complications in the United States.

occurred within the first week of presentation. Hence overall morbidity and mortality are significantly reduced only by prevention of DVT, and in-hospital mortality is decreased by prevention of a recurrence and the early initiation of effective treatment for DVT.

## Pathophysiology

***Risk factors.*** General conditions that promote deep venous thrombosis formation were first described by Virchow. These include *vascular intimal injury, blood stasis, and hypercoagulability* and are present in a number of clinical situations associated with an increased risk of DVT (see the box below). Patients can be divided according to the degree of risk and their management directed accordingly. The *low*-risk group experiences DVT less than 0.5% of the time. *Medium*-risk patients are older and may experience a DVT 2% to 10% of the time if untreated. The key individuals for whom preventive therapy has been targeted are those who fall into the *high*-risk group. DVT can occur more than 20% of the time in these individuals (see the box below). In a number of these cases significant risks converge to strongly promote the development of this disease.

A minority of patients may be predisposed to thrombotic events due to a primary or secondary imbalance in coagulation. These conditions are generally referred to as the hypercoagulable states (see the box at right). These disorders are uncommon, and diagnostic screening is best directed toward patients who are young, have a family history of thrombotic events, have had recurrent events, or have not had the normal resolution of thromboses with adequate anticoagulation. Certain disorders, such as the antiphospholipid syndrome, often lead to recurrent, devastating complications including multiple venous and arterial thrombosis, thrombocytopenia, pulmonary and systemic hypertension, and livedo reticularis. However, other individuals with the inherited disorders may not experience any significant complications. In fact, in a cohort study of asymptomatic, antithrombin III–deficient individuals, the prevalence of thrombotic events was low; researchers suggest withholding anticoagulants from these patients until they are at risk or develop a complication. If these patients are diagnosed with VTE or other thrombotic complication, lifelong intermediate to high-intensity warfarin therapy is recommended. Long-term *prophylactic* anticoagulation has not been demonstrated to be beneficial for any of these disorders.

Malignancy is well known to be associated with venous thrombosis. Trousseau first described this association in 1865. A peculiar form of migrating, superficial, venous thrombosis—*thrombophlebitis migrans*—may antedate the signs and symptoms of cancer by years. A new DVT in the common locations in an otherwise healthy individual may also be an early clue to the presence of an occult malignancy. There is no proven benefit from exhaustive diagnostic tests for occult malignancy. However, the lung, gastrointestinal tract, breast, and reproductive organs are the most common cancer sites, and directed examinations are reasonable.

***Complications.*** Noninvasive studies of the lower extremities have been reported to return to normal in the majority of patients within 3 months and in 90% of patients by 1 year. Furthermore, there is a small risk of recurrence in patients who are adequately treated and in whom the noninvasive studies have returned to normal. This does not necessarily imply a fully competent and normal vein, however. There remains well-known substantial morbidity and cost associated with the postphlebitic syndrome, particularly in patients who have had an iliofemoral thrombosis. These troublesome local complications have promoted the investigation of more aggressive treatment strategies for DVT itself.

VTE kills patients by PE, the respiratory and hemodynamic consequences of which are summarized in the box on p. 1605. Hyperventilation is almost universal and is reported to be relatively proportional to the severity of the obstruction. The exact mechanisms that lead to hyperventilation are not known, but lung mechanoreceptors (j receptors) are felt to play an important role. The embolism leads to obstruction and a decrease in perfusion. This causes an increase in alveolar dead space and increases the ventilatory requirement of the patient. The

### Patient risk groups for VTE

Low: <40 years old, no other risks, general anesthesia <30 minutes
Medium: >40 years old, general anesthesia >30 minutes
High: Clear predisposing underlying risks
- *Prolonged immobilization, conditions requiring ICU care*
- Congestive heart failure and myocardial infarction
- Prior DVT
- Inherited and acquired coagulation defects
- Malignancy
- Obesity
- Age >65 years
- Hip fracture, hip replacement, knee replacement
- Pelvic or lower extremity trauma or surgery

### Hypercoagulable states

**Primary disorders**

- Fibrinolytic defects
- Dysfibrinogenemia
- Factor XII deficiency
- Protein C deficiency (homozygous patients only)
- Protein S deficiency
- Antithrombin III deficiency
- Antiphospholipid syndrome
- Homocystinuria

**Secondary disorders**

- Nephrotic syndrome and other glomerulonephritis
- Liver disease
- Peripartum state
- Malignancy
- Estrogen therapy (varying risks with different compounds)
- Acquired platelet disorders
- Hyperviscosity syndromes

obstruction may be relieved in a matter of hours by fibrinolytic mechanisms, and the dead space may return to near normal shortly after the event. Hypoxemia is multifactorial. Causes include a decrease in mixed venous $O_2$ if there is a decrease in cardiac output, ventilation/perfusion inequality, and occasionally an increase in right-to-left shunt through a patent foramen ovale. However, the hyperventilation tends to increase the $PaO_2$ toward normal and limits the diagnostic utility of $PaO_2$ for PE, but the A-a gradient remains elevated in almost all instances. Severe hypoxemia in a patient without any underlying lung disease signals a massive embolism.

Atelectasis and infarction occur later in the course of PE. Atelectasis appears after 24 hours of obstruction and is due, in part, to the depletion of surfactant related to an interruption of the nutrient supply to the alveolar type II cells of the lung. Infarction is uncommon because of the dual arterial blood supply of the lung. Hemoptysis and other signs attributed to infarction also occur 24 to 48 hours after the acute event but may be the first signs of a PE. The hemodynamic consequences of PE can be life threatening. If the embolism causes more than 50% of the vascular bed to be acutely obstructed, right ventricular afterload increases precipitously and right ventricular failure may ensue. The normal right ventricle is only able to *acutely* sustain adequate blood flow up to a mean pulmonary artery pressure of 40 mm Hg or a systolic pressure in the range of 65 mm Hg. Compounds that lead to pulmonary vasoconstriction, such as serotonin and thromboxane $A_2$, are released by platelet aggregation and contribute to the acute elevation in pulmonary arterial pressure. The patient's ability to tolerate these acute insults largely depends on the underlying cardiopulmonary status. Hence the cardiopulmonary manifestations of pulmonary embolism are quite variable. Fortunately the thrombus begins to resolve within hours after treatment, and restoration of 25% of the luminal diameter allows sufficient flow to normalize a perfusion scan. A large percent of the obstruction is relieved within days, and resolution is maximal at approximately 8 weeks. Further resolution thereafter is unlikely.

Chronic major vessel thromboembolic pulmonary hypertension results from recurrent submassive or massive emboli that do not resolve. Many of the patients who develop this disease do not have a documented history of PE and did not receive treatment for their thromboembolism. Very few of these patients have recognized hypercoagulable states, but an intrinsic defect in fibrinolysis is strongly suspected. Under these circumstances the right ventricle adapts over time to an increased afterload. It becomes hypertrophied and can sustain systemic or suprasystemic pressures. These chronic right heart adaptations are usually documented by electrocardiogram (ECG) or echocardiogram. Patient survival has been correlated to the mean pulmonary artery pressure. Five-year survival is significantly decreased in patients with a mean pulmonary artery pressure greater than 35 mm Hg. Patients with a mean pulmonary artery pressure greater than 55 mm Hg have a very poor prognosis and are at significant risk of sudden death. Progressive right ventricular dysfunction is signaled by further increases in right atrial pressure and right-sided cardiac chamber volumes. Hypoxemia is also multifactorial in this condition and does not correlate with the degree of pulmonary hypertension. Some of these patients may be candidates for surgical thromboendarterectomy, whereas others have very limited therapeutic options (see treatment section).

## Complications of pulmonary embolism

**Respiratory consequences**

Hyperventilation, respiratory alkalosis
Hypoxemia, multifactorial
Increased alveolar dead space
Atelectasis
Pulmonary infarction
Pleural effusion

**Hemodynamic consequences**

Reduced pulmonary vascular volume
Increase in PVR: obstruction, vasoactive compounds
Acute right ventricular failure: Mean pulmonary artery pressure >40 mm Hg
Chronic pulmonary hypertension

### History

The diagnosis of PE is difficult to make on clinical grounds because the clinical signs, symptoms, and basic laboratory studies are neither very sensitive nor specific, and the only definitive diagnostic test, pulmonary angiography, is invasive and expensive. Nonetheless, aspects of the history help raise the clinical suspicion of PE and, in combination with certain objective tests, allow one to rule in or rule out the diagnosis with reasonable certainty. Although PE can occur silently, the sudden onset of dyspnea is usually the most common symptom reported. The large, multicenter Urokinase Pulmonary Embolism Trial (UPET) reported on the most common symptoms with angiographically proven PE (Table 119-1). Dyspnea, pleuritic chest pain, and cough were most common. The classic triad of dyspnea, pleuritic chest pain, and hemoptysis occurred in only 28% of cases, but two of the three symptoms were present in 65%. Dyspnea, chest pain of any quality, and a sense of apprehension were present in 44% of cases; two of these three symptoms were reported in 81% of patients. Syncope, reflecting inadequate systemic perfusion due to obstruction of the pulmonary vasculature, was seen in 13% of cases overall, usually with massive emboli.

In the more recent PIOPED study the subset of patients without prior cardiac or pulmonary disease was examined to identify symptoms that could be attributed solely to the pulmonary embolism (see Table 119-1). Dyspnea was present in 73% of cases, pleuritic chest pain in 66%, and cough in 37%. Hemoptysis occurred in only 13% of cases. The lack of specificity of these symptoms was confirmed, since the prevalence of these symptoms was not significantly different in patients proven not to have PE.

Since at least 90% of pulmonary emboli arise from the deep veins of the lower extremities, symptoms of DVT should also be elicited (Fig. 119-2). With thrombosis of the iliac, femoral, or popliteal veins unilateral leg swelling may be the only symptom. In calf vein thrombosis, pain is

**Table 119-1.** Incidence of symptoms and signs associated with acute pulmonary embolism

| Symptoms and signs | UPET ($n$ = 327) (% of patients) | PIOPED ($n$ = 117) (% of patients) |
|---|---|---|
| Dyspnea | 84 | 73 |
| Pleuritic chest pain | 74 | 66 |
| Cough | 53 | 37 |
| Hemoptysis | 30 | 13 |
| Syncope | 13 | NR |
| Tachypnea | 92 | 70 |
| Rales | 58 | 51 |
| Increased $P_2$ | 53 | 23 |
| Tachycardia | 44 | 30 |
| Fever | 43 | 7 |
| Phlebitis | 32 | 11 |
| Leg edema | 24 | NR |

Data from Bell WR, Simon TL, DeMets DL: *Am J Med* 62:355, 1977; and Stein PD et al: *Chest* 100:598, 1991.
*NR*, Not reported.

the most common symptom, but because of multiple veins and collaterals an isolated clot may be asymptomatic. In UPET symptoms of lower extremity DVT were present in only 21% of patients. In a small percentage of cases PE may arise from thrombosis of upper extremity veins, usually in association with a long-standing central line or in cases of trauma. Upper extremity thrombosis is often asymptomatic, but pain and swelling are the most common symptoms when any are present. Although nonspecific, the symptoms discussed above, in conjunction with the presence of the conditions that have been associated with increased risk for venous thrombosis, are important diagnostic clues in the investigation of thromboembolic disease.

## Physical examination

In the setting of PE the physical examination can be surprisingly unremarkable. Evidence of acute pulmonary hypertension—right ventricular heave, right-sided $S_3$, large jugular a wave, and an increased $P_2$—are seen infrequently and in the setting of massive embolism. In PIOPED where no prior cardiac or pulmonary disease existed tachypnea was present in 70% of cases, tachycardia in 30%, and rales in 51%. DVT was clinically evident in only 11% of cases. In UPET these signs were present in 92%, 44% and 58%, respectively. Phlebitis was present in 32% of patients. The greater incidence of signs in UPET may be due to selection criteria. In UPET patients were included only if the embolus involved at least one segmental artery, whereas in PIOPED the emboli could be smaller. All these findings are, however, not very specific, since patients without PE have a similar incidence of the same signs. The physical findings for lower extremity DVT are also deceptive. Two thirds of DVT are clinically silent, and in those patients with leg swelling, tenderness, or a positive Homans sign, only half actually have DVT. Therefore the physical findings alone are not particularly helpful but are additional diagnostic clues in the right circumstances.

## Laboratory studies

***General tests.*** Once again, routine laboratory studies are not particularly specific. The arterial blood gas classically demonstrates hypoxemia and hypocapnia, the latter the result of hyperventilation. These findings are supportive evidence, but they can be found in a variety of other settings. In patients without prior cardiac or pulmonary disease the arterial $Po_2$ was the same with and without PE, and 26% of those with angiogram-proven PE had a normal $Po_2$ (over 80 torr). ECG abnormalities are common with PE and are usually nonspecific. In UPET, ST segment and T wave abnormalities occurred in 64% of cases. Evidence of acute cor pulmonale ($S_1Q_3T_3$, right bundle branch block, p pulmonale, right axis deviation) was less common, but one or more of these were seen in 25% of cases. Sinus tachycardia was present in 43% of cases. Other rhythm disturbances (premature ventricular beats, premature atrial beats, and atrial fibrillation) occurred in 11% of cases, with atrial fibrillation accounting for 3%. These abnormalities persisted for 5 to 6 days. The ECG was normal in only 13% of cases.

The chest x-ray most often demonstrates findings of atelectasis, small pleural effusion, infiltrates, and an elevated hemidiaphragm, but can be normal. Other features, such as a pleural-based density (Hampton hump) and regional loss of vascularity with proximal vascular fullness or cutoff (Westermark's sign), have been associated with pulmonary embolism, but overall the chest x-ray has poor sensitivity and specificity for PE. Its main values are as an adjunct to the V/Q scan and its ability to detect an alternate cause for the patient's symptoms.

***Specific tests.*** Pulmonary angiography is the definitive study for the diagnosis of PE. A catheter is introduced, most often via the femoral vein, and advanced to the main pulmonary artery of interest. Pulmonary artery pressure is measured and then contrast injected while films from multiple views are taken. Subselective injection of smaller arteries can be done if necessary. A thrombus must be clearly outlined to make the diagnosis of PE (Fig. 119-3). Although definitive, angiography is not suitable as a routine test because it is invasive, expensive, not available at all centers, and has potential complications such as anaphylactoid reactions to intravenous contrast and worsening of renal dysfunction, particularly in the diabetic patient. Pulmonary hypertension was once believed to be a contraindication to angiography, but recent studies have demonstrated that in large centers with considerable experience the procedure can be done safely. This modality is reserved for cases in which the diagnosis of PE is uncertain after clinical evaluation and V/Q scanning.

Perfusion lung scanning has been in use for almost 30 years and is a sensitive, but nonspecific, method for evaluating pulmonary perfusion. Macroaggregated albumin labeled with $^{99m}Tc$ is injected intravenously, and anterior, posterior, lateral, and oblique views of the chest are taken. The distribution of particles in the lung reflects the distribution of blood flow. Localized defects can occur in areas of lung consolidation or collapse, with pulmonary vasoconstriction due to local alveolar hypoxia and from vascu-

A B

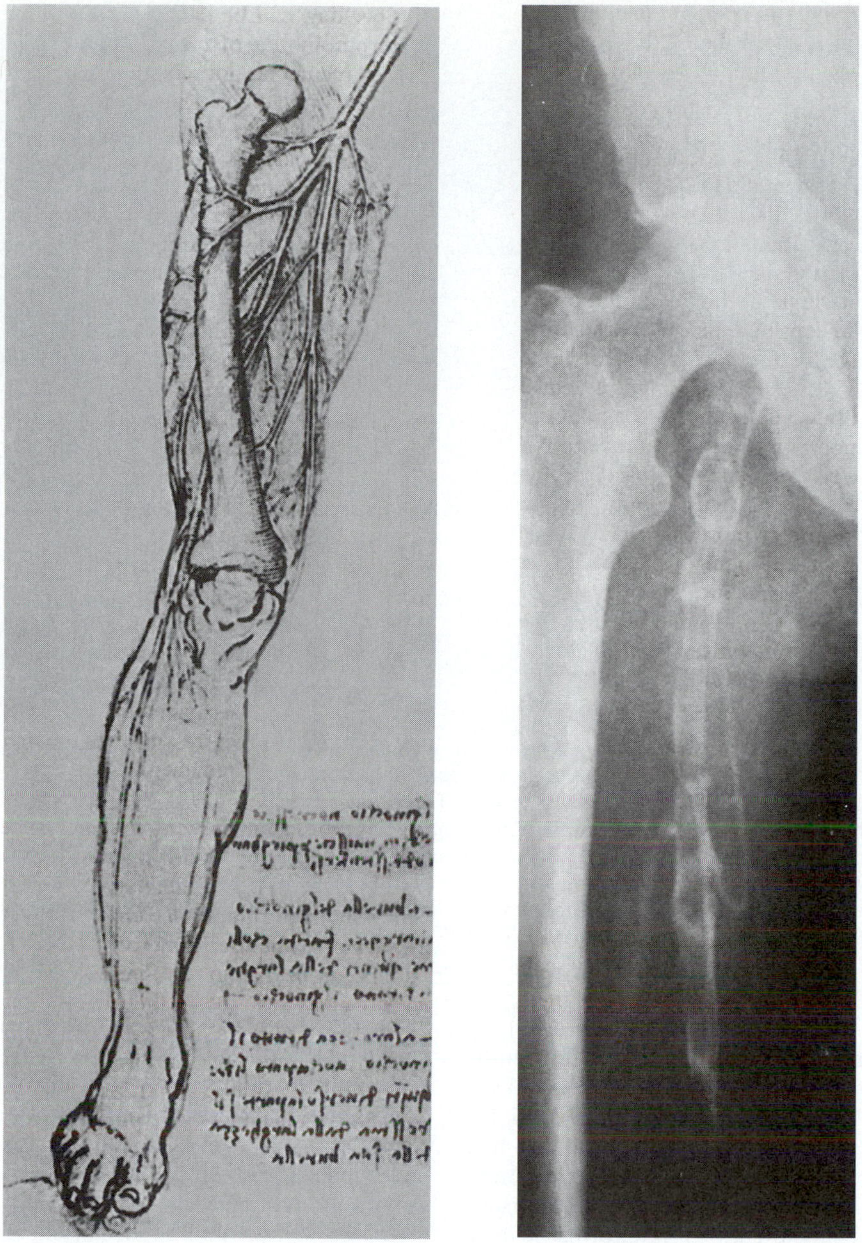

**Fig. 119-2.** **A,** Anatomic diagram of the venous drainage of the thigh, by Leonardo da Vinci. **B,** Venogram reveals contrast material flowing around extensive thrombi in the deep venous system. The superficial saphenous vein system is opacified faintly. (**A** from Corpus of the Anatomical Studies in the Collection of Her Majesty the Queen at Windsor Castle. Courtesy Boston Medical Library.)

lar obstruction. The chest x-ray is critical in evaluating lung scan perfusion defects. Abnormal perfusion without an abnormality on chest x-ray is much more specific for pulmonary vascular obstruction (embolism) than abnormal perfusion that corresponds to an area of parenchymal consolidation. Ventilation scanning is often performed after the perfusion scan to increase its specificity. A radioaerosol is inhaled for several minutes to fill all areas of the lung. The patient then breathes ambient air, and the washout of the isotope is studied. With normal ventilation the lungs clear rapidly and symmetrically. Areas of retained aerosol indicate abnormal ventilation. Areas of normal ventilation with abnormal perfusion (mismatch) are highly suggestive of PE (see the box on p. 1609).

The PIOPED trial was unique in that it combined the clinical estimate of the likelihood of PE with the findings of V/Q scanning in cases of angiographically proven PE, thus strengthening the diagnostic utility of lung scanning. The likelihood of PE based on clinical suspicion and lung scan results is shown in Table 119-2. Note that, in the setting of a high clinical suspicion, the probability of a pulmonary embolus is as high as 40% when the V/Q scan is read as low probability (see Managed Care Guide); however, when the scan is near normal or normal, the

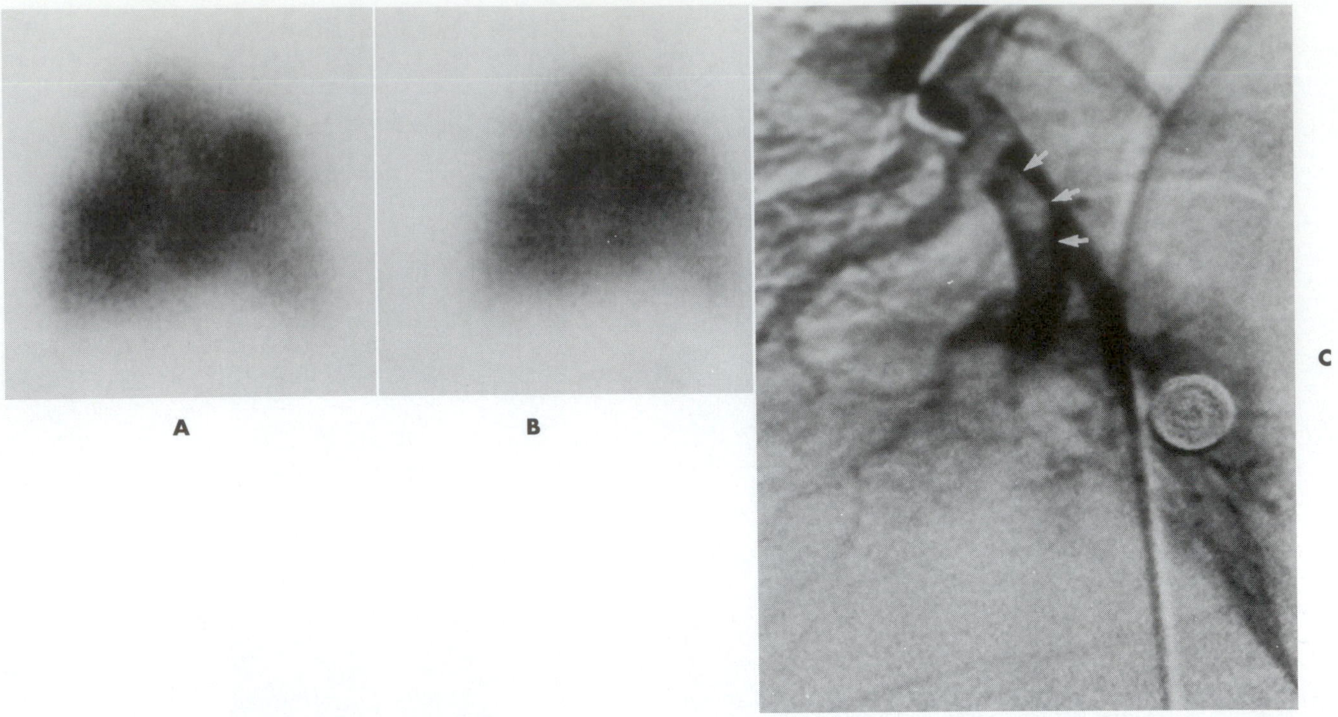


**Fig. 119-3.** Imaging studies of a 23-year-old woman with the sudden onset of pleuritic chest pain 3 days following surgery. Other risk factors included obesity and estrogen use. The chest x-ray revealed platelike atelectasis at both bases and a small right pleural effusion. The perfusion lung scan (**A**) demonstrated inhomogeneous perfusion with nonsegmental perfusion defects. The ventilation scan (**B**) showed matching non-segmental ventilation defects, therefore a low probability for PE. Because of the high clinical suspicion of PE an angiogram (**C**) was performed revealing a large thrombus in the proximal aspect of the right pulmonary artery *(arrows)*.

chance of PE is very low no matter what the level of clinical suspicion. Another important finding of this study was that the utility of the V/Q scan was not impaired by preexisting cardiac or pulmonary disease. It should be evident, however, that the diagnosis of PE is still not simple. In PIOPED near normal or normal and high-probability scans occurred in only 14% and 13% of cases, respectively, leaving most patients in categories with a significant probability of having PE.

Since most pulmonary emboli arise from the lower extremity, techniques for the detection of DVT are important modalities to consider in a PE workup. Contrast venography is the definitive test for detection of DVT, but it is invasive and requires large amounts of intravenous contrast material. Several noninvasive modalities have been studied, such as $^{125}$I- fibrinogen scanning, impedance plethysmography (IPG), and venous compression ultrasound. $^{125}$I- fibrinogen is incorporated into freshly forming thrombus and is a sensitive method for detecting thrombus formation in the calf veins, popliteal vein, and veins of the distal thigh. This test requires active thrombus formation so has little value in the immediate diagnosis of DVT; because of the potential risk of transmissible infection it is no longer available for clinical use. IPG works by assessing venous drainage from the thigh after partial release of an occlusive cuff. Using a mild electrical current the impedance of the thigh is measured after the application of an occlusive cuff; it should decrease as venous blood is allowed to drain proximally. Failure of impedance to fall suggests obstruction to venous outflow due to a thrombus. Compared to venograms, IPG has been found to be more than 90% sensitive to the presence of a proximal DVT. Calf thrombi do not usually affect venous outflow so are not detected reliably by IPG, and extrinsic compression of thigh vein(s) or elevated central venous pressure (congestive heart failure) may give false positive results. Ultrasound examination of the proximal veins of the lower extremity has been found to be another sensitive and specific test for DVT. If the vessel is adequately visualized *and* cannot be compressed, the diagnosis of DVT is confirmed. Visualization of thrombus is unreliable, and the test is somewhat operator dependent. The choice of IPG or compression ultrasound is usually based on local availability.

### Diagnostic strategies

The signs and symptoms of PE are neither very sensitive nor specific, but these findings in conjunction with one or more predisposing conditions for PE increase the degree of clinical suspicion. A chest x-ray should be taken, and if it does not reveal an alternate diagnosis, a V/Q scan should follow. If the perfusion scan is normal, PE is essentially ruled out, and therapy or further workup is unnecessary. The lack of subsequent DVT or PE in this setting has been confirmed in several prospective studies. A high-probability V/Q scan indicates an 85% to 90% probability of PE; however, if combined with a high clinical suspicion, the positive predictive value is as high as 96%. In this

## V/Q lung scan categories and criteria

**High probability of PE**

Two or more large segmental perfusion defects without corresponding ventilation or CXR abnormalities or substantially larger than either matching ventilation or CXR abnormalities

Two or more moderate segmental perfusion defects without matching ventilation or CXR abnormalities and one large mismatched segmental defect

Four or more moderate segmental perfusion defects without matching ventilation or CXR abnormalities

**Intermediate probability (indeterminate)**

Not falling into normal, very low, low, or high probability categories

Borderline high or borderline low

Difficult to categorize as low or high

**Low probability**

Nonsegmental perfusion defects

Single moderate mismatched segmental perfusion defect with normal CXR

Any perfusion defect with a substantially **larger** CXR abnormality

Large or moderate segmental perfusion defects involving no more than four segments in one lung and no more than three segments in one lung region with **matching** ventilation defects either equal to or larger in size, and CXR either normal or with abnormalities substantially smaller than perfusion defects

More than three small segmental perfusion defects with a normal CXR

**Very low probability**

Three or fewer small segmental perfusion defects with a normal CXR

**Normal**

No perfusion defects

Perfusion outlines exactly the shape of the lungs as seen on the CXR (hilar and aortic impressions may be seen, CXR and/or ventilation study may be abnormal

Modified from PIOPED Investigators: *JAMA* 263:2753, 1990.
*CXR*, Chest x-ray.

setting treatment is initiated without further evaluation.

Unfortunately, most patients do not have normal or high-probability scans and fall into more difficult categories. In PIOPED 73% of patients had low- or intermediate-probability V/Q scans. Combined with different levels of clinical suspicion, these indicate probabilities of PE from 4% to 66% (see Table 119-2). This degree of uncertainty requires further diagnostic investigation, and there are several options. The first is to perform pulmonary angiography. This is the definitive test, but it is invasive and not universally available. The alternative is to study the lower extremity for evidence of DVT. Contrast venography is an option, but for reasons previously mentioned noninvasive studies have become more prevalent. Finding a proximal DVT by IPG or compression ultrasound warrants therapy, making the diagnosis of PE unimportant, since the therapy is the same. In the setting of PE a proximal DVT is found in approximately half of cases.

Conversely, with a nondiagnostic V/Q scan and a negative noninvasive leg study the probability of PE may still be as high as 30% to 50%, and pulmonary angiography is indicated to clarify the diagnosis. A recent cost-effectiveness analysis confirmed this diagnostic plan as safe, effective, and able to reduce the need for pulmonary angiography by as much as 40%. Diagnostic strategies for the diagnosis of PE in the setting of a nondiagnostic V/Q scan are summarized in the Managed Care Guide. It should be noted that this strategy applies equally well for women and men. In a separate analysis of women enrolled in PIOPED signs, symptoms, and risk factors were essentially the same as those for men, with the exception that oral contraceptive use (not postmenopausal estrogen use) in the setting of surgery was associated with a more frequent diagnosis of PE. In addition, the sensitivity of a high-probability V/Q scan appeared to be diminished in this group, so angiography was needed more frequently to confirm the diagnosis of PE.

## Differential diagnosis

Because the symptoms associated with pulmonary embolism are nonspecific, initial evaluation of the patient through chest x-ray and general laboratory studies usually identifies alternative diagnoses. For example, chest pain and dyspnea may herald the onset of pneumococcal pneumonia, an acute myocardial infarction, or a pneumothorax. Fever, an elevated white blood cell (WBC) count, purulent sputum, and a segmental infiltrate on chest x-ray signals pneumonia. Signs of acute ischemia on the

**Table 119-2.** The likelihood of pulmonary embolism combining clinical estimate and V/Q scans in patients with angiographically proven PE

| Scan category | Clinical probability (PE positive) 80%-100% | 20%-79% | 0%-19% | All probabilities |
|---|---|---|---|---|
| High probability | 96 | 88 | 56 | 87 |
| Intermediate probability | 66 | 28 | 16 | 30 |
| Low probability | 40 | 16 | 4 | 14 |
| Near normal/normal | 0 | 6 | 2 | 4 |

Data from PIOPED Investigators: *JAMA* 263:2753, 1990.

## Managed Care Guide
## Diagnostic strategy for PE in the setting of a nondiagnostic V/Q scan

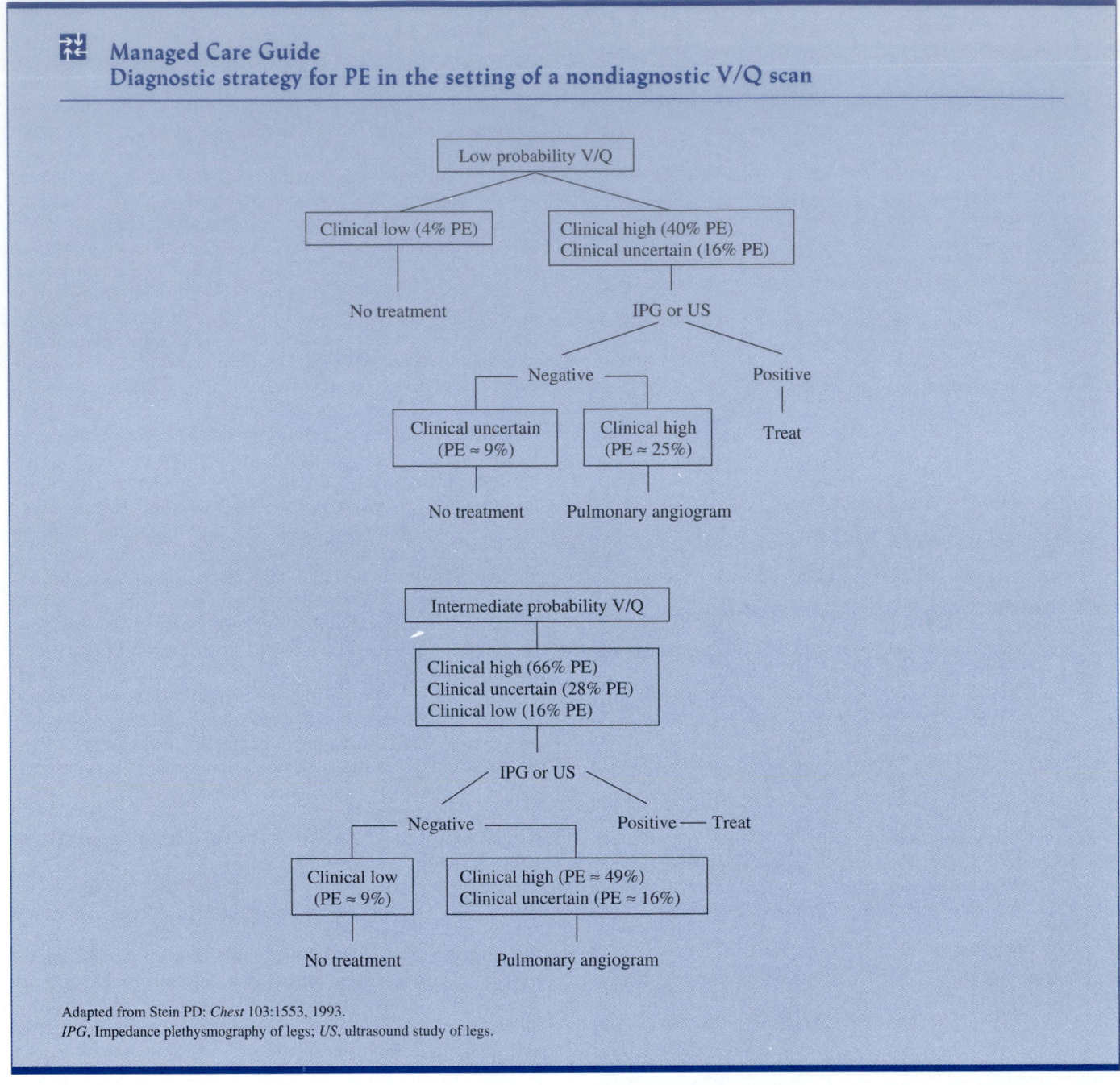

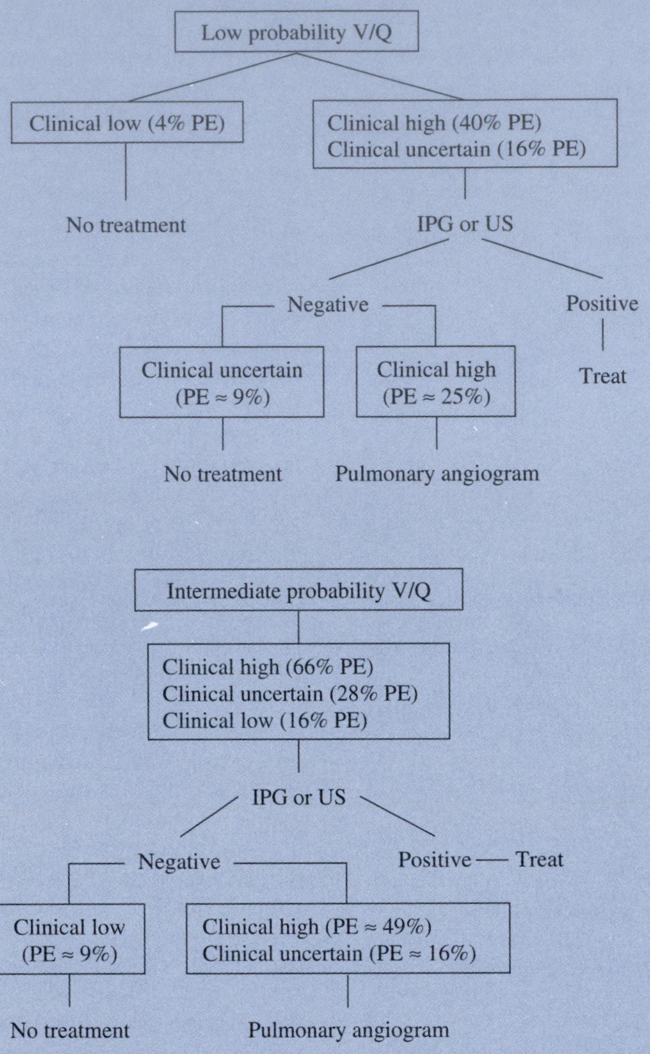


Adapted from Stein PD: *Chest* 103:1553, 1993.
*IPG*, Impedance plethysmography of legs; *US*, ultrasound study of legs.

ECG with evidence of congestive heart failure should direct the focus toward ischemic heart disease. The chest x-ray alone should confirm the presence of a pneumothorax. Irritation of the diaphragm by abdominal processes such as pancreatitis and subdiaphragmatic abscess may also produce lower chest pain and a sense of dyspnea but can usually be distinguished from PE by physical examination. The failure to find a clear alternative diagnosis and the presence of predisposing factors for thromboembolic disease are the diagnostic clues that increase the suspicion for PE and lead to the next level of investigation.

### Management

Heparin remains the initial treatment of choice for DVT and PE unless there are specific contraindications (see further), since it immediately inhibits thrombus formation. Heparin binds to antithrombin III, inducing a conformational change in its active center and allowing antithrombin III to rapidly inactivate factors IIa (thrombin), Xa, and IXa and the body's thrombolytic mechanisms to proceed unopposed. It is important to remember that, although thrombus formation is arrested, heparin does not prevent embolization of already established thrombus. The embolization risk decreases when the thrombus is either dissolved or organized; therefore thromboembolism within the first few days is not a failure of therapy. Heparin's efficacy increases with increasing dosages; however, at higher dosages the risk of bleeding becomes significant, and therapy is usually adjusted to maintain the activated partial thromboplastin time (PTT) in a therapeutic range (one and a half to two and a half times the control). It has been shown that a delay in achieving a

**Table 119-3.** Nomogram for the management of heparin therapy

Initiate therapy with a 5000-U bolus of heparin followed by continuous infusion of heparin, 20,000 U in 500 ml, at 32 ml/hour (1280 U/hour). The PTT is checked 6 hours after the initial bolus, and further dosage changes are made as follows:

| PTT (seconds) | Bolus (U) | Hold dose (minutes) | Rate change (ml/hour)* | Repeat PTT |
|---|---|---|---|---|
| <50† | 5000 | 0 | +3 | 6 hours |
| 50-59 | 0 | 0 | +3 | 6 hours |
| 60-85 | 0 | 0 | 0 | Next morning |
| 86-95 | 0 | 0 | −2 | 6 hours |
| 96-120 | 0 | 30 | −2 | 6 hours |
| >120 | 0 | 60 | −4 | 6 hours |

Modified from Cruickshank MK et al: *Arch Intern Med* 151:333, 1991.
*1 ml/hour = 40 U/hour.
†For PTT <50 seconds in the first 48 hours of therapy, bolus with 5000 U and increase rate by 5 ml/hour.

therapeutic PTT or allowing the PTT to fall into a nontherapeutic range increases the risk of recurrent thrombosis from seven to 15 times, whereas in patients with adequate anticoagulation recurrent thrombus occurs in fewer than 5% of cases. Heparin can be administered by multiple daily subcutaneous injections or be given intravenously. The intravenous route is most common and usually involves a bolus of 5000 to 10,000 U intravenously, followed by an infusion of 1000 U per hour. The dosage of heparin is adjusted according to the PTT drawn every 4 to 6 hours until a therapeutic range has been reached. Thereafter the PTT is checked daily. One published nomogram for managing heparin therapy is shown in Table 119-3. Heparin was usually administered for 7 to 10 days. However, it is now evident that 5 days of heparin therapy (with an appropriately prolonged PTT) is adequate to prevent further thrombosis.

Anticoagulation is continued for 3 months on an outpatient basis with warfarin sodium (Coumadin), maintaining the prothrombin time (PT) at approximately one and a half times control, or an international normalized ratio (INR) of 2.0 to 2.5. There has been a call to standardize the reporting of the PT because thromboplastins of varying sensitivity are in commercial use. The INR, or ratio of patient PT/control $PT^{ISI}$ (ISI is the international sensitivity index for thromboplastin), allows the reporting of therapeutic range to be universally applicable. Coumadin can be started simultaneously with heparin, so after 5 days the INR should be in therapeutic range, allowing the discontinuation of heparin. Coumadin is usually initiated at 10 mg daily for 2 days followed by 5 mg daily, with further adjustments made according to the PT or INR. Coumadin should be continued for 3 months, or indefinitely if a predisposing condition persists.

It has been clearly shown that the use of oral anticoagulants alone for the initial treatment of proximal DVT results in three times the rates of thrombus extension and PE compared with intravenous heparin therapy. When properly diagnosed and treated, recurrence and mortality for PE are 8.3% and 2.5%, respectively. The major complications of these medications must also be considered. The major complication of heparin is hemorrhage, which usually occurs when there is a coexistent disease or coagulopathy, such as uremia, unsuspected peptic ulcer disease, thrombocytopenia, or concomitant aspirin use, but it can occur with a therapeutic PTT. Reversible heparin-associated thrombocytopenia (HAT), mediated by a heparin-IgG immune complex, has been noted more frequently with bovine-derived, as opposed to porcine-derived, heparin. With porcine heparin the incidence of thrombocytopenia is 2.4% for therapeutic heparin, and 0.3% for prophylactic heparin. The usual time of onset is between 3 and 15 days from the onset of therapy. The incidence of arterial or venous thrombosis following the thrombocytopenia is approximately 0.4%. Other heparin complications include osteoporosis, alopecia, skin necrosis, and hypoaldosteronism.

As with heparin, warfarin's major complication is hemorrhage. The rare but serious complication of skin necrosis can occur with the initiation of therapy and is thought to be due to a rapid fall in protein C, a vitamin K–dependent inhibitor of coagulation factors Va and VIIIa. A fall in protein C before reduction of the other factors results in a transient hypercoagulable state with thrombosis of subcutaneous vessels. Treatment requires discontinuation of warfarin and administration of vitamin K.

The low-molecular-weight heparins (LMWH), approved for use in orthopedic DVT prophylaxis (see previously) may offer an alternative to standard unfractionated heparin in the treatment of DVT. There is experimental evidence that subcutaneous LMWH in fixed body weight–adjusted doses may be a better alternative than standard intravenous heparin in treating lower extremity DVT. Avoiding intravenous administration, not having to monitor the PTT, and the ease of outpatient therapy are major potential advantages. LMWH has not yet been evaluated in the treatment of PE. Large clinical trials need to be performed before these become standard therapy. The heparinoid ORG 10172 has been used successfully in cases of heparin-associated thrombocytopenia.

Since the greatest risk for PE occurs in patients with proximal DVT, some clinicians have questioned whether venous thrombi in the calf need to be treated at all. There are studies showing good outcomes without anticoagulation in some settings. Patients with clinically suspected DVT were not given anticoagulants unless there was evidence of proximal extension of thrombus seen on serial IPG of the lower extremities (confirmed venographically). When the IPG remained normal, there were no recurrences of DVT or episodes of symptomatic PE during the follow-up period. A similar trial in patients with clinically suspected PE was performed in which anticoagulation was not initiated as long as serial IPG studies remained negative for proximal thrombus. In 3 months of follow-up the rate of PE was as low as for patients with normal perfusion scans, supporting the belief that thrombi from the proximal veins of the lower extremities are the usual cause of significant PE. The use of serial compression ultrasound in this manner has not been evaluated. Whether serial noninvasive studies are practical, cost effective, and safe remains to be seen.

*Thromboembolic disease in pregnancy.* Pregnancy presents unique problems in thromboembolic disease and its management for a variety of reasons. During pregnancy there is an increase in clotting factors V, VII, VIII, IX, X, XII, and fibrinogen, creating a hypercoagulable state; however, this is usually balanced by an increase in baseline fibrinolytic activity. Other factors that are associated with an increased risk of PE are older maternal age, race, operative delivery, and prior thromboembolism. The diagnostic strategy is as discussed above. The total radiation dose to the fetus from a chest x-ray, V/Q scan, and pulmonary angiogram (via the brachial vein) is approximately 0.05 rad, a low dose, particularly when balanced against the potential fatal effect of a PE.

Heparin is the drug of choice during pregnancy for thromboembolic disease because its size precludes transit across the placenta. The daily requirement of intravenous heparin can be given in two or three daily doses subcutaneously, but monitoring is necessary to ensure that the PTT measured at the midpoint between doses is maintained at one and a half to two times control. The potential risk of osteoporosis with long-term heparin use becomes a problem in this setting; 20,000 U daily for more than 20 weeks is associated with an increased risk of bone demineralization, but even prophylactic heparin may result in vertebral compression fractures in as many as 1.6% of pregnant women. The demineralization is reversible with discontinuation of heparin but may be a slow process.

Warfarin is contraindicated during pregnancy because of well-known teratogenic effects. First-trimester exposure results in a characteristic set of findings including nasal hypoplasia, depressed bridge of the nose, epiphyseal stippling, and a high rate of developmental retardation. Exposure in the second trimester is associated with central nervous system and ophthalmologic abnormalities. Overall, 13% of pregnancies exposed to warfarin result in abnormal infants. The use of thrombolytic agents is reserved for life-threatening situations and carries the risk of placental abruption and fetal death; however, there are anecdotal reports of uncomplicated use of thrombolytic therapy during pregnancy.

*DVT prophylaxis.* Given the natural history of VTE, no other treatment affects patient outcome as much as preventive measures. However, recent surveys indicate that fewer than 50% of patients at high risk for VTE received acceptable DVT prophylaxis. These practice patterns are unacceptable, but education and management strategies are evolving to ameliorate this problem. Key principles for the administration of prophylactic regimens include the following: (1) the risk group has to be well defined; (2) the modality to be used needs to be simple and easily implemented by the common practitioner; and (3) the modality has to be safe for widespread use among many patients. The box above lists the most common modalities used for DVT prophylaxis. These modalities have varying efficacy among the different risk groups. Some, such as graded elastic stockings, should be limited to a few select patient groups and have little applicability to high-risk populations.

**Common prophylaxis modalities for venous thromboembolism***

Graded compression stockings
Intermittent compression devices
Anticoagulants (heparin, low-molecular-weight heparins, warfarin)
Dextran
Antiplatelet agents
(?) Inferior vena cava filter

*Modalities can be used alone or in combination.

The anticoagulant drugs—heparin, warfarin, and LMWH—are by far the most useful agents and are effective in most of the highest risk groups. The LMWH enoxaparin (Lovenox), is the only FDA-approved LMWH agent at this time. It is specifically approved for DVT prophylaxis in hip replacement surgery. All LMWH compounds have different activities and safety profiles. They need to be individually scrutinized in different clinical settings as they become available. For those patients at high risk for VTE a combination of intermittent compression devices and an anticoagulant agent should be strongly considered. Intermittent compression devices when used alone have the disadvantage that they may need to be discontinued at various times for other aspects of care. Table 119-4 summarizes recommended DVT prophylaxis regimens in some common high-risk groups along with the risk reduction afforded by each. Other less effective modalities have been studied, and the reader is referred to other sources for this detailed information.

*Thrombolysis.* Tissue plasminogen activator (TPA), streptokinase, and urokinase are all approved for treatment of PE. The only consensus indication for thrombolytic therapy in acute PE is in the setting of a patient with a submassive or massive emboli and hemodynamic compromise. Many clinicians administer this therapy only after initial resuscitative efforts have failed to restore adequate hemodynamics. Thrombolysis has been shown to accelerate clot lysis and improve hemodynamics within hours. Moreover, peripheral intravenous administration was found to be equivalent to intrapulmonary artery administration allowing for rapid administration of these drugs. At day 7, though, the effects of thrombolytics followed by heparin were equivalent to heparin alone. Furthermore, thrombolysis has not been shown to improve

**Table 119-4.** Deep venous thrombosis prophylaxis: incidence and risk reduction with the currently recommended agents

| Condition | DVT incidence | Prophylaxis | Risk reduction |
|---|---|---|---|
| General surgery | 25% | ES | 63% |
| | | ICD | 61% |
| | | LDH | 68% |
| Hip replacement | 50% | LD warfarin | 63% |
| | | Adjusted LDH | 77% |
| | | LMW | 68% |
| Spinal cord injury | 70%-90% | Adjusted LDH | >70% |
| | | (LMW) | >70% |
| Elective neurosurgery | 25% | ICD | 73% |
| Myocardial infarction | 25% | LDH | 72% |
| Ischemic stroke | 47% | LDH | 45% |
| | | (LMW) | 79% |
| ICU patients | 50% | LDH | 50% |
| Immobile medical patients | — | LDH | 31% reduction in hospital mortality |

Modified from Clagett GP et al: *Chest* 102:391S, 1992.

*ES*, Graded elastic stockings; *ICD*, intermittent calf-thigh compression devices; *adjusted LDH*, low-dose heparin adjusted to high normal or 1.5 × PTT; *LDH*, heparin, 5000 U SC q8-12 h; *LMW*, enoxaparin 30 mg SC bid, 7-10 days; *(LMW)*, unapproved low-molecular-weight heparin compound; *LD warfarin*, various protocols.

mortality in patients with PE, nor will any trial be forthcoming to study this question in a larger number of hemodynamically compromised patients. Other trials looking at the safety and efficacy of thrombolytics in patients with submassive or massive PE but without hemodynamic compromise are in progress. In addition, like other applications of thrombolytic agents, protocols are being tested with varying dosage ranges and times of administration in an attempt to increase efficacy and improve safety.

The use of thrombolytic agents in patients who have a documented DVT only and no symptoms or evidence of a PE is more controversial. Studies are in progress to evaluate the risk/benefit profile of this therapy in this setting. Many clinicians strongly consider the use of these drugs in a patient with an acute, iliofemoral thrombosis so as to prevent long-term severe disability. Data thus far have been limited. Whereas some studies have shown more complete and earlier recovery of venous flow, long-term venous competence and decreased morbidity have yet to be demonstrated. The benefits of this management approach in patients for DVT alone need to be balanced with the small, but remaining, risks of major hemorrhage, including intracranial hemorrhage. The standard of care for DVT remains heparinization followed by warfarin therapy.

### Inferior vena cava (IVC) filters

**Recommended indications***

***To prevent PE with documented VTE (common, well accepted)***

Treatment failure with anticoagulation
Patient is unable to be anticoagulated

***To prevent death from recurrent PE while also giving anticoagulation (controversial, varying practice patterns)***

After an acute, massive PE
If IVC or large proximal thrombus visualized
In chronic pulmonary hypertension from recurrent PE

***To prevent PE in patients at high risk for VTE (controversial, varying practice patterns)***

Trauma patients
Other high-risk groups

**Complications**

Incorrect placement
Hematoma at insertion site (rare with new designs)
Venous thrombosis at insertion site (2%)
Recurrent PE (2%)
Worsened symptoms of venous insufficiency (5%)
Migration compromising function (rare)
Fatal complications (<0.5%)

*None of the indications have been proven in well-designed trials.

***IVC filters.*** Inferior vena cava (IVC) ligation is a therapy that dates as far back as the late 1800s. This therapy has the untoward side effects of severe venous stasis, and the development of venous collateral flow may again lead to life-threatening PE. Therefore alternative methods of treatment were needed to prevent PE in instances where standard therapy had failed or was not feasible. Over the last 20 years IVC filters have been in use. The most widely used design has been the Greenfield filter, but newer designs have been implemented over the last 5 years. These filters can trap emboli as small as 2 mm in diameter. In addition, the filter design allows for a significant proportion of its volume to be obstructed while preserving a sufficient cross-sectional area for proximal venous flow. The recommended indications and complications of these devices are included in the box above. None of the indications has been substantiated by controlled, clinical trials. However, the decreased rate of PE reported with these devices as compared to untreated

DVT legitimizes their common application in cases where anticoagulation has failed or cannot be administered. In addition, certain clinicians have advocated more widespread use of these devices without the need for supportive data because of their low risk of complication and potential benefit. However, this view is controversial, and the use of IVC filters for other clinical circumstances is quite variable. Some of these expanded indications are also included in the box on p. 1613. In a multicenter prospective study no increased embolic risk was seen if IVC thrombosis was present, as compared with more peripheral thrombosis in anticoagulated patients. Therefore this one small study would not favor employing an IVC filter if one happened to document an IVC thrombosis. Complications from placement of these devices are now quite rare. Given the low, but remaining, risk of a venous thrombosis at the insertion site, a femoral vein approach remains the preferred route. Fortunately, worsening symptoms of venous insufficiency are also uncommon. If safe, anticoagulation is recommended concurrently with these devices to prevent filter obstruction and decrease the incidence of venous insufficiency.

***Chronic major vessel thromboembolic pulmonary hypertension.*** These patients come to medical attention because of severe, undiagnosed exertional dyspnea. Like other patients with pulmonary hypertension, the degree of symptoms is usually quite severe at presentation. Those patients with mean pulmonary artery pressures greater than 35 mm Hg who are symptomatic should have a thorough evaluation to determine if they are candidates for surgical therapy. The surgical options include pulmonary thromboendarterectomy and lung transplantation. Thromboendarterectomy does incur a 10% to 15% perioperative mortality, but survivors recover well enough to return to work or other usual activities. Candidates for this major surgery need to have a proximal, organized, pulmonary vascular thrombus demonstrated. The imaging procedures most helpful in defining the anatomic location of the thrombus are the pulmonary angiogram and the helical CT scan of the thorax with contrast. Perfusion scanning invariably shows a segmental or larger defect but usually underestimates the degree of obstruction. Those who are not candidates for endarterectomy can be considered for single- or double-lung transplantation. All patients should have oxygen therapy scrupulously administered as necessary to keep their $SaO_2$ at or above 90% at rest, with sleep, and with exertion. Most clinicians do recommend lifelong anticoagulation and an IVC filter for these patients. As shown in Fig. 119-1, only a small number of patients develop this complication. In those who do have a previous history of VTE it is not clear what predisposed them to this condition. Despite the small number of patients and unknown risk factors, some clinicians are advocating thrombolytic therapy in patients with acute, submassive, or massive PE without hemodynamic compromise to avoid this complication. Thrombolytic therapy has no proven value for this chronic condition and may also be hazardous.

## SEPTIC EMBOLISM

In several situations bacterial infections can result in vascular injury and subsequent thrombosis. If the offending organisms infect the thrombus, a friable mass of bacteria and clot develops with subsequent embolization of small particles. This results in both small vessel obstruction and delivery of infectious organisms to distal sites. This is most often seen following obstetric-gynecologic procedures, with intravenous drug abuse, infections of indwelling medical devices (e.g., central venous catheters, pacemakers), and occasionally after other infections that involve the vasculature. Patients usually have a febrile illness followed by dyspnea, a productive cough, and variable hemoptysis. Pleuritic chest pain and pleural effusions are not uncommon. The chest x-ray is characteristic, demonstrating multiple small peripheral densities with a characteristic evolution. Older lesions may cavitate as newer lesions appear. Septic pelvic thrombophlebitis is more difficult to diagnose, often presenting as a fever of unclear etiology with the onset after an obstetric-gynecologic procedure. Treatment consists of antibiotics to empirically cover the most likely bacteria, anaerobes, and staphylococci. An infected prosthetic device must be removed and cultured. If there is no response to antibiotics, anticoagulation with heparin and/or surgical ligation of the offending vessel(s) should be considered.

## FAT EMBOLISM

Fat embolism is a well-described complication of skeletal trauma, particularly in the setting of multiple long bone fractures. Intramedullary fat enters the venous circulation and embolizes to the lung. Clinical signs and symptoms range from a subclinical form to a fulminant syndrome consisting of a petechial rash, respiratory distress, and an altered sensorium. The onset of symptoms occurs most often within the first 48 hours after the trauma. The systemic signs and symptoms are felt to be secondary to the release of toxic free fatty acids from embolized fatty material. Treatment is supportive. Steroids have been effective in preventing the systemic components of the syndrome in animal studies but disappointing for treatment of patients who manifest the full clinical syndrome.

## AMNIOTIC FLUID EMBOLISM

Amniotic fluid embolism is a rare syndrome consisting of the sudden and dramatic onset of hypotension, hypoxemia, and coagulopathy (DIC) with a mortality as high as 80%. It occurs most often in the setting of labor but is also seen with placental abruption, abortion, abdominal trauma, and amniocentesis. It is felt to be the result of passage of amniotic fluid and its particulates to the systemic venous circulation, with obstruction of small pulmonary arteries. Prostaglandin and the leukotrienes produced have vasoactive properties that could account for the hemodynamic and hematologic effects. Amniotic fluid itself may be a procoagulant contributing to the coagulopathy by stimulating platelet aggregation and activation of factor X. The finding of fetal particulate debris in the venous circulation of asymptomatic pregnant women suggests that some other abnormal substance in amniotic fluid may be important. Treatment is supportive and includes supplemental oxygen, mechanical ventilation for respiratory failure, fluids and vasopressor medication guided by a pulmonary artery, catheter, and red blood cell and fresh frozen plasma transfusion.

## PULMONARY HYPERTENSIVE DISEASES

Although flow through the pulmonary circulation usually equals that through the systemic circulation, pulmonary artery pressures are normally much lower than those in the systemic arteries. This difference in arterial pressure reflects the proportionately lower resistance of the pulmonary vessels than those in the systemic counterparts. Furthermore, the pulmonary circulation has a high compliance, and nonmuscularized small vessels and capillaries are very distensible. Therefore significant increases in pulmonary blood flow are accommodated with only slight increases in pressure. According to the Poiseuille law describing flow through a tube, resistance to flow is inversely proportional to the luminal radius. Therefore, as vascular remodeling changes occur and the pulmonary arterioles are narrowed, resistance may increase precipitously, leading to significant increases in pulmonary artery pressure at normal blood flows. For obstructive vascular diseases, such as pulmonary thromboemboli, increases in pulmonary artery pressure are usually not evident unless more than 50% of the vascular bed has been lost. A diagnosis of pulmonary arterial hypertension is made when resting systolic pressures exceed 30 mm Hg, diastolic pressures exceed 15 mm Hg, and the mean pressure is greater than 18 mm Hg. Since extensive pulmonary vascular changes are often present before pulmonary arterial hypertension results, many patients develop symptoms and come to medical attention at an advanced stage of their disease.

### Etiology

As indicated in the box below, many different causes of pulmonary hypertension have been described. Wood described six general mechanisms that lead to pulmonary hypertension. These are listed in Table 119-5 with common examples of each.

Although thromboembolic disease usually involves macroscopic clots that cause a heterogenous loss of pulmonary vessels reflected by irregular perfusion scans or angiograms, multiple small emboli may occasionally result in a relatively uniform distribution of vascular obstruction, thereby complicating diagnosis. In situ thrombosis is particularly common in patients with sickle cell disease and may also occur with the hypercoagulable states. The hypertensive effects of either the obstructive or restrictive lung diseases may be related to obliteration of pulmonary blood vessels along with the primary lung destruction. Alternatively, hypoxia may be a significant contributor to the pulmonary hypertension in these individuals. Hypoxia is one of the most potent pulmonary vasoconstrictors, and administration of oxygen may acutely reverse some of the elevation in pulmonary arterial pressure. However, chronic hypoxia can lead to vascular remodeling changes that may be only partially reversed over time. Chronic exposure to high flows in patients with left-to-right shunts through atrial or ventricular septal defects results in what eventually may become irreversible changes in the pulmonary vasculature. Similarly, chronically elevated left atrial pressures associated with mitral stenosis or atrial myxomas as well as diseases that increase the resistance of the pulmonary venous system may also cause pulmonary arterial hypertension. Collagen vascular disease may cause pulmonary hypertension by interstitial lung disease or primary vascular involvement. The prognosis is quite poor in those patients who do develop pulmonary vasculitis or other primary pulmonary vascular changes. Portal hypertension from hepatic or extrahepatic origin is associated with pulmonary hypertension that can be quite severe. These patients usually do not have hepatopulmonary syndrome and therefore usually have normal $PaO_2$ values at rest. Primary pulmonary hypertension is defined by a process of exclusion when no other cause for the disorder can be found. It is more frequent among young adult women, but the pathogenesis remains obscure. A primary defect in endothelial cell function and endothelial cell–smooth muscle cell signaling is being actively investigated.

### Clinical manifestations and diagnosis

Unfortunately, most patients with pulmonary hypertension develop symptoms only after their underlying disorder is quite advanced. Dyspnea on effort and eventually dyspnea at rest are the most common complaints expressed by patients with severe pulmonary artery hypertension. Any persistent complaint of effort intolerance should be taken

### Causes of pulmonary hypertensive disorders

**Acute disorders**

- Acute pulmonary embolic diseases
- Acute lung injury
- Acute hypoxic vasoconstriction (various causes)
- Pulmonary hypertensive crisis with congenital heart or mitral valve disease

**Chronic disorders**

- Chronic embolic disorders
- Hypoventilation syndromes
- Obstructive airways diseases
- Interstitial lung diseases
- Thoracic cage deformities
- Cardiac abnormalities
- Disorders causing pulmonary venous compression or obstruction
- Idiopathic, associated with portal hypertension
- Primary pulmonary hypertension

**Table 119-5.** Pulmonary hypertension mechanisms

| Mechanism | Example |
|---|---|
| Passive | Pulmonary venous hypertension from congestive heart failure |
| Hyperkinetic | Congenital heart disease with left-to-right shunt |
| Obstructive | Pulmonary embolus |
| Obliterative | Interstitial lung disease |
| Vasoconstrictive | Hypoxic pulmonary vasoconstriction |
| Multifactorial | Primary pulmonary hypertension |

Described by Paul Wood, MD, 1958.

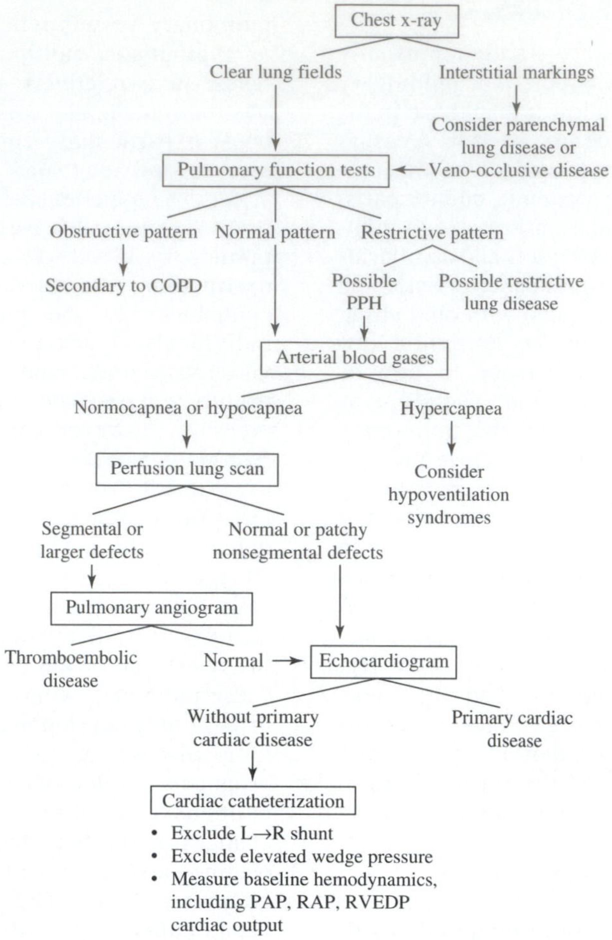


**Fig. 119-4.** Algorithm for the investigation of causes of pulmonary hypertension. (In Rich S: *Prog Cardiovasc Dis* 31:205, 1988.)

seriously. Pulmonary hypertension may be associated with substernal chest pain that can be indistinguishable from angina. However, it may be attributable to distention of the pulmonary artery rather than myocardial ischemia. As pulmonary vascular changes progress, resistance increases and cardiac output falls, leading to further limitation and occasionally syncopal episodes. Hemoptysis is uncommonly observed. As pulmonary vascular resistance becomes excessive, the right side of the heart dilates and right atrial and right ventricular end-diastolic pressures rise. Systemic venous hypertension is required for adequate venous return, and peripheral edema is apparent.

Other typical signs of pulmonary arterial hypertension and cor pulmonale include jugular venous distention, jugular venous v waves, a palpable pulmonary artery impulse, and a precordial lift from right ventricular hypertrophy and distention. On auscultation a loud pulmonic component of the second heart sound and right-sided $S_3$ or $S_4$ may be heard. Holosystolic and diastolic murmurs may be present when tricuspid or pulmonary valvular regurgitation is present, respectively. As cardiac function declines, peripheral edema, cyanosis, and other signs of hypoperfusion can be seen. Raynaud phenomenon can often be demonstrated in patients with collagen vascular disease or primary pulmonary hypertension. Flow murmurs over the lung fields have been described in patients with chronic pulmonary hypertension from PE.

The general diagnostic approach to the patient with suspected pulmonary hypertension is presented in Fig. 119-4. Chest x-rays can provide information regarding any lung disorder as well as the general vascular changes seen with these diseases. The central pulmonary vessels are often dilated, and a right descending pulmonary artery that is greater than 19 mm in diameter suggests pulmonary hypertension. Oligemia can be present in the more peripheral regions of the lungs. Disorders that raise pulmonary venous pressure, including pulmonary venoocclusive disease, may lead to pulmonary edema. Arterial $PO_2$ at rest may be normal but tends to fall with exercise, and as the $PO_2$ falls, the A-a $O_2$ gradient increases. Hypoxemia stimulates ventilation, and a compensated respiratory alkalosis is a common event. The $V_{DS}/V_T$ may be relatively high because some ventilated regions of the lungs are underperfused, and it may fail to fall in a normal fashion with exercise. Diffusing capacity ($D_LCO$) usually decreases as the pulmonary vasculature is lost. However, decreases in $D_LCO$ can be mild in patients with primary pulmonary hypertension or other diseases that primarily affect the pulmonary blood vessels alone. Serologic studies are helpful for diagnosis of the collagen vascular diseases.

### Chronic pulmonary hypertensive disease treatment options

Treat underlying pulmonary disorder
Oxygen therapy: keep $SaO_2$ >90%
Anticoagulation
Pulmonary vasodilator therapy*
  Chronic oral agents
  Continuous IV prostacyclin infusion
Surgical options
  Correction of specific cardiac lesion
  Lung or heart-lung transplantation
  Blade septostomy for recurrent syncope
  Thromboendarterectomy for chronic PE

*Vasodilators should be initiated in the ICU with adequate monitoring.

Echocardiography is quite useful because it permits evaluation of the right ventricle. Color Doppler evaluation allows estimation of pulmonary artery systolic pressure if tricuspid regurgitation is present. Furthermore, these studies can be conducted with injections of solutions that generate microbubbles, which are visible on the echocardiograms to identify the presence of shunting of blood from the right side of the heart to the left through a septal defect or patent foramen ovale. ECGs are abnormal in the majority of patients, and evidence of right axis deviation, right ventricular hypertrophy with strain, and right atrial enlargement is common. Perfusion scans and pulmonary arteriography are essential for detecting pulmonary thromboembolic disease. Infused helical CT scan of the thorax is helpful for chronic thromboembolic disease. Ultimately cardiac catheterization is frequently needed to rule out congenital heart defects and obtain accurate hemodynamics on the right side of the heart and to evaluate the efficacy of acute and chronic therapy.

### Treatment

General treatment options for pulmonary hypertension are summarized in the box above. When pulmonary artery hypertension is secondary to some known underlying disease, treatment of the primary disorder is obviously indicated. Similarly, if the pulmonary artery hypertension is due to hypoxemia (e.g., in obesity hypoventilation), then correction of hypoxemia may yield lower pulmonary artery pressures and improved right-sided heart function. On the other hand, many patients are quite ill at the time of presentation and treatment options are limited. Patients with primary pulmonary hypertension experience symptomatic benefit from vasodilator therapy if their pulmonary vascular resistance decreases by 30% or more. Moreover, recent studies have shown improved survival from titrated, high-dose calcium channel blockers or continuous intravenous prostacyclin therapy. Unfortunately, only 15% to 20% of patients with primary pulmonary hypertension respond to vasodilator therapy. Patients with secondary pulmonary hypertension are not as likely to respond to vasodilator therapy, and they need to be carefully selected for vasodilator trials. Furthermore, these agents can cause systemic hypotension, which limits their application and requires hemodynamic monitoring in the ICU when they are initiated. Warfarin also improves survival in patients with primary pulmonary hypertension independent of their response to other therapy. No convincing data are available with regard to the use of anticoagulants in the other disorders, with the exception of venous thromboembolism. Some of the patients with end-stage disease from pulmonary hypertension are candidates for lung transplantation. The need for serious consideration of transplantation is signaled by worsening right-sided heart failure with rising right atrial pressures and decreasing cardiac output. Inhaled nitric oxide has been used as a selective pulmonary vasodilator in certain patient groups. However, its value for evaluation and treatment of patients with chronic pulmonary hypertensive diseases is not defined.

## BIBLIOGRAPHY

Becker DM, Philbrick JT, Selby JB: Inferior vena cava filters: indications, safety, effectiveness, *Arch Intern Med* 152:1985, 1992.
Carson JL et al: The clinical course of pulmonary embolism, *N Engl J Med* 326:1240, 1992.
Clagett GP et al: Prevention of venous thromboembolism, *Chest* 102 (suppl):391S, 1992.
Hull RD: A noninvasive strategy for the treatment of patients with suspected pulmonary embolism, *Arch Intern Med* 154:289, 1994.
Moser KM: Venous thromboembolism, *Am Rev Respir Dis* 141:235, 1990.
Moser KM, Auger WR, Fedullo PF: Chronic major-vessel thromboembolic pulmonary hypertension, *Circulation* 81:1735, 1990.
The PIOPED Investigators: Value of the ventilation/perfusion scan in acute pulmonary embolism. Results of the prospective investigation of pulmonary embolism diagnosis (PIOPED), *JAMA* 263:2753, 1990.
Presberg KW, Wood LDH: Critical illness due to pulmonary hypertension and cor pulmonale. In Hall JB, Schmidt GA, Wood LDH, editors: *Principles of critical care,* New York, 1992, McGraw-Hill.
Urokinase Pulmonary Embolism Trial, *JAMA* 214:2163, 1970.

CHAPTER

# 120 Neoplasms of the Lung

**Akira Funahashi**

## BENIGN NEOPLASMS

Benign neoplasms of the lung account for no more than 5% of all neoplasms of the lung. Benign neoplasms include hamartoma, fibroma, leiomyoma, lipoma, and others. Among these benign neoplasms, only hamartoma is clinically important.

### Hamartoma

Hamartoma is the most common benign neoplasm of the lung. It is believed to be congenital in origin. Histologically, hamartoma contains cartilage, smooth muscle, and mucus-secreting glands. The majority of hamartomas appear as a small, peripheral nodular density on the chest radiograph and may show a popcorn-type calcification.

When there is no clear calcification on the chest radiograph, a computed tomography (CT) scan may reveal a calcification or a characteristic fat density that allows the diagnosis of hamartoma. If there is no calcification to indicate the benign nature of the lesion, it is often necessary to perform a thoracotomy for a definitive diagnosis, since commonly applied diagnostic procedures, such as fiberoptic bronchoscopy (FOB) and transthoracic needle aspiration (TNA), often do not yield a definitive diagnosis (see section on solitary pulmonary nodule). Rarely a hamartoma presents as an endobronchial mass lesion with the clinical and radiographic signs of an obstructive endobronchial lesion, such as a cough, repeated episodes of pneumonia, and atelectasis.

If the radiographic or CT scan appearance makes the diagnosis of hamartoma certain, no treatment is necessary. However, if the diagnosis is uncertain, the lesion should be excised. Generally, an endobronchial hamartoma also requires surgical resection because the diagnosis remains uncertain due to small biopsy samples obtained by FOB. If the diagnosis is certain, a local treatment with an yttrium-aluminum-garnet (YAG) laser can be considered.

### Bronchial adenoma

The term *bronchial adenoma* was once used to refer to bronchial carcinoid, bronchial cylindroma (adenoid cystic), and mucoepidermoid carcinomas. They comprise approximately 90%, 8%, and 2% of cases, respectively. Because these tumors are histologically distinct, they are no longer categorized together under the heading of bronchial adenoma. All three are low-grade malignant tumors and should be separated from bronchial adenomas (bronchial cystadenoma and mucoepidermoid adenoma), which are rare, but truly benign, neoplasms.

### Bronchial carcinoid

The majority of bronchial carcinoids occur in the larger, centrally located bronchi, and only 20% or less originate in the peripheral airways. Bronchial carcinoids are believed to originate in the neurosecretory cells of the bronchial mucosa. Histologically they are composed of small polyhedral cells grouped in nests, trabeculae, or poorly developed tubercles.

The clinical presentation and radiographic findings of bronchial carcinoid differ greatly depending on the location and size of the tumor. Centrally located bronchial carcinoids usually grow into the bronchial lumen; thus the patient commonly presents with symptoms associated with airway involvement, such as cough and dyspnea. Because bronchial carcinoids are highly vascular, nearly 50% of the patients have hemoptysis. If a tumor obstructs the bronchus, the patient may present with symptoms of pneumonia distal to the obstructed bronchus. Unlike carcinoid tumor of the gastrointestinal (GI) tract, carcinoid syndrome with bronchial carcinoid is very rare. Radiographic findings of bronchial carcinoid also vary greatly. In patients with a centrally located bronchial carcinoid without bronchial obstruction, a chest radiograph often shows a centrally located mass lesion. If bronchial obstruction is present, there is usually atelectasis or pneumonic infiltrates distal to the obstruction. If the tumor growth is limited within the bronchial lumen and there is no obstruction, the chest radiograph may be completely normal. When a relatively young individual, particularly a nonsmoker, presents with hemoptysis with a normal chest radiograph, the physician should suspect the possibility of bronchial carcinoid and an FOB should be performed. When bronchial carcinoid originates from a small peripheral airway, the patient is usually asymptomatic and the lesion is discovered as an incidental finding on the chest radiograph. Establishing the diagnosis of a centrally located bronchial carcinoid is relatively easy once the diagnosis is suspected. In the past, a forceps biopsy at the time of bronchoscopy with a rigid bronchoscope was considered to be contraindicated due to the potential of massive bleeding. With the advent of FOB and the relatively smaller size of biopsy forceps, a forceps biopsy has been performed safely in some cases. However, the danger of massive hemoptysis should be kept in mind if a biopsy is performed. A thoracotomy is often required for the definitive diagnosis of a peripherally located carcinoid.

The treatment of bronchial carcinoid is a surgical resection. The prognosis after surgical resection is generally favorable (5-year survival is 90%). However, bronchial carcinoids vary in their potential for malignancy, and metastases and death occur early in some cases.

### Bronchial cylindroma (adenoid cystic carcinoma)

Unlike bronchial carcinoid, which arises from neurosecretory cells, bronchial cylindroma arises from the bronchial mucous gland. Microscopically these consist of interlacing cylinders of tumor cells, the centers of which are often canalized to form tubular spaces.

Since this tumor grows into bronchial lumen, the clinical and radiographic presentations are those of endobronchial mass lesions that cause cough, dyspnea, and hemoptysis. Treatment is surgical excision, but there may be a local recurrence.

## CARCINOMA

### Epidemiology and etiology

Carcinoma of the lung is closely associated with cigarette smoking. As the worldwide consumption of cigarettes has increased over the past several decades, the sharp increase in the incidence of carcinoma of the lung has become an international problem. According to one estimate, approximately 2 million people will develop carcinoma of the lung annually by the year 2000. In the United States the predicted incidence of lung carcinoma in 1995 is 170,000 (100,000 males, 70,000 females) with an estimated mortality of 149,000 (93,000 males, 56,000 females). Lung carcinoma is now the leading cause of death among all types of malignancies for both sexes in the United States, although it remains less frequent than prostate carcinoma in males and breast carcinoma in females.

Most lung carcinomas are due to the use of tobacco products, notably cigarettes. It is estimated that 85% of all lung carcinomas are secondary to cigarette use. Other causes include exposure to materials such as asbestos, uranium, and radon. Chronic interstitial lung diseases, such as pulmonary fibrosis due to scleroderma, are associated with lung carcinoma. Carcinoma may also arise at the site of scarring of the lung produced by other diseases, including tuberculosis. There is clear-cut evidence that the effect of smoking and asbestos exposure are synergistic, meaning that smokers who are exposed to asbestos have a much higher incidence of lung carcinoma than smokers not exposed or than asbestos workers who do not smoke (50 to 90 times higher). There is some evidence that passive smoking is a risk factor for lung carcinoma. There is undoubtedly a genetic predisposition for lung carcinoma because only a minority of cigarette smokers develop the disease.

## Histopathology

Most lung carcinomas belong to four major cell types: squamous cell carcinoma, adenocarcinoma, large-cell carcinoma, and small-cell carcinoma. Because of the similarities in response to treatment and prognosis, the first three cell types are often grouped together as non–small-cell carcinomas to distinguish them from small-cell carcinomas, which behave quite differently. A significant number of tumors have more than one cell type in the same specimen and are classified as mixed non–small-cell carcinomas. Small-cell carcinomas mixed with non–small-cell carcinomas are uncommon, however. In the past, squamous cell carcinoma was the most common cell type. However, recent observations indicate that there has been a decline in squamous cell carcinomas and an increase in adenocarcinomas, which have become the most common cell type.

***Squamous cell carcinomas.*** Squamous cell carcinomas (30% to 35% of all lung carcinomas) often originate in the mucosa of relatively large airways (trachea, mainstem bronchi, and lobar bronchi) and less commonly in the peripheral airways. Mucosal changes progress slowly from hyperplasia to metaplasia, dysplasia, carcinoma in situ, and finally to invasive carcinoma. Characteristic features of squamous cell carcinoma are keratin formation and intercellular bridges. A chest radiograph often shows a central lesion with hilar or mediastinal involvement. Presentation as a small peripheral nodule is less common.

***Adenocarcinomas.*** Adenocarcinomas (approximately 35% to 40% of all cases) frequently originate in relatively small airways; consequently, they are often asymptomatic and found in the middle and peripheral areas of the lung on the chest radiograph. Histologically, they are characterized by gland formation and mucin production. Bronchoalveolar cell type is a subset of adenocarcinoma. This carcinoma is believed to originate from alveolar wall cells and tends to show an infiltrative pattern on chest radiograph that is indistinguishable from infectious and inflammatory processes. Early intrapulmonary metastases are common and may cause profuse bronchorrhea.

***Large-cell carcinomas.*** Large-cell carcinomas (approximately 10% of all cases) are relatively undifferentiated histologically. Giant-cell carcinoma is a subset of large-cell carcinoma and has a particularly poor prognosis. Radiographically, large-cell carcinomas tend to appear as large mass lesions in the middle and peripheral lung zones.

***Small-cell carcinomas.*** Small-cell carcinomas (approximately 20% to 25% of all cases) are histologically subdivided into oat cell and intermediate cell types. They show small hyperchromatic nuclei with little discernible internal architecture, inconspicuous nucleoli, and scant cytoplasm. They often present as a large hilar and/or mediastinal mass on the chest radiograph. Occasionally a small-cell carcinoma presents as a peripheral solitary mass.

## Clinical manifestations

***History.*** The history is often nonspecific, and the physician must have a high index of suspicion for possible lung carcinoma when faced with a middle-aged smoker who presents with respiratory complaints. In the past the male sex was emphasized, but the rapidly increasing incidence of lung carcinoma in females has made gender an irrelevant issue. Any smoker who has more than a 40-pack year history of cigarette smoking should be considered at high risk to develop lung carcinoma. Since many smokers have smoker's cough and often have chronic obstructive pulmonary disease (COPD) with dyspnea, careful questioning is necessary to identify subtle symptoms. Any change in the pattern of cough or increase in the degree of dyspnea without apparent reason is often the only clue for the presence of lung carcinoma. Blood-tinged sputum without a preceding episode of respiratory infection or frank hemoptysis warrants a chest radiograph. A word of caution is that a chest radiograph that does not exhibit an abnormality suggesting lung carcinoma does not rule out the presence of lung carcinoma. FOB is often indicated for patients at high risk for developing carcinoma of the lung who have blood-tinged sputum or hemoptysis, regardless of radiographic findings. Chest wall pain is a relatively uncommon complaint and is usually attributable to metastases to the ribs or a pleural effusion. Patients with a pneumonia that initially responds to antibiotic treatment but shows poor radiographic resolution after 4 to 6 weeks of follow-up may have bronchial narrowing or obstruction from carcinoma of the lung.

***Physical examination.*** Physical examination of patients with lung carcinoma is often unrevealing unless the carcinoma is sufficiently advanced to cause obstruction of major airways, a pleural effusion, or bone or brain metastases. Unilateral or localized wheezing is an important sign of airway narrowing. Careful examination of the neck may reveal an enlarged supraclavicular lymph node(s) or a prominent vascular pattern due to obstruction of the superior vena cava. Patients with a superior sulcus tumor that originates in the pulmonary superior sulcus often present with long-standing shoulder pain that may radiate to the arm. This tumor often invades the brachial plexus and may cause Horner's syndrome (ptosis, miosis, and loss of sweating on the forehead). Clubbing of the digits, particularly of recent onset, suggests the presence of lung carcinoma because chronic obstructive lung disease alone does not cause clubbing. Weakness of the extremities, particularly in the legs, may be due to the presence of a small-cell carcinoma of the lung. This is referred to as Eaton-Lambert syndrome. In this syndrome the chest radiograph usually shows obvious abnormalities. Occasionally, however, profound neurologic findings dominate the clinical picture with very subtle chest radiographic findings. In these situations establishing the diagnosis of lung carcinoma may be difficult and is often delayed.

***Laboratory findings.*** Laboratory studies of lung carcinoma are nonspecific and do not contribute to the diagnosis. Hypercalcemia associated with lung carcinoma is usually due to parathyroid hormone–like substances secreted by the tumor rather than to bony metastases and is usually seen in patients with squamous cell carcinoma. Hyponatremia may be associated with small-cell lung carcinoma and is often due to the syndrome of inappropriate antidiuretic hormone secretion (SIADH). There are a number of other paraneoplastic syndromes associated with lung carcinoma, but they are clinically less important.

## Diagnosis

Since history, physical examination, and laboratory findings are usually nonspecific, the key to the diagnosis of lung carcinoma is frequently the chest radiograph, which often provides the first clue to diagnosis. The decision of when to obtain a radiograph is of utmost importance. When a patient presents with a recent onset of respiratory complaints, such as a newly developed cough, a changing pattern of cough, or an insidious increase of dyspnea, a chest radiograph should be obtained. Obviously, a chest radiograph is required when a patient complains of blood-tinged sputum or of hemoptysis.

Chest radiographic findings of lung carcinoma vary. Commonly there are parenchymal infiltrates or a mass lesion with hilar or mediastinal lymph node enlargement. These changes are often associated with atelectasis or volume loss of the lung in cases of carcinoma originating in large, central airways. Signs of volume loss include displacement of the normal anatomic structure, such as the mediastinum, large airways, and an elevation of diaphragm (Fig. 120-1). These findings on the chest radiograph should raise the suspicion of an endobronchial process causing a narrowing or obstruction of the airways, even without a parenchymal abnormality. Recurrent pneumonia in the same lobe within several months or a slow resolution of infiltrates on chest radiograph also suggests a narrowed bronchial lumen. When a carcinoma arises from a small peripheral airway in the case of an adenocarcinoma or some squamous cell carcinomas, it usually appears as a relatively small nodular lesion; however, it may grow large and cavitate. If the lesion shows a cavitation, it is usually a squamous cell carcinoma (Fig. 120-2). Small-cell carcinomas tend to present as central lesions with extensive involvement of mediastinal and hilar lymph nodes (Fig. 120-3). Unusual presentations include extensive pneumonic infiltrates that may involve more than one lobe and that mimic an infectious process without clinical evidence of pneumonia. This is characteristically seen in bronchoalveolar cell carcinomas (Fig. 120-4). The key to a correct diagnosis of lung carcinoma is a high index of suspicion when the physician is faced with a middle-aged smoker whose chest radiographs are abnormal. Regardless of the chest radiographic abnormality, the diagnosis of lung carcinoma requires tissue confirmation.

***Cytopathology.*** A cytologic examination of daily morning sputum for three days should be obtained if the patient produces sputum. Various methods of sputum induction can be applied for patients who are unable to produce sputum samples. The most commonly used method is for the patient to inhale a nebulized solution of 10% to 15% saline and 15% to 20% propylene glycol heated to 110° F. The overall diagnostic yield of a cytologic examination of sputum is approximately 60% to 65%. The larger and more centrally located the lesion, the more likely it is that the cytology will be positive. In small peripheral lesions the yield is very low unless the patient has bloody sputum or the lesion shows cavitation on the chest radiograph, both of which are evidence of an endobronchial component. If the patient has a pleural effusion, thoracentesis and a cytologic examination of the fluid are essential, not only to establish the diagnosis, but also to determine if the effusion contains malignant cells. The presence of pleural effusion in association with known lung carcinoma does not necessarily mean that the carcinomatous process has extended to the pleura. For example, the fluid may be present as parapneumonic fluid secondary to pneumonia distal to an obstructed bronchus. This distinction is important, since the presence of a malignant effusion precludes surgery. Thoracentesis combined with a pleural biopsy via closed needle often increases the diagnostic yield.

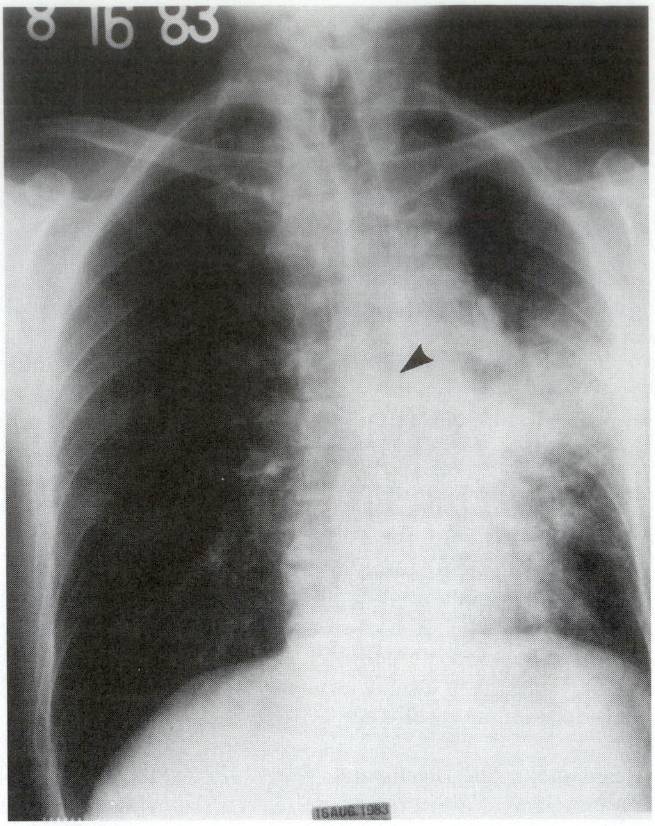


**Fig. 120-1.** Squamous cell carcinoma originating from the distal left main stem bronchus (*arrow*). Note the shifting of the mediastinum and trachea and an elevation of the left diaphragm.

***Fiberoptic bronchoscopy.*** FOB was originally developed to improve the diagnostic yield of carcinoma of the lung (see section on bronchoscopy). It is still the most important tool in the diagnosis and evaluation of carcinoma of the lung. Generally, it is performed under local anesthesia and does not require hospitalization. It can be

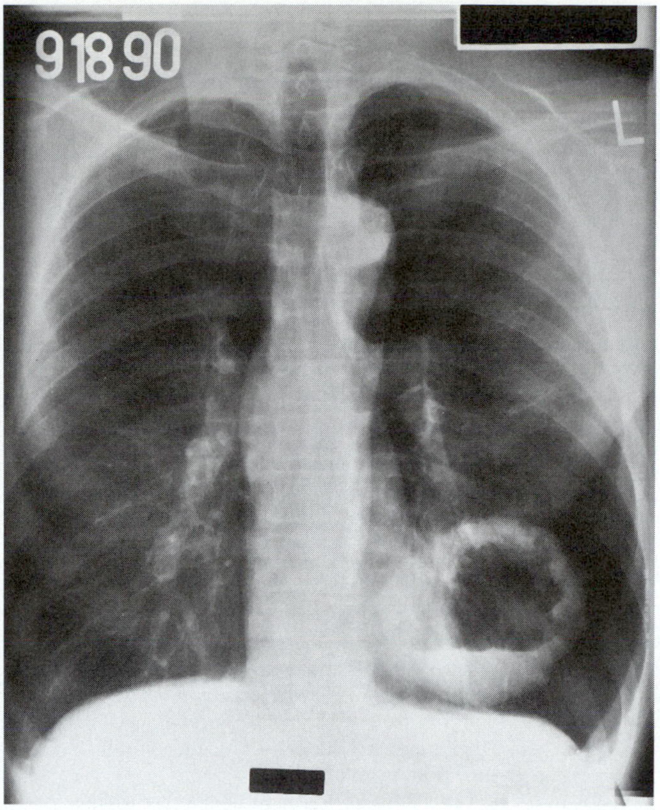


**Fig. 120-2.** Large peripheral squamous cell carcinoma. A fiberoptic bronchoscopy did not reveal an endobronchial lesion. Note a large cavity with air-fluid level.

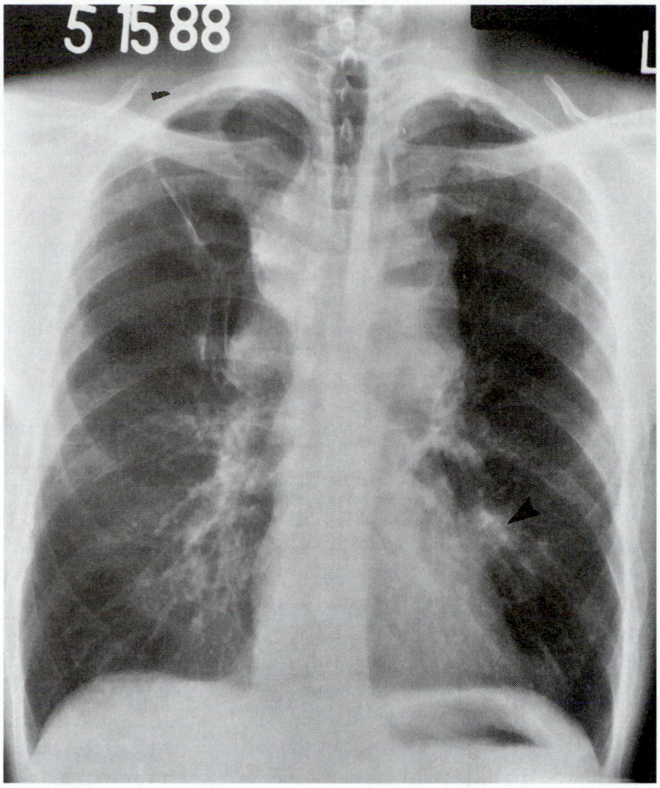


**Fig. 120-3.** Small-cell carcinoma. Note a small parenchymal lesion (*arrow*) and massive mediastinal involvement.

performed safely even when patients have limited pulmonary reserve due to previous surgery or advanced COPD. The diagnostic yield of FOB varies, depending on the location of the tumor and the skill of the physician. In cases where a lesion is visible through a bronchoscope, brushings and forceps biopsies are routinely performed. In addition, bronchial washings are frequently obtained and the diagnosis is made in more than 90% of cases. When no endobronchial lesion is visible through the bronchoscope, both brushings and biopsies are performed under fluoroscopic guidance and the diagnosis can be made in up to 60% of cases. However, FOB is a very low yield procedure for peripheral lesions that are smaller than 2 cm in diameter.

***Transthoracic needle aspiration.*** TNA has become the method of choice for peripherally located nodular lesions, particularly those that are smaller than 2 cm in diameter. If the procedure is performed by a well-trained radiologist and the specimens are examined by an experienced pathologist, the diagnostic yield is as high as 95% if the lesion is malignant. However, if the process is nonmalignant, TNA has a low yield for providing a specific diagnosis. TNA also has a high incidence of complications, primarily pneumothorax (25% to 35%), which often require a chest tube insertion. A small pneumothorax is well tolerated in patients with good pulmonary reserve but can cause a serious problem for patients with very limited pulmonary function. The choice of FOB or TNA after cytopathologic examination of sputum specimens has

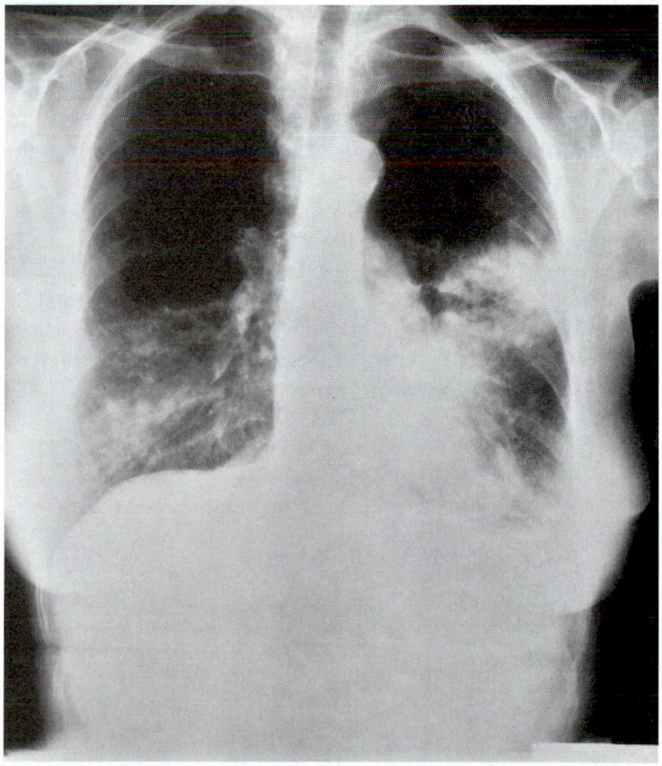

**Fig. 120-4.** Bronchoalveolar cell carcinoma, showing bilateral multiple pneumonic infiltrates.

**Table 120-1.** Transthoracic needle aspiration (TNA) versus fiberoptic bronchoscopy (FOB)

| | TNA | FOB |
|---|---|---|
| Lesion size | ≤2 cm | >2 cm |
| Clinical symptoms | None | Cough, blood-tinged sputum |
| Clinical diagnosis | Malignancy | Both malignant and benign processes |
| Airway examination (staging) | Not possible | Routine |
| Pneumothorax | 25%-30% | <5% |

failed to provide a diagnosis depends on the availability of each procedure, the type of lesion, and the condition of the patient. For example, if clinical suspicion is very high for carcinoma, the lesion is small and peripherally located, and the patient has good pulmonary reserve, TNA is the method of choice. If the history suggests bronchial mucosal involvement, such as bloody sputum, the chest radiograph shows a centrally located lesion or a peripheral lesion that shows a cavitation, and the differential diagnosis includes infectious and inflammatory diseases, FOB is the procedure of choice because it allows an examination of airways, permits staging in case of carcinoma, and frequently provides a definitive diagnosis of a nonmalignant process. FOB may be preferable even in a relatively small peripheral lesion if the patient has severely compromised pulmonary function because of FOB's very small incidence of pneumothorax (Table 120-1).

***Mediastinoscopy and thoracoscopy.*** Mediastinoscopy is usually performed to evaluate the mediastinum for the staging of carcinoma of the lung. Mediastinoscopy can also be used as a diagnostic tool when FOB has failed to make a diagnosis of a pulmonary lesion that involves the mediastinum and is relatively inaccessible to TNA. Thoracoscopy was recently revived for the examination of pleural processes, but it can also be used to perform limited lung surgery. Thoracoscopic surgery is particularly suitable for a small peripheral lesion that is located close to the pleural surface.

## Staging

Once the diagnosis of lung carcinoma has been established, staging is essential for the treatment planning and prediction of survival. Staging is also crucial to the comparison of the data generated by different institutions. The international staging system was developed for staging of non–small-cell lung carcinomas, based on a tumor, node, and metastases (TNM) classification (see the box at right and Table 120-2).

Clinical staging must be distinguished from surgical staging. Clinical staging relies on the information obtained by noninvasive methods (see the Managed Care Guide). It often underestimates the extent of disease. Surgical staging is done at the time of surgery and is more accurate.

### Tumor, node, and metastases definitions

**Primary tumor (T)**

$T_X$ Tumor proven by the presence of malignant cells in bronchopulmonary secretions but not visualized radiographically or bronchoscopically, or any tumor that cannot be assessed, as in a retreatment staging

$T_0$ No evidence of primary tumor

$T_{IS}$ Carcinoma in situ

$T_1$ A tumor that is 3 cm or less in greatest dimension, surrounded by lung or visceral pleura, and without evidence of invasion proximal to a lobar bronchus at bronchoscopy

$T_2$ A tumor more than 3 cm in greatest dimension, or a tumor of any size that either invades the visceral pleura or has associated atelectasis or obstructive pneumonitis extending to the hilar region; at bronchoscopy the proximal extent of the demonstrable tumor must be within a lobar bronchus or at least 2 cm distal to the carina; any associated atelectasis or obstructive pneumonitis must involve less than an entire lung

$T_3$ A tumor of any size with direct extension into the chest wall (including superior sulcus tumors), diaphragm, or the mediastinal pleura or pericardium without involving the heart, great vessels, trachea, esophagus, or vertebral body, or a tumor in the main bronchus within 2 cm of the carina without involving the carina

$T_4$ A tumor of any size with invasion of the mediastinum or involving the heart, great vessels, trachea, esophagus, vertebral body, or carina, or the presence of malignant pleural effusion

**Nodal involvement (N)**

$N_0$ No demonstrable metastasis to regional lymph nodes

$N_1$ Metastasis to lymph nodes in the peribronchial or the ipsilateral hilar region, or both, including direct extension

$N_2$ Metastasis to ipsilateral mediastinal lymph nodes and subcarinal lymph nodes

$N_3$ Metastasis to contralateral mediastinal lymph nodes, contralateral hilar lymph nodes, ipsilateral or contralateral scalene, or supraclavicular lymph nodes

**Distant metastasis (M)**

$M_0$ No known distant metastasis

$M_1$ Distant metastasis present—specify sites)

From Mountain CF, Greenberg SD, Fraire AE, *Chest* 99:1258, 1991.

Fig. 120-5 shows the survival curve of non–small-cell lung carcinoma by the stage of the disease. It has been hotly debated as to what constitutes adequate clinical staging for non–small-cell lung carcinoma, particularly in the current climate to limit medical expenditures.

The use of mediastinoscopy or limited left anterior thoracotomy (Chamberlain procedure) depends on the surgeon's preference and the condition of the patient. For example, if the patient is elderly or has limited pulmonary reserve and a chest CT scan shows possibly abnormal enlarged mediastinal lymph nodes, a thorough evaluation of the mediastinum by mediastinoscopy is appropriate before subjecting the patient to thoracotomy. On the other hand, a questionable ipsilateral mediastinal lymph node

**Table 120-2.** Stage grouping of TNM subsets in lung cancer

| | Tumor | Node | Metastases |
|---|---|---|---|
| Occult carcinoma | $T_X$ | $N_0$ | $M_0$ |
| Stage 0 | $T_{is}$ | | $M_0$ |
| Stage I | $T_1$ | $N_0$ | $M_0$ |
| | $T_2$ | $N_0$ | $M_0$ |
| Stage II | $T_1$ | $N_1$ | $M_0$ |
| | $T_2$ | $N_1$ | $M_0$ |
| Stage IIIa | $T_1$ | $N_2$ | $M_0$ |
| | $T_2$ | $N_2$ | $M_0$ |
| | $T_3$ | $N_0$, $N_1$, $N_2$ | $M_0$ |
| Stage IIIb | Any T | $N_3$ | $M_0$ |
| | $T_4$ | Any N | $M_0$ |
| Stage IV | Any T | Any N | $M_1$ |

## Managed Care Guide
## Pointers on clinical staging of non-small-cell lung cancer

1. A chest CT scan, including the upper abdomen for evaluation of the mediastinum and adrenal glands, is a minimal requirement.
2. A bone scan is obtained before thoracotomy in most cases, but not for small peripheral lesions.
3. A head CT scan is not indicated unless the patient is being considered for surgery, but it is often obtained in cases of adenocarcinoma before surgery.
4. If the patient has clinical evidence of distant metastases, such as palpable supraclavicular nodes, superior vena cava syndrome, vocal cord paralysis, or paralysis of the diaphragm, no scanning procedure is indicated unless the patient is clinically symptomatic with bone pain or laboratory study shows possible organ involvement, such as abnormal liver function studies.
5. The value of magnetic resonance imaging (MRI) has yet to be clearly defined.

involvement in an otherwise healthy individual does not require mediastinoscopy. It is mandatory to obtain pulmonary function studies to assess pulmonary reserve before surgery.

Staging for small-cell carcinoma is much simpler because it is believed that the majority of patients with this type of carcinoma have distant metastases at the time of diagnosis. Patients with small-cell carcinoma are divided according to limited disease or extensive disease. When a tumor is restricted to one hemithorax, with or without involvement of ipsilateral supraclavicular lymph nodes, the patient is classified as having limited disease. The workup for patients with small-cell carcinoma includes CT scans of the chest, abdomen, and head. A bone marrow biopsy and a bone scan are usually performed before the initiation of therapy.

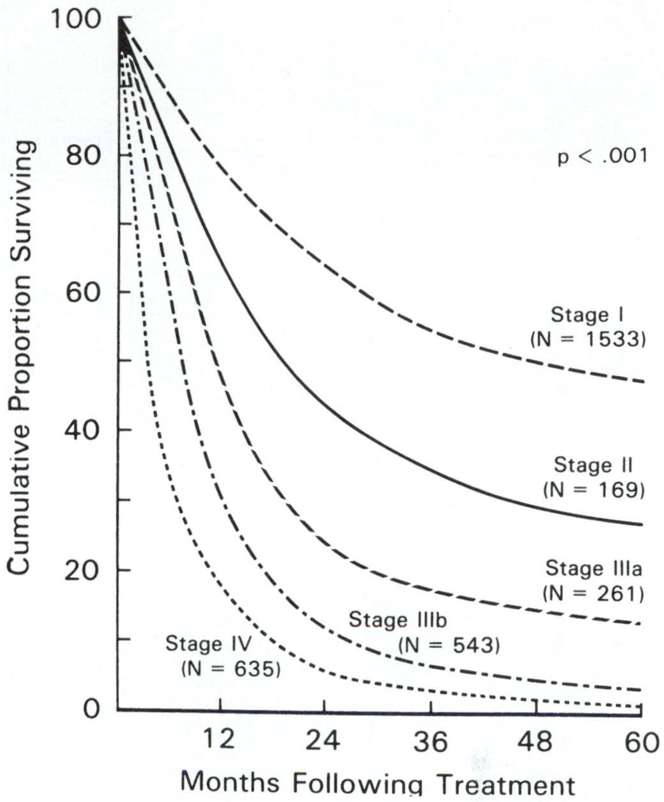


**Fig. 120-5.** Survival in non–small-cell lung cancer by clinical staging. (From Mountain CF: *Chest* 89(4):2325, 1986.)

### Solitary pulmonary nodule

Solitary pulmonary nodule (SPN) is a fairly common radiographic entity. It is usually an incidental finding on a chest radiograph and is defined as a round or oval peripheral density surrounded by aerated lung tissue with the largest diameter less than 4 cm and without associated hilar or mediastinal lymph node involvement or pleural effusion.

The etiology of an SPN differs greatly depending on geographic location. In the developing countries a large number of SPNs represent infectious processes, particularly tuberculous granuloma. In the United States and other developed countries approximately 50% of SPNs are primary carcinoma of the lung. When a carcinoma of the lung presents as an SPN and is resected early, it is potentially curable. For this reason the differentiation between a benign and malignant SPN is of utmost importance. The patient's age, smoking history, and past residency are all important clinical factors. For example, if the patient is a nonsmoker, younger than age 35, and has lived in an endemic area for histoplasmosis, the SPN seen on the chest radiograph is likely to be benign (histoplasmoma). Chest radiograph provides the most important findings to differentiate a benign lesion from a malignant one. If the diameter of the lesion is smaller than 1 cm, it is very likely to be benign. The widely accepted radiographic finding of benign lesions is the presence of a characteristic pattern of calcification (central and lamellar). A popcorn type of calcification indicates a probable benign neoplasm (hamartoma). The presence of calcifica-

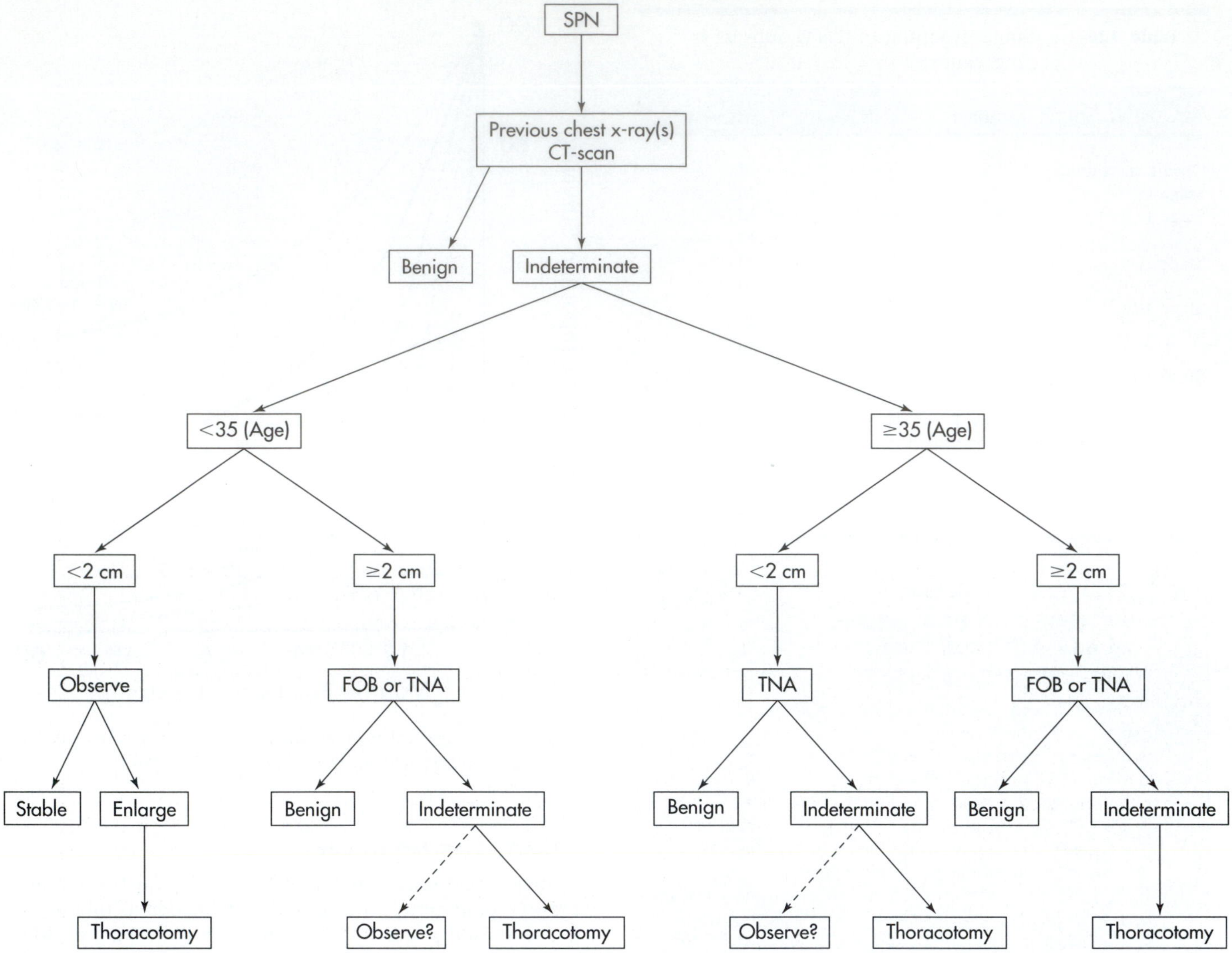


**Fig. 120-6.** Approach to solitary pulmonary nodule.

tion in the periphery of the lesion does not indicate that the lesion is benign. The importance of a previous chest radiograph cannot be overemphasized. If the lesion is stable for more than three years, it is very likely to be benign.

When a standard chest radiograph does not show these characteristic calcifications and no previous chest radiograph is available, a chest CT scan should be obtained. When a standard CT scan does not reveal a characteristic pattern of calcification, the use of a densitometer often improves the results. If the CT scan does not demonstrate the benign nature of a lesion, a more invasive approach becomes necessary. FOB or TNA should be the next diagnostic procedure. FOB is useful for patients who have clinical complaints that are suggestive of bronchial involvement, such as increased cough or blood-tinged sputum. If the lesion shows a cavitation on the chest radiograph, TNA is preferable to FOB for lesions smaller than 2 cm in diameter. Some authors advocate proceeding to a full thoracotomy for patients who have no serious medical conditions without prior FOB or TNA, since surgery is eventually required whether or not a neoplasm is found. However, many experts recommend obtaining a specific diagnosis before subjecting the patient to a full thoracotomy. If attempts do not yield a specific diagnosis, a thoracotomy should be performed unless the patient has a serious medical condition that prohibits thoracotomy. Fig. 120-6 shows the suggested approach to SPN.

## Treatment

***Surgery.*** For non–small-cell lung carcinoma, surgery is the best method to achieve long-term survival or a cure. All patients in clinical stages I and II should be offered surgery unless there is severely compromised pulmonary function or other conditions that prohibit surgery, such as advanced age or severe coronary artery disease. It is generally agreed that the patient should have a minimum predicted postoperative forced expiratory volume in 1 second ($FEV_1$) of 800 ml or greater to be considered for resection. A simple way to make a rough estimate of a postoperative

$FEV_1$ is to subtract the estimated number of segments to be removed from the total number of segments (19), divide by 19, then multiply the current $FEV_1$ by this factor. For example, if the patient requires right upper lobe resection (three segments) and the current $FEV_1$ is 1300 ml, then the estimated postoperative $FEV_1$ is:

$$1300 \text{ ml} \times 16/19 \cong 1100 \text{ ml}$$

Obviously, the size of the individual segment is not equal. Therefore, an adjustment is required depending on which segments will be removed. Also, this formula assumes that all parts of the lungs are equally contributing to the overall spirometric values. However, the lobe or the lung that will be removed is usually not fully functional due to disease process. In addition, for the patient who has uneven ventilation due to a localized disease elsewhere, such as a bullous emphysema, the difference in the regional ventilation becomes an important factor in predicting the postoperative pulmonary function. Therefore the patient who has a localized disease process in the noncarcinomatous lung or a borderline postoperative predicted $FEV_1$ should have a ventilation/perfusion scan for better assessment of the postoperative predicted pulmonary function. The value of preoperative pulmonary exercise testing has not been clearly established. When the lesion is located relatively close to the pleura, a more limited resection, such as segmentectomy or a wedge resection, can be performed in patients with borderline pulmonary function to minimize loss of functioning lung tissue. A number of surgical techniques, such as sleeve resection to preserve nondiseased lung, have also been developed. Many patients with clinical stage IIIa disease are potential surgical candidates, although the long-term survival rate for this group is poor. Patients with stage IIIb disease are generally not considered to be surgical candidates.

The therapy of small-cell carcinoma consists of chemotherapy and radiation. The value of surgery followed by chemotherapy in selected cases of limited disease has yet to be established.

***Radiation therapy.*** Patients with stage I or stage II disease who have had complete surgical resection of a lesion usually do not receive radiation. Postoperative radiation is generally given if the pathologic examination of resected lymph nodes shows metastases. Radiation therapy is also used with non–small-cell carcinoma that is found to be inoperable due to extensive disease, limited pulmonary reserve, or other reasons. Patients with stage I or stage II disease who are unwilling or unable to undergo resection should receive radiation for potential curative purposes. A 5-year survival of more than 20% may be achieved for patients with stage I disease with a small peripheral lesion. Although patients with stage III disease often receive radiation treatment with a curative dose, achieving long-term survival is uncommon. In stage IV disease radiation therapy is used for a palliative purpose, most often for the control of pain from metastases to the bones. Obstruction or narrowing of large airways, causing a distal pneumonia or significant dyspnea, as well as the obstruction of a large vessel, as in superior vena cava syndrome, are additional indications for radiation therapy. In these situations radiation treatment often provides significant symptomatic relief. Brachytherapy is a form of local radiation in which a source of radioactivity is placed in the tumor to minimize the effects on the surrounding normal lung tissue. In some situations, such as superior sulcus tumors, radiation is often given before surgery.

***Chemotherapy.*** Chemotherapy is unequivocally effective in small-cell lung carcinoma. The majority of patients show an initial, sometimes dramatic response to chemotherapy, which is often combined with radiation. Chemotherapy definitely prolongs survival, even for patients with extensive disease. Long-term survival can be achieved in a small percentage of patients with limited disease.

In contrast to patients with small-cell carcinoma, the role of chemotherapy in patients with non–small-cell carcinoma is very limited. No chemotherapy is employed for patients with stage I or stage II disease who undergo a complete resection. For patients who received a curative dose of radiation alone and had complete radiographic resolution, the value of chemotherapy is not well established. Patients with nonoperable stage III disease who have received a full dose of radiation often receive chemotherapy. A number of studies are being conducted to evaluate the value of adjuvant chemotherapy in this setting, but it is not clearly established at this time. In stage IV disease, where chemotherapy is most often employed, the benefit of treatment is marginal at best and the potential benefit must be weighed against the associated discomfort and the increased chance of infection.

***Other treatment modalities.*** Obstruction of the central airways that results from a large endobronchial mass lesion at the time of initial presentation or late in the course of the disease is a serious problem. These patients usually develop severe and rapidly progressive dyspnea. Local treatment with a YAG laser can be applied for immediate relief of symptoms. The treatment is often performed with a specially designed rigid bronchoscope while the patient is under general anesthesia, although some pulmonologists use only a FOB. Recurrence due to tumor regrowth or scarring is common. A number of stents were recently developed and are being used in conjunction with laser treatment. Clearly, these types of treatment should be performed in specialized centers.

### Early detection

By the time many patients with lung carcinoma present with symptoms, the disease is far advanced and inoperable. The prognosis of patients with stage I disease who have been treated with surgery, however, is generally favorable. Therefore, efforts have been made to detect lung cancer in its early stage with the hope of improving the prognosis of patients with lung carcinoma. The value of screening in lung carcinoma, however, is controversial. The result of a large-scale investigation to evaluate the value of screening high-risk patients with an annual chest radiograph combined with cytologic examination of sputum specimens did not demonstrate a reduction in the mortality rate. Because the study did not show an impact on the death rate, it was concluded that a good survival in patients whose carcinomas were discovered by screening was due to a lag-time effect; namely, patients achieved long-term survival because the carcinoma was found in its early stage rather than because of treatment. This conclusion assumes that, even if the early lesions found with screening were left unresected, patients would not have died earlier from their carcinomas. The current recommendation of the American Cancer Society for early detection of cancer does not include an annual chest radiograph for lung carcinoma. However, recent analysis of the follow-up data, performed by one of the groups that was involved in the original investigation, revealed that most patients with stage I disease who were not treated by surgery died from lung cancer, and the 5-year survival rates of treated patients and untreated patients were approximately 65% and 10%, respectively. This group strongly recommended that high-risk patients be screened with annual chest radiographs. In my practice many patients with stage I disease are asymptomatic and the disease is discovered by an annual chest radiograph or by a chest radiograph obtained for another reason. For these reasons, it is recommended that an annual chest radiograph be obtained in all patients who are at high risk of developing lung carcinoma and who are being followed by a physician because the chest radiograph is the only method available to the physician to detect lung carcinomas in early and potentially curable stages. High-risk patients include smokers of more than 40-pack years, patients with COPD, patients who have a chronic pulmonary interstitial process, such as progressive systemic sclerosis, and idiopathic pulmonary fibrosis, and patients with a history of exposure to known substances that increase the chance of developing lung cancer, such as asbestos and uranium.

### Prevention

The best method to prevent lung carcinoma is to never start smoking. Due to the strong antismoking campaign of the last two decades, total cigarette consumption in the United States has declined, but it will take a long time before a decline occurs in the incidence of lung carcinoma. Current smokers should be strongly urged to stop smoking. It is the physician's responsibility to advise patients to stop smoking. Indeed, many patients would like to stop but are unable to do so. Currently, the most effective method to help patients stop smoking is the use of the nicotine patch in conjunction with a multidisciplinary smoking cessation clinic. This subject is discussed in Chapter 124.

## METASTATIC CARCINOMA OF THE LUNG

Due to their anatomic location, the lungs are common sites of metastases from malignant neoplasms outside of the thorax. In patients with metastatic neoplasm of the lungs, the primary site is often known at the time of the development of lung lesions, or there is a recent history of malignancy. However, occasionally the metastatic lesion in the lung is discovered without a known primary site. Metastatic malignancy of the lung usually presents as multiple nodular lesions on the chest radiograph, although sometimes it may appear as a solitary lesion. When it appears as a solitary lesion on the chest radiograph, a CT scan of the chest often reveals other lesions that are not apparent on the chest radiograph. Careful history, physical examination, and simple laboratory tests, such as a urinalysis or stool guaiac test, usually suggest the primary site. Common primary sites are the genitourinary system (hypernephroma, transitional cell carcinoma of the urinary bladder, and germ cell tumor of the testis) in males and the breasts and reproductive system (breast cancer, cervical cancer, and choriocarcinoma) in females. GI system carcinoma (gastric, pancreatic, and colorectal) and head and neck carcinoma in smokers are frequent primary sites in both sexes. In younger individuals the primary sites include muscle, bone, cartilage, and testis (leiomyosarcoma, osteosarcoma, synovial cell sarcoma in both sexes, and germ cell tumor of the testis in males). In some cases the metastasis occurs in the bronchial submucosa and causes an endobronchial lesion, and the patient may develop symptoms and signs related to endobronchial involvement. In cases of endobronchial involvement the diagnosis can be made by FOB, whereas in patients who present with single or multiple peripheral lesions the diagnosis is often made by TNA. Occasionally it is necessary to perform a thoracotomy to establish the diagnosis. The treatment of a metastatic lesion(s) in the lung depends on the condition of the primary site. Surgery is usually not indicated after the lesions are diagnosed as metastatic neoplasms. Surgical resections have been performed occasionally, however, for highly selected patients when primary tumors have been completely resected, there is no sign of local recurrence, and the lung lesion(s) can be completely resected without serious consequence to pulmonary function.

A less common but clinically important presentation of metastatic spread is of the lymphangitic type. This type of metastatic spread is usually seen in patients with carcinoma of the stomach, the pancreas, and the lung. The patient presents with rapidly progressive dyspnea, and the chest radiograph shows linear and coarse irregular nodular infiltrates, often in the distribution of a segment or a lobe. Hilar and mediastinal lymph nodes are often enlarged. When a patient with carcinoma of the lung who underwent or is undergoing radiation treatment presents with this pattern of metastasis, a differential diagnosis for radiation pneumonitis becomes very important because this condition responds to treatment with steroids. Presumptive diagnosis of radiation pneumonitis can often be made on the basis of clinical and radiographic findings and a trial of steroids may be given. Occasionally a lung biopsy is necessary to confirm the diagnosis.

## LYMPHOMA

Lymphoma is a malignant disease of the lymphatic tissue and frequently involves the intrathoracic lymph node as well as the lung parenchyma. Lymphoma is usually divided into Hodgkin's disease and non-Hodgkin's lymphoma.

### Hodgkin's disease

Both Hodgkin's disease and non-Hodgkin's lymphoma occur in all ages; however, Hodgkin's disease is more likely in younger individuals than is non-Hodgkin's lymphoma. The peak incidence of Hodgkin's disease is the third decade, whereas non-Hodgkin's lymphoma is seen more commonly in patients over the age of 50. Involvement of the intrathoracic structures by Hodgkin's disease is usually a part of the generalized disease process, and primary pulmonary Hodgkin's disease is very rare. Patients with Hodgkin's disease usually have constitutional symptoms such as general malaise, easy fatigability, fever, and weight loss at the time of presentation. Physical examination often reveals peripheral lymph node(s) enlargement and anemia. When the disease involves the thorax, it usually presents as mediastinal and hilar lymph node enlargement on chest radiograph. The mediastinal and hilar lymph node enlargement is usually asymmetric but bilateral. The involvement of the lung parenchyma is uncommon and is almost always associated with a mediastinal mass. The lung parenchymal involvement is more often seen in patients with a nodular sclerosis type and is usually the result of direct extension of the mediastinal process. Occasionally it may cause a compression of the airway or actual invasion of the bronchus, resulting in atelectasis or distal pneumonia. The major differential diagnosis of intrathoracic Hodgkin's disease is sarcoidosis. Patients with sarcoidosis with bilateral hilar lymphadenopathy are usually asymptomatic unless there is a significant lung involvement. The diagnosis of sarcoidosis is usually made with FOB and a transbronchoscopic lung biopsy, which has a very high diagnostic yield (80% to 85%), even for patients without appreciable lung parenchymal involvement on chest radiograph. The diagnosis of Hodgkin's disease confined in the mediastinum often requires a mediastinoscopy.

Treatment of Hodgkin's disease is a combination of radiation and chemotherapy. The response to treatment and the prognosis for patients with Hodgkin's disease are generally better than for patients with non-Hodgkin's lymphoma.

### Non-Hodgkin's lymphoma

Non-Hodgkin's lymphoma is a heterogenous group of malignant diseases of lymphatic origin and frequently involves the mediastinum and the lungs. Non-Hodgkin's lymphoma is sometimes classified as primary and secondary lymphoma. In primary pulmonary lymphoma, only the lung is involved at the time of diagnosis and there is no evidence of extrathoracic dissemination for at least three months after the initial diagnosis. In secondary pulmonary lymphoma, patients are known to have disease outside of the thorax prior to the pulmonary involvement. Pathologically the most common cell type of primary pulmonary lymphoma is a small lymphocytic type. Radiographically, primary pulmonary lymphoma manifests as reticulonodular, nodular, or parenchymal consolidation. Clinically the majority of patients with primary pulmonary lymphoma are asymptomatic. The histologic diagnosis can be made by the examination of the specimens obtained by FOB but often require a thoracotomy. Secondary pulmonary lymphoma is much more common than primary pulmonary lymphoma. The most common radiographic manifestation of secondary pulmonary lymphoma is mediastinal and hilar lymph node enlargement. When the lungs are involved, the lesion may present as a solitary nodule or as multiple nodules. Cavitation may occur, but less commonly than in Hodgkin's disease. The lesion may extend to the large airway and cause an atelectasis or a distal pneumonia. Clinical presentation depends on the extent of extrathoracic disease. Constitutional symptoms, such as fever, anorexia, and weight loss, are common.

Treatment is a combination of chemotherapy and radiation. The response to treatment and the prognosis are less favorable than those of Hodgkin's disease.

## BIBLIOGRAPHY

Bains MS: Surgical treatment of lung cancer, *Chest* 100:826, 1991.

Boring C, Squires TS, Tong T: Cancer statistics, *CA* 43:7, 1993.

Chi NC, et al: Cancer of the lung, *Cancer manual,* 1990, American Cancer Society.

Flehinger BJ, Kimmel M, Melmad MR: The effect of surgical treatment on survival from early lung cancer: implication for screening, *Chest* 101:1013, 1992.

Ihde DC: Chemotherapy of lung carcinoma, *N Engl J Med* 327:1434, 1992.

Mountain CF, Greenberg SD, Fraire AE: Tumor stage in non–small-cell carcinoma of the lung, *Chest* 99:1258, 1991.

Murren JR, Buzaid AC: Chemotherapy and radiation for the treatment of non–small-cell lung cancer, *Clin Chest Med* 14:161, 1993.

# XIII Psychosocial and Behavioral Issues

CHAPTER

## 121 Psychotherapeutic Techniques of Physicians and Psychotherapies of Counselors: Uses and Guidelines

John D. Stoeckle
Sherman Eisenthal

### PSYCHOSOCIAL DISTRESS AND PSYCHIATRIC DISORDERS OF MEDICAL PATIENTS

The psychosocial distress and psychiatric disorders encountered in medical practice differ, as do their implications for treatment. Psychosocial distress consists of the emotional reactions that may accompany disease, disability, and medical treatment, or those that accompany stressful events, crises, and personal losses of everyday life. For example, family strains, marital conflicts, work/career concerns, and other reactions may be brought to the physician or to others in the patient's social network. The emotional reactions most commonly encountered are grief, anxiety, panic, somatization, and depression.

The second group consists of psychiatric disorders, of which the most commonly reported in physician surveys are anxiety, depression, alcohol/substance abuse, marital/sexual problems, psychophysiologic and pain disorders, adjustment reactions, organic brain syndromes, and psychoses.

### USING TECHNIQUES OF PSYCHOTHERAPY VS. PRACTICING PSYCHOTHERAPY

When managing patients with the *psychologic distress* of coping with disabilities and stressful life events, the physician uses psychotherapeutic techniques, deliberately or intuitively, that include communicative behaviors and rhetoric common to various psychotherapies and the medical interview. When managing patients with *psychiatric disorders,* the physician may make referrals to mental health professionals who practice psychotherapy for the disorders. The distinction between using psychotherapy techniques and practicing psychotherapy is important in defining the role of the generalist physician.

#### The generalist's role

The physician's time commitments, goals of care, practice duties, and training differ from those of counseling professionals. The physician's goals of psychosocial care are focused on (1) the support of patients with emotional reactions; (2) the facilitation of the expression and clarification of feelings and thoughts; (3) the resolution of fears associated with illness and the communication of hope; (4) the communication of information and meaning for understanding and adapting to disease, particularly the psychosocial roots of many physical complaints; (5) the encouragement of shared decision making to promote compliance with diagnosis, treatment, and prevention. The use of psychotherapeutic techniques for these focused goals is appropriate for the generalist physician whose practice duty is to be readily available to patients seeking help for many acute and chronic bodily complaints. The generalist physician realizes that patients neither expect nor contract for psychotherapy.

#### The role of the mental health practitioner

Practicing psychotherapy requires regular, frequent visits with patients that are usually longer than medical visits, for conditions that limit access to the physician and restrict his or her attention to psychosocial problems. In addition, mental health practitioners of psychotherapy may have broader goals of care than some physicians, namely, to collaborate in changing a patient's feelings, thoughts, and behavior. Special technical skills and knowledge, such as identifying psychiatric disorders and contracting over the treatment, negotiating the use of a variety of specific approaches (e.g., psychodynamic versus cognitive), and the format of therapy (e.g., individual versus group or family) are shared by psychotherapist and physician. Providing such interventions requires specialized training and continuing education and supervision. Moreover, professional responsibility and accountability for potential problems (e.g., psychosis) may be based on specialized training in psychotherapy.

#### Psychotherapeutic techniques used by the physician

***Listening.*** Listening to the patient's story (as an illness narrative) is essential to gather the necessary information to make a medical diagnosis, to learn about the patient's personality and perspective on the illness for which help is being sought, and to develop a supportive relationship. The patient's perspective includes attributions about the illness, requests for diagnosis and treatment, expectations of care, and the relationship with the physician, all of which are used by the physician in decision making and negotiation with the patient about care. Listening with patience and close attention helps the physician to establish relationships with patients.

Listening therapeutically differs from listening to gather information for a diagnosis. The former conveys the physician's interest in the patient's experience with illness and develops a supportive relationship. The process of therapeutic listening is active, receptive, and nondirective. This may entail continuing to pay close attention even when the patient is unfocused, which tends to happen particularly at the start of the interview, or when the patient becomes momentarily silent. Useful, nondirective tactics include waiting judiciously for the patient to continue (a nonverbal cue), reflective cuing (building on the patient's words; e.g., "You were saying that the pain made you. . . ."), but not controlling the patient's communication with premature diagnostic questions, (e.g., "When did the pain start?" or "How intense was the pain?"). Early, focused questions are often prompted by the physician's discomfort with the patient's silence or eagerness to quickly form or test a diagnostic hypothesis. Nondirective listening conveys the physician's interest in the patient as well as in the disease.

***Catharsis.*** Catharsis (ventilation) is the emotional release that occurs when the patient is encouraged to "talk out" feelings, such as anger, tension, guilt, humiliation, regret, and shame. The patient's relief comes from the expression of these feelings and thoughts and from the physician's empathic acknowledgment of the distress. For example, a woman in her early 40s comes to the physician's office and is distraught, reporting that she found a lump in her breast after having postponed a mammogram. She says repeatedly that she thought a mammogram was unnecessary until she reached her 50s. The physician could try reassurance, such as saying, "That was not an unreasonable approach for a woman of your age" or "There is no guarantee that a mammogram would have been positive." Reassurance, however, may not be what the patient wants and may circumvent the opportunity for the patient to ventilate her feelings, especially anger with herself or others. To facilitate ventilation, the physician might reflect the patient's feelings by saying, "I sense that you are really upset with yourself for putting the mammogram off. You feel like you have . . ." (pause, waiting for the patient to continue). This approach not only allows the physician to facilitate the expression of the patient's feelings, but also conveys an empathic understanding of the patient's situation through the language of the statement and the tone of voice. The message conveys that the physician understands the patient's feelings and does not judge the patient for postponing the mammogram.

***Abreaction.*** Abreaction is a specific type of catharsis that occurs when the patient relives repressed thoughts and feelings in an emotionally charged way. Reliving past events occurs through the exploration of intense, often traumatic experiences, such as unresolved grief, abuse, rape, or disease.

***Reassurance.*** Reassurance is a supportive technique to bolster the patient's sense of competence and worth by relieving worries, such as those about the presence, severity, and prognosis of disease. Reassurance minimizes the negative and maximizes the positive outcomes. When the patient feels overwhelmed, such communication reestablishes a sense of control and conveys hope. Premature reassurance, however, may undermine trust and therefore hope.

***Empathy.*** Empathy is an awareness of and identification with the patient's thoughts and feelings, pain and suffering, and fears and hopes, while maintaining a sense of separateness. The physician demonstrates empathy with the patient's experience by communicating understanding and goes beyond reiterating what the patient has expressed.

***Clarification.*** Clarification addresses the patient's ambiguity, confusion, misinterpretation, and uncertainty about illness and treatment. The aim is to clarify thoughts and feelings, choices, and alternative approaches that are available to reduce confusion and misinterpretation. The subject in need of clarification may be cognitive (choices, alternatives, decisions, and assumptions) or affective (feelings associated with misperception of the thoughts and feelings of others).

For example, a man in his early 60s becomes very upset when he is told that he has an enlarged prostate. He expresses confusion about the seriousness and treatment of the problem, thinking it may be cancer. Before reassuring the patient that his conclusions may be wrong, it is important for the physician to review each conclusion, one at a time, to clarify what is and is not true (e.g., are the causes of the enlargements age-related, due to prostatitis, or to cancer? What are the diagnostic steps and treatment options?).

***Reflection.*** Reflection is a nondirective method that "replays" the patient's thoughts, feelings, and actions by rephrasing, restating, or summarizing. This technique acknowledges the patient's reported experience and facilitates further exploration.

***Interpretation.*** Interpretation provides explanations of the patient's illness. The physician explains the disease, its signs and symptoms, and its diagnosis and treatment in terms that the patient can understand. The physician also elaborates on the patient's psychologic problems, diagnosis, and the patient's resistance and conflict so the patient can gain insight into his or her thoughts, feelings, and actions. In a case of depression, for example, the physician might use a psychodynamic, biologic, or cognitive/behavioral explanatory model.

***Persuasion.*** Persuasion is a directive psychotherapeutic method of influencing the patient's thoughts, feelings, and actions by appealing to evidence, authority, and suggestion. For example, providing evidence not only educates the patient about the pros and cons of treatment choices, but, within the context of persuasion, also influences the patient to comply with a particular choice that, in the physician's view, serves the patient's best interests.

***Advice and guidance.*** This technique consists of the practitioner giving explicit directions regarding what the patient should do to get better.

***Relaxation techniques.*** See the discussion of relaxation techniques on p. 1631.

***Countertransference.*** In addition to attending to patients, physicians must listen to themselves. A patient's personality and style may affect the physician and thus the physician's approach to the patient. Patients may confuse, attack, seduce, make demands on, and disturb their physicians. Both positive and negative feelings may be evoked that can distort the physician's appropriate response to the patient. Bibring and Groves addressed countertransference (emotional reactions of the physician to the projections of the patient) in medical settings, describing the types of patients who evoke such reactions: angry, dependent, ingratiating, hypercritical, self-willed, and seductive patients. The physician's reactions provide valuable clues to the patient's state of mind. For the physician, the challenge is to contain his/her emotional reactions to the patient's provocative behavior and then to decipher the message. Physicians' difficulties in dealing with provocative behaviors are normal and natural. They can be ameliorated by training and colleague support, by learning to listen to their own feelings, by acknowledging and labeling these reactions, by recognizing their impact, and by responding appropriately to the needs of the patient that are projected onto the physician. Groups for discussion of such problems and coping with patients may be useful.

## PSYCHOTHERAPIES PRACTICED BY MENTAL HEALTH PRACTITIONERS

Negotiating a psychotherapy referral requires the physician to resolve with the patient the type and the provider of psychotherapy. When the patient's problems are neither chronic nor associated with a personality disorder (axis II diagnoses) or psychosis, then short-term psychotherapies should be considered first. Several psychotherapies that counselors may use in the treatment of referred patients are summarized below, and the process of making a referral is described.

### Psychodynamic

The focus of this type of psychotherapy is on character change of patients through insight from analysis of transference, intrapsychic conflicts, and interpersonal relationships. Long-term treatments are directed primarily at self-defeating character traits (e.g., passive-dependency, obsessive-compulsiveness, and narcissism), whereas short-term treatment tends to focus on one character trait and on psychologic states, such as anxiety and depression. Long-term treatment is more appropriate for fairly well-integrated, educated, and introspective individuals who express a strong interest in self-understanding.

### Cognitive/behavioral

In recent years behavioral and cognitive approaches have become integrated. The cognitive approach focuses on modifying and replacing false and self-defeating thoughts or "cognitions" (assumptions, attitudes, and beliefs) about oneself and others with more adaptive ones. The behavioral approach focuses on replacing and modifying maladaptive behaviors (avoidant or inhibited learned responses to the environment, people, and situations) through the reinforcement of more appropriate behavior, relaxation training, modeling, and desensitization. These complementary methods are short term and oriented to the present and have been effective in treating depressive and anxiety disorders, as well as other disorders with focal symptoms that are responsive to direct intervention (e.g., sexual dysfunction).

### Interpersonal

The focus of this treatment is on current interpersonal adjustment, addressing stresses associated with changes in family or social roles (e.g., family and marital conflict, worker/supervisor conflict, interpersonal deficits associated with social isolation and withdrawal, and grieving for the loss of significant others). Klerman and colleagues developed the interpersonal psychotherapy of depression. This treatment method involves nondirective exploration and clarification of problems, exploration and ventilation of feelings, and modification of distortions in interpersonal communication (e.g., acting on false assumptions about the feelings and attitudes of significant others). It is short term, is oriented to the present, and was developed to treat depressive disorders.

### Supportive

This type of psychotherapy aims to restore impaired functioning to the patient's previous best norms (social, personal, and occupational) with a problem-solving, reassuring approach. The goals are to restore self-confidence and to minimize the impact of stress. It may be short term or long term, and is oriented to the present. Long-term therapy is appropriate for individuals with chronic and serious disabilities.

### Marital/couple/family

This method defines problems and conflicts as defective solutions to the life situations of couples or groups, rather than as individual symptoms. Treatment attempts to modify these self-defeating solutions by changing the couple's or the group's dynamics (e.g., patterns of communication and responsibility).

### Relaxation training

This training applies a set of behavioral procedures that facilitate relaxation in treating a number of disorders in which anxiety and tension are prominent, such as phobias, hypertension, cessation of cigarette smoking, and weight control. Manuals are available that describe these procedures step by step.

## MENTAL HEALTH REFERRALS FOR PSYCHOTHERAPY

To illustrate the referral process for psychotherapy, depression is used as an example considering the various psychotherapies (dynamic, cognitive, behavioral, interpersonal, and supportive) and the various formats (individual, group, and couples/family) to make decisions about diagnosis, treatment, and referral. The referral process may start with forming a therapeutic relationship, making a diagnostic evaluation, negotiating the diagnosis and treatment, and organizing a referral to a specific mental health specialist if appropriate and desired.

### Diagnostic evaluation

The first step of the diagnostic evaluation is to classify the depressive symptoms as severe, moderate, or mild (a symptom checklist for physicians is helpful), based on the American Psychiatric Association's criteria of major depression. A moderate to severe case involves at least one of the major indicators, such as a depressed mood or a loss of interest or pleasure in daily activities for a minimum of 2 weeks, and at least four of the minor indicators, such as weight loss or gain, insomnia or hypersomnia, psychomotor retardation or agitation, fatigue, guilt and/or worthlessness, poor concentration, and thoughts of death or suicide. A number of screening instruments have been developed to facilitate or confirm the clinical judgment. An empirically tested screening instrument is the five-item emotional well-being subscale of the SF-36 Health Survey. Another popular test for screening depression is the Beck Depression Inventory.

The second step of the diagnostic evaluation is to assess the comorbidity of disorders that may precipitate or be associated with the onset of depressive symptoms. These include substance abuse, medications such as glucosteroids and β-blockers, medical disorders such as myocardial infarction that may precipitate depression, and conditions such as anxiety, eating disorders, and grief reactions. Clinical practice guidelines suggest setting priorities when treating depression with associated disorders. All medical disorders and certain associated psychiatric disorders should be treated first, monitoring the beneficial effects of treatment, if any, on the depression. However, some cases require that treatment of depression begin at the same time as the treatment of the associated disorder, such as cases of anorexia, insomnia, and potential suicide, when symptoms are in need of immediate attention. Associated psychiatric disorders include substance abuse, obsessive-compulsive disorder, eating disorders, and personality disorders. If no benefit appears within a maximum of 6 weeks, treatment of the depression should be initiated. Other associated psychiatric disorders have different priorities. Cases of general anxiety require that the depression be treated first. The treatment decision regarding panic disorder with depression should be based on which condition is more severe. Setting priorities to treat associated disorders does not mean ignoring the depression, which often occurs in patients with serious medical conditions. These patients are often more comfortable with somatic explanations for their psychologic responses to medical conditions. Other practitioners do not see the benefit of deferring treatment of depressive disorders that are concurrent with medical disorders (see Chapter 133).

## Referral process: a negotiation

The physician's response to a patient's depressive symptoms entails three decision steps. The first decision is made in concurrence with the patient about the diagnosis. The negotiated approach reviews the patient's symptoms and behaviors, the causative basis of the disorder, and the implications for treatment. The second decision is made on the basis of negotiations with the patient over the kind of treatment, the indications for selecting a psychotherapist (psychiatrist, psychologist, or social worker) and information about psychotherapeutic approaches. The third decision concerns the indications for offering antidepressants on an outpatient basis.

## Making the intervention

Reaching a consensus with the patient about the diagnosis is ideally achieved before the physician proceeds with a mental health intervention. Although most patients agree with their physicians about the severity, cause, and significance of depressive symptoms, some do not. Discussing and resolving differences facilitate cooperation, enhance the working relationship, and avoid problems of compliance with treatment plans.

In negotiating a consensus about the presence of depression, patients strongly resist psychologic explanations for their headaches, sleeplessness, and loss of appetite. These resistances can be frustrating for the physician. Nonetheless, it is essential to work with them. For example, a patient may fear that his physician thinks his symptoms are being made up or that he is crazy and needs to be hospitalized. A mental health referral also may signify disengagement, if not abandonment, by the physician. The physician should therefore indicate a desire to follow the patient's progress after the referral.

After achieving consensus on the problem, the physician can proceed to a review of treatment options. The four major options for depression are (1) office-based pharmacotherapy (antidepressants); (2) referral to a mental health practitioner for psychotherapy; (3) a combination of pharmacotherapy and referral; and (4) referral to a psychiatrist, especially when there are questions about appropriate pharmacotherapy or in the presence of indications of the need for other somatic therapies, such as electroconvulsive therapy.

The negotiation process concerning treatment can start with either a nondirective or a directive approach. The nondirective scenario may begin with the physician saying, "I would like to review the treatment of your depression. There are four choices. First...." The physician can then describe each choice, inviting the patient to express a preference or to ask questions that will help to make a choice. The directive scenario could begin with the physician saying, "Given your depressive symptoms, I recommend [the method] and Dr. [name], who has been very helpful in cases like yours and gets good results." The physician then negotiates with the patient about any reservations he or she has.

Patients commonly do not follow through with referrals. The reasons are sometimes that the physician did not negotiate about the referral or that there was a disagreement about the problem or its treatment before making the referral. Many somatizing patients, for example, resist psychiatric diagnoses and do not comply with referrals to mental health specialists because they attribute their illness to a medical disease.

To negotiate with patients about a psychotherapy referral, it is essential to convey a readiness to hear reservations and to ask open-ended questions, such as "What do you think of my making arrangements with you for psychotherapy?" A question such as, "Do you have any questions?" prompts a "yes/no" answer and may cause confusion. Resistant patients may say "yes," but mean "no." As part of reaching a consensus about a treatment referral, the physician should explore the patient's preferences; for example, the physician might say, "Many patients have ideas and preferences regarding psychotherapy. How can I help you in this regard?" Many patients ask for a name; some ask for a particular treatment approach. Many patients do not know what to expect and want to be told. It is necessary to have the names of a number of therapists of both sexes, and of both generalists and specialists (e.g., those who work with children, adolescents, and adults, and those who practice family or cognitive/behavioral therapy).

Special considerations are involved in making psychiatric referrals for minorities, particularly concerning language and cultural diversity.

A problem related to making referrals is interprofessional communication. For example, in psychiatric referrals, generalist physicians have a greater difficulty in referring to and consulting with their psychiatric colleagues, since psychiatrists often have fewer consultation relationships than those in other medical specialties. Part of the difficulty also involves a failure in reciprocal communication. The generalist and the mental health specialist may not understand what each wants of the other, partly because they often do not regularly exchange concerns and information about patients. It is important for the generalist physician to frame questions in specific terms, including the need for the patient's follow-up, which is essential for coordinated care. A lack of follow-up information influences the physician's choice of referrals, including the choice to refrain from referring patients to noncommunicative colleagues.

## CHOOSING A TREATMENT OPTION

As a general guideline, office-based antidepressant pharmacotherapy is appropriate under the following conditions: mild to moderate depression, absence of psychosis, the patient's preference, no contraindicated comorbid medical or psychiatric disorders, past benefits, and infrequent relapse. It is appropriate to provide psychologic support during office-based pharmacotherapy. Referral for psychotherapy is appropriate with all the conditions listed above, the presence of significant psychosocial problems, and when antidepressants have made only limited improvement within two months. Consultation with a psychiatrist is recommended when there is only partial improvement, to review dosage adjustment, when there are disturbing side effects, and when there are questions regarding a change of medication. As a general guideline, referral to a psychiatrist for pharmacotherapy should be considered under the following conditions: moderate to severe depression, psychosis, comorbid psychiatric disorders, the patient's preference, and frequent relapse (see the clinical guidelines). The addition of psychotherapy also should be considered if there is limited improvement from pharmacotherapy within 8 weeks and/or there are significant, chronic psychosocial problems.

For the cases of mild to moderate depression or anxiety, for patients who prefer pharmacotherapy, and for cases in which there has been limited or no benefit with office-based treatment, it is appropriate to seek consultation for pharmacotherapy and for the feasibility of psychotherapy.

## SUMMARY

The care of patients with psychiatric disorders who are in the crises of illness and of everyday life requires both psychotherapeutic work by the physician and psychotherapy provided by the counselor. Distress and disorders may occur together. The physician can provide patients with relief through empathetic listening, reassurance, and direction—a therapeutic experience that, in turn, can make the referral acceptable for the counselor's psychotherapy.

## BIBLIOGRAPHY


Acosta FX, Yamamoto J, Evans LA: *Effective psychotherapy for low-income and minority patients,* New York, 1982, Plenum.

American Psychiatric Association: *Diagnostic and statistical manual of mental disorders,* ed 3, Washington, DC, 1987, American Psychiatric.

Balint M: *The doctor, his patient, and the illness,* New York, 1966, International Universities.

Beck AT et al: An inventory for measuring depression, *Arch Gen Psychiatry* 4:561, 1961.

Beck AT et al: *Cognitive therapy of depression,* New York, 1979, Guilford.

Benson H, Proctor W: *Beyond the relaxation response,* New York, 1985, Berkeley/GP Putnam's Sons.

Bibring GL: Psychiatry and medical practice in a general hospital, *N Engl J Med* 254:366, 1956.

Broadhead WE et al: Effects of medical illness and somatic symptoms on treatment of depression in a family medicine residency practice,

Depression Guideline Panel: *Depression in primary care,* Vol 1, Detection and diagnosis, clinical practices guideline, No 5, Rockville, MD: US Department of Health and Human Services, Public Health Service, Agency for Health Care Policy and Research, AHCPR Publication No 93-0550, April 1993.

Depression Guideline Panel: *Depression in primary care,* vol 2, Treatment of major depression, clinical practices guideline, No 5, Rockville, MD: US Department of Health and Human Services, Public Health Service, Agency for Health Care Policy and Research, AHCPR Publication No 93-0551, April 1993.

Groves JE: Taking care of the hateful patient, *N Engl J Med* 298:883, 1978.

Klerman GL et al: *Interpersonal therapy of depression,* New York, 1984, Basic.

Matthews DA, Suchman AL, Branch WT Jr: Making "connexions": enhancing the therapeutic potential of patient-clinician relationships, *Ann Intern Med* 118:973, 1993.

Orleans CT et al: How primary care physicians treat psychiatric disorders: a national survey of family practitioners, *Am J Psychiatry* 142:52, 1985.

Rosenbaum JF, Pollack MH: Anxiety. In Cassem N, editor: *Massachusetts General Hospital handbook of general hospital psychiatry,* St. Louis, 1991, Mosby.

Ware JE Jr: *SF-36 health survey: Manual and interpretation guide,* Boston, 1993, The Health Institute, New England Medical Center.


CHAPTER

# 122 Dealing with Difficult Patients

Martin R. Lipp

Every practitioner has difficulties with some patients, but are there some patients whom all practitioners find difficult? Research suggests there is no single type of patient whom all physicians call difficult, even though some types of difficulties are more common than others.

For example, a survey of 700 physicians in a major West Coast HMO asked respondents to identify their difficult patients. Angry patients provided a major challenge for 72% of respondents, followed by hypochondriacs (62%) and anxious patients (53%). It is interesting to note that 28% had no difficulty with angry patients, 38% reported no problems with hypochondriacs, and 47% felt comfortable with anxious patients.

Studies such as this tell what all physicians should know: difficult relationships and interactions are a function of all the parties involved and the circumstances in which they interact. The values, personalities, tolerances, experiences, training, and goals of individuals influence the kinds of behavior they desire or are willing to accept in the people with whom they are in contact.

## ORIGINS OF DIFFICULT BEHAVIOR

Why do interactions with patients become so difficult that physicians eventually label a specific patient as *difficult?* The literature provides several sets of explanations. Traditional psychiatric teaching interprets patients' misbehavior in the clinical setting in terms of psychopathology. This emphasis is a natural consequence of psychiatry's focus on individual cognitive and affective functions; but explaining interpersonal difficulties in terms of an individual's psychodynamics has far less predictive value than is commonly thought. Virtually any patient is likely to be perceived as difficult if conditions promote such perceptions. That is especially true for physicians and other knowledgeable health professionals. When *you,* for example, get sick or are hospitalized, how cooperative are you likely to be when cared for by an assortment of inexperienced medical students, rushed house officers who haven't slept in 24 hours, and nurses who are overworked and underpaid?

Although certain behavioral patterns inevitably stress the relationship between the physician and patient, this does not mean that either has a character disorder. Both may do perfectly well in other situations.

In the 1960s and 1970s, major revisionist literature emerged that explained the relationships between physicians and patients. In this literature, which continues to be written today, conflict between physicians and patients is said to stem from defects and limitations of the physician, not the patient. The problem with this, as teachers of medical students and house officers know, is that regardless of how tolerant students are in the beginning, no matter how strong the foundation in humanities, and no matter the sex or ethnicity, students become less tolerant of patients' behavioral eccentricities as education progresses, responsibilities increase, and the amount of time allotted to patients decreases.

The third principal body of literature to focus on relationships between physicians and patients (and their inherent problems) explains the friction in the clinical setting in terms of the role demands of the parties involved. Each individual is basically an actor on the stage, this view contends, acting out a role according to society's demands. The role of the patient carries certain rights and obligations, with the physician acting out an opposite and complementary role. For example, the patient is presumed not to be responsible for his or her condition and therefore can be excused from normal duties. The patient also has a right to expect care and assistance from others but in return is obliged to want to get well as soon as possible, to seek competent help, and to cooperate with treatment.

Strife develops between the doctor and the patient when either party is not accorded the rights inherent in his or her social role or fails to meet the obligations of that role. Although this sociologic formulation has provoked substantial thought and discussion, experience in clinical medicine quickly teaches that the rights and obligations of idealized social roles often bear little relation to reality. Chronic disease patients, for example, must forego the desire to get well as soon as possible and accept more restricted goals.

Difficult interactions are part of all human relationships and commerce. Anyone can become difficult under the right circumstances, depending on the highly variable aspects of individual personalities and how they are expressed at a given moment, and depending on the values, skills, and tolerance of the persons with whom individuals interact. Situational constraints also make contributions

Of course physicians prefer patients who are stoical, respectful, obedient, rational, and reliable, but people with these characteristics are easy for *everyone* to deal with, not only physicians.

Patients become a problem for the physician when their attitudes or behaviors interfere with the physician's perceived job. Patients are most likely to become difficult when they feel they have a problem in need of attention. The patient who tests the physician's tolerance is likely to be considered a problem. The physician's tolerance level depends not only on the broad aspects of personality and training, but also on the specific, current experiences of everyday life.

Emotionally charged issues, such as those concerning moral values, control, and time constraints, abound in the relationships between physicians and patients and may also cause problems. These issues are likely to be as important to patients as they are to physicians. Today's patients may be informed, wary, demanding, and desirous of collaborative relationships. For example, a woman who is concerned that she might have breast cancer may be educated on the subject and may have clear ideas about how the physician should proceed diagnostically. If her ideas differ from those of her physician, she may be perceived by the physician as demanding, difficult, and manipulative. The patient may perceive the physician as rigid, insensitive, and arrogant. Ironically, the two may be much alike—bright, responsible, organized, and caring—and each may be struggling to behave appropriately. The struggle, however, may become one for control.

Overwhelmingly, perceived misbehavior in the clinical setting does not reflect psychopathology. The physician who remembers this when emotions start to flare is better able to treat patients with respect and is more likely to be treated with respect in return.

It is useful to view problem behaviors as potentially multicausal. That is, problems may be related to the patient's personality style, disease process, and the hospital or clinic milieu. Physicians tend to assess the medical components of patients' behaviors, such as those that are expressions of underlying disease or drug side effects, and to make allowances for the patients' baseline character. Since most problems have an interpersonal component, however, the problems that arise within these relationships belong to both physicians and patients. Hence the most useful approach is to collaborate on solutions.

It is worth emphasizing that certain characteristics of physicians tend to bring out certain characteristics of patients. Rigidity in a physician tends to elicit rigidity in a patient, anger tends to elicit anger, and aloofness in response to a needy patient may result in the patient becoming even more dependent.

The most important determination to make when a patient's behavior seems to be troublesome is to whom the problem belongs. If the problem is heavily influenced by the patient's personality and the physician's response to it, then the suggestions offered in this chapter are particularly useful.

## GUIDELINES

What follows is a review of a variety of patient types and the types of interactions with patients that physicians commonly find difficult (see the box below).

Make the utmost effort to *avoid becoming defensive.* When the physician anticipates a difficult interaction with a patient, or when an interaction has already become difficult, it is important to alleviate the tension. The use of a soft voice and effective body language helps to reach an amicable solution. For example, the physical position most conducive to expressing anger is standing; therefore the physician should sit. It is also important for the physician not to become unnerved by difficult interactions that may cause problems later. The physician should do whatever is necessary to avoid an adversarial situation.

*Look for emotional issues* within the patient that might be adding to the difficulty of the situation. Many physicians are preoccupied with statistics and try to deal with difficult interactions by marshaling information and explaining data to patients. This approach rarely helps when a patient is upset. The patient does not care how much the physician knows until he or she is convinced of how much the physician cares. If the patient's circumstances are dominated by emotional considerations, that's where the physician should focus. Showing concern, such as offering the patient some coffee or facial tissue, is important. It may be difficult to express empathy when a patient is yelling, but again, the physician should avoid becoming unnerved.

*Accept the patient's emotional response* as something that is appropriate for him or her. It is unnecessary to fight the patient's emotions or to run from them. Emotions are part of the package the patient brings. The physician is not responsible for the patient's feelings and does not have to admire or feel burdened by them.

If possible, *validate the patient's emotions,* showing agreement with the patient's perceptions and interpretations. This is an external process in which the physician expresses empathy and diminishes potential strain, emotional distance, and an adversarial atmosphere. The physician might say, "Your emotions make perfect sense from your point of view," "Many people share such concerns," or, "I'm sure I might feel the same way in similar circumstances."

### Guidelines for interactions with difficult patients

- Avoid becoming defensive.
- Look for emotional issues.
- Accept the patient's emotions as valid from his or her point of view.
- Validate the patient's perceptions, interpretations, and emotions when possible.
- Clarify the intent to be a good physician and to take good care of the patient.
- When setting limits becomes necessary, physicians should set limits on themselves, not on their patients.
- Always remain the patient's ally.

If appropriate, *express the intent to be a good physician,* according to both personal standards and the patient's standards. The patient's satisfaction is an essential ingredient to professional life, including income, reputation, professional security, and personal satisfaction. Maintaining amicable relations with patients adds to personal confidence and lowers stress. Physicians who consistently fail to meet patients expectations eventually must respond to formal inquiries from hospital and department chiefs, health plan administrators, attorneys, and licensing boards. The patient who expresses concerns directly to the physician allows the opportunity to solve problems at the most desirable level.

When setting limits becomes necessary, physicians should *set limits* on themselves, not on their patients. Instead of saying, "You can't do that," it is more appropriate to say, "I don't feel comfortable doing what you requested." Few adults like being judged or told what to do by another adult. The physician should avoid being perceived as attacking the pride or dignity of the patient. A patient's request (verbal or nonverbal) for a certain type of response does not mean the physician must comply, just as the patient is not required to comply with the physician's wishes.

Traditionally, the most important function of the physician in the relationship with patients has been to *always remain the patient's ally.* This is usually important to the physician's self-esteem, to professional satisfaction, and to being held in high regard by co-workers. The most difficult patients can become the most satisfying. Nothing creates lasting bonds more successfully than surviving difficult times together. If the patient does not at first appear to be someone with whom the physician wishes to be allied, the physician should look for attractive qualities and mutual interests that may be hidden. This can be accomplished by asking about hobbies, life experiences, spouses and children, favorite sports teams, and favorite foods or recipes. Seeking common interests that enhance mutual respect and regard can be very effective.

## ANGRY PATIENTS

Anger is related to, but is not necessarily synonymous with, irritation, hostility, verbal abuse, belligerence, and a lack of cooperation. Anger is a normal part of the illness experience for many patients, and it is crucial that physicians do not get defensive when faced with such anger. A patient's anger, even when directed toward the physician, does not mean that the physician is to blame. Furthermore, the patient who expresses displeasure with a nurse or consultant may not be perceived as a hostile person by the physician. The patient who aims displeasure directly at the physician, however, is much more likely to be perceived as hostile.

The physician may foster anger in patients by being aloof, distant, defensive, insensitive, accusatory, or impolite. Furthermore, patients may respond aggressively to a physician's lack of humility, especially if the patient feels humiliated by illness or the process of seeking care.

Anger is a symptom and an indication to the physician to seek the cause. Patients seldom express anger for the purpose of punishing the people around them; their feelings are more often a response to a situation. Whether anger is kept inside or expressed verbally or physically depends on the intensity of the feeling, situational constraints, the expected outcome of exhibiting the anger, and the individual's personality style.

Anger has many positive functions. For some, anger is simultaneously scary and satisfying. Many individuals treasure their anger, and allow themselves to express rage as a rare gift to themselves. Anger endows an individual with a sense of potency, of being in charge. A man who says he is really angry, for example, tends to get attention. Anger can be intimidating to others and makes the individual expressing it feel more secure. Like a porcupine's spines, anger tends to keep people at a distance. Anger has considerable instrumental value: the power to instigate action, whether constructive or not. Finally, anger provides a means for externalizing conflict. Depression frequently results from anger turned inward; depression turned outward in the form of anger tends to put the responsibility for change on factors outside of the individual.

Anger kept inside can become a formidable barrier to amicable relations between the physician and the patient. Conversely, ventilated anger, handled with appropriate finesse by the parties involved, can provide the basis for a good relationship.

All these functions are as relevant to physicians as they are to patients. Therefore the physician's temptation to respond to a patient's anger by becoming angry in return is sometimes considerable. Anger of patients usually results in one of three responses from the medical staff: anger in return, avoidance, or an attempt to placate. No single approach is correct, but following the guidelines described earlier can help the physician to choose from a wide range of acceptable responses to resolve tensions with patients.

As mentioned earlier, the physician should avoid becoming defensive. It is not appropriate to argue or preach, or to take the patient's anger as a personal attack. Also, the physician should never take sides with the patient against another staff member as a means of redirecting the patient's anger.

The patient's anger must be accepted as appropriate from his or her point of view. This acceptance can be conveyed by the physician saying, for example, "If that's what your experience was, I can certainly understand why you are upset," or, "I'm glad you are telling me these things. People like you help us improve our service" (see the box at right).

The physician must maintain a thoroughly respectful and professional stance. Condescension is unacceptable. Humor is inappropriate unless the physician is extremely skilled because the patient may intrepret that the matter (or the patient) is not being taken seriously. Informality should be avoided. If the patient is at all suspicious, he or she may misjudge warmth as a ploy.

If an angry situation erupts and gets out of hand, attempts should be made at resolution. One unpleasant interaction should not interfere with the physician's usual standards of thoroughness and continuity of care. If the conflict occurs in the office, both the physician and the patient should have an opportunity to calm down. Later, the physician can call the patient and express his or her feelings, such as saying, "I'm sorry the situation got away from us. I'd like to work things out between us and see that your health care needs are well served. Shall we try again?" Most patients respond to such an overture and, even for those who do not, it is reassuring for the physician to make the effort.

### Suggested responses to the angry patient

"If that is what you experienced, your feelings are certainly understandable."
"I understand. Lots of people would be upset in similar circumstances."
"If that's what you feel, I'm glad you aren't keeping your feelings inside."

## COMPLAINING, DEMANDING PATIENTS

There are obvious similarities between the angry patient and the patient who complains, but there are important differences. The patient with a complaint is not unique. Every person can find plenty to complain about in life, more so during illness, and particularly when in the presence of a physician or in a complex medical center. However, only a minority of patients actually complain to the physician or staff, and a much smaller group do so with any regularity.

Complaints are usefully seen as communications of dissatisfaction or discomfort resulting from fear, anxiety, loneliness, generalized neediness, and insecurity. Complaints do not necessarily require a response in the form of a specific action. Although complaints may focus on matters of personal discomfort, medical treatment, or the hospital or clinic environs, it is useful to ask why this patient has chosen to express a complaint rather than remain passive and quiet like most patients.

Complaints occur most frequently among several specific groups of patients. The first group is composed of those who have a genuine complaint. This possibility should always be considered, even though other less reasonable factors may contribute to the complaint. Second, complaints tend to be most prominent among certain long-term and chronic patients. Commonly the patient becomes progressively more disenchanted with health care at the same time that he or she becomes increasingly knowledgeable about the ways in which his or her health care might be managed. The difference between the amount of experience the patient has had with his or her condition and the amount of experience the physician has had with the same condition tends to lessen considerably with all but the most experienced physicians.

The patient typically begins to feel that he or she knows almost as much as the physician knows about the disorder, realizing also that only the physician can mobilize medical services. The patient in this circumstance sometimes comes to resent physicians as obstacles to, rather than facilitators of, medical care. For example, a patient knows he needs his catheter irrigated, but the nurse refuses to comply unless ordered to do so by the physician. The medical environment becomes a dominant feature of chronic patients' landscape and they often seek to influence it.

### Suggested responses to the complaining patient

"It's frustrating when things don't go the way we wish."
"If that's the way you see things, I'm glad you are speaking up."
"Observations like yours keep me on my toes. Thanks for bringing that to my attention."

Some locations in medical facilities seem to be magnets for complaints, particularly those which process large numbers of patients in relatively impersonal contacts, where a patient's view of what is needed may differ significantly from that of the staff. Screening nurses often become special targets of complaints, as do drop-in clinics and emergency departments, where sick but not critically ill patients are made to wait for care.

Complaints often stem from perceived brusqueness, impersonal behavior, and insensitivity by staff members. Frequently patients do not complain about these experiences or even about individuals directly, but focus instead on seemingly trivial matters that are only marginally related to the specific staff members involved (see the box above).

Sometimes complaints have strong cultural components. Suffering with dramatic flair is highly esteemed in some cultures; indeed, it is expected. Only when this type of patient begins to brood silently should the physician become concerned. Another culturally sanctioned behavior that is sometimes perceived by physicians as criticism has to do with patients who use aggression as a method of bonding. For example, a patient may say, "Doc, you have the worst handwriting on the face of this earth," in the same way he might say to a basketball buddy, "My baby sister can hit hoops better than you."

Another type of patient prone to frequent complaints is the compulsive individual who copes with stress by mastering detail. This individual tends to be logical, self-disciplined, orderly, precise, and cost conscious. Requiring knowledge and data to cope, this patient asks a lot of questions and may become quite obstinate when information is not forthcoming. This patient can also become upset by lapses in routine. The more stressful the circumstances, the more compulsive the patient becomes, and complaints usually develop proportionately (see the boxes at right).

A series of complaints tends to elicit a progression of responses. The first complaint results in a response; the repeated complaint produces a diminished response; the complaint made yet again results in no response, and finally an aversive response.

The first task for the physician is to develop a level of frustration tolerance. It helps to keep a sense of humor and to see the patient's capacity for suffering noisily as adaptive. The challenge is to empathize without forcing a personal variety of help on the patient. Physicians should convey care about how the patient feels and appreciation for the patient's need to ventilate, but the primary focus should remain on the health concerns of the patient.

### Suggested responses to the complaining, very knowledgeable patient

"You really know a lot about your condition. How have you managed to learn so much?"
"A knowledgeable patient is a wonderful ally. Your cousin who is a nurse gave you a good overview. There is a lot he said that I agree with, but I view some things differently."
"You obviously know a lot about this topic. Perhaps we can teach one another."

### Suggested responses to the complaining patient with a list of problems

"It's frustrating to have a whole list of concerns when your doctor can only deal with a few. Let's see if we can set some priorities."
"I appreciate that you organized your concerns. An organized patient is a big help to me."
I'm glad you wrote everything down. Let me see your list."

The following statement can be very effective in coping with dissatisfied patients: "It must be frustrating for you to feel such dissatisfaction and be unable to alter our behavior to suit your needs." With some patients the physician can also acknowledge his or her own frustration: "I would really like to be of more help to you, but I have my limitations. It's frustrating for me not to be able to do things to your satisfaction."

Patients whose complaints reflect a compulsive need for control can be helped by giving them access to data that are relevant to their conditions. Physicians should understand that these patients need control over anxiety, not over the technical aspects of their care per se, although some participation in the latter may help. These patients can be given tasks that occupy their attention, such as keeping their own intake and output records, charting their own exercise records, and changing their own dressings. Physicians must always remember to ask for suggestions from colleagues and, if the breach with the patient is beyond repair, arrange for the orderly transfer of care to another physician.

## DEPENDENT, PASSIVE PATIENTS

The patient who is viewed as overly dependent appears to expect others to do all the work to change a state of relative illness into a state of relative health and seems unwilling to assist with the process. Such individuals are usually perceived as wasting vast quantities of the physician's time for reasons that make no apparent sense.

Excessive dependency occurs most often in individuals with a bona fide medical disorder, particularly older patients who are under coexistent psychologic or social stress. This latter group tends to produce feelings in physicians concerning potential dependency by their own parents. Consequently, responses are often quite personal.

Interactions between the physician and an overly dependent patient follow a pattern. The patient makes implicit or explicit needs known and the physician attempts to satisfy the patient's request. When the attempts do not satisfy the patient, the physician tries again. These attempts fail and the cycle continues until the physician or the patient can no longer tolerate it. Eventually, the frustration is likely to result in anger or withdrawal. Neither response helps the patient or satisfies the physician.

Many physicians feel annoyed with themselves and with the patients. There is often a sense of helplessness and guilt. The patient seems to defeat every effort to help. The doctor is torn between vain, repeated efforts and the desire to avoid the patient entirely. Patients who add a note of urgency to their requests, perhaps with tears, and those who present themselves as especially giving and caring persons are particularly irritating.

Dependency has many implications for both the patient and the physician. It represents general neediness, a means of maintaining human contact, and a way of controlling relationships. Being given something—a gesture, an object, an emotion, or time—can represent love, caring, or affection. Illness, to many, not only means being taken care of, but also represents stress that may exaggerate neediness in the person's character. Illness is sometimes the only situation in which a person can show dependency needs, and so needs that have been stored up erupt with a vengeance.

Physicians typically do not show their dependency needs. Indeed, many are not consciously aware of having dependency needs. Those needs, however, exist in everyone, and many people are frightened of them. Consequently dependence in patients can be particularly rankling. Only by accepting their own dependency needs can physicians come to accept the dependency needs of patients without making moral judgments.

The first step in adequate treatment of dependent patients involves the development of tolerance for dependency and feelings of comfort in its presence. If the physician can perceive dependency as something other than a personal threat, relationships with dependent patients can be greatly improved.

Dependency can be approached as a paradox: "It must be awfully difficult for an ordinarily self-sufficient person like you to be so dependent on others for so many basics of daily living." This helps patients to understand that the physician does not define them totally by their dependent needs and understands that they are complex individuals. A comment like this brings the issue out in the open in a manner that rarely arouses an objection.

Next, the physician can try to see dependency as a symptom. Why does the patient prefer to be helpless at this time rather than independent? What does the patient really want? Satisfaction of generalized neediness? To maintain human contact? To exert some control over the relationship with the physician?

The physician should try to gratify some of the patient's needs. The patient can be allowed time in which the physician asks relatively little, but gives a little extra.

**Suggested responses to the dependent patient**

"It must be awfully rough having to go through all this by yourself."

"I'm glad you are telling me all this. It helps me understand your situation so much better."

"It must be frustrating for a self-sufficient person like you to need help."

Most patients respond extremely well to small gestures: a profferred glass of water, the fluffing of a pillow, an arm to lean on while walking down the hall.

A lack of time is almost always a problem, but physicians can learn to give something other than time. For example, the physician and the patient may perceive the prescription as a symbolic gift. Rather than overprescribing chemicals, however, the same principle can be adapted by writing instructions ("Don't forget to take your orange juice with your pills for swelling"), requests ("Bring an exercise log to your next visit"), and resources (telephone numbers for support groups). An inspired gift is to help dependent patients to feel needed; for example, say, "I have a patient who is having the same problems you overcame last year. May I ask her to give you a call?"

Setting time limits for dependent patients is often necessary so that the patient's needs do not outdistance resources (see the box above). However, it is important that the physician does not appear to be impatient, unresponsive, or punitive when doing so. This can be avoided by explaining to the patient, "I'm not going to be able to spend as much time with you today as I would like, but here's what I'm going to try to do."

## MANIPULATIVE PATIENTS

All patients who want something from the physician cannot be considered manipulative, but most physicians find it difficult to assess patients who make social and economic requests without using derogatory labels. Traditionally, the terms physicians use to label such patients reflect: the degree to which organic disease is present, the degree to which the patients seem to be trying to get well, and the degree to which the patients' requests are justified. For example, if a patient who clearly has an organic disease, seems to be cooperating with the standard therapeutic regimen, and has reasonable requests, most physicians do their best to be helpful and to comply. On the other hand, if a patient has no evidence of organic disease, seems to relish being ill, and makes requests that are dramatically disproportionate to those made by comparable patients, physicians tend to regard such individuals as manipulators.

This assumption has significant limitations. First, experienced physicians know that patients who have no objective evidence of disease at one point in time may develop conditions that explain their earlier symptoms. Second, unless there is concrete evidence to the contrary, it may be difficult to know to what degree an ambulatory patient is actively participating in a treatment regimen, since patients spend most of their time outside the scrutiny of health professionals. Third, determining the degree to which a patient's requests are justified is fraught with problems. It is impossible for the physician to know how a patient feels. One challenge in clinical medicine is for physicians to maintain the integrity of their beliefs without being so judgmental that care for patients is hindered.

There is a wide range of behavior that can be described as manipulative, from disability compensation patients to professional invalids to narcotic-seeking patients.

The lives of disability compensation patients seem to be dominated by the desire for financial remuneration. Compensation tends to be more important to these patients than the technical and physical limitations imposed by their medical conditions. This group must be distinguished from the truly disabled, for whom living life despite physical limitations becomes the major concern.

Various personality types that have been identified as manipulative include the following:

- The passive, dependent, immature individual who seeks to avoid competition for fear of failure or even because the possibility of success is frightening
- The self-punishing individual who emphasizes inner flaws to atone for feelings of guilt
- The angry person, for whom disability is a weapon to punish others or society by requiring one group or another to pay financial penance
- The self-dramatizing individual, for whom disability is a way of gaining attention and providing a convenient identity and means for relating to other people
- The aging worker who has been dedicated to a job for years, but no longer feels satisfaction with work or cannot tolerate it any longer, and who has no financially secure alternative to disability compensation

Whatever the explanation, many patients have much to gain and little to lose by seeking compensation for a physical disability. There are a number of paradoxes at work here. Although there is a tradition of pride in working in this country, and although most of adolescence is spent preparing to find a satisfying job or occupation, the prime ambition for many is nonetheless to retire early on a guaranteed income. Total disability may be an individual's sole access to that goal. Partial disability offers only restricted benefit; it is difficult for the partially disabled to find employment, and benefits are often reduced or eliminated with limited employment.

These paradoxes are translated into reality by the multiple individuals concerned with the patient's disability (attorney, physician, employer, therapist, insurance agent, union representative), each of whom may have a narrow goal that works at cross purposes with those of others in the group.

It becomes natural for disabled individuals to want whatever compensation is available. There is no punishment for trying to gain disability benefits. In fact, there is a broad current in societal attitudes that fosters disability. For example, some individuals feel justified in seeking disability because they have paid taxes. The courts can sometimes be quite generous, and there has been a trend to require less obvious cause-and-effect relationships between disabilities and potential causative events or circumstances.

### Suggested responses to the manipulative patient

"From your point of view, it certainly makes sense to ask for that."

"If you see me as an obstacle to something that you want, it's understandable to be upset."

"Since I'm not comfortable giving you what you ask, let's consider alternatives."

### Suggested responses to the manipulative patient who requests pain medications

"If you think only medications will help, I can understand your wanting them so badly."

"It's frustrating for you to want pain medications and for me to say 'no.'"

"Your wishes are completely understandable, but since I don't feel comfortable writing the prescription, let's consider other alternatives."

Achievement of satisfactory treatment and relative satisfaction for the participants depends on two principles. First, avoid getting into an adversarial position. Physicians should not attempt to police patients or behave as if patients are criminals. Physicians should impose limits on themselves, not on patients (see the box above). The physician might say, "I will try to describe your disability honestly as it appears to me, but of course I am only seeing you in the office and not at your home and job." In cases where a patient wants more time off work than seems appropriate, the physician might say, "I understand that you would like a month off, but I really don't feel comfortable authorizing more than a few days." For patients requesting narcotic medications that the physician believes are unnecessary, say "I am comfortable giving you some codeine pills, but I'd feel really awkward prescribing anything stronger than that" (see the box above).

Second, don't expect significant improvement until all compensation issues are settled, if then. Physicians cannot cure patients for whom a cure means returning to an unhappy and financially precarious life.

## PATIENTS IN DENIAL

Denial makes a lot of sense when viewed from the patient's perspective. Many individuals, when forced to choose between conscious and unconscious suffering, would choose the latter. Lack of awareness might be a blessing. Denial, in fact, is a matter of day-to-day existence; for example, few people are able to face the idea of potential carcinogens in their food and water or the ever-present danger of nuclear accidents.

Physicians are most concerned with denial as a patient's response to the fact of illness. Physicians must recognize that the patient in denial has been overwhelmed by the awareness or suspicion of illness and its potential seriousness. It is an achievement for such patients simply to make an appointment with the physician, and they should not be punished by being forced to confront fate. The patient in this circumstance is saying, "I can handle some of what is happening, but I want to see myself, and I want you to see me, as healthy, intact, and able."

There are multiple levels of denial, both of degree and of the conscious acceptance of the fact of the illness, its significance, and affective significance:

*Delusion:* "This isn't me. I'm not here. This isn't happening."

*Minimization:* "This is happening. I am here, but this isn't serious."

*Repression:* "I know I am sick, but I keep forgetting the details."

*Blunted affect:* "I know I am sick. I know what is happening, but I have no feelings about it."

*Suppression:* I know what is happening, but as long as I try not to think about it, I don't feel so bad."

Denial may be adaptive for the person experiencing it, but physicians are often irritated because they see denial as an obstacle to treatment. The physician may respond emotionally with frustration, anger, and bewilderment. Many physicians feel obliged to confront the patient who is in denial. This customarily leads to greater anxiety for the patient, however, with consequent increased denial, increasingly strident confrontations between the physician and the patient, and finally either decompensation or elopement from treatment.

Denial can create problems for the physician when the patient chooses to focus on one aspect of a condition without acknowledging other, perhaps more important, aspects. For example, the terminal cancer patient may appear unwilling to accept the prognosis but nonetheless keeps asking, "Why am I losing all this weight?" Physicians often find such questions extremely frustrating. Frustration, however, may act as a guide to approaching the patient effectively. In some respects the physician's frustration reflects the patient's frustration from the lack of control over destiny. An appropriate response for the physician therefore is to say, "It must be awfully frustrating for you to want to get well and to nonetheless lose weight" (see the box below).

Physicians should focus on their own emotional responses without pitting themselves against patients. For example, the response to a severely emphysematous patient who is dyspneic and coughing but who still smokes is to say, "It upsets me to see what you are doing to yourself, but I will do my best for you, even if you can't cut down on your smoking."

### Suggested responses to the patient in denial

"Let's not worry about what we call this condition. Let's focus on helping you feel better."

"It's scary to be sick, but you have a lot of positive things going for you. Let's figure out how to make all your strengths work for you."

"I have confidence in you and in the two of us working together."

## OVERLY AFFECTIONATE PATIENTS

Relationships between physicians and patients have an enormous potential for intimacy. Intimacy represents a powerful tool for patient care, but there is also a potential for problems. Patients with whom physicians have the greatest intimacy are the source of their most dramatic successes and greatest troubles. The line between a useful amount of intimacy and too much intimacy is difficult to draw.

There are many kinds of overly affectionate patients, including those who are adoring, respectful, or seductive. The overly affectionate patient appears to want more from the relationship than simply interacting on the basis of the illness and its treatment. These patients may be flirtatious, playful, inviting, or demanding. They are highly personal in manner, forthcoming, and seem to demand a similar response from their physicians. They often have self-dramatizing or charming qualities. They may ask physicians and other medical personnel personal questions. The approach may seem sexual or, from an older patient, may seem maternal or paternal.

This behavior has an adaptive value for patients to reach out to someone else on a personal level. Flirting with female nurses, for example, results in a patient gaining a clear identity, ensuring that the staff recognizes him as an individual. A patient who approaches medical personnel as a potential friend or lover is a patient whose name is not likely to be forgotten. The patient succeeds in raising himself or herself above the level of being "the gastrectomy in room 432." Seductive patients often feel they will not *gain* special attention unless they *pay* special attention. The goal of this behavior is to win allies.

Some physicians never have trouble with overly personal patients, indicating that certain kinds of physicians tend to elicit certain kinds of behaviors from their patients. There are seductive physicians as well as seductive patients. When a sexual liaison develops between a physician and a patient, it is usually due to personal neediness of the physician, for example, when he or she is feeling depressed or lonely. The distinction between the seducer and the seduced is not always clear.

A patient's intimate or seductive behavior usually indicates a need to be noticed and a desire for a personal relationship rather than an impersonal one. Seductive behavior can easily be interpreted as bravado. If bravado is taken at face value, the physician may miss the anxiety that prompts it. Seductive behavior may hide feelings of helplessness. Occasionally the patient's seductive behavior is designed to make authority figures appear more accessible and humble, particularly during an illness that makes the patient feel defective and unattractive. Fear of decreased personal attractiveness, sexual or otherwise, that prompts seductive behavior may be a bid for approval.

Physicians struggle with their response to a patient's seductive behavior usually for fear of rejecting or hurting the patient, or of appearing stuffy. A further struggle ensues with the emotional impact on physicians' own psyches. The physician may wonder how he or she would feel as a patient under these circumstances. There may be questions about the physician's need for approval, the possibility of being seduced, and the fear these possibilities cause.

It is important to recognize that personal and intimate relations between the physician and patient are not necessarily evil or destructive. Most physicians feel a particular closeness with some of their patients. However, intimacy is a *hazard* for physicians resulting in the patient's needs becoming blurred with the physician's. Maintaining the primacy of the patient's needs is an important ethic in medicine. Physicians risk losing self-respect when they stop behaving in a way that says to the patient, "You can trust me. I will not confuse your needs with my own."

There are several guidelines for physicians in such situations. First, the seductive behavior should be viewed as a symptom, the patient is asking for a positive response, and the range of positive responses is broad (see the box below). Withholding a positive response usually causes the patient's behavior to escalate. Potential positive responses include saying, "You appear to be doing quite well," "You seem to have made quite a hit with the nursing staff," and "You may have a bum knee but there's nothing wrong with the rest of you."

Second, in general, it is appropriate to acknowledge the patient's overtures without feeling the need to respond in a specific fashion. Ignoring the overtures entirely is rarely sufficient. The physician's manner and tone are more important than what is said. The goal is to demonstrate that the patient is considered a unique, decent individual who deserves the best possible care.

Third, the limits set for seductive behavior should be comfortable for the physician, but not punitive toward the patient. Limits that are most appropriate differ among physicians, but regardless of these differences, all physicians should adhere to the limitations they have set. For example, a physician can avoid resentment or guilt by saying, "I appreciate your invitation to dinner, but I find it difficult to take good professional care of patients with whom I am socially and personally involved. Since that takes such a high priority with me, I must decline."

In addition, the physician should acknowledge that a patient who has been sick or hospitalized for a long time is likely to feel sexual neediness and a need for enhancement of self-esteem. Giving symbolic attention, reassurance, and approval is appropriate, but the physician should never become enmeshed with a patient.

Finally, discussing positive feelings openly with a patient can be very helpful, but it requires a lot of skill, sensitivity, and self-assurance. Discussing mutual attraction and maintaining a professional relationship is extremely difficult without experience, and a consultation with someone who has more experience may be in order. Whenever possible, the input and perspective of someone the physician trusts is preferable to coping alone.

**Suggested responses to the seductive, overly affectionate patient**

"You are very special. I care about you as an individual, but my duty is to you as a patient."

"It's important to me to maintain a professional manner with you and all my patients."

## BORDERLINE PATIENTS

In contrast to the types of patient discussed earlier, the borderline patient is a formal psychiatric diagnosis that is based on explicit criteria. The term was first introduced in 1938 to refer to a group of disorders that are intermediate between neuroses and psychoses. In the decades since, the concept has continued to evolve and, although the formal diagnosis seems quite scientific in the official nomenclature, the psychiatric literature reveals enormous controversy about borderline disorder. Numerous articles attack the validity of the concept, as well as the reliability and specificity of the criteria used to apply the diagnosis to individual patients.

Nonetheless, the term *borderline* is widely used among clinicians, often without regard to specific diagnostic criteria. The term often becomes a perjorative label, a pseudodiagnostic term that a growing number of health professionals prefer to less elegant terms. Thus, the focus of this section is on the kinds of difficulties physicians experience when they label a patient as a borderline personality, regardless of the accuracy of that diagnosis according to formal psychiatric criteria.

The predominant feature of patients who are most likely to be viewed as borderline by clinicians is turbulence. Borderline individuals tend to live turbulent lives and have turbulent relationships, both with the important people in their lives and with health care professionals. They are commonly regarded as demanding, contentious, impetuous, noncompliant, and manipulative. Listening to those labeled borderline personalities, however, makes it clear that they see themselves somewhat differently. Commonly, they regard themselves as adventurous people who live for the moment and hate being in a rut. They are passionate, but the objects of their passion may change regularly. Relationships have considerable importance while they last, but they do do not last, and loneliness is often preferable to relationships that no longer meet expectations. Plagued by doubts concerning their own self-worth, borderline individuals devalue everyone who gets involved with them; thus the more giving the physician is, the more the borderline patient doubts the physician's basic competency.

A behavior that a physician might regard as dangerous or potentially self-destructive the borderline views as worth it because the emotional intensity and experiential pleasure justify the risks that might frighten or repel others. Logic and objectivity tend not to be held in great esteem; courage, spontaneity, and zest for life rank high. Borderline individuals are not enthusiastic about planning and organizing their futures because they believe in chance and luck, and they want to take advantage of opportunities as they occur. Consequently, they tend to do poorly in highly organized settings, and few have patience for much formal schooling or career building, for the legal system, for complicated medical regimens, or for preventive health care. As they describe their own lives, borderline patients commonly alternate between congratulatory self-justification and profound self-criticism.

To interact comfortably with borderline patients, physicians have to make some mental shifts. The first step is to accept the patient as he or she is, including impulsive changes in priorities, compliance failures, and prolonged lapses in contact. The physician copes best with these patients by being flexible and making health care as hassle free as possible. This means being satisfied with providing episodic assistance as needed and as the patient is willing to accept it and avoiding demands that the patient make fundamental lifestyle changes. In cases of a borderline patient with a chronic illness for which compliance is important (e.g., diabetes), the physician should acknowledge frustration with the clinical realities imposed by the patient's lifestyle: "Until you are able to better control your diet, we won't be able to get your blood sugar under control. It's frustrating for both of us, but we'll have to do the best we can."

Second, while trying to be flexible, the physician must recognize his or her own limits and make them clear to the patient without being punitive. It is unnecessary to be instantly available to the patient and to meet all of the patient's requests. It suffices for the physician to stress the wish to be visibly fair to all patients and to practice medicine in a manner that is comfortable over a long period. The physician might say, "I'm here. I want to help. Try to accept what I can give without being too upset by my limitations."

Third, borderline patients develop passionate, volatile relationships that they have difficulty sustaining. Generally, physicians do best with borderline patients if they remain friendly but professional, saying in essence "I am your doctor. I care for you, and I will be here for you, but I am not your bosom buddy." The physician must provide stability and consistency without expecting the patient to do the same. Attempts by the borderline patient to intensify the doctor-patient relationship beyond the physician's level of comfort should thus be thwarted. The physician should also expect sudden bursts of criticism from the patient.

Finally, to the extent that is possible, the physician should approach borderline patients with a sense of respect and compassion rather than with a desire to confront and change (see the box below). The constant pursuit of stimulation often masks the borderline patient's considerable substrate of depressive symptoms and thoughts, and their bluster and aggressive posturing frequently represent a cover for low self-esteem.

### Suggested responses to the borderline patient

"Let's get beyond what is going wrong, and see if we can focus on what we can do right."

"I want to be a good doctor for you, but I'm only available by appointment."

"There are so many things going on in your life that it's easy to overlook some health care concerns. Let's try to figure out some ways to make it easier for you to keep track of them."

If borderline patients do not self-destruct as a result of high-risk behavior, they generally settle down and stabilize their lifestyles as they get older. Although volatility tends to dominate their early years, such frenetic activity becomes much harder to sustain into middle age. Many arrive at their middle years with a head full of memories and a life filled with dramatic experiences, but a body covered with tatoos and scars, and few enduring successes to ease their later years. Thus adult borderline patients typically need to work hard at meeting material needs for themselves and their families, and little about their lives is easy. As they evolve, they tend to be enormously grateful to individuals who had patience and understanding with them during the tumultuous years. Eventually they may be among the physician's most satisfying patients.

## PARANOID PATIENTS

Paranoia in any given individual may range from a few suspicious notions to a personality that is dominated by paranoid ideation to frank psychosis. All adults who live in contemporary society need some degree of suspiciousness to survive. To be lacking in vigilance leaves oneself and one's loved ones open to misadventure, fraud, theft, and predation. However, to be suspicious to the point of believing that civilization is organized to persecute you personally is clearly not compatible with ordinary life.

Individuals who have paranoid delusions, who think society (or significant portions of it) are conspiring against them, constitute the most extreme examples of paranoia. It is difficult to imagine living with the belief that the world is organized specifically against you. Such individuals feel they have limited choices in coping with their environment. Some withdraw completely, some attempt what they regard as crafty negotiations and maneuvering with all potential adversaries, and some attack. It is the last group who raise the most concern.

Violent attacks on health care providers by paranoid psychotic persons tend to make all health care professionals wary of paranoid individuals generally. Paranoid psychotics are patients whose health care needs must be provided by medical specialists who work with psychiatrists.

Some paranoid features of an otherwise normal individual occur frequently among patients in primary care. All health care workers need to be able to contend with patients in whom there is some degree of paranoia. Ordinary levels of paranoia range from simple and rather generalized problems of trust to highly focused suspicions about specific health care providers or institutions. Patients who harbor such concerns may or may not talk about them. Sometimes these patients withdraw from potentially threatening situations and the physician views them as shy, withdrawn, or aloof. Sometimes they pretend to participate in treatment, but quietly refrain from full cooperation, and physicians see them as noncompliant or passive-aggressive. Sometimes they become quarrelsome or accusatory and physicians regard them as hostile or frankly paranoid.

As paranoia becomes more severe, the patient becomes increasingly wary, even hypervigilant. Because these patients trust so little, they tend to believe only information and experiences that confirm their paranoid views. Paranoid patients usually have little confidence in themselves, but shield these inadequacies for fear of giving others a competitive advantage. Paranoid patients feel disliked and become overly sensitive to criticism and rejection. Feeling unjustly criticized, they in turn are critical. Perceiving no generosity of spirit around them, they have little for others. They also fear the unfamiliar and the spontaneous.

Many physicians find paranoid patients difficult to cope with because a certain amount of trust is considered an essential ingredient in the relationship between physicians and patients, and resentment can arise for patients who withhold that trust. Often, physicians respond to the hostility of paranoid patients, whether subliminal or blatant, with hostility. Physicians have been taught that paranoia can lead to violence and, paradoxically, sometimes become wary, suspicious, and paranoid themselves. Thus, if the physician becomes unaccountably wary with a patient, the feeling may have diagnostic significance: the patient may have some paranoia of which the physician was not aware.

The following are guidelines to help physicians cope with paranoid patients.

Accept the patient's wariness as an ongoing ingredient in the relationship. The patient's trust is not available for the asking. To overcome the adverse experiences and beliefs that generate the patient's paranoia, the most important contribution that the physician can make involves establishing a relationship in which continuing trustworthy behavior is a conspicuous component. Trust, if ever gained, takes a lot of time.

Be direct, honest, and straightforward. Patients should be allowed to look at x-rays, laboratory reports, and written communications. The physician should invite the patient to seek second opinions when possible. The physician should admit when he or she does not know the answer to a question. Every effort should be made toward a concrete, problem-solving approach to the patient and to his or her condition. Patients can be invited to seek additional information in books and resource material but warned when there is a range of acceptable opinions. The physician might say, "When you encounter a range of opinions, it's often difficult to know how much to trust any single one. I understand that, and I'm happy to discuss your options with you." It is appropriate to be responsive but not to haggle over details.

Typically paranoid patients (who find it difficult to trust already) become increasingly suspicious in the presence of warmth and informality, which they are inclined to see as ploys or coverups. Thus the physician should avoid trying to get close to such patients and to remain professional and respectful (see the box at right).

Finally, neither arguing with nor ignoring a patient who is suspicious of the physician's ability or intent is effective. Instead, the physician might say, "If you doubt my skill or my character, it must be very difficult for you to accept my diagnosis and treatment. Is there anything we can or should do to make it easier for us to proceed?" If there is a reasonable approach that will improve the situation, the physician can proceed. If not, the patient will want to seek other alternatives.

**Suggested responses to the paranoid patient**

"If you doubt my concern for your best interests, it will be difficult for you to trust me. How should we proceed?"

"You may feel more comfortable if you get a second opinion. What information or material can I give you to make that simpler?"

"I understand that it can be difficult to trust someone you don't know well."

## COPING SKILLS: SELF-CARE AND DIFFICULT ENCOUNTERS WITH PATIENTS

Caring for patients is hard work under any circumstances. It is even more difficult if the physician cares about his or her patients as human beings, but it is also dramatically more rewarding.

No matter how competent and experienced, all physicians have less than perfect encounters. First, it is important to remember that difficult encounters are the exception rather than the rule. Physicians should enjoy the human encounters that go well, even as they struggle with those that don't. Second, it is useful to discuss problem patients with colleagues, especially those whom the physician knows well, trusts, and considers competent. Physicians readily ask for assistance with a puzzling ECG; there is no reason to be more reticent with problems in the physician-patient relationship. Third, try to learn from difficult patient encounters. Finally, it helps to have a sense of humor. Stress between physicians and patients certainly can have serious consequences, but it can also be instructive and entertaining. Learning to get pleasure from the care of other human beings makes the practice of medicine far more emotionally rewarding.

## BIBLIOGRAPHY

Portions of this chapter were originally published in slightly different form in Lipp MR: *Respectful treatment—a practical handbook of patient care,* ed 2, New York, 1986, Elsevier.

Block B, Pristach CA: Diagnosis and management of the paranoid patient, *Am Fam Physician* 45:2634, 1992.

Gardner JW: Personal renewal, *West J Med* 157:457, 1992.

Groves JE: Taking care of the hateful patient, *N Engl J Med* 298:883, 1978.

Kahana RJ, Bibring GL: Personality types in medical management. In Zinberg NE, editor: *Psychiatry and general practice in a general hospital,* New York, 1964, International Universities.

Kroll J: *The challenge of the borderline patient,* New York, 1988, WW Norton.

Quill TE, Williamson PR: Healthy approaches to physician stress, *Arch Intern Med* 150:1857, 1990.

Redelmeier DA, Rozin P, Kahneman D: Understanding patients' decisions—cognitive and emotional responses, *JAMA* 270:72, 1993.

Schwenk TL, Romano SE: Managing the difficult physician-patient relationship, *Am Fam Physician* 46:1503, 1992.

Skodol AE, Oldham JM: Assessment and diagnosis of borderline personality disorder, *Hosp Community Psychiatry* 42:1021, 1991.

CHAPTER

# 123 Common Family Problems

David B. Seaburn
Susan H. McDaniel
Thomas L. Campbell

The primary care physician is in an excellent position to address many family problems because of the continuity of his or her relationship with patients and families over time (Fig. 123-1). Primary care physicians are part of a family's life through myriad developmental transitions, such as marriage, childbirth, childrearing, adolescence, leaving home, separation and divorce, remarriage, midlife, old age, dying, and death. Any of these family transitions can create stress that may contribute to the symptoms patients present to their physicians, from headaches and chronic pain to gynecologic problems and depression. Approximately three-fourths of all psychiatric disorders are diagnosed by primary care physicians who also are the providers for half of all visits for psychiatric problems (Schurman, Kramer, and Mitchell, 1985).

Many patient problems have roots in family distress. More often the family is a valuable resource to the physician in addressing patient difficulties. The family has great influence on how an individual thinks, feels, and behaves about his or her health. The family also has primary responsibility for individuals when they are ill. Enlisting family members involvement can be pivotal in understanding patient problems and in facilitating effective treatment.

This chapter presents common family problems that can be addressed in primary care. This chapter discusses how to involve family members when a patient is chronically ill, and other specific family difficulties that can arise during the adult life cycle, such as sexual issues, adolescent concerns, problems of aging, and end-of-life decisions. It also delineates practical considerations in making mental health referrals, as well as how to collaborate with mental health professionals.

## ENLISTING FAMILY MEMBERS' INVOLVEMENT

When family factors are part of the patient's problem, it is often difficult to assess or treat the problem without the involvement of other family members. Sometimes the physician asks the patient to invite family members in, the patient does so, and a productive meeting ensues. However, sometimes the patient is hesitant to involve family members for many reasons, and this should be discussed carefully. Ultimately the patient must agree to involve family members before they can be invited in.

A planned approach to inviting family members is best. It enables the physician to address common fears that the patient or family member may have, such as whether the family members or the patient will be blamed for the problem or whether the family members will be told they have a problem. The following are some basic guidelines for preparing patients and family members for a family visit.

*Be supportive, empathic, and impartial.* Do not take sides with the patient against other family members. Even if he or she has been critical, the patient may have a negative reaction to criticism of family and be protective of them. The patient may be reluctant to invite family members for fear of what may happen or of loss of confidentiality; or the patient may be eager to invite family

**Fig. 123-1.** Visit to the family physician. (From the Library of Congress.)

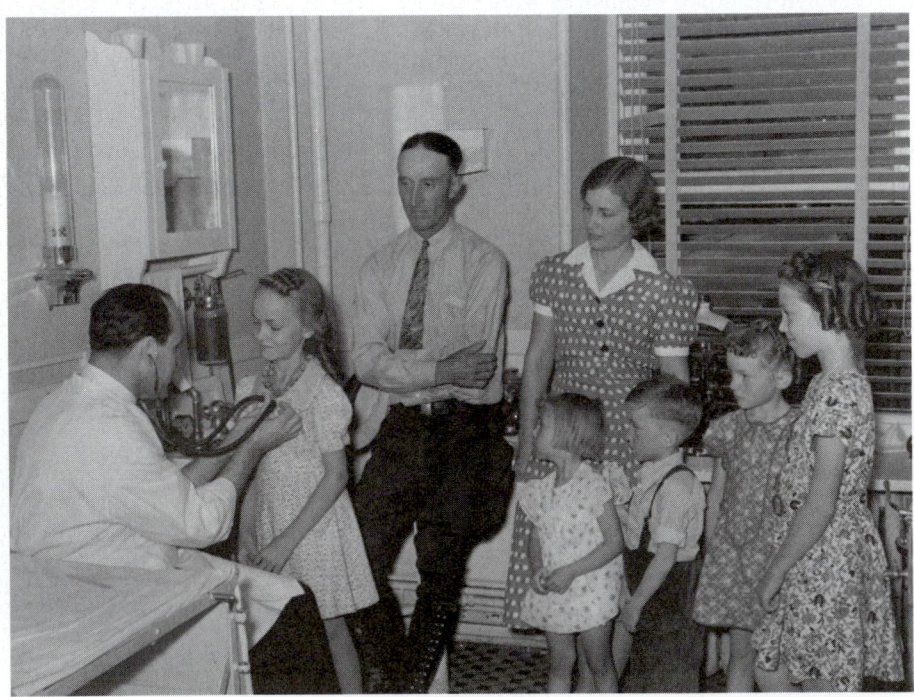

members, hoping the physician will take sides and defeat them. In any case, family members may be unlikely to come, perhaps sensing they are at risk. Neutrality in family issues should be abandoned, however, in cases of physical or sexual abuse. Here it is important to advocate for the patient at risk and to act in ways that ensures his or her safety. This may include not inviting the abusive family member to come for a visit if the physician is unsure whether such a visit could escalate conflict.

*Emphasize concern for the patient and for the family as a whole.* This involves communicating understanding of the patient's dilemma as well as sensitivity to the possible stresses of other family members.

*Involve family members* to better understand what the patient and family is facing. This communicates both sensitivity to their distress and respect for each family member's view of the situation.

*Stress the benefits of including others.* There may be greater likelihood that change can occur if the family works together.

*Clarify what the patient can expect* in a meeting with other family members. The meeting is not a time of reporting to the family everything the patient has said. Confidentiality must be maintained. Rather, it will be an opportunity for everyone to share their views and make plans for how to address any problems.

*Offer to invite family members* by phone or letter. This is effective when the physician is unsure whether the patient will be able or willing to invite the family. A phone call to a partner or other significant family member during the patient's visit has the benefit of ensuring that the patient and the family hear the same message at the same time.

With difficult patients or serious family problems, the invitation process can take several office visits with the patient to answer questions before a family visit can be arranged.

## COMMON FAMILY PROBLEMS IN PRIMARY CARE

This section presents common family problems and how to address them.

## WHEN A FAMILY MEMBER IS CHRONICALLY ILL: INCLUDING THE FAMILY

Family difficulties that can arise when a member is ill have to do with the degree and nature of other family members' involvement in treatment. This involvement can influence whether or not patients are motivated for treatment or are capable of carrying out a treatment plan. Some common patterns of involvement follow.

### Family member as customer

When a patient is unclear about the reasons for a visit, it may be because the patient has been sent to the doctor by a family member. The family member may have greater explicit concern about the patient's health than the patient and may be more motivated for treatment. This family member can be thought of as the "customer" for care. Middle-aged men who come for physical examinations are often sent by spouses who are worried their husbands are overworking or are not taking care of themselves. It is tempting to dismiss the customer's concerns because the patient seems unconcerned. It is best, though, to investigate who is concerned, and get permission from the patient to invite the partner in to better assess the situation. The customer can often be a valuable reporter on the patient's health. However, caution is advised since the patient may object and may feel intruded on.

> Mr. K., a patient with early, undiagnosed Alzheimer's disease, came for a physical. When Dr. F. asked why he decided to have a check-up, he said, "I don't know. My wife seemed to think something was wrong." Dr. F. learned that Mrs. K. was in the waiting room. He invited Mrs. K. to join them in the examination room, whereupon Mrs. K. reported that her husband had become more forgetful and irritable in the past few months.

### Overinvolved family members

The customer may be overly involved with the patient's problem for many reasons. Family member overinvolvement is often, but not necessarily, pathological. For instance, there is evidence that parental overinvolvement in some childhood chronic illnesses may have a positive influence on the course of the illness (Woods, 1993). Whether the effect is positive or negative, the overinvolvement of family members can greatly influence the course of a patient's illness and the patient's decisions about treatment.

Signs of dysfunctional family overinvolvement include patient passivity toward treatment, greater knowledge about the illness by family members than by the patient, reluctance on the part of the patient and/or family members for the patient to be seen alone, and reports of family member overfunctioning on behalf of the patient who is not incapacitated. Overinvolvement of family members can manifest itself as competitiveness with the physician over how the patient should be treated, or in prodding the patient to "do what the doctor says." The patient may respond by passively resisting one side or the other, usually the physician.

> Viola is a single mother in her mid-twenties who has IDDM. She lives with her mother who has primary responsibility for Viola's son while Viola goes to business school. Viola's sugar levels are often uncontrolled. Viola's mother called Dr. J. to say she was frustrated with her daughter and worried about her diabetes. Viola's mother had a brother who died of complications from untreated diabetes. She hoped Dr. J. could make Viola take care of herself. Dr. J. invited Viola's mother to the next appointment with Viola's consent. Dr. J. learned that Viola's mother monitors Viola's diet constantly, keeping a chart on the refrigerator and leaving notes for Viola everyday about her insulin. Viola appreciated her mother's concern and efforts to help, especially with Viola's son, but she resented her mother's effort to "control everything" Viola did.

It is best to talk directly to overinvolved family members in order to understand their concerns and to enlist their help in a different way. In the case of Viola, Dr. J. spoke with Viola's mother and learned there was a family history of diabetes that increased her worry and protectiveness. She was willing to negotiate with her daughter about the management of her diabetes. Viola's mother was relieved to interact directly with the physician and be advised how best to approach her daughter's illness.

### Underinvolved family members

Lack of comment by patients about their families can be mistaken as evidence that everything is fine. In some instances, lack of comment reflects a lack of involvement that may negatively affect the illness' course. However, lack of involvement should not always be considered lack of interest or concern. Family members may feel helpless and expect the physician to take full responsibility; they may not understand the illness and the role they might play.

> Mr. B. is in his late fifties. He is obese and has hypertension. Dr. M. has tried unsuccessfully for 6 months to encourage Mr. B. to lose weight. Mr. B. appears motivated and has met with a dietician several times, but to no avail. Dr. M. is also treating Mr. B. with an antihypertensive, but since he is concerned that Mr. B. could have a stroke, he invited Mr. B.'s wife to the next visit. At that time he learned that Mrs. B. cooks all the family meals. She uses salt in her cooking, and Mr. B.'s favorite meals are high in fat content. She did not worry about her husband's hypertension because Mr. B. always said he was doing fine after each doctor visit. Dr. M. described hypertension in detail and also discussed diet with Mrs. B., who, once she understood the role she could play in her husband's health was willing to make changes in her cooking.

The best approach with chronic illness is to involve family members early and periodically. This enables the physician to assess the degree and nature of family member involvement, its impact on the illness course, and how to enlist family members as allies in treatment. This must be accompanied by maintaining or enhancing the patients' autonomy.

## ADOLESCENT HEALTH CARE PROBLEMS: SECRETS AND CONFIDENTIALITY

In caring for adolescents it is helpful to respect both the adolescent's growing autonomy and the parents' role in the overall health and development of the adolescent. The adolescent's need to develop a sense of identity and independence has been established as important in adolescent health care. Some believe that the absence of the parent is essential to developing a relationship with the physician and that the physician can play a role in "accelerating the process of children becoming independent patients" (Cogswell, 1985).

Beyond the importance of a one-to-one relationship between the physician and adolescent, the physician must consider one context that shapes the adolescent greatly—the family. Despite the common view of adolescence as a period of rebellion against parental values, most adolescents derive much of their self-esteem from parental support and approval. It is recommended that the physician remain adolescent-focused but with a family orientation. In the end, it is important to work with adolescents and their parents in a balanced way. Three general guidelines include the following:

*1. Maintain a relationship with both the adolescent and his or her parents, provided the adolescent tolerates this.* Avoid taking sides where possible. Siding with either the adolescent or the parent may result in the physician losing the trust of either or both.

*2. Be sensitive to the emotional issues that can arise when working with adolescents.* The natural pull to side with the adolescent or the parents can reflect the physician's own issues around adolescence. These responses are normal. It is important to recognize how they may influence the physician's work with adolescent patients.

*3. Be aware of how adolescent efforts to individuate play a part in adolescent health care.* Individuation can play a part in everything from discussions about who will enter the examination room, to physical examinations for work, to requests for contraceptives, to pregnancy tests. The physician is in an excellent position to help adolescents and parents address these issues together if appropriate and helpful.

A balanced approach to adolescent health problems is challenged most when issues of confidentiality arise. The following illustrates a common dilemma that may upset the balance:

> Mrs. Dumas asked to speak with Dr. L. privately before he saw Alex, age 17. She explained that she and her husband were worried that Alex might be using drugs. A family friend reported seeing Alex smoking marijuana at a party. Mrs. Dumas hoped Dr. L. would explore this issue with Alex during his work physical to find out if he was using drugs. During the visit with Alex, Dr. L. learned that he had been smoking marijuana and had also been drinking heavily on weekends. Alex was very open about this but added, "You aren't going to tell my mother, are you?"

Physicians are often given information about patients and family members and are asked to keep the information secret. Some physicians feel that all information shared by patients must be kept as confidential, without question. Others see secrets as posing both ethical and clinical dilemmas. As Newman (1993) indicates, blanket acceptance of secrets may draw the physician into dysfunctional family patterns of relating. Furthermore, colluding in a secret may "limit our freedom to provide appropriate health care, and force us to compromise our own integrity." However, legitimate requests for confidentiality may be essential for some patients to pursue treatment for such conditions as sexually transmitted diseases, drug use, HIV, and pregnancy.

The issue again is one of balance and sensitivity to the adolescent's needs for care *and* confidentiality. The physician's task is to maintain confidentiality where appropriate without entering into bonds of secrecy that may influence the provision of health care or contribute to unhealthy family relations. This task is perhaps most daunting when working with adolescents. The adolescent's process of forming an identity may include experimentation that can pose health risks. Adolescent individuation often includes an effort to limit the information that parents have about one's behavior. On the other hand, parents are often struggling with issues of control while trying to maintain a relationship with their adolescent. An encounter with a physician offers an opportunity to facilitate communication.

In the previous case, Dr. L. is asked to keep two secrets. Mrs. Dumas does not want him to divulge their conversation, but she does want him to investigate Alex's "drug problem." Alex also wants Dr. L. to keep a secret, since he does not want his parents to know about his drug and alcohol use. This poses a dilemma for Dr. L. Both secrets influence how Dr. L. can provide care for Alex. Both secrets also reflect family issues concerning communication between Alex and his parents.

When dealing with adolescent health care problems that raise issues of confidentiality, the following guidelines may be helpful in promoting healthy communication between the adolescent, the parents, and the provider:

*1. Structure adolescent health care visits in a way that maximizes open communication, minimizes secrecy, and respects both the adolescent's autonomy and need or demand for privacy and the parent's role.* Many adolescents simply reject the doctor as their doctor if he or she is dealing with the parents. One successful format when parents accompany the adolescent, is to see the parents with the adolescent at the beginning of the visit. Explain that the visit includes time together, time alone with the adolescent, and time at the end with everyone to discuss some treatment directions (others may be confidential) and answer questions. See the adolescent alone for the majority of the visit. Negotiate with the adolescent what to share with the parents at the end of the visit. End by discussing some findings and treatment directions with the adolescent and the parents together.

With regard to Mrs. Dumas' request, Dr. L. encouraged Mrs. Dumas to share her concerns with Alex present. Mrs. Dumas did so, but had she refused, Dr. L. would have pushed for permission to share their conversation with Alex. In this way, Dr. L. could avoid keeping a binding secret and could also facilitate communication between Mrs. Dumas and her son.

*2. Discuss confidentiality with the parents and the adolescent together.* In a series of decisions between 1976 and 1983, the Supreme Court extended the adolescent's right to confidential treatment in many areas, including the purchase and use of contraception and requests for abortions (Holder, 1987). With homicidal behavior or threat of felony, confidentiality must be broken and the problem reported in most states. Finally, despite the adolescent's legal right to consent to his or her own treatment, the responsibility for judging the adolescent's capacity to make clear decisions often falls to the physician. Confidentiality remains a complex issue that is best dealt with honestly and directly.

Confidentiality should be presented as a multifaceted issue that deserves discussion and often requires negotiation. In the Dumas case, Dr. L. took the opportunity to address confidentiality with Mrs. Dumas and Alex together:

> Dr. L.: When I see adolescents with their parents I like to take the opportunity to discuss confidentiality. Patients often share information with me that they would like to keep confidential. In most cases I honor that request. In several areas I cannot extend confidentiality. For example, if either of you were at risk of hurting yourself or someone else, I would have to inform others for the sake of your safety or the safety of others. In all requests for confidentiality, I may feel as a physician that it would be better, for health reasons, if the information was shared with others, particularly family. In those instances I encourage the adolescent or family member to talk with other family members, and I offer to assist in whatever way I can. But I do not communicate confidential information to other family members without the patient's consent. And I never refuse treatment even if a patient does not want to talk with others about their problems. My main concern is to provide necessary and adequate health care for any patient.

This approach has the benefit of modeling openness, honesty, and directness. It allies the physician not only with the parents and the adolescent but with the goal of quality health care for the adolescent. Furthermore, if raised early in patient care, it avoids the problem of raising the issue after confidential information has already been shared.

Involve parents when appropriate. Parents should not be contacted when a teen is adamantly opposed to parental involvement, would not seek health care if his or her parents were notified, or would be at risk for abuse if parents knew about the treatment. Parents should be involved in any treatment, though, if the adolescent desires. Involvement of parents can help the physician understand how the adolescent's health and development both affect and are affected by the family. In cases such as pregnancy, abortion, or substance abuse, the physician should explore the possibility of including parents. Adolescents may refuse their involvement at first; but often, adolescents, though possibly apprehensive, want their parents to be included. As an example, national surveys indicate that more than half of teenagers who obtain abortions tell at least one parent.

Parental involvement also protects the physician from becoming a substitute parent for the teen. Replacing the adolescent's parents compromises the physician's capacity to treat the teen and overburdens the physician with responsibilities that are rightfully the parents. Inclusion of parents benefits both the adolescent and the physician.

> Dr. L. was concerned about Alex's substance use. Alex admitted concern as well because he had recently had a blackout that frightened him. Dr. L. supported Alex and suggested Alex be evaluated for possible treatment. He encouraged Alex to talk with his parents, but Alex refused. Dr. L. discussed a referral to a treatment facility, but added that it would be unlikely that treatment could be kept a secret from Alex's parents. Dr. L. also said Alex may need his parents' support. Alex agreed to informing his mother about his substance use, but wanted Dr. L. to do it without Alex there. Dr. L. and Alex reached a compromise in which Dr. L. would help Alex talk to his mother. Together they would discuss a possible referral.

A primary care approach to adolescent health issues involves respect for the rights and developmental needs of the adolescent as well as respect for the role and responsibility of parents in childrearing.

## SEXUAL AND RELATIONSHIP PROBLEMS: INVOLVING BOTH PARTNERS

Like adolescent problems, sexual problems often require special interviewing skill. Patients who present with low back pain, abdominal pain, urinary difficulties, and other somatic complaints may have underlying sexual complaints that they are hesitant to voice. Assessment of sexual problems in primary care depends largely on the physician's initiative in discussing the matter. Masters and Johnson (1970) have estimated that 50% of all marriages experience sexual problems at some time. Physicians who do not inquire learn about these problems only 10% of the time, while physicians who routinely inquire identify sexual problems 50% to 100% of the time (Pauly, 1971).

Problems with sexual intimacy may arise because of organic factors that, in turn, affect the couple's relationship; or they may arise because of general intimacy problems that then affect the physiology of sexual functioning. For this reason, a biopsychosocial approach should always be used when assessing sexual intimacy.

Organic causes of sexual problems, such as disease (diabetes, circulatory problems, or multiple sclerosis) or the use of medication or drugs that affect sexual functioning (alcohol, antidepressants, or antihypertensives), make up a small percentage of sexual problems. Chronic sexual problems are more likely to have an organic cause. Some evaluation questions that address the nature of the problem and its possible causes are included in the following (Kaplan, 1974; Kolodny, Masters, Johnson, 1979):

- Are you satisfied with the degree of intimacy in your relationship?
- Are you satisfied with your sex life? If not, what difficulties are you having?
- Do these problems occur all the time or just under certain circumstances?
- (to men) Do you have problems obtaining or maintaining an erection?
- (to women) Do you have difficulty becoming sexually aroused? Do you ever have pain during intercourse or difficulty achieving an orgasm?
- What do you feel is the reason for these problems?
- Have either of you been ill recently? Are you on medication? Do you drink alcohol or use drugs?
- How would you like your sexual relationship to be?

The following case illustrates how sexual and relationship problems are frequently intertwined.

Mrs. Gaudino came in complaining her marriage was stale and lifeless. Dr. C. said he'd be happy to explore this problem further, but that it would be best if her husband could join her. Mrs. Gaudino appeared apprehensive, but agreed that a session with her husband to identify the problems would be most likely to lead to improvements in the relationship. Mr. Gaudino surprised his wife by his willingness to come in. He hoped the doctor would ask about their sexual relationship, his primary concern. He wasn't sure he could bring it up himself.

Dr. C. greeted both Mr. and Mrs. Gaudino, and, after discussing some work issues, asked if their relationship stress had affected their sexual relationship. At first both were nervous and said "No." When Dr. C. asked if they were satisfied with their sexual relationship, Mrs. Gaudino said, "Not really." She said they weren't "close" often enough. When Dr. C. asked what she meant by close, Mrs. Gaudino said, "You know, we don't have sex enough." Dr. C. learned that the Gaudinos had been having sex approximately once a month during the past six months. They agreed it was more often before then but could not be specific. Mr. Gaudino said he was often too tired from his new job, and when he wasn't tired his wife sometimes "turned a cold shoulder." The last two times they tried to have intercourse, Mr. Gaudino could not maintain an erection. They had not tried again in the past six weeks. Dr. R. talked with Mr. Gaudino further and learned that he had not been ill, that he drank alcohol in moderation ("3 to 4 beers a week"), and that he was able to have erections at other times. The couple speculated that relationship problems were the cause of their sexual difficulties. Dr. C. referred them for sexual counseling.

## FAMILIES AND THE ELDERLY: CARING FOR THE CAREGIVER

The fastest growing segment of the population is the elderly (over 65 years). Contrary to popular belief, most elders are close to their families. The majority live near one of their children and visit them often. Only 5% live in nursing homes or other institutional settings.

The importance of family connections increases with age. Physical deterioration and social and financial changes often push people back to their families, despite a desire to remain independent. The majority of caregivers for the elderly are family, typically women. There are important gender differences between male and female caregivers. Because women are socialized to assume caregiving responsibilities, they are more likely to feel responsible for all the caregiving and have difficulty asking for or receiving help. Men often have more difficulty accepting caregiving responsibilities and are more likely to ask or pay for help. For example, women who are recovering from a myocardial infarction often continue household responsibilities, such as cooking and cleaning, while men are usually cared for by their wives during the post-MI period. Men are also more likely to hire a housekeeper or helper to care for a disabled family member.

Caregiving of elder family members is very demanding and often highly emotional, as the specter of death and grief highlights longstanding family processes, loyalties, obligations, and responsibilities. When there is intense involvement of family caregivers, medical care of the elderly needs to be consciously family-oriented.

The physician's role at this stage may be powerful. The physician is seen as a supporter, advisor, healer, social contact, lifeline, and guide to the patient and family. With regard to the family, one of the physician's most important roles is to involve, assess, and support any primary family caregiver(s). To overlook this can lead to a downward spiral that can greatly affect the elder family member; the caregiver becomes more distressed and is less able to meet the elder family member's needs; the elder family member may then deteriorate physically and emotionally, thus putting greater demands on the caregiver who may then burnout. For these reasons, the family caregiver(s) should be included routinely in part of patient office visits. The caregiver can be a valuable reporter on the patient's condition and has primary responsibility for implementing treatment plans. Routine involvement also makes it possible for the physician to assess the potential for caregiver burnout.

Mr. Benjamin had gradually developed serious Parkinson's disease with accompanying dementia. He came to live with his daughter and son-in-law six months ago. They were committed to caring for him. Mrs. Yolom, Mr. Benjamin's daughter, accompanied him to every visit. At one visit with Dr. F., Mrs. Yolom appeared lethargic. She had little to say and often yawned during the interview. When asked how she was doing, Mrs. Yolom said she was losing sleep because her father had been up each night for the past week. Her husband had offered to help, but she felt guilty allowing his involvement. Mr. Benjamin was her father, she said, and she should take care of him.

Depression can accompany the demands of caregiving. The risk of depressive symptoms increases when the caregiver either is isolated and has little support or refuses to accept available help. The physician should assess several aspects of the caregiver's experience (McDaniel, Campbell, & Seaburn, 1990).

***The caregiver's relationship to the patient.*** Can the caregiver express affection with the patient or must it be withheld? Does the caregiver feel solely responsible for the patient? Was the previous relationship with the patient positive or negative?

***The patient's condition.*** How impaired is the patient, physically and emotionally? Is the patient's behavior disruptive? How independent is the patient? How knowledgeable is the caregiver about the patient's condition?

***The caregiver's condition.*** How is the caregiver's physical health? Is the caregiver depressed? Does the caregiver have support? Does the caregiver take time for himself or herself? Can the caregiver delegate responsibilities to other family members? Does the caregiver have a realistic sense of his or her responsibility for the patient's health?

***Family resources.*** Can the family afford (professional) assistance with caregiving? How is the family coping with the patient's needs? Do family members maintain some degree of social activity? Can family members talk with and support each other?

***Community resources.*** Is a day care program available for the patient? Are there support groups available for the caregiver and family? Is respite care available? Are psychological and family therapy available for the patient, caregiver, and family?

By addressing how the caregiver is doing, the physician is making a powerful statement to the patient and family, that the caregiver has legitimate needs. This often results in other family members providing more support and assistance. By preventing caregiver burnout, the physician is able to help the patient remain at home with the family.

## MENTAL HEALTH REFERRAL AND COLLABORATION

Family problems that do not abate once they are identified and discussed often should be referred to a family-oriented mental health provider. Among the most common signals for a referral, in addition to a patient's request, are the following:

*Serious problems.* Sometimes the severity of the problem is not clear initially. Regardless, if the family's difficulties include a history of psychiatric problems, suicidal or homicidal ideas or intent, physical or sexual abuse, substance abuse, and most sexual problems, then a referral is warranted.

*Chronic problems.* If the family reports having problems for longer than 8 months, a mental health referral may be indicated.

*A multiplicity of problems.* Families that report more than one problem occurring at the same time may warrant a referral even if the problems are not severe or chronic. The complexity of multiple psychosocial problems may be best handled by involving a family-oriented mental health provider.

### Successful referral and collaboration

Many primary care mental health referrals are not just made, they are accomplished over time. Except when a patient or family directly requests a referral, successful referrals are usually part of a process rather than being a single event. Preparing a family for a referral may take more than one visit. The effectiveness of a mental health referral also depends on the relationship between the physician and mental health professionals. A collaborative relationship enhances both the referral and the course of treatment. A successful referral and collaboration includes the following:

*Introduce the idea of referral gradually over time.* First, help the patient identify and discuss the problem. Second, involve relevant family members. Third, introduce the idea of referral as a resource that may benefit everyone in the family.

*Refer to someone you know and trust if possible.* Patients are more likely to transfer the trust they have in you to a new person rather than a clinic or agency.

*When possible, consult early with the therapist to whom you are referring.* This sets the stage for ongoing collaboration with the therapist during treatment.

*Maximize the patient and family's motivation* by using language that is meaningful to them when presenting the idea of referral. For example, "You both have demonstrated your commitment to making things better, and are working very hard; your efforts deserve the support of someone who specializes in the issues you are addressing." It is helpful not to pathologize the patient or family when discussing referral.

*Give the patient and family time to consider the referral.* Schedule a follow-up visit to discuss the decision. When a patient and family are ambivalent, this allows them time to make their own decision while maintaining a connection with you no matter what the decision.

*Have the patient and family* decide to accept the referral, *call the therapist for an appointment before they leave the office* (Doherty & Baird, 1983).

*Do not push a family to accept a referral prematurely.* Give the process time. Be available to the family.

*Make explicit what kind of communication you want from the therapist.* The number one complaint physicians have about therapists is that physicians never hear from them once the referral is made. It is best to be direct about the communication you desire.

*Clarify your own availability regarding the case.* How can you be contacted? When is it best to call you? Will you be available?

*Negotiate and clarify areas of responsibility.* What issues are best discussed with the therapist (e.g., relationship issues)? What issues should the therapist refer back to the physician (e.g., possible physiologic factors in sexual dysfunction)? What issues should the physician and therapist discuss together (e.g., when the patient and family are somatically fixated)? In difficult cases this process can be aided by a face-to-face meeting between the physician, therapist, and family.

## SUMMARY

Family problems may be a significant factor in a patient's decision to see his or her primary care physician. Early recognition of relationship problems by the doctor may decrease the frequency of medical visits by patients whose symptoms are grounded in family stress. Engaging family members in addressing such problems can be an effective intervention. Involving family members also protects the physician from entering into exclusive individual relationships with patients that do not address the familial roots of problems.

When family-based problems require more than primary-care counseling, the physician is in a central position to prepare patients and families for working with family-oriented mental health providers. Collaboration with a family-oriented mental health provider may help mend the mind-body split and facilitate effective treatment, and can be professionally rewarding for both the therapist and physician.

## BIBLIOGRAPHY


Cogswell BE: Cultivating the trust of adolescent patients, *Fam Med* 27(6):254, 1985.

Doherty WJ, Baird WA: *Family therapy and family medicine.* New York, 1983, Guilford Press.

Holder AR: Minors' rights to consent to medical care, *JAMA* 257(24): 3400, 1987.

Kaplan HS: *The new sex therapy,* New York, 1974, Brunner/Mazel.

Kolodny RC, Masters WH, Johnson VE: *Textbook of sexual medicine.* Boston, 1979, Little, Brown.

McDaniel SH, Campbell TL, Seaburn DB: *Family-oriented primary care: a manual for medical providers.* New York, 1990, Springer-Verlag.

Masters Wm, Johnson VE: *Human sexual inadequacy,* Boston, 1970, Little, Brown.

Newman NR: Family secrets: a challenge for family physicians, *J Fam Prac* 36(5):494, 1993.

Pauly TB: Human sexuality in medical education and practice, *J Psychiatry* (Australia/New Zealand) 5:204, 1971.

Schurman RA, Kramer PD, Mitchell JB: The hidden mental health network: treatment of mental illness by nonpsychiatric physicians, *Archives of Gen Psych* 42:89, 1985.

Woods B: Beyond the "psychosomatic family": a biobehavioral family model of pediatric illness, *Fam Prac* 32(3):261, 1993.


CHAPTER

# 124 Behavior Change: The Example of Smoking Cessation


**Barrie J. Guise**
**Michael G. Goldstein**
**Matthew M. Clark**
**Ronald W. Thebarge**


Therapeutic interventions in general medicine are varied, but almost all involve patient behavior. Physicians routinely prescribe medication, suggest changes in activity or lifestyle, and recommend various self-care regimens. Each of these interventions requires that patients engage in or avoid specific behaviors. These behaviors may range from simple and temporary (e.g., antibiotics three times per day for the next 10 days) to complex and long-term (e.g., quiting smoking, eating less fat and salt, exercising regularly, and avoiding excessive exertion).

Patients are frequently unsuccessful at fully implementing even simple and short-term health behavior changes. However, medical goals are closely linked to behavioral goals; lifestyle factors significantly contribute to more than half of the annual deaths in the United States.

Behavioral medicine has its roots in behavioral psychology. Early behavioral scientists first described paradigms that applied the experimental method to the study of observable behavior, explained behavior in terms of controlled operations, and permitted the reliable prediction of behavior given particular environmental conditions. In more recent years it has been asserted that cognitions (thoughts and beliefs) can be governed by the same principles as observable behavior and that motivation is an important mediating variable for human behavior. Together these ideas comprise the foundation of behavior therapy. Behavior therapy has evolved over the past 40 years to achieve notable success in treating psychologic disorders.

In the early 1970s behavioral investigators began to explore applications of behavior therapy to medical disorders. Behavioral medicine is the interdisciplinary field that integrates the knowledge and techniques of behavioral and biomedical science and applies them to the prevention, diagnosis, and treatment of medical illness. This chapter introduces the fundamental principles and techniques of behavioral medicine and then elaborates using an example of the treatment of cigarette smoking.

## BASIC PRINCIPLES OF BEHAVIOR CHANGE

To facilitate behavior change, it is necessary to systematically formulate behavior as a target for intervention. Behavior changes that promote health range from increasing the frequency of some behaviors (e.g., aerobic exercise) to decreasing the frequency of others (e.g., cigarette smoking) to introducing new behaviors (e.g., home blood glucose testing) (Fig. 124-1).

Classical conditioning, or learning by association, accounts for the relationship that develops between unrelated experiences when they are paired, such as smoking a cigarette at the end of a meal. Operant conditioning describes the behavior that is learned as a result of its consequences or contingencies. Operant conditioning explains why individuals are likely to take antihypertensive medication regularly if doing so eliminates a headache, and less likely to do so if impaired sexual functioning is a side effect. In recent years it has become clear that cognitive variables (thoughts and beliefs) and motivation play a role in the regulation of human behavior. The transtheoretical model of change proposes that an individual's readiness to change is an important factor in predicting the response to strategies designed to modify behavior. Specifically, Prochaska and DiClemente propose the transtheoretical model in which individuals move through a series of stages of readiness to change:

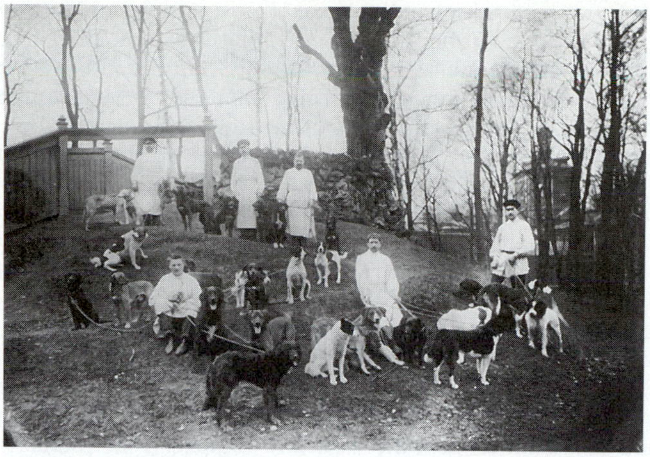

**Fig. 124-1.** Pavlov's dogs. (Courtesy The Trustee of the Wellcome Trust, London, England.)

*precontemplation* (not yet willing to consider change), *contemplation* (ambivalent but considering change), *preparation* (intending to change imminently), *action* (actively attempting to change), and *maintenance* (attempting to maintain a change). This model has important implications for the selection of interventions. For example, it stands to reason that an individual who is not yet willing to consider starting an exercise program might not make much use of specific instructions on how to begin exercising. This individual may benefit more from efforts to move him or her along to the contemplation stage, such as an effort to personalize a rationale for exercise. This implies that low motivation need not be an intractable barrier to change, but rather a legitimate target for change.

## BEHAVIOR CHANGE: CIGARETTE SMOKING

The beginning of this chapter has presented a brief exposure to the principles and techniques by which behavior may be addressed systematically in the practice of medicine. The remainder of this chapter is devoted to integrating behavioral and biomedical principles and techniques to address perhaps the most important behavioral challenge in primary care: cigarette smoking. An effort is made to translate the recommended approach into a format delivered through the most available vehicle for care in general medical practice, the encounter between the physician and the patient.

### Scope of the problem

The Surgeon General has stated that smoking is the chief avoidable cause of death in our society. Cigarette smokers have greater overall morbidity than nonsmokers, more restricted activity days, more bed disability days, more school and work absenteeism, and higher utilization of inpatient and outpatient services. An additional 53,000 nonsmoker deaths per year are attributed to the effects of environmental tobacco smoke (Fig. 124-2).

Although the prevalence of smoking among adults in the United States has fallen from 43% in 1966 to 26% in 1991, since 1974 smoking prevalence has decreased at a rate of less than 1% per year. Recent demographic trends suggest that, to have maximum impact, interventions must be targeted toward less educated, socioeconomically disadvantaged smokers as well as toward adolescents and women. Because the majority of smokers visit a physician at least once each year, primary care physicians can play a central role in reducing the morbidity and mortality associated with cigarette smoking. Although most primary care physicians report that they provide smoking cessation advice to all or almost all of their smoking patients, population-based surveys of patients indicate that only a relatively small percentage (44% to 51%) of smokers report ever having been advised to quit smoking by a physician.

Moreover, results of surveys of primary care physicians indicate that, of those who do encourage their patients to stop smoking, few are providing a significant intervention that has true impact. Fewer than 50% of physicians use a combination of strategies, including counseling; fewer than 50% counsel all smoking patients for more than 3 minutes at every visit; and only approximately 30% regularly spend 5 minutes or more counseling patients about smoking on the first visit.

In a recent survey more physicians rated smokers who are not interested in quitting as the most important barrier to smoking cessation. More than two thirds of this sample also reported that counseling about smoking is frustrating. These findings suggest that physicians feel especially unprepared and ineffective when faced with patients who are not yet ready to quit smoking. For some physicians these negative feelings are fueled by unrealistic expectations. Because even the most effective physician-delivered intervention results in 1-year abstinence rates of less than 25%, physicians become increasingly frustrated if they expect their efforts to produce abstinence rates of greater magnitude. This barrier may be overcome by helping physicians to develop more realistic expectations, by providing specific training in motivational and behavioral techniques, and by encouraging physicians to focus on intermediate outcomes, such as moving a patient who is not interested in quitting to the contemplation stage, where the patient thinks about quitting for the first time. Strategies to address these barriers are discussed in the sections below on assessment and management.

### Assessment

Biologic, psychologic, behavioral, and environmental factors all contribute to the initiation and maintenance of cigarette smoking. Therefore, according to the behavioral medicine approach, a biopsychosocial assessment of each smoker is helpful in choosing a specific intervention. The principal goals of this assessment process are to (1) characterize the patient's stage of change and motivation to quit smoking; (2) assess the severity of nicotine dependence; (3) assess the contingencies, such as triggers and perceived reasons, for smoking; and (4) identify the psychiatric comorbidity that is likely to complicate treatment.

***Assessing the patient's stage of change.*** The transtheoretical model of change described earlier can help physicians to assess and intervene more effectively with their smoking patients. Assessment of the patient's stage of change is accomplished with three questions:

1. Do you intend to quit smoking within the next 6

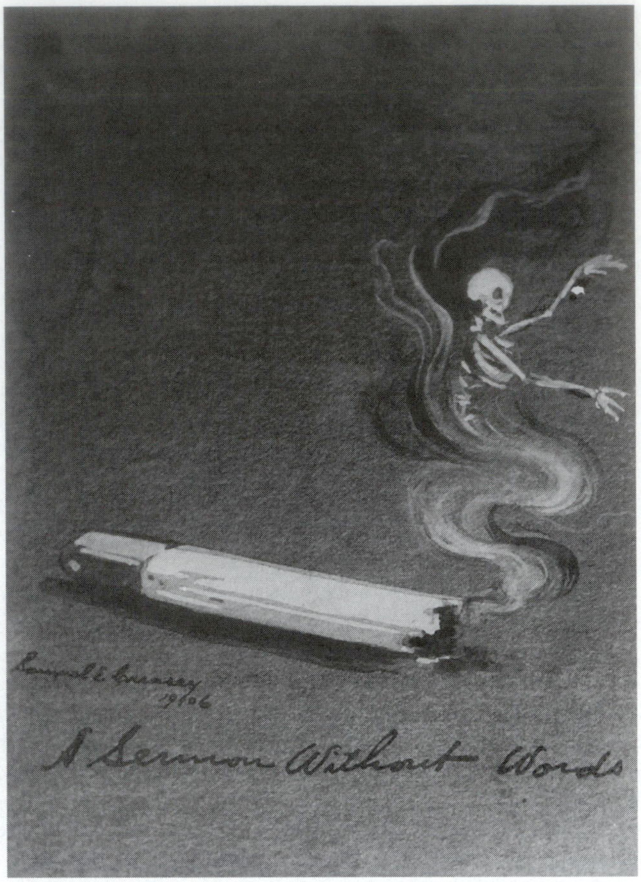


**Fig. 124-2.** "A Sermon Without Words," Samuel E. Creasey, 1906. (From the Collections of the Library of Congress.)

months? If the answer is no, the patient is in the precontemplation stage.

2. Do you intend to quit smoking within the next month? If the answer is no and the patient answered yes to the first question, the patient is in the contemplation stage.
3. Did you try to quit smoking within the past year? If the answer is yes, and the patient also answered yes to the second question, the patient is in the preparation stage. Individuals who answer yes to questions 1 and 2, but no to question 3, are in the contemplation stage.

Individuals at the precontemplation stage, who may represent as many as 40% of current smokers seen in a typical medical practice, are not likely to respond to exhortations to quit smoking or interventions that are oriented to quitting, such as nicotine replacement. These patients need motivational interventions that increase awareness and help the individual to recognize the negative aspects of smoking (the cons). (See management section below.) Another 40% of smokers seen in the medical setting are in the contemplation stage and have given serious thought to quitting but are not yet ready to do so. These individuals also benefit more from motivational counseling than from interventions oriented toward quitting. Only about 20% of smokers who seek medical care are in the preparation stage and have taken steps toward quitting, such as making recent attempts to quit, delaying their first cigarette in the morning, or cutting down on the number of cigarettes that they smoke. These individuals are most likely to respond to interventions that will help them to successfully manage a subsequent attempt to quit, such as nicotine replacement, self-help manuals, behavioral skill training, and referral to a formal treatment program or group.

After individuals have quit smoking, a single question assesses their current stage: How long ago did you quit smoking? If the answer is less than 6 months, the patient is in the action stage. If the answer is more than 6 months, the patient is in the maintenance stage. Because smokers are very likely to relapse during the action stage, especially during the first few days and weeks after quitting, these individuals benefit from interventions that are designed to prevent slips and relapses (see management section below).

An important finding by Prochaska and colleagues was that individuals frequently take several years to move through the stages of change until finally reaching a stable period of maintenance. Moreover, individuals take an average of three to four cycles through the stages before finally becoming cigarette free. By recognizing that the vast majority of smokers are not ready to quit smoking at the time of their office visit, physicians can modify their expectations and utilize strategies to attain intermediate outcomes, such as moving a patient in the precontemplation stage to the contemplation stage.

***Assessing the level of nicotine dependence.*** Because smoking may lead to the development of physical dependence on nicotine, assessment of each smoker's level of nicotine dependence is an important component of the evaluation process. Nicotine, the major psychoactive substance in cigarettes, has a wide variety of stimulant and depressant effects involving multiple physiologic systems. Nicotine has been shown to increase attention, memory, and learning in smokers. Research also suggests that nicotine has anxiolytic and antinociceptive effects, that smokers smoke more during stressful situations or in situations involving a negative mood, and that nicotine use is associated with decreases in negative affect. Each of these effects contributes to nicotine's power as a reinforcer of smoking behavior. Moreover, evidence has led to the conclusion that nicotine is an addicting or dependence-producing drug, with a well-defined abstinence or withdrawal syndrome. Several strategies can assess a patient's level of nicotine dependence (see the box on p. 1653). Self-reported smoking rates and the nicotine content of cigarettes provide some index of the degree of nicotine dependence. Individuals who smoke more than 25 cigarettes per day may be more likely to report withdrawal symptoms during abstinence than smokers consuming fewer cigarettes, although the evidence for this relationship is limited. Heavy smokers are also more likely to fail when attempting to quit smoking. Perhaps the most common, currently used measure of nicotine dependence is the Fagerstrom Tolerance Questionnaire (FTQ). This is a seven-item, self-administered form that identifies behaviors thought to reflect nicotine dependence (e.g., high smoking rate and brand nicotine level, smoking when ill or soon after awakening). Scores on the FTQ are related to withdrawal symptoms and the success of smoking

### Assessment of smokers

- Stage of change
- Level of nicotine dependence
  - Smoking rate
  - Nicotine content of cigarettes
  - Fagerstrom Tolerance Questionnaire
  - Previous attempts to quit
  - Measures of nicotine exposure
    - Cotinine
    - Carbon monoxide
- Smoking triggers and reasons for smoking
- Psychiatric comorbidity

cessation. The scale can be administered within several minutes and is easily scored. The time to the first cigarette in the morning, a specific item on the FTQ, appears to be an independent predictor of smoking cessation outcome. A response of "less than 30 minutes" is associated with poor outcome and suggests that the patient is smoking to control the withdrawal that results from overnight abstinence.

Because most smokers have made one or more unsuccessful efforts to cut down or quit smoking, inquiring about previous quit attempts is a useful assessment strategy to identify high levels of nicotine dependence. The physician should ask about withdrawal signs and symptoms during abstinence, the duration of withdrawal symptoms, and the reasons for returning to smoking. Symptoms may also have occurred when the patient switched to a low tar/nicotine cigarette, or after the patient stopped using smokeless tobacco products or nicotine gum. Nicotine withdrawal symptoms can be monitored using one of many available scales. Withdrawal symptoms, as defined by the *Diagnostic and Statistical Manual of Mental Disorders* (DSM IV), include craving, anxiety, irritability, frustration or anger, difficulty concentrating, restlessness, increased appetite or weight gain, and decreased heart rate. Disrupted sleep and depressed mood were recently added to the list of common withdrawal symptoms.

Biologic tests of nicotine exposure provide an objective, although costly, measure of nicotine dependence. Cotinine, a metabolite of nicotine, has a half-life of approximately 16 hours and can be measured in any body fluid. Higher cotinine levels are related to nicotine tolerance, regulation, and withdrawal symptoms during periods of tobacco abstinence. Price per assay may range from $10 to 60, depending on the laboratory and the type of assay conducted. Because of the relatively high cost of analysis and a turnaround time of 1 to several weeks, cotinine analysis is not a feasible method for determining nicotine intake for most physicians. Efforts are currently underway to produce inexpensive and easy-to-use cotinine screening kits that may classify individuals into gross categories of intake (i.e., low, moderate, or high).

A less expensive alternative to cotinine assays to assess nicotine exposure is analysis of expired alveolar carbon monoxide (CO). Devices to measure concentrations of CO (parts per million) in breath samples are readily available and relatively inexpensive (approximately $500). An advantage of CO measurement is that it can be used at the bedside or in an outpatient office setting to provide immediate feedback to patients.

***Assessing smoking triggers and reasons for smoking.*** A useful assessment strategy is to make a detailed functional analysis of the patient's triggers, or cues, for smoking. Patients are simply instructed to monitor their smoking for a few days, indicating the time of each cigarette, the situation in which smoking took place, their mood or affect, and their thoughts about the cigarette. The physician and patient review the self-monitoring record to make note of frequent or powerful triggers for smoking. Providing the patient with small, preprinted monitoring cards that can be kept with a pack of cigarettes facilitates this process.

Smoking typology scales, which classify individuals' reasons for smoking (e.g., management of affect, craving, habit, stimulation, or an automatic response) can also be used to assess aspects of nicotine dependence, as well as psychologic and behavioral factors (i.e., contingencies) that may contribute to smoking behavior.

***Assessment of comorbidity.*** A crucial step in assessment is to determine whether there is any evidence for psychiatric comorbidity. There is a strong association between smoking and other psychiatric disorders, especially other substance use disorders, schizophrenia, mood disorders, and anxiety disorders. The current existence or a history of any of these disorders is likely to make smoking cessation more difficult. Moreover, smoking cessation may precipitate the development of depressive symptoms in patients with a history of depression and may even precipitate a relapse of depression in susceptible patients. Smoking cessation does not appear to increase the risk of relapse of alcohol abuse or dependence.

The identification of psychiatric comorbidity has important implications for treatment. Although there are few research-based data on the treatment of nicotine dependence of patients with psychiatric comorbidity, identification, monitoring, and treatment of psychiatric comorbidity are important components of the management of such patients (see management section below).

## Management

After assessment is completed, interventions can be tailored to match each patient's needs. A step-care approach has been advocated for matching patients and treatments. The first step in management is to provide an intervention that is matched to the patient's stage of change. Since most patients are not ready for action, motivational interventions are usually most beneficial.

Once patients are ready to quit, a decision is made regarding the level, type, and intensity of smoking cessation treatment. This decision should be based on the patient's preferences, the level of nicotine dependence, the presence or absence of psychiatric comorbidity, the history of previous attempts to quit, and relevant behavioral parameters. Patients with low levels of nicotine dependence and little experience with quitting are most likely to respond to the lowest level of care: low-cost, minimal interventions, such as self-help, advice, and follow-up in the primary care setting. Those who have failed self-help approaches and those with high levels of nicotine dependence should be considered for the next level in care: brief face-to-face counseling and follow-up in the primary care setting or elsewhere (see section below on quitting strategies).

Nicotine replacement or other pharmacologic adjuncts to behavioral counseling should be considered for patients with high levels of nicotine dependence or a history of withdrawal on previous attempts to quit (see section below on pharmacologic treatment). Patients with psychiatric comorbidity, including other substance abuse, may require a specific treatment for their associated problem before, or concurrent with, treatment for nicotine dependence. These patients, as well as those who have failed despite repeated attempts to quit, are also candidates for more intensive, formal treatment programs.

Because practitioners of primary care have an opportunity to intervene with smokers repeatedly over time, results of the initial intervention can be reviewed at subsequent visits. During follow-up patients who have not successfully quit smoking can be reassessed, can be provided with another intervention at the same level, or can be advanced to a more intensive intervention. The discussion on the management of smoking cessation concludes with a section on organizational resources and aids available to primary care physicians.

### *Matching interventions to the patient's stage of change*

**Motivational interventions.** As discussed earlier, motivation is an important mediator of behavior change. Patients in the precontemplation stage respond best to motivational interventions that help them begin to think about quitting smoking. Personalized information and feedback can raise the smoker's awareness of the ways in which smoking is affecting their health, thus raising the cons of smoking. CO measurements, pulmonary function tests, and other direct physiologic evidence of smoking's health effects are useful components to feedback. Asking patients to reflect on their feelings about smoking is another useful intervention to patients in the precontemplation stage. It helps to make empathic statements, such as "I know it may be hard to quit smoking," and supportive statements, such as "When you are ready to quit, I'm willing to help." Feelings of demoralization can be addressed by informing the patient that most smokers make several attempts to quit before they are finally successful.

For patients in the contemplation stage it is especially useful to explore the reasons for smoking (pros), as well as other barriers to quitting, so that potential solutions for overcoming barriers can be discussed. For example, if a patient reports that she depends on smoking to help her to manage her weight, the offer and provision of alternative weight management strategies may tip the balance of pros and cons toward a decision to quit smoking. If a smoking patient's spouse or other family member smokes, an offer to help both of them to quit may remove another barrier to taking action.

Providing a menu of options from which the patient may choose is another effective motivational tool. Patients who become chronically stuck in the contemplation stage may benefit from encouragement to take small steps toward action, such as cutting down the number of cigarettes they smoke, delaying their first cigarette of the day, or trying to quit for only 24 hours. These patients may also be willing to monitor their smoking to identify important barriers and triggers that can be reviewed at a subsequent visit.

Patients in the contemplation stage may express negative feelings or fears about quitting. Clarification and legitimization of their feelings and expressions of support and respect may help these patients to feel heard and understood. Statements such as "I'm glad that you're thinking about quitting" are especially useful, since they reinforce patients' interest in quitting. Even if patients do not decide to quit in the near future, these interventions may help them to feel more comfortable when talking to their physicians about smoking and to feel more receptive to future interventions.

**Quitting strategies.** When the patient is finally in the preparation stage, or ready for action, appropriate action-oriented strategies can be advised or prescribed. Several reviews have described strategies in considerable detail for patients in the action or the maintenance stage. Useful interventions for patients in the action stage are listed in the box below and include setting a specific date with the patient to quit, writing a contract, providing self-help materials, prescribing nicotine replacement or other pharmacologic adjuncts, teaching behavioral skills (e.g., self-monitoring, setting goals, self-reward, stimulus control, substituting alternative behaviors, relaxation exercises, and coping skills training), and enhancing social support. If the patient has identified powerful triggers during a period of self-monitoring, the clinician can help the patient to identify specific strategies to manage these. For example, a patient who finds that the use of alcohol is a powerful trigger for smoking can choose among a wide variety of coping strategies: avoiding all use of alcohol during the first 2 weeks after quitting smoking, limiting total alcohol consumption or restricting its use to specific

#### Interventions for patients in preparation, action, or maintenance stages of change

- Set a specific date to quit
- Write a contract
- Provide self-help materials
- Prescribe nicotine replacement (when appropriate)
- Teach behavioral skills
  - Self-monitoring
  - Setting goals
  - Self-reward
  - Stimulus control
  - Substituting alternative behaviors
  - Relaxation exercises
  - Coping skills training
  - Relapse prevention skills
- Identify and treat psychiatric comorbidity
- Recommend an exercise program
- Refer to formal treatment programs
- Enhance social support

situations (e.g., with dinner, when cigarettes are not available), handling a straw or toothpick as an alternative to cigarettes, and engaging in cognitive strategies to combat craving and maladaptive thoughts (e.g., "I really don't need to have a cigarette with my drink"). Individuals are most successful when multiple cognitive and behavioral strategies are used when attempting to quit smoking. Encouraging patients to begin or to continue a program of regular exercise is another useful intervention for patients in the action or maintenance stage.

***Follow-up.*** Follow-up visits become especially important when patients are in the action or maintenance stage. Since the vast majority of patients relapse after attempted abstinence, follow-up visits can help patients to use relapse as an opportunity for learning. By exploring the circumstances that led to a return to smoking, the physician and patient can develop a revised plan that includes specific strategies to address the triggers that led to the relapse. It may become apparent that the patient experienced the development or exacerbation of an underlying psychiatric disorder. These disorders may require specific treatment or referral before the patient is able to successfully quit smoking.

At the follow-up visit the health care provider can praise the patient's efforts and reinforce the strategies that the patient used effectively. Praise and reinforcement are also useful to patients who are abstinent at follow-up. Anticipation of and planning for future problem situations and triggers for relapse is also beneficial.

***Pharmacologic interventions.*** Pharmacologic agents are effective as interventions for smoking cessation when used in conjunction with behavioral interventions. (Pharmacologic agents can be characterized using the same typology that has been developed for treating other forms of drug dependence.) The four categories of pharmacologic treatment, based on the pharmacologic strategy employed, are nicotine replacement, nonspecific pharmacotherapy (including clonidine, antidepressants, buspirone, and stimulants), blockade therapy (e.g., mecamylamine), and deterrent therapy (e.g., silver acetate). Among these therapies only nicotine replacement strategies (i.e., nicotine resin complex and nicotine transdermal patches) are clearly efficacious, especially when considering use in primary care settings. The reader is referred to recent reviews for detailed information about pharmacologic interventions.

Nicotine replacement therapy is indicated when the assessment indicates that there is evidence for significant nicotine dependence (see the box on p. 1653). Nicotine resin complex is effective when combined with formal behavioral treatment, but its use is limited when no behavior counseling is provided, especially as it is usually delivered in primary care settings. The 4 mg dose, recently released in the United States, appears to be more effective for heavily dependent smokers. However, the acceptability of nicotine resin complex is limited by the need to chew multiple pieces per day, frequent side effects, and problems associated with long-term use, which occur in up to 25% of those who use it successfully to stop smoking.

Nicotine transdermal patches are relatively safe and easy to use and have been found to be modestly effective when combined with behavior counseling. Although the patches' efficacy can be enhanced when additional behavior treatment is provided, potentially serious complications may occur if patients smoke while wearing the patch. See guidelines in the box below.

***Referral to formal treatment programs.*** Referral to a formal treatment program is indicated only when the patient is highly motivated to quit and is willing to attend such a treatment program. Patients with high levels of nicotine dependence, those who have repeatedly failed to quit using self-help methods and brief counseling, and patients with psychiatric comorbidity are most likely to benefit from formal treatment. Formal treatment programs range from volunteer-led programs that combine group support with an introduction to behavioral quitting strategies, to multidisciplinary outpatient and inpatient

## Guidelines for the use of nicotine transdermal patches in primary care

**Patient selection criteria**

- Significant nicotine dependence is present
  - Smoking rate of more than 20 cigarettes per day
  - First cigarette within 20 to 30 minutes after arising
  - Withdrawal symptoms during previous attempts to quit
- Patient is in preparation or action stage (highly motivated to quit)
- Patient is willing to use self-help materials or formal program *and* to return for follow-up

**Selection of dosage**

- Highest dosage for patients
  - Smoking more than 10 cigarettes per day
  - Weighing more than 100 pounds
- Intermediate dosage for patients
  - Smoking 10 or fewer cigarettes per day
  - Weighing 100 pounds or less
  - Elderly
  - Existence of an acute vascular disease or event
  - Pregnant women (when nonpharmacologic management has failed)

**Elements of therapy**

- Establish a date to quit; begin patch only after cessation of smoking
- Discontinue patch if patient returns to smoking
- Monitor and adjust dosage for
  - Side effects and toxicity
    - Skin reactions
    - Insomnia or vivid dreams
  - Nausea, lightheadedness, gastrointestinal symptoms
  - Breakthrough withdrawal
- Duration of therapy
  - Initial dosage for 2 to 6 weeks
  - Taper to next dosage for 2 weeks
  - Taper to lowest dosage for 2 weeks or discontinue
- Always provide
  - Office-based counseling
  - Self-help materials from the pharmaceutical company or agency
  - Follow-up visits or phone calls

treatment centers that can provide intensive behavioral and pharmacologic treatment. The success of formal treatment programs with carefully selected, motivated smokers ranges from 15% to 40%.

***Organizational resources and aids.*** Kottke, Solberg, and Brekke described the organizational components and systems that are essential to the delivery of effective and consistent counseling in primary care office settings. Because research has demonstrated that physician-delivered smoking cessation interventions are most likely to be effective when physicians are routinely reminded to intervene with all smoking patients with the use of chart stickers or similar reminder systems, these systems should be integrated into all office practices.

Resources for patients, physicians, and office staff members are important tools that enhance the capacity of health care providers to provide information and advice. Self-help manuals for smoking cessation are effective and are available through voluntary agencies.

## BIBLIOGRAPHY

American Psychiatric Association: *Diagnostic and statistical manual of mental disorders (DSM IV),* ed 3, Washington, DC, 1994, American Psychiatric Association.

Brown RA et al: Nicotine dependence: assessment and management. In *Principles of medical psychiatry,* ed 2, 1993.

Fagerstrom KO, Schneider NG: Measuring nicotine dependence: a review of the Fagerstrom Tolerance Questionnaire, *J Behav Med* 12(2):159, 1989.

Goldstein MG et al: Behavioral medicine strategies for medical patients. In Stoudemire A, editor: *Clinical psychiatry for medical patients,* Philadelphia, 1990, JB Lippincott.

Kottke TE et al: Smoking cessation strategies and evaluation, *J Am Coll Cardiol* 12(4):1105, 1988.

Miller WR, Rolnick S: *Motivational interviewing: preparing people to change addictive behavior,* New York, 1991, Guilford.

Ockene JK: Physician-delivered interventions for smoking cessation: strategies for increasing effectiveness, *Prev Med* 16(5):723, 1987.

Prochaska JO, DiClemente CC: Towards a comprehensive model of change. In Miller WR, Heather N, editors: *Treating addictive disorders: processes of change,* New York, 1986, Plenum.

Prochaska JO, Goldstein MG: Process of smoking cessation. Implications for clinicians, *Clin Chest Med* 12(4):727, 1991.

Redd WH: Management of anticipatory nausea and vomiting. In Holland JC, Rowland JH, editors: *Handbook of psychooncology,* New York, 1990, Oxford University.

Sachs DPL, Leischow SJ: Pharmacologic approaches to smoking cessation, *Clin Chest Med* 12(4):769, 1991.

CHAPTER

# 125 Obesity

**Robert H. Lerman**

Obesity is one of the most common conditions confronting the primary care physician. It is of multifactorial origin and is associated with many complications that lead patients to seek medical care. Most importantly, obesity is a chronic problem that is very upsetting to many women and men. Although all treatments can be reduced to the simple formula of producing negative caloric balance, obesity remains resistant to therapy. Unfortunately, no diet is universally effective. The tendency to regain weight after treatment has led to criticism of most weight loss approaches and to involvement of the U.S. Federal Trade Commission (FTC) in monitoring weight management practices.

The management of obesity presents a major challenge to the primary care physician. This chapter provides a comprehensive review of obesity and a foundation on which to build individualized treatment plans for each patient. The topics covered include epidemiology and etiology, pathophysiology, health implications and complications, assessment, and management. Several diets, drug therapy, and surgical procedures are described to provide the practitioner with approaches to be considered based on degree of obesity, lifestyle, and complicating medical conditions. In addition, because the treatment of the obese patient requires more than diet alone, a multimodality approach is emphasized, including exercise, nutrition education, behavior modification, and strategies for weight loss maintenance as necessary concomitants to short-term and long-term management.

## EPIDEMIOLOGY AND ETIOLOGY

### Definitions

*Obesity* is a disease manifested by excessive accumulation of adipose tissue and is defined as a weight 20% or more above desirable body weight. Table 125-1 presents a classification of obesity based on body weight and *body mass index* (BMI).

The term *colossal obesity* is introduced in view of the author's growing experience with massively obese patients meeting this criterion.

Standards for desirable body weight are generally obtained from the 1959 Metropolitan Life Insurance tables. However, a simple **rule of thumb** to estimate desirable body weights may be used:

For men, 106 pounds for first 5 feet + 6 pounds/inch above 5 feet

For women, 100 pounds for first 5 feet + 5 pounds/inch above 5 feet

BMI (weight [kg]/height [$m^2$]) is a useful parameter of extent of obesity, since obesity-related morbidity and mortality increase directly with BMI. The 1985 U.S. National Institutes of Health Consensus Panel on Obesity recommended that physicians adopt the BMI in evaluating obese patients. BMI, which at normal weight is 22, is related to risk status (Table 125-2).

Although BMI correlates with risk, the distribution of body fat may be a more important prognostic guide. Two body distributions of excess fat have been described: *central* (android, apple-shaped, abdominal, or upper-body) obesity and *peripheral* (gynoid, pear-shaped, gluteal, femoral, or lower-body) obesity (Fig. 125-1). The *waist-hip ratio* (WHR) is used to differentiate the types. A high WHR, associated with large, centrally located adipose cells, is a risk factor for ischemic heart disease, hypertension, cerebrovascular accident (CVA, stroke), diabetes

**Table 125-1.** Classification of obesity based on body weight and body mass index (BMI)

| Classification | Percent above desirable body weight | BMI (kg/m$^2$) |
|---|---|---|
| Overweight | 10 to 20 | |
| Obesity | ≥20 | ≥26.4 (men) ≥25.8 (women) |
| Morbid obesity | ≥100 (≥100 lb) | >~40 |
| Supermorbid obesity | | ≥50 |
| Colossal obesity | | ≥75 |

**Table 125-2.** BMI and health risk in obesity

| BMI (kg/m$^2$) | Risk status |
|---|---|
| 22 | Normal |
| 22-25 | Little increased risk |
| 25-30 | Low risk |
| 30-40 | Moderate risk |
| >40 | High risk |

mellitus, and death. In the male a WHR greater than 1 and in the female greater than 0.8 is associated with central obesity and steeply increasing risks for these diseases. Hernia, osteoarthrosis, and varicose veins are more common in peripheral obesity; the incidence of these disorders in persons with apple-shaped obesity is no higher than in the normal-weight population. The pear-shaped distribution of fat is thought to provide energy stores for lactation.

In central obesity, accumulation of fat in intraabdominal and extraabdominal regions is associated with increased mobilization of free fatty acids to the portal vein. Increased free fatty acid concentration decreases insulin uptake in the liver and causes hyperinsulinemia, which in turn leads to insulin resistance, glucose intolerance, and hypertriglyceridemia.

*Complicated obesity* is obesity associated with medical complications such as sleep apnea, severe arthritis, coronary artery disease, or diabetes mellitus and/or obesity of such a degree that the activities of daily living are significantly impaired. Obesity can also be characterized by age of onset, with *juvenile-onset obesity* associated with increased fat cell number (*hyperplastic obesity*) and *adult-onset obesity* associated with *hypertrophic obesity.* Adults may also develop hyperplastic obesity. Once weight reaches about 70% above desirable body weight, further weight gain is caused by hyperplasia.

Individuals of normal body weight may also develop the metabolic abnormalities characteristic of obesity, which include hypertriglyceridemia, increased plasma insulin levels, glucose intolerance, and hypertension; these abnormalities may be corrected by weight reduction. Thus, the term *normal-weight metabolic obesity* has been suggested. This group of patients probably represents a subset of central obesity, having lost lean body mass and developed increased fat mass as a result of sedentary lifestyles and aging. A physically inactive, 165-pound, 53-year-old man has approximately 15 pounds more fat than he did at age 25 because of loss in lean body mass, despite no change in body weight.

## Incidence

The incidence of obesity in Americans is increasing; 1991 data indicate that 31% of men and 35% of women are obese, compared with 24% of men and 27% of women in 1980. According to federal surveys of health practitioners, 33% to 40% of women and 20% to 24% of men are trying to lose weight at any given time. Obesity incidence is increasing most rapidly in children (see following discussion).

The prevalence of obesity is influenced by many factors, including age, gender, race, and economic status. The U.S. National Health and Nutrition Examination Survey (NHANES), conducted between 1988 and 1991, indicated that among both women and men the prevalence of obesity increased from 20 to 59 years of age, after which it declined. For women, the prevalence reached 52% by ages 50 through 59.

Obesity among white, black, and Hispanic men does not differ greatly. However, black women (49%) and Hispanic women (47%) are much more prone to obesity than white women (33%). The age-specific prevalence of obesity in Pima Indians 20 to 74 years of age ranged from 31% to 78% in men and 60% to 87% in women.

The prevalence of obesity increased between 1980 and 1991 by 9% in white females and 8% in white males and by 5% in black females and 21% in black males. Morbid obesity is present in an estimated 1% of adult Americans.

## Etiology

Many interacting factors participate in the etiology of obesity, which remains incompletely understood. Body weight generally is tightly regulated, with most people able to prevent major weight gain without conscious consideration of daily intake. Very small increments of excess caloric intake or equivalent decreases in energy expenditure may lead to significant weight gain. For example, if an individual consumes an excess of 100 calories per day above daily energy expenditure, a weight gain of approximately 10 pounds in 1 year or 100 pounds after 10 years would occur.

***Diet, lifestyle, and environmental factors.*** Sedentary lifestyles and prevalence of high-fat food items are clearly major factors in producing obesity in the United States. It has been estimated that since 1900, physical activity has decreased by 75%, dietary fat intake has increased by 31%, and complex carbohydrate intake has decreased by 43%. The availability of high-fat fast foods such as pizza, no farther away than a telephone call, provides an ideal environment for the epidemic of obesity to flourish in the United States. Dietary fat is more efficiently deposited in adipose tissue than is carbohydrate or protein. Some investigators have suggested that 1 g fat is equivalent to 11 kcal, not 9 as is generally accepted (carbohydrate and protein provide 4 kcal/g).

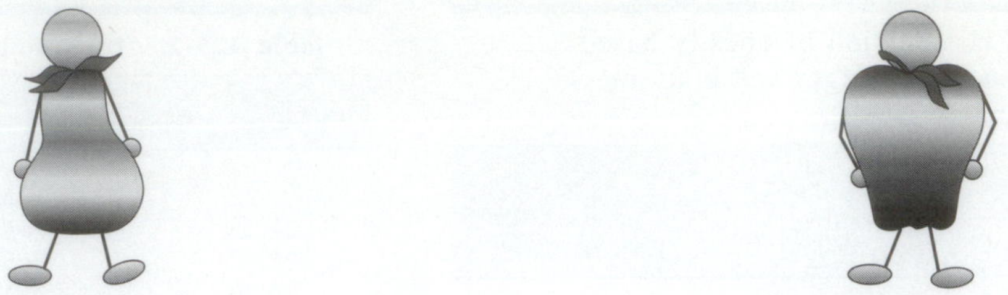
Pear-shaped obesity
↑ Heavy menstrual flow and irregularity
↑ More than 36 days in cycle
↓ Fewer children, fewer gravidities
↑ More frequently varicose veins, peripheral edema, osteoarthritis
↑ More frequently substantial weight increase in connection with pregnancy
↑ Early onset of obesity
↑ Less frequently cigarette smoking
Often depressive mood provoked by reducing regimen
↓ Poor prognosis for successful weight reduction
↓ Generally less morbidity in the past and fewer actual illnesses, but more often retired and out of work due to overweight itself
↓ Less frequently diabetes in the family
↓ Plasma C peptide
↑ Plasma insulin
↓ Low insulin removal
No change in body weight and composition after training
Apple-shaped obesity (abdominal obesity)
↑ Blood pressure
↑ Blood glucose
↑ Plasma insulin
↑ Plasma C peptide
↑ Plasma triglycerides
↑ Incidence of diabetes
↑ Diabetes in the family
↑ Spontaneous physical activity
↑ Gallbladder disease
↑ Fat cell weight
↓ Fat cell number
↑ Hirsutism
↑ Ratio of LBM/BF
↑ Higher % of FTb muscle fibers

**Fig. 125-1.** Two types of obesity. Prevalence of complications on the basis of a questionnaire given to 456 obese women. *LBM,* Lean body mass; *BF,* body fat; *FTb,* fast twitch fibers that are highly glycolytic.

A strong association has been found between television viewing and obesity in children. In preschool children, the more hours of TV watched, the greater is the increase in body fat. Many factors may be involved in this relationship. Children who watch a lot of TV are not only less physically active than other children. Their energy expenditure actually falls below resting levels during TV viewing as well.

Obesity may also be triggered by a sudden decrease in physical activity. This often occurs in physically active subjects who have sustained an injury and do not compensate by calorie restriction. Cessation of cigarette smoking is characteristically associated with modest weight gain. Other factors related to the environment include socioeconomic status and educational level attained. In contrast to an overall predominance of obesity in women compared with men, among better educated people and those of higher economic status, males tend to be more obese than females.

***Genetics.*** Animal models clearly demonstrate genetic strains that are prone to obesity. For example, investigators have cloned a receptor in fat cells of rats that controls the efficiency of fat metabolism. Levels of these receptors in adipocytes of genetically obese rats were about 70% less than those of normal rats. Recently, an obesity gene, *ob,* was characterized in mice. It is hypothesized that the *ob* gene product is secreted by adipose tissue and signals satiety. A homologue has been found in humans. Human twin studies indicate that fatness is under a high degree of genetic control. Data from an epidemiologic study of more than 500 adult adoptees showed that a strong correlation existed between the adoptees' weights and their biologic parents' weights. No such association was noted with the weights of their adoptive parents.

The influence of parental obesity may be related to heredity and/or the environment. However, if both parents are obese, there is an 80% chance of obesity in an offspring, whereas if one parent is obese, the chances are 40%. If neither parent is obese, the probability of an obese child is reduced to only 7%.

Rare genetic diseases are associated with obesity. The Prader-Willi syndrome, associated with hyperphagia, mental retardation, hypotonia, and a predilection for diabetes mellitus, appears to be caused by a lesion of the ventromedial nucleus of the hypothalamus with resultant loss of the satiety center. Recently, a specific chromosomal abnormality has been identified in persons with this

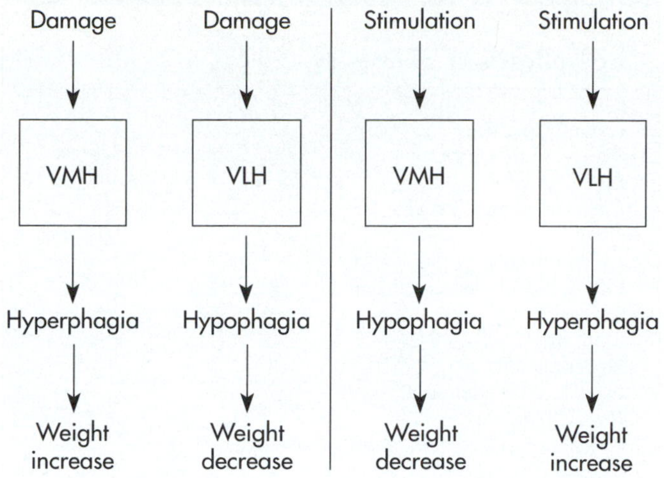


**Fig. 125-2.** Effects of the stereotactic damage or electrical stimulation of the ventromedial (*VMH*) and ventrolateral (*VLH*) hypothalamus.

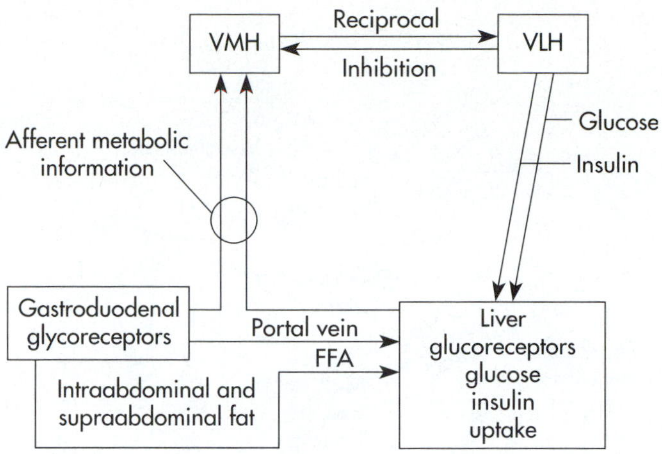


**Fig. 125-3.** Appetite and satiety are controlled centrally by the balance between the VMH and the VLH and peripherally by nutritional needs and stores. Afferent and efferent nerves link these four regions. *FFA,* Free fatty acids.

syndrome. This information may provide a clue regarding genetic areas of control in more common forms of obesity.

***Psychology.*** The importance of psychologic factors in the development of obesity cannot be overemphasized. People often turn to food when they are bored, anxious, or under stress. Obesity may protect an individual from dreaded social interactions. It has been suggested that cues for eating are external in obese persons, rather than being driven by nutritional factors (see Pathophysiology). A segment of the obese population suffers from binge eating, consuming excessive quantities of food to the point of physical discomfort. Some patients claim that they binge in an effort at self-destruction.

## PATHOPHYSIOLOGY

### Regulation of appetite and caloric intake

The hypothalamus plays a central role in appetite regulation. Electrical stimulation of the ventromedial hypothalamus (VMH) causes hungry rats to stop eating, whereas ablative stereotactic lesions of the VMH cause overeating and obesity (Fig. 125-2). However, overweight rats that overeat before the VMH lesion do not increase body weight and food intake after the lesion. This suggests the presence of a set point or "adipostat" that can be raised by lesions in the VMH or by other special conditions, such as pregnancy. If applicable to human obesity, weight reduction in an obese subject may be opposed by hypothalamic adipostat regulation. Increased food intake has also been described in patients with pituitary tumors with invasion of the VMH.

The ventrolateral hypothalamus (VLH) has been designated as the main feeding center of the brain. Electrical stimulation of the VLH elicits feeding in sated animals, and damage to the VLH leads to hypophagia. In addition, the VLH appears to be one of the most potent "reward" or pleasure centers, where endogenous opiates, endorphins, and enkephalins act as neurotransmitters. Humans and animals learn responses early in life that produce increased firing within this area. The same electrode that provides pleasure will also induce appetite and eating. Fig. 125-3 illustrates the interaction of the two hypothalamic centers with nutritional needs and stores.

The VLH center increases firing activity (hunger) under the influence of external (visual, gustatory, olfactory) stimuli. The VMH center increases firing activity (satiety) after receiving information about the nutritional state. Speculation that messengers control the nutritional state inspired the "glucostatic" (arteriovenous differences of glucose concentrations), "lipostatic" (free glycerol concentration), and "aminostatic" (amino acids) theories. However, rather than a single messenger involved in the control of appetite, multiple neural and hormonal factors appear to interact and provide this control. The pathogenesis of obesity based on these concepts assumes that in obese subjects the hypothalamic activity induced in the VLH by external cues dominates over the firing activity induced in the VMH by internal afferent information about nutritional state (Fig. 125-4). Supporting evidence for this theory is derived from studies in obese subjects who promptly elevate their plasma insulin levels after viewing and smelling food, or after only imagining that they are eating, in contrast to lean individuals whose plasma insulin levels remain unchanged after these stimuli.

The concept that the ventral hypothalamus has two separate control centers is an oversimplification. A number of other central nervous system tracts seem to be involved, as illustrated in Fig. 125-4. Lesions to these pathways alter eating behavior and weight in predictable ways.

### Other factors

Additional factors may be related to the development of obesity. They include alterations in lipoprotein lipase activity, altered sodium-potassium pump activity, reduced dietary thermogenesis, and reduced levels of brown adipose tissue. Slight lowering of resting energy expenditure also may be a factor. A study of Native Americans indicated that those with the lowest measured resting energy expenditures had the greatest incidence of weight gain over a 4-year period. Animal studies indicate that

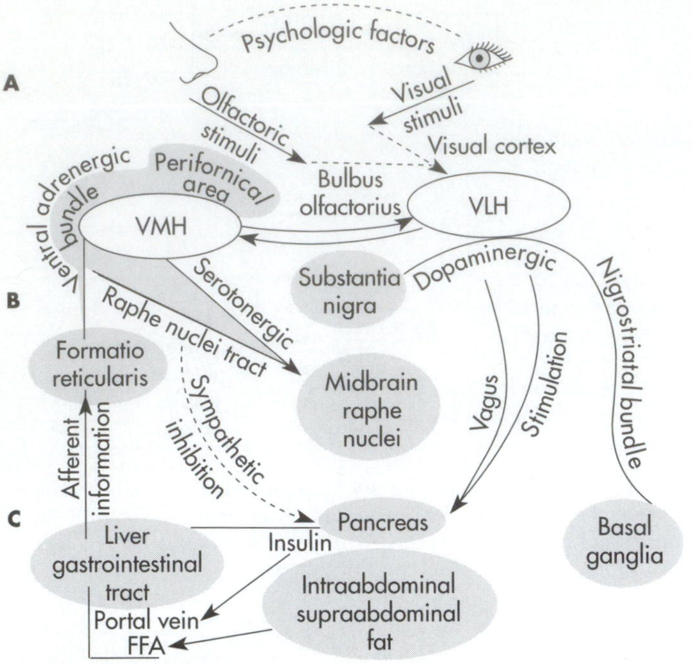


**Fig. 125-4.** Integrated illustration of different factors engaged in appetite regulation *A,* External stimulation. *B,* Hypothalamic integration. *C,* Peripheral afferent information about nutritional status. In obesity *A* > *C;* thus, VLH > VMH. *FFA,* Free fatty acids.

### Complications of obesity

Diabetes mellitus
Shortness of breath
Sleep apnea
Coronary artery disease
Gout
Cholelithiasis
Polycystic ovarian syndrome
Osteoarthritis
Skin tags
Hypertension
Pickwickian syndrome
Hyperlipidemia
Cerebrovascular accident (stroke)
Certain cancers
Hepatic steatosis
Pseudotumor cerebri
Cardiomyopathy
Intertrigo
Acanthosis nigricans
Sudden death

more adipose tissue is deposited in animals consuming one meal per day than in those consuming equivalent calories in multiple small feedings.

### Secondary obesity

Obesity may be secondary to an underlying medical condition, such as hypothyroidism, Cushing disease, insulinoma, or hypothalamic disorders. Only a minority of hypothyroid patients are truly obese, and clinical experience indicates that very few obese patients are found to be hypothyroid. Cushing disease should be considered in a patient with "buffalo hump," "moon face," and purple abdominal striae. Insulinomas rarely cause obesity. Hypothalamic disorders include Fröhlich's syndrome, found in boys and associated with hypogonadotrophic hypogonadism and variable features such as diabetes insipidus, visual impairment, and mental retardation. The pituitary gland is usually free of pathology, but in some patients, including Frölich's original subject, pituitary tumors are present.

## HEALTH IMPLICATIONS AND ASSOCIATIONS

### Relationship of obesity to disease

The box above lists conditions associated with obesity.

***Diabetes mellitus and insulin resistance.*** About 70% to 80% of subjects with non-insulin-dependent diabetes mellitus are overweight. Native Americans and Hispanics are especially susceptible to developing both obesity and diabetes. The relative risk of diabetes among Pima Indians in the American southwest is almost 11-fold that of lean counterparts. This relates to their remarkable predisposition to becoming obese. The relative risk of diabetes mellitus in overweight Americans ages 20 to 44 is 3.8, in obese people ages 20 to 75 is 2.9, and increases 10-fold in severely obese persons. The prevalence is greatly increased in morbidly obese persons; 55.9% of 515 morbidly obese subjects undergoing gastric surgery were diabetic or had glucose intolerance. According to an American Cancer Society (ACS) study, the disease associated with the highest mortality ratios with increasing body weight was diabetes mellitus.

The most characteristic feature of the metabolic disturbances in obesity is insulin insensitivity: hyperinsulinemia and impaired glucose tolerance. The body's initial response to insulin with regard to glucose and lipid metabolism remains normal at supramaximal insulin concentrations. With increased duration and severity of obesity, however, insulin resistance progresses so that even supramaximal concentrations of insulin are ineffective. The decreased responsiveness to insulin is related to fat cell size. It is also influenced by changes in nutrition. The decreased insulin sensitivity can be combined with the varying degrees of impaired insulin release, leading to overt diabetes or "diabesity" (Fig. 125-5). The tendency to develop carbohydrate metabolism abnormalities and diabetes is characteristic only of central obesity. Obese patients with pear-shaped (peripheral) obesity do not differ from the normal-weight population in the incidence of disturbances of carbohydrate metabolism. It seems likely that a variety of causes of hyperinsulinemia and insulin resistance in obesity will become evident as the various types of obesity are better defined.

Caloric restriction and weight reduction reverse hyperinsulinemia and restore tissue sensitivity and responsive-

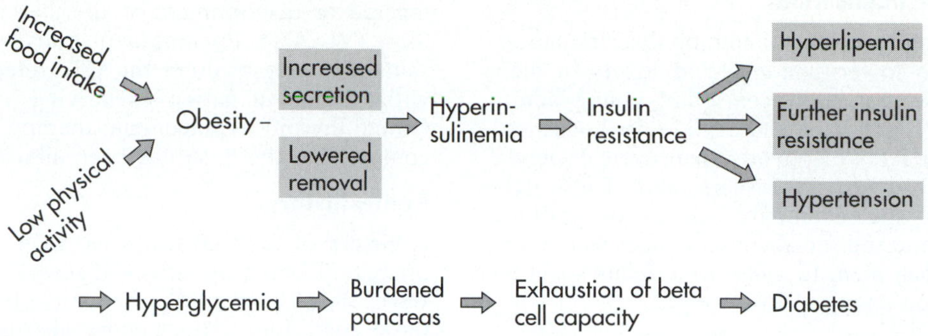


**Fig. 125-5.** Consequences of increased food intake and low physical activity leading to successive development of "diabesity." Important and recently discovered role of impaired insulin clearance in liver is one of the first stages of the developmental chain.

ness to normal. Physical training increases the glucose disposal rate and, in some patients, improves hyperinsulinemia by decreasing insulin release and increasing insulin uptake in the muscles and liver.

***Hypertension and cardiovascular disease.*** The NHANES II Study indicated a threefold relative risk for hypertension in obese people ages 20 to 75. According to the Framingham Heart Study, blood pressure increased 6.5 mm Hg for every 10% increase in relative weight. The prevalence of ventricular ectopy, a risk factor for sudden death, was 30 times more prevalent in obese hypertensive patients with eccentric left ventricular hypertrophy than in lean people.

Hypertension was found in more than 25% of a series of morbidly obese subjects undergoing gastric restrictive surgery. Blood volume and cardiac output of a 170 kg (374-pound) individual are about twice those of one weighing 70 kg (154 pounds).

Obesity is an independent risk factor for cardiovascular disease and sudden death according to the Framingham Heart Study (see Chapter 7). After exclusion of cigarette smokers, at the 26-year follow-up, each kilogram (2.2 pounds) of excess weight at the start of the study increased the risk of death from cardiovascular disease by 4%. Thus, 5 kg (11 pounds) of excess weight increased the risk of cardiac death by 20%. Much of the effect of obesity is mediated through reversible factors associated with obesity, such as hypertension, glucose intolerance, high total cholesterol and triglycerides, and low high-density-lipoprotein (HDL) levels. Therefore, reduction of excess weight is probably the most important hygienic measure available for the control of cardiovascular disease.

***Cancer.*** Mortality for cancer in the ACS study of 750,000 men and women was increased in those at least 40% overweight because of cancer of the colon, rectum, and prostate in men and the gallbladder, biliary tract, breast, cervix, endometrium, uterus, and ovary in women. Although the exact mechanism by which obesity increases cancer rates is unknown, elevated estrogen levels may be an important factor in tumors of reproductive organs and breasts of women. The adipocyte is the principal source of estrogen formation in postmenopausal females.

***Respiratory disease.*** Respiratory side effects of obesity may lead to significant disability and risk. Shortness of breath is a common complaint. Sleep apnea, although much less common, may be life-threatening. Respiration ceases with onset of stage III or IV sleep, with a fall in oxygen levels and rise in carbon dioxide levels stimulating awakening and resumption of breathing. The cycle may be repeated hundreds of times per night. Daytime sleepiness results, reducing productivity and potentially leading to motor vehicle accidents and other mishaps. In obesity, sleep apnea is usually obstructive but may be of central, peripheral, or mixed origin.

The pickwickian syndrome is typically associated with morbid obesity and is characterized by hypersomnolence, congestive heart failure, and hypertension. In a large series of subjects undergoing gastric surgery for morbid obesity, 12.5% had evidence of respiratory insufficiency. Sixty-five of 126 subjects had sleep apnea syndrome, 16 of 126 had obesity hyperventilation syndrome, and 45 had both.

***Gallstones.*** The overall incidence of gallstones is doubled to tripled with obesity and, according to the Nurses Health Study, was six times more frequent in the highest one fifth of the obesity scale. Among morbidly obese patients undergoing bariatric surgery, the incidence of gallstones was approximately 35%.

## Psychologic ramifications

Whereas little evidence indicates a relationship between mild-to-moderate obesity and mental disorders, with more severe degrees of obesity, loss of self-esteem, anxiety disorders, and depression become more prevalent. The psychologic effects of obesity are related to a large extent to the current media-driven association between leanness/ultraleanness and physical attractiveness. Common "wisdom" dictates that body weight is under voluntary control and that obese people are therefore held responsible for their condition. At the extremes of obesity, patients indicate they would prefer to be of normal weight and to have a major handicap (e.g., deafness, dyslexia, diabetes mellitus, legal blindness, bad acne, heart disease, amputated leg) than to be morbidly obese. All preferred to be a normal-weight person than be a morbidly obese multimillionaire.

### Social and economic implications

Obese people are subject to social and job discrimination. They tend to attain lower-than-expected levels in their occupations. Overweight adolescents and young adults were found to marry less often and have lower household incomes and higher rates of poverty than normal-weight individuals when followed up 7 years later. These data held regardless of socioeconomic origins or aptitude scores. Both economic and social consequences were more severe in women than men. In 1989, Americans spent an estimated $30 billion trying to lose weight.

### Mortality

Mortality increased from all causes with increasing obesity in the previously mentioned large ACS study. Nearly 50% higher mortalities were found among men and women who were 30% to 40% above normal weight. Overweight in adolescent males was associated with increased long-term mortality. Morbid obesity is associated with at least a doubling of all morbidity and mortality compared to the general population. Unexplained death occurs at least 13 times more often in morbidly obese women than in those of normal weight. Morbidly obese men 25 to 34 years of age have a twelvefold increase of mortality and a sixfold increase from ages 35 to 44.

• • •

The obese patient deserves a thorough history, physical examination, and evaluation, including dietary intake, weight history, assessment of motivation and commitment to necessary lifestyle changes, and a determination of the risks posed to the patient by obesity.

## HISTORY

### Diet and weight

The diet history is used to assess the subject's usual intake. A 3- to 7-day diet diary may be helpful, although a 24-hour dietary recall may be more practical. A food frequency questionnaire, more often used in epidemiologic research (The Willett), may be helpful. The percent calories as fat, intake of saturated fat, and polyunsaturated fatty acids can be estimated from these data.

Aspects of the history relevant to obesity management include age of onset of obesity, life events precipitating obesity, associated illnesses (e.g., hypertension, hypercholesterolemia, diabetes mellitus, osteoarthritis), previous weight loss attempts, types of diets used, other modalities attempted, magnitude of weight losses, history of binge eating, binging and purging, tobacco use, alcoholism or other substance abuse, frequency and magnitude of repeat weight gains, and exercise history, including past and present participation in physical activity.

### Medications

A complete list of both prescription and over-the-counter (OTC) medications may help identify medications associated with weight gain, such as valproic acid, oral contraceptives, insulin, and certain antidepressants. In addition, medications associated with attempts at weight loss, such as laxatives and diuretics, may be found. Adjustments in medication dosage on diet initiation may be indicated. For example, diuretics are generally discontinued and insulin and oral hypoglycemic agents are tapered or discontinued at the start of very-low-calorie diets (VLCDs). Phenothiazines and tricyclic antidepressants that may prolong the QTc interval should be used with caution in patients receiving VLCDs. In a patient taking thyroid replacement therapy, it is important to confirm that the dose has been adjusted correctly.

### Family history

A history of familial illnesses, such as diabetes mellitus, premature coronary artery disease, and hyperlipidemia, warns the physician that the patient is more likely to have these conditions. This history also may be used to help motivate the patient to lose weight, alter diet, and increase physical activity. A history of obesity in the patient's spouse and/or children is important for treatment and prevention.

### Symptoms related to obesity

Patients may not volunteer information suggestive of sleep apnea. Careful questioning about morning headaches, daytime hypersomnolence, wakenings with dyspnea, loud snoring, or observed apneic episodes may provide evidence for obstructive sleep apnea. Other symptoms of significance include shortness of breath with minimal exertion, chest pain, ankle swelling, joint pain, skin rashes, and limitations in the activities of daily living, such as inability to maintain hygiene, dress, and bathe. Additional symptoms may include depression, anxiety, or suicidal ideation.

## PHYSICAL EXAMINATION

Accurate determinations of body weight and height are necessary initial parameters and may require special scales. A hoist-type scale may be necessary in bed-bound, massively obese patients. Unless a blood pressure cuff with adequate dimensions (cuff bladder 40% to 50% of arm circumference and cuff bladder length greater than 80% of arm circumference) is used, hypertension may be incorrectly diagnosed. A satisfactory abdominal examination may be impossible, especially in patients with morbid to colossal obesity. Other aspects of the physical examination include a search for signs of thyroid deficiency (dry skin, loss of lateral aspect of eyebrows, thickened hair, sluggish deep tendon reflexes), stigmata of Cushing's disease (purple abdominal striae, truncal obesity, buffalo hump), signs of bulimia (loss of calcium from inner aspects of teeth), skinfold candidal infection or intertrigo, and presence of edema and venostasis. The practitioner should keep in mind conditions that might affect potential treatment, including exercise (flat feet, osteoarthritis).

## EVALUATION: QUANTITATIVE ASSESSMENT OF OBESITY

### Body mass index calculation

$$\text{BMI} = \text{Weight (kg)}/\text{Height (m)}^2$$

Fig. 125-6 provides a convenient nomogram for determining BMI.

### Waist-to-hip ratio

$$\text{WHR} = \text{Minimal waist circumference}/\text{Maximal hip circumference}$$

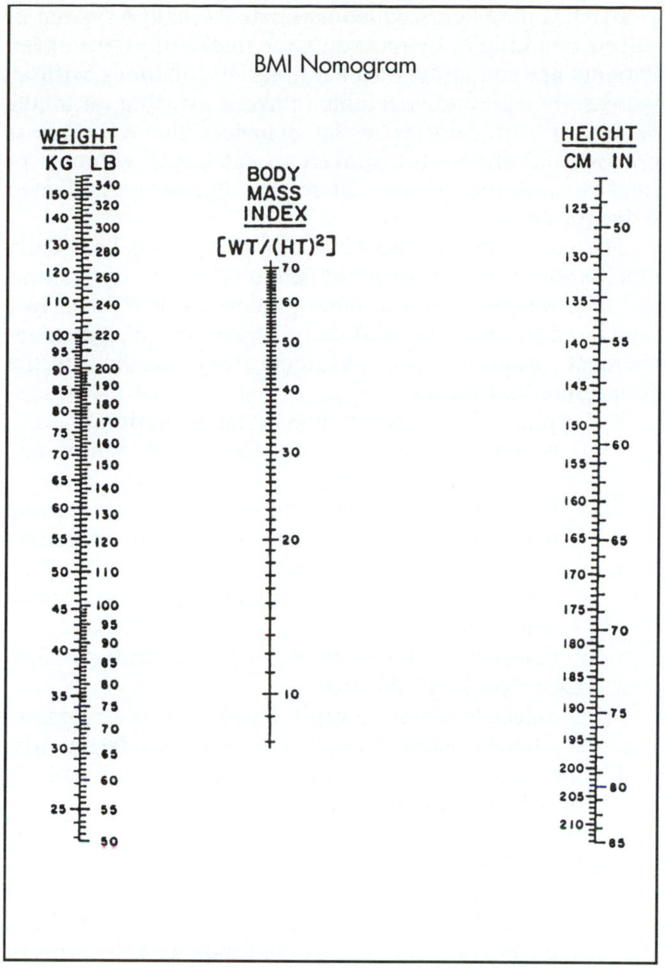


**Fig. 125-6.** Body mass index (BMI) nomogram. (From Bray GA, editor: *Obesity in America,* USDHEW, Public Health Service, National Institutes of Health, NIH pub no. 79-359, November, 1979.)

### Laboratory tests

Laboratory analyses may be done to search for an underlying etiology of a patient's obesity, to assess body composition, to evaluate possible complications, or to screen before institution of and during treatment with VLCDs. In addition, specialized laboratory testing may be needed in the workup of intercurrent illnesses.

Unfortunately, besides unusual laboratory findings indicating hypothyroidism, blood tests are unlikely to be of value. Although the yield is generally quite low, it is reasonable to obtain a thyroid-stimulating hormone (TSH) level to rule out hypothyroidism. Skull x-rays may be indicated in obese patients with headaches and visual problems.

Impedance plethysmography is a readily available test to assess percent body fat and lean body tissue. It appears to be more reliable than skinfold measurements and is certainly more easily obtainable than underwater weighing. A 24-hour urine collection for creatinine may provide baseline data related to lean body mass. The quantity of creatinine in the urine is a reflection of lean body mass.

Bloods obtained after a 14-hour fast should be sent for glucose, total cholesterol, HDL, and triglyceride determinations. When clinical suspicion of gallstones is high, a gallbladder ultrasound should be obtained.

Body size may prevent use of magnetic resonance imaging (MRI) or other specialized equipment. Rather than delay evaluation and embarrass the patient, one should confirm the capability of equipment and staff before scheduling studies.

## MANAGEMENT

### Patient recognition

Patients come to physicians with a variety of medical problems, many of which are weight related. They are often chagrined when the issue of weight is addressed rather than the concerns for which they presented. Their weight problem is no surprise to them, but their weight being an aggravating or etiologic factor to their diabetes, hypertension, or osteoarthritis often is surprising. Physicians should remember that weight reduction may be the treatment of choice for such conditions, even when body weight is at or near "normal" (see previous discussion). For this reason, although the diagnosis of obesity is generally clear by physical inspection, indices of body composition are recommended in patients not clearly obese but with clinical and metabolic derangements seen in obesity.

### Prevention

Even with the best guidance and intentions, a minority of obese individuals attain and maintain long-term weight loss. In those who do, the tendency to regain weight appears to persist indefinitely. For these reasons and because of the significant morbidity and mortality associated with obesity, every effort to prevent its development should be made. Prevention begins by learning about the family's eating and exercise habits, information that is often overlooked or considered unimportant by intervention-oriented physicians. Many cultures place an emphasis on not only eating well, but also eating large quantities. This is especially true for people who have undergone the trials of war, poverty, deprivation, and discrimination.

Based on diet and exercise history, education must be individualized. From the earliest ages, the physician may exert influence by encouraging and monitoring regular physical activity and discussing the need to limit sedentary activities such as TV viewing. The potential value of an aggressive exercise program in the prevention of adult obesity was shown in a study of the effects of a 2-year aerobic exercise program with no alteration in diet on 41 obese 11-year-old children. The children ran at approximately 70% of maximal oxygen uptake for 20 minutes seven times per week. One year later, fat mass decreased by an average of more than 9 kg (20 pounds) in both the boys and the girls, while height increased 6 cm (2.4 inches) in the boys and 7 cm (2.8 inches) in the girls. The BMI decreased significantly in both groups, and a continued improvement was noted at 2 years.

Whereas it may be unreasonable to label any food as prohibited, emphasis must be placed on limiting the intake of high-fat foods such as fried foods, mayonnaise, bacon, sausages, and red meats. Providing alternatives enhances the chance of success. A transition to low-fat cooking methods with the gradual incorporation of vegetarian entrees is encouraged. At least five servings of fruits and vegetables daily will add needed nutrients and fiber while limiting caloric intake. When physician time is not available for in-depth counseling in a busy medical practice, referral to a registered dietitian or office nurse is encouraged for preventive counseling. It is advisable to target at-risk families and populations for education or referral. This may include people with strong family histories of obesity, premature heart disease, or diabetes mellitus.

## Weight reduction

Many approaches to the medical management of obesity have been tried. Current recommendations suggest that a combination of diet, exercise, nutrition education, and behavior modification (see Chapter 124) provides the best opportunity for success. The following sections assume this combined approach unless otherwise stated.

### *Diets*

**Balanced-calorie dieting.** Balanced-calorie dieting relies on portion control and low-fat food choices. Table 125-3 outlines a sample menu providing about 1150 calories over 1 day.

Weight loss depends on the calorie deficit achieved. A 500 kcal daily deficit is translated into a 1 pound per week weight loss (3500 kcal/lb of fat).

**To determine the daily caloric needs for weight maintenance, multiply body weight in pounds by 11 for women and 12 for men.**

Whereas more sophisticated formulas may be used, the one above serves well for everyday use. For example, if a woman weighs 180 pounds, her daily energy expenditure is $180 \times 11 = 1980$ kcal/day. Therefore, a 1500 kcal daily diet would lead to a weight loss of approximately 1 pound per week and a 1000 kcal daily diet to a loss of 2 pounds per week. In general, with a standard balanced-calorie-deficit diet (BCDD), weight loss usually ranges from 1 to 2 pounds per week but may be accelerated by exercise.

**Table 125-3.** Sample menu in balanced-calorie dieting*

| Meal/snack | Sample foods |
|---|---|
| Breakfast | 1 cup flaked bran cereal |
| | ½ cup skim milk |
| | 1 fruit (½ banana) |
| Snack | Apple |
| Lunch | 2 slices bread |
| | 1 oz turkey |
| | 2 cups salad/mixed vegetables |
| | 2 tbs reduced-calorie salad dressing |
| Snack | Orange |
| Dinner | 3 oz chicken, fish, turkey, or meat |
| | ½ cup broccoli |
| | 1 small (3 oz) baked potato |
| | 2 tsp margarine or diet margarine |
| | Orange (pear) |
| Snack | ½ cup fruit cocktail |

*1157 calories: 59% carbohydrates, 23% fat, 18% protein.

BCDDs may be provided using an exchange system or calorie counting or by recording the intake of grams of fat. Patients are encouraged to eat a variety of foods with an increase in fruit and vegetable intake. Lowering fat intake below 30% of calories as fat enhances the weight loss process and allows the subject to eat larger volumes of food because the quantity of fruits, vegetables, and fiber is increased.

The use of preprinted 1200, 1500, or 1800 kcal daily diets is discouraged, as is the admonition by a physician to "lose weight" without clear guidelines or referral to a registered dietitian or medically supervised weight management program. The physician may provide initial counseling as follows:

1. Emphasize the importance of fat reduction.
   a. Avoid all added fats, fried foods, whole milk, and cheeses for 2 weeks.
   b. Limit the following to no more than one serving per week: baked desserts, ice cream, or candy.
2. Stress vegetarian selections.
   a. Can eat unlimited amounts of unadorned cooked and fresh vegetables.
   b. Eat at least three servings of fresh fruit per day.
3. Alter "protein" choices.
   a. Select moderate portion if red meat is still eaten.
   b. Choose fish and poultry dishes more frequently.
4. Encourage physical activity: recommend walking for a half hour per day.

Another approach worthy of trial in motivated patients is a very-low-fat diet providing less than 10% of calories as fat. To accomplish this, animal products (except for egg whites and nonfat yogurt) are eliminated from the diet. Patients are instructed to eat whole foods with portions of vegetables, beans, and fruits, limited only by hunger. Among nonanimal products, only oils, olives, avocados, nuts, and seeds are forbidden. Caution must be used because a very-low-fat diet improperly formulated may lead to essential fatty acid deficiency. This diet is especially advantageous for patients with coronary artery disease, since angiographically documented reversal of atherosclerotic lesions has been reported with such a diet when combined with exercise, meditation, and stress reduction.

If progress in weight reduction is made after 1 month, it is reasonable to follow the patient at monthly intervals. If progress is minimal, consider referral to a multidisciplinary, medically supervised weight management program staffed by physicians with nutrition training, registered dietitians, and other nutrition educator health professionals. The modalities used in such programs include exercise, behavior modification, nutrition education, and diet.

**Very-low-calorie diets.** All diets work by the same mechanism, caloric restriction. VLCDs are no exception. They are modified fasts providing 800 kcal or less and 0.8 to 1.5 g protein per kilogram of ideal body weight per day. VLCDs completely replace usual food intake. They include a number of commercially prepared, liquid frappé-like or soup products, including Health Management Resources (HMR), Optifast and Medifast, and the food-based Protein Sparing Modified Fast (PSMF). VLCDs lead to consistent, rapid, and sizable weight losses. They are recommended to be used as part of a comprehensive weight management program and are generally reserved for individuals at least 30% and/or 40 pounds above desirable body weight (or BMI greater than 30 kg/m$^2$). VLCDs may be used in patients with lesser degrees of obesity who have clear medical complications such as angina pectoris, diabetes mellitus, hypertension, sleep apnea, or osteoarthritis and who have been unsuccessful with BCDDs. Patients with type II diabetes are good candidates because insulin or oral hypoglycemic agents can be tapered rapidly with the institution of this dietary approach. In most patients, insulin doses may be cut in half at the start of the diet and tapered subsequently based on fingerstick blood sugar levels. Specific protocols describing the mechanisms of action of VLCDs, their dietary components, contraindications, and side effects are provided in the bibliography.

### *Exercise*

**Potential benefits.** Exercise is associated with an increase in metabolic rate, appetite suppression, changes in body composition, alterations in substrate oxidation, and psychologic effects of improved general well-being. In addition, substrate and hormone levels associated with complications of obesity are favorably altered by exercise. Unfortunately, exercise as the sole approach to weight reduction in adult obesity is rarely effective. When combined with other modalities, however, it becomes an essential component, helping to increase the loss of adipose tissue while maintaining lean tissue. The role of exercise both in the prevention of obesity and in weight loss maintenance cannot be overemphasized.

***Increase in lean body mass.*** Physical training produces a decrease in fat mass and an increase in lean body mass. Studies of physically fit middle-aged men have shown that the usual changes in body composition that occur with aging and associated with sedentary lifestyles are prevented. Indeed, lean body mass and percentage of body fat in these men have been found to be similar to those of lean men in their twenties. Weight loss with exercise alone results in a preservation of lean body mass. It has been found that with training, adipocytes decrease in size and stabilize at lower levels than those attained with diet alone.

***Change in lipids, glycogen, and metabolism.*** Exercise lowers insulin levels, increases insulin sensitivity, and improves glucose tolerance. Triglyceride levels fall, and HDL cholesterol levels increase. These changes decrease the risk of diabetes mellitus and cardiovascular complications. The respiratory quotient decreases with sustained aerobic exercise, indicating an energy source shift from carbohydrates to fat. With strenuous aerobic exertion, glycogen stores are depleted. In comparisons of food intake between middle-aged, weight-stable, physically active men and sedentary men, the drive to replete glycogen stores may lead to preferential consumption of a diet higher in carbohydrates and lower in fat in those who exercise. Because lipogenesis from carbohydrate ingestion is limited, this alteration in dietary intake may help to prevent gains in body fat.

***Calorie expenditure.*** Appetite suppression occurs in obese persons but not in lean subjects after physical activity. The thermic effect of exercise in obese subjects is increased by eating a meal after exercise. The amount of weight that can be lost quickly with exercise alone, however, is generally less than that achieved through dieting alone. A carry-over effect on metabolic rate from a bout of exercise has been debated. Data supporting this concept indicate that for such an effect to be produced, high-intensity, long-duration aerobic exercise is required. Other data indicate that energy expenditure returns to baseline levels shortly after completion of the exercise. Thus it may be concluded that in the typical obese person who cannot exercise at high intensity, caloric expenditure is limited to the exercise period itself.

***Weight maintenance.*** Regular physical activity has a particular attractiveness in efforts to maintain reduced body weight and increased lean body mass over the long term. Exercise appears to be the most important factor in maintaining long-term weight loss. In studies 18 months and 3 years after weight loss in members of the Boston Police Force, subjects who had not exercised and did not begin to exercise after the weight reduction program regained all their weight. Those who exercised for 90 minutes three times a week during the 8- or 12-week weight loss programs and continued a regular exercise regimen during the follow-up period maintained essentially all their weight loss. Interview studies with formerly obese people indicate that exercise is one of the most important factors in successful weight maintenance.

**When to prescribe.** Exercise is an essential part of a weight management program, whether for obesity prevention, weight loss, or weight maintenance. Unless specific contraindications exist, physical activity should be instituted at the start of any weight loss program.

**Regimens.** Exercise should include components of aerobic activity, flexibility, and muscle strengthening. As a first step, exercise may be incorporated into daily activities by using stairs instead of elevators, parking farther from destinations, and walking rather than driving when feasible. A walking program can be instituted gradually by most previously sedentary obese people. Most subjects are willing to begin by walking 10 minutes from their home and 10 minutes back, or about a mile at an average pace. In conjunction with dietary restriction, frequency and duration of exercise is gradually increased to a minimum expenditure of 2000 kcal per week. Weight-bearing exercises such as walking and jogging lead to a greater consumption of calories in obese than in lean individuals provided that the distances covered are comparable. The caloric expenditure of these activities is directly related to body weight. For example, a 150-pound person burns 100 kcal per mile of walking, whereas a 300-pound person expends 200 kcal. Non–weight-bearing activities such as the use of an exercise cycle do not lead to higher energy expenditures in obese than in lean people. More than one aerobic activity is encouraged because a change in weather may dissuade walking. Warming up, stretching, and cooling down are important exercise components. A weight-training program to increase lean body mass may be gradually phased in, with two or three low-intensity circuit-type sessions as part of an overall workout.

**Safeguards: when to do exercise tolerance test (ETT).** Some guidelines suggest that because of their increased risk of coronary artery disease, obese individuals should be stress-tested before entering exercise programs. Ultimately, however, the decision to order an ETT is a matter of physician judgment. Stress testing in obese patients is appropriate when they give a history of symptoms suggestive of angina or risk factors such as hypertension, hypercholesterolemia, and diabetes mellitus. When obese patients plan to begin a strenuous exercise program, stress testing should also be strongly considered to rule out coronary disease and to determine the baseline level of physical fitness. One should remember that an ETT requires exertion beyond that recommended for institution of a mild-to-moderate physical activity program. It may be threatening to and potentially poorly tolerated by obese patients, and the results may not alter the plans for institution of a gradual walking program. Therefore, the decision to order an ETT should be fitted to the patient's history and special situation.

## Behavior modification

*Goals.* The goals of behavioral therapy are to assist the obese patient to identify and modify habits of inappropriate eating and lack of exercise and attitudes that contribute to obesity (See Chapter 124 for an expanded discussion). With behavior modification, easily measurable, clear goals are set. The aim is to change behaviors rather than to determine the underlying psychopathology responsible for a particular behavior. Attention is focused on finding ways to change behavior. Traditional behavior modification focuses on the "ABCs": **A**ntecedents of behavior, the **B**ehavior itself, and the **C**onsequences of that behavior. Approaches in weight management include the control of stimuli that precede eating, the development of techniques to control eating behavior, and the provision of rewards for successful behavior or successful progress in weight loss. The circumstances eliciting overeating are monitored by carefully kept diet diaries detailing what is eaten. Some advocate also recording when, where, with whom, over what period of time, what else the subject was doing (e.g., watching TV), and how the person felt during eating.

The assumption that obesity results from faulty eating habits has been questioned. For the most part, eating habits of obese people do not differ radically from those of lean individuals. Focusing on changing eating style or habits rarely leads to lifelong change. With this in mind, it appears that the primary focus in the behavioral approach should be placed on what the person eats rather than on how eating takes place. Thus, the principal strategy of behavior therapy is to develop the knowledge and skills necessary to balance caloric intake and expenditures.

This may be accomplished by teaching self-monitoring. Patients are instructed to determine and record their daily caloric intake and expenditures. They are taught to estimate portion sizes (ounces or cups) and caloric content of foods to allow computation of caloric intake (e.g., kcal per ounce × ounces consumed). Daily energy needs are estimated (11 × body weight in pounds for females and 12 × body weight in pounds for males), and to this is added the caloric expenditure of physical activity. Thus, the caloric deficit (or excess) may be computed on a daily and weekly basis. Dividing weekly caloric deficit by 3500 gives an estimate of expected weight loss. Choices are emphasized. For example, 36 cups of air-popped popcorn provides the same number of calories as 1 cup of peanuts (860 kcal).

The preparation and consumption of meals can be structured to reduce random snacking of high-calorie foods. Refrigerators and other food sources should be localized in one place in the apartment or house and not distributed throughout the living space. Low-calorie snacks and beverages should be available if food craving is a problem.

*Group format.* Weekly group sessions lasting 1 to 1½ hours with 10 to 15 people in attendance for behavior modification instruction are an important part of a comprehensive weight loss program. The length of treatment varies from 8 weeks to several months. The sessions help patients to incorporate lifestyle changes. Behavior modification may be combined with any dietary approach. In conjunction with a VLCD program, emphasis is placed on approaches to help prevent deviations from supplemental fasting. Environmental control and exercise are stressed. Patients are encouraged to meet an expected caloric expenditure with physical activity (e.g., at least 2000 kcal by about week 6 in the program). The sessions may be provided by a registered dietitian or other health professionals trained to provide group education. Once the patient's weight goal has been attained, the patient is encouraged to enter a long-term maintenance program. The length of maintenance varies with different programs, but a minimum of 18 months is recommended. Relapse prevention and posttreatment contact by telephone and mail have been evaluated as possible approaches to improve the long-term outcome.

Relapse prevention methods include the training of subjects to identify high-risk situations that might lead to uncontrolled eating and the use of problem-solving techniques to prepare for these situations. In addition, patients receive supervised practice in actual situations, such as dinner parties. They are also trained in cognitive restructuring techniques to minimize the sense of failure often associated with a temporary lapse in eating behavior.

## Drug therapy

Currently available pharmacologic therapy for obesity is limited essentially to appetite suppressants. Anorectic agents appear to have a limited role in obesity management, leading to short-term weight loss, with a regaining of weight the rule on cessation of therapy. These agents may be justified if a short-term need exists for weight loss, for example, to qualify for elective surgery. Chronic therapy with anorectic agents appears to have produced effective long-term weight loss.

*Centrally acting anorectic agents.* Most of these agents, except for mazindol (Mazanor, Sanorex), are phenethylamine derivatives and include such drugs as fenfluramine (Pondimin), phenmetrazine (Preludin), and diethylpropion (Tenuate, Tepanil). Except for fenfluramine, which is believed to act through serotoninergic pathways, these other drugs release epinephrine and norepinephrine in the prefornical region of the brain. The anorectic drugs are generally more effective than a placebo and produce a weight loss of about 0.6 pound per week more than that achieved with placebo. Fenfluramine may lower blood pressure and improve glucose tolerance and thus may be appropriate for hypertensive and diabetic patients. Fen-

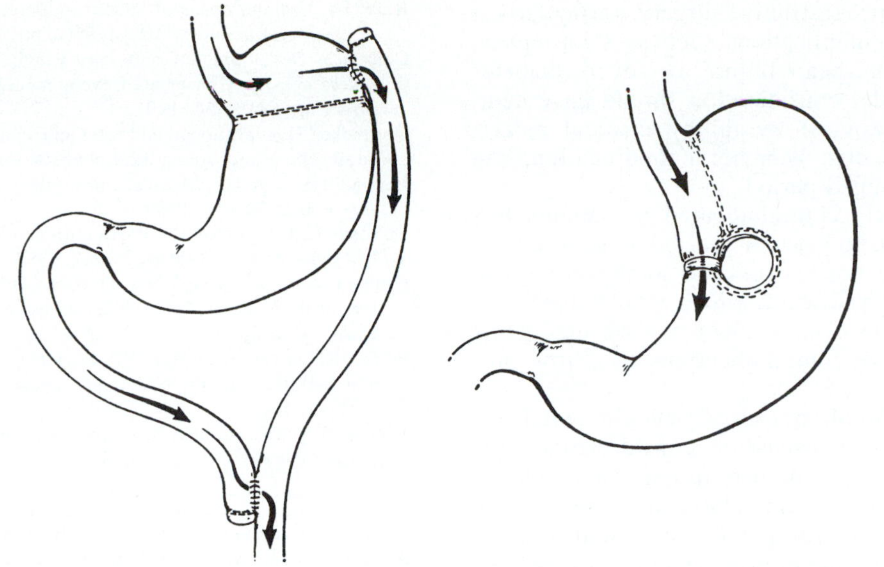

**Fig. 125-7.** *Left,* Vertical-banded gastroplasty with a 15 to 25 ml vertically placed pouch and a plastic constrainer on the exit. *Right,* Gastric bypass with creation of a fundic pouch, gastrojejunostomy, and a Roux-en-Y anastomosis. (After Lerman RH, Cave DP: *Adv Intern Med* 34:154, 1989.)

fluramine may also be advantageous in carbohydrate-craving patients by timing drug dosage to coincide with the onset of their symptoms.

The use of centrally acting anorectic agents over prolonged periods is tempered by potential adverse reactions. With fenfluramine, reversible pulmonary hypertension has been reported, and depression may develop on abrupt withdrawal.

***Seasonal affective disorder.*** Drug therapy may be helpful in seasonal affective disorder (SAD), a recurrent depressive disorder typically occurring in the winter, remitting in the spring and summer, and associated with carbohydrate craving, weight gain, and increased sleep. In some patients it is followed by hypomania. Early studies suggest that serotonin-releasing agents may be effective in resolving all symptoms in some patients with SAD. Since up to 85% of patients respond to artificial bright light administered for 2 to 6 hours a day, the role of drugs such as *d*-fenfluramine in the treatment of SAD needs to be determined.

***Antidepressants.*** Patients treated with antidepressants often gain weight. However, the antidepressant serotonin reuptake inhibitors fluoxetine (Prozac) and sertraline (Zoloft), appear to be associated with weight loss. Weight losses in general have been small, and most subjects regained weight when treatment was continued for more than 16 weeks.

***Over-the-counter agents.*** OTC appetite suppressants are widely used. Phenylpropanolamine (Acutrim) in a controlled-release formulation was associated with significantly more weight loss (13.4 pounds) than placebo (9.5 pounds) over a 14-week period. It was particularly effective in controlling appetite and intake over the holiday season. Side effects were minimal, but phenylpropanolamine has been the subject of much controversy because of cardiovascular effects, including hypertensive episodes.

***Abuse potential.*** Anorectic drugs such as amphetamines and phenmetrazine have been associated with widespread abuse and addiction in school-aged children and young adults. Therefore use of these agents has no role in the treatment of obesity. It is best to avoid fenfluramine in depressed patients and stimulants in those with hypertension.

## Surgical procedures

Vertical-banded gastroplasty and gastric bypass (Fig. 125-7) are the dominant surgical procedures for obesity currently employed in the United States. These procedures create a small gastric pouch that physically limits food intake and produces the sensation of satiety. In vertical-banded gastroplasty, the gastric pouch is constructed with a restricted outlet along the lesser curvature of the stomach. The outlet may be reinforced to prevent disruption or dilation. In the Roux-en-Y gastric bypass, a proximal gastric pouch is constructed with an outlet consisting of a Y-shaped limb of small bowel of variable length. No part of the stomach is resected in these procedures, so they are theoretically reversible. The dumping syndrome occurs with gastric bypass, leading to weakness, palpitations, and diaphoresis with excessive intake of carbohydrates. These side effects are believed to be responsible for the higher effectiveness of the gastric bypass procedure.

***Patient selection.*** The indications for surgery are not clearly defined. In general, surgical procedures are considered in morbidly obese patients (BMI greater than 40 $kg/m^2$) who have failed medical therapy. Patients with lesser degrees of obesity (BMI 35 to 40 $kg/m^2$) may also be considered for gastric restrictive surgery, particularly if they have high-risk complications such as sleep apnea, pickwickian syndrome, heart failure, or severe diabetes mellitus. Patients under consideration should have demonstrated failure to control weight by medical means, including the use of diet, behavioral modification, and exercise over a prolonged period.

Surgery is generally contraindicated in patients less than 18 or greater than 60 years of age and those who have alcoholism, overt psychosis, excessive somatization, and major cardiopulmonary disease, which would make surgery unduly dangerous. Peptic ulcer disease and reflux esophagitis are relative contraindications to gastric procedures.

Informed consent for obesity surgery should include the opportunity for prolonged discussion, consideration of the surgical options, long- and short-term risks, and complications. Exposure of the candidate to patients with successful and unsuccessful procedures should be arranged. It is also essential to inform the patient of the need for prolonged postoperative follow-up, at least for 5 years and ideally for life.

***Risks and side effects.*** Short-term problems with these gastric restrictive procedures include leakage at the anastomoses, stomal obstruction, perforation of the proximal pouch, marginal ulcer, deep vein thrombophlebitis, wound infection, pulmonary problems, and wound dehiscence. Long-term problems may include chronic vomiting, dumping syndrome, reflux esophagitis, stomal ulcerations, small-bowel obstruction, vitamin deficiencies, anemia, and neuropathies. Vitamin deficiencies, including particularly vitamin $B_{12}$, folate, and iron, occur in 15% to 30% of gastric bypass patients and are somewhat less frequent with gastroplasty. Perioperative mortality is reportedly less than 1% in centers specializing in these surgical procedures.

***Results.*** Weight loss with these procedures is considerable, amounting to 25% to 35% of preoperative weight with a weight nadir at 18 to 24 months. Some regaining of weight is common by 2 to 5 years postoperatively. Also, these procedures can be nullified if the patient consumes large quantities of high-calorie liquids. Submitting the morbidly obese patient to an expensive major surgical procedure may be justified if the risk/benefit ratio outweighs the option of remaining morbidly obese. This has not yet been proved despite some major successes; there has been inadequate follow-up for most studies.

***Other approaches.*** In addition to major interventional surgery, several temporary methods have been conceived to reduce food intake. Jaw wiring has come and largely gone. Inflatable intragastric devices have been developed, but initial enthusiasm has been replaced by skepticism, and these devices have been relegated to an investigational status.

## BIBLIOGRAPHY

Anderson JW, Hamilton CC, Brinkman-Kaplan V: Benefits and risks of an intensive very-low-calorie diet program for severe obesity, *Am J Gastroenterol* 87(1):6, 1992.

Bray GA: Use and abuse of appetite-suppressant drugs in the treatment of obesity, *Ann Intern Med* 119*(7, pt 2):707, 1993.

Consensus Development Conference Panel: Gastrointestinal surgery for severe obesity: Consensus Development Conference statement, *Ann Intern Med* 115:956, 1991.

Gortmaker SL et al: Social and economic consequences of overweight in adolescence and young adulthood, *N Engl J Med* 329:1008, 1993.

Lerman RH, Cave DP: Medical and surgical management of obesity, *Adv Intern Med* 34:127, 1989.

National Task Force on the Prevention and Treatment of Obesity: Very low calorie diets, *JAMA* 270:967, 1993.

Ornish D: *Eat more weigh less:* Dr. Dean Ornish's Life Choice Program for losing weight safely while eating abundantly, New York, 1993, Harper Collins.

Pavlou KN, Krey S, Steffee WP: Exercise as an adjunct to weight loss and maintenance in moderately obese subjects, *Am J Clin Nutr* 49:1115, 1989.

Wadden TA, Van Itallie TB, editors: *Treatment of the seriously obese patient,* New York, 1992, Guilford.

*NOTE: This supplement to the *Annals of Internal Medicine* is devoted to "Methods for Voluntary Weight Loss and Control." It presents an extensive review.

CHAPTER

# 126 Eating Disorders

**Mark Murphy**
**Douglas A. Drossman**

The eating disorders—anorexia nervosa, bulimia nervosa, and rumination syndrome—are relatively common maladies that affect up to 10% of the young female population (as well as a substantially smaller proportion of the male population, although the exact percentage is unknown). Primary care physicians usually encounter eating disorders when patients seek help with medical or psychiatric complications of malnutrition or illness-related behaviors, or when family members bring them to the physician's attention (often against the patient's wishes). It is now clear that the eating disorders are the end result of a complex interaction of biologic, psychologic, and social influences. Recognition of these components is crucial in the diagnosis and treatment of patients with eating disorders.

## ANOREXIA NERVOSA

### Epidemiology and etiology

Anorexia nervosa was once thought to be due to a decreased desire for food that had no organic basis, or the result of a hypothalamic dysfunction. It is now known that patients with anorexia nervosa are preoccupied with food; the disorder is the result of (1) an obsessive fear of becoming overweight; (2) perceptual disturbances relating to one's body size; and (3) the institution of compulsive rituals to effect weight loss.

Anorexia nervosa primarily affects women (about 95% of cases), with the overwhelming majority of those affected being young white women of at least normal intelligence. The prevalence has been estimated at 0.7% among randomly selected females, although it is higher among those in the uppermost socioeconomic strata (1% of a group of British private school students). Both American and European studies imply that the incidence may be increasing, although these data may be skewed somewhat by increased media attention.

Anorexia nervosa is not the result of a single biologic factor or psychologic aberration. It is, rather, the product of a dynamic interaction of biologic, psychologic, and social influences. Certain familial stressors play a significant role; hereditary predisposition may also be a factor.

## Pathogenesis and pathophysiology

***Biologic factors.*** Although anorexia nervosa does not have clear hereditary antecedents, there is an increased prevalence among siblings and among monozygotic twin pairs as compared to dizygotic twin pairs. Several studies have shown a high incidence of affective disorders in first-degree relatives of patients with anorexia nervosa.

Numerous neurochemical abnormalities have been described in anorectic patients, and it appears that the hypothalamic-pituitary-adrenal (HPA) axis modulates the clinical expression of the disorder. Dysregulation of this system would explain the reported abnormalities in satiety, temperature regulation, and endocrine function, as well as anorexia's coassociation with affective disorders. It is likely that, in the biologically predisposed individual, the physiologic and psychologic events that occur at adolescence may lead to alterations in neurotransmitter, endocrine, and immune function. These changes, in turn, lead to the clinical expression of anorexia nervosa.

***Sociocultural factors.*** In both anorexia nervosa and bulimia nervosa the modern cultural value for females to be thin undoubtedly plays a role. The cultural ideal for women's bodies has shifted in the last century from that of plumpness (formerly symbolic of abundance, wealth, materialism, and maturity) to a slimmer image (representing independence and assertiveness). An oft-cited study by Garner and colleagues found that the bust and hip measurements of Miss America pageant winners and *Playboy* centerfolds has decreased substantially over the past 25 years, even as the population as a whole has become heavier. Certainly, the increased prevalence of eating disorders among women who engage in certain activities and occupations (e.g., professional models, ballet dancers) is evidence of the strong influence of sociocultural phenomena in the genesis of anorexia nervosa. The higher prevalence of eating disorders among Western societies (and the development of these disorders among individuals of Eastern heritage transplanted to Western societies) is further evidence of a strong cultural influence on eating disorder pathogenesis. However, since anorexia nervosa has been described for over 300 years, it is evident that modern sociocultural ideals are not the sole cause of this disease. It is believed instead that these factors create the environment for the expression of an eating disorder in the predisposed individual.

***Psychologic factors.*** Certain familial and individual characteristics common to preanorectics have been identified. Usually the preanorectic individual is white and has older middle to upper class parents. The family is often female dominated, and high achievement, "proper" behavior, and maintenance of an acceptable outward appearance are emphasized over individual growth and development. Family members are less likely to express feelings for one another than are family members of nonanorectics. Anorectic individuals often describe growing up with the sense that they are expected to excel, but they lack the sense that they are valued and loved for themselves. Preanorectic children are often described as model children, without the usual periods of undesirable behaviors (assertiveness, rebellion) that during adolescence contribute to the development of an autonomous personality. Typically, they are hard working, eager to please, and unusually attentive to family needs—behaviors that are supported and reinforced by the child's parents. Rather than developing a sense of self-worth based on internal standards, the preanorectic girl finds herself engaged in an obsessive quest for external (parental) approval; she has a difficult time separating her goals and desires from those of her parents. The development of autonomy, which evolves from peer influences, is therefore impaired by the dependence of self-esteem upon parental approval.

Over 80% of anorectic patients develop symptoms within 7 years of menarche. The inevitable conflicts that ensue between the preanorectic girl and her parents during this period of psychologic and physical growth leave her with a feeling of being out of control. Moreover, these conflicts damage her sense of self-worth by interfering with the successful pursuit of parental approval; one study cited low self-esteem as the most important predictor of future anorexia nervosa among several risk factors for the disease. The sensation of a loss of control is heightened by the major life changes (leaving home to start school, marriage, or the death of a parent) that may occur at this time of life. Often one of these events precipitates the onset of symptoms. The conflicts and the loss of control are resolved by the anorectic through the pursuit of thinness, which allows her to control one aspect of her life absolutely. It has been proposed that the amenorrhea and the loss of body fat seen in anorexia nervosa maintain the anorectic in a prepubertal, childlike state, thereby reducing the psychosocial pressures related to her developing sexuality. Clinical improvement of anorexia nervosa has been associated with the worsening of psychoneurotic symptoms in the parents; as the focus of attention is removed from the illness, unresolved familial conflicts reemerge.

Recently several researchers have noted an association between childhood sexual abuse and the development of eating disorders. Although there are conflicting data on this subject, most studies now suggest a high prevalence of childhood sexual and physical abuse among eating disorder patients (35% to 65%). Additionally, some studies have found that, although anorectics have no greater incidence of sexual abuse than the general population, bulimics—particularly those with no history of anorexia—did have a significantly higher incidence. One author has suggested that abuse is not causative but may affect the disorder's clinical expression (i.e., the eating disorder's manifestation as anorexia nervosa or bulimia).

***Natural history.*** Typically, patients with anorexia nervosa present in the teenage years. Some have described a bimodal incidence curve, with one peak at 13 to 14 years and another at 17 to 18 years. The typical anorectic has either been somewhat overweight or has perceived herself to be so and has dieted sporadically. She is often a high achiever, with some obsessive-compulsive tendencies. The clinical syndrome of anorexia nervosa usually begins with an innocuous attempt to lose weight; however, through either restriction of food intake, purging behaviors (laxative or diuretic abuse or self-induced vomiting), excessive exercise, or a combination of these means she begins to fall below the accepted standards for weight relative to height. The onset of symptomatic anorexia is often precipitated by a major life stress; this may result in either rapid, precipitous weight loss or in an insidious, chronic illness with multiple exacerbations and remissions. The patient may become moody or withdrawn, and sexual interest wanes. However, unlike patients with organically based starvation, anorectics usually maintain their personal appearance. The medical complications, to be discussed later, are a direct result of self-imposed starvation. Although the short-term prognosis is favorable, with over 75% of patients attaining a body weight over 75% of ideal, the long-term prognosis is variable; relapses requiring hospitalization occur in about 50% of patients. There is a high comorbid association with affective illness, and the suicide rate in chronic anorexia nervosa has been estimated at 2% to 5%. The overall mortality due to the disorder is 4% to 13%, with the main causes of death being inanition, arrhythmias, and suicide. The degree of social integration (with parents and friends) as opposed to social isolation is a stronger predictor of a favorable outcome than either medical treatment or psychotherapy.

### Screening questions for patients with suspected eating disorders

1. Have you had any difficulties or concerns with controlling your weight?
2. Do others see your body size as different than you do?
3. How would you estimate your body size? Too heavy? Too thin? Too light?
4. At what weight would you feel most comfortable?
5. Have you had experiences with binge eating, that is, having an uncontrollable desire to overeat?
6. Are you satisfied with your eating patterns?*
7. Do you ever eat in secret?*

From Freund KM et al: *J Gen Intern Med* 8:236, 1993.
*These questions have been shown to have a positive predictive value of 0.36 in screening patients with suspected bulimia, based on a 5% prevalence of disease. The sensitivity and specificity of these questions were 1.00 and 0.90 for bulimic patients, respectively.

## History

For a patient suspected of having anorexia nervosa a careful history, with assessment of eating attitudes, is essential.

Obtaining a history of these disorders requires sensitivity and recognition of the patient's reluctance to disclose information that is usually regarded as shameful. A sense of trust needs to be established, and questions should be asked in a caring and nonjudgmental manner. Examples of some screening questions are shown in the box above.

Patients are often brought to the physician's attention by friends or relatives and may emphatically deny that they have a problem. Anorectics may also present with complaints such as constipation, crampy abdominal pain, abdominal bloating, or amenorrhea; a high index of suspicion is needed in such patients.

## Physical examination

A complete physical examination is likewise very important in patients suspected of having anorexia nervosa and should include a nutritional assessment. Height and weight are usually sufficient screening parameters, but other factors (e.g., serum transferrin, albumin, triceps skinfold thickness, measurement of delayed-type hypersensitivity) may be considered if weight loss is profound (i.e., greater than 20% below ideal body weight).

Findings may include a thin body habitus, increased amounts of fine, downy body hair (lanugo hair), and acrocyanosis (see the box on p. 1671). Marked diminution of subcutaneous fat may be noted. The skin of anorectic patients is often dry and scaly and may have a slightly yellow cast due to carotenemia. Mild peripheral edema, without associated hypoproteinemia, may be noted. Vital signs are frequently notable for decreased core body temperature, bradycardia, and mild hypotension. If symptoms develop before puberty, secondary sex characteristics may not have developed. Unlike patients with involuntary starvation, anorectics do not usually manifest signs and symptoms of vitamin deficiency, although there are case reports of scurvy and pellagra in some patients.

***Psychologic and behavioral features.*** Far from being truly anorectic, patients with anorexia nervosa endure a constant struggle against hunger; they are often preoccupied with food and may exhibit bizarre food preferences or prepare elaborate meals for others. Unlike patients with starvation due to organic disease, anorectics maintain their determination not to eat. Although most anorectics lose weight through dietary restriction and exercise (restrictor subgroup), up to 50% also self-induce vomiting or take purgatives (bulimic subgroup). *Perceptual disturbances* are commonly seen, as well. Anorectics frequently overestimate their body width and insist that they are overweight despite objective evidence to the contrary. Their perception of the body size of others is unimpaired, however. *Abnormalities in perception of enteroceptive stimuli* are also present; the sensation of satiety is altered, and anorectics often deny fatigue. Frequently they work or exercise to the point of exhaustion. Recognition of emotional states such as anger and depression is blunted. *Disturbances in mood,* primarily depression, are common, and upon clinical presentation major affective disorder is seen in approximately 50%. *Defects in conceptual thought and abstract reasoning* are evidenced by the anorectic's sense of being controlled by her environment and her resultant feelings of ineffectiveness. Anorectics tend to view situations in extremes; they have difficulty perceiving the "grays" in life and interpret the actions of others in a rigid and highly personalized form (Fig. 126-1).

## Medical findings in anorexia nervosa

**Physical examination**

Thin body habitus
Increased amounts of lanugo hair
Acrocyanosis
Decreased amounts of subcutaneous fat
Dry, scaly skin
Decreased body temperature
Bradycardia
Mild hypotension
Delayed development of secondary sex characteristics

**Endocrine**

Amenorrhea
Hypoestrogenemia
Mild hypothyroid symptoms (without biochemical evidence of hypothyroidism)
Decreased plasma norepinephrine levels
Increased human growth hormone levels
Decreased somatomedin C levels

**Cardiovascular**

Left ventricular wall thinning
Decreased cardiac output
Arrhythmias
ECG abnormalities
Refeeding congestive heart failure

**Gastrointestinal**

Delayed gastric emptying
Increased gastrointestinal transit times
Constipation
Crampy abdominal pain
Elevated serum transaminases and alkaline phosphatase
Hepatic steatosis
Acute gastric dilatation, acute pancreatitis, malabsorptive diarrhea with refeeding

**Renal**

Prerenal azotemia
Decreased glomerular filtration rate
Refeeding peripheral edema

**Miscellaneous**

Elevated serum carotene, cholesterol, vitamin A
Mildly decreased serum albumin, total protein
Mild leukopenia, anemia, thrombocytopenia
Hypocomplementemia

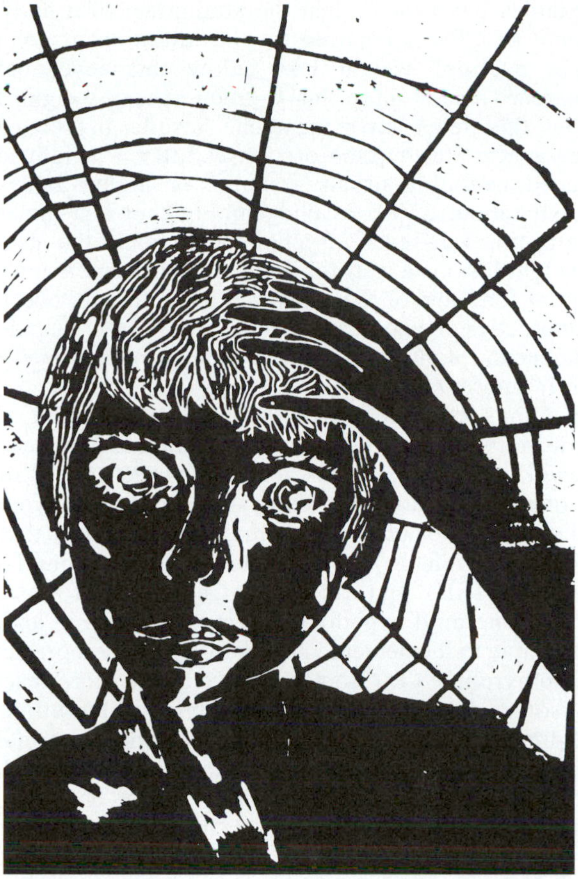

**Fig. 126-1.** Self-portrait of a patient with anorexia nervosa. (From Drossman DA, Ontjes DA, Heizer WD: *Gastroenterology* 77:1115, 1979.)

## DSM-IV criteria for anorexia nervosa

Refusal to maintain body weight over a minimal normal weight for age and height, e.g., weight loss leading to maintenance of body weight 15% below that expected; or failure to make expected weight gain during period of growth, leading to body weight 15% below that expected
Intense fear of gaining weight or becoming fat, even though underweight
Disturbance in the way in which one's body weight, size or shape is experienced, e.g., claiming to feel fat even when obviously underweight
In females, absence of at least three consecutive menstrual cycles when otherwise expected to occur (primary or secondary amenorrhea)

From *Diagnostic and statistical manual of mental disorders,* ed 4, 1994, American Psychiatric Association.

***Medical features.*** The medical findings of anorexia nervosa are primarily the result of starvation (see the box above). The progression of complications correlates with the severity of malnutrition. Measures have been developed to allow estimates of prognosis based on nutritional parameters (see Bibliography).

*Endocrine abnormalities* are among the most consistent medical findings among anorectics. Amenorrhea is, in fact, part of the DSM-IV diagnostic criteria; its onset may precede weight loss (see the box at right). The origin of amenorrhea in anorexia nervosa is due to hypothalamic-pituitary dysfunction. Serum estradiol levels in patients with anorexia nervosa are uniformly lower than in normal controls, as are serum follicle-stimulating hormone (FSH) and luteinizing hormone (LH) levels. The patterns of LH secretion in anorectics are similar to those seen in pubescent or prepubescent females. Anorectics who recover normal weight often have resumption of menses; amenorrhea may persist in up to 38% of these patients.

Studies have shown that the attainment of a body fat content of 17% is required for the initiation of gonadotropin cycling. Weight loss below this level before menarche results in primary amenorrhea; weight loss below this level after menarche results in secondary amenorrhea. Resumption of menses after a weight loss–induced cessation usually requires a higher body fat content (about 22%). Psychogenic amenorrhea (amenorrhea in times of severe psychologic stress in the absence of weight loss) is a well-recognized phenomenon and may account for some of the menstrual irregularities observed in anorectics. Hypoestrogenemia, along with nutritional deficiencies, contributes to the osteoporosis sometimes seen in anorexia nervosa.

Findings consistent with hypothyroidism (dry skin, brittle nails, coarse hair, cold intolerance, bradycardia, delayed deep tendon reflex relaxation, and constipation) are often seen; however, clinically significant hypothyroidism does not occur in anorexia nervosa, and thyroid supplementation is not indicated. Thyroid-stimulating hormone (TSH) and free thyroxin levels are usually normal. The mild hypothyroid symptoms seen in anorectics are due to the decreased availability of the more active triiodothyronine ($T_3$) isomer relative to the more inactive $rT_3$ isomer, which occurs as a response to starvation.

Adrenal hormone abnormalities include a normal or slightly increased plasma cortisol and decreased levels of urinary 17-hydroxycorticosteroids. These changes are believed to be due to decreased clearance of cortisol from the plasma and an increase in cortisol-binding capacity, since 24-hour cortisol production rate and basal adrenocorticotropic hormone (ACTH) secretion are normal. Plasma norepinephrine levels are diminished, a finding also seen in starvation; these values return to normal with weight increase.

*Cardiovascular findings* include left ventricular wall thinning, decreased left ventricular chamber size, and consequent decreased cardiac output. These are adaptive changes to decreases in circulating catecholamine levels and can lead to decreased blood pressure and peripheral edema. Electrocardiographic (ECG) abnormalities (including decreased QRS amplitude, prolongation of the QT interval, nonspecific ST segment changes, and U waves) have been reported and may be related to electrolyte abnormalities. Arrhythmias may occur, especially in the face of electrolyte abnormalities, and sudden death has been described in severely malnourished patients. Acute congestive heart failure may occur during refeeding.

*Gastrointestinal abnormalities* include delayed gastric emptying, increased gastrointestinal transit times, and constipation. Complaints of bloating and crampy abdominal pain are common and may be related to motility disturbances. Rapid refeeding in anorectics can result in acute gastric dilatation, acute pancreatitis, and malabsorptive diarrhea (which may be caused by deficiencies in pancreatic and intestinal brush border digestive enzymes). Elevations in serum transaminases and alkaline phosphatase are felt to be due to starvation-induced hepatic steatosis. Most of the gastrointestinal manifestations resolve with careful refeeding.

*Renal complications* include prerenal azotemia, which is caused by increased protein catabolism and intravascular volume depletion, resulting in decreased glomerular filtration rate (GFR). Decreased GFR can also result in an increased tendency toward nephrolithiasis. Refeeding can result in volume overload secondary to aldosterone-induced sodium retention—changes that may take months to completely reverse.

Other *miscellaneous* findings include elevation in serum carotene, cholesterol, and vitamin A levels; these are all decreased in most patients with starvation due to wasting diseases. The reason for these differences in the anorectic population is unknown, although some have postulated that the increased intake of vegetables high in β-carotene and thus vitamin A value account for their elevated levels, and that shifts in adrenocortical or thyroid metabolism account for the elevated cholesterol. Mild decreases in serum albumin and other serum proteins may be seen in anorexia nervosa; these findings are less pronounced relative to similar abnormalities seen in other starved patients. Finally, anorectics may manifest hematologic abnormalities, including leukopenia, mild anemia, and thrombocytopenia. Hypocomplementemia has been reported. However, anorectics do not have a substantially increased risk of infectious complications.

## Differential diagnosis

The diagnosis of anorexia nervosa is made via the application of the DSM-IV diagnostic criteria (see the box on p. 1671). Although definitive establishment of the diagnosis requires the exclusion of any specific diseases that produce malnutrition, such considerations should include only those for which a reasonable index of suspicion may be established as a result of historical or physical examination data. The differential diagnosis includes Addison disease, diabetes mellitus, panhypopituitarism, hyperparathyroidism, hypothyroidism or hyperthyroidism, celiac disease, Crohn disease, intestinal parasitosis, tuberculosis, AIDS, lymphoma (or other neoplastic processes), hypothalamic tumor, schizophrenia, and primary major depression.

Laboratory tests should be individualized and should be obtained only if the diagnosis is in question or to assess metabolic derangements. Some patients require very little diagnostic testing, whereas others—particularly the extremely malnourished—require more. Laboratory tests that may be valuable in patients suspected of having an eating disorder are listed in the box on p. 1673.

## Management

The treatment of anorexia nervosa must address the nutritional and medical consequences of the disorder and the psychologic and environmental factors that maintain the anorectic behavior. A multidisciplinary approach, with medical, psychologic, and nutritional support, is therefore crucial. The primary care physician is usually responsible for medical and nutritional care as well as psychologic support. Factors in the effectiveness of this ongoing care include fostering a sense of autonomy in the patient by encouraging her to take responsibility in the treatment, remaining objective and honest to maintain the patient's sense of trust, working with the family, and serving as the liaison (and patient's advocate) with consultants and counselors. The physician must help the patient to acknowledge and relate thoughts and feelings and should

### Laboratory tests for differential diagnosis in eating disorders*

Complete blood count, sedimentation rate
Serum electrolytes, blood urea nitrogen, creatinine, liver enzymes, serum amylase
Total protein, albumin
Serum cholesterol, vitamin A levels
Serum carotene
Thyroid function tests
Fasting plasma cortisol level
Sigmoidoscopy
Stool examination for occult blood, fecal fat, parasites
CT scan of brain (or MRI)
Upper GI series with small bowel follow-through
Stool and urine cathartic screens

*The decision to obtain any specific tests should be guided by historical data, physical examination results, and other clinical findings that lead one to suspect either metabolic abnormalities or the possibility of an underlying organic disease.

strive to encourage behaviors that reinforce the patient's status as a fully differentiated individual. It is essential to inform the patient that she may see treatments as undesirable and that she may feel that her control is threatened by them, and to point out that a return to better health is in her best interest. The methods and goals of treatment, and any later changes in plans, should be explained to the patient, with ample time allotted to the patient for expression of her thoughts and feelings regarding these plans. Any lack of consistency, evasiveness, or judgmental behavior by the physician will undermine the patient's sense of trust and should be avoided; such a loss of trust substantially impedes the treatment process. Involvement of the family is encouraged. Initially, therapy should be directed toward modifying the dysfunctional pattern within the family that helps maintain the patient's anorectic behavior. Later, family members can be used to aid the patient in weight gain through positive reinforcement. The primary care physician, with the input of appropriate consultants, should make all long-term treatment decisions.

***Correction of nutritional deficits.*** This is accomplished on an inpatient or outpatient basis, depending on the degree of malnutrition. Special attention should be given to the manner in which any supplemental feedings are given. Forced feedings in eating disorder patients may worsen the patient's sense of a loss of control; supplemental feedings should therefore be initiated only when medically indicated and with the integral involvement of the patient in the decision process. Patients with body weight greater than or equal to 80% of ideal may be managed on an outpatient basis, with nutritional and psychologic counseling. Patients with a body weight 65% to 80% of ideal can usually be managed on an outpatient basis but may require nutritional supplementation. Supplemental (i.e., in addition to daily food intake) oral repletion at a level of 250 to 500 kcal per day above daily basal energy requirements with a palatable, nutritionally complete formulation (e.g., Ensure Plus) is ideal, with the use of metoclopramide or cisapride to aid in patient tolerance of supplemental feedings. Severely malnourished patients (body weight less than 65% of ideal) require hospitalization and intensive nutritional repletion at an initial level of 400 to 600 kcal per day above basal daily energy requirements. The level of caloric supplementation should be gradually increased over 2 weeks to an amount that allows around 1 kg of weight gain per week (i.e., basal needs plus approximately 1100 kcal per day). Oral nutritional supplementation may be attempted, but feeding tube placement is frequently necessary. Although enteral feeding is preferable, parenteral nutrition may be needed if the patient is noncompliant or if multiple complications of malnutrition are present. When parenteral supplements are used, caloric delivery should start at half the daily requirement on day 1 to three fourths on day 2, with full repletion on day 3 and thereafter. This is to minimize the possible complications from rapid infusion of hyperosmolar solutions.

When considering involuntary feeding measures in anorectics, a balance must be struck between the patient's willingness to undergo such feedings and their medical necessity. As mentioned previously, forced feedings can enhance the anorectic's sense of loss of control and as such may exacerbate some of the psychologic symptoms of the illness. However, if the patient can be made to understand the medical need for such feedings and can be made an active participant in the decision to initiate them, the psychologic side effects may be minimized.

Care should be taken during refeeding to observe for congestive heart failure, acute gastric dilatation, and pancreatitis. Electrolytes (including potassium, magnesium, and phosphate), glucose, BUN, and creatinine should be monitored closely during refeeding (especially during the first 5 to 7 days), since all of these can be severely deranged during this period. Elevated transaminases associated with tender hepatomegaly can occur as a result of fatty infiltration of the liver during refeeding; this responds to decreasing the infusion rate. Refeeding peripheral edema is common. The goals of supplemental nutrition in anorexia nervosa are to achieve a weight that removes the patient from acute medical danger (i.e., greater than 80% of ideal body weight) and to correct overt metabolic derangements. Supplemental feedings should be discontinued when the medical and nutritional goals are achieved.

***Psychotherapy.*** This has met with variable success. Behavior modification has been useful in achieving some short-term gains; however, since it focuses on the patient's symptoms rather than the underlying problems, it is less useful over the long term. Moreover, it utilizes an external reward system, so the patient may experience a heightened sense of the loss of control. Family therapy has also been used and appears to have some success in the long term, especially in younger patients with a shorter duration of illness. Combined behavioral modification and family therapy approaches have been used, and one study has demonstrated impressive long-term positive results. There is no current consensus on a uniform method of psychotherapy in anorexia nervosa.

*Pharmacotherapy.* Drugs have no proven benefit in anorexia nervosa; numerous medications, including amitriptyline, chlorpromazine, cyproheptidine, fluoxetine, and lithium carbonate, have been of some effectiveness in small trials, but no medication appears to be consistently beneficial in all patients. The use of medications such as lithium carbonate and tricyclic antidepressants must be undertaken cautiously in anorectics; the increased incidence of suicide and the metabolic derangements caused by their disease may make these patients particularly susceptible to the potential adverse effects of these drugs. The use of a serotonin reuptake inhibitor (e.g., fluoxetine) may be preferred, since these agents do not initially produce weight gain or sedation; these factors may enhance patient compliance, although these agents can depress appetite.

## BULIMIA NERVOSA

### Epidemiology and etiology

Bulimia (from the Greek terms for "ox hunger") is a compulsive behavior defined by episodic bouts of overeating (binge eating) usually followed by acts designed to avert weight gain (self-induced vomiting, cathartic or diuretic use). This behavior can be seen in anorexia nervosa. However, patients with bulimia nervosa are distinguished by their normal body size.

Like anorexia nervosa, bulimia nervosa typically affects young (under 30 years) white women (90% to 95%). Although the point prevalence using the DSM-IV criteria is about 1% of the general population, studies of female high school and college students have found that between 4.5% and 18% have had bulimia, and that 19.6% of college-age women had binge-purge behaviors consistent with bulimia. The prevalence of bulimic behaviors among men is less than among women, although one study has estimated the prevalence of such behaviors among college-age men at up to 10%. It is believed that the majority of bulimics exercise their bulimic behaviors in secret; one British survey revealed that only a third of a group of nearly 500 women who met diagnostic criteria for bulimia had ever discussed their eating problems with a physician.

Like anorexia nervosa, bulimia nervosa is believed to have a multifaceted origin; biologic predisposition combines with psychologic and sociobehavioral determinants to yield the integrated syndrome.

### Pathogenesis and pathophysiology

*Biologic factors.* Evidence of an underlying biologic defect in bulimia nervosa is circumstantial but compelling. As noted in patients with anorexia nervosa, bulimic patients have a higher familial incidence of affective disorders than the general population. Alcoholism and major depression have the strongest correlations. Bulimics, even those of normal weight, frequently have menstrual abnormalities; a significant proportion have amenorrhea. Perhaps the strongest evidence of a biologic aberration in bulimia nervosa is seen in the neurotransmitter abnormalities noted with the disease. Evidence exists for a defect in serotonin-mediated satiety regulation in bulimia; serotonin metabolism in bulimics has been shown to be abnormal in multiple studies. Norepinephrine metabolism has also been found to be persistently altered in bulimic patients. Cholecystokinin (CCK), a gut peptide secreted in response to food intake, is also a neurotransmitter in the CNS involved in the regulation of the satiety response. One study found that postprandial serum CCK levels in bulimics were blunted relative to a group of normal controls. Satiety sensation was also blunted in this group. It is interesting to note that a subgroup of these bulimic patients was treated with antidepressants; this treated group had a significant increase in both CCK response to eating and satiety sensation. These data imply that bulimic behaviors are related in some fashion to CNS neurotransmitter and/or receptor dysregulation. This lends further credence to the use of psychopharmacologic agents in treatment of bulimia nervosa.

*Psychologic factors.* The psychologic underpinnings of bulimia nervosa are similar in many respects to those of anorexia nervosa. Like anorectics, bulimics tend to come from families with conflict resolution problems and express similar feelings of a loss of control, low self-esteem, and the use of external sources (e.g., parents) for validation of self-worth. Childhood sexual abuse, as mentioned earlier, is emerging as a risk factor for the development of bulimia nervosa.

*Sociocultural factors.* The same social pressures to be thin noted in the discussion of anorexia nervosa apply in the genesis of bulimia nervosa. Purging behavior becomes a prominent manner in which the bulimic patient attempts to control her weight to attain a perceived ideal body habitus in the face of a periodic uncontrollable urge to have an eating binge.

*Natural history.* Bulimia nervosa classically begins later in life than anorexia nervosa (usually ages 17 to 25) and may occur in an individual with a history of anorexia. The prebulimic patient is typically mildly overweight and has attempted to lose weight by dieting without success. She may be introduced to purging as a means of weight control by a friend or relative; often, purging behaviors precede binge eating. At some point the hallmark of the disorder—the uncontrollable urge to eat and the inability to stop—sets in. Subsequently, repeated cycles of binge-purge behavior ensue; the patient's sense of a lack of control intensifies after each binge episode, and her self-esteem suffers as a result. Due to the secretive nature of the bulimic's behaviors and to the fact that patients are usually of normal weight, patients often do not present for treatment until their 30s or 40s. Bulimics may be diagnosed as a result of a medical complication of the illness or as a result of major psychologic distress. By the time of presentation most bulimics are clinically depressed, and 5% have attempted suicide. Bulimics are more likely to exhibit impulsive behaviors (e.g., kleptomania, substance abuse, sexual promiscuity) than anorectics. The risk of drug and alcohol use among bulimics is three to five times greater than in nonbulimic women in the general population. Bulimia has often been characterized as a disease of stuttering course, with frequent relapses and remissions. In general, outpatients with bulimia with at least 1 year's follow-up have demonstrated recovery rates of 30% to 70%, with an average of 50%. Most recoveries have been noted within 1 year of presentation; those who fail to recover by that point are unlikely to do so. Relapse rates are high (40% to 63%). Factors predictive of a poor outcome include a history of ethanol abuse, suicide attempts, and increased depressive symptoms. Mortality per se has not been found to be increased over the general female population.

### History

Although bulimics are more distressed by their behaviors than are anorectics (and therefore are more likely to seek medical attention), they are also often embarassed by their binge-purge activities and may not be willing to reveal these activities to their health care provider. Again, a careful history with assessment of eating attitudes is essential (see the box on p. 1670). Like anorectics, bulimics may present with complaints of constipation, crampy abdominal pain, and amenorrhea; they may also have complications from their binge-purge activity.

### Physical examination

As with patients with anorexia nervosa, a complete physical examination is important in patients with bulimia nervosa and may provide clues to the diagnosis in patients suspected of having the disorder. *Physical examination findings* associated with bulimia include painless parotid or salivary gland swelling, bruised or abraded knuckles secondary to self-induction of vomiting (Russell sign), and facial ecchymoses, conjunctival hemorrhages, pharyngitis, and dental enamel erosions secondary to repeated emesis.

***Psychologic and behavioral features.*** The characteristic behavioral manifestation of bulimia nervosa is the binge-purge cycle. This is typified by episodes of compulsive eating with a failure to respond to or achieve normal satiety. Bulimics typically binge on high-calorie food rich in carbohydrates that requires little chewing. Binge episodes, during which the bulimic individual consumes between 1000 and 55,000 kcal during a relatively brief interval, usually occur in secret, after extensive planning. The binge is usually terminated by feelings of guilt or physical discomfort (nausea, abdominal pain). At this point most patients self-induce vomiting or take laxatives. Although most bulimics report feelings of excitement and anticipation while planning a binge, there are nearly universal feelings of shame afterwards. Bulimics are typically embarrassed by their symptoms and are reluctant to reveal details of their illness to family members and health care providers. The bulimic's obsession with food and binge-related activities can interfere with her social interactions with others. Unlike anorectics, however, bulimics are usually outgoing and engage in heterosexual relationships.

Bulimic behavior is viewed by the patient as an uncontrollable compulsion, so bulimics are more willing to try to stop. By contrast, anorectics go to great lengths to hide their behavior from friends and co-workers, since they are unwilling to change.

As mentioned previously, affective disorders—particularly depression—are common; estimates of the frequency of depression in bulimics range from 20% to 80%. Bulimics also have a higher incidence of anxiety disorders (45%) than either anorectics or the general population.

#### Medical complications of bulimia

**Physical examination findings**

- Parotid and salivary gland swelling
- Bruised or abraded knuckles (Russell sign)
- Facial ecchymoses
- Conjunctival hemorrhages
- Pharyngitis
- Dental enamel erosions

**Endocrine**

- Menstrual irregularity (including amenorrhea)

**Gastrointestinal**

- Esophagitis
- Esophageal erosions and ulcerations
- Mallory-Weiss tears
- Esophageal rupture
- Delayed gastric emptying
- Crampy abdominal pain
- Acute gastric dilatation (with binge)
- Constipation
- Pancreatitis
- Asymptomatic elevations in serum amylase

**Miscellaneous**

- Ipecac cardiotoxicity
- Arrhythmias
- Pneumomediastinum
- Aspiration pneumonia
- Metabolic alkalosis or acidosis
- Hypochloremia
- Hypokalemia
- Hypomagnesemia
- Hypocalcemia
- Hyponatremia
- Hypophosphatemia

Recently, some correlations between the presence of bulimia and personality disorders, particularly borderline personality disorder, have been made. It is notable that obese bulimics are less likely to use purgatives than normal-weight bulimics and are more prone to have affective disorders (91% versus 70%), especially major depression.

***Medical complications.*** The box above lists medical complications of bulimia. *Endocrine* abnormalities may include menstrual irregularity (40% to 50%), and 20% of bulimic women without a history of anorexia have amenorrhea for at least 3 months at some point during their illness. Additionally, approximately 50% of bulimics have abnormal dexamethasone suppression tests. Serum cortisol levels and secretion patterns in bulimics are normal.

*Gastrointestinal* effects of bulimia primarily related to repeated emesis may include oropharyngeal complications (dental erosions, pharyngitis, and parotid enlargement) as well as esophagitis, esophageal erosions and ulcerations, Mallory-Weiss tears, and esophageal rupture. Acid-peptic esophageal injury has been reported to be of higher incidence in bulimics than in the general population.

Delayed gastric emptying and prolonged whole-gut transit times have been documented in bulimics, as compared to age- and sex-matched controls; these findings may explain the symptoms of bloating and crampy abdominal pain reported by many bulimics. Acute gastric dilatation has been described, usually in relation to the ingestion of large meals, and gastric rupture has been reported. Constipation is a common complaint among bulimics, and degeneration of the Auerbach plexus due to chronic stimulant laxative use (cathartic colon) has been described. Asymptomatic elevations in serum amylase have been reported; fractionation reveals a predominance in the salivary isoenzyme fraction in most cases. Acute pancreatitis in bulimics may be due to either alcohol abuse or abrupt pancreatic stimulation during binge eating.

Other organ systems may be affected. *Cardiovascular* effects of bulimia may include ipecac cardiotoxicity (the result of poisoning with the alkaloid found in this proemetic agent) and arrhythmias due to hypokalemia, a common electrolyte abnormality in bulimics.

*Pulmonary* findings may include pneumomediastinum (due to pulmonary rupture caused by vigorous emesis) and aspiration pneumonia (often as a result of vomiting while under the influence of alcohol).

*Metabolic* complications may include metabolic alkalosis due to repeated emesis (the most common finding), metabolic acidosis due to laxative abuse, hypochloremia, hypokalemia, hypomagnesemia, hypocalcemia, hyponatremia, and hypophosphatemia. Dehydration can also occur, leading to secondary hyperaldosteronism and to reflex peripheral edema, an effect that can become quite pronounced with cessation of the abused diuretics or laxatives.

### Differential diagnosis

The DSM-IV diagnosis of bulimia nervosa is based upon the presence of the binge eating pattern, the persistent overconcern about body shape and size, and the exclusion of other medical concerns (see the box above). The differential diagnosis is limited and includes schizophrenia, seizure disorders, and rare neurologic disorders such as Kleine-Levin syndrome and Klüver-Bucy syndrome. Diagnostic testing is usually not necessary, except as indicated by historical and physical examination data and as needed to monitor complications of the disorder.

### Management

Because bulimic patients are cognizant of the maladaptive nature of their behaviors, they are often willing to work with their physician in therapy. The patient can usually interpret symptoms in terms of current and past emotional issues, so psychologic concerns and establishment of better coping methods should be points of discussion for the physician. The family may need to be involved. Generally, inpatient therapy is not recommended.

**Psychotherapy.** The psychotherapeutic approach to bulimia usually emphasizes controlling the abnormal behaviors. Cognitive-behavioral therapy is commonly used currently; the patient recognizes the specific abnormal behaviors and uses behavior modification techniques to control them. This technique uses a three-stage approach, beginning with a self-monitoring period (during which the patient is taught to become more aware of her eating behavior and to establish a regular pattern of eating, with conscious avoidance of binge behavior by decreasing available food for bingeing). This is followed by a recognition period (during which the patient recognizes the association between binges and stress, thereby allowing her greater control over her eating pattern) and a maintenance period (during which the patient records the tactics used to avert bingeing and purging during stress to reinforce these learned behavioral adaptations). Both individual and group approaches have been used successfully.

#### DSM-IV criteria for bulimia nervosa

Recurrent episodes of binge eating (rapid consumption of a large amount of food in a discrete period of time)
A feeling of lack of control over eating behavior during the eating binges
Self-induced vomiting, use of laxatives or diuretics, strict dieting or fasting or rigorous exercise to prevent weight gain
A minimum of two binge eating episodes per week for at least 3 months
Persistent overconcern with body shape and weight

From *Diagnostic and statistical manual of mental disorders,* ed 4, 1994, American Psychiatric Association.

**Pharmacotherapy.** Antidepressants have been very successful in the treatment of bulimia. Virtually all antidepressants have shown striking reductions in binge frequency when compared to placebo. On average, a 50% reduction in binge frequency has been seen. These findings were seen in both depressed and nondepressed bulimics. One caveat is that most of these studies were short term (6 to 8 weeks' duration); some reports indicate that long-term efficacy is not as high for all medications tested. Notably, patients taking fluoxetine seem to maintain their response as long as they take the medication, although higher dosages (e.g., 60 mg per day) may be needed in some patients. The usual tricyclic antidepressant dosage (e.g., 100 to 250 mg per day of desipramine) seems to be effective. The best candidates for pharmacotherapy are those who have failed cognitive behavioral therapy, those who are severely depressed, and (at the very least) those who are responsible and capable of communicating potential beneficial and adverse drug effects to the physician. Patients with a partial response to cognitive-behavioral therapy or pharmacotherapy may benefit from combined therapy; two studies have demonstrated that such combined therapy is more effective than either therapy alone.

## RUMINATION SYNDROME

Rumination syndrome (merycism) has been considered a medical curiosity for over 300 years, yet it is infrequently diagnosed due to a lack of physician recognition. It is an eating disorder in which the patient repetitively regurgitates small amounts of food from the stomach, rechews the food, and then reswallows it. There are three subgroups with the disorder: (1) emotionally deprived or mentally retarded children and adults; (2) persons in whom the behavior develops as a maladaptive habit, worsening in times of stress; and (3) persons in whom rumination is associated with bulimia.

The prevalence of rumination in adults is unknown. Patients who seek treatment report symptoms of weight loss, regurgitation, or vomiting and may express concern of an underlying medical disorder. The diagnosis is made by manometric or radiographic studies, which reveal that episodes are initiated by a belch or a swallow. The lower esophageal sphincter pressure is lowered to allow creation of a common channel between the stomach and esophagus. At the same time, diaphragmatic and rectus muscle contractions raise intraabdominal pressure, leading to regurgitation. Diagnosis is based on identifying the typical clinical features and excluding other medical or psychiatric disease. Extensive diagnostic testing is usually not needed. Since the disorder appears to be a learned maladaptive habit, behavioral modification and biofeedback techniques are recommended as treatment approaches.

## BIBLIOGRAPHY

Agras WS: Nonpharmacologic treatments of bulimia nervosa, *J Clin Psychol* 52(suppl):29, 1991.

Amarnath RP, Abell TL, Malagelada JR: The rumination syndrome in adults. A characteristic manometric pattern, *Ann Intern Med* 105:513, 1986.

Balaa MA, Drossman DA: Anorexia nervosa and bulimia: the eating disorders, *Dis Mon* 31:9, 1985.

Drossman DA: Approach to unexplained weight loss and the eating disorders. In Yamada T, editor: *Textbook of gastroenterology,* ed 2, 1995. In press.

Drossman DA et al: *Functional gastrointestinal disorders: diagnosis, pathophysiology, and treatment,* Boston, 1994, Little, Brown.

Harris RT: Bulimia and related serious eating disorders with medical complications, *Ann Intern Med* 99:800, 1983.

Herzog DB, Copeland PM: Eating disorders, *N Eng J Med* 313:295, 1985.

Herzog DB, Keller MB, Lavori PW: Outcome in anorexia nervosa and bulimia nervosa, *J Nerv Ment Dis* 176:131, 1988.

Kennedy SH, Garfinkel PE: Advances in diagnosis and treatment of anorexia nervosa and bulimia nervosa, *Can J Psychiatry* 37:309, 1992.

Walsh BT, Devlin MJ: The pharmacologic treatment of eating disorders, *Psychiatr Clin North Am* 15(1):149, 1992.

CHAPTER

# 127 Domestic Violence

**Margaret McHugh**
**Carol Mahon Salazar**
**John A. Rich**

This chapter includes discussion of violence from three perspectives. The first section addresses interpersonal violence (violent injury, homicide). The second focuses on domestic violence (spouse abuse, women battery). The third discusses violence involving children (child abuse and neglect). Each section provides a complementary perspective on violence and underscores the role of the primary care provider in prevention, early detection, and intervention.

## INTERPERSONAL VIOLENCE

Primary care physicians play an essential role in detecting violent victimization and its consequences. They must maintain a high level of suspicion and avoid being unduly swayed by stereotypic images of who may be at risk for violence. Treatment should be aimed at the consequences of past injury, and primary and secondary prevention strategies should be employed for those who are at risk of violence.

### Epidemiology and etiology

Interpersonal violence, an old and growing problem in American society, is defined as violence where physical force is used with the intent of causing harm, injury, or death to another person (Fig. 127-1). In 1989 there were 21,500 Americans who died as victims of violence. Every day in the United States, on average, 65 people die among the 6000 physically injured by interpersonal violence. In 1987 physical injury from violence among adults led to $23 billion in lost productivity and $145 billion in reduced quality of life. Homicide ranks as the eleventh leading cause of death overall in the United States. Violence is now the leading cause of death for young African-American males between 15 and 34. Nearly 50% of homicides occur between individuals who know one another. Of these homicides, two thirds occur between friends or acquaintances and one third between family members. About 60% of these homicides involve the use of a handgun.

Though the terms *crime* and *violence* are often used interchangeably, they are not the same. Many instances of violence go unreported to the police and thus do not appear in any crime statistics. For example, the National Crime Survey, a telephone survey of households that asks about instances of assault or criminal victimization, consistently reports a higher incidence of assault than do police statistics. Persons decline to involve the police for a number of reasons. They may fear retaliation from the person who committed the assault. They may also fear involvement with the police will yield few benefits or may uncover their own legal problems.

A number of factors have been associated with risk of violent injury. Most instances of interpersonal violence involve three factors: use of alcohol or drugs, the presence or availability of a weapon, and an argument. Under these circumstances even friends and family may become victims of injury or homicide. Other factors seem to predispose individuals toward violent injury. Chief is poverty. Although black race is frequently cited as a risk factor for involvement in violence, several studies have shown this is not true after adjustment for poverty. Poverty subjects individuals to higher levels of frustration, overcrowded living situations, and greater exposure to environments that are replete with weapons and illegal activity. Other factors associated with violence are shown in the box on p. 1678.

More recently violence has been moved to the forefront as a major *public health problem* with the view that

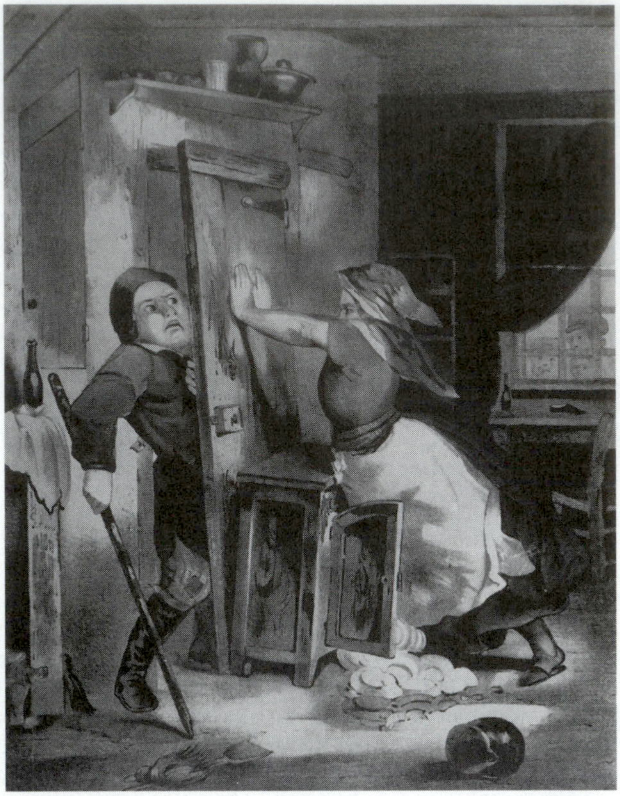

**Fig. 127-1.** "Victory Doubtful." (Currier and Ives. 1860, New York.)

### Risk factors for interpersonal violence

- History of abuse as a child
- History of witnessing violence
- Poverty
- Past head injury
- Substance use or abuse
- School failure
- Involvement with street crime or other illegal activities
- Ownership of a gun or gun kept in home
- Exposure to television violence
- Definition of masculinity as male dominance
- Racial segregation and discrimination
- Poor housing, characterized by overcrowding and lack of recreational space
- Gang involvement
- Unemployability
- Low self-esteem
- Limited social supports
- Fear
- Hopelessness

violence is preventable and involves an interaction between host, agent, and environment. The host or victim is most often male, impoverished, and more likely to be African-American or Latino. The agent is usually a handgun or knife. The environment may include drugs or alcohol, limited socioeconomic, educational, and employment opportunities, poverty, poor housing conditions, gangs, unstable families, limited community supports and services, and brutalization by the police. By treating violence as a public health problem, maintaining injury surveillance, and identifying risk factors it is possible to produce strategies for violence prevention and intervention. Because primary care physicians are likely to interact with patients at risk for violent injury, they can play an important role in prevention, detection, and intervention.

## History

When asking patients whether they have been victims of violence, physicians must do so with the assumption that violence is rampant in the patients' social context. They should begin the discussion with open-ended questions that allow patients to begin with details that are comfortable and nonthreatening.

Violence is seldom a premeditated act. Rather it is a response to a set of circumstances that may be quite outside of patients' control. Many patients therefore attribute their violent injury or threat of injury to being in the wrong place at the wrong time. It is therefore essential that physicians try to flesh out as much as possible the context in which patients live by exploring the risk factors.

Physicians should determine how patients handle anger and stress. Patients who typically have no outlet for feelings of anger, who are impulsive or given to blind rage, or who use alcohol or drugs to gain relief are at increased risk for violence. Primary care physicians should inquire about the use of alcohol and other drugs, including marijuana, cocaine, opiates, and PCP with regard to patterns of use, history of drug treatment, and complications. The CAGE and MAST questionnaires are a good way to open the discussion of substance use (see Chapter 130).

In the present epidemic of violence all patients, regardless of age, ethnicity, gender, or socioeconomic status, should be asked about violent victimization as a part of their initial evaluation and workup. For patients who reveal concerns about violence, the issue should be raised on subsequent visits. This should include questions about physical, sexual, or emotional abuse as a child or adult. Patients may present for care with symptoms that are more related to psychologic stress than to a specific injury. Psychosomatic complaints that are vague or difficult for the patient to describe should be investigated further for evidence of violence. Patients should be asked if they have ever been injured in any way by another person. It is also useful to ask if the person has ever been "cut," since many patients do not consider shallow knife wounds as stabbings. If a patient has had a serious injury in the past, as much detail should as appropriate be gathered, from the patient, from the patient's family, and from the medical record about the nature of the injury. Some patients may have undergone splenectomy or nephrectomy after a gunshot wound and may not understand the significance of these procedures. In addition, providers should inquire whether the patient has been threatened with a weapon. Patients should be asked whether they have ever witnessed violence (see the box on p. 1679).

Persons who have been victimized may display signs and symptoms of posttraumatic stress disorder (PTSD). This reaction to a distressing event outside usual human

## Questions to ask primary care patients regarding violence

**History of violence**

Have you ever been hit, kicked, or hurt in any way, either by someone you know or by a stranger?
When did this last happen?
Have you ever been shot or stabbed?
Have you ever seen someone get shot or stabbed, or badly beaten up? When and how? Tell me about it.
Has anyone ever pointed a gun at you or threatened you with a knife or other weapon?

**Anger management**

How do you deal with anger?
What do you do to someone who makes you very angry?

**Weapons**

Do you carry a weapon?
When and how often do you carry it?
Why do you carry a weapon?

**Safety**

Are you worried about someone hurting you in the near future?
Do you feel safe?

## Managed Care Guide Pointers on gun safety

1. Know where the gun is stored in the home at all times.
2. Be sure the gun is not loaded with ammunition.
3. Store the bullets in a different location.
4. When threats of gun violence are made, leave the premises immediately. Do not linger or argue.

experience is characterized by symptoms of depression or hypervigilance, reexperiencing the events in nightmares, intrusive thoughts, or flashbacks, and numbing of responsiveness or avoidance of thoughts or acts related to the trauma (see Chapter 132). A gun kept in the house is more than 40 times more likely to be used against a friend or family member in a homicide or suicide than to be used against a criminal intruder. For those who do own or carry weapons, it is essential that providers understand their reason for carrying a weapon. Many of these individuals truly feel that they are in danger and that carrying a weapon makes them feel safe. After seeking to understand the underlying issues of the patient's life, physicians may be able to suggest other ways to feel safe (see the Managed Care Guide).

The sensitive nature of the issues raised by violence demand that primary care physicians respect the confidentiality of the patient to the highest degree. Often in the discussion of violent threat or injury, patients may reveal information about their own illegal involvements or past criminal actions. This information, if treated lightly or documented in a cavalier manner, may place the patient at great risk of criminal prosecution or incarceration. Thus such discussions should begin with a clear understanding that all information obtained will be held in strictest confidence, unless information indicates that the patient intends to do harm to another person or to himself or herself.

### Physical examination

The physical examination of patients at risk of violence should focus on evidence of past injury and any residual disability. Physicians should examine the skin and note the presence of any bruises or scars, surgical or other. They should look carefully for needle tracks or other signs of substance use. Some patients may have scars that mark initiation into a gang. Do not assume this, but ask if any of the wounds were self-inflicted. Often patients do not receive care for a shallow stab wound but care for it themselves at home. These patients may have other signs of poor access to medical care, such as extensive dental caries and gingivitis or undiagnosed sexually transmitted diseases. Those who are at risk for violent injury are also at highest risk for other health problems. Young African-American males, in particular, have a high incidence of violent injury, hypertension, and sexually transmitted diseases, including HIV infection, and often lack any insurance that would provide primary care. So even though an issue related to violence may have brought these patients to the emergency room or walk-in clinic, they should be referred for health education and support on primary care.

## Differential diagnosis

When patients who have been exposed to violence display extreme hypervigilance, an exaggerated startle response, or flashbacks or hallucinations about the traumatic event, physicians must distinguish between symptoms of PTSD and a primary psychotic or paranoid disorder.

Patients who have been victims of violence may have feelings of anger and fantasies of revenge. These feelings may be quite appropriate and may dissipate over time with support and encouragement to work through the anger appropriately. Patients may also be very wary and suspicious of even close friends as they seek to reestablish their sense of safety. When patients appear obsessed with the notion of revenge or have a very clear plan for exacting this revenge, referral for psychiatric evaluation and counseling should be made immediately, if possible. This action may be required of physicians by law.

## Management

When dealing with patients who are at risk of violence, primary care physicians are responsible for detecting the problem, providing support, and facilitating effective referral to an appropriate source of care. To accomplish this they must do the following:

1. *Know and use strengths:* Provide a safe and confidential setting where patients may talk about their fears and concerns. This is an excellent opportunity to counsel patients in a sensitive manner, once the patients' life situation with regard

to violence is understood. Where appropriate, prescribe short courses of anxiolytic therapy to patients with extreme anxiety or insomnia (but not to addicts).

2. *Know resources:* Because of the broad social context and multiple causation of interpersonal violence, learn about available resources both within the health care system and in the patients' community. Numerous programs exist to address violence, ranging from mentor programs for young men and women to school-based violence prevention curricula. Physicians, nurses, social workers, mental health workers, and public health administrators must work together with community agencies.

Patients who express real concern for their safety should be taken seriously, and strategies in consultation should be formulated to provide a plan of safety for the patient. Likewise, patients insistent upon revenge, with plans to do harm to another person, should not be discharged from the office or emergency room until counseling and assessment by a psychiatrist or psychologist trained or experienced in issues of interpersonal violence have been performed. In some circumstances admission to the medical or surgical service is indicated for these patients until their anger and rage can be dealt with. Again, one must know the legalities of this situation.

Patients who are substance dependent or in whom substance use is related to their injury should be counseled about their substance use. (see Chapters 130 and 131).

Community organizations such as youth clubs and churches may be very helpful to young men and women for whom low self-esteem has led to involvement in violence or drug use. Community referral is essential if physicians are to have a real effect on interpersonal violence (see the box below).

## BATTERED WOMEN

### Etiology

The term *domestic violence* is used interchangeably with spouse abuse, partner abuse, person battering. It is a syndrome that is characterized by repeated acts of violence or the threat of violence used by the perpetrator to establish and maintain control over a mate or intimate partner. It includes violence in couples who have separated and also dating couples who may not necessarily be living together. About 85% to 90% of persons reporting abuse and two thirds of domestic murder victims are women. Men do report being victims of abuse, but they may not develop the same sequelae as women, and more research is needed in this area. In addition, more research is needed to examine partner abuse in gay and lesbian couples. This discussion focuses on data and recommendations from the work that has been done with women who have been battered.

From a medical perspective there is a progression from the initial stage of acute injury to the battered woman syndrome. Four stages are seen in battered women: (1) acute injury, (2) illness, (3) isolation, (4) severe psychosocial problems.

In the first stage the patient comes into the emergency room or office with an acute injury. It may be the first time her partner has hit or pushed her, but usually the injury is part of an ongoing pattern of abuse. Each incident is characterized by a tension-building phase, followed by the event (which often brings a release of tension, perhaps even for the woman). This is followed by promises that it will not happen again. About 25% of women leave the relationship after a single episode of abuse, but in the other 75% of couples the tension begins to rise again, and as the cycle continues, the baseline level of tension and danger rises, the sense of safety falls, and the woman may move into the next stage by symptoms of illness.

In stage 2 the woman seeks medical help with complaints such as headache, palpitations, gastrointestinal problems, anxiety, depression, insomnia, and dyspareunia. These complaints may be a result of the violence itself or from the stress of living with the violence. Often the woman receives symptomatic treatment but is not asked about the abuse. The women may repeatedly seek help for physical complaints and eventually be labeled a difficult patient. The patient becomes more and more isolated (third stage) and may become hostile or evasive, which frustrates the physician.

If the violence continues over time, the most common scenario is that it increases in intensity and severity and the woman's isolation and fear increase in parallel. The isolation may then progress into the fourth stage, which consists of serious psychosocial problems (e.g., alcoholism, drug dependence, suicide). Often at this point the abuse may be incorrectly identified as the result of mental health problems, instead of part of the cause.

### Epidemiology

Domestic violence is epidemic. The prevalence is unknown. Multiple attempts to study it have come up with similar results, and most authorities agree that these are underestimates. In 1975 a nationwide random sample of couples involving 2143 households found that 28% had experienced violence at some point in their history and 16% at some time in the past year. In a 1993 national poll 34% of adults in the United States reported having witnessed a man beating his wife or girlfriend, and 14% of women reported that a husband or boyfriend had been violent with them. According to the recent American Medical Association (AMA) guidelines on domestic violence, battered women account for 22% to 35% of women seeking care in any ambulatory care internal medicine clinic, 25% of women who attempt suicide, 25% of women utilizing a psychiatric emergency service, and 23% of women in a prenatal clinic.

Despite these alarming statistics and the fact that

#### Types of programs for referral

Mentor programs for young men or women
Parenting skills programs
Violence prevention curricula
Gang prevention programs
Alcoholics Anonymous/Narcotics Anonymous
Community-based conflict resolution programs
Rites of passage programs
Skills training for real jobs

women who are battered seek care from physicians and other health workers, the problem is rarely recognized.

### History

Who should be asked about domestic violence? Who is likely to be battered? No well-defined criteria predict who will be battered. Among women at increased risk for abuse are those who are single, divorced, or planning a separation, those between the ages of 17 and 28, those who abuse alcohol or other drugs or whose partners do, those who are pregnant, and those whose partners are excessively jealous or possessive. There are no socioeconomic or racial predictors of women at risk.

Most authorities, including the AMA in their recent guidelines on domestic violence, recommend screening all women, since the only risk factor agreed on by all is female gender. At a minimum all women between 16 and 35 should be screened, since 67% to 74% of women in abusive relationships are under 35. (This may miss a significant number of women who are victims of elder abuse, a problem that is increasingly being recognized.) Any woman, no matter what her age, who presents with facial trauma, bruises on breasts, trunk, or genitalia, chronic headaches or any chronic physical complaint without obvious physiologic cause, depression, or anxiety should be asked about abuse (current and past). Studies support the relationship of physical and sexual abuse to somatization.

What are the barriers to asking? Barriers exist for both patients and physicians. Barriers for physicians include close identification with patients, fear of offending patients, a feeling of inadequacy and frustration by not being able to control the situation (i.e., inability to make patients leave the relationship), and a fear that the issue might consume too much time. Some of these barriers can be addressed through an increased awareness of available resources and education of physicians.

Barriers for patients include fear that mentioning the violence might jeopardize their safety, shame and humiliation, thinking they deserve the abuse and do not deserve help, lack of awareness that their physical symptoms may be related to the abuse, and feeling protective of their partners, who may be the sole source of love and financial support.

However, studies consistently show that, although women may not volunteer the information initially, when asked in a nonthreatening manner about abuse they are not only willing but relieved to talk about their experience. It is critical that the patient be interviewed alone with attention to her safety. In settings where there is a need for interpreters a family member or partner should not be used as an interpreter. It is also important to elicit any history of substance abuse in patient or partner. Alcohol or drug use in the batterer may make the situation more volatile and dangerous, but it is not usually responsible for the violent behavior. When a batterer becomes sober, the battering does not stop unless specifically addressed as a problem.

In interviewing a woman about domestic violence it is important to ask in a nonthreatening, nonjudgmental way if abuse is or was present. Some examples of questions to ask are shown in the box at right.

Just by listening to the history the physician validates the patient's experience, an important part of the therapy. A physician who demonstrates no fear in talking about the violence facilitates the woman's telling of her story. In addition, it is helpful to state how common the problem is. For example, say "Two million women are beaten each year," or "Many women in your situation feel the way you do; it's difficult, but there is help available."

It is important to assess whether violence or threat of violence is ongoing. The emphasis of the treatment is different if the symptoms are due to ongoing abuse as opposed to abuse from which the woman has extricated herself.

### Physical examination and laboratory findings

An important aspect of the physical is that it be done in a sensitive and respectful manner, without the partner present. This is true if the physician suspects abuse, even if the woman has not admitted to it. During the examination the physician should pay attention to the general mood of the patient. Is she fearful, anxious? Completely examine the skin for bruises (sometimes in different stages of healing), lacerations, and scars. Be especially alert to injuries on the face, neck, breasts, trunk, and genitalia. Musculoskeletal injuries such as fractures, strains, and sprains are common. Sexually transmitted diseases and recurrent vaginitis are common. Laboratory tests such as x-rays and culture of vaginal and cervical tissue can document consequences of abuse.

## Differential diagnosis

The differential diagnosis depends on the stage of abuse. If the woman has an acute injury, the differential includes accidental trauma or intentional trauma. If the patient seems to be accident prone, careful investigation of the circumstances around each instance is warranted. When the woman denies abuse during the history but the physician still suspects it, it could be helpful to say "Many women who come in with this kind of injury have been hit or are being hit repeatedly by someone they know; could this be happening to you?" That lets the woman know the

### Questions about domestic violence

Is anyone in your family hitting you?
Has anyone hit you in the past?
Does your partner ever threaten you?
Everyone has arguments at home. Do you ever get hurt when you and your partner fight? *OR* What happens when you and your partner argue?
Do you ever get hurt?
Does your partner ever prevent you from leaving the house or going to school or work?
Does your partner threaten to hurt you when you disagree with him? *OR* What happens when you disagree with your partner?
Does your partner destroy things you care about?
Are you forced to engage in sex that makes you uncomfortable?
Does your partner watch your every word?

physician is open to hearing about the abuse, even if she is not ready to talk about it at that time.

When seen in an office, women more commonly show symptoms of one of the other three stages, with physical illness or psychologic distress. The differential then is more complex and includes major psychiatric disorders such as generalized anxiety disorder, panic disorder (see Chapter 132), major depression (see Chapter 133), PTSD (see Chapter 133), somatization (see Chapter 134), and character disorders. In addition, if the symptom is somatic, such as headache, its evaluation includes all of the appropriate medical diagnoses. The presence of a psychiatric or medical diagnosis does not exclude the possibility of abuse.

## Management

Management is interwoven in the fabric of the interview by the way in which the provider helps the woman name the abuse, lets her decide that violence is not acceptable, and provides a safe place for exploration of possibilities. Always think about the woman's safety. Initial management consists of treatment of immediate medical or psychiatric problems (fractures, lacerations, depression, vaginal infections). Also, in every visit one needs to do a safety/lethality assessment. Certain indicators, especially if clustered, should alert the physician to danger (see the box below).

It is important to warn the woman of any danger signs, but ultimately she is the best judge of her safety. If she is not safe or wants to leave, questions that need to be asked are: Does she have a safe place to go? If not, is she willing to go to a shelter? Are there children involved? It is useful to ask the woman what she needs to be safe. What would her partner do if she left? Does she have an extra set of car keys? Suggest she keep a suitcase with important papers and clothes at a neighbor's, if possible, including the children's papers and change of clothes.

Physicians, no matter how busy, can declare the violence unacceptable and help the woman name the forms of abuse. They can also help begin the next therapeutic work: empowerment. This process involves the four main ideas listed in the box below, right.

Even if there are no trained personnel or shelters available nearby, much of this therapeutic process begins with physicians. If a support group is available, physicians should urge these women to join one. They should stress that certain feelings are common: "Many women who have been beaten feel this way." Sometimes medications are appropriate to treat pain, depression, and infections. Yet physicians should communicate that the medicine will not solve the underlying problem. Assessing the risk of suicide (see Chapter 133) is essential.

It is important for physicians to help the woman see that she has options. It is useful to have the number of a battered women's shelter available and even let her call from the office. Information about shelters in the area is available from the National Coalition for Prevention of Violence. It is helpful to know state laws regarding the options for protection or to have the name and number of someone to refer the woman to.

It is also important to help the woman recognize her own strengths: How has she protected herself and her children in the past? What does she see in the future? Does she want to go back to school or get a job? Many of these steps take time, and it is ideal to use counselors of battered women and support groups in the area to help achieve success. However, if there are no such services in the area, physicians can still weave these steps into the routine patient care. This may be also true if the woman does not feel safe going anywhere else but the physician's office.

### Legal responsibilities

Because physicians may become involved in a legal process, they need to be prepared. This means simply recording everything carefully and legibly. Since the medical record is a legal document, it can be admitted in court. If there are acute injuries, physicians should take color photos, but only with the patient's written consent. Photos should include an identifying feature such as a face or hand (there may be some state-to-state variation). A description of the injury should accompany the photo. Each picture should be dated and signed by the patient, the photographer, and a witness, placed in a sealed envelope in the patient's medical record, and marked *confidential*. In most states domestic violence is not reportable without consent of the victim, unless the victim is a child or elder. Since many states mandate reporting of child abuse, if it comes up, it needs to be addressed, and the woman may be in greater danger in this situation.

A separate issue is how to treat the batterer. Couples therapy, especially at the beginning, is not recommended and may be dangerous. Whether physicians should treat both partners is controversial. Especially in rural areas physicians are the primary care providers for both, so care has to be taken to respect confidentiality and above all to consider the safety of the partner at risk.

### Attributes of the batterer indicating danger

- A history of suicide or homicide attempts (or threats or fantasies of such)
- Depression and or situational stressors (such as job loss)
- Weapons possession or past use of weapons
- Obsession about partner
- Rage over her leaving
- Drug and alcohol use, especially in a state of fury or depression
- Continual harassment of woman
- Escalation of threats and violence

### Empowerment

- Validating the woman's experience
- Exploring her options and advocating for her safety
- Building on her own strengths and avoiding blame of victim
- Respecting her right to self-determination

## CHILD ABUSE AND MALTREATMENT

Maltreatment includes physical abuse, sexual abuse, and neglect. Physical abuse is any nonaccidental injury inflicted or allowed to be inflicted by the parent or caretaker; sexual abuse is any contact between an adult and a child for the sexual gratification of the adult; and neglect is the failure to provide a minimal degree of care for the child.

### Epidemiology and etiology

In the past decade there have been 1.5 to 2 million cases of child maltreatment reported annually in the United States. In 1991 about 45 out of every 1000 children in the United States were abused. Over 1000 children died as a result of abuse. Reported cases of neglect are far more common than reports of physical or sexual abuse. In the medical setting, especially the emergency service, children who have been physically or sexually assaulted may represent a significant number of cases. Children who have been neglected may not be as readily identified in medical settings, which emphasize acute problems.

Child maltreatment is an extremely complex group of behaviors characterized by maladaptive interactions between infants and children of all ages and their caretakers. Although it may be impossible to absolutely predict which individual will become an abuser or a victim, statistics and studies have helped to identify the vulnerable family. Risk factors for caretakers include a history of abuse in childhood, social isolation of the family, excessively high expectations for the child's behavior, parental expectations inconsistent with the child's developmental abilities, lack of empathy for the child, and impaired parent-child attachment. Stressors such as drug or alcohol use, economic difficulties, early parenting (teenage pregnancies), and mental illness are associated with child abuse. Often adult caretakers lack the necessary maturity and experience for childrearing responsibilities.

Violence toward children is especially common in families where the husbands and wives resort to violence toward one another. It is estimated that more than 3 million children witness parental violence annually, resulting not only in physical abuse of some children but long-lasting psychologic problems for witnesses as well as the abused. As with the parent, there are certain characteristics that place a child at greater risk for child maltreatment (see the box below). The vulnerable child can be viewed as abnormal or different by the parents.

#### Child at risk for maltreatment

- Premature
- Child of adolescent parent(s)
- Child born with congenital anomalies or deficiencies
- Child hospitalized in the neonatal period with subsequent loss of parental bonding
- Child with exaggerated common childhood behaviors such as colic or excessive crying

### History

The medical workup can be very straightforward when a child presents with injuries and/or a history of abuse. If such symptoms or history comes to light during the course of an otherwise routine visit, it is imperative that the physician be able to initiate the appropriate evaluation and to coordinate care with other members of the primary care team. The physician should use the protocols and consultants available for such assessments. The evaluation must include the history given by the parents and caretakers, the history from the child, a thorough physical examination, laboratory tests, and radiologic studies as indicated (see the box below).

The historian in most child-related health visits is the parent or guardian. If both parents are present and there is a question of child abuse, every effort should be made to interview the parents separately. It is imperative that separate interviews be conducted if there is the possibility of spouse abuse. The interview should address the details of the presenting symptoms with careful questioning of the sequence of events. If the history is vague or conflicting, the physician should become alert to the existence of some problem and make further inquiries. The interviewer should express concern about obvious discrepancies in the history but must avoid confrontations in such situations. The parent should be asked for details of the child's growth and development. The inability to provide simple data about the child's immunizations and developmental

#### Criteria for suspecting child maltreatment

**History**

- Vague or no history to explain injury
- Explanation changes during course of interview
- Different histories given to various members of staff, triage nurse, doctor, social worker
- Parents give different histories of same episode
- Parent offers no explanation for delay in care
- Parent appears indifferent to the pain of the child
- Parent blames child for the injury
- Parent reports child to be a liar and not to be believed

**Physical examination**

- Evidence of major injuries with history of minor trauma
- Specific evidence of inflicted trauma: e.g., cord marks, pattern burns
- Injury inconsistent with the developmental age of the child
- Injury located in area not commonly associated with routine childhood trauma
- Injuries in different stages of healing when there is a history given of a single episode of trauma
- Evidence of old scars from previous injuries

**Laboratory testing**

- None of the tests reveal any medical explanation for the observed injuries
- For a child with a chronic disease there is no evidence of acute exacerbation of the disease to account for the injuries

milestones may lessen the credibility of the account given by the parent concerning the presenting symptom. If the parent volunteers the information that he or she has injured the child, the physician should ask the parent for an explanation of the behavior. If a parent accuses the other parent or caretaker, the physician must carefully attempt to identify factors that might influence such a disclosure, including a custody issue. At all times the interviewer must be nonjudgmental, recording all statements with quotation marks as needed. The interview of the child should be done by an individual who is trained in the techniques of interviewing children and has the necessary experience.

### Physical examination

The primary objectives of the medical examination are threefold: (1) medical, to assess any physical injury to the child and provide necessary treatment; (2) psychologic, to afford the child a sense of safety; and (3) legal, to provide physical documentation that may be used as evidence. The child should be fully informed of the nature and extent of the physical examination, which should be complete, including the genital area.

The examiner should document the following factors:

1. *Appearance/hygiene:* Briefly describe the general condition of the child.
2. *Behavioral assessment:* Record the child's affect (e.g., depressed, withdrawn, friendly).
3. *Age-appropriate behavior:* Assess the child's behavior and describe significant reactions to parent(s) and staff. For example, it is unusual for a 2-year-old child to have no fear of strangers and to readily separate from parents. Note whether the child is very fearful of the parent and similarly if the parent offers no support for the child during the examination.
4. *Physical examination:* Include evaluation of the child's physical development with the height and weight (statistics plotted on a growth curve to document that the child's stature is appropriate for age) and Tanner staging (the staging of pubertal growth in both males and females).
5. *Documentation of current/old physical abuse:* Clearly document bruises and scars that might indicate abuse (see the box above), using bodygrams or similar diagrams and photography as indicated, such as Polaroids.

If the diagnosis of child maltreatment is considered, the physician should use the protocols within the facility or area to obtain the necessary consultations to clarify the diagnosis. If the diagnosis is clear, the physician must begin the process of reporting to the appropriate authorities for investigation, again using established community protocols. In either situation the parent(s) or guardian should be informed of the diagnosis and the process required by law be outlined for them.

### Severe abuse

In addition to neglect and maltreatment, more severe physical and sexual abuse of children occurs. Common signs of physical abuse include bruises, welts, lacerations, burns, fractures, and abdominal and CNS injuries (see the box on p. 1685).

Sexual abuse of children encompasses a range of presentations from fondling to sexual intercourse. When clinical symptoms are questionable, the expertise and training of the physician are crucial to determine if abuse has occurred or if further assessment is necessary to reach such a diagnosis. Such evaluations should follow the protocols established in each locality as well as guidelines provided by national organizations such as the American Academy of Pediatrics.

The evaluation of children who have been sexually abused is best handled by referral to an experienced team of health professionals, who can assess the problem, document adequately for legal purposes, and provide immediate and long-term care for the child.

### Dating bruises by color

The approximate age of bruises can be categorized by assessing the color of the lesions as follows:

| | |
|---|---|
| 0-2 days: | red (swollen/tender) |
| 2-5 days: | red to blue |
| 5-7 days: | blue to green |
| 7-10 days: | green to yellow |
| 10-14 days: | brown |
| 14-28 days: | clearing |

Such color presentation and progression depend on the amount of force used, the area injured (blood supply to an area will determine the rate of clearing), the condition of the skin (degree of turgor of the skin will affect the degree of bruising and resolution of bruises), and the presence of any condition that might heighten bruising, such as a platelet disorder.

### Role of the primary care physician

The physician functions in many roles with respect to child abuse: by identifying a family at risk for maltreatment and developing a plan for primary prevention, by identifying and reporting a suspected case of child abuse, and by playing an active role in the treatment and secondary prevention of child maltreatment. Each of these tasks requires that the physician be familiar with local statutes concerning child maltreatment and community programs. Identification of abusive situations must be followed by the development of treatment plans, not just by reporting of the case to the appropriate authorities.

There are reporting requirements for health care providers in each state. It is imperative that practitioners be familiar with these regulations and laws. Within localities there may be additional procedures requiring reporting of specific offenses to specialized units.

Within this body of child abuse legislation are provisions concerning protection of reporters from liability and penalties for the failure to report. Protection of reporting sources from liability is based on the concept of good faith reporting, that is, the report was made in accordance with the mandates of the child abuse legislation and with no malice toward the family concerned. Documentation and adherence to accepted protocols offer the best proof when the good faith of a report is challenged. Failure to report a situation of suspected child abuse may result in a fine, a criminal conviction, or civil liability.

## Signs of significant physical abuse

**Examples of physical signs of child abuse by site**

Mouth: Tear of the frenulum secondary to forced feeding of an infant or toddler

Ears: Rupture of the tympanic membrane caused by a blow to the side of the head, or ecchymoses of the pinnae from being pinched

Back: Bruising consistent with a punch or kick; may present with hematuria

The injury may be identified by the pattern produced by an object such as a belt buckle, an electrical cord, or a paddle. Other recognizable patterns are hand prints from a slap, pinch or grab marks, and teeth marks.

**Burns**

Cigarette/cigar: Usually located on the face when a child walks into a cigarette dangling from someone's hand; inflicted burns are found on palms, soles, back, and buttocks in patterns not consistent with the scars secondary to varicella

Immersion burns: Glovelike or stockinglike burns of the extremities; when the child is immersed in hot water, the burn may be doughnut-shaped on the buttocks or genitals with central sparing where the buttocks contacted the bottom of the tub or basin

Patterned burns: Resemble the object used to inflict the burn, including irons, cigarette lighters, grills, or curling irons; location and extent of the burn can be useful if the burn was accidental

**Fractures**

Long bone fractures, especially in nonwalking infants
Posterior rib
Facial

**Abdominal injuries**

Range from mild discomfort to major injury from ruptured viscera
Bruises on abdominal wall
Intestinal perforation
Ruptured spleen

**Central nervous system injuries**

Violent shaking can produce subdural hematoma, retinal hemorrhage, or subarachnoid bleed

The health care provider can be the conduit for the primary prevention of child maltreatment by screening all families for risk factors that may predispose to abuse. The involved practitioner can function as an advocate for the child and the family to expand services to all families in their community.

## BIBLIOGRAPHY

Carlson BF: Children's observation of interparental violence. In Roberts A, editor: *Battered women and their families: intervention strategies and treatment programs,* New York, 1984, Springer-Verlag.

Chadwick D et al: *Color atlas of child sexual abuse,* Chicago, 1989, Year Book.

*Child sexual abuse: report of the 22nd Ross roundtable in critical approaches to common pediatric problems,* Columbus, Ohio, 1991, Ross Laboratories.

Committee on Child Abuse and Neglect: Guidelines for the evaluation of sexual abuse of children, *Pediatrics* 87:254, 1991.

Daro D, McCurdy K: *Current trends in child abuse reporting and fatalities: the results of the 1991 annual fifty state survey,* Chicago, 1992, National Committee for the Prevention of Child Abuse.

Dubowitz H: Prevention of child maltreatment: what is known, *Pediatrics* 83:570, 1989.

Garbarino J, Guttman E, Seeley JW: *The psychologically battered child,* San Francisco, 1987, Jossey-Bass.

Goins WA, Thompson J, Simpkins C: Recurrent intentional injury, *J Natl Med Assoc* 84(5):431, 1989.

Heger A, Emans SJ: *Evaluation of the sexually abused child: a medical textbook and photographic atlas,* New York, 1992, Oxford University Press.

Helfer R et al: *The battered child,* ed 4, Chicago, 1987, University of Chicago Press.

Kleinman PK, editor: *Diagnostic imaging of child abuse,* Baltimore, 1987, William & Wilkins.

Krugman RD: Child abuse and neglect: the role of the primary care physician in the recognition, treatment, and prevention, *Primary Care* 11:527, 1984.

McHugh M et al: *Suspected child abuse and maltreatment: identification and management in hospitals and clinics,* State of New York, 1991.

Oates K, editor: *Child abuse: a major concern of our times,* New York, 1986, Citadel.

Prothrow-Stith D: *Deadly consequences,* New York, 1991, HarperCollins.

Reece R, editor: Child abuse, *Pediatr Clin North Am* 37:4, 1990.

Rosenberg ML, Mercy JA: Assaultive violence. In Rosenberg M, Fenley MA, editors: *Violence in America,* New York, 1991, Oxford University Press.

Sims DW et al: Urban trauma: a chronic recurrent disease, *J Trauma* 29(7):940, 1989.

Wissow LS: *Child advocacy for the clinician: an approach to child abuse and neglect,* Baltimore, 1990, Williams & Wilkins.

CHAPTER

# 128 Death and Dying

Timothy E. Quill
Robert V. Brody

Primary care physicians make a commitment to care for their patients through sickness and health, often until the patient's death. Patients who enter the care of a subspecialist for aspects of their medical care often return to the primary care physician when that treatment stops working, or when the burdens of curative treatment become too great to continue. Many hospice programs require that patients sustain the active involvement of their primary care physician. When a physician has an intimate relationship with the patient and family, he or she is in a unique position to guide the patient through the last phases of illness. That commitment, to work through the end stages of life no matter where it takes the patient, is fundamental to primary care practice.

Against this backdrop are disturbing data that many physicians avoid talking with their patients about the possibility of death and that they often continue burdensome, unwanted fights for life using medical technology well beyond the point of any significant chance of success.

Death is frequently misperceived as a medical failure rather than a natural, inevitable part of the life cycle. Because of medical successes in prolonging life and other larger social forces, the nature of dying has profoundly changed in the United States. About 80% of deaths now occur in hospitals or chronic care facilities, often far removed from caring families and the familiar surroundings of home. The same medical technology that can save and prolong meaningful life can, paradoxically, prolong the process of dying. Physicians report that they sometime use too much medical technology at the end of life, but they often do not know how to stop. Hospice care tends to be offered late, if at all, and reports abound about physicians' undertreatment of pain and fear of opioids even when the patient is dying. In this context primary care physicians are in a unique position to take an active role informing, caring for, treating, and advocating for their severely ill and dying patients.

## BASIC ETHICAL PRINCIPLES IN THE CARE OF THE DYING

Despite a wide gap between principle and practice, enormous ethical and legal progress has increased the options for severely ill and dying patients.

### Right to refuse treatment

Patients have the right to be fully informed about potentially effective treatment options and to accept or reject them according to their own values and beliefs. Provided the patient is competent and fully informed, this includes the right to refuse effective, life-saving treatment even when death is certain without treatment. When a patient's choices are at odds with the physician's recommendations, the reasons for the discrepancies should be fully understood and explored. Final decisions, however, rest with patients.

### Right to have treatment withdrawn once started

Though clinicians are often more reluctant about stopping life-sustaining treatments once started (e.g., ventilator, feeding tube, dialysis) than they are about not starting them, there are no significant ethical or legal differences between these acts. The experience of stopping life-sustaining treatment once started may be more difficult for clinicians partly because of the proximity of the physician's action to the patient's death. Nonetheless, this option allows patients to undergo limited trials of life-sustaining treatment without being obligated to continue them indefinitely. It also allows the patient's goals, circumstances, and choices to change over time. Therefore informed, competent patients must be supported in their rights to have unwanted treatment stopped, even if that treatment is life sustaining.

### Substituted judgment for incompetent patients

The following principle should underlie all medical decision making for patients who have lost the mental capacity to make their own decisions: caregivers should try to reconstruct *incapacitated patients' values and philosophies* to make decisions as the patients would if they could comprehend their medical situation and the options available. Since only about 10% of Americans have formally expressed their end of life philosophy through an advance directive (living will or health care proxy), such determinations are often approximations at best (Figs. 128-1 and 128-2). Family members should be made aware that their role in these matters is not to express what they would want for the patient or for themselves, but what the patient would want for himself or herself. Physicians and families should try to reconstruct the patient's wishes and values as much as possible, even in the face of uncertainty, rather than letting their own values guide treatment. Only when there is no clue to what the patient would have decided can the vague notion of the patient's best interests be invoked to make medical decisions.

### Hospice care for the dying

Hospice care is a meaningful and effective alternative to continuing ineffective or excessively burdensome medical treatment of dying patients. Hospice care should be the standard of care for the dying, and primary care physicians must become skilled in its application. Hospice values differ significantly from those of usual medical care in that they emphasize a shift away from cure toward comfort and much more attention to the person and to relief of suffering than to the treatment of the underlying disease. Treatment plans should be highly individualized, allowing each person as much choice and latitude as possible given the limitations of their disease. Human contact with caring persons within and outside of the patient's family should be maximized within the limits set by the patient. Formal hospice programs usually include a multidisciplinary team, including nurses, social workers, clergy, health aides, volunteers, and others. Many offer financial and legal counseling, assistance in housing, and other services that ease the burden on dying patients and their families. As far as possible the patient's agenda with input from the family should be assessed and followed, rather than that of the caring professionals, agencies, or institutions. Offering patients the hospice philosophy of care should not depend on their being accepted into a formal program, since it can be implemented in most settings.

There should be no reluctance about the use of potent analgesics to relieve the patient's pain, even if the high dosages required inadvertently or indirectly contribute to the patient's death. In hospice care, relief of suffering is given the highest priority, and the unintended contribution to the patient's death is justified under the principle of double effect (that actions initiated with good intentions can have unintended bad consequences and still be ethically and morally appropriate.) With modern pain-relieving techniques dying patients who fear physical pain should be reassured that the physician will diligently and aggressively work with them to find a regimen that effectively manages their pain. Other uncomfortable symptoms should also be identified and relieved as much as possible.

Since the course that any individual dying patient will undergo is uncertain, the most significant commitment that a primary care physician can make is not to abandon. This implies an obligation to be there until the patient's death, to continue to problem solve, to support the caregivers (both family and professional), and to try to be helpful no matter what questions arise or what path the patient's illness takes. This commitment can take some of the

**DIRECTIVE REGARDING FUTURE USE OF EXTRAORDINARY LIFE SUPPORT PROCEDURES**
**(Equivalent to Living Will)**

To: My Family, my Physicians, my Lawyer, any Medical Facility in whose care I happen to be, any Individual who may become responsible for my Health Affairs, and All Others Whom It May Concern:

I, being of sound mind and over 18 years of age, hereby issue a directive, which I intend to be legally binding, *which shall become effective at some future time, only under the following circumstances:*

1. When I become unable to make my own decisions or express my wishes; *AND*
2. CHOOSE ALL THAT YOU WANT TO APPLY
   - ☐ If I have a terminal illness; and/or
   - ☐ I am permanently unconscious; and/or
   - ☐ If extraordinary life support procedures or "heroic measures" would be medically futile; and/or
   - ☐ Under the following circumstances (Please specify, for example, dementia, severe neurological illness or other permanent disabling condition to which you want this Directive to apply.):

   ______________________________
   ______________________________
   ______________________________
   ______________________________

Then I direct that my dying not be unreasonably prolonged; *AND*

CHOOSE *ONE*

☐ I wish to have COMFORT CARE ONLY, which is directed only toward relieving pain and suffering, regardless of the progress of my disease.

☐ I want CONSERVATIVE CARE, which is usual treatment (such as antibiotics) *but not* extraordinary treatment (such as cardiopulmonary resuscitation, mechanical ventilation, kidney dialysis, etc.)

OPTIONAL: I wish to make additional directives (about life support equipment or other matters):

______________________________
______________________________
______________________________
______________________________

PLEASE NOTE: If, at some future time, you cannot make decisions for yourself, New York State law prohibits withholding artificial nutrition and hydration from you, unless you have already made your wishes known.

If I cannot eat or drink enough because of my irreversible medical conditions: ( ☐ I DO / ☐ I DO NOT ) want

artificial nutrition (intravenous or tube feeding) and hydration (intravenous fluids).

In the absence of my ability to give directions regarding the aforementioned life sustaining procedures, it is my intention that this directive shall be honored as the final expression of my legal right to refuse medical treatment and to accept the consequences of such refusal.

I understand the full importance of this directive and I have signed it after thorough consideration of the nature and consequences of my refusal of such extraordinary life support procedures, including their benefits and disadvantages. This directive is in accordance with my strong convictions and beliefs and is made freely without any inducement or coercion from any person or institution.

______________________________ Signature

______________________________ Date

I hereby certify that I am over 18 years of age and that I have witnessed the above declarant's signature.

| | |
|---|---|
| Witness | Witness |
| Printed Witness Name | Printed Witness Name |
| Date | Date |

**Fig. 128-1.** Equivalent of a living will. (Redrawn from Genesee Hospital, Rochester, New York.)

**HEALTH CARE PROXY**

I, ______________________ hereby appoint the following person as my HEALTH CARE AGENT, to make any and all health care decisions for me except for any restrictions I have noted below. This Proxy shall take effect when and if I become unable to make my own health care decisions.

Health Care Agent Name/Address ______________________ Phone ______________

Alternate Health Care Agent Name/Address ______________________ Phone ______________

Optional instructions or limitations on the Health Care Agent's authority, if any:

______________________________________________

______________________________________________

Unless I revoke it, this proxy shall remain in effect indefinitely. (Or until the date or condition stated below, if any.)

______________________________________________

______________________________________________

PLEASE NOTE: If, at some future time, you cannot make decisions for yourself, New York State law prohibits your Health Care Agent from making decisions about withholding artificial nutrition and hydration from you, unless you have already made your wishes known.

If I cannot eat or drink enough because of my irreversible medical conditions: ( ☐ I DO / ☐ I DO NOT ) want

artificial nutrition (intravenous or tube feeding) and hydration (intravenous fluids).

Signature ______________________ Date ______________

Address ______________________

I hereby certify that I am over 18 years of age, and that the person who signed this Proxy appeared to do so willingly and free from duress and that he or she signed (or asked another to sign for him or her) this Proxy in my presence.

Witness ______________________ Witness ______________________

Printed Witness Name ______________________ Printed Witness Name ______________________

Date ______________________ Date ______________________

**Fig. 128-2.** Example of a health care proxy. (Redrawn from Genesee Hospital, Rochester, New York.)

fear out of this profound process. A continued clinical presence is at the core of providing humane care of the dying.

## COMMON TRANSITIONS WHERE DEATH IS PRESENT

### Advance directives

All adult patients should consider completing an advance directive. Both the health care proxy (naming an individual to represent the patient for health-care decisions should the patient lose mental capacity in the future) and the living will (setting out one's philosophy and specific directives toward health care should one lose mental capacity in the future) have gained substantial ethical and legal standing throughout the country. Despite passage of the Patient Self-Determination Act in 1991, requiring all patients entering a hospital, nursing facility, home health or hospice program, or health maintenance organization to be informed of their rights with regard to advance directives, only about 10% of the population have completed such a document. The reasons for this include the inherent difficulty defining an end of life philosophy and contemplating one's death, conflicts within families, the complexity of the forms and concepts, and the sustained effort needed to complete the process.

Advance directives can be invaluable to clinicians and families making complex medical decisions for patients who have lost mental competence, since they allow the patient's philosophy to remain in the foreground. Physicians should initiate discussion as part of routine care, perhaps as part of a complete physical or when considering health maintenance. These discussions can be more difficult and frightening when considered for the first time when the patient is severely ill and at immediate risk for losing mental capacity. Nonetheless, the discussion is crucial if the patient's values are to remain central to future health-care decisions.

If the patient has trusted family or friends, many favor the health care proxy over the living will because of its increased flexibility to deal with unanticipated conditions. However, proxies who are uninformed about patient wishes may have a hard time being sure they are remaining true to the patient's values. The living will has the advantage of being a direct expression of the patient's philosophy, but the disadvantage is that it may not explicitly cover the patient's actual condition. Perhaps the safest procedure is to have the patient complete both documents whenever possible. The presence of an advance directive should be clearly marked as part of the patient's medical record in case it is needed in an emergency situation. Advance directives have no relevance to the care of competent patients because these persons can directly participate in their own medical decision making. Advance directives are activated only when patients lose this capacity.

### Bad news/treatment not working/serious uncertainty about the future

Primary care physicians regularly encounter patients who are working through these crises. There is no preset formula about how to proceed, except to say that telling the truth, even in the face of uncertainty or a bad prognosis, is usually critical to informed decision making. Whenever possible the physician should follow the patient's lead about how rapidly and in what detail to convey the medical situation. Sometimes the process must be accelerated because of the immediacy of the patient's condition and the need for rapid decision making, but more often time can be allowed to enable the patient to integrate enough information to make a good decision. Attention should be paid to each patient's unique emotional responses, information needs, and support.

When the news is overwhelming (e.g., a new, unexpected diagnosis of cancer or HIV), it is prudent to initially develop a miniplan (how to tell close family members, where to go from the office, how to handle fear) before making major treatment decisions or learning all there is to know about the illness. When the patient has integrated the relevant medical information and is ready to make medical decisions, all reasonable treatment options should be explored, from the most aggressive to those that emphasize comfort and symptom relief. Physicians should not shy away from sharing their own opinions, biases, and recommendations while at the same time reinforcing that the final decision rests with the patient. At some point relatively early in the patient's course it is important for primary care physicians to convey their commitment to work with the patient through the illness no matter what choices are made or what course is followed.

Sometimes family members and even clinicians believe that telling the truth when the prognosis is poor may deprive the patient of hope. Though there is significant cultural variation on this issue, most clinicians and ethicists in the United States believe that physicians should almost always fully inform, unless there is a compelling reason not to. Most often such protective secrets tend to isolate family members from the patient and may deprive the patient of the opportunity to make informed medical decisions, to settle affairs, or to say goodbye. Since medical treatment is only one avenue for finding hope, the patient may also be deprived of the opportunity to seek it in other domains (e.g., religion). The physician should respectfully explore the reasons being suggested for collusion in not telling a patient the truth, but ultimately should follow the patient's lead in deciding whether and in what detail to inform.

### Do not resuscitate (DNR)

Though this decision technically applies only to attempting cardiopulmonary resuscitation (CPR), it often represents a complex amalgam of decisions and meanings. It may be the first open acknowledgment to the patient and the family that treatment is not working and that death is likely in the near future. Since CPR is largely ineffective in noncardiac, multisystem disease, it seems cruel to have patients and families anguish over DNR decisions as they frequently do.

Unfortunately, DNR emphasizes what will not be done and says nothing about what treatment will be tried. Therefore it is often confused by patients, families, and medical personnel with abandonment (to do nothing). To avoid this confusion, discussions about DNR must also include an explanation of what treatments will be provided. For some patients this might include all aggressive medical treatments except CPR (potentially including antibiotics, fluids, chemotherapy, blood products, radiation, and even ICU or surgery), whereas for others a hospice approach is appropriate. The treatment plan should be individualized, tailored to the patient's values, goals, and medical condition. Clearly defining what will be done, as well as the primary care physician's commitment to see the process through with the patient, should allay any fear of abandonment.

### Hospice care

Hospice care is frequently offered to patients only after all possible medical interventions have been exhausted and death is imminent. Physicians should discuss it as a possibility much earlier in the course of a patient's illness, perhaps when the odds of a treatment working become remote or when the burdens of treatment begin to grow out of proportion to the expected benefits. It should also be explored when patients raise fears about what dying might be like, reassuring them about the possibility of a more humane and less technologically dominated approach. Hospice care should in no way be equated with giving up. Instead, it is an alternative medical approach emphasizing intensive caring for the person and an explicit focus on relieving suffering and symptoms rather than treating disease.

### Wanting to die

Though relatively few severely ill patients actually choose to commit suicide, many go through periods of intense suffering when they wish for death. The physician is in a unique position to lessen the isolation and despair that often accompany such feelings and also to explore potentially unaddressed issues. When such feelings arise, the physician may be asked about his or her willingness to help the patient die. Rather than responding with a "yes" or "no" based on assumptions about what the patient might actually be asking for, the physician should explore the request in detail, including a consideration of why it is occurring at that particular time. Special attention should be paid to untreated depression, anxiety, or pain, and to the emergence of unaddressed psychologic, social, or spiritual issues.

Though treatment alternatives to a physician-assisted death can be found through this exploration, physicians may encounter patients whose suffering is intolerable, whose request is rational, and for whom hospice care alternatives are ineffective or unacceptable. Physicians' responsibilities in caring for such patients are currently under intense debate in the United States, and their potential role in actively assisting such patients to die is controversial and beyond the scope of this chapter. An open discussion of the issue, when raised by a patient, is not controversial, since most often it leads to alternatives to assisted dying. Thoroughly exploring a patient's request for a physician-assisted death does not imply an obligation for the physician to accede. Physicians must consider their own values, the status of the law, and their relationship with the patient before responding.

### Decisions on behalf of incompetent patients

When a patient loses the mental capacity to participate in personal health-care decisions, the physician should first determine if an advance directive has been completed. If it has, then that directive should guide treatment whenever possible. Physicians should not override such directives unless there is substantial evidence that they do not reflect the patient's actual wishes or, rarely, that following such directives creates unresolvable ethical dilemmas for the caregiver. If a proxy has been identified by the patient in the past, that person should be consulted and reminded that his or her job is to represent the patient using the patient's values rather than his or her own. Such a reminder keeps the surrogate focused on the task at hand and can obviate guilt if hard decisions about stopping treatment have to be made. Guilt in the surrogate decision maker can also be minimized by the physician making clear recommendations that are consistent with the patient's values and medical condition, rather than requiring a layperson to make a medical decision without the benefit of professional judgment. Similarly, if a living will has been completed that does not address the exact dilemma faced by the patient, then the physician and the family should take what has been expressed and apply it as best they can to the patient's clinical situation.

Medical decisions also have to be made on behalf of patients who have not completed an advance directive when they lose mental capacity (85% to 90% of the population). Legislation is being considered in several states to formally designate a proxy decision maker from a list of potentially close family members. Until such legislation is enacted, the principle of substituted judgment should guide such decisions. The closest caring family member (or members) should be identified and should help the physician address the potential benefits and burdens of each medical intervention using what is known or can be pieced together about the patient's wishes and values. It is an inexact process. The patient's previously stated wishes, and his or her best interests as perceived by the family and the physician, should always guide such decisions. There is legal and ethical consensus that even life-sustaining treatments can be abated if agreement is reached between the health-care providers and the family about the patient's wishes and best interests.

## ADDITIONAL COMMUNICATION ISSUES

### Listen carefully to and learn from dying patients before intervening

Dying people can become very isolated. Sometimes even close friends and family members are uncomfortable with the dying process and may shy away from intimate contact. Patients need to be listened to and understood in a caring relationship that will be there throughout the dying process until the patient's death. When such patients face a complex dilemma, it should be fully explored and understood before physicians recommend any solution. Rather than shying away from the depths of suffering, the physician should ask questions such as "What is your biggest fear?" and "What is the worst part?" Sometimes this exploration exposes physicians to forms and depths of suffering with which they are unfamiliar and uncomfortable, and which defy resolution. Remember that exploration does not necessarily imply an obligation or ability to resolve. Dying patients do not have a choice about facing such suffering, and one of the most important imperatives of a therapeutic relationship is to do our best to relieve suffering and to lessen the isolation of dying.

### Explore the patient's spirituality and the illness's meaning

Dying is a time when many choose to take a careful look at the meaning of their life and also come to grips with their spirituality and religion. Those who believe in an all-powerful God have to make sense of their becoming irreversibly ill, and all patients must consider what might happen to their families and themselves after death. For some patients there is unfinished business with family members and friends, the resolution of which might help the patient die more peacefully and help the survivors experience the loss in a more healing and less destructive way. Dying patients should be encouraged to identify and take care of such "business" earlier rather than later, since it is better to begin work on such issues prematurely than to miss the opportunity by waiting too long. It is often useful to ask patients how they make sense out of having become ill ("Why me?"), and explicitly ask how they see the future and whether they believe in an afterlife. Such discussions are very rich and meaningful for both doctors and patients and often lead to levels of understanding and connection that are rare in medical practice. Experienced clergy can also be invaluable resources in these explorations.

### Try to help families come together

The death of a patient has far-reaching effects on the family and its dynamics. For some families it is a time of coming together and healing, and for others old conflicts and issues can emerge that appear at times senseless, cruel, and insoluble. These dynamics can exert powerful positive or negative effects on the patient's final days. Family meetings, where everyone has a chance to be heard and to have their questions addressed, can often promote family growth. Though the patient remains the primary focus of the caring, many family members may also need support. Sensitive work with families can often prevent future bereavement problems with guilt, shame, or anger.

Several principles can be helpful in working with families who must help make decisions for a patient who has lost mental capacity:

1. If the patient has completed an advance directive, use it as the foremost guide for decision making.
2. Keep the decision-making focus on the patient's wishes.
3. Family members whose wishes are at apparent odds with the patient's wishes must be asked for information about why they think the patient changed his or her mind.

4. If possible, allow the family time to achieve a consensus on divisive issues rather than forcing a decision.
5. Have a family meeting including all interested parties, and choose a person whom the family trusts (doctor, nurse, clergy, social worker) to facilitate the decision making.
6. Allow family members, particularly those without intimate, longitudinal knowledge about the patient's condition, to spend considerable periods of time at the patient's bedside.
7. Involve medical or nonmedical consultants whom both the physician and the family trust.

### Do not withhold your recommendations and expertise

There is a potential to both overuse and underuse physician power and influence in the care of the dying. Though in the past there may have been excessive paternalism in the physician-patient relationship, the pendulum may have swung so far in the direction of respecting patient autonomy that many physicians are withholding their opinions and recommendations. Since physicians have experience with severe illness and with the benefits and burdens of medical intervention, it is essential that this expertise is shared with patients and families in the form of recommended courses of action. Presenting all the possibilities in a neutral fashion without guidance and direction may be closer to abandonment than it is to respecting patient autonomy. Of course, the patient has the final say after hearing about the options and the physician's recommendation. Physicians should be open about their biases and personal philosophies and should seek to understand those of the patient when there are substantial differences. Major differences should be the subject of mutual exploration and negotiation, with final emphasis on the choice of a fully informed patient.

## PAIN MANAGEMENT

Primary care physicians must become skilled at pain and symptom management if they are to care for severely ill and dying patients. Though specialized pain centers are available at many major medical centers to help with unusual or intractable problems, pain can usually be managed using basic principles and techniques. These include caregiver continuity, careful assessments over time, and individually tailored treatment regimens that often combine pharmacologic and psychosocial/behavioral techniques. The goals of pain management are outlined in the box below.

### Goals of pain management

Identify and address the cause of pain.
Prevent chronic pain.
Erase the memory and expectation of pain.
Allow the patient to remain alert and to function.
Allow patient to experience feelings other than pain.
Intervene as noninvasively as possible.

### Pain assessment

The patient's pain should be assessed thoroughly and treated respectfully. Pain is always subjective—it usually represents an integrated biologic, psychologic, and social experience, and clinicians should attempt to assess its multiple dimensions simultaneously. The patient's report of pain is the most reliable information available.

Pain has consequences. In addition to the unnecessary suffering, patients with unrelieved pain become catabolic, respond less well to other treatments, have greater complication rates, show more emotional disturbance, and sometimes die sooner. Cultural and psychologic factors influence the expression of and tolerance for pain. Factors that aggravate pain include insomnia, fatigue, nausea, anxiety, fear, misunderstanding, anger, shame, sadness, depression, the memory of past pain, and the expectation that pain will recur. Conversely, pain may be lessened with sleep, rest, sympathy, understanding, diversion, relief of other symptoms, and around-the-clock pain medication.

Acute pain has a well-defined temporal onset and may be associated with autonomic nervous system activity such as tachycardia, diaphoresis, elevated blood pressure, pallor, and pupil dilatation. It may serve as a warning or protective purpose. Acute pain is best treated by recognizing and addressing the underlying cause directly and by analgesics, which should be administered around the clock to avoid uncontrolled pain by maintaining steady analgesic blood levels. Acute, episodic pain that is associated with procedures (chest tube insertion or removal, dressing changes, bone marrow aspiration or biopsy, lumbar puncture) can be anticipated and should be treated prophylactically.

Chronic pain may not have a well-defined temporal onset, may last months to years, and may have no signs of autonomic nervous system hyperactivity. Instead, it is often associated with the signs and symptoms of depression including hopelessness, helplessness, anhedonia, appetite and weight change, sleep disturbance, and decreased social interaction. The underlying causes may not be treatable and in some circumstances not clearly identifiable. Chronic pain should always be prevented whenever possible and once identified should be treated aggressively.

The accurate assessment of pain and pain therapy requires a mechanism to facilitate communication about pain intensity between provider and patient. It is useful to ask the patient to rate the pain on a numeric scale, with 0 being no pain and 10 being the worst imaginable pain. After any therapeutic intervention, one needs to learn how much relief was achieved (i.e., where did the pain rating move on the scale) and how long the relief lasted. Intervals between analgesic dosages are adjusted so that the analgesic effect is uninterrupted. The goal of pain management is not necessarily complete absence of pain, but a maximally functional patient. The patient is the ultimate arbitrator of whether the goal has been achieved.

### Pain treatment

This almost always involves a combination of pharmacologic and psychosocial/behavioral techniques.

*Psychosocial and behavioral approaches.* Meditation, self-hypnosis, distraction, humor, psychotherapy, spiritual exploration, hobbies, biofeedback, music, art, and many others approaches can be very effective and helpful. The choice of these techniques depends on the interests and condition of the patient and the presence of skilled practitioners or partners.

***Pharmacologic treatments.*** Drugs are generally effective provided they are utilized skillfully, with knowledge of the underlying pharmacokinetics and without unnecessary fear or restraint. As shown in Table 128-1, an analgesic ladder of progressively stronger medications can be tried in the management of chronic pain. The higher the step, the more analgesic effect, while adverse reactions also become more likely. To treat any chronic pain, analgesics should be taken around the clock. Chronic pain should not be managed solely with as-needed dosing (though prn dosages should be provided for breakthrough pain in between regular dosing intervals). The initial drug dosage and interval are determined by the pharmacologic properties of the specific drug, but the final regimen of any drug should be individualized. Onset, peak effect, and duration of analgesia may vary from person to person due to differences in absorption, organ dysfunction, or tolerance.

The biologic half-life of the analgesic agent must be taken into account when adjusting the dosage and interval. The maximum effect of a given dose may not be seen until the drug has been administered over 4 to 5 half-lives. In addition, the duration of analgesia may be shorter than the half-life, and the half-life may be prolonged in renal or hepatic failure. In the latter situation one should usually administer short-acting agents at longer intervals. Details of the administration of these medications are available in the texts referenced.

Oral medications are generally preferred when possible. Physicians should also be familiar with unique routes of administration (e.g., highly concentrated oral solutions, transdermal patches, subcutaneous infusions) that may be effective in special situations. Subcutaneous, intravenous, and intramuscular injections should be avoided if possible to enhance patient comfort and to minimize the risk to caregivers. Patient-controlled analgesia (within professionally established limits) has been shown to lessen postoperative pain, decrease complications, lead to earlier discharge, and lessen the overall opiate level consumed. Though this concept has been applied most frequently to parenteral pumps, it reinforces the desirability of active patient participation in the selection, assessment, and control of analgesic regimens.

With step 2 and step 3 drugs (see Table 128-1), side effects must be anticipated. Constipation is predictable and should be treated prophylactically. Table 128-2 outlines the treatment of likely side effects.

### Special pain situations

***Parenteral opiates.*** These may be administered after failure of the oral route. Continuous subcutaneous infusion is as effective as intravenous infusion and less invasive. Adding 600 U/L of hyaluronidase allows an increase in the infusible volume to as high as 80 ml per hour (hypodermoclysis). The initial hourly dosage of a constantly infused drug should be one fourth the every 4 hour bolus dose. Boluses of the 1- to 2-hour equivalent amount may be given as a loading dose, before painful procedures, and/or every 15 minutes for breakthrough pain.

Intraspinal (epidural or intrathecal) opiates can provide analgesia at lower dosages and may reduce systemic side effects. This route may be especially useful in acute postoperative pain, particularly after thoracic, abdominal, or pelvic surgery. The equianalgesic epidural dosage of morphine is about one tenth the parenteral dosage, whereas the intrathecal dosage is about one tenth the epidural dosage. The intraspinal route is invasive, expensive, requires close monitoring, and necessitates involvement of an anesthesiologist or pain specialist. Nerve blocks, such as celiac block for the pain of pancreatic cancer, or other sympathetic or neurolytic blocks may also be useful when pain is well localized, especially when systemic analgesia fails because of unacceptable side effects.

***Neuropathic pain.*** This pain is characterized by burning, tingling, numbness, and electrical and pins-and-needles qualities. It accompanies many medical and surgical conditions and is often underdiagnosed. Neuropathic pain does not respond well to conventional analgesics. It may also coexist with other forms of pain. Tricyclic antidepressants are very useful for management, since these agents have a specific analgesic effect lacking in other classes of antidepressants. Compared to the antidepressant effect, pain relief occurs at lower dosages (for desipramine, 10 to 25 mg for pain versus 150 to 300 mg for depression) and sooner (1 to 3 days for analgesia versus 2 to 4 weeks for depression). These drugs are usually started at a low dosage and titrated up to relief of neuropathic pain or the development of side effects. Dosing at night may help with sleeplessness, and these drugs may treat coexisting depression, which can aggravate pain.

Anticonvulsants such as carbamazepine, phenytoin, valproic acid, and clonazepam have been used for the management of neuropathic pain. Carbamazepine seems to be the most predictably effective analgesic. The analgesic dosage is usually the same as the anticonvulsant dosage but may be less. Start low (200 mg twice a day of carbamazepine or even once a day) and follow blood levels until adequate analgesia or a therapeutic range is reached. Mexiletine, an orally administered form of lidocaine, and capsaicin, a topical substance P inhibitor derived from chili peppers, have also been used to treat neuropathic pain. Conventional analgesics may be utilized if these more specific approaches are neither effective nor tolerated.

***Anxiety and depressive disorders.*** These are among the most common conditions seen in the general population, and they are frequently associated with chronic pain or with terminal diseases. These disorders contribute to considerable suffering and can aggravate chronic pain. Anxiety and depression tend to be very responsive to treatment, even in the terminally ill (see Chapter 133). It is important not to overnormalize ("Of course he is depressed; he is dying"), since even depression that is secondary to an overwhelming loss (i.e., terminal illness) may respond to treatment. On the other hand, it is important to remember that not all sadness or anxiety that accompanies grief, loss, or the dying process is part of a disorder. Each patient's unique circumstances should be

**Table 128-1.** The analgesic ladder

| Drug | Equianalgesic dosage | Comments |
|---|---|---|
| **Step 1: Equivalents for mild or moderate pain** | | |
| Acetaminophen (Tylenol, Datril, Panadol) | 650 mg | No antiinflammatory effect; does not inhibit platelet function; avoid in liver failure |
| Aspirin, ASA | 650 mg | Avoid during pregnancy, in hemostatic disorders, in GI or GU bleeding, preoperatively, and in patients under age 18; may precipitate asthma |
| Nonsteroidal antiinflammatory drug (NSAID) (various) | | Like ASA; also useful with opiates for pain of bone metastases |
| Ketorolac (Toradol) | 30 mg | IM preparation with all NSAID side effects; expensive |
| Choline magnesium trisalicylate (Trilisate) | 1500 mg | Antiinflammatory; dose does not inhibit platelet function; every 12 hr dosing |
| Propoxyphene napsylate (Darvon) | 100 mg | Opiate with potentially toxic metabolite; used with acetaminophen (Darvocet-N); does not inhibit platelet function or cause GI upset or bleeding; may be habituating; not recommended |
| **Step 2: Equivalents for moderate pain** | | |
| Codeine | 30-60 mg | Often used in combination with acetaminophen or ASA (325 mg); analgesic effect plateaus in adults receiving more than 120 mg q4hr |
| Hydrocodone (Hycodan) | 5-10 mg | Combined with acetaminophen (500 mg) (Vicodin) |
| Oxycodone (Roxicodone) | 5-10 mg | Used in combination with ASA (Percodan, Roxiprin) or acetaminophen (Percocet, Tylox, Roxicet); upper limit of dosing not defined except for combination preparations |
| Meperidine (Demerol) | 50 mg | Short acting (about 2 hr); toxic metabolite causes irritability and seizures with repeated dosing; parenteral dose one-third oral dose; not recommended |
| Pentazocine (Talwin) | 50 mg | Combined with naloxone to discourage abuse; mixed antagonist, may precipitate opiate withdrawal when given subsequent to pure antagonists; not recommended |

*Continued.*

**Table 128-1.** The analgesic ladder—cont'd

| Drug | Equianalgesic dosage | Comments |
|---|---|---|
| **Step 3: Equivalents for severe pain** | | |
| Morphine | 10 mg 20-30 mg | Standard against which all other analgesics are judged; available as several different preparations:<br>2 or 4 mg/ml oral solution (MSIR oral solution) when low doses needed<br>20 mg/ml concentrated oral solution (Roxanol, OMS Concentrate, MSIR oral solution concentrate) absorbed sublingually when patient is NPO or has difficulty swallowing; used when higher doses indicated<br>Sustained-release tablet (MS Contin, Oramorph SR); 15, 30, 60, 100 mg; lasts 8-12 hr instead of 3-4 hr; titrate first with rapid acting preparations for 24 hr, then divide into 2-3 doses for ATC administration of sustained release tablet; continue short-acting preparation PRN for breakthrough pain; may be used rectally; do not crush tablet<br>Immediate release tablet (MSIR tablets), 15 and 30 mg, short acting<br>Rectal suppositories (MS/S or RMS suppositories), short acting, 5, 10, 20, 30 mg per suppository<br>Also indicated for intractable dyspnea; no upper limit to morphine dosing, but it is relatively ineffective for neuropathic pain; see text for discussion of parenteral use |
| Hydromorphone (Dilaudid) | 1.5 mg 7.5 mg | Like morphine; duration of action 3-4 hr; 2, 3, 4, 8 mg tablets, 3 mg rectal suppositories, and 1, 2, 4, 10 mg/ml parenteral solutions available |
| Methadone (Dolophine) | 10 mg 20 mg | Give q6-8hr for pain, not qd; will accumulate with repeated dosing; equianalgesic dosage may cause unacceptable persistent sedation, so should be reduced on the third or fourth day of titration |
| Levorphanol (Levo-Dromoran) | 2 mg 4 mg | Like methadone |
| Meperidine (Demerol) | 75 mg 300 mg | See step 2; not recommended |
| Fentanyl (Duragesic) | 25, 50, 75 and 100 μg patches | 25, 50, 75, and 100 μg patches (Duragesic); 25 μg patch approximates morphine 10 mg parenterally or 20-30 mg PO 4 hr; with transdermal patch, steady state reached only after 24 hr, so other analgesics needed in interim; replace q72hr at different site; fever may lead to increased levels; skin reservoir causes long half-life (50% 17 hr after removal), so careful monitoring required; most useful in stable pain situations |

*GI*, Gastrointestinal; *GU*, genitourinary.

**Table 128-2.** Anticipate opioid side effects

| Side effect | Treatment | Comments |
|---|---|---|
| Constipation | Bisacodyl (Ducolax), 250 mg 1-2 bid and/or Senna (Senekot), 1-2 bid and/or MOM 30-60 ml qd or bid | Prophylactic better than PRN for step 2 and 3 drugs<br>Avoid bulk laxatives |
| Sedation | Decrease dosage or increase interval of opiate<br>Dextroamphetamine, 2.5-7.5 mg q6hr | Tolerance to sedation usually develops in 24-72 hr<br>Sedation usually appears well before respiratory depression<br>Avoid naloxone, which will cause major withdrawal |
| Nausea | Antihistamines, phenothiazines, butyrophenones, scopolamine, metoclopramide, steroids | Trial and error<br>Be sure nausea is not secondary to constipation<br>Be aware of drug-specific side effects (e.g., dystonic reaction with phenothiazines or metoclopramide) |

*MOM,* Milk of magnesia.

thoroughly explored with the hope of finding a way to lessen suffering.

***Patients with a history of substance abuse.*** Whether the substance is opiates, alcohol, or other chemicals, this situation presents complex pain management dilemmas. History should include the drug(s) of choice, route, dosage, and frequency of use, including time of last dose. Withdrawal must be recognized and treated. Because of physiologic tolerance, regular users of opiates require stronger analgesics and larger dosages to achieve the same analgesic effect compared to those who are opiate-naive. Effective pain management cannot take place until acute substance abuse issues such as prevention and treatment of withdrawal are addressed and brought under control. However, drug rehabilitation during an acute hospitalization for other major medical or surgical problems is seldom appropriate. Including substance abuse caregivers in the plan of care is helpful.

The patient in recovery from abuse who develops a chronic pain problem requires an open discussion regarding the risks and benefits of opioid analgesics, including the potential of addiction relapse. If opioids are needed, active and recovering substance users may best be treated with a long-acting oral preparation given at scheduled times. Needles, which can be the environmental trigger for drug craving, should generally be avoided. Prescribing contracts, which include mutually agreed upon amounts and dosages renewed at fixed, relatively frequent intervals, are often helpful.

Patients without a history of abuse do not become addicted when opiates are prescribed for acute pain. Health-care providers must not allow this fear to prevent patients in their care from receiving adequate analgesia. We must also understand that some patients exhibit drug-seeking behavior because no physician has adequately assessed or provided treatment for their pain. Chronic pain in the terminally ill must not be undertreated out of physician fear or ignorance.

***Other physical symptoms.*** Nausea, vomiting, diarrhea, constipation, open wounds, confusion, incontinence, and many others symptoms may develop in dying patients, may aggravate pain or suffering, and may undermine quality of life. It is beyond the scope of this chapter to explore the treatment of each of these symptoms, but strategies for approaching them are published in the hospice literature. Experienced hospice physicians and nurses can be consulted in circumstances where a patient has developed a particularly intractable physical symptom. Though not all such symptoms can be relieved with available interventions, many can be improved or at least made tolerable.

## FINAL RECOMMENDATIONS

Caring for dying patients and their families can be a uniquely rewarding facet of primary care practice. Although dying is physiologically destructive, it may be psychologically, socially, and spiritually constructive. Facilitating this growth can be enormously gratifying. Dying patients need a knowledgeable guide, witness, and friend who will commit to facing the unknown with them through the entire process no matter where it goes. The prospect of enduring severe illness and death in our culture with all the inherent medical possibilities without a caring physician at one's side must be daunting. Having known the patient when healthy, and having weathered disease processes too, the primary care physician is often in an ideal position to take on this role.

To prepare for this responsibility, primary care physicians should undertake several activities. First, they should articulate their own personal end-of-life philosophy and put it in writing in some form of advance directive. Physicians who have not personally been through this process are often unpersuasive in encouraging their patients to complete their own advance directives, and they may be less open about their own beliefs and recommendations as they help those who are facing death. Second, primary care physicians must become expert at hospice care, including basic palliative measures used to relieve severe pain and other symptoms. Third, primary care physicians should extend themselves in the intensive caring of their dying patients and their families. This includes compassion and creative problem solving in the face of considerable uncertainty. Finally, they must commit to caring for and working with their dying patients, no matter what course their illnesses take, through to their deaths. The promise not to abandon may be the most fundamental aspect of our commitment as primary care physicians to our dying patients.

## BIBLIOGRAPHY


Annas G: The health care proxy and the living will, *N Engl J Med* 324:1210, 1991.

Foley K: The treatment of cancer pain, *N Engl J Med* 313:84, 1985.

Jacox A et al: Management of cancer pain. Clinical practice guideline No. 9. ACHPAR Publication No. 94-0592, Rockville, MD, Agency for Health Policy and Research, U.S. Department of Health and Human Services, Public Health Service, March 1994.

Meisel A: Legal myths about terminating life support, *Arch Intern Med* 151:1497, 1991.

Miranda J, Brody RV: Communicating bad news, *West J Med* 156(1):83, 1992.

Patt RB, editor: *Cancer pain,* Philadelphia, 1993, JB Lippincott.

Quill TE: Bad news: delivery, dialogue and dilemmas, *Arch Intern Med* 151:463, 1990.

Quill TE: *Death and dignity: making choices and taking charge,* New York, 1993, WW Norton.

Quill TE: "Doctor, I want to die. Will you help me?" *JAMA* 270:841, 1993.

Quill TE: Partnerships in patient care: a contractual approach, *Ann Intern Med* 98:228, 1983.

Quill TE, Brody RV: "You promised me I wouldn't die like this." A bad death as a medical emergency, *Arch Intern Med* 155:1250, 1995.

Quill TE, Cassel CK: Nonabandonment: a central obligation for physicians, *Ann Intern Med* 122:368, 1995.

Solomon MZ et al: Decisions near the end of life: professional views on life-sustaining treatment, *Am J Public Health* 83:14, 1993.

Stoddard S: Hospice in the United States: an overview, *J Palliative Care* 5:10, 1989.

Tomlinson T, Brody H: Ethics and communication in do-not-resuscitate orders, *N Engl J Med* 318:43, 1988.

Wallston KA et al: Comparing the quality of death for hospice and nonhospice cancer patients, *Medical Care* 26:177, 1986.


CHAPTER

# 129A Primary Care of Lesbians


**Jocelyn C. White**
**Wendy Levinson**


The care of lesbians has received little attention, and medical literature rarely addresses the needs of this group. Lesbians may comprise up to 10% of the female population, a large group of patients with unique medical, psychologic, and social needs. According to current theories a lesbian's sexual orientation is most likely determined by a combination of biologic and environmental factors. The dictionary definition of a lesbian is "a female homosexual," meaning a woman who is sexually attracted to other women. For practical purposes this definition is too narrow because lesbianism is not only a sexual orientation but also an identity based on emotions and psychologic responses, societal expectations, and the individual's own choices in identity formation. Therefore some women call themselves lesbians but are not sexually active with women; conversely some are sexually active with women but do not identify as lesbians. Most lesbians prefer the term lesbian as opposed to gay or homosexual because it also refers to emotions, behavior, and a cultural system.

Lesbians are a diverse group of women from all racial, economic, geographic, religious, cultural, and age populations. Despite this diversity lesbians have formed a culture of their own replete with music, art, literature, history, spiritual beliefs, ethics, and politics. In New York City in 1969, in response to police harassment and brutality directed against the gay and lesbian community, clients of a bar called Stonewall and other community members rioted. The Stonewall riot marked the beginning of the modern gay and lesbian era. Many older women who developed their lesbian identity before Stonewall feel less connected to this culture and community. These older women may be more reluctant to reveal their identity even to peers because of experiences with or fears of discrimination. The lesbian community is an important source of support to many women and often provides an alternative family or kin group to its members. Community resources may also be of use to physicians looking for lesbian-sensitive referrals for social services, counseling, or peer support.

Lesbians are also a diverse group in terms of sexual practices. They may be celibate or sexually active with women, men, or both. Most lesbians are currently either sexually active with women exclusively or are celibate, although in one study 77% of lesbians had at some point participated in heterosexual coitus. The specific sexual practices of an individual patient determine her risks of particular diseases and are important in developing individual medical recommendations.

Unfortunately there is limited scientific information about the lesbian population. The few clinical studies available are methodologically flawed by sample bias or small sample size, and clinicians may not be able to generalize from these results. In other areas, such as cancer risks and screening, specific information about lesbians is unavailable, but inferences can be drawn from larger epidemiologic studies of women.

## THE PHYSICIAN-PATIENT INTERACTION

Many lesbians are reluctant to share their sexual orientation with physicians for fear of negative judgments and homophobic responses. Some lesbians do not share this information even when asked. Negative experiences with health care professionals make lesbian patients more likely to terminate care and avoid routine screening. On the other hand, physicians may feel inexperienced in dealing with lesbian health issues or uncomfortable deciding what language to use to elicit information sensitively. Because of both patient and physician discomfort, important information is often not shared.

An effective physician-patient interaction has three functions: information gathering, rapport building, and patient education. This framework also applies to the interaction between a physician and a lesbian. The physician should ask questions of all women that will (1) elicit information needed to identify lesbian patients and provide appropriate medical care; (2) develop a nonjudgmental attitude that conveys a sense of acceptance; and (3) provide educational information, resources, and referrals sensitive to the needs of lesbians.

Gathering information from female patients about the lesbian lifestyle and sexual practices is the first stumbling block encountered by practitioners. The most commonly used patient interview questions often lead to inaccurate or incomplete information. They set up barriers for the

### Helpful questions in taking a history

**When a woman's sexual orientation is unknown**

Who do you consider to be in your immediate family?
Are you single, partnered, or married?
Are you in an intimate relationship with a man or woman?
Are your sex partners men, women, or both?
Do you have a need for contraception?
If you become ill, is there someone important to you whom I should involve in your care?

**When a woman is identified as a lesbian**

Have you told you family and friends that you are a lesbian?
Are you "out" at work?
Who do you consider part of your support system?
Do you have any questions about having or raising children?
Do you experience any stress because you're a lesbian?
Have you ever been harassed because you're lesbian?

### How to indicate acceptance of lesbian patients

Include *living with a partner* or *living as a couple* along with *married* and *single* as options on office forms.
Use the term *spouse or partner* on office forms.
Include the possibility that a partner may wish to be included in next-of-kin and advance directive discussions.
Train staff not to use "Mrs." to address all women patients.
Display brochures on lesbian health issues.
Compile and use lesbian-sensitive educational materials and community resources.
Ask patients about their preferences for documenting sexual orientation in the chart and discuss options.
Ask patients if they would like their partner to participate in the medical visit.

lesbian patient because they assume she is heterosexual: "What form of birth control do you use?" "Are you married?" and "When was the last time you had intercourse?" are common examples. Examples of questions that facilitate communication are shown in the box above and include: "Have you ever had sex with men, women, or both?" "Are you in an intimate relationship with a man or a woman?" "Who do you include in your immediate family?"

Physicians should ask these questions of all women from adolescence through old age. Not uncommonly physicians have the misperception that the sexual history is important only for patients in their reproductive years. It is important to recognize elderly lesbians because of their risk of social isolation. Physicians may be a significant source of support to these patients.

Once a physician has demonstrated a nonjudgmental approach and asked questions sensitively, a trusting relationship is more likely to develop. Sensitivity to important concerns of the lesbian patient improves rapport (see the box above, right). For example, offering to include a partner in discussions and ensuring that she has access to patient care areas such as the delivery room or intensive care unit demonstrate acceptance. The physician also builds rapport by discussing the stresses of homophobia and exploring the patient's perceptions of the health care system. In addition, physicians can ensure that all next-of-kin policies and discussions of advance directives include the possibility of a lesbian partner. Physicians may also show acceptance by ensuring that office and hospital forms use wording that recognizes alternative family structures such as "living with a partner" or "living as a couple" in addition to "spouse."

Providing education for lesbian patients involves physician self-education as well as compilation of reference materials and brochures with information specific to lesbians. Verbal instruction in preventing the transmission of sexually transmitted diseases, including HIV, should be clear and specific to lesbian sexual practices. Physicians should educate lesbians about risks for cervical cancer based on sexual history and be able to counsel or refer patients for counseling about issues including parenting, coming out, battery, and hate crimes. Referrals should include other providers and community-based resources sensitive to the needs of lesbians.* Hotlines, book stores, and bibliographies can help educate. Youth groups and senior groups, community centers, lesbian and gay religious organizations and retirement centers, and counselors who deal with lesbian issues provide support. Gay and lesbian substance abuse support groups are also available.

Finally, it is important for physicians to discuss explicitly with lesbians the documentation of sexual orientation in the chart. We suggest that if a patient does not want her lesbian identity documented, physicians may consider using a coded entry in the chart. This provides physicians with a record to remind them about the patient's sexual orientation but prevents inadvertent breaches of confidentiality through use of the chart.

## SEXUALLY TRANSMITTED DISEASES

Sexually transmitted diseases (STDs) in lesbian patients are less common than in either heterosexual women or in gay males. This may be due in part to the relative epidemiologic isolation of this population from men and the lack of penile-vaginal intercourse among lesbians. Lesbian sexual practices include kissing, breast stimulation, manual and oral stimulation of the genitals and anus, friction of the clitoris against the partner's body, and penetration of the vagina and anus with fingers and devices. There are no gynecologic problems unique to lesbians and none that occur more often in lesbians than in bisexual or heterosexual women.

Based on uncontrolled clinical and survey data, lesbians appear to have a lower incidence of syphilis and gonorrhea than any other population except those who have never been sexually active at all. Therefore routine screening forthese diseases in lesbians does not appear

*For further information and referral sources for lesbian and gay health issues contact Gay and Lesbian Medical Association, 273 Church Street, San Francisco, CA 94114, (415) 255-4547.

to be cost effective. Testing is appropriate only in the setting of other risk factors, particularly recent heterosexual exposure.

Other STDs common among heterosexual women are reported rarely related to the lesbian population. *Chlamydia* and herpes organisms are rarely found in lesbians who have been sexually active exclusively with women. Herpes can be transmitted between women, but the prevalence in the lesbian population seems to be low. Pelvic inflammatory disease (PID) also appears to be rare among lesbians. Venereal warts caused by human papillomavirus (HPV) are uncommon unless the patient has had heterosexual contact. However, because women with venereal warts may theoretically transmit them to their female partners, partners should also be evaluated. Unlike in the gay male population, enteric infections due to hepatitis A, *Amoeba, Shigella,* and helminths have a low prevalence in lesbians. Hepatitis B does not occur unless other risk factors are present.

In contrast to STDs, vaginitis commonly occurs in lesbians. Little is known about the transmission of nonspecific vaginitis, more recently called bacterial vaginosis. Physicians should inquire about vaginal discharge in lesbians and evaluate those partners of infected patients who have symptoms. Although bisexual women report vaginal candidiasis more often than do lesbians, probably because of heterosexual contact, transmission between women is possible. Partners of lesbians with vaginal candidiasis should be treated.

*Trichomonas vaginalis* bacteria have been found in women sexually active exclusively with women, women with no sexual contact at all, and lesbians with a bisexual woman as contact. This infection can be transmitted by fomites such as damp towels and underwear or possibly by hand/genital contact. Based on this information, clinicians should include *Trichomonas* infection in the differential diagnosis of vaginal discharge in lesbians. Sexual partners of lesbians diagnosed with *Trichomonas* infection should also be treated. Screening recommendations for STDs in lesbians are summarized in the box below.

## HIV AND AIDS

As of June 1991 the Centers for Disease Control (CDC) had reported 164 cases of AIDS in lesbians. About 93% of these women were intravenous drug users. To date, transmission of HIV between women as a result only of sexual contact may have occurred in up to nine cases but is not proven. Exposure to menstrual and traumatic bleeding was probably the source of transmission. However, HIV has been cultured from cervical and vaginal secretions and cervical biopsies taken throughout the menstrual cycle. Therefore HIV may theoretically be transmitted by infected women who are not bleeding. However, because of the low rate of transmission from infected women to men in the general population, the rate of transmission between women is probably also low.

Although the prevalence of HIV infection is low in lesbians without risk factors, physicians should counsel lesbians to avoid contact with cervical and vaginal secretions, menstrual blood, and blood from vaginal and rectal trauma in partners who have not been tested negative for the virus. Methods believed to protect against transmission for oral-genital contact include latex squares, known as dental dams, and latex condoms or gloves cut open and laid flat. For vaginal penetration, latex gloves used on hands and condoms on sexual toys may be appropriate.

Lesbians who undergo artificial insemination with either fresh semen from donors in the community or frozen semen from sperm banks are also at risk for HIV infection. Sperm banks routinely test donors for HIV infection at the time of donation and 6 months later before releasing the sample for use. However, because of delays in seroconversion, it is possible for lesbians to be exposed to HIV with fresh semen from a seronegative donor. Lesbians should avoid fresh semen, especially fresh semen from donors with an unknown HIV status.

In general, recommendations to test lesbians for HIV infection should therefore be based on individual risk factors. Physicians should recommend safer sex practices with partners whose HIV status is unknown and screening of all sperm donors.

### STD screening recommendations for lesbians

Syphilis, gonorrhea, chlamydial infection, and pelvic inflammatory disease are unusual in women who are sexually active only with women.

Routine screening for STDs is probably not necessary.

Partners of lesbians with STDs, herpes, HPV, and vaginosis should be evaluated.

## CANCER

There are no population-based studies of gynecologic and breast cancer risk in lesbians. As a result, cancer screening decisions in lesbians should be based on individual risk factors using standard screening guidelines for women. Based on their sexual and reproductive histories, however, the incidence of certain cancers in lesbians differs.

Cervical cancer appears less common among lesbians than among bisexual or heterosexual women as suggested by lower rates of dysplasia and abnormal Pap smears. This is most likely due to decreased exposure to risk factors for cervical cancer, such as early age of first coitus with a man, total number of heterosexual contacts, infection with HPV, and possibly herpes simplex II virus. Current American Cancer Society (ACS) recommendations and other preventive health guidelines give no information for cervical cancer screening in women who are celibate or who are sexually active with women only. In the absence of appropriate data, we recommend screening these women every 3 years, similar to the ACS maintenance screening interval. Women with a history of significant heterosexual contact or other known risk factors should be screened according to published guidelines.

There is also no specific information on breast cancer, endometrial cancer, or ovarian cancer in lesbians. Epidemiologic studies suggest an increased risk of breast cancer among nulliparous women, women who are older with their first birth, and women who have never breastfed. Many lesbians fall into these categories, and their physicians should adhere to current guidelines for breast examination and mammography.

Ovarian cancer has been reported to occur more frequently in women who have not used oral contraception and those who have not given birth. Endometrial cancer is also more common in nulliparous women. The association between nulliparity and cancers of the ovary and endometrium may be due partly, however, to infertility and the use of fertility drugs in nulliparous women. Based on these risk factors, some lesbians may be at a slightly higher risk for ovarian and endometrial cancers. Therefore physicians should follow current guidelines on screening for these cancers where available.

## PARENTING AND REPRODUCTIVE ISSUES

Parenting plays a role in the lives of many lesbians. Lesbians may have children from previous heterosexual relationships, from adoption, by artificial insemination, or by being a foster parent. Some members of society oppose motherhood for lesbians due to concerns about the sexual development and sexual orientation of the children. However, studies have not demonstrated differences between children raised by lesbians and those raised by heterosexuals. Open communication with children about parents' lesbianism appears important in family function.

Most lesbians who wish to conceive find artificial insemination, also called alternative insemination or alternative fertilization, the preferred method. Legal statutes regarding artificial insemination vary from state to state, but most refer only to married women and assume a physician will do the procedure, as opposed to a woman performing insemination at home, which is often the case. Some physicians feel uncomfortable performing artificial insemination for lesbians, and the law is unclear regarding a physician's responsibility and liability toward a lesbian who has been inseminated. We and others believe it is ethically justifiable for physicians to inseminate lesbians but should not be mandated. A physician who feels unable to comply with a patient's wishes should refer the patient to another provider for the service.

A pregnant lesbian may find it more difficult than other women to find social or family support for her pregnancy. The development of her identity as a mother may also be more complex. Primary care physicians can support the pregnant lesbian by demonstrating nonjudgmental attitudes, encouraging acceptance of lesbian motherhood among members of the obstetric team and childbearing classes, and including partners in the process of conception, prenatal care, and delivery.

## PSYCHOSOCIAL AND PSYCHOLOGIC ISSUES

The American Psychiatric Association removed homosexuality from its list of mental illnesses in 1973. In general, psychologic illness is no more common in lesbians than in heterosexual women. Lesbians do experience unique psychosocial stressors, however, that often affect their physical and emotional health. The issues most relevant for primary care physicians include homophobia, "coming out," alcohol abuse, suicide, lesbian battery, and hate crimes.

Stress experienced by lesbians may be a result of a conflict between who they really are and the identity they express to the outside world. Although lesbians' self-esteem is similar to that of heterosexual women, lesbians often find it difficult to act in accordance with their identity because of society's negative attitudes, known as homophobia. Societal attitudes may be compounded by the lesbian's own internal homophobia developed from years of living in an intolerant society.

Evaluation of a lesbian patient's support network is necessary to determine her ability to cope with these and other stressful life events. Lesbians most often derive support from partners, friends, and lesbian and gay community organizations. The quality of the relationship with a partner can be particularly important to a lesbian's psychologic well-being. Discord in a lesbian couple can be even more stressful than for a married heterosexual couple because of a lack of traditional social support.

The process of discovering one's sexual orientation and revealing it to others, known as coming out, may begin at any age and may be associated with significant emotional distress. The process of coming out has been well described. It involves a shift in core identity that takes place in four stages: (1) awareness of homosexual feelings; (2) testing and exploration; (3) identity acceptance; and (4) identity integration and disclosure to others. Prevailing social attitudes influence the experience of coming out. Internalized and societal homophobia cause the lesbian to perform a sophisticated and fatiguing cost benefit analysis for each situation in which she considers coming out. If the costs are high, she may ultimately become socially isolated or deny the identity. Lesbian adolescents are particularly vulnerable to the emotional distress of coming out, and this distress often confounds their developmental tasks. Parental acceptance during this process, especially maternal, may be the primary determinant of the development of healthy self-esteem in adolescent lesbians. Signs of sexual orientation confusion in adolescents may include depression, diminished school performance, alcohol and substance abuse, acting out, and suicidal ideation. In fact, gay and lesbian youth are two to three times more likely to attempt suicide and may account for 30% of completed youth suicides. It is important for the primary care provider to screen adolescents for these signs and to consider sexual orientation confusion in the differential diagnosis of depression and substance use.

As part of a comprehensive clinical evaluation, primary care providers should screen all women, including their lesbian patients, for alcohol abuse, depression, and violence. Alcohol use may be up to three times more common in lesbians than in heterosexual women. These figures may be artificially elevated because lesbians surveyed may not be representative of the population, and rates of alcohol abuse may have changed since these studies were conducted. A recent national mail survey from a lesbian publication reported that 59% of subjects had used alcohol to cope with stress and 42% had considered suicide. Violence is an issue in lesbians as well as heterosexual relationships. One small study reported that among lesbians aged 22 to 52 years about 38% had experienced battery by a partner, and alcohol or drug use was involved in 64% of these incidents.

Hate crimes, or bias crimes, against lesbians, including verbal abuse, threats of violence, property damage, physical violence, and murder are increasing each year. Lesbians at universities report being victims of sexual assault twice as frequently as heterosexual women. According to a study for the US Department of Justice, lesbians and gay men may be the most victimized group in the nation. Perpetrators of hate crimes often include family members and community authorities. About 25% of lesbians in a Philadelphia study reported being the victim of a crime committed by a family member. Many gay and lesbian adolescents may leave home because of abuse related to their sexual orientation. The primary care provider should be aware of the possibility that a patient has been a victim of violence, particularly when patients present with symptoms of depression or anxiety.

• • •

Many primary care providers are caring for lesbian patients without recognizing their sexual orientation or their unique medical and psychologic needs. Enhanced knowledge and skills allow these physicians to provide optimal and sensitive patient care for lesbians. Clearly, much more research on this group is needed to provide appropriate guidelines for clinicians.

## BIBLIOGRAPHY

Byne W, Parsons B: Human sexual orientation, *Arch Gen Psychiatry* 50:228, 1993.

Patterson CJ: Children of lesbian and gay parents, *Child Dev* 63:1025, 1992.

Stevens PE: Lesbian health care research: a review of the literature from 1970 to 1990, *Health Care Women Int* 13:91, 1992.

White J, Levinson W: Primary care of lesbian patients, *J Gen Intern Med* 8:41, 1993.

CHAPTER

# 129B Primary Care of Gay Men

**Michael J. Clement**

In the last decade gay men's health care issues have focused almost entirely on infection with the human immunodeficiency virus (HIV). In fact, gay men's health care and HIV and AIDS have become virtually synonymous in many major metropolitan areas. Before the HIV epidemic the medical literature had few references to the primary care of gay men, except for the treatment of sexually transmitted diseases. Therefore primary care physicians have had rare opportunities for training in the care of the non–HIV-infected gay man (Fig. 129B-1).

This chapter addresses common medical and psychologic problems seen in gay men—problems that make the provision of health care for this population somewhat different from that for the general male population. The objectives of this chapter also include providing the reader with an understanding of homophobia: how it affects access to health care by gay men and how heterosexual assumptions regarding health care can make gay men uncomfortable when seeking care.

Finally, it is emphasized that the health care concerns of gay men are really not much different from those of heterosexual men. Gay men worry about their cholesterol level, their risk for coronary artery disease, diabetes, and colon or prostate cancer. Gay men are concerned about the cost and availability of health care and the rights of their lover or partner, as expressed in the durable power of attorney.

## CREATING A SAFE ENVIRONMENT

Homophobia has been described as the irrational hatred and fear of people based solely upon their sexual orientation. This irrational fear has led to many untrue assumptions about gay men. In creating a safe environment for gay male patients, practitioners must first confront their own homophobia and assess how their own beliefs may affect the creation of a safe and friendly environment for the patient. Confronting one's own homophobia might begin with challenging some of these assumptions, for example: that something must have happened to a person to make him gay, like having a passive father or a domineering mother; that somehow gay men had a choice about whether or not they were homosexual or heterosexual; that being gay is some kind of immature or transient developmental phase; that gay people recruit other people to be gay; that gay people should not be able to be publicly affectionate; that gay people are sex crazed; or that gay people are incapable of committed, stable, relationships. Reducing these assump-

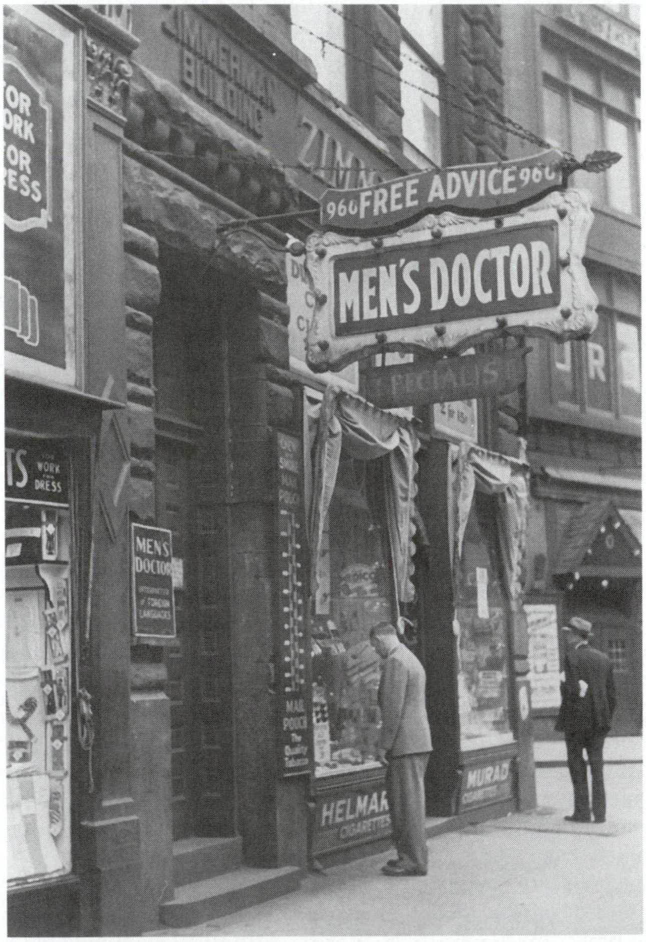


**Fig. 129B-1.** Men's clinic in the early 1900s. (Courtesy Library of Congress.)

tions and discarding them are major steps toward creating an emotionally safe environment for a gay patient.

A large health maintenance organization recently held a focus group for gay male patients and asked them questions about what was important with respect to their health care. Specifically, they were asked whether it was important that their provider be gay. None of the patients on this focus group panel said that it was important that their provider be gay. This is an important point. Gay men do not care if their providers are gay or straight, male or female. They do care that the provider provides a safe environment and that they are treated with dignity. It was also important that their partners be acknowledged and treated with dignity and respect.

## WHO IS THE GAY MALE PATIENT?

It is important to realize that behavior does not necessarily equal identity. This means that, although some men may have sex with other men, they may not consider themselves gay or bisexual. There are many men whose primary sexual partners are other men, but who are married to women. There are gay men who are celibate. There are gay men who live in monogamous, long-term relationships and others who live in nonmonogamous, nontraditional, or open, relationships. It is important to realize that the gay male population is as diverse as the straight male population. Men who have sex with men are members of every race and every culture, but these men may not identify as gay men because of their cultural or racial heritage. Therefore taking a sexual history relies upon focusing on behavior, rather than labels of sexual practice. An initial question when taking a sexual history could be: "Are your sexual partners women, men, or both?" This avoids the stigmatizing labels of gay or bisexual, labels that some cultures do not accept. Another sexual history question could be: "Do you have a partner?" or "Are you married?" The term *partner* (as opposed to wife) conveys the provider's sensitivity to the issue of sexual preference. Another strategy for taking a sexual history could be to open that part of the history with the question: "Do you consider yourself at risk for infection with HIV? For example, have you ever had a blood transfusion, or have you shared needles, or have your partners been women, men, or both?" This question conveys the provider's concern about the risk for HIV infection but also places the issue of sexual preference in the context of a legitimate health concern.

After ascertaining sexual preference, all patients should be asked whether they understand the term *safer sex* regardless of their sexual preference. Having the patients define safer sex allows the provider to immediately educate the patient on safer sexual practices. Though it is not necessarily part of the routine history to ascertain specific sexual practices of the gay male patient, it is important for the provider to understand the range of sexual expressions practiced by gay men. Sexual practices include mutual masturbation, fellatio, anal intercourse, and anilingus. Sadomasochistic and bracheopractic activities (fisting) also occur but are much less common.

## SPECIFIC MEDICAL ISSUES FOR GAY MEN

Substance abuse issues in gay male patients have most recently been studied amongst those gay men who are HIV infected. Relatively fewer studies have looked at the non–HIV-infected gay male population. Accurate estimates of the prevalence of substance abuse do not exist for alcoholism, tobacco addiction, or the use of methamphetamine or marijuana. Obtaining an appropriate history is vital for gay men and heterosexual men.

Specific medical problems that occur in gay men include proctitis, caused by *Neisseria gonorrhoeae,* herpes simplex virus, chlamydial infection, and syphilis. Human papillomavirus (HPV) can cause anogenital warts. When warts occur in the perianal area, there is believed to be an increased incidence of the development of anal cancer. Therefore all gay men should have careful inspection of their perianal area. If perianal venereal warts exist, digital rectal examination should not be done because of the risk of possible spread of the perianal warts into the anal canal. Because of the risk for anal cancer, these warts should be aggressively treated. Gastrointestinal parasites occur with increased frequency in gay men. *Entamoeba histolytica* and *Giardia lamblia* are both common parasites and can occur as asymptomatic infections in gay men. *Salmonella, shigella,* and *Campylobacter* organisms can all produce proctitis or colitis. Urethritis may be present, caused by *N. gonorrhoeae* or *Chlamydia trachomatis.* Pharyngitis in a gay man should raise the possibility of gonorrhea, herpes, or candidal infections. Hepatitis A, B, and C all occur with increased frequency in gay men. All gay men should be screened for hepatitis B, and if there is no serologic evidence of previous infection of hepatitis B, they should be vaccinated.

Any gay man who presents with a sexually transmitted disease has, by definition, engaged in unsafe sexual practices. This patient must be carefully counseled with respect to unsafe sexual practices and the risk for HIV infection. He should also probably be tested for HIV infection.

## PSYCHOLOGIC ISSUES FOR THE GAY MALE PATIENT

In major metropolitan areas it is not uncommon for non–HIV-infected gay men to have lost many friends or lovers to HIV infection. Some of these men identify themselves as the last survivor of a group of friends and may present with depression. Some may engage in self-destructive behaviors, including excessive alcohol or drug use or engaging in unsafe sexual practices.

Younger gay men moving into major metropolitan areas have also recently been identified as being at increased risk for new infections with HIV. This is primarily because young gay males do not identify themselves as being at risk for HIV disease. Instead, they consider the HIV epidemic as a problem of older gay men who had engaged in unsafe sexual practices during the early 1980s. Reiterating the risk for HIV infection to these young gay men is crucial. Providers caring for adolescent gay males should also be aware that, of adolescent males who commit suicide, an estimated one third are gay. Obviously issues around sexual preference should be addressed with any depressed adolescent male.

## SUMMARY

Effective, comprehensive primary care of the gay male begins with the creation of a emotionally safe environment by the health care provider. Our ability to provide this environment is enhanced by our willingness to confront our own heterosexual assumptions and homophobia.

Few specific medical needs differ for the gay male as opposed to the heterosexual male. Issues of substance abuse, tobacco use, safer sexual practices, sexually transmitted diseases, and psychologic well-being are obviously pertinent to all men, gay or straight. Providers should be aware, however, of HPV infection and its role in the development of anal cancer; of commonly practiced sexual activities and how they may predispose patients to pharyngitis, proctitis, urethritis; of the sometimes devastating psychologic impact of the HIV epidemic upon the non–HIV-infected sole survivor patient; and of the high risk for suicide among gay male adolescents.

**Examples of clues to alcohol problems**

Psychosocial symptoms: marital problems, drunken driving, anxiety, depression
Medical syndromes: pancreatitis, gastritis, withdrawal signs (high blood pressure, odor of alcohol, edema, jaundice)
Trauma: fall at home or elsewhere, motor vehicle accident
Alcohol talk: high quantity, intoxication, "partying"

CHAPTER

# 130 Alcohol Problems

William D. Clark

## EPIDEMIOLOGY AND ETIOLOGY

All patients who show any hint of trouble from alcohol deserve their physician's attention and possibly intervention. Too few physicians consistently attend to early, minor clues (see the box above), ignoring all but prototypical or flagrant medical problems. Intervention before onset of late medical problems not only lowers morbidity, mortality, and medical costs of patients and family members, but also prevents progressive damage to family and social relationships, self-esteem, and emotional stability (Fig. 130-1).

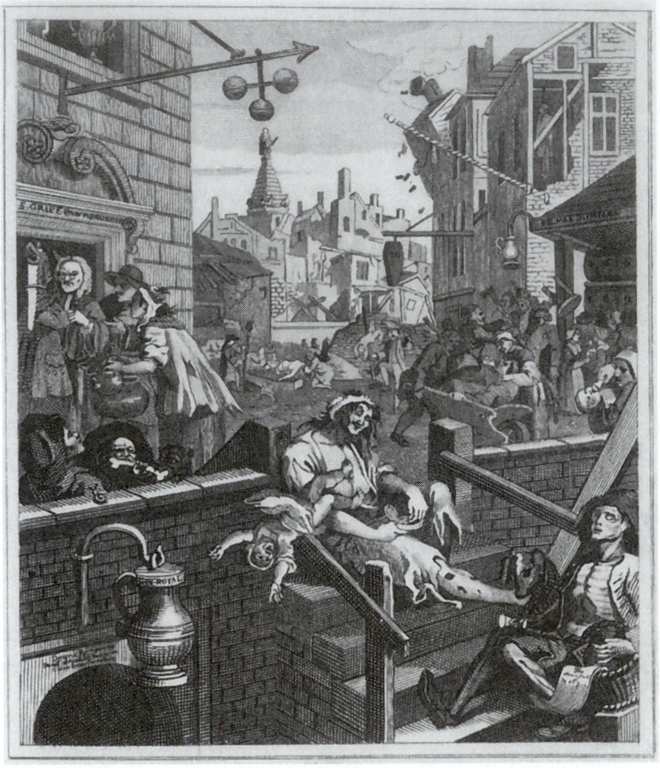

**Fig. 130-1.** *Gin Lane.* William Hogarth (1697-1764). Alcoholism: disease or moral problem; what should be the physician's role. (Courtesy Yale Center for British Art.)

Problems with description and definitions of "alcoholism" (and related terms) bog physicians down. Indeed, physicians and others become confused because the relationships among key parameters such as amount drunk, physical dependence, and medical or social problems are inconsistent. What can be agreed on for clinical purposes?

A characteristic syndrome can be described that includes consistent inability to limit drinking so as to avoid dependence and/or medical and social adverse consequences. This is usually labeled "alcoholism." Typical and recognizable defenses develop in parallel with other aspects of the syndrome, and people hide important facts, responding negatively to attempts to expose the "truth" and to promote changes in drinking behaviors. Fundamental characteristics of this syndrome are similar across cultures, for example, in France, the United States, or Russia. People who have fewer problems or problems of low severity are said to have "alcohol abuse." Experts believe that "healthy drinking" may be defined by modest amounts of alcohol, a social setting for drinking, and little intoxication.

Risk of alcoholism is genetically transmitted, and family studies show that 50% [sic] of brothers, fathers, and sons of men with alcoholism are afflicted. Considerable data indicate how genetic risk operates, and differences in blood level kinetics, tendency to hangover, and relief of anxiety have shown positive results on study. Higher problem rates are found among homeless persons, those with a major psychiatric disorder, and people in the criminal justice system. Which comes first remains uncertain.

Prevalence of alcohol problems is high; the Epidemiologic Catchment Area study, using DSM-IIIR* definitions, found a lifetime prevalence of 13.6%. The 1988 National Health Interview Survey found 10.3% of men alcohol dependent and 4.1% of women. A population-based British study found 10% of men who were CAGE (a screening test) positive, 7.6% who averaged more than 3.5 daily drinks, and 3.2% who stated they had problems with drinking. Women consistently show 30% to 50% fewer problems. From 21% to 27% of hospitalized medical-

**Diagnostic and Statistical Manual of Mental Disorders,* Third edition.

surgical patients and 50% to 70% of psychiatric patients screen positive. In 1987, 2.7 million years of potential life were lost (based on life expectancy) because of alcohol-related mortality. Yearly health care costs for people with alcoholism average 100% higher than for comparable nonalcoholic people. Total medical costs directly attributable to alcohol are estimated at $10.5 billion. This figure accounts for only 10.7% of total alcohol abuse costs (1990), with annual reduced productivity costs valued at $36.6 billion.

## PATHOPHYSIOLOGY

Alcohol problems are not equivalent to alcoholism; moreover, studies demonstrate the natural history of the spectrum of alcohol disorders. Heavy drinking poses a high risk of serious short-term or long-term negative outcomes; for example, from trauma in the short term and from addiction, cirrhosis, or full-blown alcoholism in the long term. People with light drinking or few consequences are more likely to revert to a healthy pattern, but remission from seriously disordered drinking also occurs.

No one asks to develop alcoholism. Most people drink for enjoyment or to have good times in the company of others, whether or not mediated by a chemical process that produces variants of "intoxication." People "learn to drink" from their culture and modulate drinking according to feedback from internal states (shame, hangover) and external cues (reprimands, criticism, sanctions). Some people modulate and adjust easily, whereas others fail to keep to sensible limits and respond poorly to those internal and external cues. Experiments show that physiologic, psychologic, interactional, and social factors are important in the failure to limit drinking in response to feedback. Investigations of twins and adopted siblings support the view that genetic factors mediate regulation of drinking. Other experiments suggesting genetic influences include, for example, the dysphoria (flushing and nausea, headache) that prevents many Asians from drinking; the finding that sons of alcoholic fathers predict their blood alcohol levels less accurately than men from nonalcoholic backgrounds; and the finding that intensity of anxiety during tests administered under the influence of alcohol varies with familial loading for alcoholism.

As drinking and associated activities gradually occupy more time, people tend to minimize the amounts drunk or ignore linkages between drinking and life problems. As people drink more, they must develop more effective "blinders" in order not to see the problem. They accomplish this by making excuses for their behavior and directing blame onto others; often they become isolated because they show hostility whenever alcohol is discussed. They are adept at repressing realities seen by others, successful at suppressing negative feelings, and especially clever at getting others to give advice that they can reject, becoming skillful "resisters" almost as second nature. People select friends and partners who tolerate or encourage drinking and tacitly agree to ignore consequences. The unhealthy relationship dynamics are exaggerated not only by the cognitive deficits and dysphoric aspects of intoxication, hangover, and related states, but also because others resent the apparently voluntary "having fun and being irresponsible" nature of frequent drinking.

### Effective screening for alcohol problems: CAGE

**C** Have you felt the need to CUT DOWN on your drinking?
**A** Have you felt ANNOYED BY CRITICISM of your drinking?
**G** Have you felt GUILTY (or had regrets) about your drinking?
**E** Have you felt the need for an EYE-OPENER in the morning?

People with alcohol problems are heavily stigmatized by society because they repetitively act irresponsibly despite sanctions. Stigma inhibits naming of drinking problems—by patients, families, and physicians. Clinicians are further inhibited from identifying alcoholism because they do not want to upset or anger patients, thinking "he'll come back when he is ready." They do not want to lose the patient, thinking "some care is better than none." Physicians may have personal issues about alcoholism stemming from family experiences or from encounters in training with intoxicated patients or others not yet in recovery.

## HISTORY

Because the illness seeks cover rather than exposure, frequently no clue is discernible without use of a screening strategy. Physicians now miss 60% to 80% of cases and seldom utilize one of the screening devices of documented efficacy. As with hypertension or cervical cancer, irreversible consequences will occur without screening.

Every patient who responds positively to "Do you drink alcohol?" should be screened. The CAGE test (see the box above) is sensitive and specific (70% to 90%). Questions are uncomplicated enough to use for walk-ins, in the emergency room, or during hospitalization. Do *not* proceed by asking about amounts of drinking. "How much do you drink?" is worse than inadequate. Not only does it remind people of shameful overindulgence and fail to encourage reflection, but study demonstrates that asking about amounts limits reponse to subsequent structured assessments.

In clinical practice, a positive screen (any response other than an unequivocal "no" to each question) should be pursued, as should any other clue. These clues take predictable form in primary care. In the somatic domain, gastritis, trauma, hypertension, unexplained liver function disorder, or new-onset seizure frequently is seen. In the realm of emotions, symptoms of anxiety, depression, overdose, or a request for psychotropic medications may provide the initial hint of an alcohol disorder. More specifically in relation to alcohol, virtually any spontaneous mention of drinking behavior, such as "partying" or hangover, is a sufficiently uncommon event as to alert the physician. Alcohol on the breath in any encounter is an alarming sign.

A comprehensive assessment that may require several

### Structured primary care assessment for alcohol problems

**HALT**

**H** Do you drink to get HIGH?
**A** Do you drink ALONE?
**L** Do you LOOK FORWARD to drinking (instead of the event)?
**T** Has your TOLERANCE for alcohol increased, or decreased?

**BUMP**

**B** Have you had BLACKOUTS?
**U** Is your drinking UNPLANNED (you drink when you said you would not or drink more than you thought)?
**M** Do you drink MEDICINALLY (when depressed, sad, anxious, etc.)?
**P** Do you PROTECT your supply (so you will always have enough)?

**FATAL DTs**

**F** FAMILY HISTORY of alcohol problems?
**A** ALCOHOLICS ANONYMOUS attendance?
**T** THOUGHTS or attempts at suicide?
**A** ALCOHOLISM, ever thought you might have it?
**L** LEGAL PROBLEMS, such as driving under the influence or assault?
**D** DEPRESSION, feeling DOWN, low or sad?
**Ts** TRANQUILIZER (or disulfiram) use?

long interviews may not be the primary care physician's task. However, after a positive screening question or other clue is noted, a simple search for characteristic elements of alcoholism is warranted and not time consuming if thoughtfully structured. Physicians usually ask about somatic problems just mentioned but seldom systematically inquire about other domains. Even if an early clue arises that obviates the need for screening, the CAGE questions might nevertheless be used to open a more reflective search for typical symptoms. Asking the questions in the box above can be done in a few minutes and facilitates further assessment of risk factors, tolerance, dependence, loss of control, adverse consequences, or preoccupation with drinking.

Interviews with others, including family, nurses, or social workers, enlarge the inquiry if concerns are insufficiently addressed through direct history taking. Other physicians' records or hospital records may contain unanticipated information that establishes a diagnosis.

Obtaining these data allows the physician to discuss impressions in an informed and compasssionate manner. In fact, the very action of informed inquiry effectively disrupts the pathophysiology of the illness process. Even though a formal alcohol diagnosis may not be made now, or ever, experimental data show that thoughtful diagnostic conversation itself produces beneficial therapeutic effects. Setting priorities for the pacing and vigor of subsequent discussions requires adding data from the physical and laboratory examinations.

## PHYSICAL EXAMINATION AND LABORATORY STUDIES

Physical and laboratory examinations are useful adjuncts to the critically important skills of screening and assessment through structured interviewing.

Odor of alcohol is a moderately specific finding, distinctly abnormal in medical encounters. If one easily smells alcohol in the room, the blood alcohol level (BAL) is likely greater than 0.125 g/dl, and a less dramatic, definite odor suggests a blood level between 0.075 and 0.125 g/dl. The nose is an insensitive breath analyzer. These levels are rarely present with healthy drinking.

Further, if the odor of alcohol is apparent, and if the patient manifests no evidence of intoxication (slurred speech, incoordination, emotional lability), tolerance to alcohol effect is present. Tolerance indicates a nervous system adjustment to intoxicating alcohol levels, caused by steady, heavy drinking, which is inevitably toxic. Tolerance always signals a serious alcohol disorder.

Intoxication in any encounter is worrisome. Even in the emergency situation, intoxication means a high likelihood of alcohol disorder. To underscore this important point, assume that the alcoholic 10% of the population are drunk once a week, and assume that the 60% who are healthy drinkers are intoxicated once yearly. Thus, in a year, from a population of 100, 30 abstainers yield no episodes of intoxication, 60 healthy drinkers yield 60 episodes, and 10 alcoholics yield 520! Further, healthy drinkers seldom become as intoxicated and are more likely to drink in controlled environments (e.g., where someone else can drive). Intoxicated people in the emergency situation are probably not healthy drinkers who "have had one too many." In the office, hospital, or clinic (visitors, etc.), intoxication or odor of alcohol is inappropriate and strongly suggests an alcohol disorder.

Other physical and laboratory findings are *ineffective* screening tests because of low sensitivity and specificity. Because of alcohol's broad toxicity, however, an abnormality may prove to be highly useful in an individual case. First, an unexplained finding may begin a fruitful investigatory process; for example, despite a negative CAGE test, the concerned physician of a young woman with palmar erythema continued the assessment (vide supra), allowing the patient to reveal her alcohol problem. Second, in the presence of an historic clue, characteristic physical or laboratory findings can substantially raise the "posttest probability" of an alcohol disorder. A 55-year-old man with chronic obstructive pulmonary disease (COPD) was admitted for atrial fibrillation. His wife complained about his drinking, and elevated mean corpuscular volume (MCV) and aspartate aminotransferase (AST, SGOT) confirmed not only alcoholism, but also "holiday heart" (see Chapter 7 case study).

The box on p. 1705 presents findings of high utility and underscores the value of thorough, thoughtful examination. Discussion of the pathophysiology of complications and meaning of physical and laboratory findings can be found in the specialty chapters.

### Physical and laboratory manifestations of high utility to detect alcohol problems

**General**
High blood pressure
Intoxication
Tolerance
Odor of alcohol

**Hepatic**
Icterus
Palmar erythema
Spider angiomata
Bruising
Hepatomegaly
AST (SGOT), γ-glutamyltransferase (GGT), or other enzyme elevation

**Hematopoietic**
Elevation of MCV
Anemia
Low platelets

**Skin**
Facial telangiectases
Seborrheic dermatitis
Rosacea
Skin atrophy
Distal extremity hair loss
Superficial infections

**Neuromuscular**
Agitation
Tremor
Emotional lability
Poor tandem gait (or wide-based gait)
Ankle, wrist weakness
Atrophy of shoulder, pelvic girdle muscles

**Cardiac**
Tachycardia
Atrial fibrillation
Cardiomyopathy

**Genitalia**
Testicular atrophy

## MANAGEMENT OF WITHDRAWAL AND MEDICAL COMPLICATIONS

Medical complications such as arrhythmias, hepatic failure, bleeding gastritis, and pancreatitis require immediate attention, and their treatment is covered elsewhere. Of special concern to the primary care physician is the understanding, assessment, and treatment of alcohol withdrawal.

Withdrawal is not an all-or-nothing state, and addicted patients experience symptoms whenever their BAL falls. The brain perceives any drop in BAL as potentially signaling the "last" drink and expresses its "need" for alcohol through withdrawal symptoms.

### Risk factors for severe alcohol withdrawal

Drinking around the clock
Daily consumption of a fifth of liquor, a case of beer, or more than a half gallon of wine
Heavy drinking more than 5 years
Poor nutrition
Concomitant heavy sedative, cocaine, or narcotic use
Past history of severe withdrawal

As physical dependence develops, initial manifestations of anxiety, sleep disorder, tremor, and vague discomforts are mild, sometimes not even attributed to alcohol, but easily relieved by drinking. As months pass, however, alcohol less reliably controls symptoms, and intoxication is fleeting, occurring only at high BAL (greater than 250 mg/dl). Soon the person drinks steadily to alleviate withdrawal, but relief is brief. The range of BAL at which the person feels "not sick" diminishes, little distinguishes withdrawal from nonwithdrawal, and severe symptoms, even delirium tremens, may develop despite a BAL of 300 mg/dl or more.

The uncertain predictability of alcohol withdrawal poses a dilemma because outpatient treatment is sensible in mild cases, but inpatient support is required for severe ones. Degree of tremor, anxiety, tachycardia, and stomach symptoms are poor predictors of need for inpatient care. Clouded sensorium, fever, hyperventilation, or a concomitant medical problem (hepatic failure, pancreatitis, etc.) mandate admission. In addition, the presence of three factors from the box above suggests inpatient management.

When outpatient management is feasible, pharmacologic support helps with symptom relief (see the box on p. 1706) and should be integrated with the patient education and referral options discussed subsequently.

## MANAGEMENT OF PATIENTS WITH ALCOHOL PROBLEMS

Physicians should undertake discussion and referral whenever they find a case or a potential case. The desired outcomes are a sustained change in drinking behavior (usually abstinence) and improvement in health and psychosocial functioning. Usually the achievement of these outcomes requires access to specialized assistance, so the major "work" of generalists is to initiate action and refer patients.

Physicians are reluctant to intervene and confront patients who ignore reality, suppress negative feelings, and so flawlessly, as if by second nature, reject sound advice, no matter that this is a routine part of the illness dynamic. Patients' behaviors are negative, confusing, and hurtful. Often, roles are reversed, and the physician unwittingly rejects and humiliates the patient. This fundamental distortion in physicians' experience of caring

## Outpatient withdrawal regimen

50-100 mg chlordiazepoxide PO (IM unreliably absorbed) in office; initiate referral to counseling or structured program.

Day 1: take 25-50 mg PO every 4-6 hours as needed.

Day 2: take 25 mg PO every 4-6 hours as needed; visit the office.

Day 3: take 25 mg PO once or twice as needed.

NOTE:

Give patient not more than 250 mg to take away.

Expect 200-300 mg total for average severity.

Do not exceed 250 mg day 1, 150 mg day 2, 50 mg day 3.

Lethal dose of chlordiazepoxide uncertain; exceeds 2 g.

If patient drinks, admit for detoxification.

for patients is painful and unsatisfying. The clinician comes to believe that any intervention is unwarranted interference in the patient's life. The situation becomes framed as, "Shall I now confront the patient and waste valuable time for unlikely gain, or delay until a better moment?" Problems remain unaddressed until later complications ensue.

Strategies employed to help change depend on patients' readiness to change, and five "stages" have been named: precontemplation, contemplation, preparation for action, action, and maintenance. In "precontemplation," a person is neither linking drinking with consequences nor interested in changing drinking behavior. Clinicians have pejoratively labeled this state "denial." As people notice linkages between drinking and life problems, they may begin to "contemplate" change or even "prepare for change" by imagining change strategies or a different lifestyle or quitting drinking. In "action" and "maintenance" stages, people try to make and sustain changes. Physicians' ability to assist, as well as their satisfaction, should be improved if they utilize strategies adapted to patients' "stage" of change.

Stage of change is neither fixed nor all inclusive. Patients may say, "I'll go to AA, but I'm not going to stop drinking" (or vice versa), or "My liver is sick, so I'll cut back for a time," or "I'd like to stop drinking to improve my family relationships, but I have to drink with my professional clients." The patient may take action to dry out and relieve symptoms of withdrawal but fail to understand the need for continued treatment.

When patients are in precontemplation ("denial"), they need information about how the illness works and how treatment helps in order to make better-informed choices. In precontemplation, discussion of action strategies will be met with resistance. In fact, slogans from the self-help community such as, "No one but the patient can make a diagnosis," or "He won't do anything until he hits bottom," reflect lay wisdom derived from the frustration of pressing for change when people are not ready. However, professionals who understand that recovery requires a natural progression through several stages of change can enable patients to initiate change well before they might have done so without skillful assistance.

## Techniques of brief intervention

**F** FEEDBACK, of personal risk or impairment
**R** RESPONSIBILITY, emphasis on personal responsibility for change
**A** ADVICE, clear advice to change
**M** MENU, of alternative treatment options
**E** EMPATHIC STYLE, of interviewing
**S** SELF-EFFICACY, enhance patient's optimism

Physicians can structure their confrontations using a model called *brief intervention.* Designed for primary care settings, it recognizes that patients whose problem is newly brought to light will have high levels of ambivalence and resistance, since they will be in a precontemplation or contemplation stage. Patients may benefit greatly from the physician who effectively presents information and attempts a referral, even if they do not seek formal treatment in another setting. The mnemonic FRAMES denotes the tasks and the style that research has shown to be effective for addictive disorders (see the box above).

The physician should *feedback* the pertinent data from history, physical, and laboratory examinations in understandable terms, expressing concern for health without yet naming the problem. Labels of any sort seem like name-calling to the susceptible patients, provoke resistance, and should be avoided. Helping the patient take *responsibility* for change is a complex process. Potential humiliation and misinterpretation are minimized by using language such as, "The choice is yours; no one else can decide what you should do about this." Frequent use of the question "Where does that leave you?" or "What are you thinking about this, now?" underscores the notion that the physician gives advice, while the patient makes the decisions and is in charge. *Advise* the patient that change is indicated by the data available. Let the patient know how health might improve if changes were made. Tell what other people do in this situation.

Motivation for change arises from interactions. Patients become "motivated" when the *Menu* looks hopeful and provides opportunity for success. Give the patient a *Menu* of the options available. What do experts often advise to patients at this juncture? The idea that "You must do exactly this . . ." provokes increased resistance; in comparison to, "Let's give thought to a few options . . ." which suggests that the patient wants to act responsibly.

An *empathic interview style* is more effective than confrontative, coercive, or other styles. Empathic styles include noticing and naming feelings, expressing guesses about how the patient might be feeling, and being reflective about the patient's dilemma. Accepting the patient's emotional situation and explicitly communicating an understanding of it facilitate internal reflection and motivation to change. With alcohol problems particularly, avoidance of labels helps to communicate physician understanding.

*Support for self-efficacy* provides an optimistic framework and shows respect for the patient by recognizing and

### Providing information: strategy outline

**Aim**

To provide information about substance-use in a sensitive manner.

**How not to do it**

The worst way to provide information is to "wag your finger" at the patient, for example. "You are . . . and if you are not careful, you will . . ., and then you will find that . . .". With a moralistic tone to your voice, you risk pushing the patient into a corner. He or she will have no choice but either to agree with you (or pretend to) or to disagree.

**How to do it**

1. Choose the right moment and ask permission.
   - Best when patient seems curious, actually asks for information, or is at least not in a defensive frame of mind.
   - Your voice tone should be neutral. If the patient decides not to receive information, that's their choice.
   - Ask permission, for example: "I wonder, would you be interested in knowing more about the effect of —— on ——?"
2. Provide information in a neutral and nonpersonal way, referring generally to "what happens to people" rather than to this particular person. It is also useful to refer to what experts think rather than what you think.
3. When finished, ask: "I wonder, what do you make of all this? How does it tie in with your use of ——?"

NOTE
- Take your time when discussing the personal implications in Step 3 above.
- Some people don't need or want information: because they already know the facts, or because they are not ready to receive them. That's why it's important to ask permission and gauge their reaction first.
- Giving people potentially "frightening" information does not necessarily motivate them to change. It can have the opposite effect.

From Rollnick S: *Mental Health* 1:25, 1992.

### Dr Helps CD

**D** DEPENDENCE on alcohol seems part of your current dilemma (or use the word hooked, preoccupied with, stuck, trapped, or some synonym).
**R** RETURN VISIT is important; you and I need to work together.
**H** HELP is available here and elsewhere; don't continue to go it alone.
**E** EVIDENCE convincing me that this is hurting you is . . . .
**L** LEAVE ALCOHOL BEHIND; abstain, at least for a time.
**P** PERSPECTIVE is invariably limited; affected persons can't see what is apparent to others.
**S** SNEAK UP ON people is what alcohol problems insidiously do.
**C** CONCERN for your health is paramount, and I'm worried.
**D** DOWN, DEPRESSED, or DESPAIRING feelings often result from drinking.

naming strengths needed to effect change. Statements such as, "You are courageous to discuss this difficult material, so I know you have the courage to do more," or "You have an independent mind and spirit, which gives you a good chance to stick to decisions that you make," acknowledge previous successes.

Many patients with drinking problems may have the feeling, "Something terrible may be happening; I may be acting irrationally and even immorally, but it's not something I can discuss with anyone." Linking new information to feedback about the specifics of the patient's situation is a unique physician opportunity to help reframe the situation or suggest action options. Specific strategies for the difficult task of presenting information in a sensitive manner are outlined in the box above. Choosing a moment when the patient is not defensive, asking, "Would you be interested in knowing more about . . . ?" and then giving the information in a neutral, nonpersonal way and asking what the patient thinks about it facilitates open dialogue, reflection, and exploration. "Wagging one's finger," actually or figuratively, tends to push patients into a corner, highlight any feelings of shame or stigma, and generally inhibit discussion.

Which information is of particular pertinence? Critical elements include the following: people seldom understand what is happening to them; people are not to blame for being ill or in trouble; experts know what actions facilitate recovery; and help is at hand. This amounts to a new explanatory model, and because the "stage of change" is seldom black and white, the physician should present concepts and ideas that could be relevant at various stages. The mnemonic DR HELPS CD (CD derives from chemical dependency, see the box above) may help physicians remember these ideas when slightly put off or confused by the conflict and tension of a complex encounter. The concept that drinking may get a bit out of control without recognition is central, and telling the person. "People inadvertently become DEPENDENT, or 'hooked', and have little PERSPECTIVE on this problem that SNEAKS UP on them," conveys the concepts while minimizing the stigma. Summarizing this aspect by saying, "After all, no one ever asks to get into this kind of a pickle or jam" really helps patients sense the physician understands the dilemma in a broader context than a moral one. When the physician says something such as, "I'm terribly CONCERNED about your health, and I want to HELP as much as I can; I want you to have a RETURN VISIT scheduled so we can continue to work on this together," and "I know from experience with other patients that expert HELP is available," professional and personal interest in the outcome is underscored. If the physician can say, "People often feel a bit DEPRESSED, or DOWN, or sometimes even DESPAIRING in situations like this," it expresses a willingness to tolerate and even encourage discussion of feelings and to continue the relationship despite irrational drinking activity and shameful consequences.

### Helping with decision-making: strategy outline

- Do not rush patients into decision-making.
- Present options for the future rather than a single course of action.
- Describe what other patients have done in a similar situation.
- Emphasize that "you are the best judge of what will be best for you."
- Provide information in a neutral, nonpersonal manner.
- Failure to reach a decision to change is not a failed consultation.
- Resolutions to change often break down. Make sure that patients understand this and do not avoid future contact if things go wrong.
- Commitment to change is likely to fluctuate. Expect this to happen and empathize with the patient's predicament.

From Rollick S: *J Ment Health* 1:25, 1992.

### Referral options

Alcoholics Anonymous
Physician specialist in addiction medicine (preferably certified by the American Society of Addiction Medicine, ASAM)
Licensed or certified substance abuse counselor
Family therapist specifically experienced in substance abuse
Substance abuse treatment agency (for inpatient or outpatient treatment)

After presentation of this new model and the offer of help, followed by asking the patient, "I wonder, what do you make of all this?" patients frequently ask what the doctor thinks. The physician can give further feedback and formulate a recommendation, saying, "these (a, b, c . . .) facts constitute the EVIDENCE that underlie my growing concern. In this situation, the experts recommend that a person LEAVE alcohol behind, at least for a time."

As people approach action and change, ambivalence is magnified. Deciding about important behavior change provokes inner conflicts, which the physician will experience as indecisiveness and delay. Physicians who appreciate this dynamic tension utilize several strategies (see the box above) to help patients make important decisions. Help patients look at what is better and worse about drinking. Ignoring the "good things" about drinking means that the patient will guard these as inner, secret reasons to avoid change. Making a written list while exploring concerns gives the patient a reference point and reminds one about which topics have already been covered. Discussion of the extent to which the patient's life is not progressing as he had hoped it would, or exploration of the ways in which the patient is unable to live up to his own values, develops the discrepancy between the present and the future and motivates people for change. Because many situations are life-threatening, or potentially so, physicians tend to be intolerant of delay. Perhaps paradoxically, time spent attentively listening to patients and exploring their ambivalences will help them decide and build commitment to change, whereas taking one side of ambivalence and trying to push decisions provokes more resistance and delays change.

Available options depend on competing priorities (pancreatitis, homelessness, etc.) and previous treatment experience. A list of options often includes those shown in the box above, right. Patients entrenched in precontemplation may limit action to a return visit or an agreement to consider the information the physician has given. Observing the consequences of future drinking and generating a list of pros and cons about change represent a more active step. "Treatment" requires adopting many changes in behavior and attitudes and developing the skills to maintain these changes in the face of inner (psychologic) pressures not to change, as well as external (social) forces committed to the status quo (e.g., drinking partners and family dynamics).

Physicians should refer people for treatment, and research data show that attempted referral is intrinsic to the change process, whether or not the referral is completed. This finding probably reflects the dynamics previously discussed regarding exploring ambivalence, giving choices, not rushing decisions, and clearly expressing support and concern. Patients who are cognitively impaired (intoxicated or in withdrawal) need to "dry out" before treatment referral is attempted. Patients should be referred to outpatient treatment unless they are medically ill, psychotic, or homeless or have previously failed outpatient counseling. Most communities have specialized services available, in both public and private sectors. Community mental health centers employ substance abuse specialists. Specialized licensing in substance abuse is available in all states for therapists with credentials, such as social workers and psychologists. Physicians must know local resources in order to provide quality referrals.

Alcoholics Anonymous (AA) should be part of the referral for each patient, whether the perceived problem is early or late, mild or severe; all patients can benefit. The experienced clinician presents AA attendance as a joint educational effort and suggests that talking over experiences at meetings will be important to help the physician and patient more fully understand the situation. If the problem is severe, recovery will be facilitated by participation in an abstinent subculture, where people can learn the "how to" as well as the "why" for being sober as they identify with others who formerly shared this patient's limited perspective and are now doing well. If not so severe, attendance at a minimum of six different meetings (AA meetings have distinct tenor and style, and patients find one more congenial than another) informs patients regarding the nature of problems they face and provides beneficial advice for future change. Meetings provide invaluable assistance not available from the physician or counseling, namely, nonverbal and nonrational opportunities to discover that their "alcoholic" stereotype is too narrow. Participating with recovering people who seem otherwise like themselves motivates patients.

## PHARMACOLOGIC CONSIDERATIONS IN PRIMARY CARE MANAGEMENT

The primary care physician has pharmacologic options available to assist patients in recovery. Disulfiram and naltrexone have been shown effective in certain circumstances.

Disulfiram provokes acetaldehye accumulation after the ingestion of alcohol, producing a toxic state manifest by nausea, headache, unpleasant flushing, and respiratory distress. Severity depends on dose of alcohol and blood level of disulfiram. Several doses of disulfiram are needed to reach a significant blood level, and several days without medication are needed to avoid a toxic reaction after alcohol ingestion. Theoretically, patients taking a daily dose will avoid alcohol. In practice, few maintain the medication and most relapse, but studies show that the addition of a supervisor to monitor the ingestion dramatically improves sobriety rates. The supervisor cannot take responsibility for ensuring ingestion but must observe the patient's use daily. The physician can arrange for this to be done at the office for a few days, then transfer responsibility to an appropriate person in the patient's life or to a professional treatment program. If patients using opiates or cocaine are drinking alcohol and not undergoing drug treatment, disulfiram is highly recommended to help them think clearly enough to undertake treatment. The recommended prescription is two 250 mg tablets daily for 4 days, then one 250 mg tablet daily. Anticipate use in 3-month blocks.

Randomized studies show naltrexone, an opioid antagonist, has beneficial effects in treatment of alcohol problems. Naltrexone diminishes craving, and treated patients who drank did not move into full relapse as often as control subjects. Naltrexone may be a useful addition to the menu of treatment options.

## SUMMARY

The principal goal of this chapter is to encourage case finding and present guidelines for physician action with any potential case of alcohol disorder. Conversations about drinking are painful, but physicians who apply guidelines presented here can improve their interview outcomes. Successful confrontation requires timing, persistence, and sufficient skill to structure interactions so as to encourage optimism, the choice for change, reflection, dialogue, and help seeking, while avoiding the expression of frustration or lack of interest when little motivation or change is apparent.

## BIBLIOGRAPHY


Bean M: Clinical implications of models for recovery from alcoholism, *Adv Alcohol Subst Abuse* 3:91, 1983.

Bein T, Miller W, Tonigan J: Brief interventions for alcohol problems: a review, *Addiction* 88:315, 1993.

Buchsbaum D et al: Screening for alcohol abuse using CAGE scores and likelihood ratios, *Ann Intern Med* 115:774, 1991.

Elvy G, Wells J, Baird K: Attempted referral as intervention for problem drinking in the general hospital, *Br J Addict* 83:83, 1988.

Graham A: Screening for alcoholism by life-style risk assessment in a community hospital, *Arch Intern Med* 151:958, 1991.

Holden H, Blose J: Reduction of health care costs associated with alcoholism treatment: a 14 year longitudinal study, *J Stud Alcohol* 53:293, 1992.

Johnson B, Clark W: Alcoholism: a challenging physician-patient encounter, *J Gen Intern Med* 4:445, 1989.

McLellan A et al: Private substance abuse treatments: are some programs more effective than others? *J Subst Abuse Treat* 10:243, 1993.

Miller W, Rollnick S: *Motivational interviewing: preparing people to change addictive behavior,* Guilford, NY, 1991, Guilford Press.

Miller W, Benefield G, Tonigan J: Enhancing motivation for change in problem drinking: a controlled comparison of two therapist styles, *J Consult Clin Psychol* 61:455, 1993.

Rollnick S, Heather N, Bell A: Negotiating behavior change in medical settings: the development of brief motivational interviewing, *J Ment Health* 1:25, 1992.

Steinweg D, Worth H: Alcoholism: the keys to the CAGE, *Am J Med* 94:520, 1993.

Turner R et al: Alcohol withdrawal syndromes: a review of pathophysiology, clinical presentation and treatment, *J Gen Intern Med* 4:432, 1989.

Wallace P, Cutler S, Haines A: Randomized controlled trial of general practitioner intervention in patients with excessive alcohol consumption, *Br Med J* 297:663, 1988.


CHAPTER

# 131 Drug Abuse

**Daniel Shine**

## APPROACH TO THE DRUG-ABUSING PATIENT

The pathologic use of psychoactive drugs is a common problem, usually chronic and of unknown and probably multifactorial etiologies. Successful management of patients with this problem requires medical knowledge, psychologic acumen, the ability to work with other professionals, and a steady sense of social perspective. There are, in fact, few conditions whose management so specifically calls for the skills of a primary care internist.

When evaluating symptoms or signs in a drug abuser, the physician must consider acute and chronic illnesses that result from the toxicities of one or several drugs. Routes of administration, diluents and contaminants, drug-related aberrations of laboratory tests, and syndromes of abstinence or intoxication are also among the important features of a differential diagnosis. In addition, medical illness may be unrelated to drugs but masked by the use of them or feigned by the patient seeking a prescription. With diagnostic problems of such difficulty, a close working relationship with the patient becomes important; it may be elusive. Denial, manipulation, and ambivalence are characteristics of drug abusers that can defeat the best diagnostic or therapeutic plan.

Care of drug abusers is also complicated by the involvement of courts, public assistance services, schools, and child protection agencies. This dispersion of responsibility reflects the diverse societal manifestations of drug abuse and the absence of any generally accepted etiologic hypothesis. For the physician accustomed to occupying a central role it is often difficult to function effectively in a supportive or even a subordinate position. Drug abusers may evoke in the physician feelings of pessimism, anger, disapproval, or disappointment. On the other hand, much of the gratification in taking care of these patients results

### Criteria for substance dependence

A maladaptive pattern of substance use leading to clinically significant impairment or distress as manifested by three (or more) of the following occurring at any time in the same 12-month period:

(1) Tolerance, as defined by either of the following:
  (a) A need for markedly increased amounts of the substance to achieve intoxication or desired effect
  (b) Markedly diminished effect with continued use of the same amount of the substance
(2) Withdrawal, as manifested by either of the following:
  (a) The characteristic withdrawal syndrome for the substance
  (b) The same (or a closely related) substance is taken to relieve or avoid withdrawal symptoms
(3) The substance is often taken in larger amounts or over a longer period than was intended
(4) There is a persistent desire for the substance or unsuccessful efforts to cut down or control substance use
(5) A great deal of time is spent on activities necessary to obtain the substance (e.g., visiting multiple doctors or driving long distances), on use of the substance (e.g., chain smoking), or on recovering from its effects
(6) Important social, occupational, or recreational activities are given up or reduced because of substance use
(7) The substance use is continued despite knowledge of having a persistent or recurrent physical or psychologic problem probably caused or exacerbated by the substance (e.g., current cocaine use despite recognition of cocaine-induced depression or continued drinking despite recognition that an ulcer was made worse by alcohol consumption.

Specify if:
With physiologic dependence there is evidence of tolerance or withdrawal
Without physiologic dependence

Course specifiers:
Early full remission
Early partial remission
Sustained full remission
Sustained partial remission
On agonist therapy
In a controlled environment

From *Diagnostic and statistical manual of mental disorders*, ed 4, 1994, American Psychiatric Association.

### Criteria for substance abuse*

A maladaptive pattern of substance use leading to clinically significant impairment of distress, as manifested by one (or more) of the following, occurring within a 12-month period:

(1) Recurrent substance use resulting in a failure to fulfill major role obligations at work, school, or home (e.g., repeated absences or poor work performance related to substance use; substance-related children or household)

(2) Recurrent substance use in situations in which it is physically hazardous (e.g., driving an automobile or operating a machine when impaired by substance use)

(3) Recurrent substance-related legal problems (e.g., arrests for substance-related disorderly conduct)

(4) Continued substance use despite having persistent or recurrent social or interpersonal problems caused or exacerbated by the effects of the substance (e.g., arguments with spouse about consequences of intoxication, physical fights)

*These symptoms have never met the criteria for substance dependence for this class of substance.

from the perspective gained through a successful struggle with these feelings.

Drug abuse, like many chronic conditions the physician treats, is not frequently cured. The patients can, however, be successfully managed: their lives prolonged, their morbidity minimized, and the quality of their lives dramatically improved. In order to achieve these results the primary care physician must draw on a broad range of professional skills.

## Definitions

Historically a number of terms have been used to emphasize different aspects of pathologic drug use. The word *addiction* has usually been applied to summarize concepts of physiologic tolerance, withdrawal, and compulsive drug-seeking behavior. *Abuse* implicitly emphasizes pathologic departure from the societal norms of psychoactive chemical use without a requirement for physiologic tolerance. *Dependence* has been used to suggest the central role of drug use in patients' lives; the American Psychiatric Association's *Diagnostic and Statistical Manual* (DSM IV) has emphasized this term since its third edition.

Currently *DSM IV* divides pathologic drug use into two main categories: dependence and abuse (see the boxes). Use despite adverse consequences, preoccupation with use, and evidence of physical addiction are the three salient elements of substance dependence.

Thus defined, substance dependence and abuse are typically relapsing conditions characterized by medical complications affecting many organ systems, a high rate of mortality, and severe disruptions in psychosocial functioning. *Abstinence* is used in this discussion to denote the stereotypical physical and psychologic sequelae of a cessation in drug use. *Withdrawal* (sometimes called detoxification) refers to any of several techniques for attenuating abstinence.

## Extent of drug abuse

The financial costs, direct and indirect, of substance abuse and dependence in the United States were estimated at $177 billion in 1991.

Three large, ongoing national studies of drug use incidence and prevalence are commonly quoted. The Drug Abuse Warning Network (DAWN) reports on emergency room visits at participating hospitals throughout the country. This information underestimates total use and overrepresents drugs with acute complications. From

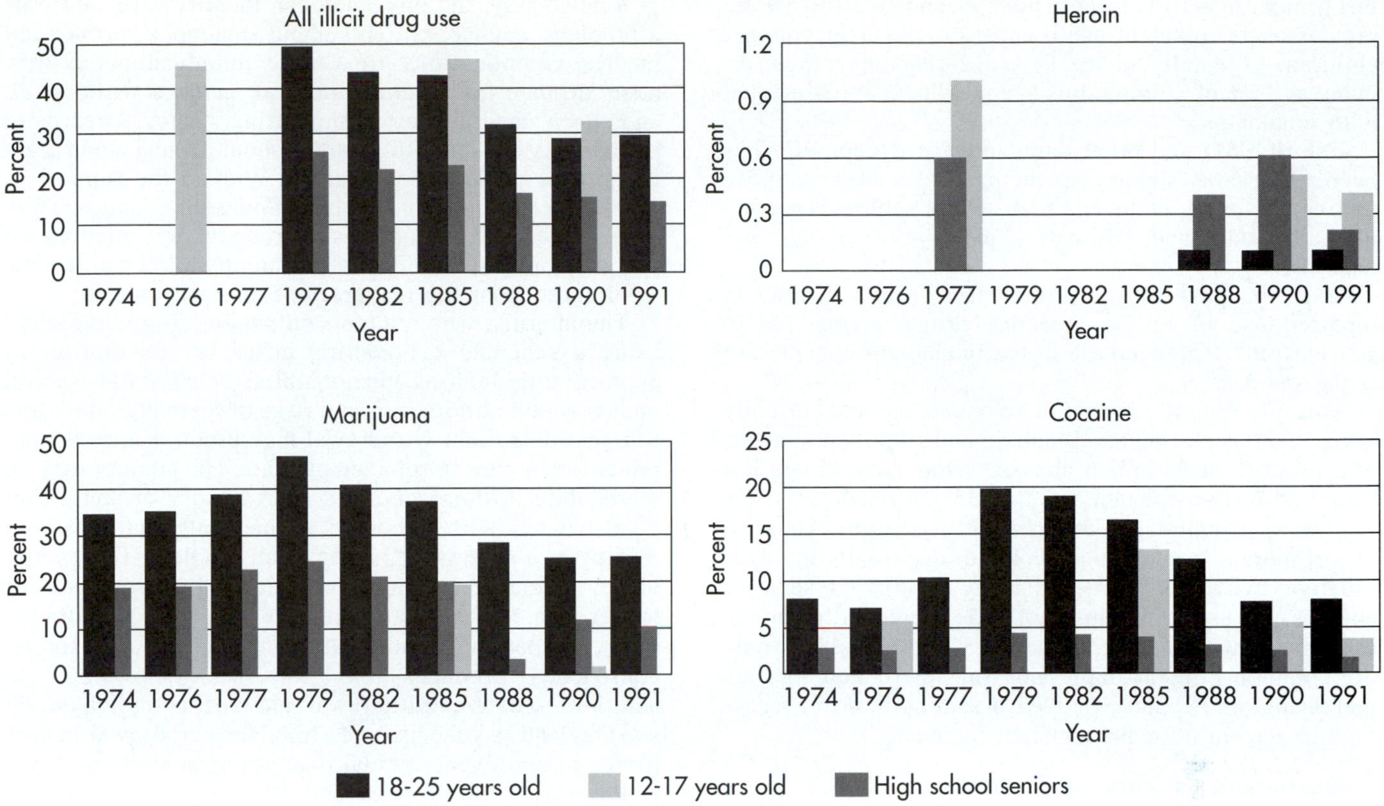


**Fig. 131-1.** Percent of respondents reporting drug use. Selected data from the National Household Survey on Drug Abuse and Drug Use Among American High School Students and Other Young Adults. (From Statistical Abstracts, 1994.)

DAWN data it is clear that a steep increase in emergency room visits throughout the 1970s stabilized in the 1980s; however, the number of visits began to climb again in 1988 and continued to increase through 1992. The data, at variance with other measures of national drug use, may represent utilization of emergency rooms by a subset of patients who became addicted earlier and are now developing complications.

The National Household Survey is an annual survey of selected households regarding recent, remote, and lifetime drug use. The High School Senior Survey reports on use by graduating seniors, without capturing students who, perhaps because of drug use, have left school. Fig. 131-1 summarizes selected recent data from these two national surveys.

Heroin use underwent a rapid increase in the 1960s, and another one in the 1970s, as well as a shift in target population from rural whites and urban bohemians to inner-city African-American young men. By 1972 there were an estimated 2 million users and 600,000 "addicts." The national population of heroin users now appears to have stabilized at about one half million. Between 0.1% and 0.3% of young adults currently report having used heroin at least once.

There are approximately one million regular users, of whom 15% are in some form of treatment, most commonly methadone maintenance.

Mortality among these young heroin abusers may be as high as 2% per year. Morbidity has not been well described. Studies suggest that the numbers and population characteristics of heroin users will not change much over the next decade. From the same studies it appears clear that the use of nonopiates does not necessarily lead to heroin use and (contrary to popular belief) may identify low-risk individuals. The tendency of heroin users to abandon opiate use with increasing age has been confirmed in several reports.

Like heroin, the popularity of cocaine has risen and fallen in discrete epidemics throughout this century. The most recent epidemic in the 1970s and 1980s was in part related to the new availability of inexpensive alkaloidal cocaine suitable for smoking ("crack"). In 1979, nearly 20% of adults in the 18 to 25 age group reported use during that year. By 1991 this proportion had fallen to 7.7%. From 1986, when use among high school seniors peaked at 16.9%, to 1991 reported use had fallen to 7.8%.

About one half of all adults middle-aged and younger have smoked marijuana at least once. About one fourth of this group use marijuana occasionally, and 10% to 15% are regular users. Inhalant use is most prevalent in younger children, especially in the 9- to 12-year age range. As many as 15% of children this age may have experimented with inhalants.

Use of LSD and other hallucinogens except PCP has been remarkably stable over the past 2 decades, with 5% to 10% of young adults and high school seniors reporting use at least once. However, phencyclidine use has declined.

Over the past 10 years there has been a decline in reported use of all psychoactive drugs among 12- to 17-year-olds. The decrease in marijuana and cocaine use is the steepest.

Multiple drug use is said to be increasing and certainly is common among opiate, sedative, and stimulant abusers. The proportion of opiate abusers using other drugs has been variously estimated at 3% to 35% for sedatives, 2% to 20% for cocaine, and 4% to 40% for alcohol. Abuse of two or more nonopiate, nonalcohol drugs usually involves sedatives with stimulants. As many as 40% of sedative abusers also use stimulants, and 40% of both hallucinogen and stimulant abusers report sedative use as well. Despite the common clinical impression that these numbers are increasing, it is unclear to what extent improved case finding accounts for the apparent increase.

## Interactions of patients and physicians

In the treatment of drug abusers a relationship of trust is both essential and difficult to establish or sustain. A number of characteristic problems arise in the formation and maintenance of this relationship.

***Confusion over the physician's role.*** The role of the physician, particularly when other agencies and professionals are involved, must be defined early, explicitly, and often repeatedly. The first interview is not too early to discuss with the patient such issues as drug prescriptions, intervention with other agencies, times of appointments, emergency phone arrangements, inpatient and withdrawal capabilities of the physician, and the nature and extent of adequate health maintenance visits. None of this need sound threatening or paternalistic.

Without such definition the physician's duties may come to include protecting a patient from the legal system or intervening repeatedly between the patient and the drug treatment program. Physicians may find themselves issuing letters to a variety of government agencies or prescribing a succession of psychoactive medications.

This sort of ever-expanding involvement comes about through patient pressure, especially when the physician feels ineffective or inadequate. Doctors may readily observe in their drug-abusing patients the unrealistic wish for immediate, magical solutions. Failure to discern their own desires to work that magic may lead physicians to extend their role inappropriately.

Overprescribing is an especially common problem of role confusion. The physician is well advised to avoid prescribing any psychoactive drug without adequate consultation from a psychiatrist or the drug treatment program in which the patient is enrolled. A policy regarding prescription should be part of the "ground rules" established with the patient at the outset.

Realistically, the physician can identify drug abuse as a problem, counsel patients about treatment options and medical complications, treat these complications as they arise, arrange for inpatient referral, manage withdrawal, and play a steadfast part in supporting whatever treatment modality is chosen. Only rarely should a physician treat drug abuse or dependence alone. Without the support of others the task is formidable. Counseling expertise is specialized, and such options as group therapy, methadone prescription, and therapeutic community exceed either the legal capacity or the resources of most physicians.

The internist who attempts outpatient drug withdrawal using a schedule of tapering doses or substitution of another drug such as phenobarbital or clonidine should understand the limitations and risks of these attempts. It is true that outpatient withdrawal may produce long-lasting remission or cure in selected patients. The attempt may be worthwhile in those giving a short history of abuse that is associated with a course of medically administered therapy or a reversible psychosocial problem. This is not, however, the usual situation. Pathologic drug use for longer than 1 month is unlikely to respond to withdrawal alone. Outpatient withdrawal from opiates, for example, consistently produces remission rates below 5%. In addition, sedative withdrawal may be complicated by seizures and psychosis, and stimulant withdrawal causes profound and even suicidal depression in some patients.

Physicians faced with the need for an immediate decrease in the patient's drug use should strongly consider hospitalization for sedative and stimulant abusers and referral to ambulatory or inpatient programs for opiate abusers. Withdrawal in a specialized drug treatment setting increases the chance that a patient will be directed to definitive therapy and minimizes the risks of abstinence.

***Testing and manipulation.*** A conspicuous feature of even the best defined physician-patient relationship is the tendency for drug abusers to test the limits and rules of that relationship. The lack of structure that usually characterizes the lives of uncontrolled drug users often leads them to desire, but at the same time to doubt, the enforcement of contracts with stated limits. In this respect drug abusers have been compared with adolescents, another group whose sense of internal controls is not fully developed.

Physicians must expect that drug abusers will seek a confrontation over the "ground rules," whatever they may be. Beyond the often trivial issue being tested is the patient's ability to trust in the consistency of the contract itself.

Patient testing often takes the form of attempted manipulation: the patient who must be seen immediately for a chronic complaint; the patient who has lost the same prescription twice and needs a third; the patient who wants a prescription and states that the alternative is a resort to street crime. These forms of testing can be upsetting, even when the basis for them is appreciated. It is important, therefore, for the physician to keep in mind the real issue behind the manipulation, to enforce the limits of the therapeutic contract gently but firmly, and to remember that exceptions, clearly identified as such, must sometimes be made. No physician can correctly identify every manipulation, and every patient sometimes "wins one." A sense of humor is an invaluable asset.

***Denial and ambivalence.*** It must be expected that patients tend to deny the seriousness of their drug use. The alcoholic who grossly underrepresents daily consumption is a familiar example. Physicians annoyed, puzzled, or even amused by their patients' apparent blindness may construe denial as an attempt to deceive.

Denial can be expressed in many ways. The patient may subtly redefine a difficult chronic problem as a simple acute one (e.g., the opiate user who needs only a prescription to tide him or her over until he or she starts the methadone program, the cocaine user who needs only a diuretic for swollen, phlebitic ankles). Denial may also appear as the suppression of important information (e.g., the patient who uses sedatives insists that the drugs "just keep me normal," but in fact has had abstinence seizures, lost work, endangered important relationships, caused several accidents, and become severely depressed).

When patients deny the extent of their problem it is usually because they are ambivalent about abandoning drug use. This is not necessarily a poor prognostic sign. The patient who solemnly admits how bad things are but who has only indefinite future plans to "get off on my own" is not likely to do well. The patient who minimizes the problem but has sought help for it often stands the better chance.

It is important for the physician to understand that in addition to the adversities of drug use there are pleasures and advantages. For the street addict it is difficult but immediately rewarding and regular work to maintain a habit. The skills brought into play are vastly more complex than those required for the usual alternative: low paid menial employment. A sense of identity and peer recognition accrue to the successful, streetwise user. In others, the use of drugs may provide a convenient explanation for and an escape from serious psychosocial problems. For many the advantages are obscure, but they undoubtedly exist.

## Legal implications of treating drug abusers

Treatment of drug abuse is tightly regulated by state and federal laws. when these laws differ, the more limiting of the two is applied. Some federal regulations are summarized below.

***Prescription of opiates.*** Physicians may *prescribe* schedule II opiates to individuals known to be opiate-dependent only under the following circumstances:

1. To treat pain in an outpatient only if the physician notifies the state department of health. Hospitalized patients may be treated without notification.
2. To continue methadone maintenance in a hospitalized patient.
3. To effect opiate withdrawal in a hospitalized patient only if there is another, primary diagnosis for which the patient is being treated. Patients may be admitted for the primary purpose of withdrawal only to specialized facilities or if opiates are not used in treating abstinence.

Physicians may *dispense* schedule II opiates to a known opiate abuser only under the following circumstances:

1. To treat opiate abstinence in an emergency room or other appropriate medical setting. Only one dose of opiate may be given per day for a maximum of 3 consecutive days, and attempts to refer the patient to a drug treatment program must be made (see the Managed Care Guide).
2. To maintain or withdraw an opiate-dependent individual in specially licensed drug treatment facilities.

***Other schedule II drugs.*** There are no federal regulations concerning the prescription or dispensing of other schedule II drugs to patients dependent on them. Most states, however, prohibit prescription to a known abuser for longer than several months.

***Confidentiality.*** Patients enrolled in drug treatment programs have a federally guaranteed right to confidentiality. Information, including the fact that the patient is in the program, can be released only after the patient gives written permission. An exception is made for medical emergencies.

Physicians are obliged to inform the state health department when they prescribe opiates to an opiate-dependent individual but must not reveal the diagnosis of opiate abuse to any other person outside the treatment setting. Information obtained by the state cannot be released except for aggregated statistical and epidemiologic studies or in response to subpoena in a criminal prosecution.

***Admission of drug abusers to hospitals.*** It may be a violation of civil rights law and may constitute malpractice to deny hospital admission to a drug abuser because of the patient's history of drug abuse.

***Treatment of abstinence.*** There is no legal obligation to treat drug abstinence syndromes except in prisons. Failure to treat or refer iatrogenically-induced dependence may, however, be considered medical abandonment (e.g., discharging a hospitalized patient without referral after methadone has been started). Failure to treat abstinence may also constitute malpractice if damage results to the patient.

### Managed Care Guide
### Requirements for admission to methadone maintenance

Because methadone maintenance is still regarded by federal law as a treatment of last resort, patients must meet the following criteria for admission:

1. A documented history of opiate dependence (by prior treatment, a medical opinion, or physical examination) for at least 1 year (2 years if the patient is under 18).
2. Current dependence documented by signs of abstinence or the opinion of a physician.
3. An exception to criterion 1 is pregnant women.
4. Exceptions to criterion 2 are patients who voluntarily left maintenance treatment within 2 years and patients who have been institutionalized within 6 months but were previously eligible.

# EXAMINATION OF DRUG ABUSERS

## History

A detailed drug use history is of importance when conducting and interpreting the physical examination, choosing among referral options, selecting appropriate laboratory tests, and estimating prognosis. Relapse is common, even among patients who have not used drugs in several years, and former drug abusers should also be questioned about their drug use histories.

Intoxicated patients are unlikely to give accurate information within a reasonable period of time, and patients undergoing abstinence are often too restless to give a thoughtful and detailed history. Therefore the history should be reviewed at a subsequent interview.

If additional information is required from a family member, the patient's permission should always be obtained. Interviewing patient and relative together is usually confusing, and both may withhold information.

## Physical examination

Drug abuse is sometimes unsuspected or underestimated from the history. Physical examination may make or confirm the diagnosis. The primary purpose of the examination, however, is to exclude drug-related and other disease.

***Skin.*** The extent of parenteral drug use can often be estimated by examining the skin. The absence of accessible, patent veins is of great prognostic significance as regular subcutaneous injection almost invariably leads to abscess formation, cellulitis, lymphedema, and venous insufficiency. The threat of gangrene and osteomyelitis is greatly increased.

Evidence of deep injections into the axillary, internal jugular, or femoral veins should be sought in patients with no other venous access. Findings in these areas greatly increase the probability that the patient has sought "expert" assistance in a shooting gallery or among friends and should prompt a search for traumatic neuropathies, fistulas, deep abscesses, hematomas, and mediastinitis.

Parallel needle marks, a single row of scars, hyperpigmentation overlying a vein, and palpably sclerotic veins are all signs of chronic intravenous use. When needle marks are many and recent, cocaine use should be suspected. When tissue damage seems out of proportion to the number of needle marks, particularly irritating drugs such as cocaine, oxycodone (Percodan), or propoxyphene are suspected.

Signs of chronic venous or lymphatic insufficiency include edema and multiple scars from old or new abscesses. When edema is limited to the hands, renal disease and heart failure are unlikely explanations; however, methadone (especially in high doses) can cause edema. Women appear to be more commonly affected.

Another consequence of drug abuse is thrombocytopenia induced by alcohol, quinine, or brown heroin and manifested by petechiae. Urticaria resulting from opiate-mediated histamine release may also be present. Dermal bullae and acne suggest barbiturate and bromide abuse, respectively; scars from cigarette burns are commonly found in opiate and sedative abusers. Excoriations can result from opiate-induced pruritus, poor hygiene, or stimulant-associated tactile hallucinations. It is rare for Kaposi's sarcoma to occur in heterosexual drug abusers with acquired immune deficiency syndrome (AIDS). Herpes zoster, however, is not infrequently seen in patients who subsequently develop AIDS-related complex (ARC) or AIDS.

***Head and neck.*** Perforation of the nasal septum is often found in nasal users, particularly of stimulants. Dental caries are also extremely common among stimulant users. Their presence is of bacteriologic importance in patients suspected of pulmonary infection. Scleral icterus should be routinely sought, and ophthalmoscopy may disclose retinal emboli and ischemia (usually due to talc particles) in parenteral users and central nervous system (CNS) disease associated with AIDS. Vertebral palpation, especially in the neck, may disclose tenderness suggestive of osteomyelitis.

***Chest.*** Right ventricular failure manifested by prominent neck veins, pedal edema, and a right ventricular heave or gallop sound can be due to cor pulmonale (from pulmonary talc granulomas or vasculitis) or to heroin-induced cardiomyopathy. If, in addition, a pulsatile liver, a murmur, or large V waves are discovered, infectious tricuspid valvular damage becomes a likely cause of failure. Irregularity of the pulse may indicate a toxic arrhythmia, sequelae of a prolonged QT interval (described in heroin users), or a chronic cardiomyopathy.

Scarring from recurrent pneumonia and bronchiectasis may be suspected from early inspiratory rales. Opiate and sedative abusers are at particular risk because of suppression of their respirations and cough reflexes.

Marijuana or methadone-induced hypogonadism are in the differential diagnosis of gynecomastia in a drug user. The possibilities of testicular and hepatic disease must, of course, also be investigated in the young population with a high prevalence of alcoholism and viral hepatitis. "Pseudogynecomastia" occurs when subcutaneous injection of drugs in breast tissue causes local fibrosis.

***Abdomen.*** Signs of hepatitis must be sought, including punch tenderness over the liver, hepatomegaly, and icterus. Splenomegaly is a relatively common finding in otherwise healthy parenteral drug users. Enlargement of the spleen should, however, prompt closer examination of the lymph nodes (AIDS-related adenopathy, chronic infection, lymphoma), mucous membranes (oral candidiasis), lungs (tuberculosis and *Pneumocystis carinii*), CNS (syphilis, opportunistic infection), and bones (osteomyelitis).

Both male and female drug abusers may be prostitutes. Genital and rectal examinations to exclude venereal disease and cervical cancer are essential. In addition to the usual considerations, the presence of blood in the stool suggests sexual trauma, chronic constipation from opiates, and gastritis or an ulcer from such irritants as alcohol, Percodan, and chloral hydrate.

***Lymph nodes.*** Adenopathy in parenteral users is common, particularly in the groin and axillae. Cervical adenopathy may be due to local intravenous injections, poor dental hygiene, AIDS-related adenopathy, lymphoma, or as part of a syndrome of benign hyperplastic adenopathy. Subcutaneous fibrosis from cervical injection is sometimes difficult to distinguish from adenopathy. Adenopathy should never be neglected because of a history of drug abuse.

*Nervous system.* Peripheral neuropathy with a predilection for the radial nerve and brachial plexus is an unexplained complication of parenteral opiate use. Hexane inhalation, lead toxicity from gasoline sniffing, and alcohol may also produce distal neuropathy. Cerebellar ataxia may indicate alcohol- or inhalant-induced atrophy as well as intoxication with opiates, sedatives, stimulants, inhalants, or hallucinogens. Necrotizing cerebral angiitis seen in stimulant abusers (parenteral or oral), may produce a variety of neurologic findings. Cocaine-related problems include focal deficits from spasm, bleeding, bland infarction, or postictally; however, the evidence for cocaine vasculitis is not so strong as for amphetamine. Opiate overdose occasionally leaves the patient with unexplained focal deficits. AIDS-associated infection or lymphoma and emboli from infective endocarditis can also cause focal findings in the CNS.

*Extremities.* In addition to the dermatologic abnormalities mentioned, arterial insufficiency resulting from repeated intraarterial injection should be sought. Cyanosis is sometimes present in nitrite abusers owing to the formation of methemoglobin; the absence of cardiopulmonary disease and failure to improve with oxygen suggests the diagnosis. Joint examination should include the sternoclavicular and sacroiliac joints, where septic arthritis is most common.

### Laboratory screening

A number of common laboratory tests are frequently abnormal in drug abusers. The choice of baseline data varies with the age and drug history of the patient. A blood count, multichannel chemical analysis of serum, an electrocardiogram, tuberculin and *Trichophyton* skin testing, and urinalysis suffice for most patients. Hepatitis B surface antigen, which is present in the serum of 10% to 40% of parenteral drug users, is an expensive test. A positive finding, however, would prompt urgent counseling about needle sharing, closer follow-up of liver function tests, and further serologic testing. At this time neither T-lymphocyte testing nor viral serology is indicated for routine screening of parenteral drug users for AIDS.

Urine toxicology is an often inaccurate guide to drugs in the body. It is possible that more harm is done to the treatment relationship than information gained by its routine use.

### Routine immunization and prophylaxis

Drug abusers are at increased risk of tetanus, pneumonia, tuberculosis, viral hepatitis, and AIDS-associated infections. Regular tuberculin skin testing and tetanus prophylaxis every 10 years are advisable. Pneumovax prophylaxis should be strongly considered in a population at risk for HIV infection. Patients who are negative for hepatitis B surface antibody (only about 10% of parenteral drug users) should be given hepatitis B vaccine, but the cost of screening may be a poor use of resources in a population where the prevalence is so high.

Positive tuberculin skin tests in young patients should certainly be treated with 1 year of isoniazid if the conversion is recent. Prophylaxis of conversion when it is of uncertain age in a population prone to liver disease and neuropathy is probably a matter for individual decision. The local prevalence of atypical mycobacterial infection and tuberculosis, the adequacy of follow-up, and the patient's compliance, age, and drug use history must be weighed.

## DRUGS OF ABUSE

### Opiates

Opiates have long been recognized as prototypical drugs of abuse and dependence. Within the past few years, observation of increased norepinephrine turnover in opiate-abstinent subjects suggested a role for the major norepinephrine brainstem locus, the locus ceruleus, in opiate dependence. The locus ceruleus appears to be supplied with opiate receptors that inhibit the firing of ascending norepinephrine neurons. These ascending neurons, however, are also inhibited by other, nonopiate substances, particularly alpha-2 agonists. Rebound hyperexcitability of locus ceruleus neurons has been shown to occur in opiate abstinence and to be reversed by alpha-2 agonists such as clonidine and lofexidine. Clinical reversal of abstinence signs and symptoms has also been accomplished with these drugs.

Current biochemical research is largely focused on the development of other alpha-2 agonists and possibly other types of locus ceruleus blocking agents. Work continues on the development of partial agonists with acceptable subjective effects, low dependence liability, and the ability to block the euphoria produced by potent opiates. (Buprenorphine is one such drug.) Finally, it appears possible that opiate receptor pharmacology will greatly clarify the physiology and biochemistry of opiate dependence in the near future.

*Opiate types.* Commonly abused opiates produce similar clinical syndromes of intoxication and abstinence. There are, however, important differences among these drugs in regard to purity, oral potency, time course in the body, and presentation in overdose.

*Heroin* (diacetyl morphine) is a synthetic derivative of opium, easily produced, illegally manufactured, and heavily diluted with adulterants. The most common of these is quinine (quinine and not heroin metabolites are most commonly assayed for evidence of recent drug use); however, the following are also encountered: mannitol, lactose, talc, baking soda, procaine, caffeine, and (with homicidal intent) nicotine or battery acid. Modal purity of street heroin (only 2% to 3% in the 1970s) has increased in response to the popularity of crack. Most heroin in the United States in recent years has come from Asian opium, although Mexican heroin is also seen. Asian heroin is a white or off-white powder or crystalline material sold on the street usually in glassine envelopes and as fractions of a gram. A heroin abuser may use up to 10 or more nominal quarter-grams ("quarters" now refers to the price, $25) daily in one to more than eight doses.

Heroin is prepared for injection by heating it with water from the nearest available source, usually in a spoon or bottle cap. Once in solution the hot heroin is strained through a cigarette filter or balled cotton (to prevent undissolved particles from blocking the needle) and drawn into a tuberculin syringe or eye dropper to which a small-gauge needle is mounted. Injection of the solution may be followed by "booting," the practice of drawing back and reinjecting blood several times before removing the needle from the vein. When heroin is unobtainable, the filter may be heated in water to release trapped particles.

Heroin can also be insufflated ("snorted") or heated in a pipe or on tinfoil while the smoke is inhaled ("chasing the dragon").

Absorption of heroin after oral ingestion is good, but first-pass hepatic metabolism greatly decreases systemic availability. Heroin itself has a half-time in the body of only 20 to 30 minutes; it is rapidly metabolized to monoacyl morphine (MAM) and morphine. These active products are in turn metabolized by the liver into inactive glucuronides. The half-times of morphine and MAM are each about 2 hours. Neither is extensively protein- or tissue-bound.

*Methadone,* diverted chiefly from maintenance and withdrawal programs, is a common street drug. It comes as a soluble 40-mg, scored orange disk with cellulose added to discourage parenteral use. Methadone is, however, easily filtered. Small white Dolophine (methadone) tablets, 5 and 10 mg, are also available ("dollies"). Methadone comes also as a syrup and a solution (each 10 mg/ml). Parenteral solutions are used in hospitals.

Orally, methadone is well absorbed and undergoes unusually little first-pass transformation in the liver. Parenterally, methadone is a slightly more potent analgesic than morphine on a weight basis. Peak plasma levels occur 2 to 4 hours after ingestion and fall with an elimination half-time of about 1 day. Tissue distribution is extensive, mainly to lung and liver, forming a large deep compartment. Plasma methadone is about 85% protein-bound. It is not dependent on high liver blood flow for clearance, nor have displacement interactions with other drugs been reported. Methadone is metabolized in the liver to inactive compounds and is also excreted unchanged in the urine, particularly in women. Urinary acidification produces a demonstrable but clinically unimportant increase in urinary excretion. Even advanced liver disease appears to have little effect on methadone kinetics.

Used as an analgesic, methadone's duration of action is no longer than that of morphine until accumulation takes place after a week or more. With chronic dosing, however, analgesia may last 8 to 12 hours.

Methadone metabolism is induced by rifampin, phenytoin, and possibly phenobarbital. Abstinence in maintenance patients has been precipitated by rifampin and phenytoin. Propoxyphene and possibly tricyclic antidepressants may decrease methadone metabolism through competitive inhibition, but clinically important effects have not been reported.

*LAAM,* α-*l*-acetylmethadol, is a synthetic derivative of methadone. It is slightly less potent than methadone on a weight basis but is metabolized with a half-time of 1.5 to 2 days. LAAM is used in a few maintenance programs and comes as a solution (10 mg/ml). The clinical effects of LAAM are similar to those of methadone, although initial hyperactivity followed after 24 hours by sluggishness seems to be a distinguishing characteristic.

*Percodan* is the trade name for a mixture of oxycodone, aspirin, and caffeine. *Percocet* contains oxycodone and acetaminophen. Both are common street opiates. Although insoluble, oxycodone in these preparations can be injected by forming a suspension in water ("cold shake"). Oxycodone is relatively bioavailable (about 50%). It is metabolized in the liver to inactive products and excreted unchanged in the urine. Elimination half-time is about 2 hours. The use of large quantities in tolerant individuals may present as salicylism, acetaminophen-induced hepatic dysfunction, gastric hemorrhage from aspirin toxicity, and severe chemical or septic phlebitis from venous irritation.

*Demerol* (meperidine) is an uncommon street opiate but is not infrequently abused by medical personnel. It comes in prefilled syringes for parenteral use containing 25, 50, or 100 mg and in multidose bottles. Tablets are 50 and 100 mg.

Meperidine is metabolized in the liver in part to the active normeperidine, which is weakly analgesic and a convulsant. Seizures have been reported in poisoning cases, in patients receiving chronic high doses, and in patients with renal insufficiency or cancer. Naloxone does not prevent seizures in normeperidine-treated animals. The half-time and duration of analgesia of meperidine are rather shorter than those of morphine.

*Darvon* (propoxyphene) is a weak opiate agonist available as the napsylate (Darvon-N, 65 mg; Darvon-N 100, 100 mg) and the more soluble hydrochloride (Darvon, 100 mg). Combination products with aspirin and acetaminophen are also available. The oral bioavailability of propoxyphene is high. It is metabolized in the liver with a variable half-time of 3 to 8 hours and is little bound to plasma proteins. Dependence, even when the intravenous route is used, usually is mild and self-limited. Intravenous use is also short-lived owing to the drug's irritating effect on veins.

Propoxyphene has been used with some success in doses up to 1200 mg daily to treat opiate abstinence. It is not, however, as effective as stronger opiates, and in high doses liver function abnormalities and behavioral changes have been noted. With overdose, cardiac conduction, disturbances, and seizures may produce an unusual picture of opiate toxicity.

*Talwin* (pentazocine) is a partial opiate antagonist developed as a nonaddicting analgesic but capable of causing mild dependence. It is available as 50-mg white tablets and in ampules containing 25 and 50 mg.

*Dihydrocodeinone,* marketed in pure form as Dicodid and Tussionex, is a highly bioavailable oral opiate used for cough suppression. Parenterally, dihydrocodeinone is equipotent with morphine on a weight basis; however, first-pass metabolism of morphine is much higher. Tablets (5 mg) and a syrup (5 mg/cc) are available. The drug is also found in combination with antihistamines, anticholinergics, and catecholamines. Marked dependence can occur in persons taking up to 1500 mg daily.

*Other opiates* that may be encountered include Dilaudid (hydromorphone), a short-acting oral and parenteral opiate of greater potency than morphine and considerable street popularity. Deodorized tincture of opium (DTO) is a 10% opium solution in water and alcohol that is equivalent to about 1% morphine. Numorphan (oxymorphone) is an orally active opiate that is rarely encountered. Codeine is an uncommon cause of opiate dependence because of its side effects at relatively low doses.

***Intoxication and overdose.*** Opiate intoxication causes drowsiness, contentment, a sense of warmth, and analgesia. The peak effect from intravenous injection ("flash" or "rush") is marked by intense euphoria lasting several seconds. Especially in novices, intoxication may cause nausea and vomiting. Pruritus also occurs commonly. Despite similar clinical effects, different opiates are reliably distinguished by experienced users.

On examination the patient may be dozing intermittently ("nodding") and scratching. Speech is infrequent and slurred, pupils are pinpoint, pulse and blood pressure are slightly decreased, and respirations are diminished in depth and frequency. In cold climates there may be hypothermia. The sensorium is clear, and neither tremor nor nystagmus is present. Miosis and the absence of nystagmus or marked ataxia distinguishes opiate intoxication from sedative, alcohol, and solvent intoxication. Combination of opiates with cocaine ("speed ball") may produce tachycardia, tremor, alertness, and fluent speech along with signs of opiate intoxication.

Despite the often dramatic picture of intoxication, overdose is surprisingly rare. Poisoning usually follows the use of pure pharmaceutical drugs or unexpectedly high grade street heroin. Overdose with street opiates is uncommon among methadone-maintained patients because of their consistently high tolerance.

Opiate overdose may present as sudden death, hypoxia from alveolar hypoventilation, pulmonary edema, or coma. Focal neurologic deficits are occasionally part of the presentation. Seizures and arrhythmias characterize propoxyphene poisoning, and seizures with mydriasis suggest meperidine overdose. Seizures may also be due to hypoxemia, mixed overdose, or overdose associated with head trauma.

There appear to be two sudden death syndromes, one resulting from arrhythmia and occurring within seconds, the other a result of respiratory depression and developing over minutes to hours. Arrhythmia deaths may be related to the observation of chronic ST-T wave changes and prolonged QT intervals in the electrocardiograms of some heroin abusers. Concomitant alcohol use may also be associated with arrhythmia deaths.

The diagnosis of opiate poisoning should be suspected from the physical examination; however, response to naloxone is definitive. Given intravenously 0.8 mg (two ampules) of naloxone reliably reverses all opiate intoxications. A possible exception is propoxyphene poisoning, which may require two such doses. All obtunded patients in whom the cause of coma is not fully understood should receive naloxone. Naloxone is a pure opiate antagonist which, unlike nalorphine, does not deepen coma in nondependent patients.

Given intravenously, naloxone reaches peak effect within 5 to 10 minutes. By the intramuscular route absorption is maximal within about 15 minutes, and this route should be used without waiting for a cutdown or deep vein cannulation to be completed. Naloxone has been reported to arouse some alcohol-intoxicated patients, but such response is unusual. Naloxone may also increase blood pressure and cardiac output in patients with septic shock. Other causes of coma do not respond to naloxone and are excluded by a complete response.

Before giving naloxone, pupil size, vital signs, and coma grade are recorded. Any response to 0.8 mg should prompt administration of 0.4 mg every 5 minutes until 10 doses have been given or coma is reversed. Rapid reversal of opiate toxicity has rarely been reported to precipitate pulmonary edema and cause hypertension. Abstinence occurs in dependent persons, with the risk of rage reaction and discharge against advice.

Lack of response to naloxone or an incomplete response raises the following considerations in known drug abusers: postictal confusion; sepsis (with or without cerebral embolism); cerebral anoxia (from hypoventilation, pulmonary edema, arrhythmia, or shock); tetanus; hypertensive stroke from stimulants; neurologic sequelae of hepatitis; cerebral angiitis associated with stimulant abuse; AIDS-related cerebral infection (including toxoplasmosis, cryptococcosis, herpes encephalitis, progressive multifocal leukoencephalopathy, and cytomegalovirus encephalitis); uremia (from heroin-induced glomerulopathy, amyloidosis, or rhabdomyolysis); gastrointestinal hemorrhage from aspirin-containing opiates such as Percodan; hemorrhagic pancreatitis masked by opiate analgesia; and internal bleeding from heroin- or quinine-induced thrombocytopenia. Mixed poisoning is another frequent cause of partial response to naloxone. The possibility of attempted homicide should not be overlooked. Strychnine, acid, or unexpectedly pure heroin are reliably fatal.

Home remedies applied by the patient's friends may complicate diagnosis and management. Salt water injections, forced ingestions of milk, and ice packs to the genitals are among the popular antidotes.

Pulmonary edema of opiate overdose presents as the rapid onset of bilateral alveolar infiltrates. Heart size is normal, and blood gases demonstrate metabolic and respiratory acidosis. The mechanism of pulmonary edema is thought to be mainly central; however, the local toxicity of heroin may also play a part.

Focal neurologic findings occasionally complicate the presentation of opiate poisoning. Middle cerebral artery syndromes, sometimes with arteriographic occlusions, are unexplained.

The treatment of opiate overdose includes naloxone, support of blood pressure and respiration, treatment of pulmonary edema, and only rarely gastrointestinal decontamination with ipecac, charcoal, and cathartics.

Induced vomiting can be helpful within 4 hours of opiate ingestions if the patient is alert or can be aroused with naloxone. Apomorphine is antagonized by naloxone and should not be used for inducing emesis when naloxone is given.

Severe cerebral hypoxia or pulmonary edema may require intubation, but an endotracheal tube is not routinely passed for the purpose of airway protection during lavage until naloxone has failed.

The duration of action of naloxone is 45 minutes, shorter than that of most opiates. Infusions or repeated doses of naloxone are therefore often required. When coma has once been completely reversed by naloxone, however, there is usually no reason to maintain complete reversal. It is a good deal easier to manage a stable, sleepy patient than an angry, obstinate one.

Treatment of pulmonary edema is with the usual means, but digoxin is not used. Infiltrates clear within 48 to 72 hours, although pulmonary function tests may be abnormal for several weeks.

Opiates produce fecal impaction and urinary retention. These conditions should be sought and corrected.

Initial work-up of the seriously poisoned patient includes a complete blood count, assays for arterial blood gases, clotting studies, hepatic and renal function tests, assays for electrolytes, blood glucose determination, an electrocardiogram, and a chest x-ray. When Percodan, Percocet, or propoxyphene combinations are suspected, blood levels of aspirin or acetaminophen are obtained. Screening of serum for poisons is not helpful. The utility of urine toxicology screening has also been questioned, although it may provide useful confirmation of a mixed overdose.

Admission of opiate-poisoned patients is considered in the following circumstances: (1) when overdose is caused by a long-acting opiate such as methadone or LAAM; (2) when multiple drugs are suspected; (3) when there is a serious medical problem related or unrelated to the overdose. No patient should be discharged until it is clear that additional naloxone is unnecessary.

***Abstinence.*** Daily administration of opiates in increasing doses for several weeks produces clinical tolerance. The extent of this tolerance may be extreme; daily use in some patients can approach 100 times the customary doses in nontolerant subjects. Upon deprivation a typical abstinence syndrome occurs. Acute, or primary, abstinence was the only recognized syndrome until the 1960s. It is clear, however, that a milder, more prolonged illness follows the acute phase. The onset of primary abstinence, its duration, and its severity are related mainly to the half-time of the particular opiate, the dose, and the dosage frequency. Abstinence is unpleasant but never life-threatening or extremely painful, and it is always self-limited. The lengths to which opiate abusers go in order to avoid the syndrome often appear disproportionate to its objective severity. Attempts to describe stages or grades of primary abstinence minimize overlapping but can be useful (Table 131-1).

Primary abstinence is characterized by hyperadrenergic signs. Delayed, or secondary, abstinence presents mainly hypoadrenergic manifestations. It has been suggested that these result from desensitization of norepinephrine receptors in structures projecting from the locus ceruleus. Miosis, sluggishness, sleep disturbances, and malaise characterize this syndrome, which emerges gradually from primary abstinence and may persist for 6 months. The occurrence of secondary abstinence provides the physiologic rationale for drug-free programs that segregate patients for up to a year. For the same reason it is the goal of most methadone programs that patients withdraw over many months. An interesting but unresolved question is whether suppression of hyperadrenergic activity with clonidine or lofexidine during primary abstinence attenuates secondary abstinence as well.

Alcohol and sedative abstinence can resemble opiate deprivation: Diaphoresis, tremor, anorexia, tachycardia, and hypertension are common to all three. Seizures and delirium, however, occur only with alcohol and sedative abstinence. If it proves difficult to differentiate a sedative-related syndrome from an opiate-related syndrome, a short-acting barbiturate (e.g., pentobarbital 400 mg orally) or opiate (e.g., morphine 10 mg subcutaneously) can usually make the distinction. Patients frequently self-medicate opiate abstinence or attempt self-directed withdrawal using alcohol, sedatives, mild opiates such as codeine and propoxyphene, or virtually any other psychoactive agent. Hence the resulting picture of intoxication with abstinence may be confusing.

The differential diagnosis of opiate abstinence also includes gastroenteritis, ketoacidosis, surgical conditions in the abdomen, and upper respiratory infection. Rhinorrhea, sometimes said to be a reliable differential sign of abstinence, is also present in viral respiratory infections and allergy. Fever may accompany abstinence but is never more than low grade.

Management of opiate abstinence should never be exclusively chemical. Only intervention that directs the patient toward long-term, definitive treatment is of long-lasting utility. Useful interventions include admission for withdrawal and consideration of options, referral to an outpatient withdrawal or maintenance program, and transfer to a specialized inpatient setting for admission. Prescription of methadone is usually unwise and in most circumstances illegal (see Approach to the Drug-Abusing Patient). Methadone and clonidine schedules used to withdraw hospitalized patients are described in the section on Management of Drug Abusers.

***Medical complications of chronic opiate abuse.*** Cardiac complications of opiate abuse include a toxic cardiomyopathy thought to be heroin-induced, abnormalities of the conduction system including QT prolongation and ST-T wave changes, cor pulmonale, and endocarditis. The dictum remains sound that any parenteral drug user with a fever should be suspected of having endocarditis. Acute bacterial endocarditis is more common than the subacute variety. Frequently isolated organisms are coagulase-positive staphylococci and (in some parts of the United States) *Pseudomonas*. The tricuspid is the most commonly affected valve unless there is preexisting damage at another site. Unlike subacute endocarditis, the acute disease presents as an explosive febrile illness of several days' duration, often with prominent pulmonary findings resulting from septic embolization. A murmur may not be present on initial examination, and immunologic findings such as splenomegaly, vasculitic skin lesions, and a positive latex fixation test are not characteristic. The infecting organism is usually found on the skin and not in the drug. Heroin itself is most often sterile or harbors a few diphtheroids and *Bacillus* species.

Pulmonary complications of opiate abuse include bronchiectasis and recurrent pneumonia, in part from chronic hypoventilation and opiate-mediated cough suppression but also perhaps from heroin toxicity and immune dysfunction. Talc or cotton granulomas in the parenchyma or vessels of the lung may be a cause of pulmonary hypertension and cor pulmonale. Asymptomatic patients may have unexplained ventilation/perfusion mismatch on lung scanning and abnormalities in pulmonary flow rates and volumes. Infectious or chemical mediastinitis is an occasional complication of injection into neck veins; computed tomography is usually diagnostic.

Immunologic and infectious complications include

**Table 131-1.** Abstinence signs in sequential appearance after last dose of narcotic in patients with well established parenteral habits

| Signs (observed in cool room, patient uncovered or under only a sheet) | Hours after last dose Morphine | Heroin | Meperidine | Dihydromorphinone | Codeine | Methadone |
|---|---|---|---|---|---|---|
| Grade 0* | 6 | 4 | 2-3 | 2-3 | 8 | 12 |
| Craving for drug | | | | | | |
| Anxiety | | | | | | |
| Grade 1 | 14 | 8 | 4-6 | 4-5 | 24 | 34-48 |
| Yawning | | | | | | |
| Perspiration | | | | | | |
| Lacrimation | | | | | | |
| Rhinorrhea | | | | | | |
| "Yen" sleep | | | | | | |
| Grade 2 | 16 | 12 | 8-12 | 7 | 48 | 48-72 |
| Increase in above signs plus | | | | | | |
| Mydriasis | | | | | | |
| Gooseflesh (piloerection) | | | | | | |
| Tremors (muscle twitches) | | | | | | |
| Hot and cold flashes | | | | | | |
| Aching bones and muscles | | | | | | |
| Anorexia | | | | | | |
| Grade 3 | 24-36 | 18-24 | 16 | 12 | — | — |
| Increased intensity of above plus | | | | | | |
| Insomnia | | | | | | |
| Increased blood pressure | | | | | | |
| Increased temperature | | | | | | |
| Increased respiratory rate and depth | | | | | | |
| Increased pulse rate | | | | | | |
| Restlessness | | | | | | |
| Nausea | | | | | | |
| Grade 4 | 36-48 | 24-36 | — | 16 | — | — |
| Increased intensity of above plus | | | | | | |
| Febrile facies | | | | | | |
| Position: curled up on hard surface | | | | | | |
| Vomiting | | | | | | |
| Diarrhea | | | | | | |
| Weight loss (5 lb daily) | | | | | | |
| Spontaneous ejaculation or orgasm | | | | | | |
| Hemoconcentration, leukocytosis, eosinopenia, increased blood glucose | | | | | | |

*Grade of abstinence.
From Blachly P: *Am J Psychiatry* 122:7, 1966.

laboratory abnormalities of uncertain significance, cotton fever, and most importantly, increased susceptibility to infections, particularly those related to AIDS. False-positive serologic tests for syphilis occur in as many as 30% of parenteral drug users, usually in low titer. Treponemal tests, however, retain specificity. Similarly, latex fixation and other immunologic tests may be abnormal. Hyperglobulinemia, eosinophilia, and increases in titer of antibody to smooth muscle antigens and to lymphocytes have been reported.

Cotton fever is an acute, self-limited, febrile illness manifested by rigors. It is caused by the injection of cotton fibers when users boil their filters to release trapped heroin. The fever, which may reach 105°F, is gone within 24 hours. Confident distinction from endocarditis is usually impossible on presentation.

Parenteral drug users are susceptible to cellulitis, septic arthritis (especially of the sternoclavicular and sacroiliac joints), pneumonia, endocarditis, osteomyelitis (particularly with *Pseudomonas* or *Serratia* species and particularly of the vertebrae), tuberculosis, tetanus, and AIDS.

New cases of AIDS are far more likely to be due to intravenous drug use now than was the case at the start of the epidemic 10 years ago. In the early 1980s approximately 20% of new AIDS cases were attributable to injection drug use; that proportion is now over 50%. Approximately three quarters of children now diagnosed with AIDS were infected as a result of drug use in one or both parents. Some 40% of women with AIDS were infected because of drug use by their sexual partners.

Data concerning the survival of patients with AIDS attributed to drug use have been inconsistent but appear to show decreased mean survival from diagnosis. Unlike homosexuals with AIDS, drug abusers usually present with opportunistic infections or constitutional and CNS symptoms and only rarely develop Kaposi's sarcoma.

The only malignancies that appear to be unusually prevalent in opiate abusers are AIDS-associated lymphomas and carcinoma of the bladder, which has been reported in opium users. The major hepatic complication of chronic opiate abuse is hepatitis B infection. The prevalence of surface antigen is 10% to 40% in asymptomatic users, and most users have demonstrable surface antibody. Transaminase elevation in healthy opiate users is common but of uncertain cause. Some studies have found viral or chronic hepatitis to be the commonest diagnosis on biopsy, whereas others report mainly alcohol-related disease. Methadone maintenance does not by itself cause hypertransaminasemia.

Renal findings may be primary or secondary. The existence of heroin-induced focal glomerulosclerosis has been established. Black men appear to be at particularly high risk. Other, older studies found a variety of renal lesions in addicts at autopsy. Secondary pathology includes renal complications of hepatitis, septicemia, endocarditis, and myoglobinuria.

Thrombocytopenia is probably the most common hematologic complication. Quinine allergy is well recognized, and a steroid-responsive thrombocytopenia has been ascribed to the use of brown heroin from Mexico.

Endocrine effects of opiates include changes in sex hormones, increases in antidiuretic hormone (ADH), and elevation of serum thyroxine. A dose-related decrease in serum testosterone and libido has been reported in methadone-maintained men and to a lesser extent in heroin users. A hypothalamic mechanism is probable, and gynecomastia is an occasional, possibly related finding. Amenorrhea and decreased libido occur among women using opiates, including methadone. The occurrence of edema in patients (usually women) using high doses of methadone cannot be wholly attributed to increases in ADH that have been observed. Slight elevations of thyroxine and serum copper are due to increases in thyroid-binding globulin and ceruloplasmin. These increases may be related to, and a marker for, concomitant chronic active hepatitis.

Surgical problems associated with opiate abuse include acute arterial insufficiency (from embolus or spasm) following arterial injection, mycotic aneurysms or arteriovenous fistulas, and necrotizing fasciitis from which mixed flora are usually isolated. Necrotizing fasciitis presents like cellulitis, but pain and fever are disproportionate to the apparent lesion. As for tetanus, extensive debridement is essential. An uncommon, apparently surgical complication of opiate use is pseudobowel obstruction. Distention, pain, obstructive bowel sounds, and air-fluid levels seen on x-ray films respond to withdrawal of opiates.

Psychiatric illnesses among opiate abusers are common and varied. Depression appears to be particularly prevalent, although this finding has been challenged. Personality disturbance manifested as high psychopathic scores on testing is a persistent finding, but the patterns of dysfunction and the degree of severity are highly variable. It is unclear if psychiatric illness is ever a toxic effect of opiates. What is probable is that a sizable and growing population uses opiates to alleviate symptoms of preexisting psychiatric disease. Opiates, even in tolerant individuals, appear to produce a variety of chronic psychotropic effects that have not yet been categorized. Even slow withdrawal in susceptible patients can precipitate decompensation.

Psychotherapeutic drugs are effective in opiate abusers when prescribed for clear indications. Monoamine oxidase inhibitors may, however, nonspecifically inhibit enzymes responsible for the metabolism of some opiates, prolonging their actions.

Neurologic sequelae of opiate abuse include postanoxic encephalopathy and unexplained focal deficits following overdose. Acute transverse myelitis and peripheral neuropathies (with a predilection for the radial nerve and brachial plexus) occur in chronic users.

Opiate-abusing women are at high risk for gynecologic infection and unwanted pregnancy because of the prevalence of prostitution. Pregnant heroin abusers rarely receive adequate prenatal care, and they develop many obstetric complications including meconium staining, anemia, premature rupture of membranes, abruption, placenta previa, and multiple births. Their infants tend to be underweight and small for dates. Perinatal mortality is higher than normal, but there is no evidence for an increase in birth defects. There are several case reports linking methadone maintenance with sudden infant death syndrome, but there is no statistical evidence of a connection.

Methadone-maintained women are more likely to attend prenatal clinics than are street heroin users, but it is unclear to what extent obstetric complications are reduced. The infants are larger, better developed, and more likely to remain in the mother's custody. These infants grow slowly during their first 4 months, but subsequently their rate of growth and development accelerates.

High dose methadone appears to produce more severe and more prolonged neonatal abstinence than does heroin or low dose methadone. Attempts to reduce methadone dosage during pregnancy, however, can induce abortion (particularly during the first and third trimesters) and may precipitate a return to heroin abuse. Placental metabolism of methadone during the third trimester may in fact require increases in dosage. Methadone is not present in breast milk in important quantities even during periods of peak plasma levels.

### Sedatives

Sedative hypnotics are a group of synthetic, chemically heterogeneous compounds that nevertheless produce many similar clinical effects. They are antispasmodics and antiepileptics, and they affect the electroencephalogram (EEG). These drugs are self-reinforcing, produce tolerance, and are associated with serious abstinence.

The first synthetic, nonopiate sedatives were the barbiturates, which gained popularity during the 1940s and 1950s. Problems with these compounds quickly became apparent. A narrow therapeutic index makes even a few too many tablets potentially toxic. Moreover, the moderate tolerance that develops to sedative doses does not much increase the threshold to toxic ingestions. With chronic use therefore the margin between hypnosis and toxicity grows even smaller. Moreover, abstinence occurs after chronic doses only two to three times greater than normal, producing a syndrome that includes seizures, delirium, and occasionally death.

Meprobamate, bromide compounds, and subsequently glutethimide, methaqualone, ethchlorvynol, carisoprodol, methyprylon, and chloral hydrate were synthesized in a series of largely unsuccessful attempts to isolate desired anxiolytic and hypnotic properties from tolerance, abstinence, and toxicity.

Benzodiazepines, developed during the 1960s, represent a considerable improvement over their predecessors. Toxicity is extremely low; and it is unlikely that many poisoning deaths are attributable to benzodiazepines taken alone.

As with other sedatives, tolerance develops to the hypnotic effect of benzodiazepines. Anxiolysis, however, is well maintained for at least 6 months without dosage adjustment. Mild abstinence syndromes occur after chronic use of normal doses for several months; however, severe benzodiazepine abstinence requires the chronic use of five to ten times the usual dose. Although self-reinforcing in animal and human experiments, benzodiazepines are less so than other sedatives except major tranquilizers.

The discovery of several types of specific benzodiazepine receptors in the central nervous system and other tissues has stimulated a search for endogenous ligands analogous to endorphins. Receptor-specific antagonists and agonists have been synthesized.

Although benzodiazepines are safe and effective anxiolytics for use in the general population, drug abusers commonly take them in high doses for their sedative effects. These and other sedatives are generally obtained in pharmaceutical form and are taken orally. Medical complications relate therefore to the toxicities of the compounds themselves rather than to their diluents or routes of administration. Complicating the diagnosis and treatment of sedative abuse is the ubiquity of these drugs in daily life. Additional difficulties are raised by the tendency of sedative abusers to take multiple drugs and to suffer from cognitive impairment and affective illnesses.

***Types of sedatives.*** Despite the similarities among sedative hypnotics there are also important kinetic and clinical differences.

*Barbiturates* of abuse are usually intermediate-acting compounds, although abuse of long-acting phenobarbital and barbital also occurs. Secobarbital (Seconal), pentobarbital (Nembutal), and amobarbital (with secobarbital in Tuinal) are white powders soluble in alcohol and hot water. Tablets or capsules contain 30 to 200 mg. Butalbital is present (50 mg) in Fiorinal. These barbiturates are well absorbed, distributed in the body water, and metabolized in the liver to inactive products. Urinary excretion is of little clinical importance and independent of pH. The duration of sleep is 6 to 8 hours in nontolerant individuals; however, effects on the performance of standard tasks are demonstrable for a day.

Half-times are as long as 40 hours, but the effects of these drugs are terminated mainly by redistribution. Tolerance to hypnosis develops over several weeks in chronic dosing, but acute tolerance to large doses is also observed. Poisoned patients, for example, may emerge from coma with blood levels that would otherwise render them unconscious. Tolerance does not develop to doses higher than 1 to 2 g daily; patients taking these doses are chronically intoxicated.

Intermediate-acting barbiturates stimulate the hepatic microsomal enzymes that metabolize them and can lower plasma levels of drugs such as phenytoin, warfarin, alcohol, and other sedatives. Plasma protein binding is slight, however, and displacement interactions do not occur.

*Benzodiazepines* are an ever-expanding group of anxiolytic and hypnotic drugs that at high concentrations also reduce muscle tone by their action on spinal interneurons. Tablet strengths vary from 2 mg (lorazepam) to 30 mg (chlordiazepoxide). Combinations with antidepressants and anticholinergics are also available. Benzodiazepines have similar effects and are best categorized by their kinetics as quickly or slowly metabolized and rapidly or slowly bioavailable (Table 131-2).

Slowly metabolized compounds are demethylated in the liver to active metabolites with half-times of several days. The half-times of these compounds are linearly related to age and importantly prolonged by liver disease or competitive enzyme inhibition (e.g., cimetidine). Quickly metabolized compounds form glucuronides, which are inactive. The half-times of these benzodiazepines are independent of age or even advanced liver disease. Slowly bioavailable benzodiazepines are either slowly absorbed or must be metabolized from an inactive parent drug to active products. Intramuscular absorption of benzodiazepines except lorazepam and the newly introduced midazolam may be erratic. Duration of benzodiazepine action varies among compounds, depending largely on the rate of redistribution, which is in turn a function of lipid solubility.

*Methaqualone* (Quaalude and others) is a fat-soluble white powder available as 150- and 300-mg tablets. It has sedative, hypnotic, and anticonvulsant properties as well as an antitussive and possibly analgesic action. Methaqualone is quickly and completely absorbed, distributed in a large volume owing to tissue binding, and metabolized by microsomal liver enzymes. Half-time is long (about 20 hours), but the drug's action is terminated by redistribution. Enzyme induction is moderate. Methaqualone has a reputation as an aphrodesiac.

*Bromide salts* are rarely abused now. They are slowly excreted by the kidney (half-time 400 hours), but saline diuresis markedly increases clearance. Skin eruptions (acneiform or bullous) are characteristic. Artifactual increases in serum chloride suggest bromide overdose.

*Chloral hydrate* (e.g., Noctec) is often considered a mild hypnotic but can produce tolerance and severe abstinence as well as serious multiorgan toxicity in overdose. It comes as a syrup (100 mg/ml) and as 500- and 1000-mg capsules. Chloral hydrate is rapidly absorbed and immediately converted in the tissues to trichloroethanol, which in turn is metabolized by the liver with a half-time of 8 hours. Both enzyme induction and displacement interactions are characteristic of trichloroethanol.

*Tricyclic antidepressants* are not sedatives; however, those with sedative properties, especially amitriptyline (Elavil), are increasingly popular drugs of abuse. Amitriptyline comes in tablets of 10 to 150 mg. It is quickly absorbed, widely distributed, and metabolized to active products, some with long half-times.

***Intoxication and overdose.*** Sedatives, like alcohol and solvent inhalants, produce disinhibition euphoria and then

**Table 131-2.** Characteristics of benzodiazepines used in the United States

| Administered drug (year introduced) | Brand name | Approved indications | Rate of appearance after oral dose | Active substances in blood* | Overall rate of elimination |
|---|---|---|---|---|---|
| Chlordiazepoxide (1960) | Librium | Anxiety<br>Alcohol withdrawal<br>Preoperative sedation | Intermediate | Chlordiazepoxide<br>Desmethylchlordiaz-epoxide<br>Demoxepam<br>Desmethyldiazepam | Slow |
| Diazepam (1961) | Valium | Anxiety<br>Alcohol withdrawal<br>Muscle spasm<br>Preoperative sedation<br>Status epilepticus | Rapid | Diazepam<br>Desmethyldiazepam | Slow |
| Oxazepam (1963) | Serax | Anxiety<br>Anxiety-depression<br>Alcohol withdrawal | Intermediate to slow | Oxazepam | Intermediate to rapid |
| Flurazepam (1970) | Dalmane | Insomnia | Rapid to intermediate | Hydroxyethyl flurazepam (flurazepam aldehyde)<br>Desalkylflurazepam | Slow |
| Clorazepate (1972) | Tranxene | Anxiety<br>Seizure disorders<br>Alcohol withdrawal | Rapid | Desmethyldiazepam | Slow |
| Clonazepam (1974) | Clonopin | Seizure disorders | Intermediate | Clonazepam | Intermediate |
| Lorazepam (1977) | Ativan | Anxiety<br>Anxiety-depression<br>Preoperative sedation | Intermediate | Lorazepam | Intermediate |
| Prazepam (1977) | Centrax | Anxiety | Slow | Desmethyldiazepam | Slow |
| Temazepam (1981) | Restoril | Insomnia | Intermediate to slow | Temazepam | Intermediate |
| Alprazolam (1981) | Xanax | Anxiety<br>Anxiety-depression | Intermediate | Alprazolam | Intermediate |
| Halazepam (1981) | Paxipam | Anxiety | Intermediate to slow | (Halazepam)<br>Desmethyldiazepam | Slow |
| Triazolam (1983) | Halcion | Insomnia | Intermediate | Triazolam | Rapid |

*Parentheses indicate compounds of minor quantitative importance.
From Greenblatt D et al: *N Engl J Med* 309:354, 1983.

depression and coma. On examination, slurred speech, marked ataxia, and horizontal nystagmus in primary gaze are evident. Miosis, scratching, tremor, vasodilatation, and disorientation are not present. Respirations are depressed, but other vital signs are usually normal. Postural hypotension occurs mainly during early abstinence.

In overdose, profound respiratory depression is characteristic of the barbiturates, whereas cardiovascular effects often predominate with other sedative poisonings. Other findings that may help identify specific sedatives include seizures, prolonged coma, extrapyramidal signs, pulmonary edema, cardiac arrhythmias, skin lesions, and anticholinergic manifestations. Seizures suggest tricyclics or glutethimide, whereas prolonged coma is associated with ethchlorvynol and glutethimide poisonings. Fluctuating coma is common with long-acting barbiturates and may also occur in meprobamate toxicity when a drug mass is present in the stomach. Methaqualone may produce hypertonicity and extrapyramidal signs in overdose. Pulmonary edema raises suspicion of ethchlorvynol or meprobamate poisoning if opiates and salicylates can be ruled out. Cardiac arrhythmia in the absence of severe circulatory compromise may be due to overdoses of chloral hydrate (ectopy), tricyclics (QRS prolongation), or ethchlorvynol (bradycardia). Dermatologic findings suggest barbiturates (bullae), or glutethimide (dermographism). Anticholinergic manifestations characterize tricyclic poisoning.

Alcohol in combination with sedatives may produce grave poisoning, which improves as the alcohol is metabolized. Because of alcohol's predictably constant rate of metabolism (10 to 15 g/h) temporizing is sometimes indicated with mixed alcohol and sedative poisonings. Benzodiazepines taken alone do not produce profound coma; a history of benzodiazepine ingestion in a deeply comatose patient should prompt the search for additional toxins.

Alert patients with a history of sedative overdose should be given ipecac (15 to 30 ml), followed after emesis by charcoal (optimally in a 10:1 proportion to the weight of ingested drug), and (if renal function is adequate) magnesium citrate in repeated doses until diarrhea is produced. For tricyclic poisoning, repeated doses of charcoal bind drug that is recycled in the bile. Obtunded patients require greater circumspection. The dangers of endotracheal intubation are weighed against the possibility of unabsorbed drug remaining in the stomach. With the exceptions of glutethimide and meprobamate, sedatives are completely absorbed within 4 to 6 hours.

Patients with acceptable alveolar ventilation, blood pressure, and cardiac rhythm can usually just be observed. If gastric lavage is performed, however, samples of gastric fluid from the first and final lavage are sent for qualitative and quantitative analysis. The presence of persistently high levels in the final lavage fluid suggests concretion requiring gastroscopy.

Routine use of physostigmine to arouse patients with overdoses of tricyclics, other anticholinergics, and possibly benzodiazepines has been advocated but may be hazardous. Arousal reactions are not specific for these drugs, and side effects can occur. Seizures, pancreatitis, and atrial arrhythmias have been reported after intravenous physostigmine. Physostigmine may, however, be useful in the treatment of tricyclic-associated arrhythmias that are resistant to bicarbonate and standard antiarrhythmics. Refractory seizures may also respond to physostigmine, but its use for arousal should probably be limited to the prevention of endotracheal intubation in patients with known anticholinergic overdose.

Serious poisoning requires attention to oxygenation, fluid balance, cardiac rhythm, acid-base status, and renal and hepatic function. Moderate diuresis helps prevent acute tubular necrosis, but fluid overload can be a problem, particularly when myocardial contractility is compromised as in ethchlorvynol and meprobamate overdose. There are no data supporting pH manipulation either of serum or urine for any of these drugs. Bicarbonate appears to be effective in tricyclic-induced arrhythmias, however, and forced saline diuresis markedly improves bromide excretion.

Charcoal or resin hemoperfusion removes most sedatives more efficiently than does hemodialysis; however, the latter is preferred when renal failure, acid-base disturbance, electrolyte abnormalities, or fluid overload is present. Tricyclics have large volumes of distribution and are not removed in important amounts by clearing the blood. Patients with sedative poisoning who are clinically deteriorating despite vigorous supportive care and who do not have a gastric drug mass are considered candidates for dialysis or perfusion.

***Abstinence.*** Sedative and alcohol abstinence syndromes are clinically similar. They range from anxiety, tremor, and insomnia to delirium, seizures, dehydration, and death.

Clinical trials have delineated the features of abstinence from intermediate-acting barbiturates. Taken in daily doses of more than 600 to 800 mg for several weeks, these drugs can be expected to cause severe abstinence.

After an initial improvement over 12 to 16 hours as intoxication resolves, anxiety, insomnia, hyperadrenergic signs, abdominal pain with vomiting, and twitching appear by the end of 24 hours. Seizures occur in a large number of these patients, most commonly between the first and second day but occasionally as late as 5 days after the last dose of sedative. EEG abnormalities persist for 2 weeks. Hallucinosis (both visual and auditory) usually follows the onset of seizures and may continue for several days or longer.

Abstinence from nonbarbiturate sedatives produces a similar clinical picture, although latency and duration vary. Minimal doses of these drugs and the duration of dosing needed to produce serious abstinence are based on case reports. Meprobamate has caused serious abstinence after 3 to 6 g taken daily for 6 weeks and 2.0 to 2.5 g taken daily for 9 months. Glutethimide in daily doses of 2.5 g taken for 3 months, ethchlorvynol in chronic daily doses of 2 g, and methyprylon in doses of 5 to 12 g daily have produced serious abstinence. Lower doses are associated with mild abstinence.

Benzodiazepines predictably cause abstinence after chronic ingestion of extremely high daily doses (chloridazepoxide 100 to 600 mg or diazepam 120 mg). There are case reports of serious abstinence after prolonged use of ordinary doses; however, systematic trials have found only mild symptoms in patients treated for longer than 2 months. These studies suggest that long-acting benzodiazepines produce milder abstinence than the short-acting variety and that the onset of symptoms may be delayed for up to a week following the last dose. Techniques and schedules for the withdrawal of sedatives in hospitalized patients are discussed in Management of Drug Abusers.

***Complications of chronic use.*** Prolonged sedative abuse is associated with cognitive impairment, particularly in older patients, which resolves only slowly. Depression is another extremely common problem. The chronic state of inebriation observed in sedative abusers differs from the cyclical intoxication seen in opiate abusers. Sedative abuse is therefore particularly associated with trauma and burns. When parenteral routes are used, local and systemic lesions resemble those of opiate abusers except that the solubility and pruity of pharmaceutical sedatives allow injection with low risk of the local chemical and thermal tissue injury seen with heroin, cocaine, and methamphetamine abuse.

The obstetric risks of sedative abuse have not been well studied. Neonatal coagulopathy in the infants of barbiturate users has been described, as have fetal malformations following maternal benzodiazepine and meprobamate use. A syndrome of neonatal abstinence similar to that seen with opiates has been reported following maternal sedative use of relatively low daily doses for longer than 3 months before delivery. Whether withdrawal of sedatives during pregnancy can adversely affect the fetus is at present unknown.

### Inhalants

Psychoactive gases and volatile liquids have been occasionally abused for many years. Organic solvents, alkyl nitrates, and nitrous oxide are the most commonly encountered inhalants. Most are easily obtained, inexpensive, and legal.

Solvent abuse among children and teenagers became widespread and highly publicized during the 1960s. Epidemiologic studies suggest that solvent abusers are usually young (under 19), inexperienced in the use of other drugs, of low intelligence, male, white or hispanic, and poor.

Practically any lipid-soluble compound with a high vapor pressure can produce intoxication. Many household products are mixtures of such compounds. Most are sniffed directly from their containers or from a saturated rag, a bowl, or a plastic or paper bag. Oral and parenteral use is rare but often fatal. Because of their lipid solubility and route of administration, solvents act quickly. Most are also quickly eliminated; however, some compounds are metabolized to active products with long half-times. The prevalence of chronic toxicity from solvents is limited by the usually brief career of abusers (1 to 2 years); more prolonged use is associated with complications.

Nitrates have gained popularity, particularly among male homosexuals, in whom their use appears to be a marker for sexual promiscuity and therefore an indirect risk factor for the acquisition of AIDS. Chronic effects of nitrate abuse have not been well described. Nitrous oxide abuse remains occasional and is usually limited to medical and dental personnel.

***Types of inhalants.*** *Organic solvents* include toluene (cements, lacquer thinner, gasoline); hexane and other aliphatic hydrocarbons (gasoline, industrial solvents); fluorocarbons such as carbon tetrachloride, dihydrodifluoromethane, and trichlorofluoromethane (aerosols, refrigerants, cleaning fluids); acetone (fingernail polish remover, cements); naphtha (lighter fluid, cleaners); and trichloroethylene (cleaners).

*Alkyl nitrates and nitrates* are neither solvents nor centrally acting intoxicants. Peripheral vasodilatation with hypotension and decreased cerebral blood flow appears to be responsible for psychoactivity. Amyl and isobutyl nitrite are sold as cannisters or cans under a variety of trade names. Cotton-wrapped ampules of 0.18 and 0.30 ml are also available.

***Intoxication and overdose.*** Intoxication has classically been thought to involve receptor-independent changes in the fluidity of axonal membranes. It now appears possible that glutamate or GABA-A receptor-mediated changes in ion channels may also mediate the neuronal effects of these compounds. Solvent intoxication produces disinhibition euphoria followed by ataxia, confusion, vomiting, tinnitus, hallucinations, and finally coma. There is a superficial resemblance to alcohol or sedative intoxication; however, the progression from excitement to depression is much more rapid, the odor is usually prominent, and hallucinosis is more typical of solvent than alcohol intoxication. Tinnitus and photophobia as well as sneezing and flushing are other characteristics of solvent use.

Sudden death may be related to suffocation from tightly fitting masks or plastic bags but has also been reported as an instantaneous event. Trichloroethylene and fluorinated hydrocarbons appear to be particularly likely to produce this syndrome, which has also been associated with stress or sudden activity.

Management of solvent intoxication includes fresh air, a restful environment, and a search for the neurologic, renal, hepatic, and hematologic disorders associated with chronic abuse. Delirium usually clears quickly, but trichloroethylene, toluene, and gasoline sniffing may present as a long-lasting delirium associated with cerebellar findings, choreiform movements, or seizures. Resuscitative efforts in hypotensive or asystolic patients probably should minimize the use of adrenergic drugs, whose arrhythmogenic actions may be potentiated by solvents.

Nitrate intoxication lasts only seconds to minutes and causes fainting, relaxation of sphincters, flushing, and headache. It is reputed to intensify sounds and to enhance orgasm. Patients who have underlying cardiovascular disorders may present with hemodynamic compromise.

Heavy nitrate use can produce clinically significant methemoglobinemia. Levels of 20% occur after recreational use. With oral use, however, and in patients with hemoglobinopathies or familial hemoglobin reductase deficiency, levels may be much higher. Patients with anemia or heart disease are at risk at lower levels. Central cyanosis unresponsive to oxygen in the absence of cardiopulmonary disease suggests the diagnosis. Cyanosis occurs at relatively low methemoglobin levels and resolves over several days. Treatment with methylene blue is therefore reserved for patients who are comatose or who have an underlying condition exacerbated by methemoglobinemia.

***Abstinence.*** It is not clear whether tolerance develops to some or all of this heterogenous group of compounds. The best evidence of tolerance has been reported in butane and toluene abuse. Abstinence syndromes with irritability, insomnia, diaphoresis and abdominal or chest pain have been described but rarely observed. Industrial exposure to nitrates at high dose has been associated with chest pain and even sudden death when the drugs were abruptly discontinued.

***Complications of chronic inhalant abuse.*** Central nervous system effects include alteration in cognitive function, cerebellar and cerebral atrophy, vascular lesions in the basal ganglia, and prolonged toxic delirium. Peripheral neuropathy is a feature of hexane and nitrous oxide abuse.

Centrilobular hepatitis with fibrosis may occur alone or in association with pancreatitis and renal tubular lesions among abusers of toluene, trichloroethylene, and carbon tetrachloride. The renal lesions, which may also occur alone, include acute tubular necrosis, distal renal tubular acidosis, and proteinuria. Lactic acidosis has also been reported in toluene abusers. A red papular rash around the mouth and nose is occasionally seen ("glue sniffer's nose").

Hematologic complications consist of aplastic anemia and myeloid metaplasia, each associated with benzene and hydrocarbon abuse. Patients with sickle cell anemia may be at increased risk.

Contaminants such as tetraethyl lead in gasoline or metal fragments in fluorocarbon aerosols can produce their own toxicities.

The effects of these inhalant compounds during pregnancy are unknown.

### Hallucinogens

Hallucinogens are drugs that impair reality testing and alter the perception of time and sense data. They may also produce hallucinations and delusions. Like other psychoactive drugs, hallucinogens frequently cause changes in mood, behavior, and thought content. Chemically, these compounds exhibit a variety of structures, including ergot alkaloids such as lysergic acid diethylamide (LSD), phenylalkylamines (mescaline), and indolealkylamines (psilocybin, dimethyltryptamine). Cannabinoids (marijuana, hashish) and phencyclidine ("PCP") are often classified as hallucinogens but in fact produce hallucinations only rarely.

The similarities between functional psychosis and states of hallucinogen intoxication have stimulated detailed inquiry into the neurochemistry of drugs such as LSD and PCP. If there is a common pharmacodynamic mechanism among these drugs, it has not yet been identified. LSD is a serotonin inhibitor and dopamine agonist that produces highly selective stimulation of limbic and forebrain structures after minute doses (0.5 to 1.0 µg/kg). There is some evidence that PCP acts on a psychotomimetic subtype of opiate receptor to produce its cognitive and perceptual effects.

Marijuana has been used by at least 10% to 15% of the American population and by 60% of young adults. Although a great deal is known about the kinetics of cannabinoids, there is little information about mechanisms of psychoactivity and no consensus about the dangers of chronic use.

***Individual hallucinogens.*** *Phencyclidine* is often referred to as PCP, which is not a chemical acronym but stands for *P*ea*C*e *P*ill. It is an illegally but easily manufactured street drug which is often sold as LSD, tetrahydrocannabinol (THC, the major active component in marijuana), and other more exotic hallucinogens. Its medical use as a short-acting, dissociative anesthetic was discontinued because of dysphoric side effects, although a derivative is still in use in veterinary practice. Phencyclidine is available as a water-soluble white powder sold in tablet form, as a liquid, or sprinkled on marijuana. The drug can be smoked, insufflated, ingested, or injected parenterally. Other names for PCP include "angel dust," "animal tranquilizer," "rocket fuel," "pig killer," and "supergrass."

Phencyclidine is lipid-soluble, rapidly absorbed by any route, concentrated in the cerebrospinal fluid and red blood cells, and probably not bound extensively to plasma proteins. The parent drug is reexcreted into gastric juice and bile. Phencyclidine is metabolized in the liver to an inactive hydroxy metabolite and excreted in urine unchanged. The half-time is about 1 hour after low doses.

Unlike some other hallucinogens, phencyclidine produces effects that are clearly proportional to dose and plasma level. Despite its short half-time, phencyclidine can cause toxicity that persists many hours.

*Marijuana* ("pot," "dope," "grass," "weed," "reefer") is the dried leaf of *Cannabis sativa,* or hemp plant; the potent resin, compressed into blocks, is hashish. Marijuana is the more common preparation in the United States. It is sold on the street as individual cigarettes ("joints"), small bags costing $5 or $10 ("nickel," "dime"), or as an ounce ("lid"), a kilogram ("key"), or more.

Cannabis contains a number of psychoactive alkaloids of which the most important is THC. Marijuana is 2% to 20% THC, and hashish 15% to 20%. Marijuana may be smoked, ingested, and rarely made into an aqueous infusion and injected. THC in marijuana smoke is about 20% absorbed, extensively bound to plasma proteins, and metabolized by the liver and lung in part to active products. Lipid solubility of THC is high, and there is extensive distribution into fat. Redistribution and not elimination is responsible for terminating psychoactivity. Metabolites can be recovered in the urine of regular users for 3 weeks after drug use is discontinued. Ingested THC is less well absorbed, but effects appear to occur at lower plasma concentrations.

Unlike phencyclidine, cannabinoids produce effects that depend a great deal on user expectation and regularity of use. The antiemetic and ocular effects of these compounds are being studied in glaucoma and cancer chemotherapy.

*LSD* ("acid," "sunshine") is an alkaloid amine of unusual potency and variable purity which is sold on the street as a liquid, on absorbent paper, or in tablets. It is usually ingested, by which route it is rapidly absorbed and reaches peak plasma levels after an hour. Psychoactivity is maximal after 2 to 5 hours and continues for about 12 hours. The half-time is short, and its metabolic fate is uncertain.

***Intoxication and overdose.*** Phencyclidine intoxication occurs at doses below 10 mg. Poisoning results from higher doses, and 100 to 200 mg has caused death. Intoxication produces euphoria and lability of mood, often combined with confusion, and distortions in body image and concrete thinking. After higher doses, marked anxiety, depersonalization, sensitivity to light and sound, and panic states occur. After doses of 100 mg or more, intoxication usually evolves into coma.

On examination the mildly overdosed patient usually presents with agitated or violent behavior, hypertension, tachycardia, and hyperpnea but with a clear sensorium. After more serious poisoning, delirium or catatonia may be seen. Catatonia, when it occurs, is characteristically accompanied by hyperreflexia and muscular rigidity. Diminished response to pain and a staring facies are also characteristic of this curious state.

A combination of cholinergic signs (diaphoresis, salivation, bronchospasm, miosis) and anticholinergic manifestations (mydriasis, urinary retention) may also be present in overdose, along with facial grimacing and purposeless or athetoid movements. Hyperthermia or hypothermia may be seen. Seizures, hypoventilation, and toxic myocardial depression are late signs.

Complications of severe poisoning include shock, hyperpyrexic myoglobinuria, and difficulties with endotracheal intubation resulting from laryngospasm. Close monitoring of blood pressure, renal function, temperature, and respiration is essential. Bloody diarrhea, when it occurs, is probably due to a by-product of drug synthesis.

Treatment of mild overdose consists in sensory deprivation. "Talking down" has no place. Ideally the patient is positioned on the floor in a quiet room with low lighting. Mild sedation may be needed. Neuroleptics should not be used, however, since they may increase the risk of seizures, augment anticholinergic manifestations, produce hypotension, and impair thermoregulation.

More serious poisoning requires consideration of urinary acidification and continuous nasogastric suction. Phencyclidine has a pKa of 8.5. Acidification has been reported to increase urine concentration and therefore clearance of the parent drug by a factor of 20 to 200. Similar clearances have been reported for continuous nasogastric suction. Poisoning with phenobarbital or salicylate should be excluded before urinary acidification, as clearance of these drugs is markedly reduced in acidic urine.

A rapidly acting benzodiazepine (e.g., diazepam) is the best therapy for seizures and muscle spasm. Hypertension is probably due to α-adrenergic hyperactivity and may therefore respond best to phentolamine. Endotracheal intubation, if required, is performed by an experienced practitioner, and care is taken with succinylcholine because phencyclidine may inhibit pseudocholinesterase and prolong paralysis. Physiologic signs and symptoms usually clear within 24 hours, but psychiatric effects may last many days.

Marijuana intoxication occurs after one or two joints (20 to 1500 mg, or 5 to 150 mg of THC). Euphoria, suggestibility, hilarity, appetite stimulation, and subtle changes in perceptions of time and stimuli occur in many. Sedation, confusion, depersonalization, and paranoia may also be seen. Toxic psychosis has been reported, particularly in patients with underlying psychiatric illness. The patient may be talkative or withdrawn on examination. Mild tachycardia, injected conjunctivae, and a slight tremor are characteristic. Postural hypotension is seen after high doses.

Except for the rare occurrence of psychosis, toxic manifestations of ingested or smoked marijuana usually are mild and transient. Cannabis-induced vascular dilatation occasionally exacerbates underlying heart disease. Intravenous injection of marijuana infusion, however, produces extreme tachycardia, hypotension, abdominal pain with vomiting, myalgia, and weakness. The patient may be febrile and hyporeflexic, although the sensorium is clear. The prognosis is usually good, despite such complications as hepatitis, pancreatitis, thrombocytopenia, transient renal failure, and arrhythmia.

Treatment of overdose consists in reassurance with or without a small dose of a benzodiazepine. Parenteral poisoning, however, requires intensive care.

LSD intoxication produces intensification and a blending of sense data, hallucinations (usually visual), altered time perception, suggestibility, and frequently depersonalization. Lability of mood, dizziness, nausea, tremor, and blurred vision may occur. Panic states are not uncommon. On examination mild muscle weakness, vasoconstriction, mydriasis, rapid change in mood, and inability to concentrate are usually found. Treatment consists in reassurance, observation, and a benzodiazepine or phenothiazine if needed. Occasionally, psychotic states persist beyond 24 hours. It is unclear if these represent unmasking of an underlying illness or an idiosyncratic reaction.

***Abstinence.*** Phencyclidine has been shown to produce mild tolerance and self-reinforcement in animals. Abstinence in the form of depression and craving has been reported but is not predictable. The use of desipramine may assist patients in abandoning PCP use, although the mechanism of action is obscure.

Marijuana produces moderate tolerance to its cardiovascular, autonomic, ocular, and behavioral effects after 1 to 3 weeks. A withdrawal syndrome similar to mild sedative abstinence has been reported, with onset after about a week and duration of a few days. Seizures and psychosis have not been reported. The acquisition of tolerance may be due to metabolic induction or tissue tolerance. Interestingly, experienced users report subjective effects at plasma levels that do not affect nonusers. It is possible that chronic users metabolize THC more quickly to products of greater potency or stability. Experienced users also excrete radioactive cannabinoids more quickly, possibly because of increased metabolism or saturation of depot sites.

LSD produces a rapidly developing acute tolerance that may even occur shortly after ingestion and account for termination of the drug's effects. Cross-tolerance with mescaline and psilocybin appears to occur. No abstinence syndrome has been reported, and tolerance is quickly lost.

***Complications of chronic hallucinogen abuse.*** The complications of chronic phencyclidine and LSD use are principally psychiatric, consisting of chronic psychosis and "flashbacks." Phencyclidine psychosis may have an insidious onset and presents with hallucinosis or delusional states, often with neurologic findings (usually nystagmus). It appears to be commoner in individuals with poor premorbid ego strength and adjustment to work, family, or school. Severity is also dose-related. The syndrome responds to neuroleptics and resolves over several weeks. LSD-precipitated psychosis is indistinguishable at the outset from toxicity. Dose relationships are less clear than for phencyclidine, and neurologic examination is unremarkable. Flashbacks are spontaneous subjective recurrences of former states of intoxication. They occur usually during times of stress and may appear several months after LSD use. Typically these episodes last several minutes or hours. Flashbacks are almost always dysphoric.

The possibility of toxicity from chronic marijuana use is of particular concern because of the drug's popularity among children. Heavy marijuana smoking, especially in combination with tobacco, has been shown to increase airway resistance, although in single doses marijuana is a bronchodilator. Carcinogenic polyaromatic hydrocarbons are more numerous in marijuana than in cigarette smoke; however, effects are similar in standard tests of carcinogenicity. Hypothalamic and possibly testicular suppression with decreased serum testosterone, oligospermia, and gynecomastia is a well-recognized complication of heavy marijuana use. Pubertal arrest has also been reported.

Early reports of cerebral atrophy in chronic users have not been confirmed; the chronic effects of marijuana on the central nervous system are unknown. An "antimotivational syndrome" characterized by a lack of energy or purpose and mental clouding has been ascribed to heavy marijuana use in children. A possible effect of marijuana on cellular immunity is also under study.

Government programs to eradicate *Cannabis sativa* have included large scale spraying with paraquat and other herbicides. Paraquat is a potent and irreversible pulmonary toxin that is largely inactivated when burned but is absorbed from the gastrointestinal tract and the skin. No poisoning related to paraquat-treated marijuana has so far been reported.

Although LSD in high concentrations is toxic to mammalian cells, there is no convincing evidence of an effect on the human fetus; nor has laboratory evidence of marijuana-induced chromosomal abnormalities been confirmed or correlated with birth defects. Case reports of microcephaly in the infants of phencyclidine-abusing mothers have also noted a prolonged (2 weeks or more) neonatal abstinence syndrome resembling opiate abstinence. Whether withdrawal from phencyclidine during pregnancy can adversely affect the fetus is not known.

## Stimulants

Cortical arousal, anorexia, sympathomimetic effects on end-organs, and (in high doses) medullary suppression with respiratory collapse are the common effects of cocaine, amphetamine, phenmetrazine, and methylphenidate. Stimulation of central norepinephrine and dopamine receptors appears to mediate these effects as well as the toxic hallucinosis that is occasionally seen.

These drugs are powerfully self-reinforcing in animal and human experiments. Animals continue to self-administer cocaine until they die from its effects. In humans, craving for cocaine and amphetamine may be intense, although a predictable abstinence syndrome does not occur. Despite strong user preference for one or another drug, subjects cannot reliably differentiate cocaine from amphetamine in experimental situations. It seems clear that cocaine is becoming increasingly popular, particularly in a newly available alkaloidal form ("crack"), which is heat-stable and can be smoked.

***Types of stimulants.*** *Cocaine* ("coke," "blow," "toot," "snow") is a white crystalline powder, soluble in cold water, that is derived by hydroxylation and benzoylation from coca leaves grown in Bolivia and Peru. It is sold in grams or by dollar amounts ("nickel," "dime," etc.) after adulteration with quinine, procaine, talc, cornstarch, or sugars.

Unlike other stimulants, cocaine is a local anesthetic. It may be insufflated, injected intravenously, ingested, or smoked ("free-based"). About 20% of an insufflated or ingested dose is ultimately bioavailable; however, ingested cocaine is only slowly absorbed from the duodenum. A usual intranasal street dose is 20 to 50 mg.

Conversion of cocaine hydrochloride to the alkaloid base facilitates smoking because of the hydrochloride's thermal instability. This conversion may be performed by the user ("free-basing") or the distributor, when the resulting crystals are sold in small vials as "crack." The process in either case involves ether extraction from an alkaline, aqueous cocaine solution. Plasma levels after smoking are similar to those after intravenous use.

The effects of cocaine are almost immediate by any route other than the oral one; however, peak plasma levels are delayed for up to an hour after insufflation. The distribution space of cocaine is not large, and the drug is concentrated in the cerebrospinal fluid. Cocaine is metabolized, with a half-time of about 1 hour. It is also excreted in urine at a rate that is independent of pH. Most cocaine is metabolized to benzoylecgonine and ecgonine ester in the serum. To a lesser extent this conversion also takes place in the liver. In the presence of ethanol, liver-metabolized cocaine also forms ethylbenzoylecronine. This compound binds to the same receptors as cocaine, although with an altered affinity profile, and remains in the serum about twice as long as cocaine. Moreover, in animals the metabolite appears to be more hepatotoxic and neurotoxic than the parent compound. The role of "cocaethylene" in the toxicology of cocaine is under active study.

Cocaine can be combined with heroin ("speedball") but is not itself an opiate despite its legal description as a narcotic.

*Amphetamine* ("speed," "uppers," "street whites," "black beauties") is a white, water-soluble powder taken via the oral, intravenous, and intranasal routes. It is available in gram or dollar quantities and as capsules containing 2.5 to 30 mg. The dextro isomer is largely responsible for racemic amphetamine's central effects. Dextroamphetamine is also available in pure form. Peak levels after ingestion occur at about 2 hours, but effects are evident more quickly. The volume of distribution is small, with peak concentrations in brain and kidney. Amphetamine is not metabolized by monoamine oxidase, which it inhibits. Liver metabolism to inactive products and renal excretion occur with a half-time of 8 to 30 hours, depending on urine pH. The pKa of amphetamine is 9.9, and elimination is greatly prolonged in alkaline urine. *Methamphetamine* is a derivative with increased central effects. "Street whites" are more often ephedrine or caffeine than amphetamine.

*Other stimulants* include methylphenidate (Ritalin), an amphetamine derivative used for treating hyperkinesis, narcolepsy, and depression; and phenmetrazine and flufenamine, both used as appetite suppressants.

***Intoxication and overdose.*** The central and peripheral effects of stimulants are dose-related; however, central effects predominate at low doses. By inhalation and the intravenous route, cocaine's central potency is 10 times greater than after nasal use. Dextroamphetamine and cocaine by the intravenous route produce similar effects after roughly the same dose, although cocaine's effects are briefer. The brevity of cocaine's action (less than one-half hour) has important implications for its pattern of use. Parenteral abusers on a cocaine "run" may inject themselves several times an hour for many hours or days. The risk of transmitting infection is thus increased, as are the local complications.

Intoxication is variously described as feelings of calm, omnipotence, clarity, energy, or euphoria. Dizziness, tremulousness, and anxiety also are reported. On examination the patient is alert, oriented, and usually talkative unless there is paranoid ideation. Mydriasis, hypertension, tachycardia, tremor, hyperreflexia, and dry mucous membranes are present. Grinding of the teeth may be observed, as well as hyperactivity. Because of nasopharyngeal anesthesia, cocaine-intoxicated patients may be sniffing and reflexly swallowing. As the effects of stimulants wear off, irritability and lethargy may be seen. Duration of action is 30 to 60 minutes for cocaine and several hours for amphetamine.

Mild overdose presents as dizziness, headache, palpitations, and tremulousness. Higher doses can cause chest pain, nausea, and vomiting. Psychiatric symptoms including hallucinations and delusions may predominate. These patients are usually oriented, their memory is intact, and they are generally disturbed by their hallucinations to a greater extent than functional schizophrenics.

Serious overdose produces ventricular arrhythmias, seizures, hyperthermia (with the risk of renal damage and consumptive coagulopathy), marked hypertension (sometimes causing stroke), and central hypoventilation. The differential diagnosis of stimulant overdose includes schizophrenia, mania, panic states, nontoxic stimulant-associated psychosis, pheochromocytoma, hyperthyroid storm, and hallucinogen toxicity.

Treatment of overdose consists of supportive care, sedation, and hastening removal of drug by gastrointestinal decontamination and/or acidification of the urine. Droperidol, chlorpromazine, diazepam, and propranolol have been used with success. Neuroleptics may be specific for psychotic manifestations and help reverse hyperthermia and hypertension. They also lower seizure thresholds, however, and prolong amphetamine elimination in some animal models. Propranolol 1 mg/min intravenously has been reported to arouse stuporous patients and to reverse tachycardia. The danger of beta blockade lies in the unopposed alpha-stimulating action of adrenergic agonists such as cocaine and amphetamine. It appears reasonable to treat anxiety with diazepam and hallucinations and paranoia with droperidol, chlorpromazine, or (if seizures are of concern) possibly thiothixene. Propranolol should probably be reserved for cardiac arrhythmias.

Ipecac, followed by charcoal and a saline cathartic, is helpful in patients with adequate renal function who are within 4 hours of stimulant ingestion. Acidification of the urine importantly increases amphetamine excretion in serious poisoning, but the presence of phenobarbital and salicylate should be ruled out, as the excretion of these drugs is markedly diminished in acidic urine. Catheterization of the bladder prevents overdistention resulting from adrenergic-mediated sphincter spasm and permits pH monitoring.

Supportive treatment of seriously poisoned patients should be administered in an intensive care setting where temperature, blood pressure, cardiac rhythm, urine pH, and neurologic status can be frequently observed. In the deteriorating patient hemodialysis effectively removes amphetamine and probably cocaine.

***Abstinence.*** Tolerance to the central and peripheral effects of amphetamine is marked, approaching that of opiates. Tolerance to cocaine has been less well described in the controlled setting but is said to be considerable and only slowly lost. In animals tolerance occurs preferentially to the peripheral actions of these drugs; indeed, a heightened sensitivity (reverse tolerance) to some behavioral effects is observed after chronic treatment.

Abstinence syndrome consists of intense craving, abnormal sleep patterns with lethargy, and depression that may be complicated by sedative abuse and even suicide. The time course and dose relationship of stimulant abstinence is not predictable, although onset is rapid.

No substitution therapy has been shown to alleviate stimulant abstinence. Tricyclic antidepressants and methylphenidate have been reported to reduce craving in some patients and lithium to antagonize the intoxication caused by cocaine. Clinical trials are not encouraging.

***Complications of chronic stimulant abuse.*** Local and systemic complications of parenteral abuse are similar to those for opiate abuse. The risk of abscess and phlebitis may be greater, however, owing to the pattern of more frequent use associated with cocaine's brief action and to the particularly irritating and vasoconstrictive effects of stimulants. Perforation of the nasal septum resulting from chronic vasoconstriction is seen in nasal users.

Major neurologic complications of sedative abuse have been described. A dose-dependent effect on brain microvasculature appears to occur after chronic use by any route. Necrotizing cerebral angiitis, cerebral hemorrhage, and microaneurysms may be related findings. A syndrome of choreiform movements has been described during intoxication, abstinence, and (rarely) for years following dextroamphetamine abuse. The etiology is uncertain. Simultaneous alcohol and stimulant use has been associated with rupture of the urinary bladder, presumably from alcohol diuresis in the presence of an unresponsive sphincter resulting from alpha stimulation.

Complications in the chest include a reduction in diffusing capacity found in cocaine smokers who have normal pulmonary volumes and flow rates. Pulmonary edema has also been associated with cocaine smoking, as have pneumomediastinum and pneumothorax.

The principle psychiatric complication is stimulant-precipitated psychosis, typically delusional, paranoid, and accompanied by tactile or visual hallucinations. It appears that a large minority of heavy stimulant users develop features of this syndrome.

Surgical complications, apart from fasciitis and rupture of the urinary bladder, include the ingestion of packaged cocaine to avoid detection. Laparotomy rather than endoscopy or emesis may be the safest method of recovery, at least when condoms are used to package the drug.

Case reports have linked maternal amphetamine abuse with cardiovascular and central nervous system malformations in the infant. A syndrome of neonatal abstinence characterized by agitation or depression and by seizures has been reported to last several days. Whether withdrawal of stimulants during pregnancy adversely affects the fetus is not known.

## MANAGEMENT OF DRUG ABUSERS

### Hospitalized patients

Drug-abusing patients may be hospitalized for elective withdrawal, medical complications of their abuse, abstinence, intoxication, and overdose, or for some unrelated condition. Whatever the admitting diagnosis, hospitalization is an ideal opportunity to address the underlying drug problem in a definitive manner. Indeed, admission may be advisable chiefly for this purpose. Decisions about the need for withdrawal, referral, or maintenance should be made early. Formulating drug abuse as a problem on the hospital chart is the first essential step in decision making. When the patient is already involved with an outpatient facility, the program should be consulted as soon as possible. Such consultation provides information about the medical history, baseline physical findings, recent laboratory values, and other test results. This is particularly true for methadone and residential programs, which are required by law to examine their patients annually. Early communication with the program also prevents the patient from being dropped because of unexplained absence.

There is an appreciable number of patients whose drug abuse represents an attempt to self-medicate underlying psychotic and affective disorders. Under the stress of withdrawal and without the chronic psychoactive properties of the abused drug, patients occasionally manifest for the first time these underlying problems. It is common for patients to notice a variety of aches and pains during withdrawal. Most of these are minor, but an underlying traumatic injury, arthritis, or even osteomyelitis may present at this time.

Before undertaking any withdrawal the patient should clearly understand and preferably have participated in formulating the plan. The following issues should be answered in advance: What the schedule is to be, what time of day to expect medication, whether the plan will be changed if it goes unexpectedly well or poorly, and whether adjunctive sedatives, hypnotics, or muscle relaxants will be used. Apparently trivial deviations from routine can create confrontations, disrupt therapeutic relationships, and precipitate possibly dangerous premature discharge.

***Opiate withdrawal.*** Opiate-dependent patients not on methadone maintenance and who are not pregnant should usually be withdrawn, even when referral to maintenance is planned. This apparent paradox is explained by the time course of referral. It is unusual for a maintenance or other program to pick up patients on the day of their hospital discharge, and it is essential that patients remain functional long enough to go through the program's screening and documentation procedures. In the ideal case, where hospital and program have close ties, maintenance may be begun during the admission. Even when this is possible, however, a drug-free period is often beneficial for patients when reviewing their treatment options.

Patients who have used short-acting opiates on at least a daily basis for 2 weeks or more and whose last dose was within 3 days may need to be withdrawn by drug substitution. There are no specific medical indications for withdrawal as opiate abstinence is neither harmful nor easily mistaken for a disease process. Factors that encourage withdrawal include a long (several months) history of parenteral abuse, self-dosing more frequently than once daily, a dose within 8 to 12 hours, abuse of long-acting opiates, anticipation of prolonged hospitalization, and a high probability of potentially dangerous discharge against advice. Obviously the wishes of the patient play a major role.

Opiates such as meperidine, hydromorphone, or morphine should not be used for withdrawal because of their short half-times and low oral bioavailability. Methadone is the opiate of choice. Treatment can be initiated empirically as 20 mg followed by 5 to 20 mg after 4 hours, depending on clinical response. It is preferable, however, to titrate the dose more precisely after the onset of withdrawal signs. An initial dose of 10 mg may be followed by 5 to 10 mg every 2 hours until signs of withdrawal abate. Piloerection, mydriasis, lacrimation, and rhinorrhea are reliable signs to follow; however, it should be understood that drug craving precedes their appearance by several hours. More than 40 mg is almost never needed to reverse abstinence from street heroin; pentazocine, propoxyphene, and codeine usually require much less.

Street methadone dependence can require high doses of methadone and prolonged hospitalization for complete withdrawal. Signs of methadone abstinence are similar to those for short-acting opiates but are less dramatic and may not appear for 2 to 3 days. Titration should be as for short-acting opiates, but the endpoint may often have to be subjective comfort or even mild intoxication. Patients are not given their self-reported maintenance or street doses until confirmation is obtained from the program or by titration to tolerance. Methadone maintenance patients are not usually encouraged to withdraw. Hospital staff must remember that withdrawal leads almost invariably to relapse, particularly when it takes place over days or weeks.

On the second day of opiate withdrawal the total given during the first 24 hours can be repeated in a single dose. Some accumulation of methadone occurs; however, the severity of abstinence is also increased on the second day. On the third and subsequent days methadone, given as a single daily dose, can be reduced by 5 mg. There is seldom a reason to give methadone parenterally. Peak effects are exaggerated by parenteral routes, and the use of needles is not desirable. Oral dosing requires a volume of only a few milliliters when syrup or solution is not further diluted. If parenteral dosing is unavoidable, 75% of the oral dose in divided intramuscular injections is a reasonable equivalent.

Clonidine and related $\alpha_2$-adrenergic agonists offer an alternate, more rapid means of withdrawal. These compounds act by presynaptic inhibition of adrenergic midbrain neurons that mediate abstinence signs and some symptoms. Unlike opiates, they act by blocking signs and symptoms rather than by attenuating abstinence through its prolongation. As for methadone, dosing strategies may be based on titration or approximation. For patients without immediate signs of abstinence 0.3 mg twice daily can be tried, but blood pressure must be closely monitored.

For an opiate abuser with signs and symptoms of abstinence, titration is probably preferable. Clonidine 0.1 mg orally every half hour can be given until one of several endpoints is reached:

1. Alleviation or substantial improvement in abstinence signs and symptoms
2. Symptomatic hypotension
3. Fall in mean blood pressure below 80 mmHg (higher in patients with vascular disease or chronic hypertension)
4. Occurrence of other severe side effects
5. Administration of 0.6 mg

If improvement occurs, the total dose can be given twice daily. A 5-day course is usually sufficient for withdrawal from short-acting opiates. A 2-week course is necessary for methadone-dependent patients, and even longer courses are needed for patients taking LAAM. Side effects may include hypotension, insomnia, extreme fatigue, dry mouth, metallic taste, and rarely hallucinations. Rebound hypertension does not appear to be a problem after short courses. Some patients complain that clonidine loses effectiveness after several days, in which case doses may be cautiously increased or schedules shortened.

Other drugs that have been used to treat and prevent abstinence include propoxyphene in divided doses of 1200 mg daily and naltrexone with clonidine. Propoxyphene may be effective for mild dependence and is probably better than nothing when methadone is not available. Doses of 1200 mg are unlikely to reverse moderate or severe abstinence, however, and have been associated with liver function abnormalities and behavioral changes. Naltrexone, an orally active derivative of naloxone, has been used to accelerate the natural course of abstinence while symptoms are controlled with clonidine. This management strategy requires experience.

Patients who should not be withdrawn include pregnant women, particularly during the first and third trimesters, patients with certain and immediate access to methadone maintenance, and gravely ill patients for whom the stress of withdrawal is contraindicated.

Some patients choose to undergo abstinence untreated. There is no reason to encourage or to deny this request; however, patients should be made aware that methadone and clonidine are available to them.

The use of anxiolytics, hypnotics, and muscle relaxants depends on the clinical state of the patient and the withdrawal plan. These adjunctive drugs are never used in unusual doses. Patients must be cautioned to expect sleep disturbances as part of the process of gradual withdrawal.

***Sedative withdrawal.*** Because the first manifestations of sedative abstinence may include seizures, decisions about withdrawal cannot await the appearance of signs and symptoms. A precise history and the results of sedative-challenge testing can be used to estimate the patient's sedative requirement. Barbiturate and nonbarbiturate sedatives are all cross-tolerant; any one agent can in theory be used to prevent and reverse abstinence from the others. In practice, however, it is often easier to estimate tolerance in terms of a single, well-studied reference drug, pentobarbital. The minimum dosage, chronicity of use, and level of tolerance necessary to produce abstinence is less well described for other, nonbarbiturate sedatives. (see Drugs of Abuse.)

Oral pentobarbital challenge followed by tapering doses of phenobarbital is the most widely used technique for sedative withdrawal. The nonintoxicated patient is given pentobarbital 200 mg orally every 2 hours until signs of mild intoxication occur: lethargy, ataxia, slurred speech, or nystagmus. If the total intoxicating dose is less than 400 to 600 mg, further barbiturates are not given. At doses above 600 mg, phenobarbital (30 mg for every 100 mg of pentobarbital) is substituted when intoxication subsides. Phenobarbital, given in divided doses to avoid peak effects, is then tapered by 10% of the original dose daily. Patients with a history of seizures or psychosis should probably be treated even if titration indicates an intoxicating dose of 400 to 600 mg.

An alternate method is to give phenobarbital 0.1 mg/kg/min intravenously until mild intoxication occurs. For most patients no further treatment is needed, as phenobarbital levels decrease slowly with a half-time of 48 to 96 hours. Unfortunately, the induction of phenobarbital metabolism by sedative abuse in some patients results in unusually short half-times for phenobarbital. Seizures have been reported in such patients, who required additional doses of phenobarbital on the second or third day.

Benzodiazepines have also been used as withdrawal agents in a limited number of patients. One method is to give diazepam 20 mg orally every 2 hours until mild intoxication occurs. Diazepam is then tapered by 10 mg each day. The main advantage claimed for this method is a reduced likelihood of sedative toxicity during the titration phase. There has, however, been a long and satisfactory experience with the pentobarbital method, and phenobarbital is a less desirable drug to most abusers than is diazepam. Moreover, peak phenobarbital levels occur about 5 days after the first dose despite tapering and therefore coincide with the peak of most severe abstinence syndromes. Unlike benzodiazepines other than lorazepam, phenobarbital is reliably absorbed after intramuscular administration.

When titrating sedatives it should be remembered that tolerance does not exceed five to ten times the usual dose of most of these drugs, far less than is seen in opiate abuse. Moreover, patients become a good deal more tolerant to the hypnotic than to the toxic effects of these compounds; in tolerant abusers, therefore, the sedative and toxic effects of pentobarbital may be separated by only one or two doses. It should also be remembered that there is no sedative antagonist to reverse overdosage. For these reasons titration is preferable to estimation when determining the correct dose of sedative.

***General management.*** Perhaps the single most important element in the successful management of a hospitalized drug abuser is the relationship between patient and staff. Many hospitalized patients are fearful or anxious, but few are as ambivalent about their admission as drug abusers. Perhaps as a result, some drug abusers choose to encourage confrontational relationships in order to justify any subsequent decision to bolt. Most hospitalized patients take their behavioral cues from professionals viewed as responsible for their lives or well-being. Physicians and nurses come to expect cheery or philosophical or at least reasonably stoic patients and communicate these expectations successfully. Drug abusers, however, often have long histories of poor relations with medical personnel. Although they follow behavioral cues erratically, they are quick to sense and respond to hostility and prejudice around them.

The nursing staff usually bears the brunt of these problems and requires support in maintaining professional attitudes. Nurses should be included in planning withdrawal schedules and should have contact with the physician on a daily basis. Involvement of nursing staff in postdischarge planning and in decisions to seek consultation from social workers or psychiatrists is beneficial to patient and staff. The night shift nurses often come to know the sleepless, anxious drug-abusing patient best but have little opportunity to contribute to decision making. Physicians who frequently admit drug abusers would do well to plan training sessions for these nursing personnel also.

***Pain.*** Hospitalized patients in general are often undermedicated for pain by both physicians and nurses. Subtherapeutic doses and dosage intervals are commonly ordered, as are low-dose combinations wrongly supposed to be synergistic (e.g., meperidine and an antihistamine). This tendency to undermedicate is especially prominent in the treatment of opiate-dependent (and particularly methadone-maintained) patients. Methadone maintenance patients, it is insufficiently appreciated, have pain thresholds and tolerances virtually indistinguishable from controls. When pain management in these patients requires opiates, at least the usual doses are needed in addition to the daily methadone.

It is probably unwise to adjust a maintenance dose to

provide pain control. The duration of methadone analgesia in maintenance patients has not been well studied; however, in naive subjects methadone's analgesia lasts no longer than that of morphine for the first week or two of dosing. Moreover, it is important to maintain the distinction between medication for pain and treatment of abuse. Perhaps surprisingly, patients can be simultaneously withdrawn using methadone and medicated for pain with short-acting opiates in usual doses.

*Sleep.* Sleep disturbance is a feature of abstinence from virtually all drugs of abuse; its treatment is usually unsuccessful. Recommended doses of common hypnotics are ineffective after several weeks even in nontolerant individuals, and patients with tolerance are not likely to respond to ordinary doses of any hypnotic. Nevertheless, it is sometimes helpful to increase the evening dose of phenobarbital or diazepam at the expense of daytime doses or even to give a single bedtime dose. Opiate-dependent patients may benefit from a nighttime sedative, but in these patients, too, a period of insomnia is usual.

Of probably greater importance than medication is enlisting the aid of the night shift nurses. These patients frequently need to talk and to be reassured. For hospital staff to accept this temporary insomnia as expected and normal greatly helps the patient to do so.

*Smuggled drugs.* The problem of extramural drugs is not uncommon but can often be prevented. Adequate medication, careful discussion of the plan for withdrawal, daily sympathetic evaluation of minor aches or pains, active postdischarge planning, and particularly a sympathetic nursing staff usually are effective deterrents. Patients admitted for elective withdrawal who are found to be using their own drugs in the hospital should be discharged promptly. Another attempt can be made later. It is disruptive, time-consuming, and destructive to therapeutic relationships for nursing staff or security to police an ambulatory drug abuser intent on smuggling in drugs.

Patients with serious illnesses who smuggle in drugs may require surveillance and limitation of visitors. Nonessential intravenous lines are discontinued. Also important is the need to review withdrawal schedules, adjunctive medications, relations with nursing and medical staff, and the patient's fears about illness or withdrawal. Even after these problems have been adequately addressed, some patients continue to use smuggled drugs. The sense of helplessness, unrequited effort, and anger that such patients bring out in hospital staff must then become the central issue.

### Outpatient management

Withdrawal, whether outpatient or inpatient, by chemical substitution, acupuncture, or "cold turkey," is almost never adequate treatment for drug abuse or dependence. Definitive treatment requires a major, prolonged, and regular commitment from the patient. The physician referring a patient for definitive drug abuse treatment should be familiar with the range of modalities, their techniques, and their results. The decision about where to refer for outpatient treatment remains one for clinical judgment. Patients with severe psychologic problems do poorly in any outpatient setting (except perhaps methadone maintenance), whereas patients with good preabuse functioning do well. For patients with intermediate functioning, the presence of family and employment problems should encourage inpatient referral.

Patients with no serious social problems or underlying psychiatric illness are candidates for outpatient group therapy. A supportive orientation is probably better if the patient is not articulate or appears psychologically fragile. An analytic or change-oriented group may be preferable if the patient is articulate and has good ego strength. Patients with more serious problems should be referred to day treatment settings with or without an affiliated halfway house. When there is good family support and a history of prolonged drug-free periods in the past, patients can be directed to Alcoholics Anonymous (AA)-style groups such as Narcotics Anonymous or Pills Anonymous. Geographic cures, sometimes regarded as impermanent, can in fact be successful, at least with opiate abusers over a several-month follow-up. Apart from these general guidelines, it is clear that even treatment programs do not select patients who do especially well in their particular forms of treatment. A trial-and-error pattern is inevitable.

*Chemical treatment.* Chemical treatment is almost entirely confined to those who abuse opiates or have severe underlying psychiatric disorders. Methadone maintenance is by far the commonest treatment modality for opiate abusers. It is legally defined as the daily dispensing of methadone for longer than 3 weeks, the usual duration of outpatient withdrawal. Methadone was first synthesized in Germany during World War II as an analgesic. It was established as the drug of choice for morphine withdrawal in 1949, and the concept of maintenance emerged during the early 1960s. Observations by Dole and Nyswander published in 1965 suggested that daily oral methadone produced a cessation of heroin use in chronic abusers, promoted employment, and encouraged patients to stabilize their lives in other ways.

In almost all methadone maintenance clinics newly enrolled patients must attend six or seven times weekly. After a period of several months, patients who are doing well and are employed can usually be given several methadone doses a week to take at home. There is no estimate of the extent to which these doses are diverted, although in some areas it is clearly appreciable. Take-home doses are defended as conducive to social rehabilitation and employment.

On average, patients spend more than 3 years in methadone maintenance. This average, however, combines a population that leaves within a few months and one that stays for many years. Unfortunately, the relapse rate is high, even after slow withdrawal over many months and even in patients who have not used street drugs for many years. In this sense methadone maintenance represents not a cure but a strategy for stabilization of opiate abuse. Favorable prognostic factors for successful withdrawal include a supportive family, several years away from opiate use, employment, and a history of long-term remissions.

The notable success of methadone maintenance is in the high rates of retention and cessation of opiate abuse. More than three fourths of patients who enroll in most programs are there a year later, and more than 90% of them abandon street opiates. Disadvantages of methadone maintenance include the many rules and regulations governing participation (including the obligation for frequent attendance), side effects of methadone, and a high rate of alcoholism and sedative or stimulant abuse.

Programs using LAAM are in other respects similar to those that undertake methadone maintenance. Because of its longer half-time, LAAM is given three times weekly.

"Methadone to abstinence" programs represent time-limited maintenance. Patients usually go through a several-month period of maintenance and then a strictly time-limited withdrawal phase and a period of drug-free counseling. There are few outcome data; however, this modality may be beneficial for the patient who needs immediate stabilization but who is hesitant to make an indefinite commitment to treatment.

Naltrexone is a pure opiate antagonist that, unlike naloxone, is orally active. Patients who take daily doses find the effects of opiate agonists such as heroin or methadone drastically curtailed or abolished. A few programs specialize in or offer this form of therapy in conjunction with counseling and other services. Rapid induction onto naltrexone in patients who are opiate-dependent can be accomplished by giving the first few doses with clonidine, which blocks the abstinence-producing properties of naltrexone. Success depends on the patient taking naltrexone daily at a time of high resolve and is similar in that respect to disulfiram treatment of alcoholism.

Early studies of naltrexone programs suggest that this treatment may work for some patients but that dropout rates are high and recruitment of patients is difficult. There do not appear to be any short-term side effects of naltrexone.

***Nonchemical treatment.*** Nonchemical treatment of drug abuse that does not involve chemical substitution or blockade includes individual counseling or psychotherapy, group therapy, day treatment programs with or without halfway house residence, AA-like organizations, and inpatient rehabilitation programs. Acupuncture has been advocated for the chronic treatment of drug abuse as well as for withdrawal, but there are few controlled data on efficacy. Each of these may be effective for selected individuals. Highly motivated, articulate patients with underlying psychiatric disorders are likely to do well in individual therapy with a psychiatrist, psychologist, or counselor. Some experts, however, consider groups to be the therapy of choice for most drug abusers.

Immediate control of life-threatening or progressive drug dependence may require inpatient or day treatment with controlled residence. Such programs, frequently called "therapeutic communities" ("TCs"), include Phoenix House, Daytop Village, Samaritan, Synanon, and many others. Such programs encourage an intense, residential experience for several years with gradually progressive responsibilities for counseling fellow clients. Such programs are as effective as methadone maintenance for patients who stay longer than several weeks and can treat drug abuse of all types. Unfortunately, the early dropout rate is high.

## BIBLIOGRAPHY


Berkowitz B: The relationship of pharmakinetics to pharmacological activity: Morphine, methadone, and naloxone, *Clin Pharmacokinet* 1:219, 1976.

Burns R et al: Phencyclidine—states of acute intoxication and fatalities, *West J Med* 123:345, 1975.

Covi et al: Length of treatment with anxiolytic sedatives and response to their sudden withdrawal, *Acta Psychiatr Scand* 49:51, 1973.

Dinwiddie S: Abuse of inhalants: A review, *Addiction* 89:925, 1994.

Ellinwood E: Amphetamine psychosis, *J Nerv Ment Dis* 144:273, 1967.

Essig C: Newer sedative drugs that can cause states of intoxication and dependence of the barbiturate type, *JAMA* 196:714, 1966.

Fauman B et al: Psychiatric sequelae of phencyclidine abuse, *Clin Toxicol* 9:529, 1976.

Greene M, Nightingale S, Dupont R: Evolving patterns of drug abuse, *Ann Intern Med* 83:402, 1975.

Harvey J: Drug related mortality in an inner city area, *Drug Alcohol Depend* 7:239, 1981.

Hollister L, Motzenbecker P, Degan R: Withdrawal reactions from chlordiazepoxide, *Psychopharmacologia* 2:63, 1961.

Isbell H et al: Chronic barbiturate intoxication, an experimental study, *Arch Neurol Psychiatry* 64:1, 1950.

Kornblith A: Multiple drug abuse involving nonopiate, nonalcoholic substances. I. Prevalence, *Int J Addict* 16:197, 1981.

Kornblith A: Multiple drug abuse involving nonopiate, nonalcoholic substances. II: Physical damage, long term psychological effects and treatment approaches and success, *Int J Addict* 16:527, 1981.

Maddox J, Desmond D: New light on the maturing out hypothesis in opioid dependence, *Bull Narc* 32:15, 1980.

Martin P: Intravenous phenobarbital therapy in barbiturate and other hypnosedative withdrawal reactions: A kinetic approach, *Clin Pharmacol Ther* 26:256, 1979.

McCarron M, Schulze B, Thompson G: Acute phencyclidine intoxication: Incidence of clinical findings in 1,000 cases, *Ann Emerg Med* 10:237, 1981.

Mclellan A et al: Certain types of substance abuse patients do better in certain kinds of treatments: Evidence for patient-program matching, *NIDA Res Monogr* 34:123, 1980.

Mclellan A et al: Is treatment for substance abuse effective?, *JAMA* 247:1423, 1982.

McClellan A, McGahan J, Druley K: Changes in drug abuse clients 1972-1978: Implications for revised treatment, *Am J Drug Alcohol Abuse* 6:151, 1979.

McLellan A, Woody G, O'Brien C: Development of psychiatric illness in drug abusers, *N Engl J Med* 301:1310, 1979.

Ohisson A et al: Plasma delta-9-tetra-hydrocannabinal concentrations and clinical effects after oral and intravenous administration and smoking, *Clin Pharmacol Ther* 28:409, 1980.

Ostor A: The medical complications of narcotic addiction, *Med J Aust* 1:410, 1977.

Ostrea E, Chavez C: Perinatal problems (excluding neonatal withdrawal) in maternal drug addiction: A study of 830 cases, *J Pediatr* 94:292, 1979.

Peak W, Fudge J, Robinowtiz R: Personality characteristics of compulsive heroin, amphetamine and barbiturate users, *J consult Clin Psychol* 47:583, 1979.

Perry P et al: Sedative hypnotic tolerance testing and withdrawal comparing diazepam to barbiturates, *J Clin Psychopharmacol,* 1:289, 1981.

Reisberg B: Infective endocarditis in the narcotic addict, *Prog Cardiovasc Dis* 23:193, 1979.

Rose J: Cocaethylene: a current understanding of the active metabolite of cocaine and ethanol, *Am J Emerg Med* 12(4):489, 1994.

Russe B, McCoy, C, Barton J: Recent findings concerning inhalant use, *Chem Depend* 4:113, 1980.

Showalter C, Thornton W: Clinical pharmacology of phencyclidine toxicity, *Am J Psychiatry* 134:11, 1977.

Simpson D, Savage L: Client types in different drug abuse treatments: Comparisons of follow-up outcomes, *Am J Drug Alcohol Abuse* 8:401, 1981-2.

Smith D, Wesson D: Phenobarbital technique for treatment of barbiturate dependence, *Arch Gen Psychiatry* 24:56, 1971.

Substance use disorders in *Diagnostic and Statistical Manual III,* 1981, Pp. 163-179.

Wilkinson P et al: Intranasal and oral cocaine kinetics, *Clin Pharmacol Ther* 27:386, 1980.

CHAPTER

# 132 Anxiety Disorders

Wendy Levinson
Mack Lipkin, Jr.

## EPIDEMIOLOGY

Anxiety has two meanings. First, anxiety is a common, normal emotion; it is the temporary sense of panic, fear, nervousness, or being overwhelmed that everyone feels on occasion. Second, anxiety may be part of a disorder, one of seven defined mental disorders in which the symptoms of anxiety are prominent, persistent, and disruptive to daily living or to a sense of well-being (see the box below).

The anxiety disorders are the second most common group of mental disorders in the general population; 16% have had an anxiety disorder sometime in their life. Anxiety disorders are twice as common in women as men. Patients with an anxiety disorder frequently seek help from a physician because they often attribute symptoms of anxiety to serious physical problems. For example, chest pain is a common symptom in an anxious young woman with "airplane phobia" just before she tries to board, even if she has no vascular disease, has low cholesterol, does not smoke, has no other risk factors, and runs the marathon.

When these patients come to physicians' offices, they create a dilemma: how much examination and testing should be done? Recognition of an anxiety disorder, based on specific defined criteria, can temper a physician's instinct to begin a series of tests on otherwise healthy-appearing people, including cardiac catheterization (chest pain), endoscopy (abdominal pain or diarrhea), vestibular testing (dizziness), and thyroid function studies (palpitations). Unfortunately, anxiety disorders are frequently unrecognized. For example, the average patient with a panic disorder sees *10*(!) physicians for her or his symptoms before the correct diagnosis is made. Table 132-1 illustrates the prevalence of panic disorder in patients with various undiagnosed physical symptoms. Early recognition of anxiety disorders is important to prevent unnecessary, expensive, and invasive diagnostic investigations; discomfort; and complications, including agoraphobia (fear of going out) or suicide.

The seven major anxiety disorders are panic disorder, generalized anxiety disorder (GAD), adjustment disorder with anxious mood, posttraumatic stress disorder (PTSD), simple phobia, social phobia, and obsessive-compulsive disorder (OCD).

### Physical symptoms experienced in anxiety disorders

Trouble swallowing or "lump in the throat"
Increased heart rate, chest pain
Sweaty palms
Weakness in the knees
"Fluttery" stomach, nausea, diarrhea
Trembling, twitching, feeling shaky
Shortness of breath
Tense, "uptight" feeling
Inability to relax
Muscle tension, aches, soreness
Dry mouth
Frequent urination
Exaggerated startle response
Difficulty concentrating or "mind going blank"
Trouble falling or staying asleep
Irritability or impatience
Faintness, dizziness

## PATHOPHYSIOLOGY

The etiology of anxiety disorders includes multiple factors. Contributors include biologic abnormalities and behavioral factors (conditioning and psychosocial stressors).

Evidence suggests that anxiety disorders are associated with specific biologic abnormalities in the central nervous system. Abnormalities are associated with receptors of the neurotransmitter $\gamma$-aminobutyric acid (GABA) and an area in the pons of the brain called the locus ceruleus. Stimulation of the locus ceruleus increases anxiety. Pharmacologic management with benzodiazepines stimulates GABA receptors and reduces anxiety symptoms. GABA receptors, found mainly in the cerebral cortex, play

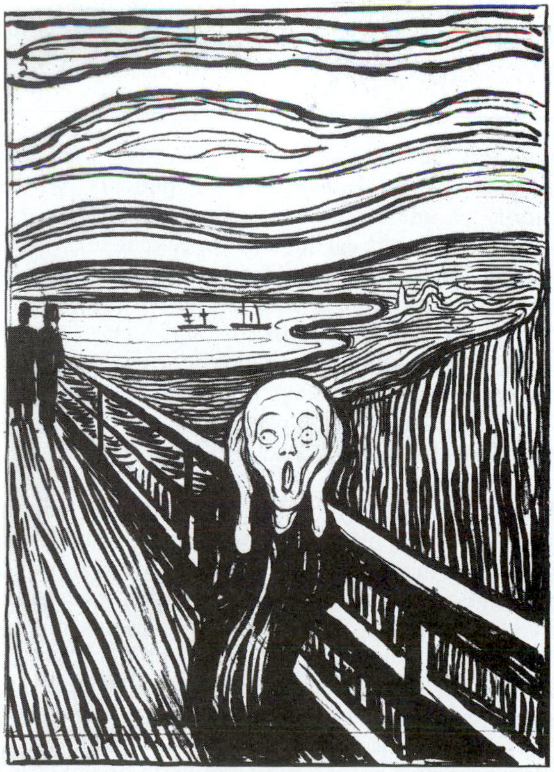

**Fig. 132-1.** *The Shriek.* Edward Munch, 1895, signed 1896. (Lithograph, printed in black, 13 15/16 × 10″. Collection, the Museum of Modern Art, New York. Matthew T. Mellon Fund.)

**Table 132-1.** Prevalence of panic disorder in patients with medically unexplained symptoms, primary care patients, and people in community

| Sample source | Panic disorder prevalence (%) |
|---|---|
| Community | 0.6-1.0 |
| Primary care | 7 |
| Chest pain and negative angiography | 33-43 |
| Hypertensive patients tested for pheochromocytoma | 35 |
| Irritable bowel syndrome | 29 |
| Unexplained dizziness or syncope | 13 |
| Migraine headaches | 5-15 |
| Chronic fatigue | 11-30 |
| Chronic pelvic pain | 8 |

Courtesy Dr. Charles Engle and Dr. Wayne Katon.

an inhibitory role. Data support a underlying genetic component of some anxiety disorders, including panic disorder, GAD, and OCD.

Conditioned responses may play a role in anxiety disorders (i.e., phobia). The development of agoraphobia in panic disorder may also be related to conditioning. Therefore an underlying biologic predisposition may be present, and then the appropriate pattern of stimulation conditions behavioral responses that are problematic for the patient.

Stressful events may also be key factors in leading to anxiety disorders such as adjustment disorder with anxious mood or PTSD. Catastrophic life events may cause PTSD.

## SPECIFIC DISORDERS

### Adjustment disorder with anxious mood

A diagnosis of an "adjustment disorder with anxious mood" should be considered in patients who have symptoms of anxiety, are experiencing or have experienced up to 2 months earlier a major psychosocial stressor, and do not meet the criteria for another anxiety disorder. The anxiety symptoms usually begin within 2 months of the onset of a major stressor and cause significant impairment in the patient's social or work functioning. If the symptoms persist longer than 6 months, another diagnosis, such as GAD, should be considered, along with chronic adjustment disorder.

***History.*** By definition, patients with an adjustment disorder have recently undergone a stressful life event. This may be a medical event, such as a surgical procedure, hospitalization, or new diagnosis. Personal events such as divorce, job change, and financial problems most often precipitate the disorder. Although most people would experience distress and some symptoms of anxiety with these events, patients with adjustment disorder experience a disruption of social or occupational function. Often, sleeplessness and autonomic symptoms of anxiety interfere, and the patient may seek care for somatic complaints. Eliciting the history of the stressful life event and ascertaining the relationship of symptoms to that event assist in this diagnosis.

**Symptoms associated with panic disorder**

- Choking sensation or "lump in the throat"
- Skipping, racing, or pounding of the heart
- Excessive sweating
- Rubbery or "jelly" legs
- Nausea or abdominal distress
- Trembling or shaking
- Difficulty in "getting one's breath," smothering sensations, overbreathing
- Chest pain, pressure, discomfort
- Faintness, lightheadedness, dizziness
- Feeling off balance or unsteady
- Tingling or numbness in parts of the body
- Hot flashes or chills
- Preoccupation with health concerns
- Feeling that objects in the environment are strange, unreal, foggy, or detached
- Feeling outside or detached from all or part of the body; having a "floating" feeling
- Fear of dying or that something terrible is about to happen
- Feeling of losing control or going insane
- Agoraphobic avoidance behavior
- Feeling frightened suddenly and unexpectedly for no immediate reason

Modified from McGlynn TJ, Metcalf HL, editors: *Diagnosis and treatment of anxiety disorders: a physician's handbook,* ed 2, New York, 1991, American Psychiatric Press.

***Management.*** The fundamental management of patients with adjustment disorder with anxious mood is individual counseling directed at helping the patient work through the feelings associated with the triggering event. Discussion of the event with a supportive person, including the primary care physician or a mental health counselor, is the most important aspect of therapy. Structured relaxation exercises and instruction in stress management may also be helpful. Support groups of patients with similar problems are useful in some situations (e.g., patients diagnosed with breast cancer). In some patients, brief use of benzodiazepines (less than 3-week course) may be needed to treat debilitating stress-related symptoms (e.g., insomnia, agoraphobia).

Patients with adjustment disorder are generally well managed by a supportive primary care physician who has learned the details of the precipitating event. Brief supportive therapy can often be incorporated into the primary care management. Referral to mental health professionals may help if patients do not respond quickly or are more severely incapacitated in their functioning.

### Panic attacks and panic disorder

Most people have experienced or will experience panic attacks. These episodes last several minutes to several hours, are not triggered by any obvious external or internal event, and consist of four or more of the symptoms listed in the box above. A sense of fear and impending doom and physical symptoms are usually prominent and often frighten patients into seeking care urgently. The physician generally can be reassuring because these panic attacks most often are infrequent, self-limited, and not related to any serious disorder.

Panic disorder is diagnosed when attacks occur more than four times in 1 month, produce persistent fear, or become significantly disruptive to the patient's life. The dilemma for the primary care physician is whether or not to evaluate the patient's specific symptoms. An appropriate strategy is to evaluate conservatively those symptoms that are potentially dangerous, consider objective findings, or present a "classic" constellation. Simultaneously the patient is treated for panic disorder, and symptoms are reevaluated periodically.

Panic disorder is often a debilitating disease with major complications. First, panic disorder leads to agoraphobia in 95% of patients, usually within 6 months of the first panic attack. We have had several patients who had not left home in the previous 3 years (the children did the shopping, etc.)! One of our patients began to develop agoraphobia after her first panic attack. This fear of a recurrent attack causes most patients to avoid important activities such as shopping, working, or socializing. Second, some evidence suggests that suicide attempts occur more frequently with panic disorder than even with major depression. Finally, since panic disorder is so frequently missed by physicians, the patients are at risk for unnecessary treatments and therefore for iatrogenic harm.

***Management.*** The principal treatment is pharmacologic with tricyclic antidepressants (especially imipramine and desipramine), some benzodiazepines (alprazolam and perhaps lorazepam and clonazepam) or with monoamine oxidase (MAO) inhibitors. These are listed here in the order we use them. Evidence for the efficacy of the serotonin reuptake inhibitors (fluoxetine and clomipramine) is preliminary but encouraging.

The antidepressants are effective and relatively safe. Usually we start at low doses (25 mg) and increase every 3 to 4 days up to full therapeutic doses, usually 150 to 300 mg but with individual variations. Treatment effects may require up to 8 weeks to peak, and exact duration of therapy is individualized. At 4 months we usually attempt to taper the dosages. Some patients may experience an exacerbation of their symptoms early in therapy and may require simultaneous benzodiazepine treatment until the antidepressants take effect.

Benzodiazepines are effective and have the advantage of a more rapid onset of controlling symptoms. Alprazolam is approved by the U.S. Food and Drug Administration (FDA) for treating panic disorder, but diazepam, lorazepam, and clonazepam are probably similarly effective. Treatment should be initiated with a low dose and increased to maximize benefit and minimize side effects (sedation). The appropriate duration of therapy is not well established, but 2 to 6 months may be required. Periodic reassessment and gradual tapering should be attempted, but most patients require longer therapy, about 2 years. The main disadvantages of benzodiazepine therapy are the potential withdrawal symptoms (increased anxiety symptoms, rebound, autonomic withdrawal symptoms) and the risk of seizures on abrupt cessation. In practice these do not occur in most patients. In addition, concerns of abuse exist, but data showing this are minimal, except in patients with a prior abuse history.

MAO inhibitors are actually the most effective. However, they are difficult medications for patients to use and physicians to explain. We use these infrequently, only if other therapies are not effective, or in consultation with a psychiatrist.

In addition to drug therapy, patients benefit from clearly understanding the nature of their problem. This eases anxiety, increases the strength of the therapeutic alliance, and increases the likelihood that the patient will follow the treatment plan. We explain that this is a biologic disorder with real physical symptoms and psychologic symptoms as well: it is not "all in their head." We explain that it is related to brain function, has a genetic component, and causes the multiple, frightening symptoms the patient has been experiencing. We underscore that it is treatable.

Cognitive therapy has recently been shown to benefit many patients and possibly to be a genuine alternative to pharmacotherapy. The best treatment may be a combination of both; however, qualified cognitive therapists may not be available. If the patient has developed agoraphobia, systematic desensitization by a suitable behavioral therapist is helpful for overcoming avoidance behaviors. Many patients with panic disorder develop secondary depression. This should improve with appropriate antidepressant therapy. Finally, good self-help books and widespread support groups are helpful to some patients.

### Phobias

Simple phobia and social phobias are characterized by episodic anxiety in response to a specific precipitant. In these situations, patients experience intense, excessive fear that makes them avoid the situation if possible. Stimuli for simple phobias are places, things, or events, typically airplane flights, heights, insects, or small animals (snakes, mice). Social phobias occur in circumstances where the person is observed by others and fears humiliation or failure, such as playing at a musical performance, delivering a speech, talking in class, or going to a party. In both simple and social phobias, patients can develop symptoms of anxiety anticipating the event, and they start avoiding the occurrence in a manner that interferes with routine functioning. For example, we noticed that one of our excellent residents never talked in conferences or attending rounds. She missed as many as possible. She told us she was terrified of being humiliated or disgraced. Behavioral therapy improved her to the point of being an effective group member.

As another example, a man in his mid-30s complained that he was developing severe palpitations, sweating, and tremulousness when he was waiting in immigration or customs lines. The symptoms were so intense that he would go back to the end of a long line after reaching the customs/immigration booth. This was a major problem for him, since his occupation was writing travel books. He started avoiding travel and began worrying about his ability to meet his writing deadlines. His symptoms were consistent with a social phobia, and he was treated successfully with behavioral therapy and brief use of β-blockers.

Most patients with simple or social phobias do not seek care for the condition. When they do, the diagnosis is usually evident from the history and does not require further testing. It is important to differentiate social phobia from panic disorder; in the former the symptoms are anticipated and occur in a predictable situation, whereas in the latter they are unpredictable and unexpected.

*Management.* Treatment of phobias is exclusively by behavioral therapy that gradually desensitizes patients to the phobia. This entails incrementally introducing a small amount of the feared stimulus or a related but less feared situation. Limited exposures while using relaxation techniques may allow the patient to become gradually closer to the object or situation, and eventually the phobia is managed. Pharmacologic therapy with β-blockers or benzodiazepines may help when the fear-provoking situation cannot or has not been desensitized (e.g., a patient with fear of flying has a death in the family far away).

### Posttraumatic stress disorder

PTSD is the syndrome occurring after a vulnerable person experiences trauma outside the range of normal human experience. The person later has flashbacks, nightmares, severe distress with or numbness to stimuli resembling (concretely or symbolically) the event or to many stimuli (generalization), anxiety, hypervigilance or other persisting signs and symptoms of autonomic arousal, and secondary depression. These patients may have subtle symptoms or a major life disruption. Some exhibit new antisocial behavior, violence, or suicidal behavior. They are at risk for alcohol and drug abuse and criminal activity.

Overall, the lifetime prevalence of PTSD is 1% to 9% of the general population. The precipitating traumatic events may include accidents, abuse, violence (especially rape), and surgery. One of our patients was a successful accountant until age 42, when he had aortic valve surgery. Subsequently, he became totally dysfunctional, losing jobs and clients. He was always angry and had flashbacks about the postoperative period of pain and confusion. He gradually became depressed, and his obnoxious angry behavior alienated friends and health care workers. Eventually, his depression and underlying PTSD were recognized and treated.

*Management.* Treatment of PTSD is multifaceted and usually best accomplished with a team approach. If present, depression needs to be treated with antidepressant medication and supportive care. It is helpful to name the problem as PTSD and legitimize the manifestations, since patients often blame themselves for these problems or see themselves as both crazy and hopeless. One might say, "Having feelings, thoughts, and problems such as yours are not uncommon among persons who have suffered a catastrophe." Aggressive treatment of substance abuse, utilizing drug or alcohol counselors or addiction specialists and residential programs, is essential because without this, such patients cannot work effectively on their other problems. Support groups are useful ways for patients to feel understood, share solutions, and problem solve. Again, benzodiazepine use should be avoided in those with a drug abuse history.

### Generalized anxiety disorder

GAD consists of constant, nonepisodic anxiety that effects the patient for more than 6 months and interferes with normal function. The symptoms are grouped into motor tension, autonomic hyperactivity, and vigilance and scanning (see the box above). The symptoms must not be attributed to other medical problems, such as hyperthyroidism, abuse of stimulant drugs, or psychiatric disorders (i.e., psychosis). Patients usually complain of feeling "uptight" or constantly nervous. These symptoms lead to problems coping with normal daily activities.

Benzodiazepine therapy is effective and allows patients to function normally. Minimum effective doses should be used, but care must be taken not to undertreat patients out of a fear of making the patient dependent. Short-term supportive psychotherapy can also be helpful.

#### Specific symptoms associated with generalized anxiety disorder (GAD)

**Motor tension**

Trembling, twitching, feeling shaky
Muscle tension, aches, soreness
Restlessness
Easy fatigability

**Autonomic hyperactivity**

Shortness of breath, smothering sensations
Palpitations, accelerated heart rate
Sweating, cold clammy hands
Dry mouth
Dizziness, lightheadedness
Nausea, diarrhea, other types of abdominal distress
Flushes (hot flashes), chills
Frequent urination
Trouble swallowing, "lump in throat"

**Vigilance and scanning**

Feeling "keyed up" or on edge
Exaggerated startle response
Difficulty concentrating or "mind going blank" because of anxiety
Trouble falling or staying asleep
Irritability

Modified from American Psychiatric Association: *Diagnostic and statistical manual of mental disorders,* ed 3, revised, Washington, DC, 1987, The Association.

### Obsessive-compulsive disorder

In OCD, patients have regular intrusive thoughts or obsessions about aggression, sex, religion, theft or loss, or other covering, mental rituals such as counting objects or letters to the extent of disrupting normal thought. The patient may also have persistent rituals or compulsions that are so frequent or complex as to interfere with normal function. Patients experience these obsessions and compulsions as intrusive, upsetting, and silly. One of our patients wrung her hands so constantly she could not cook, work, or even fall asleep. Another washed his hands every 10 to 15 minutes, interfering with normal business or social life. Some of these patients lack insight into their problems; others are desperate. These patients were refractory to psychologic or psychiatric treatment in the past. Recently, however, both behavior therapy and clomipramine (Anafranil) and other serotonin reuptake inhibitors have been of benefit in some patients, at usual doses.

## REFERRAL

In our experience, most patients with anxiety disorders can be treated by the primary care physician. Sometimes, as with patients who have panic disorder without agoraphobia, just explaining the diagnosis and providing information may help the patient significantly. Patients should be considered for referral to a psychiatrist or other mental health professional under the following circumstances:

1. The treatment does not lead to improvement in the patient's symptoms within a reasonable time frame.
2. The physician is confused about the primary diagnosis. It is particularly important to differentiate patients who have depression with symptoms of anxiety or alcoholic patients from those with anxiety disorder. Psychiatric consultation is appropriate if the primary care physician is uncertain and the distinction has therapeutic implications.
3. The patient has complicating substance abuse or suicidal behavior or thoughts.
4. The question of benzodiazepine dependence is present, and help is needed with implementing "drug holidays" in appropriate patients.

In addition, the primary care physician may be uncertain whether a patient has another organic disease and may think a specialist is necessary to consider this possibility. In these circumstances, it is helpful to choose a specialist who understands anxiety disorders and will work with the primary care physician to explain the nature of the specific anxiety disorder to the patient. It is especially important that the specialist is conservative in the approach to ordering diagnostic studies.

## TREATMENT

### Nonpharmacologic therapy

Many patients with anxiety disorders can be treated without medication. The main therapies include education, behavior therapy and systematic desensitization, psychotherapy (counseling), and cognitive therapy. In addition, hypnosis, progressive muscle relaxation, and biofeedback may be useful adjuncts.

***Education.*** Providing basic information about anxiety disorders is very helpful. Patients often think something terrible is wrong and are fearful. Physicians can explain the nature of the problem, tell patients how common the problem is ("you are not alone"), and reassure patients that treatment will improve their distress. Providing patients with appropriate written material about the problem allows them to understand more clearly and share information with their family. Good-quality lay publications are available in self-help sections of bookstores and may be useful, particularly for persons with panic disorder and PTSD.

***Behavior therapy and systematic desensitization.*** Phobias are best treated with behavior therapy. In panic disorders, this method is used to treat the secondary agoraphobia. Using this approach, patients gradually experience situations that have been associated with the unpleasant anxiety symptoms. The patient learns to relax using formal relaxation techniques. They approach a stimulus that has been anxiety provoking to them, using the relaxation methods to avoid symptoms.

This approach can be particularly helpful when used in conjunction with cognitive therapy and additional techniques, including progressive muscle relaxation and self-hypnosis.

***Psychotherapy (counseling).*** Most patients with anxiety disorders seek care from their primary care provider. As with all medical conditions, the relationship between physician and patient can play an extremely important role in the therapy. In the course of routine care, physicians listen to the patient, express empathy for the patient's feelings and concerns, and point out patterns or behaviors that may be self-defeating for the patient. In anxiety disorders, as in adjustment disorder with anxious mood, the physician can show the patient the relationship of the symptoms to the stressful event, express understanding of the patient's distress, and assist the patient in thinking of other strategies to cope with the situation. This form of brief counseling can be effective in improving the patient's symptoms. In contrast, long-term or insight-oriented psychotherapy is not beneficial to patients with anxiety disorders.

***Cognitive therapy.*** Cognitive therapy includes teaching the patient to think differently about the problem and practicing this new way of thinking. For example, patients with panic disorder think the symptoms are life-threatening and something terrible is happening. This "internal cognition" intensifies feelings of anxiety, increases autonomic stimulation, and builds a vicious cycle. To intervene in this problem, the physician can explain to patients that the symptoms are part of the panic disorder and that their life is not in jeopardy. For example, the physician might say, "When you have these symptoms, remember me saying to you, 'This is my body's reaction causing the symptoms. Nothing dangerous is happening to me. These symptoms will pass shortly. I should just relax.'" The physician then rehearses this with the patient by having her or him imagine and then react (out loud initially and then internally) in this new way. Thus the patient starts reframing the symptoms as part of a self-limited and not life-threatening situation. The patient changes the way she or he thinks about the problem.

***Relaxation techniques.*** Ways to help patients relax include hypnosis, progressive muscle relaxation, and biofeedback. These may all be helpful adjuncts in treating anxiety disorders. With all these techniques, patients learn to induce a more relaxed state and decrease the autonomic hyperstimulation associated with anxiety disorders. These techniques can then be used in conjunction with other modalities to treat the anxiety disorder.

### Pharmacologic therapy

Ideally, all patients with anxiety disorders should receive one or more of the psychotherapies just discussed. Unfortunately, resources are often scarce, and pharmacologic strategies are often the mainstay of treatment. Specifically, pharmacologic treatment is appropriate when the patient has panic disorder, when the patient's symp-

**Table 132-2.** Pharmacologic therapy for anxiety disorders

| Disorder | Appropriate class of drugs and examples | Starting dose (range) | Special concerns with class of drugs |
|---|---|---|---|
| Panic | Tricyclic antidepressants | | Anticholinergic and sedative effects |
| | Desipramine (Norpramine) | 25 mg qd | Potential risk of overdose |
| | Imipramine (Tofranil) | 25 mg qd | |
| | Nontricyclic antidepressants | | Efficacy not established |
| | Fluoxetine (Prozac) | 10-20 mg qd | |
| | Benzodiazepines | | Potential for abuse, seizures and addiction |
| | Alprazolam (Xanax) | 0.25 ml mg qd | |
| | Diazepam (Valium) | 2 mg qd | Central nervous system side effects, particularly in elderly patients |
| | MAO inhibitors | | Dietary and drug restrictions |
| | Phenelzine | 15 mg qd | |
| Phobias | β-Blockers | | Blocks symptoms only |
| | Propranolol | 10-40 mg qd | |
| | Benzodiazepines | | Brief therapy only |
| | As above | | |
| Adjustment disorder | Benzodiazepines | | Rarely necessary; if needed, brief therapy |
| | As above | | |
| Posttraumatic stress disorder | Antidepressant therapy | | Treat any accompanying substance abuse problems. |
| | As above | | |
| Obsessive-compulsive disorder | Clomipramine (Anafranil) | 25 mg qd | Therapy may require extended period of 3 months or more. |
| | Serotonin Reuptake Inhibitors (SRI) | | |
| | Fluoxetine (Prozac) | 20 mg qd | |

toms are severe enough that they are significantly interfering with the patient's routine daily functioning, and when the potential benefits outweigh the risks for an individual patient. Drug therapy is usually needed to treat the secondary depression. This decision needs to be individualized for the patient based on the particular symptoms, history of other medical illnesses (particularly drug abuse, alcoholism, etc.), and the patient's willingness to collaborate in a pharmacologic approach to symptom management.

If drug management is deemed appropriate for the individual, the proper agent should be selected based on the type of anxiety disorder. Table 132-2 indicates the most frequently used medications for each anxiety disorder and a typical starting dose. Medications should be started at a low dose and titrated gradually upward to control symptoms while minimizing side effects. Adequate doses of antidepressants need to be used for at least 4 to 6 weeks to evaluate therapeutic effectiveness, and treatment may need to be continued for months while other nonpharmacologic treatments are also used. The optimal duration of treatment for most anxiety disorders is not well established by controlled studies. If patients do not seem to be responding within a usual time frame or the benefit/side effect ratio is unfavorable, they should be referred to a specialist for assistance in therapeutic management.

## BIBLIOGRAPHY

Katon WJ: *Panic disorder in the medical setting,* Washington, DC, 1991, American Psychiatric Press.

McGlynn TJ, Metcalf HL, editors: *Diagnosis and treatment of anxiety disorders: a physician's handbook,* ed 2, New York, 1991, American Psychiatric Press.

Roy-Byrne PP: Integrated treatment of panic disorder, *Am J Med* 92(suppl 1A):49S, 1992.

Shader RI, Greenblatt DJ: Use of benzodiazepines in anxiety disorders, *N Engl J Med* 329(19):1398, 1993.

Sheehan DV: *The anxiety disease,* New York, 1983, Bantam.

CHAPTER

# 133 Mood Disorders

**Steven A. Cole**

## OVERVIEW AND DEFINITION

Five mood disorders are of importance to primary care physicians: major depression, dysthymia, adjustment disorder with depressed mood, depression caused by a general medical condition (or substance), and bipolar disorder.

Depression is one of the most painful conditions that can afflict an individual. Depressed persons generally report that their depression has caused more suffering than any other problem they have ever had. Depression is common, disabling, and often unrecognized and untreated in primary care practices. This chapter reviews the epidemiology, diagnosis, and treatment of major depression in detail and briefly discusses other mood disorders.

*Major depression* (MD) is the most severe form of depression and is associated with considerable disability, morbidity, and mortality. In several careful epidemiologic studies, MD has been demonstrated to be associated with as much disability (days in bed; days absent from work; impaired social, role, and interpersonal functioning) as eight other chronic illnesses, including arthritis and coronary artery disease. In addition, MD is also associated with considerable physical morbidity and mortality, most specifically related to the risk of suicide, but also as a risk factor for poor outcome and death in nursing home patients and in those with general medical conditions such as coronary artery disease and traumatic brain injury.

*Dysthymia* represents a milder form of depressive illness that does not meet the severity criteria of MD but is marked by considerable chronicity. Dysthymia is diagnosed when a depressed mood and at least two other symptoms of depression are present "most days" during the previous 2 years. Dysthymia can be considered a form of "minor depression" but is itself associated with significant pain and impaired functioning and may not remit spontaneously.

*Adjustment disorder with depressed mood* describes a psychiatric condition resulting from an identifiable stressor (e.g., divorce, job loss) that represents a level of impairment greater than what could normally be expected for most individuals. It can only be diagnosed within the first 6 months after a stressor has occurred. If the condition lasts longer than 6 months, the diagnosis would change to depressive disorder, NOS (not otherwise specified). It is important to recognize that a "normal" reaction to a distressing life event should not be diagnosed as an adjustment disorder. If an identifiable stressor precipitates a depressive syndrome that meets the severity criteria for MD, the diagnosis of MD is made (and not adjustment disorder).

*Mood disorders caused by a general medical condition* (or substance) refers to a psychiatric syndrome that the clinician judges to result from the direct physiologic consequence of a general medication condition or medication. Examples might include hypothyroidism or reserpine. The treatment should focus on resolution of the underlying general medical problem or withdrawal of the causative medication, but specific psychiatric treatment is also usually needed and recommended.

*Bipolar disorder,* previously called "manic-depressive" illness, occurs in about 1% of the population and represents a common and quite severe form of mental illness that has a very strong biologic and genetic substrate. About 10% of children who have one parent with bipolar disorder will develop the illness themselves.

## EPIDEMIOLOGY AND ETIOLOGY

Most epidemiologic studies indicate that the lifetime prevalence of MD is 5% to 10% in men and 10% to 20% in women. The reasons for these gender differences are unclear: numerous factors point to endocrine and biologic factors, whereas others attribute the differences to sociocultural factors. The 1-year prevalence of MD in the community is 2% to 4% for men and 4% to 8% for women. Studies of medical outpatients demonstrate similar rates, whereas studies of medical inpatients and studies in some diseases thought to predispose biologically (e.g., cerebrovascular accident [CVA, stroke], Parkinson's disease, traumatic brain injury) or psychologically (cancer) indicate much higher rates (10% to 50%).

Although clinical lore has long suggested depression is more common in elderly persons, recent epidemiologic findings demonstrate lower 1-year prevalence rates of depression in elderly persons (1% to 2%).

Many patients and physicians consider depression to be "expected" in the face of significant stress. Stressful life events certainly predispose to major depression, but MD is not the uniform outcome (either clinically or statistically) of any stressful event. In fact, studies of individuals under stress (e.g., from terminal cancer, natural disaster) show rates of MD greater than the general population rate, but almost always *less than* 50%. That is, despite the seriousness of the circumstance, *most individuals* do not develop an MD syndrome under stress.

Sad or depressed affect is an expected accompaniment of a stressful event, but the full syndrome of MD does not uniformly emerge. In this sense, no "good reasons" exist for MD. When such a syndrome develops, it is best considered a major (clinical) depression and not a "reactive depression."

Historically, the term *reactive depression* suggested (1) a mild version of the syndrome; (2) one that resulted entirely from a psychologic precipitant; (3) one that did not have a biologic substrate; and (4) one that should be treated with psychotherapy. None of these four assumptions is true about depressive syndromes precipitated by life events or physical illness. A very severe depressive syndrome can result from a stressful event (just as a myocardial infarction [MI] can result from a stress); a biologically predisposed individual may have MD in response to a life event; an MD resulting from a life stress may develop a biologic substrate; and an MD resulting from a life stress may respond as well or better to biologic therapy than to psychotherapy.

Thus, the presence or absence of identifiable precipitants (stressors) is irrelevant to the diagnosis of MD. MD may be precipitated by stressful life events, but the diagnosis should be based only on the presentation of the signs and symptoms of MD. When MD results from a life stress or general medical illness, it is best to consider the MD a dread complication of the stress (or illness) and to diagnose aggressively and treat the depression as a comorbid condition.

Many physical symptoms of MD (see following discussion), for example, fatigue, anorexia, and psychomotor retardation, can often be attributed to a comorbid general medical condition such as cancer or Parkinson's disease. This contribution of a general medical illness to the symptom profile of depression often leads clinicians to discount their relevance and thus overlook the possibility of a treatable depression. Emerging data and the revised *Diagnostic and Statistical Manual of Mental Disorders,* fourth edition (DSM-IV) criteria for MD points to the importance of *including* these symptoms in the diagnostic approach to depression in medically ill patients. Although this inclusive approach might tend to overdiagnose MD, studies of CVA, Parkinson's disease, and traumatic brain injury indicate that the problem of overdiagnosis, if it exists, is quite low (about 2%).

## PATHOPHYSIOLOGY: THE BIOPSYCHOSOCIAL MODEL OF DEPRESSION

Because MD is still a syndromal diagnosis, the illness itself probably represents a heterogenous group of disorders, many of which include a variable array of etiologic determinants.

No clear anatomic, physiologic, or biochemical lesion has been found that can explain MD. Most investigators agree that MD is a complex psychologic syndrome that, at present, can only be diagnosed on clinical criteria. Many promising studies point to possible etiologic dimensions and suggest future therapeutic interventions.

Research to date points to mixtures of environmental and biologic factors underlying severe mood disorders. Genetic and family experiences certainly play a role, but not a determining one. Even for bipolar disorder, monozygotic twins share less than a 50% concordance and dizygotic twins about 10% concordance (about the same as siblings). With respect to MD in women, recent data indicate that negative life events also play a significant etiologic role. Animal studies demonstrate that early environmental stress predisposes to biologic and behavioral abnormalities associated with depression that may not emerge until adult life.

Numerous biologic "markers" of depression have recently been identified. These factors can be said to underlie MD but not necessarily "cause" it. It is quite possible that an environmental stress leads to psychic distress, which then precipitates a biologic cascade leading to MD. Although no marker is specific enough to be able to be used diagnostically, several markers reliably and statistically differentiate groups with and without MD.

Some of these markers include endocrine factors: elevated cortisol, failure to suppress cortisol after the administration of exogenous dexamethasone (DST), blunted response of thyroid-stimulating hormone (TSH) to challenge with thyroglobulin-releasing factor (TRF), and increased growth hormone (GH) response to prolactin. Neurotransmitter levels such as norepinephrine (NE) and serotonin (5-HT) may be altered, but more likely, NE and/or 5-HT receptor function and/or number is altered during depression. One marker of altered central nervous system (CNS) 5-HT receptor function has been found to be platelet imipramine or platelet paroxetine binding. Sleep physiology is also changed in MD, with an early induction of rapid eye movement (REM) sleep and an overall increase of REM density during sleep. Finally, neuroimaging studies using positron emission tomography (PET) have demonstrated anatomically specific metabolic differences between depressed individuals and control subjects.

Loss of a parent (especially mother) is weakly predictive of future depression, whereas a low level of perceived social support (especially a wife's perception of an unsupportive husband) is predictive of future depression. Recent interpersonal, behavioral, and cognitive approaches to understanding depressive etiology and pathology have also generated important and promising therapeutic approaches, some of which have been shown to be as effective as medication for the treatment of mild but not severe depression.

### Diagnosis of major depression (MD)

Five symptoms from the following list lead to the diagnosis of MD, required. The symptoms must all have been present most of the time for the last 2 weeks.

1. Depressed mood
2. Anhedonia (lack of interest or pleasure in all or almost all activities)
3. Sleep disorder (insomnia or hypersomnia)
4. Appetite loss, weight loss, appetite gain, or weight gain
5. Fatigue or loss of energy
6. Psychomotor retardation or agitation
7. Trouble concentrating or difficulty making decisions
8. Low self-esteem or guilt
9. Recurrent thoughts of death or suicidal ideation

## HISTORY

DSM-IV criteria for MD requires five of nine symptoms (see the box above) for a 2-week period. One of the nine symptoms must be either a persistent depressed mood or a pervasive anhedonia (loss of interest or pleasure in living). "Persistent" is defined as "present most of the day, nearly every day."

Some have found it helpful to think of four hallmarks of MD for the purpose of clinical evaluation: (1) depressed mood, (2) anhedonia, (3) physical symptoms (sleep disdisorder, appetite problem, fatigue, psychomotor changes), and (4) psychologic symptoms (trouble concentrating or indecisiveness, guilt or low self-esteem, and hopelessness). The physical symptoms are important because they are predictive of a good response to biologic treatments. In particular, when middle insomnia is present (awaking at 3 or 4 AM with inability to return to sleep) and when a diurnal variation in mood is present (feeling more depressed in AM), patients are more likely to respond to biologic intervention. The psychologic symptoms are helpful in recognizing MD in patients with general medical illnesses.

### Medical interview

The medical interview is the key to making the diagnosis of MD. Although MD is diagnosed by a positive response to five of nine symptoms (see the box above), clinicians often miss the diagnosis if they are not in the habit of routine screening for this common and disabling problem. Numerous studies in primary care point to the fact that about 50% of the depressed patients are not recognized. This occurs because of time limitations for the interview, lack of knowledge and skill, fear of "opening Pandora's box," and the stigma associated with psychiatric illness.

Often, nonverbal cues can suggest depression to the busy physician. Downcast eyes, slow speech, wrinkled brow, and tearful looks all express a sad mood. However, a depressed mood is not synonymous with MD. Physicians interested in screening for MD can focus on anhedonia ("What do you do for a good time?") and/or sleep ("How is your sleep?"). When MD is present, these questions often yield positive responses, despite the patient's focus on other complaints and a tendency to deny depressed mood.

When physicians suspect a psychiatric disorder underlying a presenting physical problem, an open-ended questioning style may help reveal important data early in the interview. When patients indicate emotional distress surrounding a stressful life situation or distress related to a physical symptom, it can prove efficient for the physician to investigate the emotional issue immediately. Recognizing and treating a major depression early in the course of a general medical evaluation can save much time and expense. Physicians' clinical judgment must be fully used to investigate physical symptoms as indicated. However, concomitant recognition and treatment of MD can prove quite cost-efficient.

### Somatic presentations

The depressed patient in primary care does not present with the statement, "I have a major depression, doctor; please prescribe proper treatment." More often, the patient experiences a somatic problem such as pain (headache, backache), fatigue, insomnia, or spells. The physician should attempt to rule out significant general medical problems and assess depression simultaneously. Developing these skills to evaluate both general medical and psychiatric problems simultaneously can save much time and expense and decrease frustration of both physician and patient.

### Resistance (stigma)

Many patients are reluctant to accept the diagnosis of depression. They do not experience this illness as a psychologic problem, and they often resist their physicians' explanation of a psychiatric problem. There is a stigma to having depression, and patients often think they are to blame for this problem.

Physicians can help overcome this problem of stigma by explaining that depression is an illness, like any other. There is a biochemical derangement in depression, just as in diabetes, and proper treatment is necessary to restore function. In severe depression, proper treatment is usually biologic.

Patients should be told that depression is not their fault and that depression is common. Severe depression does not usually remit on its own, but proper treatment usually ensures a good outcome.

### Reluctance to open "Pandora's box"

Many physicians often are reluctant to pursue psychiatric or emotional problems for fear this will open "Pandora's box" and take an unreasonable amount of time. In fact, when physicians are able to respond appropriately to patients' emotions and recognize psychiatric disorders, the overall amount of time can be decreased. Lengthy extended workups of nonspecific physical complaints can be avoided. Thus, attention to emotional issues is both cost-efficient and cost-effective. Since little training has been available to most practicing physicians about communication, recent texts and workshops may be helpful.

### Suicide

Suicidal ideation needs to be evaluated in all patients with symptoms of depression. Suicide is one of the top 10 causes of death in all age groups and one of the top three causes in young adults and teenagers. Besides depression, risk factors for depression include gender (elderly white males are the highest-risk group), alcoholism, psychosis, chronic physical illness, and lack of social support. From a clinical point of view, the presence of suicidal intent, hopelessness, and a well-formulated plan all indicate high risk. Many patients who eventually commit suicide visit a primary care physician in the month before they take their lives.

#### Questions for the suicidal patient

1. How does the future look to you?
2. Do you ever feel that life is not worth living?
3. Do you sometimes feel it doesn't matter whether you live or die?
4. Have you ever considered taking your own life?
5. Have you developed a plan about how you might kill yourself?
6. Are you willing to promise me that you will call me (or this number) if you feel you cannot control an impulse to take your own life?

The topic of suicidal ideation can be approached gradually with nonspecific questions such as, "Do you ever feel so discouraged that life does not seem worth living?" Patients can be asked to elaborate on their answers. Ultimately the physician should ask a very direct question, "Do you ever feel like taking your own life?" The box above lists other questions that clarify the patient's intent and facilitate assessment of risk.

Physicians need to be aware that asking about suicide *will not* increase a patient's risk. To the contrary, inquiries about suicide can reassure the patient and enable the physician and patient together to make a plan to prevent suicide.

Once a patient has admitted to any suicidal ideation, the primary care physician must decide whether emergency psychiatric consultation and hospitalization are necessary. This is a clinical judgment for which no absolute guidelines can be set. Risk factors should be kept in mind, but the clinical evaluation should be primary. If this assessment suggests outpatient management, physicians should consider using a "no suicide contract." Although data on the effectiveness of this technique are not available, it does represent a standard clinical practice that has a high degree of face validity. Patients are simply asked to promise the physician that they will contact the physician (or alternative covering caregiver) if they think they are losing control of a suicidal impulse.

## PHYSICAL EXAMINATION

No specific signs on physical examinations indicate depression. Nonverbal cues can be helpful, however, such as furrowed brow, downcast eyes, slow speech, psychomotor retardation or agitation, hand wringing, frequent sighing, and frequent shoulder shrugging.

Some general medical conditions may also present with

depression or depressive symptoms, such as endocrine problems (hypothyroidism, Cushing's syndrome), Parkinson's disease, and cerebrovascular disease. Thus, a careful medical history and physical examination are an essential part of the evaluation of depression, at all ages, but especially in elderly persons.

## LABORATORY STUDIES AND DIAGNOSTIC PROCEDURES

A routine laboratory screen, including complete blood count (CBC), chemistry profile, and urinalysis should be part of the workup of depression because many general medical illnesses present with the symptoms of depression (e.g., fatigue, poor sleep). Thyroid studies (including TSH) and vitamin $B_{12}$ levels should also be completed on depressed patients to ensure that a metabolic derangement is not leading to depressive symptoms. Unfortunately, these studies only rule out other conditions that may mimic or exacerbate depression. No laboratory studies are yet available to "rule in" MD. In treatment of refractory cases or when indicated by medical history or physical examination, computed tomography (CT), magnetic resonance imaging (MRI), electroencephalography (EEG), or lumbar puncture (LP) can be considered, but these studies do not need to be part of the standard workup. In patients over age 40, an electrocardiogram (ECG) is usually necessary, however, to rule out conduction disturbances or bradycardia, but this does not usually add to the differential diagnosis.

Screening instruments for depressive symptoms (e.g., Zung Depression Scale, Beck Depression Scale) can be helpful to recognize potential patients and monitor changes. However, these tools rate the severity of symptoms and do not yield diagnoses.

## DIFFERENTIAL DIAGNOSIS

### Psychiatric disorders

Many other psychiatric disorders present with symptoms similar to depression and can lead to misdiagnosis. Furthermore, depression often presents in addition to another psychiatric disorder. Thus, an awareness of the other psychiatric disorders common in primary care is essential. The best way to avoid problems is to evaluate and treat MD if it is present. When another psychiatric condition is also present, treatment must be adapted to account for this comorbidity.

### Anxiety disorders

Anxiety is a ubiquitous symptom in primary care practices. Anxiety is common in MD, and depressive symptoms are common in anxiety disorders. The most important anxiety disorders of which primary care physicians should be aware include generalized anxiety disorder (GAD), panic disorder, and obsessive-compulsive disorder (OCD). Key symptoms of these disorders (discussed in other chapters) include longlasting and pervasive anxiety (GAD), discrete panic attacks, and the presence of unreasonable and disabling behaviors or thoughts (OCD). When MD occurs in a comorbid manner with GAD, panic, or OCD, a psychiatric referral is generally indicated. However, treatment of MD by itself often helps to resolve or improve these other comorbid conditions.

### Somatoform disorders

Some patients are "addicted" to their physical problems. For unclear reasons, they focus on body ailments, and reassurance from the physician often does not help. Because depression also presents frequently with unexplained body complaints, the differentiation between a depressive illness and a somatoform disorder (SD) can be quite difficult. Primary care physicians will do best by focusing on the symptoms of MD. When MD is present, despite symptoms of an SD, appropriate treatment of the MD often significantly improves the SD.

### Substance abuse

Alcoholism or other substance abuse problems are common and often disabling conditions that can present with MD. Unlike anxiety disorders or SD, treatment of the MD that is comorbid with alcoholism does not usually relieve the substance abuse problem. Physicians need to evaluate patients for substance abuse and design separate treatment programs when substance abuse is present, whether or not MD is present and treated. In general, physicians should be cautious about treating an MD by itself in the presence of a substance abuse problem. Such an action can be enabling to the substance abuser. Rather, the substance abuse needs aggressive confrontation and treatment in its own right.

### Personality disorders

Personality disorders can complicate the diagnosis and treatment of a mood disorder. Because patients with personality disorders can be difficult and demanding, physicians (as with others) often do what they can to minimize their contacts with such individuals. This may lead to avoiding emotional issues and missing the diagnosis of depression.

When MD coexists with a personality disorder, however, effective treatment of the MD often improves functioning, in general, even if the underlying personality disorder is not fundamentally changed. Thus, physicians should evaluate the basic symptoms of depression in all distressed individuals, whether or not they have a comorbid personality disorder.

### Depression caused by a generalized medical condition or other substance (including medications)

DSM-IV recognizes a diagnosis referred to as "depression due to a general medical condition." This diagnosis is meant to imply a psychiatric condition that the clinician considers to be the direct physiologic result of a general medical condition. Examples include hypothyroidism or hyperthyroidism, pancreatic cancer, Parkinson's disease, and left-sided CVAs. Table 133-1 indicates the prevalence of MD in many general physical illnesses. Of interest, the prevalence of MD is not 100% in any physical illness. Thus, the final diagnosis of "depression due to a general medical condition" is ultimately one that must be made on clinical inference alone. There are, unfortunately, no clear criteria to help guide clinicians in this endeavor. However, when five of nine of the symptoms of MD are present, the diagnosis then becomes "depression due to a general medical condition, with major depressive episode." Thus, when this diagnosis is made, clinicians should indicate the presence of a major depressive episode, whether or not it

**Table 133-1.** General medical conditions with high prevalence rates of major depression

| Condition | Prevalence (%) |
|---|---|
| Alzheimer disease | 0-27 |
| End-stage renal failure | 5-30 |
| Parkinson disease | 17-29 |
| Cerebrovascular accident (CVA, stroke) | 5-34 |
| Cancer/acquired immunodeficiency syndrome (AIDS) | 0-50 |
| Chronic fatigue | 10-77 |
| General outpatient | 2-16 |
| General inpatient | 5-22 |
| Chronic pain | 8-57 |

From Cohen-Cole SA, Kaufman K: *Depression* 1:181, 1993.

**Medications that can cause depression**

Antihypertensives
Hormones
Anticonvulsants
Steroids
Digitalis
Antiparkinsonian agents
Antineoplastic agents
Antibiotics

is presumably caused by another general medical condition. Furthermore, when this severity criterion is reached, data seem to indicate that standard treatments for MD should be used and that they are effective.

Similarly, DSM-IV recognizes that depression can be caused by exogenous medications. The prototype of this condition is reserpine, which has long been known to cause a severe depressive condition in 15% of patients. The box above lists other medications that have been reported to cause depressive syndromes. Of critical importance is the understanding that no medication has been noted to "cause" depression in all patients. Therefore, the most important clinical factors are evaluating the history and linking the initiation of depressive symptoms to the time when a new medication was started or the time the dosage of the medication was changed.

## MANAGEMENT

### Patient and family education: overcoming stigma (and resistance)

The stigma associated with depression is so common that primary care physicians should routinely assume that patients and families will resist the diagnosis and its treatment. Thus, physicians need to rely on a communication strategy to deal with this resistance.

Most resistance can be managed by pointing to several important facts about MD:

1. MD is common.
2. MD is not the patient's fault.
3. MD reflects a biologic disorder.
4. MD causes great suffering.
5. MD can exacerbate other physical complaints or illnesses.
6. MD is treatable.
7. The medication to treat MD corrects biologic disorders and is not addictive.

Enlistment of family or other supports can also be extremely important in gaining patient acceptance of the diagnosis and adherence to treatment. Patients and families can be educated about the relative benefits and costs of medication versus psychotherapy (discussed in more detail later). For mild MD, psychotherapy (including office counseling by the physician) may be effective. Mild MD may also remit on its own. However, if the MD is not better in 2 to 3 months after "watchful waiting" or after formal psychotherapy, antidepressant medication is clearly indicated. On the other hand, severe MD responds much more effectively to medication than to psychotherapy.

The distinction between mild and severe MD is a relative one for the primary care physician, and no clear-cut criteria can be counted on. However, the physician can make this clinical distinction by his or her own clinical judgment based primarily on the patient's level of functioning. If functioning remains high and suffering mild, the MD can be considered relatively mild. If suffering is great and functioning impaired, the MD should be considered severe.

Often, family, friends, or colleagues are needed to help the physician evaluate the actual extent of impairment. Patients are often reluctant to admit changes in functioning and are sometimes even unaware of such changes. Family can be asked if the patient does not seem to have as much fun anymore or if his or her sense of humor has changed. Similarly, colleagues at work (if they are available or if the patient gives consent) can be asked if productivity has been affected.

### Treatment efficacy

Physicians can point out that treatment is usually effective in more than 90% of patients. If the first treatment attempt (either psychotherapy, medication, or the combination) is not effective, switching medications, changing psychotherapy, or initiating another treatment (e.g., electroconvulsive therapy) is almost always effective. It is usually helpful to point out to patients that they deserve to feel better; that without treatment, they will probably continue to suffer the same symptoms; and that underlying general medical conditions may also have a worse outcome.

### Length of treatment and prophylaxis

Patients and physicians often wonder about the proper length of treatment and whether or not patients should receive prophylactic treatment. Most research now indicates that biologic treatment of an MD episode should last a full 6 to 9 months after it has fully remitted.

Because approximately 50% of patients with one episode of MD go on to have a recurrence, many patients deserve prophylactic medication, which has been shown to decrease the chances of recurrence. Few experts recommend that patients receive medication for life after a first depressive episode. Thus, 6 to 9 months after the first episode abates, the physician can begin gradually withdrawing the patient from his or her medication. Slow tapering over 6 to 8 weeks is preferred.

Once it is recognized that a patient clearly has recurrent major depression (i.e., at least three episodes), research now supports the concept of prophylactic antidepressant treatment to decrease the likelihood of recurrence. The data support the use of the full treatment dosage of antidepressant medication on a chronic basis.

### Role of physician support

The importance of the physician-patient relationship cannot be overemphasized for the recognition and treatment of depression. Most primary care physicians find the treatment of depression to be very satisfying because it often responds so well. However, the physician must convey a feeling of concern for the patient to be willing to discuss very personal and distressing aspects of his or her life. Since suicidal feelings are so common in depression, this dimension also becomes essential for the assessment and management of depression.

Thus, the effective primary care physician must be skilled at the recognition and management of emotional distress in his or her patients. Very few practicing primary care physicians have actually had formal communication training in their residencies. Many physicians possess some of these skills, on an intuitive basis, but literature and workshops are now available for further training in this area.

Regular visits are essential for the proper care of the depressed patient. Brief weekly visits (or biweekly) are usually indicated in the beginning of treatment to evaluate dosage, side effects, and any changes in condition that might be of concern. Instead of weekly visits, weekly phone contacts can be substituted. Patients should generally not receive more than 1 week's supply of a medication that can be lethal in overdose. Once the patient has become stabilized on a medication, monthly visits are important for support. If chronic prophylactic treatment is necessary, quarterly visits are usually appropriate, if the depression itself has remitted.

### Role of formal psychotherapy

Short-term (12 to 16 weeks) interpersonal, cognitive, and behavioral therapies have now been developed that all seem promising for the treatment and prophylaxis of depression. Some studies indicate that such treatment is as effective as medication for patients with mild MD, but generally not as effective as medication for severe MD. Psychotherapy may also help prevent recurrences.

Office counseling by the primary care physician may be helpful to many patients with milder forms of depression, including MD. When this is being offered by a primary care physician, he or she should be clear that the patient is not being offered formal psychotherapy (unless the practitioner is actually trained in such treatment modalities). Practitioners who become involved in complex interpersonal issues or notice that strong feelings (positive or negative) emerge in either the patient or themselves during office counseling should strongly consider obtaining supervision from a trained therapist or consultation from a colleague. Psychotherapeutic situations invariably arouse strong emotions in both patients and physicians, and sensitivity to these issues are helpful and often essential to good outcomes.

### Antidepressant medications

Antidepressants are indicated for the treatment of MD. About two thirds of patients with MD respond to an antidepressant medication within 3 weeks after reaching a therapeutic plasma level. This two-thirds proportion of respondees can be increased to 90% by switching initial nonrespondees to another class of antidepressants or by using augmentation strategies (e.g., addition of lithium or triiodothyronine [$T_3$]). About one third of patients with MD (usually milder forms) improve with a placebo or general support.

Patients treated for MD should keep taking medication for a minimum of 6 to 12 months after remission. Patients with recurrent MD should be considered for long-term prophylaxis with antidepressant medication (maintained at the effective treatment dose). When patients are taken off medication, it should be tapered very slowly (over 1 to 2 months or even slower) and the dose raised if prodromal symptoms of depression reappear.

Controversy exists concerning the extent to which antidepressant medication may be useful for the treatment of minor depression, such as dysthymia or adjustment disorders (including grief). Although most experts consider formal psychotherapy the most important *initial* treatment for dysthymia, emerging data from randomized clinical trials are pointing to the efficacy of antidepressants in this chronic form of minor depression. Emotional support by the physician may be sufficient for the resolution of an adjustment disorder, but clinical experience indicates that when a patient experiences significant impairment in function (e.g., poor work performance, poor sleep, distressed relationships), antidepressant medication may be helpful and should be considered.

An essential principle in using antidepressant medication lies in the understanding that there has been no demonstrated difference in efficacy among all the antidepressants on the market. Numerous comparison studies have been completed, and to date, all the agents are equally efficacious. Similarly, no particular agent(s) or class of agents has been shown to be more effective in ameliorating certain symptoms of depression, such as agitation or insomnia. No agent has been shown to improve depressive symptoms at a faster rate than other medications. Thus, the choice of antidepressant can only be made on issues other than efficacy (e.g., side effects, costs, compliance).

### Heterocyclic medications

The heterocyclic medications (Table 133-2) include the tricyclics, which have been available since the 1950s, and several other agents that are similar in structure, including maprotiline, amoxapine, and trazodone. The heterocyclic antidepressants are quite similar in side effects, dosing strategies, and efficacy. The major advantage of the heterocyclic antidepressants over newer agents is the cost.

Use of heterocyclic medications requires starting at low doses and gradually building up doses to a therapeutic level. Plasma levels can be followed, but with the exception of nortriptyline, which has a therapeutic window

**Table 133-2.** Properties of antidepressants

| Antidepressants | Sedating effect | Anticholinergic effect | Orthostatic effect | Dose range (mg) |
|---|---|---|---|---|
| **Heterocyclic antidepressants** | | | | |
| ***Tricyclics*** | | | | |
| Amitriptyline | +++ | +++ | +++ | 75-300 |
| Desipramine | + | + | + | 75-250 |
| Doxepin | +++ | +++ | +++ | 75-300 |
| Imipramine | ++ | +++ | +++ | 75-300 |
| Nortriptyline | ++ | ++ | + | 50-150 |
| Protriptyline | + | ++ | + | 10-40 |
| Trimipramine | +++ | ++ | ++ | 75-300 |
| | ++ | ++ | ++ | 150-600 |
| ***Other heterocyclics*** | | | | |
| Amoxapine | ++ | + | ++ | 150-225 |
| Maprotiline | +++ | 0 | ++ | 200-600 |
| Trazodone | | | | |
| **New agents** | | | | |
| ***Serotonin reuptake inhibitors*** | | | | |
| Fluoxetine | 0 | 0 | 0 | 20-80 |
| Paroxetine | 0 | + | 0 | 20-50 |
| Sertraline | 0 | 0 | 0 | 50-200 |
| ***Aminoketone*** | | | | |
| Buproprion | 0 | 0 | 0 | 150-450 |

0, None; +, slight; ++, moderate; +++, marked.

(i.e., levels below and above the window are less likely to lead to remission of depression), blood levels function primarily as crude indicators of whether or not the patient is taking the medication. More importantly, clinicians should treat the patient and not the blood level. Many patients with high or low blood levels may do very well clinically. For problematic situations, consultation with psychiatrists expert in psychopharmacology may be advisable. Patients may require up to 3 weeks at a therapeutic blood level to respond fully. Therefore, patients started on heterocyclic medication need to be warned that it may be many weeks before they begin to notice any positive effects of the treatment.

The heterocyclic antidepressants are characterized by varying degrees of problematic side effects that can be categorized under the rubrics of anticholinergic effects, antihistaminic effects, antiadrenergic effects (postural hypotension), and quinidine-like effects. The anticholinergic side effects include dry mouth, constipation, urinary retention, tachycardia, increased ocular pressure, and confusion.

The antihistaminic side effects are principally sedation and inhibition of gastric acid secretion. These antihistaminic effects have also led to use of some antidepressants for urticaria, especially doxepin, which seems to be the most potent.

The antiadrenergic effects cause postural hypotension, which can be quite dangerous in patients who are medically ill or elderly. Nortriptyline seems to be the safest of the heterocyclics in this regard.

All the heterocyclics (except trazodone) have quinidine-like effects. As such, they delay conduction across the bundle of His and increase the QT interval on the ECG. Patients with bundle branch block and increased conduction from other causes are at risk of higher degrees of heart block when given these medications. This side effect is probably responsible for the high lethality of these drugs in overdose. A corrected QT interval of 0.44 is considered the differentiating interval between low-risk and high-risk patients.

Among the tricyclics, desipramine (a metabolite of imipramine) and nortriptyline (a metabolite of amitriptyline) are the least anticholinergic, the least sedating, and the least likely to cause postural hypotension.

Among the heterocyclic medications, trazodone is notable because it does not cause anticholinergic or conduction problems and has very low lethality in overdose. Trazodone, however, is quite sedating and also causes postural hypotension. Table 133-2 lists many of these side effects and relative potencies.

### New agents and side effects

New agents have revolutionized psychiatric practice, especially for the treatment of depression in patients with comorbid general medical illnesses and in elderly persons. The side effects are so much less toxic and the medication so well tolerated that many patients who were too physically ill to be safely treated in the 1960s and 1970s can now receive antidepressant medication without fear of dangerous side effects. These new agents seem safe from the standpoint of overdose, with a very low therapeutic index.

The new agents include the serotonin reuptake inhibitors (SSRIs: fluoxetine, paroxetine, sertraline) and buproprion. These agents are remarkably safe for use in elderly patients and those with comorbid general medical illnesses. They do not cause postural hypotension or cardiac conduction delay. Antihistaminic side effects are nonexistent with these agents, with the exception of paroxetine (which has very mild anticholinergic effects); none of these new agents has any anticholinergic effects. Choosing among these agents can be difficult because they are all so effective.

Fluoxetine has the longest half-life (24 to 27 hours) and has a long-acting, active metabolite (half-life of 7 days). Doses can be given every other day, and when the drug is being withdrawn, the doses can eventually be given once or twice a week to allow for very smooth tapering. The other SSRIs have half-lives of about 24 hours and have no active metabolite with longer half-lives. This allows once-a-day dosing and rapid washout. Buproprion has a shorter half-life (14 hours), so it must be given at least twice a day; it also has no long-acting active metabolites.

The starting dose of the SSRIs may also be the effective treatment dose. This is most clearly the case for fluoxetine (20 mg) but may also be true for paroxetine (20 mg) and for sertraline (50 mg). Patients not responding to the starting doses of SSRIs after 1 month should be given increased doses. Frail elderly persons and patients with liver disease or other general medical illness require smaller starting doses. I generally use one-half the recommended starting dose in this population.

The SSRIs have all been shown to inhibit the cytochrome P-450 system in the liver, thus potentially leading to the buildup of other medications metabolized in the liver. Clinicians need to be aware that any of the SSRIs can cause potential problems with medications metabolized in the liver, such as anticonvulsants, digitalis, and coumadin. To avoid pharmacokinetic interactions, it may be necessary to monitor blood levels or clinical indicators of toxicity. In my clinical practice (in which I use SSRIs extensively in frail elderly persons), significant drug interactions do occur but are rare. I have occasionally had to alter digitalis or coumadin doses.

Buproprion does not seem to inhibit these enzymes. Buproprion also has been associated with a 1% to 4% prevalence of seizures, which is a very low overall risk but which is probably slightly more common than with other antidepressant medications. The medication must be given in divided doses because of its short half-life, should not be given to individuals at risk for seizures (e.g., head trauma), and should never be administered in any single dose greater than 150 mg. The starting dose (75 mg two or three times a day) should be increased slowly (once a week) to therapeutic levels of 300 to 450 mg/day to minimize the risk of seizures. The medication should also not be given to bulimic patients (patients who gorge food and often induce vomiting) because of a possible increased seizure risk.

Despite this small but potential risk, buproprion is an important and effective antidepressant that may be especially important because it does not cause the sexual problems that are often common side effects of other antidepressants.

The new agents sometimes cause side effects such as anxiety, insomnia, gastrointestinal distress, agitation, and sexual difficulties. For the most part, these occur in less than 20% of patients. When they do occur, these effects are usually mild and do not lead to discontinuation of medication. The adjunctive use of a sedating antihistamine (diphenhydramine or hydroxyzine), a sedating antidepressant (trazodone or doxepin), or an anxiolytic (e.g., clonazepam) can be helpful. These adjunctive agents can usually be discontinued after a short time, but sometimes continued treatment with two agents is indicated. If a long-acting benzodiazepine (clonazepam) is used in elderly persons, care must be exercised to avoid buildup of medication over time, which can lead to confusion, sedation, or falls after several weeks of treatment.

### Antidepressants in elderly and medically ill patients

For many of the reasons already enumerated, the new agents have generally become the agents of choice in elderly and medically ill patients. Among the heterocyclic agents, the safest agents are nortriptyline and desipramine. These agents are still widely used with some degree of safety in elderly and medically ill patients. They also seem to have a role in the treatment of refractory depression.

Dosing strategies in elderly and medically ill patients need to follow the adage "start low and go slow" for many reasons. From the pharmacokinetic point of view (i.e., absorption, metabolism, and elimination—the effect of the body on medication), these agents are metabolized more slowly in these two groups. Accumulation and toxicity can become a problem. Protein binding is also lower in elderly and medically ill patients because albumin levels are lower; this can also lead to toxic effects. Similarly, lower doses may lead to efficacious treatment. Pharmacodynamic differences (i.e., impact of the medication on the body) in elderly persons can also lead to toxicity and/or efficacy at lower-than-expected doses.

### Electroconvulsive therapy (ECT)

Primary care physicians treating depression need to know that ECT is still the most effective treatment available for the treatment of depression. Although many patients (and physicians) have developed prejudices and fears about ECT, new methodologies of administration have shown ECT to be a safe and effective treatment modality. In frail elderly persons, ECT can be safer than antidepressants. Some reversible short-term memory loss is a common side effect, but research indicates that this reverts to normal in virtually all patients. In some cases, ECT can be lifesaving and should not be denied to patients because of lack of understanding or unrealistic fear.

ECT does not lead to permanent remission of depression in patients susceptible to recurrence. Thus, patients with recurrent depression who receive ECT should receive either prophylactic medication after a course of ECT or maintenance ECT, which can now be given approximately on a once-a-month, outpatient basis.

### Referral

The clinical criteria for referral to a psychiatrist or other mental health specialist depends greatly on the experience and expertise of the primary care physician. In general, the most common reasons for referral are lack of response to initial treatment, suicidal ideation, or psychosis.

It is often helpful if primary care physicians inform patients at a very early stage of assessment and intervention that referral to a mental health specialist is sometimes needed. This early statement can make referral at a later stage much more acceptable. For example, the primary care physician can make it clear that he or she has experience treating some depressions, but that he or she wants the patient to understand that if the depression does not fully remit, a referral to a mental health specialist will be made. Because partial remission is a common occurrence, physicians should make every effort to establish clear indications of predepression functioning, and if return to baseline functioning does not occur, specialist referral should be made.

## BIBLIOGRAPHY

Brody DS, Larson DB: The role of primary care physicians in managing depression, *J Gen Intern Med* 7:243, 1992.

Cohen-Cole SA: *The medical interview,* St Louis, 1991, Mosby.

Cohen-Cole SA, Kaufman K: Major depression in physical illness: diagnosis, prevalence, and antidepressant treatment (a ten-year review: 1982-1992), *Depression* 1:181, 1993.

Depression Guideline Panel: *Depression in primary care* Vol 1. Detection and diagnosis: clinical practice guideline, no 5, Rockville, 1993, US Department of Health and Human Services.

Depression Guideline Panel: *Depression in primary care.* Vol 2. Treatment of major depression: clinical practice guideline, no 5, Rockville, 1993, U.S. Department of Health and Human Services.

Janicak PG et al: *Principles and practice of psychopharmacotherapy,* Baltimore, 1993, Williams & Wilkins.

Karasu TB: *Psychotherapy for depression,* Northvale, NJ, 1990, Jason Aronson.

Kendler KS et al: The prediction of major depression in women: toward an integrated etiologic model, *Am J Psychiatry* 150:1139, 1993.

CHAPTER

# 134 Somatization

**Charles C. Engel, Jr.**
**Wayne J. Katon**

Mention somatization, and many physicians provide animated descriptions of their most frustrating and difficult patients. These physician-patient conflicts occur in part because somatizing patients (somatizers) breach the expectation that patients with psychiatric disorders use psychologic terms to describe their emotional problems. They are ill when the "objective" biomedical data insist they are not. Despite efforts to reassure them, somatizers often challenge their physicians' opinions and competence.

These are the somatizing patients on whom physicians focus, but fortunately most are not so troublesome. This chapter emphasizes that somatization:

1. Is a ubiquitous part of human experience and medical practice.
2. Is responsible for substantial unrecognized patient morbidity, physician time, and health care costs.
3. Occurs along a continuum of severity and duration that includes acute, subacute, and chronic types. Acute and subacute types are less severe and much more common and easily treated than the chronic type.

Somatization has been defined as a psychologic defense mechanism, a bodily symptom caused by psychiatric disorder or a somatic expression of psychosocial distress. It is viewed here broadly as a pattern of excessive medical utilization of somatic symptoms that are not fully explained by medical etiology. Somatization therefore has components that are *experiential* (patients perceive symptoms), *cognitive* (they attribute the symptoms to medical origins), *behavioral* (they report them to a physician), and *medical* (a complete medical explanation is lacking).

The purpose of this chapter is to help primary care physicians recognize, diagnose, and manage somatization. To emphasize the spectrum of somatization severity, this chapter considers acute, subacute, and chronic types. *Acute somatization* occurs in the absence of a previous somatization pattern, lasts less than a few months, and is associated with an acutely stressful life event. *Subacute* or *relapsing somatization* is characterized either by persistent unexplained symptoms of several months' duration or by recurrent functional symptoms mixed with lengthy asymptomatic periods. It is usually associated with a treatable anxiety or depressive disorder. *Chronic somatization* is a pattern of persistent unexplained symptoms and excessive health care use often lasting years and is usually associated with refractory somatoform and/or personality disorders.

## EPIDEMIOLOGY

Symptom diaries show that somatizing patients record an average of one new symptom every 7 days, the most common being headaches, muscle aches, gastrointestinal (GI) and respiratory symptoms, and fatigue. One community study found that more than 4% of people had multiple, chronic, unexplained somatic complaints. Only about 5% of symptoms experienced by community respondents are ever reported to physicians. Studies of medical patients with unexplained symptoms reveal high rates of major depression and panic disorder (Table 134-1; see also Chapters 132 and 133). Patients in the community with unexplained somatic complaints and a coexisting psychiatric disorder tend to use inordinate amounts of medical care at great cost to society. In a 3-year retrospective study of 1000 ambulatory care patients, 38% had new complaints of at least 1 of 14 common symptoms. Two thirds of symptoms were evaluated diagnostically, but only 10% of evaluations yielded an organic explanation not apparent at the initial visit. The average cost per organic diagnosis was $2252. Indeed, 25% to 35% of primary care patients have current psychiatric disorders, but these are missed 50% to 80% of the time, largely because of the lack of accurate diagnosis in the more than half who complain only of medical illness or physical symptoms.

A strong relationship exists between medically unexplained symptoms and psychiatric disorders, especially anxiety and depression. Using population-based data on psychiatric disorders in more than 18,000 respondents from five U.S. communities, one study found that 49% of

The views expressed by Dr. Engel in this article are his own and do not reflect the official policy or position of the U.S. Department of the Army, the U.S. Department of Defense, or the U.S. Government.

**Table 134-1.** Prevalence of major depression and associated conditions in patients with medically unexplained symptoms compared with control subjects with explained symptoms*

| | Current major depression (%) | Lifetime major depression (%) | Associated conditions |
|---|---|---|---|
| Chronic pain | 32 | 57 | Alcoholism |
| Chest pain | 36 (4) | 64 (24) | Panic disorder |
| Pelvic pain | 28 (3) | 64 (17) | Substance abuse<br>Sexual abuse |
| Tinnitus | 60 (7) | 78 (21) | Sensorineural hearing loss |
| Fatigue | 15 (3) | 76 (42) | Somatization disorder |
| Irritable bowel | 21 (5) | 61 (16) | Panic disorder<br>Somatization disorder |
| Dizziness | 12 (5) | 42 (18) | Panic disorder |
| Migraine | 15 (7) | — | Anxiety disorders |

*Percentages in parentheses are control group proportion with the diagnosis of interest.

subjects reporting five or more functional symptoms (versus 6% of control subjects with no symptoms) had at least one current psychiatric disorder. Seventeen percent of the group with five or more symptoms had current panic disorder (versus 0.1% of controls), and 15% had current major depression (versus 1% of controls). Using self-reports from a probability sample of more than 1000 health maintenance organization enrollees, another study found that increasing number of pain complaints was strongly associated with elevated levels of anxiety, depression, and nonpain physical symptoms.

## PATHOPHYSIOLOGY

### Hereditary factors

Family studies have been completed for only the most severe forms of somatization. Somatization disorder is a chronic disorder characterized by extensive medical service use (one study found a sixfold per capita increase in hospital service expenditures, a fourteenfold increase in physician costs, and a ninefold increase in personal health costs over the national average) for recurrent, excessive, and unexplained multisystem symptoms. Patients with somatization disorder have an increased prevalence of somatization disorder in female first-degree relatives and antisocial personality disorder, alcohol abuse, and perhaps attention deficit disorder in male first-degree relatives. So far, adoption and twin studies are inconclusive regarding the relative genetic and environmental contributions to these associations.

### Neurophysiologic explanations

Evidence suggests somatization is more than a strict psychosocial phenomenon. Neurobiologic theories of somatization propose central nervous system (CNS) modulation of peripheral somatic sensations. For example, chronic pain perception is dampened centrally via the endogenous opioid system. Although less well understood, the monoamine neurotransmitters serotonin and norepinephrine also interact to alter pain perception. Research suggests that CNS alterations in monoamines also occur in patients with anxiety disorders (panic disorder, obsessive-compulsive disorder) and major depression, disorders that are typically associated with somatization. Tricyclic antidepressants reduce presynaptic reuptake of these neurotransmitters, have documented analgesic effects in both depressed and nondepressed pain patients, and reduce physical symptoms in patients with panic disorder and major depression.

Stress and emotions appear related to body symptoms via altered physiologic arousal. Autonomic arousal increases smooth muscle contractions and skeletal muscle tone. Smooth muscle contractions in the GI tract are temporally related to somatic discomfort. Painful skeletal muscles often have higher electromyographic potentials than do control muscles, and evidence exists that skeletal muscle contractions often coincide with tension headaches and perhaps back and other myofascial pain syndromes.

One study observed that fibromyalgia patients have alpha-wave intrusion into slow-wave sleep. The demonstration that experimental disruption of stage IV sleep in normal subjects results in musculoskeletal and mood symptoms has led to the postulation that fibromyalgia is a nonrestorative sleep disorder. Clinically, more than half of patients with chronic pain report sleep disturbances. Disruption of sleep patterns by anxiety and depressive disorders as well as psychosocial stress may also cause somatic symptoms.

Studies of patients with somatization disorder have revealed abnormal auditory-evoked potentials, abnormal right frontal electroencephalographic (EEG) frequencies, and bifrontal impairment and nondominant hemispheric dysfunction on neuropsychologic testing. Most unilateral conversion symptoms involve the left side of the body in right-handed individuals, and nondominant hemispheric dysfunction is one possible explanation.

### Psychologic explanations

Cognitive-behavioral, behavioral, and psychodynamic psychologic theories offer models for understanding and treating somatization. Cognitive-behavioral psychology (CBP) postulates that perceived symptoms are linked to emotions and illness behaviors (e.g., depression, grimacing, medical utilization) via underlying cognitions or *explanatory illness beliefs* (i.e., what a person believes is causing the symptom). Fig. 134-1 shows how a faulty explanatory belief might set up a worsening cycle of

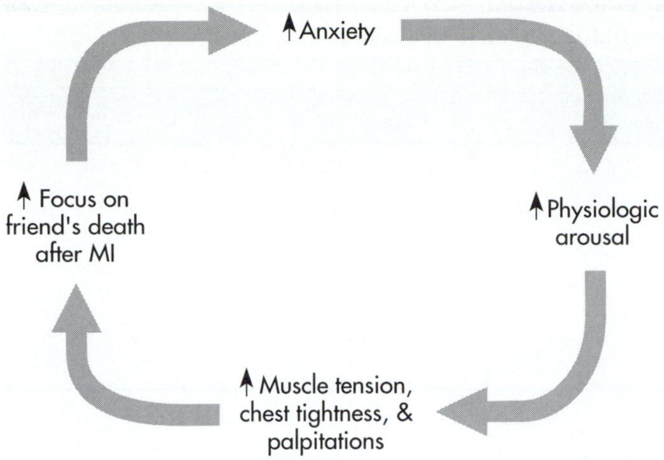


**Fig. 134-1.** Cycle of anxiety, physiologic arousal, and somatic symptoms in a person with chest pain whose friend recently had a fatal myocardial infarction (MI).

anxiety, physiologic arousal, and somatic symptoms. In the example, a man with recurrent musculoskeletal chest discomfort has recently lost a close friend who had an acute myocardial infarction. Previously unnoticed chest pain prompts worry that these transient symptoms may portend sudden death. Resulting anxiety causes psychophysiologic arousal, manifesting as sweating, shortness of breath, and more chest discomfort. Illness beliefs have diverse origins, including past experience, culture, or education. CBP treatment involves examination and alalteration of maladaptive illness beliefs and worries.

Behavioral psychology, by comparison, posits that behaviors are learned. Two ways of learning relevant to somatization are modeling (learning by imitating) and operant conditioning (learning by rewards and punishments). Modeling may partly explain why disabled or chronically ill family members often appear among somatizers. Operant conditioning explains why patients receiving illness "rewards" (e.g., worker's compensation or relief from aversive responsibilities) are prone to chronic disability. Rewards and punishments reinforcing illness behavior are called *illness maintenance systems.*

Psychodynamic psychology views somatization as a defense against conscious awareness and a verbal expression of psychologically conflicting emotions. Thus, a woman who has always subordinated her needs to those of others and fears being alone may develop sudden paralysis of her legs as she prepares to leave her abusive husband. Unconscious psychologic conflicts are thought to be the basis of conversion disorder, a relatively unusual somatoform disorder characterized by the loss or alteration of a body function.

### Sociocultural theories

Mentally ill patients are often ostracized and viewed as irresponsible and unworthy of social assistance or medical insurance coverage. Patients with physical disease, however, are seen as "victims" who are "sick" and deserving of sympathy, care, and relief from aversive responsibilities. These societal forces undoubtedly cause some distressed patients to seek the *sick role* by reporting somatic concerns to their physicians. Families are another social system that can affect symptom reporting. For example, a child may develop abdominal pain to distract parents from arguing, violence, or other family strife.

## DIFFERENTIAL DIAGNOSIS

Differential diagnosis varies according to the severity and duration of functional symptoms. Table 134-2 outlines the relative importance of various psychiatric disorders to acute, subacute, and chronic forms of somatization.

### Undiagnosed medical illness

Psychiatric and physical illness are not mutually exclusive and frequently coexist. Thus, evaluation for one should not come at the expense of the other. The primary care physician should carefully consider illnesses that often present in vague, unusual, or multisystem ways. The possibility of multiple sclerosis, collagen vascular diseases, endocrine diseases, and other conditions should be weighed as suggested by patients' specific presentations.

### Psychiatric disorders associated with unexplained symptoms

The psychiatric differential diagnosis of functional somatic complaints is wide. It is often not appreciated that most somatization is caused by common and treatable anxiety and depressive disorders. Primary care physicians must therefore be skilled at recognizing and treating these disorders. Chapters 132 and 133 describe them in detail, and only issues pertaining directly to somatization are discussed here.

***Anxiety disorders.*** Diagnostic criteria for panic disorder and generalized anxiety disorder (GAD) contain numerous somatic symptoms, including shortness of breath, muscular tension, palpitations, sweating, dizziness, GI distress, chills, hot flashes, choking, shaking, numbness, tingling, and chest pain. However, research shows that the link between anxiety and somatic symptoms persists even when scales measuring anxiety exclude somatic symptom items. Anxious patients often selectively focus on one or more physical symptoms and present them to their physician. Panic disorder occurs in 6% to 8% of primary care patients and is strongly associated with somatic symptoms, marked hypochondriasis and illness concerns, and excessive use of medical care. Typically, patients with physical complaints visit numerous providers before the diagnosis of panic is finally made. Evidence shows that somatic symptoms and hypochondriasis improve with adequate pharmacologic treatment.

***Depressive disorders.*** Depression, as with anxiety, is consistently associated with somatic symptoms across a range of study designs. Somatic complaints in depressed patients may result from (1) vegetative symptoms such as fatigue, (2) increased symptom sensitivity, (3) pessimistic symptom interpretations, (4) a mode of communicating distress, (5) a mood-state-dependent memory of past physical illness, or (6) somatic delusions (e.g., fixed, false beliefs that one's "insides are rotting") occurring during severe major depression with psychotic features. Major depression and dysthymia are easily overlooked in patients

**Table 134-2.** Length of somatization and likelihood of comorbid psychiatric disorders

| | Acute somatization | Subacute somatization | Chronic somatization |
|---|---|---|---|
| Adjustment disorders | +++ | + | 0 |
| Anxiety disorders | + | +++ | +++ |
| Depressive disorders | + | +++ | +++ |
| Substance abuse | + | + | ++ |
| Psychotic disorders | + | + | ++ |
| Personality disorders | 0 | + | +++ |
| Somatoform disorders | 0 | + | +++ |
| Factitious disorder or malingering | 0 | + | + |

0, Very uncommon; +, uncommon; ++, common; +++, very common.

with somatic complaints. A high index of suspicion is necessary, since functional symptoms in depressed individuals are often vague, multiple, inconsistently present, and seemingly unrelated to one another. The physician must look past these to assess the usual vegetative aspects of depression. The presence of a past history or family history of depression, antidepressant treatment, or psychiatric hospitalization may also suggest the diagnosis.

***Other psychiatric disorders.*** *Adjustment disorders,* maladaptive reactions to an identifiable psychosocial stressor, often result in transient episodes of functional physical symptoms. Most people describe characteristic physical symptoms such as headache or GI distress when under stress. *Uncomplicated bereavement,* the normal reaction to the loss of a loved one, is often associated with a "lump in the throat" and other physical symptoms. *Substance abuse* may cause minor physical complaints during intoxication, "hangovers," or withdrawal. Somatization is sometimes a feature of psychosis caused by *schizophrenia,* severe *mania* or major depression, or *delusional disorder.* These problems occur infrequently in primary care settings and usually are easily recognized. Somatization in a cognitively impaired patient suggests an organic mental syndrome such as *delirium* or *dementia.*

### Somatoform disorders, factitious disorder, and malingering

These are psychiatric disorders in which one or more physical symptoms are the central and defining feature.

***Somatization disorder.*** Patients with somatization disorder have a history of multiple unexplained physical complaints and often see themselves as being sickly over their entire life. This pattern begins before age 30 and persists for several years. To be diagnosed with somatization disorder, a patient must have 13 or more unexplained symptoms from a list of 35 body symptoms (see the box on p. 1751). Seven of the 35 symptoms may be used to screen for the disorder. When more than two of these screening symptoms are present, more detailed symptom assessment is advised.

Somatization disorder is unusual in the general population (0.1%) but overrepresented in medical practice (0.4% to 5%). Studies show it occurs frequently among psychosocially distressed persons with high health care use, women undergoing hysterectomy for a reason besides cancer, and patients with irritable bowel and chronic fatigue syndrome. Coexisting psychiatric disorders are the rule. As many as 80% to 90% have had major depression during their life, and more than half have anxiety disorders. Alcohol, prescription drug abuse, and personality disorders are also common. Patients with somatization disorder often relate destructively to health care systems. Their lengthy medical records often reveal "doctor shopping," prescription drug dependence, multiple unrevealing invasive procedures or surgeries, and iatrogenic injuries.

***Hypochondriasis.*** This is the nonpsychotic fear or belief that one has a serious disease, despite contrary medical evidence and reassurance. Hypochondriasis is closely associated with depression, anxiety, and psychosocial stressors, leading some to doubt if hypochondriasis ever occurs independently. Patients with panic disorder often think they are dying during attacks. Depressed patients may manifest pessimism about their health or obsessive ruminations about imagined disease. Transient hypochondriasis sometimes occurs after an acute stressor. For instance, after myocardial infarction, patients may become excessively preoccupied with minor somatic symptoms such as GI discomfort or palpitations. About 4% to 6% of medical outpatients have hypochondriasis, as defined in the *Diagnostic and Statistical Manual of Mental Disorders,* third edition—revised (DSM-III-R), independent of the severity of their medical illness. It usually starts in third decade of life, and males and females are equally affected.

***Conversion disorder.*** This is a psychologically mediated neurologic deficit or abnormality (e.g., altered motor or sensory function) that is not intentionally produced. It is estimated to have a lifetime prevalence of 0.5% in the community, up to 25% in psychiatric outpatients, and 2% to 5% of general hospital psychiatry consultation referrals. A history of somatization disorder is often found in patients with conversion disorder. Major depression, panic disorder, and substance abuse also frequently occur. Women are most often affected, but men with acute, severe stressors such as combat may also be at high risk.

Anatomic, physiologic, or other inconsistencies in the symptom presentation may cause the physician to suspect

### Unexplained symptom list for somatization disorder*

**Gastrointestinal symptoms**

1. **Vomiting**
2. Abdominal pain
3. Nausea
4. Bloating
5. Diarrhea
6. Intolerance of several different foods

**Pain symptoms**

7. **Extremity pain**
8. Back pain
9. Joint pain
10. Pain during urination
11. Other pain (exclude headaches)

**Cardiopulmonary symptoms**

12. **Shortness of breath**
13. Palpitations
14. Chest pain
15. Dizziness

**Conversion or pseudoneurologic symptoms**

16. **Amnesia**
17. **Lump in throat**
18. Loss of voice
19. Deafness
20. Double vision
21. Blurred vision
22. Blindness
23. Fainting/loss of consciousness
24. Seizure/convulsion
25. Trouble walking
26. Paralysis/muscle weakness
27. Difficult urination/retention

**Sexual symptoms**

28. **Burning sensation in genitals/rectum**
29. Sexual indifference
30. Pain during intercourse
31. Impotence

**Female reproductive symptoms**

32. **Painful menstruation**
33. Irregular menstruation
34. Excessive menstrual bleeding
35. Vomiting throughout pregnancy

From American Psychiatric Association: *Diagnostic and statistical manual of mental disorders,* ed 3, revised, Washington, DC, 1987, American Psychiatric Association.

*Screening symptoms in **bold** (two of seven suggestive).

conversion. Pseudoneurologic symptoms such as aphonia, anesthesia, paralysis, gait disturbance, pseudoseizures, and tremor account for up to 90% of cases. In about half of cases, conversion causes amplification of a symptom because of a coexisting neurologic disorder. For example, many patients with epilepsy also have intermittent pseudoseizures. Available data suggest that conversion disorder has a good prognosis. Studies in hospital inpatients show that most conversion disorders resolve before discharge. Careful medical assessment is important, however, since 13% to 30% of patients subsequently develop organic illness that explains the original symptom.

***Chronic pain.*** Somatoform pain disorder is a preoccupation with pain out of proportion to physical illness that lasts 6 months or longer. Common anatomic sites for chronic pain include low back, head, pelvis (in women), and chest pain. Psychosocial factors should be investigated if pain persists beyond the normal tissue healing time (3 months is generally adequate) or if the patient's disability exceeds that expected by objective findings. Excessive use of the health care system, failure of the patient to accept physician reassurances, or prolonged or excessive use of narcotic analgesics, sedative-hypnotics, or alcohol also suggest psychiatric complications. Symptoms of anxiety or depression are typically disabling, and routine assessment of chronic pain patients for these conditions is recommended.

***Malingering.*** Malingering is a conscious misrepresentation of symptoms that is motivated by external incentives. Malingering is often suspected but seldom "proved." It should be considered when a clear incentive exists, such as pending litigation or avoidance of military conscription; when severe disability and symptoms occur without objective findings; or when the patient is uncooperative with diagnostic evaluations or treatment efforts. Individuals with a past pattern of criminal acts, lying, stealing, cheating, gambling, or substance abuse may malinger to avoid adverse consequences from previous actions.

***Factitious disorder.*** As with malingering, factitious disorder occurs when patients deliberately misrepresent their symptoms. However, symptom production among factitious disorder patients may be quite driven and self-destructive, whereas external symptom incentives are typically absent. The medical literature contains many colorful but often morbid descriptions of this rare disorder. Factitious fever may be most common; other types include factitious diarrhea, acquired immune deficiency syndrome (AIDS), urinary tract infection, skin rash, anemia, hypoglycemia, thyrotoxicosis, pheochromocytoma, asthma, psychosis, and dementia. "Munchausen's by proxy" occurs when a mother feigns illness in her child. Most factitious patients are women less than 40 years of age. There may be a range of associated psychopathology, from mild depression or hypochondriasis to severe personality problems characterized by poor tolerance of minor stress, erratic behavior, impulsive relationships or use of substances, and history of childhood neglect or abuse leading to intense anger toward themselves and authority. Many patients have gained the medical sophistication to alter diagnostic tests through a background as a patient, nurse, physician, or technician. Diagnosis involves medical staff detective work and can result in difficult ethical dilemmas.

## HISTORY

### Chart review

Reviewing the record is usually the most efficient way to initiate a medical history in suspected somatizers. Chronic somatizers often have long, confusing medical records bearing witness to "doctor shopping," repeated visits to medical specialists for ambiguous symptom clusters (rather than clear disease states), equivocal diagnostic tests, and negative empiric treatment trials. Information must be carefully considered to avoid overlooking progressive or catastrophic disease. Clues to a psychiatric disorder often are found. Symptoms may relate temporally to relationship, occupational, family, abuse, or other stressors, or potential symptom incentives may be discovered. Recurrent urgent care or emergency room visits for sudden, ominous, episodic symptoms followed by negative evaluations suggest panic disorder. Excessive prescription drug use, elevated blood alcohol levels, macrocytic anemia, or elevated liver enzymes may suggest substance abuse.

### Present illness

Focus first on the patient's chief concern: physical symptoms. While listening to the history, strive to assume the patient's perspective of the symptoms to enhance empathy and rapport. Understanding the patient's symptoms in a biopsychosocial framework is essential. It can take several visits before many patients will entrust their psychosocial concerns to their physician, and some never do. Others, however, readily discuss psychosocial problems when asked but will not mention them otherwise. For the latter group, ask about stressors early and delay the issue without persistence if the patient is unreceptive. Confrontation in the early stages of treatment is rarely productive and almost always leads to a poor outcome.

Vague, multiple, or inconsistently presented symptoms suggest somatization. Screen all patients for recent life changes and symptoms of anxiety, depression, and substance abuse. Specifically ask about sleep disturbances, fatigue, anhedonia, impaired concentration, appetite or weight changes, hopelessness, guilt, low self-esteem, and sudden bouts of worrisome physical symptoms or anxiety. Look for changes in recent and long-term functioning, and assess their temporal relationship to physical, anxiety, and depressive symptoms as well as stressors. Physical or psychosocial dysfunction out of proportion to symptom severity often results from psychiatric illness. Important aspects of functioning to evaluate include activities of daily living and functioning in occupational, family, and other social roles.

Investigate the extent and quality of patients' support systems. Abusive relationships or well-meaning supporters that unintentionally reward symptoms by relieving responsibilities may worsen somatization. Consider how patients' disability may lead to tangible and intangible gains to their supporters. Look also for financial, legal, or other illness maintenance incentives.

### Past medical history

Elicit health care utilization over the previous 5 years, including number of visits, number of physicians, surgical procedures and indications, and chronic pain or psychophysiologic problems (e.g., GI distress, palpitations). Listen to patients' descriptions; chronic somatizers often view previous physicians with exaggerated scorn while being overly solicitous or optimistic about their new physician's ability to cure them. Clarify patients' past psychiatric history (substance abuse, hospitalizations, medications, suicide attempts, violence, criminal acts, therapy) and key elements of their developmental history, including abuse, neglect, early parental death, or chronic childhood illnesses. Inquire about family history of depression, anxiety, substance abuse, suicide, crime, violence, and somatization. Chronic illness or physical disability in the nuclear family may serve as learning models for the patient.

Many patients troubled by somatic symptoms reveal feelings of being trapped by their life situation or personal circumstances. "There is nothing I can do, doctor" is a common refrain. A major focus for the treatment of such patients is to help them to realize that over time, they can change some upsetting elements in their lives and escape from their feelings of being trapped and powerless.

## PHYSICAL EXAMINATION

A thorough initial physical examination including mental status assessment is necessary, with a brief exam performed at subsequent visits. This serves as a cost-effective screening device, validates patients' concerns, and reassures many patients. Physical stigmata of alcoholism and intravenous or intranasal substance use can confirm substance abuse. Musculoskeletal injuries, scars, burns, lacerations, bruises, and abrasions may be clues to undisclosed abuse, violence, suicide attempts, or self-injury and should always result in direct, respectful questioning about how they were obtained.

## LABORATORY AND DIAGNOSTIC ASSESSMENT

Weigh the costs and benefits of laboratory testing for each patient. Benefits include information regarding patients' physiologic status. Remember, however, that the likelihood of a false-positive result increases with the number of tests performed. Costs of testing include the monetary expense and the covert message to the patient that their physician remains concerned about undiscovered disease. Therefore, a conservative approach to testing is advised. Rely on objective examination findings or classic symptom patterns as indications for laboratory assessment. Avoid repeating normal or equivocal tests. Sometimes, reviewing the medical record or talking with past practitioners provides enough information to dispel current medical concerns. When tests or imaging studies must be done, reduce iatrogenic worries by diligently reviewing them with the patient, emphasizing normal findings when appropriate.

## MANAGEMENT OF THE SOMATIZATION SPECTRUM

There are several central principles of somatization management. Which principles are emphasized varies in important ways, depending on duration of functional somatic symptoms in each patient (Table 134-3).

### Set attainable goals

Among patients with persistent functional complaints, complete symptom eradication is rarely achieved. Consequently, setting this as a treatment goal will contribute to both physician and patient dissatisfaction. More rewarding and clinically useful goals usually involve specific improvements in patient functioning, such as

**Table 134-3.** Relative importance of principal treatment strategies across the somatization spectrum

| | Acute somatization | Subacute somatization | Chronic somatization |
|---|---|---|---|
| Primary management goals | 1. Assess acute stressors.<br>2. Provide supportive care.<br>3. Screen for mental disorders. | 1. Reduce anxiety and depression.<br>2. Increase patient functioning. | 1. Develop empathic relationship.<br>2. Avoid iatrogenesis.<br>3. Provide continuity of care.<br>4. Improve patient functioning.<br>5. Treat anxiety and depression. |
| Uncover explanatory illness model. | Extremely important | Extremely important | Extremely important |
| Assess illness maintenance systems. | Important | Very important | Extremely important |
| Ensure single primary care (PC) physician. | Usual care | Initiate treatment in PC setting. | "Doctor shopping" problematic |
| Assess pyschosocial stressors. | Acute stressors | Acute and chronic stressors* | Chronic stressors* |
| Administer sedatives. | Time-limited treatment only | Time-limited treatment; usually avoid. | Contraindicated |
| Administer anxiolytics. | Avoid; may impair coping | As indicated for anxiety disorder | Contraindicated |
| Administer antidepressants. | Not usually indicated | Depression and panic disorder | Depression and panic disorder |
| Assess activity level. | Time-limited "holiday" may be OK. | Gradually increase activity. | Structured increase (with or without physical therapy) |
| Provide follow-up arrangements. | Time contingent | Limit symptom-contingent use. | Advance pain for limit setting. |

*Chronic stressors are those with enduring consequences (e.g., abuse, assault, domestic violence, war experiences, other catastrophic events).

performance of occupational tasks or important activities of daily living.

### Provide supportive care

The importance of a supportive, caring, respectful, and empathetic relationship with somatizing patients cannot be overemphasized. Key elements of supportive care are reassurance, education, counseling, patient activity, and mobilization of family/support resources. *Reassurance* is more than simply assuring patients that their symptoms are not serious. It involves elucidating important illness beliefs and directing assurances that address these concerns when counseling, educating, predicting prognosis, and prescribing treatment plans. Examples of common maladaptive beliefs are (1) "my symptoms are a sign of disease"; (2) "when I hurt it means I am seriously injuring myself" (e.g., "pinching a nerve"); or (3) "when I have symptoms, I can't make it without rest and a break from my responsibilities."

*Education* often involves information about physiologic effects of stressors and the effect of anxiety and mood on symptom perception and interpretation. Efforts to destigmatize psychiatric and somatic symptoms through patient education can improve rapport and subsequent treatment adherence. Many somatizers have already been told their symptoms are "in their head" and are driven to find a medical explanation for them. It helps to tell some patients that aversive symptoms often are distressing and that this distress, in turn, can impair their ability to cope effectively with the symptoms. It is also useful to have one or two simple medical explanations for patients with anxiety and depressive disorders. Patients with panic disorder, for example, can be told that the disorder involves dysregulation of the "stress thermostat" that controls their "fight-or-flight" mechanism.

Other effective *primary care counseling* techniques include allowing patients time to ventilate frustrations, assisting them to delineate their problems, and suggesting realistic plans to help solve them. Convey optimism, when appropriate, that symptoms and related functional decrements will improve over time while avoiding open-ended instructions to reduce usual activities. Self-help materials such as audiotapes and books about stress reduction, relaxation techniques, depression, and anxiety are widely available. Psychiatric referral for time-limited forms of psychotherapy is frequently appropriate, especially for those who request it or who have experienced a recent stressor.

*Paced exercise* helps patients discharge stress, increase stamina, and improve function. Physical therapy programs of gradually increasing physical activity are sometimes useful for overcoming the deactivation and weight gain that occur for many patients with persistent functional symptoms. Encourage patients to remain gainfully employed, since working reduces dependence on disability compensation, thereby improving morale, self-confidence, and ability to meet expectations in social roles.

Encourage participation of available *patient support systems* in the treatment plan. These resources can help corroborate symptoms and functional deficits. They can help monitor adherence to treatment and provide information on "doctor shopping" or substance abuse. It may also be possible to learn and correct ways that well-meaning supporters are unwittingly reinforcing symptoms by relieving patients of roles and responsibilities in response to symptoms.

### Manage the process of care

Proper management of the delivery of care is both cost-effective and in the somatizer's best interest. A quality physician-patient relationship is imperative for somatizing patients. As the duration and number of unexplained somatic symptoms increase, so does the likelihood that patients will manifest persistent coping deficits, erratic behavior, relapsing mental disorders, and personality problems. Especially for chronic somatizers (somatization disorder is the prototypic example), the theme of care is construction of a trusting therapeutic alliance founded on consistent care parameters:

1. A single primary care provider
2. Appointments at regular, time-contingent intervals of about every 4 to 6 weeks
3. A brief physical examination at each visit to address new physical concerns
4. Diagnostic evaluations only for classic symptom constellations or worrisome objective signs
5. A gradual shift of focus from rehashes of "old" symptoms to discussions of current functioning, psychosocial stressors, and support structures
6. Attempts to involve social supports in the care plan

Consistency must also extend to the setting of limits on patient-initiated, symptom-contingent visits. Whenever possible, negotiate an advance plan as to how these visits will be handled. Empathic reminders of the plan can quell patient concerns about rejection when limit setting becomes necessary.

### Develop pharmacologic strategies

Psychopharmacologic interventions are often an important aspect in the treatment of somatization. They are, however, only one part of a comprehensive management plan. Care must be taken not to use psychoactive medications as a substitute for supportive care.

A brief course of a sedative-hypnotic can improve sleep and bolster patient coping during or immediately after an acute episode of functional physical symptoms precipitated by a psychologic trauma such as rape, abuse, assault, or unexpected loss. Either an antihistamine–like diphenhydramine or a benzodiazepine (e.g., temazepam) can reduce the transient stress-related insomnia that often accompanies these events. Courses of benzodiazepines lasting longer than 3 weeks are rarely appropriate, since these drugs can set up harmful illness incentives and impair function by causing sedation, depression, and rebound anxiety.

Antidepressants can reduce unexplained somatic symptoms in patients with chronic pain, panic disorder, and major depression. Generally, start with a low dose and increase slowly, since somatically focused patients tend to be more sensitive to side effects and lack of adherence can become a formidable problem. Prophylactic management of patients' treatment expectations can preserve adherence and enhance the physician-patient relationship. Offer patients a complete explanation of common medication side effects. Then, if side effects occur, the physician's expertise and trustworthiness is reinforced. Without prior knowledge of side effects, patients may prematurely discontinue medications out of discomfort or an unrealistic concern that adverse effects are harming them. Routinely instruct somatizing patients to call before discontinuing treatment on their own. The occasional brief phone conversation that results will usually carry a timely recommendation to alter a dose or switch drugs, avoiding the situation in which the patient is seen some weeks later and has made little progress taking the previously prescribed medication. With antidepressants, be sure also to inform patients that it takes 3 to 5 weeks for full antidepressant effects to occur and that side effects typically lessen over that period.

Avoid prescribing CNS depressants (e.g., sedative-hypnotics, benzodiazepine anxiolytics, most "muscle relaxants") or narcotics, especially for patients with subacute or chronic somatization problems. These agents can cause multiple adverse effects, such as dependence, cognitive impairment, depression, mood swings, insomnia, and sedation.

### Consider use of consultants

Coordination of specialty care is an essential aspect of managing somatizing patients. Chronic somatizers may require intensive collaboration with specialists to reduce "doctor shopping" and avoid unnecessary diagnostic tests and invasive procedures. It is best to know a consultant in each specialty who orders tests conservatively and understands somatization. If possible, refer somatizing patients to specialists only after informing them of the patient's propensity to experience and report medically unexplained symptoms. Avoid consultants who regularly embark on lengthy diagnostic evaluations, are uncooperative with primary care providers, or often prescribe narcotics or sedative-hypnotics. Look for consultants who recommend care rather than assuming it, since multiple providers increases the likelihood of "doctor shopping." The best psychiatric consultants usually have a subspecialty interest or training in consultation-liaison psychiatry. Unfortunately, many general psychiatrists have only infrequent exposure to somatizing patients and often do not readily appreciate the need to collaborate carefully with primary care.

Most somatizing patients are best managed in primary care settings; indeed, many will actively resist psychiatric consultation. Some, however, require or request direct psychiatric assistance. Consultation often helps to elucidate stressors in defensive patients; to confirm diagnoses of anxiety, depressive, somatoform, or other psychiatric disorders; to decide about psychopharmacologic treatment in patients with many past treatment failures or complicating medical problems; to answer questions about suicide or violence potential in those with past behaviors or current ideation; to evaluate for involuntary treatment or hospitalization; or to suggest ways of improving adherence to treatment.

Patient defensiveness, erratic style, and excessive rejection fears, as well as social stigma associated with having a mental disorder, are among the obstacles to effective psychiatric consultation for somatizing patients seen in primary care settings. When somatization is suspected during a patient's first few visits, mention consultation early rather than waiting to the completion of an exhaustive negative diagnostic evaluation. Reassure the patient that you respect that symptoms are "real," and explain that suffering caused by aversive physical symptoms can often be reduced through early mental health assistance. Later, the patient will be

## Managed Care Guide
## Algorithm for the evaluation of dizziness

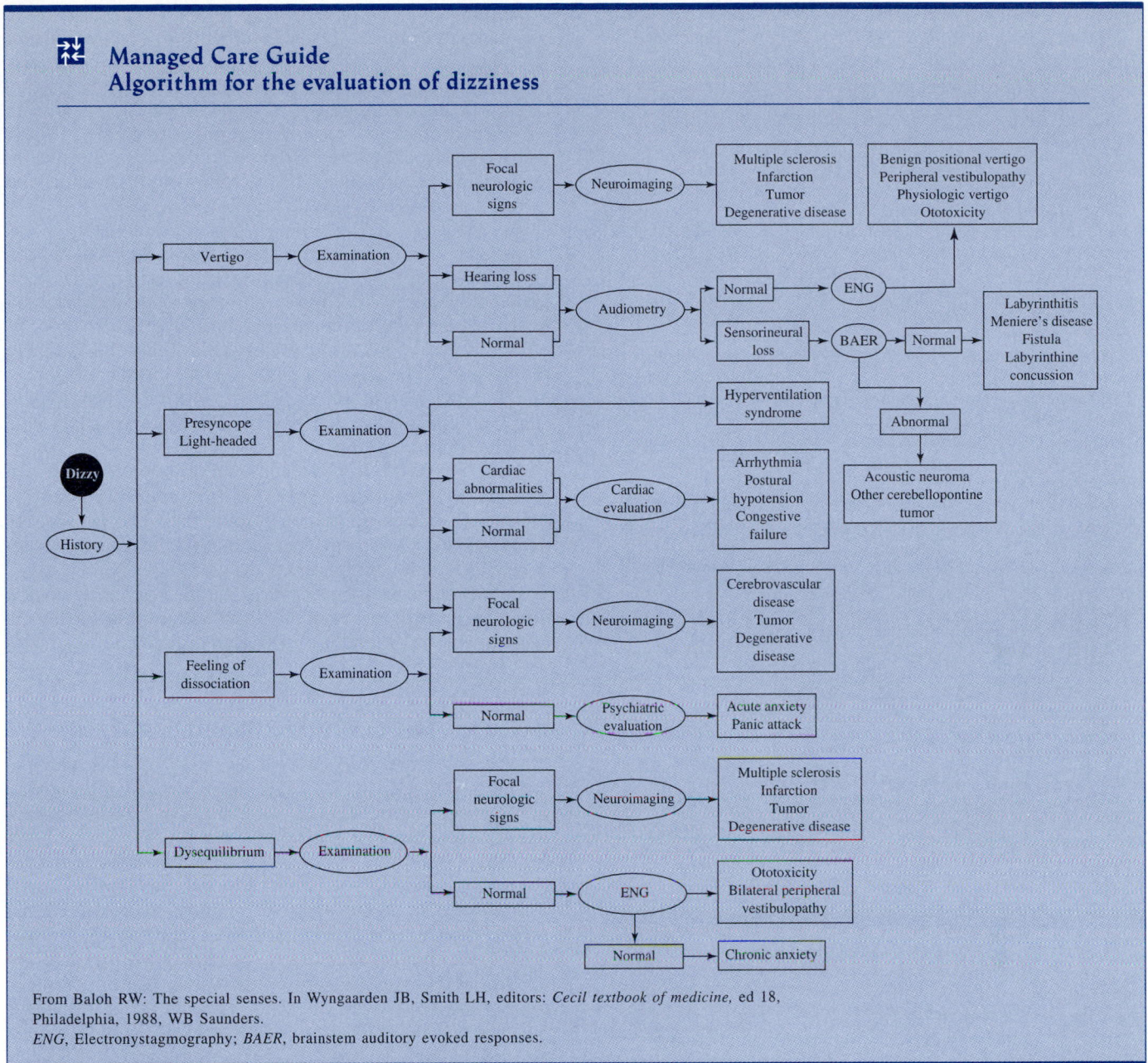

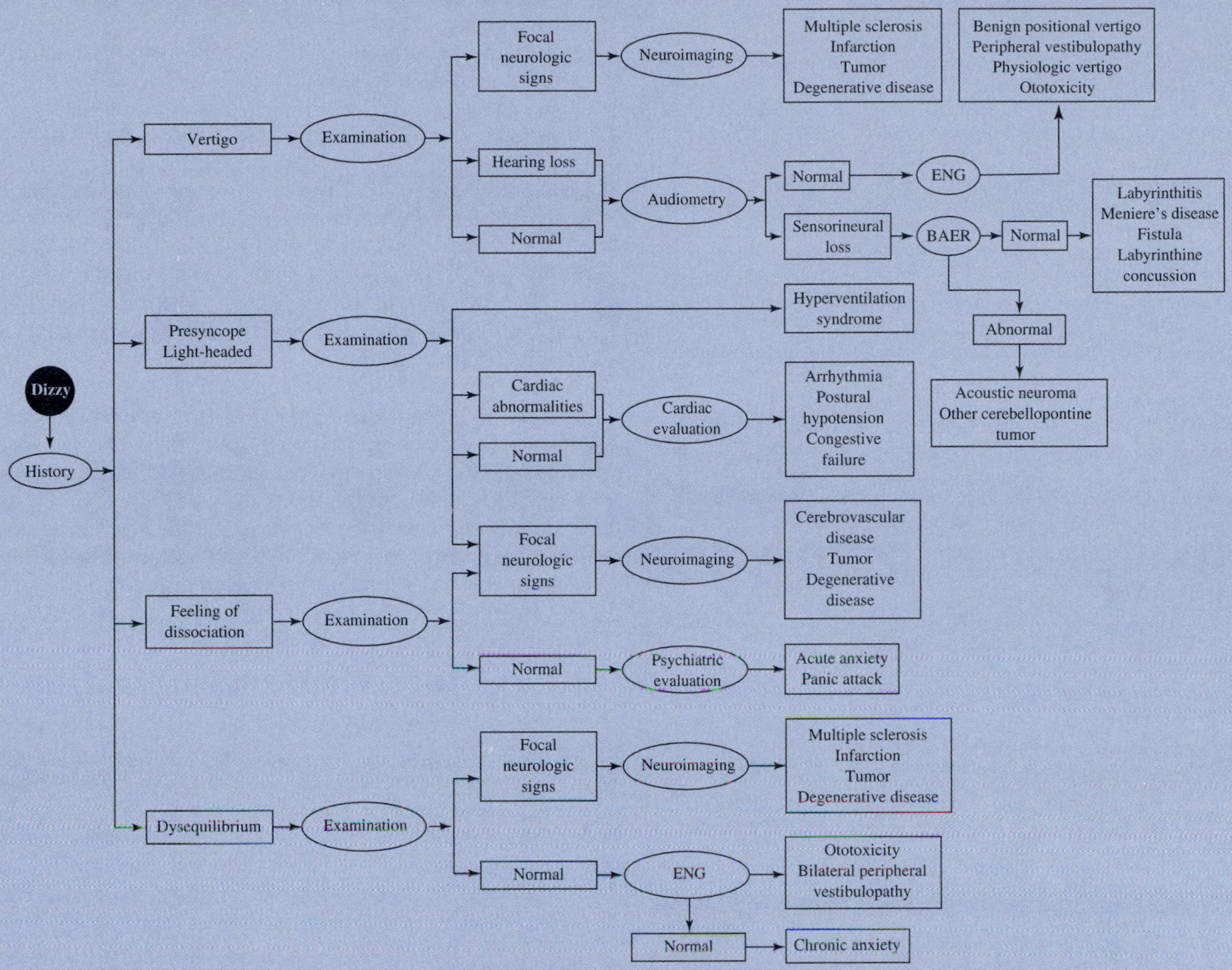


From Baloh RW: The special senses. In Wyngaarden JB, Smith LH, editors: *Cecil textbook of medicine,* ed 18, Philadelphia, 1988, WB Saunders.
*ENG,* Electronystagmography; *BAER,* brainstem auditory evoked responses.

less likely to view referral as rejection. Another strategy is routinely to schedule patients for a return primary care visit after psychiatric consultation to quell rejection concerns.

## DIZZINESS

Dizziness is a common complaint in primary care practice. It covers a broad spectrum of symptoms that range from vertigo to light-headedness, dissociation, and disequilibrium. The presentation of these symptoms may signal serious medical conditions or anxiety and stress that may be described as "falling out," swimmy head, or wooziness. The evaluation of patients complaining of dizziness requires a thorough history to assess possible neurologic, cardiac, and psychologic causes, and precipitating factors such as change in position, medications, stress, and underlying illnesses. Diagnostic assessment is summarized in the Managed Care Guide.

### Treatment

The treatment of dizziness depends on the cause of symptoms. Vertigo or spinning dizziness may respond to meclizine (25 to 50 mg q6h prn), dimenhydrinate (Dramamine 50 mg q6h prn), or a scopolamine patch. Symptoms of light-headedness may respond to low doses of benzodiazepines. The light-headedness caused by hyperventilation usually responds to rebreathing into a paper bag and antidepressants may relieve symptoms in some patients.

Patients with dizziness caused by central lesions may decrease their symptoms by performing exercises designed to produce central nervous system adaptation.

Treatment with Ativan (1 mg bid) may also lessen these symptoms. The management of vertigo is described in Chapter 27, syncope in Chapter 10, multiple sclerosis and related disorders in Chapter 100.

## BIBLIOGRAPHY


Dworkin SF, Von Korff M, LeResche L: Multiple pains and psychiatric disturbance: an epidemiologic investigation, *Arch Gen Psychiatry* 47:239, 1990.

Katon WJ: *Panic disorder in the medical setting,* Washington, DC, 1991, American Psychiatric Press.

Katon W: How does primary care address mental health needs of mentally ill and substance abusing populations? In *National Primary Care Conference Proceedings,* vol ii, p 307, U.S. Public Health Service Health Resources and Services Administration, Department of Health and Human Services, March 29-31, 1992.

Katon WJ, editor: Proceedings of a symposium: panic disorder: somatization, medical utilization, and treatment, *Am J Med* 92(suppl 1A), 1992.

Katon W, Sullivan M: Antidepressant treatment of somatic symptoms. In Mayou R, Bass C, Sharp M, editors: *The treatment of unexplained symptoms*, Oxford, 1995, Oxford University Press.

Kirmayer LJ, Robbins JM, editors: *Current concepts of somatization: research and clinical perspectives,* Washington, DC, 1991, American Psychiatric Press.

Lipowski ZJ: Somatization: the concept and its clinical application, *Am J Psychiatry* 145:1358, 1988.

Simon GE, Von Korff M: Somatization and psychiatric disorder in the NIMH Epidemiologic Catchment Area Study, *Am J Psychiatry* 148:1494, 1991.

Smith GR: *Somatization disorder in the medical setting,* Washington, DC, 1991, American Psychiatric Press.

Sullivan MD, Turner JA, Romano J: Chronic pain in primary care: identification and management of psychosocial factors, *J Fam Pract* 32:193, 1991.

Troost BT, Patton JW: Exercise therapy for positional vertigo, *Neurology* 42:1441, 1992.


CHAPTER

# 135 Psychotic Disorders

**Frank W. Brown**

## EPIDEMIOLOGY AND ETIOLOGY

*Psychosis* is a term often used to describe states of confusion, disorientation, or delirium. Psychosis is best considered a state of brain dysfunction characterized by delusions, hallucinations, and formal thought disorder (e.g., derailment, thought blocking, thought insertion). Psychosis should not be viewed as a disease but as a dynamic state induced by a neurochemical dysfunction that leads to the specific clinical presentation. Psychosis may be transient, intermittent, or continuous.

The 1-year prevalence rate of psychosis in the United States is less than 2.5%. Schizophrenia-related disorders have a 1.1% 1-year prevalence; severe cognitive impairment with superimposed psychosis accounts for approximately 1%; and other causes, such as medical illness or drug- and alcohol-induced psychosis, account for 0.5%.

Etiology may be described in terms of neurobiologic, genetic, environmental, and sociocultural factors. Brain structural and neuropathologic factors have been suspected to increase the risk of psychosis. The greatest risk factor for the development of late-life psychosis appears to be the presence of a progressive dementia. Three primary neurochemical systems (dopamine, neurotensin, and serine metabolism) have been implicated in the development of a psychotic state.

Psychosis as a result of a schizophrenic disorder has strong genetic influences, as shown from adoption, family, and twin studies. No simple pattern of inheritance has been isolated. Historic data have indicated that the risk of a person developing schizophrenia, although at 1% throughout the general population, increases if other relatives have the disorder. The risk of a patient developing schizophrenia is 10% with a schizophrenic sibling, 12% with a schizophrenic parent, and 40% to 45% if both parents have schizophrenia.

More stressful life events tend to occur before an episode of psychosis. Stressful life events cannot be viewed as causes of psychosis, but they can be seen as destabilizing factors that exacerbate a preexisting tendency to develop psychosis.

People with prolonged psychosis tend to experience a downward shift in social class. Whether this change is causative or is an effect of a prolonged psychotic state is not always clear. Most current data suggest that lower social class is a consequence of the psychosis.

## PATHOPHYSIOLOGY (NEUROBIOLOGY OF PSYCHOSIS)

Numerous theories on the neurobiology of psychosis exist, implicating neurochemical, structural, or functional factors. Most probably, multiple events (e.g., drugs, brain injury, morphologic changes) cause impairment in neurochemical pathways, which produces the expression of psychosis. Dopamine modulation through dysfunctional serine metabolism, regional neurotensin levels in the brain, and increased activity of dopamine or selected dopamine receptors in certain brain areas are important in the etiology of psychosis. There may be different trigger events, but the final common pathway would involve altered thalamic filtering.

## PSYCHIATRIC HISTORY

Symptoms of psychosis include the following:

*Delusions:* beliefs or situations not based on reality

*Hallucinations:* visual, auditory, olfactory, or tactile perceptions without external stimuli

*Thought insertion:* placement of thoughts into one's brain by an outside force, such as a patient's belief that a neighbor is putting images into the patient's head

*Derailment:* process by which one's thought processes suddenly go astray without apparent reason, such as a patient talking about one subject (e.g., his or her work), then suddenly shifting to an unrelated topic (e.g., the climate in Brazil)

*Thought blocking:* process in which one's thoughts appear to be stalled, such as when a patient who has been talking about a subject suddenly is unable to collect his or her thoughts and "goes mentally blank"

### Time course

The description of the current episode of psychosis is crucial in establishing a differential diagnosis. The knowledge that a psychosis is present does little in determining the etiology and appropriate management. Causes of psychosis can be divided into *primary* (psychosis with a concurrent psychiatric illness) and *secondary* (induced psychosis). These categories overlap because there remains a fundamental impairment in neurochemical pathways of the brain.

The length of time that the psychotic symptoms have been present needs to be established. An acute onset of visual hallucinations would heighten the suspicion of a medical illness or drug-induced psychotic process. In contrast, a 2- to 4-week history of increasing auditory and visual hallucinations may be more suggestive of a schizophrenia-related disorder. *Prodromal development of psychosis* refers to more subtle manifestations of an early psychotic process. Before the actual psychosis, the patient may have experienced social withdrawal, less attention to personal hygiene, or gradual difficulty with school or work performance. These symptoms would support the psychosis being of gradual onset. Prodromal development is most often seen in schizophrenia-related disorders and rarely in acute psychosis caused by medical illness or medications. By themselves, continuous or intermittent symptoms of psychosis add little to diagnostic clarity. Intermittent symptoms can occur in an early exacerbation of a primary psychiatric disorder (schizophrenia or major depression with psychosis), whereas continuous psychotic symptoms may indicate a greater severity of psychosis and a need for more rapid and aggressive intervention.

### Hallucinations

Visual hallucinations can occur in patients with schizophrenia; however, organic causes must be closely evaluated, such as in drug and alcohol intoxication and withdrawal. Olfactory hallucinations, which occur less frequently in schizophrenia, require careful assessment to rule out sella turcica tumors. Auditory hallucinations are often a feature of a schizophrenic type of disorder. Auditory hallucinations should be assessed as to the number of voices (one or many), whether the voices command the patient to perform some act (self-harm or violence), how often the hallucinations occur, and whether the patient perceives them as threatening or frightening. When auditory hallucinations and delusions are present, it is important to assess the patient for suicidal risk.

### Prior episodes

Previous episodes and the treatment history of psychotic symptoms provide invaluable information as to diagnosis and management techniques that will likely benefit the patient. Primary psychiatric disorders with recurrent features of psychosis include schizophrenia-related disorders, major depression with psychosis, bipolar disorder, and dementia with psychosis. The recurrence of similar psychotic features should alert the physician to explore closely the previous diagnosis and treatment. The patient with a chronic psychosis may respond well to a prior treatment plan. The patient who has major depression with psychosis requires treatment directed at the depression as well as the psychosis; attempting to treat only the psychosis without antidepressants or electroconvulsive therapy (ECT) will likely fail or delay adequate response.

### Family history

Because of the genetic "loading" of many primary psychiatric illnesses, a family history of similar psychotic symptoms or other psychiatric history provides valuable information. Effective management techniques used in the past to treat a family member are often effective in the patient with a similar psychotic presentation. This is especially important when there is a family history of schizophrenia, major depression, or bipolar disorder.

### Substance abuse

Substance abuse is known to predispose a person to develop psychosis, especially with acute ingestion of substances such as alcohol, lysergic acid diethylamide (LSD), phencyclidine (PCP), and cocaine or with acute withdrawal. Psychotic states from drugs generally have an acute onset and generally can remit with appropriate removal of the substance unless functional impairment occurs to the brain, as can happen with the use of LSD or PCP.

## EXAMINATION

### Direct examination

Although a routine physical examination is required for the patient with psychosis, a few areas of the examination should be emphasized. Possible sources of infection need to be identified. Evidence of a low-grade fever and slight tachycardia in a patient with recent onset of untreated psychosis should alert the physician to evaluate carefully for an induced psychosis. Drug intoxication with illicit or prescription drugs may present with symptoms similar to a schizophrenic disorder. Evidence of alcohol or sweet-smelling breath with tachypnea or tachycardia could indicate a psychosis caused or potentiated by alcohol or an alkaloid drug. Thyroid enlargement or thyroid nodules in the presence of acute psychosis require further study.

The office or bedside examination should include a screening mental status examination. Hallucinations may be described as to *type, complexity* (single voice or image versus multiple voices or complex visual images), and *duration.* The description of delusions should include type (paranoid, grandiose). Other psychotic symptoms should be described as to first onset, when they occur, and whether they occurred in the past. The patient's mood and affect (depressed, normal, or elevated) should be noted. Many schizophrenic patients have a flat or blunted affect with a limited range of expression. A minimal assessment for violence or suicide is necessary. Prior episodes of violence, current threats of violence, impaired judgment, and drug-seeking behavior are risk factors for recurrence of violence. If patients are hearing commanding voices, they generally acknowledge this if asked directly but rarely volunteer this information. The clinician's suspicion of psychosis should increase if the patient appears distracted or seems to be looking or responding to one part of the room, since this could indicate that the patient is responding to hallucinations. Guardedness and hyperalertness can indicate paranoia. In these cases, direct questions such as, "Do you feel safe here?" or "Are there voices that

**Table 135-1.** Laboratory tests in evaluating psychosis

| Laboratory test | Indication |
|---|---|
| Complete blood count with differential | Infection |
| Urinalysis | Infection |
| Liver enzymes | Hepatic encephalopathy |
| Serum creatinine | Uremia |
| Blood urea nitrogen | Uremia |
| Thyroid function tests | Hypothyroidism, hyperthyroidism |
| VDRL (FTA-ABS)* | Syphilis |
| Arterial blood gases (pulse oximeter) | Hypoxia |
| Electrolytes | Hyponatremia, hypernatremia |
| Glucose | Hypoglycemia |
| Urine drug screen | Drug ingestion, especially cocaine, phencyclidine, and marijuana |

*Venereal Disease Research Laboratories (fluorescent treponemal antibody absorption.)

are bothering you?" may elicit acknowledgment of the psychosis from the patient.

## Evaluation

Most routine laboratory tests that are ordered are appropriate for the patient with either acute-onset or chronic psychosis. Laboratory tests should be based on the history and physical examination; Table 135-1 provides a baseline for consideration. The goal of these evaluations is to uncover secondary causes of psychosis. Urine drug screens are most valuable at evaluating recent illicit drug use or inappropriate prescription drug use. A urine drug screen should be considered especially for acute onset of psychosis or reemergence of a previously controlled psychosis when visual hallucinations are prominent.

***Other studies.*** Chest x-rays may identify pneumonia or congestive heart failure, which could aggravate a psychotic state. An electrocardiogram (ECG) is recommended for at-risk patients to check for recent but silent myocardial infarction and arrhythmias. A lumbar puncture (LP) is not part of a normal evaluation but should be considered if infection or subarachnoid hemorrhage is suspected. An electroencephalogram (EEG) is appropriate if temporal lobe seizures are suspected. Systemic lupus erythematosus may first present as psychosis. Neuroimaging in the workup of psychosis should only be ordered when a specific reason exists, that is, signs of trauma or focal neurologic deficits. The acute onset of psychosis in a young person with a negative psychiatric history and negative family psychiatric history or new-onset psychosis in an elderly person should warrant consideration of neuroimaging. With microvascular brain disease, neurologic signs and symptoms may not always be elicited. Microvascular insults to deep white matter and the caudate nucleus may be predisposing factors in the development of psychosis in elderly persons.

***Psychologic testing.*** Psychologic tests are often misunderstood and ordered too infrequently. Comprehensive psychologic testing can be useful in evaluating selected psychotic patients who are stable enough to participate in testing. Many acutely psychotic patients simply cannot focus on this task long enough to make these tests worthwhile. The tests may be beneficial in determining how paranoid or delusional a patient is, especially if the patient does not volunteer information to direct questions. If psychologic testing is being considered, the physician must be able to formulate the specific direction of questioning, since this will determine what types of tests are performed.

## DIFFERENTIAL DIAGNOSIS

A greater sense of urgency should be shown the patient with a relatively recent onset of psychosis, the presence of a clouded sensorium, or onset of a psychotic process later in life. The patient with a recurrence of psychosis associated with a history of a schizophrenic disorder does not necessarily need to be as aggressively evaluated. Psychosis occurring with a clouded sensorium, as in delirium, signals a nonschizophrenic process; medical illnesses, metabolic abnormalities, and drug intoxication would be major considerations in causing this psychosis. Although onset in later life is often associated with dementia, the absence of memory impairment in the presence of psychosis requires close evaluation of medication side effects, vascular disease, and other physical illnesses (e.g., hypothyroidism, visual impairment, hypoxia).

### Primary causes

The most common presentation of psychosis in psychiatric illness occurs in schizophrenia-related disorders, major depression with psychotic features, bipolar disorder, and dementing disorders (see the box on p. 1759).

Schizophrenia, schizoaffective disorder, delusional disorder, and brief reactive psychosis are included together for this discussion. Typical features of each are briefly summarized; a more detailed description is available in the *Diagnostic and Statistical Manual of Mental Disorders*, fourth edition (DSM-IV).

*Schizophrenia* normally is associated with either bizarre delusions, prominent auditory hallucinations, incoherence, inappropriate or flat affect, looseness of association, or catatonia. For formal diagnosis, psychotic symptoms must be present for at least 1 week and have features lasting at least 6 weeks that do not occur entirely during an affective disorder. Although the diagnosis of schizophrenia cannot be formally made until a chronic course has been established, treatment should still be initiated with the onset of the psychosis. Associated features include a decrease in social or work performance. There may be prominent changes in activities of daily living (e.g., poor grooming), lack of drive, social withdrawal, or unusual behaviors (e.g., talking to oneself as one is walking down the street).

*Schizoaffective disorder* is a difficult diagnosis to differentiate, since it incorporates symptoms of schizophrenia and symptoms of a mood disorder while not meeting all the criteria of either. A simplified summary of schizoaffective disorder entails features of schizophrenia

**Causes of psychosis**

**Primary**

Schizophrenia related*
Major depression
Dementia
Bipolar disorder

**Secondary**

| | |
|---|---|
| Drugs† | Hypomagnesemia |
| Drug withdrawal‡ | Epilepsy |
| Drug toxicity§ | Fever |
| Charles Bonnet syndrome | Meningitis |
| Infections (pneumonia) | Encephalitis |
| Electrolyte imbalance | Brain abscess |
| Syphilis | Herpes encephalopathy |
| Congestive heart failure | Hypoxia |
| Parkinson's disease | Hypercarbia |
| Trauma to temporal lobe | Hypoglycemia |
| Postpartum psychosis | Thiamine deficiency |
| Hypothyroidism/hyperthyroidism | Postoperative states |

*Includes schizophrenia, schizophreniaform disorder, brief reactive psychosis.
†Includes hypnotics, glucocorticoids, marijuana, phencyclidine, atropine, dopaminergic agents (e.g., amantadine, bromocriptine, L-dopa), immunosuppressants.
‡Includes alcohol, barbiturates, benzodiazepines.
§Includes digitalis, theophylline, cimetidine, anticholinergic agents, glucocorticoids, catecholaminergic agents.

and affective symptoms suggesting a major depression or manic disorder at some point.

*Delusional disorder* is different from schizophrenia in several ways. The delusions are not bizarre and must be present for at least 4 weeks for diagnosis, whereas in schizophrenia, the delusions are often quite bizarre. Delusional content often focuses on paranoid themes. Delusions are generally plausible and have to be considered in context. If hallucinations are present, the hallucinations are not prominent features of the disorder.

*Brief reactive psychosis,* by definition, is less than 4 weeks' duration and remits with return to full functioning. Etiology is thought to be in response to one or multiple life stressors. Hallucinations and delusions occur but are relatively brief in duration. Other typical features include loosening of associations and disorganized or bizarre behaviors.

### Secondary causes

When psychosis results from any one of these secondary causes, the presentation may vary. Most secondary causes are seen in the context of a delirium or altered mental status. Substance abuse and drug/medication use, withdrawal, and toxicity are prime causes of delirium (see the box above). Key features to be noted may include an inability to maintain attention to a task (e.g., conversation), disorganized thought processes, visual hallucinations, labile affect, alteration in sleep-wake cycle, and impaired short-term memory. Effects of drugs/medications are more pronounced on the aging or immature brain or the brain that has previously been injured, such as with a cerebrovascular accident or head trauma. In one recent review, 83% of 177 medications were noted to have psychosis as a potential side effect.

## MANAGEMENT

Management of psychotic patients incorporates nonpharmacologic and pharmacologic interventions. Treatments depend on the severity and type of psychosis as well as the presumed etiology. Chronic psychotic patients (e.g., with schizophrenia) generally require only minor changes in their neuroleptic agents unless an acute exacerbation of the psychosis occurs. Then aggressive treatment with psychotropic drugs usually is required, along with nonpharmacologic interventions. Patients with acute onset of psychosis should always have the cause of the psychosis actively treated.

### Nonpharmacologic treatment

Any factor that could cause or potentiate a psychotic process should be eliminated. This would include the removal of suspected medications or illicit drugs as well as potential environmental stressors. A schizophrenic patient who decompensates on entering the workplace may benefit from a more structured work environment (e.g., set work hours and specific work task). The family can assist in providing a more stable home environment by simple measures such as establishing routines (meals at the same time, patient awakens at same time daily) and minimizing changes around the house (e.g., furniture not moved often).

*Behavioral intervention* and *reality orientation* are necessary for some patients. Acutely psychotic patients need to be oriented to reality (e.g., calendars/clocks in the room and reassurance from staff or family as to who they are, where they are, and the date, time, and situation). Interactions with psychotic individuals are best done from one individual at a time; psychotic patients do poorly when they must shift attention between two or more people. A better approach is for one physician or staff member to talk to and examine the patient while others remain at the patient's side (not back). With acutely psychotic patients, having a family or staff member stay with the patient may alleviate some paranoid behavior. Soft background music (no words) may also decrease the risk of potential physical agitation.

*Supportive psychotherapy (emotional management)* is a valuable technique for a psychotic patient. Calm reassurance may be offered to the patient, and the physician or staff can redirect the patient to nonpsychotic themes. Health care professionals must be alert to protect themselves from a patient who strikes out or feels threatened.

*Electroconvulsive therapy* (ECT) is appropriate in selected patients with psychosis, such as for depression with psychotic features, a manic disorder with psychosis, psychosis with catatonia, when ECT had been used with success previously, or when psychosis occurs with a strong affective component. ECT may also be beneficial when psychosis occurs from hypopituitarism or Parkinson's disease.

## Pharmacologic treatment

***Neuroleptics.*** Neuroleptic agents are the main treatment for patients with psychosis. They generally have very similar efficacy, and thus the choice of neuroleptic generally depends on the side effect profile best suited for the patient. Schizophrenic patients not treated with any form of antipsychotic drug will likely relapse within 3 years, and these relapses will have a greater intensity of psychosis and occur more often than in patients treated with antipsychotic medication. With the exception of the newer neuroleptics (e.g., clozapine, risperidone), all these medications have the potential to cause extrapyramidal side effects, tardive dyskinesia, and other anticholinergic side effects. Neuroleptic malignant syndrome (fever, muscle rigidity, altered mental status, autonomic instability) is a rare event with the use of neuroleptics but must be considered.

Tardive dyskinesia, a potentially irreversible movement disorder, can occur in up to 20% to 40% of patients treated with long-term neuroleptics. The risk of tardive dyskinesia is greater for elderly persons, women, and patients with any preexisting brain injury. Reasons for a greater risk in women is unknown. It is believed that with an increase in age and in preexisting brain injury, the changes in receptor number or sensitivity and altered homeostatic processes may increase some individuals' susceptibility to develop tardive dyskinesia. Treatment of tardive dyskinesia generally provides only partial therapeutic benefit. Neuroleptic withdrawal, especially with new-onset tardive dyskinesia, generally causes a transient increase in symptoms but a more gradual decline in abnormal movements over the next 2 to 9 months. Anticholinergic medications should be minimized because they tend to increase tardive symptoms. Patients with severe tardive dyskinesia may require treatment with reserpine (4 to 8 mg/day) or benzodiazepines. Vitamin E (α-tocopherol) at 400 IU four times a day has been successfully used in some patients with the development of tardive dyskinesia within 5 years of treatment with the vitamin E. Higher doses of neuroleptics are effective suppressors of tardive dyskinesia, but this is only a temporary measure because the tardive symptoms will reemerge.

The lower-potency neuroleptics (e.g., chlorpromazine, thioridazine) tend to have greater anticholinergic side effects and thus increase risk of falls and orthostatic blood pressure changes, especially in elderly patients. They are more sedating, which is a benefit in the younger agitated patient. Neuroleptics can also lower the seizure threshold. For these reasons, when a neuroleptic is used in a psychotic patient, the physician should obtain informed consent from the family or guardian. Table 135-2 lists the more common neuroleptics available, the haloperidol milligram equivalents, the average daily dosages, and the relative side effect profile.

***Other medications.*** Other agents have a role in the treatment of certain types of psychosis. Carbamazepine and valproic acid may be very effective if an ictal focus is thought to be contributing to the psychosis. Benzodiazepines, when combined with a neuroleptic in the severely

**Table 135-2.** Antipsychotic medications

| Medication | Equivalent to 1 mg haloperidol (approx. mg) | Average daily dosage range (mg) | Route* | Relative cumulative side effect profile† |
|---|---|---|---|---|
| 1. Butyrophenones‡ | | | | |
| Haloperidol (Haldol) | 1 | 1-25 | PO, IM, IV | 1 |
| Haloperidol decanoate | 1 | 25-200 | IM | 1 |
| 2. Thioxanthenes‡ | | | | |
| Thiothixene (Navane) | 2.5 | 15-30 | PO, IM | 1 |
| 3. Phenothiazines | | | | |
| a. Aliphatics | | | | |
| Chlorpromazine (Thorazine) | 50 | 200-1000 | PO, IM§ | 4 |
| b. Piperidines | | | | |
| Thioridazine (Mellaril) | 50 | 100-600 | PO | 3 |
| c. Phenazines | | | | |
| Fluphenazine‡ (Prolixin) | 1 | 2-20 | PO, IM | 1 |
| Fluphenazine‡ decanoate | 1 | 25-100 | IM, SC | 1 |
| d. Piperazines | | | | |
| Trifluoperazine (Stelazine) | 2.5 | 2-20 | PO, IM | 2 |
| 4. Dibenzoxazepines | | | | |
| Loxapine (Loxitane) | 5 | 60-100 | PO, IM | 2 |
| 5. Dibenzodiazepines | | | | |
| Clozapine‖ (Clozaril) | 75 | 25-700 | PO | 1 |
| 6. Risperidone (Risperdal) | 0.5 | 1-8 | PO | 1 |

*PO, Oral; IM, intramuscular; IV, intravenous; SC, subcutaneous.

†1, Minimal; 4, greatest. Lower score reflects higher potency and lower anticholinergic side effects.

‡Acute extrapyramidal reactions more common.

§Available as suppositories.

‖1% to 2% incidence of agranulocytosis. A weekly complete blood count is required. Other side effects include orthostatic blood pressure changes and lowered seizure threshold.

agitated psychotic patient, are very effective in achieving more rapid control of the agitation and psychosis. For the young to middle-aged psychotic patient, oral or intramuscular (IM) haloperidol (3 to 5 mg) and lorazepam (1 to 2 mg) may be given every 30 to 60 minutes until control is achieved. This combination can be more effective than a neuroleptic alone.

Two long-acting depot neuroleptics are readily available in the United States: haloperidol decanoate (given every 4 to 5 weeks) and fluphenazine decanoate (given every 3 to 4 weeks). Each of these long-acting IM neuroleptics is useful for the noncompliant patient or the chronic psychotic patient who will not take or is sporadic in taking oral medications. It is always recommended that before using a long-acting neuroleptic, the short-acting oral form should be given daily to ensure patient tolerance to the medication and to gauge a dosing pattern for the long-acting medication. The maximal initial dose of haloperidol decanoate is 100 mg IM; generally the decanoate is 10 to 15 times the oral haloperidol dosage. Fluphenazine decanoate, 12.5 mg IM every 3 to 4 weeks, is equivalent to about 10 mg oral fluphenazine taken daily. Initial starting dosages range from 12.5 to 25 mg, with onset of antipsychotic activity within 48 hours. Depot neuroleptics carry similar risks as oral neuroleptics, except that the depot form will continue to cause side effects for 4 to 6 weeks. If neuroleptic malignant syndrome occurs, the neuroleptic cannot be readily inactivated.

Clozapine is a dibenzodiazepine derivative and has been shown to be effective with refractory psychosis (e.g., schizophrenia) with low risk for tardive dyskinesia. Average daily doses range from 25 to more than 700 mg daily. Although clozapine is very effective, its use requires familiarity with the drug to avoid oversedation and to titrate or taper the drug depending on response and potential changes in the white blood cell count. Risperidone, the newest antipsychotic and a 5-HT2 receptor blocker and weak D2 receptor blocker, does not have the high anticholinergic properties or risk of tardive dyskinesia as other traditional neuroleptics. Dosages range from 1 to 8 mg daily.

### Family- and community-centered approaches

Most mild forms of psychosis should not require hospitalization if no major medical illness is present. Keeping the mildly psychotic patient at home in familiar surroundings may prevent further psychotic decomposition compared with hospitalization in an unfamiliar surrounding. The first-line approach to management of psychosis and especially chronic psychotic illnesses such as schizophrenia centers on family and community programs.

Family-centered approaches are ideal for a patient with a chronic or recurring psychosis, as often seen in schizophrenia. Family education about the illness, associated symptoms, treatment and management options, and prognosis provides the family with valuable information. The family who can provide a home environment with minimal change and maximal routine will have fewer problems with the psychotic patient's behaviors.

Community-centered programs are especially important because they provide assistance to the family while monitoring psychotic patients for evidence of relapse, medication compliance, or side effects and provide the patient with structured activities or employment. Day treatment programs provide 3 to 8 hours 1 to 5 days a week to assist the individual. Most states have associations for mentally ill persons that can provide a listing of resources in a specific community.

### Special patient issues

***Suicidal patients and precautions.*** Suicide occurs most often in patients with affective disorders and then in patients suffering from alcoholism. Approximately 15% of schizophrenic patients end their life by suicide. Most psychotic patients who commit suicide are young unemployed males with a high level of social functioning before the onset of the psychosis.

The early detection and treatment of psychosis especially with depressive features represents a major preventive strategy for completed suicide. The clinician who is assessing a psychotic patient for suicide risk at a minimal should address the following questions:

1. Is there a history of prior suicide atempts?
2. Is there a plan and means to commit suicide?
3. Does the patient have feelings of hopelessness or that life is not worth living?
4. Are there thoughts of death?

The presence of command hallucinations needs to be evaluated, as the commands are often for self-injury. A psychotic patient who fears mental disintegration or has not been compliant with treatment is at higher risk for completed suicide.

When a psychotic patient is identified at moderate to high suicide risk (a subjective decision), hospitalization and/or psychiatric consultation is indicated. A patient with only occasional transient suicidal ideations may be managed as an outpatient; however, the clinician must be knowledgeable about the treatment of psychosis as well as affective disorders, while realizing that a psychotic patient's judgment is generally impaired. Outpatients should be provided community services that provide linkage between treatment and recreational and occupational activities.

***Adolescents.*** When psychosis occurs in the adolescent, the physician must evaluate for primary versus secondary psychosis. Brief reactive psychosis generally is time limited and may only require supportive care and a structured environment. The use of neuroleptics in this age group requires careful consideration of whether the benefits outweigh the potential for development of tardive dyskinesia. If the psychosis necessitates a medication because of auditory or visual hallucinations, commanding voices, or delusions, risperidone or clozapine may be useful.

Adolescents require special concern regarding suicide potential. An acutely psychotic adolescent is at increased risk of self-harm because of impaired impulse control and impaired judgment as well as commanding voices. This situation would warrant hospitalization; unless the clinician is very experienced in managing young psychotic patients, it would be prudent to consult with a trusted psychiatrist.

***Pregnant and postpartum patients.*** The occurrence of psychosis during pregnancy places both the mother and the fetus at risk from the sequelae of the psychosis. Management techniques must emphasis risk versus benefit of any treatment considered. Potential causes of the psychosis must be excluded and environmental control maximized. If the pregnant patient has been taking a neuroleptic, the dosage should be kept as low as possible to control the psychosis. Any neuroleptic use requires the patient's informed consent. It is generally thought that there is minimal risk of an increased rate of physical malformation from neuroleptic use even during the first trimester. However, it is not known what potential effects neuroleptics may have on the developing fetal brain for future behavior. If a psychosis needs to be treated during pregnancy and other treatable causes have been considered, a low-dose neuroleptic (e.g., haloperidol, 2 mg daily, increased by 1-2 mg every other day up to a maximum 10 mg) should be considered. A chronic psychotic process may best be treated with a low-dose maintenance neuroleptic. Because of the potential teratogenic effect of pharmacotherapy, ECT should be considered, especially if affective or catatonic symptoms are present.

A small subset (less than 1%) of postpartum women develop a psychosis within the first weeks after delivery. These psychotic episodes may occur during a postpartum depression. Aggressive treatment to control the primary illnesses (antidepressants for the depression, neuroleptics for the psychosis) should be undertaken to maintain the bonding of mother and infant and to reduce the overall disruption caused by the psychosis. Low doses of a neuroleptic (e.g., haloperidol, 2 to 5 mg daily) should be used until the psychosis is controlled. After the psychosis has been controlled for 4 to 8 weeks, the neuroleptic can be decreased by 1 mg weekly until discontinued, with careful attention to psychotic recurrence. ECT is useful in women with postpartum psychosis with an affective component.

***Elderly patients.*** Geriatric patients with psychosis fall into four broad diagnostic groups: (1) delirium related or drug/illness induced, (2) continuation of a lifelong or chronic psychotic illness, (3) affective disorders with psychosis, and (4) dementia-related syndromes with psychosis. The first group, although likely requiring neuroleptics, should have aggressive intervention to correct the underlying deficits (e.g., hypoxia, infection, decreased cerebral blood flow) causing the delirium. Neuroleptics in elderly persons should be started at low doses and slowly titrated. Haloperidol, starting at 0.25 to 0.50 mg and increasing by 0.25 to 0.50 mg every 1 to 2 days, is appropriate. Faster titration may be needed but requires greater attention to orthostatic blood pressure monitoring. Acute episodes of psychosis with agitation may require initial doses of 1 to 2 mg haloperidol. Elderly patients show the greatest sensitivity to neuroleptic side effects, especially orthostasis, increased risk of falls, and extrapyramidal symptoms, and therefore require lower doses and slower titration. Accumulated effects of neuroleptics may require that the dose be decreased after about 3 to 4 weeks, since some patients become more sedated as the psychosis is controlled.

***Perioperative patients.*** Psychotic patients awaiting surgery must have individualized treatment recommendations. An actively psychotic patient may require a high-potency neuroleptic 2 hours before anesthesia by the oral or IM route. Stable patients with a chronic psychotic illness may safely have their neuroleptics stopped 12 to 24 hours before surgery. Psychosis generally does not reemerge immediately and normally takes weeks to reappear. Neuroleptics can then be safely restarted 24 to 48 hours postoperatively.

***Hospitalized medical patients.*** These patients have an increased risk to develop a psychotic reaction compared with people in the community. The stress of the medical illness, a different environment, and the interaction of medications can precipitate a psychosis. The medical patient who has a history of psychosis and a reemergence of psychotic symptoms can generally be treated with the same neuroleptic regimen that had been effective in the past. Medical patients who have not had previous psychotic symptoms require a careful evaluation of the causative agent(s) for the psychosis so that the agent may be removed or reduced if feasible. Short-term use of high-potency neuroleptics (e.g., oral haloperidol, 1 to 8 mg daily) would be appropriate for control of the symptoms of hallucinations, delusions, and agitation. In addition to neuroleptic use, management should incorporate a very structured, set environment and a reduction in external disrupting noise. Soft background music is appropriate, especially if agitation has been present. Potential for suicide must be assessed, and if the patient is thought to be at risk, one-to-one care should be provided until consultation is obtained.

***Stable compensated patients.*** These patients with a prior history of psychosis should be maintained with a similar treatment plan that has kept them stable in the past. The primary care physician should realize that neuroleptics are generally only one part of this treatment approach. The patient may have been in a structured home setting or group home environment, and maintaining these nonpharmacologic interventions should not be overlooked.

Neuroleptic-induced side effects (akathisia, stiffness, cogwheel rigidity) are a major reason for medication noncompliance. For patients with evidence of cogwheel rigidity or extrapyramidal symptoms, benztropine (1 to 2 mg orally twice a day) is generally effective, with 2 to 4 weeks of therapy usually sufficient. Decreasing the neuroleptic can decrease these side effects and is especially helpful in decreasing or eliminating akathisia. Tapering an antipsychotic in a patient with a history of chronic psychosis to the lowest effective dose should be attempted slowly and in small increments over several months. Recent hallucinations, delusions, bizarre behaviors, or decreased attention to grooming may indicate the reemergence of psychosis. If these symptoms emerge, an increase in the neuroleptic dose by 10% to 20% should be considered. If the patient continues to be stable for 6 months, attempts to decrease the neuroleptic by 10% to 20% is appropriate, with close follow-up to ensure that psychosis does not recur.

## INDICATIONS FOR CONSULTATION, REFERRAL, AND HOSPITALIZATION

Consultation with a psychiatric colleague for a patient with psychosis usually is recommended if any concern exists about the etiology, diagnosis, or management. Although the primary care physician is able to diagnose accurately the presence of a psychosis, evaluating the type may be difficult. Psychiatric consultation also can assist in determining the types of pharmacologic and nonpharmacologic interventions based on the patient's specific needs.

Actively psychotic patients may present such a risk of harm to themselves and others that hospitalization should be strongly considered. Disadvantages to hospitalization include (1) removing the patient from a potentially safe and structured environment; and (2) placing them on a rapidly changing hospital ward where they may become more psychotic. Psychosis in and of itself does not require hospitalization, but other features often seen with psychosis may require it; psychotic patients often have impaired judgment and impulse control. There are, however, some clear indications when hospitalization should be highly recommended. If the psychotic patient is suicidal or is hearing voices that command self-harm, or if a delusion is present that mandates self-mutilation, hospitalization with aggressive treatment is advised.

Violence or physical agitation is often a major concern of family members or health care providers. Most episodes of physical agitation are nondirected and defensive in nature, except for the delusional patient with focused paranoia who may attack a specific person. These patients are often noncompliant with outpatient management. Hospitalization provides safety and a means to gain better control of the psychosis.

Psychosis with another major mental illness (e.g., major depression, mania) is very difficult to manage in an outpatient setting and places patients at high risk from their impaired judgment and impulse control. Outpatient management of these patients should only be considered if trained 24-hour sitters are available.

## BIBLIOGRAPHY


Abramowicz MA, editor: Drugs that cause psychiatric symptoms, *Med Lett* 35:65, 1993.

American Psychiatric Association: *Diagnostic and statistical manual of mental disorders,* ed 4, Washington, DC, 1994, American Psychiatric Association.

Brown FW: The neurobiology of late-life psychosis, *Crit Rev Neurobiol* 7(3/4):275, 1993.

Carlsson A: The current status of the dopamine hypothesis of schizophrenia, *Neuropsychopharmacology* 1:179, 1988.

Davis JM et al: Dose response of prophylactic antipsychotics, *J Clin Psychiatry* 54(3, suppl):24, 1993.

Regier DA et al: The de Facto U.S. Mental and Addictive Disorders Service System: Epidemiologic Catchment Area 1-year prevalence rates of disorders and services, *Arch Gen Psychiatry* 50:85, 1993.

Wessely S: Acting on delusions. I. Prevalence, *Br J Psychiatry* 163:69, 1993.

# XIV UROLOGY

CHAPTER

# 136 Male Infertility

Robert D. Oates
Michael A. Werner

*Infertility* is defined as the inability to conceive after 1 year of unprotected intercourse. Traditionally, couples were told not to worry until a year had passed because 80% to 85% of couples would conceive within that time span. However, the increasing age of many couples, the significant psychologic burden that has prompted the question, and the ease of preliminary evaluations (including appropriate history, physical examination, and laboratory testing) makes this an untenable approach. We strongly believe that a fertility evaluation should be instituted as soon as the issue is raised by a couple. The primary care physician can often identify by history and physical examination a likely cause of male infertility. The physician can initiate a basic workup and ensure appropriate attention is directed to the male factor. Most importantly, the physician may play a preventive role in preserving a patient's fertility potential.

This chapter provides a general overview of the etiologies of male infertility and discusses what issues in a patient's history and physical examination should alert a primary care physician that a potential fertility problem exists. The chapter describes a preliminary workup and, most importantly, discusses common situations, the appropriate treatment of which may have a significant impact on the patient's fertility status. Although this chapter concerns male infertility, one must remember that infertility is a couple phenomenon, and that neither partner can be evaluated independently of the other. It is critical always to have the spouse fully evaluated in terms of ovulation status, tubal and pelvic anatomy, cervical mucus production and sperm interaction, and endometrial receptivity.

## EPIDEMIOLOGY AND ETIOLOGY OF MALE REPRODUCTIVE DYSFUNCTION

Primary infertility, the inability to conceive the first time, occurs in 15% to 20% of couples. Male factors either contribute to or are the sole cause in 30% to 50% of these couples. Many couples are delaying in their attempts to conceive, which, combined with patient awareness of the new and successful reproductive technologies, has dramatically increased visits to physicians for consultation on possible infertility.

The causes of male infertility are extremely varied. Varicocele (37%), testicular failure (9.4%), obstruction of the ductal system (6.1%), and cryptorchidism (6.1%) are the findings most frequently identified. However, no associated factors or explanations are uncovered in approximately 25% of patients. Primary endocrinopathies account for only 0.9% of cases. Sexual dysfunction occurs in 2.8% of cases, has many causes, and is often easily treated. New solutions for ejaculatory failure, present in 1.2% of patients, have recently been developed and refined. Table 136-1 summarizes the etiologies associated with male infertility found in a referral clinic.

## BASIC ANATOMY AND PHYSIOLOGY OF THE MALE REPRODUCTIVE SYSTEM

Male reproductive physiology involves the interplay between male anatomy and its hormonal milieu. The testis is composed of two major compartments: the seminiferous tubules and the interstitium. The seminiferous tubules comprise approximately 90% of the volume of the testis, and it is here that spermatogenesis takes place. Each tubule contains two main types of cells, those actually in the pathway of spermatozoa development and the Sertoli cells.

The Sertoli cells reside just off the basement membrane and envelop the developing germ cells, supporting their growth. They are essential to the blood-testis barrier. Stem cells (spermatogonia) with the normal complement of deoxyribonucleic acid (DNA) (2N) line the basement membrane of the seminiferous tubule. Spermatogonia undergo mitosis to replicate themselves but also travel a meiotic pathway on the road of spermatogenesis, the first stage being primary spermatocytes, which have twice the normal complement of DNA (4N). Primary spermatocytes undergo the first meiotic reduction division, resulting in two secondary spermatocytes, each with a 2N complement of DNA. A second meiotic reduction division of each secondary spermatocyte produces two haploid spermatids. Spermatids then undergo *spermiogenesis,* a process of morphologic transformation into spermatozoa (Fig. 136-1).

Fully formed spermatozoa enter the lumen of the seminiferous tubule, where they are passively propelled along until the tubules merge and coalesce at the rete testis. The rete testis is located underneath the encasing layer of the testis, the tunica albuginea, and gives origin to six to eight efferent ductules that exit the tunica and ramify within the head (caput) of the epididymis to form eventually one tubule. The epididymal tubule proper is highly coiled and constitutes the body (corpus) and tail (cauda) portions. The epididymal tubule gradually thickens and straightens, continuing on as the vas deferens.

The vas is a muscular tube that travels from the scrotum

**Table 136-1.** Etiology of male infertility

| Etiology | Percentage of men |
|---|---|
| Varicocele | 37.4 |
| Testicular failure | 9.4 |
| Obstruction | 6.1 |
| Cryptorchidism | 6.1 |
| Volume | 4.7 |
| Sperm agglutination | 3.1 |
| Sexual dysfunction | 2.8 |

From Greenberg SH, Lipshultz LI, Wein A: Experience with 425 subfertile male patients, *J Urol* 119:507, 1978.

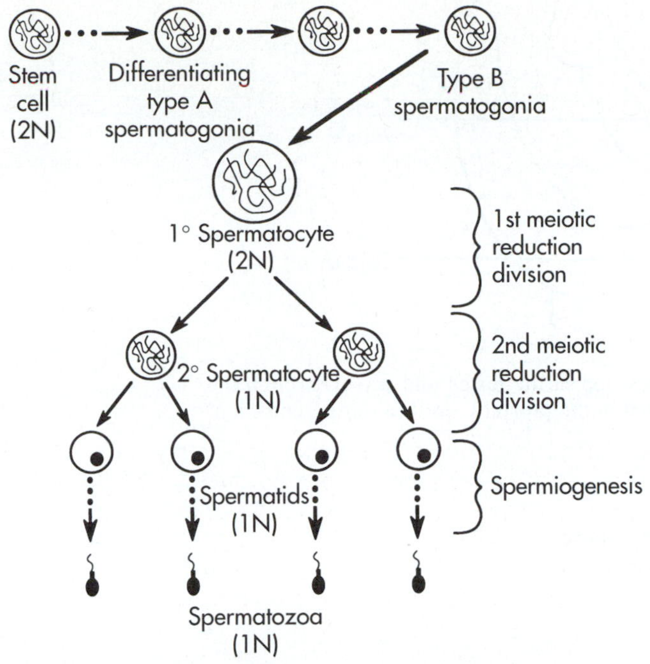


**Fig. 136-1.** Stages of spermatogenesis. Stem cells undergo mitotic division and then two meiotic divisions to become haploid. (From Oates RD, Lipshultz LI: *Ad Urol* 2:57, 1989.)

though the inguinal canal. It enters the pelvis, stays extraperitoneal, and then widens to form the ampullary region. The ampulla forms a common duct with the seminal vesicle, called the ejaculatory duct. This duct travels through the prostate and empties into the prostatic urethra (Fig. 136-2). The seminal vesicles contribute alkaline fructose-positive secretions to the ejaculate, accounting for approximately 70% of its volume. Twenty percent of the fluid is an acidic component from the prostate. The remaining 10% is spermatozoa-laden fluid from the vasal ampullae.

Semen exits the body during the complex process of ejaculation. Ejaculation consists of three phases. The first phase describes the deposition of the contents of the seminal vesicle and ampulla of the vas via the ejaculatory duct into the prostatic urethra and is termed emission. During emission the bladder neck closes, so that during ejaculation, the semen does not travel retrograde into the bladder. The bulbocavernosus muscle encircles the urethra; the ischiocavernosus muscle encircles the corporal bodies. During the third phase of antegrade ejaculation, these muscles rhythmically contract to propel the semen forward down the urethra in an antegrade direction and eventually out the penile meatus.

The processes of emission and bladder neck closure are sympathetically mediated (Fig. 136-3). These sympathetic fibers are long preganglionic neurons that travel to peripheral ganglia located near or within the adventitia of the end organs. An ejaculation coordinating center is located in the spinal cord at T12-L1 and is responsible for the initiation and coordination of the proper temporal sequence of neuronal activation driving the ejaculatory reflex.

Gonadotropin-releasing hormone (GnRH) is produced by the hypothalamus, stimulating the production by the pituitary gland of luteinizing hormone (LH) and follicle-stimulating hormone (FSH) (Fig. 136-4). LH acts on the testicular Leydig cells to stimulate the production of testosterone. Testosterone acts locally in a paracrine fashion on the seminiferous epithelium to promote spermatogenesis. Intratesticular levels of testosterone are significantly higher than the serum levels. If exogenous testosterone is given, hypothalamic GnRH and pituitary LH secretion will be inhibited, resulting in a significant or total reduction of intratesticular testosterone production and severely hampering, if not abolishing, spermatogenesis.

FSH acts on the Sertoli cell and is crucial for spermatogenesis. The Sertoli cell, when functioning appropriately, secretes inhibin, which, via a negative feedback hypothalamic/pituitary mechanism, regulates FSH secretion. If spermatogenesis is impaired at the testicular level, inhibin production is less and FSH secretion higher than normal. Therefore an elevated FSH is an indication of primary testicular dysfunction.

Male infertility may be conceptualized as having pretesticular, testicular, and posttesticular causes. Even more simply, it can be thought of as a problem with either sperm production (pretesticular and testicular) or delivery (posttesticular). Congenital or acquired hypothalamic and pituitary disease may cause decreased secretion of FSH and LH. This results in lack of stimulation of both Leydig and Sertoli cells with consequent spermatogenic deficiency. This would be an example of pretesticular or endocrinologic pathology. Testicular etiologies of male infertility include any process at the testicular level that would inhibit or preclude spermatogenesis, including androgen receptor defects, germinal cell aplasia, and various forms of deficient spermatogenesis. Posttesticular etiologies arise from any anatomic or functional obstruction of the reproductive ductal system. Testicular function is adequate, but sperm cannot make it into the ejaculate in a normal manner. A proper history and physical examination, coupled with appropriate laboratory and radiologic testing, often allow a proper categorization into one of the these three groups.

## MALE REPRODUCTIVE HISTORY

The specific history directed at male infertility can be divided into five main groups of questions: (1) Is the patient having sexual intercourse in an appropriate way, at an appropriate time in the cycle, and at an appropriate frequency? (2) Are there clearly apparent female factors? (3) Is there an endocrinopathy present? (4) Does the patient have damage, either congenital or acquired, to his genital tract? and (5) What evaluation has the couple had, and what therapeutic modalities have already been attempted? Certain factors in a patient's history may provide clues to present infertility or predict possible future difficulty in conception. Some of the more frequently seen conditions that should raise suspicion in the general practitioner's mind are briefly described next.

### Endocrinopathies

Primary endocrinopathies, although rare, are a potentially reversible cause of male infertility. Hypogonadotropic hypogonadism describes a decrease or absence of FSH and

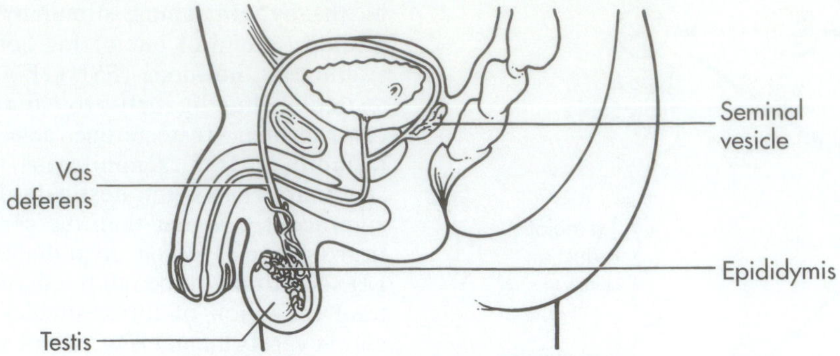


**Fig. 136-2.** Male reproductive anatomy. Sperm develop in the testes and travel through the epididymis, vas, and ejaculatory duct to be deposited in the prostatic urethra during emission.

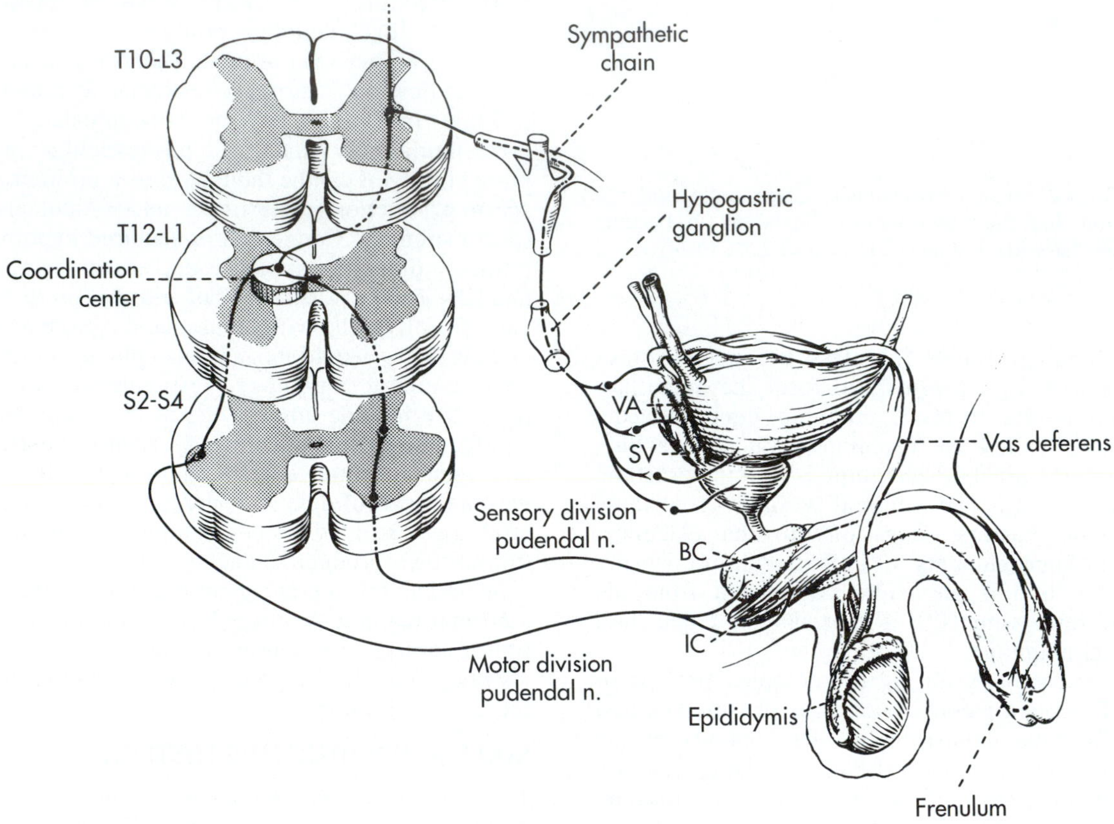


**Fig. 136-3.** Neurophysiology of ejaculation. Sensory afferent fibers travel to the coordination center. Sympathetic neurons leave from the thoracolumbar cord to innervate the vasal ampulla *(VA),* seminal vesicles *(SV),* and bladder neck. Efferent motor fibers exit the sacral cord to innervate the bulbocavernosus muscle *(BC)* and the ischiocavernosus muscle *(IC).* (From Seftel AD, Oates RD, Krane RJ: *Neurol Clin* 9:757 1991.)

LH. It is considered primary if congenital and secondary if the onset is postpubertal. It may occur at the hypothalamic or pituitary level. Kallmann's syndrome, a specific form of congenital hypogonadotropic hypogonadism, affects midline structures and may be associated with cleft lip and anosmia. These patients are typically prepubertal in appearance and may only complain of an absence of libido or lack of virilization. Secondary hypogonadotropic hypogonadism is most often caused by a prolactin-secreting pituitary adenoma. A prolactinoma may be treated surgically, medically, or with radiation and is best diagnosed with pituitary magnetic resonance imaging (MRI). Anabolic steroid abuse may be found in patients with secondary hypogonadotropic hypogonadism.

### Medications/habits/exposures

Many medications adversely affect sperm quality (see the box on p. 1767). The most important of these are sulfasalazine, colchicine, cimetidine, nitrofurantoin, and spironolactone. Excessive alchohol use, cigarette smoking, and marijuana use will negatively affect spermatogenesis. Chemotherapeutic agents may cause irreversible damage

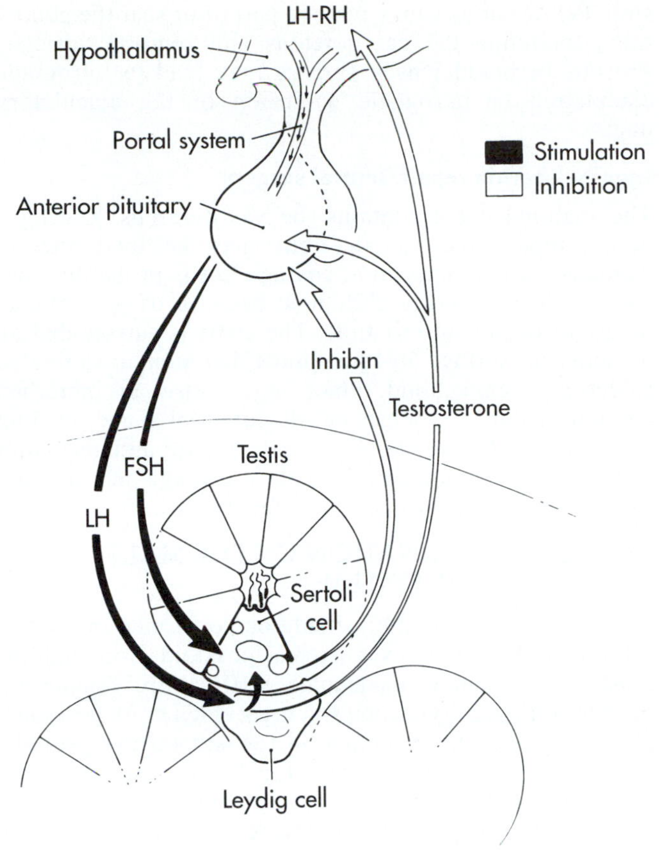


**Fig. 136-4.** Hypothalamic-pituitary-testicular axis. *LH-RH,* Gonadotrophin-releasing hormone (GnRH); *LH,* luteinizing hormone; *FSH,* follicle-stimulating hormone. (From Lipshultz LI, Kessler DL: *Monogr Urol* 7:28, April/May 1986.)

to the spermatogenic cell line by selectively destroying the more rapidly dividing germ cells. The exact agents used, the dosage regimen, and the duration of chemotherapy all play a role in the determination of ultimate spermatotoxicity. Scatter from radiotherapy may cause dose-dependent damage to the radiosensitive spermatogonia. Chemical exposures, including pesticides, pose a reproductive threat. Any environmental exposure to a chemical substance, whether it has been documented to be a reproductive hazard or not, must be curtailed as much as possible. Antihypertensives that effect $\alpha_1$ blockade, such as phenoxybenzamine hydrochloride, and antipsychotics (e.g., chlorpromazine) may cause ejaculatory dysfunction. Calcium channel blockers may impair the fertilization ability of sperm.

### Diabetes mellitus

Approximately one third of diabetic males have ejaculatory dysfunction as a consequence of sympathetic autonomic dystrophy. This may lead to failure of emission and/or retrograde ejaculation. Diabetic small-vessel vascular disease may affect the distal ampullary vas deferens, and ejaculatory ducts, resulting in ischemia and calcification that effectively blocks normal peristaltic activity during ejaculation.

### Multiple sclerosis/transverse myelitis

Multiple sclerosis (MS) and transverse myelitis may cause failure of erection and ejaculation. Both upper and lower motor neuron dysfunction occurs with MS, whereas a central cord insult is typically responsible for the suboptimal ejaculation seen in transverse myelitis.

#### Medications/habits/exposures affecting male fertility

**Medications**
Sulfasalazine
Colchicine
Cimetidine
Nitrofurantoin
Spironolactone
Chemotherapeutic agents
$\alpha_1$ Blockers
Calcium channel blockers

**Habits**
Alcohol
Cigarettes
Marijuana

**Radiotherapy**

**Chemical Exposures**
Pesticides
Lead

### Genetic diseases/syndromes

Many genetic syndromes have reproductive dysfunction as part of their pathologic spectrum. The box on p. 1768 provides an abbreviated list of the most common conditions and their basic reproductive consequences. As can be seen, all males with cystic fibrosis (CF) have bilateral absence of the vas deferens. It has recently been shown that at least 80% of patients with congenital bilateral absence of the vas deferens (a condition devoid of pulmonary and pancreatic disease) also carry mutations of the CF gene on chromosome 7. Therefore, this is a mild form of CF, with the only phenotypic manifestation being failure of proper vasal development and resultant sterility. Many other genetic syndromes, including Klinefelter's, Prader-Willi, Kallmann's, and Laurence-Moon-Bardet-Biedl, may affect spermatogenesis. Klinefelter's syndrome is the most common, occurring in 1 in 500 males. Infertility is not the chief complaint of many patients, since the reduction in libido and erectile capability secondary to low testosterone levels often first brings the patient to the attention of a physician.

### Malignancy

Testicular cancer not only leads to the loss of the affected testis (via radical orchiectomy), but is also frequently associated with reversible or irreversible impairment of spermatogenesis in the contralateral testis. Chemotherapy, radiation therapy, and retroperitoneal lymph node dissection may further impair spermatogenesis and ejaculation. Hodgkin's and non-Hodgkin's lymphomas, as well as any type of leukemia, are also associated with significant prechemotherapy and postchemotherapy decreases in spermatogenesis. Since the life expectancy of affected patients has improved, much attention has recently been focused on the reduction of chemotherapeutic gonadal toxicity while maintaining treatment efficacy. Cryopreservation should be offered before induction of chemotherapy in men desiring future fertility.

### Cryptorchidism

Seventy-four percent of patients with a history of unilateral prepubertal orchidopexy will have a normal semen analysis. If bilateral orchidopexy has been performed prepubertally, 30% of patients will have a normal semen analysis, and 39% will be azoospermic. In general, the undescended testis does not have the same overall potential for future sperm production as a normally descended gonad. With unilateral cryptorchidism, the contralateral, descended testis often has an abnormal level of spermatogenesis as well, further compounding the problem.

### Retroperitoneal/pelvic surgery

Retroperitoneal lymph node dissection as treatment for metastatic testicular carcinoma may cause damage to the sympathetic nerve pathways necessary for seminal emission. Pelvic surgery may remove part of or scar the genital tract, including the vas deferens and seminal vesicles. Prostate or bladder neck surgery may lead to retrograde ejaculation or iatrogenic occlusion of the ejaculatory ducts.

### Inguinal hernia repair/scrotal surgery

The inguinal canal contains the vas deferens. During a hernia repair, the vas deferens may be inadvertently damaged. It may happen at any age but is probably more likely to occur during childhood because of the delicate nature of the vas at this time. The testis is surrounded on its anterior surface by the fluid-filled tunica vaginalis. Infection, trauma, and tumor may cause an increased amount of fluid to collect in this potential space, leading to a clinical hydrocele. Hydrocele repair and testicular exploration for trauma may result in damage and obstruction to the epididymis or vas deferens.

## PHYSICAL EXAMINATION OF THE MALE REPRODUCTIVE SYSTEM

The physical examination should be performed in a warm room with the patient as relaxed as possible. Body habitus must be evaluated; inadequate virilization, female fat distribution, and gynecomastia are evidence of hormonal abnormalities. The examination focuses on the genitals. The penis must be observed for length and abnormal curvature; either abnormality may make intromission difficult. If the patient has severe hypospadias (penile meatus not situated on apical glans penis), the seminal fluid may not be directed toward the cervix during ejaculation. A postcoital test can screen for this.

The average testis measures 4.5 cm in length by 2.5 cm in width with an average volume of 19 ml. It has a firm consistency, similar to the thenar eminence. Ninety percent of the volume of the testis consists of the seminiferous epithelium, while only a small percentage is represented by the interstitium. Small, soft testes are a consequence of an atrophic seminiferous epithelium and predict spermatogenic deficiency. Small, firm testes may also be indicative of testicular failure in certain conditions (e.g., Klinefelter's syndrome).

The epididymis begins at the posterolateral upper pole of the testis. It courses inferiorly and gradually thickens and straightens to become the vas deferens. In general, the epididymis is soft and regular in consistency. If obstructed, it will become firm, irregular, and nodular (as can often be felt after a vasectomy). A spermatocele is a discrete, spheric nodule palpated at the upper pole of the epididymis and represents a cystic, dilated efferent duct. Unless necessary, spermatocelectomy should be delayed until procreation is no longer an issue, since the epididymis may become inadvertently obstructed.

The vas deferens can be palpated from the lower pole of the testis as the continuation of the epididymis up to the external inguinal ring. It is a firm, cordlike structure that is typically quite obvious and easy to feel. In patients with low-volume azoospermia, it is important to rule out congenital bilateral absence of the vas deferens by physical examination.

The spermatic cord should be palpated while the patient is standing to appreciate best the presence of a varicocele. A varicocele is present when the delicate group of veins

### Genetic syndromes affecting male fertility

**Y chromosomal disorders**

- Structural Y chromosomal disorders
  - XX Male (46,XX)
  - Mixed gonadal dysgenesis (45,X/46,XY)
  - XY azoospermic male
- Specific gene defects affecting azoospermia factor gene (AZF)

**Disorders of chromosomal sex**

- Klinefelter's syndrome (47,XXY or 46,XY/47,XXY)
- XYY male (47,XYY)
- Noonan's syndrome (46,XY)

**Specific gene mutations with direct reproductive consequences**

- Kallmann's syndrome
- Bioinactive luteinizing hormone
- Deficiencies of androgen synthesis
- Deficiency of 5$\alpha$-reductase
- Androgen receptor deficiency

**Specific gene mutations with indirect reproductive consequences**

- Cystic fibrosis/congenital bilateral absence of vas deferens
- Sickle cell disease
- $\beta$-Thalassemia

**Nonspecific genetic syndromes associated with male infertility**

- Prune-belly syndrome (Eagle-Barrett syndrome)
- Bladder exstrophy/epispadias complex
- Myelodysplasia
- Myotonic dystrophy
- Prader-Willi syndrome
- Laurence-Moon-Bardet-Biedl syndrome

draining the testis known as the pampiniform plexus becomes dilated. Varicoceles are graded on a scale of 1 to 3. Grade 3 varicoceles are visible without palpation. Grade 2 varicoceles are palpable without a Valsalva maneuver. Grade 1 varicoceles require a Valsalva maneuver to become palpable.

Some common abnormalities found on physical examination include the following. Abnormally small testes indicate reduced or absent spermatogenesis. Firm epididymides often signal a more distal obstruction. A tender epididymis may be seen with epididymitis. Absent vasa, either unilaterally or bilaterally, may be a finding. Bilateral vasal aplasia indicates a high probability of cystic fibrosis, and genetic evaluation is mandatory. Because of the embryologic linkage of renal and genital development, it is necessary to define renal anatomy in cases of vasal agenesis, especially in unilateral cases. Varicoceles are found in up to 40% of men attending an infertility clinic and are often associated with deficiencies of sperm production and quality.

## PRELIMINARY LABORATORY EVALUATION

### Hormonal screening

Although primary endocrine problems are present in only a small percentage of infertility patients, FSH, testosterone, and prolactin are useful screening tests. Table 136-2 lists hormonal findings in pretesticular, testicular, and posttesticular causes. FSH is produced by the anterior pituitary in response to GnRH. As mentioned earlier, FSH acts on the Sertoli cells, which line the internal basement membranes of each seminiferous tubule and are necessary in supporting sperm production. The Sertoli cells produce inhibin, which, via a negative feedback mechanism, regulates FSH secretion. FSH is thus the best preliminary screening test in the diagnosis of primary testicular problems. A significant elevation in FSH (two to three times normal) is a strong predictor that a fundamental problem exists with the seminiferous epithelium. Testosterone is the primary male androgenic hormone. The vast majority of men with infertility will have normal testosterone levels and will be well virilized. Testosterone is produced by the interstitial Leydig cells, and high intratesticular levels of testosterone are required for proper spermatogenesis. Low testosterone levels may be found in either primary or secondary hypogonadal states. Hyperprolactinemia is a rare but reversible cause of male infertility. An assay for prolactin should be included as a screening test when the semen analysis reveals impaired sperm production.

### Semen analysis

The most important test in the evaluation of male infertility is the semen analysis. It is best if the semen analysis can be performed in a laboratory with significant expertise. The semen analysis is ideally collected in the office or laboratory setting and should be maintained at room temperature. Table 136-3 outlines normal values.

It must be emphasized that as long as there are some sperm, fertility is possible. The semen analysis is not an accurate predictor of pregnancy achievement but only a rough guide to a man's fertility potential. A normal volume is 1.5 to 5 ml per ejaculate. If abnormally low, an obstruction or abnormality of the seminal vesicles or ejaculatory ducts may be present. Transrectal ultrasonography can accurately image these structures and is performed if required. However, the most common etiology of a single, isolated low-ejaculate volume is collection error or a poor overall ejaculatory event. Multiple semen analyses may be required to differentiate these causes.

Sperm density correlates with rates of spontaneous fertility achievement. The lower limit of normal is 20 million spermatozoa/ml, although the average sperm count is 60 million/ml. Sperm motility is a measure of the percentage of sperm that are moving in a given sample (normal, 60% or greater). Forward progression characterizes how fast and how straight the motile sperm fraction is moving. Sperm morphology describes the shape of the sperm. Three systems typically are used: 1987 World Health Organization (normal, greater than 60%), 1992 World Health Organization (normal, greater than 30%), and Tygerberg strict criteria (normal, greater than 14%). The latter system correlates with the ability of the sperm to fertilize during in vitro fertilization.

Patients with azoospermia (no sperm in the ejaculate) are a complex subset of patients. If the semen volume is low and the patient is azoospermic, a bilateral ejaculatory duct obstruction, bilateral vasal agenesis, retrograde ejaculation, and a severe hypogonadotropic hypogonadal state constitute the most common underlying etiologies. Physical examination, transrectal ultrasonography, hormonal assays, and a postejaculate urine analysis are all that is necessary to differentiate accurately these possible etiologies of low-volume azoospermia. If the semen volume is normal, testicular failure, inguinal vasal obstruction, and epididymal occlusion are the three likely causes. Serum FSH often suggests primary testicular dysfunction if it is in the upper ranges of normal, or even higher, in this particular scenario. Testis biopsy is often

**Table 136-2.** Hormonal profiles of infertile men based on etiology

| Etiology | LH | Testosterone | FSH | Primary defect |
|---|---|---|---|---|
| Pretesticular failure (hypogonadotropic hypogonadism) | Decrease | Decrease | Decrease | Decreased GnRH |
| Testicular (hypergonadotropic) | Normal | Normal | Increase | Reduced spermatogenesis |
| Posttesticular failure (obstructive) | Normal | Normal | Normal | |

*LH,* Luteinizing hormone; *FSH,* follicle-stimulating hormone; *GnRH,* gonadotropin-releasing hormone.

**Table 136-3.** Semen analysis: minimal standards of adequacy

| Parameter | Value |
|---|---|
| On at least two occasions | |
| Ejaculate volume | 1.5-5.0 ml |
| Sperm density | >20 million/ml |
| Motility | >60% |
| Forward progression | >2 (scale 1-4) |
| Morphology | >60% normal |
| And | |
| No significant sperm agglutination | |
| No significant pyospermia | |
| No hyperviscosity | |

From Sigman M, Lipshultz LI, Howards SS: Evaluation of the subfertile male. In Lipshultz LI, Howards SS: *Infertility in the male,* St Louis, 1991, Mosby.

necessary to gain insight into the histology of the seminiferous epithelium.

Immunologic infertility can be screened through direct detection of antisperm antibodies bound to the sperm surface using one of many commercially available kits. Disruption of the blood-testis barrier via numerous mechanisms, such as vasectomy and testicular trauma, is often a clue in the history to the presence of antisperm antibodies. They may cause sperm agglutination within the seminal fluid, decrease motility of the sperm through cervical mucus, or decrease fertilization at the sperm/oocyte level. Serum sperm antibodies are not considered clinically relevant.

### Postcoital test

The postcoital test is performed midcycle, within 12 hours of the couple having intercourse. The quality of the cervical mucus is assessed, as well as the quantity of sperm and their motility within the mucus (normal, 5 to 10 motile sperm per high-power field). This test helps assess whether the sperm are mechanically reaching the cervix, their interaction with cervical mucus, and sperm's ultimate access to the upper reproductive tract via the cervix.

## TREATMENT OF MALE REPRODUCTIVE DYSFUNCTION

### Pretesticular

*Primary* hypogonadotropic hypogonadism is treated with replacement gonadotropin therapy. If pubertal maturation is all that is desired, human chorionic gonadotropin (hCG) may be administered. hCG has LH-like action and will stimulate intratesticular testosterone production, which will induce the phenotypic changes of puberty. If fertility is a concern, FSH must be added to stimulate Sertoli cell function and spermatogenesis. Human menopausal gonadotropin (hMG) has both LH and FSH activity and will provide for both androgenic and spermatogenic stimulation. It may take up to 1 year of continued therapy before spermatogenesis has leveled off at stable values. An alternative therapy in patients with pure hypothalamic dysfunction is pulsatile GnRH therapy. This will essentially replace the hypothalamus and stimulate pituitary elaboration of FSH and LH. *Secondary* hypogonadotropic hypogonadism may be caused by a large pituitary adenoma, and it is important to image the pituitary radiographically in these circumstances. *Relative* hypogonadotropic hypogonadism (gonadotropin secretion and sperm production are both low) may be treated with clomiphene citrate, which is a nonsteroidal antiestrogen. Clomiphene competitively binds at the hypothalamic level and decreases the feedback inhibition of estradiol. This eventually leads to increased LH and FSH secretion by the pituitary. Whether clomiphene citrate actually improves testicular function is a matter of debate, but it probably has a role in those patients who have relatively low endogenous output of FSH and LH.

### Posttesticular

There are many levels at which sperm flow may be obstructed. Obviously, the exact therapy depends on the exact site at which the obstruction occurs. Briefly described here are the options undertaken by the urologic surgeon once the preliminary evaluation has been completed.

***Epididymal obstruction.*** Epididymal obstruction may often be anticipated by the history and physical examination. Normal-volume azoospermia with adequate testicular size, firm epididymides on palpation, a history of prior epididymitis, and so forth all provide clues to the existence of bilateral epididymal disease. Microsurgical reconstruction aims at bypassing the occluded epididymal site and restoring sperm flow into the vas. This is accomplished by transecting the proximal vas deferens and microsurgically reattaching it to a single epididymal tubule above the site of damage (vasoepididymostomy). Patency rates subsequent to surgery by experienced microsurgeons average 60% to 70%, and pregnancy can be expected in 30% to 40% of couples.

***Unreconstructable or absent vasa.*** Patients may have spermatogenesis but may have no pathway to transport the sperm into the ejaculate. In patients with congenital bilateral absence of the vas deferens or several failed vasal anastomoses, sperm can be microscopically harvested from the epididymis or, if present, the vas deferens. This sperm is used in conjunction with advanced reproductive techniques, including in vitro fertilization and gamete intrafallopian transfer. The technology of gamete micromanipulation is also being employed. Individual sperm are selected with the aid of delicate micromanipulators and placed either into the perivitelline space or directly into the oocyte cytoplasm.

***Ejaculatory duct obstruction.*** The ejaculatory duct(s) may be obstructed either intrinsically (secondary to scarring or a stone) or extrinsically by a cyst impinging on their lumen. The obstruction may be either complete or partial, unilateral or bilateral. A partial obstruction may allow some sperm through, but usually in greatly reduced numbers with poor motility. In both complete and partial obstructions, the seminal fluid volume is decreased. Transrectal ultrasonography not only allows a definitive diagnosis to be made, but also provides an anatomic roadmap to direct the surgery accurately and precisely. Transurethral resection of the ejaculatory ducts themselves or of an obstructing prostatic cyst is highly successful in restoring proper egress of sperm and seminal fluid into the posterior urethra.

***Vasal occlusion/interruption.*** The vas deferens is intentionally interrupted during a vasectomy to prevent sperm flow into the ejaculate. When performed by experienced microsurgeons, vasectomy reversal is a highly successful procedure, and approximately 50% of all patients will easily achieve pregnancy within 1 to 1.5 years after surgery. There is no defined cutoff point at which surgery is no longer worthwhile, as once was thought. Patients with a vasectomy for many, many years can still achieve their goals if attention is paid to the performance of the proper type of reconstruction during the reversal (often a vasoepididymostomy is required). An inguinal occlusion of the vas from a prior hernia repair can be treated with vasovasostomy at the site of vasal interruption.

***Ejaculatory dysfunction.*** Ejaculation consists of three phases: emission, bladder neck closure, and antegrade propulsion of sperm. Ejaculatory dysfunction may be psychogenic, neurogenic, or structural. In the spinal cord–injured male, both penile vibratory stimulation (PVS) and rectal probe electroejaculation (RPE) are used to obtain semen. PVS depends on an intact ejaculatory reflex center as well as functional afferents from the penis to the cord and complete sympathetic efferents from T10-L2 to the seminal vesicles and vasal ampullae. By placing a vibratory unit on the glans penis, the stimulation will activate the ejaculatory reflex, resulting in a physiologically normal antegrade ejaculate. Once the semen is obtained, any of several therapies can be employed to achieve pregnancy; the exact stategy undertaken depends on the sperm density and motility of the specimen. If PVS fails, RPE invariably allows collection of semen. Through a low level of pulsatile current, RPE directly stimulates contraction of the smooth muscle in the walls of the seminal vesicles and vasal ampullae. With each contraction, their contents are discharged via the ejaculatory duct into the posterior urethra, where the seminal fluid is able to be retrieved. Based on the count and motility of the sperm, an appropriate combined therapy (intrauterine insemination, in vitro fertilization, etc.) will be instituted to help the couple achieve conception.

### Varicocele

Varicocele is defined as a tortuous and dilated scrotal spermatic venous complex. It is the most common reversible cause of male infertility. It occurs in approximately 15% of all men, but in up to 40% of men with infertility. The mechanism by which it causes infertility is unknown, although the most common hypothesis is that it increases testicular temperature. Correction of a varicocele results in significant improvement in semen parameters in 60% of men and an improvement in baseline pregnancy rates to approximately 30%.

Most testicular growth occurs during puberty. Adolescent varicoceles are frequently associated with testicular growth retardation, much or all of which has been shown to be reversible when the varicocele is corrected. Varicoceles also cause a progressive decrease in testicular function in postadolescent males. It is clear that varicoceles in boys with ipsilateral testicular atrophy should be corrected. We believe that all patients with large varicoceles should have their semen analysis followed or their varicocele corrected, especially those who will not be trying to initiate a pregnancy for a long time.

### Cryptorchidism

Cryptorchidism is present in approximately 0.8% of boys at age 1 year. By age 2, clearly demonstrable progressive histologic damage occurs if the testis is not brought into the scrotum. Approximately 71% of boys not treated with orchidopexy will have a subfertile semen analysis, as compared to the 88% of those treated before age 2 who have a normal semen analysis. Cryptorchid testes have a slightly increased risk of developing testicular carcinoma over a normally descended testis.

## SITUATIONS WARRANTING ACUTE INTERVENTION

### Epididymitis and epididymo-orchitis

Epididymo-orchitis may cause scarring of the epididymis, leading to partial or complete obstruction. The most common etiology in men under 35 is sexually transmitted disease. If this is a bilateral occurrence, or if the other side has a separate pathology, it may lead to azoospermia or severe oligospermia. Treatment of epididymitis must be prompt and aggressive and is aimed at overcoming the infection, decreasing the inflammatory response, and providing symptomatic relief. Broad-spectrum antibiotics, antiinflammatory drugs, scrotal supports, and warm baths must be started immediately.

Viral epididymo-orchitis (most commonly mumps) is a well-known cause of postpubertal testicular atrophy and possible infertility. From 30% to 50% of affected testes will demonstrate some degree of atrophy. From 7% to 13% of patients will show impaired fertility, although azoospermia occurs infrequently. Immediate treatment with antiinflammatory agents, scrotal support, and warm baths should be instituted. Recent studies documenting treatment of mumps orchitis with interferon, by shortening the time course of inflammation and lessening the sequelae, have looked promising. Infectious disease consultation should be obtained in any man with a viral orchitis (especially bilateral) to consider institution of immunotherapy.

### Testicular torsion

The testis and cord may become twisted, thus cutting off the blood supply of the testis and leading to ischemia. This occurs most often around puberty. If detorsion does not occur within approximately 6 hours, ischemia leads to unilateral testicular infarction, resulting in loss of half the sperm-producing potential. However, the continued presence of an infarcted testis may further decrease future spermatogenesis in the remaining testis. This is probably immunologically mediated. All acute testicular pain must be treated as an emergency. Immediate urologic evaluation should be obtained.

## MEDICAL-SURGICAL INSULTS

Chemotherapy or radiation therapy may cause a transient or irreversible decrease or loss of fertility. Retroperitoneal lymph node dissection may cause damage to sympathetic nerves responsible for seminal emission and thus lead to anejaculation. Significant pelvic surgery may cause mechanical or nervous system damage, preventing proper egress of sperm. A therapy's impact on fertility must be actively considered when choosing it and in deciding how to administer it. Before any of these procedures is performed, the patient wanting to preserve his fertility must be counseled to cryopreserve his sperm. With the development of extremely sophisticated, advanced reproductive techniques, all patients should have specimens preserved no matter how poor their semen quality.

## SUMMARY

Infertility affects 15% of couples. A male factor is involved 50% of the time. Increased awareness of the male contribution to infertility has appropriately prompted earlier and more frequent questions to patients' primary physicians. Primary care physicians are in the unique position to anticipate problems from the patient's history and to discover abnormalities on physical examination (cryptorchidism, varicocele), allowing for preventive treatment. Prompt response to acute problems may help salvage a patient's fertility. This key role should not be underestimated by patients, specialists, or the primary care physicians themselves.

## BIBLIOGRAPHY

Acosta AA et al: Assisted reproduction in the diagnosis and treatment of the male factor, *Obstet Gynecol Surv* 44:1, 1989.

Allen NC et al: Intrauterine insemination: a critical review, *Fertil Steril* 44:569, 1985.

Chevall MJ, Purcell MH: Deterioration of semen parameters over time in men with untreated varicocele: evidence of progressive testicular damage, *Fertil Steril* 57:174, 1992.

Dhabuwala CB, Hamid S, Moghissi KS: Clinical versus subclinical varicocele: improvement in fertility after varicocelectomy, *Fertil Steril* 57:854, 1992.

Evans HJ, Fletcher J, Torrance M: Sperm abnormalities and cigarette smoking, *Lancet* 1:627, 1981.

Jenkins AD, Turner TT, Howards SS: Physiology of the male reproductive system, *Urol Clin North Am* 5:437, 1978.

Kass EJ, Belman AB: Reversal of testicular growth failure by varicocele ligation, *J Urol* 137:475, 1987.

Kruger TF et al: New method of evaluating sperm morphology with predictive value for in vitro fertilization, *Urology* 30:248, 1987.

Lipshultz LI, Corriere JN: Progressive testicular atrophy in the varicocele patient, *J Urol* 117:175, 1977.

Lipshultz LI, Howards SS: *Infertility in the male,* St Louis, 1991, Mosby.

Oates RD, Lipshultz LI: Azoospermia. In Resnick MI, Kursh ED, editors: *Current therapy in genitourinary surgery,* St Louis, 1992, Mosby.

Oates RD, Staskin DR: Penile vibratory stimulation in the spinal cord injured male to induce ejaculation, *J Urol* 143:344, 1990.

CHAPTER

# 137 Bladder Dysfunction and Urinary Incontinence

**Roger R. Dmochowski**
**Gary E. Leach**

Bladder dysfunction and urinary incontinence are significant health concerns, leading to substantial cost for the health care system. These entities are also associated with significant morbidity arising from infectious complications, physical debility, and psychologic stress (Fig. 137-1). The personal impact of bladder dysfunction can lead to complete social isolation and physical inactivity in an effort by the individual to compensate for these problems.

In the community population the rate of incontinence approximates 15% to 30% of those over 60 years old (U.S. National Institutes of Health). This incidence increases to approximately 50% of institutionalized elderly patients. Approximately 50% of patients experience incontinence in the acute period after cerebrovascular accident (CVA), and 14% to 20% of these patients will continue to manifest incontinence chronically. It is estimated that more than 10 million people are incontinent in the United States. The cost of caring for this group exceeded $10 billion in 1989.

Complicating the significant incidence of bladder dysfunction and incontinence are the most common treatment modalities used to deal with them. Indwelling catheters and external protective garments (diapers) not only lead to chronic infectious risks, but also are a source of urinary tract decompensation and destruction (catheters) and skin breakdown and decubiti (diapers).

Because most patients still do not complain of this incontinence, or are not asked, perhaps the greatest single problem with bladder dysfunction is the recognition of its existence so that appropriate diagnostic evaluation and therapeutic intervention may be initiated.

## NORMAL PHYSIOLOGY

An intricate control system regulates bladder function. Normal bladder physiology involves both a storage phase and an evacuation phase, which must be coordinated. Both these phases depend on interaction between the bladder and the sphincteric mechanism, which allows for low-pressure storage and the maintenance of continence. Subsequent voiding is accomplished by detrusor muscle contraction accompanied by essentially simultaneous relaxation of the sphincteric mechanism.

The detrusor is composed of smooth muscle. The sphincteric mechanism has two well-defined components in the male. The bladder neck and proximal prostatic urethra form the internal sphincteric mechanism, which is a smooth muscular structure. The external sphincter is formed by skeletal muscle contributions from the pelvic floor and a second component arising from the urethral wall. A third component of the distal mechanism is an intrinsic urethral, smooth muscular component.

In females the continence mechanism is formed predominantly by the bladder neck and proximal urethra. This mechanism is further augmented by the urethral submucosal tissues, which serve to create a "seal" effect in the urethra, thus potentiating continence. Estrogens enhance this seal by mechanisms that may involve maintenance and proliferation of the urethral submucosal vascular plexus. Estrogens further enhance this seal by promoting the function of the adrenergic receptor population that exists in this area and that is crucial to urethral mucosal closure. Failure of this seal results in intrinsic sphincteric deficiency or type III urinary incontinence.

The motor nucleus controlling detrusor function is located in the sacral spinal cord between the S2 and S4

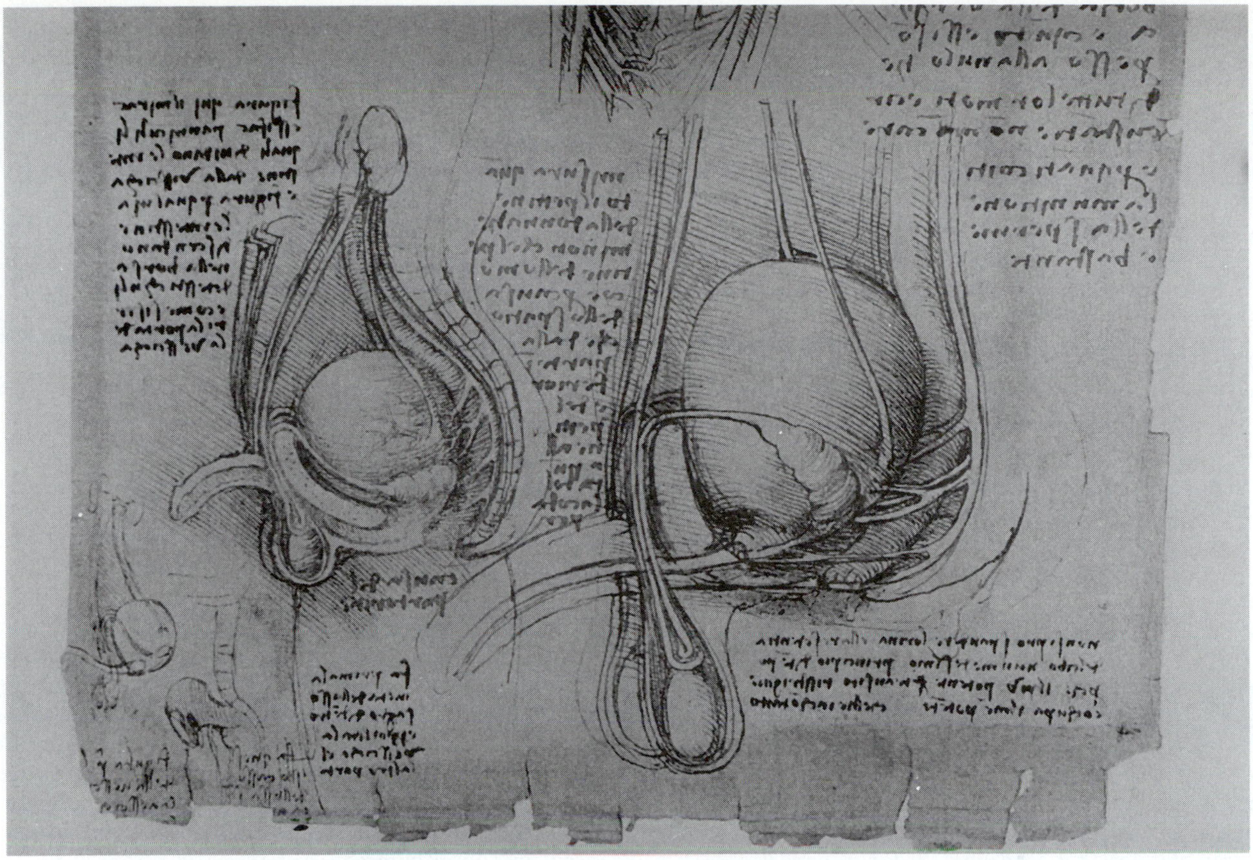

**Fig. 137-1.** Anatomic sketches of the genitourinary system. (*Quaderni Anatomica,* Leonardo Da Vinci, 1616.) (From the Collection of the Library of Congress.)

cord levels (spinal column levels T11 to L1). Parasympathetic afferents from this motor nucleus course in the hypogastric nerve to synapse with ganglia located within the detrusor wall. Postganglionic afferents carry impulses that cause detrusor excitation and bladder contraction. Receptors in the detrusor muscle are predominantly parasympathetic in mediation, with primarily muscarinic and to a lesser extent cholinergic receptors being identified. These receptors mediate detrusor contraction. Also present within the detrusor muscle are adrenergic receptors that are responsible for muscular relaxation. Efferent fibers transmit impulses from the bladder back to the detrusor nucleus. These impulses convey information, including degree of bladder distention. In the bladder base and proximal urethra, the predominant type of neuroreceptor is α-adrenergic. These receptors mediate contraction and are intimately involved in the continence mechanism.

The nucleus controlling external sphincteric function is also located in the sacral cord. Extensive neural interconnections between these two cell groupings provide continual interplay between these entities and allow coordination between them.

The sacral cord is tonically inhibited by descending impulses carried by the spinal cord that arise in the pontine mesencephalic reticular formation located in the midbrain. A specialized neural grouping that governs voiding is located in this area of the pons. This micturition center, in turn, receives descending input from the cerebral cortex, cerebellum, and limbic system.

When the detrusor reaches capacity, the higher centers cease to inhibit the sacral cord. Through descending paths, the pons potentiates the initiation of voiding and the coordination of detrusor contraction and sphincteric relaxation. Voiding is completed by a detrusor contraction, which is facilitated until emptying is complete (Fig. 137-2).

## PATHOPHYSIOLOGY

Dysfunction of any element of this mechanism will produce some loss of regulation of voiding and may result in urinary incontinence or retention. Interruption by pathology above the midbrain center will result in loss of inhibitory influences on the midbrain. This may be reflected in the appearance of uninhibited bladder contractile activity, causing urgency symptomatology and urgency incontinence. Two notable exceptions to this statement should be considered. CVAs may rarely result in retention, but only in the acute phase. Parkinson's disease often results in uninhibited and poorly sustained detrusor contractile activity. However, this activity is usually accompanied by sphincteric dysfunction, which results in poor coordination between detrusor and sphincter (sphincter bradykinesia).

Injury or disease of the midbrain or descending spinal pathways results in loss of coordination between bladder and urinary sphincter, as well as loss of descending inhibitory input on the detrusor nucleus. The resulting clinical picture is that of uninhibited detrusor contractile

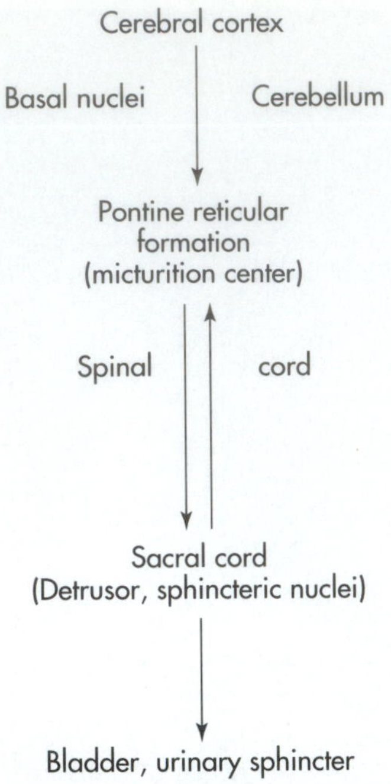


**Fig. 137-2.** Diagrammatic representation of neural pathways involved with detrusor muscle function.

activity associated with a nonrelaxing urinary sphincter. The end result of this process is a high-pressure, poorly emptying bladder that is prone to decompensation. This high pressure is subsequently transmitted to the kidneys, resulting in hydronephrosis and eventual azotemia. The most common setting for this scenario is a spinal cord injury (trauma or infection), tumor, or vascular event.

Injury or disease of the sacral cord, or peripheral neural projections from this level, results in ablation of detrusor and sphincteric nuclei function. Initially, this is manifested by an areflexic (noncontractile) detrusor. Low-pressure, large-volume urinary retention results. With chronicity, however, the characteristics of the bladder wall that produce a low-pressure, high-capacity reservoir (compliance) are altered. This alteration results in part from the loss of innervation and also from changes in the composition (increasing fibrosis) of the bladder wall. Higher pressures ensue, which may be deleterious to renal function and may also produce spontaneous urine loss.

In the discussion of any pathologic process involving the nervous system, it is important to note that the resultant clinical picture infrequently reflects a "complete" lesion. More often, an incomplete neural lesion results. Frequently, some function is preserved in the absence of other functions, which cannot be predicted by the level or degree of injury. Another aspect of importance that further obfuscates the clinical presentation is that neural lesions also may be present at multiple levels.

## EVALUATION

Data regarding an individual's bladder dysfunction should be gathered in an orderly manner so as to delineate all appropriate historic and physical examination elements crucial to establishing a diagnosis and treatment plan. These elements are supplemented by urinary evaluation and further urologic tests as indicated.

### Etiologic classification of incontinence

- Failure to store
  - Bladder dysfunction
  - Outlet dysfunction
- Failure to empty
  - Bladder dysfunction
  - Outlet dysfunction
- Combination of failure to empty and failure to store

### History

The patient history should include notation of the duration of symptoms. Whether the patient has experienced symptoms since childhood or only relatively recently yields information regarding the potential for congenital disorders. Symptoms noted only recently may indicate a potentially reversible cause of bladder dysfunction or incontinence. The presence of irritative symptoms, including nocturia and frequency, is recorded. Dysuria or pain with bladder filling may indicate infectious or inflammatory conditions. Obstructive symptoms include hesitancy, straining to void, intermittency of stream, and incomplete emptying. These symptoms may further complicate overflow incontinence. The presence of intercurrent urinary tract infection or gross hematuria is established. Diurnal and nocturnal frequency should be recorded. The volume of fluid ingested also should be evaluated. If necessary, patient home logs of intake and output should be kept to evaluate the appropriateness of fluid ingestion.

Incontinence should be classified to better define possible etiologies. The failure to store urine or the failure to empty provides an easily reproducible method by which to categorize bladder function. This system conceptualizes lower urinary tract function as depending on the interaction of bladder and bladder outlet (sphincter) for normal urine storage and expulsion. A defect in either bladder or sphincteric function can result in either failure to store or failure to empty. Mixed bladder and sphincteric dysfunction may also be responsible for the clinical scenario (see the box above).

Incontinence may be considered as fixed or transient. Transient incontinence usually has a definable, sudden onset and often has a discrete cause. A simple mnemonic summarizes the differential diagnosis of transient incontinence (see the box on p. 1775).

Fixed or established causes of incontinence may be subdivided into several broad headings with differential considerations on the basis of patient gender. These etiologic possibilities may affect either storage, emptying, or both functions of the lower urinary tract (see the box on p. 1775).

*Urge incontinence* is characterized by the patient experiencing a strong desire to void and doing so precipitously without the ability to suppress the urinary loss. This type of incontinence results from overactivity of the detrusor, resulting in uncontrollable bladder contractions. The patient may experience this loss related to a particular activity or exposure or may note no inciting etiology. This is the most common type of incontinence

### Etiologies for transient urinary incontinence: "diapers" mnemonic

**D**rugs: hypnotics, sedatives, anticholinergic agents, diuretics, adrenergic agents
**D**elirium: or altered mental status
**I**nfection
**A**trophy: of vagina or urethra
**P**sychologic disorder: functional depression
**E**ndocrine: hyperglycemia or hypercalcemia
**R**estricted mobility
**S**tool impaction

From Resnick NM, Yalla SV, Laurino E: The pathophysiology of urinary incontinence among institutionalized elderly persons, *N Engl J Med* 320:1, 1989.

noted in elderly populations. Urge incontinence frequently complicates central disorders such as Parkinson disease, Alzheimer disease, CVA, and brain tumor. Urge incontinence is also noted with local bladder disorders, such as outlet obstruction, carcinoma in situ, and infection.

*Reflex incontinence* is another category of incontinence related to urge incontinence. This type of incontinence is manifested by precipitous loss of urine with no sense of urgency. This category is most often noted in patients with suprasacral spinal cord lesions, where midbrain inhibitory influences are ablated. Failure of the storage component of bladder function ensues.

*Overflow incontinence* is caused by chronic retention of urine with small volumes being frequently voided. Overflow incontinence may result from detrusor hypocontractility, as seen in tabes dorsalis, diabetes mellitus, or vitamin $B_{12}$ deficiency. Overflow incontinence may also result from bladder outlet obstruction, caused by prostatic or urethral pathology, with subsequent bladder decompensation.

*Continuous incontinence* implies total and unabated leakage of urine, unrelated to activity. This situation is identified when a fistula of the urinary tract is present. The most common etiology for urinary tract fistula in a woman is prior hysterectomy.

*Stress incontinence* is manifested by urinary loss with physical activity or sudden increases in abdominal pressure, as encountered with coughing or lifting. This type of incontinence arises from a deficiency of the bladder outlet resulting either from hypermobility of the urethra and bladder neck in women or from intrinsic damage in either sex.

A mixed category of incontinence also should be considered because in many cases, especially those noted in elderly persons, more than one type of incontinence is present (see the box at right). An example of this situation arises in women with stress urinary incontinence. In this group of patients, a significant incidence of coexistent urge incontinence is identified, which may confuse the presenting symptomatic complaints. The need for and use of protective garments should be established.

Symptomatic history, although important in establishing the magnitude and extent of the condition, is often inaccurate in predicting the ultimate bladder or sphincter

### Types of incontinence

**Female**

***Failure to store***

- Bladder dysfunction
  - Detrusor instability/detrusor hyperreflexia
  - Decreased bladder compliance
  - Fistula
  - Urgency-related bladder decompensation
- Outlet dysfunction
  - "Typical" stress incontinence (anatomic urethral hypermobility)
  - Intrinsic sphincteric deficiency

***Failure to empty***

- Bladder dysfunction
  - Detrusor decompensation
  - Bladder denervation, resulting in absent or poorly sustained contraction
- Outlet dysfunction
  - Neurogenic sphincter dysfunction
  - Iatrogenic urethral obstruction

***Combined***

- Detrusor instability with poorly sustained contraction

**Male**

***Failure to store***

- Bladder dysfunction
  - Detrusor instability/Detrusor hyperreflexia alone
  - Detrusor instability secondary to outlet obstruction
  - Decreased bladder compliance
  - Bladder decompensation with overflow incontinence
- Outlet dysfunction
  - Stress urinary incontinence
    - Iatrogenic (after prostatectomy)
    - Neurogenic denervation

***Failure to empty***

- Bladder dysfunction
  - Bladder decompensation
  - Bladder denervation
- Outlet dysfunction
  - Benign prostatic hyperplasia with obstruction
  - Neurogenic sphincter dysfunction

***Combined***

- Detrusor hyperreflexia with poorly sustained contraction
  - DHIC (detrusor hyperreflexia with impaired contractility)
  - Parkinson disease
  - CVA (cerebrovascular accident)

dysfunction defined by more involved testing. However, in institutionalized elderly patients, simple algorithms based on patient symptoms and bedside assessment have been reported to have a diagnostic accuracy of greater than 80% when verified by urodynamic testing.

Significant neurologic symptoms are also important in the evaluation of urinary tract dysfunction. Prior cranial or spinal surgical procedures should be ascertained. Symptoms of lower extremity motor or sensory deficit are significant. Diplopia, vertigo, and gait disturbance indicate central neurologic pathology, including multiple sclerosis

(MS) and neoplasm. Voiding dysfunction associated with neurologic abnormalities noted on a screening examination may be the first indication of MS. Perineal or genital anesthesia associated with impotence indicates involvement of the cauda equina and interruption of the sacral nerves (S2 to S4) or their roots. Fecal incontinence or chronic constipation further indicates neural pathology, related either to specific nervous system lesions or to more global systemic processes such as diabetes mellitus. Any recent or chronic change in mentation or sensorium could indicate dementia, CVA, or other demyelinating disease. All will impact bladder dysfunction.

Other components of the medical history are also essential. The presence of systemic diseases such as diabetes mellitus or autonomic neuropathy should be noted. A history of cancer and therapies rendered for malignancy, including radiotherapy and chemotherapy, can give important diagnostic clues regarding metastases or injury resulting from therapy. Renal disorders may lead to neuropathy or bladder dysfunction related to increased urine production resulting from concentration defects. In women, prior gynecologic and obstetric history is crucial. Hysterectomy can cause detrusor denervation when performed for uterine or cervical carcinoma. Prior therapy for endometriosis indicates the potential for recurrent disease and associated symptoms. If the patient is perimenopausal or postmenopausal, relative lack of estrogenic supplementation can lead to vaginal atrophy and susceptibility to urinary tract infection and incontinence.

Previous surgical history is extremely important. As noted, prior neurosurgical procedures involving the back or cranium can directly contribute to bladder dysfunction. Any prior urologic or gynecologic procedure may also contribute to current symptoms.

Elucidation of the patient's current drug regimen is extremely important. Medications in many categories affect the bladder and voiding function. Antihypertensive agents, including sympatholytics, ganglionic blocking agents, and calcium channel blockers, all affect bladder physiology. $\alpha$-Adrenergic antagonists may worsen preexisting stress urinary incontinence in women. Tranquilizing agents and psychotropic drugs can result in retention because of decreased appreciation of bladder filling or parasympatholytic effects. Similarly, many medications used in the therapy of Parkinson disease can worsen bladder function as a result of anticholinergic side effects. Decongestants, as a result of sympathomimetic side effects, can exacerbate borderline voiding in men with bladder outlet obstruction due to benign prostatic hyperplasia. The recent addition or change of diuretic medication can result in substantial urinary volume increases and decompensation of a borderline obstructive situation. Opiates, including antidiarrheal agents, may inhibit detrusor contraction. Antiarrhythmic agents, such as disopyramide, may also have a negative impact on detrusor contraction. Not only should the drug and dose be noted, but also any possible relationship to the onset of the current symptoms.

### Physical examination

Physical examination includes a general examination with special attention to the genitourinary system. Blood pressure evaluation should be included.

Inspection of the back should be performed to identify overt spinal deformity such as scoliosis. Attention to the base of the spine should exclude the identification of any sacral skin discoloration or tufts of hair as well as any overt skin deformity such as a pit. These stigmata indicate the presence of spinal dysraphism and the possibility of a coexistent neurogenic bladder. The sacrum should be palpated to ensure bony integrity.

Abdominal examination should include palpation of the flanks for a mass or tenderness. The suprapubic area is evaluated for pain, and an attempt to palpate and percuss the bladder is made to identify distention.

Examination of the genitalia often indicates the presence of longstanding incontinence, with skin irritation and fungal infestation easily identifiable. Rectal examination reveals not only mucosal evaluation, but also the presence and degree of resting and augmented sphincter tone. The size and consistency of the prostate gland are evaluated at this time. The covert presence of prostatic carcinoma can be manifested by symptomatic voiding dysfunction.

Pelvic examination must be performed to evaluate the adnexal structures for mass or tenderness. Speculum examination of the vaginal vault may reveal vulvar or cervical malignancy. The presence of atrophy of the epithelial lining of the vagina is often present in postmenopausal women. Also, the presence of significant pelvic prolapse (cystocele, rectocele, uterine prolapse, vault descent) should be identified. Pelvic examination should be performed in both the supine and the standing positions to elucidate better the degree of uterine prolapse (Fig. 137-3). This prolapse may be significantly underestimated if examination is only performed while the female patient is supine. Significant bladder prolapse may result in hydronephrosis because of traction on the bladder base. Speculum examination of the vagina will document other forms of vaginal prolapse. A cystocele can be identified as a protrusion of the anterior vaginal wall that is accentuated when the patient strains. The coexistence of urinary loss associated with Valsalva maneuvers or coughing should also be identified. A cystocele represents prolapse of the bladder base and proximal urethra and is frequently seen as a component of the hypermobility associated with uncomplicated stress urinary incontinence (Fig. 137-4). This defect arises from weakness of the supporting (pubocervical) fascia of the bladder base.

A rectocele can be identified as a posterior vaginal wall protrusion composed of the rectum, which can also be accentuated by the Valsalva maneuver (Fig. 137-5). This form of prolapse arises from a defect in the pelvic floor (pubococcygeus muscles) allowing anterior "herniation" of the rectum. An enterocele represents a defect at the vaginal apex usually seen after hysterectomy. This entity contains peritoneal contents.

If a woman has previously undergone hysterectomy, the entire vaginal vault may prolapse to or through the introitus as a result of surgical damage to the supporting structures of the upper vagina (uterosacral ligaments).

Evaluation of the sacral cord can be enhanced further by eliciting the bulbocavernosus reflex (BCR), which reflects the integrity of the S2 to S4 levels of the cord. Compression of the glans penis (male) or mons pubic/clitoris (female) will produce anal sphincter contraction if the sacral cord is intact. Approximately 30% of neuro-

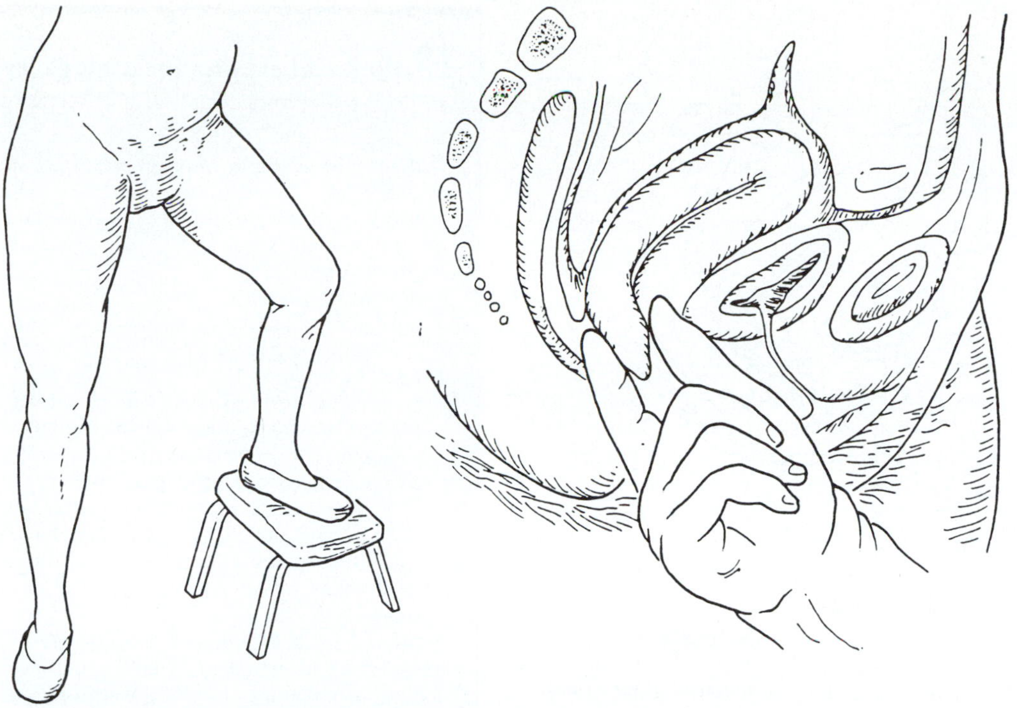

**Fig. 137-3.** Vaginal examination performed in the standing position to evaluate degree of uterine prolapse. (From Weber C et al, editors: *Reconstructive urology,* Cambridge, Mass, 1993, Blackwell.)

logically normal women and 5% of normal men will not exhibit this reflex. The sacral dermatomes in the perianal area (S2, S3) should be tested for anesthesia or diminished sensation.

Neurologic examination is crucial to the initial patient evaluation. Mental status should be documented. Gait and balance are observed. Gross abnormalities of the cranial nerves and upper extremity function can yield information regarding systemic neurologic disease. Reflex testing of the knee (L2, L3) and ankle (L5, S1) is performed. The presence of Babinski's reflexes and clonus indicating upper motor neuron disease is also identified. Sensory evaluation of the lower extremities for fine touch, pinprick, vibratory, and positional sensation is performed. Gross motor weakness of the lower extremities is documented.

Initial examination includes an assessment of postvoiding residual urine volume. Difficulty in passing a small urethral catheter for this purpose may indicate the presence of urethral stricture, prostatic enlargement, or other abnormality. The presence of overflow incontinence or large volumes of retained urine can be a significant and often overlooked etiology to the presenting symptom complex, especially in the patient with urge incontinence.

## Laboratory evaluation

Urinary examination includes urinalysis, culture, and voided cytology. Microscopic inspection of the urine will reveal hematuria, pyuria, or bacteriuria, which may coexist with pathology of the urinary system. Urinary tract infection may present with urgency or urge incontinence as the primary symptom. Voided urine cytology will identify malignant cells reflective of transitional carcinoma, which symptomatically can cause urgency and frequency.

Hematologic evaluation includes a serum creatinine to estimate renal function. Evaluation of serum glucose and calcium may be indicated in patients with large urine volumes. Other testing is determined on the basis of any specific disease entity that is identified.

## Radiographic evaluation

Radiographic evaluation should be tailored according to symptomatology. Plain films of the abdomen (KUB) will give information regarding soft tissues and any radiopaque urinary tract calculous disease. This radiograph is useful if the patient has had a history of prior stones and or has symptoms suggestive of this diagnosis. Ultrasound of the kidneys and abdomen is particularly useful in identifying hydronephrosis, calculous disease, and soft tissue pathology of the kidneys (tumor, abscess, medical renal disease). Renal ultrasound is indicated in the presence of azotemia to rule out any obstructive component. It is also indicated in the evaluation of neurogenic dysfunction of the bladder as a baseline study for longitudinal follow-up of ongoing therapy.

Further testing is predicated on diagnostic suspicions and often occurs after urologic referral. Criteria for referral have been established. This simplified system uses six categories to delineate factors that may indicate the presence of complicated urologic disease. These criteria arise from data easily obtainable from history, physical examination, and simple diagnostic tests (see the box on p. 1778).

Further radiographic imaging of the urinary tract may include an intravenous urogram (IVU) to define urinary tract anatomy or to evaluate hematuria. Voiding cystourethrography (VCUG) is selectively performed to identify

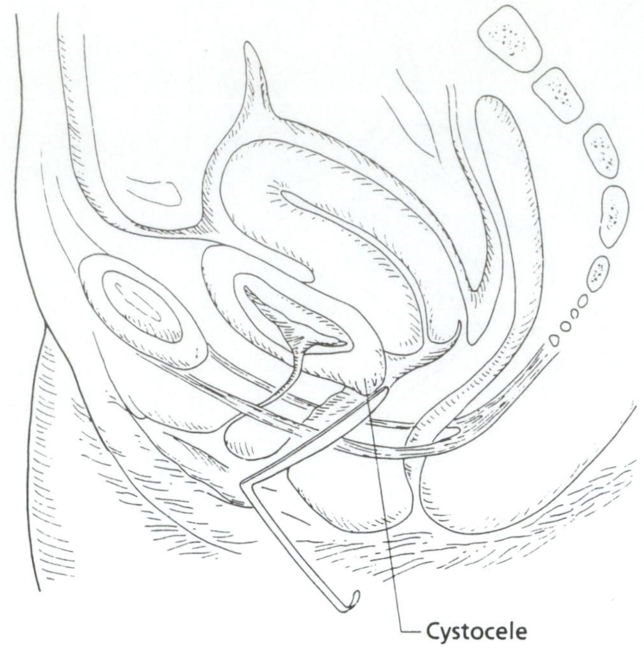


**Fig. 137-4.** Sagittal view of speculum-assisted vaginal examination showing location of a cystocele. (From Weber C et al, editors: *Reconstructive urology,* Cambridge, Mass, 1993, Blackwell.)

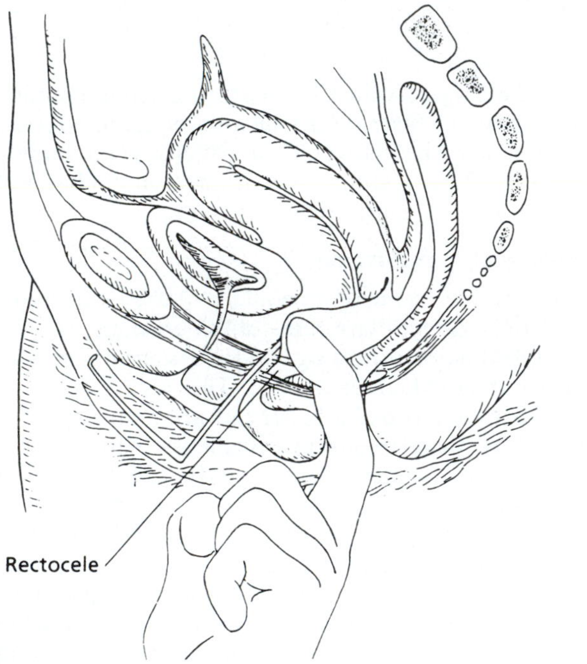


**Fig. 137-5.** Sagittal view of vaginal examination showing rectocele location. Note examiner's finger demonstrating defect. (From Weber C et al, editors: *Reconstructive urology,* Cambridge, Mass, 1993, Blackwell.)

### Referral criteria for urologic evaluation

History
- History of pelvic or lower urinary tract surgery within 6 months
- Rapid recurrence of urinary tract infection after appropriate therapy

Physical examination
- Significant pelvic prolapse
- Suspicion of prostatic carcinoma or significant enlargement of the prostate

Diagnostic tests
- Postvoiding residual urine volume greater than 100 ml
- Marked urinary hesitancy or intermittency of urine stream
- Symptomatic stress urinary incontinence in a woman who is a candidate for surgery when attempts at pharmacologic and behavioral therapy have failed
- Symptomatic stress incontinence in a man
- Obstruction to the passage of a 14 Fr. urinary catheter

Urinalysis
- Microhematuria without bacteriuria or pyuria

Lack of diagnostic certainty after initial evaluation

Failure of a therapeutic trial for urge or stress incontinence to have a response

From Ouslander J et al: Prospective evaluation of an assessment strategy for geriatric urinary incontinence, *J Am Geriatr Soc* 37:715, 1989.

vesicoureteral reflux, the presence and degree of cystocele in the standing position, postvoiding residual, and any urethral abnormality.

## Urodynamic evaluation

Bladder storage function is evaluated by cystometrogram. Cystometry may be modified in several ways. The bedside cystometrogram is the most basic form of cystometry. This involves the insertion of a 12 or 14 Fr. urinary catheter into the bladder. A 50 ml syringe, without the piston, is then attached to the end of the catheter. Sterile water is poured into the syringe in 50 ml aliquots while the syringe is held 15 cm above the symphysis pubis. Filling is continued until the column of water in the syringe rises, indicating a bladder contraction. The study is also terminated in the presence of patient discomfort or an infused volume greater than 500 ml (Fig. 137-6).

More formal cystometry involves multichannel recording of bladder and rectal pressures. The purpose of this study is to identify the compliance (volume-related pressure changes) of the bladder. Fluid is instilled through a urethral catheter at a constant rate with continuous pressure monitoring. During recording, the patient's first urgency to urinate is identified, as is the sensation of bladder fullness. Failure to store urine appropriately is identified during this stage of the study. The presence of detrusor contractions that occur involuntarily during filling are noted. If this type of activity is noted, the contractions are referred to as *detrusor instability* (in the absence of overt neurogenic disease) or *detrusor hyperreflexia* (in the presence of nervous system pathology) (Fig. 137-7). Carbon dioxide has also been used as the infusant for cystometry. However, gas cystometry is difficult to interpret and prone to artifact. Findings are also not as reproducible as with water cystometry.

Failure to store urine on the basis of outlet dysfunction is also evaluated. During this phase of the study, the patient is asked to perform Valsalva and stress maneuvers, which may identify stress incontinence. Failure to store urine as a result of combined defects in bladder storage and

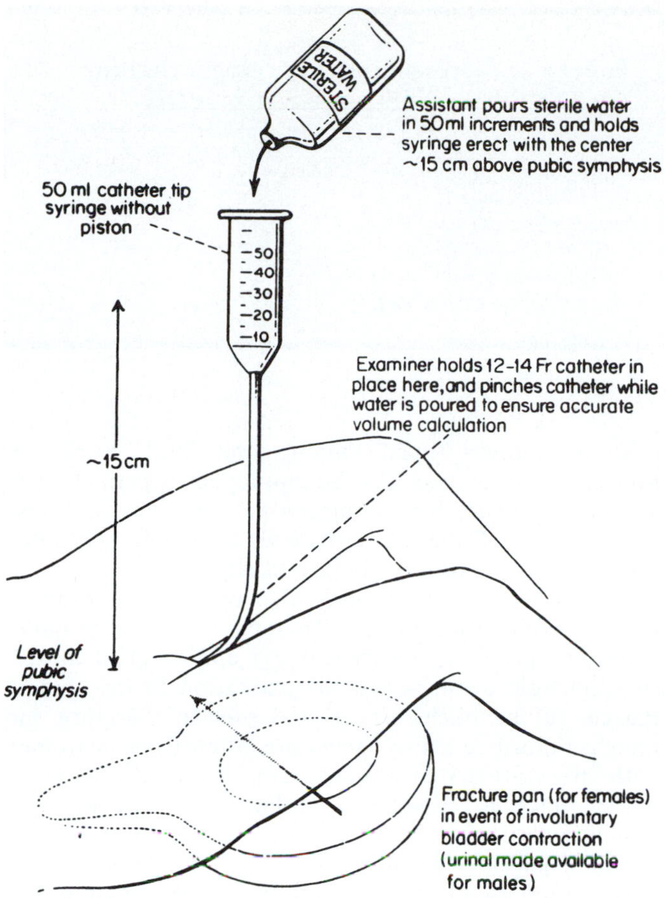


**Fig. 137-6.** Illustration of technique for performing bedside cystometrogram. Filling should be accomplished by gravity only and does not exceed 15 cm $H_2O$ water pressure. (From Ouslander JG, Leach GE, Staskin D: Simplified tests of lower urinary tract function in the evaluation of geriatric urinary incontinence, *J Am Geriatr Soc* 37:709, 1989.)

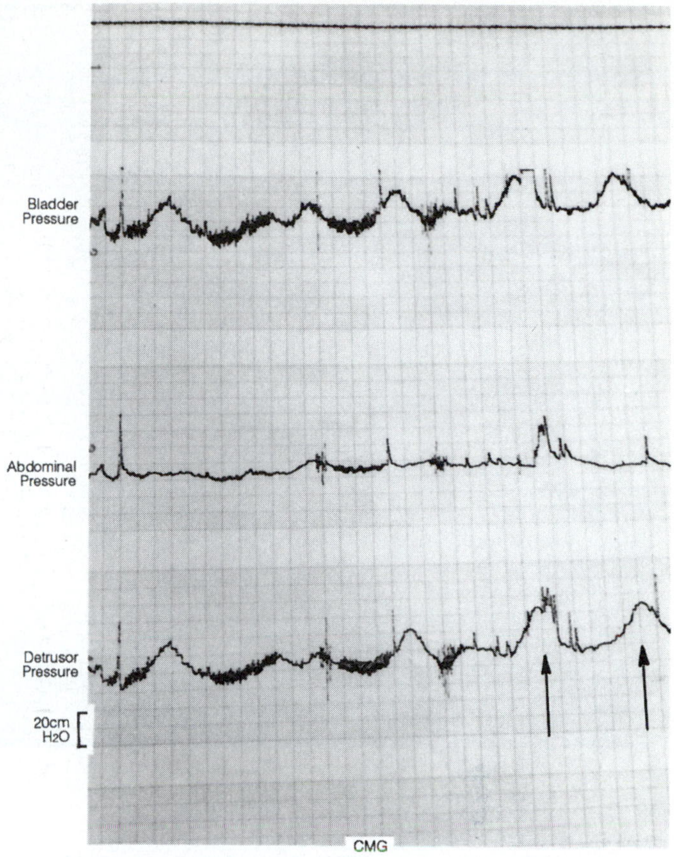


**Fig. 137-7.** Cystometrogram tracing showing low-volume bladder contractions consistent with detrusor instability/hyperreflexia.

outlet resistance will be elucidated by this simultaneous monitoring of bladder and bladder outlet events.

When the characteristics of the individual's voiding are to be determined, the patient is asked to void, and pressure/flow monitoring is continued. This simultaneous evaluation gives additive information to that obtained by uroflowmetry, which is usually performed at the same session. Failure to empty because of poor bladder contraction will be identified during this segment of the evaluation. High-pressure/low-flow voiding will identify outlet obstruction as the cause of failure to empty resulting from outlet obstruction.

Infusion with radiographic contrast allows the study to be monitored fluoroscopically, and real-time evaluation of bladder events may be made. Videourodynamics represents the most complex form of urodynamic evaluation. This type of evaluation is used to document the presence of bladder outlet dysfunction. It will also identify continuous loss of urine across the sphincteric mechanism in the absence of bladder contraction, which is seen in intrinsic sphincteric deficiency.

Outpatient urologic evaluation also includes cystoscopy. This will reveal any overt pathology of the urethra or bladder, such as tumor, stone, stricture, or foreign body.

## THERAPEUTIC INTERVENTIONS

The management of bladder dysfunction and incontinence involves a complex array of medical and surgical therapies. The primary goal of treatment of urinary tract dysfunction is preservation of renal function and control of urinary tract infection. The preservation or establishment of continence is an important consideration from the patient's viewpoint.

### Failure to store

Failure of the bladder either to store urine at low pressures with increasing intravesical volumes or to contract in a manner to completely empty indicates a failure of the reservoir function of the urinary tract. Failure of the sphincteric mechanism to remain closed during urinary storage or to open in a coordinated fashion during voiding constitutes a failure of the outlet mechanism of the lower urinary tract.

Urinary incontinence, as a manifestation of failure of the storage component of bladder function, should be managed in light of transient versus fixed etiologies. It has been estimated that 50% of new incontinence consultations during hospitalization represent remediable etiologies such as urinary tract infection, drug interactions, or mental status–related phenomena. Once transient etiologies for urinary loss have been excluded, therapy can be rendered for storage failure resulting from fixed incontinence etiologies.

### Failure to store: pharmacologic therapy for involuntary detrusor contractions

Anticholinergics
- Propantheline bromide
- Side effects: dry mouth, loss of lens ciliary muscle contraction, decreased gut motility, tachycardia, orthostatic hypotension

Musculotropics (antispasmodics)
- Oxybutynin chloride
- Flavoxate hydrochloride
- Dicyclomine hydrochloride
- Hyoscyamine sulfate
- Side effects: similar to anticholinergics

Calcium channel blockers
- Nifedipine
- Side effects: hypotensin, headache, dizziness, flushing, palpitations, dizziness, constipation

Tricyclics
- Imipramine hydrochloride
- Side effects: anticholinergic, antihistaminic (drowsiness), hypotension, cardiotoxicity

Other agents
- α-adrenergic antagonists

### Failure to store: nonpharmacologic therapy used to suppress detrusor contractility

Behavior modification, biofeedback
Electrical stimulation
Neural ablation
- Sacral rhizotomy
- Permanent subarachnoid block

Augmentation cystoplasty

Failure to store urine most often results from detrusor hyperreflexia. In elderly populations, detrusor hyperreflexia is a component of failure of storage in more than 70% of patients (see Chapter 6). However, detrusor hyperreflexia may coexist with impaired contractility (DHIC) in 20% or more of these patients, which may complicate therapy aimed at decreasing detrusor overactivity. This latter entity may be suspected when hyperreflexia is identified in the presence of significant postvoiding residual urine volumes.

Based on an understanding of the neuropharmacology of the detrusor muscle and bladder outlet, various classes of medications may be used in an effort to improve bladder storage function (see the box above). Anticholinergic medications suppress parasympathetically mediated detrusor contraction and are used for detrusor instability or detrusor hyperreflexia. Antispasmodic agents are similarly used for suppression of detrusor contractility and may offer additional local anesthetic properties. Occasionally, these agents may be combined with pure anticholinergic agents for added efficacy. Calcium channel blockers have been used for this purpose but serve a secondary role to the agents just mentioned. Tricyclic agents also serve to suppress detrusor activity on both a central and a peripheral basis. Tricyclics should be used with caution in elderly persons; the risk of orthostatic hypotension and cardiac conduction abnormalities is significantly increased in this age group. A trial of medications of this type (before urologic referral) is indicated in a patient with pure urge incontinence, minimal residual urine volume, and no obstructive symptoms.

Other modalities that have been used to control detrusor contractility have involved behavioral modification, selective electrical neurostimulation, and ablative surgical procedures (see the box above, right). Behavioral modification involves timed voiding and fluid restriction. Simple measures may also be employed in patients who are not candidates for pharmacologic intervention. These measures include the use of a bedside commode, scheduled toileting, and control of fluid intake.

Failure to store urine may also occur as a result of bladder outlet dysfunction. Therapy to augment outlet resistance also uses pharmacologic and surgical means. α-Adrenergic agonists provide excitation to the smooth muscle of the bladder neck and proximal urethra and increase closure. These agents are often used in women with stress urinary incontinence in an effort to augment outlet function. Estrogenic replacement topically and systemically improves the urethral closure mechanism in postmenopausal women. This adjunctive hormonal support is often used in combination with other modalities as an additive therapy (see the box on p. 1781). A trial of these agents in women with pure stress incontinence may be attempted before urologic referral. Adrenergic agents may also be used with caution in men who manifest postsurgical stress incontinence.

Behavioral therapy to improve outlet resistance centers on pelvic floor exercises (Kegel). This technique has efficacy both in women with incontinence secondary to urethral hypermobility and in males with incontinence after radical prostatectomy. Instructional teaching materials to assist patient education are available, (*Help for Incontinent People,* HIP). This may be augmented with electrical stimulation or other aids (vaginal cones) to allow the patient to better appreciate the pelvic floor.

Surgical management of ineffective outlet resistance involves several modalities (see the box on p. 1781). Injectable agents can be used in both sexes, with varying degrees of success. These agents have included Teflon, collagen, and autologous fat.

In women, suspension procedures can be used for stress incontinence associated with hypermobility of the proximal urethra and bladder neck. In appropriately selected patients, bladder neck suspension procedures have 1-year success rates approximating 90%. At 5 years, 75% continued success rates have been reported with these procedures. Pubovaginal slings fascia obtained from the abdominal wall or fascia lata are used for female stress incontinence associated with loss of intrinsic sphincteric function. Sling procedures offer 80% success rates for cure of stress incontinence. However, 30% of these patients will experience significant urgency-related symptomatology postoperatively. Five percent of women will experience permanent urinary retention after this procedure.

### Failure to store: pharmacologic therapy to improve outlet resistance

**Males and females**

α-Adrenergic agonists
- Ephedrine
- Pseudoephedrine
- Phenylpropanolamine hydrochloride
- Side effects: insomnia, anxiety, blood pressure elevation, tremor, palpitations, arrhythmias

**Females**

Estrogenic replacement (females)
- Vaginal
- Systemic
- Side effects: unopposed stimulation with risk of endometrial carcinoma

### Failure to store: surgical therapy for urinary incontinence from outlet dysfunction

**Females**

Urethral hypermobility
- Bladder neck suspension (retropubic, transvaginal needle suspension)

Intrinsic sphincteric deficiency
- Pubovaginal sling
- Artifical urinary sphincter
- Injection therapy (collagen, Polytef, autologous fat)

**Males**

Artifical urinary sphincter
Injection therapy

In males and females, the artificial urinary sphincter represents another option for therapy of incontinence caused by dysfunction of the intrinsic sphincteric mechanism. However, results of this procedure are much better in men than women.

In women, continuous incontinence may also represent a fistulous communication between the vagina and urinary tract (at the level of ureter, bladder, or proximal urethra). Fistulas most often are secondary to inadvertent injury to the bladder during routine hysterectomy. This diagnosis should be also considered in any woman who has had treatment for a pelvic malignancy (surgical or radiotherapeutic) or who has had a prior incontinence procedure. Diagnosis depends on thorough examination supplemented by anatomic studies.

Failure to store urine may also result from a combination of bladder and outlet dysfunction. The most common example is in women with stress incontinence who have a significant component of urgency-related urine loss. Although a trial of medical therapy directed at controlling urgency symptoms may be attempted before referral, it must be noted that mixed dysfunction can be unresponsive to medical therapy. Surgical therapy in this group of women offers a similar potential for cure of stress incontinence, as seen in women with pure stress incontinence only. Approximately 40% to 60% of women with mixed incontinence will also have resolution or improvement in concurrent urgency after surgery. Those who do not improve, however, may have persistent or de novo urgency and urge incontinence that is refractory to any therapy.

### Failure to empty: agents used to reduce outlet resistance

Adrenergic antagonists
- Prazosin
- Terazosin
- Phenoxybenzamine
- Side effects: orthostatic hypotension, fatigue, reflex tachycardia, nasal congestion

Striated muscle relaxants
- Dantrolene sodium
- Baclofen
- Diazepam
- Side effects: sedation, weakness, hepatotoxicity (dantmolene), hallucinations (baclofen)

## Failure to empty

Failure to empty may also result from detrusor or outlet dysfunction. The institution of clean, intermittent self-catheterization provides an easily learned alternative to chronic indwelling catheterization and is the primary modality for initial management of the bladder that empties poorly. Any patient or caregiver with a modicum of manual dexterity can master the technique. Once mastered, self-catheterization can be used as a foundation for the institution of additional therapies, as outlined next. If a patient is in retention, self-catheterization should be performed four to six times a day to keep bladder volumes less than 500 ml.

Unfortunately, no medication exists that has an unequivocal potentiating effect on bladder contractility. Although oral parasympathomimetic agents such as bethanechol chloride have been used, no documentation exists for their efficacy. Other avenues of enhancing bladder contractility, including selective electrical stimulation, remain experimental. The use of trigger-point reflex voiding is sometimes possible in patients with spinal cord injury.

Failure to empty on the basis of outlet dysfunction is extremely rare in women and should only be diagnosed after formal urodynamic evaluation. This is a common entity in men, especially those with obstructive prostatism. Medical options exist for the therapy of outlet dysfunction, which decrease outlet resistance and enhance detrusor emptying. α-Adrenergic antagonists block sympathetic receptors in the bladder base and proximal urethra and decrease the smooth muscular resistance to urinary outflow (see the box above). A variety of short-acting and long-acting agents have been used for this purpose. Currently, prazosin and terazosin are the most frequently

### Failure to empty: nonpharmacologic therapy for outlet obstruction

**Intermittent self-catheterization**
Urethral obstruction
- Biofeedback
- Incision of bladder neck (smooth muscle obstruction)
- Incision of urethral stricture

Prostatic obstruction
- Transurethral resection or incision (TURP)/(TUIP)
- Laser prostatectomy
- Prostatic thermotherapy (hyperthermia)
- Prostatic stenting

External sphincteric obstruction
- Intermittent catheterization
- Perineal nerve interruption
- Urethral stenting
- Surgical sphincterotomy

Iatrogenic urethral obstruction in women
- Urethrolysis

used adrenergic antagonists. Terazosin has a longer half-life but is more expensive. Studies evaluating the use of these agents in the treatment of obstructive prostatism have found statistically significant reductions in urinary symptoms associated with these medications. Also, flow rates show significant improvement. These improvements tend to be less than those associated with surgical therapy for prostatism. These agents are not used in the presence of any absolute indication for surgical intervention for obstructive prostatism, such as azotemia, urinary retention, or recurrent urinary tract infection.

Skeletal muscle relaxants have minimal efficacy in patients with hyperactivity of the striated sphincter because of spinal cord injury or neurologic illness. Most of these patients are managed with intermittent catheterization as the primary modality of therapy.

Other modalities used to decrease outlet resistance involve surgical management of obstructive prostatism or other pathologic entities (see the box above).

Failure to empty may also occur because of concomitant weak detrusor contraction and outlet obstruction. This may be seen in diabetic males with prostatic enlargement. Intermittent catheterization allows decompression of an atonic decompensated bladder, as is often found in elderly males with longstanding prostatism. Intervention to reduce outlet resistance is not indicated unless there is urodynamic evidence of adequate detrusor contractility. Intermittent catheterization may also be used with intentional pharmacologic paralyzation of the detrusor in cases of detrusor instability resulting in incontinence from high intravesical pressures, as seen in detrusor instability with impaired contractility. Chronic indwelling catheters should be avoided. Chronic bladder catheterization results in infection, loss of bladder wall compliance, and eventual upper tract decompensation.

Urinary diversion provides the last resort for management of incontinence. This may include both continent and noncontinent diversions, depending on the clinical indications.

## SUMMARY

Bladder dysfunction and urinary incontinence will continue to result in significant morbidity and social isolation, especially in light of the aging population. Often ignored or misinterpreted, both entities may result in a significant decline in quality of life. A systematic approach to evaluation will allow logical delineation of possible etiologies and subsequent treatment or referral, with the goal of improving the patient's continence status and overall quality of life.

## BIBLIOGRAPHY


Blaivas JG: The neurophysiology of micturition: a clinical study of 550 patients, *J Urol* 127:958, 1982.

Blaivas JG, Olsson CA: Stress incontinence: classification and surgical approach, *J Urol* 139:727, 1988.

Blaivas JG, Zayed AAH, Labib KB: The bulbocavernosus reflex in urology: a prospective study of 299 patients, *J Urol* 126:197, 1981.

Dula E, Leach GE: Role of urologist in diagnosis of multiple sclerosis, *Urology* 37:311, 1991.

Hu T: Impact of urinary incontinence on health care costs, *J Am Geriatr Soc* 38:292, 1990.

Lepor H: Role of long acting selective alpha-1 blockers in the treatment of benign prostatic hyperplasia, *Urol Clin North Am* 17(3):651, 1990.

Ouslander JG, Leach GE, Staskin D: Simplified tests of lower urinary tract function in the evaluation of geriatric urinary incontinence, *J Am Geriatr Soc* 37:706, 1989.

Ouslander J et al: Prospective evaluation of an assessment strategy for geriatric urinary incontinence, *J Am Geriatr Soc* 37:715, 1989.

Resnick NM, Yalla SV, Laurino E: The pathophysiology of urinary incontinence among institutionalized elderly persons, *N Engl J Med* 320:1, 1989.

Wein AJ: Lower urinary tract function and pharmacologic management of lower urinary tract dysfunction, *Urol Clin North Am* 14(2):273, 1987.


CHAPTER

# 138 Prostate Disorders—Benign and Malignant


**Ronald A. Morton**
**Herbert Lepor**


## BENIGN PROSTATIC HYPERPLASIA

Benign prostatic hyperplasia (BPH) describes a benign proliferative process of the stromal and epithelial elements of the prostate. Macroscopic enlargement of the prostate often results from the proliferative process. The macroscopic prostatic enlargement may be associated with bothersome urinary symptoms and/or bladder outlet obstruction. Until recently, the treatment options for BPH were limited to watchful waiting or prostatectomy. Medical and minimally invasive surgical strategies are presently offered for the treatment of BPH. The U.S. Food and Drug Administration (FDA) approval of two drugs with unique mechanisms of action has provided the opportunity for the primary care physician to become involved in the treatment of BPH. The diagnosis and treatment of BPH is complex and cannot be reduced to a simple flow chart. This chapter provides the primary care physician with a practical overview of the management of BPH.

## Epidemiology and natural history

The prevalence of microscopic BPH has been determined from the reported autopsy data. One study reported that microscopic BPH was rarely identified in males less than 40 years of age. The prevalence of microscopic BPH was observed to be age dependent: 50% and 90% of men developed histologic BPH by age 60 and 80 years, respectively. The prevalence of macroscopic BPH has been determined from the database of the Baltimore Longitudinal Study of Aging (BLSA). Approximately 50% of males were observed to have prostatic enlargement by age 70 based on a digital rectal examination. The clinical manifestations associated with BPH include symptoms of prostatism, incomplete bladder emptying, urinary tract infection (UTI), detrusor instability, urinary retention, bladder calculi, renal insufficiency, and hematuria. Urinary symptoms represent the most common presentation of BPH. The BLSA also revealed that the prevalence of clinical BPH is age dependent. Seventy percent of males developed symptoms of prostatism by age 70 years. Although microscopic, macroscopic, and clinical BPH are age-dependent events, no compelling evidence indicates that these phenomena are causally related.

The natural history of BPH is poorly understood. Several cohort studies have followed groups of patients with clinical BPH retrospectively and prospectively. The available natural history data strongly indicate that clinical BPH is not always a progressive process. Based on the natural history data, patients should not be encouraged to pursue intervention solely to prevent the ravages of untreated BPH. It is difficult to determine from the existing literature whether race is a determinant for the development of BPH, since a universally accepted definition of clinical BPH does not exist. Although sporadic case-controlled studies have implicated dietary factors, smoking, body habitus, sexual history, and socioeconomic status in the pathogenesis of BPH, these associations are tenuous.

## Pathogenesis

The development of BPH depends on aging and the presence of testes. The testes represent the primary source of circulating androgens. The embryologic development of the prostate and the development of BPH depends on dihydrotestosterone (DHT). The enzyme catalyzing the conversion of testosterone to DHT is 5α-reductase. Male individuals affected with a genetic deficiency of the enzyme 5α-reductase have a rudimentary prostate. BPH also rarely develops in males castrated before puberty. It is generally believed that androgens play a permissive role in the pathogenesis of BPH. The specific biochemical events initiating the hyperplastic process remain unknown. Although many growth factors have been identified in the prostate, their precise role in the pathogenesis of BPH is unknown.

### Clinical manifestations of BPH

Urinary symptoms
Incomplete bladder emptying
Detrusor instability
Urinary tract infection
Urinary retention
Bladder calculi
Hematuria

## Pathophysiology

The clinical manifestations associated with BPH include obstructive and irritative urinary symptoms, incomplete bladder emptying, detrusor instability, UTI, bladder calculi, urinary retention, renal insufficiency, and hematuria (see the box above). The most prevalent clinical manifestation of BPH is urinary symptoms. The obstructive urinary symptoms are hesitancy and straining to initiate urination, diminished caliber and interrupted urinary stream, and postmicturition dribbling. The irritative symptoms are diuria, nocturia, urinary urgency, incontinence, and dysuria. These symptoms collectively are referred to as *prostatism.* Several symptom indices have been developed to quantify the severity of prostatism. The International Prostate Symptom Score (I-PSS) has been validated and has gained the greatest level of clinical application. The I-PSS is self-administered and provides an excellent instrument to assess baseline severity, response to therapy, and disease progression (Fig. 138-1). The numeric score of symptoms provides an objective assessment of the degree of prostatism.

The pathophysiology of urinary symptoms is unclear. Since the development of prostatic enlargement and urinary symptoms are age-dependent events, it has been assumed that these phenomena are causally related. The presumed mechanism for the development of symptoms was the bladder outlet obstruction resulting from the enlarged prostate. Recent studies have challenged these assumptions. Examination of several large BPH clinical databases has demonstrated unequivocally that no direct relationship exists between prostate size and symptom severity or prostate size and degree of bladder outlet obstruction.

Incomplete bladder emptying is often attributed to bladder outlet obstruction secondary to BPH. The presumed consequences of incomplete bladder emptying include bladder calculi and UTI. Although the postvoid residual (PVR) can be measured precisely by catheterization or ultrasonography, the residual volume in a single patient is highly variable. Another limitation of PVR is that no consensus exists regarding the amount that represents a clinically or pathologically significant level. For example, no data suggest that the threshold PVR is associated with the development of irreversible bladder damage, urosepsis, or urinary retention.

Although no direct relationship exists between prostate size and bladder outlet obstruction, BPH has been implicated as a cause of obstruction. Several mechanisms

**International Prostate Symptom Score (I-PSS)**

| Patient name: | Not at all | Less than 1 time in 5 | Less than half the time | About half the time | More than half the time | Almost always | Your score |
|---|---|---|---|---|---|---|---|
| **1. Incomplete emptying** Over the past month, how often have you had a sensation of not emptying your bladder completely after you finished urinating? | 0 | 1 | 2 | 3 | 4 | 5 | |
| **2. Frequency** Over the past month, how often have you had to urinate again less than two hours after you finished urinating? | 0 | 1 | 2 | 3 | 4 | 5 | |
| **3. Intermittency** Over the past month, how often have you found you stopped and started again several times when you urinated? | 0 | 1 | 2 | 3 | 4 | 5 | |
| **4. Urgency** Over the past month, how often have you found it difficult to postpone urination? | 0 | 1 | 2 | 3 | 4 | 5 | |
| **5. Weak stream** Over the past month, how often have you had a weak urinary stream? | 0 | 1 | 2 | 3 | 4 | 5 | |
| **6. Straining** Over the past month, how often have you had to push or strain to begin urination? | 0 | 1 | 2 | 3 | 4 | 5 | |

| | None | 1 time | 2 times | 3 times | 4 times | 5 or more times | |
|---|---|---|---|---|---|---|---|
| **7. Nocturia** Over the past month, how many times did you most typically get up to urinate from the time you went to bed at night until the time you got up in the morning? | 0 | 1 | 2 | 3 | 4 | 5 | |
| Total I-PSS Score = | | | | | | | |

| **Quality of Life due to Urinary Symptoms** | Delighted | Pleased | Mostly satisfied | Mixed–about equally satisfied and dissatisfied | Mostly dissatisfied | Unhappy | Terrible |
|---|---|---|---|---|---|---|---|
| If you were to spend the rest of your life with your urinary condition just the way it is now, how would you feel about that? | 0 | 1 | 2 | 3 | 4 | 5 | 6 |

The International Prostate Symptom Score (I-PSS) is based on the answers to seven questions concerning urinary symptoms. Each question allows the patient to choose one out of five answers indicating increasing severity of the particular symptom. The answers are assigned points from 0 to 5. The total score can therefore range from 0 to 35 (asymptomatic to very symptomatic).

Furthermore, the International Consensus Committee (ICC) recommends the use of only a single question to assess the quality of life. The answers to this question range from "delighted" to "terrible" or 0 to 6. Although this single question may or may not capture the global impact of BPH symptoms or quality of life, it may serve as a valuable starting point for a doctor-patient conversation.

The ICC strongly recommends that all physicians who counsel patients suffering from symptoms of prostatism utilize these measures not only during the initial interview but also during and after treatment in order to monitor treatment response.

**Fig. 138-1.** International Prostate Symptom Score (I-PSS).

### Pertinent history in evaluation of BPH

**Urologic history**

International Prostate Symptom Score (I-PSS)
Family history of prostate cancer
History of hematuria or urinary tract infection (UTI)
Prior urologic instrumentation

**Nonurologic history**

Adult-onset diabetes mellitus (AODM)
Neurologic conditions
  Primary: Parkinson's disease
  Secondary: cerebrovascular accident (CVA)

**Medications**

Anticholinergics
$\alpha$-Adrenergic agonists

unrelated to prostate size may cause obstruction. A prominent median lobe, a noncompliant prostatic capsule, and predominantly stromal hyperplasia have been implicated as prostate-dependent factors causing bladder outlet obstruction. Bladder outlet obstruction can be measured invasively by uroflowmetry or noninvasively by multichannel urodynamics. Uroflowmetry simply measures the maximum urinary velocity. A reduced urine flow rate is indicative of bladder outlet obstruction. The primary limitation of uroflowmetry is that an acontractile bladder may also result in a decreased urine flow rate. Multichannel urodynamics allows for simultaneous determination of both bladder pressure and urine flow rate. A decreased urine flow rate at elevated detrusor pressures is pathognomonic for obstruction. Although multichannel urodynamics quantifies bladder outlet obstruction, the precise clinical and pathologic significance of these measurements is equivocal. For example, it is unknown what level of obstruction is associated with the development of irreversible bladder dysfunction or the predisposition to develop life-threatening complications of BPH.

## Evaluation of the BPH patient

***History.*** A detailed urologic history and focused general medical history are essential in the evaluation of males with BPH (see the box above). The severity of symptoms should be quantified using a validated instrument such as the I-PSS. The history should also determine the level of "bother" and the impact of the urinary symptoms on quality of life. It is not unusual for patients with identical symptom scores to have very different perceptions of the degree of bother resulting from the symptoms.

Other urologic and nonurologic conditions may masquerade as prostatism. Adult-onset diabetes mellitus (AODM) may result in diuria and nocturia because of the obligatory loss of urine associated with glucosuria. AODM may also cause neuropathic bladder dysfunction. Primary neurologic disorders such as Parkinson's disease and secondary neurologic conditions such as cerebrovascular accidents (CVAs) often cause detrusor instability, resulting in urinary frequency, urgency, and urge incontinence.

### Physical examination for BPH

Digital rectal examination
  Nodules, induration, tenderness
  Rectal tone
Percussible/palpable bladder

Prostate cancer and transitional cell carcinoma of the bladder may also cause irritative urinary symptoms.

The role of the bladder is to store urine under low pressure and empty urine in socially acceptable circumstances. Medications may affect bladder emptying and storage and therefore may interfere with bladder function and cause symptoms of prostatism. Bladder contraction is a parasympathetic event mediated by muscarinic cholinergic receptors, whereas bladder outlet resistance is a sympathetic function mediated predominantly by the $\alpha_1$-adrenoceptor. Therefore muscarinic cholinergic antagonists such as probanthine or $\alpha$-adrenergic agonists such as phenylephrine may impede bladder emptying and exacerbate or independently cause BPH-like symptoms.

***Physical examination.*** The physical examination should include careful palpation of the prostate (see the box above). The digital rectal examination of the prostate should focus on identifying stony hard nodules, induration, tenderness, or asymmetric enlargement. Although the size is often estimated, there is limited clinical significance to this observation. The rectal tone should be assessed to identify an underlying neurologic condition. The suprapubic region may be percussed for a large PVR.

***Laboratory assessment.*** A urinalysis is a simple and often informative screening test for genitourinary diseases (see the box on p. 1786). It is recommended that all men with BPH undergo this simple test. The presence of glucosuria may be the initial presentation for AODM. The presence of microscopic hematuria requires additional imaging and diagnostic studies to exclude genitourinary malignancies or benign conditions such as nephrolithiasis. The presence of pyuria or bacteriuria indicates the need for a urine culture. Additional testing is required to determine the etiology of the UTI. A serum creatinine test is often recommended to identify significant renal disease resulting from bladder outlet obstruction. This recommendation is not based on data defining the specificity and sensitivity of a serum creatinine to identify BPH-dependent renal dysfunction. If the serum creatinine is elevated, the PVR should be determined.

The role of serum prostate-specific antigen (PSA) determination for screening prostate cancer is highly controversial. The controversy does not involve whether screening will increase detection, but whether increased detection will achieve increased survival. Although the data to resolve this controversy are not available, we believe that individuals with BPH are at increased risk for developing biologically significant prostate cancer and that these individuals should routinely undergo a baseline PSA.

### Laboratory assessment for BPH

Urinalysis
  Glucosuria
  Hematuria, pyuria, bacteriuria
Serum creatinine
  Serum prostate-specific antigen (PSA)

### Optional diagnostic studies for BPH

Uroflowmetry
Postvoid residual (PVR) determination
Multichannel urodynamics
Cystoscopy
Imaging of upper urinary tracts

Uroflowmetry, multichannel urodynamics, and PVR have been discussed previously. Although these studies may provide valuable information related to the level of obstruction or the indications for intervention, the data derived from these studies are often too nonspecific to establish definitive treatment recommendations (see the box above, right). Therefore these studies should be considered options. Cystoscopy and imaging of the upper urinary tract by intravenous pyelography (IVP), ultrasound, and computed tomography (CT) should not be routinely obtained as part of the evaluation of BPH. If the history, physical examination, or laboratory studies suggest specific abnormalities, these tests may be indicated.

### Indications for intervention in BPH

**Absolute**

Urinary retention
Recurrent UTI
Refractory gross hematuria
Bladder calculi
Renal insufficiency secondary to BPH

**Relative**

Urinary symptoms
Incomplete emptying
Urodynamic obstruction

## Indications for intervention

The indications for therapeutic intervention in BPH may be stratified as absolute versus relative (see the box above, right). Absolute indications imply that the patient's overall well-being will be compromised if treatment is not rendered. Urinary retention, refractory hematuria, and UTIs secondary to BPH are widely accepted absolute indications for intervention. Only a small subset of patients with BPH have these absolute indications for intervention.

The relative indications for intervention include bothersome urinary symptoms, incomplete bladder emptying, and bladder outlet obstruction. Severe symptoms in the absence of absolute indications for intervention do not jeopardize the patient's health status. It is imperative to determine both the level of bother and the risk that the patient is willing to assume to alleviate the urinary symptoms. Physicians cannot impart their own perception of risk/benefit for patients. Although incomplete bladder emptying and urodynamic evidence of bladder outlet obstruction may exacerbate urinary symptoms and lead to UTI and irreversible bladder dysfunction, no data precisely define the clinical, physiologic, and pathologic implications of these findings. Therefore the treatment recommendations by different physicians vary and reflect individual bias.

### Surgical and minimally invasive interventions for BPH

Prostatectomy
  Open enucleation
  Transurethral resection of prostate (TURP)
Laser ablation
Transurethral incision of prostate (TUIP)
Balloon dilatation
Prostatic stents
Microwave thermotherapy

## Treatment

***Prostatectomy.*** There are several surgical and minimally invasive approaches for the treatment of BPH (see the box above, right). The prostatic tissue may be removed by open enucleation or by transurethral resection (TURP). The surgical approach is based on the size of the prostate and the surgeon's preference. Approximately 90% of prostatectomies are performed via the transurethral route. Open prostatectomy requires a lower abdominal incision and hospitalization ranging from 5 to 7 days. TURP requires no surgical incision, and the hospital stay is approximately 2 to 3 days. Table 138-1 presents the risks associated with TURP. Although the complications after prostatectomy are rarely life-threatening, the inherent risks may discourage patients with relative indications from pursuing surgical intervention. Approximately 80% to 90% of patients achieve marked/moderate symptom improvement after TURP and are very satisfied with the treatment outcome. The mean improvement in the urine flow rate is approximately 100%.

Laser energy has recently been advocated as another method for removing the obstructing prostatic tissue. The primary advantage of laser ablation over prostatectomy is that irrigation fluid is not resorbed and therefore the risks of hyponatremia and fluid overload are alleviated. Bleeding is negligible, and transfusions are rarely, if ever,

**Table 138-1.** Morbidity associated with transurethral prostatectomy (TURP)

| Complication | Incidence (%) |
|---|---|
| Epididymitis | 4.8 |
| Urinary tract infection | 8.4 |
| Impotence | 10.2 |
| Incontinence | 3.3 |
| Transfusion | 10.5 |
| Transurethral resection syndrome | — |
| Death | — |

required. Retrograde ejaculation is also a rare outcome. The patients are often discharged on the day of surgery. The preliminary data suggest that the prostatic defect following laser ablation is far less than that achieved with TURP, and that many patients experience irritative symptoms for several months. The improvements in symptom score, bladder emptying, and urine flow rate approximate but are not equivalent to those with TURP. The reduced cost from shorter hospitalization is balanced by the cost of the laser fiber and the new technology. The long-term effectiveness of laser ablation has yet to be defined. It is likely that patients will choose a less invasive and safer procedure such as laser ablation even if the level of improvement is slightly less than with TURP.

Transurethral incision of the prostate (TUIP) is an alternative surgical procedure that is less invasive than TURP. The bladder neck and prostatic adenoma are deeply incised without resecting prostatic tissue. Randomized studies have demonstrated that the effectiveness of TURP and TUIP are comparable. The intraoperative time, blood loss, and complications are less with TUIP. TUIP is not recommended if the prostate size is greater than 30 g. Approximately half the patients undergoing TURP are candidates for TUIP.

***Minimally invasive intervention.*** Balloon dilatation of the prostate (BDP) has been advocated for the treatment of BPH. Although the initial uncontrolled reports were encouraging, a randomized double-blind study reported that BDP and cystoscopy achieve equivalent therapeutic benefit. This study suggested that the observed effectiveness of BDP is likely a placebo response. BDP is rarely performed for BPH at present.

Prostatic stents and thermotherapy are other minimally invasive treatment strategies that are presently under clinical investigation in the United States for BPH. Permanent indwelling prostatic stents are endoscopically positioned in the prostatic urethra and eventually become covered by transitional epithelium. Occasional stone formation on the uncovered stent and severe irritative voiding symptoms are the primary limitations of the procedure.

Heating the prostate with microwave energy is another method to destroy prostatic tissue. The microwave energy is delivered to the prostate by a transurethral catheter. The urethra is cooled to improve patient tolerance. The cost of the microwave energy machine is approximately

### α-Blockers investigated for therapy of BPH

**Nonselective α-blockers**
Phenoxybenzamine

**Selective α-blockers**
Prazosin
Alfuzosin
Indoramin

**Selective long-acting $\alpha_1$-blockers**
Terazosin
Doxazosin
Tamsulosin

$500,000. A recent randomized sham controlled study demonstrated that the level of improvement is equivalent to α-blocker therapy. The cost of the machine, modest therapeutic benefit, and invasive nature of the procedure will likely limit the widespread acceptance of this treatment.

## Medical therapy

***Alpha blockade.*** The rational for α-blockers in BPH is based on several morphologic, physiologic, and pharmacologic observations. Double immunoenzymatic staining and color-assisted image analysis have revealed that smooth muscle accounts for 40% of the tissue volume of the prostate. In vitro isometric tension studies have demonstrated that the contractile properties of prostate smooth muscle are mediated primarily by $\alpha_1$-adrenoceptors. Radioligand receptor binding studies have shown that the human prostate contains a relative abundance of $\alpha_1$-adrenoceptors. Based on the physiologic and pharmacologic observations just mentioned, $\alpha_1$-adrenergic blockers should decrease the resistance along the prostatic urethra by relaxing the smooth muscle component of the prostate.

Several different α-blockers have been investigated for the treatment of BPH. These α-blockers can be subgrouped according to α-adrenoceptor subtype selectivity and duration of serum elimination half-lives (see the box above). Phenoxybenzamine antagonizes $\alpha_1$- and $\alpha_2$-adrenoceptors, whereas prazosin, alfuzosin, indoramin, terazosin, doxazosin, and tamsulosin are selective $\alpha_1$-antagonists. The advantage of the selective $\alpha_1$-antagonists is that the incidence and severity of adverse events are far less than with the nonselective α-blockers. Terazosin is the only α-blocker that is FDA approved for the treatment of BPH in the United States and is the α-blocker most extensively studied for BPH. The new drug application (NDA) for doxazosin's BPH indication has been submitted to the FDA. The NDA for tamsulosin's BPH indication is in preparation. The advantages of the long-acting once-a-day α-blockers are improved compliance and tolerance. The most common adverse events associated with selective $\alpha_1$-blockers include dizziness, lightheadedness, and asthenia. The administration of a once-a-day formulation

**Table 138-2.** Effectiveness of terazosin (TRZ) for BPH

| Outcome measures | Baseline | 12 weeks | %Δ* | p value† |
|---|---|---|---|---|
| Symptom score‡ | | | | |
| Placebo | 9.7 | 7.4 | −23.5 | <0.001 |
| TRZ (10 mg) | 10.1 | 5.5 | −45.1 | |
| $Q_{max}$ (ml/sec) | | | | |
| Placebo | 10.1 | 10.2 | +10.4 | |
| TRZ (10 mg) | 8.8 | 12.2 | +34.0 | 0.009 |

*Values correspond to the means of the changes from baseline in each man and therefore cannot be derived from the baseline and 12-week results.
†Comparison between mean %Δ placebo versus TRZ.
‡Boyarsky symptom score.

at bedtime appears to reduce the incidence and severity of these adverse events.

Lepor and colleagues reported the results of a Phase III multicenter, double-blind, parallel-group, randomized placebo-controlled study of once-a-day administration of terazosin to patients with symptomatic BPH. Two hundred eighty-five patients received either placebo or 2, 5, or 10 mg of terazosin once daily. The level of improvements in the symptom scores were dose dependent (Table 138-2). The percentages of patients exhibiting a greater than 30% improvement in the total symptom scores for the placebo and 2, 5, and 10 mg treatment groups were 40%, 51%, 57%, and 60%, respectively. The changes in peak urine flow rate ($Q_{max}$) were also dose dependent. The percentages of patients experiencing a greater than 30% increase in $Q_{max}$ in the placebo and 2, 5, and 10 mg treatment groups were 26%, 40%, 35%, and 52%, respectively. A significantly greater proportion of patients in the 10 mg terazosin treatment group exhibited a more than 30% improvement in symptom scores compared with the placebo group. An interim analysis of an open-label study evaluating long-term safety and effectiveness of terazosin for BPH indicates that improvements in symptom scores and urine flow rates are maintained throughout a 2½ year follow-up.

Overall, the adverse events in the four treatment groups were minor and reversible. Although a higher incidence of asthenia, flu syndrome, and dizziness were observed in the terazosin treatment groups, the differences from placebo were not statistically significant. Only one patient in the 10 mg treatment group developed syncope at the 5 mg dose.

One of the presumed limitations of α-blockers for the treatment of BPH was the consequences of lowering blood pressure in relatively elderly normotensive patients. The observed effect of terazosin on baseline systolic blood pressure in normotensive and hypertensive patients was 3 mm Hg and 14 mm Hg, respectively. These data demonstrate that terazosin lowers blood pressure in patients with BPH when it is a desired physiologic outcome.

Three multicenter randomized placebo-controlled studies have evaluated the safety and effectiveness of doxazosin for the treatment of BPH. A long-term open-label doxazosin study is in progress. The results of these studies have not been published in the peer-reviewed literature. The data recently presented at the 1994 Annual American Urological Association meeting in San Francisco demonstrated that the level of effectiveness is similar to that of terazosin.

There is a definite physiologic and pharmacologic rationale for α blockade in BPH. Multicenter randomized placebo-controlled studies have consistently and unequivocally demonstrated the ability of α-blockers to relieve symptoms of BPH and increase urine flow rates. Although no randomized double-blind studies have compared the different selective $\alpha_1$-blockers, no clinically significant differences seem to exist between the safety and effectiveness of the individual drugs. The clinical response is rapid and durable. The presumed advantages of the long-acting selective $\alpha_1$-blockers include better compliance and tolerance. Selective $\alpha_1$-blockers lower blood pressure in those patients when it is a desired clinical outcome. Since approximately 50% of men with BPH are also hypertensive, the ability to treat BPH and hypertension simultaneously and effectively with a single drug is a distinct advantage of selective $\alpha_1$-blockers.

***Androgen suppression.*** The reduction of prostate volume after castration in males with BPH was observed 100 years ago. Castration never gained widespread acceptance for the treatment of BPH because of the psychologic impact of removal of the testes and the subsequent development of impotence, loss of libido, and hot flashes resulting from the imbalance of androgens and estrogens. Medical castration can be achieved by drugs that block the action or synthesis of either testosterone (T) or DHT. The morbidity associated with the drugs lowering serum T levels often counterbalances the therapeutic benefit, especially in BPH therapy. Since the maintenance of prostate volume depends on tissue levels of DHT, a drug that selectively blocks the production or action of DHT would achieve involution of the prostate without the problematic adverse events associated with castrate levels of serum T. Finasteride, a 5α-reductase inhibitor, lowers serum and prostatic levels of DHT without lowering serum T levels. Finasteride is the only hormonal therapy that is FDA approved for the indication of BPH.

A multicenter randomized placebo-controlled double-blind study recently evaluated the safety and effectiveness of finasteride in men with BPH. A total of 895 patients were randomized to receive daily placebo or 1 or 5 mg of finasteride for 12 months. Table 138-3 summarizes the improvements in symptom scores, flow rate, and prostate

**Table 138-3.** Effectiveness of finasteride for BPH

| Outcome measures | Baseline | 52 weeks | %Δ* | *p* value† |
|---|---|---|---|---|
| Symptom score‡ | | | | |
| Placebo | 9.8 | 8.8 | −2 | <0.05 |
| Finasteride (5 mg) | 10.2 | 7.5 | −21 | |
| $Q_{max}$ (ml/sec) | | | | |
| Placebo | 9.6 | 9.8 | +8 | <0.001 |
| Finasteride (5 mg) | 9.6 | 11.2 | +22 | |
| Prostate volume | | | | |
| Placebo | 61.0 | 59.8 | −3 | <0.001 |
| Finasteride (5 mg) | 58.6 | 47.5 | −19 | |

*Values correspond to the means of the changes from baseline in each man and therefore cannot be derived from the baseline and 52-week results.
†Comparison between mean %Δ placebo versus finasteride.
‡Modified Boyarsky score.

volume. The effect of finasteride on these outcome measures was statistically significant.

Adverse events were rare in the placebo and treatment groups. The differences between decreased libido (4.7% versus 1.3%) and ejaculatory dysfunction (4.4% versus 1.7%) in the 5 mg and placebo groups were statistically significant. The percentages of patients who developed an adverse event resulting in premature withdrawal in the placebo and 5 mg treatment groups were only 6% and 5%, respectively. The short-term safety profile of finasteride is exceedingly favorable. The durability of the therapeutic response is maintained at 36 months in a subset of patients. There are insufficient data to support any claim that finasteride alters the natural history of BPH.

A definite rationale exists for androgen suppression in the treatment of BPH. Finasteride represents the only drug that has been studied in a multicenter trial with sufficient numbers of patients and adequate follow-up. Androgen suppression causes prostate involution primarily by affecting prostatic epithelium. It is not surprising that only a relatively modest reduction in prostate volume occurs, since only 10% of the prostate volume is accounted for by the epithelium. Although the differences between placebo and 5 mg of finasteride are modest, the differences are statistically significant. The adverse events associated with finasteride are minimal and reversible. Finasteride is likely to benefit a relatively small subset of patients with clinical BPH.

### Summary

Enlargement of the prostate secondary to BPH is essentially an inescapable phenomenon for the aging male population. The pathophysiology of clinical BPH is poorly understood. The evaluation of men with clinical BPH is targeted to identify other conditions that may masquerade as BPH. Prostatectomy and medical therapy represent the treatment strategies presently accepted for the treatment of clinical BPH.

Individuals with absolute indications should be offered prostatectomy. Most patients without life-threatening consequences of BPH should be offered either prostatectomy, medical therapy, or watchful waiting. The treatment decision should be based on the patient's perception of bother from the symptoms and the risks the patient is willing to incur to achieve the desired therapeutic response.

## PROSTATE CANCER

Prostate cancer is now the most frequently diagnosed cancer in American men, accounting for 32% of all diagnosed male cancers. Prostate cancer is second only to lung cancer as a cause of male cancer deaths. In 1994 there were 200,000 new cases of prostate cancer diagnosed and 38,000 deaths from prostate cancer. In addition to this critical number of clinically manifested prostate cancers, autopsy studies forecast that 11 million men in the United States over age 45 harbor histologic (clinically silent) prostate cancer. African-American men represent a particularly high-risk group. The incidence of prostate cancer in African-American men is 50% higher than in Caucasian Americans. Moreover, the 5-year survival from 1983 to 1989 for Caucasian Americans was 79% while for African Americans it was 64%. Patients with hereditary prostate cancer characterized by early age at onset and autosomal dominant inheritance represent a second high-risk group.

Two observations suggest that the clinical impact of prostate cancer will continue to expand. First, the incidence of prostate cancer increases with age more than any other malignancy. Second, the percentage of men over age 65 in the U.S. population is increasing such that there will be a 64% increase in U.S. males over age 65 by the year 2000.

At this time, the etiology of this exceedingly common cancer is unknown. Unlike other solid tumors such as colon and breast cancer, no candidate genes or genetic loci have been identified to explain the hereditary form of the disease.

### Clinical presentation

The presentation of prostate cancer depends on the stage at the time of diagnosis. In its early stages, prostate cancer is asymptomatic. Early cases are often diagnosed by digital rectal examination (DRE) during routine physical examination or during examination for another illness (see the box on p. 1790). The recent discovery of prostate-specific antigen (PSA) has had a profound impact on the clinical presentation of prostate cancer. In 1988, PSA became widely available as a serum marker for prostate cancer.

### Clinical presentation of prostate cancer

Abnormality found with screening digital rectal examination or serum prostate-specific antigen (PSA) determination
Urinary symptoms (prostatism)
Hematuria
Bony metastasis

PSA is a serine protease produced only by prostatic epithelium. Although produced by both normal and malignant cells, the contribution to serum levels differs greatly for these two cell populations. The contribution to serum PSA by BPH tissue is 0.3 ng/ml for each cubic centimeter of tissue. Elevations in PSA have been shown to correlate with increasing clinical stage and pathologic grade and stage of prostate cancer. However, wide variation in prostatic epithelial/stromal ratios among patients limits the predictive value of a single PSA measurement in a given individual. The normal reference range for serum PSA is also age dependent. Nevertheless, PSA can assist one in differentiating between benign and malignant conditions of the prostate.

The normal reference range for PSA is 0 to 4 ng/ml. Values between 4 and 10 ng/ml are difficult to interpret. Values greater than 10 ng/ml are highly suggestive but not diagnostic for prostate cancer. Three observations have provided guidelines for interpreting PSA data in the ambiguous 4 to 10 ng/ml range. Ultrasound has been used to measure prostate volume and then calculate the amount of PSA per unit volume of tissue. This value has been termed *PSA density,* or PSAD. A PSAD of 0.15 or greater in association with a PSA between 4 and 10 suggests that a needle biopsy of the prostate is indicated regardless of DRE findings. Such biopsies should be performed with transrectal ultrasound guidance. Researchers with the Baltimore Longitudinal Study of Aging (BLSA) measured the change in serial PSAs on historic samples from men with known outcomes. This has been termed *PSA velocity* (PSAV) or rate of PSA change. They were able to establish that a PSA velocity of 0.75 ng/ml/year correlated with the development and diagnosis of clinically significant prostate cancers. This value has been confirmed by two larger studies. Consequently, men with a PSA in the 4 to 10 range and serial PSA measurements demonstrating a PSAV of 0.75 ng/ml/year should undergo a full evaluation for prostate cancer. Age-associated reference ranges for PSA also have been described. The following normal values have been recommended for PSA: 0 to 2.5 ng/ml for men age 40 to 49, 0 to 3.5 ng/ml for men age 50 to 59, 0 to 4.5 ng/ml for men age 60 to 69, and 0 to 6.5 ng/ml for men age 70 and older.

Each of these concepts has certain disadvantages associated with it, and in the urologic community, no consensus has been reached concerning their application. PSAD is hampered by the inability of current radiologic techniques to measure prostate volume precisely and by the wide variance in prostatic epithelial/stromal ratios. The age-specific reference ranges were determined in a single community consisting only of Caucasians. Attempts to generalize these data to other populations have yielded inconsistent results. The optimal interval between PSA measurements necessary to calculate PSAV has yet to be determined. Until one of these practices proves useful in a prospective study, one should fully evaluate patients with PSA elevations.

There have been recent technologic improvements in radiologic techniques to image prostate cancer, such as transrectal ultrasound (TRUS), pelvic magnetic resonance imaging (MRI), and improved radionuclide bone scan. Despite these advances, approximately 40% of men thought to have clinically localized prostate cancer will not have organ-confined disease at the time of radical prostatectomy. The realization that PSA can help detect prostate cancer at an earlier stage than was previously possible has led to the use of PSA as a screening test for prostate cancer. In five large studies of screening PSA, the sensitivity ranged from 46% to 89.5% and the specificity from 59% to 91.2%. These studies encompass both office-based and community-based populations. The low sensitivity in these studies precludes the use of PSA alone as a screening test for prostate cancer. However, when combined with DRE and TRUS, PSA can lead to greater sensitivity and specificity in the early detection of prostate cancer.

Despite growing efforts to identify men with early-stage prostate cancer, 20% to 25% continue to present with advanced-stage disease. At presentation these men may have hematuria, lower urinary tract obstruction, or pain from bone metastasis. The axial skeleton is most susceptible to metastatic spread of prostate cancer, particularly the pelvis and lumbar spine. Other sites of metastasis include the seminal vesicles by local extension and lymphatic spread to the obturator and external iliac nodes.

## Diagnosing and staging

Patients identified at risk for having prostate cancer by DRE, PSA, or TRUS should undergo transrectal biopsy of the prostate. This can be performed as an outpatient procedure with oral antibiotic prophylaxis initiated the night before the procedure (fluroquinolone). Biopsies in the setting of an elevated PSA without obvious findings on DRE should be performed with transrectal ultrasound guidance. Prostate cancer sometimes appears as a hypoechoic lesion on ultrasound. The presence of a hypoechoic lesion on ultrasound is not pathognomonic for prostate cancer, and its absence does not rule out the disease. For a prostate nodule or induration that is obviously palpable, digitally guided biopsies are quite adequate. Once the presence of prostate cancer is confirmed with a biopsy specimen, the tumor is assigned a grade. The most common grading system in use today is the Gleason grading system. This system is based on the glandular architecture of the two most frequently seen patterns in the tumor. Each pattern is given a Gleason grade from 1 to 5, with a grade of 1 being the most differentiated. The sum of the two grades is the Gleason score. Therefore, the Gleason score can range from 2 to 10.

Clinical staging is used to determine the initial mode of therapy. Radiologic modalities to evaluate pelvic lymph nodes are of little benefit in the staging of prostate cancer. Clinical staging of prostate cancer can be accomplished

**Table 138-4.** Staging of prostate cancer: TNM classification

| Primary tumor stage | Clinical findings | Corresponding Whitmore classification |
|---|---|---|
| T0 | No evidence of tumor | |
| T1 | Nonpalpable disease | |
| T1a | Tumor found at TURP ≤5% of resected tissue | A1 |
| T1b | Tumor found at TURP >5% of resected tissue | A2 |
| T1c | Tumor on needle biopsy for elevated PSA only | |
| T2 | Palpable tumor confined to prostate | |
| T2a | Tumor involves half a lobe or less | B1 |
| T2b | Tumor involves more than half a lobe, not both lobes | B2 |
| T2c | Tumor involves both lobes | |
| T3 | Tumor extends through prostatic capsule | C |
| T3a | Unilateral extracapsular extension | |
| T3b | Bilateral extracapsulator extension | |
| T3c | Tumor invades seminal vesicle(s) | |
| T4 | Tumor is fixed or invades other adjacent structures | |
| T4a | Tumor invading bladder neck or rectum | |
| T4b | Tumor fixed to pelvic side wall | |

with DRE, radionuclide bone scan, PSA, and findings on transurethral prostatectomy when appropriate. Recently, a new TNM staging of prostate cancer has been adopted (Table 138-4). Organ-confined tumors are designated either T1 or T2; the ability to palpate the tumor on DRE is the feature that separates these groups. T1 tumors are nonpalpable tumors diagnosed via transurethral resection of the prostate (TURP) (T1a, T1b) or biopsy performed for an elevated PSA only (T1c). T1 tumors detected during TURP are subdivided into two groups based on the percentage of resected tissue that is cancerous: T1a is 5% or less, and T1b is greater than 5%. This distinction has prognostic significance: 16% of men with untreated T1a disease will develop metastatic disease at 10 years while 35% of men with T1b disease will have metastatic disease at 5 years and 20% will die of prostate cancer in 5 to 10 years. Palpable T2 tumors are further stratified with respect to the size of the nodule. T2a disease is tumor involving half a lobe or less, T2b disease is tumor in greater than half a lobe but not both lobes, and T2c disease is tumor involving both lobes. T3 disease encompasses local spread outside the prostate. T3a are tumors with unilateral extracapsular extension, and T3b tumors have bilateral extracapsular extension. T3c represents seminal vesicle involvement. T4 stage tumors have greater degrees of local extension with involvement of contiguous organs (see Table 138-4).

### Treatment

The treatment of prostate cancer is dictated by the clinical stage at presentation, patient's age, and patient's general health. The optimal treatment of prostate cancer is highly controversial (see the box at right). Treatment options include watchful waiting, hormonal therapy, radical prostatectomy, radiation therapy, TURP, and chemotherapy. The objectives of treatment depend on the stage and realistic expectations. The goals of therapy include cure, increased survival, relief of urinary retention and bothersome urinary symptoms, and palliation of systemic metastasis (see the box on p. 1792).

#### Treatment options for prostate cancer

Watchful waiting
Radical prostatectomy
Radiation therapy
TURP
Hormonal therapy
Chemotherapy

Radical prostatectomy and radiation therapy are offered with the intent to cure T1 and T2 disease. The limitations of treatment result in part from the limitations of clinical staging, since approximately one half of the patients with clinically localized disease do not have pathologically organ-confined disease. The morbidity of treatment also is a factor. Moreover, 60% to 75% of patients treated with radiation therapy will have positive prostate needle biopsies 18 months after treatment. The mortality associated with each treatment is similar. Less than 1% of patients will die secondary to either therapy. The major morbidities related to surgical treatment of localized prostate cancer are impotence and urinary incontinence. In patients 70 years of age or younger, 30% to 60% of those treated will be impotent regardless of the mode of therapy. The incontinence rate for radiation therapy is approximately 2%, whereas for radical prostatectomy it ranges from 2% to 10%. The incontinence rate after radical prostatectomy is likely to be reduced in academic centers where greater numbers of prostatectomies are performed.

With the widespread availability of PSA, prostate cancer is now diagnosed earlier and with greater frequency. Autopsy studies consistently show that 15% to 30% of men over age 50 harbor histologically identifiable prostate cancer cells. This percentage increases to 50% to

### Objectives of therapy for prostate cancer

Cure
Increase survival
Relieve bladder outlet obstruction
Relieve bothersome urinary symptoms
Palliation of systemic metastasis

60% of men greater than 90 years old. These types of studies document the presence of a large population of asymptomatic men with prostate cancer who never have any adverse effects from the disease. These data have prompted some to advocate that cancers diagnosed via PSA alone (T1c) may be clinically insignificant and not necessitate treatment. At present, studies imply that watchful waiting is adequate for men with stage T2 cancers or less. Although of interest, these studies have been imperfect in that some men received hormonal therapy; the mean age of patients in these studies was generally 70 or older (patients who would not be treated aggressively under standard guidelines); and the studies were biased toward patients with low-grade disease. At present, the biologic potential of a given tumor cannot be reliably predicted. Furthermore, no consistent data have been presented that suggest young healthy patients do not benefit from aggressive treatment of their prostate cancer. A recent study reviewed the pathologic findings of 157 consecutive patients with clinical stage T1c disease and found that 84% of tumors were significant and that definitive treatment was justified in most patients. The parameters suggesting that treatment may *not* be indicated include a PSAD less than 0.1 ng/ml, Gleason score of 6 or less, and tumors smaller than 3 mm on needle biopsy. Patients with tumors not meeting these criteria should receive therapy in the form of radiation or radical prostatectomy.

Stage T3 tumors extend through the prostatic capsule, and 50% to 80% of these patients will have lymph node metastases. Because there is no proven adjuvant therapy for prostate cancer, these patients do not benefit from radical prostatectomy. To achieve local control of their disease, external beam radiation therapy may be offered.

At this time, patients with known distant metastases cannot be cured, and treatment efforts for this group are largely palliative. Hormonal therapy via castration, luteinizing hormone releasing hormone (LHRH) agonist, or estrogen therapy should be administered with the development of symptoms of metastatic disease.

To date, efforts to develop chemotherapeutic regimens for prostate cancer have been disappointing. Since all tumors eventually acquire a hormonally insensitive phenotype, hormonal therapy inevitably fails. Two recent advances have increased our ability to treat hormone refractory disease. One study reported a 40% to 50% response rate using a topoisomerase II inhibitor (VP16) that acts at the level of the nuclear matrix in combination with estramustine phosphate, which binds the nuclear matrix and enhances the effects of chemotherapeutic agents at this site. Studies at the National Cancer Institute and University of Maryland have shown a 50% partial response to suramin in hormone refractory patients. The presumed mechanism of action of suramin is as a growth factor inhibitor.

## BIBLIOGRAPHY


Barry MJ: Epidemiology and natural history of benign prostatic hyperplasia, *Urol Clin North Am* 17:495, 1990.

Barry MJ et al: The Measurement Committee of the American Urological Association: The American Urological Association Symptom Index for Benign Prostatic Hyperplasia, *J Urol* 148:1549, 1992.

Benson MC et al: The use of prostate specific antigen density to enhance the predictive value of intermediate levels of serum prostate specific antigen, *J Urol* 147:817, 1992.

Berry SJ et al: The development of human benign prostatic hyperplasia with age, *J Urol* 132:474, 1984.

Boring CC et al: Cancer statistics, *CA Cancer J Clin* 44:7, 1994.

Carter HB, Pearson JD: PSA velocity for the diagnosis of early prostate cancer, *Urol Clin North Am* 20:665, 1993.

Epstein JI et al: Pathologic and clinical findings to predict tumor extent of nonpalpable (Stage T1C) prostate cancer, *JAMA* 271:368, 1994.

Gormley GJ et al: The effect of finasteride in men with benign prostatic hyperplasia, *N Engl J Med* 327:1185, 1992.

Guess HA et al: Cumulative prevalence of prostatism matches the autopsy prevalence of benign prostatic hyperplasia, *Prostate* 17:241, 1990.

Holtgrewe HL et al: Transurethral prostatectomy: practice aspects of the dominant operation in American urology, *J Urol* 141:248, 1989.

Lepor H: Medical therapy for BPH, *Urology* 42:483, 1993.

Lepor H et al: A randomized multicenter placebo controlled study of the efficacy and safety of terazosin in the treatment of benign prostatic hyperplasia, *J Urol* 148:1467, 1992.

Oesterling JE et al: Influence of patient age on the serum PSA concentration: an important clinical observation, *Urol Clin North Am* 20:671, 1993.

Pienta KJ: Novel approaches to the diagnosis, treatment, and prevention of prostate cancer and breast cancer, *J Cell Biochem Suppl* 21(18D:Y):226, 1994 (abstract).

Stein CA: Suramin: a novel antineoplastic agent with multiple potential mechanisms of action, *Cancer Res* 53:2239, 1993.


CHAPTER

# 139 Bladder and Kidney Cancer

Michael J. Droller

## BLADDER CANCER

Approximately 50,000 new cases of bladder cancer are diagnosed annually. Men are affected three to four times as often as women. Most new cases (approximately 75%) are categorized as "superficial" (see following discussion), are usually amenable to conservative treatment, and are generally not progressive or life-threatening. The remainder are deeply invasive of the bladder wall, are potentially life-threatening, and require prompt aggressive treatment that may or may not be successful.

In 1895, Rehn reported the cases of several workers in an aniline dye factory who had developed bladder cancer. Subsequent studies correlated exposure to aromatic amines with an increased risk for developing bladder cancer. Exposure to similar substances in other industries (rubber manufacturing, hairdressing, etc.) led to the institution of various guidelines and regulations designed to minimize these risks.

Cigarette smoking produces a threefold to fourfold increase in the risk for developing bladder cancer. Correlations have been made between the intensity of exposure (number of cigarettes smoked, degree of inhalation) and the increased risk of developing bladder cancer. However, these have not received widespread publicity, and public awareness of this needs to be increased.

Correlations between the use of artificial sweeteners, coffee intake, and tryptophan (as a health food additive) and the risk for development of bladder cancer have also been suggested. However, these have been called into question and remain unproved. Urinary infections with certain organisms capable of converting urinary metabolites to carcinogens have also been proposed as risk factors. Genetic risk factors have not yet been clearly identified. However, recent studies have associated several genetic changes with the development of specific types of bladder cancer. This area will undoubtedly undergo further development in the future.

### Presenting signs and symptoms

The most common presenting symptom in patients with bladder cancer is painless gross hematuria. Such hematuria is characteristically observed throughout the urinary stream. If hematuria in men occurs only at the beginning or at the end of urination, it is more likely associated with a prostatic problem. However, bladder cancer still needs to be excluded.

Patients also complain occasionally of an increasing sense of urgency or discomfort while urinating. Although these symptoms are often indistinguishable from those associated with an acute bacterial cystitis, their persistence in the absence of a positive culture should prompt an evaluation for bladder cancer.

The most common presenting sign of bladder cancer is microscopic hematuria. In many instances the patient may not have seen blood in the urine. It is important to note that no association exists between the amount of blood and the likelihood that a bladder cancer is present. Therefore, the occurrence of blood in the urine, at least the first time, should always prompt an evaluation to diagnose or exclude bladder cancer.

## Diagnostic evaluation

Standard examinations required to evaluate gross or microscopic hematuria when bladder cancer is suspected include intravenous pyelography (IVP), cystoscopy, and urinary cytology. Upper tract imaging is necessary both to exclude the possibility of upper tract disease (renal cell carcinoma, urothelial cancer, or kidney stones) and to determine whether upper tract obstruction by a bladder tumor is present. Sonography may be used instead of pyelography as an initial screen but does not permit as full a visualization of the entire collecting system. Retrograde pyelography may be performed if a patient is allergic to IV contrast.

Cystoscopy is used to examine the urothelium that lines both the urethra and the bladder. Abnormal areas can be characterized, and the type of tumor that may be present can be defined. Although the cystogram phase of the IVP can be used occasionally to visualize a bladder tumor, it is generally of insufficient sensitivity to exclude definitively the presence of a small or flat bladder cancer.

A voided urine sample should be sent for cytologic assessment. Catheterized specimens should be avoided at first, since instrumentation may produce false-positive readings. On the other hand, barbotage specimens can be obtained if a sufficiently cellular sample is needed for flow cytometry.

The definitive approach to bladder cancer diagnosis is histologic examination of tissue removed by transurethral biopsy of the bladder epithelium and resection of the bladder tumor. Biopsies should be obtained of any areas in the bladder that appear abnormal in order to assess the urothelium for the presence of epithelial dysplasia or carcinoma in situ (see next section). Bladder tumors should be fully resected so that characterization of the tumor configuration, the grade of cells that compose the tumor, and its depth of penetration into the bladder wall can be made.

### Tumor staging

A staging system has been evolved based on correlations between the depth to which a particular bladder cancer has penetrated the bladder wall and its potential behavior.

Bladder cancers have traditionally been classified as either "superficial" or "deeply invasive." "Superficial" tumors comprise those tumors that are either confined to the mucosal layer or that have penetrated through the epithelial basement membrane into the underlying connective tissue (lamina propria). "Deeply invasive" tumors comprise those tumors that have extended into the superficial or deep muscle layer or extended even more deeply into the perivesical fat. Staging is best performed by magnetic resonance imaging (MRI) as a first choice; transrectal ultrasound, especially for tumors in the bladder neck; or computed tomography (CT).

The most common form of bladder cancer is a papillary, mucosally confined tumor that generally appears as a solitary lesion resembling a clustering of raspberry-shaped fronds on a fibrovascular stalk. Even when multiple tumors are seen, they tend to be of low or moderate grade. These tumors may recur in as many as 75% of patients after the initial lesion has been resected. However, fewer than 3% of such tumor diatheses are associated with the later development of progressive disease. Although occasionally multiple, these lesions are rarely associated with atypia or frank carcinoma in situ either at their margin or at other sites in the bladder. Such tumors rarely present a life-threatening risk.

In contrast, "superficial" tumors that have infiltrated the lamina propria have been associated with later progression in as many as 30% of cases. These tumors are often of a higher grade than their mucosally confined counterparts and are often seen in association with atypia or carcinoma in situ at their margin or at other sites in the bladder. Although they may appear endoscopically to have a papillary configuration (as do the mucosally confined lesions), they may also be found to have a more solid or nodular appearance, especially when part of a more diffuse malignant diathesis.

Muscle-infiltrative bladder cancers are composed of two types: those that are invasive of only the superficial muscle and those that penetrate more deeply either into the deep muscle or into the perivesical fat. The former have been characterized as invading in a broad front and have been found to involve the bladder wall vasculature and lymphatics in approximately one third of patients. They may have a less progressive course than their more deeply infiltrative counterparts, which present with a more nodular configuration, appear to penetrate the bladder wall in a more tentacular pattern, and may involve the bladder wall vasculature and lymphatics in two thirds of cases.

The more superficial muscle-infiltrative cancers have been associated with a 40% to 65% 5-year survival, and a variety of bladder-conserving approaches have been applied with some success in treating these types of tumor (see later discussion). The more deeply muscle-infiltrative cancers have generally been associated with a 10% to 15% 5-year survival despite aggressive surgical therapies; 50% of these patients develop metastatic disease within 2 years of diagnosis despite having undergone prompt cystectomy. These forms of disease may therefore already have been systemic in most patients at the time of their initial clinical diagnosis. Deeply invasive tumors are usually already at an advanced stage at their earliest clinical presentation. Although they have undoubtedly proceeded through progressive phases of infiltration into the bladder wall, only 10% to 15% have been found clinically to arise from earlier superficial cancers. Moreover, a majority are systemic at the time of their clinical diagnosis despite our inability to detect metastases when the diagnosis is made.

*Carcinoma in situ* consists of neoplastic cells that are confined to the urothelial layer. However, in as many as 30% of cases, cells have been found to infiltrate microscopically into the lamina propria. Moreover, these cancer diatheses may ultimately demonstrate aggressive infiltration of the bladder wall at varying intervals after initial diagnosis, especially when carcinoma in situ is found in the context of papillary tumors that have penetrated the lamina propria. Nodular tumors may arise directly in areas of carcinoma in situ and infiltrate the bladder wall before any evidence of cancer is clinically evident. Whether aggressive treatments need to be applied in all these situations, or whether some can be controlled with conservative measures, requires further study.

Endoscopically, areas of carcinoma in situ may appear reddened, velvety, and "inflamed." Whereas in situ lesions are often accompanied by irritative symptoms, "superficial" or "deeply infiltrative" cancers are generally asymptomatic. The presence of carcinoma in situ generally indicates a more diffuse tumor diathesis with an often more aggressive potential behavior. Urinary cytology may be particularly useful in suggesting its existence.

The grade of a bladder cancer may also be useful in determining prognosis of a particular tumor diathesis. Grade is determined by the degree of differentiation of cells that comprise the tumor. Cells in well-differentiated (grade 1) tumors maintain a normal appearance with regularly shaped nuclei and a normal nuclear/cytoplasmic ratio. Although the number of cell layers in such tumors is often greater than in the normal epithelium, normal polarity of these cell layers is generally maintained. Cells in higher-grade tumors (grades 2 and 3) have a more irregular nuclear shape, clumped chromatin, prominent nucleoli, and a very high nuclear/cytoplasmic ratio. Cell polarity is generally lost. The higher the grade, the more deeply invasive a particular bladder cancer is likely to be. The exception is carcinoma in situ, which is generally comprised of high-grade cells that have remained confined to the epithelium without grossly penetrating the bladder wall.

### Treatment

***Superficial disease.*** Transurethral resection, which is used to obtain tissue for pathologic diagnosis, is generally successful in fully excising a tumor when it is the type that is mucosally confined and low grade. Although recurrence is frequently seen, repeat transurethral resection will again restore a normal epithelium. Transurethral resection has little morbidity, and in this setting there is minimal risk for progressive disease to occur. When rapid recurrence is seen, or a multiplicity of tumors does not permit effective resection, instillation of chemotherapeutic agents may facilitate elimination of disease.

Transurethral resection is also an effective treatment for those superficial papillary tumors that may have infiltrated the lamina propria. If extensive infiltration has occurred, however, transurethral resection may not remove all the cancer. Therefore, adjunctive intravesical agents may be instilled to eradicate any tumor cells remaining after resection. This may be especially appropriate in these situations, since many lamina propria–infiltrative tumors are high grade and are associated with carcinoma in situ elsewhere in the urothelium.

The most common intravesical agents used as adjuncts to transurethral resection for treatment of superficial disease are mitomycin-C, a chemotherapeutic agent, and bacille Calmette-Guérin (BCG), an immunotherapeutic agent. Mitomycin-C has been most effective in preventing recurrence of mucosally confined papillary transitional cell tumors and in treating some forms of carcinoma in situ. BCG has been most effective in preventing recurrence of carcinoma in situ and in the treatment of high-grade lamina propria–invasive tumors. Other agents that have been used, largely in preventing recurrence of mucosally confined tumors, include thiotepa and doxorubicin (Adriamycin). Morbidities associated with these treatments have generally been rare. Continued surveillance is necessary to detect treatment failures early and to intervene more aggressively if signs of progression are seen.

The greatest risk associated with high-grade lamina propria–infiltrative cancers, especially when accompanied by carcinoma in situ, is the possibility of rapid progression. Radical cystectomy may be important to consider in these cases, since many of these cancers, once they have progressed to the bladder wall musculature, are found to be metastatic and beyond the realm of regional cure.

***Muscle-infiltrative cancer.*** The current standard of treatment for muscle-infiltrative bladder cancer is radical cystectomy. Five-year survival rates, or "cures," have been reported to be as high as 70% to 80% when the muscle-infiltrative cancers are more superficial. Five-year survival rates for those cancers that are deeply infiltrative have been only 10% to 15%. Although occasional long-term survival rates have been described in patients with cancers that have involved one or two pelvic lymph nodes microscopically, gross involvement of pelvic lymph nodes or extension of disease beyond the pelvic lymphatics have not been associated with cure by radical surgery in most patients.

Occasionally, bladder cancers that have invaded only the superficial musculature have been amenable to treatment by transurethral resection or by partial cystectomy. Such patients, however, need to be selected carefully, and these approaches should generally be reserved for palliation rather than cure.

Additional treatments have been applied to enhance response rates. These have included preoperative radiation therapy, preoperative chemotherapy, and adjunctive chemotherapy. Although occasional long-term responders are seen, these comprise largely anecdotal events, and predictably effective regimens remain to be defined. In essence, deeply infiltrative bladder cancer in most patients is likely to represent a systemic disease. As yet, no predictably effective systemic regimen has been discovered.

Because removal of the bladder remains the standard therapy for deeply infiltrative bladder cancer, urinary diversion is an important component of treatment of patients with this condition. Major advances have been made in utilizing segments of bowel to create continent reservoirs and even to attach these reservoirs to the urethra in an attempt to retain a semblance of a good quality of existence. Generally, the ileum, or segments of colon, have been used in creating these reservoirs. Although none is perfect in replacing the normally functioning bladder, their imaginative use has led to dramatic improvement in the quality of life in patients undergoing cystectomy.

## KIDNEY CANCER

Kidney cancer, or renal cell carcinoma, is a malignancy thought to arise from the proximal tubule cells of the kidney. It is most frequently seen in patients between 40 and 60 years of age, affecting men 1.5 to 2 times more often than women. It is estimated that 28,500 new cases of renal cell cancer were diagnosed in the United States in 1994 (17,000 males; 10,500 females) and that 11,000 will die of their disease (6500 males; 4500 females).

Little is known about the carcinogenic process or epidemiologic factors that account for the development of renal cell carcinoma. Associations have been suggested between exposures to heavy metals such as mercury and cadmium and the development of kidney malignancies. Similar associations between cigarette smoking or environmental pollutants and renal cancer have not been described. Patients undergoing chronic dialysis who develop multicystic disease have been found to be at risk for the development of renal cell cancers. The mechanism underlying this phenomenon is not understood.

### Presenting signs and symptoms

The triad of hematuria, flank pain, and palpable abdominal mass that has traditionally been associated with the presence of renal cell cancer is now rarely seen. A patient may have only gross or microscopic hematuria without other symptoms. Renal colic may occur if a blood clot has obstructed the ureter. An abdominal mass rarely is palpated. Currently, renal cell cancer is most often diagnosed when imaging studies are performed in evaluation of asymptomatic microscopic hematuria. In addition, it is becoming more common for a renal mass to be diagnosed coincidentally when imaging studies are performed for unrelated symptoms (see next section).

Physical examination rarely elicits any abnormality associated with renal cell cancer. The ability to palpate a renal mass is limited by both the size of the mass and the location of each kidney under the rib cage. Flank tenderness is rarely demonstrated. Occasionally, the development or enlargement of a scrotal varicocele is observed. However, this may only be seen if the cancer has involved the renal vein on the left or has extended into the vena cava on the right.

Paraneoplastic syndromes occasionally accompany the development of renal cell cancer. Fevers of unknown origin, anemia, and polycythemia have been reported in approximately 1% to 3% of renal cell cancers.

### Diagnostic studies

Imaging studies are critical in documenting the presence of a renal mass. Previously, the most frequently used diagnostic imaging study was IVP. This has now been largely replaced by sonography. Sonography avoids the use of IV contrast materials to which patients may be allergic and permits distinctions to be made between masses that are solid and those that are cystic. In general, renal cell cancers are solid masses; it is rare to see a renal cell cancer involving a simple renal cyst. This may not be the case, however, if a cyst is multiseptated, thick-walled, and irregular or contains irregular calcifications in its wall.

The presence of a solid mass or complex cyst on ultrasound generally indicates the need for a CT scan. This should be performed both with and without IV contrast to permit determination of the character of the lesion and whether it enhances with contrast. This is generally indicative of a malignancy. The appearance of a renal cell cancer on CT scan is virtually pathognomonic. Some mass lesions, such as oncocytoma, may be indistinguishable radiographically from a renal cell cancer. Others, such as angiomyolipoma, can be distinguished easily.

CT and ultrasound studies are also useful in determining whether the renal vein and vena cava are involved by tumor thrombi. Lymph nodes at the renal hilum and around the great vessels may also be assessed for increased size and possible metastatic disease. MRI, nuclear scanning, and arteriography rarely aid in the evaluation of renal cell cancer, although the latter may occasionally be useful in planning the surgical approach when a partial nephrectomy is being considered.

It has become more and more common to diagnose kidney cancer as an incidental finding on sonograms or CT scans that have been performed for symptoms (back pain or abdominal pain) that are entirely unrelated. The tumors that are diagnosed under these circumstances are often much smaller than those that have been seen previously when imaging studies were performed for signs or symptoms associated directly with these mass lesions.

Once a diagnosis of renal cell cancer has been made, a nuclear bone scan and a pulmonary CT scan are generally performed to exclude metastases to these sites.

## Staging

A staging system for kidney cancer has evolved on the basis of correlations that have been observed between extent of the malignancy, likelihood of metastatic disease, and amenability to cure by surgical excision. Smaller lesions (those less than 3 cm in diameter) have generally been called adenomas to distinguish them from renal cell cancers on the assumption that the likelihood of these lesions metastasizing is small. Recent studies have disputed the validity of these suggestions.

Given the increased frequency with which small, solid masses are now diagnosed, these observations are important to consider in the management of these cancers. Smaller cancers are more likely to be confined within the renal capsule and appear to have the best prognosis. Once a cancer has extended beyond the renal capsule, expected 5-year survival rates are greatly reduced. Kidney cancers that have extended beyond Gerota's fascia have an even poorer likelihood of cure. Such tumors are often found to involve adjacent structures or to have metastasized to adjacent lymph nodes and distant sites. Renal cell cancers have occasionally been found to extend tumor thrombi into the renal vein and the vena cava. The prognosis for these patients is generally much better than for those who have involvement of regional lymph nodes.

## Treatment

Surgical excision is the only treatment that is predictably effective for kidney cancers. "Radical" nephrectomy involves removal of the kidney and the surrounding fat contained within Gerota's (renal) fascia. The adrenal gland, often contained in its own compartment within Gerota's fascia, is removed together with the kidney. Hilar lymph nodes are often also removed, but this largely serves a diagnostic purpose rather than one that enhances therapy.

Some have suggested that simple enucleation or segmental nephrectomy may be the appropriate approach for smaller renal masses. Earlier studies in which such procedures were performed in the setting of a solitary kidney, bilaterally poorly functioning kidneys, or multiple cancers in both kidneys (such that preservation of renal tissue was an important objective in managing the patient) documented that renal-sparing approaches were as successful as radical nephrectomy for low-stage, low-grade disease in achieving equivalent 5-year survival rates. The likelihood that microscopic disease is present at multiple sites in the affected kidney is only 10% to 15%. The risk for the development of recurrent tumor in the original cancer bed may only be as great as 10%, depending on the size and conformation of the original cancer. Each of these considerations has prompted the conclusion that radical nephrectomy should remain the standard approach in most patients with renal cell cancer, especially since the likelihood of cancer development in the contralateral kidney is small. However, the smaller size at which kidney cancers are diagnosed, in association with the increasing rate of their coincidental discovery, has prompted the suggestion that partial nephrectomy should be considered more often, especially when clinical conditions justify attempts to preserve normal renal tissue, but even in the setting of bilaterally normal-functioning kidneys. Due to the fact that increased risks may be associated with partial nephrectomy and that most patients experience minimal effects from removal of the entire kidney, radical nephrectomy remains the standard approach to treatment.

On the other hand, surgery has not been found to be an effective therapeutic modality in the setting of metastatic disease. Although nephrectomy has been associated anecdotally with resolution of metastatic lesions in 1% to 2% of patients, documentation of this, for the most part, has been inadequate, and ultimate outcome has been poor in these cases. Angioinfarction before surgery, performed to stimulate an immune response that might lead to resolution of metastatic deposits, also has not been found to be an effective approach.

In the setting of a concurrent solitary metastasis, removal of both the primary kidney cancer and the metastatic lesion has generally been followed by appearance of multiple additional metastases within a year of surgery. On the other hand, when a solitary metastasis has appeared after nephrectomy has been performed, its removal has occasionally been associated with long-term survival. This may reflect the occasionally unpredictable biology of the primary disease rather than an expression of surgical efficacy.

Radical nephrectomy in the setting of metastatic disease has largely been reserved for palliation. Flank pain seen in association with a large renal mass, uncontrollable hemorrhage (despite attempts at angioinfarction), and unremitting fever or hypercalcemia have been used as indications for radical nephrectomy even though metastatic disease may be present. Such patients ultimately succumb to their disease, often with limited survival rates.

Radiation therapy has not been effective in the treatment of renal cell cancer. Currently, no single chemotherapeutic agent or combination regimens of these agents have been found to be effective in producing lasting responses in renal cell cancer. The use of progestational agents (e.g., Megace) has produced only anecdotal responses.

Isolated reports of "spontaneous" remissions of metastatic lesions have led to suggestions that the immune response may play a role in the control of renal cell cancer. A variety of attempts have therefore been made to recruit immune response mechanisms in the design of novel approaches in the treatment of this problem.

Numerous vaccines, cytokines, lymphokines, and immune effector cells have been used to treat patients with metastatic renal cell cancer. These approaches have produced mixed results at best, with response rates ranging from 15% to 20%. These results have generally been limited.

Most recently, the efficacy of interferons, interleukin-2 (IL-2), lymphokine-activated killer cells (LAK cells), tumor-infiltrating lymphocytes (TIL cells), and various combinations of these either alone or together with cytotoxic chemotherapeutic agents has been investigated. Although some have been reported to produce variable remissions of metastatic disease at several sites, these responses have generally not been lasting, and survival rates have remained largely unimproved.

The unpredictable natural history of renal cell cancer, even when metastatic, has made interpretation of these results difficult and controversial. Because of this and because of the morbidity associated with many of these treatments, these approaches cannot be depended on to palliate or prolong survival rates predictably in patients with metastatic renal cell cancer and should remain in the realm of investigation.

## BIBLIOGRAPHY

Fleischmann J, Huntley H: Renal tumors. In Krane RJ, Siroky MB, Fitzpatrick JM, editors: *Clinical urology,* Philadelphia, 1994, JB Lippincott.

Garnick MB, Richie JP: Primary neoplasms of the kidney and renal pelvis. In Schreier RW, Gottschalk CW, editors: *Diseases of the kidney,* Boston, 1988, Little, Brown.

Novick AC et al: Conservative surgery for renal cell carcinoma: a single center experience with 100 patients, *J Urol* 141:835, 1989.

Rosenberg SA et al: Experience with the use of high-dose interleukin-2 in the treatment of 652 cancer patients, *Ann Surg* 210:474, 1989.

CHAPTER

# 140 Impotence

Michael A. Werner
Irwin Goldstein
Robert J. Krane

*Erectile dysfunction* is defined as the persistent inability to achieve and maintain an erection adequate for successful sexual intercourse. Erectile dysfunction is a significant health problem for several reasons. First, it may be a harbinger of other, even more significant health problems. Impotence is associated with hypercholesterolemia, cigarette smoking, hypertension, and diabetes. Thus previously unknown significant and treatable systemic diseases may be discovered when a patient is evaluated for erectile dysfunction. Second, impotence is widespread. Impotence is an age-related phenomenon. At age 40, approximately 40% of men will have some degree of erectile dysfunction. At age 70, the incidence is increased to approximately 70%. Third, impotence is significantly associated with poor self-esteem and increased self-destructive behavior. Men with impotence smoke, drink, and gamble significantly more, much of which they attribute to their sexual inadequacy.

Primary care physicians will encounter more and more patients with the complaint of impotence. This is secondary to both an aging population and the fact that the "last taboo" against speaking about one's sexuality is beginning to crack as patients become more aware that they are not alone and that there are significant treatment options available. This complaint should be taken seriously in terms of both helping the patient address his problem and using it as a possible insight into the existence of more threatening concurrent illness.

This chapter first discusses penile anatomy and erectile physiology and then describes the diagnostic examinations and therapeutic options for the patient with erectile dysfunction.

## PENILE ANATOMY

Erections are physiologic penile events. To understand erectile physiology, penile anatomy must be understood first.

### Corpus cavernosum

The penis contains three main chambers. The corpus spongiosum primarily contains the urethra and mushrooms out to cap the penis thereby creating the glans. The afferent sensation of the glans (as transmitted by the pudendal nerve) is responsible for initiating most erections, except for psychologically and centrally mediated erections. The erectile chambers of the penis are the paired dorsal corpora cavernosa. These tissues contain venous sinusoids that act to trap blood when filled. They are surrounded by trabeculae, consisting of connective tissue and muscle.

The corpus cavernosum is surrounded by a thick fascial investment called the tunica albuginea. The tunica has two concentric layers that, along with its elastic fibers, allow it to stretch when filled with blood. Once it has reached its maximal volume, it gains rigidity, which ultimately allows for vaginal penetration.

### Penile arterial blood supply

The main blood supply to the penis is usually the pudendal arteries, branches of the internal iliac artery. The pudendal artery eventually becomes the common penile artery, which bifurcates into the dorsal penile artery and the cavernosal artery. The cavernosal artery enters its respective corpus cavernosum at the penile hilum, then gives off helicine arteries along its course through the erectile tissue. These arteries give blood supply to the sinusoids (small pools of blood lined by smooth muscle) and the surrounding tissue matrix. Normally, communication exists between the cavernosal artery and the deep dorsal artery. This is important in understanding penile revascularization surgery, because when new blood supply is brought to the deep dorsal artery, the blood may flow retrograde into the corpora cavernosa via the cavernosal artery.

### Penile venous system

The sinusoids drain into each other, the blood moving outward toward the most peripheral sinusoids (those closest to the tunica albuginea). Small venules drain these sinusoids and travel below the tunica to coalesce into the subtunical venular plexus, which is drained by the emissary veins that pierce the tunica. During an erection, when the tunica albuginea is stretched, these veins are elongated and sheared, thus functionally closing their lumina and preventing the drainage of blood. This so-called veno-occlusive mechanism is necessary to produce penile rigidity.

### Penile neuroanatomy

The penis is innervated by autonomic nerves (the cavernous nerves) and somatic nerves (the pudendal nerve.) The parasympathetic nerve fibers originate in the second, third, and fourth sacral vertebrae (S2, S3, S4) (the erection center). The preganglionic fibers enter the pelvic plexus. They are subsequently joined by sympathetic nerves to form the cavernous nerves. These enter the hilum of the penis anterior to the bulbous urethra. Stimulation of the cavernous nerves (and pelvic plexus) will induce an erection in males. This indicates that the parasympathetic nerves are responsible for erections. However, the post-ganglionic nerves secrete nitric oxide, the neurotransmitter responsible for erectile activity by causing cavernosal smooth muscle relaxation. Stimulation of the sympathetic plexus will cause detumescence.

The sensory nerve of the penis begins as its dorsal nerve. This subsequently becomes the internal pudendal nerve. Afferent stimulation of the penis causes erection via spinal pathways. Psychogenic erections are caused by signals from the brain that are transmitted to the spinal erection center.

The pudendal nerve also carries the somatic motor innervation to the bulbocavernosus and ischiocavernosus muscles. These muscles contract during sexual excitation to compress the corpus cavernosum muscles and thus further increase the intracavernosal pressure. During ejaculation, the bulbocavernosus muscle rhythmically contracts, which pushes the semen down the urethra.

## ERECTILE PHYSIOLOGY

An erection is primarily a hemodynamic phenomenon, which has a net result of substantially increasing the amount of blood in the penis, thus giving it increased size and rigidity. Theoretically, two activities must occur: more blood must be delivered to the penis, via the arteries, and blood must be trapped by the venous sinuses. The absolute functioning of these two processes and their interaction ultimately determine the possibility for a successful erection. The psychologic and hormonal milieus as well as the intact neurologic functioning are also significant factors affecting erection. We now include a basic discussion of penile erectile physiology.

Smooth muscle relaxation is the key factor in achieving erection. Smooth muscle lines both the cavernosal sinuses and the afferent arterioles. When the smooth muscle of the arterial wall relaxes, the lumen increases in size, increasing blood flow. When the smooth muscle lining the cavernosal sinuses relaxes, they can accommodate more blood. They thus increase in size and increase the compression of the subtunical venules, causing venous trapping. If inadequate blood flow reaches the penis, inadequate rigidity will be achieved. If inadequate venous trapping occurs, even with good inflow, the penis will not become rigid.

When describing this phenomenon to our patients, we use the analogy of attempting to fill a tire that is connected to an air hose. If the tire does not become full, there can either be a kink in the air hose (an arterial problem) or a leak in the tire (a venous trapping problem). This analogy is also useful in explaining to patients why it is difficult to assess the penis in the flaccid state.

The patient must also be neurologically intact to receive afferent stimuli and transmit autonomic signals. Neurologic disorders resulting in decreased cavernosal nerve function will diminish the patient's spontaneous erections, while leaving his hemodynamic vascular system intact.

## PATIENT HISTORY

### Sexual

The patient history is especially crucial in the field of erectile dysfunction. As in many fields, the diagnosis is frequently apparent from the history. The first goal of the history is to determine exactly what the problem is. One must distinguish between problems with libido, erection, ejaculation, and orgasm. Often, patients are not clear in their own mind as to which of these aspects of erection they are having difficulty with. Next, the effects of the erectile dysfunction on the patient and his relationship must be assessed. Finally, the patient's goals in receiving treatment must be understood.

***Libido.*** Diminished libido may result from endocrine or psychologic disorders. Hypogonadism may cause a decrease in libido. However, men with low-normal testosterone are not generally treated with testosterone replacement. Patients may have a psychologic loss of libido that is a response to their erectile problems; that is, they would be interested in increasing their sexual activity if their erections were not so disappointing or unreliable.

***Erection.*** *Potency* is defined as the ability to achieve and maintain penetration until ejaculation. However, patients may not be satisfied with the quality of their erections, either in terms of absolute performance or in comparison with previous performance. The quality of the erection must be evaluated in terms of rigidity or sustaining ability.

*Rigidity* depends on the geometry of the penis (its dimensions), its biomechanical properties, and the intracavernosal pressure that can be achieved. The achievement of adequate intracavernosal pressure depends on smooth muscle relaxation and adequate hemodynamic factors.

*Sustaining capability* is best quantified by the number of minutes that rigidity can be maintained with minimal stimulation. Morning, coital, and masturbatory erections must be assessed and compared. A man who achieves a rigid erection rapidly, but loses it quickly, would most typically have a veno-occlusive problem.

The onset of the problem is also often a clue in distinguishing between organic and psychologic etiologies. If the erectile problems are of acute onset, after some traumatic event, and occur during sexual encounters but not during sleeping or masturbation, a psychologic etiology may be suspected (but is not necessarily assured.) If the change is slow in progression and not associated with a specific event or life situation, an organic etiology is more likely.

The patient must also be assessed for Peyronie's disease by asking him if he has pain with erection, penile curvature, penile bumps or lumps, or a history of penile trauma. Peyronie's disease is currently thought to be secondary to penile trauma (either chronic or acute) with resultant scarring of the tunica albuginea. This causes not only penile curvature but in many cases an inability to achieve complete veno-occlusion, and thus loss of rigidity and sustaining capability.

Finally, a psychosocial history is important in determining what psychologic factors could be affecting the patient's erections and what psychologic effects the patient's erections have had on him.

### Medical

The patient's medical history is crucial in the evaluation of organic impotence. Diabetes, atherosclerosis, neurologic disease, hypercholesterolemia, hypertension, and sickle cell disease are frequently associated with impotence. Many medications have deleterious effects on erections; it is currently thought that antihypertensive medications may have their effect not at the penile level, but by lowering systemic blood pressure and thus decreasing intracavernosal pressure. Previous pelvic surgery may have injured the innervation of the penis or its vascular supply. Previous penile or perineal trauma may cause arterial or veno-occlusive dysfunction. The patient's medical situation often reveals significant information about the etiology of the patient's impotence and helps determine the options available to him.

## IMPOTENCE EVALUATION

The purpose of an impotence evaluation is to determine the etiology of the impotence. Most importantly, the evaluation will direct the treatment. It also serves the function of filling the patient's need to know why he has developed erectile dysfunction. Most patients and their partners are very relieved to know that the problem is not psychologic. Finally, impotence may be the presenting complaint for a previously undiagnosed illness (e.g., diabetes mellitus, vascular disease).

For many patients, none of these reasons is applicable. These are older men with known risk factors who are not candidates for penile revascularization and who simply want to regain their potency. These patients need only simple screening and basic evaluation before treatment.

### Laboratory tests

Screening for systemic medical disorders, endocrine disease, and vascular risk factors is appropriate. Thus, if not done recently, complete blood counts, SMA (Sequential Multiple Analyzer) profiles (including a fasting glucose), and a cardiac profile (fasting cholesterol, low-density lipoprotein, high-density lipoprotein, triglycerides) should be obtained. If libido is diminished, serum testosterone should be measured.

*Nocturnal penile tumescence (NPT).* NPT testing may be performed at home or in a sleep laboratory. A strain gauge capable of measuring changes in penile circumference is placed around the penis. During a night of sleep, the erectile activity is measured. A portable machine able to measure both circumferential change and rigidity called the Rigiscan is available for home use.

A normal male will have three to five physiologic erections lasting approximately 25 to 35 minutes every night. Most men with psychogenic impotence have normal sleeping erections. Men with an organic etiology to their impotence usually have abnormal nocturnal erections. The most notable exception to this is patients who have neurologic impotence that affects their afferent sensory nerves. Thus, this test is a useful screen to help differentiate between psychogenic and organic impotence.

*Neurologic testing.* Neuropathology producing impotence may be present in the peripheral or central conduction pathways. Ultimately, there must be interference with the ability of the motor efferent autonomic cavernosal nerves to the penis to cause smooth muscle relaxation.

Biothesiometry, a simple test to assess the ability to sense vibration, is the usual screen for peripheral afferent abnormalities. Dorsal nerve conduction velocity or bulbocavernosus reflex latency testing can be used to test for peripheral and sacral spinal pathology. The electrical activity of the cavernosal nerve as transmitted to corporal smooth muscle can be recorded using either intracavernosal electromyographic needles or surface electrodes on the penile shaft. For evaluation of the central nervous system, a genitocerebral evoked potential study may be performed by electrically stimulating the penis and recording over the sensory cortex to determine conduction time.

*Psychogenic testing.* The psychogenic aspect of erection is obvious. Men can achieve erections without penile stimulation. Just as psychologic stimuli can create or enhance an erection, negative psychologic stimuli can inhibit them. Negative psychologic input can inhibit the sacral cord–mediated reflexogenic erections. An excessive adrenergic state may cause an increase in penile smooth muscle tone, opposing the smooth muscle relaxation needed for an erection. We have every new patient seen by a psychologist not only to help differentiate between organic and psychogenic impotence, but also to help determine how the impotence has affected the patient and his and his partner's goals in seeking treatment.

*Hormonal testing.* The role of testosterone in erections remains unclear. Thus we do not use it as a screen for men complaining of sexual dysfunction unless libido is a complaint or poor virilization is noted. Because serum testosterone varies throughout the day, early-morning specimens should be used. If these values are consistently low, we check luteinizing hormone (LH) and prolactin.

Low serum testosterone can be associated with hyperprolactinemia. However, if serum prolactin remains elevated, potency is restored in only half the patients whose testosterone is normalized by exogenous replacement. Hyperprolactinemia requires it own investigation.

Hyperthyroidism is often associated with diminished libido and occasionally with impotence. Hypothyroidism may cause impotence secondary to associated low testosterone and elevated prolactin levels.

*Vascular testing.* Erections are a complex hemodynamic process. They require both adequate blood inflow (arterial component) and adequate venous trapping (corporal venous occlusive component.) The importance of distinguishing between these two components and attempting some quantification of them is both to determine which therapy is appropriate and to help predict its outcome. Isolated blockages in the penile arterial tree (as opposed to diffuse disease) are amenable to surgical bypass therapy (Fig. 140-1). Diffuse arterial disease and venous leak, which causes the vast majority of cases of impotence, are not amenable to corrective therapy. Therapy in these patients attempts to override (penile injection therapy) or completely circumvent (prosthesis or vacuum erection devices) the problem.

*Arterial testing.* Arterial testing may be performed in the flaccid or erect state. As in any hemodynamic system,

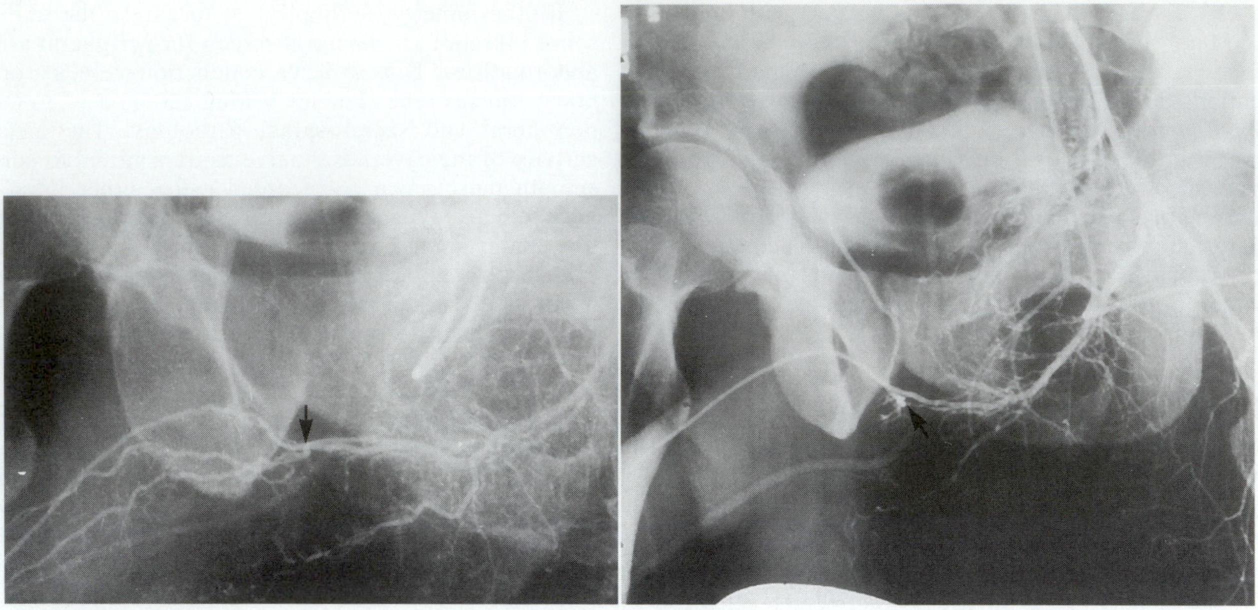


**Fig. 140-1. A,** Normal pudendal arteriogram showing a patent pudendal-penile artery bifurcating *(arrow)* into normal dorsal and corporal arteries. **B,** Arteriogram showing a diseased pudendal artery and obstruction at the takeoff of the corporal artery *(arrow).* In this case the dorsal artery is well visualized.

more accurate information will be obtained in the active state. However, the flaccid state may give some clues as to the etiology of the problem.

**Penile-brachial index (PBI).** The systolic pressure of all arteries should be approximately the same. Thus, if there is no arterial blockage, the systolic pressure in the arm (brachial pressure) should be the same as the systolic pressure in the penis. The penile pressure may be measured by placing a small cuff around the base of the penis and inflating it until the arterial pulse, as determined by Doppler ultrasound, disappears. The ratio of penile systolic pressure to brachial systolic pressure is the PBI. Normal values should be greater than 0.85.

**Duplex ultrasonography.** As discussed earlier, a more accurate picture of the arterial system's ability to deliver blood necessary for an erection will be achieved if an erection is achieved or attempted by intracavernosal injection of vasoactive agents. Medications injected intracavernosally can cause smooth muscle relaxation, which will then dilate the arterial system. The diameter changes in the cavernosal artery and the changes in blood velocity through it can be measured by duplex ultrasound. If these findings are normal, arterial insufficiency can be ruled out to the level of the vessels tested. Anxiety produced by being in the physician's office and having a needle placed in his penis may induce the patient to override the intracavernosal smooth muscle relaxation by adrenergic inhibition. If the patient can achieve an erection that closely approximates his best erections at home, however, he can be presumed to have achieved complete smooth muscle relaxation. At present, the exact values of cavernosal artery flow velocity that may be considered abnormal are not universally agreed on. Most investigators believe that velocities greater than 30 cm per second should be considered in the normal range.

**Selective pudendal arteriogram.** In patients who demonstrate focal proximal arterial obstruction but no evidence of venous leak, penile revascularization may be considered. The patient's arterial system must be evaluated before the procedure. Since this is a rather invasive and expensive test, it is almost exclusively used for patients considering revascularization.

***Corporal veno-occlusive function testing.*** The amount of water in a sink is related not only to the speed of the water being placed in it, but also to how much leaks out. No matter how good the blood supply to the penis, if there is an inadequate trapping system, difficulty obtaining an erection and holding it will be found. Corporal veno-occlusive dysfunction (CVOD) is best tested for during dynamic infusion cavernosometry and cavernosography (DICC).

During DICC two needles are placed in the penis after the intracavernosal injection of smooth muscle relaxants. One needle is attached to a pressure transducer to measure intracavernosal pressure, and the second allows fluid to be infused. During this procedure, it is possible to test the veno-occlusive function by determining the amount of flow required to maintain a given intracavernosal pressure. Normally in this study, only 2 to 3 ml per minute of flow is required to maintain a rigid erection at 120 to 150 mm Hg pressure. Leakage can be visualized by injecting contrast via one of the needles during this active test. In a normal penis with normal trapping, minimal to no contrast should be seen escaping from the corpora.

## TREATMENT

### Psychologic therapy

Traditionally, most impotence was considered secondary to psychologic causes, and therapy was directed primarily at a psychodynamic level. Psychotherapy is now mostly focused on correcting the immediate causes of the problem: to decrease performance anxiety, provide alternate methods of giving pleasure, and to deal with the secondary problems that the impotence has created. For some patients, although their impotence is psychologic, penile injections can be used as an adjunct to help them overcome otherwise unremediable performance anxiety.

### Nonhormonal medical therapies

Although significant interest exists in nonhormonal medical therapies, none has really been shown to be effective to this date. The most frequently used medication is yohimbine hydrochloride. It is an $\alpha_2$-adrenergic blocking agent and is thought to act centrally. Controlled studies have shown an improvement over placebo when yohimbine was used in patients with psychogenic impotence. For the vast majority of patients, however, it does not represent an effective solution to the problem.

Clinical trials with multiple oral agents (including trazodone and different $\alpha_2$-blockers) as well as with topically and intraurethrally administered agents continue.

### Hormonal therapy

***Testosterone.*** As men age, their serum testosterone levels decrease. Only men with hypogonadal disorders, either hypogonadotropic hypogonadism (pituitary or hypothalamic in origin) or hypergonadotropic hypogonadism (testicular failure) are candidates for testosterone replacement. The purpose of the replacement is to restore libido and improve potency. Since serum testosterone varies, only patients with consistent changes over several samplings should be treated. Since oral testosterone can be hepatotoxic, intramuscular injection of 200 to 300 mg testosterone enanthate every 2 to 3 weeks is the preferred method of testosterone replacement. Patients treated in this manner must have their serum testosterone remeasured because response is varied. Testosterone can potentially accelerate the growth of prostate carcinoma, and thus all men should be screened with a rectal examination and prostate-specific antigen (PSA) before initiating treatment. If either is abnormal, a transrectal ultrasound examination and possibly a biopsy should be performed.

***Prolactin.*** Hyperprolactinemia is usually treated by administration of bromocriptine or by surgical ablation of a pituitary prolactin-secreting tumor. Medications causing hyperprolactinemia (e.g., estrogens, $\alpha$-methyldopa) should be stopped if possible. High levels of prolactin seem to inhibit erections, since simply replacing testosterone in patients with continued hyperprolactinemia does not always restore potency.

### Vacuum constrictor devices

The components of a vacuum constrictor device (VCD) include (1) a cylindric vacuum chamber into which the penis is placed, (2) a vacuum pump attached to the chamber (this may be electric or mechanical and may have a pressure gauge), and (3) a constriction ring. The VCDs differ from a physiologic erection in several important respects. Blood is drawn into the penis by the surrounding vacuum. Once the penis is rigid, venous outflow is restricted by the rubber ring that is placed around the base of the penis. In a physiologic erection, the corpora cavernosa, and only the corpora cavernosa, are engorged with blood. Their entire length continues beyond the penoscrotal junction and into the perineum. In a VCD-created erection, all the blood distal to the constricting ring is trapped. Thus all compartments of the penis are engorged, including the corpus spongiosum (including the urethra), and the erection pivots at its base, which is the penoscrotal junction, because no blood proximal to the ring is trapped.

Because the constriction ring limits arterial inflow as well as venous outflow, the erect state is also an ischemic one. It is recommended that the ring should not be left in place for more than 30 minutes.

VCDs are part of the impotence treatment armamentarium. They can be considered in every patient except those who have significant intracorporal scarring and thus cannot fill with blood to achieve rigidity. They are specifically indicated for patients with severe venous leak who are unresponsive or poorly responsive to intracavernosal injections.

The advantages of the VCDs include their relatively low cost (about $300 to $450), which is a one-time purchase. They are clearly not invasive, and they have few long-term complications.

Patients may experience the inability to achieve adequate rigidity, difficulty with ejaculation (secondary to the constricting ring around the urethra), or penile pain, petechiae, and ecchymoses.

Patient acceptance and satisfaction with VCDs have been reported to range from 68% to 83%.

### Intracavernosal injection of vasoactive agents and penile erection program

The ability to inject drugs intracavernosally to achieve pharmacologic erections has been one of the most exciting developments in the treatment of sexual dysfunction. These drugs cause localized smooth muscle relaxation, which, as discussed earlier, increases blood flow to the penis and increases the storage of blood in the venous sinusoids. This increased blood flow begins a cascade effect by releasing local factors, which in turn increase smooth muscle relaxation.

Approximately 80% of patients will respond to intracavernosal pharmacotherapy. The patients who will have the worst response are those with severe veno-occlusive disease (venous leak). Although more blood may enter the penis, they simply cannot hold onto it.

***Medications.*** Three drugs, prostaglandin $E_1$ ($PGE_1$), phentolamine, and papaverine, are the main agents used for intracavernosal injection. Papaverine acts by relaxing the smooth muscle cells of the lacunar trabeculae and the penile arteries (primarily the helicine arteries). Thus more blood is brought into the penis via the arteries, and the trapping mechanism of the sinuses is activated. Side effects are rare but include hypotension, nausea, vomiting, weakness, flushing, dizziness, and sinus tachycardia. Rare elevations in liver transaminases have been reported. $PGE_1$ is an endogenously produced eicosanoid that also produces smooth muscle relaxation. Side effects are all local (probably because the drug is metabolized in the penis) and include penile discomfort and pain, redness, and a burning sensation of the penile skin. Phentolamine is an α-adrenergic antagonist and blocks sympathetic vasoconstrictive activity by blocking both $\alpha_1$- and $\alpha_2$-adrenergic receptors. Because it does not directly create smooth muscle relaxation, phentolamine does not work by itself to produce an erection. Rather, it is used as an adjunct to papaverine and $PGE_1$. Phentolamine's side effects include hypotension, tachycardia, cardiac arrhythmias, weakness, dizziness, nasal stuffiness, nausea, and vomiting.

***Penile erection program.*** Before being enrolled in a penile erection (injection) program (PEP), patients must be given an informed consent. They must thoroughly understand the potential side effects of the treatment. They must also understand that these medications have not been approved by the U.S. Food and Drug Administration (FDA) for penile injection, although they are approved for other uses.

The program consists of two phases. During the titration phase, the patient receives injections in the office. These are designed to approximate how much medication the patient will need and to teach the patient how to inject. During the home-trial phase, the patient is given prefilled syringes and begins to inject at home. Once a proper dosage has been achieved, the patient is given a supply of medication. He can then continue to inject at home and is required to inject each time he desires an erection.

Side effects include hematomas, penile pain with injection (which is usually because of the prostaglandin), infection, penile fibrosis, and penile curvature. Patients may develop priapism, defined as a prolonged erection lasting longer than 4 hours. Because the penis in this state is relatively ischemic, if not treated promptly, priapism may lead to severe scarring of the corpora cavernosa and subsequent impotence not responsive to intracavernosal injections. The development of priapism almost always occurs during the dosage determination phase, and patients should be instructed to call their physician if an erection following injection lasts for more than 4 hours. Patients with priapism are usually treated with an intracavernosal injection of an α-agonist to produce detumescence. Phenylephrine or ephedrine is usually employed. The second significant side effect is painless fibrotic nodules within the corpora cavernosa. These are thought to be secondary to the trauma of injection or inadequate manual compression of the injection site. They usually develop after prolonged use and rarely require cessation of therapy. On rare occasions, these nodules may lead to penile curvature.

Patient satisfaction rate with injection therapy is high, and side effects are relatively few. For these reasons, intracavernosal injections of vasoactive drugs is one of the most frequently used and successful modalities available.

### Penile prosthesis

The penile prosthesis was the first surgical innovation in the treatment of male impotence. The principle is that a device implanted within the corpora can provide sufficient rigidity for penetration and comfortable intercourse. Ideally, the prosthesis should mimic a normal penis, being erect only when desired. It should be comfortable, infection and pain free, and have no mechanical failures.

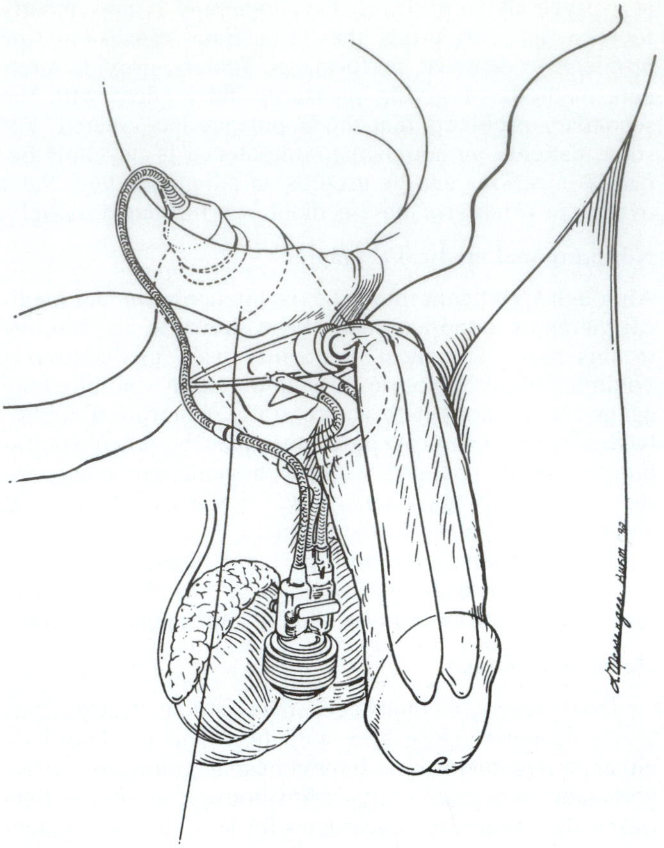

**Fig. 140-2.** After placement of an inflatable penile prosthesis, the two cylinders are within the corpora, the pump is in the scrotum, and the reservoir is in Retzius space just posterior to the pubic bone. This can all be accomplished through a scrotal incision. (From Krane RJ, Siroky MB, Fitzpatrick JM, editors: *Clinical urology,* Philadelphia, 1994, JB Lippincott.)

Penile prostheses continue to improve. With the variety of alternative methods available to achieve erection, the percentage of men with impotence wanting treatment who ultimately choose a prosthesis is rapidly decreasing, since most patients explore the nonsurgical therapies initially.

The original prostheses were semirigid. This meant that although the length of the penis was always the same, the angle of penile protrusion could be altered by bending it. Subsequently, ingenious methods have been developed, culminating in the current inflatable prosthesis (Fig. 140-2). This consists of two cylinders that are placed in the patient's corpora cavernosa. They are connected to a pump, which is placed in the scrotum. The pump in turn is connected to a reservoir, usually placed in the prevesical space. When the pump is compressed, it takes the fluid from the reservoir and pushes it into the cylinders. The cylinders fill and become rigid, making the penis around it larger and rigid. When the erection is no longer desired, the pump can be deactivated and cylinders deflated. For patients with severe erectile tissue leakage, this option may be the only viable one.

The disadvantages of the prosthesis are clear. Insertion requires a surgical procedure. A definite mechanical failure rate exists depending on the device implanted, which over time probably approaches 30%. With the invention and introduction of devices with less compliant materials and fewer connections, this rate has fallen. Prosthesis infection ranges from 1% to 8%. In these patients the prosthesis is almost always removed. The infection usually causes a severe corporitis, leading to fibrotic changes in the corpora, making a subsequent prosthesis placement, although definitely possible, more difficult. Once a prosthesis is placed, the patient's corporal tissue is no longer intact, and thus the patient may not reverse the procedure and subsequently obtain normal erections. For those patients with no other viable options, the prosthesis remains an excellent way to regain potency.

### Vascular surgery

Vascular surgery, as with vasculogenic impotence, may be divided into arterial and venous techniques. Unfortunately, venous surgery does not appear to be effective in stopping venous leak in all patients. The leak is usually secondary to a diffuse process and depends on the tissue characteristics (as opposed to the tunica albuginea.) In patients with a localized leak of small size and significant arterial disease, we simultaneously perform a microvascular bypass procedure (as described next) as well as localized vein ligation. In almost all other patients with significant leak, surgical options are not entertained.

***Arterial surgery.*** Young patients with localized lesions in the pudendal-penile arterial tree (as opposed to those with diffuse end-artery disease) are candidates for penile revascularization. Patients who are younger and have discrete lesions in the pudendal artery, the common penile artery, or both, usually caused by pelvic or perineal trauma, have the greatest chance of success. These patients may have impotence immediately after trauma, or it may be delayed, probably secondary to damage in the endothelium, which eventually causes atherosclerotic changes and discrete arterial disease. The inferior epigastric artery is the usual neoarterial source for revascularization (Fig. 140-3). The arterial blockage is bypassed by anastomosing this artery to the dorsal artery of the penis, the deep dorsal vein, or to both. Patient selection and significant surgical experience are prerequisites for performing this technique.

The preoperative patient evaluation is complex and includes DICC to ensure that venous leakage is not a significant component and to confirm that a gradient does exist between the brachial systolic pressure and the cavernosal artery pressure. Patients also must have a selective internal pudendal arteriogram to outline their arterial anatomy.

Well-selected patients have a 50% to 70% success rate with these techniques and thus may have their potency fully restored.

***Venous surgery.*** Venous surgery involves the surgical removal or ligation of the veins leaving the corpora cavernosa. This is usually accomplished by removing the deep dorsal vein and ligating the cavernosal veins with or without plication of the penile crura.

Intuitively, venous leak should also be correctable. Although in vogue for a long time, results of venous leak surgery have been poor. Venous leak may be secondary to diffuse disease affecting the erection tissue, which clearly is not amenable to surgical intervention. Focal venous leak, usually secondary to penile trauma (in the erect state), may be correctable. At this time, we reserve venous surgery for patients with a documented focal (as opposed to diffuse) leak concurrent with either arterial insufficiency or curvature secondary to Peyronie's disease, which requires surgical correction. In these patients, we perform venous leak surgery at the same time as we perform a microvascular arterial bypass procedure or a penile straightening procedure, respectively.

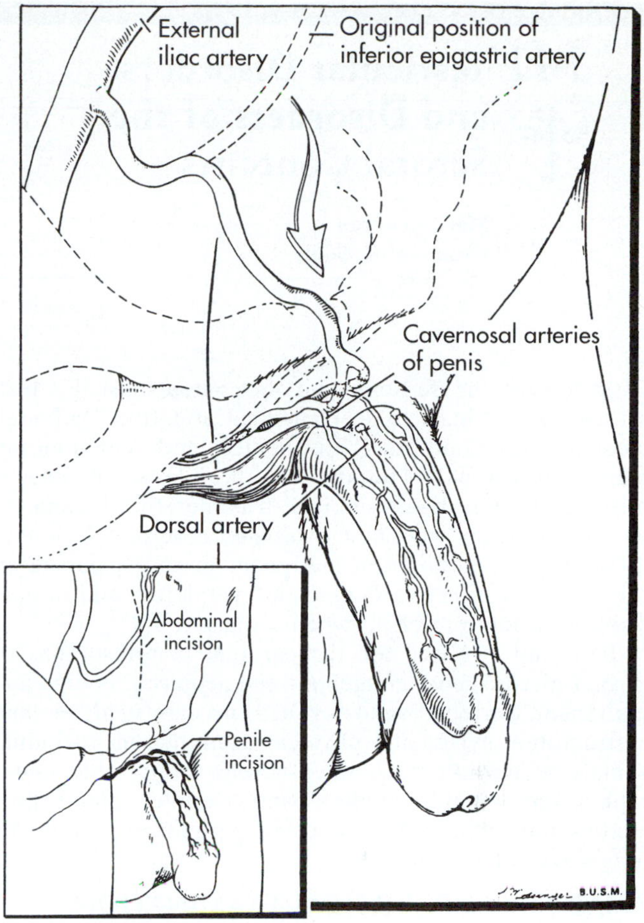


**Fig. 140-3.** Schematic representation of a penile revascularization procedure. In the inset, note that two incisions are required. Initially, the inferior epigastric artery is harvested through a vertical abdominal incision. This neoarterial source is then brought through an incision at the base of the penis. The inferior epigastric artery can then be anastomosed in a retrograde end-to-end fashion to the dorsal arteries of the penis. (From Krane RJ, Siroky MB, Fitzpatrick JM, editors: *Clinical urology*, Philadelphia, 1994, JB Lippincott.)

## SUMMARY

In the past 10 to 15 years, tremendous gains have been achieved in understanding the physiology of erections and impotence and in developing treatment modalities. Whereas once the only option was psychotherapy, it is now believed that 90% of impotence is organic. Tools have been developed to evaluate its etiology and thus target treatment appropriately. Men previously without hope now function normally; this enhancement of their life and of their health is profound.

CHAPTER

# 141 Testicular Disorders and Disorders of the Scrotal Contents

Marc Cendron
Grannum R. Sant

Disorders of the scrotum and its contents usually lead affected individuals to seek medical attention. Although most scrotal conditions are benign and self-limiting, malignant testicular tumors can be life-threatening if misdiagnosed or diagnosed late. It is therefore incumbent on the clinician who first evaluates a scrotal lesion to differentiate benign from malignant diseases, pursue an efficient cost-effective diagnostic evaluation, and initiate prompt urologic referral, when indicated.

Pain and swelling are the cardinal manifestations of scrotal disease, both congenital and acquired, benign and malignant. Correct diagnosis relies on a careful history and a structured, systematic physical examination, including urinalysis. Radiologic studies such as scrotal ultrasonography, radionuclide studies, and Doppler blood flow studies are employed in selected patients in whom the diagnosis is uncertain.

## ANATOMY AND PHYSICAL EXAMINATION

Careful examination of the scrotum and its contents is an integral part of the physical examination. Anatomically, the scrotum is a pouch situated below the penis and symphysis pubis and is partitioned into two sacs, each containing the male gonad or testis, the epididymis, and the lower portion of the spermatic cord. The scrotal wall consists of skin with the underlying dartos muscle and several thin fascial layers. The innermost layer is the tunica vaginalis, a remnant of the inner lining of the peritoneum.

Examination of the scrotum is best carried out with the patient in the standing position. A warm room and warm examining hands are encouraged because cold temperatures cause contraction of the dartos and cremaster muscles and elevation of the testis toward the external inguinal ring. The left testis frequently lies lower than the right, and the scrotal sac is usually hypoplastic when its gonad is absent. Palpation of each hemiscrotum is carried out by examining the testis for size, position, and consistency (Fig. 141-1). The epididymis is adherent to the posterolateral aspect of the testis, and the spermatic cord is palpable in the upper portion of the scrotum. Fig. 141-2 illustrates abnormalities associated with the epididymis.

The presence of an abnormal scrotal mass can be ascertained by careful palpation (see the box on p. 1805 and Fig. 141-3). The exact nature and location of the mass should be noted. Is it hard and firm or cystic and fluid filled? Does it arise from the testis or the other intrascrotal structures? How extensive is the mass? Does it change with straining or Valsalva's maneuver? Can the examining finger be inserted above it? Scrotal masses should be transilluminated with a pen light. Fluid-filled structures (e.g., hydrocele) radiate a reddish glow through the lesion. Tables 141-1 and 141-2 outline the physical signs and symptoms of mass lesions of the scrotum and the common causes of scrotal swelling.

## INFLAMMATORY DISEASES

Patients frequently seek attention for minor problems involving the external genitalia, problems that are overlooked when present in other parts of the body. Fungal skin disease is treated with topical or systemic fungicides. Furuncles of the scrotal skin and minor lacerations of the scrotum are treated as elsewhere in the body.

Purulent drainage from fistulous tracts in the scrotum requires prompt management. Causes include spontaneous urethral rupture secondary to urethral stricture disease with formation of urethrocutaneous fistulas, tuberculosis, or syphilis of the testis or epididymitis with abscess formation and fistulization. A retrograde urethrogram will document patency of the urethra. Pus should be examined and cultured for acid-fast bacilli and spirochetes. Scrotal fistulas require surgical drainage. Fistulas from the lower gastrointestinal tract (e.g., Crohn's disease) occasionally present in the perineoscrotal area.

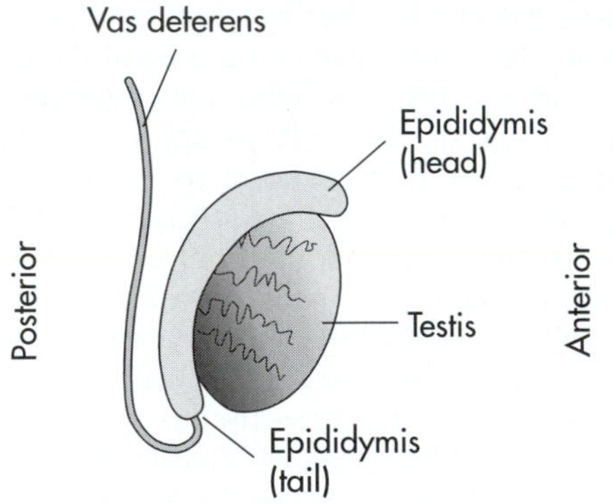


**Fig. 141-1.** Lateral view of the right testis, epididymis, and vas deferens. (From Krane RJ, Siroky MB, Fitzpatrick JM, editors: *Clinical urology,* Philadelphia, 1994, JB Lippincott.)

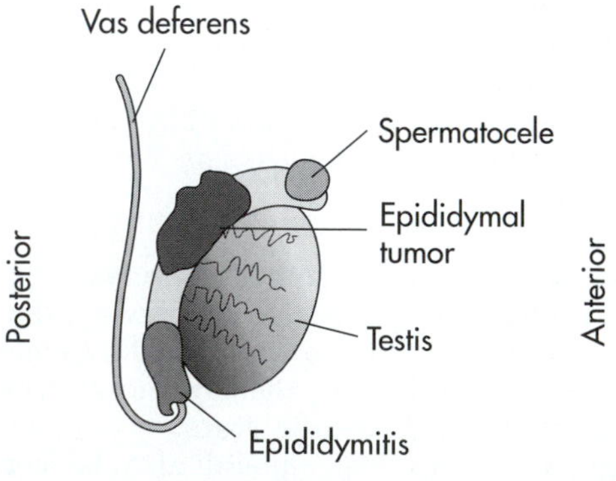


**Fig. 141-2.** Various abnormalities of the epididymis, including spermatocele, epididymal tumor, and epididymitis. (From Krane RJ, Siroky MB, Fitzpatrick JM, editors: *Clinical urology,* Philadelphia, 1994, JB Lippincott.)

### "Structured" physical examination of scrotal lesions

Cystic or solid
Tender or nontender
Confined to scrotum or extending into inguinal region
Anatomic position
- Testis, spermatic cord
- Epididymis
- Surrounding testis (hydrocele)
- Inguinoscrotal (hernias, hydroceles)

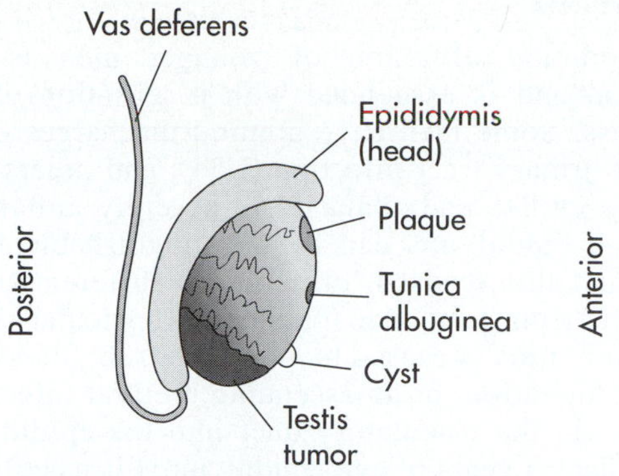


**Fig. 141-3.** Intratesticular abnormalities, including testis tumor, fibrous plaque, and cyst of the tunica albuginea. (From Krane RJ, Siroky MB, Fitzpatrick JM, editors: *Clinical urology,* Philadelphia, 1994, JB Lippincott.)

**Table 141-1.** Common intrascrotal conditions

| | Testicular torsion | Epididymitis | Testis tumor |
|---|---|---|---|
| **Age/symptoms** | | | |
| Age | Neonate through early 20s | Childhood through old age | 15 to 35 years |
| Nature of pain | Sudden | Progressive | Absent or gradual |
| Degree of pain | Severe | Variable | Absent or mild |
| Nausea/vomiting | Yes | No | No |
| **Physical examination** | | | |
| Testis | Swollen, tender | May be swollen | Hard mass |
| Epididymis | Swollen, tender | Swollen, tender | Normal |
| Spermatic cord | Shortened | Thickened, tender | Normal |
| Urinalysis | Normal | Pyuria, bacteriuria | Normal |

**Table 141-2.** Causes of scrotal swelling

| Structure | Pathology |
|---|---|
| Scrotal wall | Urinary extravasation<br>Trauma<br>Edema from cardiac, hepatic, or renal failure<br>Fungal infection |
| Testis | Carcinoma<br>Torsion of testis or appendix testis<br>Infection |
| Epididymis | Infection<br>Tumors (usually benign)<br>Torsion of appendix epididymis |
| Spermatic cord | Hydrocele<br>Hematocele<br>Hernia<br>Varicocele<br>Lipoma of cord<br>Spermatocele |

## Fournier's gangrene

This uncommon but potentially life-threatening infection of the scrotal, perineal, and inguinal skin can be a urologic emergency. It leads to tissue and fascial necrosis (necrotizing fasciitis) and is usually secondary to perirectal, ischiorectal, or periurethral infection. Initially, erythema and edema of the scrotum and a small patch of dry gangrene develop. Gangrene can extend rapidly along fascial planes into the lower abdominal wall. Diabetic patients are at increased risk for Fournier's gangrene. A complete blood count, platelet count, and Gram stain with cultures of the gangrenous area (aerobic and anaerobic) are performed.

Urgent surgical débridement and combination antibiotic therapy (high-dose penicillin, gentamicin, and clindamycin) are indicated until the causative organism(s) is (are) identified. Retrograde urethrography is performed if urinary extravasation is suspected. Prompt referral of suspected cases of Fournier's gangrene is mandatory, since these patients require hospitalization, intravenous (IV) antibiotic therapy, close monitoring and observation, and early, aggressive surgical débridement of gangrenous tissues. Significant mortality still is associated with Fournier's gangrene, especially in elderly, diabetic, and immunocompromised patients.

## Epididymitis

This common affliction of younger men is usually unilateral and is associated with a sensation of scrotal heaviness. Some men have urethral discharges or symptoms of urinary tract infection (UTI), and others develop pyrexia, chills, and malaise. A severely inflamed and indurated epididymis can be indistinguishable from the testis, and this leads to difficulty in differentiating epididymitis from testicular torsion and testicular tumor.

Epididymitis is caused by infection from bladder urine, prostate infection, or an ascending urethral infection that spreads via the ejaculatory duct into the epididymis. In men under 35 years of age, epididymitis is usually caused by chlamydial infection, and symptoms of urethritis (e.g., urethral discharge) frequently occur. In men over 35 years of age, the infection is secondary to coliform organisms from the bladder, and signs and symptoms of cystitis, prostatitis, or prostatism are frequently seen. "Sterile" epididymitis associated with vigorous physical activity can be caused by vasal reflux of sterile urine and chemical inflammation of the epididymis. Physical examination is indistinguishable from that in "infectious" epididymitis. Epididymitis may be the presenting feature of congenital urologic abnormalities in boys (e.g., ectopic ureter, posterior urethral valve). Evaluation with IV urography, cystourethroscopy, and voiding cystourethrography is indicated in all boys with epididymitis. Careful clinical and radiologic evaluation is also required to distinguish epididymitis from testicular torsion in boys.

The epididymis lies posterior to the testis, and this demarcation is preserved in all but the most severe cases of epididymitis. "Reactive" hydrocele formation may render the palpation of the intrascrotal structures difficult. Transillumination will usually confirm the presence of hydroceles. However, ultrasonography is more accurate and may be needed for confirmation. Whenever in doubt, surgical exploration is required to exclude torsion. Scrotal exploration should be done within 4 to 6 hours if testicular viability is to be preserved.

Epididymitis from syphilis, gonorrhea, or tuberculosis occurs infrequently (see the box above). Tuberculosis has now reemerged as a health care problem as a result of the increasing number of immunosuppressed patients with acquired immune deficiency syndrome (AIDS). This increased prevalence of tuberculosis will result in increased numbers of men with tuberculous epididymitis. "Chronic" epididymitis may follow acute epididymitis. However, this diagnosis most frequently represents mild, chronic, nonspecific (i.e., noninfectious) epididymitis associated with dull scrotal ache and mild induration of the epididymis.

Epididymitis is usually treated on an outpatient basis with scrotal elevation, bedrest, and appropriate antibiotics. Patients with leukocytosis and high fevers may require hospitalization for parenteral antibiotics and vigorous supportive treatment. Nonsteroidal antiinflammatory drugs (NSAIDs) (e.g., ibuprofen) and antipyretics (e.g., acetaminophen or aspirin) are usually prescribed. Severe pain may occasionally necessitate spermatic cord anesthetic block.

In younger men, epididymitis is usually caused by *Neisseria gonorrhoeae* or *Chlamydia trachomatis*. A Gram stain of the urethra may reveal the characteristic gram-negative intracellular diplococci of gonococcal urethritis. Gonococcal epididymitis is much less common, however, than chlamydial epididymitis. Nongonococcal urethritis is usually treated with doxycycline (Vibramycin), 100 mg orally twice a day, or minocycline (Minocin), 100 mg twice a day for 10 to 14 days. The new fluoroquinolones (e.g., ofloxacin) also merit consideration. In older men with pyuria and bacteriuria, third-generation quinolones such as ciprofloxacin (Cipro), 250 mg twice a day, or trimethoprim-sulfamethoxazole (Septra, Bactrim), one double-strength tablet twice a day for 10 days, are recommended. Antimicrobial therapy should be continued for 4 weeks if bacterial prostatitis is suspected. Hospitalized patients require parenteral antibiotic therapy (e.g., an aminoglycoside or cephalosporin) until they experience defervescence, at which time a longer course of oral antimicrobial therapy is instituted. The fluoroquinolones can obviate the need for parenteral antibiotics because of their broad-spectrum potency and the high tissue levels achieved after oral administration (see the box above).

Although most patients feel better within 48 hours, swelling and discomfort may persist for weeks or months after eradication of the infecting organism. Persistent enlargement or induration frequently leads to a diagnosis of "chronic" epididymitis. Persistent fever despite suitable antimicrobial therapy suggests abscess formation and is an indication for ultrasound evaluation. Surgical drainage and/or epididymo-orchiectomy is required for abcesses. Epididymitis can be complicated by testicular necrosis, testicular atrophy, or infertility. Chronic inflammation and fibrosis can block the ductal cord structures and impair sperm production, especially in severe cases of bilateral epididymitis. Swelling and edema may compromise blood flow and cause testicular atrophy (see the Managed Care Guide on p. 1807).

### Epididymitis

**Types**

"Sterile" (noninfectious)
Infectious (chlamydia, coliform bacteria)
- Acute
- Chronic (tuberculosis, syphilis)

**Physical examination**

Tender enlarged epididymis posterior to testis
Associated orchitis (minority)

**Clinical groups**

Age <35 years
- Chlamydial etiology
- Signs and symptoms of urethritis
- Pyuria
- Treatment with doxycycline/minocycline/fluoroquinolones

Age >35 years
- Enterobacteriaceae
- Signs and symptoms of cystitis/prostatitis
- Pyuria, bacteriuria
- Positive urine culture
- Treatment with trimethoprim-sulfamethoxazole (TMP-SMX), fluoroquinolones

## Managed Care Guide To epididymitis

**Presentation**
*Common*
Scrotal pain
Swelling (usually unilateral)

*Uncommon*
Urethral discharge
Fever, chills

**Baseline information required (history, screens, etc.)**
Duration symptoms
History trauma
Medical conditions–diabetes, immunosuppression
History instrumentation–Foley catheter, cystoscopy

**Recommended lab tests/diagnostic procedures**
Urinalysis, urine culture
Digital rectal examination
Urethral swab for Gram stain
Scrotal ultrasound
IVP, VCUG in selected cases (boys, elderly men)

**Approximate duration of care**
10-14 days

**Frequency of follow-up**
1 month

**Indications for consultation/referral**
Abscess formation
Nonresponse to therapy
Doubtful diagnosis

**Comments**
"Do not misdiagnose testicular tumor for epididymitis"

***Indication for consultation.*** A urologist should be consulted whenever there is intense swelling or pain and the diagnosis of torsion versus epididymitis must be considered. The question of tumor and failure to respond to therapy also indicate the need for prompt consultation.

## BENIGN SCROTAL MASSES

Most scrotal masses are benign lesions of the spermatic cord, epididymis, testis, or their coverings. Inflammation, trauma, and congenital defects are most frequent etiologies. Testicular tumors, however, must be included in the differential diagnosis of all scrotal masses.

### Hydrocele and spermatocele

Hydroceles and spermatoceles are common paratesticular lesions caused by fluid accumulation. A *hydrocele* is an abnormal collection of fluid within the tunica or processus vaginalis. It is congenital or acquired. The incidence of hydrocele in the general population is not known. Congenital or pediatric hydroceles are found in approximately 10% of boys and result from nonclosure of the processus vaginalis during embryologic testicular descent. Congenital hydroceles may vary in size during the day, becoming larger with fluid accumulation. Most resolve by 1 year of age. Surgical treatment is indicated for persistent hydroceles beyond this age. Acquired "reactive" hydroceles are secondary to intrascrotal insults, such as infection, regional or systemic disease, inguinal or scrotal surgery, trauma, or neoplasm.

Studies using injection of India ink or dye have demonstrated defects in lymphatic drainage (overproduction, underabsorption) that lead to fluid accumulation. Adult hydroceles are usually asymptomatic. Hydroceles usually enlarge slowly or remain unchanged. Occasionally, a pulling or dragging sensation is associated with large hydroceles. The hydrocele is a nontender, cystic, transilluminating mass that lies anterior to the testis. If the underlying testis cannot be palpated because of the size of the fluid-filled mass, scrotal ultrasound examination should be performed to exclude a testicular tumor.

A *spermatocele* is a cystic dilatation of the epididymis that frequently involves the upper pole or epididymal head. It is usually small and painless and may follow an episode of epididymitis. Physical examination reveals a freely movable, transilluminating cystic mass located above and separate from the testis. The cyst fluid contains dead spermatozoa in retention cysts lined by a thin layer of fibrous connective tissue and columnar epithelium. Ultrasonography easily differentiates spermatoceles from hydroceles and testicular lesions.

Surgical treatment of hydroceles and spermatoceles is reserved for men with pain and discomfort or lesions that are cosmetically embarrassing for the patients. Aspiration and sclerotherapy are used for nonsurgical management of acquired hydroceles and spermatoceles. The sclerosants used include tetracycline, minocycline, bleomycin, and sodium tetradecyl. However, aspiration may result in infection. Sclerotherapy is successful in 80% to 90% of patients, but multiple treatments may be necessary. The best results are obtained in small to moderate-sized lesions. Open surgical procedures are indicated for large hydroceles and spermatoceles, and a variety of techniques (e.g., excision, eversion) are available.

### Varicocele

A varicocele can be easily recognized by the presence of spermatic cord and/or scrotal enlargement caused by dilatation of the pampiniform venous plexus. The exact etiology of varicoceles is unknown. However, incompetent valves of the spermatic vein, especially on the left, can lead to venous stasis and varicosities. Clinically obvious varicoceles present as a "bag of worms" in the spermatic cord and are more prominent when the patient stands. The incidence of varicoceles in healthy males is approximately 15%, and the left side is involved in more than 80% (see the box on p. 1808). Varicoceles occasionally cause scrotal pain and heaviness, especially when large. They are frequently associated with male subfertility or infertility. Infertile men with varicoceles are oligospermic (low sperm counts) with "a stress pattern" on semen analysis, that is, reduced motility and abnormal morphology. A useful clinical classification of varicoceles is as follows:

*Subclinical:* nonpalpable and visible at rest or during Valsalva's maneuver but demonstrable by ultrasonography
*Grade 1:* palpable only during Valsalva's maneuver
*Grade 2:* palpable at rest but not visible
*Grade 3:* visible and palpable at rest

### Varicoceles

**Features**

Present in 15% of healthy, fertile men
Associated with:
 Infertility (80%)
 Pain (20%)
Most common treatable cause of male infertility
Dilated pampiniform venous plexus in spermatic cord

**Diagnosis**

Palpation (standing position, Valsalva's maneuver)
Ultrasound (>3 mm vein diameter)
Semen analysis ("stress" pattern: low count, low motility)

**Treatment**

Radiologic embolization
Surgical division of spermatic vein
Transperitoneal laparoscopic ligation

**Results**

Semen improvement in 60%-70%
Pregnancy in 30%-40%

Special attention should be paid to testicular size during evaluation of a varicocele because ipsilateral testicular atrophy may be present. Size is best assessed by ultrasound or calibrated orchiometers. Ultrasound evaluation of the spermatic vein and testicular volume and a semen analysis are required. A recent study of more than 9,000 male partners of infertile couples found varicoceles present in 25% of men with abnormal semen counts compared with 11% with normal semen. The exact role of the varicocele in male subfertility has not been clearly ascertained, although an elevated scrotal temperature and reflux of adrenal metabolites (steroids, etc.) may contribute to the pathogenesis.

Treatment of varicocele is variable. Asymptomatic men without a history of infertility should be observed. For patients with concomitant testicular atrophy (especially young boys) and/or infertility, various treatment modalities are available. Several techniques (e.g., retroperitoneal, inguinal, scrotal) for surgical ligation of the spermatic vein exist. A minimally invasive, transperitoneal laparoscopic approach has recently been introduced. Nonsurgical treatment can be achieved by percutaneous spermatic vein embolization. This technique provides excellent visualization of the varicocele and its collaterals. However, a skilled interventional radiologist is needed, and a small radiation risk exists. In general, improvement in semen parameters (improved motility and number of sperm) is expected in 50% to 60% of patients, and successful pregnancy occurs for 30% to 40% of couples after surgical or radiologic interruption of varicoceles.

## BENIGN TUMORS OF THE TESTIS AND EPIDIDYMIS

Benign tumors of the testis are rare (see the box above, right). Ultrasound evaluation and scrotal exploration, when indicated, ascertain the diagnosis. Paratesticular masses account for 7% of all intrascrotal tumors. Of these, 60% to 70% originate in the spermatic cord and the remainder in the epididymis. The most common paratesticular mass is a benign cord lipoma, which accounts for approximately 25% of all cord tumors. Cord lipomas arise from preperitoneal fat remnants in the spermatic cord and are easy to palpate.

### Benign solid intrascrotal tumors

Cord lipoma
Adenomatoid tumor (spermatic cord)
Cystadenoma of epididymis
Fibrous pseudotumors
Testicular cysts

Intratesticular epidermoid cysts can be confused with malignant testicular lesions on physical examination. These rare lesions can be confidently diagnosed by scrotal ultrasound. A common finding on physical examination or testicular self-examination (TSE) is tunical cysts or calcifications on the surface of the tunica albuginea of the testis. These lesions are nonmalignant, and their etiology is uncertain. Ultrasound is diagnostic, and surgical exploration can usually be avoided.

## MALIGNANT TUMORS OF THE TESTIS

Although most intrascrotal masses are benign, some are malignant. Testicular cancer is the most frequent cancer in young men (15 to 35 years of age) and is rare in African Americans. Cryptorchidism is a well-known risk factor even after orchiopexy. Testicular tumors usually present as painless lumps. However, some men (20% to 25%) develop scrotal pain as a result of bleeding caused by rapid tumor growth and necrosis. Most tumors are discovered as hard testicular lumps during TSE. Gynecomastia is an unusual manifestation associated with chorionic gonadotropin or estrogen production. An occasional patient has metastatic disease, such as retroperitoneal, mediastinal, and supraclavicular lymphadenectomy or pulmonary metastases. Unfortunately, a painful testicular tumor can be misdiagnosed as epididymitis, leading to delayed diagnosis with the risk of advanced disease and a poor prognosis.

### Diagnosis and staging

Physical examination reveals a hard mass in the testis. A small to moderate-sized "reactive" hydrocele may make palpation and identification of the lesion difficult. The testicular tumor may be small (e.g., choriocarcinoma) and not easily palpable through the thick, overlying tunica albuginea. Scrotal ultrasound is an excellent imaging modality for the assessment of testicular masses (see the box on p. 1809). Microcalcifications in the testis indicate a high propensity for developing a seminoma and patients should be screened by US every 6 months. All types of testicular cancer are typically nonhomogenous with hypoechoic areas on ultrasound (Fig. 141-4).

Lymphatic spread of testicular tumors is orderly and predictable. The first-"echelon" nodes are the paraaortic and paracaval nodes at the level of the renal vessels. The primary drainage area of right-sided tumors is the

A

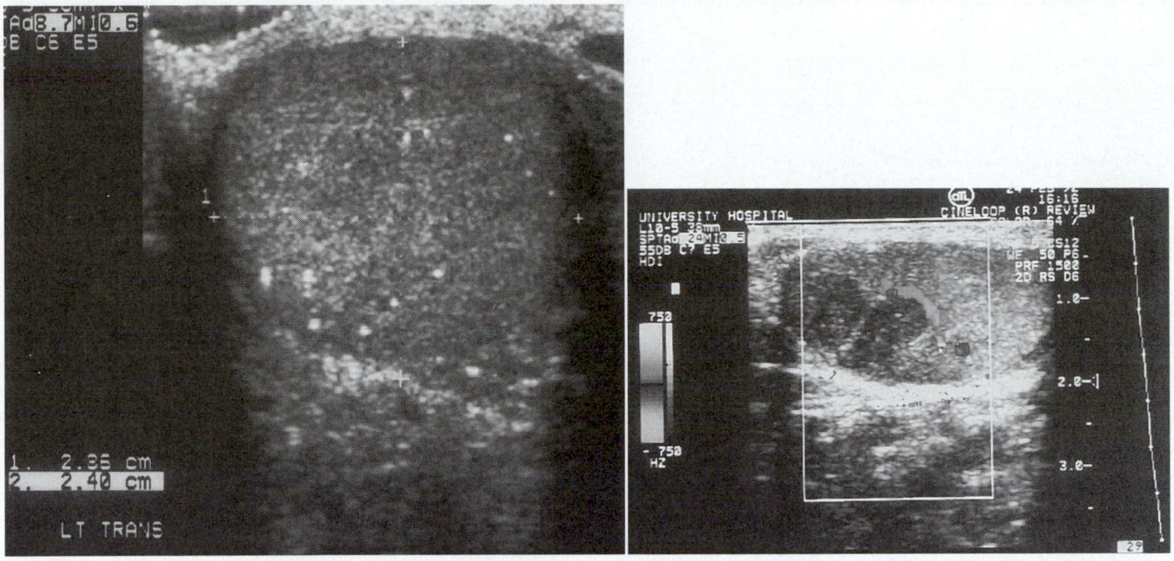


B

**Fig. 141-4. A,** Microcalcifications visualized on ultrasound of testis. This condition is often a premalignant sign of seminoma and requires ultrasound screening at 6-month to 1-year intervals. **B,** Seminoma of testis noted on ultrasound and by color Doppler.

### Treatment of testicular cancer: stage and cell type

**Clinical stage A**

Seminoma
- External beam radiation to retroperitoneum

Nonseminoma
- Retroperitoneal lymphadenectomy
  - Chemotherapy if nodes or markers positive (20%)
- Surveillance protocols
  - Meticulous follow-up (markers, CT, chest x-rays)
  - Chemotherapy for relapses (20%)

**Clinical stages B and C**

Seminoma, nonseminoma
Combination drug chemotherapy
Salvage lymphadenectomy for nonseminomas

interaortocaval nodes, and left-sided cancers spread initially to the left paraaortic nodal area. This is explained by the embryologic descent of the testis and vascular and lymphatic vessels from the abdomen into the scrotum. Avoidance of scrotal skin violation is mandatory when treating testicular tumors. The scrotal skin lymphatics drain into the inguinal nodes, and violation leads to nonretroperitoneal lymphatic dissemination of the tumor. Thus, transscrotal needle biopsy or orchiectomy is contraindicated. Suspected testicular tumors should be explored via an inguinal incision with early control of the spermatic cord to prevent vascular or lymphatic dissemination of tumor cells.

Tumor markers are helpful in the diagnosis, staging, and management of malignant testicular tumors. Alpha-fetoprotein (α-FP) and the beta subunit of human chorionic gonadotropin (β-hCG) are the clinically useful markers. α-FP is most often associated with embryonal carcinoma, whereas β-hCG elevations are seen with choriocarcinoma. However, many testicular cancers are of mixed germ cell origin (seminoma, embryonal cell carcinoma, choriocarcinoma, teratoma, etc.), and tumor marker elevation is variable. Persistent tumor marker elevation after "radical" inguinal orchiectomy suggests the presence of metastatic retroperitoneal disease or pulmonary metastases. However, there is a 25% false-negative marker elevation rate. Thus, serum tumor markers are not completely reliable for staging, especially when their levels are normal.

Computed tomographic (CT) scanning and chest x-ray are used for staging (see the box at left). Unfortunately, a 20% to 25% false-negative CT scanning rate occurs in the presence of nonenlarged (less than 1.5 cm) but microscopically involved retroperitoneal nodes. Stage A disease is confined to the testis, whereas stage B disease is associated with retroperitoneal lymphatic metastases below the diaphragm but an absence of visceral metastases. Stage B is subdivided into $B_1$, $B_2$, and $B_3$ stages according to tumor extent ($B_1$ less than 5 cm, $B_2$ greater than 5 cm, $B_3$ greater than 10 cm). Stage C disease indicates metastases (usually visceral) beyond the retroperitoneum.

## Histologic findings

Most testicular tumors are of germ cell origin—seminoma, embryonal cell carcinoma, teratoma, and choriocarcinoma—but 40% are "mixed," containing more than one cell type. A particular histologic subtype of seminoma (spermatocytic seminoma) tends to occur in older men. Choriocarcinoma is the most aggressive testicular cancer, with a propensity for rapid growth and early hematogenous spread to the lungs and other viscera.

Non–germ cell testicular tumors are rare and usually benign. Interstitial cell (Leydig cell) tumors are the most common. Leydig cell tumors in prepubertal males may secrete androgens and estrogens and cause gynecomastia.

### Initial approach to testicular cancer

**Step 1**

Suspicion on physical examination
Confirmation by scrotal ultrasound (optional)
Serum tumor markers (α-FP, β-hCG)
Chest x-ray

**Step 2**

Inguinal exploration
"Radical" inguinal orchiectomy
Histologic examination
- Pure, "mixed" tumor
- Vascular space invasion (lymphatic)
- Extension into epididymis, cord

**Step 3**

Staging
- Abdominal computed tomographic (CT) scan
- α-FP, β-hCG

Treatment selection
- Seminoma vs. nonseminoma
- Surgery vs. chemotherapy vs. radiation
- Surveillance protocol (selected patients)

### Managed Care Guide To testicular cancer

**Presentation**
*Common*
Scrotal mass or lump

*Uncommon*
Scrotal pain
Pulmonary/retroperitoneal metastases

**Baseline information required (history, screens, etc.)**
History trauma

**Recommended lab tests/diagnostic procedures**
Chest x-ray
Tumor markers (αFP, βhCG)
Scrotal ultrasound
Radical inguinal orchiectomy

**Approximate duration of care**
Variable

**Frequency of follow-up**
Every 1-3 months

**Indications for consultation/referral**
All testicular masses

**Comments**
Early diagnosis key to successful treatment
Do not confuse with epididymitis/testis torsion

Sertoli cell tumors are extremely rare and, as with Leydig cell tumors, rarely metastasize. The testis can be the site of metastatic spread from other primary tumors. In older patients (over age 50 years), infiltration by lymphoma or leukemia occurs more often than primary testicular tumors. Lung, prostate, and gastrointestinal cancers also metastasize to the testis.

## Treatment

Whenever a testicular tumor is suspected on physical examination, the next step is confirmation of the diagnosis by orchiectomy. Inguinal exploration is recommended because scrotal skin violation may alter the lymphatic spread of the tumor (see the box above). Serum tumor markers (α-FP, β-hCG) and a chest x-ray are obtained before surgical exploration. If an intratesticular lesion is noted on exploration, the spermatic cord is ligated at the level of the internal inguinal ring *(high ligation),* and the testis and its coverings are removed (*radical* inguinal orchiectomy).

Further treatment is based on histologic assessment of the tumor and staging. Microscopic examination will identify tumor type (*pure* or *mixed*), tumor extent (involvement of the epididymis or spermatic cord), and vascular space (lymphatic and venous) tumor invasion (see the Managed Care Guide above, right).

## Nonseminomatous germ cell tumors

Stage A nonseminomatous germ cell tumors are treated by retroperitoneal lymph node dissection (see the box on p. 1809). A modified, unilateral lymphadenectomy spares the sympathetic chain and preserves ejaculation. If the nodes are negative, further therapy is unnecessary, and cure rates approach 95%. Recent improvements in chemotherapy for metastatic disease have led to the emergence of surveillance protocols for selected patients with clinically localized nonseminomatous disease (stage A), that is, those with negative tumor markers, normal abdominal CT scans, and lack of vascular space invasion. However, strict selection and meticulous clinical and radiologic follow-up are needed. The overall tumor relapse rate with surveillance protocols is 20% to 30%.

Microscopic lymph node involvement or tumor marker elevation after lymphadenectomy are indications for multidrug, combination chemotherapy. Combination chemotherapy with vinblastine, bleomycin, and cisplatin has produced dramatic results. Cure rates for stages B and C testicular tumors exceed those for any other human solid-organ neoplasm. Five-year survival rates in excess of 90% are now achievable. The keys to the optimistic outlook in nonseminomatous testis cancer are early diagnosis, prompt inguinal orchiectomy, modified retroperitoneal lymphadenectomy, and combination chemotherapy.

## Seminomas

The usual treatment for testicular seminoma is radical inguinal orchiectomy and external beam irradiation to the retroperitoneum (see the box on p. 1809). Pure seminomas are exquisitely radiosensitive, and retroperitoneal lymphadenectomy is not indicated as for nonseminomatous

### Differential diagnosis of scrotal pain

- Torsion
  - Appendages
  - Spermatic cord
- Infection
  - Orchitis (mumps)
  - Abscess
  - Epididymitis
- Neoplasia
  - Benign
  - Malignant
- Incarcerated hernia
- Trauma
- Hydrocele
- Spermatocele
- Varicocele

tumors. Stage A seminoma patients undergo postorchiectomy radiation therapy with 2500 rad to the paraaortic and ipsilateral iliac nodes. Patients with stage B disease receive an additional boost of 1000 to 2000 rads to involved areas and prophylactic radiation to the mediastinal and supraclavicular nodes. Radiation therapy is less effective in "bulky" stage B or stage C disease. The outstanding success of combination chemotherapy for nonseminomatous germ cell tumors has led to its use for the treatment of "bulky" seminomas (i.e., stages B and C).

## THE ACUTE SCROTUM

Testicular pain should always be considered an emergency. Evaluation should not be delayed if testicular damage from torsion of the spermatic cord and subsequent ischemia are to be avoided. The box above outlines differential diagnosis of scrotal pain. Differentiation between testicular torsion and epididymitis can usually be made on the basis of the presentation and physical findings (see Table 141-1).

*Testicular torsion* is a surgical emergency. Testicular loss can only be avoided by prompt diagnosis and early treatment (either manual or surgical detorsion). Torsion, a disease mainly of adolescents and young adults, can be confused with epididymitis, especially in postpubertal males. A teenager with sudden onset of scrotal pain and a normal urinalysis most likely has a testicular torsion. Unrelieved torsion (longer than 6 hours) leads to testicular ischemia and atrophy, and early treatment is therefore imperative. A negative surgical exploration for torsion in the presence of epididymitis is not detrimental to testicular viability (see the box above, right). The annual incidence of torsion in males 30 to 80 years of age is 1:50,000. However, from 10 to 20 years, the incidence is 1:4,000. Ninety percent of all testicular torsions occur in patients less than 30 years of age. In contrast, the annual incidence of epididymitis in the 30 to 80 age group is 1:2,000.

A delay in the diagnosis of testicular torsion beyond 12 hours causes progressive testicular ischemia, with irreversible damage and eventual necrosis in 24 hours. A

### Testicular torsion

- Surgical emergency
- Common in pubertal boys and adolescents
- Ischemia > 6 hours irreversible
- When in doubt, exploration indicated
- Doppler/radionuclide studies in selected cases
- Early manual detorsion
- Exploration with orchiopexy/orchiectomy

technique for early manual detorsion of the spermatic cord is available. Under IV sedation, detorsion can be carried out in the emergency room by manipulating the testis and rotating it toward the respective thigh for approximately 1½ turns. Relief of pain can be dramatic, and return of testicular blood flow can be documented by color Doppler ultrasonographic examination.

Testicular torsion can be confirmed by Doppler ultrasound (greater than 90% sensitive, 70% specific) and nuclear scanning (greater than 90% sensitive, 80% specific). However, if any doubt exists, scrotal exploration and detorsion should be carried out. The common anatomic defect in testes that undergo torsion is high "investment" (or attachment) of the tunica vaginalis—the so-called bell-clapper deformity (Fig. 141-5). This inherited defect is usually bilateral and predisposes to testicular torsion. Detorsion is always followed by testicular fixation (orchiopexy) of the affected gonad as well as its contralateral mate.

If, after intraoperative detorsion, the testis remains dusky and cyanotic, irreversible ischemia is probable and an orchiectomy is indicated. Torsion of an appendix testis or an acutely incarcerated scrotal hernia may mimic the symptoms of testicular torsion. Torsion of the appendix testis can be diagnosed by the presence of localized pain in the upper pole of the testis and the presence of a "blue dot" on transillumination, caused by the ischemic appendage seen through the skin. An incarcerated hernia causes significant thickening of the spermatic cord and is associated with peritoneal signs of intestinal obstruction and the presence of bowel sounds in the scrotum (see the Managed Care Guide on p. 1812).

## SCROTAL TRAUMA

Penetrating gunshot or knife wounds can involve the scrotum. Emergency surgical débridement and exploration are required for hemostasis and testicular repair, if indicated. Severe blunt injuries of the scrotum may cause testicular dislocation or rupture. Palpation and examination of the scrotum are extremely painful, and ultrasound imaging can be misleading. Surgical exploration with repair (débridement) or orchiectomy is indicated.

Minor trauma can cause scrotal pain or hematoma formation. Testicular tumors are more likely to bleed following minor trauma compared with normal testes. Occasionally, a testicular tumor may present in this manner, with the degree of trauma not being commensurate with the degree of pain or hematoma formation.

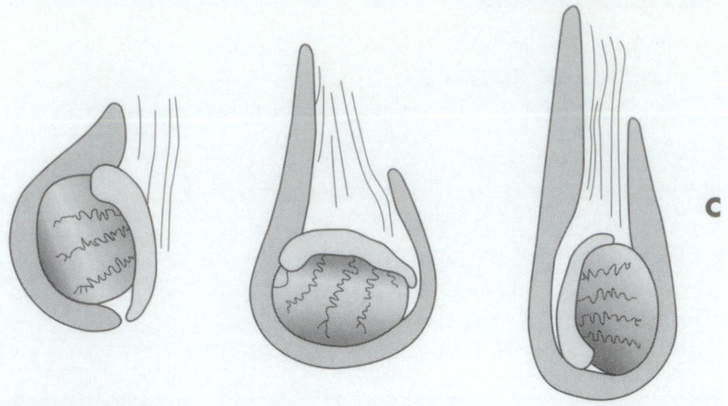


**Fig. 141-5.** Attachment of testicular mesentery to testis. **A,** The normal peritoneal disposition around the testis. **B,** Capacious tunica vaginalis surrounding the cord; the testis lies horizontally. **C,** The inverted testis, which most easily twists because of its narrow attachment, the "bell-clapper" deformity. (From Krane RJ, Siroky MB, Fitzpatrick JM, editors: *Clinical urology,* Philadelphia, 1994, JB Lippincott.)

## CONGENITAL LESIONS OF THE TESTIS

Palpation of the scrotum may reveal an absent or small testis. The absence of the testis warrants a careful search for that testis by palpation of the upper scrotum and groin. Testicular maldescent or cryptorchidism is common, affecting 0.8% of all males. Surgical repositioning of a cryptorchid testis is now routinely performed in the pediatric age group. However, patients who have not undergone such a procedure and still harbor a malpositioned testis should undergo removal of that gonad because of the high incidence of testicular tumors (usually seminomas) in cryptorchid testes (8% to 10%). If no testis can be found on physical examination, surgical exploration is indicated. Diagnostic tests such as ultrasound, CT scan, magnetic resonance imaging (MRI), and spermatic venography are not uniformaly reliable and are expensive. Laparoscopic evaluation of patients with nonpalpable testes is now being increasingly performed. Testicular absence can be confirmed and first-stage orchidopexy carried out if intraabdominal testes are discovered.

Atrophy of the testis may result from neonatal torsion or prior injury. Surgical removal of the testis is not mandatory. However, associated masses or abnormalities should be excluded by scrotal ultrasound. A number of patients will have compensatory, contralateral testicular hypertrophy.

### Managed Care Guide To testicular torsion

**Presentation**

***Common***

Scrotal pain (usually acute)
Swelling

***Uncommon***

Nausea
Vomiting
Fever

**Baseline information required (history, screens, etc.)**

History trauma
Prior history scrotal pain

**Recommended lab tests/diagnostic procedures**

Urine culture
Attempt early manual detorsion
Scrotal ultrasound
Doppler imaging } in selected patients
Radionuclide studies } in selected patients

**Approximate duration of care**

Detorsion within 6 hours

**Frequency of follow-up**

Variable

**Indications for consultation/referral**

Refer on initial suspicion

**Comments**

Early diagnosis key to testicular/fertility preservation

## BIBLIOGRAPHY

Betts JM et al: Testicular detorsion using Doppler ultrasound monitoring, *J Pediatr Surg* 18(5):607, 1983.

Blandy J: *Lecture notes on urology,* ed 4, Cambridge, Mass, 1989, Blackwell.

Hargreave TB: Varicocele—a clinical enigma, *B J Urol* 72:401, 1993.

Rowland RG, Donohue JP: Scrotum and testis. In Gillenwater JY et al, editors: *Adult and pediatric urology,* ed 2, St Louis, 1991, Mosby.

Tanagho EA, McAninch JW: *Smith's general urology,* ed 13, East Norwalk, Conn, 1992, Appleton & Lange.

# XV WOMEN'S HEALTH

CHAPTER

## 142A Primary Care of Women

Janet B. Henrich

The area of women's health has focused traditionally on reproductive issues in younger women and has been confined primarily to the discipline of obstetrics and gynecology. This concept is changing rapidly because of several societal and scientific forces including increasing life span, the increasing understanding of the pathophysiology of aging in women and the role of estrogens, increasing awareness of the behavioral and social factors that influence women's health, and the changing role of women in society.

The current interest in women's health has its basis in the women's health movement of the 1960s. This grass roots movement was fueled by the feminist movement and reflected women's discontent with the lack of accessible information about their health and the prevailing paternalistic attitude of medicine. The most important product of this movement was the publication of the book *Our Bodies Ourselves* by the Boston Women's Health Book Collaborative. This text sought to improve the health of women by teaching them how their bodies worked and how they could become active participants in their health care. Over the last three decades, this document has been the unofficial textbook for women and physicians interested in understanding the basic health needs of women.

The forces behind the current women's health movement differ markedly from those of the 1960s. In 1983, the Assistant Secretary for Health commissioned the Public Health Service (PHS) to form a task force to assess the status of women's health in the United States and identify the most important factors that influence health and disease. The task force's recommendations, published in 1985, presented a blueprint for change in the approach to women's health. The task force broadly defined women's health issues as "diseases or conditions that are unique to or more prevalent or serious in women, have distinct causes or manifest themselves differently in women, or have different outcomes or interventions." It recognized the effect of social and demographic changes on women's health status and stressed the importance of preventive health services for women. The report went further by identifying potential biases in research and clinical practice that result in inadequate care for women. In response to this report, the National Institutes of Health (NIH) established the Office of Research on Women's Health (ORWH) in 1990. This free-standing office, located within the Office of the Director of the NIH, has a threefold mandate: to enhance research in women's health and to ensure that women's health issues are addressed adequately in research conducted by the NIH, to ensure that women are appropriately represented in all studies supported by the NIH, and to increase the number of women in biomedical careers. Coincident with the establishment of the ORWH, Dr. Bernadine Healy was appointed the first woman Director of the NIH. Her strong commitment to women's health issues helped establish the strong scientific framework necessary to advance a women's health agenda.

### BASIC PRINCIPLES UNDERLYING WOMEN'S HEALTH

Although women develop most of the diseases that affect men, biologic mechanisms and psychosocial factors influence the course of disease differently in women. Unfortunately, most of the information we use to make clinical decisions in women is based on studies conducted primarily in men. Women have been excluded from research on diseases that are important to both sexes because of misconceptions about women's health, legal and ethical issues, and cultural biases. Because women, on average, live longer than men and are affected by major diseases at a later age, it is often perceived incorrectly that women are healthier than men. In fact, throughout life women experience poorer health than men, especially in the advanced years. The lack of information concerning women has important implications. Information based primarily on studies of men may be applied inappropriately to women or result in different standards of care. These concerns have been highlighted recently in the area of coronary heart disease in women.

Efforts to increase our knowledge about women's health issues require an integrated approach that acknowledges the diversity among women and considers the social factors that influence their lives. One of the important social trends over the last 50 years is the increasing participation of women in the work force. Since World War II, the number of women who work has more than doubled and is expected to exceed 80% by the end of the century. The full effects of multiple roles, work stress, and new environmental exposures on women's health and reproductive status are largely unknown, but are certain to have important health and social ramifications. Paralleling the growing numbers of women in the work force is the increasing number of single-parent families headed by women, especially minority women. Many of these families live in poverty. There is increasing evidence that socioeconomic factors are major indicators of health and that, for some health outcomes, poverty and lack of education are more important determinants of health than race. Nevertheless, important ethnic and racial differences in women's susceptibility and response to certain diseases cannot be explained wholly by socioeconomic status. For example, mortality rates for coronary heart disease, stroke, and breast cancer are higher in black than in white women, whereas death rates from lung cancer are higher in white women.

### MORBIDITY AND MORTALITY IN WOMEN

At the turn of the century the average life span of women in the United States was 48 years, compared to 46 years in men. Since then the life expectancy in women has almost doubled and is now 79 years, compared to 72 years in men. Because of the gender gap in life expectancy,

**Table 142A-1.** Age-adjusted death rates for leading causes of death: U.S. women, 1991

| Cause of death | Rate (per 100,000 population) | Total deaths (%) |
|---|---|---|
| All causes | 386.5 | 100.0 |
| Cardiovascular disease | 138.5 | 35.8 |
| Malignant neoplasms | 112.6 | 29.1 |
| Lung | 26.5 | 6.9 |
| Breast | 22.7 | 5.9 |
| Colorectal | 13.2 | 3.4 |
| Cerebrovascular disease | 24.7 | 6.4 |
| Unintentional injuries | 17.2 | 4.5 |
| Chronic lung disease | 15.5 | 4.0 |
| Diabetes | 11.1 | 2.9 |
| Pneumonia/influenza | 10.6 | 2.7 |
| Suicide/homicide | 8.8 | 2.3 |

From National Center for Health Statistics: *Advance report of final mortality statistics:* 1991, 1993, Washington, D.C., The Center.

women currently comprise close to two thirds of the population over age 65 and three fourths of the population over age 85. The fastest growing age group in the United States is the population aged 85 years and older. As a result, it is estimated that at the beginning of the next century, women will outnumber men by 2 to 1 in the age groups over 65 and 3 to 1 in the population over 85. The reasons for the dramatic increase in overall life expectancy are thought to be related to the control of infectious diseases and progress in the treatment of chronic diseases such as diabetes and cardiovascular disease. The reasons for the disparity in life expectancy in women and men are less well established but are thought to be primarily biologic (Health United States 1992 and Healthy People 2000 Review, 1993).

The leading causes of death in women of all ages and races are shown in Table 142A-1. Despite a dramatic decline in mortality rates for heart disease that has occurred in both sexes over the past two decades, heart disease remains the leading cause of death for women and accounts for one third of all deaths in women. Heart disease occurs about 10 years later in women than in men. This delayed onset is thought to be due primarily to the protective effect of estrogens in premenopausal women and accounts for the fact that 90% of heart disease mortality in women occurs after the menopause. There are significant racial and ethnic differences in mortality among women. Black women are more likely to die from heart disease than white women up to age 75; thereafter death rates are higher in white women. In contrast, Hispanic and Native American women have significantly lower rates of death from heart disease. Evidence suggests that heart disease, once it develops, is more serious in women than in men, resulting in higher mortality rates. In addition to biologic factors, the poorer survival of women may be due to the older age and increased prevalance of co-morbid conditions in women at the time of diagnosis, as well as to less well-defined social factors that influence the diagnosis and treatment of heart disease in women.

Cancer is the second leading cause of death in women and is the most common cause of premature death. The mortality rate for all cancers combined in women has changed little during the last part of this century. Major advances in the fight against cervical and uterine cancer in women have been offset by an increase in mortality rates for lung and breast cancer. Although breast cancer is still the most common cancer diagnosed in women, lung cancer is now the leading cause of cancer deaths. Unfortunately, most of these deaths can be attributed to cigarette smoking. Whereas the number of deaths from lung cancer in men has remained fairly stable as a result of a decrease in male cigarette use, the death rate for women has increased dramatically and is expected to continue to rise into the next century.

Breast cancer is the second leading cause of cancer deaths in women. Although there has been a sharp increase in the incidene of breast cancer over the past decade, mortality rates have remained relatively stable. This disparity is thought to be due partly to the widespread use of screening mammography and the detection of earlier stage cancers that have a more favorable prognosis. There are significant age and racial differences in breast cancer mortality. Declining mortality rates in younger women have been offset by an increase in breast cancer deaths in older women. Although breast cancer incidence rates are 20% lower in black women than in white women, mortality rates are 15% higher in black women. Reasons for racial differences in breast cancer incidence and mortality are unclear but may be related to socioeconomic and biologic factors, as well as certain health behaviors such as participation in screening mammography. Although it has been shown that breast cancer screening with mammography and clinical breast examination decrease mortality from breast cancer in women over age 50 by approximately 30%, less than 50% of American women 50 years and older receive regular screenings, and this figure is considerably lower in poor, minority, and elderly women (Health United States 1992 and Healthy People 2000 Review, 1993).

Cancer of the colon and rectum is the third leading cause of cancer deaths in women. Although there are no significant gender differences in the incidence and mortality rates for this disease, colorectal cancer accounts for 13% of all cancer-related deaths in women and is a significant cause of morbidity.

Although stroke-related deaths have declined by almost 60% in the United States over the past 25 years, strokes still account for approximately 6% of all deaths in women and rank third as a cause of mortality. There are striking racial differences in stroke mortality: death rates in black women are almost twice those for white women. Most of the stroke deaths in women are due to thromboembolic disease and occur in older women. However, subarachnoid hemorrhage, the least common form of stroke, is more common in women than in men and contributes to stroke mortality, particularly in younger women.

Fatal injury from unintentional acute trauma is the fourth leading cause of death in women. This category includes deaths resulting from motor vehicle accidents, drowning, poisoning, fires, and falls. Mortality rates for homicide and suicide are ranked separately from accidental deaths. Death rates as a result of these injuries are rising rapidly in both men and women and disproportionately affect younger, minority populations.

Death rates from chronic pulmonary diseases have increased steadily for both women and men during the past 25 years; however, the increase has been greater in women. Because this increase has been linked to patterns in cigarette smoking, the increase in death rates in women for pulmonary disease, as well as for lung cancer, is expected to continue into the next century. Death rates from pneumonia and influenza closely parallel pulmonary-related deaths and vary over time based on the epidemiology of these acute illnesses.

Diabetes has consistently ranked as a leading cause of death in women. Moreover, the reported death rate from diabetes most likely underestimates the impact of this disease on mortality because of its strong association with other life-threatening medical conditions such as cardiovascular disease, stroke, and kidney failure. It is estimated that diabetes affects one in seven women over age 45; however, prevalence rates are higher in black, Hispanic and Native American women. Separate from disease-related death rates, diabetes is a significant cause of morbidity and, in women of childbearing age, has important adverse effects on pregnancy outcome, resulting in an increased risk of fetal and perinatal mortality as well as congenital malformations.

HIV infection is not one of the 10 leading causes of death in women as a whole; however, of all the major causes of mortality it is responsible for the largest percentage increase in death rates. HIV-related mortality rates are nine times higher for black women than for white women. As a result, HIV infection is the fifth leading cause of death in black women ages 15 to 24, the third leading cause of death in the age group 25 to 44, and, in some geographic areas, has become the number one cause of death. With heterosexual transmission accounting for an increasing proportion of HIV cases in women, these rates are expected to continue rising.

Mortality rates alone do not provide a complete picture of women's health status. There is an interesting paradox when one compares the health of women to men. Although women live longer than men, overall measures of health status are worse in women (Table 142A-2). Based on current estimates from the National Health Interview Survey (NHIS), more women than men report symptoms or seek care for acute medical conditions such as respiratory and digestive disorders and are more disabled by these self-limited illnesses as measured by number of bed days or days lost from work. In addition, several chronic conditions occur more frequently in women and cause significant disability, such as arthritis, thyroid disease, migraine, bladder disorders, gastritis, colitis, and chronic constipation (Vital and Health Statistics: Current Estimates from the National Health Interview Survey, 1991). Although information on mental health disorders was not included in past NHIS reports, data from other sources show that affective disorders, especially major depressive episodes, and the anxiety disorders are significantly more prevalent in women. Most importantly, women's perception of their health status is lower than men's. According to estimates from the NHIS, only 36% of women describe their health as excellent, compared to 41% of men.

**Table 142A-2.** Age-adjusted selected indicators of health status and medical care utilization, 1991

| Indicator | Female | Male | Female/Male |
|---|---|---|---|
| Physician contacts (per person) | 6.6 | 4.9 | 1.3 |
| Acute conditions (per 100 persons) | 204.7 | 178.1 | 1.2 |
| Restricted activity days (per person) | 8.2 | 6.4 | 1.3 |
| Work loss days (per person ≥18 years) | 3.7 | 2.8 | 1.3 |
| Hospitalization (excluding deliveries) | 5.4% | 4.8% | 1.1 |
| Excellent health (self-report) | 35.8% | 41.4% | 0.9 |

From Vital and Health Statistics: *Current estimates from the National Health Interview Survey:* 1991.

## ROLE OF THE PRIMARY CARE PHYSICIAN

Many of the major health conditions in women can be prevented or mitigated by increased attention to lifestyle and health behaviors, a focus on the prevention and early detection of disease, and the appropriate treatment of chronic illnesses. Because of their broad-based training and outpatient focus, primary care physicians are in a unique position to provide these services. However, to provide comprehensive care to women, it is essential that primary care physicians expand their knowledge and skills to incorporate information from other disciplines, particularly gynecology, nutrition, and the behavioral sciences.

## BIBLIOGRAPHY

*Action plan for women's health.* U.S. Public Health Service Office on Women's Health. DHHS Pub. No. (PHS) 91-50214, September 1991.

Council on ethical and judicial affairs, American Medical Association. Physicians and domestic violence: ethical considerations, *JAMA* 267:3190, 1992.

Council on scientific affairs, American Medical Association. Violence against women: relevance for medical practitioners, *JAMA* 267:3184, 1992.

*Health United States 1992 and Healthy People 2000 Review* DHHS Pub. No. (PHS) 93-1232 August 1993.

Healy B: Women's health, public welfare, *JAMA* 266:566, 1991.

Report of the National Institutes of Health: *Opportunities for research on women's health.* DHHS Pub. No. (PHS, NIH) 92-3457, September 1992.

Rodin J, Ickovics JR: Women's health: review and research agenda as we approach the 21st century, *Am J Psychol* 45:1018, 1990.

U.S. Congress, Office of Technology Assessment, *"The Menopause, Hormone Therapy, and Women's Health,"* OTA-BP-BA-88 (Washington, DC: U.S. Government Printing Office, May 1992).

*Vital and Health Statistics: Current Estimates from the National Health Interview Survery, 1991.* Centers for Disease Control, National Center for Health Statistics. DHHS Pub. No. (PHS) 93-1512, December 1992.

Women's health. Report of the Public Health Service Task Force on Women's Health Issues: Volume II. DHHS Pub. No. (PHS) 85-50206, May 1985.

CHAPTER

# 142B The Clinical Management of Abnormal Menstruation

Janet B. Henrich
Wendy Levinson
Leon Speroff

The cyclic nature of the female reproductive process, expressed visibly by normal menstruation, is one of the most remarkable dynamic systems in biology. The diagnosis and management of abnormal menstrual function must be based on an understanding of the physiologic-mechanisms involved in the regulation of the normal cycle. After a brief review of normal function, this chapter describes the clinical management of abnormal bleeding, ranging from anovulation and irregular menses to amenorrhea, the total absence of menstruation.

## NORMAL MENSTRUAL FUNCTION

The clinical demonstration of menstrual function depends on visible external evidence of the menstrual discharge. This requires an intact outflow tract that connects the internal genital source of flow with the outside. The outflow tract requires patency and continuity of the vaginal orifice, the vaginal canal, and the endocervix with the uterine cavity. The presence of a menstrual flow depends on the existence and development of the endometrium lining the uterine cavity. This tissue is stimulated and regulated by the proper quantity and sequence of the steroid hormones, estrogen and progesterone. The secretion of these hormones originates in the ovary, but more specifically in the evolving spectrum of follicle development, ovulation, and corpus luteum function. This essential maturation of the follicular apparatus is guided by the stimuli provided by the sequence and magnitude of the gonadotropins, follicle-stimulating hormone (FSH) and luteinizing hormone (LH), which originate in the anterior pituitary gland. The secretion of these hormones is in turn dependent on gonadotropin-releasing hormone (GnRH), the specific peptide-releasing hormone produced in the basal hypothalamus and bloodborne via the portal vessels of the stalk to receptive cells within the anterior pituitary. The entire system is regulated by a complex mechanism that integrates biophysical and biochemical information comprised of interactive levels of hormonal signals, autocrine/paracrine factors, and target cell receptor function in the uterus, ovary, pituitary, hypothalamus, and other central nervous system (CNS) sources (Fig. 142B-1).

Just before and during menses, increased FSH is secreted by the anterior pituitary. This initial increase in FSH is essential for follicular growth and steroidogenesis. With continued growth of the follicle, autocrine/paracrine factors produced within the follicle maintain follicular sensitivity to FSH, allowing conversion from a microenvironment dominated by androgens to one dominated by estrogen, a change necessary for a complete and successful follicular life span. Continuing and combined action of FSH and activin leads to the appearance of LH receptors on the granulosa cells, a prerequisite for ovulation and luteinization. Ovulation is triggered by the rapid rise in circulating levels of estradiol. A positive feedback response at the level of the anterior pituitary (and perhaps at the hypothalamus as well) results in the midcycle surge of LH necessary for expulsion of the egg and formation of the corpus luteum. A rise in progesterone follows ovulation and, along with a second rise in estradiol, produces the 14-day luteal phase characterized by low FSH and LH levels. The demise of the corpus luteum, concomitant with

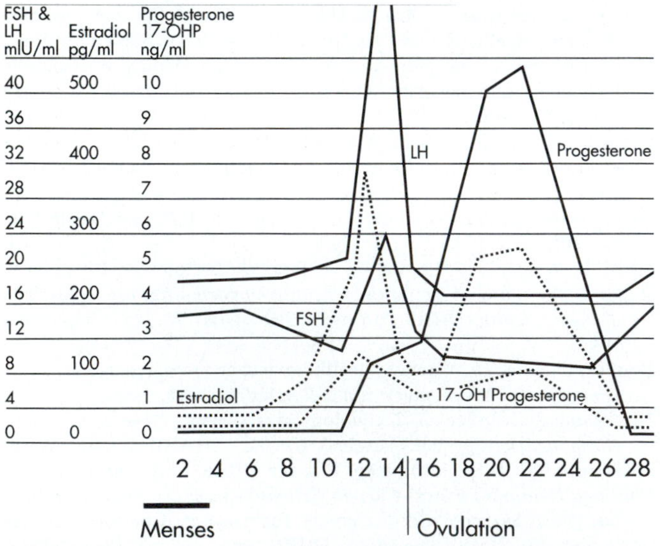


**Fig. 142B-1.** Normal hormonal fluctuations. (From Speroff L: *Clinical gynecologic endocrinology and infertility,* ed 4, Baltimore, 1994 Williams & Wilkins.)

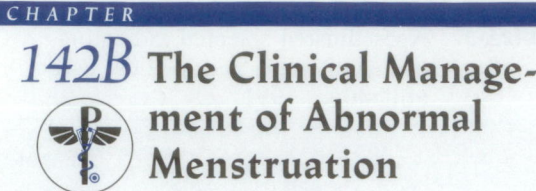

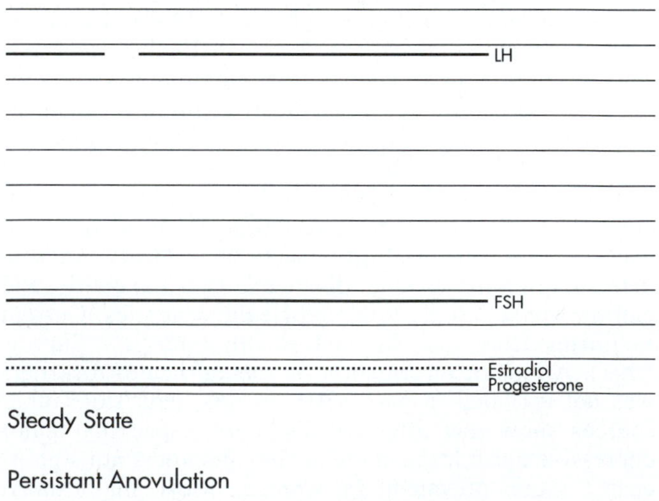


**Fig. 142B-2.** Steady state of hormonal fluctuations during persistent anovulation. (From Speroff L: *Clinical gynecologic endocrinology and infertility,* ed 4, Baltimore, 1994 Williams & Wilkins.)

**Table 142B-1.** Traditional definitions

| Term | Definition |
|---|---|
| Oligomenorrhea | Intervals more than 35 days |
| Polymenorrhea | Intervals less than 21 days |
| Menorrhagia | Regular normal intervals, excessive flow and duration |
| Metrorrhagia | Irregular intervals, excessive flow and duration |

a fall in hormone levels, allows FSH to increase again, thus initiating a new cycle.

Of all the types of hormonal-endometrial relationships, the most stable endometrium and the most reproducible menstrual function in terms of quantity and duration occur with postovulatory estrogen-progesterone withdrawal bleeding. It is so controlling that many women over the years come to expect a certain characteristic flow pattern. Any slight deviations, such as plus or minus 1 day in duration or minor deviation from expected napkin or tampon utilization, may cause women major concern.

Whereas the postovulatory phase averages 14 days, greater variability in the proliferative phase produces a distribution in the duration of a menstrual cycle. Based on normal experiences, menstrual bleeding more often than every 24 days or less often than every 35 days deserves evaluation. Flow that lasts 7 or more days also deserves evaluation. A flow that totals more than 80 ml/month usually leads to anemia and should be treated. In general, however, an effort to quantitate menstrual flow beyond historical information is not necessary because evaluation and treatment are responses to a patient's own perceptions about duration, amount, and timing of menstrual bleeding. Midcycle bleeding can be a consequence of the preovulatory fall in estrogen; however, intermenstrual bleeding is often due to pathology (Table 142B-1).

There are three reasons for the self-limited character of estrogen-progesterone withdrawal bleeding.

1. It is a universal endometrial event. Because the onset and conclusion of menses are related to a precise sequence of hormonal events, menstrual changes occur almost simultaneously in all segments of the endometrium.
2. The endometrial tissue, which has responded to an appropriate sequence of estrogen and progesterone, is structurally stable, and random breakdown of tissue due to fragility is avoided. Events leading to ischemic disintegration of the endometrium are orderly and progressive and are related to rhythmic waves of vasoconstriction of increasing duration.
3. Inherent in the events that start menstrual function following estrogen-progesterone are the factors involved in stopping menstrual flow. Just as waves of vasoconstriction initiate the ischemic events provoking menses, prolonged vasoconstriction abetted by the stasis associated with endometrial collapse enables clotting factors to seal off the exposed bleeding sites.

## DYSFUNCTIONAL UTERINE BLEEDING

Dysfunctional uterine bleeding is defined as a variety of bleeding manifestations associated with anovulatory cycles (in the absence of pathology or medical illness). It can be managed without surgical intervention by therapeutic regimens founded on sound physiologic principles.

### History/physical examination/laboratory studies

The history and physical examination include a careful menstrual and sexual history, with special attention to the amount and duration of uterine bleeding. In reproductive-aged women, the use of oral contraceptive pills and other forms of contraception is elicited and the possibility of pregnancy addressed. Symptoms suggestive of underlying endocrinopathy, coagulopathy, or systemic illness are sought. The possibility of trauma or the presence of a foreign body is raised. A complete physical examination is necessary to exclude extragenital sources of bleeding. It includes a thorough pelvic and genital examination, as well as a Papanicolaou (Pap) smear. Identification of pelvic pathology, such as polyps, uterine fibroids, and tumors of the vagina and cervix is essential. In women with active bleeding, it is important to localize the source of bleeding. Evaluation and examination should include biopsies where appropriate. Because the incidence of adenocarcinoma of the uterus increases with age, most women over the age of 40 years with abnormal bleeding are evaluated by endometrial biopsy (EMB). In addition to a complete blood count, laboratory tests include platelet count, coagulation studies, a pregnancy test, and screen for other medical disorders, including thyroid, liver, and renal function tests.

### Differential diagnosis

Dysfunctional uterine bleeding due to anovulation is a diagnosis made by exclusion. Other common causes of abnormal uterine bleeding, such as pregnancy and pregnancy-related problems including ectopic pregnancy or spontaneous abortion, should be considered. Some patients may be using medications not knowing that they affect the endometrium. For example, the use of ginseng, an herbal root, has been associated with estrogenic activity and abnormal bleeding. Pathology of the menstrual outflow tract, including cancers of the cervix and endometrium, endometrial polyps, and leiomyomata uteri, may present as uterine bleeding. Although bleeding is a common problem with various contraceptive methods and postmenopausal hormonal therapy, the clinician should make sure that another pathology is not present. Abnormal menstrual cycles occasionally are the first sign of either hypothyroidism or hyperthyroidism. One should keep in mind that as many as 20% of adolescents with dysfunctional uterine bleeding will have a coagulation defect, although the most common cause is anovulation. Bleeding secondary to a blood dyscrasia is usually characterized by a heavy flow with regular, cyclic menses (menorrhagia); this same pattern can be seen in patients being treated with anticoagulants. Irregular, serious bleeding is often associated with severe organ disease, such as renal or liver failure. In addition, genital injury or a foreign object may present with abnormal bleeding. Finally, although the effects of tubal ligation on menstrual function are uncertain, some women experience menstrual changes.

## Management of dysfunctional uterine bleeding

Once extragenital and other organic genital sources are excluded, the most common cause of abnormal uterine bleeding is anovulation. The immediate objective of medical therapy in anovulatory bleeding is to reinstate the natural controlling influences missing in this tissue. Although the treatment of anovulatory bleeding varies somewhat depending on the age of the patient and the extent of bleeding, the principles outlined below provide guidelines to the management of this condition.

***Progestin therapy.*** At sometime during their reproductive years most women will either fail to ovulate or not sustain adequate corpus luteum function or duration. This problem occurs most often during adolescence and in the decade before menopause. The usual clinical presentation is oligomenorrhea with bouts of heavy bleeding. Women usually seek medical advice promptly because these menstrual aberrations suggest unplanned pregnancy or uterine pathology. Under most circumstances, progestin therapy will control the abnormality once uterine pathology is ruled out.

In the treatment of oligomenorrhea, orderly, limited withdrawal bleeding can be accomplished by the administration of a progestin such as medroxyprogesterone acetate, 10 mg a day for 10 days every month. Absence of induced bleeding requires further workup. If menometrorrhagia or polymenorrhea is the presenting symptom, progestins are prescribed for 10 days to 2 weeks (to induce stabile endometrial stromal changes) followed by a withdrawal flow—the so-called "medical curettage." Thereafter, repeat progestin is offered cyclically the first 10 days of each month to ensure a continued therapeutic effect. Failure of progestin to correct irregular bleeding requires diagnostic reevaluation. If contraception is desired, the use of an oral contraceptive is a better choice.

***Oral contraceptive therapy.*** In young women, anovulatory bleeding may be associated with prolonged endometrial buildup, delayed diagnosis, and heavy blood loss. In these cases, combined progestin-estrogen therapy is used in the form of oral contraceptives. Any of the low-dose, oral combination monophasic tablets are useful. Therapy is administered as one pill twice a day for 5 to 7 days, even though cessation of flow usually occurs within 12 to 24 hours. If flow does not abate, other diagnostic possibilities (polyps, incomplete abortion, and neoplasia) should be considered.

During the week of treatment, attention should focus on the evaluation of causes of anovulation, investigation of hemorrhagic tendencies, and blood replacement or initiation of iron therapy. Successful therapy prevents the continued random breakdown of fragile endometrial tissue and blood loss stops; however, a large amount of tissue remains to react to estrogen-progestin withdrawal. The patient must be warned to anticipate a heavy and severely cramping flow 2 to 4 days after stopping therapy.

In successful therapy, a low-dose combination oral contraceptive medication (one pill a day) is started on the fifth day of flow. This sequence is repeated for several (usually three) 3-week treatments, punctuated by 1-week withdrawal flow intervals. A decrease in volume and pain usually occurs with each successive cycle. Birth control pills reduce menstrual flow by at least 60% in normal uteri. Early use limits growth and allows orderly regression of excessive endometrial height to normal controllable levels. If the estrogen-progestin combination is not used, abnormal endometrial height and persistent excessive flow recur.

If a patient is not sexually active, the oral contraceptive can be discontinued after 3 months and unopposed endogenous estrogen permitted to reactivate the endometrium. In the absence of spontaneous menses, the recurrence of the anovulatory state is suspected, and a brief preemptive course of an orally active progestin is administered to counter endometrial proliferation. Once pregnancy is ruled out, medroxyprogesterone acetate, 10 mg/day orally for 10 days, is given monthly. Reasonable flow (progestin withdrawal flow) will occur 2 to 7 days after the last pill is taken. If contraception is desired, routine use of oral contraception is warranted.

***Estrogen therapy.*** Intermittent vaginal spotting is frequently associated with minimal (low) estrogen stimulation (estrogen breakthrough bleeding). In this circumstance, minimal endometrium exists, and there is insufficient tissue on which the progestin can exert action. A similar situation exists in the younger anovulatory patient in whom prolonged hemorrhagic desquamation leaves little residual tissue. In these cases, when bleeding is acute and heavy, high-dose estrogen, up to 25 mg conjugated estrogen, is given intravenously every 4 hours until bleeding abates or for 12 hours. This is the sign that the "healing" events are initiated to a sufficient degree. The mechanism of action for estrogen is believed to be a stimulus to clotting at the capillary level. Progestin treatment (usually an oral contraceptive) is started at the same time. Where bleeding is less, lower oral doses of estrogen (1.25 mg of conjugated estrogens or 2.0 mg estradiol daily for 7 to 10 days) can be prescribed initially. When bleeding is moderately heavy, a more intensive oral program can be used (1.25 mg conjugated estrogen or 2 mg estradiol every 4 hours for 24 hours, followed by the single daily dose for 7 to 10 days). All estrogen therapy must be followed by progestin coverage and a withdrawal bleed.

Estrogen therapy also is useful in progestin breakthrough bleeding. These bleeding episodes occur with the use of oral contraception or with depot forms of progestational agents. In the absence of sufficient endogenous and exogenous estrogen, the endometrium shrinks and is composed almost exclusively of pseudodecidual stroma and blood vessels with minimal glands. This type of endometrium also leads to the fragility bleeding more typical of pure estrogen stimulation. The usual clinical story is a patient on long-standing oral contraception who, after experiencing marked diminution or absence of withdrawal flow in the pill-free interval, begins to see breakthrough bleeding while on medication. The use of conjugated estrogens, 1.25 mg, or estradiol, 2.0 mg a day for 7 days, during, and in addition to, the usual birth control pill administration rejuvenates the endometrium and stops the intermenstrual flow.

Another frequently encountered problem is the progestin breakthrough bleeding experienced with chronic depot administration of progestin (Depo-Provera). This agent is used for contraception and also in the treatment of endometriosis and the prevention of menses during chemotherapy. In approximately 25% of recipients, breakthrough progestin bleeding occurs. The judicious use of estrogen is effective therapy in these instances. Bleeding problems are also common with Norplant, another long-term progestin-only contraceptive. Patients with irregular bleeding from Norplant benefit from a short course of oral estrogen as outlined previously.

High doses of estrogen may precipitate a thrombotic event. More than one oral contraceptive per day and multiple doses of oral or intravenous estrogen in a 24-hour period certainly should be regarded as high dose. As a matter of clinical judgment and prudent practice, lower doses can be used in patients who are at increased risk for vascular complications.

*Use of antiprostaglandins.* Although the exact mechanism is unknown, prostaglandin synthetase inhibitors diminish menstrual bleeding in normal women, as well as in those with bleeding secondary to an intrauterine device (IUD). Excessive bleeding in women with menorrhagia can be reduced with these agents by approximately 40% to 50%. This approach should be considered as initial therapy in the absence of pathology in women who are ovulatory but bleed heavily. Side effects are unusual because treatment is limited, usually beginning with the onset of bleeding and continuing for 3 to 4 days. This treatment also may help relieve other symptoms preceding or accompanying the menstrual cycle, which when severe are referred to as the premenstrual syndrome.

*Treatment with a progestin IUD.* A progestational agent can be delivered directly to the endometrium with an IUD. The reduction in menstrual flow is significant after 12 months and some patients become amenorrheic. This option is attractive in patients with intractable bleeding associated with chronic illnesses (such as renal failure).

*Treatment with GnRH agonists.* Treatment with a GnRH agonist can achieve short-term relief from a bleeding problem, such as in a patient with renal failure or a blood dyscrasia. This option is also good for patients who experience menstrual bleeding problems after organ transplantation (especially after liver transplantation) where the toxicity of immunosuppressive drugs makes the use of sex steroids less desirable. The expense and long-term side effects, however, make this choice inappropriate for chronic therapy. If long-term GnRH agonist therapy is chosen, add-back treatment (with a daily combination of 0.625 mg conjugated estrogen or 1.0 mg estradiol and 2.5 mg medroxyprogesterone acetate or 0.35 mg norethindrone), is recommended after gonadal suppression is achieved.

*Ablation of the endometrium.* Persistent bleeding despite treatment is both aggravating and concerning. Although hysterectomy is an appropriate choice for some patients, endometrial ablation should be considered. This treatment can be accomplished with either a laser, a resectoscope with a loop or rolling ball electrode, or by radio frequency-induced thermal destruction. Approximately 90% of women with menorrhagia will improve after an ablation procedure; however, only 50% will become amenorrheic. There is concern that obliteration of segments of the uterine cavity can allow isolated, residual endometrium to progress unrecognized to carcinoma. Long-term follow-up is necessary to determine whether this risk is really a concern.

## PERSISTENT ANOVULATION AND THE POLYCYSTIC OVARY

Anovulation is a common problem that presents in a variety of clinical manifestations, including amenorrhea, irregular menses, and hirsutism. There are serious consequences of chronic anovulation such as infertility and a greater risk for developing carcinoma of the endometrium and perhaps the breast. Therefore all anovulatory patients warrant treatment.

### Pathophysiology

In 1935, Stein and Leventhal first described a symptom complex associated with anovulation. Acceptance of this syndrome as a singular clinical entity led to a rather rigid approach to this problem for many years. Only those women who had a history of oligomenorrhea, hirsutism, and obesity, together with a demonstration of enlarged, polycystic ovaries, qualified for treatment. It is far more useful clinically to consider this problem as one of persistent anovulation with a spectrum of etiologies and clinical manifestations (Fig. 142B-2).

In contrast to the characteristic picture of fluctuating hormone levels in the normal menstrual cycle, a "steady state" of gonadotropins and sex steroids is seen in association with persistent anovulation. The average daily production of estrogen and androgens is both increased and dependent on LH stimulation and results in higher circulating levels of testosterone, androstenedione, dehydroepiandrosterone (DHA), dehydroepiandrosterone sulfate (DHAS), 17-hydroxyprogesterone (17-OHP), and estrone. Testosterone, androstenedione, and DHA are secreted directly by the ovary, and the DHAS is secreted almost exclusively from the adrenal gland. Because levels of sex hormone-binding globulin (SHBG) are controlled by a balance of hormonal influences on their synthesis in the liver (testosterone is inhibitory, estrogen and thyroxine are stimulatory), there is an approximate 50% reduction in circulating levels of SHBG in response to the increased testosterone.

Compared to normal women, patients with persistent anovulation have higher mean concentrations of LH, resulting in a characteristic reversal of the LH:FSH ratio, but low or low-normal levels of FSH. The elevated LH levels are partly due to an increased sensitivity of the pituitary to releasing hormone stimulation and to increased pituitary and hypothalamic sensitivity to increased estrone and decreased SHBG levels. Although estradiol secretion does not increase, free estradiol levels are increased because of the significant decrease in SHBG. The lower FSH levels represent the sensitivity of the FSH negative feedback system to the elevated estrogen, which is comprised of both free estradiol and estrone formed from the peripheral conversion of androstenedione.

Because FSH levels are not totally depressed, ovarian follicular growth is continuously stimulated, but not to the point of full maturation and ovulation. Even though full growth potential is not realized, follicular life span may extend several months in the form of multiple follicular cysts that are 2 to 6 mm in diameter (some can be as large as 15 mm). These follicles are surrounded by hyperplastic theca cells, often luteinized in response to the high LH levels. The accumulation of follicular tissue in various stages of development allows an increased and relatively constant production of steroids in response to gonadotropin stimulation. This condition is self-sustaining. As various follicles undergo atresia, they are immediately replaced by new follicles of similar limited growth potential.

Atresia is associated with a degenerating granulosa, leaving the theca cells to contribute to the stromal compartment of the ovary. This functioning stromal tissue secretes significant amounts of androstenedione and testosterone in response to elevated LH levels. In turn, the elevated androgen levels lead to elevated estrogen levels through the process of extraglandular conversion as well as the suppression of SHBG synthesis. The elevated androgens contribute to the morphologic changes within the ovary by preventing normal follicular development and inducing premature atresia. Indeed, this local androgen block maintains the steady state of persistent anovulation. In this manner the classic picture of the polycystic ovary is attained, displaying numerous follicles in the early stages of development and atresia, and dense stromal tissue. The loss of recycling results in a hormonal steady state causing persistent anovulation and increased production of androgens. The polycystic ovary is thus the result of a "vicious cycle," which can be initiated at any one of many entry points.

The typical histologic changes of the polycystic ovary can be seen in any size ovary. A spectrum of time is involved in the development of this condition, and it is useful to view the attainment of high LH levels and large ovaries as a stage of maximal effect of persistent anovulation. Increased size of the ovaries is not a critical feature, nor is it necessary for diagnosis. The key to understanding this clinical problem is an appreciation of the disruption in ovulatory recycling function that results in increased androgen levels and failure of ovulation, whatever the reason.

### Insulin resistance, hyperinsulinemia, and hyperandrogenism

The association between increased insulin resistance and polycystic ovaries is now well recognized. In addition, there is evidence that hyperinsulinemia contributes to the hyperandrogenism in women with polycystic ovaries. Because obesity itself is associated with insulin resistance, it is important to note that this correlation of increased androgen secretion and insulin resistance has been reported in both obese and nonobese anovulatory women. However, insulin levels are higher and LH and SHBG levels are lower in obese women with polycystic ovaries than in nonobese women with polycystic ovaries.

### Clinical and laboratory findings

Regardless of the etiology, anovulation is the key feature of this condition and presents as amenorrhea in approximately 50% of cases with irregular, heavy bleeding in 30%. True virilization is rare, but 70% of anovulatory patients complain of cosmetically disturbing hirsutism. The development of hirsutism depends not only on the concentration of androgens in the blood, but on the genetic sensitivity of hair follicles to androgens. Obesity has been classically regarded as an important feature, but in view of the concept of persistent anovulation arising from many causes, its presence is extremely variable and has no diagnostic value. However, hirsutism is more common in overweight, anovulatory women. Alopecia and acne are also consequences of hyperandrogenism. Although an elevated LH value in the presence of low or low-normal FSH may be diagnostic, the diagnosis is easily made by the clinical presentation alone. About 20% to 40% of patients with this condition do not have elevated LH levels with reversal of the LH:FSH ratio.

## Management of persistent anovulation

The steady state of hormone secretion has potentially serious clinical consequences (see the box below). Besides problems of bleeding, amenorrhea, hirsutism, and infertility, the effect of unopposed and uninterrupted estrogen places the patient at considerable risk for cancer of the endometrium, and perhaps, cancer of the breast. The risk of endometrial cancer is increased threefold, and chronic anovulation during the reproductive years has been reported in some, but not all, studies to be associated with up to a fourfold increased risk of breast cancer in the postmenopausal years.

Because patients with persistent anovulation develop clinical problems, appropriate therapeutic management is essential for all anovulatory patients. The typical patient presents with anovulation and irregular menses, or amenorrhea with withdrawal bleeding after a progestational challenge. If there is no hirsutism or virilism, evaluation of androgen production is not necessary. Documentation of anovulation is usually unnecessary, especially in view of menstrual irregularity with periods of amenorrhea. In the patient who has long-standing anovulation, an endometrial biopsy (with extensive sampling) is a wise precaution based on the well-known association between this syndrome and abnormal endometrial changes. The decision to perform an endometrial biopsy should not be influenced by the patient's age because it is the duration of exposure to unopposed estrogen that is critical.

#### The clinical consequences of persistent anovulation

- Infertility
- Menstrual bleeding problems, ranging from amenorrhea to dysfunctional uterine bleeding
- Hirsutism and acne
- An increased risk of endometrial cancer and, perhaps, breast cancer
- An increased risk of cardiovascular disease
- An increased risk of diabetes mellitus in patients with hyperinsulinemia

Therapy of most anovulatory patients can be planned at the first visit. If the patient desires pregnancy, she is a candidate for the medical induction of ovulation. For the patient who does not wish to become pregnant and does not complain of hirsutism, but is anovulatory and has irregular bleeding, therapy is directed toward interruption of the steady state effect on the endometrium and breast. The use of medroxyprogesterone acetate (10 mg/day for the first 10 days of every month) is favored to ensure complete withdrawal bleeding and to prevent endometrial hyperplasia and atypia. The patient will be aware of the onset of ovulatory cycles because bleeding will occur at a time other than the expected withdrawal bleed. When reliable contraception is essential, the use of low-dose combination oral contraception in the usual cyclic fashion instead of progesterone is appropriate.

Besides contraception, there is another reason to favor continuous suppression over periodic progestational interruption. The lipoprotein profile in androgenized women with polycystic ovaries is similar to the male pattern and has an adverse impact on the risk for cardiovascular disease. Monthly periodic treatment with a progestational agent has no significant effect on androgen production by polycystic ovaries. Thus if contraception is not required and hirsutism is not an issue, assessment of the lipoprotein profile is reasonable, and in the presence of a male pattern, serious consideration should be given to suppression with oral contraceptives. However, a major contributing factor to the abnormal lipid pattern in these patients is hyperinsulinemia. Therefore a major effort must be directed to control of body weight.

Overweight, hyperandrogenic, and hyperinsulinemic anovulatory women must be cautioned regarding the risk of future diabetes mellitus. In addition, hyperinsulinemia contributes to the increased risk of cardiovascular disease, both by means of a direct atherogenic action and indirectly by adversely affecting the lipoprotein profile. Indeed, insulin resistance may be a more significant factor than androgens in determining the abnormal lipoprotein profile in overweight, anovulatory women. The only known effective therapy for these women is weight loss.

Not all women with polycystic ovaries have hyperinsulinemia; however, it is more common in overweight women and androgenic effects are more intense. Thus all obese patients with a fat distribution pattern that is associated with cardiovascular risk factors (android/central body obesity) should be tested for hyperinsulinemia.

Teenagers who present with persistent anovulation also should be tested for hyperinsulinemia, because those who fail to normalize the hyperinsulinemia associated with an increase in the growth hormone in early puberty may have an increased risk of developing diabetes mellitus.

## AMENORRHEA

Amenorrhea is defined by clinical criteria (see the box above). Primary amenorrhea refers to the lack of initiation of menses in a young woman. Secondary amenorrhea refers to women who cease menstruation after having some prior bleeding episodes. Women learn to count on regular menstrual periods and can feel anxious about missing periods. The possibility of pregnancy should always be considered first. If the patient is not pregnant, reassurance and waiting several months are often all that is needed. If amenorrhea continues or if the patient wishes to become pregnant, a cost-effective investigation of the etiology is warranted.

**Clinical criteria for amenorrhea**

1. No period by age 14 in the absence of secondary sexual characteristics.
2. No period by age 16 regardless of the appearance of secondary sexual characteristics.
3. Absence of three consecutive periods in a woman with established menstrual cycles.

### Etiology, history, and physical examination

Normal menstruation depends on the proper functioning of several discrete but interrelated organ systems. The history, examination, and investigation focus on identifying whether each system is functioning appropriately. Table 142B-2 shows the anatomic locations where problems occur, lists the possible causes of amenorrhea in each area, and provides clues to their diagnoses based on the history or physical examination. Historically, it is important to know whether patients have ever menstruated and with what pattern because patients with congenital disorders affecting the ovary or outflow tract often have never experienced menstruation. On the other hand, women who have had normal cycles and then stop are most likely to have a hypothalamic problem or ovarian failure due to immune-related disorders or menopause.

Routine physical examination of the genitals and pelvis is appropriate. Obvious physical abnormalities of the vagina and cervix can be observed, but these are rarely the causes of amenorrhea. Other manifestations of congenital abnormalities and endocrine diseases should be noted.

## Differential diagnosis

The diagnosis of amenorrhea follows the following stepwise progression.

***Step 1.*** After excluding pregnancy, the initial step in the workup of the amenorrheic patient includes a measurement of thyroid-stimulating hormone (TSH) and a prolactin level and a progestational challenge. Although only a few patients presenting with amenorrhea will have clinically inapparent hypothyroidism, treatment for hypothyroidism is simple and is rewarded by a prompt return of ovulatory cycles.

The purpose of the progestational challenge is to assess the level of endogenous estrogen and the competence of the outflow tract. Either orally active medroxyprogesterone acetate (10 mg) or parenteral progesterone in oil (200 mg) is given daily for 5 days. Within 2 to 7 days after the conclusion of progestational medication, the patient may or may not bleed. If the patient bleeds (any amount beyond a few spots), the presence of a functional outflow tract and a uterus lined by reactive endometrium sufficiently prepared by endogenous estrogen is confirmed. A diagno-

**Table 142B-2.** Etiology of amenorrhea

| Location of problem | Possible etiologies | Clue to diagnosis |
|---|---|---|
| Outflow tract | Developmental absence of vagina or uterus; obstruction of outflow tract | Physical examination (can be difficult in adolescent) |
| | Scarred uterine lining | History of curettage |
| | Cervical obstruction | History of cervical surgery |
| Ovary | Congenital chromosomal abnormality (e.g., Turner's syndrome, mosaic genetic disorders) | Primary amenorrhea<br>Characteristic physical findings |
| | Premature ovarian failure | Menopause symptoms (e.g., hot flashes) |
| Anterior pituitary | Prolactin-secreting tumors | Galactorrhea |
| | Nonfunctioning adenomas | Drugs causing elevated prolactin |
| | Empty sella syndrome | Headaches |
| CNS hypothalamus | Exercise associated | Ballet dancers, marathon runners, etc. |
| | Weight loss, anorexia, bulimia | Eating disorders |
| | Anovulation from lack of LH surge | |
| | Hypothyroidism | Clinical features of thyroid disease |
| | Hypothalamic suppression | Recent use of birth control pills |

sis of anovulation (endogenous estrogen but failure to ovulate) can then be made and the presence of estrogen and minimal function of the ovary, pituitary, and CNS established. If the prolactin level and TSH are normal, further evaluation is unnecessary. When the diagnosis of anovulation or oligoovulation is established, it is important to recognize that the patient has estrogen present without adequate progesterone for ovulation. These women are at risk for endometrial hyperplasia from the effect of unopposed estrogen on the uterus and require a progestational challenge intermittently to protect against this problem. This treatment can be administered monthly as described earlier.

***Step 2.*** If the course of progestational medication does not produce withdrawal flow, either the target organ outflow tract is inoperative or preliminary estrogen stimulation of the endometrium has not occurred. Step 2 is designed to identify which of these conditions is present. Orally active estrogen is administered in a quantity and duration certain to stimulate endometrial proliferation and withdrawal bleeding, provided that a completely reactive uterus and patent outflow tract exist. Conjugated estrogens, 1.25 mg, is administered daily for 21 days. The addition of an orally active progestational agent (medroxyprogesterone acetate, 10 mg/day for the last 5 days) is necessary to achieve maturation of the lining and subsequent withdrawal. In the absence of withdrawal flow, a validating second course of estrogen and progestin is given. As a result of this pharmacologic test, the patient will either bleed or not bleed. If there is no withdrawal flow, the diagnosis of a defect in the endometrium or outflow tract can be made with confidence.

From a practical point of view, in a patient with normal external and internal genitalia by pelvic examination and no history of infection or trauma (such as curettage), an abnormality of the outflow tract is unlikely. Outflow tract problems are due to destruction of the endometrium, generally the result of an overzealous curettage or an infection, or to discontinuity or disruption of the müllerian tube during fetal development. These abnormalities are not common, and in the absence of a reason to suspect them, Step 2 can be omitted in a patient who previously has experienced menstruation.

***Step 3.*** If the patient bleeds only after the administration of estrogen, the physiologic mechanisms responsible for the production of estrogen must be tested. To produce estrogen, sufficient pituitary gonadotropin is required to stimulate ovaries containing normal follicles. Step 3 is designed to determine whether the lack of estrogen is due to a defect in the follicle or in the CNS-pituitary axis. The level of gonadotropin (FSH) is measured first. Because Step 2 involved administration of exogenous estrogen, endogenous gonadotropin levels may be artificially and temporarily altered from their true baseline concentrations. Hence, it is necessary to wait 2 weeks before performing the gonadotropin assay.

### Elevated FSH

If the FSH is elevated, ovarian failure due to menopause is the likely explanation for amenorrhea. FSH levels begin to rise during the perimenopausal period even before bleeding has ceased, whether the perimenopausal period occurs prematurely at age 25 to 35 or at the usual time. Mildly elevated FSH levels (>15 IU/L) may indicate early ovarian failure. Rarely, elevated gonadotropin can be caused by a gonadotropin-secreting pituitary adenoma.

Amenorrhea due to premature ovarian failure can be caused by autoimmune disease. Although an autoimmune etiology is not common, evidence of abnormal thyroid function is usually present. The rest of the investigation should be based on other clinical evidence of autoimmune dysfunction.

### Normal and low FSH

FSH levels in the normal or low range are consistent with CNS failure (usually hypothalamic amenorrhea). Indeed, this is the most commonly encountered CNS cause of amenorrhea. Although the clinical history sometimes provides a clue to the etiology, the usual management is watchful waiting, correcting obvious etiologic factors if the patient wants to become pregnant, and protecting the patient against the consequences of a low estrogen state (see later). Extremely low or nondetectable FSH levels are seldom found except in anorexia nervosa and pituitary tumors. Imaging the pituitary in these cases may be indicated but conservative workup is appropriate because the majority of pituitary tumors never change and most do not require treatment.

### Management

Many patients with secondary amenorrhea will be identified as having a hypothalamic or CNS problem. If these women wish to become pregnant, they should be referred to a gynecologist for consideration of therapy to induce ovulation, such as clomiphene. Those patients who are hypoestrogenic and do not wish pregnancy, including patients with gonadal failure (menopause), hypothalamic amenorrhea, and bilateral oophorectomy, warrant hormone therapy. The long-term benefits of hormone-replacement therapy on cardiovascular disease, lipids, and bones in hypoestrogenic women are well recognized and relevant for both younger and older women. The amenorrheic exerciser should be made aware that the hypoestrogenic state is associated with a greater risk of stress fractures.

The standard program for estrogen therapy consists of 0.625 mg conjugated estrogens on days 1 through 25 of each month, with 10 mg medroxyprogesterone acetate added on days 16 through 25. Beginning medication on the first of every month establishes an easily remembered routine. Another popular method is to administer estrogen every day and progestin the first 12 days of each month. If the progestational agent causes side effects, the daily dose can be decreased to 5 mg. In a few individuals, the estrogen dose may need to be increased to 1.25 mg to achieve menstrual bleeding. Whether a flow-provoking dose of estrogen is necessary for optimal protection of the bones is likely although not proven. Menstruation generally occurs 3 days after the last day of progestin medication. Bleeding that occurs at any time other than the expected time may be a sign that endogenous function has returned. The hormone treatment program should be discontinued and the patient monitored for the resumption of ovulation.

In young women (<35 years) or older nonsmokers, low-dose birth control pills provide an alternative source of estrogen. Patients with hypothalamic amenorrhea must be cautioned that hormonal therapy will not protect against pregnancy if normal function returns. In patients who wish effective contraception, it is reasonable to use a low-dose oral contraceptive to provide the missing estrogen.

## GALACTORRHEA

Galactorrhea is the secretion of milk in a woman who is not postpartum or nursing. Galactorrhea warrants consideration in a nulliparous woman or in a woman who has stopped nursing for more than 12 months.

### Pathophysiology

An elevation in prolactin secretion from the pituitary gland is central to milk production. Multiple factors control prolactin secretion and hence several mechanisms may lead to galactorrhea (Table 142B-3). Since prolactin secretion is under continuous inhibition due to the secretion of prolactin-inhibiting factor (PIF) from the hypothalamus, factors that interfere with PIF secretion can cause galactorrhea. Examples include drugs with hypothalamic effects and hypothyroidism. The elevated levels of TRH in hypothyroidism act as a stimulus for prolactin production. In addition, microadenomas or macroadenomas of the pituitary gland may secrete excess prolactin.

**Table 142B-3.** Causes of galactorrhea

| Causes | Mechanism |
|---|---|
| Prolonged suckling | Reduction in PIF from hypothalamus |
| Drugs (isoniazid, phenothiazines, reserpine derivatives, amphetamines, and tricyclic antidepressants) | Depletion of dopamine or blocked dopamine receptors |
| Major stressors (surgery, trauma) | Inhibition of hypothalamic PIF |
| Hypothyroidism | TRH acts as prolactin releasing factor |
| Pituitary tumors | Secretion of prolactin; tumor may compress pituitary and decrease products of other hormones |

### History

History taking focuses on the identification of obvious causes (Table 142B-3). Because galactorrhea and amenorrhea share common mechanisms, the investigation of women with both conditions follows a pathway described in the preceding section on amenorrhea. Pituitary tumors that account for excess prolactin secretion are usually small and rarely progress to a larger tumor; however, under rare circumstances, larger tumors can cause symptoms of headache and visual field deficits and can interfere with the secretion of other hormones from the anterior pituitary causing endocrine abnormalities.

The investigation of galactorrhea includes thyroid function tests and a prolactin level. Prolactin levels less than 100 ng/ml are consistent with drug-induced galactorrhea, while levels higher than 100 ng/ml suggest the presence of a tumor and may warrant further investigation with imaging of the sella-turcica.

### Management

Microadenomas of the pituitary are treated medically with bromocriptine, a dopamine agonist. This agent shrinks the tumor and prevents subsequent growth. Transphenoidal microsurgery is an accepted approach in patients who fail medical treatment. In otherwise healthy women with persistent galactorrhea as an isolated symptom of hypothalamic disfunction, treatment with bromocriptine can be useful in preventing excessive milk secretion.

## BIBLIOGRAPHY

Clayton RN et al: How common are polycystic ovaries in normal women and what is their significance for the fertility of the population? *Clin Endocrinol* 37:127, 1992.

Graf MJ et al: The independent effects of hyperandrogenaemia, hyperinsulinaemia, and obesity on lipid and lipoprotein profiles in women, *Clin Endocrinol* 33:119, 1990.

Levy HL et al: Ovarian failure in galactosemia, *N Engl J Med* 310:50, 1984.

Rebar RW, Connolly HV: Clinical features of young women with hypergonadotropic amenorrhea, *Fertil Steril* 53:804, 1990.

Schlechte J et al: The natural history of untreated hyperprolactinemia: a prospective analysis, *J Clin Endocrinol Metab* 68:412, 1989.

Warren MP et al: Scoliosis and fractures in young ballet dancers, *N Engl J Med* 314:1348, 1986.

CHAPTER

# 143 Hirsutism and Hyperandrogenism in Women

Leon Speroff
James C. Shaw

Women develop a wide variability in the amount of hair growth during their lives. Genetics and androgen hormones influence hair growth and social customs influence what is considered normal or abnormal. Some increase in the quantity and coarseness of hair occurs with age in all individuals. Regardless of social acceptability, hair growth on the face and other androgen-sensitive areas is a clinical marker for increased androgen production in women.

Idiopathic hirsutism refers to increased androgen-mediated hair growth without an identifiable disease. The wide spectrum of clinical presentations within the "idiopathic" category includes acne and menstrual irregularities; laboratory testing will demonstrate increased androgens in almost all of these women.

An understanding of the pathophysiologic mechanisms that can result in hirsutism will help clinicians determine appropriate evaluation and management of these patients.

## ETIOLOGY AND PATHOPHYSIOLOGY

The primary factor in hirsutism is an increase in androgen levels (usually testosterone) that produces an initial growth stimulus to hair follicles and then acts to sustain continued growth. Essentially every woman with hirsutism has an increased production rate of testosterone or related steroids such as androstenedione.

Excess androgen production in most hirsute women usually results from the hormonal abnormalities associated with anovulatory ovaries and loss of cyclic menstrual function. Hirsutism in childhood and that associated with virilism (clitoromegaly, deepening of the voice, balding, and changes in body habitus) are usually secondary to adrenal hyperplasia or androgen-producing tumors of adrenal or ovarian origin.

Several pathophysiologic factors influence the development of clinically recognizable hirsutism. These factors include the number of hair follicles present, the degree of vellus hair conversion by androgens to terminal hair, the thickness and pigmentation of individual hairs, and the percentage of hairs in active growth phase within an androgen-sensitive area. All of these factors are genetically determined and result in individual variability in the response of hairs to circulating androgens.

## HISTORY

The most common clinical history in hirsute women is irregular menses, with the onset of hirsutism during teenage years or in the early 20s, and long, gradual worsening of the condition. Acne is frequently associated with the worsening hirsutism. The rapidity of development of hirsutism is important. A woman who develops hirsutism after the age of 25 and demonstrates very rapid progression of masculinization over several months usually has an androgen-producing tumor. Other less common causes that may be addressed in the history include Cushing's syndrome, acromegaly, and pregnancy. Drugs can stimulate hair growth by both androgen and non-androgen-mediated mechanisms—methyltestosterone, anabolic steroids, danazol, phenytoin, and diazoxide. Hypertrichosis refers to increased nonsexual hair and can be associated with porphyrias and environmental factors producing chronic irritation or reactive hyperemia of the skin.

## PHYSICAL EXAMINATION

Increased hair growth in patients with hirsutism and hyperandrogenemia ranges from fine vellus hair on the face to marked terminal (full-sized) hair on the face, breasts, genitalia, lower abdomen, and extremities. Other physical findings that suggest hyperandrogenemia include acne, increased oiliness of the skin, and male-pattern alopecia. Masculinizing features such as clitoromegaly, android muscle distribution, and a deep voice are seen in women with severe hyperandrogenemia.

## DIFFERENTIAL DIAGNOSIS

Several conditions can cause hirsutism associated with hyperandrogenemia. Idiopathic hirsutism and polycystic ovary syndrome account for more than 90% of cases, and because of the heterogeneous nature of polycystic ovary syndrome, the term *hyperandrogenism and chronic anovulation* has been coined to describe these individuals. Less common causes of hirsutism include congenital adrenal hyperplasia, late onset adrenal hyperplasia, Cushing's syndrome, androgen-producing tumors of the ovary or adrenal gland, and luteoma associated with pregnancy.

Congenital adrenal hyperplasia is caused by an enzyme defect leading to excessive androgen production. This severe condition has a prenatal onset and is inherited in an autosomal recessive fashion. A milder form of adrenal hyperplasia that causes 1% to 5% of cases of hirsutism appears later in life and has been called "late-onset," "partial," "nonclassical," "attenuated," or "acquired" adrenal hyperplasia. An asymptomatic form, cryptic adrenal hyperplasia, is revealed only with biochemical testing. Although each of the enzymatic steps in the pathway from cholesterol to cortisol can be involved in adrenal hyperplasia, a deficiency of 21-hydroxylase is the most common. This results in an excessive production of the substrate 17-hydroxy progesterone (17-OHP) (see Laboratory Evaluation).

## LABORATORY EVALUATION

Women with normal menses and mild hirsutism require little or no hormonal evaluation. In women with rapid onset of hirsutism and in those with oligomenorrhea, hormonal evaluation is indicated to rule out androgen-secreting tumors and other endocrine causes.

### The testosterone level

Plasma testosterone levels (normal 20 to 80 ng/dl [0.69 to 2.8 nmol/L]) are primarily a measure of ovarian testosterone production and are elevated in the majority of women (70%) with anovulation and hirsutism. Individual variation is great, due largely to the changes in the testosterone-binding capacity of the sex hormone-binding globulin (SHBG) in the blood. Measuring the free testosterone (a technically difficult and expensive assay) is not necessary. A routine testosterone assay adequately screens for testosterone-secreting tumors because these tumors are associated with testosterone levels in the male range and do not rely on fine discrimination of the free testosterone level. If the testosterone level exceeds 200 ng/dl (7 nmol/L), an androgen-producing tumor must be suspected.

Some women with polycystic ovaries (especially hyperthecosis) have testosterone levels greater than 200 ng/dl. In these cases, the clinical presentation should guide diagnostic decisions. A patient with an acute, rapid course of virilizing symptoms requires a full evaluation for the presence of androgen-producing tumor regardless of the testosterone level.

### The dehydroepiandrosterone sulfate (DHAS) level

DHAS is derived almost exclusively from the adrenal gland. It is a direct measure of adrenal androgen activity and correlates clinically with urinary 17-ketosteroid levels. The upper limit of normal in most laboratories is 350 μg/dl (9.5 μmol/L). A random sample of DHAS is sufficient for the evaluation of hirsutism because a slow turnover rate results in a large and stable pool in the blood with insignificant variation. Elevated levels of DHAS contribute to the clinical problem of hirsutism because DHAS is a prehormone in hair follicles, providing substrate for the hair follicle synthesis of androgens.

When the DHAS level is normal, adrenal disease is unlikely, and the source of excess androgen production is most likely the ovaries. Rare cases of adrenal tumors with normal DHAS levels have been reported; testosterone levels are elevated in these cases. Late-onset adrenal hyperplasia is not commonly associated with an increased level of DHAS (see the 17-OHP Level). Moderately elevated DHAS levels are frequently found in patients with anovulation and polycystic ovaries.

### The 17-OHP level

17 hydroxyprogesterone (17-OHP) is elevated in the setting of late-onset adrenal hyperplasia. The normal baseline 17-OHP level is less than 200 ng/dl (6 nmol/L). Levels greater than 800 ng/dl are diagnostic of 21-hydroxylase deficiency. Levels between 200 and 800 ng/dl require adrenocorticotrophic hormone (ACTH) testing to determine the degree of 21-hydroxylase deficiency (see Chapter 35).

## MANAGEMENT

Because almost all patients with hirsutism and excess androgen production are in a steady state of anovulation, treatment is directed toward interruption of this steady state. In patients in whom pregnancy is not desired, the steady state can be interrupted by suppression of ovarian steroidogenesis with oral contraceptives. Oral contraceptives provide a further benefit because they increase SHBG levels. The increase in SHBG results in a greater androgen-binding capacity with a decrease in free testosterone levels. The progestins in oral contraceptives also inhibit the activity of 5α-reductase, the enzyme that converts testosterone to the more active dihydrotestosterone (DHT). This inhibition may provide additional clinical benefit in the treatment of hirsutism.

Low-dose oral contraceptives are as effective as the higher dose formulations in treating acne and hirsutism and suppressing free testosterone levels. Multiphasic formulations appear to be equally effective.

In the patient in whom oral contraceptives are contraindicated or unwanted, good results can be achieved with the use of medroxyprogesterone acetate, either 150 mg intramuscularly every 3 months or 30 mg orally/day. The mechanism of action of medroxyprogesterone acetate is slightly different from that of the combination oral contraceptive. Suppression of gonadotropins is less intense, hence ovarian follicular activity continues. Luteinizing hormone (LH) suppression is significant, however, and testosterone production is decreased, although to a lesser degree than with combined oral contraceptives. In addition, testosterone clearance from the circulation is increased. This latter effect is due to an induction of liver enzyme activity. Although medroxyprogesterone acetate decreases SHBG, resulting in a relative increase in free testosterone, suppression of total testosterone production is so great that the net amount of free testosterone is decreased. The overall effect yields a clinical result comparable to that achieved with the combination oral contraceptive.

Hirsutism responds slowly to treatment. Because the hair growth cycle is long, change takes time. Patients should be informed that at least 6 months of hormonal suppression is necessary before reduction of hair growth can be observed.

Some patients return after a period of treatment expressing disappointment because hair is still present. The effect of treatment (prevention of new hair growth) may not be apparent unless previously established hair is removed. The use of ovarian suppression to prevent new hair growth in combination with electrolysis to remove the old hair yields the most complete and effective treatment of hirsutism.

After 1 to 2 years it is worthwhile to stop the medication and observe the patient for a return of ovulatory cycles. Even in those patients who continue to be anovulatory, testosterone suppression continues for 6 months to 2 years after discontinuing treatment. If anovulation is still present, hirsutism will eventually return.

A surgical approach should be considered in women who have no further desire for fertility or in whom hormonal therapy is contraindicated. A persistent problem of hirsutism, especially if it is progressive in severity, is a reasonable indication for hysterectomy and bilateral salpingo-oophorectomy.

## ALTERNATIVE APPROACHES

### Spironolactone

In the treatment of hirsutism, spironolactone can be used because of its antiandrogenic properties. Although spironolactone is well known for its use as an aldosterone-antagonist diuretic in hypervolemic states, it produces hormonal effects including inhibition of ovarian and adrenal steroidogenesis, inhibition of 5α-reductase activity, and competitive androgen receptor blockade in androgen-sensitive tissue such as hair follicles. The peripheral receptor blockade is responsible for most of the clinical antiandrogen effect.

Spironolactone has been successful in the treatment of hirsutism in doses ranging from 50 to 200 mg/day. Usually some response is noted within 3 months, but longer treatment may be required before any noticeable change is evident.

Side effects are usually minimal and dose related. Potential side effects include a diuresis in the first few days of use, occasional complaints of fatigue, dysfunctional uterine bleeding, and breast tenderness. Spironolactone is contraindicated in pregnancy because of a potential feminizing effect on a developing male fetus. Concomitant use of oral contraceptives prevents this potential complication, prevents menstrual irregularities, and corrects the common underlying steady state of anovulation.

### Dexamethasone

Dexamethasone suppression of endogenous ACTH secretion is used in women who have an adrenal enzyme deficiency with resultant adrenal hyperplasia. Dexamethasone is given nightly (to achieve maximal suppression of the central nervous system adrenal axis, which peaks during sleep) at a dose of 0.5 mg. The equivalent dose of prednisone is 5 to 7.5 mg. If this treatment suppresses the morning plasma cortisol level below 2.0 μg/dl (56 nmol/L), the dose should be reduced to avoid an inability to react to stress. Fortunately, adrenal androgen secretion is more sensitive to suppression by dexamethasone than is cortisol secretion. Patients with classic (congenital) adrenal hyperplasia may require higher doses to normalize the steroid blood levels. With higher doses, alternative day therapy can still accomplish significant adrenal androgen suppression without affecting cortisol secretion.

### Treatment with GnRH agonists

Because ovarian androgen production is LH-dependent, suppression of the pituitary with chronic GnRH agonist treatment improves hirsutism. A higher dose of GnRH agonist is required to suppress ovarian androgen production than that required to suppress estradiol secretion. Therefore treatment should be monitored with testosterone levels. Leuprolide, 3.75 mg/month, is effective. To avoid problems associated with estrogen deficiency, therapy with an oral contraceptive containing estrogen and progestin should be initiated after the GnRH-agonist maintenance dose has been established. This method of treatment is relatively complicated and expensive and should be reserved for severe cases of ovarian hyperandrogenism.

### Flutamide

Flutamide is a nonsteroidal antiandrogen that blocks androgen receptors at peripheral tissue, but does not influence androgen production by adrenal or ovarian tissue. Although the primary use of flutamide is in the treatment of prostate cancer, it has been used successfully in women with hirsutism. Doses ranging from 125 mg twice a day to 250 mg three times a day have been reported in the treatment of hirsutism. Flutamide is generally well tolerated, but fatal hepatotoxicity has been reported with its use in men in doses of 250 mg or more three times a day, and close monitoring of liver function is important.

## BIBLIOGRAPHY

Avgerinos PC et al: Dissociation between cortisol and adrenal androgen secretion in patients receiving alternate day prednisone therapy, *J Clin Endocrinol Metab* 65:24, 1987.

Barth JH, Cherry CA, Wojnarowaka F, Dawber RP: Spironolactone is an effective and well tolerated systemic anti-androgen therapy for hirsute women, *J Clin Endocrinol Metab* 68:966, 1989.

Kohn B et al: New MI, late-onset steroid 21-hydroxylase deficiency: a variant of classical congenital adrenal hyperplasia, *J Clin Endocrinol Metab* 55:817, 1982.

Lobo RA: Hirsutism in polycystic ovary syndrome: current concepts, *Clin Obstet Gynecol* 34:817, 1991.

Marcondes JAM et al: Treatment of hirsutism in women with flutamide, *Fertil Steril* 57:543, 1992.

Rittmaster RS: Differential suppression of testosterone and estradiol in hirsute women with the superactive gonadotropin-releasing hormone agonist leuprolide, *J Clin Endocrinol Metab* 67:651, 1988.

Rittmaster RS: Hyperandrogenism—What is normal? (editorial) *N Engl J Med* 327(3):194, 1992.

Shaw JC: Spironolactone in dermatologic therapy, *J Am Acad Dermatol* 24:236, 1991.

White PC, New MI, Dupont B: Congenital adrenal hyperplasia, *N Engl J Med* 316:1519, 1580, 1987.

Young RL, Goldzieher JW, Elkind-Hirsch K: The endocrine effects of spironolactone used as an antiandrogen, *Fertil Steril* 48:223, 1987.

CHAPTER

# 144 Epidemiology/Etiology of Chronic Pelvic Pain

Andrea J. Rapkin

## EPIDEMIOLOGY/ETIOLOGY OF CHRONIC PELVIC PAIN

Chronic pelvic pain is defined as pain that persists for greater than 6 months. Often, chronic pelvic pain presents a difficult diagnostic and management dilemma as the etiology of the pain may be obscure, and the relationship between certain types of pathology and the pain response may be inconsistent.

Laparoscopy performed for chronic pelvic pain reveals that up to 77% of patients do not have obvious gynecologic pathology (Table 144-1). More recent studies have suggested that approximately half of the patients who do not exhibit pathologic processes at the time of laparoscopy in fact do have a nonobvious, nongynecologic somatic disorder. Careful evaluation is needed to distinguish gynecologic pain from orthopedic, gastrointestinal, urologic, neurologic, and psychosomatic pain.

## PATHOPHYSIOLOGY OF CHRONIC PELVIC PAIN

The neural mechanisms underlying the transmission of chronic pelvic pain have yet to be elucidated; however, mechanisms for transmission of acute visceral pain have been delineated. The afferent nerves innervating pelvic organs are shown in Table 144-2. Painful impulses that originate in the skin, muscle, bones, joints, and parietal peritoneum travel in somatic nerve fibers, whereas those originating in the internal organs travel with visceral autonomic nerves. Visceral pain in general is diffuse, not easily localized, and often accompanied by referred pain. The referred pain is usually superficial, well localized, and appreciated within the nerve distribution or dermatome of the spinal cord segment innervating the involved viscera. Recent research has suggested that all visceral pain may in fact be "referred pain," as visceral and somatic afferents project onto the same second-order neurons in the dorsal horn of the spinal cord.

The structures of the female genital tract vary in their sensitivity to pain. The skin of the external genitalia is exquisitely sensitive. Pain sensation is variable in the vagina, because the upper segment is somewhat less sensitive than the lower. The cervix is relatively insensitive to small biopsies, but is sensitive to deep incision or to dilation. The uterus is quite sensitive. The ovaries are insensitive to many stimuli, but they are sensitive to rapid distention of the ovarian capsule or compression during physical examination.

## COMMON CAUSES OF PELVIC PAIN

As shown in the box on p. 1828, both gynecologic and nongynecologic disorders produce pelvic pain. This chapter is a guide to the diagnosis and management of pelvic pain originating from the reproductive organs. Differentiation of reproductive organ pain from pain produced by other pelvic structures and from pathologic processes tries the skills of every primary care physician. Presented here is an orderly approach to these complex diagnostic and management tasks.

**Table 144-1.** Laparoscopy for chronic pelvic pain

| | No. pts. | No path | Adhesion | Endometriosis | Other |
|---|---|---|---|---|---|
| Liston (1972) | 134 | 77% | 16% | 5% | 2% |
| Lundberg (1973) | 95 | 38% | 31% | 13% | 18% |
| Renaer (1973) | 108 | 28% | 23% | 22% | 27% |
| Kresch (1984) | 100 | 17% | 48% | 32% | 3% |
| Rapkin (1986) | 100 | 36% | 26% | 37% | 1% |

Kresch AJ et al: Laparoscopy in 100 women with chronic pelvic pain, *Obstet Gynecol* 64:672, 1984; Liston WA et al: Laparoscopy in a general gynecologic unit, *Am J Obstet Gynecol* 113:672, 1972; Lundberg WI, Wall JE, Mathers JE: Laparoscopy in the evaluation of pelvic pain, *Obstet Gynecol* 42:872, 1973; Rapkin AJ: *Obstet Gynecol* 68:13015, 1986; Rapkin A, Reading A: Current problems in obstetrics, *Gynecology and Fertility* 14(4):99, 1991; Renaer M: *Chronic pelvic pain in women,* New York, 1981, Springer-Verlag.

**Table 144-2.** Nerves carrying painful impulse from the pelvic organs

| Organ | Spinal segments | Nerves |
|---|---|---|
| Perineum, vulva, lower vagina | S2-4 | Pudendal<br>Inguinal<br>Genitofemoral<br>Posterofemoral cutaneous |
| Upper vagina, cervix, lower uterine segment, posterior urethra, bladder trigone, uterosacral and cardinal ligaments, rectosigmoid, lower ureters | S2-4 | Pelvic parasympathetics |
| Uterine fundus, proximal fallopian tubes, broad ligament, upper bladder, cecum, appendix, terminal large bowel | T11-12, L1 | Sympathetics via hypogastric plexus |
| Outer two thirds of fallopian tubes, upper ureter | T9-10 | Sympathetics via aortic and superior mesenteric plexus |
| Ovaries | T9-10 | Sympathetics via renal and aortic plexus and celiac and mesenteric ganglia |

From Hacker N, Moore JG: *Essentials of obstetrics and gynecology,* ed 2, Philadelphia, 1992, WB Saunders.

### Peripheral causes of chronic pelvic pain

- I. Gynecologic
  - A. Cyclic
    - 1. Primary dysmenorrhea
    - 2. Secondary dysmenorrhea
      - a. Structural abnormalities (imperforate hymen, transverse vaginal septum)
      - b. Cervical stenosis
      - c. Uterine anomalies (congenital malformation, bicornuate uterus, blind uterine horn)
      - d. Intrauterine synechiae (Asherman's syndrome)
      - e. Endometrial polyps
      - f. Endometriosis
      - g. Uterine leiomyoma
      - h. Adenomyosis
      - i. Pelvic congestion syndrome (varicosities)
    - 3. Atypical cyclic
      - a. Endometriosis
      - b. Adenomyosis
      - c. Ovarian remnant syndrome
      - d. Chronic functional cyst formation
  - B. Noncyclic
    - 1. Adhesions
    - 2. Endometriosis
    - 3. Salpingo-oophoritis
    - 4. Ovarian remnant syndrome
    - 5. Pelvic congestion syndrome
    - 6. Ovarian neoplasms
- II. Nongynecologic
  - A. Gastrointestinal
    - Irritable bowel syndrome
    - Ulcerative colitis
    - Granulomatous colitis (Crohn's disease)
    - Carcinoma
    - Infectious diarrhea
    - Recurrent partial small bowel obstruction
    - Diverticulitis
    - Hernia
    - Abdominal angina
    - Recurrent appendiceal colic
  - B. Genitourinary
    - Recurrent or relapsing cystourethritis
    - Urethral syndrome
    - Interstitial cystitis
    - Ureteral diverticuli or polyps
    - Carcinoma of the bladder
    - Ureteral obstruction
    - Pelvic kidney
  - C. Neurologic
    - Nerve entrapment syndrome
    - Neuroma
  - D. Musculoskeletal
  - E. Myofascial syndrome

## CYCLIC PELVIC PAIN

Pain limited to just before and during menses is considered cyclic pain. Pain occurring in a regular cyclic fashion but unrelated to menses is called atypical cyclic pain. Pain that occurs throughout the month without any particular cycle or relation to menses is termed acyclic pain. Cyclic pelvic pain can be attributed to primary or secondary dysmenorrhea. Atypical cyclic pain is usually a variant of secondary dysmenorrhea and may begin 1 week before menses and last for up to 1 week after the cessation of menstrual flow.

### Dysmenorrhea

Dysmenorrhea affects up to 50% of menstruating women. Primary dysmenorrhea refers to pain with menses without pelvic pathology, whereas in cases of secondary dysmenorrhea there is underlying pelvic pathology. Primary dysmenorrhea usually appears within 2 years of menarche. The pain begins a few hours before or just after the onset of menstrual flow and usually lasts up to 72 hours. The pain is laborlike, with suprapubic cramping accompanied by low back and interior thigh pain, nausea, vomiting, diarrhea, and occasionally syncope. Primary dysmenorrhea affects younger women with ovulatory cycles but may persist into the late reproductive years. It is associated with increased uterine prostaglandin production. Women with primary dysmenorrhea also show elevated uterine tone with high-amplitude contractions. Given that 20% to 50% of women have improvement in dysmenorrhea with placebo suggests that psychogenic factors must be taken into consideration in situations where usual treatment approaches fail.

Secondary dysmenorrhea usually occurs years after menarche and can occur even with anovulatory cycles. The most common cause of secondary dysmenorrhea is endometriosis; however, other common causes are listed in the box at left. Establishing the diagnosis of secondary dysmenorrhea entails ruling out primary dysmenorrhea and confirming the cyclic nature of the pain with a pain diary.

### Endometriosis

The incidence of endometriosis in the general female population is 1% to 2%, although, in infertile women the incidence is 15% to 25%. Endometriosis is noted in patients undergoing laparoscopy for chronic pelvic pain in 5% to 37% of the cases (see Table 144-1). Endometriosis usually presents in the third or fourth decade; however, adolescents and women in their 20s who are evaluated for chronic pelvic pain commonly have endometriosis. Rarely, postmenopausal women on hormone replacement experience pain related to the activation of preexisting endometriosis.

Endometriosis is characterized by the presence of endometrial glands and stroma located outside the uterine cavity, most commonly on the ovaries, uterosacral and cardinal uterine ligaments, rectovaginal septum and pelvic peritoneum, and, rarely, at distant locations such as the cervix, appendix, laparotomy or episiotomy scars, and pleural or pericardial cavities. Although there is a clear relationship between significant endometriosis and infertility, the relationship between endometriosis and pain can be inconsistent. Dysmenorrhea, deep dyspareunia, and pain unrelated to menses or coitus are definitely more common in women with endometriosis than in women with postinfection or postsurgical adhesions or those with a normal pelvis. Generally the extent of the endometriosis usually does not correlate with the severity of pain, possibly due to differences in depth of infiltration of disease or variations in metabolic activity of the endometriotic implants.

The most common symptoms of endometriosis are

dysmenorrhea, dyspareunia, infertility, and abnormal uterine bleeding, usually from a secretory endometrium. The patient often describes pressurelike pain and aching in the lower abdomen, back, and rectum and symptoms similar to irritable bowel syndrome. Pain with defecation (dyschezia) also may be present as a result of endometrial implants near the rectum. Signs and symptoms of an acute abdomen occur infrequently and are usually related to rupture of an endometrioma.

Examination of patients with endometriosis may reveal tender nodularity on the rectovaginal examination of the uterosacral ligaments and posterior cul-de-sac. Progressive disease results in obliteration of the cul-de-sac and fixed retroversion of the uterus. Enlarged ovaries (endometriomas) with decreased mobility may be noted. Occasionally, there is extension of rectovaginal disease into the vagina; these lesions may be noted on speculum examination. Although the intestine is involved in many patients, bowel lesions rarely extend through the mucosa. In the setting of cyclic rectal bleeding from invasion of the mucosa, colonoscopy and biopsy are necessary to rule out colonic malignancy. Endometriosis involving the peritoneum of the anterior cul-de-sac is quite common, but patients only rarely develop hematuria secondary to penetration of the bladder mucosa. Cystoscopy and biopsy are diagnostic in this setting.

### Adenomyosis or "internal endometriosis"

Adenomyosis consists of endometrial glands and stroma that penetrate into the underlying myometrium, leading to diffuse infiltration of the uterus. Adenomyosis is found in 8% to 20% of hysterectomy specimens. The incidence peaks between the ages of 40 and 50 years. The adenomyotic uterus is usually enlarged with increased vascular supply, which may account for the most common symptoms, including secondary dysmenorrhea, menorrhagia, and on occasion, polymenorrhea or premenstrual staining.

### Pelvic congestion

The role of pelvic congestion in the genesis of chronic pelvic pain has been debated. In a study of transuterine venograms in women with chronic pelvic pain, larger mean ovarian and uterine vein diameters, delayed disappearance of contrast medium, and ovarian congestion were present in a significantly greater proportion of women with chronic pelvic pain without pathology than in those with pathology or control patients. The clinical syndrome of pelvic congestion consists of secondary dysmenorrhea, low back pain, dyspareunia, and menorrhagia. The pain is usually bilateral lower pelvic in distribution and is exacerbated by the menstrual period. Many patients have coexistent irritable bowel syndrome, chronic fatigue, and anxiety. On examination, tenderness over the uterus is notable and the fundus of the uterus and cervix are often bulky. The ovaries may be enlarged with multiple functional cysts.

## NONCYCLIC PELVIC PAIN

### Adhesions

Intraperitoneal adhesions may result from previous infection, prior intraabdominal surgery, or endometriosis. Adhesions (not related to endometriosis) are present in 16% to 44% of patients undergoing laparoscopy for chronic pelvic pain (see Table 144-1). Recent studies question the role of pelvic adhesions as a common cause of chronic pelvic pain. Although adhesions may be prevalent in patients with chronic pelvic pain, these adhesions may or may not cause pain. Additionally, self-reported pain descriptions do not correlate with the degree of physical findings observed during the laparoscopy in patients with adhesions. A subset of patients with adhesions leading to intermittent partial small bowel obstruction may have pain associated with nausea, vomiting, bloating, and pain with eating. These patients should be evaluated for an acute pain process.

### Salpingo-oophoritis

Salpingo-oophoritis may cause chronic pelvic pain, although patients usually present acutely. Patients with subacute or subclinical disease may have complaints of lower abdominal pain, increased vaginal discharge, irregular bleeding, intermittent fever, dysmenorrhea, dyspareunia, and occasionally dysuria and suprapubic pain. Many women who lack the classic history noted previously may escape accurate diagnosis. Patients also may complain of having had numerous episodes of pain associated with fever and may have been given the diagnosis of pelvic inflammatory disease. When these episodes become recurrent, the patient is often considered to have chronic salpingo-oophoritis, although it is not clear that a chronic inflammatory condition exists. Instead, subacute or subclinical disease or recurrent acute infections may be present. On examination, abdominal tenderness may be accompanied by cervical motion and adnexal tenderness, and there may be purulent cervical discharge. Although fever or leukocytosis may not be present, erythrocyte sedimentation rate (ESR) may be elevated. Positive chlamydia cultures are often noted in patients whose only complaints are bloating and lower abdominal discomfort. The main reason for "reinfection" is inadequate antibiotic treatment. Approximately 20% of patients with prior acute salpingitis will suffer chronic pelvic pain; however, the specific etiology of the pain in this setting is unknown. Some may have subacute infection and others hydrosalpinx and pelvic adhesions. Because the pain is often worse with increased intraovarian pressure, anovulation therapy is often helpful.

### Ovarian remnant syndrome

Chronic pelvic pain after a hysterectomy and bilateral salpingo-oophorectomy for severe endometriosis or pelvic inflammatory disease may be caused by residual ovarian tissue that has become retroperitoneal due to scarring after difficult surgery. The patient with ovarian remnant syndrome usually complains of pelvic pain, which may be cyclic. Painful symptoms usually arise 2 to 5 years after surgery. Pelvic examination may reveal a tender mass in the lateral region of the pelvis. An ultrasonography usually confirms a mass with sonographic characteristics of ovarian tissue. In a patient who has had a bilateral salpingo-oophorectomy and is not on hormone replacement, estradiol or follicle-stimulating hormone assays may reveal a characteristic premenstrual picture.

### Tumors and cysts of the reproductive organs

Most tumors and cysts of the reproductive organs are capable of causing acute pain from adnexal torsion, rupture leading to hemoperitoneum (corpus luteum cyst), chemical peritonitis (dermoid), or degeneration of leiomyomata, and other conditions. Outside the settings of an acute event, however, vague lower abdominal discomfort may be related to pelvic tumors such as leiomyomata or ovarian neoplasms, both benign and malignant.

***Uterine leiomyoma.*** Uterine leiomyomata are the most common pelvic neoplasms. They undergo malignant transformation in approximately 2 to 3/100,000 of women and growth is usually slow. Pelvic discomfort from uterine fibroids may be present when the neoplasms encroach on adjacent bladder or rectum. This pain is not usually severe. On occasion, however, significant abdominal or pelvic pain may result from necrosis or degeneration of a myoma secondary to loss of blood supply. It is rare for a uterine leiomyoma to degenerate rapidly in the nonpregnant state. During pregnancy the leiomyomata increase rapidly in size and therefore may outgrow their arterial blood supply. Occasionally, a pedunculated subserosal leiomyoma will be torse. In these situations, examination may reveal abdominal pain with tenderness and rebound tenderness. Fever often may be present, and the white blood count may be elevated. This diagnosis is often a diagnosis of exclusion; the preferred mode of treatment is intravenous hydration and pain medication. Surgery is not recommended unless hysterectomy is warranted for abnormal bleeding or discomfort due to uterine size (usually greater than 14 cm). If the diagnosis is uncertain, a laparoscopy may be necessary.

A third type of leiomyoma that may cause acute pain and hemorrhagic vaginal bleeding is a submucous myoma. It projects from the myometrium just under the surface of the endometrium into the endometrial cavity. The pain is similar to the pain of labor, and there is usually associated heavy vaginal bleeding. Hysteroscopic resection or hysterectomy is necessary for definitive treatment.

## NONGYNECOLOGIC CAUSES OF CHRONIC PELVIC PAIN

### Gastroenterologic

Because the uterus and adnexa share the same visceral innervation with the lower ileum, sigmoid colon, and rectum, it is often difficult to determine whether lower abdominal pain is of gynecologic or enterocoelic origin. Irritable bowel syndrome is a common cause of lower abdominal pain and may account for up to 60% of referrals for chronic pelvic pain. Other gastrointestinal causes of chronic pain are listed in (see the box on p. 1828). Groin hernias are uncommon in females; however, incisional hernias and spigelian hernias (spontaneous, lateral, ventral hernias) may result in pelvic pain. Anterior and posterior perineal hernias usually are limited to cystocele, rectocele, and enterocele and may cause abdominal discomfort or perineal pressure, but usually not pain.

### Urologic causes of chronic pelvic pain

Chronic pelvic pain of urologic origin may be related to various types of pathology listed in the box on p. 1828. One of the most common causes of pain is the urethral syndrome. Symptoms include dysuria, urgency, frequency, suprapubic pain, and dyspareunia. Negative urine and urethral cultures and a negative evaluation for vulvovaginitis and contact dermatitis of the urethra should increase the suspicion of the diagnosis. *Ureoplasma, Chlamydia, Candida, Trichomonas,* as well as gonorrhea and herpes, should be ruled out. Cystoscopic evaluation should be performed to rule out urethral diverticulae, interstitial cystitis, and cancer.

### Neurologic causes of chronic pelvic pain

***Nerve entrapment.*** Abdominal cutaneous nerve entrapment always should be considered in the differential diagnosis of chronic lower abdominal pain, especially if visceral etiology is not apparent. The syndrome most commonly occurs months to years after transverse suprapubic skin incisions. The syndrome of spontaneous abdominal nerve entrapment also has been described and may involve any of the thoracic/abdominal nerves, but more commonly involves the ilioinguinal and iliohypogastric. The nerves may become trapped between the transverse and internal oblique muscles, especially when the muscles contract.

Symptoms of iliohypogastric/ilioinguinal nerve entrapment include pain elicited by exercise or hip flexion and relieved by bed rest. The pain is described as stabbing, colicky, and sudden and is judged to be coming from the abdomen and not the skin. It is located along the line of the lateral edge of the rectus muscle and may be associated with a burning pain radiating toward the linea alba and to the flank or sacroiliac region. Occasionally, pain radiates to the labia and inner aspect of the thigh. Nausea, bloating, menstruation, and a full bladder may exacerbate the pain.

On examination, the pain usually can be localized with the fingertip. The tentative diagnosis is confirmed with a diagnostic nerve block. Patients usually report immediate relief of symptoms after injection, and many patients do not require further intervention, although some patients require two or three weekly injections. After the third injection, patients should be considered for surgical removal of the involved nerves if visceral pathology can be ruled out.

### Musculoskeletal causes of chronic pelvic pain

Lower back pain without pelvic pain is rarely related to gynecologic pathology; however, lower back pain may accompany pelvic pathology. Pain localized to the sacrum is more likely to reflect pain of gynecologic origin. Nongynecologic low back pain may intensify premenstrually or menstrually.

***Myofascial pain.*** Myofascial syndrome has been found in approximately 15% of patients with chronic pelvic pain. Many additional patients, however, may have trigger points that are pathognomonic of this condition if examined carefully. A description of this syndrome and neuropathic pain is provided in Chapter 103.

Briefly, each centimeter of the abdominal wall, lower back, and vaginal area is palpated with finger tip or Q-tip (vagina), and areas that reproduce the patient's pain or cause positive jump sign are marked. Using a 22-gauge needle, 3 ml of 0.25% bupivocaine is injected at each trigger point into the fat pad just above the fascia. Pain relief is diagnostic. Permanent pain relief is usually afforded by two to three injections at weekly intervals. Anesthesia of trigger points may abolish pain by lowering the impulses from the area of referred pain, thereby diminishing the afferent impulses reaching the dorsal horn to a level below the threshold for pain transmission.

## CHRONIC PELVIC PAIN WITHOUT PATHOLOGY

The term *chronic pelvic pain without obvious pathology* refers to patients who lack pathology. These patients often have been considered to have psychogenic pain. Although the majority of patients with chronic pain have abnormal psychologic profiles, patients without recognized pathology do not appear to be psychologically different from those with organic disease.

From a psychologic perspective, various factors may promote the chronicity of pain. The meaning attached to the situation, the ability to redirect attention, personality factors, mood, and past experience amplify or attenuate pain experience. Pain and suffering tend to evoke similar behaviors, which makes it difficult to differentiate pain behaviors from those reflecting suffering. The persistence of pain or suffering over time increases the potential to affect behavior. Behaviors associated with pain, such as withdrawal, complaining, or help seeking, may more directly reflect reinforcement contingencies than the sensory experience of discomfort.

Various studies also have examined the role of prior sexual abuse as a specific risk factor for chronic pelvic pain. One study reported a significantly higher prevalence of physical or sexual abuse in childhood or adulthood in patients with chronic pelvic pain (55%) compared with patients with other types of chronic pain (36%) and a control group without pain (16%).

### History

As with the investigation of any other physical symptom, a thorough history should be obtained. The effect of menses, intercourse, exercise, work, and stress should be queried. Of these factors, the most important diagnostic feature is the presence or absence or cyclicity of pain. Pain with intercourse (dyspareunia) should be queried (location of pain, whether introital, vaginal, or pelvic). Presence and cyclicity of pain with bowel movements should be ascertained. Date of last menstrual period, the usual periodicity, duration and amount of flow, and any other abnormal vaginal bleeding, including postcoital bleeding, should be noted. The color and odor of vaginal discharge should be queried. Clear to white discharge that is not foul smelling or pruritic is usually normal. It is important to inquire about voluntary or involuntary infertility, as well as current and past methods of contraception. Other systemic symptoms should be investigated including fever, weight loss, and anorexia.

Past history, including prior evaluations for pain, should be documented. If the patient has had surgery, operative and pathology reports are important. The context in which the pain arose should be ascertained (postpartum, after abortion, after sexual assault, or an episode of pelvic infection). Inability to perform one's occupation, litigation, or workers' compensation issues should be noted.

Current and past psychologic history should include psychosocial factors, abuse, psychiatric hospitalizations, suicide attempts, and chemical dependency. The attitude and behavior of the patient and family with respect to the pain and current upheavals in the patient's life should be discussed. The part of the history addressing sensitive issues may have to be reobtained after establishing rapport with the patient.

### Examination and laboratory tests

A complete physical examination should be performed, with particular attention given to the vital signs, abdominal, back, vaginal, bimanual, and rectovaginal examinations. The patient should be examined for hernias while standing. An attempt should be made to locate by palpation the tissues that reproduce the patient's pain. A thorough evaluation for trigger points should proceed. If applicable, cervical and urethral cultures, wet mount, Pap smear, stool guaiac, and urine analysis should be obtained. A complete blood count, sedimentation rate, and pregnancy test should be performed in all patients.

## DIAGNOSIS AND MANAGEMENT OF CHRONIC PELVIC PAIN

### Cyclic gynecologic pain

It is important to distinguish between primary and secondary dysmenorrhea, because the treatment of secondary dysmenorrhea is often surgical. Because secondary dysmenorrhea (as opposed to primary dysmenorrhea) may occur with anovulatory cycles, it is important to document whether cycles are ovulatory (Chapter 142). Genital cultures for gonorrhea and *Chlamydia* and a complete blood count with ESR are usually warranted. If pelvic examination suggests the possibility of adnexal pathology, pelvic ultrasound is warranted. If no abnormalities are found, a tentative diagnosis of primary dysmenorrhea may be made.

Women with dysmenorrhea who have a normal pelvic examination should receive a trial of nonsteroidal, anti-inflammatory agents. Prostaglandin synthetase inhibitors are effective for the treatment of primary dysmenorrhea in 70% of cases. The inhibitor should be taken just before or after the onset of pain and then continuously every 6 to 8 hours to prevent reformation of prostaglandin by-products. Before confirming treatment failure, changes in doses and types of inhibitors should be attempted. Alternatively, birth control pills can be used. More than 90% of women with primary dysmenorrhea have relief with birth control pills. If the patient does not respond to prostaglandin synthetase inhibitors or is not a candidate for oral contraceptive pills, a codeine preparation can be added for 2 to 3 days.

The management of secondary dysmenorrhea involves treatment of the underlying pathology. If endometriosis is suspected, consultation with a gynecologist and laparoscopy are necessary for the definitive diagnosis.

Medical treatment of endometriosis is useful for women who do not desire fertility and for patients who develop recurrent pain after surgical treatment of endometriosis. Three forms of medical therapy are currently used: danazol (Danocrine), progestins, and chronically administered gonadotropin-releasing hormone (GnRH) agonists. Danazol is a synthetic androgen with mild antiestrogenic and antiprogestational effects. It is metabolized by the liver, and an occasional patient will have elevated liver enzymes while taking the drug. In addition, high-density lipoprotein (HDL) cholesterol may decrease with danazol use. The possible long-term effects of danazol on cardiovascular disease suggest that it should not be used for longer than 8 months at a time. The main side effects include weight gain, edema, myalgia, acne, and headaches. Danazol provides relief of pain in more than 80% of women treated, although pain often recurs within 6 to 12 months after therapy.

Gonadotropin-releasing hormone (GnRH) analog therapy for endometriosis relies on either monthly injection of depo GnRH agonist or daily nasal administration of GnRH agonist. These medications initially stimulate the pituitary with release of a burst of follicle-stimulating hormone (FSH) and luteinizing hormone (LH); however, after the first week, continuous exposure to GnRH leads to inhibition of gonadotropin production resulting in a "chemical menopause." Currently, two agonists are FDA approved for use in the United States: leuprolide acetate (Depo Lupron) monthly injection and nasal nafarelin acetate (Syneral). Because a 2% to 7% decrease in trabecular bone density occurs within 6 months after GnRH agonist usage, therapy is limited to 6 to 8 months. Side effects include hot flashes, headaches, libido decrease, atrophic vaginitis, and emotional lability. Between 40% and 60% of patients experience recurrence of pain within a year after discontinuing therapy.

Before the development of danazol or GnRH agonist, progestins alone were used for the treatment of endometriosis. Medroxyprogesterone acetate, 30 mg/day, usually produces amenorrhea and may provide relief of pain. It is particularly useful in the management of minimal to moderate endometriosis. Depo Provera (150 mg/intramuscularly every 3 months) may be used in patients who also desire contraception.

Conservative surgery is indicated for patients with moderate to severe endometriosis who desire future fertility. However, women with moderate to severe disease who do not desire future fertility are candidates for hysterectomy and bilateral salpingo-oophorectomy. Only about 30% of patients with severe endometriosis and 50% of patients with moderate endometriosis will conceive after either hormonal or surgical therapy.

Patients with secondary dysmenorrhea or atypical cyclic pain due to leiomyomata, presumed adenomyosis, or pelvic congestion can be treated with NSAIDs or oral contraception. Failure to respond to the above regimens may require laparoscopy to rule out coexistent endometriosis. Multidisciplinary pain management can be used if medical therapy fails, and if pain management fails a myomectomy or hysterectomy can be performed.

### Noncyclic chronic pelvic pain

Diagnostic laparoscopy has become a standard procedure to evaluate patients with noncyclic, chronic pelvic pain. However, laparoscopy should probably be reserved for patients with an abnormal pelvic examination, signs and/or symptoms of endometriosis or cyclic pelvic pain unresponsive to initial management who do not have other identified somatic or nongynecologic sources of pain.

### Multidisciplinary pain management

During the first visit the patient should be provided with a pain diary in which to note, on a daily basis, the onset and intensity of pain, medication intake, and aggravating and alleviating factors. A simple diary incorporates a visual analog scale from 1 (no pain) to 10 (most severe pain ever) for each morning and evening. The diary should be maintained for 1 to 2 months. Failure to comply with the pain diary is often a sign that more in-depth psychosocial evaluation is necessary.

A second visit should be scheduled in 1 to 4 weeks (depending on symptom and severity). The visit should include a review of the pain diary for cyclicity of pain. If pathology is not found during this and subsequent visits, or if pain disproportionate to pathology is noted, the patient should be evaluated by a psychologist or other mental health professional familiar with the management of chronic pelvic pain. If resolution of pain does not occur with the multidisciplinary approach, the patient should be referred to a gynecologist for possible laparoscopy.

In dealing with patients with chronic pelvic pain, a therapeutic, supportive, and sympathetic, but structured, physician-patient relationship should be established. The patient should be given regular follow-up appointments and should not be told to call only if the pain persists, as this reinforces pain behavior as a means of procuring sympathy and medical attention. A negative evaluation and laparoscopy, or the finding of pathology not amenable to therapy (for example, recurrent dense pelvic adhesions) does not mean that the patient should be discharged from care without therapy directed toward her symptoms. After initial reassurance that there is no serious underlying pathology, symptomatic therapy should be undertaken.

Multidisciplinary pain management is an excellent approach to chronic pelvic pain. Besides the primary care physician or gynecologist, the team includes a mental health professional and, occasionally, an anesthesiologist or acupuncturist. The mental health professional provides marital and sexual counseling, assertiveness training, and adaptive coping strategies. This aspect of therapy is crucial, because many of these patients have withdrawn interpersonally, sexually, and sometimes occupationally. Acupuncture, nerve blocks, and trigger point injections of local anesthetics may provide prolonged pain relief. Various studies of chronic pelvic pain have demonstrated that multidisciplinary pain management is more likely to be effective than standard approaches that address only somatic causes of pain.

## BIBLIOGRAPHY


Rapkin AJ and Reading AE: Chronic pelvic pain, *Curr Probl Obstet Gynecol Fertil* 14(4):99-137, 1991.

Rapkin AJ: Adhesions and pelvic pain: a retrospective study, *Obstet Gynecol* 68:13015, 1986.

Rapkin AJ: Neuroanatomy, neurophysiology and neuropharmacology of pelvic pain, *Clin Obstet Gynecol* 33(1):119, 1990.

Reiter RC: A profile of women with chronic pelvic pain, *Clin Obstet Gynecol* 33:130-136, 1990.

Renaer M: *Chronic pelvic pain in women,* New York, 1981, Springer-Verlag.

Slocumb JC: Neurological factors in chronic pelvic pain: trigger points and the abdominal pelvic pain syndrome, *Am J Obstet Gynecol* 149:536-543, 1984.

CHAPTER

# 145 Contraceptive Choices

**Florence P. Haseltine**
**Marguerite Perikles**

The ability to regulate fertility is an important factor in physical and mental well-being. Maternal and child health, pregnancies in high-risk women, problems arising from unwanted children, population control, improving the status of women—all are family planning issues that affect society as well as the individual. Yet, according to studies from the National Survey on Family Growth (NSFG), half of all pregnancies are unintended and one fifth occur while a family planning method is being used. The average woman who uses contraception properly is still apt to have two unplanned pregnancies during her reproductive life, and couples who use contraceptives diligently throughout their reproductive life span still have an almost 70% chance of having at least one unplanned pregnancy. Inadequate contraceptive methods play a role in a large number of induced abortions: approximately 42% of unintended pregnancies and 40% of all pregnancies in women under the age of 20 end in abortion. Thus educating people about the importance of consistent and proper use of contraceptives could greatly reduce the use of abortion as a method of family planning.

Couples who want to control their fertility are often confronted with difficult problems. They may lack the motivation or skill to use contraceptive methods consistently and correctly, or they may be unaware of the need to have access to more than one method as their life circumstances change. Many will become frustrated and discouraged by the realization that no currently available contraception method is ideal. Also, controlling fertility arouses anxieties in some people that are influenced by cultural background, family tradition, religion, and media accounts that sensationalize the pitfalls and risks associated with some methods. Health care providers can help patients make informed choices by providing them with complete, clearly understood information about what is available or feasible and advising them on the advantages and disadvantages of different methods.

## ISSUES FOR CONSIDERATION

Effectiveness and safety are the most important factors to consider. Assessing effectiveness is a problem because it is difficult to determine whether failure of the contraceptive method being evaluated occurred because of incorrect or inconsistent use or because the method itself was actually flawed. Many factors can influence outcome, including the years of use, sexual practices, and the user's ability and motivation. Although contraceptives can fail even when the user has done everything correctly, more unwanted or unplanned pregnancies occur because of user failure than method failure.

Although the medical risks of contraceptive use are few, all methods represent some type of risk—health, discomfort, unwanted pregnancy, or possible harm to the developing fetus. Most women, however, face a greater risk from an unplanned or unwanted pregnancy, or from terminating the pregnancy, than they do from using all methods of contraception, with the possible exception of oral contraceptive use in women over the age of 35 who smoke. In addition to safety and efficacy, personal issues such as cost, convenience, and ease of use are important. The need to consult with a specialist and the noncontraceptive benefits of a particular method, such as protection from sexually transmitted diseases (STDs), are also important considerations.

## CONTRACEPTIVE CHOICES

Family planning methods offer several options: temporary contraception using barrier methods or combined oral contraceptive; permanent prevention of pregnancy by voluntary sterilization; and postcoital contraception, or pregnancy interception, to prevent conception or implantation. Most available methods are targeted for women because male contraception methods are currently limited to the condom, coitus interruptus, and surgical sterilization. Safety and reversibility are important considerations for both men and women; however, concerns about libido are emphasized more heavily in men, even though women have reported changes in their libido (frequently manifested by a lowering of the libido) with every form of hormonal and most barrier methods. Unfortunately, no effort has been made to design contraceptives for women with libido as a marker for acceptability.

### Barrier methods

Barrier contraceptives include mechanical devices and chemical agents that interfere with fertilization by either preventing sperm from coming into contact with an egg or preventing the implantation of a fertilized egg. Men have used some form of mechanical device, such as the condom, for centuries. Female-controlled barriers, which are placed in the vagina to prevent sperm from entering the uterus, include the diaphragm, cervical cap, vaginal condom, vaginal sponge, and spermicides. Barrier methods are most effective if people admit that they are going to have sex, are comfortable placing the devices in the presence of their partners, and are encouraged to become familiar with the application of the device before having sexual intercourse. These methods are more challenging for people who are sexually inexperienced. All barrier methods have some risk of toxic shock syndrome (TSS). Although TSS is a rare problem, symptoms are highlighted on the products' package insert, and most women have become more careful in their use of these devices. TSS should be suspected if a woman has a fever of 101° F or higher, diarrhea, vomiting, muscle aches, or a rash that looks like a sunburn.

### The condom

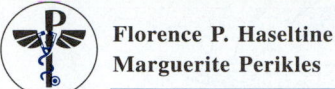

Condoms are the principal form of temporary birth control for men and are used by 10% to 15% of couples. Placed over an erect penis before ejaculation, the condom acts as barrier between the egg and the sperm. Condoms are made from a number of materials, the most effective being latex. Latex condoms are available in different sizes, shapes, textures, and thicknesses. They come with and without lubrication, spermicide, or reservoir ends. Although natural membrane condoms made from the caecum of lamb intestine are available, they do not withstand the rigors of intercourse or prevent the spread of viral infections as well as the latex condom. A new nonlatex condom made of polyurethane is being marketed and is purported to be thinner, stronger, and more comfortable than latex condoms and can be used by persons who are allergic to latex.

*Effectiveness and safety.* Condom failure is mainly due to breakage, and most of these accidents are associated with improper application. The condom's rate of effectiveness varies widely, from 98% in experienced and highly motivated users to about 70% in those who are not. Among typical users, the first year failure rate is slightly greater than 12%. Effectiveness may be enhanced if condoms are used in conjunction with a spermicidal agent, such as foam or jelly. Condoms are safe and have no side effects, except possible allergic reactions to latex in either partner.

*Advantages and disadvantages.* Condoms are readily available and relatively inexpensive; they are small, lightweight, and easily disposable. They do not require medical examination, follow-up, or prescription for use. Most important, condoms offer the best method for preventing the spread of the human immunodeficiency virus (HIV) and other STDs. Their use has apparently doubled since the awareness of HIV and acquired immune deficiency syndrome (AIDS). The effectiveness of condoms is enhanced if they are used in conjunction with contraceptive jellies or spermicides, which are both spermicidal and provide antimicrobial protection. The condom has disadvantages: It must be put on at the time of intercourse; it can leak or break at some point during or after intercourse; it can be uncomfortable because of the sensation of dryness; and some people complain that it lessens sensitivity.

*Instructions for use.* The condom should be placed on the penis after an erection has been achieved and before the penis comes in contact with the woman's genitals. It must be rolled correctly onto the penis and be held on during withdrawal. It will slip off if the penis becomes flaccid within the vagina. Extra lubrication with contraceptive foams, gels, creams or K-Y jelly can be used. Oil-based lubricants should be avoided because they can weaken latex condoms.

## The female condom

Female condoms are now being marketed. One, currently marketed under the name Reality, is available with limited clearance from the FDA. The device consists of a plastic sheath with an outer ringed opening that falls slightly outside the vagina and an inner, separate ring that is placed within the vagina and rests against the pubic bone and cervix. Because it covers the perineal area, it offers greater protection from STDs. It also permits the woman to use the method herself without having to rely on her partner using a condom. The disadvantages are that it is unattractive, noticeable to both partners and noisy during intercourse, and requires some skill to insert. User effectiveness is not clear.

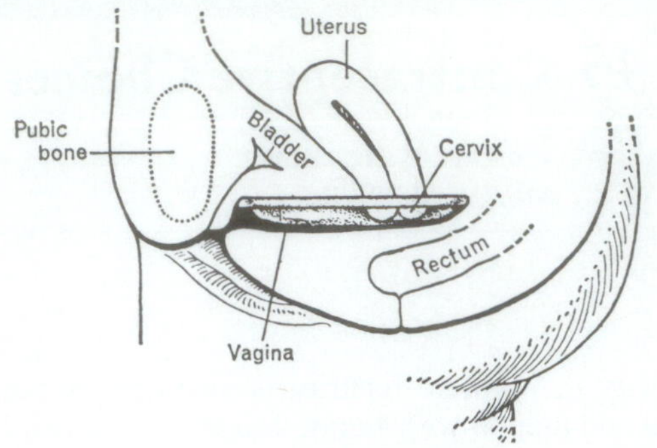


**Fig. 145-1.** The diaphragm must be sized and fitted properly to be effective. If the diaphragm is too small, it can be displaced during intercourse. If it is too large, it can cause pelvic discomfort. It must fit snugly behind the pubic bone and over the cervix into the posterior fornix. (From *Population reports,* Population Information Program, Series H, No. 4, The Johns Hopkins University, January, 1976.)

## Spermicidal agents

Spermicides are available as foams, creams, suppositories, tablets, and gels. They may be used alone or in conjunction with other barrier methods. The most widely used spermicidal contraceptives contain either nonoxynol 9 or octoxynol 9, surface-acting agents that disrupt the sperm cell membrane. Spermicides are considered safe and have not been shown to be teratogenic. Although some evidence suggests that these agents protect against most STDs, it is not clear whether they also protect against HIV infection.

## The diaphragm

The diaphragm is a rubberized dome that fits into the vagina and covers the opening of the cervix. It is designed so that sperm cannot penetrate the rubber barrier and enter the uterus after ejaculation (Fig. 145-1). To be effective, diaphragms should be used in conjunction with spermicidal agents and should remain in place for at least 6 hours after intercourse. If intercourse occurs more than once in 6 hours, spermicide should be reapplied without removing the diaphragm. For users who prefer to separate contraception from the act of intercourse, the best way to ensure that it will be in place when needed is to insert the device with spermicide each night and remove it each morning. The diaphragm's rate of effectiveness reaches 98% if it fits properly, is inserted correctly, is kept in place long enough for the spermicide to act, and is used consistently. Otherwise, its effectiveness falls to about 80%. Skin irritations or allergies and recurrent bouts of cystitis can be caused by the rubber or by the spermicidal agents used in conjunction with the device.

The primary advantage of the diaphragm is that spermicidal agents used in conjunction with it not only kill sperm, but also other microorganisms, thus reducing the likelihood of contracting STDs. Because the degree of protection from STDs has not been determined, however, the FDA will not permit labeling of the products for this purpose. The diaphragm has several relatively minor disadvantages. It can be cumbersome to use, inconvenient, or not available when needed. In addition, the vagina of some women expands greatly during intercourse, and the diaphragm can be dislodged.

The four styles of diaphragm come in a range of sizes, and women should be fitted with the one that is most comfortable for them. The diaphragm should be checked for size after each pregnancy and at least once every 4 years if a pregnancy has not occurred because of changes in the vagina from weight changes and pelvic relaxation.

### Vaginal sponge, cervical cap

The vaginal sponge and the cervical cap are similar to the diaphragm. The vaginal sponge, as its name implies, is a polyurethane sponge saturated with the spermicidal agent, nonoxynol-9. It can be purchased without a prescription at a drug store. The sponge is well moistened with water and placed inside the vagina not more than 24 hours before intercourse. It should be left in place for at least 6 hours but not longer than 24 hours, because the risk of TSS increases thereafter. The cervical cap is similar to the diaphragm, but it covers only the cervix and does not spread out to cover the upper vagina. The cervical cap must be fitted, which requires skill because of the importance of an exact fit.

The cervical cap is as effective as the diaphragm, whereas usage of the sponge is associated with a higher pregnancy rate. To be effective, the cervical cap should be used in conjunction with spermicidal agents and should remain in place for at least 6 hours after intercourse. If intercourse occurs more than once in 6 hours, the spermicide can be reapplied intravaginally. Both methods have few side effects. One nonmedical side effect of the vaginal sponge is dryness of the vagina caused by the sponges' absorptive capacities. Both devices must be used cautiously in women with a recent pregnancy or cervical surgery or a cervical lesion. Mechanical dexterity is important with either.

### Oral contraceptives

The introduction of an oral, hormonal contraceptive agent, or the "pill," changed our thinking about contraceptives and their acceptability. The birth control pill (BCP) is the most popular method of reversible contraception, particularly among young women, and has been used by over 60 million women in the United States and 150 million women worldwide (see Managed Care Guide). There are two kinds of oral contraceptives (OCs). Most common are the combined oral contraceptives (COCs), which are made up of varying doses of estrogen and progestin and comprise over 90% of the OCs in use today. The other type is the progestin-only pill, sometimes referred to as the "minipill," which contains a progestational agent only.

*Mechanism of action.* COCs interact with the hormonal receptors that promote ovulation, implantation, and fertilization of an oocyte. Principally, the pill prevents pregnancy by suppressing ovulation. It changes the pituitary pattern of gonadotrophin release so that ovulation occurs irregularly. In addition, it acts on the lining of the uterus, so that even if an oocyte is released and fertilized, implantation cannot occur. It also makes the mucus of the cervix thicker and more difficult for sperm to traverse.

*Types.* Chemically, COCs are made up of a combination of estrogen and progesterone hormones that mimic those produced normally during the menstrual cycle. The two estrogen compounds currently used in the United States are ethinyl estradiol (EE) and mestranol, which remains inactive until it is converted by the liver to EE; 30 to 35 µg of EE is equivalent to 50 µg mestranol. Six different types of progestational agents are used: norethindrone, norethindrone acetate, ethynodiol diacetate, norgestrel, levonorgenestrel, and norethynodrel. Their effectiveness is determined by their ability to prevent the onset of endometrial bleeding. Each progestational agent has variable amounts of estrogenic and androgenic activity or antiestrogen effects. At one extreme is norethindrone acetate, a compound that has little estrogenic activity or antiestrogen effects, but is very androgenic. At the other is norethynodrel, a progesterone that has a high level of estrogenic but no androgenic activity. The doses and potency of these hormonal agents determine their effectiveness and influence the side effects and complications that may occur. Lower doses, for example, are associated with more breakthrough bleeding (BTB) and higher failure rates, whereas higher doses are associated with more serious complications.

A question that always arises is how to determine which medication to use for a specific woman. Because the FDA does not recognize substantial differences among the available COCs, no company is permitted to make special claims. However, individuals may respond differently to the different formulations.

*Effectiveness and safety.* The BCPs are all effective, with an overall efficacy rate of 95% to 99%. Known side effects that are medically threatening are so rare and well known that they are not considered major health risks. The BCP is probably safer than aspirin. For these reasons, there is pressure to have the medication sold over the counter.

*Side effects and other complications.* More information is available about BCPs than any other medication on the market. Manufacturers of COCs now include in their packages lists of possible side effects of the pill. The list is long, and it is difficult to determine how common each side effect may be. The classic estrogenic effects attributed to use of the pill are nausea, breast tenderness with increase in size, fluid retention, headaches, hypertension, thromboembolic complications, pulmonary emboli, cerebrovascular accidents, hepatocellar adenomas, hepatocellular cancer, telangiectasias, and growth of fibroids. Progesterone side effects include increased appetite and weight gain, depression, fatigue, decreased libido, acne, oily skin, increased breast size, decreased carbohydrate tolerance, headaches, pruritus, increased low-density lipoproteins (LDL,) and decreased high-density lipoproteins (HDL). Lowering the dosage of the pill has reduced the risk of cardiovascular disease and thromboemboli, but not the risk of strokes.

*Contraindications.* Absolute contraindications to using the pill are thrombophlebitis or thromboembolic disease, cerebrovascular or heart disease, pregnancy, carcinoma of the breast, and liver tumors. Smoking increases the risk of

## Managed Care Guide
## Patient desires oral contraceptive

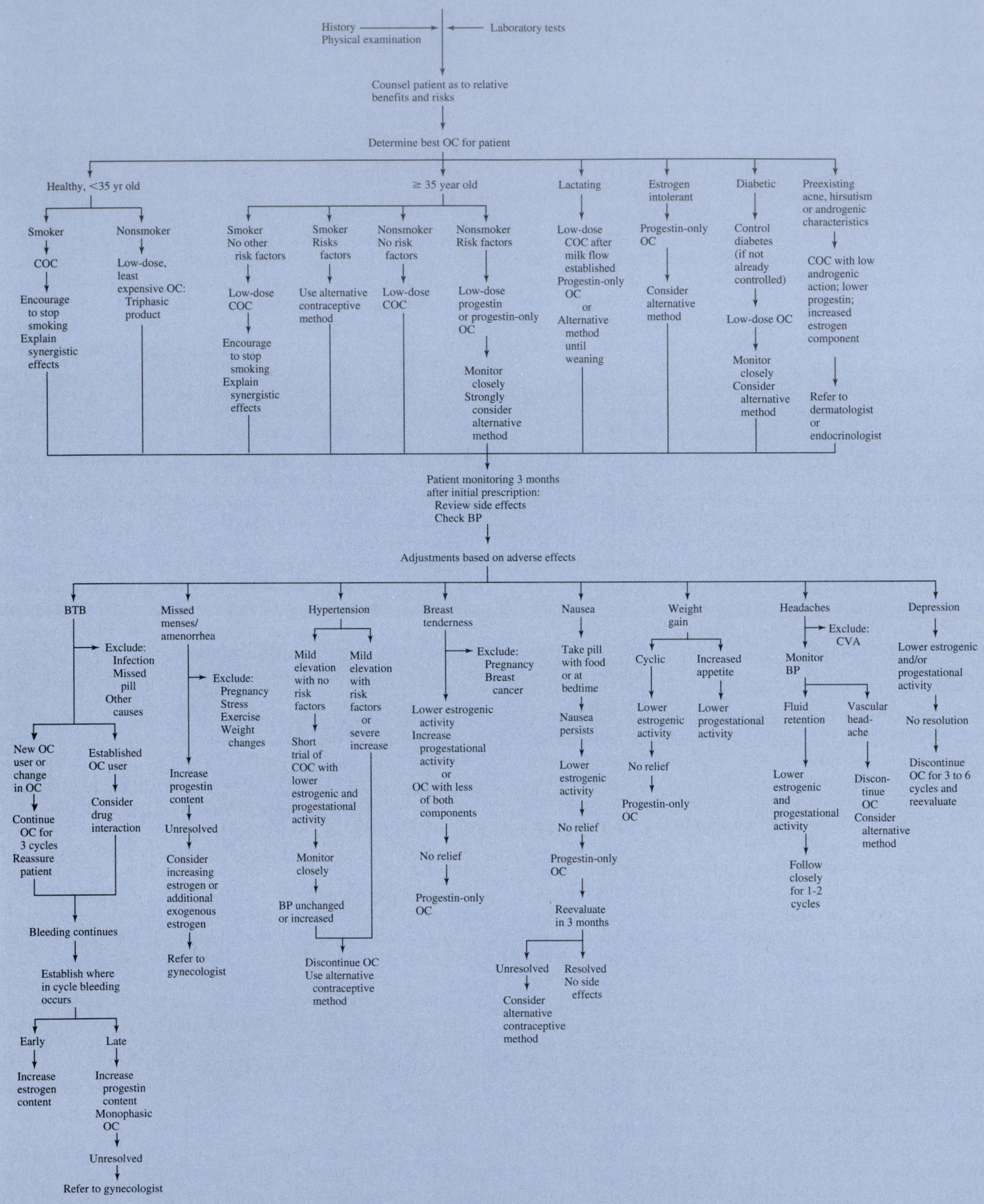


From Robles TA: Use of oral contraceptives. In Greene HL, Johnson WP, Maricic MJ, editors. *Decision making in medicine*. St. Louis, 1993, Mosby.

cardiovascular disease, and many physicians will not prescribe the pill to any woman over 35 years of age who smokes. The relative contraindications are those related to the side effects. There is no way to predict which pill will cause side effects for an individual woman.

*Advantages and disadvantages.* COCs are user friendly in that a woman takes the pill in privacy. Although the present low-dose formulations minimize side effects, they must be taken every day to be effective. Antibiotics, which interfere with the enterohepatic circulation or alter the gut flora and reduce the absorption of the steroids, lower the dose of available medication and decrease contraceptive protection. In addition, medication such as phenytoin (Dilantin), which alters the rate of degradation of steroids may decrease the effectiveness of COCs.

OCs also provide noncontraceptive benefits. Androgenic symptoms, such as acne or hirsutism, often improve while the patient takes the pill and menstrual cramps decrease. A continuous regimen of OCs can also help women who suffer from premenstrual migraines by maintaining constant hormone levels. OCs are often the first line of treatment for endometriosis and heavy uterine bleeding. Although they are not currently prescribed to decrease the risk of ovarian and uterine cancer, epidemiologic studies suggest that the use of OCs reduce the risk of these two diseases.

*Degree of monitoring and follow-up required.* Women who begin the pill should have a follow-up visit at 3 months and be monitored at yearly intervals thereafter. There is some question, however, whether this degree of follow-up and monitoring is necessary or whether OCs should be made available as an over-the-counter medication. The logic behind this debate stems from sufficient data demonstrating that OCs are safe for most women, and those who have real risk factors for not using them are well aware of those factors and would not choose to use OCs anyway. Although there may be some debate as to whether regular visits to the physician to obtain OCs are needed for safety, it does appear that a woman's interaction with her health care provider for routine preventive care is important. The most important part of the examination is measurement of blood pressure. It is not clear whether elevated lipid levels, a prediabetic condition, or heart disease are in themselves contraindications for the pill; but these conditions are important in terms of long-term care of the patient.

*Instructions for use.* COCs are packaged so that a woman takes the active hormone for 21 consecutive days followed by a placebo, iron, or nothing for the next 7 days. With this regimen, withdrawal bleeding usually occurs every month, mimicking the normal menstrual cycle. There is no medical reason, however, why a woman needs to achieve a cycle. Although the pill is used continuously to prevent all uterine bleeding in some women with endometriosis and dysmenorrhea, most women will experience irregular bleeding with continuous use.

### Progestin-only pills

These pills work mainly by their adverse effect on the lining of the uterus and cervical mucus. Although 50% of cycles in women who use progestin-only pills are ovulatory, implantation does not occur even if fertilization does. These pills are taken continuously and they are associated with irregular bleeding.

*Effectiveness.* The combined and progesterone-only pills have comparable efficacy. Both can be associated with breakthrough bleeding, although this problem is more frequent with the progesterone-only pill.

### Progestin-only contraceptive methods

In addition to the pill, progestin-only contraceptives can be delivered by injection and through implants, vaginal rings, or intrauterine devices. These approaches provide varying degrees of protection.

*Injectable progestins.* Depo-Provera. This long-acting deposition of medroxyprogesterone acetate is injected at a dose of 150 mg every 3 months. It acts by suppressing ovulation and making the uterine lining inhospitable to implantation.

*Progestin implants.* Norplant. This implantable form of progesterone (levonorgesterol) must be surgically inserted and removed. Six implants are usually placed into the anterior arm. Insertion does not usually constitute a problem, but extraction may be difficult. Once inserted, it can last as long as 5 years. The implant causes irregular uterine bleeding, and some women find this unacceptable. However, the total blood loss from vaginal bleeding on Norplant is greatly reduced compared with normal menstrual flow.

*Biodegradable implants.* Capronor (levonorgestrel). A biodegradable implant that provides protection for about 18 months is under development. It will be useful for women who want a shorter range of protection than Norplant provides and do not want an implant that must be removed by surgery. The medication has side effects similar to those of Norplant.

### IUDs

Use of the intrauterine device (IUD) decreased markedly in this country in the early 1980s after major product liability suits were filed against the makers of the Dalcon Shield because of major complications experienced by many of the women who used their product. At one point, all IUDs were removed from the US market, with the exception of one that had progesterone imbedded in it and one called Copper 7. These two are still the only IUDs available in this country.

*Mechanism of action.* The IUD device, when inserted into the uterus, causes an inflammatory reaction. Studies have shown that although ovulation occurs, the oocyte does not become fertilized, possibly as a result of the secondary inflammation in the uterus or the presence of IUD-produced spermicidal toxins.

*Effectiveness and safety.* The efficacy of the IUD is 94% to 99%. Possible complications associated with its use include expulsion from the uterus, low-grade uterine inflammation, and perforation of the uterus with migration of the IUD into the abdominal cavity. This latter complication occurs most often during insertion, but also can happen at other times. Concomitant use of antibiotics can reduce the effectiveness of the IUD by causing the low-grade uterine inflammation to subside. Women also should be instructed to check the string attached to the IUD after each menstrual period to ensure that the IUD has remained in place; if the string cannot be found, they should be examined. Finally, if an infection is suspected, the IUD should be removed immediately and antibiotics prescribed.

The IUD is not recommended for women who have never had a pregnancy. If a woman develops a pelvic infection resulting in infertility, it is considered a more serious problem. Usage in nulliparous women is discouraged because of both liability and infertility risks. The greatest advantage of an IUD is that, once inserted, it does not have to be activated when a woman has intercourse. The disadvantages are that menstrual periods tend to be heavier, irregular bleeding may occur, and there is a risk of infection with insertion. The latter can be reduced if antibiotics are taken just before insertion. The IUD should be removed immediately if a pregnancy is suspected.

Women should have a yearly pelvic examination to make sure the IUD is still located within the uterus and that the uterus is not tender. The main concern is development of infection. It is also important to check the hematocrit, because anemia will occur if bleeding is excessive.

### Vaginal ring

The vaginal ring is similar in appearance to the diaphragm. The ring releases contraceptive drugs identical to those found in the birth control pill. The medication leaches out, is absorbed by the vaginal mucosa, and delivered to the circulatory system. When these rings become available, they will be valuable alternatives to continuous oral, implanted, or injectable progesterone.

### Sterilization

A major contraceptive method in the United States, and the most popular one for persons over the age of 30, is voluntary sterilization. As of 1988, over a third of US couples had chosen this method to prevent pregnancy, relying on either ligation of the fallopian tubes in women or ligation of the vas deferens in men. These procedures are purely a mechanical means of interfering with conception and appear to have no appreciable effect on hormones. Because sterilization is meant to be permanent, however, anyone considering surgical sterilization should be counseled thoroughly to understand fully what it entails.

***Voluntary sterilization in men.*** Voluntary sterilization in men is accomplished by vasectomy, a simple surgical procedure performed on an outpatient basis using local anesthesia. Small incisions are made in the scrotum to reach and cut the vas deferens, thereby blocking the passage of sperm. Although vasectomy is both effective and safe, patients may experience some postoperative discomfort. Complications, such as infection, hematoma, epididymitis, or granuloma formation do occur but are usually minor. Vasectomy does not appear to have any long-term adverse effects, although a question has been raised about its possible relationship to prostate cancer. Despite some animal data suggesting that vasectomy may promote atherosclerosis, numerous epidemiologic studies have not found an increase in heart disease among men with vasectomies.

***Voluntary sterilization in women.*** In women, voluntary sterilization can involve ligation, electrocoagulation, or mechanical occlusion of the fallopian tubes. The fallopian tubes are reached through the abdomen either via laparoscopy or minilaparotomy. Although the laparoscopy leaves only a small scar and is quicker and less painful than minilaparotomy, it requires a fully equipped operating room and the skills of a specialist, which make it more costly. It is not recommended for postpartum women. Although laparoscopy is associated with a low rate of complications, those that do occur can be serious. The minilaparotomy is relatively easy to learn and can be performed by a general practitioner on an outpatient basis using local anesthesia. This procedure leaves a visible scar and takes longer to perform than the laparoscopy. Complications are mostly minor. It is the method of choice for postpartum women.

***Advantages and disadvantages of sterilization.*** Voluntary sterilization provides a safe and permanent method of contraception for those who do not want to risk pregnancy because of medical or genetic reasons. For persons who want no (more) children, it is an excellent option if there are contraindications to or problems using the reversible contraceptive methods. Despite its permanency, voluntary sterilization is the choice of a high percentage of couples because the failure rates of other methods are higher. The major disadvantage is that reversal of the procedure requires major surgery, and there are no guarantees for success. With the best surgical technology, the reversal rate approaches 80%.

## POSTCOITAL METHODS

Because many people in the United States consider attempts to avoid pregnancy following coitus tantamount to abortion, postcoital contraception is a politically sensitive subject. Nevertheless, because neither human behavior nor contraceptive methods are perfect, there is a place for this method of contraception. Historically, women have tried many techniques to avoid pregnancy postcoitally, such as douching or performing various physical maneuvers to remove semen from the vagina. These methods are usually ineffective because there is extremely rapid uptake of sperm by the cervical mucus.

### Oral contraceptives

The use of COCs in a different regimen is quite effective as protection against pregnancy once a woman has had a sexual exposure. Used in this manner, COCs change the lining of the uterus so that if conception occurs, the endometrium is inhospitable and implantation cannot occur. Although the use of COCs for postcoital protection has not been approved by the FDA, studies in other countries have provided physicians with information about appropriate dosages. When using low-dose pills, such as Lo/Ovral, Nordette, and Levlen, and combination pills in the Triphasil and Tri-Levlen packs, four pills should be taken as soon as possible after exposure followed by four more pills 12 hours later.

### RU 486

RU 486 is an antiprogestin that is used to produce an abortion when contraception has not been used or the method fails. Its use is based on the knowledge that the establishment and maintenance of pregnancy depend on progesterone. When used in combination with a prostaglandin, RU 486 terminates early pregnancy by preventing implantation or causing sloughing of the fertilized zygote. The drug is currently marketed only in France and is not available in this country. Its future status is not clear because of the political and legal controversies surrounding its use. RU 486 is highly effective (95%). Its side effects are minimal, the principal one being uterine bleeding. Hypertension and nausea are associated with the concomitant use of a prostaglandin.

### Abortion and pregnancy termination

An abortion can be performed at every phase of a pregnancy; however, the technique used varies depending on gestational age. Early term abortions are performed between 7 and 12 weeks of gestation. Mid-term abortions are performed between 12 and 16 weeks, and late abortions after the 16th week. No abortions are performed after the 24th week. If a pregnancy is terminated after the 24th week, it is usually because an early delivery is necessary to save the life of either the mother or the fetus.

Pregnancies less than 12 weeks gestation can usually be terminated by dilation of the cervix and evacuation of the uterus under suction. This outpatient procedure requires only one visit to the physician's office. Dilation of the cervix can be accomplished directly or more slowly using laminaria tents (compact dried seaweed sticks that are inserted into the cervix and swell slowly as they absorb water). Bleeding after an abortion is common for up to 2 weeks. Sexual activity should not resume until bleeding has stopped. Severe cramping or bleeding may indicate an incomplete abortion and the need for further treatment.

Mid-term abortions are usually performed by injecting either prostaglandin or hypertonic saline into the uterine cavity, which causes the fetus to be expelled. These terminations require hospitalization.

Most women do not experience long-term adverse medical or emotional effects after an abortion. Nevertheless, an abortion is a loss and some women may need consoling and counseling. Studies of the long-term emotional effects on women who require abortion because of maternal or fetal disorders have not been published.

## NATURAL FAMILY PLANNING

Natural family planning (NFP) is a method of birth control that involves identifying the period in a woman's cycle when she is most fertile and using this information to avoid an unwanted pregnancy. NFP is based on periodic abstinence and requires high user motivation and a great deal of understanding about the menstrual cycle for success. The method is unsuitable for women who have cycles less than 21 days or over 36 days. The effectiveness of NFP is in the same range as some barrier methods and varies from 65% to 90%.

## SELECTION OF A BIRTH CONTROL METHOD

### Basic approach

When patients who have decided to use a contraceptive ask for assistance in selecting a method, it is important to obtain information about their personal characteristics, such as their social and sexual history and degree of motivation and their medical history. Factors to be considered are the users' age and health, reproductive and menstrual history, personal lifestyle, past sexual history, current sexual practices, and concerns about convenience and cost. Patients need to think about whether and when they want children and how an unplanned pregnancy would affect their lives. The medical history should focus on a history of thrombophlebitis, cardiovascular disease, pelvic inflammatory disease, and smoking. The linkage of contraceptive dispensing to medical care is part of our health care system, and it is often the only time reproductive-aged women have contact with the medical profession. A physical examination should be performed including blood pressure and breast and pelvic examinations. A Pap smear, *Gonococcus* culture, *Chlamydia* smears, hematocrit, and lipids test are suggested.

### Special considerations

Barrier methods, such as the diaphragm or cervical cap that require mechanical dexterity, may not be appropriate for persons with certain types of physical disabilities unless the partner is willing or able to help, or they have an assistant to insert the device for them.

Oral contraceptives are not recommended for nursing mothers because of passage into the milk. Barrier methods are usually recommended in postpartum women, although an IUD can be placed at the 6-week postpartum checkup. Many women continue to use OCs until their menopause. Although the dosages of hormones in the low-dose formulations help alleviate perimenopausal symptoms, they are much higher than those used commonly in replacement therapy in postmenopausal women. Because data about the safety of long-term OC use are not available, especially in older women, it is important to know whether the patient has gone through the menopause. Periodic FSH levels should be measured; when they rise above 40 international units, menopause has occurred and contraception is not needed. Similar to hormone-replacement therapy, COCs will not fully supress FSH levels, because inhibin secretions from the ovary, which selectively inhibit the secretion of FSH, decrease at the menopause.

## BIBLIOGRAPHY

Hacker NF and Moore JG. *Essentials of obstetrics and gynecology,* Philadelphia, 1986, WB Saunders.

Hatcher RA et al: *Contraceptive technology,* 1990-1992, ed 15, Revised, New York, 1992, Irvington Publishers.

Kelsey JL and Gammon MD: The epidemiology of breast cancer, *CA Cancer J Clin* 41(3):146-65, 1991.

Schlesselman JJ: Oral contraceptives and breast cancer, *Am J Obstet Gynecol* 163 (4Pt2):1379-1387, 1990.

Trussell J and Vaughan B: Research note: aggregrate and lifetime contraceptive failure in the United States, *Fam Plann Perspect* 21:224-226, 1989.

CHAPTER

# 146 Female Infertility and Couples Counseling

Erika Goldstein
Linda D. Eckert

## EPIDEMIOLOGY

### Prevalence

Infertility is defined as the inability to conceive after at least 1 year of regular, unprotected intercourse. It may be primary (no previous conceptions) or secondary (infertility after at least one documented conception). In normal fertile couples, the chance of conception after 1 month of unprotected intercourse is 25%; after 6 months, 70%; and after 1 year, 85%. Only an additional 5% conceive after 1 to 2 years without therapy. An estimated 15% to 20% of couples desiring pregnancy in the United States experience infertility. In 1988 this translated into an estimated 5 million women, 9% of the reproductive age population. In the last decade the number of infertile couples presenting for treatment has increased. Although several factors have been postulated to account for this increase, including an older age of couples attempting pregnancy and an increase in the overall rate of sexually transmitted diseases and exposure to toxins and chemicals that may be implicated in infertility, careful demographic evaluation demonstrates that the observed increase is due to more couples seeking evaluation and treatment rather than an actual increase in the problem itself. The distribution of male and female causes of infertility is shown in Table 146-1.

## NORMAL PHYSIOLOGY

Knowledge of the female hormonal cycle, male spermatogenesis, and reproductive anatomy is important in understanding the differential diagnosis and evaluation of infertility. A detailed discussion of factors causing male infertility is presented in Chapter 136.

### Female hormonal cycle/reproductive anatomy

The female hormonal cycle consists of three phases (Figs. 146-1 and 146-2). The early follicular or proliferative phase is of variable length. During this phase follicle-stimulating hormone (FSH) released from the anterior pituitary stimulates follicle growth, estradiol production, and luteinizing hormone (LH) receptor production. One or more oocytes mature as a result of this stimulation. Estradiol produced by the ovarian follicle causes proliferation of endometrial glands and causes the cervical mucosa to produce increasing amounts of clear, watery, elastic secretions. Estradiol peaks just before ovulation. A mid-cycle surge of LH is released from the anterior pituitary in response to the pulsatile release of gonadotropin hormone-releasing hormone (GnRH) from the hypothalamus. This results in ovulation. During ovulation, the follicle ruptures, releasing an oocyte. The luteal or secretory phase lasts 12 to 16 days. During this phase the theca and granulosa cells, the follicular cells that remain after the release of the oocyte, are converted into the corpus luteum. Progesterone released by the corpus luteum prepares the endometrium for implantation of the fertilized oocyte by converting it to a secretory endometrium. Progesterone also causes an increase in basal body temperature.

In addition to these cyclic hormonal changes, several other aspects of female reproductive anatomy are necessary to ensure fertility. The fallopian tubes must be patent and function normally to pick up and move the oocyte to the uterus. The uterus must have a normal contour without any internal irregularities, polyps, inflammation, or adhesions. The cervix must be patent and cervical mucus adequate in quantity and quality to promote passage of the sperm.

**Table 146-1.** Etiology of infertility

| | Percent (%) |
|---|---|
| Female factor | 40-50 |
| Ovulatory | 30-40 |
| Uterine/tubal/peritoneal (endometriosis) | 30-40 |
| Cervical/immunologic/infectious | 15-20 |
| Male factor | 40-50 |
| Unexplained infertility | 5-10 |
| Multiple or combined female and male factors | 20-30 |

(The percentages do not equal 100% because in many cases where a female factor is involved, more than one etiology is identified, and, in 20%-30% of cases both male and female factors are involved.)

### Male spermatogenesis/reproductive anatomy

See Chapter 136.

## HISTORY

While a single woman may present to a physician requesting referral for artificial insemination or evaluation of difficulty conceiving, this discussion focuses on a female and male pair who present for evaluation of infertility. In this case, because infertility involves both partners, both should be present at the initial evaluation and throughout the entire process. Every effort should be made to ensure full disclosure of relevant information by each partner.

A helpful approach to the evaluation of infertility is to consider first the hormonal and anatomic causes in women and in men separately and then to consider possible factors related to the couple.

Of the hormonal factors in women, age is important, because fertility declines with increasing age. Fertility rates begin to decline after age 29, and after age 35 the length of time for conception doubles every 5 years. In women, information should be obtained to permit an understanding of potential menstrual irregularities. Women should be questioned about previous pregnancies, including number of live births and abortions (spontaneous or therapeutic). A detailed developmental and menstrual history includes onset of menses, regularity and length of menstrual cycles, amount and duration of menstrual bleeding, and any periods of amenorrhea. Women also should be questioned about the presence of hirsutism, galactorrhea, or hot flushes, suggesting hormonal imbalance. Previous

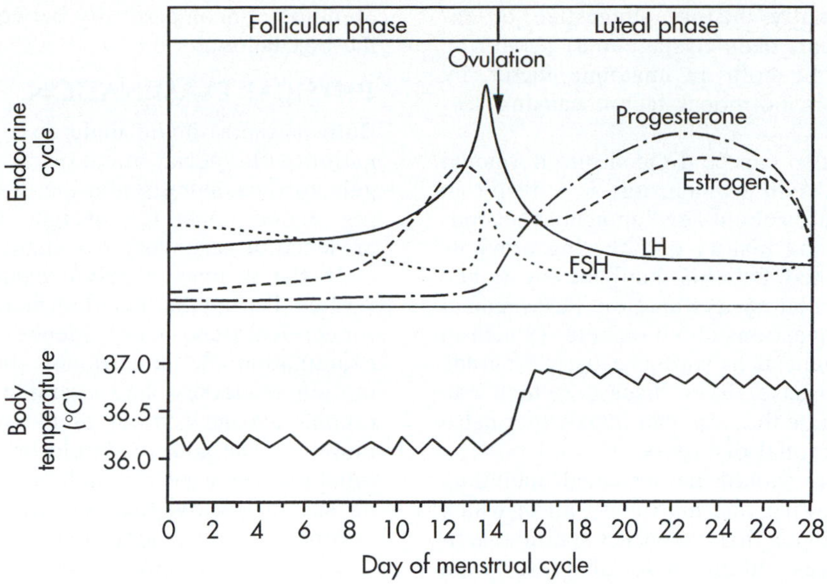


**Fig. 146-1.** The female hormonal cycle.

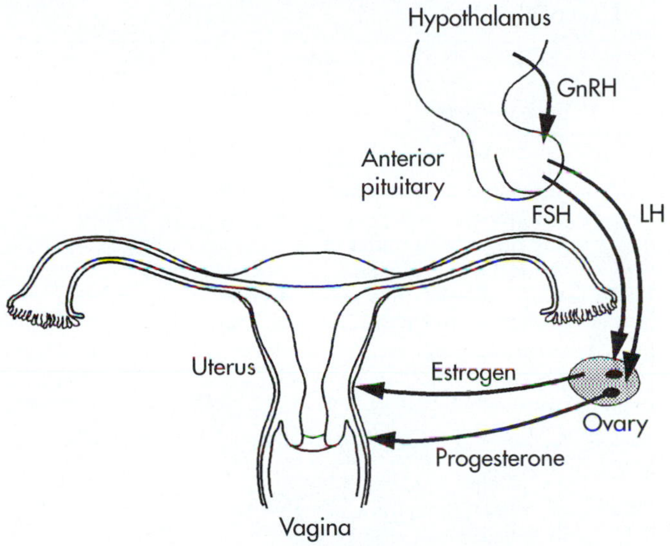


**Fig. 146-2.** Hormonal actions in the female.

contraception use should be determined, including oral contraceptives or depo forms, which may cause ovulatory disturbances for a period of time after their use. Past medical history should be obtained focusing on thyroid disease, which may cause ovulatory disorders; diabetes, which may cause anovulation; adrenal disease; or other disorders affecting the hypothalamic-pituitary-ovarian axis.

A detailed drug and medication history should be obtained. Cigarette smoking is epidemiologically related to infertility, although the pathophysiology is unknown. Both alcohol and narcotics can cause ovulatory abnormalities. Antihypertensives, tranquilizers, and tricyclic antidepressants can affect libido; antineoplastic agents can affect gametogenesis; drugs or other medical conditions that elevate prolactin (including tricyclic antidepressants, phenothiazines, reserpine, alpha-methyldopa, estrogens) can cause oligomenorrhea or amenorrhea. Although the role of occupational exposures are poorly defined, those implicated in infertility in women include noise, dry cleaning chemicals, heavy metals (mercury, cadmium), and textile dyes. Significant weight loss (especially associated with intensive exercise training or eating disorders), obesity, and psychologic stress all can cause ovulatory disturbances.

Anatomic factors affect the ability of the oocyte to be released from the ovary, picked up by the fallopian tubes, and transported to the uterus. These factors also include anything that might affect implantation of the fertilized oocyte and continued growth of the fetus. Factors affecting cervical mucus and the effective passage of sperm also can be considered in this category. From the standpoint of anatomic factors in women, anything that might cause adhesions or distort pelvic anatomy must be evaluated. A detailed surgical history should be obtained, including appendectomy (or ruptured appendix), ovarian cystectomy, tubal ligation, ectopic pregnancy, or septic abortion. Pelvic inflammatory disease (PID) can cause adhesions resulting in inability of the oocyte to be picked up by the fallopian tube. PID or pelvic tuberculosis also can cause tubal distortion. Prior use of an intrauterine device (IUD) could have caused a low-grade pelvic infection, which can result in intrauterine adhesions, or synechiae, which may prevent implantation or normal fetal development. Uterine leiomyomata or congenital uterine abnormalities can similarly affect implantation and fetal growth. A history of cervical instrumentation including conization or cryosurgery should be sought, as these can cause cervical scarring and stenosis.

In addition, factors that can affect cervical mucus include cervicitis, over-the-counter or prescription antihistamines and decongestants, and lubricants that may be toxic to sperm. Female patients should be questioned regarding in utero exposure to diethylstilbestrol (DES), which can result in anatomic abnormalities of the vagina, cervix, and uterus. Finally, history suggestive of endometriosis (in particular, deep dyspareunia) should be sought because it can be both an anatomic factor, by causing adhesions, and a hormonal factor, causing secondary amenorrhea.

In men, the history also can be divided into hormonal and anatomic factors. As in women, age is a factor in gametogenesis. Information about development of secondary sex characteristics and history of fathering previous children should be obtained. Patients should be questioned about impotence or ejaculatory dysfunction. Past medical history should include questions about diabetes (which in men can effect gametogenesis as well as cause retrograde ejaculation), thyroid disease, liver disease (which can cause a hyperestrogen state that also can impair spermatogenesis), and other hormonal disorders.

History of drug use should be obtained including cigarettes, alcohol, narcotics, and marijuana, all of which can cause hormonal changes that can affect spermatogenesis and, in some cases, libido. Use of prescription medications also should be investigated. As in women, these include antihypertensives, tranquilizers, tricyclic antidepressants, antineoplastic agents, and drugs that elevate prolactin. Postpubertal viral infections such as mumps may result in damage to sperm and permanent impairment of spermatogenesis. Men should be questioned regarding a known history of varicocele, which is thought to impair spermatogenesis, although the exact mechanism is uncertain. Evidence suggests that heat exposure such as hot tubs or saunas can impair spermatogenesis. Finally, occupational exposures, although poorly defined—including heat, vibration (e.g., jackhammering), genital radiation (either occupational or medical), and various industrial chemicals—have been implicated in male infertility (see Chapter 136 for further discussion).

Anatomically, the main concerns relate to factors that might impair sperm and seminal fluid transport and ejaculation. History of surgical procedures, including infant herniorrhaphy or hypospadias, testicular surgery or injury, and vasectomy and vasectomy reversal, should be sought. Sexually transmitted diseases, including gonococcal and chlamydial infections and possibly mycoplasma infections also may result in scarring, which can impair sperm and seminal fluid transport. Finally, men should be questioned about in utero exposure to DES, which can result in anatomic abnormalities of the vas deferens and result in male infertility.

In terms of the couple, information should be obtained from both partners about length of marriage or relationship and length of time in which conception has been attempted. This time should be dated from when the couple stopped using contraception, which may not be the same as the time at which they began attempting conception. The longer the duration of infertility, the poorer the prognosis for conception regardless of therapy. A detailed sexual history should be obtained from the couple including frequency of intercourse and problems with intercourse such as impotence, anorgasmia, and dyspareunia. A history of prior pregnancy for women or previous paternity in men with another partner raises the question of a significant factor in the other partner or an immunologic incompatibility between the two partners (see the box below).

## PHYSICAL EXAMINATION

Both partners should undergo a general physical examination with special attention to the thyroid, presence of galactorrhea, hair distribution, skin abnormalities suggesting endocrinopathies, weight and body habitus, and presence of secondary sex characteristics.

In the woman, a pelvic examination should be performed. During the speculum examination one should look for cervical stenosis or evidence of infection. On bimanual examination the practitioner should check for cervical motion tenderness and examine the uterus for size, irregular uterine contour or masses, or decreased uterine mobility. The adnexa should be examined for ovarian or tubal masses or pelvic tenderness. Examination of the cul de sac on rectovaginal examination should include assessment of uterosacral nodularity.

In the man, a genital examination should be performed to look for penile abnormalities (see Chapter 136).

### History

Female:
- Hormonal Factors
  - age
  - menstrual history
  - pregnancy and contraception history
  - past medical history
  - drug history (cigarettes, alcohol, recreational)
  - medications (prescription, over the counter)
  - occupational/environmental exposures
  - weight loss (intensive exercise, eating disorder)
- Anatomic Factors
  - surgical history
  - history of PID or cervicitis
  - leiomyomata, congenital uterine abnormalities
  - cervical instrumentation
  - use of lubricants, douches
  - in utero DES exposure
  - history of endometriosis

Male:
- Hormonal Factors
  - age
  - secondary sex development
  - previous paternity
  - past medical history
  - drug history (cigarettes, alcohol, recreational)
  - medications (prescription, over the counter)
  - postpubertal mumps
  - varicocele
  - occupational/environmental exposures
- Anatomic Factors
  - surgical history
  - history of STDs
  - sexual or ejaculatory dysfunction
  - in utero DES exposure

Couple:
- Psychologic Factors
- Immunologic Factors

## DIFFERENTIAL DIAGNOSIS/DIAGNOSTIC EVALUATION

Infertility can occur for a variety of reasons and can best be approached by systematically examining possible male and female factors. The laboratory studies and tests used in the evaluation depend on the possible factors contributing to infertility. The extent to which the evaluation is carried out by a general internist varies. Because more than one factor is involved in the etiology of infertility in up to one third of cases, all potential causes should be evaluated (Table 146-2).

### Female factors

***Ovulatory disorders.*** The first step in the evaluation of women is to determine whether ovulation is occurring. Disorders of ovulation are suspected if the history or physical examination suggests an endocrine abnormality or disruption of the hypothalamic/pituitary/ovarian axis (including evidence suggestive of polycystic ovary syndrome), and/or if there are menstrual abnormalities (amenorrhea, oligomenorrhea, or excessive bleeding). Four main techniques are used to assess follicular development and ovulation — that is, the adequate formation and release of the oocyte — and the adequacy of the luteal phase of the cycle.

1. Basal body temperature (BBT) is based on the fact that basal body temperature increases immediately before ovulation as a result of the increase in progesterone levels. In ovulating women, the normal temperature curve is biphasic (the temperature during the luteal phase is 0.3 to 1.0 degrees higher than during the follicular phase). The patient measures her temperature every morning before any activity (or when she wakes from her regular sleep, if this is not in the morning) and charts it on a graph. A 0.5 to 1 degree increase in temperature indicates that ovulation has occurred.
2. The LH surge, a twofold to threefold increase over the average of the preceding 3 days, occurs about 36 to 48 hours before ovulation. Although LH kits are available for home use, there is some question whether urinary LH offers additional information over BBT measurements alone.
3. Serum progesterone levels increase at the time of the LH surge and throughout the luteal phase. Serum progesterone is measured 5 to 9 days after ovulation (based on BBT or the LH surge). Although there is some controversy about the interpretation of these levels, a single value of less than 10 ng/ml or three levels less than 30 ng/ml suggest a luteal phase defect.
4. Endometrial biopsy is performed to determine the adequacy of the luteal phase in preparing the endometrium for implantation. The biopsy is obtained 2 to 3 days before the anticipated onset of menses. A discrepancy of more than 2 days between the dating of ovulation, based on pathology assessment of the biopsy specimen, and dating by BBT, urine LH, or serum progesterone suggests a luteal phase defect.

In patients who are anovulatory (based on BBT, urinary LH, and/or serum progesterone), prolactin levels and thyroid function tests should be performed. If signs of androgen excess are present, tests of adrenal function (specifically dihydroepiandosterone) also should be performed. If these tests are normal, the problem is likely hypothalamic in origin.

Several treatment modalities are available to induce ovulation in patients with hypothalamic or unknown causes of anovulation. Clomiphene citrate is the agent of choice. It blocks the negative feedback effect of estrogen on the hypothalamus and the pituitary with a subsequent increase in GnRH, LH, and FSH. Because there are variable degrees of hypothalamic dysfunction, clomiphene is started at a low dose (50 mg/day for 5 days starting on day 3 to 6 of the cycle). The BBT chart is followed to assess ovulation. If ovulation occurs, the medication is continued for 6 to 12 months. If ovulation is not indicated by the BBT chart, the dose is progressively increased. Side effects of clomiphene include hot flashes, pelvic discomfort, and mild ovarian overstimulation, which can result in ovarian enlargement and multiple pregnancies. Most pregnancies on clomiphene occur in the first three cycles. Therefore three to six cycles of clomiphene are given and if pregnancy does not occur, therapy is reevaluated.

**Table 146-2.** Differential diagnosis/diagnostic evaluation

| Disorder | Tests | Treatment |
|---|---|---|
| **Female factors** | | |
| Ovulatory | basal body temp<br>urinary LH<br>progesterone<br>endometrial biopsy<br>TFTs<br>prolactin | clomiphene<br>gonadotropins<br>GnRH |
| Tubal | HSG | surgery |
| Uterine | HSG<br>laparoscopy<br>hysteroscopy | surgery |
| Peritoneal | laparoscopy | GnRH agonist<br>danazol<br>surgery |
| Cervical | PCT with cervical mucous evaluation | intrauterine insemination |
| **Male factors** | | |
| Anatomic | semen analysis<br>endocrine levels<br>venogram<br>testicular biopsy<br>transrectal ultrasound | microsurgery<br>antibiotics |
| Hormonal | semen analysis<br>endocrine levels | testosterone<br>gonadotropins |
| Immunologic | semen analysis<br>antibody tests | intrauterine insemination |

*TFT,* Thyroid function tests; *HSG,* hysterosalpingogram; *PCT,* postcoital test.

If clomiphene fails to induce ovulation, human menopausal gonadotropin (HMG) may be used. This drug must be administered intramuscularly and has higher rates of ovarian hyperstimulation and multiple pregnancies. GnRH also can be used to induce ovulation. It is administered in a pulsatile fashion via a pump.

If a luteal phase defect is suspected in a patient with evidence of normal ovulation, the patient should be evaluated for thyroid disease and hyperprolactinemia. If a specific cause cannot be identified, the patient can be treated with clomiphene. Most cases of infertility due to luteal phase defects, however, are due to inadequate production of progesterone. Treatment with progesterone suppositories (vaginal or rectal) may be effective.

*Tubal factors.* Tubal abnormalities are suspected in patients with a history of PID, ectopic pregnancy, septic abortion, IUD use, ruptured appendix, or pelvic surgery. The patency of the tubes is assessed by performing a hysterosalpingogram (HSG) or laparoscopy. Treatment is surgical, although some have suggested that HSG by itself can have a therapeutic effect. Because of this possibility, a 3- to 6-month interval is suggested to see whether pregnancy occurs if HSG is normal, especially where no other cause of infertility is found.

*Uterine factors.* Uterine factors are suggested by a history of uterine instrumentation or abnormal bleeding not secondary to anovulation. To assess the anatomy of the uterus, HSG is performed followed by laparoscopy looking for intrauterine synechiae, congenital abnormalities (e.g., bicornate uterus), and uterine leiomyomata. Hysteroscopy may be performed if abnormalities are detected on HSG. Treatment is surgical.

*Peritoneal factors.* Peritoneal factors are suggested by a history consistent with the presence of pelvic adhesions (e.g., pelvic surgery, ruptured appendix) or findings consistent with endometriosis. Laparoscopy is used to evaluate the severity of endometriosis and determine the extent of adhesions. Endometriosis is treated medically with a GnRH agonist or danazol; however, in severe disease with extensive adhesions, surgery may be indicated. Pelvic adhesions due to other causes are treated surgically.

*Cervical factors.* Cervical factors are suggested in patients with a history of cervical conization or instrumentation. Cervical stenosis identified on examination can be treated by dilation. Adequacy of cervical mucus is evaluated by a postcoital test (PCT). The PCT is performed before the time of ovulation (based on a prior BBT chart or immediately after detection of the urinary LH surge) after 48 hours of sexual abstinence. The couple then has intercourse. Cervical mucus is examined 2 to 18 hours later for consistency, ferning, and the presence of white blood cells (WBC). In addition, the presence, appearance, and motility of the sperm are noted. A normal test is defined as the presence of a normal amount and consistency or cervical mucus, no WBC, and at least five motile sperm/high power field. If the PCT is abnormal, treatment depends on the results of the evaluation. If WBC are present, infection of one of the partners is suggested, and both should be cultured and treated. If cervicitis is present, cultures are often negative, and some authors suggest empiric treatment with doxycycline. Inadequate cervical mucus can be treated with low-dose estrogens in the mid to late follicular phase. Sperm antibodies, derived from either the male or female partner, can lead to an abnormal PCT with sperm agglutination or immotility. Intracervical or intrauterine insemination of the partner's sperm may be necessary in cases of hostile or inadequate cervical mucus or immunologic incompatibility.

### Male factors

See Chapter 136 for a discussion of male evaluation.

### Unexplained infertility

When both partners have undergone a complete evaluation in which no cause for infertility is identified and they remain infertile 1 year after evaluation, they are said to have unexplained infertility. This category has decreased as evaluation techniques have become more sophisticated; however, an estimated 5% to 10% of infertile couples have unexplained fertility. Many infertility experts have a regimen of empiric therapy for unexplained infertility, which may include antibiotics, clomiphene alone, clomiphene combined with intrauterine insemination, and more complex forms of assisted reproductive technology.

## MANAGEMENT

### Role of primary care physician

Primary care physicians play an important role in the evaluation and treatment of the infertile couple. A couple may present with difficulty achieving conception and not yet meet the diagnostic criteria of infertility. With a careful history, a primary care physician may uncover environmental and/or lifestyle issues that may be contributing to difficulty with conception and recommend modifications. It is also important to counsel patients that most couples achieve pregnancy within 1 year.

If the problem persists beyond 1 year, the primary care physician may initiate an infertility evaluation by obtaining a targeted history and physical examination of both partners, assessing ovulation, and ordering a semen analysis. Once a couple decides to pursue an extensive evaluation, they should be referred to an infertility specialist.

### Psychosocial aspects of evaluation and treatment

Powerful psychologic and emotional forces surround the issue of infertility. Psychologic stresses and depression can have an effect on fertility causing oligospermia and impotence in men and menstrual irregularities and amenorrhea in women. These effects are mediated through the central nervous system and eventually result in abnormal gonadotropin secretion. It is also clear that the evaluation and treatment of infertility place stresses on both partners and on their relationship.

Infertility engenders depression, anger, and guilt. It is experienced as a loss and is complicated by the fact that it is a potential and not a tangible loss. Thus it is more difficult for the patient to acknowledge and for others to understand. In addition as the evaluation proceeds, the experience of loss is delayed and made uncertain by the possibility of successful treatment.

In the course of the evaluation of infertility, issues of blame and responsibility within the relationship and feelings of guilt for past medical conditions or lifestyle behaviors may arise. Both men and women can experience feelings of being damaged or defective, which can affect self-image and identity. Men may equate the ability to father children with their masculinity; women may view their ability to conceive as a measure of their femininity, nurturing ability, or psychologic stability. Many patients describe a sense of failure or of no longer being in control of their lives. The intrusive nature of the evaluation and treatment of infertility may violate patients' sense of privacy and have a negative impact on their sexual relationship.

Psychologic screening should be part of the initial evaluation and ongoing counseling provided. Failure of treatment must be considered as a possible outcome and the implications must be discussed. In addition, a realistic end point to evaluation and treatment should be established. A nation-wide organization, RESOLVE, was founded in 1973 to help couples deal with these aspects of infertility.

## BIBLIOGRAPHY


Burger HG and Baker HWG: The treatment of infertility, *Annu Rev Med* 38:29-40, 1987.

Hammond MG: Evaluation of the infertile couple, *Obstet Gynecol Clin North Am* 14:821-830, 1987.

Hammond MG and Talbert LM: *Infertility: a practical guide for the physician,* ed 3, Boston, 1992 Blackwell Scientific Publications.

Jaffe SB and Jewelewicz R: The basic infertility investigation, *Fertil Steril* 56:599-613, 1991.

Jones HW and Toner JP: The infertile couple, *N Engl J Med* 329:1710-1715, 1993.

Mahlstedt PP: The psychological component of infertility, *Fertil Steril* 43:335-346, 1985.

Moghissi KS and Wallach EE: Unexplained infertility, *Fertil Steril* 39:5-21, 1983.

Seranfini P and Batzofin J: Diagnosis of female infertility: a comprehensive approach, *J Reprod Med* 34:29-40, 1989.

Swerdloff RS, Overstreet JW, Sokol RZ, Fajfer J: Infertility in the male, *Ann Intern Med* 103:906-919, 1985.

Taymor ML: *Infertility: a clinician's guide to diagnosis and treatment,* New York, 1990, Plenum.


CHAPTER

# 147 Obstetrics


**Urania Magriples**
**Joshua A. Copel**


## EPIDEMIOLOGY AND HIGH RISK GROUPS

The physician delivering obstetric care has the unique opportunity to provide general medical treatment and screening to a large portion of the population that might not otherwise gain access to the health care system. There are over 7 million pregnancies in the United States yearly, with over 4.1 million live births (Fig. 147-1). Although rates of infant mortality and morbidity have been drastically reduced in this century, the United States still has one of the highest rates among industrialized countries, ranking twenty-first.

Certain demographic groups are at higher risk for poor outcomes. For example, the United States has one of the highest teenage pregnancy rates, with 1 million teenagers, or 5% to 8% of the teenage population, becoming pregnant each year. Teens are more likely to register late for prenatal care, be unmarried and have less education, and have more than twice the risk of low birth weight infants, neonatal mortality, and maternal mortality compared to older mothers. Racial differences persist in both maternal and infant morbidity and mortality. Currently, the infant mortality rate of African-Americans is higher than that of impoverished nations such as Cuba. As more women and children fall below the poverty line in the United States, a concerted effort is needed to expand access to prenatal care and thereby entry into the medical system.

## PHYSIOLOGIC CHANGES OF PREGNANCY

The emerging concept that reproductive changes are a physiologic adaptation rather than a pathologic state has led internists and obstetricians to redefine their approach to the primary care of women. Although the physiologic changes during pregnancy are profound, most occur within a short period of time and are completely reversible. Those that are of primary interest to generalists are reviewed in this section.

### Hematologic

The circulating blood volume of a pregnant woman increases 45%. The expansion of plasma volume precedes and exceeds red cell volume; therefore a mild dilutional anemia is seen throughout gestation. Plasma volume expansion begins at six to eight weeks. Total red cell volume increases by 250 to 450 ml and is due to the increased production of red blood cells. This increase, as well as the sequestration of iron in the fetal compartment, creates an increased demand for iron, particularly in teenagers and multiparas who frequently have inadequate stores.

The normal white blood cell count increases from 5,000 to 12,000 cells/mm$^3$ in pregnancy. An additional dramatic rise can occur with stress and labor. These elevated counts can potentially confuse the diagnosis of infection.

Elements of the coagulation cascade are modified in pregnancy. There is increased hepatic production of fibrinogen, plasminogen, and factors VII, VIII, and X. Platelet counts decrease as pregnancy progresses toward term, and platelet turnover increases. Both activated partial thromboplastin time (aPTT) and prothrombin time (PT) are reduced in pregnancy. These changes, accompanied by diminished fibrinolysis, contribute to the increased risk for thrombotic events even in the normal gravida.

### Cardiovascular

Subtle electrocardiographic changes occur in pregnancy with slight leftward axis deviation and flattened T waves in lead three. The upward displacement of the diaphragm by the gravid uterus results in superior, lateral, and anterior displacement of the heart and the appearance of an enlarged cardiac silhouette with a straightened left border

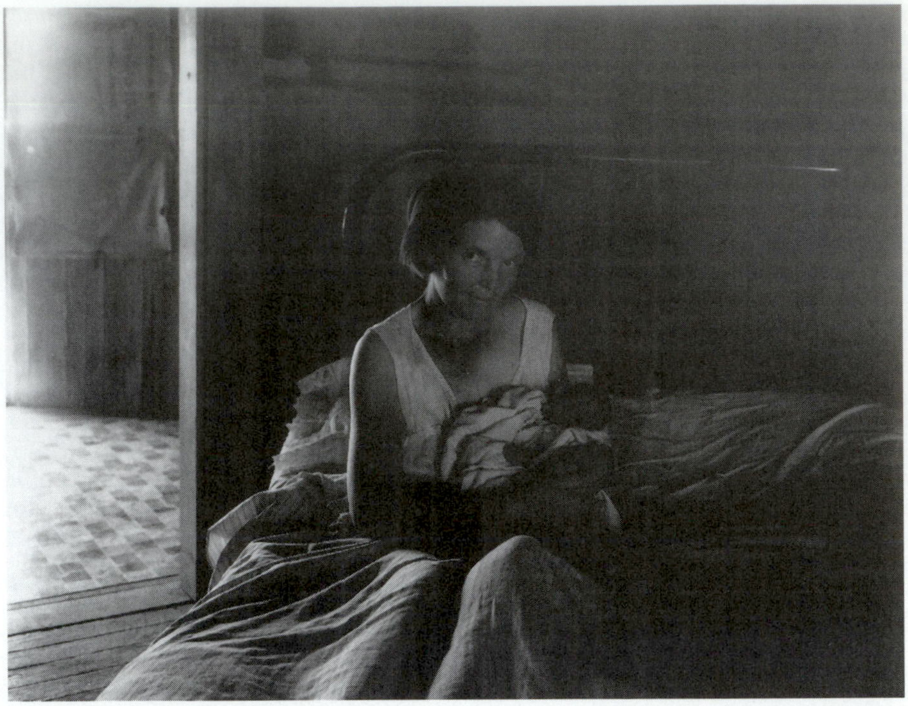

**Fig. 147-1.** Mother and her youngest child, 1937. (From Collections of the Library of Congress.)

on chest radiograph. Several auscultatory changes also occur. The first heart sound intensifies, and an exaggerated split develops between the mitral and tricuspid valve closures. Although the intensity of the second heart sound remains unchanged, physiologic splitting is sometimes lost. The appearance of a third heart sound is common, but a fourth heart sound is present in less than 5% of pregnant women and is pathologic. Almost all pregnant women have a systolic ejection murmur as a result of increased flow. It is heard best along the left sternal border from early in gestation. Diastolic murmurs are infrequent and abnormal.

Cardiac output increases by 30% to 50%, initially secondary to an increase in stroke volume and subsequently from a rise in heart rate of approximately 10 beats/minute. Most of the increase in cardiac output occurs before 20 weeks, although it continues into the third trimester and plateaus at 32 weeks' gestation. Increases in left and right ventricular end-diastolic dimensions in the second and third trimesters are due to the expanded blood volume and increased diastolic filling, as well as myocardial hypertrophy. End-systolic dimensions do not change. Blood pressure falls in the second trimester as peripheral vascular resistance decreases secondary to smooth muscle relaxation by progesterone. The increased cardiovascular demands of pregnancy can precipitate clinical symptoms in otherwise asymptomatic patients with preexisting cardiac disease.

Compression of the pelvic and iliac vessels by the gravid uterus decreases venous return, cardiac output, and placental perfusion and causes a significant increase in systolic and diastolic blood pressures. After the second trimester, women are advised to lie in the left lateral position to maximize cardiac function and avoid hypotension when rising.

In the third trimester, blood pressure normally increases to nonpregnant values. The amelioration of preexisting hypertension in the first and second trimesters can make it difficult to distinguish between chronic hypertension and pregnancy-induced hypertension, particularly in patients presenting late for prenatal care. A diastolic blood pressure higher than 90 mm Hg at any time during pregnancy is abnormal.

### Renal

Both structural and functional changes occur in the kidneys during pregnancy. Kidney length increases 1 to 1.5 cm, which is thought to be secondary to increased renal plasma flow. The collecting system expands, including the bladder, calyces, renal pelves, and the ureters; the right ureter is involved more frequently than the left. These changes are secondary to compression by the dextrorotated uterus (the left ureter is cushioned by the sigmoid colon), the position and distention of the right ovarian vein, and elevated progesterone levels. The dead space in the collecting systems may predispose to urinary tract infections and pyelonephritis in pregnancy.

Renal plasma flow increases early in the first trimester coincident with the increase in cardiac output. By mid-pregnancy, the rate is 50% greater than in the nonpregnant woman. It remains elevated until the end of pregnancy when there is a slight decrease. The glomerular filtration rate (GFR) also increases in the first trimester by 40% at 20 weeks and another 10% by the end of the second trimester. Normal values range from 120 to 160 ml/min. Because an increase in GFR may lead to accelerated excretion of medications, drug levels need to be monitored closely. Aminoaciduria, proteinuria, glucosuria and increased excretion of water-soluble vitamins also result from the increase in GFR. Glucosuria is thus a poor indicator of diabetes in pregnancy, and glucose tolerance testing is recommended.

### Alimentary tract

The combined effects of delayed gastric emptying, reduced gastric acid secretion, and decreased sphincter tone and motility cause the common pregnant symptoms of nausea, heartburn, reflux, and bloating. It has been postulated that human chorionic gonadotropin plays a role in the nausea seen in the first trimester as conditions with elevated levels such as multiple gestations and trophoblastic disease are associated with more symptoms for a longer time. Progesterone also decreases tone and motility of both the small and large bowel secondary to smooth muscle relaxation. Increased absorption of water in the large bowel and decreased tone account for the common symptom of constipation. Gastrointestinal symptoms are accentuated in the third trimester by the size of the gravid uterus.

Progesterone delays gallbladder emptying and thereby increases residual volumes to two times greater than the nonpregnant state. Estrogen, however, accounts for the increased incidence of cholestatic jaundice seen in pregnancy. Estrogen also affects hepatic production of proteins, including increases in cholesterol, clotting factors, binding proteins, globulins, transferrin, and ceruloplasmin. Serum albumin concentration is 30% lower at term, or about 3 g/dl, secondary to both decreased production and hemodilution. There is a twofold to fourfold increase in alkaline phosphatase due to an increase in the heat-stable isoenzyme originating from the placenta, making it an unreliable measure of hepatic function. There are no significant changes in serum glutamic-oxaloacetic transaminase (SGOT), serum glutamate-pyruvate transaminase (SGPT), or bilirubin levels. The increased hepatic production of binding globulins, as well as accelerated drug metabolism, leads to alterations in dosage requirements in thyroid replacement, anticonvulsant therapy, and other medications such as digoxin and theophylline.

### Respiratory

Several factors affect respiration, including the upward displacement of the diaphragm by the enlarging uterus, an increase in blood flow, and the effects of progesterone on the respiratory center. Progesterone increases sensitivity to carbon dioxide and is a direct stimulant. An increase in minute ventilation decreases the partial pressure of arterial $CO_2$ resulting in a mild respiratory alkalosis. Whereas total lung capacity and expiratory reserve volume decrease by 5% and 20%, respectively, and tidal volume increases by 30% to 40%, vital capacity, inspiratory reserve volume, and forced expiratory volume in 1 second ($FEV_1$) are unchanged. The increase in minute ventilation more than compensates for an obligatory increase in oxygen consumption. The partial pressure of arterial oxygen is essentially unchanged, and despite the common occurrence of dyspnea and breathlessness, hypoxemia is abnormal.

### Skin

Vascular changes such as palmar erythema, spider angiomata, and hyperemia of the mucous membranes are related to increased estrogen and reverse postpartum. Gingival bleeding and nasal and sinus congestion are also common. Increased pigmentation occurs in over 90% of pregnant women, with darkening of the face, areola, axilla, and linea alba. Connective tissue changes account for the appearance of striae, which occur in half of all pregnancies.

## HISTORY AND PHYSICAL EXAMINATION

The presence of pregnancy must be considered in every woman of reproductive age. Common signs and symptoms of pregnancy include amenorrhea, breast fullness and tenderness, fatigue, nausea and/or vomiting, increased appetite, and increased abdominal girth. On physical examination, the cervix appears bluish, and on bimanual palpation it is soft and flexible. The uterus increases in size with advancing gestational age and fills the pelvis at around 12 weeks. It is palpated above the pubic bone after that point and reaches the umbilicus at 20 weeks. After 20 weeks, the fundal height correlates roughly with centimeters above the pubic bone.

## LABORATORY STUDIES

Pregnancy can be rapidly ruled out using commonly available sensitive serum or urinary pregnancy tests. Human chorionic gonadotropin (hCG) is a specific marker for viable trophoblast tissue and is directly correlated with gestational age. Most urinary tests are enzyme-linked immunoadsorbent assays (ELISA), which use a color reaction produced by an enzyme that is linked to an antibody. They vary in sensitivity with the lower limits of the assays, ranging from 200 to 800 IU/ml. Urine tests are available that are positive by day 25 after the last menstrual period. Serum radioimmunoassays are sensitive and accurate if directed to the beta-subunit of the hCG molecule. In early pregnancy, hCG concentrations double approximately every 2 days, and an inadequate rise should raise the question of either a nonviable gestation or an ectopic pregnancy.

## DIFFERENTIAL DIAGNOSIS

Vaginal bleeding in the first trimester is not uncommon and occurs in about 25% of pregnancies. Implantation bleeding is common and consists of minimal bleeding around the time of the first missed menstrual period. Flow may vary from mere spotting to bleeding that is similar to a period, but is rarely heavier than a period. If bleeding is observed from a closed cervical os and there is a documented intrauterine pregnancy, the diagnosis of a threatened abortion can be made. The uterus is generally appropriate in size but may be tender to examination. Once the cervix is dilated or the bleeding is profuse, the diagnosis of an inevitable abortion is made. An incomplete abortion signifies that there is tissue still within the uterus. Incomplete abortions become more common after 6 weeks of gestation. In an anembryonic gestation, formerly referred to as a missed abortion, the pregnancy has partially resorbed but there is still viable trophoblast-secreting hCG.

Ectopic pregnancy should be suspected in any woman of reproductive age presenting with abdominal pain or vaginal bleeding. Because approximately 2% of pregnancies are ectopic, constant vigilance is necessary to make the diagnosis. Ectopic pregnancies are the most common cause of maternal mortality in the first half of pregnancy and account for up to 50 maternal deaths annually. The rates of ectopic pregnancy are two times higher for nonwhite females than white females; however, mortality rates are six times higher for African-American women, making ectopic pregnancy the single most common cause of all maternal deaths in this population. Risk factors for ectopic pregnancy include multiparity, pelvic inflammatory disease, tubal surgery, previous pelvic surgery, previous ectopic, and intrauterine device (IUD) use.

The most common presenting signs are abdominal and adnexal tenderness, which are present in nearly all patients. Vaginal bleeding is present in 90% of cases. A pelvic mass is palpable in over half of patients, and the uterus is usually not appropriately enlarged. Tachycardia, orthostasis, and shock may follow rupture. Levels of hCG over 2000 IU/ml without the presence of an intrauterine pregnancy by vaginal ultrasonography suggest an ectopic pregnancy. Ultrasonographic detection of a pelvic mass is not definitive in the diagnosis of an ectopic pregnancy, as a corpus luteum or other benign ovarian tumor may be present; therefore correlation with the quantitative hCG level is recommended.

## PRENATAL CARE

The physician taking care of women has the opportunity to have an impact not only on the lives of women, but on the lives of their children and future generations. Preconceptual care is essential in minimizing exposure to drugs and teratogens, maximizing nutritional status and identifying medical conditions that may either affect pregnancy or be influenced by it. Primary care physicians play an important role in the care of women of reproductive age who are considering pregnancy.

In the United States, 200,000 birth defects and over a half million infant deaths, spontaneous abortions, stillbirths, and miscarriages occur each year from defective fetal development. It is estimated that 1% to 5% of congenital anomalies may be drug or chemical related. Factors that determine a drug's effect on the fetus include dosage, duration, and time of exposure, as well as drug metabolism, concurrent use of other drugs, genetic susceptibility, and placental transfer. There is a critical period of embryonic development from the third through the twelfth week when the embryo is undergoing organogenesis. Before this time, exposures tend either to cause abortion or to have no effect at all (known as the "all or none phenomenon"). Beyond the twelfth week, effects are generally limited to growth and neural development. Primary care physicians often care for women in the crucial weeks of fetal organogenesis and therefore need to be aware of the effects of drugs on fetal development. Examples of recognized teratogens and their associated malformations are listed in Table 147-1.

Infectious agents also cause maldevelopment in the human (Table 147-2). The lethal or developmental effects are the result of mitotic inhibition, direct cytotoxicity, or necrosis. Inflammatory responses to infection can lead to metaplasia, scarring, or calcification, which further damages normal development.

Chronic maternal conditions also are associated with an increased risk of teratogenicity. For example diabetic mothers with hemoglobin A1C levels greater than 7.5 have a twofold increased risk of congenital malformations, and the risk is greater with increasing levels. Levels of phenylalanine greater than 20 mg/dl in mothers with phenylketonuria are associated with a 90% incidence of congenital malformations, whereas levels less than 16 mg/dl are associated with a 20% incidence. Women with seizures have a twofold to threefold increased incidence of congenital anomalies regardless of whether they are on medications.

### Nutrition

Current recommendations for nutrition in pregnancy are based on the pregnant woman's pregravid weight. For women who are within the optimal weight range for their height, the recommended weight gain is 20 to 35 pounds, with 5 pounds gained in the first trimester and approximately 1 pound per week in the second and third trimesters. For women who are overweight (20% or more above ideal body weight) the total weight gain should be about 15 to 25 pounds, with 2 pounds gained in the first trimester and about two-thirds of a pound gained per week in the second and third trimesters. For women who are underweight (10% or more below ideal body weight), the total weight gain should be 28 to 40 pounds, with 5 pounds gained in the first trimester and at least a pound a week gained in the second and third trimesters, depending on the pregravid weight. Protein, iron, and calcium requirements increase during pregnancy; but the need for supplementation depends on the pregravid nutritional status. Women with short interpregnancy intervals, teenagers, grand multiparae, and patients of low socioeconomic status are at highest risk for nutritional deficiencies. Protein requirements increase in pregnancy from 50 to 90 g/day. Iron needs average about 3.5 mg/day. Total iron demands during a singleton pregnancy average 1000 to 1100 mg and are higher for gestations with more than one fetus. Calcium requirements increase to 1200 mg/day, 50% higher than the nonpregnant recommendation. Folate requirements increase to 800 mg, and periconceptual folate supplementation decreases the incidence of neural tube defects.

### Prenatal visits

The basic laboratory tests recommended for all pregnant women are listed in the box on p. 1850. Routine visits are scheduled monthly until 30 weeks, every 2 weeks until 36 weeks, and then weekly. At each visit, weight, blood pressure, urine screening for protein and glucose, and measurement of the fundal height and auscultation of the fetal heart are performed.

Genetic testing by amniocentesis or chorionic villus sampling (CVS) is routinely offered to women who will be 35 years old at the time of delivery because they are at increased risk for fetal aneuploidy. Thorough patient and family histories will reveal other risk factors for genetically transmissable diseases. A stillborn fetus has a 6% to 11% risk of a having a chromosomal abnormality; therefore women with a history of stillborn births should be counseled. Couples with a history of three or more pregnancy losses or prolonged infertility have up to a 6% risk of a chromosomal abnormality. A previous child with a chromosomal abnormality or congenital malformation likewise puts the parents in a high risk group with future pregnancies.

**Table 147-1.** Teratogenic and fetopathic therapies and environmental agents

| Agent | Reported effects |
|---|---|
| Alcohol | FAS, IUGR, microcephaly, mental retardation, cardiac anomalies, maxillary hypoplasia, characteristic facies. (Data based on chronic, heavy use [10 to 12] drinks/day), which is associated with 30% incidence of FAS. Less known about lower amounts. |
| Aminopterin, methotrexate (antifolates) | Microcephaly, hydrocephaly, cleft palate, meningomyelocele, IUGR, abnormal cranial ossification, reduction in derivatives of first branchial a ch, mental retardation, postnatal growth retardation. |
| Androgens | Masculinization of the female embyro, clitoromegaly. |
| Angiotensin-converting enzyme inhibitors | Oligohydramnios, pulmonary hypoplasia, neonatal anuria, IUGR, skull hypoplasia, fetal and neonatal death (second and third trimester exposure). |
| Carbamazepine | Minor craniofacial defects, fingernail hypoplasia, developmental delay. |
| Cocaine | Genitourinary malformations. |
| Cyclophosphamide | IUGR, ectrodactyly, syndactyly, cardiovascular anomalies. |
| Diethylstilbestrol | Cervical and uterine anomalies. |
| Diphenylhydantoin | Microcephaly, IUGR, mental retardation, cleft lip/palate, hypoplastic nails and distal phalanges. |
| Indomethacin | Prenatal ductus arteriosus closure (reversible). |
| Iodine deficiency | Mental retardation, spastic diplegia, deafness, fetal goiter. |
| Isoretinoin | CNS, cardiovascular and ear anomalies, cleft lip/palate, branchial arch abnormalities. |
| Lead | CNS abnormalities, microcephaly. |
| Lithium carbonate | Ebstein's anomaly of the tricuspid valve and other cardiovascular anomalies. |
| Methimazole | Aplasia cutis. |
| Methyl mercury | Growth deficiency, microcephaly, poor muscle tone, deafness, blindness. |
| Nicotine | IUGR, increased incidence of sudden infant death syndrome. |
| Penicillamine | Cutis laxa, hyperflexibility of joints. |
| Quinine | Ototoxicity and vestibular damage (high dose). |
| Radiation (external) | Microcephaly, mental retardation, eye anomalies, IUGR, visceral anomalies. (No effect seen at 5 rads or less; all-or-none phenomenon seen early in gestation.) |
| Tetracycline | Bone and tooth staining. High doses can cause hypoplastic tooth enamel. |
| Thalidomide | Limb reduction defects, facial hemangioma, esophageal or duodenal atresia, cardiovascular, renal and ear anomalies. |
| Trimethadione | IUGR, V-shaped eyebrows, low set ears, high arched palate, irregular teeth, CNS anomalies, severe developmental delay. |
| Valproic acid | Neural tube defects, dysmorphic facies, IUGR, cardiac abnormalities. |
| Warfarin | Nasal hypoplasia, stippling of secondary epiphysis, IUGR, anomalies of eyes, hands and neck, CNS anomalies. |

Adapted from Brent RL, Beckman DA: Prescribed drugs, therapeutic agents, and fetal teratogenesis, *Clin Perinatol* 13:649, 1986.
*FAS,* Fetal alcohol syndrome; *IUGR,* Intrauterine growth retardation.

**Table 147-2.** Infection-induced fetopathy

| Agent | Reported effects |
|---|---|
| Cytomegalovirus | Microcephaly, chorioretinitis, deafness, mental retardation, hepatosplenomegaly, hydrocephalus, epilepsy, cerebral palsy, death. |
| Herpes simplex | Encephalitis, seizures, conjunctivitis, pulmonary disease, vesicular lesions, hepatitis, hemolytic, anemia, thrombocytopenia. |
| Parvovirus B19 | Hydrops secondary to anemia, death. |
| Rubella | IUGR, microcephaly, mental retardation, deafness, cataracts, glaucoma, cardiovascular abnormalities, hepatosplenomegaly, neonatal bleeding, purpura. |
| Syphilis | Skin rash, hepatosplenomegaly, hypotonia, rhinorrhea, periostitis. |
| Toxoplasmosis | Microcephaly, hydrocephaly, anencephaly, cerebral calcifications, hydrops, chorioretinitis, seizures, hepatosplenomegaly, growth retardation. |
| Varicella | Mental retardation, seizures, cataracts, microphthalmia, optic atrophy, chorioretinitis, growth retardation, limb hypoplasia, cutaneous scars. |
| Venezuelan equine encephalitis | Hydrocephalus, porencephaly, cataracts, microphthalmia. |

*IUGR,* Intrauterine growth retardation.

### Basic laboratory tests

Complete blood count
Blood type and antibody screen (indirect Coombs')
Hepatitis surface antigen
VDRL or RPR
Rubella
HIV
Pap smear
Cervical cultures for gonorrhea and chlamydia
Urinalysis (culture if >3 to 5 WBC/HPF)
Glucose tolerance test (at 28 weeks)
Triple screen (maternal serum alpha fetoprotein, estriol and human chorionic gonadotropin)*
Genetic testing*
Ultrasound*

**Routine visit**

Weight
Blood pressure
Urine dipstick
Estimation of fetal size by fundal height
Auscultation of fetal heart
Brief physical examination including reflexes and edema
Determination of symptoms of preterm labor (contractions, rupture of membranes and bleeding)

*Requires counseling before implementation.

Ethnicity is also important, as certain groups carry a higher risk for genetic diseases. Whites have a 1 in 20 risk of carrying the recessive gene for cystic fibrosis. Individuals of Mediterranean descent have a 1 in 12 risk of being carriers of the β-thalassemia gene. (The mean corpuscular volume [MCV] is useful as a screening test for thalassemia trait.) Ashkenazi Jews, who have a 1 in 30 risk of carrying the gene for Tay-Sachs disease, should be offered testing for the carrier state with a hexosaminidase A assay. The carrier rate for sickle cell disease is 1 in 12 in African-Americans. The chance of having an affected child when both parents are carriers of any of these autosomal recessive diseases is 25%, and prenatal testing should be offered.

Although the risk of Down syndrome (trisomy 21) is greatest in women aged 35 or over, the majority of affected infants are born to women less than 35, as they represent a larger percentage of the childbearing population. Prenatal diagnosis on the basis of age alone detects only 20% to 30% of these infants; thus screening for maternal serum markers has been used to increase detection. Alpha fetoprotein (AFP) is the major early fetal serum protein. It enters the amniotic fluid via fetal renal excretion, transudation through skin, and open lesions such as spina bifida and ventral wall defects. An elevated level is found with open neural tube and ventral wall defects, twin gestations, intrauterine fetal demise, as well as pregnancies at risk for growth retardation and fetal death. In contrast, a low level of maternal serum alpha-fetoprotein (MSAFP) has been associated with an increased risk of trisomy 21 and other trisomies. MSAFP testing in women under the age of 35 will detect an additional 25% of pregnancies affected by Down syndrome, with a 5% false-positive rate. Recent studies have shown that maternal serum concentrations of human chorionic gonadotropin (HCG) are at least two times higher than normal, and those of unconjugated estriol are 25% lower in the presence of fetal Down syndrome. The additional use of these markers improves the detection rate to 67%, with a 7.2% false-positive rate.

Ultrasound has been used as a screening tool in the detection of neural tube and ventral wall defects in women with elevated MSAFP, and in experienced hands has a very high sensitivity and specificity. Unfortunately, the detection rate of trisomies by ultrasound is variable, and therefore ultrasound is not expected to replace amniocentesis in women at high risk. Routine ultrasound in all obstetric patients is a controversial issue, but certainly if the couple desires information on prenatal diagnosis of congenital anomalies then second trimester ultrasound at a tertiary center is advisable.

A fetal karyotype can be obtained by CVS or amniocentesis. An advantage of CVS is that it can be performed in the first trimester (10 to 12 weeks) and results obtained in less than a week. Thus pregnancy termination, if desired, is a less complicated procedure. CVS has a procedure-related miscarriage rate of 0.5% to 1%. Amniocentesis can be performed after 15 weeks' gestation with a procedure-related miscarriage rate of 0.5%. Amniocytes take 10 days to 2 weeks to grow in culture. Because of these delays, termination of pregnancy requires either a dilation and evacuation, a more complex procedure than in the first trimester, or induction of labor with prostaglandin.

## MEDICAL COMPLICATIONS OF PREGNANCY

The primary care physician may intervene at two points in a high-risk pregnancy (Table 147-3). In the preconceptual patient, the physician has the opportunity to control disease and plan for its management during pregnancy. The primary care physician also may be involved in managing women who develop medical complications after conception. These patients are best cared for in close consultation with a perinatologist.

### Diabetes

Previously diagnosed diabetes complicates 0.5% of pregnancies in the United States; gestational diabetes affects an additional 4% and is predominantly diet controlled.

The hormonal changes of pregnancy cause an increased insulin response to a glucose load in normal pregnant women and worsening of control in the diabetic pregnancy. Estrogen and progesterone induce pancreatic β-cell hyperplasia and increased insulin secretion, as well as increased glycogen storage, peripheral glucose utilization, and decreased hepatic glucose production. In the late second and third trimesters, human placental lactogen, prolactin, and cortisol combine to increase insulin resistance and decrease glucose tolerance and ensure adequate levels of glucose and amino acids for fetal growth. Because of these changes, patients with insulin-dependent diabetes will commonly have frequent episodes of hypoglycemia and ketonuria in the first trimester and are more prone to ketoacidosis in the second and third trimesters.

**Table 147-3.** Medical complications of pregnancy

| Disease | Effect of pregnancy | Therapeutic considerations |
|---|---|---|
| Asthma | Unpredictable | Increased dosage of theophylline; side effects of steroids (hypertension, gestational diabetes). |
| Deep venous thrombosis | Increased risk (present in all trimesters) | Most commonly left leg thrombosis; right leg is rare. Coumadin contraindicated secondary to teratogenicity. (Can be used in breastfeeding.) |
| Diabetes | Insulin resistance increases<br>Pregnancy does not accelerate retinopathy or nephropathy | Congenital anomalies two to three times general population; correlated with Hgb A1C >7.5. Oral hypoglycemics contraindicated. Poor control correlated with fetal morbidity/mortality, macrosomia, and increased risk of C-section. Increased risk of preeclampsia. |
| Hypertension | Improvement in first trimester 30% risk of preeclampsia | Angiotensin-converting enzyme inhibitors and diuretics contraindicated (except in heart failure). |
| Nephropathy | Moderate renal insufficiency (20%-40% have decline in CrCl)<br>Proteinuria may worsen | Poor prognosis with Cr >1.5 mg/dl, proteinuria >3 g in 24 hours in first trimester or poorly controlled hypertension. |
| Rheumatoid arthritis | 75% remission (90% flare postpartum) | See systemic lupus erythematosus; teratogenicity of penicillamine; gold salts do not cross placenta. |
| Systemic lupus erythematosus | Remission 6 months before conception best prognosis. Increased risk of flare postpartum | Teratogenicity of antimalarials, nonsteroidals and alkylating agents. Main treatment steroids. Anti-Ro and La antibodies associated with congenital heart block. Lupus anticoagulant and anticardiolipin antibodies associated with recurrent abortions, IUGR, and fetal death. |
| Seizures | 50% no change<br>25% improve<br>25% worsen | Baseline malformation rate twice normal (regardless of medications). Teratogenicity of dilantin, valproic acid, tegretol, trimethadione. Depletion of folate and Vitamin K-dependent factors. Preconceptual folate recommended to decrease risk of neural tube defects. |
| Ulcerative colitis | Increased risk of flares first trimester and postpartum | If disease active at time of conception, higher risk of miscarriage, intrauterine growth retardation and fetal death. If quiescent, same as general population. |
| von Willebrand's disease | Improvement | Increased risk of bleeding with first trimester miscarriages and postpartum. |

*IUGR,* Intrauterine growth retardation.

## Gestational diabetes

Gestational diabetes is defined as the onset or recognition of glucose intolerance during pregnancy. This definition includes patients with preexisting diabetes that is first detected in pregnancy and those who develop glucose intolerance only in pregnancy. The latter group is not prone to hyperglycemia or ketosis in the first trimester and the associated increased incidence of congenital malformations.

All pregnant women should routinely be screened at 28 weeks of gestation with a 50 g oral glucose tolerance test. Those with strong risk factors (e.g., obesity, a history of gestational diabetes, or an infant with a congenital anomaly, macrosomia, or fetal demise) should be screened earlier. Women who have an abnormal screening test (1 hour serum glucose greater than 145 mg/dl) undergo a 3-hour 100 g glucose test. Criteria for diagnosing gestational diabetes vary. Many clinicians follow the guidelines developed by the National Diabetes Data Group (NDDG) in which two elevated blood glucose values greater than 105, 190, 165, and 145 mg/dl for the fasting, 1-, 2-, and 3-hour tests, respectively, are considered abnormal. Although these criteria have been criticized as being too high, the current recommendations are that the NDDG data be used until an international consensus can be obtained.

The mainstay of therapy in gestational diabetes is diet. Current recommendations call for individualized caloric intake according to the patient's weight and a dietary composition containing 50% to 60% carbohydrate, 12% to 20% protein, and approximately 25% fat, with less than 10% as saturated fatty acids, up to 10% as polyunsaturated fatty acids, and the remainder of ingested fat derived from monosaturated forms. Glucose monitoring is accomplished with daily home blood glucose monitoring of fasting and 2-hour postprandial glucose assessment. The use of insulin is recommended for those with fasting glucose values consistently greater than 100 mg/dl, or

2-hour postprandial levels greater than 120 mg/dl. Oral hypoglycemics are not recommended for use in pregnancy, as the sulfonylureas are known to cross the placenta and stimulate the fetal pancreas to secrete insulin. (Hyperinsulinemia is one of the postulated mechanisms for adverse fetal outcomes such as macrosomia.) Oral hypoglycemics also cause prolonged neonatal hypoglycemia due to slower hepatic elimination of these drugs. Teratogenetic effects have been demonstrated in animals.

Infants of gestational and overt diabetics are at an increased risk of perinatal complications, including hypoglycemia, hyperbilirubinemia, hypocalcemia, polycythemia, respiratory distress syndrome, macrosomia, and fetal trauma. Fetal demise due to poor control of gestational diabetics is rarely seen today since the implementation of glucose monitoring, diet, and antenatal testing.

Debate continues about the long-term maternal consequences of gestational diabetes. Women who have gestational diabetes are at increased risk for diabetes later in life. Longitudinal studies of women followed up to 20 years after the diagnosis of gestational diabetes report prevalence rates of diabetes requiring therapy as high as 21% and of diabetes not requiring therapy up to 54%. Individuals with persistent obesity are at highest risk for developing subsequent diabetes.

### Insulin-dependent diabetes

The leading cause of perinatal mortality in infants of mothers with insulin-dependent diabetes is congenital malformations. Major anomalies are two to three times more common and are correlated with an elevated hemoglobin A1C (glycosylated hemoglobin). Malformations are most common in the central nervous, cardiovascular, gastrointestinal, genitourinary, and skeletal systems. Preconceptual control is advocated to decrease the incidence of these malformations, as they occur in the first few weeks after conception, often before a patient presents for prenatal care. Because of these risks, a targeted ultrasound and maternal serum triple screen determinations are warranted at 15 to 16 weeks of gestation and a fetal echocardiogram at 20 weeks of gestation.

Infants of diabetic mothers are at increased risk of developing diabetes later in life. Insulin-dependent diabetes is transmitted less frequently to the offspring of diabetic women than diabetic men. Offspring with two diabetic parents have the highest risk (30%) of developing diabetes. Type II diabetes is probably inherited as an autosomal dominant trait; thus 50% of offspring with one affected parent will inherit the tendency for the disease, although other factors, such as obesity and diet, influence penetrance.

Glucose control is accomplished by one to three daily injections of insulin and glucose monitoring to maintain fasting and two hour post-prandial glucose levels less than 90 and 120 mg/dl, respectively. The addition of long-acting insulin at bedtime is often necessary to obtain euglycemia. The first trimester is characterized by episodes of hypoglycemia, whereas the second and third trimesters are characterized by increasing glucoses and insulin resistance; therefore close monitoring is necessary. Poor control, frequent insulin reactions, and new onset diabetes require hospitalization for management and education.

Pregnancies complicated by diabetes are monitored closely by ultrasound for abnormalities in fetal growth and for polyhydramnios. All diabetic pregnancies have a higher incidence of preeclampsia, pyelonephritis, and worsening of hypertension and need to be monitored closely. Patients should be seen every 2 weeks until 30 weeks, then weekly. Pregnancies with good control are allowed to progress to term, whereas pregnancies with poor control, worsening hypertension, or fetal growth derangements are delivered before term after documentation of fetal lung maturity by amniocentesis.

In addition to a careful history and physical examination, all pregnant diabetic women should be screened for end-organ complications with a baseline ophthalmologic examination, 24-hour urine collection for creatinine and protein determinations, serum electrolytes, cholesterol, and electrocardiogram. Pregnant diabetic women with preexisting nephropathy, who have a creatinine level greater than 1.5 mg/dl, proteinuria greater than 3 g in 24 hours in the first trimester, or poorly controlled hypertension have a poor prognosis in terms of pregnancy outcome. Renal function may remain stable after the pregnancy; however, in 20% to 40% of patients it declines. Pregnancy-induced hypertension occurs in 25% of diabetic pregnancies and is associated with worsening of renal function; therefore close monitoring is warranted. Proteinuria commonly increases along with the GFR, but returns to baseline after pregnancy in the majority of patients. Elevated blood pressure and a rapid decrease in creatinine clearance are the most common events leading to preterm delivery; therefore strict blood pressure control is necessary.

Most women with nephropathy have evidence of microvascular disease and atherosclerosis. The influence of pregnancy on diabetic retinopathy is not well understood. Initially, there was concern that pregnancy accelerated the process, particularly with rapid normalization of serum glucose; however, these changes may reflect the natural progression of disease and its identification in pregnancy. Close ophthalmologic follow-up is warranted. Maternal mortality rate may be as high as 67% in women with diabetes and ischemic heart disease; therefore pregnancy termination for maternal indications should be considered in these patients.

## Hypertension

Hypertension complicates 10% of pregnancies and causes significant fetal and maternal mortality and morbidity. Preeclampsia accounts for 70% of cases of hypertension in pregnancy, with chronic hypertension accounting for most of the remaining 30% of cases. The American College of Obstetrics and Gynecology defines hypertension in pregnancy as either a systolic pressure of ≥140 mm Hg or an increment of ≥30 mm Hg from the first prenatal value, or a diastolic pressure of ≥90 mm Hg or an increment of ≥15 mm Hg. The decrease in peripheral vascular resistance during pregnancy can make the diagnosis of hypertension difficult, as blood pressure normally drops in the first and second trimesters only to increase in the third trimester.

Preeclampsia is classically described as the triad of edema, proteinuria, and hypertension. Unfortunately, edema is present in up to 80% of normotensive pregnancies and is not always present in eclampsia. Mild preeclampsia is diagnosed by a blood pressure reading of 140/90 taken on two occasions 6 hours apart in the presence of proteinuria. Severe preeclampsia is diagnosed when one of the following is present: (1) blood pressure ≥160 mm Hg systolic or ≥110 mm Hg diastolic on two occasions at least 6 hours apart with the patient at bed rest, (2) proteinuria ≥5g in a 24-hour urine collection or +3 on dipstick in at least two random clean catch samples 4 hours apart, (3) oliguria (urine output <30cc/hour), (4) cerebral or visual disturbances, (5) epigastric pain, or (6) pulmonary edema or cyanosis. The appearance of preeclampsia in the first and second trimesters raises the suspicion of a molar pregnancy or maternal systemic lupus erythematosus.

Risk factors for preeclampsia include preexisting hypertension, renal disease, diabetes, multiple gestations, nulliparity, family history of preeclampsia, and a fetus with hydrops. Treatment of preeclampsia is delivery of the fetus and placenta. If the pregnancy is at or near term, delivery can be accomplished by cervical ripening and induction of labor. If the pregnancy is remote from term, then management depends on the severity of disease. Mild preeclampsia can be managed as an outpatient or inpatient, depending on patient reliability and compliance with bed rest and follow-up. Severe preeclampsia warrants admission and careful monitoring of maternal renal, hepatic, and hematologic parameters, as well as treatment of diastolic blood pressures ≥110 mm Hg. If fetal pulmonary maturity is documented, then delivery is warranted. If fetal pulmonary maturity is not present, conservative management can be considered if fetal well-being can be monitored. Steroids are given to accelerate lung maturation. These pregnancies are at high risk for intrauterine growth retardation, fetal distress, and stillbirth; therefore close fetal monitoring and consultation with maternal-fetal medicine and neonatal teams are mandatory for conservative management of severe preeclampsia.

The reported incidence of HELLP syndrome (Hemolysis, Elevated Liver enzymes, Low Platelets) in preeclampsia ranges from 2% to 12%. A severe form of preeclampsia, it can be confused with other disorders associated with liver dysfunction or hemolytic anemia.

Eclampsia is defined as the development of seizures or coma in a patient with signs and symptoms of preeclampsia. The reported incidence is up to 0.5% of all deliveries. Only about 50% of cases occur antepartum.

Magnesium sulfate is widely used in the United States in preeclampsia to prevent and control seizures. The drug is administered by continuous intravenous infusion with a 4 to 6 g load over 20 minutes followed by a maintenance rate of 2 g/hour. Serum magnesium levels are followed, and the rate of the infusion is adjusted to maintain a level between 4.8 and 9.6 mg/dl. Magnesium is excreted by the kidneys; therefore close monitoring of urine output is necessary and dose adjustment is warranted in the face of persistent oliguria. In the therapeutic range, magnesium slows neuromuscular conduction. Suppression of deep tendon reflexes, respiration, and eventually coma and asystole are seen in overdoses. Overdose can be reversed with the administration of intravenous calcium gluconate. Magnesium sulfate therapy is continued for 24 hours postpartum or after an eclamptic episode. Other anticonvulsants have been used including phenobarbital and diphenylhydantoin, but studies comparing their effectiveness with magnesum sulfate have not been conducted.

Antihypertensive drug therapy in pregnancy is limited by concerns of teratogenicity and fetal side effects. Methyldopa has been used for many years with no adverse fetal side effects. Studies on the use of calcium-channel blockers in pregnancy, are limited although adverse fetal effects are not likely. Beta-blockers also have been used widely and although initially they were thought to cause frequent fetal side effects, it is now established that side effects are due to maternal condition rather than drug effect. Angiotensin-converting enzyme inhibitors have been associated with oligohydramnios, intrauterine growth retardation, fetal renal failure, and intrauterine demise and are contraindicated in pregnancy. Diuretics are contraindicated for treatment of hypertension in pregnancy, as they decrease intravascular volume and therefore placental perfusion. Diuretics are used only in patients with congestive heart failure and pulmonary edema. Low-dose (80 mg) aspirin is recommended for women with a history of chronic hypertension, preeclampsia, or intrauterine growth retardation to decrease the risk of preeclampsia and growth retardation. Low-dose aspirin does not benefit women without a prior history of these conditions and may increase the risk for placental abruption.

Treatment of hypertension has significant maternal benefit, but it has not been proven that treatment either prolongs gestation or increases birthweight. Prevention of preeclampsia may be the primary goal of therapy.

### Thyroid disease

Several physiologic changes occur in the thyroid gland during pregnancy to maintain a euthyroid state. The thyroid increases iodine uptake and production of thyroid hormone in response to a decline in plasma iodine concentration that results from an increase in GFR and iodine clearance. Estrogen stimulates production of thyroid-binding globulin (TBG), and because 85% of circulating thyroid hormone is bound to TBG, levels of thyroxine ($T_4$) and triiodothyronine ($T_3$) increase. The $T_3$ uptake ($T_3U$), which is inversely related to thyroid hormone-binding capacity in serum, is reduced due to elevated TBG concentrations. Levels of free thyroid hormone (free thyroxine index) are in the normal range. Thyroid-stimulating hormone (TSH) levels are slightly suppressed in the first trimester and subsequently normalize; therefore they are an accurate marker for hypothyroidism.

### Hypothyroidism

Although hypothyroidism is common in reproductive-aged women, untreated hypothyroidism is not commonly seen in pregnancy, probably because of the inability of hypothyroid patients to ovulate.

Untreated hypothyroidism during pregnancy is associated with an increased incidence of spontaneous abortion, IUGR, stillbirth, and congenital anomalies, as well as preeclampsia and abruption. Autoimmune thyroiditis usually improves during pregnancy and relapses postpartum. Antimicrosomal and antithyroglobulin antibodies, if present, are rarely associated with any fetal side effects.

Treatment of hypothyroidism is with oral L-thyroxine at a starting dose of 125 to 150 mg, with follow-up determinations of serum TSH and $T_4$ levels every 3 weeks. If TSH levels remain elevated, the dose of L-thyroxine is increased by 50 mg increments. The increase in thyroid-binding globulin may necessitate higher doses than in the nonpregnant state.

### Hyperthyroidism

Hyperthyroidism occurs in about 2 of every 1000 pregnancies. Graves' disease or autoimmune thyrotoxicosis is the most common cause. Subclinical hyperthyroidism may be difficult to distinguish in early pregnancy, as an increase in heart rate, heat intolerance, skin warmth, nausea, and poor weight gain are common symptoms in the first trimester. Tachycardia, thyromegaly, exophthalmos, and failure to gain weight with normal or increased caloric intake are not normal and can be helpful clues. Thyrotoxicosis can be associated with severe vomiting and may be the cause of hyperemesis gravidarum, or result from molar gestations and choriocarcinoma. In the latter two conditions, elevated HCG levels, which stimulate thyroid hormone, and the thyroid dysfunction are completely reversible with uterine evacuation.

Hyperthyroidism is diagnosed by elevated free $T_4$ level and values of TSH below 0.1 mU/ml. Occasionally, the free $T_4$ is normal and the $T_3$ is elevated. Determination of the presence of autoantibodies (thyroid-stimulating immunoglobulins or long-acting thyroid stimulator) is necessary as they are IgG and can cross the placenta. Fetal or neonatal hyperthyroidism secondary to transfer of maternal antibodies complicates approximately 1% of pregnancies in women with a history of Graves' disease or Hashimoto's thyroiditis. In women who have undergone thyroid ablation, the presence of antibodies still must be determined.

In pregnancy, treatment of hyperthyroidism is most commonly medical. The thiourea derivatives propylthiouracil, methimazole, and carbamazole are all used. Propylthiouracil (PTU) is the most commonly used medication and is not associated with fetal abnormalities. The objective is to maintain the mother in the high normal range to avoid fetal hypothyroidism. Initially, thyroid function tests are followed every 2 weeks, but when a stable dosage is obtained, they can be followed monthly. If a drug reaction occurs, therapy is changed to methimazole (Tapazole). Methimazole is associated with reversible aplasia cutis in the fetus and therefore is kept as the second-line drug. Although both drugs are secreted in breast milk, less PTU is secreted because it is more protein-bound. Thyroidectomy is reserved for women who cannot adhere to medical therapy or who have toxic side effects to it. Radioactive iodine is contraindicated in pregnancy, as iodine is concentrated in the fetal thyroid after 10 weeks and can result in fetal goiter.

Maternal complications of hyperthyroidism in pregnancy include hyperemesis, poor weight gain, preterm labor, thyroid storm, and high-output cardiac failure. Fetal complications include fetal tachyarrhythmias, high output cardiac failure, hydrops, IUGR, and goiter.

### Cardiac disease

The physiologic changes of pregnancy, delivery, and the puerperium cause significant alteration in the maternal cardiovascular system. Increase in the myocardial workload is related to increased blood volume, metabolic demands, cardiac output, and heart rate. Increases in blood pressure and anemia also can affect cardiac output. Patients with well-compensated heart disease may thus have heart failure for the first time during pregnancy. The goal of medical management is to optimize maternal hemodynamics by changing preload, afterload, and contractility once symptomatology is present. Diuretics are reserved for pulmonary edema or right-sided heart failure. Digoxin is used to control atrial fibrillation. Afterload reduction may be beneficial in improving cardiac output.

Labor and delivery are a crucial time with increased hemodynamic load associated with contractions, pain, anesthesia, possible surgery, blood loss, and intravenous therapy. Therefore complete hemodynamic monitoring optimizes fluid management and pharmacologic manipulation of cardiac output. In labor epidural anesthesia is recommended to relieve pain and to avoid Valsalva maneuvers. Use of the lateral position is important, as it minimizes hypotension and increases preload and cardiac output. Cesarean delivery is undertaken for obstetric indications, as vaginal delivery avoids the stress and blood loss of surgery. Instrumental delivery by low forceps or vacuum extraction is recommended to avoid Valsalva maneuvers. Postpartum, intensive monitoring in the first 48 hours is necessary, as this is the period of highest risk for fluid shifts secondary to autotransfusion with placental delivery and uterine involution.

Classification of maternal mortality for various types of cardiac disease is useful in counseling patients. Mitral stenosis with atrial fibrillation or New York Heart Association classes III and IV aortic stenosis, uncorrected tetralogy of Fallot, previous myocardial infarction, and Marfan syndrome with a normal aorta are associated with a maternal mortality rate of 5% to 15%. Pulmonary hypertension, aortic coarctation, and Marfan syndrome with aortic root dilation greater than 4 cm carry a 25% to 50% maternal mortality rate and can be considered a contraindication to pregnancy.

Peripartum cardiomyopathy is characterized by the development of cardiac failure in the third trimester or within 5 months of delivery for which no other cause can be determined. The incidence of peripartum cardiomyopathy is 1 in 3000 to 4000 pregnancies. In the United States, it is more frequent among older, multiparous African-American women, twins, and patients with preeclampsia. It has a tendency to recur with subsequent pregnancies. Some investigators have implicated inadequate nutrition, viral agents, preeclampsia, or immunologic factors in its pathogenesis. Another theory suggests that viral myocarditis may be the primary inciting factor. The prognosis for dilated cardiomyopathy is poor, with progressive deterioration once symptoms occur. The mortality rate for peripartum cardiomyopathy in the United States ranges from 25% to 50%. There may be a subset of patients in whom the heart size returns to normal who have a significantly better prognosis. This group also may include patients who had stable cardiac disease before conception.

## BIBLIOGRAPHY

Briggs GG, Freeman RK, Yaffe SJ: *Drugs in pregnancy and lactation: a reference guide to fetal and neonatal risk,* ed 2, Baltimore, 1986, Williams & Wilkins.

Burrow GN, Ferris TF: *Medical complications during pregnancy,* Philadelphia, 1982, WB Saunders.

Creasy RK, Resnik R, editors: *Maternal-fetal medicine: principles and practice,* ed 3, Philadelphia, 1994, WB Saunders.

Geronimus AT, Bound J: Black/white differences in women's reproductive-related health status: evidence from vital statistics, *Demography* 27:457, 1990.

Gleicher N, editor: *Principles and practice of medical therapy in pregnancy,* ed 2, Connecticut, 1992, Appleton & Lange.

Milunsky A, editor: *Genetic disorders and the fetus,* Baltimore, 1992, Johns Hopkins University Press.

Nyberg DA et al, editors: *Transvaginal sonography,* St Louis, 1992, Mosby.

Reece EA, Coustan DR, editors: *Diabetes mellitus in pregnancy: principles and practice,* New York, 1988, Churchill Livingstone.

Reece EA et al, editors: *Medicine of the mother and fetus,* Philadelphia, 1992, WB Saunders.

Smoak IW: Embryopathic effects of the oral hypoglycemic agent chlorpropamide in cultured mouse embryos, *Am J Obstet Gynecol* 169:409, 1993.

Wegman ME: Annual summary of vital statistics—1991, *Pediatrics* 90:835, 1992.

CHAPTER

# 148 Menopause

**David L. Keefe**

More than one third of women in the United States have reached menopause, and with female life expectancy approaching 80 years, many will spend more than a third of their lives in a postmenopausal state. The first born of the baby boom generation are approaching their fifth decade, so the number of menopausal women is expected to increase further over the next 20 years. Although menopause is a natural phenomenon, the loss of ovarian estrogen production can evoke symptoms and exacerbate a number of age-related diseases, including coronary heart disease and osteoporosis. Hormone therapy alleviates menopausal symptoms and reduces the risks of coronary heart disease and osteoporosis, but may induce side effects. Thus menopausal women constitute a large and growing portion of clinicians' practices for whom recognition and treatment of hypoestrogenism may improve the quality and duration of life. The clinician must help the menopausal woman weigh potential benefits against risks of hormone therapy to decide whether hormone therapy is the right choice for her.

## DEFINITIONS, ETIOLOGY, AND PSYCHOSOCIAL PERSPECTIVES

### Definitions

Menopause is the woman's final menstrual period. Usually defined retrospectively after 6 to 12 months of amenorrhea, menopause occurs at an average age of 51. Loss of ovarian function before age 40 is termed premature ovarian failure. The transition from reproductive to nonreproductive ovarian function, a period that spans more than 10 years in most women, is the climacteric. The association of estrogen deficiency symptoms with decline in ovarian function is the menopausal syndrome.

### Etiology

Natural menopause arises as a consequence of follicular depletion, a process that begins before birth and progresses throughout the life of the woman. Oocyte mitosis ceases, and oocyte and follicle atresia begins while the female herself is still in utero. At birth, oocyte number declines from more than 8 million to fewer than 2 million. Most follicles degenerate before ovulating, which explains why decreasing or increasing the number of ovulations by oral contraceptive pills, pregnancy, lactation, or fertility drugs does not appreciably influence the onset of menopause. During the decade preceding the menopause (roughly corresponding to the climacteric), the rate of follicular loss accelerates. Nonetheless, some oocytes remain even after the cessation of menstruation. Follicular atresia probably involves apoptosis. Neuroendocrine changes precede follicular exhaustion in rodents, but neuroendocrine contributions to reproductive aging in women have been less studied.

Premature ovarian failure may result from oophorectomy, radiation, chemotherapy, autoimmune disease, chromosomal abnormalities (especially Turner mosaic), infection, metabolic abnormalities, or trauma. Menopause may begin at an earlier age in smokers. The cause of premature ovarian failure often is unclear. In some cases, ovarian biopsy can clarify the etiology of premature ovarian failure, but the associated risk and cost rarely justify its use, because the results usually do not alter clinical management.

### Psychosocial perspectives

Women from every population exhibit physiologic changes with menopause. Indeed, references to the menopause in ancient and classic texts resemble modern clinical reports; however, the incidence of menopause-associated symptoms varies greatly among cultures. Women from cultures that confer prestige and dignity on menopausal women report fewer symptoms than women from cultures that perceive the menopause more negatively. The role of menopausal women in Western culture is complex. On the one hand, Western culture increasingly deemphasizes the reproductive role of women; on the other hand, it remains emphatically youth oriented. Not surprisingly, reactions of Western women to menopause vary according to the meaning it holds for them. It should be noted that most women accept menopause as a normal stage in the cycle of life, which they share in common with their mothers, sisters, and friends. Indeed, in the Massachusetts Women's Health Study, a large community survey showed that 70% of menopausal women expressed relief or neutral feelings about the cessation of menses. For many women, the menopause years are a time of personal satisfaction and professional productivity.

The clinician may encounter women who experience difficulty with menopause. For example those who have struggled with long-term infertility may find that the finality of menopause removes their last hope of having their own child. Others see menopause as a sign of aging. Because menopause occurs at a stage of life when children may leave home, partners may become ill, or parents may die, its meaning may become entangled with the grief associated with such losses. For these women the physical nature of menopausal symptoms may be less painful to face and easier to understand than the underlying emotional turmoil. Even though clinicians can offer hormone therapy to alleviate symptoms and protect against some potentially fatal diseases, the universality of the menopause and the variability of reactions to it prompt some to caution against the "medicalization" of such a natural event. Because of this great diversity of reactions to the menopause, the clinician must help the woman place menopause within the broader context of her own life and make her a partner in every aspect of clinical decision making related to it.

## PHYSIOLOGY

After menopause the ovary becomes small and fibrotic and takes on a pitted surface. Microscopically, decreased numbers of primordial follicles and increased numbers of fibroblasts, interstitial cells, and connective tissue appear, reflecting atrophy of the ovarian cortex and hyperplasia of the medulla. Considerable variation in the degree of interstitial hyperplasia exists, which explains in part the variation in levels of ovarian steroidogenesis reported in menopausal women.

The pattern of steroidogenesis changes after the menopause. Before menopause steroidogenesis is cyclical; during the follicular phase the graafian follicle secretes 17B-estradiol; during the luteal phase the corpus luteum secretes progesterone and 17B-estradiol. After menopause ovarian estrogen and progesterone production virtually cease. Less potent estrogens, principally estrone, are produced from androgens by the enzyme aromatase, located in adipose, muscle, and brain. There are considerable differences in the extent of extraovarian estrogen formation among menopausal women, which may explain, in part, differences in the incidence of estrogen-related symptoms. High circulating levels of luteinizing hormone maintain androgen secretion from interstitial and hilar cells within the ovary, which is why oophorectomy of menopausal women reduces circulating testosterone by 50% and androstenedione by 30%, but barely affects estrogen production.

Although absolute levels of androgens also decrease, estrogen levels decrease so significantly at menopause that the ratio of circulating androgens to estrogens actually increases after menopause. Because androgens and estrogens interact at a number of levels (e.g., they downregulate each other's receptors and reciprocally influence sex hormone binding globulin levels), an increased androgen/estrogen ratio unmasks androgenic activity in some women. Women undergoing surgical menopause experience a much greater decline in androgen levels.

The manifold effects of estrogen deprivation on menopausal women should come as no surprise, because estrogen receptors appear throughout the body, where they regulate many critical functions. Estrogen receptors appear in highest concentrations in reproductive tissues, such as breast and urogenital tract, and in phylogenetically ancient parts of the brain involved in regulation of the neuroendocrine and autonomic nervous systems. Measurable levels of estrogen receptor also appear in many other tissues, including liver, blood vessels, and bone.

Estrogen receptors are part of the steroid hormone receptor superfamily. When bound to hormone, steroid receptors attach to specific DNA sequences, called hormone response elements, to regulate transcription, which creates a cascade of regulatory events within the cell. Extremely rapid effects of estrogens, especially on some tissues that lack detectable levels of estrogen receptor, suggest that sex steroids also may act independently of their receptors.

### Epidemiology

Cessation of ovarian function by the fifth or sixth decade is a universal phenomenon among women. Females of most mammalian species undergo reproductive failure by midlife, leading some sociobiologists to hypothesize that midlife loss of reproductive capacity among aging females confers survival value to species. Because of the aging world population, the number of menopausal women is increasing. Almost 60% of the U.S. population aged 65 or older, and over 70% of the population aged 85 or older are women. Improved public health and health care in developing countries have assured survival of increasingly large numbers of women into the menopausal years; globally more than 470 million women are menopausal. Because hypoestrogenism contributes to debilitating chronic diseases such as coronary heart disease and osteoporosis, the evaluation and treatment of the menopause have enormous public health and clinical implications.

Although menopause is a universal experience, only about 40% of menopausal women seek treatment for symptoms related to estrogen deficiency. As discussed earlier, reporting of menopausal symptoms depends on complex psychosociobiologic interactions. Differences in the incidence of menopausal symptoms reflect not only cultural influences on symptom reporting, but also genetic variation in body habitus, which directly affects estrogen levels by influencing rates of aromatization. Variation in dietary consumption of plant estrogens (phytoestrogens) also may influence development of symptoms, although evidence supporting this hypothesis is still preliminary.

## CLINICAL PRESENTATION

Estrogen deficiency symptoms usually begin during the climacteric, at first interspersed with symptom-free periods. As menopause approaches, symptoms may become increasingly frequent and severe. Most symptoms associated with menopause can be explained by the effects of estrogen deprivation on sensitive tissues. Hot flushes and sleep disturbance, the most common symptoms of the menopause, arise from the effects of estrogen deprivation on those parts of the brain that regulate body temperature and sleep, respectively. Hot flushes typically begin in the chest, spread to the face, and last seconds to minutes. They may be associated with anxiety and palpitations and are followed by profuse sweating and shaking. Some women experience up to 20 episodes in a 24-hour period, and for most women hot flushes increase in frequency at night. Eating, stress, or alcohol may trigger hot flushes. In at least 50% of women, they abate spontaneously within 5 years after the menopause, even without hormone therapy. Women who develop premature ovarian failure before attaining adult levels of estrogen, (e.g., Turner's syndrome patients) do not report hot flushes. Sleep disturbance is characterized by frequent nocturnal awakenings, which may be associated with hot flushes. Sleep apnea also develops after the menopause in some women.

Urogenital atrophy, manifesting as urinary frequency, dysuria, dyspareunia, genital bleeding, and occasionally stress urinary incontinence, results from the effects of estrogen deprivation on the bladder, urethra, and associated pelvic supports. Amenorrhea, which may be preceded by luteal phase defects, shortening of menstrual cycle length, or menstrual irregularity, results from loss of cyclic estrogen and progesterone effects on the endometrium. Decreased estrogen/androgen ratio contributes to mild hirsutism and breast atrophy in some women.

Decreased sex drive may arise from urogenital atrophy or psychodynamic reactions to menopause. Women who have undergone oophorectomy may experience decreased libido because of loss of ovarian androgen production. More controversial is the role of estrogen deprivation on mood and cognitive function.

Declining fertility and fecundity, which begin more than a decade before the menopause, even before detectable alterations in menstrual cyclicity, result largely from declining oocyte developmental potential and possibly from abnormal endometrial receptivity.

Some menopausal women present with symptoms associated with osteoporosis, such as back pain, kyphoscoliosis, and decreased height (first revealed by changing dress hem length). Coronary heart disease in menopausal women may present with classic angina, but atypical angina may be more common. Early detection of coronary heart disease symptoms is especially critical in menopausal women because they may have a poorer prognosis than men after myocardial infarction. Osteoporosis and heart symptoms typically appear in women only several years after menopause.

## PHYSICAL EXAMINATION

Physical examination of the menopausal woman reveals atrophy of sex steroid-dependent tissues. Skin on the vulva thins, vaginal epithelium becomes dry and loses rugations, the cervix and uterus decrease in size, and the portio of the cervix becomes friable. Breasts decrease in size and fullness. Such observations provide more reliable assessment of the state of estrogenization than measurement of circulating 17-B estradiol, because these tissues reflect overall estrogen effects, whereas the 17-B estradiol level measures only one of many bioactive estrogens. Some women develop mild hirsutism in response to declining estrogen/androgen ratio. Older postmenopausal women may have kyphoscoliosis and spinous tenderness from osteoporotic vertebral fractures.

Physical examination of the menopausal woman should include careful examination of the breasts and associated lymph nodes, cervix, vagina, uterus, adnexa, vulva, and rectum to screen for evidence of malignancy. A Pap smear and stool guaiac should be obtained.

## LABORATORY STUDIES

Although the physical examination provides a sensitive "bioassay" for the state of estrogenization, several laboratory assays can confirm the presence of hypoestrogenism. Levels of 17-B estradiol (less than 40 pg/ml), follicle-stimulating hormone (FSH) more than 40 mIU, and vaginal cytology exhibiting parabasal cells signal ovarian failure. Several accurate and reliable methods can quantify bone density. Standard radiographs reflect only late stage osteoporosis, but quantitative bone densitometry, using single or dual photon absortiometry or other methods, measures bone demineralization with greater sensitivity. The role of broad-based radiographic screening for osteoporosis is controversial at present, but most clinicians agree that bone densitometry should be restricted to patients who need osteoporosis risk assessment to weigh potential risks against benefits of hormone therapy.

Risks for several life-threatening diseases, such as coronary heart disease, stroke, breast cancer, and osteoporosis increase after the menopause. Most risks for these conditions can be determined by interview and physical examination; but cholesterol screening, mammography, and occasionally bone densitometry studies may provide additional information.

For women experiencing premature menopause, a cosyntropin (Cortrosyn) stimulation test and thyroid stimulating hormone (TSH), calcium, and phosphorus levels screen for associated hypoadrenal, hypothyroid, and hypoparathyroid states, respectively.

## DIFFERENTIAL DIAGNOSIS

The interview and physical examination must search for evidence of conditions that mimic menopause, especially in young women with premature ovarian failure. Carcinoid, pheochromocytoma, or systemic mastocytosis can present with flushing; but they usually can be differentiated by concomitant attacks of diarrhea, hypertension or hypotension, and the absence of other signs of hypoestrogenism. Hyperprolactinemia lowers estrogen levels, usually does not cause vasomotor instability, but does cause galactorrhea. Hyperandrogenic states arising from functioning adrenal or ovarian tumors produce more marked virilization, with more rapid progression than the mild and insidious hirsutism that appears in some menopausal women. Hypothalamic amenorrhea differs from menopause by its lack of hot flushes and decreased, rather than increased, FSH levels. Patients with osteoporosis should be evaluated for primary hyperparathyroidism, hyperthyroidism, or hypercortisolism.

Vulvar dermatoses or neoplasia may be mistaken for menopausal urogenital atrophy, and excoriations on atrophic vulva in menopausal women may be mistaken for neoplasia. Only biopsy can distinguish these conditions. Any white, erythematous, or raised vulvar lesions should be biopsied in women of all ages.

Sleep disturbance, decreased sex drive, and hot flushes associated with hypoestrogenism may resemble anxiety and mood disorders. A history of anxiety and mood disorders antedating the menopause may suggest a functional etiology for these symptoms. Many clinicians, however, prescribe hormone therapy if other signs and symptoms suggest hypoestrogenism. Symptoms remaining after hormonal treatment of the hypoestrogenic state may require additional psychotherapeutic and/or psychopharmacologic intervention.

## MANAGEMENT

Hormone therapy effectively treats most symptoms associated with menopause and prevents disease and prolongs life even in asymptomatic women. A major potential benefit of hormone therapy is reduced risk of cardiovascular disease. Cardiovascular disease is the leading cause of death among women in developed countries, accounting for 50% of all deaths in women over age 50. The incidence of cardiovascular disease increases fiftyfold after menopause. Consistent evidence demonstrates that unopposed estrogen reduces the risk for coronary heart disease by 35% to 50%, although only randomized, controlled clinical trials, which are still underway, can demonstrate conclusively cardioprotective effects of estrogen. Mechanisms underlying hormone therapy's cardioprotective effects are not completely understood. Hormone therapy induces favorable changes in lipid factors, but recent evidence indicates that changes in lipids account for only 20% of the cardioprotective effects of this therapy.

Addition of progestin to estrogen also probably reduces the risk of coronary heart disease, although the magnitude of risk reduction cannot be estimated with current data. Indeed, the cardioprotective effects of combined regimens may depend on the dose and chemical structure of the specific progestin administered. Because progestins that structurally resemble androgens induce androgenic side effects, they can abrogate some of the beneficial effects of estrogen.

Hormone therapy with estrogen or estrogen/progestin also reduces the risk for osteoporosis-related hip fracture by 25% and for vertebral fractures by over 50%. Osteoporosis is characterized by decreased bone mass and increased susceptibility to fractures, especially of the vertebrae, wrist, and hip. Bone mass peaks in women at age 35 to 40, declines gradually with age, and then drops precipitously in the years immediately after the menopause. The prevalence of osteoporotic fractures among menopausal women is high: Some studies estimate that 50% of 70-year-old women have had at least one osteoporosis-related fracture. Advanced age, white race, thin body habitus, smoking, family history, and lack of exercise are further risk factors for osteoporosis, which may exacerbate the effects of estrogen deficiency. Hip fractures are especially dangerous, with an associated mortality rate of almost 20%, and chronic pain and disability contribute to the morbidity associated with osteoporotic fractures (see Chapter 6). The high costs of osteoporotic fractures in the United States (more than $7 billion annually) derive from the resulting long in-patient hospitalizations and prolonged home care.

Estrogen deprivation increases osteoporosis because it increases bone turnover. Because estrogen deficiency increases bone resorption more than formation, it causes a net decrease in bone density. Hormone therapy rapidly restores normal levels of bone resorption and formation. Progestins do not counteract estrogen's protective effect on bone. The protective effects of hormone therapy are greatest when they are initiated before menopause, but even women with advanced osteoporosis may experience improvement.

These potential benefits must be weighed against possible risks and side effects of hormone therapy. The risks of hormone therapy have been overestimated by studies based on oral contraceptive pills and on unopposed estrogen. Hormone therapy provides levels of estrogenic activity close to that encountered in premenopausal women, whereas even the lowest dose of oral contraceptive pills contain estrogenic activity many times greater than that provided by hormone therapy. Furthermore, the addition of progestin to estrogen lowers the risk of endometrial cancer associated with estrogen replacement therapy to below that of women who take no hormone therapy at all (see Chapter 150). Other side effects attributed to sex steroids based on studies of oral contraceptive pill users, such as hypertension and thromboembolic disease, also generally do not apply to hormone therapy.

The most troubling, but at the same time most controversial, risk attributed to hormone therapy is increased lifetime probability of breast cancer. Data are extensive, but conclusions are inconsistent concerning the risk of developing breast cancer in women taking estrogen. That men almost never get breast cancer and that early menarche and late menopause increase the risk for developing breast cancer are consistent with the hypothesis that extending the duration of exposure to estrogens by hormone therapy may increase breast cancer risk. Data suggest, however, that women who use estrogen therapy for less than 5 years probably do not increase their risk of breast cancer. The risk for breast cancer may increase slightly among women who take estrogen for longer than 15 years but the data are not conclusive.

Contrary to early reports, progestins do not protect against breast cancer. Indeed, fundamental studies on the effects of sex steroids on breast tissue predict that combination therapy may increase the risk for developing breast cancer, and some preliminary clinical studies corroborate this theory.

For most women the most annoying side effect of hormone therapy is vaginal bleeding. In women with a uterus, estrogen therapy produces unpredictable vaginal bleeding in up to 40% of treated women per year. The addition of progestins on a monthly basis synchronizes bleeding, but often is accompanied by symptoms of irritability and depression. Other side effects associated with estrogen therapy include breast tenderness, bloating, and headache. In most women, however, these symptoms are mild and often improve after several months of therapy.

Although public health considerations dictate that most menopausal women at least consider hormone therapy, the decision to begin it ultimately must be reached only after balancing potential risks and benefits for the individual. The clinician should describe pertinent risk factors, then discuss feelings and beliefs the woman has regarding menopause and hormone therapy to help her make a rational decision about hormone therapy. For example, the clinician may counsel a woman that five times more women die of heart disease each year than from breast cancer, that hormone therapy reduces the risk of heart attack by 30% to 50%, and that the effect of hormone therapy on breast cancer is still controversial. Nevertheless, the woman who has a strong family history of breast cancer and minimal risk factors for heart disease reasonably may elect to refuse hormone therapy. Conversely, women who have coronary heart disease risks are likely to benefit from hormone therapy, even if they also are at risk for breast cancer.

Hormone therapy can be given as unopposed estrogen, unopposed progestin, or estrogen/progestin combination regimens. Women who have undergone hysterectomy do not need progestin therapy. Women who have a uterus require combined estrogen/progestin therapy. Combined regimens include estrogen plus cyclic progestin and estrogen plus continuous progestin. The continuous combined regimen may eliminate vaginal bleeding if the uterus becomes atrophic; however, usually months of irregular bleeding ensue before this goal is attained. Many varieties of hormone preparations are available (see the box below).

### Estrogen and progestin regimens

Common doses used
- Estrogens
  - 0.3 mg conjugated estrogen
  - 0.625 mg conjugated estrogen
  - 0.9 mg conjugated estrogen
  - 1.25 mg conjugated estrogen
  - 0.05 mg transdermal estrogen
  - 0.10 mg transdermal estrogen
  - 1 mg micronized 17β-estradiol
  - 2 mg micronized 17β-estradiol
- Progestins
  - 2.5 mg medroxyprogesterone acetate
  - 5 mg medroxyprogesterone acetate
  - 10 mg medroxyprogesterone acetate
  - 5 mg norethindrone acetate
  - 5 mg norethindrone

Typical regimens
- Continuous estrogen plus cyclic progestin
  - Estrogen: (0.625 mg conjugated estrogen, 1 mg micronized 17β-estradiol daily or transdermal patch changed twice a week)
  - Progestin: first 12 days of every month (5 or 10 mg)

OR
- Continuous/combined
  - Estrogen and progestin daily (0.625 mg conjugated estrogen, 1 mg micronized 17β-estradiol daily or transdermal patch changed twice a week; progestin—2.5 mg per day).

Women presenting with symptoms of hypoestrogenism and prolonged amenorrhea who elect continuous estrogen and cyclic progesterone should take estrogen alone until symptoms abate. The estrogen is then titrated to achieve the minimal effective dose, a process that may take up to 2 months. Such a short course of unopposed estrogen carries minimal risk for the endometrium in such patients and enables the clinician to adjust one hormone at a time. Furthermore, for many women the progestin creates the biggest barrier to compliance. Delaying progestin therapy until the abatement of menopausal symptoms enhances trust in the clinician-patient relationship and increases patient motivation to work through the optimization of the progestin dose. Progestin is added at a low dose for at least 12 days, beginning the first of each month (a schedule that helps the woman remember when to take progestin). If bleeding begins before day 10 of the progestin, the progestin dose is increased.

**Table 148-1.** Contraindications to estrogen use

| Absolute contraindications | Relative contraindications |
|---|---|
| Stroke | Cigarette smoking/significant nicotine abuse |
| Recent myocardial infarction | Fibrocystic breast disease |
| Breast cancer | Familial hyperlipidemia |
| Endometrial adenocarcinoma | Hypertension aggravated by estrogen therapy |
| Other estrogen-dependent tumors | Pancreatitis |
| Acute liver disease | Hepatic porphyria |
| Pancreatic disease | Endometrial hyperplasia |
| Gallbladder disease | Leiomyomata uteri |
| Chronic impaired liver function | Endometriosis |
| Recent venous thromboembolic event | Migraine headache |
| Chronic thrombophlebitis | |
| Undiagnosed vaginal bleeding | |

Adapted from Young RL, Kumar NS, Goldzieher JW, *Drugs* 40(2):220-230, 1990.

**Table 148-2.** Alternatives to estrogen therapy

| Therapy | Dose/frequency | Benefits | Side effects/risks |
|---|---|---|---|
| Medroxyprogesterone Acetate | 10 mg po qd | Relieves hot flushes, prevents osteoporosis | Worsening symptoms of urogenital atrophy<br>Depression/sedation<br>Decreased libido<br>Decreased HDL<br>Effect on breast cancer not known |
| Calcium supplementation | 1000 mg po qd | Minimal effect on osteoporosis prevention | Unmask asymptomatic hyperparathyroidism |
| Clonidine | 0.1 mg po qd or bid | Moderate relief of hot flushes | Dry mouth<br>Sedation |
| Bellergal | 1 tablet bid | Relieves hot flushes | Drowsiness<br>Paresthesias (rare) |
| Low Fat Diet | | Lower cardiac risk factors | |
| Exercise | As tolerated | Lower cardiac risk factors | Prevent osteoporosis |

Women presenting with irregular menses, even in association with evidence of hypoestrogenism, must undergo endometrial biopsy to exclude the possibility of endometrial cancer. Women who develop vaginal bleeding on hormone therapy also must undergo endometrial biopsy. The ease and accuracy of office biopsy largely have supplanted operative dilation and curettage; but suspicious histology, inadequate tissue, technical difficulty (especially in older women with a stenotic cervical os), or persistently irregular bleeding are indications for operative fractional curettage. After exclusion of neoplasia, perimenopausal, dysfunctional uterine bleeding should be treated by monthly progestin therapy.

Contraindications to hormone therapy include breast cancer, other estrogen-dependent malignancies, acute liver, pancreatic or gallbladder disease, chronically impaired liver function, or undiagnosed vaginal bleeding (Table 148-1). Relative contraindications include strong family history of breast cancer or other estrogen-dependent malignancy. For these women, clonidine or ergot preparations reduce hot flushes. Dietary supplementation with calcium reduces osteoporosis risk, although not as completely as estrogen, and exercise and restriction of dietary cholesterol and fat consumption reduce coronary heart disease risk (Table 148-2).

## BIBLIOGRAPHY


Bush TL et al: Cardiovascular mortality and noncontraceptive use of estrogen in women: results from the lipid research clinics program follow-up study, *Circulation* 75:1102-1109, 1987.

Grady D et al: Guidelines for counseling postmenopausal women about preventive hormone therapy, *Ann Intern Med* 117:1038-1041, 1992.

Grady D et al: Hormone therapy to prevent disease and prolong life in postmenopausal women, *Ann Intern Med* 117:1016-1037, 1992.

Kiel DP et al: Hip fracture and the use of estrogens in postmenopausal women. The Framingham Study, *N Engl J Med* 317:1169-1174, 1987.

Persson I et al: Risk of endometrial cancer after treatment with oestrogens alone or in conjunction with progesterones: results of a prospective study, *Br Med J* 298:147-151, 1989.

Stampfer MJ et al: Postmenopausal estrogen therapy and cardiovascular disease: ten-year follow-up from the Nurse's Health Study, *N Engl J Med* 325:756-762, 1991.

Steinberg KK et al: A meta-analysis of the effect of estrogen replacement therapy on the risk of breast cancer, *JAMA* 265:1985-1990, 1991.

US Congress, Office of Technology Assessment: *The menopause, hormone therapy, and women's health,* OTA-BP-BA-88, Washington, DC, 1992, US Government Printing Office.

Wilson PWF, Garrison RJ, Castelli WP: Postmenopausal estrogen use, cigarette smoking, and cardiovascular morbidity in women over 50. The Framingham Study, *N Engl J Med* 313:1038-1043, 1985.


CHAPTER

# 149 Breast Diseases


**Michelle Z. Schultz**
**Barbara A. Ward**
**Michael Reiss**


Breast cancer afflicts one of every eight to nine American women, an alarming statistic. Among women in the United States, it is the most commonly diagnosed malignancy and follows only lung cancer as the leading cause of death. Given the frequency of this disease, a working knowledge of breast cancer risk factors, breast anatomy, diagnostic procedures, and breast cancer treatment are paramount. Additionally, benign conditions that affect the breast are even more common and often perplexing. This chapter outlines the basic steps regarding breast evaluation and describes the options in the management of breast masses and breast cancer.

## EPIDEMIOLOGY/ETIOLOGY

### Common benign conditions

Fibrocystic disease or mastopathy refers to breast lumpiness accompanied by pain and tenderness, which is most severe in the premenstrual phase of the cycle. While the term *fibrocystic* is nonspecific, most clinicians can identify the clinical picture it represents. It is most accurate to describe fibrocystic changes based on the specific microscopic entity involved including fibroadenomas, macrocysts, periductal mastitis, papillomatosis, apocrine metaplasia, sclerosing adenosis, and hyperplastic lesions of the duct and lobule.

Fibroadenomas commonly present during the second and third decades, but they may be found at any age. Excision is generally advised because the lesions may continue to grow and may be confused with cystosarcoma phyllodes or a carcinoma. Cysts tend to appear suddenly and are much more common in the premenopausal age group. They are often tender and may be aspirated to relieve symptoms and to confirm the diagnosis. Although ultrasound is helpful in differentiating a cyst from a solid mass, needle aspiration with complete resolution of a palpable mass is the gold standard. Macrocysts generally diminish after menopause, but they may persist on estrogen replacement therapy. Periductal mastitis is a chronic condition characterized by repetitive infections that are difficult to treat. Excision of the involved duct system is the recommended treatment. Although antibiotics may temper the inflammation, they are not curative, as nests of purulent fluid remain in the undrained recesses.

### Breast cancer

In 1994, 183,000 new breast cancers were diagnosed and 46,300 women died from this disease. Over her lifetime, a woman has a 12% risk of developing breast cancer and a 3.5% risk of dying from it. The incidence and risk of developing breast cancer increase with age, and the majority of cases occur in postmenopausal women (Table 149-1). Nonetheless, even though 77% of all deaths from breast cancer occur in women over the age of 55, breast cancer is the leading cause of death in younger women between the ages of 40 and 55.

Although the incidence of breast cancer has been rising steadily over the last 60 years, the number of women who die from the disease has remained relatively constant (Fig. 149-1). These statistics appear to be the result of both earlier detection and higher cure rate. An increase in the identification of the earliest stages of disease since the introduction of film screen mammography in the early 1980s accounts for the recent, but probably temporary, surge of reported cases.

Changes in lifestyle may have contributed to the real

**Table 149-1.** Breast cancer risk by age

| Age (years) | Risk |
|---|---|
| 25 | 1 in 19,608 |
| 30 | 1 in 2,525 |
| 35 | 1 in 622 |
| 40 | 1 in 217 |
| 45 | 1 in 93 |
| 50 | 1 in 50 |
| 55 | 1 in 33 |
| 60 | 1 in 24 |
| 65 | 1 in 17 |
| 70 | 1 in 14 |
| 75 | 1 in 11 |
| 80 | 1 in 10 |
| 85 | 1 in 9 |
| Ever | 1 in 8 |

From Marshall E: *Science* 259:618-21, 1993.

increased incidence of breast cancer over the last 50 years. Prolongation of fertility periods, delayed childbearing, and pharmacologic estrogen use have all changed the hormonal environment to which the breast epithelium is exposed. Changes in nutrition and other environmental factors yet to be identified also may play a role.

Although 70% of women with breast cancer have no known predisposition, definite risk factors for the development of breast cancer include family history, early menarche, late menopause, and history of benign breast disease. Other factors, such as alcohol consumption, exposure to ionizing radiation, obesity, high dietary fat intake, and use of exogenous hormones also have been associated with increased risk. The relative risks associated with various factors are summarized in Table 149-2.

### Family history

A family history of breast cancer is among the strongest risk factors, particularly for women with premenopausal first-degree relatives who have had breast cancer. Such familial cases are more often bilateral and are often diagnosed at a younger age than sporadic cases. For example, the probability that a 30-year-old woman will develop breast cancer by age 70 approaches 50% if she has two first-degree relatives diagnosed at a young age, or one who has had bilateral breast cancers. Recent investigations have revealed that the inheritance of a dominant gene, termed BRCA-1, may be directly involved in the development of the disease. Women who have presumably inherited the allele face an 80% lifetime risk of developing breast cancer, tenfold higher than women without the allele. It is possible that acquired somatic mutations in this gene are responsible for many of the sporadic cases of breast and even ovarian cancers. If this is the case, screening for BRCA-1 mutations may become a powerful tool for early detection.

Truly hereditary breast cancers comprise fewer than 5% of all cases. The risk of developing breast cancer for patients with a second-degree relative who has had breast cancer is only slightly higher than the risk in the general population. Most patients have no family history of breast cancer.

### Benign breast disease

Epidemiologic analysis of benign (fibrocystic) breast disease has shown that nonproliferative lesions including cysts, fibroadenoma, duct ectasia, fibrosis, and metaplasia, are not associated with an increased risk for breast cancer. Hyperproliferative epithelium without atypia, including ductal hyperplasia, sclerosing adenosis, and papilloma, is associated with a mild increase in risk. Atypical hyperplasia confers a stronger increase in risk, particularly in association with a first-degree family history. At the end of the spectrum of benign breast disease is lobular carcinoma in situ (LCIS). Although not a malignant lesion in and of itself, LCIS confers the highest risk for subsequent breast cancer, in both the involved and contralateral breast.

### Hormonal factors

Estrogens promote breast cancer growth. Thus prolonged exposure to endogenous estrogens as manifested by early menarche, late menopause, delayed childbearing, or postmenopausal obesity increases breast cancer risk, whereas early menopause, without estrogen replacement, and multiple pregnancies have the opposite effect.

The association between oral contraceptive use and breast cancer has been analyzed extensively, and few studies demonstrate a clear increase in risk. Prolonged use may mildly increase risk, but the risk level returns to baseline soon after the drug is discontinued, although most of the available data that address this issue were derived from women treated with higher estrogen doses than those currently prescribed. Currently, evidence does not support the avoidance of oral contraceptive use (see Chapter 145).

Estrogen replacement therapy (ERT) also has been studied extensively; results have been contradictory (see Chapter 148).

### Environmental factors

Population studies have suggested a direct correlation between dietary fat consumption and breast cancer incidence around the world. Nonetheless, case-controlled studies have been unable to confirm this association. In a study of almost 90,000 nurses, a relation between dietary fat or cholesterol intake and breast cancer was not found. Furthermore, conclusive evidence that modifying fat intake reduces breast cancer does not exist.

Alcohol consumption has a dose-response relationship with breast cancer risk. An inverse relation between vitamin A consumption and breast cancer risk also has been observed, but no specific guidelines for supplements have been determined.

Exposure of the breast to therapeutic doses of ionizing radiation (in the range of 40 Gy), particularly during breast development between the ages of 10 and 19 years clearly increases cancer risk. Radiation exposure after age 40 carries minimal risk.

## PATHOPHYSIOLOGY

### Growth and development

Anatomically, the breast is a hormonally sensitive tissue that develops and regresses with the aging process and with monthly menstrual cycling. The mature breast is composed of epithelial and stromal elements. The stroma contains adipose tissue and fibrous connective tissue, both of which predominate in the nonlactational breast (Fig.

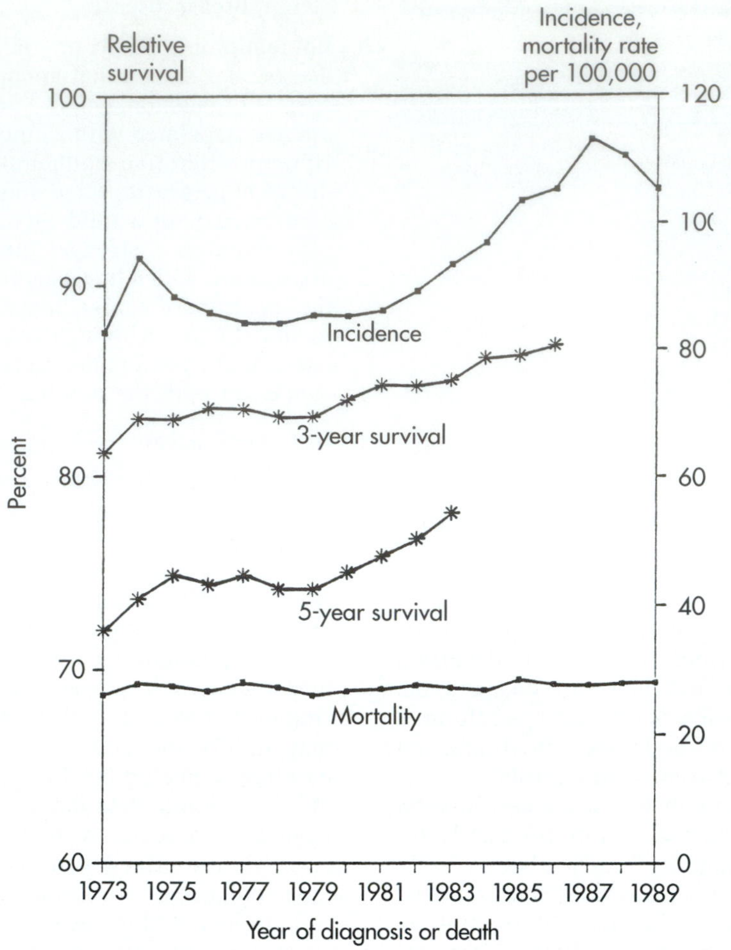


**Fig. 149-1.** Incidence, relative survival, and mortality rates of invasive breast cancer. (From Miller BA, Feuer EJ, Hankey BF, *CA Cancer J Clin* 43:27, 1993.)

149-2). The epithelial component consists of a series of 15 to 20 branching ducts that terminate in lobules with clusters of small acini. During pregnancy, this glandular component increases, so that the breast is composedmainly of epithelial elements, which persists throughout lactation. Subsequently, these changes regress, although not completely, to the virginal state. After menopause, stromal adipose tissue increases, whereas all other stromal and epithelial elements diminish.

Variations in breast anatomy are common. The majority of women have a slight asymmetry to their external breast appearance; this difference may be marked in some individuals. Accessory nipples, which are apparent at birth, are generally, but not necessarily bilateral, and occur along the midclavicular line. Breast tissue extending to the axilla may not be clinically relevant until pregnancy occurs. At this time the area becomes swollen and tender and, if this causes marked symptoms, the areas may be excised postpartum in anticipation of future pregnancies. The syndromes of virginal breast hypertrophy and Poland's syndrome, the congenital absence of the breast, nipple, and pectoralis muscles are rare. Male gynecomastia is seen commonly in the prepubertal male and is generally transient. Surgery can be performed if the patient finds significant enlargement embarrassing or painful. Gynecomastia is also common in the aging male, and is exacerbated by certain medications or hepatic dysfunction. It is characterized by classic findings on mammography.

### Histopathology of breast cancer

Most invasive breast cancers are adenocarcinomas, which can be quite heterogeneous in histologic appearance, and can be classified into several different subtypes with varying prognostic implications. Approximately 80% of adenocarcinomas are of the infiltrating ductal type. Although they vary in degree of differentiation, infiltrating ductal carcinomas have a common natural history and metastasize predominantly to the bones, lungs, liver, and brain. Infiltrating lobular carcinomas account for approximately 10% of invasive carcinomas. Although the overall prognosis is similar to that for invasive ductal carcinoma, invasive lobular carcinomas have a predilection to spread to the meninges rather than the brain parenchyma; to serosal surfaces such as the peritoneum, pleura, and ovaries; and to mediastinal and retroperitoneal lymph nodes. Less common variants of breast carcinoma, including tubular, medullary, mucinous, and papillary carcinomas, are well differentiated and carry a relatively favorable prognosis.

Noninvasive tumors confined to the lumen of the ducts are termed ductal carcinoma in situ (DCIS) or intraductal carcinomas. DCIS is the earliest form of breast cancer and

**Table 149-2.** Estimated relative risks of developing breast cancer associated with various factors

| Family history | Relative risk |
|---|---|
| 1° Relative, premenopausal | 2-3 |
| 1° Relative, postmenopausal | 1.5-2.5 |
| 1° Premenopausal relative with bilateral cancers | 9.5 |
| 1° Postmenopausal relative with bilateral cancers | 4 |
| Mother and sister | 5.6 |
| 2° Relative | 1-1.5 |
| **History of breast disease** | |
| Non-proliferative | 1 |
| Proliferative disease without atypia | 1.6-1.9 |
| Atypical hyperplasia | 4-5 |
| Atypical hyperplasia + 1° relative | 9-11 |
| LCIS | 7-10 |
| Prior breast cancer | 4 |
| **Hormonal factors** | |
| Early menarche (11 yo vs 16 yo) | 1.3 |
| Late menopause (>55 yo) | 1.5 |
| Late parity (≥30 yo vs <20 yo) | 1.9 |
| OCP use: current | 1.5 |
| >12 yrs and nulliparous | 12 |
| ERT (≥8 yrs vs. never) | 1.25 |
| **Environmental** | |
| Alcohol (3 oz/day vs. none) | 2 |
| Ionizing radiation | 1.5-4 |

*1°*, First degree; *2°*, second degree; *yo*, years old; *LCIS*, lobular carcinoma in situ; *OCP*, oral contraceptives; *ERT*, estrogen replacement therapy.

is often detected only by screening mammography. In contrast, LCIS is *not* a malignant lesion, but is a risk factor for developing an invasive breast cancer in either the ipsilateral or contralateral breast.

## EVALUATION OF A BREAST MASS

The differential diagnosis of a breast mass includes primary breast cancer; fibrocystic changes, cyst, fibroadenoma, or an associated benign mass; abscess or mastitis; phyllodes tumor; lipoma; fat necrosis; duct ectasia; sarcoma; sarcoidosis; lymphoma; metastatic cancer; skin conditions such as sebaceous cysts; costochondritis; superficial thrombophlebitis or Mondor's disease; and tumors of the chest wall. Certain lesions are most common in different age groups (Table 149-3). A new breast mass in a woman older than 50 years should be considered cancer until proved otherwise. Cancer is possible but uncommon in those less than age 35 and highly uncommon in those less than 25. The history and physical examination generally narrow this differential and ultimately pathologic examination confirms the diagnosis.

### History

The patient's age is critical in the assessment of new breast masses and helps to categorize risk. A family history of breast cancer should be noted, but because the majority of

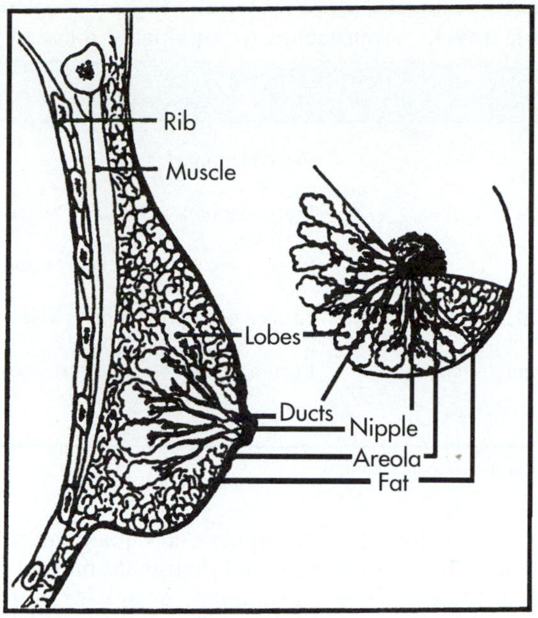


**Fig. 149-2.** Anatomy of the female breast. (Redrawn from NIH Publication No. 91-1556, October, 1990.)

women who develop breast cancer do not have a family history of this disease, a negative family history should not be designated as "protective." Duration, growth pattern, relation to menstrual cycle, spontaneous nipple discharge, pain, and tenderness are determined. The length of estrogen exposure, that is, age at menarche and menopause, are requested, as well as the use of birth control pills and estrogen replacement therapy. The number of pregnancies and live births, duration of breast feeding, a history of previous breast biopsies, timing of mammograms, and previous ultrasounds are ascertained.

Past medical history may be relevant. Previous diagnosis of colon or endometrial cancer places the patient in a higher risk category for breast cancer. Other diagnoses that may involve the breast include sarcoid, lymphoma, and metastatic melanoma. Finally, past surgery, such as oophorectomy, is important as is certain medications, such as antidepressants, which may be associated with nipple discharge.

Nipple discharge is a fairly common complaint and is generally related to a benign condition. There is increased concern if the discharge is unilateral, spontaneous, or bloody and if it emanates from one duct system alone, or occurs in a postmenopausal patient. Even with these concerns, the most common source for nipple discharge is an intraductal papilloma, a benign condition treated by excision alone. Cytologic examination of the nipple discharge may reveal malignant cells, but a negative cytologic examination does not confirm benignity. Mammography should be performed to identify any occult mass or source for the discharge followed by nipple exploration and removal. Some surgeons find ductograms helpful in delineating the anatomy of the duct system and defect.

### Physical examination

The breast is a pear-shaped structure, with the tail of Spence angled towards the axilla. The majority of active

**Table 149-3.** Approaches to a palpable mass by age

| Age | Most common lesions | Diagnostic evaluation |
|---|---|---|
| 15-25 | Fibroadenoma | Ultrasound and/or aspiration<br>Mammogram not necessary |
| 25-30 | Fibroadenoma (cyst and cancer uncommon but possible) | Ultrasound and/or aspiration<br>Mammogram if clinically suspicious |
| 35-50 | Fibrocystic changes, cancer and cysts | Mammogram (Ultrasound as recommended by mammographer) |
| Over 50 | Cancer until proven otherwise | Mammogram (Ultrasound as recommended by mammographer) |
| Pregnancy/Lactation | Lactating adenomas, cysts, mastitis, and cancer | Ultrasound, unilateral mammogram if requested by surgeon<br>Possible MRI |

*MRI,* Magnetic resonance imaging.

breast tissue is located in the upper outer quadrant, and it is in this area that most benign and malignant masses occur. When instructing breast examiners or self-examination, the breast tissue can be compared to a bunch of grapes, with the grapes signifying the lobules and the branches coalescing as the ducts at the nipple. There is a normal "lumpy" consistency to the outer breast tissue, similar to that of the outer periphery of a bunch of grapes. A true mass, however, is distinct from the bunch and possesses three dimensions. Firm masses with irregular borders are suspicious for malignancy. Normal ridges of tissue are palpable medially, where breast tissue may be accentuated by the underlying rib structure; inferiorly, where a ptotic breast forms an inframammary fold; and centrally around the edge of the nipple, where a "rim" effect may be felt. These variations should be bilateral unless surgery has altered breast symmetry.

Because of the normal cyclical changes of the breast throughout menses, the best time for examination is generally 10 to 14 days after menstruation. Immediately before the onset of menstruation, the breasts are most engorged and tender; cysts may be largest at this time and recede after menstruation. Pregnancy produces a more sustained engorgement, which is ultimately relieved with lactation. A lumpy texture results as milk is temporarily sequestered in lobules. A persistent, new mass that presents during lactation should be evaluated, however, beginning with an ultrasound evaluation. Solid masses should be biopsied, although this procedure may require a cessation of breast feeding. As the patient approaches menopause, the breast may be affected by fluctuations in hormonal levels, resulting in increased tenderness and enlarging cysts. Because the aging breast is at an increased risk for cancer, these new masses should be evaluated, aspirated if appropriate, and followed. After menopause, cysts are uncommon unless the patient is maintained on ERT. The difficulties of follow-up in the cystic breast must then be weighed against the potential benefits of ERT for a given patient.

The examination should begin with the patient disrobed in the upright position. The examiner checks for symmetry, skin thickening, nipple changes, and skin dimpling, particularly with the patient's arms raised. It is not uncommon for one breast to be slightly larger than the other, and most patients will volunteer when asked that this condition has been long-standing. The patient is then asked to lie down and raise her arm laterally above her head as each breast is examined. This maneuver is most helpful in women with large breasts. In a smaller breasted woman, the skin may be too taut with the arm raised, and the examination will be improved with the patient's arm at her side. If a patient has noted a mass herself, it is helpful to begin by asking her to point it out. The examination should then proceed, covering all four quadrants of the breast in a uniform, thorough fashion. If a patient is not familiar with self-examination, this is a good time to take her hand and repeat these steps with her hand (Fig. 149-3). Although some women find self-examination awkward, breast examination is a shared responsibility; and most patients improve with encouragement, coaching, and instructional materials.

The physical examination proceeds with an examination of the supraclavicular and axillary lymph nodes. It is common to feel small axillary lymph nodes in a thin person; however, a palpable node becomes more relevant when a coincident breast mass is also palpated. The axillary node is best examined with the patient in the upright position, with the patient's arm relaxed, resting on the examiner's forearm. The node examination may be slightly uncomfortable, as this is often a tender area in a totally benign axilla. In the unfortunate patient who presents with a highly suspicious mass, the physical examination should include a search for metastatic disease, such as hepatomegaly and points of bony tenderness.

When a breast mass is present, its physical characteristics may be helpful in determining a diagnosis. A suspicious mass is three-dimensional and firm with indistinct margins. Fibroadenomas classically are slippery smooth and easily movable within the breast. Although cysts are also smooth, they are not significantly mobile. Cysts may feel ballotable, like a water-filled balloon, or hard when they are tense with fluid. Although these characteristics are "classic," a diagnosis should not be made exclusively based on clinical characteristics. Every clinician has been fooled by a cancer that presents as a "nonsuspicious," smooth mass. Given this dilemma, it is generally safe to recommend a biopsy, which provides a definitive microscopic diagnosis.

Given the high frequency of breast cancer, every

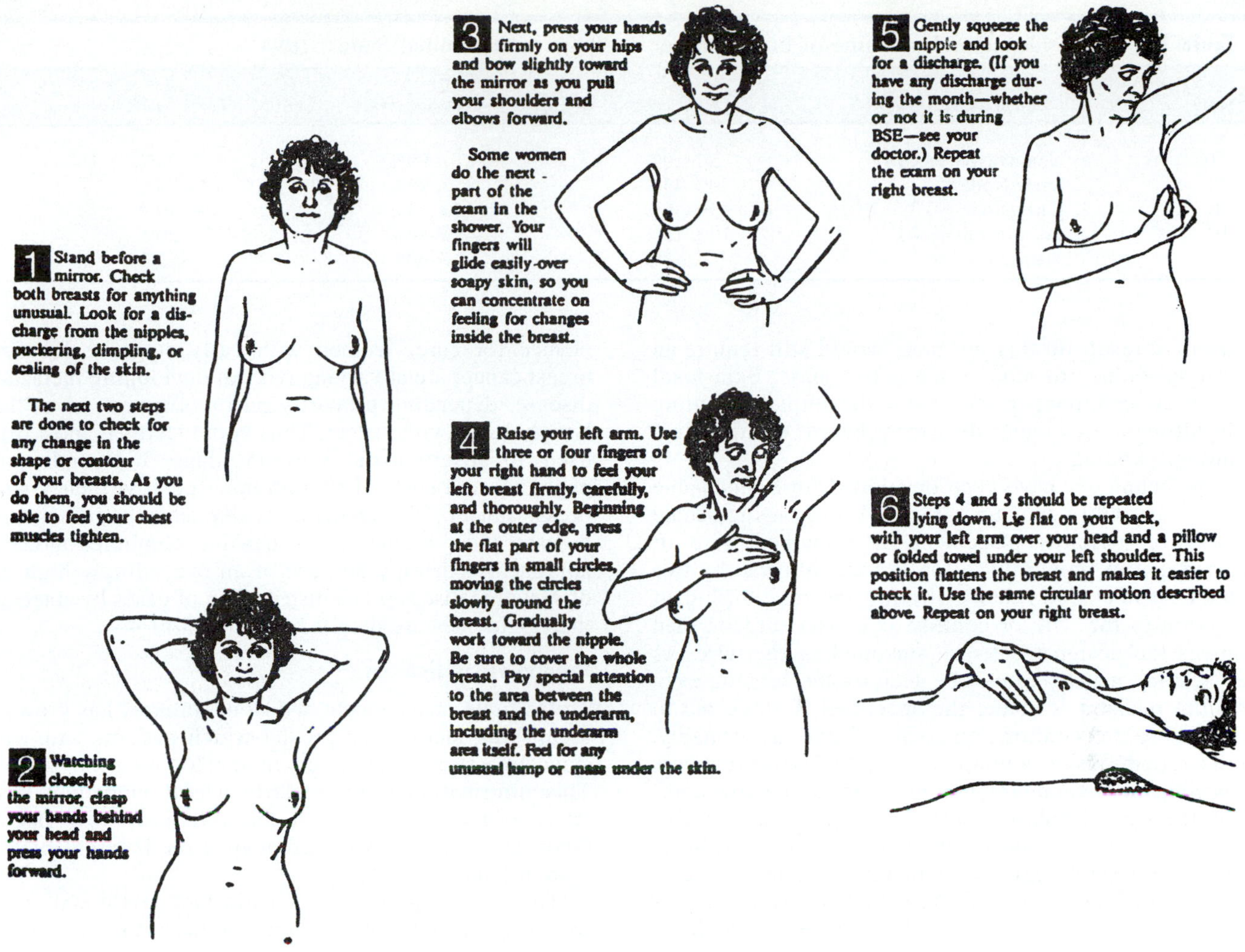

1 Stand before a mirror. Check both breasts for anything unusual. Look for a discharge from the nipples, puckering, dimpling, or scaling of the skin.
The next two steps are done to check for any change in the shape or contour of your breasts. As you do them, you should be able to feel your chest muscles tighten.
2 Watching closely in the mirror, clasp your hands behind your head and press your hands forward.
3 Next, press your hands firmly on your hips and bow slightly toward the mirror as you pull your shoulders and elbows forward.
Some women do the next part of the exam in the shower. Your fingers will glide easily over soapy skin, so you can concentrate on feeling for changes inside the breast.
4 Raise your left arm. Use three or four fingers of your right hand to feel your left breast firmly, carefully, and thoroughly. Beginning at the outer edge, press the flat part of your fingers in small circles, moving the circles slowly around the breast. Gradually work toward the nipple. Be sure to cover the whole breast. Pay special attention to the area between the breast and the underarm, including the underarm area itself. Feel for any unusual lump or mass under the skin.
5 Gently squeeze the nipple and look for a discharge. (If you have any discharge during the month—whether or not it is during BSE—see your doctor.) Repeat the exam on your right breast.
6 Steps 4 and 5 should be repeated lying down. Lie flat on your back, with your left arm over your head and a pillow or folded towel under your left shoulder. This position flattens the breast and makes it easier to check it. Use the same circular motion described above. Repeat on your right breast.


**Fig. 149-3.** Breast self-examination. (Redrawn from NIH Publication No. 91-1556, October, 1990.)

woman should be instructed regarding the three tools to early diagnosis: self examination, mammography, and examination by a health care professional. Because mammography is least helpful in the dense, lumpy breast, physical examination is an essential tool.

## Laboratory studies and diagnostic procedures

Screening mammography has led to the detection of breast cancers at earlier stages than those detected without screening. The American Cancer Society recommends that mammograms be performed every other year between the ages of 40 and 50, and every year after age 50. The benefit of screening mammography is greatest in women ages 50 to 69. In this population several studies have demonstrated a reduction of breast cancer mortality. Currently, controversy continues about the value of screening mammography in women ages 40 to 49. Results from the Canadian National Breast Screening Study showed no survival benefit from screening in this age group after 5 to 7 years. These results and others have received international attention, and the National Cancer Institute continues to examine this issue. Most clinicians believe that it is reasonable to continue to follow the recognized guidelines until sufficient evidence results in a change. Additionally, if a patient has a mother or sister who presented with premenopausal breast cancer, the screening recommendations are moved up by 10 years; at a minimum, yearly mammograms are performed after age 40. Issues about screening should not be confused with the importance of mammography in the work-up of symptomatic patients.

When mammographic abnormalities are seen on a screening study, patients may be asked to return for magnification or compression views to clarify a problem. In the case of a cancer, compression may accentuate the finding, whereas in normal dense parenchyma, the abnormality will be dispersed. Macrocalcifications are not related to cancers, but clustered microcalcifications, which are laid down within a lobule or duct, can herald an early malignant lesion. An increase in the number and density of microcalcifications is a common reason for biopsy, even though only 25% to 30% of biopsies performed for microcalcifications yield the diagnosis of cancer. If possible, it is often reassuring to show patients their mammographic abnormality. This approach gives them a real estimate of the minute size of the lesion being addressed.

Biopsies can be performed using several different methods. If a mass is palpable, a needle biopsy may be performed in the surgeon's office. This procedure is generally reserved for a mass that is suspicious for cancer.

**Table 149-4.** Incidence and outcome of breast cancer by stage in the United States, 1994

| Stage | Clinical presentation | % Total cases | 5-Year survival | "Cure" rate |
|---|---|---|---|---|
| 0 | Noninvasive (DCIS) | 5%-10% | 99% | 98% |
| I | Early/Node (–) | 40%-45% | 85%-95% | 70% |
| II | Early/Node (+) | 35%-40% | 65%-75% | 30%-40% |
| III | Locally Advanced | 10%-15% | 45%-50% | 5%-20% |
| IV | Metastatic | ~7% | 20%-30% | 0-2% |

A negative result, in this instance, would still require an excisional biopsy to remove the entire mass. Excisional biopsies are commonly performed in the outpatient setting with ultimate treatment decisions based on the final pathologic finding.

New techniques have been developed for nonpalpable masses seen only by mammography. Biopsy using needle localization requires placement of a barbed wire or contrast dye in proximity to the lesion, followed by two mammographic views demonstrating the relationship of the lesion to the wire or contrast dye. The surgeon then removes the designated tissue surrounding the wire. As the "lesion" usually cannot be seen by the surgeon even after the incision is made, the specimen is subjected to radiography to confirm removal of the abnormality. Stereotactic biopsy is a relatively new technique that uses a specialized mammographic machine to localize precisely the area of breast abnormality. Approximately five needle biopsies are taken, which provide core samples of tissue for pathologic examination. The technique is valuable in diagnosing a finding highly suspicious for cancer on mammography as well as lesions thought to be consistent with a fibroadenoma or intramammary lymph node. A core biopsy that confirms a benign lesion such as a fibroadenoma negates the need for an open biopsy. If the biopsy yields only normal breast tissue, however, an open biopsy is recommended if the lesion is highly suspicious for cancer; alternatively a 6-month follow-up mammogram may be recommended for less suspicious lesions.

The role of magnetic resonance imaging (MRI), Doppler ultrasound, and other modalities in the diagnosis of breast cancer is currently being investigated. These techniques may differentiate malignancy from benign disease based on differences in enhancement and vascular signals. More proof of clinical efficacy is needed before the techniques become part of the routine evaluation of the breast.

## BREAST CANCER MANAGEMENT

### Staging

The success of cancer treatment depends on three main variables: tumor burden, responsiveness of the tumor to treatment, and performance status of the patient. The purpose of staging is to provide an estimate of tumor burden in order to guide treatment. Patients with ductal carcinoma in situ (stage 0) have the best outcome, with nearly universal cure; patients with distant metastases (stage IV) have the worst prognosis, with essentially no chance for cure. Women with early stage or localized breast cancer are at varying risks of developing metastatic disease, depending primarily on involvement of axillary lymph nodes with cancer. Thus nodal status is most often used to discriminate between stage I (lymph node negative) and stage II (lymph node positive) early stage breast cancer. Women with locally advanced (stage III) breast cancer require an aggressive combined-modality approach to therapy because of an exceedingly high risk of systemic disease. The distribution of cases by stage and their outcomes are detailed in Table 149-4.

### Prognostic indicators

To facilitate management decisions, interest has grown in identifying factors that predict which patients with early stage breast cancer are likely to develop recurrent disease. This information is particularly useful in patients with stage I disease for whom the relatively low risk of recurrence must be balanced against the inherent risks of systemic adjuvant therapy.

The most important prognostic factor is nodal status, followed by hormone receptor status. Patients without lymph node metastases (node-negative patients) have a significantly lower risk of developing and dying from recurrent breast cancer than do patients who have nodal metastases (node-positive patients). Furthermore, the risk of recurrence and mortality increases with the number of nodal metastases. Women with tumors that express either estrogen receptors (ER-positive tumors) or progesterone receptors (PR-positive tumors) have an improved prognosis, are more likely to benefit from adjuvant hormonal therapy, and are more likely to respond to hormonal therapy for metastatic disease than women with receptor-negative tumors.

In patients with node-negative disease, indices such as the size of the primary tumor, the proliferative rate, and the DNA content are important in determining whether and how to administer adjuvant systemic therapy. Generally, tumors less than 1 cm in diameter have a low risk of recurrence. Laboratory analysis by flow cytometry detects tumors that are rapidly dividing (high fraction of cells in S-phase) and/or whose cells have an abnormal amount of DNA (aneuploid tumors). Such tumors carry a worse prognosis than those that are slowly dividing (low S-phase) and/or contain the normal (i.e., diploid) content of DNA (Table 149-5).

## TREATMENT OF DUCTAL CARCINOMA IN SITU

The use of mammography has dramatically increased the number of women diagnosed with DCIS over the last 10

**Table 149-5.** Prognostic indicators

| | Favorable | Unfavorable |
|---|---|---|
| Nodal Status | Negative | Positive |
| ER/PR Status | Positive | Negative |
| Tumor Size | <1 cm | ≥2 cm |
| Proliferative Rate | Low S-phase fraction | High S-phase fraction |
| DNA Content | Diploid | Aneuploid |

years. These lesions are most often identified on mammograms as clustered microcalcifications with or without a palpable mass. Although this lesion was traditionally treated by mastectomy in the past, recent data support the efficacy of lumpectomy and radiation for women with localized DCIS. Treatment decisions are tailored to the clinical scenario. For example, when a minute focus of DCIS is discovered, lumpectomy alone may be used. Alternatively, when mammography demonstrates extensive microcalcifications involving a large segment of the breast, simple mastectomy is the preferred treatment. Generally, axillary lymph node dissection is not required in the treatment of DCIS. Exceptions to this approach include involvement of a large area of breast in which an area of microinvasion may be missed on histology and the diagnosis of comedeocarcinoma, which is known to have a low but recognized chance of lymph node metastases. The role of tamoxifen in the treatment of DCIS is investigational.

## PRIMARY THERAPY OF INVASIVE BREAST CANCER

The standard options for the primary treatment of invasive breast cancer include lumpectomy and axillary lymph node dissection followed by radiation therapy, or modified radical mastectomy, which includes a lymph node dissection. Multiple studies have shown that equivalent survival rates are achieved with either choice. Survival rates ultimately reflect spread beyond the breast, so the primary treatment of the breast itself has little effect on metastatic potential.

The goal of lumpectomy is to achieve negative microscopic margins. If the initial biopsy demonstrating cancer resulted in positive margins, then a reexcision is performed at the time of lymph node dissection. Radiation therapy is given over 6 weeks in divided doses, sometimes supplemented by a "boost" to the lumpectomy site with x-rays, electron beam, or brachytherapy. The patient is followed by interval mammography of the treated breast and the contralateral breast. Local recurrence rates are approximately 10% to 15% over a 5-year follow-up and are generally treated by mastectomy.

Indications for modified radical mastectomy, which spares the chest wall muscles, include large tumors in a relatively small breast. If the lumpectomy will result in a distorted appearance or positive margins, then mastectomy is preferable. Traditionally, subareolar lesions were treated by mastectomy, but many patients prefer lumpectomy, which results in a breast without a nipple, to a reconstructed breast. These options must be discussed with the patient. Patients with multifocal disease, a history of prior chest irradiation, collagen vascular disease, or inability to travel for radiation also benefit from mastectomy.

Breast reconstruction can be accomplished at the time of the primary treatment or after chemotherapy. If the physician and patient are concerned about the apparent aggressiveness of a tumor with suspicious palpable axillary nodes at the time of presentation, then reconstruction should be delayed, as wound healing or implant infections could prolong the postoperative convalescent period and delay further treatment. Other than this consideration, reconstruction at the time of mastectomy has multiple benefits including one operative procedure and hospitalization, as well as the improved cosmetic results. The choice of reconstruction is decided by the patient and plastic surgeon, based on body habitus and personal choice. Common options currently include saline implant placement or a myocutaneous flap that uses an abdominal muscle (and results in a "tummy-tuck" as well) or the latissimus dorsi muscle.

## ADJUVANT THERAPY OF EARLY BREAST CANCER

Adjuvant therapy is administered to patients with early stage invasive breast cancer when there is a strong potential for relapse due to undetectable micrometastases. Because approximately 70% of patients with node-positive and 30% of patients with node-negative malignancies eventually develop metastatic breast cancer, a large cohort of women stand to benefit from adjuvant chemotherapy. In fact all women may benefit from adjuvant therapy, because the treatment delays the onset of metastatic disease, even when micrometastases are not eradicated.

An analysis of more than 130 randomized clinical trials of systemic adjuvant therapy worldwide has provided clear evidence that adjuvant therapy can enhance the survival of women with early stage breast cancer. Adjuvant therapy reduces the annual rate of recurrence of breast cancer by 25% to 28% and the annual rate of death by 16% to 25%.

### Node-positive patients

Benefits of adjuvant chemotherapy were first established in node-positive women. Combination chemotherapy regimens such as CMF (cyclophosphamide, methotrexate and 5-fluorouracil) or CAF (A=adriamycin® [doxorubicin]), administered for 6 months, reduced the risk of disease recurrence by approximately one third for all node-positive patients, especially those under the age of 50 with one to three positive lymph nodes. High-dose chemotherapy with autologous bone marrow or peripheral stem cell support is under active investigation for women who are at high risk of recurrence (i.e., those with four or more positive lymph nodes). Using this approach, 70% of patients with 10 or more involved lymph nodes have remained free of disease after 6 years, compared to 30% to 40% of historical controls treated with conventional chemotherapy.

Oophorectomy, which removes the principal source of estrogen, is a highly effective way to improve survival of premenopausal women with early stage breast cancer. Pharmacologic therapy with the antiestrogen tamoxifen prolongs disease-free and overall survival in both premenopausal and postmenopausal women, although the benefit is stronger in the latter group. Tamoxifen is most effective in cases in which the tumor is hormone-receptor positive. Overall, adjuvant tamoxifen administered for at least 5 years reduces the risk of recurrence by 25% and the risk of death by 17%. The risk of developing a contralateral second primary breast cancer is reduced by 40%. Furthermore, because tamoxifen displays estrogen-agonist properties in the cardiovascular and skeletal systems, the risk of death from vascular disease is reduced by 25% and loss of bone mineral density is slowed. Treatment with combination of chemotherapy with tamoxifen is still investigational.

### Node-negative disease

As in patients with node-positive disease, adjuvant therapy clearly improves disease-free and overall survival of women with node-negative breast cancer. However, three fourths of patients with stage I breast cancer will be cured by primary treatment with surgery and/or radiation therapy alone. The decision to administer adjuvant chemotherapy (usually CMF) or tamoxifen to node-negative patients depends on risk factors for relapse. Women whose tumors display multiple unfavorable prognostic indicators have approximately a 50% risk for recurrence within 5 years and would be more likely to benefit from adjuvant therapy (see Table 149-5). Women with only favorable prognostic indicators probably do not need adjuvant therapy because their survival approaches that of the general population. For patients with other combinations of risk factors, however, the best approach is less clear.

### Toxicity of adjuvant therapy

The benefits of adjuvant endocrine therapy and chemotherapy must be weighed against the risks of immediate and delayed toxicity. Tamoxifen is quite well tolerated in most patients and is associated with very few side effects. The major toxic effects occur in premenopausal patients and are limited to hot flashes (55%) and irregular menses (40% to 60%). One fourth of both premenopausal and postmenopausal women experience increased vaginal discharge. Phlebitis and early stage endometrial carcinoma occur infrequently. Tamoxifen has additional long-term side effects that are beneficial rather than detrimental, such as improvement in bone mineral density and serum lipid profile and a reduction in ischemic heart disease.

The major acute toxicities associated with adjuvant chemotherapy are listed in Table 149-6. Fatigue occurs in over 50% of patients, regardless of the regimen. Weight gains of 4 to 5 kg within 1 year are typical. Marked alopecia is rare with six cycles of CMF, but occurs in virtually 100% of patients receiving doxorubicin. Leukopenia occurs more frequently with doxorubicin-containing regimens as well, but life-threatening infections are rare.

Premature menopause occurs in 95% of patients over age 40 who are receiving standard adjuvant chemotherapy regimens. It is associated with all the symptoms of natural menopause, including hot flashes, atrophic vaginitis, decreased libido, infertility, osteoporosis, and increased risk of cardiovascular disease.

**Table 149-6.** Toxicities of adjuvant therapy

| | Common | Rare |
|---|---|---|
| Tamoxifen | Hot flashes<br>Irregular menses<br>Vaginal discharge | Thromboembolic events<br>Endometrial cancer |
| Chemotherapy | Fatigue<br>Weight gain<br>Myelosuppression<br>Menopausal signs and symptoms<br>Nausea and vomiting<br>Alopecia (doxorubicin)<br>Mucositis<br>Psychologic distress | Sepsis<br>Hemorrhagic cystitis<br>Conjunctivitis<br>Congestive heart failure |

## LOCALLY ADVANCED BREAST CANCER

The term *locally advanced breast cancer* (LABC) has been applied to a heterogeneous group of patients with large tumors, extensive regional lymph node metastases, or involvement of the skin or chest wall. This group composes 10% to 15% of breast cancer patients in the United States. The majority of patients with LABC will develop distant metastases and, thus, have a uniformly poor prognosis without aggressive therapy.

Current management includes neoadjuvant or induction chemotherapy before definitive treatment of the primary lesion. This strategy improves both local and distant control, with more than 90% of patients rendered free of all gross disease. Locoregional care with surgery and/or radiation follows induction therapy. Dose-intense adjuvant and neoadjuvant regimens of chemotherapy with bone marrow or stem cell support are currently under investigation, and preliminary results are encouraging. Combined-modality therapy appears to have substantially improved survival in patients with LABC, with up to 50% of patients surviving for 5 years or more.

### Inflammatory breast carcinoma

Inflammatory breast carcinoma (IBC) is often distinguished from other forms of locally advanced breast cancer because of its aggressive natural history, with almost uniform mortality within 2 years due to the rapid development of disseminated disease. Clinical diagnosis is based on diffuse enlargement of the breast with erythema and induration or peau d'orange appearance of the skin. Because there is often no discrete underlying mass, this entity is often confused with acute mastitis. The latter, however, rarely occurs in nonlactating women. Involvement of dermal lymphatics with tumor emboli is the pathologic hallmark of IBC. Treatment strategy for inflammatory carcinoma is similar to that of locally advanced breast cancer. Five-year survival ranges from 30% to 75%.

### Follow-up after treatment of early-stage breast cancer

All breast cancer patients should undergo lifetime surveillance for second primary breast cancers, as well as for recurrent disease. Although the majority of metastases occur within 5 years of diagnosis, relapses may be delayed for as long as two or three decades. Follow-up evaluations should include a history and complete physical examination, complete blood count (CBC), liver function tests, and yearly mammography. Patients are typically seen every 3 to 4 months for the first 3 years, twice a year for the next 2 years, and then yearly.

Most patients with recurrent breast cancer present with specific symptoms. There is no definitive evidence that early detection of asymptomatic metastases improves survival or palliation. Thus, although symptoms should be investigated to rule out metastatic disease, routine screening with chest radiographs, bone scans, and computed tomography (CT) scans is not indicated.

## RECURRENT BREAST CANCER

Metastatic breast cancer is a diverse disease. Its course ranges from indolent progression with a high quality of life, to rapidly disabling symptoms. Twenty percent to 30% of patients survive for 5 years, and up to 10% of patients survive for more than 10 years. The median survival is 2 to 3 years.

Metastatic breast cancer is among the few solid tumors for which effective therapy is available, but treatment is generally palliative rather than curative. Although the majority of patients are responsive to systemic therapy, few achieve a complete remission (i.e., resolution of all evidence of disease). The primary goal of systemic therapy is the relief of symptoms and improvement or maintenance of a high quality of life. In many cases, even a toxic therapy that induces tumor shrinkage is more likely to improve quality of life than a nontoxic regimen with a low probability of response.

The general approach to the management of metastatic breast cancer is similar to that of all malignancies. The patient first undergoes a staging work-up to determine the extent of disease. Treatment is administered for a given period of time, followed by restaging to assess response. Typically, a patient with breast cancer is treated for 2 to 4 months before restaging. A decision is then made whether to continue with the same therapy, change to a different therapy, or discontinue therapy altogether.

### Sites of metastases

Breast cancers can metastasize to virtually any organ, leading to a variety of symptoms and complications. Patients who eventually die of breast cancer have at autopsy widespread disease to lung, liver, and bone in 50% to 70% of cases.

Locoregional recurrence following mastectomy is a strong predictor of systemic disease. Resection, if feasible, followed by radiotherapy is the treatment of choice for isolated chest wall recurrence. If the disease involves only this area, then local therapy may be all that is warranted, particularly if the time between primary therapy and recurrence (disease-free interval) is prolonged. Radiotherapy is indicated for the palliation of localized pain from inoperable metastases to the chest wall, axilla, or brachial plexus. Hormone therapy and chemotherapy each can be effective in controlling local disease that is not amenable to surgery or radiation, or that occurs coincident with systemic disease. In addition to local therapy, most patients eventually require systemic therapy, because they develop distant metastases that lead ultimately to death.

Recurrence in the breast after lumpectomy and radiation therapy does not confer the same dire prognosis as recurrence following mastectomy. Salvage mastectomy or, in rare cases, repeated lumpectomy leads to prolonged survival in more than 50% of patients.

The most common initial site of metastasis in breast cancer is bone. Bone metastases cause significant morbidity because of pain, pathologic fractures with resultant loss of function, and hypercalcemia. Furthermore, expansion of vertebral metastases is the most common route of entry into the epidural space, leading to spinal cord compression with resultant paralysis. Ideally, pathologic fractures of long bones and spinal cord compression should be avoided by a rapid and aggressive work-up and intervention when the patient complains of skeletal pain. Radionuclide bone scanning is the most sensitive method for diagnosing skeletal metastases. Abnormalities in weight-bearing bones should be further evaluated to rule out impending fractures that may require prophylactic orthopedic intervention.

Besides bone, the lungs and pleurae are the most common sites of metastases from breast cancer. The major manifestations of pulmonary metastases include dry, irrepressible cough and dyspnea, whether from parenchymal disease, endobronchial metastases, or malignant pleural effusions. Although systemic therapy is indicated primarily, highly symptomatic patients may require interventions that provide more rapid palliation. Chest tube drainage of large pleural effusions, followed by pleurodesis produces symptomatic responses lasting longer than 1 month in 80% to 90% of patients. Endobronchial lesions that cause proximal airway obstruction can be effectively treated with laser ablation in the majority of patients. High doses of corticosteroids may provide some relief of dyspnea in patients with lymphangitic carcinomatosis refractory to chemotherapy.

The incidence of clinically manifest brain metastases is approximately 10%. Presenting symptoms include headaches, behavioral changes, seizures, and focal neurologic deficits. After diagnosis with CT or MRI scans, symptomatic brain metastases are treated with high doses of dexamethasone along with whole-brain irradiation. Surgery should be considered for the minority of patients with solitary metastases and well-controlled systemic disease. In one randomized trial, patients undergoing resection of a solitary brain metastasis followed by radiotherapy had a prolonged survival and better functional status than those who underwent radiotherapy alone.

Leptomeningeal metastasis (or carcinomatous meningitis) presents with cranial nerve palsies and spinal or nerve root symptoms, along with the less specific findings of headache, nausea, vomiting, and mental status changes. Diagnosis is made by cytologic evaluation of the cerebrospinal fluid, although meningeal enhancement on gadolinium-enhanced MRI scans is highly suggestive. Treatment involves intrathecal chemotherapy. Whole-brain irradiation may be administered for symptomatic cranial nerve palsies or other focal findings. Although the majority of patients improve with therapy, fewer than 10% of patients survive for more than 1 year.

Breast cancer is the most common cause of epidural spinal cord compression. Rapid diagnosis and treatment are crucial to prevent permanent paralysis and sphincter dysfunction. Progressive back pain is the heralding symptom and is often accompanied by radicular pain. Signs of myelopathy, weakness, and sensory loss ensue and may progress rapidly. Total spine MRI scans have supplanted myelography for rapid diagnosis and should be obtained at the first suspicion of cord compression. High doses of dexamethasone should be instituted immediately upon diagnosis, followed by spinal irradiation. The majority of patients will experience pain relief with treatment; however, impairment in ambulation or sphincter function is often irreversible and depends on the length of time the cord has been compromised. Neurosurgical intervention should be considered for rapidly progressive neurologic dysfunction.

### Staging and treatment

When metastatic disease has been documented at one site, a staging work-up is performed to determine the sites and extent of metastases. Staging typically includes laboratory evaluation (CBC, liver enzymes, calcium, and tumor markers such as carcinoembryonic antigen [CEA] and CA15-3), CT scans of the chest and liver, and a radionuclide bone scan.

The selection of systemic therapy is determined by the sites of metastatic disease, hormone receptor status of the tumor, patient age, and disease-free interval (DFI). In general, patients with disease confined to soft tissue or bone are more likely to respond to endocrine therapy and survive longer than those with visceral disease. Patients with metastases involving the liver, or with lymphangitic spread to the lungs, are poor candidates for endocrine therapy and should be considered for chemotherapy. In addition, patients whose tumors display either estrogen receptors or progesterone receptors have a better prognosis, and more than 60% respond to hormonal manipulation. Patients with a DFI longer than 2 years have a significantly longer survival and a higher probability of responding to endocrine therapy than those who have a shorter DFI.

### Endocrine therapy

Pharmacologic doses of estrogens, antiestrogens, progestins, androgens, or corticosteroids, as well as pituitary, adrenal, and ovarian blockade, have been used to treat metastatic breast cancer with nearly equivalent response rates. Tamoxifen is currently the hormonal treatment of choice because of its low toxicity profile (see Adjuvant Therapy). Approximately two thirds of hormone-receptor-positive patients respond to tamoxifen therapy.

Up to half of hormone-sensitive patients who eventually fail tamoxifen therapy respond subsequently to secondary hormonal agents. Megestrol acetate (Megace) is the progestational agent commonly used in the United States. Its principal toxicity, which occurs in 20% to 50% of patients, is weight gain due to appetite stimulation. Fluid retention may be prohibitive in patients with cardiac dysfunction. Equivalent responses can be expected with aminoglutethimide. This agent inhibits the conversion of adrenal androgens to estrogens. Androgens, high doses of estrogens, and corticosteroids are rarely used because of undue toxicity.

Five percent to 10% of patients who begin endocrine therapy experience a tumor flare, a transient worsening of pain at sites of bone metastases, within hours to weeks of treatment onset. Hypercalcemia may be induced or may worsen during this period, but can usually be managed with supportive care without discontinuing treatment.

### Chemotherapy

Combination chemotherapy results in an objective (measurable) response in approximately two thirds of patients with metastatic breast cancer. Complete remission, however, is observed in only about 20% of cases, and the median duration of response is about 1 year. Objective response rates to secondary regimens are in the range of 20% to 35%. The median survival after chemotherapy is initiated is approximately 3 years, but rare patients may survive as long as 10 years. Chemotherapy is indicated for symptomatic patients who are not good candidates for endocrine therapy. This group includes patients who have failed to respond to hormonal manipulation, are ER-negative, have had a short DFI, or have liver lesions or lymphangitic spread in the lungs.

Combinations of cyclophosphamide and fluorouracil with either methotrexate (CMF) or doxorubicin (CAF) comprise the primary regimens for most patients. Agents used mainly in salvage regimens include other alkylating agents (e.g., thiotepa or melphalan), mitomycin C, vinblastine, mitoxantrone, etoposide, cisplatin, and the novel agent, paclitaxel (Taxol).

The most frequent toxicities observed with these chemotherapeutic agents are myelosuppression, nausea, vomiting, mucositis, and alopecia. Toxicities specific to individual agents include cardiotoxicity with doxorubicin, hemorrhagic cystitis with cyclophosphamide, pulmonary toxicity with mitomycin C, neuropathy and nephrotoxicity with cisplatin, and constipation with vinblastine.

Unlike hormonal agents that are administered continuously for as long as response persists, the continuing administration of chemotherapy is not more effective than limiting the duration of therapy to about 6 months in responding patients. Patients may then be followed after therapy until symptomatic progression occurs.

### High-dose therapy

Recently, the focus of clinical research for metastatic breast cancer has shifted from palliation to cure for selected patients. Early findings indicate that the use of high-dose chemotherapy followed by autologous bone marrow transplant or peripheral blood stem cell support may improve both the disease-free and overall survival. The best candidates for this approach appear to be patients previously untreated for metastatic disease who have chemosensitive disease, with minimal residual tumor burden after standard doses of induction chemotherapy. In early clinical trials, 20% to 25% of patients have remained disease free off therapy for up to 3.5 years. Longer follow-up times are necessary to determine whether these patients have been cured.

## SPECIAL CIRCUMSTANCES

### Breast cancer prevention

The stable mortality rate of breast cancer despite advances in early diagnosis and treatment has prompted investigations into preventive measures using hormonal, dietary, and vitamin manipulations. Two nationwide clinical trials have been designed to study interventions that may reduce the incidence of breast cancers, the Breast Cancer Prevention Trial (BCPT), conducted by the National Surgical Adjuvant Breast and Bowel Project, and the Women's Health Initiative (WHI) sponsored by the National Institutes of Health. The BCPT is designed to determine whether the antiestrogen tamoxifen can prevent breast cancer in women who are at increased risk of developing the disease. The WHI is designed to test the overlapping effects of a low-fat diet, estrogen replacement therapy, and calcium supplements on the incidence of cardiovascular disease, breast cancer, colon cancer, and osteoporosis. Results of both trials will likely become available during the next decade. In addition, a clinical trial evaluating the vitamin A derivative, fenretinide, for the prevention of second primary breast cancers is underway in Europe.

Prophylactic mastectomy is reserved for highly selected patients who fall into a high-risk category. The indications for prophylactic mastectomy that are supported by the Society of Surgical Oncology include atypical hyperplasia of lobular or ductal origin, particularly if it is bilateral and multifocal; family history of premenopausal bilateral breast cancer in a mother or sister (family cancer syndrome), and fibronodular, dense breasts that are mammographically and clinically difficult to follow, coupled with either of the preceding problems.

### Breast cancer and pregnancy

Gestational breast cancer complicates approximately 1/1000 pregnancies, accounting for about 3% of all breast cancers and 7% to 14% of breast cancers in women under age 40. Historically, breast cancer diagnosed during pregnancy was thought to carry a particularly poor prognosis. More recent studies, however, in which pregnant patients were compared with age- and stage-matched controls, have not demonstrated any difference in prognosis. Nonetheless, pregnant patients generally have more advanced disease at presentation, presumably due to delayed diagnosis of up to several months.

Modified radical mastectomy is the local treatment of choice for gestational breast cancer unless the pregnancy is terminated or the diagnosis is made close to the time of delivery, because the radiotherapy necessary for breast preservation is contraindicated during pregnancy.

Pregnancy after treatment for breast cancer has not been associated with increased risk of recurrence. Nonetheless, patients should be counseled that the risk of breast cancer recurrence continues for several years after the primary diagnosis, and family planning decisions should be made accordingly.

### Estrogen replacement therapy after breast cancer

ERT decreases the morbidity and mortality of cardiovascular disease and osteoporosis in postmenopausal women. Because premature menopause is a common side effect of adjuvant therapy for early stage breast cancer, without the benefits of ERT many young women face the risks of premature heart and bone disease and other conditions related to estrogen deficiency. Although the addition of progestins to estrogen protects against the development of estrogen-dependent endometrial carcinomas, however, the effects of hormone replacement therapy on the breast are unclear. Furthermore, antiestrogen therapy with tamoxifen decreases both breast cancer recurrence rates and second primary breast cancers. For these reasons, ERT is not advisable for patients with a history of breast cancer.

### Breast cancer in the elderly

Breast cancer in the elderly generally follows a more indolent course, often presenting as a well-circumscribed mass in this unscreened population. Mammography is helpful in estimating the amount of breast involvement and thus in planning treatment. Lumpectomy followed by tamoxifen alone can be substituted for more aggressive forms of treatment, particularly when extreme old age or other medical illnesses complicate the use of conventional therapy.

### Breast cancer in men

Of the 183,000 cases of breast cancer diagnosed yearly in the United States, 1,000 (0.5%) occur in men, resulting in about 300 deaths a year. The mean age of men diagnosed with breast cancer is in the range of 60 to 70 years, approximately a decade older than that of women with breast cancer. Risk factors are similar to those in women: family history, exposure to radiation, high endogenous estrogen levels (secondary to liver disease or Klinefelter's syndrome), or exposure to exogenous estrogens. Stage for stage, survival rates are similar for men and women.

Management of male breast cancer parallels that for female breast cancer. Local treatment generally consists of mastectomy, followed by radiotherapy for locally advanced disease. The efficacy of adjuvant chemotherapy or tamoxifen for node-positive cancer in men has not been evaluated in randomized trials because of the small number of patients, but is probably similar to that in women.

## BIBLIOGRAPHY


Early Breast Cancer Trialists' Collaborative: Systemic treatment of early breast cancer by hormonal, cytotoxic or immune therapy, *Lancet* 339:1-15, 71-85, 1992.

Fisher B et al: Lumpectomy compared with lumpectomy and radiation therapy for the treatment of intraductal breast cancer, *N Engl J Med* 328:1581, 1993.

Fletcher S and Fletcher R: The breast is close to the heart, *Ann Intern Med* 117:969, 1992.

Harris JR, Hellman S, Henderson IC, Kinne DW, editors. *Breast diseases,* ed 2, Philadelphia, 1992, JB Lippincott.

Harris JR et al: Breast cancer, *N Engl J Med* 327:319-328, 390-398, 473-380, 1992.

Harris JR, Morrow M, Bonadonna G: Cancer of the breast. In DeVita VT Jr, Hellman S, Rosenberg SA, editors: *Cancer: principles and practice of oncology,* ed 4, Philadelphia, 1993, JB Lippincott.

Marshall E: Breast cancer research: a special report, *Science* 259:616, 1993.

McGuire WL and Clark GM: Prognostic factors and treatment decisions in axillary node-negative breast cancer, *N Engl J Med* 326:1756, 1992.

Shapiro CL and Henderson IC, guest editors: New directions in breast cancer. *Hematol Oncol Clin North Am* 8(1), 1994.

SSO NEWS, Newsletter of the Soc of Surg Onc, Inc. Summer, 1993.

CHAPTER

# 150 Gynecologic Neoplasms

Setsuko K. Chambers
Joseph T. Chambers

Endometrial cancer is the most common gynecologic cancer in the United States, followed by ovarian and cervical cancer (Table 150-1). In general the peak age for invasive gynecologic cancers is between 55 and 65 years (Fig. 150-1); in contrast the peak age for carcinoma in situ of the cervix is between 25 and 35 years. The mortality rate for ovarian cancers exceeds that for cancers of the cervix and endometrium combined (Fig. 150-2). The survival rates for these cancers correlate with the extent of the disease at diagnosis. Early detection is the best chance for cure. Unfortunately, except for cervical cancer screening with Pap smears, effective screening does not exist for gynecologic cancers. Endometrial cancer usually presents with abnormal bleeding in its early stages; however, ovarian cancer, the most lethal gynecologic cancer, has a vague presentation and is advanced at the time of diagnosis in most women. Lack of recognition of the correct diagnosis adds to the delay. If cancer of the gynecologic organs is suspected, a prompt referral for a gynecologic oncology consultation should be obtained.

## CERVICAL CANCER/ABNORMAL PAP SMEAR

### Epidemiology and risk factors

Although cervical cancer ranks as the third most common form of gynecologic cancer, it is the second most common cause of gynecologic cancer death. Every year 1.2 million new cases of cervical intraepithelial neoplasia (CIN), including 55,000 new cases of carcinoma in situ (CIS), are detected. These terms refer to the presence of abnormal or dysplastic cells in the squamous epithelium of the cervix; CIN 1, 2, and 3 refer to mild, moderate, or severe dysplastic changes respectively; CIS is included in the CIN 3 category.

Sexual activity is generally thought to be a prerequisite for the development of cervical neoplasia. This theory may relate to the possible etiologic, or at best strong associational, effects of certain sexually transmitted diseases, such as human papilloma virus (HPV), human immunodeficiency virus (HIV), or herpes simplex virus (HSV). Although there is strong evidence for an etiologic role HPV infection alone does not appear to constitute sufficient cause for cervical neoplasia and requires a cocarcinogen for its actions. The importance of immunosuppression in the development of malignancies is demonstrated in the association between HIV infections and CIN; nearly half of HIV-infected women demonstrate CIN on routine colposcopy, with the majority coinfected with HPV. Smoking, with its propensity for DNA damage, carries a fourfold increased risk for the development of cervical cancer. Infrequently, an unusual form of cervical cancer (such as the diethylstilbestrol [DES]-associated clear cell carcinoma) may develop in a woman who has never been sexually active.

Minority populations are at significant risk for cervical cancer; unfortunately, this population is not being effectively reached by Pap smear screening programs. Education and compliance of the general population add to the problems. A recent, large study revealed that 40% of the general population do not receive annual Pap smears; older and low-income women were least likely to have ever had a Pap smear.

### Pathophysiology

Studies of the natural history of CIN have attempted to ascertain its significance. In one large study, 70% of untreated CIS progressed to invasive cervical cancer, and no cases regressed. Although 30% to 40% of earlier stage dysplasias regressed without treatment, the rest remained

**Table 150-1.** Gynecologic cancers in the United States, 1993

| Site | New cases | Annual cancer deaths |
|---|---|---|
| All gynecologic cancer | 71,500 | 24,400 |
| Invasive cervix | 13,500 | 4,400 |
| In situ cervix | 55,000 | 0 |
| Corpus uteri | 31,000 | 5,700 |
| Ovary | 22,000 | 13,300 |
| Other gynecologic | 5,000 | 1,000 |

From American Cancer Society, CA: *Cancer Clinicians* 43(1):7-26, 1993.

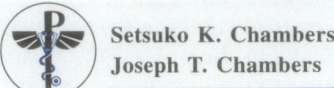

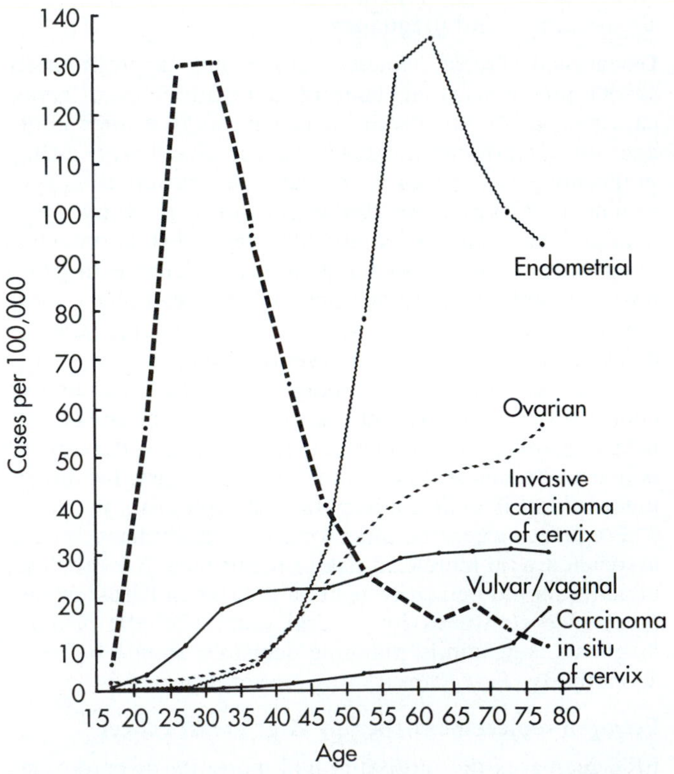


**Fig. 150-1.** Age-specific incidence curves for gynecologic cancers in the United States. (From Knapp RC, Berkowitz RS, editors: *Gynecologic oncology,* New York, 1986, Macmillan.)

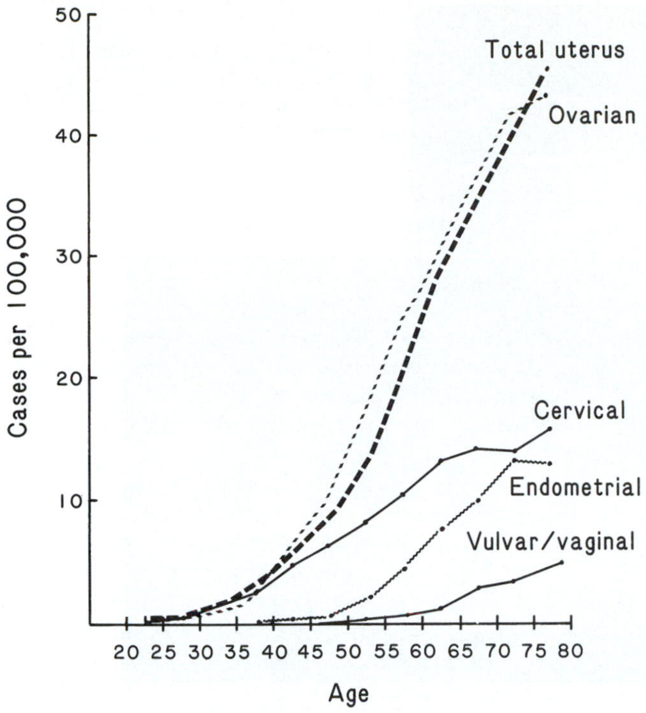


**Fig. 150-2.** Age-specific mortality curves for gynecologic cancers in the United States. (From Knapp RC, Berkowitz RS, editors: *Gynecologic oncology,* New York, 1986, Macmillan.)

stable or progressed to higher grades of dysplasia, including CIS. The problem is to identify the lesions that will progress and the time frame to progression. Recent studies seem to agree that the average transit time from the diagnosis of moderate dysplasia to CIS is 3 to 4 years. The recent reports of cancers arising in the setting of negative Pap smears suggest that transit times from a normal cervix to the diagnosis of cancer may be getting shorter. These observations, however, may relate more to false-negative Pap smears than to a more virulent form of the disease.

The role of HPV in cervical neoplasia has been the focus of research efforts for several years. HPV has long been known to cause benign anogenital infections resulting in condylomas; however, the majority of CIN and cervical cancers also contain HPV DNA. Of the many HPV subtypes that have been identified, the oncogenic subtypes are more likely to be associated with CIS and invasive cancers. The finding of HPV DNA in cervical cancer is not only an association but also causal in part. The DNA of the oncogenic subtypes is integrated into the host (patient) genome, and early viral proteins are actively expressed. The significance of the proteins lies in their ability to bind to and functionally eliminate tumor suppressor genes, allowing for the formation of cancer.

### Pap smear screening

The Pap smear is a model for a successful screening test. Its purpose is to detect premalignant conditions of the cervix. Over several decades a marked decline has occurred in the incidence of cervical cancer and its associated mortality, as well as an increase in the detection of CIN. CIN, which is asymptomatic, develops at the squamocolumnar junction (SCJ) of the cervix. The position of the SCJ varies depending on age and sexual activity. The columnar epithelium, which is positioned on the exocervix in younger women, undergoes a process of repair and formation of squamous metaplasia with aging and sexual activity. The resultant SCJ recedes into the endocervical canal, becoming invisible in the postmenopausal woman. This process of continual repair increases the opportunity for DNA mutations and the formation of dysplasia. Therefore efforts to obtain an adequate Pap smear that contains endocervical cells and to investigate an abnormal smear should be directed at this transformation zone.

Although the Pap smear is a specific test, it is only 80% sensitive. The association of necrosis and inflammation with invasive cancer makes the Pap smear a less reliable method for the detection of invasive cancer than for CIN. Some authors have reported false-negative rates for CIN as high as 40% and for cervical cancer as high as 60%. The false-negative rates are in large part due to quality control problems in cytology laboratories, although other factors, such as errors in sampling technique and interpretation, contribute. The Pap smear can detect abnormal changes associated with squamous dysplasia more easily than those associated with glandular dysplasia. Adenocarcinoma, which composes up to 20% of cervical cancers, arises in the endocervical canal and is not routinely detected by the Pap smear.

Screening for cervical cancer includes a visual examination of the cervix and a Pap smear. An endocervical brush should be used to increase the yield of endocervical cells (Fig. 150-3 for the Pap smear technique). If the patient is symptomatic (e.g., bleeding, discharge), and an ulcer or lesion is on the cervix, the diagnosis is best made promptly with a biopsy.

In an attempt to standardize Pap smear reporting among laboratories and to reduce the number of abnormal, but not clearly dysplastic, Pap smear results (previously referred to as class 2 Pap), the Bethesda system for Pap smear classification was developed (see the box on p. 1874). The major advantage of this system is that it distinguishes benign cellular changes (infection, reactive, or reparative) from truly atypical changes (atypical squamous cells or

### Managed Care Guide
### For performing routine pelvic and Pap examinations

1. The American Cancer Society and the American College of Obstetricians and Gynecologists (ACOG) recommend that annual Pap smears and pelvic examinations be obtained in all women over the age 18 who have been sexually active.
2. After at least three annual negative Pap smears, the test may be performed less frequently, depending on the patient's risk factors.
3. Due to the high prevalence of risk factors in the general population, however, most physicians recommend that women receive an annual Pap smear.

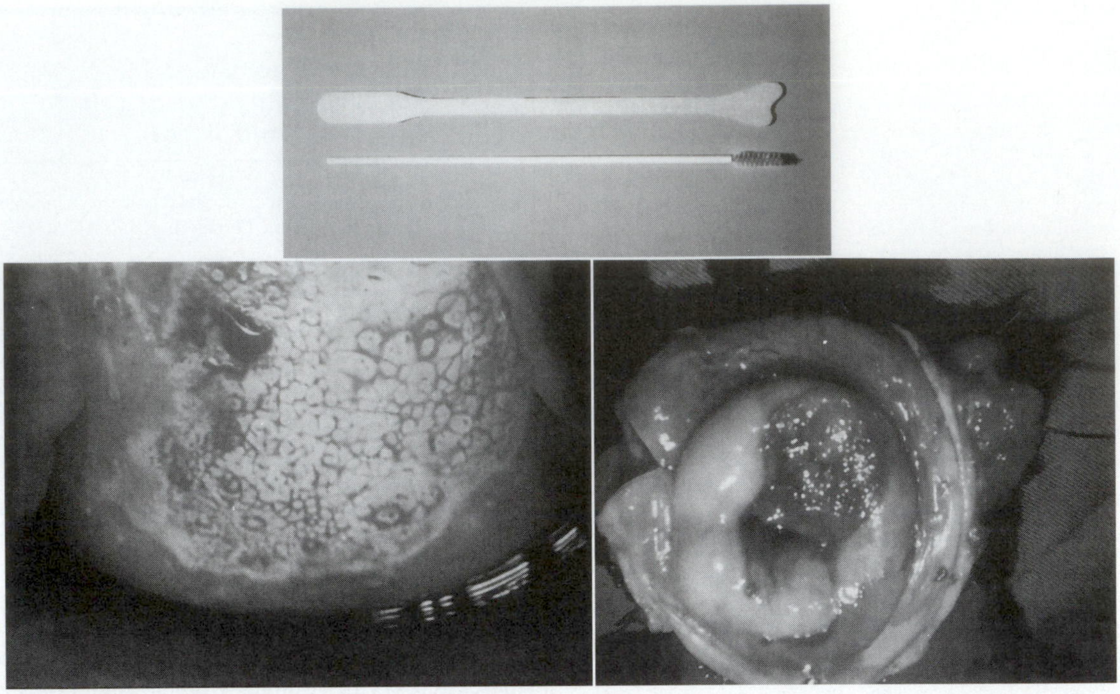

B

C

**Fig. 150-3.** **A,** Technique for obtaining a Pap smear: (1) Cells should be collected before bimanual examination and/or cultures; (2) a lubricant should not be used for insertion of the speculum; (3) the endocervical brush should be used gently, one-fourth turn only for sampling of the endocervical canal; (4) the exocervical smear, obtained by a spatula should be obtained by rotating it 360 degrees on the portio of the cervix; (5) rapid fixation is important; (6) for DES-exposed patients, the upper two thirds of the vagina should also be sampled circumferentially with the spatula. **B,** Colposcopy of CIS, highlighted by 3% acetic acid. **C,** Radical hysterectomy specimen of a stage IB invasive squamous cell cancer: gross appearance of the cervix.

atypical glandular cells of undetermined significance [ASQUS or AGUS]). The Bethesda system also replaces the categories of CIN 2 and 3 with the term high-grade *squamous intraepithelial lesion* (SIL), and morphologic changes that occur with HPV infection and CIN 1 with low-grade SIL, in the belief that the behavior of those lesions grouped together is similar. Because of changing terminology, it is imperative that physicians communicate with the cytologist frequently and understand the means of reporting.

### Causes of an abnormal Pap smear

Cervical causes of an abnormal Pap smear include both dysplasias and invasive cancers of squamous or glandular origin. Nondysplastic causes include inflammation, infection, reaction, and repair. The causes of an abnormal Pap smear are not limited to pathologies of the cervix. Lower genital tract dysplasias and cancer, upper genital tract lesions, and, rarely, urologic malignancies all have been implicated as causes of an abnormal Pap smear.

### Work-up of an abnormal Pap smear

The flow chart depicted in the Managed Care Guide on p. 1875 outlines the steps to follow in the work-up of an abnormal Pap smear. The first step is to distinguish those Pap smears that require prompt work-up (true ASQUS or AGUS, or suggestive of dysplasia or cancer) from those related to benign changes. If the Pap smear indicates a benign inflammatory change, it may also identify an

## The 1991 Bethesda System

- Statement on specimen adequacy
- General categorization
  - Within normal limits
  - Benign cellular changes
  - Epithelial cell abnormality
- Descriptive diagnosis
  - Benign cellular changes
    - Infection
    - Reactive
  - Epithelial cell abnormalities
    - Squamous cell
      - ASQUS
      - Low-grade SIL
      - High-grade SIL
      - Squamous cell carcinoma
    - Glandular cell
      - Benign endometrial cells
      - AGUS
      - Adenocarcinoma
  - Other malignant neoplasm
  - Hormonal evaluation

### Managed Care Guide
### Algorithm for the work-up of an abnormal pap smear

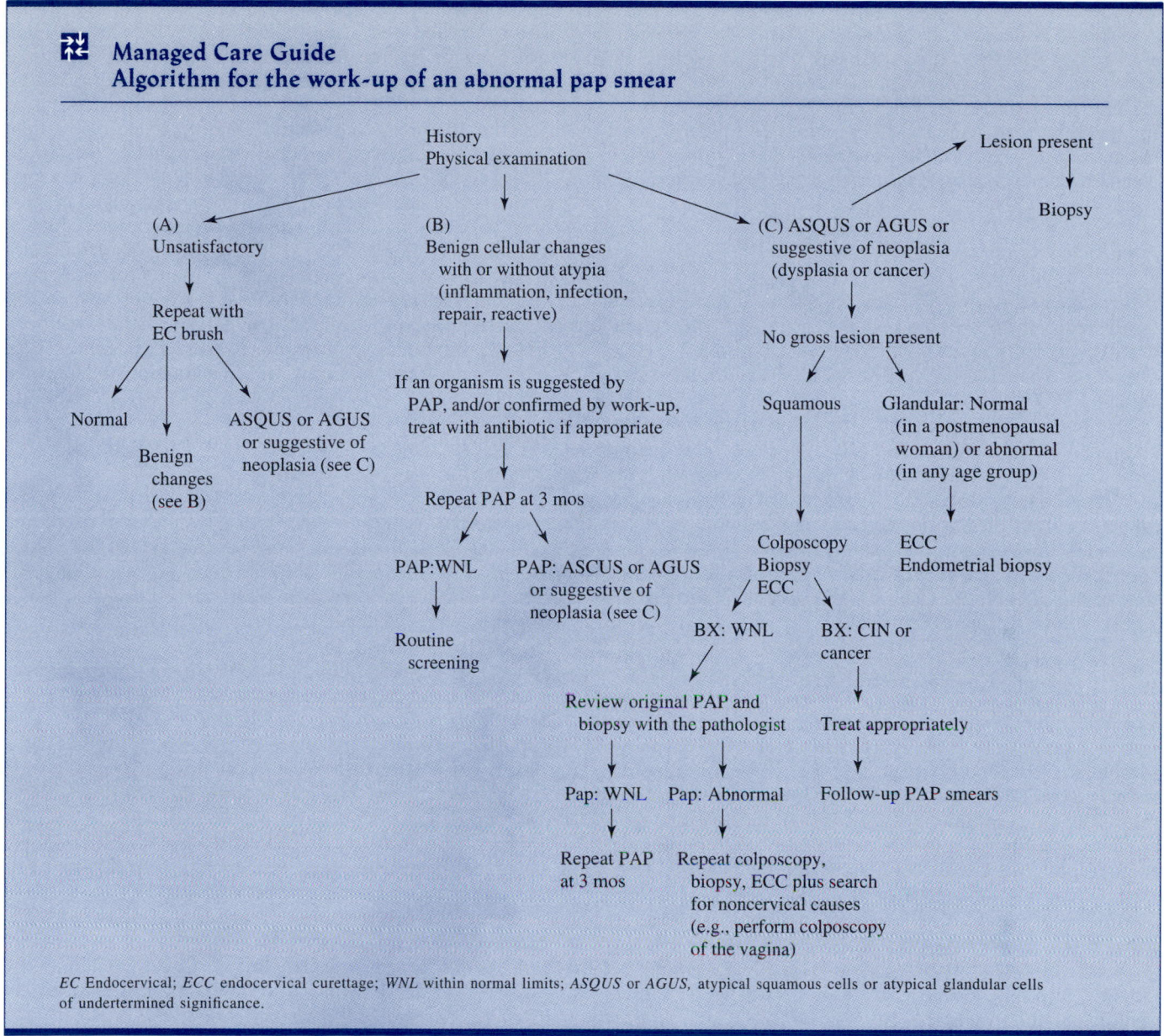

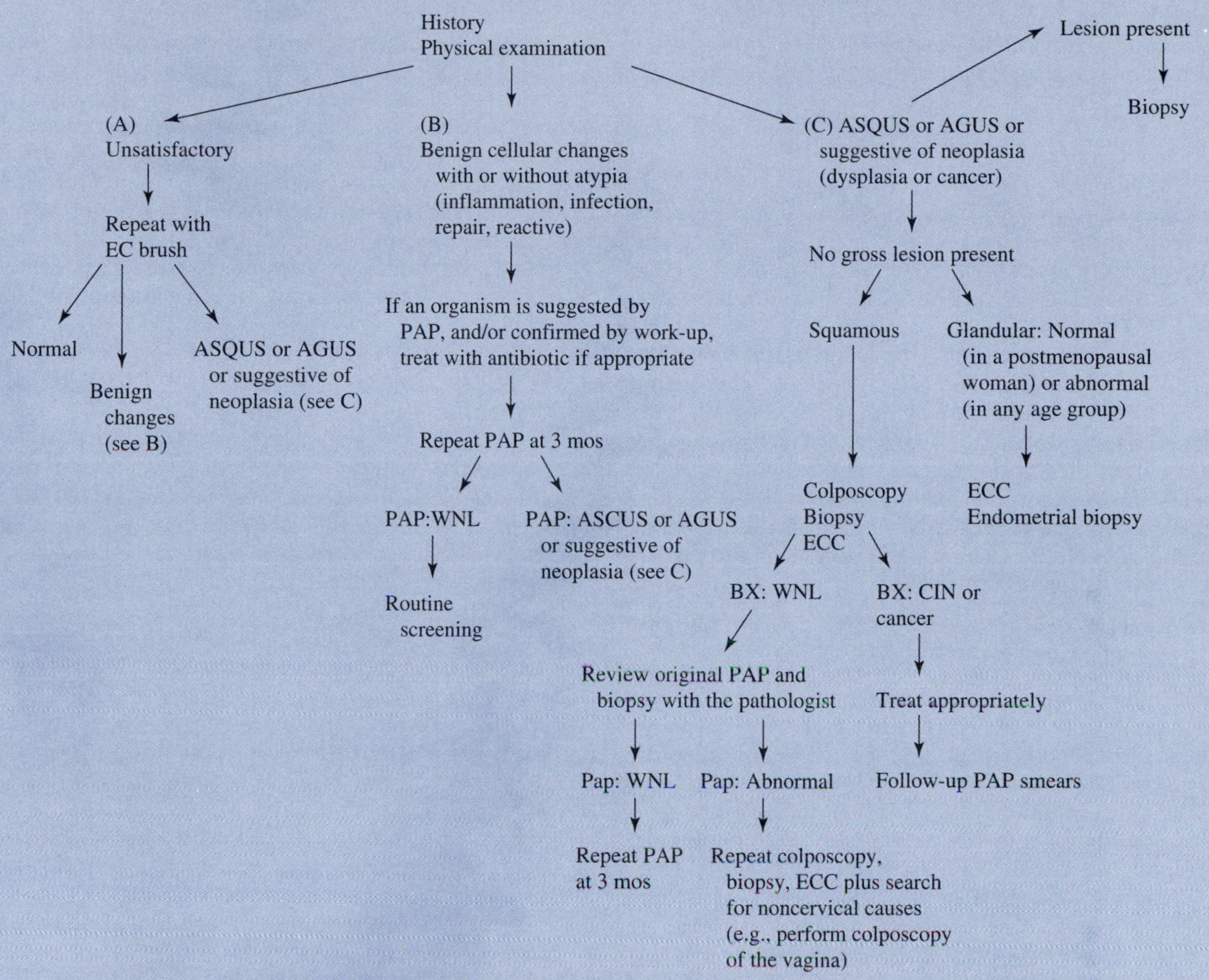


*EC* Endocervical; *ECC* endocervical curettage; *WNL* within normal limits; *ASQUS* or *AGUS,* atypical squamous cells or atypical glandular cells of undertermined significance.

infectious agent. Appropriate treatment usually results in resolution of the mild inflammatory or reactive abnormality. Routine bacterial cultures rarely yield useful information because of the preponderance of normal bacterial colonization in the vagina. Occasionally, empiric treatment with a vaginal gel or cream (e.g., metronidazole or sulfur based) or an antibiotic such as doxycycline resolves the abnormality associated with an unidentified infection. Other reparative atypical changes may not resolve except with time (e.g., those associated with radiation injury are likely to be longstanding). A follow-up Pap smear at 3 months is important to assess both the efficacy of the treatment and to rule out more serious underlying causes.

Work-up of an abnormal Pap smear showing ASQUS or AGUS, or one suggestive of neoplasia, requires the use of colposcopy. If a lesion or ulcer is readily visible (Fig. 150-3), then colposcopy is unnecessary, and prompt biopsy should be performed.

Colposcopy is an office procedure that uses a microscope to magnify the cervical epithelium after the application of a 3% acetic acid solution. The acetic acid directs biopsies to highlight areas of abnormal vascular patterns or thickened epithelium. After careful visualization, biopsies are performed, along with an endocervical curretage (ECC) in the nonpregnant patient.

### Treatment of CIN

Treatment of CIN depends on several factors, including the desire to preserve the transformation zone for ease of future follow-up, future fertility, need to know the pathology, and efficacy in the case of multifocal severe dysplasia or CIS. Uncertainty about the pathologic diagnosis or suspicion of invasive cancer should indicate the use of an excisional, rather than an ablative technique to reach a diagnosis, such as conization of the cervix using either a cold knife or laser technique, or more recently, a large loop excision. These approaches should include a separate endocervical evaluation above the excisional biopsy. Whatever the treatment modality, follow-up Pap smears are crucial to assess the success of the therapy. In general, a hysterectomy should be reserved for those women who have completed childbearing and for those in whom other procedures have failed (e.g., when the cone biopsy has positive margins, or there is a positive ECC).

### Symptoms and physical findings of invasive cervical cancer

If Pap smear screening fails, or if the cancer is not detected by the Pap smear (such as adenocarcinoma), the patient usually presents with symptoms of abnormal vaginal discharge, bleeding, or pelvic pain in more advanced cases.

On physical examination, the cervix may have an erosion or ulcer or may be partially replaced by a fungating tumor. If the tumor has arisen in the endocervix, the exocervix may occasionally appear normal; however, on palpation, it will feel indurated and may balloon out. Both bimanual and rectovaginal examinations should be performed to assess the local extent of spread. Induration of the parametria and uterosacral ligaments or fixation to the pelvic sidewalls should raise the suspicion for invasive cancer.

### Work-up of invasive cervical cancer

Cervical cancer spreads by direct penetration into the lateral parametria or by lymphatic spread to the pelvic lymph nodes. Involvement of the common iliac or paraaortic nodes is associated with systemic spread and poor survival. Once the diagnosis is confirmed by biopsy, a chest radiograph and abdominal/pelvic computerized tomography (CT) scan should be obtained. Other diagnostic imaging studies such as nuclear scans or barium enemas, are not routinely indicated unless dictated by clinical findings or an advanced presentation. Cystoscopy, with or without proctoscopy, is usually performed for staging purposes. Because accurate pretreatment clinical staging is important, the patient should be referred for formal staging.

### Prognostic factors for survival

Five-year survival rates correlate with stage and range from 85% for stage IB disease clinically confined to the cervix to minimal survival for disease that has spread beyond the pelvis. Fortunately, 50% of cervical cancers present as stage IB disease. Adenocarcinomas tend to have a worse prognosis than squamous cell cancers (SCC), stage for stage. Increased tumor size, a measure of tumor bulk, and lymph node involvement impart a significantly worse prognosis.

### Treatment of cervical cancer

Stage IB or early stage IIA (involvement of upper vagina) disease is treated by radical hysterectomy or radiation therapy. Radiation therapy results in castration of the premenopausal patient, and the possibility (usually less than 5%) of severe long-term effects on the vagina, bladder, and rectum. Mild changes, such as a decreased bladder capacity with urinary urgency and dyspareunia, are more common. The use of vaginal dilators or sexual activity during and after radiation therapy and estrogen replacement, if appropriate, helps prevent dyspareunia. Alternatively, radical hysterectomy can be performed with translocation of the ovaries in the event postoperative radiation therapy is necessary. There is a small (less than 1%) acute operative complication rate and larger (up to 30% in some studies) long-term bladder and/or rectal dysfunction rates. These problems can be obviated in most cases with careful attention during postoperative regimens to restore bladder and rectal functions. Primary radiation therapy is still the standard treatment for advanced disease. The use of chemotherapy in most centers is restricted to the treatment of advanced or recurrent disease, although some centers are using adjuvant or neoadjuvant chemotherapy in an attempt to improve survival.

## ENDOMETRIAL CANCER/ABNORMAL VAGINAL BLEEDING

### Epidemiology and risk factors

Endometrial cancer is the most common gynecologic malignancy and can be associated with prolonged or excessive estrogen states. Exogenous estrogens in postmenopausal women are firmly established as a risk factor for endometrial cancer. In general, this risk increases twofold to fourfold in estrogen users compared with nonusers. The use of combination oral contraceptive pills (OCPs) has been associated with a 50% decreased risk of developing endometrial cancer. The duration of use is important in providing the protection, which persists for at least 5 years after OCP use is discontinued.

Other conditions that can be associated with excessive estrogen states include chronic anovulation, as seen in polycystic ovarian or thyroid disease; hyperandrogenic states; delayed menopause; and hormone-producing ovarian tumors (e.g., granulosa cell tumors).

Obesity is a constitutional factor that frequently has been associated with the development of endometrial cancer, presumably due to the increased production of estrone from the peripheral aromatization of androstenedione (of adrenal origin) in fat tissue.

### Pathophysiology

During the normal menstrual cycle, the endometrium is exposed to changing levels of hormones. The mitogenic effects of estradiol that predominate during the early proliferative phase of the cycle are down-regulated by the opposing effect of progesterone during the late secretory phase. Disruptions in these cyclic influences on the endometrium may lead to a hyperplastic state, and subsequent unknown factors may cause the development of atypical hyperplasia and, eventually, endometrial carcinoma. Because hyperplasia develops in women who have had prolonged exposure to unopposed estrogen and is frequently associated with cancer, estrogen is considered to be a causative agent in the development of endometrial cancer. In a recent study, 29% of women with complex glandular patterns and cytologic atypia developed endometrial cancer, whereas only 1% with simple glandular patterns and no atypia developed cancer. Thus the finding of complex atypical hyperplasia must be considered a premalignant state.

**Managed Care Guide**
**Algorithm for the work-up of abnormal vaginal bleeding**

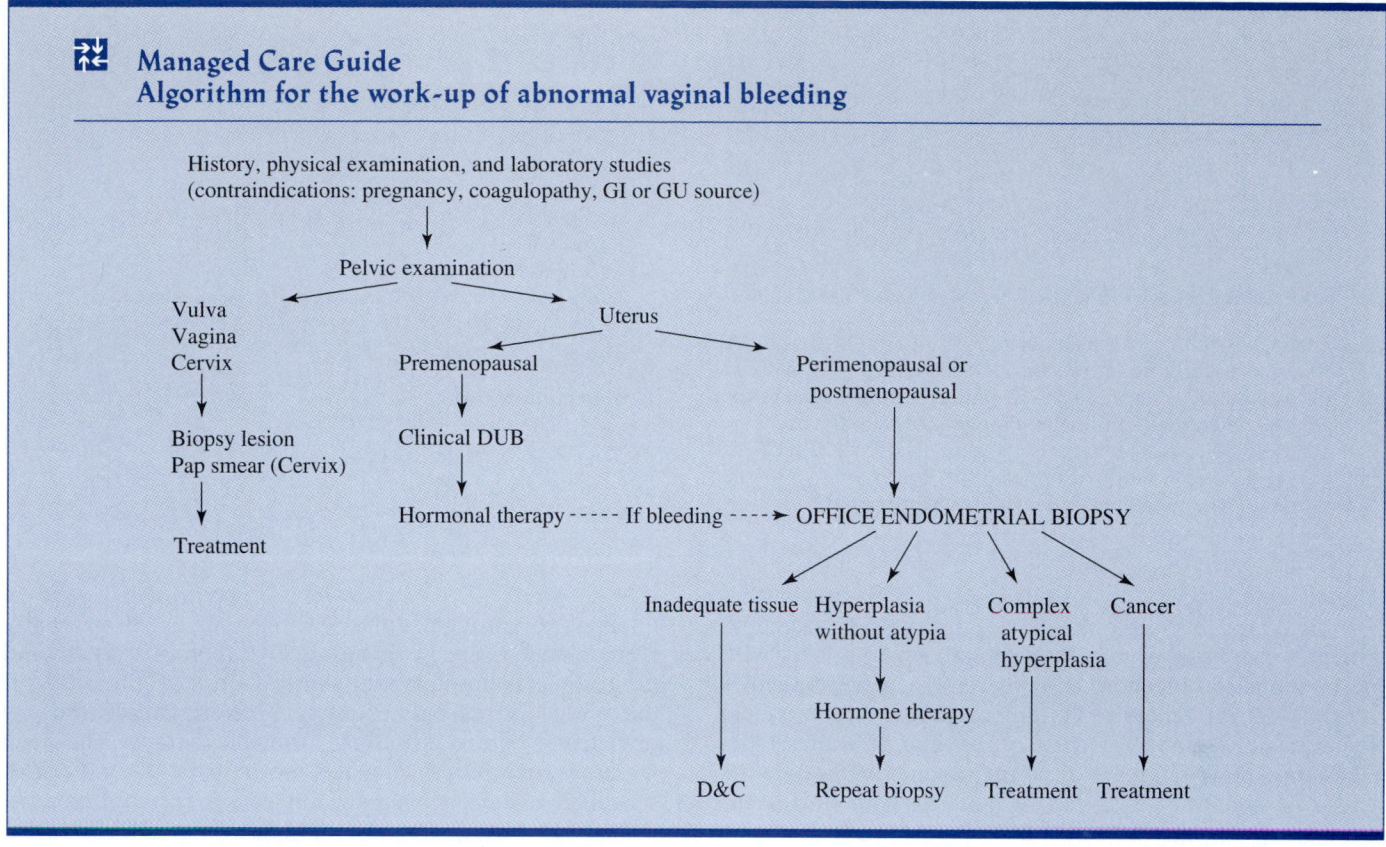

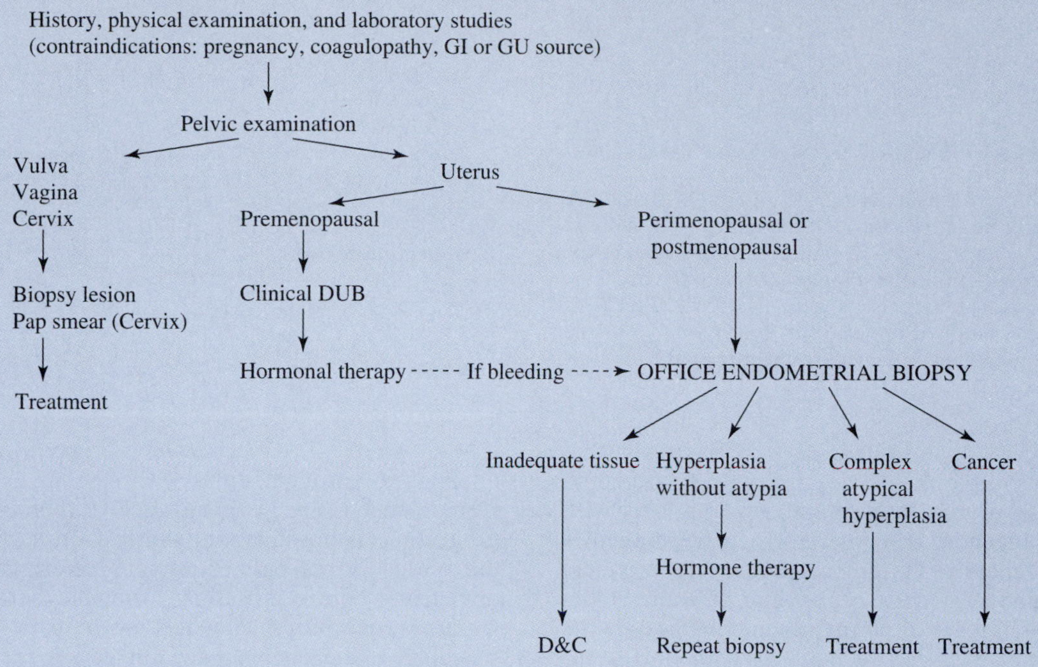


## Symptoms and physical findings of endometrial cancer

Endometrial cancer generally occurs in postmenopausal women who present with abnormal vaginal bleeding. Although only 20% of all women who present with vaginal bleeding have a gynecologic malignancy, this risk increases with age.

Premenopausal women diagnosed with endometrial cancer often have a history of heavy irregular menstrual bleeding. During the perimenopausal period, the pattern of bleeding should become lighter and less frequent. Significant deviations from this pattern suggest underlying pathology. Symptoms related to pelvic pressure, uterine enlargement, or extrauterine spread may be part of the initial presentation in patients with advanced disease.

Examination of women with abnormal bleeding should begin with inspection of the vulva, vagina, and cervix. If gross lesions are seen, a biopsy should be obtained. If no lesion is apparent, a Pap smear of the cervix should be performed. The uterus may be normal sized or enlarged, irregular, firm, or even soft. The presence of an adnexal mass is less likely to represent a metastasis from an endometrial primary than a benign condition, such as a pedunculated fibroid or a functional ovarian cyst.

## Differential diagnosis and work-up of abnormal vaginal bleeding

Abnormal vaginal bleeding could stem from pathology of any of the reproductive organs or from the gastrointestinal or urologic tracts (see the Managed Care Guide on p. above). Involvement of the latter two can generally be excluded by the lack of supporting symptoms and a negative stool or catheterized urine specimen. An ectopic or molar pregnancy or miscarriage must be considered in the premenopausal patient and a serum pregnancy test should be performed. Thyroid or liver function tests, or coagulation studies to rule out blood dyscrasias, may be indicated. In addition to these conditions, abnormal bleeding frequently signals a benign endometrial or myometrial cause, (e.g., fibroids or dysfunctional uterine bleeding) (see Chapter 142B). In perimenopausal and postmenopausal women, an evaluation of the endometrial cavity is imperative to rule out a malignancy.

## Technique of endometrial sampling and other modalities to assess abnormal vaginal bleeding

Until the early 1980s, a fractional dilatation and curettage (D&C) was the definitive diagnostic procedure for evaluating the endometrium. Today, an office endometrial biopsy is the starting point. Many instruments are commercially available for sampling the endometrium. One of the new cost-effective devices, the Pipelle (Unimar, Wilton, Conn), is a flexible, 3.1 mm diameter, plastic tube, which has gained patient acceptance because it is less painful (Fig. 150-4). The indications and few contraindications for this procedure are listed in the box on p. 1878. When bacterial endocarditis is a risk, antibiotic prophylaxis is indicated.

Several series have shown that the diagnostic accuracy of an office biopsy is 80% to 95%. If the biopsy specimen

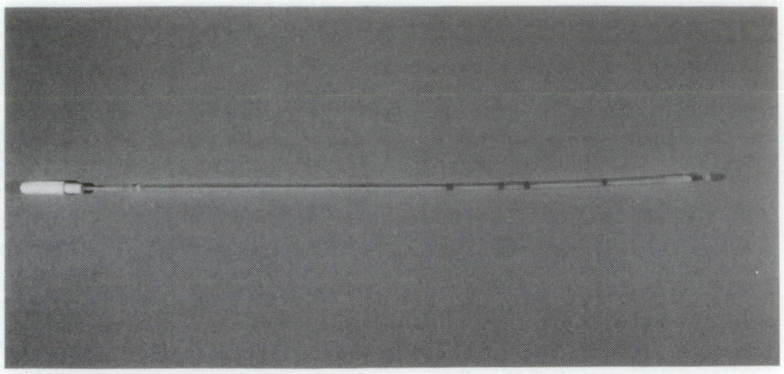

Fig. 150-4. Technique for endometrial sampling: (1) this device (Pipelle) can usually be passed through the endocervix without dilation or use of a tenaculum; (2) while pulling back on the plunger to generate suction, the Pipelle is rotated within the endometrial cavity to obtain a core specimen; (3) the Pipelle is not used as a curette, but held in place and gently rotated in one dimension; (4) the specimen is ejected by pushing on the plunger, and placed into fixative.

## Endometrial sampling

**Indications**

Dysfunctional uterine bleeding
Postmenopausal bleeding
Unanticipated bleeding on hormonal replacement therapy
Tamoxifen therapy
Abnormal endometrial cytology
Normal endometrial cytology in a postmenopausal woman
Follow-up of medical therapy for endometrial hyperplasia
Evaluation of infertility

**Contraindications**

Pregnancy
Acute pelvic inflammatory disease
Coagulopathy
Cervical stenosis

shows atypical cells or is insufficient for diagnosis (that 6% incidence in symptomatic patients), a D&C should be performed. A review of a large number of patients with perimenopausal bleeding demonstrates that the diagnosis of endometrial cancer or its precursor, complex atypical hyperplasia, is made 8% to 9% of the time. In contrast, the likelihood that malignant or premalignant changes are the cause of abnormal bleeding in patients with postmenopausal bleeding is more than 20%.

Complications from endometrial sampling can occur; however, the incidence is significantly less than from D&C. Perforation of the uterus can occur in patients with cervical stenosis, severely flexed uteri, or a necrotic uterus caused by endometrial cancer.

Although several studies have indicated that one third to one half of patients with endometrial cancer will have abnormal cervical cytology, the routine use of a Pap smear to evaluate the endometrium is inappropriate. However, endometrial cells found on a Pap smear in a postmenopausal woman, even if normal, should alert the clinician to the possibility of underlying endometrial pathology.

Newer modalities used in the evaluation of the endometrium include hysteroscopy and transvaginal ultrasound. Ultrasound findings in a postmenopausal woman that warrant further work-up with endometrial sampling include a fluid-filled endometrial cavity or a thickened endometrial stripe.

Hysteroscopy provides a direct visualization of the endometrial cavity. Although hysteroscopy can consistently identify endometrial polyps and submucosal fibroids better than an endometrial biopsy, the necessity of this approach to work-up abnormal uterine bleeding in all patients has not been documented. However, in a woman who has persistent uterine bleeding and who has undergone a D&C that is negative for a malignancy, or in a woman who has failed to respond to medical therapy for a hyperplastic state, a hysteroscopic evaluation may help identify the source of the problem.

### Hormonal replacement therapy and endometrial sampling

Because the risk of endometrial hyperplasia and/or endometrial cancer is increased in women receiving unopposed estrogen replacement therapy, it is generally recommended that women receive both estrogen and progestin (given sequentially or low-dose continuously) if the uterus is present. Physicians often sample the endometrium before initiating hormonal therapy. The need for a baseline biopsy depends on the patient's pattern of bleeding. If she has been amenorrheic for several months, a baseline biopsy may be optional. In postmenopausal women receiving daily estrogen and at least 12 days of progestins (medroxyprogesterone [Provera], 10 mg) monthly, withdrawal bleeding on day 11 or later after the addition of progestins is associated with a predominantly secretory endometrium or lack of endometrial tissue, and routine sampling is not necessary. Endometrial sampling is recommended for those women whose bleeding occurs earlier than day 11. Many women cannot tolerate the side effects that occur with this dose of Provera and receive lower doses for a shorter duration. In these circumstances, the subsequent bleeding pattern cannot be reliably taken to correlate with endometrial histology, and the recommendation for routine sampling on a yearly basis is reasonable.

Continuous low-dose estrogen and progestin therapy frequently results in endometrial atrophy and amenorrhea after 3 to 6 months. Routine endometrial sampling is not recommended for those amenorrheic women. Any unanticipated or heavy bleeding, however, signals the need for endometrial sampling. Optimal endometrial sampling for women receiving unopposed estrogen has not been determined, but should be performed routinely and often.

### Prognostic factors

Ninety percent of endometrial carcinomas are adenocarcinomas, which can be mixed with a benign or malignant squamous component.

The degree of histologic differentiation of endometrial cancer is an important prognostic feature; well-differentiated (grade 1) types have a significantly better prognosis than poorly differentiated types (grade 3). Deep myometrial tumor invasion or the presence of tumor outside the uterus, including lymph node metastases, are poor prognostic factors. For example, 5-year survival rates approach 97% in women less than age 60 with low-grade histologic lesions confined to the uterus. In contrast, 5-year survival rates may be as low as 7.5% in older patients with undifferentiated carcinomas, or with aggressive variants including clear cell, papillary serous, and adenosquamous carcinoma.

### Treatment of endometrial cancer

Endometrial cancer is treated surgically with total abdominal hysterectomy and bilateral salpingo-oophorectomy. Use of adjuvant radiation therapy to the vaginal apex, pelvic external beam radiation therapy, or a combination of both depends on the final pathologic staging. A significant decrease in vaginal apex recurrence has been documented with the use of radiation therapy. Pelvic external beam radiation therapy decreases pelvic recurrence in those who are at risk (e.g., deep myometrial invasion, positive lymph nodes, or endocervical involvement). Patients who are unacceptable anesthetic risks or refuse surgery may be treated with radiation therapy alone. Survival rates however, are lower than surgery and radiation therapy combined.

The management of advanced disease spread outside the pelvis is individualized. Radiation therapy often is used to palliate symptoms. Cytoxic chemotherapy in patients with metastatic disease has response rates of 15% to 35%. Unfortunately, complete responses are uncommon and disease-free intervals are short, although occasional patients with low-grade tumors have prolonged responses.

### Estrogen replacement therapy after successful endometrial cancer treatment

Definitive studies to guide recommendations for estrogen replacement therapy (ERT) in women with a history of endometrial cancer are not available. Common sense dictates that estrogens are contraindicated in anyone with a history of a hormonally sensitive cancer. Recently, however, the ACOG concluded that in selected women with a history of endometrial cancer, estrogens could be used for the usual indications. Eligible women should be completely informed about alternatives and the potential risks involved. If the patient is truly free of cancer, ERT should not increase the likelihood of recurrent disease. On the other hand, estrogen can be a potential mitogen for patients whose cancer cells are viable but quiescent after treatment. In general, it would be prudent to wait approximately 3 years after treatment before considering ERT for women who would benefit.

## OVARIAN CANCER/ADNEXAL MASS

### Epidemiology and risk factors

Epithelial ovarian cancer accounts for 90% of all ovarian cancers and is responsible for more deaths than all other gynecologic cancers combined (see Fig. 150-2). It is a disease of industrialized nations, and environmental and dietary factors likely play a role. The lifetime risk in the general population for the development of epithelial ovarian cancer is 1 in 70 (1.4%). Genetic factors are an important risk factor; the lifetime risk increases to 39% in the presence of two first-degree relatives with ovarian cancer. These patients constitute a recognized high-risk group. It should be noted, however, that familial ovarian cancer is rare and accounts for less than 5% of all cases. Other risk factors, such as nulliparity, infertility, prior history of breast cancer, a high-fat diet, and possibly, perineal talc exposure, increase the lifetime risk to approximately 2%.

### Pathophysiology

It is unclear whether epithelial ovarian cancer arises from cells derived from the ovarian surface epithelium or the peritoneal mesothelium. That more than 70% of women present with tumor involving multiple peritoneal surfaces suggests the presence of metachronous peritoneal tumors.

The association of ovarian cancer with incessant ovulation, however, points to an ovarian origin. Ovulation results in a major wound at the ovarian surface, which is repaired by growth and invasion of the ovarian surface epithelium, resulting in the formation of inclusion cysts. The observed protective effect of OCPs on ovarian cancer risk, coupled with the reduced risk seen in women who have multiple pregnancies, may be due to suppression of ovulation and to the decreased potential for DNA mutations (and thus initiation of neoplasia) that arise during repair of the surface of the ovulating ovary.

Although it has been suggested that early detection by screening may improve the prognosis for ovarian cancer, the benefits of screening in the general population have not been established. Studies are underway to assess the efficiency of screening, especially in high-risk women.

Several modalities can be used to screen for ovarian cancer. Transvaginal ultrasonography (TVS) is used to detect early morphologic changes associated with ovarian cancer. The ultrasonographic characteristics of an ovarian mass that are reported to correlate with malignancy include overall increased size or wall thickness, or the presence of intracystic papillary formations, septation, or solid areas. In one study, TVS had a sensitivity of 90% and specificity of 87% for detection of ovarian cancer among women undergoing surgery for an adrenal mass. To help reduce the false-positive findings, color Doppler flow studies that detect areas of neovascularization associated with malignancy have greatly improved the sensitivity of transvaginal ultrasound for diagnosing ovarian carcinoma.

CA-125 is a widely used serum tumor marker that is valuable in detecting small tumor burdens in patients with a known history of ovarian cancer. Although more than 80% of women with clinically apparent ovarian cancer have an elevated CA-125, the CA-125 is elevated in only 50% of women with stage I disease (disease confined to the ovary). In addition, 0.5% to 1% of normal women, as well as those with a variety of physiologic conditions, including endometriosis, salpingitis, pregnancy, fibroids, and menstruation, have an elevated level. The calculated positive predictive value for the detection of ovarian cancer by this modality alone is only 2.3%. Thus isolated CA-125 screening in the general population is not appropriate.

Combined use of CA-125 and TVS has increased the specificity for detection of ovarian cancer in postmenopausal women; however, guidelines for screening premenopausal women at high risk are not yet available. Because women with a family history of ovarian cancer develop the disease at a younger average age than those with the sporadic form (49 versus 59 years) and those with the Lynch II syndrome (a rare hereditary disorder in which family members are at increased risk for endometrial, colon, and ovarian cancer) develop disease at an average

age of 45 years, it would seem prudent to start screening family members at risk in their reproductive years.

### Symptoms and physical findings of an adnexal mass

The etiology and resulting symptoms and findings of an adnexal mass depend on patient age. Most neoplasms in the premenarchal age group are benign or malignant germ cell tumors. In this young age group, pain from a rapidly growing cyst or neoplasm or adnexal torsion is the most common presenting symptom. Frequently, the preoperative diagnosis is appendicitis. The diagnosis of an adnexal mass usually is made by palpation of an abdominal mass or by imaging studies rather than by pelvic examination.

Most adnexal masses are diagnosed in women of reproductive age; fortunately they usually are benign. In this age group, pelvic masses are found frequently on routine pelvic examination, as well as from a work-up of a specific symptom. The presentation depends on the underlying pathology and can include acute abdominal/pelvic pain or chronic discomfort, fever, abnormal menses, dysmenorrhea, symptoms of pregnancy, change in bowel or urinary habits, or back pain. Other than rapidly growing tumors, the majority of early ovarian cancers are asymptomatic. The most common symptom is vague abdominal swelling or discomfort. Findings of bilaterality, firmness, fixation, nodularity, and lack of tenderness on pelvic examination suggest a malignant process, as does the concomitant presence of ascites or cul-de-sac nodules. In the postmenopausal patient, any pelvic mass (other than known stable fibroids), or even a palpable ovary, are cause for concern and dictate further work-up.

### Work-up of an adnexal mass

The work-up depends on patient age, clinical presentation, and physical findings. Directed blood work includes a complete blood count (CBC) and erythrocyte sedimentation rate (ESR) for an inflammatory process, CA-125 for a malignancy, and a serum pregnancy test if indicated. Pelvic ultrasound should be used as the screening imaging modality. Magnetic resonance imaging (MRI) scans can help differentiate fibroids or endometriosis from ovarian neoplasms or simple functional cysts but are very expensive.

The use of laparoscopy not only for diagnosis but also for surgical extirpation of pelvic masses has become increasingly popular; however, the criteria for safe and appropriate use of this procedure have not been developed.

## Differential diagnosis of an adnexal mass and histology of ovarian neoplasms

The adnexa consist of the ovaries, fallopian tubes, and embryologic remnants in the broad ligament. Masses that are palpated or imaged in this area, however, may arise from many other organs, and their origin may be difficult to identify (Table 150-2). The differential diagnosis of an adnexal mass varies considerably with age.

Fibroids, the most common uterine neoplasms, are usually clearly related to the body of the uterus. However, they may be located in the broad ligament or attached to the uterus by a thin stalk, and feel like an adnexal mass. They are generally solid, but may become partially cystic with degeneration, infarction, or torsion. In the United States, at least 10% of white and 30% to 40% of black women over the age of 35 have fibroids. These estrogen-dependent neoplasms should shrink in the absence of hormonal replacement after the menopause. Sarcomatous elements are associated with fibroids only 0.1% of the time. Thus fibroids should be considered benign unless they are solitary and rapidly growing.

**Table 150-2.** Differential diagnosis of an adnexal mass

| Site | Mass |
|---|---|
| Ovary | Functional cyst |
| | Benign neoplasm |
| | Malignant neoplasm |
| | Endometriosis |
| Fallopian tube | Tuboovarian abscess |
| | Hydrosalpinx |
| | Paratubal cyst |
| | Ectopic pregnancy |
| | Benign neoplasm (rare) |
| | Malignant neoplasm |
| Uterus | Fibroid (pedunculated, interligamentous) |
| Gastrointestinal tract | Bowel loops with feces |
| | Diverticular disease |
| | Appendicitis |
| | Inflammatory bowel disease |
| | Benign small bowel neoplasm (leiomyoma) |
| | Colon cancer |
| Urinary tract | Distended bladder |
| | Pelvic kidney |
| | Urachal cyst |
| Retroperitoneum | Benign neoplasm (myxoid tumor) |
| | Sarcoma, lymphoma, or teratoma |
| | Abdominal wall hematoma or abscess |

Functional ovarian cysts are the most common cause of ovarian enlargement in the reproductive age group and include both follicular and corpus luteum cysts, theca lutein cysts, pregnancy luteomas, sclerocystic ovaries, and endometriotic cysts. These cysts usually are asymptomatic and are a function of normal ovarian activity. They can cause pain and abnormal menses. Some will respond to OCP suppression; others will regress without intervention.

Endometriosis results from implantation of endometrial glands and stroma outside the endometrial cavity. The diagnosis is most common in white and infertile women aged 35 to 45 years. The most common presenting symptom is pelvic pain. When the ectopic location of the implants includes the uterosacral ligaments, nodularity and tenderness can be found on rectovaginal examination.

Tuboovarian abscess can occur with prior or concomitant pelvic inflammatory disease. Symptoms of acute pelvic infection such as pelvic pain, fever, vaginal discharge, and abnormal bleeding, along with findings of an exquisitely tender pelvic mass, suggest this diagnosis. These findings may be absent with a chronic tuboovarian abscess. Shrinkage and resolution of the mass with intense antibiotic treatment confirm the clinical impression.

The differential diagnosis of an adnexal mass includes the benign, borderline, and malignant ovarian neoplasms. The most common ovarian neoplasms are the benign

A

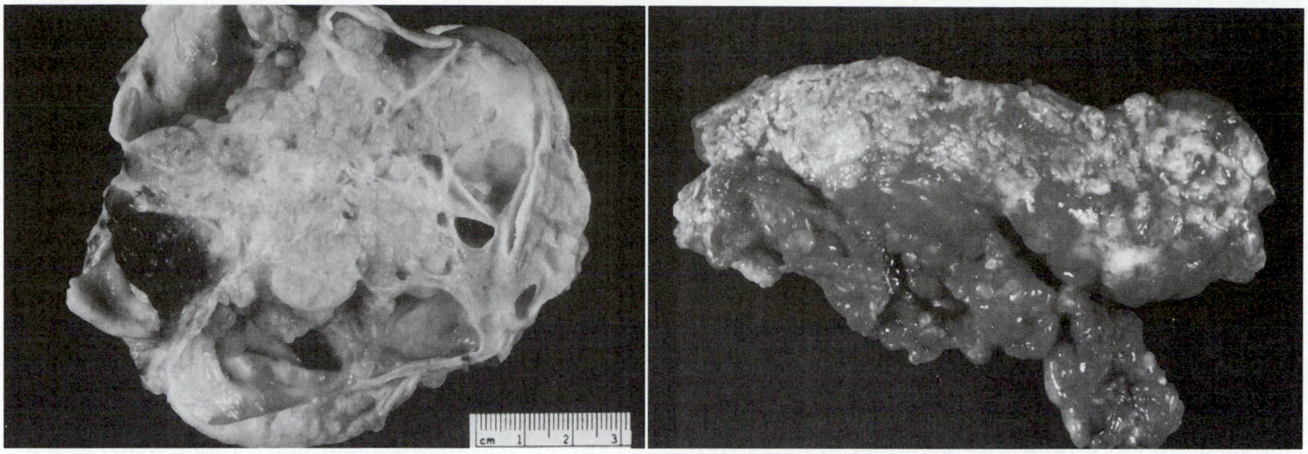


B

**Fig. 150-5.** **A,** Appearance of a primary epithelial ovarian cancer (papillary serous cystadenocarcinoma), with excrescences, an irregular surface, septae, and intracystic papillations. **B,** Classic appearance of an omental cake (common metastasis from ovarian cancer).

serous and mucinous cystadenomas and the dermoids (mature cystic teratomas). In contrast to functional cysts, these neoplasms do not regress with observation or use of OCP suppression.

### Symptoms and physical findings of advanced ovarian cancer

Because approximately 70% of all ovarian cancers present with advanced stage disease, primary care physicians must be able to recognize these findings promptly and refer patients without delay. Patients can present with abdominal swelling or bloating, generalized abdominal discomfort, dyspepsia and early satiety, lack of appetite, malaise, urinary frequency, and weight change (either gain or loss). A fixed nodular pelvic mass may be found on pelvic examination. Diffuse peritoneal implants are readily seen on TVS and almost always involve the omentum, which becomes enlarged and firm and presents as a large ballotable mass (omental cake) (Fig. 150-5). Importantly, ovarian cancer should be considered foremost in women with unexplained ascites, with or without confirmation of a pelvic mass.

### Work-up of advanced ovarian cancer

After a TVS screening examination for diagnosis, CT scan is used to image the retroperitoneum, urologic structures, rectum, pancreas, and liver and confirm a clinical diagnosis of ascites. This information is important in determining treatment approach and prognosis. Paracentesis is not indicated in the usual work-up of women with suspected ovarian cancer because of the risk of rupture of a large encapsulated early stage neoplasm.

### Surgical staging of ovarian cancer

Ovarian cancer is staged surgically through a midline abdominal incision. Ascites or washings are taken for cytologic analysis. A thorough exploration of the entire peritoneal cavity is undertaken with removal of the primary neoplasm and resection of all metastases. In addition a generous sampling of the omentum, retroperitoneal lymph nodes, peritoneal and diaphragmatic surfaces is performed, even if these structures appear normal. With a few exceptions in a reproductive-aged woman who wishes to preserve childbearing potential, the procedure includes removal of the contralateral ovary and hysterectomy. If conservative surgery is planned, complete staging includes a biopsy of the normal contralateral ovary because some neoplasms, such as serous tumors, are frequently bilateral.

### Prognosis and treatment of ovarian cancer

The prognosis of invasive epithelial ovarian cancer is dismal and relates to stage and residual disease after completion of initial debulking surgery. The 5-year survival of stages III and IV disease (extrapelvic spread) is 18%; unfortunately, 70% of patients have extrapelvic spread. They usually die from progressive inanition resulting from small bowel entrapment by tumor. The prognosis of early stage invasive ovarian cancers, as well as the borderline malignant tumors of all stages, is significantly better. The prognosis of germ cell tumors, if treated promptly with aggressive chemotherapy in a cancer referral center, is excellent. Similarly, sex-cord stromal tumors are responsive to chemotherapy.

The primary treatment of epithelial ovarian cancer is aggressive surgical tumor debulking. Treatment of remaining small or microscopic tumor burdens depends on the sensitivity of these tumors to platinum-based combination chemotherapy or, in selected cases, to whole abdominal radiation therapy. Although the original response to chemotherapy is 80%, the majority of patients relapse and go on to receive multiple regimens, which inevitably fail. Research is ongoing to understand the mechanisms of drug resistance and to develop new effective second-line agents.

Support for terminal care in the community is important; the establishment of effective hospice networks and team approaches including home nursing services are helpful. Moreover, improved techniques are available for placement of a percutaneous gastrostomy for palliation of refractory nausea and vomiting, and improved routes, such as transdermal approaches and continuous infusion pumps, for the administration of narcotics for effective pain control (see Chapters 59 and 60).

## VULVAR DISEASE

### Differential diagnosis of vulvar pruritus

Vulvar and perineal pruritus are common symptoms in women. It is important to remember that pruritus is a symptom, not a disease, and the underlying cause must be determined to treat it effectively.

Pruritus of the vulva may be caused by epithelial changes in the vulvar skin or to irritation of the nerve endings that richly supply the genital area. The primary causes of the condition include the vulvar dystrophies, (e.g., squamous cell hyperplasia or lichen sclerosis), vulvar intraepithelial neoplasms (VIN), candidiasis, and dermatologic conditions (e.g., psoriasis, seborrheic or contact dermatitis). They may present as multiple or single, white or red lesions that are raised or flat. Careful inspection of the vulva and vagina, using either a magnifying glass or a colposcope, followed by a biopsy, is the best method to establish a specific diagnosis. The glabrous skin must also be inspected because many of the dermatoses (e.g., psoriasis or lichen planus) that affect the vulva also affect this area. The work-up of vulvar disease includes an evaluation for possible systemic causes, such as diabetes mellitus in a woman with vulvar candidiasis.

### Treatment of vulvar dystrophies

Vulvar dystrophy is a benign set of conditions associated with cellular atypia in approximately 10% of cases. The progression of vulvar dystrophies to malignancy is low, but is frequently associated with vulvar cancer. Treatment is usually medical using corticosteroid creams. Lichen sclerosis is best treated with 2% testosterone mixed in petroleum. Progesterone (1%) in petroleum also may be effective. In refractory cases, it may be necessary to use subcutaneous injections of absolute alcohol in a gridlike fashion across the vulva for persistent pruritus. This procedure is performed in the operating room under general anesthesia.

### VIN and vulvar cancer

VIN is increasing in incidence, especially in younger women, and may be HPV-related. The presenting symptom is usually pruritus of varying intensity. The multicentric lesions are flat, with mild to moderate changes in pigmentation; 20% to 40% of patients with VIN have had or will have similar lesions of the anogenital tract. Multiple condylomata may be associated with VIN in some cases. Because the invasive potential of VIN has not been established, conservative management is appropriate. Wide, local excision of the specific areas involved is usually performed. For extensive and multifocal lesions, a partial skinning vulvectomy may be necessary. Laser ablation also may be used. The use of topical chemotherapy with 5% 5-fluorouracil cream can produce responses in 50% of patients, but is associated with significant morbidity due to local irritation. Unfortunately, because the area at risk is extensive and cannot be treated adequately with any of these modalities, recurrences are frequent.

Vulvar cancer is uncommon and accounts for only 1% to 5% of all female cancers. Over 75% of all patients with this disease are age 55 or older. The etiology remains unknown, but the association of squamous cell cancer of the vulva with other premalignant neoplasms of the anogenital mucosa suggest a role for HPV.

Invasive squamous cell cancer accounts for 85% to 90% of vulvar malignancies and usually presents as a vulvar mass causing discomfort after a long history of vulvar pruritus. On gross examination the lesion is raised, fleshy, ulcerative, or warty; multiple sites are involved in 5% of cases. The importance of a biopsy with appropriate early referral for surgery must be stressed. The spread of invasive disease is usually orderly after lymphatic drainage; hence the inguinal nodes should be palpated. Radical surgery is the treatment of choice and includes removal of the primary lesion with adequate margins. A bilateral inguinal lymphadenectomy is indicated depending on the location and size of the primary lesion. Small lesions with minimal stromal invasion have led to the use of more conservative surgical approaches, but these must be highly individualized.

## GESTATIONAL TROPHOBLASTIC NEOPLASIA

Gestational trophoblastic disease is a rare gynecologic malignancy that may present after a normal, ectopic or molar pregnancy, or miscarriage. Any reproductive-aged woman with abnormal vaginal bleeding, even without a recognized antecedent pregnancy, should be considered a candidate for this entity. A sensitive tumor marker produced by the tumor, human chorionic gonadotropin (HCG), correlates with the number of viable cells present and can be measured simply by obtaining a sensitive serum pregnancy test. The malignancy is exquisitely sensitive to chemotherapeutic regimens and is curable if promptly recognized, even when metastatic.

## BIBLIOGRAPHY


American Cancer Society: Cancer statistics 1993, *CA Cancer J Clin* 43(1):7, 1993.

Chambers JT, Chambers SK: Endometrial sampling: When? Where? Why? With what? *Clin Obstet Gynecol* 35(1):28, 1992.

DiSaia PJ, Creasman WT, editors: *Clinical gynecologic oncology,* ed 3, St Louis, 1989, Mosby.

Hamilton TC: Ovarian cancer, Part I: Biology, *Curr Probl Cancer* 16(1):5, 1992.

Herbst AL: The Bethesda system for cervical/vaginal cytologic diagnoses, *Clin Obstet Gynecol* 35(1):22, 1992.

Hoskins WJ, Perez CA, Young RC, editors: *Principles and practice of gynecologic oncology,* Philadelphia, 1992, JB Lippincott.

Knapp RC, Berkowitz RS, editors: *Gynecologic oncology,* ed 2, New York, 1993, McGraw-Hill.

Kurman RJ, Kaminski PF, Norris HJ: The behavior of endometrial hyperplasia. A long-term study of "untreated" hyperplasia in 170 patients, *Cancer* 56:403, 1985.

Ozols RF: Ovarian cancer, Part II: Treatment, *Curr Probl Cancer* 16(2):67, 1992.

Padwick M, Pryse-Davies J, Whitehead M: A simple method for determining the optimal dosage of progestin in postmenopausal women receiving estrogens, *N Engl J Med* 315(15):930, 1986.

Rulin MC, editor: Controversies in the management of adnexal masses, *Clin Obstet Gynecol* 36(2):361, 1993.

Sherman ME et al: The Bethesda system. A proposal for reporting abnormal cervical smears based on the reproducibility of cytopathologic diagnoses, *Arch Path Lab Med* 116:1155, 1992.

Wetchler SJ: Treatment of cervical intraepithelial neoplasia with the $CO_2$ laser: laser versus cryotherapy. A review of effectiveness and cost, *Obstet Gynecol Surv* 39(8):469, 1984.

# Index

## C

## H

**N**

**Q**



**R**

## X



## Y



## Z

## HEMATOLOGIC NORMAL VALUES—cont'd.

| | | |
|---|---|---|
| Acid hemolysis test (Ham) | No hemolysis | |
| Carboxyhemoglobin | | |
| Nonsmoker | <1% | |
| Smoker | 2.1%-4.2% | |
| Cold hemolysis test (Donath-Landsteiner) | No hemolysis | |
| Complete blood count (see Table 3) | | |
| Erythrocyte life span | | |
| Normal | 120 days | |
| $^{51}$Cr-labeled half-life | 28 days | |
| Erythropoietin by radioimmunassay | 9-33 mU/dl | |
| Ferritin, serum | | |
| Male | 15-200 μg/L | |
| Female | 12-150 μg/L | |
| Folate, RBC | 120-670 ng/ml | |
| Fragility, osmotic | | |
| Hemolysis begins 0.45%-0.38% NaCl | | |
| Hemolysis completed 0.33%-0.30% NaCl | | |
| Haptoglobin, serum | 100-300 mg/dl | |
| Hemoglobin | | |
| Hemoglobin $A_{1c}$ | 0%-5% of total | |
| Hemoglobin $A_2$ by column | 2%-3% of total | |
| Hemoglobin, fetal | <1% of total | |
| Hemoglobin, plasma | 0%-5% of total | |
| Hemoglobin, serum | 2-3 mg/ml | |
| Iron, serum | | |
| Male | 75-175 μg/dl | |
| Female | 65-165 μg/dl | |
| Iron-binding capacity, total serum (TIBC) | 250-450 μg/dl | |
| Iron turnover rate (plasma) | 20-42 mg/24 hr | |
| Leukocyte alkaline phosphatase (LAP) score | 30-150 | |
| Methemoglobin | <1.8% | |
| Reticulocytes (see Table 3) | | |
| Schilling test (urinary excretion of radiolabeled vitamin $B_{12}$ after "flushing" intramuscular injection of $B_{12}$) | 6%-30% of oral dose within 24 hr | |
| Sedimentation rate | *Male* | *Female* |
| Wintrobe | 0-5 mm/hr | 0-15 mm/hr |
| Westergren | 0-15 mm/hr | 0-20 mm/hr |
| Transferrin saturation, serum | 20%-50% | |
| Volume | *Male* | *Female* |
| Blood | 52-83 ml/kg | 50-75 ml/kg |
| Plasma | 25-43 ml/kg | 28-45 ml/kg |
| Red cell | 20-36 ml/kg | 19-31 ml/kg |

**Table 3.** Complete blood count

| Parameter | Male | Female |
|---|---|---|
| Hematocrit (%) | 40-52 | 38-48 |
| Hemoglobin (g/dl) | 13.5-18.0 | 12-16 |
| Erythrocyte count (× $10^{12}$ cells/L) | 4.6-6.2 | 4.2-5.4 |
| Reticulocyte count (%) | 0.6-2.6 | 0.4-2.4 |
| MCV (fL) | 82-98 | 82-98 |
| MCH (pg) | 27-32 | 27-32 |
| MCHC (g/dl) | 32-36 | 32-36 |
| WBC (× $10^9$ cells/L) | 4.5-11.0 | 4.5-11.0 |
| Segmented neutrophils | 1.8-7.7 | 1.8-7.7 |
| Average (%) | 40-60 | 40-60 |
| Bands (cells) | 0-0.3 | 0-0.3 |
| Average (%) | 0-3 | 0-3 |
| Eosinophils (cells × $10^9$/L) | 0-0.5 | 0-0.5 |
| Average (%) | 0-5 | 0-5 |
| Basophils (cells × $10^9$/L) | 0-0.2 | 0-0.2 |
| Average (%) | 0-1 | 0-1 |
| Lymphocytes (cells × $10^9$/L) | 1.0-4.8 | 1.0-4.8 |
| Average (%) | 20-45 | 20-45 |
| Monocytes (cells × $10^9$/L) | 0-0.8 | 0-0.8 |
| Average (%) | 2-6 | 2-6 |
| Platelet count (cells × $10^9$/L) | 150-350 | 150-350 |

## Coagulation Normal Values

| | |
|---|---|
| Template bleeding time | 3.5-7.5 min |
| Clot retraction, qualitative | Apparent in 30-60 min; complete in 24 hr, usually in 6 hr |
| Coagulation time (Lee-White) | |
| Glass tubes | 5-15 min |
| Siliconized tubes | 20-60 min |
| Euglobulin lysis time | 120-240 min |
| Factors II, V, VII, VIII, IX, X, XI, or XII | 100% or 1.0 unit/ml |
| Fibrin degradation products | <10 μg/ml or titer ≤1.4 |
| Fibrinogen | 200-400 mg/ml |
| Partial thromboplastin time, activated | 20-40 sec |
| Prothrombin time (PT) | 11-14 sec |
| Thrombin time | 10-15 sec |
| Whole blood clot lysis time | >24 hr |

## PULMONARY FUNCTION TESTS

Abbreviations

$P_B$ = barometric pressure (mm Hg)
$F_IO_2$ = inspired oxygen fraction (0.21 = room air)
$PaCO_2$ = partial pressure of carbon dioxide in arterial blood (mm Hg)
$P_ACO_2$ = partial pressure of carbon droxide in alveolar gas (mm Hg)
$PaO_2$ = partial pressure of oxygen in arterial blood (mm Hg)
$P_AO_2$ = partial pressure of oxygen in alveolar gas (mm Hg)

Alveolar-arterial oxygen gradient ($F_IO_2$ = 0.21)
P(A-a) in adolescents = <10 mm Hg
adults <40 years = 10 mm Hg
>40 years = 10-15 mm Hg

Alveolar oxygen partial pressure (sea level, $F_IO_2$ = 0.21)
$P_AO_2 = 150 - (1.2 \times PaCO_2)$

Blood gases ($F_IO_2$ = 0.21)

| | *Arterial* | *Alveolar* |
|---|---|---|
| $PO_2$ | 80-105 mm Hg | 90-115 mm Hg |
| $PCO_2$ | 38-44 mm Hg | 38-44 mm Hg |
| pH | 7.35-7.45 | |

Spirometric volumes and lung volumes are size-dependent. Typical normal values for adults are provided.

| *Lung volumes* | *Male* | *Female* |
|---|---|---|
| Total lung capacity (TLC) | 6-7 L | 5-6 L |
| Functional residual capacity (FRC) | 2-3 L | 2-3 L |
| Residual values (RV) | 1-2 L | 1-2 L |
| *Measures of air flow* | | |
| Forced vital capacity (FVC) | 4.0 L | 3.0 L |
| 1 sec forced vital capacity ($FEV_1$) | >3.0 L | >2.0 L |
| Pulmonary resistance (RL) | <3.0 cm $H_2O$/sec/L | |
| Airway resistance (Raw) | <2.5 cm $H_2O$/sec/L | |
| *Other* | | |
| Pulmonary compliance (CL) | 0.2 L/cm $H_2O$ | |
| Diffusing capacity (DLCO) | 25 ml CO/min/mm Hg | |

## RENAL FUNCTION TESTS

**Anion gap**

$Na^+ - HCO_3^- + Cl^- = 12 \pm 2$ mEq/L

**Osmolality**

$$\text{Osmolality (serum)} = 2\ \text{Na (mEq/L)} + \frac{\text{BUN (mg/dl)}}{2.8} + \frac{\text{glucose (mg/dl)}}{18}$$

**Bicarbonate deficit**

$HCO_3^-$ deficit = body weight (kg) × 0.4 (desired $HCO_3^-$ − observed $HCO_3^-$)

Glomerular filtration rate

$$\text{GFR} = \frac{\text{Ucr} \times \text{V}}{\text{Pcr}}$$

$$= 130 \pm 20 \text{ ml/min in males}$$

$$= 120 \pm 15 \text{ ml/min in females}$$

$$\cong \frac{\text{Ucr}}{\text{Pcr}} \times 70$$

where
Ucr = urine creatinine (mg/dl)
Pcr = plasma creatinine (mg/dl)
V = urine volume/24 hr (ml/min)

**Renal plasma flow**

$$\text{RPF} = \frac{\text{Upah} \times \text{V}}{\text{Ppah}}$$

$$= 700 \pm 130 \text{ ml/min in males}$$

$$= 600 \pm 100 \text{ ml/min in females}$$

where
Upah = urine para-aminohippuric acid (mg/dl)
V = urine volume/24 hr (ml/min)
Ppah = plasma para-aminohippuric acid (mg/dl)

## SEMEN NORMAL VALUES

| | |
|---|---|
| Liquefaction | Complete in 15 min |
| Morphology | >50% normal forms |
| Motility | >75% motile forms |
| pH | 7.2-8.0 |
| Spermatocrit | 10% |
| Spermatocyte count | >50 million/ml |
| Volume | 2.0-6.6 ml |

## SERUM NORMAL VALUES

| | |
|---|---|
| Acetoacetate | 0.3-2.0 mg/dl |
| Acid phosphatase | 0-0.8 U/ml |
| Acid phosphatase, prostatic | 2.5-12.0 IU/L |
| Albumin | 3.0-5.5 g/dl |
| Aldolase | 1-6 IU/L |
| Alkaline phosphatase | |
| 15-20 years | 40-200 IU/L |
| 20-101 years | 35-125 IU/L |
| Alpha-1 antitrypsin | 200-500 mg/dl |
| ALT | 0-40 IU/L |
| Ammonia | 11-35 μmol/L |
| Amylase, serum | 2-20 U/L |
| Anion gap | 8-12 mEq/L (mmol/L) |
| Ascorbic acid | 0.4-1.5 mg/dl |
| AST | 5-40 IU/L |
| Bilirubin | |
| Total | 0.2-1.2 mg/dl |
| Direct | 0-0.4 mg/dl |
| Calcium, serum | 8.7-10.6 mg/dl |
| Carbon dioxide, total | 18-30 mEq/L (mmol/L) |
| Carcinoembryonic antigen, serum | <2.5 μg/L |
| Carotene (carotenoids) | 50-300 μg/dl |
| C3 complement | 55-120 mg/dl |
| C4 complement | 14-51 mg/dl |
| Ceruloplasmin | 15-60 mg/dl |
| Chloride, serum | 95-105 mEq/L (mmol/L) |
| Cholesterol, total | |
| 12-19 years | 120-230 mg/dl |
| 20-29 years | 120-240 mg/dl |
| 30-39 years | 140-270 mg/dl |
| 40-49 years | 150-310 mg/dl |
| 50-59 years | 160-330 mg/dl |
| Copper | 100-200 μg/dl |
| Creatine kinase, total | 20-200 IU/L |
| Creatine kinase, isoenzymes | |
| MM fraction | 94%-95% |
| MB fraction | 0%-5% |
| BB fraction | 0%-2% |
| Normal values in | |
| Heart | 80% MM, 20% MB |
| Brain | 100% BB |
| Skeletal, muscle | 95% MM, 2% MB |
| Creatinine, serum | |
| Female adult | 0.5-1.3 mg/dl |
| Male adult | 0.7-1.5 mg/dl |
| Delta-aminolevulinic acid (ALA) | <200 μg/dl |
| α-Fetoprotein, serum | <40 μg/L |
| Folate, serum | 1.9-14.0 ng/ml |
| Gamma glutamyl transpeptidase | |
| Male | 12-38 IU/L |
| Female | 9-31 IU/L |
| Gastrin | 150 pg/ml |
| Glucose, serum (fasting) | 70-115 mg/dl |
| Glucose-6-phosphate dehydrogenase | 5-10 IU/g Hb |
| G6PD screen, qualitative | Negative |
| Haptoglobin | 100-300 mg/dl |
| Hemoglobin $A_2$ | 0%-4% of total Hb |
| Hemoglobin F | 0%-2% of total Hb |
| Immunoglobulin, quantitation | |
| IgG | 700-1500 mg/dl |
| IaA | 70-400 mg/dl |
| IgM | |
| Male | 30-250 mg/dl |
| Female | 30-300 mg/dl |
| IgD | 0-40 mg/dl |
| Insulin, fasting | 6-20 μU/ml |
| Iron-binding capacity | 250-400 μg/dl |
| Iron, total, serum | 40-150 μg/dl |
| Lactic acid | 0.6-1.8 mEq/L |
| LDH, serum | 20-220 IU/L |
| LDH isoenzymes | |
| $LDH_1$ | 20%-34% |
| $LDH_2$ | 28%-41% |
| $LDH_3$ | 15%-25% |
| $LDH_4$ | 3%-12% |
| $LDH_5$ | 6%-15% |
| Leucine aminopeptidase (LAP) | 30-55 IU/L |
| Lipase | 4-24 IU/dl |
| Magnesium, serum | 1.5-2.5 mEq/L |
| 5′-Nucleotidase | 0.3-3.2 Bodansky units |
| Osmolality, serum | 278-305 mOsm/kg serum water |
| Phenylalanine | 3 mg/dl |
| Phosphorus, inorganic, serum | 2.0-4.3 mg/dl |
| Potassium, plasma | 3.1-4.3 mEq/L |
| Potassium, serum | 3.5-5.2 mEq/L |
| Protein, total, serum | |
| 2-55 years | 5.0-8.0 g/dl |
| 55-101 years | 6.0-8.3 g/dl |
| Protein electrophoresis, serum | |
| Albumin | 3.2-5.2 g/dl |
| Alpha-1 | 0.6-1.0 g/dl |
| Alpha-2 | 0.6-1.0 g/dl |
| Beta | 0.6-1.2 g/dl |
| Gamma | 0.7-1.5 g/dl |
| Sodium, serum | 135-145 mEq/L |
| Sulfate | 0.5-1.5 mg/dl |
| $T_3$ uptake | 25%-45% |
| $T_4$ | 4-11 μg/dl |
| Triglycerides | |
| 2-29 years | 10-140 mg/dl |
| 30-39 years | 20-150 mg/dl |
| 40-49 years | 20-160 mg/dl |
| 50-59 years | 20-190 mg/dl |
| 60-101 years | 20-200 mg/dl |